Clinical
Anesthesia

Clinical Anesthesia

Edited by

Paul G. Barash, M.D.
Professor and Chairman, Department of Anesthesiology
Yale University School of Medicine
Chief, Department of Anesthesiology
Yale-New Haven Hospital
New Haven, Connecticut

Bruce F. Cullen, M.D.
Professor
University of Washington School of Medicine
Anesthesiologist-in-Chief, Department of Anesthesiology
Harborview Medical Center
Seattle, Washington

Robert K. Stoelting, M.D.
Professor and Chairman, Department of Anesthesia
Indiana University School of Medicine
Indianapolis, Indiana

With 86 Contributors

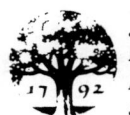

J. B. Lippincott Company
Philadelphia
London   Mexico City   New York
St. Louis   São Paulo   Sydney

Acquisitions Editor: Susan Gay
Sponsoring Editor: Richard Winters
Indexer: Maria Coughlin
Design Coordinator: Michelle Gerdes
Cover Designer: Joe Netherwood
Production Manager: Carol A. Florence
Compositor: Circle Graphics, Inc.
Printer/Binder: Murray Printing Co.

3 5 6 4 2

LIBRARY OF CONGRESS
Library of Congress Cataloging-in-Publication Data

Clinical anesthesia/edited by Paul G. Barash, Bruce F. Cullen, Robert K. Stoelting; with 86 contributors.
    p. cm.
  Includes bibliographies and index.
  ISBN 0-397-50836-0
  1. Anesthesiology. 2. Anesthesia. I. Barash, Paul G.
II. Cullen, Bruce F.   III. Stoelting, Robert K.
  [DNLM: 1. Anesthesiology.   WO 200 C6398]
RD81.C58 1989
617'.96—dc19
DNLM/DLC
for Library of Congress   88-12887
                                                          CIP

The authors and publisher have exerted every effort to ensure that drug selection and dosage set forth in this text are in accord with current recommendations and practice at the time of publication. However, in view of ongoing research, changes in government regulations, and the constant flow of information relating to drug therapy and drug reactions, the reader is urged to check the package insert for each drug for any change in indications and dosage and for added warnings and precautions. This is particularly important when the recommended agent is a new or infrequently employed drug.

*For All Students
of Anesthesiology*

Contributors

STEPHEN E. ABRAM, M.D.
Professor of Anesthesiology
Medical College of Wisconsin
Milwaukee, Wisconsin

J. JEFF ANDREWS, M.D.
Assistant Professor, Department of Anesthesiology
The University of Texas Medical Branch
Galveston, Texas

PETER G. ANDRIAKOS, M.D.
Instructor in Anesthesiology
New York University School of Medicine
New York, New York

JEFFREY ASKANAZI, M.D.
Associate Professor of Anesthesiology
Albert Einstein College of Medicine;
Director of Research, Department of Anesthesiology
Division of Critical Care Medicine
Montefiore Medical Center
Bronx, New York

MICHAEL J. AVRAM, PH.D.
Associate Professor of Anesthesia
Northwestern University School of Medicine;
Affiliated Professional Staff
Northwestern Memorial Hospital;
Research Consultant
Veterans Administration Lakeside Medical Center
Chicago, Illinois

STEVEN J. BARKER, M.D.
Associate Professor of Anesthesiology
University of California, Irvine;
Vice-Chairman
University of California, Irvine Medical Center
Irvine, California

M. LAWRENCE BERMAN, M.D., PH.D.
Professor of Anesthesiology
Associate Professor of Pharmacology
Vanderbilt University School of Medicine;
Attending Anesthesiologist
Vanderbilt University Hospital
Nashville, Tennessee

ARNOLD J. BERRY, M.D.
Associate Professor of Anesthesiology
Emory University School of Medicine
Emory University Hospital
Atlanta, Georgia

FREDERIC A. BERRY, M.D.
Professor of Anesthesia and Pediatrics
Children's Medical Center of the University of Virginia
Charlottesville, Virginia

SUSAN BLACK, M.D.
Instructor in Anesthesiology
Mayo Medical School;
Consultant in Anesthesiology
Mayo Clinic
Rochester, Minnesota

CASEY D. BLITT, M.D.
Clinical Associate, Department of Anesthesiology
University of Arizona Health Science Center;
Chairman, Department of Anesthesiology
Tucson Medical Center;
Chief of Anesthesia
El Dorado Hospital
Tucson, Arizona

EDWIN A. BOWE, M.D
Associate Professor, Department of Surgery/Anesthesiology
University of South Carolina School of Medicine
Columbia, South Carolina

MORRIS BROWN, M.D.
Department of Anesthesiology
Wayne State University School of Medicine;
Director of Critical Care Services
Vice-Chairman, Department of Anesthesiology
Sinai Hospital of Detroit
Detroit, Michigan

F. PETER BUCKLEY, F.F.A.R.C.S
Associate Professor, Department of Anesthesiology
University of Washington School of Medicine
Seattle, Washington

ROD K. CALVERLEY, M.D.
Clinical Professor of Anesthesiology
University of California, San Diego;
Attending Anesthesiologist
Veterans Administration Medical Center
University of California, San Diego Medical Center
San Diego, California

FREDERICK W. CAMPBELL, M.D.
Assistant Professor of Anesthesia
University of Pennsylvania School of Medicine
Philadelphia, Pennsylvania

RANDALL L. CARPENTER, M.D.
Staff Anesthesiologist
Virginia Mason Hospital
Seattle, Washington

FREDERICK W. CHENEY, M.D.
Professor, Department of Anesthesiology
University of Washington School of Medicine;
Professor of Anesthesiology
University Hospital
Seattle, Washington

EDMOND COHEN, M.D.
Assistant Professor of Anesthesiology
Mount Sinai School of Medicine
New York, New York

D. RYAN COOK, M.D.
Professor of Anesthesiology and Pharmacology
Children's Hospital of Pittsburgh
Pittsburgh, Pennsylvania

BENJAMIN G. COVINO, PH.D., M.D.
Professor of Anesthesia
Harvard Medical School;
Chairman, Department of Anesthesia
Brigham and Women's Hospital
Boston, Massachusetts

ROY F. CUCCHIARA, M.D.
Professor of Anesthesiology
Mayo Medical School;
Consultant in Anesthesiology
Mayo Clinic
Rochester, Minnesota

SUKUMAR P. DESAI, M.B., B.S., M.S.
Assistant Professor of Anesthesia
Harvard Medical School;
Brigham and Women's Hospital
Boston, Massachusetts

STEPHEN F. DIERDORF, M.D.
Associate Professor of Anesthesiology
Indiana University School of Medicine;
Staff Anesthesiologist
Indiana University Hospitals
Indianapolis, Indiana

LENARD R. DURRETT, PH.D., M.D.
Assistant Professor of Anesthesiology
University of Texas Medical Branch
John Sealy Hospital
Galveston, Texas

JAN EHRENWERTH, M.D.
Associate Professor, Department of Anesthesiology
Yale University School of Medicine;
Attending Anesthesiologist
Yale-New Haven Hospital
New Haven, Connecticut

JAMES B. EISENKRAFT, M.D.
Associate Professor of Anesthesiology and Director of Anesthesia Research
Mount Sinai School of Medicine
New York, New York

NORIG ELLISON, M.D.
Professor of Anesthesiology
University of Pennsylvania School of Medicine
Philadelphia, Pennsylvania

ROBERT FEINSTEIN, M.D., PH.D.
Assistant Professor of Anesthesiology
Washington University School of Medicine
St. Louis, Missouri

MIECZYSLAW FINSTER, M.D.
Professor of Anesthesiology, Obstetrics and Gynecology
College of Physicians and Surgeons
Columbia University;
Attending Anesthesiologist
The Presbyterian Hospital
New York, New York

ARTHUR S. FOREMAN, M.D.
Assistant Professor, Department of Anesthesia
Wake Forest University Medical Center
Bowman Gray School of Medicine
North Carolina Baptist Hospital
Winston-Salem, North Carolina

ROBERT J. FRAGEN, M.D.
Professor of Clinical Anesthesia
Northwestern University School of Medicine;
Director of Anesthesia
Northwestern Memorial Hospital
Chicago, Illinois

SIMON GELMAN, M.D., PH.D.
Professor of Anesthesiology
Vice-Chairman for Research, Department of Anesthesiology
The University of Alabama at Birmingham
University Hospital
Birmingham, Alabama

GEORGE GRAF, M.D.
Assistant Professor of Anesthesiology and Medicine
Yale University School of Medicine;
Attending Physician
Yale-New Haven Hospital
New Haven, Connecticut

BETTY L. GRUNDY, M.D.
Professor of Anesthesiology
University of Florida College of Medicine;
Chief, Anesthesiology Service
Veterans Administration Medical Center
Gainesville, Florida

RONALD A. HARRISON, M.D.
Associate Professor of Clinical Anesthesia
Northwestern University Medical School;
Attending Staff Physician
Northwestern Memorial Hospital
Chicago, Illinois

WILLIAM E. HOFFMAN, PH.D.
Associate Professor of Anesthesiology
Michael Reese Hospital and Medical Center
Chicago, Illinois

DUNCAN A. HOLADAY, M.D.
Professor of Anesthesiology
Vanderbilt University School of Medicine
Nashville, Tennessee

ROBERT J. HUDSON, M.D., F.R.C.P.(C)
Associate Professor of Anesthesia
Faculty of Medicine
University of Manitoba;
Attending Anesthetist
St. Boniface General Hospital
Winnipeg, Manitoba, Canada

CINDY W. HUGHES, M.D.
Assistant Professor of Anesthesiology
Yale University School of Medicine;
Attending Anesthesiologist
Yale-New Haven Hospital
New Haven, Connecticut

TAMAS KALLOS, M.D.
Clinical Associate Professor of Anesthesiology
University of Miami School of Medicine;
Anesthesiologist
South Miami Hospital
Miami, Florida

JOEL A. KAPLAN, M.D.
Horace W. Goldsmith Professor and Chairman, Department of Anesthesiology
Mount Sinai School of Medicine
New York, New York

JONATHAN D. KATZ, M.D.
Associate Professor of Clinical Anesthesiology
Yale University
New Haven, Connecticut;
Attending Anesthesiologist
St. Vincent's Medical Center
Bridgeport, Connecticut

HOSHANG J. KHAMBATTA, M.D.
Associate Professor of Clinical Anesthesiology
College of Physicians and Surgeons
Columbia University;
Associate Attending in Anesthesiology
Columbia-Presbyterian Medical Center
New York, New York

HARRY G. G. KINGSTON, M.B., B.CH. F.F.A.R.C.S.
Associate Professor, Department of Anesthesiology
Oregon Health Sciences University;
Operating Room Director, Department of Anesthesiology
University Hospital
Portland, Oregon

ELMER F. KLEIN, JR., M.D.
Professor and Chief of Anesthesia, Department of Surgery/Anesthesia
University of South Carolina School of Medicine
Columbia, South Carolina

DONALD A. KROLL, M.D., PH.D.
Assistant Professor, Department of Anesthesiology
University of California, Los Angeles School of Medicine;
Assistant Professor, Department of Anesthesiology
University of California, Los Angeles Medical Center
Los Angeles, California

CAROL LEE LAKE, M.D.
Associate Professor, Department of Anesthesiology
University of Virginia;
Clinical Staff
University of Virginia Medical Center
Charlottesville, Virginia

DONALD H. LAMBERT, PH.D., M.D.
Associate Professor of Anesthesia
Harvard Medical School;
Anesthesiologist
Brigham and Women's Hospital
Boston, Massachusetts

NOEL W. LAWSON, M.D.
Professor of Anesthesiology
University of Texas Medical Branch
John Sealy Hospital
Galveston, Texas

PHILIP W. LEBOWITZ, M.D.
Assistant Professor of Anesthesia
Harvard Medical School;
Anesthesiologist-in-Chief
Cambridge Hospital;
Associate Anesthetist
Massachusetts General Hospital
Boston, Massachusetts

JERROLD H. LEVY, M.D.
Assistant Professor of Anesthesiology
Emory University School of Medicine
Division of Cardiothoracic Anesthesiology
Emory Clinic
Associate Director, Cardiothoracic Intensive Care Unit
Emory University Hospital
Atlanta, Georgia

WEN-SHIN LIU, M.D.
Professor of Anesthesiology
Northeastern Ohio University College of Medicine
Rootstown, Ohio

KATHRYN E. McGOLDRICK, M.D.
Associate Professor of Anesthesiology
Yale University School of Medicine;
Attending Anesthesiologist
Yale-New Haven Hospital
New Haven, Connecticut

DAVID C. MACKEY, M.D.
Fellow in Regional Anesthesia
Virginia Mason Memorial Center
Seattle, Washington

CHARLES H. McLESKEY, M.D.
Associate Professor of Anesthesiology
University of Colorado Health Sciences Center
Denver, Colorado

JOHN T. MARTIN, M.D.
Professor and Chairman, Department of Anesthesiology
Medical College of Ohio at Toledo;
Director, Division of Anesthesiology
Medical College of Ohio Hospital
Toledo, Ohio

ROGER S. MECCA, M.D.
Assistant Clinical Professor, Department of Anesthesiology
Yale University School of Medicine;
Chairman, Department of Anesthesiology
Director, Recovery Services
Danbury Hospital
Danbury, Connecticut

JOHN R. MOYERS, M.D.
Associate Professor of Anesthesia
University of Iowa College of Medicine;
Chief, Cardiovascular Anesthesia
University of Iowa Hospitals and Clinics
Iowa City, Iowa

MICHAEL F. MULROY, M.D.
Staff Anesthesiologist
Virginia Mason Medical Center
Seattle, Washington

MICHAEL R. MURPHY, M.D.
Associate Professor of Anesthesiology
Emory University;
Director, Anesthesia for Surgical Specialists
Emory University Hospital
Atlanta, Georgia

WILLIAM D. OWENS, M.D.
Professor and Chairman, Department of Anesthesiology
Washington University School of Medicine;
Anesthesiologist-in-Chief
Barnes Hospital
St. Louis, Missouri

NATHAN L. PACE, M.D.
Professor of Anesthesiology
Adjunct Professor of Bioengineering
Department of Anesthesiology
University of Utah School of Medicine;
Attending Anesthesiologist
University Hospital
University of Utah Health Sciences Center
Salt Lake City, Utah

HILDA PEDERSEN, M.B., C.L.B., F.F.A.R.C.S
Associate Professor of Clinical Anesthesiology
College of Physicians and Surgeons
Columbia University;
Associate Attending Anesthesiologist
The Presbyterian Hospital
New York, New York

LAWRENCE L. PRIANO, M.D., PH.D.
Associate Professor of Anesthesiology
Oregon Health Sciences University
Portland, Oregon

DONALD S. PROUGH, M.D.
Associate Professor of Anesthesia and Neurology
Head, Section on Critical Care
Bowman Gray School of Medicine;
Associate Chief of Professional Services
North Carolina Baptist Hospital
Winston-Salem, North Carolina

FREDERIC M. RAMSEY, M.D.
Assistant Professor of Anesthesia
Harvard Medical School;
Chief of Anesthesiology
Massachusetts Eye and Ear Infirmary
Boston, Massachusetts

JAMES J. RICHTER, M.D., PH.D.
Director, Department of Anesthesiology
Hartford Hospital
Hartford, Connecticut

MICHAEL F. ROIZEN, M.D.
Professor of Anesthesia and Critical Care
Professor of Medicine
Chairperson, Department of Anesthesia and Critical Care
Pritzker School of Medicine
University of Chicago
Chicago, Illinois

STANLEY H. ROSENBAUM, M.D.
Associate Professor of Anesthesiology and Medicine
Yale University School of Medicine;
Attending Physician
Yale-New Haven Hospital
New Haven, Connecticut

HENRY ROSENBERG, M.D.
Professor and Chairman, Department of Anesthesiology
Hahnemann University Hospital
Philadelphia, Pennsylvania

ALAN C. SANTOS, M.D.
Assistant Professor of Anesthesiology
State University of New York, Stony Brook
Attending Anesthesiologist
University Hospital
Stony Brook, New York

MARK S. SCHELLER, M.D.
Assistant Professor of Anesthesiology
University of California, San Diego;
Attending Anesthesiologist
University of California, San Diego Medical Center
San Diego, California

ALAN JAY SCHWARTZ, M.D., M.S. ED.
Associate Dean for Academic Affairs
School of Medicine
Professor of Anesthesiology
Hahnemann University School of Medicine
Philadelphia, Pennsylvania

DAVID T. SEITMAN, M.D., M.S.B.M.E., B.S.E.E.
Assistant Professor of Anesthesiology
Hahnemann University;
Staff Anesthesiologist
Director of Anesthesiology
Hahnemann University Hospital
Philadelphia, Pennsylvania

B. SKEIE, M.D.
Department of Anesthesiology
Oslo University;
Ullevaal Hospital
Oslo, Norway

THEODORE C. SMITH, M.D.
Professor of Anesthesiology and Pharmacology
Loyola University;
Chief of Anesthesiology
EA Hines Jr, Veterans Administration Hospital
Maywood, Illinois

LINDA C. STEHLING, M.D.
Professor, Department of Anesthesiology
SUNY Health Sciences Center at Syracuse
University Hospital
Syracuse, New York

JEFFREY A. STEINKELER, M.D.
Assistant Professor of Anesthesiology
Oregon Health Sciences University
Portland, Oregon

WENDELL C. STEVENS, M.D.
Professor and Chairman, Department of Anesthesiology
Oregon Health Sciences University;
University Hospital
Portland, Oregon

STEPHEN J. THOMAS, M.D.
Associate Professor of Anesthesiology
New York University School of Medicine;
Director of Cardiac Anesthesia
New York University Medical Center
New York, New York

KEVIN K. TREMPER, PH.D., M.D.
Associate Professor and Chairman, Department of Anesthesiology
University of California, Irvine Medical Center
Irvine, California

LEROY D. VANDAM, PH.D., M.D., M.A. (HON)
Professor of Anesthesia Emeritus
Harvard Medical School;
Anesthesiologist
Brigham and Women's Hospital
Boston, Massachusetts

BERNARD V. WETCHLER, M.D.
Director, Department of Anesthesiology
Medical Director, Ambulatory SurgiCare
The Methodist Medical Center of Illinois;
Clinical Professor and Chief, Division of Anesthesia
University of Illinois College of Medicine at Peoria
Peoria, Illinois

K. C. WONG, M.D., PH.D.
Professor and Chairman of Anesthesiology
Professor of Pharmacology
University of Utah School of Medicine
Salt Lake City, Utah

JAMES R. ZAIDAN, M.D.
Associate Professor of Anesthesiology
Division of Cardiothoracic Anesthesia
Emory University School of Medicine
Atlanta, Georgia

Preface

The discovery and application of anesthesia has been the single most important contribution of American medicine to mankind. The major achievements of modern surgery would not have taken place without the accompanying vision of the pioneers of anesthesiology. Yet anesthesia was originally considered a technique with little scientific merit, and anesthesiology did not become a distinct academic discipline until 100 years after Dr. Crawford Long administered the first ether anesthetic.

Today, the boundaries of anesthesiology extend far beyond the operating room. As a consequence, the information needs of both the veteran practitioner and the resident in the speciality have increased dramatically, and a comprehensive reference for our discipline must now encompass significant new areas of knowledge as well as the traditional subject areas. Just as important, however, is the accessibility of the information. A truly modern textbook must support efficient, *rapid* use if it is to meet the demands of those in practice or training today. It has been the goal of the editors of *Clinical Anesthesia* to create such a comprehensive, usable book in a single volume.

The table of contents shows how we have attempted to meet this goal. The book begins with a discussion of the development of anesthesia—we have a proud heritage, and this chapter eloquently describes the exciting events that form the history of our speciality. Each of the subspecialities is discussed in subsequent chapters, with the scientific basis of each subject described in proximity to the clinical aspects. In addition, there are numerous chapters not found in traditional anesthesia textbooks. For example, the impact of modern genetics is discussed in the chapter entitled "Pharmocogenetics." Because environmental hazards continue to be a topic of great concern, "Hazards of Working in the Operating Room" eloquently examines the relationship of the anesthesiologist to the operating room setting and documents the importance of the OR environment to physical and mental well-being. This is complemented by a subsequent chapter, "Electrical Safety," which details the protection of both the patient and the operating room staff. The dilemmas confronting the anesthesiologist in the management of the elderly patient are addressed in the chapter "Anesthesia for the Geriatric Patient," which focuses on the implications of the aging process in clinical practice.

Certain topics require amplification because of their impact on daily practice. Orthopedics, the genitourinary system, and the gastrointestinal system merit the greater detail found in separate chapters. Finally, certain areas that are clinically relevant but problematic are also presented. These include the positioning of the patient, the allergic response, and the special considerations arising with the traumatized patient.

The contributors of all these chapters form a remarkable blend of 86 outstanding authorities from 48 institutions. They have provided us with a truly nationwide perspective on our specialty. Each of them, whether up and coming or long-established, is a physician actively involved in the advancement of anesthesiology.

As editors, we have tried to envision the specialty of the future, and we feel that the presentation of the material should be unique. In this regard, we chose not to contribute chapters in our own areas of expertise. Instead, we extended our energies in the editorial process, in developing themes to be used in individual chapters, encouraging contributors to prioritize various clinical options, integrating each of the chapters within appropriate sections of the book, and, finally, avoiding the duplication so often seen in multi-authored volumes. On occasion, however, we felt it important to have some redundancy, and even disagreement, in the management of a given clinical problem, because this in fact reflects the realities of consultant practice of anesthesiology.

The editors wish to acknowledge and express their gratitude to a number of individuals whose hard work not only expedited this book, but also added quality and authority to its pages: first, each of the contributors, who not only completed their chapters in a timely fashion, but also offered numerous suggestions which we feel will enhance the value of *Clinical Anesthesia* to the resident and practitioner; next, our secretaries, Gail Norup, Sue Perkins, and Deanna Walker, whose unflagging devotion to the project was a continued source of support; and finally, a special word of thanks is due to our colleagues at the J. B. Lippincott Company: Susan Gay, Executive Editor; Richard Winters, Basic Books Editor; Carol Florence, Production Manager; and Jody DeMatteo and Janet Greenwood, Production Editors. Their vision and constructive comments continually demonstrated their commitment to the highest standard of medical publishing.

Paul G. Barash, M.D.
Bruce F. Cullen, M.D.
Robert K. Stoelting, M.D.

Contents

Contents

Clinical Anesthesia

Part I

Introduction

Anesthesia as a Specialty: Past, Present, and Future

As the body of medical knowledge relevant to anesthesiology expands at a rapid pace, students and residents sometimes confine their studies to material that they believe will be immediately applicable in the operating room or the examination hall. By limiting their reading so narrowly, they fail to learn that it is only by knowledge of the past that we can appreciate our present situation and anticipate future developments. This chapter is not designed to be "commercially" valuable as a means to satisfy examiners; it has been created to help the reader understand important elements of our history, to learn how anesthesiology came to its present situation, and to recognize some of the forces that will shape both our immediate future and the more distant days to follow.

A reading of history overcomes an unfortunate tendency to accept the practice of anesthesia as having always been just what it was on the day of one's introduction to the specialty. To do so is to ignore the achievements of those who discovered all that is known and whose energies brought anesthesiology to its present attractive position. We have all received a magnificent endowment from our predecessors—machines, drugs, and techniques that we use to bring comfort to our patients every day.

This chapter provides an overview of selected elements of our history to illustrate several important segments of the evolution of anesthesia, including the development of anesthetic agents, regional techniques, anesthesia machines, monitoring equipment, and endotracheal devices. This review of technical and pharmacologic landmarks is followed by a discussion of the development of North American and British professional practice and professional societies. The chapter will close with a look ahead, an attempt to forecast the future of anesthesiology.

SURGERY BEFORE INHALATIONAL ANESTHESIA

Before the introduction of anesthesia with diethyl ether, many surgeons believed that pain was, and would always be, an inevitable consequence of surgery. In those "dark" days, many patients approached surgery as though facing execution, an often appropriate assessment of uncontained risks, including pain, hemorrhage, shock, and postoperative infection. While awaiting even a minor elective procedure, patients often put their estate and personal affairs in order in the anticipation that their wealth would soon be passed on to the next of kin. Curiously, as there was little that could be done to alleviate pain, and, as it seemed an inevitable component of injury and most disease, philosophers ennobled pain as "providential." Scholars, debating issues from the comfort of their couches, assessed the courage of less fortunate persons before declaring that the ability to withstand pain ranked among the noble virtues. In ancient as well as in modern times, there is truth to the aphorism, "The easiest pain to bear is someone else's."

The Roman writer Celsus encouraged "pitilessness" as an essential character of the surgeon, an attitude that prevailed for centuries. Although some surgeons confessed that they found elements of their work intensely disturbing, most became inured to their patient's agony. Medical students emulated their teachers and often omitted to record any appraisal of the patient's distress while taking notes of the operations that they witnessed. Even the authors of leading surgical texts often ignored surgical pain as a topic of discussion. Just before the advent of anesthesia, Robert Liston's 1842 edition of *Elements of Surgery* contained detailed descriptions of *elective* and

3

emergency procedures on the extremities, head and neck, breast, and genitals but neglected a significant discussion of any technique to make the patient comfortable. In Liston's time, pain was considered primarily a symptom of importance in differential diagnosis.

Before the discovery of surgical anesthesia, Europeans attempted to relieve pain by hypnosis, by the ingestion of alcohol, herbs, and extracts of botanical preparations, as well as through the local application of pressure or ice. The topical anesthetic created by chewing coca leaves was known only to the Incas of South America before Pizarro's conquest. A Japanese physician, Seishu Manaoke, may have used drugs to render surgery painless in 1835, but before 1846 Western surgeons could only offer their patients oral concoctions of opium in wine or whiskey and the hollow promise of hasty surgery. As late as 1839, the French surgeon, Louis Velpeau, said, "To obviate pain in operations is a chimera which it is today no longer permissible to seek after."[1] Within a decade, his gloomy pronouncement was reversed. Velpeau became an enthusiastic supporter of anesthesia and pronounced it the most important discovery yet achieved.

ANESTHETIC ANTECEDENTS

Historic chronologies frequently memorialize the date of a discovery and relate the event to the actions of one person; it is, however, inappropriate to view the development of anesthesiology from such a confined perspective. William T.G. Morton is honored as the man who, in Boston, on October 16, 1846, showed the world that ether could work, but his historic public demonstration succeeded through the prior efforts of less-celebrated men who made Morton's triumph possible.

Morton's demonstration of ether caught the world's attention in part because it took place in a public place, the surgical amphitheater of a public institution, the Massachusetts General Hospital. Surgical amphitheaters, and the charitable hospitals of which they were a part, were then a relatively recent addition to American medical teaching. During the early 19th century, large hospitals had been erected in North America and Europe as an expression of the evolving social philosophy of the time. The privileged of the community accepted a responsibility to attempt to provide shelter and medical care for the sick and injured of the poorer classes. As a result, large numbers of patients could be attended in a single location. Their medical care, however, was often of an indifferent and uncertain nature. The course of the patient's disease might be observed by medical students who "walked the wards" informally, but who would not yet profit from the techniques of bedside instruction that William Osler and his late 19th century colleagues brought to American medical practice. A few students might act as "dressers" to established surgeons, but most students only observed surgery when they sat or stood on the benches of the amphitheater where the poor underwent operations in public.

Medical school curricula were nonstandardized and highly variable. The most pronounced disparities were observed among American proprietary medical schools, as a consequence of the influence of contending philosophies of medical care, which included homeopathy, hydropathy, allopathy, and eclectic healing—all vying for a dominant role in therapeutics. As a result, Americans were accustomed to hearing of new claims that ensured a cure. Experimental procedures received attention that might be denied in more orthodox medical societies. As a consequence, nitrous oxide and ether, chemicals discovered in Europe, whose general properties were already known on both sides of the Atlantic, found their historic application in America.

A lost opportunity to discover anesthesia occurred two decades before the demonstration of ether in Boston. An English physician searched intentionally in 1823 and 1824 for an inhaled anesthetic to relieve the pain of surgery. Henry Hill Hickman (1800–1830) might have succeeded if he had used either of the drugs whose actions were later discovered in America, but the mice and dogs he studied inhaled neither ether nor nitrous oxide but high concentrations of carbon dioxide. Carbon dioxide has some anesthetic properties, as shown by the absence of response to an incision in the animals of Hickman's study, but carbon dioxide is not an appropriate clinical anesthetic. Hickman's concept was magnificent; his choice of agent, regrettable. His work was ignored both by surgeons and by the scientists of the Royal Society. Despite Hickman's earnest efforts, his research was never appreciated during his brief life. Ironically, a contemporary member of the Royal Society, Sir Humphry Davy, was familiar with the analgesic qualities of another inhaled gas, nitrous oxide. If Davy had encouraged Hickman, the younger man might have repeated his study with a more appropriate agent. Surgical anesthesia might then have been celebrated as a British rather than an American discovery.

EARLY USE OF ETHER AND NITROUS OXIDE

The first inhaled agents that would have a place in anesthesia were of different origins but had found a similar application as drugs for social entertainment in the years immediately before their use as anesthetics.

DIETHYL ETHER

Diethyl ether had been known for centuries. Although it may have been compounded first by an 8th century Arabian philosopher, Jabir ibn Hayyam, or by Raymond Lully, an alchemist of the 13th century, it was certainly known in the 16th century to both Valerius Cordus and Paracelsus, who prepared it by distilling sulfuric acid (oil of vitriol) with fortified wine to produce an "oleum vitrioli dulce" (sweet oil of vitriol). Paracelsus observed that it caused chickens to fall asleep and awaken unharmed. He must have been aware of its analgesic qualities, because he reported that it could be recommended for use in painful illnesses, but there is no record that his suggestion was followed. In 1540, Valerius Cordus recommended it as a medication to be taken in wine for the relief of whooping cough and other respiratory diseases.

For three centuries thereafter, this simple compound remained a therapeutic agent with only occasional use. Some of its properties were examined by distinguished British scientists, including Robert Boyle, Isaac Newton, and Michael Faraday, but without sustained interest. Its only routine application came as an inexpensive "recreational drug" among the poor of Britain and Ireland who sometimes drank an ounce or two of ether when taxes made gin prohibitively expensive. An American variation of this practice was conducted by groups of medical students who held ether-soaked towels to their faces at nocturnal "ether frolics."

NITROUS OXIDE

Nitrous oxide was inhaled from gas-tight bags by celebrants seeking an exhilarating experience. It was not used as frequently as was ether because it was more complex to prepare and was awkward to store. It was commonly produced by heating ammonium nitrate in the presence of iron filings. The evolved gas was passed through water to eliminate toxic oxides of nitrogen before being stored.

Nitrous oxide was first prepared in 1773 by Joseph Priestley (1733–1804), an English clergyman–scientist, who ranks among the great pioneers of chemistry. During his years of study, Priestley prepared and examined several gases, including nitrous oxide, ammonia, sulfur dioxide, oxygen, carbon monoxide, and carbon dioxide. Most of his work consisted primarily of scientific observation, but he also created the first carbonated beverage by charging water with carbon dioxide.

Even though his discovery of nitrous oxide would be sufficient to give Priestley a place in the history of anesthesia, he is also remembered for his recognition of the pure gas now known as oxygen. Priestley heated mercuric oxide to release a gas that caused greater beauty and intensity of a flame and that allowed a mouse to survive longer when breathing it than would be expected if the jar were filled with air. He identified many properties of the new gas, but, handicapped by his adherence to the phlogiston theory of combustion, termed it *dephlogisticated air*. It is a remarkable reflection of Priestley's genius that within a few months, he isolated both oxygen and nitrous oxide, the only pure gases still used routinely in anesthesia.

Other contributions might have followed if Priestley's career had remained undisturbed, but, in 1791, his home, scientific apparatus, and library were burned by a mob angered by his sympathies for the revolution in France. He later left England and migrated to Pennsylvania where his friends and correspondents included three great American revolutionaries, Benjamin Franklin, John Adams, and Thomas Jefferson.

If the French Revolution was to result in an interruption of Joseph Priestley's research, its effect upon a French scientist of exceptional genius was catastrophic. Antoine Lavoisier (1743–1794) examined Priestley's work with gases, recognized the fallacy of the phlogiston theory, and dispelled its confusion. He named Priestley's vital gas, *oxygen*. Lavoisier later proved that respiration was equivalent to combustion as the oxygen inhaled into the lungs combined with carbon and hydrogen to produce carbon dioxide and water. Lavoisier erroneously believed that the process took place in the lungs. He might have overcome that error and extended his understanding of chemistry and physiology even further, but he was imprisoned on trivial charges during the Reign of Terror. Lavoisier went to the guillotine on May 8, 1794, after a sham trial during which Robespierre, the president of the tribunal snarled, "The republic has no need for chemists."

Priestley's preparation of nitrous oxide drew the attention of other investigators on both sides of the Atlantic Ocean. A physician and chemist of New York, Samuel Latham Mitchell, recognized some of the cerebral effects of nitrous oxide while performing research on the influences of gases as factors in the transmission of disease. Although his conclusion that nitrous oxide might be a contagious influence in epidemics was erroneous, his comments on nitrous oxide were among the reports that would stimulate the attention of Thomas Beddoes and Humphry Davy of the Pneumatic Institute in Bristol, England.

At the end of the 18th century in England, there was a strong interest in the salubrious effects of mineral waters and healthful airs. This led to the development of spas, which were sought out by people of society. Particular waters and gases were believed to prevent and treat disease. A dedicated interest in the potential use of gases as remedies of scurvy, tuberculosis, and other diseases led Thomas Beddoes (1760–1808)

to open his Pneumatic Institute close to the small spa of Hotwells, in the city of Bristol, where he hired Humphry Davy to conduct research projects.

Humphry Davy (1778–1829) was a young man of ability and drive. He performed a brilliant series of investigations of several gases but focused much of his attention upon nitrous oxide, which he and his associates inhaled from cylinders through facemasks designed for the Institute by James Watt, the distinguished inventor of the steam engine. Davy used this equipment to measure the rate of uptake of nitrous oxide—its effect upon respiration and other central nervous system actions. These results were combined with research on the physical properties of the gas in a 580-page book published in 1800, *Nitrous Oxide*. This impressive treatise is now best remembered for a few incidental observations: Davy's comments that nitrous oxide transiently relieved a severe headache, obliterated a minor headache, and briefly quenched an aggravating toothache. The most frequently quoted passage was a casual entry, "As nitrous oxide in its extensive operation appears capable of destroying physical pain, it may probably be used with advantage during surgical operations in which no great effusion of blood takes place."[2]

Although Davy did not pursue this prophecy—perhaps because he was set upon a career in basic research—he did use nitrous oxide to entertain the young men of quality who visited the Pneumatic Institute, including Dr. Peter Mark Roget, later to become the author of Roget's Thesaurus, and two poets, Samuel Taylor Coleridge and the Poet Laureate, Robert Southey, who after inhaling nitrous oxide was said to exclaim that the atmosphere of the highest of all possible heavens must be composed of this gas. After one of these episodes, Davy coined the persisting sobriquet for nitrous oxide, "laughing gas."

Following Davy's researches, the only application of nitrous oxide for the next four decades was to produce hilarity and disinhibited behavior at parties and public entertainments. Nitrous oxide capers and ether frolics would eventually introduce the concept of inhaling a vapor for the transient relief of pain to the first Americans to experiment with surgical anesthesia, William Clarke of Rochester, New York, and Crawford W. Long of Jefferson, Georgia.

An anesthesia text written by Henry Lyman in 1881 provides evidence that William E. Clarke gave the first ether anesthetic in Rochester, New York, in January 1842. From techniques learned as a chemistry student in 1839, Clarke entertained his companions with nitrous oxide and ether. Lyman reported, " . . . Clarke diligently propagated this convivial method among his fellow students. Emboldened by these experiences, in January, 1842, having returned to Rochester, he administered ether, from a towel, to a young woman named Hobbie, and one of her teeth was then extracted without pain by a dentist named Elijah Pope."[3] Another indirect reference to Clarke's anesthetic suggested that it was believed that her unconsciousness was due to hysteria. Clarke was advised to conduct no further anesthetic experiments. Regrettably, no statements by Clarke, Pope, or Miss Hobbie have been found.

CRAWFORD W. LONG (1815–1878). There is no doubt that 2 months later, on March 30, 1842, Crawford Williamson Long did give ether with a towel for surgical anesthesia in Jefferson, Georgia. His patient, James M. Venable, was a young man who already knew ether's exhilarating effects, for he reported in a certificate that he had previously inhaled it frequently and was fond of its use. Venable had two small tumors on his neck but refused to have them excised, because he dreaded the cut of the knife. Knowing that Venable was familiar with ether's action, Dr. Long proposed that ether might alleviate pain and gained his patient's consent to proceed. After inhaling ether from the towel, Venable reported that he was unaware of the removal of the tumor. In determining the world's first fee for anesthesia, Long settled on a surgical charge of $2.00, plus $.25 for the ether.[4]

As a rural physician with a very limited surgical practice, Crawford Long had few opportunities to give ether anesthesia, but he did conduct the first comparative trial of an anesthetic. He wished to prove that insensibility to pain was caused by ether and not simply by a reflection of the individual's pain threshold or self-hypnosis. When ether was withheld during amputation of the second of two toes, his patient reported great pain and proclaimed a strenuous preference for ether.

For Long to gain an unrivaled position as the discoverer of anesthesia, all that remained for him to do would have been to announce his historic work in the medical literature. Long, however, remained silent until 1849, when ether anesthesia was already well known. He explained that he practiced in an isolated environment and had few opportunities for surgical or dental procedures. From our perspective, it is difficult to understand why he was so reluctant to publish his work. This remarkable man might have changed the course of the history of medicine, but, because of his failure to publish, the public introduction of anesthesia was achieved by more assured and bolder persons.

THE CRUCIAL EXPERIMENT

In contrast to the limited opportunities for surgery presented to rural practitioners in the mid-19th century, urban dentists regularly met patients who refused restorative treatment for fear of the pain that would be inflicted by the dentist. From a dentist's perspective, pain was not so much life threatening as it was livelihood threatening. A few dentists searched for new techniques of effective pain relief. Pasteur's yet-to-be-delivered aphorism that chance only favors the prepared mind, would have provided an apt description of one of these men, Horace Wells, of Hartford, Connecticut. Wells recognized what others had ignored, the analgesic potential of nitrous oxide.

HORACE WELLS (1815–1848). Horace Wells' great moment of discovery came on December 10, 1844, when he attended a lecture–exhibition by an itinerant "scientist," Gardner Quincy Colton, who prepared nitrous oxide and encouraged members of the audience to inhale the gas. Wells observed that a young man, Samuel Cooley (later Colonel Cooley of the Connecticut militia), was unaware that he had injured his leg while under the influence of nitrous oxide. Sensing that nitrous oxide might also relieve the pain of dental procedures, Wells contacted Colton and boldly proposed an experiment. The following day, Colton gave Wells nitrous oxide before a fellow dentist, William Riggs, extracted a tooth. When Wells awoke, he claimed that he had not felt any pain and declared the experiment a great success. Colton taught Wells to prepare nitrous oxide, which the dentist administered with success in his practice. His apparatus probably resembled that used by Colton. The patient placed a wooden tube in his mouth through which he rebreathed nitrous oxide from a small bag filled with the gas.

A few weeks later, in January 1845, Wells attempted a public demonstration in Boston at the Harvard Medical School. He had planned to anesthetize a patient for an amputation, but, when the patient refused surgery, a dental anesthetic for a medical student was substituted. Wells, perhaps influenced by a large and openly critical audience, began the extraction without an adequate level of anesthesia, and the trial was judged a failure.

The exact circumstances of Wells' lack of success are not known. His less-than-enthusiastic patient may have refused to breathe the anesthetic. Alternatively, Wells might have lost part of his small supply of nitrous oxide, which could have happened if the patient involuntarily removed his lips from the mouthpiece or if the patient's nostrils were not held shut. It might be that Wells did not know that nitrous oxide lacks sufficient potency to serve predictably as an anesthetic without supplementation. In any event, the student cried out, and Wells was jeered by his audience. The disappointment disturbed him deeply, and, although he continued his dental practice for some time, his life became unsettled. While profoundly distressed, Wells committed suicide in 1848. Despite his personal failure, Wells remains an important pioneer of anesthesia, for he was the first person to recognize the anesthetic qualities of the only 19th century drug still in routine use, nitrous oxide.

WILLIAM THOMAS GREEN MORTON (1819–1868). Another New Englander, William Thomas Green Morton, briefly shared a dental practice with Horace Wells in Hartford. Wells' daybook shows that he gave Morton a course of instruction in anesthesia, but Morton apparently moved to Boston without paying for his lessons. In Boston, Morton continued his interest in anesthesia and, after learning from Charles Jackson that ether dropped on the skin provided analgesia, began experiments with inhaled ether. After anesthetizing a pet dog, he became confident of his skills and anesthetized patients in his dental office. Encouraged by that success, Morton gained an invitation to give a public demonstration in the Bullfinch amphitheatre of the Massachusetts General Hospital.

The diethyl ether that Morton was to use would prove to be much more versatile than nitrous oxide. Professor Nicholas Greene has made a detailed examination of social and medical circumstances surrounding the discovery of anesthesia.[5] Greene has demonstrated that before the invention of the hollow needle and an awareness of aseptic technique, the only class of potential anesthetics that could offer a prompt, profound, and temporary action were the inhaled drugs. Of the available drugs, ether was a superb first choice. Bottles of liquid ether were easily transported, and the volatility of the drug permitted effective inhalation. The concentrations required for surgical anesthesia were so low that patients did not become hypoxic when breathing air. It also possessed what would later be recognized as a unique property among all inhaled anesthetics: the quality of providing surgical anesthesia without causing respiratory or cardiovascular depression. These properties, combined with a slow rate of induction, gave the patient a great margin of safety when physicians were attempting to master the new art of administering an inhaled anesthetic.

PAIN PUT TO SLEEP

On Friday, October 16th, 1846, William T. Morton secured permission to provide an anesthetic to Edward Gilbert Abbott before the surgeon, John Collins Warren, excised a vascular lesion from the left side of Abbott's neck. Morton was late in

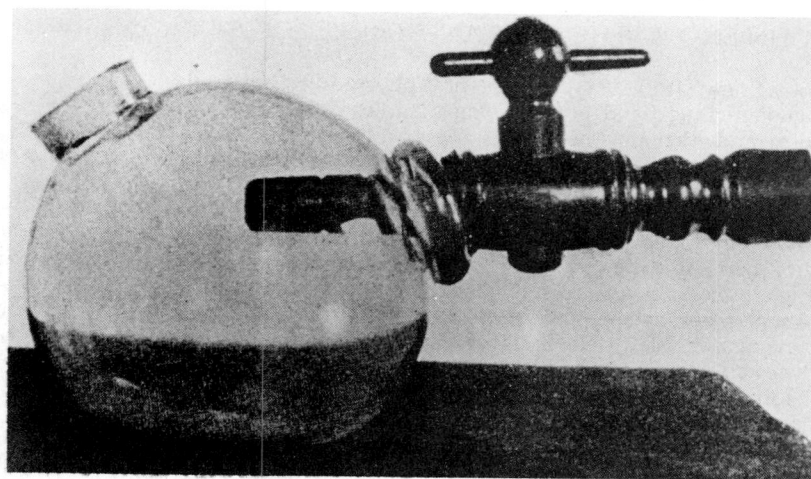

FIG. 1-1. Morton's ether inhaler (1846).

arriving, so Warren was at the point of proceeding when Morton entered. The dentist had been obliged to wait for an instrumentmaker to complete his inhaler (Fig. 1-1). It consisted of a large glass bulb containing a sponge soaked with colored ether and a spout, which was to be placed in the patient's mouth. An opening on the opposite side of the bulb allowed air to enter and to be drawn over the ether-soaked sponge with each breath.

The conversations of that morning were not accurately recorded; however, popular accounts state that the surgeon responded testily to Morton's apology for his tardy arrival by remarking, "Sir, your patient is ready." Morton directed his attention to his patient and first conducted a very abbreviated preoperative evaluation. He inquired, "Are you afraid?" Abbott responded that he was not and took the inhaler in his mouth. After a few minutes, Morton is said to have turned to the surgeon to respond, "Sir, your patient is ready." Gilbert Abbott later reported that he was aware of the surgery but had experienced no pain. At the moment that the procedure ended, Warren turned to his audience and announced, "Gentlemen, this is no humbug."[6] Oliver Wendell Holmes promptly suggested the term *anaesthesia* to describe the state of temporary insensibility.

What would be recognized as America's greatest contribution to 19th century medicine had been realized, but the immediate prospect was clouded, unfortunately, by subterfuge and argument. Some weeks passed before Morton admitted that the active component of the colored fluid that he had called "Letheon" was the familiar drug, diethyl ether. Morton, Wells, Jackson, and their supporters soon became caught up in a contentious, protracted, and fruitless debate over priority for the discovery.

When the details of Morton's anesthetic technique became public knowledge, the information was transmitted by train, stagecoach, and coasting vessels to other North American cities and by ship to the world. Anesthetics were performed in Britain, France, Russia, South Africa, Australia, and other countries almost as soon as surgeons heard the welcome news of the extraordinary discovery. Even though surgery could now be performed with "pain put to sleep," the frequency of operations did not rise rapidly. Several years would pass before anesthesia was even universally recommended. Many American surgeons believed that anesthesia was not appropriate for all procedures in all classes of patients, but the "American invention" excited interest everywhere.

BRITISH CONTRIBUTIONS

Although Americans discovered inhalation anesthesia, British doctors initiated most of the noteworthy advances of the following decades. In the years after James Y. Simpson discovered chloroform anesthesia, John Snow, Joseph T. Clover, and Frederic Hewitt were earnest advocates of improved anesthetic care. Their publications directed the attention of the medical profession to significant advances and earned greater respect for the emerging discipline of anesthesia. In succession, Snow, Clover, and Hewitt were each the leading London anaesthetist* of the day and gave anesthetics for members of the royal family. Their work not only established the principle that the administration of anesthetics was an appropriate activity for a medical doctor but also encouraged the understanding in Britain and the Commonwealth that anesthetics could be administered only by physicians.

J.Y. SIMPSON CHAMPIONS CHLOROFORM

James Young Simpson, a successful obstetrician of Edinburgh, Scotland, had been among the first to use ether for the relief of the pain of labor. He became dissatisfied with ether and sought a more pleasant, rapid-acting anesthetic. He and a few junior associates conducted a bold search for a new inhaled anesthetic by inhaling samples of several volatile chemicals collected for Simpson by British apothecaries.

David Waldie suggested chloroform, which had first been prepared in 1831. Simpson and his friends inhaled it at a dinner party in Simpson's home on the evening of November 4, 1847. They promptly fell unconscious from self-induced anesthesia. They awoke delighted at their success. Simpson quickly set about encouraging chloroform anesthesia. Within 2 weeks, he had dispatched his first account of its use to the Lancet. Although Simpson introduced chloroform with celerity, boldness, and enthusiasm and was later to become a vocal defender of the use of anesthesia for women in labor, he gave few anesthetics himself. His goal was simply to improve a patient's comfort during his operative or obstetric activities.

* Nineteenth century "anaesthetists" in America became 20th century "anesthesiologists," but their British and Canadian counterparts (unchallenged by competetion from nurses) remained "anaesthetists." The author of this chapter has adhered to this distinction.

JOHN SNOW—THE FIRST ANESTHESIOLOGIST

John Snow (1813–1858) was the first physician to undertake detailed clinical and pharmacologic studies of ether, chloroform, and other anesthetics. His mastery of clinical techniques made him the most respected anaesthetist of his time. Snow's scholarly analyses of the action of anesthetics were unequaled by any other author of the 19th century. Some concepts that Snow developed before 1852 were not extended until a century later. Although he never restricted his practice solely to anesthesia, Snow is rightfully recognized as the first anesthesiologist, because he was a masterful clinician and dedicated investigator. Many elements of his work warrant detailed review.

John Snow (Fig. 1-2) was already a respected physician who had presented papers on physiologic subjects when the news of ether anesthesia reached England in December 1846. He took an interest in anesthetic practice and was soon invited to work with many of the leading surgeons of the day. He was not only facile at providing anesthesia but was also a remarkably keen observer. His innovative description of the stages or degrees of ether based on the patient's responsiveness were not improved upon for 70 years.

He soon realized the inadequacies of ether inhalers into which the patient rebreathed through a mouthpiece. After practicing anesthesia for only 2 weeks, Snow designed the first of his series of ingenious ether inhalers. His best-known apparatus featured unidirectional valves within a malleable, well-fitting mask of his own design, which closely resembles the form of a modern facemask (Fig. 1-3). The facepiece was connected to the vaporizer (Fig. 1-4) by a breathing tube, which

FIG. 1-2. John Snow—the first anesthesiologist.

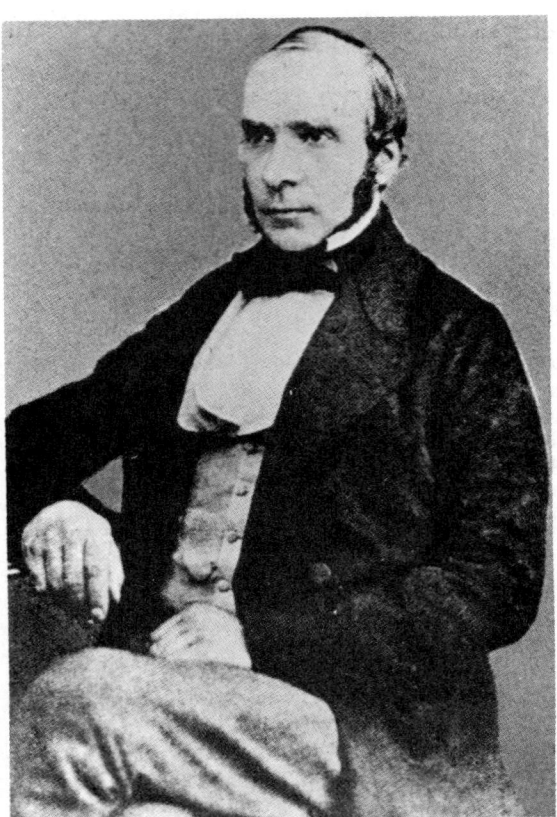

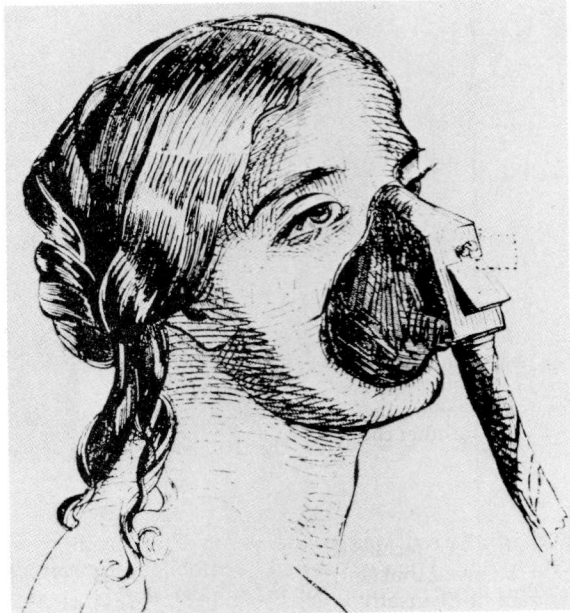

FIG. 1-3. John Snow's facemask (1847). The expiratory valve can be tilted to the side to allow the patient to breathe air.

Snow deliberately designed to be wider than the human trachea so that even rapid respirations would not be impeded. A metal coil within the vaporizer ensured that the patient's inspired breath was drawn over a large surface area to promote the uptake of ether. The device also incorporated a warm water bath to maintain the volatility of the agent. Snow did not attempt to capitalize on his creativity; he closed his account of its preparation with the very generous observation, " . . . there is no restriction respecting the making of it."[7]

The following year, John Snow introduced a chloroform inhaler; he had recognized the versatility of the new agent and came to prefer it in his practice. At the same time, he initiated what were to become an extraordinary series of experiments that were remarkable in both their scope and in the manner in which they anticipated sophisticated research performed a century later. Snow realized that successful anesthetics must not only abolish pain but also prevent movement. He anesthetized several species of animals with varying concentrations of ether and chloroform to determine the concentration required to prevent movement in response to a sharp stimulus. Despite the limitations of the technology of 1848, this element of his work anticipated the concept of minimum alveolar concentration (MAC).[8]

He assessed the anesthetic action of a large number of potential anesthetics, and, although he did not find any to rival chloroform or ether, he determined a relationship between solubility, vapor pressure, and anesthetic potency that was not fully appreciated until after World War II. He also created an experimental closed circuit device in which the subject (Snow himself) breathed oxygen while the exhaled carbon dioxide was absorbed by potassium hydroxide.

Snow's investigations were not confined to anesthesia. His memory is also respected by specialists in infectious and tropical diseases for his proof through an epidemiologic study in 1854 that cholera was transmitted by water. At that time, before the development of microbiology by Louis Pasteur and Robert Koch, most physicians in North America and Europe attributed the mysterious recurring epidemics of cholera to

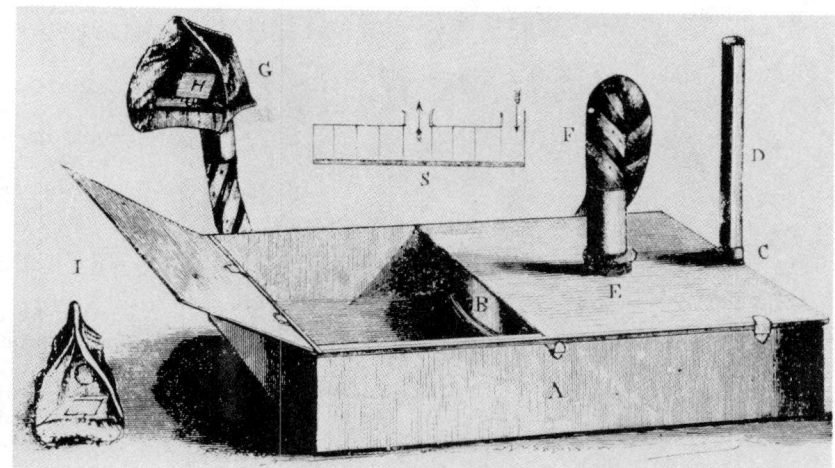

FIG. 1-4. John Snow's ether inhaler (1847). The ether chamber (*B*) contained a spiral coil so that the air entering through the brass tube (*D*) was saturated by ether before ascending the flexible tube (*F*) to the facemask (*G*). The ether chamber rested in a bath of warm water (*A*).

the contagion of "fecalized air." For many years, however, Snow had believed that since the disease affected the gastrointestinal tract, the causative agent must be ingested rather than inhaled. In 1854, he found an opportunity to prove his thesis when cholera visited his section of London and caused the deaths of more than 500 people near his residence. Snow determined that the water supply for these persons had been the Broad Street Pump. He prepared what would come to be appreciated as the first epidemiologic survey to prove his contention. With that information, he was able to encourage the parish authorities to remove the pump handle so that residents were obliged to find other sources of water. The prompt resolution of the epidemic was attributed to his action.

One hundred years later, a unique celebration commemorated Snow's action, the public house at the site of the Broad Street Pump was named "The John Snow" to mark Snow's role as a pioneer of epidemiology. It is located at 39 Broadwick Street and is among the most popular pubs of Soho; it is visited by physicians from many countries. Whether John Snow would have approved of this unique memorial is uncertain, for he abstained from spirits except for medicinal and experimental purposes.

Snow was a highly respected clinician and author as well as investigator. These qualities are reflected in his books, *On the Inhalation of the Vapour of Ether* (1847) and *On Chloroform and other Anaesthetics* (1858), which was almost completed when he died at the age of 45 years of a stroke. His books have been reprinted by the American Society of Anesthesiologists.

His opinions were respected not only by his medical contemporaries but were also sought out by prominent people with an interest in science. Queen Victoria's consort, Prince Albert, interviewed John Snow before he was called to Buckingham Palace at the request of the Queen's obstetrician to give chloroform for the Queen's last two deliveries. During the monarch's labor, Snow gave analgesic doses of chloroform on a folded handkerchief, a technique that was soon termed *chloroform a la reine*. Victoria had abhorred the pain of labor and enjoyed the relief that chloroform provided; she wrote in her Journal, "Dr. Snow gave that blessed chloroform and the effect was soothing, quieting and delightful beyond measure."[9] After the monarch's positive opinion became known, an ongoing debate over the appropriateness of the use of anesthesia in labor was abruptly quenched. Four years later, Snow was to give a second anesthetic to the Queen who was again determined to have chloroform. Snow's daybook states that by the time he arrived, Prince Albert had begun the anesthetic and

had given his wife "a little chloroform." This may be the only time in history that a Queen had a Prince as her anaesthetist.

JOSEPH THOMAS CLOVER (1825–1882)

Joseph Clover was the leading anaesthetist of London after the death of John Snow in 1858. Clover was a talented clinician and facile inventor, but he never performed research or wrote to the extent achieved by Snow. If he had written a text, he might be better remembered, but most physicians have little knowledge of Clover beyond identifying the familiar photograph in which he is seen anesthetizing a seated man while palpating his patient's pulse (Fig. 1-5).

The photograph deserves our attention, because it introduces important qualities of the man who maintained the advancement of anesthesia from 1860 until 1880. Anesthesiologists now accept Clover's monitoring of the pulse as a simple routine of prudent practice, but, in Clover's time, this was a contentious issue. Prominent Scottish surgeons scorned Clover's emphasis upon the action of chloroform on the heart. Baron Lister and others preferred that senior medical students give anesthetics and urged them to " . . . strictly carry out certain simple instructions, among which is that of never touching the pulse, in order that their attention may not be distracted from the respiration."[10] Lister also counseled, " . . . it appears that preliminary examination of the chest, often considered indispensable, is quite unnecessary, and more likely to induce the dreaded syncope, by alarming the patients, than to avert it."[11] Little progress in anesthesia could come from such reactionary statements. In contrast, Clover had observed the effect of chloroform upon animals and urged other anaesthetists to monitor the pulse at all times and to discontinue the anesthetic temporarily if any irregularity or weakness was observed in the strength of the pulse. He earned a loyal following among London surgeons, who accepted him as a dedicated specialist.

Clover was the first anaesthetist to administer chloroform in known concentrations through his construction of the Clover bag, which is seen over his shoulder in Figure 1-5. He filled it by pumping air from a bellows over a warmed evaporating vessel containing a known volume of liquid chloroform to obtain a 4.5% concentration of chloroform in air. The apparatus had inspiratory and expiratory valves of ivory supported by springs. A flap valve in the facemask permitted the dilution of the anesthetic with air. In 1868, Clover reported no deaths

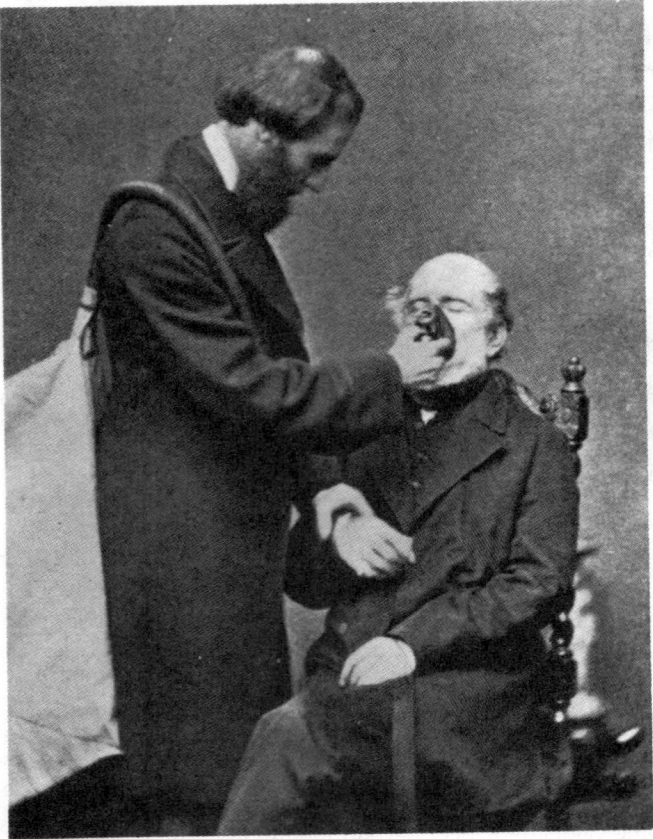

FIG. 1-5. Joseph Clover anesthetizing a patient with chloroform and air passing through a flexible tube from a Clover bag.

among 1802 applications of his device, but he later reviewed a fatality in searching detail. He attributed the death to his undetected error in calculating the volume of air diluting the chloroform.[12] After 1870, Clover favored a nitrous oxide/ether sequence. The portable anesthesia machines that he designed were in popular use for decades after his death.

In Figure 1-5, Clover projects the image of attentiveness, but there is no evidence of the resuscitative equipment, which he also had available, to control the airway. In that regard, Clover was exceptional, for he practiced at a time when other anaesthetists could only administer gases and vapors but lacked any means to care for the patient if any difficulty occurred. Clover's prudence and foresight allowed him to anticipate potential problems and to be ready to respond rapidly when a complication threatened his patient. In that regard, he was an exemplary model for the modern anesthesiologist.

Clover was very facile in maintaining the airway. He was the first to urge the now universal practice of thrusting the patient's jaw forward to overcome obstruction of the upper airway by the tongue. Despite the limitation of working before the first endotracheal tube was used in anesthesia, Clover published a landmark case report in 1877. At that time, his patient had a tumor of the mouth that obstructed the airway completely once the anesthetic was begun. Clover averted disaster by inserting a small curved cannula of his own design through the cricothyroid membrane. The anesthetic was continued through the cannula until the tumor was excised. Clover, the model of the prepared anesthesiologist, remarked, " . . . I have never used the cannula before although it has

been my companion at some thousands of anaesthetic cases."[13]

Every element of Clover's records and his published accounts reflect a consistent dedication to patient safety coupled with a prudent ability to anticipate potential difficulties and to prepare an effective response beforehand. In that way, his manner was very much like that of his successor, the first English anaesthetist to be knighted, Sir Frederick Hewitt.

SIR FREDERICK HEWITT (1857–1916)

Frederick Hewitt gained the first of his London hospital anesthesia appointments in 1884. He earned a reputation as a superb and inventive clinician and came to be considered the leading British practitioner of the next 30 years. Hewitt engineered modifications of portable ether and nitrous oxide inhalers and, recognizing that nitrous oxide and air formed an hypoxic mixture, designed the first anesthetic apparatus to deliver oxygen and nitrous oxide in fixed proportions. He also was influential in ensuring that anesthesia was taught in all British medical schools. His book, *Anaesthetics and Their Administration*, which first appeared in 1893 and continued through five editions, is considered the first true textbook of anesthesia.

Hewitt's most famous patient was King Edward VII, whose coronation in 1902 was canceled when the monarch's life was threatened by an appendiceal abscess. Hewitt anesthetized the King by mask while the surgeon, Frederick Treves, drained the abscess. Hewitt accepted the greater responsibility by anesthetizing an obese, bearded, febrile, dehydrated man with a well-developed and protracted affection for alcohol and tobacco. Following the patient's recovery and coronation, both men were honored but at different levels. Although the reasons for the awarding of honors by the court are not announced, readers wonder why the surgeon was knighted and Hewitt received a lesser honor then but was eventually knighted 7 years later.

In 1908, Hewitt developed an important appliance that would assist all anesthesiologists in managing an obstructed upper airway. He called his oral device an *air-way*. After several modifications, and with the hyphen now deleted, all anesthesiologists insert airways routinely.

NINETEENTH CENTURY ANESTHESIA IN AMERICA

American anesthesiologists of the second half of the 19th century failed to achieve the lasting recognition gained by their British colleagues. Several factors contributed to this disparity. Snow, Clover, and Hewitt were men of such genius that they would have been exceptional in any period of history. They all had mastered the demands of chloroform, an agent that demanded greater skill in its administration than did diethyl ether, which remained the dominant anesthetic in America, where the provision of anesthesia was often a service relegated to medical students, junior house officers, nurses and nonprofessionals. The subordinate status of anesthesia was even reflected in American art. Thomas Eakins' great studies, "The Gross Clinic" of 1876 and "The Agnew Clinic" of 1889, both present the surgeon as the focus of attention, while the person administering the anesthetic is found among the supporting figures.

In that period, however, Americans led the revival of nitrous oxide. Gardner Q. Colton, the "professor," who had first demonstrated the use of nitrous oxide to Horace Wells, developed the Colton Dental Association after he returned from the California gold rush. In several eastern cities, he opened offices equipped with nitrous oxide generators and, perhaps profiting by Wells' unhappy experience, larger breathing bags of 30 l capacity. By 1869, his advertisements carried the intriguing slogan "31½ Miles Long." Colton had asked each patient to sign his name to a scroll, which then contained the names of 55,000 patients who had experienced painless extractions of teeth without hazard. He proposed that if this great number of patients were to march past in single file, the line would be extend for 31½ miles.[14]

Colton gave brief exposures of nitrous oxide undiluted with air or oxygen, which raised concern that the gas was acting as an asphyxiant. The following year, a Chicago surgeon, Edmund Andrews, experimented with an oxygen/nitrous oxide mixture and proved that nitrous oxide does not cause anesthesia by depriving the brain of oxygen. While the oxygen-nitrous oxide mixture was safer, he identified a handicap to its use which was unique to that time when anesthetists attended many patients in their homes. The large bag would be conspicuous and awkward to carry as he walked along busy streets. He observed "In city practice, among the higher classes, however, this is no obstacle as the bag can always be taken in a carriage, without attracting attention."[15] Four years later, Andrews was delighted to report the availability of liquefied nitrous oxide compressed under 750 lb of pressure, which allowed a supply sufficient for three patients to be carried in a single cylinder. Despite Andrew's early enthusiasm, few American surgeons relied on nitrous oxide until it was used in combination with regional anesthesia, the last important contribution to inhaled anesthetic practice achieved in the late 19th century.

REGIONAL ANESTHESIA

Several 19th century physicians experimented with the local application of drugs to relieve pain. In 1853, Alexander Wood invented the hollow metal needle in order to inject morphine directly into a painful area. Morphine did not act locally but relieved pain only by its systemic action, but the invention of the needle would allow the successful administration of another locally acting alkaloid three decades later.

Cocaine, an extract of the coca leaf, was the first effective local anesthetic. Its property of numbing mucous membranes and exposed tissues had been known for centuries in Peru, where folk surgeons performing trephinations chewed coca leaves and allowed their saliva to fall onto the surfaces of the wound. This was a unique situation in anesthesia; there are no other instances in which both the operator and his patient routinely shared the effects of the same drug. After Albert Niemann refined the active alkaloid and named it *cocaine*, it was used in experiments by a few investigators. It was noted that cocaine provided topical anesthesia and even produced local insensibility when injected, but these observations were not applied in clinical practice before 1884, when the significance of the action of cocaine was realized by Carl Koller, a Viennese surgical intern.

CARL KOLLER (1857–1944)

Carl Koller appreciated what others had failed to recognize because of his past experience and his ambition to practice ophthalmology at a time when many operations on the eye were still being performed without anesthesia. Almost four decades after the discovery of ether, general anesthesia by mask still had several limitations. The anesthetized patient could not cooperate with his surgeon. The anesthesiologist's apparatus interfered with surgical access. More importantly, the high incidence of vomiting following the administration of either chloroform or ether threatened extrusion of internal contents of the globe with the risk of the permanent loss of sight. At that time, surgical incisions on the globe were left unclosed; fine ophthalmic sutures were not yet available.

While he had been a medical student, Koller had worked in a Vienna laboratory in a search for a topical anesthetic that would overcome the limitations of general anesthesia. Unfortunately, the suspensions of morphine, chloral hydrate, and other drugs that he had used had been ineffectual.

In 1884, his friend, Sigmund Freud, became interested in the cerebral stimulating effects of cocaine and gave Koller a small sample in an envelope, which he placed in his pocket. When the envelope leaked, a few grains of cocaine stuck to Koller's finger, which he casually licked with his tongue. It became numb. Koller realized that he had found the object of his search. That same afternoon, he dashed to the laboratory where he had worked as a student and made a suspension of the cocaine crystals. He and Gustav Gartner, a laboratory associate, observed its anesthetic effect upon the eyes of a frog, a rabbit, and a dog before they dropped the solution onto their corneas. To their amazement, their eyes were insensitive to the touch of a pin.[16]

Carl Koller could not afford to attend the Congress of German Ophthalmologists in Heidelberg on Sept 15, 1884, but, after his paper was read by a friend, a revolution in ophthalmic surgery and other surgical disciplines was underway. Within the next year, more than 100 articles supporting the use of cocaine appeared in European and American medical journals. Despite this gratifying success, Koller was not able to pursue his goal of gaining a residency position in Vienna. After a duel provoked by an anti-Semitic slur, Koller left Austria and, after studying briefly in Holland and Britain, migrated in 1888 to New York where he practiced ophthalmology for the remainder of his career.

American surgeons quickly developed new applications for cocaine. Its efficacy in anesthetizing the nose, mouth, larynx, trachea, rectum, and urethra were described in October 1884. The next month, the first reports were published of its subcutaneous injection. In December 1884, two young surgeons, William Halsted and Richard Hall, described blocks of the sensory nerves of the face and arm. Richard Hall may have been the first person to undergo dental surgery under local anesthesia when Halsted blocked his mandibular nerve. Halsted also performed a block of the brachial plexus under direct vision following a dissection of the plexus. As a consequence of their self-experimentation, both men became addicted to cocaine. Cocaine addiction was an ill-understood, but frequent problem in the late 19th century, when it was easily obtained and was offered in scores of patent medicines that were freely available.

SPINAL ANESTHESIA

In 1885, Leonard Corning, a neurologist who had observed Hall and Halsted performing nerve blocks, coined the expression "spinal anaesthesia." Corning wanted to assess the action of cocaine, not for surgery, but as a specific therapy for neurologic problems. After first assessing its action in a dog, producing a blockade of rapid onset that was confined to the animal's rear legs, he administered cocaine to a man "addicted to masturbation." He received a proportionally larger dose, but the blockade had a much slower onset. Although Corning does not refer to the escape of cerebrospinal fluid in either case, it is likely that the dog had a spinal anesthetic and that the man had an epidural anesthetic. No therapeutic benefit was described, but Corning closed his account and his attention to the subject by suggesting that cocainization might in time be " . . . a substitute for etherization in genito-urinary or other branches of surgery."[17]

Fourteen years passed before spinal anesthesia was performed for a surgical operation. In the interval, Heinrich Quincke of Kiel, Germany, described lumbar puncture. He proposed that the technique was most safely performed at the level of the third or fourth lumbar interspace, because an entry at that level would be below the termination of the spinal cord. Quincke's technique was used for the first deliberate cocainization of the spinal cord in 1899 by August Bier, a surgical colleague of Quincke. Six patients received small doses of cocaine intrathecally, but, because several of the patients cried out during surgery and some vomited and had postoperative headaches, Bier felt it necessary to conduct a clinical experiment.

Professor Bier permitted his assistant, Dr. Hildebrandt, to perform a lumbar puncture, but, after the needle penetrated the dura, Hildebrandt could not fit the syringe to the needle and a large volume of the professor's spinal fluid escaped. They were at the point of abandoning the study when Hildebrandt volunteered to be the subject of a second attempt. They had an astonishing success. Twenty-three minutes later, Bier noted: "A strong blow with an iron hammer against the tibia was not felt as pain. After 25 minutes: Strong pressure and pulling on a testicle were not painful."[18] They celebrated their success with wine and cigars. That night, both developed violent headaches, which they attributed at first to their celebration. Bier's headache was relieved after 9 days of bedrest. The house officer did not have the luxury of continued rest; Bier reported that while Hildebrandt " . . . felt very poor the next morning but with great physical effort he was able to do his work, which consisted mainly in operating and dressing of wounds."[19] Bier believed that their headaches were caused by the loss of large volumes of cerebrospinal fluid and urged that this be avoided if possible. The high incidence of complications following lumbar puncture with wide-bore needles and the toxic reactions attributed to cocaine explain Bier's later loss of interest in spinal anesthesia.

Surgeons of several other countries soon started practicing spinal anesthesia. Many of the observations found in their descriptions are still relevant. The first series from France of 125 cases was published by Theodor Tuffier, who later counseled that the solution should not be injected before cerebrospinal fluid was seen. The initial American report was by Dr. Rudolph Matas of New Orleans, whose first patient developed postanesthetic meningismus, a then-frequent complication that was overcome by the use of sterile gloves as advocated by Halsted and the hermetically sealed sterile solutions recommended by E.W. Lee of Philadelphia.

During 1899, Dudley Tait and Guidlo Caglieri of San Francisco performed experimental studies in animals and therapeutic spinals for orthopedic patients.[20] They encouraged the use of fine needles to lessen the escape of cerebrospinal fluid and urged that the skin and deeper tissues be infiltrated beforehand with local anesthesia, as had been urged earlier by William Halsted and the foremost advocate of infiltration anesthesia, Carl Ludwig Schleich of Berlin. An early American specialist in anesthesia, Ormond Goldan, published an anesthesia record appropriate for recording the course of "intraspinal cocainization" in 1900. In the same year, Heinrich Braun learned of a newly described extract of the adrenal gland,

epinephrine, which he used to prolong the action of local anesthetics with great success. Braun developed several new nerve blocks, coined the term *conduction anesthesia*, and is remembered by European writers as the "father of conduction anesthesia." Braun was the first person to use procaine, which, along with stovaine, was one of the first synthetic local anesthetics produced to reduce the toxicity of cocaine. Further advances in spinal anesthesia followed the introduction of these and other synthetic local anesthetics.

Before 1907, several anesthesiologists had been disappointed to observe that their nerve blocks were incomplete. Most believed that the drug spread solely by local diffusion before incomplete nerve blocks were investigated by Arthur Barker, a London surgeon.[21] Barker constructed a glass tube shaped to follow the curves of the human spine and used it to demonstrate the limited spread of colored solutions that he had injected through a T-piece in the lumbar region. Barker applied this observation to use solutions of stovaine made hyperbaric by the addition of 5% glucose, which worked in a more predictable fashion. After the injection was complete, Barker placed his patient's head upon pillows to contain the anesthetic below the nipple line. Lincoln Sise acknowledged Barker's work in 1935 when he introduced the use of hyperbaric solutions of pontocaine. John Adriani advanced the concept further in 1946 when he used a hyperbaric solution to produce "saddle block" or perineal anesthesia. Adriani's patients were obliged to remain in the seated position for almost a minute after injection while the drug descended to bathe the sacral nerves.

Tait, Jonnesco, and other early masters of spinal anesthesia used a cervical approach for thyroidectomy and thoracic procedures, but this radical approach was supplanted in 1928 by the lumbar injection of hypobaric solutions of "light" nupercaine by G.P. Pitkin in America and E. Etherington–Wilson of Britain 5 years later. Although hypobaric solutions are now virtually limited to patients in the jackknife position, their former use for thoracic procedures demanded skill and precise timing. The enthusiasts of hypobaric anesthesia devised formulae to attempt to predict the time in seconds needed for a warmed solution of hypobaric nupercaine to spread in patients of varying size from its site of injection in the lumbar area to the level of the fourth thoracic dermatome. At this time, the patient was suddenly tipped head down so that the drug would not involve the innervation of the diaphragm and larynx. Among the accepted risks of the hypobaric technique was a prompt and total sympathetic blockade, which occurred so predictably that wise clinicians advised their residents, "Don't bother taking the blood pressure! I know that it will be down." Even the most expert practitioners of this now-abandoned approach identified some limitations. Etherington–Wilson observed that cranial surgery under spinal anesthesia should be left in the hands of an expert.

The recurring problem of inadequate duration of single-injection spinal anesthesia led a Philadelphia surgeon, William Lemmon, to report an apparatus for continuous spinal anesthesia in 1940.[22] Lemmon's procedure began with the patient in the lateral position. The spinal tap was performed with a malleable silver needle, which was left in position. As the patient was turned supine, the needle was positioned through a hole in the mattress and table. Additional injections of local anesthetic could be performed as required. Lemmon's malleable silver needles also found a less cumbersome and more common application in 1942 when Waldo Edwards and Robert Hingson encouraged the use of Lemmon's needles for continuous caudal anesthesia in obstetrics.

After his military service, the Mayo Clinic's Edward Tuohy

introduced two important modifications of the continuous spinal technique. He developed the now-familiar Tuohy needle as a means of improving the ease of passage of lacquered silk ureteral catheters through which he injected incremental doses of local anesthetic.[23] In 1949, Martinez Curbelo of Havana, Cuba, used Tuohy's needle and an ureteral catheter to perform the first continuous epidural anesthetic. Silk and gum elastic ureteral catheters were difficult to sterilize and sometimes caused infections before they were superseded by disposable plastic catheters.

EPIDURAL ANESTHESIA

Deliberate single injection peridural anesthesia had been practiced occasionally for decades before continuous techniques brought it greater popularity. At the beginning of this century, two French clinicians experimented independently with caudal anesthesia. The neurologist, Jean Athanase Sicard, applied the technique for a nonsurgical purpose, the relief of back pain. Fernand Cathelin used caudal anesthesia as a less dangerous alternative to spinal anesthesia for hernia repairs. He wrote a thesis on epidural anesthesia in which he demonstrated the upper limit of the epidural space in the neck of a dog after injecting a solution of India ink into its caudal canal.

The lumbar approach was first used for multiple paravertebral nerve blocks before the Pages–Dogliotti single-injection technique became accepted. The technique is identified with both names, as they worked separately. Captain Fidel Pagés prepared an elegant demonstration of segmental single-injection peridural anesthesia in 1921, but his paper appeared only in a Spanish military journal.[24] Pagés died in the line of duty before he could prepare additional reports. Ten years later, Achille M. Dogliotti of Turin, Italy, wrote a classic study that made the epidural technique well known.[25] Whereas Pagés used a tactile approach to identify the epidural space, Dogliotti identified it by the loss-of-resistance technique still taught today.

NERVE BLOCK OF THE EXTREMITIES

Surgery on the extremities lent itself to other regional anesthesia techniques. At first, they were often combined with general anesthesia. In 1902, Harvey Cushing coined the phrase "regional anesthesia" for his technique of blocking either the brachial or sciatic plexus under direct vision during general anesthesia in order to reduce anesthesia requirements and provide postoperative pain relief.[26] Fifteen years before his publication, a similar approach had been energetically advanced to reduce the stress and shock of surgery by George Crile who was another dedicated advocate of the use of regional and infiltration techniques during general anesthesia.

An intravenous technique of applying procaine peripherally was described in 1908 by August Bier, the surgeon who had pioneered spinal blockade. Bier injected procaine into a vein of the upper limb between two tourniquets. Even though the technique is termed the Bier block, it was not used for many decades until it was reintroduced 55 years later by C.McK. Holmes, who modified the technique by exsanguination before applying a single cuff. Holmes used lidocaine, the very successful amide local anesthetic synthesized in 1943 by Lofgren and Lundquist of Sweden.

Several investigators achieved upper extremity anesthesia by percutaneous injections of the brachial plexus. In 1911, based on his intimate knowledge of the anatomy of the axillary area, Hirschel promoted a "blind" axillary injection. In the same year, Kulenkampff described a supraclavicular approach in which the operator sought out paresthesias of the plexus while keeping the needle at a point superficial to the first rib and the pleura. The risk of pneumothorax with Kulenkampff's approach led Mulley to attempt blocks more proximally by a lateral paravertebral approach, the precursor of what is now popularly known as the *Winnie block*. An excellent historic review of brachial plexus anesthesia is presented in Professor Winnie's fine text, *Plexus Anesthesia*.

TEXTBOOKS OF REGIONAL ANESTHESIA

Heinrich Braun wrote the earliest text of local anesthesia, which appeared in its first English translation in 1914. Although many books appeared in the next decade, one text dominated the American market for 20 years after 1922. This classic was Gaston Labat's *Regional Anesthesia*. When Labat arrived from France to begin a brief period of service as a surgeon with a special interest in regional anesthesia at the Mayo Clinic, he was already familiar with writing on the subject, as he had served as a coeditor of Pauchet's French text on regional anesthesia. Labat soon took a permanent position at the Bellevue Hospital in New York, where he worked with Hippolite Wertheim and an eager younger anesthesiologist from the University of Wisconsin, Emery Rovenstine. They formed the first American Society for Regional Anesthesia. Rovenstine developed the first American clinic for the treatment of chronic pain. He and his associates refined techniques of therapeutic injections for the relief of pain, an important element of the treatment provided in a modern pain clinic.

The development of the multidisciplinary pain clinic has been one part of the many contributions to anesthesiology made by John J. Bonica, a renowned teacher of regional techniques. During his periods of military, civilian, and university service, John Bonica formulated a series of improvements in the management of patients with chronic pain. His classic 1500-page text of 1953, *The Management of Pain*, was a monumental achievement of its time and is still regarded as a classic of the literature of anesthesia. Professor Bonica was also a pioneer in the development of obstetric anesthesia. He served with extraordinary dedication to establish, almost singlehandedly, 24-hour coverage for the obstetric patients of his hospital. When he wrote a text of obstetric anesthesia, it was not only directed to practitioners serving in well-equipped institutions but was also designed to help anesthesiologists serving in the less-privileged countries. As the first American President of the World Federation of Societies of Anaesthesiologists, Professor Bonica received honors from the professional societies of many nations for his advancement of regional and obstetric anesthesia in all countries.

ANESTHESIA EQUIPMENT

THE ANESTHESIA MACHINE

During the past few decades, the anesthesia machine has grown to become one of the most imposing objects in the operating room. Physicians of 60 years ago who practiced anesthesia with just a "rag and bottle" would be amazed to observe modern techniques in which fresh gas flows are metered precisely before a predetermined fraction is diverted through a calibrated vaporizer. The gas and vapor mixture then enters a circuit where it may be humidified and warmed en route to the patient. Ventilators permit the mechanical control of respiration. Automated monitors continuously flash numeric and oscilloscopic signals to reflect the well-being of the patient and the performance of the apparatus. A deviation in any of several monitored variables may excite a strident alarm.

Modern medical practice demands that the patient be attended in a well-equipped surgical suite. In the 19th century, however, medical services were often provided in the patient's home. With the exception of the devices created by John Snow, Joseph Clover, Edmund Andrews, Paul Bert, and a few others, almost every early practitioner carried his simple pieces of equipment in a coat pocket, and, if a manufactured mask was not available, they learned to fabricate a substitute from household objects such as a towel, a newspaper, or a Derby hat. At that time, patient monitoring was limited to the observation of physical signs. Since chloroform was known to be hazardous in excessive concentrations, a series of cunningly contrived chloroform inhalers were used in Britain and Europe after 1867. After 1870, a few practitioners favored the use of tiny metal containers of compressed nitrous oxide and oxygen, but the application of the technique was limited by the cost of renting the cylinders and purchasing the gases. The cylinders had originally been designed to receive illuminating gas for theatrical companies who created an early spotlight, the "limelight," by directing the light of a flame through a cylinder of lime. Early anesthetists followed the practice of theatrical personnel, who had to have both hands free to direct the spotlight by placing the cylinders on the floor and controlling flow by simple foot-operated valves. Anesthesiologists did not have multistaged reducing valves, so the gas escaped at cylinder pressure to be collected in a reservoir bag from which the patient breathed.

After 1900, free-standing anesthesia machines began to appear in America and in Germany. Some of the most sophisticated of these were created by Heinrich Draeger and his son, Bernhaard, who adapted compressed gas technology originally developed for rescue apparatus used by miners. In the United States, a dentist, Charles Teter, developed a continuous-flow nitrous oxide/oxygen/ether machine in 1900 that lacked flowmeters. Jay Heidbrink modified Teter's machine by adding reducing valves. Water-bubble flowmeters produced by Frederick Cotton and Walter Boothby of Harvard University in 1912 allowed the proportion and flow rates of gases to be determined for the first time. The Cotton and Boothby apparatus was modified into a practical portable machine by James Tayloe Gwathmey of New York. Gwathmey used his machine in France during World War I, where its features were admired by a British anesthesiologist, Henry E.G. "Cockie" Boyle, who incorporated them in the design of the first of the long series of "Boyle" machines that were marketed by the Coxeter and British Oxygen Corporations for many years.

After 1910, American manufacturers continued to bring forward many new innovations, which were widely admired. Some entrepreneurs, including Charles Teter and Elmer McKesson, were anesthesiologists, and others were surgeons, such as Karl Connell and Elmer Gatch. Richard von Foregger was an engineer who was unusually receptive to anesthesiologists' suggestions about additional features, which were subsequently added to his Foregger anesthesia machines.

The machines reflected the practices of the times in which they were created. For many years, a Yale physiologist, Yandell Henderson, argued that high concentrations of carbon dioxide were beneficial. He encouraged rebreathing or the addition of supplemental carbon dioxide to stimulate respiration during either anesthesia or resuscitation. He argued that hypercapnia prevented shock. As a consequence, many early machines featured supplemental cylinders of carbon dioxide. In an era of inflammable anesthetics, Elmer McKesson carried nonflammable nitrous oxide anesthesia to its therapeutic limit by performing inductions with 100% nitrous oxide and thereafter adding small volumes of oxygen. If the resultant cyanosis became too profound, McKesson depressed a valve on his machine that flushed a small volume of oxygen into the circuit. Even though his techniques of primary and secondary saturation with nitrous oxide are no longer used, the oxygen flush valve is part of McKesson's legacy.

CARBON DIOXIDE ABSORBERS

The first use of carbon dioxide absorbers in anesthesia came in 1906 from the work of Franz Kuhn, a German surgeon. His use of cannisters developed for mine rescues was a bold innovation, but his circuit had unfortunate limitations: exceptionally narrow breathing tubes and a large deadspace, which might explain its very limited use. A few years later, the first American machine with a carbon dioxide absorber was fabricated by Dennis Jackson.

While working as a physiologist and pharmacologist in St. Louis, Missouri, in 1915, Dennis Jackson (1878–1979) developed an early technique of carbon dioxide absorption that permitted the use of a closed anesthesia circuit. His laboratory was located in an area heavily laden with coal smoke; thus, Professor Jackson reported that the apparatus allowed him the first breaths of absolutely fresh air he had ever enjoyed in St. Louis. He used solutions of sodium and calcium hydroxide to absorb carbon dioxide. The complexity of the apparatus limited its use in hospital practice, but his pioneering work in this field encouraged Ralph Waters to introduce a simpler device using soda-lime granules 9 years later.

Ralph Waters (1882–1979) positioned a soda-lime cannister between a facemask and an adjacent breathing bag to which was attached the fresh gas flow. As long as the mask was held against the face, only small volumes of fresh gas flow were required and no valves were needed. When the soda lime near the mask could absorb no more carbon dioxide, the cannister was reversed to present a fresh supply close to the patient.

When Waters made his first "to-and-fro" device, he was attempting to develop a specialist practice in anesthesia in Sioux City, Iowa, and was achieving only limited financial success. Waters believed that his device had advantages for both the clinician and the patient.[27] Economy of operation was an important advance at a time when private patients and insurance companies were reluctant to pay not only for professional services but even for the drugs and supplies that had been purchased by the anesthesiologist. Waters estimated that his new cannister would reduce his costs for gases and soda lime to less than $.50 per hour. Waters' apparatus was very portable. The cannister was easy to carry to the patient's home and, in any setting, prevented the pollution of the operating environment with the malodorous vapors of the anesthetics then used. His report recognized other advantages. The patient's body heat was conserved. The inspired gases were automatically humidified. Finally, he stated that his clinical observations showed that there was no need for carbon dioxide rebreathing as advocated by Yandell Henderson.

An awkward element of Waters' device was the position of the cannister by the patient's face. Brian Sword overcame this limitation in 1930 with a circle system that featured unidirectional valves and an in-circuit carbon dioxide absorber (Fig. 1-6).[28] The circle system popularized by Sword nearly 60 years ago remains the most common anesthesia circuit.

Concern over the resistance to gas flow within the circuit caused by sticking inspiratory and expiratory valves led to modifications of equipment in Canada and Britain. Daniel Revell of Victoria, British Columbia, introduced the Revell Circulator, whose spinning blades kept the gases moving continuously around the circle system at a rate that eliminated valve-induced resistance to respiration.[29]

A second valveless device, the Ayre's T piece has found wide application in the management of intubated patients. Phillip Ayre practiced anesthesia when the limitations of equipment for pediatric patients produced what he termed " . . . a protracted and sanguine battle between surgeon and anaesthetist with the poor unfortunate baby as the battlefield."[30] In 1937, Ayre introduced his valveless T piece to reduce the effort of breathing in neurosurgical patients, but the T piece found a much broader application in cleft palate repairs. This ingenious, lightweight, valveless, nonrebreathing method has passed through more than 100 modifications for a variety of special situations. A significant alteration was Gordon Jackson Rees' modification, which permitted improved control of ventilation by substituting a breathing bag on the outflow limb for the simple expiratory tube of the original T piece that was periodically obstructed by the anesthesiologist's thumb to produce inspiration at what could be an erratic rate.[31]

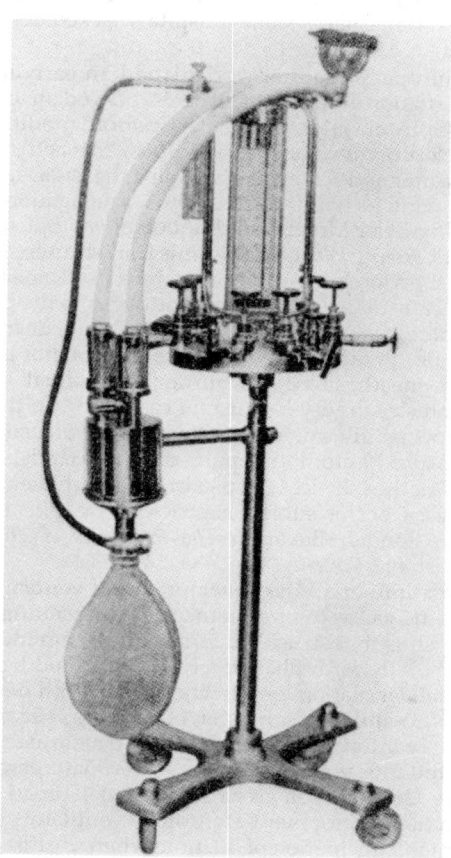

FIG. 1-6. Brian Sword's closed circle anesthesia machine (1930).

Another method to reduce the amount of equipment near the patient is that provided by the coaxial circuit of the Bain–Spoerel apparatus.[32] This lightweight tube-within-a-tube has served very well in many circumstances since its Canadian innovators at the University of Western Ontario described it in 1972, but, as in other situations, the Bain–Spoerel circuit has not been the first application of coaxial circuitry in anesthesia. Some late 19th century inhalers, including Hewitt's 1890 chloroform apparatus, used a tube-within-a-tube to lead air into the vaporizer and then back within a smaller tube to the patient.

A second precursor of the modern coaxial circuit was that developed during World War II by Richard Salt and Edgar Pask for tests undertaken by the Royal Air Force of different types of life jackets. This work was prompted by the loss of airmen who had "ditched" without injury in the waters off England and whose drowned bodies were discovered face down, even though they were wearing a life jacket. Their flotation devices had failed to hold their face above water once they lost consciousness from hypothermia. In order to mimic the motions of an unconscious person, Dr. Pask was given ether anesthesia while intubated, then placed in a swimming pool while wearing one of a series of experimental jackets. Even if the jacket failed and his body sank, the coaxial circuit continued to perform safely as the expiratory valve was above water at the level of the anesthesia machine. Once the Pask–Salt experiments were completed, the coaxial circuit passed from use until other applications were recognized by Drs. Bain and Spoerel.

FLOWMETERS

As closed and semiclosed circuit anesthesia became practical after 1930, there was a need to measure gas flow with greater accuracy. Wet flowmeters were replaced with dry bobbins and ball-bearing flowmeters, which, although they did not leak or spill, could cause inaccurate measurements if they adhered to the wall of the surrounding glass column. After World War II, freely moving rotameters provided greater accuracy for British and North American machines, but this technology had already been well developed in Germany by Deutsche Rotawerke decades before in 1908. At about the same time that all American manufacturers accepted rotameters of European origin, they also accepted metric measurements of gas flow. Before that time, only Connell and Foregger machines had displayed liters of gas flow.

VAPORIZERS

Uncalibrated glass vaporizers could be used with confidence for the administration of ether but were inadequate for more potent agents. Skilled practitioners gave ethyl chloride and chloroform with safety, but their success was built upon their expertise. Their approach was based primarily on subjective observations that were difficult to communicate to neophytes. When the inspired concentration of a potent anesthetic was unknown, the art of a smooth induction was a greater challenge.

This was particularly true for halothane; an excessive rate of administration produced lethal degrees of cardiovascular depression. The clinical introduction of halothane after 1956 might have been thwarted except for a fortunate coincidence: the prior development of calibrated vaporizers. Two types of calibrated vaporizers designed for the administration of other anesthetics had become available in the half decade before halothane was marketed. The initial prompt acceptance of the drug was in part due to the clinician's ability to provide it in carefully titrated concentrations.

The first of these was the copper kettle vaporizer, which had been developed by Lucien Morris at the University of Wisconsin in response to Professor Ralph Waters' desire to give chloroform in carefully controlled concentrations.[33] Morris achieved this by passing a metered flow of oxygen through a vaporizer chamber that contained a porex disk to separate the oxygen into tiny bubbles, which became fully saturated with anesthetic vapor as they percolated through the liquid. The concentration of the anesthetic inspired by the patient could be easily calculated through knowledge of the vapor pressure of the anesthetic, the gas flow through the vaporizer, and the total volume of gas from all sources entering the anesthesia circuit. Although experimental models of Morris' vaporizer used a water bath to maintain stability, the excellent thermal conductivity of copper was substituted in later models to maintain a more stable pressure—a suggestion that Dr. Morris recognized was first proposed by John Snow in January 1847. When first marketed, the copper kettle did not feature a thermometer to indicate changes in the temperature (and vapor pressure) of the liquid. Shuh–Hsun Ngai proposed the addition of a thermometer, a suggestion that was later incorporated in all vaporizers of that class.

Copper kettle (Foregger Company) and Vernitrol (Ohio Medical Products) vaporizers were universal vaporizers—a property that remained a distinct advantage as newer anesthetics were marketed. They could be charged with any anesthetic liquid, and, provided that the vapor pressure and temperature were known, the inspired concentration could be calculated quickly and with confidence. This feature gave an advantage to American investigators of newer anesthetics, for they were not dependent upon the construction of an agent-specific vaporizer.

Halothane was first marketed in Britain, where an effective temperature-compensated, agent-specific vaporizer had recently been placed in clinical use. It had been developed for obstetric analgesia, as many women were delivered at home by midwives who needed a safe portable machine with which to give their patients an inhaled analgesic. The TECOTA (TEmperature COmpensated Trichloroethylene Air) vaporizer had been created by two engineers who had become frustrated by a giant corporation's unresponsiveness to their proposals and who had set about starting a new company, Cyprane Limited. The TECOTA featured a bimetallic strip composed of brass and a nickel–steel alloy—two metals with different coefficients of expansion. As the anesthetic vapor cooled, the strip moved away from an orifice, thereby permitting more fresh gas to enter the vaporizing chamber. This maintained an unchanging inspired concentration of anesthetic despite changes in temperature and, as a consequence, vapor pressure. After their TECOTA vaporizer was accepted by the Central Midwives Board, their company soon gained a much greater success by adapting their technological advance to create the "Fluotec," the first of a series of agent-specific "tec" vaporizers for use in the operating room. All major manufacturers now offer a similar instrument.

VENTILATORS

Mechanical ventilators are now an integral part of the anesthesia machine. Patients are ventilated during general anesthesia by electrical or gas-powered devices that are simple to control yet sophisticated in their function. These casually employed devices were created by men and women of many countries who were responding to a variety of clinical problems.

The history of mechanical positive pressure ventilation begins with attempts to resuscitate animals or humans by a pump or bellows attached to a mask or tracheal tube, but these experiments had no place in anesthetic care for many years. At the beginning of this century, several other modalities were explored before intermittent positive pressure machines evolved.

One of these processes began as a result of the first thoracic surgeons being frustrated by the collapse of the lungs when they opened the pleura of spontaneously breathing patients. Between 1900 and 1910, sophisticated artificial environments were created in which the thoracic patient's lungs were kept in an inflated position by utilizing one of two ambitious alternatives: the positive and negative pressure techniques. The patient's head and neck could be placed in a box maintaining pressure in excess of atmospheric, or the head might project through a gas-tight hole in the wall of a subatmospheric chamber, which enclosed his body below the neck and the entire surgical team. With the first of these options, the anesthesiologist attended a patient whose head was hidden in a box; with the second option, the anesthesiologist had free access to the patient's head only; the rest of his body was sequestered in the chamber.

After World War I, intermittent automatic positive pressure devices were developed that rhythmically inflated the lungs such as the Dräger "Pulmotor" and the E & J Resuscitator. These were used almost exclusively for resuscitation by firemen and other rescue workers. There are legends dating from before 1940 that, in some small communities, doctors occasionally called for the fire department to assist in the ventilation of patients who had suddenly stopped breathing in the operating room. Many small hospitals lacked resuscitation equipment.

A few European medical workers had an early interest in rhythmic inflation of the lungs. In 1934, a Swedish team developed the "Spiropulsator," which C. Crafoord modified for use during cyclopropane anesthesia by 1938.[34] Its action was controlled by a magnetic control valve called the *flasher*, a type first used to provide intermittent gas flow for navigational marker buoys. When Trier Morch could not obtain a "Spiropulsator" in Denmark during World War II, this Danish anesthesiologist fabricated the Morch "Respirator," which used a piston pump to rhythmically deliver a fixed volume of gas to the patient. At the same time, a motorcycle engineer in Britain developed the prototype of the motor-driven Blease Pulmoflator in order to lessen the anesthesiologist's burden of manual ventilation during thoracic surgery for air raid casualties. In those days, when purpose-built miniature motors were unavailable, mechanics adapted automotive parts such as windshield blade motors and other devices for use in their early ventilators. A superb review of this subject is provided by William Mushin and Leslie Rendell–Baker in *The Principles of Thoracic Anaesthesia Past and Present.*

A major stimulus to the development of ventilators in Europe came in 1952 as a consequence of a devastating epidemic of poliomyelitis that struck Copenhagen, Denmark. The only effective therapy for bulbar paralysis that could be provided was manual ventilation by a tracheostomy with devices such as Waters' "to-and-fro" cannister, but this was successful only through the continuous efforts of scores of volunteers. Danish medical students served in relays to ventilate paralyzed patients. The Copenhagen crisis stimulated a broad European interest in the development of portable ventilators to prepare equipment in anticipation of the time when the disease would strike again in epidemic proportions.

At this time, the practice in North American hospitals was to place polio patients with respiratory involvement in "iron lungs"—large metal cylinders that encased the body below the neck. Inspiration was caused by intermittent negative pressure created by an electric motor acting on a piston-like device occupying the foot of the chamber. After an epidemic, as many as ten or 12 "iron lungs" might be operated in a single room.

One now-distinguished consultant recalls that he became irrevocably committed to the development of better ventilators as an intern when he found himself alone with a dozen patients in "iron lungs" at the moment of a power failure. Before help arrived, he was exhausted by repeated urgent circuit of the room as he manually pumped the lever of each iron lung for a few life-sustaining breaths. His frantic efforts were rewarded by his helpless patients, who whispered their appreciation, "Way . . . to go . . . Wally!" Then they lay apneic until he could once again give them another mechanical breath.

Many early American ventilators were adaptations of respiratory-assist machines originally designed for the delivery of aerosolized drugs for respiratory therapy. Two of these were the Bennett and Bird "flow-sensitive" valves. The Bennett valve was designed during World War II when a team of physiologists at the University of Southern California encountered difficulties in separating inspiration from expiration in an experimental apparatus for positive pressure breathing designed for high-altitude aviators. An engineer, Ray Bennett, visited their laboratory, observed their problem, and resolved it with a mechanical flow-sensitive automatic valve. A second valving mechanism was later designed by an aeronautical engineer, Forrest Bird, whose Bird ventilators still find wide applications.

The use of the Bird and Bennett valves gained an anesthetic application when the gas flow from the valve was directed into a plastic or glass jar containing a breathing bag or bellows as part of an anesthesia circuit. These "bag in bottle" devices mimicked the action of the anesthesiologist's hand as the gas flow compressed the bag providing positive pressure inspiration. Passive exhalation was promoted by the descent of a weight on the bag or bellows. The function of the components of some of the first machines to use these principles could be examined with ease through clear plastic, whereas now they are hidden in the interior of the instrument. It is currently possible to operate an anesthesia machine and ventilator for years without becoming aware of the principles that direct its action and protect against malfunction.

OPERATING ROOM MONITORS

The use of equipment to promote the safety of patients in the operating room has evolved since 1900. Early clinicians concentrated on physical signs—the patient's color, the briskness of capillary refill, the dilation and position of the pupil, the regularity and depth of respiration, as well as the force and regularity of the pulse. These signs were subjective and difficult to teach and required experience to interpret.

Two American surgeons, George W. Crile and Harvey Cushing, developed a strong interest in measuring blood pressure during anesthesia. Both men wrote thorough and detailed examinations of blood pressure monitoring; however, Cushing's contribution is better remembered because he was the first American to apply the Riva Rocci cuff, which he saw while visiting Italy. Cushing introduced the concept in 1902 and had blood pressure measurements recorded on anesthesia records.[26] These improved records were the successor to

those that Cushing and a colleague at Harvard Medical School, Charles Codman, had first used in their attempt to assess the course of the anesthetics they administered as students.

Anesthesiologists began to auscultate blood pressure after 1905 when Nicholai Korotkoff, a surgeon-in-training in St. Petersburg, Russia, gave an abbreviated report of the sounds that he heard distal to the Riva Rocci cuff as it was deflated. Although his one-paragraph account does not explain why he came to listen over a normal vessel—a novel approach now used universally for the clinical measurement of blood pressure—it may be that his commitment to vascular surgery caused him to auscultate vessels in the assessment of masses that might be vascular and produce a bruit. Perhaps he happened to have his stethoscope positioned over a vessel as a cuff was deflated and fortuitously heard sounds never appreciated before. Cuffs and stethoscopes are now often replaced by automated blood pressure devices, which first appeared in 1936 and which operate on an oscillometric principle. The recent development of inexpensive microprocessors has promoted the routine use of these automatic cuffs in clinical settings. A detailed review of other elements of cardiovascular monitoring can be found in Leslie Geddes, *Cardiovascular Devices and Their Applications*.

Anesthesiologists routinely auscultate breath and heart sounds with precordial or esophageal stethoscopes. The first precordial scope was believed to have been used by S. Griffith Davis at Johns Hopkins University.[35] He adapted a technique favored by Harvey Cushing in the animal laboratory in which dogs with surgically induced valvular lesions had stethoscopes attached to their chest wall so that medical students might listen to bruits characteristic of a specific malformation. Davis' technique was forgotten but was rehabilitated by Robert Smith, an energetic pediatric anesthesiologist in Boston. A Canadian contemporary, A. Codesmith, of the Hospital for Sick Children, Toronto, soon became frustrated by the repeated dislodging of his chest piece under the surgical drapes and fabricated his first esophageal stethoscope from urethral catheters and Penrose drains. His brief report heralded its clinical role as a monitor of both normal and adventitious respiratory and cardiac sounds.[36] An additional benefit was that the stethoscope could serve as a monitor to protect against the risk of disconnection of the patient from the anesthesia circuit. The patient's survival could depend upon an alert anesthesiologist's recognition of the sudden disappearance of breath sounds.

ANESTHESIA MACHINE MONITORS

The introduction of safety features is coordinated by the American National Standards Committee Z79, which has been sponsored since 1956 by the American Society of Anesthesiologists. Representatives from industry, government agencies, and health care professions meet to establish voluntary guidelines, which become accepted standards for the safety of anesthesia equipment.

Ralph Tovell (1901–1967) was the first anesthesiologist to urge standards during World War II while he was the Senior Army Consultant in Anesthesiology in Europe. Tovell learned that supplies dispatched to field hospitals might not fit their anesthesia machines, since there were no standard dimensions for connectors, tubes, or breathing bags. As Tovell observed, " . . . when a sudden need for accessory equipment arose, nurses and corpsmen were likely to respond to it by bringing parts that would not fit."[37] Although Tovell's reports did not gain an immediate response, two anesthesiologists,

Vincent Collins and Hamilton Davis, took up his concern and formed Committee Z79 in 1956.

One of the Committee's most active members, Professor Leslie Rendell–Baker, has prepared an interesting account of its domestic and international achievements.[38] Ralph Tovell, an early member, encouraged all manufacturers to select a uniform orifice of 22 mm for all adult and pediatric facemasks and to make every endotracheal tube connector 15 mm in diameter so that any mask–tube elbow adapter will fit every mask and endotracheal tube connector. Through the cooperative spirit fostered by the Z79 Committee, the anxieties encountered by Tovell and his military colleagues of World War II have been overcome.

Several other hazards have been eliminated by the Z79 Committee. Touch identification of oxygen flow control reduced the risk of the wrong gas being turned up before internal mechanical controls prevented the selection of an hypoxic mixture. These devices were helpful only if the gas in the line was oxygen. For many years, errors committed by plumbers or technicians in reassembling hospital oxygen supply lines led to a series of tragedies before "pin indexing" of connectors was introduced and polarographic oxygen analyzers were added to the inspiratory limb of the anesthesia circuit.

PATIENT MONITORS

Safer machines only assured the clinician that an appropriate gas mixture was delivered to the patient. As the practice of anesthesia evolved from being simply the administration of an anesthetic to become the assumption of professional responsibility for the care of patients during and after surgery, other monitors were required that would give an early warning of hazardous conditions before the patient suffered irrevocable damage. Every anesthesiologist who has remained in practice during the past 30 years has witnessed a great series of advances in monitoring with the advent of clinically employable forms of electrocardiography, arterial blood gas analysis, mass spectrometry, computer-processed electroencephalography, and oximetry.

Electrocardiography

Electrocardiography became practical with Willem Einthoven's application of the string galvanometer in 1903. Within 2 decades, Thomas Lewis had described its role in the diagnosis of disturbances of cardiac rhythm, while James Herrick and Harold Pardee had drawn attention to the changes produced by myocardial ischemia. After 1928, cathode ray oscilloscopes were available, but the risk of explosion owing to the presence of inflammable anesthetics forestalled the introduction of the ECG into routine anesthetic practice until after World War II. The tiny screen of the heavily shielded "bullet" oscilloscope displayed only 3 seconds of data, but that information came to be highly prized. In some hospitals, priorities were established to determine where the expensive monitor was to be used. When an assistant was dispatched to bring the "bullet" scope, everyone knew that a major anesthetic enterprise was about to begin. In modern practice, the ECG is a normal routine offered to all patients.

Arterial Blood Gas Analysis

Before 1955, the estimation of the tension of gases of the blood was a delicate activity performed best by skilled research technicians who conducted their intricate art in laboratories far removed from the operating room. Within a few years, however, the contributions of Astrup, Siggaard–Anderson, Stow, Bradley, Severinghaus, and Clark brought radical improvements in patient care through the creation of rapidly responding electrodes. Time-consuming multistaged analyses gave way to instruments whose complex functions were automated to a degree that allowed them to be operated at any hour. Many practitioners recall the historic impact of arterial blood gas analysis upon their professional practice as information of vital importance returned to the clinician within minutes.

The series of discoveries that led to the clinical application of arterial blood gas analysis have been brilliantly recounted in two volumes by Poul Astrup and John Severinghaus, *The History of Blood Gases, Acids and Bases* and its companion from the International Anesthesiology Clinics series Volume 25, Number 4, *History of Blood Gas Analysis*. Both books captivate the reader and should be enjoyed by all students of anesthesiology.

Mass Spectrometry

Although arterial blood gas determinations could be performed within minutes, anesthesiologists have recognized a need for breath by breath measurement of respiratory and anesthetic gases. After 1954, infrared absorption techniques gave immediate displays of the exhaled concentration of carbon dioxide. Clinicians quickly learned to relate abnormal concentrations of carbon dioxide to threatening situations such as the inappropriate placement of an endotracheal tube in the esophagus, abrupt alterations in pulmonary blood flow, and other factors.[39] These devices have been supplanted by mass spectrometers that display not only carbon dioxide but also the inspired and expired concentrations of other gases and anesthetic vapors. Mass spectrometry had only industrial applications before Albert Faulconer of the Mayo Clinic first used it to monitor the concentration of an exhaled anesthetic in 1954.

Electroencephalography

Dr. Faulconer was also a pioneer in the use of the electroencephalograph (EEG) in anesthesia. In 1946, Faulconer and a colleague, John W. Pender, began to work with an exceptionally gifted neurologist, Reginald Bickford, in studies of the effects of a variety of anesthetics on the EEG.[40] They related changes in anesthetic depth to alterations in the pattern of the EEG tracing and even extended their observations to include the hyperbaric administration of nitrous oxide and oxygen. Immediate application of their observations was limited by the technology of that time, but, after moving to the University of California, San Diego, Professor Bickford returned to his interest in anesthesia as a practical application of the computer-generated Compressed Spectral Array, which he had been instrumental in developing. Professor Bickford maintains an active involvement in anesthetic applications of the processed EEG more than 40 years after he and his Mayo Clinic colleagues first took up this study.

Pulse Oximetry

The pulse oximeter is the most recent addition to the anesthesiologist's array of routine monitors. This application of the optical measurement of oxygen saturation in tissues has been, by John Severinghaus' assessment, of exceptional importance. In a fine history of pulse oximetry, Severinghaus states, "Pulse oximetry is arguably the most important technological advance ever made in monitoring the well-being and safety of patients during anesthesia, recovery and critical care."[41]

Severinghaus wrote that although research in this area began in 1932, its first practical application came during World War II. An American physiologist, Glen Millikan, responded to a request from British colleagues in aviation research. Millikan set about preparing a series of devices to improve the supply of oxygen that was provided pilots flying at high altitude in unpressurized aircraft. In order to monitor oxygen delivery and to prevent the pilot from succumbing to an unrecognized failure of his oxygen supply, Millikan created an oxygen-sensing monitor worn on the pilot's earlobe, and coined the name *oximeter* to describe its action. Before his tragic death in a climbing accident in 1947, Millikan had begun to assess anesthetic applications of oximetry.

For the next 3 decades, oximetry was rarely used by anesthesiologists, and then primarily in research studies such as those of Faulconer and Pender. Recent refinements of oximetry by a Japanese engineer, Takuo Aoyagi, led to a new departure, the development of *pulse oximetry*. As Severinghaus recounted the episode, Aoyagi had attempted to eliminate the changes in a signal caused by pulsatile variations when he realized that this fluctuation could be used to measure both the pulse and oxygen saturation. Professor Severinghaus observed this was " . . . a classic example of the adage that 'one man's noise is another man's signal'."[42]

INTUBATION IN ANESTHESIA

All anesthesiologists are expected to be adept in the art of endotracheal intubation. They are assisted in this complex task by a variety of instruments that allow them to intubate the trachea of patients with severe anatomic abnormalities that would have been beyond the skill of all but the most expert (or fortunate) practitioner of past decades. The development of techniques and instruments for intubation ranks among the major advances in the history of the specialty. We are supported by a magnificent heritage of innovation and discovery that has come to us through the efforts of scores of persons of whom only a few are remembered through the eponyms attached to the Guedel airway, Magill forceps, and Macintosh blade.

The landmark advances in intubation form a fascinating history filled with episodes of brilliant observation, forgotten or unappreciated invention, rediscovery, and clinical advance. When possible, the first discoverer of an instrument will be identified, but, in other instances, the person who successfully brought it into regular use will receive greater attention. Although most of the achievements related to intubation have been realized in this century, a few date from Victorian times.

Nineteenth-Century Intubation

The first endotracheal tubes were developed for the resuscitation of the newborn and victims of drowning but were not used in anesthesia until 1878. Although John Snow and others had already anesthetized patients by means of a tracheostomy, the first use of elective oral intubation for an anesthetic was undertaken by a Scottish surgeon, William Macewan. He had practiced passing flexible metal tubes through the larynx of a cadaver before attempting the maneuver on an awake patient with an oral tumor at the Glasgow Royal Infirmary on July 5, 1878.[43] Since topical anesthesia was not yet known, the experience must have demanded fortitude by Macewan's patient, because his airway was unanesthetized. Once the tube was correctly positioned, an assistant gave a chloroform anesthetic through the tube, and the patient soon stopped coughing. Macewan's interest in intubation of the trachea was only transient. Even though he performed successful awake intubations for at least two other patients with severe obstructions of the upper airway, one owing to infection and the other to the too-rapid ingestion of a hot potato, he abandoned the practice following an unusual fatality. His last patient had been intubated while awake but had removed the tube before the anesthetic could begin and had later died while receiving chloroform by mask.

JOSEPH O'DWYER (1841–1898). Although there was a sporadic interest in endotracheal anesthesia in Edinburgh and other European centers, a contemporary American surgeon is remembered for his extraordinary dedication to the advancement of tracheal intubation. Joseph O'Dwyer had witnessed the distressing death by asphyxiation of children from diphtheria and sought an alternative to the mutilation of a hasty tracheotomy. In 1885, O'Dwyer designed a series of metal laryngeal tubes, which he inserted between the vocal cords of children during a diptheretic crisis. His humanitarian efforts were applauded by colleagues. Three years later, O'Dwyer designed a second rigid tube with a conical tip that occluded the larynx so effectively that it could be used for artificial ventilation when applied with the bellows and T-piece tube of George Fell's apparatus.[44] The Fell–O'Dwyer apparatus was used during thoracic surgery by Rudolph Matas of New Orleans, who was so pleased with it that he predicted, "The procedure that promises the most benefit in preventing pulmonary collapse in operations on the chest is . . . the rhythmical maintenance of artificial respiration by a tube in the glottis directly connected with a bellows."[45] This principle would be occasionally rediscovered by other surgeons for several decades before Matas' prophetic description would become routine.

FRANZ KUHN (1866–1929). After O'Dwyer's death, the outstanding pioneer of tracheal intubation was Franz Kuhn, a surgeon of Kassel, Germany. From 1900 until 1912, Kuhn wrote a series of fine papers and a classic monograph, "Die Perorale Intubation," which were not well known in his lifetime but have since become widely appreciated.[46] Kuhn described techniques of oral and nasal intubation that he performed with flexible metal tubes similar to the coiled tubing used for the spout of metal gasoline cans. Kuhn's tubes were introduced over a curved metal stylet and directed toward the larynx with his left index finger (Fig. 1-7). While he was aware of the subglottic cuffs that had been used briefly by Victor Eisenmenger, Franz Kuhn preferred to seal the larynx by positioning a supralaryngeal flange near the tube's tip before packing the pharynx with gauze. His writings reflect a mastery of intubation techniques unequaled for many years.

Kuhn's work might have had a much more immediate impact if it had been translated into English. Many of his principles were only appreciated after they had been rediscovered by others. His patients were made more comfortable through the use of topical cocaine, a practice that he was the first to use. He was among the first to recommend an inhalation technique through a large tube over the continuous insufflation of gases through narrow tubes that failed to protect the airway. He was the first to suggest that tracheal secretions or blood could be suctioned from the airway through a flexible catheter. He recommended the nasal route for long-term intubation, be-

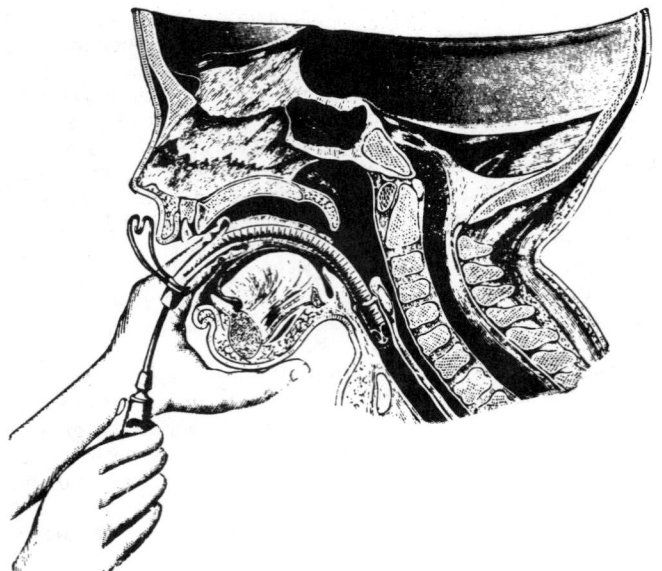

FIG. 1-7. Kuhn's endotracheal tube. The tube and introducer were guided to the trachea by the fingers of the operator's left hand.

cause a nasal tube was more easily tolerated and did not require a dental guard to prevent it from being crushed by a restless patient. Kuhn even monitored the patient's breath sounds continuously through a monaural earpiece that was connected to an extension of the endotracheal tube by a narrow rubber tube.

Early Laryngoscopes

Intubation of the trachea by palpation was an uncertain and sometimes traumatic act. Even though the use of a mirror for indirect laryngoscopy antedated Macewan's intubations, the technique could not be adapted for use in anesthesia. For some years, many surgeons believed that it would be anatomically impossible to visualize the vocal cords directly. This misapprehension was overcome in 1895 by Alfred Kirstein in Berlin who devised the first direct-vision laryngoscope.[47] Kirstein was motivated by a friend's report that a patient's trachea had been accidentally intubated during esophagoscopy. Kirstein promptly fabricated a hand-held instrument that at first resembled a shortened cylindrical esophagoscope. He soon substituted a semicircular blade open inferiorly. Kirstein could now examine the larynx while standing behind his seated patient whose head was placed in an attitude approximating the "sniffing position" later recommended by Ivan Magill. Although Alfred Kirstein's "autoscope" was not used by anesthesiologists, it was the forerunner of all modern laryngoscopes.

Endoscopy was refined by Chevalier Jackson in Philadelphia, who designed a U-shaped laryngoscope by adding a hand grip that was parallel to the blade. The Jackson blade has remained a standard instrument for endoscopists but was not favored by anesthesiologists. Two laryngoscopes that closely resembled modern L-shaped instruments were designed in 1910 and 1913 to facilitate intubation by two American surgeons, Henry Janeway and George Dorrance, but neither instrument achieved lasting use despite their excellent designs.

These clever innovations may have failed to capture wide

attention because intubating laryngoscopes lacked a wide market at a time when there were fewer than 100 anesthesiologists active in the United States. Many of these practitioners had never attempted intubation and might never learn the skill. Even after 1940, it was routine in some hospitals to call a laryngologist to the operating room for every intubation while the attending anesthesiologists confined their attention to providing the anesthetic. In time, however, all anesthesiologists would learn the skills of atraumatic nasal and oral intubation by using the instruments and techniques that would be developed by a few British and North American specialists.

SIR IVAN MAGILL (1888–1986). The most distinguished pioneer of endotracheal intubation was a self-trained British anaesthetist, Ivan (later Sir Ivan) Magill.[48] In 1919, when serving in the Royal Army as a general medical officer with no special interest in anesthesia, Magill was assigned to a military hospital near London that received large numbers of injured men. Although previously untrained in anesthesia, Magill accepted an assignment in the anesthesia service, where he was joined by another neophyte anaesthetist, Stanley Rowbotham.[49] They attended casualties disfigured by severe facial injuries who underwent repeated restorative operations that would be successful only if the surgeon, Harold Gillies, had almost unrestricted access to the face and airway. Some patients were formidable challenges, but both men became competent quickly and, because they were adept and able to appreciate the significance of fortuitous observations, soon extended the scope of early oral and nasal endotracheal anesthesia.

Magill and Rowbotham's expertise with blind nasal intubation began after they learned to soften semirigid insufflation tubes that they passed through the nose after the nostril had been dilated with a series of lubricated tubes. Even though they originally planned to position the tips of the tubes in the posterior pharynx only, the slender tubes sometimes passed directly into the trachea. Stimulated by these chance experiences, Magill developed techniques of deliberate nasotracheal intubation and, as an aid to manipulating the catheter tip, devised the Magill angulated forceps in 1920, which are still manufactured according to Magill's original design of 68 years ago.

He continued to practice anesthesia after he was released from military service. Some time later, Magill set out to develop a wide-bore tube that could be curved into a form resembling the contours of the upper airway but that would also resist kinking. In a hardware store, he found several sizes of mineralized red rubber tubing, which he cut, beveled, and smoothed to produce tubes that clinicians in all countries would come to call "Magill tubes." His tubes remained the standard for universal use for more than 40 years, until rubber products were replaced with inert plastics. Magill also rediscovered the advantages of cocainization of the airway, a technique that he perfected in developing his mastery of awake blind nasal intubation.

Magill's success in performing awake blind nasal intubation of the trachea excited the curiosity of other anaesthetists. Magill shared his principles at meetings attended by the few specialists in anesthesia, but, since his colleagues were also his competitors for the limited private practice opportunities available in London, he sometimes omitted a pertinent point from his review. As a consequence, few members of his audience could match his success.

A few determined men visited Magill to study his craft. He carefully pointed out the advantages of a tube of the correct length and the appropriateness of the "sniffing position," which he described as placing the patient's head in the posture of a man standing before his open bedroom window sniffing the morning air. They marveled at his dexterity and speed at passing the tube, not always realizing that the patient had received topical cocaine before entering the induction area.

Magill soon allowed his small secrets to become public knowledge, but few colleagues ever matched his control of the airway in the time period before muscle relaxants were introduced. Throughout his distinguished and long career, he continued to create new devices for the advantage of all concerned. His innovations included endotracheal tubes for children, an L-shaped laryngoscope, a tracheoscope, and a wire-tipped endotracheal tube for thoracic surgery. The "Magill Circuit," now catalogued as the Mapleson A Circuit, was noted for its simplicity and economy. After a distinguished career, Magill was knighted for his services to anesthesiology. Until his death in his 99th year on November 28, 1986, Sir Ivan Magill was universally recognized as "The Master" of British anesthesiology.

ARTHUR GUEDEL (1883–1956). Arthur Guedel's name is linked to the Guedel airway, but this classic device is only one of several important contributions made by this self-trained pioneer of American anesthesia.[50] The cuffed endotracheal tube is another reflection of his genius. In 1926, unaware of the prior work of Eisenmenger and Dorrance, Guedel began a series of experiments that would lead to the reintroduction of the cuffed tube. His goal was to combine the safety of endotracheal anesthesia with the economy of the closed-circuit technique, which had been recently refined by his friend, Ralph Waters.

Guedel transformed the basement of his Indianapolis home into a small laboratory, where he subjected each step of the preparation and application of his cuffs to a vigorous review.[51] He fashioned cuffs from the rubber of dental dams, condoms, and surgical gloves that were glued onto the outer wall of tubes. Using animal tracheas donated by the family butcher as his model, he considered whether the cuff should be positioned above, below, or at the level of the vocal cords. He recommended that the cuff be positioned just below the vocal cords. In that position, it not only sealed the airway and reduced the risk of the tube becoming dislodged but also prevented the accumulation of fluid below the cords in a position where it might be impossible to remove by suctioning before extubation. Ralph Waters later recommended that cuffs

be constructed of two layers of soft rubber cemented together along the edge so that a ruptured cuff might be readily replaced. The detachable cuffs were first manufactured by Professor Waters' children, who earned money for college by selling the cuffs to the Foregger Company.

Guedel demonstrated the safety and utility of his cuff in his hospital. He filled the mouth of an anesthetized and intubated patient with water and showed that the cuff sealed the airway. Even though this exhibition was successful, he searched for a more dramatic technique to capture the attention of an audience unfamiliar with the advantages of intubation. He reasoned that if the cuff would prevent water from entering the trachea of an intubated patient, it should also prevent an animal from drowning, even it if were to be submerged under water.

In order to encourage others to use endotracheal techniques, Guedel prepared the first of several "dunked dog" demonstrations (Fig. 1-8). An anesthetized and intubated dog, Guedel's own pet, Airway, was immersed in an aquarium. After the demonstration was complete, the anesthetic was discontinued and the animal removed from the water. Airway awoke promptly, shook water over the onlookers then exited the hall to the applause of the audience. With this novel demonstration, the cuffed tube gradually gained wide use.

Endobronchial Tubes

Talented observers can recognize a therapeutic opportunity when presented with what at first appears to be only a complication. This principle was demonstrated in 1931 by an episode at the University of Wisconsin. After a patient experienced an accidental endobronchial intubation, Ralph Waters realized that a very long cuffed tube could be used to ventilate the dependent lung while the upper lung was being resected.[52] On learning of his friend's success with intentional one-lung anesthesia, Arthur Guedel proposed an important modification for chest surgery, the double-cuffed single-lumen tube, which was introduced by Emery Rovenstine. These tubes could be positioned easily, which was a definite advantage over the best-known alternative, bronchial blockers, which had to be inserted by a skilled bronchoscopist.

Following World War II, several double-cuffed single-lumen tubes were used for thoracic surgery, but after 1953, these were supplanted by double-lumen endobronchial tubes. The double-lumen tube that is currently used was designed by

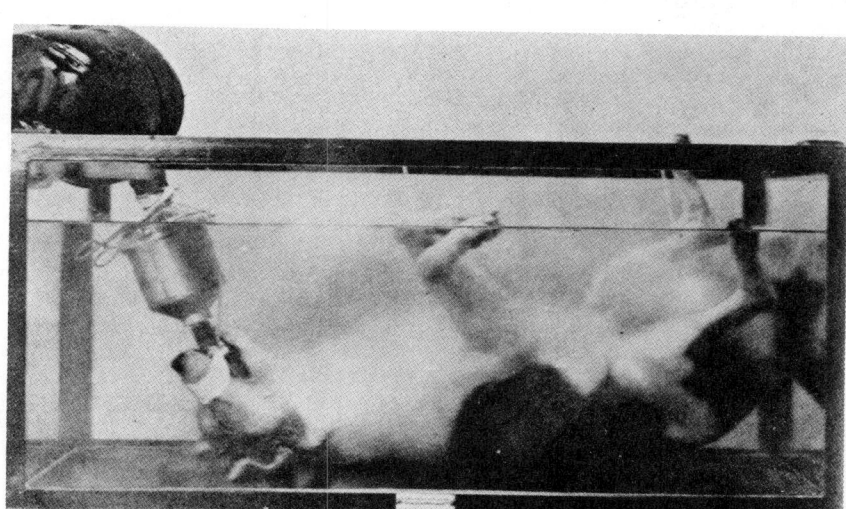

FIG. 1-8. "The dunked dog." Arthur Guedel demonstrated the safety of endotracheal intubation with a cuffed tube by submerging his anesthetized pet, Airway, in an aquarium while the animal breathed an ethylene/oxygen anesthetic through an underwater Waters' "to and fro" anesthesia circuit.

Frank Robertshaw of Manchester, England, and is prepared in both right- and left-sided versions. Robertshaw tubes were first manufactured from mineralized rubber but are now made of extruded plastic, a technique refined by Mr. David Sheridan. Sheridan was also the first person to embed centimeter markings along the side of all endotracheal tubes—a safety feature that has reduced the risk of the tip of the tube being incorrectly positioned within the trachea.

Miller and Macintosh Laryngoscopes

Early practitioners of tracheal intubation were frustrated by laryngoscopes that were cumbersome, were ill designed for prevention of dental injury, and offered only a very limited exposure of the larynx. Before the introduction of muscle relaxants, intubation of the trachea was often a severe challenge. It was in that period, however, that two blades were invented, which have become the classic models of the straight and curved laryngoscope. Robert Miller of San Antonio, Texas, and Professor Robert Macintosh of Oxford University created blades that have maintained lasting popularity.

Both blades appeared within 2 years. In 1941, Miller brought forward a slender, predominantly straight blade with a slight curve near the tip to ease the passage of the tube through the larynx. Although Miller's blade was a refinement, the technique of its use was identical to that of earlier models, as the epiglottis was lifted to expose the larynx.[53] The Macintosh blade was unique in that the tip of the blade passed in front of the epiglottis.

The event that promoted the invention of the Macintosh blade was a routine tonsillectomy, an operation that was performed at that time without intubation. Years later, Sir Robert Macintosh wrote a note to describe the circumstances of its discovery in an appreciation of the career of Mr. Richard Salt, the Chief Technician of his department who had constructed the blade. Sir Robert recalled, " . . . A Boyle–Davis gag, a size larger than intended, was inserted for tonsillectomy, and when the mouth was fully opened the cords came into view. This was a surprise since conventional laryngoscopy, at that depth of anaesthesia, would have been impossible in those pre-relaxant days. Within a matter of hours, Salt had modified the blade of the Davis gag and attached a laryngoscope handle to it; and streamlined, the end result came into widespread use."[54] Sir Robert's observation of widespread use was an understatement; more than 800,000 Macintosh blades have been produced, and many special-purpose versions have been marketed.

The variations of the Macintosh blade are representative of the diversity of equipment now available for intubation of the trachea. Prisms and fiberoptic bundles provide anesthesiologists with images beyond the expectations of early masters of tracheal intubation. A host of special-purpose plastic tubes have overcome the limitations of the metal and rubber products used 2 decades ago. Through the efforts of our predecessors, we have gained a vital skill—the ability to perform intubation of the trachea safely.

DRUGS IN ANESTHESIA

THE EVOLUTION OF INHALED ANESTHETICS

The first inhaled anesthetics were chemicals of simple preparation that had had prior application before their anesthetic action was discovered. Throughout the second half of the 19th century, many compounds were examined for their anesthetic potential, but these random searches uniformly ended in failure. The pattern of fortuitous discovery that brought nitrous oxide, diethyl ether, and chloroform forward between 1844 and 1847 continued for decades. The next inhaled anesthetics to be used routinely, ethyl chloride and ethylene, were also discovered as a result of unexpected observations.

Ethyl chloride and ethylene were first formulated in the 18th century, and both had been tested as anesthetics in Germany soon after the discovery of ether's action but were then ignored for decades. Ethyl chloride retained some use as a topical anesthetic and counterirritant, because it was so volatile that the skin "froze" after ethyl chloride was sprayed on it. Its rediscovery came after 1894, when a Swedish dentist used this technique to "freeze" a dental abscess. Carlson was surprised to discover that his patient suddenly, but briefly, lost consciousness. Ethyl chloride became a commonly used inhaled anesthetic in several countries. Because of its rapid action, it remained in routine use and was particularly favored for pediatric inductions until after 1960, when its inflammability caused it to be banned from operating rooms.

The rediscovery of ethylene in 1923 also came from an unlikely observation. After learning that ethylene gas had been used in Chicago greenhouses to inhibit the opening of carnation buds, it was speculated that a gas that put flowers to sleep might also have an anesthetic action on humans. Arno Luckhardt was the first to publish his clinical report in February 1923, but, within a month, two other independent studies were presented by Isabella Herb in Chicago and W. Easson Brown in Toronto. Ethylene was not a very successful anesthetic because it was explosive. It also had a particularly unpleasant smell, which, even though this could be partially disguised with the use of oil of orange or a cheap perfume, is still recalled with distaste by older patients and operating room personnel. A final limitation was its low potency. It had to be administered in high concentrations. Ethylene was abandoned 10 years later when cyclopropane was introduced.

There was even a fortuitous element in the discovery of cyclopropane's anesthetic action in 1929.[55] W. Easson Brown and Velyien Henderson had previously shown that propylene had desirable properties as an anesthetic when freshly prepared, but, after storage in a steel cylinder, it partially deteriorated to create a toxic material that caused humans to experience nausea and cardiac irregularities. Henderson, a professor of pharmacology at the University of Toronto, later suggested to a chemist, George Lucas, that the toxic product be identified. After Lucas found cyclopropane in the tank, the chemist prepared a sample, which he administered in a low concentration with oxygen to two kittens who had been placed in a bell jar. The animals fell asleep quietly and, after their removal from the chamber, recovered rapidly. The investigators saw that rather than being a toxic contaminant, cyclopropane was a very potent anesthetic. After studying its effects in other animals and proving that cyclopropane was stable after storage, human experimentation began. Professor Henderson was the first volunteer; George Lucas followed. They arranged a public demonstration in which Frederick Banting, already a Nobel laureate for his discovery of insulin, was anesthetized in the presence of a group of physicians. Despite this promising beginning, further research was abruptly halted for an illogical reason. It was argued that since there had been three anesthetic deaths in Toronto under ethyl chloride, no clinical trials of cyclopropane would be allowed despite its apparent safety. Rather than abandon the study, Velyien Henderson encouraged an American friend, Ralph Waters, to use cyclopropane at the University of Wisconsin. The Wisconsin group investigated the drug thoroughly and reported their clinical success in 1933. The slow pace of their studies was due to the extreme paucity of research funding during the Great Depression.

By coincidence external interference also frustrated the clinical trials of the first anesthetic to be created deliberately from a pharmacologist's knowledge of structure–activity relationships. In 1930, Chauncey Leake and MeiYu Chen performed successful laboratory trials of vinethene (divinyl ether) but were thwarted in its further development by a Professor of Surgery at the University of California, San Francisco. Ironically, Canadians, who had lost cyclopropane to Wisconsin, learned of vinethene from Leake and Chen in California and conducted the first human study in 1932 at the University of Alberta, Edmonton.

All potent anesthetics of this time period were explosive except for chloroform, whose hepatic and cardiac toxicity limited its use in America. Anesthetic explosions were a rare, but devastating risk to both the anesthesiologist and the patient. To reduce the danger of explosion during the incendiary days of World War II, many British anesthesiologists turned to trichlorethylene, a noninflammable anesthetic of limited application; it decomposed to release phosgene when warmed in the presence of soda lime. By the end of that great conflict, the first of another class of noninflammable anesthetics was being prepared for laboratory trials. After another decade, fluorinated hydrocarbons would revolutionize inhalation anesthesia.

Fluorinated Anesthetics

Fluorine, the lightest and one of the more reactive halogens, produces exceptionally stable bonds that, although sometimes created with explosive force, resist separation by chemical or thermal means. For that reason, many early attempts to fluorinate hydrocarbons in a controlled manner were frustrated by the extreme chemical activity of fluorine. In 1930, the first commercial application of fluorine chemistry was made in the production of a refrigerant, Freon. This was followed by the first attempt to prepare a fluorinated anesthetic by Harold Booth and E. May Bixby in 1932. Although their drug, monochlorodifluoromethane, was devoid of anesthetic action, as were all other drugs produced by other investigators during that decade, their report accurately forecast future developments; it began, "A survey of the properties of 166 known gases suggested that the best possibility of finding a new noncombustible anesthetic gas lay in the field of organic fluoride compounds. Fluorine substitution for other halogens lowers the boiling point, increases stability, and generally decreases toxicity."[56]

The secret demands of the Manhattan Project for refined uranium 235 were the next impetus to an improved understanding of fluorine chemistry. Researchers learned that the isotopes of uranium might be separated from uranium oxide through the creation of an intermediate compound, uranium hexafluoride. Part of this work was undertaken by Professor Earl T. McBee of Purdue University, who had had a long-standing interest in the fluorination of hydrocarbons. McBee also held a grant from the Mallinckrodt Chemical Works, a manufacturer of ether and cyclopropane, to prepare new fluorinated compounds, which were to be tested as anesthetics. By 1945, the Purdue team had created minute amounts of 46 fluorinated ethanes, propanes, butanes, and an ether.

The value of these chemicals might never have been appreciated, however, if Mallinckrodt had not also provided financial support for pharmacology research at Vanderbilt University. At that time, the Vanderbilt anesthesia department was unique in that its first chairman was a pharmacologist, Benjamin Robbins, who could assess the drugs more effectively than could any other anesthesiologist of that period. Robbins tested McBee's compounds in mice and selected the most promising for evaluation in dogs. Although none of these compounds found a place as an anesthetic, Robbins' conclusions on the effects of fluorination, bromination, and chlorination in his landmark report of 1946 encouraged later studies that would prove to be successful.[57]

A team at the University of Maryland under Professor of Pharmacology, John C. Krantz, Jr, investigated the anesthetic properties of dozens of hydrocarbons over a period of several years; only one hydrocarbon, ethyl–vinyl ether, entered clinical use in 1947. Because it was inflammable, Krantz requested that it be fluorinated. In response, Julius Shukys prepared several fluorinated analogs. One of these, trifluorethyl vinyl ether, fluroxene, became the first fluorinated anesthetic. Fluroxene was marketed from 1954 until 1974. As the drug was marginally inflammable, fluroxene had already been supplanted by more potent agents when it was withdrawn as a consequence of the delayed discovery of the action of a metabolite that was toxic to lower animals. Fluroxene is important not only for its historic interest as the first fluorinated anesthetic but also as a reminder of the importance of the continual surveillance of a drug's action—a process in which all clinicians play a significant role each day.[58]

While American researchers were conducting a rather random search for new anesthetics, a British team of researchers was applying a more direct approach. In 1951, Charles Suckling, a chemist of Imperial Chemical Industries (ICI) who already had an expert understanding of fluorination, was asked to create a new anesthetic. Suckling began by asking anaesthetists to describe the properties of an ideal anesthetic; he learned from this inquiry that his search must consider several limiting factors, including the volatility, noninflammability, stability, and high potency of the compounds. Within 2 years, Charles Suckling created halothane. As a reflection of the degree of planning that he carried out beforehand, halothane, the most successful of all fluorinated anesthetics, was among the first six compounds synthesized.

The limited number of chemicals produced for testing reflected Suckling's expert knowledge of the pharmacology of halogens and his ability to appreciate important physical relationships that apply to all anesthetics. His achievement was an extension of a principle that had been recognized in 1939 by his superior, James Ferguson, which Ferguson later learned had first been considered by John Snow in 1848. The principle was to relate the opioid actions of known anesthetics along a thermodynamic scale—the ratio of the partial pressure producing anesthesia over the saturated vapor pressure of the drug at the temperature of the experiment. The resulting ratios fall within a very narrow range, as opposed to the more than 200-fold variations seen when anesthetics are graphed by the inspired concentration required for anesthesia.[59]

After Suckling had verified halothane's purity by the new technique of gas chromatography and had determined that it had an anesthetic action by anesthetizing houseflies, it was forwarded to a pharmacologist, James Raventos, along with Suckling's accurate prediction, based on Ferguson's principles, of the concentration that would be required for anesthesia during testing in higher animals. After Raventos completed a favorable review, halothane was offered to Michael Johnstone, a respected anesthesiologist of the nearby city of

Manchester, England, who recognized its great advantages over the other anesthetics available in 1956.

Halothane was followed in 1960 by methoxyflurane, an anesthetic that was popular until 1970. At that time, a rare dose-related nephrotoxicity following methoxyflurane anesthesia was found to be due to the action of inorganic fluoride, a metabolite released by the enzymatic cleavage of a mono-fluoro carbon bond. As a consequence of that observation and a persisting concern that rare cases of hepatitis following anesthesia might be due to a metabolite of halothane, the search for newer inhaled anesthetics focused on the stability of the molecule and its resistance to metabolitic degradation.

The most recent fluorinated anesthetics to be accepted for clinical use have been enflurane and its isomer, isoflurane, which were synthesized by Ross Terrell in 1963 and 1965, respectively. Because enflurane was much easier to manufacture, it preceded isoflurane but became limited in its application after it was shown to be a marked cardiovascular depressant and to have convulsant properties in some situations. Isoflurane was nearly abandoned because of difficulties in its purification, but, after this problem was overcome by Louise Speers, a series of successful trials were published in 1971. The release of isoflurane into clinical use was delayed for more than half a decade by calls for increased testing in lower animals owing to an inappropriately raised concern that the drug might be a carcinogen. As a consequence, isoflurane was more thoroughly assessed before being offered to anesthesiologists than any other drug used in anesthesia. The era when an anesthetic could be introduced following a single fortuitous observation has given way to a cautious program of assessment and reassessment before a new drug can be used in routine practice.

INTRAVENOUS ANESTHETICS

Less than 3 decades after 1628, when William Harvey described the circulation of the blood, the first intravenous (iv) administration of a drug was undertaken by two leaders of 17th century science. In 1657, Sir Christopher Wren and his assistant, Robert Boyle, ligated a dog's vein, pierced it with a quill, and infused an opium-containing solution, which, they observed, caused the animal to become stuporous. Although they made no practical application of that observation, there is a fragmentary account that 8 years later, Sigasmund Elsholtz made the first successful iv injection of opium into a patient with the goal of producing anesthesia. No further work was reported until the mid-19th century, when several inventors prepared hollow metal needles and glass syringes. Two decades later, a French surgeon, Pierre Cyprien Oré, experimented with iv injections of chloral hydrate in animals before initiating a small clinical series. He reported his work with great enthusiasm, but, because chloral hydrate caused prolonged unconsciousness, his technique was not followed by others. In 1909, a German, Ludwig Burkhardt, produced surgical anesthesia by injecting the volatile anesthetics, chloroform and ether, iv. Seven years later, Elisabeth Bredenfeld of Switzerland reported the use of iv morphine and scopolamine. These attempts failed to show a significant improvement over inhaled techniques. None of the drugs had an action that was both sufficiently prompt or abbreviated.

The first barbiturate, barbital, was synthesized in 1903 by Fischer and von Mering. Phenobarbital and all other immediate successors of barbital had very protracted action and, thus, found little use in anesthesia. After 1929, oral pentobarbital was used as a sedative before surgery, but, when the drug was given in higher concentrations for its anesthetic effect, long periods of unconsciousness followed. The first short-acting oxybarbiturate was hexobarbital (Evipal), which was used clinically in 1932.

Hexobarbital was enthusiastically received in Britain and America because its abbreviated induction times were unrivaled by any other technique. A London anaesthetist, Ronald Jarman, found that it gave a dramatic advantage over inhalation inductions for minor procedures. Jarman developed the "falling arm" sign of anesthesia described by Terence Steen. Immediately before induction, the patient was instructed to raise one arm above him while Jarman injected hexobarital into a vein of the opposite forearm. As soon as the upraised arm fell, indicating the onset of anesthesia, the surgeon was permitted to make the incision. Steen observed that the list of cases was completed at an astonishing pace. Although today this technique would be recognized as being unsafe, it was welcomed in 1933. Patients were also pleased by barbiturate anesthesia, because the onset of its action was so abrupt that many patients awoke unable to believe that they had been anesthetized.*

Even though hexobarbital's prompt action had a dramatic effect on the conduct of anesthesia, it was soon replaced by two thiobarbiturates. In 1932, Donalee Tabern and Ernest H. Volwiler of the Abbott Company synthesized thiopental (Pentothal) and thiamylal (Surital). The sulfated barbiturates proved to be much more potent and rapid acting than their oxybarbiturate analogs. Thiopental was first given to a patient at the University of Wisconsin in March 1934, but the successful introduction of thiopental into anesthetic practice was due to the energy of John S. Lundy and colleagues at the Mayo Clinic, who began their intense and protracted assessments of thiopental during June 1934.

When first introduced, thiopental was often given in repetitive increments as the primary anesthetic for protracted procedures. Its hazardous side-effects came to be appreciated over time. At first, its depression of respiration was sometimes monitored by the simple expedient of placing a wisp of cotton over the nose and observing its motion. Only a few skilled practitioners were prepared to pass an endotracheal tube if the patient stopped breathing. These men also realized that thiopental without supplementation did not suppress airway reflexes and, thus, encouraged topical anesthesia of the airway beforehand. The depressant cardiovascular effects were appreciated only later. When the powerful vasodilating effect of

---

* Soon after Evipal was introduced, Robert Macintosh administered it to Lord Nuffield, a wealthy industrialist. Macintosh secured a result that later changed the course of anesthesia in Great Britain.[60] When Lord Nuffield awoke, he glanced at his watch and inquired as to why the operation had been postponed. On learning that his surgery was completed, Lord Nuffield was amazed by this "magic experience," which he contrasted with his vivid recollections of the terror of undergoing a mask induction as a child in a dentist's office. So impressed was Lord Nuffield with the quality of anesthetic he had received that he insisted, over the objections of Oxford's medical establishment, on endowing a university department of anesthesia for the university as a precondition of his support for a postgraduate medical center. In 1937, Robert (later Sir Robert) Macintosh became Oxford's first professor of anesthesiology and led the growth of the first university department of anesthesia in Europe from the first fully endowed Chair of Anaesthesia in the world. Fifty years later, on July 24, 1987, when the Nuffield Department of Anaesthetics celebrated its Golden Jubilee, Sir Robert greeted alumni who had returned from scores of countries. Lord Nuffield's "magic experience" of barbiturate anesthesia had led to a result beyond his imagining—the creation of one of the world's most distinguished anesthesia centers.

thiopental caused a series of fatalities among hypovolemic military casualties in the early stages of World War II, fluid replacement came to be used more aggressively, whereas thiopental was given with greater caution.

MUSCLE RELAXANTS

Many anesthesiologists regard the introduction of curare as the most important advance in anesthesia since the discovery of ether's action in 1846. Men and women who practiced without muscle relaxants recall the terror they felt when a premature attempt to intubate the trachea under cyclopropane caused persisting laryngospasm. Before 1942, abdominal relaxation was possible only if the patient tolerated high concentrations of an inhaled anesthetic that might lead to immediate and persisting problems, a profound respiratory depression, and a protracted recovery.

Curare and the drugs that followed it transformed anesthesia profoundly. Before this time, endotracheal anesthesia was an art reserved for the expert; now it was a skill that all anesthesiologists could achieve. Intubation of the trachea could be taught in a deliberate manner, as the neophyte could fail on a first attempt without placing the patient in a hazardous situation. Abdominal relaxation could be attained with light planes of inhaled agents or by a combination of iv agents providing "balanced anesthesia." The sedated and paralyzed patient could now undergo the major physiologic trespasses of cardiopulmonary bypass and deliberate hypothermia or might receive long-term respiratory support after surgery.

The curares are alkaloids prepared from plants native to equatorial rainforests. The refinement of the harmless sap of several species of vines into toxins that were lethal only when injected was an extraordinary triumph introduced by paleo-pharmacologists in loinclaths. Their discovery was the more remarkable, because it was independently repeated in South America, Africa, and Southeast Asia. These jungle tribesmen on three separate continents also achieved nearly identical methods of delivering the toxin by darts, which, after being dipped in curare, maintained their potency indefinitely until they were propelled through blowpipes to strike the flesh of monkeys and other animals of the treetops.

Europeans observed (and a few suffered) the actions of curare during explorations of South America. Some specimens of the drug were taken back to Europe. In 1780, the Abbe Felix Fontana determined that although curare had no action upon a nerve and spared the heart, it destroyed the irritability of voluntary muscles.[61] Early in the 18th century, the action of curare was examined by Squire Waterton, Francis Sibson, and Sir Benjamin Brodie in British experiments. They showed that animals injected with curare would recover unharmed if artificial ventilation were maintained. Waterton recognized that curare might have a role in the treatment of tetanus but did not have an opportunity to test his hypothesis. Seventy years after Fontana's study, Claude Bernard used curare to identify the neuromuscular junction. For the next 60 years, it was used only in the physiology laboratory, where animals were paralyzed, intubated, and ventilated.

Curare was first used in surgery in 1912, but the report was ignored for decades. Arthur Lawen, a physiologist/physician of Leipzig, had used curare in his laboratory before producing abdominal relaxation at a light level of anesthesia in a surgical patient. His German language report was not appreciated for decades, nor could it have been until his fellow clinicians learned the skills of intubation of the trachea and controlled ventilation of the lungs.

Curare remained a curiosity of laboratory practice. In 1938, Richard and Ruth Gill returned to New York from South America with 11.9 kg of crude curare, which they had collected near their Ecuadorian ranch for the Merck Company. The Gills' motivation for this unusual expedition was a mixture of personal and altruistic goals. Some months before, while on a visit to the United States from Ecuador, Richard Gill had been told by Dr. Walter Freeman that he had multiple sclerosis. Freeman mentioned that curare could have a therapeutic role in the management of spastic disorders. When the Gills returned to America with a large supply of crude curare, they were initially disappointed to learn that Merck's researchers had lost interest, but, they were later able to share some of it with E. R. Squibb & Co. The pharmaceutical company offered a semirefined curare to two groups of American anesthesiologists, who assessed its action but soon abandoned their studies when it caused total respiratory paralysis in two patients and the death of laboratory animals.

Curare entered clinical medicine through the actions of midwestern psychiatrists. In 1939, A. R. McIntyre refined a portion of Gill's curare that A. E. Bennett of Omaha, Nebraska, first injected into children with spastic disorders and, after observing no persisting benefit, next gave it to psychiatric patients about to receive Metrazol, a shock treatment that was a precursor to electroconvulsive therapy. Curare was termed a "shock absorber," because it eliminated seizure-induced fractures. By 1941, other groups of psychiatrists were following this practice and even used neostigmine as an occasional antidote when the action of curare was too protracted.

Some months later, Harold Griffith, the chief anaesthetist of the Montreal Homeopathic Hospital, learned of Bennett's successful use of curare and resolved to try it in anesthesia. Griffith was already a master of cyclopropane anesthesia and was among Canada's foremost pioneers of tracheal intubation. He was much better prepared than most of his contemporaries to attend to complications that might follow an excessive response. On January 23, 1942, Griffith and his resident, Enid Johnson, anesthetized and intubated the trachea of a young man before injecting curare early in the course of his appendectomy. Satisfactory abdominal relaxation was obtained as the surgery proceeded without incident. Griffith and Johnson's report of the successful use of curare in their series of 25 patients launched a great revolution in anesthetic care.[62]

The successful use of curare prompted several pharmacologic studies that led to the introduction of other nondepolarizing and depolarizing relaxants. Gallamine and decamethonium were synthesized by 1948. Metubine, a relaxant "rediscovered" in the past decade, was first used clinically in the same year. The most successful depolarizing relaxant, succinylcholine, was prepared by the Nobel laureate, Daniel Bovet, in 1949 and was in wide international use before historians noted that the drug was much older and that earlier investigators had not observed its primary action. In 1906, Hunt and Taveaux had prepared succinylcholine and other choline esters, which they had injected into rabbits to observe their effects upon the heart. If their rabbits had not been paralyzed with curare, the depolarizing action of succinylcholine might have been known decades earlier.

Research in relaxants was rekindled in 1960, when researchers became aware of the action of maloetine, a relaxant from the Congo basin, which was remarkable in that it had a steroidal nucleus. Investigations of maloetine led to pancuronium and vecuronium. As these drugs have provided new avenues for investigation, the pace of research has accelerated. There is every expectation that by 1992, when the Golden Jubilee of the Griffith–Johnson paper will be recognized, new families of muscle relaxants will have caused succinylcholine and curare to be set aside.

NEWER DRUGS

During the first 2 decades following World War II, other classes of drugs were developed. Anesthesiologists learned a new vocabulary as words were coined to describe the actions of novel compounds. "Lytic cocktails," "dissociative anesthesia," and "neuroleptanalgesia" became common expressions. Intravenous mixtures concocted from a succession of analgesics and anxiolytics produced a state of euphoria, tranquility, and indifference when provided with care, or profound respiratory depression when presented carelessly. "Dissociative" anesthesia was a neologism invented in 1966 by Guenter Corrsen and Edward Domino to describe the trance-like state of profound analgesia produced by ketamine. "Neuroleptanalgesia" was pioneered by J. de Castro, a Belgian anesthesiologist, who performed the first clinical investigations of many compounds synthesized under the direction of Paul Janssen.

Although many pharmacologists are remembered for the introduction of a single drug, since 1953 Paul Janssen has brought more than 60 agents forward from among 70,000 chemicals created in his laboratory. His products have had profound effects on disciplines as disparate as parasitology and psychiatry. The pace of productive innovation in Janssen's research laboratory has been astonishing. Chemical R4263 (fentanyl) synthesized in 1960 was followed only a year later by R4749 (Inapsine). Although the fixed combination (Innovar) in which they were introduced in America is now less popular, new applications of fentanyl and its successors excite attention.

THE EVOLUTION OF THE PROFESSIONAL ANESTHESIOLOGIST

The preceding segments of this survey have provided an overview of the evolution of many of the drugs, instruments, and techniques used in anesthesia. As this armamentarium began to expand at the beginning of this century, a few men and women of vision recognized that a distinct body of knowledge was being created and sought to encourage its growth by forming organizations to foster their common interests. In time, regional societies grew to attract national, and, in some cases, international representation. The charter members of these societies, most of whom were entirely self-trained, pressed for recognition of the need for formal training in anesthesiology at both the undergraduate and postgraduate levels. Dr. Ralph Waters and a few other anesthesiologists gained university posts where they performed studies in collaboration with pharmacologists and physiologists. Their basic research extended the range of articles appearing in the first journals of anesthesia, which had begun publication after World War I. With the development of a body of knowledge unique to anesthesia and with the recognition of the talents of able physicians, anesthesiology slowly became recognized as a separate specialty in clinical practice and as an appropriate discipline for research. As a consequence, a separate organization that was granted powers to establish examinations for the specialty, the American Board of Anesthesiology, was formed in 1938.

THE BEGINNINGS OF SPECIALIZATION

One of the first physicians to declare himself a specialist in anesthesia was Sydney Ormond Goldan of New York, who published seven papers in 1900, including an early description of the use of cocaine for spinal anesthesia. After studying Goldan's early career, Professor Raymond Fink recognized in him some of the qualities of many modern anesthesiologists; he declared, "He was brimful of enthusiasm for anesthesia, an excellent communicator and a prolific writer, a gadgeteer and the owner of several patents of anesthesia equipment."[63] At a time when some surgeons considered that spinal anesthesia did away with their need for an anesthesiologist, Goldan was particularly bold in his written opinions. He called for equality between surgeon and anesthesiologist and was among the first to state that the anesthesiologist had a right to establish and collect his own fee. Goldan regarded the anesthesiologist as being more important than the surgeon to the welfare of the patient. His forthright pronouncements may not have been well received, for he was not listed among the nine founding members of the Long Island Society of Anesthetists when the nation's first specialty society was founded on October 6, 1905, with annual dues of $1.00.

After 1911, the annual fee rose to $3.00 when the Long Island Society became the New York Society of Anesthetists. Although the new organization still carried a local title, it drew members from several states and, by 1915, had a membership of 70 physicians. A second society with roots in the mid-west merged in 1912 as the brief-lived American Association of Anesthetists, which, by 1915, became the Interstate Association of Anesthetists. Most of the approximately 100 professional anesthesiologists in America belonged to both medical societies.

Two years later, several specialists volunteered to serve with American forces in France. Major James T. Gwathmey, the highest ranking American anesthesiologist, taught his British counterparts the advantages of his anesthesia machine and, as the result of his service in France, gained an international audience for the first American text, Gwathmey and Baskerville's *Anesthesia*. Captain Arthur Guedel from Indianapolis gained the title of "the motorcycle anesthesiologist," because he dashed between hospitals to supervise orderlies and nurses whom he had trained to give anesthetics to the thousands of casualties evacuated from the war front.

Francis Hoeffer McMechan (1879–1939)

Accounts of the dramatic experiences of American, British, and Canadian military anesthesiologists were collected by a remarkable man, Dr. Francis Hoeffer McMechan, who reported them in the quarterly anesthesia supplements of the American Journal of Surgery, which he later republished as "The American Yearbook of Anesthesia and Analgesia." Francis McMechan had been a practicing anesthesiologist in Cincinnati until 1911, when he suffered a severe first attack of rheumatoid arthritis, which was to leave him confined to a wheelchair. Despite this limitation, McMechan, with the assistance of his devoted wife, Laurette, became a strong force in the development of anesthesia.[64] He supported himself through editing the Quarterly Supplement from 1914 until August 1922, when he became editor of the first journal devoted to anesthesia, "Current Researches in Anesthesia and Analgesia," the precursor of "Anesthesia and Analgesia," the oldest journal of the specialty. As well as fostering the organization of the International Anesthesia Research Society in

1925, Francis and Laurette McMechan became international ambassadors of American anesthesia. With Laurette's assistance, Dr. McMechan was able to travel and lecture in Britain, Europe, Cuba, Australia, and New Zealand before his death in 1939. After his passing, Ralph Waters wrote a fine appreciation of McMechan's contributions in a note entered on the inside cover of my copy of McMechan's first "American Yearbook of Anesthesia," "Frank McMechan revived anesthesia in America in the 20th century and left it for others to carry on."

Ralph M. Waters (1883–1979)

Professor Ralph Waters ranks among the most respected founding fathers of academic anesthesiology.[65] After completing his internship in 1913, he entered medical practice in Sioux City, Iowa, and, because he liked to give anesthetics, gradually limited his practice until, by 1916, his work was completely limited to anesthesia. His personal experience and extensive reading were supplemented by the only postgraduate training available—a 1-month course conducted in Ohio by E. I. McKesson. At that time, the custom of becoming a self-proclaimed specialist in medicine and surgery was not uncommon. Ralph Waters, who was frustrated by low standards and who would eventually have a great influence on establishing both anesthesia residency training and the formal examination process recalled that before 1920, "The requirements for specialization in many midwestern hospitals consisted of the possession of sufficient audacity to attempt a procedure and persuasive power adequate to gain the consent of the patient or his family."[66]

In his effort to improve anesthetic care, Waters exchanged correspondence with Professor Dennis Jackson and other scientists. He lectured regularly at medical meetings both before and after he moved to Kansas City in 1925 with the goal of gaining an academic post at the University of Kansas, but the Department of Surgery did not support his proposal. The larger city did allow him to expand his concept of the outpatient surgical facility, the "Downtown Surgical Clinic," which featured one of the first post-anesthetic recovery rooms. He continued in private practice until 1927.

Erwin Schmidt, the Professor of Surgery at the University of Wisconsin's new medical school, encouraged Dean Charles Bardeen to recruit Waters. In accepting the first American academic position in anesthesia, Waters described four objectives that have been adopted by all other academic departments. His goals were: "(1) to provide the best possible service to patients of the institution; (2) to teach what is known of the principles of Anesthesiology to all candidates for their medical degree; (3) to help long-term graduate students not only to gain a fundamental knowledge of the subject and to master the art of administration, but also to learn as much as possible of the effective methods of teaching; (4) to accompany these efforts with the encouragement of as much cooperative investigation as is consistent with achieving the first objectives."[67]

Ralph Waters' personal and professional qualities impressed many talented young men and women who sought residency posts in his department. He encouraged his residents to initiate research interests. They joined enthusiastically in studies with two pharmacologists Waters had known previously, Arthur Loevenhart and Chauncey Leake, as well as others with whom he became associated at Madison, Arthur Tatum, W. J. Meek, and H. R. Hathaway. Clinical concerns were also pursued. Anesthesia records were entered on punch cards and coded to form a data base that was used to analyze departmental activities.

Morbidity and mortality meetings, now a requirement of all training programs, originated in Madison. They were attended by all members of the department and by distinguished visitors from other cities. As a consequence of their critical reviews of the conduct of anesthesia and its outcome, responsibility for a tragedy passed from the patient to the physician. In former times, a practitioner could complain, "The patient did not take a good anesthetic." Alternatively, he might attribute the death to "status lymphaticus," of which Arthur Guedel, a master of sardonic humor, observed, "Certainly status lymphaticus is at times a great help to the anesthetist. When he has a fatality under anesthesia with no other cleansing explanation he is glad to recognize the condition as an entity."[68] Through the instruction received from Ralph Waters and his colleagues, anesthesiologists in training learned to accept responsibility for their actions by realizing that the fault lay not in the patient, but in their assessment or actions.

The University of Wisconsin became a popular destination for visiting specialists. In 1929, Ralph Waters helped organize the Anesthesia "Travel Club," whose members were leading American or Canadian teachers of anesthesia. Each year one member was the host for a group of 20 to 40 anesthesiologists who gathered for a program of informal discussions. There were demonstrations of new innovations for the operating room and laboratory, which were all subjected to what is remembered as a "high spirited, energetic, critical review." Even during the lean years of the Great Depression, international guests visited occasionally. To Geoffrey Kaye of Australia, Torsten Gordth of Sweden, Robert Macintosh and Michael Nosworthy of England, and others, Waters' department was always the "Mecca of anesthesia." It became the model for other academic departments in Europe, South America, and Asia.

Ralph Waters trained 60 residents during the 22 years he was "The Chief." From 1937 onward, the alumni, who called themselves the "Aqualumni" in his honor, returned for an annual professional and social reunion. Thirty-four "Aqualumni" took academic positions, and, of these, 14 became chairmen of departments of anesthesia. They maintained Professor Waters' professional principles and encouraged teaching careers for many of their own graduates. Sixty years after Waters' arrival at Madison, more than 80 chairmen or former chairmen of academic departments could trace their professional lineage back to Ralph Waters. Each of the 114 departments of anesthesia with residency programs in the United States has faculty members who were trained in a department led by a 2nd, 3rd, 4th, or 5th generation professional descendant of Ralph Waters. Charles Bardeen, the Dean who had recruited him in 1927, once recognized Waters' enduring legacy when he observed, "Ralph Waters was the first person the University hired to put people to sleep, but, instead, he awakened a world-wide interest in anesthesia."

Ralph Waters energetically supported the growth of physician anesthesia organizations. He supported Paul Wood's drive to give the pre-eminent New York Society of Anesthetists a title reflecting its national role. In 1936, the American Society of Anesthetists was formed, with annual dues increased to $5.00. A few years later, the officers of the American Society of Anesthetists were challenged by Dr. M. J. Seifert, who wrote, "An Anesthetist is a technician and an Anesthesiologist is the specific authority on anesthesia and anesthetics. I cannot understand why you do not term yourselves the American Society of Anesthesiologists?"[69] Ralph Waters was declared the first President of the newly named American

Society of Anesthesiologists (ASA) in 1945. In that year, when World War II ended, 739 of 1,977 ASA members were in the armed forces. In the same year, the Society's first Distinguished Service Award was presented to Paul M. Wood for his tireless service to the specialty, one element of which can be examined today in the extensive archives of anesthesiology preserved in the Society's excellent Wood Library–Museum in Park Ridge, Illinois.

WOMEN IN ANESTHESIA

Female Physicians

The first woman physician of modern times, Elizabeth Blackwell, graduated in 1849. For some years, this courageous lady was followed by only a few others, but many women entered the profession as medical colleges for women were established. Although it is not possible to determine when the first anesthetic was given by a female physician, a woman was the first American resident in anesthesia. Mary A. Ross of the University of Iowa was awarded her certificate on June 5, 1923. When Dr. Ross entered the specialty, other women physicians were already among its leaders. Before the beginning of the 20th century, Mary Botsford and Isabella Herb had been among the first Americans to become specialists in anesthesia. Both ladies were highly regarded as clinicians and were influential in the formation of professional societies.

Dr. Botsford is believed to be the first lady to establish a practice as a specialist in anesthesia. In 1897, she became anesthesiologist to a children's hospital in San Francisco. Following her example, several other California women doctors joined the specialty. She later received the first academic appointment in anesthesia in the western United States when she became Clinical Professor of Anesthesia at the University of California, San Francisco. She was active in medical affairs and became a leader of state and national anesthesia organizations. Botsford served as the president of the Associated Anesthetists of the United States and Canada.

Dr. Isabella Herb took training in anesthesia at the Augustana Hospital in Chicago before working as an anesthesiologist at the Mayo Clinic from 1900 until 1904. After further study in Europe, she became an Associate Professor of Rush Medical College and Chief Anesthetist at the Presbyterian Hospital, Chicago, where she established a widely respected clinical department. Her colleagues elected her to positions of leadership in both the American Medical Association and anesthesia societies. One of Dr. Herb's residents and colleagues was Huberta Livingstone. Livingstone was among the first to use positive pressure ventilation, which she described in several of the 150 articles she wrote between 1928 and 1952.

After World II, other female anesthesiologists gained international reputation. Kathleen Belton was a superb pediatric specialist. In 1948, while working in Montreal, Belton and her colleague, Digby Leigh, wrote the classic text, *Pediatric Anesthesia*. At the same time, another pediatric anesthesiologist, Margot Deming, was the Director of Anesthesia at the Children's Hospital of Philadelphia. Pediatric anesthesia also figured in the career of Doreen Vermeulen–Cranch, who had earlier initiated thoracic anesthesia in the Netherlands and, together with the surgeon, Boerema, pioneered hypothermic anesthesia. In 1958, the University of Amsterdam appointed Dr. Vermeulen–Cranch to the first Chair of Anesthesia in Europe. For many years, the emerging discipline of obstetric anesthesia was led in America by Professor Gertie F. Marx.

Obstetric anesthesia also figured prominently in the career of the only female anesthesiologist to receive the ASA Distinguished Service Award. After encountering severe financial and professional frustrations while serving as Director of the Division of Anesthesia at Columbia University, Virginia Apgar turned to obstetric anesthesia in 1949. She dedicated a decade of her multifaceted career to the assessment and support of mothers and their newborn infants.

One of the earliest expressions of her concern was the Apgar score. She formulated it during an informal morning conference immediately after a medical student requested a method of evaluating the newborn's need for resuscitative support. Although it was created in a few minutes, the Apgar score was substantiated by careful study before it was published in 1952. It has since found universal application as a method of neonatal assessment during the first minutes after delivery. After the Apgar score was accepted, Virginia Apgar continued her research and, with her associates, Frank James and Duncan Holladay, was among the first to recognize the impact of acidosis and hypoxia on the newborn.[70]

Nurse Anesthetists

Anesthesiology evolved slowly as an American medical specialty in part because of the presence of a second group of anesthesia care providers, nurse anesthetists. During the last decades of the 19th century, small communities were often served by a single physician, who was obliged to assign a nurse to drop ether under his direction. In larger towns, most doctors practiced independently and would not necessarily welcome being placed in what they perceived to be the subordinate role of anesthetist while their competitor enhanced his surgical reputation and collected the larger fee. Many American surgeons recalled the simple techniques they had practiced as junior house officers and regarded the administration of any anesthetic as just a technical art that could be left to a nurse in any circumstance. Some hospitals preferred to pay a salary to an anesthetist while reducing their deficit from the fees charged for anesthesia. The most compelling argument to be advanced in favor of nurse anesthesia was that of skill; a trained nurse who administered anesthetics every working day was to be preferred to a physician who practiced this skill rarely.

Religious communities of the Roman Catholic Church played a major role in building hospitals in frontier America. Sisters entering their Order first trained in metropolitan hospitals before traveling to isolated communities. Many joined small classes in hospital-based schools of nurse anesthesia. I, and tens of thousands of members of my and earlier generations, received our first anesthetic under the skilled care of a now anonymous nun.

By the first years of this century, the surgeons of many surgical clinics preferred nurse anesthesia and personally trained the most able candidates they could recruit. The Mayo brothers personal anesthetist was Alice Magaw. George W. Crile relied on the skills of Agatha Hodgins. During World War I, Agatha Hodgins, Geraldine Gerrard, Ann Penland, and Sophie Gran were among the more than one hundred nurse anesthetists who attended many thousands of American and Allied casualties in France.

The extraordinary demands of wartime service were repeated during World War II. The nation had a desperate lack of trained physicians; at the beginning of 1940, the American Board of Anesthesiologists had recognized only 87 Diplomates. Scores of nurses and young physicians were selected each year for abbreviated training. The "90 day wonders" served with distinction in arduous conditions. After the end of hostilities, many members of both professional groups elected to remain in anesthesia, a specialty into which they had been catapulted in an abrupt and involuntary fashion. In 1988, the American Association of Nurse Anesthetists (AANA) reported 20,728 members, of whom 16,806 were currently recertified.

ANESTHESIA IN CANADA

The development of anesthesia as a specialty in Canada is in many ways comparable to the American experience; the major difference is that only physicians are allowed to administer anesthetics. Only in recent decades has there been a requirement that the physician giving the anesthetic have formal training. The progress of the specialty in Canada has been closely linked to its growth in America, particularly in its earliest years. The first meeting of a short-lived Canadian Society of Anaesthetists on June 1–3, 1921, was a joint gathering with both the Interstate Association of Anesthetists and the New York Society of Anesthetists. William Webster of Winnipeg, the author of the first text by a Canadian, *The Science and Art of Anesthesia*, became the first president; Wesley Bourne of Montreal, who would later become the only Canadian to serve as president of the ASA, was the Secretary Treasurer. Seven years later, the infant organization disappeared only to re-emerge in 1943 as the Canadian Anaesthetists Society (CAS). A detailed history of Canadian anesthesia is being prepared by Professor Emeritus Roderick Gordon.[71]

Although there were three 1-year training positions as "Senior Interne" before World War II, dozens of Canadian doctors entering medical service took short courses in Montreal, Toronto, and Quebec City and remained in specialist practice thereafter. Norman Parks was assigned to a British plastic surgery unit and, like Ivan Magill before him, returned with an incomparable mastery of intubation that amazed all those he trained at The Hospital for Sick Children, Toronto.

For many years, any physician with sufficient temerity could announce that he was a "Specialist," but, in 1939, a process of Certification was begun by the Royal College of Physicians and Surgeons (Canada), which has been superseded by the creation of the higher demands of a Fellowship examination. Canadian specialists in anesthesia are obliged to complete a residency equal in length to those taken by surgical specialists before entering an examination process assumed to be as demanding as that of any other specialty. These requirements have gained the Canadian specialist a status equal to that of all other medical and surgical specialists.

In January 1988, the Canadian Anaesthetists Society had 1,535 active and Canadian Associate members and 400 student members. Since Canada's population is approximately one tenth that of the United States, the representation of anesthesiologists in the population is nearly equal. At the beginning of 1988, the American Society of Anesthesiologists reported a total of 24,900 members, of whom 16,733 held active memberships and 4,344 were resident members.

THE SCOPE OF MODERN ANESTHESIOLOGY

This overview of the development of anesthesiology could be extended almost indefinitely by an exploration of each of the anesthetic subspecialty areas, but an assessment of its present situation can be undertaken in a simple fashion by considering the areas in which anesthesiologists are involved in hospital and university service. A comparable tour could be undertaken in any university training department.

The operating room and obstetric delivery suite remain the central interest of most members of the specialty. Aside from being the location where the techniques described previously find regular application, service in these areas bring anesthesiologists into regular contact with new departures in pharmacology and bioengineering.

After surgery, patients are transported to the post-anesthesia care unit or recovery room, an area that is now considered the anesthesiologist's hospital ward. Fifty years ago, most patients returned immediately to their own bed to be attended by a junior nurse, who lacked the skills or equipment to intervene when complications occurred. After the experiences of World War II had taught anesthesiologists the value of centralized care, anesthesiologists and the nursing staff worked together to manage complex problems. Recovery rooms were soon mandated for all hospitals. By 1960, patients requiring several days of intensive medical and nursing management were often attended in a curtained corner of the recovery room. In time, drawn curtains gave way to partitions and the relocation of those areas as intensive care units. The principles of resuscitative and supportive care established by anesthesiologists were expanded in the growth of critical care medicine. From the operating room or intensive care unit, anesthesiologists make their rounds as they attend patients requiring an expert's support in controlling acute or chronic pain. At other locations within the hospital and in the classrooms and laboratories of the university campus, anesthesiologists teach undergraduates and residents and explore unproven hypotheses that may bring further progress to anesthesiology.

THE FUTURE OF ANESTHESIOLOGY*

As we have seen, the "face" of anesthesiology has changed remarkably in the 50 years since the beginning of World War II. Like most other medical specialties, anesthesiology has progressed primarily by quantum leaps made possible by numerous lesser technical and theoretical advancements, many of which have been directly attributable to the scientists working in industry. Examples that readily come to mind are the discoveries and applications of halothane and synthetic narcotics. At the same time, however, as it was not possible to separate the social, political, and economic exigencies of the past 50 years from scientific advancement, so, too, will it be necessary to examine these forces when anticipating the future.

Much of what anesthesiologists do today would not seem unusual to anesthesiologists of 50 years ago. Although anesthesiologists have expanded the scope of their practice to include intensive care work and pain management, the primary focus of anesthesiology is still to provide a motionless surgical field and maintain optimal physiologic function during surgical procedures.

Clearly, the surgical procedures performed today are vastly different from those of 50 years ago, and it is likely that the surgical procedures in which anesthesiologists will find themselves participating 50 years from now will bear little resemblance to those of today. Specifically, the field of transplant surgery will expand tremendously. Not only will virtually all

---

*This section was contributed by Mark S. Scheller, M.D., Assistant Professor of Anesthesiology at the University of California, San Diego.

organs be subject to allographic replacement, but microsurgical techniques will make possible transplantation of genetically engineered tissue to cure many medical conditions such as Parkinson's disease or Huntington's chorea. It is quite likely that mental illnesses such as schizophrenia, depression, or addiction may be treated by surgical transplantation of cultured tissues, producing either natural products such as neurotransmitters or synthetically created drugs. These transplanted tissues may also act to remove substances from the microenvironment or process these substances in some way as to effect therapeutic change. These approaches are just starting to be pursued but will likely occupy a greater place in mid-21st century practice.

Microprocessor advances may make exogenous reinervation of skeletal muscle a distinct possibility in the near future. These procedures would require surgical implantation of electrodes in various muscle groups connected to processing units in some way controlled by the patient. This has already been somewhat accomplished by applying external stimulating electrodes to lower extremity muscle groups to produce artificial gain in paraplegic patients.

Another possibility for anesthetic administration may arise if therapeutic applications for anesthetics are discovered. For example, anesthetic agents toxic only to viruses (or other infectious agents) could play a part in the treatment of acute infectious illnesses but require, of course, the administration of an anesthetic. Similarly, might there be mental disorders effectively treated or controlled acutely by anesthetic administration? There is already some precedent for immediately anesthetizing patients undergoing acute myocardial infarction to rest the myocardium and allow for expeditious management of clot lysis or angioplasty.

Nuclear war, even conducted on a limited scale, could potentially adversely affect progress in many areas of human endeavor; this would be likely to include anesthesiology. Even if the researchers and/or their institutions were not directly harmed, progress could be indirectly halted by forcing resources to be channeled exclusively to patient care. All medical specialties could similarly be affected. Many have pointed out for over a decade that the only possible rational treatment of such an epidemic is prevention, and physicians from all specialties in both the Soviet Union and the United States have participated in efforts to educate the political and general population as to the possible global devastation of even limited nuclear war. Physicians in general and anesthesiologists in particular may be able to influence proliferation or use policies by virtue of their current economic and, hence, political power.

However horrible the thought of nuclear war, the reality facing us in the next 50 years is that the probability of nuclear war occurring is greater than zero. In anticipation of this, anesthesiologists will need to be involved in research detailing the logistics and effects of anesthetic administration in patients suffering from radiation poisoning, radiation burns, and other diseases unique to the aftermath of nuclear explosions. This area has not yet been explored by anesthesiologists but could potentially yield invaluable information if nuclear war were to occur.

It is unlikely that anesthesiologists will need to organize on an international scale for the purposes of changing international or national law regarding the regulation of anesthesiology in the foreseeable future. What will become vitally important to the preservation of anesthesiology as a medical specialty within the United States are organized national and state lobbies that inform anesthesiologists about pending legislation and amass funds to support candidates whose views are consistent with the tenets that, 1) anesthesiology is the practice of medicine, which requires *medical training*; 2) As physicians, anesthesiologists must be allowed free access to hospitals' medical staffs; and 3) as physicians, anesthesiologists must be allowed to prescribe the conduct of anesthetics free from regulation by administrators or other non-anesthesiologist physicians.

Anesthesiologists have not built a positive public image over the last 50 years. As an example, the head of the Health Care Financing Administration, who controls virtually all governmental medical spending, once made the public statement that "anesthesiologists don't even say hello to their patients." This demonstrates how awareness about anesthesiology is lacking, even among other physicians. These public attitudes will need to be challenged if anesthesiologists are to remain independent medical practitioners and not become simply employees of the hospital akin to technicians and nurses. To the extent that anesthesiologists will organize and support and educate candidates for national and state office, anesthesiologists will have a chance of existing as independent practitioners. If their efforts fall short, it is likely that their services will become the property of others.

A strongly related issue relating to services rendered by anesthesiologists is that of compensation for those services. Third-party payers such as health plans, county, state, and even the federal government have (unfairly) targeted anesthesiologists as physicians who will have to accept payment based on whatever political or economic cost-cutting plan happens to be popular, with little regard for quality of care. At the extreme, these payers would prefer to simply employ the physician or contract directly with the physician's employer, that is, the hospital. Hospital-based physicians such as anesthesiologists, pathologists, and radiologists are clearly the most vulnerable, because the third-party payers, hospital administrators, and, perhaps, more sadly, the public believe that these physicians are strictly technicians and therefore employable as such. The patient/physician relationship thus changes to a patient/hospital relationship or a patient/health plan relationship. The economic implications of this to those employed are obvious, as the hospital, like any business, would be attempting to turn a profit on physician services. Anesthesiologists have been somewhat protected by their relatively high cost of malpractice insurance and liability exposure, which has made them, as a group, unattractive to hospitals or health plans to employ directly. If this changes, either because of legislation limiting liability or because it will ultimately be more lucrative for the hospital or health plan to assume the liability of the physician, economic remuneration for anesthesiologists' services will be greatly curtailed. If this occurs on a widespread basis, other physicians such as surgeons and internists will very likely find themselves in the midst of similar arrangements. Again, firm and constant political pressure at the national and state level will be the anesthesiologist's major defensive weapon of the next half century.

Changes will undoubtedly occur in the education of anesthesiologists. The American Board of Anesthesiology has increased the anesthesiology residency requirement to 4 years from 3 years following graduation from medical school. The educational requirements for anesthesiologists in the next 50 years will depend to a great extent upon their success in remaining independent practitioners and supply and demand in the marketplace. If they are successful and if the demand for anesthesiologists' services continue to remain high, it is almost certain that the educational requirements for board certification will increase. At the extreme, this would result in anesthesiology training programs accepting only physicians board certified in another specialty such as internal medicine or pediatrics. There are already precedents for this in the medical and surgical subspecialties.

On the other hand, if nonphysician practitioners are successful in winning concessions from government agencies with regard to the scope of their practices and liability, the educational requirements for anesthesiologists may actually need to expand to include areas traditionally taught in nursing school. This would be primarily a defensive maneuver by anesthesiologists to demonstrate that their training is over and above that of nonphysician practitioners and not merely of a different focus as has been the contention of some. The politics involved are obviously difficult to predict, but it is not outside the realm of possibilities that future practitioners would need to be duly certified in both disciplines.

Research done by anesthesiologists in the next 5 decades will be more closely aligned with the needs of industry and other medical specialties. Simply performing physiology experiments on normal animals or humans will be neither fundable nor interesting. Academic anesthesiology departments have traditionally performed poorly in securing significant national grant support compared with medicine or surgery departments. As funding becomes tighter, as it inevitably will, anesthesiologists will be forced to compete with other medical specialists and basic scientists for funds. This will force physician researchers to gain additional training, such as a doctoral degree. The anesthesiologist with advanced training will be in a unique position to adequately design and monitor experiments requiring the administration of an anesthetic. At the present time, the effects of anesthesia per se are frequently either ignored or poorly controlled by non-anesthesiologist investigators.

Tackling problems such as acquired immunodeficiency syndrome (AIDS), Alzheimer's disease, coronary artery disease, and cancer will become bigger priorities for anesthesiologist researchers if they are to survive the funding wars. Another avenue to secure funding, however, will be through liaisons with private industry. Competition in the marketplace will force entrepreneurs to have new products evaluated as quickly as possible in an evermore regulated society. Anesthesiologists will find themselves taking products from the laboratory to the operating room for evaluation more frequently in the years to come.

Monitoring of the patient will also become more rigorous. If there is any question or worry about a patient's well-being or status during an anesthetic, monitoring is by definition inadequate. With the recent widespread availability of noninvasive and reliable measures of oxygenation (pulse oximetry), ventilation, and anesthetic depth (end-tidal gas analysis), it is clear that "beat to beat" or "breath to breath" monitoring capabilities are a new standard of practice. With this new technology, however, comes the problem of accurately recording the ever-increasing amount of data. This problem will be solved quickly with completely automated recordkeeping. Advances in artificial intelligence, speech recognition, and data storage and retrieval will make manual recordkeeping obsolete within 15 years. All information about a patient will be instantly accessible by the anesthesiologist and permanently recorded. These systems will become as familiar to the anesthesiologist of the 21st century as clipboards are to present-day practitioners.

Noninvasive measures of tissue well-being will evolve quickly. For example, edema formation, particularly in the lungs and brain, but probably in other organs as well, is, at the present time, recognized too late in its course. Likewise, currently, we have only limited abilities to recognize local tissue ischemia, substrate deficiency, or other metabolic disturbance. On-line, noninvasive measurement techniques, which will probably require technology we cannot yet imagine, may be a reality by the year 2040.

Our understanding of the etiology, function, and treatment of pain has evolved very slowly over the last 50 years. The rather recent discoveries of the participation of specific spinal pathways in the expression of pain may be the quantum leap upon which a more complete appreciation of the physiology of pain can be built. If this is so, it is conceivable that pain as it relates to surgery or disease could be of historic interest midway into the 21st century. Research along a number of very different lines will need to intersect to eventually make this happen. Presumably, drugs with the potential to selectively block the propagation of afferent pain impulses might be developed, or, alternatively, methods of interfering with afferent pain impulses at more central locations will need to be refined (e.g., gating). At the present time, the complete understanding and control of pain is perhaps the greatest scientific challenge facing anesthesiologists.

It is likely that the number of scientific and technical breakthroughs or innovations in the next 50 years will exceed that of the previous 50 years by orders of magnitude, as a direct result of the burgeoning worldwide demand for biomedical products. These advances will impact every clinical specialty, anesthesiology included.

In the near future, newer drugs will be developed, such as volatile anesthetics with very low blood/gas solubility ratios, which will be used as nitrous oxide is used today. In fact, with the introduction of these agents, nitrous oxide will permanently be dropped from the pharmacopoeia of the anesthesiologist. Likewise, extremely short-acting nondepolarizing muscle relaxants will be used routinely within 15 years and will completely displace succinylcholine. Although fentanyl, alfentanil, and sufentanil will serve us well to the end of this century and perhaps a bit beyond, they too will be replaced by even shorter-acting, more potent compounds with no side-effects such as rigidity, nausea, hypotension, or pruritis. Along with these drugs, our understanding and ability to apply kinetic principles to clinical practice will increase, such that we will be able to deliver truly predictable iv anesthetics. It is likely that the anesthesia machine of the 21st century will have calibrated dispensers for all available iv anesthetic agents, muscle relaxants, and vasoactive drugs built into them, much like present-day machines have vaporizers attached. These delivery systems would be interfaced directly with physiologic data, including on-line plasma or possibly tissue levels of drug and require little or no hands-on attention.

The manipulation of gene expression in eukaryotic organisms may be a reality in the next 50 years. Thus, it may be possible to implant genes that can be turned on and off in humans. These genes could code for proteins that would either act directly at some site, for example, beta-endorphin, or the genes could code for proteins that would assemble compounds from normal cellular pools of components or from substances introduced by the anesthesiologist. For example, it may be possible to induce a state of prolonged hibernation (? anesthesia) by turning on a gene that produces a peptide hibernation factor. Hibernation factors have already been isolated and shown to include hibernation-like states in non-hibernating animals.

As artificially produced human insulin and erythropoietin will change clinical practice during the remainder of this century, so too will artificial blood components be an advance of the next century. All clotting factors, platelets, and oxygen-carrying compounds will be produced in the laboratory and be commercially available.

A mission to Mars is planned for the mid-21st century. The length of interplanetary trips, that is, years, will initially necessitate the availability of surgical and hence anesthetic capabilities onboard the spacecraft. This alone will open an entirely new area of scientific inquiry within the field of anesthesiology.

SUMMARY

Political, economic, and scientific developments will shape the practice of medicine in the next 50 years. Anesthesiology, as a medical specialty, will likewise be influenced by these forces. Anesthetic practice will very likely change tremendously as new surgical procedures are applied and new areas of medical endeavor are explored.

REFERENCES

1. Duncum BM: The Development of Inhalation Anaesthesia, p 86. London, Oxford University Press, 1947
2. Davy H: Researches Chemical and Philosophical Chiefly Concerning Nitrous Oxide or Dephlogisticated Nitrous Air, and Its Respiration, p 533. London, J. Johnson, 1800
3. Lyman HM: Artificial Anaesthesia and Anaesthetics, p 6. New York, William Wood, 1881
4. Long CW: An Account of the first use of sulphuric ether by inhalation as an anaesthetic in surgical operations. South Med Surg J 5:705, 1849
5. Greene NM: A consideration of factors in the discovery of anesthesia and their effects on its development. Anesthesiology 35:515, 1971
6. Duncum BM: The Development of Inhalation Anaesthesia, p 110. London, Oxford University Press, 1947
7. Snow J: On the Inhalation of the Vapour of Ether, p 23. London, J Churchill, 1847
8. Snow J: On Chloroform and Other Anesthetics, pp 58–74. London, J Churchill, 1858
9. Journal of Queen Victoria. In Strauss MB (ed): Familiar Medical Quotations, p 17. Boston, Little, Brown and Co, 1968
10. Duncum BM: The Development of Inhalation Anaesthesia, p 540. London, Oxford University Press, 1947
11. Duncum BM: The Development of Inhalation Anaesthesia, p 538. London, Oxford University Press, 1947
12. Calverley RK: J. T. Clover: A giant of victorian anaesthesia. In Rupreht J, van Lieburg MJ, Lee JA and Erdmann W (eds): Anaesthesia Essays on its History, p 21. Berlin, Springer-Verlag, 1985
13. Clover JT: Laryngotomy in chloroform anaesthesia. Br Med J i:132, 1877
14. Colton Dental Association (advertisement from the Public Ledger and Transcript, Philadelphia, December 4, 1869 Reynolds Historical Library, University of Alabama in Birmingham)
15. Andrews E: The oxygen mixture, a new anaesthetic combination. Chicago Medical Examiner 9:656, 1868
16. Becker HK: Carl Koller and cocaine. Psychoanal Q 32:332, 1963
17. Corning JL: Spinal anaesthesia and local medication of the cord. NY Med J 42:485, 1885
18. Bier AKG: Experiments in cocainization of the spinal cord, 1899. In Faulconer A, Keys TE (trans): Foundations of Anesthesiology, p 854. Springfield, Illinois, Charles C Thomas, 1965
19. Bier AKG: Experiments in cocainization of the spinal cord, 1899. In Faulconer A, Keys, TE (trans): Foundations of Anesthesiology, p 855. Springfield, Illinois, Charles C Thomas, 1965
20. Tait D, Caglieri G: Experimental and clinical notes on the subarachnoid space. JAMA 35:6, 1900
21. Lee JA: Arthur Edward James Barker, 1850–1916; British pioneer of regional anaesthesia. Anaesthesia 34:885, 1979
22. Lemmon WT: A method for continuous spinal anesthesia, a preliminary report. Ann Surg 111:141, 1940
23. Tuohy EB: Continuous spinal anesthesia: Its usefulness and technic involved. Anesthesiology 5:142, 1944
24. Pages F: Metameric anesthesia, 1921. In Faulconer A, Keys TE (trans): Foundations of Anesthesiology, p 927. Springfield, Illinois, Charles C Thomas, 1965
25. Fink BR: History of local anesthesia. In Cousins MJ, Bridenbaugh PO (eds): Neural Blockade, p 12. Philadelphia, J. B. Lippincott, 1980
26. Cushing H: On the avoidance of shock in major amputations by cocainization of large nerve trunks preliminary to their division. With observations on blood-pressure changes in surgical cases. Ann Surg 36:321, 1902
27. Waters RM: Clinical scope and utility of carbon dioxide filtration in inhalation anesthesia. Curr Res Analg Anesth 3:20, 1923
28. Sword BC: The closed circle method of administration of gas anesthesia. Curr Res Analg Anesth 9:198, 1930
29. Revell DG: An improved circulator for closed circle anesthesia. Can Anaesth Soc J 6:104, 1959
30. Obituary of T. Philip Ayre. Br Med J 280:125, 1980
31. Rees GJ: Anaesthesia in the newborn. Br Med J ii:1419, 1950
32. Bain JA, Spoerel WE: A stream-lined anaesthetic system. Can Anaesth Soc J 19:426, 1972
33. Morris LE: A new vaporizer for liquid anesthetic agents. Anesthesiology 13:587, 1952
34. Mushin WW, Rendell–Baker L: The Principles of Thoracic Anaesthesia Past and Present. p 89. Springfield, Illinois, Charles C Thomas, 1953
35. Shephard DAE: Harvey Cushing and anaesthesia. Can Anaesth Soc J 12:431, 1965
36. Codesmith A: An endo-esophageal stethoscope. Anesthesiology 15:566, 1954
37. Tovell RM: Problems in supply of anesthetic gases in the European theater of operations. Anesthesiology 8:303, 1947
38. Rendall-Baker L: History of standards for anesthesia equipment. In Rupreht J, van Lieburg MJ, Lee JA and Erdmann W (eds): Anaesthesia Essays on Its History, pp 161–165. Berlin, Springer-Verlag, 1985
39. Leigh DM, Jenkins LC, Belton MK: Continuous alveolar carbon dioxide analysis as a monitor of pulmonary blood flow. Anesthesiology 18:878, 1954
40. Faulconer A, Pender JW, Bickford RG: The influence of partial pressure of nitrous oxide on the depth of anesthesia and the electro-encephalogram in man. Anesthesiology 10:601, 1949
41. Severinghaus JC, Honda Y: Pulse oximetry. Int Anesthesiol Clin 25(4):212, 1987
42. Severinghaus JC, Honda Y: Pulse oximetry. Int Anesthesiol Clin 25(4):206, 1987
43. Macewan W: Clinical observations on the introduction of tracheal tubes by the mouth instead of performing tracheotomy or laryngotomy. Br Med J ii:122–124, 163–165, 1880
44. Mushin WW, Rendall–Baker L: The Principles of Thoracic Anaesthesia Past and Present, pp 44–45. Springfield, Illinois, Charles C Thomas, 1953
45. Mushin WW, Rendall–Baker L: The Principles of Thoracic Anaesthesia Past and Present, p 44. Springfield, Illinois, Charles C Thomas, 1953
46. Kuhn F: Nasotracheal intubation (trans): In Faulconer A, Keys TE (eds): Foundations of Anesthesiology, pp 677–680. Springfield, Illinois, Charles C Thomas, 1965
47. Hirsch NP, Smith GB, Hirsch PO: Alfred Kirstein pioneer of direct laryngoscopy. Anaesthesia 41:42, 1986

48. Thomas KB: Sir Ivan Whiteside Magill, KCVO, DSc, MB, BCh, BAO, FRCS, FFARCS (Hon), FFARCSI (Hon), DA. A review of his publications and other references to his life and work. Anaesthesia 33:628, 1978
49. Condon HA, Gilchrist E: Stanley Rowbotham twentieth century pioneer anaesthetist. Anaesthesia 41:46, 1986
50. Calverley RK: Arthur E Guedel (1883–1956). In Rupreht J, van Lieburg MJ, Lee JA, and Erdmann W (eds): Anaesthesia Essays on Its History, pp 49–53. Berlin, Springer-Verlag, 1985
51. Calverley RK: Classical file. Surv Anesth 28:70, 1984
52. Gale JW, Waters RM: Closed endobronchial anesthesia in thoracic surgery: preliminary report. Curr Res Anesth Analg 11:283, 1932
53. Miller RA: A new laryngoscope. Anesthesiology 2:317, 1941
54. Macintosh RR: Richard Salt of Oxford, anaesthetic technician extraordinary. Anaesthesia 31:855, 1976
55. Lucas GHW: The discovery of cyclopropane. Curr Res Anesth Analg 40:15, 1961
56. Calverley RK: Fluorinated anesthetics. I. The early years. Surv Anesth 29:170, 1986
57. Robbins BH: Preliminary studies of the anesthetic activity of the fluorinated hydrocarbons. J Pharmacol Exp Therap 86:197, 1946
58. Calverley RK: Fluorinated anesthetics. II. Fluroxene. Surv Anesth 30:126, 1987
59. Suckling CW: Some chemical and physical factors in the development of Fluothane. Br J Anaesth 29:466, 1957
60. Macintosh RR: Modern anaesthesia, with special reference to the chair of anaesthetics in Oxford. In Rupreht J, van Lieburg MJ, Lee JA, and Erdmann W (eds): Anaesthesia Essays on Its History, pp 352–356. Berlin, Springer-Verlag, 1985
61. Knoefel PK: Felice Fontana Life and Works, pp 284–285. Trento, Societa de Studi Trentini, 1985
62. Griffith HR, Johnson GE: The use of curare in general anesthesia. Anesthesiology 3:418, 1942
63. Fink BR: Leaves and needles: The introduction of surgical local anesthesia. Anesthesiology 63:77, 1985
64. Seldon TH: Francis Hoeffer McMechan. In Volpitto PP, Vandam LD (eds): Genesis of American Anesthesiology, pp 5–20. Springfield, Illinois, Charles C Thomas, 1982
65. Bamforth BJ, Siebecker KL: Ralph M. Waters. In Volpitto PP, Vandam LD (eds): Genesis of American Anesthesiology, pp 51–68. Springfield, Illinois, Charles C Thomas, 1982
66. Waters RM: Pioneering in anesthesiology. Postgrad Med 4:265, 1968
67. Waters RM: Pioneering in anesthesiology. Postgrad Med 4:267, 1968
68. Guedel AE: Inhalation anesthesia: a fundamental guide. New York, Macmillan, 1937, p 129
69. Little DM Jr, Betcher AM: The Diamond Jubilee 1905–1980, p 8. Park Ridge, American Society of Anesthesiologists, 1980
70. Calmes SH: Development of the Apgar score. In Rupreht J, van Lieburg MJ, Lee JA, and Erdmann W (eds): Anaesthesia Essays on Its History, pp 45–48. Berlin, Springer-Verlag, 1985
71. Gordon RA: A capsule history of anaesthesia history in Canada. Can Anaesth Soc J 25:75, 1978

Chapter 2

Frederick W. Cheney
Donald A. Kroll

Medicolegal Aspects of Anesthetic Practice

The legal aspects of medical practice have become increasingly important as the American public has turned to the courts for economic redress when the realities of medical treatment do not meet their expectations. In 1982, an AMA opinion survey of U.S. physicians cited cost of medical care as the number 1 problem facing American medicine, while professional liability was not even mentioned. By 1986, professional liability was cited as the number 1 problem by U.S. physicians, with cost of medical care and government regulation in second and third place. Although the cost of liability insurance premiums for anesthesiologists is in the middle range of all specialists, the average cost of a professional liability policy in 1987 was about $25,000. There were wide geographic differences, with premiums ranging from under $10,000 in some states to over $60,000 in others for the same coverage. It is little consolation to the anesthesiologist that some other specialists, such as cardiac surgeons, vascular surgeons, orthopedic surgeons, obstetricians, and neurosurgeons, have higher premiums. The purpose of this chapter is to provide a background for the practitioner about how the legal system handles malpractice claims and the steps that should be taken when one is the target of a malpractice action. Risk management and liability insurance options are also discussed. More extensive texts are available for more detailed information.[1]

THE TORT SYSTEM

Physicians more commonly become involved in the legal system of civil laws, which may be broadly divided into contract

Portions of the text are based on copyrighted materials of the American Society of Anesthesiologists, Inc. The American Society of Anesthesiologists takes no responsibility for the accuracy of the extracts. A copy of the full text of "Professional Liability and the Anesthesiologist" can be obtained from the American Society of Anesthesiologists, 515 Busse Highway, Park Ridge, Illinois 60068.

law and tort law. A tort may be loosely defined as a civil wrongdoing. The majority of medical malpractice lawsuits are pursued on the basis of negligence theories, but there are occasional cases where contract law theories are utilized. Malpractice actually refers to any professional misconduct, but its use in legal terms typically refers to professional negligence. To be successful in a malpractice suit, the patient-plaintiff must prove four things:

Duty: that the anesthesiologist owed him or her a duty.
Breach of Duty: that the anesthesiologist failed to fulfill his or her duty.
Causation: that a reasonably close causal relationship exists between the anesthesiologist's acts and the resultant injury.
Damages: that actual damage resulted because of the acts of the anesthesiologist.

Failure to prove any one of these four elements will result in a decision for the defendant anesthesiologist.

DUTY

As a physician, the anesthesiologist establishes a duty to the patient when a doctor-patient relationship exists. When the patient is seen preoperatively and the anesthesiologist agrees to provide anesthesia care for the patient, a duty to the patient has been established. In the most general terms, the duty the anesthesiologist owes to the patient is to adhere to the "standard of care" for the treatment of the patient. Since it is virtually impossible to delineate specific standards for all aspects of medical practice and all eventualities, the courts have created the "reasonable and prudent" physician. For all specialties, there is a national standard which has displaced the local standard.

There are certain general duties which all physicians have to their patients, and breaching these duties may also serve as the basis for a lawsuit. One of these general duties is that of obtaining an informed consent. Consent may be written, verbal, or implied. Oral consent is just as valid, albeit harder to prove years after the fact, than written consent. Implied consent for anesthesia care may be present in circumstances in which the patient is unconscious or unable, for any reason, to give his or her consent, but where it is presumed that any reasonable and prudent patient would give consent if they were able. Although there are exceptions to the requirement that consent be obtained, as a general rule, anesthesiologists should be sure to obtain consent whenever possible. Failure to do so exposes the anesthesiologist to possible prosecution for assault and battery. The requirement that the consent be "informed" consent is somewhat more obtuse. The guideline is determining whether or not the patient received a fair and reasonable account of the proposed procedures and the risks inherent in these procedures. The duty to disclose risks is not limitless, but it does extend to those risks that are reasonably likely to occur in any patient under the circumstances, and to those that are reasonably likely to occur in particular patients because of their condition.

Other general duties include the maintenance of medical records, the performance of an appropriate examination of the patient, and the use of consultations and referrals to other physician specialists. Although these duties are more applicable to the primary care specialties, anesthesiologists may be held liable for the failure to perform these general duties as they are applied to the specialty. For example, if an anesthesiologist performs a preoperative examination for another anesthesiologist or a CRNA and fails to provide adequate documentation in the medical record or to report a significant condition by direct consultation, he or she will be liable for any injury that results.

BREACH OF DUTY

Expert witnesses will review the medical records of the case, and will determine whether or not the anesthesiologist acted in a reasonable and prudent manner in the specific situation and fulfilled his or her duty to the patient. If they find that the anesthesiologist either did something that should not have been done, or failed to do something that should have been done, then the duty to adhere to the standard of care has been breached, and the second requirement for a successful suit will have been met.

CAUSATION

Judges and juries are interested in determining whether the breach of duty was the "proximate cause" of the injury. If the odds are better than even that the breach of duty led, however circuitously, to the injury, then this requirement is met.

There are two common tests employed to establish causation. The first is the "but for" test, and the second is the "substantial factor" test. If the injury would not have occurred but for the action of the defendant anesthesiologist, or the act of the anesthesiologist was a substantial factor in the injury despite other causes, then proximate cause is established.

While the burden of proof of causation ordinarily falls on the patient-plaintiff, it may, under special circumstances, be shifted to the physician-defendant under the doctrine of *res ipsa loquitur*. Applying this doctrine requires proving that:

- The injury is of a kind that typically would not occur in the absence of negligence.
- The injury must be caused by something under the exclusive control of the anesthesiologist.
- The injury must not be due to any contribution on the part of the patient.
- The evidence for the explanation of events must be more accessible to the anesthesiologist than the patient.

Because anesthesiologists render patients insensible to their surroundings and unable to protect themselves from injury, this doctrine may be invoked in anesthesia malpractice cases. All that needs to be proven is that the injury typically would not occur in the absence of negligence, and the anesthesiologist is put in the position of having to prove that he or she was *not* negligent.

DAMAGES

The law allows for three different types of damages. *General damages* are those such as pain and suffering which directly result from the injury. *Special damages* are those actual damages which are a consequence of the injury, such as medical expenses, lost income, funeral expenses, etc. *Punitive damages* are intended to punish the physician for negligence which was reckless, wanton, fraudulent, or willful. Occasionally, exemplary damages are awarded to make an example of the case to prevent any other physician from doing the same thing again.

Determining the dollar amount of damages is the job of the jury, and the determination is usually based upon some assessment of the plaintiff's condition *versus* the condition they would have been in if there had been no negligence. Plaintiffs' attorneys generally charge a percentage of the damages, and will, therefore, seek to maximize the award given.

Since medical malpractice usually involves issues beyond the comprehension of lay jurors and judges, the court establishes the standard of care in a particular case by the testimony of "expert witnesses." Expert witnesses differ from factual witnesses mainly in that they may give opinions. The trial court judge has sole discretion in determining whether or not a witness may be qualified as an expert. Although any licensed physician may be an expert, information will be sought regarding the witness's education, training, nature and scope of practice, memberships and affiliations, and publications. The purpose in gathering this information is not only to establish the qualifications of the witness to provide expert testimony, but also to determine the weight to be given to that testimony by the jury. In many cases, the success of a suit depends primarily on the stature and believability of the expert witnesses.

In certain circumstances, the standard of care may also be determined from published societal guidelines, written policies of a hospital or department, or textbooks and monographs. Some medical specialty societies have carefully avoided applying the term "standards" to their guidelines, in the hope that no binding behavior or mandatory practices have been created. In the past, the American Society of Anesthesiologists has published a number of guidelines relating to the practice of anesthesia. In 1986, the ASA, for the first time, published "Standards for Basic Intraoperative Monitoring" (Table 2-1).[3] These are more binding than guidelines. Essentially, guidelines *should* be adhered to and standards *must* be adhered to.

TABLE 2-1. Standards For Basic Intra-Operative Monitoring

(Approved by House of Delegates of The American Society of Anesthesiologists on October 21, 1986)

These standards apply to all anesthesia care although, in emergency circumstances, appropriate life support measures take precedence. These standards may be exceeded at any time based on the judgement of the responsible anesthesiologist. They are intended to encourage high quality patient care, but observing them cannot guarantee any specific patient outcome. They are subject to revision from time to time, as warranted by the evolution of technology and practice. This set of standards addresses only the issue of basic intra-operative monitoring, which is one component of anesthesia care. In certain rare or unusual circumstances, 1) some of these methods of monitoring may be clinically impractical, and 2) appropriate use of the described monitoring methods may fail to detect untoward clinical developments. Brief interruptions of continual† monitoring may be unavoidable. *Under extenuating circumstances, the responsible anesthesiologist may waive the requirements marked with an asterisk (*); it is recommended that when this is done, it should be so stated (including the reasons) in a note in the patient's medical record.* These standards are not intended for application to the care of the obstetrical patient in labor or in the conduct of pain management.

STANDARD I

Qualified anesthesia personnel shall be present in the room throughout the conduct of all general anesthetics, regional anesthetics and monitored anesthesia care.

OBJECTIVE

Because of the rapid changes in patient status during anesthesia, qualified anesthesia personnel shall be continuously present to monitor the patient and provide anesthesia care. In the event there is a direct known hazard, e.g., radiation, to the anesthesia personnel which might require intermittent remote observation of the patient, some provision for monitoring the patient must be made. In the event that an emergency requires the temporary absence of the person primarily responsible for the anesthetic, the best judgement of the anesthesiologist will be exercised in comparing the emergency with the anesthetized patient's condition and in the selection of the person left responsible for the anesthetic during the temporary absence.

STANDARD II

During all anesthetics, the patient's oxygenation, ventilation, circulation and temperature shall be continually evaluated.

OXYGENATION

OBJECTIVE

To ensure adequate oxygen concentration in the inspired gas and the blood during all anesthetics.

METHODS

1) Inspired gas: During every administration of general anesthesia using an anesthesia machine, the concentration of oxygen in the patient breathing system shall be measured by an oxygen analyzer with a low oxygen concentration limit alarm in use.*

2) Blood oxygenation: During all anesthetics, adequate illumination and exposure of the patient is necessary to assess color. While this and other qualitative clinical signs may be adequate, there are quantitative methods, such as pulse oximetry, which are encouraged.

VENTILATION

OBJECTIVE

To ensure adequate ventilation of the patient during all anesthetics.

METHODS

1) Every patient receiving general anesthesia shall have the adequacy of ventilation continually evaluated. While qualitative clinical signs such as chest excursion, observation of the reservoir breathing bag and auscultation of breath sounds may be adequate, quantitative monitoring of the CO_2 content and/or volume of expired gas is encouraged.

2) When an endotracheal tube is inserted, its correct positioning in the trachea must be verified. Clinical assessment is essential and end-tidal CO_2 analysis, in use from the time of endotracheal tube placement, is encouraged.

3) When ventilation is controlled by a mechanical ventilator, there shall be in continuous use a device that is capable of detecting disconnection of components of the breathing system. The device must give an audible signal when its alarm threshold is exceeded.

4) During regional anesthesia and monitored anesthesia care, the adequacy of ventilation shall be evaluated, at least, by continual observation of qualitative clinical signs.

CIRCULATION

OBJECTIVE

To ensure the adequacy of the patient's circulatory function during all anesthetics.

METHODS

1) Every patient receiving anesthesia shall have the electrocardiogram continuously displayed from the beginning of anesthesia until preparing to leave the anesthetizing location.*

(Continued)

TABLE 2-1.   Standards For Basic Intra-Operative Monitoring (*continued*)

STANDARD II

METHODS

2) Every patient receiving anesthesia shall have arterial blood pressure and heart rate determined and evaluated at least every five minutes.*

3) Every patient receiving general anesthesia shall have, in addition to the above, circulatory function continually evaluated by at least one of the following: palpation of a pulse, auscultation of heart sounds, monitoring of a tracing of intraarterial pressure, ultrasound peripheral pulse monitoring, or pulse plethysmography or oximetry.

BODY TEMPERATURE

OBJECTIVE

To aid in the maintenance of appropriate body temperature during all anesthetics.

METHODS

There shall be readily available a means to continuously measure the patient's temperature. When changes in body temperature are intended, anticipated or suspected, the temperature shall be measured.

†Note that "continual" is defined as "repeated regularly and frequently in steady rapid succession" whereas "continuous" means "prolonged without any interruption at any time."

WHAT TO DO WHEN SUED

A lawsuit begins when the patient-plaintiff's attorney files a complaint and demand for jury trial with the court. The anesthesiologist is then served with the complaint and a summons requiring an answer to the complaint. Until this happens, no lawsuit has been filed. Insurance carriers must be notified immediately after receiving the complaint. The anesthesiologist will need assistance in answering the complaint, and there is a time limit placed upon the response.

Specific actions at this point include:

- Do not discuss the case with *anyone*, including colleagues who may have been involved, operating room personnel, or friends.
- *Never* alter any records.
- Gather together all pertinent records, including a copy of the anesthetic record, billing statements, and correspondence concerning the case.
- Make notes recording all events recalled about the case. It may be necessary to review the medical record. Some attorneys will recommend that physicians establish a separate file for all documents pertinent to the case, making certain that the file is marked as confidential.
- Cooperate fully with the attorney provided by the insurer in answering the complaint.

If a physician believes that the attorney provided by an insurance carrier is not representing his or her interests fully, then one of several options may be exercised. The insurance company may be requested to provide another attorney, or the physician may consider retaining private counsel. If the estimated damage settlement is greater than the limits of the insurance coverage, the physician may be personally liable for the difference. A second reason to obtain private counsel is if there is a potential impact on retaining the ability to practice. If there is a possibility that practice privileges will be limited or revoked, then there is reason enough to hire someone to represent the physician's interests independent of the malpractice claim. A third reason to retain separate counsel is if the physician does not have confidence in the attorney pro-

vided by the insurance carrier, and if an alternative cannot be provided. Since the physician will be working closely with the attorney, it is of some importance that the physician have confidence in his or her abilities.

The first task the anesthesiologist must perform with an attorney is to prepare an answer to the complaint. The complaint contains certain facts and allegations with which the defense may either agree or disagree. Denial of facts or allegations constitutes a negative defense. There may also be affirmative defenses, which, if proven, would exonerate the anesthesiologist, even if the facts alleged in the complaint were true. For example, the statute of limitations may have run out before the complaint was filed, the patient may be alleged to have assumed the risk, or another physician might have contributed to the injury. Defense attorneys rely upon the frank and totally candid observations of the physician in preparing an answer to the complaint. Physicians should be willing to educate their attorneys about the medical facts of the case, although most medical malpractice attorneys will be surprisingly knowledgeable and medically sophisticated.

The next phase of the malpractice suit is called "discovery." The purpose of discovery is the gathering of facts and clarification of issues in advance of the trial. Another purpose of discovery is to assess or harass the defendant to determine how good a witness he or she will make. This occurs at several points in the discovery process, and by several mechanisms.

The anesthesiologist will, in all likelihood, receive a written interrogatory which will usually be filed through the defense attorney. Written interrogatories requesting factual information about training, experience, and qualifications are perfectly legitimate. However, if the anesthesiologist receives an interrogatory which appears to contain many irrelevant or personal questions, it is a good idea to consult with the defense attorney before spending time answering unnecessary or irrelevant questions. The interrogatory should be answered in writing, in consultation with the defense attorney, because carelessly or inadvertently misstated facts can become troublesome at a later date.

Depositions are a second mechanism of discovery. The defendant anesthesiologist will be deposed as a fact witness, and depositions will be obtained from other anesthesiologists who will act as expert witnesses. The defendant anesthesiologist may be asked to suggest other anesthesiologists who will review the medical records. A nationally recognized expert in the area in question who is not a personal friend, but agrees with the defense position, may be very valuable. Generally speaking, an acquaintance or a partner is not as believable as a stranger. Other than making a recommendation about who will serve as the expert for the defense, the defendant anesthesiologist has little control over the selection of experts. The conduct of the defendant anesthesiologist during deposition may have a profound impact on the outcome of the suit, however.

The anesthesiologist will be deposed by the plaintiff's attorney, not the defense attorney. Physicians may receive a subpoena demanding their presence at an inconvenient time or place in an attempt to harass them or make them angry. If this happens, the defense attorney will probably be able to take care of the matter for the physician. Most often, the arrangements for the deposition will be made amicably by both sides, and the deposition will occur at a place and time convenient for the anesthesiologist, typically in the defense attorney's office. As a general rule, it is best that physicians avoid having the deposition taken in their own offices. The reason for this is that the plaintiff's attorney will very carefully note such things as the medical books on the shelves, the diplomas on the walls, and the general state of disarray of the office. Information may be provided which the plaintiff's attorney may find a way to use against the anesthesiologist. A second reason to avoid pleasant and familiar surroundings is that the physician will tend to lower his or her guard if comfortable, and fall prey to certain common traps in deposition. *Despite the apparent informality of the deposition, the anesthesiologist must be constantly aware that what is said during the deposition carries as much weight as what would be said in court.*

The anesthesiologist should meet with his or her attorney prior to the deposition for the sole purpose of being coached on how to give the deposition. The defense attorney should be experienced in both taking and giving deposition testimony, and he or she should be able to advise anesthesiologists on what to expect and how to conduct themselves. There are some general guidelines to follow, and there may be specific points which the attorney will ask the anesthesiologist to make during his or her testimony.

It is important to be factually prepared for the deposition. A review of notes, the anesthetic record, and the medical record is necessary. The defendant anesthesiologist will be asked some specific questions about the dates and places of medical training and whether or not he or she has published any articles or papers, or written any chapters in textbooks. Physicians may also be asked details about their practice, the size of their group, or possibly details about their relationship to the hospital in which they practice. Defendant anesthesiologists should be sure about these details, update their curriculum vitae, and be familiar with such information before the deposition.

For the deposition, the physician should dress conservatively and professionally, as appearance and image are very important. The opposition is assessing the physician to see how he or she will appear to a jury. Answers to questions should be brief and concise. Being evasive or hostile is not helpful. Answer only the question asked, and do not volunteer information. The plaintiff's attorney may pause for long periods of time after a question in an attempt to procure an expanded answer. Silence is awkward, and there is a natural tendency to say something during a pause. Physicians should avoid this temptation, and look to their attorney for clues

about answers. If the defense attorney raises an objection, stop talking immediately, and allow the attorney to voice his or her objections. Most often, the physician will be expected to complete his or her answer after the objection, but the answer may be tempered somewhat by what the defense attorney is objecting to.

Occasionally, physicians will be asked leading questions which are impossible to answer without qualifications. In this case, the physician may qualify his or her answer, but should avoid giving lengthy opinion answers. The defendant anesthesiologist is being deposed as a witness of facts, not opinions. Experts may give opinions, but the defendant should try to avoid doing so.

Another common ploy is to try to get a physician to admit something which is apparently benign, but opens up a line of questioning which the attorney could otherwise not pursue. Questions about insurance coverage, personal assets, contractual relationships with the hospital, or anything else for which there is no obvious connection to the case are suspect. Physicians should not admit that there are any "definitive" or "authoritative" textbooks upon which they rely in their practice. Doing so may make them responsible for everything that is said in the book, whether they agree with it or not. The defense attorney should advise the anesthesiologist on how to respond to this type of questioning. Do not underestimate the plaintiff's attorney, no matter how friendly or inept he or she may seem. Taking a deposition is a finely honed skill for which the plaintiff's attorney is much better trained and more experienced than the defendant anesthesiologist. Physicians must not become cocky or overconfident, and allow themselves to be led into a trap by relaxing their guard.

The best answers are those which are responsive to the question without volunteering additional information. The answers should be given in the simplest possible terms. Technical medical terms, medical jargon, pejorative terms, and slang should be avoided. Do not try to be humorous or make a joke, as these do not translate well on paper. Court reporters will record exactly what is said, so it is important to speak clearly. Speaking slightly more slowly than normal will facilitate an accurate transcription, and will also give the defense attorney the opportunity to interrupt if the physician is headed into unfriendly territory.

The plaintiff's attorney may try to intimidate the anesthesiologist or make him or her angry. This serves two purposes. First, the anesthesiologist may say something he or she will later regret. Second, if the attorney knows that the defendant anesthesiologist is a volatile person, he or she will welcome the opportunity to make the defendant look foolish in front of a jury. Do not get angry or become emotional. Remember that the goal of the plaintiff's attorney in taking defendants' depositions is to try to get them to admit to facts which will be helpful to the plaintiff's case, and to size them up for a possible courtroom trial. The defense attorney already knows what is going to be said and what the defense position will be. If the case against an anesthesiologist is weak or doubtful, a favorable performance in deposition will serve to greatly reduce the likelihood of a jury trial and a high award. On the other hand, if there is a reasonably good case against the anesthesiologist, a poor deposition performance might make the plaintiff's attorney unwilling to consider settlement at all.

There will be depositions from expert witnesses, both for the plaintiff and for the defense. The anesthesiologist should work with his or her attorney to suggest questions and rebuttals. The better educated the attorney is about the medical facts, the reasons why the anesthesiologist did what was done, and alternative approaches, the better able he or she will be to conduct these expert depositions. The presence of the defendant anesthesiologist during the depositions of plaintiff's experts may be crucial.

There will probably be much posturing, jockeying for position, and negotiating among the various attorneys involved in the case during the discovery phase. Anesthesiologists may find that they are in an adversarial relationship with not only the plaintiff's attorney, but also the hospital's attorney, and the attorneys for other defendants. It is important not to personalize these procedures. Anesthesiologists must realize that the only issue of importance is getting out of the suit with the minimum dollar cost. If the case against them is without merit, it will probably be dropped early in the discovery process. Sometimes, lawsuits are filed by plaintiffs' attorneys before they have actually had the case reviewed by an expert. An example of this would be when the statute of limitations is about to run out at the time the attorney is consulted. If there is some merit in the case, but the damages are minimal, or if proof will be difficult, there will probably be a settlement offer. There is a high cost incurred by both plaintiffs and defendants in pursuing a malpractice claim up through a jury trial. Unless there is a strong probability of a large dollar award, reputable plaintiffs' attorneys are not likely to pursue the claim. Thus, even if physicians believe that they are totally innocent of any wrongdoing, they should not be offended or angered about settling the case. This is solely a matter of money, not medicine. The only reason for physicians to fight the settlement of an unmeritorious claim early in the discovery process is if such a settlement will have some repercussions which affect their ability to practice or impose a financial burden upon them.

A settlement may be offered because the claim is likely to be successful and result in a larger award in the event of a jury trial. In this situation, the insurer presumes that the evidence will show that the insured anesthesiologist was negligent, and is attempting to limit its losses. They will be quite uninterested in whether the defendant anesthesiologist wishes to settle or not. Fighting the settlement will probably not be advantageous. The best the physician may hope for is that his or her practice will not be affected, personal assets affected, or licensure questioned.

If a settlement is not reached during the discovery phase, a trial will occur. Only about one in 20 malpractice cases ever reaches the point of a jury trial. The reason for this is that both plaintiffs' and defendants' attorneys are aware of the strengths of the case, and it usually becomes clear during discovery whether or not the suit will be successful. Preparing for and conducting a jury trial is expensive for both sides, and there is, therefore, economic pressure to reach a settlement, especially for the side that is likely to lose. Only those cases in which both sides feel they can win, and which are likely to have significant financial impact, will proceed to trial. The jurisdiction in which a case is tried, and the composition of the jury, may have a profound impact on the eventual outcome. Juries tend to become sympathetic to one side or the other during the trial. The more pathetic and helpless the patient-plaintiff, the more likely it is that the anesthesiologist will lose. Alternatively, the more reasonable and professional the physician seems, the more likely it is that he or she will win. Whether or not the jury trusts the physician and the defense side of the story depends on the physician's ability to communicate with the jury, his or her appearance, and the jury's belief in the physician's skills and competence.

The discussion of deposition testimony also applies to testimony in court, but there are a few additional points to consider during the trial. The members of the jury will not be as medically sophisticated as the attorneys who deposed the anesthesiologist during discovery. The anesthesiologist should review his or her discovery deposition. A tendency to overuse specific medical terms should be corrected by learning to explain answers in lay terms for the benefit of the jury. Do not underestimate the intelligence of the jury, however, because talking down to them will create an unfavorable impression. Physicians should pay attention to the jury as they speak, and try to estimate whether the members of the jury are understanding the answers. It is best to speak clearly, using understandable terms. Physicians should be confident in their answers without seeming smug or pompous. If the answer to a question is not known, avoid guessing. If specific facts cannot be remembered, say so. Nobody expects total recall of events which may have occurred years before.

The defendant physician should be present during the trial, even when not testifying, and should dress conservatively, neatly, and professionally. Displays of anger, remorse, relief, hostility, etc., will hurt the physician in court. Unnecessary consultation with defense counsel while others are testifying creates a bad impression with the jury, but the defendant anesthesiologist should not appear bored or disinterested. When giving testimony, the anesthesiologist must give clear answers to all questions asked. If a question is poorly phrased and imprecise, clarification should be requested. Defendant physicians should answer only the question asked, and should not volunteer information, except when it is necessary to qualify an answer. The physician should be able to give his or her testimony without using notes or documents. When it is necessary to refer to the medical record, it will be admitted into evidence. If there are misleading or damaging statements in the medical record, the defense attorney may have gone to great lengths to try to avoid having the record admitted in evidence; admitting any part of the record may lead to having to admit the entire record.

The anesthesiologist's goal is to convince the jury that he or she behaved in this case as any other competent and prudent anesthesiologist would have behaved. Specifying the reasons for selecting a procedure or technique, or excluding alternative methods, will help the defendant anesthesiologist, assuming that the reasons were valid. This is true even if the anesthesiologist disagrees with the expert who is testifying for the plaintiff. Creating the impression that there were several possible approaches, and that the defendant anesthesiologist selected the one which was the best for the patient at the time, will tend to enhance credibility of the defense to a greater extent than trying to convince the jury that the defendant anesthesiologist's decisions were based upon 100% certainty, and, hence, that the opposing expert is 100% wrong.

It is important to keep in mind that "proof" in a malpractice case means only "more likely than not." The patient-plaintiff must "prove" the four elements of negligence, not to absolute certainty, but only to a probability greater than 50%. On the positive side, this means that the defendant anesthesiologist must only show that his or her actions were, more likely than not, within an acceptable standard of care.

CAUSES OF SUITS

The major cause of suits against anesthesiologists is patient injury. In a nationwide analysis of 624 closed claims against anesthesiologists conducted by the American Society of Anesthesiologists Committee on Professional Liability, the leading injuries for which suit was filed were: death (35%), nerve damage (16%), and brain damage (12%).[2] The causes of death and brain damage were predominantly due to inadequate ventilation, esophageal intubation, and other airway problems. Nerve damage was related to positioning, regional anesthesia, and central venous catheter placement. As death and brain damage are high-cost injuries, anesthesia practice is clearly a high-risk endeavor. Anesthesiologists use complex equipment which can fail, and potent drugs with which mistakes in dose or labelling can lead to disastrous results. Vigilance, which is the highest priority in anesthesia practice, is often difficult to maintain at all times of the day and night through long, tedious surgical procedures. The anesthesiologist is more likely to be the target of a suit, if an untoward outcome occurs, because the physician-patient relationships are usually tenuous at best. The patient rarely chooses the anesthesiologist, the preoperative visit is brief, and the anesthesiologist who sees the patient preoperatively may not actually anesthetize the patient. Communication between anesthesiologists and surgeons about complications is often lacking, and the tendency is for the surgeon to "blame anesthesia."

Supervision of nurse anesthetists is another endeavor that puts the anesthesiologist in a high-risk category. The more nurse anesthetists supervised by any one anesthesiologist, the greater the exposure to the possibility of patient injury. At the present time, there are no national standards as to the number of nurse anesthetists who can be legally supervised by one anesthesiologist. However, some professional liability insurance companies specify a staffing ratio of 1 : 2 or 1 : 3, and charge higher rates for supervision of more than this amount. Anesthesiologists are liable not only for nurse anesthetists who they employ, but also for those they supervise who are employed by the hospital. Due to the fact that anesthesiologists are employed in the care of patients undergoing high-risk surgical procedures, they are often sued along with the surgeon in the case of an adverse outcome. This may occur even if the outcome was in no way related to the anesthetic care. Finally, since anesthetic injuries are high-cost injuries, anesthesiologists have been targeted by plaintiffs' attorneys. There are frequent seminars for plaintiffs' attorneys, held throughout the country, which specifically address anesthetic injuries.

RISK MANAGEMENT

The primary goal of any risk management program is the prevention of patient injury. If a patient injury from anesthesia does not occur, the likelihood of a lawsuit is minimized. The nature of anesthetic practice, however, is such that some patient injury will inevitably occur. Therefore, the second phase of risk management is the practice of defensive medicine, the performance of which is hard to separate from good medicine.

The key factors in the prevention of patient injury are vigilance, up-to-date knowledge, and adequate monitoring.[7] Physiologic monitoring of cardiopulmonary function, combined with monitoring of equipment function, might be expected to reduce anesthetic injury to a minimum. Equipment monitors are designed to detect serious equipment failure before patient injury results. In any analysis of anesthetic mishaps, it is common to see that many could have been prevented by the use of appropriate monitors. While everyone would agree that adequacy of oxygenation, ventilation, and circulation should be monitored during all anesthetics, the means may leave some room for controversy. Clearly, the American Society of Anesthesiologists "Standards for Basic Intraoperative Monitoring" should be adhered to.[3] Basically, these "standards" call for the presence of qualified anesthesia personnel in the room at all times, and for monitoring of oxygenation, ventilation, and circulation. During general anesthesia, an oxygen analyzer should be used, and there should be adequate illumination and exposure of the patient to assess blood oxygenation. The ASA standards call for monitoring of ventilation during anesthesia, which may include such qualitative clinical signs as chest excursion, observation of the reservoir breathing bag, and auscultation of breath sounds, with the use of quantitative devices such as end-tidal CO_2 monitors and pulse oximeters encouraged. When an endotracheal tube is inserted, its correct position in the trachea must be verified by auscultation or the use of end-tidal CO_2 analysis. When a mechanical ventilator is in use, there should be a disconnect alarm with an audible signal. During regional anesthesia and monitored anesthesia care, the adequacy of ventilation should be evaluated by continual observation of the aforementioned qualitative clinical signs. In order to ensure adequacy of circulation, the standards call for continuous EKG monitoring, with arterial blood pressure and heart rate evaluated at least every 5 min. In addition to the above, each patient should have circulatory function continually evaluated by at least one of the following: palpation of the pulse, auscultation of heart sounds, monitoring of intraarterial pressure, or some other device, such as a pulse oximeter. Body temperature should be monitored when changes are "intended, anticipated, or suspected."

Although the ASA standards "encourage" the use of pulse oximeters and end-tidal CO_2 monitoring, information is emerging which indicates the use of these instruments will significantly reduce the incidence of patient injury. A study of closed malpractice claims conducted by the ASA's Committee on Professional Liability indicates that a significant portion of the high-cost injuries (e.g., brain damage and death) would have been prevented if these monitors had been in use.[2] In this study, there were 41 esophageal intubations which resulted in brain damage and death, and, in 23 instances, auscultation of the chest was documented in the record.[2] This implies that auscultation of the chest is not a completely accurate method of ensuring proper endotracheal tube placement. Clearly, end-tidal CO_2 is a more accurate method of assuring tracheal intubation and, perhaps, should be adopted as a "standard" of practice. Similarly, it seems likely that pulse oximetry would give an earlier warning of intra-anesthetic hypoxemia than more qualitative methods of diagnosis. Monitoring of respiration during regional or local anesthesia when sedation is administered is especially critical. Although not ideal, at the present time, the pulse oximeter is possibly the best monitor of respiration in any patient who is sedated beyond the point of spontaneous verbalization. Another safety-related activity is the careful checking of anesthesia equipment prior to its use. The use of checklists prior to each case, or at least daily, should reduce equipment-related mishaps.[4, 5, 8]

The practice of "defensive medicine" includes making of pre- and postoperative rounds, developing good patient relationships, and maintaining up-to-date practice habits. Good records can form a strong defense if they are adequate, and can be disastrous if inadequate. Informed consent should be documented with a general consent, which should include a statement to the effect that "I understand that all anesthetics involve risks of complications, serious injury, or, rarely, death from both known and unknown causes." In addition, there should be a note in the patient's record that the risks of anesthesia and alternatives were discussed, and that the patient accepted the proposed anesthetic plan. A brief documentation in the record that the common complications of the proposed technique were discussed is helpful. If it is necessary to significantly change the agreed-upon anesthesia plan after the patient is premedicated or anesthetized, the reasons for the change should be documented in the record.

The anesthesia record itself should be as accurate, complete, and neat as possible. In addition to vital signs every 5 min, special attention should be paid to ensure that the patient's ASA classification, the monitors utilized, fluids administered, and the doses and times of all drugs administered are accurately charted. As the major causes of hypoxic brain damage and death during anesthesia are related to respiration, all respiratory variables that are monitored should be accurately documented. It is important to note when there is a change of anesthesia personnel during the conduct of a case. Sloppy, inaccurate anesthesia records, enlarged and placed before a jury, can be quite damaging to the defense. If a critical incident occurs during the conduct of an anesthetic, the anesthesiologist should document, in narrative form in the patient's progress notes, what happened, which drugs were used, the time sequence, and who was present. A catastrophic intra-anesthetic event cannot be adequately summarized in a small amount of space on the usual anesthesia record. The critical incident note should be written as soon as possible, while all details are still fresh in the anesthesiologist's mind. The report should be as consistent as possible with concurrent records, such as the anesthesia, operating room, recovery room, and cardiac arrest records. If inconsistencies exist, they should be explained in the critical incident note. Records should never be altered after the fact. If an error is made in recordkeeping, a line should be drawn through the error, leaving it legible, and the correction should be initialed and timed. Litigation is a lengthy process, and a court appearance to explain the incident to a jury may be years away, when memories have faded. In the event of a sudden, unexpected intra-anesthetic cardiac arrest for which there is no readily apparent explanation, blood and urine should be obtained for drug screening. With the increasing frequency of surgery on an outpatient basis, some patients may be tempted to relieve their anxiety with the use of recreational drugs, which may interact adversely with drugs used for anesthesia.

If anesthetic complications occur, the anesthesiologist should be honest with both the patient and family about the cause. Whenever an anesthetic complication becomes apparent postoperatively, appropriate consultation should be obtained quickly, and the departmental or institutional risk management group should be notified. If the complication is apt to lead to prolonged hospitalization or permanent injury, the liability insurance carrier should be notified. The patient should be followed closely while in the hospital, with telephone follow-up, if indicated, after discharge. Also, the anesthesiologist and surgeon should be consistent in their explanations to the patient as to the cause of any complication.

While it may seem obvious, qualified anesthesia personnel should be in continuous attendance during the conduct of all anesthetics. The only exception should be those which lay people (i.e., judge and jury) can understand, such as radiation hazards, x-ray, or an unexpected life-threatening emergency elsewhere. Even then, provisions should be made for adequately monitoring the patient. Anesthetic complications occurring while anesthesia personnel have left the room without urgent reason are indefensible, and command high financial settlements or court awards. Adequate supervision of nurse anesthetists and residents, and good communication with surgeons when adverse anesthetic outcomes occur, are also important.

On a departmental level, an ongoing process of concurrent record review based on established standards of care criteria and anesthesia-related morbidity and mortality should be reviewed regularly.[9] A regular schedule of equipment maintenance and procedures to follow in cases in which equipment malfunction is suspected of contributing to patient injury should be established. If equipment malfunction is suspected to have contributed to a complication, the device should be impounded and examined by representatives of the hospital and manufacturer. Extensive information on anesthesia departmental quality assurance activities is available in the Joint Commission on Accreditation of Hospitals guidelines and the ASA's quality assurance manual.[6]

LIABILITY INSURANCE

Throughout the above discussion, there has been frequent reference to the role of the insurer in the defense of malpractice claims. The publicized "malpractice crisis" is, perhaps, better characterized as a crisis in insurance, rather than a crisis in medical practice, with the most important issues being the availability and cost of liability insurance.

Traditional malpractice coverage has been issued on an occurrence basis. As long as the anesthesiologist was insured at the time of the incident, coverage was provided continuously for that occurrence thereafter. This type of coverage was favorable for the physician, but insurers recognized the actuarial problem of being unable to predict the likelihood of a claim or the amount of expected losses. Most insurers no longer provide coverage on a per-occurrence basis, and have replaced this type of policy with "claims made" coverage. With claims made policies, the anesthesiologist must be insured at the time of the loss and at the time of reporting. Typically, the insurance rates start at a lower level, then increase to the mature policy rate and level off. This then makes coverage affordable to new specialists. The rates will vary with the limits of coverage, which are usually expressed as a pair of numbers indicating the limits in millions of dollars per occurrence and an annual total. A policy for $0.5/1.5 million indicates that the limit is $500,000 for any single claim, and that the total annual claims cannot exceed $1.5 million. Claims made coverage is typically available with limits of 0.5/1.5 , 1/3 , or 2/4 millions of dollars. The usually recommended coverage is $1 million/3 million. When purchasing coverage, it is important to know whether or not the policy is assessible. Assessibility means that, if the yearly premium is not adequate to cover losses, then the policy holder is "assessed" an extra amount in subsequent years to make up the difference.

Since the anesthesiologist must be insured both at the time of the loss and at the time the loss is reported, a problem arises when one type of policy or company is converted to another policy or company. This has led to two types of conversion coverage. When the new company agrees to provide coverage for claims which occurred under the previous policy, but have not yet been reported, it is referred to as "nose" coverage. If the old company provides such coverage, it is called "tail" coverage. Tail coverage also applies when the anesthesiologist leaves practice.

A third type of malpractice insurance is the "umbrella," or excess coverage, policy. This type of coverage is applied only when the limits of the primary policy are exceeded. The intent of excess coverage is to protect the physician in the event of a major catastrophic loss.

In addition to changing the types of malpractice insurance coverage available, insurers are also instituting practice guidelines as conditions for insurability. Several companies will only insure anesthesiologists if certain minimal patient monitoring criteria are met. Anesthesiologists who contract with their insurers to follow such guidelines may be financially responsible for damages which occur when the guidelines are not followed.

SPECIAL SITUATIONS

JEHOVAH'S WITNESSES

It is important to recognize that patients have well-established rights, and that among these is the right to refuse specific treatments because of religious beliefs. In the case of Jehovah's Witnesses, the treatment refused is the administration of blood or blood products. This refusal may seem irrational to some physicians, but it is a central part of their religious beliefs, which hold that they will be forbidden the pleasures of the afterlife if they receive blood or blood products. Thus, for them to receive a transfusion is a mortal sin, and many Jehovah's Witnesses would actually rather die in grace, as they see it, than live with no possibility of salvation. Anesthesiologists recognize and respect these beliefs, but are also cognizant that these convictions may conflict with the physicians' personal religious or ethical codes. Not all Jehovah's Witnesses share identical beliefs regarding blood transfusions, or which methods of blood preservation or sequestration will be allowed.

Minor children of Jehovah's Witness parents represent a special group for consideration. Although the U.S. Supreme Court has upheld the right of an adult to become a martyr by refusing treatments based upon religious convictions, no court has extended to parents the right to make their children martyrs. States have upheld the overriding interest in protecting children, and most states have provisions for the guarantee of access to medical treatment for children. This involves making the child a ward of the court for the purpose of rendering medical treatment. If the patient is an older child, the court may consider his/her wishes in reaching a decision. It must be stressed that obtaining a proper court order is of major importance in the care of a minor child with Jehovah's Witness parents, when the parents refuse to authorize a blood transfusion.

As a general rule, physicians are not obligated to treat all patients who apply for treatment in elective situations. It is well within the rights of a physician to decline to care for any patient who wishes to place burdensome constraints upon the physician or to unacceptably limit the physician's ability to provide optimal care. When presented with the opportunity to provide elective care for a Jehovah's Witness, the physician may decline to provide any care, or may limit, by mutual consent with the patient, his or her obligation to adhere to the patient's religious beliefs. If such an agreement is reached, it must be documented clearly in the medical record, and it is desirable to have the patient cosign the note. Some patients will not allow any blood which has left the body to be reinfused. Yet others will accept autotransfusion if their blood remains in constant contact with the body (*via* tubing). Therefore, it is important to reach a clear understanding of which techniques for blood preservation are to be used, and document this plan in the record. In some cases, parents may indicate that they wish a court order to be obtained, or that they want blood to be administered in life-threatening situations. There are many possible agreements which may be reached, and the physician must be able to delineate what his or her duty to the patient encompasses if he or she elects to provide care.

Emergency medical care imposes greater constraints upon the treating physician. There is no opportunity to decline the care of a patient with an immediately life-threatening condition. If the patient is an adult, and is conscious and mentally competent, then he/she has the right to refuse blood transfusion. A physician providing emergency on-call coverage may find that his/her desire to provide complete care is in conflict with the patient's religious beliefs. In this case, the patient's rights must be given precedence. The physician's duty to provide care within this framework is clear, and there is, thus, no opportunity to refuse to care for the patient in an emergency. The exceptions to patients' rights in this regard include pregnant women and adults who are the sole support of minor children. In these circumstances, the interests of the fetus in surviving may supercede the rights of the mother, as may the interests of the state in not being obligated to provide for the welfare of dependent children. In either case, obtaining a court order is the best plan if time permits. If the problem concerns blood products, and there is insufficient time to obtain a court order, pregnant women should be transfused to save the life of the fetus, but parents of minor children should not receive transfusions against their wishes unless the dependency of the children is obvious.

Unless there is ample prior notice, the anesthesiologist may not have an opportunity to communicate with the patient. The opportunity for dialogue with the patient is lost, as is the possibility of reaching a mutually agreeable compromise. Without this discussion of issues and alternatives, any ability to formulate a plan of action is lost. The extent of the patient's beliefs must be assessed, since not all Jehovah's Witnesses actually do prefer to die rather than receive blood. Some may allow the use of a cell-saver, while others may not. Some may not consider albumin to be in the same category as blood. This variation in beliefs makes the preoperative consultation with the patient essential, especially considering the importance of obtaining and documenting the informed consent.

When the patient is a minor, it is important to ascertain the true wishes of the parents. Some parents know that a court order can be obtained, and view this as a relief from the onerous burden of having to decide whether or not they are willing to let their child die. Some parents are adamant that blood not be given, and there have been cases where children have been ostracized by their parents and religious community for having received a court-ordered transfusion. Reaching an understanding about the consequences for the child who receives a court-ordered transfusion is, therefore, vital for the determination of what risks will be taken before ordering a transfusion.

The procedure for obtaining a court order may vary, depending upon the specific state laws. Typically, a court order may be obtained over the telephone. The initial contact may be with a social worker who will put the physician in contact with a judge. Details of the case will be ascertained, and the judge will issue an informal order declaring the patient a ward of the court for the purposes of receiving medical treatment only. This call initiates the issue of a written order, which will arrive several days later. Although not a totally automatic procedure, it would be very rare for a judge to deny this order for a minor.

Anesthesiologists concerned about the care of Jehovah's Witnesses should familiarize themselves with the details of the procedure in their practice locations.

IMPAIRED PHYSICIANS

Physicians may become impaired in their abilities to practice medicine skillfully and safely for a variety of reasons, but the most common impairment among anesthesiologists is chemical dependence. There are two primarily legal issues of importance: the first issue is the duty to report suspected substance abuse, and the second is the potential liability imposed by reporting.

There is considerable variability among the states in defining the legal responsibilities of a physician in reporting suspected substance abuse. In some states, the licensing authority must be notified, while in others there is no requirement. The ethical mandate to limit or restrict the practice of impaired physicians is clearly established. Furthermore, vicarious liability for the acts of an incompetent or impaired physician may be imposed upon physicians who either knew, or should have known, of the impairment. Since the hospitals which grant practice privileges may be vicariously liable for the acts of the physicians, and since the state has an inherent interest in protecting its citizens from incompetent medical care, it is likely that an impaired physician program of some sort currently exists for most practice locations. Since liability may be imposed for *not* reporting suspected chemical dependency, and there is an ethical obligation to help the impaired physician, suspicions that a colleague may be impaired should not be ignored.

Physicians are constitutionally protected by the same due process provisions as any other citizens. This has led to the fear that reporting the suspicion of an impairment, or acting as a member of an impaired physician committee in recommending restriction of privileges, may lead to a lawsuit for defamation, deprivation of livelihood, or restraint of trade. In most states, immunity from such prosecution is granted to groups or committees whose purpose is to review the quality of medical care, and to physicians who provide information to such committees. There is, however, the provision that such individuals and groups are acting reasonably and without malice or for personal gain. The issue of immunity for peer review groups has been raised at the federal level, and it is likely that federal legislation will someday clarify the issues.

REFERENCES

1. Peters JD, Fineberg KS, Kroll DA *et al:* Anesthesiology and the Law. Ann Arbor, Health Administration Press, 1983
2. Cheney FW: Anesthesia: Potential risks and causes of incidents. In Gravenstein JS, Holzer JF: Safety and Cost-Containment in Anesthesia, pp 13–16. Stoneham, MA, Butterworth, 1988
3. American Society of Anesthesiologists Directory of Members 1987:565
4. Petty C: The Anesthesia Machine, p 213. New York, Churchill Livingstone, 1987
5. Spooner RB, Kirby RR: Equipment-related anesthetic incidents. In Analysis of Anesthetic Mishaps, International Anesthesiology Clinics, 22:133, 1984
6. Duberman S: Quality Assurance in the Practice of Anesthesiology. Park Ridge, American Society of Anesthesiologists, 1986
7. Gaba DM, Maxwell M, DeAnda A: Anesthetic mishaps: Breaking the chain of accident evolution. Anesthesiology 66:670, 1987
8. U.S. Food and Drug Administration: Anesthesia Apparatus Checkout Recommendations, August 1986
9. Pierce EC: Reducing preventable anesthesia mishaps: A need for greater risk management. ASA Newsletter, American Society of Anesthesiologists, June 1985

Chapter 3

Nathan L. Pace

Research Design and Statistics

It is said that we live in a world of numbers. Our medical journals are replete with numbers which we are supposed to understand. These numbers include weights, lengths, pressures, volumes, flows, concentrations, counts, temperatures, rates, currents, energies, forces, etc. For over 30 years, our anesthesia journals have exhorted the researcher to more carefully collect, analyze, and interpret these numbers.[1-3] The analysis and interpretation of these numbers requires the use of statistical techniques; the design of the experiment to acquire the numbers is also part of statistical competence. The need for these statistical techniques is not an intellectual affectation, but is mandated by the nature of our universe, which is both ordered and random at the same time.

> The word "stochastic," strange sounding but currently very popular in scientific circles, means random, chancy, chaotic. . . . The stochastization of the world . . . means the adoption of a point of view wherein randomness or chance or probability is perceived as a real, objective and fundamental aspect of the world. It refers as well to the utilization of those methods of the theory of mathematical statistics and probability which are intended to reduce the chaos of the single unpredictable event to a less wild and more predictable pattern. The "opposite" of stochastic is deterministic; but we have learned to live simultaneously in a world that is both stochastized and deterministic . . . [4]

The elements of randomness are ubiquitous in the operating room. For example, the anesthesiologist knows that the greater the inhaled concentration of halothane, the greater the effect; a sufficiently high concentration will anesthetize; even higher concentrations will kill. Yet, for any individual patient,

only a guess can be made in advance as to the necessary concentration to produce anesthesia. Possibly, if everything was known about the function of the body, the necessary anesthetic concentration could be predicted. But, for the moment, we must rely on MAC (minimum alveolar anesthetic concentration), which roughly characterizes the expected required halothane concentration for a group of patients. It allows only an initial guess as to the amount required for any individual patient.

Regardless of differing opinions about why the concept of probability emerged when it did,[5] the initial developments occurred to solve very practical problems—the laws of probability were formulated to help gamblers in Renaissance Italy increase their winnings at dice and cards. Continuing since then, new statistics have been created to solve practical problems.[6] In the 19th century, regression and correlation were originated by Francis Galton to aid in the understanding of biological inheritance. At the beginning of this century, William Sealy Gosset worked for the Guinness brewery in Dublin, Ireland; he developed the Student's *t* test to understand variations in strains of barley to make the best brew. The greatest statistician of the 20th century, Ronald Fisher, developed the analysis of variance to help produce better agricultural crops. Even studies in anesthesia have inspired new statistics; for example, the National Halothane Study prompted new advances in the analysis of frequency tables.[7] The continuing development of statistical techniques is manifest in the increasing use of more sophisticated research designs and statistical tests in anesthesia journal articles.[8, 3]

Many anesthesiologists seem to have an aversion to mathematics and statistics; this aversion impedes the willingness to use numeric skills. The greater the time elapsed from training, the greater the decrease in skills.[9] Yet, if any physician is to be a practitioner of scientific medicine, he must read the language of science so that he can independently assess and interpret the scientific report; and, without exception, the language of the medical report is increasingly statistical. Readers of the anesthesia literature, whether in a community hospital or a university environment, cannot and should not depend on the editors of journals to banish all errors of statistical analysis and interpretation.

"The conduct of a scientific study requires a good design, appropriate measurement technology, proper execution of the study design, sound statistical analysis and appropriate interpretation."[10] This chapter will briefly scan these subjects.

DESIGN OF RESEARCH STUDIES

The investigator should view himself as an experimenter, and not as a naturalist. The naturalist literally or figuratively goes out into the field ready to capture and report the numbers which flit into view; this is a worthy activity, typified by the case report. Case reports engender interest, suspicion, doubt, wonder, and, one hopes, the desire to experiment; however, the case report is not sufficient evidence to advance scientific medicine. The experimenter attempts to constrain and control, as much as possible, the environment in which he collects numbers to test a hypothesis. Yet, the investigator may be enticed to function as a naturalist. Marvelous advances in technology and instrumentation have provided the medical researcher with ingenious devices to collect more and more numbers about previously unmeasured and unmeasurable biological events. It is tempting to simply turn these devices on and use them to collect numbers, hoping that serendipity will bless this mindless number gathering. Thought must be invested in research design before numbers are harvested. Discovery will not come by applying statistical tests one after another to a pile of numbers until the right way of extracting information is found.

In undertaking a research project, the investigator is implicitly accepting the statistical concept that the results in a group of subjects can be applied to an individual subject. Especially as applied to the therapy of disease, this idea has engendered controversy for centuries.[11] On the one side is the argument that the individuality of the organism makes the approach to therapy unique. The probabilities and results of a research report may not apply to an individual patient. A patient cannot be 4/5ths alive, but either alive or dead. For the single patient, a treatment is either a failure or a success. Thus, it is argued that treatment should be individualized to each patient, and that any type of therapy which might be possible should be allowed. On the other side is the position that no therapeutic agent can be employed with discrimination unless the general efficacy of the agent has been confirmed in analogous cases. While accepting that each patient is autonomous and that therapy should be adapted to his circumstances, this position accepts the difficulty of choosing wisely in a stochastic world; the most likely choice to benefit a patient will be that which is supported by experimental evidence.

SAMPLING, CONTROL GROUPS, RANDOM ALLOCATION, BLINDING, THE ETHICS OF ALTERNATIVE THERAPY, AND THE TYPES OF RESEARCH DESIGN

Two words of great importance to statisticians are "population" and "sample." In statistical conversation, each has a specialized meaning. Instead of referring only to the count of individuals in a geographical or political region, population refers to any target group of things (animate or inanimate) in which there is interest. For anesthesia researchers, a typical target population would be mothers in the first stage of labor or head trauma victims undergoing craniotomy. A target population could also be cell cultures, isolated organ preparations, or hospital bills. A sample is a subset of the target population. Samples are taken because of the impossibility of observing the entire population; it is generally not affordable, convenient, or practical to examine more than a relatively small fraction of the population. Nevertheless, the researcher wishes to generalize from the results of the small sample group to the entire population.

Although the subjects of a population are alike in at least one way, these population members are generally quite diverse in other ways. Since the researcher can only work with a subset of the population, he hopes that the sample of subjects in his experiment is representative of the population's diversity. Head injury patients can have open or closed wounds, a variety of coexisting diseases, normal or increased intracranial pressure, etc. Often the researcher will wish to increase the homogeneity of the target population by redefining it; perhaps only closed, and not open, head injuries will be included. Restricting the target population to eliminate too much diversity must be balanced against the desire to have the results be applicable to the broadest possible population of patients. The researcher should clearly identify to himself the target population; unfortunately, this is often overlooked.

The best hope for a representative sample would be realized if every subject in the population had the same chance of being in the experiment; this is called random sampling. Unfortunately, in most clinical anesthesia research, we are restricted to using those patients who happen to show up at our respective hospitals; this is called convenience sampling. Convenience sampling is also subject to the nuances of the surgical schedule, the good will of the referring physician and attending surgeon, and the amenability of the patient. At best, the convenience sample is representative of patients at that institution, with no assurance that these patients are similar to those elsewhere. Convenience sampling is also the rule in studying new anesthetic drugs in volunteers; most such studies are performed on healthy, young, male medical students and male anesthesia residents. Arguments about the definition of the population and the adequacy of the sampling can challenge the validity of a published study.[12, 13]

The researcher must define the conditions to which the sample members will be exposed. Particularly in clinical research, one must decide whether these conditions should be rigidly standardized, or whether the experimental circumstances, which always include treatment as well, should be adjusted or individualized to the patient. In anesthetic drug research, should a fixed dose be given to all members of the sample, or should the dose be adjusted to an effect or endpoint? Standardizing the treatment groups simplifies the research work, and will usually be helpful in distinguishing treatment effects. There are risks to this standardization: 1) a fixed dose may produce excessive numbers of side effects in some patients, and 2) a treatment standardized for the experimental protocol may be so artificial that it has no broad clinical relevance, even if demonstrated to be superior.

Even if a researcher is studying only one experimental group, the results of the experiment are usually not interpreted solely in terms of those conditions, but are also contrasted and compared with other experimental groups. Examining the effects of a new drug on blood pressure during anesthetic induction is important, but what is most important is comparing it to the effects of one or more standard drugs commonly used in the same situation. Where can the researcher obtain this comparative data? There are several possibilities: 1) each patient could receive the standard drug under identical experimental circumstances at another time; 2) another group of patients receiving the standard drug could be studied simultaneously; 3) a group of patients could have been studied previously with the standard drug under similar circumstances; and 4) literature reports of the effects of the drug under related, but not necessarily identical, circumstances could be used. Under the first two possibilities, the patient either serves as his own control (self control) or there is a so-called parallel control group. The second two possibilities are examples of historical controls.

Since historical controls already exist, they are convenient and, seemingly, cheap to use. Unfortunately, the history of medicine is littered with the debris of therapies enthusiastically accepted on the basis of comparison with past experience, but later found to be worthless. A classic example was operative ligation of the internal mammary artery for the treatment of angina pectoris. There is now firm empirical evidence that studies using historical controls usually show a favorable outcome for a new therapy, while studies with concurrent controls, i.e., parallel control group or self control, usually fail to show a benefit.[14] Nothing seems to increase the enthusiasm for a new treatment as much as the omission of a concurrent control group. If the outcome with an old treatment is not studied simultaneously with the outcome of a new treatment, one cannot know if any differences in results are a consequence of the two treatments, or of unsuspected and unknowable differences between the patients or of other changes over time in the general medical environment. One possible exception would be in studying a disease which is uniformly fatal (100% mortality) over a very short time interval.

Having accepted the necessity of an experiment with a control group, the question arises as to the method by which each subject should be assigned to the possible experimental groupings. Should it depend on the whim of the investigator, the day of the week, the preference of a referring physician, the wish of the patient, the assignment of the previous subject, the availability of a study drug, a hospital chart number, or some other arbitrary criterion? All such methods have been used, and are still used, but all can ruin the purity and usefulness of the experiment. It is important to remember the purpose for sampling: by exposing a small number of subjects from the target population to the various experimental conditions, one hopes to make conclusions about the entire population. Thus, the experimental groups should be as similar as possible to each other in reflecting the target population; if the groups are different, this introduces a bias into the experiment. Although randomly allocating subjects of a sample to one or another of the experimental groups requires additional work, this principle: 1) prevents selection bias by the researcher, 2) minimizes (but cannot always prevent) the possibility that important differences exist among the experimental groups, and 3) disarms the critics' complaints about research methods. Originally, random allocation was performed by throwing die or by using a random number table; today, computer programs can create the random allocation scheme. There are many nuances to the actual process of random allocation.[15] While random allocation does not guarantee that the experimental groups are alike, there is no better strategy for attempting to do so.

Blinding refers to masking from view the experimental group to which the subject has been, or will be, assigned. In clinical trials, the necessity for blinding starts even before a patient is enrolled in the research study. There is good evidence that, if the process of random allocation is accessible to view, either the referring physicians, the research team members, or both, are tempted, and will be tempted, to manipulate the entrance of specific patients into the study to influence their assignment into a specific treatment group; they do so having formed a personal opinion about the relative merits of the treatment groups and desiring to get the "best" for someone they favor. This creates bias in the experimental groups.[16]

Each subject should remain, if possible, ignorant of his or her assigned treatment group after entrance into the research protocol. The patient's expectation of improvement, a placebo effect, is a real and useful part of clinical care. But, when studying a new treatment, one must ensure that the fame or infamy of the treatments does not induce a bias in outcome by changing expectations. Such a study, in which the subject is unaware of the treatment given, is called single blind. A researcher's knowledge of the treatment assignment can bias his ability to administer the research protocol and to observe and record data faithfully; this is true for clinical, animal, and in vitro research. If the treatment group is known, those who observe data cannot trust themselves to impartially and dispassionately record the data. A double blind study, with both subject and data collector ignorant of the treatment group, is the best way to test a new therapy.

Enrolling patients into a randomized controlled trial (RCT) can engender considerable physician anxiety because it requires him to admit and discuss uncertainty. "The randomized clinical trial highlights the conflict of having to say, 'We don't know,' rather than the more familiar, 'I think this is the best thing to do.'"[17] Also, considerable debate on ethics has ensued since the realization of the absolute superiority of the RCT. These arguments usually revolve around the perceived conflict between the physician's ethical imperative to do the "best" for each patient and the need for random allocation of patients to both old and new therapies since there is usually some preliminary evidence to suggest the superiority of the new therapy. It is argued that the patient must be given that therapy to which the physician's affection and allegiance has been attracted.[18, 19] Of course, this preliminary evidence has often not been confirmed by a definitive therapeutic trial. What is required to resolve these qualms is the candor to recognize that, in spite of one's personal opinions about the comparative merits, a randomized controlled clinical trial is the only ethical way to solve conflicting claims about which the expert medical community is genuinely uncertain.[19]

Ultimately, research design consists of choosing what subjects to study, choosing what experimental conditions and constraints to enforce, and choosing which observations to collect at what intervals. A few key features in this research design will largely determine the strength of scientific inference on the collected data. These key features allow the classification of research reports into a scheme.[20] Such a scheme exposes the variety of experimental approaches and reveals strengths and weaknesses of the same design applied to many research problems (Table 3-1).

The first distinction is between longitudinal and cross-sectional studies. The former has as object the study of changes over time, while the latter describes a phenomenon at a certain point in time. "Generally, longitudinal designs require patient followup, documentation of intervening events, and analysis of a series of measurements. These features are less important in cross-sectional studies, so that other kinds of problems—such as errors of measurement, the interpretation of transient effects, and definitions of disease states—become relatively more prominent."[20] Reporting the frequency with which certain drugs are used during anesthesia is a cross-sectional study, while investigating the hemodynamics of different drugs during anesthesia is longitudinal.

TABLE 3-1.   Classification of Biomedical Research Reports

I. Longitudinal studies
  A. Prospective (cohort) studies
    1. Studies of deliberate intervention
      a. Concurrent controls
        (1) Parallel control group
        (2) Self-control
      b. Historical controls
        (1) Previous experiment
        (2) Literature
    2. Observational studies
  B. Retrospective (case-control) studies
II. Cross sectional studies

Longitudinal studies are, next, classified by the method with which the research subjects are selected. These methods for choosing research subjects can be either prospective or retrospective; these two approaches are also known as cohort (prospective) or case-control (retrospective). A prospective study assembles groups of subjects by some input characteristic which is thought to change an output characteristic; a typical input characteristic would be the primary drug used for anesthetic induction, *e.g.*, alfentanil and sufentanil. A retrospective study groups subjects by an output characteristic; that is the status of the subject afterwards, *e.g.*, the occurrence of a myocardial infarction. A prospective (cohort) study would be one in which a group of patients undergoing heart surgery were divided in two groups, given two different anesthetic inductions (alfentanil or sufentanil), and followed for the development of a perioperative myocardial infarction. In a retrospective (case-control) study, patients suffering a perioperative myocardial infarction would be identified from hospital records; a group of subjects of similar age, gender, and disease who did not suffer a perioperative myocardial infarction would be chosen, and the two groups would then be compared for the relative use of the two anesthetic induction drugs (alfentanil or sufentanil). Retrospective studies are a primary tool of epidemiology. A case-control study can often identify an association between an input and output characteristic, but the causal link or relationship between the two is more difficult to specify.

Prospective studies are further divided into those in which the investigator performs a deliberate intervention and those in which the investigator merely observes. In a study of deliberate intervention, the investigator would choose several anesthetic maintenance techniques and compare the incidence of postoperative nausea and vomiting. If performed as an observational study, the investigator would observe a group of patients receiving anesthetics chosen at the discretion of each patient's attending anesthesiologist, and compare the incidence of postoperative nausea and vomiting among the anesthetics used. Obviously, in this example of an observational study, there has been an intervention; an anesthetic has been given. The crucial distinction is whether the investigator controlled the intervention. An observational study may reveal differences between treatment groups, but whether such differences are the consequence of the treatments or of differences between the patients receiving the treatments will remain obscure.

With the availability of large computer databases of patient treatment information, some researchers have argued that observational studies can be performed by using advanced multivariable statistical techniques on these large data pools,

and that these observational studies will have equal merit with RCTs.[21, 22] These suggestions include the claim that decisions about treatment efficacy are possible by such observational studies. Although such observational studies may be useful in suggesting hypotheses for further study, there are tremendous methodologic problems which prevent the inferences of such an observational study from being generally accepted. The problems include: 1) bias in assignment to treatment groups, 2) nonstandard definitions in the database, 3) changing definitions over time, and 4) missing data.[23, 24]

Longitudinal studies are further subdivided into those with concurrent controls and those with historical controls. Concurrent controls are either a simultaneous parallel control group or a self-control study; historical controls include previous studies and literature reports. A randomized controlled trial is, thus, a longitudinal, prospective study of deliberate intervention with concurrent controls.

Although most of this discussion about experimental design has focused on human experimentation, the same principles apply, and should be followed, in animal experimentation. The randomized, controlled clinical trial is the most potent scientific tool for evaluating medical treatment; randomization into treatment groups is relied upon to equally weight the subjects of the treatment groups for baseline attributes which might predispose or protect the subjects from the outcome of interest.

HYPOTHESIS FORMULATION, THE LOGIC OF PROOF, AND SAMPLE SIZE CALCULATIONS

Whether his research subjects are tissue preparations, animals, or people, the researcher is constantly faced with finding both similarities and differences among the diversities of a group of subjects. The researcher starts his work with some intuitive feel for the phenomenon to be studied. Whether stated explicitly or not, this is the biological hypothesis; it is a statement of experimental expectations to be accomplished by the use of experimental tools, instruments, or methods accessible to the research team. An example would be the hope that isoflurane would produce less myocardial ischemia than fentanyl; the experimental method might be the electrocardiographic determination of ST segment changes. The biological hypothesis of the researcher becomes a statistical hypothesis during research planning. In a statistical hypothesis, statements are made about the relationship among parameters of one or more populations; a parameter is a number describing a population. The statistical hypothesis can be established in a somewhat rote fashion for every research project, regardless of the methods, materials, or goals.

The most frequently used method of setting up the algebraic formulation of the statistical hypothesis is to create two mutually exclusive statements about some parameters determined from the study population (Table 3-2); estimates for the values for these parameters will be acquired by sampling data. In the hypothetical example comparing isoflurane and fentanyl, ϕ_1 and ϕ_2 would represent the ST segment changes with

TABLE 3-2.   Algebraic Statement of Statistical Hypotheses

H_0: $\phi_1 = \phi_2$ (Null hypothesis)
H_a: $\phi_1 \neq \phi_2$ (Alternative hypothesis)

ϕ_1 = Parameter describing population 1
ϕ_2 = Parameter describing population 2

isoflurane and with fentanyl. The null hypothesis is the hypothesis of no difference of ST segment changes between isoflurane and fentanyl. The alternative hypothesis is nondirectional, i.e., either $\phi_1 < \phi_2$ or $\phi_1 > \phi_2$; this is known as a two-tail alternative hypothesis. This is a more conservative alternative hypothesis than assuming that the inequality can only be either < or >. Only the conservative, nondirectional, two-tail tests will be used in this chapter.

The statisticians Neyman and Pearson have provided the decision strategy used almost universally to choose between the null and alternative hypothesis. The decision strategy is similar to a method of indirect proof used in geometry called "reductio ad absurdum." If a theorem cannot be proved directly, assume that it is not true; show that the falsity of this theorem will lead to contradictions and absurdities; thus, reject the original assumption of the falseness of the theorem. For statistics, the approach is to assume that the null hypothesis is true even if the goal of the experiment is to show that there is a difference. One examines the consequences of this assumption by examining the actual sample numbers obtained. This is done by calculating what are called sample statistics; associated with a sample statistic is a probability. One also chooses the level of significance; the level of significance is the probability level considered too low to warrant support of the null hypothesis being tested. If sample values are sufficiently unlikely to have occurred by chance (the probability of the test statistic is less than the chosen level of significance), the null hypothesis is rejected; otherwise the null hypothesis is not rejected.

Since the statistics deal with probabilities, and not certainties, there is a chance that the decision concerning the null hypothesis is erroneous. These errors are best displayed in table form (Table 3-3); condition one and condition two could be different drugs, two doses of the same drug, different patient groups, etc. Of the four possible outcomes, two are clearly undesirable. The error of wrongly rejecting the null hypothesis (false positive) is called the Type I or alpha error. The experimenter should choose a probability value for alpha before collecting data; the experimenter decides for himself how cautious to be about falsely claiming a difference. The most common choice for the value of alpha is 0.05. What are the consequences of choosing an alpha of 0.05? Assuming that there is, in fact, no difference between the two conditions, and that the experiment is to be repeated 20 times, then, during one of these experimental replications (5% of 20), a mistaken conclusion that there is a difference would be made. The

probability of a Type I error depends on only two factors: the chosen level of significance, and the existence or nonexistence of a difference between the two experimental conditions. The smaller the chosen alpha, the smaller will be the risk of a Type I error. There is a trend recently for the research report to include the actual probability values of test statistics, rather than just a statement of whether or not the alpha probability was or was not exceeded. This allows the reader to use his own judgment in deciding the plausibility or implausibility of the experimental result.

The error of failing to reject a false null hypothesis (false negative) is called a Type II or beta error. The power of a test is 1 minus beta. The probability of a Type II error depends on four factors. Unfortunately, the smaller the alpha, the greater will be the chance of a false negative conclusion; this fact keeps the experimenter from automatically choosing a very small alpha. Second, the more variability there is in the populations being compared, the greater the chance of a Type II error. This is analogous to listening to a noisy radio broadcast; the more static there is, the harder it will be to discriminate between words. Next, increasing the number of subjects will lower the probability of a Type II error. The fourth and most important factor is the magnitude of the difference between the two experimental conditions. The probability of a Type II error goes from very high, when there is only a small difference, to extremely low, when the two conditions produce large differences in population parameters.

Discussion of hypothesis testing has always included mention of both Type I and Type II errors, but, usually, the researcher has effectively ignored the latter. The practical importance of worrying about Type II errors reached the consciousness of the medical research community with the appearance of the much quoted report of Freiman et al.[25] This work showed that the majority of controlled clinical trials which claimed to find no advantage of new therapies compared to standard therapies, in fact, lacked sufficient statistical power to discriminate between the experimental groups, would have missed an important therapeutic improvement, and did not give the new therapies a fair test. There are four options for increasing power: 1) raise alpha, 2) reduce population variability, 3) make the sample bigger, and 4) make the difference between the conditions greater. Under most circumstances, only the sample size can be varied. Sample size planning has become an important part of research design for controlled clinical trials; there are a variety of tables and formulas for these calculations which depend on specific research design circumstances.[26]

DATA COLLECTION AND DATA MANAGEMENT

The observations that are collected for anesthesia research are of all types, and include demographics, physical examination, medical history, laboratory results, hemodynamic variables, questionnaires, intraoperative events, etc. There is a tendency for the researcher to try to collect all possible observations on the experimental subject for fear that some crucial item will be left out which will impair analysis; with the aid of computers, the amount of research data being collected per experiment does seem to be increasing. Yet, the biological hypothesis and its associated statistical hypothesis should determine what to observe. There are real disadvantages in collecting excessive observations: 1) it costs more money, 2) it requires more research personnel, 3) data entry becomes more cumbersome, 4) there are more errors in data storage, 5) more data storage space is required, and 6) data analysis is bogged down by

TABLE 3-3.   Errors in Hypothesis Testing:
The Two-Way Truth Table

CONCLUSION FROM OBSERVATIONS (SAMPLE STATISTICS)	ACTUAL SITUATION/REALITY (POPULATION PARAMETERS)	
	Condition one and two equivalent	Condition one and two not equivalent
Condition one and two equivalent*	Correct conclusion	False negative Type II error (beta error)
Condition one and two not equivalent†	False positive Type I error (alpha error)	Correct conclusion

* Accept null hypothesis: Condition one = Condition two.
† Reject null hypothesis: Condition one ≠ Condition two.

extraneous variables. Guidelines to follow in data collection include: 1) minimize the collected variables to those relevant to the study question, 2) establish explicit, rigid, totally unambiguous rules about where data are found and how they are recorded, 3) define precisely how nonnumeric observations will be categorized and scored, 4) design and use a data collection record, also called a case record form, instead of collecting data on scratch paper, 5) don't expect observations in the hospital medical record to be consistently defined or consistently entered, 6) distinguish a missing value from a zero value or an uncompleted data field, and 7) make provision on the data collection record for the entry of unanticipated, but relevant, data. The investigator must continually determine that the experimental protocol is not being violated. Murphy's law seems to apply to data collection. It is always more time consuming and more expensive than expected to collect data; there are also always more mistakes than expected in the data record.

Data collection is only one of several steps in the process of data management; next in the sequence are data entry, data editing, and data storage.[10] All of these steps are sequential operational components in the process of moving numbers intact and incorruptible from their collection point onwards to statistical analysis. A failure at any step can ruin the basic integrity of the research protocol.

The second step in data management is entry of data into a permanent record, usually a computer storage device. The use of electronic data processing has become ubiquitous in even small scale research projects. A small, personal computer, as opposed to larger machines, allows the investigator greater flexibility and greater control over his data, but also puts the burden of responsibility for hardware and software maintenance upon him. After data entry, the data must be verified and edited for errors. Such errors may have been made during recording onto the case record form, or may be transcription errors during electronic entry; some entries will clearly be illogical or impossible, while others will merely be improbable. Once detected, some will be corrected by comparison with the case record form; other, probably erroneous, entries will remain, and difficult decisions about what effort to spend backtracking into other primary records must be made. Eventually, the validity of some entries will remain undecided, and these data will be rejected from analysis. The last stage in data management is data storage. There are four basic formats for electronic data storage: 1) text file, 2) spreadsheet, 3) database management system, and 4) statistical analysis software data storage. The choice of format will depend on study size (number of patients and amount of data), computer resources (equipment, budget, personnel), and confidentiality considerations. Regardless of storage method, plans to back up the electronic data are crucial. The original electronic data record must be archived, and only electronic copies used for statistical analysis.

INSTITUTIONAL REVIEW BOARDS AND THE FDA

The liberation of survivors from Nazi concentration camps in 1945, and the discovery of the criminal experiments performed by some physicians upon camp inmates, shocked the world. The trial of some of these physicians prompted the Nuremburg Military Tribunal to enunciate a set of principles on permissible human experimentation. In 1964, the World Medical Association made the Declaration of Helsinki—recommendations concerning biomedical research in humans.

Against this background of the Nazi camp medical murders and the statements of principles and guidelines at Nuremburg and Helsinki, media reports during the 1960s and 1970s of certain experiments in the United States created a furor, and made medical experimentation a suspect activity. Scientists, such as the anesthesiologist Henry K. Beecher, M.D., reviewed research protocols and found many to be ethically deficient.[27] Beginning in the mid-1970s, laws have been passed, commissions have been established, and regulations have been promulgated to control the ethical aspects of human research.[28–30]

Biomedical research with human subjects is distinguished from clinical care by the focus of attention; during ordinary clinical care, the attention is on the individual patient; during research, the acquisition of knowledge describing and generalizable to a group of patients or subjects is pursued. Obviously, during research involving patients, clinical care must continue even as generalizable knowledge is acquired. Three ethical principles have been seen as fundamental to guide human behavior in clinical research; these are: 1) respect for persons, 2) beneficence, and 3) clinical justice. Respect for people acknowledges the autonomy of each individual, and demands his consent before beginning any treatment. Beneficence includes the classic prescription to do no harm, and the obligation to maximize benefits. Justice requires that all people are treated fairly, that burdens and benefits are fairly shared, and that vulnerable groups (the poor, minorities) be particularly safeguarded from exploitation.

The application of these ethical principles during research proceeds from the fundamental premise that the investigator should not have sole responsibility for ensuring the fulfillment of ethical standards; disinterested outsiders, not involved with the research, should share the burden of this responsibility. By federal regulation, this responsibility is to be placed on a committee at the research institution or hospital; this committee is known generically as the Institutional Review Board, or IRB.

During IRB review, research proposals are judged for the presence of 1) good research design, 2) competent investigators, 3) a favorable balance of benefit to risk, 4) an adequate informed-consent form and procedure, 5) equitable selection of research subjects, and 6) provision for compensation for injury. A good research design includes optimizing the sample size and using proper statistical techniques for analysis. IRBs can have difficulty judging and recognizing poor statistical design.[31] IRBs are required to perform an ongoing review of active research protocols at least yearly; there is great variation in the application of this review. Investigators are also required to maintain their research files, data sheets, etc., for at least 3 years following the completion of the project.

The IRB is constituted and functions according to federal guidelines from the National Institutes of Health, Department of Health and Human Services, and is subject to oversight by the federal government. Although the federal government only requires IRB approval of federally funded research, at most universities, hospitals, and research institutions, IRB review and approval has been mandated for all human research, regardless of the source of research funding. This requirement for approval of all human research is generally made by the executive authority of the governing body of the research site to enforce similar standards and a consistency of approach. The Food and Drug Administration has its own set of regulations concerning human research with new drugs and new medical devices. These are essentially similar to those under which the IRB have been established.

The investigator must work flexibly with the IRB of his own institution to satisfy the slightly different requirements of different federal agencies and the local interpretations and implementations of the regulations. Penalties for failure to follow the IRB procedure to obtain protocol approval and for violations of approved protocols can be very severe, and can include prohibition of future federal research funding and of IRB approval of future research protocols. Submission of manuscripts to scientific journals and of abstracts to scientific society meetings almost uniformly must be accompanied by a statement that human research projects have been reviewed by an IRB, and that informed consent has been obtained.

ANIMAL WELFARE

In the 1980s a furor arose in the United States concerning the use of animals for research. Self-described animal activists and animal liberationists sought publicity, broke into laboratories, stole research animals, stole and destroyed research records, and made threats against medical researchers. The proclaimed goal of these anonymous groups was to stop the use of animals in scientific investigation; other traditional animal organizations seem to have accepted, at least in part, the same goal of banning animal research. Some experiments were described by the press as being "subsidized sadism," "ghoulish," and "baboon brain-bashing."[32] As a consequence, federal, state, and local legislative and regulatory action was intensified. Federal legislation and regulation has established a system of review for animal research that is comparable to that for the supervision of human research.[33]

The Public Health Service (PHS) has mandated that each institution doing research supported by the PHS must establish an Institutional Animal Care and Use Committee (IACUC). The IACUC has jurisdiction over all research involving live vertebrate animals; non-vertebrates can be used without supervision. The Department of Agriculture (USDA) has its own regulations concerning the use of animals for research; for the scientific investigator, the PHS and USDA regulations are both fulfilled by working with the IACUC. The IACUC is established by the authority of the chief executive of the institution; as with the IRB, most institutions have chosen to require review of all live vertebrate animal research by the IACUC, regardless of funding source.

Every 6 months, the IACUC is charged with reviewing the institution's program for the humane care and use of animals, and with inspecting the institution's animal facilities; a federal guide has been published that must be used for this evaluation.[34] This guide is very specific concerning recommendations for physical restraint, multiple major surgical procedures, housing systems, minimal space allowances, activity, etc.

The IACUC reviews all live vertebrate animal research projects, and may require protocol modification; without IACUC approval, research cannot be initiated. The following requirements are emphasized during IACUC review: 1) avoidance and minimization of animal pain, distress, and discomfort through the use of analgesia and anesthesia by qualified personnel; 2) appropriate euthanasia; 3) good living conditions; and 4) the availability of veterinary care for the animals. The investigator must work carefully to observe the approved research protocol, as the IACUC may suspend ongoing research projects for violations of their standards. With increasing frequency, research reports involving animals submitted to scientific journals and to scientific society meetings must be accompanied by a statement that animal research projects have been reviewed by an IACUC, and that animal care conformed to humane guidelines.

PRINCIPLES AND APPLICATIONS OF STATISTICS

Statistics are methods for working with sets of numbers, a set being a group of objects. Statistics involves the description of number sets, the comparison of number sets with theoretical models, comparison between number sets, and the comparison of number sets with the past. A typical scientific hypothesis asks which of two methods, X and Y, is better. A statistical hypothesis is formulated concerning the set of numbers collected for X and collected for Y. If set $X = [100, 95, 87, 113, 112, 75]$ and set $Y = [105, 90, 90, 85, 110, 99]$, then statistics provides methods for deciding if the values of set X are bigger than the values of set Y. Statistical methods are necessary because there are three sources of variation in any data: biological error, temporal error, and measurement error. These errors in the data cause difficulties in avoiding bias and in being precise. Bias keeps the true value from being known; precision deals with the problem of the data scatter. These statistical methods are relatively independent of the particular field of study. Regardless of whether the numbers in sets X and Y are systolic pressures, body weights, serum chlorides, or some other value, the approach for comparing sets X and Y is usually the same.

Statistical analysis consists of four broad phases. These are: 1) initial data manipulation, 2) preliminary analysis, 3) definitive analysis, and 4) presentation of conclusions. Data manipulation begins by assembling the data into a form suitable for analysis, whether this be tables of numbers on paper, or electronic files in a computer; it also includes examination of the data for logically inconsistent values, missing observations, etc. During preliminary analysis, several statistical methods may be tried on the same data to clarify the structure of the data and to specify the direction for the more elaborate definitive analysis; simple tables and graphs are often helpful during preliminary analysis. Definitive analysis then provides the basis for conclusions. Considerable thought should be given to the final phase, which is the presentation of results in a lucid fashion adapted to the statistical competence of the listener and the reader; simpler methods consistent with data complexity are to be preferred.

DATA STRUCTURE

Data collected in an experiment include the defining characteristics of the experiment and the values of events or attributes that vary over time or conditions; these latter data are called variables. The researcher records his observations on data sheets or case record forms, which may be one to many pages in length, and assembles them together for statistical analysis. However, the data are most profitably assembled by placing them into a matrix or spread sheet form. Such a matrix reveals the data structure of the experiment (Table 3-4). All research observations must be in numeric form for statistical analysis. If first obtained as a code or as text, it must be encoded as a number. This encoding of observations generally takes place as the data matrix is created. The data structure includes the number of subjects, the grouping or classification of subjects, and the number and nature of variables measured

TABLE 3-4.   Typical Data-Structure Matrix

GROUP	GROUP NUMBER	SUBJECT NUMBER	VARIABLE 1	VARIABLE 2	TIME 1 VARIABLE 3	TIME 1 VARIABLE 4	TIME 2 VARIABLE 3	TIME 2 VARIABLE 4	. . .
1	1	xxx	xxx	xxx	xxx	xxx	xxx	xxx	. . .
1	2	xxx	xxx	xxx	xxx	xxx	xxx	xxx	. . .
•	•	xxx	xxx	xxx	xxx	xxx	xxx	xxx	. . .
1	n_1	xxx	xxx	xxx	xxx	xxx	xxx	xxx	. . .
2	1	xxx	xxx	xxx	xxx	xxx	xxx	xxx	. . .
2	2	xxx	xxx	xxx	xxx	xxx	xxx	xxx	. . .
•	•	xxx	xxx	xxx	xxx	xxx	xxx	xxx	. . .
2	n_2	xxx	xxx	xxx	xxx	xxx	xxx	xxx	. . .
•	•	xxx	xxx	xxx	xxx	xxx	xxx	xxx	. . .
•	•	xxx	xxx	xxx	xxx	xxx	xxx	xxx	. . .
k	1	xxx	xxx	xxx	xxx	xxx	xxx	xxx	. . .
k	2	xxx	xxx	xxx	xxx	xxx	xxx	xxx	. . .
•	•	xxx	xxx	xxx	xxx	xxx	xxx	xxx	. . .
k	n_k	xxx	xxx	xxx	xxx	xxx	xxx	xxx	. . .

on each individual. Most experiments have identifiable subjects on which a number of variables are recorded. Each row of the matrix is the data for only one subject. A subject is not necessarily a person or animal, but might be a tissue preparation, a laboratory instrument, etc. For a large experiment, the data structure may include thousands of rows (subjects) and hundreds of columns (variables).

Each column of the matrix is a variable recorded for each subject. The columns include explanatory and response variables and a subject identification code. The subject identification code is necessary to always allow each row of the data matrix to be identified with its data sheets or case record form. One or more columns classify or group subjects together. Some grouping variables are part of the experimental plan. If a different dose of an opioid was given to five groups of subjects, then the codes in the group column might be 1 to 5. There would be n_1 subjects receiving dose 1, n_2 receiving dose 2, and so on. Other grouping columns, which might include gender, age, doses of accompanying drugs, etc., reflect the variability of the experimental subjects. Those variables which group or classify subjects are also known as explanatory variables. Explanatory variables, it is hoped, will explain the systematic variations in the response variables. In a sense, the response variables are dependent on explanatory variables.

Response variables are also called dependent variables. Response variables reflect the primary properties of experimental interest in the subjects. In our experiment with five doses of an opioid, variable 1 might be blood loss, and variable 2 might be apnea duration. Research in anesthesiology is particularly likely to have repeated measurement variables, *i.e.*, a particular measurement recorded more than once for each individual. Systolic blood pressure (variable 3) and heart rate (variable 4) might be measured at Time 1, Time 2, etc., after receiving the opioid test drug. Some variables can be both an explanatory and a response variable; these are called intermediate response variables. For example, in our hypothetical experiment with five doses of opioids, two other variables might be intraoperative maximum ST segment depression and postoperative death. One might analyze how ST segments depended on the dose of opioids; here, maximum ST segment depression is a response variable. Maximum ST segment depression might also be used as an explanatory variable to address the more subtle question of the extent to which the effect of an opioid dose on postoperative deaths can be accounted for by ST segment changes.

The mathematical characteristics of the possible values of a variable fit into five classifications (Table 3-5). Properly assigning a variable to the correct data type is essential for choosing the correct statistical technique. For interval variables, there is equal distance between successive intervals; the difference between 15 and 10 is the same as the difference between 25 and 20. Discrete interval data can only have integer values, *e.g.*, ages in years, number of live children, or papers rejected by a journal. Continuous interval data is measured on a continuum, and can be a decimal fraction; for example, blood pressure can be described as accurately as desired, 136, 136.1, or 136.14 mmHg. The same statistical techniques are used for discrete and continuous data.

Categorical variables are derived by putting observations into two or more discrete categories; for statistical analysis, numeric values are assigned as labels to the categories. Dichotomous data allows only two possible values, *e.g.*, male *versus* female. Ordinal data has three or more categories which can logically be ranked or ordered; however, the ranking or ordering of the variable indicates only relative, and not absolute, differences between values; there is not necessarily the same difference in ASA Physical Status between I and III as there is between III and V. Although ordinal data are often

TABLE 3-5.   Data Types

DATA TYPE	DEFINITION	EXAMPLES
INTERVAL		
Discrete	Data measured with an integer-only scale	Age, parity
Continuous	Data measured with a constant scale interval	Blood pressure, temperature
CATEGORICAL		
Dichotomous (existential)	Binary data	Alive versus dead, gender
Nominal	Qualitative data that cannot be ordered or ranked	Eye color, drug category
Ordinal	Data order, ranked or measured without a constant scale interval	ASA physical status, pain score

treated as interval data in choosing a statistical technique, such analysis may be suspect; alternative techniques for ordinal data are available. Nominal variables are placed into categories which have no logical ordering. The eye colors blue, hazel, and brown might be assigned the numbers 1, 2, and 3, but it is nonsense to say that blue < hazel < brown.

DESCRIPTIVE STATISTICS

After the experimental observations are double checked and entered into the data matrix, there will be one or more sets of numbers. A typical hypothetical set could be $W = [29, 32, 27, 28, 26, 27, 28, 29, 30, 32, 35, 31]$ representing a sample of ages of 12 residents in an anesthesia training program. While the results of a particular experiment might be presented by repeatedly showing the entire set of numbers, there are concise ways of summarizing the information content of the set W into a few numbers. These numbers are called sample or summary statistics; summary statistics are calculated using the numbers of the sample. By convention, the symbols of summary statistics are Roman letters. The two summary statistics most frequently used for interval variables are the central location or central tendency and the variability, but there are other summary statistics in use. Other data types have analogous summary statistics.

Although the initial purpose of descriptive statistics is to describe the sample of numbers obtained, there is also the desire to use the summary statistics from the sample to characterize the population from which the sample was obtained. For example, what can be said about the age of all anesthesia residents from the information in set W? The population also has measures of central location and variability which are called the parameters of the population; population parameters are denoted by Greek letters. Usually, the population parameters cannot be directly calculated, because data from all population members cannot be obtained. The beauty of properly chosen summary statistics is that they are the best possible estimators of the population parameters.

These sampling statistics can be used in conjunction with a theoretical probability distribution to provide additional descriptions of the sample and its population. A theoretical probability distribution is an algebraic equation, $f(x)$, which gives a theoretical percentage distribution of x. Each value of x has a probability of occurrence given by $f(x)$. The percentage is merely $100 \cdot f(x)$. If $f(x)$ is summed or integrated for all possible values of x, the percentage must total 100%, and the probability must total 1.0. The most important probability distribution is the normal or Gaussian function:

$$f(x) = (1/(\sigma \cdot (2\pi)^{0.5})) \cdot \exp(-0.5 \cdot ((x - \mu)/\sigma)^2).$$

μ and σ are two constants in the equation. The normal equation can be plotted and produces the familiar bell-shaped curve. Why are the mathematical properties of this curve so important to biostatistics? First, it has been empirically noted that, when a biologic variable is sampled repeatedly, the pattern of the numbers plotted as a histogram resembles the normal curve; thus, most biologic data is said to follow or to obey a normal distribution. Second, if it is reasonable to assume that one's sample is from a normal population, then the mathematical properties of the normal equation can be used with the sampling statistic estimators of the population parameters to describe the sample and the population. Third, a mathematical theorem (the Central Limit Theorem) allows the use of the assumption of normality for certain purposes, even if the population is not normally distributed.

Central Location

The three most common summary statistics of central location for interval variables are the arithmetic mean, the median, and the mode; these summary statistics are calculated for the hypothetical set W (Table 3-6). The mean is merely the average of the numbers in the data set. Statistical formulae use a summation notation which considerably reduces the ink needed to print mathematical equations. The summary notation for the arithmetic mean is:

$$\bar{x} = \Sigma x_i/n.$$

TABLE 3-6. Central Location and Variability of a Hypothetical Data Set of Anesthesia Resident Ages

SUBJECT i	AGE x_i	MEAN $\bar{x}$	DEVIATION $(x_i - \bar{x})$	ABSOLUTE DEVIATION $\|x_i - \bar{x}\|$	DEVIATION SQUARED $(x_i - \bar{x})^2$
1	26	29.5	−3.5	3.5	12.25
2	27	29.5	−2.5	2.5	6.25
3	27	29.5	−2.5	2.5	6.25
4	28	29.5	−1.5	1.5	2.25
5	28	29.5	−1.5	1.5	2.25
6	29	29.5	−0.5	0.5	0.25
7	29	29.5	−0.5	0.5	0.25
8	30	29.5	+0.5	0.5	0.25
9	31	29.5	+1.5	1.5	2.25
10	32	29.5	+2.5	2.5	6.25
11	32	29.5	+2.5	2.5	6.25
12	35	29.5	+5.5	5.5	30.25
12	354	354.0	0.0	25.0	75.00

Sample median: 29
Sample Mode: Polymodal
Sample mean: $\bar{x} = \Sigma x_i/n = 354/12 = 29.5$
Sample standard deviation: $s = (\Sigma(x_i - \bar{x})^2/(n-1))^{0.5} = (75/11)^{0.5} = 2.61$
Sample standard error: $SE = s/(n)^{0.5} = 2.61/(12)^{0.5} = 0.75$

Capital sigma (Σ) is the summation operator; its purpose is to add up all values of x from x_1 to x_n; the sum is then divided by the count of individuals (n) in the sample. Being a summary statistic of the sample, the arithmetic mean is denoted by the Roman letter $\bar{x}$. If all values in the population could be obtained, then the population mean could be calculated:

$$\mu = \Sigma x_i / N.$$

As these values cannot be obtained, the sample mean is the unbiased, consistent, minimum variance, sufficient estimator of the population mean; thus, $\bar{x} = \mu$ where μ is the population mean and N is the population count. The μ in the normal equation is the population mean.

The median is the middlemost number, or that number which divides the sample into two equal parts. The median is obtained by, first, ranking the sample values from lowest to highest, and then counting up halfway. The concept of ranking will be used in nonparametric statistics. A virtue of the median is that it is little affected by a few extremely high or low values. The mode is the most popular number of a sample, *i.e.*, that number which occurs most frequently. A sample may have ties for the most common value, and be bi- or polymodal; these modes may be widely separated or adjacent. The raw data should be inspected for this unusual appearance. The mode is always mentioned in discussions of descriptive statistics, but is rarely used in statistical practice.

Spread or Variability

Any set of interval data has variability unless all the numbers are identical. The range of ages from lowest to highest expresses the largest difference within set W. This spread, diversity, and variability can also be expressed in a concise manner. Variability is specified by calculating the deviation or deviate of each individual x_i from the center (mean) of all the $x_i s$ (Table 3-6). Two derivatives of the deviate are used, the absolute deviate and the squared deviate. These individual deviates are totalled; the sum of the deviates is always zero, while the sum of either the absolute or the squared deviates will always be positive unless all set values are identical. This sum is then divided by the number of individual measurements. The result is the average absolute deviation and the average squared deviation; they can be considered as average distances from each data point to the center of the data. While the mean absolute deviation is little used, the average squared deviation is ubiquitous in statistics.

The concept of describing the spread of a set of numbers by calculating the average distance from each number to the center of the numbers applies to both a sample and a population; this average squared distance is called the variance. For a population, the variance is a parameter, and is represented by σ^2; its formula is:

$$\sigma^2 = (\Sigma(x_i - \mu)^2)/N.$$

As with the population mean, the population variance is not usually known, and cannot be calculated. The sample has a sample variance, s^2, given by:

$$s^2 = (\Sigma(x_i - \bar{x})^2)/(n-1).$$

Statistical theory demonstrates that, if the divisor in the formula for s^2 is $n-1$ rather than n, then the sample variance is an unbiased estimator of the population variance. While the variance is used extensively in statistical calculations, the units

of variance are squared units of the original observations. The square root of the variance will have the same units as the original observations; the square root of the sample and population variances are called the sample and population standard deviations, s and σ, respectively. Along with μ, the population standard deviation (σ) is the other constant in the normal equation.

It was previously mentioned that most biological observations appear to come from populations with normal or Gaussian distributions. By accepting this assumption of a normal distribution, further meaning can be given to the sample summary statistics that have been calculated. This involves the use of the expression $\bar{x} \pm k \cdot s$, where $k = 1, 2, 3, \ldots$ If the population from which the sample is taken is unimodal and roughly symmetric, then:

- $\bar{x} \pm 1 \cdot s$ encompasses roughly 68% of the sample and population members;
- $\bar{x} \pm 2 \cdot s$ encompasses roughly 95% of the sample and population members;
- $\bar{x} \pm 3 \cdot s$ encompasses roughly 99% of the sample and population members.

In our example of hypothetical resident ages (Table 3-6), $29.5 \pm 1 \cdot 2.61$ includes ten of 12 observations, $29.5 \pm 2 \cdot 2.61$ includes 11 of 12 observations, and $29.5 \pm 3 \cdot 2.61$ includes all 12 values. The standard deviation will usually give a fairly good approximation of the spread of the sample data.

Confidence Intervals

A confidence interval describes how likely it is that the population parameter is guessed by any particular sample statistic. Confidence intervals are a range of the form: parameter = summary statistic $\pm$ (confidence factor) $\cdot$ (precision factor).

The precision factor is derived from the sample itself, while the confidence factor is taken from a theoretical probability distribution, and also depends on the specific confidence level chosen. For a sample of interval data taken from a normally distributed population for which confidence intervals are to be chosen for μ, the precision factor is called the standard error of the mean (SE), and is obtained by dividing the sample standard deviation by the square root of the sample size. The confidence factors are the same as used for the dispersion or spread of the sample, and are obtained from the normal distribution. The confidence interval is read as follows:

- $\bar{x} \pm 1 \cdot SE$ has roughly a 68% chance of containing the population mean;
- $\bar{x} \pm 2 \cdot SE$ has roughly a 95% chance of containing the population mean;
- $\bar{x} \pm 3 \cdot SE$ has roughly a 99% chance of containing the population mean.

For the example of Table 3-6, there is a 95% chance that 29.5 ± 1.5 years will include the mean age of the anesthesia residents in the population sampled. The coefficients given above for confidence intervals are not exact; the 95% interval should use the coefficient 1.96. But 1, 2, and 3 are easier to remember and use. These confidence intervals are also calculated, assuming that the population σ is known. In actuality, the sample s was substituted for σ. Strictly speaking, when σ is not known, the coefficients should be taken from the t distribution, another theoretical probability distribution. These coefficients will be larger than those used above. This is usually ignored if the sample size is of reasonable size; for example, $n \geq 25$. Even when the sample size is only five or greater, the use of the coefficients 1, 2, and 3 is simple and sufficiently accurate for quick mental calculations of parameter confidence intervals.

Almost all research reports include the use of the standard error of the mean, regardless of the probability distribution of the populations sampled. This use is a consequence of the Central Limit Theorem previously mentioned; it is considered one of the most remarkable theorems in all of mathematics. The Central Limit Theorem states that the sample SE can always be used, if the sample size is sufficiently large, to specify confidence intervals on the population mean. These confidence intervals are calculated as described above. This is true even if the population distribution is so different from normal that the sample s cannot be used to characterize the dispersion of the population members. Only rough guidelines can be given for the necessary size of n; for interval data, certainly, $n = 25$ and above is large enough, and $n = 4$ and below is too small.

Although the standard error is discussed here in the section on descriptive statistics, it is really an inferential statistic. The standard deviation and standard error are mentioned together because of their similarities of computation, and because of the confusion of their use in research reports. This use is most often of the form "mean ± number;" some confusion results from the failure of the author to specify whether the number after the ± sign is the one or the other. More important, the choice between using s and SE has become controversial;[35] because SE is always less than s, it has been argued that authors seek to deceive by using SE to make the data look better than it really is. The choice is really simple. When describing the spread, scatter, or dispersion of the sample, use s; when describing the precision with which the population center is known, use SE.

Bivariate Data

Some of the data collected in an experiment seem to naturally pair off because of a relationship or dependency between two variables; these paired variables are known as (x, y) pairs, or bivariate data. Typical examples found in anesthesia journals are (time, plasma concentration) and (dose, effect). Regression and correlation constitute the statistical techniques for investigating such relationships. There are considerable computational similarities between the two, but the approaches are different. In regression, one variable (the x, or independent variable) is considered as having been picked or specified; the analysis focuses on the variation of the y or dependent variable with changes in x. In correlation, there is no such distinction between a dependent and an independent variable; both x and y are considered to be dependent. If five doses of an opioid are administered and blood pressure is measured after each dose, regression analysis to describe the dose-response relationship is appropriate. If intracranial pressure and cerebral blood flow are measured simultaneously, correlation analysis is used to describe their interrelationship. Sometimes it is difficult to make the choice between the two methods; the formulas for both are easily applied, regardless of the source of the data. One of the distinctions between regression and correlation is in assumptions about the nature of x and y. In regression, x is considered a fixed, or precisely known, variable, while y is a random variable; in correlation, both x and y are random variables. From a practical point of view, x is never really a precisely known variable; however, as long as the uncertainty in the measurement of x is small, the usual regression analysis is used. There is also a distinction between regression and correlation concerning other assumptions necessary for interpretation. Regardless of these differences, most frequently, experimenters apply both techniques to all data sets.

The concept of a model is used extensively in statistics. A model is a mathematical equation which expresses a relationship among variables and parameters; it is an algebraic expression of one's belief about the nature and relationship of experimental measurements. A model is held tentatively, and is critically examined during analysis; if a model doesn't agree with the facts, *i.e.*, the numbers of the sample, it is rejected. The idea of a model is inherent in linear regression analysis. Linear regression is the fitting of a straight line through a set of (x, y) pairs (Fig. 3-1). Assuming that such a straight-line relationship exists between x and y is a model. The regression relationship is usually written $y = a + b \cdot x$, where b is the slope of the line and a is the intercept or intersection of the line at the y axis. Both a and b are summary statistics that are calculated from the sample; a and b are estimates of α, the population intercept, and β, the population slope, which are the parameters of the model. If all possible (x, y) pairs from the target population could be sampled, then α and β could be calculated directly. In the equation $y = a + b \cdot x$, y actually means the value of y predicted by the regression equation; this predicted y value is not necessarily a value of y actually measured in the sample. For this reason, statisticians write the equation as $\hat{y} = a + b \cdot x$, where $\hat{y}$ reads "the predicted y." This distinction is usually overlooked in biomedical research reports.

The most common, but not the only, method to calculate a and b is that of least squares. To any line drawn through the points of a data set, a vertical line can be drawn to connect every (x, y) pair with the regression line. The least squares regression line will have the property that the sum of the squared distances of all these vertical lines will be minimized.

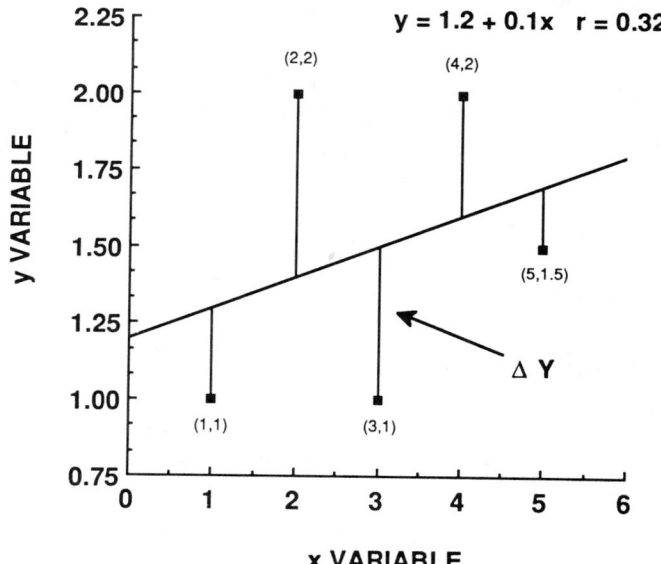

FIG. 3-1. Descriptive regression analysis. Five hypothetical data points are plotted. The line fitted by least squares regression makes the sum of the squared vertical deviations of the observed points about the line as small as possible. For the pair (3,1), large delta **Y** denotes the deviation.

By differential calculus, equations for the unique determination of both a and b can be derived; these equations use the values of the (x, y) pairs of the sample (Table 3-7). Much as $\bar{x}$ is the central location of the x_is, the linear regression line is a descriptive statistic for all the (x, y) points; it approximately divides the points into two equal groups. Other than a set of points whose x values are identical, a regression equation can always be calculated. The ability to calculate and plot a regression line does not necessarily imply that there is actually a relationship between x and y. The more nearly the regression line is either perfectly vertical or perfectly horizontal, the less important is the relationship between x and y. Also, even though the regression line can be extended beyond the minimum and maximum of the x values (Fig. 3-1), this regression relationship may well have no biologic meaning outside the range of the sample; the intercept value describes the regression line, but does not necessarily exist in reality.

Assuming that x and y are now both random variables, the same hypothetical data can be used in calculations of correlation (Table 3-7). The correlation coefficient, denoted r, is also known as the product moment correlation, or Pearson's coefficient of correlation. Inspection of the formula for r shows it to be a dimensionless ratio whose possible values extend from -1 to $+1$. There is a perfect correlation between x and y if r is either -1 or $+1$; for perfect correlation, all the points lay on the regression line. The intimate computational relationship between correlation and regression is shown by the relationship $b = r \cdot s_y/s_x$, where s_y and s_x are the standard deviations of y and x. If all (x, y) pairs of the target population were measured, the population correlation coefficient ρ could be calculated; r is the summary statistic estimate of ρ. Unless all the values of x in a sample are 0, r can always be calculated. There are certain cautions about the use of r. The correlation coefficient applies only to linear relationships. If r is 0, there is no linear relationship, but some other mathematical model may be appropriate. Most important is the warning that "correlation does not imply causation." Just because the height of skirts and the height of the stock market rise and fall together does not mean that one causes the other.

Proportions

Categorical binary data, also called enumeration data, provide counts of subject responses. Given a sample T of n subjects of whom x have a certain characteristic (death, female gender, etc.), a ratio of responders to the number of subjects can be easily calculated as $p = x/n$; this can also be expressed as a percentage, $100 \cdot p$. The ratio p is a descriptive or summary statistic of the sample T. Assume that $n = 15$ subjects and $x = 10$ deaths for sample T, then $p = 10/15 = 0.67$ and $100 \cdot p = 67\%$. If each subject who dies is given the score 1 and the others are given the score 0, the calculation of p is seen to be exactly the same as the calculation of $\bar{x}$ (Table 3-8); p is a measure of central location of the sample in the same way that $\bar{x}$ is. In the population from which the sample is taken, the ratio of responders to total subjects is a population parameter, denoted π; π is the measure of central location for the population. This population parameter, π, is not related to the geometry constant $\pi = 3.1415926. \ldots$ As with other data types, π is usually not known, but must be estimated from the sample. The sample ratio p is the best estimate of π.

The probability of binary data is provided by the binomial distribution, another theoretical probability distribution. The chance of x occurrences in a sample of n subjects from a population with an occurrence rate of π is:

$$(n!/(x! \cdot (n-x)!)) \cdot (\pi^x) \cdot ((1-\pi)^{(n-x)}).$$

If the π of a population is known, then the probability of the observed response rate p is easily calculated. For example, if there are 10 deaths in 15 subjects and the population death rate is 50% ($\pi = 0.5$), then the probability is:

$$(15!/(10! \cdot (15-10)!)) \cdot (0.5^{10}) \cdot ((1-0.5)^{(15-10)}) = 0.09.$$

This would be expressed as follows: if the population death rate was 50%, then, in a sample of 15 individuals, there would be about a 9% chance of observing ten deaths.

Since the population π is not generally known, the experimenter usually wishes to estimate π by the sample statistic p, and specify with what confidence π is known. Although computationally involved, this can be done by using the binomial distribution. Instead, advantage may be taken of the Central Limit Theorem. As previously mentioned in discussing interval data, the sampling distribution of the mean of the binomial distribution resembles the normal distribution if n is sufficiently large. This may be said in another way: as n increases, the binomial and the normal probability distributions become

TABLE 3-7. Descriptive Statistics for a Hypothetical Bivariate Data Set

x_i	y_i	$(x_i - \bar{x})$	$(x_i - \bar{x})^2$	$(y_i - \bar{y})$	$(y_i - \bar{y})^2$	$(x_i - \bar{x}) \cdot (y_i - \bar{y})$
1.0	1.0	-2.0	4.00	-0.5	0.25	$+1.0$
2.0	2.0	-1.0	1.00	$+0.5$	0.25	-0.5
3.0	1.0	0.0	0.00	-0.5	0.25	0.0
4.0	2.0	$+1.0$	1.00	$+0.5$	0.25	$+0.5$
5.0	1.5	$+2.0$	4.00	0.0	0.00	0.0
15.0	7.5	0.0	10.00	0.0	1.00	1.0

$\bar{x} = 15.0/5 = 3.0 \qquad \bar{y} = 7.5/5 = 1.5 \qquad n = 5$
$s_x = (10/4)^{0.5} = 1.58 \qquad s_y = (1/4)^{0.5} = 0.5$
$SE_x = 1.58/5^{0.5} = 0.71 \qquad SE_y = 0.5/5^{0.5} = 0.22$

Slope $\quad b = (\Sigma(x_i - \bar{x}) \cdot (y_i - \bar{y}))/(\Sigma(x_i - \bar{x})^2) = 1.0/10.0 = 0.1$
Intercept $\quad a = \bar{y} - b \cdot \bar{x} = 1.5 - 0.1 \cdot 3.0 = 1.2$
Equation $\quad y = 1.2 + 0.1x$

Correlation coefficient
$\qquad r = [\Sigma(x_i - \bar{x}) \cdot (y_i - \bar{y})]/\{[\Sigma(x_i - \bar{x})^2] \cdot [\Sigma(y_i - \bar{y})^2]\}^{0.5}$
$\qquad = 1.0/(10.00 \cdot 1.00)^{0.5}$
$\qquad = 0.32$

increasingly similar; n is said to be sufficiently large if both $n \cdot p >= 5$ and $n \cdot (1-p) >= 5$ are true. Even though the probability distribution of the population from which the sample was taken is not normally distributed, a sample standard deviation and standard error may be calculated analogously to that calculated for interval data (Table 3-8). The most compact form of these formulas is:

$$\text{Sample Standard Deviation} = s = (p \cdot (1-p))^{0.5}$$
$$\text{Sample Standard Error} = SE = s/(n)^{0.5} = (p \cdot (1-p)/n)^{0.5}.$$

The sample standard deviation is the best estimate of the population standard deviation $(\pi \cdot (1-\pi))^{0.5}$; since the population is binomial and not normal, the properties of the normal distribution cannot be used to give estimates of the spread or variability of the sample and population. However, the sample standard error is exactly analogous to the sample standard error of the mean for interval data, except that it is a standard error of the proportion. It also estimates the population standard error of the proportion, which is denoted $(\pi \cdot (1-\pi)/N)^{0.5}$. Just as a 95% confidence limit of the mean was calculated, so may a confidence limit on the proportion be obtained. Using the data of ten deaths in 15 subjects, the summary statistic $p = 10/15 = 0.67$. Since $15 \cdot 0.67 = 10$ and $15 \cdot (1-0.67) = 5$, then n is sufficiently large. The sample standard error is:

$$(0.67 \cdot (1-0.67)/15)^{0.5} = 0.12.$$

The 95% confidence interval on π will be:

$$p \pm 2 \cdot SE = 0.67 \pm 2 \cdot 0.12 = 0.67 \pm 0.24.$$

Thus, the best guess of the population death rate is 67%, and one has a 95% certainty that, in the population sampled,

the death rate is in the range of 43%–91%. The approximate nature of this calculation is reflected by the exact 95% confidence interval (36%–86%) derived for these data from the binomial equation. Larger ns and ps closer to 0.5 will have even greater precision. This simple equation can be used when the authors do not calculate confidence intervals on rates and proportions.

DISPLAY OF DATA AND STATISTICS

The research report must justify its conclusions by displaying the raw data, parameters of the raw data (descriptive statistics), and statistical test results; the presentation of raw data is encouraged to allow the reader to perform his own numerical and statistical tests. Three display methods are available: 1) text descriptions, 2) tables, and 3) graphs. Text descriptions are most commonly used to cite descriptive and inferential statistics. Descriptive statistics include means, variances, standard deviations, standard errors, frequency counts (proportions), and linear regression equations. Any listing of the form number 1 $\pm$ number 2 must clarify whether number 2 is a standard deviation or a standard error of the parameter. The listing of more than three to five data items and descriptive statistics in a text list is an awkward, difficult to read, and uninformative method of display. There are a variety of ways of listing inferential statistics; the most complete would include: 1) null hypothesis, 2) statistical test, 3) value of test statistic, 4) degree(s) of freedom, and 5) associated probability value. The inclusion of this level of detail is cumbersome in text form; text listings of inferential statistics more commonly include only items 3–5. Without giving any detail (items 1–5), authors frequently make sweeping statements in the results section of their papers concerning the presence or absence of

TABLE 3-8. Central Location and Variability for Hypothetical Data Set of Patient Mortality

SUBJECT i	OUTCOME* x_i	MEAN p	DEVIATION $(x_i - p)$	ABSOLUTE DEVIATION $|x_i - p|$	DEVIATION SQUARED $(x_i - p)^2$
1	1	0.67	+0.33	0.33	0.11
2	1	0.67	+0.33	0.33	0.11
3	1	0.67	+0.33	0.33	0.11
4	1	0.67	+0.33	0.33	0.11
5	1	0.67	+0.33	0.33	0.11
6	1	0.67	+0.33	0.33	0.11
7	1	0.67	+0.33	0.33	0.11
8	1	0.67	+0.33	0.33	0.11
9	1	0.67	+0.33	0.33	0.11
10	1	0.67	+0.33	0.33	0.11
11	0	0.67	−0.67	0.67	0.44
12	0	0.67	−0.67	0.67	0.44
13	0	0.67	−0.67	0.67	0.44
14	0	0.67	−0.67	0.67	0.44
15	0	0.67	−0.67	0.67	0.44
15	10	10.00	0.00	5.00	3.33

Sample rate or proportion
$$p = \Sigma x_i/n = 10/15 = 0.67$$
Sample standard deviation
$$s = (p \cdot (1 - p))^{0.5} = (0.67 \cdot (1 - 0.67))^{0.5} = 0.47$$
or
$$s = (\Sigma(x_i - p)^2/n)^{0.5} = (3.33/15)^{0.5} = 0.47$$
Sample standard error of the proportion
$$SE = (p \cdot (1 - p)/n)^{0.5} = s/(n)^{0.5} = 0.47/(15)^{0.5} = 0.12$$

* Patient dead = 1; Patient not dead = 0.

statistical significance for a list of variables. Unless the methods section of a paper is very clear, there will be confusion about the statistical test(s) used.

A table is a list with two or more adjacent columns characterized by descriptive headings. The use of tables is a very efficient way of displaying small raw data sets. Larger sets of raw data can be listed in a table by showing the number of subjects (frequency distribution) at each value or range of values. Tables are also used to display large numbers of means ± standard errors; generally, the table is organized with different experimental groups on each row, while each column represents a different variable or repeated measurement on the same variables.

Two or more proportions or rates are most commonly presented in table form. If the proportions or frequency data represent a comparison of classifications for the sample(s), a contingency table is used. In a contingency table, data is entered at each intersection of a row and column; each intersection is called a cell. The descriptive headings of the rows and of the columns cross classify data into cells of subjects having similar characteristics. Contingency tables are described by the number of rows and columns they contain; a contingency table with three rows and three columns would be a 3 · 3 contingency table. Thus, in a 3 · 3 contingency table, there are nine cells. The data entered in a cell are either a count of subjects or the proportion of the total subjects having the property of the intersecting row and column. The investigator must specify whether a cell entry is a frequency count or a proportion.

Tables are preferred for descriptive statistics and larger data sets, as it makes possible a future analysis using the displayed summary statistics. Complete details of inferential statistics can also be presented in tabular form; there is no more efficient way of detailing an analysis of variance output. More commonly, in the anesthesia literature, inferential statistics in tables are limited to superscripted notations (e.g., *, #, ¶) of probabilities. Unfortunately, these superscripts with their footnoted explanation can be rather ambiguous in specifying the statistical test and statistical hypothesis being used for the probability value displayed.

A graph is a visual display of measured quantities (either raw data or summary statistics) by the combined use of geometric elements (a coordinate system, points, lines, circles, etc.), text elements (numbers, symbols, words), and art elements (shading, colors, patterns). Graphs are most suitable for showing broad qualitative features of the data. The most common graph formats used in biomedical literature are the bar graph, scatter plot, and line plot. Bar graphs can be used to show large raw data sets as a frequency histogram, and to allow group comparisons of summary statistics; vertical bar graphs are also known as column graphs. Scatter plots are used to display bivariate data ((x, y) pairs). Line plots can be used for either raw data or descriptive statistics. As with tables, inferential statistics are generally limited to notations of probability values. The text elements of a graph are available to list regression equations and correlation coefficients.

INFERENTIAL STATISTICS

There are two major areas of statistical inference: the estimation of parameters and the testing of hypotheses. The use of the standard error to create confidence intervals is an example of parameter estimation. The testing of hypotheses or significance testing is the main focus of inferential statistics. Hypothesis testing allows the experimenter to use data from the sample to make inferences about the population. Statisticians have created formulas that use the values of the samples to calculate test statistics. Statisticians have also explored the properties of various theoretical probability distributions. Depending on the assumptions about how data are collected, the appropriate theoretical probability distribution is chosen as the source of critical values to accept or reject the null hypothesis; if the value of the test statistic calculated from the sample(s) is greater than the critical value, the null hypothesis is rejected. The critical value is chosen from the appropriate probability distribution after the magnitude of the Type I error is specified.

There are parameters within the equation that generates any particular theoretical probability distribution; for the normal probability distribution, the parameters are μ and σ. For the normal distribution, each set of values for μ and σ will generate a different shape for the bell-like normal curve. All theoretical probability equations contain one or more parameters, and can also be plotted as curves; these parameters may be discrete (integer only) or continuous. Each value or combination of values for these parameters will create a different curve for the probability distribution being used. Thus, each theoretical probability distribution is actually a family of probability curves. Some parameters have been given the special name, degrees of freedom, and are represented by the letters m, n, p, and s.

Associated with the formula for computing a test statistic is a rule for assigning integer values to one or more degrees of freedom. The number of degrees of freedom and the value for each degree of freedom depend on: 1) the number of subjects, 2) the number of experimental groups, 3) the specifics of the statistical hypothesis, and 4) the type of statistical test. The correct curve of the theoretical probability distribution from which to obtain a critical value for comparison with the value of the test statistic is obtained with the one or more degrees of freedom of the sample.

To accept or reject the null hypothesis, the following steps are performed: 1) confirm that experimental data conforms to the assumptions of the intended statistical test; 2) choose a significance level (alpha); 3) calculate the test statistic; 4) determine the degrees of freedom; 5) find the critical value for the chosen alpha and the degrees of freedom from the appropriate theoretical probability distribution; 6) if the test statistic exceeds the critical value, reject the null hypothesis; and 7) if the test statistic does not exceed the critical value, do not reject the null hypothesis.

Interval Data

Parametric statistics are the usual choice in the analysis of interval data, both discrete and continuous. The purpose of such analysis is to test the hypothesis of a difference between population means. The population means are unknown, and are estimated by the sample means. A typical example would be the comparison of the mean heart rates of patients receiving and not receiving atropine. Parametric test statistics have been developed by using the properties of the normal probability distribution and two related theoretical probability distributions, the t and the F distribution. In using such parametric methods, the assumption is made that the sample or samples is/are drawn from population(s) with a normal distribution. The parametric test statistics that have been created for interval data all have the form of a ratio. In general terms, the numerator of this ratio is the variability of the means of the samples; the denominator of this ratio is the variability among all the members of the samples. These variabilities are similar to the variances developed for descriptive statistics. The test statistic is, thus, a ratio of variabilities or variances. All parametric test statistics are used in the same fashion; if the test statistic ratio becomes large, the null hypothesis of no difference is rejected. The critical values against which to compare the test statistic are taken from tables of the three relevant probability distributions.

By definition, in hypothesis testing, at least one of the population means are unknown, but the population variance(s) may or may not be known. Parametric statistics can be divided into two groups by whether or not the population variances are known. If the population variance is known, the test statistic used is called the z score; critical values are obtained from the normal distribution. In most scientific applications, the population variance is rarely known; the use of z score test statistics for interval data will not be discussed further in this chapter.

t Test

An important advance in statistical inference came early in the 20th century, with the creation of the Student's t test statistic and the t distribution which allowed the testing of hypotheses when the population variance is not known. The most common use of the Student's t test is to compare the mean values of two populations. This use is further subdivided by a particular aspect of experimental design. If each subject has two measurements taken, for example, one before and one after a drug, then the one sample or paired t test procedure is used; each control measurement taken before drug administration is paired with a measurement in the same patient after drug administration. Of course, this is a self-control experiment. This pairing of measurements in the same patient reduces variability and increases statistical power. There are two target populations in such an experiment: subjects before and subjects after the study drug. For purposes of statistical analysis, the problem is converted into a one-population test (Table 3-9). The difference d_i of each pair of values is calculated; $\bar{d}$ is a

sample statistic estimator of δ. In our example, the target population has become the difference in values of blood pressure before and after a study drug; δ is the parameter of central location for this new population of blood pressure differences. Our null hypothesis is one of no drug effect, i.e., $\delta = 0$. In the formula for the Student's t statistic, the numerator is $\bar{d} - 0$, while the denominator is the standard error of d. All t statistics are created thus; the numerator is the difference of two means, while the denominator is the standard error of the two means. If the difference between the two means is large compared to their variability, then the null hypothesis of no difference is rejected. The critical values for the t statistic are taken from the t probability distribution. The t distribution is symmetrical and bell shaped, but more spread out than the normal distribution. The t distribution has a single integer parameter; for a paired t test, the value of this single degree of freedom is the sample size minus one. There can be some confusion about the use of the letter t. It refers both to the value of the test statistic calculated by the formula $t_{(df)} = \bar{d}/\mathrm{SE}_d$ and to the critical value from the theoretical probability distribution. The critical t value is determined by looking in a t table after a significance level is chosen and the degrees of freedom are computed.

More commonly, measurements are taken on two separate groups of subjects. For example, one group could receive the blood pressure treatment, while no treatment is given to a control group. The number of subjects in each group might or might not be identical; regardless of this, in no sense is an individual measurement in the first group matched or paired with a specific measurement in the second group. An unpaired or two-sample t test is used to compare the means of the two groups (Table 3-10). The obvious null hypothesis of no difference between the groups is used; thus, the numerator of the t statistic is $\bar{x} - \bar{y}$. The denominator requires extra work. It is necessary to assume that the population variance of x equals the population variance of y; under that assumption, a pooled estimate of s (s_p) can be calculated. The standard error of the difference of x and y is s_p divided by a weighted average of the

TABLE 3-9. Inferential Statistics for Hypothetical Paired Interval Data of Systolic Blood Pressure Before and After Treatment

SUBJECT i	CONTROL x_{i1}	TREATED x_{i2}	DIFFERENCE $d_i = x_{i2} - x_{i1}$	DEVIATION $(d_i - \bar{d})$	DEVIATION SQUARED $(d_i - \bar{d})^2$
1	190	170	−20	0	0
2	180	150	−30	−10	100
3	180	160	−20	0	0
4	170	170	0	+20	400
5	190	170	−20	0	0
6	160	170	+10	+30	900
7	200	150	−50	−30	900
8	190	160	−30	−10	100
8	1460	1300	−160	0	2400

$H_0 : \delta = 0$
$H_a : \delta \neq 0$

$\bar{d} = \Sigma d_i / n = -160/8 = -20$
$s_d = ((\Sigma(d_i - \bar{d})^2)/(n-1))^{0.5} = (2400/7)^{0.5} = 18.5$
$\mathrm{SE}_d = s_d/(n)^{0.5} = 18.5/(8)^{0.5} = 6.55$

Paired t test $= t_{(df)} = (\bar{d} - 0)/SE_d$ \qquad df $= n - 1$

$t_{(7)} = -20/6.55 = -3.05$ \qquad\qquad Critical Value $= t_{(0.05, 7)} = 2.37$

Reject null hypothesis, since $|t_{(7)}| = 3.05 >$ critical value $= 2.37$

TABLE 3-10. Inferential Statistics for Hypothetical Unpaired Interval Data of Systolic Blood Pressure With and Without Treatment

CONTROL x_i	TREATED y_i	DEVIATION $(x_i - \bar{x})$	SQUARED DEVIATION $(x_i - \bar{x})^2$	DEVIATION $(y_i - \bar{y})$	SQUARED DEVIATION $(y_i - \bar{y})^2$
190	170	+7.5	56.25	+7.5	56.25
180	150	-2.5	6.25	-12.5	156.25
180	160	-2.5	6.25	-2.5	6.25
170	170	-12.5	156.25	+7.5	56.25
190	170	+7.5	56.25	+7.5	56.25
160	170	-22.5	560.25	+7.5	56.25
200	150	+17.5	306.25	-12.5	156.25
190	160	+7.5	56.25	-2.5	6.25
1460	1300	0.0	1150.00	0.0	550.00

H_0: $\mu_x = \mu_y$
H_a: $\mu_x = \mu_y$

$n_x = 8 \qquad \bar{x} = \Sigma x_i/n_x = 1460/8 = 182.5$
$n_y = 8 \qquad \bar{y} = \Sigma y_i/n_y = 1300/8 = 162.5$
$s_x = ((\Sigma(x_i - \bar{x})^2)/(n_x - 1))^{0.5} = (1150/7)^{0.5} = 12.8$
$s_y = ((\Sigma(y_i - \bar{y})^2)/(n_y - 1))^{0.5} = (550/7)^{0.5} = 8.9$

Pooled $s = s_p = \{[(n_x-1) \cdot s_x^2 + (n_y-1) \cdot s_y^2]/(n_x+n_y-2)\}^{0.5}$
$\qquad\qquad\quad = \{(7 \cdot 12.8^2 + 7 \cdot 8.9^2)/14\}^{0.5} = 11.0$

SE of difference $= SE_{(x-y)} = s_p \cdot (1/n_x + 1/n_y)^{0.5} = 11.0 \cdot (1/8 + 1/8)^{0.5} = 5.5$

unpaired t test $= t_{(df)} = (\bar{x} - \bar{y})/SE_{(x-y)} \qquad df = n_x + n_y - 2$

$t_{(14)} = (182.5 - 162.5)/5.5 = 3.63 \qquad$ Critical value $= t_{(0.05, 14)} = 2.15$

Reject null hypothesis, since $t_{(14)} = 3.63 >$ critical value $= 2.15$

count of subjects in x and the count of subjects in y. The degrees of freedom for an unpaired t test are calculated as the sum of the subjects of the two groups minus two. As with the paired t test, if the t ratio becomes large, the null hypothesis is rejected.

Multiple Comparisons and Analysis of Variance

Experiments in anesthesia, be they with humans or with animals, are rarely limited to only one or two groups of data for each variable. It is very common to follow a variable longitudinally; heart rate might be measured five times before and during anesthetic induction. These are also called repeated measurement experiments; the experimenter will wish to compare changes between the initial heart rate and those taken during induction. The experimental design might also include several groups receiving different induction drugs; i.e., comparing heart rate immediately after laryngoscopy. Researchers have commonly handled these analysis problems with the t test. With heart rate being collected five times, these collection times could be labelled as A, B, C, D, and E. Then, in a paired sense, A could be compared with B, C, D, and E: B could be compared with C, D, and E: and so forth. There are a total of ten possible pairings; thus, ten paired t tests could be calculated for all the possible pairings of A, B, C, D, and E. A similar approach can be used for comparing more than two groups for unpaired data.

The use of t tests in this fashion is inappropriate. In testing a statistical hypothesis, the experimenter sets the level of Type I error; this is usually chosen to be 0.05. When using many t tests, as in the example above, the chosen error rate for performing all these t tests is much higher than 0.05, even though the Type I error is set at 0.05 for each individual comparison. In fact, the Type I error rate for all t tests simultaneously, i.e., the

chance of finding at least one of the multiple t test statistics significant merely by chance, is given by the formula $\alpha = 1 - 0.95^k$. If 13 t tests are performed, then the real error rate is 49%. This problem can be simulated by generating mock data on a computer; simply applying t tests over and over again to all the possible pairings of a variable will misleadingly identify statistical significance when there is, in fact, no statistical significance.

The most versatile approach for handling comparisons of means among more than two groups is called analysis of variance; frequently cited by the acronym ANOVA. Analysis of variance consists of rules for creating test statistics on means when there are more than two groups. These test statistics are called F ratios, after Ronald Fisher; the critical values for the F test statistic are taken from the F theoretical probability distribution which Fisher derived.

Suppose that data for three groups are obtained (Table 3-11). What can be said about the mean values of the three target populations? The null hypothesis for such comparisons is more complex, as it contains three identities. The F test is actually asking several questions simultaneously: is group 1 different from group 2, is group 2 different from group 3, and is group 1 different from group 3? As with the t test, the F test statistic is a ratio; in general terms, the numerator expresses the variability of the mean values of the three groups, while the denominator expresses the average variability or difference of each sample value from the mean of all sample values. The formulas to create the test statistic (Table 3-12) are computationally elegant, but are rather hard to appreciate intuitively. The F statistic has two degrees of freedom, denoted m and n; the value of m is a function of the number of experimental groups; the value for n is a function of the number of subjects in all experimental groups.

Enormous effort has been expended to develop different

TABLE 3-11. Inferential Statistics on Hypothetical Data
With Three Groups:
One-Way Analysis of Variance (Part I)

SUBJECT NUMBER	GROUP 1	GROUP 2	GROUP 3	GROUPS COMBINED
1	3	3	2	
2	5	0	1	
3	4	4	2	
4	2	3	3	
5	4	4	4	
6	3	1	4	
7	4	4	3	
8	7	1	6	
9	2	1	0	
10	6	6	4	
n	$10 = n_1$	$10 = n_2$	$10 = n_3$	$30 = N$
Σx_i	$40 = T_1$	$27 = T_2$	$29 = T_3$	$96 = G$
Σx^2_i	184	105	111	400
$\bar{x}$	4.0	2.7	2.9	
s	1.63	1.89	1.70	
SE	0.27	0.36	0.30	

$H_0: \mu_1 = \mu_2 = \mu_3$
$H_a: \mu_1 \neq \mu_2 \neq \mu_3$

types of ANOVA. For example, there are at least three ANOVA techniques for analyzing repeated measurement data; these are the two-way ANOVA for repeated measurements, the multivariate ANOVA for repeated measurements, and the maximum likelihood mixed-model ANOVA. Very complex experimental designs are difficult to analyze statistically without the flexibility of ANOVA methods for developing test statistics. The analysis of multigroup data is not necessarily finished after the ANOVAs are calculated. If the null hypothesis is rejected and one accepts that there are differences among the groups tested, how does one decide where the differences are? A variety of techniques are available to make what are called multiple comparisons after the ANOVA test is performed. These include tests by Bonferroni, Tukey, Scheffé, and Dunnett; there is also the Duncan's and Newman-Keuls multiple range test. All these multiple comparison tests tend to be variations on the t test statistic. The reader should refer to a text on statistics for a more comprehensive review of ANOVA.

Transformations, Robustness, and Non-Parametric Tests

As mentioned several times above, most statistical tests depend on certain assumptions about the nature of the distribution of values in the underlying populations from which experimental samples are taken. For the parametric statistics, i.e., t tests and analysis of variance, it is assumed that the populations follow the normal distribution; if one were to plot the population values in a histogram, the shape of the leading edge of the data would be the bell-shaped curve. There is a further assumption when dealing with samples from two or more populations. The variances of the populations are assumed to be equal and common; this is also described as homogeneity of variance. Usually, the experimenter cannot discern the population distributions of his data. However, for some data, there is experience or historical reasons to believe that these assumptions of a normal distribution and homogeneity of variance do not hold; some examples include proportions, percentages, and response times. Many other instances of poorly conditioned data exist. What should the experimenter do if he fears that his data are not normally distributed?

One possibility would be to engage a statistician to create new test statistics and new theoretical probability distributions. This would be expensive and inefficient; many years of work by many statisticians have been invested in the creation of parametric statistics. It is more desirable to use existing statistical techniques to save money and to avoid explaining these new methods to editors and readers. Another possibility would be to transform the data before analysis. In transforming data, a function is applied to a raw value; a common transformation is the use of logarithms. If the raw value is 10, the transformed value is log (10) or 1. These transformations can be thought of as changing the scale of measurement; it is as if the ruler by which a measure is obtained is stretched and compressed along its length. The most frequently used transformations are the logarithmic, the square root, the inverse sine function, and the reciprocal. Under appropriate circumstances, these transformations can be shown to create either normally distributed data and/or homogeneity of variance. The usual parametric statistics can then be used with confidence. Using data transformations does have its complication. What is the inherent meaning of these transformed data? How should model and population parameters (mean, standard deviation, slope) of transformed data be retransformed to the original scale of measurement after analysis? Data transforma-

TABLE 3-12.   Inferential Statistics on Hypothetical Data with Three Groups:
One-Way Analysis of Variance (Part II)

SOURCE	SUM OF SQUARES	DEGREES OF FREEDOM	MEAN SQUARE
Between treatments	SST = 9.8	$k - 1 = 2$	SST/$(k - 1)$ = 9.8/2 = 4.90
Within treatments (error)	SSE = 83.0	$N - k = 27$	SSE/$(N - k)$ = 83.0/27 = 3.07
Total	S = 92.8	$N - 1 = 29$	

Sum of squares total = $S = \Sigma x_i^2 - G^2/N = 400 - 96^2/30 = 92.8$
Sum of squares between treatments = $SST = \Sigma(T_i^2/n_i) - G^2/N = [(40^2 + 27^2 + 29^2)/10] - 96^2/30 = 9.8$
Degrees of freedom between treatments = $k - 1 = 3 - 1 = 2$
Sum of squares within treatments = $SSE = S - SST = 92.8 - 9.8 = 83.0$
Degrees of freedom within treatments = $N - k = 30 - 3 = 27$
$F_{(2, 27)}$ ratio = $[SST/(k - 1)]/[SSE/(N - k)] = 4.90/3.07 = 1.59$
Critical ratio = $F_{(2, 27; 0.05)} = 3.37$

Do not reject null hypothesis, since $F_{(2, 27)} = 1.59 < F_{(2, 27; 0.05)} = 3.37$

tion is not as widely practiced now as it was several decades ago.

The experimenter might also choose to ignore the problem of non-normal data and inhomogeneity of variance, hoping that everything will work out. Such insouciance is actually a very practical and reasonable approach to the problem. Parametric statistics are called "robust" statistics; they stand up to much adversity. To a statistician, robustness implies that the magnitude of Type I errors is not seriously affected by ill-conditioned data. Parametric statistics are sufficiently robust that the accuracy of decisions reached by means of t tests and analysis of variance remain very credible, even for moderately severe departures from the assumptions.

A fourth possibility would be to use existing statistics which do not require any assumptions about probability distributions of the populations. Such statistics are known as nonparametric tests; these statistics can be used whenever there is very serious concern about the shape of the data. Nonparametric statistics are also the tests of choice for ordinal data. The basic concept behind nonparametric statistics is the ability to rank or order the observations; nonparametric tests are also called order statistics. If there are sample values from two populations, all values are thrown into a common list and arranged or ranked in value from lowest to highest; each sample value is assigned the new value from lowest to highest; each sample value is assigned the new value of its place in line or rank in the list; for each group, these rank values are summed. A test statistic is calculated that is a function of the rank score and of the count of subjects for each group; if the test statistic is sufficiently large, the null hypothesis of no difference is rejected.

Most nonparametric statistics still require the use of theoretical probability distributions; the critical values which must be exceeded by the test statistic are taken from the binomial, normal, and chi-square distributions, depending on the nonparametric test being used. The nonparametric sign test, Mann-Whitney rank sum test, and Kruskal-Wallis one-way analysis of variance are analogous to the paired t test, unpaired t test, and one-way analysis of variance, respectively. The currently available nonparametric tests are not used more commonly because they do not adapt well to complex statistical models, and because they are less able to distinguish between the null and alternative hypotheses than parametric tests if the data are, in fact, normally distributed. Using the data of Table 3-10, the probability of the hypothesis comparing the two groups is $P = 0.003$ by unpaired t test and $P = 0.009$ by the Mann-Whitney rank sum test. Statistical significance is detected by both tests, but the nonparametric is less powerful.

Regression and Correlation

After calculating a regression line, what inferences can be made about the regression equation? Recall that this calculation required the assumption of a model relating variables and model parameters, and that the model needed reexamination during analysis. One of the crucial features of the least squares linear model is the slope of the straight line; the sample statistic b is an estimate of the population slope β. If the slope of the line is 0, then there is no relationship between x and y, and the model must be rejected. The most commonly performed statistical test during regression analysis compares b to a slope value of 0. Although no assumptions were required to calculate a regression equation, inferential statistics concerning regression assume that y is normally distributed, and that the variability of y is the same regardless of the value of x; this later property is called homoscedasticity. These assumptions are

usually reasonable, even if the values of y aren't quite normally distributed; the Central Limit Theorem also applies to regression analysis.

The test statistic for inferences about β is a t test (Table 3-13). Critical values are obtained from the t distribution; the degrees of freedom are the sample size minus two. The numerator is the difference between the two estimates of the population slope, $b-0$. The denominator is the standard error of the sample slope b (SE_b); a previously unmentioned sample statistic is used to calculate this denominator. Similar to a sample standard deviation, the standard deviation from regression ($s_{y \cdot x}$) estimates deviations of sample points about the fitted regression line. Both the standard error of the intercept and SE_b are estimated by the use of $s_{y \cdot x}$. One cannot reject the null hypothesis of $\beta = 0$ in our hypothetical data set; thus, the model of a linear relationship must be abandoned. Even when this t test is significant, the data must often be examined more closely to confirm the model. This is most frequently done by examining the residuals. In regression analysis, residuals are the difference between the sample y and the predicted y for each (x, y) pair. Other inferential statistics include confidence limits on the slope b and on the values of y predicted by the regression equation.

Inferential statistics for correlation tend to be more complicated computationally. The assumptions are more rigorous also; in general, x and y must be bivariate normally distributed. However, these assumptions are not necessary for the most commonly used test on r, which is the null hypothesis that $\rho = 0$, i.e., the hypothesis of no dependency between x and y. This hypothesis is also tested by a t test statistic. As is clear in the hypothetical example (Table 3-13), the statistical test for $\beta = 0$ and for $\rho = 0$ give identical results and are, in fact, equivalent. This equivalence again shows the close ties between regression and correlation. The form of the test statistic for correlation does give some additional insight as to the effects of sample size on significance. Notice that t increases as n increases. Suppose that 100 points had been sampled with the same calculated r. Then the value of $t = (r^2/(1-r^2))^{0.5} \cdot (n-2)^{0.5} = (0.32^2/(1-0.32^2))^{0.5} \cdot 98^{0.5} = 3.34$. This value exceeds the critical value of $t_{(0.05, 98)} = 1.99$. Besides deciding whether there is a statistically significant association

TABLE 3-13.   Inferential Statistics for a Hypothetical Bivariate Data Set*

REGRESSION

$H_0 : \beta = 0$
$H_a : \beta \neq 0$
$s_{y \cdot x} = [\{[\Sigma(y_i - \bar{y})^2] - [\Sigma(x_i - \bar{x}) \cdot (y_i - \bar{y})]^2/[\Sigma(x_i - \bar{x})^2]\}/(n-2)]^{0.5}$
$\quad\quad = [(1 - 1/10)/3]^{0.5} = 0.55$
$SE_b = s_{y \cdot x}/(\Sigma(x_i - \bar{x})^2)^{0.5} = 0.55/(10)^{0.5} = 0.17$
$t_{(df)} = (b - 0)/SE_b = b/SE_b \quad\quad df = n - 2$
$t_{(3)} = 0.1/0.17 = 0.58 \quad\quad$ Critical value $t_{(0.05, 3)} = 3.18$

Do not reject null hypothesis, since $t_{(3)} = 0.58 <$ critical value $= 3.18$

CORRELATION

$H_0 : \rho = 0$
$H_a : \rho \neq 0$
$t_{(df)} = [r^2/(1 - r^2)]^{0.5} \cdot [n - 2]^{0.5} \quad\quad df = n - 2$
$t_{(3)} = [0.32^2/(1 - 0.32^2)]^{0.5} \cdot 3^{0.5} = 0.58 \quad\quad$ Critical value $t_{(0.05, 3)} = 3.18$

Do not reject null hypothesis, since $t_{(3)} = 0.58 <$ critical value $= 3.18$
Coefficient of determination $= r^2 = 0.32^2 = 0.10$

*The data set used is that given in Table 3-7

between x and y, the degree of this association should be found. The square of r, the coefficient of determination, provides this measure of association. Roughly speaking, $100 \cdot r^2$ is the percent of the variation in y explained by the regression of y on x. For $r = 0.32$, $100 \cdot r^2$ is 10%. Thus, even though there is a significant relationship between x and y when 100 points are sampled, this relationship is very weak. Whenever an author reports a correlation coefficient, this strength of association can be mentally calculated by the reader; a remarkable number of the correlations reported to be significant have very weak associations between the two variables.

Contingency Tables

In a hypothetical experiment comparing performance on an examination, about 83% of the anesthesia faculty passed, while less than 38% of anesthesia residents passed (Table 3-14); is this difference real? This question is also stated as whether there is a dependency or association between the rows and the columns of the $2 \cdot 2$ contingency table. There are a variety of statistical techniques to compare this pass/fail rate in the underlying populations of all anesthesia faculty and all anesthesia residents. This section will discuss two test statistics: 1) the most commonly used, the chi-square test, and 2) the z score test based on an approximation to the normal distribution. These methods are used for both ordinal and nominal variables.

Just as the normal approximation of the binomial distribution was used for descriptive statistics of rates and proportions, a comparison of the relative frequencies of two groups can be created using the normal distribution if the sample sizes are sufficiently large. Under the assumption of null hypothesis, the frequencies of the two groups are identical, i.e., $\pi_1 = \pi_2$. The best estimate for the differences of the means of the two samples is the difference of the proportions, $p_1 - p_2$; $p_1 - p_2$ is a summary statistic which estimates the population parameter, $\pi_1 - \pi_2$. There is a standard error for $p_1 - p_2$, giving the precision with which $\pi_1 - \pi_2$ is known; this standard error uses a weighted average of p_1 and p_2:

$$SE(p_1 - p_2) = (p \cdot (1-p) \cdot (1/n_1 + 1/n_2))^{0.5}$$
$$\text{where } p = (n_1 \cdot p_1 + n_2 \cdot p_2)/(n_1 + n_2).$$

The z score test statistic is literally a ratio; the numerator consists of the difference between the means of the samples, while the denominator is the standard error of this difference:

$$z \text{ score} = (\mid p_1 - p_2 \mid)/SE(p_1 - p_2).$$

If the difference in proportions increases ($\mid p_1 - p_2 \mid$ larger), and/or if the precision of the difference decreases ($SE(p_1 - p_2)$ smaller), then the z score increases. The greater the z score, the greater the likelihood of a difference between the two populations from which samples were taken. If each of the quantities $n_1 \cdot p$, $n_1 \cdot (1-p)$, $n_2 \cdot p$, $n_2 \cdot (1-p)$ has a value greater than or equal to 5, the normal approximation may be used; these conditions are met in the hypothetical example (Table 3-14). The critical values against which the z score test statistic is compared are found in the tables of the normal probability function; there are no degrees of freedom for the z score test statistic or the normal probability curve. As with other test statistics, if the z score value exceeds the predetermined critical value, the null hypothesis is rejected. It has been discovered that the z score test statistic, being a continuous approximation of the discrete binomial distribution, slightly overestimates the probability of a difference; for this reason, a z score with a smaller numerator is used because it more closely approximates the exact probabilities:

$$\text{corrected } z \text{ score} = \frac{(\mid p_1 - p_2 \mid - 0.5) \cdot (1/n_1 + 1/n_2))}{SE(p_1 - p_2)}$$

The chi-square test is a more frequently used alternative to the z score; it is also known as the Pearson chi-square statistic. When used with $2 \cdot 2$ contingency tables, it is equivalent to the z score test (Table 3-15). The chi-square test offers the advantage of being computationally simpler, and can also analyze contingency tables with more than two rows and two columns. The chi-square test statistic is a sum of ratios. For each cell of the contingency table, the observed value has been recorded. Using the assumption that there is no association between the rows and the columns, the expected value for each cell is the row total multiplied by the column total divided by the total number of subjects. For each cell, the squared difference between the observed and expected value divided by the expected value expresses the variability of the observed value away from the expected value. The test statistic is the sum of these difference ratios. The formula is written:

$$X^2_{(df)} = \Sigma((\mid \text{observed} - \text{expected} \mid - 0.5)^2/\text{expected}).$$

If the difference between observed and expected cell values grows larger, it is more likely that there is an association between the rows and columns. The critical values used with the chi-square test statistic are from the X^2 or chi-square continuous theoretical probability distribution. A distinction must be made between the chi-square test statistic, which is denoted X^2, and the chi-square probability distribution, which is denoted X^2. The X^2 distribution has a single integer parameter or degree of freedom. The value of this degree of freedom is the product of the number of rows minus one times the number of columns minus one. As with the z score, a continuity correction is used, and certain restrictions concern-

TABLE 3-14.   Contingency Table of Hypothetical Data Comparing Pass/Fail Rates on Standardized Board Examination for Anesthesia Personnel

	PASS	FAIL	TOTAL
Anesthesia Residents	15 (37.5%)	25 (62.5%)	40
Anesthesia Faculty	33 (82.5%)	7 (17.5%)	40
Total	48 (60.0%)	32 (40.0%)	80

DESCRIPTIVE STATISTICS
$n_1 = 40$ $x_1 = 15$ $n_2 = 40$ $x_2 = 33$
$p_1 = x_1/n_1 = 15/40 = 0.375$ $p_2 = x_2/n_2 = 33/40 = 0.825$

INFERENTIAL STATISTICS
$H_0: \pi_1 = \pi_2$
$H_a: \pi_1 \neq \pi_2$

$p_2 - p_1 = 0.825 - 0.375 = 0.45$
Combined proportion $= \bar{p} = (x_1 + x_2)/(n_1 + n_2)$
$\qquad\qquad = (15 + 33)/(40 + 40) = 0.6$
$SE_{(p_2-p_1)} = [\bar{p} \cdot (1 - \bar{p}) \cdot (1/n_1 + 1/n_2)]^{0.5}$
$\qquad = [0.6 \cdot (1 - 0.6) \cdot (1/40 + 1/40)]^{0.5} = 0.11$
Test statistic $= z = (\mid p_2 - p_1 \mid)/SE(p_2 - p_1) = 0.45/0.11 = 4.11$
Corrected test statistic $= z_c = [\mid p_2 - p_1 \mid - 0.5 \cdot (1/n_1 + 1/n_2)]/SE_{(p_2-p_1)}$
$\qquad = [0.45 - 0.5 \cdot (1/40 + 1/40)]/0.11 = 3.88$
Critical value $= z_{(0.05)} = 1.96$

Reject null hypothesis, since $z_c = 3.88 >$ critical value $= 1.96$

ing cell size are recommended. For 2 · 2 tables, the smallest expected cell value should be at least 5, or the test statistic will be biased. The method shown in table 3-14 can be used to calculate a chi-square statistic for any size contingency table. For 2 · 2 contingency tables, there is an even simpler formula for the calculation of the chi-square test statistic (Table 3-16).

There is a third alternative to the z score and chi-square test which is coming into greater use now that computations are cheap. It is known as the Fisher exact test, and gives the exact probability of a 2 · 2 contingency table; the Fisher exact test uses the hypergeometric probability distribution, which is related to the binomial distribution. The Fisher exact test should be used if any expected cell value is less than five. As the total count of frequencies in a contingency table increase, the Fisher exact test and X^2 test give almost identical probabilities. In our example, the exact probability for table 3-15 is $P = 0.00008$, while the probability for $X^2 = 15.05$ is $P = 0.00010$. That is truly a good approximation.

In the hypothetical example (Table 3-14), the X^2 test statistic showed a statistically significant difference between the faculty and resident examination pass rate. A common mistake is to stop the analysis of contingency tables after testing for statistical significance. While X^2 is excellent as a measure of the significance of association, it is not at all useful as a measure of the degree of association. The basic measure of association is the odds ratio or cross-product ratio (Table 3-16). If the odds ratio is one, there is no association between rows and columns; if the odds ratio is not one, there is an association or dependency between rows and columns. In the sample problem, the odds ratio shows that faculty members are over seven times more likely to pass the examination than residents. X^2 is a function of both the cell proportions and the total number of subjects, while the odds ratio is only a function of the cell proportions. If a large number of subjects are used, the X^2 test may reveal statistical significance, even when there is little dependency between rows and columns. The odds ratio is easily calculated, and can be used to check the importance of a contingency table result.

Interpretation of Results

Scientific studies do not end with the statistical inference. The experimenter must commit an opinion as to the generalizability of his work to the rest of the world. Even if there is a

TABLE 3-15.   Calculation of Chi Square Test Statistic for Data Given in Table 3-14

	OBSERVED COUNTS			EXPECTED COUNTS		
	Pass	Fail	Total	Pass	Fail	Total
Residents	15	25	40	48 · 40/80 = 24	32 · 40/80 = 16	40
Faculty	33	7	40	48 · 40/80 = 24	32 · 40/80 = 16	40
Total	48	32	80	48	32	80

INFERENTIAL STATISTICS

$X^2_{(df)} = \Sigma[(|\text{observed} - \text{expected}| - 0.5)^2/\text{expected}]$

Degrees of freedom = df = (rows − 1) · (columns − 1)

Degrees of freedom = df = (2 − 1) · (2 − 1) = 1

$X^2_{(1)} = (|15 − 24| − 0.5)^2/24 + (|25 − 16| − 0.5)^2/16 + (|33 − 24| − 0.5)^2/24 + (|7 − 16| − 0.5)^2/16$

    $= (8.5)^2/24 + (8.5)^2/16 + (8.5)^2/24 + (8.5)^2/16 = 15.05$

Critical value = $X^2_{(0.05, 1)} = 3.84$

Reject null hypothesis, since $X^2_{(1)} = 15.05 >$ critical value = 3.84

TABLE 3-16.   Calculation of Chi Square Test Statistic for Data Given in Table 3-14 with Alternative Formula

	OBSERVED COUNTS			ALGEBRAIC NOTATION		
	Pass	Fail	Total	Pass	Fail	Total
Residents	33	7	40	a	b	a + b
Faculty	15	25	40	c	d	c + d
Total	48	32	80	a + c	b + d	n = a + b + c + d

INFERENTIAL STATISTICS

$X^2_{(df)} = n \cdot (|a \cdot d − b \cdot c| − n/2)^2/((a + c) \cdot (b + d) \cdot (a + b) \cdot (c + d))$

Degrees of freedom = df = (rows − 1) · (columns − 1)

Degrees of freedom = df = (2 − 1) · (2 − 1) = 1

$X^2_{(1)} = 80 \cdot (|33 \cdot 25 − 7 \cdot 15| − 80/2)^2/((33 + 15) \cdot (7 + 25) \cdot (33 + 7) \cdot (15 + 25)) = 15.05$

Critical value = $X^2_{(0.05, 1)} = 3.84$

Reject null hypothesis, since $X^2_{(1)} = 15.05 >$ critical value = 3.84

Cross product ratio = odds ratio = (a · d)/(b · c) = (33 · 25)/(7 · 15) = 7.86

statistically significant difference, one must decide if this difference is medically or physiologically important. Statistical significance does not always equate with biological relevance. The questions an experimenter should ask himself about the interpretation of results are highly dependent on the specifics of the experiment. Three examples are given. First, even small, clinically unimportant differences between groups can be detected if the sample size is sufficiently large. On the other hand, if the sample size is small, one must always worry that identified or unidentified confounding variables may explain any difference; as the sample size decreases, randomization is less successful in assuring homogenous groups. Second, if the experimental groups are three or more doses of a drug, do the results suggest a steadily increasing or decreasing dose-response relationship? Suppose the observed effect for an intermediate dose is either much higher or much lower than that for both the largest and smallest dose; a dose-response relationship may exist, but some skepticism about the experimental methods is warranted. Third, for clinical studies comparing patient outcome from different drugs, devices, and operations, are the patients, clinical care, and studied therapies sufficiently like those of other locations to be of interest to a wide group of practitioners. This last point is so important that it is now receiving editorial attention in anesthesia journals.[36] In comparing alternative therapies, the experimenter will have more or less confidence that a claim for a superior therapy is true depending on the study design. The strength of the evidence concerning efficacy will be least for an anecdotal case report; next in importance will be a retrospective study, then a prospective series of patients compared to historical controls, and, finally, a randomized, controlled clinical trial. The greatest strength for a therapeutic claim will be a series of randomized, controlled clinical trials confirming the same hypothesis.[24]

RESOURCES FOR STATISTICAL METHODS: TEXTS, JOURNALS, SOFTWARE, AND STATISTICIANS

Many materials are available to guide both the researcher and the journal reader into the depths of simple and sophisticated statistics. There are journal articles that present specific recommendations concerning common statistical problems and research design goals.[14, 37, 38] Several journals are totally devoted to research methods and statistical analysis in biological fields: *Statistics in Medicine* and *Controlled Clinical Trials* are clinically oriented, while *Biometrics* and *Biometrika* are journals for the professional statistician. Particularly interesting is a regular section in *Controlled Clinical Trials* featuring an annotated bibliography of publications regarding statistics.[39] Other authors have published reading lists with comments for self-education.[40] Besides the textbooks of statistical theory, there are many books of applied biomedical statistics. Excellent introductory textbooks are available by Glantz,[41] Phillips,[42] Colton,[43] and Mattson;[44] more advanced textbooks include those by Snedecor and Cochran,[45] Cox and Snell,[46] and Winer.[47] A variety of monographs and texts address specific subjects. These include: 1) regression analysis: Edwards[48] and Draper and Smith;[49] 2) graphical displays: Schmid,[50] Tufte,[51] and Cleveland;[52] 3) contingency table analysis: Fleiss[53] and Fienberg;[54] 4) experimental measurement: Barford;[55] 5) multivariate analysis of variance: Morrison[56] and Tabachnick and Fidell;[57] 6) research design and analysis: Marks,[58] Marks,[59] Feinstein,[60] Silverman,[61] and Gore and Altman;[62] 7) the epidemiology of anesthetic practice: Lunn;[63] 8) the ethics of hu-

man experimentation: Greenwald et al.[29] and Levine;[30] and 9) application of statistics to clinical practice: Sackett et al.[64] and Ingelfinger et al.[65]

Unless the data sets become large, all the statistical tests described in this chapter can be done by manual calculation; handheld scientific calculators can assist in this analysis and reduce computational errors. With the spread of computers into every laboratory and office, statistical software has made the process even more convenient. Also, more advanced statistical techniques are not computationally feasible without computer assistance. Whether data storage is on the investigator's desktop computer or in a large shared computer, the data can be moved, electronically, anywhere for statistical analysis. Traditionally, the analysis has been done by large, all-inclusive statistical software packages available only on mainframe and departmental computers; the most well-known of these packages include SAS, BMDP, SPSS, MINITAB, and STAT80. The users manuals for this software are not statistical textbooks, but the manuals do contain sample problems to help explain the software command language. These examples, which often involve rather advanced problems, can be followed in a cookbook fashion to analyze related problems. Besides the basic descriptive statistics available in most spreadsheet packages, an increasing variety of statistical software is now available for the personal computer.[66, 67] Choosing from all this statistical wealth should be guided by: 1) the types of analysis required, 2) the availability of computer hardware, 3) the number of subjects and number of variables, 4) the need for data management by the statistical software, 5) the experience of the user, 6) the production of finished reports with merging of text, statistics, and graphics, and 7) the budget. Although programming errors in the software can generate erroneous computer output, these packages are increasingly free of "bugs."

Biostatisticians can make available the richness of better research design and advanced statistical techniques to every researcher. For large clinical trials, the participation of a biostatistician has become mandatory from the inception of research planning. The biostatisticians also provide trained data enterers, data storage facilities, and access to large statistical software packages. Unfortunately, most researchers don't have the budget to pay for this help on all projects, but should attempt to get consultations on research design, analysis, and interpretation as new research areas are entered.

RESEARCH REPORTS: WRITING AND EDITING

When published scientific reports are evaluated for the correctness of their statistical techniques, the majority of papers are found to have errors in the application of the statistics. This is true for both general and specialty medical journals, including anesthesia journals.[8, 68, 69] These errors include all aspects of study design, analysis, and interpretation, the omission of pertinent study design details, and the presentation of results.[70, 71] Although it is not possible to assess the seriousness of these statistical errors in misrepresenting and misinterpreting the experimental results, they should be viewed as severe offenses against the scientific method, and not as trivial violations of unimportant and arbitrary rules.[72] The ethical consequences of this misuse of statistics can be serious: 1) research subjects have been put at risk or have been inconvenienced for no benefit; 2) for future patients, inferior treatment may be chosen or superior treatment may be delayed; 3) resources have been squandered; and 4) each generation of researchers will copy the substandard statistical methods reported by their predecessors.[70] The abolition of these usually unintentional statistical sins will require a long-term commitment of interest and effort.

For several decades, there has been a commonly accepted structure to the research report; this is the IMRAD format, *i.e.*, Introduction, Methods, Results (and) Discussion. To further the standardization of the editorial process, editors of major biomedical journals have promulgated "uniform requirements" for manuscripts.[73] These "uniform requirements" ask that the experimental design and statistical methods be described with sufficient detail to enable another researcher who is given access to the raw data to verify the reported results. The editorial instructions for anesthesia journals generally give few specifics about the use of statistics. Although not all anesthesia journals have accepted the use of the "uniform requirements," these requirements could be used profitably by an author preparing a manuscript for any journal.

The need for more explicit and detailed statistical guidelines for authors has been debated among professional statisticians.[74] The 1988 revision of the "uniform requirements" prompted two North American statisticians to write guidelines amplifying the requirements on statistical reporting.[75] Another outstanding set of such guidelines has been published by four English medical statisticians.[76] An international *ad hoc* group has also formulated guidelines for a more structured and informative abstract for clinical research reports;[77] this proposed abstract format includes considerable detail on research design and statistical methods, and has already been adopted by one journal.[78] It is to be hoped that journal editors will accept and mandate these detailed guidelines. It is also to be hoped that journal editors will put into practice suggested guidelines for the statistical review of papers[79] that have been demonstrated to improve the quality of published articles.[80]

RESEARCH REPORTS: READING

Medical journals are mainly written by medical school doctors. Besides their obvious interest in improving medical care, authors may also be motivated by concerns about obtaining faculty tenure, establishing a reputation, getting research grants, etc. Regardless of these disparate motives, how should the clinician determine which is useful? As suggested previously, the anesthesiologist must have some basic skills and understanding of research design and statistics to be able to critique the research report; these skills can be acquired or refreshed through the study of texts and other publications. Yet, additional skills are required. There are tens of hundreds of thousands of words each year in journal articles relevant to anesthesia. No one can read it all, even if reading to the exclusion of other activities; the physician will probably never have more time for journal reading than he already spends to peruse the literature. All that is possible is to learn to rapidly skip over most articles and concentrate on the few. Those few should be chosen by their relevance and credibility. Relevance is determined by the specifics of one's anesthetic practice. Credibility is a function of the merits of the research methods, the experimental design, and the statistical analysis; the more proficient are one's statistical skills, the more rapidly it is possible to accept or reject the credibility of a research article.

Six easily remembered appraisal criteria for clinical studies can be fashioned from the words WHY, HOW, WHO, WHAT, HOW MANY, and SO WHAT:[81] 1) WHY: Is the biologic hypothesis clearly stated? 2) HOW: What is the research design? 3) WHO: Is the target population clearly defined? 4) WHAT:

How was the therapy administered and data collected? 5) HOW MANY: Are the test statistics convincing? and 6) SO WHAT: Is it clinically relevant to my patients? There are some superb references which explore in detail how to read many types of clinical research articles.[64, 82, 83] In particular, Sackett *et al.* provide flow diagrams and question lists for this purpose.[64] These skills of critical appraisal of the literature can be learned,[84] and will tremendously increase the efficiency and benefit of journal reading.

THE FUTURE OF STATISTICS IN ANESTHESIOLOGY

What of the future? Research presentations, both oral and written, will continue to follow the trend of ever-increasing statistical rigor that has been evident for several decades. This statistical rigor will be obvious, both by the quantity of descriptive and test statistics that will be reported, and by the complexity of the methods that will be used. More advanced statistical tests will provide greater power in understanding complex phenomenon; this also suggests the prospect of even less comprehension of the scientific article by the typical journal reader. To counterbalance this complexity, better graphical data displays will become more common to provide an intuitive grasp of results.

Statistics and probability will be increasingly used in the actual practice of anesthesia. As in all other areas of medicine, there is an "information explosion" in anesthesiology. A new field, "medical informatics," has been created by those interested in the computer use and management of medical information;[85] medical informatics include research, education, and patient care. One of the creations of medical informatics has been medical expert systems; expert systems are computational tools designed to capture and make available the knowledge of experts.[86] Some of the most noted expert systems have been designed for medical diagnosis,[87] but there is also work by Miller on an expert system to provide advice for anesthetic management planning.[88, 89] Statistical methods, including linear discriminant analysis, Bayesian probability theory, and logistic regression, are used extensively, although not exclusively, in the design of some of these medical expert systems.[90] A parallel development has been the use of formal decision analysis for medical applications. Using the tools of decision trees, Bayesian probability theory, sensitivity analysis, and utility assessment, decision analysis is a logically consistent way of reasoning and choosing therapy in the face of uncertainty.[91] Although little has been developed for anesthesiology, there is some acceptance of decision analysis for other fields of medical practice.[92] Finally, there are attempts at the use of techniques of randomized controlled clinical trials to determine optimal therapy for individual patients.[93]

Statistical theory will continue to develop with great practical applications for medicine. Two examples will suffice. Using inexpensive computers, computationally intensive methods will replace the use of theoretical probability distributions with massive numbers of calculations; a billion arithmetic operations might be used to analyze 500 data points.[94] Smart statistical software will be developed that will provide: 1) a computerized statistical reference source, 2) expert guidance for the use of statistical tests, and 3) an expert system to consult on the design and analysis of experiments.[95, 96]

The intent of this chapter was to present the breadth of assistance that the discipline of statistics can provide to anesthesia research. Although an intuitive understanding of certain basic principles was emphasized, these basic principles are not necessarily simple, and have been developed by statisticians with great mathematical rigor. Academic anesthesia needs more workers to immerse themselves into these statistical fundamentals; having done so, these statistically knowledgeable academic anesthesiologists will be prepared to improve their own research projects, to assist their colleagues in research, to efficiently seek consultation from the professional statistician, to strengthen the editorial review of journal articles, and to expound to the clinical reader the whys and wherefores of statistics. The clinical reader also needs to expend his own effort to acquire some basic statistical skills.

One of the originators of the use of statistics in medicine was Francis Galton; living from 1822 to 1911, he studied the inheritance of physical and mental characteristics. Galton believed that "The object of statistical science is to discover methods of condensing information concerning large groups of allied facts into brief and compendious expressions suitable for discussion."[97] A contrary, somewhat cynical, but rather humorous point of view is: "Medical statistics are like a bikini. What they reveal is interesting but what they conceal is vital."[98] Anesthesiologists must be convinced of Galton's wisdom. They should not perceive statistics as being deceptions and obfuscations.

REFERENCES

1. Editorial: Clinical investigation. Anesthesiology 12:114, 1951
2. Longnecker DE: Support *versus* illumination: Trends in medical statistics. Anesthesiology 57:73, 1982
3. Pace NL: Ever more statistics. Anesth Analg 64:561, 1985
4. Davis PJ, Hersh R: Descartes' Dream: The World According to Mathematics, p 18. San Diego, Harcourt Brace Jovanovich, 1986
5. Hacking I: The Emergence of Probability: A Philosophical Study of Early Ideas About Probability, Induction and Statistical Inference. Cambridge, Cambridge University Press, 1975
6. Box GEP: The importance of practice in the development of statistics. Technometrics 26:36, 1984
7. Bishop YMM, Fienberg SE, Holland PW et al: Discrete Multivariate Analysis: Theory and Practice, p ix. Cambridge, The MIT Press, 1975
8. Avram MJ, Shanks CA, Dykes MHM et al: Statistical methods in anesthesia articles: An evaluation of two American journals during two six-month periods. Anesth Analg 64:607, 1985
9. Berwick DM, Fineberg HV, Weinstein MC: When doctors meet numbers. Am J Med 71:991, 1981
10. Marinez YN, McMahan CA, Barnwell GM et al: Ensuring data quality in medical research through an integrated data management system. Stat Med 3:101, 1984
11. Armitage P: Controversies and achievements in clinical trials. Controlled Clin Trials 5:67, 1984
12. Sundt TM Jr: Was the international randomized trial of extracranial-intracranial arterial bypass representative of the population at risk? N Engl J Med 316:814, 1987
13. Barnett HJM, Sackett D, Taylor DW et al: Are the results of the extracranial-intracranial bypass trial generalizable? N Engl J Med 316:820, 1987
14. Louis TA, Mosteller F, McPeek B: Timely topics in statistical methods for clinical trials. Ann Rev Biophys Bioeng 11:81, 1982
15. Kalish LA, Begg CB: Treatment allocation methods in clinical trials: A review. Stat Med 4:129, 1985
16. Chalmers TC, Celano P, Sacks HS et al: Bias in treatment assignment in controlled clinical trials. N Engl J Med 309:1358, 1983
17. Taylor KM, Margolese RG, Soskolne CL: Physicians' reasons for not entering eligible patients in a randomized clinical trial of surgery for breast cancer. N Engl J Med 310:1363, 1984
18. Spodick DH: The randomized controlled clinical trial: scientific and ethical bases. Am J Med 73:420, 1982
19. Freedman B: Equipoise and the ethics of clinical research. N Engl J Med 317:141, 1987
20. Bailar JC III, Louis TA, Lavori PW et al: A classification for biomedical research reports. N Engl J Med 311:1482, 1984
21. Hlatky MA, Lee KL, Harrell FE Jr et al: Tying clinical research to patient care by use of an observational database. Stat Med 3:375, 1984
22. Califf RM, Pryor DB, Greenfield JC Jr: Beyond randomized clinical trials: Applying clinical experience in the treatment of patients with coronary artery disease. Circulation 74:1191, 1986
23. Byar DP: Why data bases should not replace randomized clinical trials. Biometrics 36:337, 1980
24. Green SB, Byar DP: Using observational data from registries to compare treatments: The fallacy of omnimetrics. Stat Med 3:361, 1984
25. Freiman JA, Chalmers TC, Smith H Jr et al: The importance of beta, the type II error and sample size in the design and interpretation of the randomized control trial: Survey of 71 "negative" trials. N Engl J Med 299:690, 1978
26. Donner A: Approaches to sample size estimation in the design of clinical trials: A review. Stat Med 3:199, 1984
27. Beecher HK: Ethics and clinical research. N Engl J Med 274:1354, 1966
28. Beecher HK: Research and the Individual: Human Studies. Boston, Little, Brown and Company, 1970
29. Greenwald RA, Ryan MK, Mulvihill JE (eds): Human Subjects Research: A Handbook for Institutional Review Boards. New York, Plenum Press, 1982
30. Levine RJ: Ethics and Regulation of Clinical Research. Baltimore, Urban & Schwarzenberg, 1986
31. Giammona M, Glantz SA: Poor statistical design in research on humans: The role of committees on human research. Clin Res 31:572, 1983
32. Government, media, and the animal issue. Fed Proc 45:7A, 1986
33. Office for Protection from Research Risks (OPRR), National Institutes of Health. Public health service policy on humane care and use of laboratory animals. Washington, DC, Government Printing Office, 1986
34. Public Health Service, National Institutes of Health. Guide for the care and use of laboratory animals (NIH Publication No. 85-23). Washington, DC, Government Printing Office, 1985
35. Brown GW: Standard deviation, standard error: Which "standard" should we use? Am J Dis Child 136:937, 1982
36. McPeek B: Inference, generalizability, and a major change in anesthetic practice. Anesthesiology 66:723, 1987
37. Glantz SA: Biostatistics: How to detect, correct and prevent errors in the medical literature. Circulation 61:1, 1980
38. Wallenstein S, Zucker CL, Fleiss JL: Some statistical methods useful in circulation research. Circ Res 47:1, 1980
39. Hawkins BS: Perusing the literature. Controlled Clin Trials 7:332, 1986
40. Sacks ST, Glantz SA: Introduction to biostatistics: An annotated bibliography for medical researchers. West J Med 139:723, 1983
41. Glantz SA: Primer of Biostatistics. New York, McGraw-Hill, 1981
42. Phillips JL Jr: Statistical thinking, 2nd ed. San Francisco, WH Freeman, 1982
43. Colton T: Statistics in Medicine. Boston, Little, Brown and Company, 1974
44. Mattson DE: Statistics: Difficult Concepts, Understandable Explanations. St Louis, CV Mosby, 1981
45. Snedecor GW, Cochran WG: Statistical Methods, 7th ed. Ames, Iowa State University Press, 1980
46. Cox DR, Snell EJ: Applied statistics: Principles and examples. New York, Chapman and Hall, 1981

47. Winer BJ: Statistical Principles in Experimental Design, 2nd ed. New York, McGraw-Hill, 1971

48. Edwards AL: An Introduction to Linear Regression and Correlation. San Francisco, WH Freeman, 1976

49. Draper N, Smith H: Applied Regression Analysis, 2nd ed. New York, John Wiley & Sons, 1981

50. Schmid CF: Statistical Graphics: Design Principles and Practices. New York, John Wiley & Sons, 1983

51. Tufte ER: The Visual Display of Quantitative Information. Cheshire, Graphics Press, 1983

52. Cleveland WS: The Elements of Graphing Data. Monterey, Wadsworth Advanced Books and Software, 1985

53. Fleiss JL: Statistical Methods for Rates and Proportions, 2nd ed. New York, John Wiley & Sons, 1981

54. Fienberg SE: The Analysis of Cross-Classified Categorical Data. Cambridge, The MIT Press, 1977

55. Barford NC: Experimental Measurements: Precision, Error and Truth, 2nd ed. New York, John Wiley & Sons, 1985

56. Morrison DF: Multivariate Statistical Methods, 2nd ed. New York, McGraw-Hill, 1976

57. Tabachnick BG, Fidell LS: Using Multivariate Statistics. New York, Harper & Row, 1982

58. Marks RG: Analyzing Research Data: The Basics of Biomedical Research Methodology. Belmont, Lifetime Learning Publications, 1982

59. Marks RG: Designing a Research Project: The Basics of Biomedical Research Methodology. Belmont, Lifetime Learning Publications, 1982

60. Feinstein AR: Clinical Biostatistics. St Louis, CV Mosby, 1977

61. Silverman WA: Human Experimentation: A Guided Step Into the Unknown. New York, Oxford University Press, 1985

62. Gore SM, Altman DG: Statistics in Practice. Devonshire, Torquay, 1982

63. Lunn JN: Epidemiology in Anaesthesia: The Techniques of Epidemiology Applied to Anaesthetic Practice. Baltimore, Edward Arnold, 1986

64. Sackett DL, Haynes RB, Tugwell P: Clinical Epidemiology. Boston, Little, Brown and Company, 1985

65. Ingelfinger JA, Mosteller F, Thibodeau LA et al: Biostatistics in Clinical Medicine. New York, Macmillan, 1983

66. Carpenter J, Deloria D, Morganstein D: Statistical software for microcomputers: A comparative analysis of 24 packages. Byte 9:234, 1984

67. Lehman RS: Statistics on the Macintosh. Byte 12:207, 1987

68. Gore SM, Jones IG, Rytter EC: Misuse of statistical methods: Critical assessment of articles in BMJ from January to March 1976. Br Med J 1:85, 1977

69. DerSimonian R, Charette LJ, McPeek B et al: Reporting on methods in clinical trials. N Engl J Med 306:1332, 1982

70. Altman DG: Statistics in medical journals. Stat Med 1:59, 1982

71. Vaisrub N: Manuscript review from a statistician's perspective. JAMA 253:3145, 1985

72. Altman DG: Misuse of statistics is unethical. In Gore SM, Altman DG (eds): Statistics in Practice, p 1. Devonshire, Torquay, 1982

73. International Committee Of Medical Journal Editors: Uniform requirements for manuscripts submitted to biomedical journals. Ann Intern Med 108:258, 1988

74. Johnson T: Statistical guidelines for medical journals. Stat Med 3:97, 1984

75. Bailar JC III, Mostellar F: Guidelines for statistical reporting in articles for medical journals: Amplifications and explanations. Ann Intern Med 108:266, 1988

76. Altman DG, Gore SM, Gardner MJ et al: Statistical guidelines for contributors to medical journals. Br Med J 286:1489, 1983

77. Ad Hoc Working Group for Critical Appraisal of The Medical Literature: A proposal for more informative abstracts of clinical articles. Ann Int Med 106:598, 1987

78. Huth EJ: Structured abstracts for papers reporting clinical trials. Ann Intern Med 106:626, 1987

79. Altman DG: Statistics and ethics in medical research: VIII: Improving the quality of statistics in medical journals. Br Med J 282:44, 1981

80. Gardner MJ, Altman DG, Jones DR et al: Is the statistical assessment of papers submitted to the "British Medical Journal" effective? Br Med J 286:1485, 1983

81. Schechter MT, LeBlanc FE: Critical appraisal of published research. In Troidl H, Spitzer WO, McPeek B et al (eds): Principles and Practices of Research: Strategies for Surgical Investigators. New York, Springer-Verlag, 1986

82. Haynes RB, Sackett DL, Tugwell P: Problems in the handling of clinical and research evidence by medical practitioners. Arch Intern Med 143:1971, 1983

83. Kronick DA: The Literature of the Life Sciences: Reading, Writing, Research. Philadelphia, ISI Press, 1985

84. Bennett KJ, Sackett DL, Haynes RB et al: A controlled trial of teaching critical appraisal of the clinical literature to medical students. JAMA 257:2451, 1987

85. Collen MF: Origins of medical informatics. West J Med 145:778, 1986

86. Shortliffe EH: Medical expert systems: Knowledge tools for physicians. West J Med 145:830, 1986

87. Banks G: Artificial intelligence in medical diagnosis: The INTERNIST/CADUCEUS approach. CRC Crit Rev Med Inf 1:23, 1986

88. Miller PL: Critiquing anesthetic management: The "ATTENDING" computer system. Anesthesiology 53:362, 1983

89. Miller PL: A critiquing approach to expert computer advice: ATTENDING. Boston, Pitman Advanced Publishing Program, 1984

90. Begg CB: Statistical methods in medical diagnosis. CRC Crit Rev Med Inf 1:1, 1986

91. Pauker SG, Kassirer JP: Decision Analysis. N Engl J Med 316:250, 1987

92. Kassirer JP, Moskowitz AJ, Lau J et al: Decision analysis: A progress report. Ann Intern Med 106:275, 1987

93. Guyatt G, Sackett D, Taylor DW et al: Determining optimal therapy: Randomized trials in individual patients. N Engl J Med 314:889, 1986

94. Efron B: Computers and the theory of statistics: Thinking the unthinkable. SIAM Review 21:460, 1979

95. Hahn GJ: More intelligent statistical software and statistical expert systems: future directions. Am Stat 39:1, 1985

96. Gale WA (ed). Artificial intelligence and statistics. Reading, Addison-Wesley, 1986

97. Galton F: Quotation. In Strauss MB (ed). Familiar Medical Quotations, p 568. Boston, Little, Brown and Company, 1968

98. Anonymous. Quotation. In Strauss MB (ed): Familiar Medical Quotations, p 569. Boston, Little, Brown and Company, 1968

Chapter 4

Arnold J. Berry
Jonathan D. Katz

Hazards of Working in the Operating Room

Anesthesia personnel spend long hours, in fact, a majority of their waking day, in an environment which is filled with many hazards—the operating room. This setting is unlike the usual workplace in that, in addition to potential exposure to vapors from chemicals, to ionizing radiation, and to infectious agents, there is the psychological stress resulting from the constant vigilance required for quality care of patients and from the interactions with other members of the surgical and operating room teams. Although some hazards, such as fires and explosions from flammable anesthetic agents, are no longer a concern, others, including alcohol and drug abuse, are now being recognized as significant within the anesthesia community. Some hazards, like exposure to trace levels of waste anesthetic gases, have been extensively studied, while others, like suicide, have been recognized but not pursued. Only within the past 20 years have epidemiologic surveys been conducted to assess the health of anesthesia personnel. In general, the health risks to those working in the operating room may be significant, but, with awareness of the problems and the use of proper precautions, they are not formidable. In the following chapter, we will cover the suspect and proven hazards associated with this curious environment in which we work—the operating room.

PHYSICAL HAZARDS

ANESTHETIC GASES

Although the inhalation anesthetics, diethyl ether, nitrous oxide, and chloroform, were first used in the 1840s, the biologic effects of occupational exposure to these agents were not investigated for many years. There were early reports in the German literature of headaches and fatigue in personnel who had been exposed to chloroform and ether in the operating rooms. In 1949, Werthmann reported three persons who had fatigue, headaches, memory loss, and ECG abnormalities with chronic exposure to ether.[1] Not until the 1960s were studies of the effects of chronic environmental exposure to anesthetics undertaken. It has been estimated that over 60,000 anesthesiologists, nurse anesthetists, and operating room nurses and technicians, 100,000 dentists and dental assistants, and 50,000 veterinarians and their employees work in environments with potential exposure to anesthetic gases.[2, 3]

Reports on the effects of chronic environmental exposure to anesthetics have included epidemiologic surveys, *in vitro* studies, cellular research, and studies in laboratory animals and humans. These reports have addressed the areas of fertility and spontaneous abortion; incidence of congenital malformations; mortality rate, incidence of cancer, hematopoietic diseases, liver disease, and neurologic disease; and psychomotor and behavorial changes produced by anesthetic exposure. There have been many reviews of these earlier studies.[4-8] In the following section, relevant reports will be reviewed to provide an understanding of the current evidence in each of these areas. Also, suggested standards for waste anesthetic gas levels in the operating room are reviewed. Scavenging systems for the reduction of anesthetic concentrations in the operating room are discussed elsewhere.

Anesthetic Levels in the Operating Room

Early investigators established that significant levels of ether were present in the operating room when the open drop technique was used, but the first report of occupational exposure to modern anesthetics was by Linde and Bruce in 1969.[9] They sampled air at various distances from the pop-off valve of anesthesia machines and noted an average concentration of halothane of ten parts per million (ppm) and nitrous oxide of 130 ppm (parts per million is a volume per volume unit of measurement; 10,000 ppm equals 1%). These investigators found from 0 to 12 ppm of halothane in end-expired air samples taken from 24 anesthesiologists after work. Others reported similar levels of halothane around semiclosed and non-rebreathing circuits and showed that the environmental levels could be reduced significantly with scavenging equipment.[10] Higher concentrations of nitrous oxide (1100 to 9700 ppm) were found in the workspace of anesthesiologists when 5L min^{-1} flows were used to deliver a 60% concentration to the patient.[11]

In spite of the characteristic odors of volatile anesthetics, smell is not a reliable method for detecting trace levels of halothane in the operating room air. Only 50% of volunteers could detect 33 ppm of halothane by smell, and 75% could not detect 15 ppm.[12]

In a criteria document, the National Institute for Occupational Safety and Health (NIOSH) has proposed standards of less than 25 ppm nitrous oxide (time-weighted average during use) and 0.5 ppm for halogenated anesthetics, or 2 ppm (1 h ceiling) for halogenated agents when used alone.[13] Methods for reducing and monitoring waste gases in the operating room have been suggested.[5, 14–17] Through the use of scavenging equipment, equipment maintenance procedures, altered anesthetic work practices, and efficient operating room ventilation systems, the environmental anesthetic concentration can be reduced more than tenfold. Monitors to detect leaks in the high- and low-pressure systems of anesthetic machines, contamination due to faulty anesthetic technique, and scavenging system malfunction should be incorporated in programs to insure reduced occupational exposure. Environmental levels of anesthetics can be measured using instantaneously collected samples, continuous air monitoring, or time-weighted average. Methods and equipment for these monitoring techniques have been well described.[5, 15, 16]

With appropriate care, environmental levels of anesthetics in the operating room can be reduced to comply with those suggested by NIOSH. The waste anesthetic concentrations in operating rooms where these practices are followed are less than those noted prior to the 1960s and are often less than those found in the studies conducted to assess the effects of occupational exposure. This raises the question as to whether chronic exposure to these low levels of waste anesthetic gases actually constitutes a significant occupational hazard and whether results from studies performed in unscavenged operating rooms are now applicable.

Epidemiological Studies

Epidemiological surveys were among the first studies to suggest the possibility of the hazard of trace levels of anesthetics. Although epidemiologic studies may be useful in assessing problems of this type, there exists the potential for errors associated with the collection of data and their interpretation. In his review on the potential of trace anesthetic gases to produce disease, Ferstandig outlined the necessary design strategies found in good epidemiologic studies.[4] First, there should be an appropriate control group for the cohort being studied. Second, the use of questionnaires to obtain personal medical information may be misleading, since individuals may knowingly or unknowingly give incorrect information.

The use of medical records provides more reliable data. Third, retrospective epidemiologic studies rely on recorded or remembered data. In prospective studies, the anticipated, significant information can be collected temporally. Fourth, cause-and-effect relationships cannot be documented by epidemiologic data unless all other possible etiologies can be ruled out or other lines of evidence are used for substantiation. Fifth, most epidemiologic studies use a P of 0.05 for determination of statistical significance. Walts *et al*, in reviewing one epidemiological study, have argued that this level of statistical significance is too high.[18] Since a false positive conclusion may have profound implications, even a P level of 0.01 may be too large for epidemiologic data. And, sixth, percentage increases in the incidence of disease are sometimes reported. Large changes in percentage may imply significance, even when the findings are not statistically significant. There are few epidemiologic studies on the effects of occupational exposure to waste anesthetic gases that fulfill these criteria.

REPRODUCTIVE OUTCOME. Vaisman, in 1967, surveyed 303 Russian anesthesiologists (193 men and 110 women) by questionnaire.[19] The majority used diethyl ether and nitrous oxide in their practice without scavenging waste anesthetic gases. These anesthesiologists reported a high incidence of headache, irritability, and increased fatigability. There were 18 spontaneous abortions among the 31 pregnant women in the survey. Although this was an extremely small study and there was no control population, Vaisman concluded that these occurrences were due to factors in the working environment, including chronic exposure to anesthetics, a high level of emotional stress, irregular work hours, and the excessive workload.

After the early study by Vaisman, others began to perform epidemiologic surveys to assess the effects of trace anesthetics on reproductive outcome. One of the largest studies was conducted by an *Ad Hoc* Committee of the American Society of Anesthesiologists (ASA).[2] Questionnaires were sent to 49,585 operating room personnel with potential exposure to waste anesthetic gases (members of the ASA, American Association of Nurse Anesthetists, Association of Operating Room Nurses, and Association of Operating Room Technicians). A non-exposed group of 23,911 from the American Academy of Pediatrics and the American Nurses Association served as controls. The Committee concluded that there was an increased risk of spontaneous abortion and congenital abnormalities in children of women who worked in the operating room, and an increased risk of congenital abnormalities in offspring of unexposed wives of male operating room personnel. Several reviews have identified inconsistencies in the data comparing exposed and unexposed groups and within groups, which indicated that expected levels of anesthetic exposure did not correlate with reproductive outcome.[4, 5, 18, 20]

A Swedish study clearly demonstrates the inaccuracies encountered when using mailed questionnaires.[21] Women working at one hospital were surveyed to determine the relationship between anesthetic exposure and spontaneous abortion rate and the confounding effects of age, smoking habits, and working site during the first trimester of pregnancy. All spontaneous abortions in the exposed group were accurately documented in the responses to the questionnaire, but a review of hospital records revealed that one-third of spontaneous abortions went unreported in the unexposed group. When verified data were analyzed, there was no statistically significant difference between reproductive outcome in the exposed and non-exposed groups.

The American Society of Anesthesiologists commissioned a

group of epidemiologists and biostatisticians to evaluate the many epidemiologic surveys that had been published in the literature to provide an assessment of the conflicting data.[6] The group used the relative risk (the ratio of the rate of disease among those exposed to that found in those not exposed) as a measure of the strength of the association between exposure to the operating room environment and several disease processes. In considering studies on spontaneous abortion and congenital abnormalities in offspring of anesthesia personnel, the data from all but five studies were excluded from analysis because of errors in study design or statistical analysis.[2, 21–24] The relative risk of spontaneous abortion for female physicians working in the operating room was 1.4, and, for female nurses, was 1.3 (A relative risk of 1.3 represents a 30% increase in risk when compared with the control population). The increased relative risk for congenital abnormalities was of borderline statistical significance only for exposed physicians. In considering these findings, Mazze and Lecky[25] note that the epidemiological studies assessing the association of cigarette smoking and lung cancer have established a value for relative risk of 8–12 for men in the United States. The high relative risks found in smoking studies contrast to the values of less than 2 in most of the well-designed reproductive studies (Table 4-1). Relative risks of less than 2–3 may occur solely from incorrect classification of subjects. Although Buring et al[6] found a statistically significant relative risk of spontaneous abortion and congenital abnormalities in women working in the operating room, the relative risk was small compared to other more well-documented enviromental hazards. They also point out that duration and level of anesthetic exposure were not measured in any of the studies, and that other factors, such as stress, infections, and radiation, were not considered.

The majority of the existing epidemiologic data purporting to show a cause-and-effect relationship between trace anesthetic gas exposure in the operating room and reproductive complications is fraught with problems. There appears to be a slight increase in the relative risk of spontaneous abortion and congenital abnormalities in offspring of female physicians working in the operating room. Whether this is due to anesthetic exposure cannot be determined from this type of investigation. Well-designed surveys of large numbers of personnel will be necessary for definitive answers. The routine use of scavenging techniques has lowered environmental anesthetic levels in the operating room, and may make it more difficult to provide any adverse effects using epidemiologic data.

MORTALITY AND NON-REPRODUCTIVE DISEASES. One of the first surveys enumerating causes of death among anesthesiologists was reported by Bruce et al in 1968.[26] The authors compared the death rates of members of the American Society of Anesthesiologists from 1947 to 1966 with those for U.S. males and male policyholders of a large insurance company. There was a higher death rate in male anesthesiologists from malignancies of the lymphoid and reticuloendothelial tissues and from suicide, but a lower incidence of lung cancer and coronary artery disease.

In a subsequent, prospective study, Bruce et al compared the causes of death in ASA members during the years 1967–1971 with those of males insured by one company.[27] The overall death rate for ASA members was lower than for the controls, and, contrary to the previous results, there was no increase in death rates from malignancies of lymphoid and reticuloendothelial tissues. The authors concluded that their data provided no evidence to support the speculation that lymphoid malignancies were an occupational hazard for anesthesiologists because of their exposure to anesthetic agents.

Because of the interest in the effect of trace anesthetics on the health of operating room personnel, NIOSH and an *Ad Hoc* Committee of the ASA agreed to a national study to address the problem[2] (data on reproductive outcomes from this study were reviewed above). In 1972, the two groups

TABLE 4-1.   Epidemiologic Studies of Spontaneous Abortion Among Females

REFERENCE	EXPOSED POPULATION*	CONTROL	RATE OF SPONTANEOUS ABORTION (PER 100 CASES) Exposed	RATE OF SPONTANEOUS ABORTION (PER 100 CASES) Control	RELATIVE RISK†
Cohen et al[22]	OR nurses (n = 67) Anesthetists(n = 50)	General duty nurses(n = 92) Non-anesth. MDs(n = 81)	30 38	9 10	3.4‡ 3.7‡
Knill-Jones el al[23]	Anesthetists(n = 563)	Non-anesth. MDs(n = 828)	18	15	1.2‡
Rosenberg & Kirves[24]	OR nurses(n = 124) Nurse anesth.(n = 58)	Nurses(n = 75) ICU nurses(n = 48)	20	11	1.7‡
ASA Ad Hoc Committee[2]	MD anesthetists (n = 1059)	Pediatricians (n = 639)	17	9	1.9‡
	Nurse anesth. (n = 7136)	General nurses (n = 6560)	17	15	1.1
	OR nurses/tech. (n = 12,272)	General nurses (n = 6560)	20	15	1.3‡
Axelsson & Rylander[21]	OR personnel (n = 288)	Hospital personnel (n = 322)	15	11	1.2

* n is the number of responders in the survey.
† Incidence in exposed group *vs.* incidence in control.
‡ Statistically significant with P<0.05.

planned a two-phase study, with the initial survey being conducted primarily in 1973, and a second phase which had been planned for 1978. Data from the first questionnaire would not allow the investigators to prove a direct cause-effect relationship between trace concentrations of anesthetic gases and any demonstrated health hazards. By the time of the second survey, it was hoped that the introduction of scavenging and other techniques would reduce the levels of waste anesthetic gases in the operating room. If a lower incidence of health problems were demonstrated in the second phase, it could more safely be assumed that waste anesthetic gases were the causative agents. Because NIOSH believed that it had sufficient information to incriminate waste anesthetic gases as a health hazard after the initial study, it withdrew its support of the planned second phase of the study, and the follow-up survey was never conducted.[28]

The national study conducted by the ASA found no differences in cancer rates between exposed and unexposed males.[2] For women who responded to the survey, there was approximately a 1.3- to twofold increase in the occurrence of cancer in the exposed group, resulting predominantly from an increase in leukemia and lymphoma. Buring's analysis of these data confirmed an increase in relative risk of cancer in exposed women (1.4), but attributed the increase solely to cervical cancer (2.8).[6] They also noted that the ASA study did not assess the effect of confounding variables, such as sexual history or smoking, that may have contributed to the findings. It is doubtful that the carcinogenic effect of anesthetics would be sex related, and the conflicting results for men and women, especially in light of the low statistical significance of the data, cast doubt that anesthetics were the causative agent.

The data from the ASA Ad Hoc Committee noted a statistical increase in hepatic disease for female anesthesiologists and nurse anesthetists and male anesthesiologists, but not for other exposed groups.[2] Again, it is difficult to explain that male anesthetists did not experience the same results from exposure to trace anesthetic gases as their female nurse anesthetist counterparts. Although the investigators tried to exclude infectious hepatitis as a cause of hepatic disease, hepatitis B is asymptomatic in approximately 50% of infected individuals. At the time that this survey was conducted, the serum markers to identify hepatitis B had not been elucidated. From the information collected for this study, it cannot be determined whether the hepatic disease was due to anesthetic exposure, or to hepatitis B or another viral infection acquired from frequent exposure to blood.

In a survey of mortality among British doctors from 1951 through 1971, the overall mortality rate and incidence of death caused by ischemic heart disease, chronic bronchitis, and lung cancer was less for anesthesiologists than the average for all medical specialists.[29] There was a slightly increased risk of other cancers (107% of expected) due to cancer of the pancreas in anesthesiologists. These mortality data were confirmed in members of the ASA in a survey published in 1979.[30] ASA membership lists from 1954, 1959, 1967, and 1976 were obtained, so that the population studied included those exposed to both older anesthetics and to halogenated volatile agents. Mortality from all causes in anesthesiologists remained below that of the general population since 1954. Specifically, there was no evidence for an increased rate of cancer, hepatic, or renal disease.

Epidemiologic studies are useful tools to assess adverse effects of the operating room environment, including exposure to many substances, only one of which is waste anesthetic gases. The data from epidemiologic surveys can, at best, suggest relationships, but can never prove cause-and-effect

associations between exposure to some condition or substance and a disease process. In this chapter, other physical and emotional factors in the operating room environment are explored. One must realize that all of these have an impact on operating room personnel. The individual also brings hereditary, nutritional, and psychological factors that interact with the environment and may play a role in any disease process.

There are shortcomings in many surveys attempting to assess the effects of waste anesthetic gases, and these have resulted in conflicting conclusions. Overall, there appears to be some evidence that the operating room environment produces a slight increase in the rate of spontaneous abortion and cancer in women anesthesiologists and nurses.[6] There is also a statistically significant increase in liver disease in both men and women, but this is consistent with the proven risk of infectious hepatitis (see below). Overall mortality rates remain lower in anesthesiologists than for the general population and for other medical specialists.

Laboratory Studies

Concurrent with the epidemiologic studies, investigators were active in the laboratory assessing the effect of anesthetic agents on cell, tissue, and animal models. It was hoped that this work would provide the scientific evidence linking anesthetics to the adverse effects that had been reported in the epidemiologic surveys.

CELLULAR EFFECTS. At clinically useful concentrations, volatile anesthetics interfere with cell division in a reversible manner, possibly due to a reduction in oxygen uptake by mitochondria.[31] There have been no cellular studies to indicate that trace levels of volatile anesthetics have a similar effect.

Nitrous oxide administered in clinically useful concentrations affects hemopoietic and neural cells. After exposure to 0.8 atm nitrous oxide for 30 min, liver methionine synthetase activity decreased by more than 50% in mice.[32] Although 0.05 atmosphere of nitrous oxide did not affect methionine synthetase activity after 4 h, exposure to 1,100 ppm for 8–22 days produced a significant reduction in enzyme activity. Nitrous oxide oxidizes the cobalt atom of vitamin B_{12} from an active to inactive state, which inhibits methionine synthetase. This prevents the conversion of methyltetrahydrofolate to tetrahydrofolate, which is required for DNA synthesis.[32] This suggests that inhibition of methionine synthetase in patients and abusers who are exposed to high concentrations of nitrous oxide is related to anemia and polyneuropathy, but chronic exposure to trace levels does not appear to produce these effects.[33, 34]

Many studies have been performed in animals to assess the carcinogenicity of anesthetics. Corbett's pilot work indicated that isoflurane produced hepatic neoplasia when administered to mice during gestation and early life.[35] A subsequent well-controlled study failed to reproduce these results.[36] Other studies in mice and rats found no carcinogenic effect of halothane, nitrous oxide, or enflurane.[37–39] In an attempt to simulate environmental exposure to waste anesthetics, rats were exposed to low levels of halothane and nitrous oxide for 7 h per day, 5 days per week for 104 weeks.[37] This degree of exposure produced no effect on body weight, behavior, survival, or incidence of tumors.

Several investigators have used the Ames bacterial assay system for studying the mutagenicity of anesthetics.[40–42] This assay is popular in evaluating carcinogens, because it is rapid, inexpensive, and has a high true positive rate when compared with other *in vivo* tests.[43] Halothane, enflurane, methoxy-flurane, isoflurane, and urine from patients anesthetized with these agents were not mutagenic using this assay.[40, 41] Urine from individuals working in scavenged or unscavenged operating rooms was also negative using this bacterial system for analysis.[42]

There have been reports of structural changes in cells brought about by prolonged exposure of animals to subclinical levels of anesthetics. Chang and Katz reviewed a series of relevant studies from their laboratory.[44] Exposure to halothane, 10–500 ppm, for 4–8 weeks produced ultrastructural changes in hepatic, renal, and neuronal tissue. Changes included the degeneration of the mitochondria, endoplasmic reticulum, and bile canaliculi in hepatocytes. From these reports, the extent of the changes cannot be ascertained and, since control animals were not used, the effects of tissue preparation and other factors are unknown. It is also possible that the ultra-structural changes were reversible, and resulted from the administration of the xenobiotic.[45] There is no proof that there is a relationship between anesthetic exposure, cellular ultrastructural changes, and functional abnormalities.

REPRODUCTIVE OUTCOME. Because of the suggestion from epidemiologic data that occupational exposure to waste anesthetic gases resulted in an increase in spontaneous abortion and congenital abnormalities in children of female operating room personnel, numerous studies have been performed in laboratory animals to assess reproductive outcome. In one report that suggested anesthetics have an adverse effect, Coate *et al.* exposed male and female rats to combinations of halothane and nitrous oxide for 60 days prior to mating.[46] The anesthetic levels used in this experiment were similar to those that may be found in unscavenged operating rooms. Exposed females had increased ovulation and implantation efficiency, especially in the groups receiving higher concentrations of anesthetics. There were no major teratologic effects. Chromosomal aberrations were observed in both bone marrow and spermatogonial cells in the male rats.

Prolonged exposure of pregnant rats to 1,000 ppm nitrous oxide resulted in smaller litter size, increased frequency of fetal resorption, and reduced fetal crown rump measurements.[47] Lower concentrations of nitrous oxide had no effect on reproductive outcome. Similarly, daily exposure of mice to 4,000 ppm isoflurane before and during pregnancy produced no adverse effect on their litters.[48]

Sperm collected from men working in operating rooms where scavenging devices were used showed no morphologic changes when compared to specimens from physicians who practiced in other environments.[49] Low concentrations of nitrous oxide also fail to alter spermatogenesis in the mouse.[50] Analysis of sister chromatid exchanges is another method of assessing the mutagenic effect of anesthetics. Nitrous oxide and volatile anesthetic agents did not increase the sister chromatid exchange values in hamster ovary cells.[51] When this test was performed on lymphocytes taken from nurses before and during training as anesthetists, there was no indication of mutagenicity for the anesthetics in current use.[52]

The majority of animal experiments fail to demonstrate alterations in female or male fertility or reproduction with exposure to subanesthetic concentrations of the currently used anesthetic agents. It is important to realize that data from laboratory investigations in animals may not be directly applicable to humans. There is little from the animal studies to confirm that the slight increase in relative risk of spontaneous abortions and congenital abnormalities in children of female operating room personnel is due to exposure to trace amounts of anesthetic gases. Although it is easy to measure and quantify the levels of anesthetic in the operating room air, it is harder to measure and assess the effect of other possible factors, such as stress, alterations in working schedule, and fatigue.

Effects of Trace Anesthetic Levels on Psychomotor Skills

When individuals working in the operating room are exposed to trace concentrations of anesthetics, do the low levels interfere with the psychomotor skills required for providing quality care? Several studies have been conducted to attempt to clarify the effects of low concentrations of anesthetics. Student volunteers were exposed to 4 h of 500 ppm nitrous oxide with or without 15 ppm halothane in air, and were then given tests of perceptual, cognitive, and motor skills.[53] After exposure to halothane and nitrous oxide, their performance was impaired on four of 12 tests, while nitrous oxide alone produced decreased performance on only one.

A subsequent study assessed the effect of nitrous oxide (500, 50, or 25 ppm) alone or with halothane (10, 1.0, or 0.5 ppm) by using psychomotor tests.[54] After exposure to the highest concentrations of nitrous oxide and halothane, subjects' performance declined on four of the seven tests. Interestingly, there was a decrease in ability in six of seven tests after exposure to the same level of nitrous oxide alone. Exposure to the lowest concentrations studied, 25 ppm nitrous oxide and 0.5 ppm halothane, produced no effects in this group as measured by this battery of tests. These investigators suggested that attempts be made to lower anesthetic concentrations in the operating room air to levels no higher than those which were without effect in their study.

Others have found no effect on psychomotor test performance after 3–4 h of exposure to halothane, 15 ppm, with nitrous oxide, 500 ppm.[55] The reasons for difference in outcome between the latter study and the others are unclear.

NIOSH Recommendations

In 1970, the Occupational Safety and Health Act was legislated by Congress, and created NIOSH, the federal agency that was responsible for assuring that workers had a safe and healthy working environment. NIOSH was to meet these goals through the conduct and funding of research, through education of employers and employees about occupational illnesses, and through establishing occupational health standards. A second federal agency, the Occupational Safety and Health Administration (OSHA), was responsible for enacting job health standards, investigating work sites to detect violation of standards, and enforcing the standards by citing violators.[28, 56] In 1977, NIOSH published a criteria document that recommended that waste anesthetic exposure should not exceed 2 ppm of halogenated anesthetic agents when used alone, or 0.5 ppm of a halogenated agent and 25 ppm of nitrous oxide.[13] In addition, it stated that operating room employees should be advised of the potential harmful effects of anesthetics. The guidelines proposed that annual medical and occupational histories be obtained from all personnel, and that abnormal outcome of pregnancies should be documented. The publication also included information on scavenging procedures and equipment, and methods for monitoring concentrations of waste anesthetic gases in the air. For the NIOSH criteria document to become a federal standard, the proposal would have to be published in the *Federal Register*, and, following a public hearing, OSHA would finalize the text of the standard to be adopted. At present, NIOSH's criteria document has not gone through this process. The NIOSH recommendations are still included in a recent publication summarizing occupational and health standards.[57]

It is intersting to examine the rationale given for the selection of NIOSH's standards for waste anesthetic gases. According to the criteria document, "Based on the available health information a safe level of exposure to the halogenated agents cannot be defined. Since a safe level of occupational exposure to halogenated anesthetic agents cannot be established by either animal or human investigations, NIOSH recommends that exposure be controlled to levels no greater than the lowest level detectable using the sampling and analysis techniques recommended by NIOSH in this document."[13] Based on this, the recommendations for halogenated agents were set for 2 ppm. The recommendations for nitrous oxide were based on the studies of Bruce, who noted that, after exposure to levels of 25 ppm nitrous oxide with 0.5 ppm halothane, there was no impairment of subjects' performance on psychomotor tests.[54]

In view of the conflicting scientific data, it is reasonable to ask what is an acceptable exposure level for waste anesthetic gases. Although it may be difficult to be certain of a threshold concentration below which chronic exposure is "safe," it is prudent to institute scavenging techniques and anesthetic practices that reduce waste anesthetic levels in the operating room environment without compromising patient safety. Monitoring of the operating room air for nitrous oxide and halogenated agents at regular intervals is a necessary part of any program to insure the adequacy of machine servicing, to prevent leakage of anesthetics from improper seals and fittings, and to confirm appropriate practice techniques. The implementation of a well-designed program with periodic assessment should result in environmental levels of waste gases within the limits suggested by NIOSH.

CHEMICALS

Methylmethacrylate

Methylmethacrylate is commonly used to cement prostheses to bone or for repairing bone defects. The cardiovascular effects of methylmethacrylate in patients have been thoroughly studied and reviewed, but there is less data on the effects of occupational exposure. OSHA has established an 8-h, time-weighted average allowable exposure of 100 ppm. Factory workers exposed to methylmethacrylate complained of respiratory, cutaneous, and genitourinary problems after exposure to levels less than those allowed by OSHA.[58] When the Ames test was used to assess the mutagenic potential of methylmethacrylate, it was found that the compound alone was toxic to the bacteria, but, when methylmethacrylate was incubated with a rat-liver enzyme metabolizing system, mutagenesis was induced.[59]

When the substance is prepared to be used in the operating room, concentrations up to 90 ppm have been measured during the time required for polymerization. Scavenging devices for venting methylmethacrylate vapor have been described,[60] and are now commercially available. With use of these venting devices, peak concentrations of the vapor can be decreased by 75%.

Allergic Reactions

In addition to concerns about toxic effects of methylmethacrylate vapor and waste anesthetic gases, allergic reactions to these substances have been reported. Occupational asthma after exposure to methylmethacrylate in orthopedic operating rooms has been described in at least two cases.[61, 62] One anesthesiologist reproducably had asthma 8–12 h after administering enflurane to his patients.[63]

A thoroughly documented case report of an anesthesiologist who developed recurrent hepatitis after exposure and challenge with halothane was interpreted to indicate that halothane was a sensitizing agent in some individuals.[64] Repeated bouts of hepatitis in this anesthesiologist were attributed to hypersensitivity reactions, rather than to a direct toxic effect of halothane. Occupationally related effects such as this may be severe enough to require a change in practice in these individuals to remove the offending agent.

RADIATION

Occupational radiation exposure in anesthesia practice has had only limited study.[9] Anesthesiologists received an average of 13 milliroentgens per week, which was well below the acceptable limit, at the time, of 100 milliroentgens per week.[9] Since anesthesia personnel are now requested to care for patients in many areas of the hospital, there are numerous situations in which radiation exposure may occur. Diagnostic radiographs are made in the operating room, post-anesthetic care units, and intensive care units. Some patients undergoing diagnostic or therapeutic procedures, such as angiography, angioplasty, biliary dilatation, or extracorporeal shock wave lithotripsy or radiation therapy, may require care by anesthesiologists. Anesthesia personnel may also be exposed to radionuclides given to patients for diagnostic procedures or for therapy.

Hospital personnel have generally been uninformed about the effects of radiation exposure. Oncogenesis, teratogenesis, and long-term genetic effects may occur with sufficient doses of radiation. For policies on radiation safety, regulatory agencies divide workers into two classes: those who are only occasionally exposed to radiation (i.e., anesthesia personnel), and radiation workers whose normal duties require them to be in areas with large potential exposure.[65] The nonoccupational limit of exposure is set at less than 500 mrem (milliroentgen equivalent, man) per year. Implementation of radiation protection policies which include education and monitoring programs can reduce maximum exposure to this limit.[66]

Technologic advances in imaging equipment and radiation handling have reduced the risk of radiation exposure to most hospital personnel. Measurements of radiation doses to radiologists and nursing personnel provide a worst case example for estimating radiation exposure to anesthesiologists involved in the care of patients having diagnostic and therapeutic procedures.[67–72] These studies documented only minimal exposure levels that were well within the recommended limits.

Film badges or pocket dosimeters should be used by personnel for monitoring radiation exposure. Monthly documentation of exposure allows for recognition of personnel with high levels of exposure, so that their work practices can be evaluated and reassignment to work areas with less radiation exposure can be considered. Educational programs on the effects of radiation and techniques for preventing exposure are important parts of radiation safety programs.

NOISE POLLUTION

A health hazard which is virtually uncontrolled in the modern operating room is noise pollution. Noise pollution is quantified by determining both the intensity of the sound in decibels (dBA) and the time interval of the sounds. The Occupational Safety and Health Administration has established a maximum level for safe noise exposure of 90 decibels for 8 h.[57] Furthermore, each increase in noise of 5 dBA halves the permissible exposure time, so that 100 dBA is permitted for only 2 h per day. The maximum permissible exposure in an industrial setting is 115 dBA.

The noise level which constitutes a health hazard is surprisingly close to that which we routinely endure in our daily practice. As pointed out by Shapiro,[73] noise in the operating room usually exceeds that of a freeway, and sporadically approaches levels as those from a rock-and-roll band. The predicted results of excessive exposure to noise have been well documented in the literature of industrial hygiene. At the very least, noise pollution is an important factor in decreased worker productivity. At higher levels, workers are likely to show signs of irritability and demonstrate elevated blood pressures. Ultimately, hearing loss may ensue.

MAINTAINING VIGILANCE

The seal of the American Society of Anesthesiologists bears, as its only motto, "Vigilance"* (Fig. 4-1). The official motto of the Australian Society of Anaesthetists is *"Vigila et Ventila."* These serve as formal recognition of the critical importance of this function among the many tasks performed by the anesthesiologist. As stated by Gaba, "Vigilance is thus a necessary, but not sufficient condition for averting (anesthetic) accidents."[75] Surprisingly, relatively little work has been done to examine the factors in our work environment that affect our ability to maintain "vigilance."

Several components of the vigilance task, as it applies to the work of the anesthesiologist, deserve attention. First, it is important to recognize that this particular function is repetitive and monotonous. However, there are major differences that distinguish vigilance from other monotonous tasks (such as production line sorting or assembling) and promote the early onset of boredom in the former. One is the unpredictable nature and timing of the changes in the parameters being monitored. The individual is unable to establish his own pace but, rather, must respond to the cues from his monitors. Lack of automaticity is also a detriment, because the task does not fully occupy his mental activity, but neither does it leave him free to perform other mental functions. And, lastly, the task is complex, requiring visual attention, as well as manual dexterity, and the ability to perform a vigilance task varies inversely with the complexity of that task.[76]

Vigilance tasks are generally performed at the level of 90% accuracy.[77] Obviously, in a setting where the stakes are as high as that of anesthesia, this leaves an unacceptable margin of error. The current profusion of monitoring devices and alarms is an attempt to incrementally improve this performance factor.

A number of factors at work in the operating room environment may serve to diminish the ability of the operator to perform his task of vigilance. One obvious factor is sleep loss and fatigue. Several studies have documented the deleterious effect of sleep loss on work efficiency.[78, 79] Performance does not return to normal levels until 24 h of rest and recovery have occurred. An interesting phenomenon is the "end-spurt," in which previously deteriorated performance shows improvement when the subject realizes that his task is 90% com-

*Vigilance task-one which requires the detection of changes in a stimulus during long monitoring periods when the subject has little or no prior knowledge of the sequence of the changes.[74]

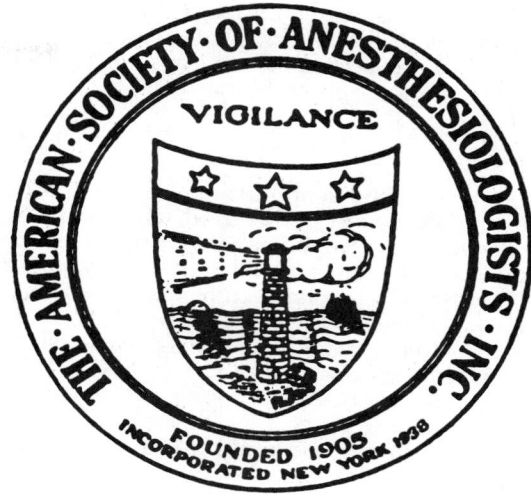

FIG. 4-1. Official Seal of the American Society of Anesthesiologists. "VIGILANCE" has always been recognized as the most critical of the tasks of the anesthesiologist.

pleted.[80] The converse undoubtedly also occurs, a "let-down" with additional deterioration in performance when the procedure is unexpectedly delayed.

Poor design in the monitor displays and the various other sources of information input can adversely affect the vigilance task. Engineering details, such as signal frequency and signal strength, as well as the mode of presentation of the input, significantly influence the operator's ability to maintain the task of vigilance. For example, if the signal rate is slow, observers tend to produce more false positive alarms.[81] On the other hand, when confronted with a fast event rate, especially when the signal is of low intensity, the observer tends toward more frequent false negative findings.[82] Interestingly, monitoring complex displays and the need to "time share" attention between several vigilance tasks is not associated with a performance decrement.[83]

Even the alarms which have been developed with the specific goal of supplementing the task of vigilance have considerable drawbacks. Alarms used in the operating room are susceptible to artifacts and transients (true readings of no significance). Frequent false positive alarms may distract the observer from more clinically significant information. One depiction of a commercial airline accident, with more than 150 fatalities, describes all three officers in the cockpit completely immersed in concern over a flashing light. The alarm indicated that the landing gear was still down, a trivial concern at that particular time. In contrast, the altimeter, which indicated that the aircraft was currently losing altitude, went unnoticed until too late. Analogous situations occur in the operating room. It is not unusual for frequently distractive alarms to be inactivated.

Noise may have a detrimental influence upon the observer attempting to perform a vigilance task. In general, various intrusive noises, such as loud talking, excessive clanging of instruments, and "broadband" noise, are all associated with decrements in performance.[84] On the other hand, certain types of background music produce the least decrement in vigilance.[85]

Exposure to trace anesthetic gases may adversely affect the performance of the vigilance task. Several studies have shown decrements in performance of various psychomotor functions after prolonged exposure to trace anesthetic gases.[86, 87] However, others have failed to corroborate these findings, and have suggested that a tolerance develops to these adverse affects in individuals exposed on a daily basis.[88]

Ergonomics

A fertile area for research and development lies within the discipline of "ergonomics," the consideration of the human factors of equipment design. The configuration of the typical machinery in most anesthetic locations is the end-product of a series of "add-ons" to existing equipment. In fact, the basic "anesthesia machine" in use today, upon which all of these embellishments and monitors are hung, varies little from Boyle's original apparatus.

However, this historical evolution of equipment has not produced an optimal product by ergonomic standards. A sample of poor equipment design is the usual placement of electrocardiogram (ECG) and O_2/CO_2 monitors on a shelf above the flow meters. This places the display well above the visual field of a tall and seated, or short and standing, anesthesiologist (Fig. 4-2).[89]

Probably worse than inappropriate placement of visual displays in the vertical plane is the positioning of machinery and displays out of the view of the anesthesiologist in the horizontal plane. In McIntyre's study of this problem, he reported situations where the machine was squarely at the back of the anesthesiologist as he viewed the patient (Fig. 4-3).[90]

This problem appears to be getting worse. We are currently experiencing a dramatic proliferation of monitoring equipment resulting from the recent introduction of oximeters and real-time gas analyzers. It is not unusual to have four or more analog displays, along with digital readouts and alarms, at each anesthetizing location. These are usually "add-ons" to the existing equipment, and often are mounted on top of a vacant shelf or cart surface.

One obvious result of such haphazard placement of equipment is distraction of the anesthesiologist from his primary task of vigilance. Indeed, nearly half of the anesthesiologist's time is spent with his attention diverted away from the patient-surgeon field.[91] In this circumstance, unnecessary energy is expended to perform routine work, and fatigue occurs prematurely. Fatigue produces a measurable decrement in the ability to concentrate on a task, such as vigilance, that requires sustained attention.[92]

Any factor that requires the expenditure of excessive energy to perform a given task contributes to fatigue. Even the most trivial aspect of an operator's performance plays a significant role over the course of time. For example, if the anesthesiologist must make frequent, rapid changes in observation from a dim distant to a bright nearby screen, the continuous muscular activity required for pupil dilation and constriction and lens accommodation will promote fatigue.

Excessive energy expenditure need not be entirely physical. As we monitor more functions in the operating room and are required to process more data during the course of a surgical procedure, we are expending increasingly larger amounts of mental work. The mental work varies directly with the difficulty encountered in extracting the information from the various displays competing for the attention of the anesthesiologist. Sustained mental alertness hastens fatigue, and fatigue adversely affects vigilance.

The importance of the people-system interface has long been recognized by industry. In fact, design and engineering standards for certain military installations and for applications in the aero-space industry are analogous, in many ways, to requirements in the operating room.[93] With this in mind,

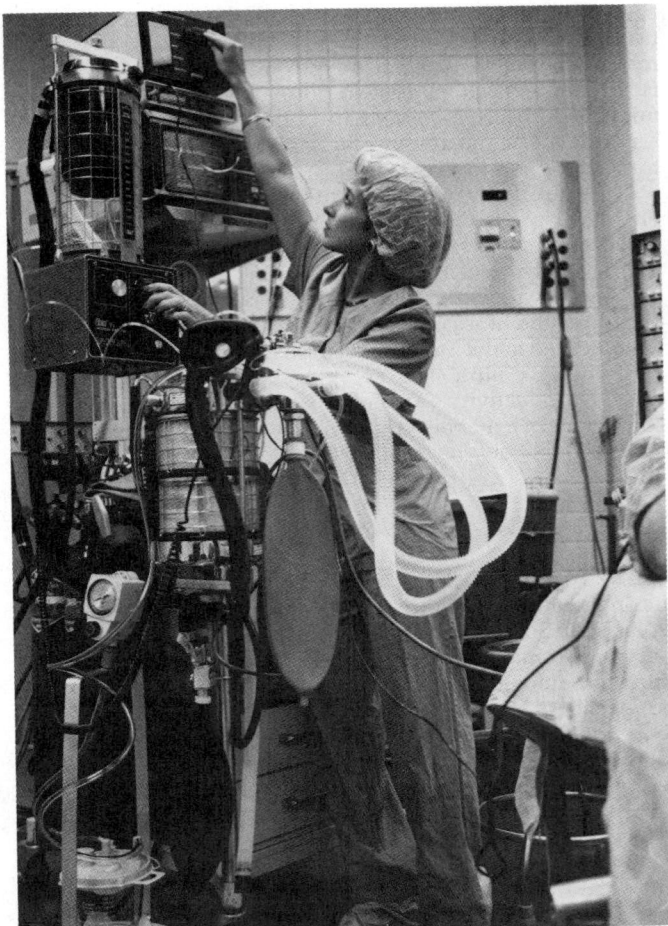

FIG. 4-2. An example of an older anesthesia machine with modern "add-on" monitors and alarms. When sitting, this anesthesiologist is unable to see or reach any of the monitors on the top shelf of the machine. Even when standing, she must take extraordinary efforts to visualize the display on the pulse oximeter and blood pressure monitor (Courtesy of Alexandra Pousoula Pappas).

preliminary reports have begun to appear documenting work directed toward modernizing anesthetic equipment to ergonometric standards.[94, 95] Most promising is the application of microprocessors to enhance the integration of data from various sources, and to provide trend information, as well as "intelligent" warnings of potential difficulties.[96] There is also progress in the application of computer technology to servo-control systems that will introduce automation into the delivery of anesthetics.[97, 98]

Work Hours and Night Call

A less subtle determinant of fatigue, well known to all clinicians, relates to "on-call" schedules and work hours. For practicing anesthesiologists, 10–12-h work days are not at all unusual. Emergency and "on-call" coverage is usually tacked onto the end of one of these days, resulting in a 24–32-h shift.

It is not surprising to find that fatigue following an "on-call" rotation is associated with a measurable deterioration in psychomotor performance. Gravenstein et al[99] reported on the performances of anesthesiology residents who viewed a simulated case scenario. The subjects were studied in a rested

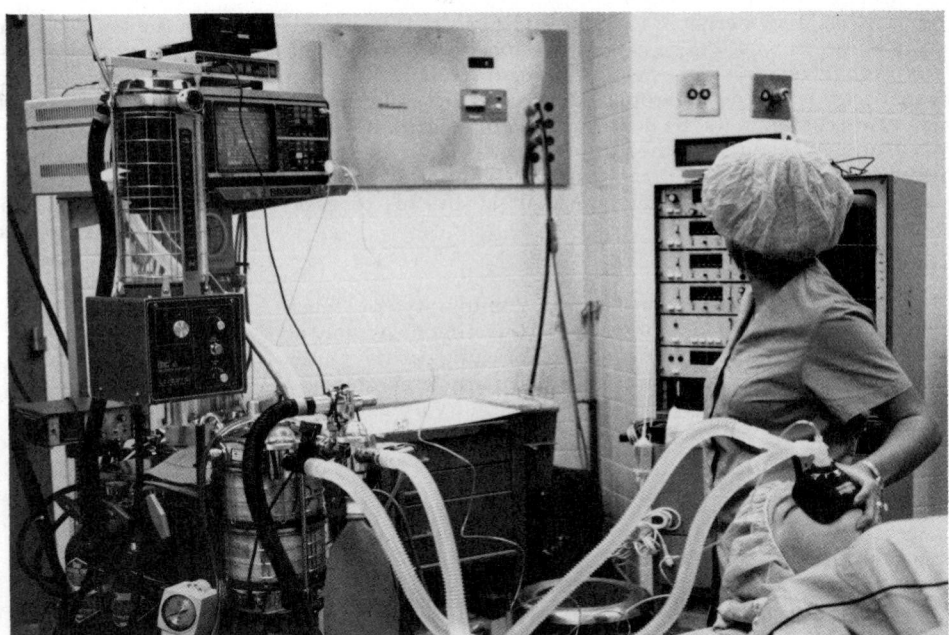

FIG. 4-3. In order to view the display of the electrocardiogram and the transduced arterial and central blood pressures, the anesthesiologist must turn fully 180° from the patient-surgical field (Courtesy of Alexandra Pousoula Pappas).

condition and after a 24-h "on-call" rotation (fatigued). The fatigued group had a lower percentage of correct answers to questions about clinical management compared with the rested group.

Similar results were reported by Narang et al,[100] who used a Leeds psychomotor tester to measure critical flicker fusion frequency and choice reaction time. Their subjects were anaesthetists who were studied between 2:00 and 4:00 PM, and between 11:00 PM and 2:00 AM. They observed a generalized impairment of arousal levels, but relative preservation of psychomotor performance in the later hours. There was a very wide range among the subjects with regard to the exact effect of late hours, with several individuals showing absolutely no change, and several manifesting extreme deterioration in both measured functions.

Others have confirmed that continuous wakefulness has a deleterious effect on performance of the vigilance task.[78, 101] What is more troubling is the suggestion that this deterioration in psychomotor functioning may contribute directly to anesthetic mishaps. In a survey of serious anesthetic-related accidents, fatigue was one of the two major sources of human error ("confusion" with anesthetic equipment was the other).[102] Together, these two sources of error accounted for greater than 96% of the lethal or near-lethal human errors reported. Similarly, in Cooper's critical incidence analysis of anesthetic mishaps, fatigue was among the most frequently reported of "associated factors" contributing to these potentially serious incidents.[103] This potential problem obviously deserves more attention.

An additional area of concern is the potential effect of sleep deprivation on health and psychosocial adjustment. Work schedules that thoroughly disrupt circadian rhythms are associated with impaired health, emotional problems, and a decline in performance.[104] Manpower considerations in all but the largest practices prohibit the utilization of a "night float system," which is probably the best scheduling plan for late-night coverage. Fortunately, most anesthesiologists work in a situation that provides enough recuperative time (24 h) after a

day and night "on-call" to avoid circadian disruption, and the associated risk of chronic fatigue and its complications.

Various state legislators had begun to focus on the problem of sleep deprivation among physicians. A well-publicized New York malpractice case, the Libby Zion Case, claims that fatal mistakes were made by exhausted, unsupervised house officers. Many states have planned, or are planning to draft legislation that would limit work shifts for hospital physicians.

INFECTIOUS HAZARDS

Hospital personnel are at risk for acquiring infections from both patients and other personnel. Viral infections reflecting the prevalence in the community are the most serious threat to healthy personnel. Hospital-acquired bacterial infection is uncommon in workers without compromised immune systems.

Nosocomial infections are transmitted in three ways: patient-to-patient, hospital personnel to patient, and patient to hospital personnel. The majority of this section will deal with the third sequence. The mechanisms for transmission of many infectious agents are now understood, and rational strategies for infection control precautions have been formulated. Although hepatitis B and herpetic whitlow are the only infections that have been documented as work-related in anesthesiologists, there are many others that are potential hazards which have not been specifically studied. Hospitals have an Infection Control Officer or other individual who can provide information on methods for preventing occupationally transmitted infection.

RESPIRATORY VIRUSES

Respiratory viruses, responsible for many community acquired infections, are usually transmitted by two routes. Small particle aerosols produced by coughing, sneezing, or talking may propel infectious viruses over a large distance. The influenza virus, and, perhaps, varicella and measles viruses, are spread in this way.[105] The other mechanism for transmitting viral agents requires close person-to-person contact. Infection can occur when large droplets produced by coughing or sneezing contaminate the donor's hands or an inanimate surface, and, subsequently, the virus is transferred to the skin or mucous membranes of a susceptible individual. Rhinovirus and respiratory syncytial virus are spread by this process.

Influenza Viruses

Because of their ease of transmission, community epidemics of influenza A and B virus infections are common. Acutely ill patients shed large amounts of virus for as long as 5 days after the onset of symptoms through small particle aerosols by coughing or sneezing. Appropriate respiratory isolation precautions should be used for the duration of the clinical illness. Because of their contact with nasopharyngeal secretions, anesthesiologists may play a central role in the spread of influenza virus within hospitals.[106]

Hospital staff with patient contact should consider annual immunization against influenza. Antigenic variation of influenza viruses occurs over time, so that new viral strains are selected for inclusion in each year's vaccine. Vaccination programs for personnel should be conducted in October or November, since the number of cases of influenza in the community begins to increase in December.[107] During hospital outbreaks of influenza A, amantadine may be effective in preventing nosocomial infection in unvaccinated hospital personnel.[107, 108] Amantadine has not been useful for prophylaxis against influenza B. Because of possible morbidity of influenza in hospitalized patients with chronic illnesses, it is recommended that, during community epidemics, elective hospital admissions and surgery should be limited.[105]

Respiratory Syncytial Virus

During periods when respiratory syncytial virus (RSV) is prevalent in the community (usually late December through February), many hospitalized infants and children may carry the virus. Large numbers of virus are present in respiratory secretions from infected children, and virus can be recovered for up to 7 h on contaminated environmental surfaces.[109] Infection occurs when RSV is transferred from these to the hands, which then contact the mucous membranes of the eyes or nose. Although most children have been exposed to RSV early in life, immunity is not permanent, and reinfection is common.

RSV is shed for approximately 7 days after infection. Hospitalized patients with RSV should be isolated in a single room, or in a ward with other infected patients. Careful handwashing between patient contact and use of gowns and gloves is recommended to prevent spread of the disease.

Parainfluenza Virus

Parainfluenza viruses are another important cause of lower respiratory disease in children. They are extremely infectious, and, like RSV, can be transmitted by close person-to-person contact. Infection control measures for parainfluenza are identical to those listed for RSV.

Rhinovirus

Approximately one-third of common colds are caused by the rhinovirus. The transmission of this virus usually occurs when the hands of the infected individual are contaminated by virus present in nasal secretions. Hand-to-hand contact or hand-to-surface contact then allows the recipient to inoculate himself by touching the mucous membranes of the nose or eyes. This process is facilitated by viral characteristics that allow its survival on surfaces for long periods.

Thorough handwashing is effective in preventing transmission of rhinovirus. Iodine-containing solutions, sodium hypochlorite, 70% ethyl alcohol, and activated glutaraldehyde are effective disinfectants for contaminated surfaces.

Adenovirus

Although adenoviruses have an affinity for lymph glands, they may also be found in the respiratory tract, the gastrointestinal tract, and the conjunctiva. Pharyngoconjunctival fever and keratoconjunctivitis caused by adenovirus have occurred among hospital personnel. Usual infection control techniques, such as handwashing and use of gloves, are effective in preventing the spread of adenovirus.

HERPES VIRUSES

Varicella-zoster virus (VZV), herpes simplex virus (HSV) types I and II, cytomegalovirus (CMV), and Epstein-Barr virus (EBV) are members of the herpetoviridine family. Close personal contact is required for transmission of all of the herpes viruses, except for VZV, which is spread by direct contact or small particle aerosols. After the primary infection with herpes viruses, the organism becomes latent, but may reactivate at a later time. Most individuals in the United States have been infected with all of the herpes viruses by middle age. Therefore, nosocomial transmission is uncommon, except in the pediatric population and in immunosuppressed patients.

Varicella-Zoster Virus

Both chicken pox and herpes zoster (shingles) are caused by VZV, which is highly contagious *via* small particle aerosols. Respiratory isolation is recommended for patients with chicken pox until all skin lesions are completely crusted. The minimum incubation period for chicken pox is 10 days, and patients may shed VZV for 4 days prior to the onset of the rash. Serologic testing can be performed to determine immunity in health care workers without a history of chicken pox. Susceptible personnel who have been exposed should be given varicella-zoster immune globulin.

Although VZV can be transmitted from patients with shingles, it is less likely than with chicken pox. The majority of American adults have detectable antibodies to VZV, and should be immune to new infection.[110] Shingles results from a reactivation of latent VZV infection, and spread to susceptible individuals is usually by direct contact. Dressings from infected patients should be considered infectious, since vesicles contain large numbers of viruses.

Herpes Simplex

Herpes simplex infection is quite common in adults. After entry through the mucous membranes, the primary illness with herpes simplex type I usually presents as a cold sore (herpes labialis). In healthy individuals, the primary infection subsides, and the virus persists in a latent state within the sensory nerve ganglion innervating the site of infection. Any of several mechanisms can reactivate the virus to produce recurrent infection, which usually manifests in the vicinity of the primary infection.

A second herpes simplex virus, type II, is usually associated with genital infection, and is a sexually transmitted disease. Although type II herpes simplex is usually associated with genital infection and type I with oral or conjunctival infections, both viruses may be responsible for infections in either area.

Herpes simplex type I is usually spread by contact with oral secretions, and type II by contact with genital fluids. Asymptomatic individuals can unknowingly transmit herpes virus type I because intraoral lesions may not be present during reactivated infection. The fingers of health care personnel may be inoculated by direct contact with oral secretions from infected patients. Herpetic infection of the finger, herpetic whitlow, is a well-recognized occupational hazard for anesthesia personnel.[111, 112]

The symptoms and course of herpetic whitlow have been well described. The infection usually begins at the site on the distal finger where the integrity of the skin has been broken. Initially, there may be itching and pain at the site of infection, followed by the appearance of a vesicle surrounded by erythema (Fig. 4-4). There may be constitutional symptoms, such as fever, malaise, and lymphadenopathy. Satellite vesicles appear near the primary lesion over several days. Within 3 weeks, the throbbing pain lessens, and the lesions begin to heal. A diagnosis of herpes simplex infection can be made by demonstrating multinucleated giant epithelial cells or nuclear inclusion bodies in smears (Tzank technique) taken from the vesicle. Although the process may resemble a bacterial paronychia, treatment should be conservative, and surgical drainage is not indicated.[113]

To prevent herpes simplex infection, personnel should wear gloves when contacting oral secretions.[114] Skin and wound precautions should be followed when caring for patients with genital infections of herpes simplex type II. Anesthetists who have active herpetic whitlow may infect susceptible patients, and should not be allowed to participate in direct patient care until all lesions have dried and crusted. Acyclovir, an antiviral drug which inhibits herpes simplex type I and II replication, is an effective treatment for primary viral infection.

FIG. 4-4. Herpetic whitlow on the index finger near the site of minor trauma in the cuticle. Erythema surrounds the blister formed from the coalescence of individual vesicles. (Reproduced with permission from Orkin FK: Herpetic whitlow. In Orkin FK, Cooperman LH (eds): Complications in Anesthesiology. Philadelphia, JB Lippincott, 1983:709.)

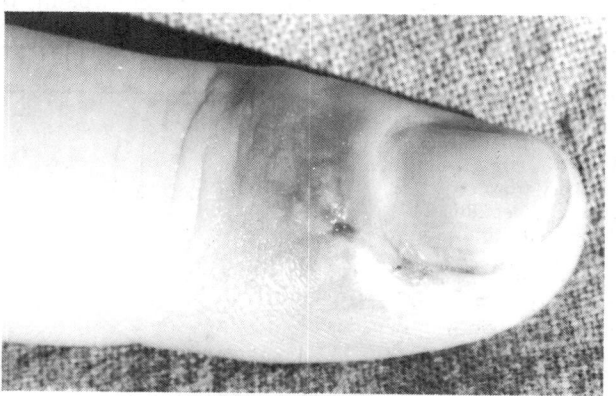

Cytomegalovirus

Cytomegalovirus (CMV), one of the herpes viruses, is spread by close contact, but the precise epidemiology is unknown. The transmission of CMV to pregnant hospital personnel is a serious concern because of its potential as a cause of congenital malformations. Women who are, or may become, pregnant should be advised not to care for patients carrying CMV. Infants and immunosuppressed transplant and oncology patients are the most likely to have active CMV infections. Gloves should be used for direct contact with patients, secretions, body fluids, or contaminated articles.

RUBELLA

There have been multiple outbreaks of rubella in hospital personnel, resulting in significant losses in employee working time, employee morbidity, and cost to the hospital.[115, 116] Although the majority of adults in the United States are immune to rubella, up to 20% of women of child-bearing age are still susceptible. Rubella infection during the first trimester of pregnancy is associated with congenital malformations or fetal death. A vaccine is available to produce immunity in susceptible adults. Many hospitals require employees to document immunity to rubella by serologic testing. Susceptible women of childbearing age, and personnel who might transfer rubella to pregnant patients, should be vaccinated.[117]

VIRAL HEPATITIS

There are three common types of viral hepatitis: type A, or infectious hepatitis; type B, or serum hepatitis; and non-A, non-B hepatitis. The viruses responsible for type A and type B have been clearly defined, but the etiology of non-A, non-B hepatitis remains to be identified.

Hepatitis A

About 20% of viral hepatitis in adults in the Unites States is due to the type A virus. Hepatitis A is usually a self-limited illness without a chronic carrier state. It is spread predominantly by the fecal-oral route, and is usually found in institutions or other closed groups where there has been a breakdown in normal sanitary conditions. Hospital personnel do not appear to be at increased risk for hepatitis A, because the majority of patients with the form of hepatitis are rarely hospitalized. When the patient with hepatitis A becomes jaundiced, there is little fecal excretion of the virus. Jaundiced patients should be placed on enteric precautions when hospitalized until a viral etiology has been ruled out.

In spite of this, there have been occasional hospital outbreaks of hepatitis A when patients were admitted during the prodromal stage of infection. The use of gloves and meticulous handwashing during contact with feces or contaminated linens or clothing prevents viral spread to hospital personnel.[118]

Antibodies to the hepatitis A virus (anti-HAV) become detectable after the onset of clinical symptoms. Initially, the antibodies consist almost entirely of the IgM class, but, after several months, anti-HAV IgM declines and IgG antibody titer rises. Acute hepatitis A is diagnosed from anti-HAV IgM, which is found in the serum for 4–6 weeks after infection. Individuals exposed to patients with hepatitis A should receive immune serum globulin to lessen the likelihood of infection.[119]

Hepatitis B

Hepatitis B is a significant occupational hazard for medical personnel who contact blood and blood products.[120, 121] The prevalence (a proportion of persons affected with a condition at the particular time when the survey of the population was performed) of hepatitis B in the general population of the United States is 3%–5% based on serologic screening of volunteers donating blood. Surveys conducted in the United States and several other countries indicate a significantly increased prevalence in anesthesiologists and anesthesia personnel (Table 4-2). The range of seropositivity in anesthesia personnel across the world probably reflects the prevalence of hepatitis B carriers in the local population. Within the United States, the prevalence in anesthesia personnel varied from 19% in one multicenter study[122] to 49% in the anesthesia department of an inner-city hospital.[125] Anesthesia residents from seven university centers had an increased seropositivity (13%).[124] In a survey of anesthesia personnel in one department, the prevalence of serum markers for hepatitis B increased with time since graduation from medical or nursing school.[122] It appears that the risk of hepatitis B infection begins in training, when patient contact is initiated, and continues throughout practice in physicians and hospital personnel who contact blood and blood products.

Acute hepatitis B infection resolves without significant hepatic damage in about 90% of cases. Less than 1% of acutely infected patients will develop fulminant hepatitis, but, with this, there is a mortality rate of greater than 60%, despite maximum medical therapy. The remaining 10% of infected individuals will become chronic carriers of the hepatitis B virus. Within 2 years, half of those chronically carrying the hepatitis B virus (HBV) resolve their infection without significant hepatic impairment. Chronic active hepatitis is likely to develop in those individuals with chronic infection for more than 2 years. Chronic HBV infection may produce cirrhosis, and has been linked as a cause of hepatocellular carcinoma.

The diagnosis of HBV infection can be made on the basis of serologic testing (Table 4-3). Hepatitis B surface antigen (HBsAg) can be detected in the serum within 3–4 weeks after infection with HBV.[132] At this time, the patient is asymptomatic, but is capable of infecting others with the virus. Within 8–12 weeks after infection, symptoms of hepatitis, jaundice, and elevated liver function tests will occur. With resolution of acute hepatitis B, HBsAg disappears from the serum and is followed by the appearance of antibody to the surface antigen (anti-HBs). Anti-HBs is the antibody which confers lasting immunity against subsequent HBV infections. During the "window" period, in which HBsAg has declined to undetectable levels and anti-HBs is not measurable, antibody to the core antigen (anti-HBc) is detectable. With resolution of infection, anti-HBc and anti-HBs persist. After many years, one of these antibodies may no longer be detectable in the serum. Chronic HBV carriers are likely to have HBsAg and anti-HBc present in serum samples.

There are several modes of transmission of HBV that put anesthesia personnel at risk for accidental infection. Percutaneous transmission can occur with contact with blood, blood products, or body fluids from patients carrying HBV. HBV is a hardy virus that may be infectious for at least 1 week in dried blood on environmental surfaces.[133] Several groups with a very high prevalence of HBV carriers have been identified, and include immigrants from endemic areas, such as Southeast Asia, users of illicit parenteral drugs, homosexual males, and patients on hemodialysis. Often, hospitalized HBV carriers not in these high-risk groups go unrecognized.[134] The clinical history and routine preoperative laboratory tests will rarely be useful in identifying undiagnosed chronic HBV carriers.

The Centers for Disease Control have formulated guidelines for hospital personnel to reduce accidental occupational infection with HBV; these are presented below in the section on AIDS. The use of these strategies to prevent transmission of HBV have been particularly successful in dialysis units, and should be adopted by others who are at high risk for occupational HBV infection.

Despite efforts to educate personnel about correct needle handling and disposal techniques, injuries from contaminated needle sticks are still very common.[135] In one multicenter study of anesthesia personnel, 94% remembered having been stuck with a previously used needle.[123] When susceptible employees have been exposed to a contaminated needle

TABLE 4-2.   Prevalence of Hepatitis B Seropositivity in Anesthesia Personnel

REFERENCE	STUDY POPULATION	PREVALENCE
Denes et al[120]	MDs at AMA meeting	17%
Berry et al[122]	MDs and non-MD anesthetists in one U.S. department	23%
Berry et al[123]	MDs and non-MD anesthetists in four U.S. departments	19%
Berry et al[124]	Residents in seven U.S. departments	13%
Fyman et al[125]	NY inner-city hospital	49%
Malm et al[126]	Anesthetists in teaching hospitals in Vancouver, Canada	12%
Chernesky et al[127]	Anesthetists in Ontario, Canada	17%
Siebke and Degre[128]	MD and non-MD anesthesia personnel in Norway	4%
Carstens et al[129]	South African anesthetists	18%
Sinclair et al[130]	Anesthetists in Oxford, UK	3%
Janzen et al[131]	Anesthesia personnel at Medical School of Hannover (West Germany)	31%

TABLE 4-3.   Patterns of Serologic Markers of Hepatitis B Virus (HBV) Infection

STAGE OF INFECTION	HBsAg	Anti-HBc	Anti-HBs
Early acute hepatitis B or chronic carrier state	+	−	−
Acute* or chronic hepatitis B	+	+	−
Recovery from acute* or chronic hepatitis B	−	+	+
Distant HBV infection, early recovery stage of hepatitis B*, or chronic carrier state	—	+	−
Distant HBV infection or after immunization with hepatitis B vaccine	−	−	+

* Anti-HBc of IgM type should be present.

or to blood from an HBsAg-positive patient, post-exposure prophylaxis with hepatitis B immune globulin (HBIG) is recommended.[136] The initial dose of immune globulin should be given as soon as possible after the exposure (within 7 days), and a second dose should be given 1 month later. It is recommended that the hepatitis B vaccine be administered simultaneously with HBIG, since this will initiate lasting immunity in personnel at high risk for repeat exposure.

Because many exposures to HBV go unrecognized, it is recommended that susceptible health-care personnel working in high-risk specialties be given the hepatitis B vaccine.[137] Administration of the three-dose vaccine in the deltoid muscle resulted in protective antibodies (anti-HBs) in more than 90% of hospital workers.[138, 139] The initial hepatitis B vaccine that was available for use in the United States is composed of HBsAg spheres prepared from the plasma of chronic carriers. The antigen particles are purified by ultracentrifugation, and undergo three separate biochemical inactivation steps. Because the population of chronic HBV carriers from whom plasma was taken for preparation of the vaccine are also at high risk for acquired immunodeficiency syndrome, there was a concern that the AIDS virus might be transmitted through the vaccine. Extensive serological, virological, and epidemiologic evaluation found no evidence that AIDS was transmitted by the plasma-derived vaccine.[140] The primary side effect of this vaccine has been local reaction around the injection site. No long-term adverse effects have been observed. It appears that protective antibodies may persist for up to 5 years after vaccination, and that the duration of protection relates to the maximal antibody response.[141, 142]

A second hepatitis B vaccine has been made available in the United States. It is composed of HBsAg produced by bread yeast, in which the genetic code for the antigen has been inserted by recombinant technology.[143] This vaccine appears to be safe and effective for providing immunity to HBV.[144] Hospitals or departments should have policies for screening and counseling personnel about their risk of acquiring hepatitis B virus infection, and should make vaccination available for susceptible individuals.[145, 146]

Non-A, Non-B Hepatitis

Non-A, non-B hepatitis can be transmitted through blood from an infected individual. Chronic hepatitis may result from acute non-A, non-B hepatitis infection, and it is estimated that up to 8% of the population of the United States may be carriers. There are no specific diagnostic tests available and, therefore, determining the epidemiology of the disease has been difficult.[147] Non-A, non-B hepatitis has been passed serially through experimental animals by innoculation with contaminated serum, and, presumably, accidental infection may occur in humans with blood exposure.[148] The agent responsible for the disease has not been identified, and the clinical diagnosis is made by exclusion. Although studies have been equivocal, it is reasonable to administer immune globulin to personnel with percutaneous exposure to blood from a patient with non-A, non-B hepatitis.[149]

ACQUIRED IMMUNODEFICIENCY SYNDROME

A retrovirus, now called the human immunodeficiency virus (HIV), has been demonstrated to be the etiology of the acquired immunodeficiency syndrome (AIDS).[150, 151] Infection with HIV is spread by intimate sexual contact, perinatally from mother to child, and through infected blood (transfusion

or shared needles) and blood products or, possibly, through infected body secretions. Those at the highest risk for HIV infection include homosexual/bisexual men, intravenous drug users, heterosexual contacts of individuals with HIV infection, and patients who have received blood or blood products infected with HIV. An antibody detectable using an enzyme-linked immunosorbent assay (ELISA test) is present in the majority of individuals infected with HIV. The antibody does not provide immunity nor lead to eradication of the virus. Not all individuals infected with HIV will develop AIDS or the AIDS-related complex.[152]

Although it appears that the modes of transmission of HBV and HIV are similar, in contrast to hepatitis B, retrospective and prospective studies have demonstrated that health-care workers have a very low risk of HIV infection even after parenteral exposure.[153–155] The risk of occupationally acquired HIV infection is not zero, since documented infection has occurred in individuals who provided care to AIDS patients.[156] Because many patients may carry the AIDS virus and not officially carry the diagnosis, particularly victims of trauma,[157] anesthesiologists should consider all patients to potentially have the disease.

The Centers for Disease Control have formulated recommendations for preventing transmission of HIV to health-care workers.[158, 159] The guidelines were based on the epidemiology of hepatitis B as a worse case model for transmission of blood-borne infections. In many instances, patients in the health-care system who are capable of transmitting HIV infections are not recognized, and infection control recommendations should be used during all patient contact.[157] The CDC strategies for infection control are based on appropriate handling of blood, body fluids, and items soiled with contaminated fluids. The CDC guidelines are summarized below.

1. All needles, blades, and sharp instruments should be handled to prevent accidental injuries, and all should be considered potentially infected. Disposable sharp items should be placed in puncture-resistant containers located as close as is practical to the area in which they are used. Needles should be recapped, bent, broken, or removed from disposable syringes prior to placing them in appropriate disposable recepticles.
2. Gloves should be worn when touching mucous membranes or open skin of all patients. When the possibility exists of exposure to blood, body fluids, or items soiled with these, gloves should be used. With some procedures, such as endoscopy, when aerosolization or splashes of blood or secretions are likely to occur, masks, eye coverings, and gowns are indicated. Gloves and body coverings should be removed and disposed of properly after patient contact.
3. Frequent handwashing, especially between patient contacts, should be encouraged. If hands are accidentally contaminated with blood or other body fluids, they should be washed as soon as possible.
4. Ventilation devices for resuscitation should be available to prevent the need for emergency mouth-to-mouth resuscitation.
5. Although pregnant health-care workers are not known to have an increased risk of contracting HIV infection, the infant is at risk of infection from perinatal transmission. Pregnant women should be counseled on the precautions for preventing HIV transmission in the health-care setting.
6. Health-care workers who have exudative lesions or

weeping dermatitis should not participate in direct patient care activities, which include performing or assisting with invasive procedures or handling contaminated equipment.

7. Health-care workers with evidence of any illness which compromises their ability to safely perform invasive procedures should be evaluated to determine whether they are both physically and mentally competent to perform these.
8. Routine serologic testing of health-care personnel for HIV infection is not recommended.
9. HIV is inactivated by sterilization and disinfection procedures currently recommended for use in health-care facilities. Contaminated instruments should undergo routine sterilization or disinfection, and surfaces exposed to blood and body fluids should be cleaned with an appropriate germicide.
10. Potentially infective wastes should be transported in clearly identified plastic bags. If the outside of a bag is contaminated, a second outer bag should be used. Current recommended practices for the disposal of infected material are adequate to handle HIV.

Recapping of needles can be associated with inadvertent skin puncture. For that reason, it may be preferable not to recap needles,[159] or to inject drugs through a stopcock.[160]

SLOW VIRUSES

Creutzfeldt-Jakob disease, caused by a slow virus, may be unsuspected in patients presenting with dementia. Although the risk of transmission to hospital personnel seems low, care must be taken in handling specimens from patients with suspected Creutzfeldt-Jakob disease. Gloves should be used when handling spinal fluid, blood, or tissue specimens. Ethylene oxide or steam sterilization or disinfection with 0.5% sodium hypochlorite or iodine are effective, but formalin and 70% ethanol fail to eradicate the virus.

BACTERIAL INFECTION

Tuberculosis

Although the incidence of tuberculosis in the United States has declined and most infected patients are treated on an outpatient basis, undiagnosed patients with the disease may be hospitalized for initial workup. Hospital personnel are especially at risk for infection from unrecognized cases.[161] Tuberculosis may not be suspected until a routine culture report is returned, or may be first recognized at autopsy.

Respiratory isolation should be used for hospitalized patients with active tuberculosis. Personnel who may have been infected by an unrecognized contagious patient should be followed by skin testing. Recent converters should be counseled on the need for isoniazid therapy. Routine periodic screening of employees for tuberculosis may be indicated as part of a hospital's employee health policy.

Recent concern over occupationally acquired hepatitis B and AIDS has resulted in heightened attention to the use of infection-control procedures in anesthesia practice. Although there had been only infrequent reports of work-related infections in anesthesiologists, in 1974, Walter suggested that "the mouth must be recognized as a microbiologic hazard that warrants the use of gloves for manipulations involving the oropharynx."[162] A survey of anesthesia residents published in 1985

demonstrated that use of gloves during patient contact was more common in recent graduates.[124]

Strategies for reducing the spread of infectious agents are based on the use of physical barriers, such as glove, gowns, masks, and eye glasses, and immunologic protection using active or passive immunization. It is essential to have regular educational programs for all employees contacting patients, laboratory specimens, or contaminated instruments or supplies. There should be a system in place for maintaining immunization records, and for follow-up of workers with accidental exposures. Programs such as these should result in less worker morbidity and absenteeism due to occupationally acquired infections.

EMOTIONAL CONSIDERATIONS

STRESS

Among the potential health hazards of working in the operating room, stress is well recognized.[163] However, despite this wide recognition, there is very little objective information specifically directed toward understanding the nature of job-related stresses among anesthesiologists.

The problem of stress has been well studied among air traffic controllers,[164, 165] and this may provide some close analogies for understanding the problem and relating it to anesthesiologists. This context also permits refining definitions, as the general concept of stress can be obscure. It may be helpful to consider the concept of *stress*, as used in engineering—the objective demands placed on an individual—and *strain*—the subjective response to these demands. Psychological *stress* occurs when an individual must deal with a situation in which his typical response pattern promises to be inadequate, and the consequences of not responding appropriately will be serious. The *strain* on an individual is a direct result of the stresses in conjunction with variables such as experience, aptitude, skills, age, and personality. The response of an individual to these stresses and strains is a consequence of defense mechanisms, which serve to alter the individual's perception of the situation, and coping mechanisms, which attempt to modify the objective nature of the situation.

What are the conditions in the anesthesiologists' workplace that account for stress in their professional life? Many are shared by both anesthesiologists and air traffic controllers, and these include: an excessive workload, the process of making difficult decisions, night duty, fatigue, increasing reliance on technology, and interpersonal tensions.[166, 167] Those areas that are very specific to the practice of anesthesiology are the anesthetic induction, overlapping areas of responsibility with the surgeon, and dealing with the critically ill or dying patient.

It is not surprising to note that the process of inducing anesthesia produces a great deal of stress on the practitioner. Although this observation is self-evident to any anesthesiologist, documentation is limited. Two reports have demonstrated changes in heart rate[168] and blood pressure[169] in the anesthesiologist during the anesthetic induction. Individual observations from these studies included cardiac arrhythmias (premature ventricular contractions), ischemic changes on the (ECG), and a blood pressure elevation to as high as 193/137 mm Hg.

Interpersonal relationships impose a unique set of demands that may serve as stressors to the anesthesiologist. In most locations within a hospital or clinic setting (i.e., radiology, pathology laboratory, during evaluation and treatment from a consultant), the direct responsibility for a patient is temporarily transferred to the consulting physician. The operating room is probably the only arena where two co-equal physicians simultaneously share ultimate responsibility for the well-being of a patient.[170] To many anesthesiologists and surgeons, the overlapping of realms of responsibility produces the highest degree of stress in their clinical practices.

The level of training and degree of experience play a role in determining the amount of strain perceived by an anesthesiologist. It has been shown that an inverse relationship exists between the duration of clinical experience and the level of anxiety[171] and hemodynamic changes[169] occurring in the anesthesiologist during the anesthetic induction.

Several factors determine the nature of the individual anesthesiologist's response to these strains. To a large extent, personality characteristics dictate which defense and coping mechanisms will be employed, and how successfully these will function. Several studies have focused on personality characteristics, some identifiable prior to entering medical school, which appear to predispose the individual toward maladaptive responses to stress.[172, 173] Prominent among these traits is the obsessive-compulsive, dependent character structure. These individuals typically manifest pessimism, passivity, self-doubt, and feelings of insecurity, and commonly, they respond to stress by internalizing anger and becoming hypochondriacal and depressed. In work reported by Vaillant, undergraduate students who demonstrated these characteristics were more likely than controls to have their medical careers disrupted by alcoholism or drug abuse, psychiatric illness, and marital disturbances.[173]

Commonly employed defense mechanisms include denial, intellectualization, reaction formation, and repression. Humor, denial, displacement of affect (anger), and projection are examples of coping mechanisms which are frequently utilized. The success of these defense and coping mechanisms depends upon the degree of the individual's personality integrity, the range of his defense repertory, and the level of his coping abilities. When the degree of strain exceeds his threshold, the individual's defenses become exaggerated and inappropriate. It is this situation that gives rise to maladaptive behavior and the personal and professional deterioration that leads to such disorders as drug addiction and impairment.

SUBSTANCE USE, ABUSE, AND ADDICTION

Illicit drug use and the risk of addiction are an ever-increasing concern in Western society. It has been estimated that as many as 22 million Americans have experimented with cocaine, and 4–5 million are regular users of cocaine. Drugs have now become a $110-billion-per-year habit for Americans. Estimates of the prevalence of alcoholism in the population run as high as 10%. Recently, the problem of addiction has drawn the attention of the national media, and has prompted the President of the United States to declare a "war on drugs."

Epidemiology

The abuse of drugs by physicians has gained considerable media attention and notoriety. However, recognition of the problem of substance abuse among physicians is not new. In the first edition of *The Principles and Practice of Medicine*, edited by Sir William Osler and published in 1892, it is stated, "The habit [morphia] is particularly prevalent among women and physicians who use the hypodermic syringe for the alleviation of pain, as in neuralgia or sciatica."[174] And, 2 years later, Mattison commented, "It is a fact—striking though sad—that

more cases of morphinism are met with among medical men than in all other professions combined."[175.]

Whether or not substance abuse is more prevalent among physicians than the general population is a subject worthy of debate. There is a large body of literature that attempts to support the notion that drug problems are more frequent among physicians.[176–178] The reported figure for drug and/or alcohol addiction among physicians varies from 10% to 40%.[179, 180] Certainly, the smaller estimate is not far out of line with that estimated for the adult population at large. However, if drug addiction alone is examined, the reported incidence of 1%–2% among physicians is 30–100 times that seen in the general public.[180]

The data from which these estimates are drawn are notoriously difficult to collect and interpret. Bias in reporting technique alone can account for extremes in under- or overestimating the actual prevalence of this disease.[181] In her extensive review of the English-language literature, Brewster finally concluded, "no one really knows how many practicing physicians are having problems with alcohol and other drugs."[180]

It is more clearly documented that substance abuse is a significant problem, specifically among anesthesiologists. At the present time, there are more addictive diseases among anesthesiologists than among any other medical speciality.[182] To some observers, addiction represents the number-one occupational hazard for the speciality of anesthesiology.

These conclusions are drawn from a number of studies that examine the problem from various vantage points. One of the most easily accessed and frequently quoted sources of information on drug abuse comes from statistics on the number of individuals who are in drug treatment programs. However, there are major flaws inherent in this system of data collection. Before a physician is entered into any treatment program, he must first identify that he has a drug problem. Unfortunately, denial is typically the first, and most tenaciously maintained, defense mechanism for the physician-substance abuser.

Even after recognition that a drug-related problem exists, physicians are less likely than the population in general to seek professional assistance.[183] Again, denial plays a major role in this reluctance to undergo counseling or therapy. Medical students learn early in their education to employ denial mechanisms to enable them to endure long, sleepless nights and the personal shortcomings inevitable in clinical medicine. These well-honed denial mechanisms encourage the physician-addict to conclude that his problem is minor, and that he can essentially treat himself. Physicians typically enter programs for treatment only after they have reached the end stages of their illness.

With these caveats in mind, it is still informative to look at the statistics pertaining to the number of anesthesiologists who are involved in treatment programs for drug-related illness. Probably the most extensive experience comes from the Medical Association of Georgia Disabled Doctors' Program.[182] Their study population includes 1000 disabled physicians, 920 of whom were treated for chemical dependence. One hundred and twenty-one of these patients were anesthesiologists (12%), although anesthesia only accounts for 3.9% of the U.S. physician population. Even more troubling is the fact that anesthesia residents constitute 33.7% of the resident population in their treatment group, despite their representation as only 4.6% of the U.S. resident population. Anesthesia residents have a 7.4 times excess prevalence in the treatment population.

Another approach towards uncovering the prevalence of drug abuse among anesthesiologists is the directed survey. Again, as with the statistics drawn from the drug treatment programs, there are major weaknesses inherent in this form of data collection. Most obvious is the willingness of the respondent to honestly and completely detail his experience in an area as sensitive as drug abuse.

One of the most extensive surveys was conducted by Ward et al.[184] They reported on the results of a questionnaire completed by 247 U.S. anesthesia training programs. Sixty-four percent of the respondents identified at least one of their personnel as an abuser of drugs. In ten programs (4%), there were five or more such individuals identified during the 10-year study period (1970–1980). The overall incidence of suspected abuse was 1.3%, and confirmed abuse was 1.1%. The two most favored chemicals for abuse were reported to be meperidine and fentanyl, with a definite tendency toward the latter in the most recent half-decade of the study. This preference had previously been observed by Talbott, who had treated 105 fentanyl addicts among the 125 anesthesiologists admitted to his facility at the time.[185] The most recent report from Talbott's group indicates a growing preference for cocaine (28% of physicians presenting for treatment in 1986) and parenteral drugs (39%).[182] Compared to other physician-patients in Talbott's study group, anesthesiologists were more likely to be poly-drug addicted, and more likely to abuse substances intravenously.

Similar results were obtained by Gravenstein et al.[186] In their study, questionnaires regarding substance abuse were completed by chairmen of academic anesthesia departments, clinical personnel from these departments, and a group of third-year medical students. Seventy-six percent of the responding chairmen reported that one or more of their staff members had been affected by substance abuse during the period of study (1974–1979). Overall, 1%–2% of the anesthesia personnel suffered from substance abuse and required some action from the chairman (Table 4-4).

Drug Addiction as a Disease

What accounts for this disproportionally high incidence of drug addiction among anesthesiologists? In order to answer this, it is best to view drug addiction as a psychosocial, biogenetic disease.[187] As such, the addiction 1) is a primary condition (not a symptom), 2) is associated with specific anatomic and physiologic changes, 3) has a set of recognizable signs and symptoms, 4) has a predictable, progressive course (if left untreated), and 5) has established etiologies.

It is important to recognize that the causative factors in this

disease process involve genetics, as well as the environment. The disease results from a dynamic interplay between a susceptible host and a "favorable" environment. Vulnerability in the host is an important factor. What constitutes an instigating exposure to a drug in one individual may have absolutely no effect on another. Unfortunately, there is no good predictive tool to identify the susceptible individual until he gets the disease.

There are causative factors specific to the environment of the anesthesiologist. These include: job stress, an orientation towards self-medication, lack of external recognition and self-respect, the availability of addicting drugs, and a susceptible pre-morbid personality.[188]

Self-prescription is commonly seen as a prelude to more extensive drug abuse and addiction. Similarly, recreational use of drugs may proceed to drug dependence, with the drug used for recreation usually becoming the primary drug of dependence.[189] Of concern is the increasing recreational use of drugs among younger physicians and medical students, and the choice of more potent drugs with enhanced potential for addiction, such as cocaine and the newer synthetic opioids, fentanyl and sufentanil.[190] As a result, recreational drug use is becoming a leading source of impairment among younger physicians.[191]

The general public's image of the anesthesiologist frequently falls short of that of other physicians. In a recent report from Australia, only 66% of the patients knew that anesthesiologists needed medical qualifications, and less than 10% could remember their anesthesiologist's name.[192] It is even more distressing when co-workers in the medical field fail to recognize special skills and contributions of anesthesiologists. In another study from Australia, only 83% of hospital nurses realized that anesthesiologists were medically qualified.[193]

Positive reinforcement and a sense of a job "well done" are important components of job satisfaction.[194] It is more difficult for the anesthesiologist than the surgeon to achieve recognition from patients and medical colleagues for a successful outcome. The "Rodney Dangerfield Syndrome—'I don't get no respect' " has been cited by several authors as an instigating event for drug experimentation.[188]

Anesthesiologists live in a climate in which a large quantity of powerful psychoactive drugs is freely available. From the experience of the U.S. Army in Vietnam, it is apparent that, when there is easy access to narcotics, alcohol use declines in favor of the opiates.[195] As each new synthetic opioid becomes available for clinical use, it also becomes the drug of choice of abusing anesthesiologists. Currently, fentanyl is seen most frequently as the abused drug, but sufentanil is rapidly increasing in popularity.[185] Cocaine and its derivatives are also popular among medical students and young practicing physicians.[182]

Since availability of drugs does play a role in the onset of this disease, it is logical that programs to better audit the distribution of drugs within the operating room setting should be a valuable preventive measure. Two university affiliated anesthesiology departments have published their protocols for better controlling the distribution of these medications.[196, 197] Talbott acknowledges that the strategies advocated within the anesthesia community are better than those of our colleagues in other medical specialties.[182] However, these are currently limited to academic centers, and require wider dissemination to be effective.

There is an apparent link between behavior prior to entering medical school and subsequent development of drug abuse.[198] At least one study examining personality profiles of anesthe-

TABLE 4-4. Number of Drug and Alcohol Abusers Among Clinical Personnel in Gravenstein's Survey of Selected Academic Departments. Of Concern is the Increasing Prevalence of Drug Abusers Noted in the More Recent Years of the Survey

YEAR	TOTAL PERSONNEL	DRUG ABUSERS	ALCOHOLICS	TOTAL
1974	358	3	3	6
1975	443	4	2	6
1976	583	5	5	10
1977	641	5	3	8
1978	763	13	1	14
1979	814	11	3	14

(Reproduced with permission from Gravenstein JS, Kory WP, Marks RG: Drug abuse by anesthesia personnel. Anesth Analg 62:467, 1983)

siologists revealed a disturbingly high proportion with a predisposition towards maladaptive behavior.[199] Talbott has observed that many of the anesthesia residents in his treatment program specifically chose the specialty of anesthesiology because of the known availability of powerful drugs.[182] It is apparent that residency selection committees must begin to screen for personality disorders as an important part of the admissions process.

The consequences of substance abuse to the practicing anesthesiologist are ultimately devastating. If left untreated, addiction is a fatal illness. In the study reported by Ward, among the 334 confirmed drug abusers, 27 died of "drug overdose," and, in another three, "abuse was discovered at death."[184] Gravenstein reported seven deaths among 44 confirmed drug abusers.[186] It is interesting to note that, in this small series, there were no deaths among narcotics abusers.

Intentional or inadvertent drug-related death is, of course, only one of the potential consequences of substance abuse (Table 4-5). More common is a gradual and inexorable deterioration in family and social relationships. The substance abuser becomes increasingly withdrawn and isolated, first in his personal life, and ultimately, in his professional existence. Every attempt is made to maintain a facade of normalcy at work, because discovery here means isolation from the source of the abused drug. When professional conduct is finally impaired such that it is apparent to the physician's colleagues, the disease is approaching its end stage.

Ward's report does ring one relatively optimistic note.[184] Approximately 55% of the confirmed drug abusers underwent rehabilitation, and half of these were offered reemployment in their original department. This rate of rehabilitation is consistent with other reports of 65%–75% successful treatment among physician-patients.[200] Left untreated, less than 30% of

addicted physicians will be practicing at 10 years, and some 10% will have died from their disease.

These results highlight the importance of early and aggressive intervention and rehabilitation. Physicians are generally highly motivated, and rehabilitation rates are higher than those seen in the general public.[201] Anesthesiologists appear to have a recovery rate approximating that of other physicians.[179] The Anesthesiology Department at the University of Pennsylvania[202] has reported its policy for dealing with the problem of substance abuse. It is important that an intervention process and referral arrangements be in place, and that confrontation of suspected abusers be handled by trained individuals with appropriate skills.[202]

IMPAIRMENT

Substance abuse probably accounts for some 85% of the cases of impairment* among physicians.[203] Other factors that may lead to impairment include physical or mental illness and deterioration due to the aging process. Some authorities include unwillingness or inability to keep up with current literature and techniques as a form of disability.

Data regarding the prevalence of these disabling disorders are more difficult to obtain than are those on drug abuse. Statistics derived from the admitting diagnoses to various psychiatric facilities indicate that close to 1% of those admitted are physicians.[204] Admission is required for (in the order of increasing frequency): organic psychoses, personality disorders, schizophrenia, neuroses, and affective disorders—particularly depression.[205]

It is not surprising that depression should figure prominently among the personality characteristics of emotionally impaired physicians. Indeed, many of the personality traits which are adaptive and assure success in the physician's world may also serve as risk factors for depression when exaggerated. These character traits include self-sacrifice, competitiveness, achievement orientation, denial of feelings, and intellectualization of emotions.[206] Two studies on alcoholic physicians provide some insight into this link between achievement orientation and emotional disturbance. Bissell and Jones reported that more than half of their group of alcoholic physicians graduated in the upper one-third of their medical school class, 23% were in the upper one-tenth, and only 5% were in the lower one-third of their class.[207] Similarly, a recent report on alcohol use in medical school demonstrated better first-year grades and higher scores on Part I—National Board of Medical Examiners among those students identified as alcohol abusers.[208] Alcohol abuse clearly does not enhance the learning process. Rather, the alcohol abuse is a manifestation of psychological disturbance resulting from excessive degrees of stress among some students most determined to have flawless records.

When all of these forms of impairment are considered, it is estimated that as many as 10% of practicing physicians are seriously impaired.[209] Fortunately, in recent years, most state legislatures and medical societies have formally recognized this problem, and have enacted laws and formed committees that address the impaired physician. These programs are generally therapeutic and non-punitive in nature. Ideally, the committees provide a non-threatening environment for iden-

TABLE 4-5. Signs of Substance Abuse and Addiction

Social

Withdrawal from leisure activities, friends, family
Uncharacteristic or inappropriate behavior in social gatherings
Impulsive behavior, *e.g.,* overspending, gambling
Domestic turmoil, *e.g.,* separation from spouse, child abuse, sexual problems
Change in behavior of spouse or children
Legal problems, *e.g.,* arrest for driving while intoxicated

Health

Deterioration in personal hygiene
Accidents
Numerous health complaints; frequent need for medical attention for unrelated illnesses

Professional

Unreliability, *e.g.,* missed appointments, inappropriate response to emergency calls, absences, poor record keeping
Complaints by patients or staff, subject of hospital gossip
Overprescription of medicines, excessive ordering of drugs from mail-order houses
Unstable employment history, *e.g.,* several relocations
Working at a level below qualifications

(Reproduced with permission from Spiegelman WG, Saunders L, Mazze RI: Addiction and anesthesiology. Anesthesiology 60:335, 1984)

* An impaired physician is defined as one "whose performance as a professional person and as a practitioner of the healing arts is impaired because of alcoholism, drug abuse, mental illness, senility, or disabling disease."[74]

tification and intervention of the impaired physician. Only in cases where there exists a real risk to the public welfare, and where the involved physician is unwilling to voluntarily suspend practice and accept assistance, is the license-suspension power of the State Board of Medical Examiners exercised. Management protocols for dealing with the impaired physician are covered in a series of articles by Canavan.[210]

SUICIDE

Perhaps one of the most alarming of the occupationally associated hazards for anesthesiologists is the extraordinarily high rate of suicide. In a recent review of mortality among American anesthesiologists, suicide was identified as the *only* major health problem.[30] A high suicide rate among anesthesiologists was first reported by Bruce et al in their 20-year retrospective study of mortality among members of the American Society of Anesthesiologists.[26] Suicide accounted for 35 of the 441 deaths in their report. This is three to four times the suicide rate expected among a contemporary, otherwise comparable socioeconomic group, and exceeds that of all but one or two other medical specialties.[211] Subsequently, Bruce reported similar findings in a larger, prospective study,[27] while others have confirmed these alarming observations.[30, 212]

The high incidence of suicide has also been observed among residents in anesthesiology training programs. A report from England has identified five deaths from suicide over a recent 5-year period.[213] Their ratio of one suicide per 500 residents compares unfavorably to the approximately one suicide per 12,000 in the general population, and one suicide in 4000 for doctors per year.[214]

Why should there be such a high rate of suicide among anesthesiologists? A partial explanation lies with the high degree of stress which is an integral part of the job. The relationship between generalized stress and suicide is not direct. But, clearly, in susceptible individuals, feelings of inability to cope resulting from overwhelming stress may give way to despair and suicide ideation.

Extensive personality profiles have been collected from suicide-susceptible individuals that indicate characteristics such as high anxiety, insecurity, low self-esteem, impulsiveness, and poor self-control. It is disturbing to note that, in Reeve's study of personality traits of a sample of anesthesiologists, some 20% manifested psychological profiles that reflected a predisposition to behavioral disintegration and attempted suicide when placed under extremes of stress.[199] His study raises the discomforting notion that "pre-morbid" personality characteristics that exist prior to entering speciality training are not being identified in the admissions process.[215]

One specific type of stress, that resulting from a malpractice lawsuit, may have a direct etiologic association with suicide among physicians in general and anesthesiologists in particular. Two recent anecdotal reports have described, in tragic detail, the emotional deterioration and ultimate suicide of experienced and previously healthy physicians involved in malpractice suits.[216, 217] One study specifically identified the anesthesiologist involved in a legal suit as being at particularly high risk for suicide.[218] In this report, four of 185 anesthesiologists being sued attempted or committed suicide.

Another potential etiologic basis for the observed high suicide rate is the high incidence of drug abuse found among anesthesia personnel. A self-administered lethal overdose occurred in as many as 16% of confirmed drug abusers in Gravenstein's study.[186] Physicians who are impaired, and whose privileges to practice medicine are removed by the licensing authority, are at heightened risk to attempt suicide. Crawshaw reported eight successful, and two near-miss, suicide attempts among 43 physicians placed on probation for drug-related disability.[219] Other occupational factors that may contribute to the high incidence of suicide include isolation and lack of colleague support at work, and the ready access to various means to complete the act of suicide.

The basis for the alarmingly high rate of suicide among anesthesiologists is complex and multi-factoral. Some of the causative factors may be the same as those that result in substance abuse. It is encouraging to see that the problem of addiction in anesthesiologists is being addressed. Likewise, there is a need for additional study of suicide and the development of programs for its prevention.

REFERENCES

1. Werthmann H: Chronic ether intoxication in surgeons. Beitr Klin Chir 178:149, 1949, Ger
2. American Society of Anesthesiologists Ad Hoc Committee on the Effect of Trace Anesthetics on the Health of Operating Room Personnel: Occupational disease among operating room personnel: A national study. Anesthesiology 41:321, 1974
3. Cohen EN, Brown BW, Bruce DL et al: A survey of anesthetic health hazards among dentists. J Am Dent Assoc 90:1291, 1975
4. Ferstandig LL: Trace concentrations of anesthetic gases: A critical review of their disease potential. Anesth Analg 57:328, 1978
5. Lecky JH: Problems of trace anesthetic levels. In Orkin FK, Cooperman LH (eds). Complications in Anesthesiology, p 715 Philadelphia, JB Lippincott, 1983
6. Buring JE, Hennekens CH, Mayrent SL et al: Health experiences of operating room personnel. Anesthesiology 62:325, 1985
7. Vessey MP: Epidemiological studies of the occupational hazards of anaesthesia—A review. Anaesthesia 33:430, 1978
8. Spence AA, Knill-Jones RP: Is there a health hazard in anaesthetic practice? Br J Anaesth 50:713, 1978
9. Linde HW, Bruce DL: Occupational exposure of anesthetists to halothane, nitrous oxide and radiation. Anesthesiology 30:363, 1969
10. Whitcher CE, Cohen EN, Trudell JR: Chronic exposure to anesthetic gases in the operating room. Anesthesiology 35:348, 1971
11. Corbett TH: Retention of anesthetic agents following occupational exposure. Anesth Analg 52:614, 1973
12. Flemming DC, Johnstone RE: Recognition thresholds for diethyl ether and halothane. Anesthesiology 46:68, 1977
13. National Institute for Occupational Safety and Health (NIOSH): Criteria for a recommended standard . . . Occupational exposure to waste anesthetic gases and vapors. DHEW (NIOSH) Publication No. 77-140
14. Lecky JH: The mechanical aspects of anesthetic pollution control. Anesth Analg 56:769, 1977
15. Whitcher C, Piziali RL: Monitoring occupational exposure to inhalation anesthetics. Anesth Analg 56:778, 1977
16. The American Society of Anethesiologists Ad Hoc Committee on Effects of Trace Anesthetic Agents on Health of Operating Room Personnel: Waste anesthetic gases in operating room air: A suggested program to reduce personnel exposure. Park Ridge, American Society of Anesthesiologists
17. Lecky JH: Anesthetic pollution in the operating room: A notice to operating room personnel. Anesthesiology 52:157, 1980
18. Walts LF, Forsythe AB, Moore JG: Critique: Occupational disease among operating room personnel. Anesthesiology 42:608, 1975
19. Vaisman AL: Working conditions in surgery and their effect on the health of anesthesiologists. Eksp Khir Anesteziol 3:44, 1967

20. Fink BR, Cullen BF: Anesthetic pollution: What is happening to us? Anesthesiology 45:79, 1976
21. Axelsson G, Rylander R: Exposure to anaesthetic gases and spontaneous abortion: Response bias in a postal questionnaire study. Int J Epidemiol 11:250, 1982
22. Cohen EN, Bellville JW, Brown BW: Anesthesia, pregnancy, and miscarriage: a study of operating room nurses and anesthetists. Anesthesiology 35:343, 1971
23. Knill-Jones RP, Moir DD, Rodrigues LV et al: Anaesthetic practice and pregnancy: Controlled survey of women anaesthetists in the United Kingdom. Lancet 2:1326, 1972
24. Rosenberg P, Kirves A: Miscarriages among operating theatre staff. Acta Anaesthesiol Scand (Suppl) 53:37, 1973
25. Mazze RI, Lecky JH: The health of operating room personnel. Anesthesiology 62:226, 1985
26. Bruce DL, Eide KA, Linde HW et al: Causes of death among anesthesiologists: A 20-year survey. Anesthesiology 29:565, 1968
27. Bruce DL, Eide KA, Smith NJ et al: A prospective survey of anesthesiologist mortality, 1967–1971. Anesthesiology 41:71, 1974
28. Mazze RI: Waste anesthetic gases and the regulatory agencies. Anesthesiology 52:248, 1980
29. Doll R, Peto R: Mortality among doctors in different occupations. Br Med J 1:1433, 1977
30. Lew EA: Mortality experience among anesthesiologists, 1954–1976. Anesthesiology 51:195, 1979
31. Jackson SH: Anesthetics and cell multiplication. Clin Anesth 11:75, 1975
32. Nunn JF, Sharer N: Inhibition of methionine synthetase by trace concentrations of nitrous oxide. Br J Anaesth 53:1099, 1981
33. Koblin DD, Watson JE, Deady JE et al: Inactivation of methionine synthetase by nitrous oxide in mice. Anesthesiology 54:318, 1981
34. Nunn JF, Sharer N: Serum methionine and hepatic enzyme activity in anaesthetists exposed to nitrous oxide. Br J Anaesth 54:593, 1982
35. Corbett TH: Cancer and congenital anomalies associated with anesthetics. Ann NY Acad Sci 271:58, 1976
36. Eger EI, White AE, Brown CL et al: A test of the carcinogenicity of enflurane, isoflurane, halothane, methoxyflurane and nitrous oxide in mice. Anesth Analg 57:678, 1978
37. Coate WB, Ulland BM, Lewis TR: Chronic exposure to low concentrations of halothane-nitrous oxide: Lack of carcinogenic effect in the rat. Anesthesiology 50:306, 1979
38. Baden JM, Mazze RI, Wharton RS et al: Carcinogenicity of halothane in Swiss/ICR mice. Anesthesiology 51:20, 1979
39. Baden JM, Egbert B, Mazze RI: Carcinogen bioassay of enflurane in mice. Anesthesiology 56:9, 1982
40. Baden JM, Brinkenhoff M, Wharton RS et al: Mutagenicity of volatile anesthetics: Halothane. Anesthesiology 45:311, 1976
41. Baden JM, Kelley M, Wharton RS et al: Mutagenicity of halogenated ether anesthetics. Anesthesiology 46:346, 1977
42. Baden JM, Kelley M, Cheung A et al: Lack of mutagens in urines of operating room personnel. Anesthesiology 53:195, 1980
43. Tennant RW, Margolin BH, Shelby MD et al: Prediction of chemical carcinogenicity in rodents from in vitro genetic toxicity assays. Science 236:933, 1987
44. Chang LW, Katz J: Pathologic effects of chronic halothane inhalation: An overview. Anesthesiology 45:640, 1976
45. Ross WT: Are effects of halothane on hepatocytes "pathologic"? Anesthesiology 47:76, 1977
46. Coate WB, Kapp RW, Lewis TR: Chronic exposure to low concentrations of halothane-nitrous oxide: Reproductive and cytogenetic effects in the rat. Anesthesiology 50:310, 1979
47. Vieura E, Cleaton-Jones P, Austin JC, et al: Effects of low concentrations of nitrous oxide on rat fetuses. Anesth Analg 59:175, 1980
48. Mazze RI: Fertility, reproduction and postnatal survival in mice chronically exposed to isoflurane. Anesthesiology 63:663, 1985
49. Wyrobek AJ, Brodsky J, Gordon L et al: Sperm studies in anesthesiologists. Anesthesiology 55:527, 1981
50. Land PC, Owen EL: Nitrous oxide does not alter spermatogenesis in the mouse. Anesthesiology 53:S255, 1980
51. White AE, Takehisa S, Eger EI et al: Sister chromatid exchanges induced by inhaled anesthetics. Anesthesiology 50:426, 1979
52. Husum B, Wulf HC, Niebuhr E: Monitoring of sister chromatid exchanges in lymphocytes of nurse-anesthetists. Anesthesiology 62:475, 1985
53. Bruce DL, Bach MJ, Arbit J: Trace anesthetic effects on perceptual, cognitive and motor skills. Anesthesiology 40:453, 1974
54. Bruce DL, Bach MJ: Effects of trace anaesthetic gases on behavioural performance of volunteers. Br J Anaesth 48:871, 1976
55. Smith G, Shirley AW: Failure to demonstrate effects of low concentrations of nitrous oxide and halothane on psychomotor performance. Br J Anaesth 48:274, 1976
56. Geraci CL: Operating room pollution: Governmental perspectives and guidelines. Anesth Analg 56:775, 1977
57. NIOSH recommendations for occupational safety and health standards. MMWR 35:33S, 1986
58. Cromer J, Kronoveter K: A study of methylmethacrylate exposure and employee health. DHEW Publication No. 77-119 (NIOSH). Washington DC. U.S. Government Printing Office, 1976
59. Poss R, Thilly WG, Kaden DA: Methylmethacrylate is a mutagen for salmonella typhimurium. J Bone Joint Surg 61A:1203, 1979
60. Taylor G: A scavenging device for venting methylmethacrylate monomer vapor. Anesthesiology 41:612, 1974
61. Pickering CAC, Bainbridge D, Birtwistle IH et al: Occupational asthma due to methyl methacrylate in an orthopaedic theatre sister. Br Med J 292:1362, 1986
62. Lee CM: Unusual reaction to methyl methacrylate monomer. Anesth Analg 63:371, 1984
63. Schwettmann RS, Casterline CL: Delayed asthmatic response following occupational exposure to enflurane. Anesthesiology 44:166, 1976
64. Klatskin G, Kimberg DV: Recurrent hepatitis attributable to halothane sensitization in an anesthetist. N Engl J Med 280:515, 1969
65. National Council on Radiation Protection and Measurements. Radiation Protection for Medical and Allied Health Personnel. Report No 48. Washington, DC; 1977
66. Laughlin JS: Experience with a sustained policy of radiation exposure control and research in a medical center. Health Physics 5:709, 1981
67. Giachino AA, Cheng M: Irradiation of the surgeon during pinning of femoral fractures. J Bone Joint Surg 62-B:227, 1980
68. Poznanski AK, Kanellitsas C, Roloff DW et al: Radiation exposure to personnel in a neonatal nursery. Pediatric 54:139, 1974
69. Kan K, Santen BC, Velthuyse HJM et al: Exposure of radiologists to scattered radiation during radiodiagnostic examinations. Radiology 119:455, 1976
70. Santen BC, Kan K, Velthuyse HJM et al: Exposure of radiologists to scattered radiation during angiography. Radiology 115:447, 1975
71. Burks J, Griffith P, McCormick K et al: Radiation exposure to nursing personnel from patients receiving diagnostic radionuclides. Heart Lung 11:217, 1982
72. Liu J, Edwards FM: Radiation exposure to medical personnel during iodine-125 seed implantation of the prostate. Radiology 132:748, 1979
73. Shapiro RA, Berland T: Noise in the operating room. N Engl J Med 287:1236, 1972
74. Olmeda EL, Kirk RE: Maintenance of vigilance by non-task re-

lated stimulation in the monitoring environment. Perceptual and Motor Skills 44:715, 1977

75. Gaba DM, Maxwell M, DeAnda A: Anesthetic mishaps: Breaking the chain of accident evolution. Anesthesiolgy 66:670, 1987

76. Baker RA, Ware JR: The relationship between vigilance and monotonous work. Ergonomics 9:109, 1966

77. Paget NS, Lambert TF, Sridhar K: Factors affecting an anaesthetist's work: Some findings on vigilance and performance. Anaesth Intensive Care 9:359, 1981

78. Friedman RL, Bigger JT, Kornfield DS: The intern and sleep loss. N Engl J Med 285:201, 1971

79. Morgan BB, Brown BR, Alluisi EA: Effects on sustained performance of 48 hours of continuous work and sleep loss. Human Factors 16:406, 1974

80. Catalano JF: Effect of perceived proximity to end of task upon end spurt. Perceptual and Motor Skills 36:363, 1973

81. Mackworth JF: The effect of signal rate on performance in two kinds of vigilance task. Human Factors 10:11, 1968

82. Guralnick MJ: Effects of event rate and signal difficulty on observing responses and detection measures in vigilance. J Exper Psych 99:261, 1973

83. Gould JD, Schaffer A: The effects of divided attention on visual monitoring of multi-channel displays. Human Factors 9:191, 1967

84. Davenport WG: Vigilance and arousal: Effects of different types of background stimulation. J Psych 82:339, 1972

85. Wolf RH, Weiner FF: Effects of four noise conditions on arithmetic performance. Perceptual and Motor Skills 35:928, 1972

86. Bruce DL, Bach MJ: Psychological studies of human performance as affected by traces of enflurane and nitrous oxide. Anesthesiology 42:194, 1975

87. Gamberale F, Svensson G: The effect of anaesthetic gases on the psychomotor and perceptual functions of anaesthetic nurses. Work Environment Health 11:108, 1974

88. Kortilla K Pfaffli P, Linnoila M et al: Operating room nurses' psychomotor and driving skills after occupational exposure to halothane and nitrous oxide. Acta Anaesthesiol Scand 22:33, 1978

89. Kendall J: Vision considerations for the anesthesia machine operator. J Assoc Nurse Anesth 54:225, 1986

90. McIntyre JWR: Man-machine interface: The position of the anaesthesia machine in the operating room. Can Anaesth Soc J 29:74, 1982

91. Drui AB, Behm RJ, Martin WE: Predesign investigation of the anesthesia operational environment. Anesth Analg 52:584, 1973.

92. Jerison HJ, Pickett RM: Vigilance: A review and reevaluation. Human Factors 5:221, 1963

93. Human engineering design criteria for military systems. US Army Missile Command Standard MIL-STD-1472C

94. Boquet G, Bushman JA, Davenport HT: The anaesthetic machine—A study of function and design. Br J Anaesth 52:61, 1980

95. Cooper JB, Newbower RS, Moore JW et al: A new anesthesia delivery system. Anesthesiology 49:310, 1978

96. Arnell WJ, Schultz DG: Computers in anesthesiology—A look ahead. Med Instr 17:393, 1983

97. Smith NT, Quinn ML, Flick J: Automatic control in anesthesia: A comparison in performance between the anesthetist and the machine. Anesth Analg 63:715, 1984

98. Kraft HH, Lees DE: Closing the loop: How near is automated anesthesia? South Med J 77:7, 1984

99. Denisco RA, Drummond JN, Gravenstein JS: Effect of fatigue on performance of a simulated anesthetic task. Anesthesiology 61:A467, 1984

100. Narang V, Laycock JRD: Psychomotor testing of on-call residents. Anaesthesia 41:868, 1986

101. Wallace-Barnhill GL, Florex G, Turndoff H et al: The effect of 24 hour duty on the performance of anesthesiology residents on vigilance, mood, and memory tasks. Anesthesiology 59:A460, 1983

102. McDonald JS, Peterson S: Lethal errors in anesthesiology. Anesthesiology 63:A497, 1985

103. Cooper JB, Newbower RS, Long CD et al: Preventable anesthesia mishaps: A study of human factors. Anesthesiology 49:399, 1978

104. Friedmann J, Globus G, Huntley A et al: Performance and mood during and after gradual sleep reduction. Psychophysiology 14:245, 1977

105. Valenti WM, Betts RF, Hall CB et al: Nosocomial viral infections: II. Guidelines for prevention and control of respiratory viruses, herpesviruses, and hepatitis viruses. Infect Control 1:165, 1980

106. Hoffman DC, Dixon RE: Control of influenza in the hospital. Am Intern Med 87:725, 1977

107. Immunization Practices Advisory Committee: Prevention and control of influenza. MMWR 36:373, 1987

108. O'Donoghue JM, Ray CG, Terry DW et al: Prevention of nosocomial influenza with amantadine. Am J Epidemiol 97:276, 1973

109. Hall CB: The shedding and spreading of respiratory syncytial virus. Pediatr Res 11:236, 1977

110. Gershon AA, Kalter ZG, Steinberg S: Detection of antibody to varicella-zoster virus by immune adherence hemagglutination. Proc Soc Exp Biol Med 151:762, 1976

111. Orkin FK: Herpetic whitlow. In Orkin FK, Cooperman LH (eds). Complications in Anesthesiology, p 706. Philadelphia, JB Lippincott Co., 1983

112. Juel-Jensen BE: Herpetic whitlows: An occupational risk. Anaesthesia 28:324, 1973

113. Rosato FE, Rosato EF, Plotkin SA: Herpetic paronychia—An occupational hazard of medical personnel. N Engl J Med 283:804, 1970

114. DeYoung GG, Harrison AW, Shapley JM: Herpes simplex cross infection in the operating room. Can Anaesth Soc J 15:394, 1968

115. Edell TA, Howard C, Ferguson SW et al: Rubella in hospital personnel and patients—Colorado. MMWR 28:325, 1979

116. Polk BF, White JA, DeGirolami PC et al: An outbreak of rubella among hospital personnel. N Engl J Med 303:541, 1980

117. Advisory Committee on Immunization Practices: Rubella prevention. MMWR 33:301, 315, 1984

118. Goodman RA, Carter CC, Allen JR et al: Nosocomial hepatitis A transmission by an adult patient with diarrhea. Am J Med 73:220, 1982

119. Favero MS, Maynard JE, Leger RT et al: Guidelines for the care of patients hospitalized with viral hepatitis. Ann Intern Med 91:872, 1979

120. Denes AE, Smith JL, Maynard JE et al: Hepatitis B infection in physicians. Results of a nationwide seroepidemiologic survey. JAMA 239:210, 1978

121. Dienstag JL, Ryan DM: Occupational exposure to hepatitis B virus in hospital personnel: Infection or immunization? Am J Epidemiol 115:26, 1982

122. Berry AJ, Isaacson IJ, Hunt D et al: The prevalence of hepatitis B viral markers in anesthesia personnel. Anesthesiology 60:6, 1984

123. Berry AJ, Isaacson IJ, Kane MA et al: A multicenter study of the prevalence of hepatitis B viral serologic markers in anesthesia personnel. Anesth Analg 63:738, 1984

124. Berry AJ, Isaacson IJ, Kane MA et al: A multicenter study of the epidemiology of hepatitis B in anesthesia residents. Anesth Analg 64:672, 1985

125. Fyman PN, Hartung J, Weinberg S et al: Prevalence of hepatitis B markers in the anesthesia staff in a large inner-city hospital. Anesth Analg 63:433, 1984

126. Malm DN, Mathias RG, Turnbull KW et al: Prevalence of hepatitis B in anaesthesia personnel. Can Anaesth Soc J 33:167, 1986

127. Chernesky MA, Browne RA, Rondi P: Hepatitis B virus antibody prevalence in anesthetists. Can Anaesth Soc J 31:239, 1984

128. Siebke JC, Degre M: Prevalence of viral hepatitis in the staff in Norwegian anaesthesiology units. Acta Anaesthesiol Scand 28:549, 1984

129. Carstens J, Macnab GM, Kew MC: Hepatitis B virus infection in anaesthetists. Br J Anaesth 49:887, 1977

130. Sinclair ME, Ashby MW, Kurtz JB: The prevalence of serological markers for hepatitis B virus infection amongst anaesthetists in the Oxford region. Anaesthesia 42:30, 1987

131. Janzen J, Tripatzis I, Wagner U et al: Epidemiology of hepatitis B surface antigen (HBsAg) and antibody to HBsAg in hospital personnel. J Infect Dis 137:261, 1978

132. Ahtone J, Maynard JE: Laboratory diagnosis of hepatitis B. JAMA 249:2067, 1983

133. Bond WW, Favero MS, Peterson NJ et al: Survival of hepatitis B virus after drying and storage for one week. Lancet 1:550, 1981

134. Linnemann CC, Hegg ME, Ramundo N et al: Screening hospital patients for hepatitis B surface antigen. Am J Clin Pathol 67:257, 1977

135. McCormick RD, Maki DG: Epidemiology of needle-stick injuries in hospital personnel. Am J Med 70:302, 1981

136. Immunization Practices Advisory Committee: Postexposure prophylaxis of hepatitis B. MMWR 33:285, 1984

137. Immunization Practices Advisory Committee: Inactivated hepatitis B virus vaccine. MMWR 31:317, 327, 1982

138. Dienstag JL, Werner BG, Polk BF et al: Hepatitis B vaccine in health care personnel: Safety, immunogenicity and indicators of efficacy. Ann Intern Med 101:34, 1984

139. Centers for Disease Control: Suboptimal response to hepatitis B vaccine given by injection into the buttock. MMWR 34:105, 1985

140. Francis DP, Feorino PM, McDougal S et al: The safety of the hepatitis B vaccine. Inactivation of the AIDS virus during routine vaccine manufacture. JAMA 256:869, 1986

141. Hadler SC, Francis DP, Maynard JE et al: Long-term immunogenicity and efficacy of hepatitis B vaccine in homosexual men. N Engl J Med 315:209, 1986

142. Immunization Practices Advisory Committee: Update on Hepatitis B protection. MMWR 36:353, 1987

143. Scolnick EM, McLean AA, West DJ et al: Clinical evaluation in healthy adults of a hepatitis B vaccine made by recombinant DNA. JAMA 251:2812, 1984

144. Brown SE, Stanley C, Howard CR et al: Antibody responses to recombinant and plasma derived hepatitis B vaccines. Br J Med 292:159, 1986

145. Mulley AG, Silverstein MD, Dienstag JL: Indications for use of hepatitis B vaccine based on cost-effectiveness analysis. N Engl J Med 307:645, 1982

146. Baker CH, Brennan JM: Keeping health-care workers healthy: Legal aspects of hepatitis B immunization programs. N Engl J Med 311:684, 1984

147. Dienstag JL: Non-A, non-B hepatitis. I. Recognition, epidemiology, and clinical features. Gastroenterology 85:439, 1983

148. Dienstag JL: Non-A, non-B hepatitis. II. Experimental transmission, putative viral agents and markers, and prevention. Gastroenterology 85:743, 1983

149. Immunization Practices Advisory Committee: Recommendations for protection against viral hepatitis. MMWR 34:313, 329, 1985

150. Gallo RC, Salahuddin SZ, Popovic M et al: Frequent detection and isolation of cytopathic retroviruses (HTLV-III) from patients with AIDS and at risk of AIDS. Science 224:500, 1984

151. Barré-Sinoussi F, Chermann JC, Rey F et al: Isolation of a T-lymphotropic retrovirus from a patient at risk for acquired immune deficiency syndrome (AIDS). Science 220:868, 1983

152. Curran JW, Morgan WM, Hardy AM et al: The epidemiology of AIDS: Current status and future prospects. Science 229:1352, 1985

153. Henderson DK, Saah AJ, Zak BJ et al: Risk of nosocomial infection with human T-cell lymphotropic virus type III/lymphadenopathy-associated virus in a large cohort of intensively exposed health care workers. Am Intern Med 104:644, 1986

154. Weiss SH, Saxinger WC, Rechtman D, et al: HTLV-III infection among health-care workers: Association with needle-stick injuries. JAMA 254:2089, 1985

155. The Cooperative Needlestick Surveillance Group: Occupational risk of the acquired immunodeficiency syndrome among health care workers. N Engl J Med 314:1127, 1986

156. Centers for Disease Control: Update: Human immunodeficiency virus infections in health-care workers exposed to blood of infected patients. MMWR 36:285, 1987

157. Baker JL, et al: Unsuspected human immunodeficiency virus in critically ill emergency patients. JAMA 257:2609, 1987

158. Centers for Disease Control: Recommendations for preventing transmission of infection with human T-lymphotropic virus type III/lymphadenopathy-associated virus in the workplace. MMWR 34:681, 691, 1985

159. Centers for Disease Control: Recommendations for prevention of HIV transmission in health-care settings. MMWR 36(suppl #2S): 3S-18S, 1987

160. Arden J: Managing patients with AIDS—Update. Anesthesiology 68:164-165, 1988

161. MacGregor RR: A year's experience with tuberculosis in a private urban teaching hospital in the post-sanitorium era. Am J Med 58:221, 1975

162. Walter CW: Cross-infection and the anesthesiologist: Twelfth annual Baxter-Travenol lecture. Anesth Analg 53:631, 1974

163. McCue JD: The effects of stress on physicians and their medical practice. N Engl J Med 306:458, 1982

164. Crump JH: Review of stress in air traffic control: Its measurement and effects. Aviat Space Environ Med 50:243, 1979

165. Melton CE, Smith RC, McKenzie JM, et al: Stress in air traffic personnel: Low density towers and flight service stations. Aviat Space Environ Med 49:724, 1978

166. Clarke TZ, Maniscalco WM, Taylor-Brown S et al: Job satisfaction and stress among neonatologists. Pediatrics 74:52, 1984

167. Mawardi BH: Satisfactions, dissatisfactions, and causes of stress in medical practice. JAMA 241:1483, 1979

168. Toung TJK, Donham RT, Rogers MC: The stress of giving anesthesia on the electrocardiogram (ECG) of anesthesiologists. Anesthesiology 61:A465, 1984

169. Azar I, Sophie S, Lear E: The cardiovascular response of anesthesiologists during induction of anesthesia. Anesthesiology 63:A76, 1985

170. Modell JH: Who is captain of the anesthesia ship? Arch Surg 121:753, 1986

171. Pinnock CA, Elling AE, Eastley RJ et al: Anxiety levels in junior anaesthetists during early training. Anaesthesia 41:258, 1986

172. Vaillant GE, Sobowale NC, McArthur C: Some psychological vulnerabilities of physicians. N Engl J Med 287:372, 1972

173. Vaillant GE, Brighton JR, McArthur C: Physician's use of mood-altering drugs. N Engl J Med 282:365, 1970

174. Osler W: The Principles and Practice of Medicine p 1005. New York, D. Appleton & Co., 1892

175. Mattison JB: Morphinism in medical men. JAMA 23:186, 1894

176. Keeve JP: Physicians at risk: Some epidemiologic considerations of alcoholism, drug abuse and suicide. J Occup Med 26:503, 1984

177. American Medical Association Council on Mental Health: The sick physician: Impairment by psychiatric disorders, including alcoholism and drug dependence. JAMA 223:684, 1973

178. McAuliffe WE, Rohman M, Fishman P et al: Psychoactive drug

use by young and future physicians. J Health Soc Behav 25:34, 1984

179. Spiegelman GS, Saunders L, Mazze RI: Addiction and anesthesiology. Anesthesiology 60:335, 1984

180. Brewster JM: Prevalence of alcohol and other drug problems among physicians. JAMA 255:1913, 1986

181. Jones RE: Do psychiatrists cover up addiction of physicians? Psychiatr Opinion 12:31, 1975

182. Talbott DG, Gallegos KV, Wilson PO et al: The Medical Association of Georgia's impaired physicians program. JAMA 257:2927, 1987

183. Talbott GD: Elements of the impaired physician program. J Med Assoc Ga 73:747, 1984

184. Ward CG, Ward GC, Saidman LJ: Drug abuse in anesthesia training programs. JAMA 250:922, 1983

185. Gallagher W: The looming menace of designer drugs. Discover (Aug): 24, 1986

186. Gravenstein JS, Kory WP, Marks RG: Drug abuse by anesthesia personnel. Anesth Analg 62:467, 1983

187. Talbott GD: Alcoholism and other drug addictions: A primary disease entity. J Med Assoc Ga 75:490, 1986

188. Farley WJ, Talbott GD: Anesthesiology and addiction. Anesth Analg 62:465, 1983

189. Lewis DC: Doctors and drugs. New Engl J Med 315:826, 1986

190. McAuliffe WE, Rohman M, Santangelo S et al: Psychoactive drug use among practicing physicians and medical students. New Engl J Med 315:805, 1986

191. McAuliffe WE: Nontherapeutic opiate addiction in health professionals: A new form of impairment. Am J Drug Alcohol Abuse 10:1, 1984

192. Burrow BJ: The patient's view of the anaesthetist in an Australian teaching hospital. Anaesth Intens Care 10:20, 1982

193. Salmon NS: The role of the anaesthetist as seen by nurses in training. Anaesthesia 38:801, 1983

194. Linn LS, Yager J, Cope D et al: Health status, job stress, and life satisfaction among academic and clinical faculty. JAMA 254:2775, 1985

195. Goodwin DW, Davis DH, Robins LN: Drinking amid abundant illicit drugs: The Vietnam case. Arch Gen Psychiatry 32:230, 1975

196. Moleski RJ, Easley S, Barash PG et al: Control and accountability of controlled substance administration in the operating room. Anesth Analg 64:989, 1985

197. Adler GR, Potts FE, Kirby RR et al: Narcotics control in anesthesia training. JAMA 258:3133, 1985

198. Vaillant GE, Sobowale NC, McArthur C: Some psychologic vulnerabilities of physicians. N Engl J Med 287:372, 1972

199. Reeve PE: Personality characteristics of a sample of anaesthetists. Anaesthesia 335:559, 1980

200. Herrington RE, Benzer DG, Jacobson GR et al: Treating substance-use disorders among physicians. JAMA 247:2253, 1982

201. Morse RM, Martin MA, Swenson WM et al: Prognosis of physicians treated for alcoholism and drug dependence. JAMA 251:743, 1984

202. Lecky JH, Aukburg SJ, Conahan TJ et al: A departmental policy addressing chemical substance abuse. Anesthesiology 65:414, 1986

203. Canavan DJ: The impaired physician program: The subject of impairment. Med Soc NJ 80:47, 1983

204. Roeske NCA: Stress and the physician. Psych Annals 11:245, 1981

205. Duffy JC, Litin EM: Psychiatric morbidity of physicians. JAMA 189:989, 1984

206. Bittker TE: Reaching out to the depressed physician. JAMA 236:1713, 1976

207. Bissell L, Jones R: The alcoholic physician: A survey. Am J Psychiatry 133:1142, 1976

208. Clark DC, Eckenfels EJ, Daugherty SR et al: Alcohol-use patterns through medical school. JAMA 257:2921, 1987

209. Council on Mental Health: The sick physician; Impairment by psychiatric disorders, including alcoholism and drug dependence. JAMA 223:684, 1973

210. Canavan DI: The impaired physicians program. J Med Soc NJ 79:980, 1982

211. DeSole DE, Singer P, Aronson S: Suicide and role strain among physicians. Int J Soc Psychiatry 15:294, 1969

212. Cohen EN: Mortality among anesthesiologists. Anesthesiology 51:193, 1979

213. Helliwel PJ: Suicides amongst anaesthetists-in-training. Anaesthesia 38:1097, 1983

214. Council on Scientific Affairs: Results and implication of the AMA-APA physicians mortality project-Stage II. JAMA 257:2949, 1987

215. Crisp AH: Selection of medical students—Is intelligence enough? J Royal Soc Med 77:35, 1984

216. Wohl S: Death by malpractice. JAMA 255:1927, 1986

217. May C: Doctor facing suit is found dead. New York Times Bl, November 26, 1986

218. Birmingham PK, Ward RJ: A high risk suicide group: The anesthesiologist involved in litigation. Am J Psychiatry 142:1225, 1985

219. Crawshaw R, Bruce JA, Eraker PL et al: An epidemic of suicide among physicians on probation. JAMA 243:1915, 1980

Chapter 5

Steven J. Barker
Kevin K. Tremper

Physics Applied to Anesthesia

Applications of the fundamental laws of physics are seen in every aspect of anesthesiology. An understanding of some of these basic principles facilitates the study of anesthesiology and makes clinical practice more rewarding, enjoyable, and safe. Classical physics is not difficult to understand—it is only the mathematical modeling of physical laws that may become complex. In this chapter, we will stick to the basics, explaining important principles both in words and in the language of mathematics. The mathematics will be kept as simple as possible, but they are the price we must pay to apply our basic principles to the solution of practical problems.

Each physical principle will be illustrated with examples related to the practice of anesthesiology. We hope readers will find these applications useful, both for their own sake and as aids in clarifying the underlying physics. Some examples are mathematically more complicated than others; the reader may wish to pass over some of the details of the more difficult ones. On the other hand, these details are presented so that the mathematically oriented reader can see fairly complete derivations of solutions to physics problems. Previous texts and chapters aimed at physicians suffer from an almost phobic avoidance of mathematics, making the physics seem unscientific or arcane. The only earlier physics text for anesthesiologists that we recommend is that of Macintosh,[1] which is limited mainly by being 30 years out of date.

It is traditional for physics texts or chapters to begin with a rather dull section on units and dimensions, running the risk of spoiling the reader's taste for the whole subject. Instead, we shall handle units and dimensions as they are needed with each topic, hopefully making their discussion more palatable by dilution.

CLASSICAL MECHANICS

BASIC PRINCIPLES—NEWTON'S SECOND LAW

The term *classical mechanics* is used by physicists to distinguish this field from quantum mechanics and relativity, neither of which has many applications in anesthesiology. Classical mechanics describes the motions of all types of matter (solids, liquids, gases) acted upon by various forces (gravity, electromagnetic, pressure). It becomes inaccurate for very small bits of matter (*i.e.*, atoms) and for objects with velocities close to the speed of light. Classical mechanics is subdivided into the mechanics of solids (particles, rigid bodies, vibrations) and the mechanics of fluids (liquids and gases). The early history of classical mechanics has been described by Dugas.[2]

All of classical mechanics is based on a single physical principle: Newton's Second Law of Motion.[3] In its simplest terms, this law is given by the equation:

$$\underline{F} = m\underline{a}, \qquad (5\text{-}1)$$

where $\underline{F}$ is the force vector acting on mass m to produce the acceleration vector $\underline{a}$. Acceleration is the time derivative of the velocity vector $\underline{v}$, that is, the rate of change of velocity. Force and mass, although well understood intuitively, are not so easily defined mathematically. One of Newton's contributions to physics was to define these terms using his law of motion in the form of Equation 5-1. Note that force and acceleration are vectors, that is, they have both magnitude and direction. They each require three numbers to describe them, such as x, y, and z components in the Cartesian coordinate system. Mass is a scalar and is described by only one number.

Each time that we encounter a new physical quantity, we will define its units in the Système International (SI), or meters–kilograms–seconds system. English units and "practical units," such as millimeters of mercury, will also be used when appropriate. Hence, the SI unit of force is the newton, and the English unit is the pound. (Note that pound is a unit of force, not mass. This is one of many reasons why the English system is being replaced.) The SI unit of mass is the kilogram, and the English unit is the slug. Acceleration, the time derivative of velocity, has units of meters per second per second, abbreviated as m/sec^2. The English units are ft/sec^2. Note from Equation 5-1 that one newton equals one kg-m/sec^2.

There is frequent confusion between the terms *units* and *dimensions*, and the two are often inappropriately used interchangeably. A dimension describes the measure by which a physical variable is quantitatively expressed. For example, length is the dimension used to describe distance, height, and width. Units are specific ways of measuring a given dimension; meters, feet, furlongs, and light-years are all units of length. In mechanics, all dimensions can be expressed in terms of the three "fundamental" dimensions: mass (M), length (L), and time (T). In problems involving energy transport, a fourth dimension of temperature or heat must be added. Getting back to Newton's Second Law in Equation 5-1, the dimensions of acceleration are L/T^2, and the dimensions of force are ML/T^2.

Another common source of confusion in mechanics arises from the terms *mass* and *weight*, particularly in the English system of units. Mass is the property of matter that resists being put into motion, as expressed in Equation 5-1. Weight is the force exerted by gravity on a given mass. Weight is proportional to mass, with the proportionality constant being 9.8 newtons/kg on the earth's surface (32.2 lb/slug in English units). An object in outer space may have no weight, but its mass is the same as on the surface of the earth.

MECHANICS OF PARTICLES

The simplest applications of Newton's Second Law are those of known forces acting on particles, which are simply objects whose mass can be represented as being concentrated at one point. A particle's location at a given time (t) can be fully described by three numbers: the Cartesian coordinates x, y, and z. This may seem like an oversimplification in dealing with the motions of large objects, but Newtonian particle mechanics is accurate enough that it is used in virtually all problems of orbital mechanics. This includes predicting the trajectories of planets as well as spacecraft.

We begin with the simplest of all particle problems: one-dimensional motion of a particle of mass m. Suppose that the particle starts at x = 0 with velocity v = 0 at time t = 0 and is free to move in the x-direction under the influence of a constant force F. The particle's position (which we are trying to find) is given by x(t) at a given time t. Its velocity is v = dx/dt, and its acceleration is the second derivative of x(t):

$$a = \frac{dv}{dt} = \frac{d^2x}{dt^2}.$$ (5-2)

If F is a constant, then Equation 5-1 simply reduces to

$$F = m\frac{d^2x}{dt^2}$$

or

$$\frac{d^2x}{dt^2} = \frac{F}{m}.$$

Since F/m is constant, we can integrate twice with respect to time:

$$\frac{dx}{dt} = \frac{F}{m}t + A$$

$$x = \frac{1}{2}\frac{F}{m}t^2 + At + B.$$ (5-3)

Now, if we apply the two "boundary conditions" that at t = 0 we must have x = 0 and v = 0, Equation 5-3 requires that the integration constants A and B must both be zero. The solution to our simple one-dimensional problem is thus

$$x = \frac{1}{2}\frac{F}{m}t^2.$$ (5-4)

This solution by itself may not help us practice better anesthesia, but it illustrates the technique used for solving all problems in classical mechanics. First, we must write an "equation of motion" in the form of Equation 5-1, which requires a mathematical description of all the forces involved. Second, we must integrate this equation to obtain an expression for the particle's location. Finally, we must use the specified boundary conditions (usually the initial position and velocity) to assign values to the integration constants that arise in the second step. In complicated problems, the second and third steps may consist of millions of calculations performed by a digital computer.

It is convenient to use the aforementioned example to introduce the concepts of momentum and kinetic energy. Newton defined momentum as the product of an object's mass and its velocity, or

$$\underline{P} = m\underline{v}.$$ (5-5)

The dimensions of momentum are ML/T, and the SI units are kg-m/sec. Note that the momentum $\underline{P}$ is a vector quantity, as is the velocity $\underline{v}$. Newton's Second Law (Eqn. 5-1) can be rewritten in terms of momentum as

$$\underline{F} = \frac{d\underline{P}}{dt}.$$ (5-6)

The kinetic energy E of a particle is given by

$$E = \frac{1}{2}mv^2.$$ (5-7)

The dimensions of energy are ML^2/T^2. The SI unit is the kg-m^2/sec^2, which is called the *joule*. E is a scalar quantity; it has a magnitude but no direction. This distinction between E and $\underline{P}$ is important when we consider systems of particles or bodies. For example, two particles of equal mass and equal speed moving in opposite directions have a total momentum of zero, because the vectors cancel. However, their total kinetic energy is twice the kinetic energy of either one. Thus, the total momentum of all the molecules of gas in a stationary box is zero, but the total energy is the sum of all the E's of the individual molecules. This total energy defines a new variable, which we call temperature, to be discussed subsequently.

Another important concept in mechanics is that of *work*,

defined as force times the distance over which the force acts:

$$W = Fd. \qquad (5\text{-}8)$$

(F is used without underscore here to designate the magnitude of the force rather than the force vector.) The dimensions of work are force times length, which from $\underline{F} = m\underline{a}$ is equivalent to ML^2/T^2—the same dimensions as energy! Let us look back at the example of linear motion under a constant force. We found that in time t, the particle reaches a velocity of $v = Ft/m$ and moves a distance of $(\frac{1}{2})(F/m)t^2$, so the work done in that time is:

$$\begin{aligned} W = Fd &= F \cdot \frac{1}{2}\frac{F}{m}t^2 \\ &= \frac{1}{2}\frac{F^2t^2}{m} = \frac{1}{2}m\left(\frac{Ft}{m}\right)^2 \\ &= \frac{1}{2}mv^2. \end{aligned} \qquad (5\text{-}9)$$

Thus, we have shown for this example that the work done on the particle is equal to the kinetic energy acquired by the particle. This statement is true for all forces, constant or not, and is a direct consequence of $\underline{F} = m\underline{a}$.*

Now that we understand work and kinetic energy, we will introduce another important form of energy: the potential energy. The simplest illustration of this concept is gravitational potential energy. In a uniform gravitational field such as that at the earth's surface, the force of gravity on any object is proportional to its mass:

$$F = mg. \qquad (5\text{-}10)$$

The gravitational constant g equals 9.8 newtons/kg (32.2 lb/slug) at the earth's surface. If we lift an object of mass m to a height z above its origin, we must do work given by

$$W = Fd = mgz. \qquad (5\text{-}11)$$

What happens to the energy represented by this amount of work? It is stored in the form of "gravitational potential energy," which can be converted into kinetic energy simply by letting the mass fall back to its origin; that is, when the mass falls to $z = 0$, its velocity will be such that the kinetic energy (E) equals the previous potential energy (U):

$$E = U$$
$$\frac{1}{2}mv^2 = mgz,$$
$$v = \sqrt{2gz}. \qquad (5\text{-}12)$$

The same result could be obtained by applying $F = ma$ directly to this problem.

Potential energy is thus a form of stored energy that can be exchanged for kinetic energy or used to do work. In systems in which energy cannot be lost in other forms, such as heat or radiation, the sum of the kinetic and potential energies will be constant:

total energy $= U + E =$ constant. $\qquad (5\text{-}13)$

Potential energy can be found in the operating room in many forms. For example, a great deal of energy is stored in a cylinder filled with oxygen at a pressure of 2,100 lb/sq inch. Relatively little energy would be stored in the same cylinder filled with water at the same pressure. Why?

EXAMPLE: THE HARMONIC OSCILLATOR AND ARTERIAL PRESSURE MEASUREMENT

Now we shall use simple particle dynamics to investigate a problem of practical importance to all anesthesiologists: How to interpret intraarterial pressure waveforms. The moving particle, just discussed, was acted upon by a constant force $\underline{F}$. Suppose instead that this particle is acted on by an oscillating external force given by

$$F = A \sin(\omega t).$$

Furthermore, suppose that the particle is tethered by a spring and its motions are resisted by a damper (Fig. 5-1). The spring force, assuming a linear "Hooke's Law" spring, is given by

$$F_s = -kx.$$

The damping force is assumed to be proportional to the particle velocity:

$$F_d = -c\left(\frac{dx}{dt}\right).$$

The spring and damping forces are both negative, because both forces tend to restore the particle to its equilibrium position at $x = 0$. Now we can write the equation of motion ($\underline{F} = m\underline{a}$) for this system by summing the three forces:

$$A \sin(\omega t) - kx - c\left(\frac{dx}{dt}\right) = m\left(\frac{d^2x}{dt^2}\right)$$

or, by transposing the terms:

$$m\left(\frac{d^2x}{dt^2}\right) + c\left(\frac{dx}{dt}\right) + kx = A \sin(\omega t). \qquad (5\text{-}14)$$

---

*In the case of a force that varies with x, the expression for work $W = Fd$ is replaced by the integral expression:

$$W = \int F(x)dx,$$

where the limits of integration are defined by the distance over which the force acts.

FIG. 5-1. The forced simple harmonic oscillator. Mass M is acted upon by driving force $F = A \sin(\omega t)$, spring force $F_s = -kx$, and damping force $F_d = -c(dx/dt)$.

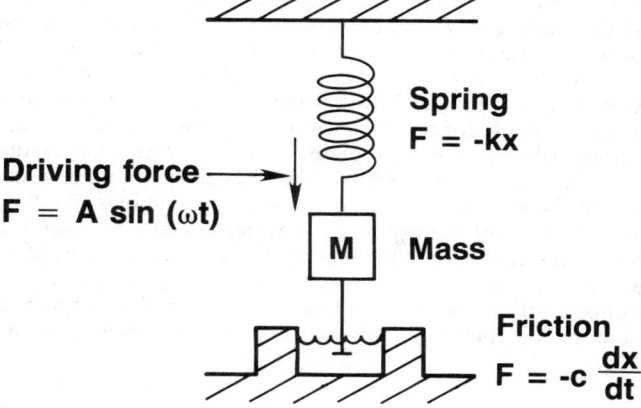

This differential equation is called the *forced harmonic oscillator equation*. It is a second-order (it contains a second derivative), linear (the unknown x appears only once in each term), ordinary differential equation. The solution is:

$$x(t) = D \sin(\omega t + \phi), \qquad (5\text{-}15)$$

where the motion amplitude D is given by

$$D = \frac{A/k}{\sqrt{\left(1 - \frac{\omega^2}{\omega_0^2}\right)^2 + 4\zeta^2 \omega^2/\omega_0^2}}. \qquad (5\text{-}16)$$

In Equation 5-16, ω_0 is the "resonant angular* frequency," given by

$$\omega_0 = \sqrt{\frac{k}{m}} \qquad (5\text{-}17)$$

and ζ is the "damping coefficient," given by

$$\zeta = \frac{c}{\sqrt{2km}}. \qquad (5\text{-}18)$$

The phase angle ϕ in Equation 5-15 is given by another complicated expression that is not important to us here. Figure 5-2 shows a series of plots of the motion amplitude D as a function of the driving frequency ω for various values of the damping coefficient ζ. Note that if there is no damping ($\zeta = 0$), the amplitude of oscillation will become infinite when the driving frequency equals the resonant frequency. As the damping is increased, the amplification that occurs at resonance decreases. The "amplification ratio," given by D/A, is approximately $1/(2\zeta k)$ at resonance (see Eqn. 5-16).

What does this have to do with arterial waveforms? A fairly accurate analogy exists between the forced harmonic oscillator and the commonly used arterial pressure monitoring system using fluid-filled tubing and an extracorporeal transducer. The mass m of the oscillator represents the mass of the fluid in the pressure tubing (from cannula to transducer) as well as the mass of the transducer diaphragm. The spring constant k represents the elasticity of the tubing itself and the compliance of the transducer, whose diaphragm has its own spring constant. The damping constant c is a measure of the friction in the system, which is mainly viscous friction from the fluid moving to and fro in the pressure tubing.

Using this forced oscillator model, we can characterize a catheter–transducer system by two quantities: the resonant frequency f_0 ($f_0 = \omega_0/2\pi$) and the damping coefficient ζ. Gardner has measured these quantities for various systems; some of his results are presented in Table 5-1.[4] Typical clinical systems have damping coefficients of 0.2 to 0.3 and resonant frequencies as low as 10 Hz. This implies a maximal amplification factor of about 2.0 at resonance (Fig. 5-2). If resonance occurs at 10 Hz (or 600 cycles/min), one might conclude that amplification is not a problem. However, arterial pressure waveforms are not sinusoids. Fourier analysis, or representation of the waveforms as a sum of sinusoids, shows that they have significant energy at frequencies up to ten times the heart rate. It is these "higher harmonics" that are amplified by the catheter–transducer system, producing severe distortion of the waveform. Depending upon the shape and frequency of the "true" arterial waveform, this distortion can

* Angular frequency ω is related to ordinary frequency f by $\omega = 2\pi f$.

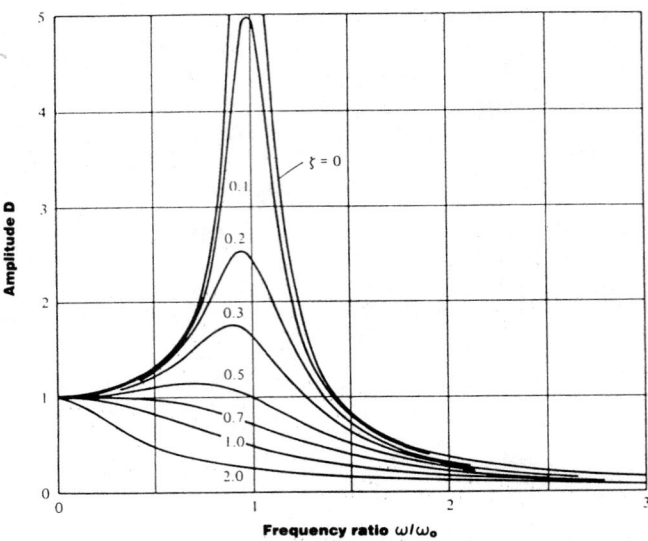

FIG. 5-2. Amplitude D of the forced harmonic oscillator *versus* ratio of driving frequency ω to resonant frequency ω_0. Curves shown are for different values of damping coefficient ζ. Note that for $\zeta = 0.2$ (clinical transducer systems), the maximal amplification factor is greater than two.

result in 20%–30% "overshoot" error in systolic blood pressure readings. Furthermore, the error is dependent upon heart rate, so that an error determined for a given patient at the beginning of a case may not remain constant.

What characteristics of the transducer system determine the f_0 and ζ values given in Table 5-1? Obviously, these are related to system mass, elasticity, and damping as previously described. A system with a longer length of fluid-filled tubing will have more mass and a lower resonant frequency f_0. Softer, more compliant tubing adds elasticity (lower spring constant k), which also lowers f_0. The presence of air bubbles in the tubing strongly affects both f_0 and ζ. Bubbles add elasticity in proportion to their total volume, thus lowering f_0. Large bubbles will also increase friction and thereby increase ζ. Both large and small bubbles must be carefully eliminated in order to obtain the f_0 and ζ values given in Table 5-1.

In the clinical setting, it is easy to determine the approximate resonant frequency of a transducer system. If the high pressure flush is turned on and then rapidly turned off while the pressure wave form is displayed at a high chart speed (50 mm/sec), the resulting tracing will oscillate through several cycles at a frequency near f_0. The damping coefficient can also be determined by the ratio of amplitudes of successive oscillations in this tracing. Thus, the solution of a basic problem in particle mechanics has provided us with a quantitative method to evaluate the performance of catheter–transducer pressure monitoring systems.

There are many intermediate and advanced texts on the mechanics of particles and rigid bodies.[5-8] In addition to Newton's *In Principia*,[3] the historically inclined reader should also see the works of Lord Kelvin.[9]

MECHANICS OF FLUIDS

The field of fluid mechanics has numerous applications in physiology, anesthesiology, and critical care. Here, we shall discuss some basic principles of fluids and illustrate each of

TABLE 5-1. Catheter–Tubing–Transducer System Characteristics*

NO.	DESCRIPTION	NATURAL FREQUENCY (Hz) f_0	DAMPING COEFFICIENT ζ
1	5-Fr two-lumen pulmonary artery HP transducer; dyne diaphragm dome	9.5	0.32
2	5-Fr two-lumen pulmonary artery HP transducer; HP diaphragm dome	10.0	0.30
3	4-Fr two-lumen pulmonary artery (47 cm); Bell & Howell transducer and diaphragm dome	12.0	0.30
4	6-Fr two-lumen pulmonary artery HP transducer; no diaphragm dome	13.0	0.15
5	5-Fr two-lumen pulmonary artery HP transducer; no diaphragm dome	14.0	0.25
6	7-Fr four-lumen thermodilution pulmonary artery (#1)	14.5	0.20
7	CAP† 18-ga with 24″ pressure tubing	15.0	0.72
8	7-Fr pulmonary artery (#2) (see #6)	15.5	0.20
9	7-Fr pulmonary artery (#3) (see #6)	14.0	0.32
10	Vinca‡ + 84″ pressure tube (#1)	16.0	0.10
11	Vinca + 84″ pressure tube (#2) (see #10)	16.0	0.20
12	CAP 18-ga direct	20.0	0.30
13	48″ pressure tubing direct	24.0	0.28
14	7-Fr pulmonary artery	25.0	0.15
15	Vinca + 24″ PVC pressure tubing	38.0	0.10
16	Vinca + 48″ PVC pressure tubing	45.0	0.13
17	Vinca + 24″ polyethylene pressure tubing	48.0	0.14

*Unless otherwise specified, runs were made with Bentley Model 800 Transducer without a diaphragm dome.
†CAP = 18-gauge CAP catheter—Sorenson.
‡Vinca = 2″, 18-gauge over-the-needle arterial catheter.

these with an application related to anesthesia. First of all, what is a fluid? By definition, a fluid is matter that "deforms continuously when subjected to a shearing stress." Visualize two flat, parallel walls with fluid contained between them (Fig. 5-3). If we exert a tangential (parallel to the surface) force on the upper wall while holding the lower wall stationary, we are creating a shearing stress in the fluid. Our definition states that the upper wall will continue to move, thereby deforming or "straining" the fluid, for as long as we continue to exert the force. This behavior is in contrast to solid matter, which, when stressed in this way, will deform a given amount and reach a fixed equilibrium shape. The amount of deformation is referred to as a "strain." In other words, shearing stress is related to strain in solids, whereas in fluids, it is related to "rate of strain." From this definition, we see that both liquids and gases are fluids. The difference between the two is that gases can be compressed by external pressure, while liquids are nearly incompressible. This should correct a misuse of terminology that is common in anesthesiology. We often say "fluid" when what we really mean is "liquid." For example, "Do you use air or fluid to test for loss of resistance in an epidural?" Air is a fluid, which makes this question irrational.

There are numerous texts, both old and recent, on the subject of fluid mechanics; only a few will be cited here. The reader who wishes a rigorous yet broad coverage at the intermediate to advanced level is referred to Landau and Lifshitz[10] or Batchelor.[11] Somewhat easier and more applied general texts include those of Streeter and Wylie[12] and Sabersky and Acosta.[13] For an excellent and very readable coverage of viscous flows, we strongly recommend Schlichting's book.[14] For

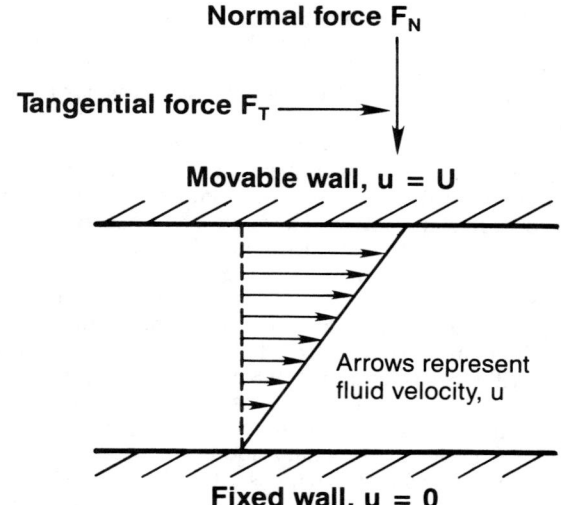

FIG. 5-3. Flow between two parallel plane walls. The upper wall is moving to the right at speed U; the lower wall is stationary. Arrows represent fluid velocity vectors at points between the walls.

the historically inclined reader, we suggest Sir Horace Lamb's *Hydrodynamics*.[15] The best introductory text in the field of compressible flow is that of Liepmann and Roshko[16]; we also recommend the works of Thompson[17] and Zucrow and Hoffman.[18]

INCOMPRESSIBLE FLUIDS

Incompressible fluids can include not only liquids but also gases in situations in which compressibility is not important. For example, the flow of air in and out of the lungs and through an anesthesia circuit can be considered incompressible for practical purposes, because the pressure variations in this flow are small relative to the total pressure of one atmosphere. We have not yet defined the term *pressure*; for this purpose we will consider nonmoving fluids, or the field of hydrostatics.

We defined a fluid as matter that deforms continuously as long as a shearing or tangential force is exerted. This means that if the fluid is not deforming, there must be no shear stress present. Therefore, a stationary fluid can have only "normal forces," that is, forces applied perpendicular to plane areas such as shown in Figure 5-3. If we divide this normal force by the area of the plane surface, we obtain the normal stress, or pressure. Pressure (p) is defined at a point by letting the area of the imaginary surface approach zero. Pressure thus has dimensions of force/area, which in terms of mass–length–time is M/LT^2. The SI unit of pressure is the Newton/meter^2, called the *pascal* (Pa). Since this is a rather small unit of pressure, we usually prefer to deal in kilopascals, or kPa. The English unit of pressure is the pound per square foot (lb/ft^2), although lb/inch^2 is often used for convenience. It is of value to remember that atmospheric pressure at sea level (called 1 *atmosphere* of pressure) equals 101.3 kPa, or 2116 lb/ft^2.

To complete our formulation of Newton's Second Law in fluids, we define the "density" (ρ) as the mass per unit volume of fluid. The dimensions of density are mass/volume, or M/L^3. The SI units of density are kg/m^3, and the English units are slugs/ft^3. Since liquids are nearly incompressible, their density is virtually constant except for a dependence upon temperature. (There are exceptions to this statement, called stratified liquids, that will not be discussed here). The density of water at room temperature is 997.8 kg/m^3, or 1.936 slugs/ft^3. A more practical unit of density in liquids is the gram/centimeter^3 (gm/cm^3), because the density of water is nearly 1.0 gm/cm^3.

The force exerted by gravity on an object is proportional to the object's mass, as shown above in Equation 5-10: F = mg. The direction of this force is usually chosen as the −z direction in a Cartesian system. The units of g are force/mass, or L/T^2 (use Eqn. 5-1 to convince yourself that these units are equivalent). At the earth's surface, g is equal to 9.8 newtons/kg, or 9.8 m/sec^2. If gravity is the only force acting on an object, from Equations 5-1 and 5-10 we have: mg = ma, or g = a. Thus, any object in "free fall" near the earth's surface will fall with an acceleration of 9.8 m/sec^2, as long as there are no other forces acting. For this reason, the gravitational constant g is also called the *acceleration of gravity*. Consider now a vertical cylinder of stationary liquid whose cross-sectional area (A) in the horizontal plane is 1 m^2 (Fig. 5-4). The height of this cylinder is z, and the volume of fluid within it is V = zA = z (because A = 1). Since ρ is the mass per unit volume of liquid, the total mass of liquid in the cylinder is m = ρV = ρz. The gravitational force on this mass (*i.e.*, its weight) is just mg, or ρgz. If the cylinder is resting on its bottom surface as in Figure 5-4, this weight is balanced by the pressure force p acting on that surface. (Pressure force = pA; A = 1 in this case.) Thus, the "balance of forces" in this statics problem is pressure force = weight, or

$$p = \rho g z. \tag{5-19}$$

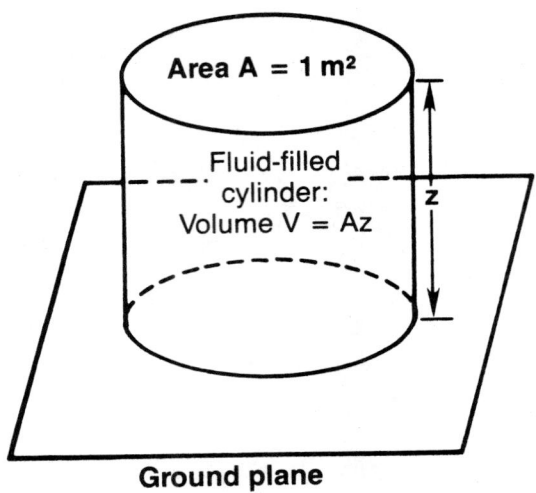

Ground plane

FIG. 5-4. Hydrostatics of a fluid-filled cylinder resting on a horizontal plane (gravity directed downward). The cylinder has height z and cross-section A = 1 m^2. It is filled with incompressible fluid of density ρ.

This equation is the basis of hydrostatics, the determination of pressures and forces in liquids at rest.

EXAMPLE: THE MANOMETER

A manometer is simply a vertical (or inclined) column of liquid used to measure an opposing pressure or force. Examples in medicine include the sphygmomanometer for blood pressure measurement and the water manometer for measurement of central venous or intracranial pressures. Equation 5-19 is a formula for manometer pressures. If the manometer contains mercury, the density ρ is 13,600 kg/m^3 in SI units (13.6 gm/cm^3, or 13.6 times the density of water). The manometer pressure is then

$$p[Pa] = 13{,}600 \times 9.8 \times z[m] = 1.333 \times 10^5 \times z[m]. \tag{5-20}$$

Remember that p is in pascals, and z is in meters here. We often use the millimeter of mercury, or torr, as a convenient unit of pressure. If we convert meters to millimeters and pascals to kPa, Equation 5-20 becomes p[kPa] = 0.1333 z[mm]; that is, 1 torr equals 0.1333 kPa (one atmosphere = 760 torr = 101.3 kPa). Manometer pressures using any liquid can be calculated from Equation 5-19 by substituting the appropriate value for the density ρ.

We will now discuss incompressible fluids in motion, or incompressible fluid dynamics. As noted previously, all equations of motion in classical physics are expressions of Newton's Second Law, $\underline{F} = ma$. In fluids, these equations can appear complex because of the coordinate systems used and the various forces that can come into play. Fluid forces can usually be divided into three categories: gravity, pressure, and friction. We have already considered gravity force and seen that the force per unit volume is simply ρg, acting in the vertical (−z) direction. Pressure forces on fluids are actually caused by *differences* in pressure, expressed mathematically as the negative of the pressure gradient. This gradient is a vector in the direction of the maximal rate of increase of pressure whose magnitude is the pressure derivative in that direction.

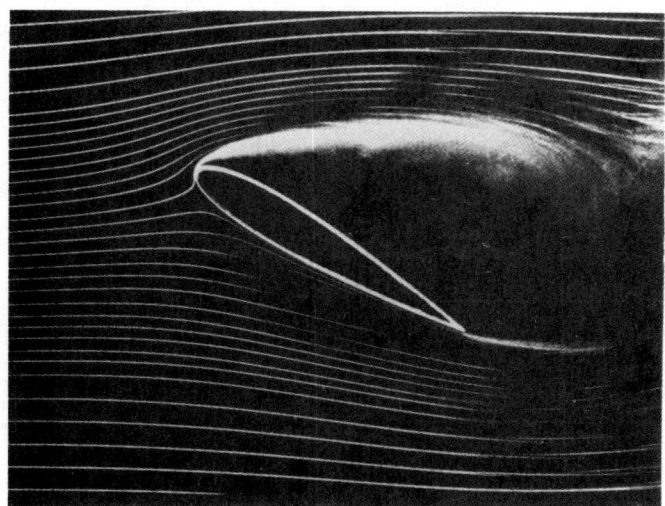

FIG. 5-5. Streamlines of flow approaching an airfoil at a high angle of attack, illustrating separation of flow from the upper surface, or "stall."

Cross-section #1:
Area A_1, Velocity U_1

Cross-section #2:
Area A_2, Velocity U_2

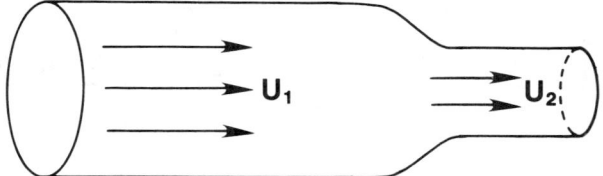

FIG. 5-6. Flow into a contraction. At #1, the cross-sectional area is A_1, and the mean velocity is U_1; at #2, the area is A_2, and the mean velocity is U_2.

If, for example, the fluid can move only in the x-direction (one-dimensional motion), then the pressure gradient is simply dp/dx.

Before we examine friction (viscous) forces in fluids, let us consider flow of an "ideal" or frictionless fluid, one that has zero viscosity. We define *streamlines* as lines in a moving fluid that are everywhere parallel to the velocity vector, as shown in Figure 5-5. For steady flow of an incompressible, inviscid fluid, the equation of motion can be integrated to yield:

$$p_0 = p + \frac{1}{2}\rho U^2 + \rho g z, \qquad (5\text{-}21)$$

where p_0, called the *stagnation pressure,* is constant along streamlines. U is the magnitude of the fluid velocity. Even though there is no such thing as an inviscid fluid, this Bernoulli equation can be applied to many flows in which viscosity does not play an important role.

EXAMPLE: FLOW THROUGH A VENTURI

Consider steady flow through a horizontal pipe of changing diameter as shown in Figure 5-6. Given the pressure p and velocity U at cross-section #1, find the values of p and U at cross-section #2. First, we can neglect gravity in this problem, since the pipe is horizontal, so the Bernoulli equation becomes:

$$p_1 + \frac{1}{2}\rho U_1^2 = p_2 + \frac{1}{2}\rho U_2^2. \qquad (5\text{-}22)$$

We also know that the volume of flow or "flux" (Q) at each cross-section must be the same, since no fluid is entering or leaving through the walls of the pipe. Fluid flux has SI units of m³/sec (dimensions L³/T) and is given at each cross-section by the velocity U times the cross-sectional area A:

$$U_1 A_1 = U_2 A_2. \qquad (5\text{-}23)$$

Now use Equation 5-23 to solve for U_2 in terms of U_1, and plug this expression into Equation 5-22, which we solve for $p_2 - p_1$:

$$p_2 - p_1 = \frac{1}{2}\rho U_1^2 \left[1 - \left(\frac{A_1}{A_2} \right)^2 \right]. \qquad (5\text{-}24)$$

Note some features of this result: 1) since A_1 is greater than A_2, the pressure falls as we enter the narrowing of the pipe; 2) for large A_1/A_2, the pressure drop is proportional to the *square* of the area ratio, or the fourth power of the diameter ratio; and 3) the pressure drop is proportional to the square of the velocity. We could just as easily make A_2 greater than A_1; then p_2 would be greater than p_1. Thus, pressure falls as pipe diameter decreases and rises as pipe diameter increases. This last statement violates some people's intuition—pressure does not always fall in the direction of flow!

This Venturi effect of lower pressure in areas of smaller diameter and higher velocity has many practical applications. It is used in an automobile carburetor to draw liquid fuel through a small orifice and atomize it. It can contribute to airway closure by creating lower pressures in regions of narrowing where velocities are higher. As expiratory flow velocity increases, the Venturi effect moves the equal pressure point, the point at which the pressures inside and outside of an airway are equal, more distally into smaller airways. These smaller airways are less well tethered and hence more likely to collapse, particularly in the emphysematous patient. We could also solve Equation 5-24 for U_1 in terms of $p_1 - p_2$ and thus use the Venturi as a flow meter; we can measure $p_1 - p_2$ with a simple liquid manometer.

The technique of jet ventilation (*e.g.,* during rigid bronchoscopy) makes use of a flow principle related to the Venturi effect. The high-velocity, small-diameter jet "entrains" the surrounding gas and sets it into motion in the direction of the jet. As we travel downstream in the jet flow, more and more of the moving fluid is entrained fluid that did not originate from the jet orifice but rather came from the gas surrounding the orifice. Hence, the gas mixture (in particular, the oxygen fraction) of the downstream flow in the trachea can be considerably different (*i.e.,* lower FI_{O_2}) than the mixture in the original jet at the orifice.

If fluids were really inviscid, we could use Bernoulli's equation on every problem, and fluid mechanics would be greatly simplified. However, friction exists in all real fluids and is manifested by the physical property termed *viscosity*. This important fluid property was defined by Newton,[3] using the same flow geometry shown in Figure 5-3. The upper wall in

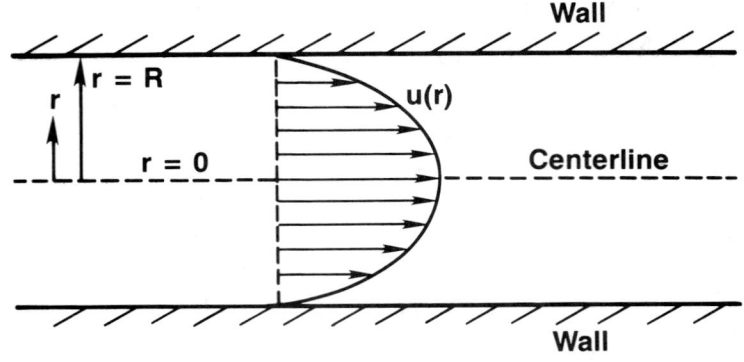

FIG. 5-7. Poiseuille flow in a tube of circular cross-section. The tube radius is R; the fluid velocity, at distance r from the centerline is u(r). At the tube wall, u(R) = 0. Arrows represent velocity vectors within the tube.

this figure has surface area A, is moving with speed U, and is separated from the lower wall by distance d. If the force required to move the wall is F, then Newton found

$$F = \mu \frac{UA}{d}. \qquad (5\text{-}25)$$

The force is directly proportional to velocity and area, and inversely proportional to the distance between the parallel walls. The constant of proportionality μ is called the *dynamic viscosity*. If we define shear stress τ as F/A in Equation 5-25, and replace U/d with the derivative of fluid velocity in the y-direction, we obtain

$$\tau = \mu \frac{du}{dy}. \qquad (5\text{-}26)$$

Fluids that obey this linear relation between shear stress and rate of strain (du/dy) are called *Newtonian fluids*. Note from Equation 5-25 that μ has dimensions of FT/L^2, or M/LT. The units of μ are kg/m-sec in SI, or slug/ft-sec in the English system. Viscosity is a function of temperature. In general, it increases with temperature in gases and decreases with temperature in liquids. Here are some sample viscosity values (in kg/m-sec):

air (20°C)	1.8×10^{-5}
water (20°C)	1.0×10^{-3}
SAE 30 oil (20°C)	0.26
glycerin (20°C)	1.5
blood (37°C)	$3 - 6 \times 10^{-3}$*

Now that we understand viscosity as a proportionality between shear stress and rate of strain in fluids, we shall consider a viscous flow of great physiologic importance: flow through a circular tube. The equation of motion for an incompressible, viscous fluid (called the *Navier–Stokes equation*) has a simple solution if we assume a straight, circular tube of infinite length (Fig. 5-7). We must also assume here that the flow is steady and "laminar," a distinction we will subsequently discuss in detail. Under these precise conditions, we can show that the flow velocity u at a distance r from the center of a tube of radius R is given by:

$$u(r) = -\frac{1}{4\mu} \frac{dp}{dx} (R^2 - r^2). \qquad (5\text{-}27)$$

Note that the velocity is proportional to the pressure gradient

*The viscosity of blood depends upon the shear rate, which means that blood is a non-Newtonian fluid.

dp/dx, is maximum at the centerline (r = 0), and is zero at the wall of the tube (r = R). The shape of this velocity profile (Fig. 5-7) is that of a parabola. To find the volume flow or flux Q through the tube, we simply integrate this velocity profile over the cross-sectional area of the tube (velocity × area = volume flow). The result is the so-called Hagen–Poiseuille Law of Friction:

$$Q = \frac{\pi R^4}{8\mu} \left(-\frac{dp}{dx} \right). \qquad (5\text{-}28)$$

This famous "R to the fourth law" is often incorrectly applied in medicine, as we will see subsequently. Note some characteristics of this formula: flow is directly proportional to the pressure drop along the tube (the negative pressure gradient); it is proportional to the fourth power of tube radius; and it is inversely proportional to the viscosity.

EXAMPLE: FLOW THROUGH AN INTRAVENOUS CANNULA

Consider a 20-gauge (inside radius = 3.81×10^{-4} m) 2-inch long (0.0508 m) cannula connected to a bag of normal saline, which is at a height of 0.8 m above the end of the cannula. The viscosity of saline is very near that of water, 1.0×10^{-3} kg/m-sec. We neglect the pressure loss through the supply tubing, because the diameter of this tubing is much greater than that of the cannula. The pressure at the upstream (proximal) end of the cannula is thus given by our manometer formula [Eqn. 5-19]:

$$p = \rho g z = (1{,}000 \text{ kg/m}^3)(9.8 \text{ m/sec}^2)(0.8 \text{ m})$$
$$= 7{,}840 \text{ pa} = 7.84 \text{ kPa}.$$

This pressure would be measured relative to a pressure of one atmosphere (the pressure exerted on the upper surface of the saline solution); thus, we refer to it as a *gauge pressure*. The pressure gradient along the cannula is simply the pressure drop along its length divided by the length:

$$dp/dx = (7{,}840 \text{ Pa})/(0.0508 \text{ m}) = 1.54 \times 10^5 \text{ Pa/m}.$$

We have assumed atmospheric pressure at the downstream (distal) end of the cannula. Now we can apply the Hagen–Poiseuille Law (Eqn. 5-28) to predict the flow Q:

$$Q = (3.142)(3.81 \times 10^{-4} \text{ m})^4/(8 \times 1.0 \times 10^{-3} \text{ kg/m-sec})$$
$$\times (1.54 \times 10^5 \text{ Pa/m})$$
$$= 1.27 \times 10^{-6} \text{ m}^3/\text{sec} = 1.27 \text{ ml/sec} = 76 \text{ ml/min}.$$

Comparing this with experimental data, we find that the actual flow is about one-third less than our prediction. Equation 5-28 assumes ideal conditions: a perfectly round, straight tube with a smooth entrance, smooth walls, steady flow, and no turbulence (discussion follows). This formula will usually underestimate friction and thereby overestimate flow by amounts that depend upon the actual conditions.

The Hagen–Poiseuille Law says that flow will increase in direct proportion to the pressure gradient. However, if we continue increasing the supply pressure in a Poiseuille flow, we eventually find that the actual flow is increasing more slowly than we predict. From experiment, we know that above a certain "critical velocity," the flow will become "turbulent" (Fig. 5-8). Turbulence is characterized by a very erratic, unsteady motion of fluid particles with much mixing in directions perpendicular to the direction of mean motion. This is in sharp contrast to "laminar" flow, in which fluid streamlines are steady and there is very little mixing. The transition from laminar to turbulent flow usually appears fairly abrupt, so that any region of flow can be characterized as one or the other, as seen in Figure 5-8.

In 1883, Osborne Reynolds showed that transition from laminar to turbulent flow in a given flow geometry (e.g., flow through a circular tube) is determined by the value of a non-dimensional parameter called the *Reynolds Number*.[19] In general, this number is given by

$$Re = \frac{\rho UL}{\mu},$$ (5-29)

where U and L are a characteristic velocity and length for the flow in question. Note that this number is dimensionless, that is, the units in the formula all cancel out. For the Poiseuille flow that we have been considering, Re is given by $\rho UD/\mu$, where U is the mean velocity in the tube, and D is the diameter. Reynolds showed that for tubes of any size, transition to turbulence occurs when Re reaches a value of about 2,100. Once transition has taken place, the Hagen–Poiseuille "R to the fourth" Law is invalid and cannot be used. This is a common reason for the misuse of this law in medicine. In the 20-gauge cannula example given previously, the Reynolds number at our predicted flow rate is 2,111—roughly equal to the transition value of 2,100. This is another reason why the Hagen–Poiseuille prediction of the flow through the cannula is higher than experimental result. If disturbances are very carefully minimized, much higher transition Reynolds numbers can be achieved, up to 100,000 in tube flow. However, most flows in physiologic or anesthetic applications are not low in disturbance levels.

The exact equations of motion have never been successfully solved for any turbulent flow. We are forced to rely on experi-

FIG. 5-8. Laminar flow approaching a cylinder (visualized by dye streak) from the left, becoming turbulent in the wake on the right.

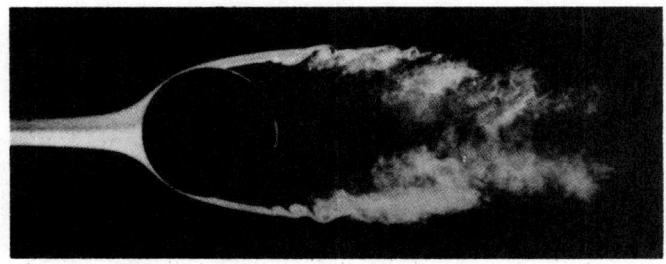

mental data and semiempirical laws to predict turbulent flow behavior. Let us consider again flow through a circular tube as an example. Suppose that we wish to predict the frictional pressure loss through an intravenous (iv) cannula for Reynolds number values at which the flow is likely to be turbulent. First we must express everything in a nondimensional form, so that we can use experimental results obtained in tubes whose sizes are different from our cannula. Since pressure has the same dimensions as density times velocity squared (see Eqn. 5-21), we can "normalize" the pressure drop per unit length of tube with the formula:

$$\frac{p_1 - p_2}{L} = \frac{\lambda}{D}\left(\frac{1}{2}\rho U^2\right).$$ (5-30)

Here, L is the length of the tube, D is its diameter, U is the mean velocity, and λ is called the *friction factor*. Note that λ is dimensionless.

According to Reynolds' principle of "dynamical similarity," any dimensionless coefficient in an incompressible flow is a function only of the flow geometry and the Reynolds number.[19] Thus, the friction factor λ for flow through a circular tube depends only upon the Reynolds number, Re. The relationship, as determined from experimental data, is shown in Figure 5-9. Also shown in this figure is the Hagen–Poiseuille Friction Law for laminar flow, which, when expressed in this form, becomes simply λ = 64/Re. It is often stated that friction in turbulent flow is proportional to the square of velocity. We can see in Figure 5-9 that this statement is incorrect for the circular tube. Although pressure appears proportional to U^2 in Equation 5-30, the friction factor λ decreases with increasing velocity, so that friction actually varies roughly as $U^{7/4}$ in this case.

As an example of a turbulent flow calculation, suppose that we wish to increase the flow Q in the 20-gauge cannula discussed previously from 76 to 200 ml/min. The cross-section A of the cannula is 4.56×10^{-7} m², which means that the required mean velocity from U = Q/A is 7.31 m/sec. This works out to a Reynolds number (Eqn. 5-29) of 5,570, well over the 2,100 value for transition to turbulence. From the experimental data shown in Figure 5-9, we predict a friction factor of 0.037. Using this value of λ in Equation 5-30, we find a pressure loss through the cannula of 65.05 kPa, or 6.65 m of water! We have had to increase supply pressure by a factor of 8.3 over the original value to produce 2.6 times the original flow rate.

EXAMPLE: ORIFICE FLOWMETERS

Most flowmeters used in anesthesia are based on known relationships between pressure and flow rate through an orifice, such as that depicted in Figure 5-10. The flow in the vicinity of such an orifice is almost always turbulent, because the transition Reynolds number for this flow geometry is less than 100. (Remember, the transition Reynolds number value of 2,100 is only for flow in straight, smooth tubes!) For the orifice, we use a formulation for pressure loss similar to that of Equation 5-30:

$$p_1 - p_2 = \frac{1}{2}\rho\frac{U^2}{C_d^2},$$ (5-31)

where U is the mean velocity in the orifice, and C_d is a constant called the *discharge coefficient*. We really want this equa-

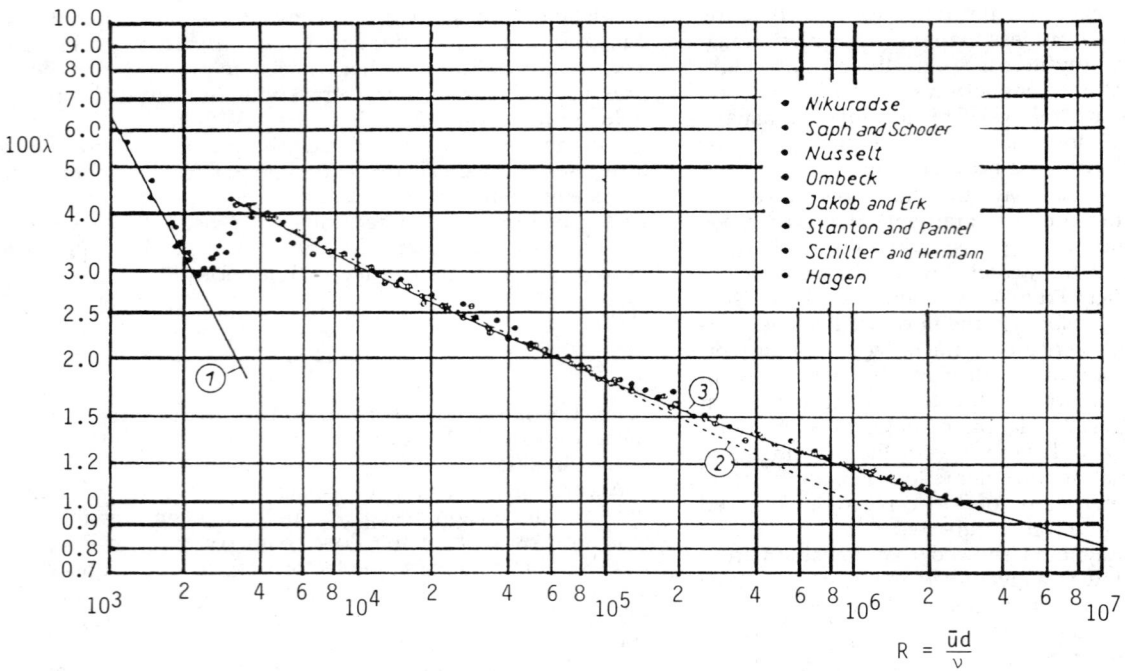

FIG. 5-9. Friction factor λ *versus* Reynolds number (Re) for flow through a tube. Experimental data from several investigators are shown. Curve #1: laminar friction predicted by Hagen-Poiseuille law ($\lambda = 64/Re$). Curve #2: Blasius' law for turbulent friction ($\lambda = 0.3164/Re^{.25}$). Curve #3: Prandtl's "universal" law of turbulent friction. Curves #2 and #3 are purely empirical best-fit relationships. (Schlichting H: Boundary Layer Theory. New York, McGraw-Hill, 1968.)

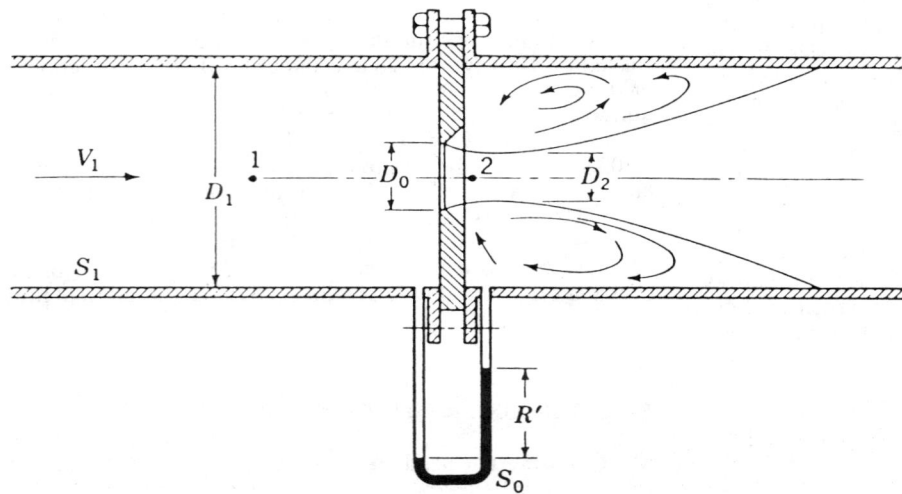

FIG. 5-10. Schematic of a fixed-orifice flowmeter. Orifice of diameter D_0 is located in tube of diameter D_1. The manometer height R' is related to the square of the flow rate Q (see text). Jet leaving orifice contracts to diameter D_2 (which is less than D_0); therefore, the discharge coefficient C_d is less than one.

tion to be solved for the flow Q, so we substitute U = Q/A and obtain:

$$Q = C_d A \sqrt{\frac{2(p_1 - p_2)}{\rho}}. \qquad (5\text{-}32)$$

As you might guess, the dimensionless coefficient C_d is a function of the diameter ratio D_0/D_1 (Fig. 5-10) and the Reynolds number. C_d is roughly 0.59 for D_0/D_1 less than 0.2 and Re greater than 10^5. Note from Equation 5-32 that Q is indeed proportional to the square root of p at high Re values where C_d is constant.

If we measure the pressure loss across the orifice of Figure 5-10, we have from Equation 5-32 a "fixed orifice flowmeter"; that is, the orifice area A is fixed, and the pressure is a measure of the flow. Another alternative using the same principle is the "variable orifice flowmeter," shown schematically in Figure 5-11. Here, the pressure difference $p_1 - p_2$ is fixed by the weight of the bobbin, and the orifice area A varies according to the bobbin height in the tapered tube. Gas flow meters currently used on anesthesia machines are the variable orifice type. As the flow through the meter increases, the pressure loss through the orifice (in this case, an annular space between the bobbin and the tube) increases and the bobbin rises. As it rises, the orifice area increases owing to the gradual widening of the tube, which in turn causes the pressure loss to decrease (Eqn. 5-32). An equilibrium is reached when the height of the bobbin is such that the pressure force on the bobbin is equal to its weight. Thus, each value of bobbin height corresponds to a specific value of flow Q.

The only physical fluid property appearing in Equation 5-32 is the density ρ; therefore, the calibration of the flow-

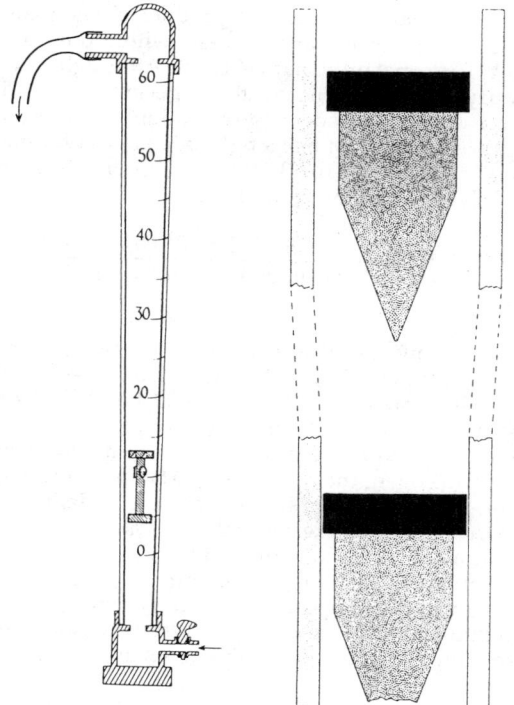

FIG. 5-11. Schematic of a variable-orifice flowmeter. Orifice area is proportional to bobbin height in tapered tube. (Macintosh R (Sir), Mushin WW, Epstein HG: Physics for the anesthetist. Springfield, Illinois, Charles C Thomas, 1958.)

meter should depend only upon density. However, remember that at lower Reynolds numbers (*i.e.*, low flow rates through the meter) the discharge coefficient C_d also varies with Re, which in turn depends upon the fluid viscosity μ. Thus, the meter calibration will depend upon both the density and viscosity of the working fluid at low flow rates, but only upon density at higher flow rates. A good example of this effect is seen with carbon dioxide and cyclopropane (Fig. 5-12). These gases have nearly the same density, but the viscosity of cyclopropane is 0.6 that of carbon dioxide. Thus, if we produce a flow of 1,000 ml/min of CO_2 through a cyclopropane flowmeter, the meter will indicate 1,180 ml/min, or a 12% error. However, if we reduce the flow to 100 ml/min of CO_2 (low flow and low Re), the meter will indicate 200 ml/min, or a 100% error.[1]

In our discussion of incompressible fluid flow, we have emphasized the use of the Reynolds number, because this dimensionless parameter enables us to compare flows that are of very different physical scales. In this way, the results of an experiment done in a tube that is 1 cm in diameter, for example, can be used to predict flow behavior in a tube that is 0.01 cm in diameter. Equations or formulae that can be expressed with nondimensional coefficients, such as the discharge coefficient C_d in Equation 5-32, are universally applicable because dimensionless coefficients do not depend upon which system of units is used. There are other dimensionless flow parameters that become important in types of flows other than those we have considered here. For example, in high-speed gas flows, we must consider the Mach number, which is the ratio of the flow velocity to the speed of sound.[16] In physiologic flows, and even in an anesthesia machine, Mach number is usually unimportant and the fluid behaves as though it were incompressible.

COMPRESSIBLE FLUIDS—THERMODYNAMICS

The term *compressible fluids* generally refers to gases, since liquids are usually considered incompressible. With incompressible fluids, the only variables we were concerned with were pressure and velocity. Since velocity has three compo-

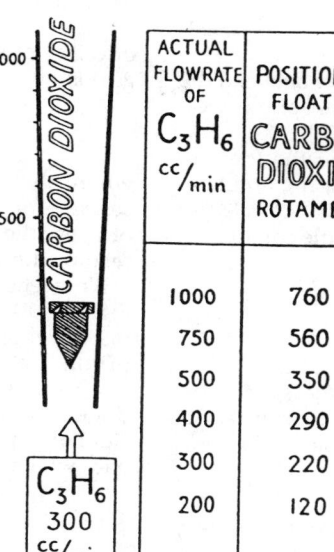

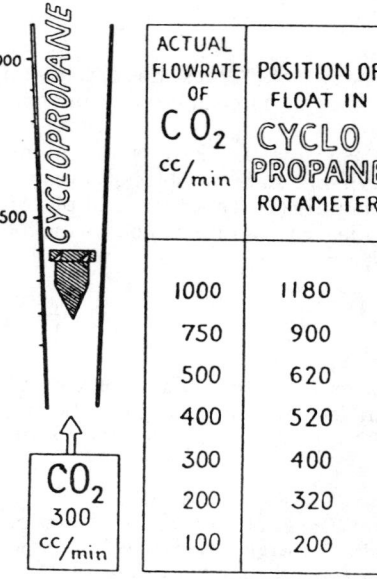

FIG. 5-12. Illustration of the effects of flowing C_3H_6 through a CO_2 flowmeter and *vice versa*. The two gases have nearly the same density, but the viscosity of cyclopropane is 0.6 that of carbon dioxide. (Macintosh R (Sir), Mushin WW, Epstein HG: Physics for the anesthetist. Springfield, Illinois, Charles C Thomas, 1958.)

ACTUAL FLOWRATE OF C_3H_6 cc/min	POSITION OF FLOAT IN CARBON DIOXIDE ROTAMETER
1000	760
750	560
500	350
400	290
300	220
200	120

ACTUAL FLOWRATE OF CO_2 cc/min	POSITION OF FLOAT IN CYCLO PROPANE ROTAMETER
1000	1180
750	900
500	620
400	520
300	400
200	320
100	200

nents (x, y, and z), we had a maximum of four variables. Now, with compressible fluids, we must also consider temperature, density, and "heat," which we shall define subsequently. Although these quantities all exist in incompressible fluids, they usually do not affect the motion. In gas flows, these quantities vary in both space and time, and they most definitely affect the motion. The study of heat and its interactions with other variables constitutes the subject of thermodynamics. Much of the original work in this field is found in the works of Carnot[20] and Planck.[21] A very readable if not recent short text is that of Fermi.[22] Several good intermediate and advanced texts are also available.[23–28]

Temperature and the Equation of State

Let us start with temperature: What is it? We already have an intuitive concept of temperature (T), but thermodynamics makes it a precisely defined quantity. According to the "zeroeth law of thermodynamics,"

> "There exists a variable of state, the temperature T. Two systems that are in thermal contact; i.e., separated by an enclosure that transmits heat, are in equilibrium only if T is the same in both."[16]

In other words, equal temperature is the condition that two systems in thermal contact will eventually reach if left alone long enough. By simple analysis, we find that this "equilibrium" means that the average kinetic energy of the molecules in both systems is the same. Thus, the temperature is really a measure of the mean kinetic energy of random molecular motions. We arbitrarily define an absolute temperature scale by

$$E = \frac{1}{2}kT, \tag{5-33}$$

where E is the mean kinetic energy per degree of freedom* per molecule, T is absolute temperature in degrees Kelvin (°K), and k is "Boltzman's constant" (1.38×10^{-23} joule/°K). Note that there is no thermal kinetic energy at 0°K, which corresponds to −273°C or −460°F. The "size" of a °K is the same as a °C, so that

$$T(°K) = T(°C) + 273. \tag{5-34}$$

The size of 1°C was chosen so that the difference between the boiling and freezing points of water at one atmosphere pressure is 100°.

For any gas, there is a relationship between the thermodynamic state variables of pressure (p), density (ρ), and temperature (T). This relationship is called an *equation of state*. An "ideal gas" is one that obeys the following simple equation of state:

$$pV = \frac{m}{M}RT, \tag{5-35}$$

where V is the volume of the gas, m is the mass, M is the molecular weight, and R is the "universal gas constant": R = 8317 joule/kg-mole-°K (8.317×10^7 erg/gm-mole-°K in c.g.s.)

*Degrees of freedom are modes of molecular motion that can carry kinetic energy. These modes can be translational (motion in the x, y, or z direction), rotational, or vibrational. The number of degrees of freedom depends upon the number of atoms in the gas molecule.

units). The number of gram-moles (n) of a gas is defined as the mass in grams divided by the molecular weight. One mole of anything contains 6.023×10^{23} molecules (Avogadro's number). Note from Equation 5-35 that 1 mole of any ideal gas at atmospheric pressure and 0°C temperature occupies the same volume, and that volume turns out to be 22.4 l (0.0224 m³).

Equation 5-35 gives us some important features of ideal gas behavior. For any isothermal process, that is, a change in which T is held constant, the product pV is a constant (Boyle's Law). For an isobaric process, where p is constant, the ratio V/T is constant (Charles' Law). Although real gases do not obey Equation 5-35 exactly, especially at low T and high p, it is usually a good approximation. As an example, let's calculate the mass of oxygen (M = 32) in a cubic meter at atmospheric pressure (101.3 kPa) and room temperature (293°K). Solving Equation 5-35 for m:

$$m = MpV/RT = \frac{(32)(101.3 \times 10^3 \text{ Pa})(1.0 \text{ m}^3)}{(8317. \text{ joule/kg} - \text{mole} - °K)(293° K)}$$
$$= 1.33 \text{ kg}.$$

By this same law, at 10 atmospheres pressure, our cubic meter would contain 13.3 kg of oxygen. Do this same calculation for an H-cylinder at 13,800 kPa (2,000 lb/in²), and you will find that the cylinder contains 9 kg of oxygen.

If we have a mixture of more than one gas, for example, oxygen and nitrogen, the concept of partial pressure becomes important. The partial pressure of each gas is defined as the pressure that would be exerted if that gas alone occupied the entire volume at the same temperature. Dalton's Law states that "the pressure exerted by a mixture of gases is equal to the sum of the partial pressures of all the components present in the mixture." Thus, partial pressures are additive, and they also obey Equation 5-35 if the gases are ideal.

Work, Energy, Heat: The First Law of Thermodynamics

We have seen that work and energy are related in mechanics; now we must understand this relationship in gases. We know that all matter has an internal "thermal" energy related to random molecular motions. This form of energy has been used previously in the definition of temperature; therefore, it can be thought of as a function of temperature. For a "calorically perfect gas," the thermal energy e (per unit mass of gas) is given by

$$e(T) = c_v T, \tag{5-36}$$

where the constant c_v is called the *specific heat at constant volume*. For real gases, the specific heat c_v is itself a function of T, and Equation 5-36 becomes a more complicated integral relationship.

Now let us consider the work done by an expanding gas in Figure 5-13. The gas in the cylinder exerts a pressure p on the piston whose area is A, thus applying a force F = pA to the piston. If the piston moves to the right by a small amount dx (dx is very small so that p remains constant), then the gas has done an amount of work dW = Fdx (work = force × distance). But Fdx = pAdx, and Adx is the change in the volume of the gas, which we shall call dV. Therefore,

$$dW = Fdx = pAdx = pdV, \tag{5-37}$$

or the work done by a gas on its surroundings is equal to the gas pressure times the change in gas volume.

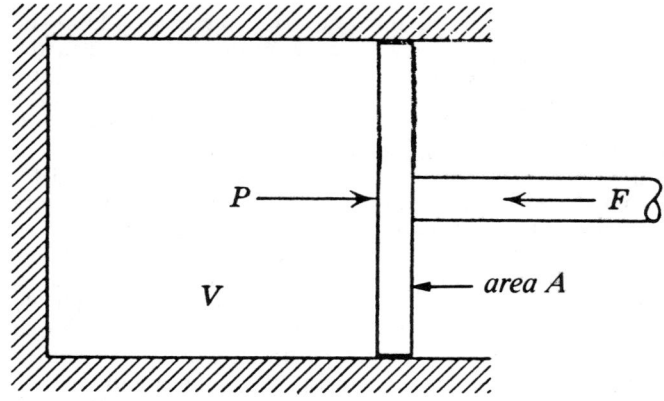

FIG. 5-13. Piston and gas-containing cylinder. Force F applied to piston of area A is opposed by pressure P (F = PA) in gas having volume V.

If the cylinder and piston in Figure 5-13 are thermally insulated, then no heat (which we are about to define) can get in or out, and the change in internal energy is equal to the work:

$$de = -dw = -pdV. \tag{5-38}$$

The minus sign is needed because dw is work done *by* the gas, which obviously results in a *decrease* in internal energy. We now define *heat* as thermal energy that can pass through the cylinder walls if they are not well insulated, and thus add another term to our energy conservation equation:

$$de = dq - dw. \tag{5-39}$$

This is the first law of thermodynamics, which in words says: "The increase in internal energy equals the heat absorbed by the gas minus the work done by the gas." Heat has the same dimensions as energy (ML^2/T^2) and can thus be measured in joules. However, it is more commonly measured in calories: One calorie is the heat required to raise the temperature of 1 gm of water from 14.5°C to 15.5°C. (1 calorie = 4.185 joules.)

An adiabatic, reversible process is one in which there is no heat conduction (dq = 0), and changes are made slowly.* If a gas expands or is compressed adiabatically, then de = $-$dw = $-$pdV. If that gas is also "calorically perfect" (see Eqn. 5-36), then

$$de = c_v dT = -pdV. \tag{5-40}$$

Now consider 1 mole (m/M = 1) of gas, and divide Equation 5-40 by the equation of state RT = pV (Eqn. 5-35):

$$(c_v /R)dT/T = -dV/V.$$

Recalling how to take derivatives of logarithms, we know that this equation implies

$$T^{-c_v/R} = (constant) \times V. \tag{5-41}$$

*Reversible means that local thermodynamic equilibrium is maintained during the change. Some authors include reversible as part of their definition of adiabatic,[22] whereas others refer to a process that is both adiabatic and reversible as being "isentropic."[16]

We can use pV = RT again to eliminate T from this equation, yielding

$$pV^\gamma = constant, \tag{5-42}$$

where $\gamma = (R/c_v) + 1$. If we define another specific heat c_p as "specific heat at constant pressure," it is easily shown that $R = c_p - c_v$ and, therefore, $\gamma = c_p/c_v$.

Why is this important? We all know that as a gas expands, it cools, but now we can see the difference between an isothermal expansion (which is hard to do) and an adiabatic expansion (which is much more common). In the isothermal case, pV = constant, so, if we double the volume, we would halve the pressure. In the adiabatic case, using oxygen ($\gamma = 1.4$) as an example, doubling the volume would multiply the pressure by 0.38. The pressure drops more in an adiabatic expansion than in an isothermal one, which is obvious because, in the latter, we must supply heat from the outside. In this same adiabatic volume doubling, the absolute temperature would be reduced by a factor of 0.76. Thus, if we started at 20°C (293°K), we would finish at −51°C (222°K)!

Phase Changes

Matter can exist in three forms: solid, liquid, or gas. Many elements and compounds can exist in all three of these states, depending upon the temperature and pressure. The different forms of the same material are called *phases*. Water is the most familiar example: It can exist as ice, liquid water, or steam. We know that at 1 atmosphere pressure, water changes from ice to liquid at 0°C, and from liquid to gas (steam) at 100°C.

What happens at pressures other than 1 atmosphere? The easiest way to understand this is through a pressure *versus* volume graph, in which we plot isotherms, or lines of constant temperature. A family of such isotherms is shown in Figure 5-14. Consider first the isotherm labeled g, corresponding to the highest temperature. As the gas is compressed (decreasing volume V), pressure p increases smoothly and continuously, and the substance stays in its gaseous phase throughout. If our substance were an ideal gas, curve g

FIG. 5-14. Isotherms on a pressure *versus* volume plot for a real gas. Region G—gas only is present; region V—vapor; region L, V—liquid and vapor in equilibrium; region L—liquid only. Isotherm "e" is at critical temperature.

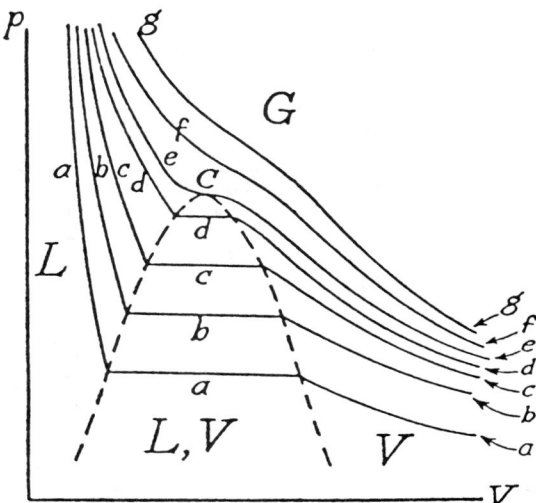

would be a hyperbola (pV = constant), as given by Equation 5-35. Now look at the isotherm labeled a, starting from the right at high volume and low pressure. As V decreases on this isotherm, p increases until we reach the area bounded by the dashed curve. At this point, some of the gas turns into liquid, so that we have both gas and liquid phases at the same temperature and pressure. The bottom of our container will hold liquid, while the rest will still be filled with gas, which in this type of equilibrium is referred to as a *vapor*. As we continue to reduce the volume V, the pressure does not increase (Fig. 5-14). Instead, we continue changing more of the substance from gas to liquid phase. As we move leftward on the isotherm in this region, visualize a steadily shrinking container filled more and more with liquid. When we reach the dashed curve again on the left side of Figure 5-14, the whole container is filled with liquid; there is no vapor left. We have "condensed" all the vapor to the liquid phase. As we try to further reduce volume, the pressure rises very steeply, because we are now attempting to compress a liquid.

The area labeled L,V in Figure 5-14 is thus a region in which liquid and vapor exist together in equilibrium. As we increase temperature (move to higher isotherms on Fig. 5-14), this equilibrium region becomes smaller until at the isotherm labeled e it disappears. This temperature is called the *critical temperature*, T_c, and it is the highest temperature at which the substance can be liquified by any amount of pressure. In other words, in the isotherms above e, the substance stays in gaseous phase at all pressures. Critical temperatures and other parameters for some common substances are shown in Table 5-2. Note that nitrous oxide (N_2O) has a T_c of 36°C, which means that at room temperature, N_2O can be liquified if we can apply the 51 atmospheres pressure required for the task. Oxygen, on the other hand, has a T_c of −119°C, which means that oxygen cannot be liquified at room temperature by any amount of pressure. Whenever a substance is in the gaseous phase at a temperature at which it could be liquified by sufficient pressure, we call this substance a *vapor* (region "V" in Fig. 5-14). The same substance at any temperature above T_c is then referred to as a *gas* (region "G" in Fig. 5-14).

In any liquid–vapor equilibrium (region "L,V" in Fig. 5-14), there is only one value of pressure possible for a given temperature. This is called the *vapor pressure*, p_v, and it always increases with temperature. For example, the vapor pressure of water at 20°C is 2.4 kPa (18 torr). At 37°C $p_v(H_2O)$ is 6.3 kPa

(47 torr), and, at 100°C, it is 1 atmosphere, or 101.3 kPa. The temperature at which Pv equals 1 atmosphere is called the *boiling point*. If we try to further increase T without raising pressure, the liquid will rapidly change to vapor, or "boil," until there is no liquid left. The boiling point of N_2O is −89°C (Table 5-2). The vapor pressure *versus* temperature relationships of some common substances are shown in Figure 5-15.

When we convert liquid to vapor at a constant temperature (moving to the right along an isotherm in the L,V region of Fig. 5-14), we increase the volume of our container while maintaining constant pressure. This means that the gas is doing work on the environment (dw = pdV, Eqn. 5-37). By the first law of thermodynamics (Eqn. 5-39), we know that heat (dq) must be added to the gas to accomplish this volume increase (de = 0 in this case, so dq = dw). The amount of heat that must be added per unit mass vaporized is called the *latent heat of vaporization*. It is a function of the temperature and the substance being vaporized. For water at 20°C, the latent heat is 580 cal/gm, whereas at 100°C, it is 540 cal/gm. If the latent heat is not supplied by the surroundings, then it must be supplied by the liquid itself. This is why open liquids become cooler as they evaporate. The rate of evaporative cooling is proportional to the vapor pressure (because higher p_v means faster evaporation) and the latent heat.

For the same reason, vaporizers for the volatile anesthetics tend to cool as they are used. They are therefore designed to conduct heat from the environment into the liquid to minimize the fall in liquid temperature. If the liquid temperature falls, the vapor pressure will decrease, as shown in Figure 5-15, thus reducing the amount of anesthetic being vaporized. Modern "variable bypass" vaporizers are temperature-compensated to correct for this effect, but older vaporizers such as the Copper Kettle and Vernitrol are not. During administration of ether by the open drop method (which a few of us remember), it is common to see ice crystals forming on the mask—an excellent illustration of the importance of latent heat of vaporization.

EXAMPLE: OXYGEN AND NITROUS OXIDE STORAGE

Now that we thoroughly understand gases, vapors, and latent heat, let us consider the storage of a gas and a vapor: oxygen and N_2O (Fig. 5-16). Oxygen is a gas at 20°C. It cannot

TABLE 5-2.   Critical Temperatures and Other Parameters for Common Substances

	MOLECULAR WEIGHT	DENSITY AT 20°C (gm/ml)	VAPOR PRESSURE PV AT 20°C (torr)	LATENT HEAT AT 20°C (Cal/gm)	BOILING POINT (°C)	CRITICAL TEMP T_c (°C)
Chloroform	119	1.49	160	64	61	260
Ethyl alcohol	46	0.79	44	220	78	240
Diethyl ether	74	0.71	440	87	35	190
Halothane	197	1.86	243	35	50.2	
Isoflurane	184.5	1.51*	239	41*	48.5	
Water	18	1.0	18	580	100	370
Carbon dioxide	44	0.00184	56 Atm.	35		31
Nitrous oxide	44	0.00184	51 Atm.	41	−89	36
Air	29	0.0012				−141
Oxygen	32	0.00133				−119
Nitrogen	28	0.00117				−147

* Values at 25°C.

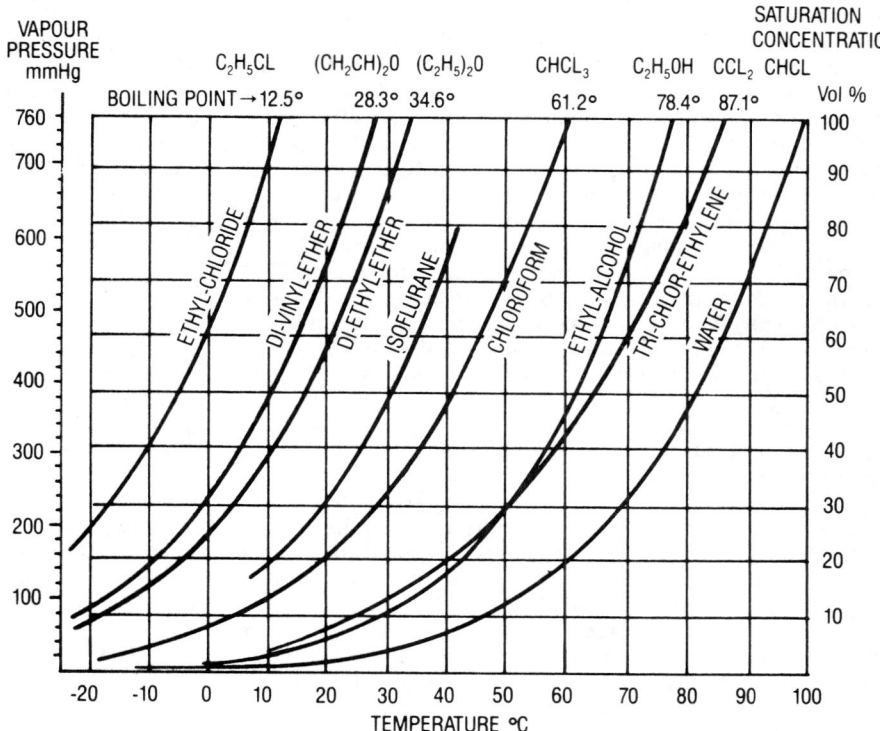

FIG. 5-15. Vapor pressure *versus* temperature curves for volatile anesthetics and other liquids. The temperature at which Pv = 760 mm Hg is the boiling point.

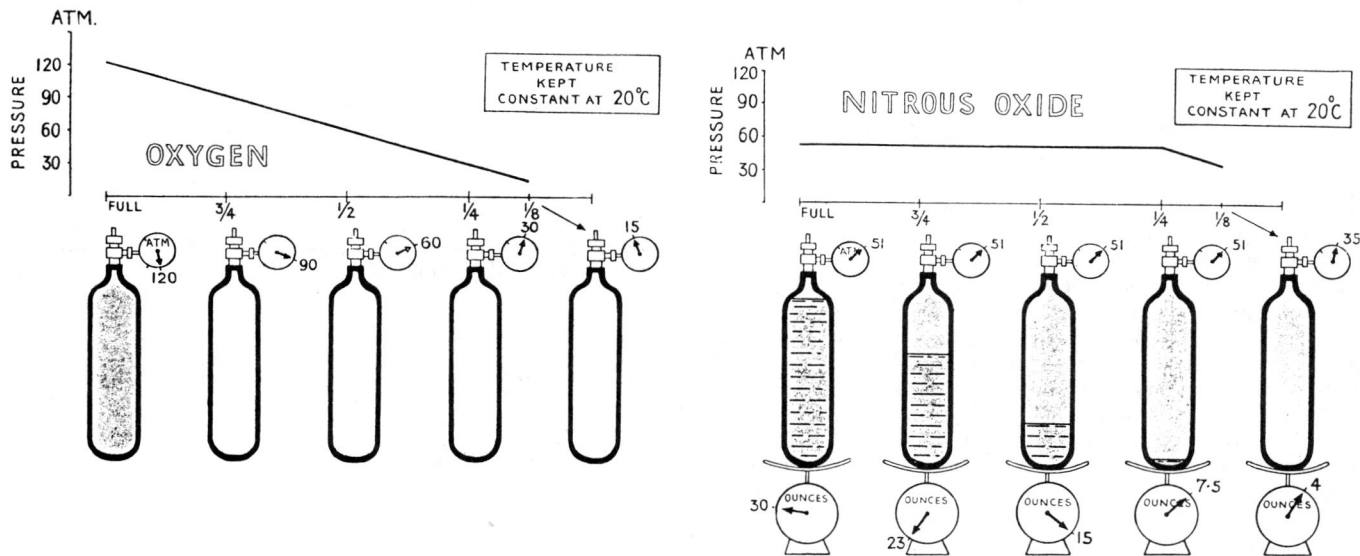

FIG. 5-16. Pressure cylinders containing oxygen and nitrous oxide at 20°C. The oxygen is a gas at all pressures at this temperature; the pressure falls steadily as gas is removed. The nitrous oxide is liquefied at 51 atmospheres pressure; as N₂O is removed from a full cylinder, the pressure remains constant until there is no more liquid in the cylinder. (Macintosh R (Sir), Mushin WW, Epstein HG: Physics for the anesthetist. Springfield, Illinois, Charles C Thomas, 1958.)

be liquified by any amount of pressure, because it is above its critical temperature. Thus, when the oxygen cylinder is "full" at 136 atmospheres (13,777 kPa, or 2,000 lb/in²) pressure, it contains twice as many grams of oxygen as it would at 68 atmospheres, and four times what it would contain at 34 atmospheres. In other words, the oxygen follows ideal gas behavior: pV = (m/M)RT. In contrast, N₂O is a vapor at 20°C;

it can be liquified by a pressure of 51 atmospheres (5,166 kPa, or 750 lb/in² at this temperature. Consider a tank filled to the top with liquid N₂O (Fig. 5-16, *lower left*). If we remove some N₂O from the tank, some of the remaining liquid will vaporize, and the tank will be filled partially with liquid and partially with vapor. The pressure in the tank will remain at 51 atmospheres as long as any liquid remains; we are simply moving to the right along one of the "L,V" isotherms of Figure 5-14. When the pressure does begin to fall, it means that there is no longer any liquid in the tank. Since the density of N_2O vapor at 51 atmospheres is less than one fourth the density of liquid N_2O, the tank is actually less than one-quarter full before the pressure begins to fall. A pressure gauge is not a good indicator of how much N_2O is in a tank, but, if the gauge reads less than 51 atmospheres, the tank is nearly empty. There is one exception to this behavior: If we rapidly take off some N_2O from the tank, the remaining liquid will be cooled by the effect of latent heat of vaporization. This cooling decreases the vapor pressure, thus lowering the tank pressure below 51 atmospheres while there is still liquid remaining. Of course the pressure would return to 51 atmospheres as the tank warmed up to room temperature again.

EXAMPLE: HALOTHANE STORAGE AND VAPORIZATION

How much halothane gas can we get from 1 ml of halothane liquid? Like nitrous oxide, halothane is a vapor at room temperature, but unlike N_2O, the vapor pressure of halothane at 293°K is less than 1 atmosphere (243 torr, 32.4 kPa, 0.32 atm.). This means that to vaporize all the liquid halothane in a closed container, we must lower the pressure in that container to 0.32 atmospheres. (Similarly, we had to raise the pressure in our N_2O container to 51 atm. in order to liquify the N_2O.) One milliliter of liquid halothane (293°K) has a mass of 1.86 gm, or 0.00186 kg. The molecular weight of halothane is 197. The ideal gas law (Eqn. 5-35) tells us the volume occupied by this mass of halothane at the given volume and temperature (SI units):

$$V = (m/M)RT/p$$
$$= (0.00186/197)8317 \times 293/32,392$$
$$= 7.10 \times 10^{-4} \text{ m}^3 = 710 \text{ ml.}$$

One milliliter of liquid halothane becomes 710 ml of vapor at room temperature and $p_v = 0.32$ atm.

If we mix this 710 ml of halothane with oxygen to obtain a gas–vapor mixture with a total pressure of 1 atm., we must supply 0.68 atmosphere (68.9 kPa, 517 torr) of oxygen to make up the difference (see Dalton's Law of Partial Pressure, stated previously). The gas–vapor mixture will occupy a volume of 710 ml at a pressure of 1 atmosphere and will consist of 1.86 gm of halothane and 0.642 gm of oxygen. (The last number is from Eqn. 5-35). We say that such a mixture consists of one-third halothane and two-thirds oxygen, because those are the proportions of their partial pressures and of the numbers of molecules of each species. Thus, if 100 ml of oxygen at 1 atmosphere passes through a vaporizer and becomes fully saturated with halothane, the mixture that emerges will have a volume of 147 ml, and the partial pressures of halothane and oxygen will be 0.32 and 0.68 atmospheres, respectively. Although it is often said that the oxygen has "picked up" 47 ml of halothane vapor, the halothane actually occupies the entire 147-ml volume, as does the oxygen.

Sound Transmission and Doppler Effect

Sound waves are small disturbances in pressure, density, and velocity that can propagate through all types of matter: solids, liquids, and gases. Sound waves cannot propagate through a vacuum. They are called *longitudinal waves* because

the motions of the fluid particles are in the same direction as the wave propagation, as shown in Figure 5-17. By contrast, surface waves on the ocean are "transverse waves" because the particle motions are mostly perpendicular to the direction of wave propagation. In gases, if the disturbances in pressure and density are small relative to their mean values, then sound waves of all frequencies will propagate at the same speed. For an ideal gas, as previously defined, it is easy to show that this "speed of sound" is given by

$$a = \sqrt{\frac{\gamma p}{\rho}}. \qquad (5\text{-}43)$$

We can use the ideal gas equation of state (Eqn. 5-35) to obtain another useful form of this expression:

$$pV = (m/M)RT$$
$$p = (m/V)(R/M)T = \rho R'T. \qquad (5\text{-}44)$$

Here we have used the fact that m/V is by definition the density ρ, and we have defined a new "gas constant" by $R' = R/M$. (Note that R' is gas species-dependent; it is not a universal constant.) Substituting Equation 5-44 into Equation 5-43, we have:

$$a = \sqrt{\frac{\gamma p}{\rho}} = \sqrt{\gamma R'T}. \qquad (5\text{-}45)$$

In other words, the speed of sound in an ideal gas depends only upon the gas properties γ and R' and the temperature T. For example, in air at room temperature (molecular weight 28.8, $\gamma = 1.4$):

$$a = \sqrt{1.4 \times \frac{8317.}{28.8} \times 293}$$
$$= 344 \text{ m/sec} = 1,129 \text{ ft/sec} = 770 \text{ miles/hr.}$$

FIG. 5-17. Sound waves generated by movement of a piston in a straight tube. The gas movement is in the same direction as the wave propagation, making this a "longitudinal wave."

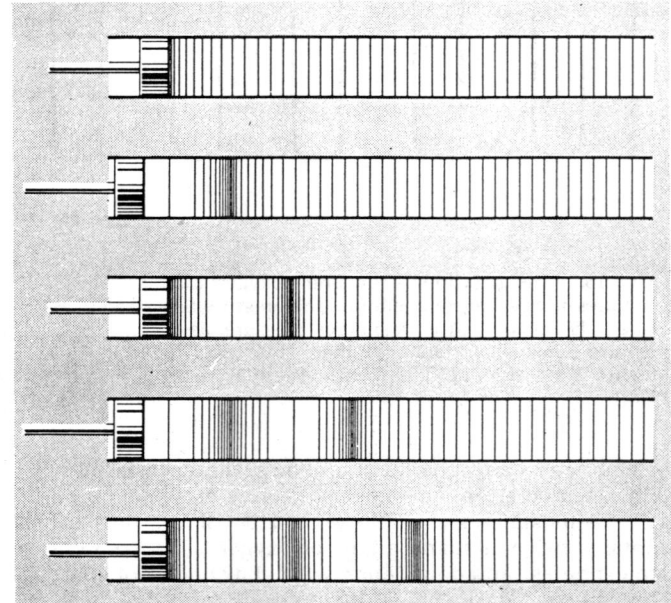

By comparison, at an altitude of 13,000 m (40,000 ft), the temperature is −57°C (216°K), and the speed of sound is only 295 m/sec (661 miles/hr). Speeds of sound in some common substances are given in Table 5-3.

We measure the amplitude of sound waves according to the root–mean–square (rms) value of the pressure fluctuation p′, which is called *sound pressure level*, or SPL. Since a very wide range of SPL values is common in everyday life, we use a logarithmic scale defined by:

$$SPL = 20 \log\left(\frac{p'}{p_0}\right). \quad (5\text{-}46)$$

The units of this scale are called *decibels*, and the reference pressure p_0 is chosen as the lowest sound pressure detectable by the human ear. This hearing threshold, at a frequency of about 2 kHz (kHz = kiloHertz; 1 kHz = 1,000 cycles/sec) is an rms pressure of 2×10^{-8} kPa (0.0002 dyne/cm²). Thus, a sound pressure of 2×10^{-8} kPa corresponds to an SPL of zero decibels (0 db), because $p'/p_0 = 1$ and $\log(1) = 0$. The threshold of pain to the human ear is an SPL of about 120 db, a level that has been measured frequently at rock concerts. Prolonged exposure to an SPL greater than 90 db will eventually result in permanent hearing impairment. Note that 100 db is a pressure 100,000 times that of the hearing threshold.

In 1842, Christian Johann Doppler described how the color of a luminous body and the pitch of a sound source are changed by a relative motion of the source and observer or listener. This "Doppler effect" has many applications in modern medicine and is worthy of a brief discussion here. If the source of sound is stationary (Figure 5-18A) and is radiating sound of frequency f, it is clear that the wavelength λ is given by

$$\lambda = a/f, \quad (5\text{-}47)$$

because the time between wavefronts is 1/f, and these fronts are traveling at the speed of sound a. Now if the listener is moving *toward* this stationary source at speed v_0 (Fig. 5-18A), he will be crossing more wavefronts per unit time than if he were standing still. His velocity relative to the moving wavefronts is $a + v_0$, so the number of wavefronts he crosses per unit time is

f′ = relative velocity/distance between waves = $(a + v_0)/\lambda$.

Since the sound frequency for the stationary listener (Eqn.

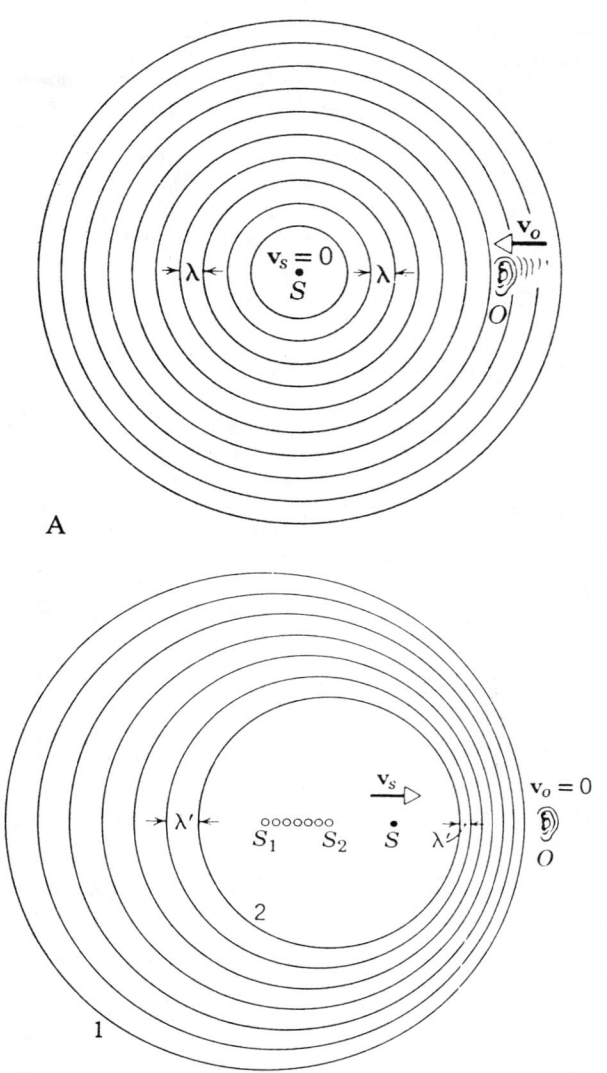

FIG. 5-18. (*A*) A stationary source "S" of sound being heard by a moving listener "0." The wavefronts are concentric circles separated by a constant wavelength λ. (*B*) A moving source of sound being heard by a stationary listener. The circular wavefronts are not concentric, and the wavelength λ′ depends upon the direction from the source.

5-47) is f = a/λ, the frequency f′ heard by the moving listener is

$$\begin{aligned} f' &= (a + v_0)/\lambda = f + v_0/\lambda = f + v_0 f/a \\ &= f\{1 + v_0/a\}. \quad (5\text{-}48) \end{aligned}$$

Thus, the listener's frequency increases by the factor $1 + v_0/a$. For example, if he is moving toward the source at one half the speed of sound, the listener hears a frequency 1.5 times that of a stationary listener. Similarly, if the listener is moving *away* from the source at this same speed, he will hear a frequency one half that of the stationary listener.

Now, suppose that the listener is stationary and the source is moving toward him at speed v_s. The wavefronts now have the pattern of Figure 5-18B, in which the wavefront labeled 1 was emitted when the source was at S1, and wavefront 2 was

TABLE 5-3. Speed of Sound

MEDIUM	TEMPERATURE (°C)	SPEED	
		Meters/sec	*Ft/sec*
Air	20	344	1,129
Air	0	331.3	1,087
Hydrogen	0	1,286	4,220
Oxygen	0	317.2	1,041
Water	15	1,450	4,760
Lead	20	1,230	4,030
Aluminum	20	5,100	16,700
Copper	20	3,560	11,700
Iron	20	5,130	16,800
Extreme Values			
Granite		6,000	19,700
Vulcanized rubber	0	54	177

emitted when the source was at S2. The source is following the rightward-moving waves, so that these waves become closer together. If the source frequency is f and the source speed is v_s, then during each vibration, the source moves a distance of v_s/f. (Remember, the time between vibrations is $1/f$.) Hence, each wavelength will be shortened by the distance v_s/f, so that the wavelength at the listener is $\lambda' = a/f - v_s/f$. The waves themselves are still traveling at speed a, so the frequency heard by the stationary listener is

$$f' = \frac{a}{\lambda'} = \frac{a}{(a - v_s)/f} = f\frac{a}{a - v_s}$$
$$= f\left[\frac{1}{1 - v_s/a}\right]. \tag{5-49}$$

If the source is moving at one half the speed of sound toward the listener, the apparent frequency will double. Yet, when the listener is moving at the same speed toward a stationary source (Eqn. 5-48), the frequency increases by only 50%. What happens if the source is moving faster than the speed of sound in Equation 5-49? The answer is that the small disturbance analysis of linear acoustics is no longer valid. However, one can intuitively predict the end result of all these wavefronts piling on top of each other near the source: a sonic boom!

In the Doppler systems used in medicine, we usually have a slightly different geometry. Here the source is a stationary transducer, the sound is reflected from a moving "target" (e.g., red blood cells) from which it returns to a stationary listener (the receiving transducer). This can be analyzed as a two-stage process in which the target is first a moving listener to sound from a stationary source. The target then re-radiates this sound as a moving source transmitting to a stationary listener. The result is thus a combination of Equations 5-48 and 5-49:

$$f' = f\left[\frac{1 + v/a}{1 - v/a}\right]. \tag{5-50}$$

Note that now if the target is moving at one half the speed of sound toward the detector, the observed frequency f' will be increased by a factor of three! Changes in the frequency of sinusoidal sound waves can be measured very precisely. In fact, the human ear can detect even a 1-Hz frequency change at 1,000 Hz. The Doppler principle is thus a potentially very accurate means of measuring the velocity of any moving object that will reflect sound. If relatively high frequencies (10 megaHertz or more) are used, objects as small as red blood cells will scatter enough sound for detection. The same principle can be applied to reflection of light, as in laser–Doppler velocimeters used to detect skin blood flow.

Example: Echocardiography

Modern echocardiography uses measurements of both amplitude and frequency of reflected sound waves to visualize cardiac structures and blood flow velocity. Sound waves in the frequency range from 1 to 10 megahertz are transmitted into the heart in short bursts from a piezoelectric transducer, which then "listens" to the reflected echoes between signal bursts. The speed of sound in the heart and surrounding tissues is a fairly constant 1540 m/sec, so that the time of flight between the signal burst and the received echo can be used to derive the distance to the reflecting structure. Strong echoes come from large changes in tissue density; lung (low density) and bone (high density) will therefore reflect most of the sound waves and must be kept out of the signal path. The sound beam is a very narrow "searchlight" pattern, so that the exact direction of the reflecting structures is known. If the beam is aimed in a fixed direction and the echo strength is displayed *versus* distance from the transducer and time, then the result is called an *M-mode* or one-dimensional ultrasound. Since M-mode only looks in one direction, it provides very limited information. On the other hand, it can sample roughly 1,000 times per second, thus providing excellent time resolution of rapidly moving objects (*e.g.*, a mitral valve leaflet).

If we vary the direction of the ultrasound beam by sweeping it through an arc, we can develop a two-dimensional echocardiogram (2-D echo) that shows the reflecting structures in an entire plane. The 2-D echo technique obviously shows us much more of the heart at a given time, but its time resolution is more limited in that it can produce only 15 to 100 pictures per second.[29-31] A new development in 2-D echo technology is the addition of doppler analysis of the echo.[32] Moving sound reflectors shift the frequency of the echo (as derived in Eqn. 5-50), resulting in a change in color on the display screen.

HEAT TRANSPORT

As previously discussed, heat is energy in the form of random molecular motions in matter. Heat transfer occurs from a point of higher temperature to one of lower temperature. Heat is transferred from one body to another by three mechanisms: conduction, convection, and radiation. Conduction requires that the two bodies be in contact, and convection requires fluid motion, whereas radiation can take place through a vacuum.

Heat can be conducted through solids, liquids, and gases. Illustrations of heat conduction are usually chosen with an opaque solid as the conducting substance, because, in such materials, conduction is the only method by which heat can be transferred. The basic equation for one-dimensional heat conduction is Fourier's equation:

$$q = -KA\frac{dT}{dx} \tag{5-51}$$

where

q = heat conduction rate in the x-direction (joule/sec or watt);
A = cross-sectional area for heat transport;
$\frac{dT}{dx}$ = temperature gradient (x-component);
K = thermal conductivity of the conducting medium.

The thermal conductivity K is relatively independent of temperature until the material changes phase. Conductivity decreases significantly as a substance changes from solid to liquid to gas, as shown in Table 5-4.[33]

For heat conduction through a layer of thickness ΔX, the rate of heat conduction is proportional to the temperature difference:

$$q = \frac{KA}{\Delta X}(T_1 - T_2) \tag{5-52}$$

TABLE 5-4.   Thermal Conductivities,
K at 300°K

MATERIAL		K WATTS/m-°K
SOLIDS		
	Silver	429
	Steel	15
	Skin	0.37
	Wool	0.04
WATER		0.60
AIR		0.026

(Reprinted with permission from Incropera FP, DeWitt DP: Fundamentals of
Heat and Mass Transfer, Appendix A, 2nd
ed, p 752. New York, John Wiley & Sons,
1985.)

Thermal Conducting Layers

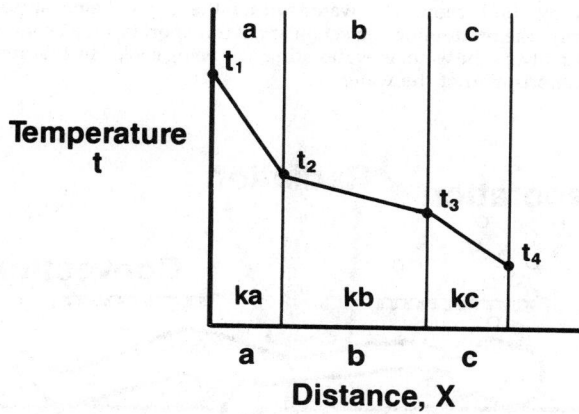

FIG. 5-19. Illustrated above is the temperature gradient for steady-
state heat conduction through three layers, a, b, and c, with three
different thermal conductivities, K_a, K_b, and K_c. Owing to conservation of energy, the heat conducted through each layer will be equal;
therefore, the temperature drop from T_1 to T_4 can be solved by writing
Fourier's Law of Heat Conduction for each layer and equating the
amount of heat transferred, q. Note above that layer b has the highest
thermal conductivity, as noted by the least rate of temperature decrease across that layer.

where

T_1 and T_2 are the temperatures on both sides of a layer
of thickness ΔX.

This one-dimensional, steady-state heat conduction equation
can be applied to a series of thermal conducting layers as in
Figure 5-19:

$$q = \frac{K_a A}{\Delta X_a}(T_1 - T_2) = \frac{K_b A}{\Delta X_b}(T_2 - T_3) = \frac{K_c A}{\Delta X_c}(T_3 - T_4). \quad (5\text{-}53)$$

The heat conduction (q) through layers a, b, and c must be
equal. Solving each of these equations for the temperature
difference and adding the equations produces the following
result:

$$q = \frac{T_1 - T_4}{\dfrac{\Delta X_a}{K_a A} + \dfrac{\Delta X_b}{K_b A} + \dfrac{\Delta X_c}{K_c A}}. \quad (5\text{-}54)$$

This equation can be used to solve for the temperature drop
across a series of thermal conducting layers, just as the voltage drop across a series of electrical resistors is calculated
(discussed subsequently). The term $\Delta X/KA$ is the thermal
resistance of the layer. The mathematics becomes more complex as the geometry becomes three dimensional instead of
one dimensional and as unsteady-state (time response to
temperature changes) solutions are required.[34]
    The heat transport associated with fluid motion is called
convective heat transport. If the fluid motion is caused by the
heat itself, it is referred to as natural convection. Heating a fluid
causes it to expand and rise, producing fluid motion and
carrying heat with the motion. If the fluid motion is produced
by an external energy source (a fan or a pump), it is called
forced convection. The equation used to describe convective
heat transport is similar to Fourier's equation for conduction.

$$q = HA(T_s - T_m) \quad (5\text{-}55)$$

where T_s is the surface temperature, T_m is the moving fluid
mean temperature, and A is the contact area. Because convective heat transport occurs at a phase interface (i.e., solid–
liquid, solid–gas, or liquid–gas), the thickness ΔX is not easily
measured, so it is incorporated into the heat-transfer coefficient H. The resistance owing to convective heat transport
(1/HA) is thus similar to the conductive resistance ($\Delta X/KA$).
Because convective heat transport can involve complex geometric and fluid dynamic problems, the determination of the
heat transfer coefficient is a mixture of theoretical and empirical effort. Table 5-5 gives some example values of heat transfer coefficients.
    Conductive and convective heat transport can be combined
into an overall heat transport coefficient, U.[35,36] Following is
an example of the use of an overall heat transfer coefficient to
describe the heating of water in a pot.

$$q = U(T_{air} - T_{water}) \quad (5\text{-}56)$$

where

$$U = \frac{1}{\dfrac{1}{H_{air} A} + \dfrac{\Delta Xa}{KaA} + \dfrac{1}{H_{water} A}};$$

H_{air} = convective heat transfer coefficient from air to pot;
H_{water} = convective heat transfer coefficient from pot to water;
Ka = thermal conductivity of pot, whose thickness is ΔXa.

TABLE 5-5.   Typical Values of Convective Heat Transfer
Coefficients, H

PROCESS	H WATTS/m²-°K
Natural convection	5–25
Forced convection	
Gases	25–250
Liquids	50–20,000
Convection with phase change	
Boiling or condensation	2,500–100,000

(Reprinted with permission from Incropera FP, DeWitt DP: Fundamentals of Heat and Mass Transfer, 2nd ed, chapter 1, p 8. New York,
John Wiley & Sons, 1985.)

Radiant heat energy is emitted by every body having a temperature greater than 0°K (−273°C). This does not mean that the amount of thermal radiation is always significant compared with the other forms of heat transfer. In most situations in which objects are below room temperature, thermal radiation is small. When the temperature of an object exceeds 500°C, radiation is usually the predominant mechanism of heat transport. Because thermal radiation is electromagnetic (see following section), it requires no medium for transport. The sun radiates energy at a temperature of 5,000°C to the earth through 93,000,000 miles of vacuum. All radiant energy hitting a surface is either absorbed, transmitted, or reflected. The fractional contributions of these three processes must total one:

$$\alpha + \tau + \rho = 1 \qquad (5\text{-}57)$$

where

$$\alpha = \text{absorptivity;}$$
$$\tau = \text{transmissivity;}$$
$$\rho = \text{reflectivity.}$$

These fractions usually vary with the wavelength of the radiant energy. If the absorptivity α is one, the object will gain the maximal possible amount of heat. Such an object is called a *black body*. By contrast, if all radiant energy is either reflected or transmitted (*i.e.*, $\rho + \tau = 1$), the object will gain no heat. The equation for radiant heat transfer to a black body ($\alpha = 1$) is called the Stefan–Boltzmann Law:

$$q_{12} = \sigma \times A \times F_{12}(T_1^4 - T_2^4) \qquad (5\text{-}58)$$

where q_{12} is the net heat transferred between objects 1 and 2 at temperatures T_1 and T_2, respectively. σ is the Stefan–Boltzmann constant ($\sigma = 4.8 \times 10^{-8}$ Kcal/hr-M²-K⁴ or 5.6×10^{-8} watts/M²-°K⁴). A is the area being irradiated, and F_{12} is the *view factor*. The view factor is the fraction of the radiation from object 1 "seen" by object 2. It is a complex function of geometric considerations. Since radiant heat transport depends upon temperature to the fourth power, we expect this form of heat transport to dominate at high temperature differences.

Figure 5-20 illustrates all three of these mechanisms of heat transport. In this example, water is being heated in a pot by a flame. The flame transfers heat to the pot by natural convection and by radiation. Heat is conducted through the metal of the bottom of the pot and then heats the water predominantly by forced convection because the water is being stirred. Ultimately much of the heat transported into the water will be dissipated by the latent heat of vaporization of the water (see previous discussion of latent heat of vaporization).

Analyzing the heat transport to and from a patient in the operating room is a complex problem involving all the aforementioned mechanisms of heat transport. To maintain a constant temperature, the patient must dissipate an amount of heat equal to his metabolic heat production. A 70-kg adult will generate approximately 85 kilocalories or the same as a 100-watt light bulb.[37, 38] Figure 5-21 illustrates the four mechanisms of heat loss for a patient in the operating room: conduction, convection, radiation, and latent heat of vaporization. The following example will illustrate how each mechanism participates in the dissipation of metabolic heat. Note that many assumptions and approximations are made in attempting to model the real situation, and the accuracy of the

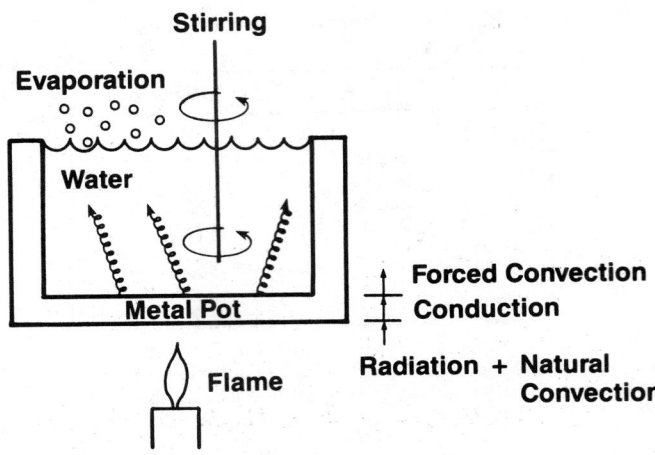

FIG. 5-20. This illustration demonstrates that several types of heat transport are simultaneously involved in the process of heating a pot of water. The flame transmits heat to the metal pot by radiant heat transport and natural convection owing to the rising hot gases from the hot flame. Heat is transported through the metal bottom of the pot purely by conduction. The water within the pot is being stirred; therefore, the predominant mechanism of transport is forced convection. Finally, as the water is evaporating, it is being cooled by the latent heat vaporization of the water.

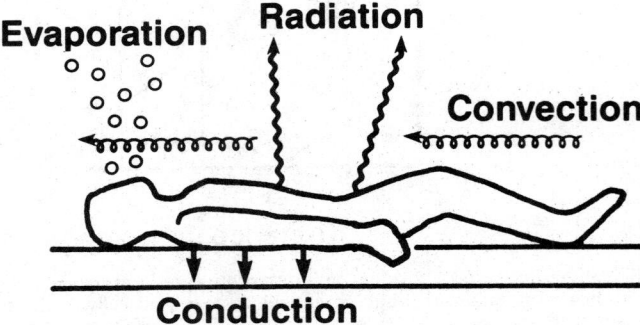

FIG. 5-21. This figure illustrates the major mechanisms of heat loss for a patient in the operating room. Although it is often written that 50% or more of heat loss is due to radiation, any of the four forms of heat loss illustrated above can be substantial, depending upon the surrounding conditions. See the text for several examples of calculations for each mechanism of heat loss.

calculations is dependent upon the validity of these assumptions. For this reason, several assumptions will be made to demonstrate how these changes will affect the amount of heat lost by each mechanism.

EXAMPLE: HEAT LOSS FOR A PATIENT IN THE OPERATING ROOM

Mechanism I. Heat Loss by Conduction

For a patient lying on an operating table uncovered, heat is lost by conduction through contact with the operating table itself. If the patient is covered with a blanket, heat will also be conducted through the blanket. The conductive heat loss will be calculated using equation 5-51 for three conditions: the patient 1) lying on a cold metal table, 2) on an insulated table, and 3) on a heating blanket.

Heat Loss to the Operating Room (OR) Table

Assuming 1) patient skin temperature = 37°C,
2) table temperature = 20°C,
3) table thickness = 1 cm,
4) body surface area (BSA) in contact = 0.5 m²

CASE 1. Steel table without insulation:

$$q = (0.5 \text{ m}^2)\left(15 \frac{\text{watt}}{\text{m°C}}\right)\left(\frac{37-20}{0.01\text{m}}\right)°C$$
$$q = 12,750 \text{ watts!}$$

CASE 2. OR table with 2 cm of insulation with a thermal conductivity of 0.04 $\frac{\text{watt}}{\text{m°C}}$ (e.g., wool, foam):

$$q = (0.5 \text{ m}^2)\left(0.4 \frac{\text{watt}}{\text{m°C}}\right)\left(\frac{37-20}{0.02\text{m}}\right)°C$$
$$q = 170 \text{ watts}$$

CASE 3. OR table with a 1-cm heating blanket maintained at 37°C:

$$q = (0.5 \text{ m}^2)\left(0.60 \frac{\text{watt}}{\text{m°C}}\right)\left(\frac{37-37}{0.01}\right)°C$$
$$q = 0 \text{ watts}$$

Conductive Heat Loss to 20°C Room When Covered

CASE 4. A wool blanket of 0.3 cm thickness. The contact area is assumed to be 1 m²:

$$q = (1.0 \text{ m}^2)\left(0.04 \frac{\text{watt}}{\text{m°C}}\right)\left(\frac{37-20}{0.003\text{m}}\right)°C$$
$$q = 227 \text{ watts}$$

CASE 5. Two wool blankets with a 0.5-cm air space between the patient and the blanket. Using Equation 5-54:

$$q = \frac{(37-20)°C}{\dfrac{0.006 \text{ m}}{(0.5 \text{ m}^2)\left(0.04 \frac{\text{watt}}{\text{m°C}}\right)} + \dfrac{0.005 \text{ m}}{(0.5 \text{ m}^2)\left(0.026 \frac{\text{watt}}{\text{m°C}}\right)}}$$
$$q = 25 \text{ watts}$$

Cases 4 and 5 assume that the outer surface of the blanket is maintained at 20°C.

The previously given calculations illustrate the dramatic dependence of conductive heat loss on the insulation of the patient and operating table. All these calculations assume that the patient skin temperature is 37°C, which is too high for skin in contact with a cold operating table. Nonetheless, it is evident that even a small amount of good insulating material can dramatically reduce the heat loss to the operating table by conduction. Because air is a fluid, the analysis of heat transport from the patient to the air (whether covered with a blanket or not) involves convection, which will be discussed subsequently.

Mechanism II. Heat Loss by Convection

Wherever the body surface is in contact with a fluid, natural or forced convection is involved. A standard OR is ventilated with 10 to 15 room volume changes per hour. Reducing this to a linear air velocity for a standard-sized OR yields an air speed over the body of approximately 3 cm/sec. Using this velocity and assuming the patient to be a cylinder 30 cm in diameter, the flow Reynolds number can be estimated. This fluid dynamic effect on heat transport (forced convection) is then weighed against the heat transport from natural convection. The result of a fairly involved analysis is an estimate of a heat transfer coefficient (Eqn. 5-55) for the convective heat loss. The details of this calculation are beyond the scope of this chapter; readers are referred to engineering texts on the subject.[39, 40] This type of analysis predicts a natural convective heat transfer coefficient of approximately 4 watts/m²-°C, and a forced convective heat transfer coefficient of 1 watt/m²-°C. An increase in air velocity owing to patient or personnel movement would increase the forced convective heat transfer coefficient. A "rule of thumb" is that the heat transport will go up in proportion to the square root of the air velocity. Using this heat transfer coefficient, the heat loss resulting from convection in our patient would be as follows:

$$q = AH(T_b - T_r)$$

CASE 6. Assuming that the patient is not covered, has a temperature of 37°C, and has an exposed area of 1 m²:

$$q = (1 \text{ m}^2)\left(4 \frac{\text{watt}}{\text{m}^2 \text{ °C}}\right)(37-20)°C$$
$$q = 68 \text{ watts}$$

CASE 7. If the patient is covered with a blanket as in Case 5, the blanket surface temperature must be calculated. This is done by equating the heat conducted in and convected out of the blanket.

$$q_{in} = \frac{(37 - T_{blanket})°C}{0.685°C/\text{watt}}$$

$$q_{out} = \frac{(T_{blanket} - 20)°C}{\left[\dfrac{1}{(1 \text{ m}^2)\left(4 \frac{\text{watt}}{\text{m}^2 \text{ °C}}\right)}\right]}$$

$$0.685 (T_b - 20) = 0.25(37 - T_b)$$
$$T_b = 24.5°C$$

With a blanket surface temperature of 24.5°C, the convective heat loss can be calculated:

$$q = (1 \text{ m}^2)\left(4 \frac{\text{watt}}{\text{m}^2 \text{ °C}}\right)(24.5 - 20)°C$$
$$q = 18 \text{ watts}$$

Mechanism III. Radiant Heat Loss from a Patient in the Operating Room

Assuming that the patient in the OR acts as a black body absorber ($\alpha = 1$), the following calculations can be made:

Heat Losses by Radiation

$$q = A\sigma(T_{body} - T^4_{room}) \text{(Stefan–Boltzmann; Eqn. 5-58)}$$

where

$$\sigma = 5.6 \times 10^{-8} \text{ watts/m}^2\text{-°K}$$

CASE 8. Assuming

1) skin temperature = 37°C = 310°K;
2) room wall temperature = 20°C = 293°K;
3) BSA involved = 1 m²:

$$q = (1 \text{ m}^2)\left(5.6 \times 10^{-8} \frac{\text{watt}}{\text{m}^2 \text{ }^\circ K^4}\right)(310^4 - 293^4)^\circ K^4$$

$$q = 104 \text{ watts}$$

CASE 9. Assuming skin temperature = 35°C = 308°K:

$$q = (1 \text{ m}^2)\left(5.6 \times 10^{-8} \frac{\text{watt}}{\text{m}^2 \text{ }^\circ K^4}\right)(308^4 - 293^4)^\circ K^4$$

$$q = 91 \text{ watts}$$

CASE 10. Assuming a blanket temperature = 24.5°C = 297.5°K (radiation from blanket to walls):

$$q = (1 \text{ m}^2)\left(5.6 \times 10^{-8} \frac{\text{watt}}{\text{m}^2 \text{ }^\circ K^4}\right)(297.5^4 - 293^4)^\circ K^4$$

$$q = 26 \text{ watts}$$

Mechanism IV. Heat Loss by Evaporation

Heat loss by evaporation in the form of perspiration is the body's predominant mechanism of cooling when the body temperature is over 37°C. When the patient becomes cold, the evaporative loss from the skin is minimized. Evaporative heat losses from the respiratory tract are a side-effect of ventilation and therefore are an obligate heat loss. If a patient inspires 100% humidified gases at body temperature, there will be no heat loss due to respiratory evaporation, but, as seen in the following calculations, if the patient inspires dry gases, there can be a significant heat loss resulting from respiratory evaporation.

Heat Loss by Respiratory Evaporation (Latent Heat)

$$q = M \times LH$$
M = rate of water loss (mg/min)
LH = latent heat of vaporization of water (at 37°C)
    $= 2.43 \times 10^3$ joule/gm

Assuming

1) minute ventilation = 7 l/min,
2) inspired air is dry,
3) expired air is 100% saturated at 37°C (34 mg H_2O/l),

mass of water evaporated will be:

$$M = (7 \text{ l/min})(34 \text{ mg } H_2O/l)$$
$$= 238 \text{ mg/min};$$
$$q = \left(238 \frac{\text{mg}}{\text{min}}\right)(2.43 \times 10^3 \text{ joule/gm})\left(10^{-3} \frac{\text{gm}}{\text{mg}}\right);$$
$$q = 578 \text{ joule/min} = 9.6 \text{ joule/sec}$$
$$q = 9.6 \text{ watts}.$$

The preceding example illustrates the basic mechanisms of heat loss for a patient in the OR. In this example, each mechanism is treated independently to simplify calculating the heat loss. In reality, these processes are occurring in series and in parallel simultaneously, and therefore should be analyzed in that fashion (analogous to series and parallel resistors in an electrical circuit analysis). It is evident from these calculations that the heat loss by each mechanism can be dramatically altered by the assumed boundary conditions. Conduction to the operating table can be completely eliminated by a heating blanket, whereas convective and radiative losses can be substantially reduced by covering the patient with a blanket.[41, 42] Finally, the loss by evaporation can be eliminated by using heated, humidified inspired gases. When heat loss in the OR is discussed, it is generally stated that radiation is the predominant mechanism followed by convective and evaporative losses.[41–44] As can be seen from this example, there can be wide variation in heat loss by each mechanism, depending upon the specific conditions. Radiation can be a major source of heat loss, which is less controllable than some of the other losses. In the real situation, there are also potential heat losses from the surgical field by evaporation, convection, and radiation. Furthermore, the skin temperature will probably be somewhat less than body core temperature, and the patient will be well insulated from the operating table.[43, 44] Some of these predicted heat losses will therefore be reduced, whereas an open surgical field will allow dramatic increases in evaporative and radiative heat losses.

MASS TRANSPORT AND KINETIC THEORY

Matter is transported by bulk flow, forced or natural convection, and molecular diffusion. In this section, we will discuss molecular diffusion. The other two mechanisms, which are much more efficient, have been discussed in previous sections.

Molecular diffusion is a process described by what is called the *kinetic theory*.[45] Kinetic theory assumes that all matter is composed of particles (atoms or molecules) that are in continuous, random motion. This motion only stops when the temperature is lowered to absolute zero (0°K, −273°C). When kinetic theory is applied to gases, it assumes that the particles are small and that all collisions between particles and walls of the container are completely elastic (*i.e.*, no energy is lost). With these assumptions, the ideal gas laws previously discussed can be derived from kinetic theory.

Diffusion occurs because of the random motion of fluid (gas or liquid) particles. In Figure 5-22A, the container is filled with particles of nitrogen (N). Since all the N's are in constant random motion, on the average, equal numbers of particles will be going east and west. Consequently, the container is homogeneously filled with N's, and there is no net transport of N's in either direction, in spite of the fact that constant diffusion of N's is occurring in all directions. Now we add a second type of particle, which we call oxygen (O), on the west side of the container in Figure 5-22B. The O particles will be randomly moving east and west, but since initially there are no O's on the east side, there will be a net movement of O's from west to east. The opposite will happen with the N's that were initially on the east side until the N's and the O's are homogeneously filling the container. This is the process of *molecular diffusion*. For a net mass transport to take place in one direction, there must be a concentration difference or gradient in that direction. This net transport by diffusion in the presence of a concentration gradient is described by Fick's Law of Diffusion:[45]

$$J = D_{o,N} \frac{dC_o}{dx} \qquad (5-59)$$

where

J = mass flux or net transport across a plane (molecules/sec-cm^2);

$D_{o,N}$ = diffusivity (diffusion constant) for component O diffusing in N (cm^2/sec);

$\dfrac{dCo}{dx}$ = concentration gradient of O in the X-direction (molecules/cm^3/cm).

If component O was constantly removed as it reached the east side of the container, there would be a steady diffusion of O from the west to the east. In biologic systems, it is common that diffusion takes place through a membrane, for example, oxygen diffusing through the alveolar cell wall and the pulmonary capillary wall into the blood stream. Oxygen diffuses from a high concentration (or partial pressure) in the alveoli to a low concentration in the blood stream. Concentration can be replaced by partial pressure if the solubility (the ratio of concentration to partial pressure) is entered into Fick's equation. Solubility will be discussed subsequently. In biological systems, it is difficult to determine the actual partial pressure gradient through a membrane, so the partial pressure difference across the membrane is used. For oxygen diffusing in the lung (Fig. 5-22C):

$$J = \frac{\alpha D}{\Delta X}(P_{alv_{O_2}} - P_{cap_{O_2}}) \qquad (5\text{-}60)$$

where

D = diffusivity;
α = solubility constant for oxygen;
ΔX = membrane thickness;
$P_{alv_{O_2}}$ = alveolar oxygen partial pressure;
$P_{cap_{O_2}}$ = pulmonary capillary oxygen partial pressure.

In biologic systems D, α and ΔX are combined and called the permeability constant, P:

$$P = \frac{\alpha D}{\Delta X}$$

As shown in Equation 5-60 and Figure 5-22C, the rate of diffusion J of a substance through a membrane is directly proportional to the partial pressure difference, the solubility of the substance in the membrane, and the molecular diffusivity constant. It is inversely proportional to the thickness of the membrane. The molecular diffusivity D of a substance is inversely proportional to the square root of the molecular weight and directly proportional to the temperature.[45]

Molecular diffusion of gases through gases is a slow process; diffusion of gases through liquids is a very slow process; and the diffusion of gases through solids is an extremely slow process (Table 5-6).[46] For this reason, in sites where the body depends upon molecular diffusion for transport, the distances are very short. For example, in oxygen delivery, diffusion is the only mechanism involved in transport from the alveolus to the blood and again from the tissue capillary wall to the mitochondria. These diffusion distances are 5 to 20 μ.

It is interesting that carbon dioxide (CO_2) has a slightly smaller diffusivity than oxygen (O_2), even though it is often stated that CO_2 diffuses more quickly in the lung than does O_2. The diffusivity of CO_2 is lower because it is a larger mole-

TABLE 5-6. Diffusivities of Oxygen and Carbon Dioxide @ 25°C

	O_2	CO_2 cm^2/sec
Air	0.21	0.16
Water	2.40×10^{-5}	2.0×10^{-5}
Rubber	2.1×10^{-6}	1.1×10^{-6}

(Reprinted with permission from Incropera FP, DeWitt DP: Fundamentals of Heat and Mass Transport, Appendix A-8, p 777. New York, John Wiley & Sons, 1985.)

cule, but since its solubility in water is approximately 20 times greater than O_2, CO_2 has a larger permeability constant P for lung transport, (Eqn. 5-60). Solubility's ability to increase the permeability constant and thereby increase mass flux is used in "facilitated" diffusion. This is a process whereby a freely diffusible carrier substance in the membrane attaches to the diffusing molecule, which may by itself have a very low solubility in the membrane. The molecule plus carrier will have a lower diffusivity (because of the larger molecular weight) but a much larger permeability owing to the effect of increased solubility in the membrane.

OSMOTIC PRESSURE, ONCOTIC PRESSURE, AND THE NERNST EQUATION. Two other phenomena involving diffusion of particles through membranes are important in biological systems: 1) diffusion through semipermeable membranes (osmotic pressure and oncotic pressure); and 2) diffusion of charged substances through semipermeable membranes (Nernst equation and membrane potential).

In Figure 5-22C, if there is neither production nor consumption of either substance, equal concentrations on both sides of the membrane will eventually result. What will happen if the membrane separating the two compartments is permeable to one type of particle but not to the other, as in Figure 5-22D? For example, in Figure 5-22D, let W represent water, which freely passes through the entire container and equilibrates on both sides. The P's represent protein molecules, which are nonpermeable to the membrane and thus remain on the west side of the container. Consequently, there are more total particles (W's and P's) on one side, which causes the pressure to be greater on that side of the membrane (see Dalton's Law, in the section entitled Thermodynamics). This pressure difference is called the *osmotic pressure* and is related to the number of particles or moles of nonpermeable solute, that is, the number of P's. When this principle is applied to the vascular space whose capillary walls are permeable to water and electrolytes but not to plasma proteins, the pressure developed is referred to as *oncotic pressure*.

When a semipermeable membrane separates solutions for which one ion is permeable and the oppositely charged ion is not, a charge imbalance can be produced, as shown in Figure 5-22E. This imbalance produces a transmembrane potential difference, which can be calculated by the Nernst equation:[47]

$$\text{EMF (millivolts)} = -61 \log \frac{K^+ \text{ (east)}}{K^+ \text{ (west)}}. \qquad (5\text{-}61)$$

Nerve cells use this diffusion mechanism to re-establish their transmembrane potential after depolarization and impulse transmission. The original concentration gradient between the inside and outside of the cell is produced by a sodium–

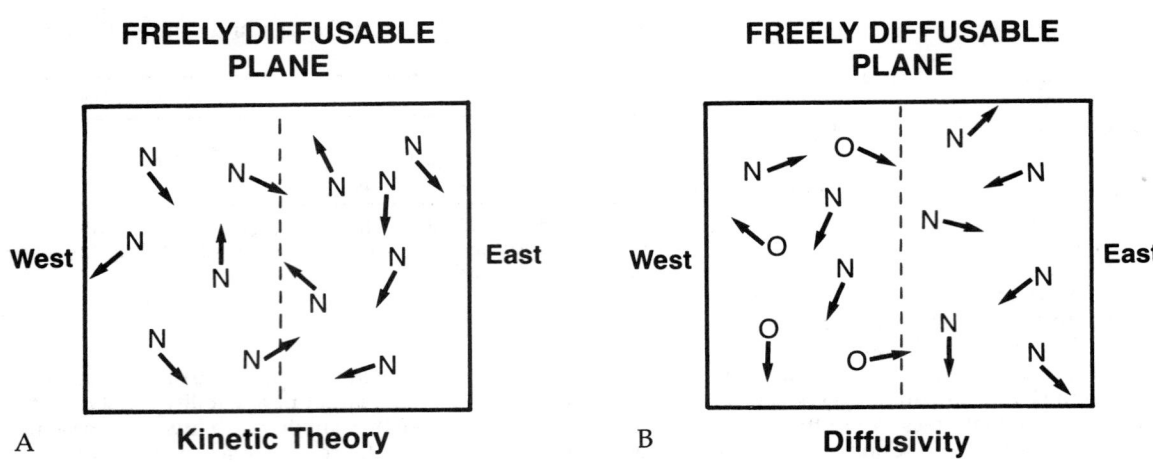

A Kinetic Theory

B Diffusivity

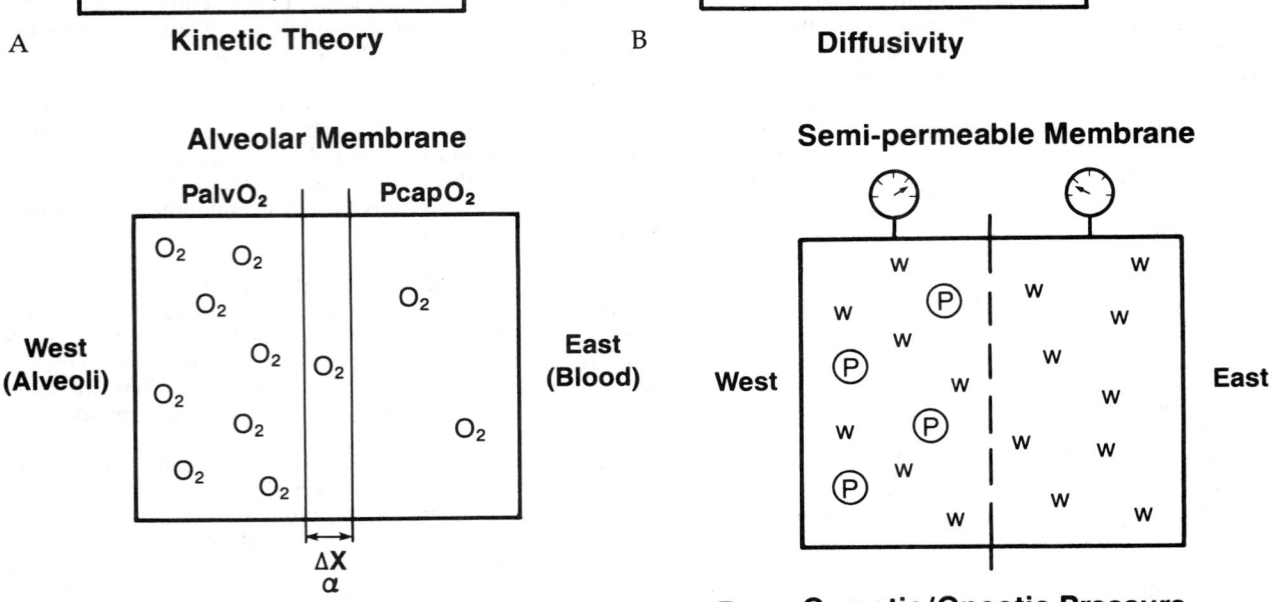

C Permeability

D Osmotic/Oncotic Pressure

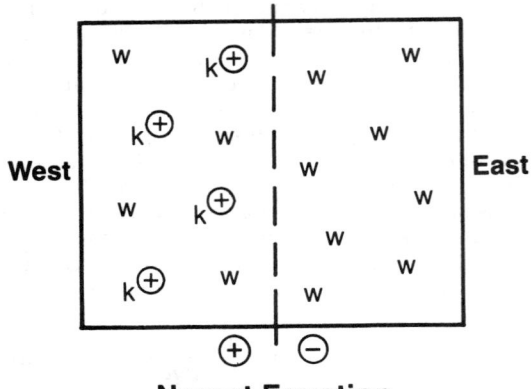

E Nernst Equation
(Membrane Potential)

potassium pump. This pump is an active process, pumping ions against a concentration gradient.

SOLUBILITY

VAPORS AND GASES. When a pure, solid substance reaches its melting point, it becomes a liquid; when it reaches its boiling point, it becomes a vapor; and when it reaches its critical temperature, it becomes a gas. It is easy to distinguish a solid from a liquid from a vapor, but vapors and gases are not as easily discriminated. By definition, when a substance reaches its critical temperature, it is a gas. The difference between a vapor and a gas is that a vapor can be compressed at constant temperature into a liquid, whereas a gas cannot. (See Thermodynamics.) When a liquid is placed in a container, some of the molecules will evaporate, forming a vapor phase above the liquid. Eventually, an equilibrium state will be reached between molecules leaving and entering the liquid phase. At this point, the pressure of the vapor is called the *equilibrium vapor pressure*, as discussed previously (Table 5-2 and Fig. 5-15).

SOLUBILITY. When a pure liquid is enclosed in a container, the vapor above that liquid will produce a pressure (the vapor pressure at that temperature), which is also the total pressure. When a second vapor or gas is added to the container, it will produce an additional pressure; the sum of these pressures will be the total pressure (Dalton's Law of Partial Pressures,

discussed previously). Some of the molecules of this second gas will dissolve in the primary liquid, and the amount dissolved is directly proportional to the partial pressure of the gas above the liquid. This proportionality is known as Henry's Law of Solubility:

$$P_i = H_{i,1} \times X_i \qquad (5\text{-}62)$$

where

P_i = partial pressure of substance i in the gas phase;
$H_{i,1}$ = Henry's law constant for i in l;
X_i = mole fraction of i in the liquid phase.

The Henry's law constant $H_{i,1}$ is specific for a solute (gas) and solvent (liquid) pair and is a function of temperature. Almost all gases and vapors become more soluble in liquids as temperature decreases, that is, they become closer to being liquids themselves. The specific solubility constant depends upon the molecular weight, size, and intermolecular forces between solvent and solute molecules. These constants are determined experimentally. Because the partial pressure in the gas phase and the concentration in the liquid phase are directly proportional (Eqn. 5-62), it is common to express the concentration of a gas in a liquid in terms of its equilibrium partial pressure or tension.

In Henry's Law, the concentration of the solute is expressed in terms of mole fraction X_i, which is not convenient for medical calculations. Solubility coefficients may also be

◀ FIG. 5-22. (*A*) The container above is filled with molecules N moving randomly. Because of the random motion, the particles will eventually be homogeneously distributed throughout the container, and, at any one time, an equal number of particles will be passing through a plane in both directions. (*B*) This container is similar to the one shown in Figure 5-22*A* except that there are two types of molecules, N and O. Initially, the O molecules are only on the west side of the container. Owing to random motion of both the N's and the O's, an equal number of molecules will be moving in both directions. Because there are initially no O molecules on the east side of the container, there will be no O molecules moving from the east, and, therefore, there will be a net movement of O molecules from west to east until the container is homogeneously filled with both N's and O's throughout. This process of net movement of one type of molecule through space as a result of random motion is called *diffusion*. (*C*) This figure is divided into two sections by a permeable membrane of thickness ΔX. Oxygen molecules are in higher concentration on the west side, which represents an alveolus, than on the east side, which represents a capillary blood. Because of the higher concentration on the west side, oxygen molecules will randomly diffuse eastward. The amount of oxygen in the membrane is related to the concentration of oxygen on the alveolar side and the solubility of the oxygen in the membrane material. If the capillary blood is moving and continuously removing oxygen from the east side, there will be a continuous flux of oxygen molecules from the west side to the east side by diffusion. (*D*) This container is similar to that shown in Figure 5-22*B* except that the membrane dividing the east and the west side of the container is a semipermeable membrane. Semipermeable membranes are permeable to some components but not to others. In this container, the W's, which represent water, are freely permeable to the membrane and, therefore, homogeneously distributed throughout the container. The P molecules, which represent protein, are semipermeable and do not freely diffuse through the membrane; therefore, they remain on the west side of the container. The water molecules diffuse in both directions through the membrane randomly, unaffected by the presence of the P molecules on the west side. For this reason, the water molecules try to distribute evenly throughout the entire container, thus producing more total molecules on the west side. This results in a higher pressure on the west side of the container. Note that the pressure on the west side is higher than the pressure on the east side; this pressure is known as *osmotic pressure*. If the semipermeable membrane is a capillary wall and the osmotic pressure is produced by plasma proteins, this pressure is referred to as *oncotic pressure*. (*E*) This container is similar to that in Figure 5-22*D* except that the semipermeable component on the west side of the container is a charged particle, K+. The semipermeable membrane thus maintains a difference in charged concentrations between the west side and the east side of the container. This potential difference maintained by the membrane can be calculated by an equation known as the Nernst Equation (see text equation 5-61) if the difference in concentrations of ions is known.

expressed in terms of the volume of gas that dissolves into a given volume of liquid. The international scientific community uses the Bunsen coefficient (α), defined as the volume of gas corrected to standard temperature and pressure ($0°C$ and 1 atmosphere), which dissolves in a unit volume of liquid at the temperature concerned. A more useful way of expressing solubility for anesthetic practice is the *Ostwald solubility coefficient*, which is defined as the volume of gas that dissolves in a unit volume of liquid at the temperature concerned. In the Ostwald coefficient, the gas volume is not corrected to standard temperature and pressure. In Table 5-7, the Ostwald coefficients for several anesthetic agents in water, blood, and oil are listed.[48]

Another way of describing solubility is in terms of the distribution of a substance between two phases. The partition coefficient is defined as the ratio of the amount of substance present in equal volumes of two phases at a stated equilibrium temperature. If one of the phases is gaseous, then the partition coefficient is the same as the Ostwald coefficient. The partition coefficient is most frequently used when the two phases are both solid or liquid (*e.g.*, oil–water or tissue–blood). The partition coefficient can be calculated as the quotient of the Ostwald (liquid–gas) coefficients for each of the liquid phases. For example, a tissue–blood partition coefficient may be obtained by dividing the Ostwald tissue–gas coefficient by the blood–gas coefficient, that is, $T/b = (T/g)/(b/g)$. Thus, from Table 5-7, the muscle–blood partition coefficient for halothane would be $6/2.4 = 2.5$. It is said that solubility coefficients and partition coefficients are a function of temperature but not of pressure or concentration. This is not exactly true, because these coefficients do vary slightly over wide ranges of pressure. In the clinical range, however, we can assume that the coefficients are independent of pressure and concentration.

MEASUREMENT TECHNIQUES FOR OXYGEN, CARBON DIOXIDE, AND HEMOGLOBIN SATURATION

Ensuring adequate oxygenation and ventilation may be the most important aspect of monitoring critically ill and anesthetized patients. To this end, several techniques have been developed to measure oxygen, carbon dioxide, and hemoglobin saturation over the past 30 years. More recently, techniques have been developed for the continuous monitoring of oxygenation and ventilation. In this section, we will describe the theoretical principles on which these techniques are based.

OXYGEN MEASUREMENT. Blood oxygen content is usually defined as the number of milliliters of oxygen contained in 100 ml of blood (volume%). Since oxygen is both dissolved in

plasma and bound to hemoglobin, the calculation of oxygen content has two terms:

$$\overset{\text{bound}}{}\qquad\overset{\text{dissolved}}{}\qquad(5\text{-}63)$$
$$CaO2 = (1.37 \times Hb \times Sa_{O_2}) + (0.003 \times Pa_{O_2})$$

where

the subscripted ''a'' = an arterial value;
Hb = hemoglobin in grams per 100 ml of blood;
Sa_{O_2} = (oxyhemoglobin/total hemoglobin) × 100%, or fractional hemoglobin saturation;
1.37 = the number of milliliters of oxygen bound to 1 gm of fully saturated hemoglobin;
Pa_{O_2} = arterial oxygen partial pressure;
0.003 = the solubility coefficient of oxygen in plasma.

Equation 5-63 contains three variables and two constants, the variables being Hb, Sa_{O_2}, and Pa_{O_2}. Hemoglobin can be measured directly or estimated as one third of the hematocrit. To determine Ca_{O_2}, we must therefore be able to measure Sa_{O_2} and Pa_{O_2}. For this reason, oxygen-measuring devices can be divided into two groups: 1) those that measure oxygen partial pressure (P_{O_2}), and 2) those that measure hemoglobin saturation (S_{O_2}).

Oxygen partial pressure can be measured in the gas phase by polarographic electrode, paramagnetic analyzer, oxygen fuel cell, mass spectrometer, and, most recently, by fluorescence quenching optode. Two of these methods, polarographic electrode and optode, can just as easily be used to measure oxygen tension in a liquid and therefore are used to measure the P_{O_2} of blood. By far the most common method in medicine today is the polarographic "Clark" oxygen electrode.[45] The Clark electrode is composed of a platinum cathode and a silver anode in an electrolyte solution covered with an oxygen-permeable membrane (Fig. 5-23). When an electric potential is maintained between these electrodes, a current flows in proportion to the P_{O_2}. Oxygen is consumed at the cathode according to the following reaction:

$$O_2 + 2\ H_2O + 4e^- \rightarrow 4\ OH^-$$

This electrode was developed by Leland Clark in 1956 and is currently used in all blood gas analyzers.[49] It is also used for the measurement of inspired oxygen tension and has been miniaturized to create an *in vivo* continuous Pa_{O_2} monitor. Oxygen tension can also be measured at the heated skin surface with a Clark electrode, which continuously and noninvasively monitors oxygenation (transcutaneous P_{O_2}).[50]

Recently, the phenomenon of fluorescence quenching by oxygen has been used to create new P_{O_2} measurement devices.[51, 52] The ability of oxygen to absorb energy from excited states in certain fluorescent dyes and thus prevent this energy from being radiated as light is illustrated in Figure 5-24. In theory, a fluorescence quenching probe is relatively simple, requiring only a fiberoptic light transmission path and the fluorescent dye. For this reason, these devices can be made much smaller than Clark electrodes. Another theoretical advantage of the optode over the Clark electrode is that its sensitivity is highest at lower P_{O_2} values.

HEMOGLOBIN SATURATION MEASUREMENTS. In the 1930s, Matthes used spectrophotometry to determine hemoglobin oxygen saturation. This method of measuring oxyhemoglobin concentration, known as oximetry, is based on the Lambert–Beer Law. This law relates the concentration of

TABLE 5-7.   Ostwald Solubility Coefficients at 37°C

	WATER	BLOOD	OIL	MUSCLE
Nitrogen	0.014	0.015	0.07	—
Nitrous oxide	0.47	0.47	1.4	1.1
Halothane	0.80	2.4	220	155
Enflurane	0.78	1.9	98	70
Forane	0.62	1.4	97	68

(Reprinted with permission from Hill DW: Physics Applied to Anesthesia, 3rd ed, p 177. London, Butterworths, 1976.)

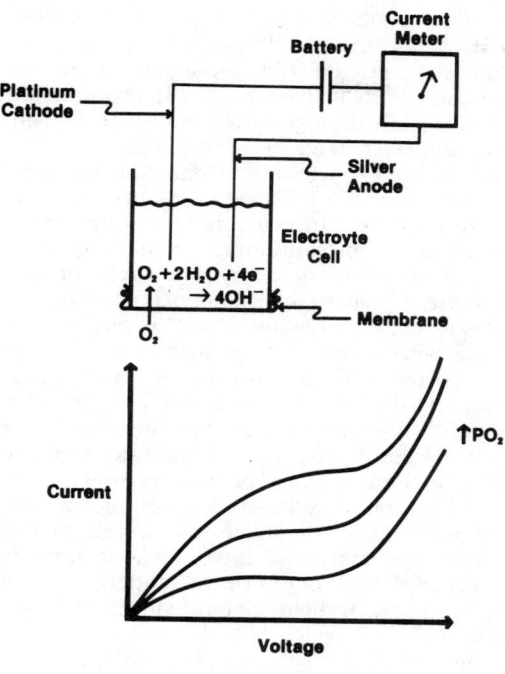

Polarogram

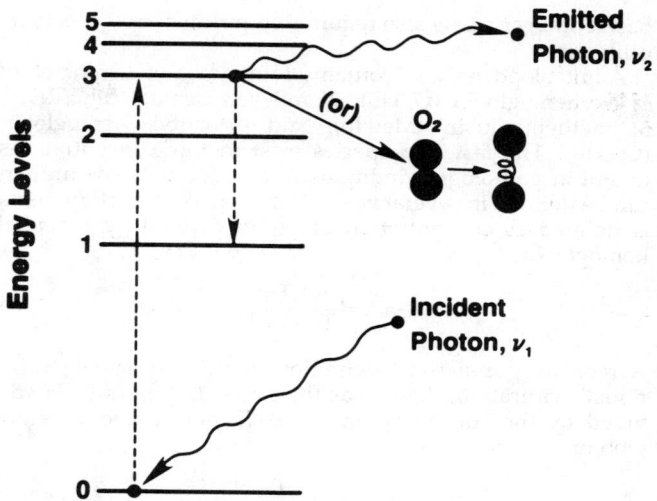

FIG. 5-24. The fluorescence quenching phenomenon. An electron of the fluorescent dye is excited to a higher energy level by an incident photon (ν_1). This excited electron can return to a lower energy level either by emitting a photon (ν_2) or by interacting with an oxygen molecule and raising the latter to a higher vibrational energy level. (Reprinted with permission from Barker SJ, Tremper KK, Hyatt J et al: Continuous fiberoptic arterial oxygen measurement in dogs. J Clin Monitoring 3:48, 1987.)

FIG. 5-23. The upper diagram is a schematic of a Clark polarographic oxygen electrode. The circuit consists of a voltage source (battery) and a current meter connecting platinum and silver electrodes. The electrodes are immersed in an electrolyte cell. A membrane permeable to oxygen, but not to the electrolyte, covers one surface of the cell. Oxygen diffuses through the membrane and reacts at the platinum cathode with water to produce hydroxyl ions. The current meter measures the current produced by the electrons consumed in the reaction at the cathode. The lower diagram is a plot of current produced as a function of the voltage between the two electrodes (polarizing voltage). This plot is called a *polarogram*. In the range of 600 mV, there is a plateau in the polarogram. The plateau occurs at higher currents as the P_{O_2} in the cell is increased. Most polarographic oxygen electrodes use a 600-mV polarizing voltage to obtain a stable current at each P_{O_2}.

BEER'S LAW

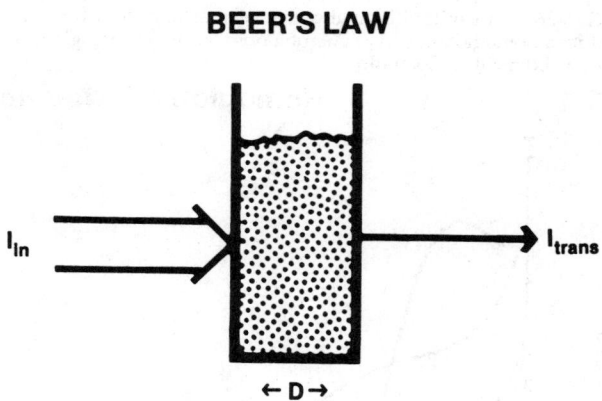

a solute in suspension to the intensity of light transmitted through the solution (Fig. 5-25):

$$I_{trans} = I_{in}\, e^{-(DC\alpha)} \qquad (5\text{-}64)$$

where

I_{trans} = intensity of transmitted light;
I_{in} = intensity of incident light;
D = distance light is transmitted through the liquid;
C = concentration of solute (hemoglobin);
α = extinction coefficient of the solute (a constant for a given solute at a specified wavelength).

As illustrated schematically in Figure 5-25, if a known solute is in a clear solution in a cuvette of known dimensions, the solute concentration may be calculated from measurements of the incident and transmitted light intensity at a known wavelength.

Laboratory oximeters use this principle to determine hemoglobin concentration by measuring the intensity of light

FIG. 5-25. The concentration of a solute dissolved in a solvent can be calculated from the logarithmic relationship between the incident and transmitted light intensity and the solute concentration. (From Tremper KK, Barker SJ: Pulse oximetry and oxygen transport. In Payne JP, Severinghaus JW [eds]: Pulse Oximetry, Chapter 2, p 23. Berlin, Springer-Verlag, 1986, with permission.)

transmitted through a cuvette filled with a hemoglobin dispersion produced from lysed red blood cells. For Beer's Law to be valid, both the solvent and the cuvette must be transparent at the wavelength used, the light path length must be known exactly, and no other absorbing species can be present in the solution. It is difficult to fulfill all these requirements in clinical devices; therefore, each device theoretically based on Beer's Law also requires empirical corrections to its calibration.

Adult blood usually contains four types of hemoglobin: 1) oxyhemoglobin (O_2Hb); 2) reduced hemoglobin (RHb); 3) methemoglobin (MetHb); and 4) carboxyhemoglobin (COHb). The last two species exist in low concentrations except in pathologic conditions. The hemoglobin saturation can be defined in several ways. "Fractional" saturation (Sa_{O_2}) is defined as concentration of O_2Hb divided by the total hemoglobin.[53]

$$Sa_{O_2} = \frac{O_2Hb}{Total\ Hb} \qquad (5-65)$$

A recently popularized definition of Sa_{O_2} is that of "functional" saturation, defined as the concentration of O_2Hb divided by the concentration of O_2Hb plus reduced hemoglobin:

$$Func.\ Sa_{O_2} = \frac{O_2Hb}{RHb + O_2Hb} \qquad (5-66)$$

In this definition, MetHb and COHb are ignored because they do not contribute to oxygen transport. When using oximetry to measure hemoglobin saturation, each wavelength of light will produce one equation (Eqn. 5-64) to solve for one unknown concentration. If either fractional or functional saturation is to be determined in the presence of significant levels of MetHb and COHb, a minimum of four wavelengths of light are required. Even though only two hemoglobin species appear in the definition of functional Sa_{O_2} (Eqn. 5-66), four equations are required to solve for the four unknowns:

RHb, O_2Hb, MetHb, and COHb. If there were two wavelengths at which both MetHb and COHb had zero absorbance while HbO_2 and RHb did not, then functional Sa_{O_2} could be determined with a two-wavelength oximeter. Unfortunately, this is difficult in practice because of the behavior of the absorption coefficients, as seen in Figure 5-26.

Invasive *in vivo* oximeters can estimate hemoglobin saturation by analyzing light reflected from intact red cells. These devices use fiberoptics incorporated into catheters placed in the vascular space for continuous monitoring of mixed venous saturation in the pulmonary artery or arterial saturation in a major artery.[54] These reflectance oximeters use either two or three wavelengths. Owing to extraneous reflectances in the vascular space from red cell membranes, vascular wall artifacts, and other blood constituents, empirical data have been required to calibrate these devices. Little is known about the effect of dyshemoglobins on these invasive oximeters. A recent animal study investigated the effects of methemoglobinemia on the accuracy of pulmonary artery oximeters. In this study, the monitored mixed venous saturation values increased with rising MetHb levels in spite of decreasing values of *in vitro* measured mixed venous saturation and P_{O_2}.[55] Because of their empirical calibration, it is difficult to predict *a priori* how dyshemoglobins will affect these invasive oximeters.

Over the past 40 years, noninvasive oximeters have been developed for continuous monitoring of arterial hemoglobin saturation (Sa_{O_2}). These devices measure red and infrared light transmitted through a tissue bed (*e.g.*, finger or ear). They effectively use the finger or ear as a cuvette containing the hemoglobin. There are several problems in estimating

FIG. 5-26. Transmitted light absorbance spectra of four hemoglobin species: oxyhemoglobin, reduced hemoglobin, carboxyhemoglobin, and methemoglobin. (Courtesy of Ohmeda Corporation, Louisville, Colorado.)

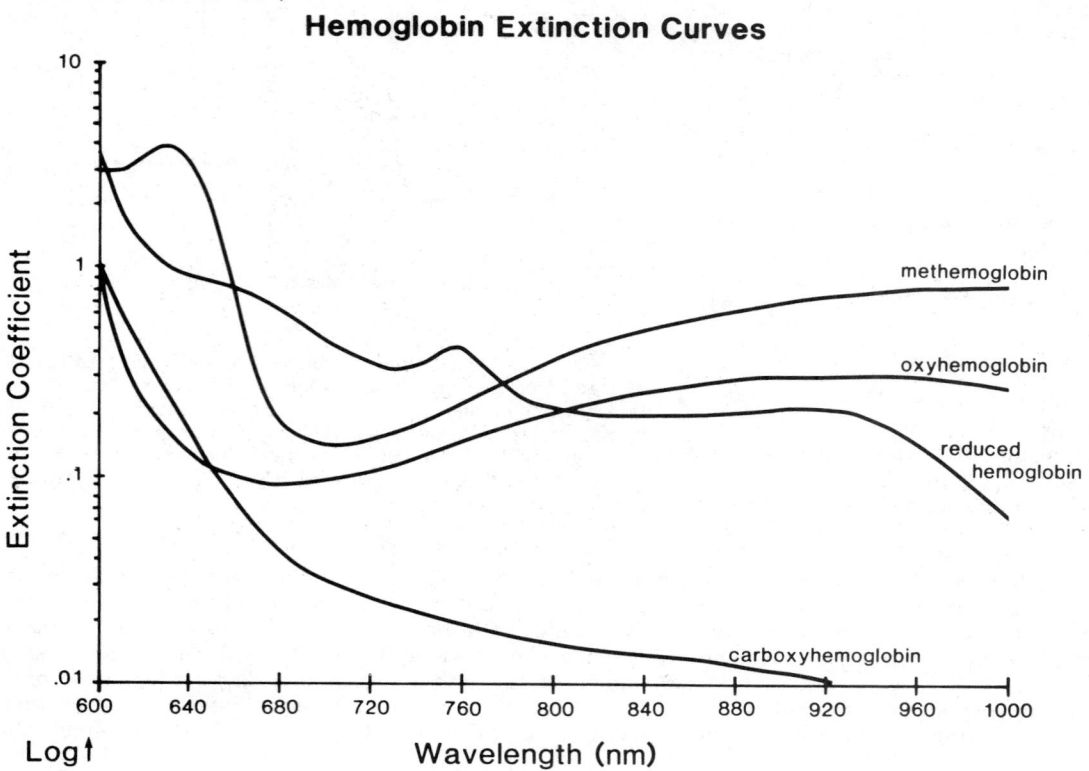

Hemoglobin Extinction Curves

Sa_{O_2} by this method. There are many absorbers in the light path other than arterial hemoglobin, including skin, soft tissue, and venous and capillary blood.

The early oximeters eliminated the effect of tissue absorbance by first compressing the tissue to eliminate all the blood and using the absorbance of bloodless tissue as the zero point. Next, to obtain a signal that is related to arterial blood without interference by venous and capillary blood, the oximeter heated the tissue. Heating produced hyperemia beneath the sensor, which was assumed to "arterialize" the blood in that tissue bed. Devices of this type were developed during World War II for use in aviation research.[56]

Later, in the 1950s, these oximeters were used in the OR, where they detected significant arterial desaturation during routine anesthetics.[57] In spite of their recognized utility by early users, these oximeters were not clinically accepted because they were cumbersome to calibrate and apply and had the potential of burning tissue.[57]

Two technological advances and one bright idea in the late 1970s allowed the development of a new generation of noninvasive oximeters. The two technological advances were the development of small inexpensive light emitting diodes (LEDs) as monochromatic light sources and miniature microprocessors, which could handle complex empirical algorithms. The bright idea was that of a Japanese engineer named Takuo Aoyagi.[58] He found that the pulsatile component of light absorbance is sensitive chiefly to changes in Sa_{O_2}. Because these new oximeters estimate Sa_{O_2} by analyzing the pulsatile component of absorbance, they are referred to as *pulse oximeters*. Figure 5-27 illustrates a pulse-added Beer's Law absorber. The baseline, or DC, component represents the absorbances of the tissue bed, including venous blood, capillary blood, and nonpulsatile arterial blood. The pulse-added, or AC, component is from the pulsatile arterial blood. All pulse oximeters assume that the only pulsatile absorbing component is the arterial blood. They use two wavelengths of light: 660 nm (red), and 940 nm (infrared). The pulse oximeter analyzes the AC component of absorbance at both wavelengths and produces a ratio of the pulse-

PULSE OXIMETERY

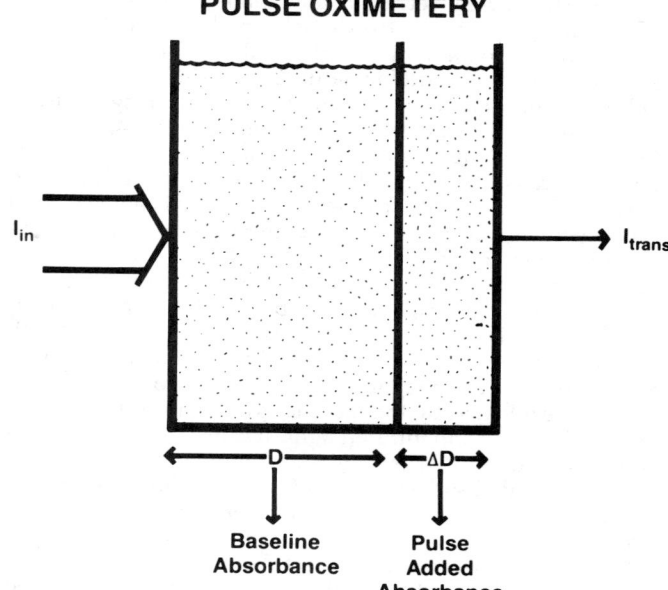

FIG. 5-27. Application of Beer's law to a "pulse-added" signal. The diastolic tissue absorbance represented by D is used as a "zero" point. The pulse-added signal ΔD is empirically correlated to Sa_{O_2}. (From Tremper KK, Barker SJ: Pulse oximetry and oxygen transport. In Payne JP, Severinghaus JW [eds]: Pulse Oximetry, Chapter 2, p 26. Berlin, Springer-Verlag, 1986, with permission.)

added absorbances, which is empirically related to Sa_{O_2}. Figure 5-28 is an example of a pulse oximeter calibration curve.[59] The actual curves used in commercial devices are developed from experimental studies in human volunteers. Note in Figure 5-28 that when the ratio of red to infrared absorbance is one, the saturation is approximately 85%.

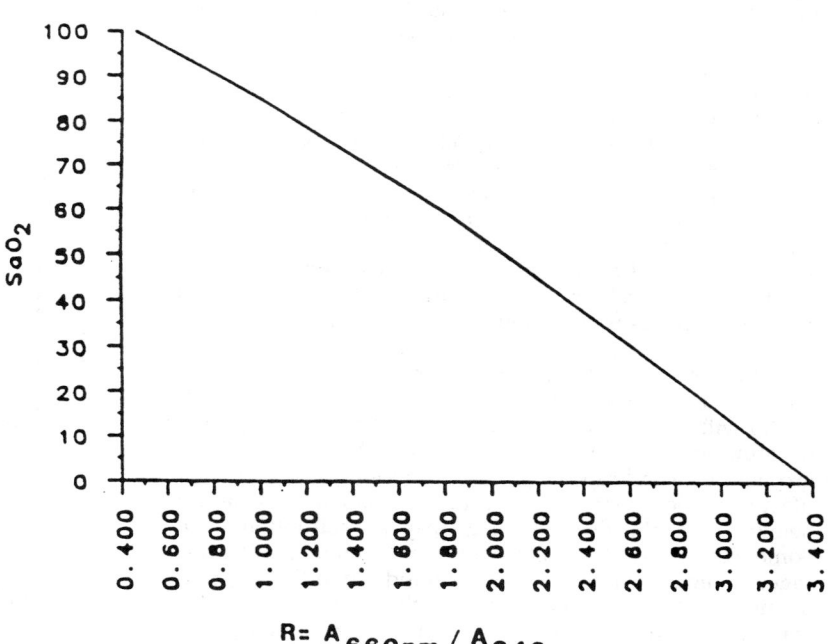

FIG. 5-28. Calibration curve used by the oximeter to calculate arterial oxygen saturation (Sa_{O_2}) from the ratio (R) of the light absorbed (A) by the tissue being monitored. (Courtesy of Ohmeda Corporation, Louisville, Colorado.)

There are several technical limitations inherent in pulse oximeters. First, being two-wavelength devices, they can identify only two unknowns. This would be adequate to measure functional hemoglobin saturation if MetHb and COHb did not absorb red or infrared light at the wavelengths used. Unfortunately, as can be seen in Figure 5-26, MetHb and COHb do absorb at 660 nm and 940 nm; therefore, if present, they will cause errors in the pulse oximeter reading. The effect of COHb on pulse oximeter values has been evaluated experimentally. It was noted that the pulse oximeter reads approximately the sum of O_2Hb plus COHb.[60] This is due to the fact that both O_2Hb and COHb are red and absorb red light similarly. The effect of MetHb on pulse oximeter readings has also been measured. It was found that as MetHb increased, the pulse oximeter tended toward 85% saturation and eventually became almost independent of Sa_{O_2}.[55] This has been explained by the fact that MetHb is very dark and absorbs both red and infrared light. It causes a large pulsatile absorbance at both wavelengths and thus forces the ratio of red to infrared absorbance toward one. As illustrated in Figure 5-28, an absorbance ratio of one corresponds to a saturation of 85%.

Intravenous dyes can also affect the accuracy of pulse oximeters.[61, 62] Scheller *et al*[61] evaluated the effects of methylene blue, indigo carmine, and indocyanine green on pulse oximeters in human volunteers. They found that methylene blue caused a drop in saturation to approximately 65% for 1 to 2 minutes. Indigo carmine produced a very small drop in saturation, whereas indocyanine green had an intermediate effect.

There are two engineering problems in pulse oximeter design that may affect clinical use.[59] The first is light interference. The photodiodes used as light sensors cannot discriminate one wavelength of light from another. Therefore, the sensor does not know whether a light signal is from the red LED, the infrared LED, or the room lights. This problem is solved by alternating the red and infrared LED, that is, the red LED is turned on first, and the photodiode produces a current resulting from the red LED plus the room lights. Next, the red LED is turned off and the infrared LED is turned on, and the photodiode signal represents the infrared LED and the room lights. Finally, both LEDs are turned off, and the photodiode measures a signal from just the room lights. This sequence is repeated 480 times per second. In this way, the oximeter subtracts out light interference, even in a quickly changing background of room light.[59] Some light sources can cause problems in spite of this clever design.

Another problem that is difficult to overcome is that of low signal to noise ratio and motion artifact. When a low pulse-added absorbance signal is seen by the photodetector, the pulse oximeter will amplify that signal and then estimate the saturation from the ratio of amplified absorbances. The pulse oximeter can thereby estimate saturation values from a wide range of patients with various pulse-added absorbance amplitudes. Unfortunately, as with a car radio, when a weak signal is amplified, the background noise (static) is also amplified. If amplified enough, it is possible that the pulse oximeter will analyze this noise signal and interpret it as a value of saturation. To prevent the oximeter from amplifying background noise and reporting false saturation values, the manufacturers incorporate cutoff values for signal to noise ratio below which the device will display no saturation value. Some oximeters also display a low signal strength error message. A similar problem is encountered when there is noise owing to patient motion artifact. In this situation, the pulse oximeter may not be able to determine an appropriate ratio of absorbances.

One of the main clinical advantages of a pulse oximeter is that it does not require calibration. In reality, a pulse oximeter cannot be calibrated, since the calibration curve is set in the factory, using data gathered from a small number of adult volunteers. Therefore, it is important that these devices be tested to ensure their accuracy under the conditions of their actual clinical use. We have already discussed how dyshemoglobins, dyes, and motion artifact can alter the output of a pulse oximeter. Severinghaus and Naifeh[63] evaluated the response of pulse oximeters from six manufacturers to an acute hypoxic plateau of 40%–70% saturation in adult volunteers. In this study, significant variability was found between the various pulse oximeters in both response time and accuracy in determining the low saturation value. It was noted that sensors placed on the ears responded more quickly than finger sensors. The accuracies were in the range of ±5%–10% compared with the manufacturers' stated accuracies of ±2%–3%.

CARBON DIOXIDE MEASUREMENT. The polio epidemic of the 1950s spurred the development of a rapid method for measuring arterial blood carbon dioxide tension (Pa_{CO_2}). In 1958, John Severinghaus presented the first blood gas analyzer using a Clark electrode for measuring P_{O_2} and a new P_{CO_2} electrode of his own design.[64] The Severinghaus P_{CO_2} electrode consists of a pH-sensitive glass electrode in an electrolyte cell surrounded by a CO_2-permeable membrane (Fig. 5-29). CO_2 diffuses through the membrane into the cell and reacts with water to produce carbonic acid, which changes the pH within the cell. The pH electrode is then calibrated to measure P_{CO_2}. This "secondary" sensing P_{CO_2} electrode is currently used in all blood gas analyzers. Like the oxygen electrode, the Severinghaus CO_2 electrode has also been used to

FIG. 5-29. A schematic of the Stow–Severinghaus P_{CO_2} electrode. It consists of a pH-sensitive glass electrode, referenced to a silver/silverchloride electrode. The glass electrode is immersed in an electrolyte cell with a CO_2 permeable membrane covering on the surface. CO_2 diffuses into the cell, reacts with water in the cell, producing carbonic acid, and the pH electrode detects the pH change.

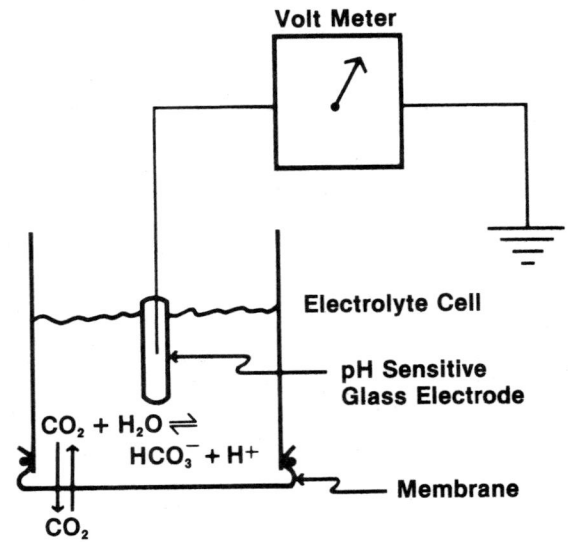

Stow-Severinghaus P_CO_2 Electrode

continuously monitor carbon dioxide from heated skin (transcutaneous P_{CO_2}).[65]

The hydrogen ion concentration in SI units is given in nanomoles per liter, although it is more frequently expressed as the negative logarithm of the hydrogen ion concentration, in "pH units." pH is usually measured with a glass pH electrode, which, when placed in solution, will develop a voltage relative to a reference electrode that is proportional to the hydrogen ion concentration. This electrode will produce approximately 60 millivolts for each pH unit. As noted previously, the carbon dioxide electrode in Figure 5-29 incorporates a pH electrode as its sensing device. A pH-sensitive optode has also been developed using a dye whose fluorescence is quenched in the presence of hydrogen ion. This pH optode has also been used to produce a CO_2 measuring device using the same secondary sensing principle as the Severinghaus CO_2 electrode.

Infrared analyzers for measuring CO_2 in the gas phase were developed in Germany during World War II. CO_2 absorbs infrared light at a wavelength of about 4.3 μ (4.3×10^{-6} m).[66] The height of this absorption peak is proportional to the CO_2 concentration. Infrared absorption systems used for monitoring carbon dioxide in the airway are known as capnometers, and they usually display a P_{CO_2} versus time waveform known as a capnogram. The mass spectrometer described later in this chapter can measure CO_2 and O_2 concentration as well as the concentrations of anesthetic agents in the airway.

ELECTRICITY, MAGNETISM, AND CIRCUITS

Electricity and magnetism affect every aspect of our existence, both in and out of the OR. Much of physiology is based on electrical phenomena, as is most of the modern technology that we apply to anesthesia and critical care. Electromagnetic waves are so important that they deserved special mention in Genesis: "Let there be light." One modern physicist has paraphrased this quotation: "Let there be electricity and magnetism, and there is light!"[67] In this section, we survey this field superficially, but hopefully with enough depth to provide an understanding of the laws of electromagnetics and their importance in medicine. The reader interested in original sources should consult the republished works of Faraday,[68] Priestley,[69] Thompson,[70] and Maxwell,[71] who were some of the pioneers in this field. Good histories of electrical science have been written by Meyer,[72] Benjamin,[73] and Bordeaux.[74] There are many good textbooks of electricity and magnetism for the reader in need of more detail.[75-81]

ELECTROSTATICS: CHARGE AND FIELDS

Benjamin Franklin (1706-1790) is credited with being the first person to understand that there are two (and only two) types of electric charge, which he named positive and negative. His early experiments, in which glass and rubber rods were charged by rubbing them, led to the conclusion that "like charges repel and unlike charges attract." Franklin also realized that, in some materials, the charge is free to move within the material, whereas in others, it is not. We call the former materials conductors and the latter materials insulators, or dielectrics. From other experiments, we know that in metallic conductors, only the negative charges (electrons) are free to move, while the positive charges are immobile. In electrolyte conductors, on the other hand, both positive and negative charges can move.

Coulomb, in 1785, determined that the force between two point charges is proportional to the magnitude of charge and

the inverse square of the separating distance r, thus leading to Coulomb's Law:

$$F = \frac{1}{4\pi\varepsilon_0} \frac{q_1 q_2}{r^2}. \qquad (5\text{-}67)$$

Here, q_1 and q_2 are the magnitudes of the two charges, and ε_0 is called the permittivity constant. The dimensions of charge are somewhat of a problem, because charge was initially defined in two different ways. In one system (electrostatic units, or esu), the dimensions are length × (force)$^{1/2}$, and the units of charge are called statcoulombs. In the other system (electromagnetic units, or emu), charge has dimensions of time × (force)$^{1/2}$, and the units are called abcoulombs. The conversion is one abcoulomb = 2.998×10^{10} statcoulombs. It is no coincidence that this conversion factor equals the speed of light in centimeters per second. Along with most modern texts, we use so-called rationalized emu here, in which 1 (rationalized) coulomb = 0.1 abcoulomb. In these units, the permittivity constant ε_0 is 8.854×10^{-12} coul^2/newton-meter^2, and the charge of an electron is -1.60×10^{-19} coulomb.

The electrostatic force exerted on a charged particle has a magnitude and a direction, that is, it is a vector. If we measure this force vector on a small "test charge," which we move around to determine the force everywhere in space, then we have defined an electrostatic field (or electric field). This field $\underline{E}$ is simply the vector force exerted on a unit charge at any point in space (x, y, z) and time (t). The force on any charged particle is proportional to its charge q and the field strength:

$$\underline{F} = q\underline{E}. \qquad (5\text{-}68)$$

A related concept invented by Faraday is that of lines of force.[68] These lines are everywhere parallel to the direction of the field vector, and the number of lines per unit cross-section is proportional to the magnitude of $\underline{E}$. Lines of force between two point charges of opposite sign are shown in Figure 5-30.

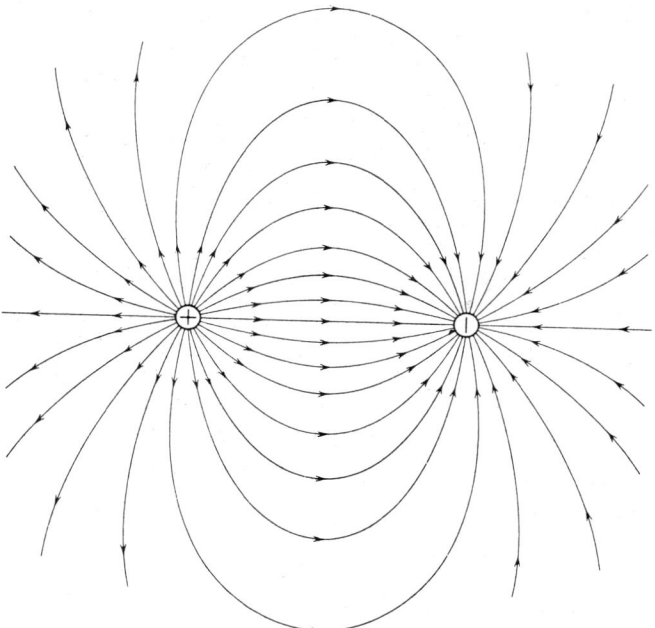

FIG. 5-30. The electric "lines of force" from a dipole, or two point charges of equal strength and opposite sign. The lines are everywhere parallel to E, and they are more closely spaced where E is stronger.

Suppose that we have two flat, parallel plates carrying equal and opposite charges, separated by distance d as shown in Figure 5-31. If the plates are large in area, the field between them will have uniform strength and direction. The force on a charged particle in that field is qE, and the work required to move the particle from the bottom plate to the top plate is:

$$W = \text{force} \times \text{distance} = qEd. \qquad (5\text{-}69)$$

(E without underscore refers to the magnitude of the vector E.) We now define the work required to move a unit charge from point A to point B as the *potential difference* V between these two points. In our parallel plate example, the potential difference is simply

$$V = W/q = Ed. \qquad (5\text{-}70)$$

Since field strength E has dimensions of force/charge (Eqn. 5-68), the dimensions of potential difference are (force × distance)/charge or work/charge. The SI unit of potential difference is the joule/coulomb or volt.

Electric fields obey a *superposition principle*, whereby the field created by any number of point charges is simply the vector sum of the individual fields from each particle. Therefore, the strength of the field between the two plates in Figure 5-31 will be directly proportional to the total charge Q on either plate. This means that the potential difference V must also be proportional to Q (Eqn. 5-70), so that:

$$Q = CV. \qquad (5\text{-}71)$$

The constant of proportionality C is called the *capacitance*, and the two plates are said to be a *capacitor* (in older terminology, a *condenser*). The dimensions of capacitance from Equation 5-71 are charge^2/(force × distance), and the SI unit of capacitance is the coulomb per volt, or *farad*. (A farad is such a large capacitance that we usually deal in microfarads, μf, where $1 \mu f = 10^{-6}$ f.) The capacitance of the two flat plates in Figure 5-31 is directly proportional to their area and inversely pro-

portional to the distance between them. Think of a capacitor as something that accumulates charge in response to a potential difference. The mechanical analog of a capacitor is a spring, which stores mechanical potential energy as the capacitor stores electrical potential energy.

Groups of capacitances are often combined in series or in parallel (Fig. 5-32). In Figure 5-32A, parallel connection, the total accumulated charge is $Q = q_1 + q_2 + q_3$; the potential difference V is the same across all three capacitors; therefore, the total capacitance C_t is simply the sum of the individual values:

$$C_t = C_1 + C_2 + C_3. \qquad (5\text{-}72)$$

In other words, capacitances in parallel are additive. This has important implications in the combination of leakage capacitances from several OR devices, as we shall see subsequently. In Fig. 5-32B, series connection, we note that the charge q on each capacitor must be the same. The potential differences across the three capacitors are not the same but are related by Equation 5-71:

$$V_1 = q/C_1, \qquad V_2 = q/C_2, \qquad V_3 = q/C_3,$$

and, since potential differences in series are additive,

$$\begin{aligned} V &= V_1 + V_2 + V_3 \\ &= q/C_1 + q/C_2 + q/C_3 = q[1/C_1 + 1/C_2 + 1/C_3]. \end{aligned}$$

The equivalent capacitance of the three is given by $V = q/C_t$, so

$$\frac{1}{C_t} = \frac{1}{C_1} + \frac{1}{C_2} + \frac{1}{C_3}. \qquad (5\text{-}73)$$

FIG. 5-32. (A) Capacitors connected in parallel. The voltage V is the same across all three capacitors. (B) Capacitors in series. The charge on each capacitor must be the same (the net charge inside the dotted line must be zero). (Halliday D, Resnick R: Physics, Part II. New York, John Wiley & Sons, 1962.)

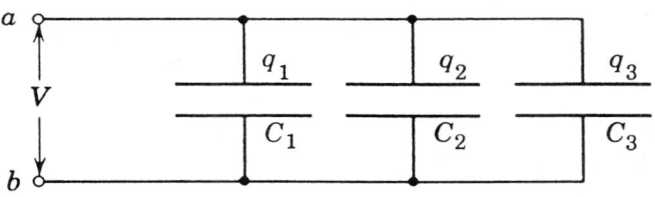

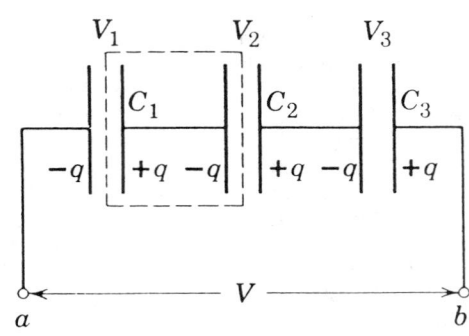

FIG. 5-31. The parallel plate capacitor. Plates P_1 and P_2, separated by distance d, have equal and opposite charges distributed on them, resulting in a uniform electric field E between the plates.

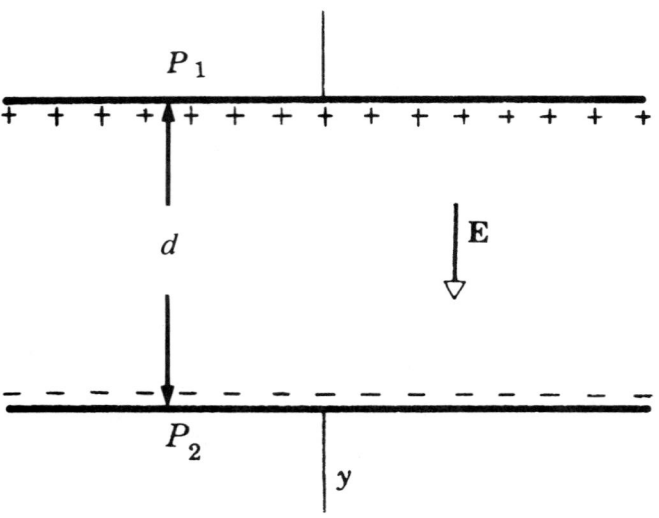

Capacitors in series thus add reciprocally, so that the equivalent capacitance is less than the smallest capacitance in the chain.

CURRENT, RESISTANCE, AND CIRCUITS

A *battery* is an electromechanical device that generates a potential difference between two points called the *battery terminals*. A battery is thus a source of voltage or electromotive force (EMF), as it is also called. If we connect the two battery terminals by a conductor, an electric field will be set up within the conductor, causing charges to move. This motion of charge through the conductor is called an *electric current* I, and it has dimensions of charge/time. The SI unit of current is the coulomb/second, or *ampere*. Although the electrons in a metal conductor flow in the *opposite* direction of the electric field (because they are negatively charged), the electric current is defined to be in the same direction as the field, that is, current is in the direction that positive charges would flow if they were free to move.

Now suppose that we connect a particular conductor to several batteries having different EMF values. For most metals at constant temperature, we obtain a linear relationship between the voltage and current:

$$V = IR. \qquad (5\text{-}74)$$

The proportionality constant R is called *resistance*. Its dimensions are length/time (which is the same as force × length × time/charge^2), and the SI units are volts/amperes, or ohms. Equation 5-74 is called Ohm's Law. Although it is valid for most metals, there are many materials that do not obey Ohm's Law.

When considering properties of conductors, an important quantity is the current density, or current per unit cross-sectional area of conductor (Fig. 5-33). Current density J has dimensions of charge/second/length^2, and the SI units are

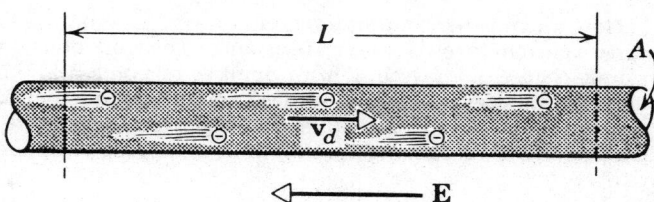

FIG. 5-33. A metallic conductor of length L and cross-section A. The electron drift velocity v_d is in the direction opposite to the electric field E.

amperes/meter^2. If A is the cross-sectional area of the conductor, then J = I/A. Another useful form of Ohm's Law is:

$$E = \rho J, \qquad (5\text{-}75)$$

where E is the electric field, J is current density (defined previously), and ρ is the resistivity, which is a property of the conducting material rather than of a particular specimen (not to be confused with ρ the fluid density). ρ has units of ohm-meters and is related to R by:

$$R = \rho L / A, \qquad (5\text{-}76)$$

where L and A are the length and cross-section of the specimen, respectively. (To show that Eqns. 5-74 and 5-75 are equivalent, use V = EL, I = JA, and Eqn. 5-76 in Eqn. 5-74.) Values of resistivity of common metals at room temperature are shown in Table 5-8. Note that the resistivity of metals increases with temperature (second column), whereas that of carbon decreases. Materials that develop extremely low resistivities at low temperatures are called *superconductors*. Low temperature superconductors are used in magnetic resonance imaging (MRI) to generate the intense magnetic fields required (see following paragraphs).

TABLE 5-8.   Properties of Metals as Conductors

	RESISTIVITY (at 20°C), ohm-m	TEMPERATURE COEFFICIENT OF RESISTIVITY,* α, per C°	DENSITY gm/cm^3	MELTING POINT, °C
Aluminum	2.8×10^{-8}	3.9×10^{-3}	2.7	659
Copper	1.7×10^{-8}	3.9×10^{-3}	8.9	1080
Carbon (amorphous)	3.5×10^{-5}	-5×10^{-4}	1.9	3500
Iron	1.0×10^{-7}	5.0×10^{-3}	7.8	1530
Manganin	4.4×10^{-7}	1×10^{-5}	8.4	910
Nickel	7.8×10^{-8}	6×10^{-3}	8.9	1450
Silver	1.6×10^{-8}	3.8×10^{-3}	10.5	960
Steel	1.8×10^{-7}	3×10^{-3}	7.7	1510
Wolfram (tungsten)	5.6×10^{-8}	4.5×10^{-3}	19	3400

*This quantity, defined from

$$\alpha = \frac{1}{\rho} \frac{d\rho}{dT}$$

is the fractional change in resistivity (dρ/ρ) per unit change in temperature. It varies with temperature, the values here referring to 20°C. For copper (α = 3.9 × 10^{-3}/C°), the resistivity increases by 0.39% for a temperature increase of 1 C° near 20°C. Note that α for carbon is negative, which means that the resistivity *decreases* with increasing temperature.

(Reprinted with permission from Halliday D, Resnick R: Physics, part II. New York, John Wiley & Sons, 1962.)

How much work per unit time, or "power," is required to drive a current through a given resistance? The work done on a unit charge in moving it from point A to point B is the potential difference V between these points. The number of charges being moved per unit time is the current I. Therefore, the total work being done per unit time is the product of the two:

$$P = VI. \qquad (5\text{-}77)$$

If we combine Equation 5-77 with Ohm's Law, V = IR, we obtain two other important power relationships:

$$P = I^2 R; \qquad P = V^2/R. \qquad (5\text{-}78)$$

Power has dimensions of force × distance/time, and the SI unit is the joule/sec, or watt. The power required to drive current through a resistance is dissipated as heat. Any fixed resistance through which current flows will generate heat in proportion to the square of the current (Eqn. 5-78). For example, a resistance of 1 ohm carrying a current of 1 ampere will dissipate 1 watt of power. The same resistance carrying 2 amperes will dissipate 4 watts. In terms of common heat units, 1 watt = 0.239 cal/sec = 0.860 Kcal/hr. Another unit of power is the horsepower, which equals 746 watts.

EXAMPLE: ELECTROCAUTERY

Electrocautery units use the resistive or joule heating described previously to generate high temperatures near a cauterizing electrode. High-frequency electrical current is used (10^5 to 10^6 Hertz range) to minimize the incidence of ventricular fibrillation. The total heat generated is $I^2 R$ (Eqn. 5-78), and the local rate of heating is proportional to the square of the current density J, as defined previously. J is far greater near the cauterizing electrode than in the surrounding tissue, because the current "spreads out" as it leaves the small electrode. (J falls as $1/r^2$, where r is distance from the electrode.) Under normal circumstances, then, the tissue heating is significant only very near the electrode.

In a "unipolar" electrocautery system, the current from the single cauterizing electrode travels through the body and leaves by means of the "grounding pad," which makes good electrical contact (*i.e.*, low resistance contact) with a large area of the skin. There are two factors that can cause skin burns in the area of the grounding pad. First, if only a small area of the pad is in actual contact with the skin, the current density J becomes large in this area in the same way that it becomes large near the cautery electrode. Second, if the ground pad is not well covered with conducting gel, it will make a high resistance contact with the skin. Even though the contact area may be large and the current density small in this case, $I^2 R$ is increased (by increasing R), and a very large burn can result. The electrocautery circuitry is designed to supply a fixed current through the electrode no matter what the resistance between the electrode and ground. In cases of defective grounding pads, patients have been burned at ECG electrode sites and other grounding pathways. We know of one anesthesiologist who was burned while touching the patient with one hand and his anesthesia machine with the other.

In the "bipolar" electrocautery system, the current flows between two small electrodes that are held a millimeter or so apart in the tissue. This geometry not only reduces the risk of skin burns but is also less likely to cause unwanted tissue damage or interfere with cardiac pacemakers. Bipolar devices are used exclusively in intracranial neurosurgery and are strongly recommended in all patients with pacemakers.

We have found that capacitances connected in a parallel circuit are additive, whereas in a series circuit, they combine reciprocally (Eqns. 5-72 and 5-73). Resistances connected in series (Fig. 5-34A) will be additive, because the same current I must pass through all three resistors:

$$V = IR_1 + IR_2 + IR_3 = I(R_1 + R_2 + R_3),$$
$$R_t = R_1 + R_2 + R_3. \qquad (5\text{-}79)$$

For resistors connected in parallel (Fig. 5-34B), the voltage will be the same across all three, so that:

$$I_1 = V/R_1, \qquad I_2 = V/R_2, \qquad I_3 = V/R_3.$$

The total current flowing through the battery is the sum of the three branch currents:

$$I = I_1 + I_2 + I_3 = V(1/R_1 + 1/R_2 + 1/R_3) = V/R_t,$$
$$1/R_t = 1/R_1 + 1/R_2 + 1/R_3. \qquad (5\text{-}80)$$

Resistors in parallel thus combine in a reciprocal fashion in the same way as capacitors in series.

FIG. 5-34. (*A*) Resistors connected in series to a source of EMF (V). The current I is the same through all three resistors. (*B*) Resistors connected in parallel. The voltage V is the same across all three resistors.

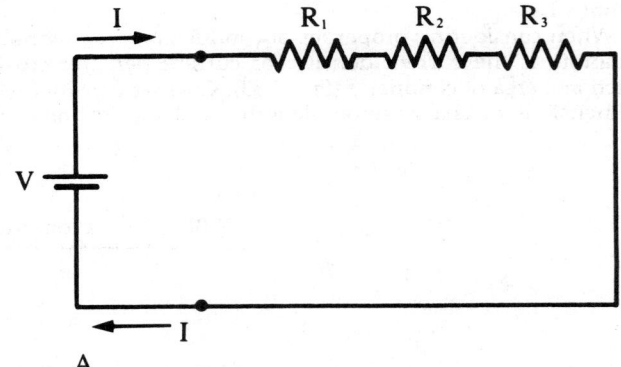

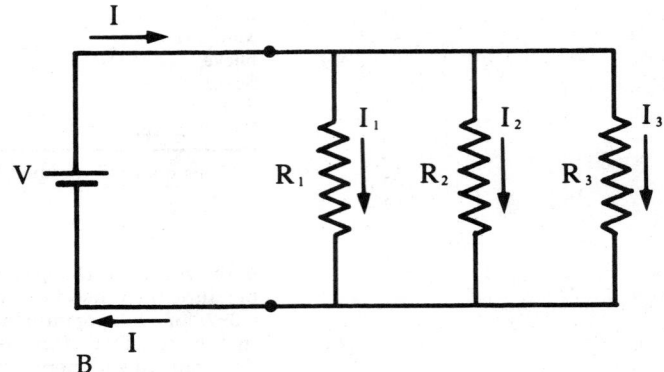

The preceding discussion and examples of resistive circuits are valid whether the voltage supply is a direct current battery or an alternating current generator, such as that of the commercial electricity supply. Alternating current implies a supply voltage that varies sinusoidally with time:

$$V(t) = A \sin(2\pi ft), \qquad (5-81)$$

where A is the amplitude, and f is the frequency (60 Hz in the United States, 50 Hz in Europe). When we speak of AC voltage, we usually mean the root–mean–square (rms) value of V(t), which is equal to 0.707 times the peak value (A) for a sinusoidal waveform.

EXAMPLE: THE RC-CIRCUIT

Let us consider a circuit involving both resistance and capacitance, a so-called RC-circuit (Fig. 5-35). When the switch is thrown from position b to a at time t = 0, the battery will drive a current I through the resistor and thereby charge the capacitor. As the charge Q builds up on the capacitor, the potential difference across the capacitor will increase (V = Q/C) until it is equal to the EMF from the battery. At this point, the current will reach zero. At any time during this process, the EMF from the battery equals the sum of the voltage drop across the resistor and the potential difference across the capacitor (Q/C):

$$V = IR + Q/C. \qquad (5-82)$$

The variables I and Q are related, since I = dQ/dt. We can thus rewrite Equation 5-82 as a differential equation for the charge Q:

$$R\frac{dQ}{dt} + \frac{Q}{C} - V = 0. \qquad (5-83)$$

The solution to this equation is:

$$Q = CV[1 - \exp(-t/RC)],$$

and

$$I = \frac{dQ}{dt} = (V/R)\exp(-t/RC). \qquad (5-84)$$

Figure 5-36 shows the charge Q and current I plotted versus time for R = 1,000 ohms, C = 1.0 microfarad, and V = 10

FIG. 5-35. Schematic of an RC circuit. Switch S moves from b to a at t = 0, which begins charging of capacitor C through resistor R.

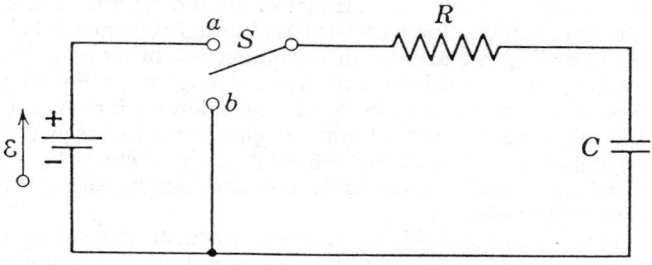

volts. Note that at t = 0, the current is V/R, which is the value it would have if the capacitor were not present. At t = RC (please verify that RC has the dimensions of time), Equation 5-84 yields:

$$I = (V/R) \exp(-1) = 0.37 \text{ V/R}.$$

The quantity RC is called the *capacitive time constant*, or *RC time constant*, of the circuit, and it is the time required for the current to fall to 37% of its initial value. During this same period, the charge Q rises to 63% of its final value of CV. The RC time constant is analogous to the time constants used in any physical process that can be represented by an exponential function, such as the "wash-in time" of fresh gas introduced into an anesthesia circuit. In one time constant, an exponential function will change by 63% of the amount that it would change over a very long period of time. In two time constants, it will change by 86%, and, in three time constants, by 95%.

MAGNETISM

Observations of magnetic phenomena date back for centuries, but it was Oersted in 1820 who first noted that an electric current in a wire can produce magnetic effects, namely, movement of a compass needle.[81] Just as electrostatic forces can be represented by the electric field vector $\underline{E}$, magnetic forces can be represented by a vector field $\underline{B}$, called the *magnetic induction*. By analogy to the lines of force shown for an electric field in Figure 5-30, we define magnetic lines of induction. These lines are everywhere parallel to the induction vector $\underline{B}$, and their density is proportional to the magnitude of $\underline{B}$.

We have not yet stated what a magnetic field is. If a particle carrying charge q moving at velocity $\underline{v}$ is deflected by a sideways force, we say that a magnetic field is present. The magnetic deflecting force is proportional to the field strength, the charge, and the velocity of the particle. Mathematically, this magnetic force is given by

$$\underline{F} = q\underline{v} \times \underline{B}. \qquad (5-85)$$

The product indicated here is the vector product, or *cross-product* of the two vectors $\underline{v}$ and $\underline{B}$. This is a vector of magnitude vB sin (θ), where θ is the angle between $\underline{v}$ and $\underline{B}$, and direction perpendicular to both $\underline{v}$ and $\underline{B}$ (Fig. 5-37). Since the cross-product is perpendicular to the velocity $\underline{v}$, magnetic force is always at right angles to the direction of motion. Although only one direction is required to determine the electrostatic force (the direction of $\underline{E}$), we need two directions ($\underline{v}$ and $\underline{B}$) to determine magnetic force.

From Equation 5-85, $\underline{B}$ has dimensions of force/charge/velocity. The SI unit of induction is the (newton/coulomb)/(meter/sec), defined as the *tesla*. Since one coulomb/sec is an ampere, the tesla is also equivalent to the newton/ampere-meter. An older unit of magnetic induction still commonly used is the gauss, given by 1 tesla = 10^4 gauss. The earth's magnetic induction is roughly 0.5 gauss in most parts of the United States. The direction of $\underline{B}$ is about 60 degrees downward from horizontal, so that the horizontal component is 0.2 to 0.3 gauss. The field generated in a MRI is one to two tesla (1 to 2×10^4 gauss).

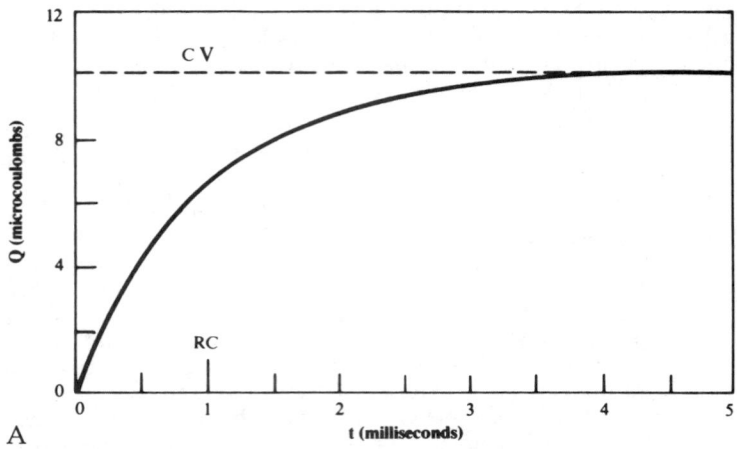

A

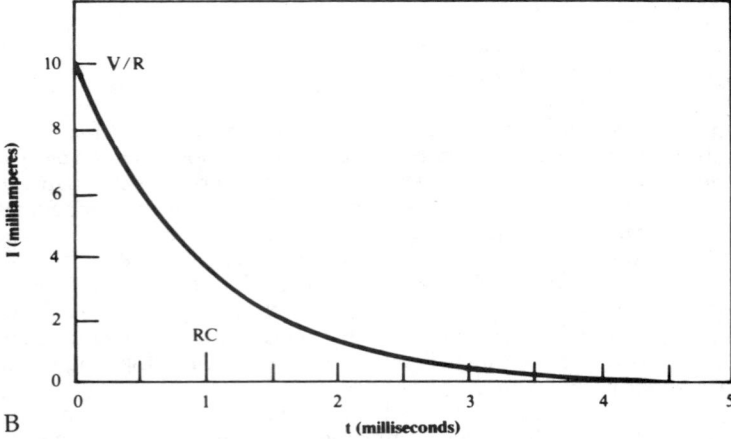

B

FIG. 5-36. The RC circuit (R = 1,000 ohms, C = 1 microfarad, V = 10 volts): Charge Q on the capacitor and current I through the resistor as functions of time t after switch closure. As t increases, Q approaches CV, and I approaches zero.

FIG. 5-37. Illustration of the vector relationships between a charged particle's velocity $\underline{v}$, the magnetic field $\underline{B}$, and the magnetic force $\underline{F}$ acting upon the particle.

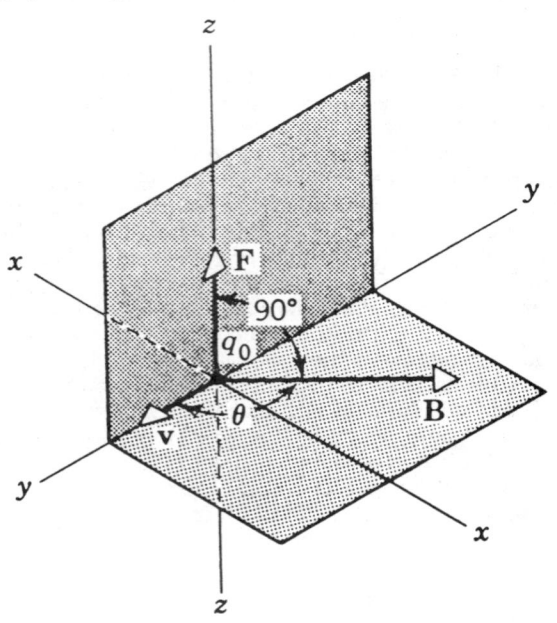

EXAMPLE: MASS SPECTROMETRY

The mass spectrometer is useful for measurement of anesthetic and respiratory gases in a mixture. The mass spectrometer determines the charge to mass ratio (q/m) of charged molecules or "ions" by making use of both magnetic and electrostatic forces. For a particle under the influence of both types of force, Equations 5-68 and 5-85 can be combined:

$$\underline{F} = q\underline{E} + q\underline{v} \times \underline{B}. \qquad (5-86)$$

The spectrometer is able to identify the ions by their characteristic q/m values and thus determine how much of each species is present. As shown in Figure 5-38, the spectrometer first accelerates the ions through a known electric field $\underline{E}$. Once accelerated, the particles pass through a magnetic field $\underline{B}$ oriented perpendicular to their direction of motion. The ions experience a sideways magnetic force given by Equation 5-86, and their trajectories bend. The sideways force is proportional to q, and the sideways acceleration is inversely proportional to m, so that the deflection angle α (Fig. 5-38) is a function of q/m. α is measured by the detectors, and q/m is thus determined.

From Equation 5-85, we can also calculate the magnetic force exerted on a wire carrying a current through a magnetic field. If a length L of wire carrying current I is placed in a field

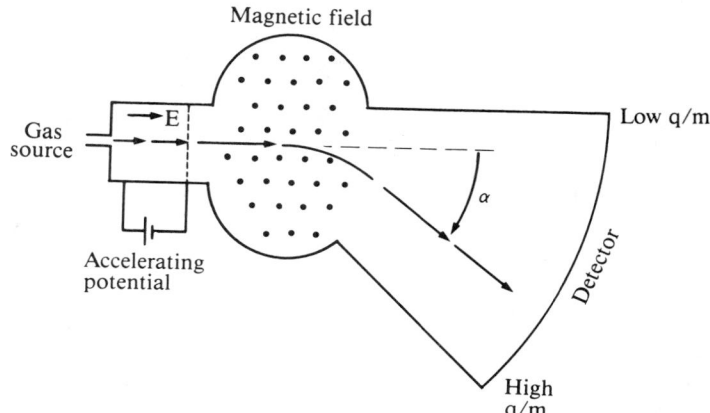

FIG. 5-38. Schematic of the mass spectrometer principle. Gas ions at left are accelerated by electric field E; their trajectories are then bent by the magnetic field (shown directed out of page). Deflection angle is proportional to charge/mass ratio (q/m).

of strength B and direction perpendicular to the wire, it is easy to show from Equation 5-85 that the force on the wire is

$$F = ILB. \qquad (5\text{-}87)$$

The direction of this force is perpendicular to both the wire and the field.

Just as a magnetic field exerts a force on any moving charged particle, any moving charge or electric current will itself generate a magnetic field. For a current I passing through a long, straight wire, the induction at a distance r from the wire is given by:

$$B = \frac{\mu_0 I}{2\pi r}. \qquad (5\text{-}88)$$

(μ_0, the permeability constant, is $4\pi \times 10^{-7}$ in SI units.) The direction of the magnetic field is in a series of concentric circles around the wire. This direction is easy to determine by the "right-hand rule": grasp the wire with the right hand, the thumb pointing in the direction of the current. The fingers will then curl around the wire in the direction of $\underline{B}$. With this rule and Equation 5-85, you should be able to predict the direction of the magnetic force between two parallel wires carrying current in the same direction (Fig. 5-39). The two wires will attract each other with a force proportional to the product of the two currents. Obviously, if the currents are in opposite directions, the wires will repel. These facts were discovered by both Ampere and Oersted in 1820, and Equation 5-88 is a form of "Ampere's Law."

MAGNETIC INDUCTION AND INDUCTANCE

Faraday[68] discovered another important link between electricity and magnetism in 1831: A moving magnet will generate an electric current in a stationary wire (Fig. 5-40A). As long as the magnet in Figure 5-40A is moving, a current will flow through the wire loop causing a deflection of the galvanometer. If the direction of motion or the polarity of the magnet is reversed, the current will reverse. Similarly, in Figure 5-40B, when the switch is closed and a current begins to flow through wire loop A, an induced current will flow through loop B until the current through A reaches a constant value. When this occurs, the induced current through B will fall to zero. In other words, it is the *rate of change* of the magnetic field that is responsible for the induced current in both cases.

The quantitative form of this physical law, called *Faraday's Law of Induction*, is the basis for all electric generators and transformers. A generator is simply an apparatus that moves loops of wire through a fixed magnetic field, or *vice versa*—it does not matter which element is moving and which is fixed. An induced current is generated in the wires, and the energy required to turn the generator is thereby converted into electricity. The current generated in this manner can be AC or DC, depending upon the switching connections to the moving wires. A transformer is an arrangement of two sets of wire coils that operates on the principle of Figure 5-40B. The changing magnetic field caused by the varying current through the "primary coil" induces a current in the "secondary coil." Because it is the rate of change of the magnetic field of the primary coil that induces current in the secondary coil, transformers will work only for AC power. Transformers are used to change the voltage of an AC source while maintaining constant power (remember: P = VI, Eqn. 5-77). The ratio of the secondary voltage to the primary voltage is equal to the

FIG. 5-39. Two parallel wires "a" and "b" carrying currents i_a and i_b in the same direction. The magnetic field from wire a (B_a) is directed downward at wire b, causing a magnetic force F attracting wire b toward wire a.

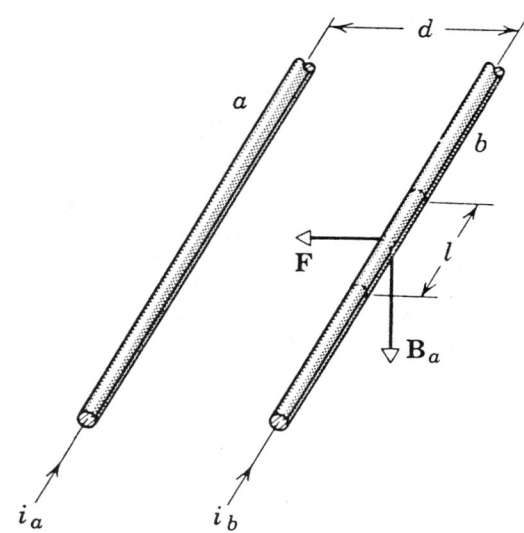

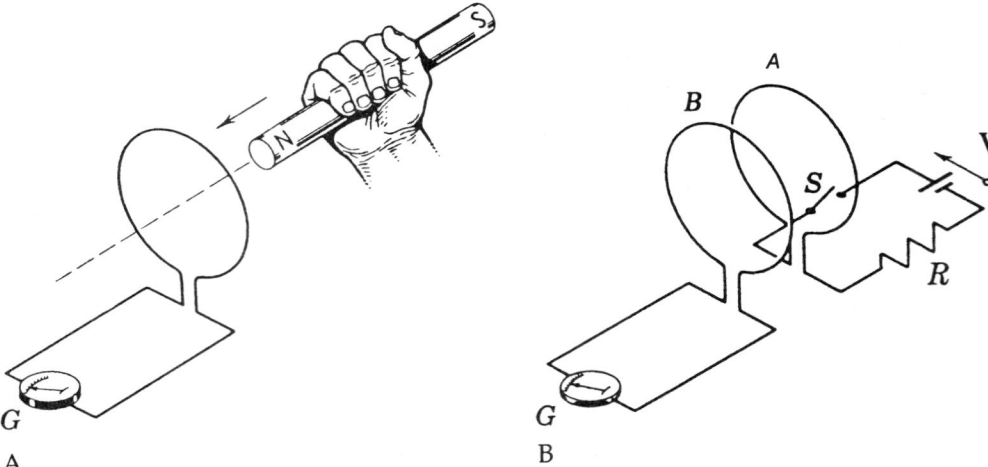

FIG. 5-40. Current induced by a changing magnetic field (Faraday's Law). (*A*) A magnet moving through a wire loop induces current through galvanometer G. (*B*) When switch S is thrown, the time-varying current through loop A causes a time-varying magnetic field in loop A, which induces a current in loop B. (Halliday D, Resnick R: Physics, Part II. New York, John Wiley & Sons, 1962.)

ratio of the numbers of loops in the secondary and primary coils. We shall discuss the use of transformers in the OR subsequently.

When a changing current passes through a coil of wire as in the primary coil of a transformer, the resulting varying magnetic field will also induce an EMF *in the same coil* that produces the field. This phenomenon is called *self-induction,* and the induced EMF opposes the EMF that produced the original current. This self-induced EMF is proportional to the rate of change of the current through the coil:

$$V = L \frac{dI}{dt}. \qquad (5\text{-}89)$$

The proportionality constant L is called the *inductance* of the coil. The SI unit of inductance is the volt-sec/ampere, which is called the *henry.* The henry is a rather large unit (like the farad in capacitance), so we commonly use the millihenry (10^{-3} henry).

With the addition of inductance, we now have three types of "reactance," or voltage change resulting from current or charge:

REACTANCE TYPE (UNITS)	SYMBOL	FORMULA
Resistance (ohm):	—⟋⟍⟋⟍⟋—	V = IR
Capacitance (farad):	—⊣ ⊢—	V = Q/C
Inductance (henry):	⟀⟀⟀⟀⟀	V = L(dI/dt)

Since current is the time derivative of charge ($I = dQ/dt$), the three reactances are proportional to charge and its first- and second-time derivatives. From these formulas, we see that the ratio of voltage to current for an AC source will depend upon the source frequency for capacitors and inductors. This ratio, called the *reactance,* for a sinusoidally varying voltage of angular frequency ω is given by:

Capacitive reactance $R_c = \dfrac{1}{\omega C}$

Inductive reactance $R_L = \omega L$. $\qquad (5\text{-}90)$

Capacitive reactance decreases with increasing frequency, whereas inductive reactance increases. For a frequency of

zero (DC source), the capacitive reactance is infinite (open circuit), whereas the inductive reactance is zero (short circuit).

EXAMPLE: THE L-R-C CIRCUIT

If we combine all three reactances with a time-varying voltage source V(t) as shown in Figure 5-41, Ohm's law for this circuit can be written as:

$$V(t) = L \frac{d^2Q}{dt^2} + R \frac{dQ}{dt} + \frac{Q}{C}. \qquad (5\text{-}91)$$

Comparing this equation with Equation 5-14 for the forced harmonic oscillator problem, we see that they are essentially the same equation. We can therefore draw an analogy between the mass-spring oscillator and the L-R-C circuit of Figure 5-41, in which the displacement x is analogous to the electrical charge Q. Mass m corresponds to inductance L; the spring constant k corresponds to reciprocal capacitance 1/C; and friction c corresponds to resistance R. The solution for the L-R-C circuit shows the same resonance behavior (Eqn. 5-16 and Fig. 5-2) as the mass-spring oscillator. This analogy between mechanics and electrical circuits is useful in studying many physical phenomena, such as the arterial pressure waveform discussed previously.

FIG. 5-41. The L-R-C circuit. An oscillating source of EMF, V(t) drives current through inductance L, resistance R, and capacitance C.

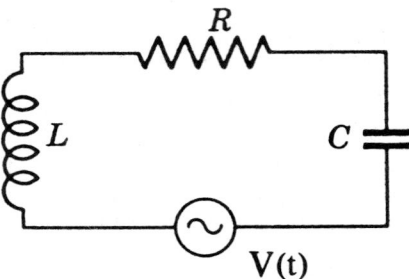

EXAMPLE: ELECTRICAL SAFETY, ISOLATION TRANSFORMERS

The human body is not very tolerant of electrical current; in fact, as little as 50 μA (μA = microampere = 10^{-6} ampere) passing through the heart can cause ventricular fibrillation. Current that is delivered directly to the heart is called *microshock*, whereas current passing through the skin or tissue remote from the heart is called *macroshock*. While a microshock current of 50 μA can fibrillate the heart, the required macroshock is in the range of 0.1 to 2.5 ampere. Thus, the distinction between the two is of practical importance in electrical safety. The threshold of sensation of a 60-Hz macroshock current is 300 to 500 μA; pain is felt at 1 to 2 mA (mA = milliampere = 10^{-3} ampere). Sustained muscle contraction occurs at 8 to 20 mA, the so-called cannot let-go current. (Above this value, a subject who grasps a "hot" wire will not be able to release it.) Shocks also pose other hazards in the OR: fires, tissue burns, nerve stimulation or damage, and pacemaker interference are only a few.[82–85]

Figure 5-42 illustrates the danger of macroshock from electrical equipment. In Figure 5-42A, we depict a 60-Hz power supply connected directly at points A and B to a piece of equipment shown as resistance R. Side B of the power supply is connected to "ground," which is simply an infinite source (or sink) for electrons, always maintained at zero electrical potential no matter what current is flowing. We see that one

side of the equipment circuitry is grounded (through B), as is the metal case around the equipment. If a grounded patient (or anesthesiologist) comes into contact with part of the equipment circuitry connected to side A of the power supply, he will receive a macroshock of up to 120 volts (the assumed supply voltage). This will yield a current well above the "cannot let-go" value, even if the contact is with dry skin. The line isolation monitor (LIM) shown in Figure 5-42A would indicate a current of 120 mA in this case (see following).

The dangers of the circuit in Figure 5-42A led to the use of the isolation transformer, shown in Figure 5-42B. Side B of the power supply is still grounded, but the equipment power leads C and D are both ungrounded. Neither lead makes contact with the equipment case, which is generally grounded. The isolation transformer creates a potential between leads C and D, but there is no potential between either C or D and ground. Thus, the equipment receives its power (current flows through R), but the grounded patient touching any part of the equipment circuitry will not receive a macroshock. The line isolation monitor reads zero current, because it does not complete a circuit between power leads C and D, or between A and ground. The LIM thus tests the safety of all circuits connected to the transformer at C, D by indicating their degree of isolation from ground.

In practice, electrical circuits are never perfectly isolated from ground. There is always some capacitive coupling to

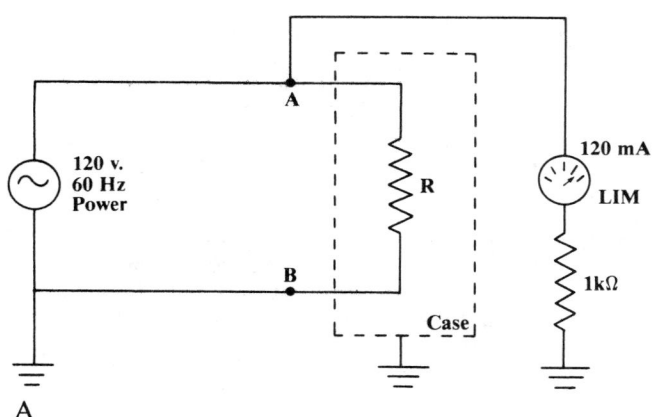
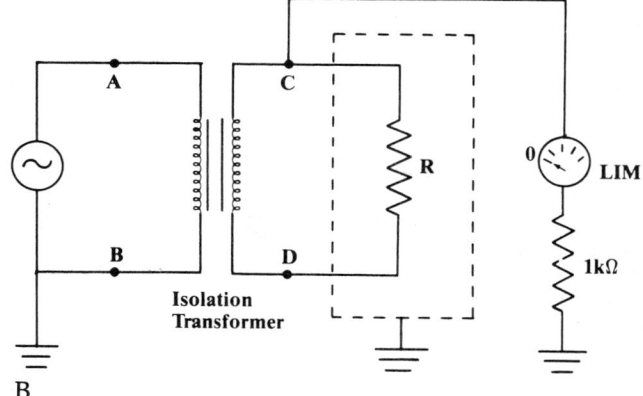
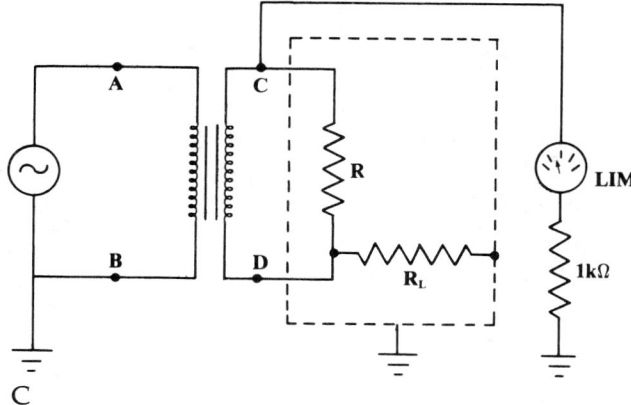

FIG. 5-42. Electrical isolation and leakage currents. (A) No isolation: circuitry (R) is "hot" relative to electrical ground, resulting in serious macroshock hazard. LIM reads 120 mA. (B) Isolation: Neither C nor D is "hot" relative to ground. LIM reads zero. (C) Isolation with leakage in equipment (R_L). D is now partially grounded through R_L, making C "hot" relative to ground. LIM reads leakage current inversely proportional to R_L.

ground—remember the parallel plate capacitor example discussed previously (Fig. 5-31). Recall also that capacitances connected in parallel are additive (Eqn. 5-72), so that the capacitive leakage from multiple devices will be cumulative. If equipment is faulty, there may also be a resistive connection to ground, or even a short-circuit to one side (C or D). This is illustrated in Figure 5-42C by the "leakage" resistance R_L. The LIM now reads a nonzero leakage current, because it completes a circuit (through R_L) between C and D. In the OR, the LIM actually monitors both sides of the power supply (C and D) and is usually set to alarm at a current of 2 to 4 mA. The LIM will not warn of leakage currents in the microshock range (50 μA). Additional precautions should therefore be taken with equipment that is in contact with the heart or major blood vessels (e.g., ECG measured through a central venous line). Blood is a fairly good electrical conductor, and leakage currents into large vessels must be considered as microshock hazards.

ELECTROMAGNETIC WAVES

If we combine all the relationships between $\underline{E}$, $\underline{B}$, I, and q, we obtain a set of four equations called *Maxwell's Equations*,[71] which govern the behavior of all electromagnetic fields. Through Maxwell's Equations, we can demonstrate the existence of electromagnetic waves of the type shown in Figure 5-43, in which the $\underline{E}$ and $\underline{B}$ fields are oriented at right angles to one another, and both are perpendicular to the direction of wave propagation. This is called a *transverse electromagnetic wave*, and it propagates to the right in Figure 5-43 at the speed of light, c. The oscillating electric and magnetic fields are given by

$$E = E_m \sin k(x - ct)$$
$$B = B_m \sin k(x - ct). \qquad (5-92)$$

(k is called the *wavenumber* and is related to wavelength by $k = 2\pi/\lambda$.) Numerous experiments have determined c to be 2.9979×10^8 m/sec (186,400 miles/sec or 7.5 times around the earth's circumference in 1 sec). Foucalt measured c with three-digit accuracy as early as 1862, using a rotating mirror apparatus.

There are some important differences between electromagnetic waves and sound waves. The particle motions in sound waves are in the same direction as the wave propagation (longitudinal wave), whereas in electromagnetic waves, the $\underline{E}$ and $\underline{B}$ fields are both perpendicular to the direction of propagation (transverse wave). Sound waves can only propagate through matter, whereas electromagnetic waves will propagate through a vacuum without attenuation. The speed of light is about one million times faster than the speed of sound in air. If an observer is moving relative to a sound source, he can measure a speed of sound that depends upon his own motion, but the speed of light is the same to any observer in any frame of reference. This statement is the basic premise of Einstein's special theory of relativity.

Electromagnetic radiation spans a very wide frequency spectrum, as shown in Figure 5-44. Frequency and wavelength are related by $c = f\lambda$, so that one is easily found from the other. The visible light spectrum is centered at a wavelength of 5.55×10^{-7} meter. For historical reasons, three different units are used to measure light wavelengths:

$$
\begin{aligned}
1 \text{ micron } (\mu) &= 10^{-6} \text{ meter} \\
1 \text{ nanometer (nm)} &= 10^{-9} \text{ meter} \\
1 \text{ angstrom (A)} &= 10^{-10} \text{ meter.}
\end{aligned}
$$

The visible spectrum extends from 4300 A (violet) to 6900 A (red). The corresponding frequency range ($c = f\lambda$) is from 4.3 to 7×10^{14} Hz. Note that visible light covers a very small fraction of the total electromagnetic spectrum shown in Figure 5-44.

EXAMPLE: ELECTROMAGNETIC RADIATION IN THE OPERATING ROOM

We know from Ampere's Law (Eqn. 5-88) that any electric current in a wire will create a magnetic field. If this current is oscillating, electromagnetic (EM) radiation will be emitted from the wire. This is the principle of all radio antennas. Unshielded wires or other sensing devices in the vicinity of the radiating source will then "receive" the signal. It can be shown from Maxwell's Equations that the radiated power from a wire is proportional to the square of the frequency.[80] This has important implications for two sources of EM radiation in the OR: the 60-Hz (wall) power supply and the elec-

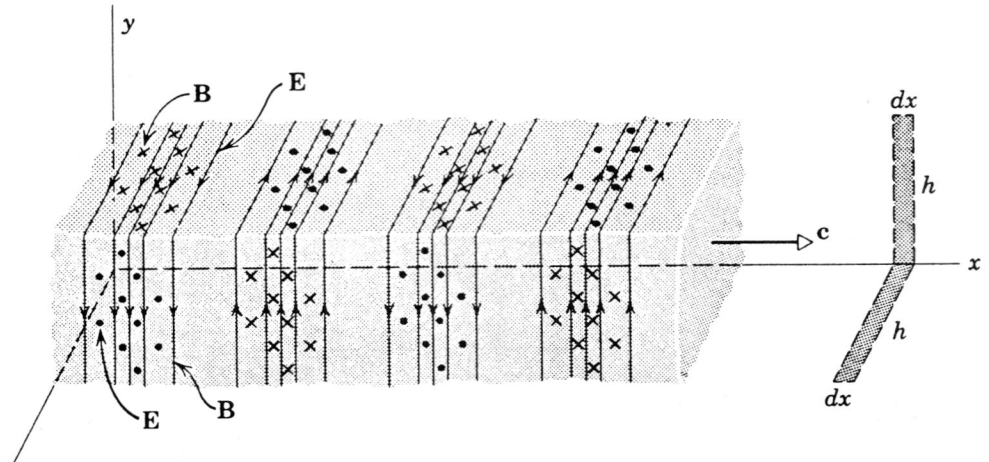

FIG. 5-43. A transverse electromagnetic wave. The E field is in the z-direction; the B field is in the y-direction; and the wave propagates in the x-direction at speed c.

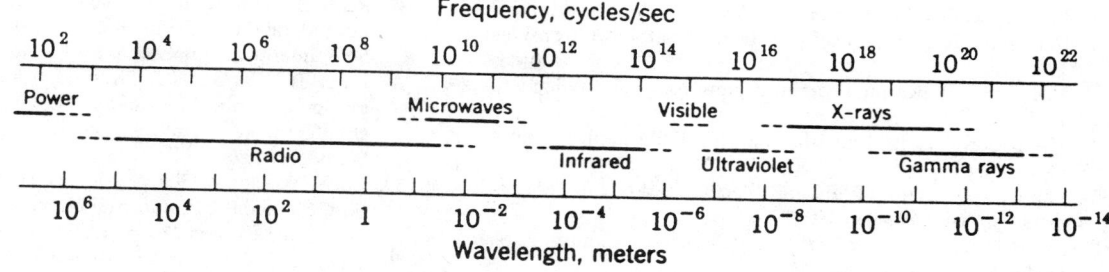

FIG. 5-44. The electromagnetic wave spectrum (frequency above, wavelength below). Visible light represents a small fraction of this spectrum. (Halliday D, Resnick R: Physics, Part II. New York, John Wiley & Sons, 1962.)

trocautery. If the electrocautery current frequency is 500 kHz, then its efficiency relative to the common household current is 7×10^7. That is, a given length of wire carrying a given current will emit 7×10^7 times more EM radiation at 500 kHz than it will at 60 Hz! Thus, while 60-Hz interference from the usual electrical sources may be significant for unshielded ECG leads, it is relatively easy to eliminate from shielded circuits. On the other hand, electrocautery interference or "Bovie artifact" is a constant problem that has required thousands of engineering man-hours to eliminate.

Ionizing Radiation

At the high-frequency end of the EM radiation spectrum in Figure 5-44, we see two forms of ionizing radiation: x-rays and gamma-rays. These high-frequency EM waves are capable of knocking electrons out of their orbits and can thereby cause cell injury, cell death, or oncogenesis. Gamma-rays are commonly emitted by decaying radioactive nuclei, along with two other types of ionizing radiation: alpha and beta particles. Alpha particles are helium nuclei (two protons, two neutrons) and are relatively heavy and slow moving. Although they can injure tissue with prolonged exposure close to a source, they do not travel very far in air, and most are stopped by a sheet of paper. Beta particles are high-energy electrons emitted from unstable nuclei. They can damage tissue but are blocked by a thin sheet of almost any metal. Gamma-rays are the most penetrating of the nuclear emissions; they can travel any distance through air and require lead or other heavy shielding to block them. Radiation not originating from nuclear decay can also be hazardous, as exemplified by the proton accelerators now used to treat cancer. Both high-energy x-rays and particle beams may not be blocked by lead aprons.

Ionizing radiation is quantified in four ways: activity, exposure, absorption, and biological damage. The activity of a radioactive substance is simply the number of disintegrations per second and is measured in Curies (1 Curie = 3.7×10^{10} disintegrations/sec). Exposure is a measure of radiation ionization at a particular location and is defined by the number of free electrons released from a kilogram of exposed air. The unit of exposure is the Roentgen (1 R = 2.58×10^{-4} coulomb/kg of air). Absorption refers to the radiation energy dissipated in each kilogram of tissue, given in units of rads (1 rad = 0.01 joule/kg). Biological damage or dose-equivalent depends upon the type of radiation as well as the absorption; thus, it equals absorption times a quality factor Q. The unit is the *rem*, or Roentgen-equivalent-man. The maximal "safe" occupational whole-body radiation dose per year is now set at 5 rem. For comparison, a patient having a chest x-ray receives 20 to 30 millirem (mrem) of radiation. The dose for a CT scan is about 1 rem per cross-section. The obligate radiation dose from cosmic rays in the United States is about 80 mrem per year.[86-90]

Radiation exposure of OR personnel depends upon the source intensity or activity, the directionality of the radiation (*e.g.*, for x-ray or proton beam), and the distance from the source. Radioactive substances, such as iridium implants, emit equally in all directions. The exposure is then directly proportional to the activity and inversely proportional to the square of the distance from the source. In other words, the exposure 10 m from the source is only 1% of that at 1 m. For x-rays, the exposure will depend upon the direction as well as distance from the source. In general, the back-scattered radiation (in the direction opposite that of the gun) is more intense than the forward-scattered radiation.

CONCLUSION

We have only scratched the surface of the fields discussed in this chapter, and there are many important fields of physics not even mentioned here. Concepts that start as simple as $\underline{F} = m\underline{a}$ can lead to considerable mathematical complexity when applied to practical problems, as we have seen. Although this complexity may discourage some readers, as physicians we should at least be familiar with the basic concepts and with the types of approaches used to apply these to the "real world." Only with some understanding of the mathematics of physics can we make use of the many physical analogies that apply to anesthesia. For example, how can we speak of the time constant of a circle system without knowing how a time constant is defined for an exponential process (such as the RC-circuit) or why such a process should occur? The more we know of basic physics, the better we shall be able to understand, practice, and teach anesthesiology.

REFERENCES

1. Macintosh R (Sir), Mushin WW, Epstein HG: Physics for the anesthetist. Springfield, Illinois, Charles C Thomas, 1958
2. Dugas R: A history of mechanics. Switzerland, Editions Du Griffon, 1955
3. Newton I: In Principia. Translation by Motte, University of California Press, Berkeley, 1934
4. Gardner RM: Direct blood pressure measurement—dynamic response requirements. Anesthesiology 54:227, 1981
5. Goldstein H: Classical Mechanics. Cambridge, Massachusetts, Addison-Wesley, 1953

6. Lindsay R: Physical Mechanics. New York, Van Nostrand, 1961
7. Symon K: Mechanics. Reading, Massachusetts, Addison-Wesley, 1960
8. Meriam JL: Statics and Dynamics. New York, John Wiley & Sons, 1978
9. Thompson W (Lord Kelvin): Principles of Mechanics. New York, Dover, 1962
10. Landau LD, Lifshitz EM: Fluid Mechanics. Reading, Massachusetts, Addison-Wesley, 1959
11. Batchelor GK: Introduction to Fluid Dynamics. Cambridge, Cambridge University Press, 1970
12. Streeter VL, Wylie EB: Fluid Mechanics. New York, McGraw-Hill, 1979
13. Sabersky R, Acosta A: Fluid Flow. New York, Macmillan, 1971
14. Schlichting H: Boundary Layer Theory. New York, McGraw-Hill, 1968
15. Lamb H (Sir): Hydrodynamics. New York, Dover, 1945
16. Liepmann HW, Roshko A: Elements of Gas Dynamics. New York, John Wiley & Sons, 1967
17. Thompson P: Compressible-Fluid Dynamics. New York, McGraw-Hill, 1972
18. Zucrow MJ, Hoffman JD: Gas Dynamics. New York, John Wiley & Sons, 1976
19. Reynolds O: On the experimental investigation of the circumstances which determine whether the motion of water shall be direct or sinuous, and the law of resistance in parallel channels. Philos Trans R Soc Lond 174:935, 1883
20. Carnot S: Reflexions on the Motive Power of Fire. New York, Lillian Barber Press, 1986 (Orig. 1830)
21. Planck M: Treatise on Thermodynamics. New York, Dover, 1945
22. Fermi E: Thermodynamics. New York, Dover, 1936
23. Sabersky R: Elements of Engineering Thermodynamics. New York, McGraw-Hill, 1957
24. Beattie JA, Oppenheim I: Principles of Thermodynamics. New York, Elsevier, 1979
25. Black WZ, Hartley JG: Thermodynamics. New York, Harper & Row, 1985
26. Guggenheim EA: Thermodynamics. New York, John Wiley & Sons, 1967
27. Lewis GN, Randall M: Thermodynamics. New York, McGraw-Hill, 1961
28. Sears FW: Thermodynamics, the Kinetic Theory of Gases, and Statistical Mechanics. Reading, Massachusetts, Addison-Wesley, 1953
29. Riba A, Berger HJ: Echocardiography. In Glenn WWL, Baue AE, Geha AS et al (eds): Thoracic and Cardiovascular Surgery, 4th ed. Norwalk, Connecticut, Appleton-Century-Crofts, 1983
30. Gramiak R, Nanda NC: New techniques in cardiac imaging with ultrasound: State of the art. Radiology 6:1, 1981
31. Popp RL, Rubenson DS, Tucker CR et al: Echocardiography: M-mode and two-dimensional methods. Ann Intern Med 93:844, 1980
32. Ludomirsky A, Huhta JC, Vick GW et al: Color doppler detection of multiple ventricular septal defects. Circulation 74(6):1317, 1986
33. Incropera FP, DeWitt DP: Fundamentals of Heat and Mass Transfer, Appendix A, 2nd ed, p 752. New York, John Wiley & Sons, 1985
34. Incropera FP, DeWitt DP: Fundamentals of Heat and Mass Transfer, 2nd ed, Chapter 1, Introduction, p 8. New York, John Wiley & Sons, 1985
35. Incropera FP, DeWitt DP: Fundamentals of Heat and Mass Transfer, 2nd ed, Chapter 3, One-dimensional steady-state conduction, p 66. New York, John Wiley & Sons, 1985
36. Bennett CO, Myers JE: Momentum, Heat and Mass Transport, Chapter 19, Conduction and thermal conductivity, p 242. New York, McGraw-Hill, 1962
37. Ruch TC, Patton HD: Physiology and Biophysics, vol 3, Digestion, Metabolism, Endocrine Function and Reproduction, Chapter 4, Energy metabolism, p 85. Philadelphia, WB Saunders, 1973
38. Ruch TC, Patton HD: Physiology and Biophysics, vol 3, Digestion, Metabolism, Endocrine Function and Reproduction, chapter 5, Temperature regulation, p 105. Philadelphia, WB Saunders, 1973
39. Ruch TC, Patton HD: Physiology and Biophysics, vol 3, Digestion, Metabolism, Endocrine Function and Reproduction, chapter 9, Free convection, p 417. Philadelphia, WB Saunders, 1973
40. Edwards DK, Denny VE, Mills AF: Transfer Processes, an Introduction to Diffusion, Convection and Radiation, 2nd ed, chapter 5, Convective transfer rates, p 140. New York, McGraw-Hill, 1979
41. Morley PK: Unintentional hypothermia in the operating room. Can Anaesth Soc J 33:516, 1986
42. Chang KS, Farrell RT, Snellen JW et al: Calorimetrical comparison of insulative properties of metalized plastic, clear polyethylene, and polyester blanket. Can Anaesth Soc J 31(6):690, 1984
43. Parbrook GD, Davis PD, Parbrook EO: Basic Physics and Measurement in Anesthesia, 2nd ed, chapter 9, Temperature, p 119. Norwalk, Connecticut, Appleton-Century-Crofts, 1986
44. Guyton AC: Textbook of Medical Physiology, 6th ed, chapter 72, Body temperature, temperature regulation, and fever, p 886. Philadelphia, WB Saunders, 1981
45. Bird RB, Stewart WE, Lightfoot EN: Transport Phenomena, chapter 16, Diffusivity and the mechanisms of mass transport, p 495. New York, John Wiley & Sons, 1960
46. Incropera FP, DeWitt DP: Fundamentals of Heat and Mass Transport, Appendix A-8, p 777. New York, John Wiley & Sons, 1985
47. Guyton AC: Textbook of Medical Physiology, 6th ed, chapter 10, Membrane potentials, action potentials, excitation and rhythmicity, p 104. Philadelphia, WB Saunders, 1981
48. Hill DW: Physics Applied to Anesthesia, 3rd ed, p 177. London, Butterworths, 1976
49. Clark LC: Monitor and control of blood and tissue oxygen tension. Trans Am Soc Artif Intern Organs 2:41, 1956
50. Tremper KK: Transcutaneous P_{O_2} measurement. Can Anaesth Soc J 31:664, 1984
51. Barker SJ, Tremper KK, Hyatt J et al: Continuous fiberoptic arterial oxygen measurement in dogs. J Clin Monitoring 3:48, 1987
52. Optiz N, Lubbers DW: Theory and development of fluorescence-based optochemical oxygen sensors: Oxygen optodes. In Tremper KK, Barker SJ (eds): IAC, Advances in Oxygen Monitoring, p 177. Boston, Little, Brown and Co, 1987
53. Payne JP, Severinghaus JW (eds): Pulse Oximetry. p xxi. Berlin, Springer-Verlag, 1986
54. Schweiss JF: Mixed venous hemoglobin saturation: Theory and applications. In Tremper KK, Barker SJ (eds): IAC, Advances in Oxygen Monitoring, p 113. Boston, Little, Brown and Co, 1987
55. Barker SJ, Tremper KK, Hyatt J, Zaccari J: Effects of methemoglobinemia on pulse oximetry and mixed venous oximetry. Anesthesiology 67(3A):A171, 1987
56. Severinghaus JW, Astrup PB: History of blood gas analysis, oximetry. Int Anesthesiol Clin 25(4):167, 1987
57. Stephen CR, Slater HM, Johnson AL et al: The oximeter—a technical aid for the anesthesiologist. Anesthesiology 12:541, 1951
58. Severinghaus JW, Astrup PB: History of blood gas analysis, pulse oximetry. Int Anesthesiol Clin 25(4):205, 1987
59. Pologe J: Pulse oximetry: Technical aspects of machine design. Int Anesthesiol Clin 25(4):137, 1987
60. Barker SJ, Tremper KK: The effect of carbon monoxide inhalation on pulse oximetry and transcutaneous P_{O_2}. Anesthesiology 66:677, 1987
61. Scheller MS, Unger RJ, Kelner MJ: Effects of intravenously administered dyes on pulse oximeter readings. Anesthesiology 65:550, 1986

62. Kessler MR, Eide T, Humayun B et al: Spurious pulse oximeter desaturation with methylene blue injection. Anesthesiology 65:435, 1986

63. Severinghaus JW, Naifeh KH: Accuracy of response of six pulse oximeters to profound hypoxia. Anesthesiology 67:551, 1986

64. Severinghaus JW, Bradley AF: Electrodes for blood P_{O_2} and P_{CO_2} determination. J Appl Physiol 13:515, 1958

65. Severinghaus JW: A combined transcutaneous P_{O_2}–P_{CO_2} electrode with electrochemical H_{CO_3} stabilization. J Appl Physiol 51:1027, 1981

66. Parbrook GD, Davis PD, Parbrook EO: Basic Physics and Measurement in Anesthesia, 2nd ed, chapter 19, Measurement of pH and CO_2, p 262. Norwalk, Connecticut, Appleton-Century-Crofts, 1986

67. Feynman RP, Leighton RB, Sands M: The Feynman lectures on physics. Reading, Massachusetts, Addison-Wesley, 1966

68. Faraday M: Experimental Researches in Electricity. New York, Dover, 1966

69. Priestley J: The History and Present State of Electricity. New York, Johnson Reprint Corp, 1966

70. Thompson JJ: Electricity and Matter. New York, Charles Scribner's Sons, 1904

71. Maxwell JC: A Treatise on Electricity and Magnetism. London, Oxford University Press, 1955

72. Meyer HW: A History of Electricity and Magnetism. Norwalk, Connecticut, Burndy Library, 1972

73. Benjamin P: A History of Electricity. New York, Arno Press, 1975

74. Bordeaux S: Voltz to Hertz, the Rise of Electricity. Minneapolis, Burgess Publishing Co, 1982

75. Sears FW: Electricity and Magnetism. Reading, Massachusetts, Addison-Wesley, 1958

76. Bleaney BI, Bleaney B: Electricity and Magnetism. London, Oxford University Press, 1976

77. Lorrain P, Carson DR: Electromagnetic Fields and Waves. San Francisco, WH Freeman, 1970

78. Rojansky V: Electromagnetic Fields and Waves. Englewood Cliffs, New Jersey, Prentice-Hall, 1971

79. Kip AF: Fundamentals of Electricity and Magnetism. New York, McGraw-Hill, 1968

80. Jackson JD: Classical Electrodynamics. New York, John Wiley & Sons, 1962

81. Halliday D, Resnick R: Physics, Part II. New York, John Wiley & Sons, 1962

82. Bruner JMR: Hazards of electrical apparatus. Anesthesiology 28:396, 1967

83. Bruner JMR: Common abuses and failures of electrical equipment. Anesth Analg 51(5):810, 1972

84. Ward CS: On electrical safety. Anaesthesia 35(9):921, 1980

85. Titel JH, El Etr AA: Fibrillation resulting from pacemaker electrodes and electrocautery during surgery. Anesthesiology 29:845, 1968

86. Prasad KN: Human Radiation Biology. Hagerstown, Maryland, Harper & Row, 1974

87. Whalen JP, Balter S: Radiation Risks in Medical Imaging. Chicago, Year Book Medical Publishers, 1984

88. Noz ME, Maguire GQ: Radiation Protection in the Radiologic and Health Sciences. Philadelphia, Lea & Febiger, 1985

89. Meredith WJ, Massey JB: Fundamental Physics of Radiology. Chicago, Year Book Medical Publishers, 1977

90. Feldman KL (ed): Radiological Quality of the Environment in the United States, 1977. EPA 520/1–77–009. Washington, DC, U.S. Environmental Protection Agency, Office of Radiation Programs, 1977

Part II

Pharmacology

Chapter 6   *Robert J. Hudson*

Basic Principles of Pharmacology

Twenty-five years ago, Dr. E. M. Papper opened a symposium on inhalational anesthetics with a paper in which he stressed the importance of understanding the basic pharmacology of anesthetics:[1]

> Clinical anaesthetists have administered millions of anaesthetics during more than a century with little precise information of the uptake, distribution, and elimination of inhalational and non-volatile anaesthetic agents. Considering how serious is the handicap of not knowing those fundamental and important facts about the drugs they have used so often, the record of success and safety in clinical anaesthesia is an extraordinary accomplishment indeed. It can in some measure be attributed to the accumulated experience and successful teaching of a highly developed sense of intuition from generation to generation of anaesthetists. It can also be attributed in part to the ability to learn by error after observing patients come uncomfortably close to injury and even to death.
>
> In the last few years, however, sufficient fundamental information has become available to explain these clinical successes. The empirical process of giving an anaesthetic can be better understood because of the specific data provided by the studies reported in this symposium and by the work of others which has preceded them.

Understanding the principles of pharmacology and knowledge of the specific properties of individual drugs is probably even more important today. In the last twenty-five years, new anesthetics, narcotics, and neuromuscular blockers have been introduced. We do not have the benefit of decades of experience with these new drugs, and so we must depend on carefully conducted investigations to provide the information needed to use them safely. As Dr. Papper wrote:

> If the anaesthetist studies the pharmacology of these agents and understands their pharmacokinetic properties, he can with reasonable certainty predict which of these newer anaesthetic agents will hold promise for clinical utility . . . the clinician can spare his patients much danger and his own work many hardships if he is aware of the physicochemical and pharmacological [properties] of new agents.

Our patients have also changed over the last twenty-five years. Many present for surgery with concomitant disease states that were once considered contraindications to anesthesia and surgery. Therefore, we have to consider the impact of chronic diseases, and the drugs used to treat those diseases, on the response to drugs administered during the anesthetic. Clearly, comprehensive knowledge of clinical pharmacology is a prerequisite to the current practice of anesthesiology.

The first sections of this chapter discuss the biologic and pharmacologic factors that influence drug absorption, distribution, and elimination. The quantitative analysis of these processes is discussed in the section on pharmacokinetics. The next section presents the fundamentals of pharmacodynamics—those factors that determine the duration and intensity of pharmacologic effects. The applications of pharmacokinetics and pharmacodynamics in clinical anesthesiology are then discussed. The final section briefly presents the mechanisms of drug interactions. Although specific properties of some drugs have been used to illustrate basic pharmacologic principles, detailed information regarding the pharmacology of drugs used in anesthesiology is presented in succeeding chapters.

TRANSFER OF DRUGS ACROSS MEMBRANES

Absorption, distribution, metabolism, and excretion of drugs require that they be transferred across cell membranes. Most drugs must also traverse cell membranes to reach their sites of action. Biologic membranes consist of a lipid bilayer with a non-polar core and polar elements on the intracellular and extracellular surfaces of the membrane. Proteins are embedded in the lipid bilayer, and are similarly oriented with ionic and polar groups on the membrane surfaces and hydrophobic groups in the membrane interior. The non-polar core limits the passage of water-soluble molecules, and only lipid-soluble molecules easily traverse cell membranes.

TRANSPORT PROCESSES

Drugs can cross membranes either by passive processes or by active transport through the membrane. *Passive diffusion* occurs when a concentration gradient exists across a membrane. Passive transfer is directly proportional to the magnitude of the concentration gradient and the lipid solubility of the drug. The passage of water-soluble drugs is largely restricted to small aqueous channels through the membrane. These channels are generally so narrow that only molecules having molecular weights less than 200 can pass through them. Capillary endothelial membranes, except those in the central nervous system, have larger aqueous channels that permit transfer of very large molecules, such as albumin (molecular weight 67,000). There are also large intercellular gaps in capillary endothelium. Because of these unique features, diffusion of drugs across capillary membranes outside the central nervous system is limited by blood flow, and not by lipid solubility.[2]

Some drugs are transferred through cell membranes of hepatocytes, renal tubular, and other cells by *active transport*. This is an energy-requiring process that is both specific and saturable. Active transport can pump compounds across membranes against their concentration gradients. *Facilitated diffusion* shares some characteristics with active transport. It is also carrier-mediated, specific, and saturable, but does not require energy and cannot work against a concentration gradient.[2]

EFFECTS OF MOLECULAR PROPERTIES

Most drugs are too large to pass through cellular membrane channels, and must traverse the lipid component of membranes. Almost all drugs are either weak acids or weak bases, and are present in solution in both the ionized and non-ionized forms at physiologic pH. Generally, it is the non-ionized form which is more lipid soluble and able to easily traverse cell membranes. The non-ionized fraction of weak acids, such as salicylates and barbiturates, is greater at low pH values, so these drugs become more lipid soluble as pH decreases. The non-ionized fraction of weak bases like narcotics and local anesthetics increases as the pH becomes more alkaline. The pK_a is the pH at which exactly 50% of a weak acid or base is present in each of the ionized and non-ionized forms. The closer the pK_a is to the ambient pH, the greater the change in the degree of ionization for a given change in pH. If there is a

pH gradient across a membrane, drug will be trapped on the side that has the higher ionized fraction, because only the non-ionized drug is diffusible. This phenomenon is known as *ion trapping*. The total drug concentration is greater on the side of the membrane with the higher ionized fraction. However, at equilibrium, the concentration of non-ionized drug will be the same. In most situations, the range of pH values is too small to cause major changes in the degree of ionization. However, there are major pH changes in the upper gastrointestinal tract. In the stomach, weak acids are mostly non-ionized, which facilitates their absorption. In contrast, basic drugs are highly ionized at low pH, so they cannot cross the gastric mucosa, and are "trapped" in the stomach. This situation is reversed in the proximal small intestine, where the more alkaline pH hinders the absorption of acidic drugs, while enhancing uptake of basic drugs.[2]

DRUG ABSORPTION

Except for intravenous injections, drugs must be absorbed into the circulation before they can be delivered to their sites of action. The manner in which drugs are absorbed is an important determinant of both the intensity and duration of drug action. Incomplete absorption limits the amount of drug reaching the site of action, reducing the peak pharmacologic effect. Rapid absorption is a prerequisite for rapid onset of action. In contrast, slow absorption permits a sustained duration of action because of the "depot" of drug at the absorptive site. The speed of absorption depends on the solubility and concentration of drug. All drugs must dissolve in water to reach the circulation. Consequently, drugs in aqueous solutions are absorbed faster than those in solid formulations, suspensions, or organic solvents, such as propylene glycol. A high concentration of drug facilitates absorption. Local blood flow also affects absorption. Increased circulation to the absorptive site increases the rate of absorption. Decreased blood flow, secondary to hypotension, vasoconstrictors, or other factors, slows drug absorption.[2] Vasoconstrictors are often added to local anesthetics to delay absorption after subcutaneous injection. This prolongs the duration of action at the site of injection, and lessens the chance of systemic toxicity.

ROUTE OF ADMINISTRATION

In general medical practice, oral administration of drugs is the most commonly used method. Its advantages are convenience, economy, and safety. Disadvantages include the requirement for a cooperative patient, incomplete absorption, and metabolism of the drug in gastrointestinal tract or liver before it reaches the systemic circulation.[2] In anesthesia, the intravenous and inhalational routes are the most frequently used methods of drug administraton. Both permit rapid attainment of the desired blood concentration of drug in a reasonably predictable manner.

Oral Administration

Drug absorption occurs mainly from the upper part of the small intestine, and, to a lesser extent, from the stomach. Absorption from the gastrointestinal tract is highly variable because of the multiple factors involved. Tablets and capsules must disintegrate, so that the drug can dissolve in the gastrointestinal lumen. The drug must then cross the lipid membranes of the gastrointestinal epithelial cells before it can be absorbed into the portal circulation. The non-ionized fraction of weak acids, such as barbiturates, is higher at low pH values, so these drugs tend to be more readily absorbed from the stomach. The relative ease of absorption of acidic drugs from the stomach is offset, to some extent, by the small surface area of the gastric mucosa and the rapidity of gastric emptying. Weak bases, such as narcotics, are more easily absorbed from the intestine, because the more alkaline pH increases the non-ionized fraction of these drugs. The larger surface area of the intestinal mucosa also facilitates drug absorption. Even though the higher pH in the small intestine increases the ionized, less-readily-absorbed fraction of weakly acidic drugs, such as salicylates, this is still an imporant site for absorption of these drugs because of the large surface area of the small intestine and the prolonged exposure of drugs to the intestinal mucosa.[2]

Once the drug has entered the portal circulation, it must pass through the liver before reaching the systemic circulation. A considerable proportion of certain drugs is metabolized during this initial pass through the liver, so that only a small fraction of the absorbed drug reaches the systemic circulation. This phenomenon is called the *first-pass effect*. Depending on the magnitude of this effect, the oral dose has to be proportionally larger than the intravenous dose to achieve the same pharmacologic response.[3] Metabolism of some drugs by the gastrointestinal mucosa may also contribute to the first-pass effect.[4]

Sublingual Administration

Drug absorbed from the oral mucosa passes directly into the systemic circulation, eliminating the possibility of the first-pass effect. Because of the small surface area for absorption, this route is only efficacious for nonionized, highly lipid-soluble drugs, such as nitroglycerin.[2]

Rectal Administration

The first-pass effect is less evident after rectal administration, because much of the drug is absorbed into the systemic circulation. Unfortunately, absorption from the rectum is often irregular and incomplete.[2]

Transcutaneous Administration

Only lipid-soluble drugs penetrate intact skin to the extent that systemic effects result. Nitroglycerin ointment is probably the most widely used transcutaneous medication. Recently, sophisticated systems for transcutaneous delivery of drugs have been developed. They consist of an adhesive patch containing a reservoir of drug that is slowly released after application to the skin. This produces a stable pharmacologic effect which can last for several days. Drugs currently administered in this fashion include scopolamine (for motion sickness), the antihypertensive clonidine, and nitroglycerin. Transcutaneous administration of narcotics for postoperative analgesia is under investigation.[5]

Intramuscular and Subcutaneous Injection

Absorption of drugs from subcutaneous tissue is relatively slow, which permits a sustained effect. Also, the rate of absorption can be altered by changes in the drug formulation. Examples of such manipulations are the various types of insulin, and the addition of vasoconstrictors to local anesthetic solutions.

Uptake of drugs after intramuscular injection is more rapid than after subcutaneous administration, because of greater blood flow. Drugs in aqueous solution are very readily absorbed. The effect of drugs in non-aqueous solutions, such as diazepam in propylene glycol, is less predictable because of erratic absorption.[6]

Intravenous Injection

Intravenous injection bypasses absorption processes, so that the desired blood concentration is rapidly attained. This is especially advantageous when rapid onset of drug action is desired. It also facilitates titration of dosage to individual patients' responses. Unfortunately, the rapidity of onset also has its hazards. Should an adverse drug reaction or overdose occur, the effects are immediate and, frequently, severe.[2]

Inhalational Administration

Uptake of inhalational anesthetics from the pulmonary alveoli to the blood is exceedingly rapid because of the large total surface area of the alveoli and the fact that alveolar blood flow is almost equal to cardiac output. The low molecular weight and high lipid solubility of these drugs also facilitate their absorption from the alveoli.

Drugs are also given by inhalation when local, as opposed to systemic, effects are desired. Inhaled bronchodilators are delivered directly to their site of action, minimizing the risk of adverse effects from high blood levels.

Intrathecal and Epidural Injection

Spinal anesthesia is produced by intrathecal injection of local anesthetics. Injection close to the sites of action in the spinal cord permits the use of very low doses, reducing the risk of adverse systemic drug effects. This advantage is lessened with epidural injections, because a much greater total dose is required. The major disadvantage of these routes of injection is the expertise that they require.

BIOAVAILABILITY

Bioavailability is an important concept that describes the fraction of the dose that reaches the systemic circulation. Bioavailability is reduced by factors such as incomplete absorption from the gastrointestinal tract, the first-pass effect, and poor absorption from the site of injection.

Even after intravenous injection, the bioavailability of drugs formulated in lipid suspensions may be less than 100%. These suspensions contain small lipid droplets similar to endogenous chylomicra. Some, but not all, of the drug diffuses from the lipid droplets into the plasma. These droplets are taken up by the liver and metabolized. Presumably, some of the drug is also metabolized before it is released back into the circulation. Compared to diazepam in propylene glycol, the bioavailability of the lecithin suspension of diazepam is 30% less, even with direct intravenous injection.[7]

DRUG DISTRIBUTION

After absorption or injection into the systemic circulation, drugs are distributed throughout the body. The first step in drug distribution is delivery to various organs. The pattern of distribution depends on regional blood flow. Highly perfused organs, such as the brain, heart, lungs, liver, and kidneys, receive most of the drug soon after injection. Delivery to muscle, skin, fat, and other tissues with lower blood flows is slower, and equilibration of distribution into these tissues may take several hours or even days.[2]

Capillary membranes are freely permeable in most tissues except the brain, so that drugs quickly pass into the extracellular space. Subsequent distribution depends on the physicochemical properties of the drugs. The distribution of highly polar, water-soluble drugs such as the neuromuscular blocking agents is largely limited to the extracellular fluid. Lipid-soluble drugs, such as thiopental, easily cross cell membranes and are, therefore, distributed much more extensively.[2]

Distribution of drugs into central nervous system is unique. Brain capillaries do not have the large aqueous channels typical of capillaries in other tissues. Consequently, diffusion of water-soluble drugs into the brain is severely restricted. In contrast, distribution of highly lipid-soluble drugs into the central nervous system is limited only by cerebral blood flow. For more polar compounds, the rate of entry into the brain is proportional to the lipid solubility of the non-ionized drug.[2]

Drugs can accumulate in tissues because of binding to tissue components, pH gradients, or uptake of lipophilic drugs into fat. These tissue stores can act as reservoirs which prolong the duration of drug action, either in the same tissue or by delivery to the site of action elsewhere after reabsorption into the circulation.[2]

It is intuitively obvious that degree of binding of drugs to plasma proteins and erythrocytes influences distribution to other tissues. Drugs that are highly bound to blood constituents cannot be distributed extensively because only the free, unbound drug can cross the capillary membrane.

REDISTRIBUTION

The rapid entry and equally rapid egress of lipophilic drugs from richly perfused organs, such as the brain and heart, is referred to as *redistribution*. This phenomenon is illustrated by the events that follow an injection of the intravenous anesthetic thiopental. The brain concentration of thiopental peaks within 1 min, because of high blood flow to the brain and the high lipid solubility of thiopental. As the drug is taken up by other, less well-perfused tissues, the plasma level rapidly decreases. This creates a concentration gradient from cerebral tissue to the blood, so that thiopental quickly diffuses back into the blood, where it is redistributed to the other tissues that are still taking up drug. Ultimately, adipose tissue takes up most of the drug because of the high lipid solubility of thiopental. However, recovery from a single dose of thiopental is predominantly dependent upon redistribution of thiopental from the brain to muscle, because of the larger mass and greater perfusion of muscle compared to adipose tissue.[8, 9]

A single moderate dose of thiopental (5–6 mg/·kg^{-1}) has a very short duration of action because of redistribution. If repeated injections are given, the concentration of thiopental builds up in the peripheral tissues, and termination of drug action becomes increasingly dependent on the much slower process of drug elimination.

PLACENTAL TRANSFER

Most drugs cross the placenta by simple diffusion, so that thiopental, fentanyl, and other lipid-soluble drugs with low molecular weights are most readily transferred. Highly polar, water-soluble compounds such as the neuromuscular blocking drugs do not cross the placenta to a significant extent. Fetal pH is normally slightly lower than maternal pH, and this difference increases with fetal distress. This pH gradient causes the ionized fraction of weak bases, such as narcotics and local anesthetics, to be higher in the fetus. Therefore, the fetal total drug level may be higher than predicted from the maternal total drug level because of "ion trapping."[10] Different total drug concentrations can also be due to differences between mother and fetus in the degree of binding to plasma proteins and erythrocytes. However, regardless of the effects of pH and protein binding, the concentration of free, non-ionized drug will be the same on both sides of the placenta once equilibrium is reached. For most drugs, this is the most important form, because it has the most pharmacologic activity. Therefore, although ion trapping may increase total fetal drug levels, it is of little clinical significance.

DRUG ELIMINATION

Elimination is an inclusive term referring to all the processes that remove drugs from the body. Elimination can occur by excretion of unchanged drug or by metabolism (biotransformation) and subsequent excretion of metabolites. The liver and the kidney are the most important organs for drug elimination. The liver eliminates drugs primarily by metabolism to less active compounds, and, to a lesser extent, by hepatobiliary excretion of drugs or their metabolites. The primary role of the kidneys is the excretion of water-soluble, polar compounds. Drugs such as the nondepolarizing neuromuscular blockers d-tubocurarine and metocurine undergo renal excretion intact.[11] The kidneys are also the primary route for excretion of water-soluble metabolites of drugs that initially undergo hepatic biotransformation. Pulmonary excretion is the major route for elimination of anesthetic gases and vapors. Drugs can also be eliminated *via* tears, saliva, sweat, and breast milk, but these routes are quantitatively unimportant.

The term *drug clearance* describes the ability of an individual organ, or the whole body, to remove drug from the blood. Drug clearance is the theoretical volume of blood from which drug is completely removed in a given time interval. It is analogous to creatinine clearance, which quantitatively describes the ability of the kidneys to eliminate creatinine. Like creatinine clearance, drug clearance has units of flow, $ml \cdot min^{-1}$. Many drugs are cleared by more than one means, and multiple elimination pathways have additive effects. As a result, total drug clearance is equal to the sum of the clearances of all of the elimination pathways.

Total drug clearance can be calculated with pharmacokinetic models of blood concentration *versus* time data. However, clearance by individual organs and the biologic factors influencing drug elimination cannot be estimated from blood concentration data alone. Additional data, such as the hepatic arteriovenous drug concentration difference or the rate of urinary excretion of the drug, are needed to determine the contribution of a specific organ to total drug clearance.

HEPATIC DRUG CLEARANCE

Drug clearance by the liver is dependent on three biologic factors: 1) hepatic blood flow, 2) the intrinsic ability of the liver to irreversibly eliminate the drug from the blood, and 3) the degree to which the drug is bound to plasma proteins or other blood constituents. The interrelationships between these factors have been described with the perfusion-limited model of hepatic drug clearance.[12–14] According to this model, drug in the liver cells is in equilibrium with drug in the blood leaving the liver. Therefore, the unbound concentration of drug in hepatic venous blood is equal to the unbound concentration in hepatocytes. The unbound drug within the liver is the drug that can be eliminated by biotransformation and biliary excretion.

The perfusion-limited model is based on the assumptions that hepatic drug clearance is limited by delivery of drug to the liver, and that elimination is a first-order process.[13] By definition, "first-order" means that a constant fraction of the drug is eliminated per unit time. The fraction of the drug removed from the blood passing through the liver is the hepatic extraction ratio, E:

$$E = \frac{(C_a - C_v)}{C_a}, \qquad (6\text{-}1)$$

where C_a is the mixed hepatic arterial-portal venous drug concentration, and C_v is the mixed hepatic venous drug concentration. The total hepatic drug clearance, Cl_H, is:

$$Cl_H = QE, \qquad (6\text{-}2)$$

where Q is the hepatic blood flow. Therefore, hepatic clearance is a function of hepatic blood flow and the ability of the liver to extract drug from the blood perfusing the liver. The ability to extract drug depends upon the activity of hepatic drug-metabolizing enzyme systems and other elimination processes, such as hepatobiliary excretion.

The concept of intrinsic clearance was developed to overcome the modifying effects of blood flow and drug binding in the blood on elimination processes.[13] Intrinsic clearance represents the overall ability of the liver to remove drug from the blood in the absence of any limitations imposed by blood flow and drug binding. The relationship of total hepatic drug clearance to the extraction ratio and intrinsic clearance, Cl_I, is:

$$Cl_H = QE = Q \times \frac{(Cl_I)}{Q + Cl_I} \qquad (6\text{-}3)$$

The right-hand side of Equation 6-3 indicates that if intrinsic clearance is very high (many times larger than hepatic blood flow), then total hepatic clearance will approach hepatic blood flow. This is intuitively obvious. On the other hand, if intrinsic clearance is very small, hepatic clearance will be similar to intrinsic clearance. These relationships are shown in Figure 6-1.

The preceding discussion indicates that hepatic drug clearance and extraction are determined by two independent biologic variables, intrinsic clearance and hepatic blood flow. Changes in either will change hepatic clearance. However, the extent of the change depends upon the initial intrinsic clearance.

If the inherent ability of the liver to eliminate a drug (intrinsic clearance) is doubled, then the extraction ratio will also increase, but not necessarily to the same extent. The extraction ratio and intrinsic clearance do not have a simple, linear relationship:

$$E = \frac{Cl_I}{Q + Cl_I} \qquad (6\text{-}4)$$

If the initial intrinsic clearance is small (in relation to hepatic blood flow), then the extraction ratio is also small, and Equation 6-4 indicates that doubling intrinsic clearance will produce an almost proportional increment in the extraction ratio, and, consequently, clearance. However, if intrinsic clearance is much greater than hepatic blood flow, a twofold change in intrinsic clearance has a negligible effect on the extraction ratio and drug clearance. In non-mathematical terms, high intrinsic clearance indicates efficient hepatic elimination. It is hard to enhance an already efficient process, whereas it is relatively easy to improve upon inefficient drug clearance due to low intrinsic clearance.

The effect of changes in hepatic blood flow also depends on the magnitude of intrinsic clearance (Figs. 6-2, 6-3). If extraction and intrinsic clearance are high, a decrease in hepatic blood flow causes a small increase in the extraction ratio (Fig. 6-2) that is insufficient to offset the effects of reduced hepatic

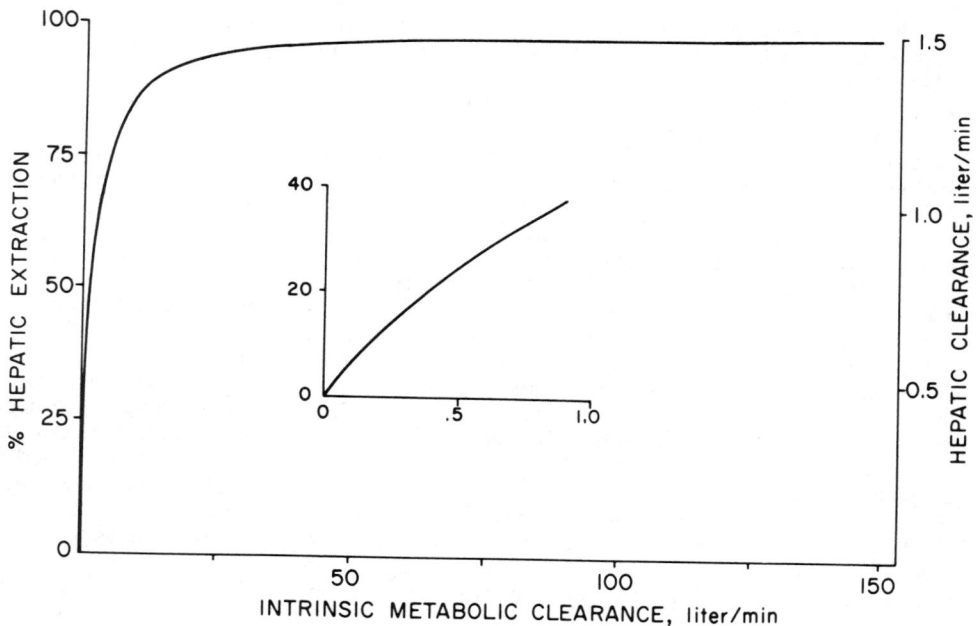

FIG. 6-1. The relationship between hepatic extraction ratio, intrinsic clearance, and hepatic clearance at the normal hepatic blood flow of $1.5 \ l \cdot min^{-1}$. For drugs with high intrinsic clearance ($>25 \ l \cdot min^{-1}$), increases in intrinsic clearance have little effect on hepatic extraction and total hepatic clearance. The inset demonstrates the relationship at low values of intrinsic clearance on an expanded scale. (Reprinted with permission from Wilkinson GR, Shand DG: A physiologic approach to hepatic drug clearance. Clin Pharmacol Ther 18:377–390, 1975.)

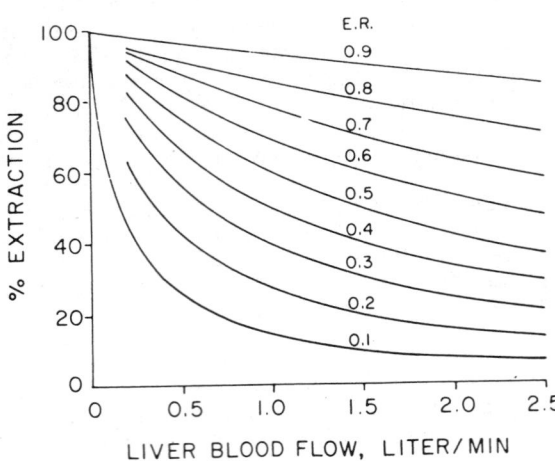

FIG. 6-2. The effect of changes in hepatic blood flow on extraction of drugs with different extraction ratios. The extraction ratios at the normal hepatic blood flow of $1.5 \, l \cdot min^{-1}$ are above the corresponding curves. (Reprinted with permission from Wood AJJ: Drug disposition and pharmacokinetics. In Wood M, Wood AJJ [eds]: Drugs and Anesthesia—Clinical Pharmacology for Anesthesiologists, p 36. Baltimore, Williams and Wilkins, 1982. After Wilkinson GR, Shand DG: A physiologic approach to hepatic drug clearance. Clin Pharmacol Ther 18:377–390, 1975.)

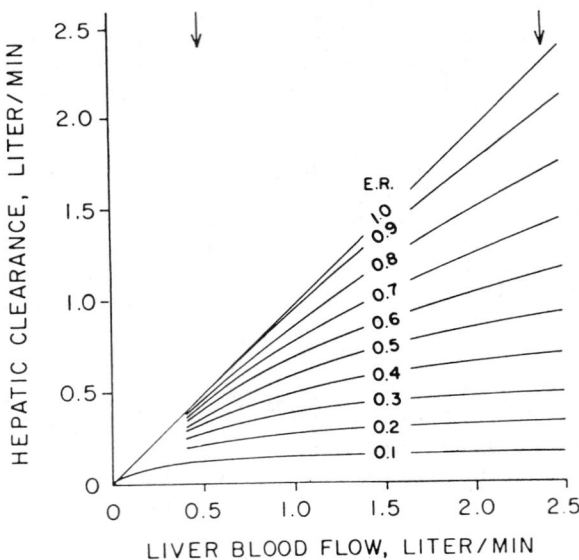

FIG. 6-3. The effect of changes in hepatic blood flow on hepatic clearance of drugs with different extraction ratios. The extraction ratios for each curve are indicated at $1.5 \, l \cdot min^{-1}$ flow. The arrows indicate the normal physiologic range of hepatic blood flow. (Reprinted with permission from Wood AJJ: Drug disposition and pharmacokinetics. In Wood M, Wood AJJ [eds]: Drugs and Anesthesia—Clinical Pharmacology for Anesthesiologists, p 37. Baltimore, Williams and Wilkins, 1982. After Wilkinson GR, Shand DG: A physiologic approach to hepatic drug clearance. Clin Pharmacol Ther 18:377–390, 1975.)

flow (Equation 6-4). Consequently, changes in hepatic blood flow produce virtually proportional changes in clearance of drugs with high extraction ratios (Fig. 6-3). For a drug with a low intrinsic clearance, a decrease in hepatic blood flow is associated with a larger, almost proportional increase in the extraction ratio (Fig. 6-2). This largely offsets the effects of changes in blood flow, so that clearance of drugs with low extraction ratios is essentially independent of hepatic blood flow (Fig. 6-3).

Under some circumstances, binding of drugs to plasma proteins and other blood constituents can also affect hepatic drug clearance. Only free drug can enter hepatocytes and subsequently be eliminated. However, in many cases, the intrinsic ability of the liver to eliminate drugs is so high that free drug is reduced to very low concentrations early during passage through the liver. When this happens, more drug dissociates from binding sites, and some of this newly released drug is extracted. Therefore, two types of extraction can be described. If both free and bound drug can be eliminated, then extraction is *nonrestrictive*.[13] This applies to drugs having high extraction ratios, so that their clearance is independent of the degree of binding in the blood.[13, 15] If extraction is limited to the free drug, it is termed *restrictive*.[13] This situation is typical of drugs with low extraction ratios. Depending on the fraction of the drug that is bound, clearance of these drugs may be altered by changes in binding. If the free fraction is already very high, then a given absolute change in the degree of binding has a small relative effect on the free drug concentration, and clearance is minimally affected. In contrast, if the free fraction is low, the same absolute change in binding produces a greater relative change of the free drug concentration, and results in a proportional change in extraction and drug clearance.

The ultimate extraction ratio reflects not only the intrinsic ability of the liver to eliminate a drug, but also takes into account the influence of blood flow and drug binding. Drugs can be classified as having either high, intermediate, or low

TABLE 6-1. Classification of Some Drugs Encountered in Anesthetic Practice According to Hepatic Extraction Ratios

LOW	INTERMEDIATE	HIGH
diazepam	alfentanil	alprenolol
lorazepam	methohexital	bupivicaine
phenytoin	midazolam	fentanyl
theophylline	vecuronium	ketamine
thiopental		lidocaine
warfarin		meperidine
		metoprolol
		morphine
		naloxone
		propranolol
		sufentanil

Drugs eliminated primarily by other organs have not been included in this table.

extraction ratios (Table 6-1). Comparing drugs with high *versus* low extraction ratios reveals easily discernible differences in disposition.[13]

A low extraction ratio is due to an intrinsic clearance that is small in relation to hepatic blood flow. Hepatic clearance of drugs with extraction ratios of 30% or less is independent of changes in liver blood flow, but very sensitive to the liver's ability to metabolize the drug, which can vary as a result of pathologic conditions, inhibition or induction of drug-metabolizing enzymes, or interindividual differences. Increased intrinsic clearance causes a parallel increase in total hepatic clearance, which, in turn, decreases the elimination half-time.

Decreased intrinsic clearance produces the opposite effects. After oral administration of a drug with a low hepatic extraction ratio, the first-pass effect is minimal and most of the drug reaches the systemic circulation, and variations in intrinsic clearance will not significantly change the bioavailability.[13]

For drugs with high extraction ratios (greater than 70%), hepatic clearance is determined primarily by liver blood flow rather than the activity of drug-metabolizing enzymes. Accordingly, clearance and elimination half-time will be affected by changes in hepatic blood flow, but not by changes in metabolic activity. These drugs undergo considerable first-pass elimination, so their bioavailability after oral administration is small, and it is significantly affected by changes in intrinsic clearance.[13] Drugs with intermediate extraction ratios, between 30% and 70%, share characteristics with both the other groups. The relative importance of intrinsic clearance and hepatic blood flow in determining hepatic drug clearance varies according to extraction ratio.

The effect of the unbound drug concentration is complex because it depends on the magnitude of intrinsic clearance. Three classes of hepatic clearance can be defined by integrating the effects of drug binding in the blood and the extraction ratio (Fig. 6-4).[15] Clearance of drugs with high extraction ratios is *flow-limited*, because it depends only on hepatic perfusion, and is not affected by changes in drug binding or intrinsic clearance. The combination of a low extraction ratio and a high free fraction results in *capacity-limited, binding-insensitive* clearance, which is affected by changes in intrinsic clearance, but is not significantly influenced by binding or hepatic perfusion. Drugs with low extraction ratios and low free fractions have *capacity-limited, binding-sensitive* clearance, which is not greatly affected by changes in hepatic blood flow, but depends upon both intrinsic clearance and the free drug concentration. Elimination of drugs with intermediate extraction ratios and binding will be influenced by all three biologic factors—hepatic blood flow, intrinsic clearance, and the free drug concentration in the blood. The relative importance of these three factors cannot be predicted unless the precise values of the extraction ratio and the unbound fraction in the blood are known.

Physiologic, Pathologic, and Pharmacologic Alterations in Hepatic Drug Clearance

At rest, approximately 30% of total cardiac output perfuses the liver. The hepatic artery provides roughly 25% of total hepatic flow, with the remainder supplied *via* the portal vein. Many physiologic and pathologic conditions alter hepatic blood flow, but there is little information regarding the effect of these changes in blood flow on hepatic drug clearance. The splanchnic circulation responds to a variety of stimuli, and splanchnic flow is often sacrificed to meet the demands of other tissues.

Moving from the supine to the upright position decreases cardiac output, which results in a reflex increase in systemic vascular resistance. The splanchnic circulation participates in this generalized vasoconstriction, which, in turn, results in a 30%–40% decrease in hepatic blood flow.[14] The clearance of aldosterone, which has a high hepatic extraction ratio, is decreased in the upright position.[14] Postural changes probably also influence clearance of drugs with high hepatic extraction ratios, but this has not been systematically investigated.

Exercise, heat stress, and hypovolemia all decrease splanchnic blood flow in proportion to the associated increase in heart rate, suggesting that these responses are mediated by the

FIG. 6-4. Classification of drugs according to factors affecting hepatic drug clearance. The closer a drug comes to one of the apices of the triangle, the more its clearance will be affected by the factors indicated on the graph. (Reprinted with permission from Blaschke TF: Protein binding and kinetics of drugs in liver diseases. Clin Pharmacokinet 2:32–44, 1977.)

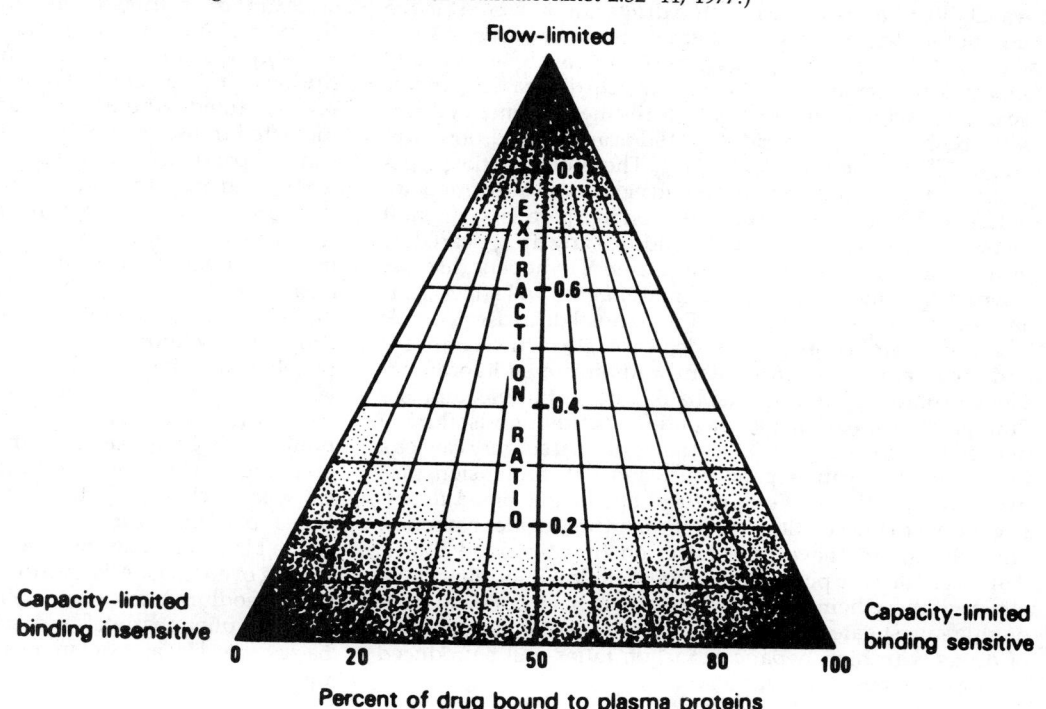

sympathetic nervous system.[14] As expected, these conditions decrease clearance of indocyanine green, which has a high hepatic extraction ratio. In contrast, the clearance of antipyrine, a low extraction ratio drug, is not affected by these same conditions.[16]

Pathologic conditions that decrease cardiac output produce reflex splanchnic vasoconstriction, which, in turn, reduces hepatic blood flow. Congestive heart failure decreases liver blood flow in proportion to the reduction in cardiac output.[17] Clearance of lidocaine is reduced in patients with congestive cardiac failure.[18] During a continuous intravenous infusion, the steady-state blood level of a drug is inversely proportional to drug clearance. Consequently, if usual doses of lidocaine are given to patients with congestive heart failure, the incidence of lidocaine toxicity is increased. This demonstrates that decreased liver blood flow can produce clinically important changes in the clearance of lidocaine and other drugs with high hepatic extraction ratios. Marked reduction of hepatic blood flow can result in hepatocellular dysfunction. Therefore, severe congestive heart failure can decrease drug clearance by reducing both intrinsic clearance and hepatic blood flow.[19]

Regardless of the etiology, cardiovascular collapse with shock severely compromises both liver blood flow and hepatocellular function.[14] In experimental hemorrhagic shock, clearance of lidocaine was decreased by 40%, while hepatic blood flow declined by 30%.[20] The reduction in clearance is too large to be attributed to only decreased hepatic perfusion, implying a concomitant reduction in intrinsic clearance secondary to hepatic ischemia.

Liver disease can decrease drug clearance due to both hepatocellular dysfunction and altered hepatic blood flow.[14] Cirrhosis reduces the clearance of many drugs with high extraction ratios, including lidocaine,[18] meperidine,[21, 22] and propranolol.[23] This is a consequence of decreased hepatic perfusion, which can be due to reduced total liver blood flow, intrahepatic shunting, or extrahepatic shunting of portal venous blood.[14] Any shunting will greatly increase the bioavailability of high extraction ratio drugs administered *via* the oral route.[14] Cirrhosis also decreases clearance of some drugs with low extraction ratios, such as diazepam,[24, 25] because of impaired hepatocellular function, which decreases intrinsic clearance. Acute viral hepatitis reduces the clearance of drugs with both high (meperidine,[26] lidocaine[27]) and low (diazepam[24]) hepatic extraction ratios. These observations suggest that both acute and chronic liver disease affect hepatocellular function and hepatic perfusion in a parallel fashion. It follows that, as a general rule, the dose of any drug cleared by the liver should be reduced in the presence of hepatic disease.

Drugs that alter splanchnic hemodynamics will affect clearance of highly extracted drugs. Propranolol decreases hepatic blood flow, and consequently decreases its own clearance,[14] and the clearance of concomitantly administered lidocaine.[28] The volatile anesthetic agents, halothane, enflurane, and isoflurane, all decrease hepatic blood flow, although isoflurane does so to a lesser extent.[29, 30] Intraabdominal surgery causes a further decrease in hepatic perfusion.[29] Hypotension produced by spinal anesthesia reduces splanchnic blood flow.[31] In contrast to the volatile anesthetics, nitrous oxide, narcotics, and barbiturates have little effect on hepatic blood flow.[14] Although they are potentially of great clinical importance, the effects of these hemodynamic alterations have not been thoroughly investigated. It is logical to assume that the clearance of drugs with high hepatic extraction ratios will be reduced during anesthesia and surgery.

RENAL DRUG CLEARANCE

Although the kidneys can metabolize drugs, their major function in drug elimination is the excretion of drugs and metabolites produced elsewhere (primarily the liver) into the urine. The renal clearance of a drug is determined by the net effects of three processes: glomerular filtration, tubular secretion, and tubular reabsorption.[32, 33]

Glomerular filtration is a relatively inefficient means of drug elimination. The glomerular filtration rate is approximately 20% of renal plasma flow.[33] Consequently, even if none of the drug was bound to plasma proteins, only about 20% of the total amount in the plasma could be removed by glomerular filtration. Drug binding in the blood reduces the amount that can be filtered, because only drug not bound to plasma proteins and erythrocytes can be passed through the glomerular membrane into the renal tubule.[33] If a drug is neither secreted nor reabsorbed by the renal tubules, then renal drug clearance will be equal to glomerular clearance. Drugs and metabolites excreted in this fashion have low renal extraction ratios, and their renal clearance depends upon the degree of binding to blood constituents. Therefore, protein binding is a major determinant of both hepatic and renal clearance of drugs with low extraction ratios.

Proximal renal tubular cells have two discrete mechanisms for secreting acidic and basic organic compounds.[32, 33] These processes are carrier-mediated, so they are saturable. Drugs with similar physicochemical characteristics witll compete for available carrier molecules and interfere with each other's secretion. Although this has the potential to cause toxicity, it can also be advantageous. For example, probenicid is used to delay excretion of penicillin and prolong the duration of effective antimicrobial levels. If a drug is very avidly secreted by the tubular cells, and not subsequently reabsorbed, it will have a high renal extraction ratio. Renal clearance of such drugs is largely determined by the magnitude of renal blood flow.[32] This is analogous to the importance of liver blood flow in clearance of drugs with high hepatic extraction ratios.

Clearance of drugs filtered by the glomeruli or secreted by the proximal renal tubule may be decreased by subsequent reabsorption from the renal tubule. If this is extensive, the drug will have a very low renal extraction ratio and negligible renal clearance. Tubular reabsorption occurs by active, carrier-mediated transport that is similar to active secretion.[33] Drugs can also passively diffuse across the tubular epithelium and be reabsorbed into the circulation. The progressive, extensive reabsorption of water from the renal tubule facilitates passive reabsorption of drugs by creating a tubule-to-plasma concentration gradient for free drug. Consequently, oliguria can decrease renal drug clearance.[33] Passive reabsorption is determined by the lipid solubility and the degree of ionization of a drug. Highly lipophilic drugs like thiopental are almost completely reabsorbed, and have virtually no renal clearance. For less lipophilic drugs, the degree of ionization is major determinant of the extent of passive reabsorption because only the nonionized drug readily diffuses across the renal tubular epithelium. Urine pH can range from 4.5 to 8.0, which can cause large changes in the ionized fraction of weak acids and bases, particularly if the pK_a is close to or within this range. Urine pH can be manipulated to increase renal clearance following overdoses. Alkalinizing the urine by intravenous injection of sodium bicarbonate increases excretion of weak acids, such as phenobarbital and salicylates.[34] Renal excretion of basic drugs like amphetamines can be enhanced by acidifying the urine.

Physiologic, Pharmacologic, and Pathologic Alterations in Renal Drug Clearance

In the adult human, renal blood flow is approximately 1200 ml·min^{-1}, so that renal plasma flow is approximately 700 ml·min^{-1}. About one-fifth of the plasma is filtered by the glomerulus, resulting in an average glomerular filtration rate of 125 ml·min^{-1}. Renal blood flow and glomerular filtration rate are autoregulated, so that they remain fairly constant as long as mean arterial pressure is between 70–160 mm Hg.[35] Consequently, renal drug clearance is more constant than hepatic clearance, which can be affected by a variety of physiologic stimuli. Although renal blood flow can be increased with dopamine, or decreased by alpha-adrenoceptor agonists,[32] drugs such as probenicid that alter tubular function have a greater effect on renal drug clearance.[36]

The ability of the kidneys to excrete endogenous and exogenous compounds depends on the number of functionally intact nephrons. A decrease in glomerular filtration rate is accompanied by a parallel loss of renal tubular functions. Therefore, the clearance of endogenous creatinine, which is essentially equivalent to the glomerular filtration rate, can be used to estimate overall renal function. It follows that renal drug clearance is proportional to creatinine clearance, even for drugs eliminated primarily by tubular secretion. This principle has been used to develop nomograms for reducing drug doses according to the creatinine clearance in the presence of renal dysfunction.[33, 34] Many drugs, including lidocaine,[37] pancuronium,[38] and meperidine,[39] have pharmacologically active metabolites than are excreted by the kidneys. Therefore, both parent drugs and their metabolites can contribute to drug toxicity in patients with renal failure.

Renal function decreases progressively with age, so that by age 80 years, creatinine clearance is reduced by about 50%. Creatinine is produced by metabolism of muscle creatine. Despite the age-related decrease in glomerular filtration rate, serum creatinine is not elevated in healthy elderly patients because skeletal muscle mass also decreases progressively with age. Therefore, even if serum creatinine is normal, renal clearance of drugs is reduced in elderly patients.[40]

Many drugs encountered in anesthetic practice are eliminated primarily by the kidneys (Table 6-2). In the presence of renal failure, doses of these drugs must be reduced to avoid adverse effects. In addition to renal disease, other pathologic processes can impair kidney function. Circulatory shock and severe congestive heart failure reduce renal flood flow, glomerular filtration, and, consequently, renal drug clearance.[32] Advanced hepatic cirrhosis also interferes with renal function,[32] and this combination, termed the hepatorenal syndrome, will reduce the elimination of virtually any drug.

DRUG METABOLISM

It is obvious that, unless tolerance* develops, termination of drug action is dependent upon elimination of the drug, and any pharmacologically active metabolites, from the body. As discussed earlier, drugs must usually cross cell membranes to reach their sites of action. Consequently, most pharmacologically active compounds are lipid soluble to some extent. This property makes excretion of drugs difficult, because lipophilic compounds are readily reabsorbed from the gut and the distal renal tubule after hepatobiliary or renal excretion. Metabolism, or *biotransformation* of drugs to more polar, water-soluble compounds facilitates the ultimate excretion of metabolites in the bile and urine. Therefore, the rate of biotransformation of drugs is a primary determinant of the duration and intensity of their pharmacologic effects. Teleologically, biotransformation can be regarded as a protective mechanism for preventing the accumulation, and resultant toxic effects, of various lipophilic compounds acquired from the environment.

Metabolites are usually less active pharmacologically than the parent drug. However, this is not always true. Many benzodiazepines have metabolites that have similar pharmacologic effects.[6] The biotransformation of codeine to morphine produces a metabolite that is more potent than the parent compound. Metabolites can also be toxic. The major metabolite of meperidine is normeperidine, which can cause seizures.[39] If metabolites are active or toxic, further biotransformation or excretion is required for termination of pharmacologic effect.

Metabolism of drugs and other exogenous compounds (known collectively as xenobiotics) occurs primarily in the liver. Other organs, including the kidneys, lungs, gut, and skin, also metabolize drugs. However, the contribution of these extrahepatic sites to biotransformation is, in most instances, quantitatively unimportant.

BIOTRANSFORMATION REACTIONS

The biochemical reactions responsible for biotransformation have classically been divided into two groups. Phase I reactions consist of processes that alter the molecular structure of xenobiotics by modifying an existing functional group of the drug, by adding a new functional chemical group to the compound, or by splitting the original molecule into two fragments. These changes in molecular structure result from either oxidation, reduction, or hydrolysis of the parent compound. Phase II reactions consist of the coupling, or conjuga-

TABLE 6-2. Drugs with Significant Renal Excretion Encountered in Anesthetic Practice

acetazolamide
aminoglycosides
atenolol
cephalosporins
metocurine
cimetidine
digoxin
d-tubocurarine
edrophonium
nadolol
neostigmine
pancuronium
penicillins
procainamide
pyridostigmine

---

* Tolerance is defined as decreasing pharmacologic effect with sustained exposure to a drug. It results in higher doses (or concentrations) being required to maintain a given effect. The mechanisms responsible for tolerance are diverse. They include adaptive or reflex responses to drug effects which alter the observed effects, as well as such mechanisms as alterations in the number or sensitivity of receptors.

tion, of a variety of endogenous compounds to polar chemical groups. The polar functional group at which conjugation occurs is frequently the result of a previous phase I reaction, hence the phase I-phase II nomenclature. However, not all drugs are eliminated by this sequential pathway of biotransformation. The oxidation of thiopental produces its major metabolite thiopental carboxylic acid,[41] which undergoes renal excretion without undergoing further (phase II) biotransformation. Morphine already has polar functional groups, so it can be directly conjugated to form its major metabolite, morphine glucuronide, without first undergoing a "phase I" reaction.[42] Because of the many exceptions to the phase I-phase II sequence of biotransformation, the term "functionalization reactions" has been proposed as an alternative to "phase I reactions" to describe those reactions which result in the creation or modification of functional chemical groups.[43] Similarly, phase II reactions are often termed "synthetic" or "conjugation reactions."

Phase I Reactions

Phase I reactions are processes that result in either the hydrolysis, oxidation, or reduction of the parent compound. Hydrolysis is defined chemically as the insertion of a molecule of water into another molecule that results in the formation of an unstable compound that splits apart. Thus, hydrolysis cleaves the original substance into two separate molecules. Hydrolytic reactions are the primary way in which amides, such as lidocaine and other amide local anesthetics, and esters, such as succinylcholine, are metabolized. Amide hydrolysis is catalyzed by amidases that are primarily located in the cytoplasm of hepatocytes.[44] Ester hydrolysis is catalyzed by esterases found in the liver and many other tissues; for example, the hydrolysis of succinylcholine by plasma pseudocholinesterase.[44]

Many drugs are biotransformed by some type of oxidative reaction. Oxidations are defined as reactions that result in the removal of electrons from a molecule. The electrons are transferred from the biochemical electron donor, reduced nicotinamide adenine dinucleotide phosphate (NADPH), to one of the oxygen atoms in molecular oxygen (O_2), reducing that atom to form a molecule of water (H_2O). The other oxygen atom is inserted into the drug molecule. The common element of most, if not all, oxidations is the enzymatically mediated insertion of a hydroxyl ($-OH$) group into the drug molecule.[44] In some instances, this produces a chemically stable, more polar hydroxylated metabolite. However, hydroxylation often creates an unstable compound which spontaneously splits into two separate molecules. Many different biotransformations are effected by this basic mechanism. Dealkylation (removal of a carbon-containing group), deamination (removal of nitrogen-containing groups), oxidation of nitrogen-containing groups, desulfuration, dehalogenation, and dehydrogenation all follow an initial hydroxylation.[44] It is evident that hydrolysis and hydroxylation are analogous processes. Both have an initial, enzymatically mediated step which produces an unstable compound that rapidly dissociates into two separate molecules.

Some drugs are metabolized by reductive reactions; that is, reactions that add electrons to a molecule. In contrast to oxidations, where electrons are transferred from NADPH to an oxygen atom, the electrons are transferred to the drug molecule. Oxidative metabolism of xenobiotics requires oxygen, but reductive biotransformation is inhibited by oxygen, so it is facilitated when the intracellular O_2 tension is low.[45]

THE CYTOCHROME P-450 SYSTEM. The complex of enzymes and pigmented hemoproteins that catalyzes most oxidative and some reductive biotransformations is known collectively as the *cytochrome P-450 system*. This term is derived from the fact that the heme-containing pigments, when reduced by carbon monoxide, have an absorption spectrum with a peak at the 450 nm wavelength. This system is incorporated into the smooth endoplasmic reticulum of hepatocytes. Other tissues, including the kidneys, lungs, gut, and skin, also contain cytochrome P-450, but in much smaller amounts.[42] The endoplasmic reticulum is an intracellular network of tubules similar in ultrastructure to cellular membranes. When liver cells are homogenized, the fragments of the endoplasmic reticulum form vesicles called *microsomes* that can be separated from other cellular constituents by centrifugation. The cytochrome P-450 complex is capable of metabolizing hundreds of compounds, including endogenous substances, such as steroids and biogenic amines, as well as drugs and other exogenous compounds acquired from the environment.[46] The cytochrome P-450 system oxidizes its substrates primarily by the insertion of an atom of oxygen in the form of a hydoxyl ($-OH$) group, while another oxygen atom is reduced to water. Because of these various properties, other terms have been used to describe the cytochrome P-450 complex, such as microsomal hydroxylase, monooxygenase, mixed-function oxidase, and polysubstrate monooxygenase.

The sequence of events involved in the oxidation of drugs and other substrates by the cytochrome P-450 system is shown in Figure 6-5. The drug molecule binds to the oxidized form of cytochrome P-450, designated as Fe^{3+} in Figure 6-5. This drug-cytochrome P-450 complex is then reduced by cytochrome P-450 reductase, which requires a reduced flavoprotein as a cofactor. The reduced drug-cytochrome complex then binds a molecule of oxygen. The reaction is completed with the addition of a second electron and two hydrogen ions (H^+), which reduces one of the oxygen atoms to water while the drug is oxidized. The oxidized drug-cytochrome complex then dissociates, regenerating the oxidized form of cytochrome P-450. The reduced flavoprotein is regenerated by the acquisition of an electron from NADPH, which is, in turn, regenerated by intermediary metabolism of carbohydrates.

It is now apparent that cytochrome P-450 is not a single entity with a unique and invariant molecular structure. Rather, cytochrome P-450 is a family of *isoenzymes* that have polypeptides with slightly different amino acid sequences.[46, 47] Isoenzymes are enzymes that catalyze the same reaction in spite of slight differences in their own molecular structures. There are "constitutive" forms of cytochrome P-450 that are involved in the metabolism of various endogenous compounds, such as steroids, thyroxine, prostaglandins, and biogenic amines. It has been suggested that there may be as many as 100 cytochrome P-450 isoenzymes that catalyze reactions with endogenous substrates.[46]

INDUCTION AND INHIBITION OF CYTOCHROME P-450 ACTIVITY. Cytochrome P-450 drug-metabolizing activity increases after exposure to various exogenous chemicals, including some drugs. Early research demonstrated two distinct patterns of altered drug-metabolizing enzyme activity after exposure to two different inducing agents—phenobarbital and polycyclic hydrocarbons. Consequently, compounds were originally classified as belonging to one of these two prototypical classes of cytochrome P-450 inducers.[46] However, it now seems that this two-tiered classification is an oversimplification. In addition to the constitutive forms of cytochrome

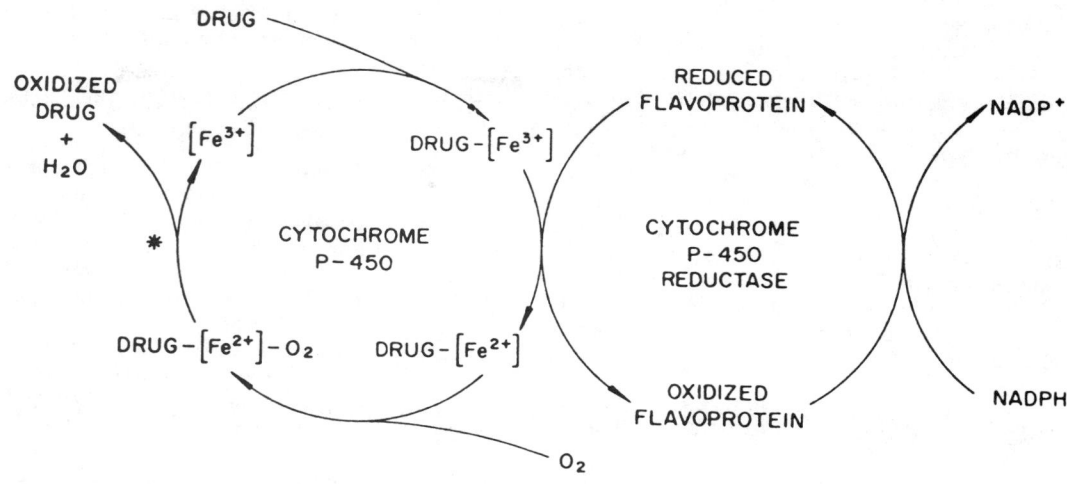

FIG. 6-5. The cytochrome P-450 drug-metabolizing enzyme system. The asterisk indicates the contribution of a second electron and two hydrogen ions from NADPH-flavoprotein or from NADPH-flavoprotein-cytochrome b_5. Cytochrome b_5 is another electron transfer system located in the endoplasmic reticulum.[42] (Reprinted with permission from Mayer SE, Melmon KL, Gilman AG: Introduction: The dynamics of drug absorption, distribution and elimination. In Gilman AG, Goodman LS, Gilman A [eds]: The Pharmacological Basis of Therapeutics, p 15. New York, Macmillan, 1980.)

P-450, multiple "inducible" isoenzymes with a wide variety of inducing agents have been isolated.[46, 47] It has been suggested that there is the genetic capacity to produce hundreds of inducible isoezymes of cytochrome P-450, and that the number and type of different isoenzymes present at any one time would vary according to exposure to different xenobiotics.[46] If this hypothesis is true, then induction of cytochrome P-450 isoenzymes would be analogous to the synthesis of specific immunoglobulins after exposure to different antigenic substances.[46]

After a single injection of phenobarbital, cytochrome P-450 activity peaks after 24 h.[42] With continued exposure to an inducing agent, cytochrome P-450 increases until a new steady-state is reached, usually within 3–5 days. The degree of enzyme induction is dependent on the dose of the inducing agent. After removal of the enzyme inducer, the amount of cytochrome P-450 decreases with a half-time of approximately 24 h. This appears to be the usual half-time for turnover of hepatic cytochrome P-450.[42]

The cytochrome P-450 system is able to protect the organism from the deleterious effects of accumulation of exogenous compounds because of its two fundamental characteristics—wide substrate specificity and the capability to adapt to exposure to different substances.

Biotransformations mediated by cytochrome P-450 can also be inhibited under certain circumstances. This can occur when different substrates compete for the same enzyme. The effects of two competing substrates on each others' metabolism depend upon their relative affinities for the enzyme. Generally, metabolism of the compound with the lower affinity will be inhibited to a greater degree. Inhibition can also occur if the drug-binding site on the cytochrome is blocked. This is the mechanism by which the widely used histamine$_2$-receptor antagonist, cimetidine, inhibits the metabolism of many drugs, including meperidine, propranolol, and diazepam.[48–50] The newer H$_2$-antagonist, ranitidine, has a different structure, and has been shown to cause fewer clinically significant problems related to decreased biotransformation.[51]

Other drugs, including the calcium channel blockers verapamil and diltiazem, also bind to cytochrome P-450, and diltiazem inhibits oxidative drug metabolism in humans.[52] Because so many drugs are metabolized by the cytochrome P-450 system, it is likely that more clinically significant interactions affecting drug metabolism will become evident in the future.

Induction and inhibition of hepatic drug-metabolizing enzyme systems will result in changes in the intrinsic hepatic clearance of drugs. This is most important for drugs that have low hepatic extraction ratios, because intrinsic clearance is a primary determinant of their hepatic clearance. Alterations in drug-metabolizing enzyme activity have little effect on drugs with high hepatic extraction ratios, because their clearance is primarily dependent on hepatic blood flow.

Phase II Reactions

Phase II reactions are also known as *conjugation* or *synthetic* reactions. The end products of these reactions result from the enzymatically mediated combination of various endogenous compounds with parent drugs or metabolites.[44] Conjugation reactions can occur only at susceptible functional groups. Many drugs do not have a suitable functional group, and the site at which conjugation occurs is a result of a previous phase I reaction. Other drugs, such as morphine, already have a functional group that can serve as a "handle" for conjugation, and they undergo these reactions directly.[42]

Various endogenous compounds can be attached to parent drugs or their phase I metabolites to form different conjugation products. The endogenous substrates include glucuronic acid, acetate, and amino acids. Mercapturic acid conjugates result from the binding of exogenous compounds to glutathione. Other conjugation reactions produce sulfated or methylated derivatives of drugs or their metabolites. The enzymes that catalyze glucuronide conjugations are part of the drug-metabolizing complex that is bound to the endoplasmic reticulum.[44] The other enzymes are located in the cytoplasm.[44]

Like the cytochrome P-450 system, the enzymes that catalyze phase II reactions are also inducible.[53]

Phase II reactions produce conjugates that are polar, water-soluble compounds. This facilitates the ultimate excretion of the drug from the body *via* either the kidneys or, to a lesser extent, by hepatobiliary secretion. Conjugates that enter the gut after hepatobiliary secretion may be hydrolyzed by bacterial or mucosal enzymes. This regenerates a more lipid-soluble drug moiety, which can then be reabsorbed into the portal circulation and returned to the liver. This process is termed *enterohepatic circulation*, and it limits the excretion of conjugates *via* the gastrointestinal tract. Because not all of the reabsorbed drug is extracted by the liver, some will reenter the systemic circulation, prolonging the duration of action of the drug.

FACTORS AFFECTING BIOTRANSFORMATION

Drug metabolism varies substantially between individuals. To a large extent, this variability stems from differences in the genes that control the numerous enzymes responsible for biotransformation. For most drugs, individual subjects' rates of metabolism are normally distributed. However, inherited differences in rates of biotransformation do not always conform to this type of unimodal distribution (see Chapter 17). Distinct subpopulations with different rates of elimination of some drugs have been identified. This results in a multimodal distribution of individual rates of metabolism, a phenomenon known as *polymorphism*. For example, different genotypes result in either normal, low, or (rarely) absent plasma pseudocholinesterase activity, and account for the well-known differences in individuals' responses to succinylcholine and procaine, which are hydrolyzed by this enzyme.[44] Several acetylation reactions also exhibit polymorphism.[44]

Drug metabolism also varies with age. The fetus and neonate have less capacity for some biotransformations, especially hydroxylations[44] and conjugations.[42] The latter deficiency also causes "physiologic jaundice," which is due to impaired conjugation of bilirubin. Metabolism of some drugs may also be decreased in geriatric patients, although it is difficult to separate the effects of age *per se* from other factors, such as pathologic processes.[40, 44]

Exposure to various foreign compounds can alter drug-metabolizing enzyme activity. Barbiturates, rifampin, and phenytoin are frequently implicated as the cause of drug interactions secondary to induction of hepatic drug-metabolizing enzymes.[53] Chronic ethanol consumption induces enzyme activity, but acute intoxication inhibits the biotransformation of some drugs.[53] Smoking increases the metabolism of some drugs, probably because of enzyme induction by the polycyclic hydrocarbons in tobacco smoke.[54]

Liver disease profoundly affects drug disposition. However, because of the normal degree of variability in drug metabolism and variations in the severity and type of pathologic processes, it is often very difficult to demonstrate significant changes in patients with hepatic diseases. It is also difficult to separate the effects of altered biotransformation *per se* from other effects of liver disease, such as altered binding of drugs to plasma proteins and decreased liver blood flow. Nonetheless, hepatic disease has been shown to decrease clearance of drugs with low hepatic extraction ratios,[15, 55] which implies impaired biotransformation.

Congestive heart failure has been shown to decrease the metabolism of lidocaine and theophylline.[19] Renal failure has different effects on different biotransformation reactions. The rates of hydrolytic and acetylation reactions are decreased, but conjugations are usually not affected, and some oxidations may actually be enhanced.[56]

Effects of Anesthesia and Surgery on Biotransformation

Recent research indicates that drug disposition is altered in the perioperative period. Although many other factors are probably also involved, biotransformation reactions are affected by anesthesia and surgery. In dogs anesthetized with halothane, the intrinsic hepatic clearance of propranolol is decreased, which implies that hepatic drug-metabolizing ability is impaired.[57] Animal studies indicate that halothane inhibits demethylation of aminopyrine in a dose-dependent fashion.[58] The same study showed that isoflurane is a less potent inhibitor, and that enflurane did not affect this biotransformation.

Many investigators have studied the effects of anesthesia and surgery on antipyrine clearance. Antipyrine, an antipyretic that is no longer used clinically, does not bind to plasma proteins, has a low hepatic extraction ratio, and is not cleared by the kidneys. Therefore, clearance of antipyrine is independent of changes in protein binding and hepatic blood flow, and is solely dependent on the activity of hepatic drug-metabolizing enzymes. This permits the use of antipyrine clearance as an indicator of overall hepatic drug metabolizing activity.[59] Clearance of antipyrine is generally increased after surgery conducted with a wide variety of general anesthetic techniques,[60-62] although there are exceptions to this rule. General anesthesia with enflurane does not appear to increase antipyrine clearance.[63] After operations lasting more than 4 h, antipyrine clearance is decreased.[60] Presumably, major surgical trauma interferes with drug metabolism, although the precise mechanisms are not known. Antipyrine clearance is also increased after spinal anesthesia.[62] Therefore, general anesthesia is not a prerequisite for increased rates of biotransformation in the postoperative period, and other perioperative factors also affect drug metabolism. For example, the caloric source of intravenous nutritional regimens influences antipyrine clearance. It is decreased when the only caloric source is 5% dextrose, and increased when amino acids are substituted for dextrose.[64] Occupational exposure to halothane increased antipyrine clearance in anesthesiologists working in operating theaters without equipment for scavenging excess anesthetic gases.[65] The implications of this finding for operating room personnel are not known.

In addition to altered rates of biotransformation, other factors, such as decreased hepatic blood flow during surgery,[29, 30] also affect drug elimination in the perioperative period. In many patients, the magnitude of these changes will be too small to cause any clinically evident problems. However, in some patients, clinically significant changes in drug elimination will occur. Decreased drug clearance can result in higher concentrations of drugs and increase the risk of adverse effects, especially during and after prolonged surgery. The clinician must be vigilant in looking for signs of excessive pharmacologic effects, and tailor doses according to individual patients' responses. Increased drug clearance after surgery could theoretically decrease the effectiveness of usual doses of drugs, necessitating increased doses.

BINDING OF DRUGS TO PLASMA PROTEINS

After injection or ingestion, drugs are transported to their sites of action and to the eliminating organs *via* the blood. Drugs are present in the blood in two fractions. Some of the drug is simply dissolved in plasma water; the rest is bound to various components of whole blood, such as plasma proteins and red blood cells. Usually, only the total drug concentration is measured. However, knowledge of the degree of binding is critical to the correct interpretation of therapeutic implications of the total drug concentration. If binding is decreased, then the free drug concentration will be higher for any given total drug concentration. This increases the risk of adverse effects, although the total concentration is the same.

Drug levels are generally measured in plasma or serum. Ideally, drug concentrations should be measured in whole blood, because drugs are transported in blood, not plasma, and drugs equilibrate between erythrocytes and plasma very quickly.[66] Unfortunately, measurement of total drug levels and drug binding in whole blood is technically much more difficult than in plasma, and very few investigators have directly measured whole blood binding. As a compromise, the blood : plasma concentration ratio can be used to estimate whole blood binding.

Drugs bind to plasma proteins in a reversible fashion that obeys the law of mass action:

$$[\text{unbound drug}] + [\text{protein}]$$
$$\xrightarrow[k_2]{k_1} [\text{drug-protein complex}] \qquad (6\text{-}5)$$

The rate constant of the forward (association) and reverse (dissociation) reactions are k_1 and k_2, respectively. These reactions are very rapid, having half-times of a few milliseconds.[67] Binding of drugs to blood constituents other than proteins, such as erythrocytes, proceeds in an analogous fashion. The equilibrium association constant, K_a, quantifies the affinity of drug-protein binding:

$$K_a = \frac{k_1}{k_2} = \frac{[\text{drug-protein complex}]}{[\text{unbound drug}] \times [\text{protein}]} \qquad (6\text{-}6)$$

Binding can also be described with the dissociation constant, K_d, which is the reciprocal of the association constant, and is equal to k_2/k_1. The dissociation constant has units of moles · liter^{-1}, and is the drug concentration at which 50% of the binding sites are occupied.[67] It is evident from equations 6-5 and 6-6 that the degree of binding is dependent upon the protein concentration, the affinity of the protein for the drug, and the unbound drug concentration, which is, in turn, dependent on the total drug concentration.

The extent of plasma drug binding can be expressed as the *percent of drug bound*, which is the percent of the total drug present that is bound to plasma proteins. Alternatively, the *free fraction*, which is the percent of drug not bound to plasma proteins, can be used. For example, approximately 83% of fentanyl is bound to plasma proteins. Therefore, the free fraction of fentanyl is about 17%.[68, 69]

The degree of drug binding to plasma proteins is determined by one of two methods—equilibrium dialysis or ultrafiltration.[70] In equilibrium dialysis, drug-containing plasma is separated from a protein-free buffer by a membrane that is permeable to the drug, but does not allow passage of protein molecules. After equilibration, the drug concentration on the protein-free side will be identical to the free drug concentration in the plasma. Ultrafiltration uses centrifugation to create a protein-free filtrate across a similarly semipermeable membrane. In both techniques, the drug concentration in the protein-free solution is measured, and the free fraction in plasma is then calculated. Protein binding is affected by many factors,

including temperature and *p*H.[66, 67] At high drug concentrations, binding sites become saturated, and the free fraction increases.[67] There are also qualitative differences between species in plasma proteins that affect drug binding, and binding to purified human albumin may not correlate with binding in plasma.[66, 67] Consequently, to provide clinically useful information, studies of drug binding must be conducted at physiologic temperature and *p*H with human plasma, and at concentrations within the usual therapeutic range.

The extent of drug-protein binding has important pharmacologic implications, because only unbound drug can cross cell membranes to reach its sites of action. Also, free drug is more readily available for elimination processes. This has led to the frequently held misconception that drug bound to plasma proteins and other blood constituents is pharmacologically inert. This is not the case. As soon as unbound drug leaves circulation, the law of mass action dictates that some drug will dissociate from binding sites, which tends to restore the free drug concentration. This occurs almost instantaneously,[67] so that the binding of drugs to plasma proteins constitutes a dynamic reservoir which tends to buffer acute changes in the free drug concentration.

As discussed earlier, the rate of elimination of some drugs is dependent on the degree of protein binding. The extent of distribution of drugs throughout the body also depends on the degree of binding. At equilibrium, the proportion of drug in the body that is in extravascular sites is determined by the relative affinity of blood binding *versus* binding to other tissues. A drug that is highly bound to plasma proteins or erythrocytes cannot be extensively distributed. The exceptions to this rule are drugs that have even greater affinity for extravascular binding sites. Protein binding also affects drug action. Drugs' interactions may result from competition for the same binding site. These pharmacokinetic and pharmacodynamic consequences of altered drug-protein binding will be discussed in detail in succeeding sections of this chapter.

BINDING PROTEINS

The two plasma proteins primarily responsible for drug binding are albumin and alpha$_1$-acid glycoprotein (AAG). Drugs also bind other plasma proteins, such as globulins and lipoproteins,[71] and to erythrocytes. Many drugs bind to more than one protein. For example, fentanyl and sufentanil bind to albumin, AAG, and globulins, and also to red blood cells.[69]

Albumin comprises over half of the total plasma protein content, and is the most important drug binding protein. In addition to a wide range of drugs, including barbiturates, benzodiazepines, and penicillins, albumin binds endogenous compounds, such as bilirubin. Many drugs bind to more than one site on the albumin molecule, and most drugs have one, or perhaps two, high-affinity (primary) binding sites, and a variable number of secondary, low-affinity sites.[66] Studies with radioactively labelled drugs indicate that albumin has at least three discrete, high-affinity drug binding sites.[72] Diazepam, digitoxin, and warfarin each bind to a different site, so they can be used as markers to identify and characterize these three distinct binding sites. The sites at which other drugs bind to albumin and the affinity of the drug-albumin bond can be determined using these three markers.[72] This permits prediction of the likelihood of one drug displacing another. Drugs that compete for the same binding site are more likely to displace one another than drugs that bind at different sites, and the drug with the lower affinity for the binding site will be more easily displaced.

TABLE 6-3.   Drugs Binding to alpha$_1$-
Acid Glycoprotein

alfentanil
alprenolol
bupivicaine
disopyramide
etidocaine
fentanyl
lidocaine
meperidine
methadone
propranolol
quinidine
sufentanil
verapamil

TABLE 6-4.   Plasma Protein Binding of Some Drugs Used
in Anesthetic Practice

	PERCENT BOUND	REFERENCE
ANTIARRHYTHMICS AND β-BLOCKERS		
Digoxin	25	105
Esmolol	55	106
Propranolol	89	96
Verapamil	91	107
BENZODIAZEPINES		
Diazepam	97–99	108
Lorazepam	88–92	109
Midazolam	96	86
INTRAVENOUS ANESTHETICS		
Methohexital	73	110
Thiopental	85	93
LOCAL ANESTHETICS*		
Bupivicaine	95	111
Etidocaine	95	111
Lidocaine	70	111
Mepivicaine	80	111
NARCOTICS		
Alfentanil	92	69
Fentanyl	84	69
Meperidine	53–63	73, 85
Morphine	35	90
Sufentanil	92	69
NEUROMUSCULAR BLOCKERS		
d-Tubocurarine	49–56	11, 112
Metocurine	65	11
Pancuronium	11–29	112, 113
Vecuronium	30	112

*At nontoxic concentrations. At toxic total plasma concentrations,
binding of local anesthetics decreases, leading to a marked increase in
the free drug concentration.

Albumin is the major binding protein for organic acids, such
as penicillins and barbiturates. Basic drugs also bind to albumin, but to a lesser extent. The primary binding protein for
many basic drugs, such as the amide local anesthetics,
meperidine and propranolol, is alpha$_1$-acid glycoprotein.[71, 73]
Some drugs known to bind to alpha$_1$-acid glycoprotein are
listed in Table 6-3. Basic drugs also bind to lipoproteins and
globulins.[71] Alpha$_1$-acid glycoprotein is an acute phase reactant, and its plasma concentration increases in a variety of
acute and chronic illnesses.

FACTORS AFFECTING DRUG BINDING

The physicochemical properties of drugs influence binding to
plasma proteins. As discussed earlier, organic acids tend to
bind to albumin, and basic drugs are more inclined to bind to
alpha$_1$-acid glycoprotein. As a rule, drugs that are lipid soluble
are highly bound to plasma proteins. It is evident from Table
6-4 that water-soluble drugs, such as the neuromuscular
blocking agents d-tubocurarine, pancuronium, and vecuronium, are bound to a lesser extent than lipid-soluble drugs,
such as sufentanil and thiopental. This is also true for drugs
that belong to the same class. The degree of binding of narcotics parallels their lipid solubility. Morphine is the least
bound, fentanyl and its derivatives are highly bound, and
meperidine is intermediate. Similarly, bupivicaine is bound to
a greater extent than lidocaine.

Many physiologic and pathologic states result in quantitative and qualitative changes in the primary drug-binding
plasma proteins, albumin and alpha$_1$-acid glycoprotein. Drug
binding may also be affected by acid-base disturbances that
alter the degree of ionization of drugs and proteins, and by
accumulation endogenous compounds that compete for drug
binding sites.

Maternal and Neonatal Drug Binding

The binding of drugs in pregnancy and in the fetus or neonate
has received much attention because of its impact on placental
drug transfer. Pregnant women have reduced levels of albumin, and the binding of many organic acids, such as phenytoin, is decreased at term.[74–76] Thiopental, another organic
acid, is widely used in obstetrical patients for induction of
anesthesia. However, unlike phenytoin, the free fraction of
thiopental is not increased in patients undergoing cesarean
section,[77] so usual doses of thiopental do not result in excessive free drug levels. This is fortunate, because high free drug
levels would increase the risk of side effects and enhance
placental transfer of the drug. The free fraction of diazepam,
which binds primarily to albumin, is increased at term.[78] Al-
pha$_1$-acid glycoprotein levels are not changed during pregnancy.[78] However, the free fractions of lidocaine and propranolol are, nonetheless, increased at term.[78]

Neonates have decreased levels of albumin and levels of
alpha$_1$-acid glycoprotein that are only about one-third the
adult level.[78, 79] In addition to these quantitative defects, neonatal albumin may have less affinity for some drugs.[79] Consequently, the free fraction of many drugs, especially those that
bind to alpha$_1$-acid glycoprotein, is higher in the neonate than
in the mother.[66] Although binding of many drugs is decreased
in neonates, this does not affect the unbound concentration of
drugs transferred across the placenta. Under near steady-state
conditions, maternal and fetal free drug concentrations will be
the same, although the total fetal level will be lower. Because
the free drug is the more pharmacologically active species, the
decrease in maternal plasma protein drug binding is of greater
consequence as far as placental transfer of drugs is concerned.
Obviously, decreased drug binding must be considered in
neonatal therapeutics.[80]

Age and Sex

The plasma concentrations of the primary drug-binding proteins change with increasing age, with albumin decreasing

slightly, while alpha$_1$-acid glycoprotein tends to increase.[81–83] However, these changes are generally too small to produce clinically important effects on drug binding. The free fractions of lidocaine, meperidine, and propranolol, which all bind to alpha$_1$-acid glycoprotein, are not changed in the elderly.[81–85] Similarly, binding of drugs to albumin is minimally altered. The binding of midazolam does not change,[86] and diazepam binding may decrease slightly.[24, 81, 87] The typical magnitude of age-associated decreases in drug binding is illustrated by thiopental. The average free fraction of thiopental increases from about 18% in young adults to only 22% in geriatric patients.[88] Clinically significant changes in drug binding are much more likely to be due to various pathologic conditions than to the effects of age *per se*.

Studies comparing drug binding in men and women have generally not found any differences between the sexes. For example, the free fractions of diazepam, lidocaine, meperidine, phenytoin, and propranolol in men and women are similar.[78, 82] The absence of sex-related differences in binding is not surprising, because the concentrations of albumin an alpha$_1$-acid glycoprotein in men and women do not differ significantly.[78, 82]

Hepatic Disease

Liver disease often causes decreased plasma albumin levels. Drug binding may also be affected by qualitative changes in the albumin molecule that decrease affinity for drugs, and by accumulation of endogenous substances, such as bilirubin, that compete for drug binding sites.[15] Although hepatic diseases vary widely in pathophysiology and severity, it is possible to make some generalizations regarding their impact on drug binding. The free fractions of drugs that bind primarily to albumin are typically increased. This is true for diazepam,[24, 89] morphine,[90] and for the organic acids phenytoin[90] and thiopental.[91, 92] The free fractions of basic drugs, such as lidocaine[27] and meperidine,[26] are not increased in patients with acute viral hepatitis, suggesting that drug binding to alpha$_1$-acid glycoprotein is minimally affected in patients with liver disease.

Renal Disease

Renal disease is also often associated with decreased albumin concentrations. However, even when albumin levels are normal, the binding of thiopental[93] and phenytoin[90] is decreased. The free fraction of phenytoin is correlated with both the albumin concentration and the severity of renal dysfunction.[90] These observations indicate that renal failure produces a qualitative defect of the albumin molecule that reduces its affinity for organic acids. Dialysis does not restore the affinity of albumin for thiopental or phenytoin.[90, 93] The plasma protein binding of many other organic acids is also decreased in renal failure.[94]

The effect of renal disease on the binding of basic drugs depends on whether the drug binds primarily to albumin or alpha$_1$-acid glycoprotein, and the type of renal disease. Albumin levels tend to decrease in all types of renal disease. The free fraction of diazepam, which binds primarily to albumin, is increased in the nephrotic syndrome, renal failure, and after renal transplantation.[95] Similarly, the binding of morphine is decreased in uremia.[90] The binding of other basic drugs varies according to the changes in alpha$_1$-acid glycoprotein in different types of renal disease.[66] Lidocaine binding increases in renal failure and after renal transplantation, conditions associated with increased alpha$_1$-acid glycoprotein levels.[95] Like-

wise, propranolol binding is increased in patients with renal disease and elevated concentrations of alpha$_1$-acid glycoprotein.[96] Lidocaine binding is not altered in the nephrotic patients, who have normal levels of alpha$_1$-acid glycoprotein.[95]

Other Diseases

Patients with a variety of inflammatory diseases, such as rheumatoid arthritis, Crohn's disease, and ulcerative colitis, have increased levels of alpha$_1$-acid glycoprotein and decreased free fractions of drugs that bind to this protein.[96] Malignant disease is also associated with elevated levels of alpha$_1$-acid glycoprotein, and increased binding of lidocaine has been demonstrated in patients with cancer.[97] In contrast, albumin tends to decrease in patients with malignancies, which can decrease binding of acidic drugs.[97]

After acute myocardial infarction, alpha$_1$-acid glycoprotein levels double, and remain elevated for about 3 weeks.[98] Consequently, the binding of lidocaine and propranolol is increased in these patients.[98, 99]

Surgery and Trauma

The catabolic state that follows surgery and trauma decreases plasma albumin levels.[100] In contrast, the concentrations of alpha$_1$-acid glycoprotein increase after trauma[101] and surgery,[102] and remain elevated for several weeks. These changes result in alterations in drug binding to plasma proteins after surgery and trauma. The free fraction of phenytoin increases after surgery, probably secondary to decreased levels of albumin, although the contemporaneous increase in free fatty acids may result in competetion for binding sites.[100] The increase in alpha$_1$-acid glycoprotein levels results in increased binding of basic drugs, such as lidocaine and propranolol, after trauma[101] and surgery.[103, 104]

PHARMACOKINETIC PRINCIPLES

Clearly, the concentration of a drug at its site, or sites, of action is a primary determinant of its pharmacologic effects. Because drugs are transported to and from their sites of action in the blood, the concentration at the active site is, in turn, a function of the concentration in the blood. Changes in drug concentration over time in the blood, at the site of action, and in other tissues are a result of the complex interaction of various biologic factors with the physicochemical characteristics of the drug. Together, these factors determine the rate, extent, and pattern of drug absorption, distribution, metabolism, and excretion. The term *pharmacokinetics*, which is derived from the Greek words for "drug" and "moving," applies to the study of these factors. In its broadest sense, pharmacokinetics is the quantitative analysis of the relationship between the dose of a drug and the ensuing changes in drug concentration in the blood and other tissues.

Some early studies of the pharmacokinetics of intravenous anesthetics used physiologic, or perfusion models. In these models, body tissues are classified according to similarities in perfusion and affinity for drugs.[114] Highly perfused tissues, including the brain, heart, lungs, liver, and kidneys, make up the vessel-rich group. Muscle and skin comprise the lean tissue group, and fat is considered as a separate group. The vessel-poor group, which has minimal effect on drug distribution and elimination, is composed of bone and cartilage.

Physiologic pharmacokinetic models made major contributions to understanding the factors influencing recovery from thiopental. They demonstrated that awakening after a single dose was primarily due to redistribution of thiopental from the brain to muscle and skin.[8, 9] Distribution to other tissues and metabolism played minor roles. This fundamental concept, redistribution, also applies to other lipophilic drugs, such as fentanyl. Physiologic models have also contributed greatly to the understanding of the uptake and distribution of inhalational anesthetics.[115]

Physiologic pharmacokinetic models provide much insight into factors affecting drug action. They can predict the effects of physiologic changes, such as altered regional blood flows or reduced cardiac output, on drug distribution and elimination.[116] The disadvantage of perfusion-based models is their complexity. Verification of these models requires data regarding concentrations in many different tissues, which is rarely available, and sophisticated mathematical analyses.[114] Because of these disadvantages, simpler pharmacokinetic models have been developed. In these models, the body is envisaged as being composed of one or more compartments. Drug concentration data from blood is used to define the relationship between dose and the time course of changes of the drug concentration.[117] It is important to understand that the "compartments" that make up a compartmental pharmacokinetic model cannot be equated with the tissue groups used in physiologic pharmacokinetic models. Compartments are theoretical entities that are used to derive pharmacokinetic parameters, such as clearance, volume of distribution, and half-times. This provides a quantitative analysis of drug distribution and elimination.

Although compartmental models are simpler than physiologic pharmacokinetic models, they also have some disadvantages. For example, cardiac output is not a parameter of compartmental models. Therefore, compartmental models cannot be used to predict the effects of congestive heart failure on drug disposition. In spite of lacking such predictive capabilities, compartmental models can still quantify the effects of reduced cardiac output on the disposition of a drug if a group of patients with cardiac failure is compared to a group of normal subjects.

The discipline of pharmacokinetics is, to the despair of many, mathematically based. In the succeeding sections, the number of equations has been kept to the minimum required to develop the concepts needed to understand and interpret pharmacokinetic studies.

PHARMACOKINETIC CONCEPTS

Rate Constants and Half-times

The elimination of most drugs follows *first-order* kinetics. A first-order kinetic process is one in which a constant fraction of the drug is removed during a finite period of time. This fraction is equivalent to the *rate constant* of the process. Rate constants are usually denoted by the letter k, and have units of inverse time, such as min^{-1} or $hours^{-1}$. If 10% of the drug is eliminated per minute, then the rate constant is $0.1 \ min^{-1}$.

Because a constant fraction is removed per unit time in first-order kinetics, the absolute amount of drug eliminated is proportional to the concentration of the drug. It follows that, in first-order kinetics, the rate of change of the concentration at any given time is proportional to the concentration present at that time. When the concentration is high, it will fall faster than when it is low. First-order kinetics apply not only to elimination processes, but also to absorption and distribution of drugs.[117]

Rather than using rate constants, the rapidity of pharmacokinetic processes are usually described with half-times, which is the time required for the plasma concentration to change by a factor of two. Half-times are calculated directly from the corresponding rate constants with this simple equation:

$$t \ 1/2 = \frac{(\text{natural logarithm of 2})}{k} = \frac{0.693}{k} \quad (6\text{-}7)$$

Thus, a rate constant of $0.1 \ min^{-1}$ translates into a half-time of 6.93 min. The half-time of any first-order kinetic process, including drug absorption, distribution, and elimination, can be calculated.

In theory, first-order processes, such as drug elimination, can never be completed because a constant fraction of the drug, not an absolute amount, is removed per unit time. Therefore, first-order processes continually approach completion. However, after five half-times, the process will be almost 97% complete (Table 6-5). For practical purposes, this is close enough to 100%, and can be considered as such.

Volumes of Distribution

The volume of distribution is the pharmacokinetic parameter that quantifies the extent of drug distribution. The physiologic factor that governs the extent of drug distribution is the overall capacity of tissues for a drug, relative to the capacity of the blood for that drug. Overall tissue capacity for uptake of a drug is, in turn, a function of the total volume of the tissues into which a drug distributes and their average affinity for the drug. In compartmental pharmacokinetic models, drugs are envisaged as distributing into one or more "boxes," or compartments. These compartments cannot be equated with tissues. Rather, they are hypothetical entities that permit analysis of drug distribution and elimination.

The volume of distribution is an "apparent" volume because it represents the size of these hypothetical boxes, or compartments, that is necessary to explain the concentration of drug in a reference compartment, usually the so-called central or plasma compartment. The volume of distribution, Vd, relates the total amount of drug present to the concentration observed according to this equation:

$$Vd = \frac{\text{total amount of drug present}}{\text{concentration}} \quad (6\text{-}8)$$

Putting the arithmetic aside, this formula is logical. If a drug is extensively distributed, then the concentration will be lower, which equates to a larger volume of distribution. For example, if a total of 10 mg of drug is present and the concentration is 2 $mg \cdot l^{-1}$, then the apparent volume of distribution is 5 l. On the

TABLE 6-5.   Elimination Half-times and Percent of Drug Eliminated

NUMBER OF ELIMINATION HALF-TIMES	PERCENT OF DRUG REMAINING	PERCENT OF DRUG ELIMINATED
0	100	0
1	50	50
2	25	75
3	12.5	87.5
4	6.25	93.75
5	3.13	96.87

other hand, if the concentration was 4 mg·l^{-1}, then the volume of distribution would be 2.5 l.

Simply stated, the apparent volume of distribution is a numeric index of the extent of drug distribution that does not have any relationship to the actual volume of any tissue or group of tissues. It may be as small as plasma volume, or, if overall tissue uptake is extensive, the apparent volume of distribution may greatly exceed the actual total volume of the body (Fig. 6-6). Because the volume of distribution is a mathematical approximation, it cannot be directly correlated with the anatomic and physiologic factors that influence drug distribution. Determination of the volume of distribution from a compartmental model does not provide any information regarding the tissues into which the drug actually distributes or the concentrations in those tissues. Despite these limitations, knowledge of the volume of distribution is often very useful. For example, if a drug has a larger apparent distribution volume than another drug with similar pharmacologic activity, then a larger loading dose will be required to "fill up" the "box" and achieve the same concentration. Various pathologic conditions also alter the volume of distribution, necessitating therapeutic adjustments.

Total Drug Clearance

In compartmental pharmacokinetic models, the ability of the system as a whole to irreversibly eliminate a drug is quantified

FIG. 6-6. The volume of distribution of various drugs. (Reprinted with permission from Stanski DR, Watkins WD: Drug Disposition in Anesthesia, p 19. New York, Grune and Stratton, 1982. After Rowland M: Drug absorption and disposition. Melmon KL, Morelli HF [eds]: Clinical Pharmacology, p 40. New York, Macmillan, 1978.)

Volume of Distribution

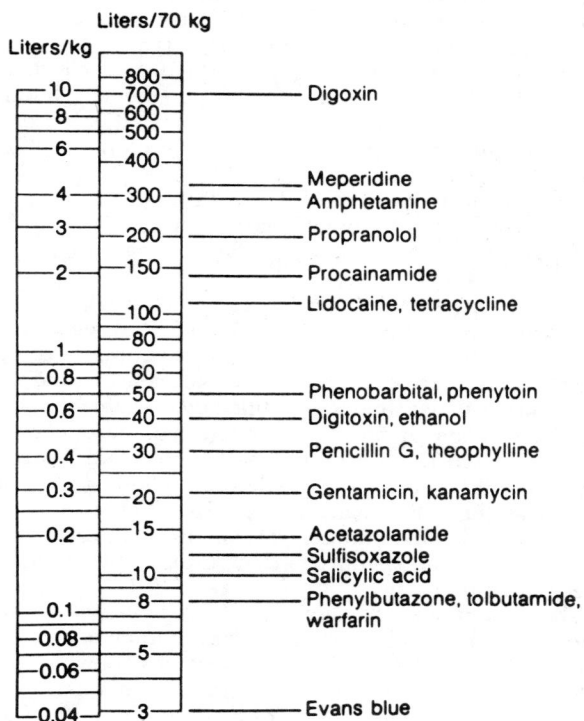

by the *total drug clearance*. Drug clearance is the portion of the volume of distribution from which drug is completely removed in a given time interval. It is analogous to creatinine clearance, which measures the ability of the kidneys to eliminate creatinine, and, like creatinine clearance, drug clearance has units of flow. Multiple elimination pathways are additive, so total drug clearance is the sum of the clearances of the various routes of elimination. Drug clearance is often corrected for weight or body surface area, in which case the units are ml·min^{-1}·kg^{-1} or ml·min^{-1}·m^{-2}, respectively.

Total drug clearance, *Cl*, can be calculated from the declining blood levels observed after an intravenous injection as follows:

$$Cl = \frac{dose}{\text{area under the } concentration \text{ } versus \text{ } time \text{ curve}} \quad (6\text{-}9)$$

Again, this formula is intuitively logical. If a drug is rapidly removed from the plasma, its concentration will fall more quickly than the concentration of a drug that is less readily eliminated. This results in a small area under the concentration *versus* time curve, which equates to greater clearance.

There are limitations to the calculation of total drug clearance from pharmacokinetic models of concentration *versus* time data. If drug levels are measured in plasma, then only total *plasma* clearance can be derived, whereas drug elimination is actually a function of total *blood* clearance. The relative contribution of different organs to drug elimination cannot be determined from blood concentration data alone. Nonetheless, estimation of drug clearance with these models has made important contributions to clinical pharmacology. In particular, these models have provided a great deal of clinically useful information regarding altered drug elimination in various pathologic conditions.

COMPARTMENTAL PHARMACOKINETIC MODELS

One-Compartment Model

In this model, the body is envisaged as a single homogeneous compartment. Drug distribution after injection is assumed to be instantaneous, so that there are no concentration gradients within the compartment. The concentration can decrease only by elimination of drug from the system. The plasma concentration *versus* time curve for a hypothetical drug that instantly distributes throughout the body is shown in Figure 6-7. The initial plasma concentration is 100 μg·ml^{-1}, and the concentration decreases with time as a result of first-order elimination. The tangents at 10 and 50 min reflect the instantaneous rates of decline of the concentration at those times. They illustrate that the rate of change of the concentration is proportional to the concentration, a fundamental characteristic of first-order processes. If the concentration is plotted on a logarithmic scale, then the concentration *versus* time curve becomes a straight line (Fig. 6-8). The slope of this line is equal to the first-order elimination rate constant.

Immediately after injection, before any drug can be eliminated, the amount of drug present is equal to the dose. Therefore, by modifying Equation 6-8, the volume of distribution can be calculated:

$$Vd = \frac{dose}{\text{initial concentration}} \quad (6\text{-}10)$$

Although, for most drugs, the one-compartment model is an over-simplification, it does serve to illustrate the basic

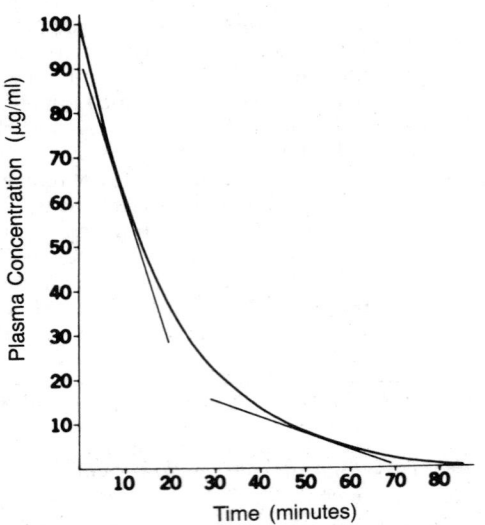

FIG. 6-7. A plasma concentration *versus* time curve for a hypothetical drug with single compartment kinetics. The plasma concentration is plotted on a linear scale. The tangents at 10 and 50 min indicate the instantaneous rates of decline of the concentration at those times. (Reprinted with permission from Stanski DR, Watkins WD: Drug Disposition in Anesthesia, p 7. New York, Grune and Stratton, 1982.)

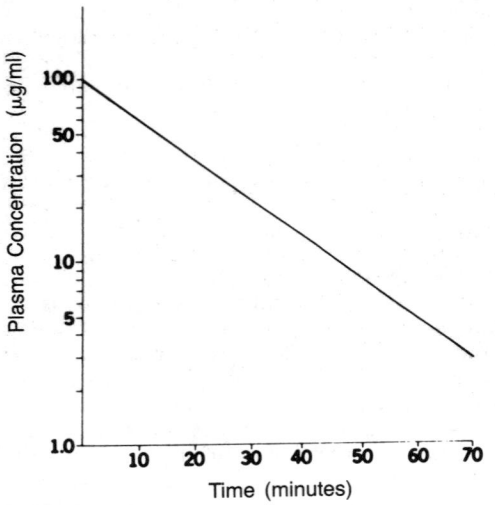

FIG. 6-8. The plasma concentration, plotted on a logarithmic scale, *versus* time for the same drug as in figure 6-7. (Reprinted with permission from Stanski DR, Watkins WD: Drug Disposition in Anesthesia, p 7. New York, Grune and Stratton, 1982.)

relationship between clearance, volume of distribution, and the elimination half-time. In the one-compartment model, drug clearance, Cl, is equal to the product of the elimination rate constant and the volume of distribution:

$$Cl = k\ (Vd) \qquad (6\text{-}11)$$

Combining equations 6-7 and 6-11 yields:

$$Cl = \frac{0.693\ (Vd)}{t\ 1/2} \quad \text{thus:} \quad t\ 1/2 = \frac{0.693\ (Vd)}{Cl} \qquad (6\text{-}12)$$

Therefore, the greater the clearance, the shorter the elimination half-time, which is easy to understand. Less obvious is the impact of the volume of distribution on the elimination half-time. It is easiest to understand if the physiologic correlate of a large volume of distribution is considered. A large volume of distribution reflects extensive tissue uptake of a drug, so that only a small fraction of the total amount of drug is in the blood and accessible to the organs of elimination. Consequently, the greater the volume of distribution, the longer the elimination half-time. These interrelationships between clearance, volume of distribution, and the elimination half-time are the same for drugs that exhibit multicompartment pharmacokinetics.

Although the elimination half-time is important, it is not a truly fundamental pharmacokinetic parameter. Rather, the elimination half-time is dependent on two independent variables, clearance and volume of distribution, that characterize the independent processes of drug distribution and drug elimination.

Two-Compartment Model

For many drugs, a graph of the logarithm of the plasma concentration *versus* time after an intravenous injection is similar to the schematic graph shown in Figure 6-9. There appear to be two discrete phases of the decline of the plasma concentration. The first phase after injection represents drug distribution, and is characterized by a very rapid decrease in concentration. The rapid decrease in concentration during this "distribution phase" is largely due to passage of drug from the plasma into tissues. The distribution phase is followed by a slower decline of the concentration due to drug elimination. Elimination also begins immediately after injection, but its contribution to the drop in plasma concentration is initially masked by the much greater fall in concentration due to drug distribution.

To account for this biphasic behavior, one must consider the body to be made up of two compartments—a central (or plasma) compartment and a peripheral compartment (Fig. 6-10). In the two-compartment model, it is assumed that it is the central compartment into which the drug is injected and from which the blood samples for measurement of concentration are obtained, and that drug is eliminated only from the central compartment (Fig. 6-10). Drug distribution within the central compartment is considered to be instantaneous. In reality, this last assumption cannot be true. However, drug uptake into some of the highly perfused tissues is so rapid that it cannot be detected as a discrete phase on the plasma concentration *versus* time curve.

Immediately after intravenous injection, all of the drug is in the central compartment. Simultaneously, three processes begin. Drug moves from the central to the peripheral compartment. This intercompartmental transfer is a first-order process, and its magnitude is quantified by the rate constant k_{12}. As drug builds up in the peripheral compartment, some passes back to the central compartment, a process characterized by the rate constant k_{21}. Drug is eliminated from the system *via* the central compartment. The elimination rate constant is k_e. The fall in the central compartment concentration following intravenous injection is a result of the net effects of these three processes.

The distribution and elimination phases can be separated and then individually characterized by graphic analysis of the plasma concentration *versus* time curve, as shown in Figure 6-9. The elimination phase line is extrapolated back to time zero (the time of injection). At any time, the difference be-

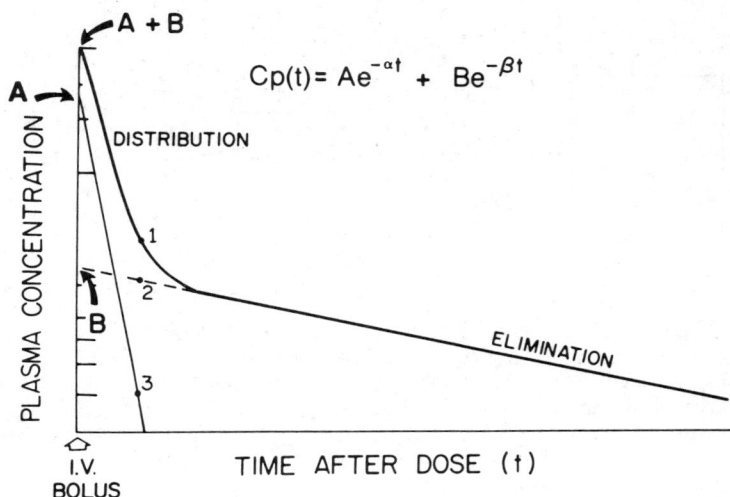

FIG. 6-9. A schematic graph of the plasma concentration *versus* time for a drug with a distribution phase preceding the elimination phase (two-compartment or biexponential kinetics). See text for explanation. (Reprinted with permission from Stanski DR, Watkins WD: Drug Disposition in Anesthesia, p 13. New York, Grune and Stratton, 1982.)

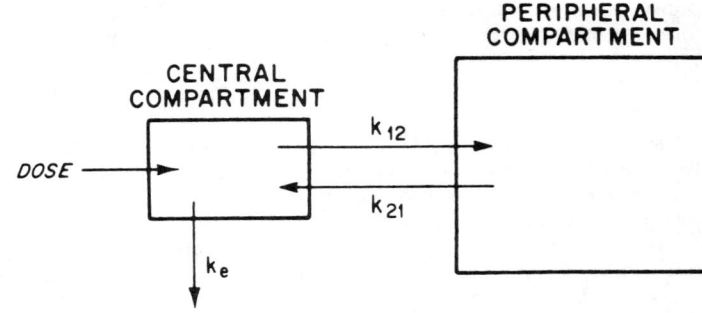

FIG. 6-10. A two-compartment pharmacokinetic model. (Reprinted with permission from Stanski DR, Watkins WD: Drug Disposition in Anesthesia, p 13. New York, Grune and Stratton, 1982.)

tween the total concentration (indicated by point 1 on the graph) and the value on the extrapolated elimination phase line (indicated by point 2) is the corresponding value on the distribution phase line (point 3). This process is repeated at several times to construct the distribution phase line. In Figure 6-9, the zero time intercepts of the distribution and elimination lines are points A and B, respectively. The distribution and elimination rate constants are determined from the slopes of the two lines, and then used to calculate the distribution and elimination half-times. Therefore, at any time after an intravenous injection, the plasma concentration of drugs with two-compartment kinetics is equal to the sum of two exponential terms:

$$Cp_{(t)} = Ae^{-\alpha t} + Be^{-\beta t}, \qquad (6\text{-}13)$$

where $Cp_{(t)}$ = plasma concentration at time t; A = intercept of the distribution phase line; α = rate constant of the distribution phase; B = intercept of the elimination phase line; β = rate constant of the elimination phase; and t = time. The first term characterizes the distribution phase, and the second term characterizes the elimination phase. Immediately after injection, the first term is much larger fraction of the calculated plasma concentration than the second term. After several distribution half-times, the value of the first term approaches zero, and the plasma concentration is essentially equal to the value of the second term.

In multicompartment models, the drug is initially distributed only within the central compartment. Therefore, the initial apparent volume of distribution is the volume of the central compartment. Immediately after injection, the amount of drug present is the dose, and the concentration is the extrapolated concentration at time = 0, which is equal to the sum of the intercepts of the distribution and elimination lines. The volume of the central compartment, Vc, is calculated by modifying Equation 6-8:

$$Vc = \frac{\text{dose}}{\text{initial plasma concentration}} = \frac{\text{dose}}{A + B} \qquad (6\text{-}14)$$

The volume of the central compartment is important in clinical anesthesiology, because it is the pharmacokinetic parameter that determines the peak plasma concentration after an intravenous bolus injection. Hypovolemia, for example, might reduce the volume of the central compartment. If doses are not correspondingly reduced, the higher plasma concentrations will increase the incidence of adverse pharmacologic effects.

At equilibrium, the drug is distributed among the central and the peripheral compartment, and by definition, the concentrations in the compartments are equal. Therefore, the ultimate volume of distribution, termed the volume of distribution at steady-state (Vd_{ss}), is the sum of the central and peripheral compartment volumes. Extensive tissue uptake of a drug is reflected by a large volume of the peripheral compartment. Consequently, the Vd_{ss} can greatly exceed the actual volume of the body. The Vd_{ss} can be calculated directly from the intercepts and rate constants of the exponential equation.[118]

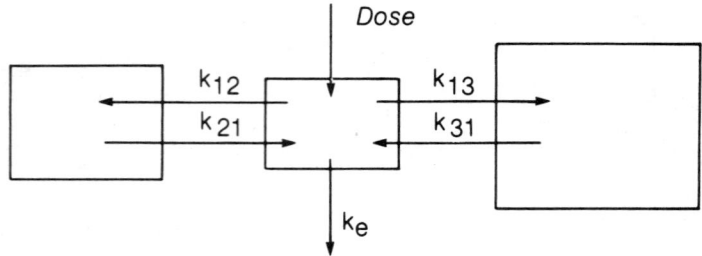

FIG. 6-11. A three-compartment pharmacokinetic model. (Reprinted with permission from Stanski DR, Watkins WD: Drug Disposition in Anesthesia, p 16. New York, Grune and Stratton, 1982.)

Like the single compartment model, in multicompartment models, the total drug clearance is equal to the dose divided by the area under the concentration *versus* time curve. This area, and, hence, clearance, can also be directly calculated from the intercepts and rate constants.[118]

Three-Compartment Model

After intravenous injection of some drugs, the initial, rapid distribution phase is followed by a second, slower distribution phase before the elimination phase becomes evident. Therefore, the plasma concentration is sum of three exponential terms:

$$Cp_{(t)} = Pe^{-\pi t} + Ae^{-\alpha t} + Be^{-\beta t}, \qquad (6\text{-}15)$$

where $Cp_{(t)}$ = plasma concentration at time t; P = intercept of the rapid distribution phase line; π = rate constant of the rapid distribution phase; A = intercept of the slower distribution phase line; α = rate constant of the slower distribution phase, B = intercept of the elimination phase line, β = rate constant of the elimination phase; and t = time. This triphasic behavior is explained by a three-compartment pharmacokinetic model (Fig. 6-11). As in the two-compartment model, the drug is injected into and eliminated from the central compartment. Drug is reversibly transferred between the central compartment and two peripheral compartments, which accounts for two distribution phases. Drug transfer between the central compartment and the more rapidly equilibrating, or "shallow," peripheral compartment is characterized by the first-order rate constants k_{12} and k_{21}. Transfer in and out of the more slowly equilibrating, "deep" compartment is characterized by the rate constants k_{13} and k_{31}.

The pharmacokinetic parameters of interest to clinicians, such as clearance, volumes of distribution, and distribution and elimination half-times, are determined by calculations analogous to those used in the two-compartment model. Accurate estimates of these parameters depend on accurate characterization of the measured plasma concentration *versus* time data. A frequently encountered problem is that the duration of sampling is not long enough to accurately define the elimination phase.[119] Similar problems arise if the assay cannot detect low concentrations of the drug. Whether a drug exhibits two- or three-compartment kinetics is of no clinical consequence. In fact, some drugs have two-compartment kinetics in some patients and three-compartment kinetics in others.[87, 120] Generally, the model with the smallest number of compartments or exponents that accurately reflects the data is used.

EFFECTS OF HEPATIC AND RENAL DISEASE ON PHARMACOKINETIC PARAMETERS

A common element of both renal and hepatic disease is reduced binding of drugs to plasma proteins. Consequently, the effects of alterations in protein binding on pharmacokinetic parameters must be considered independently of the effects of impaired organ function to fully understand the pharmacokinetic effects of hepatic and renal disease.

The extent of drug distribution depends on the relative affinity of blood and tissues for the drug. Therefore, if the free fraction in plasma increases, the volume of distribution will also increase. The magnitude of the change depends upon the initial free fraction and volume of distribution. An increase in the free fraction will produce the greatest increase in the volume of distribution for drugs that are highly bound to plasma proteins and have small volumes of distribution. In contrast, changes in plasma protein binding of drugs with initially large volumes of distribution have minimal effects on the volume of distribution, because so little of the total amount of drug is in the plasma.[121]

In theory, a parallel change in tissue binding would cancel the effect of changes in plasma binding. However, this appears to be uncommon. Increased volumes of distribution of propranolol[122] and diazepam[24] associated with increased free fractions have been observed in patients with hepatic disease. Decreased binding of thiopental in patients with renal failure also increases the volume of distribution.[93]

The effect of changes in protein binding on total drug clearance also depends on the initial magnitude of the clearance. Increases in the free fraction of drugs with low hepatic extraction ratios and drugs eliminated primarily by glomerular filtration cause a proportional increase in clearance. In contrast, altered protein binding has little effect on drugs with high hepatic or renal clearance.

The effect of an increased free fraction on the elimination half-time depends on the balance of the changes in clearance and volume of distribution.[121] The elimination half-time will increase if increased volume of distribution is the paramount change, or decrease if increased clearance predominates. The elimination half-time may not change if clearance and volume of distribution change in parallel fashion. The increase of the free fraction of thiopental in renal failure increases both clearance and volume of distribution to a similar extent. Consequently, the elimination half-time is unchanged.[93]

Differences in pathophysiology preclude prediction of the pharmacokinetics of a given drug in individual patients with hepatic or renal disease. However, some generalizations of use to the clinician can be made. Binding of drugs to albumin is decreased, so doses of drugs given as an intravenous bolus, such as thiopental, must be reduced. In patients with hepatic disease, the elimination half-time of drugs metabolized or excreted by the liver will often be increased because of decreased clearance and, possibly, increased volume of distribution. Large doses of such drugs as benzodiazepines, narcotics, and barbituates may have a greatly prolonged duration of action, and should be avoided. Recovery from small doses of drugs such as thiopental and fentanyl is largely due to redistribution, so the response to conservative doses will be minimally affected. In patients with renal failure, similar concerns apply to the administration of drugs excreted by the kidneys. It is almost always better to underestimate a patient's dose requirement, observe the response, and give additional drug if necessary.

NONLINEAR PHARMACOKINETICS

The physiologic and compartmental models that have been discussed thus far are based on the assumption that drug distribution and elimination are first-order processes. Therefore, their parameters, such as clearance and elimination half-time, are independent of the dose or concentration of the drug. However, the rate of elimination of a few drugs is dose-dependent, or *nonlinear*.

The elimination of most drugs involves interactions with protein molecules, either enzymes of biotransformation reactions, or carried-mediated secretion. If sufficient drug is present, the capacity of the drug-eliminating systems can be exceeded. When this occurs, it is no longer possible to excrete a constant fraction of the drug present to the eliminating system. Consequently, the extraction ratio decreases as the concentration increases. Decreased extraction decreases total drug clearance. Phenytoin is a well-known example of a drug that exhibits this type of nonlinear elimination. If the concentration is high enough to completely saturate the system, then a constant amount, as opposed to a constant fraction, of the drug is eliminated per unit time. This is known as *zero-order* elimination. Ethanol is metabolized in a zero-order fashion at usual "therapeutic" concentrations. In theory, all drugs are cleared in a nonlinear fashion. In practice, the capacity to eliminate most drugs is so great that this is not evident at usual, or even toxic, doses.

Nonlinear clearance has important clinical implications. The plasma concentration is the arithmetic product of clearance and the infusion rate. Therefore, the concentration will progressively increase unless the dose is adjusted. This sets up a positive-feedback loop whereby decreased extraction leads to even higher concentrations, which further decreases extraction and clearance, and so on. The other consequence of nonlinear clearance is that the elimination half-time gets progressively longer as the concentration increases. Clearance of thiopental is nonlinear at high concentrations.[123] This may be partly responsible for the delayed awakening of patients given thiopental for prophylaxis of neurologic complications during open-heart surgery.[124]

PHARMACODYNAMIC PRINCIPLES

In its broadest sense, *pharmacodynamics* can be defined as the study of the effects of drugs on the body. Classically, pharmacologic effects have been examined with dose-response

studies. Advances in drug assay techniques and methods of data analysis have made it possible to define the relationship between the drug concentration and the associated pharmacologic effect *in vivo*. As a result, the term *pharmacodynamics* has acquired a more specific definition. It is now considered to be the quantitative analysis of the relationship between the drug concentration in the blood, or at the site of action, and the resultant effects of the drug on biochemical or physiologic processes.[116, 125]

DOSE-RESPONSE RELATIONSHIPS

Dose-response studies determine the relationship between increasing doses of a drug and the ensuing changes in pharmacologic effects. A schematic dose-response curve, beginning with a dose that produces a barely measurable effect, is shown in Figure 6-12A. There is a curvilinear relationship between dose and the intensity of response, and, at near-maximal response, large increases in dose produce little change in effect. Usually, the dose is plotted on a logarithmic scale (Fig. 6-12B), which expands the part of the curve where a small increase in dose produces a large change in response. Between 20% and 80% of the maximum effect, there is a linear relationship between the logarithm of the dose and the intensity of the response.

Dose-response curves provide information regarding four aspects of the relationship of dose and pharmacologic effect. The *potency* of the drug, that is, the dose required to produce a given effect, is determined. Potency is usually expressed as the dose required to produce a given effect in 50% of subjects, the ED50. The *slope* of the curve between 20% and 80% of the maximal effect indicates the rate of increase in effect as the dose is increased. The maximum effect is referred to as the *efficacy* of the drug. Finally, the *variability* in potency, efficacy, and the slope of the dose-response curve can be estimated.

For drugs that produce graded responses, dose-response curves can be constructed with either single-dose or cumulative-dose techniques. In the former method, the effect of a single dose in each subject is measured. By giving a range of doses to different subjects, the dose-response curve can be defined for the group as a whole. In the cumulative-dose technique, small, incremental doses are given and the effect is plotted against the cumulative dose. The two methods generally yield equivalent results. However, if the drug has a very short duration of action, the ED50 of a cumulative dose-response curve will be higher than the ED50 of a single-dose response curve, because the effects of the initial doses wane during the course of the study. This has been demonstrated for the short-acting nondepolarizing neuromuscular blockers.[126] Some drugs produce all-or-none, or quantal, responses. For example, after a dose of thiopental, a patient is

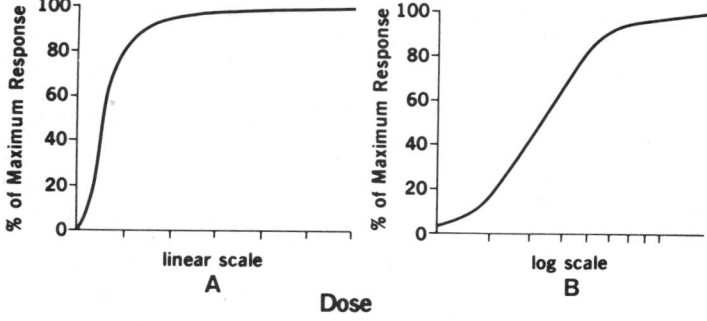

FIG. 6-12. (*A*) A schematic graph of the effect of a drug plotted against the dose, starting with a dose that produces a barely measureable response. (*B*) The same curve as in figure 6-12A, replotted with dose on a logarithmic scale. This yields the familiar sigmoid curve, which is essentially linear between approximately 20% and 80% of the maximal effect. (Reprinted with permission from Stanski DR, Watkins WD: Drug Disposition in Anesthesia, p 39. New York, Grune and Stratton, 1982.)

either asleep or awake. Dose-response curves for these drugs must be constructed with the single-dose technique.

In anesthesiology, the usual therapeutic objectives are to maintain a given pharmacologic effect, such as unconsciousness or neuromuscular blockade, for a finite period, and then to have rapid recovery. Attaining these objectives is made difficult by the wide range of individual patients' sensitivity to drugs. This variability in response is a result of differences between individuals in the relationship between drug concentration and pharmacologic effect, superimposed upon differences in pharmacokinetics. Dose-response studies have the disadvantage of not being able to determine whether variations in pharmacologic response are due to differences in pharmacokinetics, pharmacodynamics, or both.

CONCENTRATION-RESPONSE RELATIONSHIPS

Ideally, the concentration of drug at its site of action should be used to define the concentration-response relationship. Unfortunately, these data are rarely available, so the relationship between the concentration of drug in the blood and pharmacologic effect is studied instead. This relationship is easiest to understand if the changes in pharmacologic effect that occur during and after an intravenous infusion of a hypothetical drug are considered (Fig. 6-13). If a drug is infused at a constant rate, the plasma concentration initially increases rapidly, and asymptotically approaches a steady-state level after approximately five elimination half-times have elapsed. The effect of the drug initially increases very slowly, then more rapidly, and, eventually, also reaches a steady-state (Fig. 6-13). When the infusion is discontinued, indicated by point C in Figure 6-13, the plasma concentration immediately decreases because of drug distribution and elimination. However, the effect stays the same for a short period, and then also begins to decrease. It is evident that there is a time lag between changes in plasma concentration and changes in pharmacologic response. Figure 6-13 also demonstrates that the same concentration can produce different responses if the concentrations in the plasma and at the site of action are changing. At points A and B in Figure 6-13, the plasma concentrations are the same, but the effects at each time differ. When the concentration is increasing, there is a concentration gradient from blood to the site of action. When the infusion is discontinued, the concentration gradient is reversed. Therefore, at the same plasma concentration, the concentration at the site of action is higher after, compared to during, the infusion. This is associated with a correspondingly greater effect.

FIG. 6-13. The changes in plasma drug concentration and pharmacologic effect during and after an intravenous infusion. See text for explanation. (Reprinted with permission from Stanski DR, Sheiner LB: Pharmacokinetics and pharmacodynamics of muscle relaxants. Anesthesiology 51:103–105, 1979.)

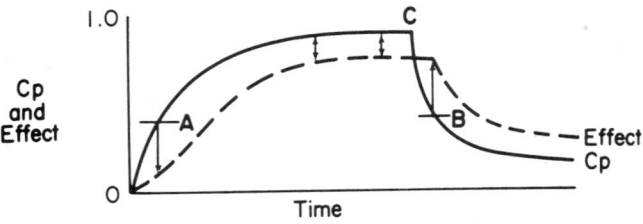

In theory, there must be some degree of temporal disequilibrium between plasma concentration and drug effect for all drugs with extravascular sites of action. However, for some drugs, the time lag may be so short that it cannot be demonstrated. The magnitude of this temporal disequilibrium depends on several factors:

1. perfusion of the organ on which the drug acts,
2. the rate of diffusion or transport of the drug from the blood to the cellular site of action,
3. the tissue:blood partition coefficient of the drug,
4. the rate and affinity of drug-receptor binding, and
5. the time required for processes initiated by the drug-receptor interaction to produce the pharmacologic effect.

The consequence of this time lag between changes in concentration and changes in effects is that the plasma concentration will only have an unvarying relationship with pharmacologic effect under steady-state conditions. At steady-state, by definition, the concentration in the plasma is in equilibrium with the concentrations in all tissues, including the site of action. Accordingly, the steady-state plasma concentration is directly proportional to the steady-state concentration at the site of action that is actually causing the observed pharmacologic effect. A plot of the logarithm of the steady-state plasma concentration *versus* percent maximal response will be identical in appearance to the dose-response curve shown in Figure 6-12B. From the concentration-response curve, the average steady-state plasma concentration producing 50% of the maximal response ($Cp_{ss}50$) can be determined. Like the ED50, the $Cp_{ss}50$ is a measure of sensitivity to a drug, but the $Cp_{ss}50$ has the advantage of being unaffected by pharmacokinetic variability. Because it takes five elimination half-times to approach steady-state conditions, it is rarely practical to directly determine the $Cp_{ss}50$. For drugs that have long elimination half-times, the pseudoequilibrium that exists during the elimination phase can be used to approximate steady-state conditions, because the concentrations in plasma and at the site of action are changing very slowly.

From the foregoing discussion, it is evident that the onset and duration of pharmacologic effects depends not only on pharmacokinetic factors, but also on the pharmacodynamic factors governing the degree of temporal disequilibrium between changes in concentration and changes in effect. The magnitude of the pharmacologic effect is a function of the amount of drug present at the site of action, so that increasing the dose will increase the peak effect. Larger doses have a more rapid onset of action because the rate at which drug is delivered to the site of action increases. The duration of action also increases because pharmacologically effective concentrations will be maintained for a longer time.

Integrated pharmacokinetic-pharmacodynamic models have been developed by several investigators.[125, 127] These models fully characterize the relationships between time, dose, plasma concentration, and pharmacologic effect. This is accomplished by adding an "effect compartment" to a standard compartmental pharmacokinetic model. Transfer of drug between central (plasma) compartment and the effect compartment is assumed to be a first-order process, and the pharmacologic effect is assumed to be directly related to the effect compartment concentration. By quantifying the time lag between changes in plasma concentration and changes in pharmacologic effect, these models can also define the $Cp_{ss}50$, even if steady-state conditions have not been attained. These models have contributed greatly to our understanding of factors influencing the response to intravenous anesthetics,[128, 129] narcotics,[130] and nondepolarizing muscle relaxants[127, 131, 132] in man.

Dose-response and concentration-response relationships can be altered by many factors, such as interactions with other concomitantly administered drugs or pathologic conditions. They are also affected by the development of tolerance to the drug's effects, which increases the ED50 and $Cp_{ss}50$. When tolerance develops after only a few doses of drug, it is usually referred to as *tachyphylaxis*.

DRUG-RECEPTOR INTERACTIONS

The biochemical and physiologic effects of many drugs, neurotransmitters, and hormones are due to the binding of these compounds to receptors, which initiates changes in cellular function. In addition to the well-known muscarinic and nicotinic cholinergic receptors, and alpha- and beta-adrenoceptors, there are specific receptors for histamine, serotonin, dopamine, opiates, benzodiazepines, and calcium-channel blockers, to name a few.[133] Most receptors are protein molecules situated on the cell membrane, although some are located within the cell.

Binding of drugs to receptors, like binding to plasma proteins, is generally reversible, and follows the law of mass action:

$$[drug] + [receptor] \leftrightarrow [drug\text{-}receptor\ complex] \quad (6\text{-}16)$$

The higher the concentration of free drug or unoccupied receptor, the greater the tendency for drug-receptor binding. Plotting the percentage of receptors occupied by a drug against the logarithm of the concentration of the drug yields a sigmoid curve, as shown in Figure 6-14.

It is often assumed that the percent of the maximal effect observed at any given drug concentration is equal to the percent of receptors occupied by the drug. However, there are exceptions to this rule. At the neuromuscular junction, only 20%–25% of the receptors need to bind acetylcholine to produce contraction of all the fibers in the muscle.[134] Thus, 75%–80% of the receptors can be considered as "spare receptors." There are two important consequences of the presence of spare receptors. As indicated by Equation 6-16, the higher the concentration of unoccupied receptors, the greater the tendency to form the drug-receptor complex. Therefore, spare receptors permit near-maximal effects at very low concentrations of drugs or neurotransmitters.[135] The other corollary of the existence of spare receptors is that most of the receptors must be occupied by an antagonist before transmission is affected. This accounts for the "margin of safety" of neuromuscular transmission.[134]

The binding of drugs to receptors and the resulting changes in cellular function are the last two steps in the complex series of events between administration of the drug and production of its pharmacologic effects. These two processes contribute to the delay between changes in the plasma concentration of the drug and changes in the intensity of its effects.

Receptors are not static entities. Rather, they are dynamic cellular components that adapt to their environment. For example, administration of beta-adrenergic agonists leads to desensitization of beta-adrenoceptors. This occurs by "down regulation," which is the removal of receptors from the cell membrane, and also by alterations in the functional state of the receptor.[136] Administration of adrenoceptor antagonists

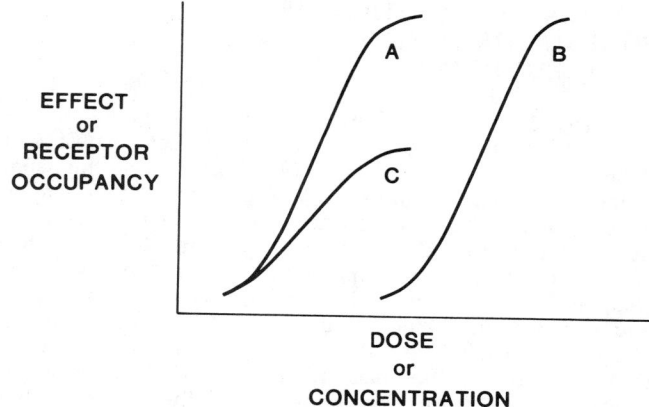

FIG. 6-14. Schematic dose-response curves representing various conditions. Either dose or concentration is plotted on the x-axis, and either effect or number of receptors occupied is plotted on the y-axis. Curve A is a typical dose-response curve. Curve B is a parallel rightward shift of the curve, and could represent a drug that is less potent than the drug depicted by curve A, but that is a full agonist and, thus, can produce the same maximal effect. Curve B would also result if the same drug used to generate curve A was studied in the presence of a competitive antagonist. Curve C is shifted to the right, the slope is decreased, and the maximal effect is decreased. This is the curve observed with partial agonists, and also seen when a full agonist (curve A) is studied in the presence of a noncompetitive antagonist.

increases the number of receptors.[136] Other hormones, and various disease states, also influence the number of adrenergic receptors.[136]

Agonists, Partial Agonists, and Antagonists

Drugs which bind to receptors and produce an effect are called *agonists*. Many drugs may be capable of producing the same maximal effect. If this results from binding to same receptors, then the dose-response curves will parallel (curves A and B in Fig. 6-14). Differences in potency of agonists reflect differences in affinity for the receptor. *Partial agonists* are drugs that are not capable of producing the maximal effect, even at very high concentrations (curve C in Fig. 6-14).

Compounds that bind to receptors without producing any changes in cellular function are referred to as *antagonists*. Binding of agonists to receptors is inhibited by antagonists. *Competitive antagonists* bind reversibly to receptors, and their blocking effect can be overcome by high concentrations of an agonist. Competitive antagonists produce a parallel shift in the dose-response curve (Fig. 6-14, curves A and B). *Noncompetitive antagonists* bind irreversibly to receptors. This has the same effect as reducing the number of receptors, and shifts the dose-response curve downward and to the right (curves A and C in Fig. 6-14). The effect of noncompetitive antagonists is reversed only by synthesis of new receptor molecules.

The underlying mechanisms by which different compounds that bind to the same receptor act as agonists, partial agonists, or antagonists are not fully understood. Presumably, agonists produce a structural or functional alteration of the receptor molecule that initiates changes in cellular function. Partial agonists may produce a qualitatively different change in the receptor, while antagonists bind without producing a change in the receptor that results in altered cellular function.

CLINICAL APPLICATION OF PHARMACOKINETICS AND PHARMACODYNAMICS

Pharmacokinetics and pharmacodynamics are not merely abstract mathematical games. Rather, they permit the design of dosing regimens in a logical fashion. In anesthesia, the usual therapeutic objectives are to rapidly produce pharmacologic effects, such as unconsciousness or muscle relaxation, to maintain the optimal intensity of these effects during the anesthetic, and to have the patient recover rapidly upon conclusion of surgery. Knowledge of pharmacokinetic principles and of the pharmacokinetic and pharmacodynamic properties of the drugs used in anesthesiology makes it easier to attain these objectives. If the pharmacokinetics and the therapeutic concentration of a drug are known, then the average doses required to achieve and maintain the desired pharmacologic effect can be calculated. The steady-state plasma concentration (Cp_{ss}) is a function of the rate of infusion of the drug and drug clearance:

$$Cp_{ss} = \frac{\text{infusion rate}}{\text{clearance}} \qquad (6\text{-}17)$$

Infusion of the drug for five elimination half-times is required to reach steady-state conditions. Therefore, for most drugs used in anesthesia, it would take 24 h or more to reach a stable plasma concentration by merely infusing the drug at a constant rate. This is obviously impractical, and it does not meet the first of the above-stated objectives.

The volume of distribution must be rapidly "filled up" by giving a loading dose to achieve a more rapid onset of action. The loading dose can be calculated by multiplying the volume of distribution (Vd) by the desired concentration:

$$\text{Loading Dose} = Cp_{ss} \times Vd \qquad (6\text{-}18)$$

Almost all drugs, including those used in anesthesia, have multicompartment pharmacokinetic properties. Therefore, their initial volume of distribution, which is equal to the volume of the central compartment, gets progressively larger until the ultimate volume of distribution, the volume of distribution at steady state (Vd_{ss}), is reached. Consequently, the loading dose can vary according to specific therapeutic objectives.

A minimal loading dose is the amount of drug required to "fill up" the central compartment:

$$\text{Minimal Loading Dose} = Cp_{ss} \times Vc \qquad (6\text{-}19)$$

This rapidly achieves the desired concentration and effect, satisfying the first of the three therapeutic objectives. However, the concentration will decrease very quickly because of drug distribution and elimination, even if the loading dose is followed by an infusion, as calculated with Equation 6-17. This means that the desired effect will be maintained for a very short period.

A full loading dose can be defined as the amount of drug needed to provide the desired concentration once distribution has been completed, and it is calculated as follows:

$$\text{Full Loading Dose} = Cp_{ss} \times Vd_{ss} \qquad (6\text{-}20)$$

Figure 6-15 demonstrates the plasma concentration profile if a full loading dose is followed by a maintenance infusion. The concentration is initially much higher than desired, and it eventually falls to the optimal concentration. The disadvantage of this combination is obvious. The high initial concentra-

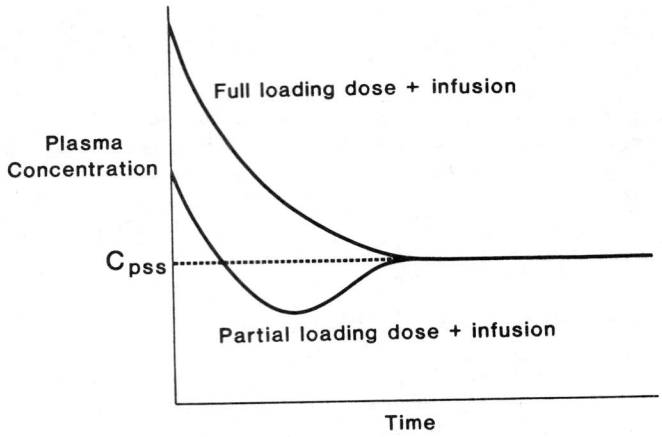

FIG. 6-15. Plasma concentration *versus* time curves after administration of a full or partial loading dose followed by a maintenance infusion at a constant rate.

tion may produce adverse effects, and there may still be a higher than optimal concentration at the conclusion of surgery, preventing rapid recovery.

As a compromise, a partial (more than the minimal, but less than the full) loading dose can be given. If this is followed by a maintenance infusion, the concentration will initially be higher than desired, and will then fall below the optimal concentration before increasing toward the steady-state value. Figure 6-15 demonstrates that the discrepancy between the desired and actual concentrations is less after the partial loading dose-infusion combination than with the full loading dose-maintenance infusion combination. The lower initial concentration is less prone to produce adverse effects, and there is also less likelihood of having an excessive concentration at the conclusion of the operation. Therefore, the partial loading dose-maintenance infusion combination comes closest to fulfilling the three therapeutic objectives. If the nadir of the concentration results in an inadequate effect, then a supplementary loading dose can be given. This principle can be extended by giving a minimal loading dose, followed by many progressively smaller supplementary doses, so that the concentration is close to the desired level virtually all the time.

Pharmacokinetic and pharmacodynamic principles have been used to develop computer-controlled drug infusion systems.[137, 138] The desired concentration is rapidly reached by giving enough drug to fill up the central compartment as a loading dose, and the concentration is maintained by continuously infusing the drug at an exponentially decreasing rate to replace drug lost from the blood by distribution and elimination. This technology will also allow the anesthesiologist to change the concentration more precisely than is possible with manual methods of administering intravenous drugs. The use of computer-assisted infusions will likely become more widespread in clinical anesthesiology, because these systems will facilitate attainment of the usual therapeutic objectives in anesthesiology—rapid onset and maintenance of the optimal effect, followed by rapid recovery at the end of surgery.

DRUG INTERACTIONS

Taking into account premedication, perioperative antibiotics, intravenous agents used for induction of anesthesia, inhalational anesthetics, narcotics, muscle relaxants, and the drugs used to restore neuromuscular transmission, ten or more drugs may be given during a relatively "routine" anesthetic. Consequently, a thorough understanding of the basic mechanisms of drug interactions and knowledge of specific interactions with drugs used in anesthesia is essential to the safe practice of anesthesiology. Indeed, anesthesiologists often deliberately take advantage of drug interactions to achieve the desired effect. For example, reversal of the effects of nondepolarizing neuromuscular blockers is accomplished by giving cholinesterase inhibitors, such as edrophonium or neostigmine, which increases the concentration of acetylcholine at the nicotinic receptors of the motor end-plate. Unfortunately, the concentration of acetylcholine is also increased at muscarinic receptors, leading to undesirable side effects, such as bradycardia, so antimuscarinic agents such as atropine are administered concomitantly. Therefore, the reversal of neuromuscular blockade involves interactions between three drugs at two different receptors. The basic principles of drug interactions, illustrated by a few examples, will be covered in this section. Specific interactions are discussed in succeeding chapters.

Drugs' interactions due to physicochemical properties can occur *in vitro*. Mixing acidic drugs, such as thiopental, and basic drugs, such as narcotics or muscle relaxants, results in the formation of insoluble salts which precipitate out of solution.[139] Another type of *in vitro* reaction is the absorption of drugs by plastics. Examples include the uptake of nitroglycerine by polyvinylchloride infusion sets,[140] and the absorption of fentanyl by the apparatus used for cardiopulmonary bypass.[141]

Drugs can alter each others' absorption, distribution, and elimination. Absorption from the gastrointestinal tract can be altered by drugs like ranitidine, which alters gastric pH,[51] and metoclopramide, which speeds gastric emptying.[142] Vasoconstrictors are added to local anesthetic solutions to prolong their duration of action at the site of injection and to decrease the risk of systemic toxicity from rapid absorption.

Drugs that compete for binding sites on plasma proteins have complex interactions.[66] Displacement of a drug from plasma proteins affects its distribution. The increase in the free drug concentration increases tissue uptake of the drug, increasing the volume of distribution. The extent of the effect on drug distribution depends on the fraction of the total drug in the body that is bound to plasma proteins. The change in distribution will be greatest when drugs with small volumes of distribution that are extensively bound to plasma proteins are displaced. Displacement of one drug by another may acutely produce toxin-free drug concentrations. When a steady-state is reestablished, the effect of decreased binding on total and free drug concentrations depends on the rate of clearance of the drug. For drugs with low extraction ratios, clearance varies with the degree of binding, and clearance will increase proportionately to the increase in free fraction. Therefore, when a steady state is reestablished, the total drug concentration will be lower, but the free drug level will be the same as the level prior to displacement. Clearance of drugs with high extraction ratios is not restricted to the free fraction, and is not affected by changes in binding. Consequently, when a new steady state is reached, the total drug concentration is unchanged, and the higher free drug level will persist. Adverse interactions are, thus, most likely to occur if the displaced drug has high (nonrestrictive) clearance, a small volume of distribution, and is extensively bound to plasma proteins.

As discussed earlier, drugs which inhibit or induce the enzymes that catalyze biotransformation reactions can affect clearance or other concomitantly administered drugs. Clearance can also be affected by drug-induced changes in hepatic blood flow. Drugs cleared by the kidneys that have similar physicochemical characteristics compete for the transport mechanisms involved in renal tubular secretion.

Pharmacodynamic drug interactions fall into two broad classifications. Drugs can interact, either directly or indirectly, at the same receptors. Narcotic antagonists *directly* displace narcotics from opiate receptors. Cholinesterase inhibitors *indirectly* antagonize the effects of neuromuscular blockers by increasing the amount of acetylcholine at the motor end-plate, which displaces the blocking drug from the nicotinic receptor. Pharmacodynamic interactions can also occur if two drugs affect a physiologic system at different sites. This is presumed to be the mechanism by which premedication increases sensitivity to inhalational anesthetics,[143] and is also the reason for increased sensitivity to neuromuscular blocking drugs in the presence of volatile anesthetics, such as halothane.[131]

REFERENCES

1. Papper EM: The pharmacokinetics of inhalation anaesthetics: clinical applications. Br J Anaesth 36:124, 1964
2. Mayer SE, Melmon KL, Gilman AG: Introduction: The dynamics of drug absorption, distribution and elimination. In Gilman AG, Goodman LS, Gilman A (eds): The Pharmacological Basis of Therapeutics, p 1. New York, Macmillan, 1980
3. Stanski DR, Watkins WD: Drug Disposition in Anesthesia, p 24. New York, Grune and Stratton, 1982
4. George CF: Drug metabolism by the gastrointestinal mucosa. Clin Pharmacokinet 6:259, 1981
5. Holley FO, van Steennis C: Transdermal administration of fentanyl for postoperative analgesia. Anesthesiology 65:A548, 1986
6. Greenblatt DJ, Shader RI, Abernethy DR: Current status of benzodiazepines. N Engl J Med 309:354, 410, 1983
7. Fee JPH, Collier PS, Dundee JW: Bioavailability of three formulations of intravenous diazepam. Acta Anaesthesiol Scand 30:337, 1986
8. Price HL, Kovnat PJ, Safer JN et al: The uptake of thiopental by body tissues and its relationship to the duration of narcosis. Clin Pharmacol Ther 1:16, 1960
9. Saidman LJ, Eger EI II: The effect of thiopental metabolism on duration of anesthesia. Anesthesiology 27:118, 1966
10. Brown WU Jr, Bell GC, Alper MH: Acidosis, local anesthetics and the newborn. Obstet Gynecol 48:27, 1976
11. Meijer DFK, Weitering JG, Vermeer GA et al: Comparative pharmacokinetics of d-tubocurarine and metocurine in man. Anesthesiology 51:402, 1979
12. Rowland M, Benet LZ, Graham GG: Clearance concepts in pharmacokinetics. J Pharmacokinet Biopharm 1:123, 1973
13. Wilkinson GR, Shand DG: A physiological approach to hepatic drug clearance. Clin Pharmacol Ther 18:377, 1975
14. Nies AS, Shand DG, Wilkinson GR: Altered hepatic blood flow and drug disposition. Clin Pharmacokinet 1:135, 1976
15. Blaschke TF: Protein binding and kinetics of drugs in liver diseases. Clin Pharmacokinet 2:32, 1977
16. Swartz RD, Sidell FR, Cucinell SA: Effects of physical stress on the disposition of drugs eliminated by the liver in man. J Pharmacol Exp Ther 188:1, 1974
17. Stenson RE, Constantino RT, Harrison DC: Interrelationships of hepatic blood flow, cardiac output, and blood levels of lidocaine in man. Circulation 43:205, 1971
18. Thomson PD, Melmon KL, Richardson JA et al: Lidocaine pharmacokinetics in advanced heart failure, liver disease, and renal failure in humans. Ann Int Med 78:499, 1973
19. Benowitz NL, Meister W: Pharmacokinetics in patients with cardiac failure. Clin Pharmacokinet 1:389, 1976

20. Benowitz NL, Forsyth RP, Melmon KL et al: Lidocaine disposition kinetics in monkey and man II. Effects of hemorrhage and sympathomimetic drug administration. Clin Pharmacol Ther 16:99, 1974

21. Klotz U, McHorse TS, Wilkinson GR et al: The effect of cirrhosis on the disposition and elimination of meperidine in man. Clin Pharmacol Ther 16:667, 1974

22. Neal EA, Meffin PJ, Gregory PB et al: Enhanced bioavailability and decreased clearance of analgesics in patients with cirrhosis. Gastroenterology 77:96, 1979

23. Wood AJJ, Kornhauser DM, Wilkinson GR et al: The influence of cirrhosis on steady-state blood concentrations of unbound propranolol after oral administration. Clin Pharmacokinet 3:478, 1978

24. Klotz U, Avant GR, Hoyumpa A et al: The effects of age and liver disease on the disposition and elimination of diazepam in adult man. J Clin Invest 55:347, 1975

25. Klotz U, Antonin KH, Brugel H et al: Disposition of diazepam and its major metabolite desmethyldiazepam in patients with liver disease. Clin Pharmacol Ther 21:430, 1977

26. McHorse TS, Wilkinson GR, Johnson RF et al: Effect of acute viral hepatitis in man on the disposition and elimination of meperidine. Gastroenterology 68:775, 1975

27. Williams RL, Blaschke TF, Meffin PJ et al: Influence of viral hepatitis on the disposition of two compounds with high hepatic clearance: Lidocaine and indocyanine green. Clin Pharmacol Ther 20:290, 1976

28. Branch RA, Shand DG, Wilkinson GR et al: The reduction of lidocaine clearance by dl-propranolol. An example of hemodynamic drug interaction. J Pharmacol Exp Ther 184:515, 1973

29. Gelman S: Disturbances in hepatic blood flow during anesthesia and surgery. Arch Surg 111:881, 1976

30. Gelman S, Fowler KC, Smith LR: Liver circulation and function during isoflurane and halothane anesthesia. Anesthesiology 61:726, 1984

31. Cooperman LH: Effects of anaesthetics on the splanchnic circulation. Br J Anaesth 44:967, 1972

32. Duchin KL, Schrier RW: Interrelationship between renal haemodynamics, drug kinetics, and drug action. Clin Pharmacokinet 3:58, 1978

33. Garrett ER: Pharmacokinetics and clearances related to renal processes. Int J Clin Pharmacol 16:155, 1978

34. Fabre J, Balant L: Renal failure, drug pharmacokinetics and drug action. Clin Pharmacokinet 1:99, 1976

35. Guyton AC: Textbook of Medical Physiology, 5th ed p 468. Philadelphia, WB Saunders, 1976

36. Mudge GH: Drugs affecting renal function and metabolism. In Gilman AG, Goodman LS, Gilman A (eds): The Pharmacological Basis of Therapeutics, p 885. New York, Macmillan, 1980

37. Collinsworth KA, Strong JM, Atkinson AJ et al: Pharmacokinetics and metabolism of lidocaine in patients with renal failure. Clin Pharmacol Ther 18:59, 1975

38. Miller RD, Agoston S, Booij LHDJ et al: The comparative potency and pharmacokinetics of pancuronium and its metabolites in anesthetized man. J Pharmacol Exp Ther 207:539, 1978

39. Szeto HH, Inturrisi CE, Houde R et al: Accumulation of normeperidine, an active metabolite of meperidine, in patients with renal failure or cancer. Ann Int Med 86:738, 1977

40. Craig DB, McLeskey CH, Mitenko PA et al: Geriatric anaesthesia. Can J Anaesth 34:156, 1987

41. Stanski DR, Watkins WD: Drug Disposition in Anesthesia, p 76. New York, Grune and Stratton, 1982

42. Remmer H: The role of the liver in drug metabolism. Am J Med 49:617, 1970

43. Testa B, Jenner P: Novel drug metabolites produced by functionalization reactions: Chemistry and toxicology. Drug Metab Rev 7:325, 1978

44. Tucker GT: Drug metabolism. Br J Anaesth 51:603, 1979

45. Wood AJJ: Drug metabolism. Drugs and Anesthesia Clinical Pharmacology for Anesthesiologists, p 59. In Wood M, Wood AJJ (eds): Baltimore, Williams and Wilkins, 1982

46. Nebert DW, Eisen HJ, Negishi M et al: Genetic mechanisms controlling the induction of polysubstrate monooxygenase (P450) activities. Ann Rev Pharmacol Toxicol 21:431, 1981

47. Coon MJ: Drug metabolism by cytochrome P-450: Progress and perspectives. Drug Metab Dispos 9:1, 1981

48. Guay DRP, Meatherall RC, Chalmers JL et al: Cimetidine alters pethidine disposition in man. Br J Clin Pharmacol 18:907, 1984

49. Feely J, Wilkinson GR, Wood AJJ: Reduction of liver blood flow and propranolol metabolism by cimetidine. New Engl J Med 304:692, 1981

50. Klotz U, Reimann I: Delayed clearance of diazepam due to cimetidine. N Engl J Med 302:1012, 1980

51. Kirch W, Hoensch H, Janisch HD: Interactions and non-interactions with ranitidine. Clin Pharmacokinet 9:493, 1984

52. Carrum G, Egan JM, Abernethy DR: Diltiazem treatment impairs hepatic drug oxidation: Studies of antipyrine. Clin Pharmacol Ther 40:140, 1986

53. Park BK, Breckenridge AM: Clinical implications of enzyme induction and enzyme inhibition. Clin Pharmacokinet 6:1, 1981

54. Alvares AP: Interactions between environmental chemicals and drug biotransformation in man. Clin Pharmacokinet 3:462, 1978

55. Williams RL, Mamelok RD: Hepatic disease and drug pharmacokinetics. Clin Pharmacokinet 5:528, 1980

56. Reidenberg MM: The biotransformation of drugs in renal failure. Am J Med 62:482, 1977

57. Reilly CS, Wood AJJ, Koshakji RP et al: The effect of halothane on drug disposition: Contribution of changes in intrinsic drug metabolizing capacity and hepatic blood flow. Anesthesiology 63:70, 1985

58. Wood M, Wood AJJ: Contrasting effects of halothane, isoflurane, and enflurane on in vivo drug metabolism in the rat. Anesth Analg 63:709, 1984

59. Vesell ES: The antipyrine test in clinical pharmacology: Conceptions and misconceptions. Clin Pharmacol Ther 26:275, 1979

60. Pessayre D, Allemand H, Benoist C et al: Effect of surgery under general anaesthesia on antipyrine clearance. Br J Clin Pharmacol 6:505, 1978

61. Duvaldestin P, Mazze RI, Nivoche Y et al: Enzyme induction following surgery with halothane and neurolept anesthesia. Anesth Analg 60:319, 1981

62. Loft S, Boel J, Kyst A et al: Increased hepatic microsomal enzyme activity after surgery under halothane or spinal anesthesia. Anesthesiology 62:11, 1985

63. Duvaldestin P, Mauge F, Desmonts JM: Enflurane anesthesia and antipyrine metabolism. Clin Pharmacol Ther 29:61, 1981

64. Pantuck EJ, Pantuck CB, Weismann C et al: Effects of parenteral nutrition regimens on oxidative drug metabolism. Anesthesiology 60:534, 1984

65. Duvaldestin P, Mazze RI, Nivoche Y et al: Occupational exposure to halothane results in enzyme induction in anesthetists. Anesthesiology 54:57, 1981

66. Wood M: Plasma drug binding—Implications for anesthesiologists. Anesth Analg 65:786, 1986

67. Koch-Weser J, Sellers EM: Binding of drugs to serum albumin. N Engl J Med 294:311, 526, 1976

68. McLain DA, Hug CC: Intravenous fentanyl kinetics. Clin Pharmacol Ther 28:106, 1980

69. Meuldermans WEG, Hurkmans RMA, Heykants JJP: Plasma protein binding and distribution of fentanyl, sufentanil, alfentanil and lofentanil in blood. Arch Int Pharmacodynam 257:4, 1982

70. Bowers WF, Fulton S, Thompson J: Ultrafiltration vs equilibrium

dialysis for determination of free fraction. Clin Pharmacokinet 9(Suppl. 1):49, 1984

71. Piafsky KM: Disease-induced changes in plasma binding of basic drugs. Clin Pharmacokinet 5:246, 1980
72. Sjoholm I, Ekman B, Kober A et al: Binding of drugs to serum albumin: XI. Mol Pharmacol 16:767, 1979
73. Nation RL: Meperidine binding in maternal and fetal plasma. Clin Pharmacol Ther 29:472, 1981
74. Chen S-S, Perucca E, Lee J-N et al: Serum protein binding and free concentration of phenytoin and phenobarbitone in pregnancy. Br J Clin Pharmacol 13:547, 1982
75. Dean M, Stock B, Patterson RJ et al: Serum protein binding of drugs during and after pregnancy in humans. Clin Pharmacol Ther 28:253, 1980
76. Perucca E, Crema A: Plasma protein binding of drugs in pregnancy. Clin Pharmacokinet 7:336, 1982
77. Morgan DJ, Blackman GL, Paull JD et al: Pharmacokinetics and plasma binding of thiopental. II: Studies at Cesarean section. Anesthesiology 54:474, 1981
78. Wood M, Wood AJJ: Changes in plasma drug binding and alpha₁-acid glycoprotein in mother and newborn infant. Clin Pharmacol Ther 29:522, 1981
79. Wallace S: Factors affecting drug-protein binding in the plasma of newborn infants. Br J Clin Pharmacol 3:510, 1976
80. Morselli PL, Franco-Morselli R, Bossi L: Clinical pharmacokinetics in newborns and infants. Clin Pharmacokinet 5:485, 1980
81. Davis D, Grossman SH, Ketchell BB et al: The effects of age and smoking on the plasma protein binding of lignocaine and diazepam. Br J Clin Pharmacol 19:261, 1985
82. Verbeeck RK, Cardinal J-A, Wallace SM: Effect of age and sex on the plasma binding of acidic and basic drugs. Eur J Clin Pharmacol 27:91, 1984
83. Wallace S, Whiting B: Factors of affecting drug binding in plasma of elderly patients. Br J Clin Pharmacol 3:327, 1976
84. Herman RJ, McAllister CB, Branch RA et al: Effect of age on meperidine disposition. Clin Pharmacol Ther 37:19, 1985
85. Holmberg L, Odar-Cederlof I, Nilsson JLG et al: Pethidine binding to blood cells and plasma proteins in old and young subjects. Eur J Clin Pharmacol 23:457, 1982
86. Greenblatt DJ, Abernethy DR, Locniskar A et al: Effect of age, gender, and obesity on midazolam kinetics. Anesthesiology 61:27, 1984
87. Greenblatt DJ, Allen MD, Harmatz JS et al: Diazepam disposition determinants. Clin Pharmacol Ther 27:301, 1980
88. Jung D, Mayersohn M, Perrier D et al: Thiopental disposition as a function of age in female patients undergoing surgery. Anesthesiology 56:263, 1982
89. Thiessen JJ, Sellers EM, Denbeigh P et al: Plasma protein binding of diazepam and tolbutamide in chronic alcholics. J Clin Pharmacol 16:345, 1976
90. Olsen GD, Bennett WM, Porter GA: Morphine and phenytoin binding to plasma proteins in renal and hepatic failure. Clin Pharmacol Ther 17:677, 1975
91. Ghoneim MM, Pandya H: Plasma protein binding of thiopental in patients with impaired renal or hepatic function. Anesthesiology 42:545, 1975
92. Pandale G, Chaux F, Salvadori C et al: Thiopental pharmacokinetics in patients with cirrhosis. Anesthesiology 59:123, 1983
93. Burch PG, Stanski DR: Decreased protein binding and thiopental kinetics. Clin Pharmacol Ther 32:212, 1982
94. Reidenberg MM, Drayer DE: Alteration of drug-protein binding in renal disease. Clin Pharmacokinet 9(Suppl. 1):18, 1984
95. Grossman SH, Davis D, Kitchell BB et al: Diazepam and lidocaine plasma protein binding in renal disease. Clin Pharmacol Ther 31:350, 1982
96. Piafsky KM, Borga O, Odar-Cederlof I et al: Increased plasma protein binding of propranolol and chlorpromazine mediated by

disease-induced elevations of plasma alpha₁-acid glycoprotein. N Engl J Med 299:1435, 1978
97. Jackson PR, Tucker GT, Woods HF: Altered plasma drug binding in cancer: Role of alpha₁-acid glycoprotein and albumin. Clin Pharmacol Ther 32:295, 1982
98. Routledge PA, Stargel WW, Wagner GS et al: Increased alpha₁-acid glycoprotein and lidocaine disposition in myocardial infarction. Ann Int Med 93:701, 1980
99. Routledge PA, Stargel WW, Wagner GS et al: Increased plasma protein binding in myocardial infarction. Br J Clin Pharmacol 9:438, 1980
100. Elfstrom J: Drug pharmacokinetics in the postoperative period. Clin Pharmacokinet 4:16, 1979
101. Edwards DJ, Lalka D, Cerra F et al: Alpha₁-acid glycoprotein concentration and protein binding in trauma. Clin Pharmacol Ther 31:62, 1982
102. Fremstad D, Bergerud K, Haffner JFW et al: Increased plasma binding of quinidine after surgery: A preliminary report. Eur J Clin Pharmacol 10:441, 1976
103. Feely J, Forrest A, Gunn A et al: Influence of surgery on plasma propanolol levels and protein binding. Clin Pharmacol Ther 28:579, 1980
104. Holley FO, Ponganis KV, Stanski DR: Effects of cardiac surgery with cardiopulmonary bypass on lidocaine disposition. Clin Pharmacol Ther 35:617, 1984
105. Hoffman BF, Bigger JT Jr: Digitalis and allied cardiac glycosides. In Gilman AG, Goodman LS, Gilman A (eds): The Pharmacological Basis of Therapeutics, p 729. New York, Macmillan, 1980
106. Lowenthal DT, Porter RS, Saris SD et al: Clinical pharmacology, pharmacodynamics and interactions with esmolol. Am J Cardiol 56:14F, 1985
107. McGowan FX, Reiter MJ, Pritchett ELC et al: Verapamil plasma binding: Relationship to alpha₁-acid glycoprotein and drug efficacy. Clin Pharmacol Ther 33:485, 1983
108. Mandelli M, Tognoni G, Garattini S: Clinical pharmacokinetics of diazepam. Clin Pharmacokinet 3:72, 1978
109. Greenblatt DJ: Clinical pharmacokinetics of oxazepam and lorazepam. Clin Pharmacokinet 6:89, 1981
110. Brand L, Mark LC, Snell MM et al: Physiologic disposition of methohexital in man. Anesthesiology 24:331, 1963
111. Tucker GT, Mather LM: Pharmacokinetics of local anaesthetic agents. Br J Anaesth 47:213, 1975
112. Duvaldestin P, Henzel D: Binding of tubocurarine, fazadinium, pancuronium, and Org NC45 to serum proteins in normal man and in patients with cirrhosis. Br J Anaesth 54:513, 1982
113. Wood M, Stone WJ, Wood AJJ: Plasma binding of pancuronium: Effects of age, sex, and disease. Anesth Analg 62:29, 1983
114. Himmelstein KJ, Lutz RJ: A review of the application of physiologically based pharmacokinetic modelling. J Pharmacokinet Biopharm 7:127, 1979
115. Eger EI II: Anesthetic Uptake and Action, p 79. Baltimore, Williams and Wilkins, 1974
116. Hull CJ: Pharmacokinetics and pharmacodynamics. Br J Anaesth 51:579, 1979
117. Gibaldi M, Perrier D: Pharmacokinetics, 2nd ed, p 45. New York, Marcel Dekker, 1982
118. Wagner JH: Linear pharmacokinetic equations allowing direct calculation of many needed pharmacokinetic parameters from the coefficients and exponents of polyexponential equations which have been fitted to the data. J Pharmacokinet Biopharm 4:443, 1976
119. Gibaldi M, Weintraub H: Some considerations as to the determination and significance of biologic half-life. J Pharm Sci 60:624, 1971
120. Hudson RJ, Stanski DR, Burch PG: Pharmacokinetics of methohexital and thiopental in surgical patients. Anesthesiology 59:215, 1983

121. Rowland M: Protein binding and drug clearance. Clin Pharmacokinet 9(Suppl 1): 10, 1984

122. Branch RA, James J, Read AE: A study of factors influencing drug disposition in chronic liver disease, using the model drug (+)-propranolol. Br J Clin Pharmacol 3:243, 1976

123. Stanski Dr, Mihm FG, Rosenthal MH et al: Pharmacokinetics of high-dose thiopental used in cerebral resuscitation. Anesthesiology 53:169, 1980

124. Nussmeier NA, Arlund C, Slogoff S: Neuropsychiatric complications after cardiopulmonary bypass: Cerebral protection by a barbiturate. Anesthesiology 64:165, 1986

125. Holford NHG, Sheiner LB: Understanding the dose-effect relationship: Clinical application of pharmacokinetic-pharmacodynamic models. Clin Pharmacokinet 6:429, 1981

126. Fisher DM, Fahey MR, Cronnelly et al: Potency determination for vecuronium (Org NC45). Anesthesiology 57:309, 1982

127. Hull CJ, Van Beem H, McLeod K et al: A pharmacodynamic model for pancuronium. Br J Anaesth 50:1113, 1978

128. Stanski DR, Hudson RJ, Homer TD et al: Pharmacodynamic modelling of thiopental anesthesia. J Pharmacokinet Biopharm 12:223, 1984

129. Homer TD, Stanski DR: The effect of increasing age on thiopental disposition and anesthetic requirement. Anesthesiology 62:714, 1985

130. Scott JC, Ponganis KV, Stanski DR: EEG quantitation of narcotic effect: The comparative pharmacodynamics of fentanyl and alfentanil. Anesthesiology 62:234, 1985

131. Stanski DR, Ham J, Miller RD et al: Pharmacokinetics and pharmacodynamics of d-tubocurarine during nitrous oxide-narcotic and halothane anesthesia in man. Anesthesiology 51:235, 1979

132. Fisher DM, O'Keeffe C, Stanski DR et al: Pharmacokinetics and pharmacodynamics of d-tubocurarine in infants, children, and adults. Anesthesiology 57:203, 1982

133. Snyder SH: Drug and neurotransmitter receptors in the brain. Science 224:22, 1984

134. Waud BE, Waud DR: The margin of safety of neuromuscular transmission in the muscle of the diaphragm. Anesthesiology 37:417, 1972

135. Norman J: Drug-receptor reactions. Br J Anaesth 51:595-601, 1979

136. Lefkowitz RJ, Caron MG, Stiles GL: Mechanisms of membrane receptor regulation. N Engl J Med 310:1570, 1984

137. Alvis JM, Reves JG, Govier AV et al: Computer-assisted infusions of fentanyl during cardiac anesthesia: Comparison with a manual method. Anesthesiology 63:41, 1985

138. Shafer SL, Siegel LC, Cooke JE et al: Testing computer-controlled infusion pumps by simulation. Anesthesiology 68:261, 1988

139. Cullen BF, Miller MG: Drug interactions in anesthesia: A review. Anesth Analg 58:413, 1979

140. Mutch WAC, Thomson IR: Delivery systems for intravenous nitroglycerin. Can Anaesth Soc J 30:98, 1983

141. Koren G, Goresky G, Crean P et al: Pediatric fentanyl dosing based on pharmacokinetics during cardiac surgery. Anesth Analg 63:577, 1984

142. Rawlins MD: Drug interactions and anaesthesia. Br J Anaesth 50:689, 1978

143. Quasha AL, Eger EI II, Tinker JH: Determinations and applications of MAC. Anesthesiology 53:315, 1980

Chapter 7

Lenard R. Durrett
Noel W. Lawson

Autonomic Nervous System Physiology and Pharmacology

Neither the old, nor the new by itself is interesting: the absolutely old is insipid, the absolutely new makes no appeal at all. The old in the new is what claims attention.

William Jones
(1842–1910)

Claude Bernard (1878–1979) stated that "the constancy of the 'Milieu Interieur' is the condition of a free and independent existence." In 1932 Walter Cannon referred to the biologic responses necessary to maintain a steady state in the internal environment as homeostasis. Bernard suspected, and Cannon proved, that the autonomic nervous system (ANS) is in large measure responsible for maintaining constant conditions within the body.[1]

Anesthesiology is the practice of ANS medicine. The drugs that produce anesthesia also produce potent ANS side-effects. For example, most vasoactive drugs in clinical use either alter or mimic effects of the ANS system. The greater part of our training and practice is spent acquiring skills in averting or using the ANS side-effects of anesthetic drugs under a variety of pathophysiologic conditions. The success of any anesthetic adventure depends on how well we maintain homeostasis. The numbers we generate and faithfully record during the course of anesthesia often reflect ANS function and homeostasis. Numbers, such as heart rate and blood pressure measurements, do not necessarily indicate the presence of surgical anesthesia.[2] A knowledge of the anatomy, physiology, and biochemistry of the ANS, particularly its junctional sites and receptors, is a prerequisite to an understanding of its pharmacology.

AUTONOMIC NERVOUS SYSTEM PURPOSE

The ANS includes that part of the central and peripheral nervous system that concerns the involuntary regulation of cardiac muscle, smooth muscle, and glandular and visceral function throughout the body. ANS activity refers to visceral reflexes that function essentially below the conscious level.[3] The term *autonomic* remains the best description of this ubiquitous nervous system as opposed to *automatic*. Autonomic implies self controlling, whereas automatic infers nonreflexic or intrinsic responses; however, the use of "autonomy" to describe this nervous system is also illusory. The ANS is exquisitely responsive to changes in somatic motor and sensory activities of the body.[4] The physiologic evidence of visceral reflexes as a result of somatic events is abundantly clear.[5] Psychosomatic disease is an expression of this connection and has long interested those concerned with disease related to emotional behavior. The ANS is therefore not as distinct an entity as the term suggests because neither somatic nor ANS activity occurs in isolation.[6] The ANS organizes visceral support for somatic behavior and adjusts body states in anticipation of emotional behavior or responses to the stress of disease, *i.e.*, fight or flight.

Traditionally, the ANS has been viewed as strictly a peripheral, efferent (motor) system.[4] This concept is no longer tenable.[3,7,8] Afferent fibers from visceral structures are the first link in the reflex arcs of the ANS whether relaying visceral pain or changes in vessel stretch. Most ANS efferent fibers are accompanied by sensory fibers that are now commonly recognized as components of the ANS. The afferent components of the ANS however, cannot be as distinctively divided as can the efferent nerves.

Historically, many investigators have refused to classify any afferent fibers within the ANS because visceral sensory nerves are anatomically indistinguishable from somatic sensory nerves.[9,10] Visceral afferent pathways are like afferent somatic nerves in that they are unipolar. ANS efferents are bipolar (Fig. 7-1). Furthermore, afferent fibers that are anatomically aligned with ANS efferents do not differ by design, function, or drug response from somatic afferents.[11] In addition, both somatic and visceral sensory nerves are able to initiate ANS reflexes. However, the argument is functional rather than anatomic because visceral pain can be attenuated by sympathectomy. ANS afferent fibers that arise from the baroreceptors and chemoreceptors of the carotid arteries and aorta are carried by the glossopharyngeal (IX) and vagus (X) nerves to the medulla. These reflexes are important in the control of cardiac output and ventilation but do not involve any somatic nerve.[3] Four-fifths of vagal nerve fibers are sensory.[6] The clinical importance of visceral afferent fibers is more closely associated with chronic pain management.

FUNCTIONAL ANATOMY

From the anatomic, physiologic, and pharmacologic viewpoints, the ANS naturally falls into two divisions.[3] Willis in 1665 recognized the sympathetic nervous system (SNS) and carefully distinguished it from the vagus (L. wandering) nerve. He designated this ganglion chain the intercostal nerve. In 1732 Winslow studied the intercostal nerve and renamed it the grand sympathetic nerve. Stimulation or injury to one part of the body was accompanied by reactions in other organs as though sympathetic relationships existed. It was in 1921 that Langley divided this nervous system into two parts. He retained the term *sympathetic* for the first part and introduced the term *parasympathetic nervous system* (PNS) for the

second. The term *autonomic nervous system* was adopted as a comprehensive name for both. Ordinarily, activation of the SNS produces expenditure of body energy, whereas stimulation of the PNS produces conservation or accumulation of resources.[7] Table 7-1 lists the complementary effects of SNS and PNS activity of organ systems.

CENTRAL AUTONOMIC ORGANIZATION

No purely central ANS or somatic centers are known, and extensive overlap of function occurs.[12] Integration of ANS activity occurs at all levels of the cerebrospinal axis. Efferent ANS activity can be initiated locally and by centers located in the spinal cord, brain stem, and hypothalamus. The cerebral cortex is the highest level of ANS integration. Fainting at the site of blood is an example of this higher level of somatic and ANS integration. ANS function has also been successfully modulated through conscious,[13] intentional efforts demonstrating that somatic responses are always accompanied by visceral responses and *vice versa*.

The principal site of ANS organization is the hypothalamus. SNS functions are controlled by nuclei in the posterolateral hypothalamus. Stimulation of these nuclei result in a massive discharge of the sympathoadrenal system (Table 7-2). PNS functions are governed by nuclei in the midline and some anterior nuclei of the hypothalamus. Regulation of temperature is involved with the anterior hypothalamus. The supraoptic hypothalamic nuclei are involved in water metabolism and are anatomically and functionally associated with the posterior lobe of the pituitary (see the sections on interactions).[1] This hypothalamic-neurohypophyseal connection represents a central ANS mechanism that affects the kidney by means of the antidiuretic hormone (ADH). Long-term blood pressure control, reactions to physical and emotional stress, sleep, and sexual reflexes are regulated through the hypothalamus.

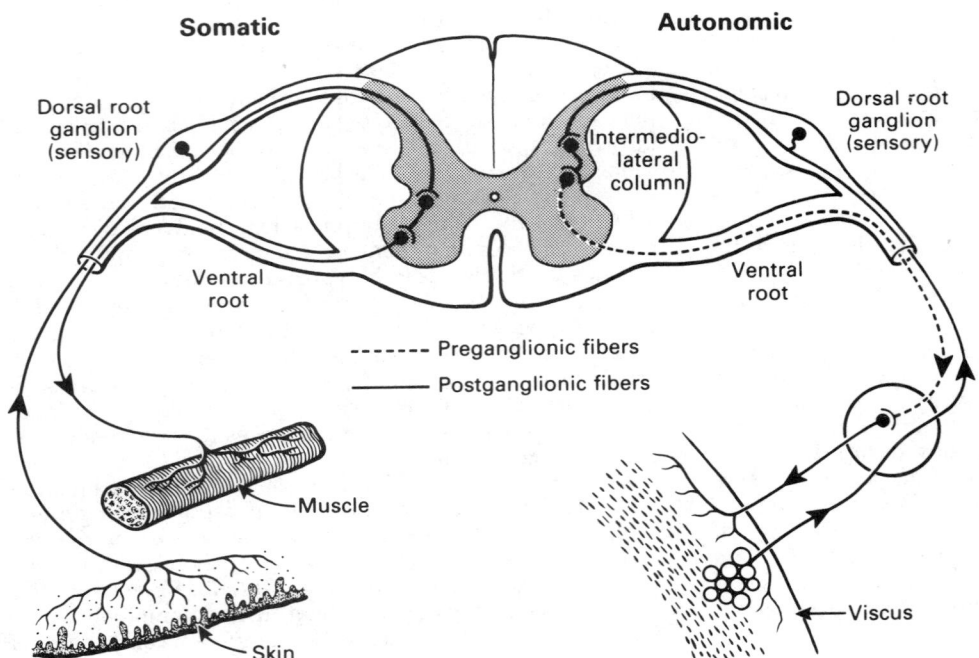

FIG. 7-1. Comparison of somatic and autonomic reflex arcs. Somatic arcs are unipolar and autonomic arcs are bipolar.

TABLE 7-1.   Homeostatic Balance Between Adrenergic and Cholinergic Effects

ORGAN SYSTEM	RESPONSE	
	Adrenergic	*Cholinergic*
HEART		
SA Node	Tachycardia	Bradycardia
AV Node	Increased conduction	Decreased conduction
His-Purkinje	Increased automaticity and conduction velocity	Minimal
Myocardium	Increased contractility, conduction velocity, automaticity	Minimal decrease in contractility
Coronary vessels	Constriction (α_1) and dilation (β_1)	Dilation and constriction?*
BLOOD VESSELS		
Skin and mucosa	Constriction	Dilation
Skeletal muscle	Constriction (α_1) > dilation (β_2)	Dilation
Pulmonary	Constriction	? Dilation
BRONCHIAL SMOOTH MUSCLE	Relaxation	Contraction
GASTROINTESTINAL TRACT		
Gall bladder and ducts	Relaxation	Contraction
Gut motility	Decreased	Increased
Secretions	Decreased	Increased
Sphincters	Constriction	Relaxation
BLADDER		
Detrusor	Relaxes	Contracts
Trigone	Contracts	Relaxes
GLANDS		
Nasal	Vasoconstriction and reduced secretion	Stimulation of secretions
Lacrimal		
Parotid		
Submandibular		
Gastric		
Pancreatic		
SWEAT GLANDS	Diaphoresis (cholinergic)	None
APOCRINE GLANDS	Thick, odiferous secretion	None
EYE		
Pupil	Mydriasis	Miosis
Ciliary muscle	Relaxation for far vision	Contraction for near vision

* See Interaction of Autonomic Nervous System Receptors.

TABLE 7-2.   Hypothalamic Nuclei

ANTERIOR	POSTERIOR
PARAVENTRICULAR NUCLEUS (oxytocin release) (water conservation)	POSTERIOR HYPOTHALAMUS (increased blood pressure) (pupillary dilation) (shivering) (corticotropin)
MEDIAL PREOPTIC AREA (bladder contraction) (decreased heart rate) (decreased blood pressure)	DORSOMEDIAL NUCLEUS (GI stimulation)
SUPRAOPTIC NUCLEUS (water conservation)	PERIFORNICAL NUCLEUS (hunger) (increased blood pressure) (rage)
POSTERIOR PREOPTIC AND ANTERIOR HYPOTHALAMIC AREA (body temperature regulation) (panting) (sweating) (thyrotropin inhibition)	VENTROMEDIAL NUCLEUS (satiety)
	MAMMILLARY BODY (feeding reflexes)
	LATERAL HYPOTHALAMIC AREA (thirst and hunger)

The medulla oblongata and pons are the vital centers of acute ANS organization. Together, they integrate momentary hemodynamic adjustments and maintain the sequence and automaticity of ventilation (Fig. 7-2). Integration of afferent and efferent ANS impulses at this central nervous system (CNS) level is responsible for the tonic activity exhibited by the ANS.[4, 6] Control of peripheral vascular resistance, and thus blood pressure, is a striking example of this tonic activity. Tonicity holds visceral organs in a state of intermediate activity that can be either diminished or augmented by altering the rate of nerve firing. The nucleus tractus solitarius, located within the medulla, is the primary area for relay of afferent chemoreceptor and baroreceptor information from the glossopharyngeal and vagus nerves. Increased afferent impulses from these two nerves inhibit peripheral SNS vascular tone, producing vasodilatation, and increase efferent vagal tone, producing bradycardia. High spinal cord transection eliminates the medulla and results in severe hypotension.[8] Unwanted ANS side-effects of drugs may be produced at medullary sites and thus overshadow their desired peripheral effects.[14]

Reflex ANS centers within segments of the spinal cord are capable of producing complex, organized responses to afferent stimuli. Studies of patients with high spinal cord lesions show that a number of reflex changes are mediated at the spinal or segmental level. ANS hyperreflexia is an example of spinal cord mediation of ANS reflexes without integration of function from higher inhibitory centers.[15, 16]

PERIPHERAL AUTONOMIC NERVOUS SYSTEM ORGANIZATION

The peripheral ANS is the efferent (motor) component of the ANS and consists of two complementary parts: the SNS and PNS. Most organs receive fibers from both divisions (Fig. 7-3). In general, activities of the two systems produce opposite but complementary effects (Table 7-1). Actions of the two subdivisions are supplementary in some tissues such as the salivary glands. A few tissues such as sweat glands and spleen are innervated by only SNS fibers.

Although the anatomy of the somatic and ANS sensory pathways are identical, the motor pathways are characteristically different. The efferent somatic motor system, like somatic afferents, is composed of a single (unipolar) neuron with its cell body in the ventral gray matter of the spinal cord.[5] Its myelinated axon extends directly to the voluntary striated

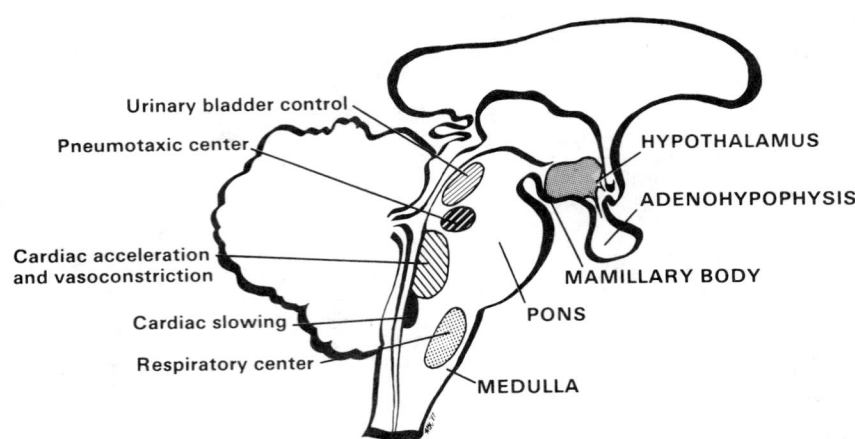

FIG. 7-2. Central vital centers of the medulla oblongata and pons.

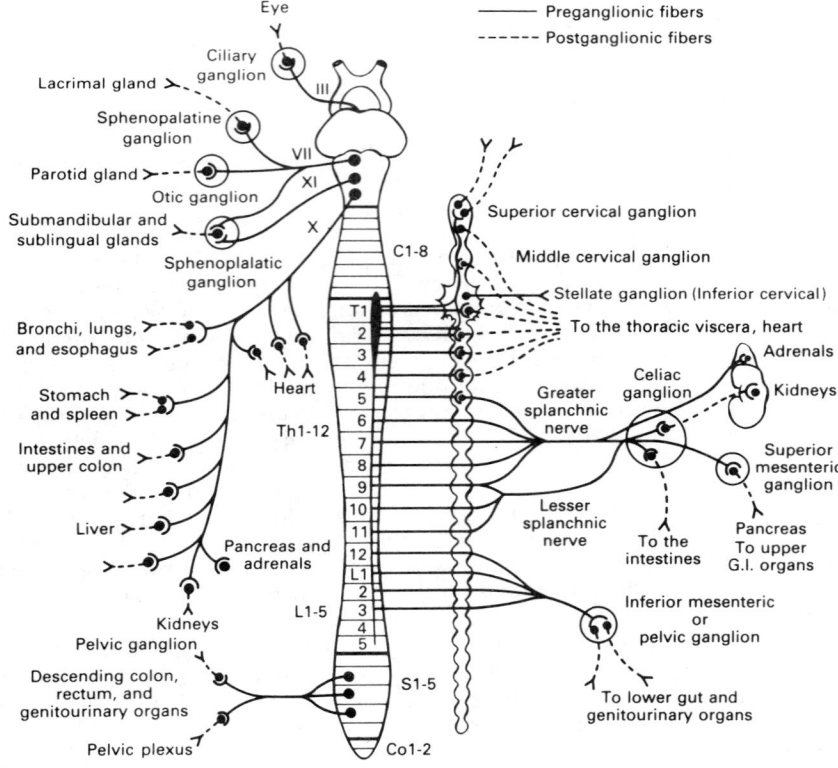

Parasympathetic nerve distribution
(Craniosacral outflow)

Sympathetic nerve distribution
(Thoracolumbar outflow)

FIG. 7-3. Schematic distribution of the craniosacral (parasympathetic) and thoracolumbar (sympathetic) nervous system. Parasympathetic preganglionic fibers pass directly to the organ that is innervated. Their postganglionic cell bodies are situated near or within the innervated viscera. This limited distribution of parasympathetic postganglionic fibers is consistent with the discrete and limited effect of parasympathetic function. The postganglionic sympathetic neurons originate in either the paired sympathetic ganglia or one of the unpaired collateral plexi. One preganglionic fiber influences many postganglionic neurons. Activation of the sympathetic nervous system produces a more diffuse physiologic response rather than discrete effects.

muscle unit. In contrast, the efferent (motor) ANS is a two-neuron (bipolar) chain from the CNS to the effector organ (Fig. 7-1). The first neuron of both the SNS and PNS originates within the CNS but does not make direct contact with the effector organ. Instead, it relays the impulse to a second station known as an autonomic ganglion, which contains the cell body of the second autonomic (postganglionic) neuron. Its axon contacts the effector organ. Thus, the motor pathways of both divisions of the ANS are schematically a serial, two-neuron chain consisting of a preganglionic and a postganglionic effector neuron (Fig. 7-4).

Preganglionic fibers of both subdivisions are myelinated with diameters of less than 3 μm.[3, 4, 6] Impulses are conducted at a speed of 3–15 m·s^{-1}. The postganglionic fibers are unmyelinated and conduct impulses at slower speeds of less than

2 m·s^{-1}. They are similar to unmyelinated visceral and somatic afferent C fibers (Table 7-3). Compared with the myelinated somatic nerves, the ANS conducts impulses at speeds that preclude its participation in the immediate phase of a somatic response.

Sympathetic Nervous System, or Thoracolumbar Division

The efferent SNS is also referred to as the thoracolumbar nervous system. The origin of its preganglionic fibers provides the anatomic basis for this designation. Figure 7-3 demonstrates the distribution of the SNS and its innervation of visceral organs.

The preganglionic fibers of the SNS (thoracolumbar divi-

BIPOLAR AUTONOMIC NERVES

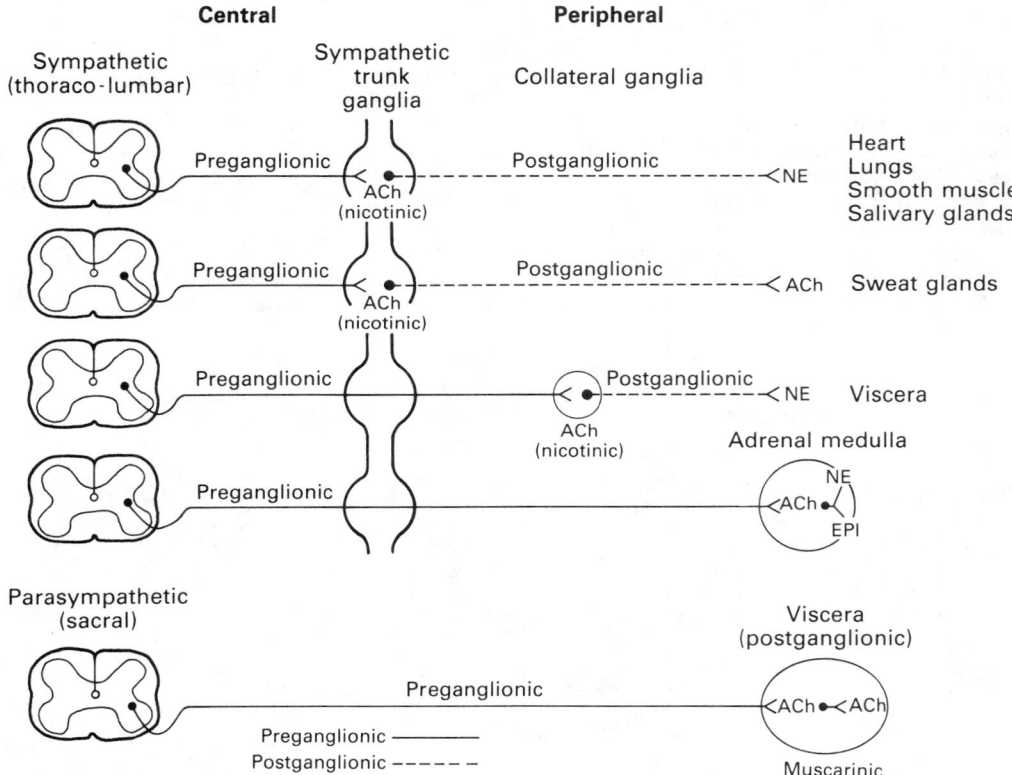

FIG. 7-4. Schematic diagram of the efferent autonomic nervous system. Afferent impulses are integrated centrally and sent reflexly to the adrenergic and cholinergic receptors. Sympathetic fibers ending in the adrenal medulla are preganglionic and acetylcholine (ACh) is the neurotransmitter. Stimulation of the chromaffin cells, acting as postganglionic neurons, release epinephrine (EPI) and norepinephrine (NE).

TABLE 7-3.   Classification of Nerve Fibers

DESCRIPTION OF NERVE FIBERS	GROUP	DIAMETER (μm)	CONDUCTION VELOCITY
Myelinated somatic	A { Alpha α	20	120 m·s^{-1}
	Beta β		
	Gamma δ		5–40 (pain fibers)
	Delta Δ	3–4	5–40 (pain fibers)
	Epsilon ε*	2	5
Myelinated visceral (preganglionic autonomic)	B	< 3	3–15
Unmyelinated somatic	C*	< 2	0.5–2 (pain fibers)

sion) originate in the intermediolateral gray column of the twelve thoracic (T1–12) and first three lumbar segments (L1–3) of the spinal cord. The myelinated axons of these nerve cells leave the spinal cord with the motor fibers to form the white (myelinated) communicating rami (Fig. 7-5). The rami enter one of the paired 22 sympathetic ganglia at their respective segmental level. Upon entering the paravertebral ganglia of the lateral sympathetic chain, the preganglionic fiber may follow one of three courses: (1) synapse with postganglionic fibers in ganglia at the level of exit; (2) course upward or downward in the trunk of the SNS chain to synapse in ganglia at other levels; or (3) track for variable distances through the SNS chain and exit without synapsing to terminate in an outlying, unpaired, SNS collateral ganglion (Fig. 7-5). The adrenal gland is an exception to the rule. Preganglionic fibers pass directly into the adrenal medulla without synapsing in a ganglion (Fig. 7-4). The cells of the medulla are derived from neuronal tissue and are analogous to postganglionic neurons.[4, 6, 12]

The SNS postganglionic neuronal cell bodies are located in ganglia of the paired lateral SNS chain or unpaired collateral ganglia in more peripheral plexi. Collateral ganglia, such as the celiac and inferior mesenteric ganglia (plexi), are formed by the convergence of preganglionic fibers with many postganglionic neuronal bodies. SNS ganglia are almost always located closer to the spinal cord than to the organs they innervate. The SNS postganglionic neuron can therefore originate in either the paired lateral paravertebral SNS ganglia or one of the unpaired collateral plexi. The unmyelinated postganglionic fibers then proceed from the ganglia to terminate within the organs they innervate.

Many of the postganglionic fibers pass from the lateral SNS chain back into the spinal nerves, forming the gray (unmyelinated) communicating rami at all levels of the spinal cord (Fig. 7-5). They are distributed distally to sweat glands, pilomotor muscle, and blood vessels of the skin and muscle. These nerves are unmyelinated C-type fibers (Table 7-3) and are carried within the somatic nerves. Approximately 8% of the fibers in the average somatic nerve are sympathetic.[6]

The first four or five thoracic spinal segments generate preganglionic fibers that ascend in the neck to form three special paired ganglia. These are the superior cervical, middle cervical, and cervicothoracic ganglia. The last is known as the stellate ganglion and is actually formed by the fusion of the inferior cervical and first thoracic SNS ganglia. These ganglia provide SNS innervation of the head, neck, upper extremities, heart, and lungs. Afferent pain fibers also travel with these nerves, accounting for chest, neck, or upper-extremity pain with myocardial ischemia.

Activation of the SNS produces a diffused physiologic response (mass reflex) rather than discrete effects. Function follows design. SNS postganglionic neurons outnumber the preganglionic neurons in an average ratio of 20:1 to 30:1.[4, 5, 17] One preganglionic fiber influences a larger number of postganglionic neurons, which are dispersed to many organs. In addition, the SNS response is augmented by the hormonal release of epinephrine from the adrenal medulla.

Parasympathetic Nervous System, or Craniosacral Division

The PNS, like the SNS, has both preganglionic and postganglionic neurons. This division is sometimes called the craniosacral outflow because the preganglionic cell bodies origi-

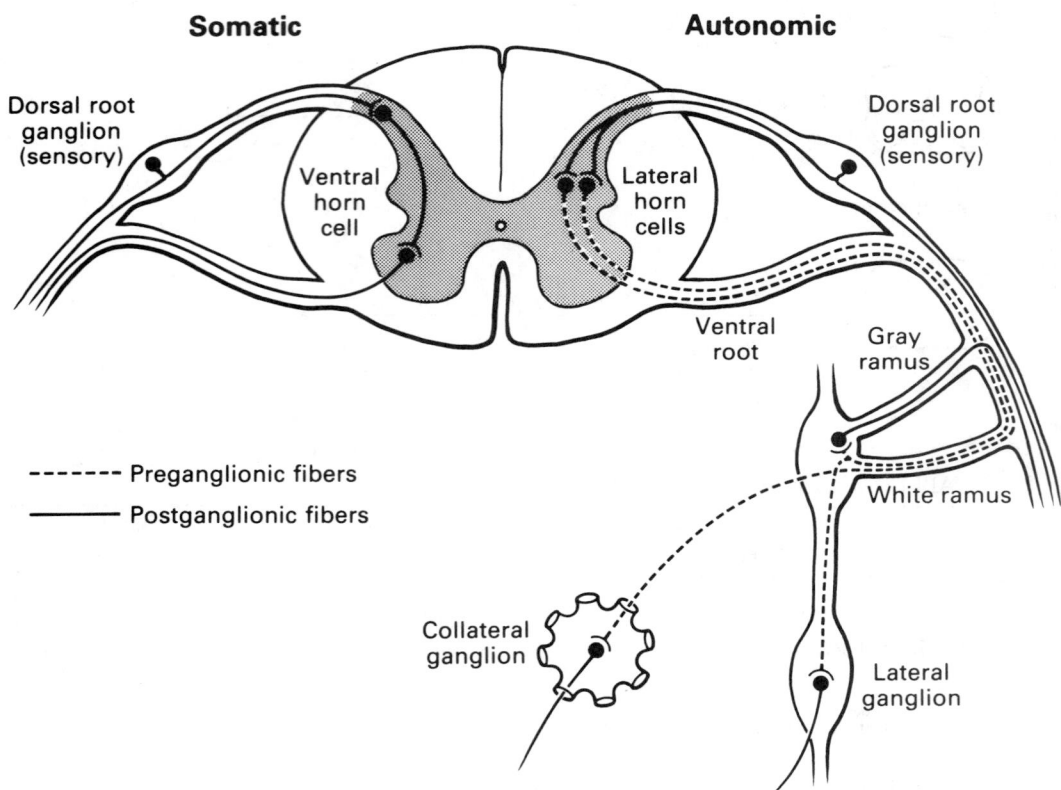

Somatic   **Autonomic**

Dorsal root ganglion (sensory)

Ventral horn cell

Lateral horn cells

Dorsal root ganglion (sensory)

Ventral root

Gray ramus

------- Preganglionic fibers
——— Postganglionic fibers

White ramus

Collateral ganglion

Lateral ganglion

FIG. 7-5. The spinal reflex arc of the somatic nerves is shown on the left. The different arrangements of neurons in the sympathetic system are shown on the right. Preganglionic fibers coming out through white rami may make synaptic connections following one of three courses: (1) synapse in ganglia at the level of exit; (2) course up or down the sympathetic chain to synapse at another level; or, (3) exit the chain without synapsing to an outlying collateral ganglion.

nate in the brain stem and sacral segments of the spinal cord. PNS preganglionic fibers are found in cranial nerves III (oculomotor), VII (facial), IX (glossopharyngeal), and X (vagus). The sacral outflow originates in the intermediolateral gray horns of the second, third, and fourth sacral nerves. Figure 7-3 shows the distribution of the PNS and its innervation of visceral organs.

The vagus (X) nerve has the most extensive distribution of all the PNS, accounting for more than 75% of PNS activity.[6] The paired vagus nerves supply PNS innervation to the heart, lungs, esophagus, stomach, small intestine, proximal half of the colon, liver, gallbladder, pancreas, and upper portions of the ureters. The sacral fibers form the pelvic visceral nerves, or nervi erigentes. These nerves supply the remainder of the viscera not innervated by the vagus. It supplies the descending colon, rectum, uterus, bladder, and lower portions of the ureters and is primarily concerned with emptying. Various sexual reactions are also governed by the sacral PNS. The PNS is responsible for penile erection, but SNS stimulation governs ejaculation.

In contrast to the SNS, PNS preganglionic fibers pass directly to the organ that is innervated. The postganglionic cell bodies are situated near or within the innervated viscera and generally are not visible. The proximity of PNS ganglia to, or within, the viscera provides a limited distribution of postganglionic fibers. The ratio of postganglionic to preganglionic fibers in many organs appears to be 1 : 1 to 3 : 1 compared with the 20 : 1 found in the SNS.[4, 5] Auerbach's plexus in the distal colon is the exception, with a ratio of 8000 : 1. The fact that PNS preganglionic fibers synapse with only a few postganglionic neurons is consistent with the discrete and limited effect of PNS function. For example, vagal bradycardia can occur without a concomitant change in intestinal motility or salivation. Mass reflex action is not a characteristic of the PNS. The effects of organ response to PNS stimulation are outlined in Table 7-1.

Autonomic Nervous System Innervation

HEART. The heart is well supplied by the SNS and PNS. These nerves affect cardiac pumping in three ways: (1) by changing the rate (chronotropism); (2) by changing the strength of contraction (inotropism); and (3) by modulating coronary blood flow. The PNS cardiac vagal fibers approach the stellate ganglia and then join the efferent cardiac SNS fibers; therefore, the vagus nerve to the heart and lungs is a mixed nerve containing both PNS and SNS efferent fibers. The PNS fibers are distributed mainly to the sinoatrial (SA) and atrioventricular (AV) nodes and to a lesser extent to the atria. There is little or no distribution to the ventricles.[5, 18] Therefore, the main effect of vagal cardiac stimulation to the heart is chronotropic. Vagal stimulation decreases the rate of SA node discharge and decreases excitability of the AV junctional fibers, slowing impulse conduction to the ventricles. A very strong vagal discharge can completely arrest SA node firing and block impulse conduction to the ventricles. Vagal stimulation or vagotonic drugs such as methacholine reduce the vulnerability of the heart to ventricular fibrillation, decrease the frequency of premature ventricular beats, and can abolish ventricular tachycardia (see Interactions of Autonomic Nervous System Receptors).[19]

The physiologic importance of the PNS effect on myocardial contractility is not as well understood as that for the SNS. Cholinergic blockade can double the heart rate without altering contractility of the left ventricle. Vagal stimulation of the heart can reduce left ventricular maximum rate of tension development (dP/dT) and decrease contractile force by as much as 10–20%; however, PNS stimulation is relatively unimportant in this regard compared with its predominant effect on heart rate.

The SNS nerves have the same supraventricular distribution as the PNS, but with stronger representation to the ventricles. SNS efferents to the myocardium funnel through the paired stellate ganglia. The right stellate ganglion distributes primarily to the anterior epicardial surface and the interventricular septum.[20, 21] Right stellate stimulation decreases systolic duration and increases heart rate. The left stellate supplies the posterior and lateral surfaces of both ventricles. Left stellate stimulation increases mean arterial pressure and left ventricular contractility without causing a substantial change in heart rate. Normal SNS tone maintains contractility approximately 20% above that in the absence of any SNS stimulation.[22] Therefore, the dominant effect of the ANS on myocardial contractility is mediated primarily through the SNS. Intrinsic mechanisms of the myocardium, however, can maintain circulation quite well without the ANS, as evidenced by the success of cardiac transplants[23, 24] (see Denervated Heart).

Early investigations, performed in anesthetized, open-chest animals, demonstrated that cardiac ANS nerves exert only slight effects on the coronary vascular bed; however, more recent studies on chronically instrumented, intact, conscious animals show considerable evidence for a strong SNS regulation of the small coronary resistance and larger conductance vessels.[25–27] This information is important, but the anesthesiologist must be careful to place this new information into context. As in the older studies, our patients are anesthetized and often with their thorax open. The new studies refute the old concept that there is minimal ANS coronary influence, but instead demonstrate that anesthesia minimizes the contribution of the ANS to the regulation of coronary blood flow as compared with the conscious state. These data have already proven useful in anesthetizing patients during acute myocardial infarction.[28]

Different segments of the coronary arterial tree react differently to various stimuli and drugs. Large conductance vessels, the primary location for atheromatous plaques, are found on the epicardial surface, whereas the small, precapillary resistance vessels are found within the myocardium. Normally, the large conductance vessels contribute little to overall coronary vascular resistance. Fluctuations in resistance primarily reflect changes in lumen size of the small, precapillary vessels. Blood flow through the resistance vessels is regulated primarily by the local metabolic requirements of the myocardium. The larger conductance vessels, however, can constrict markedly with neurogenic stimulation. Neurogenic influence also assumes a greater role in the resistance vessels when they become hypoxic and lose autoregulation. There is a strong interaction between SNS and PNS nerves in organs with dual, antagonistic innervation. The tone of the coronary arteries is under this interacting control in a manner that is only now becoming understood (see Interaction of Autonomic Nervous System Receptors).[29]

PERIPHERAL CIRCULATION. The SNS nerves are by far the most important regulators of the peripheral circulation.[30] The PNS nerves play only a minor role in this regard.[6] PNS stimulation dilates vessels, but only in certain limited areas such as the genitals. SNS stimulation produces both vasodilatation and vasoconstriction with vasoconstrictor effects predominating. The effect is determined by the type of receptors on which the SNS fiber terminates (see Receptors). SNS constrictor receptors are distributed to all segments of the circulation. This distribution is greater in some tissues than others. Blood vessels in the skin, kidneys, spleen, and mesentery have an extensive SNS distribution, whereas those in the heart, brain, and muscle have less SNS innervation. SNS stimulation of the coronary arteries may produce vasoconstriction or vasodilation, depending on the predominant receptor activity at the time of stimulation (Table 7-1). Vagal stimulation may also produce coronary vasoconstriction (see β-Adrenergic Receptors).[27] However, local autoregulatory factors usually have the predominant influence on coronary vascular tone.

Vascular tone is the sum of the muscular forces in the walls of blood vessels that oppose an increase of vessel diameter. Vasomotor tone denotes that portion of vascular tone controlled by the ANS vasomotor nerves. Thus, vascular tone can be influenced by local and circulating substances as well as the vasomotor nerves. Blood vessels have differing sensitivities to the influence of local or neurogenic control. Arterioles and venules are under strong neurogenic control and have vasomotor tone. Local autoregulation is the predominant force at the precapillary and postcapillary sphincters.[31, 32]

Basal vasomotor tone is maintained by impulses from the lateral portion of the vasomotor center in the medulla oblongata that continually transmits impulses through the SNS, maintaining partial arteriolar and venular constriction. Circulating epinephrine from the adrenal medulla has additive effects. This basal ANS tone maintains arteriolar constriction at near half-maximum diameter.[4] The arteriole, therefore, has the potential for either further constriction or dilatation. If the basal tone were not present, the SNS could only effect vasoconstriction and not vasodilatation.[6, 33] The SNS tone in the venules produces little resistance to flow as compared with the arterioles and the arteries. The importance of SNS stimulation of veins is to reduce or increase their capacity. By functioning as a reservoir for approximately 80% of the total blood volume, small changes in venous capacitance will produce large changes in venous return and, thus, cardiac preload.

LUNGS. The lung is innervated by both the SNS and PNS.[4] Postganglionic SNS fibers from the upper thoracic ganglia (stellate) pass to the lungs to innervate the smooth muscle of the bronchi and pulmonary blood vessels. PNS innervation of these structures is from the vagus nerves.

SNS stimulation produces bronchodilatation and pulmonary vasoconstriction.[34] Little else has been proven conclusively about the vasomotor control of the pulmonary vessels other than they adjust to accommodate the output of the right ventricle. The effect of stimulation of the pulmonary SNS nerves on pulmonary vascular resistance is not very great but may be quite important in maintaining hemodynamic stability during stress and exercise by balancing right and left ventricular outputs.[35, 36] This response is likely mediated *via* the hypothalamus. Stimulation of the vagus, on the other hand, produces almost no vasodilation of the pulmonary circulation. The recently described phenomenon of hypoxic pulmonary vasoconstriction (HPV) appears to be a more important force in regulation of pulmonary blood flow.[37, 38] HPV, however, does not appear to be mediated through the ANS, but rather is a local phenomenon capable of providing a faster adjustment to needs.

Both the SNS and vagus nerves provide active bronchomotor control. SNS stimulation causes bronchodilatation, whereas vagal stimulation produces constriction. PNS stimulation may also increase secretions of the bronchial glands. Vagal receptor endings in the alveolar ducts also play an important role in the reflex regulation of the ventilation cycle.[39] The lung has important nonventilatory activity as well. It serves as a metabolic organ that removes local mediators, such as norepinephrine (NE), from the circulation and converts others, such as angiotensin I, to active compounds[40–43] (see Interaction with Other Regulatory Systems).

AUTONOMIC NERVOUS SYSTEM NEUROTRANSMISSION

Transmission of excitation across the terminal junctional sites (synaptic clefts) of the peripheral ANS occurs through the mediation of liberated chemicals (Fig. 7-6). These chemical transmitters interact with a receptor on the end organ to evoke a biologic response. The ANS can be pharmacologically subdivided by the neurotransmitter secreted at the effector cell. Pharmacologic parlance designates the SNS and PNS as adrenergic and cholinergic, respectively. The terminals of the PNS postganglionic fibers release acetylcholine (ACh). With the exception of sweat glands, NE is the neurotransmitter

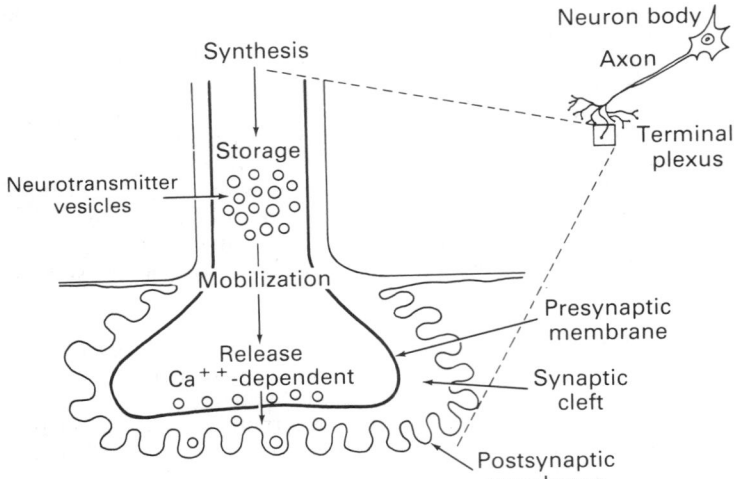

EFFECTOR CELL

FIG. 7-6. The anatomy and physiology of the terminal postganglionic fibers of sympathetic and parasympathetic fibers are similar.

released at the terminals of the sympathetic postganglionic fibers (Fig. 7-4). The preganglionic neurons of both systems secrete ACh.

The termination of the postganglionic fibers of both ANS subdivisions are anatomically and physiologically similar. The terminations are characterized by multiple branchings called terminal effector plexi, or reticula. These filaments surround the elements of the effector unit "like a mesh stocking."[44] Thus, one SNS postganglionic neuron, for example, can innervate some 25,000 effector cells, e.g., vascular smooth muscle.[12, 17] The terminal filaments end in presynaptic enlargements called varicosities. Each varicosity contains vesicles, approximately 500 A in diameter, in which the neurotransmitters are stored (Fig. 7-6). The varicosities are also heavily populated with mitochondria, which relates to the increased energy (adenosine triphosphate [ATP]) requirements of ACh and NE synthesis. The rate of synthesis depends on the level of ANS activity and is regulated by local feedback. The distance between the varicosity and the effector cell (synaptic or junctional cleft) varies from 100 A in ganglia and arterioles to as much as 20,000 A in large arteries. This distance determines the amount of transmitter required to stimulate and the time it takes to diffuse to the effector cell. The time for diffusion is directly proportional to the width of the synaptic gap. Depolarization releases the vesicular contents into the synaptic cleft by exocytosis.

PARASYMPATHETIC NERVOUS SYSTEM NEUROTRANSMISSION

Synthesis

ACh is the neurotransmitter that mediates the PNS. It is formed in the presynaptic terminal by acetylation of choline with acetyl coenzyme A. This step is catalyzed by choline acetyl transferase (Fig. 7-7). ACh is then stored in a concentrated form in presynaptic vesicles containing approximately 10,000 molecules of ACh. A continual release of small amounts of ACh, called quanta, occurs during the resting state. Each quantum results in small changes in the electrical potential of the synaptic end-plate without producing depolarization. These are known as miniature end-plate potentials (MEPP). Arrival of an action potential causes a synchronous release of hundreds of quanta, resulting in depolarization of the end-plate (Fig. 7-6). Release of ACh from the vesicles is dependent on influx of calcium (Ca^{++}) from the interstitial space.[45] Drugs

that alter Ca^{++} binding or influx may decrease ACh release and affect end-organ function.[46] ACh is not reused as is NE and therefore must be synthesized constantly.

Metabolism

The ability of a receptor to modulate function of an effector organ is dependent on rapid recovery to its baseline state after stimulation. For this to occur, the neurotransmitter must be rapidly removed from the vicinity of the receptor. In the case of ACh, removal occurs by rapid hydrolysis by acetylcholinesterase (AChE) (Fig. 7-7). This enzyme is found in neurons, at the neuromuscular junction, and in various other tissues of the body. A similar enzyme, butyrocholinesterase (pseudocholinesterase or plasma cholinesterase), is also found throughout the body but only to a limited extent in nervous tissue. It does not appear to be physiologically important in termination of the action of ACh. Both AChE and pseudocholinesterase hydrolyze ACh as well as other esters (such as the ester-type local anesthetics), but they may be distinguished by specific biochemical tests.[19, 47]

ACh is a quarternary ammonium compound that possesses a cationic moiety joined by a chain of two carbon atoms to an ester grouping. ACh binds to AChE at two sites. One site is specific for the positively charged quarternary ammonium moiety, the anionic site. The other is specific for the esteratic moiety. These binding sites stereospecifically orient ACh correctly as the substrate for hydrolysis. The esteratic site forms a covalent bond with the enzyme, thus acetylating the enzyme that ruptures the ester linkage of ACh (Fig. 7-7). The acetylated enzyme reacts with water to produce regenerated active enzyme and acetic acid. Thus, the products of ACh hydrolysis are free choline, acetic acid, and the enzyme regenerated for further use.

SYMPATHETIC NERVOUS SYSTEM NEUROTRANSMISSION

The SNS is mediated peripherally by the catecholamines, epinephrine, and NE. NE is the exclusive neurotransmitter released from localized postganglionic, presynaptic vesicles. IT is released directly into the site where it acts. The SNS fibers ending in the adrenal medulla are preganglionic and ACh is the neurotransmitter (Fig. 7-4). It interacts with the chromaffin cells in the medulla, causing the release of epinephrine

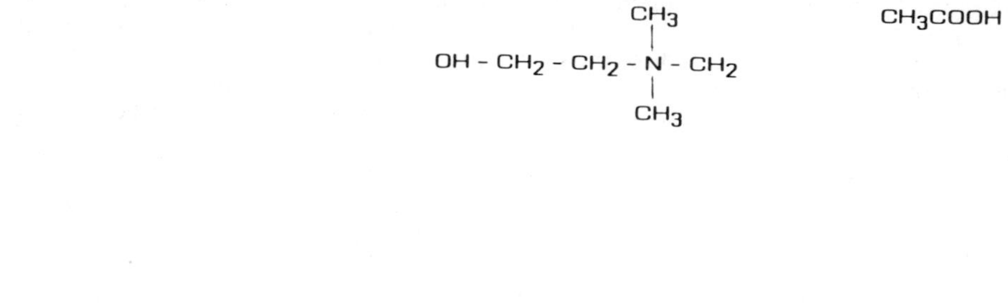

FIG. 7-7. Synthesis and metabolism of acetylcholine.

and NE. The chromaffin cells take the place of the post-ganglionic neurons.[12, 23] Stimulation of the SNS nerves to the adrenal medulla, however, causes the release of large quantities of a mixture of epinephrine and NE into the circulation to become neurotransmitter hormones. The greater portion of this hormonal surge is normally epinephrine.[6, 12, 48] Epinephrine and NE, when released into the circulation, are classified as hormones in that they are synthesized, stored, and released from the adrenal medulla to act at distant sites.

Hormonal epinephrine and NE have almost the same effects on effector cells as those caused by local direct sympathetic stimulation; however, the hormonal effects, although brief, last about ten times as long as those caused by direct stimulation.[4, 49] Epinephrine has a greater metabolic effect than NE. It can increase the metabolic rate of the body by as much as 100%.[6] It also increases glycogenolysis in the liver and muscle with glucose release into the blood. These functions are all necessary to prepare the body for fight or flight.

The normal resting state of secretion by the adrenal medulla is about $0.2\ \mu g \cdot kg^{-1} \cdot min^{-1}$ of epinephrine and about $0.02\ \mu g \cdot kg^{-1} \cdot min^{-1}$ of NE.[6, 48, 49] Some of the overall vascular tone results from the basal resting secretion of the adrenal medulla in addition to the tone that is maintained directly through stimulation from central vasomotor centers in the medulla.

Catecholamines—The First Messenger

The endogenous catecholamines in humans are dopamine, NE, and epinephrine.[12, 24] Dopamine is a neurotransmitter in the CNS. It is primarily involved in coordinating motor activity in the brain. In addition, it is the precursor of NE.[17] NE is synthesized and stored primarily in nerve endings of postganglionic SNS neurons. It is also synthesized in the adrenal medulla and is the chemical precursor of epinephrine. Stored epinephrine is located chiefly in chromaffin cells of the adrenal medulla. Eighty to eighty-five percent of the catecholamine content of the adrenal medulla is epinephrine, and 15–20% is NE. The brain contains both noradrenergic and dopaminergic (DA) receptors, but circulating catecholamines do not cross the blood–brain barrier.[29] The catecholamines present in the brain are synthesized there. Endogenous catecholamines are unique in that several intermediates in the synthesis function as neurotransmitters.

A catecholamine is any compound composed of a catechol nucleus (a benzene ring with two adjacent hydroxyl groups) and an amine-containing side chain.[50] The chemical configuration of five of the more common catecholamines in clinical use are demonstrated in Fig. 7-8. A true catecholamine must possess this basic structure. Catecholamines are often referred to as adrenergic drugs because their effector actions are mediated through receptors specific for the SNS. Synthetic catecholamines can activate these same receptors because of their structural similarity. Drugs that produce sympathetic-like effects but lack the basic catecholamine structure are defined as sympathomimetics. All clinically useful catecholamines are sympathomimetics, but not all sympathomimetics are catecholamines (Table 7-4). In addition, not all sympathomimetic drugs are adrenergic. Many are capable of producing a sympathomimetic effect by acting at sites exclusive of adrenergic receptors.

The effects of endogenous or synthetic catecholamines on adrenergic receptors can be direct or indirect (Table 7-4).[51, 52] Indirect-acting catecholamines have little intrinsic effect on adrenergic receptors, but produce their effects by stimulating release of the stored neurotransmitter from SNS nerve terminals. Some synthetic and endogenous catecholamines stimu-

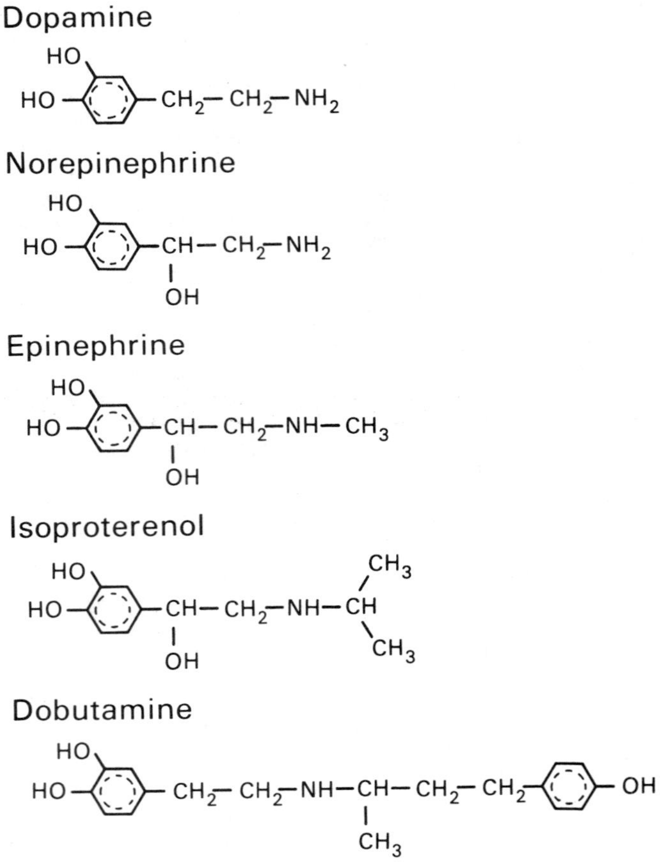

FIG. 7-8. The chemical configurations of five common catecholamines are shown. Sympathomimetic drugs differ in their hemodynamic effects largely because of differences in substitution of the amine group on the catechol nucleus (a benzene ring with two hydroxyl groups).

late adrenergic receptor sites directly, while others have a mixed mode of action. The actions of direct-acting catecholamines are independent of endogenous NE stores; however, the indirect-acting catecholamines are totally dependent on adequate neuronal stores of endogenous NE.

SYNTHESIS. The main site of NE synthesis is in or near the postganglionic nerve endings.[3] Some synthesis does occur in vesicles near the cell body that pass to the nerve endings.[53] Phenylalanine or tyrosine is taken up into the axoplasm of the nerve terminal and synthesized into either NE or epinephrine.[6, 12, 17] Figure 7-9 demonstrates this synthesis cascade. Tyrosine hydroxylase catalyzes the conversion of tyrosine to dihydroxyphenylalanine (DOPA). This is the rate-limiting step at which NE synthesis is controlled through feedback inhibition.[12, 54, 55] DOPA and the subsequent compounds in this cascade are catecholamines.

Dopamine is formed from DOPA by DOPA decarboxylase. Synthesis to this point occurs in the cytoplasm of the neuron. Dopamine then enters the storage vesicles. In the brain, synthesis stops at this point where dopamine is the neurotransmitter. The vesicles of peripheral postganglionic neurons contain the enzyme dopamine-β-hydroxylase, which converts dopamine to NE. The adrenal medulla additionally contains phenylethanolamine-N-methyltransferase (PNMT),

TABLE 7-4. Sympathomimetic Drugs

Adrenergic Amines

CATECHOLAMINES	TRADE NAME
Epinephrine	Adrenalin
Norepinephrine	Levophed
Dopamine*	Intropin
Dobutamine	Dobutrex
Isoproterenol	Isuprel

NONCATECHOLAMINES	
Metaraminol*†	Aramine
Mephentermine†	Wyamine
Ephedrine†	Ephedrine
Methoxamine	Vasoxyl
Phenylephrine	Neosynephrine

Nonadrenergics

Xanthines	Aminophylline
Glucagon	Glucagon
Digitalis	Lanoxin
Calcium Salts	—
Naloxone	Narcan
Amrinone	Inocor

* Direct-acting catecholamine with some in-direct action.

† Primarily indirect-acting with some direct action. Adrenergic amines produce sympathomimetic effects *via* adrenergic receptors. Nonadrenergics produce sympathomimetic effects exclusive of the adrenergic receptor.

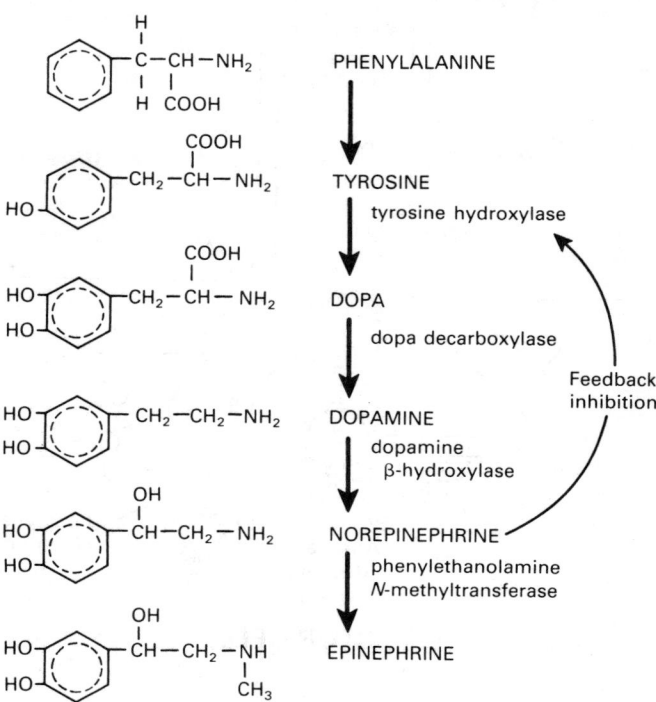

FIG. 7-9. Schematic of the synthesis of catecholamines. The conversion of tyrosine to DOPA by tyrosine hydroxylase is inhibited by increased NE synthesis. Epinephrine is shown in these steps but is primarily synthesized in the adrenal medulla.

which converts NE to epinephrine. This reaction takes place outside the medullary vesicles, and the newly formed epinephrine then enters the vesicle for storage (Fig. 7-10). All the endogenous catecholamines are stored in presynaptic vesicles and released on arrival of an action potential. Excitation-secretion coupling in sympathetic neurons is Ca^{++} dependent.[45, 56]

REGULATION. Increased SNS, as in congestive heart failure or chronic stress, stimulates the synthesis of tyrosine hydroxylase and dopamine-β-hydroxylase.[12, 57] Glucocorticoids from the adrenal cortex pass through the adrenal medulla and stimulate an increase in PNMT that methylates NE to epinephrine.[3]

The mechanism of NE release by nerve stimulation is not completely understood, but the release of NE is dependent on depolarization of the nerve and an increase in calcium ion permeability. Calcium may cause microfilaments in the prejunctional membrane to contract and trigger exocytosis of NE granules.[45, 55, 56] This release is inhibited by colchicine and prostaglandin E2, suggesting a contractile mechanism. Blockade of prostaglandin synthesis enhances NE release. NE inhibits its own release by stimulating presynaptic (prejunctional) α_2 receptors. Phenoxybenzamine and phentolamine, α-receptor antagonists, increase the release of NE by blocking inhibitory presynaptic α_2 receptors (Fig. 7-11). Other receptors may also be important in NE regulation and are discussed later (see Other Receptors).

INACTIVATION. As with the PNS, the ability of the adrenergic receptor to modulate function of the end-organ is dependent on rapid recovery to its baseline state after stimulation. The neurotransmitter must therefore be rapidly inactivated. Unlike ACh, the catecholamines are removed from the synaptic cleft by three mechanisms (Fig. 7-10).[12] These are (1) reuptake into the presynaptic terminals; (2) extraneuronal

uptake; and (3) diffusion. Termination of NE at the effector site is almost entirely by reuptake of NE into the terminals of the presynaptic neuron (uptake 1). Once NE is back in the nerve terminal, it is stored in the varicosities for reuse. A small amount is deaminated in the cytoplasm of the neuron by monoamine oxidase (MAO) to form dihydroxymandelic acid (DOMA), which diffuses out of the nerve terminal and into the interstitial fluid. Uptake 1 is an active, energy-requiring, temperature-dependent process that can be inhibited pharmacologically.

The reuptake of NE in the presynaptic terminals is also a stereo-specific process. Structurally similar compounds (guanethidine, metaraminol) may enter the vesicles and displace the neurotransmitter. Tricyclic antidepressants and cocaine inhibit the reuptake of NE, resulting in high synaptic NE concentrations and accentuated receptor response. In addition, recent evidence suggests that NE reuptake is mediated by a presynaptic β-adrenergic mechanism because β blockade causes marked elevations of epinephrine and NE[55, 58] (Fig. 7-10 and 7-11). Alpha blockade does not. The clinical significance of this presynaptic β receptor is unknown at this time.

Extraneuronal uptake (uptake 2) is a minor pathway for inactivating NE. NE is taken up by effector cells and other extraneuronal tissues. The NE that is taken up by the extraneuronal tissue is metabolized by MAO and by catechol-O-methyltransferase (COMT) to form vanillylmandelic acid (VMA) (Fig. 7-12).[9, 59] The minute amount of catecholamine that escapes uptake 1 and uptake 2 diffuses into the circulation (uptake 3)* where it is similarly metabolized in the liver and

* "Uptake 3" is used as a clinical term to describe uptake of exogenous drug administration.

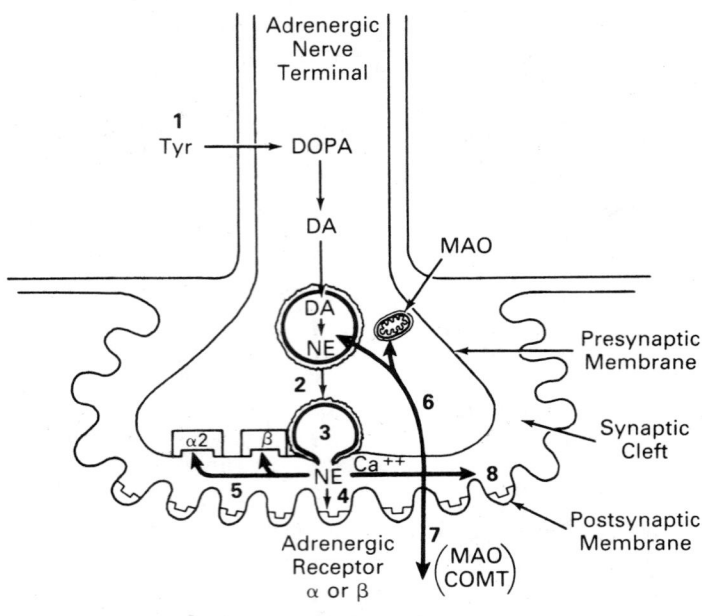

FIG. 7-10. Schematic of the synthesis and disposition of NE in adrenergic neurotransmission. (1) synthesis and storage in neuronal vesicles; (2) action potential permits calcium entry with (3) exocytosis of NE into synaptic gap. (4) Released NE reacts with receptor on effector cell. NE (5) may react with presynaptic α_2 receptor to inhibit further NE release or with presynaptic β receptor to enhance reuptake of NE (6) (uptake 1). Extraneuronal uptake (uptake 2) absorbs NE into effector cell (7) with overflow occurring systemically (8). MAO = monoamine oxidase; COMT = catechol-O-methyltransferase; Tyr = tyrosine; DOPA = dihydroxyphenylalanine; NE = norepinephrine.

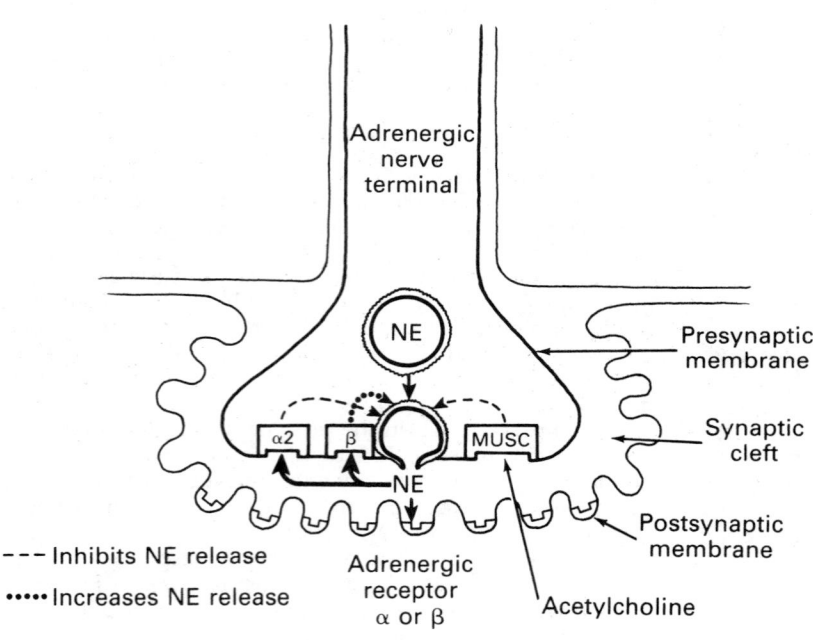

FIG. 7-11. This schematic demonstrates just a few of the presynaptic adrenergic receptors thought to exist. Agonist and antagonist drugs are clinically available for these receptors (Table 7-5). The α_2 receptors serve as a negative feedback mechanism whereby NE stimulation inhibits its own release. Presynaptic β stimulation increases NE uptake, augmenting its availability. Presynaptic muscarinic (MUSC) receptors respond to ACh diffusing from nearby cholinergic terminals. It inhibits NE release and can be blocked by atropine.

kidney. The importance of uptake 1 and uptake 2 is diminished when sympathomimetics are given exogenously. Epinephrine is inactivated by the same enzymes. Whereas uptake 1 is the predominant pathway for inactivation of the endogenous catecholamines, uptake 3 is the predominant pathway for catecholamines given exogenously and is clinically important. This accounts for the longer duration of action by exogenous catecholamines than that noted at the local synapse.

The former is slow (liver metabolism) and the latter is fast (uptake 1).

The final metabolic product of the catecholamines is VMA. VMA constitutes the major metabolite (80–90%) of NE found in the urine. Less than 5% of released NE appears unchanged in the urine.[9] The metabolic products excreted in the urine provide a gross estimate of SNS activity and can facilitate the clinical diagnosis of pheochromocytoma.

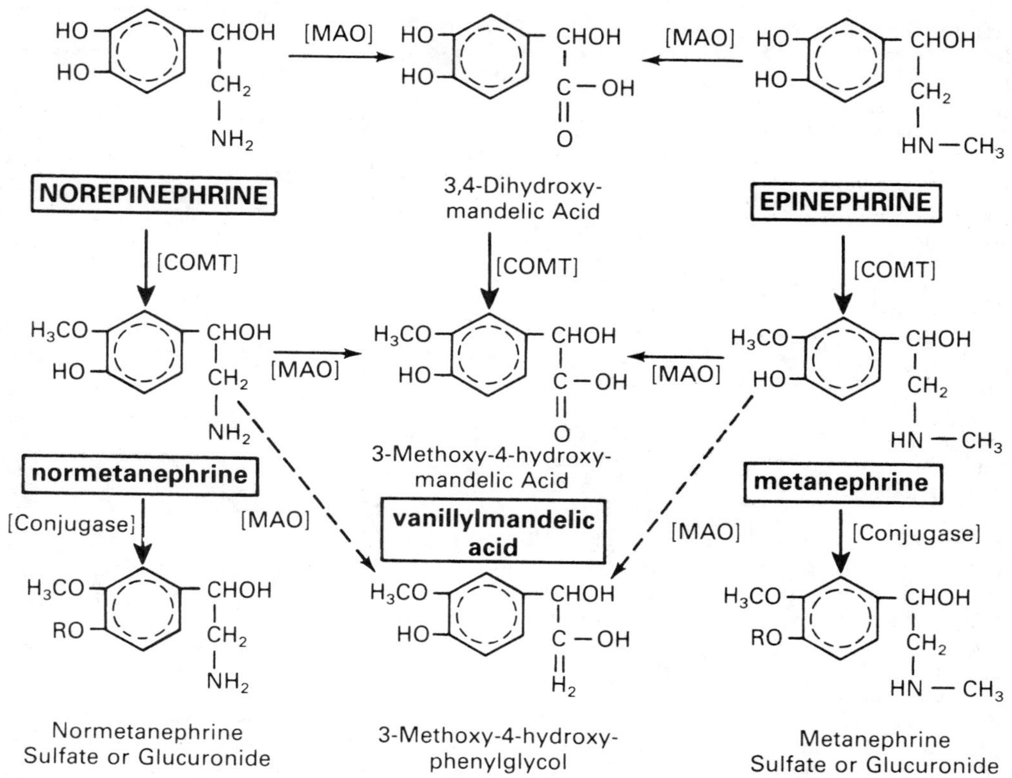

FIG. 7-12. Catabolism of nor-epinephrine and epinephrine.

NOREPINEPHRINE · [COMT] · [MAO] · **normetanephrine** · [Conjugase]

3,4-Dihydroxy-mandelic Acid · [COMT] · [MAO]

3-Methoxy-4-hydroxy-mandelic Acid · **vanillylmandelic acid**

EPINEPHRINE · [COMT] · [MAO] · **metanephrine** · [Conjugase]

Normetanephrine Sulfate or Glucuronide

3-Methoxy-4-hydroxy-phenylglycol

Metanephrine Sulfate or Glucuronide

RECEPTORS

The concept that receptors are the initial decoders of extracellular messengers has guided research on hormones and neurotransmitters for many years. An agonist is a substance that interacts with a receptor to evoke a biologic response. ACh and NE are the agonists of the ANS. An antagonist is a substance that interferes with the evocation of a response at a receptor site by an agonist. Receptors are therefore regarded as target sites on a cell that, when activated by an agonist, will lead to a response by the effector cell. Receptors have never been identified as precise anatomic structures; rather, their existence has been demonstrated biochemically and on the basis of biologic response.[24] Receptors are macromolecules that appear to be proteins and are located in the plasma membrane. Several thousand receptors have been demonstrated in a single cell.[12, 60] The enormity of this network is realized when one considers that some 25,000 single cells can be innervated by a single neuron.[17, 61]

CHOLINERGIC RECEPTORS

ACh is the neurotransmitter at three distinct classes of receptors. These receptors can be differentiated by their anatomic location and their affinity to bind various agonists and antagonists.[62] ACh mediates the "first messenger" function of transmitting impulses in the PNS, the ganglia of the SNS, and the neuroeffector junction of striated, voluntary muscle (Fig. 7-4). The receptors are referred to as choliceptive or cholinergic receptors. The PNS is often referred to as the cholinergic system.

Cholinergic receptors are further subdivided into muscarinic and nicotinic receptors because muscarine and nicotine stimulate them selectively.[3, 19] However, both muscarinic and nicotinic receptors respond to ACh (see Cholinergic Agonists). Muscarine, derived from the poisonous mushroom *Amantia muscaria*, stimulates cholinergic receptors at the postganglionic PNS junctions of cardiac and smooth muscle throughout the body. Muscarinic stimulation is characterized by bradycardia, decreased inotropism, bronchoconstriction, miosis, salivation, gastrointestinal hypermotility, and increased gastric acid secretion (Table 7-1). Muscarinic receptors can be blocked by atropine without effect on nicotinic receptors (see Cholinergic Antagonists).

Muscarinic receptors are known to exist in sites other than PNS postganglionic junctions. Muscarinic receptors are found on the presynaptic membrane of sympathetic nerve terminals in the myocardium, coronary vessels, and peripheral vasculature (Fig. 7-11).[20, 24] These are referred to as adrenergic muscarinic receptors because of their location; however, they are stimulated by ACh. Stimulation of these receptors inhibits release of NE in a manner similar to α_2-receptor stimulation.[27, 63] Muscarinic blockade removes inhibition of NE release, augmenting SNS activity. Atropine, the prototypical muscarinic blocker, may produce sympathomimetic activity in this manner as well as vagal blockade. Neuromuscular blocking drugs that cause tachycardia are thought to have a similar mechanism of action.

ACh acting on presynaptic adrenergic muscarinic receptors is a very potent inhibitor of NE release.[20, 58] The prejunctional muscarinic receptor may play an important physiologic role because several autonomically innervated tissues (*e.g.*, the heart) possess ANS plexi in which the SNS and PNS nerve terminals are closely associated.[19] In these plexi, ACh, released from the nearby PNS nerve terminals (vagus), can inhibit NE release by activation of presynaptic adrenergic muscarinic receptors (Fig. 7-11).

Nicotinic receptors are found at the synaptic junctions of both SNS and PNS ganglia. Because both junctions are cholinergic, ACh or ACh-like substances such as nicotine will excite postganglionic fibers of both systems (Fig. 7-4). Low doses of nicotine produce stimulation of ANS ganglia, whereas high doses produce blockade. This dualism is referred to as the nicotinic effect (see Ganglionic Drugs). Nicotinic stimulation of the SNS ganglia will produce hypertension and tachycardia by causing the release of epinephrine and NE from the adrenal medulla. Adrenal hormone release is mediated by ACh in the chromaffin cells, which are analogous to postganglionic neurons (Fig. 7-4).[6] A further increase in nicotine concentration will produce hypotension and neuromuscular weakness as it becomes a ganglionic blocker. The cholinergic neuroeffector junction of skeletal muscle also contains nicotinic receptors, although not identical to the nicotinic receptors in ANS ganglia. For example, PNS transmission is not "all or nothing" as at the neuromuscular junction.[3] Postganglionic cholinergic transmission appears to be graded. The magnitude of response is related to the number of active units and their frequency of firing. Continuous, small amounts of ACh are released from the cholinergic nerve endings without nerve stimulation. This results in random, small, spontaneous depolarization of the postganglionic membrane known as MEPPs. ACh is not taken up by the presynaptic nerve terminals and, in contrast to NE, must be continuously synthesized.

ADRENERGIC RECEPTORS

Von Euler differentiated the physiologic effects of epinephrine and NE in 1946.[64] The adrenergic receptors were termed adrenergic or noradrenergic depending on their responsiveness to adrenaline (epinephrine) or noradrenaline (NE). The dissimilarities of these two drugs led Ahlquist in 1948 to propose two types of opposing adrenergic receptors termed alpha (α) and beta (β).[65] This postulation further implied that selective antagonism of these receptors was possible. The receptors can be classified according to the order of potency by which they are affected by SNS agonists and antagonists.[66] Receptors that respond with an order of potency of NE $\geq$ epinephrine > isoproterenol are called α receptors. Those responding with an order of potency of isoproterenol > epinephrine $\geq$ NE are called β receptors (Table 7-5). The development of new agonists and antagonists with relatively selective activity allowed Lands to subdivide the β receptors into β_1 and β_2 in 1967[67, 68] Then Langer (1973) subdivided α receptors into α_1 and α_2. The concept of relative selective activity arises from differential potencies among tissue groups to the same drug such that two dose–response curves are obtained (Fig. 7-13). The sympathomimetic adrenergic drugs in current use differ from one another in their effects largely because of differences in substitution on the amine group, which influences the relative α or β effect (Fig. 7-8).[50] Figure 7-14 demonstrates the spectrum of actions of catecholamines on α and β receptors, with methoxamine representing a pure α drug and isoproterenol a pure β drug.

Further studies have revealed not only subsets of the α and β receptors, but also the DA receptors.[31, 69] These DA receptors have been identified in the CNS and in renal, mesenteric, and coronary vessels. The physiologic importance of these recep-

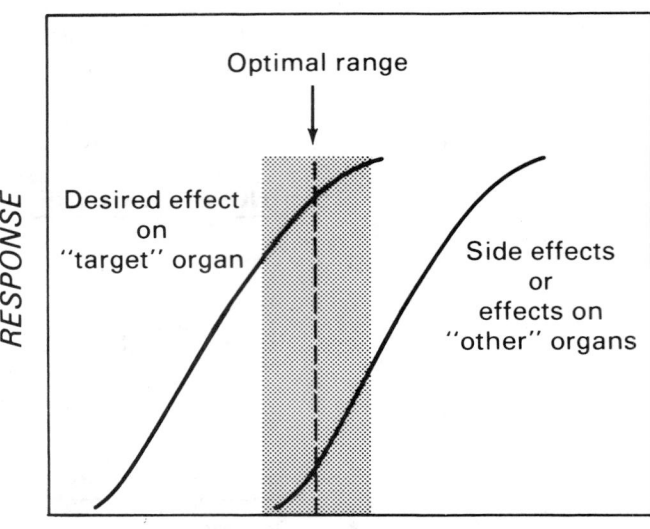

FIG. 7-13. Relative dose–response relationship on target and other organs. Relative selectivity is illustrated by showing the relationship between two dose–response curves. The curve on the left represents the desired response of bronchodilatation using a relatively selective β_2 agonist. The unwanted effects on other organs that occur at higher doses are represented by the curve on the right. For example, an increased heart rate (β_1 effect) may occur with higher doses of a relatively select β_2 agonist. The *optimal range* is that concentration of drug that will give the maximum desired response with minimal effects on other organs. The size of the optimal range is dependent on the *therapeutic index*, or the distance between the two curves (see Chapter 3). These are usually established *in vitro* where drug concentration can be precisely controlled. For many cardiovascular drugs the optimal range is small and wide fluctuations in serum level of the drug are common; therefore, secondary or side-effects are often seen during drug therapy.

FIG. 7-14. The differential effects of the catecholamines on adrenergic receptors range from the pure α drug, methoxamine, or the pure β drug, isoproterenol. (Reprinted with permission. Lawson NW, Wallfisch HK: Cardiovascular pharmacology: A new look at the "pressors." In Stoelting RK, Barash PG, Gallagher TJ [eds]: Advances in Anesthesia, p 195. Chicago, Year Book Publishers, 1986)

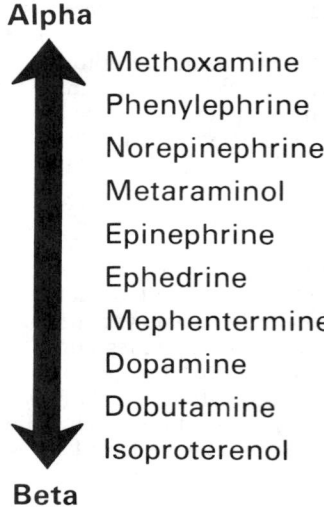

TABLE 7-5. Adrenergic Receptors: Order of Potency of Agonists and Antagonists

RECEPTOR	AGONISTS*	ANTAGONISTS	LOCATION	ACTION
α_1	$++++$ Norepinephrine $+++$ Epinephrine $++$ Dopamine $+$ Isoproterenol	Phenoxybenzamine† Phentolamine† Ergot alkaloids† Prazosin Tolazoline† Labetolol†	Smooth muscle (vascular, iris, radial, ureter, pilomotor, uterus, trigone, gastrointestinal, and bladder sphincters) Brain Smooth muscle (gastrointestinal) Heart Salivary glands Adipose tissue Sweat glands (localized) Kidney (proximal tubule)	Contraction Vasoconstriction Neurotransmission Relaxation Glycogenolysis Increased force $^+$, glycolysis Secretion (K^+, H_2O) Glycogenesis Secretion Gluconeogenesis Na^+ reabsorption
α_2	$++++$ Clonidine $+++$ Norepinephrine $++$ Epinephrine $++$ Norepinephrine $+$ Phenylephrine	Yohimbine Piperoxan Phentolamine† Phenoxybenzamine† Tolazoline† Labetolol†	Adrenergic nerve endings Presynaptic—CNS Platelets Adipose tissue Endrocrine pancreas Vascular smooth muscle—? Kidney Brain	Inhibition norepinephrine release Aggregation, granule release Inhibition lypolysis Inhibition insulin release Contraction Inhibition renin release Neurotransmission
β_1	$++++$ Isoproterenol† $+++$ Epinephrine $++$ Norepinephrine $+$ Dopamine	Acebutolol Practolol Propranolol† Alprenolol† Metoprolol Esmolol	Heart Adipose tissue	Increased rate, contractility, conduction velocity Coronary vasodilatation Lipolysis
β_2	$++++$ Isoproterenol* $+++$ Epinephrine $+++$ Norepinephrine $+$ Dopamine	Propranolol† Butoxamine Alprenolol Esmolol Nadolol Timolol Labetalol	Liver Skeletal muscle Smooth muscle (bronchi, uterus, vascular, gastrointestical, detrusor, spleen capsule) Endocrine pancreas Salivary glands	Glycogenolysis, gluconeogenesis Glycogenolysis, lactate release Relaxation Insulin secretion Amylase secretion
DA_1	$++++$ Dopamine $+++$ Epinine $+++$ Apomorphine $+$ Metaclopromide	Haloperidol Droperidol Phenothiazines	Vascular smooth muscle Renal and mesentery	Vasodilatation
DA_2	$++$ Dopamine $+$ Bromocriptine	Domperidone	Presynaptic—adrenergic nerve endings	Inhibits norepinephrine release

* Listed in decreasing order of potency.
† Nonselective.
$^+$ β_1 = Adrenergic responses are greater.
Pluses indicate strength of potency.

tors is a matter of controversy because there are no identifiable peripheral DA neurons. Dopamine measured in the circulation is assumed to result from spill-over from the brain.

Dopamine not only stimulates α and β receptors in a dose-related manner, but it also dilates renal and mesenteric vessels, unlike the other catecholamines. This action has been found to be independent of α or β blockade, but is modified by DA antagonists such as haloperidol and the phenothiazines.[30] Thus, the necessity of adding the DA receptor to the Ahlquist classification is explained. The DA receptor has also been subdivided according to action. Thus, there are three types of receptors (six subtypes) that respond to the catecholamines: α, β, and DA. Table 7-5 lists the types, locations, and actions of adrenergic receptors now thought to exist.

α-Adrenergic Receptors

Two classes of α receptors have been demonstrated, α_1 and α_2. The α_1-adrenergic receptors are found in the smooth muscle cells of the peripheral vasculature of the coronary arteries, skin, uterus, intestinal mucosa, and splanchnic beds[30] (Table 7-5). The α_1 receptors serve as postsynaptic activators of vascular and intestinal smooth muscle as well as endocrine glands. Their activation results in either decreased or increased tone, depending on the effector organ. The response in resistance and capacitance vessels is constriction, whereas in the intestinal tract it is relaxation. The myocardium is usually described as being void of α receptors; however, α-receptor–mediated effects have been reported.[52] The physiologic and clinical significance of these myocardial α receptors is not yet clear.[70, 71]

The α receptors are found in both presynaptic and postsynaptic positions at the adrenergic neuroeffector junction. They are also found on platelets where they mediate platelet aggregation.[72] Stimulation of presynaptic α_2 receptors mediates inhibition of NE release, serving as a negative feedback mechanism.[73–75] NE acts on both α_1 and α_2 receptors. Thus, it activates smooth muscle vasoconstriction (α_1) and at the same time inhibits its own release *via* presynaptic α_2 receptors.[58]

Postsynaptic α_2 receptors, like the α_1 receptor, affect vasoconstriction. The distinction between the two is based on differences in order of potency for a series of agonists and antagonists (Table 7-5).[66, 68] Stimulation of the presynaptic α_2 receptor by an agonist could produce a beneficial reduction of peripheral vascular resistance. Unfortunately, most known α_2 agonists also stimulate the postsynaptic α_2 receptors, causing vasoconstriction. Vasodilatation occurs with the blockade of α_1 and α_2 postsynaptic receptors. Blockade of α_2 presynaptic receptors, however, ablates normal inhibition of NE, causing vasoconstriction (Fig. 7-11).

β-*Adrenergic Receptors*

The β-adrenergic receptors, like the α receptors, have been subdivided into two categories.[67, 68] The β_1 receptors predominate in the myocardium, the SA node, the ventricular conduction system, and adipose tissue. Also, the β_1 receptors mediate the effects of the sympathomimetic amines on myocardium. This receptor is equally sensitive to epinephrine and NE, which distinguishes it from β_2 receptors. Effects of β_1 stimulation are outlined in Table 7-5.

The β_2 receptors are located in smooth muscle of the blood vessels in the skin, muscle, and mesentery and in bronchial smooth muscle. Stimulation produces vasodilation and bronchial relaxation. The β_2 receptors are more sensitive to epinephrine than NE.[30, 76] The β_1 receptors are suggested to be innervated receptors responding to neuronally released NE, whereas β_2 receptors are "hormonal" receptors responding primarily to circulating epinephrine.

Dopaminergic Receptors

Dopamine was recognized in 1959, not only as a precursor in the synthesis of epinephrine and NE, but also as an important neurotransmitter. DA receptors have been localized on blood vessels and postganglionic sympathetic nerves (Table 7-5). There are two subdivisions of DA receptors. The DA_1 receptors are found on vascular smooth muscle and mediate vasodilatation of the renal and mesenteric vessels. The DA_2 receptors, like the α_2 receptors, are presynaptic and inhibit norepinephrine release.[58, 73] Stimulation of the presynaptic DA_2 receptor results in vasodilatation.[78] Unlike the α_2 receptor, DA_2 receptors have not been found postsynaptically.[79] DA receptors have been identified in the hypothalamus where they are involved in prolactin release, and they are also found in the basal ganglia where they coordinate motor function.[80, 81] Another central action of dopamine is to stimulate the chemo-

receptor trigger zone of the medulla, producing nausea and vomiting. Dopamine antagonists such as haloperidol or droperidol are clinically effective in countering this action. There is evidence for existence of DA receptors in the esophagus, stomach, and small intestine. These receptors enhance secretions and diminish intestinal motility when stimulated.[82] Metaclopromide, a dopamine antagonist, is useful in aspiration prophylaxis by promoting gastric emptying.[83]

Defining specific DA receptors has been difficult because dopamine also exerts an effect on the α and β receptors.[84, 85] This effect is weak in the cardiovascular system. Its action on adrenergic receptors is only 1/35 and 1/50 as potent as epinephrine and NE respectively.[82, 84]

OTHER RECEPTORS

There are a number of receptors on the presynaptic sympathetic nerve ending in addition to the α_2 receptor and muscarinic receptor. These receptors, when activated, mediate inhibition of NE release in a manner similar to the α_2 presynaptic receptor. The clinical significance of these receptors remains to be defined.

Adenosine Receptors

Adenosine produces inhibition of NE release.[58, 73] The effect of adenosine is blocked by caffeine and other methylxanthines.[86, 87] The physiologic and pharmacologic roles of adenosine-mediated inhibition of NE release are not clearly defined. The physiologic function of these receptors may be the reduction of sympathetic tone under hypoxic conditions when adenosine production is enhanced. As a consequence of reduced NE release, cardiac work would be decreased and oxygen demand reduced. Recently, adenosine has been effectively used to produce controlled hypotension.[88]

Serotonin

Serotonin (5-hydroxytryptamine [5-HT]) depresses the response of isolated blood vessels to SNS stimulation and decreases release of labeled NE in these preparations.[89] This inhibitory action of serotonin is antagonized by raising the external calcium ion concentration. Thus, serotonin may inhibit neuronal NE release by a mechanism that limits the availability of calcium ions at the nerve terminal.

Prostaglandin E2, Histamine, and Several Opioids

Prostaglandin E2, histamine, and several opioids have been reported to act on prejunctional receptor sites to inhibit NE release in certain sympathetically innervated tissue;[58] however, these inhibitory receptors are unlikely to play a physiologic role in limiting NE release because inhibitors of cyclo-oxygenase, histamine antagonists, and naloxone, respectively, produce no increase in NE release.

Histamine acts in a manner similar to the neurotransmitters of the SNS.[90] It has membrane receptors specific for histamine, with the individual response being determined by the type of cell being stimulated. Two receptors for histamine have been determined. These have been designated H_1 and H_2, for which it has been possible to develop specific agonists and antagonists. Stimulation of the H_1 receptors produce bronchoconstriction and intestinal contraction. The major role of the H_2 receptor is related to acid production by the parietal cells of the stomach; however, histamine is present in relatively high concentrations in the myocardium and cardiac conducting tissue where it exerts a positive inotropic and chronotropic effect while depressing dromotropism. The positive inotropic and chronotropic effects of histamine is an H_2-receptor effect that is not blocked by β antagonism. It is blocked by H_2 antagonists, such as cimetidine, which accounts for the occasional report of cardiovascular collapse following the use of cimetidine.[91] The negative dromotropic effect and that of coronary spasm caused by histamine is an H_1-receptor effect.

ADRENERGIC-RECEPTOR NUMBERS OR SENSITIVITY

The number or sensitivity of adrenergic receptors can be influenced by hormonal, genetic, and developmental factors.[67, 68, 92, 93] Changes in the number of receptors will alter the response to catecholamines. Alterations in the number of receptors is referred to as either *up* or *down regulation*.[94] As a rule, there is an inverse relationship between the ambient concentration of the catecholamines and the number of receptors.[95] Extended exposure of receptors to their agonists markedly reduces, but does not ablate, the biologic response to the agonist. This phenomenon has been demonstrated for a large number of hormones and drugs. There appears to be a reduction in numbers or sensitivity of β receptors in hypertensive patients who also have elevated plasma catecholamines. Down regulation is reversible because resensitization occurs on termination of the agonist. Down regulation is the presumptive explanation for the lack of correlation between plasma catecholamine levels and the blood pressure elevation in patients with pheochromocytoma. Chronic use of β agonists such as terbutaline, isoproterenol, or epinephrine for the treatment of asthma can result in tachyphylaxis because of down regulation in receptor numbers.[96] Even short-term use (1–6 h) of β-adrenergic agonists may cause down regulation of receptor numbers.

When blood and tissue levels of catecholamines are lowered, the number of receptor sites increases. Sympathetic denervation of an organ increases both α- and β-adrenergic receptor concentrations. Chronic depletion of catecholamines in animal studies results in a 50–100% increase in β receptors.[93] Likewise, chronic treatment of animals with the β-adrenergic antagonist propranolol causes a 100% increase in the number of β receptors.[97] This might account for the propranolol withdrawal syndrome. The discontinuation of β antagonists leaves unopposed a greater number of sensitive β receptors. This phenomenon may also account for the clonidine withdrawal syndrome.[98, 99] Inhibition of vasodilatation by antagonists, however, does not increase the sensitivity of α receptors to α agonists.[100]

The pharmacologic factors affecting up or down regulation of the α and β receptors are similar. Humoral influences known to regulate α-receptor numbers include estrogen (up), progesterone (down), and thyroxin (up).[101] The effects of dopamine on receptor number and binding affinity remain largely unknown, but estrogen does increase dopamine receptor numbers centrally.[61]

MOLECULAR PHARMACOLOGY AND EFFECTOR RESPONSE

Receptors are only the first link in a series of reactions that summate in the cellular response. The β-adrenergic receptor is the best-delineated ANS receptor at the present time. This is largely due to the pioneering work of Sutherland, who re-

vealed that, for the β receptor, cyclic adenosine monophosphate (cAMP) serves as the intracellular mediator of the first messenger—the catecholamines.[102–104] cAMP is often referred to as the *second messenger*. Recently, receptor complexes have been isolated that consist of distinctive components, each of which affect the cellular response.

The β-adrenergic receptor consists of three distinct components: (1) a specific hormone receptor that interacts with the chemical messenger: (2) two regulatory proteins that bind guanosine triphosphate (GTP) and regulate the interaction of the receptor protein with adenyl cyclase; and (3) the catalytic moiety of adenyl cyclase.[105] The guanine nucleotide regulatory components are important moderators of the receptor complex (Fig. 7-15). Both inhibitory (N_i) and stimulatory (N_s) components have been isolated. These appear to be two of a large group of guanine nucleotide regulatory proteins that may function in the coupling of various receptors to different physiologic effector systems.[106] As such, they may be important in modulating the response of the ANS or the effects of certain sympathomimetic drugs.

The receptor itself is actually a bifunctional protein situated on the superficial surface of the plasma membrane. It interacts specifically with a chemical messenger and then undergoes a conformational change to activate some other response mechanism. In the case of the β receptor, this effector mechanism is the adenyl cyclase–cAMP system.[107]

The first messenger, the catecholamine, binds to the receptor and stimulates adenyl cyclase (Fig. 7-15). Adenyl cyclase catalyzes the conversion of ATP to cAMP, which, in cascade fashion, phosphorylates multiple cellular components, altering cellular function. The cellular response is tissue specific. The positive inotropic and chronotropic actions of the catecholamines in the heart are the result of augmented cAMP concentrations that, in turn, enhance the mobilization and availability of ionized calcium within the myocardial cell. The transmembrane flux of calcium is also an important regulator of contractility in vascular smooth muscle. Here, however, β-receptor stimulation activates the adenyl cyclase system, but cellular components are activated that enhance removal of calcium from the cytosol, resulting in relaxation rather than contraction; therefore, drugs that augment cAMP levels will have opposite effects in cardiac and smooth muscle.

The final mediator of the effects of β-receptor stimulation in cardiac muscle is Ca^{++}. The concentration of CA^{++} in the cytosol during systole regulates not only strength of myocardial contraction, but also ion fluxes across the sarcolemma and, therefore, impulse conduction. Cytosolic Ca^{++} is derived from several cellular sources, including the sarcoplasmic reticulum and the superficial surface of the sarcolemma. Ca^{++} derived from the sarcolemma enters *via* channels in the membrane called slow Ca^{++} channels, so named due to their action potential characteristics. These membrane calcium channels are thought to be double gated. The outer gate is dependent on depolarization for Ca^{++} influx, whereas phosphorylation of a cAMP-dependent protein kinase is necessary to open the inner gate. β-Receptor stimulation is therefore intimately involved in regulation of Ca^{++} influx.[108] Increased cAMP activates myocardial sarcolemmal calcium channels, resulting in an increase in the rate and degree of tension development. Phosphorylation of components of the sarcoplasmic reticulum also enhances Ca^{++} uptake and causes more rapid relaxation.[109] Augmented cAMP in cardiac nodal and conduction tissues increases the slope of diastolic depolarization (phase 4) and the rate of rapid depolarization (phase 0), effecting an increase in both heart rate and conduction.

Transmembrane calcium influx can be blocked at two points: (1) blockade of depolarization; and (2) inhibition of

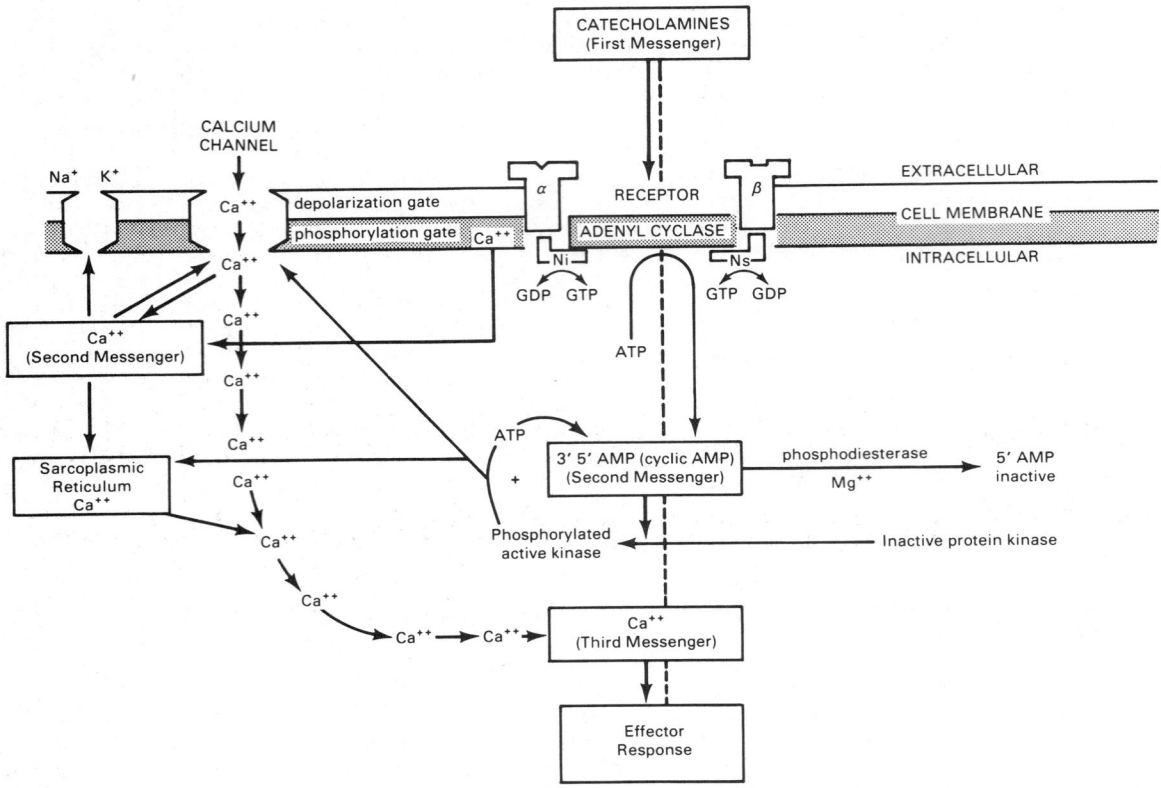

FIG. 7-15. The putative cascade from the first messengers to effector response. The activated α receptor (1) inhibits, whereas the activated β receptor (2) stimulates the enzyme adenyl cyclase, which catalyzes the conversion of ATP to the second messenger cyclic adenosine monophosphate (cyclic AMP). Interactions of the receptor–enzyme complex are regulated by guanine nucleotide regulatory proteins (Ns, Ni). Cyclic AMP regulates many cellular functions, including opening of membrane Ca^{++} channels (6), which allows the third messenger Ca^{++} into the cell. Ca^{++} channels are further regulated by an intracellular membrane-bound receptor (5), which is stimulated by Bay K 8644 and inhibited by the calcium-entry blockers nifedipine and verapamil. It is also postulated that in some tissues α stimulation releases adjacent membrane-bound Ca^{++}, which also acts as a second messenger, releasing more Ca^{++}. Intracellular free Ca^{++} is the third messenger, which is the final link in initiating the effector response. Nonadrenergic sympathomimetic drugs enhance the effector response by either stimulating the formation of cyclic AMP (forskolin [3] or glucagon [4], inhibition of phosphodiesterase (xanthines [7], or enhancing Ca^{++} entry (Bay K 8644 [5]).

enzymatic reduction of ATP to cAMP. β-Blocking drugs interfere with agonist binding to the receptor and, therefore, the formation of cAMP. Verapamil, a calcium channel blocker, is thought to interact with a receptor on the inner surface of the sarcolemma, which regulates activation of the calcium channel. Thus, β blockers and calcium channel blockers, working at different steps in the receptor cascade, have a final common pathway—the calcium channel. The potentiating effect of β blockers and verapamil in humans is well known, and historically, verapamil was originally thought to be a β blocker.

The cellular responses to β-receptor activation cannot be totally ascribed to cAMP, however. Activation of sarcolemmal Ca^{++} transport systems may occur directly by β-receptor stimulation. Increased cytosolic Ca^{++} also results in activation of another intracellular second messenger called calmodulin.[110] It is a protein that binds Ca^{++} and activates a variety of enzymes and cellular processes via a calmodulin-dependent protein kinase. These are usually different than

those acted on by cAMP-dependent protein kinase. The result in cardiac muscle is enhanced contractility. In smooth muscle of blood vessels, the esophagus, and ureters, the Ca^{++}–calmodulin complex activates myosin kinase and increases tone. In this case, the primary target is via the α receptor, however, illustrating how the same second messenger can be activated by two different receptors and cause opposite physiologic effects in different organs (Fig. 7-16).

Other intracellular messengers have been proposed, but their physiologic roles are as yet incompletely characterized. Cyclic GTP may be important in mediating the relaxant effects of nitroglycerin and nitroprusside, but earlier suggestions that it mediates cholinergic or α-adrenergic responses are no longer accepted.[110, 111] Hormones that use Ca^{++} as an intracellular mediator, such as epinephrine and ACh, also appear to trigger changes in a family of membrane lipids.[112, 113] Phosphatidyl inositol (PI) is acted on by a PI kinase and broken down to a series of lipid compounds with cellular activity. One

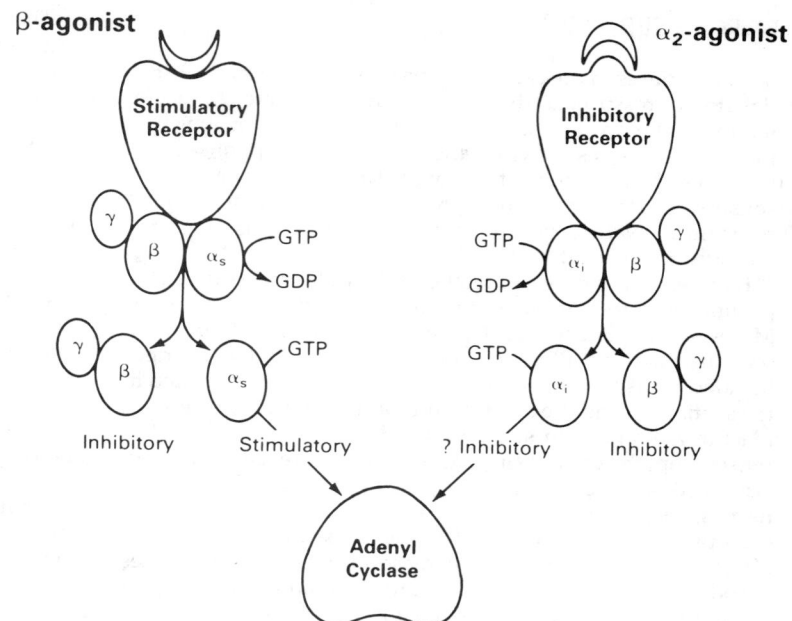

FIG. 7-16. The molecular mechanisms involved in regulating the formation of cAMP are shown schematically. The β-adrenergic agonist stimulates whereas the α_2-adrenergic agonist inhibits the enzyme adenyl cyclase that catalyzes the formation of cAMP. Guanine-nucleotide–binding proteins influence the response not only by mediating the hormone–receptor interaction, but also by modulating the coupling of the agonist–receptor complex to adenyl cyclase. (Reproduced with permission. Exton EH: Mechanisms involved in α-adrenergic phenomena. Am J Physiol 248:E633, 1985)

of these, inositol triphosphate, appears to be important in triggering Ca^{++} release from intracellular stores. The physiologic significance of the inositols is not well understood, but they appear to be important second messengers that may mediate cellular responses of the ANS.

Each signal must be transient in nature for the adenylate–cyclase system to be an effective modulator of cell activity. This is assured by the rapid hydrolysis of cAMP to inactive metabolites by phosphodiesterase enzymes. Three phosphodiesterases have been isolated and characterized. Their activity may be inhibited pharmacologically, resulting in elevated cAMP levels and a cellular response that mimics that of β-receptor stimulation.[114] These phosphodiesterases appear to be selectively inhibited by different drugs (see Non-adrenergic Sympathomimetic Drugs).

A similar enzyme second-messenger system has not been substantiated for α receptors. In general, stimulation of α_1 receptors results in increased cytosolic Ca^{++} levels and enhanced tone.[93] However, α_1 activation in gastrointestinal smooth muscle causes relaxation. In either case, the mechanism is thought to involve release of Ca^{++} from the internal membrane surface adjacent to the α_1 receptor.[110] This event triggers the release of more Ca^{++} from the sarcoplasmic reticulum. In blood vessels, the internal release of Ca^{++} is responsible for the initial phasic contraction that is succeeded by a slower tonic component, which is dependent on extracellular Ca^{++}. Calcium is regarded as the *third messenger*, but it may also function as a second messenger in mediating its own membrane flux (Fig. 7-15).

The transmembrane flux of Ca^{++} is an important commonality to the function of both α and β receptors.[24] Adequate ionized calcium is a prerequisite for the function of the catecholamines regardless of either α or β properties. The Ca^{++} messenger system promises to be one of the most exciting areas of clinical pharmacology of this decade. It has become evident that the Ca^{++} messenger system is more complex than the cAMP messenger system. Rasmussen and Barret summarize the four major attributes of messenger Ca^{++}:

(1) Calcium is a nearly universal messenger in animal cells; (2) It is a minatory messenger in that excess cellular Ca^{++} leads to cellular death; (3) It is a mercurial messenger in that its rise in concentration in the cell is transient even in those cells displaying a sustained response; (4) It is a synarchic messenger in that it nearly always regulates cell function in concert with other intracellular messengers, such as cAMP.[31]

We can conclude that the response of a receptor to a catecholamine can be regulated by: (1) the concentration of the catecholamine agonists; (2) the activity of phosphodiesterase; (3) factors affecting coupling of the receptor to the activated kinases; (4) receptor numbers and binding affinity; and (5) calcium availability.[61] We can medically manipulate all of these factors with the possible exception of receptor numbers. However, guanine nucleotides have been shown to reverse quickly α- and β-receptor insensitivity due to down regulation and may soon be available clinically.[24]

AUTONOMIC NERVOUS SYSTEM REFLEXES

ANS reflexes have been compared with the computer circuit.[115] This control system, as in all reflex systems, has: (1) sensors; (2) afferent pathways; (3) CNS integration; and (4) efferent pathways to the receptors and efferent organs. Fine adjustments are made at the local level according to positive and negative feedback mechanism. The baroreceptor is an example. The variable to be controlled (blood pressure) is sensed (carotid sinus), integrated (medullary vasomotor center), and adjusted through specific effector receptor sites. Drugs or disease can interrupt this circuit at any point. A β blocker may attenuate the effector response, whereas clonidine may alter both the effector and the integrator functions of blood pressure control[98] (see Antihypertensive Drugs).

BARORECEPTORS

Several reflexes in the cardiovascular system help control arterial blood pressure, cardiac output, and heart rate. An examination of the cardiovascular ANS reflexes reveals an anachronism. The business of circulation is the production of blood flow. Yet, the most important controlled variable to which the sensors are attuned is blood pressure, a product of flow and resistance. "Nature, like the human engineer, finds it easier to measure pressure than flow."[116]

Etienne Marey noted in 1859 that the pulse rate is inversely proportional to the blood pressure, and this is known as Marey's law.[22] Subsequently, Hering, Koch, and others demonstrated that the alterations in heart rate evoked by changes in blood pressure were dependent on baroreceptors located in the aortic arch and the carotid sinuses. These pressure sensors react to alterations in stretch caused by blood pressure. Impulses from the carotid sinus and aortic arch reach the medullary vasomotor center by the glossopharyngeal and vagus nerves, respectively. Increased sensory traffic from the baroreceptors, due to increased blood pressure, inhibits SNS effector traffic. The relative increase in vagal tone produces vasodilatation, slowing of the heart rate, and a lowering of blood pressure.[117] Real increases in vagal tone occur when blood pressure exceeds normal limits.[115, 118]

The arterial baroreceptor reflex can best be demonstrated by using the Valsalva maneuver as an example (Fig. 7-17). The Valsalva maneuver raises the intrathoracic pressure by forced expiration against a closed glottis. The arterial blood pressure will rise momentarily as the intrathoracic blood is forced into the heart (preload).[17] Sustained intrathoracic pressure diminishes venous return, reduces the cardiac output, and drops the blood pressure. Reflex vasoconstriction and tachycardia ensue. Blood pressure returns to normal with release of the forced expiration, but then briefly "overshoots" because of the vasoconstriction and increased venous return. A slowing of the heart rate accompanies the overshoot in pressure, according to Marey's law.

The cardiovascular responses to the Valsalva maneuver require an intact ANS circuit from peripheral sensor to peripheral adrenergic receptors. The Valsalva maneuver has been used to identify patients at risk for anesthesia due to ANS instability (Fig. 7-17). This was once a major concern in patients receiving drugs that depleted catecholamines, such as reserpine. Dysfunction of the SNS is implicated if exaggerated and prolonged hypotension develops during the forced expiration phase (more than 50% from resting mean arterial pressure).[22, 115] In addition, the overshoot at the end of the Valsalva maneuver is absent. Dysfunction of the PNS can be assumed if the heart rate does not respond appropriately to the blood pressure changes. The Valsalva maneuver may still be a valid clinical preoperative test of ANS reserve, but such data are lacking.

The ready availability of blood pressure and heart rate measurements serves to emphasize the importance of the arterial baroreceptors; however, venous baroreceptors may be more dominant in the moment-to-moment regulation of cardiac output. Baroreceptors in the right atrium and great veins produce an increase in heart rate when stretched by increased right atrial pressure.[31, 119] Reduced venous pressure decreases heart rate. Unlike the arterial baroreceptors, venous sensors are not thought to alter vascular tone; however, venoconstriction is postulated to occur when atrial pressures decline.[120] Nevertheless, stretch of the venous receptors produces changes in heart rate opposite to those produced when the arterial pressure sensors are stimulated. The pressure receptors, arterial and venous, are separately monitoring two of the four major determinants of cardiac output—afterload and preload. Venous baroreceptors sample preload by the stretch of the atrium produced by venous pressure. Arterial baroreceptors survey resistance, or afterload, as reflected in the arterial pressure. Afterload and preload produce opposite effects on cardiac output; thus, one should not be surprised that the venous and arterial baroreceptors produce opposite effects to a similar stimulus, pressure.

Bainbridge described the venous baroreceptor reflex and

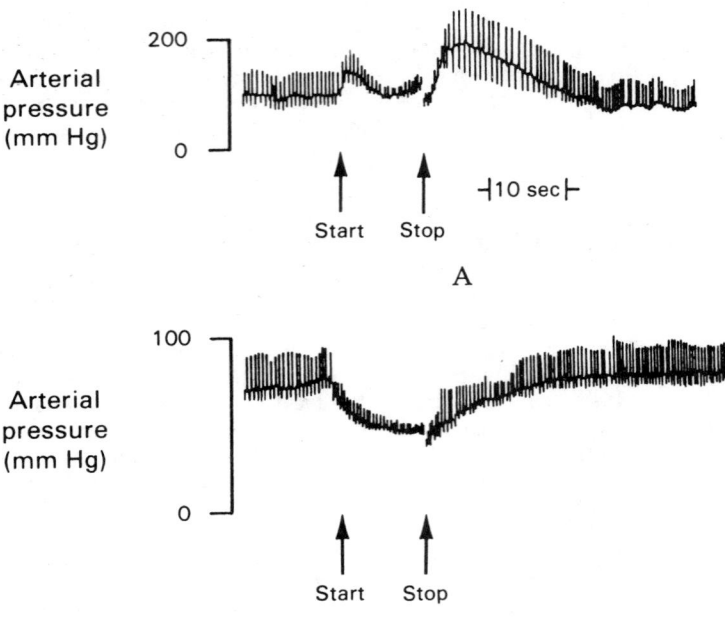

FIG. 7-17. (A) The normal blood pressure response to the Valsalva maneuver is demonstrated. Pulse rate moves in a reciprocal direction according to Marey's "law of the heart." (B) An abnormal Valsalva response is shown in a patient with C-5 quadriplegia.

demonstrated that it can be abolished by vagal resection. Numerous investigators have confirmed the acceleration of the heart rate in response to volume.[22] However, the magnitude and direction of the heart rate response is dependent on the prevailing heart rate at the time of stimulation. The exact mechanism of the Bainbridge reflex remains in doubt and controversy. It is of interest to note that the denervated, transplanted mammalian heart also accelerates in response to volume loading.[121] Heart rate, like cardiac output, can be adjusted to the quantity of blood entering the heart.[122, 123]

Greene relates the Bainbridge reflex to the characteristic, but paradoxical slowing of the heart seen with spinal anesthesia.[124] Blockade of the SNS levels of T_{1-4} ablates the efferent limb of the cardiac accelerator nerves. This source of cardiac deceleration is obvious as the vagus nerve is unopposed. Close study, however, reveals that bradycardia during spinal anesthesia is more related to the development of arterial hypotension than to the height of the block. The primary defect in the development of spinal hypotension is a decrease in venous return. Theoretically, the arterial hypotension should reflexly produce a tachycardia through the arterial baroreceptors. Instead, bradycardia is more common. Greene feels that in the unmedicated person, the venous baroreceptors are dominant over the arterial. A reduced venous pressure therefore slows heart rate.[125] In contrast, humorally mediated tachycardia is the usual response to hypotension or acidosis from other causes.

DENERVATED HEART

Reflex modulation of the adrenergic agonists is best seen in the denervated transplant heart, which retains the recipient's innervated SA node and the donor's denervated SA node. Knowledge derived from these studies is assuming great importance, not only because of the reemergence of cardiac transplants on a national scale, but also because we are treating an increasing population of patients whose intact hearts are being selectively denervated with adrenergic and calcium channel blockade. Table 7-6 is a summary of drug effects on

the transplanted heart.[121, 126, 127] It was derived from several sources, which were not always complete because the studies were limited by the delicate condition of the volunteer patients.[128–132] NE simultaneously activates α and β receptors of the intact heart and vessels. NE infusion in the transplanted heart produces a slowing of the recipient's atrial rate through vagal feedback as the blood pressure rises. In the unmodulated donor heart, atrial rate increases. Methoxamine-induced hypertension and nitrite-induced hypotension fail to induce deceleration and acceleration of the donor atrial rate. The baroreceptors are therefore not operant in the transplanted heart. Isoproterenol, a pure β agonist, increases the discharge rate of both the recipient and donor node by direct action, with the donor rate near doubling that of the recipient node. Atropine accelerates the recipient's atrial rate, whereas no effect is seen on the donor rate, which now controls heart rate. Hypersensitivity to β-cardiac stimulation in denervated dog hearts has been demonstrated.[20] Whether or not this occurs in the human heart remains unclear. Patients who have undergone chemical sympathectomy with bretylium or guanethidine are known to be hyperreactive to usual doses of catecholamines. A β blockade produces comparable slowing of the SA node of both recipient and donor. The exercise capability of the denervated heart is conspicuously reduced by β blockade, presumably because of its reliance on circulating catecholamines. Propranolol has also been demonstrated to reduce the β response to chronotropic effects of NE and isoproterenol in the transplanted heart. The cardiac output of the transplanted heart varies appropriately with changes in preload and afterload.

INTERACTION OF AUTONOMIC NERVOUS SYSTEM RECEPTORS

Recently, strong interactions have been noted between peripheral SNS and PNS nerves in organs that receive dual, antagonistic innervation. Release of NE at the presynaptic terminal is modified by the PNS. For example, vagal inhibition of left ventricular contractility is accentuated as the level of

TABLE 7-6. Drug Effects on the Denervated Heart

DRUG	SINUS RATE Recipient	SINUS RATE Donor	AV CONDUCTION VELOCITY	INTRAVENTRICULAR CONDUCTION VELOCITY	BLOOD PRESSURE	CARDIAC OUTUT	SYSTEMIC VASCULAR RESISTANCE
Resting	Normal	↑*	Normal	Normal	Normal	Normal or low	Normal
Exercise	↑	Slow ↑			↑	↑	
Atropine	↑	—	—				
Norepinephrine	↓	↑ ↑*	↑	—	↑	— or ↑	↑ ↑
Methoxamine	↓	—			↑	↓	↑ ↑
Isoproterenol	↑	↑ ↑	↑		↓	↑ ↑	↓
Glucagon	↑	↑					
Propranolol	↓	↓	↓	—	— or ↓	↓	↑
Amyl nitrite	↑	—			↓		↓
Digoxin							
Acute	↓	—	—*	—	—	— or ↑†	
Chronic	↓	—	↓				
Quinidine	↑	↓*	↓*	↓			
Edrophonium	↓	—*	—*				
Increased preload		↑				↑ or ↓†	

↑ = Increase; ↓ = Decrease; — = No change; * = Opposite from normals; † = Response depends on contractile state related to rejection.
(Reprinted with permission. Lawson NW, Wallfisch HK: Cardiovascular pharmacology: A new look at the "pressors." In Stoelting RK, Barash PG, Gallagher TJ [eds]: Advances in Anesthesia, p 195. Chicago, Year Book Medical Publishers, 1986)

SNS activity is raised.[19] This interaction is termed *accentuated antagonism* and is mediated by a combination of presynaptic and postsynaptic mechanisms.[20] The coronary arteries present an example of this phenomenon and deserve special attention.

The myocardium and coronary vessels are abundantly supplied with adrenergic and cholinergic fibers.[133] Strong activity of both α and β receptors has been demonstrated in the coronary vascular bed. The predominant adrenergic receptor in the coronary arteries is the β_1 receptor.[22, 134] Normally, the tone of these arteries favors relaxation because tonic stimulation of these receptors by endogenous NE produces vasodilatation (Table 7-6). This action is like the vasodilatation produced by stimulation of β_2 receptors in peripheral vessels; however, exogenous NE, usually given in exponentially higher concentrations, causes coronary vasoconstriction and a reduction of blood flow, which can be reversed to vasodilatation in the presence of α_1-adrenergic blockade. Selective stimulation of both the α_1 and postsynaptic α_2 receptors increases coronary vascular resistance, whereas selective α blockade eliminates this effect. Therefore, both β_1 and α_1 adrenoreceptors are present on coronary arteries and accessible to NE from sympathetic nerves.[25, 133]

The close anatomic proximity of the postganglionic vagal and SNS nerve endings in coronary arteries provides the morphologic basis for strong interaction.[19, 32, 66] SNS and PNS nerve terminals are found in such close proximity that transmitter from one can easily reach the other and affect transmitter release. In addition, the presynaptic adrenergic terminals of the myocardium and coronary vessels, like all blood vessels examined, contain muscarinic receptors.[33, 58, 135] Recent observations confirm that muscarinic drugs and vagal stimulation, acting on the presynaptic, SNS muscarinic receptor, inhibit the release of NE in a manner similar to the presynaptic α_2 and DA_2 receptors (Fig. 7-11). Conversely, blockade of the muscarinic receptors with atropine markedly augments the positive inotropic responses to catecholamines.[20] Suppression of the NE release explains, in part, vagal-induced attenuation of the inotropic response to strong SNS stimulation (accentuated antagonism) and only a weak negative inotropic effect of vagal stimulation when there is low-background SNS activity. This may also explain why vagal activity reduces the vulnerability of the myocardium to fibrillation during infusions of NE.

ACh may cause coronary spasm during periods of high SNS tone.[27, 136] Inhibition of NE release by presynaptic adrenergic muscarinic receptors of the smooth muscle of coronary vessels would lessen the coronary relaxation normally produced by NE on the β_1 receptor (Fig. 7-11). In anesthetized dogs, the rate of NE outflow into the coronary sinus blood, evoked by cardiac SNS stimulation, is markedly diminished by simultaneous vagal efferent stimulation.[137, 138] This action is known to be prevented by atropine, which also causes coronary vasodilatation. Metacholine, a muscarinic parasympathomimetic, has been reported to cause coronary vasoconstriction.[139] It simultaneously reduces ventricular irritability, however, by reducing NE release in myocardial fibers.[19]

The concept of accentuated antagonism has yet to be clearly defined because it is unusual for high SNS and PNS activity to coexist—except during anesthesia. Its important in the intact, conscious human has yet to be demonstrated; however, it may explain the clinical observation that angina in myocardial infarction due to coronary spasm in humans is not often related to cardiac work as is angina due to sclerotic coronary disease. Attacks of the former usually occur at rest, often waking the patient from sleep. This diurnal variation also corresponds to

the greatest activity of the PNS. The mechanism by which coronary arterial spasm occurs remains unknown, but continues to be an exciting area of investigation.

INTERACTION WITH OTHER REGULATORY SYSTEMS

The ANS is integrally related with several endocrine systems that ultimately summate to control blood pressure and regulate homeostasis. These include the renin–angiotensin system, ADH, glucocorticoids, and insulin.

ADH, or vasopressin, is formed in the hypothalamus and released from nerve endings in the posterior pituitary gland. It causes vasoconstriction and increased reabsorption of water in the distal collecting ducts of the kidney. It therefore affects not only central blood volume but plasma osmolality. The primary regulator of ADH release is plasma osmolality; however, several other stimuli may outweigh this control in stressful situations.[140] Release is also triggered by decreased central blood volume *via* low-pressure atrial receptors and hypotension *via* the carotid baroreceptors. Stress, pain, hypoxia, anesthesia, and surgery also stimulate ADH release. Infusion of catecholamines may alter ADH release, but these effects appear to be mediated by the carotid baroreceptors. ANS drugs that induce hypotension or decreased cardiac filling may induce ADH release and thus affect plasma osmolality.

Both α and β receptors have been found in the endocrine pancreas and modulate insulin release (Table 7-5). β-Stimulation increases insulin release, whereas α stimulation decreases it. The overall importance of this interaction is not entirely clear, but decreased glucose tolerance has been noted in subjects taking β-blocking drugs.[141]

The renin–angiotensin system is a complex endocrine system that modulates both blood pressure and water–electrolyte homeostasis (Fig. 7-18). Renin is a proteolytic enzyme contained within the cells of the juxtaglomerular apparatus of the renal cortex. When released, it acts on plasma angiotensinogen to form angiotensin I. Angiotensin I is then converted to angiotensin II by converting enzyme in the lung. Angiotensin II is a very powerful, direct arterial vasoconstrictor. It also acts on the adrenal cortex to release aldosterone and the adrenal medulla to release epinephrine. In addition to its direct effects on vascular smooth muscle, angiotensin II augments NE release *via* presynaptic receptors, thus enhancing peripheral SNS tone. Several antihypertensive drugs act by interfering with the formation or function of angiotensin II. Captopril and enalopril inhibit the action of converting enzyme, thus preventing the conversion of angiotensin I to angiotensin II.[142, 143] Saralasin is a direct angiotensin-II receptor antagonist that is useful as an antihypertensive drug, but is not in common clinical use.[144]

Renin is released in response to hyponatremia, decreased renal perfusion pressure, and ANS stimulation *via* β receptors on juxtaglomerular cells. Changes in SNS tone may thus alter renin release and affect homeostasis in a variety of ways. The mechanism of action of some antihypertensive drugs is thought to involve alterations in activity of the renin–angiotensin system in parallel with the ANS.

The ANS is also intimately related to adrenocortical function. As outlined above, glucocorticoid release modulates PNMT formation and thus synthesis of epinephrine. Glucocorticoids are also important in regulating the response of peripheral tissues to changes in SNS tone. Thus, the ANS is intimately related to other homeostatic mechanisms.[1]

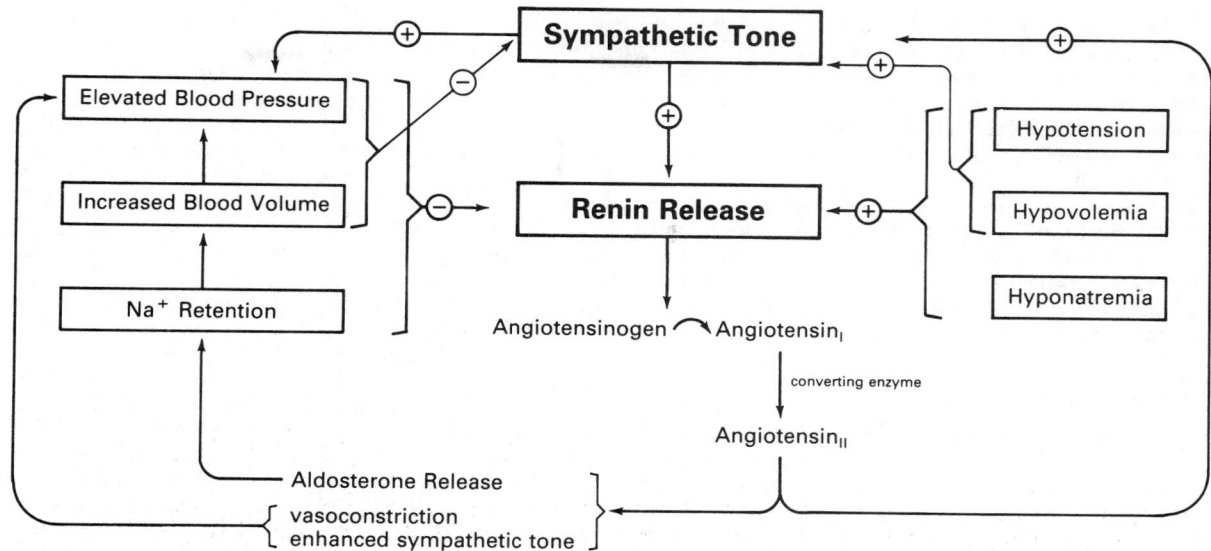

FIG. 7-18. The interactions of the renin–angiotensin and sympathetic nervous systems in regulating homeostasis are shown schematically along with the physiologic variables that modulate their function. *Arrows* with a [+] represent stimulation, and those with a [−] represent inhibition. See text for details.

CLINICAL AUTONOMIC NERVOUS SYSTEM PHARMACOLOGY

The clinical application of ANS pharmacology is based on knowledge of ANS anatomy, physiology, and molecular pharmacology. Drugs that modify ANS activity can be classified by their (1) site of action; (2) mechanism of action; or (3) pathology for which they are most commonly used. Antihypertensive drugs are an example of the third category.

SITE OF ACTION

ANS drugs may be broadly categorized as working on the CNS or at peripheral nerve sites. This classification is a matter of degree because considerable functional overlap occurs. An example of classification by site relates to the ganglionic agonists or blocking agents.[7] ANS drugs can be further categorized as those that act at the prejunctional membrane and those acting postjunctionally. They can then be more specifically classified by the predominant receptor or receptors on which they act.

MODE OF ACTION

ANS drugs may be broadly classified by mode of action according to their mimetic or lytic actions. This may also be termed agonism or antagonism. A sympathomimetic, such as ephedrine, mimics SNS activity by stimulation of adrenergic receptor sites both directly and indirectly. Sympatholytic drugs cause dissolution of SNS activity at these same receptor sites. β-Receptor blockers are examples of sympatholytic drugs. The terms *parasympathomimetic* and *parasympatholytic* are self explanatory and may be further divided by their site of action on the muscarinic or nicotinic receptors.

Several modes of ANS drug action become evident when one follows the cascade of neurotransmission. The mode is related to site. Drugs that act on prejunctional membranes may therefore: (1) interfere with transmitter synthesis (α-methyl paratyrosine); (2) interfere with transmitter storage (reserpine); (3) interfere with transmitter release (clonidine); (4) stimulate transmitter release (ephedrine); or (5) interfere with reuptake of transmitter (cocaine). Drugs may also (6) modify metabolism in the neurotransmitter in the synaptic cleft (anticholinesterase). Drugs acting at postjunctional sites may: (7) directly stimulate postjunctional receptors; and (8) interfere with transmitter agonist at the postjunctional receptor.

The ultimate response of an effector organ to an agonist or antagonist depends on (1) the drug; (2) its plasma concentration; (3) number of receptors in the effector organ; (4) binding by the receptor; and (5) reflex adjustments by the organism. This is the source of conflicting results for drugs used in differing clinical circumstances.

GANGLIONIC DRUGS

SNS and PNS ganglia are pharmacologically similar in that transmission through these ANS ganglia is effected by ACh (Fig. 7-4). Most ganglionic agonists and antagonists are not selective and affect SNS and PNS ganglia equally.[145] This nonselective property creates many undesirable and unpredictable side-effects that have limited the clinical usefulness of this category of drug.

Agonists

There are essentially no clinically useful ganglionic agonists. Nicotine is the prototypical ganglionic agonist.[3] In low doses, it stimulates ANS ganglia and the neuromuscular junction of striated muscle. High doses produce ganglionic and neuromuscular blockade. Low-dose stimulation and high-dose blockade are referred to as nicotinic effects in describing any drug with similar effects. Most ganglionic agonists and antagonists produce their effects through their nicotinic effects. The protean side-effects of nicotinic stimulation render it useful only as an investigative tool.

Despite its lack of clinical usefulness, nicotine is widely used in the form of tobacco. The novice tobacco user can often describe the overlap of SNS and PNS side-effects of nicotinic stimulation, which appear as nausea and vomiting, tachycardia, bradycardia, diarrhea, and sometimes fainting as a result of high-dose ganglionic blockade.[19]

Antagonists

Drugs that interfere with neurotransmission at ANS ganglia are known as ganglionic blocking agents. Nicotine, in high doses, is the prototypical ganglionic blocking agent also; however, early stimulatory nicotinic activity can be blocked at the ganglia and muscle end-plates with other ganglionic blockers and muscle relaxants, respectively, without blocking muscarinic effects.[146] Ganglionic blockers produce their nicotinic effects by competing, mimicking, or interfering with ACh metabolism. Hexamethonium, trimethaphan, and pentolinium produce a selective nondepolarizing blockade of neurotransmission at ANS ganglia without producing nicotinic neuromuscular blockade. They compete with ACh in the ganglia without stimulating the receptors. Decamethonium, a depolarizing muscle relaxant, selectively produces neuromuscular blockade in a manner similar to nicotine, but possesses no ganglionic effect.[19] The depolarization produced is initially associated with increased excitability, but depolarization persists. The neuron, therefore, cannot be excited and block exists. d-Tubocurarine (dTC), on the other hand, produces a competitive nondepolarizing block of both motor endplates and ANS ganglia. The action of motor paralysis predominates, but the concomitant ganglionic blockade at higher doses explains part of the hypotensive effect often seen with the use of dTC for muscle relaxation. Histamine release is the major hypotensive factor that is common to dTC and other ganglionic blockers. Anticholinesterase drugs may produce nicotinic-type ganglionic blockade by competition with ACh as well as by persistent depolarization via accumulated ACh.

The overall effects of ganglionic blockers on particular organ systems depend on whether the ANS activity of the system is predominantly sympathetic or parasympathetic (Table 7-1). The overall effect on peripheral vessels is vasodilatation due to release from SNS ganglionic constrictor control. The effect on the gastrointestinal tract may produce ileus. Although these drugs have a paraganglionic effect, blockade of the SNS ganglia and vascular dilatation is the property for which they were first used. They were initially used to treat chronic hypertension, but their lack of selectivity and global side-effects denied popularity. The introduction of drugs that produce vasodilatation directly or by action on the SNS vasomotor center has made the ganglionic blockers obsolete. They continue to have limited acute use in anesthesia to produce controlled hypotension and to treat hypertensive crisis.

Trimethaphan is the only ganglionic blocker available in the United States. Trimethaphan produces blockade by competition with ACh for receptors, thus stabilizing the postsynaptic membrane. However, side-effects and rapid-onset tachyphylaxis have markedly reduced its used in anesthesia.[147] The pupils become fixed and dilated during administration, which obscures eye signs, and important consideration for neuro-

surgery. In this regard, it is distinctly inferior to nitroprusside. The major advantage of trimethaphan is its short duration of action, which is the result of pseudocholinesterase hydrolysis.

Trimethaphan is mixed in a concentration of 500 mg in 250–500 ml of diluent. The dosage to produce a given blood pressure is extremely variable. A starting dose of 10–20 $\mu g \cdot kg^{-1} \cdot min^{-1}$ by infusor with invasive arterial monitoring is recommended. Doses higher than 1 g are not recommended because ganglionic blockade may persist, direct vasodilatation develops, histamine is released, and nicotinic neuromuscular blockade may appear.

Pentolinium is a ganglionic-blocking drug available in the United Kingdom.[146] Its mechanisms of action are similar to that of trimethaphan, but it is devoid of muscle-relaxant properties. The main disadvantage of pentolinium is its relative lack of controllability compared with trimethaphan or nitroprusside. Pentolinium is given in intermittent intravenous doses after anesthesia and position are established. The dose is 2.5–10 mg, with the effect lasting up to 45 min. One-fourth of the initial amount is repeated if needed. Pupillary dilatation, as with trimethaphan, will occur. Hypotension and vasomotor instability may outlast the procedure.

CHOLINERGIC DRUGS

Cholinergic drugs may be classified by the following outline, which follows physiologic response and site of action. Neuromuscular transmission is discussed in detail in Chapter 16. Nicotinic agonists and antagonists have been discussed as ganglionic drugs.

I. Cholinergic Drugs—Agonists[19]
   A. Nicotinic
      1. ANS ganglionic transmission
      2. Neuromuscular transmission
   B. Muscarinic
      1. Direct-acting
      2. Indirect-acting

II. Cholinergic Agents—Antagonists
   A. Nicotinic
      1. ANS ganglionic transmission
      2. Neuromuscular transmission
   B. Muscarinic

Muscarinic Agonists

The cholinergic muscarinic drugs act at sites in the body where ACh is the neurotransmitter of the nerve impulse. These drugs may be divided into three groups, of which the first two are direct muscarinic agonists.[148, 149] The third group acts indirectly. These groups are choline esters (ACh, methacholine, carbamylcholine, bethanechol); alkaloids (pilocarpine, muscarine, arecoline); and anticholinesterases (physostigmine, neostigmine, pyridostigmine, edrophonium, echothiophate).

DIRECT CHOLINOMIMETIC. ACh has virtually no therapeutic applications because of its diffuse action and rapid hydrolysis by cholinesterase (Fig. 7-7).[148] One may encounter the use of topical ACh (1%) drops during cataract extraction when a rapid miosis is desired. Systemic effects are not usually seen because of the rapidity of ACh hydrolysis.

Other choline esters have been synthesized, mostly derivatives of ACh, that possess more selective muscarinic activity than ACh. They differ from ACh in being more resistant to inactivation by cholinesterase and thus having a more prolonged and useful action. They also differ from ACh in their relative muscarinic and nicotinic activity.[149] The best studied of these drugs are methacholine, bethanechol, and carbamylcholine.[19] The chemical structures of ACh and these choline esters are shown in Figure 7-19. Their pharmacologic actions are compared with ACh in Table 7-7. These are not important drugs in anesthesiology, but they deserve discussion because anesthesiologists may encounter patients who are receiving them, and they may be useful in the postoperative period to alleviate cardiac tachydysrhythmias, urinary retention, and ileus.[150]

ACh is a quarternary ammonium compound that interacts with postsynaptic receptors, causing conformational membrane changes. This results in increased permeability to small ions and thus, depolarization. All the receptors translate the reversible binding of ACh into openings of discrete channels in excitable membranes allowing Na^+ and K^+ ions to flow along their electromechanical gradients. Structure–activity relationships point to the presence of two important binding sites on the receptor, an esteratic site that binds the ester end of the molecule, and an ionic site that binds the quarternary amine portion (Fig. 7-7). Subtle changes in the structure of the compound can markedly alter the responses among different tissue groups. The degree of muscarinic activity falls if the acetyl group is replaced, but this confers a resistance to enzymatic hydrolysis. Carbamylcholine is synthesized by replacing the acetyl group with carbamyl (Fig. 7-19). It possesses both muscarinic and nicotinic actions but is virtually resistant to esterase hydrolysis (Table 7-7). Bethanechol is also resistant to hydrolysis but possesses mainly muscarinic activity. β-Methyl substitution produces methacholine, which is less resistant to hydrolysis but is primarily a muscarinic agonist.

Methacholine is destroyed by cholinesterase less rapidly than ACh and is potentiated by anticholinesterase drugs. Its muscarinic effects are predominantly cardiovascular. Methacholine slows the heart and dilates peripheral blood vessels. It is used to terminate supraventricular tachydysrhythmias, especially paroxysmal tachycardia, when other measures have failed. Intestinal tone is also increased. Methacholine should not be given to patients with asthma. Hypertensive patients may also develop marked hypotension. Side-effects are those of PNS stimulation such as nausea, vomiting, and flushed sweating. Methacholine dosage is 100–200 mg orally or 10–25 mg subcutaneously. Overdose is treated with atropine.

Bethanechol has predominantly muscarinic actions that are relatively select for the gastrointestinal and urinary tracts. It does not slow the heart or lower the blood pressure like methacholine in usual doses. Bethanechol is of value in treating postoperative abdominal distention (nonobstructive paralytic ileus), gastric atony following bilateral vagotomy, congenital megacolon, nonobstructive urinary retention, and some cases of neurogenic bladder. The optimal oral dose is between 30 and 60 mg daily in divided doses. It is not a parenteral drug. Precautions are as for methacholine.

The use of carbamylcholine has largely been supplanted by better drugs because of its dual nicotinic and muscarinic ef-

TABLE 7-7. Comparative Muscarinic Actions of Direct Cholinomimetic Agents

	SYSTEMIC				
	Acetylcholine	Methacholine	Carbamylcholine	Bethanechol	Pilocarpine
ESTERASE HYDROLYSIS	+ + +	+	0	0	0
EYE (TOPICAL)					
Iris	+ +	+ +	+ + +	+ + +	+ + +
Ciliary	+ +	+ +	+ + +	+ + +	+ +
HEART					
Rate	– – –	– – –	–	–	?
Contractility	–	–	–	–	
Conduction	– –	– – –	–	–	
SMOOTH MUSCLE					
Vascular	– –	– – –	–	–	– –
Bronchial	+ +	+ +	+	+	+ +
G.I. Motility	+ +	+ +	+ + +	+ + +	+ +
G.I. Sphincters	– –	–	– – –	– – –	+ +
Biliary	+ +	+ +	+ + +	+ + +	+ +
Bladder					
detrusor	+ +	+ +	+ + +	+ + +	+ +
sphincter	– –	–	– – –	– – –	– –
EXOCRINE GLANDS					
Respiratory	+ + +	+ +	+ + +	+ +	+ + + +
Salivary	+ +	+ +	+ +	+ +	+ + + + +
Pharyngeal	+ +	+ +	+ +	+ +	+ + + +
Lacrimal	+ +	+ +	+ +	+ +	+ + + +
Sweat	+ +	+ +	+ +	+ +	+ + + + +
G.I. acid and secretions	+ +	+ +	+ +	+ +	+ + + +
NICOTINIC ACTIONS	+ + +	+	+ + +	–	+ + +

+ = Stimulation; – = Inhibition.
(Compiled from reference sources with permission.)

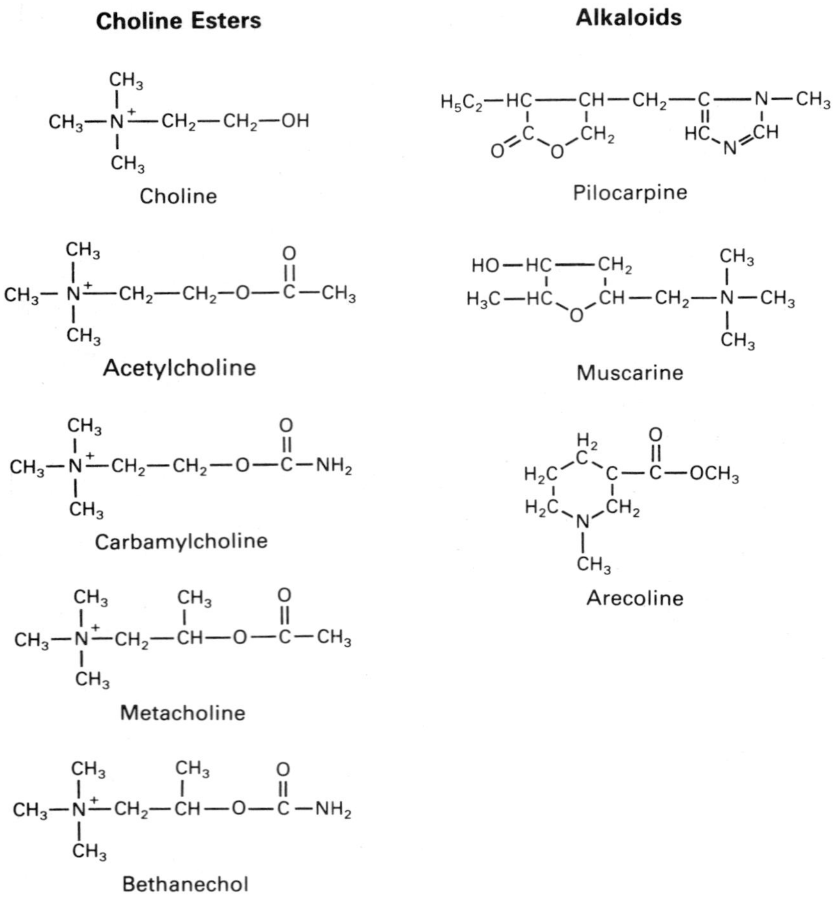

Choline Esters

Choline

Acetylcholine

Carbamylcholine

Metacholine

Bethanechol

Alkaloids

Pilocarpine

Muscarine

Arecoline

FIG. 7-19. Chemical structures of direct-acting cholinomimetic esters and alkaloids.

fects. It is a long-acting agent because it is completely resistant to hydrolysis. Atropine will block the muscarinic actions but unmask its nicotinic effects. In this case, blood pressure will rise as sympathetic ganglia are stimulated and catecholamines are released. Carbamylcholine is currently limited to topical ophthalmologic drops to produce miosis and for the treatment of wide-angle glaucoma.[148]

Direct-acting cholinomimetic alkaloids include muscarine, pilocarpine, and arecoline. They act at the same sites as ACh, and their effects are similar to the effects of ACh as described in Table 7-7. There are no uses in anesthesiology for these drugs. Pilocarpine is the only drug of this group used therapeutically in the United States. Its sole use is for the treatment of glaucoma, for which it is the standard. It is used as a topical miotic drug in ophthalmologic practice to reduce intraocular pressure in glaucoma. Pilocarpine has primary muscarinic effects with minimal nicotinic effects unless given systemically, in which case hypertension and tachycardia may result. Toxicity with topical application is rare.

Muscarine acts almost exclusively at muscarinic receptor sites, but it has no therapeutic application. Arecoline stimulates nicotinic receptors in addition to muscarinic receptors when given systemically. Its use has been limited to topical application in ophthalmology. Acelidine is a synthetic compound resembling arecoline that is used for the treatment of glaucoma in Europe.

The benefits of muscarinic agonists must be carefully considered when one or more of its actions is likely to be dangerous (Table 7-7). They are rarely given intravenously because of side-effects. Common side-effects are those of intense PNS stimulation, which include gastrointestinal cramping, hypotension, diaphoresis, salivation, diarrhea, and bladder pain.[19] Muscarinic agonists are particularly dangerous in patients with myasthenia gravis (who are receiving anticholinergics), bulbar palsy, cardiac disease, asthma, peptic ulcer, progressive muscular atrophy, or mechanical intestinal obstruction or urinary retention.[151]

INDIRECT CHOLINOMIMETICS. The indirect-acting cholinomimetic drugs are of greater importance to the anesthesiologist than are the direct drugs. These drugs produce cholinomimetic effects indirectly as a result of inhibition or inactivation of the enzyme AChE, which normally destroys ACh by hydrolysis.[47] These are referred to as cholinesterase inhibitors or anticholinesterases. Table 7-8 lists therapeutic cholinesterase inhibitors and their major indications. Most of these drugs inhibit both AChE and pseudocholinesterase. Inhibition of AChE permits the accumulation of ACh transmitter in the synapse resulting in intense PNS activity similar to that of the direct cholinomimetic drugs. The action of ACh is therefore potentiated and prolonged. Their effects can be predicted from a knowledge of ANS pharmacology previously presented (Table 7-7). Some of the AChE drugs (i.e., edrophonium) may also stimulate cholinergic receptors by direct action.[152] The accumulation of ACh produced by anticholinesterases potentially can produce all of the following:

TABLE 7-8. Cholinesterase Inhibitors

DRUG	TRADE NAME	ROUTE	DURATION	INDICATIONS
REVERSIBLE				
Physostigmine	Eserine	Topical	6–12 h	Glaucoma
Pyridostigmine	Mestinon Regonol	Oral, iv, im	4 h	Myasthenia gravis Reversal of neuromuscular blockade
Neostigmine	Prostigmine	Oral, iv	4–6 h	Myasthenia gravis Reversal of neuromuscular blockade
Edrophonium	Tensilon Enlon	iv	1–2 h	Reversal of neuromuscular blockade Diagnosis of myasthenia gravis
Demecarium	Humorsol	Topical	3–5 days	Glaucoma
Ambenonium	Mytelase	Oral	4 h	Myasthenia gravis
NONREVERSIBLE				
Echothiopate	Phospholine	Topical	3–14 days	Glaucoma
Isoflurophate		Topical	3–7 days	Glaucoma research
Malathione		Topical		Insecticide—relatively safe for mammals because of rapid hepatic metabolism
Parathion		Topical		Insecticide—highly toxic to higher animals; frequent accidental poisoning
Sarin (GB)	Nerve gas	Topical and gas		
Tabun	Nerve gas	Topical and gas		There are no indications for the use of nerve gas
Soman	Nerve gas	Topical and gas		

Note: Atropine should always be given prior to or with intravenous cholinesterase inhibitors and when only nicotinic effects are desired; muscarinic effects are dangerous when excessive

(1) stimulation of muscarinic receptors at ANS effect organs; (2) stimulation, followed by depression of all ANS ganglia and skeletal muscle (nicotinic); and (3) stimulation, with later depression of cholinergic receptor sites in the CNS. All of these effects may be seen with lethal doses of anticholinesterase drugs, but therapeutic doses only produce the first two.

Actions of therapeutic significance to the anesthesiologist concern the eye, the intestine, and the neuromuscular junction. The effects of anticholinesterases are useful in the treatment of myasthenia gravis, glaucoma, and atony of the gastrointestinal and urinary tracts. AChE drugs are used routinely in anesthesia to reverse nondepolarizing neuromuscular block. A detailed discussion of their use for this purpose is covered in Chapter 13 ("Muscle Relaxants").

The most prominent pharmacologic effects of the anticholinesterase drugs are their muscarinic effects. The most useful actions are their nicotinic effects.[19] Muscarinic activity is evoked by lower concentrations of ACh than are necessary to produce the desired nicotinic effect. For example, the anticholinesterase neostigmine reverses neuromuscular blockade by increasing ACh concentration at the muscle end-plate, a nicotinic receptor. Nicotinic reversal of neuromuscular blockade can usually be produced safely only when the patient has been protected by atropine or other muscarinic blockers. This prevents the untoward muscarinic effects of bradycardia, hypotension, bronchospasm, or intestinal spasm. Conversely, neuromuscular paralysis can be produced or increased if excessive anticholinesterase is used. Excess accumulation of ACh at the motor end-plates produces a depolarization block similar to that produced by succinylcholine or nicotine. This is characteristic of the nicotine receptors.

Reversal of neuromuscular blockade in patients who have had bowel anastomosis was at one time a major controversy. Some felt that the muscarinic effects of anticholinesterase drugs (hypermotility) increased the risk of anastomotic leakage,[153, 154] whereas others found no association between their use and subsequent breakdown.[155, 156] National experience has favored the latter opinion.

The interactions between ACh and the anticholinesterases is complex.[157] Anticholinesterase drugs inhibit hydrolysis of ACh by binding to either, or both, the anionic or esteratic sites of AChE forming inhibitor–enzyme complexes that are more stable than ACh–enzyme complexes. These complexes prevent proper stereotactic access of ACh to the active enzyme sites; thus, hydrolysis is delayed and ACh accumulates.

Anticholinesterase drugs may be clinically divided into two types. These are the reversible and nonreversible cholinesterase inhibitors.[62, 149] Reversible cholinesterase inhibitors delay the hydrolysis of ACh from 1 to 8 h. Nonreversible drugs are so named because their inhibitory effects may last from days to weeks. The differences in duration of various anticholinesterases apparently depend on whether they inhibit the anionic or esteratic site of AChE.[152] Therefore, the anticholinesterase drugs have also been pharmacologically subdivided. Drugs that inhibit the anionic site are called prosthetic, competitive inhibitors. Their action is due to competition between the anticholinesterase and ACh for the anionic site. These drugs tend to be short acting. Edrophonium is an example of this type. Those drugs that inhibit the esteratic site are called acid-transferring inhibitors. These drugs include the longer-acting neostigmine, pyridostigmine, and physostigmine. Thus, the differences in mechanism of inhibition produced by prosthetic inhibitors (edrophonium) and acid-transferring inhibitors (neostigmine) account for the longer duration of action associated with the latter.

Most of the reversible cholinesterase inhibitors are quarternary ammonium compounds and do not cross the blood–brain barrier. Physostigmine is a tertiary amine that readily passes into the CNS (Fig. 7-20). It produces central muscarinic stimulation and, thus, is not used to reverse neuromuscular blockade but can be used to treat atropine poisoning. Conversely, atropine is used to treat physostigmine poisoning. Physostigmine has also been found to be a specific antidote in the treatment of postoperative delirium (see Central Anticholinergic Syndrome).[19]

The irreversible cholinesterase inhibitors are mostly organ-

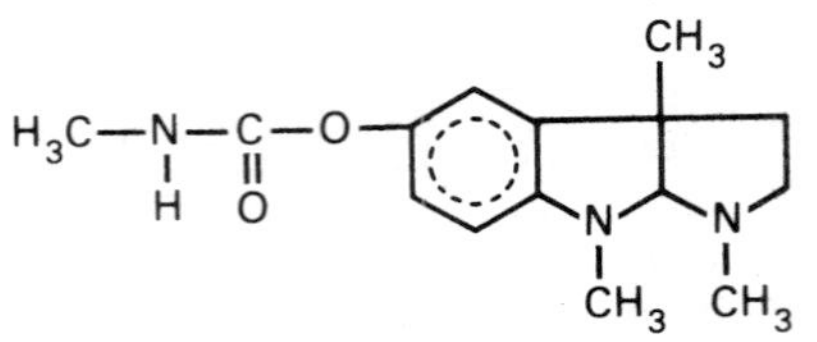

Physostigmine

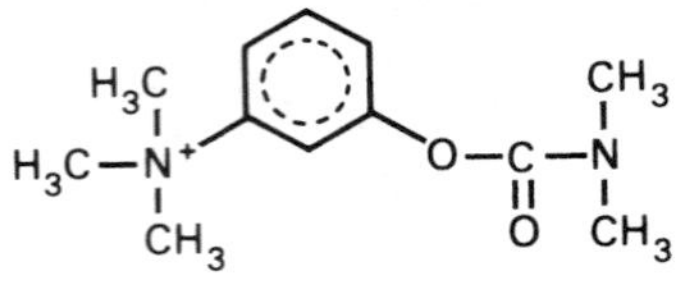

Neostigmine

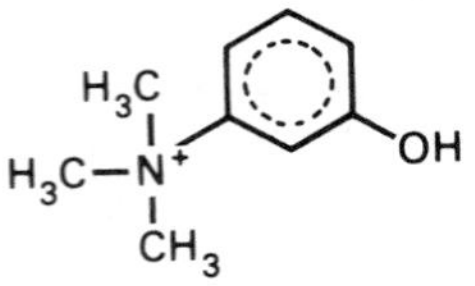

Edrophonium

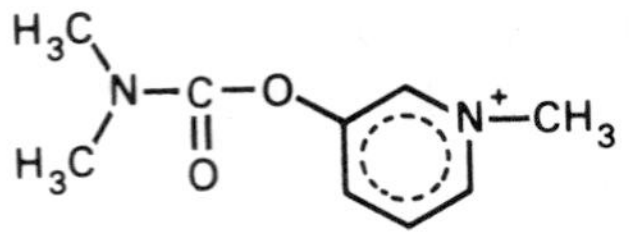

Pyridostigmine

FIG. 7-20. Structural formulas of clinically useful reversible anticholinesterase drugs. Physostigmine is a tertiary amine and crosses the blood–brain barrier. It is useful in treating the central anticholinergic syndrome.

ophosphate compounds. These are also considered acid-transferring inhibitors that form a phosphorylated enzyme resistant to attack by water. The phosphorylated enzyme cannot hydrolyze ACh to any measurable degree. In addition, the organophosphate compounds are highly lipid soluble; they readily pass into the CNS and are rapidly absorbed through the skin. They are used as the active ingredient in potent insecticides and chemical warfare agents known as nerve gases. Table 7-8 lists some of these agents.

The only therapeutic drug of this group is echothiophate, which is available as topical drops for the treatment of glaucoma. Its primary advantage is its prolonged duration of action. Topical absorption is variable but considerable. Echothiophate can remain effective for 2 or 3 weeks following cessation of therapy.[158] History of use is important in avoiding prolonged action of succinylcholine, which requires pseudocholinesterase for its hydrolysis.

Organophosphate poisoning presents all the signs and symptoms of excess ACh.[159] The antidote cartridges dispensed to troops to counter the effects of anticholinesterase nerve gases contain only atropine, which would effectively counter the muscarinic effects of the gas; however, atropine does little for the high-dose nicotinic muscle paralysis or the

central ventilatory depression that contributes to death from nerve gases. Treatment requires large doses of atropine, 35–70 $\mu g \cdot kg^{-1}$ intravenously every 3–10 min until muscarinic symptoms abate. Smaller doses at less frequent intervals may be required for several days. Central ventilatory depression and nicotinic paralysis or weakness require ventilatory support and specific therapy of the cholinesterase lesion. Pralidoxime has been reported to reactivate cholinesterase activity by hydrolysis of the phosphate–enzyme complex. It is particularly effective with parathion poisoning and is the only cholinesterase reactivator available in the United States.[149]

Muscarinic Antagonists

Muscarinic antagonist refers to a specific drug action for which the term anticholinergic is widely used. Any drug that interferes with the action of ACh as a transmitter can be considered an anticholinergic drug. The term *anticholinergic* refers to a more broad classification that would include nicotinic antagonists already discussed.

ATROPINIC DRUGS. Atropine, scopolamine, and glycopyrrolate are the most commonly used muscarinic antagonists in anesthesia (Fig. 7-21). The use of antimuscarinic drugs for premedication is outlined in Chapter 18.

FIG. 7-21. Structural formulas of the clinically useful antimuscarinic drugs.

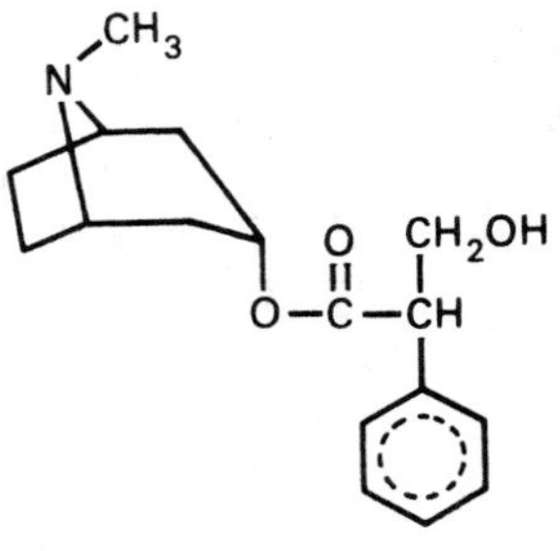

Atropine

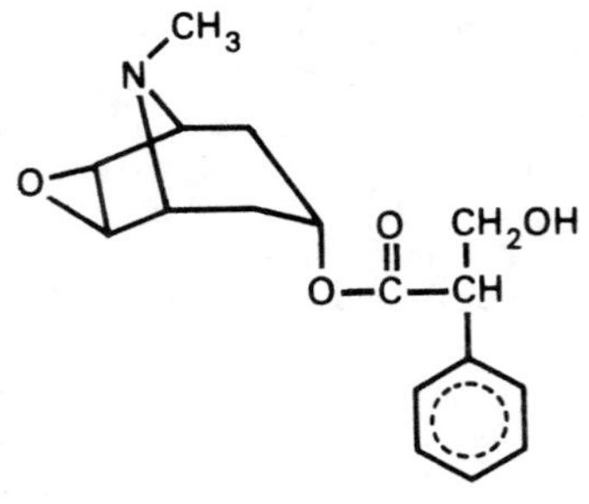

Scopolamine

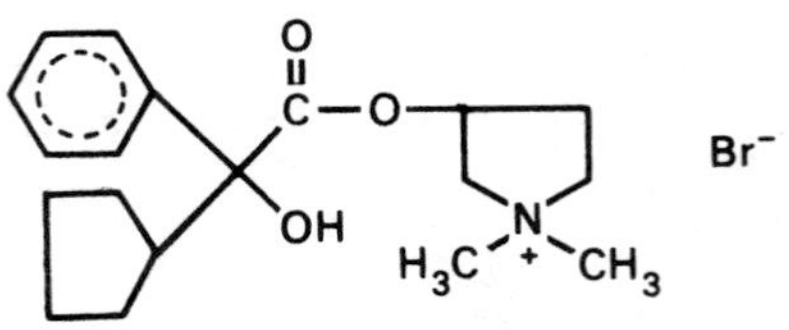

Glycopyrrolate

The actions of these drugs include inhibition of salivary, bronchial, pancreatic, and gastrointestinal secretions. Historically, atropine was introduced to anesthesia practice to prevent excessive secretions during ether anesthesia and to prevent vagal bradycardia during the administration of chloroform. Atropine-like drugs increase heart rate, relax bronchial and tracheal smooth muscle, and act as a gastrointestinal relaxant.[160] Atropine and scopolamine also possess antiemetic action. Scopolamine skin patches are now used to control motion sickness and perhaps could be useful in controlling nausea on an outpatient basis.[161] Atropine, however, reduces the opening pressure of the lower esophageal sphincter, which theoretically increases the risk of passive regurgitation.[162] Atropinic drugs also produce dilatation of the pupil (mydriasis) and paralysis of accommodation (cycloplegia).

Antimuscarinic agents do not inhibit transmission equally, and there are marked variations in sensitivity at different muscarinic sites due to differences in penetration and affinities of the various receptors.[163] Differences in relative potency among the different antimuscarinics are outlined in Table 7-9. For example, glycopyrrolate produces less tachycardia than atropine and is a more potent antisialogogue. They are also used to counter unwanted muscarinic actions of anticholinesterases when these are required for their nicotinic effect (see Chapter 13, "Muscle Relaxants").

The antimuscarinic effects of the atropinic drugs are due to competitive inhibition of ACh at the receptors of organs innervated by cholinergic postganglionic nerves. The antagonism can be overcome by sufficient concentrations of cholinomimetic drugs or anticholinesterases that increase ACh levels at the receptor site. This explains most of the therapeutic actions of atropinic drugs; however, they are neither purely antimuscarinic nor purely antagonist.[19]

The belladonna alkaloids (atropine and scopolamine) also block ACh transmission to sweat glands, which, although cholinergic, are innervated by the SNS. Antimuscarinic agents produce antinicotinic actions at higher doses and produce important actions on CNS transmission that are pharmacologically similar to that at the postganglionic cholinergic junction.[164] Atropine and scopolamine are tertiary amines (Fig. 7-21) and easily penetrate the blood–brain barrier and placenta. Glycopyrrolate is a quarternary amine that, like the reversible anticholinesterase drugs, does not easily penetrate these barriers. Glycopyrrolate, a synthetic antimuscarinic, has gained popularity because it avoids the central effects of the other two drugs.

Atropine and scopolamine have notable CNS effects that are dissimilar. Scopolamine differs from atropine mainly in having central depressant effects that produce sedation, amnesia, and euphoria. Such properties are widely used for premedication for cardiac cases in combination with morphine and a major tranquilizer. Atropine, as a premedicant, has slight effects on the CNS, including a mild stimulation. Higher doses such as those given for reversal of muscle relaxants (1–2 mg) may produce restlessness, disorientation, hallucinations, and delirium (see Central Anticholinergic Syndrome). Excessive stimulation may be followed by depression and paralysis of respiration. Atropine is closely related chemically to cocaine. Occasionally, scopolamine in low doses may cause restlessness and delirium. This syndrome is more frequently seen in the elderly and patients experiencing pain, as in obstetrics.

Atropine and scopolamine are noted to produce a paradoxical bradycardia when given in small doses. Scopolamine (0.1–0.2 mg) usually causes more slowing than atropine, but likewise produces less cardiac acceleration at higher doses. The usual intramuscular premedicant doses of scopolamine cause either a decrease or no change in heart rate, which is another advantage in cardiac anesthesia. The paradoxical bradycardia was once thought to be due to an early central inhibition of the medullary cardioinhibitory center. However, this phenomenon occurs in animals that have had total vagotomy. Flacke and Flacke conclude that atropine must have a weak peripheral cholinergic agonist effect at low doses superceded by high-dose antimuscarinic effects.[19] Atropine may also produce sympathomimetic effects by blocking presynaptic muscarinic receptors found on adrenergic nerve terminals.[20, 27, 58] ACh stimulation of these receptors inhibits NE release, and blockade by atropine releases this inhibition (see Cholinergic Receptors: Muscarinics).

The antimuscarinic drugs are used in anesthesia to diminish salivary and bronchial secretions during anesthesia, to protect heart rate from vagal inhibition, and to antagonize the muscarinic side-effects of anticholinesterases during reversal of muscle relaxants. Atropine is useful in increasing cardiac output with sinus bradycardia due to vagal stimulation if hypoxia is ruled out. It has many uses outside of anesthesia for the treatment of renal colic, gastrointestinal spasm, gastric secretion, and asthma.

Atropinic drugs are widely used in ophthalmology as mydriatics and cycloplegics. Atropine is contraindicated in patients with narrow-angle glaucoma. Pupillary dilatation thickens the peripheral part of the iris, which narrows the irido–corneal angle. Drainage of aqueous humor is impaired and intraocular pressure increases. Doses of atropine used for premedication have little effect in this regard, whereas equal doses of scopolamine will cause mydriasis. Prudence would avoid either in narrow-angle glaucoma. The need for antimuscarinic premedication is questionable in this situation.[162]

Atropine is best avoided where tachycardia would be harmful as may occur in thyrotoxicosis, pheochromocytoma, or obstructive coronary artery disease. Theoretically, antimuscarinic drugs should benefit coronary spasm, but the

TABLE 7-9. Comparison of Antimuscarinic Drugs

	DURATION		CNS	GI TONE	GASTRIC ACID	AIRWAY SECRE- TIONS*	HEART RATE
	iv	im					
Atropine	15–30 min	2–4 h	+ +	– –	–	–	+ + +‡
Scopolamine	30–60 min	4–6 h	+ + + +†	–	–	– – – –	– 0‡
Glycopyrrolate	2–4 h	6–8 h	0	– – –	– – –	– – –	+ 0

* Secretions may be reduced but inspissated.
† CNS effect often manifest as sedation before stimulation.
‡ May decelerate initially.

benefit may be offset by the oxygen cost of the ensuing tachycardia. Atropine should be avoided in hyperpyrexial patients because it inhibits sweating.

CENTRAL ANTICHOLINERGIC SYNDROME. The belladonna alkaloids have long been known to produce undesirable side-effects ranging from stupor (scopolamine) to delirium (atropine). This syndrome has otherwise been called postoperative delirium and atropine toxicity. The central anticholinergic syndrome (CAS) appears to involve the muscarinic receptors.[19] Biochemical studies have demonstrated abundant muscarinic ACh receptors in the brain that can be affected by any drug possessing antimuscarinic activity and capable of crossing the blood–brain barrier. Hundreds of drugs exist that meet these criteria with which this syndrome has been associated. Table 7-10 lists some of those drugs.[19, 164] One is surprised that this syndrome is not more prevalent.

Patients receiving high doses of atropinic alkaloids rapidly develop dryness of the mouth, blurred vision with photophobia (mydriasis), hot and dry skin (flushed), and fever.[164] Mental symptoms range from sedation, stupor, and coma to anxiety, restlessness, disorientation, hallucinations, and delirium. They may have convulsions and ventilatory arrest if lethal poisoning has occurred. This is not the usual case encountered in anesthesiology. Although an alarming reaction may occur, fatalities are rare. Intoxication is usually short lived and followed by amnesia. These reactions can be controlled by the intravenous injection of physostigmine.[165] Physostigmine is an anticholinesterase that, by virtue of being a tertiary amine, readily passes into the CNS to counter antimuscarinic activity. It should be given slowly in 1 mg doses, not exceeding 3 mg, to avoid producing peripheral cholinergic activity. Neostigmine, pyridostigmine, and edrophonium are not effective because they cannot pass into the CNS. Likewise, atropine is an effective antidote for physostigmine overdose.[19] The duration of physostigmine action may be shorter than that of the offending antimuscarinic drug and require repeated injection should symptomatology recur. Physostigmine appears safe when used within dose recommendations and indications are established. Central disorientation alone does not establish a diagnosis.[163] Peripheral signs of antimuscarinic activity should also be present in addition to a central anticholinergic syndrome.

Physostigmine has been reported to reverse the CNS effects of many of the drugs listed in Table 7-10. This includes antihistamines, tricyclic antidepressants, and tranquilizers. Reversal of the sedative effects of opioids and benzodiazepines has also been reported.[166, 167] However, anticholinesterase agents potentiate cholinergic synaptic transmission and increase neuronal activity, even if no receptor antagonist is present. Thus, arousal may not be a function independent of its cholinesterase activity and claims that physostigmine is a nonspecific CNS stimulant may not be warranted, and could, in fact, be dangerous.[19] These phenomena require more study.

ADRENERGIC DRUGS

Adrenergic Agonists

Since the isolation of epinephrine by Abel in 1899, the naturally occurring catecholamines and synthetic sympathomimetic amines have attracted considerable attention and enjoyed popular use as vasopressors. A vasopressor is a drug that is used to elevate arterial blood pressure above the exist-

TABLE 7-10. Antimuscarinic Compounds Associated with Central Anticholinergic Syndrome

Belladonna Alkaloids
Atropine sulfate
Scopolamine hydrobromide

Synthetic and Natural Tertiary Amine Compounds
Dycyclomine (Bentyl)—antispasmodic with local anesthetic activity
Thiphenalmil (Trocinate)—antispasmodic with local anesthetic activity
Procaine
Cocaine
Cyclopentalate (Cyclogyl) mydriatic

Quarternary Derivatives of Belladonna Alkaloids
Methscopolamine bromide (Pamine)—antispasmodic
Homatropine methylbromide (Ru-spas, Sed-tense)—sedative, antispasmodic
Homatropine hydrobromide—ophthalmic solution—mydriatic

Synthetic Quarternary Compounds
Methantheline bromide (Banthine)
Propantheline bromide (Probanthine)

Antihistamines
Chlorpheniramine (Ornade)
Diphenhydramine (Benadryl)

Plants
Deadly nightshade (atropine)
Bittersweet
Potato leaves and sprouts
Jimson or loco weed
Coca plant (cocaine)

Over-the-counter
Asthma-Dor—atropine-like
Compoz—scopolamine sedation
Sleep Eze—scopolamine sedation
Sominex—scopolamine sedation

Antiparkinson Drugs
Benztropine (Cogentin)
Trihexphenidyl (Artane)
Biperiden (Akineton)
Ethopropazine (Parsidol)
Procyclidine (Kemadrin)

Antipsychotic Drugs
Chlorpromazine (Thorazine)
Thioriazine (Mellaril)
Haloperidol (Haldol)
Droperidol (Inapsine)
Promethazine (Phenergan)

Tricyclic Antidepressants
Amytriptyline (Elavil)
Imipramine (Tofranyl)
Desipramine (Norpramine, Pertofrane)

Synthetic Opioids
Demerol
Methadone

ing level because the pressure is "too low." Until recently, sympathomimetics were the most common means of treating shock, or the low-output syndrome, because of the associated hypotension.[57] Elevation of arterial blood pressure has been repeatedly demonstrated to be an insufficient goal in the treatment of the low-output syndrome.[31] The goal instead is to reestablish blood flow to vital organs. There is no definite evidence that the adrenergic amines increase survival from shock states, with the exception of epinephrine for anaphylaxis.[168] The outcome of cardiogenic shock treated with the "pressors" alone shows mortality rate of 90% or greater.[169, 170] The sympathetic amines do not remove the cause of the shock or hypotension; they are temporary drugs to be used only until more definite therapy is instituted or the pathologic process abates.

Today, shock is simply defined as tissue perfusion inadequate to meet metabolic demands. Shock can be present with "normal" blood pressures, and hypotension can be produced without shock. Hence, blood pressure is no longer the *sine qua non* in defining shock.[31] Recognition of the importance of volume therapy brought an end to the "age of the vasopressor" and ushered in a more rational approach to vasoactive drugs used with adequate hydration. It is now apparent that the problems associated with the use of vasopressors were caused, in large part, by an insufficient understanding of clinical cardiovascular physiology and the inability to monitor critically ill patients. We can now selectively detect and manipulate the weak links in the chain of cardiovascular events that produce blood flow rather than just pressure. A clinical appreciation of the differential effects of the vasopressors as inotropes, as chronotropes, or as pressors has developed.

SELECTION OF ADRENERGIC EFFECT. The selection of vasoactive drugs requires a knowledge of both the hemodynamic disturbance and pharmacology of the available drugs. The principal hemodynamic effects include changes in heart rate (chronotropism), contractility (inotropism), myocardial conduction velocity (dromotropism), rhythm, and peripheral vascular dilatation or constriction. The last effect influences preload and afterload.

Most commonly used adrenergic amines activate both α and β receptors (Table 7-11). The exceptions are phenylephrine and methoxamine, which are predominately α agonists, and isoproterenol, which is exclusively a β agonist. Each catecholamine has a distinctive effect, qualitatively and quantitatively, on the myocardium and peripheral vasculature. The relative effects of the adrenergic amines on inotropism, chronotropism, and arteriolar-resistance vessels have long been recognized. Table 7-11 demonstrates the relative potencies of the adrenergic amines on the various myocardial and arteriolar adrenergic receptors. This relative potency is often dose dependent, adding still another variable.

The net effect of a sympathomimetic drug is usually defined as the algebraic sum of its relative action on the α, β, and DA receptors.[52] This traditional pharmacologic statement requires further physiologic definition. For many years, the emphasis on catecholamines was focused almost entirely on their actions on the myocardium and on arteriolar resistance vessels. This was in keeping with the preoccupation for maintaining blood pressure. Changes in venous resistance contribute little to total vascular resistance and blood pressure. However, small changes in venous capacitance make large changes in venous return because most of the circulating blood volume is in the venous circulation.[119] Venous return (preload) has repeatedly been demonstrated to be of paramount importance in supporting cardiovascular function, yet the effect of the vasoactive amines on venous capacitance has largely been ignored.[171] The effect of the sympathomimetic amines on the venous circulation appears to be distributive in that acute venular constriction increases the central blood volume (preload), whereas dilatation decreases venous return by the promotion of peripheral pooling.[172, 173] The distributive effect of a catecholamine may be as important as its inotropic action and more important than its arteriolar effect.[43, 174, 175]

Zaimis[51] and Smith and Corbascio[52] reviewed the effect of catecholamines on the venous circulation, but until recently few data have been available. Further definition should elucidate some of the complex and confusing data in the literature generated when clinical observations are limited solely to adrenergic effects on the myocardium and arteriolar vasculature.

TABLE 7-11.   Actions of Catecholamines

CATECHOLAMINES	RECEPTORS						DOSE DEPENDENCE (α, β, or DA)	COMMENTS
	α_1	α_2	β_1	β_2	DA_1	DA_2		
Methoxamine	+ + + + +	?*	0	0	0		0	Vasoconstriction only
Phenylephrine	+ + + + +	?	±	0	0		+ +	Primarily vasoconstriction
Norepinephrine	+ + + + +	+ + + + +	+ + +	0	0		+ + +	β_2 effect *present* but not seen clinically
Metaraminol	+ + + + +	?	+ + +	0	0		+ + +	Releases norepinephrine
Epinephrine	+ + + + +	+ + +	+ + + +	+ +	0		+ + + +	
Ephedrine	+ +	?	+ + +	+ +	0		+ +	Direct and indirect
Mephentermine	0 to + +	?	+ + + +	+ ?	0		+ +	Cerebral stimulation
Dopamine	+ to + + + + +	?	+ + + +	+ +	+ + +	?	+ + + + +	
Dobutamine	0 to +	?	+ + + +	+ +	0		+ +	Inotropism greater than chronotropism
Prenalterol	+		+ + + +	+ +			+	
Isoproterenol	0	0	+ + + + +	+ + + + +	0		0	

* Clinical significance of the effects of agonism and antagonism are not yet known.

The catecholamines exert potent constrictor effects on the resistance and capacitance vessels in addition to their effects on capillary sphincters.[176, 177] Intravenous and intraarterial infusions of epinephrine in humans has been shown to cause marked constriction of the veins.[178] Arteriolar vasoconstriction precedes venoconstriction; however, stroke volume does not increase until the onset of venoconstriction.[120] Sharpey-Shafer and Ginsburg have concluded that the initial increase in cardiac output seen with the infusion of epinephrine is more an effect of increased preload than an arteriolar or direct cardiac effect.[179] NE produces a similar effect, but the onset of venoconstriction is slower.

Zimmerman et al.[180] noted a differential ability of the amines to constrict veins. The data are expressed as the average percentage contribution of venous resistance to total change in vascular resistance (Table 7-12). Note in Table 7-11 that methoxamine and NE are considered equipotent α_1-arteriolar vasoconstrictors; however, these effects differ dramatically from their effects on venoconstriction shown in Table 7-12. Venoconstriction contributes little to the overall increase in total resistance with methoxamine, whereas NE produces a marked venoconstriction. The lack of venoconstrictor response to methoxamine has been demonstrated in humans.

Schmid et al.[181] performed a similar study in humans and found similar results. Table 7-13 is the result of their study of the relative potencies of several catecholamines on resistance versus capacitance vessels. These data represent only the relative potencies of the amines within either resistance or capacitance vessels and are not a comparison of potency ratios between the two. Nevertheless, the data point out the marked differences between the agents. NE is the most potent amine with respect to arteriolar and venous constriction. Metaraminol is 1.5 times more potent than phenylephrine in constricting resistance vessels; however, phenylephrine is 1.5 times more effective on capacitance vessels than metaraminol. NE proved to be 12 times more potent than metaraminol in constricting resistance vessels and 24 times more effective in constricting capacitance vessels.

Marino et al.[182] reported the responses of resistance and capacitance vessels to catecholamines in humans while on cardiopulmonary bypass (Table 7-14). This is a unique method of examining hemodynamic drug response because flow rate (cardiac output) is fixed, excluding the myocardial effects of the drugs. Changes in resistance or capacitance are reflected as either changes in pressure or reservoir volume, respectively. The α agonist phenylephrine produced a marked decrease in venous capacitance (venoconstriction). Arteriolar resistance increased also, but to a lesser degree, confirming the study by Schmid et al. Isoproterenol reduced arteriolar and venous resistance in a manner similar to the α antagonist phentolamine. Surprisingly, dopamine produces significant venoconstriction at doses that produce no direct arteriolar or cardiac effect, confirming studies of dopamine in animals.[175, 183, 184]

An in vitro study by DeMay and Vanhoutte[185] compared the effects of sympathetic agonists on rings of arterial and venous vessels from dogs. Their data were similar to that in Table 7-13. NE was the most potent arterial and venous constrictor, and relative sensitivity of the arterioles to phenylephrine and methoxamine was also similar. Their data, however, indicated that methoxamine had greater venoconstrictor effect than that demonstrated in humans. Nevertheless, their study demonstrated that the differences in response between veins and arteries lay in the uneven distribution of postjunctional α_1 and α_2 receptors. Their results indicate the presence of both receptors on venous smooth muscle, whereas arterial smooth muscle cells contain mainly postjunctional α_1 receptors.

Arterial or venous vasoconstriction (α_1) influences cardiac output in several ways that may be antagonistic.[31] An acute increase in arteriolar adrenergic (α_1) tone increases peripheral vascular resistance, imposes additional afterload, and may reduce cardiac output. Arteriolar vasodilatation produces opposite effects. Venous return can be increased by increasing volume or reducing venous capacitance. Therefore, acute venoconstriction, also an α_1 effect, increases preload and increases cardiac output within the limits of the contractile state of the myocardium, an effect opposite that of α_1-arteriolar constriction. Acute venodilation, a β_2 effect, reduces venous return and may reduce cardiac output, as does venous pooling following α blockade.

The ratio of arteriolar resistance to venous resistance is important in adjusting cardiac output. Each catecholamine has a distinctive effect, qualitatively and quantitatively, on each vascular region.[43] Therefore, a knowledge of each drug's action in altering the ratio of arteriolar to venous resistance is of great importance in drug selection. A drug that increases preload, even though it possesses good inotropic properties, may not be appropriate in the treatment of cardiac failure with high filling pressures. It might be more appropriately used in a distributive shock syndrome such as sepsis. Venoconstriction and arteriolar constriction are both α_1 effects, but have

TABLE 7-12.   Average Percentages of Contributions of Increments in Venous Resistance to Increments in Total Resistance ($\Delta VR/\Delta TR \times 100$)

AGENT	$\Delta VR/\Delta TR \times 100$
Norepinephrine	13.8
Tyramine	8.0
Metaraminol	7.2
Ephedrine	3.3
Mephentermine	1.9
Phenylephrine	1.8
Methoxamine	1.4

(After Zimmerman BG, Abboud FN, Eckstein JW: Comparison of the effects of sympathomimetic amines upon venous and total vascular resistance in the foreleg of the dog. J Pharmacol Exp Ther 139:290, 1963)

TABLE 7-13.   Relative Potencies of Several Sympathomimetic Amines in Humans with Respect to Constrictor Effects on Resistance Vessels and Capacitance Vessels

RESISTANCE VESSELS		CAPACITANCE VESSELS	
Drug	Relative Potency	Drug	Relative Potency
Norepinephrine	1.0000	Norepinephrine	1.0000
Metaraminol	0.0874	Phenylephrine	0.0570
Phenylephrine	0.0684	Metaraminol	0.0419
Tyramine	0.0148	Methoxamine	0.0068
Mephentermine	0.0049	Ephedrine	0.0025
Ephedrine	0.0020	Tyramine	0.0023
Methoxamine	0.0018	Mephentermine	0.0023

(After Schmid PG, Eckstein JW, Abboud FM: Comparison of the effects of several sympathomimetic amines on resistance and capacitance vessels in the forearm of man. Circulation 34:III-209, 1966)

widely divergent effects on cardiac output. Proper drug selection, therefore, cannot be made solely on the basis of the net α and β effect.

Table 7-15 is a summary of the available data on the relative potencies of the amines on the α_1 receptors of the resistance and capacitance vessels. Scant data permit inaccuracies, but the table is derived from sources that demonstrate remarkable consistency. It is offered as a clinical guide to drug selection. The peripheral α receptors of both resistance and capacitance vessels subserve vasoconstriction, but with divergent effects on afterload and preload; therefore, the α_1 receptors have been subdivided into α_1 arterial (α_{1a}) and α_1 venous (α_{1v}). Note that methoxamine and phenylephrine, both pure α drugs, are equipotent arterial vasoconstrictors. Phenylephrine, however, is a potent venous constrictor, but methoxamine has virtually no effect on the capacitance vessels. Dopamine has a potent venoconstrictor (α_{1v}) effect at doses where few α_{1a} or β_1 effects are noted.

DRUG DOSAGE AND ADVERSE EFFECTS. The major adverse effects of the sympathomimetic amines are related to excessive α or β activity. The potential for harm can be understood in terms of receptor characteristics. Excessive β_1 activity may increase contractility but increase heart rate and myocar-

TABLE 7-14. Effects of Drugs Administered Intraarterially on Perfusion Pressure and Oxygenator Blood Volume During Cardiopulmonary Bypass (Mean $\pm$ SD and Range)

DRUG	NUMBER OF PATIENTS	CHANGE IN PERFUSION PRESSURE (mm Hg)	CHANGE IN VOLUME IN OXYGENATOR RESERVOIR (ml)
Controls	10	-0.1 ± 4.0 (-8 to $+5$)	$+20 \pm 133$ (-200 to $+300$)
Phenylephrine, 0.3 mg	12	$+23 \pm 7.0$† ($+7$ to $+38$)	$+247 \pm 149$† (-50 to $+550$)
Isoproterenol, 0.08 mg	11	-13 ± 6.0† (-5 to -22)	-25 ± 139 (-250 to $+250$)
Dopamine, 0.2 mg	8	$+0.13 \pm 0.9$ (-2 to $+3$)	$+444 \pm 76$† (0 to $+750$)
Dopamine, 4 mg	5	$+15 \pm 5.0$* ($+9$ to $+23$)	$+687 \pm 102$† ($+600$ to $+850$)
Phentolamine, 10 mg, and dopamine, 0.2 mg	5	$+0.2 \pm 2.2$ (-3 to $+2$)	-20 ± 33 (-50 to $+25$)
Phentolamine, 10 mg, and phenylephrine, 0.3 mg	5	0.0 ± 2.0 (-3 to $+2$)	$+20 \pm 76$ (-100 to $+100$)

* Significant, $P < 0.005$ by t test for paired replicates.
† Significant, $P < 0.001$.
(Reprinted with permission. Marino RJ, Alexander R, Keats AS: Selective vasoconstriction by dopamine in comparison with isoproterenol and phenylephrine. Anesthesiology 43:570, 1975)

TABLE 7-15. Comparison of Relative α_1 Catecholamine Responses on Peripheral Resistance and Capacitance Vessels*

VASOCONSTRICTION			
Alpha₁ Arterial (α_{1a})		Alpha₁ Venous (α_{1v})	
Norepinephrine	$+ + + + +$	Norepinephrine	$+ + + + +$
Metaraminol	$+ + + + +$	Phenylephrine	$+ + + + +$
Phenylephrine	$+ + + +$	Metaraminol	$+ + + +$
Methoxamine	$+ + +$	Dopamine	$+ + +$
Epinephrine	$0 - + + + +$†	Epinephrine	$0 - + + + +$†
Dopamine	$0 - + + + +$‡	Ephedrine	$+ + +$
Ephedrine	$+ +$	Mephentermine	$+ ?$
Mephentermine	$+ +$	Methoxamine	$0 - + ?$
Dobutamine	$0?$	Dobutamine	$?$
Isoproterenol	0	Isoproterenol	0

* Drugs are listed in descending order of potency within each vascular region.
† Dose dependent; β effects of epinephrine predominate at low doses.
‡ Dose dependent; DA and β effects predominate at low doses.
(Reprinted with permission. Lawson NW, Wallfisch HK: Cardiovascular pharmacology: A new look at the "pressors." In Stoelting RK, Barash PG, Gallagher TJ [eds]: Advances in Anesthesia, p 195. Chicago, Year Book Medical Publishers, 1986)

dial oxygen consumption beyond supply. Severe cardiac dysrhythmias are a frequent companion of excess β_1 activity as a result of increased conduction velocity, automaticity, and ischemia. The β_2 activity has the potential to increase cardiac output by reducing resistance (afterload) while reducing blood pressure. An excessive decrease in diastolic pressure, however, reduces coronary perfusion and may further aggravate myocardial ischemia. The β_1 and β_2 effects of adrenergic agonists are more useful clinically than α_1 effects and can be used for longer periods of time. Unfortunately, it is difficult to separate the inotropic, dromotropic, and chronotropic effects in the clinical setting. The characteristics of the ideal positive inotropic agent are listed in Table 7-16 for comparison with each drug as it is discussed.[31]

Drugs with prominent α_1-agonist effects may produce a desirable increase in blood pressure, but reduce total flow due to increases in arteriolar resistance. A more prominent α_1-venous constriction may improve cardiac output by increasing preload or precipitate failure if preload exceeds the contractile limits of the myocardium. An increase in afterload increases myocardial oxygen consumption, produces ischemia of other organs, reduces renal blood flow, and produces dangerous increases in coronary artery resistance.[186]

In general, the α effects of the sympathomimetics are of benefit only when used for specific indications and for the briefest possible time. Other measures are usually more effective in improving flow and are indicated before a pressor should be used. The only time an adrenergic amine should be used as a pressor or in pressor-dose-range without consideration of flow is when arterial perfusion pressure must be increased immediately to prevent imminent death or morbidity.[187] Cardiopulmonary resuscitation is the primary example where a pressor effect is necessary to create diastolic coronary perfusion during closed- or open-heart massage. Any drug with strong α-agonist properties seems equally effective in this regard. Epinephrine, with its added β properties, is the first-line drug for this situation. Drugs that vasodilate, such as isoproterenol, have little use in this setting even if they possess inotropic properties.[7] Another situation in which a vasoconstrictor may be justified as a temporary measure is hypotension when cerebral, coronary, or extracorporeal bypass perfusion pressure is the prime consideration.

The prolonged use of adrenergic agonists with strong α properties commonly results in tachyphylaxis. This phenomenon is probably due to increasing plasma volume loss through ischemic capillaries and "down regulation" of the adrenergic receptors. Precapillary sphincters are under local

myogenic control and relax when hypoxic and acidotic, despite strong α stimulation. Postcapillary sphincters are more functional in a hypoxic and acidotic milieu, but are under stronger central neurogenic control. Continued postcapillary tone in the face of precapillary relaxation increases hydrostatic pressure with a net loss of intravascular volume. These events are just a few of the explanations for the once-mysterious "levophed shock," in which cases patients were unable to be weaned from NE infusions.[51, 55]

Dopamine is the only clinically available example of a DA agonist. This property has been put to effective clinical use in reducing resistance in the mesenteric and renal beds, mediating an improvement in perfusion of these regions in the low-flow state. Few complications have been ascribed to dopamine when used solely for this purpose.[85]

LOW-OUTPUT SYNDROME. Cardiac output is dependent on the integration of synchrony, heart rate, contractility, afterload, and preload. Synchrony of atrioventricular contraction is an additional determinant when cardiac dysrhythmias develop (Fig. 7-22). Note that blood pressure is not among the factors that determine cardiac output; rather, it is the product of cardiac output and not the cause.

Patients with the low-cardiac-output syndrome have abnormalities of either the heart, the blood volume, or the blood flow distribution.[188] Those remaining in this state for more than 1 h usually have dysfunction of all three components. Modern hemodynamic monitoring has pinpointed hypovolemia, relative or absolute, as the most common cause of the low-output syndrome, regardless of the etiology.[188, 189] The use of a vasopressor or vasoconstrictor drug is rarely, if ever, warranted in absolute hypovolemia. Initial treatment with adrenergic amines in this setting is likely to delay volume repletion and potentiate the shock state. The proper hemodynamic management of septic shock, the most commonly seen distributive abnormality, remains controversial, but volume repletion is the primary consideration. Likewise, the initial treatment of cardiac dysfunction is optimum volume replacement because hypovolemia is a frequent accompaniment of impaired myocardial performance. Ventricular performance may be improved solely on the basis of increased preload and the Frank-Starling mechanism.

The treatment of cardiogenic shock is an excellent example of the low-flow state that requires multiple ANS interventions common to other forms of the low-output syndrome. Figure 7-23 demonstrates the cascade of events following the loss of ventricular contractility due to myocardial infarction with left ventricular dysfunction.[190] As depicted, the condition worsens in a cyclic manner. One could draw this same cascade of dysfunction beginning with any of the five determinants of cardiac output (Fig. 7-22). The ideal drug for the condition depicted in Figure 7-23 would improve inotropism and reduce afterload without increasing chronotropism. Figure 7-24 depicts the theoretical reversal of this cascade with the ideal agent.

Table 7-17 presents one approach to the management of cardiogenic shock listed in order of relative importance. The use of sympathomimetic support is placed in proper perspective. It emphasizes the essential role that invasive hemodynamic monitoring and volume management play in confirming a diagnosis of cardiogenic failure.[31] Although volume expansion and reduction of afterload may improve cardiac output, other pharmacologic interventions may still be necessary to optimize cardiac output and its distribution. Invasive monitoring is a prerequisite for the rational use of the vasoactive drugs to (1) establish that a sympathomimetic is neces-

TABLE 7-16.   Characteristics of the Ideal Positive Inotropic Agent

Enhances contractile state by increasing velocity and force of myocardial fiber shortening
Lacks tolerance
Does not produce vasoconstriction
No cardiac dysrhythmias
Does not affect heart rate
Controllability—immediate onset and termination of action
Elevates perfusion pressure by raising cardiac output rather than systemic vascular resistance
Redistributes blood flow to vital organs
Direct acting—not dependent on release of endogenous amines
Compatible with other vasoactive drugs
Effective orally or parenterally

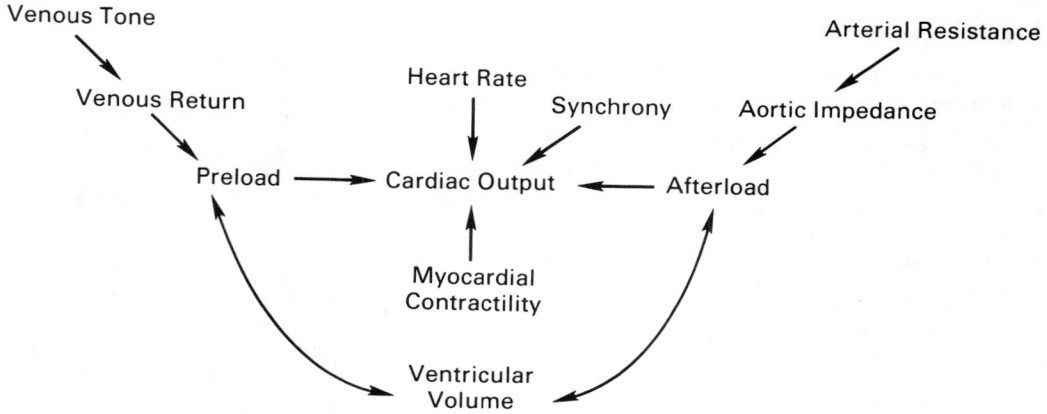

FIG. 7-22. The four principal factors determining cardiac output are demonstrated. Synchrony of atrioventricular contraction is an additional factor becoming important with the development of cardiac dysrhythmias. (Reprinted with permission. Lawson NW, Wallfisch HK: Cardiovascular pharmacology: A new look at the "pressors." In Stoelting RK, Barash PG, Gallagher TJ [eds]: Advances in Anesthesia, p 195. Chicago, Year Book Publishers, 1986)

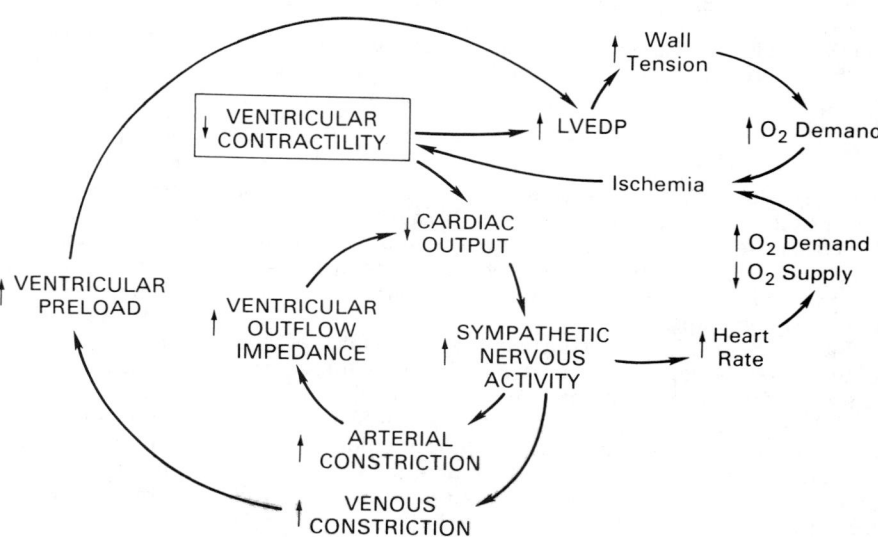

FIG. 7-23. The low-cardiac-output syndrome may be precipitated by a reduction in myocardial contractility. This example depicts the cascade of events following decreased contractility secondary to a myocardial infarction. The primary insult produces a reduction in cardiac output, increased left ventricular end-diastolic pressure, and a host of reflex responses. Any dysfunction of the five determinants of cardiac output could be entered in this same cascade. As depicted, the failure worsens in a cyclic manner. (Redrawn with permission. Evans DB, Weishaar RE, Kaplan HR: Strategy for the discovery and development of a positive inotropic agent. Pharmacol Ther 16:303, 1982)

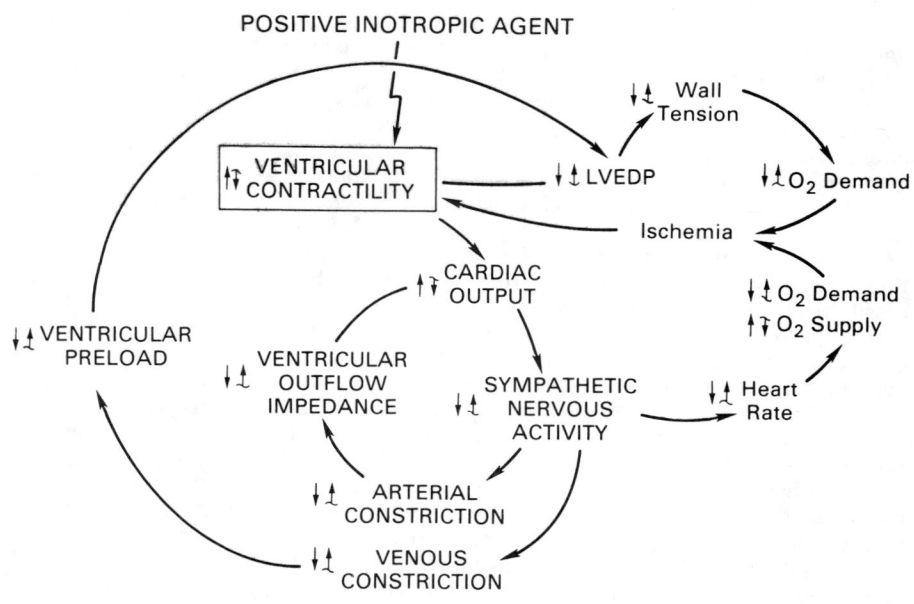

FIG. 7-24. Reversal of heart failure by intervention ($\updownarrow$) with the ideal positive inotropic agent is depicted. (Reprinted with permission. Evans DB, Weishaar RE, Kaplan HR: Strategy for the discovery and development of a positive inotropic agent. Pharmacol Ther 16:303, 1982)

TABLE 7-17.   Management of Low-Output Syndrome Due to Myocardial Dysfunction

1. Assure adequate ventilation and oxygenation
2. Relieve pain and symptoms of recurrent ischemia
3. Hemodynamic monitoring (pulmonary artery, pulmonary capillary wedge, and arterial pressures; urine output; cardiac output)
4. Optimize left ventricular filling pressure
5. Correct metabolic abnormalities
6. Control dysrhythmias (#2. priority if life threatening)
7. Pharmacologic support
   a. Diuretics
   b. Inotropic drugs
   c. Vasodilators
8. Rule out "correctable" causes of shock (septal or left-ventricle rupture, mitral regurgitation, acute aneurysm)
9. Mechanical support of circulation
10. Surgical correction if possible

Note: Hemodynamic monitoring is essential in confirming a diagnosis, optimizing filling pressures and cardiac output, selecting pharmacologic support, and avoiding complications. Adjustment of left ventricular filling pressure may require additional volume or a relative volume reduction with vasodilators. The diagnostic criteria for cardiogenic shock are not met until step 4 is accomplished.

sary; (2) select drugs for the hemodynamic condition; (3) follow resultant hemodynamic changes, because many of the beneficial effects of the catecholamines are hidden to the clinical eye; and (4) avoid complications of pressor therapy that are visible to all. Drug selection for the low-output state remains the most enigmatic.

Table 7-18 is a summary of the hemodynamic effects of some of the currently popular and once popular sympathomimetic drugs.[31] Many of the hemodynamic effects are dose related. The dose ranges are listed and a standard infusion rate is cited. Standard rates of infusion are simply guidelines, and the actual dose administered should be determined by patient response. The doses are calculated assuming the use of calibrated infusors in which 60 drops equals 1 ml.

METHOXAMINE AND PHENYLEPHRINE. Methoxamine is the prototype pure vasoconstrictor, or α-stimulating drug. Phenylephrine produces similar actions, but there are important clinical differences. Table 7-11 demonstrates that methoxamine possesses only α_1 properties, and Table 7-15 demonstrates that it produces almost no venoconstriction (α_{1v}). Its only pharmacologic effects are to increase arterial resistance, increase afterload, and reduce flow even though blood pressure is elevated. Few clinical uses for methoxamine remain. It has been useful for treating paroxysmal atrial tachycardias (PAT). A single intravenous dose of methoxamine can break a PAT reflexly through baroreceptor stretch, obviating the necessity for digitalis or countershock (see Table 7-18). Carotid massage produces similar results by a similar mechanism. The calcium channel blockers will likely displace methoxamine even further in this regard.

Table 7-15 demonstrates that phenylephrine, considered a pure α drug, increases venous more than arterial constriction.[181, 182] Venous constriction may be its most redeeming feature when compared with the purely arteriolar effect of methoxamine. Acutely, this favors venous return (preload), even though arterial resistance (afterload) also increases. The net effect may produce an increase in pressure and flow. Phenylephrine, like methoxamine, does not change cardiac output in normal individuals but does cause a decreased output in patients with ischemic heart disease.[55] It is rarely necessary to give a pure α pressor for extended periods, but phenylephrine has continued to receive favor in operating rooms to sustain pressure during cardiopulmonary bypass as well as during cerebral and peripheral vascular procedures.[191] It does not produce cardiac dysrhythmias as a direct effect. Phenylephrine is also useful in reversing right-to-left shunt in tetralogy of Fallot when patients are having "spells" during anesthesia.[31, 43] A dose of 2 $\mu g \cdot kg^{-1}$ iv "push" may be used. The arterial vasoconstrictors may produce favorable effects on the size of an ischemic injury when used in conjunction with intraaortic balloon pumping or nitroglycerin.[192]

NOREPINEPHRINE AND METARAMINOL. NE and metaraminol produce hemodynamic effects that are similar. Both have been widely used for the treatment of cardiogenic shock. NE is the naturally occurring mediator of the SNS and the immediate precursor of epinephrine. It produces direct-acting hemodynamic effects on the α and β receptors in a dose-related manner when given in an exogenous infusion. Metaraminol possesses direct action but acts primarily by causing release of stored endogenous NE. Both drugs produce increases in cardiac output and blood pressure when given in small doses (Table 7-18), primarily as a result of predominant β action at this level.[193] Larger doses reduce flow as α-arteriolar constriction supersedes the β effects. Reflex bradycardias may occur, as with methoxamine and phenylephrine, despite active β_1 stimulation.

Objections to the use of NE (or metaraminol) for the treatment of cardiogenic shock are based on two considerations: (1) vasoconstriction increases the pressure work of the left ventricle, with an adverse effect on the oxygen economy of the already ischemic pump; and (2) these drugs cause further vasoconstriction and organ ischemia in a syndrome in which intense constriction may have already occurred.[55] The use of NE or metaraminol requires the use of invasive monitoring; otherwise, complications are to be expected. It is not usually necessary to elevate the systolic blood pressure above 90–100 mm Hg. At this level of infusion, the cardiac output will normally be increased as a β effect without excessive peripheral vasoconstriction. Both drugs are potent venoconstrictors, which should alter interpretation of venous filling pressures as a guide to adequate volume repletion.

NE remains a useful agent because its effects are predictable, prompt, and potent. Metaraminol is neither as prompt nor as potent as NE. Metaraminol can be given im or iv without causing necrosis, which is commonly seen with the continued use of NE. Benefits of metaraminol are limited, however, because it is thought to depend on tissue NE levels for its efficacy. It loses its effectiveness during prolonged use as it displaces NE and replaces it as a false transmitter. It may also not be effective initially in patients who are receiving catechol depleters. Other undesirable effects associated with the use of NE and metaraminol include renal arteriolar constriction and aggravation of oliguria. In addition, prolonged therapy may produce a reduction in plasma volume as a result of fluid transudation at the capillary level. Indeed, in some instances, cardiogenic shock requiring continuous NE infusions has been reversed by fluid infusions.[55] The use of the minimal effective dose of these drugs in combination with careful invasive monitoring and attention to fluid management is the only way to avoid iatrogenic disasters.

EPINEPHRINE. Epinephrine is the prototypical endogenous catecholamine. It is synthesized, stored, and released from

TABLE 7-18. Dose Schedule and Hemodynamic Effects of the Sympathomimetic Amines

HEMODYNAMICS: ↑ = Increase; ↓ = Decrease; − = No change

DRUG Listed From α to β	DOSAGES IV Push Adults	DOSAGES IV Infusion*	α₁art	α₁ven	β₁	β₂	DA	CO	Inotrop	HR	VR	TPR	RBF
Methoxamine / Phenylephrine	5–10 mg / 50–100 μg	Not Recommended (N/R); a. 10 mg/250 ml; b. 40 μg·ml⁻¹; c. 0.15–0.75 μg·kg⁻¹·min⁻¹; d. 0.15 μg·kg⁻¹·min⁻¹	++++	0-+?	0	0	0	−→	−	Reflex ↓	−	↑	↓
Norepinephrine	(N/R)	a. 4 mg/250 ml; b. 16 μg·ml⁻¹; c. 0.1–0.4 μg·kg⁻¹·min⁻¹; d. 0.1 μg·kg⁻¹·min⁻¹	++++	+++++	0	0	0	−↓	−	Reflex ↓	↑↑↑	↑↑	−↓
Metaraminol	(N/R)	a. 100 mg/250 ml; b. 400 μg·ml⁻¹; c. 0.5–7 μg·kg⁻¹·min⁻¹; d. 0.5 μg·kg⁻¹·min⁻¹	+++	+++	++++	?+	0	↑−↓	↑	Reflex ↓	↑↑↑	↑↑↑	↓↓
Epinephrine	0.3–0.5 ml 1:1000 (0.3 to 0.5 mg) SubQ—Asthma; IV—Anaphylaxis; 5 ml 1:10,000 (0.5 mg) Cardiac arrest Q 5 min.	a. 1 mg/250 ml; b. 4 μg·ml⁻¹; c. 0.01–0.03 μg·kg⁻¹·min⁻¹; 0.03–0.15 μg·kg⁻¹·min⁻¹; 0.15–0.30 μg·kg⁻¹·min⁻¹; d. 0.015 μg·kg⁻¹·min⁻¹	+ / +++ / +++++ / +	+ / +++ / +++++ / +	++++ / ++++ / +++	++++ / ++++	0	−→	↑	Reflex ↓	↑↑	↑↑↑	↑↑↑
Ephedrine / Mephentermine	5–10 mg / 15–30 mg	(N/R); a. 500 mg/250 ml; b. 2000 μg·ml⁻¹; c. 4–8 μg·kg⁻¹·min⁻¹	++	+++	+++	++	0	↑	↑	↑	↑−	↑	↑→
Dopamine**	(N/R)	a. 200 mg/250 ml; b. 800 μg·ml⁻¹; 0.5–5 μg·kg⁻¹·min⁻¹; c. 2–10 μg·kg⁻¹·min⁻¹; 10 μg·kg⁻¹·min⁻¹†	0-++ / +?	+?	++++	+?	0 / +++++ / +++++	↑	↑	↑	↑?	↑	↓−↑
Dobutamine**	(N/R)	d. 2 μg·kg⁻¹·min⁻¹; a. 250 mg/250 ml; b. 1000 μg·ml⁻¹; c. 2–30 μg·kg⁻¹·min⁻¹	+ / +++++	+++	+++ / +++++ / +	++ / +++++ / +++++	0 / +++++	↑↑−↓	−−↑−↑	−↑−↑−	↑−↓−	−↑−↑−	↑−↓−
Isoproterenol	0.4 mg (0.2 ml of 2 μg·ml⁻¹ solution) Third Degree Heart Block	c. 0.15 μg·kg⁻¹·min⁻¹ to desired effect; d. 0.015 μg·kg⁻¹·min⁻¹; a. 1 mg/250 ml; b. 4 μg·ml⁻¹	0-+	?	+++++ +++++	+++++ +++++	0	↑↑ −↓	↑↑ ↑↑↑	−↑ ↑↑↑	? ↓	− ↓	−↑

*a. Mixture
b. Concentration μg·ml⁻¹
c. Dose range μg·kg⁻¹·min⁻¹
d. Standard rate infusion
†"Rule of Six"

**Dopamine and Dobutamine employ the same doses. Dosage of either may quickly be calculated by multiplying patients' weight (kg) × 6 = Mg added to 100 ml D5%W. The number of drops delivered through a calibrated infusor (60 drops = 1 ml) will be the number of μg·kg⁻¹·min⁻¹ infused into the patient. Example: 70 kg × 6 = 420; 420 mg/100 ml = 4200 μg·ml⁻¹ or 70 μg/gtt; 5 μg·kg⁻¹·min⁻¹ = 5 gtts/min.

CO = cardiac output; INOTROP = contractility; HR = heart rate; VR = venous return (preload); TPR = peripheral resistance (afterload); RBF = renal blood flow.

(Reprinted with permission. Lawson NW, Wallfisch HK: Cardiovascular pharmacology: A new look at the "pressors." In Stoelting RK, Barash PG, Gallagher TJ [eds]: Advances in Anesthesia, p 195. Chicago, Year Book Medical Publishers, 1986)

the adrenal medulla and is the key hormonal element in the fight-or-flight response. It is the most widely used catecholamine in medicine. Epinephrine is used to treat asthma, anaphylaxis, cardiac arrest, and bleeding and to prolong regional anesthesia. The cardiovascular effects of epinephrine, when given systemically, result from its direct stimulation of both α and β receptors. This is dose dependent and is outlined in Table 7-18.

The effect of epinephrine on the peripheral vasculature is mixed.[195] It has predominantly α-stimulating effects in some beds (skin, mucosa, and kidney) and β-stimulating actions in others (skeletal muscle). These effects are also dose dependent. At therapeutic doses, β-adrenergic effects predominate on the peripheral vessels, and total resistance may be reduced. Constriction, however, is maintained in the renal and cutaneous areas because of its dominant α effect in these areas. An increase in cardiac output with epinephrine may therefore be due to a redistribution of blood to low-resistance vessels in the muscle, but with further reduction in flow to vital organs. Cardiac dysrhythmias are a prominent hazard, and the strong chronotropic effects of epinephrine have limited its use or systematic investigation in the treatment of cardiogenic shock. In contrast, it is frequently used for cardiac failure after open-heart surgery.

Some volatile anesthetics sensitize the myocardium to circulating catecholamines and induce cardiac dysrhythmias. This is especially true in the presence of hypoxia and hypercarbia. Halothane has the most pronounced cardiac-sensitizing action of the volatile anesthetics in use today. The mechanism has been thought to be related to the stimulation of α- and β-adrenergic receptors, since blockade of these receptors consistently abolishes these cardiac dysrhythmias.[196, 197] However, Kapur and Flacke demonstrated that calcium channel blockade is equally effective.[198] This is not surprising if the shared final pathway of β and calcium-entry blockade proves to be correct (see Fig. 7-15).[199] The exact mechanism is further confused by studies showing that the myocardial depression produced by the volatile anesthetics is related to blockade of the slow-calcium current.[200] These findings are compatible with the observations that β blockade, calcium blockade, and general anesthetics produce myocardial depression.[201]

Intravenous and locally infiltrated adrenergic drugs should be used cautiously during inhalational anesthesia, especially with halothane. The following schedule has been found relatively safe during halothane anesthesia.[196]

1. Epinephrine concentrations no greater than 1 : 100,000 to 1 : 200,000 (1 : 200,000 = 5 μg·ml^{-1})
2. Adult dose should be no greater than 10 ml of 1 : 100,000 or 20 ml of 1 : 200,000 within 10 min
3. Total should not exceed 30 ml of 1 : 100,000 (60 ml of 1 : 200,000) within 1 h.

In another report, the dose of submucosally injected epinephrine necessary to produce ventricular cardiac dysrhythmias in 50% of patients anesthetized with a 1.25 MAC concentration of a volatile anesthetic was 2.1, 3.4, and 6.7 μg·kg^{-1} during administration of halothane, enflurane, and isoflurane, respectively.[201] The incidence of cardiac dysrhythmias was abolished when this dose was halved in patients anesthetized with halothane or isoflurane. In contrast with adults, children seem to tolerate higher doses of subcutaneous epinephrine without developing cardiac dysrhythmias.[202]

EPHEDRINE. Ephedrine is one of the most commonly used noncatecholamine, sympathomimetic agents in the practice of anesthesia. It is used extensively for treating hypotension following spinal or epidural anesthesia. Ephedrine stimulates both α and β receptors by direct and indirect actions. It is predominately an indirect-acting pressor, producing its effects by causing NE release.[55] Tachyphylaxis develops rapidly and is probably related to the depletion of NE stores with repeated injection.[195] The cardiovascular effects of ephedrine (Table 7-18) are nearly identical to those of epinephrine, but less potent.[51, 52] Its effects are sustained about ten times longer than epinephrine.

Ephedrine remains the pressor of choice in obstetrics because uterine blood flow improves linearly with blood pressure.[124, 125] This effect is probably not related to its arteriolar vasoconstriction but rather its venoconstrictive action. Ephedrine is a weak, indirect-acting sympathomimetic agent that produces venoconstriction to a greater degree than arteriolar constriction[172, 174] (Table 7-15). This may be its most important and unappreciated effect. It causes a redistribution of blood centrally, improves venous return (preload), increases cardiac output, and restores uterine perfusion. The mild β action restores heart rate simultaneously with improved venous return. An increased blood pressure is noted as a result, rather than a cause, of these events. Mild α$_1$-arteriolar constriction does occur, but the net effect of improving venous return and heart rate is increased cardiac output. Uterine blood flow is spared. This response, however, is dependent on the patient's state of hydration.

Dopamine is an attractive alternate vasopressor for obstetrics for similar reasons. It produces strong α$_1$ venoconstriction and volume redistribution at infusion rates at which α$_{1a}$ or β effects are minimal (Table 7-14). The primary disadvantage of dopamine is its lack of immediate availability as an "iv push" drug. It requires more careful titration than ephedrine. The prophylactic administration of ephedrine before spinal blockade in obstetrics can produce misleading clinical estimates of volume status because of its effects on venous return and arterial pressure.

MEPHENTERMINE. Mephentermine is a rarely used, direct- and indirect-acting sympathomimetic agent similar to metaraminol. Agonists with these properties are unpredictable and have largely been replaced by new and more selective agents.[55] Mephentermine has a direct, positive inotropic action on the heart with prolonged action (see Tables 7-11 and 7-18). The peripheral α effects of mephentermine appear to be the result of an indirect release of NE. Its peripheral effects are complex and unpredictable. Discrepancies between experimental and clinical observations are in part due to important differences in the physiologic status of experimental subjects and patients. Mephentermine increases cardiac output, heart rate, and peripheral vascular resistance in normal subjects; however, large doses result in decreases in peripheral resistance in patients in shock. This is presumably a direct vasodilating effect. A pronounced increase in venous return has been noted with mephentermine.[52] This is disputed by the studies of Zimmerman et al.[180] and Schmid et al.,[181] who indicate that mephentermine is a relatively weak venoconstrictor. Table 7-18 indicates its unknown status in this regard.

DOPAMINE. Dopamine is the immediate precursor of NE. The actions of dopamine as a neurotransmitter in the CNS have been well defined. It is also found in high concentrations of the postganglionic nerve terminals of the SNS and in the adrenal gland. Dopamine offers distinct advantages over many sympathomimetics in treating the low-output syndrome.[57] Dopamine is an agonist to all three types of adrenergic receptors, depending on the dosage used (see Table 7-18). This advantageous spectrum of activity is the reason it has become a drug of choice, after volume expanders, in managing shock in the surgical intensive care units.[79, 168] One can select the desired action by alteration of the infusion rate. Dopamine is primarily a direct-acting drug but causes some NE release in its β-dose range. Renal and mesenteric vascular dilatation, mediated through the DA receptors, is produced at infusion rates of 0.5–5 $\mu g \cdot kg^{-1} \cdot min^{-1}$.[85, 92] An increase in cardiac output may be noted at this dose level without a change in blood pressure or heart rate.[203] Improved perfusion is the result of a reduced afterload in the mesenteric vessels and an increased venous return. Note in Table 7-14 that venoconstriction (α_{1v}) occurs at doses at which direct cardiac and peripheral arterial effects are minimal.[182] Increasing doses stimulate β effects, which begin at approximately 2 $\mu g \cdot kg^{-1} \cdot min^{-1}$. The onset of α activity begins around 7 $\mu g \cdot kg^{-1} \cdot min^{-1}$. Infusion rates of 10 $\mu g \cdot kg^{-1} \cdot min^{-1}$ or greater produce more intense α vasoconstriction and may override any beneficial DA or β effects. When vasoconstriction predominates, dopamine behaves as NE.[187]

The distributive effects of dopamine are useful in the surgical patient, in whom sepsis is the most common distributive abnormality.[204] Dopamine can sustain cardiac output and renal and mesenteric function until definitive therapy is successful.[194, 195] Dopamine is a proven cardiotonic drug after open-heart surgery. It facilitates management of patients with heart failure who have had surgery and helps avoid problems related to excessive infusion of intravenous fluids by support of cardiac output and urine excretion.[85, 205] Dopamine increases mean pulmonary artery pressure and is not recommended for patients in right heart failure.[186, 206, 207] Although dopamine is frequently given to patients in cardiogenic shock, its positive inotropic, chronotropic, and vasoconstrictive effects may increase myocardial oxygen demand. Increased venous return may not be desirable in the situation. Adverse effects of dopamine are tachycardia, nausea and vomiting, headache, and angina pectoris. Ventricular cardiac dysrhythmias may become troublesome, although the incidence is less than that with isoproterenol, epinephrine, or NE.[195] Excessive infusion can cause distant gangrene similar to that produced by NE. Dopamine inhibits insulin secretion and may contribute to hyperglycemia in the critically ill.[57] This drug's beneficial effects are best titrated by using invasive monitoring.

DOBUTAMINE. Dobutamine is a synthetic catecholamine that is a modification of isoproterenol, which is derived from dopamine.[55] It is an example of pharmacologic engineering in which modification of a basic molecular structure produces a useful drug. Variations in chemical structure among isoproterenol, dopamine, and dobutamine can be seen in Fig. 7-8. Dobutamine has some clear advantages in certain clinical situations. It acts directly on β-adrenergic receptors, but exerts a much weaker β₂-adrenergic action than isoproterenol.[191] It does not cause NE release or stimulate DA receptors. It produces a positive inotropic effect with minimal changes in heart rate or vascular resistance at standard rates of infusion (see Table 7-18).[56] A positive inotropic effect without a correspondingly strong chronotropic effect is an obvious advantage over isoproterenol. It is not totally devoid of chronotropic action. Dobutamine increases automaticity of the SA node and increases conduction through the AV node and ventricles. Troublesome tachycardias can occur in sensitive individuals, and caution should be exercised in giving dobutamine to patients with established atrial fibrillation and other tachydysrhythmias. Increases in heart rate may be seen at infusion

rates exceeding 10–15 $\mu g \cdot kg^{-1} \cdot min^{-1}$. Increases in cardiac output are primarily through its positive inotropic action and secondarily through reduction in afterload. Changes in arterial blood pressure may not occur. Dobutamine possesses very weak α properties, which can be unmasked by β blockade. Administration of propranolol will produce a prompt and dramatic increase in blood pressure. In the absence of adrenergic blockade, dobutamine increases coronary blood flow by reducing resistance.

With a half-life of 2 min, the controllability of dobutamine is superb. Tachyphylaxis is rare, but may be noted if dobutamine is given for more than 72 h. This drug is to the cardiologist what dopamine is to the surgical intensivist. Dobutamine is of most value in patients with acute or chronic congestive failure from ischemic disease. It has proved to be as effective as dopamine and nitroprusside combined in the treatment of myocardial failure with infarction. Dobutamine is contraindicated in the patient with idiopathic hypertrophic subaortic stenosis.

Like isoproterenol, it seems to inhibit hypoxic pulmonary vasoconstriction.[57, 206, 208] It may, therefore, be useful in managing right ventricular failure following surgery for congenital heart disease or cor pulmonale. This observation requires confirmation.

ISOPROTERENOL. Isoproterenol is a potent balanced β₁- and β₂-receptor agonist with no vasoconstrictor effects. It increases heart rate and contractility while decreasing systemic vascular resistance. Although it can increase cardiac output, it is not useful in shock because it redistributes blood to nonessential areas by its preferential effect on the cutaneous and muscular vessels.[203] As a result, it produces variable and unpredictable results on cardiac output and blood pressure in patients with cardiogenic shock. Isoproterenol is a potent cardiac dysrhythmogenic drug and extends myocardial ischemic areas. Deleterious effects on an evolving ischemic process include cardiac dysrhythmias, tachycardia, and reduced diastolic coronary perfusion pressure and time. Increased myocardial oxygen demand and only modest hemodynamic improvement make it an unattractive drug for patients in shock, especially after acute myocardial infarction.

Isoproterenol helps in cardiac failure associated with bradycardia, asthma, and cor pulmonale. It is also a useful chemical pacemaker in third-degree heart block until either an artificial pacemaker can be inserted or the cause is removed.[195] Chernow et al.[57] and Zaritsky[55] suggest that isoproterenol might be useful in treating both idiopathic and secondary pulmonary hypertension. It has also been reported as useful in improving the forward flow in patients with regurgitant aortic valvular disease, but should not be used if there is an accompanying stenosis.[203, 209]

COMBINATION THERAPY. Many combinations of vasoactive drugs are useful in making fine hemodynamic adjustments in the critically ill.[187] One of the first such combinations was used to prevent tissue necrosis caused by NE that could occur with or without extravasation.[52] Phentolamine, an α blocker (5–10 mg/4 mg of NE), was added to the infusion bottle to prevent the intense vasoconstriction of NE. No hemodynamic data are available from this era describing other possible benefits from the α blockade and afterload reduction of phentolamine.

The available sympathomimetic agents provide a wide range of hemodynamic effects. An even greater spectrum of activity can be achieved by combining different sympathomimetic drugs, or sympathomimetics, with vasodilators. For example, if a larger positive inotropic action and less vasoconstriction are desired, isoproterenol can be added to either dopamine or dobutamine. If an increase in afterload is desirable, the addition of NE to dopamine or dobutamine might be helpful.[210] Combinations are also useful in redistributing blood flow to vital organs despite adequate cardiac output. One of the advantages of dopamine in the surgical patient is its dose-related effect on vascular tone and cardiac contractility. Dopamine improves renal and mesenteric blood flow. Dobutamine may be used to increase global cardiac output, and dopamine can be added to the low-dose range to distribute a higher percentage of the increased cardiac output to the renal bed. Many combinations have been advocated.[123, 140, 193, 210]

α-Adrenergic blocking agents (phenoxybenzamine and phentolamine) have been used in the treatment of shock when intense vasoconstriction prevents the administration of adequate volume for resuscitation.[187, 205] This was often balanced with an inotropic agent to support cardiac output and diastolic blood pressure. Animal studies have shown that cardiac output and renal blood flow increase when dopamine-induced vasoconstriction is attenuated by α blockers. On this basis, vasodilators have been beneficially used in patients experiencing vasoconstriction who did not respond adequately to dopamine alone.[193] Recently, the short-acting vasodilators, sodium nitroprusside and nitroglycerin, have been successfully combined with dopamine or dobutamine. The use of nitroprusside or nitroglycerin improves these patients by reducing afterload. Nitroglycerin is a more potent venodilator than nitroprusside and appears more efficacious in reducing preload. Dobutamine and nitroprusside produce comparable increases in cardiac output in patients with congestive heart failure. When they are infused together, the increase in cardiac output is greater than when either drug is used alone.[193] In addition, there is a greater reduction in pulmonary wedge pressure and pulmonary vascular resistance. This combination improves cardiac output by providing both inotropism and afterload reduction.

During combination therapy, standard rates of infusion as outlined in Table 7-18 no longer apply, and invasive monitoring is mandatory for success. Obviously, it would be simpler to use one drug. Side-effects of combinations must be weighed in terms of the economy of myocardial oxygen balance. A reduction of pressure work by the myocardium and better coronary perfusion may be offset by an increase in inotropic or chronotropic myocardial oxygen consumption.[211]

OTHERS

TOCOLYTICS. The term *tocolytic* simply means to stop labor. Eighty-five per cent of early neonatal deaths that are not related to lethal abnormalities are associated with premature labor.[212] Various pharmacologic agents have been used to: (1) decrease stimulus to the myometrium (alcohol); or (2) prevent myometrial response to stimuli. Drugs belonging to the latter category include opioids, magnesium sulfate, prostaglandin inhibitors, and calcium channel inhibitors. β agonists have now become the focus of research in this area. The principal action of these drugs is to stimulate β_2 receptors of the myometrium and produce relaxation (Table 7-5).[213]

Metaproterenol and isoxsuprine were the first β agonists used successfully. Unfortunately, these drugs are equipotent β_1 and β_2 agonists and the side-effects of tachycardia and hypotension were unacceptable.[214] A second generation of β-adrenergic drugs were applied in which the predominant action is β_2. Ritodrine and terbutaline are receiving widespread use as tocolytic agents because of their predominate β_2

agonism, which minimizes the undesirable β_1 effects. Ritodrine is the only β-agonist tocolytic currently approved in the United States. It was specifically synthesized for this purpose and is structurally related to epinephrine.

All β-agonist tocolytic drugs have both β_1 and β_2 properties, but in different proportions. The circulatory effects will vary from one drug to another depending on the degree of β_1 stimulation. Table 7-19 compares the β_1 cardiovascular effects of ritodrine and terbutaline while being used as tocolytics in humans. The side-effects of these drugs may result in maternal complications that are serious. Predictable complications in pregnant women include hyperglycemia with resultant hypokalemia (Table 7-5).[50] All manner of cardiac dysrhythmias have been described that may be associated with ischemia and chest pain. The occurrence of pulmonary edema following the use of β-agonist tocolytics with and without corticosteroids has been described, although the mechanism is not clear.[215, 216] Table 7-20 outlines contraindications for the use of β drugs for inhibiting labor.[217]

NONADRENERGIC SYMPATHOMIMETIC DRUGS. Table 7-4 classifies the drugs that mimic the SNS into two broad categories, adrenergic or nonadrenergic. Adrenergic agonists exert their action through adrenergic receptors either by direct stimulation or indirectly *via* release of NE. Adrenergic agonists may be catecholamines or noncatecholamines by chemical configuration. Nonadrenergic sympathomimetic drugs also act indirectly by influencing the cAMP–calcium cascade, exclusive of the receptors (see Fig. 7-15). The function of the second messenger (cAMP) and the third messenger (Ca^{++}) nearly always go together.[218, 219] This concept reinforces the recent appreciation of the homogeneity of action of a wide variety of drugs that were previously thought to be unrelated. Sympathomimetics have more pharmacologic similarities than differences.

Xanthines. The clinically important xanthine is theophylline–ethylenediamine (aminophylline).[192] Caffeine is a

TABLE 7-19. Cardiovascular Effects of Ritodrine and Terbutaline[212–214, 217]

HEMODYNAMICS	% CHANGE FROM BASELINE	
	Ritodrine (%)	Terbutaline (%)
Systolic blood pressure	+12	+6
Diastolic blood pressure	−7	−7
Total peripheral resistance	−33	−23
Cardiac output	+50	52
Heart rate	+33	+28
Stroke volume	+20	+15

TABLE 7-20. Contraindications for β Tocolytic Therapy

Eclampsia or severe preeclampsia
Intrauterine infection
Maternal hyperthyroidism
Maternal cardiac disease
Uncontrolled maternal diabetes mellitus
Significant vaginal bleeding
Severe anemia or hypovolemia
Fetal anomaly incompatible with extrauterine life
Death *in utero*

socially important xanthine. Aminophylline has been the mainstay in the treatment of asthma and bronchospasm since 1902 because of its strong β_2-mimetic effect. Epinephrine, isoproterenol, and ephedrine are used for asthma for the same reason. Levels of cAMP in the cell are governed by a magnesium-dependent phosphodiesterase (PDE) (Fig. 7-15). This enzyme catalyzes the second messenger 3'5' cAMP to the less active 5'AMP. Three major PDE enzymes have been discovered that have been designated as PDE I, PDE II, and PDE III.[220] The xanthines are nonspecific PDE inhibitors that interact with all three types. Inhibition of PDE results in increased levels of cAMP and β response (Fig. 7-25). Increases in cAMP by this mechanism are important when reviewing the many complicated interactions of the xanthines in the clinical setting.

Catecholamines influence the accumulation of cAMP by activating adenyl cyclase. Increased catecholamine levels, combined with the xanthines, may lead to synergistic adrenergic activity by increasing production and reducing breakdown of cAMP. Cardiac dysrhythmias are common in such circumstances and are further potentiated during general anesthesia with halothane.[221] Serious cardiac dysrhythmias and arrest have been produced with this combination when not carefully controlled.

Intravenous aminophylline produces an increase in cardiac output as a result of its positive inotropic and chronotropic effects. It also reduces afterload by its β_2-vasodilating effect.[194, 195] The cardiac-stimulating effects are still manifest in the presence of β blockade because the xanthines are not receptor-dependent for their agonism. Thus, they may be temporarily useful in those situations where excessive β blockade has been produced.[50] The inotropic effects are short-lived, lasting 20–30 min. Care must be taken during infusion because common side-effects include hypotension and cardiac dysrhythmias. Seizures have also been reported.[221]

Phosphodiesterase Inhibitors. A new group of drugs has been developed that have pharmacologic properties approaching the characteristics of the ideal inotropic drug (Table 7-16).[190] They are the product of a search for a nonglycosidic, noncatecholamine inotropic agent. These drugs combine positive inotropism with vasodilator activity; like the xanthines, they are PDE inhibitors, but differ in that they selectively inhibit PDE III.[220] PDE I and II hydrolyze all cyclic nucleotides; PDE III acts specifically on cAMP. Amrinone apparently interacts with PDE III at the cell membrane and impedes the breakdown of cAMP by inhibition of PDE III. cAMP levels increase and protein kinases are activated to promote phosphorylation

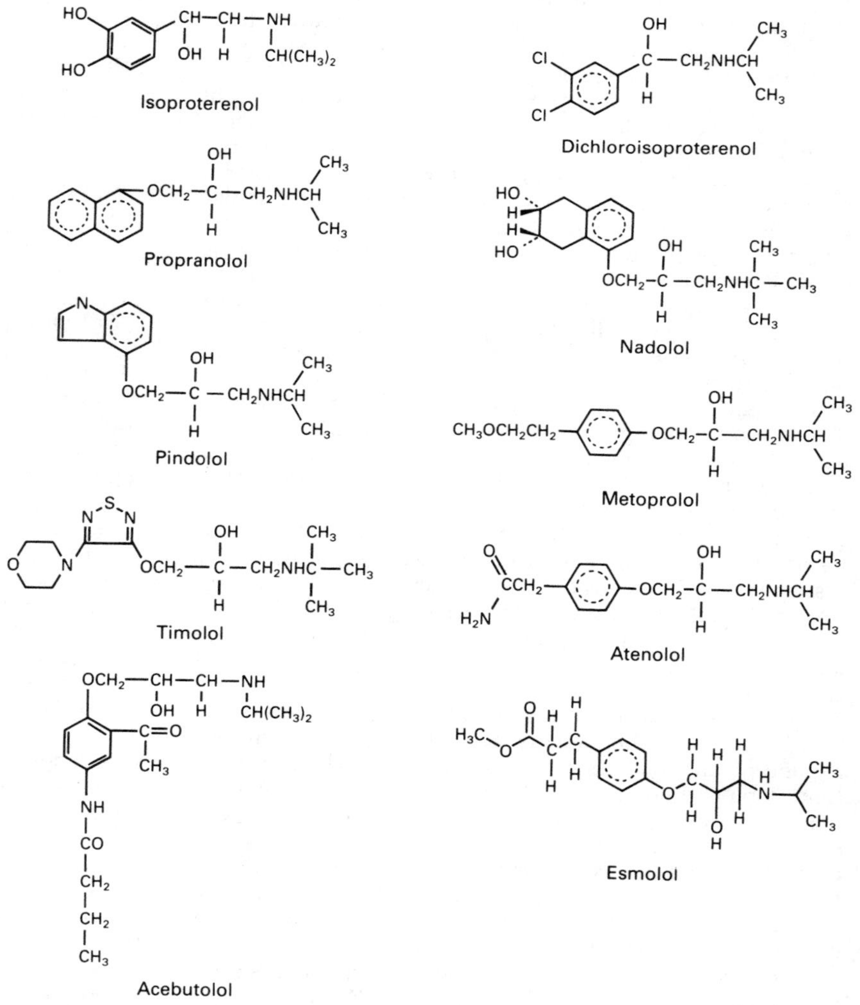

FIG. 7-25. The structures of the commonly used β blockers are compared with the pure β agonist, isoproterenol, and the partial agonist, dichloroisoproterenol.

of the sarcoplasmic reticulum in a cascade manner similar to the adrenergic drugs (Fig. 7-25). In cardiac muscle, phosphorylation increases the slow inward movement of calcium current, promoting increased intracellular calcium stores. Thus, inotropism increases. In vascular smooth muscle, increased cAMP activity accounts for the vasodilatation and decreased peripheral vascular resistance.

A variety of PDE inhibitors are undergoing clinical trials.[222, 223] The relative contribution of inotropism and vasodilatation differs with each. Amrinone is the only PDE inhibitor released for clinical use in the United States. It is the prototypical PDE III inhibitor. The degree of hemodynamic effect of these drugs depends on dose, degree of inotropic reserve, and state of cAMP depletion.

Amrinone is a bipyridine derivative that produces strong inotropic activity and weak vasodilatory effects. The relative contribution of these factors remains a matter of conjecture in congestive heart failure. Amrinone was released in the United States in the fall of 1984 and has had limited clinical usage outside of controlled clinical trials. Clinical experience has been relatively short term and limited to patients with severe congestive heart failure refractory to conventional therapy.

The characteristics of amrinone, compared with those of the ideal inotropic agent (see Fig. 7-24, Table 7-16), rank it very near the ideal drug. It is the first oral inotrope available since the introduction of digitalis.[224] Single-dose and short-term oral and intravenous studies show dose-related improvements at rest in cardiac index and left ventricular stroke index (40–80% increase); left ventricular end-diastolic pressure (40% decrease); pulmonary capillary wedge pressure (16–44% decrease); pulmonary artery pressure (17–33% decrease); right atrial pressure (16–44% decrease); left ventricular ejection fraction (50% increase); and systemic vascular resistance (23–50% decrease). Significantly, heart rate and mean arterial pressure are not affected. Hemodynamic improvement is also noted when amrinone is used in combination with hydralazine. The improvement is greater than with either drug alone. Peak response with an intravenous dose occurs after 5 min and reveals no evidence of tolerance over short-term trials (24 h). It is an effective inotropic agent in patients receiving β blockers. Its efficacy in the patient who has been digitalized has been demonstrated.

Intravenous amrinone therapy should be initiated with a $0.75 \text{ mg} \cdot \text{kg}^{-1}$ bolus given over 2 or 3 min. It is continued with a maintenance infusion of $5-10 \text{ μg} \cdot \text{kg}^{-1} \cdot \text{min}^{-1}$, adjusted by hemodynamic monitoring. An additional bolus dose of $0.75 \text{ mg} \cdot \text{kg}^{-1}$ may be given 30 min after initiation of therapy. Care must be taken not to give the bolus too quickly because sudden decreases in peripheral vascular resistance may occur and result in severe hypotension. The infusion should not exceed a total daily dose of $10 \text{ mg} \cdot \text{kg}^{-1}$, including the bolus doses. Amrinone has the same range of infusion rates as dopamine and dobutamine, and dose calculation follows the "rule of six," described in Table 7-18.

Amrinone has two uncommon side-effects. Thrombocytopenia occurs in some patients, but it has not been clinically significant and has responded to dose reduction.[222, 223, 225] Centrilobular hepatic necrosis occurs in dogs given large doses of amrinone for periods exceeding 3 months. There is no evidence of such an effect in humans, but the implications of using halothane in a patient taking amrinone are obvious. If the side-effects do not prove troublesome, this will be a valuable drug. It has a therapeutic index of approximately 100:1 as compared with 1.2:1 with the digitalis glycosides.

Milrinone is an experimental bipyridine inotropic agent that is a derivative of amrinone.[226] It has nearly 20 times the inotropic potency of the parent compound. Milrinone is active both intravenously and orally and has beneficial short-term hemodynamic effects in patients with severe refractory congestive heart failure. Improvement of cardiac output appears to result from a combination of enhanced myocardial contractility and peripheral vasodilatation. Treatment with oral milrinone for up to 11 months has been effective and well tolerated without evidence of fever, thrombocytopenia, or gastrointestinal effects.

Forskolin and BAY K 8644. Forskolin is an experimental drug with actions similar to the PDE inhibitors.[227, 228] It produces marked positive inotropic and vasodilatory properties *in vitro* and *in vivo*. Forskolin acts directly on the catalytic unit of adenyl cyclase to cause stimulation of this enzyme. This results in increases in cardiac cAMP production, calcium influx into the myocardium, and increased contractility.

BAY K 8644 is an experimental drug that promotes calcium influx and increased myocardial contractility.[227, 228] Unfortunately, it also promotes peripheral and coronary artery vasoconstriction. Although Forskolin and BAY K 8644 are not yet clinically useful, their mechanism of action is included in Figure 7-25 to demonstrate mechanisms by which sympathomimetic drug action may be engineered to function exclusive of the adrenergic receptors. BAY K 8644, a calcium agonist, is structurally similar to nifedipine, a calcium-entry blocker.

Glucagon. Glucagon is a single-chain polypeptide of 29 amino acids that is secreted by pancreas α cells in response to hypoglycemia. The liver and kidney are responsible for its degradation. Known effects of this hormone in humans include[194, 195, 209, 229]:

1. Inhibition of gastric motility
2. Enhanced urinary excretion of inorganic electrolytes
3. Increased insulin secretion
4. Hepatic glycogenolysis and gluconeogenesis
5. Anorexia
6. Inotropic and chronotropic cardiac effects

Little attention was given to glucagon until 1968, when it was demonstrated to produce positive inotropic and chronotropic effects in the canine heart. Glucagon enhances the activation of adenyl cyclase in a manner similar to NE, epinephrine, and isoproterenol, but with an important difference. These cardiac actions of glucagon are not blocked by β blockade or catecholamine depletion. Glucagon, in contrast to the xanthines, rarely causes cardiac dysrhythmias even in the face of ischemic heart disease, hypokalemia, and digitalis toxicity. Glucagon may, in fact, possess cardiac anti-dysrhythmic activity in digitalis toxicity because it has been shown to enhance AV nodal conduction in patients with varying degrees of AV block. It should be used carefully in patients with atrial fibrillation. In humans, an intravenous dose of 1–5 mg of glucagon increases cardiac index, mean arterial pressure, and ventricular contractility, even in the presence of digitalis therapy.

Glucagon can be mixed in 5% dextrose in water and is stable for long periods. After a bolus dose, its action dissipates in approximately 30 min. A continuous infusion of $5 \text{ μg} \cdot \text{kg}^{-1} \cdot \text{min}^{-1}$ is augmented by an initial bolus of $50 \text{ μg} \cdot \text{kg}^{-1}$. Onset of action occurs in 1–3 min and peaks at 10–15 min.

Nausea and vomiting are common side-effects in the awake patient, especially following a bolus dose. Hypokalemia, hypoglycemia, and hyperglycemia are also seen. Despite the obvious benefits of glucagon in cardiac patients, its use has not become popular.[227] This may be related to expense and the multiple metabolic and physiologic effects that are common after its administration.

This pancreatic hormone may be of benefit when more conventional approaches have proved refractory in the following settings: (1) low-cardiac-output syndrome following cardiopulmonary bypass; (2) low-cardiac-output syndrome with myocardial infarction; (3) chronic congestive heart failure; and (4) excessive β-adrenergic blockade.

Digitalis Glycosides. The most important actions of the digitalis glycosides are those affecting myocardial contractility, conduction, and rhythm. The glycoside most likely to be used by the anesthesiologist is digoxin.

The principal uses of digoxin are for the treatment of congestive heart failure and to control supraventricular cardiac dysrhythmias such as atrial fibrillation. Digoxin is one of the few positive inotropes that does not increase heart rate. Digoxin enhances myocardial inotropism and automaticity, but slows impulse propagation through the conduction tissues.[230] Despite nearly 2 centuries of use, the mechanism of action is only modestly certain. Digitalis reciprocally facilitates calcium entry into the myocardial cell by blocking the Na^+-K^+ adenosine triphosphatase (ATPase) pump.[231] This calcium influx may account for its positive inotropic action because this inotropic response is not catecholamine- or β-receptor-dependent and is therefore effective in patients taking β-blocking drugs. The inhibition of this enzyme transport mechanism also results in a net K^+ loss from the myocardial cell. This contributes to digitalis toxicity with hypokalemia. Calcium potentiates the toxic effects of digitalis. Extreme caution should be observed when calcium is given to a patient taking digitalis or when digitalis administration is contemplated in the patient with hypercalcemia.

A common indication for the glycosides is the chronic management of cardiac tachydysrhythmias. Cardiac dysrhythmias are, paradoxically, their most common side-effect. Synchrony of the cardiac beat is an important determinant of cardiac output, and digoxin can be beneficial when heart failure is due to a cardiac tachydysrhythmia, even in ischemic myocardial disease. However, the use of β- or calcium-channel blockers is increasing in this regard because they concomitantly reduce overall myocardial oxygen consumption.

The positive inotropic effects of digoxin are potentially beneficial in selected cases of the low-cardiac-output syndrome. It produces a dose-related increase in contractility in both normal and failing hearts. Limits are imposed on the upper reaches of inotropism by the development of serious cardiac dysrhythmias.

Confusion has risen in the past about whether digitalis increases or decreases myocardial oxygen consumption. This was based on the observation that the increased inotropism of digoxin increases myocardial oxygen consumption (MVO_2) in patients with normal hearts but decreases it in patients with heart failure. The tension developed within the ventricular wall is a prime determinant of oxygen consumption. By augmenting contractility, wall tension and MVO_2, at any given afterload, will be decreased with a reduction in ventricular radius and heart rate.[206, 211] This may underlie the clinical observation that angina is often decreased by digoxin in patients with cardiomegaly, whereas angina may be increased markedly by digitalis in patients with ischemic disease without cardiomegaly.

Digitalis tends to increase the tone of the peripheral resistance vessels in normal subjects by a direct vasoconstrictor effect. Untreated congestive heart failure is accompanied by high peripheral vascular resistance due to compensatory SNS activation. Successful treatment by digitalis usually reduces resistance as increased contractility improves cardiac output. This is the result of SNS release associated with improved cardiac function. Caution must be exercised, however, in giving intravenous digoxin or ouabain in a setting where an increase in afterload would be deleterious. An immediate peripheral vasoconstrictor effect can occur, producing a transient worsening of congestive heart failure. Inconsistent hemodynamic benefit has occurred with digitalis in congestive heart failure following myocardial infarction. It has been of no benefit in cardiogenic shock and has proved potentially injurious in patients with uncomplicated myocardial infarction because of its vasoconstrictive properties and effects on myocardial oxygen consumption in the absence of cardiomegaly.

Digoxin is of potential value in patients with signs and symptoms of congestive heart failure due to ischemic, valvular, hypertensive, or congenital heart disease.[207] Patients with cardiomyopathies or cor pulmonale may also benefit. Care must be taken to rule out conditions in which the use of digitalis is of no benefit and potentially harmful. These include mitral stenosis with normal sinus rhythm and constrictive pericarditis with tamponade. Signs and symptoms of idiopathic hypertrophic subaortic stenosis are often exacerbated with digitalis. With increased strength of contraction, the muscular obstruction can be markedly increased. The same is true for the use of digitalis in patients with infundibular pulmonic stenosis as occurs with tetralogy of Fallot. Any augmentation of contractility may further reduce an already diminished pulmonary blood flow. Beware of digitalis toxic reactions in the older age group; in patients suffering from arterial hypoxemia, acidosis, renal compromise, hypothyroidism, hypokalemia, or hypomagnesemia; and in patients receiving quinidine or calcium channel blockers.

The issue of prophylactic digitalization of patients with diminished cardiac reserve about to undergo major surgical procedures remains controversial.[195, 230] Meyer reviewed indications for preoperative digitalis and concluded that clinical settings in which the prophylactic administration of digoxin should be considered include: (1) previous heart failure; (2) increased heart size; (3) coronary flow disturbances by ECG; (4) age over 60 years; (5) age over 50 years before lung surgery; (6) anticipated massive blood loss; (7) atrial flutter or atrial fibrillation; (8) cardiovascular surgery; (9) rheumatic valvular lesions.[232] The negative inotropic effects of anesthesia can be effectively antagonized, and postoperative cardiac stress and fluid fluxes are better tolerated with the administration of digitalis. The opinion of many clinicians who pay compulsive attention to extracellular potassium levels is that the risk of toxicity is low and the benefits to be gained by prophylactic digitalis administration are worthwhile.[233]

When entertaining the possibility of perioperative digitalis administration, the following points must be considered[31]:

1. Myocardial oxygen balance is threatened in the non-failing, nondilated heart.
2. The therapeutic to toxic ratio of digitalis is narrow.
3. Inotropic drugs that are less toxic and may be stopped immediately are readily available.
4. Verapamil or β blockers are more efficacious for supraventricular tachydysrhythmias not initiated by heart failure.
5. Digitalis in the unstable patient may cause serious cardiac dysrhythmias.

6. Serum potassium concentrations may fluctuate in the surgical patient who is critically ill.
7. Any cardiac dysrhythmia that occurs in the presence of digitalis must be considered a toxic phenomenon.
8. Digitalis-induced cardiac dysrhythmias are difficult to treat.
9. Renal compromise will result in toxic effects with standard maintenance doses.
10. Cardioversion may be dangerous after digitalis administration.
11. After initiation of digitalis therapy, the administration of alternative drugs becomes more complicated.

Digitalization is not an all-or-none state, and improved contractility is dose related. Even a small dose will strengthen myocardial contractility. Within 10 min following an intravenous injection of 0.25–1 mg of digoxin, a marked improvement in presystolic ejection period can be seen. It is not necessary, once the desired effect has been gained, to continue administering the drug just because a digitalizing dose has not been reached. The goal, therefore, is to correct heart failure with the minimum effective dose necessary. The amount of digitalis administered should be guided by the clinical improvement of the patient. Control of the ventricular response provides a relatively straightforward end-point in patients with atrial flutter or atrial fibrillation. Toxic symptoms should be searched for when digitalis is administered for rate control. Toxic concentrations of digoxin that produce serious cardiac dysrhythmias are usually higher than doses required for a substantial inotropic effect. When evaluating for digitalis toxic effects, the useful maneuver of carotid sinus pressure can give some clue to potential digitalis excess. Cardiac rhythm disorders such as second-degree AV block, accelerated AV junctional rhythm, or bradycardia may emerge in response to carotid sinus stimulation before they occur spontaneously. There has been an increased effort in recent years to use serum assays in an effort to define end-points for digitalis administration. Serum levels, however, may not correlate with heart rate, tissue-bound levels, or toxicity.

Calcium Salts. Ringer established the importance of calcium in cardiac contraction more than 150 years ago. It is of great importance in the genesis of the cardiac action potential and is the key to controlling intracellular energy storage and utilization. Movement of extracellular calcium across membranes also governs the function of uterine smooth muscle as well as the smooth muscle of the blood vessels. Only recently have we begun to appreciate the critical role that calcium plays in a wide spectrum of biologic processes from coagulation to neuromuscular transmission. The sympathomimetic drugs promote the transmembrane influx of calcium, whereas the β blockers and calcium-channel blockers inhibit such movement.

Despite its molecular simplicity, calcium is one of the least understood drugs.[234] Calcium chloride is often part of the treatment of ventricular fibrillation, yet the published data to support this indication are scarce. There are data confirming its capability to initiate ventricular fibrillation in a manner similar to epinephrine. Although many of the effects of epinephrine are mediated by calcium, the two drugs are clearly not identical. The fact that epinephrine can improve defibrillation success by strengthening the fibrillatory pattern is the apparent basis for the use of calcium salts in this setting. This assumption has not been experimentally or clinically documented.[235] The American Heart Association has recommended against the use of calcium during cardiac arrest except when hyperkalemia, hypocalcemia, or calcium-entry inhibitor toxicity is present.[236]

Traditionally, calcium gluconate has been preferred in pediatric patients and calcium chloride for use in adult patients. Previous data held that calcium chloride produced consistently higher and more predictable levels of ionized calcium than an equivalent dose of the other preparations.[237] Recent studies have shown, however, that ionization of any of the preparations is immediate and equally as effective.[238, 239] Intravenous calcium appears effective for the transient reversal of hypotension thought to be the result of myocardial depression from the potent volatile anesthetic drugs. Some clinicians feel that recurrent intraoperative hypotension response to calcium chloride may be an indication for the administration of digoxin. Calcium chloride is also given at the termination of cardiopulmonary bypass to offset the myocardial depression associated with hypothermic potassium cardioplegia.[195] The use of calcium salts is clearly indicated during rapid or massive transfusions of citrated blood.[240] Citrate binds calcium, and rapid infusion rates of citrated blood result in myocardial depression that is reversible by calcium.

Three forms of calcium salts are available: calcium chloride, gluconate, and gluceptate. Calcium chloride produces only transient (10–20 min) increases in cardiac output.[230] If inotropic effects are needed for a longer period of time, other inotropic agents should be selected. Bolus doses of 2–10 mg·kg^{-1} (1.5 mg·kg^{-1}·min^{-1}) of calcium chloride can produce moderate improvement in contractility. The rapid administration of calcium salts, if the heart is beating, can produce bradycardia and must be used cautiously in the patient who is digitalized because of the hazard of producing toxic effects.

Calcium gluceptate can be given in a dose of 5–7 ml (4.5–6.3 mEq) and calcium gluconate in a dose of 10–15 ml (4.8–7.2 mEq). These doses are approximately equivalent to that suggested for calcium chloride. Calcium gluconate is unstable and no longer in frequent use. All of the calcium salts will precipitate as calcium carbonate if mixed with sodium bicarbonate.

ANTIDEPRESSANT DRUGS. *Monoamine Oxidase Inhibitors.* MAO inhibitors and the tricyclic antidepressants (TAD) are used to treat psychotic depression. These drugs are not used in the practice of anesthesia, but are a source of potentially serious interactions in patients who are receiving them chronically. chronically.

MAO inhibitors (Table 7-21) block the oxidative deamination of endogenous catecholamines into inactive vanillylmandelic acid (VMA) (Fig. 7-12). They do not inhibit synthesis.[241] Thus, blockade of MAO would produce an accumulation of NE, epinephrine, dopamine, and 5-HT in adrenergically active tissues, including the brain. Alleviation of depression may be related to elevations of the endogenous catecholamines. Overdose with MAO inhibitors is expressed as SNS hyperactivity. They may produce agitation, hallucinations, hyperpyrexia, convulsions, hypertension, and hypotension. Orthostatic hypotension is a common complaint in patients taking MAO inhibitors.[242]

The action of sympathomimetic amines is potentiated in patients taking MAO inhibitors. Indirect-acting sympathomimetics (ephedrine, tyramine) will produce an exaggerated response as they trigger the release of accumulated catecholamines. Foods with a high tyramine content, such as cheese, red Italian wine, and pickled herring, can likewise precipitate hypertensive crisis.[242] SNS reflex stimulation is also intensified. Meperidine has been reported to produce hypertensive crisis, convulsions, and coma. Hepatotoxicity

TABLE 7-21. Antidepressant Drugs

NONPROPRIETARY NAME	TRADE NAME
Monoamine Oxidase Inhibitors	
Isocarboxazid	Marplan
Pargyline	Eutonyl
Phenelzine	Nardil
Tranylcypromine	Parnate
Tricyclic Antidepressants	
Imipramine	Imavate, Janimine, Presamine, SK-Pramine, Tofranil
Desipramine	Norpramin, Pertofrane
Amitriptyline	Amitril, Elavil, Endep
Nortriptyline	Aventyl, Pamelor
Doxepin	Adapin, Sinequan
Protriptyline	Vivactyl

has been reported that does not seem to be related to dosage or duration of treatment. The incidence is low but remains a factor in selecting anesthesia.

The MAO inhibitors produce long-lasting, irreversible enzyme inhibition unrelated to duration of treatment. Regeneration of MAO may, therefore, take weeks. This is much the same effect on adrenergic metabolism that organophosphates have on the cholinesterase system. MAO inhibitors are known to intensify CNS depression due to ethanol, analgesics, and general anesthesia. The depressive mechanism is not known.

The anesthetic management of patients taking MAO inhibitors remains controversial and essentially undefined. Current recommendations for management include discontinuation of the drugs for at least 2 weeks before surgery; however, this recommendation is not based on controlled studies, but rather is the result of limited case reports that suggest potent drug interactions.[241] A small number of studies found few adverse effects in humans given analgesics, opioid anesthesia, or regional blocks. However, opioids that cause release of catecholamines (meperidine) or histamine (morphine) may be avoided in these patients.

Symptoms of SNS overdose or interactions due to MAO inhibitors can be treated effectively with either α blockers, ganglionic blockers, or direct-acting vasodilators.

TADs should not be substituted for the MAO inhibitors in the perioperative period. Adverse CNS interactions similar to those encountered with the indirect sympathomimetic amines have been reported. A 2-week wash-out period is recommended before introducing TADs into a patient taking an MAO inhibitor.

Tricyclic Antidepressants. This group of antidepressant drugs is referred to as TADs because of their structure. The important TADs are listed in Table 7-21. These drugs have almost replaced the use of the MAO inhibitors because there are fewer side-effects.[241] The manner in which the TADs relieve depression is not clear, but all TADs block uptake of NE into adrenergic nerve endings. Just as with the MAO inhibitors, high doses of the TADs can induce seizure activity that is responsive to diazepam.

There is a tendency for patients taking TADs to develop tachycardia and cardiac dysrhythmias. This may be related to high concentrations of NE in cardiac tissues. Other reported cardiovascular effects have included orthostatic hypotension, myocardial infarction, and precipitation of congestive heart failure.[243] Imipramine may cause hypotension and bradycardia due to direct cardiac depression. Death from TAD overdose is usually due to cardiac failure or the development of cardiac dysrhythmias that are refractory to treatment. TAD can also cause a CAS, which is responsive to physostigmine.

Neuroleptic drugs may potentiate the effects of TADs by competition with metabolism in the liver. Chronic barbiturate use increases metabolism of the TAD by microsomal enzyme induction. Other sedatives, however, potentiate the TAD in a manner similar to that which occurs with the MAO inhibitors. Atropine has an exaggerated effect also because of the anticholinergic effect of TADs. Prolonged sedation from thiopental has been reported. Ketamine may also be dangerous in patients taking TADs by producing acute hypertension and cardiac dysrhythmias. Cardiac arrest has been reported. Likewise, muscle relaxants that produce tachycardia (pancuronium, gallamine) have been observed to produce serious ventricular cardiac dysrhythmias in humans and dogs pretreated with imipramine.

Despite these serious interactions, discontinuation of these drugs before surgery is probably not necessary. The latency of onset of these drugs is from 2 weeks to 5 weeks; however, the excretion of TADs is rapid, with approximately 70% of a dose appearing in the urine during the first 72 h. One might consider a discontinuation of the drug for 72 h, but the risk of recurrent depression may be greater than that of any untoward drug reaction. The long latency period for resumption of treatment militates against interrupted treatment. A thorough knowledge of the possible drug interactions and autonomic countermeasures obviates postponement.

Adrenergic Antagonists

Drugs that bind selectively to α-adrenergic receptors block the action of endogenous catecholamines at effector sites and alter the ANS response. The resultant effects may be ascribed to unopposed β-adrenergic receptors and are dependent on the prevailing adrenergic tone. In the vasculature, for example, the response to the α-blocker phenoxybenzamine may vary over a wide range in a single vascular bed, depending on its intrinsic state of constriction. Vessels with higher initial tone have a greater response to α blockade. Classically, α *blockers* are defined as drugs that convert the vascular response to epinephrine from constriction to vasodilatation.[244] Prominent clinical effects of α blockers include hypotension, tachycardia, and miosis. Nasal stuffiness, diarrhea, and inhibition of ejaculation are common side-effects.

The α blockers may be divided into two groups according to binding characteristics (Table 7-22). Phenoxybenzamine is a drug that binds covalently to receptors and produces an irreversible blockade. It is relatively nonspecific and has antagonistic activity at several other receptor types as well.[245] They are not used widely now that more specific, shorter-acting drugs are available. Phentolamine, tolazoline, and prazosin

TABLE 7-22. α-Adrenergic Blocking Drugs

	TYPE OF ANTAGONISM	SELECTIVITY
Phenoxybenzamine	Noncompetitive	$\alpha_1 > \alpha_2$
Phentolamine	Competitive	$\alpha_1 = \alpha_2$
Tolazoline	Competitive	$\alpha_1 = \alpha_2$
Prazosin	Competitive	$\alpha_1 >> \alpha_2$
Yohimbine	Competitive	$\alpha_2 >> \alpha_1$

comprise the second group and are characterized by reversible binding and antagonism.

There are also important differences among the drugs with regard to relative receptor specificity. As with the β blockers, some show greater affinity for one subset of α receptors than another. Phenoxybenzamine, for example, is 100 times more potent on α_1 than α_2 receptors. Prazosin is also markedly specific for α_1 receptors, whereas phentolamine has nearly equal blocking activity on both subsets. Phentolamine, therefore, by blocking presynaptic inhibitory α_2 receptors, causes greater NE release from the presynaptic terminal. The tachycardia as well as the reflex response to hypotension seen commonly with phentolamine is thought to be secondary to this enhanced NE release.

PHENOXYBENZAMINE. Phenoxybenzamine is a haloalkylamine with predominantly α_1-antagonist activity. Because of the noncompetitive nature of the block, as discussed above, it has a relatively long duration of 24 h. In the past it was the drug of choice for treating patients with pheochromocytoma in preparation for surgery. It has now been replaced with shorter-acting, more specific drugs such as phentolamine or prazosin.

PHENTOLAMINE. Phentolamine is an imidazoline, which is a competitive antagonist at α_1 and α_2 receptors. The imidazolines also have some antihistaminic and cholinomimetic activity. The cholinomimetic activity may result in abdominal cramping and diarrhea, both of which are blocked by atropine. Tachycardia and hypotension are also common side-effects.[244] It also is commonly used in the diagnosis and treatment of pheochromocytoma. It is usually given in 2–5 mg iv boluses until adequate control of blood pressure is obtained.

TOLAZOLINE. Tolazoline is also an imidazoline derivative and acts much like phentolamine. It is less potent on peripheral α receptors, however, and some of its vasodilatory action has been ascribed to histamine-like activity. It effectively decreases pulmonary vascular resistance and has been used in neonates with respiratory distress syndrome to improve pulmonary blood flow. The effects, however, were detrimental and inconsistent.[246, 247]

PRAZOSIN. Prazosin is a piperazine derivative that has relative selectivity for α_1 receptors and, as a result, does not cause the tachycardia seen with phentolamine. Cardiovascular effects include decreased peripheral vascular resistance and venous return with little change in heart rate or cardiac output. When used alone, it is not remarkably effective in treatment of essential hypertension resulting from fluid retention. When combined with a diuretic, however, it is a quite effective antihypertensive drug. It should not be used with clonidine or α methyldopa (discussed below) as it appears to decrease their effectiveness. Prazosin also may bronchodilate, and it decreases serum cholesterol and triglyceride levels.[248]

YOHIMBINE. Yohimbine is an α_2 antagonist (Table 7-5). It blocks the action of clonidine on presynaptic receptors and increases NE release. It is mostly used as a research tool, but has been used in the treatment of impotence and orthostatic hypotension.[249]

Beta Antagonists

The use of β-blocking drugs has markedly escalated in the last 10 years as more indications for their use have been found and more compounds have been developed.[250] They are among the most common drugs used in the treatment of cardiovascular disease, and frequently the anesthesiologist must deal with their effects and side-effects during anesthesia. There are now a variety of drugs available with β-blocking activity that may be distinguished by differing pharmacokinetic and pharmacodynamic characteristics.[251, 252] Examples of drugs available for clinical use in the United States and their characteristics are listed in Table 7-23. Their structures are shown in Figure 7-25.

Several of these drugs are marketed on the basis of cardioselectivity, i.e., antagonist activity is greater at β_1 than β_2 receptors in an isolated muscle preparation. Theoretically, this implies that these would be of greater benefit in treatment of patients with obstructive airway disease, diabetes mellitus, or peripheral vascular disease.[253] The practitioner must keep in mind, however, that this means relative selectivity, not specificity, and that β-blocking effects may be seen in all tissues if higher blood levels are reached (Fig. 7-13). Clinical studies have not shown greater effectiveness of cardioselective β blockers in the treatment of hypertension[254] or diabetes mellitus,[255] and the relative effectiveness in the treatment of peripheral vascular disease is still controversial.[253]

The use of β_1-selective blockers in patients with obstructive airway disease is also controversial. The degree of bron-

TABLE 7-23.   β-Adrenergic Blocking Drugs

	RELATIVE β_1 SELECTIVITY	MEMBRANE STABILIZING ACTIVITY	INTRINSIC SYMPATHOMIMETIC ACTIVITY	PLASMA HALF-LIFE (H)	ORAL AVAILABILITY	LIPID SOLUBILITY	ELIMINATION	PREPARATIONS
Propranolol	0	+	0	3–4	36	+ + +	Hepatic	Oral, iv
Nadolol	0	0	0	14–24	34	0	Renal	Oral
Timolol	0	0	0	4–5	50	+	Hepatic and renal	Oral, eye drops
Pindolol	0	+	+ +	3–4	86	+	Hepatic and renal	Oral
Esmolol	+ +	0	0	0.16	—	?	Blood esterase	iv
Acebutolol	+	+	+	3–4	37*	0	Hepatic*	Oral
Atenolol	+ +	0	0	6–9	57	0	Renal	Oral
Metoprolol	+ +	0	0	3–4	38	+	Hepatic	Oral

* Primarily hepatic, but active metabolites are formed that must be renally excreted.

choreactivity present is an important consideration in their use. Patients with reactive airway disease may develop serious reductions in ventilatory function even with β_1-selective drugs.[256] No β blocker can be considered safe in patients with obstructive airway disease, and other types of drugs are available for treatment of supraventricular arrhythmias and hypertension.

Some β antagonists have partial agonist activity at low doses. This is referred to as intrinsic sympathomimetic activity (ISA). Drugs with ISA decrease resting heart rate less than those without ISA.[257] In the presence of similar degrees of β blockade, however, all β blockers blunt exercise-induced increases in heart rate to a similar extent.[255] The clinical relevance of this is unclear, but it has been implied that ISA would be advantageous in patients treated with nonselective β blockers who are troubled by bradycardia or worsening ventricular failure.[258] A distinct advantage to ISA in β blockers has not been clearly shown in clinical studies.

Several of the β blockers listed in Table 7-23 also have a local anesthetic-like effect on myocellular membranes at high doses. It is similar to that of quinidine in that phase 0 of the cardiac action potential is depressed, slowing conduction. This membrane-stabilizing activity (MSA) is caused by the d-isomer, whereas the l-isomer is responsible for β-blocking activity. The clinical significance of MSA is also unclear.[252]

PROPRANOLOL. Propranolol is the prototype β-blocking drug against which all others are compared. It is nonselective, has no ISA, but does have MSA at higher doses. It is available in both iv and oral forms. It is highly lipophilic and is metabolized by the liver to more water-soluble metabolites, one of which, 17-OH propranolol, has weak β-blocking activity. There is a significant first-pass effect by the liver after oral administration of the drug. It is highly protein bound, and the free drug level may be altered by other highly bound drugs. The elimination half-life is approximately 4 h, but the pharmacologic half-life is approximately 10 h.

Hemodynamic effects include decreased heart rate and contractility. The major factors contributing to the decrease in blood pressure by propranolol are decreased cardiac output and renin release. Systemic vascular resistance may increase on acute administration due to blockade of β_2 receptors in the peripheral vasculature. With chronic administration, however, peripheral vascular resistance decreases. This is thought to be secondary to decreased renin release and, possibly, decreased central SNS outflow.[249, 259] Complications with the use of propranolol include bradycardia, heart block, worsening of congestive heart failure, bronchospasm, and sedation. During anesthesia with halothane, it may cause severe bradydysrhythmias.

NADOLOL. Nadolol is a noncardioselective β blocker with no MSA or ISA. It is approximately equipotent to propranolol, but its effects are prolonged due to slower elimination. It is relatively lipid insoluble and is excreted 70% unchanged in urine and 20% unchanged in the feces. The elimination half-life is 24 h. Because it is lipid insoluble, it does not cross the blood–brain barrier, and sedation is less a problem than with propranolol. Hemodynamic effects are the same as for propranolol. The main advantage with the drug is capability for once-per-day dosing.

TIMOLOL. Timolol is also noncardioselective with little ISA and no MSA. It is the only β blocker used as the l-isomer rather than the racemic mixture. It is 5–10 times as potent as propranolol. Hepatic metabolism accounts for approximately 66%

of its elimination, and another 20% is found unchanged in the urine. The elimination half-life is 5.6 h and pharmacologic half-life is approximately 15 h. It was first used topically for treatment of glaucoma but is now used in hypertension and has been shown to decrease the risk of reinfarction and death following myocardial infarction.[260] The hemodynamic effects and side-effects are similar to those of other β blockers. The anesthesiologist should also be aware that timolol eye drops may be absorbed systemically and cause bradycardia and hypotension that are refractory to treatment with atropine.[261]

PINDOLOL. Pindolol is a nonselective β blocker with MSA and ISA. It is 10–40 times as potent as propranolol. It is lipid soluble and metabolized by the liver, but not as avidly extracted; therefore, biologic availability after oral administration is more predictable. It is excreted 40% unchanged in the urine. The elimination half-life is 3.5 h. It is useful in the treatment of angina pectoris, cardiac dysrhythmias, and hypertension. As discussed above, the clinical usefulness of the ISA property is unclear.

OXPRENOLOL. Oxprenolol is similar to pindolol except for less ISA and lower potency.

METOPROLOL. Metoprolol is a relatively selective β_1-blocking drug with β_2-blocking effects at moderate and high doses. It has neither ISA or MSA. It has a possible advantage in patients with reactive airway disease at oral doses up to 100 $mg \cdot day^{-1}$.[262] In this case, it should probably be used with a β_2-mimetic drug. It is mostly metabolized in the liver with only about 5% excreted unchanged in the urine. The elimination half-life is 3.5 h. It has recently become available in iv as well as oral form, so it may be useful during anesthesia.

ATENOLOL. Atenolol is similar to metoprolol in that it is relatively cardioselective and has no ISA or MSA. It is less lipophilic, however, and is eliminated primarily by renal excretion. The elimination half-life is 6–7 h. The lack of first-pass metabolism results in more predictable blood levels after oral dosing.

ACEBUTOLOL. Acebutolol is a cardioselective β blocker with ISA and MSA.[263] It is metabolized in the liver and is subject to extensive first-pass metabolism. The primary metabolite is diacetolol (Fig. 7-26), which has a similar pharmacologic profile to the parent drug and is excreted renally.[264] The pharmacologic effects by the drug, therefore, are dependent on both hepatic transformation and renal excretion. The elimination half-life of acebutolol is 3–4 h and diacetolol 8–13 h. Elimination is prolonged in the elderly and patients with renal disease. For acebutolol, like pindolol, having ISA may be more advantageous than the other β blockers in patients with cardiac bradydysrhythmias or myocardial failure.

ESMOLOL. Esmolol is the most recently released β blocker and shows considerable promise for use in the perioperative period.[265–269] The most unique feature of the drug is the ester function incorporated into the phenoxypropanolamine structure (Fig. 7-26). This allows for rapid degradation by esterases in the blood and a resultant pharmacologic half-life of 10–20 min.[270]

Esmolol is cardioselective and appears to have little effect on bronchial or vascular tone at doses that decrease heart rate in humans. It has been used successfully in low doses in patients with asthma,[271] but caution is again advised when using β blockers in these patients.[253]

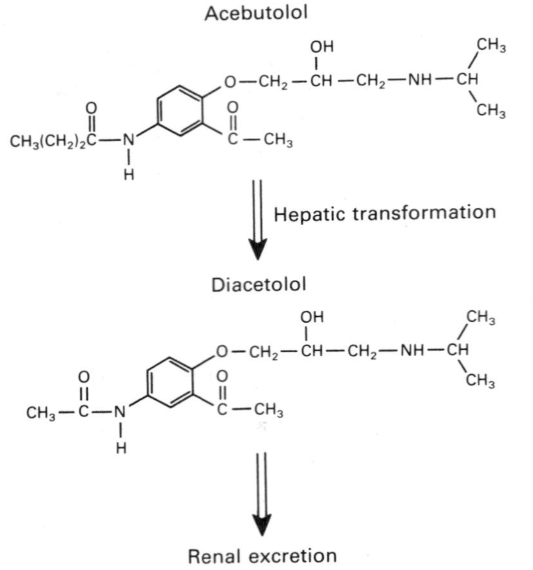

Acebutolol

Hepatic transformation

Diacetolol

Renal excretion

FIG. 7-26. Acebutolol is metabolized in the liver to diacetolol, which has a potency similar to the parent drug. Diacetolol is eliminated by renal excretion. The pharmacologic half-life of acebutolol, therefore, depends on both hepatic and renal function.

Esmolol is metabolized rapidly in the blood by an esterase located in the red blood cell cytoplasm. It is different from the plasma cholinesterase and is not inhibited to a significant degree by physostigmine or echothiophate, but is markedly inhibited by sodium fluoride. There are no apparent important clinical interactions between esmolol and other ester-containing drugs. At the highest infusion rates (500 $\mu g \cdot kg^{-1} \cdot min^{-1}$), esmolol does not prolong neuromuscular blockade by succinylcholine.[270]

Esmolol may prove to be quite useful in the perioperative period because of its capability to be administered intravenously and its short half-life.[272] It has been shown to blunt the response to intubation of the trachea[269] and is moderately effective in treating postoperative hypertension.[265] Most reported studies in humans have used doses of 50–500 $\mu g \cdot kg^{-1} \cdot min^{-1}$. The most beneficial approach seems to be a loading dose of 500 $\mu g \cdot kg^{-1}$ over 1 min, followed by continuous infusion of 50–300 $\mu g \cdot kg^{-1} \cdot min^{-1}$. Peak blockade appears to occur within 5 min. On discontinuation of the infusion, serum levels decline with an elimination half-life of 9 min. The heart rate response to isoproterenol returns to control in 20 min.

Mixed Antagonists

LABETALOL. Labetalol is an antihypertensive drug with blocking activity at both α and β receptors. The relative α/β blocking effects are dependent on the route of administration. After oral administration, the ratio of α/β effectiveness is 1:3; however, when given intravenously, it is 1:7 (*i.e.*, it is 3 and 7 times more potent on β than α receptors, respectively). The α effects are primarily on α_1 receptors, whereas the β effects are nonselective.

Hemodynamic effects consist primarily of decreased peripheral resistance and decreased or unchanged heart rate with little change in cardiac output.[272] Serum renin activity is decreased. Maintenance of lower heart rates in the presence of decreased systemic blood pressure is beneficial in controlling the myocardial oxygen supply/demand ratio and is a major benefit of labetalol in patients with coronary artery disease.[273]

Labetalol is eliminated by hepatic glucuronide conjugation. The elimination half-life after intravenous administration is 5.5 h and 6–8 h after oral use. Elimination is not markedly prolonged in patients with hepatic or renal failure. Another advantage with the drug is the ability to convert from iv to oral forms of the same drug after the patient is stable.[274]

For treatment of hypertension when used as a bolus, the initial dose is 0.25 mg $\cdot$ kg^{-1} iv over 2 min, then repeat every 10 min to a total of 300 mg. When used as a continuous infusion, it is usually started at 2 mg $\cdot$ min^{-1} and titrated to effect. There is an enhanced effect by inhalation anesthetics, so these doses should be decreased when used intraoperatively.

Complications and contraindications are similar to those of the β blockers. It should be used with caution in patients with compromised myocardial function as it may worsen heart failure. Also, due to β_2-blocking activity, it may induce bronchospasm in patients with asthma. As with other β blockers, abrupt withdrawal is not recommended.

CALCIUM ENTRY BLOCKERS

Calcium is regarded as the universal messenger in cells and plays a critical role in a number of biologic processes.[218, 219] It is involved in blood coagulation; a broad array of enzymatic reactions; the metabolism of bone; neuromuscular transmission; the electrical activation of various excitable membranes as well as endocrine secretion; and muscle contraction. Calcium initiates several physiologic events in the specialized automatic and conducting cells in the heart.[276] It is involved in the genesis of the cardiac action potential; it links excitation to contraction and controls energy stores and utilization. Movement of extracellular calcium across membranes also governs the function of smooth muscle in the bronchi, the uterus, and coronary, pulmonary, and systemic arterioles. Its role in adrenergic effector response has been outlined in detail in Molecular Pharmacology and Effector Response.

Membrane calcium channels are known to exist that provide a pathway for calcium influx across cell membranes that differs from calcium efflux movements associated with active pumps or exchange.[277] The inward calcium channel exhibits two distinguishing properties: (1) it exhibits selectivity in that it has the ability to distinguish between ion species; and (2) it demonstrates excitability in that it has the property of responding to changes in membrane potential.[278]

Separate, ion-specific channels for sodium and calcium influx are thought to exist. The status of these channels can vary to produce three kinetic states: resting, activated, and inactivated. Sodium channels are referred to as fast channels because the transition among resting, activated, and inactivated states is more rapid than the calcium channels. Thus, calcium channels are often referred to as membrane "slow channels".[200]

Classification of calcium entry blockers has been difficult since their discovery. They were initially thought to be β-adrenergic blocking drugs because of their sympatholytic action. Later they were called calcium antagonists. It is clear, however, that these drugs are not true pharmacologic antagonists of calcium. Instead, they interact with the cell membrane to control the intracellular concentration of calcium. The correct terminology for this group of drugs appears to be *calcium-entry blockers* (CEBs).[279] *Slow-channel inhibitors* or *calcium channel blockers* would also suffice.

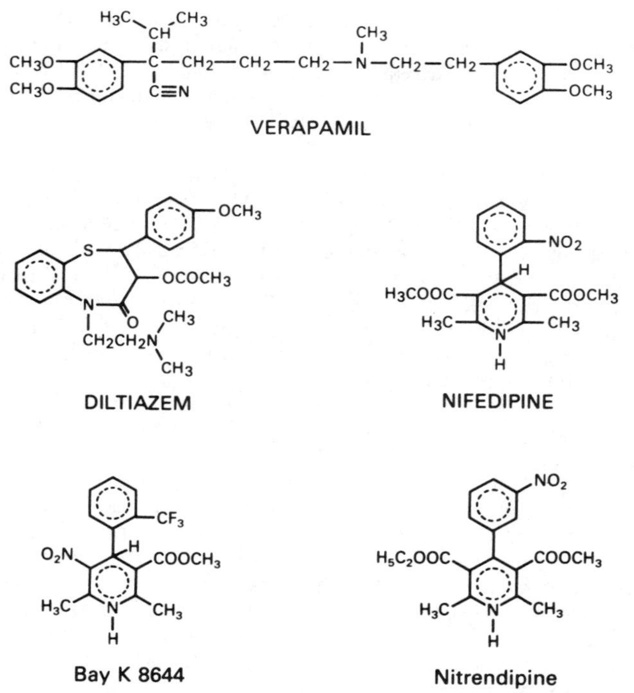

FIG. 7-27. Structural formulas of the calcium-entry blockers demonstrate dissimilar structures consistent with their dissimilar electrophysiologic and pharmacologic properties. They also share some similarities but cannot be considered therapeutically interchangeable. Nifedipine and nitrendipine are structurally similar and are both potent vasodilators; however, Bay K 8644 is also similar but is a calcium-channel agonist.

CEB drugs that are useful include verapamil, nifedipine, and diltiazem. Their molecular structures are seen in Figure 7-27.

CEBs are a heterogenous group of drugs with dissimilar structures and electrophysiologic and pharmacologic properties.[199] Despite structural dissimilarities, this group shares some important actions, which are consistent with the known importance of extracellular calcium and adrenergic function. Any drug that alters slow-channel kinetics could be expected to produce vasodilatation, depress cardiac conduction velocity (dromotropism), depress contractility (inotropism), and decrease heart rate (chronotropism). All CEBs do this, but with varying degrees of potency in the intact human and in vitro (Table 7-24).[280, 281] Thus, despite their similarities, these drugs cannot be considered therapeutically interchangeable. Clinically, nifedipine is a potent coronary artery vasodilator with little direct effect on cardiac conduction. It may reduce cardiac dysrhythmias secondarily when increased coronary

blood flow is of benefit. Verapamil is valued for its specific cardiac antidysrhythmic activity, but it is a myocardial depressant with little vasodilator activity. Verapamil also has local anesthetic activity (fast-channel inhibition) slightly greater than that of procaine on an equimolar basis.[282] The significance of this observation in humans has not been established.

The structural heterogenicity of this group of drugs also suggests more than one site and mechanism of action. Although the molecular basis of the action of these compounds is unknown, they are lipophilic, and it appears likely that they work by producing conformational changes in the cell membranes (see Molecular Pharmacology and Effector Response).

The useful pharmacologic effects of the CEBs have been confined almost solely to the cardiovascular system, although the list of uses will likely grow.[200] Table 7-25 lists some of the areas of investigation in which they appear to be of clinical benefit.[283-286] CEBs have been described, perhaps erroneously, as selective slow-channel blockers. A review of the literature, however, suggests that these drugs are not selective, but rather the slow-channel effects on the cardiovascular system are just more apparent. Their lack of selectivity should not be surprising considering the critical role calcium plays in a wide variety of biologic processes. The sensitivity of a given tissue to the CEBs is related to that tissue's dependence on extracellular calcium for its function. This would explain the sensitivity of the calcium-dependent myocardium and smooth muscle on the one hand, and the apparent insensitivity of striated muscle on the other.[287] Extracellular calcium is relatively insignificant in the function of striated muscle where the sarcoplasmic reticulum is the major storage organelle of calcium. Striated muscle can recycle intracellular calcium for prolonged periods, which is in keeping with its function of sustained contraction as opposed to the rhythmic or cyclic contraction of the myocardium and smooth muscle.

The drugs are all absorbed via the gastrointestinal tract, but the extensive first-pass hepatic extraction of verapamil limits its bioavailability orally (Table 7-26). Onset of action is equivalent for all three drugs and is consistent with rapid membrane transport. All three drugs are extensively protein bound and subject to the effect of changes in plasma protein concentration and competition from other protein-bound drugs. Hepatic metabolism is active for all the drugs and metabolites, but final elimination of verapamil and nifedipine is primarily renal.

Verapamil

Verapamil is a CEB that is administered intravenously for terminating supraventricular tachydysrhythmias.[288-291] Nearly all forms of supraventricular tachydysrhythmias are caused by reentry using either the SA or AV node as part of the circuit. Verapamil will terminate these cardiac dysrhythmias by decreasing nodal conductivity, converting the unidirectional block of reentry to a bidirectional block. In this

TABLE 7-24.   Autonomic Effects of Calcium Entry Blockers in Intact Humans

	VERAPAMIL	DILTIAZEM	NIFEDIPINE	LIDOFLAZINE
Negative inotropic	+	0/+	0	0
Negative chronotropic	+	0/+	0	0
Negative dromotropic	+ + + +	+ + +	0	0
Coronary vasodilatation	+ +	+ + +	+ + + +	+ + + +
Systemic vasodilatation	+ +	+ +	+ + + +	+ + +
Bronchodilatation	0/+		0/+	

regard, its action on supraventricular cardiac dysrhythmias is similar to that of quinidine on ventricular reentry cardiac dysrhythmias.

Verapamil does not alter the action-potential upstroke in fibers whose resting membrane potential (RMP) is more negative than -60 mV, *i.e.*, fast-action potentials.[292] It does slow or prevent depolarization in cardiac tissue with an RMP less negative than -50 mV, *i.e.*, calcium-dependent upstroke. Verapamil, therefore, has profound effects on pacemaker cells, which depend on the calcium current for depolarization.[293] It depresses the rate of sinus discharge, reduces conduction velocity, and increases refractoriness of the AV node. A dose-dependent increase in the P-R and AV interval is produced on the ECG. This has been described as a quinidine-like effect similar to that produced by class 1A antidysrhythmic drugs (procainamide), which are also effective for supraventricular cardiac dysrhythmias. In contrast to the procainamide, verapamil does not increase the QRS or Q-T interval because it lacks activity on the sodium-dependent action potentials.

Verapamil is becoming the first-line drug for supraventricular tachydysrhythmias (Table 7-27). The incidence of successful termination of PAT with verapamil in adults has approached 90%.[290] It is also effective in treating atrial fibrillation and atrial flutter by either converting to a sinus rhythm or slowing the ventricular response. The ventricular rate will slow as a result of decreased conduction velocity through the AV node even when conversion is not produced. Caution must be exercised in treating patients when the underlying cause of the atrial tachycardia, atrial fibrillation, or atrial flutter is the Wolff-Parkinson-White syndrome.[294] An accessory bypass tract lies near the AV node, which participates in the reentry of these tachydysrhythmias. Verapamil may terminate the tachydysrhythmia by its specific depressant effects on the AV node, which is one limb of the reentrant pathway. It may also increase conduction velocity in the accessory tract, however, in which case the heart rate may actually increase.

Verapamil has no adverse effects in bronchial asthma or obstructive lung disease and may be selected over propranolol in patients with these conditions.[283] It should be avoided in patients with sick sinus syndrome or AV block and in the presence of heart failure unless the heart failure is the result of a supraventricular tachycardia.

Recent studies further support the hypothesis that Ca^{++} participates directly in the genesis of ventricular dysrhyth-

TABLE 7-25.   Uses of Calcium Channel Blockers

Vascular disorders
Systemic hypertension
Pulmonary hypertension
Cerebral arterial spasm
Raynaud's phenomenon
Migraine

Nonvascular disorders
Bronchial asthma
Esophageal spasm
Dysmenorrhea
Premature labor

TABLE 7-26.   Comparative Pharmacology of Calcium Entry Blockers

	VERAPAMIL	DILTIAZEM	NIFEDIPINE
Dose			
Oral	80–160 mg tid	60–90 mg tid	10–20 mg tid
IV	75–150 µg·kg^{-1}	75–150 µg·kg^{-1}	5–15 µg·kg^{-1}
Absorption			
Oral (%)	> 90%	> 90%	> 90%
Bioavailability			
Oral (%)	< 20%	? < 20%	60–70%*
Onset			
Oral	15–20 min	20–30 min	15–20 min
IV	1 min	?	1 min
Sublingual	—	—	3 min
Peak Effect			
Oral	5 h	30 min	1–2 h
IV	5–30 min	?	1–3 h
Elimination half-life	2–7 h	4 h	4–5 h
Plasma protein binding	90%	80%	90%
Metabolism	70% 1st-pass hepatic	deacetylated	80% to lactone
Elimination			
Renal	75%	35%	70%
GI (liver)	15%	75%	< 15%
Side-Effects	Constipation, headache, vertigo, hypotension, AV conduction disturbances	Headache, dizziness, flushing, AV conduction disturbances, constipation	Headache, hypotension, flushing, digital dysesthesias, leg edema

* Light-sensitive.

TABLE 7-27.

Verapamil
Vasodilator
  ↓ systemic vascular resistance → ↑ heart rate
  → ↑ ejection fraction and cardiac output
Small decrease in LV dP/dt
Little or no change in coronary resistance
↓ conduction through AV node (↑ P-R interval)
Should not be given with digitalis or β blockers

Diltiazem
More like verapamil than nifedipine
Dilates coronary more than systemic vessels and has less marked
  hemodynamic effects than nifedipine or verapamil
Little effect on cardiac output
Does not cause tachycardia
Similar effects on conduction system as verapamil
Less inotropic effect than verapamil

Nifedipine
Rapid onset of action, may be used sublingually
Potent peripheral vasodilator, may be useful in HTN
Has little clinically important negative inotropic activity
Less tendency to produce cardiac decompensation than verapamil
Little effect on nodal activity and no antiarrhythmic activity, therefore
  causes no ECG changes
Increases coronary blood flow in normal and ischemic myocardium

mias (Fig. 7-28).[294] When sodium channels are inactivated by hypoxia, stretch, or hyperkalemia, the remaining Ca^{++} current can produce a depolarizing current in these abnormal cells, especially in the presence of catecholamines. The conversion of a fast-response cell to a cell with slow-response characteristics presents all the necessary ingredients for the reentry phenomenon: slow depolarization and delayed conduction. The resulting ventricular dysrhythmias can usually be terminated with one of the class I drugs as long as the RMP of the slow response is between −80 and −60 mV. Verapamil has been effective in terminating ventricular tachycardias and premature depolarizations in about two-thirds of the treatment trials when other drugs have failed. The RMP of these abnormal "slow-response" foci has been postulated to be less negative than −60 mV, a range where lidocaine would be ineffective on the calcium current conduction and depolarization. More information is needed before recommendations can be made for verapamil in treating dysrhythmias other than supraventricular tachydysrhythmias. Other drugs are significantly more effective for the initial treatment of ventricular dysrhythmias.

The important side-effects of verapamil are directly related

to its predominant pharmacologic action (Table 7-27). It may produce unwanted AV conduction delays and bradycardia, resulting in cardiovascular collapse. Verapamil must be used very carefully, if at all, in the presence of propranolol. The combined effect has produced complete heart block in animals and humans. It must be used carefully in patients who are digitalized for the same reason. No such interactions exist with nifedipine. The combination of β blockade and nifedipine may be beneficial in patients with ischemic heart disease because the reflex tachycardia seen with nifedipine can be countered with β blockade.

Nifedipine

Nifedipine is the most potent CEB when tested in isolated tissue preparations. It is an equipotent cardiac depressant and vasodilator. Depression of inotropism and cardiac conduction, however, is not evident in the intact human. It does not affect baroreflex mechanisms and, as a result, the marked vasodilatation is accompanied by increased SNS tone and after 1–1 load reduction (Table 7-27).[200] A compensatory tachycardia may result and cardiac output may actually increase as a result of the afterload reduction.

The most specific therapeutic application for nifedipine is coronary vasospasm (variant or Prinzmetal's angina).[199, 281] It has been more successful than nitroglycerin for this purpose because it produces a more profound and predictable coronary vasodilatation. It has also been extremely useful in other types of ischemic heart disease ranging from unstable angina to myocardial infarction. The decrease in myocardial oxygen demands that result from the reduced afterload and reduced left ventricular volume appears to be the mechanism for the relief of angina. Coronary vasodilatation is another factor, but it is not known if this is the antianginal effect in patients with coronary artery disease. The dilating effect may last only 5 min, but the antianginal effect may last more than 1 h.

Nifedipine is not available for intravenous use, but clinical practice has demonstrated that sublingual nifedipine is an effective therapeutic application with a nearly immediate onset of effect.[199, 200] One need only puncture the end of a nifedipine capsule and squirt it under the patient's tongue. Use of this technique is particularly applicable for the anesthesiologist in situations where oral medication cannot be given. We have also used sublingual nifedipine effectively in those situations where perioperative hypertension and evidence of acute coronary ischemia coexist. In these circumstances, a reduction in afterload, coronary vasodilatation, and reduced blood pressure are all achieved with the same drug.[296] Reflex tachycardia, if it occurs, can be managed with β blockers without significant interaction with nifedipine.

FIG. 7-28. Verapamil may be useful in treating ventricular dysrhythmias when first-line drugs are ineffective. The source of the cardiac dysrhythmia has been speculated to have inoperative fast sodium channels and thus to be susceptible to a calcium-entry blocker in terminating reentry.

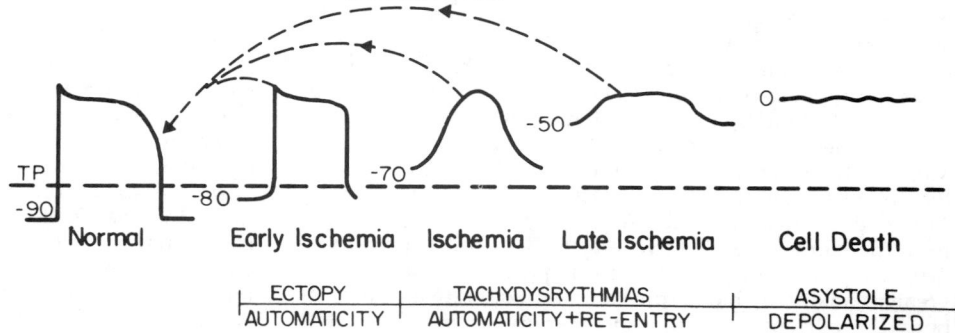

Diltiazem

The hemodynamic effects of diltiazem lie somewhere between verapamil and nifedipine.[200] It is less potent than either.[297] Diltiazem is a good coronary artery dilator but a poor peripheral vasodilator. It often produces bradycardia and delayed conduction, and reflex tachycardia is not a problem.[298] It appears to be an effective oral drug for the treatment of coronary disease in which cardiac dysrhythmias are troublesome. Cardiac dysrhythmias are noticeably a part of the clinical picture in patients suffering coronary spasm.

Calcium Entry Blockers and Anesthesia

Recent evidence indicates that halothane depresses slow-channel kinetics. All of the potent inhalational anesthetics behave in a similar fashion in that they depress myocardial contractility and vascular tone in a dose-related manner.[299, 300] Most studies indicate that the CEBs and inhalational anesthetics exert additive effects on the inward calcium current.[199, 281] Opioids do not appear to add anything to the effects of the CEBs.

Several recent studies indicate an interaction between the CEBs and the neuromuscular blocking drugs similar to that seen with the mycin antibiotics.[200] This interaction is not well defined, but in vitro and in vivo studies indicate a reduced margin of safety with these drug combinations. CEBs appear to augment the effects of both depolarizing and nondepolarizing muscle relaxants.[301] These observations serve as a word of caution because the clinical significance has not been defined. Prolonged apnea and relaxation have been reported when verapamil was used to treat a supraventricular tachycardia in a patient with Duchenne's muscular dystrophy.[302]

CEBs should be continued until the time of surgery to maintain control of angina pectoris, hypertension, or cardiac dysrhythmias.[200] One could anticipate that sudden discontinuation of these drugs theoretically could produce a rebound of symptoms, although this phenomenon has not been reported. Up regulation of calcium receptors would likely occur during periods of entry blockade.[303]

Verapamil may increase the toxicity of digoxin, benzodiazepines, carbamazepine, oral hypoglycemics, and possibly quinidine and theophylline.[304] Cardiac failure, AV conduction disturbances, and sinus bradycardia may be more frequent with concurrent use of β blockers, and severe hypotension and bradycardia may occur with bupivicaine. Decreased lithium effect and lithium neurotoxicity have both been reported with the concurrent use of verapamil.[305] The effects of verapamil may also be increased by cimetidine.[304]

ANTIHYPERTENSIVES

Increased awareness and treatment of hypertension over the last 20 years has resulted in increasing numbers of patients presenting for anesthesia and surgery who are taking one or more antihypertensive medications. These drugs are numerous, affect multiple organ systems, and have the potential for many deleterious interactions in the perioperative period. Most antihypertensive drugs either blunt the ANS or its effector organs or cause reflex increases in ANS outflow. Most anesthetic agents also inhibit ANS tone to some degree[306] and may therefore have additive effects with antihypertensive drugs. In addition, patients with hypertension may exhibit greater lability in blood pressure intraoperatively and rebound hypertension in the postoperative period.[307, 308] The

anesthesiologist should therefore maintain a thorough understanding of the commonly used antihypertensive drugs. A rational approach to their perioperative use includes decisions as to holding or continuing them preoperatively, interactions with anesthetic drugs, and resumption of treatment postoperatively. The commonly used antihypertensive drugs are grouped below according to their primary mechanism of action and discussed briefly with emphasis on considerations for the anesthesiologist.

Diuretics

Diuretics are the most commonly prescribed drugs for hypertension. The basic mechanism of action is decreased plasma and extracellular volume. Although the thiazides and furosemide have been shown to have vasodilating properties, the clinical significance of this effect is unclear. Chronic diuretic therapy results in decreased intravascular volume. The cardiovascular response to induction of anesthesia may therefore be accentuated, resulting in hypotension and tachycardia. Other problems associated with diuretic use include hypokalemia, hyponatremia, hypocalcemia, and hyperglycemia. Chronic hypokalemia is quite common with diuretic therapy and may predispose to cardiac dysrhythmias.[309] The clinical relevance of perioperative hypokalemia is unclear and has stirred considerable debate among anesthesiologists as to whether surgery should be postponed until plasma potassium levels are treated.[310, 311]

Adrenergic-Receptor Antagonists

BETA BLOCKERS. β-Adrenergic-receptor blockers are also commonly used now in the treatment of hypertension. They have been discussed in detail above, but certain comments about their perioperative use are pertinent here (Table 7-23). Following the introduction of propranolol, several deleterious interactions (in particular, the enhanced negative inotropic and chronotropic effects of halothane) were noted with anesthetics. This resulted in a debate over whether or not the blocker should be discontinued preoperatively. β-blocker therapy should be continued up to the time of operation. A withdrawal syndrome has been noted after acute discontinuation of chronic β-blocker therapy.[312, 313] Also, the control of heart rate and blood pressure perioperatively is easier if chronic medications are continued and one alters the anesthetic plan rather than acutely stopping the chronic medications and administering a routine anesthetic plan. Heart rate is a major determinant of myocardial oxygen demand. Tachycardia has recently been shown to increase the risk of poor outcome in patients with ischemic heart disease.[211, 314] The control of heart rate, therefore, as well as blood pressure, is important perioperatively, and β-blocker therapy should be continued to maximize this control.

ALPHA BLOCKERS. The α blockers in use today include prazosin and phentolamine (Table 7-22). Phentolamine is used almost exclusively in the diagnosis and treatment of pheochromocytoma. Prazosin is now commonly used to treat essential hypertension. When patients taking these drugs are to undergo anesthesia, it should be borne in mind that the normal ANS responses to stress and inhalational anesthetic drugs may be blocked at the vascular effector site; therefore, elevations of catecholamines will not reflexly increase peripheral vascular resistance and may actually decrease it if vascular β receptors are left unopposed. In the presence of α blockade we suggest preloading with intravenous fluids to assure adequate central volume and careful titration of halogenated anesthetic drugs.

Sympatholytics

Sympatholytic drugs include those that block central SNS outflow or NE release from the presynaptic neuron at the effector site. Currently included in this group are α methyldopa, clonidine, and guanabenz.

α-Methyldopa is a catechol derivative that is enzymatically converted to active compounds by enzymes in the catecholamine synthesis chain (Fig. 7-9). α-Methyldopamine and α methylnorepinephrine (αMNE) are the primary metabolites. The precise mechanism responsible for decreased SNS tone is unclear, but it is thought that αMNE, which is stored in presynaptic vesicles, is released and stimulates presynaptic α_2 receptors, thereby inhibiting NE release.[249] Because of the unique metabolism of α methyldopa to the active compound and the storage of the metabolite in presynaptic vesicles, both the time to onset and duration of action are long. Even after intravenous administration, the peak effect may not be seen for several hours. Although the elimination half-life is 2 h, the effect of an oral dose may last up to 24 h.

Clonidine stimulates presynaptic α_2 receptors and inhibits NE release from both central and peripheral adrenergic terminals. It also has some α_1-agonist activity and in high oral doses may cause paradoxical hypertension by stimulating vascular α_1 receptors. Under normal circumstances, the α_2 effects predominate. The prominent antihypertensive effect is thought to be secondary to stimulation of α_2 receptors in the vasomotor centers of the medulla oblongata.[249] Whether these are presynaptic or postsynaptic remains controversial;[244] however, the end result is decreased SNS and enhanced vagal tone. Peripherally, there is decreased plasma renin activity as well as decreased epinephrine and NE levels.

Cardiovascular effects of clonidine include decreased peripheral vascular resistance and heart rate. The cardiovascular response to exercise is usually maintained. Prominent side-effects include hypotension, sedation, and dry mouth. One of the more worrisome complications of clonidine use is the occurrence of a withdrawal syndrome on acute discontinuation of the drug. This usually occurs approximately 18 h after discontinuation and consists of hypertension, tachycardia, insomnia, flushing, headache, apprehension, sweating, and tremulousness. It lasts 24–72 h and is most likely to occur in patients taking more than $1.2 \text{ mg} \cdot \text{day}^{-1}$ of clonidine. The withdrawal syndrome has been noted postoperatively in patients who had clonidine held for surgery.[315] This can be confused with anesthesia emergence symptoms, particularly in a patient with uncontrolled hypertension. Clonidine is not available for intravenous use, but symptoms of the withdrawal syndrome, as well as routine postoperative hypertension, can be treated with clonidine administered transdermally or rectally.[316] We do not recommend holding clonidine prior to surgery. Guanabenz is an α_2 agonist that is thought to act like clonidine.

Converting-Enzyme Inhibitors

The renin–angiotensin system is integrally related to the ANS in controlling blood pressure (Fig. 7-18). Captopril and enalapril inhibit converting enzyme and thereby prevent the conversion of angiotensin I to the active angiotensin II.[317] These two drugs are extremely effective in controlling renovascular and malignant hypertension. Cardiovascular effects normally involve only decreased peripheral resistance with no change in cardiac output or filling pressures. In patients with congestive heart failure, however, cardiac output may increase markedly in response to decreased afterload. There is usually not an increase in SNS tone in response to the lowered blood pressure, and postural hypotension is uncommon.[249]

Side-effects from captopril treatment are numerous and include hypotension on initiation of therapy, drug rash, fever, eosinophilia, neutropenia, and proteinuria. For this reason other drugs are preferred as first-line agents, and these are used only in patients refractory to other therapy.

Vasodilators

The drugs that directly relax smooth muscle to cause vasodilation reflexively increase ANS tone and are included here for the sake of a complete discussion of antihypertensive drugs.[147] These will be discussed with emphasis on perioperative use.

HYDRALAZINE. Hydralazine is the most commonly used vasodilator and can be given by im, iv, and oral routes (Table 7-28). It relaxes smooth muscle tone directly, without interacting with adrenergic or cholinergic receptors. The mechanism of action is unknown. It is most potent on coronary, splanchnic, renal, and cerebral vessels, causing increased blood flow in each of these organs. The decrease in cardiac afterload is beneficial but, unfortunately, there is usually a reflex tachycardia that may be severe. It is commonly combined with a β blocker such as propranolol. It may also cause fluid retention and is usually given chronically with a diuretic.[249]

Hydralazine is metabolized by hepatic acetylation, and oral bioavailability may be low due to first-pass metabolism. The elimination half-life is about 4 h, but the pharmacologic half-life is much longer due to avid binding of the drug to smooth muscle. The effective half-life is approximately 100 h.[318] Side-effects include a lupus-like syndrome, drug fever, skin rash, pancytopenia, and peripheral neuropathy. The iv dose we recommend for perioperative use is 5–10 mg iv bolus every 15–20 min until blood pressure control is achieved. It may also be given 10–40 mg im, but the response is slower.

SODIUM NITROPRUSSIDE. Sodium nitroprusside (SNP) is an extremely potent vasodilator that is available only for iv administration. It acts directly on smooth muscle, causing both arterial and venous dilatation.[147, 319] The mechanism of action is not entirely clear but appears to involve binding to a receptor on the surface of the myocyte, then activation of an intracellular vasodilator intermediate.

The action of SNP on both venous and arterial sides of the circulation causes decreases in cardiac preload as well as afterload. This results in decreased cardiac work; however, it has been suggested that SNP may further compromise ischemic myocardium in the presence of occlusive coronary artery disease by shunting blood away from the ischemic zone.[320]

SNP is very useful during the perioperative period. It lowers blood pressure within 1–2 min, with the effect dissipating within 2 min after infusion is stopped. It is extremely potent and should be administered through a central venous line by infusion pump while continuously monitoring arterial pressure. The starting dose is 0.25 to 0.5 $\mu g \cdot kg^{-1} \cdot min^{-1}$. It can be increased slowly as needed to control blood pressure, but chances for toxicity are greater if the dose of 10 $\mu g \cdot kg^{-1} \cdot min^{-1}$ is exceeded. The dose required for steady-state–induced hypotension is variable.

Chemically, SNP consists of a ferrous iron atom bound with five cyanide molecules and one nitric group. The ferrous iron

TABLE 7-28.   Antihypertensive Drugs for Perioperative Use

DRUG	DOSE	LATENCY	DURATION	SIDE-EFFECTS*
Diuretics				
Furosemide	20–40 mg iv	5–10 min	4 h	Hypokalemia, hypovolemia
Sympatholytics				
α-methyldopa	250–500 mg siv	20 min	24 h	Sedation, hepatitis, hemolytic anemia
Clonidine	0.2 mg in 10 ml NS per rectum	20 min	12–24 h	Sedation, dry mouth, withdrawal syndrome
Vasodilators				
Hydralazine	5–10 mg iv	15–20 min	4–6 h	Lupus-like syndrome, drug fever, rash
	10–40 mg im	20–40 min		
Nifedipine	10 mg siv	5–10 min	7 h	Headache, fluid retention
Verapamil	5 mg iv	2–5 min	4–6 h	Heart block, myocardial failure
Diazoxide	300 mg siv	3–5 min	5–12 h	Decreased cerebral blood flow, hyperuricemia
Sodium nitroprusside	0.25–0.5 $\mu g \cdot kg^{-1} \cdot min^{-1}$	1–2 min	2–5 min	Cyanide toxicity, increased cerebral blood flow
Nitroglycerin		2–5 min	3–5 min	Headache, fluid retention
Adrenergic Blocking Drugs See Tables 22 and 23				

Doses shown are for 70-kg adult. iv = intravenous push; siv = slow intravenous infusion; im = intramuscular; sl = sublingual.
*All of the drugs listed may also cause hypotension. All possible side-effects are not listed. The ones shown are the most common.

reacts with sulfhydryl groups in red blood cells and releases cyanide.[321] Cyanide is reduced to thiocyanate in the liver and excreted in the urine. The half-life of thiocyanate is 4 days, and it will accumulate in the presence of renal failure.[322] There is no evidence, however, that preexisting hepatic or renal failure increases the likelihood of cyanide toxicity. Administration of high doses of SNP can result in cyanide toxicity. The cyanide molecule binds to cytochrome oxidase, interfering with electron transport and causing cellular hypoxia. This can be recognized by increasing tolerance to the drug, elevated mixed venous P_{O_2}, and metabolic acidosis. The treatment of cyanide toxicity is (1) administration of amyl nitrate (by inhalation or directly into the anesthesia circuit); (2) infusion of sodium nitrite 5 mg $\cdot$ kg^{-1} over 4–5 min; and (3) sodium thiosulfate 150 mg $\cdot$ kg^{-1} in 50 ml water over 15 min.

The hypotensive effects of SNP may be potentiated by inhalation anesthetics and blood loss, so close perioperative monitoring is essential. It is commonly used to induce hypotension for decreasing blood loss in cases predisposed to major hemorrhage. Administration of SNP causes a reflex increase in SNS tone and renin release.[323] Drugs that blunt these reflexes markedly enhance the effects of SNP. Preoperative treatment with propranolol or captopril decreases the amount of SNP required for hypotension and thus decreases the potential for toxicity.[324, 325]

GLYCERIL TRINITRATE. Glyceril trinitrate, or nitroglycerin, is a venodilator used to treat myocardial ischemia (see Chapter 35). Its predominant action is on venules, causing increased venous capacitance and decreased cardiac preload. Effects on the arterial side are minimal except at very high doses. Upon iv administration, effects can be seen within 2 min, and they usually resolve within 5 min of discontinuing the drug. Side-effects are minimal, and there is no potential for cyanide toxicity as with SNP. Use of nitroglycerin for control of perioperative hypertension has been reported[326] but, due to its relatively weak arteriolar action, it is not as useful as other drugs as an antihypertensive agent. In obstetric patients with preeclampsia, however, it may be chosen over SNP to circumvent potential cyanide toxicity to the fetus.[327]

DIAZOXIDE. Diazoxide is a directly acting vasodilator that may be given iv and is useful in hypertensive emergencies. It has a greater effect on resistance than capacitance vessels, thus decreasing cardiac afterload with little effect on preload. It also causes fluid retention and induces a reflex SNS response.[249] The hypotensive effect is potentiated by diuretics, sympatholytics, and hypovolemia.

It is usually administered as an iv bolus of 300 mg for an adult weighing 70 kg. It is 90% bound to serum albumin so a substantial portion of the initial bolus may not reach the site of action. Rapid boluses (less than 30 s) of 100 mg every 5 min are often recommended as an alternative to allow more free drug to reach the arterioles.[249] The hypotensive effect is usually obtained in 5–10 min and lasts 5–12 h.

Calcium Entry Inhibitors

The CEBs verapamil and nifedipine may also be useful for treating hypertension in the perioperative period.[328, 329] They are discussed in detail above.

Treatment of Postoperative Hypertension

The wide variety of antihypertensive drugs discussed above makes the treatment of hypertension in the recovery room easier because we can now choose from multiple routes of administration and variable onsets and duration of action of the different drugs;[330, 331] however, treatment may become confusing unless the basic pharmacology of each of the drugs is understood. Those drugs available only for oral administration are not routinely used due to unreliable gastrointestinal function during this period. The etiology of postoperative hypertension in each case should be considered. A determination should be made if this requires emergency therapy or is just urgent. Pain should be eliminated by assurance of adequate analgesia prior to therapy with antihypertensive drugs. Also, due to the complex pathophysiology of hypertension, a thorough knowledge of each patient is mandatory in choosing a regimen. The medications required for preoperative control may provide the most information in determining what will be necessary postoperatively. In particular, the use of drugs that may have an associated withdrawal syndrome, such as clonidine or β blockers, as well as whether they were held prior to surgery, should be noted. The volume status of the patient is important. Fluid overload may require diuretic therapy. Volume depletion or hemorrhage may predispose to severe hypotension in response to routine doses of sympatholytics or vasodilators.

For severe elevations of blood pressure that require immediate treatment, we feel SNP is the drug of choice. Diazoxide and nifedipine (sublingual) are also useful but may take 5–10 min to work. In the presence of ischemic heart disease, sublingual nifedipine is quite effective as a result of its beneficial effects on coronary blood flow as well as blood pressure. Also, if nifedipine is readily available, it can usually be given and start to work before an SNP infusion can be prepared. Central line placement may also be circumvented in choosing nifedipine over SNP. If control of blood pressure requires SNP, several of the slower-acting drugs may be used to wean the patient. Hydralazine 5–10 mg iv and propranolol 0.2–0.5 mg iv in repeated doses is a commonly used approach. Propranolol can be titrated to maintain heart rate below 100 beats/min, then hydralazine can be used to lower blood pressure to the desired level with boluses every 20–30 min. Labetalol, metoprolol, and esmolol may also be used iv. Esmolol has the advantage of being rapidly titratable.[267] α methyldopa may be used iv but takes much longer to work. Clonidine can be given rectally and begins to act in 10–20 min.[316] If conditions permit, it is helpful to use the drugs the patient was taking preoperatively to ease transition in the postoperative period. Caution must be exercised if the hypertension is the result of excessive exogenous catecholamines, pheochromocytoma, or thyrotoxicosis. α blockade should be started before β blockade. The hypertension may, in fact, worsen if β receptors are blocked first, leaving the α receptors unopposed.

REFERENCES

1. Axelrod J, Reisine TD: Stress hormones: Their interaction and regulation. Science 224:452, 1984
2. Pinsker MC: Anesthesia: A pragmatic construct. Anesthesiology 65:819, 1986
3. Weiner N, Taylor P: Neurohumoral transmission and the autonomic nervous system. In Gilman AG, Goodman LS, Rall TW et al (eds): The Pharmacological Basis of Therapeutics, p 66. New York, Macmillan, 1985
4. Koizumi K, Brooks CC: The autonomic nervous system and its role in controlling visceral activities. In Mountcastle VB (ed): Medical Physiology, p 783. St Louis, CV Mosby, 1974
5. Warwick R, Williams PL: The autonomic nervous system. In Warwick R, Williams PL (eds): Gray's Anatomy, 35th ed, p 1065. Philadelphia, WB Saunders, 1973
6. Guyton AC: The autonomic nervous system: The adrenal medulla. In Guyton AC (ed): Textbook of Medical Physiology, p 686. Philadelphia, WB Saunders, 1986
7. Bevan JA: Introduction. In Bevan JA (ed): Essentials of Pharmacology, p 108. New York, Harper & Row, 1976
8. Everett NB: The autonomic nervous system. In Everett NB (ed): Functional Neuroanatomy, p 242. Philadelphia, Lea & Febiger, 1971
9. Davson H, Eggleton MG: The autonomic nervous system. In Davson H, Eggleton MG (eds): Principles of Human Physiology, p 1131. Philadelphia, Lea & Febiger, 1962
10. White JC, Smithwick RH, Simeone FA: Physiology of visceral pain. In White JC, Smithwick RH, Simeone FA (eds): The Autonomic Nervous System, p 126. New York, Macmillan, 1952
11. Willis WD: The pain system: The neural basis of nociceptive transmission in the mammalian nervous system. In Gildenberg PL (ed): Pain and Headache, vol 8. New York, Karger, 1985
12. Lake CR, Chernow B, Feuerstein G et al: The sympathetic nervous system in man: Its evaluation and the measurement of plasma NE. In Ziegler MG, Lake CR (eds): Norepinephrine, p 1. Baltimore, Williams & Wilkins, 1984
13. Miller NE: Biofeedback and visceral learning. Ann Rev Psychol 29:373, 1972
14. Davies DS, Reid JL (eds): Central Action of Drugs in Blood Pressure Regulation. Baltimore, University Park Press, 1975
15. Lambert DH, Deane RS, Mazuzan JE: Anesthesia and the control of blood pressure in patients with spinal cord injury. Anesth Analg 61:344, 1982
16. Kewalrami LS: Autonomic dysreflexia in traumatic myelopathy. Am J Phys Med 59:1, 1980
17. Axelrod J, Weinshilboum R: Catecholamines. N Engl J Med 287:237, 1972
18. Guyton AC: Rhythmic excitation of the heart. In Guyton AC (ed): Textbook of Medical Physiology, p 165. Philadelphia, WB Saunders, 1986
19. Flacke WE, Flacke JW: Cholinergic and anticholinergic agents. In Smith NT, Corbascio AN (eds): Drug Interaction in Anesthesia, p 160. Philadelphia, Lea & Febiger, 1986
20. Fugii AM, Vatner SF: Autonomic mechanisms regulating myocardial contractility in conscious animals. Pharmacol Ther 29:221, 1985
21. Yanowitz F, Preston JB, Abildskov JA: Functional distribution of right and left stellate innervation to the ventricles. Circ Res 18:416, 1966
22. Berne RM, Levy MN: Control of the heart. In Berne RM, Levy MN (eds): Cardiovascular Physiology, p 221. St Louis, CV Mosby, 1977
23. Bexton RS, Milne JR, Cory-Pearce R et al: Effect of beta blockade on exercise response after cardiac transplantation. Br Heart J 49:584, 1983
24. Manger WM: Catecholamines in normal and abnormal cardiac function. In Kellerman JJ (ed): Advances in Cardiology, p 30. New York, Karger, 1982
25. Vatner SF: Regulation of coronary resistance vessels and large coronary arteries. Am J Cardiol 56:16E, 1985
26. Hillis LD, Braunwald E: Coronary-artery spasm. N Engl J Med 299(13): 695, 1978
27. Shepard JT, Vanhoutte PM: Spasm of the coronary arteries: Causes and consequences (the scientist's viewpoint). Mayo Clin Proc 60:33, 1985
28. Kates RA, Stack RS, Hill RF et al: General anesthesia for patients undergoing percutaneous transluminal coronary angioplasty during acute myocardial infarction. Anesth Analg 65:815, 1986
29. Braunwald E: A symposium: Experimental and clinical aspects of coronary vasoconstriction. Am J Cardiol 56:(9), 1985
30. Osswald W, Guimaraes S: Adrenergic mechanisms in blood vessels: Morphological and pharmacological aspects. Rev Physiol Biochem Pharmacol 96:54, 1983
31. Lawson NW, Wallfisch HK: Cardiovascular pharmacology: A new look at the "pressors." In Stoelting RK, Barash PG, Gallagher TJ (eds): Advances in Anesthesia, p 195. Chicago, Year Book Medical Publishers, 1986
32. Bevan JA: Some basis of differences in vascular response to sympathetic activity: Variations on a theme. Circ Res 45:161, 1979

33. Guyton AC: Local control of blood flow by the tissues, and nervous and humoral regulation. In Guyton AC (ed): Textbook of Medical Physiology, p 230. Philadelphia, WB Saunders, 1986

34. Nandiwada PA, Hyman AL, Kadowitz PJ: Pulmonary vasodilator responses to vagal stimulation and acetylcholine in the cat. Circ Res 53:86, 1983

35. Guyton AC: The pulmonary circulation. In Guyton AC (ed): Textbook of Medical Physiology, p 287. Philadelphia, WB Saunders, 1986

36. Benumof JL: The pulmonary circulation. In Kaplan JA (ed): Thoracic Anesthesia, p 249. New York, Churchill-Livingstone, 1983

37. Benumof JL: One-lung ventilation and hypoxic pulmonary vasoconstriction: Implications for anesthetic management. Anesth Analg 64:821, 1985

38. Carlsson AJ, Bindslev L, Hedenstierna G: Hypoxia-induced pulmonary vasoconstriction in the human lung. Anesthesiology 66:312, 1987

39. Comroe JH: Reflexes from the lungs. In Comroe JH (ed): Physiology of Respiration, p 72. Chicago, Year Book Medical Publishers, 1979

40. Junod AF: Metabolism of vasoactive agents in lung. Am Rev Respir Dis 115:51, 1977

41. Youdim MBH, Bakhle YS, Ben-Harari RR: Inaction of monoamines by the lung. In Metabolic Activities of the Lung, p 105. Amsterdam, Ciba Foundation Symposium 78, Excerpta Medica, 1980

42. Halter JB, Pflug AE, Tolas AG: Arterial-venous differences of plasma catecholamines in man. Metabolism 29:9, 1980

43. Pearl RG, Maze M, Rosenthal MH: Pulmonary and systemic hemodynamic effects of central venous and left atrial sympathomimetic drugs administration in the dog. J Cardiothorac Anesth 1:29, 1987

44. Bevan JA: Some basis of differences in vascular response to sympathetic activity. Circ Res 45:161, 1979

45. Miller R: Multiple calcium channels and neuronal function. Science 235:46, 1987

46. Carpenter RL, Mulroy MF: Edrophonium antagonizes combined lidocaine-pancuronium and verapamil-pancuronium neuromuscular blockade in cats. Anesthesiology 65:506, 1986

47. Wood M: Cholinergic and parasympathomimetic drugs. Cholinesterases and anticholinesterases. In Wood M, Wood AJJ (eds): Drugs and Anesthesia, p 111. Baltimore, Williams & Wilkins, 1982

48. Thomas J, Fouad FM, Tarazi RC et al: Evaluation of plasma catecholamines in humans: Correlation of resting levels with cardiac responses to beta-blocking and sympatholytic drugs. Hypertension 5:858, 1983

49. Lake CR, Ziegler MG, Kopin IJ: Use of plasma norepinephrine for evaluation of sympathetic neuronal function in man. Life Sci 18:1315, 1976

50. Stoelting RK: Sympathomimetics. In Stoelting RK (ed): Pharmacology and Physiology in Anesthetic Practice, p 251. Philadelphia, JB Lippincott, 1987

51. Zaimis E: Vasopressor drugs and catecholamines. Anesthesiology 29:732, 1968

52. Smith NT, Corbascio AN: The use and misuse of pressor agents. Anesthesiology 8:58, 1970

53. Shepard JT, Vanhoutte PM: Neurohumoral Regulation. The Human Cardiovascular System, p 368. New York, Raven Press, 1984

54. Zsigmond EK: Catecholamines and anesthesia. In Oyama T (ed): Endocrinology and the Anaesthetist, p 225. New York, Elsevier, 1983

55. Zaritsky AL, Chernow B: Catecholamines, sympathomimetics. In Ziegler MG, Lake CR (eds): Frontiers of Clinical Neuroscience, vol 2 (Norepinephrine), p 481. Baltimore, Williams & Wilkins, 1984

56. Kopin IJ: Catecholamine metabolism and the biochemical assessment of sympathetic activity. Clin Endocrinol Metab 6:525, 1977

57. Chernow B, Rainey TG, Lake CR: Catecholamines in critical care medicine. In Ziegler MG, Lake CR (eds): Frontiers of Clinical Neuroscience, vol 2 (Norepinephrine), p 368. Baltimore, Williams & Wilkins, 1984

58. Fuder H: Selected aspects of presynaptic modulation of noradrenaline release from the heart. J Cardiovasc Pharmacol 7 (Suppl 5):S2, 1985

59. Kopin IJ: Metabolic degradation of catecholamines and relative importance of different pathways under physiological conditions and after the administration of drugs. In Blaschko H, Muscholl E (eds): Catecholamines: Handbook of Experimental Pharmacology, p 270. New York, Springer Verlag, 1972

60. Lefkowitz RJ: Beta-adrenergic receptors: Recognition and regulation. N Engl J Med 295:323, 1976

61. Maze M: Clinical implications of membrane receptor function in anesthesia. Anesthesiology 55:160, 1981

62. Wood M: Cholinergic and parasympathomimetic drugs. Cholinesterases and anticholinesterases. In Wood M, Wood AJJ (eds): Drugs and Anesthesia, p 111. Baltimore, Williams & Wilkins, 1982

63. Reardon DP, Bailey JC: Parasympathetic effects on electrophysiologic properties of cardiac ventricular tissue. J Am Coll Cardiol 2:1200, 1983

64. Von Euler US: A specific sympathomimetic ergone in adrenergic nerve fibers (sympathin) and its relation to adrenaline and noradrenaline. Acta Physiol Scand 12:73, 1946

65. Ahlquist RP: A study of the adrenotropic receptors. Am J Physiol 153:586, 1948

66. Exton JH: Mechanisms involved in α-adrenergic phenomena. Am J Physiol 248:E633, 1985

67. Lands AM, Arnold A, McAnliff JP et al: Differentiation of receptor systems activated by sympathomimetic amines. Nature 214:597, 1967

68. Ariens EJ, Simonis AM: Physiological and pharmacological aspects of adrenergic receptor classification. Biochem Pharmacol 32:1539, 1983

69. Kebabian JW, Calne DB: Multiple receptors for dopamine. Nature 277:93, 1979

70. Dresel PE: Cardiac alpha receptors and arrhythmias. Anesthesiology 63:582, 1985

71. Maze M, Hayward E, Gaba EM: Alpha$_1$-adrenergic blockade raises epinephrine-arrhythmia threshold in halothane-anesthetized dogs in a dose-dependent fashion. Anesthesiology 63:611, 1985

72. Steer ML, Wood A: Regulation of human platelet adenylate cyclase by epinephrine, prostaglandin E and guanine nucleotides. J Biol Chem 254:10791, 1979

73. Langer SZ: Presynaptic regulation of catecholamine release. Biochem Pharmacol 23:1793, 1974

74. Hoffman BB, Lefkowitz RJ: Alpha-adrenergic receptor subtypes. N Engl J Med 302:1390, 1980

75. Berthelesen S, Pettinger WA: A functional basis for classification of alpha adrenergic receptors. Life Sci 21:595, 1977

76. Bryan LJ, Cole JJ, O'Donnell SR et al: A study designed to explore the hypothesis that the beta$_1$ adrenoceptors are 'innervated' receptors and beta$_2$ adrenoceptors are 'hormonal' receptors. J Pharmacol Exp Ther 216:395, 1981

77. Carlsson A: The occurrence, distribution and physiological role of catecholamines in the nervous system. Pharmacol Rev 11:493, 1959

78. Goldberg LI: Dopamine receptors and hypertension. Am J Med 77(4A):37, 1984

79. Rajfer SI, Goldbert LI: Dopamine in the treatment of heart failure. Eur Heart J 3(suppl. D):103, 1982

80. Peringer E, Jenner P, Donaldson IM *et al*: Metoclopramide and dopamine receptor blockade. Neuropharmacology 15:463, 1976

81. Yahr JD: Levodopa. Ann Intern Med 83:677, 1975

82. Goldberg LI, Volkman PH, Kohli JD: A comparison of the vascular receptor with other dopamine receptors. Ann Rev Pharmacol Toxicol 18:57, 1978

83. Solanki DR, Suresh M, Ethridge HC: The effects of intravenous cimetidine and metaclopramide on gastric volume and pH. Anesth Analg 63:599, 1984

84. Thorner MD: Dopamine is an important neurotransmitter in the autonomic nervous system. Lancet 1:662, 1975

85. Hilberman M, Maseda J, Stinson EB *et al*: The diuretic properties of dopamine in patients following open heart operations. Anesthesiology 61:489, 1984

86. Daly JW, Bruns RF, Snyder SH: Adenosine receptors in the central nervous system: Relationship to the central actions of methylxanthines. Life Sci 28:2083, 1981

87. Barrett JE, Tessel RE: Behavioral pharmacology of drugs affecting norepinephrine transmission. In Ziegler MG, Lake CR (eds): Frontiers of Clinical Neuroscience, vol 2 (Norepinephrine), p 160. Baltimore, Williams & Wilkins, 1984

88. Owall A, Gordon E, Lagerkranser M *et al*: Clinical experience with adenosine for controlled hypotension during cerebral aneurysm surgery. Anesth Analg 66:229, 1987

89. Engel G, Gothert M, Muller-Schweinitzer E *et al*: Evidence for common pharmacological properties of 5-hydroxy-tryptamine binding sites; presynaptic 5-hydroxytryptamine auto-receptors in CNS and inhibitory presynaptic 5-hydroxytryptamine receptors on sympathetic nerves. Naunyn Schmiedebergs Arch Pharmacol 324:116, 1983

90. Manchikanti L, Kraus JW, Fields SP: Cimetidine and related drugs in anesthesia. Anesth Analg 61:595, 1982

91. Lineberger AS, Sprague DH, Battaglini JW: Sinus arrest associated with cimetidine. Anesth Analg 64:554, 1985

92. Goldberg LI: The dopamine vascular receptor: New areas for biochemical pharmacologists. Biochem Pharmacol 24:651, 1975

93. Williams LT, Lefkowitz RJ: Receptor Binding Studies in Adrenergic Pharmacology. New York, Raven Press, 1979

94. Motulsky JH, Insel PA: Adrenergic receptors in man. N Engl J Med 302:18, 1982

95. Tell GP, Haour F, Saez JM: Hormone regulation of membrane receptors and cell responsiveness: A review. Metabolism 27:1566, 1978

96. Galant SP, Duriseti L, Underwood S *et al*: Decreased beta-adrenergic receptors on polymorphonuclear leukocytes after adrenergic therapy. N Engl J Med 299:933, 1978

97. Glaubiger G, Lefkowitz RJ: Elevated beta-adrenergic number after chronic propranolol treatment. Biochem Biophys Res Commun 78:720, 1977

98. Hoefke W: Clonidine. In Scriabine A (ed): Pharmacology of Antihypertensive Drugs, p 55. New York, Raven Press, 1980

99. Johnston RV, Nicholas DA, Lawson NW *et al*: The use of rectal clonidine in the perioperative period. Anesthesiology 64:288, 1986

100. Myers MG: Beta adrenoreceptor antagonism and pressor response to phenylephrine. Clin Pharmacol Ther 36:57, 1984

101. Williams LT, Lefkowitz RJ: Thyroid hormone regulation of β-adrenergic receptor number. J Biol Chem 252:2787, 1977

102. Sutherland EW, Robison GA: The role of cyclic-3′5′ AMP in response to catecholamines and other hormones. Pharmacol Rev 18:145, 1966

103. Sutherland EW, Robison GA, Butcher RW: Some aspects of the biological role of adenosine 3′5′ monophosphate. Circulation 37:279, 1968

104. Schramm M, Selinger Z: Message transmission: Receptor controlled adenylate cyclase system. Science 225:1350, 1984

105. Lefkowitz RJ, Cerione RA, Codina J *et al*: Reconstitution of the β-adrenergic receptor. J Membr Biol 87:1, 1985

106. Gilman AG: Proteins and dual control of adenylate cyclase. Cell 36:577, 1984

107. Sutherland EW, Oye I, Butcher RW: The action of epinephrine and the role of adenyl cyclase system in hormone action. Recent Prog Hor Res 21:623, 1965

108. Tomlinson S, MacNeil S, Brown BL: Calcium, cyclic AMP and hormone action. Clin Endocrinol 23:595, 1985

109. Lamers JM: Calcium transport systems in cardiac sarcolemma and their regulation by the second messenger cyclic AMP and calcium-calmodulin. Gen Physiol Biophys 4:143, 1985

110. Exton JH: Mechanisms involved in α-adrenergic phenomena. Am J Physiol 258:E633, 1985

111. Ignarro LJ, Kadowitz PJ: The pharmacological and physiological role of cyclic GMP in vascular smooth muscle relaxation. Ann Rev Pharmacol Toxicol 25:171, 1985

112. Berridge MJ: Inositol triphosphate and diaglycerol as second messengers. Biochem J 22:345, 1984

113. Marx JL: Polyphosphoinositide research updated. Science 235:974, 1987

114. Kariya T, Wille L, Dage R: Biochemical studies on the mechanism of cardiotonic activity of MDL 17,043. J Cardiovasc Pharmacol 4:509, 1982

115. Krieger EM: Time course of baroreceptor resetting in acute hypertension. Am J Physiol 218:486, 1970

116. Flacke WE, Flacke JW: Cardiovascular physiology and circulatory control. Semin Anesth 1:185, 1982

117. Takeshima R, Dohi S: Circulatory responses to baroreflexes, valsalva maneuver, coughing, swallowing, and nasal stimulation during acute cardiac sympathectomy by epidural blockade in awake humans. Anesthesiology 63:500, 1985

118. Berne RM, Levy MN: Coronary circulation and cardiac metabolism. In Berne RM, Levy MN (eds): Cardiovascular Physiology, p 221. St Louis, CV Mosby, 1977

119. Guyton AC: Cardiac output, venous return, and their regulation. In Guyton AC (ed): Textbook of Medical Physiology, p 272. Philadelphia, WB Saunders, 1986

120. Sharpey-Schafer EP: Venous tone: Effects of reflex changes, humoral agents and exercise. Br Med Bull 19:115, 1963

121. Blinks JR: Positive chronotropic effect of increasing right atrial pressure in the isolated mammalian heart. Am J Physiol 196:299, 1956

122. Baron JF, Decauz-Jacolot A, Edouard A *et al*: Influence of venous return on baroreflex control of heart rate during lumbar epidural anesthesia in humans. Anesthesiology 64:188, 1986

123. Kotrly KT, Ebert TJ, Vucins E *et al*: Baroreceptor reflex control of heart rate during isoflurane anesthesia in humans. Anesthesiology 60:173, 1984

124. Greene NM: The cardiovascular system. In Greene NM (ed): Physiology of Spinal Anesthesia, p 43. New York, Kreiger Publishing, 1976

125. Greene NM: Perspectives in spinal anesthesia. Reg Anesth 7:55, 1982

126. Bexton RS, Milne JR, Cory-Pearce R *et al*: Effect of beta blockade on exercise response after cardiac transplantation. Br Heart J 49:584, 1983

127. Orlick AE, Ricci DR, Alderman EL *et al*: Effects of alpha adrenergic blockade upon coronary hemodynamics. J Clin Invest 62:459, 1978

128. Fowles RE, Reitz BA, Ream AK: Drug actions in a transplanted or artificial heart. In Kaplan JA (ed): Cardiac Anesthesia, vol 2 (Cardiovascular Pharmacology), p 641. New York, Grune & Stratton, 1983

129. Cannom DS, Rider AK, Stinson EB *et al*: Electrophysiologic studies in the denervated transplanted human heart. II. Re-

sponse to norepinephrine, isoproterenol and propranolol. Am J Cardiol 36:859, 1975

130. Leachman RD, Cokkinos DVP, Cabrera R et al: Response of the transplanted, denervated human heart to cardiovascular drugs. Am J Cardiol 27:273, 1971

131. Bexton RS, Milne JR, Cory-Pearce R et al: Effect of beta blockade on exercise response after cardiac transplantation. Br Heart J 49:584, 1983

132. Wallace AC, Schaal SF, Sugimoto G et al: Electrophysiological effects of beta-adrenergic blockade in cardiac denervation. Bull NY Acad Med 43:1119, 1967

133. Shepard JT, Vanhoutte PM: Why nerves to coronary vessels? Symposium—Autonomic control of coronary tone: Facts, interpretations, and consequences. Fed Proc 43:2855, 1984

134. Moreland RS, Bohr DF: Adrenergic control of coronary arteries. Fed Proc 43:2858, 1984

135. Vanhoutte PM, Cohen RA: Effects of acetylcholine on the coronary artery. Fed Proc 43:2878, 1984

136. Feigl EO: Parasympathetic control of coronary blood flow. Fed Proc 43:2881, 1984

137. Loffelholz K, Muscholl E: Muscarinic inhibition of the noradrenaline release evoked by postganglionic sympathetic nerve stimulation. Naunyn Schmiedebergs Arch Pharmacol 265:1, 1969

138. Levy MN, Blattberg B: Effect of vagal stimulation on the overflow of norepinephrine into the coronary sinus during cardiac sympathetic nerve stimulation in the dog. Circ Res 107:508, 1976

139. Yasue H, Touyama M, Shimamoto M et al: The role of the autonomic nervous system in the pathogenesis of Prinzmetal's variant form of angina. Circulation 50:534, 1984

140. Schrier RW, Berl T, Anderson RJ: Osmotic and nonosmotic control of vasopressin release. Am J Physiol 236(4):F321, 1979

141. Coore HG, Randle PJ: Regulation of insulin secretion studied with pieces of rabbit pancreas incubated in vitro. Biochem J 93:66, 1964

142. Case DB, Atlas SA, Laragh JH et al: Clinical experience with blockade of the renin-angiotension-aldosterone system by an oral converting enzyme inhibitor (SQ 14, 225; captopril) in hypertensive patients. Prog Cardiovasc Dis 21:195, 1978

143. Todd PA, Heel RC: Enalapril: A Review. Drugs 31:198, 1986

144. MacGregor GA, Dawes PM: Agonist and antagonist effects of Sar¹-Ala⁸-angiotensin II in salt-loaded and salt-depleted normal man. Br J Clin Pharmacol 3:483, 1976

145. Taylor P: Ganglionic stimulating and blocking agents. In Gilman AG, Goodman LS, Rall TW et al (eds): The Pharmacological Basis of Therapeutics, p 315. New York, Macmillan, 1985

146. Vickers MD, Wood-Smith FG, Stewart HC: Cardiovascular drugs. In Vickers MD, Wood-Smith FG, Stewart HC (eds): Drugs in Anesthetic Practice, p 337. Boston, Butterworth, 1979

147. Stoelting RK: Peripheral vasodilators. In Stoelting RK (ed): Pharmacology and Physiology in Anesthetic Practice, p 307. Philadelphia, JB Lippincott, 1987

148. Taylor P: Cholinergic agonists. In Gilman AG, Goodman LS, Rall TW et al (eds): The Pharmacological Basis of Therapeutics, p 100. New York, Macmillan, 1985

149. Stoelting RK: Anticholinesterase drugs and cholinergic agonists. In Stoelting RK (ed): Pharmacology and Physiology in Anesthetic Practice, p 207. Philadelphia, JB Lippincott, 1987

150. Vickers MD, Wood-Smith FG, Stewart HC: Parasympathomimetic and cholinergic agents: Anticholinesterases. In Vickers MD, Wood-Smith FG, Stewart HC (eds): Drugs in Anesthetic Practice, p 306. Boston, Butterworth, 1979

151. Westfall TC: Muscarinic agents. In Bevan JA (eds): Essentials of Pharmacology, p 116. New York, Harper & Row, 1976

152. Westfall TC: Cholinesterase inhibitors. In Bevan JA (eds): Essentials of Pharmacology, p 120. New York, Harper & Row, 1976

153. Bell CMA, Lewis CB: Effect of neostigmine on integrity of ileorectal anastomoses. Br Med J 3:587, 1968

154. Wilkins JL, Hardcastle JD, Mann CV et al: Effects of neostigmine and atropine on motor activity on ileum, colon, and rectum of anesthetized subjects. Br J Med 1:793, 1970

155. Brown EN, Daugherty MJ, Petty WC: Integrity of intestinal anastomoses muscle relaxant reversal with neostigmine. Anesth Analg 1:117, 1973

156. Child CS: Prevention of neostigmine-induced colonic activity. Anesthesia 39:1083, 1984

157. Taylor P: Anticholinesterase agents. In Gilman AG, Goodman LS, Rall TW et al (eds): The Pharmacological Basis of Therapeutics, p 110. New York, Macmillan, 1985

158. De Roetth A, Wong A, Dettbarn WD et al: Blood cholinesterase activity of glaucoma patients treated with phospholine iodide. Am J Ophthalmol 62:834, 1966

159. Milby TH: Prevention and management of organophosphate poisoning. JAMA 216:2131, 1971

160. Stoelting RK: Anticholinergic drugs. In Stoelting RK (ed): Pharmacology and Physiology in Anesthetic Practice, p 232. Philadelphia, JB Lippincott, 1987

161. Price NM, Schmitt LG, McGuire J et al: Transdermal scopalamine in the prevention of motion sickness at sea. Clin Pharmacol Ther 29:414, 1981

162. Wood M: Anticholinergic drugs: Anesthetic premedication. In Wood M, Wood AJJ (eds): Drugs and Anesthesia: Pharmacology for Anesthesiologists, p 141. Baltimore, Williams & Wilkins, 1982

163. Weiner N: Atropine, scopalamine, and related antimuscarinic drugs. In Gilman AG, Goodman LS, Rall TW et al (eds): The Pharmacological Basis of Therapeutics, p 110. New York, Macmillan, 1985

164. Westfall TC: Antimuscarinic agents. In Bevan JA (ed): Essentials of Pharmacology, p 128. New York, Harper & Row, 1976

165. Duvoisin RC, Katz RL: Reversal of central anticholinergic syndrome in man by physostigmine. JAMA 206:1963, 1968

166. Spaulding BC, Choi SD, Gross JB et al: The effect of physostigmine on diazepam-induced ventilatory depression: A double-blind study. Anesthesiology 61:551, 1984

167. Snir-Mor I, Weinstock M, Davidson JT et al: Physostigmine antagonizes morphine-induced respiratory depression in human subjects. Anesthesiology 59:6, 1983

168. Ruiz CE, Weil MH, Carlson RW: Treatment of circulatory shock with dopamine: Studies on survival. JAMA 242:165, 1979

169. Resnekov L: University of Chicago Myocardial Infarction Research Unit, Comprehensive Clinical and Laboratory Research. Washington, DC, US Public Health Service PH43-68-1334-A73, 1975

170. Resnekov L: Cardiogenic shock. Chest 83:893, 1983

171. Rothe CF: Physiology of venous return. Arch Intern Med 146:977, 1986

172. Stanton-Hicks M, Hock A, Stuhmeier K et al: Venoconstrictor agents mobilize blood from different sources and increase intrathoracic filling during epidural anesthesia in supine humans. Anesthesiology 66:317, 1987

173. Lundberg J, Norgren L, Thomson D et al: Hemodynamic effects of dopamine during thoracic epidural analgesia in man. Anesthesiology 66:641, 1987

174. Ramanathan S, Grant G, Turndorf H: Cardiac preload changes with ephedrine therapy for hypotension in obstetrical patients. Anesth Analg 65:S125, 1986

175. Butterworth JF, Austin JC, Johnson MD et al: Effect of total spinal anesthesia on arterial and venous responses to dopamine and dobutamine. Anesth Analg 66:209, 1987

176. Cubbold A, Folkow B, Kjellmer I et al: Nervous and local chemical control of pre-capillary sphincters in skeletal muscle as measured by changes in filtration coefficient. Acta Physiol Scand 57:180, 1963

177. Folkow B, Mellander S: Veins and venous tone. Am Heart J 68:309, 1964
178. Coffman JD, Lempert JA: Venous flow velocity, venous volume and arterial blood flow. Circulation 52:141, 1975
179. Sharpey-Schafer EP, Ginsburg J: Humoral agents and venous tone. Effects of catecholamines, 5-hydroxytryptamine, histamine and nitrites. Lancet 2:1337, 1962
180. Zimmerman BG, Abboud FM, Eckstein JW: Comparison of the effects of sympathomimetic amines upon venous and total vascular resistance in the foreleg of the dog. J Pharmacol Exp Ther 139:290, 1963
181. Schmid PG, Eckstein JW, Abboud FM: Comparison of the effects of several sympathomimetic amines on resistance and capacitance vessels in the forearm of man. Circulation 34:209, 1966
182. Marino RJ, Romagnoli A, Keats A: Selective venoconstriction by dopamine in comparison with isoproterenol and phenylephrine. Anesthesiology 43:570, 1975
183. Guimaraes S, Osswald W: Adrenergic receptors in the veins of dogs. Eur J Pharmacol 5:133, 1969
184. McNay JL, McDonald RA, Goldberg LI: Direct renal vasodilatation produced by dopamine in the dog. Circ Res 16:510, 1965
185. DeMay J, Vanhoutte PM: Uneven distribution of postjunctional alpha$_1$- and alpha$_2$-like adrenoreceptors in canine arterial and venous smooth muscle. Circ Res 48(6):875, 1981
186. Rude RE: Pharmacologic support in cardiogenic shock. Adv Shock Res 10:35, 1983
187. Rajfer SI, Goldberg LI: Sympathetic amines in the treatment of shock. In Shoemaker WC, Thompson WL, Holbrook RP (eds): Textbook of Critical Care, p 490. Philadelphia, WB Saunders, 1984
188. Houston MC, Thompson WL, Robertson D: Shock diagnosis and management. Arch Intern Med 144:1433, 1984
189. Shoemaker WC: Fluid management. Semin Anesth 2:251, 1983
190. Evans DB, Weishaar RE, Kaplan HR: Strategy for the discovery and development of a positive inotropic agent. Pharmacol Ther 16:303, 1982
191. Hug CC, Kaplan JA: Pharmacology—Cardiac drugs. In Kaplan JA (ed): Cardiac Anesthesia, p 39. New York, Grune & Stratton, 1979
192. Bourdaris JP, Dubourg O, Gueret P et al: Inotropic agents in the treatment of cardiogenic shock. Pharmacol Ther 22:53, 1983
193. Makabali C, Weil MH, Henning RJ: Dobutamine and other sympathomimetic drugs for the treatment of low cardiac output failure. Semin Anesth 1:63, 1982
194. Glass DD: Cardiovascular drugs. In Civetta JM (ed): Intensive Care Therapeutics, p 199. New York, Appleton-Century-Crofts, 1980
195. Waller JL: Inotropes and vasopressors. In Kaplan JA (ed): Cardiac Anesthesia, vol 2 (Cardiovascular Pharmacology), p 273. New York, Grune & Stratton, 1983
196. Wood M: Drugs and the sympathetic nervous system. In Wood M, Alistair JJ (eds): Drugs and Anesthesia, Baltimore, Williams & Wilkins, 1982
197. Maze M, Smith CM: Identification of receptor mechanism mediating epinephrine-induced arrhythmias during halothane anesthesia in the dog. Anesthesiology 59:322, 1983
198. Kapur PA, Flacke WE: Epinephrine-induced arrhythmias and cardiovascular function after verapamil during halothane anesthesia in the dog. Anesthesiology 55:218, 1981
199. Reves JG, Kissin I, Lell WA et al: Calcium entry blockers: Uses and implications for anesthesiologist. Anesthesiology 57:504, 1982
200. Stoelting RK: Calcium entry blockers. In Stoelting RK (ed): Pharmacology and Physiology in Anesthetic Practice, p 335. Philadelphia, JB Lippincott, 1987
201. Johnston RR, Eger EI, Wilson C: A comparative interaction of epinephrine with enflurane, isoflurane, and halothane in man. Anesth Analg 55:709, 1976
202. Karl HW, Swedlow DB, Lee KW et al: Epinephrine-halothane interactions in children. Anesthesiology 58:142, 1983
203. Boudaris JP, Duborg O, Gueret P et al: Inotropic agents in the treatment of cardiogenic shock. Pharmacol Ther 22:53, 1983
204. Houston MC, Thompson WL, Robertson D: Shock diagnosis and management. Arch Intern Med 144:1433, 1984
205. Goldberg LI, Hsieh Y, Resnekov L: Newer catecholamines for treatment of heart failure and shock: An update on dopamine and a first look at dobutamine. Prog Cardiovasc Dis 19:327, 1977
206. Pank JR, Tinker JH: Cardioactive drugs and their monitorable effects. Semin Anesth 11:268, 1983
207. Lappas DG, Powell WMJ, Daggett WM: Cardiac dysfunction in the perioperative period, pathophysiological diagnosis and treatment. Anesthesiology 47:117, 1977
208. Furman WR, Summer WR, Kennedy TP et al: Comparison of the effects of dobutamine, dopamine, and isoproterenol on hypoxic pulmonary vasoconstriction in the pig. Crit Care Med 10:371, 1982
209. Hug CC, Kaplan JA: Pharmacology—Cardiac Drugs. In Kaplan JA (ed): Cardiac Anesthesia, p 39. New York, Grune & Stratton, 1979
210. Lipman J, Plit M: A guide to the rational use of dopamine, dobutamine, and isoprenaline in patients who need inotropic support. S Afr Med J 65:506, 1984
211. Tinker JH: Perioperative myocardial infarction. Semin Anesth 1:253, 1982
212. Ferguson JE, Hensleigh PA, Kredenster D: Adjunctive use of magnesium sulfate with ritodrine for preterm labor tocolysis. Am J Obstet Gynecol 148:166, 1984
213. Schwarz R, Retzke U: Cardiovascular effects of terbutaline in pregnant women. Acta Obstet Gynecol Scand 62:419, 1983
214. Beneditti TJ: Maternal complications of parenteral β-sympathetic therapy for premature labor. Am J Obstet Gynecol 145:1, 1983
215. Pou-Martinez A, Kelly SH, Newel FD et al: Postpartum pulmonary edema after ritodrine and betamethason use. J Reprod Med 27:428, 1982
216. Semchyshyn S, Zuspan FP, O'Shaughnessy R: Pulmonary edema associated with the use of hydrocortisone and a tocolytic agent for the management of premature labor. J Reprod Med 28:47, 1983
217. Spielman FJ: Maternal effects and complications of beta-adrenergic therapy for premature labor. Resident and Staff Phys 32:102, 1986
218. Rasmussen H: Cell communication, calcium ion and cyclic adenosine monophosphate. Science 170:404, 1970
219. Rasmussen H, Barret PO: Calcium messenger system: An integrated view. Pharmacol Rev 64:938, 1984
220. Rutman HI, LeJemtel, Sonnenblick EH: Newer cardiotonic agents: Implications for patients with heart failure and ischemic heart disease. J Cardiothor Anesth 1:59, 1987
221. Stirt JA, Sullivan SF: Aminophylline. Anesth Analg 60:587, 1981
222. Braunwald E: A symposium: Amrinone. Am J Cardiol 56:1B, 1985
223. Braunwald E: Newer positive inotropic agents. Circulation (Suppl), P2, 73(3) 1986
224. Benotti JR, Grossman W, Braunwald E et al: Effects of amrinone on myocardial energy metabolism and hemodynamics in patients with severe congestive heart failure due to coronary artery disease. Circulation 68:28, 1980
225. Ward A, Brogden RN, Heel RC et al: Amrinone—A preliminary review of its pharmacological properties and therapeutic use. Drugs 26:468, 1983
226. Baim DS, McDowell AV, Cherniles J et al: Evaluation of a new bipyridine inotropic agent—milrinone—in patients with severe congestive heart failure. N Engl J Med 309:748, 1983

227. Colucci WS, Wright RF, Braunwald E: New positive inotropic agents in the treatment of congestive heart failure. P 1. N Engl J Med 314:290, 1986

228. Colucci WS, Wright RF, Braunwald E: New positive inotropic agents in the treatment of congestive heart failure. P 2, N Engl J Med 314:349, 1986

229. Zaloga GP, Chernow B: Insulin, glucagon and growth hormone. In Chernow B, Lake CR (eds): The Pharmacologic Approach to the Critically Ill Patient, p 562. Baltimore, Williams & Wilkins, 1983

230. Stoelting RK: Digitalis and related drugs. In Stoelting RK (ed): Pharmacology and Physiology in Anesthetic Practice, p 269. Philadelphia, JB Lippincott, 1987

231. Haustein KO: Digitalis. Pharmacol Ther 18:1, 1983

232. Meyer J: Concerning the question of pre-, intra, and postoperative digitalis administration. Surv Anesthesiol 16:9, 1972

233. Pinaud MLJ, Yvonnick AG, Blanoeil YAG et al: Preoperative prophylactic digitalization of patients with coronary artery disease—randomized echocardiographic and hemodynamic study. Anesth Analg 62:865, 1983

234. Silverberg RA, Weil MH: Cardiopulmonary resuscitation. In Chernow B, Lake CR (eds): The Pharmacologic Approach to the Critically Ill Patient, p 140. Baltimore, Williams & Wilkins, 1983

235. Blecic S, De Backer D, Huynh CH et al: Calcium chloride in experimental electromechanical dissociation: A placebo-controlled trial in dogs. Crit Care Med 15:324, 1987

236. Montgomery WH, Donegan JD, McIntyre KM: Standards and guidelines for cardiopulmonary resuscitation (CPR) and emergency cardiac care (ECC). Pt III Adult advanced cardiac life support. JAMA 255:2933, 1986

237. White RD, Goldsmith RS, Rodriguez R et al: Plasma ionic calcium levels following injection of chloride, gluconate, and gluceptate salts of calcium. J Thorac Cardiovasc Surg 71:609, 1976

238. Bull J, Band DM: Calcium and cardiac arrest. Anesthesiology 35:1006, 1980

239. Cote CJ, Drop LJ, Daniels AL et al: Calcium chloride versus calcium gluconate: Comparison of ionization and cardiovascular effects in children and dogs. Anesthesiology 66:465, 1987

240. Marquez J, Martin D, Virji MA et al: Cardiovascular depression secondary to ionic hypocalcemia during hepatic transplantation in humans. Anesthesiology 64:457, 1986

241. Wong KC, Everett JD: Sympathomimetic drugs. In Smith NT, Corbascio AN (eds): Drug Interactions in Anesthesia, p 71. Philadelphia, Lea & Febiger, 1986

242. Stoelting RK: Drugs used in treatment of psychiatric disease. In Stoelting RK (ed): Pharmacology and Physiology in Anesthetic Practice, p 347. Philadelphia, JB Lippincott, 1987

243. Kosanin R: Anesthetic considerations in patients on chronic tricyclic antidepressant therapy. Anesth Review 8:38, 1981

244. Weiner N: Drugs that inhibit adrenergic nerves and block adrenergic receptors. In Gilman AG, Goodman LS, Rall TW (eds): The Pharmacological Basis of Therapeutics, p 181. New York, Macmillan, 1985

245. Nickerson M, Goodman LS: Pharmacological properties of a new adrenergic blocking agent: N, N-dibenzyl-β-chloroethylamine (dibenamine). J Pharmacol Exp Ther 89:167, 1947

246. Hickey PR, Hansen DD: Anesthesia and cardiac shunting in the neonate: Ductus arteriosus, transitional circulation, and congenital heart disease. Semin Anesth 3(2):106, 1984

247. Grover RF, Reeves JT, Blount SG: Tolazoline hydrochloride (Priscoline) and effective pulmonary vasodilator. Am Heart J 61:5, 1961

248. Graham RM, Pettinger WA: Drug therapy: Prazosin. N Engl J Med 300:232, 1979

249. Ziegler MG: Antihypertensives. In Chernow B, Lake CR (eds): The Pharmacologic Approach to the Critically Ill Patient, p 303. Baltimore, Williams & Wilkins, 1983

250. Lowenthal DT, Saris SD, Packer J et al: Mechanisms of action and the clinical pharmacology of beta-adrenergic blocking drugs. Am J Med 77(4A): 119, 1984

251. Wood A: Pharmacologic differences between beta blockers. Am Heart J 108:1070, 1984

252. Shand DG: Comparative pharmacology of the β-adrenoreceptor blocking drugs. Drugs 25(Suppl):92, 1983

253. McDevitt DG: Clinical significance of cardioselectivity. State of the art. Drugs 25:211, 1983

254. Clausen N, Damsgaard T, Mellemgaard K: Antihypertensive effect of a nonselective and cardioselective (Metoprolol) beta adrenergic blocking agent at rest and during exercise. Br J Clin Pharmacol 7:379, 1979

255. Woods LL, Wright AD, Kendall MJ: Lack of effect of propranolol and metoprolol on glucose tolerance in maturity-onset diabetes. Br Med J 281:1321, 1980

256. Chang LCT: Use of practolol in asthmatics: A plea for caution. Lancet 2:321, 1971

257. Silke B, Verma SP, Ahuja RC et al: Is the intrinsic sympathomimetic activity (ISA) of beta-blocking compounds relevant in acute myocardial infarction? Eur J Clin Pharmacol 27:509, 1984

258. Taylor SH, Silke MB, Lee PS: Intravenous beta-blockade in coronary heart disease. Is cardioselectivity or intrinsic sympathomimetic activity hemodynamically useful? New Engl J Med 306:631, 1982

259. Reid JL, Dean CR, Jones DH: Central actions of anti-hypertensive drugs. Cardiovasc Med 2:1185, 1977

260. Frishman WH: Atenolol and timolol, two new systemic β-adrenoceptor antagonists. New Engl J Med 306:1456, 1982

261. Mishra P, Calvey TN, Williams NE et al: Intraoperative bradycardia and hypotension associated with timolol and pilocarpine eye drops. Br J Anaesth 55:897, 1983

262. Formgren H: The effects of metoprolol and practolol on lung function and blood pressure in hypertensive asthmatics. Br J Clin Pharmacol 3:1007, 1976

263. Wollman GL, Cody RJ, Tarazi RC et al: Acute hemodynamic effects and cardioselectivity of acebutolol, practolol and propranolol. Clin Pharmacol Ther 25:813, 1979

264. Basil B, Jordan R: Pharmacological properties of diacetylol, a major metabolite of acebutolol. Eur J Pharmacol 80:47, 1982

265. Gray RJ, Bateman TM, Czer LSC et al: Esmolol: A new ultra-short-acting beta-adrenergic blocking agent for rapid control of heart rate in postoperative supraventricular tachyarrhythmias. J Am Coll Cardiol 5:1451, 1985

266. Girard D, Shulman BJ, Thys DM et al: The safety and efficacy of esmolol during myocardial revascularization. Anesthesiology 65:157, 1986

267. Reves J, Flezzani P: Perioperative use of esmolol. Am J Cardiol 56:57F, 1985

268. Gray R, Bateman TM, Czer LSC et al: Use of esmolol in hypertension after cardiac surgery. Am J Cardiol 46:49F, 1985

269. Menkhaus P, Reves JG, Kissin I et al: Cardiovascular effects of esmolol in anesthetized humans. Anesth Analg 64:327, 1985

270. Gorczynski R: Basic pharmacology of esmolol. Am J Cardiol 56:3F, 1985

271. Steck J, Sheppard D, Byrd R et al: Pulmonary effects of esmolol. Clin Res 33:472A, 1985

272. de Bruihn NP, Reves JG, Croughwell N et al: Pharmacokinetics of esmolol in anesthetized patients receiving chronic beta blocker therapy. Anesthesiology 66:323, 1987

273. Wilson DJ, Wallin JD, Vlachakis ND et al: Intravenous labetalol in the treatment of severe hypertension and hypertensive emergencies. Am J Med 95, 1983

274. Gagnon RM, Morissette M, Priesant S et al: Hemodynamic and coronary effects of intravenous labetalol in coronary artery disease. Am J Cardiol 49:1267, 1982

275. Weidmann P, De Chiatel R, Ziegler WH et al: Alpha and beta

adrenergic blockade with orally administered labetalol in hypertension. Am J Cardiol 41:570, 1978

276. Atlee JA: Normal electrical activity of the heart. In Atlee JA (ed): Perioperative Cardiac Dysrhythmias, p 16. Chicago, Year Book Medical, 1985

277. Nayler WG, Poole-Wilson P: Calcium antagonists: Definition and mode of action. Basic Res Cardiol 76:926, 1981

278. Triggle DJ: Calcium antagonists: Basic chemical and pharmacological aspects. In Weiss GB (ed): New Prospectives on Calcium Antagonists, p 1. Baltimore, Williams & Wilkins, 1981

279. Henry PD: Comparative pharamacology of calcium antagonists: Nifedipine, verapamil, and diltiazem. Am J Cardiol 46:1047, 1980

280. Millard RW, Lathrop DA, Grupp G et al: Differential cardiovascular effects of calcium channel blocking agents: Potential mechanisms. Am J Cardiol 49:499, 1982

281. Reves JG: The relative hemodynamic effects of CA^{++} entry blockers: Uses and implications for anesthesiologists. Anesthesiology 61:3, 1982

282. Kraynack BJ, Lawson NW, Gintautas J: Local anesthetic effect of verapamil in vitro. Reg Anesthesia 7:114, 1982

283. So SY, Ip M, Lam WK: Calcium channel blockers and asthma. Lung 164:1, 1986

284. Schwartz ML, Rotmench HH, Vlasses PH et al: Calcium blockers in smooth muscle disorders. Arch Intern Med 144:1425, 1984

285. Solomon GD, Steel JG, Spaccavento LJ: Verapamil prophylaxis of migraine. JAMA 250:2500, 1983

286. McLeod AA, Jewitt DE: Drug treatment of primary pulmonary hypertension. Drugs 31:177, 1986

287. Fleckenstein A: Specific pharmacology of calcium in myocardium, cardiac pacemakers, and vascular smooth muscle. Ann Rev Pharmacol Toxicol 17:149, 1977

288. Atlee JA: Drugs used for treatment of cardiac dysrhythmias. In Atlee JA (ed): Perioperative Cardiac Dysrhythmias, p 272. Chicago, Year Book Medical, 1985

289. Hwang MH, Danoviz J, Pacold I et al: Double blind crossover randomized trial of intravenously administered verapamil. Arch Intern Med 144:491, 1984

290. Klein HO, Kaplinsky E: Digitalis and verapamil in atrial fibrillation and flutter. Is verapamil now the preferred agent? Drugs 31:185, 1986

291. Haft JI, Habbab MA: Treatment of atrial arrhythmias—effectiveness of verapamil when preceded by calcium infusion. Arch Intern Med 146:1085, 1986

292. Antman EM, Stone PH, Muller JE et al: Calcium channel blocking agents in the treatment of cardiovascular disorders. Part I. Basic and clinical electrophysiologic effects. Ann Intern Med 93:875, 1980

293. Morad M, Tung L: Ionic events responsible for the cardiac resting and action potential. Am J Cardiol 49:584, 1982

294. Atlee JA: Management of specific cardiac dysrhythmias. In Atlee JA (ed): Perioperative Cardiac Dysrhythmias, p 380. Chicago, Year Book Medical, 1985

295. Clusin WT, Bristow MR, Karaguezian HS et al: Do calcium-dependent currents mediate ischemic ventricular fibrillation? Am J Cardiol 49:606, 1982

296. Given BD, Lee TH, Stone PH et al: Nifedipine in severely hypertensive patients with congestive heart failure and preserved ventricular systolic function. Arch Intern Med 145:281, 1985

297. Kapur PA, Campos JH, Buchea OC: Plasma diltiazem blood levels, cardiovascular function and coronary hemodynamics during enflurane anesthesia in the dog. Anesth Analg 65:918, 1986

298. Reves JG, Kissin I, Lell WA, et al: Calcium entry blockers. Uses and implications for anesthesiologists. Anesthesiology 57:504, 1982

299. Merin RG, Basch S: Are the myocardial functional and metabolic effects of isoflurane really different from those of halothane and enflurane? Anesthesiology 53:398, 1981

300. Hysing ES, Chelly JE, Doursout MF et al: Cardiovascular effects of and interaction between calcium blocking drugs and anesthetic in chronically instrumented dogs. III. Nicardipine and isoflurane, Anesthesiology 65:385, 1986

301. Carpenter RL, Mulroy MF: Edrophonium antagonizes combined lidocaine-pancuronium and verapamil-pancuronium neuromuscular blockade in cats. Anesthesiology 65:506, 1986

302. Zalman F, Perloff JK, Durant NN et al: Acute respiratory failure following intravenous verapamil in Duchenne's muscular dystrophy. Am Heart J 105:510, 1983

303. Snyder SH, Reynolds IJ: Calcium-antagonist drugs. New Engl J Med 313:995, 1985

304. Abramowicz M: Verapamil for hypertension. The Medical Letter on Drugs and Therapeutics 29:37, 1987

305. Price WA, Giannini AJ: Neurotoxicity caused by lithium-verapamil synergism. J Clin Pharmacol 26:717, 1986

306. Roizen MF, Moss J, Muldoon SM: The effects of anesthesia, anesthetic adjutant drugs, and surgery on plasma norepinephrine. In Ziegler MG, Lake CR (eds): Frontiers of Clinical Neuroscience, vol 2 (Norepinephrine), p 227. Baltimore, Williams & Wilkins, 1984

307. Goldman L, Caldera DL: Risks of general anesthesia and elective operation in the hypertensive patient. Anesthesiology 50:285, 1979

308. Prys-Roberts C: Hypertension, ischemic heart disease and anesthesia. Int Anesthesiol Clin 18:3, 1980

309. Holland DB: Diuretic-induced hypokalemia and ventricular arrhythmias. Drugs 28(Suppl):86, 1984

310. Vitez T, Soper L, Wong KC et al: Chronic hypokalemia and intraoperative dysrhythmias. Anesthesiology 63:130, 1986

311. McGovern B: Hypokalemia and cardiac arrhythmias. Anesthesiology 63:127, 1985

312. Boudoulas H, Lewis RP, Kates RE et al: Hypersensitivity to adrenergic stimulation after propranolol withdrawal in normal subjects. Ann Intern Med 86:433, 1977

313. Stoelting RK: Alpha- and beta-adrenergic receptor antagonists. In Stoelting RK (ed): Pharmacology and Physiology in Anesthetic Practice, p 280. Philadelphia, JB Lippincott, 1987

314. Slogoff S, Keats AS: Does perioperative myocardial ischemia lead to postoperative myocardial infarction? Anesthesiology 62:107, 1985

315. Brodsky JB, Brave JJ: Acute postoperative clonidine withdrawal syndrome. Anesthesiology 44:519, 1976

316. Johnston FV, Nicholas DA, Lawson NW et al: The use of rectal clonidine in the perioperative period. Anesthesiology 64:288, 1986

317. Stoelting RK: Antihypertensive drugs. In Stoelting RK (ed): Pharmacology and Physiology in Anesthetic Practice, p 294. Philadelphia, JB Lippincott, 1987

318. O'Malley K, Segal JL, Israili ZH et al: Duration of hydralazine action in hypertension. Clin Pharmacol Ther 18:581, 1975

319. Cohn JN, Burke LP: Nitroprusside. Ann Intern Med 91:752, 1979

320. Chiarello M, Gold HK, Leinback RC: Comparison between the effects of nitroprusside and nitroglycerin on ischemic injury during acute myocardial infarction. Circulation 54:766, 1976

321. Tinker JH, Michenfelder JD: Sodium nitroprusside: Pharmacology, toxicology and therapeutics. Anesthesiology 45:340, 1976

322. Tinker JH, Michenfelder JD: Increased resistance to nitroprusside-induced cyanide toxicity in anuric dogs. Anesthesiology 50:40, 1980

323. Miller ED, Ackerly JA, Vaughn ED et al: The renin-angiotensin system during controlled hypotension with sodium nitroprusside. Anesthesiology 47:257, 1977

324. Khambatta HJ, Stone JG, Khan E: Propranolol alters renin release during nitroprusside-induced hypotension and prevents hyper-

tension on discontinuation of nitroprusside. Anesth Analg 60:569, 1981

325. Woodside J, Garner L, Bedford RT *et al:* Captopril reduces the dose requirement for sodium nitroprusside-induced hypotension. Anesthesiology 60:413, 1984

326. Fremes SE, Weisel RD, Mickle D *et al:* A comparison of nitroglycerin and nitroprusside. I. Treatment of postoperative hypertension. Ann Thorac Surg 39:53, 1985

327. Hood D, Dewan D, James F *et al:* The use of nitroglycerin in preventing the hypertensive response to tracheal intubation in severe preeclampsia. Anesthesiology 63:399, 1985

328. Goa KL, Sorkin EM: Nitrendipine—A review of its pharmacodynamic and pharmacokinetic properties and therapeutic efficacy in the treatment of hypertension. Drugs 33:123, 1987

329. Guazzi M, Olivari MT, Polese A *et al:* Nifedipine, a new antihypertensive with rapid action. Clin Pharmacol Ther 22:528, 1977

330. Ferguson RK, Vlasses PH: Hypertensive emergencies and urgencies. JAMA 255(12):1607, 1986

331. Abramowicz M: Drugs for hypertension. Medical Letter on Drugs and Therapeutics. 29(Issue 730):1, 1987

Chapter 8

Robert J. Fragen
Michael J. Avram

Nonopioid Intravenous Anesthetics

The dictionary defines *anesthesia* as a loss of sensation in a part of the body or in the body generally, induced by administration of a drug.[1] Anesthesiologists usually expand this definition in line with the concept of Woodbridge.[2] In 1957, he proposed four components of general anesthesia for drugs of limited or specific action comparable to Guedel's signs for general anesthesia with diethyl ether. His components are blockades of sensory, reflex, mental, and motor functions. Adequate sensory blockade results in minimal response to painful stimuli and is indicated by stability of the cardiovascular and respiratory systems. Troublesome cardiovascular, respiratory, and gastrointestinal reflexes are prevented by adequate reflex blockade. Sedation, amnesia, and unarousable deep sleep are produced by mental blockade. Motor blockade provides muscle relaxation and a quiet surgical field. No single intravenous anesthetic drug is yet available that can produce all the components of adequate anesthesia. Because the drugs available have relatively selective blocking actions, it is necessary to use a combination of drugs that together provide the desired effect.

Excluding ketamine, nonopioid intravenous (iv) anesthetics generally provide only the mental component of the anesthetic state, requiring the addition of analgesics, inhaled anesthetics, and/or muscle relaxants to provide the other components. Thus, the drugs discussed in this chapter are mainly amnestic, sedative (anxiolytic, ataraxic), and hypnotic. The terms *sleep, hypnosis,* and *unconsciousness* are used interchangeably in anesthesia literature to refer to the state of artificially induced (*i.e.*, drug-induced) sleep.

Nonopioid iv drugs can be used initially as anesthetic induction drugs to produce the unconscious state, or they can be given by repeated injection or by infusion to maintain the mental component of the anesthetic state.

There has been an expanded research effort in recent years to discover more specific, controllable compounds that can be injected iv to provide selective hypnotic, analgesic, or muscle relaxant actions; or that can be injected in combination to provide all the components of general anesthesia. Total iv anesthesia refers to general anesthesia administered only with injectable drugs, avoiding inhaled anesthetics entirely. The potential advantage of total iv anesthesia is its facility to provide each component of anesthesia with a dose of a specific drug sufficient to meet the particular needs of the patient and surgeon. When volatile inhalation anesthetics are administered, all the components of anesthesia are increased or decreased in intensity at the same time, as are their side-effects. Research must still determine whether currently there are hypnotics, analgesics, and muscle relaxants with appropriate pharmacokinetic-pharmacodynamic profiles to provide successful iv anesthesia with recovery as rapid as that following inhalation anesthetics.

HISTORY

The iv route of drug administration became possible only after the careful descriptions of the vascular system by William Harvey in 1628 in *De Motu Cordis* and the introduction of the syringe by Rynd (1845) and Pravaz (1853) and of the hypodermic needle by Wood (1855). The first monograph on iv anesthesia was published by Ore, a Frenchman, at the University of Bordeaux in 1874. Unfortunately, he used chloral hydrate, which had a long duration of action and a very narrow margin of safety. At the end of the 19th century and early in the 20th century, hedonal, a derivate of urethane, was used for iv anesthesia, but it caused prolonged drowsiness, respiratory failure, tachycardia, and phlebitis. The use of procaine was reported by August Bier in 1909. All the early barbiturates were long-acting and unsatisfactory for anesthesia. In 1933, Hellmuth Weese described the first ultra-short-acting barbiturate, hexobarbital. The untoward effects he reported were respiratory depression, phlebitis, allergy, and convulsions.[3]

The most important barbiturate is thiopental, introduced in 1934. It was first described by Dr. Ralph Waters and coworkers at the University of Wisconsin, although some give credit for its introduction to Dr. John S. Lundy at Mayo Clinic.[4] When thiopental was used as the sole anesthetic for battle casualties in World War II, it was termed the "ideal form of euthanasia" because of the many deaths associated with its administration to patients in shock.[5] Thiopental could have fallen into disuse as a result of this experience, but, instead, it became a major component of the concept of the narcosis-relaxant-analgesic anesthesia proposed by Reese and Gray in the United Kingdom.[6] They realized that drugs administered by the iv route bypassed the absorption and first-pass variable of drugs given orally or intramuscularly (im). Thus, modern iv anesthesia was born with the introduction of thiopental. However, it soon became apparent that this was not an ideal iv agent, neither as a sole anesthetic, nor as an anesthetic induction agent, nor as a maintenance anesthetic; it could not fulfill Reese and Grays' concept of the anesthetic triad.

It was not until 1952 that another successful iv anesthetic was discovered. Since that time, nine new agents have appeared (Table 8-1), all attempting to improve upon the major drawbacks of thiopental—slow recovery, respiratory depression, and cardiovascular depression. Of these drugs, gamma hydroxybutric acid was never studied in the United States but is still used in some countries of Europe. Both propanidid and althesin were recently withdrawn from the market because of an unacceptably high incidence of anaphylactoid reactions to their solvent, cremophor El (about 1/1,000). Propofol was originally dissolved in cremophor El and caused anaphylactoid reactions,[7] but it is now produced with a safer solvent.

Before comparing the pharmacology of currently used iv anesthetic drugs, it is important to review the "ideal" properties of an iv anesthetic agent (Table 8-2).

For more than 50 years, anesthesiologists have circumvented thiopental's deficiencies, while investigators have continued to pursue the goal of finding a more ideal drug. Currently, there are no approved or investigational iv anesthetics that fulfill all the criteria for the ideal drug.

TABLE 8-1. Intravenous Anesthetics and Their First Year of Clinical Administration

1934 — Thiopental
1952 — Thiamylal
1957 — Methohexital
1957 — Ketamine
1960 — Gamma OH-butyric acid
1961 — Propanidid
1964 — Diazepam
1971 — Althesin
1973 — Etomidate
1977 — Propofol
1978 — Midazolam

TABLE 8-2. Properties of an "Ideal" Intravenous Anesthetic Agent

I. Physicochemical and pharmacokinetic
   A. Water soluble
   B. Long shelf life (> 1 year)
   C. Stable on exposure to light (> 1 day)
   D. Small volume (± 10 ml) required for anesthetic induction
II. Pharmacodynamic
   A. Small interindividual variation
   B. Safe therapeutic ratio
   C. Onset in one arm–brain circulation time
   D. Short duration of effect
   E. Inactivated by rapid metabolism to nontoxic metabolites
   F. Rapid recovery
III. Hypersensitivity
   A. No anaphylaxis
   B. No histamine release
IV. Side-effects
   A. No local toxicity
   B. No alterations in body organ function, except primary CNS effects
      1. Central nervous system
      2. Cardiovascular system
      3. Respiratory system
      4. Gastrointestinal system

CHEMISTRY AND FORMULATION

The thiobarbiturates, thiopental [5-ethyl-5-(1-methylbutyl)-2-thiobarbituric acid] and thiamylal [5-allyl-5-(1-methylbutyl)-2-thiobarbituric acid], and the methylated oxybarbiturate methohexital [α-dl-1-methyl-5-allyl-5-(1-methyl-2-pentynyl) barbituric acid] (Fig. 8-1) are the barbiturate induction drugs used in the practice of anesthesia. The sodium salts of these drugs, plus 6% by weight anhydrous sodium carbonate, must be reconstituted with either water or 0.9% sodium chloride, providing 2.5%, 2.0%, or 1.0% solutions of thiopental, thiamylal, or methohexital, respectively. The moderate alkalinity (pH 10 to 11) of the barbiturate solutions is maintained by the buffering action of the sodium carbonate in the presence of atmospheric carbon dioxide. Ringer's lactate solution should not be used to reconstitute any of the barbiturates, nor should the reconstituted barbiturates be mixed with acidic solutions of other drugs, because the decrease in alkalinity will result in the precipitation of the barbiturates as the free acids. Properly reconstituted solutions of the thiobarbiturates are stable for up to 1 week if refrigerated; sterile water solutions of methohexital can be used up to 6 weeks after reconstitution.

The parenteral formulations of the benzodiazepine induction agents, diazepam (7-chloro-1,3-dihydro-1-methyl-5-phenyl-2H-1,4-benzodiazepin-2-one) and midazolam [8-chloro-6-(2'fluorophenyl)-1-methyl-4H-imidazo[1,5α][1,4]benzodiazepine] (Fig. 8-1), are quite different from each other owing to the availability of water-soluble salts of midazolam but not of diazepam. Diazepam is marketed as a 5 mg·ml^{-1} solution in a 50% organic (40% propylene glycol and 10% ethanol) vehicle that also contains a buffer and a preservative. Although diazepam is stable in solution, it cannot be mixed with solutions of other drugs; if it is, its solubility will be reduced. The midazolam formulation, on the other hand, contains 1 or 5 mg·ml^{-1} of the hydrochloride salt in a buffered, pH 3.5, aqueous solution that is stable and compatible with saline, Ringer's lactate solution, and formulations of acidic salts of other drugs.

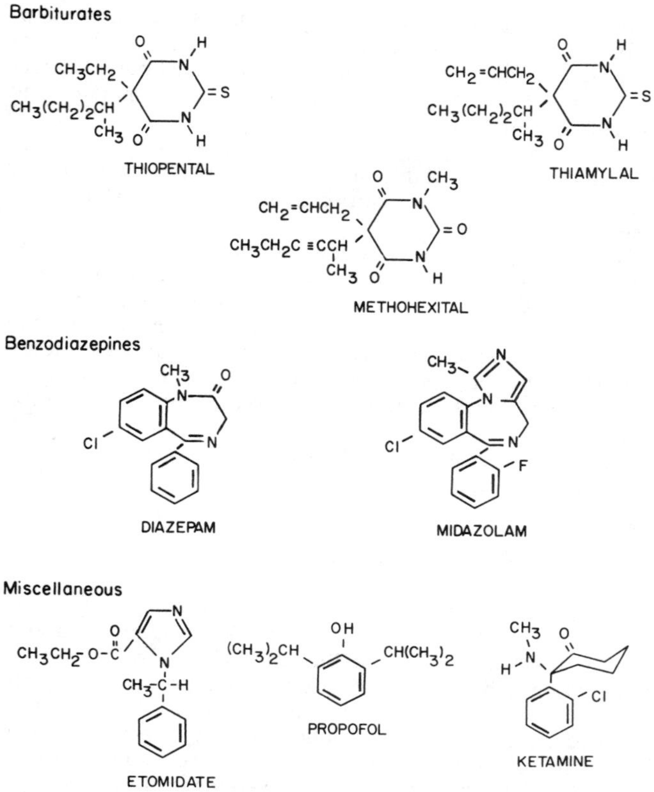

FIG. 8-1. Agents used for the induction of general anesthesia. (Reprinted with permission from Fragen RJ, Avram MJ: Comparative pharmacology of drugs used for the induction of anesthesia. In Stoelting RK, Barash PG, Gallagher TJ [eds]: Advances in Anesthesia, p 103. Chicago, Year Book Medical Publishers, Inc, 1986.)

Although water-soluble salts and a 10% ethanolic formulation of etomidate [R-(+)-ethyl 1-(α-methylbenzyl)-1H-imidazole 5-carboxylate] (Fig. 8-1) exist, the only formulation available in the United States is a $2\,mg \cdot ml^{-1}$ solution in a 35% propylene glycol vehicle. While etomidate is stable in solution in this vehicle, it should not be diluted or mixed with other drug formulations.

Propofol (2,6-diisopropylphenol) (Fig. 8-1) is a hydrophobic liquid at room temperature. It is formulated as a 1% aqueous emulsion, containing 10% soybean oil, 2.25% glycerol, and 1.2% egg phosphatide,[8] and is stable at room temperature. This formulation should not be mixed with other solutions.

The iv formulation of ketamine[(d1-2-(o-chlorophenyl)-2-(methyl-amino)-cyclohexanone] (Fig. 8-1) contains 10, 50, or $100\,mg \cdot ml^{-1}$ of the hydrochloride salt in a moderately acidic (pH 3.5 to 5.5) solution with a preservative. Ketamine is stable in solution but should not be mixed with solutions of the moderately alkaline barbiturates or with diazepam, with which it is commonly coadministered.

STRUCTURE–ACTIVITY RELATIONSHIPS

Structure–activity relationships are descriptions of the way in which modifications of the chemical structure of prototypical drugs affect their pharmacologic activities. The addition, modification, or removal of functional groups on the fundamental structure of a drug lend it physicochemical properties that affect the drug's ability to gain access to its site of action and to interact with its presumed receptor; they also determine the effect it will have on the receptor when interacting with it.[9] The structure–activity relationships for the anesthesia induction drugs are reasonably well described.

Modification of the structure of barbituric acid (Fig. 8-2A), 2, 4, 6-trioxohexahydropyrimidine, can convert the inactive compound into a hypnotic with a variety of pharmacologic activities.[10] The addition of aliphatic side chains in positions 5 and 5' introduces hypnotic activity to the molecule, particularly if at least one of the side chains is branched. The length of the side chains in the 5 and 5' positions can influence the duration of action of the barbituric acid derivatives as well as their potency; both pentobarbital and secobarbital contain relatively long (i.e., branched 5 carbon) side chains in position 5' and have a relatively short duration of action, whereas secobarbital is slightly more potent than pentobarbital because of the slightly longer (3 vs. 2 carbon) side chain in position 5. Replacement of the oxygen atom in position 2 of an active barbiturate with a sulphur atom produces a drug with a faster onset of action and a shorter duration of action; the thiobarbiturates, thiopental and thiamylal (Fig. 8-1) have a more rapid onset and shorter duration of action than their oxybarbiturate analogs, pentobarbital and secobarbital. Methylation of an active barbiturate in the 1 position produces a barbiturate, like methohexital (Fig. 8-1), with a rapid onset and short duration of action at the expense of an increased incidence of excitatory side-effects. Thus, given basic hypnotic activity, any chemical modification of a barbiturate that increases its lipophilicity will generally increase both its potency and rate of onset while shortening its duration of action.

The pharmacologic activity of the classical 5-phenyl-1,4 benzodiazepin-2-one ring system (Fig. 8-2B) can be affected by substitution in a number of positions.[11] The introduction of an electronegative group in position 7 on ring A, such as the

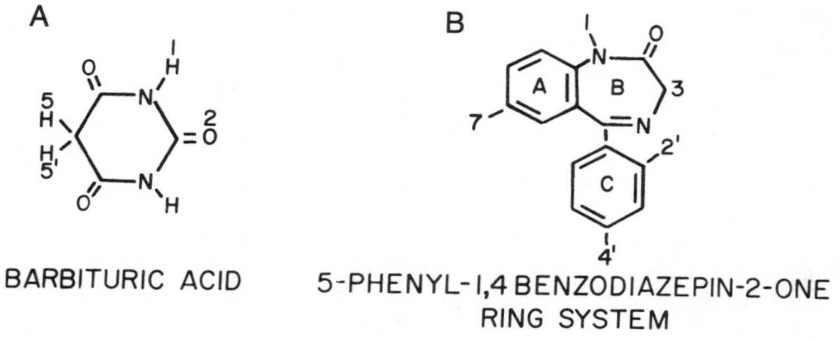

FIG. 8-2. (A) Barbituric acid, (B) 5-phenyl-1,4 benzodiazepin-2-one ring system.

chloro group in diazepam and midazolam (Fig. 8-1), is nearly essential for typical benzodiazepine activity. A methyl group in position 1 on ring B, as in diazepam, increases biological activity, whereas larger substituents in that position decrease it.

A halogen in position 2' of ring C, as in midazolam, increases pharmacologic activity, whereas any substituent in the 4' position very strongly decreases it. The fused imidazole ring contributes unique properties to midazolam (Fig. 8-1).[12] The basicity of the imidazole nitrogen (pK_a 6.15) allows the preparation of salts that are both soluble and stable in acidic aqueous solution (pH of approximately 3.5) yet lipophilic at physiologic pH. In addition, the methyl group in position 1 of the fused imidazole ring is metabolized rapidly by hepatic oxidation (hydroxylation), contributing, with redistribution, to its shorter duration of action; the methylene group in position 3 of the classical diazepine ring (Fig. 8-2B) is metabolized more slowly.

Imidazole derivatives have classically been used as antimycotic agents. Several 1-(1 aralkyl)-imidazole-5-carboxylic acid esters such as etomidate (Fig. 8-1) are potent hypnotic drugs with good therapeutic indices.[13] Hypnotic activity in such a molecule requires the presence of both an alkyl branched carbon atom between the aryl moiety and the imidazole nitrogen and an ester moiety.

Propofol (Fig. 8-1) is one of a series of di-ortho-substituted phenols with moderate to high hypnotic potencies and therapeutic ratios.[14] Sleeping time increases with increasing side chain length. Potency increases and induction time decreases with increasing length of the side chains up to a total of 7 to 8 carbon atoms. With side chains longer than this, potency is decreased, induction is slowed, and recovery is prolonged. The 2,6-di-sec-alkylphenols are generally more potent and have higher therapeutic ratios than the 2,6-di-n-alkylphenols, because potency and therapeutic ratios increase with increased steric compression of the phenolic hydroxyl group.

The cyclohexane ring geminally substituted with an aromatic ring and a basic nitrogen is essential to the PCP-like activity of the arylcycloalkylamines, of which ketamine (Fig. 8-1) is a member.[15] The potency of these compounds is influenced by substitutions on the nitrogen, but their pharmacologic activity is unaffected. An electron withdrawing group on the aromatic ring, such as the o-chloro group in ketamine, decreases the psychotropic activity of the molecule.

An important but often overlooked aspect of structure–activity relationships is the relationship of stereoisomerism to biological activity. Many important molecules in biology and medicine contain one or more asymmetric carbon atoms. Except for the presence of the asymmetric centers, the stereoisomers of a given molecule are physically and chemically identical. Nonetheless, biological activity is often predicated on the active stereoisomer of a given neurotransmitter, hormone, or drug interacting with the chiral active center of a receptor or enzyme.[16] Because side-effects are often due to the nonspecific action of drugs (i.e., they are often not receptor- or enzyme-mediated), the inactive stereoisomers can contribute significantly to the side-effects of the racemic mixture. Some isomers have been shown to even have effects at the receptor or enzyme opposite that of the active isomer. The "inactive" isomer, therefore, should be considered an impurity.[17]

Many barbiturates, including thiopental, thiamylal, and methohexital, have asymmetric carbon atoms in one of the side chains attached to carbon 5 of the barbiturate ring.[18] The (−) isomers of both thiopental and thiamylal are the most potent isomers in mice.[18, 19] Methohexital, on the other hand, has not only an asymmetric carbon atom on one of the side chains attached to carbon 5 but also an asymmetric site at carbon 5 itself. It therefore has four stereoisomers, the most active of which, the β-1, is four to five times as potent as the least active, the α-1.[18, 20] All the barbiturates are marketed as the racemic mixture.

The (+) isomer of etomidate is the only stereoisomer with hypnotic activity.[21] Etomidate is the only anesthetic induction drug with an asymmetric carbon atom that is marketed as the most active isomer.

The stereoisomers of ketamine have been tested in humans. The (+) isomer was reported to be 3.4 times as potent a hypnotic as the (−) isomer and, "at equianesthetic doses," to be an even more potent analgesic.[22] The (−) isomer, on the other hand, at an equally hypnotic dose, had more clinically important side-effects, including disturbing emergence reactions.[22] Nonetheless, ketamine is marketed as a racemic mixture.

Neither propofol nor the benzodiazepines contain asymmetric carbon atoms.

MECHANISMS OF ACTION

Given the enormous complexity of the central nervous system (CNS), it is hardly surprising that neither neurotransmission nor the mechanisms of anesthetic induction drugs are fully understood. There are many theories purporting to explain the mechanisms of various anesthetic agents. Some of these theories suggest that anesthetics directly affect cell membranes (biophysical theories), whereas others suggest direct interaction with neurotransmitter systems (transmitter theories).[23–26] Although no drug has a single action and many drugs have a variety of actions, some of which are concentration-dependent, there is a substantial body of evidence suggesting that most of the anesthetic induction drugs exert many of their effects by modulating GABAminergic transmission.[27–29] Such an action is consistent with the GABA (gamma-aminobutyric acid) transmitter theory of anesthetic action.[30]

GABA is the most common inhibitory neurotransmitter in the mammalian CNS. Activation of the postsynaptic GABA receptor increases chloride conductance through the ion channel, hyperpolarizing and, as a result, inhibiting the postsynaptic neuron. The GABA receptor is actually an oligomeric complex (Fig. 8-3) consisting of the GABA receptor and its associated chloride ion channel, the benzodiazepine receptor, the barbiturate receptor, and the picrotoxin binding site.[32] Both barbiturates and benzodiazepines, by activating distinct receptors on the GABA receptor complex, increase chloride ion flux initiated by the interaction of GABA with its receptor, thereby enhancing GABA-induced postsynaptic inhibition. Benzodiazepines bind to their receptor (possibly displacing an endogenous modulator of GABA function), producing an allosteric modification of the GABA receptor and increasing the efficiency of GABA receptor/effector (i.e., chloride ion channel) coupling. As a result, benzodiazepines increase the frequency of chloride ion channel openings produced by GABA.[26, 27, 29, 33] Barbiturates, on the other hand, by binding to their receptor, decrease the rate of dissociation of GABA from its receptor and increase the duration of GABA-activated chloride ion channel openings.[24, 28, 29, 33] There is evidence that the benzodiazepines and the barbiturates exert their anticonvulsant and anxiolytic actions through their interactions with the GABA receptor complex, but it is less certain that they produce their sedative/hypnotic effects by this mechanism.[31, 34–36]

Etomidate may also modulate GABAminergic neuro-

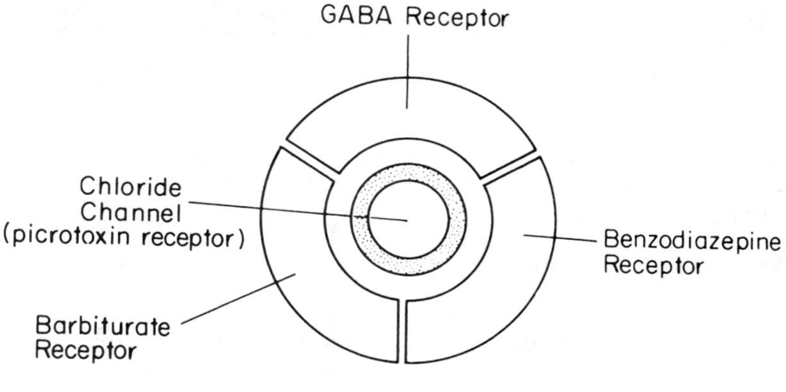

FIG. 8-3. Representation of the hypothetical GABA receptor oligomeric complex. (Reprinted with permission from Olsen RW, Fischer JB, Dunwiddie TV: Barbiturate enhancement of γ-amino-butyric acid receptor binding and function as a mechanism of anesthesia. In Roth SH, Miller KW [eds]: Molecular and Cellular Mechanisms of Anesthetics, p 165. New York, Plenum, 1986.)

transmission. In contrast to the increased affinity of the GABA receptor produced by barbiturates, etomidate appears to increase the number of GABA receptors, possibly by displacing endogenous inhibitors of GABA binding.[37]

Just as the dissociative anesthetic ketamine has actions that are significantly different from the other iv anesthetic induction drugs, it also has different effects on neurotransmission within the CNS. Although their effects on neurotransmission are not as well described as the effects of barbiturates and benzodiazepines, arylcycloalkylamines have been reported to interact with CNS muscarinic acetylcholine receptors as antagonists and opioid receptors as agonists.[38] The interaction of ketamine with the sigma opioid receptor may produce the dysphoric reactions to this drug.[39]

The effects of propofol on neurotransmission in the CNS have not been described.

Until recently, there were no specific antagonists for the CNS effects of the iv anesthetic induction drugs. Physicians have attempted to antagonize their effects nonspecifically with drugs such as the anticholinesterase physostigmine because of its ability to produce relatively nonspecific cortical activation and arousal.[40] Flumazenil and Ro 15–3505 are specific benzodiazepine receptor antagonists. Flumazenil is a pure benzodiazepine receptor antagonist, whereas Ro 15–3505 is a more potent benzodiazepine receptor antagonist that may have very weak partial inverse agonist properties (i.e., it may behave slightly like the hypothetical endogenous modulator of GABA function at the benzodiazepine receptor).[41, 42]

PHARMACOKINETICS

GENERAL

Selected pharmacokinetic parameters for the iv anesthetic induction drugs are listed in Table 8-3.

Because the various studies may have different pharmacokinetic models and sampling times, it is difficult to compare the initial or central volumes of distribution (V_c) of these drugs. However, the V_cs for all of them appear to exceed intravascular space. The rapid onsets of effects of most of these drugs suggest that the brain is part of their initial volumes of distribution.

The action of these drugs is terminated through "dilution" in the body by redistribution from the relatively small V_c (including the brain) to the much larger total apparent volume of distribution Vd_{ss} (see below); this is taking place during the rapidly declining portions of the plasma concentration versus

time relationship (Fig. 8-4). Vd_{ss} for benzodiazepines is approximately a $1 \cdot kg^{-1}$, suggesting relatively uniform distribution of the drugs throughout the body, whereas Vd_{ss}s for the other induction agents are 2 to 3 $1 \cdot kg^{-1}$, implying extensive uptake by some tissues of the body (Table 8-3).

Elimination clearance, the irreversible removal of drug from the body, begins the moment that a drug reaches the clearing organs (e.g., liver, kidneys) but becomes a dominant influence on the plasma drug concentration versus time relationship only after the end of the rapid decline in plasma drug concentrations characterizing the distribution phase (Fig. 8-4). The elimination clearances of these hepatically eliminated drugs range from very low to very high, whether expressed in $ml \cdot min^{-1}$ [50, 59] or $ml \cdot min^{-1} \cdot kg^{-1}$ (Table 8-3). The low, restrictive elimination clearances of diazepam and thiopental reflect their low hepatic extraction ratios. The fact that the extraction ratios of diazepam and thiopental are equal to the unbound fractions of these drugs suggests that their restrictive elimination is due to extensive protein binding (Table 8-3). The other induction drugs have much higher hepatic extraction ratios and elimination clearances despite the extensive protein binding of some of these drugs. This implies that the rate of their dissociation from plasma proteins does not limit their rate of elimination. The extremely high elimination clearance of propofol suggests that there is a significant extrahepatic contribution to its clearance. Because of their high elimination clearances, etomidate and propofol are well suited pharmacokinetically for use by continuous iv infusion for sedation or hypnosis.

Elimination half-life ($T_{1/2\beta}$) is a pharmacokinetic variable depending directly on volume of distribution (Vd_β, which is useful only for calculating $T_{1/2\beta}$) and inversely on elimination clearance. The wide range of half-lives of these drugs, from less than 1 hour for propofol to over 40 hours for diazepam, is more a reflection of the large differences in the elimination clearances of the drugs than it is of the small differences in their volumes of distribution.

Pharmacodynamic modeling of the effects of the anesthetic induction drugs is extremely difficult, because there is no unequivocal measure of their effects. Stanski and colleagues have begun work in this complex area using changes in the processed EEG as measures of effect.[44]

TERMINATION OF HYPNOTIC EFFECT

The classic physiologic pharmacokinetic studies of the disposition of thiopental demonstrated that redistribution of drug from the brain to other, less well perfused, tissues is the

TABLE 8-3.   The Pharmacokinetics of Intravenous Anesthesia Induction Drugs (x ± SD)*

DRUG	V_c (l·kg^{-1})	Vd$_{ss}$ (l·kg^{-1})	Vd$_\beta$ (l·kg^{-1})	Cl$_e$ (ml·min^{-1})	Cl$_e$ (ml·min^{-1}·kg^{-1})	$t_{1/2\beta}$ (hr)	ESTIMATED HEPATIC EXTRACTION RATIO	PLASMA PROTEIN BINDING (%)	MINIMAL EFFECTIVE PLASMA CONCENTRATION (μg·ml^{-1})
Thiopental[43]	0.53 ±0.18	2.34 ±0.75	3.46 ±1.54†	247†	3.4 ±0.4	12.0 ±5.5	0.15	83.4 ±1.4	19.2 ±6.3[44]‡
Methohexital[47]	0.35 ±0.10	2.2 ±0.7	3.68†	835†	10.9 ±3.0	3.9 ±2.1	0.50	73[48]	10[49]
Etomidate[50]	0.15 ±0.03	2.52 ±0.90	4.46 ±2.26	1210 ±303	17.9 ±5.6	2.9 ±1.1	0.90	76.9 ±1.0†[51]	0.307 ±0.076
Propofol[52]	0.63†	2.83†	4.66†	3454§ ±202	59.4§	0.9	Nearly 1.0?	96.8– 98[53]	1.05 ±0.09
Ketamine[54]	1.7†	3.1 ±0.9	5.1 ±0.7	1429†	19.1 ±2.5	3.1†	Nearly 1.0?	12[55]	0.640 ±0.213[56]
Diazepam[57]	0.31 ±0.12	1.13 ±0.28	1.53†	26.6 ±4.1	0.4†	46.6 ±14.2	0.03†	97.8 ±1.0	N.A.¶
Midazolam[59]	0.17 ±0.03	1.09 ±0.18	1.60 ±0.31	436 ±127	7.5 ±2.4	2.7 ±0.8	0.51†[59, 60]	94 ±1.9[60]	0.157 ±0.079

  * These data are not available for thiamylal.
  † These values have been calculated by the present authors from data in the sources cited.
  ‡ Pentobarbital is either an artifact encountered in the measurement of thiopental[45] or such a minor metabilite[46] that it cannot be considered to contribute to the CNS effects of thiopental.
  § Whole blood clearance.
  ¶ Not applicable because diazepam has several clinically important pharmacologically active metabolites, one of which has a half-life that is longer than that of diazepam.[58]
  (Reprinted with permission from Fragen RJ, Avram MJ: Comparative pharmacology of drugs used for the induction of anesthesia. In Stoelting RK, Barash PG, Gallagher TJ (eds): Advances in Anesthesia, p 103. Chicago, Year Book Medical Publishers, 1986)

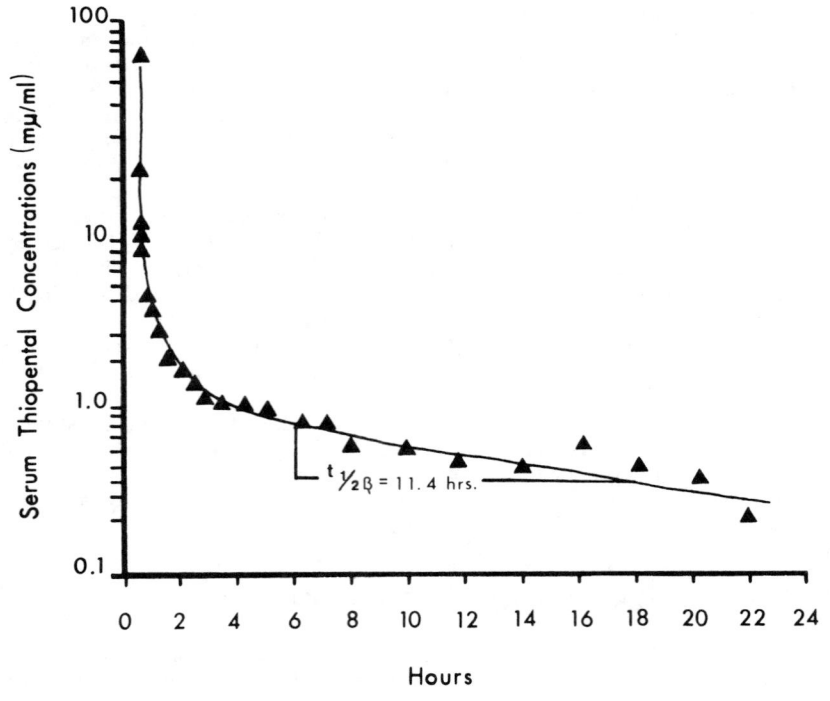

FIG. 8-4. Serum thiopental concentrations versus time relationship after a rapid intravenous (bolus) administration of the drug. The triangles represent measured serum concentrations, and the line represents a computer-generated fit to a triexponential equation. (Modified with permission from Burch PG, Stanski DR: The role of metabolism and protein binding in thiopental anesthesia. Anesthesiology 58:146, 1983.)

primary mechanism for the termination of the effects of anesthetic induction drugs after rapid iv administration (Fig. 8-5).[62–64] Although never a principal factor, elimination clearance plays a more important role in terminating the effects of drugs with intermediate or high hepatic extraction ratios (*e.g.*, methohexital; Table 8-3)[47] than it does with drugs having low extraction ratios (*e.g.*, thiopental; Table 8-3).[43] When drugs such as the iv anesthetic induction drugs are administered in large doses, in multiple doses, or by continuous iv infusion, the importance of elimination clearance to the termination of drug effect increases as the size of the dose or duration of infusion increases. As an extreme example, the effect of thiopental administered for 42 to 89 hours by continuous iv infusion in cerebral resuscitation was terminated by nonlinear (*i.e.*, Michaelis–Menten) elimination, with no contribution from redistribution (Fig. 8-6).[46]

VOLATILE ANESTHETICS AND PHARMACOKINETICS

There is a growing body of literature on the effects of anesthetics, particularly volatile anesthetics, on the absorption and disposition of drugs.[65] Most of these studies have examined the effects of volatile anesthetics on elimination clearance of drugs administered perioperatively.

Few studies have directly assessed the effects of volatile anesthetics on the elimination clearance of iv anesthetic induction drugs in humans. Nonetheless, there are suggestions that volatile anesthetic drugs decrease the elimination clearance of such high and intermediate extraction ratio drugs as etomidate,[50, 66, 67] ketamine,[68] and methohexital.[69] The elimination

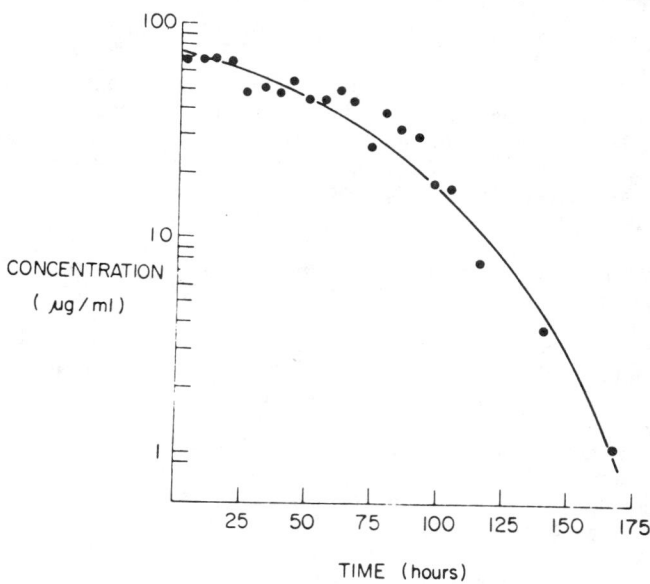

FIG. 8-6. Plasma thiopental concentration versus time relationship after a 42-hour infusion of a total dose of 40,200 mg of the drug in cerebral resuscitation, illustrating nonlinear (Michaelis–Menten) elimination clearance. Note the difference between this postdrug administration relationship and that illustrated in Figure 8-4 for a standard dose of the same drug, which has typical distributional phases followed by linear elimination clearance. (Modified with permission from Stanski DR, Mihm FG, Rosenthal MH *et al:* Pharmacokinetics of high-dose thiopental used in cerebral resuscitation. Anesthesiology 53:169, 1980.)

clearance of high extraction ratio drugs is usually reduced by a decrease in hepatic blood flow; the clearance of low extraction ratio drugs is reduced by a decreased hepatic extraction ratio, resulting from enzyme inhibition; the clearance of intermediate extraction ratio drugs is affected by changes in both hepatic blood flow and extraction ratio.[70] Most volatile anesthetics decrease hepatic blood flow.[71] There is also evidence from studies in rats,[72] dogs,[73] and sheep[74] that volatile drugs can effect a decrease in hepatic clearance by decreasing not only hepatic blood flow but also hepatic metabolism. Regardless of the mechanism, decreases in the clearances of induction agents by volatile anesthetics would prolong their elimination half-lives. Because the effects of standard doses of the induction drugs are largely terminated by redistribution, decreased elimination clearance and the resultant prolongation of elimination half-life would result in a prolonged effect only after very large doses, multiple doses, or continuous iv infusions. The nonspecific stimulation of drug-metabolizing enzymes by volatile anesthetic drugs[75] is unlikely to be an acute effect and is, therefore, unlikely to affect the clearance of the anesthetic induction drugs.

The effects of the volatile anesthetics on the distribution of ketamine have been studied in the rat,[72] and propranolol in the dog.[76] Further studies on the effects of anesthetics on drug distribution, including studies in humans, must be conducted before it is possible to speculate on the implications of alternations in the distribution of the induction drugs. Nonetheless, clinical experience suggests that any effect seldom has profound consequences.

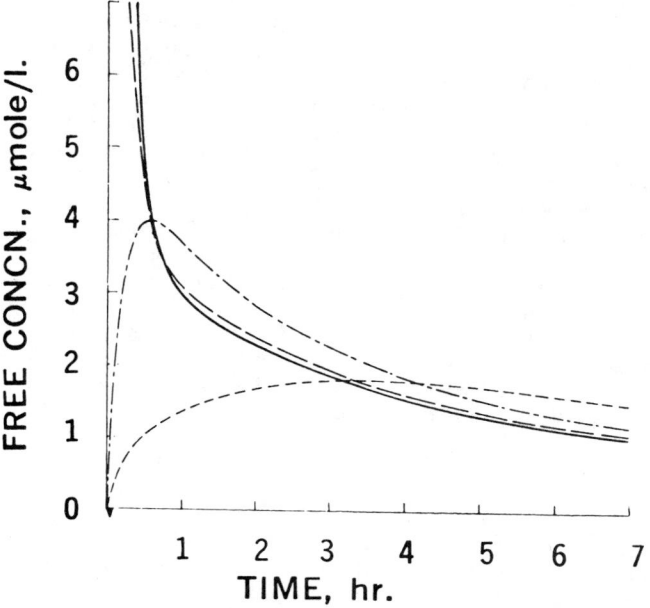

FIG. 8-5. Free thiopental concentrations in blood (– – –), viscera (———), adipose (- - - - -), and lean (— · —) body tissues after a rapid intravenous (bolus) administration of the drug. (Reprinted with permission from Bischoff KB, Dedrick RL: Thiopental pharmacokinetics. J Pharm Sci 57:1346, 1968.)

234   PHARMACOLOGY

AGE AND PHARMACOKINETICS

Elderly patients require significantly lower induction doses of the iv anesthetic drugs, including thiopental,[77-80] diazepam,[81] midazolam,[82, 83] etomidate,[84] and propofol[85] than do young patients. There are suggestions in the literature that the increased reactivity of elderly patients to the iv induction drugs has a pharmacokinetic rather than a pharmacodynamic basis.[77, 80, 84, 86, 87]

Anatomic and physiologic changes with aging could have important effects on the pharmacokinetics of the iv induction drugs. There is a decrease in the proportion of body weight represented by total body water and in lean body mass;[88] this could result in an increase in the total apparent volume of distribution of lipophilic drugs like the induction drugs. An age-related decrease in cardiac output with a concomitant alteration in the distribution of systemic flow,[89] usually at the expense of drug-clearing organs, may decrease the elimination clearance of high clearance drugs in the elderly. These changes could prolong the half-lives of drugs but cannot provide a pharmacokinetic explanation for the increased reactivity of the elderly to the iv induction drugs.

The change in the disposition of thiopental with aging has been the subject of several investigations. One group reported a correlation between age and both the total volume of distribution and the elimination half-life of thiopental. They could find no change in the early distribution of the drug and, thus, could not explain the need to reduce the induction dose of thiopental for the elderly.[90] In addition to an age-related increase in both the volume of distribution and half-life of thiopental, Christensen and colleagues found a decrease in the rate at which the drug is transferred from the central to the fast compartment in the elderly.[86] Homer and Stanski found that the initial distribution volume of thiopental decreased with age,[80] resulting in less initial dilution of a dose of thiopental. Since thiopental equilibrates very rapidly between plasma and the brain,[63] either a slower rate of drug transfer from the central to the fast compartment[86] or a decreased central volume of distribution[80] would explain the increased CNS and cardiovascular sensitivity of elderly patients to standard doses of thiopental. While these observations are both interesting and appealing, recent reports suggest that there may be no simple answer to this long-standing question.[80, 91, 92]

EFFECTS ON ORGAN SYSTEMS

CENTRAL NERVOUS SYSTEM EFFECTS

Intravenous anesthetics primarily modify activity within the CNS, alter consciousness, produce anti-recall effects, and, in the case of ketamine, produce analgesia as well. These agents also affect the electroencephalogram (EEG), intracranial pressure (ICP), cerebral blood flow (CBF), cerebral metabolic rate for oxygen ($CMRO_2$), and intraocular pressure (IOP). Clinically, desirable effects include reductions in blood flow, metabolism, and pressures within the CNS as well as a sleep pattern on the EEG; these are especially important for patients with intracranial pathology and increased ICP.

Thiopental causes an increase in the amplitude and a slowing in the frequency of the EEG.[93] If the dose is high enough, burst suppression, then a flat EEG will appear. Etomidate produces EEG effects similar to those exhibited after use of thiopental.[94] There is an initial increase in alpha amplitude followed by a progressive decrease in activity and, in some cases, periods of burst suppression. The myoclonic movements that occasionally occur during induction of anesthesia with etomidate are not associated with specific EEG changes of epileptiform activity, but convulsions have been reported following the use of etomidate.[95, 96]

Anesthetic induction doses of midazolam cause the awake alpha rhythm to change to a beta rhythm. After about 30 minutes, alpha activity returns, but some EEG effects are still seen an hour after drug administration.[97] This is not the classical sleep pattern but is similar to the EEG changes following the use of diazepam and other benzodiazepines. Ketamine anesthesia leads to increases in alpha, delta, and theta waves but results in no change in beta activity.[98]

Another index of CNS activity is evoked potential monitoring, commonly used since the mid-1980s. This monitoring is useful in detecting abnormalities of neural transmission in the spinal cord or intracranial structure. Anesthetics that could blunt the evoked response during the monitoring period would be detrimental. There is a scarcity of reports in the medical literature of well-controlled studies of the effects of iv anesthetics on the somatosensory evoked potentials (SSEP). Thiopental can be used safely for anesthetic induction and, in small doses, during anesthetic maintenance, because it elicits minimal alteration in SSEP. Etomidate, on the other hand, increases the amplitude of SSEP transiently, sometimes mimicking the pattern at the onset of ischemia. It also alters the waveform, making the diagnosis of neurologic injury more difficult.[99]

Other CNS effects of etomidate, however, are beneficial for the neurosurgical patient. CBF, $CMRO_2$, and ICP are reduced in a dose-related fashion by etomidate,[100, 101] the barbiturates,[102, 103] the benzodiazepines,[104] and propofol.[105, 106] An exception was described in a study in which ICP was unchanged after midazolam, 0.32 mg · kg^{-1} was given to patients with brain tumors, and ICP was over 20mm Hg.[107] Because etomidate has the least effect on systemic blood pressure, it is more successful than other drugs in maintaining cerebral perfusion pressure. The one drug that is inappropriate for patients with intracranial pathology is ketamine, because it increases CBF, ICP, and cerebrospinal fluid pressure (CSFP).[98]

Many iv hypnotics have been used clinically and experimentally for brain protection against seizures caused by epilepsy[108-110] or by local anesthetic overdose.[111] Methohexital, however, would be an inadvisable choice for brain protection, as high doses (24 mg · kg^{-1}), which suppress EEG activity, can cause refractory postoperative seizures.[112] There is also a report of ketamine inducing seizures in epileptics.[113]

Among the factors that may affect IOP are systemic arterial pressure (SAP), central venous pressure (CVP), patency of the drainage system for the aqueous humor, and diseases of the eyes themselves. All the nonopioid iv anesthetics except ketamine, by themselves, reduce IOP. This has been demonstrated with thiopental, diazepam, and midazolam (Table 8-4),[114] as well as with etomidate[115] and propofol.[116] If normal doses of these induction drugs are followed by succinylcholine and tracheal intubation, however, IOP rises above control values. When a second dose of propofol, 1 mg · kg^{-1}, was given just before succinylcholine administration, it offered protection against the usual rise in IOP in such circumstances; a second dose of thiopental offered no such protection.[116] Etomidate, 0.3 mg · kg^{-1},[117] and propofol, 2.1 mg · kg^{-1},[116] caused a sharper decrease in IOP than thiopental, 4 to 5 mg · kg^{-1}. Possible mechanisms for this decrease in IOP are an increase in the outflow of aqueous humor, relaxation of extraocular muscles, and peripheral vasodilation. Thus, all the drugs except ketamine can be used safely to induce anesthesia for ophthalmologic surgery, even for the emergency patient with an open globe. Ketamine, however, can be safely administered to children for tonometry.[118] Although most of the reported studies concerning the effects of induction drugs on IOP used succinylcholine as the muscle relaxant, a nondepolarizing relaxant may be a more appropriate companion to iv induction agents for patients with open eye injuries.

The beneficial cerebral effects of the barbiturates, benzodiazepines, etomidate, or propofol are useless if the patient is allowed to cough, breathhold, or strain or if hypercarbia is present. The cerebral vasculature is still capable of responding after induction doses of these hypnotic drugs. Because hypercarbia is the most important cerebral vasodilator, hypocarbia is the goal during intracranial surgery. Although benzodiazepines may be used to ameliorate the stimulatory effects of ketamine, midazolam does not protect against the rise in ICP caused by ketamine.[109]

Table 8-5 summarizes the relative CNS effects of these drugs. Other possible CNS effects will be discussed under induction and recovery side-effects of these drugs.

RESPIRATORY EFFECTS

Nonopioid iv anesthetics are always given with other drugs such as opioids, volatile anesthetics, or skeletal muscle relaxants, all of which cause respiratory depression. Under general anesthesia, ventilation of the lungs can be assisted or controlled to maintain normocarbia, but if iv anesthetics are used as sedatives or hypnotics in spontaneously breathing patients, their respiratory depression may adversely affect the patients. Thus, it is important to know the effects of these iv anesthetics on respiratory rate, tidal volume, bronchial smooth muscle, and respiratory reflexes. None of these drugs produce long-term respiratory depression or cause bronchoconstriction.

At one time, thiopental was blamed for causing airway spasm and increased sensitivity of airway reflexes, but it is more likely that these were due to the introduction of artificial airways or endotracheal tubes in inadequately anesthetized patients. Methohexital is associated with a higher incidence of hiccup and coughing.

Intravenous induction drugs can reduce tidal volume and respiratory rate until apnea occurs. Respiratory depression is greater when opioid premedication is administered[119, 120] or when the drug is injected rapidly. When propofol is given alone, the respiratory rate increases for the first 30 seconds, then rapidly decreases to apnea in most patients,[120] producing a more profound respiratory depression than does thiopental. Its main effect is on tidal volume rather than rate;[121] the rate returns to control values by 4 minutes after injection of 2.5 mg · kg^{-1}. When fentanyl is given before propofol induction, apnea occurs within 30 seconds after propofol is injected. When thiopental is used, tidal volume is depressed more than respiratory rate.[122] Etomidate causes a brief period of hyperventilation with a small increase in both tidal volume and respiratory rate toward the end of induction; this is followed by a period of short-lived respiratory depression or apnea.[123] Apnea following etomidate is less common than after barbiturate or propofol induction, but more frequent than after midazolam, diazepam, or ketamine induction. It is also more

TABLE 8-4.   IOP Changes in mm Hg (Mean ± SEM)

DRUG	CONTROL	1 MIN	3 MIN	AFTER SUCCINYLCHOLINE	AFTER TUBE
Midazolam	16.3 ± 1.0	11.8 ± 0.9*	9.6 ± 1.0*	21.6 ± 1.0†	24.9 ± 1.9*
Diazepam	17.5 ± 0.8	12.1 ± 0.7*	11.5 ± 0.6*	23.7 ± 1.5*	26.6 ± 1.8*
Thiopental	17.8 ± 1.4	13.4 ± 1.4*	12.4 ± 1.7*	23.7 ± 2.3†	26.9 ± 2.6*

* P < 0.001 compared with control
† P < 0.01 compared with control
(Reprinted with permission from Fragen RJ, Hauch T: The effects of midazolam maleate and diazepam in intraocular pressure in adults. In Aldrete JA, Stanley TH [eds]: Trends in Intravenous Anesthesia, p 245. Chicago, Year Book Medical Publishers, 1980.)

TABLE 8-5.   Cerebral Effects (Healthy Adults)*

	CBF	CPP	CMRO$_2$	ICP	IOP
Thiopental	− −	− −	− −	− −	−
Thiamylal	− −	− −	− −	− −	−
Methohexital	− −	− −	− −	− −	−
Etomidate	− −	0	− −	− −	−
Propofol	− −	− −	− −	− −	−
Ketamine	+ +	+	+	+	+
Diazepam	−	−	−	−	−
Midazolam	−	−	−	−	−

* + + to − − is a five-point scale qualitatively describing the relative increase (+, + +) or decrease (−, − −) or no effect (0) among the induction agents for each cerebral effect. (CBF = cerebral blood flow; CPP = cerebral perfusion pressure; CMRO$_2$ = cerebral metabolic rate of oxygen; ICP = intracranial pressure; and IOP = intraocular pressure) (Reprinted with permission from Fragen RJ, Avram MJ: Comparative pharmacology of drugs used for the induction of anesthesia. In Stoelting RK, Barash PG, Gallagher TJ [eds]: Advances in Anesthesia, p 103. Chicago, Year Book Medical Publishers, 1986.)

frequent and of longer duration with opioid premedication and in older patients.

When midazolam was given to volunteers, tidal volume decreased about 40%, respiratory rate increased about 40%, but minute ventilation was unchanged. This effect was not dose related over the dose range of 0.05 to 0.2 mg·kg^{-1} (Fig. 8-7). The highest dose, 0.2 mg·kg^{-1}, reduced oxygen saturation as a result of a longer duration of apnea.[124] Specific benzodiazepine antagonists will reverse the respiratory depressant effects of the benzodiazepines; these effects are not reversed by the opioid antagonist, naloxone.[124]

Midazolam, given for anesthetic induction to patients with chronic obstructive pulmonary disease, produced a more profound and longer-lasting respiratory depression than it did in normal patients or than equivalent doses of thiopental produced in patients with pulmonary disease.[125]

Ketamine generates few respiratory effects. Its effect ranges from mild respiratory stimulation to mild depression,[126] de-

pression being more common in spontaneously breathing elderly patients[127] or related to rapid administration of the drug.[128] Although, all these induction drugs can be used safely for asthmatic patients, ketamine can be beneficial in relieving bronchospasm because of its sympathomimetic effect. After ketamine induction, cough and laryngospasm are rare and laryngeal reflexes are intact, but, when a belladonna alkaloid is excluded from premedication, excess secretions can develop in the respiratory tract. The respiratory response to CO_2 continues during ketamine anesthesia.[129]

Table 8-6 summarizes the relative respiratory effects of equivalent doses of nonopioid iv drugs administered to induce general anesthesia. Slower injection times and lower doses, such as might be used for continuous infusion, result in less respiratory depression for each agent. For safety, one should be prepared to maintain the airway artificially and assist or control ventilation of the lungs when any of them are used.

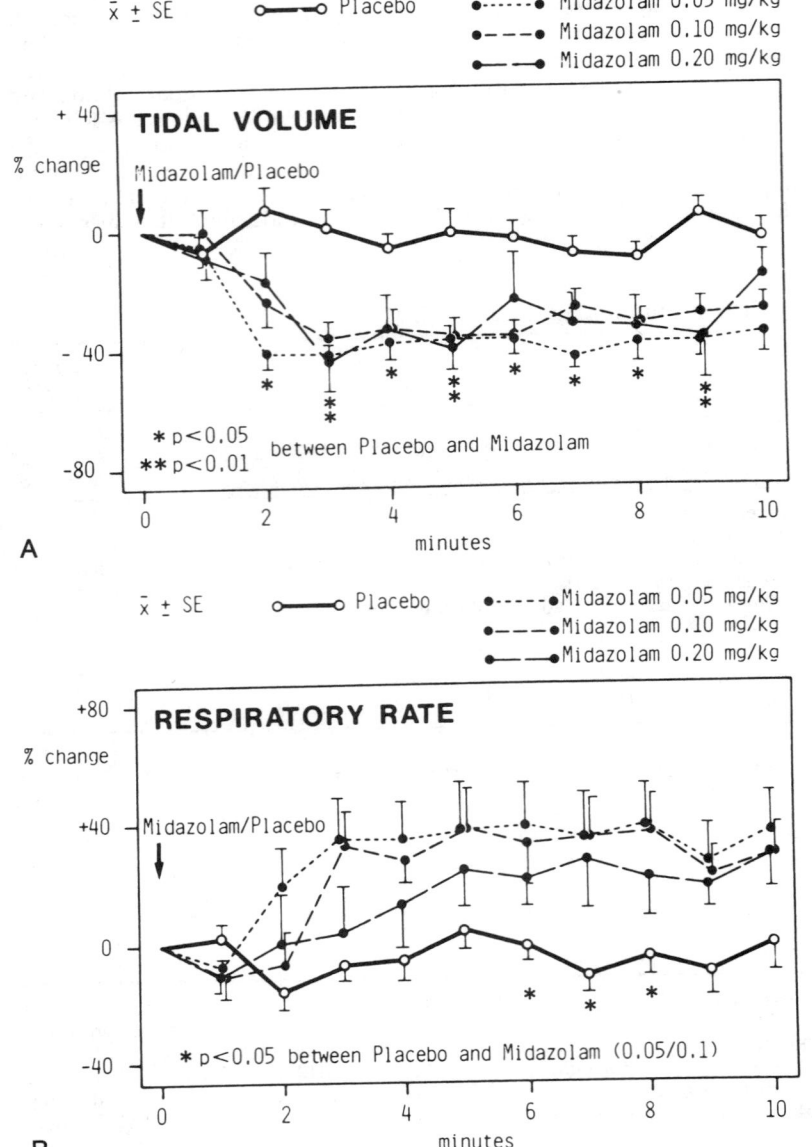

FIG. 8-7. The A and B figures show the per cent changes in tidal volume and respiratory rate, respectively, for 10 minutes after the injection of three different doses of midazolam or a placebo. These doses of midazolam are within the therapeutic range for intravenous (iv) sedation to anesthetic induction. There were significant differences in respiratory effects between midazolam and placebo, but the effects were not different between the three midazolam doses. (Reprinted with permission from Forster A, Morel D, Bachmann M et al: Respiratory depressant effect of different doses of midazolam and lack of reversal with naloxone. A double-blind randomized study. Anesth Analg 62:920, 1983.)

TABLE 8-6.   Comparative Respiratory Effects

	RESPIRATORY DEPRESSION	BRONCHOMOTOR TONE
Thiopental	+ +	0
Thiamylal	+ +	0
Methohexital	+ +	0
Etomidate	+	0
Propofol	+ +	0
Ketamine	0	+
Diazepam	+	0
Midazolam	+	0

Note: 0 to + + + represents a scale of increasing severity of respiratory depression or beneficial effect on bronchomotor tone. They represent only a qualitative comparison of each drug.

CARDIOVASCULAR EFFECTS

The effects of iv anesthetics on the cardiovascular system are more important than their effects on the respiratory system; there is no simple maneuver to counteract temporary cardiovascular depression in the way that artificial ventilation of the lungs is used to reverse temporary respiratory depression. Unfortunately, all iv anesthetics are either cardiovascular depressants or stimulants. A number of factors that can influence the cardiovascular system of patients undergoing general anesthesia are listed in Table 8-7.

These factors can have multiple effects on hemodynamics. As a person goes from the awake to the unconscious state, blood pressure and heart rate decrease about 10%. This degree of change is expected after anesthetic induction. Resting sympathetic tone is high in nervous and hypertensive patients. Anesthetics causing vasodilation will, therefore, have a more profound effect in these patients. Hypercarbia causes vasodilation and stimulates release of catecholamines. The more rapid the injection, the greater the concentration of drug that reaches the heart and the more profound the cardiac effect of the induction drugs. Cardiovascular depression after anesthetic induction is greater in the hypovolemic patient. Restoration of blood volume is the aim of good patient care prior to surgery, but, when hypovolemia exists in the emergency patient, the barbiturates, benzodiazepines, and propofol must be used with extreme care, if at all.

Diseases of the cardiovascular system or autonomic nervous system may exaggerate the cardiovascular response to anesthetic drugs, or they may blunt the compensatory reflexes to drug-related cardiovascular changes. Premedicants and other drugs seldom produce cardiovascular effects except in the elderly and in patients with pre-existing cardiovascular disease; in such cases, changes in blood pressure or heart rate may occur. For example, morphine can cause bradycardia, and meperidine can cause tachycardia. Atropine increases heart rate. Slow heart rates are found in patients on digitalis, calcium channel blockers, and beta blockers. Because many of these factors may exist prior to iv induction of anesthesia, studies reporting different cardiovascular effects of the same iv induction drug may be misleading unless the modifying factors are considered.

The general effects of midazolam on circulation are shown schematically in Fig. 8-8.[130] This pattern of drug action and body reaction pertains to most of the other induction drugs as well, except for etomidate and ketamine. Induction drugs may cause dilation of the capacitance or resistance vessels or may directly depress the myocardium, blunt compensatory cardiovascular reflexes, affect the autonomic nervous system di-

TABLE 8-7.   Factors Influencing the Cardiovascular System at the Time of Anesthetic Induction

1. Change from awake to unconscious state
2. Resting sympathetic tone
3. Ventilatory status
4. Speed of injection
5. Vascular volume
6. Pathophysiology of diseases affecting the autonomic nervous system or the cardiovascular system directly
7. Cardiovascular effects of ancillary drugs
8. Residual effects of cardiovascular drugs
9. Cardiovascular effects of premedicants

rectly or centrally, or affect the conduction system. Other than sinus bradycardia or tachycardia, dysrhythmias are not produced by the induction drugs discussed here unless someone fails to counteract their respiratory depressant effects by ventilatory assistance.

Ketamine produces tachycardia by central sympathetic stimulation[98], but concomitant administration of diazepam,[98] droperidol,[98] thiopental,[131] midazolam,[132] volatile anesthetics,[131] or labetalol blunts this response. This chronotropic effect is partially responsible for the rise in blood pressure that occurs after ketamine administration. Tachycardia is exaggerated if pancuronium is given with ketamine. Other physiologic alterations that ketamine may produce include an adrenergic constriction of capacitance vessels with an increased venous return,[131] direct autonomic nervous system stimulation, and baroreceptor depression.[133] In another study, the baroreceptor mechanism remained intact after both ketamine and etomidate induction.[134] Ketamine actually has a direct vasodilating effect, but this is overcome by sympathetic stimulation[134] resulting in little change in systemic vascular resistance. In critically ill patients, the autonomic nervous system response may be absent, and the catecholamines may be depleted. In such patients, ketamine can be a cardiovascular depressant.[135] Ketamine is not recommended for patients with coronary artery disease, because intraventricular pressures are elevated and contractility is increased,[133] resulting in increased myocardial oxygen demand.

Ketamine may be advantageous for some conditions. It is antidysrhythmogenic and counteracts both epinephrine-induced ventricular dysrhythmias and digitalis-induced dysrhythmias.[136] It is beneficial for patients in cardiogenic shock[98] or hypovolemic shock, as perfusion of the myocardial, renal, hepatic, and cerebral circulations improve with the rise in arterial pressure.[135] After ketamine induction in patients with

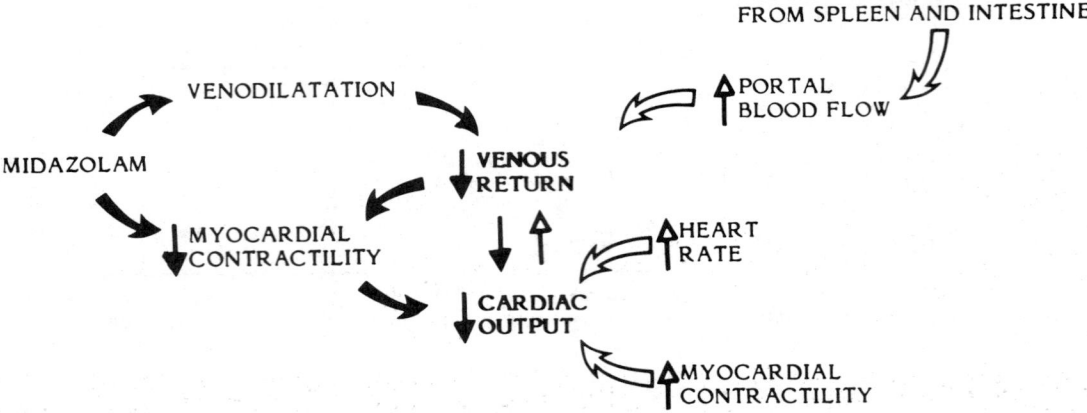

FIG. 8-8. The hemodynamic changes that occur after midazolam are illustrated by the solid arrows on the left side of the figure. They evoke compensatory changes that attempt to return circulation toward normal and are depicted by the open arrows in the right side of the figure. This illustration is probably also correct for some of the other induction agents. (Reprinted with permission from Gelman S, Reves JG, Harris D: Circulatory responses to midazolam anesthesia: Emphasis on canine splanchnic circulation. Anesth Analg 62:135, 1983.)

pericardial effusion, either with or without constrictive pericarditis, cardiac index remained stable; blood pressure, systemic vascular resistance, and right atrial pressure increased; and heart rate was unchanged from the usual tachycardia found in these patients.[132] Although ketamine is recommended for induction in such patients, it sometimes causes a decrease in cardiac output.[132] Children with congenital heart disease who were given ketamine, 2 mg·kg⁻¹, for anesthetic induction had preserved myocardial function. Although blood pressure and heart rate rose, there was no change in ejection fraction and no change in wall motion as determined by M-mode echocardiography.[137] Ketamine is the only iv induction drug that usually stimulates the cardiovascular system. It is thought to have a more pronounced effect on the right heart and pulmonary circulation than on the left heart and systemic vascular bed.[138]

Another induction drug that is nonstimulating and causes minimal cardiovascular depression is etomidate. In 1974, German investigators demonstrated the minimal changes in cardiovascular and coronary hemodynamics associated with its use. Bruckner found that etomidate, 0.3 mg·kg⁻¹, produced a slight increase in cardiac index and a slight decrease in heart rate, arterial blood pressure, and systemic vascular resistance. The changes were maximal 3 minutes after injection, returned to control values over the next 5 minutes, and were of lesser magnitude than demonstrated by other iv hypnotics.[139] Kettler et al showed that the same dose of etomidate increased coronary blood flow 19% with no increase in myocardial oxygen consumption. Coronary vascular resistance decreased 19% with no change in coronary perfusion pressure (Fig. 8-9).[140] This was interpreted as a mild nitroglycerin-like effect, suggesting that etomidate is a good anesthetic induction drug for patients with coronary artery disease who undergo either coronary artery bypass grafting or noncardiac procedures. Patients with valvular heart disease displayed a decrease of 10%–20% in systemic arterial pressure, pulmonary artery pressure, and pulmonary capillary wedge pressure[132] without change in CVP, heart rate, or electrocardiogram (ECG). Colvin et al demonstrated that etomidate caused less hypotension than did thiopental when each was given to patients with mild

hypovolemia.[141] In one study of etomidate, an unchanged dP/dT with no change in preload or afterload implied unimpaired myocardial function. Of all the rapidly acting iv hypnotics, etomidate produces the least detrimental cardiovascular changes[142]; this may be the main reason for its use.

Diazepam and midazolam rarely produce cardiovascular changes when used in small doses for premedication or iv sedation provided that precautions are taken against ventilatory depression. In induction doses, these benzodiazepines usually cause mild cardiovascular changes but may cause significant cardiovascular effects.

In one study, both diazepam and midazolam transiently depressed baroreflex function and reduced norepinephrine plasma concentrations from awake levels. Epinephrine levels were only reduced by midazolam. None of these changes were as significant as those occurring after anesthetic maintenance concentrations of volatile anesthetic drugs.[143]

Results of a number of studies comparing diazepam with other hypnotic induction drugs illustrate its vascular and myocardial effects. Used for patients with coronary artery disease, diazepam, 0.1 to 0.5 mg·kg⁻¹, caused a decrease in mean arterial pressure of 7%–18% but no change in heart rate, cardiac index, systemic vascular resistance, stroke index, or left ventricular stroke work index (LVSWI) despite this fivefold difference in dose.[132] In another study, 5 to 8.5 mg of diazepam reduced left ventricular end diastolic pressure (LVEDP), tension time index, and myocardial oxygen consumption for at least 20 minutes after injection.[144] There was no change in either coronary blood flow or coronary vascular resistance. The reduction in LVEDP could be due to a preload or afterload reduction; a nitroglycerine-like action on the circulation is unlikely. These changes resulted in improved cardiac function. In dogs, diazepam caused both active sympathetic and cholinergic vasodilation by acting as a specific ganglion stimulant.[145]

When diazepam, 5 mg, was given after morphine anesthesia, 2 mg·kg⁻¹, systolic blood pressure and heart rate decreased; cardiac output, stroke volume, and diastolic blood pressure decreased very slightly; and peripheral vascular resistance increased. A second dose of diazepam caused only a

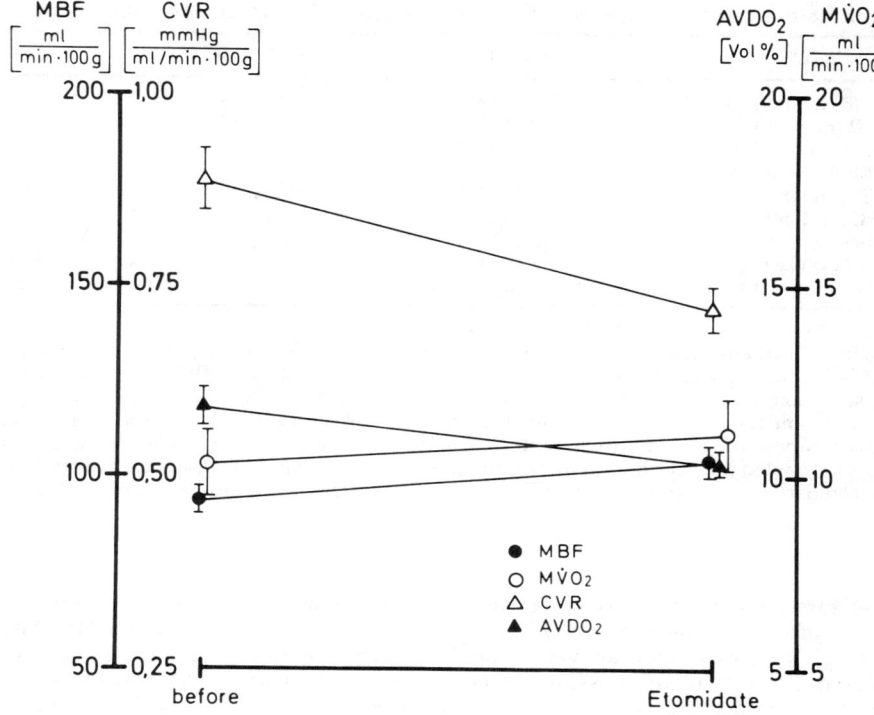

FIG. 8-9. This figure illustrates the effect of 0.12 mg·kg^{-1}·min^{-1} of etomidate on coronary hemodynamics and myocardial oxygen consumption in a healthy patient. There was a mild decrease in coronary vascular resistance (CVR) and a corresponding increase in myocardial blood flow (MBF). Myocardial oxygen consumption (MVO$_2$) was unchanged because of a simultaneous decrease in the arteriocoronary venous oxygen difference (AVDO$_2$). (Reprinted with permission from Kettler D, Sonntag H, Donath V et al: Haemodynamics, myocardial function, oxygen requirements and oxygen supply to the human heart after administration of etomidate. Anaesthesist 23:116, 1974.)

further decrease in systolic pressure and a further increase in peripheral resistance.[146]

Diazepam was also more cardiovascularly depressing for patients with LVEDP more than 15 mm Hg and with mean ejection fractions less than 0.38 than it was for patients with LVEDP less than 15 mm Hg. Blood pressure decreased in both groups of patients. The pre-ejection period (PEP) lengthened and the PEP/LVET (left ventricular ejection time) increased, suggesting that hypotension coincided with a reduction in myocardial performance.[147] Diazepam should be used with care in patients with coronary artery disease and elevated LVEDP.

Diazepam, 0.4 mg·kg^{-1}, caused a more profound decrease in peripheral resistance and arterial pressure than did thiopental, 3 mg·kg^{-1}, when either drug was given iv to healthy patients undergoing dental procedures in the semisupine position.[148] Thiopental is usually more depressant in supine patients. Tilting 12 volunteers before and after administering diazepam, 10 mg, caused no change in their measured hemodynamics.[149] Diazepam proved superior to thiopental as a hypnotic for cardioversion in an experiment in which premature ventricular contractions (PVCs) occurred in 11 of 18 patients who received thiopental, but none who received diazepam. When cardioversion was performed in patients with mitral stenosis, cardiac output remained nearer to control values after diazepam.[149] When compared with methohexital for electroshock therapy anesthesia, diazepam was associated with more cardiac dysrhythmias.[150]

These studies show that diazepam has both peripheral vascular and direct myocardial effects, but the degree of these effects is mild compared with that of most hypnotic induction drugs.

Midazolam was originally considered twice as potent as diazepam on a milligram basis, but further experience suggested that it is probably even more potent. Differences in the cardiovascular effects produced by the two benzodiazepines in earlier studies may be attributed to the effects of nonequivalent doses as much as to real differences between them.

After midazolam induction, a small decrease in blood pressure and an increase in heart rate occur in patients with normal cardiovascular function. In premedicated patients with coronary artery disease, changes in these measurements are usually less than 20% of control values.[151] When midazolam was given for sedation to patients with coronary artery disease undergoing cardiac catheterization, no significant changes in hemodynamic measurements occurred.[152]

In another group of patients with stable coronary artery disease who were asleep after receiving iv midazolam, 0.2 mg·kg^{-1}, for cardiac catheterization, mean arterial pressure (MAP) decreased 15%, and LVEDP decreased 44%. Cardiac index, stroke index, and heart rate of these patients changed less than 15%, whereas systemic vascular resistance (SVR) and V$_{max}$ were unchanged.[153] In the same study, effects of midazolam on coronary circulation were measured (Table 8-8). There were no ECG changes or changes in myocardial lactate extraction; nor was there an equivalent reduction in coronary blood flow and myocardial metabolism. When control pulmonary artery occlusion pressure (PAOP) exceeded 18 mm Hg and when cardiac index was less than 2.2 l·min^{-1}·m^{-2}, induction of anesthesia with midazolam caused a significant reduction in PAOP toward normal; and, at the same time, cardiac index and heart rate increased, whereas LVSWI, SVR, and MAP decreased. The 40% decrease in SVR in this group was about twice that which occurred in patients with PAOP less than 17 mm Hg.[154] It, therefore, can be concluded that midazolam can be used safely in patients with coronary artery disease.

However, midazolam, 0.075 or 0.15 mg·kg^{-1}, cannot be

TABLE 8-8. Cardiovascular and Coronary Effects of Midazolam (x ± SD)

	CONTROL	5 MIN	15 MIN
HR (beats·min^{-1})	81 ± 17	87 ± 16†	87 ± 15†
MAP (mm Hg)	109 ± 20	93 ± 15‡	92 ± 13‡
LVEDP (mm Hg)	7.7 ± 2.7	4.9 ± 2.4†	4.2 ± 2.6†
CSBF (ml·min^{-1})	134 ± 58	104 ± 38†	104 ± 30†
CVR (units)	0.84 ± 0.2	0.92 ± 0.2	0.91 ± 0.2
MVO$_2$ (ml·min^{-1})	16.8 ± 10.1	11.4 ± 4.4†	11.1 ± 3.6†
C(a-cs)O$_2$ (ml·dl^{-1})	12.1 ± 1.4	10.9 ± 1.5†	10.8 ± 1.3
Lact (a-cs)/lact a	0.45 ± 0.15	0.52 ± 0.15	0.44 ± 0.2
P$_{cs}$O$_2$ (mm Hg)	22 ± 3	25 ± 0.4*	25 ± 4*

* = $P < 0.05$; † = $P < 0.01$; ‡ = $P < 0.001$

(HR = heart rate; MAP = mean arterial pressure; LVEDP = left ventricular end diastolic pressure; CBSF = coronary sinus blood; CVR = coronary vascular resistance; MVO$_2$ = myocardial oxygen consumption; C(a-cs)O$_2$ = aorta-coronary sinus oxygen-content difference; Lact(a-cs)/lact a = aorta-coronary sinus lactate concentration divided by aortic lactate concentration; P$_{cs}$O$_2$ = oxygen tension in the coronary sinus. These measurements were made before and 5 and 15 min after midazolam, 0.2 mg/kg, iv) (Adapted with permission from Marty J, Nitenberg A, Blanchet F et al: Effects of midazolam in the coronary circulation in patients with coronary artery disease. Anesthesiology 64: 206, 1986.)

given safely to patients with coronary artery disease breathing oxygen after high-dose fentanyl, 75 µg·kg^{-1}. After high-dose fentanyl, there was significant venous pooling and both stroke index and systolic blood pressure decreased, the latter about 30%.[155] In contrast to diazepam, midazolam caused a decrease in cardiac index without a reduction in SVR. Midazolam also decreased coronary sinus blood flow and coronary perfusion pressure without altering coronary vascular resistance.

When midazolam was used to induce anesthesia for adults with valvular heart disease, pump function was maintained and there was a decrease in SVR.[156]

When flow was held constant during cardiopulmonary bypass, diazepam 0.3 mg·kg^{-1}, caused a transient decrease in SVR, whereas SVR remained stable after midazolam, 0.2 mg·kg^{-1}. Venodilation was greater after midazolam, however.[157]

As suggested by Figure 8-8, midazolam would be a more cardiovascularly depressing drug without the compensatory mechanisms. It should, therefore, be used cautiously, if at all, in patients who are hypovolemic or beta-blocked, have a blunted baroreflex, or have myocardial disease severe enough to prevent improvement in contractility. Tracheal intubation performed shortly after midazolam induction also returns blood pressure toward control values; there is less tachycardia than when tracheal intubation follows shortly after thiopental induction.[151, 158]

Barbiturates have more effects on the cardiovascular system than do benzodiazepines. Thiopental's main effects are to decrease cardiac output and increase heart rate. A decrease in cardiac output can be caused by 1) less ventricular filling (preload) owing to dilation of the capacitance vessels; 2) a direct negative inotropic effect; or 3) a decrease in central catecholamine outflow. The baroreceptor reflex is probably responsible for increased heart rate. Standard induction doses of thiopental usually produce an unchanged, or slightly decreased, mean arterial pressure and cardiac index in healthy patients, as well as in patients with compensated heart disease.[132] However, cardiovascular depression is exaggerated if the patients have valvular heart disease, either left or right heart failure, cardiac tamponade, or hypovolemia or are elderly. Thiopental must be used cautiously, if at all, in these cardiovascular conditions. It is particularly dangerous for patients with "compensated shock"[159] and for those with a fixed

cardiac output. (Digitalis reduces the depressant effect of thiopental on the heart.[160]) Methohexital, 1 mg·kg^{-1}, and thiopental, 3 mg·kg^{-1}, produce a similar decrease in myocardial contractility in healthy adults.[161] Methohexital induction is associated with a greater increase in heart rate than occurs after induction of anesthesia with equivalent doses of thiopental. Although methohexital dilates capacitance vessels and has a direct myocardial effect, it may also cause some change in total peripheral resistance by either a central or peripheral effect.[162] In most studies in healthy patients, thiopental had little effect on the resistance vessels. Regional blood flow is usually reduced. Thiopental decreases cerebral, hepatic, and renal blood flow and reduces central blood volume, because blood is pooled in the splanchnic circulation. Although baroreceptor function is intact in healthy patients, thiopental may markedly decrease baroreceptor activity in hypersensitive patients.[163] Thiopental's myocardial depressant effects will be more obvious when the baroreflex is blunted by volatile anesthetics, when there is beta-adrenergic blockade, or when insufficient myocardial reserve exists to sustain an increased heart rate.

When high doses of thiopental or methohexital were given to neurosurgical patients, both drugs caused decreases of about 15% in blood pressure, stroke volume index, and SVR; heart rate increased.[112, 164] The ventricular stroke work indices were decreased, and other hemodynamic measurements remained stable. These were tolerable changes in patients with normal cardiovascular systems.[112, 165] When thiopental, 6 mg·kg^{-1}, was given to patients with coronary artery disease, there was a parallel decrease in myocardial oxygen consumption and coronary blood flow.[166]

The most significant adverse cardiovascular effect of propofol is hypotension. Although the other induction agents may also cause hypotension, they concomitantly generate a greater degree of compensatory increase in heart rate. After propofol induction of anesthesia, blood pressure returns toward control values after a few minutes. The temporary 15%-20% decrease in systolic blood pressure, although not important for healthy patients, is a slightly greater decrease than occurs after barbiturate induction in healthy patients, patients with coronary artery disease, or those with valvular heart disease.[167-171]

After receiving propofol, 2.5 mg·kg^{-1}, for coronary artery bypass grafting, patients who had no myocardial infarct for at least 3 months and an ejection fraction over 30% had a significant decrease in MAP, SVR, and LVSWI; their heart rate increased. Table 8-9 shows the changes in hemodynamic variables after propofol induction of anesthesia as well as further changes that occurred when halothane was added. The changes were transient and without sequelae in these patients, but the changes probably represent both vasodilation and direct myocardial depression.[172] In an earlier study, propofol caused a 25% decrease in MAP and a significant decrease in SVR; two of 10 patients had a systolic blood pressure decrease of more than 70 mm Hg.[173] After intubation of the trachea, there was less cardiovascular stimulation than after thiopental induction, but propofol does not suppress the hemodynamic response to laryngoscopy and tracheal intubation.[173] It is the authors' opinion that propofol should be used with utmost caution, if at all, in patients who cannot tolerate temporary significant decreases in blood pressure.

The effects of propofol on coronary circulation were addressed in one study[174]; an induction dose of 2 mg·kg^{-1} was followed by a 200 μg·kg^{-1}·min^{-1} continuous infusion.

Myocardial blood flow decreased 26%, myocardial oxygen consumption decreased 31%, and coronary vascular resistance increased 19% without change in arterial-coronary sinus oxygen content difference.[174] A few patients had some myocardial lactate production, suggesting possible imbalance of regional myocardial oxygen demand and supply associated with propofol. In another study, there was no difference in the degree of hypotension between a rapid (5-sec) injection and a slower (60-sec) injection when propofol was given for anesthetic induction in young, healthy patients.[175] A slower injection time will usually result in less hypotension. Elderly patients have more hypotension after propofol than younger patients; the degree of hypotension seems dose related in the elderly (Table 8-10).[85]

The condition of patients when they enter a given study may influence their cardiovascular changes on induction of anesthesia. When propofol was used to induce anesthesia in patients with good ventricular function, right-sided pressures such as the CVP, PAP pressure, and PAOP, as well as the SVR and pulmonary vascular resistance (PVR) were unchanged.[176] When similar induction was performed on patients with im-

TABLE 8-9. Cardiovascular Effects of Propofol vs. Thiamylal in Patients with Coronary Artery Disease

		CONTROL	T_1	T_3	T_4
MAP	(P)	97±11	83±18#	75±16^{+}*	66±9*
	(T)	95±13	93±10	95±8	77±11*
HR	(P)	60±14	72±19*	68±12#	71±10*
	(T)	67±12	75±11#	67±8	71±8
CI	(P)	2.4±0.4	2.4±0.4	2.4±0.5	2.6±0.6
	(T)	2.8±1	2.8±0.8	2.5±0.6	2.4±0.9
PAOP	(P)	16±5	15±5	14±5	12±4#
	(T)	18±3	18±3	17±3	15±4
SVR	(P)	1565±262	1246±328#	1146±227^{+}*	987±291^{+}*
	(T)	1426±450	1379±442	1522±349	1307±358
LVSWI	(P)	45±10	28±9*	30±10*	28±8*
	(T)	44±15	37±10	39±9	29±14

$^{+}P < 0.01$ between groups; *$P < 0.01$ within groups; #$P < 0.05$ within groups; $\bar{x} \pm 1$ SD
T_1 = 1 minute after injection; T_3 = 3 minutes after injection; T_4 = 1 minute after halothane
(P = propofol; T = thiamylal; MAP = mean arterial pressure; HR = heart rate; CI = cardiac index; PAOP = pulmonary artery occlusion pressure; SVR = systemic vascular resistance; LVSWI = left ventricular stroke work index) (Reprinted with permission from Profeta JP, Guffin A, Mikula S et al: The hemodynamic effects of propofol and thiamylal sodium for induction in coronary artery surgery. Anesth Analg 66:5142, 1987.)

TABLE 8-10. Induction Characteristics of Propofol in Older vs. Younger Patients

DOSE mg·kg^{-1}	% INDUCED		SYSTOLIC BLOOD PRESSURE DECREASED >40 mm Hg	>40 mm Hg	APNEA >1 min	
	−60	+60	−60	+60	−60	+60
1.5	53	96	3	12	3	0
1.75	83	100	0	8	3	4
2	87	96	0	20	10	20
2.25	97	100	0	45	13	25

(Reprinted with permission from Dundee JW, Robinson FP, McCollum JSC et al: Sensitivity to propofol in the elderly. Anaesthesia 41:482, 1986.)

paired cardiac function, the reductions in cardiac index and MAP were primarily related to a marked decrease in CVP (16%–29%) and PAOP (35%–44%). Neither SVR nor PVR changed in these patients.[177]

Table 8-11 compares the relative hemodynamic effects of the various induction agents in healthy patients. All these agents can be used safely in healthy patients, but the data presented in this section should help the anesthesiologist make appropriate choices for patients with compromised cardiovascular function.

HEPATORENAL EFFECTS

None of these anesthetic induction drugs have adverse effects on the hepatic system,[130, 178, 179] even though those that cause hypotension can reduce hepatic blood flow. Most of the drugs decrease urine output because of an increase in antidiuretic hormone. Glomerular filtration and effective plasma flow decrease, and water and electrolyte reabsorption increase. Unlike opioids, the nonopioid induction drugs do not increase intrabiliary pressure. The barbiturates cause slight hyperglycemia and reduce carbohydrate metabolism.

ENDOCRINE EFFECTS

The suppression or release of central catecholamines by these drugs was discussed in the section concerning cardiovascular effects. None of these drugs appears to affect the anterior pituitary, thyroid, or adrenal medulla. Etomidate suppresses adrenal cortical function; its duration is dose related. In anesthetic induction doses, it can suppress adrenocortical response to stress for 5 to 8 hours[67], whereas an infusion produces a longer effect.[180] Etomidate causes a decrease in cortisol, 17-hydroxyprogesterone, aldosterone, and corticosterone production. It inhibits 17-α- and 11-β-hydroxylase and the cholesterol side-chain cleavage enzyme.[180] Clinical doses of propofol and thiopental did not suppress the adrenocortical response to the stress of surgery or to ACTH stimulation (Fig. 8-10).[181] However, in large doses, in vitro thiopental acts on 11-β-hydroxylase, and propofol acts at the first stage of cholesterol synthesis.[182] Midazolam does not suppress adrenocortical function either; ACTH and β-endorphin increase at the end of surgery after etomidate or methohexital anesthesia[183] but are suppressed by midazolam. In this study, etomi-

date given by bolus and infusion to a mean dose of 63 mg suppressed the cortisol response to ACTH stimulation for 6 hours and the aldosterone response to ACTH stimulation for 20 hours, but without electrolyte changes.[183]

ALLERGIC EFFECTS

None of the recently introduced anesthetic induction drugs are associated with histamine release.[184] Histamine release has been reported after the use of barbiturates, and anaphylactoid reactions have been reported occasionally after the use of thiopental.[185–187] Histamine release is increased by high dosage and rapid injections.

OTHER EFFECTS

None of these induction drugs have adverse effects on the reproductive system, and they can all cross the placenta to depress the fetus. Most drugs can be used safely for pregnant patients in normal induction doses. The benzodiazepines are discouraged for cesarean section anesthesia because diazepam in large doses is associated with hypotonic babies with low Apgar scores.[188] Midazolam is a poor choice for sedation with regional anesthesia because its amnestic effect may prevent the mother from remembering the birth of her baby.[189] The same may also be true of diazepam.

Propofol and the benzodiazepines can produce muscle relaxant effects in an in vitro model,[190, 191] but neither propofol, thiopental, nor midazolam produced significant clinical effects on concomitantly administered muscle relaxants.[192, 193] Propofol may affect muscles directly, and the benzodiazepines act through the spinal cord. Barbiturates, ketamine, and etomidate have no direct effects on skeletal muscles, nor do they interact with the commonly used muscle relaxant drugs.[193]

USES DURING CLINICAL ANESTHESIA

INDUCTION OF ANESTHESIA

Intravenous induction drugs, with the exception of the benzodiazepines, are used primarily by anesthesiologists to induce general anesthesia. Table 8-12 lists the drugs and the

TABLE 8-11. Cardiovascular Effects (Healthy Adults)*

	MAP	HR	CO	SVR	VENODILATION	dP/dT
Thiopental	−	+	−	0 to +	+	−
Thiamylal	−	+	−	NR	+	−
Methohexital	−	+ +	−	NR	+	−
Etomidate	0	0	0	0	0	0
Propofol	−	+	0	−	+	NR
Ketamine	+ +	+ +	+	+	0	0
Diazepam	0 to −	− to +	0	− to +	+	0
Midazolam	0 to −	− to +	0 to −	0 to −	+	0

* + + to − − is a five-point scale qualitatively describing the relative increase (+, + +) or decrease (−, − −) or virtually no effect (0) among the induction agents for each cardiovascular effect. (MAP = mean arterial pressure; HR = heart rate; CO = cardiac output; SVR = systemic vascular resistance; dP/dT = myocardial contractility; NR = not reported) (Reprinted with permission from Fragen RJ, Avram MJ: Comparative pharmacology of drugs used for the induction of anesthesia. In Stoelting RK, Barash PG, Gallagher TJ [eds]: Advances in Anesthesia, p 103. Chicago, Year Book Medical Publishers, 1986.)

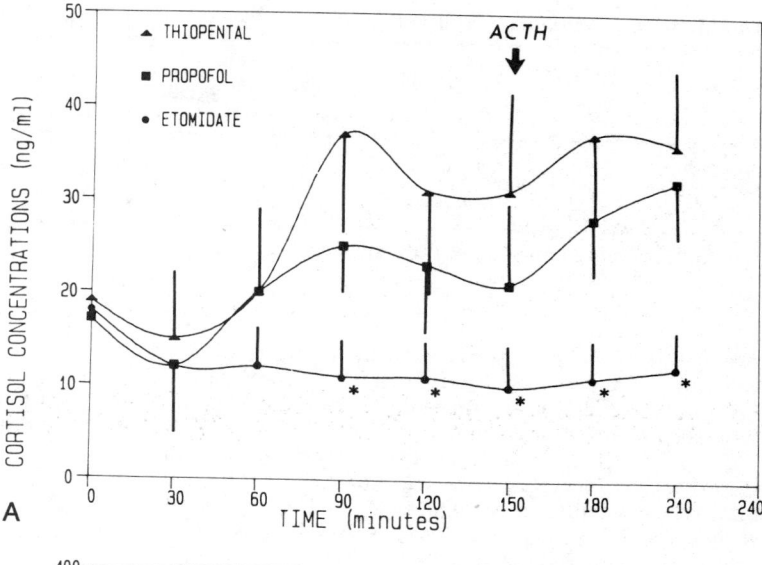

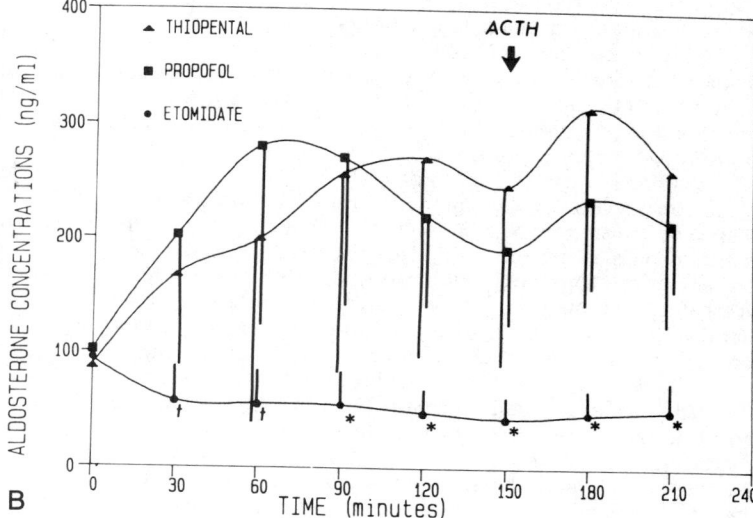

FIG. 8-10. The *A* and *B* figures show the blood cortisol (*A*) and aldosterone (*B*) concentration before and after anesthetic induction with thiopental, propofol, and etomidate and after an ACTH stimulation test administered 150 minutes after injection of the hypnotic drug. Asterisks (*) show significant differences ($P < 0.05$) between blood concentrations of cortisol or aldosterone after etomidate and those after either thiopental or propofol at the same time. There were no significant differences between the hormone concentrations in patients receiving propofol or thiopental. (Reprinted with permission from Fragen RJ, Weiss HW, Molteni A: The effect of propofol on adrenocortical steroidogenesis: A comparative study with etomidate and thiopental. Anesthesiology 66:839, 1987.)

TABLE 8-12. Drug Doses (Healthy Adults)

Thiopental	3–5 mg·kg^{-1}
Thiamylal	3–5 mg·kg^{-1}
Methohexital	1–1.5 mg·kg^{-1}
Etomidate	0.3 mg·kg^{-1}
Propofol	1.5–2.5 mg·kg^{-1}
Ketamine	0.5–1.5 mg·kg^{-1}
Diazepam	0.3–0.6 mg·kg^{-1}
Midazolam	0.15–0.4 mg·kg^{-1}

ranges of commonly recommended induction doses. To identify persons who might be particularly sensitive to these drugs, one can inject approximately 25% of the calculated dose initially and then observe the patient's level of consciousness, respiration, and cardiovascular response. If there is much effect from this small dose, the calculated dose based on population averages should be reduced. Differences in rapidity of the onset of effect for comparable induction doses depend upon the speed of injection, the central volume of distribution, and cardiac output. Most of these drugs act in one

arm–brain circulation time. The exceptions are the benzodiazepines and ketamine. To reduce ketamine's side-effects, a 60-second injection time is recommended. Opioid premedication or opioids given iv shortly before the anesthetic induction drug also speed onset, especially with the benzodiazepines. When midazolam was titrated during early dose-ranging studies,[194] or given slowly over 20 to 30 seconds,[195] induction times were longer than after thiopental but shorter than after diazepam. Usually, when midazolam is administered over 5 seconds and preceded by iv fentanyl, 100 μg, for an adult, patients lose consciousness in about 1 minute. Normal induction doses of the barbiturates, etomidate, and propofol last 3 to 5 minutes when given alone and slightly longer if other sedative drugs or opioids are given beforehand. Action of the benzodiazepines lasts 6 to 15 minutes, and ketamine lasts 10 to 15 minutes. The duration of effect can be prolonged by a larger initial dose, repeated fractional doses, or a continuous infusion.

Routes other than iv can be used to provide basal hypnosis or unconsciousness. Midazolam, thiamylal, and methohexital can induce unconsciousness with deep intramuscular (im) injection; midazolam is the least irritating. Any of these three

TABLE 8-13. Incidence (% of Patients) of Excitatory Effects After Three Anesthetics

	N	ANY EXCITATORY EFFECTS	SPONTANEOUS MOVEMENTS	TWITCHING	TREMOR	HYPERTONUS	HICCUP
Propofol	1459	13.9	8.7	3.0	0.8	1.9	2.3
Methohexital	86	41.9	10.5	17.4	2.3	1.2	26.7
Thiopental	123	7.3	4.1	1.6	0	0	1.6

(Reprinted with permission of ICI Pharmaceuticals.)

drugs can be used to provide basal hypnosis in children. Ketamine, 4 to 6 mg·kg^{-1}, has been used successfully by the im route for pediatric anesthesia. Thiopental and midazolam have also been administered rectally in children.

For all drugs, the anesthetic induction dose should be reduced for hypovolemic patients. Adequate time should be allowed for the initial dose to take effect when circulation time is slowed; otherwise an overdose may be given. As previously mentioned, elderly patients normally have increased reactivity to standard doses of these drugs.

The incidence and severity of induction side-effects are usually related to dose, rate of injection, initial distribution volume, and the amount and type of premedication. A slower injection time may reduce induction side-effects but will also prolong induction. Opioids reduce the incidence and severity of side-effects caused by etomidate.

Pain on injection can occur whether the induction agents are dissolved in water or organic solvents, although patients who mention pain at the time of induction of anesthesia seldom remember or complain about it postoperatively. Its incidence is greater and more severe when the drug is injected into small hand veins rather than larger arm or antecubital veins. Opioid premedication given either iv or im before the induction agent or lidocaine mixed with the induction drug can decrease both the incidence and severity of pain.[196] Midazolam, ketamine, and thiopental are the least irritating to the vein, whereas a disturbing incidence of pain on injection (up to 40%) accompanies use of methohexital, etomidate, propofol, and diazepam. Injected into the hand or wrist veins, propofol caused pain in all patients, and methohexital caused pain in 80% of patients, whereas thiopental was injected without pain.[197] Because injectable diazepam is associated with a relatively high incidence of venous sequelae, it virtually has been replaced by midazolam for anesthetic use.

Excitement phenomena, which include fine skeletal muscle tremors, twitching, hiccup, or coughing, may accompany induction of anesthesia. They are low in incidence and severity following induction of anesthesia with midazolam, thiopental, ketamine, diazepam, and propofol. Myoclonus is reported after induction of anesthesia with etomidate, and any of these phenomena can be present when methohexital is used. Stark et al compared the incidence of excitatory effects after propofol to those following the barbiturates.[198] The data were published in tabular form by the manufacturer (Table 8-13). Propofol and thiopental were associated with fewer excitatory effects than was methohexital. The methyl group on the barbiturate molecule may be responsible for the higher incidence of excitement reactions to methohexital than to thiopental.[199] Mackenzie and Grant reported a 75% incidence of excitatory movements after methohexital induction compared with 20% following propofol induction.[200] When Doze et al compared propofol and methohexital in outpatient anesthesia, they, too, found a lower incidence of excitement after propofol induc-

tion.[201] Excitement phenomena occur after loss of consciousness, so they are not perceived by the patient. Usually, their duration of effect is less than 1 minute, and they are a mild annoyance.

MAINTENANCE

Ketamine can be used by infusion to maintain both unconsciousness and analgesia, but the other drugs may only be suitable to maintain hypnosis (unconsciousness) in a balanced anesthesia technique or for sedation with regional or local anesthesia. This can be accomplished by using a continuous infusion or an intermittent bolus technique in which about 20%–25% of the initial induction dose is given whenever further doses are necessary. Drugs with the highest elimination clearances are least likely to cause prolonged drowsiness when given by infusion, depending, of course, upon the dose administered. Exponential infusion rates that follow the plasma decay curves are most likely to achieve and maintain a target blood concentration. They must be correlated with the clinical picture, and appropriate adjustments must be made in the infusion rate.

In the future, propofol is likely to be used by infusion because of rapid patient recovery after the infusion is terminated. Used in one study for iv sedation with regional anesthesia, the mean infusion rate was 3 mg·kg^{-1}·hr^{-1} in patients over age 65 years, and 4.1 mg·kg^{-1}·hr^{-1} in younger patients. Recovery occurred approximately 4 minutes from the end of the infusion when the mean infusion time was 98 minutes.[202] For total iv anesthesia, Camu et al recommend an initial infusion of 6 to 9 mg·kg^{-1}·hr^{-1} for about 30 minutes following induction with propofol, 2 mg·kg^{-1}; followed by a maintenance infusion of 3 mg·kg^{-1}·hr^{-1}.* Willaert recommends an infusion rate of 9 mg·kg^{-1}·hr^{-1} for 30 minutes, then 4.5 mg·kg^{-1}·hr^{-1} when propofol is given with alfentanil, oxygen, and air.*

Patients recovered more quickly from propofol than from methohexital when a maintenance dose of methohexital, 0.1 to 0.3 mg·kg^{-1}·min^{-1} after a 1.5 mg·kg^{-1} induction dose, was compared with a maintenance dose of 0.1 to 0.2 mg·kg^{-1}·min^{-1} of propofol after a 2 mg·kg^{-1} induction dose in patients breathing 67% nitrous oxide in oxygen.[203] Thiopental infusions must be used cautiously, because they can be associated with prolonged recovery. Some authorities advocate using ketamine infusions for general surgical cases,[204] or for thoracic surgery using one-lung ventilation.[205] Midazolam, used by intermittent bolus for hypnosis in a balanced anesthetic technique with fentanyl and nitrous oxide, proved superior to thiopental, because fewer supplemental

* Oral presentation at European Anaesthesia Congress, Vienna, 1986.

drugs were needed to maintain an adequate depth of anesthesia.[206] Midazolam was associated with fewer emergence complications and more amnesia for early postoperative events.[206, 207]

Etomidate is not the best choice for prolonged infusion unless supplemental steroids are administered, but after a 1- to 2-hour infusion, no harmful effects have been reported.[50] Diazepam is also not a good choice for infusions because of its long half-life, active metabolites, and venous irritation.

The side-effects during maintenance infusions are fewer than those seen during induction of anesthesia because a low dose is given per unit of time compared with that of an induction dose. However, an overdose can produce prolonged drowsiness.

Recent reports describe the successful use of a midazolam infusion to sedate children requiring artificial ventilation after cardiac surgery.[208, 209] A blood level of 250 ng $\cdot$ ml^{-1} was necessary for adequate sedation, achieved with a 2 μg $\cdot$ kg^{-1} $\cdot$ min^{-1} infusion combined with morphine, 0.33 μg $\cdot$ kg^{-1} $\cdot$ min^{-1}. When controlled ventilation was changed to continuous positive airway pressure (CPAP), morphine was discontinued and the rate of midazolam administration was increased to a mean of 4 μg $\cdot$ kg^{-1} $\cdot$ min^{-1} (range 2 to 5 μg $\cdot$ kg^{-1} $\cdot$ min^{-1}). When hepatic function was impaired, recovery was longer.[208] When midazolam or propofol was given by infusion to sedate patients after cardiac surgery, patients recovered consciousness more rapidly after propofol infusion.[210] Sedation following propofol infusion was easily controlled, and there was little cardiovascular depression.[210]

Midazolam is the most versatile of the nonopioid induction drugs. It can be used for children[211] as well as for adults for im premedication and iv sedation for surgical and diagnostic procedures,[109] as well as for sedation in intensive care units and for induction of anesthesia. Benzodiazepines are also the only sedatives for which there is a specific antagonist. Flumazenil is a specific benzodiazepine antagonist that can reverse all the CNS effects of the benzodiazepines, including sedative-hypnotic, amnestic, muscle relaxant, and EEG effects. Titrating flumazenil to effect is a useful method of administration. It has been used in this way to reverse sedation produced by flunitrazepam,[212] diazepam,[213] and midazolam.[214] When flumazenil is used to reverse long-acting benzodiazepines, resedation is possible because the half-life of the antagonist is 0.7 to 1.8 hours, owing to its high hepatic clearance.[215] In one study, some patients appeared to be asleep after receiving flumazenil but were wide awake when addressed.[214] An increase in delta activity on the EEG could explain this phenomenon. Physostigmine, 2 mg, combined with glycopyrolate, 0.2 mg, produces nonspecific reversal of hypnosis produced by benzodiazepines as well as other hypnotic drugs.[216] Aminophylline, 60 mg iv, can also counteract deep diazepam sedation, apparently by an adenosine blockade of GABA-receptors in the CNS. Aminophylline given to patients during benzodiazepine anesthesia could result in patient awareness.[217]

IMPACT OF PRE-EXISTING DISEASE

Ketamine is considered to be the preferred induction drug for children with tetralogy of Fallot or transposition of the great vessels. It should not be used in patients with Wolff-Parkinson-White syndrome.[218]

Acute intermittent porphyria and some other types of porphyria may be triggered by the barbiturates; they are contraindicated for patients with these diseases. There is some ques-

tion about the safety of the benzodiazepines and ketamine for patients with porphyria, although ketamine has been used safely in such patients. Etomidate can be used for induction in the presence of this disease, but propofol has not undergone investigation in humans with porphyria.[218]

Although etomidate temporarily suppresses adrenocortical function, there is no contraindication to its use for any disease states. Patients with adrenocortical insufficiency, regardless of the etiology, are on maintenance cortisone therapy, usually with a boost in dose at the time that they come to surgery, which provides added protection against the stress of surgery and anesthesia.

Only the few disease states previously mentioned are currently known to contraindicate these induction drugs. None of these drugs trigger malignant hyperpyrexia.

RECOVERY

The time required for initial awakening, orientation to time and place, and return of normal psychomotor performance should be as short as possible after administration of the anesthetic drugs ceases. The quickest possible return of the patient's homeostatic mechanisms is the goal after any anesthetic. Every recovery is especially important in the expanding outpatient surgical population. Early discharge is not only desirable from the patient's viewpoint but may also be cost-saving. Adequate analgesia in the early postoperative period must also be provided. Because the anesthetic drug or maintenance hypnotic is usually only one of a number of drugs that constitute the anesthetic regimen, it is not the only drug that affects the duration of recovery. A number of studies have been performed in which short anesthetics differed from each other only in the induction drugs used.[95, 171, 202, 203, 219–223] In many of these studies, different induction drugs caused differences of only 5 to 10 minutes in time to awakening and orientation. Although some of the differences are statistically significant, they are not clinically important. Assuming that equivalent doses of the iv anesthetics are given to an ideal patient, time to recovery will increase in the following order, from most rapid to slowest: propofol, methohexital, etomidate, thiopental, midazolam, ketamine, and diazepam. Thus, propofol, having the fastest recovery, may become the induction drug of choice for healthy outpatients.

Mackenzie and Grant showed that psychomotor performance was impaired for 30 minutes following propofol administration, 60 to 90 minutes after methohexital administration, and up to 2 hours or longer after thiopental administration in outpatient anesthesia.[223] Patients undergoing ambulatory surgery who received propofol could walk 14 minutes sooner than those who received methohexital.[202] After propofol administration, awakening usually occurs at a blood concentration of about 1 μg $\cdot$ ml^{-1} and orientation at about 0.6 μg $\cdot$ ml^{-1}.[203]

Patients receiving midazolam became oriented 20 minutes later than those receiving thiopental. They also had a slower return of hand coordination, vigilance, spatial concepts, and short-term learning.[224] Return of these functions was slow enough for these authors to recommend that midazolam be avoided as an anesthetic induction drug for outpatients. Some investigators believe that midazolam induction is satisfactory for outpatients, even though some patients did not fully recover until 3 hours or more after surgery.[207, 225] Patients should be eligible for discharge from an outpatient surgical facility by 2 hours after surgery or sooner. Recovery from midazolam usually takes twice as long as from thiopental. Its amnestic properties are another negative factor for use of midazolam as an induction drug for outpatients: Outpatients may seem quite alert but be unable to remember instructions given to them in the early postoperative period. After midazolam anesthesia, outpatient instructions should be in writing. Because the duration of amnesia is dose related, amnesia is less prolonged with the smaller doses of midazolam used for iv sedation. A 5-mg dose of midazolam produces amnestic effects in 1 to 2 minutes lasting for at least 32 minutes.[226]

Recovery after methohexital administration is perceived to be faster than after thiopental administration, but comparisons of the two do not always give consistent results.[200] Recovery after etomidate induction is similar to that after thiopental.[219] When ketamine is used in outpatients, they are usually ready for discharge by 2 hours, but, occasionally, recovery is prolonged.[128]

Recovery after continuous infusions may be prolonged when the redistribution sites are saturated, and recovery depends upon elimination clearance. Active metabolites, such as N-desmethyldiazepam, can prolong recovery. Drugs that have relatively low elimination clearances (hence, long elimination half-lives), can leave prolonged residual effects. Small doses of sedatives or opioids given postoperatively can have additive effects with the residual anesthetic drugs, causing resedation.

The early recovery period will be pleasant if the anesthetic drugs leave no emergence side-effects and if there is sufficient analgesia to obtund the pain of surgery.

Recovery side-effects are important, because they may interfere with a patient's recovery and persist well into the postoperative period. Recovery side-effects are least common after propofol and are compared to the effects of the barbiturates in Table 8-14.[198] Patients return to a clear-headed state sooner after propofol induction than after other induction agents. Because it also results in the lowest incidence of nausea and vomiting, propofol is well-suited to induce anesthesia for outpatients. Nausea and vomiting are also acceptably low in incidence following use of the benzodiazepines, barbiturates, and ketamine. After midazolam induction, the incidence of nausea and vomiting ranges from none to 15%; 15% is the incidence after other induction drugs. Of 1,130 patients, the overall incidence of vomiting after midazolam was 3% during the investigational period.[109] Nausea and vomiting are frequent side-effects following induction of anesthesia with etomidate, especially when it is used for short anesthetics.[219]

Other factors in the perioperative period contribute to postoperative nausea, including the presence of pain, use of opioids, surgical site, and use of volatile anesthetics. Some authorities claim that nitrous oxide contributes because it dilates the bowel and increases middle ear pressure. However, one study claims that 60% nitrous oxide did not play a major role, but predisposing factors such as female gender, young adults, and a prior history of postoperative nausea are important.[227]

Emergence excitement following etomidate and ketamine induction has been reported. When etomidate was used by bolus plus infusion as part of a total iv anesthetic technique, restlessness and disorientation occurred from early awakening until full orientation.[50] This has not been reported when etomidate was given only for induction of anesthesia. After ketamine induction, patients should recover in a quiet place without being disturbed. They may experience mood alterations, feelings of estrangement or isolation, negativism, hostility, apathy, drowsiness, and repetitive motor behavior. Diplopia or other visual disturbances sometimes occur on return of consciousness. Patients may have difficulty speaking or experience severe emergence delirium. These unpleasant emergence phenomena can be ameliorated or avoided by giving lorazepam, midazolam, diazepam, or thiopental before or with ketamine; or they can be used to treat the symptoms postoperatively. Because these drugs can prolong recovery from ketamine, midazolam, with its shorter duration of effect, may be the best of the benzodiazepines for this function. Droperidol may increase the incidence of vivid dreams when it is used to treat emergence reactions. Preoperative discussion with patients about the possibility of these symptoms occurring also reduces their incidence and severity.[128] If excitement occurs following administration of the other iv drugs, the anesthesiologist should consider other causes, such as pain or hypoxia.

Venous sequelae such as venous thrombosis, thrombophlebitis, or phlebitis may occur up to the 10th day after irritant iv drugs have been injected. There is less than a 5% incidence after most drugs, including midazolam, propofol, ketamine, and the barbiturates. Because both etomidate and diazepam are dissolved in propylene glycol, the incidence of venous sequelae is 10%-20% following etomidate induction and up to 40% following diazepam induction.[178] Venous reactions usually involve a small segment of vein, are treated symptomatically, and rarely result in permanent damage.

If thiopental or thiamylal is extravasated, it is irritating, and tissue slough may occur. This is treated by heat to increase absorption of barbiturate. If injected intraarterially, vascular spasm and gangrene can occur.[228] Local injection of vascular dilators or stellate ganglion blockade has been used to treat this unfortunate circumstance and should be performed as soon as possible.

Other postoperative side-effects include a low incidence of headache after all the drugs, prolonged drowsiness (usually dose related), and prolonged amnesia after midazolam is given in high doses or to the elderly.

If both induction and recovery side-effects are considered, midazolam appears to be the best induction drug, because it is associated with the fewest side-effects. Methohexital causes a high incidence of induction side-effects, and the barbiturates are associated with a low incidence of recovery side-effects. Etomidate has both induction and recovery side-effects. Ketamine is pleasant for induction, but excitement on recovery can be troublesome. Propofol causes some induction side-

TABLE 8-14. Incidence (% of patients) of Recovery Side-Effects

	N	HEADACHE	NAUSEA	VOMITING	RESTLESSNESS
Propofol	1223	2.2	2.0	2.5	1.6
Methohexital	86	9.3	12.8	10.5	3.5
Thiopental	79	1.3	10.1	10.1	2.5

(Reprinted with permission of ICI Pharmaceuticals.)

effects, but recovery after its use is more rapid and pleasant than that following any of the other drugs described here.

DRUG INTERACTIONS

There is considerable potential for drug interactions during anesthesia and surgery for three reasons: 1) patients requiring anesthesia and surgery are often receiving other drugs; 2) the anesthetic frequently takes the form of polypharmacy; and 3) most drugs used during anesthesia acutely depress the CNS and inhibit protective reflexes.[229] Therefore, the possibility of drug interactions must always be on the mind of the vigilant anesthesiologist. However, the anesthesiologist need not memorize the long lists of drug interactions in books,[230] review articles, and compendia, because many of the drug interactions in those lists are either inaccurate or clinically unimportant and of purely academic interest.[229, 231-233] Most clinically important adverse drug interactions can be avoided by understanding the pharmacology of the drugs being used and the mechanisms of interactions. Drug interactions can generally be classified as pharmaceutical, pharmacokinetic, or pharmacodynamic.[229, 231-234]

Pharmaceutical interactions result from physicochemical incompatibilities of drug formulations with each other or with iv fluids. An acidic drug, such as a barbiturate, is dissolved in a basic medium and will precipitate as the free acid if the pH is lowered; a basic drug, such as ketamine, is dissolved in an acidic medium and will precipitate as the free base if the pH is raised. On the other hand, some drugs, such as diazepam, have limited solubility in aqueous media and will precipitate if there is an increase in the water:organic solvent ratio of their vehicle (see Chemistry and Formulation). Additionally, some drugs are unstable in acidic or basic media; mixing a barbiturate with atracurium is likely to result not only in precipitation of the barbiturate but also in inactivation of atracurium by the Hofmann reaction, which occurs at basic pH. Pharmaceutical interactions are easily avoided by neither mixing drugs nor diluting them with iv fluids unless they are known to be compatible.

Pharmacokinetic drug interactions result from one drug interfering with the absorption or disposition of another. Since the anesthetic induction drugs are administered iv, the process of absorption is avoided. Because investigation into the interference of drugs with drug distribution is only beginning, the potential clinical implications of such interference remain speculative. Most research on pharmacokinetic drug interactions has focused on the effect of drugs on the elimination clearance of other drugs. Because the iv anesthetic induction drugs are eliminated almost exclusively by hepatic metabolism, potential pharmacokinetic interactions affecting hepatic drug clearance are the most relevant to this discussion.

One drug can affect the elimination clearance of another by altering the rate at which the other drug is delivered to the liver (*i.e.*, hepatic blood flow) or the ability of hepatic enzymes to metabolize the drug (*i.e.*, enzymatic induction or inhibition). The elimination clearance of high hepatic extraction ratio drugs (Table 8-3) can be decreased by the lowered hepatic blood flow produced by drugs such as propranolol or the volatile anesthetics. Chronic treatment with drugs such as phenobarbital or rifampin will induce hepatic microsomal enzyme activity, resulting in increased elimination clearance of drugs metabolized by these enzymes. Enzyme induction, however, is a slow process and is unlikely to occur after the acute administration of barbiturates during anesthesia. On the other hand, cimetidine therapy or the volatile anesthetics

can inhibit enzymes, decreasing the hepatic elimination of drugs metabolized by various oxidative enzymes. Because the effects of single doses of the iv anesthetic induction drugs are terminated primarily by redistribution, drug interactions affecting the elimination clearance of these drugs are unlikely to alter their duration of action unless they are given in very large doses, in multiple doses, or by continuous infusion. In such cases, elimination clearance can play a significant role in the termination of drug effect.

Pharmacodynamic interactions occur when one drug increases or decreases the reactivity to another drug as a result of their action at the same receptor or in the same physiologic system. Pharmacodynamic interactions involving CNS depressant drugs such as the anesthetic induction drugs are the most common serious interactions reported. Nonetheless, the pharmacodynamic interactions of these drugs is quite predictable because of the well-defined pharmacologic actions of these drugs and the drugs with which they interact. Thus, the induction dose requirement is decreased in the patient acutely intoxicated with alcohol but is increased in the sober chronic alcoholic. Chronic abusers of amphetamines or cocaine may be more sensitive to the depressant effects of the anesthetic induction drugs, whereas those acutely intoxicated with amphetamine or cocaine may require larger than standard doses for the induction of anesthesia. Caution in the administration of these powerful depressant drugs is always recommended when the potential for a pharmacodynamic drug interaction may exist.

TOXICITY

One need look no further than the tragic consequences of administering thiopental to the hypovolemic casualties of the Japanese attack on Pearl Harbor[5] to realize the tremendous potential toxicity of the iv anesthetic induction drugs. New induction agents that will have less toxicity are constantly being sought; the failure of newly developed drugs, such as propanidid, althesin, and minaxolone, to achieve and maintain a position in the armamentarium of the anesthesiologist is often due to their unacceptable toxicity or "adverse effects."

The toxicity or "adverse effects" of the anesthetic induction drugs can be classified as: 1) the effects of the drugs when administered in relative or absolute overdose, 2) side-effects of standard doses of the drugs, 3) abnormal or unpredictable responses to standard doses, and 4) drug interactions.[235] Several reviews have been devoted exclusively to the subject.[236-238] The "adverse effects" of these agents can be minimized by administering doses appropriate for the patient's physiologic condition at the slowest rate practical for the clinical situation.

SUMMARY

Although thiopental is not the ideal iv anesthetic induction drug, the fact that it has no major disadvantages accounts for its long-standing position as the standard drug for this application. Few of the drugs developed to displace thiopental as the standard are used today. Those that have survived have properties that make their use in specific clinical situations advantageous, whereas other properties preclude their use as routine induction drugs. The important clinical properties of these drugs are summarized in Table 8-15.

The older induction drugs are not generally better than thiopental. Although not extensively studied, thiamylal ap-

TABLE 8-15.   Summary of the Important Clinical Properties of the IV Sedative/Hypnotics Used for Anesthetic Induction*

	PREDICTABILITY OF INDUCTION	INDUCTION PAIN AND EXCITEMENT	CEREBRAL EFFECTS	RESPIRATORY EFFECTS	CARDIOVASCULAR EFFECTS	RECOVERY CHARACTERISTICS
Thiopental	+	0	+	−	−	+
Thiamylal	+	0	+	−	−	+
Methohexital	+	−	+	−	+	−
Etomidate	+	− −	+ +	0	−	+ +
Propofol	+	−	+	−	−	− −
Ketamine	+	0	−	+	0	+
Diazepam	−	− −	+	0	0	+
Midazolam	0	0	+	0	0	+

* + + to − − is a five-point qualitative scale describing the relative positive (+, + +), neutral (0), or negative (−, − −) effect of each agent in each category. (Reprinted with permission from Fragen RJ, Avram MJ: Comparative pharmacology of drugs used for the induction of anesthesia. In Stoelting RK, Barash PG, Gallagher TJ [eds]: Advances in Anesthesia, p 103. Chicago, Year Book Medical Publishers, 1986.)

pears to be similar to thiopental. Methohexital is associated with faster recovery after induction of anesthesia than is thiopental, but it also produces tachycardia and more excitatory effects on induction. Ketamine's advantages are its ability to produce somatic analgesia, bronchodilation, and cardiovascular stimulation, although, in some situations, the latter may be a disadvantage. Disadvantages of ketamine are its adverse cerebral effects and psychotomimetic effects on recovery. When used for induction of anesthesia, diazepam produces less cardiovascular and respiratory depression than does thiopental, but induction of anesthesia is less predictable, recovery is slower, and venous complications are associated with its use.

The newer drugs, etomidate, midazolam, and propofol, are clearly superior to some of the older induction drugs for specific clinical applications but not to thiopental for routine induction of anesthesia. Etomidate causes less respiratory and cardiovascular depression than does thiopental and has more beneficial cerebral effects, but these advantages are often offset by induction and recovery side-effects. Midazolam has the advantages of diazepam, less cardiovascular and respiratory depression than thiopental, but results in a more prolonged recovery than that associated with thiopental induction. However, midazolam causes less frequent venous irritation than does diazepam and has a shorter elimination half-life. Propofol causes cardiovascular and respiratory depression equivalent to that produced by thiopental but appears to have a shorter recovery time.

REFERENCES

1. Stedman's Medical Dictionary, p 73. Baltimore, Williams & Wilkins, 1953
2. Woodbridge PD: Changing concepts concerning depth of anesthesia. Anesthesiology 18:536, 1957
3. Frost EAM: Essays on the History of Anesthesia, p 31. Georgetown, McMahon Publishing, 1985
4. Pratt TW, Tatum AL, Hathaway HR et al: Sodium ethyl (1-methyl butyl) thiobarbiturate, preliminary experimental and clinical study. Am J Surg 31:464, 1935
5. Halford FJ: A critique of intravenous anesthesia in war surgery. Anesthesiology 4:67, 1943
6. Dundee JW: Historical vignettes and classification of intravenous anesthetics. In Aldrete JA, Stanley TH (eds): Trends in Intravenous Anesthesia, p 1. Chicago, Year Book Medical Publishers, 1980

7. Briggs LP, Clarke RSJ, Watkins J: An adverse reaction to the administration of disoprofol (Diprivan). Anaesthesia 37:1099, 1982
8. Glen JB, Hunter SC: Pharmacology of an emulsion formulation of ICI 35 868. Br J Anaesth 56:617, 1984
9. Albert A: Relations between molecular structure and biological activity: States in the evolution of current concepts. Ann Rev Pharmacol 21:13, 1971
10. Dundee JW: Molecular structure–activity relationships of barbiturates. In Halsey MJ, Millar RA, Sutton JA (eds): Molecular Mechanisms in General Anesthesia, p 16. New York, Churchill Livingstone, 1974
11. Sternbach LH: The benzodiazepine story. J Med Chem 22:1, 1979
12. Gerecke M: Chemical structure and properties of midazolam compared with other benzodiazepines. Br J Clin Pharmacol 16:11S, 1983
13. Godefroi EF, Janssen PAJ, Van der Eycken CAM et al: DL-1 (1-arylalkyl) imidazole-5-carboxylate esters. A novel type of hypnotic agent. J Med Chem 8:220, 1965
14. James R, Glen JB: Synthesis, biological evaluation, and preliminary structure–activity considerations of a series of alkylphenols as intravenous anesthetic agents. J Med Chem 23:1350, 1980
15. Cone EJ, McQuinn RL, Shannon HE: Structure–activity relationship studies of phencyclidine derivatives in rats. J Pharmacol Exp Ther 228:147, 1984
16. Simonyi M: On chiral drug action. Med Res Rev 4:359, 1984
17. Ariëns EJ: Stereochemistry, a basis for sophisticated nonsense in pharmacokinetics and clinical pharmacology. Eur J Clin Pharmacol 26:663, 1984
18. Andrews PR, Mark LC: Structural specificity of barbiturates and related drugs. Anesthesiology 57:314, 1982
19. Christensen HD, Lee IS: Anesthetic potency and acute toxicity of optically active disubstituted barbituric acids. Toxicol Appl Pharmacol 26:495, 1973
20. Gibson WR, Doran WJ, Wood WC et al: Pharmacology of stereoisomers of 1-methyl-5-(1-methyl-2-pentynyl)-5-allyl-barbituric acid. J Pharmacol Exp Ther 125:23, 1959
21. Heykants JJP, Meuldermans WEG, Michiels LJM et al: Distribution, metabolism and excretion of etomidate, a short-acting hypnotic drug, in the rat. Comparative study of (R)−(+) and (S)−(−)−etomidate. Arch Int Pharmacodyn Ther 216:113, 1975
22. White PF, Ham J, Way WL et al: Pharmacology of ketamine isomers in surgical patients. Anesthesiology 52:231, 1980
23. Ueda I, Kamaya H: Molecular mechanisms of anesthesia. Anesth Analg 63:929, 1984
24. Miller KW: General anesthetics. In Feldman SA, Scurr CF, Paton W (eds): Drugs in Anaesthesia: Mechanisms of Action, p 133. Baltimore, Edward Arnold, 1987

25. Nimmo WS: Hypnotics. In Feldman SA, Scurr CF, Paton W (eds): Drugs in Anaesthesia: Mechanisms of Action, p 125. Baltimore, Edward Arnold, 1987
26. Stone TW: Drugs interfering with synaptic transmission in the central nervous system. In Feldman SA, Scurr CF, Paton W (eds): Drugs in Anaesthesia: Mechanisms of Action, p 234. Baltimore, Edward Arnold, 1987
27. Costa E, Guidotti A: Molecular mechanisms in the receptor action of benzodiazepines. Ann Rev Pharmacol Toxicol 19:531, 1979
28. Ho IK, Harris RA: Mechanism of action of barbiturates. Ann Rev Pharmacol Toxicol 21:83, 1981
29. Olsen RW: Drug interactions at the GABA receptor–ionophore complex. Ann Rev Pharmacol Toxicol 22:245, 1982
30. Cheng SC, Brunner EA: The effects of anesthetic agents on GABA metabolism in rat brain synaptosomes. In Hertz L, Kvamme E, McGeer EG et al (eds): Glutamine, Glutamate, and GABA in the Central Nervous System, p 653. New York, Alan R Liss, 1983
31. Olsen RW, Fischer JB, Dunwiddie TV: Barbiturate enhancement of γ-amino-butyric acid receptor binding and function as a mechanism of anesthesia. In Roth SH, Miller KW (eds): Molecular and Cellular Mechanisms of Anesthetics. New York, Plenum, p 165. 1986
32. Olsen RW: GABA-benzodiazepine-barbiturate receptor interactions. J Neurochem 37:1, 1981
33. Study RE: Barker JL: Diazepam and (−)-pentobarbital: Fluctuation analysis reveals different mechanisms for potentiation of γ-aminobutyric acid responses in cultured central neurons. Proc Natl Acad Sci 11:7180, 1981
34. Roth SH, Tan K-S, MacIver MB: Selective and differential effects of barbiturates on neuronal activity. In Roth SH, Miller KW (eds): Molecular and Cellular Mechanisms of Anesthetics, p 43. New York, Plenum, 1986
35. Macdonald RL, Skerritt JH, Werz MA: Barbiturate and benzodiazepine actions on mouse neurons in cell culture. In Roth SH, Miller KW (eds): Molecular and Cellular Mechanisms of Anesthetics, p 17. New York, Plenum, 1986
36. Ticku MK, Rastogi SK: Barbiturate-sensitive sites in the benzodiazepine-GABA receptor–ionophore complex. In Roth SH, Miller KW (eds): Molecular and Cellular Mechanisms of Anesthetics, p 179. New York, Plenum, 1986
37. Willow M: A comparison of the actions of pentobarbitone and etomidate on [³H] GABA binding to crude synaptosomal rat brain membranes. Brain Res 220:427, 1981
38. Vincent JP, Cavey D, Kamenka JM et al: Interaction of phencyclidines with the muscarinic and opiate receptors in the central nervous system. Brain Res 152:176, 1978
39. Sircar R, Zukin SR: Further evidence of phencyclidine/sigma opioid receptor commonality. In Clouet DH (ed): Phencyclidine: An Update, p 14. Rockville, Maryland, National Institute on Drug Abuse, 1986
40. Friedman J: Physostigmine: The universal antagonist. In Aldrete JA, Stanley TH (eds): Trends in Intravenous Anesthesia, p 509. Chicago, Year Book Medical Publishers, 1980
41. Martin IL: The benzodiazepine receptor: Functional complexity. Trends Pharmacol Sci 5:343, 1984
42. Haefely W, Kyburz E, Gerecke M et al: Recent advances in the molecular pharmacology of benzodiazepine receptors and in the structure–activity relationships of their agonists and antagonists. In Testa B (ed): Advances in Drug Research, Vol 14, p 165. New York, Academic Press, 1985
43. Burch PG, Stanski DR: The role of metabolism and protein binding in thiopental anesthesia. Anesthesiology 58:146, 1983
44. Stanski DR, Hudson RJ, Homer TD et al: Pharmacodynamic modeling of thiopental anesthesia. J Pharmacokinet Biopharm 12:223, 1984
45. Furano ES, Greene NM: Metabolic breakdown of thiopental in man determined by gas chromatographic analysis of serum barbiturate levels. Anesthesiology 24:796, 1963
46. Stanski DR, Mihm FG, Rosenthal MH et al: Pharmacokinetics of high-dose thiopental used in cerebral resuscitation. Anesthesiology 53:169, 1980
47. Hudson RJ, Stanski DR, Burch PG: Pharmacokinetics of methohexital and thiopental in surgical patients. Anesthesiology 59:215, 1983
48. Brand L, Mark LC, Snell MMcM et al: Physiologic disposition of methohexital in man. Anesthesiology 24:331, 1963
49. McMurray TJ, Robinson FP, Dundee JW et al: A method for producing constant plasma concentrations of drugs. Applications to methohexitone. Br J Anaesth 58:1085, 1986
50. Fragen RJ, Avram MJ, Henthorn TK et al: A pharmacokinetically designed etomidate infusion regimen for hypnosis. Anesth Analg 62:654, 1983
51. Meuldermans WEG, Heykants JJP: The plasma protein binding and distribution of etomidate in dog, rat and human blood. Arch Int Pharmacodyn Ther 221:150, 1976
52. Adam HK, Briggs LP, Bahar M et al: Pharmacokinetic evaluation of ICI 35 868 in man: Single induction doses with different rates of injection. Br J Anaesth 55:97, 1983
53. Major E, Verniquet AJW, Waddell TK et al: A study of three doses of ICI 35 868 for induction and maintenance of anaesthesia. Br J Anaesth 53:267, 1981
54. Clements JA, Nimmo WS: Pharmacokinetics and analgesic effect of ketamine in man. Br J Anaesth 53:27, 1981
55. Wieber J, Gugler R, Hengstmann JH et al: Pharmacokinetics of ketamine in man. Anaesthesist 24:260, 1975
56. Idvall J, Ahlgren I, Aronsen KF et al: Ketamine infusions: Pharmacokinetics and clinical effects. Br J Anaesth 51:1167, 1979
57. Klotz U, Avant GR, Hoyumpa A et al: The effect of age and liver disease on the disposition and elimination of diazepam in adult man. J Clin Invest 55:347, 1975
58. Greenblatt DJ, Shader RI, Divoll M et al: Benzodiazepines: A summary of pharmacokinetic properties. Br J Clin Pharmacol 11:11S, 1981
59. Avram MJ, Fragen RJ, Caldwell NJ: Midazolam kinetics in women of two age groups. Clin Pharmacol Ther 34:505, 1983
60. Allonen H, Ziegler G, Klotz U: Midazolam kinetics. Clin Pharmacol Ther 30:653, 1981
61. Fragen RJ, Avram MJ: Comparative pharmacology of drugs used for the induction of anesthesia. In Stoelting RK, Barash PG, Gallagher TJ (eds): Advances in Anesthesia, p 103. Chicago, Year Book Medical Publishers, 1986
62. Brodie BB, Bernstein E, Mark LC: The role of body fat in limiting the duration of action of thiopental. J Pharmacol Exp Ther 105:421, 1952
63. Price HL, Kovnat PJ, Safer JN et al: The uptake of thiopental by body tissues and its relation to the duration of narcosis. Clin Pharmacol Ther 1:16, 1960
64. Bischoff KB, Dedrick RL: Thiopental pharmacokinetics. J Pharm Sci 57:1346, 1968
65. Runciman WB, Mather LE: Effects of anaesthesia on drug disposition. In Feldman SA, Scurr CF, Paton W (eds): Drugs in Anaesthesia: Mechanisms of Action, p 87. Baltimore, Edward Arnold, 1987
66. Van Hamme MJ, Ghoneim MM, Ambre JJ: Pharmacokinetics of etomidate, a new intravenous anesthetic. Anesthesiology 49:274, 1978
67. Fragen RJ, Shanks CA, Molteni A et al: Effects of etomidate on hormonal response to surgical stress. Anesthesiology 61:652, 1984
68. Nimmo WS, Clements JA: Ketamine. In Prys-Roberts C, Hug CC, Jr (eds): Pharmacokinetics of Anaesthesia, p 235. Boston, Blackwell Scientific, 1984

69. Stanski DR: Pharmacokinetics of barbiturates. In Prys-Roberts C, Hug CC, Jr (eds): Pharmacokinetics of Anaesthesia, p 112. Boston, Blackwell Scientific, 1984

70. Wilkinson GR, Shand DS: A physiological approach to hepatic drug clearance. Clin Pharmacol Ther 18:377, 1975

71. Larson CP, Mazze RI, Cooperman LH et al: Effects of anesthesia on cerebral, renal, and splanchnic circulation: Recent developments. Anesthesiology 41:169, 1974

72. White PF, Marietta MP, Pudwill CR et al: Effects of halothane anesthesia on the biodisposition of ketamine in rats. J Pharmacol Exp Ther 196:545, 1976

73. Reilly CS, Wood AJJ, Koshakji R et al: The effect of halothane on drug disposition: Contribution of changes in intrinsic drug metabolizing capacity and hepatic blood flow. Anesthesiology 63:70, 1985

74. Runciman WB, Mather LE, Ilsley AH et al: A sheep preparation for studying interaction between blood flow and drug disposition. II. Experimental applications. Br J Anaesth 56:1117, 1984

75. Linde HW, Berman ML: Nonspecific stimulation of drug-metabolizing enzymes by inhalation anesthetic agents. Anesth Analg 50:656, 1971

76. Gordon L, Wood AJJ, Koshakji RP et al: Acute effects of halothane on arterial and venous concentrations of propranolol in the dog. Anesthesiology 67:225, 1987

77. Dundee JW: The influence of body weight, sex and age on the dosage of thiopentone. Br J Anaesth 26:164, 1954

78. Christensen JH, Andreasen F: Individual variation in response to thiopental. Acta Anaesth Scand 22:303, 1978

79. Dundee JW, Hassard TH, McGowan WAW et al: The 'induction' dose of thiopentone: A method of study and preliminary illustrative results. Anaesthesia 37:1176, 1982

80. Homer TD, Stanski DR: The effect of increasing age on thiopental disposition and anesthetic requirement. Anesthesiology 62:714, 1985

81. Giles HG, MacLeod SM, Wright JR et al: Influence of age and previous use on diazepam dosage required for endoscopy. Can Med Assoc J 118:513, 1978

82. Gamble JAS, Kawar P, Dundee JW et al: Evaluation of midazolam as an intravenous anaesthetic induction agent. Anaesthesia 36:868, 1981

83. Dundee JW, Halliday NJ, Loughran PG: Variation in response to midazolam. Br J Clin Pharmacol 17:645P, 1984

84. Arden JR, Holley FO, Stanski DR: Increased sensitivity to etomidate in the elderly: Initial distribution versus altered brain response. Anesthesiology 65:19, 1986

85. Dundee JW, Robinson FP, McCollum JSC et al: Sensitivity to propofol in the elderly. Anaesthesia 41:482, 1986

86. Christensen JH, Andreasen F, Jansen JA: Pharmacokinetics and pharmacodynamics of thiopentone: A comparison between young and elderly patients. Anaesthesia 37:398, 1982

87. Sear JW, Cooper GM, Kumar V: The effect of age on recovery: A comparison of the kinetics of thiopentone and althesin. Anaesthesia 38:1158, 1983

88. Bruce A, Andersson M, Arvidsson B et al: Body composition. Prediction of normal body potassium, body water and body fat in adults on the basis of body height, body weight and age. Scand J Clin Lab Invest 40:461, 1980

89. Bender AD: The effect of increasing age on the distribution of peripheral blood flow in man. J Am Geriatr Soc 13:192, 1965

90. Jung D, Mayersohn M, Perrier D et al: Thiopental disposition as a function of age in female patients undergoing surgery. Anesthesiology 56:263, 1982

91. Henthorn TK, Krejcie TC, Avram MJ: Age and intravascular mixing during induction with thiopental. Anesthesiology 67:A663, 1987

92. Krejcie TC, Henthorn TK, Avram MJ et al: Thiopental kinetics and age: A reassessment. Anesthesiology 67:A664, 1987

93. Kiersey DK, Bickford RG, Faulkner A: Electroencephalographic patterns produced by thiopental sodium during surgical operations: Description and classification. Br J Anaesth 23:141, 1951

94. Ghoneim MM, Yamada T: Etomidate: A clinical and electroencephalographic comparison with thiopental. Anesth Analg 56:479, 1977

95. Lees NW, Hendry JGB: Etomidate in urological outpatient anaesthesia. Anaesthesia 32:592, 1977

96. Gancher S, Laxer KD, Krieger W: Activation of epileptogenic activity by etomidate. Anesthesiology 61:616, 1984

97. Brown CR: Clinical electroencephalographic and pharmacokinetic studies of a water-soluble benzodiazepine, midazolam maleate. Anesthesiology 50:467, 1979

98. Silvay G: Ketamine. Mt Sinai J Med 50:300, 1983

99. McPherson RW, Sell B, Traystman RJ: Effects of thiopental, fentanyl, and etomidate on upper extremity somatosensory evoked potentials in humans. Anesthesiology 65:584, 1986

100. Moss E, Powell D, Gibson RM et al: Effect of etomidate on intracranial pressure and cerebral perfusion pressure. Br J Anaesth 51:347, 1979

101. Renou AM, Vernheit J, Macrez P et al: Cerebral blood flow and metabolism during etomidate anaesthesia in man. Br J Anaesth 50:1047, 1978

102. Astrup J, Rosenorn J, Cold GE et al: Minimum cerebral blood flow and metabolism during craniotomy. Effect of thiopental loading. Acta Anaesthesiol Scand 28:478, 1984

103. Bendtsen AO, Cold GE, Astrup J et al: Thiopental loading during controlled hypotension for intracranial aneurysm surgery. Acta Anaesthesiol Scand 28:473, 1984

104. Nugent M, Artru AA, Michenfelder JD: Cerebral effects of midazolam and diazepam. Anesthesiology 53:S8, 1980

105. Stephan H, Sonntag H, Schenk HD et al: Einfluss von Disoprivan (Propofol) auf die Durchblutung und den Sauerstoffverbrauch des Gehirns und die CO_2—Reaktivität der Hirngefasse bein Menschen. Anaesthesist 36:60, 1987

106. Hartung HJ: Beeinflüssung des Intrakrahiellendrukes durch Propofol (Disoprivan). Anaesthesist 36:66, 1987

107. Dundee JW, Halliday NJ, Harper KW: Midazolam: A review of its pharmacological properties and therapeutic uses. Drugs 28:519, 1984

108. Giese JL, Stanley TH: Etomidate: A new intravenous anesthetic induction agent. Pharmacotherapy 3:251, 1983

109. Reves JG, Fragen RJ, Vinik MR et al: Midazolam: Pharmacology and uses. Anesthesiology 62:310, 1985

110. Helrich M, Papper EM, Rovenstine EA: Surital sodium: A new anesthetic for intravenous use. Preliminary clinical evaluation. Anesthesiology 11:33, 1950

111. deJong RH, Bonin JD: Benzodiazepines protect mice from local anesthetic convulsion and deaths. Anesth Analg 60:385, 1981

112. Todd MM, Drummond JC, U HS: The hemodynamic consequences of high-dose methohexital anesthesia in humans. Anesthesiology 61:495, 1984

113. Bennett DR, Madsen JA, Jordan WS et al: Ketamine anesthesia in brain-damaged epileptics: Encephalographic and clinical observations. Neurology 23:449, 1973

114. Fragen RJ, Hauch T: The effects of midazolam maleate and diazepam on intraocular pressure in adults. In Aldrete JA, Stanley TH (eds): Trends in Intravenous Anesthesia p 245. Chicago, Year Book Medical Publishers, 1980

115. Famewo CE, Adugbesian CO, Osuntakum OD: Effect of etomidate on intraocular pressure. Can Anaesth Soc J 24:712, 1977

116. Mirakhur RK, Shepherd WFI, Darrah WC: Propofol or thiopentone: Effects on intraocular pressure associated with induction of anaesthesia and tracheal intubation (facilitated with suxamethonium). Br J Anaesth 59:431, 1987

117. Calla S, Gupta A, Sen N et al: Comparison of the effects of

etomidate and thiopentone on intraocular pressure. Br J Anaesth 59:437, 1987

118. Ausinsch B, Rayburn RL, Munson ES et al: Ketamine and intraocular pressure in children. Anesth Analg 55:773, 1976

119. Helrich M, Eckenhoff JE, Jones RE: Influence of opiates on the respiratory response of man to thiopental. Anesthesiology 17:459, 1956

120. Streisand JB, Nelson P, Bubbers S et al: The respiratory effect of propofol with and without fentanyl. Anesth Analg 66:S171, 1987

121. Taylor MB, Grounds RM, Mulrooney PD et al: Ventilatory effects of propofol during induction of anesthesia. Anaesthesia 41:816, 1986

122. Guerra F: Thiopental forever after. In Aldrete JA, Stanley TH (eds): Trends in Intravenous Anesthesia, p 143. Chicago, Year Book Medical Publishers, 1980

123. Kalenda K: Etomidate as an induction agent. Lancet 2:1143, 1976

124. Forster A, Morel D, Bachmann M et al: Respiratory depressant effect of different doses of midazolam and lack of reversal with naloxone. A double-blind randomized study. Anesth Analg 62:920, 1983

125. Gross JB, Zebrowski MB, Carel WD et al: Time course of ventilatory depression after thiopental and midazolam in normal subjects and in patients with chronic obstructive pulmonary disease. Anesthesiology 58:540, 1983

126. Corssen G, Gutierrez J, Reves JG: Ketamine in the anesthetic management of asthmatic patients. Anesth Analg 51:588, 1972

127. Stefansssen T, Wickerstrom I, Haljamae H: Haemodynamic and metabolic effects of ketamine anesthesia in the geriatric patient. Acta Anaesthesiol Scand 26:371, 1982

128. White PF, Way WL, Trevor AJ: Ketamine—Its pharmacology and therapeutic uses. Anesthesiology 56:119, 1982

129. Soliman MG, Brinale GF, Kuski G: Response to hypercapnia under ketamine anaesthesia. Can Anaesth Soc J 22:486, 1975

130. Gelman S, Reves JG, Harris D: Circulatory responses to midazolam anesthesia: Emphasis on canine splanchnic circulation. Anesth Analg 62:135, 1983

131. Johnstone M: The cardiovascular effects of ketamine in man. Anesthesia 31:873, 1976

132. Reves JG, Kissen I: Intravenous anesthetics. In Kaplan J (ed): Cardiac Anesthesia, p 3. New York, Grune & Stratton, 1983

133. Tweed WA, Minuckm, Mymin D: Circulatory responses to ketamine anesthesia. Anesthesiology 37:613, 1972

134. Altura BM, Altura BT, Carella A et al: Vascular smooth muscle and general anesthesia. Fed Proc 39:1584, 1981

135. Pedersen T, Engback J, Klausen NO et al: Effects of low-dose ketamine and thiopentone on cardiac performance and myocardial oxygen balance in high risk patients. Acta Anaesth Scand 26:235, 1982

136. Corssen G, Reves JG, Carter JR: Neuroleptanesthesia, dissociative anesthesia, and hemorrhage. Int Anesth Clin 12(1):145, 1974

137. Bini M, Reves JG, Berry D et al: Ejection fraction during ketamine anesthesia in congenital heart diseased patients. Anesth Analg 63:186, 1984

138. Gooding JM, Dimick AR, Tavakoki M: A physiologic analysis of cardiopulmonary response to ketamine anesthesia in non-cardiac patients. Anesth Analg 56:813, 1977

139. Bruckner JB: Investigations in the effects of etomidate in the human circulation. Anaesthesist 23:322, 1974

140. Kettler D, Sonntag H, Donath V et al: Haemodynamics, myocardial function, oxygen requirements and oxygen supply to the human heart after administration of etomidate. Anaesthesist 23:116, 1974

141. Colvin MP, Savege TM, Newland PE et al: Cardiorespiratory changes following induction of anesthesia with etomidate in patients with cardiac disease. Br J Anaesth 51:551, 1979

142. Kettler D, Sonntag H, Donath V et al: Haemodynamics, myocardial function, oxygen requirements and oxygen supply of the human heart after administration of etomidate. In Doenicke AE (ed): Etomidate—An Intravenous Hypnotic Agent, p 81. New York, Springer, 1977

143. Marty J, Gauzit R, Lefebre P et al: Effects of diazepam and midazolam on baroreflex control of heart rate and on sympathetic activity in humans. Anesth Analg 65:113, 1986

144. Cote P, Guenet P, Bourossa M: Systemic and coronary hemodynamic effects of diazepam in patients with normal and diseased coronary arteries. Circulation 50:1210, 1974

145. Abel RM, Reis RL, Starosik RN: The pharmacologic basis of coronary and systemic vasodilator actions of diazepam (Valium). Br J Pharmacol 39:261, 1970

146. Stanley TH, Bennett GM, Loeser EA et al: Cardiovascular effects of diazepam and droperidol during morphine anesthesia. Anesthesiology 44:255, 1976

147. Douchot PJ, Staub F, Berzina L et al: Hemodynamic response to diazepam-dependence on prior left ventricular and diastolic pressure. Anesthesiology 60:499, 1984

148. Rubin A, Allen GD, Everett GB: Induction of general anesthesia with diazepam or thiopental. A comparison of the cardiorespiratory effects. Anesthesia Progress 39, 1978

149. Dundee JW, Haslett WHK: The benzodiazepines. Br J Anaesth 42:217, 1970

150. Allen RE, Pitts FN Jr, Summers WK: Drug modification of ECT: Methohexital and diazepam II. Biol Psychiatry 15:257, 1980

151. Samuelson PN, Reves JG, Kouchoukos NT et al: Hemodynamic responses to anesthetic induction with midazolam or diazepam in patients in ischemic heart disease. Anesth Analg 60:802, 1981

152. Fragen RJ, Myers SN, Baressi V et al: Hemodynamic effects of midazolam in cardiac patients. Anesthesiology 51:S103, 1979

153. Marty J, Nitenberg A, Blanchet F et al: Effects of midazolam in the coronary circulation in patients with coronary artery disease. Anesthesiology 64:206, 1986

154. Reves JG, Samuelson PN, Lewis S: Midazolam maleate induction in patients with ischaemic heart disease. Haemodynamic observations. Can Anaesth Soc J 26:402, 1979

155. Heikkila H, Jalonen J, Arola M et al: Midazolam as adjunct to high-dose fentanyl anesthesia for coronary artery bypass grafting operation. Acta Anaesthesiol Scand 28:683, 1984

156. Schulte-Sasse U, Hess W, Tarnow J: Haemodynamic responses to induction of anaesthesia using midazolam in cardiac surgical patients. Br J Anaesth 54:1053, 1982

157. Samuelson PN, Reves JG, Smith LR et al: Midazolam versus diazepam. Different effects on systemic vascular resistance. Arzneimittelforsch 31:2268, 1981

158. Boralessa H, Senior DF, Whitwam JG: Cardiovascular response to intubation. Anaesthesia 38:623, 1983

159. Graves CL: Management of general anesthesia during hemorrhage. Int Anesth Clin 12(1):1, 1974

160. List WF: Digitalis—thiopentone effects on myocardial function. Anaesthesia 30:624, 1975

161. Blackburn JP, Conway CM, Leigh M et al: The effects of anaesthetic induction agents upon myocardial contractility. Anaesthesia 26:93, 1971

162. Bernhoff A, Eklund B, Kaijser L: Cardiovascular effects of short-term anaesthesia with methohexitone and propanidid in normal subjects. Br J Anaesth 44:2, 1972

163. Bristow JD, Prys-Roberts C, Fisher A et al: Effects of anesthesia on baroreflex control of heart rate in man. Anesthesiology 31:422, 1969

164. Filner BE, Karliner JS: Alteration of normal left ventricular performance by general anesthesia. Anesthesiology 45:610, 1976

165. Todd MM, Drummond JC, U HS: The hemodynamic consequences of high-dose thiopental anesthesia. Anesth Analg 64:681, 1985

166. Reiz S, Balfors E, Freedman A et al: Effects of thiopentone on cardiac performance, coronary haemodynamics and myocardial

oxygen consumption in chronic ischemic heart disease. Acta Anaesthesiol Scand 25:103, 1981

167. Al-Khudairi D, Gordan G, Morgan M et al: Acute cardiovascular changes following disoprofol: Effects in heavily sedated patients with coronary artery disease. Anaesthesia 37:1007, 1982

168. Aun C, Major E: The cardiorespiratory effects of ICI 35 868 in patients with valvular heart disease. Anaesthesia 39:1006, 1984

169. Coates DP, Prys-Roberts C, Spelina RR et al: Propofol ('Diprivan') by intravenous infusion with nitrous oxide: Dose requirement and haemodynamic effects. Postgrad Med J 61(suppl 3):76, 1985

170. Fahy L, van Maurik GA, Utting JE: A comparison of the induction characteristics of thiopentone and propofol (2,6 di-isopropyl phenol). Anaesthesia 40:939, 1985

171. Rolly G, Versechelin L: Comparison of propofol and thiopentone for induction of anaesthesia in premedicated patients. Anaesthesia 40:945, 1985

172. Profeta JP, Guffin A, Mikula S et al: The hemodynamic effects of propofol and thiamylal sodium for induction in coronary artery surgery. Anesth Analg 66:S142,1987

173. Patrick MR, Blair IJ, Feneck RO et al: A comparison of the hemodynamic effects of propofol ('Diprivan') and thiopental in patients with coronary artery disease. Postgrad Med J 61(suppl 3):23, 1985

174. Stephan H, Sonntag H, Schenk HD et al: Effects of propofol on cardiovascular dynamics, myocardial blood flow and myocardial metabolism in patients with coronary artery disease. Br J Anaesth 58:969, 1986

175. Rolly G, Versechelin L, Hughes L et al: Effects of speed of injection on induction of anaesthesia using propofol. Br J Anaesth 57:743, 1985

176. Lippman M, Paicius R, Gingerich S et al: A controlled study of hemodynamic effect of propofol vs. thiopental during anesthesia induction. Anesth Analg 65:S89, 1986

177. Williams JP, McArthur JD, Walker WE et al: The cardiovascular effects of propofol in patients with impaired cardiac functions. Anesth Analg 65:S166, 1986

178. Dundee JW: Intravenous Anesthetic Agents. Chicago, Year Book Medical Publishers, 1979

179. Kawar P, Briggs LP, Bahar M et al: Liver enzyme studies with disoprofol (ICI 35 868) and midazolam. Anaesthesia 37:305, 1982

180. Wagner RL, White PF: Etomidate inhibits adrenocortical function in surgical patients. Anesthesiology 61:647, 1984

181. Fragen RJ, Weiss HW, Molteni A: The effect of propofol on adrenocortical steroidogenesis: A comparative study with etomidate and thiopental. Anesthesiology 66:839, 1987

182. Robertson WR, Reader SCJ, Davidson B et al: On the biopotency and site of action of drugs affecting endocrine tissues with specific reference to the antisteroidogenic effect of anesthetic agents. Postgrad Med J 61(suppl 3):145, 1985

183. Crozier TA, Beck D, Schlaeger M et al: Endocrinological changes following etomidate, midazolam or methohexital for minor surgery. Anesthesiology 66:628, 1987

184. Doenicke A, Lorenz W, Stenworth D et al: Effects of propofol 'Diprivan' on histamine release, immunoglobulin levels and activation of complement in healthy volunteers. Postgrad Med J 61(suppl 3):15, 1985

185. Doenicke A, Lorenz W, Beigl R: Histamine release after intravenous application of short-acting hypnotics. Br J Anaesth 45:1097, 1973

186. Westacott P, Ramachandran PR, Jancelewicz Z: Anaphylactic reaction to thiopentone: A case report. Can Anaesth Soc J 31:434, 1984

187. Clarke RSJ: Hypersensitivity Reactions. In Dundee JW (ed): Intravenous Anesthetic Agents, p 87. Chicago, Year Book Medical Publishers, 1979

188. Flowers CE, Rudolph AJ, Desmond MM: Diazepam (Valium) as an adjunct in obstetric analgesia. Obstet Gynecol 36:68, 1969

189. Camann W, Cohen MB, Ostheimer GW: Is midazolam desirable for sedation in parturients. Anesthesiology 65:441, 1986

190. Fragen RJ, Booij LHDJ, van der Pol F et al: Interactions of disopropyl phenol (ICI 35 868) with suxamethonium, vecuronium and pancuronium in vitro. Br J Anaesth 55:433, 1983

191. Driessen JJ, Vree TB, Booij LHDJ et al: Effect of some benzodiazepines on peripheral neuromuscular function in the rat in vitro hemidiaphragm preparation. J Pharm Pharmacol 36:244, 1984

192. Robertson EN, Fragen RJ, Booij LHDJ et al: Some effects of disopropyl phenol (ICI 35 868) on the pharmacodynamics of atracurium and vecuronium in anaesthetized man. Br J Anaesth 55:723, 1983

193. Nightingale P, Retts NV, Healy TN et al: Induction of anesthesia with propofol (Diprivan) or thiopentone and interaction with suxamethonium, atracurium and vecuronium. Postgrad Med J 61(suppl 3):31, 1985

194. Fragen RJ, Gahl F, Caldwell N: A water-soluble benzodiazepine Ro 21-3981, for induction of anesthesia. Anesthesiology 47:41, 1978

195. Berggren L, Erickson I: Midazolam for induction of anesthesia in outpatients. A comparison with thiopentone. Acta Anaesth Scand 25:492, 1981

196. Redfern N, Stafford MA, Hull CJ: Incremental propofol for short procedures. Br J Anaesth 57:1178, 1985

197. Hynynen M, Kortilla K, Tammisto T: Pain on I.V. injection of propofol (ICI 35868) in emulsion formulation. Acta Anaesth Scand 29:651, 1985

198. Stark RD, Binks, SM, Dutka VN et al: A review of the safety and tolerance of propofol ('Diprivan'). Postgrad Med J 61(suppl 3):152, 1985

199. Thornton JA: Methohexitone and its application in dental anaesthesia. Br J Anaesth 42:255, 1970

200. Mackenzie N, Grant IS: Comparison of propofol with methohexitone in the provision of anaesthesia for surgery under regional block. Br J Anaesth 57:1167, 1985

201. Doze VA, Westphal LM, White PF: Comparison of propofol with methohexital for outpatient anesthesia. Anesth Analg 65:1189, 1986

202. Mackenzie N, Grant IS: Propofol for intravenous sedation. Anaesthesia 42:3, 1987

203. Vinik HR, Shaw B, MacKrell T et al: A comparative evaluation of propofol for the induction and maintenance of general anesthesia. Anesth Analg 66:S189, 1987

204. Aldrete JA, McDonald JS: Low dose ketamine-diazepam prevents adverse reactions. In Aldrete JA, Stanley TH (eds): Trends in Intravenous Anesthesia, p 331. Chicago, Year Book Medical Publishers, 1980

205. Silvay G, Weinrich AI, Lumb P et al: Continuous infusion of ketamine for thoracic surgery using one-lung ventilation. In Aldrete JD, Stanley TH (eds): Trends in Intravenous Anesthesia, p 355. Chicago, Year Book Medical Publishers, 1980

206. Reves JG, Vinik R, Hirschfield AM et al: Midazolam compared with thiopentone as a hypnotic component in balanced anaesthesia: A randomized double-blind study. Can Anaesth Soc J 26:42, 1979

207. Crawford ME, Carl P, Andersen RS et al: Comparison between midazolam and thiopentone-based balanced anaesthesia for day care surgery. Br J Anaesth 56:165, 1984

208. Booker PD, Beechey A, Lloyd-Thomas AR: Sedation of children requiring artificial ventilation using an infusion of midazolam. Br J Anaesth 58:1104, 1986

209. Lloyd-Thomas AR, Booker PD: Infusions of midazolam in

paediatric patients after cardiac surgery. Br J Anaesth 58:1109, 1986

210. Grounds RM, Lalor JM, Lumley J et al: Propofol infusion for sedation in the intensive care unit: Preliminary report. Br Med J 294: 397, 1987

211. Rita L, Seleny FL, Mazurek A et al: Intramuscular midazolam for pediatric preanesthetic sedation: A double-blind controlled study with morphine. Anesthesiology 63:528, 1985

212. Bello CN, Mathias L, Torres MA et al: Evaluation of the effects of Ro 15-1788 in clinical anesthesia. Anesth Analg 66:S11, 1987

213. Kirkegaard I, Knudsen I, Jensen S et al: Benzodiazepine antagonist Ro 15-1788. Antagonism of diazepam sedation in outpatients undergoing gastroscopy. Anaesthesia 41:1184, 1986

214. Freye E, Fournell A: The benzodiazepine antagonist Ro 15-1788 reverses midazolam-induced EEG changes postoperatively. Anesth Analg 66:S60, 1987

215. Klotz U, Ziegler G, Ludwig L et al: Pharmacodynamic interaction between midazolam and a specific benzodiazepine antagonist in humans. J Clin Pharmacol 25:400, 1985

216. Caldwell CB, Gross JB: Physostigmine reversal of midazolam-induced sedation. Anesthesiology 57:125, 1982

217. Kanto J, Aaltonen L, Himberg JJ et al: Midazolam as an intravenous induction agent in the elderly: A clinical and pharmacokinetic study. Anesth Analg 65:15, 1986

218. Stoelting RK, Dierdorf SF (eds): Anesthesia and Co-existing Disease. New York, Churchill Livingstone, 1983

219. Fragen RJ, Caldwell NJ: Comparison of a new formulation of etomidate with thiopental—side effects and awakening times. Anesthesiology 50:242, 1979

220. Vinik R, Shaw B, Harris C et al: Randomized evaluation of induction and recovery from anesthesia with diprivan or thiopental sodium. Anesth Analg 65:S162, 1986

221. Jessup E, Grounds RM, Morgan M et al: Comparison of infusions of propofol and methohexitone to provide light general anaesthesia during surgery with regional block. Br J Anaesth 57:1173, 1985

222. Milligan KR, Howe JP, O'Toole DP et al: Outpatient anesthesia: Recovery after propofol, methohexital and thiopental. Anesth Analg 66:S118, 1987

223. Mackenzie N, Grant IS: Comparison of the new emulsion formulation of propofol with methohexitone and thiopentone for induction of anaesthesia in day cases. Br J Anaesth 57:725, 1985

224. Reitan JA, Porter W, Braunstein M: Comparison of psychomotor skills and amnesia after induction with midazolam or thiopental. Anesth Analg 65:933, 1986

225. Fragen RJ, Caldwell NJ: Awakening characteristics following anesthesia induction with midazolam for short surgical procedures. Arzneimittelforsch (Drug Res) 31:2261, 1981

226. Connor JT, Katz RL, Pagano RR et al: RO 21-3981 for intravenous surgical premedication and induction of anesthesia. Anesth Analg 57:1, 1978

227. Muir JJ, Warner MA, Offord KP et al: Role of nitrous oxide and other factors in postoperative nausea and vomiting: A randomized and blinded prospective study. Anesthesiology 66:513, 1987

228. Dohi S, Naito H: Intraarterial injection of 2.5% thiamylal does cause gangrene. Anesthesiology 59:154, 1983

229. Halsey MJ: Drug interactions in anaesthesia. Br J Anaesth 59:112, 1987

230. Smith NJ, Corbascio AN: Drug Interactions in Anesthesia. Philadelphia, Lea & Febiger, 1986

231. Gibb D: Drug interactions in anaesthesia. Clinics in Anaesthesiology 2:485, 1984

232. Greenblatt DJ, Shader RI: Pharmacokinetics in Clinical Practice. Philadelphia, WB Saunders, 1985

233. Prescott LF: Clinically important drug interactions. In Avery GS (ed): Drug Treatment, Principles and Practice of Clinical Pharmacology and Therapeutics, p 236. New York, Adis Press, 1980

234. Soni N: Mechanisms of drug interactions. In Feldman SA, Scurr CF, Paton W (eds): Drugs in Anesthesia: Mechanisms of Action, p 408. Baltimore, Edward Arnold, 1987

235. Halsey MJ: Adverse effects of drugs used in anesthesia. Br J Anaesth 59:1, 1987

236. Clarke RSJ, Dundee JW: Adverse reactions to intravenous induction agents. In Thornton JE (ed): Adverse Reactions to Anaesthetic Drugs, p 29. New York, Excerpta Medica/Elsevier, 1981

237. Whitwam JG: Intravenous induction agents. Clinics in Anesthesiology 2:515, 1984

238. Sear JW: Toxicity of I.V. anaesthetics. Br J Anaesth 59:24, 1987

Chapter 9

Michael R. Murphy

Opioids

The term *opioids*, as it is presently used, is an all inclusive term that distinguishes those drugs, natural or synthetic, that have morphine-like qualities as well as drugs that bind at morphine receptor sites.[1] The term is even applied to the sites themselves. Therefore, the term *opioid* may refer to drugs that are agonists (*e.g.*, morphine, fentanyl), agonist–antagonists (*e.g.*, butorphanol, nalorphine), antagonists (*e.g.*, naloxone), or the receptor sites for these drugs in the body. (Fig. 9-1). The term *opiate* is often used interchangeably with *opioid*, but historically *opiate* designates drugs derived from opium (*e.g.*, morphine, codeine). The term *narcotic* often refers to opioids. However, this term is actually nonspecific, having been derived from the Greek word for stupor and describes any drug that produces sleep. Today *narcotics* may be used to describe any number of drugs that are used illegally, whether or not they possess true opioid characteristics.

HISTORY

Opium comes from the milky exudate of the unripe seed capsule of the poppy (*Papaver somniferum*), and the term is a derivative of the Greek word for juice. Although the psychological effects of opium apparently were known as far back as the ancient Sumerians, the first known recorded reference to poppy juice was Theophrastus in the 3rd century, B.C.[1] Opium is comprised of more than 20 distinct alkaloids. It was not until 1806 that Surturner isolated one of these alkaloids, morphine, which he named for the Greek god of dreams, Morpheus. Further alkaloids, including codeine (Robiquet, 1832) and papaverine (Merck, 1848), were derived from opium over the next several years.

The syringe was invented by Rynd (1845) and Pravaz (1853), and the hollow needle by Wood (1855), opening the door for the use of parenteral morphine. Claude Bernard used morphine as a premedication in 1869. By 1900, morphine, 2 mg·kg^{-1}, plus scopolamine, 1 to 3 mg, was described by Schneiderlein for surgical anesthesia. Despite the patients' lack of recall of the surgical events, these episodes predated the use of muscle relaxants or controlled ventilation, necessitating the restraint of the patients during the procedure. Furthermore, a number of the patients died postoperatively, probably secondary to respiratory depression.[2-4] Opioids fell into disfavor following these deaths.

In 1938, the first synthetic opioid, meperidine, was introduced by Eisleb and Schaumann.[1] In 1947, Neff *et al* reported that "Nitrous oxide and oxygen, plus intravenous (iv) Demerol, plus curarization, afford good anesthesia and excellent muscular relaxation."[5] Nitrous oxide plus various opioids became popular. In 1958, Bailey *et al* reported anesthesia for cardiac surgery with meperidine and oxygen alone following induction with thiopental.[6] High-dose morphine (0.5 to 1.0 mg·kg^{-1})and 100% oxygen became popular following a report by Lowenstein and coworkers in 1969.[7] Despite the relative stability of the patients in this study, a number of patients in subsequent uses of this technique were deemed to have inadequate depth of anesthesia. Stanley *et al*, in an effort to overcome the problem of inadequate anesthesia, increased the morphine dose to 8 to 11 mg·kg^{-1} but encountered unacceptable side-effects, including increased fluid requirements and generalized edema.[8]

Whereas the continued search for more efficacious opioids for anesthesia has resulted in the introduction of a number of new synthetic agonists (the fentanyl family) in the last 20

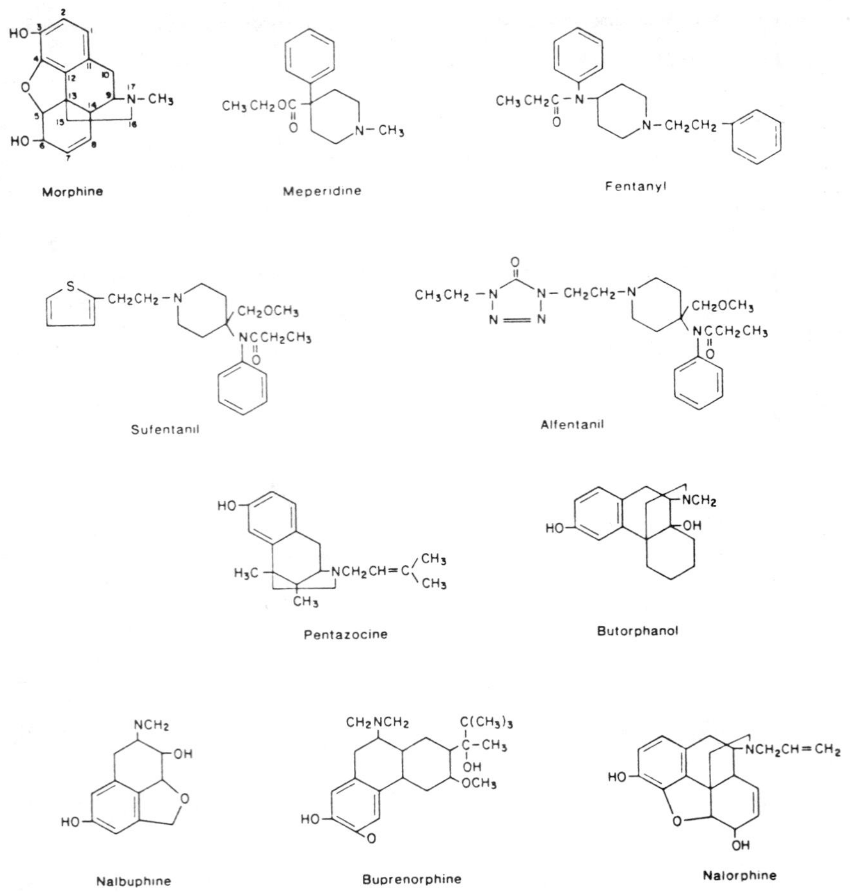

FIG. 9-1. Chemical structures of opioid agonists (morphine, meperidine, fentanyl, sufentanil, alfentanil) and opioid agonist–antagonists (pentazocine, butorphanol, nalbuphine, buprenorphine and nalorphine.)

years, the earlier search for a potent, nonaddicting analgesic produced an n-allyl derivative of morphine, nalorphine. Nalorphine antagonized the effects of morphine, precipitated acute abstinence in addicts, and, importantly, also had analgesic actions.[1, 9] This discovery led to the development of other agonist–antagonist compounds (e.g., pentazocine, butorphanol) and the relatively pure antagonist naloxone.

PHARMACOLOGY

RECEPTORS AND ENDOGENOUS OPIOID PEPTIDES

The importance of the mixed actions of nalorphine was not so much its clinical usefulness as the fact that it increased the evidence for and aided the search for opioid receptors in the body. It was known that morphine-like drugs were structurally similar and exhibited stereospecificity, which suggested opioid receptor sites on the surface of or within cells. When it was demonstrated that the opioid antagonist nalorphine also had analgesic (agonist) properties, the homogenous receptor theory was replaced by a heterogenous receptor theory, originally proposing two receptors and eventually several.[10–14]

Martin et al identified three distinct opioid receptors.[1, 12] Morphine and morphine-like drugs interact with the morphine or mu receptor to produce supraspinal analgesia, respi-

ratory depression, indifference to environmental stimuli, bradycardia, miosis, hypothermia, physical dependence, and tolerance (Table 9-1). Ketacyclazocine is the prototype agonist for the kappa receptors, which are characterized by spinal analgesia, miosis, and sedation. The sigma receptors mediate dysphoric effects, hallucinations, tachypnea, tachycardia, and mydriasis; the typical agonist is N-allylnormetazocine (SKF–10,047). A delta and an epsilon receptor have been proposed to explain the relative potencies of opioid peptides and drugs to inhibit contraction of the isolated guinea pig ileum and mouse vas deferens.[13, 14] More recently, the mu receptor has been subdivided. Analgesia has been associated with the mu_1 but not with the mu_2 receptor, whereas respiratory depression is probably mediated by mu_2 or delta receptors but not by mu_1.[1, 15–17] The possibility of separating analgesia from respiratory depression apparently exists.

The realization of specific receptors in the mammalian central nervous system (CNS) and nerve plexi of intestines for chemicals derived from plants, started a search for endogenous opioid receptor ligands. A number of opioid peptides have been identified. A review by Akil et al divides these into three opioid peptide families according to precursor.[18] The precursor for the first family is beta-endorphin/ACTH (also known as Proopiomelanocortin, or POMC). These peptides are primarily produced in the pituitary. The second group is from the enkephalin precursor (known as proenkephalin or proenkephalin A). These peptides include [Met]enkaphalin and [Leu]enkephalin, and their opioid neuronal pathways

TABLE 9-1. Interactions of Morphine and Morphine-like Drugs With Opioid Receptors

	RECEPTOR TYPES		
	μ	κ	σ
Effects	Supraspinal analgesia	Spinal analgesia	Dysphoria
	Respiratory depression	Respiratory depression	Hallucinations
	Euphoria	Sedation	Vasomotor stimulation
	Physical dependence	Miosis	
Drugs			
Morphine	Ag	Ag	0
Buprenorphine	pAg	—	0
Nalorphine	Ant	pAg	Ag
Pantazocine	Ant	Ag	Ag
Butorphanol	0	Ag	Ag
Nalbuphine	pAg/Ant	Ag	Ag
Naloxone	Ant	Ant	Ant

Abbreviations: Ag, agonist; pAg, partial agonist; Ant, antagonist; 0, no interaction. (Used with permission from Hug CC Jr: Seminars in Anesthesia 1:14, 1982.)

include endocrine and CNS distributions. The enkephalins are also found in the adrenal medulla, gastrointestinal tract, and other structures; in the CNS, they are widely spread from cells in the cortex to cells in the spinal cord. The most recently described dynorphin/neo-endorphin precursor (also known as prodynorphin or proenkephalin B) family is found primarily in gut, posterior pituitary, and brain.

The location of the opioid receptors and the endogenous ligands are related to their functions. For instance, those receptors and peptides involved in mediating analgesia are found in greater density in areas of the brain and spinal cord involved with pain sensation. The significance of a number of peptides, their locations, and the sites of the opioid receptors are not clearly understood. Continuing studies will provide answers to many questions and further explain the mechanism of actions of opioid drugs.

CENTRAL NERVOUS SYSTEM EFFECTS

Discussion of the CNS effects of opioids will focus on analgesia, drowsiness–consciousness, mood alteration, electroencephalographic (EEG) changes, and emetic effects. Other effects with a CNS component such as respiratory depression, cardiovascular responses, and endocrine responses will be addressed later.

Analgesia is generally the primary reason that the opioids are given. The analgesia produced is a complex effect with components of suppression of transmission of noxious stimulation, reflex depression of afferent stimuli, and altered mental responses. There is minimal evidence of peripheral nervous system involvement in the analgesia produced by the opioids, but most of the effects are mediated by the receptors found in the spinal cord and brain.[19] The analgesia is unlike that produced by local anesthetic agents, which may block all sensation and motor ability by blocking neuronal transmission. The opioids are more selective for painful stimuli, leaving other sensory and motor modalities intact. A patient may be aware of the stimulus but may describe it as less or not painful at all.

Several areas (tracts/laminae) of the spinal cord are known to contain opioid receptors. The substantia gelatinosa, which serves as the main termination of the small afferent nerve fibers thought to be involved with pain, has the highest concentration of opioid receptors in the spinal cord.[19] The trans-

mission of noxious stimuli is suppressed when the spinal cord opioid receptors are activated. Opioids applied locally by intrathecal or epidural techniques diminish pain.

Analgesia results when nociceptive stimuli to higher centers of the brain are depressed in the spinal cord. However, there are many supraspinal opioid receptor sites that act to modulate the sensory input from the spinal cord by descending neuronal pathways, and it has been suggested that the primary sites of analgesic actions of opioids are supraspinal. For instance, focal stimulation of the periaqueductal gray area of the midbrain will produce profound analgesia similar to that seen after the injection of large doses of morphine; naloxone will reverse both the focal stimulation or morphine-induced analgesia.[19] The actual mechanisms involved in opioid analgesia are complex and involve the modulation of painful stimuli by an intricate system of receptors in both afferent and efferent neuronal pathways.

Opioids are mood-altering drugs. Patients in distress report diminished pain, feelings of warmth and well-being, drowsiness, and, occasionally, euphoria. In normal, pain-free persons, the experience may not be pleasant but may produce feelings of lethargy and mental clouding. Alterations in mood and perception of surroundings are apparently mediated through the limbic system.[1, 19]

Morphine-like drugs may produce drowsiness or sleep in some patients (especially the old or very ill), but, even at very high doses, unconsciousness is not ensured. Occasionally, in patients in whom "anesthetic" doses of opioids have induced sleep, arousal may be elicited by noxious stimulation.[20] Morphine-like drugs do not produce amnesia without unconsciousness; the risk of awareness during surgery is present unless other CNS depressant drugs (e.g., nitrous oxide, scopolamine, barbiturates, benzodiazepines) are combined with the opioid as part of the anesthetic or preoperative medications.[21, 22]

Constriction of the pupils (miosis) is produced by morphine and most mu and kappa opioid agonists in humans, presumably by an excitatory action on the autonomic segment of the nucleus of the oculomotor nerve.[1] The constriction is probably dose related and considered "pathognomonic" of opioid toxicity but may be altered by other factors such as other drugs or asphyxia.

Opioids depress the cough reflex in part by a direct effect on the cough center in the medulla.[1] This suppression decreases the incidence and severity of cardiovascular stimulation with intubation of the trachea and improves tolerance of an endotracheal tube in ventilated patients.[23]

All the opioid analgesics in sufficient dosage will produce excitatory or convulsive activity in lower animals and probably humans. There are considerable interspecies differences in the dosage required to produce seizures.[1, 24, 25] In humans, clinically useful, high doses of commonly used opioids producing profound analgesia ("anesthesia") do not produce seizures. Myoclonic and myotonic seizure-like movements reported in the literature are produced with no evidence of cortical seizure activity on the EEG. The exception to this is meperidine. Very large doses of meperidine (>5 mg $\cdot$ kg^{-1}) may induce excitation and seizures. Meperidine is biotransformed to normeperidine, which is a potent CNS stimulant responsible for the excitatory symptoms.[1]

Opioids produce nausea and vomiting by stimulating the chemoreceptor trigger zone for emesis in the area postrema of the medulla.[1] The emetic effects are more common in ambulatory than in recumbent patients, suggesting a vestibular component. Morphine-like drugs have been shown to increase vestibular sensitivity. All clinically useful opioids will produce nausea and vomiting, and, at equianalgesic doses, the incidence is not significantly lower than that of morphine. Opioids also depress the vomiting center, and higher plasma concentrations of opioids may overcome the chemoreceptor trigger zone (CTZ) stimulating effect. Nausea is less common with higher "anesthetic" doses or subsequent doses following an initial therapeutic dose.

CARDIOVASCULAR EFFECTS

The relative stability of cardiovascular and myocardial responses found when high doses of morphine are used as the primary anesthetic lead to the increased use of the opioids in patients in whom the cardiovascular depression produced by the potent inhalational agents is particularly detrimental.[7] However, there are cardiovascular changes produced by the opioids. Opioids produce a dose-dependent bradycardia, probably by stimulation of the vagal nucleus in the medulla.[26, 27] Since the resultant bradycardia is mediated by the vagus nerve, it can be attenuated or blocked by atropine.[28] Experimentally, morphine has a direct effect on the sinoatrial node, but, with clinically useful doses, no effect on the sinoatrial node is seen.[29, 30] Although bradycardia is the usual effect of opioids, large iv doses of meperidine and its congener alphaprodine have been associated with tachycardia, presumably related to their atropine-like structure.

Sufficiently large doses of all opioids will produce direct depression of the myocardium.[23, 31, 32] However, the concentrations of opioids necessary to produce depression are hundreds to thousands of times greater than the peak plasma concentrations found clinically, even after very large "anesthetic" doses of opioid drugs. Except for meperidine, the opioids do not directly depress myocardial contractility at clinically useful doses. At doses as low as 2 to 2.5 mg $\cdot$ kg^{-1}, meperidine may produce decreases in cardiac output and arterial pressure secondary to a significant negative ionotropic effect.[32, 33] The use of meperidine as a primary anesthetic is limited.

The usual effect of morphine on the peripheral vasculature is arteriolar and venous dilation. Morphine is reported to have a direct action on vascular smooth muscle and to selectively block the venous vascular response to alpha-adrenergic stimulation; however, the primary mechanism for vasodilation is

apparently histamine release (Fig. 9-2).[34-36] Meperidine and codeine also evoke the release of histamine, whereas fentanyl and sufentanil do not.[36, 37]

VENTILATORY EFFECTS

All the agonist opioids produce a dose-dependent respiratory depression. It is likely that equianalgesic concentrations of the various available agonists produce equivalent respiratory depression. The differences occasionally noted by clinical observation generally have to do with the pharmacokinetics and pharmacodynamics of the different drugs as well as their relative potencies. The peak ventilatory effect of fentanyl injected iv will be within 5 to 10 minutes, whereas that of morphine may be as late as 30 to 60 minutes and therefore not as obvious to someone who has injected the morphine but may no longer be observing the patient as carefully.[38-40] Furthermore, it is difficult to compare relative potencies of drugs that have radically different pharmacokinetic and pharmacodynamic timetables.

Codeine is an opioid commonly used in place of morphine because it is alleged to produce less respiratory depression

FIG. 9-2. Intravenous administration of morphine, but not fentanyl, evokes declines in blood pressure (*BP*) and systemic vascular resistance (*SVR*) that parallel increases in the serum concentration of histamine (Mean $\pm$ SE; *$P < 0.05$; **$P < 0.005$). (Reprinted with permission from Rosow CE, Moss I, Philbin DM *et al*: Histamine release during morphine and fentanyl anesthesia. Anesthesiology 56:93, 1982.)

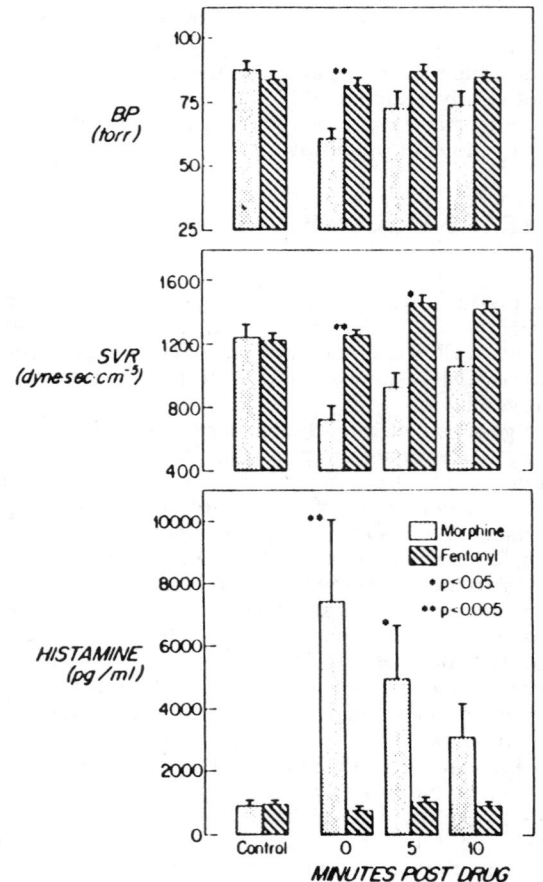

than morphine. Unfortunately, at the doses used, it also does not produce as much analgesia as morphine. In the same context, fentanyl is more acceptable as an intraoperative opioid because it does not produce as much (prolonged) respiratory depression postoperatively. Again, this is purely a kinetic-dynamic phenomenon related to the duration of action of fentanyl and morphine in the doses used.

Opioids decrease the response of the respiratory centers in the brain stem to increases in CO_2. In normal subjects, when ventilatory response to increasing CO_2 is plotted with CO_2 on the abscissa of the graph, there is a relatively steep response (Fig. 9-3). When opioids are added in the awake subject, the response is shifted (displaced) to the right, but the slope of the line is not significantly changed.[41] The respiratory centers are reset for a higher CO_2 threshold, but the sensitivity of the centers is not changed. If the subject goes to sleep, the line is shifted further to the right, and the slope of the response line is also depressed.[42] Much greater depression of ventilation is produced with loss of consciousness.

Lower doses of opioids tend to decrease breathing rate while maintaining tidal volume. As the dose is increased, tidal volume as well as breathing rate usually decreases. Irregular or periodic breathing may be induced as the pontine and medullary centers, which regulate rhythmicity of respiration, are depressed.[1] Large enough doses may produce apnea even in an awake subject; however, the subject can still breathe on command or if he makes his own conscious effort.

Other CNS depressant drugs such as the potent inhaled anesthetics, barbiturates, sedative-hypnotics, and alcohol, as well as sleep, will increase the respiratory depressant action of the opioids. Pain, on the other hand, is a natural antagonist to the respiratory depressant action of opioids. Again, pain/analgesia and breathing are intertwined.

It has been suggested that depression of ventilation may outlast the analgesic properties of the opioids. This assumption is probably not true and is most likely related to the mechanisms of measurement as well as the effects of other CNS depressant drugs and sleep. Furthermore, a biphasic depression of ventilation has been proposed for fentanyl and possibly meperidine (Fig. 9-4).[43, 44] The biphasic response noted in the study by Becker and colleagues in surgical patients is most likely related to exogenous stimuli (or the lack thereof) in the postoperative period rather than to any inherent drug action or pharmacokinetic phenomenon.[38]

Older patients have lower dose requirements for depressants in general, and this includes the opioids. The increased sensitivity of older patients is probably related to pharmacokinetics.

HEPATORENAL AND GASTROINTESTINAL EFFECTS

The renal effects of opioids have been somewhat confusing because of the multitude of factors involved in urine formation.[45] Early animal experiments demonstrated a release of antidiuretic hormone (ADH) by opioids. Studies in humans suggested that opioids do not release ADH but that surgical stimulation does. In fact, higher doses of opioids may tend to decrease the stress-related release of ADH.

A decrease in glomerular filtration rate (GFR) with a subsequent decrease in urine output has been noted with opioids. However, if cardiovascular dynamics are unchanged, morphine does not decrease GFR, urine osmolarity, or urine output. When nitrous oxide is added as an anesthetic agent, significant decreases in GFR (40%–60%) and urine output are

FIG. 9-3. Respiratory response curves obtained before and 1 hour after 10 mg morphine sulfate was administered intramuscularly. The end-expiratory P_{CO_2} is plotted against the alveolar ventilation. (Used with permission of Bellville JW, Seed JC: The effect of drugs on the respiratory response to carbon dioxide. Anesthesiology 21: 727, 1960.)

FIG. 9-4. Carbon dioxide response slopes as percentages of control slope at the time of the last dose of fentanyl or Innovar (time = 0) and subsequently. Recurrence of depression of ventilation (flattest postoperative) corresponds to a time when external stimulation was reduced (Mean ± SE). (Reprinted with permission from Becker L, Paulson B, Miller R et al: Biphasic respiratory depression after fentanyl-droperidol or fentanyl alone used to supplement nitrous oxide anesthesia. Anesthesiology 44:291, 1976.)

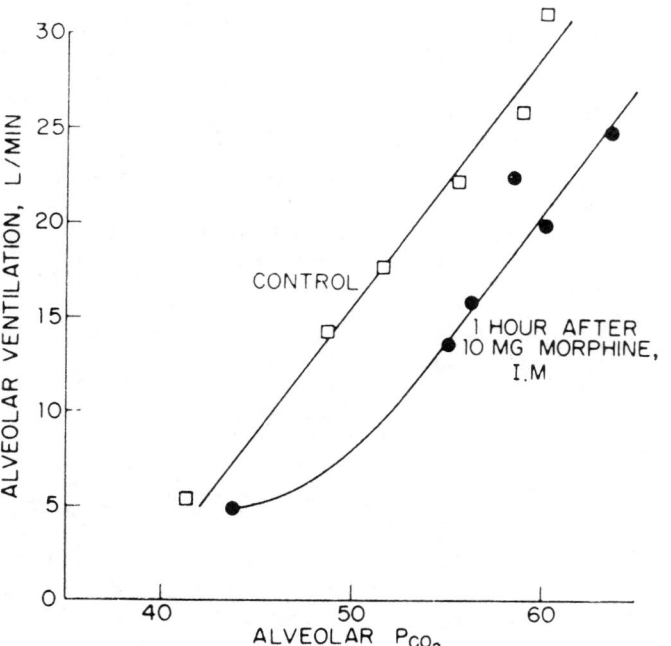

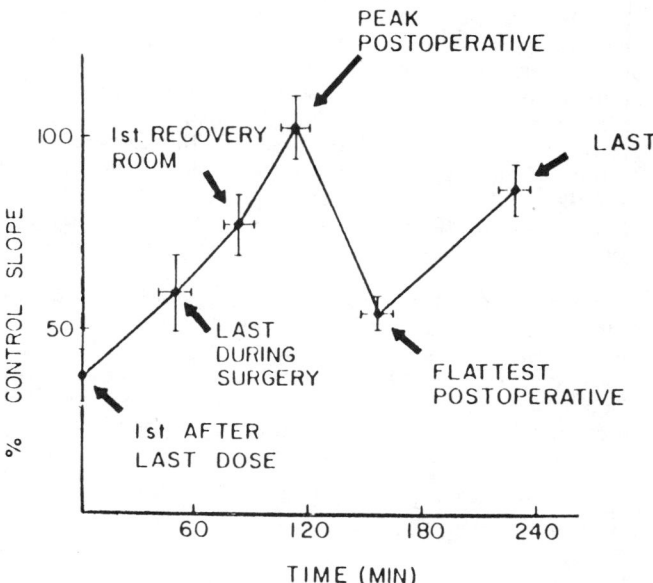

seen, even with minimal alterations in systolic and diastolic blood pressure.[45]

The diminution of urine output associated with opioids is probably not a result of direct opioid effects, but, rather surgical stresses that increase pituitary ADH secretion or alter renal hemodynamics as a result of sympathetic stimulation and vasoconstriction. It should also be noted that opioids increase ureteral and detrusor muscle tone, which may result in urinary retention requiring catheterization or reversal with naloxone.

There is no substantial evidence that the opioids themselves produce direct liver dysfunction in humans. However, morphine can produce symptoms of biliary colic owing to spasm of the sphincter of Oddi and the resulting rise of pressure in the biliary tract. Other agonist and agonist–antagonist opioids have also been implicated in sphincter pressure changes, and all probably obstruct flow through the ampulla.[46] Clinical manifestation of the spasm is inconsistent. In surgical patients requiring cholangiography, opioid-induced obstruction can result in unnecessary exploration of the common bile duct.[46] These situations may require reversal of the spasm. Reversal can be consistently accomplished with naloxone, but naloxone will also reverse beneficial opioid effects. Other drugs that have been suggested to reverse the biliary spasm include nitroglycerin, glucagon, and atropine. The effect of these drugs is considerably less reliable.

Occasionally, in awake patients, the epigastric distress associated with biliary colic may mimic angina peotoris. In these patients, a differentiation must be made. If naloxone reverses the pain, it is probably biliary colic; if the pain increases or remains the same, it may be angina. Nitroglycerin may relieve both angina and colic and, therefore, may not be helpful in differentiation. Electrocardiographic changes usually indicate angina. The treatment of angina may include repeated doses of opioids, whereas this approach would accentuate biliary colic.

The antidiarrheal effects of opium were used centuries before its analgesic effects were appreciated. Opioids decrease the motility of the gastrointestinal tract. Decreased gastric motility coupled with increased tone of the antrum may slow passage of gastric contents through the duodenum for up to 12 hours following morphine and retard absorption of orally administered drugs.[1] The danger of pulmonary aspiration in patients having general anesthesia who have eaten since, or just prior to, a dose of opioid is obvious. Throughout the rest of the intestine, there is an increase in resting tone with periodic spasms but a decrease in propulsive activity. The decrease in propulsive activity in the large intestine leads to desiccation of the feces and constipation. The effects of opioids on the intestine appear to be both peripherally (locally) and centrally mediated.[1] A number of opioid receptors have been identified in the gut and are a source for the study of opioids. Central actions on the intestines have been shown to be mediated by the vagus.

Clinical observations suggest that meperidine, compared with other opioids, has a less intense spasmogenic effect on smooth muscle relative to its analgesic action. Meperidine tends to cause less constipation when given over prolonged periods of time. After equianalgesic doses, the increases in common bile duct pressures produced by meperidine are less than morphine but greater than codeine.[1]

ENDOCRINE EFFECTS

Opioids inhibit the release of the hypothalamic releasing factors, gonadotropin-releasing hormone (GnRH) and corticotropin-releasing factor (CRF), with the ultimate result of decreased plasma concentrations of luteinizing hormone (LH), follicle-stimulating hormone (FSH), adrenocorticotropic hormone (ACTH), beta-endorphin, testosterone, and cortisol. Concentrations of prolactin and growth hormone (GH) in plasma are increased by opioids, although they probably do not directly affect the release of ADH.[1, 45]

The stress of surgery or trauma results in metabolic changes in the body designed to repair the damage. Generally, there are increases in the plasma concentrations of a number of substances, including cortisol, ADH, GH, aldosterone, thyroid hormone, renin, glucose and the catecholamines (epinephrine and norepinephrine).[47] In recent years, it has been noted that higher doses of opioids used for surgical anesthesia (especially the fentanyl drugs) modify or block the metabolic stress response to surgery ("stress-free anesthesia"). Generally, high-dose fentanyl–family drugs plus oxygen will either decrease or not alter plasma concentrations of the catecholamines, cortisol, ADH, glucose, insulin, and GH while increasing prolactin concentrations. If patients in whom these agents are administered are further stressed by cardiopulmonary bypass, the opioids are unable to block the release of ADH, GH, glucose, and the catecholamines during or after bypass.[47, 48]

REPRODUCTIVE EFFECTS

The opioid agonist analgesics are generally considered to be nonteratogenic and are considered safe for use in women in early pregnancy. The placenta does not act as a barrier to opioid analgesics, and chronic or addictive use of opioids by the mother can addict her fetus/neonate. Neonates born of addicted mothers must be carefully observed and treated for signs of withdrawal.

Several different opioid agonist analgesics have been used for the pain of labor. Morphine was originally popularized in combination with scopolamine as "twilight sleep." The sedation and amnesia produced by scopolamine are less popular today, and the technique has fallen into disuse.[49] Morphine produces more neonatal depression than does meperidine.[1] Part of this depression is related to the pharmacokinetics of morphine (a long-acting drug) versus meperidine (a short-acting drug). One study noted that babies delivered between 1 and 6 hours after the mother was given morphine showed signs of narcosis, with a peak incidence of depression at approximately 3.5 hours following maternal administration.[50] Neonates appear to be more sensitive to morphine than do adults. This is probably related to increased permeability of the blood-brain barrier in the fetus/neonate. When morphine and meperidine directly administered are compared in the neonate, there is a greater shift of the ventilation–CO_2 response curve to the right with morphine than with meperidine.[49, 50] Morphine has also been implicated in the prolongation of labor.[1]

Meperidine is more popular than morphine as an analgesic during labor. Therapeutic doses given once labor is well established do not appear to delay delivery, significantly alter rhythmic uterine contractions, interfere with normal postpartum contraction or with involution of the uterus.[1, 49]

Meperidine can obviously produce neonatal depression. The degree of depression is related to the total dose and time interval between maternal administration and delivery. Greater concentrations of meperidine are achieved in the fetus following iv rather than intramuscular (im) administration to the mother owing to higher peak plasma concentrations in the mother with iv injection and the subsequent increased concentration gradient between the maternal and fetal blood. It has been suggested that meperidine doses of not more than 50 to 75 mg given im more than 3 hours before delivery, or 25 to 50 mg given iv more than 2 hours before delivery, coupled with a regional block for delivery, will ensure significant maternal pain relief with little or no detrimental neonatal effect.[49]

Some studies noting minor opioid depression of infants delivered within 1 hour of maternal administration of meperidine describe an increasing depression with time.[49, 50] This apparent contradiction has been attributed to the accumulation of meperidine metabolites, particularly normeperidine, in the fetus. The higher pK_a of the metabolites makes them more likely to be trapped in the more acidotic fetus. Normeperidine has a longer half-life and is possibly a more potent respiratory depressant than is meperidine in the fetus.

Alphaprodine (Nisentil) is less commonly used in obstetrics than in the past, when it was popular because of its good sedative properties and supposedly lower incidence of nausea and vomiting than meperidine.[49, 50] The onset of analgesia with alphaprodine is rapid, within 5 minutes following subcutaneous administration or 1 to 2 minutes after iv administration, and its duration of action is short (approximately 2 hours). Its propensity to cause apnea, even at therapeutic doses, has made alphaprodine less popular. (Respiratory depression is a dose-related response—smaller doses at more frequent intervals might be more useful.) Alphaprodine has also been associated with a decrease in fetal heart variability and a high incidence of sinusoidal fetal heart rate pattern.[50]

NEUROMUSCULAR JUNCTION AND SKELETAL MUSCLE EFFECTS

In clinical dosing, the opioids do not appear to have an effect on the neuromuscular junction of skeletal muscle or directly on skeletal muscle itself. However, all opioids given iv in high doses have the ability to produce rigidity of skeletal muscles, particularly in the chest and abdomen, but also in the extremities and jaw. Although rigidity is reported with morphine (2 $mg \cdot kg^{-1}$ plus nitrous oxide), it is more commonly seen with fentanyl and its analogs. Rigidity has been reported following iv doses of fentanyl as low as 80 to 200 μg (8% incidence) or with infusion rates as slow as 35 $\mu g \cdot min^{-1}$.[25] The incidence of rigidity following 8 $\mu g \cdot kg^{-1}$ of fentanyl given iv was 100% in one study. In patients pretreated with small doses of nondepolarizing relaxants, rigidity is usually noted at approximately 15 $\mu g \cdot kg^{-1}$ of fentanyl.[25] Sufentanil and alfentanil in comparable doses act like fentanyl. There are reports of recurrence both intra-and postoperatively with fentanyl and sufentanil.[25, 51]

The incidence and severity of rigidity may be increased by rapid infusion of the drug or the addition of nitrous oxide. Alternatively, the incidence and severity can be decreased by slower administration of opioids, deepening of anesthesia with potent inhalational agents or thiopental, or pretreatment with small doses of nondepolarizing muscle relaxants.[25] Jaffe and Ramsey reported a decreased incidence of rigidity in patients pretreated with metocurine (50 $\mu g \cdot kg^{-1}$) but not those pretreated with pancuronium (12.5 $\mu g \cdot kg^{-1}$) when compared with a nontreated group.[52] Other studies suggest that pancuronium is effective.

In severe cases, truncal rigidity may make ventilation of the patient's lungs difficult or impossible. Unconsciousness usually occurs before or with development of rigidity, but this is not always true. Severe rigidity may necessitate the use of a muscle relaxant to produce paralysis in an awake patient. Truncal rigidity can also create hemodynamic problems. If high airway pressures are used in an attempt to expand a rigid chest, the increased intrathoracic pressures may impede venous return and decrease cardiac output.

The mechanism of opioid-induced muscle rigidity is not clear. Even the site of the source of inability to ventilate the lungs has been called into question. Glottic rigidity and glottic closure as well as supraglottic airway obstruction have been described.[53, 54] The mechanism is not at the neuromuscular junction and probably not at the spinal cord level but most likely related to mμ receptors in the caudate nucleus.[25, 54]

TOXICOLOGY

In general, the opioid agonists are very safe drugs with high margins of safety. Coma, pinpoint pupils, and depression of ventilation suggest overdosage. In most cases of overdosage or poisoning with opioids, the common factor determining sequelae is depression of ventilation and hypoxia. If overdosage is noted early and breathing is maintained before hypoxic damage, patients will usually survive. Treatment is based on support of failing systems—ventilation, pulmonary edema, shock, tonic-clonic seizures. Initial treatment is support of respiration and iv doses of naloxone (0.2 to 0.4 mg, or 0.01 $mg \cdot kg^{-1}$ for children) repeated every 2 to 3 minutes until the patient is breathing and responsive or up to a total dose of about 10 mg. Doses of naloxone greater than 10 mg suggest an inaccurate diagnosis or a missed nonopioid drug overdose.[1]

Toxicologic studies in dogs using low to massive doses of differing opioids have resulted in several conclusions. There is an inverse relationship between analgesic potency and toxic activity.[24] Weak opioids (meperidine, piritramide) may produce cardiac depression, seizures, and metabolic acidosis in doses that would be considered "anesthetic." Medium potency drugs (morphine, phenoperidine, and alfentanil) given in high doses, much greater than clinically used "anesthetic" doses, and high potency drugs (fentanyl and sufentanil) given in massive doses produce cardiovascular hyperactivity, seizures, and metabolic acidosis. The less potent the drug, the more severe the toxic manifestation. The higher the potency, the less severe the toxicity and the higher the dose at which it appears. For the more potent opioids, the toxic dose may be thousands of times greater than high therapeutic doses.[24]

ALLERGIC REACTIONS

Allergic reactions to opioid analgesics are uncommon and usually consist of urticaria or skin rashes. Anaphylactoid reactions to codeine and morphine have been reported and have been suggested as a mechanism for sudden death in iv heroin users.[1] It is not uncommon to see flushing, urticaria, or wheals at the site of injection in patients given morphine or codeine, which are known histamine releasers.[1, 36] Meperidine, in a recent study, appears to be a more potent histamine releaser than morphine.[37] More potent opioids, fentanyl and sufentanil, do not release histamine.[36, 37]

PHARMACOKINETICS AND PHARMACODYNAMICS

Pharmacokinetics is the study of drug disposition in the body and includes the processes of absorption, distribution, biotransformation, and excretion (Table 9-2). Pharmacokinetic

TABLE 9-2. Pharmacokinetics of Opioid Agonists

	RAPID DISTRIBUTION HALF-TIME (min)	SLOW DISTRIBUTION HALF-TIME (min)	ELIMINATION HALF-TIME (hr)	VOLUME OF DISTRIBUTION $(l \cdot kg^{-1})$	CLEARANCE $(ml \cdot kg^{-1} \cdot min^{-1})$	PROTEIN BINDING (%)	pK_a
Morphine	1.2–2.5	9–13.3	1.7–2.2	3.2–3.4	15–23	26–36	7.93
Meperidine	4–17		3.2–4.1	2.8–4.2	10–17	64–82	8.5
Fentanyl	1.4–1.7	13–28	3.1–4.4	3.2–5.9	11–21	79–87	8.43
Sufentanil	1.4	17.7	2.7	2.86	13	92.5	8.01
Alfentanil	1–3.5	8.2–16.8	1.2–1.7	0.5–1	5–7.9	89–92	6.5

data are usually derived from measurement of concentrations of a drug in plasma. Opioids have no effect in plasma but have sites of action called receptors in certain specified tissues. It is the combination of the drug with its receptors that initiates an effect.

$$\text{drug} + \text{receptor} \leftrightarrows \text{drug–receptor complex} \approx \text{effect}$$

The intensity of the effect is the result of the number of receptors occupied by the opioid. The drug–receptor interaction is reversible, and the effect may be increased or decreased by increasing or decreasing the receptor occupancy. The concentration of the drug at the receptor is more imporant than the concentration of the drug in plasma, but direct measurement of the concentration at the receptor is difficult or impossible in an intact patient or animal. Since plasma is the vehicle of transport of drugs to and from their sites of action, storage, biotransformation, and excretion, the concentration of drug in the plasma is generally proportional to (but not necessarily equal to) the concentration at these sites. Factors that influence the concentration of opioids in plasma will affect their concentration at the receptors.

With iv administration of a drug, there is no delay from absorption. Peak concentrations in plasma occur almost immediately following bolus administration of opioids and then decrease rapidly as the drug is distributed to tissues of action, storage, biotransformation, or excretion. The onset and duration of action is related to the rise and fall of the number of action receptors occupied. The uptake of the drug by a tissue is determined by its rate of delivery and the capacity of the tissue to accumulate the drug. Rate of delivery is primarily determined by blood flow, the concentration gradient between plasma and the tissue, and the permeability coefficient of the drug. For an opioid to reach a tissue, it must cross a biological membrane, generally by dissolution and diffusion in the lipoprotein matrix of the membrane. For opioid drugs, the most important physiochemical properties that influence the rate of diffusion across biological membranes (the permeability coefficient) are molecular size, ionization, and lipid solubility. Opioids are all relatively small molecules, and permeability is not significantly limited by size. Ionization is important, because non-ionized drugs cross membranes more readily. The lower the pK_a of the opioid, the greater the percentage of the drug that will be non-ionized at a particular pH (generally 7.4 in plasma) and the greater percentage of the drug available to cross membranes. Due to the lipoprotein matrix of biological membranes, the more lipid soluble a drug, the faster it crosses.

The capacity of a tissue is determined by the affinity of the drug for the particular tissue (the tissue–plasma partition

upon drug binding, dissolution, active transport into the tissue, and pH-dependent partitioning of the drug between plasma and the tissue.

The concentration of the opioid in plasma is determined by its distribution and redistribution to its sites of action (receptors), storage (inactive sites), and tissues or organs of elimination. Elimination is the result of biotransformation and/or excretion. For the opioids, biotransformation is primarily in the liver. Biotransformation of the opioids is usually to an inactive metabolite or to a metabolite with considerably less activity than the parent drug. The most important exception to the rule is meperidine, which biotransforms in part to normeperidine, a drug with considerable activity. Biotransformation of the opioids usually facilitates excretion of the drug from the body at one or more sites—generally the kidneys.

MORPHINE

When morphine is administered iv, the decrease in the plasma concentration can be described by a biexponential or triexponential equation. Following an iv dose of 0.05 to 0.2 $mg \cdot kg^{-1}$, there is an initial rapid distribution of the drug to tissues and organs. By 10 minutes, 96%–98% of the drug is cleared from plasma.[55] The initial rapid distribution phase has a half-time of 1.2 to 2.5 minutes in adults and children 1 to 15 years of age.[55–58] In those studies demonstrating triexponential curves, the slower distribution half-time is also relatively short (9 to 13.3 min). A morphine dose of approximately 1.0 $mg \cdot kg^{-1}$, given at a rate of 5.0 $mg.min^{-1}$ to elderly adult males, resulted in similar values of 1.3 and 19.8 minutes for the rapid and slow distribution phases.[56] The half-time of the terminal elimination phase for morphine using analytical methods specific for unchanged morphine is 1.7 to 2.2 hours.[55, 57] Other studies have reported terminal elimination half-times as high as 2.9 to 4.5 hours.[56] The discrepancies among the studies are probably related to the employment of radioimmunoassay antibodies in the latter studies, which cross-react with morphine metabolites. This cross-reactivity will result in falsely high estimates of the concentration of morphine (especially at the later times when the concentration of metabolites is higher) and produce exaggerated elimination half-times.

Estimates of the volume of distribution for analgesic doses of morphine (0.05 to 0.2 $mg \cdot kg^{-1}$) administered iv in adults are 3.2 to 3.4 $l \cdot kg^{-1}$.[55, 56, 58] Whereas the volume of distribution for analgesic doses in children 1 to 15 years of age is 1.2 $l \cdot kg^{-1}$, the estimated volume of distribution in elderly adults is 4.7 $l \cdot kg^{-1}$.[56, 57] The variabilities noted may be the result of many factors, including age, physical status, and anesthetic and surgical conditions. Nonetheless, the volume of distribution of morphine is relatively large, suggesting extensive tissue uptake. Since morphine is somewhat lipid insoluble, the sequestration is most probably in non–fat tissues, with skeletal muscle containing the greater fraction because of its mass.

The clearance of morphine from the body is primarily the result of hepatic metabolism to morphine–glucuronide and other minor metabolites that are ultimately removed by the kidneys (Fig. 9-5). Less than 15% of a morphine dose is eliminated unchanged in the urine.[59, 60] The clearance of morphine (15 to 23 ml·kg⁻¹·min⁻¹) is very high (approaching hepatic blood flow), indicating a high hepatic extraction ratio.[55, 56] Because extraction of morphine from plasma is relatively complete, the elimination of morphine is dependent upon blood flow to the liver and the re-uptake of morphine from its sites of storage in the body. The large volume of distribution for morphine tends to keep the concentrations of morphine in plasma low, making re-uptake the rate-limiting step in elimination. The high hepatic extraction ratio also ensures that little orally administered morphine reaches the circulation owing to enterohepatic first-pass metabolism.

Stanski *et al* reported that 10 mg of morphine given im had an absorption half-life of 7.7 (range 3 to 15) minutes with a 100% systemic availability.[56] Peak plasma concentrations were reached between 7.5 and 20 minutes after injection. Brunk and Delle found that 10 mg·kg⁻¹ doses of morphine given im or subcutaneously (sc) resulted in higher plasma concentrations than those seen after iv dosing in the period from 15 minutes to 3 hours after administration.[60] The iv doses are rapidly distributed out of the plasma, whereas the im or sc sites continue to release morphine into the plasma for distribution.

At physiologic *p*H (7.40), 23%–36% of morphine is bound to plasma proteins—primarily albumin.[61, 62] Only the unbound fraction (approximately 70%) would be available for distribution across membranes. Also, only non-ionized drugs will readily distribute (cross) into the lipid phase of the membrane. The *p*K$_a$'s for morphine (7.93/9.63 at 37°C) mean that only a small fraction (less than 10%) of morphine is normally non-ionized in plasma.[63, 64] Furthermore, morphine is relatively lipid insoluble with an octanol/water partition coefficient of 1.0.[64] The result is that only a small portion of the morphine found in plasma at any particular time will readily cross into the CNS. Acute changes in the concentration of morphine in plasma do not result in immediate changes in the levels in the CNS, and equilibrium between plasma and CNS levels of morphine is found only after prolonged steady-state levels of morphine in plasma.

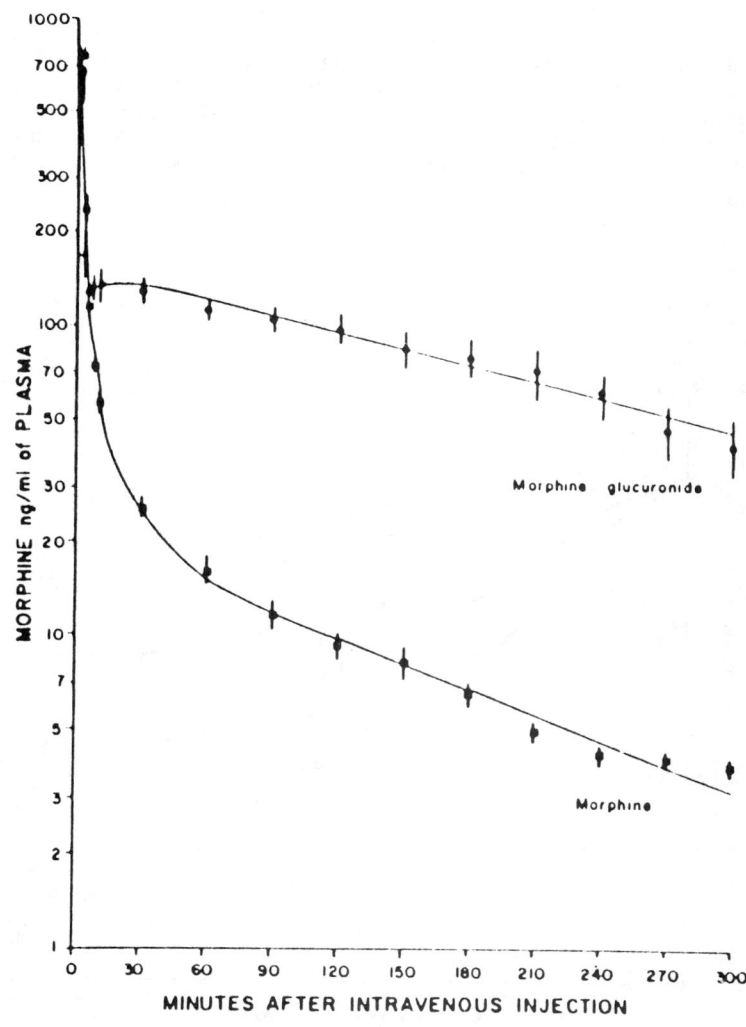

FIG. 9-5. Plasma concentrations of morphine and its principal metabolite, morphine glucuronide, following intravenous administration of morphine. (Mean ± SE) Reprinted with permission from Murphy MR, Hug CC: Pharmacokinetics of intravenous morphine in patients anesthetized with enflurane-nitrous oxide. Anesthesiology 54:187, 1981.

It is interesting that morphine is considered to be a relatively long-acting opioid with analgesic effects lasting 4 to 5 hours while its elimination half-time is actually less than that for the reportedly shorter-acting drug fentanyl. And, although patients are aware of the effects of an iv dose of morphine within minutes of its injection, the peak effect of the dose may be delayed for over 15 minutes. A few reports in the literature have attempted to correlate plasma levels of morphine with analgesic intensity, but the studies show only crude and indirect comparisons. The studies have not been able to demonstrate a direct relationship between plasma concentrations of morphine and intensity of analgesia or respiratory depression.

Studies in animals also suggest that the blood–brain barrier is a significant impediment to the movement of morphine both into and away from its sites of analgesic and respiratory effects in the CNS. In dogs given an iv dose of 0.3 mg·kg^{-1} of morphine and allowed to breathe spontaneously, peak concentrations of morphine in the cerebral spinal fluid (CSF) did not occur until 15 to 30 minutes following injection (Fig. 9-6).[40] The delay probably reflects the low lipid solubility of morphine and the limitations imposed by biological membranes on less lipid soluble drugs. Diffusion of morphine from brain to CSF to plasma may occur and result in a concentration in CSF between that of plasma and brain. But once in the CSF, the elimination of morphine did not parallel its elimination from plasma.[40] These observations have been confirmed in other studies. One study that reported a delayed elimination of morphine from the brain in relation to that in plasma suggested that the slowed elimination was the result of a greater portion of the morphine existing in the ionized state in the relatively acid milieu of the brain.[65]

Ventilatory depression demonstrated by changes in the end-tidal CO_2 of spontaneously breathing dogs (Fig. 9-6) did not correlate with the concentration of morphine in either the plasma or CSF.[40] Ventilatory depression is the pharmacodynamic effect of morphine measured in this study and probably most directly reflects the concentration of morphine at its receptors or sites of action. Plasma concentrations of morphine do not adequately reflect the intensity of effect of morphine, but the pharmacokinetic data do help explain the pharmacodynamics of the drug.

The literature suggests that a 10-mg dose of morphine is equivalent to approximately 20% nitrous oxide. The efficacy of a number of opioids to act as anesthetics or reduce the concentration of potent inhalational agents necessary to maintain MAC (minimal alveolar concentration) have been performed. In dogs given increasing iv doses of morphine, the end-tidal concentration of enflurane necessary to prevent movement to an applied tail-clamp can be reduced in a linear fashion up to a morphine dose of 5 mg·kg^{-1}.[20] A dose of 0.5 mg·kg^{-1} reduced the MAC of enflurane by 17%, 1.5 mg·kg^{-1} reduced MAC 32%, and 5 mg·kg^{-1} produced a 63% reduction in MAC. A fourfold increase in the dose of morphine to 20 mg·kg^{-1} reduced MAC to a maximum of 67%, which was not statistically different from the 63% reduction of the 5 mg·kg^{-1} dose. The effectiveness of morphine as an anesthetic appears to plateau at about 65% of a total MAC, suggesting that it does not provide complete anesthesia.

Similar studies in rats given sc doses of morphine found linear reductions of cyclopropane and halothane MAC up to a dose of 8 mg·kg^{-1}, in which the reductions were 55% and approximately 68%, respectively.[66] In the halothane study, further doses of 12 and 20 mg·kg^{-1} produced reductions of approximately 70% and 84%, demonstrating a response approaching plateau.

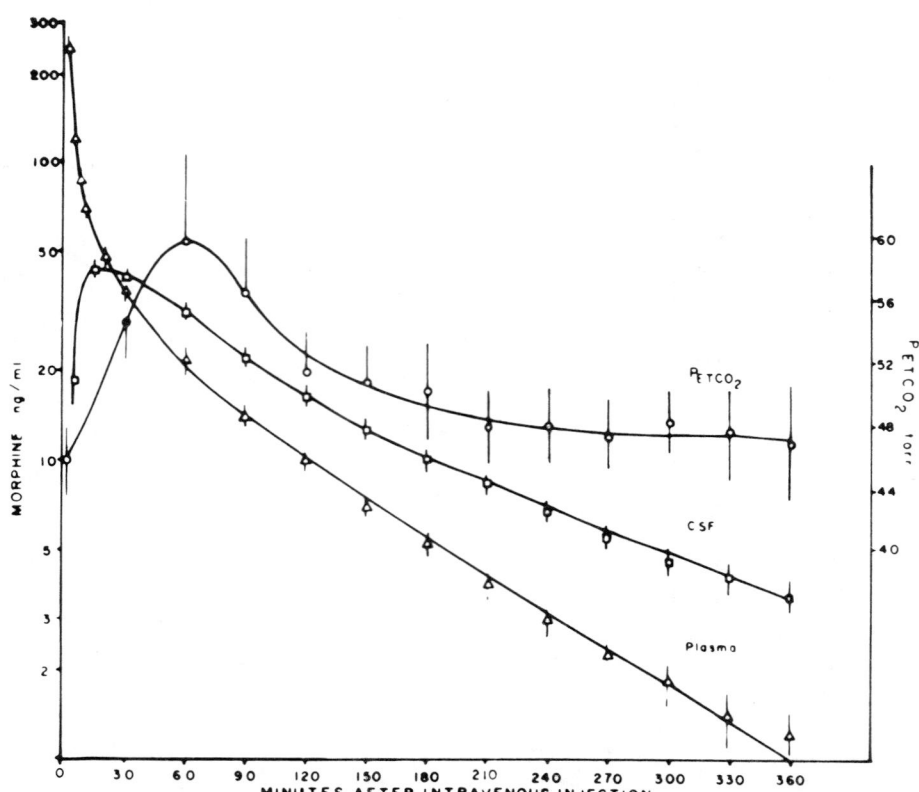

FIG. 9-6 Cerebrospinal fluid (*CSF*) and plasma levels of morphine and end-tidal CO_2 (PET$_{CO_2}$) in six dogs given a 0.3 mg·kg^{-1} dose intravenously and allowed to ventilate spontaneously. Each point and vertical line represents the mean ± SEM. There is a lack of correlation between the concentrations of morphine in plasma, CSF, and the receptors for ventilatory depression as represented by the PET$_{CO_2}$. (Adapted with permission from Hug CC Jr, Murphy MR, Rigel EP et al: Pharmacokinetics of morphine injected intravenously into the anesthetized dog. Anesthesiology 54:38, 1981.)

MEPERIDINE

Intravenous injection of meperidine in normal subjects results in a biexponential decline of the concentration of meperidine in plasma. Meperidine has a relatively rapid tissue distribution half-time of 4 to 17 minutes.[67-70] The volume of distribution of meperidine is 2.8 to 4.2 $l \cdot kg^{-1}$, indicating extensive tissue distribution similar to that seen with morphine.[67-70] Meperidine also has a high clearance rate (10 to 17 $ml \cdot kg^{-1} \cdot min^{-1}$), which is slightly less than that of morphine.[67-71] The elimination half-time for meperidine is 3.2 to 4.1 hours greater than that of morphine. Sampling for 24 hours, rather than the 6 to 7 hours, sampled in the previous studies, Verbeeck et al found an even longer terminal half-life (6 to 7 hours) and smaller clearance (7.6 $ml \cdot kg^{-1} \cdot min^{-1}$).[72] Despite the longer elimination half-time for meperidine in relation to morphine, meperidine is a shorter-acting drug.

Meperidine's high clearance is indicative of a high hepatic extraction ratio. Meperidine is readily metabolized in the liver, and a number of metabolites are possible—the major ones being normeperidine, meperidinic acid, and normeperidinic acid. Normeperidine is found in plasma after repeat doses of meperidine and is eliminated much more slowly than is meperidine.[73] Normeperidine is an active metabolite, possessing twice the convulsive properties of meperidine with only half the analgesic effect.[73] Stambaugh et al found only 3.9% of an iv dose of meperidine excreted unchanged in the urine by 48 hours, whereas 4.2% was excreted as normeperidine.[68] The urinary excretion rate was 4.5% and 5.5% for meperidine and normeperidine, respectively, following im administration, and 3.3% and 6.2% after oral administration.

Absorption of an im dose of meperidine in postsurgical patients is extremely variable. Peak concentrations in plasma following 100-mg doses given at 4-hour intervals varied over a fivefold range among the patients. The peak concentrations were also associated with wide variations in the times to reach those peaks following im injection. The mean time to reach peak concentrations among the patients was 44 minutes but varied from 15 to 110 minutes.[74]

The free fraction of meperidine in plasma is 18% to 36%, meaning that it is much more protein bound than is morphine. Meperidine is primarily bound to alpha$_1$-acid glycoprotein (and, to a lesser extent, albumin). Meperidine protein binding can be affected by surgery and/or disease states that alter alpha$_1$-acid glycyprotein. Meperidine is also considerably more lipid soluble than is morphine, with an octanol/water partition coefficient of 11.5 (morphine's is 1.0). The onset of action of meperidine is somewhat faster than that of morphine after both iv and im dosing. The duration of effect (2 to 3 hours) for analgesic doses is shorter than that of morphine, despite a longer elimination half-time for meperidine. The prolongation of morphine's pharmacodynamic effects has been examined.

Unlike morphine, there is a reasonable correlation between the plasma concentration of meperidine and the intensity of its effects. Austin et al found that the minimal effective analgesic concentration of meperidine in postsurgical patients was independent of the route of delivery (im vs iv) and ranged between 0.24 and 0.76 $\mu g \cdot ml^{-1}$, with a mean of 0.46 $\mu g \cdot ml^{-1}$.[75] The maximal blood concentration still associated with severe pain ranged from 0.10 to 0.98 $\mu g \cdot ml^{-1}$, with a mean of 0.41 $\mu g \cdot ml^{-1}$. These researchers concluded that concentrations of meperidine less than 0.10 $\mu g \cdot ml^{-1}$ did not alter the perception of pain. With gradual increases in blood concentrations, a critical point is reached, at which very small increases in concentration (0.05 $\mu g \cdot ml^{-1}$) can produce complete analgesia. Although the variation of minimal analgesic concentrations was large among patients, the concentrations were stable and consistent for any individual. In practice, a meperidine concentration of 0.6 $\mu g \cdot ml^{-1}$ would produce suppression from severe pain 84% of the time, whereas 0.7 $\mu g \cdot ml^{-1}$ would produce relief from severe pain 95% of the time.[75] In another study, healthy volunteers given 50 mg of meperidine iv had a maximal serum concentration of 0.52 $\mu g \cdot ml^{-1}$ observed in the first sample at 1 minute.[68] By 5 minutes, the concentration of meperidine in serum had decreased by one half to 0.25 $\mu g \cdot ml^{-1}$. At 30 minutes, it was 0.14 $\mu g \cdot ml^{-1}$ and thereafter decreased more slowly. By 3 hours, the level was 0.11 $\mu g \cdot ml^{-1}$ and, at 8 hours, 0.07 $\mu g \cdot ml^{-1}$. If the volunteers had been surgical patients, adequate analgesia would have been nonexistent or very short-lived following a single 50-mg bolus of meperidine.

The aforementioned data have added significance when it is noted that in patients given 100 mg of meperidine im every 4 hours postoperatively, the concentration of meperidine in the blood of the patients was above the minimal analgesic concentration only about 35% of each 4-hour im dosing interval.[74] Variable pain control was the result of inadequate and unpredictable blood concentrations owing to unpredictable absorption from im sites of injection. The fact that there is a good correlation between blood concentration and pharmacodynamics (analgesia) allows the use of pharmacokinetic data to create a treatment regimen that produces satisfactory analgesia without significant toxicity. Just such a treatment plan was summarized in an editorial by Hug utilizing previously published data (Fig. 9-7) and was proved by Stapleton et al in patients.[76, 77] An infusion of 0.4 $mg \cdot min^{-1}$, preceded by loading infusion of 1.0 $mg \cdot min^{-1}$ for 45 minutes followed by 0.53 $mg \cdot min^{-1}$ for 28 minutes, resulted in the abolition of severe pain after 3 hours and in continued analgesia for the 2-day study in post–abdominal hysterectomy patients.[77]

FENTANYL

Much has been written about the variability of the pharmacokinetics of fentanyl in humans.[78, 79] Excluding studies in which duration of sampling (less than 6 hours) was inadequate (too few samples were obtained at crucial times) or in which aortic cross-clamping or cardiopulmonary bypass intervened, the pharmacokinetic data are not quite so varied. Five studies, two in volunteers and three in surgical patients, appear to represent reasonable pharmacokinetic studies of fentanyl. The iv doses ranged from 5 to 10 $\mu g \cdot kg^{-1}$ and were given either as rapid bolus doses or as rapid infusions of up to 2.5 minutes, depending upon the study.[38, 80-83]

When fentanyl is injected iv, there is a very rapid decline in plasma concentration. In dogs given 10 or 100 $\mu g \cdot kg^{-1}$ of fentanyl iv, 98% of the dose was eliminated from plasma at 5 minutes, and 99% by 30 minutes.[84] In volunteers, 98.6% of the injected dose has been eliminated from plasma by 60 minutes.[38] The concentration–time curve for fentanyl is described by either a biexponential or triexponential equation, depending upon the rate of injection or sampling times immediately following injection. In those studies in which fentanyl is given rapidly and sufficient numbers of samples are obtained early in the study, a triexponential decline in plasma concentrations is found.[38, 80] In patients and volunteers, the rapid distribution half-time for fentanyl is 1.4 to 1.7 minutes, whereas the slower distribution phase is 13 to 28 minutes in the studies in which three phases are apparent.[38, 80] Although there is no direct evidence in humans, animal studies suggest that the rapid

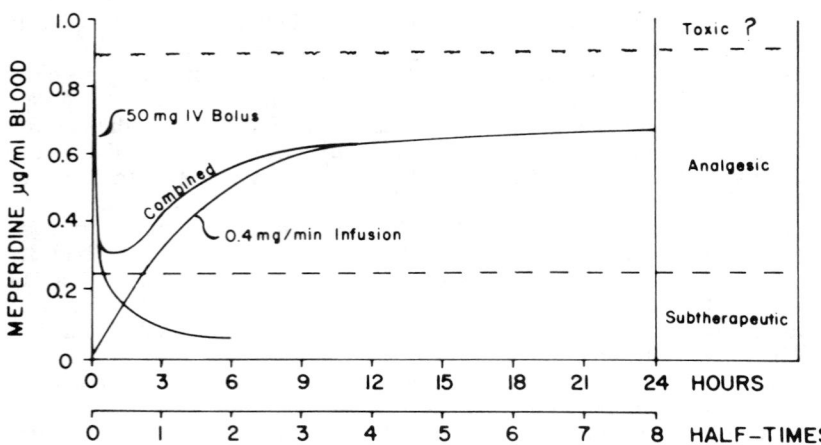

FIG. 9-7. Simulation of blood levels of meperidine resulting from the combination of an intravenous bolus dose of 50 mg and a continuous infusion of 0.4 mg·min^{-1} begun at time zero. After the bolus dose alone, blood levels would initially be higher than necessary (near toxic?) and would fall into the subtherapeutic range after 20 to 40 minutes. With the continuous infusion of 0.4 mg·min^{-1}, it would take slightly more than 2 hours to reach the lowest analgesic concentrations. By combining the two methods of administration, blood levels of meperidine remain within the analgesic range; an additional bolus dose might be useful after about 20 minutes. An even better method would involve the use of a priming infusion to limit the peak concentration and to minimize the depth of the concentration trough. The toxic level of meperidine has not been defined; a concentration of 0.7 μg·ml^{-1} was estimated to provide relief of pain in 95% of cases and gave no evidence of clinically significant respiratory depression (or toxicity). (Used with permission from Hug CC Jr: Improving analgesic therapy. Anesthesiology 53:441, 1980.)

distribution phase represents the equilibration of the vessel-rich group of tissues (*e.g.*, brain, lung, heart) and plasma with skeletal muscle (Fig. 9-8).[85] The slower distribution (and redistribution) phase is the equilibration of the plasma/vessel-rich group of tissues and skeletal muscle with fat (Fig. 9-8).[85] The elimination half-time for fentanyl is 3.1 to 4.4 hours.[38, 80-83]

The pharmacokinetics and pharmacodynamics of fentanyl are very much influenced by its extreme lipid solubility, which allows it to cross biological membranes very rapidly. Following iv injection in the rat, the uptake of fentanyl by the highly perfused (vessel-rich) group of tissues, heart, lung, and brain, reached a maximum at or before the first sampling at 1.5 minutes (Fig. 9-8).[85] The concentrations in these tissues paralleled the concentration of fentanyl in plasma and were therefore indistinguishable from plasma pharmacokinetically and are designated as part of the central compartment. The actual concentrations in these tissues were higher: two to three times greater in brain and heart than in plasma, and ten times greater in lung. The uptake of fentanyl by skeletal muscle was somewhat slower than that for the central group of tissues and reached a maximum at about 5 minutes—the actual concentrations being two to four times greater than that in plasma. Maximal concentrations were found at 30 minutes in fat and were 35 times greater than those in plasma. Both skeletal muscle, because of its mass in relation to body size, and fat, because of its high partition coefficient for highly lipid soluble drugs, act as storage sites for fentanyl. As the concentration of fentanyl in plasma decreases following its initial equilibration with adipose tissues, the fat, acting as a reservoir to maintain plasma concentrations, slowly releases the fentanyl back into the plasma for transport to the liver for biotransformation to excretable metabolites. This slow release maintains plasma

concentrations and produces the relatively prolonged elimination half-time of 3.1 to 4.4 hours.[38, 80-83]

Very little of a dose of fentanyl is eliminated by renal excretion as fentanyl. Only about 6.5% is eliminated as unchanged drug in the urine.[38] Fentanyl's high lipid solubility allows it to be readily reabsorbed from the renal tubules. Most of the fentanyl excreted by the kidneys is excreted as metabolites. Fentanyl metabolism is rapid and extensive in the liver. (Undefined extrahepatic sites appear to contribute to fentanyl metabolism in anhepatic dogs but are of little significance in the presence of a functioning liver.[86]) By 30 minutes after iv injection, the concentration of metabolites of fentanyl in plasma exceed the concentration of fentanyl and the metabolites are eliminated at a much slower rate.[38] The primary route of metabolism is by N-dealkylation to norfentanyl and by hydroxylation of both fentanyl and norfentanyl to hydroxypropionyl fentanyl and hydroxypropionyl norfentanyl.[79, 85] The pharmacologic activity, if any, of the fentanyl metabolites is not known.

The clearance of fentanyl is high, between 11 and 21 ml·kg^{-1}·min^{-1}.[38, 80-83] These rates approach hepatic blood flow and indicate a high hepatic extraction ratio approaching 100%. With this high extraction ratio, hepatic metabolism is perfusion-dependent. The large volume of distribution, 3.2 to 5.9 l·kg^{-1}, reflects the great tissue affinity of fentanyl. The slow release of fentanyl from muscle and fat keeps the plasma concentration relatively low and is the rate-limiting step in the elimination of fentanyl from the body.

The pK_a of fentanyl is 8.43. At pH 7.4, 91% of fentanyl is ionized.[79] Protein binding is approximately 79%–87% at pH 7.4 and is consistent over large ranges of drug concentrations (100-fold or more).[38, 79, 83] The free fraction of fentanyl is there-

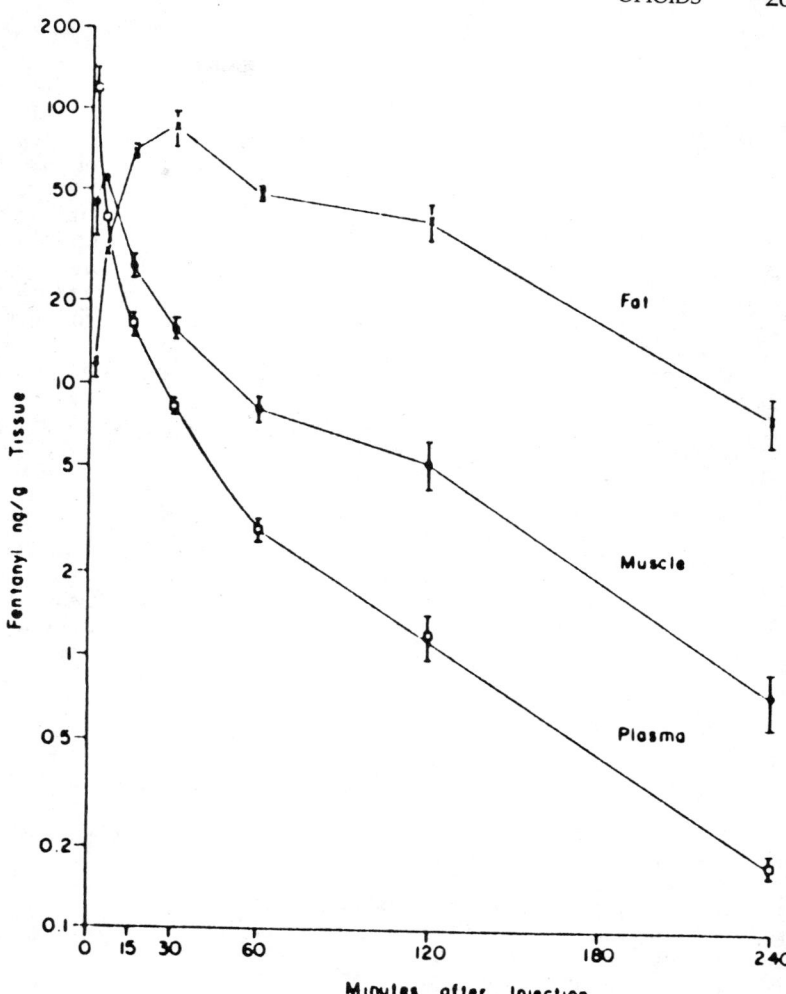

FIG. 9-8. The short duration of a single dose of fentanyl reflects its rapid redistribution to inactive tissue sites such as fat and skeletal muscle with an associated decline in the serum concentration of drug. Reprinted with permission from Hug CC, Murphy RR: Tissue redistribution of fentanyl and termination of its effects in rats. Anesthesiology 55:369, 1981.)

fore 13%–21%. Changes in pH will affect protein binding; pH's as low as 6.2 were associated with 38% bound drug, whereas increasing the pH increased binding to 90% at pH 7.6.

The pharmacodynamics of fentanyl, especially as related to ventilation, have been fairly well studied. Unlike morphine, there appears to be a fair correlation between the concentration of fentanyl in plasma and its pharmacologic effects on ventilation and probably analgesia. The onset of the effects of fentanyl is rapid. There is marked depression of ventilation within 2 minutes following iv injection of analgesic doses. In 7 volunteers injected over 90 seconds with iv doses of 3.2 or 6.4 $\mu g \cdot kg^{-1}$ of fentanyl base (equivalent to 5 or 10 $\mu \cdot kg^{-1}$ of fentanyl citrate, which is the commercially available form), decreases in the sense of awareness and concern occurred during the injection of fentanyl.[38] By 2 minutes, the subjects were relaxed. These feelings were maximal between 5 and 10 minutes. Onset of ventilatory depression was as rapid, and apnea occurred in four subjects. A previous study in healthy subjects also noted the greatest ventilatory depression between 2 and 5 minutes following 6 $\mu g \cdot kg^{-1}$ of fentanyl administered iv.[87] Comparison of the pharmacokinetic study with the ventilatory study revealed a close correlation between plasma levels of fentanyl and ventilatory depression as measured by increases in end-tidal CO_2 (Fig. 9-9).[38, 87]

This same correlation has been demonstrated in dogs lightly anesthetized with enflurane/oxygen and breathing spontaneously. A 10 $\mu g \cdot kg^{-1}$ dose of fentanyl administered iv over 30 seconds produced an immediate onset of ventilatory depression; apnea occurred within 1.5 minutes.[39] Concentrations of fentanyl in CSF increased rapidly, with near maximal concentrations in the earliest sample taken at 2 to 3 minutes postinjection. Following equilibration between plasma and CSF, there was a linear relationship between the log concentration of fentanyl in plasma and CSF and its effect (ventilatory depression) as measured by changes in end-tidal CO_2. This contrasts with the lack of correlation noted earlier with morphine (Fig. 9-6). Ventilatory depression is an indirect measure of the concentration of the drug at its sites of action in the CNS.

The concentration of fentanyl in plasma and brain is proportional to dose.[84, 85] When small doses are used, the concentration of drug in plasma and at its receptors rapidly falls below a threshold for effect. Increasingly larger doses will produce increasingly prolonged effects. Repetition of the same dose of fentanyl at set intervals produces accumulation of fentanyl in the body. Not only are there higher peak plasma concentrations following each injection, but there are also proportional increases in end-tidal CO_2 and a more prolonged effect.[39]

When the pharmacodynamics of fentanyl were measured

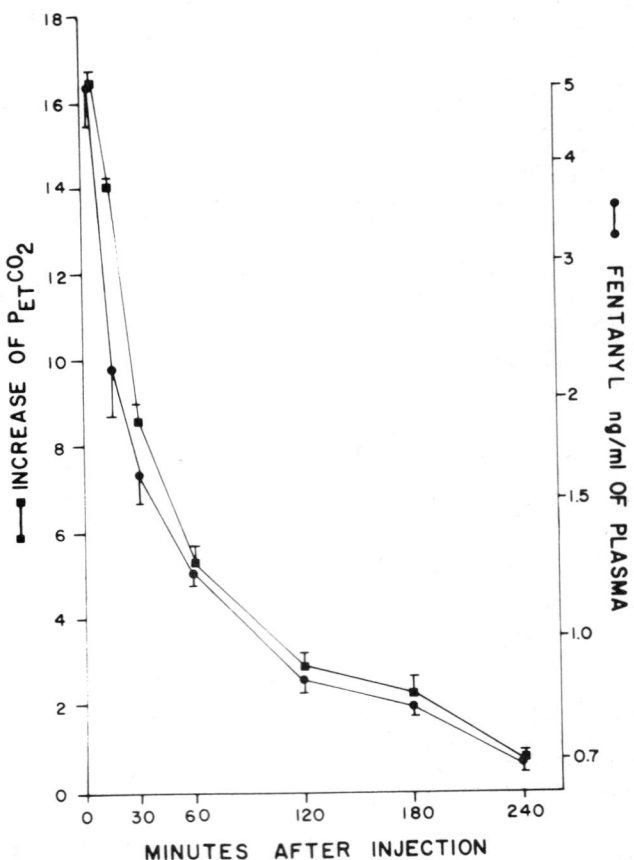

FIG. 9-9. Comparison of the decline in log of ^{3}H-fentanyl plasma level in five subjects given 6.4 $\mu g \cdot kg^{-1}$ with the recovery from ventilatory depression (PET_{CO_2}) in ten subjects given 6 $\mu g \cdot kg^{-1}$ intravenously. A very close correlation between the plasma concentration and the ventilatory depression produced by fentanyl is evident. Ventilatory depression is an indirect measure of the concentration of fentanyl at its receptors. (Adapted with permission from McClain DA, Hug CC Jr: Intravenous fentanyl kinetics. Clin Pharmacol Ther 28:106, 1980.)

by EEG spectral edge analysis in patients, there was a measurable lag between fluctuations in plasma concentrations of fentanyl and its EEG slowing effects.[88] A time lag exists between the peak plasma concentration of fentanyl and its peak spectral edge effect; thereafter, the spectral edge changes and plasma concentrations parallel each other, but with a time lag of approximately 6 minutes. It is suggested that the onset of the peak effect of fentanyl in patients is not quite as rapid as previously thought and that dosing should be 5 to 10 minutes before intense stimulation is anticipated. Clinically, this lag may not be as noticeable, since relatively larger than needed doses of fentanyl may raise the receptor levels of fentanyl beyond the threshold for pain or unconsciousness at some time earlier than the peak effect is seen. The lag between peak serum concentrations and peak effect (dynamics) has been attributed to the partitioning of fentanyl between serum and brain.[88] Because of fentanyl's great lipid solubility, it moves rapidly across the blood-brain barrier into the brain, but then must fill a great number of nonreceptor storage sites. The suggestion is that fentanyl must fill a large depot before the concentration of drug at the receptor sites is adequate to produce the opioid effect.

Fentanyl has also been reported to produce a biphasic respiratory response noted as an increasing ventilatory depression in the recovery room following a apparent recovery from fentanyl, nitrous oxide anesthesia (Fig. 9-4).[43] A number of pharmacokinetic studies have noted secondary increases in plasma concentrations of fentanyl in volunteers and patients.[38] These bumps in the concentration curves have been attributed to mobilization of fentanyl away from tissue storage areas back into the plasma secondary to increased perfusion of the storage areas. The most likely explanation is increased perfusion of skeletal muscles associated with movement in volunteers or during awakening from anesthesia in patients. In the report noted previously, the biphasic ventilatory depression is probably a result of the increased intensity of noxious stimulation and its antagonism of ventilatory effects immediately after surgery when the patients were awakened and transported to the recovery room. Later, when the patients were unstimulated, the residual respiratory depression produced by the remaining fentanyl was not antagonized by the stimulation and became more obvious.[38, 43] Again, this report simply demonstrates that noxious stimulation is a natural antagonist to the effects of opioids and that unstimulated patients may become severely depressed postoperatively if the intensity of the stimulation is much less than it is intraoperatively.

Studies similar to those described for morphine to determine the ability of opioids to reduce the MAC concentration of potent inhalational agents have been performed with fentanyl. In dogs, infusion of fentanyl produced stable plasma concentrations at which MAC determinations could be made. There is a dose–plasma concentration-related reduction in enflurane MAC with increasing concentrations of fentanyl up to a maximal reduction of approximately 66% at a plasma concentration of 30 $ng \cdot ml^{-1}$ (Fig. 9-10).[89] The maximal reduc-

FIG. 9-10. Per cent reduction of enflurane MAC as a function of the logarithm of the plasma fentanyl concentration. Each point represents the mean concentration ($\pm$SEM) of fentanyl in plasma and the average per cent ($\pm$SEM) reduction of enflurane MAC in the number of dogs indicated below the vertical standard error bar. Similar curves are produced by morphine, sufentanil, and alfentanil in the dog and may represent saturation of opioid receptors. (Adapted with permission from Murphy MR, Hug CC Jr: The anesthetic potency of fentanyl in terms of its reduction of enflurane MAC. Anesthesiology 57:485, 1982.)

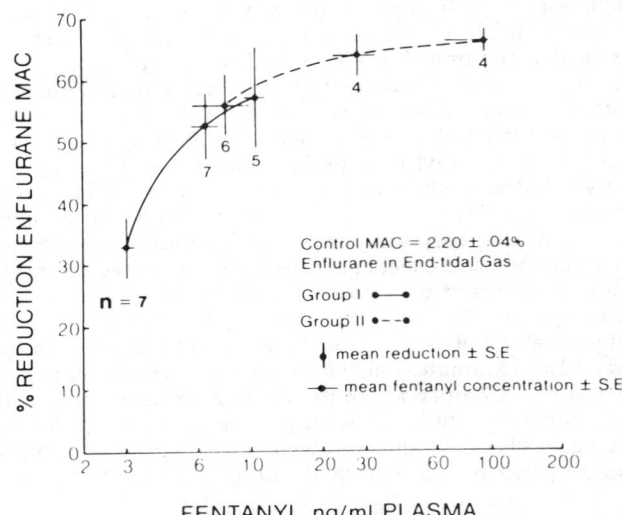

tion of isoflurane MAC in dogs is the same at 67%.[90] These reductions are similar to those seen with high doses of morphine (63%) and suggest saturation of opioid receptors.

In another study using awake dogs, fentanyl was injected in increasing doses from 2.5 up to 100 $\mu g \cdot kg^{-1}$ at 5-minute intervals.[91] Plasma concentrations were then compared with the effects on pain responses, ventilation, and circulation. It is of interest that the analgesic effects could not be separated from the ventilatory or circulatory effects and that all these receptor-mediated effects were maximal at the same plasma concentration of fentanyl, 30 $ng \cdot ml^{-1}$—the same maximal concentration noted in the enflurane MAC reduction study previously cited.

Although these studies were performed in dogs, and there certainly are species differences from humans, the differences may not be that great. In patients having cardiac surgery, plasma fentanyl levels of 15 $ng \cdot ml^{-1}$ were necessary for suppression of hemodynamic responses to noxious stimuli in 50% of subjects (EC_{50}).[92] Extrapolation of the data in this study suggests that the EC_{90} (the effective concentration in 90% of the patients) would be approximately 30 $ng \cdot ml^{-1}$. The 15 $ng \cdot ml^{-1}$ concentration in plasma was achieved by the administration of 50 $\mu g \cdot kg^{-1}$ fentanyl as a loading dose followed by an infusion of 0.5 $\mu g \cdot kg^{-1} \cdot min^{-1}$. It is probably not rational to give patients increasing doses of fentanyl once all opioid-effect receptors are occupied, because this will prolong the effect but not increase its intensity.

SUFENTANIL

Plasma levels of sufentanil for pharmacokinetic studies (and most opioid studies) are determined by radioimmunoassay (RIA). The sufentanil RIA is accurate to a plasma concentration of 0.1 to 0.5 $ng \cdot ml^{-1}$. Owing to the extreme potency of sufentanil (about ten times greater than fentanyl), smaller amounts of drug are given to attain the same clinical response as equally effective doses of fentanyl. Since fewer molecules are given, the plasma concentrations are low and may become undetectable before sufficient time has elapsed after administration to obtain enough concentration–time points for pharmacokinetic analysis.

The pharmacokinetics of sufentanil in animals are similar to those of fentanyl, and most pharmacokinetic properties of fentanyl can be applied to sufentanil. In a clinical study of sufentanil pharmacokinetics in ten surgical patients not scheduled for cardiac surgery or bypass, the sufentanil concentration–time curve was best described by a triexponential equation where 98% of the drug was cleared from plasma by 30 minutes.[93] The rapid distribution half-time was 1.4 minutes, whereas the slower distribution phase was 17.7 minutes. These times are similar to those seen with fentanyl. The elimination half-time for sufentanil is 2.7 hours (164 minutes), which is somewhat less than that of fentanyl (3.1 to 4.4 hours). The volume of distribution for sufentanil is 2.86 $l \cdot kg^{-1}$, which is somewhat less than that for fentanyl. This smaller volume of distribution coupled with a clearance of 13 $ml \cdot kg^{-1} \cdot min^{-1}$ for sufentanil (similar to that of fentanyl) accounts for the shorter elimination half-time of sufentanil compared with that of fentanyl.

Sufentanil is highly protein bound. At pH 7.40, 92.5% is protein bound.[79] This large protein binding and sufentanil's volume of distribution suggest that sufentanil is highly lipophilic and extensively bound to tissues. As with fentanyl, the rate-limiting step for elimination from the body is reuptake from peripheral tissues. The pK_a for sufentanil is 8.01, and 80% of sufentanil is ionized at pH 7.4.[79]

The pharmacodynamics of sufentanil are not as well studied as those of fentanyl. However, the similarities of the pharmacokinetics would suggest that the dynamics of fentanyl and sufentanil will be similar. This assumption generally holds true, with sufentanil having a slightly more rapid onset of effect and a slightly shorter duration of action.

Sufentanil is the most potent opioid available for clinical use, being approximately five to ten times more potent than fentanyl. Studies in rats showed a reduction of halothane MAC of 90% with an infusion of $1 \cdot 10$ $mg \cdot kg^{-1} \cdot min^{-1}$, suggesting the possibility of complete anesthesia with sufentanil as opposed to what has been observed with fentanyl.[94] Even though 90% MAC was achieved to tail-clamp response, the rats still opened their eyes or lifted their heads in response to loud noises or jarring, suggesting that complete anesthesia was not achieved.

In dogs, the reduction of enflurane MAC by sufentanil is essentially the same as that for fentanyl. At a sufentanil concentration in plasma of 48 $ng \cdot ml^{-1}$, produced by an infusion of 1.2 $\mu g \cdot kg^{-1} \cdot min^{-1}$, the MAC of enflurane was maximally depressed by 70%.[95] Despite its increased potency, sufentanil is probably not more efficacious as a complete anesthetic and requires adjuvant drugs (N_2O, benzodiazepines, other depressants) to produce complete anesthesia.

ALFENTANIL

Alfentanil has pharmacokinetic and pharmacodynamic properties that permit newer, more refined methods of administration. In pharmacokinetic studies when alfentanil is administered iv in patients as a bolus dose (50 to 200 $\mu g \cdot kg$), the decline in plasma concentration is described by either a bi- or triexponential equation. Where found, the initial rapid distribution half-time is 1.0 to 3.5 minutes.[96, 97] The slower distribution half-time is 8.2 to 16.8 minutes.[96–99] In one study, 90% of the dose had disappeared from plasma by 30 minutes, whereas in another study, 96.4% was gone by 60 minutes.[96, 97] The terminal elimination half-time for alfentanil is very short in these surgical patients. It varies between 70 and 103 minutes (1.2 to 1.7 hours).[96–99] In volunteers, the elimination half-time is very similar at 97 minutes.[83] The terminal elimination half-times for alfentanil are considerably shorter than those of fentanyl (3.1 to 4.4 hours).[38, 80–83]

The volume of distribution is 0.5 to 1.0 $l \cdot kg^{-1}$ in surgical patients, and 0.4 $l \cdot kg^{-1}$ in volunteers.[83, 96–99] The volume of distribution for fentanyl is considerably larger at 3.2 to 5.9 $l \cdot kg^{-1}$.[38, 80–83] The clearance for alfentanil is 5.0 to 7.9 $ml \cdot kg^{-1} \cdot min^{-1}$ in surgical patients, and 3.4 $ml \cdot kg^{-1} \cdot min^{-1}$ in volunteers.[83, 96–99] The clearance for fentanyl is 11 to 21 $ml \cdot kg^{-1} \cdot min^{-1}$.[38, 80–83]

The pharmacokinetics of alfentanil and fentanyl were compared in an editorial by Stanski and Hug (Figs. 9-11 and 9-12).[100] The following points were made:

1. Fentanyl (as do most opioids) has a high clearance, approaching that of hepatic blood flow.
2. The elimination half-time of a drug is directly proportional to the volume of distribution and inversely proportional to clearance. Fentanyl's large volume of distribution limits the amount of drug available in plasma for elimination by the liver. Release of drug by the tissues (the rate-limiting step) keeps the plasma concentration low; thus, fentanyl has a relatively long terminal elimination half-time.
3. Fentanyl's short duration of action after a single dose results from redistribution rather than elimination. Af-

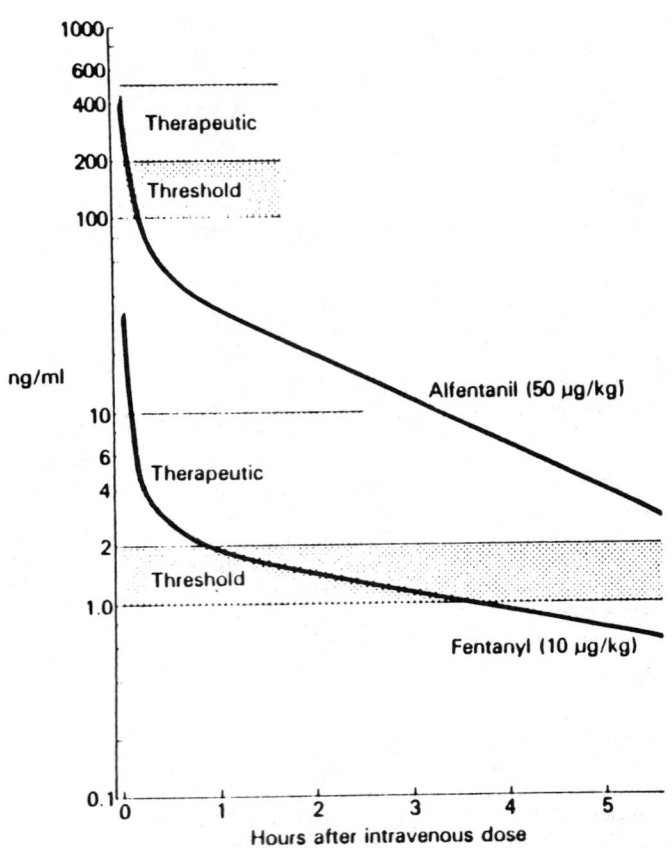

FIG. 9-11. A comparison of serum decay curves following intravenous administration of fentanyl or alfentanil. Despite equivalent doses, the serum concentration of alfentanil greatly exceeds that of fentanyl owing in part to the small volume of distribution of alfentanil. (Reprinted with permission from Stanski DR, Hug CC Jr: Alfentanil—a kinetically predictable narcotic analgesic. Anesthesiology 57:435, 1982.)

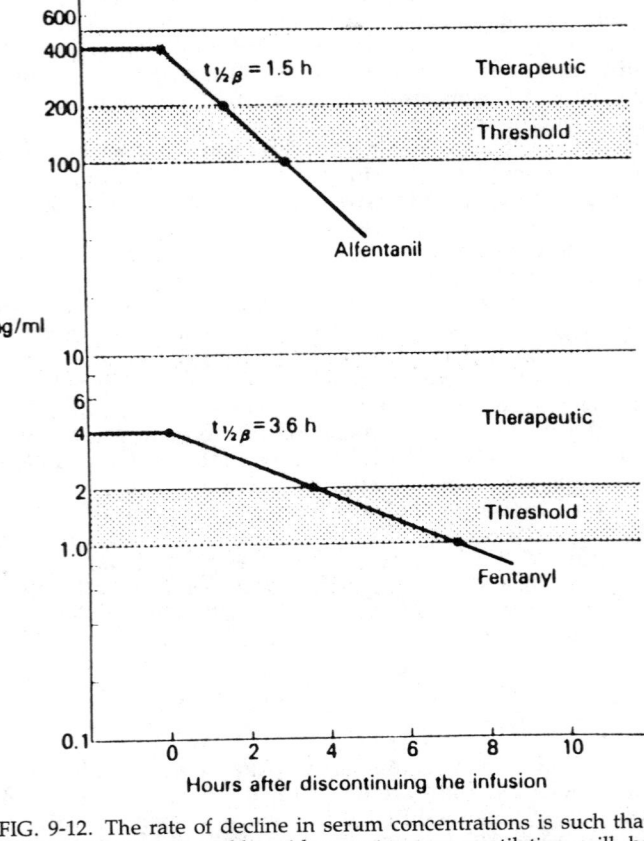

FIG. 9-12. The rate of decline in serum concentrations is such that concentrations compatible with spontaneous ventilation will be reached in about 3 hours after discontinuation of alfentanil and after about 7.2 hours after discontinuation of fentanyl. (Reprinted with permission from Stanski DR, Hug CC Jr: Alfentanil—a kinetically predictable narcotic analgesic. Anesthesiology 57:435, 1982.)

ter very large or multiple smaller doses, accumulation of fentanyl occurs as a result of its long half-time, and redistribution is less effective in removing fentanyl from its sites of action in the brain.

4. The smaller volume of distribution of alfentanil (about one fourth to one sixth of fentanyl's) means that there is more alfentanil in the plasma for elimination by the liver (as opposed to being stored in tissues).

5. The clearance of alfentanil is approximately one half that of fentanyl. However, "the greater decrease of alfentanil's distribution volume relative to the decrease in its clearance results in a significantly shorter terminal elimination half-time."[100]

Alfentanil is relatively lipid soluble but considerably less so than fentanyl. The heptane:water coefficients at pH 7.4 and 37°C for alfentanil and fentanyl are 2.5 and 9.0, respectively.[83] The lower lipid solubility probably accounts for alfentanil's small volume of distribution. Alfentanil has a higher percentage of protein binding than does fentanyl. Approximately 89%–92% of alfentanil is protein bound.[83, 98, 101] However, with a pK_a of 6.5, 89% of alfentanil is non-ionized at pH 7.4. Since the non-ionized molecule moves more rapidly across

biological membranes, alfentanil's pK_a, coupled with its moderate lipid solubility, accounts for alfentanil's rapid onset of action.[100, 101]

Only about 0.4% of alfentanil is excreted unchanged in the urine at 24 hours following an iv bolus injection.[98] The high degree of protein binding of alfentanil decreases its glomerular filtration, while its prevalent non-ionized form favors reabsorption from the renal tubules.[102]

Alfentanil's small volume of distribution and short elimination half-time preclude significant accumulation of the drug in the body and render alfentanil a useful drug for continuous infusion. The rapid onset (1 to 2 min) and rapid equilibration between the plasma concentration of alfentanil and its CNS receptors also make alfentanil an excellent drug for titration to response.[88] There is a good correlation between plasma concentration and effect. Furthermore, plasma concentrations can be rapidly altered, either increased with boluses or increasing infusion doses, or decreased by decreasing infusion rates, because of alfentanil's lack of accumulation and short elimination time.

Excellent data have been collected that demonstrate the plasma concentrations necessary to suppress responses to varying surgical stimuli. Although there is a 1.6- to 3.3-fold variability of concentration to suppress responses among patients anesthetized with alfentanil and 66% nitrous oxide, the response curves for individual patients is steep.[103] The plasma concentration of alfentanil that is necessary, along with 66% nitrous oxide, to obtund response to tracheal intubation in 50% of surgical patients studied (Cp_{50}) was 475 ng · ml^{-1}. The concentration necessary for skin closure was much less at 150 ng · ml^{-1}. The intensity of surgical stimulation varied considerably between these extremes. The important point is that stimulation does vary, and the amount of drug necessary to produce adequate analgesia needs to be frequently altered to meet this variation.

Alfentanil given by infusion with small bolus doses for rapid increases in plasma levels can be used as effectively as an inhalational agent and actually probably more efficiently. Large iv doses for induction (150 µg · kg^{-1}) in combination with nitrous oxide rapidly establishes levels sufficient for intubation of the trachea. Infusions of alfentanil can then maintain the plasma level. If the patient demonstrates no signs of light anesthesia (e.g., increases in blood pressure, heart rate, skeletal muscle movement), the infusion can progressively be decreased. If light anesthesia is noted, increases in the infusion rate and small bolus doses of alfentanil will quickly restore adequate levels of analgesia. Because alfentanil does not accumulate to any significant degree in the body, the infusion can be turned off 15 to 20 minutes before the end of the procedure, with the likely expectation of recovery adequate for the patient to be safely taken to the postanesthesia care unit. This whole procedure is analogous to the use of a potent inhalational agent such as isoflurane.

Just as seen with other agonist opioids, alfentanil produces a concentration-dependent reduction in the MAC of enflurane. Again, the effect plateaus at 70% reduction in enflurane MAC.[104] It is of interest that the concentration of alfentanil that produced the maximal reduction of MAC in response to tail-clamp (223 ng · ml^{-1}) is similar to that required in combination with nitrous oxide to provide adequate anesthesia to skin incision in patients (279 ng · ml^{-1}).[103, 104] This fact suggests that the anesthetic efficacy of alfentanil in humans and dogs is similar.

DRUG INTERACTIONS

Since opioids are not complete anesthetics, they are often used in combination with other drugs (e.g., hypnotics, inhalational agents, muscle relaxants) to achieve the required anesthetic effects (unconsciousness, analgesia, skeletal muscle relaxation, and suppression of stress responses). It is known that increasing concentrations of opioids will produce a progressive decrease in the concentration of inhalational agents necessary to maintain anesthesia.[89, 90, 94, 95] The potent inhalational agents (halothane, enflurane, isoflurane) are known dose-dependent cardiovascular depressants. Exaggerated cardiovascular depressive effects may be expected when they are added to a primarily opioid anesthetic or when opioids are added to a primarily inhalational anesthetic.[105, 106] Doses of both agents may have to be significantly decreased when used in combination.

More commonly, nitrous oxide has been used in combination with the opioids to produce unconsciousness and amnesia and to potentiate analgesia in the so-called balanced anesthesia technique. In volunteers, nitrous oxide appears to produce a small negative inotropic and chronotropic cardiac effect combined with alpha stimulation of the peripheral vasculature.[107] Nitrous oxide in combination with opioids in patients has been associated with decreases in cardiac output, stroke volume, and heart rate, with variable effects on systemic vascular resistance.[108, 109] These effects are measurable when nitrous oxide is added to opioids but may not be pronounced in patients with good left ventricular function. However, these myocardial depressant effects can be very significant in patients with poor left ventricular function and appear not to be the result of the opioid but primarily the nitrous oxide.[109, 110] At least part of the depressant effects of nitrous oxide in the impaired heart may be related to the reduction of the inspired oxygen concentration with the high concentrations of nitrous oxide generally needed.[111]

Just as nitrous oxide is often used in combination with opioids to produce anesthesia, other hypnotics, primarily benzodiazedines and barbiturates, have been used to increase depth of anesthesia (unconsciousness) and amnesia. These combinations appear to be additive in their anesthetic-related effects.[112, 113] Smaller doses of both the opioid and hypnotic are needed to produce the desired state of anesthesia. Thiopental in combination with morphine or fentanyl appears to antagonize some of the analgesic effect of the opioids.[113]

When benzodiazepines (diazepam, midazolam) are given alone in hypnotic (sleep-producing) doses, little or no changes in hemodynamics are seen. The same is true for large doses of fentanyl. However, the addition of small doses of a hypnotic to large doses of opioids may result in falls in blood pressure.[114] Occasionally, the effect may be profound and is characterized by decreases in blood pressure, systemic vascular resistance, and cardiac output. The hemodynamic effects are accompanied by decreases in circulating epinephrine and norepinephrine levels, but with no change in histamine with the fentanyl drugs. The mechanism appears to be an indirect centrally mediated decrease in vasoregulatory (mainly sympathetic) outflow from the CNS.[115] The reverse is also true. The addition of small doses of opioids to a benzodiazepine may result in hypotension. More frequently, the hemodynamic changes are not great when benzodiazepines and opioids are combined, and the changes produced are readily treatable. This combination is still clinically useful and commonly used to ensure amnesia.

Droperidol and scopolamine have been used as adjuvants to opioid anesthesia with insignificant hemodynamic changes. However, both have the potential for hemodynamic changes of their own, which are apparent when they are given in larger doses. Droperidol used alone occasionally produces unpleasant feelings of anxiety or excitement, even though the individual may appear very calm. These feelings are not noted when droperidol is used in combination with an opioid.

It has been suggested that the choice of muscle relaxant in combination with high-dose opioids may be important. The actions observed are an extension of the pharmacologic effects of the drugs. Opioids have a vagotonic effect and produce bradycardia. Pancuronium has a vagolytic effect and produces tachycardia. The combination may minimize or prevent changes in heart rate. The bradycardia produced by opioids may be beneficial to patients with ischemic heart disease, whereas tachycardia may increase ischemia. Vecuronium and metocurine either do not alter or may even potentiate the vagotonic effects of the opioids; lower heart rates are seen when these muscle relaxants are used.[116, 117]

Drugs that affect metabolism of opioids, either directly or indirectly by decreasing liver blood flow, will decrease the clearance of the opioid. Cimetidine, for instance, was shown to alter the elimination of fentanyl in dogs. Even acute administration of cimetidine, 10 mg·kg^{-1} im the night before and 5 mg·kg^{-1} im 90 minutes prior to 100 µg·kg^{-1} of fentanyl, resulted in an increase in the terminal elimination half-time of fentanyl from 155 to 340 minutes in these animals (Borel *el al*, personal communication).

Phenothiazines, monoamine oxidase (MAO) inhibitors, and tricyclic antidepressants may exaggerate and prolong the depressant effects of opioids.[1] Severe reactions of excitation, delirium, hyperpyrexia, convulsions, and severe respiratory depression have been reported in patients on MAO inhibitors given meperidine. Clonidine, a centrally acting preferential alpha$_2$-adrenergic agonist, primarily used as an antihypertensive agent, has been shown to decrease opioid requirements for surgery.[118] Amphetamines enhance the analgesic effects of opioids.[1]

IMPACT OF PRE-EXISTING DISEASES

AGE

Pre-existing diseases may alter responses to any drug. Choice of anesthesia-related drugs is generally determined following an evaluation of the patient's medical status and history. Many of the alterations in response (pharmacodynamics) are the result of pharmacokinetic changes produced by the disease.

Old age technically is not a disease but does produce changes in physiology and organ function that affect pharmacokinetics and pharmacodynamics. Furthermore, the elderly patient tends to have more ailments requiring drug intervention, thereby increasing the likelihood for drug interactions.

In general, increasing age is associated with decreasing ability to the kidneys and liver to clear drugs. Plasma concentrations of drugs, dependent upon clearance by these routes, may be increased in the elderly. This results in higher concentrations of the drug at sites of action. This increased action may be viewed as an increased sensitivity, because the intensity of the effect of a dose of drug seems to be greater than normal. In reality this is simply a concentration effect phenomenon. Generally, opioids are dependent upon liver blood flow for clearance. Liver blood flow may be reduced by as much as 40%–45% in the elderly.[119] Furthermore, enzyme function may be reduced; thus, lower doses and less frequent doses of opioids are needed in the elderly.

The elderly also tend to undergo changes in body composition. There is an increased proportion of adipose tissue in relation to body weight. Lean body mass is reduced. Lipid-soluble drugs will tend to be more widely distributed with an increase in the volume of distribution.[119] There is also a decline of plasma albumin in the elderly, which may increase the free fraction for highly protein bound drugs. Furthermore, it is possible that the blood–brain barrier is not as efficient in the elderly as in younger people, allowing more of a drug to cross from plasma to its sites of action in the CNS. This is apparently true in the fetus and newborn, in whom an immature blood–brain barrier is blamed for the apparent increased sensitivity of the neonates to certain drugs.

Studies of the pharmacokinetics and pharmacodynamics of opioids in the elderly tend to demonstrate decreases in clearance of the opioids and increased intensity and prolongation of effects of these drugs.[80] However, variability is great, and dosages are not predicable based on age alone. It is suggested that cautious titration to the desired opioid effect, beginning with lowered initial doses, is appropriate.

RENAL DISEASE

Only a small percentage of most opioids is excreted unchanged by the kidneys. Most of the opioids are first metabo-lized in the liver to metabolites that are readily excretable. Renal failure should not alter tremendously the dosage requirements, but few studies are available for confirmation. Renal failure does not appear to significantly affect the clearance of fentanyl, and it would be expected that this would also be true of the fentanyl derivatives. Renal failure will result in increased concentrations of fentanyl metabolites in the plasma, but none is known to produce pharmacologic effects.

In contrast, both morphine and meperidine are metabolized to active metabolites. The major metabolite of meperidine, normeperidine, may readily accumulate to significant levels and result in prolonged respiratory depression and convulsions.[73] Meperidine is not a good choice for patients with renal failure.

The morphine–glucuronide metabolites are generally much less active than morphine, primarily because of their severely decreased ability to cross the blood–brain barrier; however, they are known to have opioid effects when injected directly into the CNS. It is possible that continued high plasma concentrations of these metabolites would result in some of the morphine–glucuronide crossing into the CNS, with resultant opioid effects. Naloxone reversible opioid toxicity has been reported as much as 1 week following the last dose of morphine in renal failure patients.[120]

LIVER DISEASE

Because clearance of the opioids is heavily dependent upon the liver, it would be anticipated that decreases in liver function or liver failure would significantly decrease the clearance of opioids. This is, in fact, the case. Pharmacokinetic studies in patients with liver failure, cirrhosis, and viral hepatitis who are given morphine, meperidine, or alfentanil usually demonstrate a tremendously smaller clearance than in normal subjects, a prolonged elimination half-time with a relatively normal initial distribution. In these patients the volume of distribution is not significantly different from those of normal subjects.[69, 121] Initial doses of opioids will usually produce the expected intensity of effect, but it may be somewhat prolonged. Subsequent doses should be considerably smaller or delayed, since clearance of the drug is delayed and significant accumulation will result.

It is interesting that in patients with cirrhosis who were given fentanyl, 5 μg·kg^{-1} iv, no significant changes in clearance, volumes of distribution, or elimination half-time were seen.[82] However, none of the patients in this study had severe liver disease; thus, some liver function was present. Fentanyl, unlike alfentanil, has a very large volume of distribution. Fenatanyl's ultimate clearance is its re-uptake from these peripheral compartments to the liver, where it is metabolized. In this instance, the amount of drug taken up from these storage areas was not great enough to saturate the liver's metabolizing systems, and no significant pharmacokinetic changes were noted. If, however, large or repeated doses of fentanyl are given or if the patient has negligible liver function, more rapid accumulation of fentanyl will occur and a prolonged duration of effects will be found.

OBESITY

Because of the excessive adipose tissue of obese patients, it might be expected that highly lipophilic drugs such as fentanyl would have an increased volume of distribution and prolonged elimination half-time, whereas less lipophilic drugs, such as morphine, would be less affected. There are no studies to confirm the effect of obesity on morphine, but it is suggested that the dose be given according to ideal rather than actual body weight.

There were no significant differences of clearance, volume of distribution, or elimination half-time between normal controls and obese patients given 10 $\mu g \cdot kg^{-1}$ iv.[122] It might still be assumed that accumulation of large or multiple doses will occur and prolong anesthesia, whereas responses to initial doses will be normal.

In a similar study of alfentanil (100 $\mu g \cdot kg^{-1}$ of lean body weight) in obese versus nonobese patients, it was found that the elimination half-time was double but the clearance was approximately one half the normal in the obese patients, and the volume of distribution was similar.[123] The reason for this reversal of expected results is not clear.

NEUROLOGIC PROBLEMS

It is a commonly held belief that opioids are inappropriate in patients with head trauma. The rationale is that respiratory depression and concomitant increases in CO_2 may further increase an already high intracranial pressure. Opioids may aggravate the effects of cerebral and spinal ischemia. The opioid effects of miosis, vomiting, and mental clouding may mask the important clinical signs of increasing CNS pathology.[1] In those patients in whom increased intracranial pressure is not a problem or in whom ventilation is mechanically supported, opioids are not specifically contraindicated.

CLINICAL USES OF OPIOIDS

Opioids have a number of clinical uses for the anesthesiologist. Opioids are commonly used for premedication for surgical procedures. The feeling of well-being, warmth, and drowsiness, as well as the analgesia, make opioids a good choice for preoperative medications. These are frequently used in combination with sedatives or tranquilizers. The choice, dose, and route of administration of the opioid is dependent upon several factors, including whether the drug is given to the patient on the ward, in a preoperative holding area, or in the operating room itself. In general, longer-acting opioids such as morphine or meperidine, given im, are used when the patient is medicated on the ward. These drugs may be given 1 to 3 hours prior to coming to the operating room with the expectation of a continuous, significant effect upon arrival. Shorter-acting drugs such as fentanyl or sufentanil are less useful as ward premedicants, because much of their activity will have dissipated by the time that the patient reaches the surgical suite. These shorter-acting drugs are very useful in the holding area or operating room where they can easily be titrated to effect by incremental iv dosing. Alfentanil is probably not useful as a premedicant because of its extremely short action.

Opioids are also useful to aid induction of anesthesia. Smaller doses reduce the amount of other induction agents necessary to induce anesthesia, whereas large doses may be used as the primary induction agent. The more rapid-acting fentanyl drugs are especially useful because they decrease the time necessary for induction when compared with morphine. Morphine must be given more slowly (5 $mg \cdot min^{-1}$ to avoid histamine release) and has a much slower onset of action. Meperidine has a relatively fast onset of action but cannot be used in large doses because of detrimental cardiac side-effects.

Maintenance of anesthesia is aided by opioid drugs. Again, they may be used as the primary anesthetic or in combination with the potent inhalational agents and/or nitrous oxide. The higher the dose of opioid, the less of the other anesthetic agents needed. Because of the significant myocardial depressant effects of the potent inhalational agents, opioids are frequently used in higher doses in patients with severe myocardial disease.

Most of the opioids used for clinical anesthesia have been given by infusion. Pharmacokinetic and pharmacodynamic considerations suggest that of the opioids commonly used in anesthesia, morphine is the least useful by infusion, whereas alfentanil would be the most useful, especially in shorter procedures. Fentanyl and sufentanil are often given by infusion and can be titrated such that they are fairly predictable. Alfentanil, because of its even more rapid onset and short duration, is more predictable and can be administered in a manner comparable to that in which the inhalational agents are administered.

Opioid analgesics are especially useful postoperatively for the relief of surgical pain. The choice of drugs and routes of administration are varied. For immediate control of severe pain, iv administration of rapid-acting drugs (fentanyl, sufentanil) are practical but will probably have to be repeated. Meperidine has a fairly rapid effect that will persist longer. Morphine is also excellent for postoperative pain, because it lasts longer but its onset is slower.

When patients return to the wards, most opioids are no longer given by iv route but rather im because of the fear of respiratory depression from the high initial concentrations seen after iv injection. As discussed earlier, postoperative analgesia is frequently intermittent and inadequate. Other routes or techniques for analgesia are being increasingly used, including patient controlled analgesia (PCA) pumps and epidural or intraspinal opioids. Spinally administered opioids are also used intraoperatively alone or in combination with general anesthesia. Spinal opioids have been beneficial for the relief of chronic pain syndromes.

Opioid analgesics have a role in the critical care unit, where they are used not only for relief of pain but also to help maintain patient comfort while on mechanical ventilation. The pharmacologic effects of the opioids make them excellent drugs for the mechanically ventilated patient. Depression of the cough reflex increases tolerance of the endotracheal tube; depression of ventilation helps prevent the patient from "fighting the ventilator"; sedation decreases anxiety; and analgesia increases patient comfort. No other single class of drugs will produce all these benefits for the mechanically ventilated patient.

OPIOID AGONIST–ANTAGONISTS AND PARTIAL AGONISTS

The agonist–antagonists and partial agonist drugs are characterized by their binding to opioid receptors, and the various effects produced reflect this binding (Table 9-1). The morphine-like drugs (agonists) are noted for their mu receptor activity—supraspinal analgesia, dose-dependent respiratory depression, and euphoria. Agonists–antagonists are thought to bind to mu receptors and can compete with the agonist for these sites. At mu receptors, they may either exert no action (competitive antagonist), or they may exert limited actions (partial agonists).[1] Buprenorphine (and the investigational drugs meptazinol, profodol, and propiram) have a high affinity for mu receptors but a low intrinsic activity (partial agonists). Nalorphine, pentazocine, nalbuphine, and butorphanol are competitive antagonists at mu receptors (and block the effects of morphine-like drugs) but have agonistic activity at other receptors (kappa and sigma). These drugs are classified as agonist–antagonists. It is believed that these drugs produce their analgesic and respiratory depressant effects by interaction with kappa receptors and that their psychomimetic and dysphoric effects are mediated by actions at the sigma receptors (Table 9-1). Agonist–antagonist opioid drugs are useful for the study of the opioid receptors and have stimulated the search for opioids with high analgesic potency, absent or limited respiratory depression, and low abuse potential.

PENTAZOCINE

Pentazocine appears to produce its analgesic effects primarily by its agonistic activity at the kappa receptors. Parenterally, pentazocine is approximately one fourth as potent as morphine but exhibits a ceiling to both its respiratory depressant and analgesic effects. Doses beyond 30 to 50 mg do not produce proportionate increases in respiratory depression or analgesia. However, as the dose is increased, there is a high incidence of dysphoric, psychomimetic, and hallucinatory effects.

Pentazocine-related cardiovascular changes may be particularly significant to patients with reduced myocardial reserve. Pentazocine produces increases in systemic and pulmonary artery pressures, left ventricular end-diastolic pressure and cardiac work.[124] It increases plasma epinephrine and norepinephrine concentrations unrelated to respiratory depression or carbon dioxide accumulation.[1]

Pentazocine has limited use for the anesthesiologist because of its dysphoric and cardiovascular effects as well as its limited analgesic effects. It also has significant abuse potential and can produce physical dependency. If given in sufficient doses to subjects dependent upon agonist analgesics, pentazocine produces withdrawal symptoms as a result of its mu antagonistic actions.[1]

BUTORPHANOL

Butorphanol is a moderately potent analgesic that appears to have weak antagonistic effects at the mu receptors. It can be used before or after morphine-like drugs without tremendously altering their analgesic or anesthetic properties. However, butorphanol has been demonstrated to improve ventilation and the response to carbon dioxide following fentanyl, nitrous oxide, isoflurane anesthesia.[125]

Butorphanol is approximately five times more potent than morphine. A parenteral dose of 2 to 3 mg produces respiratory depression and analgesia equivalent to approximately 10 mg of morphine with an onset, peak, and duration of action similar to that of morphine.[1] Like pentazocine, its ventilatory depressant, analgesic, and anesthetic sparing effects do not increase proportional to dose and are limited. In dogs, butorphanol decreases the MAC for enflurane by 11% at a dose of 0.1 mg·kg^{-1}.[20] Doses 40 times larger do not further decrease MAC. Patients given 0.15 or 0.3 mg·kg^{-1} are easily aroused and follow commands appropriately (Moldenhauer CC et al, personal communication). Although butorphanol is limited as a primary anesthetic, it has successfully been used in conjunction with nitrous oxide or the potent inhalational agents in a balanced technique. Its cardiovascular effects are similar to those of pentazocine. The adjuvant agents used to produce balanced anesthesia in combination with butorphanol will increase myocardial depression, which

could be significant in cardiovascularly impaired patients, but is probably not significant in healthy patients.

The psychomimetic effects of butorphanol are similar to those of pentazocine at equianalgesic doses, but the incidence is somewhat less.[1] Since butorphanol has minimal mu receptor actions, it does not suppress or produce a withdrawal syndrome in patients dependent upon morphine-like drugs. Its abuse potential is considered minimal.

NALBUPHINE

Nalbuphine is structurally related to the mu agonist oxymorphone and the antagonist naloxone.[1] It produces its analgesic effects at kappa receptors and is a moderately potent antagonist at mu receptors. It is considered equipotent to morphine at analgesic doses; 10 mg of im nalbuphine is approximately equivalent to 10 mg of im morphine. Nalbuphine has a similar onset, peak, and duration of effect to morphine. However, like other agonist–antagonist opioids, nalbuphine is limited in its effects. A dose of 0.5 mg·kg^{-1} of nalbuphine given iv in dogs reduced enflurane MAC by 8%.[20] Doses as high as 20 mg·kg^{-1} did not further decrease MAC. A ceiling effect for analgesia and ventilatory depression by nalbuphine has also been demonstrated in volunteers given nalbuphine or morphine in successive 0.15 mg·kg^{-1} doses.[126] Successive doses of morphine produced increasing ventilatory depression and analgesia to experimental pain. The initial dose of nalbuphine resulted in similar pain reduction and ventilatory depression as seen with morphine. However, further doses did not increase analgesia or ventilatory depression, and the authors concluded that the ceiling effect for respiratory depression of nalbuphine is paralleled by its limited analgesic effects. This study confirmed an earlier study that demonstrated a ceiling effect for respiratory depression by nalbuphine at 30 mg·70 kg^{-1}, which was equivalent to a morphine dose of 20 mg·70 kg^{-1}.[127] In surgical patients, nalbuphine doses as high as 3 mg·kg^{-1} were not sufficient to produce anesthesia and required the addition of diazepam, nitrous oxide, or halothane.[128] The P$_{CO_2}$ remained at 45 mm Hg or less. Unlike pentazocine or butorphanol, nalbuphine does not appear to produce deleterious hemodynamic effects when given to patients with stable coronary artery disease or acute myocardial infarction.[1, 128]

Nalbuphine produces fewer psychic side-effects than other agonist–antagonists at analgesic doses. It may produce an abstinence syndrome in subjects dependent upon morphine-like drugs.[1] The abuse potential is similar to that of pentazocine.

Because of the lower incidence of psychic side-effects and the hemodynamic stability noted with even large doses of nalbuphine, it has proved to be an effective drug to reverse the ventilatory depression of mu agonist–type drugs while maintaining reasonable analgesia. Nalbuphine has been shown to antagonize ventilatory depression produced by moderate and large doses of fentanyl.[129, 130] Large doses (0.1 to 0.3 mg·kg^{-1} iv) of nalbuphine have been used to antagonize opioid-induced ventilatory depression in noncardiac patients without adverse sequelae. In post–cardiac surgery patients, incremental doses (15 µg·kg^{-1}) of nalbuphine up to a total of 1 to 10 mg effectively decreased P$_{CO_2}$ below 50 mm Hg, allowing extubation of the trachea of patients in the intensive care unit following fentanyl doses as high as 120 µg·kg^{-1}.[130] Adequate analgesia was maintained. Although the hemodynamic effects produced by nalbuphine are minimal, the rapid, partial reversal of the analgesia produced by mu agonists could result in significant catecholamine release. Titration to response is therefore recommended, especially in patients with limited cardiac reserve. Furthermore, respiratory depression will be produced by the nalbuphine itself. There is a ceiling to the depression, but, nonetheless, it is significant. The analgesia also has a ceiling, and, in cases of severe pain, nalbuphine may not be adequate for pain control. Finally, renarcotization is a possibility, especially when lower doses of nalbuphine are titrated to minimal reversal of ventilatory depression.

BUPRENORPHINE

Buprenorphine is a partial mu agonist that is highly lipophilic and can be administered sublingually, im, or iv. Buprenorphine is 25 to 50 times more potent than morphine and produces analgesia and other CNS effects that are qualitatively similar to those of morphine.[1] Intramuscular doses of 0.4 mg, equivalent to about 10 mg of morphine, have a slower onset of effect and a prolonged duration of action. Peak respiratory depression may not occur for 3 hours. There is little relationship between the plasma concentration and duration of effect.

Depression of ventilation and other effects of buprenorphine can be prevented by prior administration of naloxone. However, because buprenorphine dissociates very slowly from mu receptors, even large doses of naloxone will not readily reverse the effects of buprenorphine once they have been produced.[1, 131] Antagonism of ventilatory depression has been elicited by the stimulant effects of doxapram, but an infusion may be necessary because of the prolonged effect of buprenorphine.[131] Although there is probably a ceiling effect to the ventilatory depression produced by buprenorphine (it has been used to reverse fentanyl and sufentanil depression), significant clinical ventilatory depression has been reported.[131, 132]

Buprenorphine is not useful as a sole anesthetic but is a satisfactory supplement for balanced anesthesia and is useful for postoperative pain management.[131–133] Because it is only a partial mu agonist but dissociates slowly from the receptor, buprenorphine may limit the effect of morphine-like drugs when given in conjunction with them. Buprenorphine may not be a good premedicant drug if mu agonists are to be used for anesthesia. It will also decrease the ability of mu agonists to relieve severe pain.

Hemodynamic effects are mild, even in cardiovascularly impaired patients. Usually, decreases in heart rate are seen along with slight decreases in blood pressure.[131] The incidence of psychomimetic effects is low. A withdrawal syndrome, similar to that produced by morphine abstinence, can be seen when chronically administered buprenorphine is discontinued, with a delayed onset of up to 15 days. Buprenorphine can block or attenuate the subjective and physiologic effects of subcutaneous morphine (in doses of up to 120 mg) and has been suggested as a methadone substitute for the treatment of opioid addiction.[1] Buprenorphine has also been used as an epidural analgesic with effects similar to those of morphine.

DEZOCINE

Dezocine is an agonist–antagonist opioid that is as potent as, or slightly more potent than, morphine on a milligram per milligram basis. It has a more rapid onset and slightly shorter duration of action than morphine. Side-effects are similar, although dezocine does not appear to release histamine, at least in lower doses.[1, 134] Studies in dogs suggest that dezocine may be more efficacious as an anesthetic supplement than are other agonist–antagonists. A 58% reduction of enflurane MAC was produced in dogs with an iv dose of 20 mg·kg^{-1} of dezocine. This reduction is almost equal to the maximal reduction produced by the opioid agonists morphine and fentanyl (65%) studied under the same experimental conditions.[20, 89, 135] The upward slope of the dose–response curve at the 20 mg·kg^{-1} dose of dezocine suggested that greater reductions might be achieved at higher doses; however, this and larger doses were accompanied by severe hypotension or death in the enflurane anesthetized dog, primarily as a result of myocardial depression.[135] Dezocine is considerably more effective than other opioid agonist–antagonists as an anesthetic supplement, but further clinical studies are needed to determine its safety in large clinical doses.

ANTAGONISTS

Naloxone and naltrexone are oxymorphone derivatives that are generally considered to be "pure" antagonist opioids. Both drugs are competitive antagonists at mu, delta, kappa, and sigma opioid receptors. In moderate doses, they demonstrate no discernible activity except in the presence of stimulation of the opioid agonist receptors, either by drugs with agonist opioid effects or when the endogenous opioid systems are stimulated.[1] At very high doses, special effects of little clinical importance have been reported. Naloxone, at doses in excess of 0.3 mg·kg^{-1}, produces increases in systolic blood pressure and decreases performance on tests of memory.[1] Naltrexone, at high doses, may have produced mild dysphoria in one study, but no subjective effects were found in several other studies.[1]

Naloxone is used clinically to reverse unwanted opioid agonist effects (generally, ventilatory depression and sedation). Remember that all opioid effects will be reversed in parallel, including analgesia. The initial injection of large doses of naloxone postoperatively to patients given opioids for surgical procedures not only will rapidly reverse respiratory depression but will also suddenly unmask pain, which may result in significant sympathetic and cardiovascular stimulation that may be detrimental to the patient. Intravenous bolus injections of naloxone, 0.1 to 0.4 mg, have resulted in reports of hypertension, atrial and ventricular dysrhythmias, pulmonary edema, and cardiac arrest.[136] It is suggested that, where possible, ventilation should be supported and naloxone titrated in incremental iv doses of 20 to 40 μg until the patient is appropriately ventilating but still comfortable.

Naloxone is readily titrated to response because it has a very rapid onset of effect. Peak effects are seen within 1 to 2 minutes after iv injection, since naloxone rapidly enters the brain.[137] The pharmacologic duration of effect is dose-dependent, but, at appropriate doses, it can be expected to be approximately 1 to 4 hours.[1] The plasma half-time of naloxone is 60 to 90 minutes.[1, 137, 138] The concentration of naloxone in the brain parallels that in the plasma. Naloxone is primarily cleared by metabolism in the liver.[1, 138] The major metabolite is naloxone-3-glucuronide.

Because of naloxone's short half-time, there is a chance that renarcotization of patients may occur when naloxone has been used to reverse longer-acting opioids. Patients should be closely monitored for renarcotization. In one study, it was found that 5 to 10 μg·kg^{-1} of naloxone would readily reverse the ventilatory depression of 1.25 to 1.5 mg·kg^{-1} of morphine, but all the patients became renarcotized.[139] Satisfactory and prolonged reversal of morphine's ventilatory depression was achieved by a single 5 $\mu g \cdot kg^{-1}$ iv dose of naloxone followed 15 minutes later by a 10 $\mu g \cdot kg^{-1}$ im dose.

A more efficient method for titrating reversal is the use of a naloxone infusion. Intravenous infusions of naloxone in the range of 3 to 10 $\mu g \cdot kg^{-1} \cdot hr^{-1}$, following initial loading doses of 1.5 to 3.5 $\mu g \cdot kg^{-1}$ have successfully been used to reverse the ventilatory depression of high doses of morphine (2 $mg \cdot kg^{-1}$) and fentanyl (> 100 $\mu g \cdot kg^{-1}$).[140, 141] These infusion rates are also useful to suppress the side-effects of spinal opioids, especially ventilatory depression and pruritus.[142] Infusion rates should be increased or decreased according to patient response.

Naloxone has been reported to be useful in the treatment of overdosages of alcohol, benzodiazepines, barbiturates, and clonidine; diagnosing physical dependence; and treating opioid addicts. Naloxone can be used to reverse agonist–antagonist opioids, but, generally, higher doses of naloxone are necessary since it has a greater affinity for mu receptors than for kappa and sigma receptors. Animal studies indicate that naloxone may be beneficial in the treatment of endotoxic and hypovolemic shock.

Naltrexone is a longer-acting competitive mu receptor antagonist, which is available for oral administration. Naloxone is not used orally, because most is rapidly metabolized in its first passage through the liver.[1] Naltrexone is used in oral doses of 100 mg or greater to prevent the euphoric effects of opioids in addicted patients.[1] Peak plasma concentrations are found within 1 to 2 hours, and the plasma half-time is 10 hours. Naltrexone has also been used to counteract the side-effects of spinal opioids used for chronic pain therapy.

REFERENCES

1. Jaffe JH, Martin WR: Opioid analgesics and antagonists. In Gilman AG, Goodman LS, Rall TW et al (eds): The Pharmacological Basis of Therapeutics, 7th ed, p 491. New York, Macmillan, 1985
2. Foldes FF, Swerdlow M, Siker ES: Narcotics and Narcotic Antagonists, p 3. Springfield, Illinois, Charles C Thomas, 1964
3. Smith RR: Scopolamine-morphine anesthesia, with report of two hundred and twenty-nine cases. Surg Gynecol Obstet 7:414, 1908
4. Sexton JC: Death following scopolamine-morphine injection. Lancet 55:582, 1905
5. Neff W, Mayer EC, Perales M: Nitrous oxide and oxygen anesthesia with curare relaxation. Calif Med 66:67, 1947
6. Bailey P, Gerbode F, Garlington L: An anesthetic technique for cardiac surgery which utilizes 100% oxygen as the only inhalant. Arch Surg 76:437, 1958
7. Lowenstein E, Hallowell P, Levine FH et al: Cardiovascular response to large doses of intravenous morphine in man. N Engl J Med 281:1389, 1969
8. Stanley TH, Gray NG, Stanford W et al: The effects of high-dose morphine on fluid and blood requirements in open-heart operations. Anesthesiology 38:536, 1973
9. Lasagna L, Beecher HK: The analgesic effectiveness of nalorphine and nalorphine–morphine combinations in man. J Pharmacol Exp Ther 122:356, 1965
10. Martin WR: Opioid antagonists. Pharmacol Rev 10:452, 1967
11. Gilbert PE, Martin WR: The effects of morphine- and nalorphine-like drugs in the nondependent, morphine-dependent and cyclazocine-dependent chronic spinal dog. J Pharmacol Exp Ther 198:66, 1976
12. Martin WR, Eades CG, Thompson JA et al: The effects of mor-

phine- and nalorphine-like drugs in the nondependent and morphine-dependent chronic spinal dog. J Pharmacol Exp Ther 197:517, 1976
13. Lord JAH, Waterfield AA, Hughes J et al: Endogenous opioid peptides: Multiple agonists and receptors. Nature 267:495, 1977
14. Schultz R, Wuster M, Herz A: Pharmacological characterization of the epsilon receptor. J Pharmacol Exp Ther 216:604, 1981
15. Pasternak GW: High and low affinity opioid binding sites: Relationship to mu and delta sites. Life Sci 31:1302, 1982
16. Ling GSF, Spiegel K, Nishimura SL et al: Dissociation of morphine's analgesic and respiratory depressant actions. Eur J Pharmacol 86:487, 1983
17. Ward SJ, Takemori AE: Determination of the relative involvement of μ-opioid receptors in opioid-induced depression of respiratory rate, by use of β-funaltrexamine. Eur J Pharmacol 87:1, 1983
18. Akil H, Watson SJ, Young E et al: Endogenous opioids: biology and function. Ann Rev Neurosci 7:223, 1984
19. Kitahata LM, Collins JG, Robinson CJ: Narcotic effects on the nervous system. In Kitahata LM, Collins JG (eds): Narcotic Analgesics in Anesthesiology, p 57. Baltimore, Williams & Wilkins, 1982
20. Murphy MR, Hug CC Jr: The enflurane sparing effect of morphine, butorphanol, and nalbuphine. Anesthesiology 57:489, 1982
21. Lowenstein E: Morphine "anesthesia"—A perspective. Anesthesiology 35:563, 1971
22. Mummaneni N, Rao TLK, Montoya A: Awareness and recall with high-dose fentanyl–oxygen anesthesia. Anesth Analg 59:948, 1980
23. Barash P, Kopriva C, Giles R et al: Global ventricular function and intubation: Radionuclear profiles. Anesthesiology 53:S109, 1980
24. de Castro J, van de Water A, Wouters L et al: Comparative study of cardiovascular, neurological and metabolic side-effects of eight narcotics in dogs. Acta Anaesthesiol Belg 30:5, 1979
25. Moldenhauer CC, Hug CC Jr: Use of narcotic analgesics as anaesthetics. Clinics in Anaesthesiology 2(1): 1984
26. Reitan JA, Stengert KB, Wymore MC et al: Central vagal control of fentanyl induced bradycardia during halothane anesthesia. Anesth Analg 57:31, 1978
27. Laubie M, Schmitt H, Vincent M: Vagal bradycardia produced by microinjections of morphine-like drugs into the nucleus ambiguus in anesthetized dogs. Eur J Pharmacol 59:287, 1979
28. Liu WS, Bidwai AV, Stanley TH et al: Cardiovascular dynamics after large doses of fentanyl and fentanyl plus N_2O in the dog. Anesth Analg 55:168, 1976
29. Urthaler F, Isobe JH, Gilmour KE et al: Morphine and autonomic control of the sinus node. Chest 64:203, 1973
30. Urthaler F, Isobe JH, James TN: Direct and vagally mediated chronotropic effects of morphine studied by selective perfusion of the sinus node of awake dogs. Chest 68:222, 1975
31. Goldberg AH, Padget CH: Comparative effects of morphine and fentanyl on isolated heart muscle. Anesth Analg 48:978, 1969
32. Strauer BE: Contractile responses to morphine, piritramide, meperidine and fentanyl: A comparative study of effects on the isolated ventricular myocardium. Anesthesiology 37:304, 1972
33. Freye E: Cardiovascular effects of high doses of fentanyl, meperidine and naloxone in dogs. Anesth Analg 53:40, 1974
34. Lowenstein E, Whiting RB, Bittar DA: Local and neurally mediated effects of morphine on skeletal muscle vascular resistance. J Pharmacol Exp Ther 180:359, 1972
35. Ward JW, McGrath RL, Weil JV: Effects of morphine on the peripheral vascular response to sympathetic stimulation. Am J Cardiol 29:656, 1972
36. Rosow CE, Moss I, Philbin DM et al: Histamine release during morphine and fentanyl anesthesia. Anesthesiology 56:93, 1982

37. Flacke JW, Flacke WE, Bloor BC et al: Histamine release by four narcotics: A double-blind study in humans. Anesth Analg 66:723, 1987

38. McClain DA, Hug CC Jr: Intravenous fentanyl kinetics. Clin Pharmacol Ther 28:106, 1980

39. Hug CC Jr, Murphy MR: Fentanyl disposition in cerebrospinal fluid and plasma and its relationship to ventilatory depression in the dog. Anesthesiology 50:342, 1979

40. Hug CC Jr, Murphy MR, Rigel EP et al: Pharmacokinetics of morphine injected intravenously into the anesthetized dog. Anesthesiology 54:38, 1981

41. Bellville JW, Seed JC: The effect of drugs on the respiratory response to carbon dioxide. Anesthesiology 21:727, 1960

42. Forrest WH, Bellville JW: The effect of sleep plus morphine on the respiratory response to carbon dioxide. Anesthesiology 25:137, 1964

43. Becker L, Paulson B, Miller R et al: Biphasic respiratory depression after fentanyl-droperidol or fentanyl alone used to supplement nitrous oxide anesthesia. Anesthesiology 44:291, 1976

44. Kaufman RD, Agleh KA, Bellville JW: Relative potencies and duration of action with respect to respiratory depression of intravenous meperidine, fentanyl and alphaprodine in man. J Pharmacol Exp Ther 208:73, 1979

45. Ruskis AF: Effects of narcotics on the gastrointestinal tract, liver, and kidneys. In Kitahata LM, Collins JG (eds): Narcotic Analgesics in Anesthesiology, p 143. Baltimore, Williams & Wilkins, 1982

46. Radnay PA, Brodman E, Mankikar D et al: The effect of equianalgesic doses of fentanyl, morphine, meperidine and pentazocine on common bile duct pressure. Anaesthetist 29:26, 1980

47. de Lange S, Stanley TH, Boscoe JM et al: Catecholamine and cortisol responses to sufentanil-O_2 and alfentanil-O_2 anaesthesia during coronary artery surgery. Can Anaesth Soc J 30:248, 1983

48. Bovill JG, Sebel PS, Fiolet JWT et al: The influence of sufentanil on endocrine and metabolic responses to cardiac surgery. Anesth Analg 62:391, 1983

49. Clark RB, Seifen AB: Systemic medication during labor and delivery. In Wynn RM (ed): Obstetrics and Gynecology Annual, Vol 12, p 165. Norwalk, Connecticut, Appleton-Century-Crofts, 1983

50. Brooks GZ, Ngeow YF: Narcotics: mother, fetus, and neonate. In Kitahata LM, Collins JG (eds): Narcotic Analgesics in Anesthesiology, p 157. Baltimore, Williams & Wilkins, 1982

51. Goldberg M, Ishak S, Garcia C et al: Postoperative rigidity following sufentanil administration. Anesthesiology 63:199, 1985

52. Jaffe TB, Ramsey FM: Attenuation of fentanyl-induced truncal rigidity. Anesthesiology 58:562, 1983

53. Scamman FL: Fentanyl-O_2-N_2O rigidity and pulmonary compliance. Anesth Analg 63:332, 1983

54. Benthuysen JL, Smith NT, Sanford TT et al: Physiology of alfentanil-induced rigidity. Anesthesiology 64:440, 1986

55. Murphy MR, Hug CC Jr: Pharmacokinetics of intravenous morphine in patients anesthetized with enflurane-nitrous oxide. Anesthesiology 54:187, 1981

56. Stanski DR, Greenblatt DJ, Lowenstein E: Kinetics of intravenous and intramuscular morphine. Clin Pharmacol Ther 24:52, 1978

57. Dahlström B, Bolme P, Feychting J et al: Morphine kinetics in children. Clin Pharmacol Ther 26:354, 1979

58. Stanski DR, Paalzow L, Edlund PO: Morphine pharmacokinetics: GLC assay versus radioimmunoassay. J Pharm Sci 71:314, 1982

59. Yeh SY: Urinary excretion of morphine and its metabolites in morphine-dependent subjects. J Pharmacol Exp Ther 192:201, 1975

60. Brunk SF, Delle M: Morphine metabolism in man. Clin Pharmacol Ther 16:51, 1974

61. Olsen GD: Morphine binding to human plasma proteins. Clin Pharmacol Ther 17:31, 1975

62. Höllt V, Teschemacher H-J: Hydrophobic interactions responsible for unspecific binding of morphine-like drugs. Naunyn Schmiedebergs Arch Pharmacol 288:163, 1975

63. Kaufmann JJ, Semo NM, Koski WS: Microelectrometric titration measurement of the pK_a's and partition and drug distribution coefficients of narcotics and narcotic antagonists and their pH and temperature dependence. J Med Chem 18:647, 1975

64. Herz A, Teschemacher H-J: Activities and sites of antinociceptive action of morphine-like analgesics. In Harper NJ, Simmonds AB (eds): Advances in Drug Research, p 79. New York, Academic Press, 1971

65. Nishitateno K, Ngai SH, Finck AD et al: Pharmacokinetics of morphine: Concentrations in the serum and brain of the dog during hyperventilation. Anesthesiology 50:520, 1979

66. Lake CL, DiFazio CA, Moscicki JC et al: Reduction in halothane MAC: Comparison of morphine and alfentanil. Anesth Analg 64:807, 1985

67. Mather LE, Tucker GT, Pflug AE et al: Meperidine kinetics in man: Intravenous injections in surgical patients and volunteers. Clin Pharmacol Ther 17:21, 1975

68. Stambaugh JE, Wainer IW, Sanstead JK: The clinical pharmacology of meperidine—Comparison of routes of administration. J Clin Pharmacol 16:245, 1976

69. Klotz U, McHorse TS, Wilkinson GR et al: The effect of cirrhosis on the disposition and elimination of meperidine in man. Clin Pharmacol Ther 16:667, 1974

70. Fung DL, Asling JH, Eisele JH et al: A comparison of alphaprodine and meperidine pharmacokinetics. J Clin Pharmacol 20:37, 1980

71. Dunkerley R, Johnson R, Schenker S et al: Gastric and biliary excretion of meperidine in man. Clin Pharmacol Ther 20:546, 1976

72. Verbeeck RK, Branch RA, Wilkinson GR: Meperidine disposition in man: Influence of urinary pH and route of administration. Clin Pharmacol Ther 30:619, 1981

73. Szeto HH, Inturrisi CE, Houde R et al: Accumulation of normeperidine, an active metabolite of meperidine, in patients with renal failure or cancer. Ann Intern Med 86:738, 1977

74. Austin KL, Stapleton JV, Mather LE: Multiple intramuscular injections: A major source of variability in analgesic response to meperidine. Pain 8:47, 1980

75. Austin KL, Stapleton JV, Mather LE: Relationship between blood meperidine concentrations and analgesic response: A preliminary report. Anesthesiology 53:460, 1980

76. Hug CC Jr: Improving analgesic therapy. Anesthesiology 53:441, 1980

77. Stapleton JV, Austin KL, Mather LE: A pharmacokinetic approach to postoperative pain: Continuous infusion of pethidine. Anaesth Intensive Care 7:25, 1979

78. Reilly CS, Wood AJJ, Wood M: Variability of fentanyl pharmacokinetics in man. Computer predicted plasma concentrations for three intravenous dosage regimens. Anaesthesia 40:837, 1984

79. Mather LE: Clinical pharmacokinetics of fentanyl and its newer derivatives. Clin Pharmacokinet 8:422, 1983

80. Bentley JB, Borel JD, Nenad RE et al: Age and fentanyl pharmacokinetics. Anesth Analg 61:968, 1982

81. Koska AJ, Romagnoli A, Kramer WG: Effect of cardiopulmonary bypass on fentanyl distribution and elimination. Clin Pharmacol Ther 29:100, 1981

82. Haberer JP, Schoeffler P, Couderc E et al: Fentanyl pharmacokinetics in anaesthetized patients with cirrhosis. Br J Anaesth 54:1267, 1982

83. Bower S, Hull CJ: Comparative pharmacokinetics of fentanyl and alfentanil. Br J Anaesth 54:871, 1982

84. Murphy MR, Olson WA, Hug CC Jr: Pharmacokinetics of ³H-fentanyl in the dog anesthetized with enflurane. Anesthesiology 50:13, 1979

85. Hug CC Jr, Murphy MR: Tissue redistribution of fentanyl and termination of effect in rats. Anesthesiology 55:369, 1981

86. Hug CC Jr, Murphy MR, Sampson JF et al: Biotransformation of morphine and fentanyl in anhepatic dogs. Anesthesiology 55:A261, 1981

87. Harper MH, Hickey RF, Cromwell TH et al: The magnitude and duration of respiratory depression produced by fentanyl and fentanyl plus droperidol in man. J Pharmacol Exp Ther 199:464, 1976

88. Scott JC, Ponganis KV, Stanski DR: EEG quantitation of narcotic effect: The comparative pharmacodynamics of fentanyl and alfentanil. Anesthesiology 62:234, 1985

89. Murphy MR, Hug CC Jr: The anesthetic potency of fentanyl in terms of its reduction of enflurane MAC. Anesthesiology 57:485, 1982

90. Murphy MR, Hug CC Jr: Efficacy of fentanyl in reducing isoflurane MAC; antagonism by naloxone and nalbuphine. Anesthesiology 59:A338, 1983

91. Arndt JO, Mikat M, Parasher C: Fentanyl's analgesic, respiratory, and cardiovascular actions in relation to dose and plasma concentration in unanesthetized dogs. Anesthesiology 61:355, 1984

92. Sprigge JS, Wynands JE, Whalley DG et al: Fentanyl infusion anesthesia for aortocoronary bypass surgery: Plasma levels and hemodynamic response. Anesth Analg 61:972, 1982

93. Bovill JG, Sebel PS, Blackburn CL et al: The pharmacokinetics of sufentanil in surgical patients. Anesthesiology 61:502, 1984

94. Hecker BR, Lake CL, DiFazio CA et al: The decrease of the minimum alveolar anesthetic concentration produced by sufentanil in rats. Anesth Analg 62:987, 1983

95. Hall RI, Murphy MR, Hug CC Jr: The enflurane sparing effect of sufentanil in dogs. Anesthesiology 67:518, 1987

96. Camu F, Gepts E, Rucquoi M et al: Pharmacokinetics of alfentanil in man. Anesth Analg 61:657, 1982

97. Bovill JG, Sebel PS, Blackburn CL et al: The pharmacokinetics of alfentanil (R39209). A new opioid analgesic. Anesthesiology 57:439, 1982

98. Schüttler J, Stoeckel H: Alfentanil (R39209) a new, short-action opiate: Pharmacokinetics and preliminary clinical experience. Anaesthesist 31:10, 1982

99. McDonnell TE, Bartkowski RR, Bonilla FA et al: Nonuniformity of alfentanil pharmacokinetics in healthy adults. Anesthesiology 57:A236, 1982

100. Stanski DR, Hug CC Jr: Alfentanil—A kinetically predictable narcotic analgesic. Anesthesiology 57:435, 1982

101. Meuldermans WEG, Hurkmans RMA, Heykants JJP: Plasma protein binding and distribution of fentanyl, sufentanil, alfentanil and lofentanil in blood. Arch Int Pharmacodyn Ther 257:4, 1982

102. Hug CC Jr, Chaffman M: Alfentanil: Pharmacology and Uses in Anesthesia, p 1. Auckland, New Zealand, ADIS Press, 1984

103. Ausems ME, Hug CC Jr, Stanski DR et al: Plasma concentrations of alfentanil required to supplement nitrous oxide anesthesia for general surgery. Anesthesiology 65:362, 1986

104. Hall RI, Szlam F, Hug CC Jr: The enflurane-sparing effect of alfentanil in dogs. Anesth Analg 66:1287, 1987

105. Stoelting RK, Creasser CW, Gibbs PS: Circulatory effects of halothane added to morphine anesthesia in patients with coronary-artery disease. Anesth Analg 53:449, 1974

106. Bennett GM, Stanley TH: Cardiovascular effects of fentanyl during enflurane anesthesia in man. Anesth Analg 58:179, 1979

107. Eisele JH, Smith NT: Cardiovascular effects of 40 percent nitrous oxide in man. Anesth Analg 51:956, 1972

108. Stoelting RK, Gibbs PS: Hemodynamic effects of morphine and morphine–nitrous oxide in valvular heart disease and coronary-artery disease. Anesthesiology 38:45, 1973

109. Moffitt EA, Scovil JE, Barker RA et al: The effects of nitrous oxide on myocardial metabolism and hemodynamics during fentanyl or enflurane anesthesia in patients with coronary disease. Anesth Analg 63:1071, 1984

110. Eisele JH, Reitan JA, Massumi RA et al: Myocardial performance and N₂O analgesia in coronary-artery disease. Anesthesiology 44:16, 1976

111. Michaels I, Kay H, Barash P: Does nitrous oxide or a reduced FIO₂ alter hemodynamic function during high-dose fentanyl anesthesia? Anesthesiology 57:A44, 1982

112. Hall RI, Hug CC Jr: A quantitative description of the interaction of fentanyl and midazolam in reducing enflurane MAC in dogs. Can J Anaesth 1988 (in press)

113. Kissin I, Mason JO, Bradley EL Jr: Morphine and fentanyl hypnotic interactions with thiopental. Anesthesiology 67:331, 1987

114. Tomicheck RC, Rosow CE, Philbin DM et al: Diazepam–fentanyl interaction—Hemodynamic and hormonal effects in coronary artery surgery. Anesth Analg 62:881, 1983

115. Flacke JW, Davis LJ, Flacke WE et al: Effects of fentanyl and diazepam in dogs deprived of autonomic tone. Anesth Analg 64:1053, 1985

116. Salmenpera M, Peltola K, Takkunen O et al: Cardiovascular effects of pancuronium and vecuronium during high-dose fentanyl anesthesia. Anesth Analg 62:1059, 1983

117. Starr NJ, Sethna DH, Estafanous FG: Bradycardia and asystole following the rapid administration of sufentanil with vecuronium. Anesthesiology 64:521, 1986

118. Flacke JW, Bloor BC, Flacke WE et al: Reduced narcotic requirements by clonidine with improved hemodynamic and adrenergic stability in patients undergoing coronary artery bypass. Anesthesiology 67:11, 1987

119. Greenblatt DJ, Sellers EM, Shader RI: Drug disposition in old age. N Engl J Med 306:1081, 1982

120. Don HF, Dieppa RA, Taylor P: Narcotic analgesics in anuric patients. Anesthesiology 42:745, 1975

121. Ferrier C, Marty J, Bouffard Y et al: Alfentanil pharmacokinetics in patients with cirrhosis. Anesthesiology 62:480, 1985

122. Bentley JB, Borel JD, Gillespie TJ et al: Fentanyl pharmacokinetics in obese and nonobese patients. Anesthesiology 55:A117, 1981

123. Bentley JB, Finley JH, Humphrey LR et al: Obesity and alfentanil pharmacokinetics. Anesth Analg 62:251, 1983

124. Alderman EL, Barry WH, Graham AF et al: Hemodynamic effects of morphine and pentazocine differ in cardiac patients. N Engl J Med 287:623, 1972

125. Bowdle TA, Greichen SL, Bjurstrom RL et al: Butorphanol improves CO₂ response and ventilation after fentanyl anesthesia. Anesth Analg 66:517, 1987

126. Gal TJ, DiFazio CA, Moscicki J: Analgesic and respiratory depressant activity of nalbuphine: A comparison with morphine. Anesthesiology 57:367, 1982

127. Romagnoli A, Keats AS: Ceiling effect for respiratory depression by nalbuphine. Clin Pharmacol Ther 27:478, 1980

128. Lake CL, Duckworth EN, DiFazio CA et al: Cardiovascular effects of nalbuphine in patients with coronary or valvular heart disease. Anesthesiology 57:478, 1982

129. Latasch L, Probst S, Dudziak R: Reversal by nalbuphine of respiratory depression caused by fentanyl. Anesth Analg 63:814, 1984

130. Moldenhauer CC, Roach GW, Finlayson CD et al: Nalbuphine antagonism of ventilatory depression following high-dose fentanyl anesthesia. Anesthesiology 62:647, 1985

131. Heel RC, Brogden RN, Speight TM et al: Buprenorphine: A

review of its pharmacological properties and therapeutic efficacy. Drugs 17:81, 1979

132. Cook PJ, James IM, Hobbs KEF et al: Controlled comparison of i.m. morphine and buprenorphine for analgesia after abdominal surgery. Br J Anaesth 54:285, 1982

133. Kay B: A double-blind comparison between fentanyl and buprenorphine in analgesic-supplemented anesthesia. Br J Anaesth 52:453, 1980

134. Pandit SK, Kothary SP, Pandit UA et al: Double-blind placebo-controlled comparison of dezocine and morphine for postoperative pain relief. Can Anaesth Soc J 32:583, 1985

135. Hall RI, Murphy MR, Szlam F et al: Dezocine MAC reduction and evidence for myocardial depression in the presence of enflurane. Anesth Analg 66:1169, 1987

136. Smith G, Pinnock C: Naloxone—Paradox or panacea? Br J Anaesth 57:547, 1985

137. Ngai SH, Berkowitz BA, Yang JC et al: Pharmacokinetics of naloxone in rats and in man. Anesthesiology 44:398, 1976

138. Fishman J, Roffwarg H, Hellman L: Disposition of Naloxone-7,-8,-^{3}H in normal and narcotic-dependent men. J Pharmacol Exp Ther 187:575, 1973

139. Longnecker DE, Grazis PA, Eggers GNN: Naloxone for antagonism of morphine-induced respiratory depression. Anesth Analg 52:447, 1973

140. Johnston RE, Jobes DR, Kennell EM et al: Reversal of morphine anesthesia with naloxone. Anesthesiology 41:361, 1974

141. Shupak RD, Harp JR: Reversible narcotic coma for neuroanesthesia. Anesthesiology 55:A230, 1981

142. Rawal N, Schött U, Dahlström B et al: Influence of naloxone infusion on analgesia and respiratory depression following epidural morphine. Anesthesiology 64:194, 1986

Chapter 10   *James J. Richter*

Mechanisms of General Anesthesia

General anesthesia is the result of reversible changes in neurologic function caused by drugs that modulate synaptic communication. Intravenous agents interfere with membrane protein receptors and volatile agents interact with the hydrophobic regions of membrane lipids and proteins. This chapter summarizes the major work that supports the neurophysiologic and molecular theories about the action of anesthetics.[1,2] Dluzewski et al[3] focus on membrane actions of anesthetic molecules. These reviews[1,3] and their exhaustive bibliographies are good points of entry to the basic science literature. The intent of this chapter is to give a brief overview of the current theories of the mechanisms of both intravenous and volatile anesthetics, including a discussion concerning memory and amnesia.

Exhaustive reviews and critical analysis of the experimental evidence are available to satisfy the basic scientist or the anesthesiologist with research interests. Two recent volumes devoted to anesthetic mechanisms give thorough reviews of the many theories and approaches to mechanisms of action of anesthetics.[1,2] Dluzewski et al[3] focus on membrane actions of anesthetic molecules. These reviews[1,3] and their exhaustive bibliographies are good points of entry to the basic science literature. The intent of this chapter is to give a brief overview of the current theories of the mechanisms of both intravenous and volatile anesthetics, including a discussion concerning memory and amnesia.

The elements of general anesthesia that are frequently described include amnesia, analgesia, inhibition of noxious reflexes, and skeletal muscle relaxation.[4] Reversible changes in neurologic function cause loss of perception and reaction to pain, unawareness of immediate events, and loss of memory of those events.[5] The pharmacologic mechanisms for such reversible neurologic events include effects of drugs on synaptic communication and the physical-chemical behavior of volatile hydrocarbons in biologic membranes.

SYNAPTIC COMMUNICATION

Discussion of synaptic communication begins by reviewing the work of Sherrington,[6] who established that communication between neurons occurs at synaptic junctions and is the physiologic basis for central nervous system (CNS) function. The classic explanation states that a chemical neurotransmitter is released from the presynaptic ending, traverses the synaptic cleft, and binds to a receptor on the postsynaptic membrane. When occupied by a neurotransmitter molecule, the receptor complex induces electrochemical changes in the postsynaptic cell. Figure 10-1 is a generalized scheme to illustrate the concept of synaptic function. The neuropharmacologic basis for these concepts is reviewed by Cooper et al.[7]

Neurotransmitters can have either inhibitory or excitatory properties. Gamma-amino butyric acid (GABA) is the major inhibitory neurotransmitter in the brain and glycine is the major inhibitory neurotransmitter in the spinal cord.[8–10] Glutamate is the major excitatory neurotransmitter in the brain.

DRUG–RECEPTOR INTERACTIONS

Drug–receptor interactions have been described for most of the intravenous drugs used in anesthesia practice. Neuromuscular blockers bind to receptors and modulate (inhibit) the function of acetylcholine (ACh) on the motor end-plates of skeletal muscle cells. It was well established in 1975 that opioids work by occupying opiate receptors in the brain and

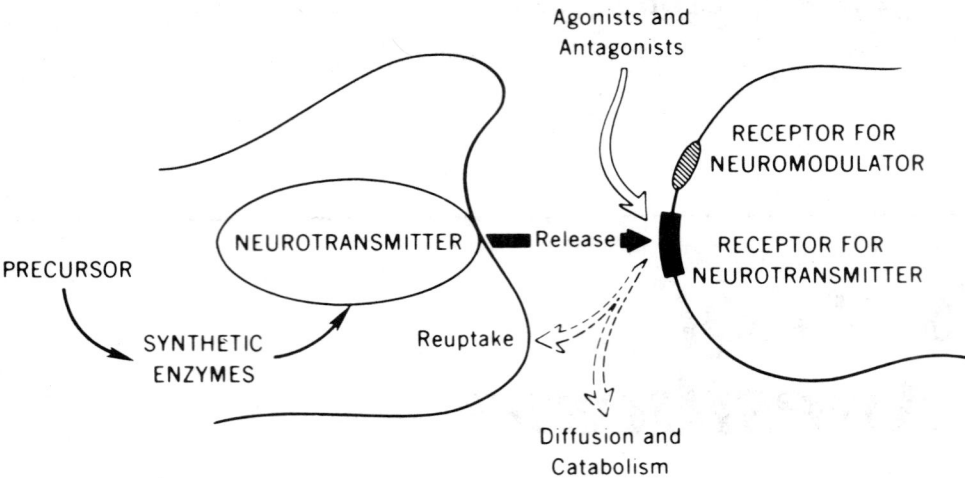

FIG. 10-1. Generalized schematic diagram of neurotransmitter function. (Reprinted with permission. Richter JJ: Current theories about the mechanisms of benzodiazepines and neuroleptic drugs. Anesthesiology 54:66, 1981.)

spinal cord. Analgesia results from the modulation of peptide function (endorphins and enkephalins), which are endogenous ligands for the opiate receptors.[5] Receptor mechanisms are recognized also for other drugs commonly used in intravenous anesthesia techniques, including benzodiazepines, barbiturates, and neuroleptic drugs.[4, 9]

MODULATION OF GABA FUNCTION

Data are accumulating that support the concept that several aspects of anesthesia may result from modulation of GABA function. Intravenous drugs such as benzodiazepines and barbiturates,[4] and even inhalation drugs,[11] have been shown to enhance inhibitory tone mediated by GABA. The inhibitory properties of GABA, a major neurotransmitter in mammalian brain, have been deduced from data about the metabolic turnover and receptor binding of the compound. Some convulsive drugs work by inhibiting the synthesis of GABA.[8] The consequent decreased tissue concentration of GABA results in a decrease in inhibitory tone of upper motor neurons, which leads to myoclonic seizure activity.[8] Other convulsants, such as picrotoxin and bicuculline, are GABA antagonists and bind directly to GABA receptors. The antagonistic action of these drugs prevents the normal inhibitory influence of GABA and results in seizure activity.[8, 9]

Systems other than motor activity are inhibited by the neurotransmitter function of GABA. Gillis et al[12] showed that GABA-mediated mechanisms are important in the CNS control of autonomic and cardiovascular function. Control of serotonin-releasing neurons may also be influenced by GABA.[13] In 1982 Antonaccio[14] suggested that GABA inhibits the flow of autonomic stimulation from the CNS. In 1987 Sample and DiMiccio[15] localized forebrain sites where GABA agonists and antagonists mediated cardiovascular function. They demonstrated that GABA-ergic centers in the brain stem modulate sympathetic tone and that GABA agonists depress sympathetic activity (blood pressure and heart rate). Their data suggest that sympathetic effects of GABA arise from sites in the caudal periventricular hypothalamus and that vagal effects of GABA arise from rostral periventricular hypothalamic regions.[15] Because the hypothalamus and limbic region of the brain is associated with emotional changes in humans, the authors speculate that decreased GABA-ergic tone may be responsible for cardiovascular changes that accompany emotional arousal.[15]

The potential role of GABA-mediated mechanisms for control of sympathetic activity could be quite significant in the development of drugs useful in anesthesia practice. Certainly, the control of sympathetic activity is of central importance in the administration of general and regional anesthesia.

As a neurotransmitter, GABA mediates inhibition of neurons by binding to a receptor protein in postsynaptic membranes. Benzodiazepines bind to specific receptors that are contingent to the GABA receptor. The GABA–benzodiazepine receptor complex has been designated the GABA$_A$ receptor.[16] When occupied by drug molecules, the benzodiazepine receptor reacts allosterically with the adjacent GABA receptor in a fashion that enhances the inhibitory tone. The GABA$_A$ receptor causes neural inhibition by opening a transmembrane channel for conducting chloride ions.

Very recent and exciting research has outlined much of the detail of the macromolecular structure and function of the GABA$_A$ receptor in membrane action.[16] Using bovine cerebral cortex, Sigel and Barnard[17] purified the receptor complex and Casalotti et al[18] identified α and β subunits. The α subunit binds benzodiazepines and the β subunit binds GABA. Schofield et al[16] have described the amino acid sequences of the α and β subunits of the GABA$_A$ receptor. Although the receptor macromolecule is too large and complex for direct-sequencing studies, the amino acid sequences of peptide fragments were determined. Synthetic DNA probes were prepared to match the templates of the peptide amino acid chains. The synthetic DNA probes were then used to screen libraries of DNA from bovine brain. These steps allowed the identification of hybridizing clones of DNA where the probe DNA matched up with fragments of nucleic acids representing brain tissue. The resulting DNA was subsequently used to deduce the code and the amino acid sequence of the entire receptor macromolecule.

Analysis of the amino acid sequence of the receptor subunits yields information about the structural and functional details of the membrane proteins. Specific sequences of hydrophobic amino acids are identified as the transmembrane portion of the receptor. Branches of the protein that project into the intracellular and extracellular environments are also described (Fig. 10-2). In addition to the transmembrane structure, functional aspects of the receptor proteins begin to emerge from analysis of the amino acid sequence. A unique proline residue in the transmembrane portion of the protein causes a flexure in the structure that might change and thereby control the transport of chloride ion when neurotransmitters bind to the receptor portion of the macromolecule.

Furthermore, Schofield et al[16] have recognized remarkably similar domains in the structures of GABA$_A$ receptors and nicotinic receptors for acetylcholine (nAChR). Transmembrane portions of the two receptors have very similar amino acid sequences, as do some parts of the extracellular portions of the molecules. These structural similarities imply that common mechanisms are responsible for functional aspects of binding receptors and activation of ion channels across membranes. Schofield et al suggest that the structural similarities between GABA$_A$ and ACh receptors indicate that they may both belong to a " . . . super family of chemically gated ion channel receptors."[18]

An elegant confirmation of the authenticity of the receptor structure is the synthesis and function of the GABA$_A$ complex in Xenopus oocyte membranes. Cloned DNA encoding the receptor structure was inserted into plasmids and in vitro transcription produced appropriate messenger RNA. Purified RNA was then injected into Xenopus oocytes that subsequently synthesized and inserted GABA$_A$ receptors into the cell membrane. With the intact GABA$_A$ receptor, the oocyte demonstrated an appropriate current response to GABA, indicating correct functional assembly of the membrane protein complex.[18]

Detailed explanations of membrane structure and function will provide a framework for the development of new and more specific drugs that will modulate synaptic communication and improve the specificity and safety of general anesthesia.

BENZODIAZEPINES AND GABA FUNCTION

It is well established that most properties of benzodiazepines result from drug–receptor interactions that modulate GABA function. The properties of benzodiazepines are (1) antianxiety; (2) anticonvulsant; (3) sedation; (4) centrally mediated muscle relaxation; and (5) amnesia. Costa and Guidotti[19] proposed that anticonvulsant and sedative properties result from enhanced inhibitory effects of GABA caused by benzodiazepines bound to receptors that are contingent with, but separate from, GABA receptors.

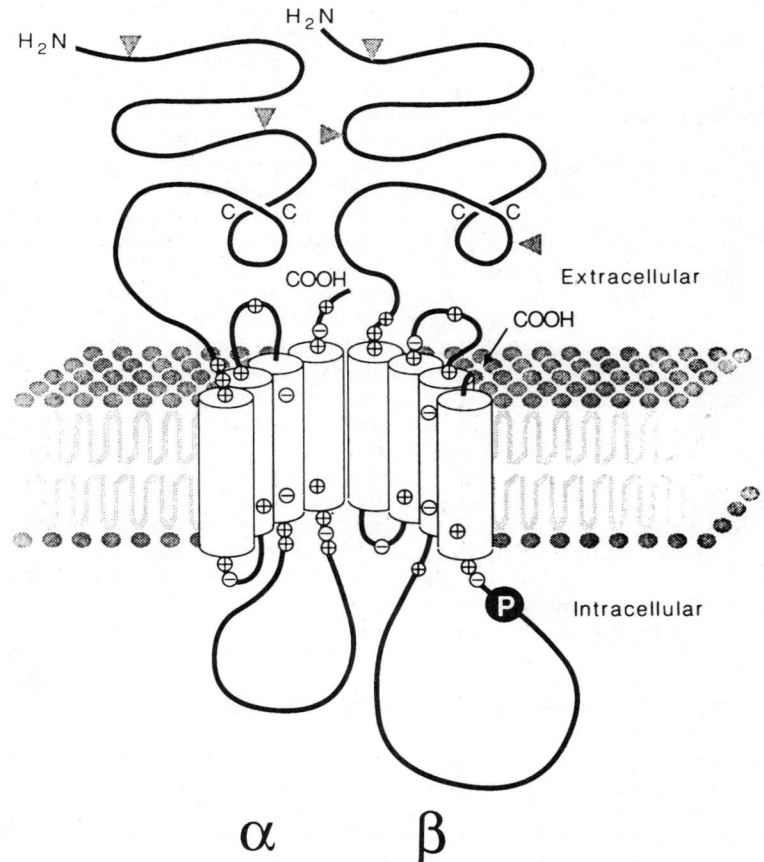

FIG. 10-2. Schematic diagram of the GABA$_A$ receptor in the lipid matrix of a membrane. The binding site for GABA is the extracellular portion of the β subunit. The binding site for benzodiazepines is the extracellular portion of the α subunit. The generalized structure may be similar for other types of membrane receptor complexes. (Reprinted with permission. Schofield PR et al: Sequence and functional expression of the GABA$_A$ receptor shows a ligand-gated receptor super-family. Nature 328:221, 1987. © 1987 Macmillan Magazines Limited.)

The muscle relaxation and anti-anxiety properties of benzodiazepines have been attributed to glycinemimetic effects.[10] The drugs have been shown to bind to glycine receptors, mimicking the inhibitory tone of glycine neurotransmission in the brain stem and spinal cord.[9, 10]

Benzodiazepine antagonists have been identified recently. An imidazobenzodiazepine, flumazenil, antagonizes the sedative and hypnotic effects of midazolam in human volunteers.[20] During infusions to maintain constant plasma concentrations of midazolam, flumazenil promptly caused all seven subjects to become fully oriented within 2 min after administration.[20] The antagonist did not induce anxiety or agitation in the subjects. The antagonist data are even further support for the concept of benzodiazepine–receptor interactions as the basis for pharmacologic activity of this class of drugs.

BARBITURATES AND GABA FUNCTION

Although barbiturates have been used much longer, it has only been since the discovery of benzodiazepine receptors that similar mechanisms have been demonstrated for barbiturate mechanisms. Receptors for barbiturates are adjacent to GABA receptors, and the barbiturate-occupied receptor is thought to enhance the inhibitory tone of GABA and thereby exert the anticonvulsant and sedative effects of these drugs.[21] Olsen has summarized the experimental data suggesting that a GABA receptor–ionophore complex of proteins exists in synaptic membranes, with associated receptors for benzodiazepines and barbiturates.[22] GABA-occupied receptors produce inhibitory actions by increasing membrane conductance to chloride ion. When associated receptors are occupied by benzodiazepine or barbiturate molecules, the chloride conductance is increased further, enhancing the effect of GABA.

Experimental evidence cited above suggests strongly that benzodiazepines and barbiturates modulate synaptic function by enhancing the inhibitory effects of GABA. There are, however, probably many other neurochemical mechanisms that might be involved in the pharmacologic mechanisms of sedative and hypnotic drugs. Richards and Strupinski have shown recently that pentobarbital depressed miniature end-plate synaptic potentials but did not change resting membrane potentials in guinea pig olfactory cortex neurons.[23] These investigators found no evidence for a GABA-mediated change in membrane potential from barbiturate action using drug concentrations that span the effective anesthetic range.[23] In a subsequent report, Pocock and Richards[24] described the inhibition of catecholamine release from bovine adrenal chromaffin cells by pentobarbital. Pentobarbital inhibited competitively the action of nicotinic agonists that stimulate release of catecholamines. They also showed that pentobarbital decreased calcium ion influx, and they speculated that such a mechanism could inhibit release of neurotransmitters, thereby causing CNS depression.[24] Both of these articles illustrate that the mechanisms of action of CNS-active drugs are much more complex and subtle than merely enhancing GABA-mediated inhibition.

STEROID ANESTHETICS AND GABA FUNCTION

Steroid anesthetic molecules were shown to interact with the GABA receptor complex by Harrison *et al* in 1987.[25] In an experimental preparation of rat hippocampal neurons, they showed that steroid anesthetic molecules caused a marked prolongation of postsynaptic inhibitory currents mediated by GABA. In this preparation, synaptically released GABA nor-

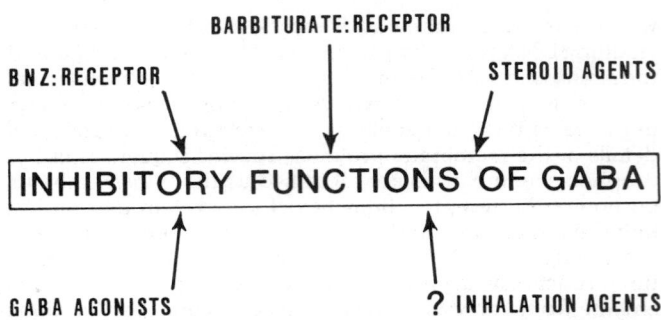

FIG. 10-3. Drugs that modulate GABA. Several drugs used in anesthesia practice have been shown to depress some CNS functions by enhancing the inhibitory effects of this endogenous neurotransmitter.

mally binds to receptors and causes an increased chloride conductance in the postsynaptic membrane. The steroid molecules prolong this chloride conductance and thereby enhance the inhibitory actions of GABA. Whereas barbiturates and benzodiazepines bind to specific receptors contingent to the GABA-receptor–chloride-channel complex of proteins, they have not identified such specific binding of steroid anesthetic molecules to membrane proteins. Specific binding of steroids might be masked from experimental detection by nonspecific interaction of the steroids with membrane sites. Nevertheless, this report[25] does strongly suggest that the mechanism of steroid-induced anesthesia may involve modulating GABA function.

Cheng and Brunner[26] have proposed that volatile anesthetics act by potentiating the inhibitory effects of GABA-mediated neurotransmission. Intravenously administered GABA does not induce general anesthesia or act as an anticonvulsant because the molecule does not cross the blood–brain barrier and is also subject to metabolic transformation. In 1985, however, Cheng and Brunner[26] described the use of a GABA analog that does induce general anesthesia. This report is strong evidence for a GABA-mediated mechanism as a central aspect of general anesthesia. It also suggests the possibility of synthesizing prospectively designed molecules that might be more specific anesthetics without undesirable side effects. Figure 10-3 is a summary of drugs that have been shown to modulate the inhibitory functions of GABA.

NEUROLEPTIC DRUGS AND DOPAMINE RECEPTORS

The effects of neuroleptic drugs (*e.g.*, droperidol) are thought to result from interaction with dopaminergic receptors. Although the details are complex, the general concept is that neuroleptic drugs bind to receptors and modulate the neurotransmitter effects of dopamine.[27]

The common element in the mechanisms of intravenous anesthetic agents is the modulation of synaptic function that results from drug–receptor interactions as summarized in Table 10-1.

CURRENT THEORIES FOR MECHANISMS OF VOLATILE ANESTHETICS

Volatile agents probably cause general anesthesia by modulating synaptic function from within cell membranes rather than direct binding to receptors in the fashion of intravenous

TABLE 10-1   Summary of Drug–Receptor Interactions for Intravenous Agents Used to Produce General Anesthesia*

CLASS OF DRUGS	RECEPTOR	NEUROTRANSMITTERS MODULATED
Narcotics	Opiate	Enkephalins
Muscle relaxants	Motor end plate	Acetylcholine
Benzodiazepines	Benzodiazepine	GABA
Barbiturates	Barbiturate	GABA
Steroid anesthetics	Specific membrane site†	GABA
Neuroleptics	Dopaminergic	Dopamine

* Drug–receptor interactions modify normal physiologic processes caused by "endogenous ligands" or neurotransmitters.
† Specific membrane receptors for steroid molecules have not been identified.
(Modified from Richter JJ: Neuropharmacologic mechanisms of general anesthesia. In Barash PG [ed]: Refresher Courses in Anesthesiology, vol 14, p 199. Philadephia, JB Lippincott, 1986.)

TABLE 10-2   Theories of Anesthetic Mechanisms

EXPERIMENTAL OBSERVATIONS	MOLECULAR THEORIES	NEURORPHYSIOLOGIC EFFECTS
Lipid solubility/potency correlations	Meyer-Overton hypothesis	
Pressure reversal data	Membrane expansion	Modulation of synaptic communication
	Membrane disordering	
Physicochemical changes of lipid bilayers	Lipid perturbation	
	Lipid phase transitions	
	Lipid protein interactions	
Luciferace inhibition	Direct protein actions	

Detailed explanations of the experimental data and the molecular theories are presented in recent reviews by Dluzewski, et al[3] and Miller.[1]

agents. In recent reviews[1, 2] Miller discussed the major details of the theories of molecular mechanisms of action of anesthetics. Because anesthesia can be produced by a wide range of chemically distinct compounds (e.g., inert gases, alcohols, volatile hydrocarbons, steroids, and so forth), it is unlikely that a unique "receptor" exists for anesthetic drugs. The potency of various anesthetic drugs has been correlated with their physical properties.[28] Lipid solubility and pressure reversal studies have characterized the physical theories about anesthetic action. Such studies have implicated the lipid matrix of cell membranes as the most important site for the pharmacologic effects of anesthetics.[1] The various physical and chemical theories of anesthetic mechanisms are outlined in Table 10-2.

NEUROPHYSIOLOGIC EFFECTS OF VOLATILE ANESTHETICS

Five steps of synaptic communication have been identified as possible sites for the action of anesthetics.[29]

1. Synthesis and transport of neurotransmitters
2. Release of neurotransmitter from the presynaptic cell
3. Removal of neurotransmitter from the synaptic cleft
4. Binding of neurotransmitter to the postsynaptic receptor
5. Electrochemical changes at the postsynaptic membrane

Many observations have suggested that volatile anesthetics depress excitatory transmission regardless of the specific neurotransmitter. Sodium and chloride ion channels in post-synaptic membranes are affected by volatile agents.[29] There have been little data to suggest that volatile anesthetics affect the synthesis, release, or binding of neurotransmitters.[29]

Richards has suggested that general anesthesia results from the disruption of information transfer at a synaptic level of organization in the CNS.[30] Although basic processes of synaptic function are similar in all systems, the susceptibilities of various synaptic groups to volatile agents are different. Richards suggests that the specific nature of channel structure or the activation mechanisms determines the sensitivity of each synapse to volatile agents.[30] In a brief review, Halsey notes that synapses in the region of the ventrobasal thalamus may be particularly sensitive to manipulation by volatile anesthetics.[31] However, a single brain region for the control of consciousness or the anesthetic state has not been identified. The brain stem reticular activating system has been implicated in the control of wakefulness, and a variety of anesthetics are known to alter the neurophysiologic activity of the region.[32] It is clear that there is no exclusive brain region for the pharmacologic control of consciousness or all of the CNS elements of general anesthesia.

MOLECULAR MECHANISMS OF VOLATILE ANESTHETICS

The dominant theories of the molecular mechanisms by which volatile agents affect membrane function are based on the lipid solubility of the drugs and on experimental demonstrations of pressure reversal of anesthesia. An excellent detailed review appeared in 1983 by Dluzewski et al.[3]

All discussions of anesthetic mechanisms acknowledge the early observations of the Meyer-Overton lipid solubility theory[1-3]. The anesthetic potency of volatile agents correlates directly with the relative solubility of each drug.[28] The conclusion is that the primary molecular actions of anesthetics occur in the lipid portion of cell membranes. Potential membrane regions for anesthetic actions include hydrophobic areas of proteins and protein–lipid interface regions, as well as the phospholipid matrix.

VOLUME EXPANSION THEORIES

In the 1950s it was demonstrated that high pressures (100–200 atmospheres) reverse the anesthetic effects of several drugs.[1, 33] The conclusion was that the high pressure could be compressing the volume of cell membranes. If membrane compression reverses anesthesia, the drugs could be causing anesthesia by increasing membrane volume at normal atmospheric pressure. Miller[33 34] has generated much data to support the concept, and it has been expanded to a "critical-volume theory" for the mechanism of action of anesthetics.

Pressure reversal experiments have also led to a "multisite" expansion hypothesis from Halsey's laboratory.[35] Anesthetic potencies of drug mixtures were shown to be additive in some cases, but other mixtures were not additive. The interpretation of such data is consistent with the concept that general anesthesia is caused by membrane expansion at several types of molecular sites and that different drugs may be acting at different sites.[35] The studies included intravenous as well as inhalation drugs.[36] Halsey's summary of the concept describes several critical hydrophobic sites that are susceptible to expansion caused by different drugs. The sites of anesthetic action must have varying sensitivity to drugs. Such sites could include hydrophobic portions of proteins as well as membrane lipids.[35] Expansion of critical hydrophobic sites would modify protein activity and thereby modulate synaptic function.[29, 35]

The effects of anesthetic agents on pressure-reversible binding of ACh to cholinergic membranes prepared from the electric eel have been studied.[33] Firestone et al[37] found that most agents did increase ACh binding, but the drug concentrations required were about four times greater than the amounts sufficient to cause signs of anesthesia (loss of righting reflex) in experimental animals. They furthermore noted some paradoxical results where the most potent anesthetics did not have similar effects on the binding assay. Their conclusion is that the electroplaque model does not reflect all of the properties of the unidentified CNS sites of action of anesthetics.[37]

Dodson and Miller[38] showed that anesthesia (loss of righting reflex in amphibians) could be reversed with pressure when anesthesia was produced by either an alcohol (octanol) or by a peptide, the leucine-enkephalin analog BW831C. The octanol-induced anesthesia was unaffected by naloxone, but the peptide-induced anesthesia was reversed by the opiate antagonist. They interpret their data to reveal distinct sites for the action of the different anesthetic molecules.[38] Although the sites of action are different, they share the properties of hydrophobic environments and susceptibility to pressure reversal.

THEORIES ABOUT FLUIDITY OF MEMBRANE LIPIDS

In the lipid matrix of cell membranes, individual molecules have well-defined, limited motion that has been described as *fluidity*. Measured by physicochemical changes (*e.g.*, order

parameter) of probe molecules inserted into experimental membranes, changes in fluidity caused by anesthetics have been described by several investigators, including Trudell.[39] Such observations have suggested that anesthetics caused "disordered" (*i.e.*, more fluid) motions of membrane lipids and possibly lateral separation of fluidity phases within membranes that indirectly alter protein behavior; however, it has also been argued that such fluid changes are caused by anesthetics only at very high concentrations (partial pressures).

In contrast, Veda et al use a different manifestation of lipid fluidity to suggest that anesthetics weaken lipid–water interactions rather than lipid–lipid interactions.[40] They showed that halothane decreased the surface viscosity (i.e., increased fluidity) of an artificial monolayer of phospholipid spread on a water surface.[40] Consequently, these investigators suggest that the primary effect of anesthetics is to weaken lipid–water interfaces. At this point there are no direct biologic models to relate the postulated effect to membrane functional changes.

ANESTHETIC–PROTEIN INTERACTIONS

Franks and Lieb have described details of the effects of anesthetics on the enzyme luciferase, a soluble protein isolated from fireflies.[41-43] The enzyme activity is inhibited by clinically effective concentrations of anesthetics. They have shown that anesthetics appear to participate in competitive inhibition by preventing the substrate (luciferin) from binding to a specific site on the enzyme macromolecule.[42] They suggest that despite the structural and chemical diversity of general anesthetic agents, the drugs might act by preventing endogenous ligands from binding to specific protein sites.

Franks and Lieb have also shown that the luciferase model is consistent with the "cut off" effect associated with certain types of anesthetics.[43] In a homologous series of some compounds (n-alkanes, h-alcohols), anesthetic potency stops at a specific point as larger molecules in the series are tested. They have demonstrated that the same cut-off effect is exhibited when homologous series of anesthetic compounds are tested for inhibition of luciferase activity. They claim that the cut-off effect is a consequence of drug molecules binding to an amphiphilic protein site with fixed dimensions. The implication is that the critical site cannot accommodate molecules above a certain size, rendering such larger compounds ineffective as inhibitors of the enzyme (and therefore presumably ineffective as anesthetics at some structurally similar site of anesthetic action).[43]

SATURABLE BINDING OF HALOTHANE

New evidence in 1987 by Evers et al[44] that rat brains have saturable binding sites for halothane may have dramatic effects on the future direction of research and theories of anesthetic mechanisms. So far in this chapter, proposed mechanisms of volatile anesthetics can be grouped into theories of nonspecific, general membrane perturbations (volume expansion, *etc.*) or direct effects of anesthetics on specific membrane proteins. Evers et al[44] presented data suggesting specific membrane sites that become saturated with anesthetic molecules. By using nuclear magnetic resonance ^{19}F-NMR labeling of halothane, they measured both the brain concentration and the molecular environments of halothane in anesthetized rats. *In vitro* and *in vivo* experiments showed that brain tissue became saturated with halothane at inspired concentrations of 2.5%. Half-maximal brain concentration was observed with 1.2% halothane-inspired concentration, which is the ED_{50} for halothane in rats.[44]

Specialized calculations from NMR spectroscopy data give information about the rotational motion of the labeled molecule (^{19}F-halothane) and thereby suggest features of the chemical environment of the labeled compound. "Spin-lattice relaxation time" and "spin-spin relaxation time" are indicators of molecular motion that can be determined from NMR spectroscopy data. Observations of these parameters exhibited by ^{19}F-halothane led the authors to suggest that brain halothane resides in two chemically distinct microenvironments. One site of brain halothane is probably nonspecific accumulation in membrane lipids. The second site, however, represents halothane molecules that are relatively immobile halothane, and therefore in an environment other than the lipid matrix. They caution that their data cannot distinguish between either separate sites within membranes or separate cell types altogether.[44] Nevertheless, this shows that the immobilized halothane binding becomes saturated at 2.5% inspired concentration and that the other site continues to accumulate halothane as a linear function of inspired concentration up to 4% (Fig. 10-4). The saturable location becomes 50% occupied by halothane at 1.2% inspired concentration, suggesting that occupancy of this site is associated with the anesthetic effect. Evers et al point out that the saturable, immobile halothane binding locus might represent drug interaction with a family of membrane proteins that shares similar macromolecular characteristics.[44]

In an editorial accompanying the report about NMR studies of halothane binding, Franks and Lieb comment about the potential significance of this approach to the study of anesthetic mechanisms.[45] They emphasize the surprising data of Evers et al that with the rapid induction of inhalation anesthesia, only a small amount of halothane appears in the general lipid portion of membranes and that, in fact, most of the halothane is in a saturable environment, specialized at least to the point where the bound anesthetic molecules are relatively immobile. The implication is that the saturable site might be lipid–protein interface regions or direct-binding regions of membrane proteins.[45] Confirmation of the halothane binding

sites and further development of these observations will need to be performed in brain slices and tissue homogenates.[45] Nevertheless, this approach to studying halothane activity in brain may open up an entirely new and more sophisticated theory of synaptic function and anesthetic mechanisms.

ANESTHESIA AND AMNESIA

Amnesia, or the absence of awareness of stimuli and events, is an essential element of general anesthesia; however, clinical episodes and case reports of awareness during general anesthesia are not uncommon. Estimates are that from 1% to as high as 3.8% of patients have some psychologic manifestation of memory or recall during an anesthetic.[46, 47] Robinson et al[48] reported a 2% incidence of intraoperative awareness during cardiac surgery with high-dose fentanyl, lorazepam, and isoflurane anesthesia. They speculated that supplemental doses of lorazepam might have prevented the awareness in those particular patients. Knowledge about the biochemical and physiologic mechanisms of memory and learning would allow future development of anesthetics that could modulate more predictably the amnesia component of general anesthesia. Anesthesia and amnesia have been discussed in two recent reviews,[49, 50] so only a brief summary is included here.

From a clinical point of view, the highest incidence of awareness during general anesthesia is associated with cesarean section and cardiac surgery.[46, 47, 50] Most prospective studies have not been able to document conscious recall when patients have been tested for memory of stimuli delivered during anesthesia. Eich et al[51] distinguish between the awareness of recall and the unconscious acquisition of learned behavior, but they were unable to demonstrate that either type of memory developed during a prospective study of patients receiving general anesthesia; however, Bennett et al[52] have reported that patients do demonstrate nonverbal behavior in response to intraoperative suggestions. Goldmann et al[53] have recently confirmed similar observations about patients exhibiting non-

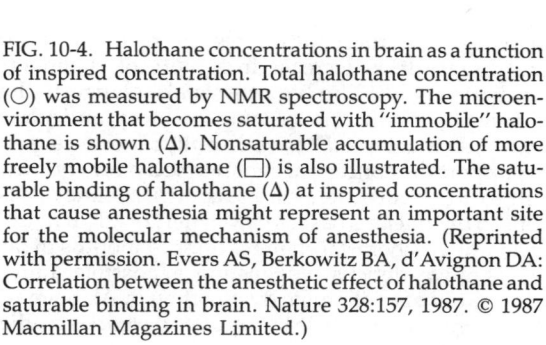

FIG. 10-4. Halothane concentrations in brain as a function of inspired concentration. Total halothane concentration (O) was measured by NMR spectroscopy. The microenvironment that becomes saturated with "immobile" halothane is shown (Δ). Nonsaturable accumulation of more freely mobile halothane (□) is also illustrated. The saturable binding of halothane (Δ) at inspired concentrations that cause anesthesia might represent an important site for the molecular mechanism of anesthesia. (Reprinted with permission. Evers AS, Berkowitz BA, d'Avignon DA: Correlation between the anesthetic effect of halothane and saturable binding in brain. Nature 328:157, 1987. © 1987 Macmillan Magazines Limited.)

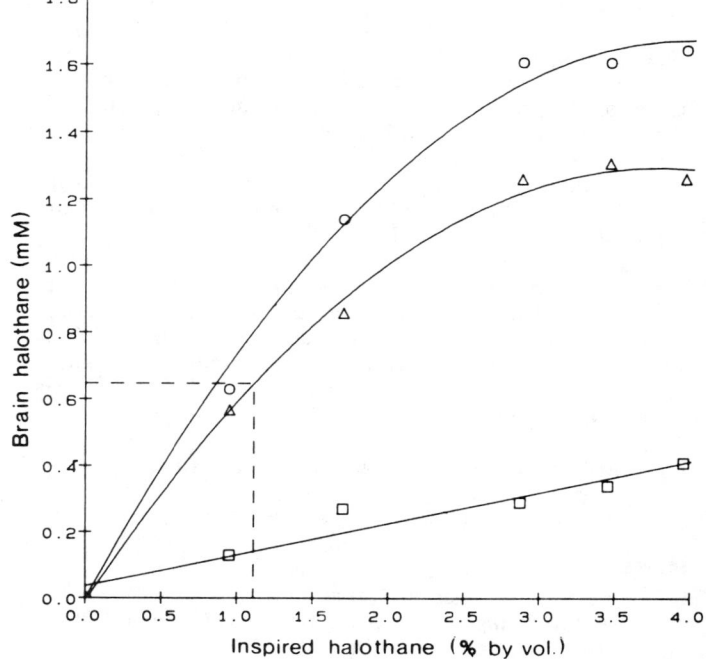

verbal manifestations of intraoperatively acquired suggestions.

The fundamental clinical dilemma is whether awareness occurs during otherwise adequate general anesthesia, or whether it is merely the consequence of inadequate or "too light" anesthesia. This issue reflects the most basic problem, which is the lack of definitive parameters for monitoring the depth of general anesthesia when muscle relaxants preclude movement as a clinical sign. The few prospective studies that reported that patients did learn nonverbal responses to intraoperative suggestions did not control for depth of anesthesia.[52] In 1987, Woo et al[54] reported "the lack of response to suggestion under controlled surgical anesthesia." Their subjects were in four groups, all of whom underwent the identical surgical procedure with identical anesthetic techniques where depth was judged to be stable by vital signs, end-tidal anesthetic concentrations, and compressed spectral array of EEG signals.[54] Postoperative evaluation showed that none of the patients had conscious recall, nor did they have behavioral or emotional characteristics that might be attributed to acquiring subliminal intraoperative information.[54] The researchers conclude that awareness does not occur during adequately controlled depth of general anesthesia.

A recent editorial by Mori[55] offers exceptionally good insight into the difficulties of measuring physiologic indicators (EEG signals) that reflect the transition of brain functioning from awareness to unawareness. He defines depth of anesthesia as the " . . . efficiency of performance of brain functions. . . . " He points out that slowing of EEG signals has only an empirical correlation with brain function and may not be sensitive enough to indicate the transition from awareness to unawareness. Mori states that our present knowledge of EEG signals and neurophysiologic function of the cerebral cortex is still rather primitive.[55]

In a short, speculative article, Crick suggested a model for memory formation by subtle changes (e.g., phosphorylation) of synaptic proteins.[56] Schwartz and Greenberg[57] have recently reviewed the literature supporting Crick's generalized idea. The suggestion is that the short-term phase of memory is represented by synaptic events such as second messenger-mediated changes in synaptic ion channels or receptors (membrane proteins). Long-term memory retention is thought to require durable changes in protein structure secondary to changes in gene expression.[57, 58]

Lynch and Baudry proposed a calcium-activated mechanism for changes in synaptic protein structure and function that could be associated with memory formation.[59] Their proposal incorporates several observations about electrical activity and receptor function in hippocampus-to-cortex pathways.[50, 59] It has been established that memory formation and retrieval involve pathways in the hippocampus of the human brain, with communication to the cerebral cortex for memory storage. During memory formation, intense electrical activity occurs in pathways of the hippocampus and cortex. Long-term potentiation (LTP) is a particular type of electrical activity that occurs in the hippocampus during memory formation. Lynch and Baudry have therefore suggested the following sequence of events as a hypothesis:[59]

1. Memory formation begins with electrical activity associated with LTP;
2. Binding of glutamate (an excitatory neurotransmitter) is increased in association with LTP;
3. Associated with LTP and initial glutamate binding is an intracellular release of calcium ion;
4. Within synaptic terminals, the free calcium activates a proteinase called calpain;

5. Activated calpain degrades a structural protein (fodrin) at the synaptic membrane; and
6. Changes in fodrin result in an ultrastructural change in the membrane that enables even further binding of glutamate.

According to this scheme, memory is associated with changes in the actual structure of synaptic membranes and consequent remodeling of the receptors exposed at the surface of the membranes (Fig. 10-5).

Further support for the concept of calcium-activated changes of synaptic proteins is emerging from current work on spectrin, a cytoskeletal protein found in erythrocytes and neurons.[60, 61] A protein involved in the structure and shape of red blood cells, spectrin has been identified and studied in the brain tissue as well. In the red blood cell model, spectrin is a tetramer of 2-α and 2-β subunits that binds to actin filaments and is attached to the membrane by interactions with membrane proteins (protein 4.1, ankyrin).[60] With characteristics similar to the red blood cell protein, two isoforms of brain spectrin have been identified in nerve cell membranes. One of the spectrin types has been named fodrin (see above). It has been suggested that the protein lends structure to neural membranes and may be involved in the placement and movement of vesicles.[60]

Lynch and Baudry[61] reviewed evidence that calpain activation can result in partial degradation of cytoskeletal protein (spectrin), causing changes in the availability of receptors and the shape of red blood cell and platelet membranes. The blood cell phenomena are models for the proposed sequence of long-term potential changes releasing intracellular calcium, which activates calpain. Activated calpain could then break down brain spectrin, resulting in altered ultrastructure and receptor availability in synaptic membranes.[61]

It is also well established that cholinergic mechanisms are important in memory formation. Bartus et al have summarized the cholinergic hypothesis based on the effects of cholinergic drugs and on measurements of cholinergic dysfunction in brain tissues of patients with Alzheimer's disease.[50, 62]

1. *Cholinergic Markers.* The activity of choline acetyl-transferase (CAT) is reduced in the brain tissue of patients with Alzheimer's disease. CAT is the enzyme that catalyzes the synthesis of ACh in presynaptic cells.
2. *Loss of Cholinergic Function at the Neuronal Level.* The density of postsynaptic cholinergic receptors decreases in brain tissue with normal aging.
3. *Pharmacologic Evidence.* Scopolamine is a cholinergic drug well known to cause amnesia. The CNS effects of scopolamine can be reversed by physostigmine, and acetylcholinesterase inhibitor. Also, cholinemimetic drugs (e.g., arecoline) have been shown actually to improve the acquisition of memory in experimental situations.

The cholinergic hypothesis attributes the memory loss of Alzheimer's disease to a decrease in activity of cholinergic synapses in brain tissue. The hypothesis also suggests that cholinergic function is critical to learning, memory, and amnesia in general.[62] Arendash et al[63] have recently reported experiments that support the concept of cholinergic dysfunction as a key element in the neurochemical basis of Alzheimer's disease. Lesions to the nucleus basalis of Meynert result in neuropathologic and neurochemical changes after 14 months in rats that show cognitive deficits, suggesting a possible animal model for the study of cholinergic dysfunction in Alzheimer's disease.[63] A recent review article by Squire[64] describes studies

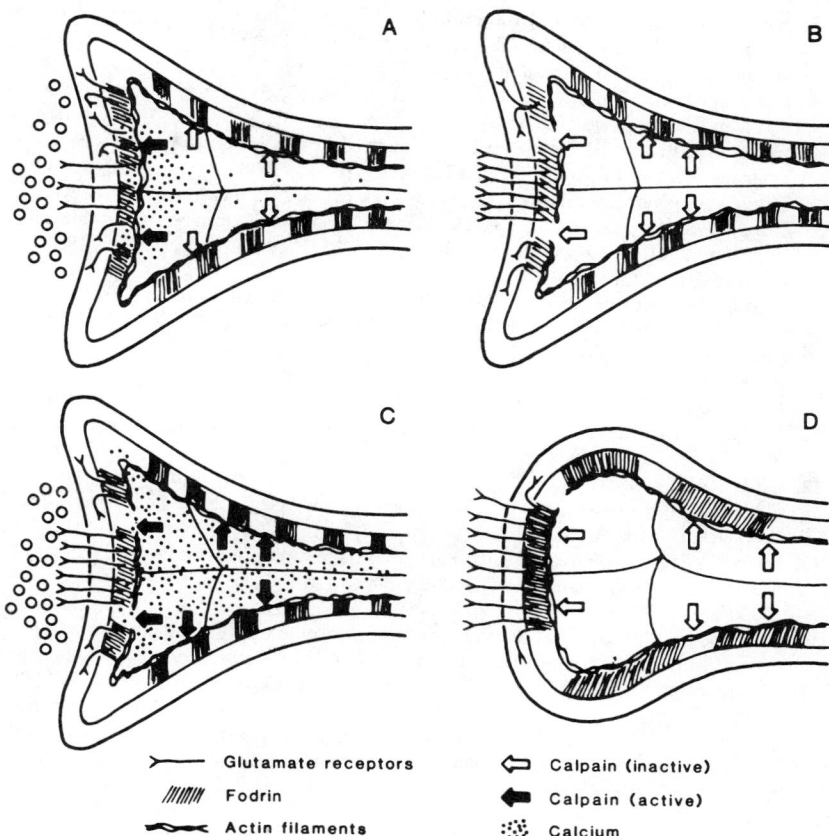

Glutamate receptors
Fodrin
Actin filaments

Calpain (inactive)
Calpain (active)
Calcium

FIG. 10-5. Diagram illustrating a proposed calcium-activated mechanism for changes in synaptic protein structure and function that could be associated with memory formation. Intracellular calcium activates calpain, an enzyme that degrades a membrane structural protein called fodrin. With partially degraded fodrin, glutamate receptors and membrane structure change. (Reprinted with permission. Lynch GA, Baudry M: The biochemistry of memory: A new and specific hypothesis. Science 224:1057, 1984. © 1984 by the AAAS.)

FIG. 10-6. Anesthesia results from the reversible modulation of synaptic communication between neurons. Most intravenous agents bind to receptors and influence the effects of neurotransmitters. Volatile agents influence membrane function by causing physicochemical changes within membrane lipids and proteins.

SYNAPTIC MECHANISMS OF GENERAL ANESTHESIA

INTRAVENOUS AGENTS

BIND TO RECEPTORS

MODULATE SYNAPTIC FUNCTION

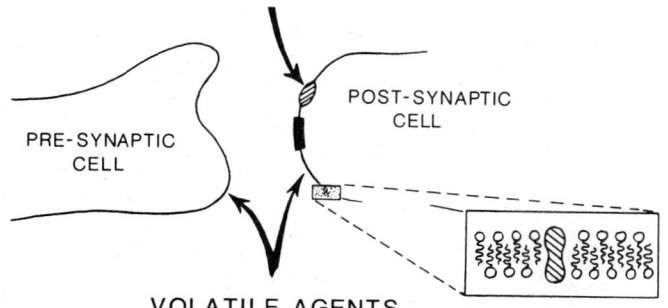

PRE-SYNAPTIC CELL

POST-SYNAPTIC CELL

VOLATILE AGENTS

DISSOLVE IN MEMBRANE

MODIFY BEHAVIOR OF MEMBRANE PROTEINS (RECEPTORS?)

MODULATE SYNAPTIC FUNCTION

of memory and learning that focus on brain processes and systems at a "neuropsychological level of analysis." Obviously, cellular and molecular actions of anesthetics and amnesia-producing drugs are likely to influence neurophysiologic processes and the integrative functions of neuroanatomic regions in the brain.

Whereas the details of the current theories of memory mechanisms do not easily reconcile with the pharmacologic mechanisms of anesthetics, elements common to all aspects are in fact emerging. The broad, general principle is that synaptic communication is the basis of CNS function. Amnesia, analgesia, and control of sympathetic responses are features of anesthesia that result from drug-induced, reversible modulation of synaptic communication. Figure 10-6 is a summary of anesthetic actions on synaptic activity. This discussion has been a simplistic overview of neuropharmacologic mechanisms of general anesthesia.

REFERENCES

1. Miller KW: General anaesthetics. In Feldman SA, Scun CF, Paton W (eds): Drugs in Anaesthesia: Mechanisms of Action, p 133. London, Edward Arnold, 1987
2. Roth SH, Miller KW (eds): Molecular and Cellular Mechanisms of Anesthetics, p 490. New York, Plenum, 1986
3. Dluzewski AR, Halsey MJ, Simmonds AC: Membrane interactions with general and local anaesthetics: A review of molecular hypotheses of anaesthesia. Molec Aspects Med 6:459, 1983
4. Richter JJ: Neuropharmacologic mechanisms of general anesthesia In Barash PG (ed): Refresher Courses in Anesthesiology, vol 14, p 199. Philadelphia, JB Lippincott, 1986

5. Finck AD: Opiate receptors and endorphins: Significance for anesthesiology. In Hershey SG (ed): Refresher Courses in Anesthesiology, vol 7, p 103. Philadelphia, JB Lippincott, 1979

6. Sherrington CS: The Integrative Action of the Nervous System, p 80. New Haven, Yale University Press, 1986

7. Cooper JR, Bloom FE, Roth RH: The Biochemical Basis of Neuropharmacology. New York, Oxford University Press, 1978

8. Tapia R: Biochemical pharmacology of GABA in CNS. In Iverson LL, Iverson SD, Snyder SH (eds): Handbook of Psychopharmacology, vol 4. Amino Acid Transmitters, p 1. New York, Plenum Press, 1975

9. Richter JJ: Current theories about the mechanisms of benzodiazepines and neuroleptic drugs. Anesthesiology 54:66, 1981

10. Snyder SH, Enna SJ: The role of central glycine receptors in the pharmacologic actions of benzodiazepines. Adv Biochem Psychopharmacol 14:81, 1975

11. Cheng S-C, Brunner EA: Inducing anesthesia with a GABA analog, THIP. Anesthesiology 63:147, 1985

12. Gillis RA, DiMiccio JA, Williford DJ et al: Importance of CNS GABA-ergic mechanisms in the regulation of cardiovascular function. Brain Res Bull 5:suppl 2, 303, 1980

13. Stein L, Wise CD, Beluzzi JD: Effect of benzodiazepines on central serotonergic mechanisms. Adv Biochem Psychopharmacol 14:29, 1975

14. Antonaccio MJ: GABA and inhibition of autonomic outflow: A central transmitter role. In Kalsner S (ed): Trends in Autonomic Pharmacology, vol 2, p 217. Baltimore, Urban and Schwarzenberg, 1982

15. Sample RHB, DiMiccio JA: Localization of sites in periventricular forebrain mediating cardiovascular effects of Y-aminobutyric acid agonists and antagonists in anesthetized cats. J Pharmacol Exper Therap 240:498, 1987

16. Schofield PR, Darlison MG, Fujita N et al: Sequence and functional expression of the GABA$_A$ receptor shows a ligand-gated receptor super-family. Nature 328:221, 1987

17. Sigel E, Barnard EA: A gamma-aminobutyric acid/benzodiazepine receptor complex from bovine cerebral cortex. Improved purification with preservation of regulatory sites and their interactions. J Biol Chem 259:7219, 1984

18. Casalotti SO, Stephenson FA, Barnard EA: Separate subunits for agonist and benzodiazepine binding in the gamma-aminobutyric acid A receptor oligomer. J Biol Chem 261:15013, 1986

19. Costa E, Guidotti A: Molecular mechanisms in the receptor action of benzodiazepines. Annu Rev Pharmacol Toxicol 19:531,1979

20. Lauven DM, Schwilden H, Stoeckel H et al: The effects of benzodiazepine antagonist Ro 15-1788 in the presence of stable concentrations of midazolam. Anesthesiology 63:61, 1985

21. Hoik: Mechanism of action of barbiturates. Annu Rev Pharmacol Toxicol 21:83, 1983

22. Olsen RW: Drug interactions at the GABA receptor–ionophore complex. Annu Rev Pharmacol Toxicol 22:245, 1982

23. Richards CD, Strupinski K: An analysis of the action of pentobarbitane on the excitatory postsynaptic potentials and membrane properties of neurones in the guinea-pig olfactory cortex. Br J Pharmacol 89:321, 1986

24. Pocock G, Richards CD: The action of pentobarbitone on stimulus–secretion coupling in adrenal chromaffin cells. Br J Pharmacol 90:71, 1987

25. Harrison NL, Majewska M, Harrington JW et al: Structure–activity relationships for steroid interaction with the Y-aminobutyric acid$_A$ receptor complex. J Pharmacol Exper Therap 241:346, 1987

26. Cheng S-C, Brunner EA: Effects of anesthetic agents on synaptosomal GABA disposal. Anesthesiology 55:34, 1981

27. Seeman P, Titeler M, Tedesco J et al: Brain receptors for dopamine and neuroleptics. Adv Biochem Psychopharmacol 19:167, 1978

28. Firestone LL, Miller JC, Miller KW: Tables of physical and pharmacological properties of anesthetics. In Roth SH, Miller KW (eds): Molecular and Cellular Mechanisms of Anesthetics, p 453. New York, Plenum Medical, 1986

29. Judge SE: Effect of general anaesthesia on synaptic ion channels. Br J Anaesth 55:191, 1983

30. Richards CD: Actions of general anaesthetics on synaptic transmission in the CNS. Br J Anaesth 55:201, 1983

31. Halsey MJ: Anaesthetic mechanisms. Br J Hosp Med 36:445, 1986

32. Winters WD: Effects of drugs on the electrical activity of the brain: Anesthetics. Annu Rev Pharmacol Toxicol 16:413, 1976

33. Sauter JF, Braswell LM, Miller KW: Action of anesthetics and high pressure on cholinergic membranes. In Fink BR (ed): Progress in Anesthesiology, vol 2. Molecular Mechanisms of Anesthesia, p 199. New York, Raven Press, 1980

34. Miller KW: The pressure reversal of anesthesia and the critical volume hypothesis In Fink BR (ed): Progress in Anesthesiology, vol 1. Molecular Mechanisms of Anesthesia, p 341. New York, Raven Press, 1975

35. Wardley-Smith B, Halsey MJ: Mixtures of inhalation and IV anaesthetics at high pressure. A test of the multi site hypothesis of general anaesthesia. Br J Anaesth 57:1248, 1985

36. Halsey MJ, Wardley-Smith B, Wood S: Pressure reversal of alphaxalone/alphadolone and methohexitone in tadpoles: Evidence for different molecular sites for general anaesthesia. Br J Pharmacol 89:299, 1986

37. Firestone LL, Sauter JF, Braswell LM et al: Actions of general anesthetics on acetylcholine-receptor-rich membranes from Torpedo californica. Anesthesiology 64:694, 1986

38. Dodson BA, Miller KW: Evidence for a dual mechanism in the anesthetic action of an opioid peptide. Anesthesiology 62:615, 1985

39. Trudell JR: A unitary theory of anesthesia based on lateral phase separation in nerve membranes. Anesthesiology 46:5, 1977

40. Veda I, Hirakawa M, Arakawa K et al: Do anesthetics fluidize membranes? Anesthesiology 64:67, 1986

41. Franks NP, Lieb WR: Molecular mechanisms of general anesthesia. Nature 300:487, 1982

42. Franks NP, Lieb WR: Do general anesthetics act by competitive binding to specific receptors? Nature 310:599, 1984

43. Franks NP, Lieb WR: Mapping of general anaesthetic target sites provides a molecular basis for cut-off effects. Nature 316:349, 1985

44. Evers AS, Berkowitz BA, D'Avignon DA: Correlation between the anaesthetic effect of halothane and saturable binding in brain. Nature 328:157, 1987

45. Franks NP, Lieb WR: Neuron membranes: Anesthetics on the mind. Nature 328:113, 1987

46. Mummaneni N, Rao TLK, Montoya A: Awareness and recall with high-dose fentanyl-oxygen anesthesia. Anesth Analg 59:948, 1980

47. Abuleish E, Taylor FH: Effect of morphine-diazepam on signs of anesthesia, awareness and dreams of patients under nitrous oxide for cesarean section. Anesth Analg 55:702, 1976

48. Robinson RJS, Boright WA, Ligier B et al: The incidence of awareness and amnesia for perioperative events, after cardiac surgery with lorazepam and fentanyl anesthesia. J Cardiothorac Anesth 1:524, 1987

49. Breckenridge JL, Aitkenhead AR: Awareness during anaesthesia: A review. Ann Roy Coll Surg 65:93, 1983

50. Richter JJ: Anesthesia, amnesia, and alchemy. Semin Anesth 6:128, 1987

51. Eich E, Reeves JL, Katz RL: Anesthesia, amnesia, and the memory/awareness distinction. Anesth Analg 64:1143, 1985

52. Bennett HL, Davis HS, Giannini JA: Non-verbal response to intraoperative conversation. Br J Anaesth 57:174, 1985

53. Goldmann L, Shah MV, Hebden MW: Memory of cardiac anaesthesia. Anaesthesia 42:596, 1987
54. Woo R, Seltzer JL, Marr A: The lack of response to suggestion under controlled surgical anesthesia. Acta Anaesthesiol Scand 31:567, 1987
55. Mori K: The EEG and awareness during general anaesthesia. Anaesthesia 42:1153, 1987
56. Crick F: Memory and molecular turnover. Nature 312:101, 1984
57. Schwartz JH, Greenberg SM: Molecular mechanisms for memory: Second messenger induced modifications of protein kinases in nerve cells. Annu Rev Neurosci 10:459, 1987
58. Goelet P, Castellucci VF, Shacher S et al: The long and the short of a long-term memory—a molecular framework. Nature 322:419, 1986
59. Lynch G, Baudry M: The biochemistry of memory: A new and specific hypothesis. Science 224:1057, 1984
60. Goodman SR, Zagon IS: Brain spectrin: Structure, location, and function. A symposium overview. Brain Res Bull 18:773, 1987
61. Lynch G, Baudry M: Brain spectrin, calpain and long-term changes in synaptic efficacy. Brain Res Bull 18:809, 1987
62. Bartus RT, Dean RL, Beer R et al: The cholinergic hypothesis of geriatric memory dysfunction. Science 217:408, 1982
63. Arendash GW, Millard WJ, Dunn AJ et al: Long-term neuropathological and neurochemical effects of nucleus basalis lesions in the rat. Science 238:952-956, 1987
64. Squire LS: Mechanisms of memory. Science 232:1612, 1986

Chapter 11

Wendell C. Stevens
Harry G. G. Kingston

Inhalation Anesthesia

The role of the inhalation drugs in general anesthesia is changing: the number of patients who receive only inhalation drugs following induction of general anesthesia with an intravenous drug is decreasing; the use of intravenous drugs as adjuvants is increasing. The combination of intravenous and potent inhaled drugs might be called the new *balanced anesthesia*. A variety of drugs are chosen to derive the specific benefits of each. Thus, tachycardia occurring during isoflurane anesthesia may lead the anesthesiologist to administer an opioid to take advantage of the specific vagal actions of the opioid and to reduce the dose of isoflurane. Many anesthesiologists now prefer to decrease the total dose of a potent inhaled drug that a patient receives with any one of a number of intravenous drugs.

The inhaled anesthetics of greatest importance today are enflurane, halothane, and isoflurane, the potent drugs, and nitrous oxide, the weaker drug. Discussion of these four drugs will provide the major emphasis of this chapter. Although methoxyflurane is still available commercially, it is used infrequently. A new compound, sevoflurane, is under clinical trial but as yet is not commercially available. Some of the physical characteristics of these compounds are given in Table 11-1. Their chemical structures are shown in Figure 11-1.

HISTORY

The recent introduction of sevoflurane as an inhaled anesthetic drug represents the latest of the group of drugs whose lineage goes back to nitrous oxide, diethyl ether, and chloroform, which were introduced into clinical practice almost si-

multaneously. The search for new inhaled drugs continues because they offer at least two general advantages over drugs administered by routes other than ventilatory. These are the ability to increase and decrease drug levels in the body at will and easy estimation of the concentration of anesthetic at the sites of action once the alveolar concentration is known. Since instruments of reasonable cost are now available to measure accurately and promptly the alveolar concentration of anesthetic gases, control of anesthetic dose can be done with great precision. Of course, we do not imply that anesthetics should be administered "by number" without close attention to the patient and the drugs' pharmacologic effects.

Advances in fluorine chemistry associated with nuclear research in the 1940s that allowed cost-effective incorporation of fluorine into molecules was pivotal to the development of modern anesthetics.[1] Prior to that time, the mainstays of inhalation anesthesia, cyclopropane, diethyl ether, and divinyl ether, were flammable. The nonflammable halogenated compounds chloroform and trichlorethylene were associated with hepatotoxicity or neurotoxicity and also were highly soluble in tissue.

In 1946 Robbins[2] reported studies of a series of fluorinated hydrocarbons. He showed that agents of a lower boiling point were more likely to produce convulsions than anesthesia. Halogenated aliphatic hydrocarbons and short-chain ethers with boiling points in the range of 50–100° C and containing a large proportion of fluorine as the halogen proved to be the best anesthetics. Some compounds with these components either have not withstood the test of practice or have been replaced by better drugs.

Fluroxene, the first of the new fluorinated anesthetics to be

293

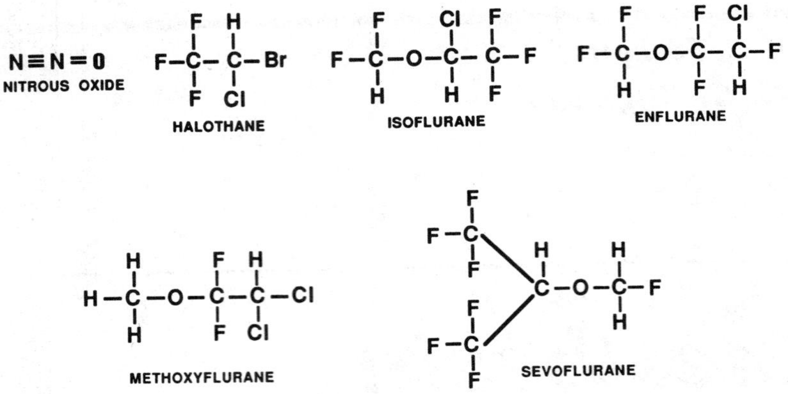

FIG. 11-1. Molecular structures of inhaled anesthetics.

TABLE 11-1.   Physical Characteristics of Anesthetics

AGENT	MOLECULAR WEIGHT (g)	BOILING POINT (760 mm Hg °C)	VAPOR PRESSURE (mm Hg @ 20°C)	LIQUID DENSITY	VAPOR/ LIQUID (ml)	CHEMICAL STABILIZER NECESSARY	FLAMMABILITY LIMITS
Enflurane	184.5	56.5	175	1.517(25° C)	198	No	None
Halothane	197.4	50.2	241	1.86 (20° C)	227	Yes	None
Isoflurane	184.5	48.5	238	1.496(25° C)	196	No	None
Methoxyflurane	165	104.7	22.5	1.43 (20° C)	208	Yes	7% in air 5.4% in O_2
Nitrous oxide	44	−88.0	39,000	—	—	—	None in air
Sevoflurane	200	58.5	160	1.505(20° C)	181	—	11% in O_2 10% in N_2O

(Physical data are from manufacturer's literature; Wallin WF, Regan BM, Napoli MD et al: Sevoflurane: A new inhalational anesthetic agent. Anesth Analg 54:758, 1975; Vitcha JF: A history of Forane. Anesthesiology 35:4, 1971; Halsey JM: Physiochemical properties of inhalational anesthetics. In Gray TC, Nunn JF, Utting JE [eds]: General Anaesthesia, p 45. London, Butterworths, 1980.)

widely used clinically, was synthesized by Shukys in 1951 and evaluated by Krantz et al[3] and Sadove et al.[4] The requirements for testing drugs at that time were minimal, and rapid introduction of a new drug into clinical practice was common. Because fluroxene maintained cardiorespiratory function at near awake values, it maintained some popularity for nearly 2 decades, but several features limited its popularity.[5] These included flammability, some danger of ventricular arrhythmias, a high incidence of nausea and vomiting, and the threat of hepatotoxicity.[6]

Halothane was synthesized by Suckling in England in 1951,[7] tested in animals shortly thereafter, and introduced into clinical practice by 1956.[8, 9] Halothane was readily accepted by the anesthesia community.[10] Its nonflammability, favorable solubility characteristics, tolerance by patients at high inspired concentrations (overpressure), rapid induction, capacity to provide muscle relaxation, and an acceptably low incidence of nausea and vomiting made it a far superior drug to other available anesthetics.

Methoxyflurane, synthesized before either fluroxene or halothane, was evaluated in humans by Artusio et al[11] in 1960. Perhaps it was tested because certain drawbacks became apparent for halothane. These drawbacks included sensitization of the heart to the arrhythmic effects of epinephrine, cardiorespiratory depression, and the suspicion that halothane shared, along with other halogenated compounds such as chloroform, the danger of being a hepatotoxin.[12] Methoxyflurane's favorable characteristics proved to be nonflammability, adequate muscle relaxation, and effective analgesia at low concentrations. Its high blood and tissue solubility, however, led to slow induction of anesthesia and exceedingly prolonged recovery. Even greater drawbacks proved to be nephrotoxicity[13] and reports of hepatotoxicity.[14]

The disadvantages of halothane listed above, including hepatotoxicity,[15, 16] encouraged the search for better inhaled anesthetics.[17] Out of hundreds of compounds tested by Terrell et al,[18, 19] the two compounds enflurane and isoflurane have become important anesthetic drugs in current clinical practice. Terrell centered his developmental work on the methyl-ethyl series of compounds because they tended to be stable, nonflammable, and excellent anesthetics.[19] The clinical trials of these two compounds proceeded nearly in parallel[20] involving patients[21, 22] and human volunteers.[23, 24]

The extent of studies completed with each drug was far reaching compared to requirements with earlier compounds.[20, 25–27] This was especially true for isoflurane where putative carcinogenicity,[28] subsequently unsubstantiated, delayed the drug's introduction into clinical practice.[29]

A number of other drugs have either had only a brief trial clinically or are still in the evaluation process.[27] Among the former, halopropane ($CHF_2 CF_2 CH_2 Br$) required prolonged time for induction of anesthesia and was excessively arrhythmogenic.[30-32] Teflurane (CF_3 CHBrF) was associated with a high incidence of cardiac arrhythmias even in low concentrations.[33-35] Sevoflurane is still in the evaluative process and shows promise, particularly because of its low solubility in blood,[36] a property that may make it an excellent drug for use in outpatients. Finally, aliflurane has been administered to a few patients[37] and the MAC determined in dogs,[38] but it is not yet commercially available.

PHARMACOKINETICS OF INHALED ANESTHETICS

UPTAKE, DISTRIBUTION, AND ELIMINATION

The inhaled drugs are distributed in the body according to the same principles which apply to other drugs. (see Chapter 6) The gas anesthetics differ from most other drugs in that they enter the body through the lungs *via* ventilation. Thereafter, their absorption by blood and distribution to other tissues are determined by the solubility of the drug in blood (blood : gas partition coefficient), blood flow through the lungs, the subsequent distribution of blood to individual organs, solubility of anesthetics in the tissue (tissue : blood partition coefficient), and mass of the tissue.[39] Table 11-2 lists solubility characteristics of the inhaled anesthetics described in this chapter.

The goal of inhalation anesthesia is to develop and maintain a satisfactory partial pressure or tension of anesthetic at the site of anesthetic action, the brain. Partial pressure, or tension, is related to concentration of anesthetic in the gas phase by the following formula:

Concentration = (Tension ÷ Barometric Pressure) × 100.

Induction of anesthesia is achieved, in a pharmacodynamic sense, when an anesthetizing partial pressure of anesthetic has been achieved in the brain. The brain or any individual tissue under consideration can be considered as the final site for a series of gradients in anesthetic partial pressure, which begins at the delivery hose exiting from the anesthetic machine. The gradients in gas tension may be arranged as follows: delivered > inspired > alveolar > arterial > tissue. In a purely pharmacokinetic interpretation, induction of anesthesia is complete when all tissues attain the same anesthetic tension as the alveolar tension. Until equilibrium is achieved, the gradients noted above will continue to exist. This discussion of uptake and distribution of the inhaled drugs will consider each gradient in succession.

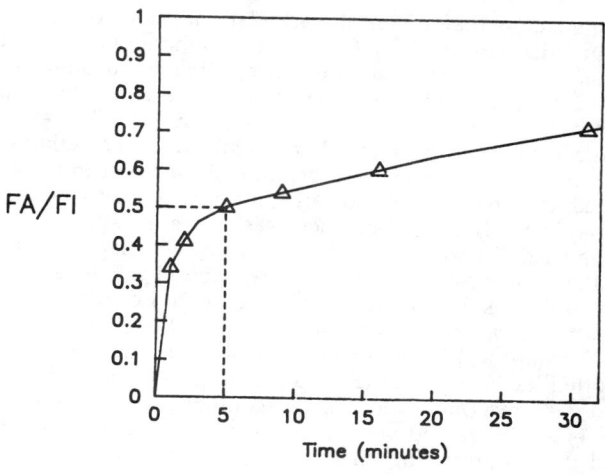

FIG. 11-2. Depiction of the manner in which the alveolar concentration (FA) of an inhaled anesthetic approaches the inspired concentration (FI) over time. Presumptions include normal ventilation and cardiac output and blood : gas partition coefficient ~2.

First, a difference between delivered and inspired tension exists as long as uptake of anesthetic continues unless a nonrebreathing delivery system is being used. By definition, with a nonrebreathing system there is no difference between delivered and inspired tension. Use of high inflow rates to a circle system approximates a nonrebreathing system.[40, 41] Anesthetic-system components can be arranged to favor preferential loss of anesthetic-poor gases during induction,[42, 43] and the components of the anesthetic system can absorb anesthetics to widen a delivered-to-inspired tension difference.[44, 45]

At the circuit–patient interface there can exist an inspired-to-alveolar tension difference (Fig. 11-2). During induction of anesthesia, blood returning to the lung from tissues has an anesthetic tension lower than that in the alveoli. As a result, uptake of anesthetic drugs will occur from alveoli and will cause an inspired-to-alveolar tension difference. The alveolar anesthetic concentration is of great importance during anesthesia with an inhaled drug because the arterial blood quickly equilibrates with the alveolar tension of the anesthetic[46] and, in turn, there is quick equilibration with the brain; therefore, the ability to measure or control the alveolar tension of an anesthetic provides an indirect but reliable method to measure and control the brain tension (partial pressure) of an anesthetic.

TABLE 11-2.   Partition Coefficients at 37° C

AGENT	BLOOD: GAS	BRAIN: BLOOD	LIVER: BLOOD	MUSCLE: BLOOD	FAT: BLOOD	OIL: GAS	RUBBER: GAS	OTHER
Enflurane	1.91	1.4	2.1	1.7	36	98.5	74(25° C)	Polyvinyl:gas 120 (25° C)
Halothane	2.3	2.9	2.6	3.5	60	224	120(23° C)	Polyethylene:gas 26.3
Isoflurane	1.4	2.6	2.5	4.0	45	90.8	62(25° C)	Soda lime:gas 1 Polyethylene:gas 2 (25° C)
Methoxyflurane	12	2.0	1.9	1.3	49	970	630(23° C)	Polyvinyl:gas 110 (25° C)
Nitrous oxide	0.47	1.1	0.8	1.2	2.3	1.4	1.2(23° C)	
Sevoflurane	0.60	—	—	—	—	53.4	—	

(Physical data are from manufacturer's literature; Eger EI II, Larson CP Jr, Severinghaus JW: The solubility of halothane in rubber, soda lime and various plastics. Anesthesiology 23:356, 1962; Wallin WF, Regan BM, Napoli MD *et al:* Sevoflurane: A new inhalational anesthetic agent. Anesth Analg 54:758, 1975; Eger RR, Eger EI II: Effects of temperature and age on the solubility of enflurane, halothane, isoflurane, and methoxyflurane in human blood. Anesth Analg 57:224, 1978.)

The factors that govern the alveolar anesthetic tension are summarized in detail by Eger.[39] Achievement of an alveolar tension results from a balance between delivery of anesthetic to the lung and uptake of anesthetic from the lung by blood and tissues. The inspired concentration and alveolar ventilation control delivery of anesthetic to the lung. The higher the inspired concentration, the more rapid the increase in alveolar concentration (concentration effect).[47] As alveolar (but not necessarily total) ventilation increases, more anesthetic molecules are delivered to the lung. Increasing alveolar ventilation will make alveolar gas more like the inspired gas, that is, will lessen the inspired-to-alveolar concentration difference.

Administration of high concentrations of one gas (e.g., nitrous oxide) will facilitate the rise in alveolar concentration of another gas (e.g., halothane); a phenomenon called the second-gas effect (Fig. 11-3). The two components of the second-gas effect, increased ventilation (increased tracheal in-flow) and the concentrating effect,[48] are operative at the alveolar level. Although a second-gas effect will exist for nearly any combination of inhaled drugs given simultaneously, it is most pronounced when nitrous oxide is used with a more potent drug like halothane (the second gas). Despite nitrous oxide's relatively low blood solubility, the volume taken up early in anesthesia is large, as much as 1500 ml·min^{-1} or more, because it is delivered in high concentrations.[49]

The increase in alveolar concentration caused by delivery of anesthetic to the lung is opposed by uptake of anesthetic by the pulmonary capillary blood. Pulmonary capillary blood and alveolar anesthetic tensions are equal for any one alveolus–capillary unit; therefore, the next step in the tension gradient chain, the alveolar-to-arterial difference, will ordinarily be small. This is particularly true when only minor ventilation/perfusion abnormalities exist.[46, 50] Factors governing uptake include the anesthetic blood : gas partition coefficient, pulmonary blood flow, and the alveolar-to-mixed-venous tension difference. The higher the blood solubility of the anesthetic, the greater the uptake. Anesthetics act as ideal gases, so their solubility is not influenced by their partial pressure.[51, 52] Their solubilities in blood and other tissues increase as temperature decreases but are not influenced by the patient's age.[53] Blood solubility of anesthetics increases soon after a meal[54] and the blood : gas solubility of enflurane is lower in obese than nonobese patients.[55]

The last link in the chain of gradients, the blood-to-tissue tension difference, leads to uptake of anesthetic by tissues. Factors governing tissue uptake include the anesthetic tissue : blood partition coefficient, tissue blood flow, and the arterial-to-venous tension difference. Except for adipose tissue, the tissue : blood coefficients are generally quite similar to the blood : gas coefficients (Table 11-2). Blood flow in relation to tissue mass is therefore of crucial importance in determining the capacity of the tissue for the anesthetic. A pertinent example of the importance of these factors in determining the rate of tissue anesthetic uptake is the rapid rise of alveolar and, therefore, myocardial concentration, of anesthetics in infants.[56] A small amount of anesthetic is lost via the skin and must, of course, be replaced by further uptake at the lung.[57]

When administration of an inhaled anesthetic is discontinued, removal of anesthetic from the body proceeds in a fashion that is nearly the reverse of induction. Emergence from anesthesia is more rapid with low blood or tissue anesthetic solubility,[58] increased ventilation,[58] and replacement of nitrous oxide with nitrogen.[59] The higher the concentration of nitrous oxide when elimination begins, the greater the effect in elimination of halothane.[60]

Emergence from anesthesia differs from induction in that anesthetic metabolism will affect the rate of decrease of the alveolar anesthetic concentration. Although anesthetics are quite inert, as with other drugs they are metabolized, usually to more polar compounds.[61] The amount of anesthetic removed from the body by metabolism is small compared with the amount exhaled. The amount metabolized is governed primarily by hepatic enzyme activity plus the amount and duration of availability of the anesthetic drug to the liver. The alveolar concentration of an anesthetic during induction and maintenance of anesthesia is influenced little by anesthetic metabolism because the amount of anesthetic administered or supplied to the patient far exceeds its uptake. During emergence, however, as the alveolar concentration falls below the Km for metabolism of the drug (the partial pressure of anesthetic at which the rate of metabolism is one-half the maximum rate of metabolism), a large fraction of the anesthetic presented to the liver will be metabolized. As a result, the venous and alveolar concentrations decrease.[62, 63] During the first few minutes of emergence, when the alveolar concentra-

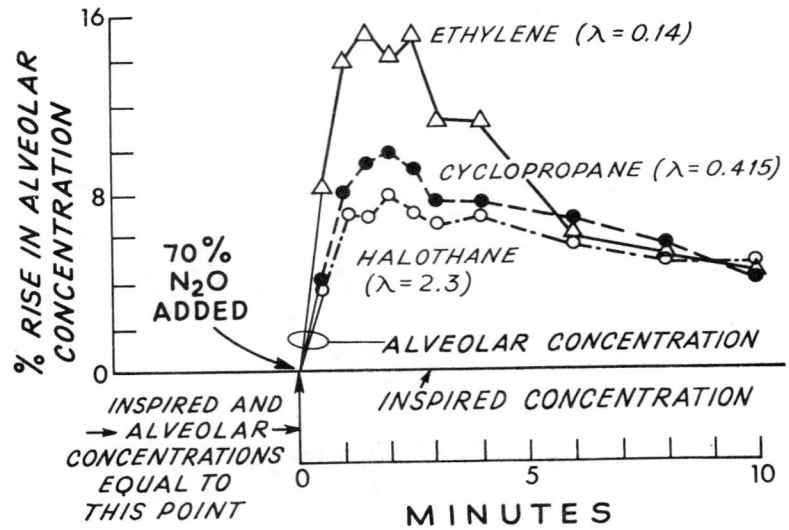

FIG. 11-3. Average per cent rise of the alveolar concentration of a second gas with the addition of 70% nitrous oxide. (Reprinted with permission. Stoelting AK, Eger EI: An additional explanation for the second gas effect. Anesthesiology 30:273, 1969.)

TABLE 11-3. Minimum Alveolar Concentrations (MAC) in Humans as Per Cent of 1 Atmosphere

	MAC				MAC		
	With Oxygen	Reference Number	Age in Yr	With N₂O	Reference Number	% N₂O	Age in Yr
Enflurane	1.7	419	39±3 SE	0.60	420	70	38±2 SE
Halothane	0.77	66	42±7 SD	0.29	75	66	
Isoflurane	1.15	421	44.2±1.3 SE	0.50	421	70	46.3±1.2 SE
Methoxyflurane	0.16	66	38±9 SD	0.07	422	56	30–55
Nitrous oxide	104	68	21–35				
Sevoflurane	1.71	416	30–59	0.66	416	64	30–59

tion is relatively large, drugs of lowest solubility exhibit the most rapid decline of alveolar concentration. Once the alveolar concentration decreases to the range of 0.01 MAC, drugs that undergo considerable metabolism may be removed more rapidly than those resistant to metabolism, even though the former possess greater blood solubility. This factor accounts at least in part for the failure of the alveolar concentration of anesthetics to fall in strict accordance with their blood solubilities.

THE REQUIREMENT FOR ANESTHETICS— MINIMUM ALVEOLAR CONCENTRATION (MAC)

The pharmacokinetics of anesthetics (uptake and distribution) can be linked to pharmacodynamics (effect of the drug on the body) by consideration of anesthetic potency. The linkage exists because the desired alveolar concentration is what one strives to achieve and maintain during anesthesia. For the inhaled drugs, potency is commonly referred to as the minimum alveolar concentration (MAC) of the anesthetic. This is the alveolar concentration of anesthetic at 1 atmosphere that prevents movement in 50% of subjects in response to a painful stimulus (Table 11-3).[64–67] Various noxious stimuli have been used to provoke the response, including skin incision or electrical current.[66, 68] End-points of response other than skeletal muscle movement have been proposed.[69] The 95% confidence limits for MAC are approximately 25% of the MAC value. A suggestion has been made that the dose of anesthetic preventing response to noxious stimuli in 95% of subjects, AD₉₅, more nearly approximates clinical anesthetic requirement.[70] In practice, the conventional MAC must be exceeded by a factor of 1.25–1.3 to assure surgical anesthesia in most patients.

MAC has been used when comparing the effects of equipotent doses of anesthetics on various organ functions. The relative effects for anesthetics can be defined by calculating anesthetic or therapeutic indices, the dose producing a given effect divided by the MAC. For example, the dose of an anesthetic producing apnea when divided by the MAC defines its respiratory anesthetic index,[71] an index of the anesthetic's margin of safety.[72, 73] The MAC has also been useful in quantifying the effect of other drugs or pathophysiologic states on anesthetic requirement. Factors increasing, decreasing, or not changing anesthetic requirement are summarized in Tables 11-4–6. A single explanation for the effect of these factors on MAC has not been found. Many seem to act through influences on central nervous system (CNS) catecholamine levels[74] and CNS depression such as by opioids[75] or hypoxia.[76, 77] Some drugs both increase and decrease the MAC, depending on dose or duration of administration. The acute administration of dextroamphetamines may increase the MAC, but

TABLE 11-4. Physiologic or Pharmacologic Factors That Increase MAC

Increased central neurotransmitter levels (monoamine oxidase [MAO] inhibitors, acute dextroamphetamine administration, cocaine, ephedrine, levodopa)
Hyperthermia
Chronic ethanol abuse*
Hypernatremia

* Determined in humans.

TABLE 11-5. Physiologic or Pharmacologic Factors that Decrease MAC

Metabolic acidosis
Hypoxia (Pa₀₂ < 38 mm Hg)
Induced hypotension (AP < 50 mm Hg)
Decreased central neurotransmitter levels (α methyldopa, reserpine, chronic dextroamphetamine administration, levodopa)
Clonidine
Hypothermia
Hyponatremia
Lithium
Hypo-osmolality
Pregnancy
Acute ethanol administration
Ketamine
Pancuronium*
Physostigmine (10 times clinical doses)
Neostigmine (10 times clinical doses)
Lidocaine
Opioids
Opioid agonist–antagonist analgesics
Barbiturates*
Chlorpromazine*
Diazepam*
Hydroxyzine*
Δ-9-Tetrahydrocannabinol
Verapamil

* Determined in humans.

chronic administration may decrease the MAC.[78] Levodopa may initially increase and then decrease the MAC when large doses are used, but smaller doses may decrease the MAC.[79] Some opioids exhibit a ceiling effect—an effect more prominent for agonist–antagonist compounds than for agonists alone.[80, 81] The inhaled drugs are considered to be nearly additive in their effects on MAC.[82, 83] The most common interaction, that of nitrous oxide with a potent inhaled drug, provides a predictable reduction in requirement for the potent drug. The reduction is approximately equal to 1% of the MAC value for each volume-per cent alveolar nitrous oxide concentra-

TABLE 11-6. Physiologic or Pharmacologic Factors Not Altering MAC

Duration of anesthesia*
Type of stimulation*
Gender*
Hypocarbia (Pa_{CO_2} to 21 mm Hg)*
Hypercarbia (Pa_{CO_2} to 95 mm Hg)
Metabolic alkalosis
Hyperoxia
Isovolemic anemia (hematrocrit to 10%)
Systemic arterial hypertension *per se*
Thyroid function
Magnesium
Hyperkalemia
Hyperosmolality
Propranolol
Isoproterenol
Promethazine
Naloxone
Aminophylline

* Determined in humans.

tion.[75] For example, 66% nitrous oxide will decrease halothane requirement in middle-aged adults to $0.77 - (0.77 \times 0.66) = 0.26\%$.

Pregnancy decreases the MAC when a sheep model is used,[84] but a decrease[67] or no change in the MAC is seen in the rat.[85] MAC is also influenced by age. In the near-term sheep fetus, the MAC is approximately one-half what it is in the adult sheep.[86] In humans the MAC is highest in the first 6 months of life[87] and is slightly lower in neonates.[88] Beyond adolescence, anesthetic requirement decreases with age so that an 80-yr-old patient requires only three-fourths the alveolar concentration for anesthesia as a young adult.[89]

At least two additional MAC values have been determined. One is MAC-awake, the dose at which response to the command "open your eyes" occurs.[90] The alveolar concentration at this point is approximately one-half the standard MAC value. MAC-BAR is the alveolar concentration required to block the adrenergic response to noxious stimuli.[91] This value is approximately 1.5 times the standard MAC value.

EFFECTS OF INHALED ANESTHETICS ON ORGANS AND SYSTEMS

CENTRAL NERVOUS SYSTEM

Inhaled anesthetics produce significant changes in mental function, cerebral oxygen consumption, cerebral blood flow (CBF), cerebrospinal fluid (CSF) dynamics, and CNS electrophysiology.

The changes in mental function, which so obviously are a necessary part of anesthesia, persist beyond the period of anesthetic administration and the immediate postoperative period. Following prolonged anesthesia, volunteers exhibit decreased intellectual function and an increased incidence of subjective symptoms. In one study, the effects of halothane exceeded those of isoflurane; the effect was greatest at 2 days following anesthesia and returned to near normal by 8 days.[92] In another study, neither halothane nor isoflurane consistently altered intellectual, visual, motor function, or personality characteristics.[93] Anesthesia with halothane or enflurane, when combined with nitrous oxide, led to altered

psychomotor performance and driving skills.[94] The persistent mental effects of halothane may be due in part to its biodegradation to bromide,[95] an ingredient in nonprescription sleeping pills. Studies have also shown that trace concentrations of anesthetics can significantly impair perceptual, cognitive, and motor skills[96] or learning.[98] Other studies examining trace concentrations have failed to confirm impairment of psychomotor function.[97] It is probably safe to assume that concentrations of anesthetics in the brain several hours after surgery or present in the ambient air of an operating room are too low to impair most tests of mental function.

Each of the potent inhaled anesthetics decreases cerebral metabolic rate (CMR_{O_2}), with the order of effect from greatest to least being isoflurane > enflurane $\geq$ halothane. The decrease in CMR_{O_2} is closely linked to cerebral electrical activity. With isoflurane it has been shown that once an isoelectric electroencephalogram is achieved, further increases in isoflurane concentration do not lead to further decreases in CMR_{O_2}.[99] Enflurane results in decreased CMR_{O_2} at a time when the EEG demonstrates a spike-suppression pattern.[100] If seizure activity occurs, however, CMR_{O_2} may increase.[101] Brain hypoxia does not result from enflurane-induced seizures despite increased CMR_{O_2}, most likely because CBF increases proportionately. The greatest decrease in CMR_{O_2} occurs during the transition from wakefulness to loss of consciousness.[102] With the inhaled anesthetics, decrease in CMR_{O_2} *per se* does not result in decrease in cerebral energy stores.[103] The decrease in CMR_{O_2} produced by isoflurane may provide some cerebral protection during periods of oxygen deprivation if the oxygen deprivation itself has not abolished electrical activity.[104] Other workers have not reached the same conclusion.[105] Isoflurane-induced hypotension may produce sufficient cerebral vasodilation to maintain CBF at the prehypotensive levels, but during this time CMR_{O_2} decreases. Thus, cerebral O_2 supply–demand relationships may be somewhat better preserved by isoflurane than halothane.[106–108]

Each of the inhaled agents, including nitrous oxide, produce cerebral vasodilation and an increase in CSF pressure. The order of potency for this effect is halothane > enflurane > isoflurane (Fig. 11-4).[109] This cerebral vasodilation will cause

FIG. 11-4. Cerebral blood flow measured in volunteers when awake and when anesthetized at varying MAC levels during controlled ventilation and normocapnea. (Reprinted with permission. Eger EI: Isoflurane: A review. Anesthesiology 55:559, 1981.)

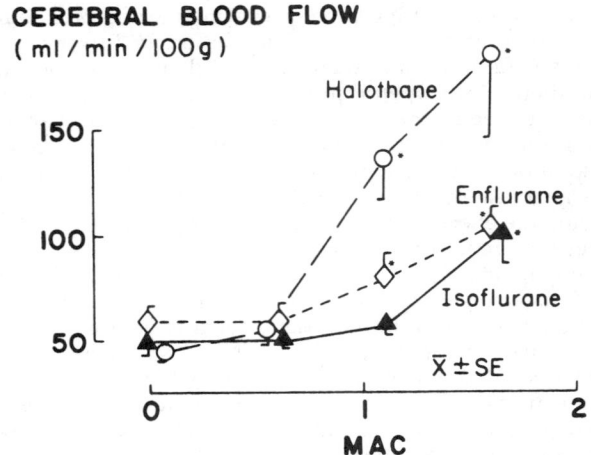

CEREBRAL BLOOD FLOW
(ml / min /100g)

increased CBF and cerebral blood volume. Nitrous oxide, either by itself or when added to one of the more potent drugs, can also produce cerebral vasodilation, but only to a modest degree. In the awake state, CBF is closely linked to CMR_{O_2}; if CMR_{O_2} decreases, CBF decreases. Isoflurane may preserve this relationship better than the other anesthetics and may explain the smaller increase in CBF produced by isoflurane. The increase in CBF with anesthetics tends to attenuate with time. With halothane, Albrecht et al[110] demonstrated the normalization of CBF within 2 h after induction of anesthesia.

Cerebrovascular responses to carbon dioxide are preserved when low concentrations of volatile anesthetics are used. Differences in the pattern of response exist, however. Hypocapnia will lead to a greater reduction in CBF during isoflurane than halothane;[111] that is, the effect of isoflurane on regional CBF appears to be highly CO_2-dependent. In humans, critical regional CBF, the blood flow at which EEG evidence of cerebral ischemia occurs, is significantly lower with isoflurane than with halothane, approximately 10 ml $\cdot$ 100 g^{-1} $\cdot$ min^{-1} and 18–20 ml $\cdot$ g^{-1} $\cdot$ min^{-1}, respectively.[112]

Recent studies in laboratory animals show that each of the potent inhaled drugs has important effects on CSF volume as well as effects on brain and cerebral blood volume. Anesthetics can affect both the production and reabsorption of CSF. Enflurane increases CSF production and decreases its reabsorption; that is, it increases the resistance to reabsorption of CSF.[113, 114] Isoflurane results in no significant change in CSF production or reabsorption.[113, 115] Halothane decreases the rate of CSF production but increases resistance to reabsorption.[116, 117] As with the effects of anesthetics on CBF, these effects on CSF dynamics tend to return toward normal values with time, except for enflurane. Both the cerebrovascular and CSF dynamic effects of the anesthetics contribute to an effect on CSF pressure. In the presence of modest hypocapnia, isoflurane appears less likely to produce potentially dangerous increases in CSF pressure than enflurane or halothane.[118, 119] Isoflurane may not be totally benign in this regard, however, because significant increases in CSF pressure have been reported in patients with brain tumors.[120] All evidence seems to indicate enflurane is the least favorable drug with respect to control of CSF pressure.

The pattern of EEG changes with the various inhaled anesthetics is quite similar in that increased anesthetic concentration decreases EEG wave frequency and increases voltage. At high concentrations, the anesthetics may produce electrical silence, sometimes passing through a burst-suppression pattern.[121, 122] The pattern of EEG dominance shifts from a posterior to an anterior location as anesthetic depth increases.[123] Unlike the other drugs, enflurane can produce high-voltage, repetitive-spiking activity.[124] This activity can be attenuated or abolished by decreasing enflurane dose or increasing the arterial carbon dioxide partial pressure (Pa_{CO_2}).[124–126] Enflurane does not increase the risk of seizures in patients with epileptic foci.

Anesthetics also produce significant changes in sensory-evoked potentials[127, 128] and must be considered along with many other factors in interpreting these responses.[129] The magnitude of the effect differs depending on the type of evoked responses being recorded. Cortical responses are more affected than subcortical responses. Enflurane, halothane, and isoflurane produce a dose-related decrease in the amplitude and increase in the latency of cortical components of somatosensory-evoked potentials.[130] Nitrous oxide decreases somatosensory responses[131] and may produce greater attenuation of these responses than low concentrations of enflurane or isoflurane.[132, 133] With respect to brain stem auditory-evoked potentials, enflurane,[134] halothane,[135, 136] and isoflurane[137] each increase the latencies of certain peaks. Nitrous oxide can increase latency and decrease amplitude of both visual- and auditory-evoked potentials.

RESPIRATORY SYSTEM

Inhaled anesthetics, including nitrous oxide, all have similar effects on breathing. Although these properties are similar, they need to be clearly understood in order to prepare safely for and manage the patient's ventilation in the perianesthetic period. Although this section emphasizes the effects of the drugs on breathing, the anesthetic state, per se, also alters other aspects of the respiratory system. Examples of the latter effects include the decrease of lung volume associated with induction of anesthesia and the change in the way gravitational factors affect diaphragm function.[138, 139]

Ventilatory Volumes and Frequency of Breathing

All inhaled anesthetics cause respiratory depression, with an elevation of Pa_{CO_2}, in a dose-related manner (Fig. 11-5). Most inhaled anesthetics increase frequency of breathing and decrease tidal volume as anesthetic concentration increases.[24, 140–142] These two changes counteract each other so that minute volume decreases less than one might expect from the decrease in tidal volume alone.[143] The increase in frequency as anesthetic depth increases is not a general property of all anesthetics because isoflurane tends not to increase frequency.[142] Nitrous oxide tends to increase respiratory frequency when added to isoflurane.[144] Adding 60% N_2O to 1 MAC halothane increases frequency to the same degree as an increase in the alveolar concentration of halothane alone, from 0.8% to 1.5%.[145] If minute volume is changed minimally, one would expect Pa_{CO_2} to change minimally unless other factors occur. Other factors do occur, however, including significant

FIG. 11-5. Pa_{CO_2} in spontaneous breathing volunteers when awake and anesthetized with enflurane, halothane, isoflurane, or nitrous oxide in oxygen. (Reprinted with permission. Eger EI: Isoflurane: A review. Anesthesiology 55:559, 1981.)

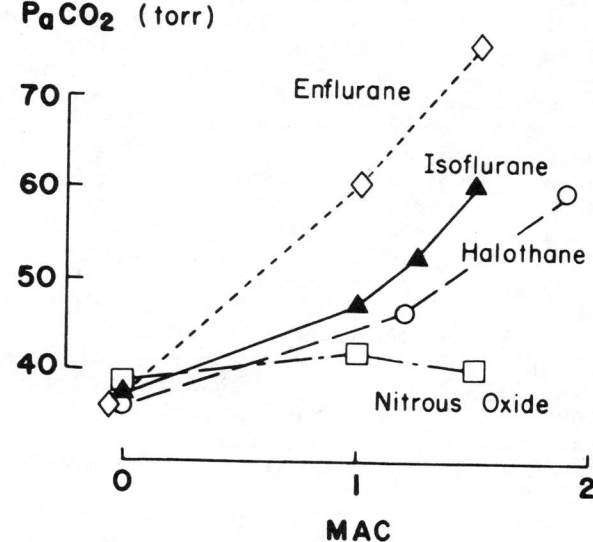

increases in wasted ventilation and small but consistent decreases in oxygen consumption and carbon dioxide production.

Effects on the Intercostal Muscle and Diaphragm

It is estimated that approximately 40% of normal tidal exchange is contributed by intercostal activity and 60% by the diaphragm.[146] In children and adolescents, halothane anesthesia decreases thoracic excursions but awake-state abdominal excursions persist, presumably because the phrenic motor-neuron pool is more resistant to depression than the intercostal motor-neuron pool. The clinical result is a loss of intercostal function as depth of anesthesia increases. Recruitment of intercostals does not occur in response to increased chemical drive. Also, especially in children, active stabilization of the rib cage cannot occur to resist any inward motion that might occur in response to negative intrathoracic pressure. Diaphragm function is also depressed by anesthetics.[147] Phrenic nerve activity is more resistant to depression by anesthetic drugs than is activity in the hypoglossal nerve.[148] There can be an end-inspiratory increase in thoracic volume that leads to the rocking appearance so characteristic of a deepening level of anesthesia.

Chemical Control of Breathing

The effects of anesthetics on the chemical control of breathing have probably received more emphasis than other respiratory effects. These effects certainly are important, for it is the loss of normal responses to chemical stimuli such as hypercarbia and hypoxia that so jeopardize the patient in the perianesthetic period. The ventilatory response to carbon dioxide is depressed more or less proportionately to anesthetic dose,[24, 140–142] except for diethyl ether,[141] but the hypoxic ventilatory response is blocked nearly completely by low concentrations of anesthesia.[149] Accordingly, during spontaneous breathing, as anesthetic concentration is increased, Pa_{CO_2} also increases. Duration of anesthesia does not affect the response, except with enflurane, where Pa_{CO_2} returns toward normal values as anesthesia is prolonged.[24]

Complete apnea will result if the anesthetic dose is high enough. The margin between the anesthetizing concentrations (MAC) and the concentration producing apnea (the respiratory anesthetic index) is least for enflurane. If apnea occurs, the apneic point is approximately 4 or 5 mm Hg below the Pa_{CO_2} maintained during spontaneous breathing, regardless of depth of anesthesia.[150] There are several clinical implications from these data. First, Pa_{CO_2} will be increased somewhat above normal during anesthesia if spontaneous breathing is allowed. The magnitude of the increase will depend on the anesthetic dose. Second, one is limited in how low the Pa_{CO_2} can be maintained and still preserve spontaneous breathing as a guide to depth of anesthesia. One should anticipate the Pa_{CO_2} will be 50–55 mm Hg at surgical planes of anesthesia when the most potent inhaled anesthetics are used. Surgical stimuli will decrease this level by 4–5 mm Hg at an equivalent level of anesthesia.[151] Assisting ventilation just to the apneic point will only decrease the Pa_{CO_2} an additional 4 or 5 mm Hg. Nitrous oxide, when studied under hyperbaric conditions at 1–1.25 times MAC, does not increase the Pa_{CO_2} during spontaneous breathing.[152] N_2O is less depressant than the potent inhaled drugs but is not free of a significant effect.[153, 154]

If the respiratory system is challenged by imposed increases of CO_2 during anesthesia, tidal volume increases but there are relatively minor changes in frequency of breathing. Although some do more so than others, all of the anesthetics produce an anesthetic dose-related depression of the ventilatory response to carbon dioxide (Fig. 11-6).[24, 140–143, 157] Large doses can obliterate the response.

Potentially more harmful is anesthetic depression of the ventilatory response to hypoxia. In dogs, isoflurane is somewhat less depressant than halothane or enflurane.[155–157] Knill et al.[158–161] performed a number of elegant studies to show that anesthetics also depress the hypoxic ventilatory drive in humans. Unlike the situation with anesthetic depression of the ventilatory CO_2 response, even subanesthetic concentrations of halothane, enflurane, and isoflurane markedly depress the hypoxic response in humans, with the depression maximal at anesthetizing concentrations. N_2O, too, significantly depresses the hypoxic response.[149] The normal augmentation of breathing produced by adding hypercarbia to hypoxia in the awake state is not observed during anesthesia.[156, 161] The ventilatory response to metabolic acidemia is also depressed by anesthesia.[161] The absence of hyperpnea during hypoxemia means that a useful clinical sign of hypoxia cannot be relied on during anesthesia.

Responses to Mechanical Loading

EXTERNAL. Another important aspect of ventilatory function is the response to mechanical loading such as might be seen with partial occlusion of an endotracheal tube or the presence of a weight on the chest or abdomen.[162] In general, the ability of the anesthetized patient to respond to external (extrinsic) loads is better than to internal (intrinsic) ones. In an early report Beecher[163] concluded that endotracheal tubes with internal diameters of 5–7 mm can be tolerated adequately by anesthetized, spontaneously breathing adults; that is, patients can maintain normal ventilation despite increased resistance to breathing. More recently, a number of workers

FIG. 11-6. Per cent change from awake values in the slope of the curve relating an increase in ventilation to imposed increases in Pa_{CO_2} in anesthetized volunteers. (Reprinted with permission. Eger EI: Isoflurane: A review. Anesthesiology 55:559, 1981.)

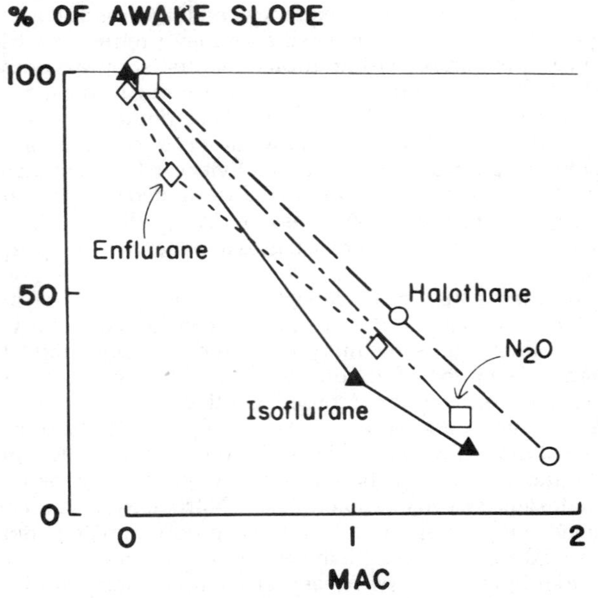

have shown that the anesthetized patient is less able to compensate for an increase in resistive loads than the awake patient. Behrakis et al[164] found that the anesthetized patient is better able than the awake patient to compensate for a first loaded breath (the first breath after a resistance is placed in the airway). Thereafter, however, the compensation is less complete in the anesthetized subject. Even subanesthetic concentrations of nitrous oxide may inhibit the normal response to resistive loads.[165] Moote et al[166] demonstrated in adults anesthetized with halothane at 1.1% that both resistive and elastic loads can be compensated for to a point but, if the loads are large enough, the loads may exceed the compensatory ability. Lindahl et al[167] imposed resistive loads in children during N_2O/halothane anesthesia. They found a negligible effect on frequency of breathing and an initial decrease in tidal volume that returned toward control levels in a fairly short time. In their study the larger the child, the poorer the compensation, presumably because of the larger tidal volume and flow rates prior to the addition of resistance.

What happens when weights (such as a surgeon's elbow) are placed on the chest or abdomen? Recall that with anesthesia, the intercostal component of inspiration is decreased to a greater extent than the diaphragmatic component.[146] As a result there is a more profound effect of abdominal weights than chest weights on breathing.[162] No compensation occurs with time, nor does an overshoot occur when the weights are removed.

INTERNAL. An example of a major internal load is the increased expiratory resistance encountered in a patient with chronic obstructive pulmonary disease. Pietak et al[168] found a rough correlation between the degree of abnormality of forced expiratory volume in 1 s and the increase in Pa_{CO_2} during anesthesia. If spontaneous ventilation is allowed, inordinate hypoventilation may occur in such patients.

Responses to Surgery

Surgery and presumably the attendant pain stimulate breathing so that average Pa_{CO_2} values are lower than without surgery.[151, 153] The effect of surgery in lowering Pa_{CO_2} is about the same over a modest range of anesthetic concentrations. The decrease in Pa_{CO_2} is less than one might have expected from the increase in minute ventilation because CO_2 production increased. Rosenberg et al[169] measured 2-point ventilatory responses to CO_2 in patients receiving N_2O–enflurane anesthesia and found that ventilation was increased at each CO_2 level. The slopes of the ventilatory-response curves were roughly parallel so that no change in sensitivity occurred. Lam et al[170] also showed that surgery increased ventilation but did not alter the sensitivity to CO_2 or improve the hypoxic ventilatory response.

Airway Caliber

It appears that the potent inhaled agents do not differ markedly in their effects on bronchomotor tone. They all will increase airway resistance to some degree because of loss of lung volume.[138] On the other hand, the potent inhaled drugs decrease airway resistance by causing bronchodilation.[171–174] Heneghan et al[175] showed in humans that halothane decreases airway resistance to a greater extent than isoflurane. Halothane and isoflurane both attenuate increased airway resistance caused by hypocapnia.[176] Hirshman et al[177, 178] studied the effects of anesthetics on both antigen-induced bronchoconstriction and bronchoconstriction resulting from topi-

cal stimulation and methylcholine. In each instance, all potent agents blocked bronchoconstriction to a similar extent. She showed, too, that the anesthetics did not block histamine release but rather blocked the bronchoconstrictor response to the mediator. All of the potent inhaled anesthetics are effective for the patient with asthma, although halothane may be somewhat preferable to isoflurane because the latter has a pungent odor that can cause airway irritation.

Hypoxic Pulmonary Vasoconstriction

The phenomenon of diversion of blood away from atelectatic lung has been known for many years.[179] The relation of this diversion to hypoxia-induced pulmonary arterial constriction and the effect of anesthetic drugs on the response are more recent findings.[180–182] There is general agreement that the inhaled anesthetics do depress the response in animals in a dose-related manner, but results with laboratory models may not apply under clinical conditions. Rees and Gaines[183] compared shunt fraction in patients undergoing one-lung anesthesia with ketamine or enflurane, drugs with differing effects on hypoxic pulmonary vasoconstriction in laboratory models, and found no differences in gas exchange in the patients. Neither halothane nor isoflurane decreased arterial oxygen tension (Pa_{O_2}) during one-lung ventilation of patients under opioid anesthesia,[184] and Carlsson et al[185] demonstrated no important clinical effect of isoflurane anesthesia on pulmonary vessel responses to hypoxia. These findings do not mean that selection of anesthetics is unimportant with regard to their effects on hypoxic pulmonary vasoconstriction. Rather, they mean that under clinical conditions with relatively low doses of inhaled drugs, the disease status of the lung and other effects of the anesthetics are of relatively greater importance.

Tracheal Ciliary Activity

Tracheal activity and mucociliary flow[186–188] are inhibited by the inhaled anesthetics. This effect, when combined with a similar inhibition found with endotracheal intubation, inhalation of dry gases, and others, may contribute to postoperative pulmonary infections.

CIRCULATORY SYSTEM

Hemodynamics

HALOTHANE, ENFLURANE, AND ISOFLURANE. The circulatory effects of halothane,[189] enflurane,[190] isoflurane,[23] and nitrous oxide[204] have been determined in human volunteers not undergoing operations. Results from these studies are important starting points in the consideration of the circulatory effects of these drugs because the study methods were similar for all agents, the general physical status of the volunteers was similar and normal, and no surgical events affected the results. Knowing how the drugs affect healthy humans provides a basis for understanding how diseases or other events change the effects. To a large degree the findings from the studies in volunteers have been substantiated by studies in patients.

All of the potent drugs decrease arterial pressure in a dose-related manner (Fig. 11-7). The mechanism of the decrease in blood pressure includes vasodilation, decreased cardiac output due to myocardial depression, and decreased sympathetic nervous system tone. With halothane, decreased cardiac out-

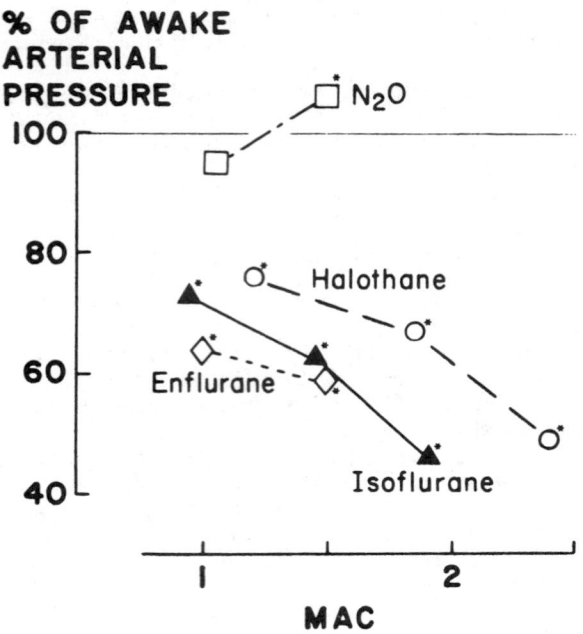

FIG. 11-7. Per cent change from awake values of mean arterial blood pressure in anesthetized, normocapnic volunteers. (Reprinted with permission. Eger EI: Isoflurane: A review. Anesthesiology 55:559, 1981.)

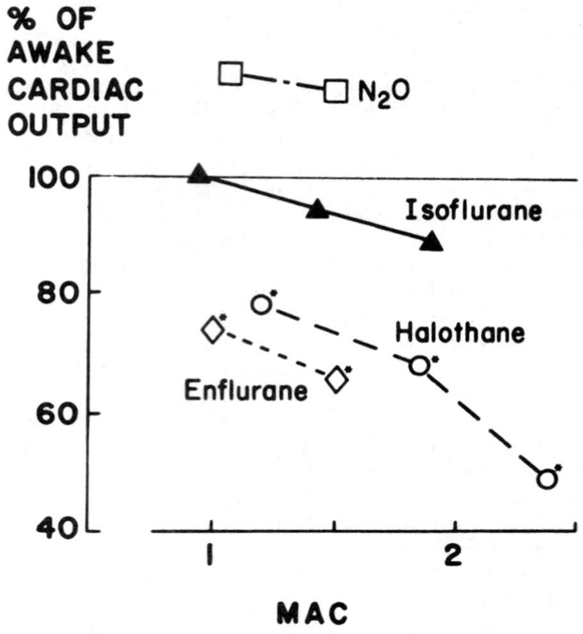

FIG. 11-8. Per cent change from awake values of cardiac output in anesthetized, normocapnic volunteers. (Reprinted with permission. Eger EI: Isoflurane: A review. Anesthesiology 55:559, 1981.)

put is the predominant cause (Fig. 11-8).[189] Halothane also increases venous compliance[191] and in patients who have high sympathetic tone, such as those with heart failure, halothane decreases systemic vascular resistance.[192] With enflurane both vasodilation and decreased myocardial contractility are important.[190] With isoflurane, a low peripheral resistance is the major cause of hypotension. Evidence of the relatively greater myocardial depression with halothane and enflurane is the greater increase in right atrial pressure seen with these drugs than with isoflurane.[193] Nevertheless, isoflurane also fits the criteria for a myocardial depressant in that cardiac output may not increase despite increased left ventricular filling pressure and decreased systemic vascular resistance.[194, 195]

The inhaled anesthetics differ in their effects on heart rate.[196] The heart rate changes least with halothane and increases most with isoflurane. Because arterial pressure decreases and cardiac output is either stable or decreased, myocardial work is decreased with all the inhaled anesthetics.

Oxygen consumption is decreased approximately 10%–15% below awake values in the anesthetized subject. As anesthetic dose is increased, the main reason for further decreases in O_2 consumption is decreased myocardial oxygen consumption.[197]

Anesthetics alter the distribution of cardiac output. Blood flow to the liver, kidneys, and gut is decreased, whereas blood flow to the brain, muscle, and skin is increased. Increases in muscle blood flow are most prominent with isoflurane.[23]

The findings in human volunteers obtained during controlled ventilation and normocarbia are altered when breathing is spontaneous. The resultant increase in Pa_{CO_2} and decrease in mean airway pressure cause heart rate and cardiac output to increase and systemic vascular resistance to decrease. Mean arterial pressure differs little from values obtained during controlled ventilation at comparable MAC levels.[198–200]

In the awake subject, when Pa_{CO_2} is increased by adding CO_2 to the breathing system and ventilation is held constant, cardiac output increases, systemic vascular resistance decreases, and blood pressure changes little. The potent inhaled anesthetics attenuate this response to CO_2 in a dose-related manner.[200] Circulatory changes therefore may not provide a reliable clue that hypercarbia or hypoxemia are occurring intraoperatively as might occur from a nonfunctioning anesthetic system valve, for example.[201]

As duration of anesthesia increases, there is recovery from the circulatory depressant effects of the anesthetics. This is especially true with halothane, to a lesser degree with enflurane, and to a yet smaller degree with isoflurane. The mechanism may involve β-adrenergic stimulation[202] leading to increased cardiac output, stroke volume, and decreased systemic vascular resistance.[189, 203]

NITROUS OXIDE. Nitrous oxide does not have a consistent hemodynamic effect. When given alone in a 40% concentration, it can decrease cardiac output.[204] When nitrous oxide is added to halothane in healthy volunteers, it lowers cardiac output and appears to stimulate the sympathetic nervous system, leading to increased systemic vascular resistance and increased arterial pressure.[154, 205] For enflurane, the addition of nitrous oxide produces no change or small decreases in arterial pressure and cardiac output. Reduction of the enflurane concentration and substitution of some of the required enflurane with nitrous oxide lead to less depression of circulatory variables than seen with enflurane alone.[206] For isoflurane at equivalent MAC levels, a nitrous oxide–isoflurane combination yields higher blood pressure than isoflurane alone, due mainly to greater systemic vascular resistance.[207] When nitrous oxide is given to patients with heart disease,[208, 209] particularly in combination with opioids,[210] it will cause hypotension and a decrease in cardiac output.

The pulmonary vascular effects of nitrous oxide are also variable. Patients with already-high pulmonary artery pressure may have further increases when nitrous oxide is added.[211] There is a significant correlation between the initial level of pulmonary vascular resistance and the further increases produced by nitrous oxide.[212] Whereas nitrous oxide can increase pulmonary vascular resistance in adults, a study in infants failed to show further increases of pulmonary vascular resistance with the addition of nitrous oxide.[213] It is of interest that the decrease in pulmonary vascular resistance with isoflurane is less than the decrease in systemic vascular resistance.[214]

INTESTINAL CIRCULATION. Splanchnic blood flow usually is decreased by anesthetics, an effect that is produced in two ways.[215] One is a decrease in hepatic perfusion that is due to decreases in arterial pressure or cardiac output. The other is an increase in splanchnic vascular resistance due to sympathetic stimulation such as occurs with surgical stimulation or increased Pa_{CO_2}. The anesthetics also may have a direct effect on the hepatic circulation. Laboratory studies show that halothane and isoflurane have differing effects on hepatic vascular resistance.[216, 217] Isoflurane produces hepatic arterial vasodilation and halothane does not. With both drugs, total hepatic blood flow decreases but oxygen delivery to the liver is better preserved with isoflurane. The hepatic oxygen supply/consumption ratio is higher during exposures to hypoxia with subanesthetic isoflurane than equivalent doses of enflurane or halothane.[218] When nitrous oxide is added to halothane anesthesia, splanchnic blood flow decreases further.[219] Isoflurane may protect against renal and splanchnic vasoconstriction from somatic and visceral nerve stimulation.[220]

REFLEX CONTROL OF THE CIRCULATION. Several studies have quantified the effects of the various inhaled anesthetics on these responses. Although the magnitude of the effect differs among the studies, it is clear that all of the inhaled agents,[221–224] including nitrous oxide,[225] attenuate baroreflex responses. Halothane attenuates both the pressor and depressor baroreflex responses.[226] Kotrly et al.[224] found that the depression is less pronounced with isoflurane than others had shown for halothane or enflurane. Infants who become hypotensive during halothane anesthesia do not show an increase in heart rate, perhaps in part because of the undeveloped baroreflexes in this age group.[227]

In addition to effects on reflex changes in heart rate, vasomotor reflex responses are also attenuated by the anesthetics. In humans, application of lower-body negative pressure and the resulting decrease in central blood volume does not result in as great an increase in peripheral resistance during halothane anesthesia as it does in awake subjects.[228]

The attenuation of cardiovascular reflexes by anesthetics is important in determining the anesthetized patient's response to hemorrhage. Dogs anesthetized with halothane, enflurane, or isoflurane and subjected to graded hemorrhage showed no change in heart rate despite gradual decreases in arterial pressure.[229] In another study, nitrous oxide and halothane given at equal multiples of their MAC had similar depressant effects on the circulation of hypovolemic swine.[230]

CARDIAC ARRHYTHMIAS, CONDUCTION, AND DRUG INTERACTIONS. Susceptibility of the heart to the arrhythmic effects of epinephrine differs among these anesthetics. Both enflurane and isoflurane are significantly less sensitizing than halothane (Fig. 11-9).[231–233] Epinephrine sensitivity is not closely related to the anesthetic dose.[234] Cardiac arrhythmias due to interactions of the anesthetics and other vasoactive drugs also are less likely with isoflurane than with halothane.[235] There is a relationship between responsiveness of the α-adrenergic system and epinephrine sensitivity.[236] The greater the degree of α-adrenergic responsiveness, the greater the epinephrine sensitivity during halothane anesthesia. Children are less likely than adults to exhibit ventricular arrhythmias from epinephrine during halothane anesthesia.[237]

Arrhythmias may occur during halothane anesthesia in the

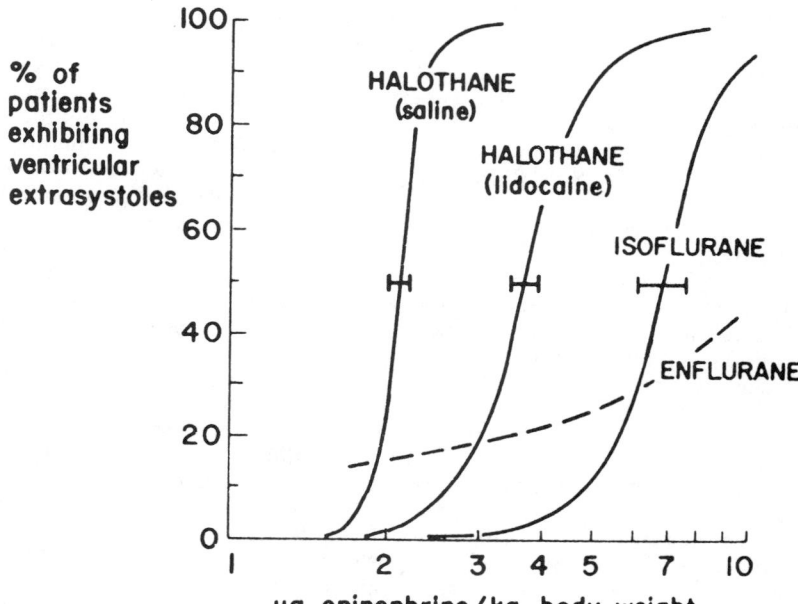

FIG. 11-9. Per cent of patients exhibiting three or more ventricular extrasystoles in response to a subcutaneous injection of epinephrine. (Reprinted with permission from the International Anesthesia Research Society from Johnston RR, Eger EI, Wilson C: A comparative interaction of epinephrine with enflurane, isoflurane and halothane in man. Anesth Analg 55:709, 1976.)

presence of hypercarbia. The threshold for arrhythmias is high, over 80 mm Hg.[238] During surgery the threshold decreases significantly. The tolerance for carbon dioxide is somewhat greater when nitrous oxide is added to halothane. Thiopental given prior to the potent inhaled drugs enhances epinephrine sensitivity, initially decreasing the arrhythmic dose of epinephrine by approximately 50%.[239, 240] Aminophylline is less likely to produce arrhythmias during anesthesia with enflurane or isoflurane than during halothane.[241, 242]

Enflurane, halothane, and isoflurane exert a direct negative chronotropic effect at the sinoatrial (SA) node.[243] Cardiac conduction is preserved *via* normal pathways better by isoflurane than by enflurane or halothane.[244] Conduction changes are believed to be a necessary part of the etiology of ventricular arrhythmias caused by reentry of excitation. The volatile anesthetics do not appear to alter cardiac-pacing stimulation thresholds.[245] Atrioventricular junctional rhythms are common with all anesthetics, but more so with enflurane and nitrous oxide.[246]

The cardiovascular effects of the inhaled anesthetics can be altered by other drugs. For example, the myocardial depression with isoflurane is enhanced by the calcium channel-blocking drug, verapamil, and is related to doses of each drug.[247–250] Some reversal of depression can be achieved by calcium administration. The data of Kapur et al[247] suggest that tolerance to verapamil is least with enflurane, next best with isoflurane, and best with halothane. In their study the primary problem seen in halothane-treated animals was prolongation of the P-R interval; however, the interaction depends on both the halothane and verapamil doses. Anesthetics alter verapamil pharmacokinetics so that higher plasma levels of verapamil are achieved during anesthesia than in the awake state.[248, 249] Diltiazem, another calcium channel blocker, has been used to treat premature ventricular contractions and tachyarrhythmias during halothane anesthesia.[251] It increases the threshold for epinephrine-induced arrhythmias. Isoflurane interacts to prevent the reflex tachycardia that occurs with nicardipine.[252] Halothane and propranolol have similar cardiovascular-depressant effects and they appear to be additive.[253]

CORONARY CIRCULATION. Coronary autoregulation links coronary blood flow to myocardial oxygen demand. This relationship persists in the normal heart during anesthesia but may be perturbed by the inhaled anesthetics. In patients with normal coronary vessels the effects of the drugs on coronary vessels are of minor importance compared with the influence of the major metabolic determinants of coronary blood flow and resistance. Differences in drug effects are more obvious and clinically relevant in the presence of coronary stenosis or occlusion.

Bollen et al[254] determined in isolated coronary vessels that halothane, more than isoflurane, relaxes coronary arteries that constrict in response to potassium or a prostaglandin compound. Using a dog model with coronary-vessel stenosis or occlusion to produce a zone of myocardial blood-flow deprivation, studies have shown that isoflurane is a potent coronary vasodilator and that it can steal blood away from ischemic zones of the myocardium.[255, 256] It appears isoflurane uncouples the generally close relationship between coronary blood flow and myocardial oxygen demand more than the other potent inhaled drugs. It produces greater dilation of intramyocardial arterioles than epicardial arteries.[257]

In patients with coronary artery disease receiving iso-

flurane, coronary blood flow is maintained despite decreased arterial pressure. At the same time, coronary sinus O_2 levels increase and, in some patients, lactate production occurs.[195] When hypotension is produced by isoflurane, animals with critical coronary stenosis may develop myocardial ischemia.[258] On the other hand, isoflurane was shown to increase the tolerance to pacing-induced myocardial ischemia in humans.[259]

Enflurane also has prominent coronary vasodilating properties.[260, 261] Nitrous oxide, when added to the potent inhaled agents, may have deleterious effects on the distribution of coronary blood flow.[208] When nitrous oxide is added to isoflurane, there is a further decrease in heart rate and arterial pressure.[209] Despite unchanged coronary flow, addition of nitrous oxide decreases myocardial oxygen extraction. Patients anesthetized with nitrous oxide and isoflurane may show large increases in coronary blood flow with only small decreases in oxygen consumption, suggesting autoregulation has been impaired. A similar effect occurs when nitrous oxide is added to enflurane anesthesia.

RENAL CIRCULATION. The primary effect of inhaled anesthetics on the kidney is mediated through their effects on the renal circulation. Renal blood flow generally decreases during anesthesia either because cardiac output or arterial pressure decrease or renal vascular resistance increases.[262–267] Bastron et al[268] showed that autoregulation of blood flow in the kidney is preserved during halothane anesthesia. Priano[269] chronically implanted ultrasonic flow probes on a renal artery of dogs and found that halothane did not decrease renal blood flow. He also found that the administration of halothane to acutely hypovolemic dogs did not decrease renal blood flow.

Blood

Inhaled agents can have effects on hemopoiesis, individual cell elements, and coagulation. Anesthetics also can alter the function of elements of the immune response, but this subject is covered in Chapter 51.

HEMOPOIESIS. Much of our concern about inhalation anesthetics and hemopoiesis involves a consideration of the potential toxic effects of nitrous oxide on the bone marrow and other tissues with rapidly dividing cells. Green and Eastwood noted dose-dependent depression on bone marrow in rats exposed to nitrous oxide.[270] Prolonged exposure to nitrous oxide will produce an anemia similar to pernicious anemia. Subsequently, it has been shown that nitrous oxide inhibits methionine synthetase, an enzyme involved in the metabolism of vitamin B_{12}.[271, 272] Exposure of rats to 1% nitrous oxide for 1 week to 6 months is not associated with bone marrow depression[273] but sensitive tests of DNA biosynthesis such as deoxyuridine suppression[274, 275] indicate that megaloblastic changes can occur after exposure of patients to nitrous oxide for as little as 1 h. Nunn et al[276] reported megaloblastic bone marrow changes in a seriously ill patient after 105 min of nitrous oxide anesthesia. Interestingly, the same patient required another anesthetic some 7 h after the first, and on this occasion, 30 mg of folinic acid was given prior to the anesthetic. This anesthetic was not associated with bone marrow changes. The effect of nitrous oxide on the bone marrow is apparently transitory and the white blood cell count increases again after withdrawal of the nitrous oxide.[277] The commonly used halogenated agents do not appear to have an adverse effect on hemopoiesis at concentrations used clinically.[278, 279]

WHITE BLOOD CELLS. Halothane is known to inhibit polymorphonuclear leukocyte chemotaxis[280, 281] and has little or no effect on phagocytic engulfment of bacteria.[282] Halothane and enflurane do, however, consistently inhibit the killing activity of polymorphonuclear leukocytes, an effect that appears to be transient.[283] Isoflurane and nitrous oxide do not appear to inhibit the microbicidal function of polymorphonuclear cells.[284] The clinical consequences of these findings have not been established.

RED BLOOD CELLS. There has been speculation about the effect of inhaled drugs on the oxygen–hemoglobin dissociation curve. Studies have been contradictory, showing either a small rightward shift of the curve[285] or a shift to the left.[286] Using a technique of automatic hemoglobin-dissociated curve plotting, Shah et al[287] found no shift in the oxygen dissociation curve in patients receiving nitrous oxide. In contrast to conclusions from an earlier study,[288] these authors additionally demonstrated that the measurement of blood gases using a polarographic technique was not influenced by the presence of nitrous oxide.

PLATELETS. Volatile anesthetic drugs have been imputed as a cause of increased bleeding during surgery, either because of the effect on vascular smooth muscle[289] or because of an interaction with platelets. A slight prolongation of bleeding time has been observed during halothane anesthesia, and halothane can inhibit platelet aggregation.[290] Nevertheless, vast clinical experience suggests this effect is more of a theoretical than practical concern. Isoflurane and enflurane do not change the bleeding time.[291, 292]

The inhalation anesthetics have been shown to have a variety of other potentially harmful side-effects. For a complete discussion the reader is referred to Chapter 12, on anesthetic toxicity.

NEUROMUSCULAR SYSTEM

The potent inhaled anesthetic agents have muscle-relaxant properties by themselves, but also potentiate the action of neuromuscular blocking drugs. The mechanism by which inhaled agents potentiate neuromuscular blocking drugs is not clear, but may involve desensitization of the postjunctional membrane[295] or changes in muscle blood flow, such as occurs with isoflurane.[199]

Although there are minor differences between them, all of the potent inhaled anesthetics potentiate the depolarizing relaxants. Isoflurane has a greater potentiating effect on succinylcholine block than halothane.[296] The transition from Phase I to Phase II block occurs at a lower dose of succinylcholine when halothane or enflurane is used than when a nitrous oxide–narcotic technique is used.[297] Donati et al[298] suggested that enflurane did not potentiate succinylcholine block but did accelerate the onset of Phase II block, as described with halothane. In a similar manner, isoflurane appears to accelerate the transition from Phase I to Phase II block when succinylcholine infusion is used.[299]

In general, the potent inhaled anesthetics have an even more profound potentiating effect on the nondepolarizing muscle relaxants. Isoflurane is more effective than halothane. Approximately three times as much d-tubocurarine is required to produce equivalent neuromuscular blockade in patients receiving halothane compared with those receiving isoflurane (Fig. 11-10).[300] Because both halothane and isoflurane

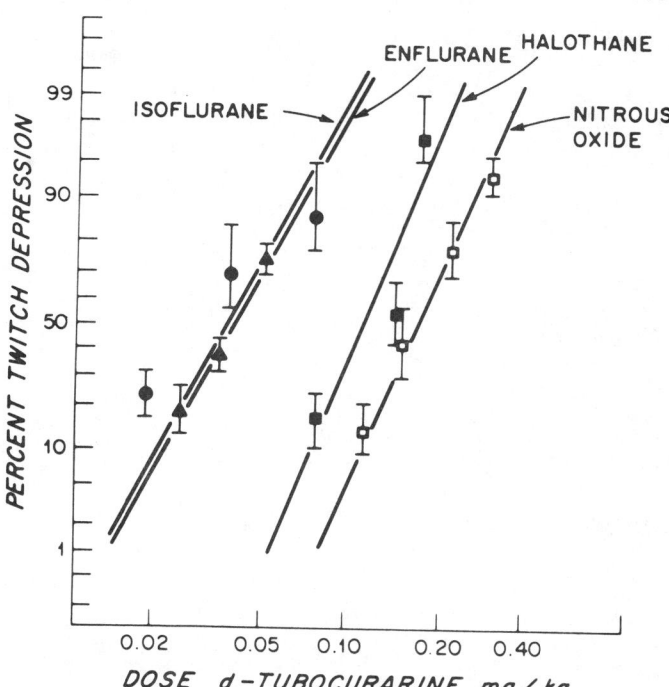

FIG. 11-10. Interaction of 1.25 MAC isoflurane, enflurane, halothane, and 66% nitrous oxide with d-tubocurarine. (Reprinted with permission. Ali HH, Savarese JJ: Monitoring of neuromuscular function. Anesthesiology 45:216, 1976.)

produce a similar degree of neuromuscular blockade in vitro, Vitez et al[301] suggested that the greater potentiation of neuromuscular blockade produced with isoflurane in vivo may be explained by the increase in muscle blood flow produced by this agent. Pancuronium and metocurine, like d-tubocurarine, are potentiated more by isoflurane than by halothane.[302, 303]

Enflurane has effects on neuromuscular function similar to those of isoflurane.[304] Rupp et al.[305] demonstrated that enflurane potentiated the neuromuscular-blocking effect of vecuronium to a greater extent than occurred with isoflurane or halothane. They concluded that the mechanism by which volatile anesthetic drugs enhance neuromuscular blockade was different in the case of vecuronium. More specifically, vecuronium, when compared with other neuromuscular blockers, appeared to be least affected by inhaled halogenated drugs; therefore, in circumstances where the end-tidal anesthetic concentration is not known, vecuronium would be of clinical advantage in that the neuromuscular blockade produced by vecuronium would be more predictable than that produced by other relaxants.

The action of atracurium is also potentiated by the inhaled drugs. A smaller dose of atracurium is necessary to produce a given level of neuromuscular blockade in the presence of halothane.[306] Less atracurium is necessary when isoflurane is administered than when a nitrous oxide–opioid anesthetic technique is used.[307] In a comparison of the effect of halothane and isoflurane on atracurium dose requirement when administered by infusion, Brandom et al.[308] showed that halothane and isoflurane equally reduced the atracurium infusion requirement in children undergoing surgery.

ENDOCRINE SYSTEM

Islet Cell Function and Glucose Metabolism

During anesthesia, the blood glucose level is usually elevated, and there is a diminished plasma insulin response to glucose administration.[309] The increase in blood glucose levels during anesthesia is due either to a reduction in insulin release from islet cells or decreased peripheral metabolism of glucose. Gingerich et al.,[310] using isolated rat pancreatic cells, showed that halothane caused a marked reduction in pancreatic insulin excretion that was not associated with a significant change in glucose oxidation. Ewart et al.[311] demonstrated a similar finding for enflurane and speculated that the effect of anesthetic drugs on insulin secretion by the pancreas may be due to alteration in calcium availability or to microtubular or microfilament function or even be a result of an effect of the halogenated drug on the plasma membrane itself.

Antidiuretic Hormone

It has been suggested that all opioids and inhaled anesthetic drugs affect antidiuretic hormone (ADH) release[312] and this may or may not affect intraoperative renal function.[313] With more accurate assessment of ADH by radioimmunoassay and more frequent sampling, it has been shown that while neither opioid nor "light" halothane anesthesia, per se, stimulates ADH release, surgical stimulation results in a massive release of ADH, which is part of a stress response.[314, 315] Higher concentrations of anesthetics, i.e., a "deeper" level of anesthesia, can modify the response.

Renin

Plasma renin activity varies very little as a result of anesthesia but is influenced by catecholamine release in the perioperative period and by the fluid status of the patient.[313, 315]

Serotonin

Inhaled anesthetic drugs, per se, do not protect against the effects of the carcinoid syndrome.[316, 317] While mechanical ventilation has been shown to be associated with more effective removal of serotonin by the lungs, halothane appears to have no effect on this mechanism.[318]

Testosterone

Halothane has been shown to reduce significantly the level of testosterone in the blood.[319] The level of testosterone not only was reduced intraoperatively, but continued to decrease well into the postoperative period. No explanation was offered for this.

Surgical Stress and Endocrine Response

Surgical stress causes increased activity of the hypothalamus and the pituitary and adrenal glands. This stress response is both a result of anesthesia and the noxious stimuli of a surgical procedure. Extent of the stress can be quantified by measurement of serum adrenocorticotropic hormone (ACTH), cortisol, and catecholamine levels.

Induction of anesthesia by mask with inhaled anesthetics is more stressful than when intravenous anesthetics are used. Induction of halothane–oxygen anesthesia by mask, without the use of thiopental, caused plasma norepinephrine levels to increase 15 min after the induction of anesthesia, but they returned to control levels some 45–60 min later.[320] This was attributed to increased norepinephrine release rather than to alteration in the mechanism of reuptake. Sumikawa et al[321] demonstrated that halothane inhibits the reuptake of norepinephrine into chromaffin granules. ACTH, β lipoprotein, cortisol, aldosterone, and dehydroepiandrostenedione levels are all elevated in patients anesthetized for elective orthopedic procedures.[322] The rise of aldosterone may be the result of elevated ACTH and serum renin levels. In a study of patients undergoing hysterectomy, Lacoumenta et al.[323] noted that hormonal changes were similar in two groups of patients who received either 1.2 or 2.1 MAC of halothane, respectively, suggesting that a higher concentration of halothane does not reliably suppress the endocrine response to surgery. This contradicts earlier work that suggested that the endocrine response could be attenuated with deeper levels of anesthesia.[91] Comparing the stress response to surgery during either halothane or balanced anesthesia with fentanyl, it was found that halothane was less effective than fentanyl in preventing an increase in plasma norepinephrine concentrations.[324] Enflurane is more effective than neurolept anesthesia in blocking sympathoadrenal responses to surgical stress.[325]

A rise in catecholamines occurs with the onset of surgery during isoflurane anesthesia when the anesthetic concentration equals 1 MAC.[326] Increasing the level of isoflurane to a concentration of greater than 1 MAC does not have any advantage in this regard over a technique of inhaled anesthesia supplemented by opioids. Enflurane inhibits the secretion of both epinephrine and norepinephrine from the adrenal medulla,[327] apparently because of an effect of enflurane on the cell membrane.[328]

Direct comparison between halothane and enflurane when used to anesthetize children for adenoidectomy showed that although the catecholamine levels increased with both drugs, the levels were greater with halothane than with enflurane.[329]

Adrenal Medulla

In addition to information learned from the studies just noted, our knowledge of the effect of anesthetic drugs on the hormones of the adrenal medulla has been enhanced by experience gained in the management of pheochromocytoma.[330] Halothane is known to sensitize the myocardium to the arrhythmic effects of epinephrine, and the dose of epinephrine needed to produce premature ventricular contractions is lower during halothane anesthesia than isoflurane or enflurane.[232] Enflurane and isoflurane are therefore of theoretical advantage for resection of pheochromocytoma, and both have given satisfactory results.[331, 332]

Thyroid Gland

Anesthetic agents can exert an effect on thyroid function either by influencing secretion of thyroid-stimulating hormone (TSH) by the anterior pituitary gland, by a direct effect on the thyroid gland, or by attenuating the peripheral activity of the thyroid hormone. By measuring TSH and serum thyroxine levels simultaneously, Oyama et al[333] were able to show that neither the stress of surgery nor anesthesia with halothane or methoxyflurane anesthesia influenced TSH release. In patients receiving halothane there was a significant increase in serum thyroxine but no significant change when patients were anesthetized with methoxyflurane. It would seem that TSH does not play a significant role in modulating the serum thyroxine level during anesthesia or surgery.

Hyperthyroidism has been shown to be associated with an enhancement of halothane-induced hepatotoxicity in rats.[334] This appears to be due to a new balance between cytochrome P450 bioactivation and glutathione. Servin et al[335] showed that hyperthyroid patients metabolize more halothane and enflurane than do euthyroid patients. The percentage decrease in oxygen uptake produced by halothane in hyperthyroid animals is significantly greater than in the euthyroid control animals.[336] The clinical significance of these data is not known.

There are no data on the anesthetic requirement of hypothyroid humans,[337] but there is a clinical impression that the hypothyroid state is associated with an increased sensitivity to anesthesia.

UTERINE AND FETAL EFFECTS

The inhaled anesthetics can have effects on both uterine muscle and the fetus.

Uterine Muscle

Volatile anesthetic drugs cause myometrial relaxation[338] and can contribute to perinatal blood loss. Enflurane, isoflurane, and halothane are equally depressant to uterine smooth muscle at similar MAC values.[339, 340] This relaxation results in greater blood loss when an abortion is performed under halothane anesthesia than when a nitrous oxide–opioid technique is used.[341] Although the MAC of pregnant patients is reduced, even 70% nitrous oxide in oxygen is associated with a high incidence of intraoperative maternal awareness; therefore, adding low doses of inhaled halogenated drugs is indicated. While this practice could potentially result in increased blood loss at the time of cesarean section as a result of myometrial relaxation, 0.5% halothane, 1% enflurane, or 0.75% isoflurane can be used safely.[342]

Fetal Effects

Inhaled drugs delivered to the mother do, of course, cross the placenta and therefore affect the fetus.[343] Halothane (1 MAC) has been shown to cause fetal hypotension even when this level of anesthesia results in little change in maternal blood pressure and pulse rate. Blood flow to fetal organs remained unchanged despite a 27% decrease in mean fetal blood pressure. Thus, although 1 MAC halothane anesthesia is associated with fetal hypotension as a result of decreased fetal peripheral vascular resistance, this does not appear to affect adversely the fetal regional blood flow.[344] When the fetus is acidotic, however, the addition of an anesthetic drug can further depress the cardiovascular system and result in a reduction in CBF and a potential decrease in oxygen delivery.[345]

Enflurane and isoflurane have favorable cardiovascular and metabolic effects on the fetus during anesthesia for cesarean section. Because enflurane is partially metabolized to inorganic fluoride, the potential exists for a toxic effect of this ion on the fetus. The total dose is small, however, and follow-up studies of infants delivered by cesarean section under enflurane anesthesia have not demonstrated any renal function impairment.[346] Isoflurane augmented fetal acidosis in an animal model when the anesthetic was continued for a period of greater than 90 min.[347] Although this duration of isoflurane anesthesia during cesarean section is not common in clinical practice, Biehl et al[347] suggested that halothane may be a more appropriate drug for obstetric anesthesia.

Because nitrous oxide can interfere with methionine syn-

thetase and cell division, there is concern that the use of nitrous oxide during pregnancy may be associated with an increased incidence of fetal abnormalities. Evidence to date suggests that this is not the case.[348–351]

SIGNS OF ANESTHESIA

In the days when diethyl ether was nearly the only anesthetic available, assessment of anesthetic depth was relatively easy. With anesthetic induction, the patient passed through stages of anesthesia that could be monitored by observation of pupils, muscle activity, tearing, respiratory patterns, muscle relaxation, and so forth.[352] With the onset of the modern era of anesthesia, however, that era which began when fluorinated inhaled drugs and muscle relaxants appeared, there began a problem in determining what constitutes adequate anesthesia.[353] For example, in an effort to provide adequate conditions for surgery, muscle relaxants were given and one important sign of anesthesia, lack of movement, was removed.[354] The problem of assessing adequately the depth of anesthesia has persisted to the present time, especially when nitrous oxide is used as the primary anesthetic and is supplemented with other drugs to provide complete anesthesia.[355–358] Guedel's[352] description of observable and reproducible physical signs for ether anesthesia no longer apply when anesthesiologists use a barbiturate for induction, inhaled drugs with low blood solubility for maintenance, and muscle relaxants. In addition, misinterpretation of respiratory signs can confuse deep anesthesia with airway obstruction because the pattern of chest movement can be similar in both instances. Finally, pupillary dilation can reflect not only deep anesthesia but also sympathetic stimulation from hypercarbia or surgical stimulation.

Woodbridge[359] described well the concepts or components that comprise "general anesthesia." Although somewhat different terms are used in more recent literature, e.g., attenuation of the stress response rather than Woodbridge's depression of reflexes, the ideas are quite similar if not identical. The elements of the nervous system that are depressed during anesthesia include sensory (afferent), motor (efferent), reflex, and mental components. How does depression of each of these components contribute to clinical signs as a patient is anesthetized? What follows is a description of phenomena that occur as one might anesthetize a patient with nitrous oxide combined with one of the potent inhaled drugs, or with a potent drug used with oxygen alone.

Although it applied to diethyl ether, Artusio[360] was the first to describe the "lightest" or first stage of anesthesia, a stage of sensory and gentle mental depression virtually not used today except when providing analgesia with nitrous oxide. Patients in this state will open their eyes on command, breathe normally, and tolerate mild painful stimuli such as suturing of skin, superficial debridement, and so forth. In general, airway and other reflexes remain intact.

Increasing the dose of anesthetic further may cause the patient to enter a stage of excitement. This stage is marked by muscle movement, retching, heightened laryngeal reflexes, disconjugate pupils, tachycardia, hypertension, and hyperventilation. Because many of these signs are unwanted, the goal should be to pass through this stage quickly by increasing the inspired concentration of the inhaled drug or by eliminating excitement altogether by use of an intravenous barbiturate. An excitement stage is quite likely to occur when nitrous oxide is used in concentrations exceeding 50% (vol/vol) because that closely approaches the estimated MAC awake[90] for this drug.[361, 362] MAC awake, although described as the anesthetic dose at which subjects begin to respond to commands, also defines a dose of anesthetic at which most patients lose consciousness and recall.

The next deeper level of anesthesia is notable by the absence of movement in response to a surgical incision. The MAC is that concentration at which 50% of patients do not move when a skin incision is made[64, 65] and when the MAC is exceeded by a factor of 1.25–1.3, the vast majority of patients will not move in response to an incision.[70] This level of anesthesia is associated with depression of each of the four elements of nervous system function. Sensory loss will allow surgery to proceed without the patient experiencing pain. There will be loss of recall, although there are a few reports of recall occurring even at the deeper levels of anesthesia.[363, 364] The incidence of recall is greatest when only low concentrations of anesthetics are used and neuromuscular blocking drugs are relied on to provide relaxation.[365] Evidence of reflex depression at this level of anesthesia is the absence of an increase of blood pressure or heart rate with surgical stimulation. A very pronounced autonomic response is indicative of a light level of surgical anesthesia. Finally, although the patient may not move when the incision is made, there may be insufficient motor relaxation for operations in the abdomen or thorax.

As anesthesia with the inhaled drugs deepens beyond the MAC, further respiratory, cardiovascular and CNS depression occurs. It may be difficult or impossible to predict accurately the alveolar concentration of the anesthetic from assessment of clinical signs. This is because a given clinical sign, such as a change in blood pressure, is not affected by all anesthetics in the same way.[366, 367] Furthermore, the impact of other drugs, age, debility, and surgical stimulation on clinical signs is unpredictable. Another mitigating factor is the alteration of circulatory effects of some anesthetics with time. For example, with halothane, the dose–response relationship between halothane and blood pressure that exists during the first hour of anesthesia is eliminated when anesthesia is prolonged.[366, 368] Some recovery from the respiratory depression of enflurane occurs as anesthesia continues.[24] Monitoring the depth of anesthesia requires familiarity with the properties of each anesthetic and evaluation of the response of each patient to the anesthetic drug alone and to surgical stimulation.[367]

With further increases in alveolar concentration a level of anesthesia can be achieved at which the autonomic response to noxious stimuli is totally blocked. This conforms to MAC-BAR, the MAC required to block the adrenergic and cardiovascular response to incision.[91] At this dose one would not expect tachycardia or hypertension in response to surgical stimulation or other interventions such as endotracheal intubation.

As the concentration of potent inhaled anesthetics is deepened still further, the clinical picture is one of increasing depression of circulation and respiration. Although precise dose–response relationships may not exist,[366] arterial pressure and cardiac output will be progressively reduced as the anesthetic dose is increased. Hypotension can be profound.

Changes in breathing are probably the most sensitive indices of depth of anesthesia, probably because breathing is less intimately under autonomic control. Movement of the diaphragm persists at levels of anesthesia that block intercostal muscle function.[146] For most drugs ventilatory frequency increases as anesthetic dose increases over a clinically useful range.[142] This change is accompanied by loss of active intercostal activity, leading to loss of thoracic expansion and persistence of only diaphragmatic descent.[369] A rocking breathing pattern results, often with a lower rib cage flaring, leading to

an out-of-phase pattern of chest wall movement.[369] Unfortunately, liberal use of muscle relaxants, opioids, and controlled ventilation has prevented respiration from being a common monitor of anesthetic depth.

Pupillary and other eye signs of anesthetic depth do not follow a reliable dose–response relationship.[366, 367] Eye movement is a somewhat better guide to depth than pupillary diameter, and presence of eye movement ordinarily is a sign of light anesthesia. Change of the eyes from conjugate to disconjugate positions with onset of surgery can usually be relied on as an indicator of the lightening level of anesthesia. Although lacrimation occurs even with deep levels of cyclopropane and ether, it is not apparent during deep enflurane, halothane, and isoflurane anesthesia. Conversely, the occurrence of lacrimation where it did not previously exist suggests a lightening level of anesthesia with all drugs. Of the eye signs, pupillary diameter changes may be the least reliable indicator of anesthetic depth. This is because pupillary caliber is under sympathetic control.[366] A variety of variables can influence sympathetic activity, including drugs and Pa_{CO_2}. As with newly appearing eye movement, acute pupillary enlargement with onset of surgery may be a sign of relatively light anesthesia, but one must remember that dilated pupils may also be a sign of cerebral hypoxia.

Some consideration of motor or efferent blockade is warranted. Muscle tone decreases as anesthetic depth increases.[370] The active abdominal muscle expiratory effort that occurs as anesthesia is induced gradually becomes less intense and the abdomen becomes soft[369] as a surgical plane of anesthesia is achieved. Expiratory contraction of the rectus abdominis and other abdominal muscles gradually decreases as depth of anesthesia increases. The prominence of the recti is enhanced by contraction of the oblique and transverse abdominal muscles because their contraction makes the semilunar line more prominent. Stout patients with diastasis recti or with thin, incompetent recti often show paradoxical abdominal motion as consciousness is lost. This results from oblique and transverse muscle contraction during expiration that increases the intraabdominal pressure during expiration, leading to protrusion of abdominal contents under or between the recti. Even profound levels of anesthesia will not obliterate muscle contraction from an electrocautery stimulus.

Although misjudgments about the level of anesthesia can occur, with practice and experience one can ordinarily estimate the adequacy of anesthesia from clinical signs.[356, 369] Accurate assessment is most difficult in the period after induction of anesthesia and before surgical stimulation begins. Tolerance of anesthesia may be poor so that even very lightly anesthetized patients may be hypotensive at this time. If the concentration of anesthetic is reduced too much, these patients may move and exhibit hypertension, tachycardia, pupillary dilation, and salivation when surgery begins. Anesthetic depth should be viewed as a continuum, with patients maintained at various levels of the continuum depending on surgical requirements.[369] It is somewhat gratuitous, although true, to state that constant vigilance is necessary and that, when in doubt about the level of anesthesia, one should decrease the delivered concentration and closely observe the patient for changes in clinical signs. This will allow one to determine whether this initial safest change in concentration, a decrease, was also the most appropriate change. We especially support the concept of tailoring the administered dose to the needs of the patient. This will often include light, deep, and in-between levels in the same patient at various stages of the anesthetic.

CLINICAL USES AND TECHNIQUES

Several features about the clinical use of inhaled anesthetics lead to continued enthusiasm for these drugs by many anesthesiologists. These features, not all of which are unique to the inhaled drugs, nonetheless when taken in combination make these drugs versatile mainstays of the practice of anesthesia. These include the ability to induce and maintain anesthesia regardless of age or habitus of the patient; presence of clinical signs that give an indication of depth of anesthesia; ability to increase or decrease depth of anesthesia at will; a predictable pattern of recovery from anesthesia; provision of all of the components of the anesthetic state in many patients without the use of adjuvants; knowledge of the concentration of the drug at the site of action; and the ability to deliver a broad range of oxygen concentrations. In the absence of outcome studies that allow us to know whether one technique of anesthesia is better than another, we believe the inhaled drugs will continue to be important parts of our armamentarium.

INDUCTION OF ANESTHESIA

Patient comfort and speed of induction lead many anesthesiologists to begin anesthesia with intravenous drugs and then to add inhaled agents. In these instances consideration must be given to the safety and smoothness of the transition from anesthesia provided by the intravenous drugs to the maintenance state provided by the inhaled agents. Anesthesia provided by a single dose of a thiobarbiturate and depolarizing relaxant is brief due to their redistribution from brain and metabolism, respectively. There are four methods for introducing an inhaled anesthetic in a concentration sufficient for the patient to tolerate the endotracheal tube or not to move when an incision is made, after such a brief time. One is for the anesthesiologist to provide both high inspired anesthetic concentrations (over pressure) and controlled alveolar hyperventilation. Reference to the rate of rise of alveolar concentration toward the inspired concentration of an inhaled anesthetic is appropriate at this point. A typical pattern of the rate of rise of alveolar concentration toward the inspired concentration for a drug of intermediate blood solubility, such as isoflurane, is shown in Figure 11-2. In this example, it is assumed that alveolar ventilation maintains eucapnia. In order for a surgical level of anesthesia to be achieved within 5 min, the inspired concentration must be twice the desired alveolar concentration. For instance, when using isoflurane in a young adult, the inspired concentration required for induction to occur in 5 min or less with normal alveolar ventilation would be approximately 3%. It should also be recalled that the small influence of the second-gas effect accompanying the use of nitrous oxide may further aid induction.

A second approach to achieving an anesthetizing concentration of the inhaled drug during an intravenous induction is to administer supplemental doses of the sedative and relaxing drugs or to select intravenous drugs with more than ultrashort duration of action. This approach will allow more time for inhaled induction to occur.

A third approach is to rely on a mixture of intravenous and inhaled drugs not only for induction, but also for maintenance of anesthesia. Only a portion of the anesthetizing conditions are provided by the inhaled drugs. For example, one might combine intravenous opioids with a drug of low potency such as nitrous oxide, or subanesthetic concentrations of a potent agent such as enflurane. Because in the one instance a drug of low solubility is chosen and in the other only a low alveolar concentration of the anesthetic is needed, induction should be rapid.

A fourth approach is to use a potent drug of low blood solubility such as sevoflurane. This will allow achievement of inhaled induction before loss of effect from the intravenous induction drugs occurs.

An inhaled induction with spontaneous breathing can be achieved with any of the potent drugs in oxygen alone or with nitrous oxide and oxygen. This can be done with or without a dose of thiobarbiturate or other injected drug. When thiobarbiturates are used, they will cause some decrease in ventilation, thereby decreasing the speed of induction. The principles governing appropriate delivered and inspired anesthetic concentrations are similar to those noted above. Nitrous oxide speeds induction with potent drugs slightly (second-gas effect). A novel approach to rapid induction is the inspiration of a single breath of a high concentration of potent drug followed by a brief period of breath-holding to allow redistribution of the gas molecules taken up by pulmonary capillary blood.[371]

It is tempting to perform an inhaled induction by controlled ventilation once the patient has received a thiobarbiturate and neuromuscular-blocking drugs for an endotracheal intubation. A danger exists in attempting to achieve a rapid rise of alveolar concentration of the potent drugs by this method. A very rapid increase of brain and cardiac anesthetic concentrations can occur. Profound depression of both organs may occur rapidly even with drugs of high blood solubility that are ordinarily associated with slow induction of anesthesia. Reversal of the profound depression may be impeded by slow removal of drug from tissues due to low organ blood flow, low flow abetted further by zealous hyperventilation, and resultant additional decreases in cardiac output. If spontaneous ventilation is preserved until surgical levels of anesthesia are achieved, less dependence is placed on circulatory parameters as the only signs of depth of anesthesia. Also, the respiratory depression of the anesthetic inhibits further uptake of the drug.[372] Ordinarily, apnea, the most profound respiratory depression, occurs before cardiac failure, the most profound circulatory depression.[373] A margin of safety is preserved when one avoids "pumping potent drugs into paralyzed patients."

The ease of induction with the inhaled drugs is influenced by features other than potency and tissue solubility. Patient acceptance depends in part on pungency of the drug and the airway irritability that accompanies its use.[374, 375] Although experience and familiarity with a drug lead one to accommodate to or even overlook its drawbacks, it appears that isoflurane is accompanied by a greater incidence of breath-holding and coughing on induction than halothane.[374–376] Each of the three commonly used potent drugs can produce hypotension and slow heart rates on induction in children.[377]

MAINTENANCE OF ANESTHESIA

Maintenance anesthesia can be provided with inhaled anesthetics alone without the use of adjuvants. On the other hand, some anesthesiologists prefer to add adjuvants to a primary inhaled technique. The weights given to factors governing this choice depend on personal experience, the significance one attaches to dangers of one drug compared with another, individual interpretation of results of experiments, and degree of concern about maintaining simplicity as opposed to polypharmacy in anesthesia care.

Unfortunately, relatively few results are available about outcome from anesthesia and surgery in relation to choice of anesthesia.[378] This represents an area of investigation in which pioneering studies such as those of Beecher et al,[379] Dripps et al[380] and Shnider er al[381] were followed by a significant hiatus until workers including Gold et al[382] and Warren et al[342] stimulated new interest in outcome studies. The simplicity accompanying the use of only an inhaled drug to provide all of the anesthetic components required for an intraabdominal or intrathoracic procedure is attractive, but this approach may require deep levels of anesthesia, levels accompanied by systemic hypotension. This hypotension may be tolerated well by some patients and not by others. In such a situation, some anesthesiologists would prefer to use lower concentrations of the inhaled drugs and provide the needed relaxation with neuromuscular-blocking drugs. This preference carries with it a decision to cope with the side-effects and complications of muscle relaxants. Similarly, one might elect to supplement inhaled drugs with opioids, but these, too, are not devoid of problems. One must be guided by the needs of the individual patient and apply knowledge of the specific pharmacology of the drugs.

There are a number of situations in which selection of an inhaled drug for maintenance anesthesia is particularly indicated. The prominent vasodilating effects of enflurane and isoflurane or the myocardial effects of halothane may be advantageous in providing deliberate hypotension.[106, 383–386] They are also effective for reversal of hypertension in the circumstance of cardiac surgery prior to and during cardiopulmonary bypass.[387, 388] Finally, the potent inhaled anesthetics are excellent for patients with bronchospastic disorders. Unfortunately, one cannot prove safety of one approach over another, but only the absence of complications.

Surgery in outpatients requires prompt induction of and emergence from anesthesia. It may also require complete suppression of airway reflexes or profound muscle relaxation. The inhaled drugs will provide these conditions. Rapid induction is limited by the pungency of isoflurane and enflurane, a limitation that is overcome by an intravenously administered drug. The rapid increase in alveolar concentration may produce profound circulatory depression. After brief operations recovery from anesthesia is rapid with all of the inhaled drugs, but especially so with nitrous oxide and sevoflurane. All of the drugs tested thus far have detrimental effects on mental functions that persist beyond the time of overt wakefulness.[389, 390]

Although outcome studies are not available, there is a body of experimental evidence that anesthesia for neurosurgery can be provided safely with inhaled drugs, among which isoflurane appears to produce more favorable conditions than the other drugs, including nitrous oxide.[119] Isoflurane preserves well the dependence of cerebral vessel caliber on Pa_{CO_2},[111] decreases cerebral oxygen requirement,[106] and has favorable effects on CSF dynamics.[115] One can have the advantage of precise control of anesthetic dose that an inhaled anesthetic provides and still preserve cerebral welfare. These comments do not mean that CSF pressure will not increase in any circumstances during isoflurane anesthesia.[120]

The inhaled drugs produce muscle relaxation by themselves and potentiate the effects of neuromuscular-blocking drugs administered intravenously.[300, 304] In some patients the muscle relaxation provided by the inhaled drug will be sufficient. When neuromuscular-blocking drugs are used with inhaled drugs, several issues need to be considered. One, the degree of potentiation of neuromuscular block depends on the anesthetic and the relaxant being used. Enflurane and isoflurane produce a similar degree of potentiation of d-tubocurarine

blockade,[391] but enflurane produces greater potentiation of vecuronium blockade than do isoflurane or halothane.[305] The potent inhaled drugs produce greater potentiation of neuromuscular blockers than do combinations of nitrous oxide and intravenous drugs.[307] One therefore should adjust the doses of relaxant drugs downward when using the potent inhaled agents. Decreasing the concentration of inhaled drug effectively decreases the effect of the neuromuscular-blocking drug.[392] Finally, there is the potential for detrimental cardiac arrhythmias when combining inhaled anesthetics[393] with drugs that inhibit norepinephrine reuptake. The relaxants by themselves do not necessarily affect epinephrine sensitization produced by inhaled drugs.[394]

INHALED DRUGS AS PART OF BALANCED-ANESTHESIA TECHNIQUES

Little has been written about the popular current practice of balanced anesthesia, that is, the practice of combining inhaled drugs with sedatives, opioids, and other drugs possessing effects on the central nervous system. The term balanced anesthesia when first coined by Lundy in 1925[395] referred to the use of a mixture of drugs, a "diet" of compounds, to provide the anesthetic state. A mixture was used with an eye to utilizing the advantages of small amounts of each drug, hopefully without having to contend with the disadvantages of larger doses of any one drug. The term balanced anesthesia took on a different connotation when muscle relaxants were developed. The emphasis shifted to augmenting the effects of nitrous oxide. Nitrous oxide was the basic anesthetic, and its deficiencies as a complete anesthetic were overcome by adjuvants: sedation and amnesia by barbiturates or scopolamine; reflex suppression by belladonna drugs or opioids; analgesia by opioids; and muscle relaxation by neuromuscular-blocking drugs. Deficiencies in a particular response were detected by clinical signs and the appropriate adjuvant was given.

In our opinion, the new era and scope of balanced anesthesia began when the cardiovascular benefits of morphine were described by Lowenstein et al.[396] Opioids became the favorite drugs of many to provide anesthesia for patients with advanced cardiovascular disease. But, as inadequate suppression by opioids of reflex and motor responses (or even wakefulness) became apparent, the potent inhaled drugs were added to the anesthetic regimen. The concept of the new (or, revival of the old) balanced anesthesia has matured further as the potential disadvantages of nitrous oxide have come more clearly into focus.[397] These include not only its cellular toxic effects but also its effects on breathing and on the circulation. We have returned more nearly to the original concept of balanced anesthesia described by Lundy.[395] Thus, sedation and amnesia are provided by barbiturates, benzodiazepines, or butyrophenones; reflex suppression and some portion of the anesthetic requirement are provided by an opioid, barbiturate, benzodiazepine, or butyrophenone; rapid induction of unconsciousness and relaxation for intubation is offered by the barbiturate–relaxant combination; the remainder of the anesthetic requirement and reflex suppression is achieved by an inhaled anesthetic. Muscle relaxation is provided by a neuromuscular-blocking drug given intravenously. Even when large doses of opioids are used to provide anesthesia, supplemental inhaled drugs often are given to attenuate hypertension, the dose being governed by the amount of drug needed to achieve the desired arterial pressure.[387] When the major component of the anesthetic is one of the inhaled drugs, an opioid may be used to decrease heart rate[398] or a benzodiazepine to assure amnesia. These patterns of use of the inhaled agents reflect the variety of new drugs that are now available and the increased acceptance of polypharmacy. In addition, greater knowledge of pharmacokinetics and pharmacodynamics allows us to tailor several anesthetic drugs to clinical needs.

RECOVERY

Rate of recovery from anesthesia with an inhaled drug is quite predictable. The decrease in alveolar concentration is related to blood solubility of the anesthetic, alveolar ventilation, and duration of anesthesia.[399] The speed of recovery after short operations is not greatly dependent on solubility of the anesthetic. As anesthesia is prolonged, however, drugs of greater blood solubility will be associated with significantly slower recovery. The more rapid the recovery from anesthesia, the earlier the need for analgesic drugs because the commonly used inhaled agents provide little analgesia in low, subanesthetic concentrations. Despite this drawback, there may be an advantage to early return of protective airway and circulatory reflexes.

METHOXYFLURANE

As recently as 1983, one writer stated that "methoxyflurane is virtually no longer used in clinical anesthesia."[400] Rather, methoxyflurane now serves as a drug model of fluoride-related nephrotoxicity, one with which new and older drugs are compared because methoxyflurane provides such predictable effects. Introduced into clinical practice by Artusio et al[11] in 1960, methoxyflurane was used and acclaimed because one of its greatest drawbacks, high blood solubility, was also a strength. The drug persisted in the body to provide ongoing sedation and pain relief following surgery. Another advantage of the drug was its prominent analgesic property leading to a role in providing analgesia for labor via self-administration devices.[401] The clinical impression was that methoxyflurane was an excellent muscle-relaxing drug.

The report of putative methoxyflurane nephrotoxicity by Crandell et al[13] in 1966, however, set in motion a series of elegant studies by Mazze et al,[402, 403] studies that in our view have provided standards for assessment of the toxic effects of anesthetics on the kidney for the subsequent 2 decades. Although methoxyflurane could be administered safely if rigid limits to the total administered dose, e.g., MAC-h of anesthesia, were followed,[403] advantages of methoxyflurane over the other drugs did not warrant its continued use. Furthermore, reports of possible hepatotoxicity related to the use of methoxyflurane appeared.[14, 404] For all of these reasons, although still available, methoxyflurane appears to be used rarely if at all in the United States.

SEVOFLURANE

The first report on sevoflurane (fluoromethyl-1,1,1,3,3,3-hexafluoro-2-propyl ether) by Wallin et al[405] appeared in 1971 and was followed by a more thorough analysis of the chemical, pharmacologic, and toxicologic properties of the agent.[406] Interest in the compound stemmed especially from its very low solubility in blood (the blood : gas partition coefficient is near that of N_2O), leading to rapid induction and emergence from anesthesia and to the ability to change anesthetic levels rapidly. It is remarkable among current anesthetics in the combination of potency and blood solubility that it offers. As another of the new anesthetics evaluated during and after the late 1960s it, too, has had to undergo extensive testing similar to that described by Stevens et al.,[20] so that progress toward introduction into clinical practice has been slow. The progression of studies of sevoflurane reflects the primary concerns of the recent era of development of new inhaled anesthetics: metabolism and toxicity.[27] Understandably, only after a drug has been shown to be less or at least no more toxic than available compounds will its other pharmacologic properties be explored.

Among the first studies to be done with sevoflurane were tests of its metabolism to produce fluoride ions and possible renal injury.[407] In the Fischer 344 rat model, peak serum inorganic fluoride levels of $29.1 \ \mu M \cdot l^{-1}$ occurred 4 h following 4 h of anesthesia with 1.4% delivered sevoflurane. These levels were short lived, probably because of the rapid removal of sevoflurane from the body. Interestingly, the defluorinase-specific activity of sevoflurane is nearly identical to methoxyflurane; therefore, it is not the susceptibility to metabolism but other factors, in this instance the rapid pulmonary excretion, that account for much lower and more transient increases in serum fluoride with sevoflurane than methoxyflurane.

Another study of the metabolism of sevoflurane has produced an estimate that 2%–3% of sevoflurane taken up by humans during a 1-h anesthetic is metabolized, an amount similar to enflurane.[408] Its metabolism is induced by isoniazid[409] and ethanol,[410] but phenobarbital has been reported to increase[411] or not change[410] the rate of sevoflurane metabolism. Strum et al[412] performed toxicity studies with several anesthetics, combining prolonged administration of anesthesia with hypoxia. Halothane was associated with greater hepatic injury than sevoflurane and isoflurane. The latter drugs had similar effects. Of particular significance is the observation that sevoflurane is more unstable in soda lime than other inhaled anesthetics; however, Strum et al.[412] delivered the sevoflurane through soda lime and did not detect a detrimental effect on rats. No mutagenic effect was found with sevoflurane by Baden et al.[413] Sevoflurane can trigger malignant hyperthermia.[414]

Holaday et al.[408] anesthetized humans for 1 h with 2% or 3% inspired sevoflurane. Respiratory frequency and Pa_{CO_2} increased in a manner similar to that produced by other potent inhaled drugs, an effect corroborated recently by Doi et al.[415] Systolic blood pressure decreased slightly and pulse rate did not change significantly. Holaday et al.[408] did not detect detrimental effects on liver, kidney, or hematologic systems in their volunteers. Katoh et al.[416] determined the MAC for sevoflurane in ASA physical status I patients aged 30–59 yr (Table 11-3). The value for the sevoflurane–oxygen group was 1.71 + 0.07% (SE) and for the sevoflurane–63.5% nitrous oxide group was 0.66 + 0.06% (SE). Kikuchi et al[36] have gained considerable experience with sevoflurane and favor it especially for its induction and emergence characteristics. Inhaled induction appears to be pleasant and prompt. Manohar et al[417] studied the circulatory effects of sevoflurane in pigs. They found decreased cardiac output, aortic pressure, and left ventricular work. Their data indicate that sevoflurane may not increase CBF to the degree other potent inhaled drugs do. Sevoflurane does not sensitize the myocardium to the arrhythmic effects of epinephrine.

Although sevoflurane has not yet received approval by the U.S. Food and Drug Administration nor been released for routine use, one would predict it will be of special use for procedures of relatively short duration.

CONCLUSION

The list of characteristics of an ideal anesthetic is long.[20] A drug should provide rapid onset of action with predictable and, in most instances, rapid recovery from its effects. It should not have an effect on the brain or other organs that appears or persists after the time of anesthesia. It should be easy to administer, and its administration should be guided by clear signs of depth of anesthesia. The drug should possess a high safety margin in patients of all ages and physiognomy.

The search continues for drugs that approach these ideals. It appears that various anesthetic drugs may provide one or more of these ideal properties to a greater extent than other anesthetic agents but offer no benefit in other areas. For example, sevoflurane's solubility characteristics are of great advantage in terms of onset of action of anesthesia, alteration of depth of anesthesia, and recovery from anesthesia. Its respiratory effects, however, are not superior to those of other drugs, and the significance of its interactions with soda lime needs further clarification. We anticipate that future research for anesthetic drugs will be directed at the development of drugs with a high degree of specificity of action. As this research continues, anesthesia will likely be provided by a combination of drugs that the anesthesiologist believes will offer the patient as ideal anesthetic care as can be administered.

REFERENCES

1. Vitcha JF: A history of Forane. Anesthesiology 35:4, 1971
2. Robbins JH: Preliminary studies of the activity of fluorinated hydrocarbons. J Pharmacol Exp Ther 86:197, 1946
3. Krantz JC Jr, Carr J, Lu G et al: Anesthesia: Anesthetic action of trifluoroethyl vinyl ether. J Pharmacol Exp Ther 108:488, 1953
4. Sadove MS, Balagot RC, Linde HW: Trifluoroethyl vinyl ether (Fluoromar): Preliminary clinical and laboratory studies. Anesthesiology 17:591, 1956
5. Cullen BF, Eger EI et al: Cardiovascular effects of fluroxene in man. Anesthesiology 32:218, 1970
6. Tucker WK, Munson ES, Holaday DA et al: Hepatorenal toxicity following fluroxene anesthesia. Anesthesiology 39:104, 1973
7. Suckling CW: Some chemical and physical factors in development of fluothane. Br J Anaesth 29:466, 1957
8. Johnstone M: Human cardiovascular response to Fluothane anaesthesia. Br J Anaesth 28:392, 1954
9. Raventos J: Action of fluothane—New volatile anaesthetic. Br J Pharmacol 11:394, 1956
10. Johnstone M: Halothane: The first five years. Anesthesiology 22:591, 1961
11. Artusio JF Jr, Van Poznak A, Hunt RE et al: Clinical evaluation of methoxyflurane. Anesthesiology 21:512, 1960
12. Virtue RW, Payne KW: Postoperative death after Fluothane. Anesthesiology 19:562, 1958
13. Crandell WB, Pappas SG, Macdonald A: Nephrotoxicity associated with methoxyflurane anesthesia. Anesthesiology 27:591, 1966
14. Rubinger D, Davidson JT, Melmed RN: Hepatitis following the use of methoxyflurane in obstetric anesthesia. Anesthesiology 43:593, 1975
15. Brody GL, Sweet RB: Halothane anesthesia as a possible cause of massive hepatic necrosis. Anesthesiology 24:29, 1963
16. Subcommittee on the National Halothane Study: Summary of the National Halothane Study. JAMA 197:775, 1978
17. Burns THS, Hall JM, Bracken A et al: Fluorine compounds in anaesthesia. Anaesthesia 19:167, 1964
18. Terrell RC, Speers L, Szur AJ et al: General anesthetics. I. Halogenated methylethyl ethers as anesthetic agents. J Med Chem 14:517, 1971
19. Terrell RC: Physical and chemical properties of anaesthetic agents. Br J Anaesth 56:38, 1984
20. Stevens WC, Eger EI II: Comparative evaluation of new inhalation anesthetics. Anesthesiology 35:125, 1971
21. Virtue RW, Lund LO, Phelps M Jr et al: Difluoromethyl 1,1,2-trifluoro-2-chlorethyl ether as an anaesthetic agent: Results with dogs and a preliminary note on observations with man. Can Anaesth Soc J 13:233, 1966
22. Dobkin AB, Nishioka K, Gengaje DB et al: Ethrane (Compound 347) anesthesia: A clinical and laboratory review of 700 cases. Anesth Analg 48:477, 1969
23. Stevens WC, Cromwell TH, Halsey MJ et al: The cardiovascular effects of a new inhalation anesthetic, Forane, in human volunteers at constant arterial carbon dioxide tension. Anesthesiology 35:3, 1971
24. Calverley RK, Smith NT, Jones CW et al: Ventilatory and cardiovascular effects of enflurane during spontaneous ventilation in man. Anesth Analg 57:610, 1978
25. Raventos J, Spinks A: Methods of screening volatile anesthetics. Manchester Med Gaz 37:55, 1958
26. Burn JH: Pharmacological screening of anaesthetics. Proc Roy Soc Med 52:95, 1959
27. Halsey MJ: Investigations on isoflurane, sevoflurane and other experimental anaesthetics. Br J Anaesth 53:43S, 1981
28. Corbett TH: Cancer and congenital anomalies associated with anesthetics. Ann NY Acad Sci 271:58, 1976
29. Eger EI II, White AE, Brown CL et al: A test of the carcinogenicity of enflurane, isoflurane, halothane, methoxyflurane, and nitrous oxide in mice. Anesth Analg 57:678, 1978
30. Fabian LW, Gee HL, Dowdy EA et al: Laboratory and clinical investigations of a new fluorinated anesthetic compound, halopropane (CHF₂CF₂CH₂Br). Anesth Analg 41:707, 1962
31. Virtue RW, Young RV, Lund LO et al: Halopropane anesthesia in man: Laboratory and clinical studies. Anesthesiology 24:217, 1963
32. Stephen CR, North WC: Halopropane—a clinical evaluation. Anesthesiology 25:600, 1964
33. Artusio JF Jr, Van Poznak A: Laboratory and clinical investigations of teflurane, 1,1,1,2-tetrafluoro-2-bromethane (DA-708). Fed Proc 20:312, 1961
34. Artusio JF Jr: Clinical investigation of teflurane, 2-bromo-1,1,1,2-tetrafluoroethane—DA 708. Fed Proc 22:186, 1963
35. Warner WA, Orth OS, Weber DL et al: Laboratory investigations of teflurane. Anesth Analg 46:32, 1967
36. Kikuchi H, Morio M, Fujii K et al: Clinical evaluation and metabolism of sevoflurane in patients. Hiroshima J Med Sci 36:93, 1987
37. Holaday DA, Jardines MC, Greenwood WH: Uptake and biotransformation of aliflurane (1-chloro-2-methoxy-1,2,3,3-tetrafluorocyclopropane, compound 26-P) in man. Anesthesiology 51:548, 1979
38. Munson ES, Schick LM, Chapin JC et al: Determinations of the minimum alveolar concentration (MAC) of aliflurane in dogs. Anesthesiology 51:545, 1979
39. Eger EI II: Anesthetic Uptake and Action, pp 77–94. Baltimore, Williams & Wilkins, 1974
40. Hamilton WK, Eastwood DW: A study of denitrogenation with some inhalation anesthetic systems. Anesthesiology 16:861, 1955
41. Eger EI II: Factors affecting the rapidity of alteration of nitrous oxide concentration in a circle system. Anesthesiology 21:348, 1960
42. Brown ES, Seniff AM, Elam JO: Carbon dioxide elimination in semiclosed systems. Anesthesiology 25:31, 1964
43. Eger EI II, Ethans CT: The effects of inflow, overflow and valve

placement on economy of the circle system. Anesthesiology 29:93, 1968

44. Eger EI II, Larson CP Jr, Severinghaus JW: The solubility of halothane in rubber, soda lime and various plastics. Anesthesiology 23:356, 1962

45. Grodin WK, Epstein MA, Epstein RA: Soda lime absorption of isoflurane and halothane. Anesthesiology 62:60, 1985

46. Eger EI II, Bahlman SH: Is end-tidal anesthetic partial pressure an accurate measure of the arterial anesthetic partial pressure? Anesthesiology 35:301, 1971

47. Epstein RM, Rackow H, Salanitre E et al: Influence of the concentration effect on the uptake of anesthetic mixtures: The second gas effect. Anesthesiology 25:364, 1964

48. Stoelting RK, Eger EI II: An additional explanation for the second gas effect. Anesthesiology 30:273, 1969

49. Severinghaus JW: Role of lung factors. In Papper EM, Kitz RJ (eds): Uptake and Distribution of Anesthetic Agents, p 59. New York, McGraw-Hill, 1963

50. Cromwell TH, Eger EI II, Stevens WC et al: Forane uptake, excretion, and blood solubility in man. Anesthesiology 35:401, 1971

51. Coburn CM, Eger EI II: The partial pressure of isoflurane or halothane does not affect their solubility in blood: Inhaled anesthetics obey Henry's Law. Anesth Analg 65:672, 1986

52. Steward A, Allott PR, Cowles AL et al: Solubility coefficients for inhaled anaesthetics for water, oil and biological media. Br J Anaesth 45:282, 1973

53. Eger RR, Eger EI II: Effect of temperature and age on the solubility of enflurane, halothane, isoflurane, and methoxyflurane in human blood. Anesth Analg 64:640, 1985

54. Munson ES, Eger EI II, Tham MK et al: Increase in anesthetic uptake, excretion, and blood solubility on man after eating. Anesth Analg 57:224, 1978

55. Miller MS, Gandolfi AJ, Vaughan RW et al: Disposition of enflurane in obese patients. J Pharmacol Exp Ther 215:292, 1980

56. Brandom BW, Brandom RB, Cook DR: Uptake and distribution of halothane in infants: *In vivo* measurements and computer simulations. Anesth Analg 62:404, 1983

57. Stoelting RK, Eger EI II: Percutaneous loss of nitrous oxide, cyclopropane, ether and halothane in man. Anesthesiology 30:278, 1969

58. Stoelting RK, Eger EI II: The effects of ventilation and anesthetic solubility on recovery from anesthesia: An *in vivo* and analog analysis before and after equilibrium. Anesthesiology 30:290, 1969

59. Masuda T, Ikea K: Elimination of nitrous oxide accelerates elimination of halothane: Reversed second gas effect. Anesthesiology 60:567, 1984

60. Masuda T, Ikeda K: Effect of inspired nitrous oxide concentrations on the rate of fall of alveolar concentrations: Reversed concentration effect. Acta Anaesthesiol Scand 30:164, 1986

61. Cohen EN, Van Dyke RA: Biochemical aspects. In Cohen EN, Van Dyke RA (eds): Metabolism of Volatile Anesthetics, p 8. Reading, MA, Addison-Wesley, 1977

62. Cahalan MK, Johnson BH, Eger EI II: Relationship of concentrations of halothane and enflurane to their metabolism and elimination in man. Anesthesiology 54:3, 1981

63. Carpenter RL, Eger EI II, Johnson BH et al: Pharmacokinetics of inhaled anesthetics in humans: Measurements during and after the simultaneous administration of enflurane, halothane, isoflurane, methoxyflurane and nitrous oxide. Anesth Analg 65:575, 1986

64. Merkel G, Eger EI II: A comparative study of halothane and halopropane anesthesia. Anesthesiology 24:346, 1963

65. Eger EI II, Saidman LJ, Brandstater B: Minimum alveolar concen-

tration: A standard of anesthetic potency. Anesthesiology 26:756, 1965

66. Saidman LJ, Eger EI II, Munson ES et al: Minimum alveolar concentrations of methoxylflurane, halothane, ether and cyclopropane in man: Correlation with theories of anesthesia. Anesthesiology 28:994, 1967

67. Quasha AL, Eger EI II, Tinker JH: Determination and applications of MAC. Anesthesiology 53:315, 1980

68. Hornbein TF, Eger EI II, Winter PM et al: The minimum alveolar concentration of nitrous oxide in man. Anesth Analg 61:553, 1982

69. Kissin I, Morgan PL, Smith LR: Anesthetic potencies of isoflurane, halothane and diethyl ether for various end points of anesthesia. Anesthesiology 58:88, 1983

70. de Jong RH, Eger EI II: MAC expanded: AD_{50} and AD_{95} values of common inhalation anesthetics in man. Anesthesiology 42:384, 1975

71. Regan MJ, Eger EI II: Effect of hypothermia in dogs on anesthetizing and apneic doses of inhalation agents. Determination of the anesthetic index (apnea/MAC). Anesthesiology 28:689, 1967

72. Wolfson B, Kielar CM, Lake C et al: Anesthetic index—A new approach. Anesthesiology 38:583, 1973

73. Wolfson B, Hetrick WD, Lake CL et al: Anesthetic indices—further data. Anesthesiology 48:187, 1978

74. Miller RD, Way WL, Eger EI II: The effects of alpha-methyldopa, reserpine, guanethidine, and iproniazid on minimum alveolar anesthetic requirement (MAC). Anesthesiology 29:1153, 1968

75. Saidman LJ, Eger EI II: Effect of nitrous oxide and of narcotic premedication on the alveolar concentration of halothane required for anesthesia. Anesthesiology 25:302, 1964

76. Cullen DJ, Eger EI II: The effects of hypoxia and isovolemic anemia on the halothane requirement (MAC) of dogs. I. The effect of hypoxia. Anesthesiology 32:28, 1970

77. Cullen DJ, Cotev S, Severinghaus JW et al: The effects of hypoxia and isovolemic anemia on the halothane requirement (MAC) of dogs. II. The effects of acute hypoxia on halothane requirement and cerebral surface P_{O_2}, P_{CO_2}, pH, and HCO_3. Anesthesiology 32:35, 1970

78. Johnston RR, Way WL, Miller RD: Alteration of anesthetic requirement by amphetamines. Anesthesiology 36:357, 1972

79. Johnston RR, White PF, Way WL et al: The effect of levodopa on halothane anesthetic requirements. Anesth Analg 54:178, 1975

80. Murphy MR, Hug CC Jr: The enflurane sparing effect of morphine, butorphanol and nalbuphine. Anesthesiology 57:489, 1982

81. Lake CL, DiFazio CA, Moscicki JC et al: Reduction in halothane MAC: Comparison of morphine and alfentanil. Anesth Analg 64:807, 1985

82. Miller RD, Wahrenbrock EA, Schroeder CF et al: Ethylene–halothane anesthesia: Addition or synergism? Anesthesiology 31:301, 1969

83. Cullen SC, Eger EI II, Cullen BF et al: Observations on the anesthetic effect of the combination of xenon and halothane. Anesthesiology 31:305, 1969

84. Palahniuk RJ, Shnider SM, Eger EI II: Pregnancy decreases the requirement for inhaled anesthetic agents. Anesthesiology 41:82, 1974

85. Mazze RI, Rice SA, Baden JM: Halothane, isoflurane, and enflurane MAC in pregnant and non-pregnant female and male mice and rats. Anesthesiology 62:339, 1985

86. Gregory GA, Wade JG, Beihl DR et al: Fetal anesthetic requirement (MAC) for halothane. Anesth Analg 62:9, 1983

87. Cameron CB, Robinson S, Gregory GA: The minimum anesthetic concentration of isoflurane in children. Anesth Analg 63:418, 1984

88. Lerman J, Robinson S, Willis MM et al: Anesthetic requirement

for halothane in young children 0–1 month and 1–6 months of age. Anesthesiology 59:421, 1983

89. Gregory GA, Eger EI II, Munson ES: The relationship between age and halothane requirement in man. Anesthesiology 30:488, 1969

90. Stoelting RK, Longnecker DE, Eger EI II: Minimum alveolar concentrations in man on awakening from methoxyflurane, halothane, ether and fluroxene anesthesia: MAC awake. Anesthesiology 33:5, 1970

91. Roizen MF, Horrigan RW, Frazer BM: Anesthetic doses blocking adrenergic (stress) and cardiovascular responses to incision—MAC BAR. Anesthesiology 54:390, 1981

92. Davison LA, Steinhelber JC, Eger EI II et al: Psychological effects of halothane and isoflurane anesthesia. Anesthesiology 43:313, 1975

93. Storms LH, Stark AH, Calverley RK et al: Psychological functioning after halothane or isoflurane anesthesia. Anesth Analg 59:245, 1980

94. Korttila K, Tammisto T, Ertama P et al: Recovery, psychomotor skills, and simulated driving after brief inhalational anesthesia with halothane or enflurane combined with nitrous oxide and oxygen. Anesthesiology 46:20, 1977

95. Tinker JH, Gandolfi AJ, Van Dyke RA: Elevation of plasma levels in patients following halothane anesthesia: Time correlations with total halothane dosage. Anesthesiology 44:194, 1976

96. Bruce DL, Bach MJ, Arbit J: Trace anesthetic effects on perceptual, cognitive and motor skills. Anesthesiology 40:453, 1974

97. Ghoneim MM, Mewaldt SP, Petersen RC: Memory effects of subanesthetic concentrations of nitrous oxide. Anesth Analg 59:540, 1980

98. Cook TL, Smith M, Winter PM et al: Effect of subanesthetic concentrations of enflurane and halothane on human behavior. Anesth Analg 57:434, 1978

99. Newberg LA, Milde JH, Michenfelder JD: The cerebral metabolic effects of isoflurane at and above concentrations that suppress cortical electrical activity. Anesthesiology 59:23, 1983

100. Sakabe T, Maekawa T, Fujii S et al: Cerebral circulation and metabolism during enflurane anesthesia in humans. Anesthesiology 59:532, 1983

101. Wollman H, Smith AI, Neigh JL et al: Cerebral blood flow and oxygen consumption in man during electroencephalographic seizure patterns associated with enflurane anesthesia. In Brock M, Fieschi C, Ingvar D et al (eds): Cerebral Blood Flow, p 246. Berlin, Springer-Verlag, 1969

102. Stullken EH, Milde JH, Michenfelder JD et al: The non-linear responses of cerebral metabolism to low concentrations of halothane, enflurane, isoflurane and thiopental. Anesthesiology 46:28, 1977

103. Brunner EA, Passonneau JV, Molstad C: The effect of volatile anaesthetics on levels of metabolites and on metabolic rate in brain. J Neurochem 18:2301, 1971

104. Newberg LA, Michenfelder JD: Cerebral protection by isoflurane during hypoxemia or ischemia. Anesthesiology 59:29, 1983

105. Nehis DG, Todd MM, Spetzler RF et al: A comparison of the cerebral protective effects of isoflurane and barbiturates during temporary focal ischemia in primates. Anesthesiology 66:453, 1987

106. Newberg LA, Milde JH, Michenfelder JD: Systemic and cerebral effects of isoflurane-induced hypotension in dogs. Anesthesiology 60:541, 1984

107. Newman B, Gelb AW, Lam AM: The effect of isoflurane-induced hypotension on cerebral blood flow and cerebral metabolic rate for oxygen in humans. Anesthesiology 64:307, 1986

108. Seyde WC, Longnecker DE: Cerebral oxygen tension in rats during deliberate hypotension with sodium nitroprusside, 2-chloroadenosine, or deep isoflurane anesthesia. Anesthesiology 64:480, 1986

109. Adams RW, Cucciara RF, Gronert GM et al: Isoflurane and cerebrospinal fluid pressure in neurosurgical patients. Anesthesiology 54:97, 1981

110. Albrecht RF, Miletich DJ, Madala LR: Normalization of cerebral blood flow during prolonged halothane anesthesia. Anesthesiology 58:26, 1983

111. Scheller MS, Todd MM, Drummond JC: Isoflurane, halothane, and regional cerebral blood flow at various levels of Pa_{CO_2} in rabbits. Anesthesiology 64:598, 1986

112. Messick JM, Casement B, Milde LN et al: Correlation of regional cerebral blood flow (rCBF) with EEG changes during isoflurane anesthesia for carotid endarterectomy: Critical rCBF. Anesthesiology 66:344, 1987

113. Artru AA: Effects of enflurane and isoflurane as resistance to reabsorption of cerebrospinal fluid in dogs. Anesthesiology 61:529, 1984

114. Artru AA, Nugent M, Michenfelder JD: Enflurane causes a prolonged and reversible increase in the rate of CSF production in the dog. Anesthesiology 57:255, 1982

115. Artru AA: Isoflurane does not increase the rate of CSF production in the dog. Anesthesiology 60:193, 1984

116. Artru AA: Effects of halothane and fentanyl on resistance to reabsorption of CSF. J Neurosurg 60:252, 1984

117. Artru AA: Effects of halothane and fentanyl on the rate of CSF production in dogs. Anesth Analg 62:581, 1983

118. Campkin TV: Isoflurane and cranial extradural pressure: A study in neurosurgical patients. Br J Anaesth 56:1083, 1984

119. Adams RW, Cucchiara RF, Gronert GA et al: Isoflurane and cerebrospinal fluid pressure in neurosurgical patients. Anesthesiology 54:97, 1981

120. Grosslight K, Foster R, Colohan AR et al: Isoflurane for neuroanesthesia: Risk factors for increases in intracranial pressure. Anesthesiology 63:533, 1985

121. Stockard J, Bickford R: The neurophysiology of anaesthesia. In Gordon EA (ed) Basis and Practice of Neuroanaesthesia, p 3. Amsterdam, Excerpta Medica, 1975

122. Eger EI II, Stevens WC, Cromwell JH: The electroencephalogram in man anesthetized with Forane. Anesthesiology 35:504, 1971

123. Tinker JH, Sharbrough FW, Michenfelder JD: Anterior shift of the dominant EEG rhythm during anesthesia in a Java monkey. Anesthesiology 46:252, 1977

124. Neigh JL, Garman JK, Harp JR: The electroencephalographic pattern during anesthesia with enflurane: Effects of depth of anesthesia, Pa_{CO_2} and nitrous oxide. Anesthesiology 35:482, 1971

125. Joas TA, Stevens WC, Eger EI II: Electroencephalographic seizure activity in dogs during anaesthesia. Br J Anaesth 43:739, 1971

126. Lebowitz MH, Blitt CD, Dillon JB: Enflurane-induced central nervous system excitation and its relation to carbon dioxide tension. Anesth Analg 51:355, 1972

127. Clark DL, Rosner BS: Neurophysiologic effects of general anesthetics. I. The electroencephalogram and sensory evoked responses in man. Anesthesiology 38:564, 1973

128. Domino EF: Effects of preanesthetic and anesthetic drugs on visually evoked responses. Anesthesiology 28:184, 1967

129. Grundy BL: Intraoperative monitoring of sensory-evoked potentials. Anesthesiology 58:72, 1983

130. Peterson DO, Drummond JC, Todd MM: Effects of halothane, enflurane, isoflurane, and nitrous oxide on somatosensory evoked potentials in humans. Anesthesiology 65:35, 1986

131. Sloan TB, Koht A: Depression of cortical somatosensory evoked potentials by nitrous oxide. Br J Anaesth 57:849, 1985

132. McPherson RW, Mahla M, Johnson R et al: Effects of enflurane, isoflurane, and nitrous oxide on somatosensory evoked potentials during fentanyl anesthesia. Anesthesiology 62:626, 1985

133. Sebel PS, Flynn PJ, Ingram DA: Effect of nitrous oxide on visual

auditory and somatosensory evoked potentials. Br J Anaesth 56:1403, 1984

134. Dubois MY, Sato S, Chassy J et al: Effects of enflurane on brainstem auditory evoked responses in humans. Anesth Analg 61:898, 1982

135. Uhl RR, Squires KC, Bruce DL et al: Effect of halothane anesthesia on the human cortical visual evoked response. Anesthesiology 53:273, 1980

136. James FM, Thornton C, Jones JG: Halothane anaesthesia changes the early components of the auditory evoked responses in man. Br J Anaesth 54:787, 1982

137. Manninen PH, Lam AM, Nicholas JF: The effects of isoflurane and isoflurane–nitrous anesthesia on brainstem auditory evoked potentials in humans. Anesth Analg 64:43, 1985

138. Rehder K, Mallow JE, Fibuch EE et al: Effects of isoflurane anesthesia and muscle paralysis on respiratory mechanics in normal man. Anesthesiology 41:477, 1974

139. Froese AB, Bryan AC: Effects of anesthesia and paralysis on diaphragmatic mechanics in man. Anesthesiology 41:242, 1974

140. Munson ES, Larson CP Jr, Babad AA et al: The effect of halothane, fluroxene and cyclopropane on ventilation: A comparative study in man. Anesthesiology 27:716, 1966

141. Larson CP Jr, Eger EI II, Muallem M et al: The effects of diethyl ether and methoxyflurane on ventilation. II. A comparative study in man. Anesthesiology 30:174, 1969

142. Fourcade HE, Stevens WC, Larson CP Jr et al: The ventilatory effects of Forane, a new inhaled anesthetic. Anesthesiology 35:26, 1971

143. Devine JC, Hamilton WK, Pittinger CB: Respiratory studies in man during fluothane anesthesia. Anesthesiology 19:11, 1958

144. Murat J, Saint-Maurice JP, Beydon L et al: Respiratory effects of nitrous oxide during isoflurane anesthesia in children. Br J Anaesth 58:1122, 1986

145. Wren WS, Meeke R, Davenport J et al: Effects of nitrous oxide on the respiratory pattern of spontaneously breathing children during anaesthesia. Br J Anaesth 56:881, 1984

146. Tusiewicz K, Bryan AC, Froese AB: Contributions of changing rib cage–diaphragm interactions to the ventilatory depression of halothane anesthesia. Anesthesiology 47:327, 1977

147. Clergue F, Viires N, Lemesle P et al: Effect of halothane on diaphragmatic muscle function in pentobarbital-anesthetized dogs. Anesthesiology 64:181, 1986

148. Nishino T, Shirahata M, Yonezawa T et al: Comparison of changes in the hypoglossal and the phrenic nerve activity in response to increasing depth of anesthesia in cats. Anesthesiology 60:19, 1984

149. Knill RL, Clement JL: Variable effects of anaesthetics on the ventilatory response to hypoxaemia in man. Can Anaesth Soc J 29:93, 1982

150. Hickey RF, Fourcade HE, Eger EI II et al: The effects of ether, halothane and Forane on apneic thresholds in man. Anesthesiology 35:32, 1971

151. Eger EI II, Dolan WM, Stevens WC et al: Surgical stimulation antagonizes the respiratory depression produced by Forane. Anesthesiology 36:544, 1972

152. Eger EI: Respiratory effects of nitrous oxide. In Eger EI (ed): Nitrous Oxide, p 109. New York, Elsevier, 1985

153. France CJ, Plumer MH, Eger EI II et al: Ventilatory effects of isoflurane (Forane) or halothane when combined with morphine, nitrous oxide and surgery. Br J Anaesth 46:117, 1974

154. Hornbein TF, Martin WF, Bonica JJ et al: Nitrous oxide effects on the circulatory and ventilatory responses to halothane. Anesthesiology 31:250, 1969

155. Hirshman CA, McCullough RE, Cohen PJ et al: Depression of hypoxic ventilatory response by halothane, enflurane and isoflurane in dogs. Br J Anaesth 49:957, 1977

156. Weiskopf RB, Raymond LW, Severinghaus JW: Effects of halothane on canine respiratory responses to hypoxia with and without hypercarbia. Anesthesiology 41:350, 1974

157. Duffin J, Triscott A, Whitman JG: The effect of halothane and thiopentone on ventilatory responses mediated by the peripheral chemoreceptors in man. Br J Anaesth 48:975, 1976

158. Knill RL, Gelb AW: Ventilatory responses to hypoxia and hypercapnia during halothane sedation and anesthesia in man. Anesthesiology 49:244, 1978

159. Knill RL, Manninen PH, Clement JL: Ventilation and chemoreflexes during enflurane sedation and anaesthesia in man. Can Anaesth Soc J 26:353, 1979

160. Knill RL, Kieraszewicz HT, Dodgson BG et al: Chemical regulation of ventilation during isoflurane sedation and anaesthesia in humans. Can Anaesth Soc J 30:607, 1983

161. Knill RL, Clement JL: Ventilatory responses to acute metabolic acidemia in humans awake, sedated, and anesthetized with halothane. Anesthesiology 62:745, 1985

162. Nunn JF, Ezi-Ashi TI: The respiratory effects of resistance to breathing in anesthetized man. Anesthesiology 22:174, 1961

163. Beecher HK: A note on the optimal size of endotracheal tubes based upon studies of blood gases. Anesthesiology 11:730, 1950

164. Behrakis PK, Higgs BD, Baydur A, Zin WA, Milic-Emili J: Active inspiratory impedance in halothane-anesthetized humans. J Appl Physiol 54:1477, 1983

165. Royston D, Jordan C, Jones JG: Effect of subanaesthetic concentrations of nitrous oxide on the regulation of ventilation in man. Br J Anaesth 55:449, 1983

166. Moote CA, Knill RL, Clement J: Ventilatory compensation for continuous inspiratory resistive and elastic loads during halothane anesthesia in humans. Anesthesiology 64:582, 1986

167. Lindahl SGE, Charlton HJ, Hatch DJ et al: Ventilatory responses to inspiratory mechanical loads in spontaneously breathing children during halothane anaesthesia. Acta Anaesthesiol Scand 30:122, 1986

168. Pietak S, Weenig CS, Hickey RF et al: Anesthetic effects on ventilation in patients with chronic obstructive pulmonary disease. Anesthesiology 42:160, 1975

169. Rosenberg M, Tobias R, Bourke D et al: Respiratory responses to surgical stimulation during enflurane anesthesia. Anesthesiology 52:163, 1980

170. Lam AM, Clement JL, Knill RL: Surgical stimulation does not enhance ventilatory chemoreflexes during enflurane anaesthesia in man. Can Anaesth Soc J 27:22, 1980

171. Colgan FJ: Performance of lungs and bronchi during inhalation anesthesia. Anesthesiology 26:778, 1965

172. Coon RL, Kampine JP: Hypocapnic bronchoconstriction and inhalation anesthetics. Anesthesiology 43:635, 1975

173. Hickey RF, Graf PD, Nadel JA et al: The effects of halothane and cyclopropane on total pulmonary resistance in the dog. Anesthesiology 31:334, 1969

174. Kingston HGG, Hirshman CA: Perioperative management of the patient with asthma. Anesth Analg 63:844, 1984

175. Heneghan CPH, Bergman NA, Jordan C et al: Effect of isoflurane on bronchomotor tone in man. Br J Anaesth 58:24, 1986

176. Alexander CM, Chen L, Ray R et al: The influence of halothane and isoflurane on pulmonary collateral ventilation. Anesthesiology 62:135, 1985

177. Hirshman CA, Edelstein G, Peetz S, Wayne R et al: Mechanism of action of inhalational anesthesia on airways. Anesthesiology 56:107, 1982

178. Hirshman CA, Bergman NA: Halothane and enflurane protect against bronchospasm in an asthma dog model. Anesth Analg 57:629, 1978

179. Bjork VO, Carlens E, Friberg O: Endobronchial anesthesia. Anesthesiology 14:60, 1953

180. Bjertnaes L, Mundal R, Honje A et al: Vascular resistance in

atelectatic lungs: Effects of inhalation anaesthetics. Acta Anaesthiol Scand 24:109, 1980

181. Marshall C, Lindgren L, Marshall BE: Effects of halothane, enflurane and isoflurane on hypoxic pulmonary vasoconstriction in rat lungs *in vitro*. Anesthesiology 60:304, 1984

182. Domino KB, Borowec L, Alexander CM et al: Influence of isoflurane on hypoxic pulmonary vasoconstriction in dogs. Anesthesiology 64:423, 1986

183. Rees DI, Gaines GY III: One-lung anesthesia—A comparison of pulmonary gas exchange during anesthesia with ketamine or enflurane. Anesth Analg 63:521, 1984

184. Rogers SN, Benumof JL: Halothane and isoflurane do not decrease Pa_{O_2} during one-lung ventilation in intravenously anesthetized patients. Anesth Analg 64:946, 1985

185. Carlsson AJ, Bindslev L, Hedenstierna G: Hypoxia-induced pulmonary vasoconstriction in the human lung. Anesthesiology 66:312, 1987

186. Forbes AR: Halothane depresses mucociliary flow in the trachea. Anesthesiology 45:59, 1976

187. Forbes AR, Horrigan RW: Mucociliary flow in the trachea during anesthesia with enflurane, ether, nitrous oxide, and morphine. Anesthesiology 46:319, 1977

188. Lee KS, Park SS: Effect of halothane, enflurane, and nitrous oxide on tracheal ciliary activity *in vitro*. Anesth Analg 59:426, 1980

189. Eger EI II, Smith NT, Stoelting RK: Cardiovascular effects of halothane in man. Anesthesiology 32:396, 1970

190. Calverley RK, Smith NT, Prys-Roberts C et al: Cardiovascular effects of enflurane anesthesia during controlled ventilation in man. Anesth Analg 57:619, 1978

191. Caffrey JA, Eckstein JW, Hamilton WK et al: Forearm venous and arterial responses to halothane and cyclopropane. Anesthesiology 26:786, 1965

192. Reiz S, Bälfors E, Gustavsson B et al: Effects of halothane on coronary haemodynamics and myocardial metabolism in patients with ischaemic heart disease and heart failure. Acta Anaesthiol Scand 26:133, 1981

193. Wade JG, Stevens WC: Isoflurane: An anesthetic for the eighties? Anesth Analg 60:666, 1981

194. Merin RG, Basch S: Are the myocardial functional and metabolic effects of isoflurane really different from those of halothane and enflurane? Anesthesiology 55:398, 1981

195. Moffitt EA, Barker RA, Glenn JJ et al: Myocardial metabolic and hemodynamic responses with isoflurane anesthesia for coronary arterial surgery. Anesth Analg 65:53, 1986

196. Eger EI II: The pharmacology of isoflurane. Br J Anaesth 56:71S, 1984

197. Theye RA, Michenfelder JD: Whole body and organ V_{O_2} changes with enflurane, isoflurane and halothane. Br J Anaesth 47:813, 1975

198. Bahlman SH, Eger EI II, Halsey MJ et al: The cardiovascular effects of halothane in man during spontaneous ventilation. Anesthesiology 36:494, 1972

199. Cromwell TH, Stevens WC, Eger EI II et al: The cardiovascular effects of compound 469 (Forane) during spontaneous ventilation and CO_2 challenge in man. Anesthesiology 35:17, 1971

200. Cullen DJ, Eger EI II: Cardiovascular effects of carbon dioxide in man. Anesthesiology 41:345, 1974

201. Manninen P, Knill RL: Cardiovascular signs of acute hypoxaemia and hypercarbia during enflurane and halothane anaesthesia in man. Can Anaesth Soc J 26:282, 1979

202. Price HL, Skovsted P, Pauca AL et al: Evidence for B-receptor activation produced by halothane in normal man. Anesthesiology 32:389, 1970

203. Ritter JW, Shigezawa GY, Roe SD et al: Increasing myocardial oxygen demand during prolonged halothane anesthesia in dogs. Anesth Analg 62:788, 1983

204. Eisele JH, Smith NT: Cardiovascular effects of 40 percent nitrous oxide in man. Anesth Analg 51:956, 1972

205. Smith NT, Eger EI II, Stoelting RK et al: The cardiovascular and sympathomimetic responses to the addition of nitrous oxide to halothane in man. Anesthesiology 32:410, 1970

206. Smith NT, Calverley RK, Prys-Roberts C et al: Impact of nitrous oxide on the circulation during enflurane anesthesia. Anesthesiology 48:345, 1978

207. Dolan WM, Stevens WC, Eger EI II et al: The cardiovascular and respiratory effects of isoflurane–nitrous oxide anaesthesia. Can Anaesth Soc J 21:557, 1974

208. Moffitt EA, Sethna DH, Gary RJ et al: Nitrous oxide added to halothane reduces coronary flow and myocardial oxygen consumption in patients with coronary disease. Can Anaesth Soc J 30:5, 1983

209. Reiz S: Nitrous oxide augments the systemic and coronary haemodynamic effects of isoflurane in patients with ischaemic heart disease. Acta Anaesthesiol Scand 77:464, 1983

210. Lappas DG, Buckley MJ, Laven MB et al: Left ventricular performance and pulmonary circulation following addition of nitrous oxide to morphine during coronary-artery surgery. Anesthesiology 43:61, 1975

211. Hilgenberg JC, McCammon RL, Stoelting RK: Pulmonary and systemic vascular responses to nitrous oxide in patients with mitral stenosis and pulmonary hypertension. Anesth Analg 59:323, 1980

212. Schulte-Sasse U, Hess W, Tarnow J: Pulmonary vascular responses to nitrous oxide in patients with normal and high pulmonary vascular resistance. Anesthesiology 57:9, 1982

213. Hickey PR, Hansen DD, Stratford M et al: Pulmonary and systemic hemodynamic effects of nitrous oxide in infants with normal and elevated pulmonary vascular resistance. Anesthesiology 65:374, 1986

214. Priebe HJ: Differential effects of isoflurane on regional right and left ventricular performances, and on coronary, systemic and pulmonary hemodynamics. Anesthesiology 66:262, 1987

215. Epstein RM, Deutsch S, Cooperman LH et al: Splanchnic circulation during halothane anesthesia and hypercapnia in normal man. Anesthesiology 27:654, 1966

216. Gelman S, Fowler KG, Smith LR: Regional blood flow during isoflurane and halothane anesthesia. Anesth Analg 63:557, 1984

217. Gelman S, Fowler KC, Smith LR: Liver circulation and function during isoflurane and halothane anesthesia. Anesthesiology 61:726, 1984

218. Matsumoto N, Rorie DK, VanDyke RA: Hepatic oxygen supply and consumption in rats exposed to thiopental, halothane, enflurane, and isoflurane in the presence of hypoxia. Anesthesiology 66:337, 1987

219. Seyde WC, Ellis JE, Longnecker DE: The addition of nitrous oxide to halothane decreases renal and splanchnic flow and increases cerebral blood flow in rats. Br J Anaesth 58:63, 1986

220. Ostman M, Biber B, Martner J et al: Influence of isoflurane on renal and intestinal vascular responses to stress. Br J Anaesth 58:630, 1986

221. Duke PC, Hill K, Trosky S: The effect of isoflurane and isoflurane with nitrous oxide anesthesia on baroreceptor reflex control of heart rate in man. Anesthesiology 57:A41, 1982

222. Hageman W, Pietsch D, Arndt JO: The effect of halothane and enflurane as well as propanidid and ketamine on the aortic baroreceptor discharge of decerebrated cats. Anaesthetist 25:331, 1976

223. Morton M, Duke PC, Ong B: Baroreflex control of heart rate in man awake and during enflurane and enflurane–nitrous oxide anesthesia. Anesthesiology 52:221, 1980

224. Kotrly KJ, Ebert TJ, Vucins E et al: Baroreceptor reflex control of heart rate during isoflurane anesthesia in humans. Anesthesiology 60:173, 1984

225. Bagshaw RJ, Cox RH: Nitrous oxide and the baroreceptor reflexes in the dog. Acta Anaesthesiol Scand 26:31, 1982
226. Duke PC, Fownes D, Wade J: Halothane depresses baroreflex control of heart rate in man. Anesthesiology 46:184, 1977
227. Gregory GA: The baroresponses of preterm infants during halothane anaesthesia. Can Anaesth Soc J 29:105, 1982
228. Ebert TJ, Kotrly KJ, Vucins EJ et al: Halothane anesthesia attenuates cardiopulmonary baroreflex control of peripheral resistance in humans. Anesthesiology 63:668, 1985
229. Weiskopf RB, Townsley MI, Riordan KK et al: Comparison of cardiopulmonary responses to graded hemorrhage during enflurane, halothane, isoflurane, and ketamine anesthesia. Anesth Analg 60:481, 1981
230. Weiskopf RB, Bogetz MS: Cardiovascular actions of nitrous oxide or halothane in hypovolemic swine. Anesthesiology 63:509, 1985
231. Joas TA, Stevens WC: Comparison of the arrhythmic doses of epinephrine during Forane, halothane and fluroxene anesthesia in dogs. Anesthesiology 35:48, 1971
232. Johnston RR, Eger EI II, Wilson C: A comparative interaction of epinephrine with enflurane, isoflurane, and halothane in man. Anesth Analg 55:709, 1976
233. Horrigan RW, Eger EI II, Wilson C: Arrhythmias under enflurane anesthesia in man: A non-linear dose–response relationship and dose-dependent protection from lidocaine. Anesth Analg 57:547, 1978
234. Metz S, Maze M: Halothane concentration does not alter the threshold for epinephrine-induced arrhythmias in dogs. Anesthesiology 62:470, 1985
235. Tucker WK, Rackstein AD, Munson ES: Comparison of arrhythmic doses of adrenaline, metaraminol, ephedrine and phenylephrine during isoflurane and halothane anaesthesia in dogs. Br J Anaesth 46:392, 1974
236. Spiss CK, Maze M, Smith CM: Alpha-adrenergic responsiveness correlates with epinephrine dose for arrhythmias during halothane anesthesia in dogs. Anesth Analg 63:297, 1984
237. Karl HW, Swedlow DB, Lee KW et al: Epinephrine–halothane interactions in children. Anesthesiology 58:142, 1983
238. Robertson BJ, Clement JL, Knill RL: Enhancement of the arrhythmogenic effect of hypercarbia by surgical stimulation during halothane anaesthesia in man. Can Anaesth Soc J 28:342, 1981
239. Atlee JL III, Malkinson CE: Potentiation by thiopental of halothane-epinephrine-induced arrhythmias in dogs. Anesthesiology 57:285, 1982
240. Atlee JL III, Roberts FL: Thiopental and epinephrine-induced dysrhythmias in dogs anesthetized with enflurane or isoflurane. Anesth Analg 65:437, 1986
241. Stirt JA, Berger JM, Ricker SM et al: Arrhythmogenic effects of aminophylline during halothane anesthesia in experimental animals. Anesth Analg 59:410, 1980
242. Stirt JA, Berger JM, Sullivan SF: Lack of arrhythmogenicity of isoflurane following administration of aminophylline in dogs. Anesth Analg 62:568, 1983
243. Bosnjak ZJ, Kampine JP: Effects of halothane, enflurane and isoflurane on the SA node. Anesthesiology 58:314, 1983
244. Atlee JL III, Brownlee SW, Burstrom RE: Conscious-state comparisons of the effects of inhalation anesthetics on specialized atrioventricular conduction times in dogs. Anesthesiology 64:703, 1986
245. Zaidan JR, Curling PE, Craver JM Jr: Effect of enflurane, isoflurane, and halothane on pacing stimulation thresholds. PACE 8:32, 1985
246. Roizen MF, Plummer GO, Lichtor JL: Nitrous oxide and dysrhythmias. Anesthesiology 66:427, 1987
247. Kapur PA, Bloor BC, Flacke WE et al: Comparison of cardiovascular responses to verapamil during enflurane, isoflurane or halothane anesthesia in dogs. Anesthesiology 61:156, 1984

248. Chelly JE, Rogers K, Hysing ES et al: Cardiovascular effects of and interaction between calcium blocking drugs and anesthetics in chronically instrumented dogs. I. Verapamil and halothane. Anesthesiology 64:560, 1986
249. Rogers K, Hysing ES, Merin RG et al: Cardiovascular effects of and interaction between calcium blocking drugs and anesthetics in chronically instrumented dogs. II. Verapamil, enflurane, and isoflurane. Anesthesiology 64:568, 1986
250. Kates RA, Kaplan JA, Guyton RA et al: Hemodynamic interaction of verapamil and isoflurane. Anesthesiology 59:132, 1983
251. Iwatsuki N, Katoh M, Ono K et al: Antiarrhythmic effect of diltiazem during halothane anesthesia in dogs and in humans. Anesth Analg 64:964, 1985
252. Hysing ES, Chelly JE, Doursout MF et al: Cardiovascular effects of and interaction between calcium blocking drugs and anesthetics in chronically instrumented dogs. III. Nicardipine and isoflurane. Anesthesiology 65:385, 1986
253. Slogoff S, Keats AS, Hibbs CW et al: Failure of general anesthesia to potentiate propranolol activity. Anesthesiology 47:504, 1977
254. Bollen BA, Tinker JH, Hermsmeyer K: Halothane relaxes previously constricted porcine coronary artery segments more than isoflurane. Anesthesiology 66:748, 1987
255. Buffington CW, Ranson JL, Levine H et al: Isoflurane induces coronary steal in a canine model of chronic coronary occlusion. Anesthesiology 66:280, 1987
256. Reiz S, Balfors E, Sorensen MP et al: Isoflurane—A powerful coronary vasodilator in patients with coronary artery disease. Anesthesiology 59:91, 1983
257. Sill JC, Bove AA, Nugent M et al: Effects of isoflurane on coronary arteries and coronary arterioles in the intact dog. Anesthesiology 66:273, 1987
258. Priebe HJ, Föex P: Isoflurane causes regional myocardial dysfunction in dogs with critical coronary artery stenoses. Anesthesiology 66:293, 1987
259. Tarnow J, Markschies-Hornung A, Schulte-Sasse U: Isoflurane improves the tolerance to pacing-induced myocardial ischemia. Anesthesiology 64:147, 1986
260. Saito T, Tanaka Y, Tonogai R et al: Enflurane-induced hypotension modified transmural blood flow distribution in the canine left ventricle. Tohoku J Exp Med 126:273, 1978
261. Rydvall A, Häggmark S, Nyhmon H et al: Effects of enflurane on coronary haemodynamics in patients with ischaemic heart disease. Acta Anaesthesiol Scand 28:690, 1984
262. Mazze RI, Schwartz FD, Slocum HC et al: Renal function during anesthesia and surgery. I. Effects of halothane anesthesia. Anesthesiology 24:279, 1963
263. Deutsch S, Goldberg M, Stephen GW et al: Effects of halothane anesthesia on renal function in normal man. Anesthesiology 27:793, 1966
264. Theye RA, Maher FT: The effects of halothane on canine renal function and oxygen consumption. Anesthesiology 35:54, 1971
265. Bastron RD, Deutsch S: Anesthesia and the kidney, p 29. New York, Grune and Stratton, 1976
266. Mazze RI, Cousins MJ, Barr GA: Renal effects and metabolism of isoflurane in man. Anesthesiology 40:536, 1974
267. Tranquilli WJ, Manohar M, Parks CM et al: Systemic and regional blood flow distribution in unanesthetized swine and swine anesthetized with halothane and nitrous oxide, halothane, or enflurane. Anesthesiology 56:369, 1982
268. Bastron RD, Perkins FM, Pyne JL: Autoregulation of renal blood flow during halothane anesthesia. Anesthesiology 46:142, 1977
269. Priano LL: Effect of halothane on renal hemodynamics during normovolemia and acute hemorrhagic hypovolemia. Anesthesiology 63:357, 1985
270. Green CD, Eastwood DW: Effects of nitrous oxide inhalation on hemopoiesis in rats. Anesthesiology 24:341, 1963

271. Nunn JF: Clinical aspects of the interaction between nitrous oxide and vitamin B_{12}. Br J Anaesth 59:3, 1987

272. Chanarin I: Cobalamins and nitrous oxide: A Review. J Clin Pathol 33:909, 1980

273. Cleaton-Jones P, Austin JC, Banks D et al: Effect of intermittent exposure to a low concentration of nitrous oxide on haemopoiesis in rats. Br J Anaesth 49:223, 1977

274. Skacel PO, Hewlett AM, Lewis JD et al: Studies of the haemopoietic toxicity of nitrous oxide in man. Br J Haematol 53:189, 1983

275. Nancekievill DG, Amess JAL: The effects of folinic acid on patients who have received nitrous oxide. In Boulton, Atkinson (eds): Sixth European Congress of Anaesthesiology, p 18. New York, Grune and Stratton, 1982

276. Nunn JF, Chanarin I, Tanner AG et al: Megaloblastic bone marrow changes after repeated nitrous oxide anaesthesia. Br J Anaesth 58:1469, 1986

277. Lassen HCA, Kristensen HS: Remission in chronic myeloid leukaemia following prolonged nitrous oxide inhalation. Dan Med Bull 6:252, 1959

278. Baden JM, Egbert B, Rice SA: Enflurane has no effect on haemopoiesis in mice. Br J Anaesth 52:471, 1980

279. Coate WB, Kapp RW, Lewis TR: Chronic exposure to low concentrations of halothane–nitrous oxide. Reproductive and cytogenic effects in the rat. Anesthesiology 50:310, 1979

280. Duncan PG, Cullen BF: Anesthesia and immunology. Anesthesiology 45:522, 1976

281. Moudgil GC, Allan RB, Russell RJ et al: Inhibition by anaesthetic agents of human leukocyte locomotion towards chemical attractants. Br J Anaesth 49:97, 1977

282. Nunn JF, Sturrock JE, Jones AJ et al: Halothane does not inhibit human neutrophil function in vitro. Br J Anaesth 51:1101, 1979

283. Welch WD: Halothane reversibly inhibits human neutrophil bacterial killing. Anesthesiology 55:650, 1981

284. Welch WD: Effect of enflurane, isoflurane and nitrous oxide on the microbicidal activity of human polymorphonuclear leukocytes. Anesthesiology 61:188, 1984

285. Smith TC, Colton ET, Behar MG: Does anesthesia alter hemoglobin dissociation? Anesthesiology 32:5, 1970

286. Fournier L, Major D: The effect of nitrous oxide on the oxyhaemoglobin dissociation curve. Can Anaesth Soc J 31:173, 1984

287. Shah MV, Anderson LK, Bergman NA: The influence of nitrous oxide on oxyhaemoglobin dissociation and measurement of oxygen tension. Anaesthesia 41:586, 1986

288. Evans MC, Caneren IR: Oxygen electrodes sensitive to nitrous oxide. Lancet 2:1371, 1978

289. Black GW, McArdle L: The effects of halothane on peripheral blood vessels. Anaesthesia 17:82, 1961

290. Dalsgaard-Nielsen J, Risbo A, Simmelkjaer P et al: Impaired platelet aggregation and increased bleeding time during general anaesthesia with halothane. Br J Anaesth 53:1039, 1981

291. Fyman PN, Triner L, Schranz H et al: The effect of volatile anaesthetics and nitrous oxide–fentanyl anaesthesia on bleeding time. Br J Anaesth 56:1197, 1984

292. Gotta AW, Gould P, Sullivan CA et al: Effect of enflurane and fentanyl anaesthesia on human platelet aggregation in vitro. Can Anaesth Soc J 27:319, 1980

293. Nunn JF, O'Mordin C: Nitrous oxide decreases motility of human neutrophils in vitro. Anesthesiology 56:45, 1982

294. Edwards AE, Gammell LW, Mankin PP et al: The effects of three differing anaesthetics on the immune response. Anaesthesia 39:1071, 1984

295. Gissen HA, Karis JG, Nastuk WL: The effect of halothane on neuromuscular transmission. JAMA 197:770, 1966

296. Miller RD, Way WL, Dolan WM et al: Comparative neuromuscular effects of pancuronium, gallamine and succinylcholine during Forane and halothane anesthesia in man. Anesthesiology 35:509, 1971

297. Hilgenberg JC, Stoelting RK: Characteristics of succinylcholine-produced phase II neuromuscular block during enflurane, halothane and fentanyl anesthesia. Anesth Analg 60:192, 1981

298. Donati F, Bevan DR: Effect of enflurane and fentanyl on the clinical characteristics of long-term succinylcholine infusion. Can Anaesth Soc J 29:59, 1982

299. Donati F, Bevan DR: Long-term succinylcholine infusion during isoflurane anesthesia. Anesthesiology 58:6, 1983

300. Miller RD, Eger EI II, Way WL et al: Comparative neuromuscular effects of Forane and halothane alone and in combination with d-tubocurarine in man. Anesthesiology 35:38, 1971

301. Vitez TS, Miller RD, Eger EI II et al: Comparison in vitro of isoflurane and halothane potentiation of d-tubocurarine and succinylcholine neuromuscular blockades. Anesthesiology 41:53, 1974

302. Miller RD, Way WL, Dolan WM et al: The dependence of pancuronium and d-tubocurarine-induced neuromuscular blockades on alveolar concentrations of halothane and Forane. Anesthesiology 37:573, 1972

303. Bennett MJ, Hahn JF: Potentiation of the combination of pancuronium and metocurine by halothane and isoflurane in humans with and without renal failure. Anesthesiology 62:759, 1985

304. Fogdall RP, Miller RD: Neuromuscular effects of enflurane, alone and combined with d-tubocurarine, pancuronium and succinylcholine, in man. Anesthesiology 42:173, 1975

305. Rupp SM, Miller RD, Gencarelli PJ: Vecuronium-induced neuromuscular blockade during enflurane, isoflurane and halothane anesthesia in human. Anesthesiology 60:102, 1984

306. Stirt JA, Murray AL, Katz RL et al: Atracurium during halothane anesthesia in humans. Anesth Analg 62:207, 1983

307. Sokoll MD, Gergis SD, Mehta M et al: Safety and efficacy of atracurium (BW 33A) in surgical patients receiving balanced or isoflurane anesthesia. Anesthesiology 58:450, 1983

308. Brandom BW, Cook R, Wolfel SK et al: Atracurium infusion requirements in children during halothane, isoflurane and narcotic anesthesia. Anesth Analg 64:471, 1975

309. Merin RG, Samuelson PN, Schalch DS: Major inhalation anesthetics and carbohydrate metabolism. Anesth Analg 50:625, 1971

310. Gingerich R, Wright PH, Paradise RR: Effect of halothane on glucose-stimulated insulin secretion and glucose oxidation in isolated rat pancreatic islets. Anesthesiology 53:219, 1980

311. Ewart RBL, Rusy BF, Bradford MW: Effects of enflurane on release of insulin by pancreatic islets in vitro. Anesth Analg 60:878, 1981

312. Oyama T, Sato K, Kimura K: Plasma levels of antidiuretic hormone in man during halothane anaesthesia and surgery. Can Anaesth Soc J 18:614, 1971

313. Moran WH Jr, Mittenberger FW, Shuayb WA et al: The relationship of antidiuretic hormone secretion to surgical stress. Surgery 56:99, 1964

314. Philbin DM, Coggins CH: Plasma antidiuretic hormone levels in cardiac surgical patients during morphine and halothane anesthesia. Anesthesiology 49:95, 1978

315. Robertson D, Michelakis AM: Effect of anesthesia and surgery on plasma renin activity in man. J Clin Endocrinol Metab 34:831, 1971

316. Dery R: Theoretical and clinical considerations in anaesthesia for secreting carcinoid tumors. Can Anaesth Soc J 18:245, 1971

317. Miller R, Boulukos PA, Warner RRP: Failure of halothane and ketamine to alleviate carcinoid syndrome-induced bronchospasm during anesthesia. Anesth Analg 59:621, 1980

318. Tarkka M: Effects of mechanical ventilation and halothane on

pulmonary serotonin removal in dogs. Acta Anaesthesiol Scand 29:300, 1985

319. Oyama T, Aoki N, Kudo T: Effect of halothane anesthesia and of surgery on plasma testosterone levels in man. Anesth Analg 51:130, 1971

320. Joyce JT, Roizen MF, Gerson JI et al: Induction of anesthesia with halothane increases plasma norepinephrine concentrations. Anesthesiology 56:286, 1982

321. Sumikawa K, Amakata Y, Yoshikawa K et al: Catecholamine uptake and release in isolated chromaffin granules exposed to halothane. Anesthesiology 53:385, 1980

322. Seitz W, Luebbe N, Bechstein W et al: A comparison of two types of anaesthesia on the endocrine and metabolic responses to anaesthesia and surgery. Eur J Anaesth 3:283, 1986

323. Lacoumenta S, Paterson JL, Burrin J et al: Effects of two differing halothane concentrations on the metabolic and endocrine responses to surgery. Br J Anaesth 58:844, 1986

324. Campbell BC, Parikh RK, Naismith A et al: Comparison of fentanyl and halothane supplementation to general anaesthesia on the stress response to upper abdominal surgery. Br J Anaesth 56:257, 1984

325. Hamberger B, Jarnberg PO: Plasma catecholamines during surgical stress: Difference between neurolept and enflurane anaesthesia. Acta Anaesthiol Scand 27:307, 1983

326. Gelman S, Rivas JE, Erdemir H et al: Hormonal and haemodynamic responses to upper abdominal surgery during isoflurane and balanced anaesthesia. Can Anaesth Soc J 31:509, 1984

327. Göthert M, Wendt J: Inhibition of adrenal medullary catecholamine secretion by enflurane. I. Investigation in vivo. Anesthesiology 46:400, 1977

328. Göthert M, Wendt J: Inhibition of adrenal medullary catecholamine secretion by enflurane. II. Investigations in isolated bovine adrenals—Site and mechanism of action. Anesthesiology 46:404, 1977

329. Sigurdsson GH, Lindahl SGE, Norden NE: Catecholamine and endocrine response in children during halothane and enflurane anaesthesia for adrenoidectomy. Acta Anaesthiol Scand 28:47, 1984

330. Desmonts JM, LeHouelleur J, Remond P et al: Anaesthetic management of patients with phaeochromocytoma: A review of 102 cases. Br J Anaesth 49:991, 1977

331. Roizen MF, Horrigan RW, Koike M et al: A prospective randomized trial of four anesthetic techniques for resection of pheochromocytoma. Anesthesiology 57:A43, 1982

332. Suzukawa M, Michaels IAL, Ruzbarsky J et al: Use of isoflurane during resection of pheochromocytoma. Anesth Analg 62:100, 1983

333. Oyama T, Matsuki A, Kudo T: Effect of halothane, methoxyflurane anaesthesia and surgery on plasma thyroid-stimulating hormone (TSH) levels in man. Anaesthesia 27:2, 1972

334. Smith AC, Burman ML, James RC et al: Characterization of hyperthyroidism enhancement of halothane-induced hepatotoxicity. Biochem Pharmacol 32:3531, 1983

335. Servin FF, Nivoche Y, Desmonts JM et al: Biotransformation of halothane and enflurane in patients with hyperthyroidism. Anesthesiology 64:387, 1986

336. Babad AA, Eger EI II: The effects of hyperthyroidism and hypothyroidism on halothane and oxygen requirements in dogs. Anesthesiology 29:1087, 1968

337. Murkin JM: Anesthesia and hypothyroidism: A review of thyroxine physiology, pharmacology and anesthetic implications. Anesth Analg 61:371, 1982

338. Marx GF, Kim YI, Lin C et al: Post-partum uterine pressures under halothane or enflurane anesthesia. Obstet Gynecol 51:695, 1978

339. Munson ES, Embro WJ: Enflurane, isoflurane and halothane and isolated uterine muscle. Anesthesiology 46:11, 1977

340. Paull J, Ziccone S: Halothane, enflurane, methoxyflurane and isolated human uterine muscle. Anaesth Intensive Care 8:397, 1980

341. Cullen BF, Margolis AJ, Eger EI II: The effects of anesthesia and pulmonary ventilation on blood loss during therapeutic abortions. Anesthesiology 32:108, 1971

342. Warren TM, Datta S, Ostheimer GW et al: Comparison of the maternal and neonatal effects of halothane, enflurane, and isoflurane for cesarean delivery. Anesth Analg 62:516, 1983

343. Biehl DR, Cote J, Wade JG et al: Uptake of halothane by the fetal lamb in utero. Can Anaesth Soc J 30:24, 1983

344. Biehl DR, Tweed WA, Cote J et al: Effect of halothane on cardiac output and regional flow in the fetal lamb in utero. Anesth Analg 62:489, 1983

345. Palahniuk RJ, Doig GA, Johnson GN: Maternal halothane anesthesia reduces cerebral blood flow in the acidotic sheep fetus. Anesth Analg 59:35, 1980

346. Khristianson B, Magno R, Wickstrom I: Anesthesia for cesarean section. VI. Late effects on the infant of enflurane anesthesia for cesarean section. Acta Anaesthiol Scand 24:187, 1980

347. Biehl DR, Yarnell R, Wade JG et al: The uptake of isoflurane by the fetal lamb in utero: Effect on regional blood flow. Can Anaesth Soc J 30:581, 1983

348. Mazze RI, Fujinaga M, Rice SA et al: Reproductive and teratogenic effects of nitrous oxide, halothane, isoflurane, and enflurane in Sprague-Dawley rats. Anesthesiology 64:339, 1986

349. Mazze RI: Nitrous oxide during pregnancy. Anaesthesia 41:897, 1986

350. Shnider SM: Maternal and fetal hazards of surgery during pregnancy. Am J Obstet Gynecol 92:891, 1965

351. Duncan PG, Pope WDB, Cohen MM et al: Fetal risk of anesthesia and surgery during pregnancy. Anesthesiology 64:790, 1986

352. Guedel AE: Inhalation anesthesia: A fundamental guide, p 16. New York, Macmillan, 1951

353. Winterbottom EH: Insufficient anesthesia. Br Med J 1:247, 1950

354. Neff W, Mayer EC, Perales ML: Nitrous oxide and oxygen anesthesia with curare relaxation. Calif Med 66:67, 1947

355. Brotman M, Cullen SC: Supplementation with demerol during nitrous oxide anesthesia. Anesthesiology 10:696, 1949

356. Mushin WW: Analgesics as supplements during anaesthesia. Proc Roy Soc Med 44:840, 1951

357. Siker ES: Analgesic supplements to nitrous oxide anesthesia. A review. Br Med J 2:1326, 1956

358. Utting JE: Awareness in anaesthesia. Anaesth Intensive Care 3:334, 1975

359. Woodbridge PD: Changing concepts concerning depth of anesthesia. Anesthesiology 18:536, 1957

360. Artusio JF Jr: Diethyl ether analgesia: A detailed description of the first stage of ether anesthesia in man. J Pharmacol Exp Ther 111:343, 1954

361. Wise RP: Pain clinic and operative nerve blocks. In Churchill-Davidson HC (ed): A Practice of Anesthesia, p 893. Chicago, Year Book Medical Publishers, 1984

362. Baskett PJF: The use of Entonox in the ambulance service. Proc Roy Soc Med 65:7, 1972

363. Saucier NS, Walts LF, Moreland JR: Patient awareness during nitrous oxide, oxygen and halothane anesthesia. Anesth Analg 62:239, 1983

364. Bahl CP, Wadwa S: Consciousness during apparent surgical anaesthesia. Br J Anaesth 40:289, 1968

365. Manizar J: Awareness, muscle relaxants and balanced anaesthesia. Can Anaesth Soc J 26:386, 1979

366. Cullen DJ, Eger EI II, Stevens WC et al: Clinical signs of anesthesia. Anesthesiology 36:21, 1972

367. Eger EI II: Monitoring the depth of anesthesia. In Saidman LJ, Smith NT (eds): Monitoring in Anesthesia, p 1. Boston, Butterworths, 1978

368. Eger EI II, Smith NT, Cullen DJ et al: A comparison of the cardiovascular effects of halothane, fluroxene, ether and cyclopropane in man: A resume. Anesthesiology 34:25, 1971

369. Evaluation of anesthetic depth. In Cullen SC, Larson CP Jr (eds): Essentials of Anesthetic Practice, p 77. Chicago, Year Book Medical Publishers, 1974

370. Miller RD: Monitoring of neuromuscular blockade. In Saidman LJ, Smith NT (eds): Monitoring in Anesthesia, p 193. Boston, Butterworths, 1978

371. Ruffle JM, Snider MT, Rosenberger JL et al: Rapid induction of halothane anaesthesia in man. Br J Anaesth 57:607, 1985

372. Munson ES, Eger EI II, Bowers DL: Effects of anesthetic-depressed ventilation and cardiac output on anesthetic uptake: A computer nonlinear simulation. Anesthesiology 38:251, 1973

373. Wolfson B, Hetrick WD, Lake CL et al: Anesthetic indices—further data. Anesthesiology 48:187, 1978

374. Fisher DM, Robinson S, Brett CM et al: Comparison of enflurane, halothane, and isoflurane for diagnostic and therapeutic procedures in children with malignancies. Anesthesiology 63:647, 1985

375. Kingston HGG: Halothane and isoflurane anesthesia in pediatric outpatients. Anesth Analg 65:181, 1986

376. Buffington CW: Reflex action during isoflurane anaesthesia. Can Anaesth Soc J 29:S35, 1982

377. Friesen RH, Lichtor JL: Cardiovascular effects of inhalation induction with isoflurane in infants. Anesth Analg 62:411, 1983

378. Keats AS: What do we know about anesthetic mortality? Anesthesiology 50:387, 1970

379. Beecher HK, Todd DP: A study of the deaths associated with anesthesia and surgery. Ann Surg 140:2, 1954

380. Dripps RD, Lamont A, Eckenhoff JE: The role of anesthesia in surgical mortality. JAMA 178:261, 1961

381. Shnider SM, Pappas EM: Anesthesia for the asthmatic patient. Anesthesiology 22:886, 1961

382. Gold MI, Schwam SJ, Goldberg M: Chronic obstructive pulmonary disease and respiratory complications. Anesth Analg 62:975, 1983

383. Green DW, Verner IR, Fahmey NR: Techniques for deliberate hypotension. In Enderby GEH (ed): Hypotensive Anaesthesia, p 109. Edinburgh, Churchill-Livingstone, 1985

384. Lam AM, Gelb AW: Cardiovascular effects of isoflurane-induced hypotension for cerebral aneurysm surgery. Anesth Analg 62:742, 1983

385. Firn S: Enflurane for controlled hypotension. Postgrad Med J 59:608, 1983

386. Fairbairn ML, Eltringham RJ, Young PN et al: Hypotensive anaesthesia for microsurgery of the middle ear. A comparison between isoflurane and halothane. Anaesthesia 41:637, 1986

387. Hess W, Arnold B, Shulte-Sasse U et al: Comparison of isoflurane and halothane when used to control intraoperative hypertension in patients undergoing coronary artery bypass surgery. Anesth Analg 62:15, 1983

388. Eckenhoff JE: Observations during hypotensive anesthesia. Proc Roy Soc Med 55:942, 1962

389. Herbert M, Healy TEJ, Bourke JB et al: Profile of recovery after general anesthesia. Br Med J 286:1539, 1983

390. Azar I, Karambelkar DJ, Lear E: Neurologic state and psychomotor function following anesthesia for ambulatory surgery. Anesthesiology 60:347, 1984

391. Ali HH, Savarese JJ: Monitoring neuromuscular function. Anesthesiology 45:216, 1976

392. Gencarelli PJ, Miller RD, Eger EI II et al: Decreasing enflurane concentrations and d-tubocurarine neuromuscular blockade. Anesthesiology 56:192, 1982

393. Edwards RP, Miller RD, Roizen MF et al: Cardiac responses to imipramine and pancuronium during anesthesia with halothane or enflurane. Anesthesiology 50:421, 1979

394. Schick LM, Chapin JC, Munson ES et al: Pancuronium, d-tubocurarine, and epinephrine-induced arrhythmias during halothane anesthesia in dogs. Anesthesiology 52:207, 1980

395. Lundy JS: Balanced anesthesia. Minnesota Med 8:399, 1925

396. Lowenstein E, Hallowell P, Levine FH et al: Cardiovascular response to large doses of intravenous morphine in man. N Eng J Med 281:1389, 1969

397. Eger EI II: Should we not use nitrous oxide? In Eger EI II (ed): Nitrous Oxide/N₂O, p 339. New York, Elsevier, 1985

398. Cahalan MK, Lurz FW, Beaupre PH et al: Narcotics alter the heart rate and blood pressure response to inhalation anesthesia. Anesthesiology 59:A26, 1983

399. Eger EI II: Recovery from anesthesia. In Eger EI II (ed): Anesthetic Uptake and Action, p 228. Baltimore, Williams & Wilkins, 1974

400. Rice SA, Dooley JR, Mazze RI: Metabolism by rat hepatic microsomes of fluorinated ether anesthetics following ethanol consumption. Anesthesiology 58:237, 1983

401. Major V, Rosen M, Mushin WM: Methoxyflurane as an obstetric analgesic: A comparison with trichloroethylene. Br Med J 2:1554, 1966

402. Mazze RI, Trudell JR, Cousins MJ: Methoxyflurane metabolism and renal dysfunction: Clinical correlations in man. Anesthesiology 35:247, 1971

403. Cousins MJ, Mazze RI: Methoxyflurane nephrotoxicity. A study of dose–response in man. JAMA 225:1611, 1973

404. Lischner MW: Fatal hepatic necrosis following surgery. Possible relation to methoxyflurane anesthesia. Arch Intern Med 120:225, 1967

405. Wallin RF, Napoli MD: Sevoflurane (fluoromethyl-1,1,1,3,3,3-hexafluoro-2-propyl ether): A new inhalational anesthetic agent. Fed Proc 30:442, 1971

406. Wallin WF, Regan BM, Napoli MD et al: Sevoflurane: A new inhalational anesthetic agent. Anesth Analg 54:758, 1975

407. Cook TL, Beppu WJ, Hitt BA et al: Renal effects and metabolism of sevoflurane in Fischer 344 rats: An in-vivo and in-vitro comparison with methoxyflurane. Anesthesiology 43:70, 1975

408. Holaday DA, Smith FR: Clinical characteristics and biotransformation of sevoflurane in healthy human volunteers. Anesthesiology 54:100, 1981

409. Rice SA, Sbordone L, Mazze RI: Metabolism by rat hepatic microsomes of fluorinated ether anesthetics following isoniazid administration. Anesthesiology 53:489, 1980

410. Rice SA, Dooley JR, Mazze RI: Metabolism by rat hepatic microsomes of fluorinated ether anesthetics following ethanol consumption. Anesthesiology 58:237, 1983

411. Martis L, Lynch S, Napoli MD et al: Biotransformation of sevoflurane in dogs and rats. Anesth Analg 60:186, 1981

412. Strum DP, Eger EI II, Johnson BH et al: Toxicity of sevoflurane in rats. Anesth Analg 66:769, 1987

413. Baden JM, Kelley M, Mazze RI: Mutagenicity of experimental inhalational anesthetic agents: Sevoflurane, synthane, dioxychlorane, and dioxyflurane. Anesthesiology 56:462, 1982

414. Shulman M, Braverman B, Ivankovich AD et al: Sevoflurane triggers malignant hyperthermia in swine. Anesthesiology 54:259, 1981

415. Doi M, Ikeda K: Respiratory effects of sevoflurane. Anesth Analg 66:241, 1987

416. Katoh T, Ikeda K: The minimum alveolar concentration (MAC) of sevoflurane in humans. Anesthesiology 66:301, 1987

417. Manohar M, Parks CM: Porcine systemic and regional organ blood flow during 1.0 and 1.5 minimum alveolar concentrations of sevoflurane anesthesia without and with 50% nitrous oxide. J Pharmacol Exp Ther 231:640, 1984

418. Halsey JM: Physiochemical properties of inhalational anesthetics. In Gray TC, Nunn JF, Utting JE (eds): General Anaesthesia, p 45. London, Butterworths, 1980

419. Gion H, Saidman LJ: The minimum alveolar concentration of enflurane in man. Anesthesiology 35:361, 1971

420. Torri G, Damia G, Fabian ML: Effect of nitrous oxide on the anaesthetic requirement of enflurane. Br J Anaesth 46:468, 1974

421. Stevens WC, Dolan WM, Gibbons RT et al: Minimum alveolar concentrations (MAC) of isoflurane with and without nitrous oxide in patients of various ages. Anesthesiology 42:197, 1975

422. Stoelting RK: The effect of nitrous oxide on the minimum alveolar concentration of methoxyflurane needed for anesthesia. Anesthesiology 34:353, 1971

Chapter 12

M. Lawrence Berman
Duncan A. Holaday

Inhalation Anesthetic Metabolism and Toxicity

For many years it was thought that the volatile anesthetics, with the exception of tricholoroethylene, were taken up and eliminated unchanged *via* the lungs. This concept of anesthetic inertness was irreparably invalidated by reports in the early 1960s demonstrating that animals metabolize chloroform, diethyl ether, halothane, and methoxyflurane to volatile and nonvolatile metabolites.[1-7] Subsequent research has established that all the clinically useful inhaled anesthetics undergo metabolism.

Volatile anesthetics are metabolized by an enzyme system known as the *mixed-function oxidases,* or *monooxygenases.* The mixed-function oxidases also metabolize endogenous compounds such as corticosteroids, sterols, thyroid hormones, prostaglandins, leukotrienes, and fatty acids.[8] The liver, because of its large mass and abundant supply of mixed-function oxidases, is the principal site for the metabolism of many xenobiotics, including the volatile anesthetics. Metabolism of inhaled anesthetics has significance for hepatotoxicity, nephrotoxicity, mutagenicity, and teratogenicity (see Toxicity).

PRINCIPLES OF DRUG METABOLISM

Before describing the metabolism of the inhaled anesthetics, it is important to ask: Why is drug metabolism necessary? To have therapeutic value, a drug must be absorbed, gain access to its site of action, and be eliminated in a reasonable period of time. Renal excretion terminates the action of drugs that are relatively lipid insoluble and fully ionized at body pH. Such drugs are excreted unchanged by the kidney because they cannot be reabsorbed from the glomerular filtrate. The tubular epithelium is a lipoid barrier preventing back diffusion of lipid-insoluble compounds. The lipophilic nature of the tubular epithelium, however, permits the reabsorption of highly lipid-soluble non-ionized drugs from the glomerular filtrate into the peritubular capillaries. Drug metabolism converts these highly lipid-soluble drugs into lipid-insoluble and ionized metabolites. It has been speculated that the mixed-function oxidases evolved to provide animals with a means of eliminating xenobiotics like hydrocarbons, sterols, terpines, and alkaloids that are ingested with food and would accumulate to dangerous levels unless they were biotransformed to polar metabolites readily excreted by the kidneys. Also, it has been suggested that synthetic drugs are biodegraded because they mimic xenobiotics to which the animals have always been exposed. For example, a liposoluble drug such as thiopental would have a half-time of more than 100 years if it were not for the metabolic conversion to a more water-soluble and excretable metabolite.[9]

The mixed-function oxidases are remarkable for their lack of substrate specificity, attracting types of molecules rather than specific compounds. A substrate for this enzyme system need only to be lipophilic and non-ionized at body pH. Liposoluble xenobiotics can be converted to a more polar metabolite by acquiring a carboxylic, alcoholic, phenolic, sulfhydryl, or amino group. These groups can be formed by oxidation, oxidative deamination, hydroxylation, epoxidation, dealkylation, dehalogenation, or reduction reactions. Acquisition of a polar group by a liposoluble compound is called a *Phase I reaction.* If a Phase I metabolite is sufficiently polar, it may be easily excreted by the kidneys. A Phase I metabolite, however, may be only slightly water soluble and not readily eliminated. Solubility of a Phase I metabolite may be enhanced by a subsequent reaction in which an endogenous substrate such as glucuronic acid, sulfuric acid, acetic acid, or amino acid conjugates with the newly formed functional group to form a highly polar compound. Formation of a conjugated synthetic compound is called a *Phase II reaction.*

A number of enzymes not related to the mixed-function oxidases can perform Phase I reactions. Examples of some of these enzymes are the esterases found in plasma that hydrolyze succinylcholine and the ester-type local anesthetics. Alcohol dehydrogenase, localized in the soluble fraction of liver, lung, and kidney cells, converts alcohols to their corresponding aldehydes. Xanthine oxidase, also found in the soluble fraction of cells, metabolizes xanthine-containing drugs like caffeine and theophylline to the corresponding uric acid derivatives. These enzymes are not involved in the metabolism of the inhaled anesthetics.

In most instances, the metabolism of a xenobiotic by the mixed-function oxidases is the method the body uses to terminate drug action and to increase its rate of clearance. In other instances, the xenobiotic substrate may be converted to a metabolite that is more or less active pharmacologically than the parent compound, or the product may be unchanged in its activity, or the substrate may be converted to highly reactive intermediate(s) that can adduct to cellular macromolecules like DNA, RNA, lipids, and proteins. Such interaction may lead to a variety of detrimental consequences: cellular necrosis, mutagenesis, carcinogenesis, and teratogenesis.

The mixed-function oxidases are localized in the endoplasmic reticulum. In the cell, the endoplasmic reticulum consists of a continuous network of filamentous membrane-bound canals extending from the plasma membrane to the nucleus. The endoplasmic reticulum has a rough, granular appearance because its surface is studded with ribosomes. The rough-surfaced reticulum synthesizes proteins and is the site for the synthesis of the smooth-surface (no ribosomes) reticulum. Mixed-function oxidases are imbedded in the lipophilic membranes of the smooth-surfaced reticulum. The rough or smooth reticulum can be isolated by differential gradient centrifugation of homogenized cells. Isolated endoplasmic reticulum forms small vesiculated bodies called *microsomes.* The term *microsomal fraction* refers to the vesiculated fragments of endoplasmic reticulum that contain mixed-function oxidase activity.

The term mixed-function oxidase, or monooxygenase, is used because it describes the mechanism, reactants, and products of the reaction:

$$DH + O_2 \rightarrow DOH + HOH$$

where DH represents an oxidizable drug substrate and DOH the hydroxylated drug metabolite. Both atoms of oxygen, derived from air, not from water, enter into the reaction, one being inserted into the substrate while the other is reduced to water.

The mixed-function oxidases require a coenzyme, reduced nicotinamide adenine dinucleotide phosphate (NADPH), which is an electron transport chain consisting of a flavin-containing enzyme (a flavoprotein), NADPH, cytochrome P-450 reductase, and a family of hemoprotein isozymes, cytochromes P-450. Cytochromes P-450 are the terminal oxidases in the electron transport system present in the endoplasmic reticulum and are classified as heme-containing enzymes (hemoproteins), with iron protoporphyrin IX as the prosthetic group. The heme is noncovalently bound to the apoproteins.

The name cytochrome P-450 (P stands for "pigment") is derived from the spectral properties of the heme portion of the enzyme. In its ferrous (reduced) form, carbon monoxide binds to the iron to yield a ferrocarbonyl adduct that exhibits a spectral maximum at 450 nm. The hemoproteins function as both the oxygen- and substrate-binding sites for the mixed-function oxidase reactions.

A simplified scheme of the cytochrome P-450 catalytic cycle is presented in Figure 12-1. Oxidized (Fe^{+3}) cytochrome P-450 combines with a drug substrate to form cytochrome P-450 drug complex; NADPH donates an electron to cytochrome P-450 reductase, which, in turn reduces the cytochrome P-450 drug complex (Fe^{+2}). The complex is oxygenated. A second electron, which reduces molecular oxygen to form activated oxygen–cytochrome P-450 drug complex, is introduced from NADPH cytochrome P-450 reductase. (Although not shown in Fig. 12-1, the second electron can be provided by cytochrome b_5 *via* a NADPH–microsomal flavoprotein cytochrome b_5 reductase.) The activated oxygen–cytochrome P-450 drug complex transfers the activated oxygen to the drug substrate to form the oxidized product.

ENZYME INDUCTION

The mixed-function oxidases can be stimulated by repeated administration of certain drugs and by exposure to a variety of chemicals in the environment. Substances that stimulate the mixed-function oxidases do so by increasing the rate of enzyme synthesis relative to their normal rate. This increased rate of synthesis is called *enzyme induction.* Although the molecular basis of enzyme induction is not fully understood, there are data to suggest that inducing agents increase messenger RNA by augmenting transcription. The result is an increase in the rate of synthesis of several isozymes of cytochrome P-450 and suppression of other cytochrome P-450 isozymes. These isozymes differ from each other in their inducibility by drugs and chemicals and in their substrate specificity, molecular weights, and spectral and immunologic properties. Agents that stimulate the mixed-function oxidases have been loosely classified into two groups, based on their similarities to the enzyme-inducing characteristics of either phenobarbital or the polycyclic aromatic hydrocarbons. Phenobarbital induces the synthesis of a cytochrome P-450 isozyme called *cytochrome P-450b,* or *cytochrome LM₂* (liver microsomal form 2), whereas the isozyme induced by the polycyclic aromatic hydrocarbons is called *cytochrome P-448* (also called P_1-450, or P-450c, or LM₄). Because each isozyme is encoded by a specific gene, different genes are likely to be involved in the induction by these two groups of agents. Induction by phenobarbital results in altered metabolism of a wide spectrum of substrates; an increased rate of synthesis of cytochrome P-450 reductase; a proliferation of the smooth-surfaced endoplasmic reticulum; an increased accumulation of phospholipids (a component of the endoplasmic reticulum); and an increase in liver weight, in microsomal and other liver proteins, as well as an increase in liver blood and bile flow. Induction by the polycyclic aromatic hydrocarbons results in an increased rate of drug metabolism of only a few substrates, and there is no induction of cytochrome P-450 reductase and no proliferation of the endoplasmic reticulum.

Enzyme induction occurs almost exclusively in the liver, the site of greatest mass of mixed-function oxidases. However, induction can also occur to some extent in the placenta, kidneys, adrenal glands, small intestine, pancreas, skin, and lungs.

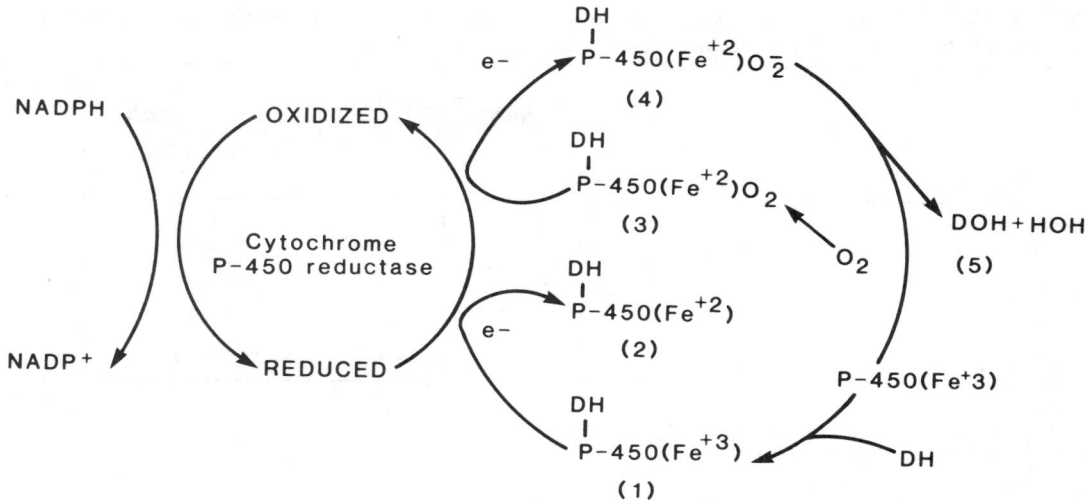

FIG. 12-1. A simplified scheme of cytochrome P-450 catalytic cycle in drug oxidation. A drug substrate (DH) complexes with oxidized cytochrome P-450 (Fe^{+3}) (1) and is reduced by an electron (e^-) donated from NADPH *via* cytochrome P-450 reductase, which reduces oxidized cytochrome P-450 (Fe^{+2}) drug complex (2). The complex is oxygenated (3). A second e^- is introduced from NADPH by way of cytochrome P-450 reductase to produce an oxygen radical–activated oxygen cytochrome P-450 drug complex (4), which transfers activated oxygen to DH to form oxidized drug (DOH) (5).

The direct consequence of enzyme induction is an acceleration of metabolism. This usually results in a decrease in the intensity and duration of action of the inducing agent and of a variety of coadministered drugs that are substrates for mixed-function oxidases. If the drug substrate requires metabolic activation before it can exert its pharmacologic action, however, enzyme induction accelerates the formation of the active metabolite. Drug-mediated tissue toxicity can also be enhanced by enzyme induction. This can occur if there is an increase in the formation of a reactive intermediate that, in the absence of induction, would normally be present in trace amounts, have a fleeting existence, and exert no biologic action. Enzyme induction also enhances the metabolism of normal body constituents (cortisol, male and female sex hormones, and vitamin D), all of which are substrates for mixed-function oxidases.

It is not known why some substances are inducers and others are not. The inducers are usually substrates for the mixed-function oxidases. Common features of chemically dissimilar inducers are high solubility in lipids and moderately long half-times. In animals, several hundred drugs are capable of inducing the mixed-function oxidases. Pharmacologically, they represent almost every type of drug action. Exposure to chemicals in the environment, such as herbicides, pesticides, industrial chemicals, (*e.g.*, polychlorinated biphenyls), and carcinogens, such as benzapyrene, (which is present in tobacco smoke and other organic pyrolysis products [*e.g.*, charcoal-broiled meats]) induce the microsomal drug-metabolizing enzymes. Much of the data on enzyme induction has been obtained from animal studies and may not be completely applicable to humans.

Some of the same drugs and chemicals that induce the mixed-function oxidases (Phase I drug metabolism) also induce glucuronyl transferase and glutathione-s-transferase. Both of these enzymes exist in multiple forms and catalyze conjugation reactions (Phase II drug metabolism). Glucuronyl transferase is localized in the endoplasmic reticulum, and

there are data that some forms of the glutathione-s-transferases are also found in the endoplasmic reticulum. These enzymes are positioned to conjugate products of the mixed-function oxidase reactions.

METABOLISM

With the aid of isotopic labeling, metabolites of halothane, chloroform, diethyl ether, and methoxyflurane were identified by Van Dyke et al[1] in urine of dogs exposed to these drugs. Studies of metabolic degradation of the fluorinated anesthetics in humans have been facilitated by the presence in the anesthetic molecules of atoms having a usually low concentration and constant turnover in the body. Stier et al[2] traced rising concentrations of bromide ion in urine of patients, and Holaday et al[10] quantitated inorganic fluoride (F^-) and organic fluorine to define the pharmacokinetics of methoxyflurane, enflurane, isoflurane, sevoflurane, and other experimental inhalational drugs in patients and in normal volunteers. Mass balance studies, based on the difference between estimates of quantities of anesthetic absorbed during exposure and anesthetic exhaled unaltered following exposure, have consistently given higher estimates of the fraction of absorbed drug that is metabolized than comparisons of accumulated uptake and collections of excreted metabolites (Table 12-1).[3–7]

Volatile anesthetics are metabolized principally by enzymes (mixed-function oxidases or cytochrome P-450–mediated monooxygenases) located mainly in the endoplasmic reticulum (microsomes) of hepatocytes. These enzymes are responsible for oxidation reactions characterized as dehalogenation and O-dealkylation, which account for the greatest proportion of anesthetic metabolism. Dehalogenation is the result of oxidation of the halogen-containing carbon producing a chemically unstable compound that decomposes to carboxylic acid and thus liberates halogens. Two halogens on the terminal carbon represent the optimal condition for deha-

TABLE 12-1.   Uptake and Metabolism of Anesthetics as Assessed by Mass Balance in Nine Patients Compared with the Results of Previous Mass Balance and Metabolic Recovery Studies

ANESTHETIC	TOTAL UPTAKE (ml)	TOTAL RECOVERY (ml)	PER CENT RECOVERY	RECOVERY NORMALIZED TO ISOFLURANE (%)	NORMALIZED METABOLISM (%)	RESULTS OF PREVIOUS STUDIES		
						Per Cent Recovery	Metabolites as a Per Cent of Total Uptake	References
Isoflurane	381 ± 24	354 ± 28	92.8 ± 4.0	100	0*	95	0.2	(7)
Enflurane	682 ± 43	579 ± 48	84.9 ± 3.8	91.5 ± 1.0	8.5 ± 1.0	85	2.4	(3)
						90–91		(10)
Halothane	356 ± 22	179 ± 13	50.2 ± 2.3	53.9 ± 0.9	46.1 ± 0.9	37	11–25	(6)
							17–20	(1)
						41–45		(10)
Methoxyflurane	127 ± 12	29 ± 2	23.1 ± 1.9	24.7 ± 1.6	75.3 ± 1.6	29–35	48	(2)

Values are mean ± SE.
*Metabolism of isoflurane was assumed to be 0 for this calculation.
(Reprinted with permission.)

logenation, while a terminal carbon with three halogens (trifluoro) is oxidized to a limited extent. O-dealkylation is the result of hydroxylation of an alkyl group (ether cleavage) adjacent to the oxygen of an ether bond. The resulting hemiacetyl is a relatively unstable intermediate that rapidly decomposes to an alcohol and an aldehyde. Halothane is the only volatile anesthetic known to undergo reductive metabolism. Hydrolysis of inhaled anesthetics does not occur because none of these drugs possesses an ester bond. Overall, genetic factors, more than environmental conditions (enzyme induction, diet, pollutants), determine the overall rate of anesthetic metabolism.

The pharmacokinetics of metabolism of each anesthetic and the fate of its metabolites are determined by its chemical stability and susceptibility to enzymatic attack; its solubilities in blood and fat; the concentrations used during exposure; the previous drug history of the subject; the solubilities of the drug's metabolites; and the blood flow and ventilation patterns of the subject during the period of excretion of the drug and metabolites.

NITROUS OXIDE

Nitrous oxide is not metabolized to any demonstrable extent by rat liver microsomes or liver homogenates, nor in vivo in mice or infused swine liver.[11] It is metabolized to nitrogen, however, by intestinal bacteria (Fig. 12-2).[12] The authors of this meticulous study incubated intestinal contents of rats and humans with ^{15}N–N_2O in several concentrations of oxygen from 0 to 20%. They estimated that 1 ml or 0.004% of the N_2O absorbed during 3 hr of anesthesia could be converted to gaseous nitrogen by reductive metabolism. They warn, however, that during this process, carcinogenic and teratogenic free radical intermediates may be produced, absorbed, and transported to other organ systems. Metabolism of nitrous oxide by intestinal bacteria is inhibited by both antibiotics and increasing (above 10%) concentrations of oxygen.

HALOTHANE

Halothane is degraded as a result of oxidative metabolism of the carbon containing two halogen atoms to Br, trifluoroacetic acid (TFA), and Cl^{-1}.[3] Reductive metabolism results in

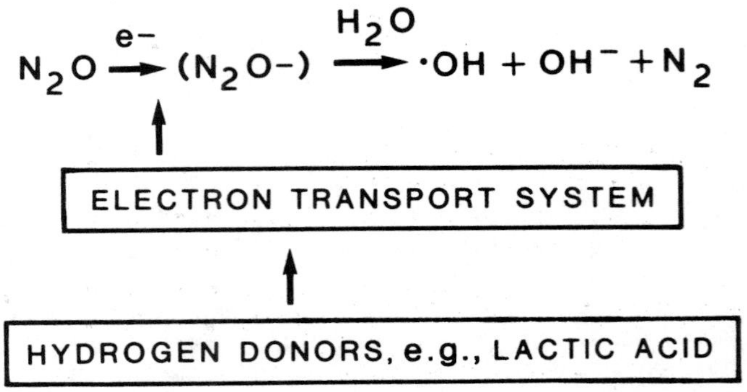

$$N_2O \xrightarrow{e-} (N_2O-) \xrightarrow{H_2O} \cdot OH + OH^- + N_2$$

ELECTRON TRANSPORT SYSTEM

HYDROGEN DONORS, e.g., LACTIC ACID

FIG. 12-2. Nitrous oxide may be metabolized to nitrogen by intestinal bacteria. (Reprinted with permission. Hong K, Trudell JR, O'Neil JR et al: Metabolism of nitrous oxide by human rat and intestinal contents. Anesthesiology 52:16, 1980.)

2-chloro-1,1,1-trifluoroethane (CTE) and 2-chloro-1,1,1-difluoroethylene (CDE), two volatile metabolites, and F^- (Fig. 12-3).[13–15] To a limited extent, mammalian enzymes can degrade halothane to CO_2.[16] All of these metabolites, except Cl^- and CO_2 (which must be derived from radioactive halothanes), have been identified directly in human urine or exhaled air following exposure to halothane. In addition, Cohen et al have isolated and identified two conjugated metabolites of ^{14}C–halothane in urine of heart donors: N-trifluoroacetylaminoethanol, a possible derivative of a condensation of a trifluoroacetyl radical with phosphatidylethanolamine in the lipid portion of the cell membrane, and N-acetyl-S-(2-bromo-2-chloro-1,1-difluoroethyl)-L-cysteineate, a possible product of a condensation of bromochlorodifluoroethylene, a potent alkylating agent derived from halothane, and glutathione (Fig. 12-4).[17] Later studies by the same group revealed that formation of bromochlorodifluoroethylene requires passage of halothane through a closed breathing system containing soda lime.[14]

The last two urinary metabolites listed above demonstrate the existence of mechanisms that can account for irreversible binding of halothane metabolites to fixed macromolecular structures of cells, as has been reported by several investigators.[19–29] The metabolic pathway responsible for the production of free radicals and other highly reactive intermediate metabolites of halothane depends on NADPH for electron transfer and a microsomal enzyme, P-450.[19] Binding is diminished by higher oxygen concentrations and in the presence of glutathione and other antioxidants, and is increased by induction of microsomal enzymes. Reductive dehalogenation producing free radicals is believed to be responsible for the acute hepatic toxicity that can follow exposure to halothane but not enflurane or isoflurane.[30, 31]

Cytochrome P-450 activity of liver microsomes is inducible by a large number of drugs, notably phenobarbital; polychlorinated biphenyls; isoniazid; 3-methylcholanthrene (3-MC); a number of tranquilizers, including chlorpromazine; and a

number of insecticides, including DDT and chlordane. Among the anesthetics, halothane, methoxyflurane, and enflurane are also capable of induction.[32] Cytochrome P-450 is not a single enzyme, but a group of isozymes having different substrate specificities. Similarly, the inducers exhibit specificity for the isozymes. For instance, 3-MC induces a closely related enzyme, P-448, which acts rapidly to increase the weight of the liver but not its protein concentration nor its defluorination activity.[31] Phenobarbital, on the other hand, increases the total liver protein and the amount of protein per g, but requires several days of treatment to achieve maximum effect. Phenobarbital induction stimulates both the oxidative and reductive metabolism of halothane and the dechlorination and ether cleavage of methoxyflurane, whereas 3-MC has little or no effect on these activities.[32]

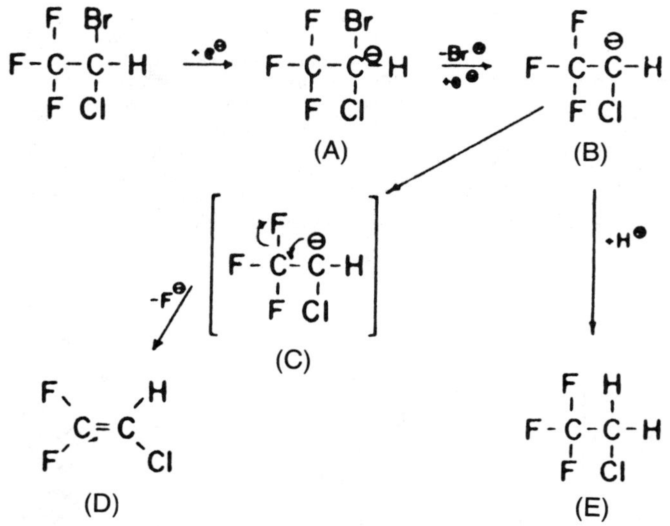

Studies in perfused swine liver[33] and rats[34] have supported the view that the fraction of absorbed halothane that undergoes metabolism is inversely related to exposure concentration (Fig. 12-5).[33] In the study by Sawyer et al,[33] clinically effective anesthetic concentrations of halothane appeared to block metabolism, while exposure to concentrations between 0.1% and 0.5% produced a constant rate of metabolism. At lower concentrations the fraction removed increased progressively.[32] This experiment suggests that the enzymes that metabolize halothane are saturable. Mass balance studies in humans supported a greater fraction of halothane being removed by metabolism at an inspired concentration of 0.1% than at 0.4% (Table 12-1).[3-7] On the other hand, the same fraction of enflurane taken up was metabolized at an inspired concentration of 0.87% as at 0.21%. This suggests that halothane saturates microsomal enzymes to a greater extent and at lower MAC values than enflurane.

Rehder et al[3] estimated that humans metabolized 17%–20% of halothane by determining the fraction of absorbed drug excreted as urinary bromide. Carpenter et al[7] found the extent of metabolism to average 46% when measured by mass balance in healthy adults. Individuals differ in the extent to which they metabolize halothane; those who have been exposed to enzyme inducers tend to metabolize at a higher rate than those not normally exposed.[4]

FIG. 12-3. Reductive metabolism of halothane may result in formation of fluoride (C), 2-chloro-1, 1-difluoroethylene (D) and 2-chloro-1, 1-trifluoroethane (E). (Reprinted with permission. Sharp JH, Trudell JR, Cohen EN: Volatile metabolites and decomposition products of halothane in man. Anesthesiology 50:2, 1979.)

FIG. 12-4. Urinary metabolites of halothane include trifluoroacetic acid (C), N-trifluoroacetyl-2 aminoethanol (A), and 2-bromo-2 chloro-1, 1-defluoroethylene (B). (Reprinted with permission. Cohen EN, Trudell JR, Edmunds HN et al: Urinary metabolites of halothane in man. Anesthesiology 43:392, 1975.)

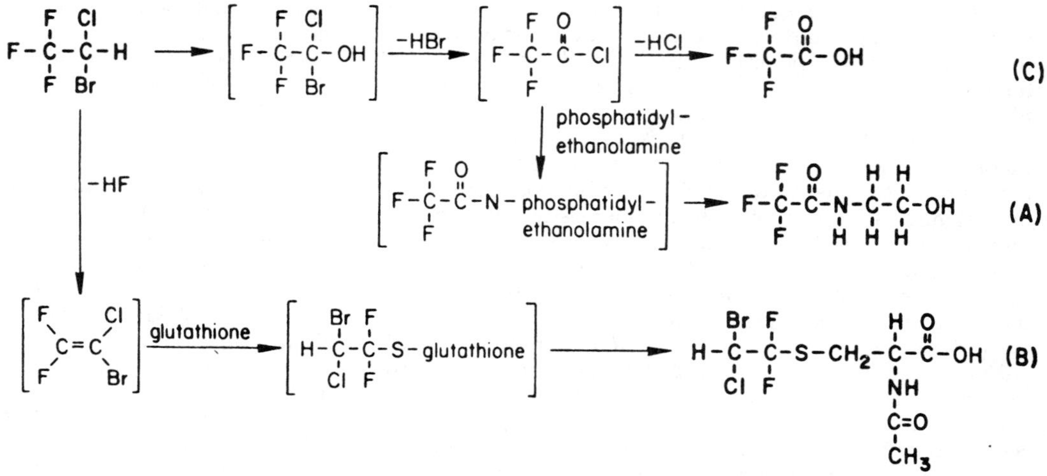

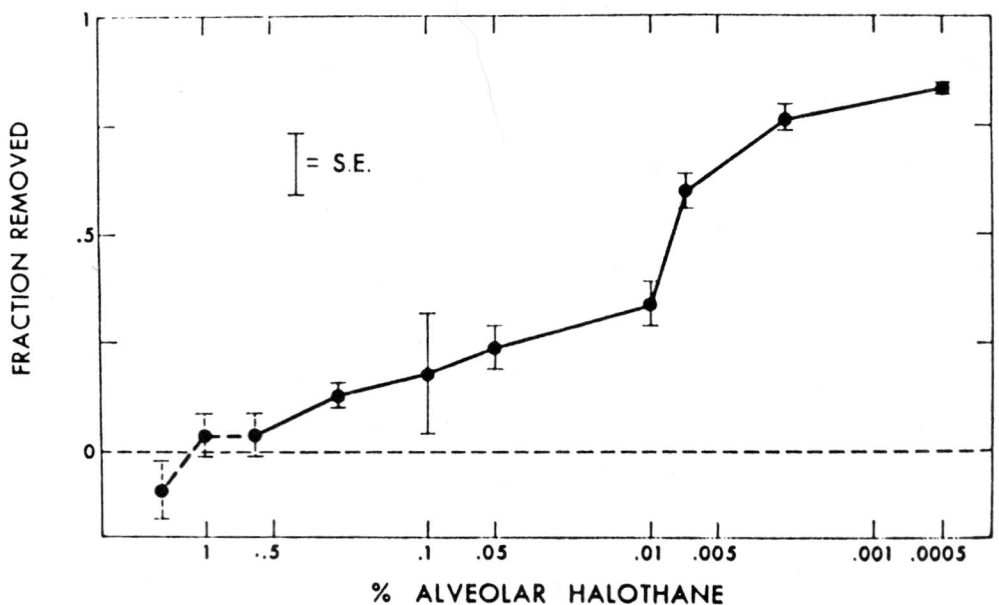

FIG. 12-5. The fraction of halothane removed by the liver increases as the calculated alveolar concentration decreases. (Reprinted with permission. Sawyer DC, Eger EI, Bahlman SH *et al:* Concentration dependence of hepatic halothane metabolism. Anesthesiology 34:230, 1971.)

Obesity and female gender have been suspected of increasing the metabolism of halothane[35, 36] because the potential for fulminant hepatic necrosis seems to be favored by these factors. Solid evidence is lacking in humans, however, for either contention. In the enzyme-induced hypoxic rat model, the female rat metabolizes halothane by the oxidative pathway to the same extent as the male rat, but less by the reductive pathway, the latter being held more responsible for liver necrosis (Fig. 12-6).[37] Furthermore, the female rat is less susceptible than the male rat to halothane hepatotoxicity. The finding that obesity may increase metabolism of halothane rests on somewhat firmer ground.[38] Increased F^- and bromide levels in morbidly obese patients have been demonstrated after halothane anesthesia, suggesting an increase in both reductive and oxidative metabolism.[39, 40] Also, increased F^- formation has been observed in obese patients following methoxyflurane and enflurane anesthesia.[38, 41]

Drugs commonly administered to surgical patients in the perioperative period can influence halothane metabolism. Cimetidine, a powerful inhibitor of drug metabolism and an H_2-receptor antagonist, was found by Plummer *et al*[42] to inhibit significantly the reductive, but not the oxidative, metabolism of halothane and to protect against hepatic necrosis in the phenobarbital-hypoxic rat model. Wood *et al*[43] confirmed the protection against hepatic necrosis but observed a nonsignificant reduction of reductive and oxidative metabolism in the phenobarbital-hypoxic model (Fig. 12-7).[43] They did note a modest but statistically significant reduction of oxidative metabolism in the phenobarbital-air and phenobarbital-hyperoxic rat models. When ranitidine, another H_2-receptor antagonist, was given to the phenobarbital-hypoxic Fischer 344 rat model, reductive metabolism of halothane was not affected, nor was there protection against liver injury; however, oxidative metabolism was slightly reduced.[42]

Dithiocarb is the sodium salt of a half-molecule of disulfuram and shares the latter's chelating activity and antidotal action against heavy metal poisoning. It also is protective against experimental carbon tetrachloride hepatotoxicity. Siegers *et al*[44] found it protective against other hepatotoxic drugs. They postulated that it inhibited the microsomal mono-

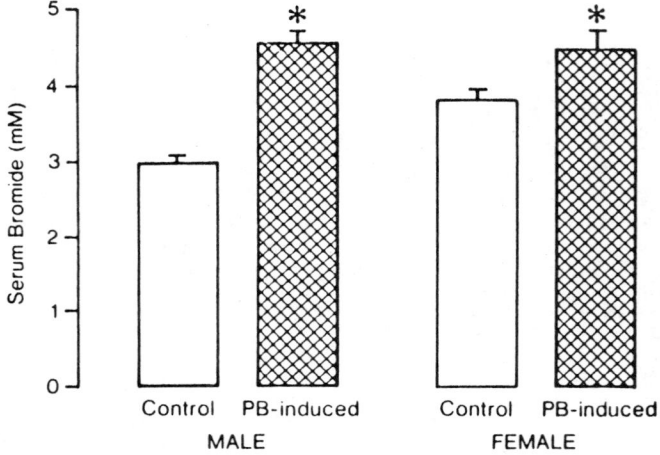

FIG. 12-6. In the enzyme-induced hypoxic rat model, the female metabolizes halothane by the oxidative pathway to the same extent as the male, as confirmed by similar changes in serum bromide concentrations. (Reprinted with permission. Plummer JL, Hall PM, Jenner MA *et al:* Sex differences in halothane metabolism and hepatotoxicity in a rat model. Anesth Analg 64:563, 1985.)

oxygenase system and determined its effect on the elimination of a number of solid and volatile drugs, including halothane. Treatment with dithiocarb before exposure prolonged the metabolic elimination half-life of halothane in rats 7.6 times. Eckes and Buch[45] confirmed this inhibition and concluded that CS_2, a metabolite of both dithiocarb and disulfuram, was responsible for the inhibition.

Other factors that may affect the extent or rate of metabolism of the anesthetics include the extremes of age, during which P-450 activity is reduced; the destruction of P-450 by chemicals, the metabolites of which bind irreversibly with the enzymes, *e.g.*, carbon tetrachloride[46] and chloroform; and a host of different compounds that can reversibly inhibit with variable specificity the metabolism of a number of drugs. Included in the latter category are SKF 525A,[47] metyrapone,[48] chloramphenicol,[49] and contraceptive agents.[50] The prior or simultaneous exposure to an anesthetic that interacts with the microsomal mixed-function oxidase system can modify the metabolism of another. Fiserova-Bergerova[51] demonstrated that isoflurane inhibited the metabolism in rats of halothane in a dose-dependent manner when mixed with a trace amount of halothane. Similarly, Fish and Rice were able to inhibit the metabolism of enflurane dose-dependently by prior exposure to halothane (Fig. 12-8).[52] Another way to limit metabolism of a drug is to decrease its chemical reactivity. The carbon–deuterium (^{2}H-C) bond is considerably stronger than the carbon–hydrogen (H-C) bond. By substituting ^{2}H for H in halothane, Sipes et al[53] were able to demonstrate a 65% reduction in the oxidative metabolism, but no change in its reductive metabolism. This is consistent with an attack by activated oxygen on the hydrogen, but with the C–H bond remaining intact in the products of reductive metabolism.

ENFLURANE

Chase et al[5] recovered 82.7% of the amount of enflurane absorbed by 7 healthy gynecologic patients as unaltered drug in exhaled air, and 2.4% in urine as F^- (0.5%) and organic fluorine (1.9%). A mass balance study of 9 healthy patients, based on the assumption that isoflurane undergoes no metabolism, indicated that enflurane metabolism, normalized to isoflurane recovery, amounts to 8.5% of uptake (Table 12-1).[3-7] The half-time for excretion of F^- was 37 h, and for RF was 89 h.[5] Serum F^- rose progressively from the beginning of exposure in 20 ASA Class I and Class II male patients, peaked between 1.5 h and 8 h after anesthesia at 22 $\mu M \cdot l^{-1}$, and fell gradually over 48 h to below 10 $\mu M \cdot l^{-1}$.[54] Hitt el al[55] observed that equimolar amounts of F^- and organic fluorine are produced in vitro by microsomes from rats and humans. Burke et al[56] corroborated the observations by Hitt et al and identified the single organic metabolite as difluoromethoxydifluoroacetic acid. They also noted that no formaldehyde was formed, and concluded that cytochrome P-450 catalyzed the oxidation of the C–H bond on the β carbon. In rats exposed to enflurane labeled with ^{14}C in the methoxy group, it was demonstrated by collection of $^{14}CO_2$ that 9% of that which was metabolized resulted from cleavage of the ether linkage (Holaday DA, personal communication). Enflurane undergoes oxidative metabolism by one or more pathways (Fig. 12-9).

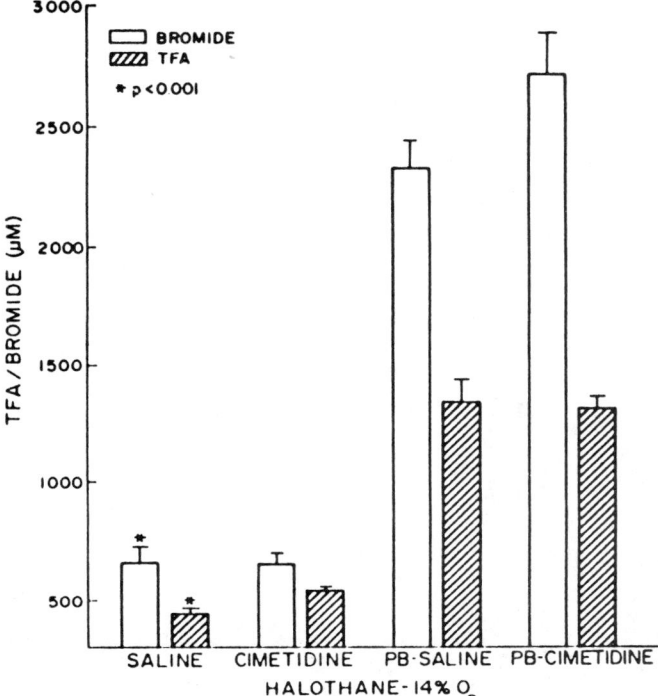

FIG. 12-7. The effect of cimetidine on the oxidative metabolism of halothane to bromide and trifluoroacetic acid (TFA) in the phenobarbital (Pb)-hypoxia rat model. (Reprinted with permission. Wood M, Uetrecht J, Phythyon JM et al: The effect of cimetidine on anesthetic metabolism and toxicity. Anesth Analg 65:481, 1986.)

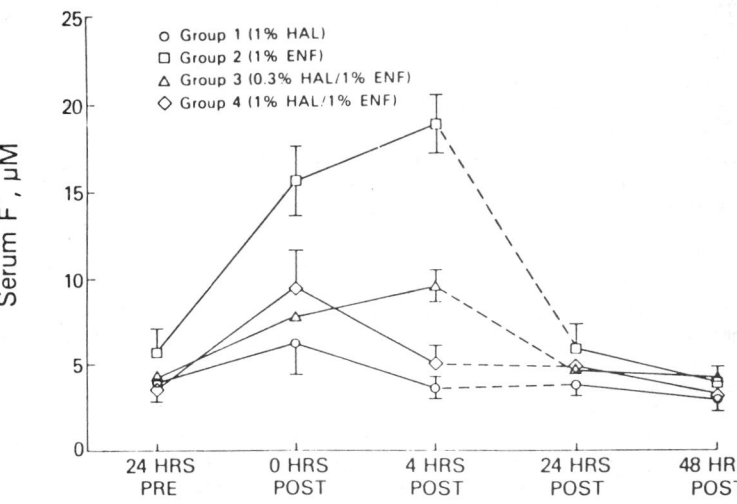

FIG. 12-8. Metabolism of enflurane (ENF), as reflected by serum fluoride (F^-) concentrations, is inhibited by low concentrations of halothane (HAL). (Reprinted with permission. Fish KJ, Rice SA: Halothane inhibits metabolism of enflurane in Fischer 344 rats. Anesthesiology 59:417, 1983.)

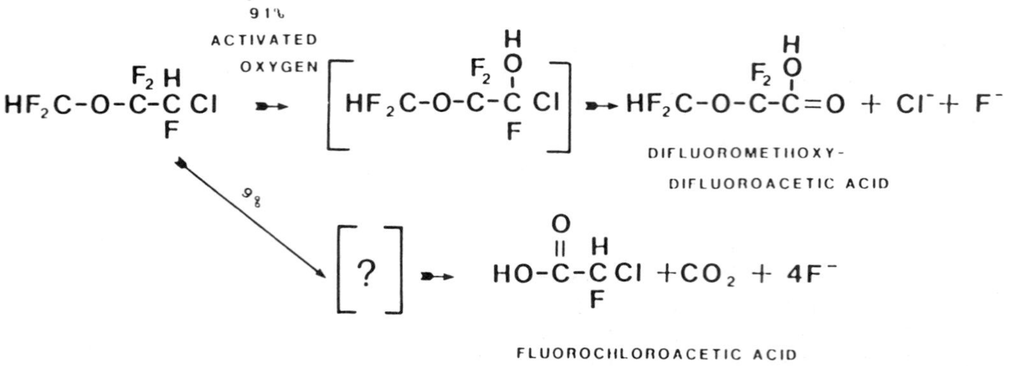

$$HF_2C-O-\overset{\overset{\displaystyle F_2}{\displaystyle |}}{C}-\overset{\overset{\displaystyle H}{\displaystyle |}}{\underset{\displaystyle F}{C}}Cl \xrightarrow{\overset{\displaystyle 91\%}{\text{ACTIVATED}}\atop\text{OXYGEN}} \left[HF_2C-O-\overset{\overset{\displaystyle F_2}{\displaystyle |}}{C}-\overset{\overset{\displaystyle OH}{\displaystyle |}}{\underset{\displaystyle F}{C}}Cl \right] \rightarrow HF_2C-O-\overset{\overset{\displaystyle F_2}{\displaystyle |}}{C}-\overset{\overset{\displaystyle H}{\displaystyle |}}{C}=O + Cl^- + F^-$$

DIFLUOROMETHOXY-
DIFLUOROACETIC ACID

$$\xrightarrow{9\%} \left[? \right] \rightarrow HO-\overset{\overset{\displaystyle O}{\displaystyle \|}}{C}-\overset{\overset{\displaystyle H}{\displaystyle |}}{\underset{\displaystyle F}{C}}Cl + CO_2 + 4F^-$$

FLUOROCHLOROACETIC ACID

FIG. 12-9. Oxidative pathways of metabolism of enflurane.

Metabolism of enflurane by rat microsomes can be increased by pretreatment with phenobarbital, but not with 3-MC.[55] On the other hand, in vivo induction of enflurane by Fischer 344 rats did not occur,[57] and patients who had been taking barbiturate medication chronically developed peak serum levels of F^- not different from those of patients known not to have been exposed to enzyme-inducing drugs.[58] A comparison of four groups of patients, distinguished by their respective histories of drug exposure, showed no significant differences with regard to dose-related peak serum F^- levels following enflurane anesthesia between those who served as controls, those who had received phenobarbital or phenytoin, those who had regularly consumed alcohol, and those who had been exposed to miscellaneous drugs (Fig. 12-10).[59] A small fraction of patients, however, developed serum F^- levels four times or five times that of average uninduced patients.[54, 57] Some of these patients were obese, but the highest levels occurred in a patient who had been under treatment with isoniazid,[54] and who subsequently suffered from high-output renal failure. Studies in rats have since shown that isoniazid (isonicotinic acid hydrazide)[60, 61] and other hydrazide-containing drugs and drug metabolites[62] strongly induce the defluorination rate of enflurane and other fluorinated ether anesthetics, namely methoxyflurane, isoflurane and sevoflurane. A comparison of peak serum F^- levels versus MAC-h of enflurane anesthesia was conducted between 20 patients who had been treated with isoniazid and 36 patients who were not treated with any drugs or enzyme inducers (Fig. 12-11).[63] Eleven of the isoniazid patients showed no difference from the control group; the remaining nine showed very high F^- levels. This difference in behavior was thought to be related to the known existence of fast and slow acetylators,[64] which produces a four-fold difference in the rate of acetylation of isoniazid.

Rice and Fish observed significant differences between the peak serum F^- levels and urinary F^- excretions of obese versus nonobese rats (Fig. 12-12).[65] Following enflurane anesthesia, Miller et al[41] measured an approximately two-fold increase in the urinary excretion of F^- and peak serum F^- levels in obese over nonobese patients.

Chronic alcohol ingestion increases the metabolism of enflurane by rat hepatic microsomes three-fold to four-fold without increasing the levels of cytochrome P-450.[66, 67] This is in apparent contrast to the report cited above,[59] in which mostly male surgical patients who regularly consumed 40–105 ml of alcohol per day defluorinated enflurane no differently than a similar group who had a history of no prior drug exposure.

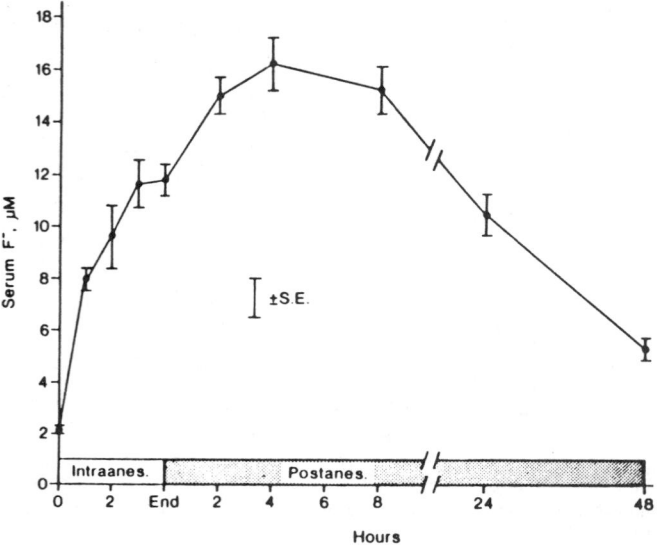

FIG. 12-10. Serum fluoride (F^-) concentrations as a reflection of metabolism of enflurane are not influenced by drugs that produce enzyme induction. (Reprinted with permission. Dooley JR, Mazze RI, Rice SA et al: Is enflurane defluorination inducible in man? Anesthesiology 50:213; 1979.)

Pantuck et al[68] demonstrated in Fischer 344 rats that alcohol, whether ingested chronically or acutely, increased the enflurane defluorinating activity of hepatic microsomes rapidly, within 1 h, and that the defluorinating activity fell rapidly, within 24 h. Increased in vitro activity following chronic exposure to alcohol was accompanied by an increase of microsomal protein that coincided with a band of the same molecular weight and same mobility on polyacrylamide gels as a band induced by isoniazid. In the presence of elevated serum levels of alcohol in vivo, defluorinating activity was severely inhibited, despite the presence of increased levels of microsomal protein. Hence, whether alcohol inhibits, increases, or has no effect on defluorinating activity depends on how long after alcohol ingestion exposure to enflurane occurs.

Among the factors that can influence the rate of defluorination of enflurane is streptozotocin-induced diabetes, which increases the defluorination of enflurane in the rat by 350%,[69]

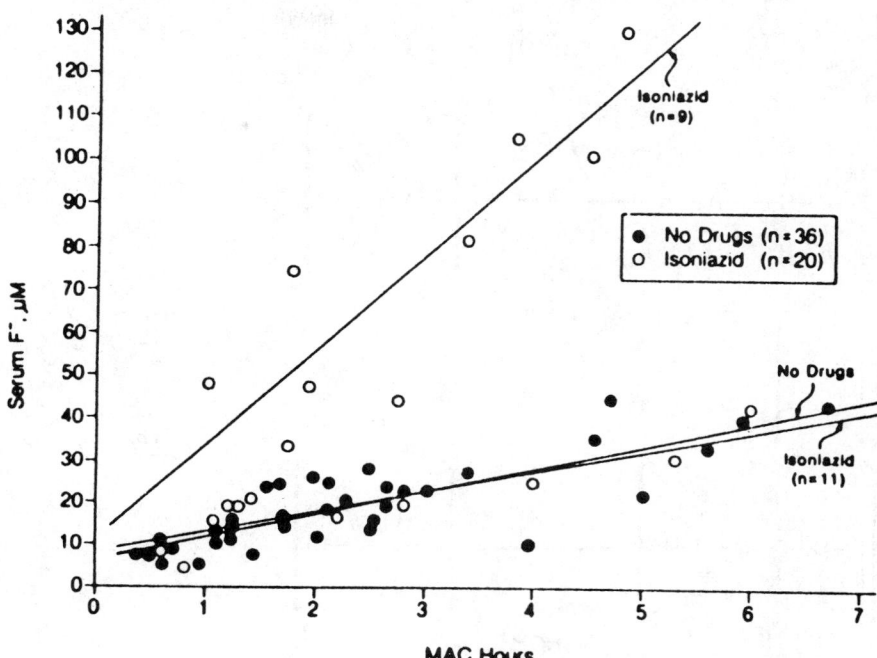

FIG. 12-11. Isoniazid enhances defluorination of enflurane in patients who are presumed to be rapid acetylators. (Reprinted with permission. Mazze RI, Woodruff RE, Heerdt ME: Isoniazid-induced enflurane defluorination in humans. Anesthesiology 57:5, 1982.)

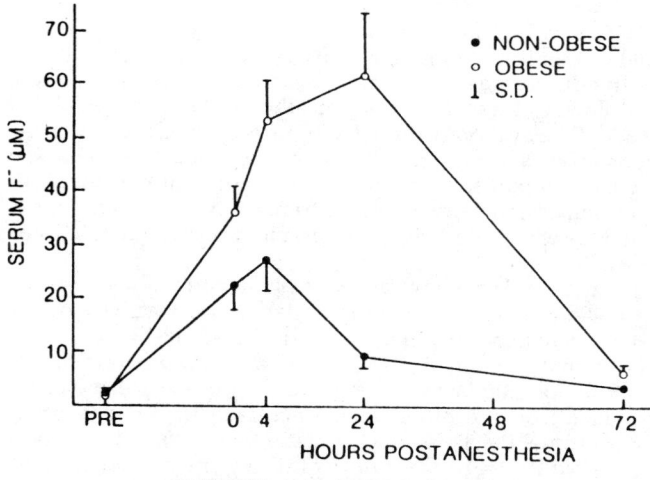

FIG. 12-12. Defluorination of isoflurane is greater in obese than nonobese rats. (Reprinted with permission. Rice SA, Fish KJ: Anesthetic metabolism and renal function in obese and nonobese Fischer 344 rats following enflurane or isoflurane anesthesia. Anesthesiology 65:28, 1986.)

and *in vitro* defluorination by 270%. This enhancement of *in vitro* defluorination was shared by diabetic rats exposed to isoflurane, but not those exposed to methoxyflurane, or hypoxia and halothane. Enhanced defluorination activity was reversed by control of diabetes with insulin. Microsomal cytochrome P-450 content was not increased in the diabetic rats. The authors of this study point out the possibility that the

isozyme responsible for this reaction could be the same as that which is induced by alcohol and isoniazid.

Destruction of the P-450 mixed-function oxidase system by carbon tetrachloride (CC14) resulted in similar reductions in the metabolic disappearance rates of enflurane, halothane, and methoxyflurane.[46] These three drugs are metabolized at very different rates and are oxidized, in part at least, by different isozymes, suggesting that CC14 depletes a number of P-450 isozymes.

Deuteration of the β carbon, $CF_2H-0-CF_2-CFC1-D$, resulted in a 65% reduction of metabolic defluorination of enflurane, whereas deuteration of the methoxyl carbon caused little or no detectable change of defluorination from the original compound, confirming that the major pathway of oxidation is through attack on the β carbon–hydrogen bond.[70] Exploitation of the much greater strength of the carbon–deuterium bond as compared with the carbon–hydrogen bond has been helpful in identifying metabolic pathways and determining which pathways are responsible for toxic reactions that result from drug metabolism.

ISOFLURANE

Isoflurane undergoes very limited metabolism in humans (Fig. 12-13).[71, 72] Less than 0.2% appeared as urinary metabolites.[73] Two mass balance studies indicated that 95% and 92.8%, respectively, of the measured amount of anesthetic absorbed by patients was reclaimed in exhaled air (Table 12-1).[3–7] Liver perfusion studies in swine indicated a removal fraction of 0 ± 0.02, *i.e.*, no metabolism of isoflurane.[74] Serum F^- rose negligibly during and following isoflurane anesthesia (Fig. 12-14).[72] F^- and an organic fluorine compound appear in the urine during the first 48–72 h following exposure.[72] The organic fluorine has been tentatively identified as TFA.[71] Lim-

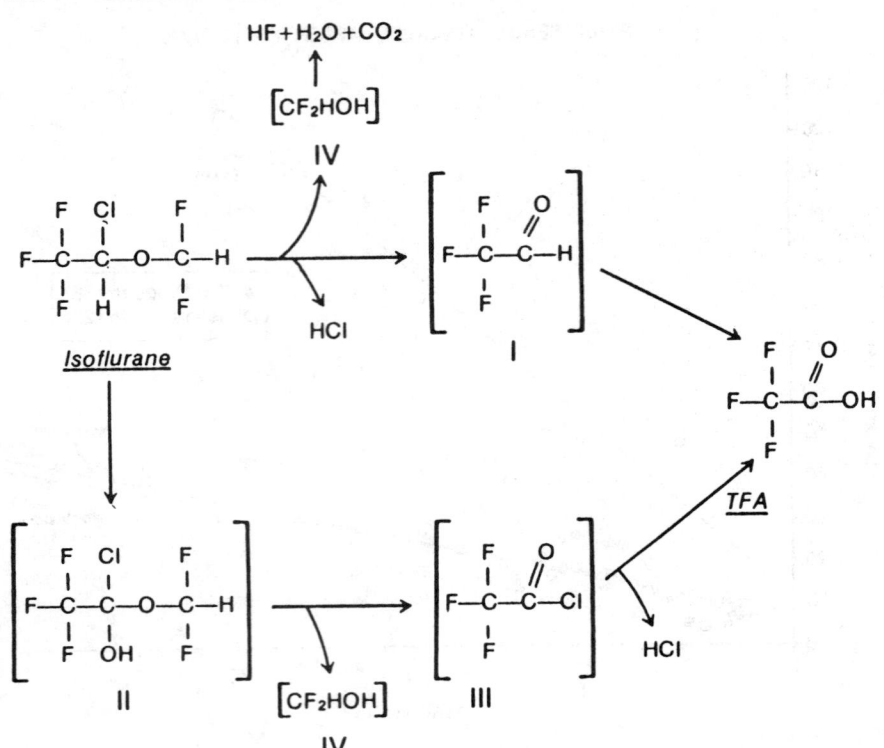

FIG. 12-13. Minimal oxidative metabolism of isoflurane results principally in the formation of trifluoroacetic acid (TFA). A small amount of ionic fluoride is also formed. (Reprinted with permission. Hitt BA, Mazze RI, Cousins MJ *et al:* Metabolism of isoflurane in Fisher 344 rats and man. Anesthesiology 40:62, 1974.)

FIG. 12-14. Serum fluoride elevations following administration of isoflurane are insufficient to cause renal dysfunction. (Reprinted with permission. Mazze RI, Cousins MJ, Barr GA: Renal effects and metabolism of isoflurane in man. Anesthesiology 40:536, 1974.)

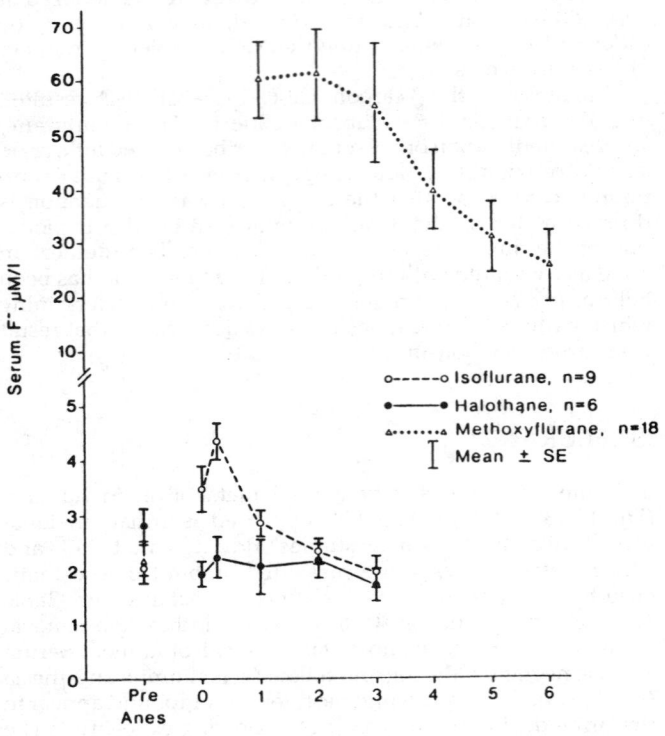

ited metabolism is most likely due to oxidation of the α carbon, as the difluoromethyl carbon is resistant to dehalogenation.

Following 4 h of isoflurane anesthesia, obese rats exhibited serum F^- elevations to 27 $\mu M \cdot l^{-1}$ and increased urinary excretions of F^- as compared with nonobese rats. These changes were accompanied by a mild reduction of creatinine and urea nitrogen clearance, but no overt renal failure.[65] Alterations of renal function following anesthesia in humans have not been seen.[75]

Enzyme induction in rats with phenobarbital resulted in a three-fold increase in isoflurane defluorinase activity of isolated microsomes *in vitro*, but no demonstrable increase of *in vivo* activity in rats.[76] 3-MC failed to induce isoflurane defluorination, similar to its effect on enflurane metabolism.[77] Isoniazid, on the other hand, increased the activity of rat cytochrome P-450 isoflurane defluorinase *in vitro* activity three-fold.[60] Obesity, as with enflurane, increased serum F^- levels and urinary F^- excretion, and postanesthesia creatinine and urea nitrogen clearances were decreased in obese rats as compared with nonobese rats. Isoflurane defluorination is increased 2.5 times in the rat rendered diabetic by treatment with streptozotocin.[69]

METHOXYFLURANE

A consideration of the metabolism of methoxyflurane is included here because of its unusually high solubility characteristics and the importance of solubility on the extent of drug metabolism of volatile drugs. As a result of the extensive metabolism of methoxyflurane and the renal toxicity associated with its metabolitie, F^-, it has fallen into disuse clinically except as an occasional self-administered analgesic for use during obstetric labor.

Carbon dioxide derived from the methoxy moiety of methoxyflurane was identified in exhaled air of patients within 5 min after onset of exposure.[6] Maximum excretion rates occurred between 1–3 h later. Other metabolites include methoxydifluoroacetic acid, dichloroacetic acid, Cl^-, and oxalate.[6, 78] Formaldehyde necessarily occurs as an intermediate in the conversion of the methoxyl moiety to CO_2.

An illustration of the influence of anesthetic solubility on duration and extent of metabolism is the correlation of lipid solubility with half-time for urinary excretion, total F^- excretion, and peak serum F^- concentration. The half-time of excretion of ingested fluoride in humans is 4 h. The half-time for excretion of F^- in patients following methoxyflurane, enflurane, and sevoflurane (lipid/gas partition coefficients of 885, 132, and 55, respectively) were 48,[78] 37[5] and 16.3[79] h, respectively. Average peak serum F^- concentrations were 58, 33.6[80] and 22[79] $\mu M \cdot l^{-1}$, and average total F^- excretions were 7.7%, 0.5%[10] and 1.6%,[79] respectively.

Methoxyflurane is metabolized *via* two pathways; both require a cytochrome P-450 enzyme and oxygen (Fig. 12-15).[81–83] Oxidative dehalogenation of methoxyflurane occurs on the carbon atom carrying two chlorine atoms, resulting in methoxydifluoroacetic acid, which breaks down under acidic conditions to fluoride, oxalic acid, and formaldehyde, which is further oxidized to carbon dioxide. Oxidative cleavage of the ether linkage of methoxyflurane also occurs.

Methoxyflurane is more extensively metabolized than other fluorinated anesthetics. From 29% to 44% of the amount absorbed by humans is excreted as metabolites,[6, 78] and only 19%–35% of uptake was excreted unchanged in exhaled air; an average of 37% could not be accounted for. This latter amount can be assumed to have been metabolized as well, and either bound permanently to tissues or excreted by routes or in time frames not detectable by the methods used. Carpenter *et al* estimated that an average of 75% of methoxyflurane is metabolized by normal humans (Table 12-1).[7] How much is metabolized is dose related, and the elevation of serum F^- is dependent on the duration and concentration of exposure.[84] Obesity more than doubled peak serum F^- concentrations[39] as compared with nonobese subjects.[85] The authors suggest that the high incidence of fatty infiltration of the liver that accompanies obesity is responsible for larger collections of lipid-soluble anesthetics in the liver and, hence, greater quantities of drug being metabolized.[39]

Methoxyflurane causes a nonspecific induction of microsomal enzymes,[86] which includes enhancement of the dechlorinating system of its own β carbon,[87] similar to the induction resulting from isoniazid and alcohol.

SEVOFLURANE

Sevoflurane is an experimental inhalational anesthetic under development in Japan and the United States. It exhibits relative chemical stability. It is stable without preservative in amber glass bottles for more than 1 y. It hydrolyzes slowly in water, and produces up to five reaction products in contact with soda lime,[88] most of which occur in trace amounts only, and the most plentiful, fluoromethyl 2,2-difluoro-1-(trifluoromethyl) vinyl ether ($CF_2C[CF_3]-OCH_2F$), peaked at 15 ppm and has a therapeutic index (anesthetic/toxic index) of 2.84.

Sevoflurane is metablized in humans and experimental animals to F^- and hexafluoroisopropyl alcohol, the latter of which is excreted in urine as a glucuronide conjugate.[79, 89–91] Peak serum F^- levels in studies in humans ranged from 13.7 ± 8.2 $\mu M \cdot l^{-1}$ to 22.1 ± 6.1 $\mu M \cdot l^{-1}$; the highest serum F^- recorded from among 12 healthy adult volunteers and 9 patients was 38.3 $\mu M \cdot l^{-1}$, well below the minimal concentration associated with signs of nephrotoxicity.[92]

When humans are presented with a constant inspired concentration of sevoflurane, end-expired tracheal concentrations plateau in 4 min, and at the end of exposure, blood concentrations decreased in 5 minutes to 20% of plateau concentrations sustained during exposure.[91, 92] The blood/gas partition coefficient of sevoflurane is 0.6, closer to that of N_2O than that of isoflurane. The rapid increase and decrease of blood concentrations can be ascribed to this property. Serum F^- increased progressively for 2 h during anesthesia, lasting from 2 h to 5 h, leveling off at 2 h, but continuing to increase after the end of exposure for 2–4 h, then gradually returning toward baseline by 72 h. Urinary excretion of F^- and organic fluorine peaked between 24 h and 48 h and decreased with half-times of 16 and 14 h, respectively, in volunteers,[79] and with half-times of 34 h and 30 h, respectively, in patients. Reported quantities of organic and inorganic fluoride metabolites excreted range between 1.5 $\mu M \cdot l^{-1}$ and 2 μM and represent approximately 1.5%–2% of uptake.[79] This small fraction of drug metabolized

FIG. 12-15. Oxidative pathways of methoxyflurane metabolism.

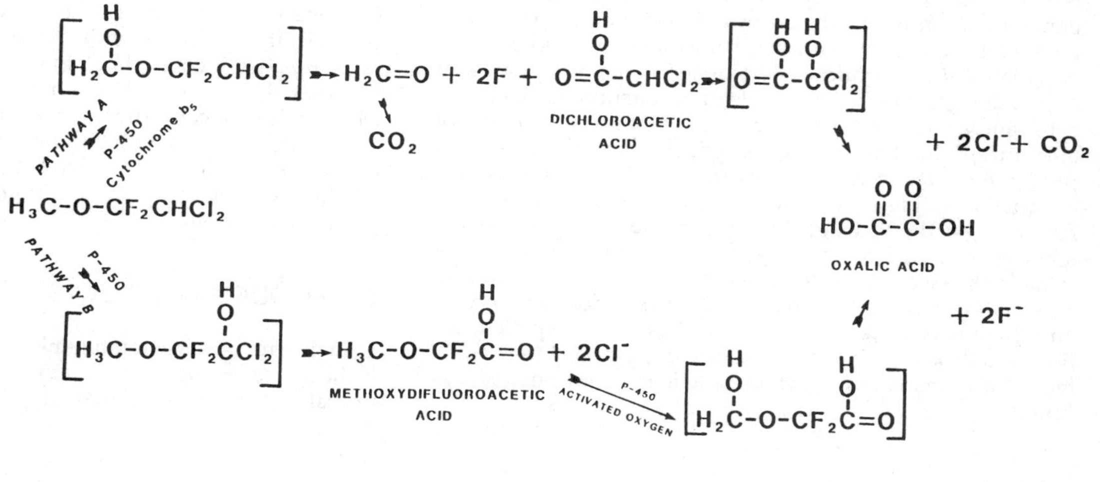

is owing, in part at least, to the rapid excretion of the parent drug in exhaled air.

The extent of metabolism of sevoflurane in the rat can be increased 3.3 times by pretreatment with phenobarbital and 2.2 times with isoniazid.[93] Deuteration of the single C—H bond reduced metabolism 79% and 70%, respectively, in the two induced groups. Cimetidine failed to effect the rates of metabolism of sevoflurane in either noninduced rats or induced rats, whereas simultaneous exposure of induced rats to 0.2% isoflurane reduced excretion of F^- and organic flurine 25% and 22% respectively.

I-653

I-653 (CF_2H-0-CFH-CF_3) is a new, experimental, volatile anesthetic that is of interest because of its low blood/gas partition coefficient of 0.42,[94] which promises rapid induction of and recovery from anesthesia. It is of particular interest in the present context, drug metabolism, because it is reported to be completely stable in moist soda lime,[95] as well as nontoxic to hypoxic enzyme-induced rats[96] and to rats following repeated anesthesia using a closed, rebreathing circuit containing drug soda lime.[97]

TOXICITY

Toxicity of inhaled anesthetics most often reflects direct effects of the parent molecule or metabolites on the liver, kidneys, or reproductive system. There is no evidence that any inhaled anesthetic acts as a mutagen or carcinogen.[98, 99] Unique toxic effects of nitrous oxide most likely reflect the ability of this drug to inhibit vitamin B12-dependent enzymes. Inhaled anesthetics, particularly nitrous oxide, produce dose-dependent inhibition of polymorphonuclear leukocytes and their subsequent migration (chemotaxis) for phagocytosis, which is necessary for the inflammatory response to infection.[100] Nevertheless, decreased resistance to bacterial infection owing to inhaled anesthetics seems unlikely, considering the duration and dose of these drugs that are administered.

HALOTHANE-ASSOCIATED HEPATIC DYSFUNCTION

The mechanism responsible for halothane-associated hepatic dysfunction (estimated incidence 1 in 35,000 administrations) is unknown but may reflect intermediate metabolites or a cell-damaging immune-mediated hypersensitivity response (i.e., an allergic reaction). With respect to toxic metabolites, it is speculated that products of reductive metabolism can bind irreversibly (covalently) to intracellular constituents of hepatocytes and cause their destruction. Halothane is the only volatile anesthetic that undergoes reductive metabolism in the presence of low oxygen partial pressures with the possible production of highly reactive intermediate metabolites. The fact that anesthetic drugs that do not undergo reductive metabolism can also cause hepatic necrosis in the hypoxic rat model has cast doubt on the role of toxic intermediary metabolites in the production of liver injury.[101] The ability of inhaled anesthetics, particularly halothane, to reduce hepatic blood flow and thus jeopardize hepatocyte oxygenation may be the more likely explanation for anesthetic-induced hepatic dysfunction.[102]

An allergic response as the mechanism for halothane-associated hepatic dysfunction is suggested by eosinophilia and accelerated liver dysfunction following repeat exposures to halothane. Conversely, it is difficult to accept the likelihood of antibody production evoked by a small nonprotein molecule such as halothane. Nevertheless, reductive metabolites of halothane that bind covalently to hepatocytes could act as haptens.[103] A possible genetic role is suggested by variations in the susceptibility of the liver to toxic metabolites of halothane in different strains of rats as well as the occurrence of hepatitis following administration of halothane to three pairs of closely related females.[104] Genetic factors could be important in determining the likelihood that susceptible patients will form antibodies or utilize reductive pathways of metabolism for halothane.

FLUORIDE-INDUCED NEPHROTOXICITY

Metabolism of methoxyflurane, and to a lesser extent enflurane, to F^- may result in nephrotoxicity. F^--induced nephrotoxicity is characterized by an inability to concentrate urine. The resulting polyuria leads to dehydration with hypernatremia and increased serum osmolarity. Inability to concentrate urine may reflect F^--induced inhibition of adenylate cyclase activity necessary for the normal action of antidiuretic hormone on distal convoluted renal tubules. Alternatively, F^- may produce intrarenal vasodilation with increased medullary blood flow that interferes with the counter current mechanism in the kidneys necessary for optimal concentration of urine.

Detectable renal dysfunction is likely when the administered dose of methoxyflurane results in serum F^- concentrations that exceed 50 $\mu M \cdot l^{-1}$.[54] This level of F^- elevation is likely when the duration of methoxyflurane administration to adults exceeds 2.5 MAC hr.

Metabolism of enflurane to F^-, although much less than with methoxyflurane, is potentially great enough to produce transient decreases in urine concentrating ability, particularly after prolonged administration (1 MAC for 9.6 hr) (Fig. 12-16).[80] Nevertheless, short administration (1 MAC for 2.7 hr) does not reveal a difference between enflurane or halothane with respect to urine concentrating ability (Fig. 12-17).[54] Indeed, the likelihood of F^--induced nephrotoxicity due to metabolism of enflurane seems remote because serum F^- concentrations after clinical use of this drug are about one-half the speculated toxic level of 50 $\mu M \cdot l^{-1}$.

F^--induced nephrotoxicity depends on the duration of the exposure of the renal tubules to F^- as well as on the absolute increase in the serum F^- concentration. As a result, it is possible that patients with decreased glomerular filtration rates are at an increased risk in the presence of F^- concentrations usually considered to be nontoxic (i.e., below 50 $\mu M \cdot l^{-1}$). Despite this concern, there is no detectable reduction in renal function in patients with chronic renal disease who undergo elective operations and receive enflurane or halothane.[105] Metabolism of halothane or isoflurane to F^- is insufficient to produce nephrotoxicity.

REPRODUCTIVE EFFECTS

Evidence for possible teratogenic effects of inhaled anesthetics is the increased incidence of spontaneous abortions in women operating room personnel (1.3–2 times) compared with

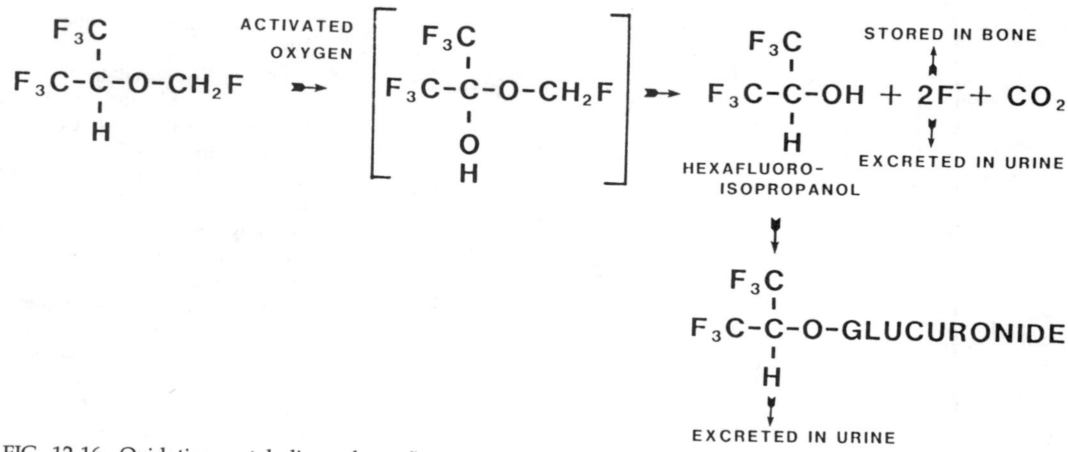

FIG. 12-16. Oxidative metabolism of sevoflurane.

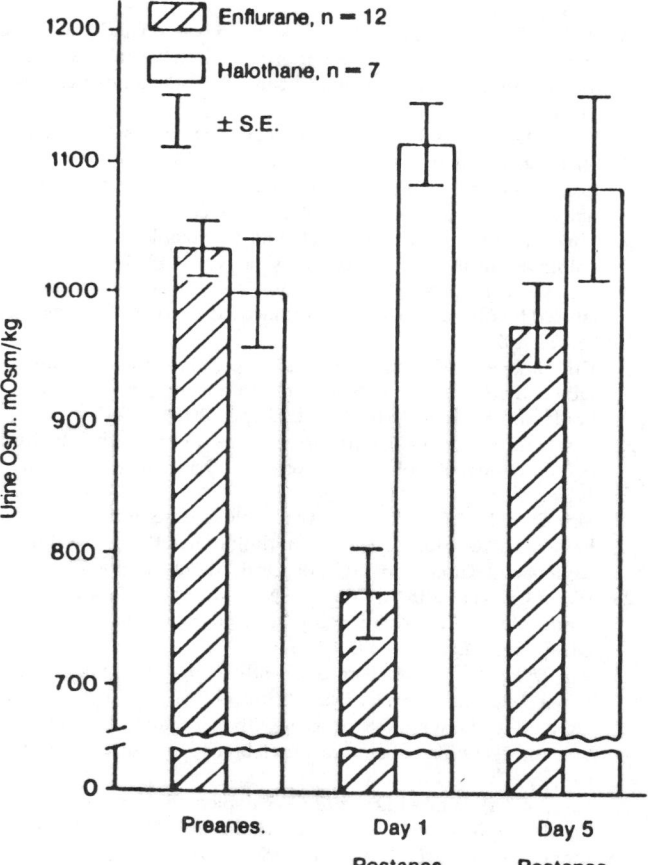

FIG. 12-17. Prolonged administration (9.6 MAC h) of enflurane may transiently impair the ability of patients to concentrate urine. (Reprinted with permission. Mazze RI, Calverley RK, Smith NT: Inorganic fluoride nephrotoxicity: Prolonged enflurane and halothane anesthesia in volunteers. Anesthesiology 46:265, 1977.)

matched controls but not working in the operating rooms.[106] Less well-documented than the increased incidence of spontaneous abortion is an increased incidence of congenital malformations in the offspring of women operating room personnel. The cause of the increased incidence of teratogenic responses observed in women operating room personnel is not known, but chronic exposure to trace concentrations of inhaled anesthetics, paticularly nitrous oxide, has received much attention. Indeed, the teratogenic effects of nitrous oxide are supported by the ability of this inhaled anesthetic to cause fetal resorptions (i.e., spontaneous abortions), congenital anomalies, and growth retardation in rodents exposed during gestation.[107]

It is the concern about possible teratogenic effects from chronic exposure to trace concentrations of inhaled anesthetics that has led to the use of scavenging systems to reduce the trace concentrations of anesthetic gases in the operating room atmosphere and hopefully reduce any toxic effects associated with chronic exposure to these gases. Nevertheless, animal studies employing intermittent exposure to trace concentrations of nitrous oxide, halothane, enflurane, and isoflurane have not revealed harmful reproductive effects.[108]

NITROUS OXIDE

Nitrous oxide is unique among the inhaled anesthetics with respect to its ability to inhibit methionine synthetase activity by oxidizing the cobalt atom in vitamin B_{12} from an active to inactive state.[109, 110] Inhibition of enzyme activity results in decreased availability of tetrahydrofolate, which is necessary for the synthesis of DNA (Fig. 12-18). Interference with synthesis of DNA is consistent with development of bone marrow depression and polyneuropathy resembling pernicious anemia in individuals chronically exposed to high concentrations of nitrous oxide.[111-114] Nevertheless, onset of nitrous oxide-induced inhibition of methionine synthetase activity seems to be much slower in humans than in animals (Fig. 12-19). For example, the mean half-time of inactivation of methionine synthetase while breathing 70% nitrous oxide was 46 min in patients and 5.4 min in rats.[115] The absence of changes in activity of methionine synthetase during chronic exposure to trace concentrations of nitrous oxide does not support a role

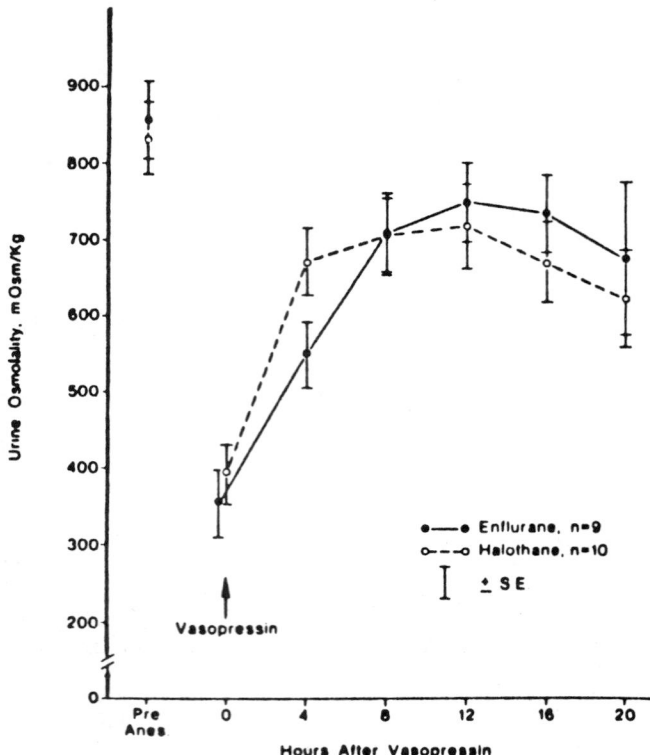

FIG. 12-18. Short-term administration of enflurane (2.7 MAC h) does not alter the ability of vasopressin to increase urine osmolarity as compared with halothane. (Reprinted with permission. Cousins MJ, Greenstein LR, Hitt BA *et al*: Metabolism and renal effects of enflurane in man. Anesthesiology 44:44, 1976.)

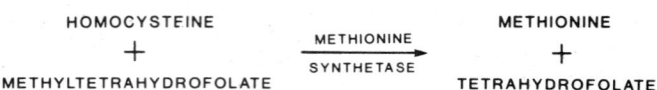

FIG. 12-19. Nitrous oxide inhibits methionine synthetase activity.

for this mechanism in the production of spontaneous abortion or birth defects.

REFERENCES

1. Van Dyke RA, Chenoweth MB, VanPosnak: Metabolism of volatile anesthetics. I. Conversion *in vivo* of several anesthetics to $^{14}CO_2$ and chloride. Biochem Pharmacol 13:1239, 1964
2. Stier A, Alter H, Hessler O, *et al*: Urinary excretion of bromide in halothane. Anesth Analg 43:723, 1964
3. Rehder K, Forbes J, Alter H *et al*: Halothane biotransformation in man: A quantitative study. Anesthesiology 28:711, 1967
4. Cascorbi HF, Blake DA, Helrich M: Difference in the biotransformation of halothane in man. Anesthesiology 32:119, 1970
5. Chase RE, Holaday DA, Fiserova-Bergerova V *et al*: The biotransformation of Ethrane in man. Anesthesiology 35:261, 1971
6. Holaday DA, Rudofsky S, Truehaft PS: The metabolic degradation of methoxyflurane in man. Anesthesiology 33:579, 1970
7. Carpenter RL, Eger EI II, Johnson BH *et al*: The extent of metabolism of inhaled anesthetics in humans. Anesthesiology 65:201, 1986
8. Brommer RR: Metabolism of endogenous substrates by microsomes. Drug Metab Rev 6:155, 1977
9. Brodie BB, Marckel RP: Comparative biochemistry of drug metabolism. In Bridie BB, Erclos EG (eds): Proceedings of the First International Pharmacological Meeting, p 299. New York, Macmillan, 1962
10. Holaday DA, Fiserova-Bergerova V: Fate of fluorinated metabolites of anesthetics in man. Drug Metab Rev 9:61, 1979
11. Trudell JR: Metabolism of nitrous oxide. In Eger EI II (ed): Nitrous Oxide, p 204. New York, Elsevier, 1985
12. Hong K, Trudell JR, O'Neil JR *et al*: Metabolism of nitrous oxide by human and rat intestinal contents. Anesthesiology 52:16, 1980
13. Uehleke H, Hellmer KH, Tabarelli-Poplawski S: Metabolic activation of halothane and its covalent binding to liver endoplasmic proteins *in vitro*. Naunyn Schmiedebergs Arch Pharmacol 279:39, 1973
14. Sharp TH, Trudell JR, Cohen EN: Volatile metabolites and decomposition products of halothane in man. Anesthesiology 50:2, 1979
15. Widger LA, Gandolfi AJ, Van Dyke RA: Hypoxia and halothane metabolism *in vivo*: Release of inorganic fluoride and halothane metabolite binding to cellular constitutents. Anesthesiology 44:197, 1976
16. Van Dyke RA, Chenoweth MB, Larsen ER: Synthesis and metabolism of halothane-1-C^{14}. Nature 204:471, 1964
17. Cohen EN, Trudell JR, Edmunds HN *et al*: Urinary metabolites of halothane in man. Anesthesiology 43:392, 1975
18. Mukai S, Morio M, Fujii K, Hanaki C: Volatile metabolites of halothane in the rabbit. Anesthesiology 47:248, 1977
19. Van Dyke RA, Wood CL: Binding of radioactivity from ^{14}C-labeled halothane in isolated perfused rat livers. Anesthesiology 38:328, 1973
20. Van Dyke RA, Gandolfi AJ: Studies on irreversible binding of radioactivity from [^{14}C]halothane to rat hepatic microsomal lipids and protein. Drug Metab Dispos 2:469, 1974
21. Van Dyke RA, Wood CL: *In vitro* studies on irreversivle binding of halothane metabolite to microsomes. Drug Metab Dispos 351, 1975
22. Van Dyke RA, Gandolfi AJ: Anaerobic release of fluoride from halothane: Relationship to the binding of halothane metabolites to hepatic cellular constituents. Drug Metab Dispos 4:40, 1976
23. Wood CL, Gandolfi AJ, Van Dyke RA: Lipid binding of a halothane metabolite: Relationship to lipid peroxidation *in vitro*. Drug Metab Dispos 4:305, 1976
24. Van Dyke RA: Metabolism of anesthetic agents: Toxic implications. Acta Anaesthesiol Scand [Suppl] 7:57, 1982
25. Topham JC, Longshaw S: Studies with halothane I. The distribution and excretion of halothane metabolites in animals. Anesthesiology 37:311, 1972
26. Gandolfi AJ, White RD, Sipes IG *et al*: Bioactivation and covalent binding of halothane *in vitro*: Studies with [^{3}H]- and [^{14}C]halothane. J Pharmacol Exp Ther 214:721, 1980
27. Trudell JR, Bosterling B, Trevor AJ: Reductive metabolism of halothane by human and rabbit cytochrome P-450: Binding of 1-chloro-2,2,2-trifluoroethyl radical to phospholipids. Mol Pharmacol 21:710, 1982
28. Muller R, Stier A: Modification of liver microsomal lipids by halothane metabolites: A multinuclear NMR spectroscopic study. Naunyn Schmiederbergs Arch Pharmacol 321:234, 1982
29. Cohen EN, Hood N: Application of low temperature autoradiography to studies of uptake and metabolism of volatile anesthetics in the mouse. III. Halothane. Anesthesiology 31:553, 1969

30. Van Dyke RA: Hepatic cellular necrosis in rats after exposure to halothane, enflurane or isoflurane. Anesth Analg 61:812, 1982

31. Plummer JL, Beckweth ALJ, Bastin FN et al: Free radical formation in vivo and hepatotoxicity due to anesthesia with halothane. Anesthesiology 57:160, 1982

32. Mazze RI: Metabolism of the inhaled anaesthetics: Implications of enzyme induction. Br J Anaesth 56:27S, 1984

33. Sawyer DC, Eger EI II, Bahlman SH et al: Concentration dependence of hepatic halothane metabolism. Anesthesiology 34:230, 1971

34. Fiserova-Bergerova V, Kawiecki RW: Effects of exposure concentration on distribution of halothane metabolites in the body. Drug Metab Dispos 12:98, 1984

35. Brown BR: Halothane hepatitis revisited. N Engl J Med 313:1347, 1985

36. Stuck JGL, Strunin L: Unexplained hepatitis following halothane. Anesthesiology 63:424, 1985

37. Plummer JL, Hall P, Jenner MA et al: Sex differences in metabolism and hepatotoxicity in a rat model. Anesth Analg 64:563, 1985

38. Abernathy DR, Greenblatt DJ: Pharmacokinetics of drugs in obesity. Clin Pharmacokinet 7:108, 1982

39. Young SR, Stoelting RK, Petersen C et al: Anesthetic biotransformation and renal function in obese patients during and after methoxyflurane or halothane anesthesia. Anesthesiology 42:451, 1975

40. Vaughan RW: Biochemical and biotransformation alterations in obesity. Contemp Anesth Pract 5:55, 1982

41. Miller MS, Gandolfi AJ, Vaughan RW et al: Disposition of enflurane in obese patients. J Pharmacol Exp Ther 215:292, 1980

42. Plummer JL, Wanwimolruk S, Jenner MA et al: Effects of cimetidine and ranitidine on halothane metabolism and hepatotoxicity in an animal model. Drug Metab Dispos 12:106, 1984

43. Wood M, Uetrecht J, Phythyon JM et al: The effect of cimetidine on anesthetic metabolism and toxicity. Anesth Analg 65:481, 1986

44. Siegers CP, Biltz H, Pentz R: Effect of diethyldithiocarbamate on the metabolic elimination of hexobarbitone, phenazone, tolbutamide and four halogenated hydrocarbons. Eur J Drug Metab Pharmacokinet 6:141, 1981

45. Eckes L, Buch HP: Influence of diethyldithiocarbamate and carbon disulfide on the metabolic formation of trifluoracetic acid from halothane in the rat. Arzneimittelforschung 35:1447, 1985

46. Siegers CP, Mackenroth T, Wachter S et al: Effects of liver injury and cholestasis on microsomal enzyme activities and metabolism of halothane, enflurane and methoxyflurane in vivo in rats. Xenobiotica 11:293, 1981

47. Kato R, Chiesara E, Vassanelli P: Further studies on the inhibition and stimulation of microsomal drug-metabolizing enzymes of rat liver by various compounds. Biochem Pharmacol 13:69, 1964

48. Liebman KC, Ortiz E: Metyrapone and other modifiers of microsomal drug metabolism. Drug Metab Dispos 1:184, 1973

49. Halbert JC, Balfour C, Miller NE et al: Isozyme selectivity of the inhibition of rat liver cytochromes P450 by chloramphenicol in vivo. Mol Pharmacol 28:290, 1985

50. Jori A, Bianchetti A, Prestini PE: Effect of contraceptive agents on drug metabolism. Eur J Pharmacol 7:196, 1969

51. Fiserova-Bergerova V: Inhibitory effect of isoflurane upon oxidative metabolism of halothane. Anesth Analg 63:399, 1984

52. Fish KJ, Rice SA: Halothane inhibits metabolism of enflurane in Fischer 344 rats. Anesthesiology 59:417, 1983

53. Sipes IG, Gandolfi AJ, Pohl LR et al: Comparison of the biotransformation and hepatotoxicity of halothane and deuterated halothane. J Pharmacol Exp Ther 214:716, 1980

54. Cousins MJ, Greenstein LR, Hitt BA et al: Metabolism and renal effects of enflurane in man. Anesthesiology 44:44, 1976

55. Hitt BA, Mazze RI, Beppu WJ et al: Enflurane metabolism in rats and man. J Pharmacol Exp Ther 203:193, 1977

56. Burke TR Jr, Branchflower RV, Lees DE et al: Mechanism of defluorination of enflurane: Identification of an organic metabolite in rat and man. Drug Metab Dispos 9:19, 1981

57. Barr GA, Cousins MJ, Mazze RI et al: A comparison of the renal effects and metabolism of enflurane and methoxyflurane in Fischer 344 rats. J Pharmacol Exp Ther 188:257, 1974

58. Maduska AL: Serum inorganic fluoride levels in patients receiving enflurane anesthesia. Anesth Analg 53:351, 1974

59. Dooley JR, Mazze RI, Rice SA et al: Is enflurane defluorination inducible in man? Anesthesiology 50:213, 1979

60. Rice SA, Talcott RE: Effects of isoniazid treatment on selected hepatic mixed-function oxidases. Drug Metab Dispos 7:260, 1979

61. Rice SA, Sbordone L, Mazze RI: Metabolism by rat hepatic microsomes of fluorinated ether anesthetics following isonizaid administration. Anesthesiology 53:489, 1980

62. Fish MP, Rice SA: Isooniazid metabolites and anesthetic metabolism. Anesthesiology 51:256, 1979

53. Mazze RI, Woodruff RE, Heerdt ME: Isoniazid-induced enflurane defluorination in humans. Anesthesiology 57:5, 1982

64. Clark DWJ: Genetically determined variability in acetylation and oxidation: Therapeutic implications. Drugs 29:342, 1985

65. Rice SA, Fish KJ: Anesthetic metabolism and renal function in obese and nonobese Fischer 344 rats following enflurane or isoflurane anesthesia. Anesthesiology 65:28, 1986

66. Rice SA, Dooley JR, Mazze RI: Metabolism by rat hepatic microsomes of fluorinated ether anesthetics following ethanol consumption. Anesthesiology 58:237, 1983

67. Van Dyke RA: Enflurane, isoflurane, and methoxyflurane metabolism in rat hepatic microsomes from ethanol-treated animals. Anesthesiology 58:221, 1983

68. Pantuck EJ, Pantuck CB, Ryan DE et al: Inhibition and stimulation of enflurane metabolism in the rat following a single dose or chronic administration of alcohol. Anesthesiology 62:255, 1985

69. Pantuck EJ, Pantuck CB, Conney AH: Effect of streptozotocin-induced diabetes in the rat on the metabolism of fluorinated volatile anesthetics. Anesthesiology 66:24, 1987

70. Pohl LR, Gillette JR: Determination of toxic pathways of metabolism by deuterium substitution. Drug Metab Rev 15:1335, 1984–1985

71. Hitt BA, Mazze RI, Cousins MJ et al: Metabolism of isoflurane in Fischer 344 rats and man. Anesthesiology 40:62, 1974

72. Mazze RI, Cousins MJ, Barr GA: Renal effects and metabolism of isoflurane in man. Anesthesiology 40:536, 1974

73. Holaday DA, Fiserova-Bergerova V, Latto IP et al: Resistance of isoflurane to biotransformation in man. Anesthesiology 43:325, 1975

74. Halsey MJ, Sawyer DC, Eger EI II et al: Hepatic metabolism of halothane, methoxyflurane, cyclopropane, Ethrane, and Forane in miniature swine. Anesthesiology 35:43, 1971

75. Eger EI II: Isoflurane: Its place in anesthesia. Contemp Anesth Pract 7:113, 1983

76. Mazze RI, Hitt BA, Cousins MJ: Effect of enzyme induction with phenobarbital on the in vivo and in vitro defluorination of isoflurane and methoxyflurane. J Pharmacol Exp Ther 190:523, 1974

77. Mazze RI, Hitt B: Effects of phenobarbital and 3-methylcholanthrene on anesthetic defluorination in Fischer 344 rats. Drug Metab Dispos 6:680, 1978

78. Yoshimura N, Holaday DA, Fiserova-Bergerova V: Metabolism of methoxyflurane in man. Anesthesiology 44:372, 1976

79. Holaday DA, Smith FR: Clinical characteristics and biotransformation of sevoflurane in man. Anesthesiology 54:100, 1981

80. Mazze RI, Calverley RK, Smith NT: Inorganic fluoride nephro-

toxicity: Prolonged enflurane and halothane anesthesia in volunteers. Anesthesiology 46:265, 1977

81. Adler L, Brown BR Jr, Thompson MF: Kinetics of methoxyflurane biotransformation with reference to substrate inhibition. Anesthesiology 44:380, 1976

82. Biermann JS, Rice SA, Gallagher EJ et al: Effect of diazepam treatment on hepatic microsomal anesthetic defluorinase activity. Arch Int Pharmacodyn Ther 283:181, 1986

83. Canova-Davis E, Chiang JYL, Waskell L: Obligatory role of cytochrome b₅ in the microsomal metabolism of methoxyflurane. Biochem Pharmacol 34:1907, 1985

84. Cousins MJ, Nishimura TG, Mazze RI: Renal effects of low dose methoxyflurane with cardiopulmonary bypass. Anesthesiology 36:286, 1972

85. Creasser C, Stoelting RK: Serum inorganic fluoride concentrations during and after halothane, fluroxene, and methoxyflurane anesthesia in man. Anesthesiology 39:537, 1973

86. Berman ML, Bochantin JF: Nonspecific stimulation of drug metabolism in rats by methoxyflurane. Anesthesiology 32:500, 1970

87. Van Dyke RA: The metabolism of volatile anesthetics. III. Induction of microsomal dechlorinating and ether-cleaving enzymes. J Pharmacol Exp Ther 154:364, 1966

88. Wallin RF, Regan BM, Napoli MD et al: Sevoflurane: A new inhalational anesthetic agent. Anesth Analg 54:758, 1975

89. Martis L, Lynch S, Napoli MD et al: Biotransformation of sevoflurane in dogs and rats. Anesth Analg 60:186, 1981

90. Fujii K, Morio M, Kikuchi H et al: Pharmacokinetic study on excretion of inorganic fluoride ion, a metabolite of sevoflurane. Hiroshima J Med Sci 36:89, 1987

91. Kikuchi H, Morio M, Fujii K et al: Clinical evaluation and metabolism of sevoflurane in patients. Hiroshima J Med Sci 36:93, 1987

92. Cousins MJ, Mazze RI: Methoxyflurane nephrotoxicity: A study of dose–response in man. JAMA 225:1611, 1973

93. Holaday DA, England R: Deuteration reduced significantly the biotransformation of sevoflurane. Anesthesiology 57:A246, 1982

94. Eger EI II: Partition coefficients of I-653 in human blood, saline and olive oil. Anesth Analg 66:971, 1987

95. Eger EI II: Stability of I-653, in soda lime. Anesth Analg 66:983, 1987

96. Eger EI II, Johnson BH, Strum DP et al: Studies of the toxicity of I-653, halothane, and isothane in enzyme-induced, hypoxic rats. Anesth Analg 66:1227, 1987

97. Eger EI II, Johnson BH, Ferrell LD: Comparison of the toxicity of I-653 and isoflurane in rats: A test of the effect of repeated anesthesia and use of dry soda lime. Anesth Analg 66:1230, 1987

98. White AE, Takehisa S, Eger EI et al: Sister chromatid exchanges induced by inhaled anesthetics. Anesthesiology 50:426, 1979

99. Coate WB, Ulland BM, Lewis TR: Chronic exposure to low concentrations of halothane–nitrous oxide: Lack of carcinogenic effect in the rat. Anesthesiology 50:306, 1979

100. Duncan PG, Cullen BF: Anesthesia and immunology. Anesthesiology 45:522, 1976

101. Fassoulaki A, Eger EI, Johnson BH et al: Nitrous oxide, too, is hepatotoxic in rats. Anesth Analg 63:1076, 1984

102. Gelman S, Fowler KC, Smith LR: Liver circulation and function during isoflurane and halothane anesthesia. Anesthesiology 61:726, 1984

103. Vergani D, Tsantoulas D, Eddleston ALWF et al: Sensitization to halothane-altered liver components in severe hepatic necrosis after halothane anesthesia. Lancet 2:801, 1978

104. Hoft RH, Bunker JP, Goodman HI et al: Halothane hepatitis in three pairs of closely related women. N Engl J Med 304:1023, 1981

105. Mazze RI, Sievenpiper TS, Stevenson J: Renal effects of enflurane and halothane in patients with abnormal renal function. Anesthesiology 60:161, 1984

106. American Society of Anesthesiologists. Report of an ad hoc committee on the effect of trace anesthetics on the health of operating room personnel. Occupational disease among operating room personnel. A national study. Anesthesiology 41:32, 1974

107. Lane GA, DuBoulay PM, Tait AR et al: Nitrous oxide is teratogenic, halothane is not. Anesthesiology 55:A252, 1981

108. Mazze RI, Fujinaga M, Rice SA et al: Reproductive and teratogenic effects of nitrous oxide, halothane, isoflurane and enflurane in Sprague-Dawley rats. Anesthesiology 64:339, 1986

109. Spence AA: Environmental polution by inhalation anaesthetics. Br J Anaesth 59:96, 1987

110. Koblin DD, Watson JE, Deady JE et al: Inactivation of methionine synthetase by nitrous oxide in mice. Anesthesiology 54:318, 1981

111. Treatment of tetanus. Severe bone-marrow depression after prolonged nitrous oxide anaesthesia. Lancet 1:527, 1956

112. Brodsky JB, Cohen EN, Brown BW et al: Exposure to nitrous oxide and neurologic disease among dental professionals. Anesth Analg 60:297, 1981

113. Layzer RB, Fishman RA, Schafer JA: Neuropathy following abuse of nitrous oxide. Neurology 28:504, 1978

114. Layzer RB: Myeloneuropathy after prolonged exposure to nitrous oxide. Lancet 2:1227, 1978

115. Nunn JF, Weinbren HK, Royston D et al: Rate of inactivation of human and rodent hepatic methionine synthetase by nitrous oxide. Anesthesiology 68:213, 1988

Chapter 13

Philip W. Lebowitz
Frederic M. Ramsey

Muscle Relaxants

CLINICAL REQUIREMENTS FOR MUSCLE RELAXATION

The modern-day anesthesiologist, in providing patient comfort, patient safety, and optimal surgical conditions, uses a variety of drugs to produce the desired pharmacologic effect termed *general anesthesia*. Intravenous (iv) muscle relaxants serve this triad well by permitting surgical conditions to be achieved with lesser doses or at lower concentrations of potentially toxic anesthetic drugs than would otherwise be required. Because the patient can be maintained at lighter levels of general anesthesia, more rapid recovery to the preanesthetic state can occur, and, theoretically, fewer anesthesia-related side-effects will be seen. Understanding muscle relaxants enables the clinician to incorporate these drugs into a rational anesthetic plan individualized for each patient.

Clinical muscle relaxation can be provided by direct central nervous system (CNS) depression achieved with general anesthetics, which decrease firing of upper motor neurons. In addition, blockade of axonal conduction along motor nerves can occur either centrally at the spinal cord level or peripherally with the application of local anesthetics along motor nerves. Neuromuscular transmission can be blocked by neuromuscular blocking drugs and other factors that act at the neuromuscular junction, whereas the muscle contractile response can be depressed by either general anesthetics or drugs such as dantrolene, which affect the muscle membrane distal to the neuromuscular junction. The clinical production of muscle relaxation undoubtedly involves a complex interplay of such factors as the patient's body habitus, the degree of surgical stimulation, the depth of general anesthesia, and the influence of neuromuscular blocking drugs given specifically to facilitate muscle relaxation.

HISTORICAL CONTEXT

Diethyl ether exemplifies a complete inhalational anesthetic. At deep levels of ether anesthesia, relaxation of the abdominal musculature is sufficient to permit exploratory laparotomy. Following the introduction of *d*-tubocurarine (*d*Tc) into clinical practice by Griffith in 1942,[1] doses as small as 6 mg were seen to amplify muscle relaxation during ether anesthesia and allow reduction of anesthetic depth. However, prolonged respiratory depression after *d*Tc use, reflected in the Beecher–Todd mortality figures of 1:370 for "curare" (including gallamine and succinylcholine) anesthetics, compared to 1:2100 in anesthetics given without muscle relaxants, led many anesthesiologists to reject *d*Tc use.

As halogenated anesthetics replaced diethyl ether in common practice, a greater need to rely on curare-type drugs to block neuromuscular transmission developed, since the muscle relaxing properties of the halogenated anesthetics were not adequate for abdominal surgery unless high (and toxic) anesthetic concentrations were used. Better understanding of relaxant action and the use of anticholinesterase drugs to antagonize persistent neuromuscular blockade at the conclusion of surgery became incorporated into anesthetic practice and improved patient safety.

Succinylcholine (SCh) had been introduced in 1951 as a

short-acting depolarizing muscle relaxant that was ideal for facilitating tracheal intubation. However, complications associated with its use became apparent over a period of time.[3] As anesthesiologists gained experience with iv relaxants, it became obvious that the ideal agent should be nondepolarizing yet have a time course of action similar to that of SCh, that is, a short-acting nondepolarizer. Great efforts and research dollars were expended in the 1970s leading to the development of atracurium and vecuronium, both intermediate-duration nondepolarizing relaxants.

Also during the 1970s, monitoring techniques were promulgated to provide the clinician with a quantitative means of determining a particular patient's response to muscle relaxants, a subject of great individual variability. Anesthesiologists can now measure an individual's initial dose response, as well as the rate and adequacy of recovery of neuromuscular function; this real-time analysis permits a greater degree of precision in titrating muscle relaxant use for individual patients. A detailed discussion of monitoring neuromuscular function is provided in Chapter 21.

INTRAOPERATIVE USES OF MUSCLE RELAXANTS

Muscle relaxants are not a necessary element in every general anesthetic. The decision to include a relaxant in the anesthetic plan is based on many factors (Table 13-1); the interplay between surgical needs and the patient's response to the anesthetic is perhaps the most important factor.

Muscle relaxants are not anesthetic agents. Rather, they are adjunctive drugs intended to be used with appropriate doses of sedative, hypnotic, and analgesic medications to promote ideal surgical and anesthetic conditions. Too great a reliance on muscle relaxants risks patient awareness. The reported incidence of awareness during anesthesia, approximately 1%, appears highest in the setting of N_2O/opioid/muscle/relaxant use, when potent inhalational agents are not added.[4]

Patient movement generally dictates the need for deeper anesthesia. Exceptions to this rule include patients who manifest intolerance of deeper anesthetic levels by becoming hypotensive (e.g., patients with hypovolemia secondary to hemorrhage). Patients undergoing stimulating procedures in parts of the body where sudden movement could cause catastrophic damage, for example, patients operated upon for laser excision of a laryngeal tumor, also require temporary motor paralysis, as well as anesthesia.

TABLE 13-1.   Factors Involved in the Decision to Use a Muscle Relaxant as Part of the Anesthetic

I. Surgical procedure
  A. Anatomic location
  B. Intensity and duration
  C. Patient position
II. Anesthetic technique
  A. Primary agent (inhalational vs. N_2O opioid)
  B. Airway management (mask vs. endotracheal)
  C. Ventilatory pattern (spontaneous/assisted vs. controlled)
III. Patient factors
  A. Body habitus (lean vs. obese)
  B. ASA status
    1. Respiratory
    2. Cardiovascular
    3. Neuromuscular
    4. Neurologic
  C. Age

Intravenous muscle relaxants have contributed to advances in modern anesthesia and surgery by improving two components of the anesthetic triad: 1) promoting patient safety; and 2) optimizing surgical conditions. Knowledge of neuromuscular physiology and pharmacology, as well as surgical needs, allows rational decision making with respect to the management of muscle relaxation during general anesthesia.

PHYSIOLOGY OF NEUROMUSCULAR TRANSMISSION

NEUROMUSCULAR JUNCTION

The process of muscle contraction originates at the neuromuscular junction (Fig. 13-1).[5] There, striated muscle is innervated by myelinated, fast-conducting Group A axons of somatic efferent nerve fibers; these lower motor neurons arise from cell bodies in the anterior horns of spinal cord gray matter and synapse with upper motor neurons arising in the cerebral cortex. A motor unit, which consists of a single nerve fiber and its branches innervating many muscle fibers, serves to organize muscle contraction in a coordinated rather than in a random fashion. Graded muscle responses result from recruitment of as few as ten or as many as one thousand or more motor units in a single muscle.

NERVE DEPOLARIZATION

The nerve's electrochemical balance in the resting state, with Na^+ ions in high concentration outside the cell and K^+ ions intracellular, is maintained by an active transport mechanism, the Na^+/K^+ pump. This mechanism utilizes cellular ATP and the Na^+/K^+ ATPase enzyme system to keep the intracellular transmembrane potential polarized at about -90 mV, reflecting the membrane's greater permeability for K^+ relative to that for Na^+ in the resting state.

When the nerve is stimulated, Na^+ channels open and the nerve membrane becomes suddenly and selectively permeable to Na^+ ions. As the transmembrane potential becomes less negative intracellularly, a threshold for depolarization is achieved, and an action potential is generated (Fig. 13-2). Local electrical currents flowing further along the nerve membrane are created by this process and result in a membrane potential drop of about 15 mV in adjoining regions of the membrane, which is sufficient to initiate opening of corresponding Na^+ channels and propagate the action potential along the membrane.

Reversal in polarity of the action potential occurs when the Na^+ channels close and the transmembrane potential is restored to its resting level by the opening of K^+ channels and the loss of K^+ ions extracellularly. During this period of time, the nerve membrane is refractory to additional excitement from stimulation. Until the Na^+/K^+ pump effects repolarization by extruding Na^+ and returning K^+, the membrane remains relatively refractory and is difficult to excite.

NEUROMUSCULAR TRANSMISSION

Motor nerve endings develop in intimate proximity to motor end-plates of muscle—the junctional gap between them being on the order of only 50 nm. When the propagated action potential reaches a nerve ending, the neurotransmitter acetylcholine (ACh) is released into the junctional gap near

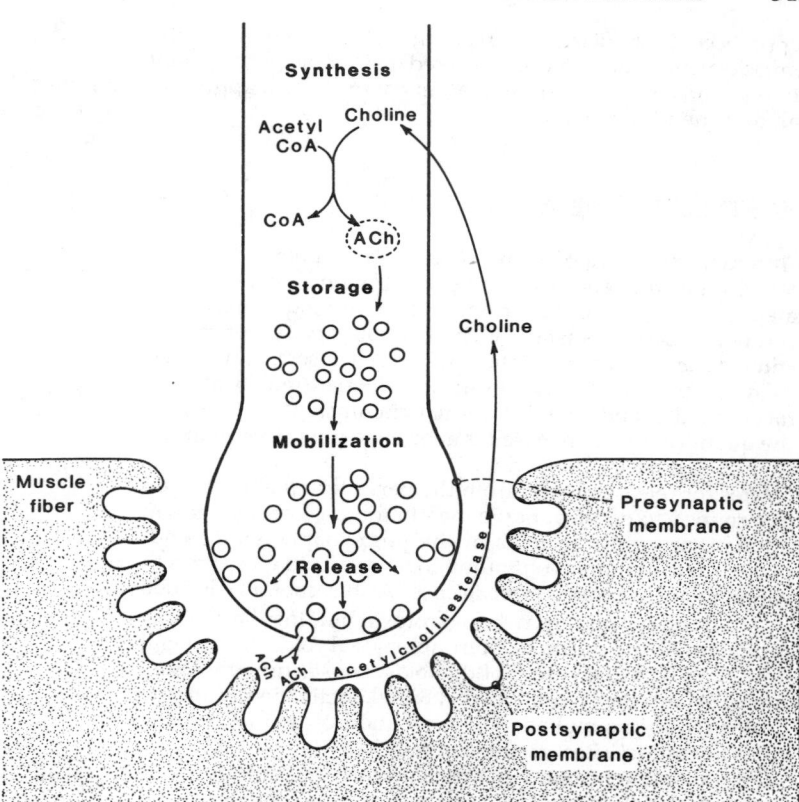

FIG. 13-1. Schematic representation of a neuromuscular junction. Acetylcholine (ACh) is synthesized, stored, mobilized, and released by a motor nerve terminal; ACh subsequently stimulates motor end-plate receptors and is eventually metabolized in the synaptic cleft by acetylcholinesterase.

nicotinic cholinergic receptors on motor end-plates in sufficient quantities as to produce an action potential in muscle and induce muscle contraction.[6] Catalyzed by the enzyme choline acetylase, ACh is synthesized from choline and acetyl-coenzyme A in the axoplasm of the nerve terminal. About 80% of this ACh is stored within synaptic vesicles at the nerve terminal near the cell membrane; the remainder is stored in more deeply situated nonvesicular reserve.

The storage and release of ACh in vesicular packets is evidenced by the presence of small electrical potentials (0.5 to 1.0 mV), termed *miniature end-plate potentials (mepps)*, recorded postsynaptically as a result of induced Na^+ muscle membrane permeability, even in the absence of a nerve impulse. When a nerve is stimulated, many vesicles of ACh are released exocytotically in integral quantae. The total voltage change (approximately 40 mV) generated postsynaptically by the resultant Na^+ muscle membrane permeability is termed the *end-plate potential (epp)*. Epps are graded according to the quantity of ACh released and can be summated. A further, sudden voltage change can be recorded when the amplitude of the

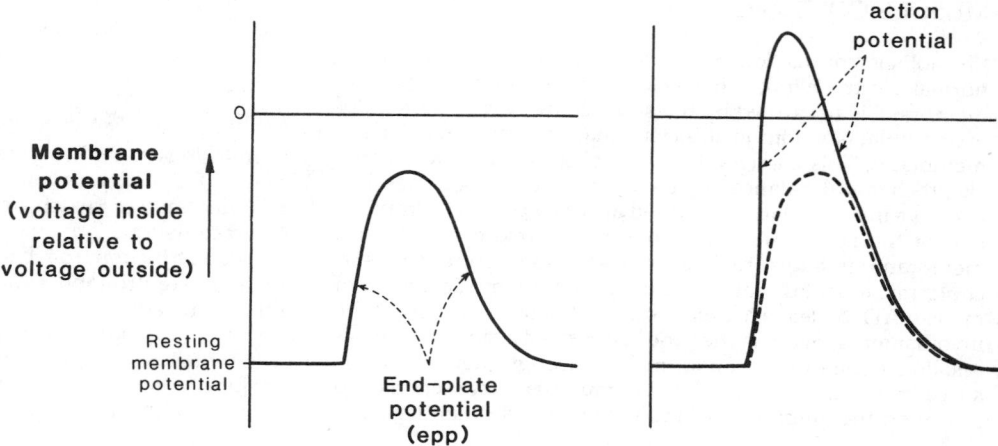

FIG. 13-2. Diagram depicting both an end-plate potential and the action potential that it triggers in adjacent electrically excitable membrane. In actuality, generation of an action potential following production of an end-plate potential obscures all but the initial portion of the end-plate potential, yielding the sketch illustrated on the right. Modified from Waud BE, Waud DR (In Katz RL (ed): Muscle Relaxants. New York, American Elsevier, 1975.)

epps become sufficient to create an action potential at the muscle membrane. Reflecting altered membrane permeability to Na$^+$ ions, the action potential, in contrast to an epp, is an all-or-none phenomenon.

ACETYLCHOLINE AVAILABILITY

Although synthesis of ACh proceeds in tandem with its release, high frequencies of nerve stimulation require accelerated mobilization of ACh from reserve to readily releasable positions. During sustained, high frequency, experimental stimulation (tetanic stimulation of 200 Hz × 5 sec), diminished ACh output will occur as a result of inadequate mobilization to meet the demand.[7] Under normal circumstances, however, the quantity of ACh released is about five times that required to induce muscle contraction.

Sites for release of ACh from the nerve terminal have been determined to occur in nerve membrane projections lying in intimate proximity to folds in the postsynaptic motor end-plate. Their anatomic configuration favors rapid receptor activation following transmitter release. ACh receptors,[8] located by studying specific alpha-bungarotoxin binding, lie in a ring formation at the crests of these junctional folds and extend only slightly into the neck of the folds, constituting the outer rim of an internally contained channel. Activation of the receptor requires simultaneous occupation of two ACh molecules at distinct sites on the receptor.

Physiologic neuromuscular transmission depends upon the presence of axoplasmic Ca^{++}, to aid both in ACh release and in receptor activation. Cyclic AMP also serves as a cofactor in the synthesis, storage, and mobilization of ACh in the nerve terminal, and possibly plays a part in ACh release. Drugs, such as theophylline, which increase intracellular concentrations of cyclic AMP, tend to promote neuromuscular transmission. The significance of ACh release is underscored by the muscle weakness produced by botulinum toxin and tetanus toxin, which prevent ACh release from cholinergic nerve endings.

Once released from the nerve terminal, ACh is exposed in the junctional cleft between nerve and muscle to the enzyme acetylcholinesterase (AChE), which inactivates ACh by hydrolyzing it to choline and acetate. The choline is then efficiently drawn back within the nerve terminal for use in synthesis of new ACh.

MUSCLE CONTRACTION

Physiologic contraction of striated muscle occurs when the normal electrochemical balance across the muscle's plasma membrane is perturbed by the sudden, inward movement of extracellular Na$^+$ ions in sufficient quantities to depolarize the membrane. This change in the muscle cell's transmembrane electrochemical balance, whereby the muscle becomes less negative intracellularly, is termed an *action potential*. Propagation of the action potential along the course of the muscle membrane initiates release of Ca^{++} ions from the sarcoplasmic reticulum into the sarcoplasm, where activation of myosin ATPase leads to excitation–contraction coupling of the myofilaments. Because the production of an action potential is an all-or-none phenomenon, muscle strength depends upon successive, summated, and fused muscular contractions and not upon the amplitude of individual action potentials.

NEUROMUSCULAR BLOCKING DRUGS

Drugs that primarily and specifically interfere with the physiologic sequence of neuromuscular transmission are classified pharmacologically as neuromuscular blocking drugs.[9] The clinical result of their use, namely weakness of skeletal muscle, has allowed the term *muscle relaxants* to be used almost interchangeably among anesthesiologists. Such drugs are classified as either depolarizing or nondepolarizing, according to their effects upon the motor end-plate.

DEPOLARIZING BLOCKING DRUGS

In order for release of ACh into the synaptic cleft to produce an action potential at the muscle membrane, the transmitter–receptor activation must depolarize the motor end-plate. The flux of ACh from the receptor takes place in milliseconds and allows the muscle membrane to repolarize in preparation for additional ACh stimulation. However, in the absence of AChE, multiple transmitter–receptor interactions may occur as ACh stimulates the motor end-plate, comes off the receptor, then stimulates it again. Consequently, epps will be prolonged and the muscle maintained in a state of persistent depolarization. In the absence of repolarization, the muscle cannot contract again, and clinical weakness results.

Depolarizing blocking drugs possess quaternary ammonium moieties (Fig. 13-3) that closely resemble ACh and initially stimulate the cholinergic receptor at the motor end-plate, then slowly separate from it. During the period of attachment to the receptor, persistent depolarization (channels remain open) of the muscle membrane prevents propagation of action potentials and, similarly, results in decreased muscle strength.

Succinylcholine

Succinylcholine (SCh), the prototypical depolarizing blocking drug, consists of two ACh molecules joined together.[10] The positively charged choline moieties mimic ACh and form strong attachments to cholinergic receptors, depolarizing the motor end-plate and initially causing muscular contraction. Because multiple muscle fibers are stimulated more or less simultaneously, rippling and uncoordinated contractions (fasciculations) may be observed in various muscle groups. Subsequently, depolarizing neuromuscular blockade, typified by SCh, causes motor weakness through stimulation of postjunctional cholinergic receptors, causing depolarization of the muscle membrane. Block persists because the half-life of SCh, measured in milliseconds, is substantially longer than that of ACh, which is measured in microseconds.

Monitoring Depolarizing Blockade

Monitoring of evoked muscle strength produced by single twitch (0.15 Hz) nerve stimulation after SCh shows progressive decrease of twitch height with increasing drug dose.[11] Characteristically, tetanic (50 Hz × 5 sec) stimulation also shows a reduction from baseline in twitch amplitude, which is maintained throughout the period of contraction (*i.e.*, there is little or no fade). Train-of-four (four 2-Hz impulses over 2 sec) nerve stimulation similarly shows an equal reduction of all four twitches in the trains. These findings are explained by the prejunctional effect of depolarizing neuromuscular blocking drugs to accelerate the mobilization and release of ACh from

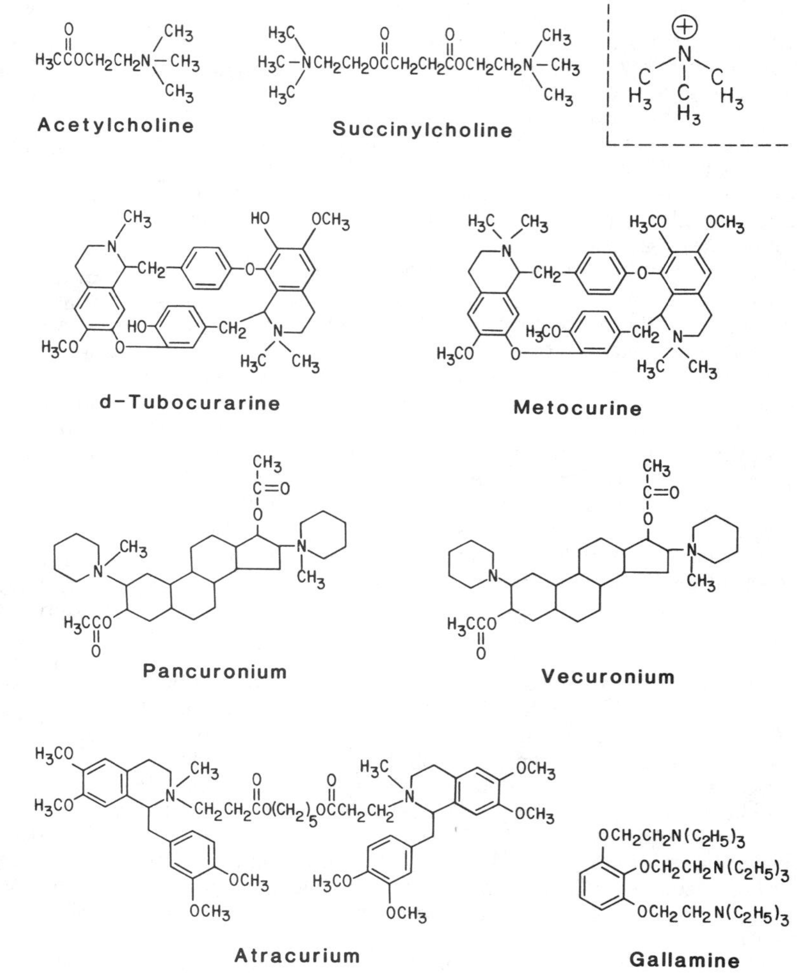

FIG. 13-3. Chemical structures of acetylcholine and neuromuscular blocking drugs in current use. Common to all these quaternary ammonium compounds is the presence of one or more positively charged nitrogen atoms (*inset*), which fosters binding to cholinergic receptors. (Modified from Stoelting RK: Pharmacology and Physiology in Anesthetic Practice, p 171. Philadelphia, JB Lippincott, 1987.)

the nerve terminal.[12] Consequently, tetanic or train-of-four nerve stimulation results in maintenance of repetitive nerve fiber firing and a muscle contractile response limited by the degree of postjunctional receptor blockade.

Furthermore, because ACh mobilization and release proceed apace with each other, single twitch stimulation of the nerve following tetanic stimulation does not result in a sudden augmented release of ACh (*i.e.*, there is no post-tetanic potentiation). Other characteristics of depolarizing neuromuscular blockade include antagonism by nondepolarizing relaxants and augmentation by AChE inhibitors.

Succinylcholine Metabolism

Normally, SCh is rapidly hydrolyzed to relatively inactive metabolites, succinylmonocholine and choline, by the enzyme plasma cholinesterase (also called pseudocholinesterase to distinguish this enzyme from AChE, which has no effect on SCh) in plasma. The same enzyme also acts in plasma, but more slowly, to break down succinylmonocholine into succinic acid and choline. Plasma cholinesterase has an enormous capacity to hydrolyze SCh, thus limiting, to a small fraction of the original iv dose, that drug which reaches the neuromuscular junction. There is minimal plasma cholinesterase present

at the neuromuscular junction, emphasizing the importance of diffusion of SCh away from its site of action for termination of neuromuscular blockade. Therefore, plasma cholinesterase influences duration of SCh by determining the size of the fraction of the initial dose that reaches the neuromuscular junction.

Plasma cholinesterase is synthesized in the liver. Consequently, altered hepatic synthetic activity, as occurs in cirrhosis of the liver, pregnancy, and the first 6 months of life, is associated with low plasma cholinesterase activity. In these situations, SCh-induced neuromuscular blockade, which normally lasts approximately 10 minutes from injection of a 1 $mg \cdot kg^{-1}$ dose to full recovery of twitch height, may be slightly prolonged.[13] On the other hand, drug-induced inhibition of plasma cholinesterase may result in prolongation of muscle weakness for several hours following administration of SCh. In contrast, hyperthyroid patients display increased plasma cholinesterase activity and may be relatively resistant to SCh.

Despite having diminished plasma cholinesterase activity, patients may have entirely normal enzyme. Approximately 4% of the population are heterozygous for the normal gene, which controls the production of plasma cholinesterase; these persons elaborate an atypical form of plasma cholinesterase and show slightly reduced SCh hydrolysis. One person in 2,500, however, is homozygous for the atypical esterase and will show respiratory inadequacy for 2 to 3 hours after an intubating dose of SCh.[14]

Because of the finding that serum with a full complement of normal plasma cholinesterase is inhibited *in vitro* by the local anesthetic dibucaine to a greater degree than serum lacking the normal enzyme, determination of an individual's dibucaine number (the percentage of inhibition of enzyme by dibucaine) may elucidate that person's ability to elaborate normal plasma cholinesterase. Normal people have dibucaine numbers between 70 and 85. Heterozygotes for atypical enzyme have dibucaine numbers between 30 and 65, whereas people who produce only atypical enzyme have dibucaine numbers between 16 and 25. Persons with rarer allelic variants also have markedly abnormal enzymic activity: Those with the fluoride resistant type have a mean dibucaine number of 34, and those with the silent type have a dibucaine number of 0. Persons with no plasma cholinesterase activity must depend upon glomerular filtration to eliminate SCh, resulting in prolonged SCh activity. These persons metabolize nondepolarizing relaxants normally and respond to their administration without prolonged duration.[15]

Phase II Blockade

Infusion of SCh in large doses over a prolonged period of time or to patients with atypical plasma cholinesterase may result in a Phase II blockade also called desensitizing SCh neuromuscular blockade.[16] To distinguish it from Phase I blockade, or classical depolarizing neuromuscular blockade, Phase II blockade is characterized by a nonsustained response (fade) to tetanic or train-of-four stimulation, as well as post-tetanic potentiation of single twitch response. The blockade can be antagonized by AChE inhibition, suggesting a mechanism similar, but not identical, to competitive nondepolarizing blockade.

Dual blockade refers to the simultaneous existence of both Phase I- and Phase II-type neuromuscular blockade during SCh administration after nondepolarizing characteristics have developed.[17] The onset of dual blockade is commonly denoted by tachyphylaxis during inhalational anesthesia[18] (in contrast to N_2O/opioid anesthesia[19]) and SCh infusion (*i.e.*, the rate of infusion must be increased to maintain the same degree of twitch suppression, reflecting mixed agonist [depolarizing] and self-antagonist [nondepolarizing] effects from SCh).

The development of tachyphylaxis and the lower SCh dose requirement to produce Phase II blockade during inhalational anesthesia, which contributes to neuromuscular blockade through effects on the muscle membrane, provide evidence for Phase II blockade having a postjunctional basis. Although the mechanisms underlying Phase II blockade remain uncertain, it is believed that SCh causes conformational changes in the cholinergic receptor, perhaps by occluding part of the Na^+ channel, and renders it inexcitable (desensitized) beyond the time course of usual SCh attachment, receptor activation, and release.[20]

In addition to these post junctional effects, Phase II blockade may result from reduced ACh mobilization and release when SCh, given in large and protracted dosings, exhausts the nerve terminal's capacity. The fact that there may be an element of competitive receptor blockade is supported by the ability to antagonize a Phase II blockade with AChE inhibitors.[19] However, since antagonism is not as predictable from Phase II blockade as it is from nondepolarizing blockade, an element of Na^+ channel blockade may also be present.

Autonomic Effects

Structurally resembling ACh, SCh can stimulate autonomic ganglia and increase transmission in both sympathetic and parasympathetic limbs of the autonomic nervous system. SCh principally affects heart rate by accentuating transmission to a relatively greater degree in the nondominant side. Therefore, children, who are generally sympathotonic, will be prone to bradycardia after a single dose of SCh,[21] whereas adults, who are relatively vagotonic, will be more likely to experience an increase in heart rate.[22] Atropine should be given iv to infants and small children prior to SCh and administered immediately to any child who becomes bradycardic after SCh.

Additionally, successive bolus doses of SCh given 2 to 10 minutes apart (with a peak effect at an interval of 4 to 5 minutes) in adults or children can result in sinus bradycardia, junctional rhythms, ventricular escape beats, and even sinus arrest. Vagal stimulation, for unclear reasons, appears to be the cause, perhaps as a result of myocardial sensitization by succinylmonocholine and choline.[23] Intravenous administration of atropine or gallamine immediately prior to SCh administration can prevent the sinus slowing; intramuscular (im) administration of atropine for premedication, however, is not effective.[24] Intravenous atropine is promptly curative if bradycardia occurs.

Similarly, the combined administration of SCh and vagotonic drugs may result in marked heart rate slowing. Sherman et al[25] reported a case of sinus arrest following SCh during anesthesia in a healthy patient given sufentanil; iv administration of atropine promptly restored sinus rhythm.

Hyperkalemia

Because of its depolarizing activity upon muscle membrane, SCh may cause complications not encountered with use of nondepolarizers. SCh-induced depolarization of normal muscle results in serum K^+ elevation in the range of 0.5 to 1.0 $mEq \cdot l^{-1}$. However, when SCh depolarizes muscle that has been traumatized or denervated, sufficient potassium may extrude from the cell as to produce systemic hyperkalemia, sometimes to the point of ventricular standstill and cardiac arrest. Goldhill et al[26] have raised the possibility that SCh-induced serum K^+ elevation is enhanced by beta-adrenergic blockade or alpha-adrenergic stimulation, which prevent K^+ from entering cells.

Although SCh ($1\ mg \cdot kg^{-1}$) maximally increases serum potassium by 11% in normal persons, Mazze et al[27] found that mean arterial potassium rose 84% in patients with massive bone and soft tissue wounds of the extremities. When K^+ increased by 2.5 $mEq \cdot l^{-1}$, peaked T waves, widened QRS complexes, and the absence of P waves were noted on the ECG. In three of five patients with $K^+ > 9.0\ mEq \cdot l^{-1}$, ventricular fibrillation and cardiac arrest occurred. The risk of SCh-induced hyperkalemia was seen in the third week postinjury and continued until all the wounds were healed. On the theory that hyperkalemia in this situation results from a progressive loss of muscle membrane integrity and consequent inability to return potassium intracellularly, Kopriva et al[28] found that SCh does not cause hyperkalemia during the acute phase of massive trauma.

A similar risk of hyperkalemia following SCh use in burned patients was reported by Birch et al,[29] noting heightened K^+ release from the third week after massive thermal injury. Since the precise point at which SCh induces hyperkalemia following burns and other muscle trauma cannot be known with certainty, it is advisable not to administer SCh to such patients beyond the first 24 hours postinjury.[30]

The mechanism for SCh-induced hyperkalemia in patients with denervation injury is better understood.[31] In this situation, extrajunctional cholinergic receptors develop along the muscle membrane in response to the lack of neural stimulation. When SCh is given, depolarization of the entire muscle mass may occur simultaneously with large K^+ efflux. Patients with encephalitis or severe Parkinson's disease or those who have suffered recent cerebrovascular accidents or head injury and have resultant upper motor neuron deficit are at risk for developing hyperkalemia after SCh as long as the nerve dysfunction remains progressive or unresolved. Tong,[32] for example, reported hyperkalemia-associated ventricular tachycardia following administration of SCh 2 weeks after a 2-year-old child had suffered near-drowning with hypoxic brain damage.

Cooperman[33] found that SCh ($1\ mg \cdot kg^{-1}$) produced rises > $1\ mEq \cdot l^{-1}$ in 13 of 28 paraplegics and hemiplegics. The highest susceptibility was noted within the first 6 months after upper motor neuron denervation; after 12 months, the K^+ release decreased unless the disease was progressive. He also reported elevated K^+ levels following SCh administration to one patient with multiple sclerosis and to another with muscular dystrophy. Similarly, Roth and Wuthrich[34] observed patients with tetanus develop hyperkalemia and cardiac arrest following SCh.

Tobey et al[35] showed that denervation hypersensitivity to SCh also occurs with lower motor neuron lesions by demonstrating increased K^+ levels following SCh in the venous blood from a limb paralyzed by peripheral nerve injury, as compared to the non-paralyzed limb. Single extremity paralysis, or even disuse atrophy of an extremity, according to Gronert and Theye,[36] represent possible contraindications to SCh, the period of risk ranging from the third week postinjury to 6 months or longer. Additional examples of lower motor neuron disease considered to promote hyperkalemic responses to SCh include myelomeningocele,[37] amyotrophic lateral sclerosis, syringomyelia, poliomyelitis, polyneuropathy,[38] and proximal muscle atrophy.[39] In contrast, SCh does not appear to cause hyperkalemia in patients with cerebral palsy.[40] Severe intraabdominal infection has also been associated with a hyperkalemic response to SCh.[41]

Hyperkalemia has also been alleged to occur during SCh used in patients with renal failure. Although these patients have elevated baseline K^+ levels, Koide and Waud[42] showed that serum potassium increased no more in uremic patients than in normal patients. However, when SCh is considered for a patient with a resting $K^+ > 5.5\ mEq \cdot l^{-1}$, dysrhythmias may result from an acute $0.5\ mEq \cdot l^{-1}$ rise following SCh.

Other Complications of SCh Use

Rarely, SCh can cause an allergic reaction.[43] Release of histamine and other vasoactive substances in such persons produces tachycardia and hypotension; treatment to restore circulation and maintain oxygenation is paramount. There may be cross-sensitivity between SCh and nondepolarizing muscle relaxants, especially in patients with circulating antibodies to quaternary ammonium groups of succinylcholine. Another source of tachycardia following SCh use is malignant hyperthermia.[44] Because this syndrome can be triggered in susceptible persons during anesthesia, particularly in association with SCh, persistent and unexplained tachycardia, particularly when associated with jaw rigidity, must be evaluated with malignant hyperthermia in mind.

Patients with myotonia may also develop jaw rigidity along with myotonic muscle contractures following SCh,[45] undesirable events in themselves, but unrelated to malignant hyperthermia. Since nondepolarizing neuromuscular blocking drugs are not considered to trigger malignant hyperthermia, they may be used during N_2O/opioid anesthesia when susceptible patients must receive general anesthesia. An additional aberrant response to SCh is seen in the "Stiff Baby syndrome,"[46] in which patients are SCh-resistant but respond normally to nondepolarizers.

SCh-induced depolarization and the resulting stretch of muscle spindles may cause postanesthetic myalgias, notably across the shoulders, back, and neck, which particularly bother patients who have undergone surgical procedures from which the patients would not have expected postoperative pain. Muscle fasciculations may also be caused prejunctionally by repetitive motor nerve firing.[47] Giving small doses of nondepolarizing neuromuscular blocking drugs such as dTc, which acts prejunctionally to suppress these repetitive discharges, several minutes prior to SCh appears to be the most effective means of eliminating muscle fasciculations. Just the same, prevention of fasciculations does not necessarily eliminate SCh-induced muscle aches. Although pretreatment with atracurium before SCh reduced the incidence of fasciculations from 85% to 30% and decreased the incidence of postoperative myalgias from 45% to 10% in a study by Manchikanti et al,[48] there was little correlation between fasciculations and myalgias.

Intraocular pressure (IOP) rises as a consequence of SCh-induced contracture of multiply innervated fibers of the extraocular muscles, which, in turn, causes contraction of the smooth muscle of the globe.[49] Although patients with treated glaucoma are at little risk, SCh administration to patients with penetrating eye injuries may result in vitreous expulsion and loss of vision. Miller et al[50] stated that pretreatment with dTc or gallamine could prevent dangerous rises in IOP, whereas Meyers et al[51] found no protection afforded by prior nondepolarizer administration.

Debate continues as to the value of nondepolarizer pretreatment before SCh, the use of nondepolarizing blockade alone, and the provision of deep levels of anesthesia prior to intubation of the trachea in preventing increased IOP.[52] Libonati et al[53] described their experience with 2,000 cases of open eye injury, in which anesthesia included dTc pretreatment (3 to 6 mg) and SCh (60 to 160 mg). They reported no instances of vitreous expulsion or pulmonary aspiration of gastric contents. Schneider et al[54] found that neither atracurium nor vecuronium affected IOP, but tracheal intubation consistently caused IOP elevation. The use of nondepolarizers in high doses with priming to expedite suitable conditions for intubation of the trachea has been advocated in order to obviate the use of SCh, but Donlon[55] maintains that smooth, rapid induction of anesthesia with controlled tracheal intubation provides the safest means of dealing with the problem.

Continued preference for SCh in patients with a "full stomach" stems from SCh's unmatched speed in providing excellent conditions for tracheal intubation; a $1\ mg \cdot kg^{-1}$ dose yields complete twitch suppression in 60 to 90 seconds. However, Miller and Way[56] found that SCh $1\ mg \cdot kg^{-1}$ caused intragastric pressure elevation to 40 cm H_2O, presumably as a result of abdominal muscle contraction, and increased the risk of esophageal regurgitation and potential pulmonary aspiration. Pretreatment with a nondepolarizer limited the rise in intragastric pressure following SCh. Other investigators[57] have pointed out that lower esophageal sphincter pressure also rises following SCh, even without pretreatment, resulting in maintained barrier pressure to esophageal regurgitation and little added risk.

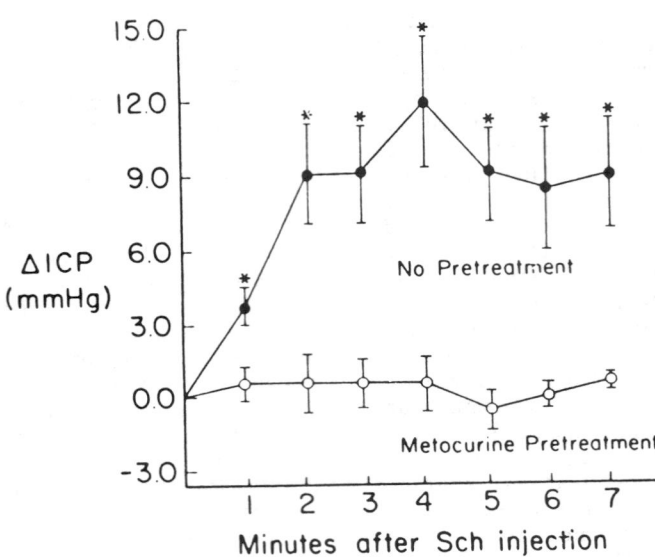

FIG. 13-4. Changes in intracranial pressure (*ICP*) following administration of succinylcholine 1 mg·kg^{-1} (*no pretreatment*) or metocurine 0.03 mg·kg^{-1} followed by succinylcholine (*metocurine pretreatment*) to patients with brain tumors (Mean ± SE; *$p < 0.05$ compared to baseline prior to injection of succinylcholine). (Reprinted with permission from Stirt JA, Grosslight KR, Bedford RF *et al*: "Defasciculation" with metocurine prevents succinylcholine-induced increases in intracranial pressure. Anesthesiology 67:50, 1978.)

SCh appears to cause intracranial pressure (ICP) to increase. Although the mechanism has been presumed to be neck muscle contraction leading to jugular venous compression, recent evidence points to a SCh-induced increase in afferent muscle spindle activity, as causative of increased cerebral blood flow.[58] Administration of subparalyzing doses of nondepolarizing muscle relaxants (pretreatment) prevents SCh-induced increases in ICP (Fig. 13-4).[59] Thus, the responses to tracheal intubation during light anesthesia is more likely responsible for ICP elevation than is SCh itself.

The relative value of expeditious tracheal intubation using SCh in these patients, compared with ensuring deep levels of anesthesia and using nondepolarizing relaxants in a slower, more controlled fashion, continues to be debated.[60] However, when the need for immediate airway control assumes precedence, SCh may be used, provided that deep levels of anesthesia have been produced and that hyperventilation is ensured. Because atracurium[61] and vecuronium[62] have no effect on ICP, either may be used in patients with increased ICP, when the need for airway control is not as acute.

NONDEPOLARIZING BLOCKING DRUGS

This group of muscle relaxants is considered to act principally by binding to the postsynaptic cholinergic receptor on the motor end-plate and competitively preventing transmitter ACh from activating Na$^+$ channels and initiating action potentials at muscle membrane.[8] These drugs do not depolarize the motor end-plate upon binding. Inasmuch as current theory holds that two ACh molecules must bind simultaneously to corresponding sites on a given receptor, even one molecule of nondepolarizer at that receptor effectively blocks neuromuscular transmission for as long as the nondepolarizer main-

tains its covalent attachment (Fig. 13-5). Similarly, nondepolarizer receptor binding prevents SCh from depolarizing that particular area of motor end-plate. At high doses, these muscle relaxants may enter the ion channel to produce channel blockade. Nondepolarizing muscle relaxants may also act at presynaptic sites to block Na$^+$ channels. As a result, presynaptic mobilization of ACh from synthesis sites to release sites is impaired.

Like ACh or SCh, all nondepolarizing neuromuscular blocking drugs are quaternary ammonium compounds and contain at least one positively charged amine group, which attaches to an anionic component of the receptor. In contrast to the relatively simple linear structure of depolarizing muscle relaxants, the nondepolarizing drugs are bulky and have rigid ring structures that conceal the presence of the ACh moiety (Fig. 13-3). Whereas dTc has only one charged nitrogen ion but can reversibly develop a second, most neuromuscular blocking drugs possess two, and gallamine has three. The stereospecific attachment of nondepolarizers to receptors favors prolonged binding, with detachment and reattachment by diffusion, until mass action of ACh molecules gradually restores physiologic neuromuscular transmission.

Neuromuscular Margin of Safety

Through the work of Paton and Waud[63] as well as that of Waud and Waud,[64] it has been established that a margin of safety exists to maintain neuromuscular transmission. Accordingly, 75%–80% of receptors must be blocked before any interference with twitch response can be seen, and 90%–95% of receptors must be occluded before neuromuscular transmission fails in all muscle fibers. Similarly, tetanic stimulation at 30 Hz produced fade only after 75%–80% of receptors were blocked, whereas tetanus at 100 Hz and 200 Hz faded with 50% and 30% receptor occlusion, respectively. Train-of-four stimulation showed fade with 70%–75% of receptors blocked.[65] Furthermore, the diaphragm has even a greater margin of safety for maintaining function, in that it has been shown to have twice as many free receptors as does peripheral musculature at corresponding points of twitch suppression.[66] The fact that the diaphragm continues to function with an estimated 90% of receptors occupied is evidenced by its spontaneous recovery of function at a significantly faster rate than that of the adductor pollicis.[67]

Monitoring Nondepolarizing Blockade

Monitoring nondepolarizer activity by evoked muscle strength following single twitch (0.15 Hz) nerve stimulation shows progressive reduction in twitch height with increasing dose of relaxant.[11] In contrast to SCh, tetanic (50 Hz × 5 sec) and train-of-four (four 2-Hz impulses over 2 sec) nerve stimulation during nondepolarizer blockade show a decrement in twitch height over the course of the stimulation (*i.e.*, fade).

Lee[68] determined that the visual return of the first twitch in a train-of-four following dTc block during halothane anesthesia could be seen with less than 75% recovery of single twitch control height, whereas visual return of the second, third, and fourth twitches in a train-of-four correlated with 75%, 80%, and 90% recovery, respectively. O'Hara *et al*[69] found that reappearance of the first, second, third, and fourth twitches in a train-of-four during recovery from vecuronium blockade occurred at approximately 60%, 70%, 80%, and 90% of single twitch control height, respectively, during either enflurane or N$_2$O/opioid anesthesia.[70] The fact that recovery of single twitch and train-of-four responses are not parallel suggests

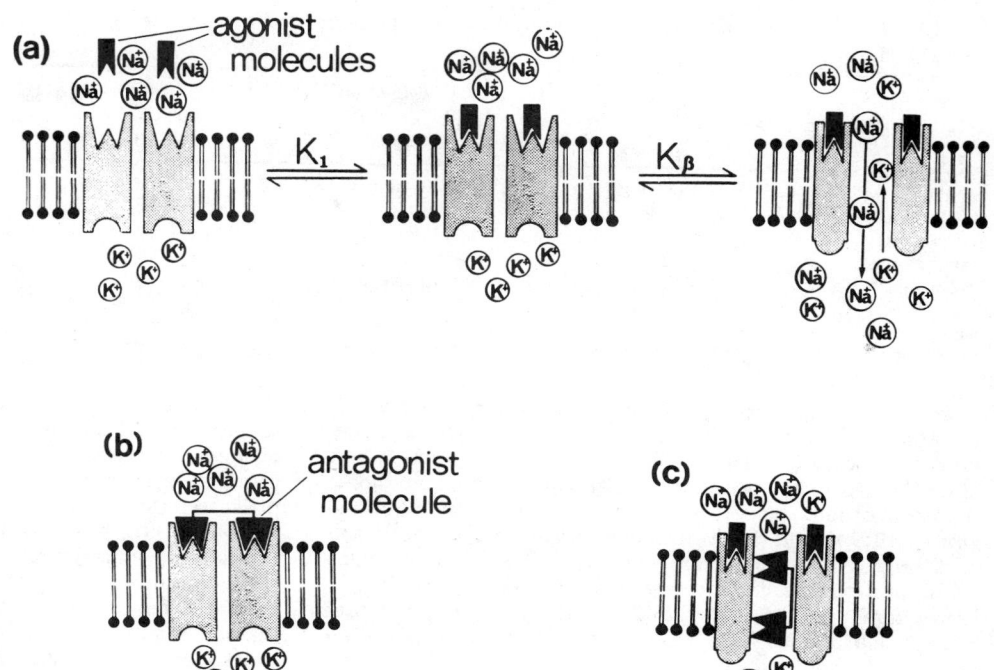

FIG. 13-5. Diagrammatic representation of the interaction of an agonist (acetylcholine) and an antagonist (*e.g.*, d-tubocurarine) with motor end-plate cholinergic receptors. (*A*) Agonist molecules combine with recognition sites of the receptor and induce a conformational change in the ion conductance modulator protein. Ion channels open, allowing the diffusion of Na^+ and K^+ ions down their concentration gradients. (*B*) Antagonist molecules, having already combined with recognition sites of the closed channel form of the receptor, prevent agonist-induced conformational change. (*C*) After agonist molecules have opened the ion channel, antagonist molecules enter and block the open channel. (Reprinted with permission from Bowman WC. Anesth Analg 59:942, 1980.)

that nondepolarizing muscle relaxants have effects at two different sites of action.[71]

Prejunctional effects of nondepolarizing drugs inhibit ACh mobilization from adequately meeting the demand of sustained, rapid nerve stimulation, causing fade to tetanic or train-of-four stimulation.[72] Post-tetanic potentiation occurs when single twitch nerve stimulation takes place following tetanus; increased availability of ACh owing to high-frequency stimulation, though lagging during tetanus, allows augmented ACh release and facilitation of transmission.[73] Characteristically, nondepolarizing neuromuscular blockade is antagonized by the administration of AChE-inhibiting drugs.

Nondepolarizers in Clinical Use

The nondepolarizing neuromuscular blocking drugs in clinical use today include dTc, metocurine, gallamine, and pancuronium, which have roughly equal, moderately long durations of action, and atracurium and vecuronium, which have similar intermediate durations of action. The selection of a nondepolarizing muscle relaxant logically depends upon the intended duration of neuromuscular blockade, the autonomic and cardiovascular effects of a given drug, and the health or disease of the patient with respect to specific organ function. The dose chosen likewise depends upon these same factors, as well as upon the onset time and depth of muscle relaxation desired (Table 13-2).

For example, increasing the dose of pancuronium from its ED_{95} (0.07 mg·kg^{-1}) to that of $2 \times ED_{95}$ shortens the onset of block from 4.2 minutes to 1.8 minutes, produces intense neuromuscular blockade, and lengthens the time to spontaneous 5% recovery of control twitch height from 43 minutes to 129 minutes. A dose-related increase in heart rate is also observed.[74]

Autonomic and Histamine-Releasing Side-Effects

Because they are quaternary ammonium compounds, like ACh, neuromuscular blocking drugs can, to greater or lesser

TABLE 13-2.   Suggested Muscle Relaxant Doses (mg·kg^{-1}) for Clinical Use

DRUG	ED_{95}	INTUBATING DOSE	SUPPLEMENTAL DOSES	
			N_2O/Opioid	Inhalational
d-Tubocurarine	0.51	0.60	0.10	0.05
Metocurine	0.28	0.40	0.07	0.04
Pancuronium	0.07	0.10	0.015	0.007
Vecuronium	0.05	0.08–0.10	0.02	0.015
Atracurium	0.20	0.40–0.50	0.10	0.07
Gallamine	2.8	3.5	0.60	0.30
Pancuronium–metocurine combination	0.018 + 0.072	0.025 + 0.10	0.004 + 0.016	0.003 + 0.012
Pancuronium–*d*-tubocurarine combination	0.024 + 0.144	0.03 + 0.18	0.005 + 0.03	0.004 + 0.025

TABLE 13-3. Autonomic and Histamine-Releasing Effects of Neuromuscular
Blocking Drugs

DRUG	AUTONOMIC GANGLIA	PARASYMPATHETIC RECEPTORS (VAGUS)	HISTAMINE RELEASE
Succinylcholine	Stimulates	Stimulates	Rare
d-Tubocurarine	Blocks++	No effect	+++
Metocurine	Blocks+	No effect	++
Pancuronium	No effect	Blocks++	None
Vecuronium	No effect	No effect	None
Gallamine	No effect	Blocks+++	None
Atracurium	No effect	No effect	+

degrees, stimulate or block other cholinergic receptors throughout the body (Table 13-3).[75] Cholinoceptive sites may be either nicotinic, such as the neuromuscular junction and autonomic ganglia, or muscarinic, including postganglionic parasympathetic receptors in bowel, bladder, bronchi, the sinoatrial (SA) and atrioventricular (AV) nodes of the heart, and the pupillary sphincter. The active sites of the enzymes AChE and plasma cholinesterase are also cholinoceptive.

In examining the autonomic effects on nondepolarizing muscle relaxants in cats, Hughes and Chapple[76] established dose–response curves for the four longer-acting relaxants by measuring tibialis anterior muscle twitch, vagus-induced heart rate change, and nictitating membrane contraction (an indicator of sympathetic ganglionic activity) against graded doses of each drug. Within the clinical dose range for neuromuscular blockade, dTc exhibited both sympathetic and ganglionic parasympathetic (vagal) blockade. Corresponding doses of gallamine and pancuronium did not block sympathetic transmission but did produce muscarinic vagal blockade. Within the dose range for neuromuscular blockade, metocurine yielded neither sympathetic nor vagal blocking effects, though both effects were seen at high doses.

In addition to their vagolytic effects, pancuronium[77] and gallamine[78] stimulate adrenergic autonomic activity by blocking muscarinic receptors located in sympathetic ganglia[79] and on postganglionic sympathetic nerve endings.[80] Pancuronium also blocks re-uptake by adrenergic nerves of released norepinephrine.[81]

Histamine release by muscle relaxants[82] does not have an immunologic basis, but rather occurs as a nonspecific displacement of histamine and possibly other vasoactive substances from vascular mast cells, particularly when certain relaxants are given in large doses (Table 13-3).[83] Effects include decreased systemic vascular resistance (SVR) and hypotension, tachycardia, erythema, edema from increased capillary permeability, and bronchospasm.

Because of its H_2 histamine–blocking properties, cimetidine has been shown to block histamine-induced vasodilation following dTc administration.[84] Scott et al[85] have further shown that a dose of atracurium, which, when given over 5 seconds, releases histamine, fails to do so when given over 75 seconds. When that same dose is given over 5 seconds but following cimetidine and chlorpheniramine pretreatment, the increase in serum histamine concentration is blunted and hemodynamic changes are not seen. In addition, histamine release after dTc administration appears to be blunted by inhalational anesthetics.[86]

Structure–Activity Relationships

Bisquaternary compounds generally lack significant ganglionic blocking or histamine-releasing properties.[5] The ganglionic blockade and histamine release seen with dTc are consistent with the fact that dTc is monoquaternary. Methylation of the dTc molecule at its tertiary amine and at its hydroxyl groups yields metocurine, which, as a bisquaternary drug, possesses three times weaker ganglionic blocking and histamine-releasing properties than the parent compound. The bisquaternary structure of pancuronium, ACh-like on a rigid steroidal nucleus gives pancuronium its vagal blocking property and its plasma cholinesterase-inhibiting activity. The marked vagolytic property of gallamine appears to be related to its three positively charged nitrogen atoms. Neither pancuronium nor gallamine cause histamine release.

Cardiovascular Side-Effects

The hemodynamic consequences of administering each of these muscle relaxants derive from their autonomic and histamine-releasing effects. In patients anesthetized with N_2O/halothane, Stoelting[87] determined that dTc (0.4 mg · kg^{-1}) administration resulted in decreased mean arterial pressure (MAP), cardiac output (CO), and SVR, whereas heart rate (HR) increased slightly (Fig. 13-6). Longnecker et al[88] found that vasodilation was the primary event. The degree of reduction in SVR depends upon the depth of anesthesia, pre-existing sympathetic tone, intravascular volume status, as well as the dose of dTc given and its rate of administration. Hypotension is more likely to occur when large doses are given in bolus fashion to hypovolemic patients during deep levels of anesthesia.[89] Giving the dose incrementally over 5 to 10 minutes can minimize the hemodynamic change.

In a similar group of patients, Stoelting[90] found that metocurine (0.2 mg · kg^{-1}) caused little change from control with respect to CO, SVR, and HR (Fig. 13-6). The 10% drop in MAP was less then the 25% reduction encountered with equipotent doses of dTc. Savarese et al[91] found that giving metocurine (0.3 mg · kg^{-1}) during N_2O/opioid anesthesia resulted in little hemodynamic change, whereas higher-dose metocurine (0.4 mg · kg^{-1}) caused a 6% drop in MAP and an 18% increase in HR (Fig. 13-7). These cardiovascular effects probably result from histamine release, since sympathetic and vagal blockade do not occur in the clinically useful dose range.

In patients given pancuronium (0.08 mg · kg^{-1}) under N_2O/halothane anesthesia, Stoelting[87] found that MAP, CO, and HR increased, whereas SVR remained the same (Fig. 13-6). Kelman and Kennedy[92] noted even greater increases in MAP, CO, and HR in patients anesthetized with N_2O/opioid technique. Tachycardia is both dose related and cumulative; furthermore, the increase from baseline is proportionately greater when the resting HR is low.[93]

As a result of its sympathotonic and vagolytic effects, pancuronium was associated with a higher incidence of myocardial ischemia, compared with metocurine or a pancuronium–

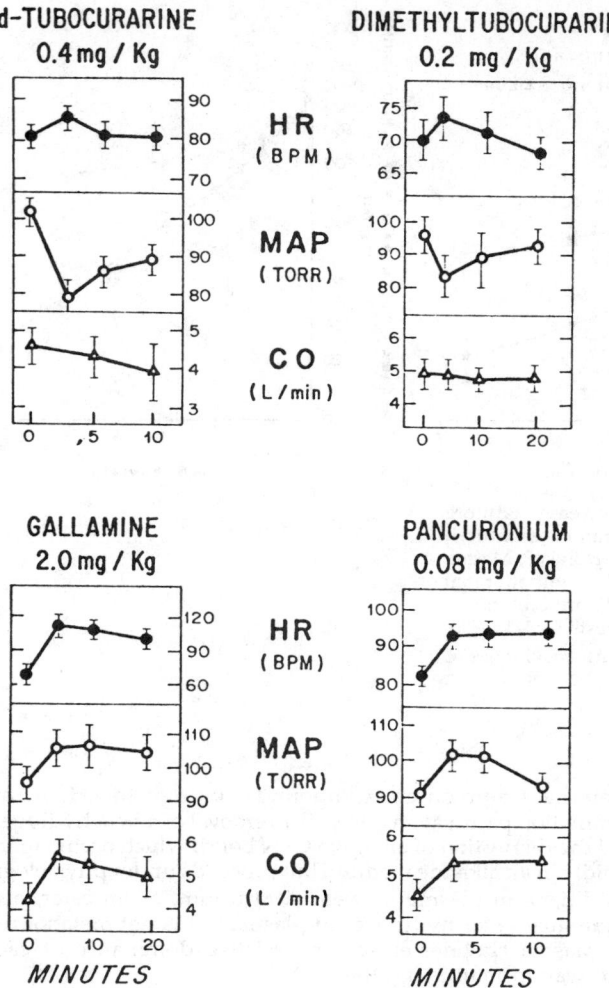

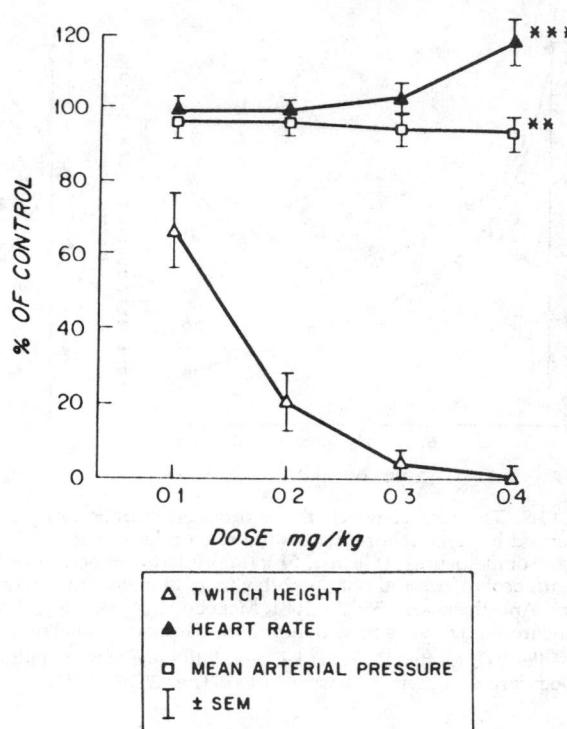

FIG. 13-6 Comparative cardiovascular effects in humans of dTc, metocurine (dimethyltubocurarine), gallamine, and pancuronium administration in approximately equipotent doses during halothane-nitrous oxide anesthesia. (Reprinted with permission from Lebowitz PW, Savarese JJ: ASA Refresher Course in Anesthesiology, vol 8, 1980. Data from Stoelting RK: The hemodynamic effects of pancuronium and d-tubocurarine in anesthetized patients. Anesthesiology 36:612, 1972; Stoelting RK: Hemodynamic effects of dimethyltubocurarine during nitrous oxide-halothane anesthesia. Anesth Analg 53:513, 1974; and Stoelting RK: Hemodynamic effects of gallamine during halothane-nitrous oxide anesthesia. Anesthesiology 39:645, 1973.)

FIG. 13-7. Neuromuscular and cardiovascular effects of increasing doses of metocurine administered intravenously to adult patients anesthetized with nitrous oxide-morphine-thiopental (**$P < 0.01$; ***$P < 0.001$). (Reprinted with permission from Savarese JJ, Ali HH, Antonio HP: The clinical pharmacology of metocurine: Dimethyltubocurarine revisited. Anesthesiology 47:277, 1977.)

metocurine combination, in patients undergoing coronary artery bypass surgery during fentanyl/O_2 anesthesia.[94] Pancuronium enhances AV conduction and promotes the occurrence of premature ventricular contractions (PVCs).[95] In the presence of imipramine, a tricyclic antidepressant, and halothane-enhanced AV conduction, and accentuated catecholamine release owing to pancuronium, Edwards[96] found a high incidence of ventricular arrhythmias, which did not occur when enflurane or dTc were substituted, respectively.

Gallamine (2.0 mg·kg^{-1}) given by Stoelting[97] to patients during N_2O/halothane anesthesia consistently produced a sustained increase in HR; MAP and CO also rose, whereas SVR declined, perhaps secondary to the increase in CO. Because of gallamine's[98] predictable proclivity toward causing tachycardia, it should be avoided in patients who cannot tolerate an elevation in HR (Fig. 13-6).

Nondepolarizer Metabolism

As quaternary ammonium compounds, nondepolarizing muscle relaxants are highly ionized and are readily excreted by the kidneys. Increasing urine volume, as can be achieved with an osmotic diuretic such as mannitol, has no effect on relaxant elimination, which depends upon the rate of glomerular filtration.[99]

Studied in dogs by Cohen et al,[100] 75% of a 0.3 mg·kg^{-1} dose of dTc was measured in urine over the first 24 hours, and 10%–15% of the dTc was recovered in bile. In the presence of renal dysfunction, hepatic conjugation of dTc becomes more important. When the same dose was given to nephrectomized dogs, hepatic dTc excretion increased three-to fourfold. Miller et al[101] drew similar conclusions after measuring elimination pathways for dTc in man (Fig. 13-8).

Although pancuronium can be excreted in bile, the kidneys bear primary responsibility for removal of unchanged drug from the body. Agoston et al[102] measured 37%–44% of a 6-mg dose of pancuronium in urine within 30 hours, compared with 11% in bile. Furthermore, pancuronium is unique among the longer-acting nondepolarizers, in that it is broken down into less active metabolites in the liver. Nonetheless, renal failure patients accumulate pancuronium, even when used in small doses. As McLeod et al[103] have shown, the elimination half-life of pancuronium is increased about five times in anephric persons (Fig. 13-8). In addition, Miller et al[104] found that the duration of pancuronium-induced neuromuscular blockade is prolonged in patients with renal failure, reflecting a lack of adequate hepatic compensation.

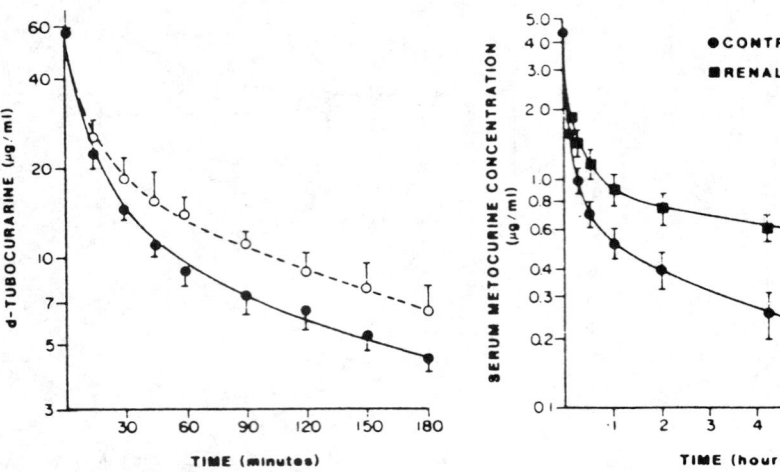
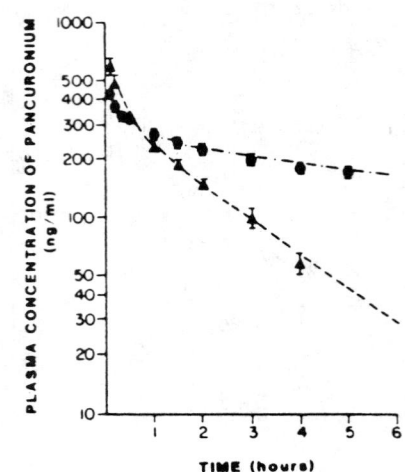

FIG. 13-8. The rate at which the serum concentration of pancuronium decreases is more influenced by renal failure than is the rate of decline in the serum concentrations of d-tubo-curarine or metocurine (Mean ± SE). (Reprinted with permission from Brotherton WP, Matteo R: Pharmacokinetics and pharmacodynamics of metocurine in humans with and without renal failure. Anesthesiology 55:273, 1981; McLeod K, Watson MJ, Rawlings MD: Pharmacokinetics of pancuronium in patients with normal and impaired renal function. Br J Anaesth 48:341, 1976; and Miller RD, Matteo R, Benet LZ et al: Influence of renal failure on the pharmacokinetics of d-tubocurarine in man. J Pharmacol Exp Ther 202:1, 1977.)

Gallamine[105] and metocurine[106] each depend heavily upon renal excretion for their elimination and have poorly developed alternative excretory pathways. When these drugs are used in patients with renal failure, prolonged paralysis should be expected. Because these drugs, like dTc and pancuronium, are ionized, they may be removed from the body by dialysis.

Liver disease affects the metabolism of nondepolarizing muscle relaxants in several different ways. In comparing patients before and after splenorenal anastomosis for cirrhosis, Dundee and Gray[107] noted resistance to dTc prior to improvement of liver function. Baraka[108] suggested that such resistance was due to binding of dTc by gamma globulin, whose levels are increased in cirrhosis. Such binding is unique to dTc among neuromuscular blocking drugs.

Duvaldestin et al[109] also found that patients with cirrhosis required higher than expected doses of pancuronium, a phenomenon explainable by the 50% increase in drug volume of distribution found in such patients. These patients also required less supplemental pancuronium to maintain a constant degree of blockade. Reduced hepatic biotransformation of pancuronium in these persons may contribute to a slower than normal decline in serum drug levels. Patients with complete biliary tract obstruction were found by Somogyi et al[110] to be relatively resistant to pancuronium, also likely as a result of a higher than normal volume of distribution. Maintenance relaxant requirements are decreased because serum drug levels remain higher than normal, secondary to reduced biliary clearance.

INTERMEDIATE-DURATION NONDEPOLARIZERS

Atracurium

Atracurium[111, 112] is a bisquaternary ester nondepolarizing neuromuscular blocking drug that was synthesized specifically to take advantage of the spontaneous degradation of quaternary ammonium compounds through the Hofmann elimination pathway, namely, the removal of a beta hydrogen and the disruption of an alpha C–N bond, which occurs more rapidly in an alkaline medium but proceeds under physiologic conditions in plasma as well. Atracurium, as an ester, also undergoes ester hydrolysis in plasma but is not metabolized by plasma cholinesterase. The relative dominance of each pathway in man is unclear.

In animal studies, atracurium was seen to be highly specific for neuromuscular blockade with minimal sympathetic blocking effects and vagal blockade only at doses well beyond the clinical range. Atracurium appears to have both prejunctional and postjunctional neuromuscular blocking effects.[113] Histamine release, though less marked than with dTc or even with metocurine, did occur and had a greater likelihood of occurring at higher atracurium doses.[83] Lavery et al[114] reported a case of severe bronchospasm caused by atracurium at a dose of 1 mg·kg⁻¹. Rash, hypotension, and tachycardia may also result from histamine release.[115] Scott et al[116] found that at 0.8 mg·kg⁻¹ given over 5 seconds, caused a 25% reduction in blood pressure; administering this dose over 75 seconds or antihistamine pretreatment limited the drop in blood pressure.

A dose of atracurium producing 95% neuromuscular blockade (0.2 mg·kg⁻¹) results in an onset time of 4.0 minutes, spontaneous recovery to 95% of control first twitch height in 44.1 minutes, and a recovery index (return from 25% to 75% of control first twitch height) of 12.3 minutes.[111] In contrast to longer-acting drugs, once recovery has begun for atracurium, the recovery index appears independent of the administered dose. Lennon et al[117] found that atracurium, administered in a dose of 1.5 mg·kg⁻¹ produced onset of block in 56 seconds, yet allowed recovery of the second twitch of a train-of-four by 71 minutes. With repeated doses, there appears to be little or no cumulation of effect.

Atracurium has advantage for use in patients with renal or

hepatic failure, since its metabolism proceeds independently of both kidney and liver. The elimination half-life of atracurium in patients with renal[118] or hepatic[119] failure does not differ from that in normal persons.

One of the breakdown products of atracurium, laudanosine, is a tertiary amine that can cross into the brain and, at high plasma concentrations, has caused seizures in dogs.[120] Even when infused over 38 to 219 hours to intensive care unit (ICU) patients,[121] however, atracurium did not cause evidence of cerebral excitation; laudanosine concentrations, though elevated, were substantially below the seizure threshold determined in dogs. Animal studies have suggested that laudanosine is responsible for EEG "arousal" responses,[122] as well as a concentration-dependent increase in anesthetic requirement.[123] Another breakdown product of atracurium, acrylate, has been implicated in damage to rat hepatocytes.[124] However, no evidence of toxicity during extensive animal testing or clinical use has been reported to date.

Vecuronium

Vecuronium,[112, 125] a monoquaternary steroidal nondepolarizer, resembles pancuronium except that one nitrogen has been demethylated, rendering it uncharged. Nonetheless, the compound has high specificity for the neuromuscular junction, is virtually devoid of sympathetic blocking or vagal blocking effects, and does not release histamine. There is experimental evidence for both prejunctional and postjunctional neuromuscular blocking activity.[126] The virtual absence of autonomic side-effects, although usually advantageous, has led to vecuronium's association with bradycardia and asystole in situations in which vagotonic, beta-blocking, or Ca^{++} channel-blocking drugs are given without autonomic opposition.[127]

Administration of vecuronium in a dose equal to its ED_{95} (0.05 mg·kg^{-1}) results in an onset time of approximately 4 minutes,[128] whereas giving doses $3 \times ED_{95}$ and $5 \times ED_{95}$ shortened onset time to 2.8 minutes and 1.1 minutes, respectively.[117] Vecuronium is relatively noncumulative and exhibits rapid spontaneous recovery from doses used clinically; the recovery index ranges from 9 to 12 minutes. Vecuronium's duration of action is similar to that of atracurium. Increasing the dose of vecuronium to $5 \times ED_{95}$ resulted in recovery of the second twitch of a train-of-four by 83 minutes.[117] Because these two drugs are intermediate-acting, care must be taken not to allow premature loss of adequate conditions for surgical relaxation.

Vecuronium is unique among neuromuscular blocking drugs in its dependence upon hepatic metabolism.[129] Patients with cirrhosis[130] and those with biliary tract obstruction[131] display prolongation of recovery. In cases of mild hepatic dysfunction, however, the lengthened extent of block is not clinically important. About 15%–25% of a vecuronium dose is normally excreted by the kidney; increased hepatic metabolism and biliary excretion can compensate in the absence of renal function to avoid prolongation of block. Vecuronium may be used safely in patients with renal failure.[132]

RELAXANTS AND UNUSUAL DISORDERS

Patients with neuromuscular disease frequently respond abnormally to neuromuscular blocking drugs. The myotonias constitute a triad of disorders (myotonia dystrophica, myotonia congenita, and paramyotonia) characterized by delayed muscle relaxation following contraction. Typically, SCh can induce contractures severe enough to impede ventilation;

such abnormal muscle reactions may not easily be reversed by nondepolarizer administration. In the absence of depolarization, the response to nondepolarizers is normal.[45, 133, 134]

Patients with myasthenia gravis are extraordinarily sensitive to nondepolarizing blockade. Doses of dTc as small as 3 mg may be sufficient to block neuromuscular transmission completely and cause apnea. Since anticholinesterase drugs constitute primary maintenance therapy for such patients, the interaction of muscle relaxants, anticholinesterase drugs, and anesthesia may be complex and unpredictable. Consequently, myasthenic patients are often anesthetized without the use of any muscle relaxants. However, patients known to have this disorder, caused by an autoimmune-induced depletion of cholinergic receptors at the neuromuscular junction, may be given nondepolarizers provided that appropriate neuromuscular monitoring is performed and that adequacy of ventilation is ensured before extubation. Atracurium[135] and vecuronium,[136] because of their shorter durations, offer greater control of relaxation in myasthenics than do longer-acting drugs.

Myasthenic patients tend to be resistant to SCh, in contrast to patients with myasthenic syndrome owing to bronchial carcinoma, who are sensitive to both depolarizers and nondepolarizers. Baraka[137] has also reported that patients with Von Recklinghausen's disease or neurofibromatosis, like myasthenics, are sensitive to dTc but resistant to SCh.

Patients with collagen disorders, such as systemic lupus erythematosus, polymyositis, dermatomyositis, and polyarteritis nodosa, tend to be sensitive to both nondepolarizers and SCh, depending upon the degree of muscle involvement by the underlying condition.[138] Lower motor neuron disorders, such as amyotrophic lateral sclerosis, syringomyelia, poliomyelitis, and Duchenne-type proximal muscle atrophy, are likely to be associated with sensitivity to nondepolarizers; SCh use may result in hyperkalemia, an issue of overriding importance. On the other hand, patients with thyrotoxic myopathy, muscular dystrophies, and porphyria do not display unusual sensitivity to dTc; the safety of SCh use in these conditions is unpredictable.[39]

Hemiplegic patients have been shown to have less twitch suppression by nondepolarizing blockade on their weaker side, compared with their normal side.[139, 140] As Brett et al[141] have postulated in the case of multiple sclerosis, a greater number of cholinergic motor receptors develop on affected parts of the body because of diminished efferent neural input. Shayevitz and Matteo[142] have further found that, in addition to these effects, the contralateral, unaffected side is relatively resistant to nondepolarizer blockade, perhaps owing to increased receptor generation, compared with normal persons. A similar peripheral resistance to dTc-induced neuromuscular blockade has been seen experimentally with disuse atrophy in dogs.[143] However, since the diaphragm is not affected, it is conceivable that it can be blocked at a time that limb response is normal, thus decreasing the margin of safety for neuromuscular transmission.[144]

Patients undergoing excision and grafting of major burns have an increased requirement for nondepolarizing muscle relaxants.[145] Although initially thought to be due to pharmacokinetic factors, such as increased protein-binding, a larger volume of distribution, or increased drug clearance, Matteo et al[146] have demonstrated a much higher plasma concentration for dTc or metocurine to produce a given degree of neuromuscular blockade in burned patients, compared with that in normal controls. Dwersteg et al[147] have confirmed this pharmacodynamic effect in burned patients for atracurium, as well. The need for higher relaxant doses may be caused by an increase in the number of extrajunctional cholinergic receptors on burned muscle cells, a phenomenon that could also explain the propensity of SCh to produce hyperkalemia in these patients.

RELAXANT PHARMACODYNAMICS AND PHARMACOKINETICS

Drugs create pharmacologic effects by producing physical or chemical changes at their sites of action. The traditional dose–response relationship suggests that the magnitude of the response is directly related to the dose of drug, that the relationship is nonlinear (sigmoid), and that there is a maximal effect that cannot be exceeded by even an infinite dose of drug. These relationships describe a drug's pharmacodynamic effects—what the drug does to the body. These effects are best measured at a steady state and are generally time-independent (Table 13-4).

DOSE–RESPONSE (PHARMACODYNAMIC) CURVES

The dose response to muscle relaxants is quantified by the degree of muscle twitch suppression (expressed as a percentage of baseline twitch height) observed following stimulation of a motor nerve. Although the dose–response curve is sigmoid-shaped, it is relatively linear over its midportion (20%–80% twitch suppression) (Fig. 13-9A). Dose–response relationships are, therefore, best defined at doses that produce responses in this range. Generally, doses producing 20%, 50%, and 80% inhibition define a line of best fit, which can be interpolated over the range studied to predict the response to any dose.

A log-dose probit transformation straightens the sigmoid curve and expands the range of linearity from approximately 1% to 99% of baseline response.[148] The use of log-dose *versus* probit curves permits determination of the ED95 for a given drug, that is, the mean dose that produces a maximal effect of 95% twitch suppression (Fig. 13-9B). Log-dose probit curves also allow comparisons of drug potencies and interpretation of interactions of added drugs or changed conditions, represented as shifts in the curve. A parallel shift to the left of the curve for a given relaxant relative to another indicates increased potency, whereas a shift to the right represents opposite effects. Drugs acting in similar ways should have curves with equal slopes, whereas drugs with different mechanisms of action may have markedly different slopes.

A given drug's dose–response curve for neuromuscular blockade can also be compared to its dose–response curve for other activities, such as autonomic side-effects. The greater

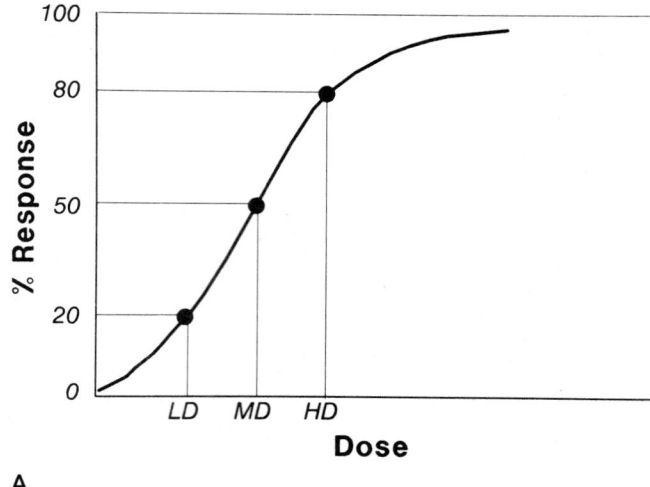

A

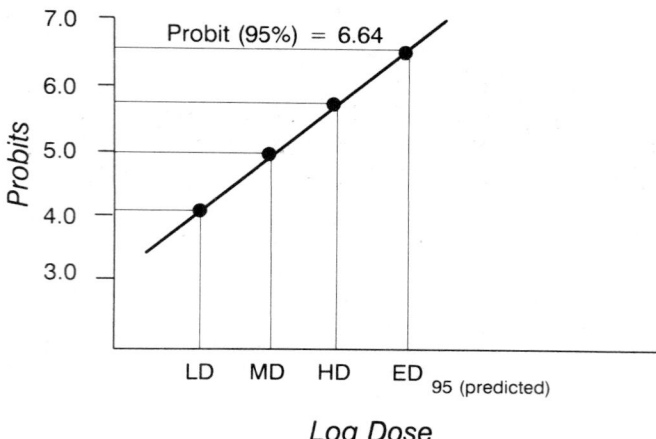

B

FIG. 13-9. (A) Sigmoid dose–response relationship. The linear portion of the curve is defined by measuring the response to three doses of relaxant (LD = low dose, MD = middle dose, HD = high dose). These doses are best selected to cover a range encompassing 20%–80% of the full measurable response. (B) Creating a log-dose versus probit transformation extends the linearity to encompass 1%–99% of the full measurable response. This allows extrapolation of the predicted ED95 from the straight line of best fit through three or more data points.

TABLE 13-4.   Pharmacokinetic and Pharmacodynamic Parameters for Intravenous Muscle Relaxants

RELAXANT	Vdss $(l \cdot kg^{-1})$	$T_{1/2}\alpha$ (min)	$T_{1/2}\beta$ (min)	Cl $(ml \cdot kg^{-1} \cdot min^{-1})$	$Cp_{ss(50)}$ $(mg \cdot ml^{-1})$	REFERENCES
d-Tubocurarine	0.30–0.60	6.2–23.8	120–348	0.9–2.7	0.22–0.60	9–14
Metocurine	0.42–0.57	16.5–28.6	216–348	1.2–1.8	0.25–0.31	12, 15, 16–18
Gallamine	0.21	6–35	138–144	1.2	5.8	19, 20
Pancuronium	0.13–0.38	5.2–13.2	102–144	1.0–1.9	0.14–0.30	21–27
Atracurium	0.13–0.19	1.3–3.4	18–25	4.4–6.5	0.65	28–31
Vecuronium	0.19–0.27	7.4–13	58–80	3.0–5.2	0.09–0.25	32–34

the separation between the curves, the freer that drug is from unwanted side-effects.

Dose–response studies can be performed using either single dosing or cumulative dosing techniques. With the latter, the maximal response to a first dose is quantified, then followed by additional doses, whose responses are quantified sequentially in cumulative fashion. For long-acting relaxants, either technique suffices.[149] However, cumulative dose measurements are less accurate for atracurium or vecuronium, since effects from a first dose are waning by the time that the second and third doses are given.[150]

A more accurate description of dose response would relate the concentration of a drug at its effector site to measurable graded responses. Although the concentration of drug at the neuromuscular junction is inaccessible *in vivo*, the drug concentration in plasma, which produces 50% twitch suppression at steady-state conditions [$Cp_{ss(50)}$], provides a means of comparing drug potencies and the factors that affect them. For example, vecuronium $Cp_{ss(50)}$ in infants is lower than that in children and adults,[151] reflecting immaturity of the neuromuscular junction; a lesser drug concentration in plasma is required in infants to produce the same degree of neuromuscular blockade.

RELAXANT PHARMACOKINETICS

In addition to a drug's producing an effect on the body, the body has effects on the drug (Table 13-4). Pharmacokinetics deals with the time-dependent fate of a drug as it is distributed throughout the body, metabolized, and eliminated. As drug concentrations decline in plasma, a concentration gradient develops, which favors removal of drug from its site of action back into plasma. Because muscle relaxants are polar, ionized compounds, they are highly soluble in water and relatively insoluble in fat. Consequently, the volume of distribution (Vd_{ss}) of muscle relaxants approximates that of extracellular fluid.[152] Although relaxants might be expected to be just as soluble in intracellular fluid, the lipid composition of cellular membranes acts as a barrier to their inward transport and limits their access to this space.

Pharmacokinetics for a given drug are determined by measuring drug concentration in plasma over time. Although the drug concentration should ideally be measured at its effector site, the drug level in plasma is assumed to reflect this concentration and is used for pharmacokinetic calculations.

TWO-COMPARTMENT MODEL

Drug concentration, as a function of time, following initial bolus injection of a muscle relaxant, is often described by a two-compartment pharmacokinetic model.[153] Two hypothetical compartments are chosen because the data points obtained from serial sampling are best fitted by a summation of two exponential functions, each decaying with a measurable half-life (Fig. 13-10). The more rapidly decaying exponential represents the reduction in plasma concentration owing to drug distribution shortly after the bolus injection. Its half-life, designated alpha (α), is generally several minutes. As time progresses, the curve is noted to flatten; the half-life, designated beta (β), is much longer, reflecting the slower decline in plasma drug concentration related to metabolism and excretion.

Immediately following a bolus injection of relaxant, the alpha phase predominates, and drug levels decline rapidly. Redistribution of drug is more than 95% complete within 5 half-lives (20 to 30 min). Henceforth, the beta phase predominates, and plasma levels decrease slowly. Measured pharmacokinetic values for the commonly used relaxants are grouped together in Table 13-4.[99, 103, 105, 106, 130, 146, 154–173]

EXPONENTIAL DECAY (PHARMACOKINETIC) CURVES

Precisely how fast the clinical effects of a particular relaxant dissipate depend upon the shape of the drug's pharmacokinetic curve where it crosses the band of drug concentrations associated with measurable levels of blockade (Fig. 13-11). Hypothetical Curve A shows association of a drug's range of clinical activity with plasma level decay along the steep portion of the curve during the distribution (α) phase. This type of pharmacokinetic curve is typical of a drug having a relatively

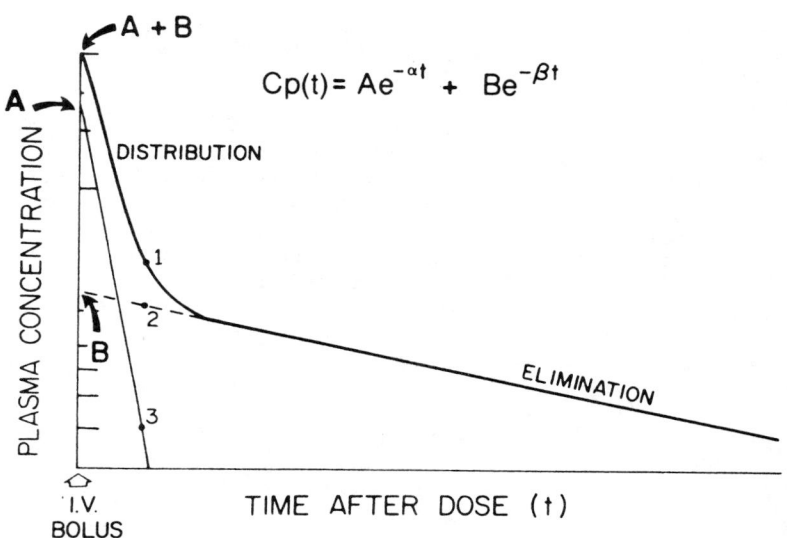

FIG. 13-10. The plasma concentration Cp(t) versus time curve for a drug with distribution (α) and elimination (β) phases. (Reprinted with permission from Stanski DR, Watkins WD: Drug Disposition in Anesthesia, p 13. New York, Grune & Stratton, 1982.)

$$Cp(t) = Ae^{-\alpha t} + Be^{-\beta t}$$

Dependence of Spontaneous Recovery Time (SRT) on Slope of Pharmacokinetic Curve

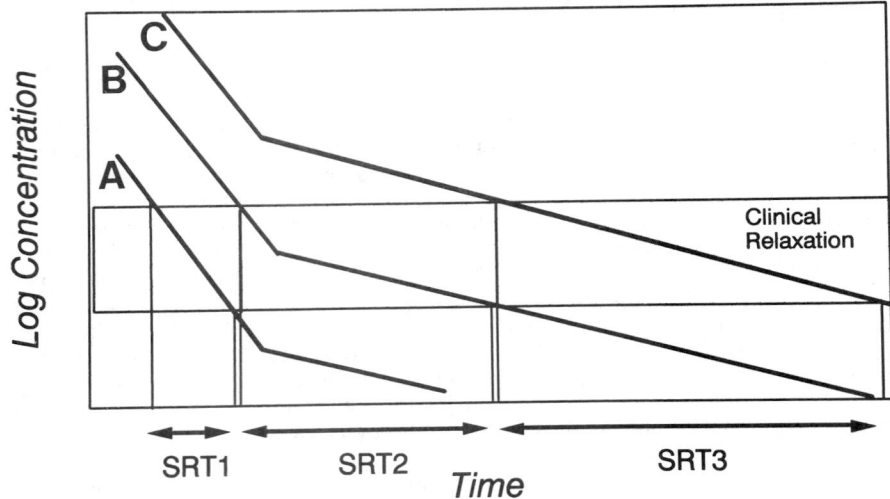

FIG. 13-11. Dependence of spontaneous recovery time (*SRT*) on the slope of a pharmacokinetic curve as it passes through the range of drug concentrations associated with clinical muscle relaxation. See text for details.

short duration of action. The other extreme is portrayed by Curve C, which shows the range of clinical activity occurring entirely during the elimination phase—a long-acting drug. Most clinical situations are represented by Curve B, where the initial decline is primarily alpha, but where a transition (the knee of the curve) to the slower beta phase occurs within the clinical range.

The higher the position of the knee of the curve in the clinical range, the greater the dependence of the drug on its terminal elimination half-life ($T_{1/2}\beta$) for recovery from the drug's clinical effect. Thus, a drug has a relatively short duration if its dose is limited, so that a substantial portion of recovery occurs during the distributive phase. At higher doses, recovery depends more upon its elimination characteristics. Drugs with the shortest and most predictable durations will have the shortest $T_{1/2}\beta$.

In distinction to the curves in Figure 13-11, the pharmacokinetic curve for atracurium does not have a sharp knee. Its $T_{1/2}\beta$ is relatively short, and the slope of the curve remains relatively steep throughout the elimination phase. Consequently, increasing the dose of atracurium does not cause a significant change in the slope of its curve passing through the concentration range associated with clinical neuromuscular blockade. The recovery index is not prolonged, even though the duration of complete block, associated with drug concentrations above the band of clinical relaxation, is lengthened.

Although plasma levels of relaxants are not measured for clinical purposes, these concepts help explain the cumulative action of muscle relaxant drugs. With either a large initial bolus or with repeated smaller doses, the knee of the pharmacokinetic curve can become elevated above the clinical range. Increasing plasma levels will change the decay characteristics for a given drug from Curve B to Curve C, and clinical activity is prolonged. Fisher and Rosen[174] demonstrated this effect by computer simulation using pharmacokinetic data available for pancuronium, vecuronium, and atracurium. Their predicted results confirm what is obvious clinically: that pancuronium is more cumulative than vecuronium, and that atracurium essentially shows no cumulative effects.

RELAXANT CLEARANCE

The clearance (Cl) of a drug can be measured in a fashion analogous to that for creatinine clearance. A drug's Cl is proportional to its V_d divided by its $T_{1/2}\beta$. For relaxants dependent upon renal or hepatic function for their excretion, decreased Cl owing to renal or hepatic disease is associated with a prolongation in $T_{1/2}\beta$ and lengthened clinical activity. This effect is represented by a flattening of that portion of the pharmacokinetic curve representing terminal elimination and has been demonstrated for gallamine,[105] metocurine,[106] dTc,[101] and pancuronium[103] in the presence of renal failure, and for vecuronium[130] in hepatic failure (Fig. 13-8).

AGE-RELATED EFFECTS

Relaxant Effects in Children

Neonates have traditionally been considered sensitive to nondepolarizing neuromuscular blocking agents, an effect ascribed to the immature status of the neuromuscular junction at birth.[175] In addition to the greater sensitivity of the myoneural junction of infants to nondepolarizing relaxants, pharmacokinetic differences, particularly their larger volume of distribution and reduced relaxant clearance, may affect the dose requirement and pattern of recovery observed.[176–178] The opposite relationship has been observed with depolarizing relaxants, that is, on a weight basis, infants require more SCh than do adults.[179] With careful monitoring of neuromuscular function, both depolarizing and nondepolarizing relaxants can be used safely in all age groups.

Relaxant Effects in the Elderly

Although pharmacodynamic studies show similar dose–response relationships in the elderly as in younger adults, that is, $Cp_{ss(50)}$ determinations are similar in both groups, pharmacokinetic studies clearly show $T_{1/2}\beta$ to increase with advancing age (Fig. 13-12).[160] Relaxants that require renal or hepatic

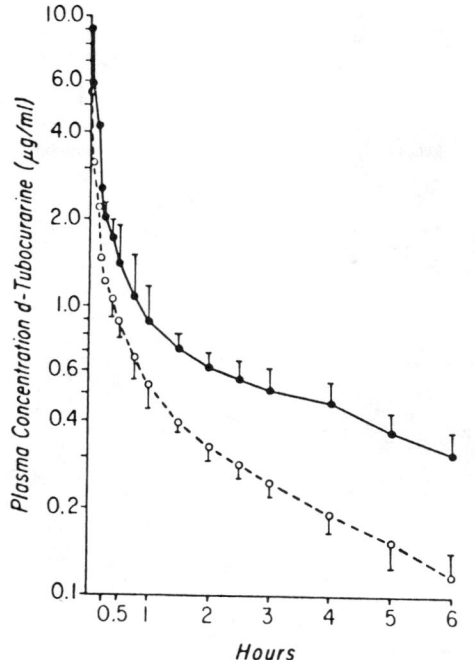

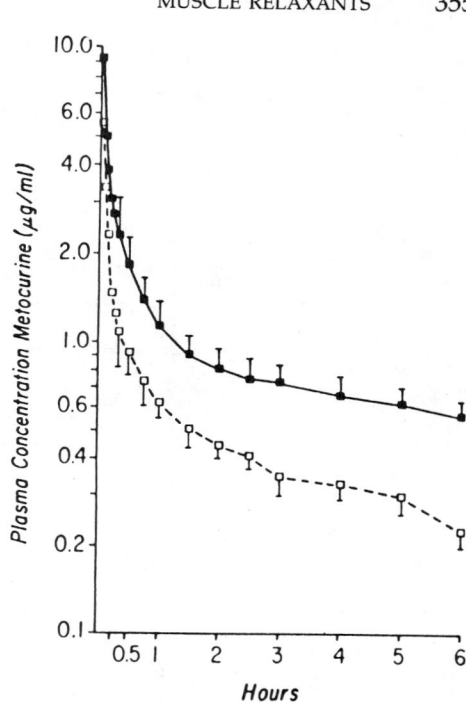

FIG. 13-12. Plasma concentration–time course curves for elderly (*solid symbols*) and young (*clear symbols*) adults receiving intravenous injection of d-tubocurarine (0.3 mg·kg⁻¹) or metocurine (0.3 mg·kg⁻¹) (Mean ± SD). (Reprinted with permission from Matteo RS, Backus WW, McDaniel DD *et al*: Pharmacokinetics and pharmacodynamics of d-tubocurarine and metocurine in the elderly. Anesth Analg 64:23, 1985.)

function for elimination can have prolonged effects when kidney or liver function is impaired. With advancing age, deteriorating renal and hepatic function commonly result in reduced maintenance dose requirements for the nondepolarizing relaxants.

Atracurium is unique as a nondepolarizing relaxant in this regard. Since it does not depend upon the kidneys or liver for its elimination, dose requirements are similar in the elderly, in younger adults, and in children, independent of renal or hepatic function (Fig. 13-13).[180] Vecuronium, on the other hand, as a result of its reliance on the liver for metabolism, is used in smaller doses in the elderly for maintenance of relaxation. (Fig. 13-13).[180, 181]

FACTORS AFFECTING RELAXANT PHARMACOKINETICS

Consider the fate of a muscle relaxant administered iv. A bolus dose is initially diluted by the patient's blood volume and distributed to highly perfused tissues, depicted as the central compartment in Figure 13-14. Some of the drug remains dissolved in its free ionized form, while part of the injected dose binds to plasma proteins, principally albumin. Drug in its bound form is inactive. Thus, the higher the degree of protein-binding, the less drug available in the active form and, all else being equal, the lower the potency of the injected dose. Binding proteins act, therefore, as a sink, draining potentially effective drug away from the site of action. Later, as plasma drug levels decline because of redistribution, metabolism, and excretion, proteins release bound drug into plasma, thus retarding the drop in free plasma level and prolonging the duration of action. Once dissolved in plasma, free drug is available to be distributed to its effector site at the neuromuscular junction, located in the peripheral compartment in

FIG. 13-13. Comparison of ORG NC 45 (vecuronium) and atracurium dose requirements and rate of recovery (*TH 10-25* and *TH 25-75*) at the completion of drug administration to patients of increasing age. (Reprinted with permission from D'Hollander AA, Luyckx C, Barvais L *et al:* Clinical evaluation of atracurium besylate requirement for a stable muscle relaxation during surgery: Lack of age-related effects. Anesthesiology 59:237, 1983.)

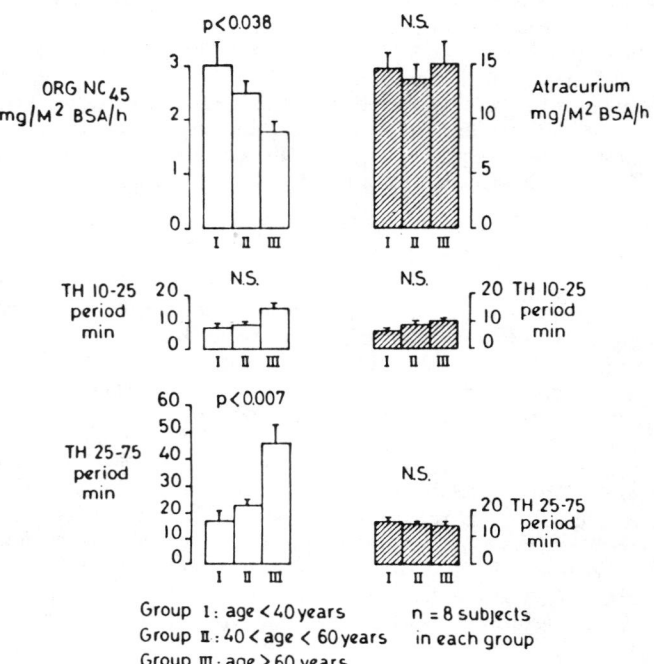

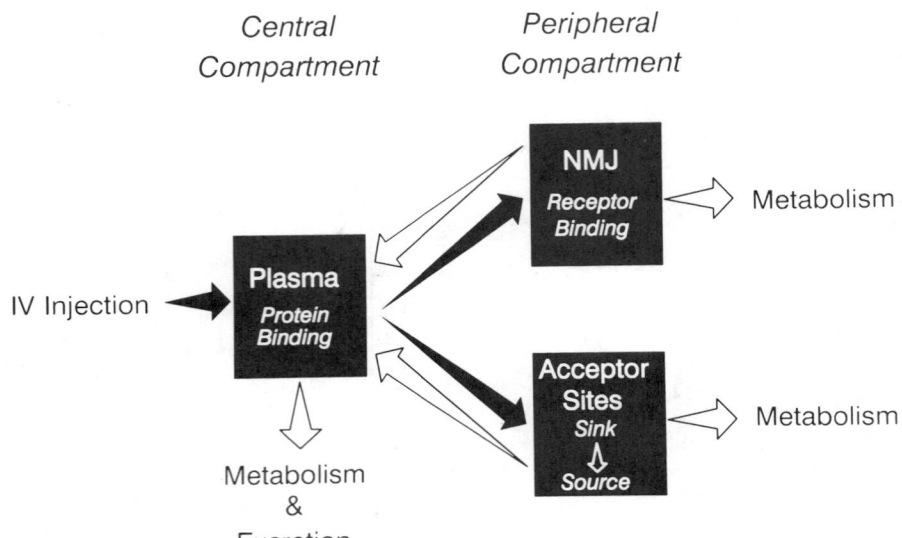

FIG. 13-14. Pharmacokinetic model of drug distribution, metabolism, and excretion. Although all other relaxants require redistribution back into plasma prior to metabolism, atracurium, uniquely, is metabolized at all sites in the body.

Figure 13-14. However, it may also be distributed to other acceptor sites where further dilution occurs.

With the exception of atracurium, nondepolarizing relaxants are eliminated by renal or biliary excretion of the unchanged drug. Additionally, hepatic metabolism of the parent compound to partially active or inactive metabolites, which are then excreted, is significant for pancuronium and vecuronium. Relaxants that have been distributed throughout the body return to the central blood volume for redistribution to the organs of elimination. Therefore, receptors at the neuromuscular junction and other acceptor sites that act initially as a sink later become a source of drug, which retards the drop in plasma concentration, analogous to the effect of protein-binding.

Pharmacokinetic modeling is further complicated in the case of atracurium because of its unique organ-independent breakdown pathways. The atracurium molecule is metabolized at all sites in the body, and therefore, need not return through the central compartment for redistribution to an organ of elimination. Although organ-independent elimination complicates the model, it is clinically relevant to the short $T_{1/2}\beta$ (21 min) determined for atracurium.

THE PRIMING PRINCIPLE

The onset of action of a muscle relaxant depends upon delivery of an effective concentration of the drug to the neuromuscular junction. In the case of nondepolarizing blockade, approximately 90%–95% of the receptors must be occupied in order to produce complete suppression of evoked twitch response.[63] Such blockade can be achieved more rapidly by giving an intentional overdose, but this carries the disadvantage of prolonged duration. Atracurium and vercuronium, as intermediate-acting drugs with short $T_{1/2}\beta$, pose less of a problem than longer-acting relaxants in this regard. Succinylcholine is particularly advantageous because of its very short $T_{1/2}\beta$. A massive overdose of SCh to effect a rapid onset does not routinely lead to a prolonged period of muscle weakness.

The priming principle has been advocated to overcome the problem of slow onset seen with nondepolarizing relaxants.[182, 183] According to the priming principle, giving a small subtherapeutic dose of a nondepolarizing relaxant prior to induction of anesthesia with subsequent administration of a full "intubating" relaxant dose hastens the onset of neuromuscular blockade. Although no clinical effect may be apparent, the priming dose may block as many as 50%–70% of receptors at the neuromuscular junction. When the rest of the relaxant dose is given, an additional 20%–40% of available receptors are blocked more rapidly than can be achieved by single bolus administration.

In addition to a more rapid onset of blockade, priming offers the possibility of using a lower total dose of relaxant with fewer side-effects and more rapid spontaneous recovery. Disadvantages include the potential for dangerously weakening awake patients and the unpredictability of individual patient response.[184–186] Priming with a drug synergistic with the relaxant used to induce neuromuscular blockade may potentially provide a more rapid onset of blockade; recovery under these circumstances, however, may be delayed because of the combination's synergism.[187]

Although Kunjappan et al[188] reported onset times using priming with vecuronium (0.015 mg · kg^{-1}) not significantly different from that following SCh (1.5 mg · kg^{-1}), other investigators have been unable to reliably shorten the onset of complete twitch suppression to less than 2 minutes. In determining the ideal priming dose and time interval before giving the remainder of the relaxant, Taboada et al[189] recommended a 0.01 mg · kg^{-1} priming dose of vecuronium, followed 4 minutes later by the remainder (0.09 mg · kg^{-1}) of an intubating dose of vecuronium. For atracurium, Naguib et al[113] suggested a priming dose of 0.06 to 0.08 mg · kg^{-1}, followed 3 minutes later by the remainder of 0.5 mg · kg^{-1} dose.

Consequently, because of its reliably rapid onset, SCh remains the relaxant of choice in situations demanding rapid sequence induction of anesthesia. However, if SCh is contraindicated and nondepolarizing relaxants are chosen instead, the priming principle can be used in an attempt to facilitate the onset of neuromuscular blockade. Atracurium or vecuronium are the preferred relaxants in this setting because of their relatively shorter durations of action. Under these circumstances, ventilation of the lungs with mask oxygen and positive pressure may be required while cricoid pressure is ap-

TABLE 13-5. Loading Doses (mg · kg^{-1}) and Continuous Infusion Doses (μg · kg^{-1} · min^{-1}) to Maintain Approximately 90% Neuromuscular Blockade

DRUG	LOADING DOSE	INFUSION DOSE	
		N$_2$O/Opioid	Inhalational
Succinylcholine	1.0–1.5	60–100	30–50
Atracurium	0.3–0.5	5–10	3–6
Vecuronium	0.06–0.10	1–2	0.6–1.2

plied, until the degree of blockade is sufficient for tracheal intubation to proceed.

MAINTENANCE OF NEUROMUSCULAR BLOCKADE

To maintain a clinically effective degree of muscle relaxation, the serum level of relaxant must be maintained in a therapeutic range. As the T$_{1/2}$β of a relaxant decreases, so does the interval between the required supplemental relaxant doses. Intermediate-acting relaxants such as atracurium and vecuronium require supplementation at shorter intervals (10–20 min) than do longer-acting relaxants (30–60 min).

Drugs with a very short T$_{1/2}$β, such as SCh are conveniently given as a continuous infusion to maintain a steady degree of blockade (rather than as intermittent boluses). A continuous infusion may be considered an infinite number of miniscule doses injected at very short intervals. Because newly infused relaxant molecules take the place of those removed from the neuromuscular junction, plasma drug level fluctuation becomes diminishingly small.

Both atracurium[190] and vecuronium[191] have been given as continuous infusions throughout surgery to provide constant levels of relaxation, which is then easily reversible soon after the drug's discontinuation. Recommended doses[152] are shown in Table 13-5. Neuromuscular blockade is generally established from an initial bolus dose, and an infusion is started once recovery has been documented. From a practical standpoint, one or two twitches of the train-of-four should remain visible during maintenance relaxation. Reappearance of the third and fourth twitches suggests the need for augmenting the infusion rate, whereas the persistent absence of all four twitches risks drug overdose and block irreversibility.

As new drugs (mivacurium) with even shorter half-lives become introduced, infusion techniques are expected to replace the traditional technique of intermittent bolus dosing. Although mechanically controlled infusion pumps have been used, steady-state relaxation can be achieved using intermediate-duration relaxants with simple gravity drip devices.

ANTAGONISM OF NEUROMUSCULAR BLOCKADE

At the conclusion of surgery, residual neuromuscular blockade may put the patient at risk for developing potentially life-threatening hypoxia or respiratory acidosis owing to inadequate ventilation. Even when muscular strength is sufficient to sustain normal minute ventilation, the patient's ability to maintain an unobstructed airway and produce an effective secretion-clearing cough may be compromised. Whereas some degree of respiratory depression resulting from residual opioid or sedative effects can be tolerated in the early postoperative recovery phase because of their therapeutic benefit, any degree of residual neuromuscular blockade is unwarranted and must be avoided.

ASSESSMENT OF NEUROMUSCULAR RECOVERY

It is the anesthesiologist's responsibility to ensure complete clinical recovery of neuromuscular function before withdrawing ventilatory support and airway protection. Appraisal of recovery is best accomplished by monitoring the depth of neuromuscular blockade throughout the procedure, so that only appropriate relaxant doses are given and that antagonism of residual blockade, if it exists, can be facilitated. In addition to confirming return to control of the single twitch, complete recovery of the train-of-four and a sustained tetanus at 50 to 100 Hz stimulation, the anesthesiologist should look for clinical evidence of complete recovery. Clinical signs include adequate respiratory efforts, a sustained hand grip, the ability to sustain limb or head movement against gravity, and the absence of discoordinated movements during voluntary muscular activity.

RECOVERY FOLLOWING SUCCINYLCHOLINE

Recovery from SCh-induced depolarizing blockade is generally spontaneous and does not require pharmacologic antagonism. Because of its rapid hydrolysis by plasma cholinesterase, the plasma half-life of SCh is 3.5 minutes;[153] complete recovery from a profound SCh-induced blockade occurs in 10 to 15 minutes. In patients with atypical cholinesterase, a routine dose of SCh causes profound, prolonged paralysis with delayed spontaneous recovery. With routine twitch monitoring, those patients with genotypically abnormal plasma cholinesterase can be clinically detected before additional relaxants are given.

The normal pattern of recovery of the train-of-four response following a depolarizing blockade exhibits equal amplitude of all four twitches (T$_4$/T$_1$ = 1). Following repeated SCh doses or a prolonged SCh infusion, even in normal persons, depolarizing blockade may change to resemble characteristic nondepolarizing blockade by monitoring criteria.

The transition from SCh-induced depolarizing blockade to Phase II blockade is best detected by the development of fade in the train-of-four response (T$_4$/T$_1$ < 0.5). In the setting of a Phase II blockade, the anesthesiologist must be alert to the possibility of delayed clinical recovery (Fig. 13–15). Lee[18] associated the development of Phase II blockade with tachyphylaxis to SCh infusion and found the transition during halothane anesthesia to occur at a fairly low total SCh dose of 2 to 5 mg · kg^{-1}.

Ramsey et al[19] found a more variable response over a wide dosage range during balanced anesthesia; a correlation between tachyphylaxis and the transition to Phase II blockade was not evident. Although 50% of their patients exhibited a prolonged recovery, it was not possible to predict, based on dose alone, which patients would recover slowly.

In slowly recovering patients, anticholinesterase drugs can effectively accelerate recovery once a plateau in recovery has been reached. A 5-mg test dose of edrophonium with 0.4 mg of atropine should be used to ensure an effective response and, if successful, followed by additional edrophonium or neostigmine to effect reversal. (Fig. 13-16 depicts effective

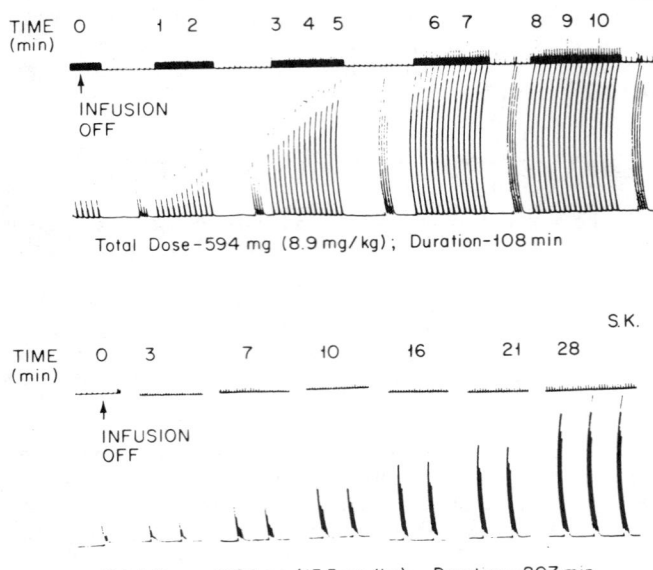

FIG. 13-15. Spontaneous recovery from Phase II blockade induced during infusion of succinylcholine. *Upper trace:* rapid spontaneous recovery in less than 10 minutes. *Lower trace:* prolonged recovery, showing evidence of train-of-four fade 28 minutes after the infusion had been discontinued. (Reprinted with permission from Ramsey FM, Lebowitz PW, Savarese JJ et al: Clinical characteristics of long-term succinycholine neuromuscular blockade during balanced anesthesia. Anesth Analg 59:110, 1980.)

antagonism of residual train-of-four fade resulting from SCh infusion.)

An anticholinesterase drug should not be given during the early recovery phase because it may inhibit plasma cholinesterase and further slow the breakdown of SCh. However, Donati et al[192] were able to antagonize Phase II blockade successfully as soon as 10 minutes after discontinuing a SCh infusion. Although antagonism of Phase II blockade is possible in patients who metabolize SCh normally, it is not recommended in the setting of a patient with atypical plasma cholin-

esterase. In such a patient, anticholinesterase drugs may contribute to prolongation of SCh-induced blockade.

RECOVERY FOLLOWING NONDEPOLARIZERS

Owing to its competitive nature, nondepolarizing neuromuscular blockade may be antagonized by anticholinesterase drugs (Fig. 13-17). Acetylcholine and nondepolarizing relaxants exist in dynamic equilibrium, competing for the same binding sites at the neuromuscular junction. Anything that increases the concentration of ACh or decreases the concentration of a nondepolarizing muscle relaxant in the synaptic cleft will favor reversal of the blockade and restoration of neuromuscular transmission. AChE-inhibiting agents extend the half-life of ACh, raise its concentration, and allow ACh to displace nondepolarizing relaxants from their binding sites at the postjunctional membrane. Following displacement by mass action from cholinergic receptors by the increased concentration of ACh, unbound drug is washed away from its site of action, as it flows along a concentration gradient from the synaptic cleft back into plasma.

Anticholinesterase drugs also act prejunctionally to increase neuromuscular transmission. These drugs induce stimulus-bound repetitive axonal firing of nerve terminals and facilitate CA^{++} uptake into nerve terminals;[7] through the latter mechanism, mobilization and release of ACh are enhanced. Although antagonism of nondepolarizing neuromuscular blockade appears to be predominantly postjunctional, prejunctional effects may play a significant role in the effectiveness of anticholinesterase drugs.

Reversal of nondepolarizing neuromuscular blockade is due to redistribution of relaxant away from its site of action. At steady-state conditions, a given plasma concentration is associated with a given degree of blockade. However, patients are rarely in steady-state, and any depth of block may be associated with a range of plasma concentrations. If the plasma concentration is high, the gradient for relaxant washout will be low and antagonism may be difficult. This clinical situation may occur if reversal is attempted closely following supplemental relaxant administration. Katz[193] demonstrated this effect in four patients in whom neuromuscular blockade was more difficult to antagonize from 80%–90% twitch suppression after they had received a supplemental bolus dose of

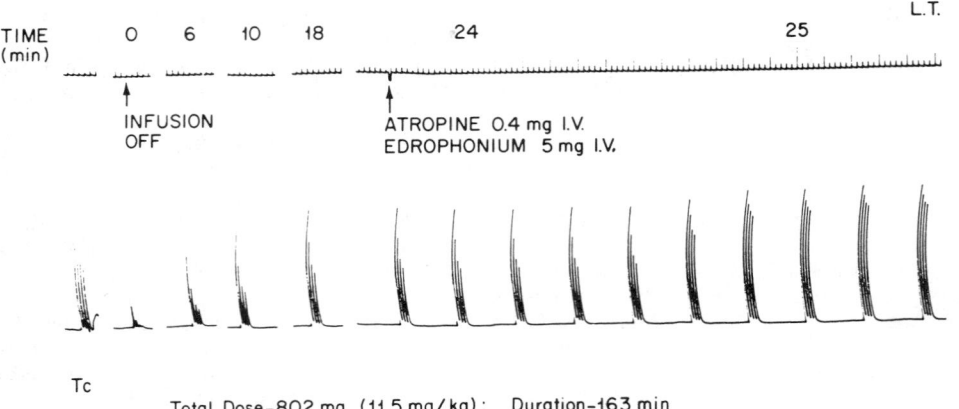

FIG. 13-16. Antagonism of residual Phase II block with edrophonium. Spontaneous recovery over 23 minutes to T_1 = 70% of control, and T_4 = 50% of T_1. Within 1.5 minutes following edrophonium administration, T_4 = 85% of T_1. (Reprinted with permission from Ramsey FM *et al:* Anesth Analg 59:110, 1980.)

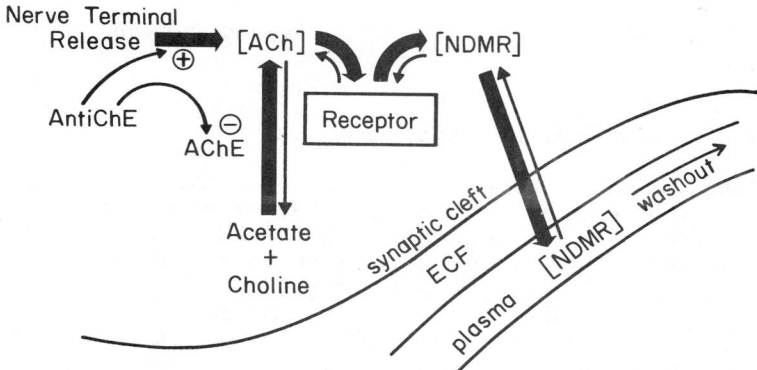

FIG. 13-17. Pharmacodynamics of antagonism of neuro-muscular blockade. Anticholinesterase (Anti ChE) administration causes increased concentration of acetylcholine (ACh) to accumulate at receptor sites. Nondepolarizing muscle relaxant (NDMR) is displaced from receptors and flows from the vicinity of the receptor along a concentration gradient back into plasma, thus clearing the relaxant from the neuromuscular junction.

relaxant than it was from a similar degree of blockade following spontaneous recovery subsequent to a single large dose given much earlier.

ANTICHOLINESTERASE (ACETYLCHOLINESTERASE-INHIBITING) DRUGS

Clinically useful anticholinesterase drugs include neostigmine, pyridostigmine, and edrophonium.[194] Neostigmine and pyridostigmine bind covalently with AChE to form an inactive carbamylated complex, which ultimately is hydrolyzed to form regenerated AChE. Edrophonium, on the other hand, binds electrostatically and reversibly with the enzyme. Since covalent bonds are not formed or broken, the magnitude and duration of the inhibition are less with edrophonium than with neostigmine or pyridostigmine.

For many years, edrophonium was not considered useful for reversing a nondepolarizing blockade because of edrophonium's short duration of action compared with that of dTc-type drugs. Potentially, recurarization could occur. However, a dose of edrophonium, sufficiently large as to maintain an effective concentration throughout the period of reversal, securely antagonizes the block.[195, 196] The pharmacokinetics of edrophonium at this dose range are similar to those of neostigmine, that is, its $T_{1/2}\beta$ is longer than that of dTc.[197] Therefore, given an adequate dose of edrophonium, recurarization should not occur. Furthermore, in the absence of renal function, plasma clearance of AChE drugs is delayed as long, if not longer, than nondepolarizing muscle relaxants, making the occurrence of recurarization unlikely.

Anticholinesterase drugs have potent muscarinic stimulating properties on the heart (SA and AV node slowing), bronchi (bronchoconstriction and secretion production), and gut (peristalsis). These cholinergic side-effects can be blocked by either prior or simultaneous administration of an anticholinergic drug. Ramamurthy et al[198] recommend the use of glycopyrrolate in place of atropine when antagonizing residual neuromuscular blockade with neostigmine or pyridostigmine. The time course of action in terms of onset and duration of these drugs is more synchronous with that of glycopyrrolate than that of atropine, which has a more rapid onset and shorter duration of action. The simultaneous administration of glycopyrrolate with either neostigmine or pyridostigmine leads to minimal changes in HR,[199] which may be important in patients with ischemic or valvular heart disease, where wide swings in HR could pose a hazard. Atropine is better suited for

combination with edrophonium because of their better matched, more rapid onsets of action.[200]

A high incidence of transient arrhythmias occurs following administration of reversal agents. These electrocardiographic (ECG) effects vary from innocuous changes in the atrial pacemaker to junctional rhythms, ectopic ventricular foci, and high-grade heart block, including complete heart block and cardiac arrest. It is imperative that the anesthesiologist monitor the ECG during the reversal process in order to detect these arrhythmias and treat the more serious ones. No combination of anticholinergic/AChE or pattern of administration guarantees a stable cardiac rhythm.

The anesthetic technique may also play a role in determining the incidence and severity of cardiac dysrhythmias following reversal. For example, Urquhart et al[201] found cardiac dysrhythmias to be more frequent and more serious following reversal with a mixture of edrophonium and atropine during N_2O/fentanyl anesthesia than during isoflurane/N_2O anesthesia. They concluded that the combined vagotonic effects of fentanyl and edrophonium on AV conduction may have precipitated a greater degree of heart block than was seen with edrophonium following inhalational anesthesia.

Although it is not the drug of choice for antagonism of a profound neuromuscular blockade,[202–207] edrophonium possesses several advantages over neostigmine and pyridostigmine for reversal of light or intermediate blockade. Its onset of action peaks in less than 5 minutes, compared with 7 to 10 minutes for neostigmine and 12 to 15 minutes for pyridostigmine. Consequently, edrophonium yields information regarding reversibility more quickly than do the other two drugs.

In addition, Cronnelly et al[207] have demonstrated that edrophonium possesses less potent muscarinic side-effects than does neostigmine or pyridostigmine. Thus, the dose of anticholinergic drug can be reduced by one half with edrophonium under usual circumstances and need not be increased when the dose of edrophonium is increased. Because of edrophonium's very rapid onset, atropine is the preferred accompanying anticholinergic drug. Although anticholinergic drugs may be administered simultaneously with neostigmine or pyridostigmine, atropine administration preceding edrophonium diminishes the risk of bradycardia or heart block.

Glycopyrrolate, in comparison with atropine, is also associated with more rapid patient arousal when combined with neostigmine for reversal of neuromuscular blockade.[208] Since glycopyrrolate does not cross the blood-brain barrier as readily as does atropine, it has less proclivity for inducing CNS depression.

FACTORS AFFECTING REVERSIBILITY

When a nondepolarizing neuromuscular blockade is antagonized with anticholinesterase drug, the dose selected for any given drug depends upon the depth of blockade at the point of reversal. Larger doses are required at greater degrees of blockade (Table 13-6). Furthermore, neostigmine has been shown to be more effective than edrophonium for antagonism of profound neuromuscular blockade.[202-207] Edrophonium is not recommended for antagonism of neuromuscular blockade when fewer than all four twitches are visible with train-of-four stimulation.[209]

The time to effective recovery is directly related to the intensity of the blockade at the point of reversal.[193] Thus, whereas modest blockade may recover in several minutes, profound blockade may take 20 to 30 minutes or more for adequate antagonism. The time to effective recovery following reversal from atracurium- or vecuronium-induced neuromuscular blockade is similar to that of dTc or pancuronium for a given depth of blockade at the point of reversal. The advantage of atracurium or vecuronium in this regard is not that the blockade is easier to reverse, but that patients will recover spontaneously to a reversible degree of blockade sooner than occurs following use of longer-acting relaxants. Thus, the enhanced recovery achieved with anticholinesterase drugs and the spontaneous recovery rate are both important in determining the clinical recovery time.

The ability to antagonize nondepolarizing neuromuscular blockade can be affected by temperature, metabolic factors, and other drugs that potentiate neuromuscular blocking agents. Profound hypothermia to less than 30°C, as occurs in the setting of cardiopulmonary bypass, has pharmacodynamic and pharmacokinetic effects on neuromuscular transmission,[210] leading to lesser or greater relaxant requirements, depending upon the relaxant used.[211] In the more usual clinical setting, antagonism can be difficult when core temperature approaches 32°C, probably secondary to pharmacokinetic factors affecting drug redistribution. Blood flow to the neuromuscular junction may be reduced by cold-induced vasoconstriction, limiting delivery of anticholinesterase drugs to the neuromuscular junction and making washout of relaxant difficult.

Respiratory acidosis and metabolic alkalosis,[212, 213] as well as hypokalemia,[214] and hypermagnesemia,[215] are associated with difficulty in antagonizing neuromuscular blockade. The effect of acute changes in pH, Pa_{CO_2}, and electrolytes may differ significantly from those caused by chronic changes. Acute hypokalemia, for example, produces a state of hyperpolarization, that is, the muscle's resting potential is more negative intracellularly and the skeletal muscle is harder to depolarize. Consequently, hypokalemia tends to potentiate nondepolarizing relaxants and make reversal more difficult. In chronic hypokalemia, both extracellular and intracellular K^+ decrease, so that, theoretically, there may be no change in the resting transmembrane potential.

Consistent with the findings for acutely produced hypokalemia, Miller et al[213] noted that metabolic alkalosis made dTc blockade difficult to reverse. Respiratory acidosis, but not respiratory alkalosis or metabolic acidosis, also accentuated the blockade in this setting. Miller and Roderick[212] showed these acid–base relationships to be true for pancuronium as well.

Since Ca^{++} plays important roles in the mobilization and release of ACh from motor nerve terminals, concentrations of Mg^{++} sufficient to antagonize these effects can be clinically significant in the setting of parenteral magnesium therapy for eclampsia or preeclampsia.[215] Theoretically, hypocalcemia may augment nondepolarizing neuromuscular blockade, but clinical significance has not been well established.

Consequently, when difficulty is encountered in attempting reversal, additional AChE-inhibitor can be administered up to the maximal doses shown in Table 13-6. If the maximal recommended doses are not sufficient, additional doses are unlikely to further augment recovery and may lead to heightened side-effects. In this setting, where relative overdose of relaxant, metabolic abnormality, or drug interaction at the neuromuscular junction lead to incomplete reversal of blockade, the patient's airway should be protected with an endotracheal tube, and ventilatory support should be provided until full clinical recovery ensues.

PRACTICAL ISSUES IN REVERSAL

Recommendations regarding antagonism of nondepolarizing neuromuscular blockade are given in Table 13-7. The most important consideration is to avoid overdosing the patient with a muscle relaxant in temporal proximity to antagonism. Appropriate dosing is best accomplished by carefully monitoring neuromuscular function with train-of-four stimulation throughout the anesthetic.

A current controversy exists regarding the routine need to

TABLE 13-6.   Anticholinesterase (and Anticholinergic) Drug Doses ($\mu g \cdot kg^{-1}$) Recommended for Antagonism of Residual Nondepolarizing Neuromuscular Blockade

DEPTH OF BLOCK	TRAIN-OF-FOUR	NEOSTIGMINE (Glycopyrrolate)	PYRIDOSTIGMINE (Glycopyrrolate)	EDROPHONIUM (Atropine)
Shallow	4 of 4 twitches visible (with fade)	25 (5)	100 (5)	500 (10)
Intermediate	2–3 of 4 twitches visible (with fade)	50 (10)	200 (10)	1000 (10)
Deep	0–1 twitches visible	75 (15)	300 (15)	Not recommended

TABLE 13-7.   Recommendations for Muscle Relaxant Reversal

1. Monitor neuromuscular function throughout the course of anesthesia.
2. Maintain some level of measurable function by train-of-four monitoring.
3. Strive to have three or four twitches of the train-of-four visible by the time of anticipated relaxant reversal.
4. Adjust doses of reversal agents according to the depth of block, as listed in Table 13-6.
5. Monitor train-of-four during the recovery period.
6. Support ventilation during the recovery period.
7. Assess recovery by clinical criteria before discontinuing ventilatory support.

antagonize residual nondepolarizing neuromuscular blockade. Administering an anticholinesterase drug to free subclinically occupied receptors from competitive blockade, even when monitoring criteria suggest complete spontaneous recovery, theoretically increases the margin of safety of neuromuscular transmission. Pharmacologic antagonism of longer-acting relaxants has become the standard of care. Nevertheless, many anesthesiologists believe that use of atracurium and vecuronium allows room for clinical judgment regarding the necessity of routinely administering AChE drugs.

To date, there have been no reports of "recurarization" following adequate recovery from atracurium or vecuronium. Their shorter half-lives reflect an enhanced rate of receptor freeing, which increases the margin of safety of neuromuscular transmission, in and of itself. Just the same, clinical criteria, as well as monitoring criteria, for recovery must be met. Allowing some time, perhaps a drug half-life, to elapse following documentation of complete spontaneous recovery before extubating the patient's trachea provides additional security.

Proponents of routine reversal aruge that the neuromuscular margin of safety is improved by administering a relaxant antagonist, even though the clinical benefit may not be measurable. Those who argue for relying on clinical judgment cite the pharmacologic risks of reversal. If a clinician elects not to administer reversal drugs, full recovery should be ensured and documented in the patient's record.

An additional, different approach to achieving reversal of competitive blockade is exemplified by use of 4-aminopyridine, which does not inhibit AChE but, rather, selectively blocks K^+ channels located at motor nerve terminals. As a result, repolarization of the nerve terminal is delayed after it has been depolarized. Increased Ca^{++} influx at the nerve terminal consequently leads to marked enhancement of ACh release, which competitively displaces nondepolarizing relaxant from receptors at the neuromuscular junction.

Although 4-aminopyridine can antagonize competitive neuromuscular blockade alone or in combination with anticholinesterase drugs, it has not gained acceptance in clinical practice because of CNS side-effects. Its ability to cross the blood–brain barrier results in CNS excitability, possibly leading to seizure activity.[216]

CLINICALLY IMPORTANT MUSCLE RELAXANT/DRUG INTERACTIONS

Prominent among the drug interactions that affect the clinical activity of muscle relaxants are those between one type of relaxant and another.

SUCCINYLCHOLINE AND NONDEPOLARIZERS

Because SCh behaves as an agonist at the neuromuscular junction, it is opposed by the antagonist function of nondepolarizing relaxants. This interaction has found clinical application in the administration of a small, subclinical dose of a nondepolarizing relaxant several minutes before giving SCh to aid in tracheal intubation.[217] Such pretreatment is intended to minimize side-effects from the depolarizing action of SCh, primarily reducing SCh-induced muscle fasciculations. Whether pretreatment effectively decreases the incidence or severity of postoperative muscle pain, however, is controversial.[218, 219] Nevertheless, it is clear that the effectiveness of a given dose of SCh is reduced by the competitive action of nondepolarizing relaxants at the neuromuscular junction and that the SCh dose should generally be increased following pretreatment in order to reach the same depth of depolarizing blockade.[220]

Erkola et al[217] found that dTc was more effective than gallamine, pancuronium, or vecuronium in preventing fasciculations and that dTc also interfered more with the depth of depolarizing blockade. The best intubating conditions and the longest duration of depolarizing blockade were seen with pancuronium, which exhibits mild anticholinesterase activity.

In contrast, SCh potentiates the effects of subsequently administered nondepolarizing relaxants.[221] Following recovery of neuromuscular blockade induced by SCh, a lower dose of nondepolarizing relaxant is required to re-establish neuromuscular blockade; residual SCh effects make the neuromuscular junction more vulnerable to blockade by competitive relaxants. This activity probably represents an early manifestation of Phase II-type blockade. In the presence of Phase II blockade following repeated or prolonged use of SCh by infusion, documented by fade to train-of-four stimulation, a small dose of a nondepolarizing relaxant can exert an unusually profound degree of blockade.

Some anesthesiologists have advocated that SCh be added to a recovering nondepolarizing blockade near the conclusion of surgery to aid in peritoneal closure. However, the agonist action of SCh can antagonize a competitive blockade in a fashion similar to that seen after administration of an anticholinesterase drug (Fig. 13-18A–D).[222] In the presence of nondepolarizing neuromuscular blockade, a small dose of SCh (20 mg) accelerates reversal of blockade, which is then reestablished with administration of an additional nondepolarizing relaxant. Subsequently, a larger dose of SCh (100 mg) causes transient partial reversal, followed by complete twitch suppression. Following SCh metabolism, neuromuscular function recovers to a level greater than that which existed prior to SCh administration. In this setting, SCh exerts dual effects: It partially antagonizes the nondepolarizing blockade, and it induces depolarizing blockade. It is possible that some Phase II blockade also contributes to the residual blockade that persists after the SCh is metabolized.

SUCCINYLCHOLINE AND ANTICHOLINESTERASE DRUGS

Plasma cholinesterase, which hydrolyzes SCh, is inhibited by the same anticholinesterase drugs that act on AChE. Therefore, giving SCh following anticholinesterase drug administration, as may occur in the setting of laryngospasm treatment after extubation of the trachea, can be expected to cause pro-

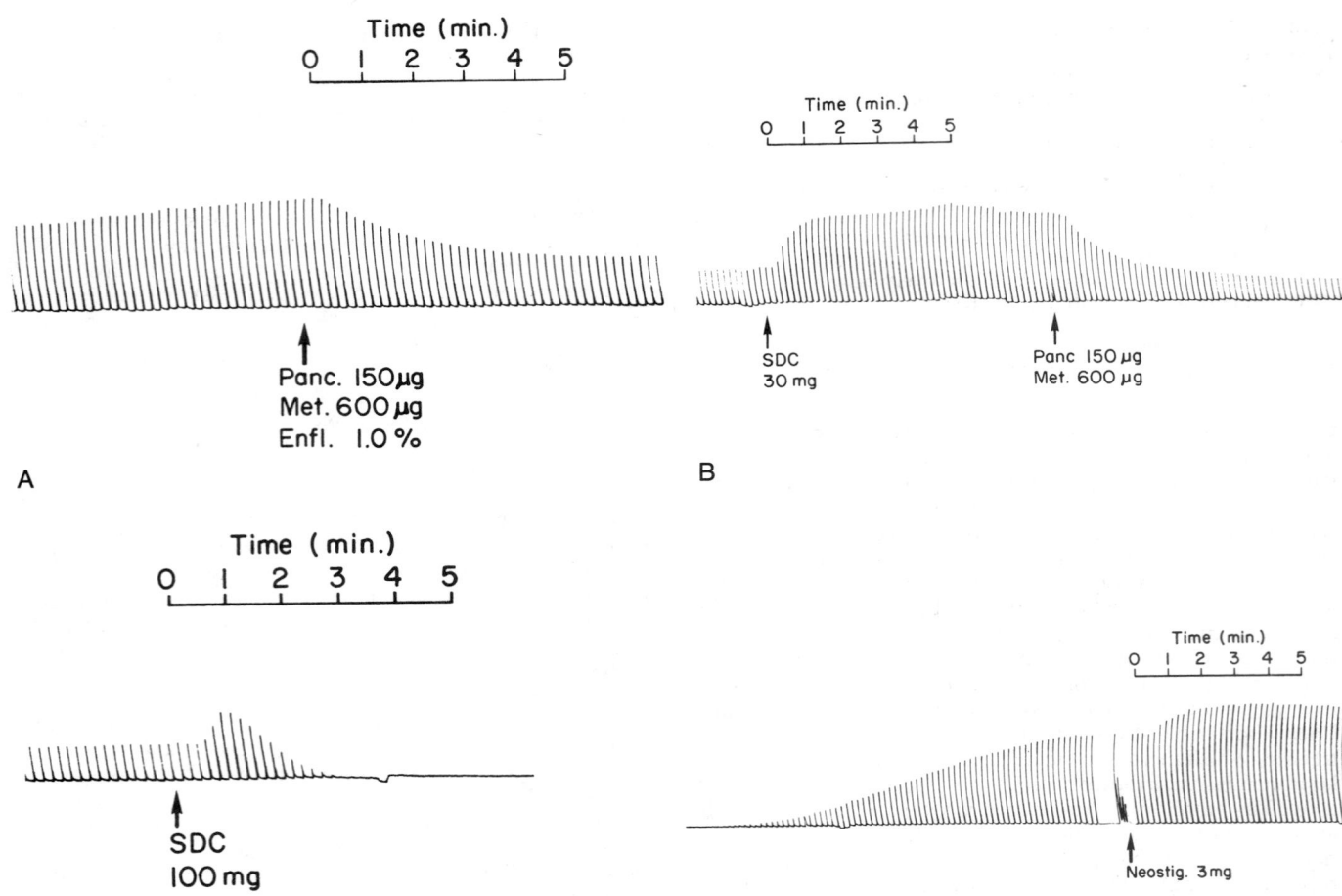

FIG. 13-18. Interaction of depolarizing and nondepolarizing relaxants. (*A*) Nondepolarizing blockade is produced by pancuronium and metocurine during enflurane anesthesia. (*B*) Partial reversal of nondepolarizing blockade occurs after giving succinylcholine (SDC), which acts as an agonist compound, displacing nondepolarizing muscle relaxant from receptors in a fashion similar to that of acetylcholine (ACh). The blockade is then reinstituted following additional pancuronium and metocurine administration. (*C*) A larger dose of succinylcholine begins to antagonize the nondepolarizing blockade but, because of the dose size, proceeds to depolarize the membrane instead. (*D*) Relatively rapid recovery from succinylcholine-induced blockade, showing residual fade, indicative of the pre-existing nondepolarizing blockade from pancuronium and metocurine, and possibly some Phase II effects from succinylcholine as well. Neostigmine easily antagonizes the residual blockade.

longed depolarizing blockade with the potential for development of Phase II blockade.

Chronic therapy with anticholinesterase drugs such as echothiophate can have long-lasting effects.[223] Functional quantities of plasma cholinesterase may be deficient for several weeks following cessation of these eyedrops. Although SCh is not absolutely contraindicated in such patients, most clinicians would avoid it or use much reduced doses and carefully monitor neuromuscular function.

NONDEPOLARIZER COMBINATIONS

Nondepolarizing muscle relaxants are not interchangeable in terms of their effects at the neuromuscular junction. Lebowitz et al[224] demonstrated a synergistic relationship between pancuronium and metocurine, as well as between pancuronium and *d*Tc, while combined doses of metocurine and *d*Tc were only additive. Because individual nondepolarizing relaxants possess both presynaptic and postsynaptic effects, a possible explanation for synergism between nondepolarizing relaxant pairs could relate to differing affinities of each drug for pre- and postsynaptic receptors. The clinical application of such synergism permits small equipotent doses of two drugs to produce a degree of neuromuscular blockade that would otherwise require four times the dose of either drug alone. Monitoring neuromuscular function is particularly important in this setting to avoid an unintentional overdose.

The authors further demonstrated two significant advantages of intentionally mixing paired combinations of nondepolarizing relaxants.[74] Utilizing mixtures of pancuronium and metocurine, they showed that recovery from a given degree of measured blockade occurred sooner and that hemodynamic side-effects of pancuronium were lessened by using reduced doses of both drugs. Although they were unable to demonstrate a significant reduction in onset time with combination therapy when the doses were reduced to compensate for the synergism, they did find faster onset if the doses were not reduced. Similar to the situation achieved by increasing the dose of a single agent to several times the ED_{95} for neuromuscular blockade, the blockade produced by normal dose combination therapy was deeper and was more prolonged than that resulting from a combination of low doses.

RELAXANTS AND OTHER DRUGS

In addition to muscle relaxants themselves, other drugs used during anesthesia can have profound effects on muscle relaxation. The potent inhalational agents significantly potentiate the neuromuscular blocking effects of muscle relaxants and thereby reduce their dose requirements (Fig. 13-19).[11, 225] This action has been demonstrated for diethyl ether,[226] halothane,[227] enflurane,[226, 228] and isoflurane.[226, 227] Waud and Waud,[229] investigating the site of inhalational anesthetics' suppression of neuromuscular function, concluded it to be postsynaptic, at a stage subsequent to the interaction of ACh and the cholinergic receptor. Fogdall and Miller[228] compared equi-MAC concentrations of halothane, enflurane, and isoflurane and determined their effect on the ED_{50} for inhibition of thumb twitch by dTc or pancuronium. The doses of long-acting relaxants may be reduced by about one third for halothane and by about one half to two thirds for enflurane and isoflurane, compared with doses required during N_2O/opioid anesthesia. With atracurium and vecuronium, the degree of potentiation by inhalational agents is not as great, and relaxant doses should be reduced only by about one fourth (Fig. 13-20).[230, 231]

FIG. 13-19. Volatile anesthetics cause dose-dependent and anesthetic drug-specific enhancement of neuromuscular blockade produced by long-acting nondepolarizing muscle relaxants (Mean ± SE). (Reprinted with permission from Ali HH, Savarese JJ: Monitoring of neuromuscular function. Anesthesiology 45:216, 1976.)

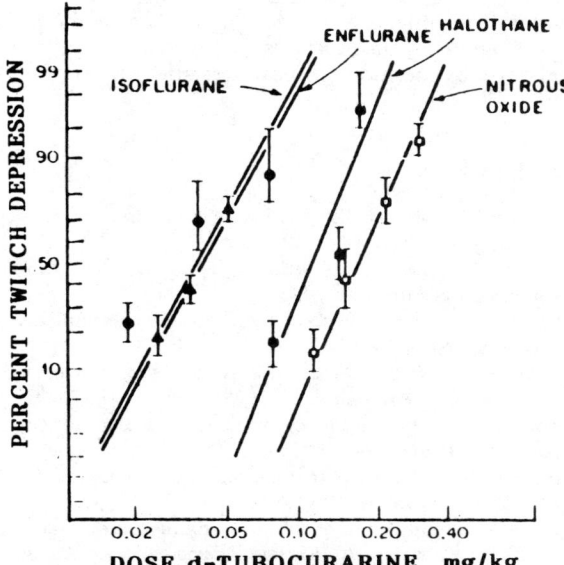

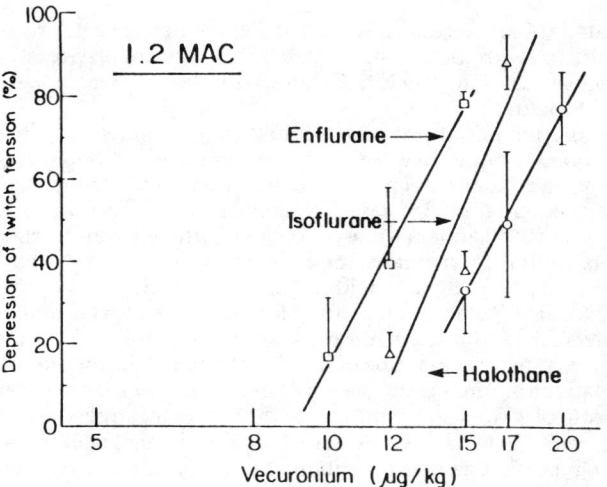

FIG. 13-20. The impact of volatile anesthetics on the required dose of vecuronium (Mean ± SD). (Reprinted with permission from Rupp SM, Miller RD, Gencarelli PJ: Vecuronium-induced neuromuscular blockade during enflurane, isoflurane, and halothane anesthesia in humans. Anesthesiology 60:102, 1984.)

Stanski et al[155] demonstrated a time-dependent effect of enflurane on pancuronium-induced neuromuscular blockade, so that in long anesthetics, the degree of potentiation progressively increases. At the beginning of anesthesia, when the end-tidal concentration of an inhalational agent is low, potentiation may not be manifest. Therefore, the dose of relaxant needed to establish blockade at this time is the same, regardless of the type of anesthesia used. However, with monitoring of neuromuscular function as a guide, supplemental relaxant doses should be reduced or the interval between them lengthened when potent inhalational anesthetics are used. Furthermore, a reduction in the plasma concentration of an inhalational anesthetic, as occurs during emergence, is associated with enhanced recovery of neuromuscular function, even during constant relaxant infusion.[232]

Therapeutic levels of antibiotics such as streptomycin or other aminoglycosides have neuromuscular blocking effects that potentiate nondepolarizing relaxants.[233] This potentiation has been attributed to both Mg^{++}-like prejunctional effect, inhibiting release of ACh from nerve terminals, and a postjunctional membrane stabilizing action. Although some reversal is observed with anticholinesterase drugs or administration of Ca^{++}, antagonism may be incomplete. Polymyxin-induced blockade, in fact, appears not to be pharmacologically reversible. Irrigation of the abdominal or thoracic cavities with neomycin has been associated with profound neuromuscular blockade.[234] However, neomycin given through the alimentary tract for bowel preparation prior to surgery is not absorbed in sufficient quantities as to affect neuromuscular transmission. Fortunately, the penicillins and cephalosporins do not have significant effects on clinical muscle relaxation.

The neuromuscular blocking properties of procaine have been known for many years. Local anesthetics inhibit transmission at the neuromuscular junction, either by reducing the ACh content of the quanta or by decreasing the sensitivity of the postjunctional membrane to ACh by blocking Na^+ channels. Matsuo et al[235] found potentiation of dTc or pancuronium by cocaine, procaine, lidocaine, and etidocaine. Quinidine, related pharmacologically to local anesthetics, acts synergistically with both depolarizers and nondepolarizers, as much as doubling the intensity and duration of neuromuscular blockade.

Although barbiturates and opioids have no measurable effect on neuromuscular transmission, a number of claims have been made that diazepam enhances nondepolarizing blockade. Dretchen et al[236] failed to confirm this effect and suggested that diazepam's site of action in reducing muscle rigidity is central, particularly the reticular activating system and polysynaptic pathways within the spinal cord.

Likewise, ketamine fails to gain a consensus regarding its effects on neuromuscular transmission. Johnston et al[237] found that in humans, ketamine enhances dTc blockade, but not that of pancuronium. Furthermore, Amaki et al[238] observed potentiation of dTc, pancuronium, and SCh with large doses of ketamine in the rat. It is doubtful, however, that ketamine has any important clinical potentiating effect on the action of neuromuscular blockers.

Borden et al[239] presented a case of prolonged blockade following pancuronium in a patient receiving lithium therapy for a manic-depressive state. Since Li^+ can displace Na^+ and K^+ from the body, hypokalemia and augmentation of nondepolarizing blockade may result. Hill et al[240] found that, in dogs, lithium potentiated blockade from pancuronium and SCh but not from dTc or gallamine.

Anticonvulsant therapy is associated with resistance to nondepolarizing neuromuscular blockade. This effect has been demonstrated for pancuronium, metocurine, and vecuronium when administered to patients receiving chronic phenytoin treatment[241]; dTc and atracurium, however, were unaffected. Roth and Ebrahim[242] also showed resistance to pancuronium-induced neuromuscular blockade in patients chronically receiving carbamazepine. The interaction between nondepolarizing relaxants and anticonvulsants appears to be due to pharmacodynamic rather than pharmacokinetic effects, for example, the $Cp_{ss(50)}$ for metocurine is approximately 50% higher in patients who are taking phenytoin compared with controls.[159]

Dantrolene, which acts directly on muscle by interfering with Ca^{++} uptake or release by the sarcoplasmic reticulum, should be anticipated to potentiate nondepolarizing muscle relaxants. Driessen et al[243] have reported prolonged duration of vecuronium-induced neuromuscular blockade in a malignant hyperthermia-susceptible patient pretreated with dantrolene prior to surgery. Flewellen et al[244] further determined a dose–response relationship for twitch suppression resulting from iv dantrolene administered to awake patients. This study suggested that patients receiving dantrolene are likely to be sensitive to the effects of nondepolarizing relaxants.

Nitroglycerin has been reported by Glisson et al[245] to prolong the duration of pancuronium-induced neuromuscular blockade in cats. However, a similar study by Schwarz et al[246] failed to substantiate any such interaction between nitroglycerin and pancuronium or vecuronium. There is no evidence for a clinically important relationship in humans.

Theophylline facilitates neuromuscular transmission by increasing intracellular cyclic AMP, which is important in the synthesis, storage, mobilization, and release of ACh at motor nerve terminals. Thus, patients receiving theophylline or its derivatives may have an increased requirement for competitive relaxants.[247]

Furosemide has also been reported to potentiate the action of dTc in humans.[248] In addition to potentiation caused by producing metabolic alkalosis through kaliuresis, furosemide probably acts through a mechanism opposite to that of theophylline, namely inhibition of cyclic AMP–mediated effects on presynaptic ACh release.

Calcium channel blockers exert their effects predominantly on slow calcium channels, as opposed to fast calcium channels, which are more important in skeletal muscle contraction. Therapeutic levels of these drugs do not generally affect the vigor of skeletal muscle contraction. In contrast, cardiac and smooth muscles have smaller endoplasmic Ca^{++} stores, are more reliant on CA^{++} influx, and are more sensitive to calcium channel blockers. However, verapamil has been shown to have prejunctional effects that can become manifest in the setting of partial nondepolarizing or depolarizing blockade in the rabbit.[249] In addition, a postjunctional effect on the muscle contractile response may explain the report of acute respiratory failure following verapamil administration in a patient with Duchenne's muscular dystrophy.[250]

Although Durant et al[251] demonstrated steroid-induced potentiation of pancuronium neuromuscular blockade in cats, Schwartz et al[252] failed to show any effect of hydrocortisone or dexamethasone on the indirectly elicited muscle twitch response in humans. For different reasons, steroids and ACTH have been shown to improve neuromuscular function in the treatment of myasthenia gravis.

Drugs that inhibit plasma cholinesterase may prolong recovery from SCh.[253, 254] This group includes trimethaphan, cyclophosphamide, mechlorethamine, and triethylenethiophosphoramide. Chemotherapeutic agents that act as alkylating agents inhibit plasma cholinesterase by alkylating the enzyme.

SUMMARY

Muscle relaxants assume an essential role in everyday anesthetic practice. These drugs offer the anesthesiologist the option of reducing the requirement for inhalational or iv anesthetics, thereby increasing patient safety.

The logical selection of a particular muscle relaxant is based on its desired pharmacologic characteristics, which are weighed against its potential for causing unwanted side-effects. The selection of drug, dose, and method of administration is further determined by the complex interrelationship of the patient's health, the surgical procedure, the anesthetic technique, and other drugs given to or taken by the patient. Safe, intelligent practice dictates that relaxants be titrated to clinical effect by monitoring neuromuscular function in every patient.

REFERENCES

1. Griffith HR, Johnson GE: The use of curare in general anesthesia. Anesthesiology 3:418, 1942
2. Beecher HK, Todd DP: A study of deaths with anesthesia and surgery. Ann Surg 140:2, 1954
3. Hunter JM: Adverse effects of neuromuscular blocking drugs. Br J Anaesth 59:46, 1987
4. Mainzer J: Awareness, muscle relaxants and balanced anaesthesia. Can Anaesth Soc J 26:386, 1979
5. Bowman WC: Pharmacology of Neuromuscular Transmission. Baltimore, University Park Press, 1980
6. Standaert FG: Release of transmitter at the neuromuscular junction. Br J Anaesth 54:131, 1982
7. Riker WF: Prejunctional effects of neuromuscular and facilitatory drugs. In Katz RL (ed): Muscle Relaxants, p 59. Amsterdam, Excerpta Medica, 1975

8. Dreyer F: Acetylcholine receptor. Br J Anaesth 54:115, 1982

9. Donati F, Bevan JC, Bevan DR: Neuromuscular blocking drugs in anaesthesia. Can Anaesth Soc J 31:324, 1984

10. Durant NN, Katz RL: Suxamethonium. Br J Anaesth 54:195, 1982

11. Ali HH, Savarese JJ: Monitoring of neuromuscular function. Anesthesiology 45:216, 1976

12. Blaber LC: The effect of facilitatory concentrations of deca-methonium on the storage and release of transmitter at the neuromuscular junction of the cat. J Pharmacol Exp Ther 175:664, 1970

13. Viby-Mogensen J: Clinical assessment of neuromuscular transmission. Br J Anaesth 54:209, 1982

14. Kalow W: Pharmacogenetics and anesthesia. Anesthesiology 25:377, 1964

15. Baraka A: Nueromuscular blockade of atracurium versus succinylcholine in a patient with complete absence of plasma cholinesterase activity. Anesthesiology 66:80, 1987

16. Katz RL, Ryan JF: The neuromuscular effects of suxamethonium in man. Br J Anaesth 41:381, 1969

17. Churchill-Davidson HC, Christie TH, Wise RP: Dual neuromuscular block in man. Anesthesiology 21:144, 1960

18. Lee C: Dose relationships of Phase II, tachyphylaxis and train-of-four fade in suxamethonium-induced dual neuromuscular block. Br J Anaesth 47:841, 1975

19. Ramsey FM, Lebowitz PW, Savarese JJ et al: Clinical characteristics of long-term succinylcholine neuromuscular blockade during balanced anesthesia. Anesth Analg 59:110, 1980

20. Bowman WC: Prejunctional and postjunctional cholinoceptors at the neuromuscular junction. Anesth Analg 59:935, 1980

21. Leigh MD, McCoy DD, Belton MK et al: Bradycardia following intravenous administration of succinylcholine chloride to infants and children. Anesthesiology 18:698, 1957

22. Williams CH, Deutsch S, Linde HW et al: Effects of intravenously administered succinyldicholine on cardiac rate, rhythm, and arterial blood pressure in anaesthetized man. Anesthesiology 22:947, 1961

23. Schoenstadt DA, Whitcher CE: Observations on the mechanism of succinycholine-induced cardiac arrhythmias. Anesthesiology 24:358, 1963

24. Stoelting RK, Peterson C: Heart-rate slowing and junctional rhythm following intravenous succinycholine with and without intramuscular atropine preanesthetic medication. Anesth Analg 54:705, 1975

25. Sherman EP, Lebowitz PW, Street WC: Bradycardia following sufentanil-succinylcholine. Anesthesiology 66:106, 1987

26. Goldhill DR, Martyn JAJ, Hoaglin DC: Beta-adrenoceptor blockade, alpha-stimulation and changes in plasma potassium concentration after suxamethonium administration in dogs. Br J Anaesth 59:611, 1987

27. Mazze RI, Escue HM, Houston JB: Hyperkalemia and cardiovascular collapse following administration of succinylcholine to the traumatized patient. Anesthesiology, 31:540, 1969

28. Kopriva C, Ratliff J, Fletcher JR et al: Serum potassium changes after succinylcholine in patients with acute massive muscle trauma. Anesthesiology 34:246, 1971

29. Birch AA, Mitchell GD, Playford GA et al: Changes in serum potassium response to succinylcholine following trauma. JAMA 210:490, 1969

30. Tolmie JD, Joyce TH, Mitchell GD: Succinylcholine danger in the burned patient. Anesthesiology 28:467, 1967

31. Azar I: The response of patients with neuromuscular disorders to muscle relaxants: A review. Anesthesiology 61:173, 1984

32. Tong TK: Succinylcholine-induced hyperkalemia in near-drowning. Anesthesiology 66:720, 1987

33. Cooperman LH: Succinylcholine-induced hyperkalemia in neuromuscular disease. JAMA 213:1867, 1970

34. Roth F, Wuthrich H: The clinical importance of hyperkalaemia following suxamethonium administration. Br J Anaesth 41:311, 1969

35. Tobey RE, Jacobsen PM, Kahle CT et al: The serum potassium response to muscle relaxants in neural injury. Anesthesiology 37:332, 1972

36. Gronert GA, Theye RA: Pathophysiology of hyperkalemia induced by succinylcholine. Anesthesiology 43:89, 1975

37. Dierdorf SF, McNiece WL, Rao CC et al: Failure of succinylcholine to alter plasma potassium in children with myelomeningocele. Anesthesiology 64:272, 1986

38. Fergusson RJ, Wright DJ, Willey RF et al: Suxamethonium is dangerous in polyneuropathy. Br Med J 282:298, 1981

39. Wise RP: Muscle disorders and the relaxants. Br J Anaesth 35:558, 1963

40. Dierdorf SF, McNiece WL, Rao CC et al: Effect of succinylcholine on plasma potassium in children with cerebral palsy. Anesthesiology 62:88, 1985

41. Kohlschutter B, Baur H, Roth F: Suxamethonium-induced hyperkalaemia in patients with severe intra-abdominal infections. Br J Anaesth 48:557, 1976

42. Koide M, Waud BE: Serum potassium concentrations after succinylcholine in patients with renal failure. Anesthesiology 36:142, 1972

43. Harle DG, Baldo BA, Fisher MM: Cross-reactivity of metocurine, atracurium, vecuronium and fazadinium with IgE antibodies from patients unexposed to these drugs but allergic to other myoneural blocking drugs. Br J Anaesth 57:1073, 1985

44. Gronert GA: Malignant hyperthermia. Anesthesiology 53:395, 1980

45. Mitchell MM, Ali HH, Savarese JJ: Myotonia and neuromuscular blocking agents. Anesthesiology 49:44, 1978

46. Cook WP, Kaplan RF: Neuromuscular blockade in a patient with stiff-baby syndrome. Anesthesiology 65:525, 1986

47. Hartman GS, Fiamengo SA, Riker WF: Succinylcholine: Mechanism of fasciculations and their prevention by d-tubocurarine or diphenylhydantoin. Anesthesiology 65:405, 1986

48. Manchikanti L, Grow JB, Colliver JA et al: Atracurium pretreatment for succinylcholine-induced fasciculations and postoperative myalgia. Anesth Analg 64:1010, 1985

49. Murphy DF: Anesthesia and intraocular pressure. Anesth Analg 64:520, 1985

50. Miller RD, Way WL, Hickey RF: Inhibition of succinylcholine-induced increased intraocular pressure by non-depolarizing muscle relaxants. Anesthesiology 29:123, 1968

51. Meyers EF, Krupin T, Johnson M et al: Failure of nondepolarizing neuromuscular blockers to inhibit succinylcholine-induced increased intraocular pressure: A controlled study. Anesthesiology 48:149, 1978

52. Badrinath SK, Vazeery A, McCarthy RJ et al: The effect of different methods of inducing anesthesia on intraocular pressure. Anesthesiology 65:431, 1986

53. Libonati MM, Leahy JJ, Ellison N: The use of succinylcholine in open eye surgery. Anesthesiology 62:637, 1985

54. Schneider MJ, Stirt JA, Finholt DA: Atracurium, vecuronium, and intraocular pressure in humans. Anesth Analg 65:877, 1986

55. Donlon JV: Succinylcholine and open eye injury. II. Anesthesiology 64:525, 1986

56. Miller RD, Way WL: Inhibition of succinylcholine-induced increased intragastric pressure by nondepolarizing relaxants and lidocaine. Anesthesiology 34:185, 1971

57. Smith G, Dalling R, Williams TIR: Gastro-oesophageal pressure gradient changes produced by induction of anaesthesia and suxamethonium. Br J Anaesth 50:1137, 1978

58. Lanier WL, Milde JH, Michenfelder JD: Cerebral stimulation following succinylcholine in dogs. Anesthesiology 64:551, 1986

59. Stirt JA, Grosslight KR, Bedford RF et al: "Defasciculation" with metocurine prevents succinylcholine-induced increases in intracranial pressure. Anesthesiology 67:50, 1987

60. Minton MD, Stirt JA, Bedford RF et al: Intracranial pressure after atracurium in neurosurgical patients. Anesth Analg 64:1113, 1985

61. Rosa G, Orfei P, Sanfilippo M et al: The effects of atracurium besylate (Tracrium) on intracranial pressure and cerebral perfusion pressure. Anesth Analg 65:381, 1986

62. Rosa G, Sanfilippo M, Vilardi V et al: Effects of vecuronium bromide on intracranial pressure and cerebral perfusion pressure. Br J Anaesth 58:437, 1986

63. Paton WDM, Waud DR: The margin of safety of neuromuscular transmission. J Physiol (London) 191:59, 1967

64. Waud BE, Waud DR: The relation between tetanic fade and receptor occlusion in the presence of competitive neuromuscular block. Anesthesiology 35:456, 1971

65. Waud BE, Waud DR: The relation between the response to "train-of-four" stimulation and receptor occlusion during competitive neuromuscular block. Anesthesiology 37:413, 1972

66. Waud BE, Waud DR: The margin of safety of neuromuscular transmission in the muscle of the diaphragm. Anesthesiology 37:417, 1972

67. Chauvin M, Lebrault C, Duvaldestin P: The neuromuscular blocking effect of vecuronium on the human diaphragm. Anesth Analg 66:117, 1987

68. Lee C: Train-of-four quantitation of competitive neuromuscular block. Anesth Analg 54:649, 1975

69. O'Hara DA, Fragen RJ, Shanks CA: Reappearance of the train-of-four after neuromuscular blockade induced with tubocurarine, vecuronium or atracurium. Br J Anaesth 58:1296, 1986

70. O'Hara DA, Fragen RJ, Shanks CA: Comparison of visual and measured train-of-four recovery after vecuronium-induced neuromuscular blockade using two anaesthetic techniques. Br J Anaesth 58:1300, 1986

71. Graham GG, Morris R, Pybus DA et al: Relationship of train-of-four to twitch depression during pancuronium-induced neuromuscular blockade. Anesthesiology 65:579, 1986

72. Hubbard JI, Wilson DF, Miyamoto M: Reduction of transmitter release by d-tubocurarine. Nature 223:531, 1969

73. Galindo A: The role of prejunctional effects in myoneural transmission. Anesthesiology 36:598, 1972

74. Lebowitz PW, Ramsey FM, Savarese JJ et al: Combination of pancuronium and metocurine: Neuromuscular and hemodynamic advantages over pancuronium alone. Anesth Analg 60:12, 1981

75. Bowman WC: Non-relaxant properties of neuromuscular blocking drugs. Br J Anaesth 54:147, 1982

76. Hughes R, Chapple DJ: Effects of nondepolarizing neuromuscular blocking agents on peripheral autonomic mechanisms in cats. Br J Anaesth 48:59, 1976

77. Segarra Domenech J, Carlos Garcia R, Rodriguez Sasiain JM et al: Pancuronium bromide: An indirect sympathomimetic agent. Br J Anaesth 48:1143, 1976

78. Gardier RW, Tsevdos EJ, Jackson DB: Effects of gallamine and pancuronium on inhibitory transmission in cat sympathetic ganglia. J Pharmacol Exp Ther 204:46, 1978

79. Clark AL, Mitchelson F: The inhibitory effect of gallamine on muscarinic receptors. Br J Pharmacol 58:323, 1976

80. Brown BR, Crout JR: The sympathomimetic effect of gallamine on the heart. J Pharmacol Exp Ther 172:266, 1970

81. Docherty JR, McGrath JC: Sympathomimetic effect of pancuronium bromide on the cardiovascular system of the pithed rat: A comparison with the effects of drugs blocking neuronal uptake of noradrenaline. Br J Pharmacol 64:589, 1978

82. Moss J, Roscow CE, Savarese JJ et al: Role of histamine in the hypotensive action of d-tubocurarine in humans. Anesthesiology 55:19, 1981

83. Basta SJ, Savarese JJ, Ali HH et al: Histamine-releasing potencies of atracurium, dimethyltubocurarine, and tubocurarine. Br J Anaesth 55:105S, 1983

84. Philbin DM, Moss J, Akins CW et al: The use of H$_1$ and H$_2$ histamine antagonists with morphine anesthesia: A double-blind study. Anesthesiology 55:292, 1981

85. Scott RP, Savarese JJ, Basta SJ et al: Atracurium: Clinical strategies for preventing histamine release and attenuating the haemodynamic response. Br J Anaesth 57:550, 1985

86. Kettlekamp NS, Austin DR, Downes H et al: Inhibition of d-tubocurarine-induced histamine release by halothane. Anesthesiology 66:666, 1987

87. Stoelting RK: The hemodynamic effects of pancuronium and d-tubocurarine in anesthetized patients. Anesthesiology 36:612, 1972

88. Longnecker DE, Stoelting RK, Morrow AG: Cardiac and peripheral vascular effects of d-tubocurarine in man. Anesth Analg 49:660, 1970

89. Munger WL, Miller RD, Stevens WC: The dependence of d-tubocurarine-induced hypotension on alveolar concentration of halothane, dose of d-tubocurarine, and nitrous oxide. Anesthesiology 40:442, 1974

90. Stoelting RK: Hemodynamic effects of dimethyltubocurarine during nitrous oxide-halothane anesthesia. Anesth Analg 53:513, 1974

91. Savarese JJ, Ali HH, Antonio RP: The clinical pharmacology of metocurine: Dimethyltubocurarine revisited. Anesthesiology 47:277, 1977

92. Kelman GR, Kennedy BR: Cardiovascular effects of pancuronium in man. Br J Anaesth 43:335, 1971

93. Miller RD, Eger EI, Stevens WC et al: Pancuronium-induced tachycardia in relation to alveolar halothane, dose of pancuronium, and prior atropine. Anesthesiology 42:352, 1975

94. Thomson IR, Putnins CL: Adverse effects of pancuronium during high-dose fentanyl anesthesia for coronary artery bypass grafting. Anesthesiology 62:708, 1985

95. Geha DG, Rozelle BC, Raessler KL et al: Pancuronium bromide enhances atrioventricular conduction in halothane-anesthetized dogs. Anesthesiology 46:342, 1977

96. Edwards RP, Miller RD, Roizen MF et al: Cardiac responses to imipramine and pancuronium during anesthesia with halothane or enflurane. Anesthesiology 50:421, 1979

97. Stoelting RK: Hemodynamic effects of gallamine during halothane-nitrous oxide anesthesia. Anesthesiology 39:645, 1973

98. Eisele JH, Marta JA, Davis HS: Quantitative aspects of the chronotropic and neuromuscular effects of gallamine in anesthetized man. Anesthesiology 35:630, 1971

99. Matteo RS, Nishitateno K, Pua EK et al: Pharmacokinetics of d-tubocurarine in man: Effect of an osmotic diuretic on urinary excretion. Anesthesiology 52:335, 1980

100. Cohen EN, Corbascio A, Fleischli G: The distribution and fate of d-tubocurarine. J Pharmacol Exp Ther 147:120, 1965

101. Miller RD, Matteo RS, Benet LZ et al: The pharmacokinetics of d-tubocurarine in man with and without renal failure. J Pharmacol Exp Ther 202:1, 1977

102. Agoston S, Vermeer GA, Kersten UW et al: The fate of pancuronium bromide in man. Acta Anaesthesiol Scand 17:267, 1973

103. McLeod K, Watson MJ, Rawlins MD: Pharmacokinetics of pancuronium in patients with normal and impaired renal function. Br J Anaesth 48:341, 1976

104. Miller RD, Stevens WC, Way WL: The effect of renal failure and hyperkalemia on the duration of pancuronium neuromuscular blockade in man. Anesth Analg 52:661, 1973

105. Agoston S, Vermeer GA, Kersten UW et al: A preliminary investi-

gation of the renal and hepatic excretion of gallamine triethiodide in man. Br J Anaesth 50:345, 1978

106. Brotherton WP, Matteo RS: Pharmacokinetics and pharmacodynamics of metocurine in humans with and without renal failure. Anesthesiology 55:273, 1981

107. Dundee JW, Gray TC: Resistance to *d*-tubocurarine chloride in the presence of liver damage. Lancet 2:16, 1953

108. Baraka A: Nondepolarizing relaxants and liver disease. Br J Anaesth 50:635, 1978

109. Duvaldestin P, Agoston S, Henzel D *et al*: Pancuronium pharmacokinetics in patients with liver cirrhosis. Br J Anaesth 50:1131, 1978

110. Somogyi AA, Shanks CA, Triggs EJ: Disposition kinetics of pancuronium bromide on patients with total biliary obstruction. Br J Anaesth 49:1103, 1977

111. Basta SJ, Ali HH, Savarese JJ *et al*: Clinical pharmacology of atracurium besylate (BW 33A): A new non-depolarizing muscle relaxant. Anesth Analg 61:723, 1982

112. Miller RD, Rupp SM, Fisher DM *et al*: Clinical pharmacology of vecuronium and atracurium. Anesthesiology 61:444, 1984

113. Naguib M, Abdulatif M, Gyasi HK *et al*: The pattern of train-of-four fade after atracurium: Influence of different priming doses. Anesth Analg 66:427, 1987

114. Lavery GG, Boyle MM, Mirakhur RK: Probable histamine liberation with atracurium. Br J Anaesth 57:811, 1985

115. Siler JN, Mager JG, Wyche MQ: Atracurium: Hypotension, tachycardia and bronchospasm. Anesthesiology 62:645, 1985

116. Scott RP, Savarese JJ, Basta SJ *et al*: Clinical pharmacology of atracurium given in high dose. Br J Anaesth 58:834, 1986

117. Lennon RL, Olson RA, Gronert GA: Atracurium or vecuronium for rapid sequence endotracheal intubation. Anesthesiology 64:510, 1986

118. deBros FM, Lai A, Scott R *et al*: Pharmacokinetics and pharmacodynamics of atracurium during isoflurane anesthesia in normal and anephric patients. Anesth Analg 65:743, 1986

119. Bell CF, Hunter JM, Jones RS *et al*: Use of atracurium and vecuronium in patients with oesophageal varices. Br J Anaesth 57:160, 1985

120. Chapple DJ, Miller AA, Ward JB *et al*: Cardiovascular and neurological effects of laudanosine. Br J Anaesth 59:218, 1987

121. Yate PM, Flynn PJ, Arnold RW *et al*: Clinical experience and plasma laudanosine concentrations during the infusion of atracurium in the intensive therapy unit. Br J Anaesth 59:211, 1987

122. Lanier WL, Milde JH, Michenfelder JD: The cerebral effects of pancuronium and atracurium in halothane-anesthetized dogs. Anesthesiology 63:589, 1985

123. Shi W, Fahey MR, Fisher DM *et al*: Laudanosine (a metabolite of atracurium) increases the minimum alveolar concentration of halothane in rabbits. Anesthesiology 63:584, 1985

124. Nigrovic V, Klaunig JE, Smith SL *et al*: Potentiation of atracurium toxicity in isolated rat hepatocytes by inhibition of its hydrolytic degradation pathway. Anesth Analg 66:512, 1987

125. Fahey MR, Morris RB, Miller RD *et al*: Clinical pharmacology of ORG NC45 (Norcuron): A new nondepolarizing muscle relaxant. Anesthesiology 55:6, 1981

126. Baker T, Aguero A, Stanec A *et al*: Prejunctional effects of vecuronium in the cat. Anesthesiology 65:480, 1986

127. Starr NJ, Sethna DH, Estafanous FG: Bradycardia and asystole following the rapid administration of sufentanil with vecuronium. Anesthesiology 64:521, 1986

128. Krieg N, Crul JF, Booij LHDJ: Relative potency of ORG NC45, pancuronium, alcuronium and tubocurarine in anaesthetized man. Br J Anaesth 52:783, 1980

129. Bencini AF, Houwertjes MC, Agoston S: Effects of hepatic uptake of vecuronium bromide and its putative metabolites on their neuromuscular blocking actions in the cat. Br J Anaesth 57:789, 1985

130. Lebrault C, Berger JL, D'Hollander AA *et al*: Pharmacokinetics and pharmacodynamics of vecuronium. (ORG NC45) in patients with cirrhosis. Anesthesiology 62:601, 1985

131. Lebrault C, Duvaldestin P, Henzel D *et al*: Pharmacokinetics and pharmacodynamics of vecuronium in patients with cholestasis. Br J Anaesth 58:983, 1986

132. Bencini AF, Scaf AHJ, Sohn YG *et al*: Disposition and urinary excretion of vecuronium bromide in anesthetized patients with normal renal function or renal failure. Anesth Analg 65:245, 1986

133. Stirt JA, Stone DJ, Weinberg G *et al*: Atracurium in a child with myotonic dystrophy. Anesthesiology 64:369, 1985

134. Nightingale P, Healy TEJ, McGuinness K: Dystrophica myotonia and atracurium. Br J Anaesth 57:1131, 1985

135. Vacanti CA, Ali HH, Schweiss JF *et al*: The response of myasthenia gravis to atracurium. Anesthesiology 62:692, 1985

136. Buzello W, Noeldge G, Krieg N *et al*: Vecuronium for muscle relaxation in patients with myasthenia gravis. Anesthesiology 64:507, 1986

137. Baraka A: Myasthenic response to muscle relaxants in Von Recklinghausen's disease. Br J Anaesth 46:701, 1974

138. Flusche G, Unger-Sargon J, Lambert DH: Prolonged neuromuscular paralysis with vecuronium in a patient with polymyositis. Anesth Analg 66:188, 1987

139. Moorthy SS, Hilgenberg JC: Resistance to non-depolarizing muscle relaxants in paretic upper extremities of patients with residual hemiplegia. Anesth Analg 59:624, 1980

140. Iwasaki H, Namiki A, Omote K *et al*: Response differences of paretic and healthy extremities to pancuronium and neostigmine in hemiplegic patients. Anesth Analg 64:864, 1985

141. Brett RS, Schmidt JH, Gage JS *et al*: Measurement of acetylcholine receptor concentration in skeletal muscle from a patient with multiple sclerosis and resistance to atracurium. Anesthesiology 66:837, 1987

142. Shayevitz JR, Matteo RS: Decreased sensitivity to metocurine in patients with upper motoneuron disease. Anesth Analg 64:767, 1985

143. Gronert GA: Disuse atrophy with resistance to pancuronium. Anesthesiology 55:547, 1981

144. Waud BE, Waud DR: Tubocurarine sensitivity of the diaphragm after limb immobilization. Anesth Analg 65:493, 1986

145. Martyn JAJ, Szyfelbein SK, Ali HH *et al*: Increased *d*-tubocurarine requirement following major thermal injury. Anesthesiology 52:352, 1980

146. Matteo RS, Brotherton WP, Nishitateno K *et al*: Pharmacokinetics and pharmacodynamics of metocurine in humans: Comparison to *d*-tubocurarine. Anesthesiology 57:183, 1982

147. Dwersteg JF, Pavlin EG, Heimbach DM: Patients with burns are resistant to atracurium. Anesthesiology 65:517, 1986

148. Tallerida RJ, Jacob LS: Construction of dose–response curves: Statistical considerations. In Tallerida RJ, Jacob LS (eds): The Dose–Response Relation in Pharmacology, p 85. New York, Springer Verlag, 1979

149. Donlon JV, Savarese JJ, Ali HH *et al*: Human dose–response curves for neuromuscular blocking drugs. Anesthesiology 53:161, 1980

150. Fisher DM, Fahey MR, Cronnelly R *et al*: Potency determination for vecuronium (ORG NC45): Comparison of cumulative and single-dose techniques. Anesthesiology 57:309, 1982

151. Fisher DM, Castagnoli K, Miller RD: Vecuronium kinetics and dynamics in anesthetized infants and children. Clin Pharmacol Ther 37:402, 1985

152. Shanks CA: Pharmacokinetics of the nondepolarizing neuromuscular relaxants applied to calculation of bolus and infusion dosage regimens. Anesthesiology 64:72, 1986

153. Stanski DR, Watkins WD: Drug disposition in anesthesia. New York, Grune & Stratton, 1982

154. Stanski DR, Ham J, Miller RD et al: Pharmacokinetics and pharmacodynamics of d-tubocurarine during nitrous oxide-narcotic and halothane anesthesia in man. Anesthesiology 51:235, 1979

155. Stanski DR, Ham J, Miller RD et al: Time-dependent increase in sensitivity to d-tubocurarine during enflurane anesthesia in man. Anesthesiology 52:483, 1980

156. Ramzan MI, Shanks CA, Triggs EJ: Pharmacokinetics of tubocurarine administered by combined iv bolus and infusion. Br J Anaesth 52:893, 1980

157. Meijer DKF, Weitering JG, Vermeer GA et al: Comparative pharmacokinetics of d-tubocurarine and metocurine in man. Anesthesiology 51:402, 1979

158. Gibaldi M, Levy G, Hayton W: Kinetics of the elimination and neuromuscular blocking effect of d-tubocurarine in man. Anesthesiology 36:231, 1972

159. Ornstein E, Matteo RS, Young WL et al: Resistance to metocurine-induced neuromuscular blockade in patients receiving phenytoin. Anesthesiology 63:294, 1985

160. Matteo RS, Backus WW, Dudley DM et al: Pharmacokinetics and pharmacodynamics of d-tubocurarine and metocurine in the elderly. Anesth Analg 64:23, 1985

161. Ramzan MI, Triggs EJ, Shanks CA: Pharmacokinetic studies in man with gallamine triethiodide: Single and multiple clinical doses. Eur J Clin Pharmacol 17:135, 1980

162. Miller RD, Agoston S, Booij LHDJ et al: The comparative potency and pharmacokinetics of pancuronium and its metabolites in anesthetized man. J Pharmacol Exp Ther 207:539, 1978

163. Shanks CA, Somogyi AA, Triggs EJ: Dose–response and plasma concentration–response relationships of pancuronium in man. Anesthesiology 51:111, 1979

164. Hall CJ, English MJM, Sibbald A: Fazadinium and pancuronium: A pharmacodynamic study. Br J Anaesth 52:1209, 1980

165. Duvaldestin P, Demetriou M, Henzel D et al: The placental transfer of pancuronium and its pharmacokinetics during caesarian section. Acta Anaesthesiol Scand 22:327, 1978

166. Somogyi AA, Shanks CA, Triggs EJ: Clinical pharmacokinetics of pancuronium bromide. Eur J Clin Pharmacol 10:367, 1976

167. Agoston S, Feldman SA, Miller RD: Plasma concentrations of pancuronium and neuromuscular blockade after injection into the isolated arm, bolus injection, and continuous infusion. Anesthesiology 51:119, 1979

168. Ward S, Neill EAM: Pharmacokinetics of atracurium in acute hepatic failure (with acute renal failure). Br J Anaesth 55:1169, 1983

169. Fahey MR, Rupp SM, Fisher DM et al: The pharmacokinetics and pharmacodynamics of atracurium in patients with and without renal failure. Anesthesiology 61:699, 1984

170. Fisher DM, Canfell PC, Fahey MR et al: Elimination of atracurium in humans: Contribution of Hofmann elimination and ester hydrolysis versus organ-based elimination. Anesthesiology 65:6, 1986

171. Weatherly BC, Williams SG, Neill EAM: Pharmacokinetics, pharmacodynamics and dose–response relationships of atracurium administered iv. Br J Anaesth 55:395, 1983

172. Fahey MR, Morris RB, Miller RD et al: Pharmacokinetics of ORG NC45 (Norcuron) in patients with and without renal failure. Br J Anaesth 53:1049, 1981

173. Cronnelly R, Fisher DM, Miller RD et al: Pharmacokinetics and pharmacodynamics of vecuronium (ORG NC45) and pancuronium in anesthetized humans. Anesthesiology 58:405, 1983

174. Fisher DM, Rosen JI: A pharmacokinetic exploration for increasing recovery time following larger or repeated doses of nondepolarizing muscle relaxants. Anesthesiology 65:286, 1986

175. Goudsouzian NG, Standaert FG: The infant and the myoneural junction. Anesth Analg 65:1208, 1986

176. Fisher DM, Miller RD: Neuromuscular effects of vecuronium (ORG NC45) in infants and children during N₂O–halothane anesthesia. Anesthesiology 58:519, 1983

177. Goudsouzian N, Liu LMP, Gionfriddo M et al: Neuromuscular effects of atracurium in infants and children. Anesthesiology 62:75, 1985

178. Brandom BW, Woelfel SK, Cook DR et al: Clinical pharmacology of atracurium in infants. Anesth Analg 63:309, 1984

179. Cook DR: Muscle relaxants in infants and children. Anesth Analg 60:335, 1981

180. D'Hollander AA, Luyckx C, Barvais L et al: Clinical evaluation of atracurium besylate requirement for a stable muscle relaxation during surgery: Lack of age-related effects. Anesthesiology 59:237, 1983

181. D'Hollander AA, Massaux F, Nevelsteen M et al: Age-dependent dose–response relationship of ORG NC45 in anaesthetized patients. Br J Anaesth 54:653, 1982

182. Schwarz S, Ilias W, Lackner F et al: Rapid tracheal intubation with vecuronium: The priming principle. Anesthesiology 62:388, 1985

183. Mehta MP, Choi WW, Gergis SD et al: Facilitation of rapid endotracheal intubations with divided doses of nondepolarizing neuromuscular blocking drugs. Anesthesiology 62:392, 1985

184. Musich J, Walts LF: Pulmonary aspiration after a priming dose of vecuronium. Anesthesiology 64:517, 1986

185. Sosis M, Larijani GE, Marr AT: Priming with atracurium. Anesth Analg 66:329, 1987

186. Ramsey FM, Weeks DB, Morell RC et al: The priming principle: Ineffectiveness of atracurium pretreatment. Anesthesiology 63:A431, 1985

187. Ramsey FM, Morell RC, Gerr P: The priming principle: Pretreatment with metocurine prior to vecuronium neuromuscular blockade. Anesthesiology 65:A298, 1986

188. Kunjappan VE, Brown EM, Alexander GD: Rapid sequence induction using vecuronium. Anesth Analg 65:503, 1986

189. Taboada JA, Rupp SM, Miller RD: Refining the priming principle for vecuronium during rapid sequence induction of anesthesia. Anesthesiology 64:243, 1986

190. Eagar BM, Flynn PJ, Hughes R: Infusion of atracurium for long surgical procedures. Br J Anaesth 56:447, 1984

191. D'Hollander AA, Czerucki R, DeVille A et al: Stable muscle relaxation during abdominal surgery using combined intravenous bolus and demand infusion: Clinical appraisal with ORG NC45. Can Anaesth Soc J 29:136, 1982

192. Donati F, Bevan DR: Antagonism of Phase II succinylcholine block by neostigmine. Anesth Analg 64:773, 1985

193. Katz RL: Clinical neuromuscular pharmacology of pancuronium. Anesthesiology 34:550, 1971

194. Taylor P: Anticholinesterase agents. In Gilman AG, Goodman LS, Rall TW et al (eds): Goodman and Gilman's The Pharmacological Basis of Therapeutics, 7th edition, p 110. New York, Macmillan, 1985

195. Kopman AF: Edrophonium antagonism of pancuronium-induced neuromuscular blockade. Anesthesiology 51:139, 1979

196. Bevan DR: Reversal of pancuronium with edrophonium. Anaesthesia 34:614, 1979

197. Morris R, Cronnelly R, Miller RD et al: Pharmacokinetics of edrophonium and neostigmine when antagonizing d-tubocurarine neuromuscular blockade in man. Anesthesiology 54:399, 1981

198. Ramamurthy S, Shaker MH, Winnie AP: Glycopyrrolate as a substitute for atropine in neostigmine reversal of muscle relaxants. Can Anaesth Soc J 19:4, 1972

199. Salem MG, Richardson JC, Meadows GA et al: Comparison between glycopyrrolate and atropine in a mixture with neostigmine for reversal of neuromuscular blockade. Br J Anaesth 57:184, 1985

200. Mirakhur RK: Antagonism of the muscarinic effects of edrophonium with atropine or glycopyrrolate: A comparative study. Br J Anaesth 57:1213, 1985

201. Urquhart ML, Ramsey FM, Royster RL et al: Heart rate and rhythm following an edrophonium/atropine mixture for antagonism of neuromuscular blockade during fentanyl/N2O/O2 or isoflurane/N2O/O2 anesthesia. Anesthesiology 67:561, 1987

202. Kopman AF: Recovery times following edrophonium and neostigmine reversal of pancuronium, atracurium and vecuronium steady-state infusions. Anesthesiology 65:572, 1986

203. Hennart D, D'Hollander A, Plasman C et al: Importance of the level of paralysis recovery for a rapid antagonism of atracurium neuromuscular blockade with moderate doses of edrophonium. Anesthesiology 64:384, 1986

204. Rupp SM, McChristian JW, Miller RD et al: Neostigmine and edrophonium antagonism of varying intensity neuromuscular blockade induced by atracurium, pancuronium, or vecuronium. Anesthesiology 64:711, 1986

205. Caldwell JE, Robertson EN, Baird WL: Antagonism of vecuronium and atracurium: Comparison of neostigmine and edrophonium administered at 5% twitch height recovery. Br J Anaesth 59:478, 1987

206. Mirakhur RK, Gibson FM, Lavery GG: Antagonism of vecuronium-induced neuromuscular blockade with edrophonium or neostigmine. Br J Anaesth 59:473, 1987

207. Cronnelly R, Morris RB, Miller RD: Edrophonium: Duration of action and atropine requirement in humans during halothane anesthesia. Anesthesiology 57:261, 1982

208. Sheref SE: Pattern of CNS recovery following reversal of neuromuscular blockade: Comparison of atropine and glycopyrrolate. Br J Anaesth 57:188, 1985

209. Lavery GG, Mirakhur RK, Gibson FM: A comparison of edrophonium and neostigmine for the antagonism of atracurium-induced neuromuscular block. Anesth Analg 64:867, 1985

210. Buzello W, Pollmaecher T, Schluermann D et al: The influence of hypothermic cardiopulmonary bypass on neuromuscular transmission in the absence of muscle relaxants. Anesthesiology 64:279, 1986

211. Buzello W, Schluermann D, Pollmaecher T et al: Unequal effects of cardiopulmonary bypass-induced hypothermia on neuromuscular blockade from constant infusion of alcuronium, d-tubocurarine, pancuronium, and vecuronium. Anesthesiology 66:842, 1987

212. Miller RD, Roderick LL: The influence of acid-base changes on neostigmine antagonism of a pancuronium neuromuscular blockade. Br J Anaesth 50:317, 1978

213. Miller RD, Van Nyhuis LS, Eger EI et al: The effects of acid-base balance on neostigmine antagonism of d-tubocurarine-induced neuromuscular blockade. Anesthesiology 42:377, 1975

214. Miller RD, Roderick LL: Diuretic-induced hypokalaemia, pancuronium neuromuscular blockade and its antagonism by neostigmine. Br J Anaesth 50:541, 1978

215. Ghoneim MM, Long JP: The interaction between magnesium and other neuromuscular blocking agents. Anesthesiology 32:23, 1970

216. Miller RD, Booij LHDJ, Agoston S et al: 4-Aminopyridine potentiates neostigmine and pyridostigmine in man. Anesthesiology 50:416, 1979

217. Erkola O, Salmenpera A, Kuoppamaki R: Five nondepolarizing muscle relaxants in precurarization. Acta Anaesthesiol Scand 27:427, 1983

218. Brodsky JB, Brock-Utne JG, Samuels SI: Pancuronium pretreatment and post-succinylcholine myalgias. Anesthesiology 51:259, 1979

219. Jansen EC, Hansen PH: Objective measurement of SCh-induced fasciculations and the effect of pretreatment with pancuronium or gallamine. Anesthesiology 51:159, 1979

220. Miller RD: The advantages of giving d-tubocurarine before succinylcholine. Anesthesiology 37:568, 1972

221. Katz RL: Modification of the action of pancuronium by succinylcholine and halothane. Anesthesiology 35:602, 1971

222. Feldman SA: Rational use of muscle relaxants and anticholinesterase in clinical practice. In Feldman SA (ed): Muscle Relaxants, p 219. Philadelphia, WB Saunders, 1979

223. Pantuck EJ: Ecothiopate eyedrops and prolonged response to suxamethonium. Br J Anaesth 38:406, 1966

224. Lebowitz PW, Ramsey FM, Savarese JJ et al: Potentiation of neuromuscular blockade in man produced by combinations of pancuronium and metocurine or pancuronium and d-tubocurarine. Anesth Analg 59:604, 1980

225. Ngai SH: Action of general anesthetics in producing muscle relaxation: Interaction of anesthetics with relaxants. In Katz RL (ed): Muscle Relaxants, p 279. Amsterdam, Excerpta Medica, 1975

226. Waud BE, Waud DR: The effects of diethyl ether, enflurane and isoflurane at the neuromuscular junction. Anesthesiology 42:275, 1975

227. Miller RD, Way WL, Dolan WM et al: The dependence of pancuronium and d-tubocurarine-induced neuromuscular blockade on alveolar concentrations of halothane and forane. Anesthesiology 37:573, 1972

228. Fogdall RP, Miller RD: Neuromuscular effects of enflurane alone and in combination with d-tubocurarine, pancuronium and succinylcholine in man. Anesthesiology 42:173, 1975

229. Waud BE, Waud DR: Comparison of the effects of general anesthetics on the end-plate of skeletal muscle. Anesthesiology 43:540, 1975

230. Rupp SM, McChristian JW, Miller RD: Neuromuscular effects of atracurium during halothane-nitrous oxide and enflurane-nitrous oxide anesthesia. Anesthesiology 63:16, 1985

231. Rupp SM, Miller RD, Gencarelli PJ: Vecuronium-induced neuromuscular blockade during enflurane, isoflurane, and halothane anesthesia in humans. Anesthesiology 60:102, 1984

232. Gencarelli P, Miller RD, Eger EI et al: Decreasing enflurane concentrations and d-tubocurarine neuromuscular blockade. Anesthesiology 56:192, 1982

233. Sokoll MD, Gergis SD: Antibiotics and neuromuscular function. Anesthesiology 55:148, 1981

234. Benz JH, Lunn JN, Foldes FF: Recurarization by intraperitoneal antibiotics. Br Med J 2:241, 1961

235. Matsuo S, Rao DBS, Chaudry I et al: Interaction of muscle relaxants and local anesthetics at the neuromuscular junction. Anesth Analg 57:580, 1978

236. Dretchen K, Ghoneim MM, Long JP: The interaction of diazepam with myoneural blocking agents. Anesthesiology 34:463, 1971

237. Johnston RR, Miller RD, Way WL: The interaction of ketamine with d-tubocurarine, pancuronium, and succinylcholine in man. Anesth Analg 53:496, 1974

238. Amaki Y, Nagashima H, Radnay PA et al: Ketamine interaction with neuromuscular blocking agents in the phrenic nerve-hemidiaphragm preparation of the rat. Anesth Analg 57:238, 1978

239. Borden H, Clarke MT, Katz H: The use of pancuronium bromide

in patients receiving lithium carbonate. Can Anaesth Soc J 21:79, 1974

240. Hill GE, Wong KC, Hodges MR: Lithium carbonate and neuromuscular blocking agents. Anesthesiology 46:122, 1977

241. Plotkin CN, Ornstein E: Resistance to pancuronium: Adult respiratory distress syndrome or phenytoin. Anesth Analg 65:820, 1986

242. Roth S, Ebrahim ZY: Resistance to pancuronium in patients receiving carbamazepine. Anesthesiology 66:691, 1987

243. Driessen JJ, Wuis EW, Gielen MJM: Prolonged vecuronium neuromuscular blockade in a patient receiving orally administered dantrolene. Anesthesiology 62:523, 1985

244. Flewellen EH, Nelson TE, Jones WP et al: Dantrolene dose–response in awake man: Implications for management of malignant hyperthermia. Anesthesiology 59:275, 1983

245. Glisson SN, EI-Etr AA, Lim R: Prolongation of pancuronium-induced neuromuscular blockade by intravenous infusion of nitroglycerin. Anesthesiology 51:47, 1979

246. Schwarz S, Agoston S, Houwertjes MC: Does intravenous infusion of nitroglycerin potentiate pancuronium- and vecuronium-induced neuromuscular blockade? Anesth Analg 65:156, 1986

247. Standaert FG, Dretchen KL: Cyclic nucleotides in neuromuscular transmission. Anesth Analg 60:91, 1981

248. Miller RD, Sohn YJ, Matteo RS: Enhancement of d-tubocurarine neuromuscular blockade by diuretics in man. Anesthesiology 45:442, 1976

249. Durant NN, Nguyen N, Katz RL: Potentiation of neuromuscular blockade by verapamil. Anesthesiology 60:298, 1984

250. Zalman F, Perloff JK, Durant NN et al: Acute respiratory failure following intravenous verapamil in Duchenne's muscular dystrophy. Am Heart J 105:510, 1983

251. Durant NN, Briscoe JR, Katz RL: The effect of acute and chronic hydrocortisone treatment on neuromuscular blockade in the anesthetized cat. Anesthesiology 61:144, 1984

252. Schwartz AE, Matteo RS, Ornstein E et al: Acute steroid therapy does not alter nondepolarizing muscle relaxant effects in humans. Anesthesiology 65:326, 1986

253. Dillman JB: Safe use of succinylcholine during repeated anesthetics in a patient treated with cyclophosphamide. Anesth Analg 66:351, 1987

254. Zgismond EK, Robins G: The effect of a series of anti-cancer drugs on plasma cholinesterase activity. Can Anaesth Soc J 19:75, 1972

Chapter 14

Randall L. Carpenter
David C. Mackey

Local Anesthetics

Local anesthetics may be defined as drugs which block the generation and propagation of impulses in excitable tissues. Although the anesthesiologist is primarily concerned with the blocking effects of local anesthetic solutions upon the spinal cord, spinal nerve roots, and peripheral nerves, these compounds also affect other excitable tissues, such as cardiac muscle,[1-3] skeletal muscle,[4, 5] and brain;[6, 7] this is an important consideration in local anesthetic toxicity. Local anesthetics are usually administered topically or by local infiltration, though they may also be delivered intravenously for regional anesthesia or for their systemic effects. A wide variety of substances, such as certain alpha and beta receptor blocking agents, volatile general anesthetics, alcohols, opioids, barbiturates, tranquilizers, and plant and animal toxins may exhibit local anesthetic activity.[8-14] This discussion will be limited to those local anesthetics utilized in clinical anesthesia; principally, the aminoesters and the aminoamides.

Acupuncture, hypnotism, refrigeration, and nerve compression are known to have been used for many years to alleviate surgical pain prior to the development and utilization of local anesthetic drugs, and the anesthetic and central nervous system stimulant effect derived from the leaves of the *erythroxylon coca* bush had been recognized by Peruvian natives. In 1860, the alkaloid cocaine was isolated from the coca leaf by Niemann. In 1884, Koller reported the first use of a local anesthetic for surgery when he described the topical application of cocaine for ophthalmologic surgery. However, cocaine was found to be extremely toxic and addictive, and the search for a suitable substitute culminated in the synthesis of procaine, in 1904, by Einhorn. Procaine, the prototype aminoester local anesthetic, was first used clinically in 1905. Numerous other aminoester local anesthetics have been subsequently introduced, including tetracaine, in 1932, and 2-chloroprocaine, in 1955. In 1943, lidocaine was synthesized by Lofgren, and its clinical introduction 1 year later marked the first use of a new class of local anesthetics, the aminoamides. Several additional amide local anesthetics have been developed, including mepivacaine (1956), bupivacaine (1957), prilocaine (1959), and etidocaine (1971), and have subsequently been placed into clinical use, where they remain today. There are several excellent reviews of the development of local anesthetics and local anesthesia for those who desire greater detail.[15-21]

CHEMISTRY OF LOCAL ANESTHETICS

THE LOCAL ANESTHETIC MOLECULE

In order to understand and predict the differences in biological activity of local anesthetic agents, it is necessary to appreciate both the general structure of the local anesthetic molecule and the properties of each of its subunits. The typical, clinically employed, local anesthetic molecule is weakly basic in nature, containing an amine residue which contributes water solubility in its quaternary form and which is separated from a lipophilic domain by an intermediate alkyl chain (Fig. 14-1). The intermediate chain connecting the lipophilic head and the hydrophilic tail contains either an ester or an amide linkage, thus subdividing the clinically useful local anesthetics into two main groups: the aminoesters, which are metabolized by plasma cholinesterase; and the aminoamides, which are metabolized in the liver. The lipophilic portion of the molecule is usually an aromatic residue, contributed by a derivative of

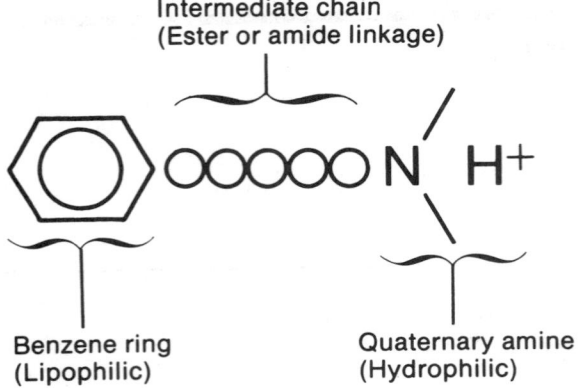

Intermediate chain
(Ester or amide linkage)

Benzene ring
(Lipophilic)

Quaternary amine
(Hydrophilic)

FIG. 14-1. General structure of a local anesthetic molecule.

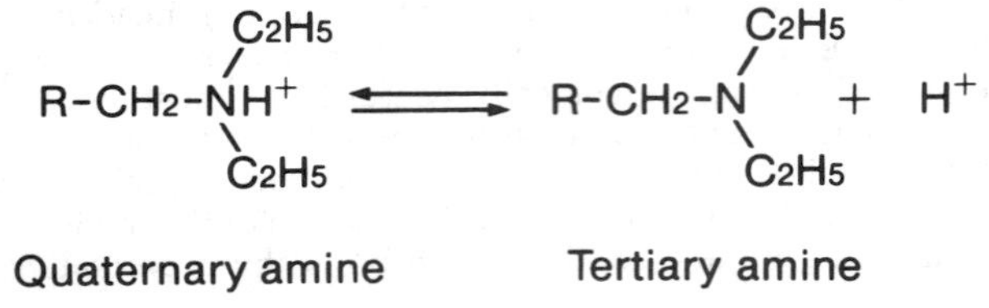

TABLE 14-1.   Effect of pH on Local Anesthetic Base Dissociation

AGENT	pK_a	PERCENTAGE OF TOTAL DRUG IN BASE FORM		
		$pH = 7.0$	$pH = 7.4$	$pH = 7.8$
Benzocaine	3.5	100	100	100
Mepivacaine	7.6	20	39	61
Lidocaine	7.9	11	24	44
Etidocaine	7.7	17	33	56
Bupivacaine	8.1	7	17	33
Tetracaine	8.6	6	14	28
Procaine	8.9	1	3	7
2-Chloroprocaine	9.1	0.8	2	5

Adapted from: Tucker GT, Mather LE: Absorption and disposition of local anesthetics: Pharmacokinetics. In: Cousins MJ, Bridenbaugh PO (eds): Neural Blockade in Clinical Anesthesia and Management of Pain, pp 48–49. Philadelphia, JB Lippincott, 1980. With permission from the publisher.

benzoic acid, in the case of the aminoester anesthetics; or by a derivative of aniline, in the case of the aminoamides.

STRUCTURE-ACTIVITY RELATIONSHIPS

In its tertiary form, the local anesthetic molecule is poorly soluble in water, but, because of its basic nature, it combines readily with acids to form water-soluble salts. Thus, for clinical utility, local anesthetics are usually prepared as their salt form, most often as hydrochlorides. In aqueous solution, the hydrochloride salt ionizes to yield a positively charged quaternary amine and a chloride anion. The charged, quaternary amine exists in solution in equilibrium with its uncharged, free-base, tertiary amine form (Fig. 14-2). The exact percentage of local anesthetic molecules in each of the two forms depends upon the pK_a, or dissociation constant, of the local anesthetic and the pH of the surrounding medium (Table 14-1). For example, as the pH is decreased, the equilibrium is shifted to favor the protonated form, and, thus, a relatively larger percentage of the local anesthetic will exist as positively charged, cationic molecules.

The degree of ionization is important, as it is the uncharged, free-base form which is most lipid soluble, and, thus, most able to traverse the lipid milieu of the axon membrane, its myelin sheath (if present), and the surrounding connective tissue coverings of the nerve fiber bundles and nerve.[22, 23] As will be seen, both the lipophilic, neutral (free-base) form, and the hydrophilic, charged (cationic) form of the local anesthetic molecule are involved in the blockade of the nerve impulse. Charged molecules probably gain access to specific receptors on the interior of the neuronal sodium channel *via* the aqueous pathway of the sodium channel pore, while neutral, un-

charged forms interact with sodium channels through the lipid environment of the axon membrane (Fig. 14-3).[22, 24–29]

Basic properties of a local anesthetic can be manipulated through alterations in its molecular structure.[30–33] For example, increasing the degree of alkyl substitution on the aromatic ring or on the tertiary amine increases lipid solubility and produces greater local anesthetic potency. Lengthening the intermediate chain increases anesthetic potency, but at the expense of increasing toxicity. Compounds containing ethyl esters, such as procaine and chloroprocaine, are more easily metabolized and produce less systemic toxicity. Finally, molecular changes which lead to increased protein binding result in prolongation of the duration of local anesthetic action.

COMMERCIAL PREPARATIONS

Because the free base form of most local anesthetics is poorly soluble in aqueous solution, they are prepared as hydrochloride salts dissolved in sterile water or normal saline. The solution is acidified to a pH of 4.40–6.40 to favor existence of

FIG. 14-3. Local anesthetic access to the sodium channel. The uncharged molecule diffuses most easily across lipid barriers and interacts with the channel through the axolemma interior. The charged species formed in the axoplasm gains access to a specific receptor *via* the sodium channel pore.

FIG. 14-2. The dissociation equilibrium of charged, quaternary amine and uncharged, tertiary amine local anesthetic molecules in an aqueous solution.

$$R-CH_2-NH^+ \rightleftharpoons R-CH_2-N + H^+$$

Quaternary amine   Tertiary amine

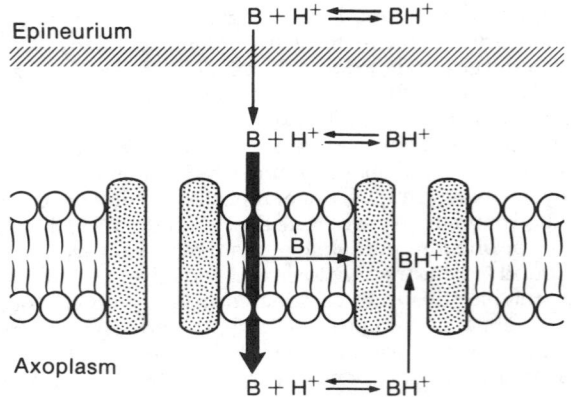

Epineurium

$$B + H^+ \rightleftharpoons BH^+$$

$$B + H^+ \rightleftharpoons BH^+$$

Axoplasm

$$B + H^+ \rightleftharpoons BH^+$$

the water soluble, cationic, quaternary amine form of the local anesthetic molecule.[34, 35] Unfortunately, this decreases the local anesthetic potency, and, although it has been suggested that increasing the pH of the local anesthetic solution may shorten the onset and increase the duration of the blockade,[36, 37] this also increases the risk of precipitation of the local anesthetic out of solution. The action of local anesthetics may also be potentiated by carbonation, with the suggested mechanism of action being a direct depressant effect of carbon dioxide on the axon, an increased conversion of the local anesthetic to the active cation form at the site of action inside the axon, or diffusion trapping of the local anesthetic inside the axon.[38-40]

Commercially prepared epinephrine-containing solutions must also be acidified, because alkaline solutions promote oxidation of catecholamines.[41] However, recent evidence suggests that epinephrine-containing solutions can be alkalinized to a pH range of 7.0–8.0 for a time period of at least 2–6 h without significant oxidation.[42, 43] Antioxidants have also been added to epinephrine-containing solutions, as well as to some local anesthetic solutions, to retard their breakdown. The antioxidant sodium metabisulfite has been implicated in the reported neurotoxicity of 2-chloroprocaine, although this antioxidant has now been replaced with sodium EDTA in 2-chloroprocaine solutions.

Because of their antibacterial and antifungal activity, antimicrobial preservatives are added to local anesthetic solutions contained in multidose vials. Preservative-containing local anesthetic solutions should not be used in spinal, epidural, or caudal anesthesia, due to their potentially cytotoxic effects. The most frequently used antimicrobials are the paraben derivatives of para-hydroxybenzoate, such as methylparaben, ethylparaben, and propylparaben. The paraben derivatives are potent allergens, and have been implicated in allergic reactions initially attributed to the local anesthetic.[44, 45] Because of this, preservative-containing local anesthetics are not recommended for intravenous use.

Proper handling and storage of local anesthetics is important. Because of the possibility of small pieces of glass falling into single-dose ampules when they are opened, some manufacturers prefer to prepare their single-dose local anesthetic solutions in rubber-stoppered vials. However, it must be remembered that these containers do not contain antimicrobial preservatives, and should not be used to disperse multiple doses of local anesthetic. Local anesthetic solutions that contain glucose may caramelize with prolonged heat. These solutions should be autoclaved only one time, and they should not remain in the autoclave any longer than necessary. Ampules of local anesthetic should never be sterilized by soaking in an antiseptic solution, because of the potential for contamination of the local anesthetic through unnoticed cracks in the ampule. Any local anesthetic solution containing a free aromatic amino group, such as 2-chloroprocaine and procaine, may be discolored by prolonged exposure to light. Similarly, epinephrine will oxidize with prolonged exposure to light.

MECHANISM OF ACTION OF LOCAL ANESTHETICS

ANATOMY OF THE PERIPHERAL NERVE

The basic unit of the peripheral nerve is the nerve fiber, composed of an axon which is enclosed almost its entire length by a sheath of Schwann cells. The axolemma of the axon is the continuation of the neuronal cell membrane, and it

surrounds the axoplasm, the contents of the axon. Schwann cells, like neurons, are ectodermally derived, and are vitally important in supporting the life and function of the axons they envelop.[46] The Schwann sheath of the larger peripheral axons contains concentric layers of myelin, a lipoid material which is composed of spiral wraps of the Schwann cell membrane itself.[47] Because of this, nerve fibers are often designated as myelinated or unmyelinated (Fig. 14-4; Table 14-2). Between successive Schwann cells along the length of the axon, there are small, non-myelinated junctional regions, the nodes of Ranvier. Although the nodal regions of the nerve axon were originally thought to be entirely uncovered and uninsulated, investigators have more recently noted, in these areas, an array of microvillous interdigitations between the adjacent Schwann cells (Fig. 14-4).[48] A polyanionic ground substance matrix is found between the microvilli, and this organization of microvilli and negatively-charged ground substance may serve as a barrier to limit the access of local anesthetic molecules to the nodal axolemma.[49-52]

The nerve fibers of the peripheral nerve vary in thickness from less than 1μm to greater than 20μm. Delicate connective tissue layers around each fiber form the endoneurium. Groups of nerve fibers are bundled together by concentric layers of connective tissue, the perineurium, to form fascicles, and an additional outer layer of connective tissue cells and fibers, the epineurium, holds the fascicles together to form the peripheral nerve (Fig. 14-5).[53] These concentric coverings may be important in limiting the diffusion of local anesthetic into the nerve fibers.[54]

PHYSIOLOGY OF THE NERVE FIBER

The purpose of peripheral nerves and their constituent nerve fibers is to carry information, and this is accomplished through electrical signals generated and conducted by neu-

FIG. 14-4. Unmyelinated and myelinated nerve fibers, with the microvillous interdigitations of two adjacent Schwann cells at a node of Ranvier.

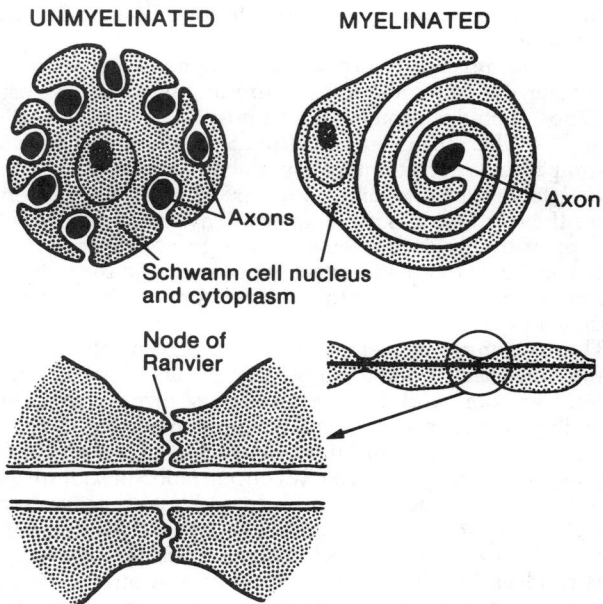

TABLE 14-2. Classification of Nerve Fibers

CONDUCTION/ BIOPHYSICAL CLASSIFICATION	ANATOMIC LOCATION	MYELIN	DIAMETER (μ)	RATE ($m \cdot s^{-1}$)	FUNCTION
A-FIBERS A-alpha A-beta	Afferent to and efferent from muscles and joints	Yes	6–22	30–85	Motor and Proprioception
A-gamma	Efferent to muscle spindles	Yes	3–6	15–35	Muscle Tone
A-delta	Sensory roots and afferent peripheral nerves	Yes	1–4	5–25	Pain Temperature Touch
B-FIBERS	Preganglionic sympathetic	Yes	<3	3–15	Vasomotor Visceromotor Sudomotor Pilomotor
C-FIBERS sC	Postganglionic sympathetic	No	0.3–1.3	0.7–1.3	Vasomotor Visceromotor Sudomotor Pilomotor
drC	Sensory roots and afferent peripheral nerves	No	0.4–1.2	0.1–2.0	Pain Temperature Touch

rons.[55] Although electrical potentials exist across the membranes of essentially all cells of the body, nerve cells possess the property of excitability; that is, they respond to stimuli by undergoing transient physicochemical changes which may alter the resting electrical potential of the cell and initiate a nerve impulse. Through the property of conductivity, the action potential, which is a rapid change in membrane potential, is propagated along the axolemma to its end. At the neuron terminal, a neurotransmitter is released, causing excitation of succeeding neurons or of effector cells, such as skeletal muscle.

The axolemma is typical of other cell membranes, in that it is a fluid or dynamic mosaic structure of alternating oligosaccharides, globular proteins, and phospholipid bilayers (Fig. 14-6).[56, 57] The molecular constituents of the membrane are amphipathic, or structurally asymmetric, with one polar, or hydrophilic, end and one nonpolar, or hydrophobic, end. Since the membrane is in an aqueous environment, the polar groups of the lipids, proteins, and oligosaccharides are oriented so that they are in contact with water, and the nonpolar regions are sequestered within the membrane, away from the aqueous phase.

The axolemma is metabolically active, controlling transmembrane electrochemical potential by active transport in either direction and by controlling its own relative permeability to various ions. ATP-dependent active transport results in the intracellular fluid containing a high concentration of potassium ions and a low concentration of sodium ions relative to the extracellular fluid. In addition to active transport, the membrane is specifically permeable to potassium ions, and allows them to leak out of the cell faster than sodium ions can leak in. The difference in ionic concentration across the membrane results in an electrical potential, or charge, with the interior negative to the exterior in the resting state. The magnitude of the potential inside the membrane relative to the outside is determined by the ratio of the tendency for the ions to diffuse in one direction or the other, and the contribution of a particular ion is quantitated by the Nernst equation:

$$\text{Membrane Potential} = \text{(millivolts)}$$
$$-61 \log \frac{\text{intracellular ion concentration}}{\text{extracellular ion concentration}}$$

The degree of importance of each of the ions in determining the voltage is proportional to the membrane permeability for that particular ion. Since, in the resting state, the neuronal membrane is very permeable to potassium and only slightly permeable to sodium, it is potassium, with its Nernst potential of −94 mV, that contributes the most to the membrane potential. However, because there is some contribution to the resting membrane potential by sodium and chloride ions, the membrane resting potential is more accurately calculated from the more complicated Goldman-Hodgkin-Katz equation, and averages −60 to −70 mV, with the cell interior negative relative to the exterior.[58]

Although electrical potentials exist across the cell membranes of most of the cells of the body, it is the development and propagation of rapid changes in membrane potential, the action potential, which allows nerve fibers to carry signals. This electrical excitability is possible because of the presence in the axolemma of voltage-sensitive ion channels that are specific for sodium, potassium, or calcium ions.[59-64] In response to voltage fluctuation, these channels sequentially open and close in gate-like fashion to allow the rapid diffusion of specific ions down their concentration gradients across the axolemma,

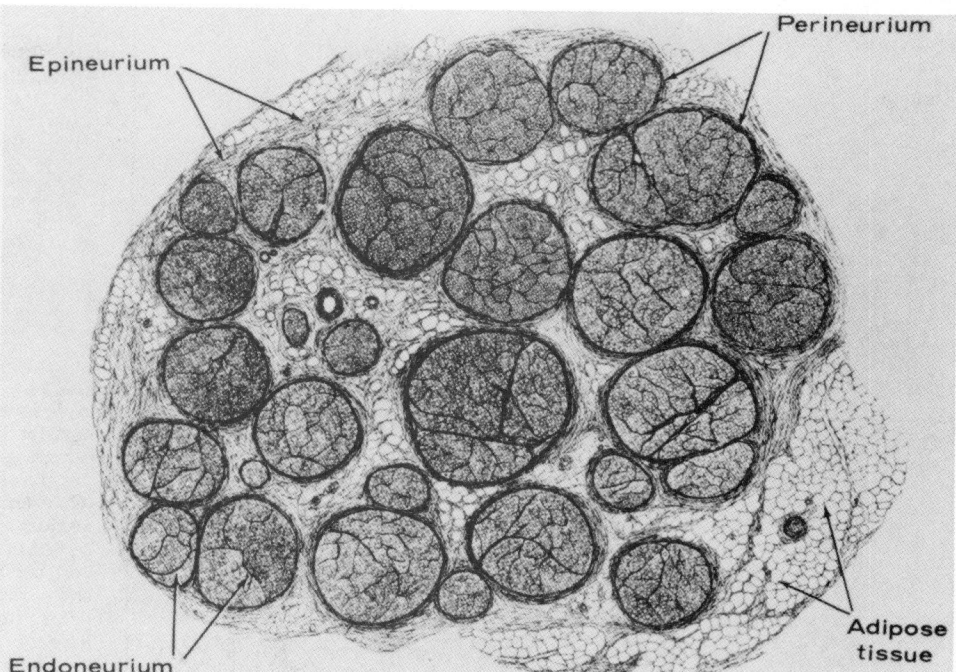

FIG. 14-5. Drawing of a cross-section of a human ulnar nerve at very low magnification, illustrating the endoneurium, perineurium, and epineurium, as well as the perineural vascular and adipose tissue. (Reprinted with permission from Angevine JB: The nervous tissue. In Fawcett DW [ed]: A Textbook of Histology, p 336. Philadelphia, WB Saunders, 1986.)

so that the resultant ionic current flux across the cell membrane depolarizes and repolarizes it (Fig. 14-7).

Although the sodium, potassium, and calcium ion channels are each important for initiation and propagation of the action potential in neurons, the properties of the sodium channel and its contribution to the action potential are the most important and best understood. Sodium channels exist in one of three states: closed (or resting), open, and inactivated (Fig. 14-8). When the membrane transiently becomes less negative relative to the resting potential (*i.e.*, increases from the resting voltage of −70 mV toward zero), and the magnitude of the change is sufficient to reach a triggering value or initial threshold potential, which is approximately −55 mV, a voltage-dependent conformational change in the closed, or resting, sodium channel is induced, so that the sodium permeability of the membrane is increased 500- to 5,000-fold, and the sodium ions are free to move down their electrochemical gradient into the cell. The sodium channel then closes to an inactivated state by voltage- and time-dependent mechanisms, resulting in the membrane once again becoming impermeable to sodium ions.[65–71] Once inactivated, the sodium channel cannot reopen again until the membrane potential returns to a value near that of the original resting membrane potential, which allows the channel to first return to its closed, or resting, state. The voltage-dependent permeability changes, or gatings, of ion channels result from intrinsic electrical properties of the macromolecules that compose the channel.[72]

Sequential opening and closing of the ion-specific channels allows passive ion fluxes down electrochemical gradients. These ion fluxes change the transmembrane electrical potential and produce an action potential. Because the sodium channels open at the beginning of the action potential, a far greater amount of sodium ions are entering the axon than potassium ions are exiting it. This results in the membrane potential becoming positive. Shortly after the onset of the action potential, the sodium channels close and voltage gating

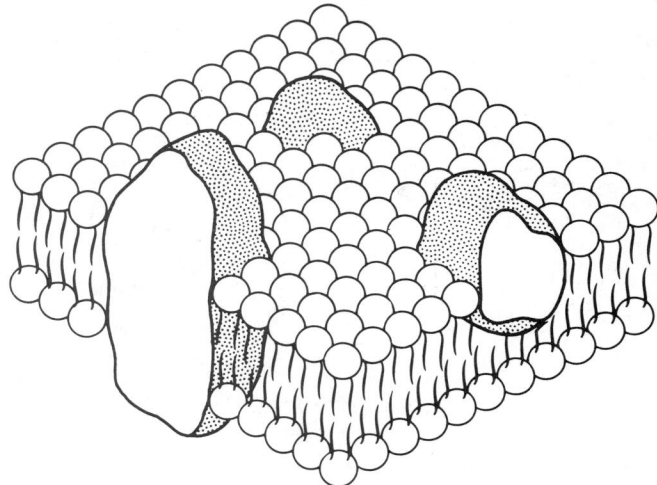

FIG. 14-6. The fluid mosaic model of the structure of a typical cell membrane. Globular proteins are partially embedded in a fluid bilayer of phospholipid molecules. The polar groups of the protein molecules protrude from the membrane into the aqueous phase, and their nonpolar groups are buried in the hydrophobic membrane interior. Certain proteins extend entirely through the membrane, and these include those functioning as the ionic channels responsible for the electrical properties of cell membranes. (Redrawn with permission from Singer SJ, Nicolson GL: The fluid mosaic model of the structure of cell membranes. Science 175:723, 1972. Copyright 1972 by the AAAS.)

of the potassium channels occurs, resulting in greatly increased transmembrane permeability to potassium ions. At that point, the membrane potential returns to its baseline negative resting potential of approximately −70 mV after first undergoing a transient hyperpolarization (positive after-po-

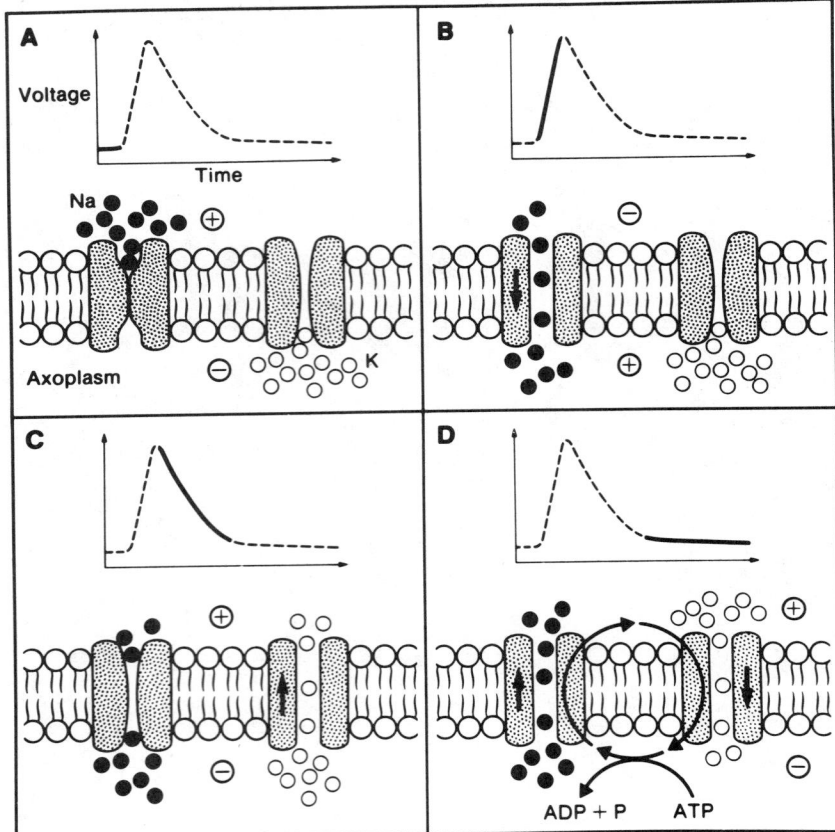

FIG. 14-7. Sodium and potassium ion flux across the axolemma *via* specific channels, and the resultant nerve action potential. At rest (*A*) an ATP-dependent pumping mechanism creates ionic gradients across the axolemma, with a relative excess of sodium ions (●) exterior to the cell and a relative excess of potassium ions (○) in the cell interior. During depolarization of the neuron (*B*), sodium channel pores open and sodium ions flow freely down their electrochemical gradient into the cell. During repolarization (*C*), sodium channels close and the axolemma is no longer permeable to sodium ions, but potassium ion channels open and potassium ions flow down their electrochemical gradient out of the cell. Upon completion of the action potential (*D*), sodium and potassium ions are actively transported back to the cell exterior and interior, respectively. (Redrawn from Covino BG, Scott DB: Handbook of Epidural Anaesthesia and Analgesia, p 58. Orlando, Grune and Stratton, 1985, by permission.)

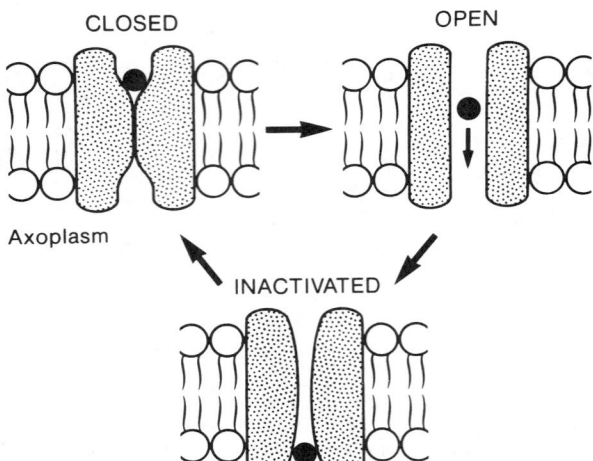

FIG. 14-8. The three sodium channel states: closed or resting, open, and inactivated. Once inactivated, a sodium channel cannot reopen until the original resting membrane potential is re-established, allowing the channel to first return to its closed, or resting, state.

tential), because some of the potassium channels remain open after the repolarization process is completed (Fig. 14-9).

For a signal to be transmitted by a nerve, it is necessary for an action potential to be conducted along a nerve fiber. If a local membrane depolarization is of sufficient magnitude to reach the critical threshold potential and trigger an action

potential, the resultant voltage changes are usually of adequate strength to reach the initial threshold of the adjacent membrane segments and result in propagation of the action potential along the nerve fiber. This is called an "all-or-none phenomenon," because either the local depolarization reaches the initial threshold potential of adjacent membrane segments and propagates itself over the entire axolemma, or it does not reach the necessary initial threshold voltage potential and the spread of depolarization stops.[73]

Once an action potential is initiated in an unmyelinated nerve fiber, it is propagated as a wave of depolarization that spreads at a constant speed, activating the sodium channels of each successive membrane segment as it travels along the axon. The larger the diameter of the fiber, the greater the speed of this impulse traveling along it.[73, 74] Myelinization of nerve fibers is an adaptation which greatly increases the speed and efficiency of impulse transmission when compared to unmyelinated nerve fibers of equal diameter. Myelin is an excellent insulator, increasing the resistance to ion flow through the axolemma approximately 5,000-fold. However, between successive Schwann cells along the length of the axon are the small, unmyelinated, junctional regions, the nodes of Ranvier, where ions can flow in relatively unimpeded fashion between the axoplasm and the extracellular fluid during an action potential. In addition, the nodal regions of the axolemma contain dense concentrations of sodium channels, which is in contrast to the internodal and perinodal regions, where few, if any, sodium channels exist.[67] Because of these factors, in myelinated nerve fibers, the action potential can occur only at the nodes of Ranvier, so the nerve impulse is forced to jump from node to node. This process, called salta-

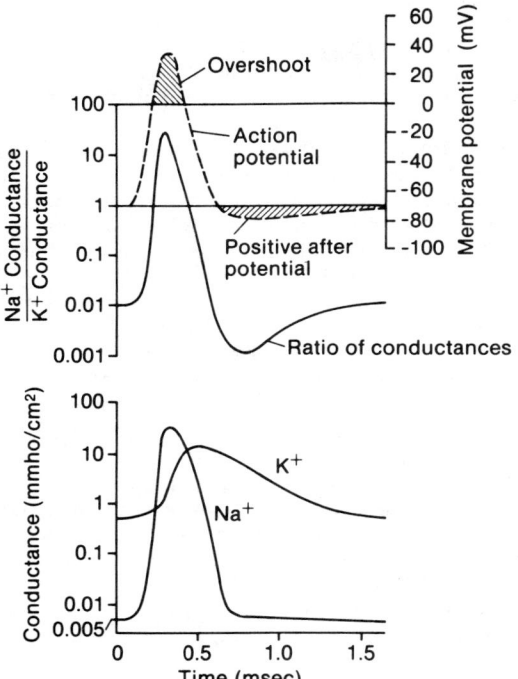

FIG. 14-9. Sodium and potassium ion flux across the axolemma during an action potential. Note that sodium conductance increases several thousand-fold during the early stages of the action potential, yet potassium conductance increases only approximately 30-fold during the latter phase of the action potential. (Redrawn from Guyton AC: Textbook of Medical Physiology, p 109. Philadelphia, WB Saunders, 1986, by permission.)

tory conduction, contributes to increased speed and efficiency of neural transmission through several mechanisms. Because the nerve impulse jumps from node to node instead of spreading directly to adjacent axolemma segments, the velocity of conduction is increased an average of five to seven times. Since only the nodal regions of the axons depolarize, the total ion flux across the entire neural membrane is greatly decreased, and the energy expenditure needed to re-establish cationic gradients across the membrane after a series of depolarizations is less. Lastly, because conduction of the nerve impulse is an "all-or-none phenomenon," propagation of the action potential may be more likely in myelinated fibers, because the higher density of sodium channels in the nodal regions reduces the threshold for excitation by allowing generation of an action potential when a smaller percentage of the channels are activated.[67]

ELECTROPHYSIOLOGIC EFFECTS OF LOCAL ANESTHETICS

Inhibition of sodium ion influx across the neuronal cell membrane is the common mechanism of action through which all local anesthetic agents produce blockade of the nerve impulse.[75] To block the generation and conduction of the action potentials, local anesthetics must interfere with the function of the ion channels that specifically conduct sodium ions across the membrane.[76–80] The ionic gradients and resting membrane potential of the nerve are unchanged, but the increase in sodium permeability associated with the nerve impulse is inhibited. Since a wide variety of chemical compounds exhibit local anesthetic activity, it is unlikely that they all block sodium conductance in the same manner. Several theories regarding the mechanism of action of local anesthetics include: calcium-mediated local anesthetic inhibition of sodium flux; interference with membrane permeability by expansion of membrane volume; local anesthetic-induced changes in the surface charge of the axolemma; and local anesthetic interaction with a specific receptor in the neuronal membrane.

Displacement of calcium from a membrane site that controls sodium permeability has been advanced as a mechanism of local anesthetic activity.[81] A low calcium ion concentration outside the neuron enhances local anesthetic activity, and an increasing external calcium concentration antagonizes the blocking action of local anesthetics. However, the direct actions of calcium and local anesthetics appear to be independent of each other.[82, 83] Thus, it is unlikely that calcium directly mediates the activity of local anesthetic agents.

A second theory regarding the mechanism of local anesthetic activity involves an application of the Meyer-Overton rule of anesthesia. It postulates that diffusion of the relatively lipophilic anesthetic molecules into the lipid component of the neuronal membrane expands the membrane to a critical volume and interferes with sodium conductance. Decreased sodium permeability could occur either through an increase in the lateral pressure in the membrane, which would directly compress the sodium channels, or through a conformational change in the proteins of the sodium channels brought about by an increase in the degree of the disorder of the membrane lipid molecules.[84–86] Local anesthetic agents have been shown to both increase the volume of lipid membranes and to increase their degree of disorder and, thus, fluidity.[87–91] High-pressure antagonism of the anesthetic activity of certain uncharged local anesthetic molecules, such as benzyl alcohol and benzocaine, has been shown to occur by some investigators, and may be evidence for the applicability of the membrane expansion theory to the mechanism of action of these compounds.[92, 93] However, pressure reversal has not been shown to occur in the case of charged local anesthetics, and there is no direct evidence that membrane expansion is important in their activity. These findings, as well as others, indicate that charged and uncharged local anesthetic molecules may have separate sites of action, and that membrane expansion may be more important for the action of only the uncharged local anesthetics.[94]

A third proposal for the mechanism of action of local anesthetics involves the induction of alterations in the membrane surface charge. Because some of the neuronal membrane molecules contain hydrophilic, anionic tails that are arrayed so that they protrude outward from the membrane lipid to both the external (extracellular) and internal (axoplasmic) surfaces of the membrane, both surfaces of the axolemma are negatively charged relative to the membrane interior.[95, 96] These fixed negative charges attract cations such as sodium and calcium, and these charge interactions add to the electrochemical resting potential to yield the net transmembrane potential.[97] The fixed negative charges of the membrane's two surfaces may also attract cationic local anesthetic molecules, aligning the charged local anesthetic molecule at the membrane-water interface with its nonpolar, aromatic domain in the membrane lipid, and its hydrophilic, charged portion in the adjacent aqueous phase.[98] The cationic local anesthetic molecule thus neutralizes to a variable degree the fixed negative charges on the membrane surface and alters the trans-

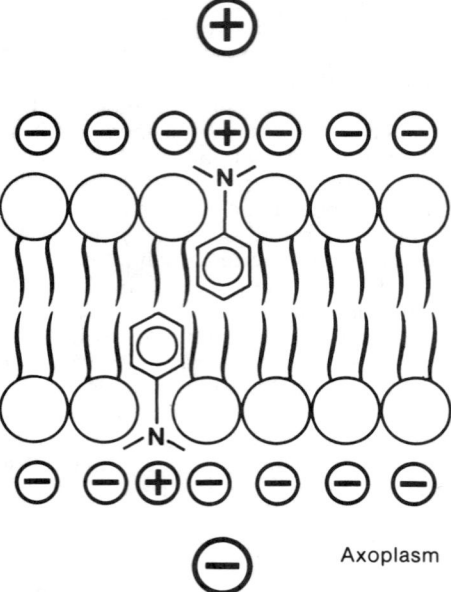

Axoplasm

FIG. 14-10. Neutralization of membrane surface fixed negative charges by cationic local anesthetic molecules, according to the surface charge theory. The additional positive charges on the relatively positive-charged extracellular surface of the axolemma may hyperpolarize the membrane. The additional positive charges on the relatively negative-charged intracellular surface of the axolemma may prevent sufficient membrane repolarization for reactivation of sodium channels. Thus, additional positive charges provided by local anesthetic molecules at either axolemma surface could interfere with the development of action potentials. (Redrawn from Scurlock JE: The mechanism of action of local anesthetics. Reg Anesth 2:5, 1977, with permission.)

membrane potential (Fig. 14-10).[99] If the local anesthetic molecule is absorbed to the extracellular side of the axonal membrane, the extra positive charges there could add to the already relatively positive extracellular charge and hyperpolarize the membrane, resulting in it being more difficult for an approaching nerve impulse to raise the transmembrane potential to depolarization threshold. On the other hand, if the local anesthetic molecule is absorbed into the intracellular side of the axonal membrane, the increase in positive charge could prevent sufficient repolarization of the membrane interior to allow for reactivation of sodium channels inactivated by a previous action potential. If sufficient sodium channels remain in the inactivated state, a subsequent action potential could not occur. Either mechanism could produce neural blockade.

The surface charge theory has the support of several investigators, and also accounts for the antagonism between divalent cations, such as calcium, and local anesthetic compounds.[98–101] Although the surface charge hypothesis may account for the action of charged local anesthetics, it does not explain the ability of uncharged local anesthetics, such as benzyl alcohol and benzocaine, to block nerve impulse. However, the failure of a single theory to satisfactorily explain the actions of all local anesthetic types does not necessarily invalidate it. Different local anesthetic molecules may have different mechanisms of action.

The fourth and most popular theory regarding the mechanism of action of local anesthetics proposes that they interact directly with specific receptors in the neuronal membrane.[102, 103] These receptors, in turn, would affect specific ion channels of the neuronal membrane in such a fashion that the ionic flux needed for initiation and propagation of the action potential is inhibited.

The structure of the sodium channel is apparently that of a lipoglycoprotein that spans the neuronal membrane and contains an aqueous pore that is able to discriminate between sodium and other ions, being selectively more permeable to sodium.[104–107] Intrinsic electrical properties of the macromolecules that compose the channel allow it to change configuration in response to changes in membrane potential, thus determining conductance of sodium ions across the axolemma. The distribution of the population of sodium channels between the resting and inactivated states, as previously described, is an important determinant of the refractory behavior of neurons. Immediately following an action potential, many of the sodium channels are in the inactivated state, and cannot be reopened by a subsequent voltage change.[107] Therefore, once an excitable membrane has been depolarized by an action potential, it cannot conduct a second impulse until it has first repolarized and thereby allowed inactivated sodium channels to return to the resting state. If an adequate number of sodium channels are not present in the resting state, sodium current sufficient for a second action potential cannot be generated.

The property of use- or frequency-dependent blockade, in which neuronal blockade by charged local anesthetic molecules increases with repetitive, brief membrane depolarizations, is one phenomenon that suggests direct interaction between sodium channel receptors and the charged local anesthetic molecule.[108, 109] It is postulated that frequency dependence develops because charged, hydrophilic anesthetic molecules inhibit sodium ion conductance through the sodium channel by gaining access to a channel receptor, located within the channel itself, while the sodium channel pore is in the open state. Reversal of the local anesthetic inhibitory effect would also require an open channel pore to facilitate the dissociation of the local anesthetic molecule, and, thus, a closed channel containing a local anesthetic molecule would be slow to return to its uninhibited state. In contrast to charged anesthetics, neutral anesthetic compounds exhibit much less frequency-dependent blockade, and this may be the result of these molecules not being restricted to the aqueous phase, gaining access to a channel binding site through the lipid milieu of the membrane interior.[110, 111] Local anesthetics may also shift the sodium channel population to a non-conducting state by binding preferentially to channels that have already been inactivated, preventing their return to the resting, depolarization-susceptible configuration.

In addition to interacting with sodium channels that are in the open and in the inactivated state, it appears that local anesthetics can also produce a tonic, or resting, block by binding with the channels in the resting state to prevent their voltage-induced activation.[107] This third type of local anesthetic sodium channel association appears to be much weaker. The discovery that the blocking potency of local anesthetic molecules is much greater when the interaction is with receptors of open or inactivated channels, as compared to those of resting channels, has led to the modulated receptor hypothesis of local anesthetic-receptor binding.[110, 112–115] The variable state of the local anesthetic receptor determines the strength of its interaction with the local anesthetic molecule, and an excitable membrane with a higher depolarization frequency will be more sensitive to the blocking effects of local anesthetics. The charged local anesthetics interact with all three sodium channel states, and the resultant variable drug potency is manifested as frequency-dependent blockade. Use- or frequency-dependence may be a mechanism by which a local anesthetic solution causes a differential blockade of the fibers within a given nerve.

At this time, it is uncertain as to where exactly the local anesthetic receptors of the sodium channel are located, and there may be at least three sites of local anesthetic binding (Fig. 14-11). One is located near the interior opening of the sodium pore, and has a higher affinity for the more charged local anesthetic molecules, and one is located at the interface between the sodium channel structure and the surrounding membrane lipid, being more easily accessed by uncharged, lipophilic local anesthetic molecules.[107, 116, 117] In addition, there are a variety of other sodium channel sites where certain pharmacologic compounds and toxins specifically combine.[106] Tetrodotoxin, produced by several species of puffer fish, frogs, and newts; and saxitoxin, produced by a marine dinoflagellate, are examples of other molecules that specifically bind to sodium channels. They directly interact with the outer aspect of the sodium channel to block sodium conductance.[118, 119] Although chemicals such as these are not clinically important as local anesthetics, modification of their structures may lead to new classes of anesthetics in the future.

MINIMUM BLOCKING CONCENTRATION (C_m)

The minimum blocking concentration, or C_m, of a local anesthetic is the lowest concentration of anesthetic that blocks impulse conduction along a given nerve fiber or nerve within a specified time. The concept of C_m is analogous to the minimum alveolar concentration (MAC) of inhalational anesthetics, and is a direct indication of the relative potency of a given anesthetic.[120] However, this value is determined *in vitro*, and is extremely influenced by minor variations in experimental conditions.[121] For example, minor variations in the temperature, *p*H, or calcium ion concentration of the solution

FIG. 14-11. Sites of action of different types of local anesthetics. Aminoesters and aminoamides act at the axoplasmic surface of the sodium channels in their charged form (BH$^+$), or, to a lesser extent, at the intramembrane portion of the sodium channels in their base form (B). Uncharged local anesthetics, such as benzocaine, also act from within the membrane interior. Tetrodotoxin (TTX) and other biotoxins have sites of action at the external aspect of the sodium channels. (Redrawn from Covino BG, Scott DB: Handbook of Epidural Anaesthesia and Analgesia, p 64. Orlando, Grune and Stratton, 1985, with permission.)

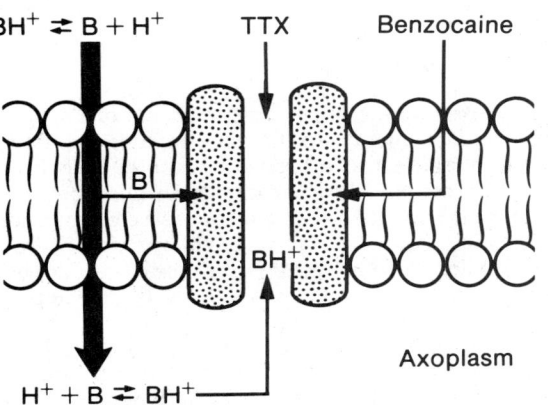

bathing the nerve will alter the value of C_m.[121–123] Similarly, the frequency of nerve stimulation also affects the apparent potency of the local anesthetic.

Despite the determination of differential potencies of local anesthetics *in vitro* (different C_ms), these relationships may not be directly applicable to clinical practice. Differences in diffusion, local tissue binding, systemic absorption, and nerve penetration will all affect the concentration of local anesthetic that ultimately develops in a nerve after injection of a given dose. Because intraneural concentrations of local anesthetics are rarely measured, clinical use is based on a dose-response relationship.

Dose-response relationships, in humans, suggest that pregnancy reduces the anesthetic requirement necessary to achieve a given level of epidural anesthesia.[124] *In vitro* comparison of nerve fibers from pregnant and nonpregnant rabbits suggests that pregnancy may increase the sensitivity of nerve membranes to local anesthetics.[125, 126]

DIFFERENTIAL BLOCK

It has long been a clinical observation that all neuronal functions are not affected by local anesthetics in equal fashion. For example, blockade of the components of a peripheral nerve may proceed at different rates, with loss of sympathetic function first, followed by pin-prick sensation, touch and temperature, and, lastly, motor function, or there may be relative sparing of one neuronal function over another, as in the low-dose bupivacaine labor epidural with its relatively intact motor tone. Clinical findings such as these have given rise to the concept of differential blockade of the various nerve fiber types, and there are currently several potential explanations for the existence of this phenomenon. No uniformly accepted theory exists at present because of conflicting data generated by investigations performed under differing laboratory conditions, and because of the difficulty of designing a suitable laboratory model. Also, there may very well be several independent mechanisms for differential blockade.

Peripheral nerve fibers have been classified according to size and function (Table 14-2).[127, 128] Myelinated somatic nerve fibers, or A fibers, are largest in diameter and conduct impulses the most rapidly. These are further divided according to progressively decreasing size into alpha, beta, gamma, and delta fibers. The alpha and beta fibers convey motor and proprioception information, the gamma fibers control muscle spindle tone, and the delta fibers, which are the smallest in diameter of the A fibers, transmit messages concerning pain, temperature, and touch. In contrast to the A fibers, which, as a group, are quite variable in diameter, ranging from 6 to 22 μm, the B and C fibers are much more uniform in size. The thinly myelinated B fibers are smaller in diameter than A fibers, and have a preganglionic autonomic function. The unmyelinated C fibers are the smallest-diameter nerve fibers, have the lowest rate of impulse conduction velocity, and contain postganglionic autonomic axons, as well as axons conveying pain, temperature, and touch information.[129]

For many years, it was felt that differential blockade could be explained on the basis of relative vulnerability of various neuronal fiber types to the blocking activity of local anesthetic solutions, with fiber diameter inversely proportional to susceptibility to local anesthetic blockade. Thus, the larger A fibers were thought to be less susceptible to blockade, whereas the small C fibers should be the most easily blocked.[130] This inverse relationship between fiber size and susceptibility to local anesthetic blockade was drawn from *in vitro* data obtained using differently sized myelinated fibers only,[128] and it was subsequently shown that its application to the small C fibers did not hold true once C fibers were actually studied.[131–138] A-delta and B fibers were found to be more susceptible to local anesthetic blockade than the relatively smaller C fibers, and, later, the largest A fibers were noted by some investigators to actually be the most susceptible of all to local anesthetic block. Thus, nerve fiber vulnerability to local anesthetic action would vary directly with fiber size, the largest A fibers being the most sensitive, and the small C fibers being the least sensitive.[139–141]

One explanation for the relative susceptibilities of different nerve fiber types to local anesthetic block involves the concept of conduction safety. A voltage change substantially greater than the action potential threshold of the adjacent membrane provides a margin of safety for continued conduction of the action potential. This ratio of the values of the nerve impulse voltage change to the adjacent membrane action potential threshold is termed the safety factor, and impulse propagation will fail if this value falls below 1, such as in local anesthetic blockade.[130, 142, 143] The conduction safety factor of smaller myelinated fibers may be less than that of larger myelinated fibers, making the smaller fibers more vulnerable to the effects of local anesthetics. Since local anesthetics must block at least three adjacent nodes of Ranvier to halt impulse propagation,[144] and since internodal distance is directly proportional to fiber size,[145] a relatively small distribution of local anesthetic solution may be sufficient to differentially block the smaller fibers (Fig. 14-12).[133, 134] The conduction safety factor may be greater for non-myelinated fibers, since only the immediately adjacent area of the axonal membrane must reach depolarization threshold for propagation of the action potential, whereas, in myelinated fibers, the current generated at one node must be sufficient to depolarize the membrane of the next node some distance away. This may explain the relative *in vitro* resistance of non-myelinated fibers to local anesthetic blockade.[146–149] An additional finding is that the safety factor of an individual nerve fiber is variable, depending on the location along the fiber itself, the degree of impulse activity, the CO_2 tension, and the local ionic gradients.[150–153] Because of the interaction of these factors, the relative effects of a local anesthetic upon different nerve fibers may be a dynamic phenomenon.

Although the large, fast-conducting A fibers have been found by some to be intrinsically the most sensitive to blockade by local anesthetics, and the small, slow-conducting C fibers the least sensitive, this fact is not always immediately apparent in clinical situations involving nerve blocks. This may be a reflection of the relative rate of onset of block in different fiber types, in contrast to the relative susceptibility of different fibers to local anesthetic blockade in the setting of a steady-state local anesthetic concentration. Because of the decreased ability of local anesthetic molecules to cross the multilayered lipoprotein membranes of the myelin sheath, the rate of onset of block will be slower in A fibers when compared to the unmyelinated C fibers. Therefore, in contrast to the rapid onset of block in C fibers due to the relatively unimpeded local anesthetic access to the axon, the slower local anesthetic blockade of A fibers depends upon the pK_a and lipid partition coefficient of the local anesthetic molecule.[140, 141, 149, 154] The lower the pK_a (and, thus, the greater the percentage of lipophilic, uncharged molecules at physiologic pH) and the greater the lipid partition coefficient of the local anesthetic molecule, the more rapid the onset of block in the A fibers. However, in high concentrations, even a relatively hydrophilic local anesthetic will produce a rapid block of A fibers, because the greater diffusion gradient will cause a more rapid transit across the myelin sheath. Thus, the use of a lower concentration of a less lipid-soluble local anesthetic would be most likely to result in a differential blockade of A-delta and C fibers at the onset of the nerve block.

The exact mechanism of differential blockade has not been conclusively demonstrated, and there may very well be more than one factor involved. Despite the general agreement that the unmyelinated C fibers are less sensitive to local anesthetics than the larger A and B fibers, the concepts of size-related differential susceptibility of myelinated nerve fibers to local anesthetic blockade, as well as that of the myelin sheath as a barrier to local anesthetic diffusion, are not universally accepted.[155–161] It has been suggested that differential blockade may be the manifestation of a frequency-dependent process, with more rapidly firing fibers, such as those conveying sensory information, being more susceptible to blockade than slower-firing fibers, such as somatic motor efferents.[151, 162–165] Differential block may also be a reflection of the geographical arrangement of the nerve fibers within the peripheral nerve, with the outermost fibers blocked preferentially if the local anesthetic solution bathing the nerve is dilute enough so that there is a concentration gradient of local anesthetic extending from the outermost layers of the nerve to its center.[166, 167]

FIG. 14-12. Differential blockade of myelinated nerve fibers of differing diameters. Internodal distance is proportional to axon diameter, and conduction blockade occurs when at least three adjacent nodes of a nerve fiber are exposed to blocking concentrations of the local anesthetic agent. Thus, equivalent spread of local anesthetic may produce conduction blockade of a thin axon, but not the adjacent thick axon. (Redrawn from Franz DN, Perry RS: Mechanisms for differential block among single myelinated and non-myelinated axons by procaine. J Physiol 236:207, 1974, with permission.)

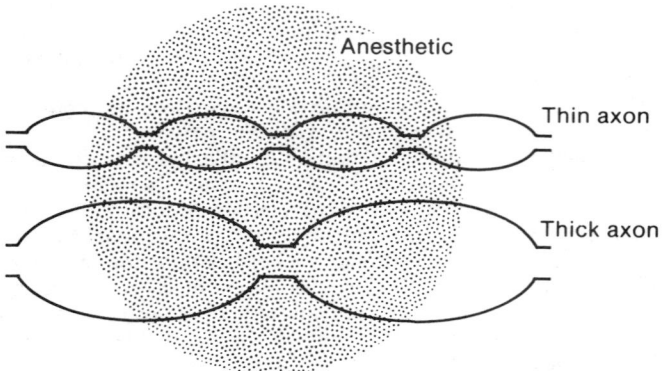

Anesthetic

Thin axon

Thick axon

PHARMACOKINETICS

Pharmacokinetics describes the movement of a drug through the body: movement into the bloodstream, movement from blood into tissues, and movement out of the body by metabolism and excretion. Pharmacodynamics describes the drug's effect on the body (usually expressed as a concentration-effect relationship). An understanding of pharmacokinetics enables anesthesiologists to predict the concentration of drug that will develop at the desired organ, and thus, be able to predict the effect that will be produced.

For regional anesthesia, local anesthetic is injected in close proximity to the site of desired effect so that local, physical factors become much more important than systemic pharmacokinetic factors for predicting the desired pharmacodynamic effect (*i.e.*, neural blockade) (Fig. 14-13). The goal in regional anesthesia is to use just enough local anesthetic to provide adequate anesthesia, but less than the amount that will produce toxicity. Ideally, the minimum dose required would be determined by the minimum concentration of local anesthetic in the nerve necessary to produce the desired degree of neural blockade. However, the concentration that develops in neural tissue is difficult to predict due to the complex interaction of multiple factors, including: 1) the proximity of the injected anesthetic to the nerve tissue; 2) the flow of anesthetic around the neural tissue; 3) diffusion across the tissue barriers and into neural tissue; 4) binding of anesthetic to local non-neural tissues; and 5) absorption into the vascular and lymph system.

Thus, identical doses of local anesthetic used for the same block may result in markedly different concentrations of local anesthetic in the nerves, and dose-response relationships are extremely variable. Appreciation of this variability of effect, combined with the fact that many regional anesthetic techniques are performed with a single injection of drug, with no titration to effect, causes most anesthesiologists to use maximal doses of local anesthetic for regional blockade in an attempt to reduce the incidence of inadequate blocks. An understanding of pharmacokinetics allows us to predict peak blood levels resulting from a given dose of drug, and, it is hoped, define the maximum dose that can be administered and still avoid systemic toxicity.

FIG. 14-13. This figure depicts the factors determining the distribution of local anesthetic near the site of injection and within the body. A relatively high concentration of local anesthetic is injected in close proximity to a nerve bundle. Non-ionized anesthetic (**B**) diffuses into the axon and provides neural blockade. Nonspecific tissue binding (*e.g.*, to fat muscle or connective tissue) and absorption into the blood stream reduces the mass of drug available to diffuse into neural tissue. Once absorbed into the blood stream, the local anesthetics are distributed to systemic tissues, and are metabolized in the liver to compounds which are primarily excreted by the kidney.

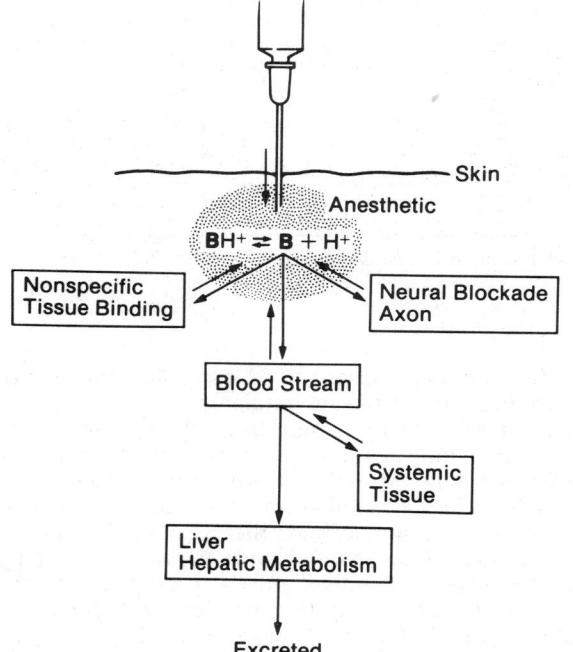

In this section, we will address local disposition of anesthetic, which is determined by bulk flow, diffusion, and systemic absorption. Then we will examine systemic distribution and elimination of absorbed anesthetic, interactions with other commonly used drugs, and the effects of coexistent disease.

LOCAL DISPOSITION

Bulk Flow

Because intraneural injection is painful and may result in nerve damage, local anesthetic should always be injected near the nerve.[168] The amount of anesthetic that reaches the nerve depends, to a large extent, on the proximity of injection to the nerve. The drug then needs to diffuse through connective tissue and past fat to reach the nerve (Fig. 14-13). The barriers to diffusion and the amount of adipose tissue vary considerably among different nerves in the body. For example, spinal nerve roots are floating free in cerebrospinal fluid, and the application of small amounts of local anesthetic produces profound blockade. In contrast, brachial plexus and sciatic nerves are surrounded by fascial sheaths and adipose tissue, and the application of large amounts of drug is necessary to provide reliable anesthesia.

It seems obvious that a larger volume of local anesthetic solution will spread by bulk flow to a greater extent, and should, therefore, produce a greater spread of nerve block. However, bulk flow and spread of anesthesia are not synonymous. For example, physical spread of local anesthetic solution in the epidural space is not directly correlated with the resulting clinical spread of anesthesia.[169, 170] Concentration, or total mass of drug, also affects the spread, probably by influencing diffusion gradients. Separating the effects of volume, concentration, and mass is difficult.[171, 172] It is likely that both factors are important: a minimum volume is necessary to provide adequate spread of local anesthetic around the nerves, and a minimum concentration is necessary to provide an adequate diffusion gradient for penetrance into the nerve. Furthermore, once above these minimum values, the total mass of drug becomes most important.[172]

Diffusion

After the local anesthetic is injected near the nerve, it must then move to the nerve, into the nerve, and within the nerve. These movements occur through the process of diffusion. During this process, the anesthetic is diluted by absorption into tissues, blood, and lymph. Although smaller compounds diffuse faster, the small range of differences in molecular weights of local anesthetics should not produce clinically significant differences in diffusion rates. Therefore, the rapidity and extent of diffusion depends in largest extent upon the pK_a of the local anesthetic, the concentration of anesthetic injected, and, possibly, the lipid solubility.

Because the pK_a of all local anesthetics are higher than physiologic pH, and higher than the pH of all commercially available local anesthetic solutions, most of the injected anesthetic is in the ionized, less lipid-soluble, form (Tables 14-1, 14-3). The ionized form of the drug diffuses poorly, whereas the non-ionized (free base) form is thought to be freely diffusible (Fig. 14-2). Consequently, the relatively high pK_a of tetracaine and procaine may, in part, explain these agents' relatively poor ability to spread and penetrate tissues. However,

TABLE 14-3. Chemical Structure, Physio-Chemical Properties, and Maximum Dose of Selected Local Anesthetic Agents

	CHEMICAL STRUCTURE			RELATIVE LIPID SOLUBILITY	PROTEIN BINDING (%)	pK_a	EQUIEFFECTIVE CONCENTRATION (%)	MAXIMUM DOSE (mg)
	Aromatic End	Intermediate Chain	Amine End					
AMINO ESTERS								
Procaine	H_2N–⬡–	$COOCH_2CH_2$	$-N(C_2H_5)_2$	1	5	8.9	2	1000
2-Chloroprocaine	H_2N–⬡(Cl)–	$COOCH_2CH_2$	$-N(C_2H_5)_2$	1	—	9.1	2	1000
Tetracaine	H_9C_4(NH)–⬡–	$COOCH_2CH_2$	$-N(CH_3)_2$	80	85	8.6	0.25	200
AMINO AMIDES								
Lidocaine	⬡($CH_3)_2$	$NHCOCH_2$	$-N(C_2H_5)_2$	4	65	7.9	1	500
Prilocaine	⬡(CH_3)	$NHCOCH(CH_3)$	$-N(C_3H_7)H$	1.5	55	7.7	1	900
Mepivacaine	⬡($CH_3)_2$	$NHCO$	piperidine $N-CH_3$	1	75	7.6	1	500
Bupivacaine	⬡($CH_3)_2$	$NHCO$	piperidine $N-C_4H_9$	30	95	8.1	0.25	200
Etidocaine	⬡($CH_3)_2$	$NHCOCH(C_2H_5)$	$-N(C_2H_5)(C_3H_7)$	140	95	7.7	0.25	300

Adapted from: Bonica JJ: Principles and Practice of Obstetric Analgesia and Anesthesia, p 476. Philadelphia, FA Davis, 1967. With permission from the publisher.

tetracaine is very effective when injected into the subarachnoid space, where diffusion barriers are minimal.

Alkalinization of the injected solution will increase the proportion of non-ionized drug and should facilitate diffusion.[37] In contrast, ampules of local anesthetic with epinephrine added have lower pH values than plain local anesthetic solutions, and might, therefore, diffuse less readily.[35] Similarly, any factor that lowers extracellular pH, such as acidosis from local infection, will retard diffusion of local anesthetics because of increased ionization.

Higher concentrations, or greater total mass, of local anesthetic will penetrate thicker nerve fibers, intensify the blockade, and may speed onset.[173, 174] Presumably, this occurs because of increased diffusion gradients.

Local anesthetics with high lipid solubility would be expected to penetrate membranes more readily, and have higher potency and longer duration. However, the ability to spread will be offset by increased penetration into, and nonspecific binding with, fat, muscle, and other tissues. Thus, high lipid solubility might impede diffusion to the nerve receptor sites through nonspecific binding, and delay the onset of anesthesia. Finally, local tissue binding may serve as a depot, slowly releasing local anesthetic to the nerve and prolonging duration. In conclusion, diffusion is affected by multiple factors whose ultimate interaction must often be observed and explained rather than predicted.

Kinetics of Nerve Block

In isolated nerve preparations, the sensitivity to local anesthetics is found, by some authors, to vary depending on nerve diameter. Thus, in a clinical situation, the order of neural blockade might be expected to be analgesia, anesthesia, paresis, and, finally, paralysis. However, when the onset of neural blockade is critically examined for the brachial plexus, paresis occurs prior to analgesia.[166] Although these results at first appear to be inconsistent, this discrepancy can be easily explained by anatomical factors.

When local anesthetic is deposited near the brachial plexus, it must diffuse to the nerves before blockade results. Because the local anesthetic concentration at the outside of the nerve trunk is initially higher than in the center, the nerve bundles at the outside (mantle bundles) of the nerve trunk are blocked first, and onset of anesthesia is proximal to distal (Fig. 14-14). Motor nerve fibers are usually at the periphery of the nerve trunk, and sensory fibers in the center (or core). Consequently, if the concentration of local anesthetic injected is sufficient to produce motor blockade, the onset of motor blockade precedes the onset of sensory blockade.[166] Similar results would not be expected for regional anesthetic techniques where diffusion barriers are minimal, such as spinal anesthesia.

SYSTEMIC ABSORPTION

The rate of systemic absorption is an important factor in determining the peak blood level (C_{max}) that results from injection of local anesthetic, the amount of local anesthetic remaining at the site of injection, and, thus, the duration of anesthesia. The most important factors affecting C_{max} are: 1) the total dose of local anesthetic, 2) the site of injection, 3) the physiochemical properties of the local anesthetic, and 4) the addition of vasoconstrictors.

The greater the total dose of local anesthetic administered, the greater the peak blood level that results (Fig. 14-15). This relationship between dose and maximum blood level is almost linear.[175, 176] The effects of anesthetic concentration and the speed of injection on absorption rates are small.[175–177] Consequently, once the maximum safe total dose is identified, the concentration and volume used should be determined by anesthetic needs, rather than by pharmacokinetic concerns.

Different sites of anesthetic injection have considerable differences in local blood flow and tissue binding. Absorption will be rapid from highly vascular sites, and slower from sites with large amounts of fat and tissue that will bind the local anesthetic. In general, these effects are independent of the agent used.[178] Consequently, the rates of absorption differ between sites of injection to a greater extent than between anesthetic agents (Fig. 14-16).

The rate of absorption of local anesthetic from various sites decreases in the order: intercostal > caudal > epidural > brachial plexus > sciatic/femoral. Rapid absorption is evidenced by high maximum blood levels and a relatively shorter time to reach maximum levels.[177] Absorption is also rapid after paracervical, pudendal, and subcutaneous infiltration of the vagina, while subcutaneous infiltration of the abdomen results in low levels.[175, 178] Similarly, lidocaine sprayed on various parts of the respiratory tract results in concentrations similar or lower than those expected for epidural injection.[178, 179]

The interaction of local blood flow and tissue binding is apparent when looking at the above order. Although the epidural space is highly vascular compared to the intercostal

FIG. 14-14. Representation of the somatotopic arrangement of fibers in the trunks of the brachial plexus. Nerve fibers in the mantle (or peripheral) bundles innervate the proximal arm and fibers in the core (or central) bundles innervate the distal arm. The concentration gradient that develops during initial diffusion of local anesthetic into the nerve trunk causes onset of anesthesia to proceed from proximal to distal. (Modified from de Jong RH: Physiology and Pharmacology of Local Anesthesia, p 66. Springfield, Charles C Thomas, 1977, with permission.)

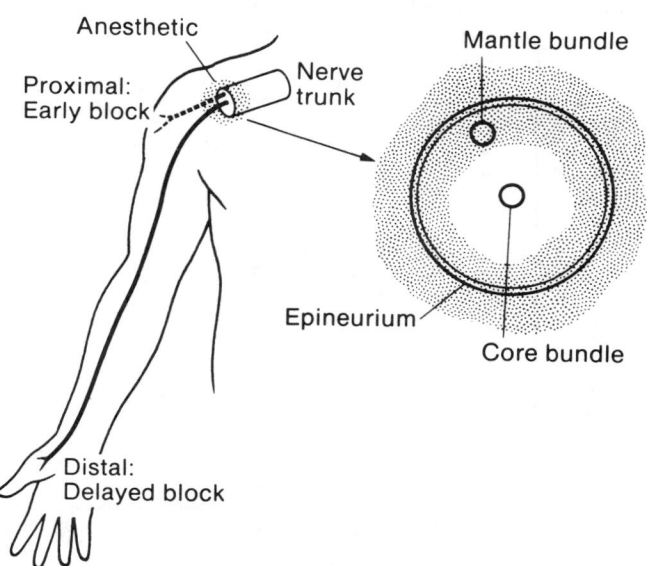

FIG. 14-15. Mean plasma concentrations of lidocaine, resulting from epidural injection, increases with increasing doses. (From Braid DP, Scott DB: Dosage of lignocaine in epidural block in relation to toxicity. Br J Anaesth 38:596, 1966, with permission.)

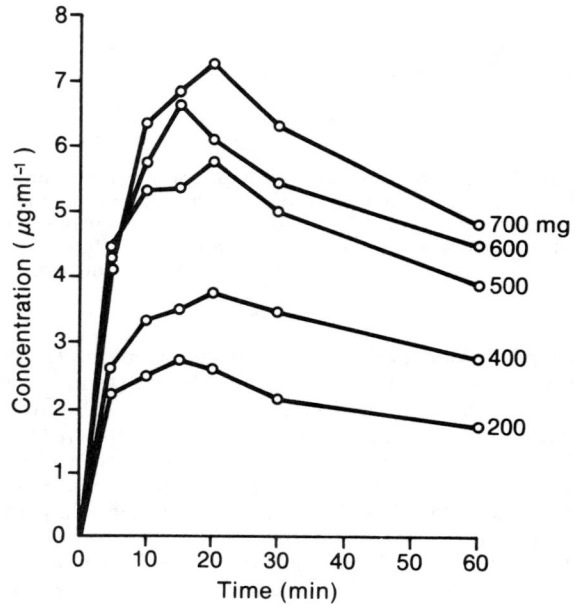

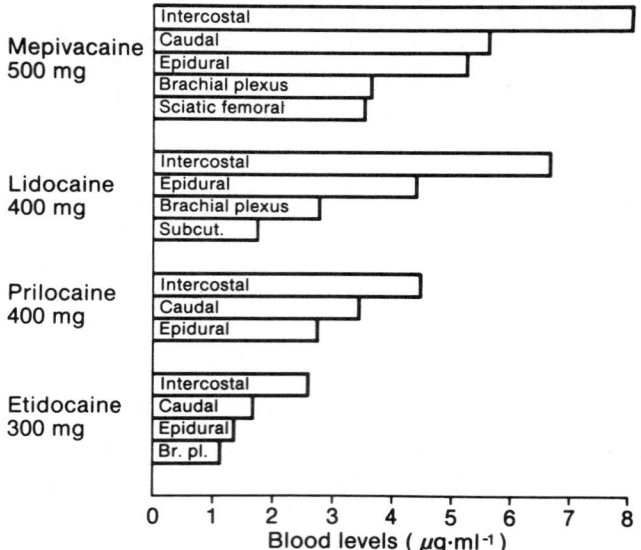

FIG. 14-16. Peak serum levels of several local anesthetics resulting from various types of regional anesthetic procedures. (Covino BG, Vassallo HG: Local Anesthetics: Mechanism of Action and Clinical Use, p 97. New York, Grune & Stratton, 1976, with permission.)

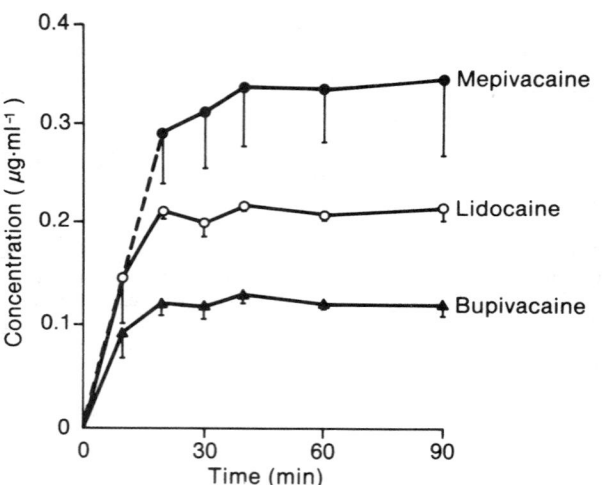

FIG. 14-17. Blood concentrations of local anesthetic resulting from epidural injection of a mixture of equal mg dosages of the three anesthetics (mean ± SE). (Reynolds F: A comparison of the potential toxicity of bupivacaine, lignocaine, and mepivacaine during epidural blockade for surgery. Br J Anaesth 43:567, 1971, with permission.)

space, peak blood levels are lower following epidural blockade than after intercostal blockade, probably as a result of greater fat binding in the epidural space. Similarly, although the epidural space has much greater vascularity than the subarachnoid space, the maximum blood levels seen after epidural or subarachnoid injection are not significantly different, probably as a result of greater nonspecific binding in the epidural space to fat and tissue.[180]

Physiochemical differences between local anesthetics also significantly affect C_{max}. For example, bupivacaine and etido-

caine appear to produce greater vasodilation than lidocaine or mepivacaine.[181] Greater vasodilation should increase the rate of absorption of local anesthetic. However, the increment in C_{max} for each 100 mg of bupivacaine or etidocaine injected into the epidural space is about half that observed for lidocaine and mepivacaine.[178] Furthermore, when equal doses of lidocaine, mepivacaine, and bupivacaine are injected together into the epidural space, the systemic blood levels that result are significantly different (Fig. 14-17).[182] Because local blood flow has to be the same when these drugs are injected together into the same space, the difference in systemic absorption must reflect differences in local tissue binding, and, indeed, parallels the differences in lipid solubility (Table 14-3).

Vasoconstrictors may be added to local anesthetic solutions to reduce systemic absorption, and prolong duration.[183] These agents have variable effects, yet seem to be the most effective for reducing peak blood levels when administered with the shorter-acting local anesthetics (lidocaine, mepivacaine, and prilocaine). From the above data, it appears that local tissue and nerve binding is more important than tissue blood flow in determining systemic absorption of etidocaine and bupivacaine. Perhaps this helps to explain why epinephrine is more effective at reducing C_{max}, and at prolonging the duration of lidocaine and mepivacaine than for bupivacaine or etidocaine (Table 14-4).

Physical and Pathophysiological Factors

Although the maximum safe dose of a local anesthetic is frequently stated in terms of mg · kg, there is no correlation between weight and peak plasma levels in adult patients (Fig. 14-18).[175, 176] Acute hypovolemia slows the absorption of lidocaine after peridural injection, probably by decreasing cardiac output.[184] In contrast, increasing the cardiac output appears to increase absorption of local anesthetic.[185, 186] Surprisingly, age and pregnancy do not appear to affect the rate of systemic absorption.[175, 176, 187–189]

FIG. 14-18. This scattergram illustrates the lack of correlation between body weight and the peak plasma concentration of lidocaine that results from epidural injection of 400 mg of lidocaine. (From Braid DP, Scott DB: Dosage of lignocaine in epidural block in relation to toxicity. Br J Anaesth 38:596, 1966, with permission.)

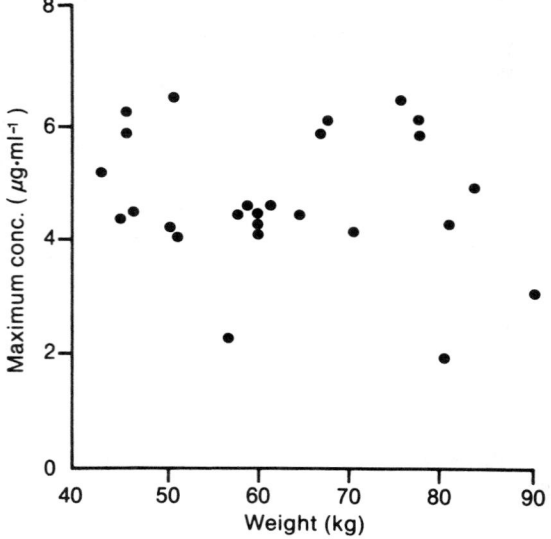

TABLE 14-4. Comparative Onset Times and Analgesic Durations of Various Local Anesthetic Agents and Effects of Addition of Epinephrine (5 $\mu g \cdot ml^{-1}$) on Duration and Peak Plasma Levels (C_{max})

ANESTHETIC TECHNIQUE	ANESTHETIC AGENT	USUAL CONC.(%)	AVERAGE ONSET TIME (MIN ± SE)	AVERAGE ANALGESIC DURATION (min ± SE)	ADDITION OF EPI % CHANGE	
					Duration	C_{max}
Brachial plexus block (40–50 ml)	Lidocaine	1.0	14 ± 4	195 ± 26	+ 50	− 20 − 30
	Mepivacaine	1.0	15 ± 6	245 ± 27	—	− 20 − 30
	Bupivacaine	0.25–0.5	10 − 25	575	—	− 10 − 20
	Etidocaine	0.5	9	572	—	− 10 − 20
Epidural anesthesia (20–30 ml)	Lidocaine	2.0	15	100 ± 20	+ 50	− 20 − 30
	Mepivacaine	2.0	15	115 ± 15	+ 50	− 20 − 30
	Bupivacaine	0.5	17	195 ± 30	+ 0 − 30	− 10 − 20
	Etidocaine	1.0	11	170 ± 57	+ 0 − 30	− 10 − 20
Local infiltration	Lidocaine	0.5		75 (35–340)	+ 200	− 50
	Mepivacaine	0.5		108 (15–240)	+ 120	—
	Bupivacaine	0.25		200 ± 33	+ 115	—

(Adapted from Covino BG, Vassallo HG: Local Anesthetics: Mechanism of Action and Clinical Use, pp 63, 81. New York, Grune & Stratton 1976; and Tucker GT, Mather LE: Absorption and disposition of local anesthetics. In Cousins MJ, Bridenbaugh PO [eds]: Neural Blockade in Clinical Anesthesia and Management of Pain, p 45. Philadelphia, JB Lippincott, 1980, with permission.)

DISTRIBUTION AND ELIMINATION

Once local anesthetic is absorbed into the blood, it is usually distributed first to the lung. Local anesthetics have high solubilities in the lung, leading to a large uptake in lung tissue (Fig. 14-19).[190, 191] This uptake of local anesthetic reduces the amount of drug that reaches the systemic circulation during accidental intravascular injection, and, thus, could be considered protective.

Upon reaching the systemic circulation, distribution is determined by tissue blood flow and the relative blood and tissue solubilities of the local anesthetic. Most of the local anesthetic is initially delivered to tissue groups with a high relative perfusion, the so-called vessel rich group (e.g., heart, brain, kidneys) (Fig. 14-19). Redistribution then occurs into tissues with lower relative perfusion, such as muscle and fat. Finally, local anesthetic is eliminated by metabolism and excretion.

Several factors have an important effect on distribution and elimination, including: 1) protein binding, 2) clearance and metabolism, 3) physiologic effects of absorbed local anesthetic or peripheral blockade, and 4) other physical and pathophysiological factors.

Protein Binding

Pharmacologic activity is generally related to unbound, or free, drug levels. The extent of protein binding, therefore, determines the amount of drug in the blood that is free, or available, to produce pharmacologic effect. The extent of protein binding varies considerably among the local anesthetics (Table 14-3). Furthermore, as the concentration of local anesthetic increases, the percentage that is bound to protein decreases, probably as a result of saturation of binding sites (Fig. 14-20).[192]

Amide local anesthetics are primarily bound to alpha$_1$-acid glycoprotein (AAG) and, to a lesser extent, albumin.[190] The extent of protein binding varies considerably between patients. For example, the unbound lidocaine fraction may vary up to eightfold, being relatively low in patients with cancer and relatively high in neonates (Fig. 14-21).[193] Thus, differences in protein binding would lead to differences in the

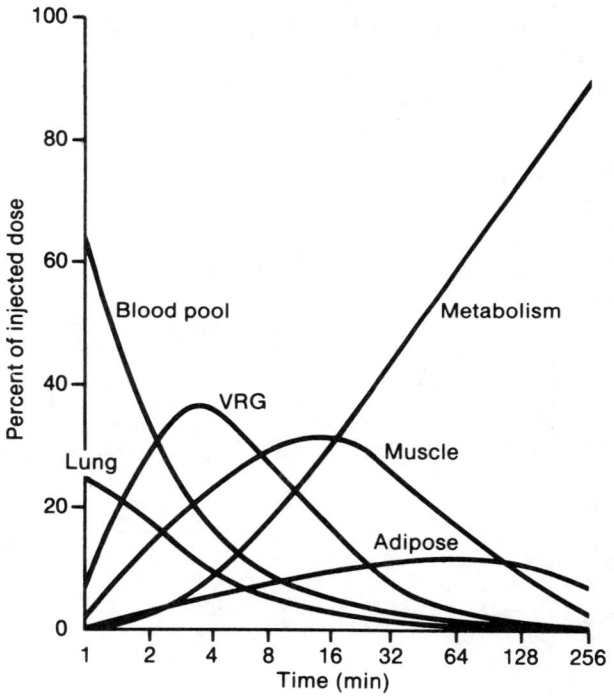

FIG. 14-19. A perfusion model of the distribution of lidocaine in various tissues and its elimination from humans following an intravenous infusion for 1 min (VRG = vessel rich group: different tissues grouped together because of relatively similar high tissue blood flows). Note the use of a logarithmic scale for time. (From Benowitz N, Forsyth RP, Melmon KL et al: Lidocaine disposition kinetics in monkey and man. I. Prediction by a perfusion model. Clin Pharmacol Ther 16:87, 1974, with permission.)

unbound drug fraction, and could result in differences in the effects produced by the same total blood level of local anesthetic.

Another situation in which protein binding is important is in the understanding of placental transfer of drugs. The rela-

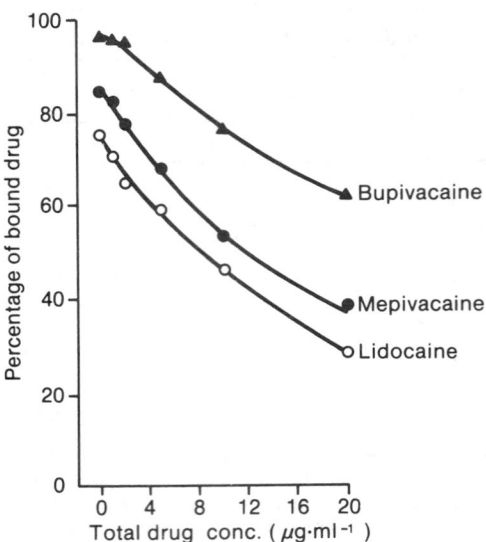

FIG. 14-20. As the plasma concentration of local anesthetic increases, the percentage that is bound to plasma proteins decreases, and the percentage that is unbound, or free, increases. (From Tucker GT, Boyes RN, Bridenbaugh PO *et al:* Binding of anilide-type local anesthetics in human plasma: I. Relationships between binding, physiochemical properties, and anesthetic activity. Anesthesiology 33:287, 1970, with permission.)

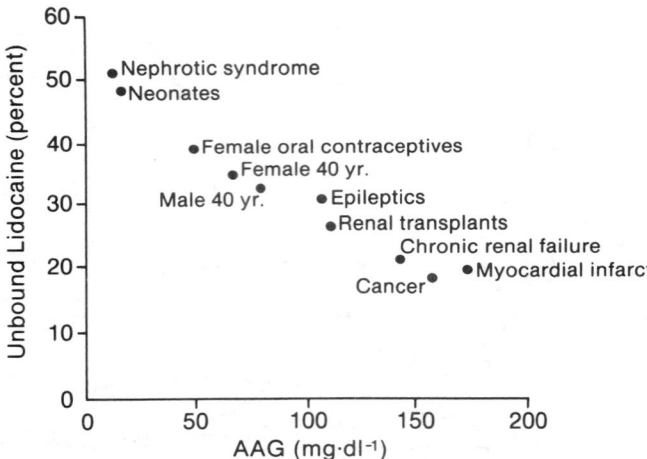

FIG. 14-21. Relationship between the mean percentage of unbound, or free, lidocaine in plasma and the mean alpha$_1$-acid glycoprotein concentration in various groups of patients. (Modified from Routledge PA, Stargel WW, Barchowsky A *et al:* Control of lidocaine therapy: New perspectives. Ther Drug Monit 4:265, 1982, with permission.)

tively low fetal:maternal plasma concentration ratio of bupivacaine, compared to that of the shorter-acting amides, is assumed to imply that bupivacaine is safer for the baby. However, maternal plasma proteins bind approximately twice as much bupivacaine as fetal proteins.[194] Thus, the principal reason for differences in cord:maternal total anesthetic concentrations is this difference in protein binding.[194, 195] It is likely that the concentration of unbound, pharmacologically active drug is the same in fetal and maternal blood. Indeed,

intersubject variations in the fetal:maternal ratio are related, in large part, to individual variations in the extent of protein binding in maternal and fetal blood.[196] Consequently, the increased safety of bupivacaine may only be apparent.

Clearance

Clearance of a drug is defined as the volume of blood that is completely cleared of drug during a specific time period. Aminoamide local anesthetics are primarily cleared from the bloodstream by metabolism in the liver, with only prilocaine having any significant extrahepatic metabolism.[197, 198] Because local anesthetics are highly extracted by the liver, the rate of clearance is largely determined by hepatic blood flow.[199] The net balance of distribution and clearance is such that the terminal elimination half-lives and mean body residence times of all amides are similar (Table 14-5).[190] Mean body residence time represents the average time that drug molecules are present in the body.

Since the rate of clearance is similar for all amides, but the duration of anesthesia is much different, lidocaine and mepivacaine tend to accumulate during continuous techniques, whereas bupivacaine only minimally accumulates.[200]

Aminoester local anesthetics are primarily cleared from the blood by plasma and liver cholinesterases. The pharmacokinetic parameters for 2-chloroprocaine have not been well defined because of its relatively rapid degradation in plasma. The *in vitro* blood half-life ranges from 7 to 20 s.[201] However, after epidural analgesia, the apparent half-life ranges from 1.5 to 6.4 min. This discrepancy probably results from the continuous uptake of anesthetic from the epidural space, even while chloroprocaine is being metabolized in the blood. This continued uptake makes it appear that chloroprocaine is being cleared from the blood more slowly. In this situation, where absorption is slower than elimination, as it is after epidural anesthesia, the half-life reflects the absorption rate, rather than the clearance rate. Thus, usual pharmacokinetic formulas, which are designed to describe intravenous administration of drugs, may not be entirely accurate for describing the pharmacokinetics of local anesthetics used for regional anesthesia.[190]

Although the aminoester local anesthetics are rapidly metabolized in normal patients, patients with abnormal or deficient plasma cholinesterases can exhibit signs of toxicity from usual dosages of 2-chloroprocaine.[202]

Finally, some metabolites of local anesthetics have been shown to be pharmacologically active. Monoethylglycinexylidide (MEGX), the metabolite that arises from N-deethylation of lidocaine, is near equipotent with lidocaine, and can contribute to the occurrence of central nervous system toxicity.[203, 204] Fortunately, MEGX levels are usually 1/6 to 1/4 of lidocaine levels, and the half-life of MEGX is comparable to lidocaine. However, MEGX accumulates in blood of patients in congestive heart failure, and could contribute to toxicity even when plasma levels of lidocaine are in the therapeutic range.[203] Other metabolites may also have important pharmacologic effects; however, none have been identified to date.

Effects of Absorbed Local Anesthetic or Neural Blockade

The systemic effects of neural blockade, or of the absorbed local anesthetic itself, can alter the pharmacokinetics of the local anesthetics. Peripheral regional block techniques, and local anesthetic blood levels commonly associated with regional anesthesia, have minimal effects on blood flow.[204, 208] In

TABLE 14-5. Pharmacokinetic Parameters Describing the Disposition Kinetics of Amide Local Anesthetics

	PRILOCAINE	LIDOCAINE	MEPIVACAINE	BUPIVACAINE	ETIDOCAINE
Vd_{ss} (l)	191	91	84	73	134
$T_{1/2}$ (h)	1.6	1.6	1.9	2.7	2.7
Cl (l·min^{-1})	2.37	0.95	0.78	0.58	1.11
MBRT (h)	1.3	1.6	1.8	2.1	2.0

Vd_{ss} = volume of distribution (steady state); $T_{1/2}$ = terminal elimination half-life; Cl = systemic clearance; MBRT = mean body residence time. (Modified from Tucker GT: Pharmacokinetics of local anaesthetics. Br J Anaesth 58:717, 1986.)

contrast, high thoracic levels of spinal or epidural anesthesia, or high local anesthetic blood levels, may significantly alter blood flow.[204, 205, 208, 209]

Although these interactions initially seem to be straightforward and obvious, the effects are often surprising. For example, intravenous administration of lidocaine or bupivacaine decreases splanchnic resistance and increases hepatic blood flow.[207] One might expect that systemic absorption of local anesthetic during epidural blockade would produce the same effect. However, epidural blockade reduces hepatic blood flow, largely as a result of increased splanchnic vascular resistance.[210] Similarly, epidural anesthesia may produce significantly different systemic effects than spinal anesthesia, despite similar levels of sympathetic block, as a result of the higher blood levels of local anesthetic that occur with epidural anesthesia.[205, 208, 210]

Local anesthetics can directly reduce placental blood flow by vasoconstricting placental vascular beds and by stimulating myometrial contractility.[211, 212] This effect is usually insignificant during routine peridural analgesia, but can become significant after paracervical blockade or intravascular injection.

Physical and Pathophysiological Factors

A reduction in cardiac output reduces the volume of distribution and plasma clearance of local anesthetics.[213, 214] Reductions in clearance most likely result from a reduction in total hepatic blood flow.[215, 216] As a result, a relatively low rate of lidocaine infusion can produce potentially toxic blood levels in some patients with cardiac failure.[213] However, plasma levels after peridural anesthesia are lower in the presence of decreased cardiac output, probably due to decreased absorption.[184] The ultimate result depends on the physiologic response of the patient to the particular regional technique and local anesthetic, and is difficult to predict. To be safe, the total dose should be reduced when regional anesthesia is used in patients with cardiac failure.

Liver disease reduces plasma clearance and prolongs the half-life of lidocaine (Table 14-6) and, probably, all local anesthetics.[214, 217] In contrast, renal disease has minimal effect.[214, 218] Cholinesterase activity is reduced in newborns, pregnancy, renal or liver disease, and in patients who are debilitated or produce abnormal or insufficient amounts of enzymes.[219] Usually, enough cholinesterase activity remains, and the rate of absorption from the site of injection is slow enough that minimal accumulation of drug results. However, for patients with severely abnormal cholinesterase activity, or in situations of accidental intravascular injection, these impairments of cholinesterase activity may lead to toxicity.[202]

Physiologic changes associated with old age would be expected to reduce the volume of distribution, the degree of protein binding, and the rate of elimination of local anesthetics, each contributing to increased plasma levels. Although some studies support this expectation,[177, 220] numerous others do not.[175, 187, 188] However, the aged patient may accumulate higher plasma levels of local anesthetic with repeated dosages. Thus, the initial dose of local anesthetic need not necessarily be reduced in the elderly, but subsequent doses should.[187, 188] Pharmacologic changes at the other end of the age spectrum are much more dramatic. The elimination half-life of a local anesthetic may be prolonged two to three times in neonates.[221, 222] Yet, children over 6 months of age distribute and eliminate intravenous lidocaine in a manner similar to adults.[223, 224]

The effect of acid-base changes is complicated. Lactic acid produced in tissue could increase the total concentration of local anesthetic in that tissue. The non-ionized form of the drug crosses the cell membrane and becomes ionized to a greater extent in the acidic intracellular medium than it was in extracellular fluid, and the ionized local anesthetic is trapped (i.e., ion-trapping), producing a higher total concentration within the cell. The effect that this higher concentration of ionized local anesthetic would have is purely speculative. However, the ionized form of the local anesthetic is thought to be active intracellularly. If so, there should be an increased pharmacologic effect that may be quite prolonged.

Similarly, fetal acidosis appears to result in greater transfer of local anesthetic from the mother to the fetus.[225] However, peak blood levels are not higher than for the non-acidotic fetus, perhaps because the local anesthetic is taken up and trapped in the acidotic fetal tissues.[226] In any case, there is no evidence that the acidotic fetus is more susceptible to local anesthetic-induced toxicity.

Acidosis of the plasma decreases protein binding, so that the free fraction of local anesthetic increases with decreasing

TABLE 14-6. Effect of Disease on Lidocaine Pharmacokinetics.

	$T_{1/2}$ (h)	Vd_{ss} (l·kg^{-1})	Cl (ml·kg^{-1}·min^{-1})
Normal	1.8	1.32	10.0
Renal Disease	1.3	1.2	13.7
Heart Failure	1.9	0.88	6.3
Liver Disease	4.9	2.31	6.0

$T_{1/2}$ = terminal elimination half-life; Vd_{ss} = volume of distribution (steady state); Cl = systemic clearance. (Thomson PD, Melmon KL, Richardson JA et al: Lidocaine pharmacokinetics in advanced heart failure, liver disease, and renal failure in humans. Ann Intern Med 78:499, 1973.)

pH.[227] Since there is less bound drug at a given total concentration of anesthetic, acidosis should increase the systemic effects of absorbed local anesthetics.

DRUG ACTIONS AND INTERACTIONS

Concomitant administration of vasoactive drugs can affect cardiac output and modify the pharmacokinetics of local anesthetics through mechanisms previously discussed.[186, 228] Halothane, cimetidine, and propranolol lower the clearance of lidocaine through inhibition of mixed function oxidases and/or decreased hepatic blood flow.[198, 229, 230] Most of the general anesthetics, except nitrous oxide, probably also lower clearance.[230] However, the mechanisms of action and relative effects may vary significantly among general anesthetics and patients.[198] These interactions suggest that toxic concentration of local anesthetics could occur if any of these drugs are used concomitantly.

Because bupivacaine and diazepam are both highly protein bound, it is possible that one might displace the other. Thus, diazepam was suggested to have the potential to increase bupivacaine toxicity.[231] However, diazepam does not appear to be able to displace bupivacaine from serum binding sites.[232] Consequently, the use of diazepam to treat a toxic reaction will not increase the unbound fraction of bupivacaine.

Addition of epinephrine or phenylephrine to local anesthetics for regional blockade can decrease absorption, alter distribution, and increase the elimination rate of local anesthetics (see section on Adjuvants and Combinations).[228, 233, 234] Similarly, beta-adrenergic agents increase clearance and volume of distribution of lidocaine.[186, 235]

COMBINATIONS OF LOCAL ANESTHETICS

Mixtures of aminoester and aminoamide local anesthetics have been reported to combine the best characteristics of the individual agents.[236] For example, mixing chloroprocaine and bupivacaine is reported to produce a block with rapid onset and long duration.[237] In theory, combinations of local anesthetics may result in synergistic toxicity through competition for binding sites or metabolic enzymes, or through inhibition of metabolic enzymes.[238, 239] However, the systemic toxicity of local anesthetics appears to be merely additive, indicating that a mixture of bupivacaine and chloroprocaine might be less cardiotoxic than an equivalent dose of bupivacaine alone.[240] Despite the potential benefits of combining local anesthetics, clinical and laboratory evidence suggests that neural blockade produced by mixtures of local anesthetics is unpredictable, and may not be any different than blockade produced by the individual agents.[241, 242] Furthermore, prior administration of chloroprocaine reduces the ability of bupivacaine to produce neural blockade.[243] Thus, the clinical utility of anesthetic combinations remains to be clarified.

TOXICITY OF LOCAL ANESTHETICS

ALLERGIC REACTIONS

True allergic reactions to local anesthetics are rare.[244] However, adverse reactions (*e.g.*, local anesthetic overdose, fainting) appear to be common.[245–247] Differentiating between allergic and adverse reactions is often difficult because of the similarity of symptoms that may be produced.[246] Unlike most adverse reactions, however, allergic reactions are potentially fatal.

Thus, many physicians are conservative, and label patients as "allergic" to all "-caine" drugs, even when the signs and symptoms are consistent with an adverse reaction. This label can prove to be a problem in patients where the use of local anesthetics would be desirable.

Provocative skin testing has been advocated as a safe and effective procedure to differentiate between patients with adverse and true allergic reactions to local anesthetics.[245, 246, 248] If the local anesthetic skin test and progressive challenge is negative, these authors maintain that it is safe to use the local anesthetic. However, the concept of skin testing with local anesthetics may not be scientifically sound, and the reliability of skin testing is questionable.[246, 249] For example, local anesthetic compounds are too small to directly evoke an allergic response without prior conjugation to a carrier molecule. The immunologic response is initiated by, and directed against, this local anesthetic-carrier conjugate. Because appropriate local anesthetic-carrier conjugates are not available for skin testing, the reliability of skin testing is questionable. Finally, provocative testing engenders the risk of producing severe and potentially fatal reactions in patients who are truly allergic.[247, 250]

Paraben esters have excellent bacteriostatic and fungistatic properties, and are widely used in multidose local anesthetic preparations, other drugs, cosmetics, and foods. Despite the fact that a large percentage of the population has been exposed to parabens, the incidence of immediate toxicity to parenterally administered parabens is rare.[45] However, some patients thought to be allergic to local anesthetics, after more careful examination, were found to be allergic to the preservative methylparaben.[44, 45, 245] Finally, the potential for cross sensitivity with some of the aminoester local anesthetics and p-aminobenzoic acid (PABA) exists.[45] True allergy to aminoamide local anesthetics is exceedingly rare.

It is hoped that patients will not be denied the use of local anesthetics because of a wrong diagnosis of local anesthetic drug allergy. Cautious testing with local anesthetic drugs may be useful at the time they present for surgery. If skin testing is negative, it should probably be followed by provocative challenge with an alternate local anesthetic, based on the history. Resuscitation equipment and trained individuals must be available when performing these tests, since severe systemic toxicity can be provoked by small quantities of local anesthetic.[247] The mechanism and treatment of allergic reactions to drugs is discussed in greater detail in Chapter 51.

LOCAL TISSUE TOXICITY

When careful technique is utilized, and when proper concentrations of local anesthetics are used, tissue toxicity is rare. However, serious neurotoxicity may result from the unintentional injection of large volumes or high concentrations of local anesthetic, from chemical contamination of the local anesthetic solution, or from neural ischemia produced by local pressure or hypotension.[251–255] Similarly, intraneural injection and direct trauma from the injection needle may produce neural deficit.[168]

Accidental subarachnoid injection of large doses of 2-chloroprocaine during the performance of epidural anesthesia has been reported to produce persistent, and possibly permanent, neurologic deficit.[251, 252] Although animal models have produced conflicting results, it appears that both sodium bisulfite (the preservative) and a low pH are necessary to produce neurotoxicity.[254, 256–258] 2-Chloroprocaine itself does not appear to be neurotoxic at clinical concentrations.[257, 259] The new formulation of nesacaine (Nesacaine-MPF[R]) does not contain bisulfite and does not appear to possess neurotoxic properties.

SYSTEMIC TOXICITY

Systemic blood levels of local anesthetic produce a concentration-dependent continuum of effects ranging from therapeutic to toxic (Fig. 14-22). The appropriate use of local anesthetics for regional nerve blockade may occasionally result in minor signs of systemic toxicity, but should rarely result in overt toxicity. Systemic toxicity most frequently results from one of two causes: 1) accidental intravascular injection, or 2) administration of an excessive dose of local anesthetic. The toxic effects of local anesthetics are primarily directed at the central nervous system and cardiovascular system, with the cardiovascular system being considerably more resistant. For example, four to seven times the dose of local anesthetic necessary to produce convulsions is required to produce cardiovascular collapse.[7]

Central Nervous System Toxicity

The toxic effects of local anesthetics on the central nervous system (CNS) are concentration dependent (Fig. 14-22). Low concentrations produce sedation, whereas higher concentrations produce seizures.[7, 260] The convulsant activity of local anesthetics probably results from selective depression of inhibitory fibers or centers in the CNS, allowing excessive excitatory input.[261] Seizures appear to originate in the subcortical brain structures, probably in the amygdala, with subsequent spread leading to grand-mal seizures.[260, 262] In general, CNS toxicity parallels anesthetic potency (Table 14-7).[7, 263] Thus, the toxic:therapeutic ratios of local anesthetics are quite similar after intravenous administration.

Central nervous system toxicity is increased by raising the P_{CO_2}, decreasing the pH, or prior administration of a drug such as cimetidine that will slow elimination.[264–267] Ranitidine does not appear to increase CNS toxicity of local anesthetics, perhaps because it does not decrease hepatic blood flow.[267] Increasing arterial P_{CO_2} could increase CNS toxicity by increasing cerebral blood flow and increasing local anesthetic

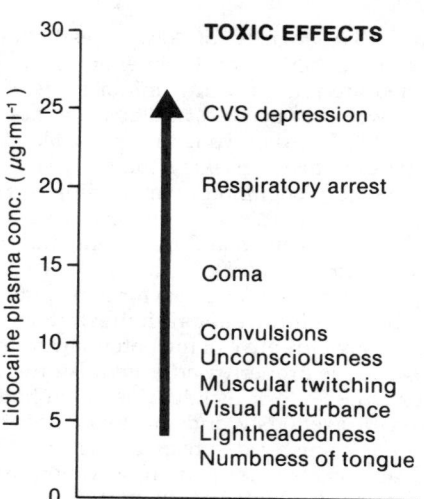

FIG. 14-22. Continuum of toxic effects produced by increasing lidocaine plasma concentrations. (CVS = cardiovascular system)

delivery to the brain, by increasing the concentration of ionized drug in the brain, or by a direct excitatory effect on subcortical structures.[264] Similarly, a decrease in pH may increase the concentration of ionized drug in the brain or may increase systemic distribution of local anesthetic to the brain.

Increasing the rate of intravenous drug administration produces systemic toxicity at a lower total dose of local anesthetic.[268] Similarly, electroencephalographic changes occur within one circulation after intravenous injection, indicating that the concentration of local anesthetic may also be an important determinant of the toxic effect.[260]

Central nervous system toxicity of local anesthetics is decreased by barbiturates, benzodiazepines, and inhalation anesthetics.[264, 269–272] The effect of barbiturates and benzodiazepines is not surprising, as both are clinically useful for treating and preventing seizures. Inhalational anesthetics depress the central nervous system, and probably raise the seizure threshold in a nonspecific manner.

TABLE 14-7.   Threshold for Production of CNS Toxicity by Local Anesthetics in Man and Monkeys

AGENT	RELATIVE ANESTHETIC POTENCY	CONVULSIVE THRESHOLD IN MONKEY		THRESHOLD FOR CNS SYMPTOMS IN MAN: DOSE (mg·kg⁻¹)
		Dose (mg·kg⁻¹)	Arterial Blood Level (μg·ml⁻¹)	
Procaine	1	—	—	19.2
Chloroprocaine	1	—	—	22.8
Lidocaine	2	14–22	18–26	6.4
Mepivacaine	2	18	22	9.8
Prilocaine	2	18	20	>6
Bupivacaine	8	4.3	4.5–5.5	1.6
Etidocaine	8	5.4	4.3	3.4
Tetracaine	8	—	—	2.5

(Modified from Covino BG, Vassallo HG: Local Anesthetics: Mechanism of Action and Clinical Use, p 126. New York, Grune & Stratton, 1976, with permission.)

Decreasing CNS toxicity of local anesthetics could be viewed as either beneficial or detrimental. If the peak blood levels obtained are relatively low, minor signs of local anesthetic toxicity would be masked, and this might be considered a beneficial effect. In the event that peak blood levels will eventually become toxic, masking the early signs of toxicity may interfere with recognition of impending seizures or cardiovascular collapse. In this scenario, raising the CNS threshold would delay recognition and treatment, and, thus, might be considered detrimental.[269]

Although toxic:therapeutic ratios for most local anesthetics are comparable after intravenous administration, these ratios are not necessarily indicative of the potential for toxicity when regional blockade is properly performed. For example, etidocaine is four times as toxic as lidocaine when both drugs are administered intravenously, and only two times as toxic when the drugs are administered subcutaneously.[273] This discrepancy is probably explained by the observation that the more potent, more lipid-soluble anesthetics (*e.g.*, bupivacaine, etidocaine) are absorbed into the systemic circulation much more slowly than the less potent agents (*e.g.*, lidocaine, mepivacaine) (Fig. 14-17). Thus, the toxic:therapeutic ratios for etidocaine or bupivacaine after properly performed regional anesthesia may be much greater than for lidocaine or mepivacaine.

Intraarterial Injection

Accidental injection of a very small dose of local anesthetic into an artery can result in central nervous system toxicity. For example, grand mal seizures can occur after the injection of only 2.5 mg of bupivacaine into the vertebral artery during the performance of stellate ganglion block.[274] More worrisome, though, is the finding that small doses of local anesthetic injected into peripheral arteries, such as the brachial or femoral artery, can produce retrograde flow in the arterial system. This retrograde flow could allow direct access of local anesthetic to the cerebral circulation.[275] Thus, direct arterial injection may account for reports of systemic toxicity after the injection of small doses of local anesthetic.

Cardiovascular System (CVS) Toxicity

Local anesthetics produce dose-related decreases in myocardial contractility and the rate of conduction of cardiac electrical impulses, and either contract or dilate vascular smooth muscle. Low concentrations may produce beneficial effects, such as prevention or treatment of arrhythmias.[276, 277] In contrast, higher concentrations may produce refractory arrhythmias and cardiovascular collapse. Although the cardiovascular system (CVS) is more resistant to local anesthetic toxicity than the CNS, CVS toxicity can be severe and difficult, if not impossible, to treat.[278]

Initially, the ratio of cardiac toxicity of local anesthetics was thought to parallel anesthetic potency.[279] Recent reports, however, suggest that bupivacaine and etidocaine may be relatively more cardiotoxic than would be predicted by their potency.[280, 281] This relative increase in cardiotoxicity appears to result from more potent electrophysiologic effects.

Local anesthetics produce a dose-dependent delay in the transmission of impulses through the cardiac conduction system by their action on the cardiac sodium channels.[282, 283] Sodium channel blockade develops during systole and dissipates during diastole. Both bupivacaine and lidocaine can block sodium channels rapidly during systole; however, bupivacaine dissociates from the sodium channel much more slowly during diastole.[282] Bupivacaine dissociates so slowly that the duration of diastole at physiologic heart rates (60–150 beats·min^{-1}) is insufficient for complete recovery of all sodium channels, and sodium channel block accumulates (Fig. 14-23). In contrast, diastolic time during physiologic heart rates is sufficient for lidocaine to dissociate from the sodium channel before the next heart beat, and little accumulation of block results. Because sodium channel block accumulates with bupivacaine, it is much more potent in depressing traffic through the cardiac conduction system than would be predicted on the basis of local anesthetic potency. Thus, bupivacaine is approximately 70 times more potent than lidocaine in blocking cardiac conduction, at heart rates of 60–150 beats·min^{-1}, yet it is only four times more potent in blocking conduction in nerve tissues.[282] Bupivacaine and etidocaine also impair myocardial performance by producing a frequency-dependent block of sodium channels in myocardial muscle cells.[284] The interaction of these two effects appears to further compound myocardial depression.

Cardiac arrhythmias and hypotension can also result from local anesthetic effects on the central nervous system.[285, 286] Furthermore, bupivacaine and etidocaine are also relatively more cardiotoxic than lidocaine or mepivacaine through this indirect mechanism of action. Thus, the increased cardiac toxicity of etidocaine and bupivacaine, most likely, results from both direct actions on the heart and indirect actions on the central nervous system.[283, 287, 288]

Cardiovascular toxicity of local anesthetics is increased by hypoxia, acidosis, pregnancy, and hyperkalemia, and is possibly increased in neonates.[289–294]

Local anesthetics produce direct vasoconstriction or vasodilation of vascular smooth muscle, and indirect effects through central stimulation of the autonomic nervous system and endocrine system.[288, 295–297] The typical response at low concentrations is a minimal increase in mean arterial pressure due to increased total peripheral resistance.[206] At high concentrations, local anesthetics can either vasodilate or cause vasoconstriction.[212, 295–297]

FIG. 14-23. The effect of lidocaine (10 μg·ml^{-1}) and bupivacaine (1 μg·ml^{-1}) on maximum upstroke velocity (V_{max}) of the action potential at different rates of stimulation (values are mean ± SD, *values significantly different from control, $P < 0.01$). Bupivacaine produced a progressive decrease in V_{max} at stimulation rates above 3 beats·min^{-1}. Lidocaine did not significantly reduce V_{max} until the stimulation rate increased to 150 beats·min^{-1}. (From Clarkson CW, Hondeghem LM: Mechanism for bupivacaine depression of cardiac conduction: Fast block of sodium channels during the action potential with slow recovery from block during diastole. Anesthesiology 62:396, 1985.)

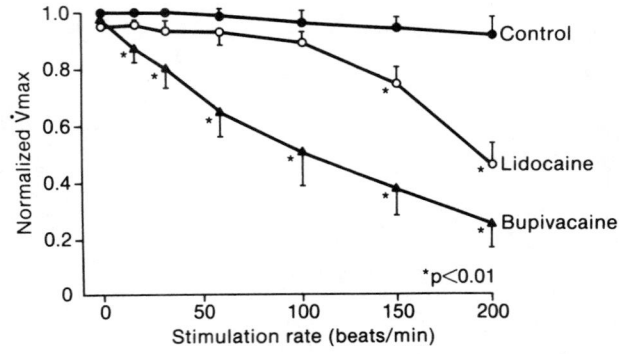

TREATMENT OF SYSTEMIC TOXICITY

When local anesthetic-induced seizures occur, hypoxia, hypercarbia, and acidosis develop rapidly.[263, 298] Furthermore, these metabolic changes greatly increase the toxicity of local anesthetics.[290] At the first signs of toxicity, oxygen must be delivered immediately. Administration of oxygen alone, by bag and mask, is often all that is necessary to treat seizures.[299] However, if seizure activity interferes with ventilation, or is prolonged, anticonvulsant drug therapy is indicated.

The optimal drug for the initial treatment of local anesthetic-induced seizures is controversial. Because local anesthetic-induced seizures are usually of short-duration, succinylcholine has been advocated as the treatment of choice.[299] Succinylcholine is rapid in onset and effectively facilitates ventilation. It also abolishes muscular activity, which decreases the severity of metabolic acidosis. However, neuronal seizure activity is not inhibited, and, thus, cerebral metabolism and oxygen requirements remain increased. Although muscle relaxation and ventilation with oxygen can prevent global cerebral ischemia, focal cerebral ischemia may not be prevented.[300, 301] Consequently, succinylcholine may not be sufficient as a sole treatment.

Diazepam has been reported to be an effective anticonvulsant, with minimal side effects.[302] However, diazepam is relatively slow acting and may not stop seizures for 2–3 min after administration.[303] Thiopental acts more rapidly, yet may produce greater cardiorespiratory depression than that produced with benzodiazepines.[270, 303] Furthermore, administration of barbiturates may decrease cardiac output and blood pressure to a greater extent than usual due to a synergistic interaction with local anesthetics.[304]

Our suggestion would be to administer oxygen at the first sign of systemic toxicity. Then, use succinylcholine to facilitate ventilation. Finally, administer either a barbiturate or benzodiazepine, as tolerated by the cardiovascular system, to reduce CNS metabolic demands. The need to have oxygen, resuscitation equipment, and airway management skills when using local anesthetics should be obvious.

There is little information regarding the treatment of cardiovascular toxicity of local anesthetics in man.[305, 306] Animal data suggest that: 1) large doses of epinephrine may be necessary to support the heart rate and blood pressure; 2) atropine may be useful for bradycardia; 3) DC cardioversion is often successful; and 4) ventricular arrhythmias are probably better treated with bretylium than with lidocaine.[307–311]

The best treatment for toxic reactions is prevention. Do not administer excessive doses of local anesthetic. Use meticulous technique, and utilize test doses whenever possible. It is also necessary to have knowledge of those doses of local anesthetic that should not be exceeded (Table 14-3). If toxic reactions occur, early detection and prompt support of ventilation and circulation are necessary.

Inhibition of Catecholamine Uptake by Cocaine

In addition to the CNS and CVS toxicities described above, cocaine causes norepinephrine and dobutamine to accumulate at neuronal synapses by blocking the normal re-uptake of these neurotransmitters. This explains the local vasoconstriction observed with this drug, and why it is often preferred for use in vascular areas. Excess neurotransmitter acts on postsynaptic terminals in the CNS to produce a myriad of effects, ranging from euphoria and alertness to delirium, dysphoric agitation, and seizures. Excess neurotransmitters act through the sympathetic nervous system to cause hypertension, tachycardia, ventricular arrhythmias, myocardial infarction, and death.[311–315] Because cocaine is detoxified by plasma and liver cholinesterases, persons with cholinesterase deficiencies may be at increased risk for sudden death if they use cocaine.

Methemoglobinemia

Regional blockade performed with more than 500 mg of prilocaine is associated with methemoglobinemia.[316] It appears that prilocaine does not directly cause methemoglobinemia; rather, one of its metabolites is responsible. Thus, peak methemoglobin levels may not occur until 4–8 h after administration, and are directly related to the total dose of prilocaine administered.[316, 317] Despite the finding that methemoglobinemia rarely reaches dangerous levels, the potential for cyanosis has surely limited the use of this drug. Prilocaine should probably not be used in obstetrics, because fetal cyanosis interferes with newborn assessment, and fetal blood is deficient in enzymes necessary to reduce methemoglobin.[316]

Methemoglobinemia is easily treated, and rapidly reduced to hemoglobin, by the administration of methylene blue ($1-5 \text{ mg} \cdot \text{kg}^{-1}$) or, less successfully, with ascorbic acid ($2 \text{ mg} \cdot \text{kg}^{-1}$).[317, 318]

CLINICAL USES OF LOCAL ANESTHETICS

FEATURES OF AN IDEAL LOCAL ANESTHETIC

Because anesthetic requirements vary considerably, no single set of local anesthetic properties can be considered ideal in all situations. For example, the ideal local anesthetic for laboring parturients would provide analgesia with no motor blockade. In contrast, many orthopedic surgeries require intense motor blockade.

In contrast to the clinical needs, the pharmacokinetic characteristics of an ideal anesthetic should be fairly uniform, and would include slow systemic absorption (hence, low peak concentrations in the blood) and a high clearance from the blood leading to a short half-life. Additionally, the local anesthetic, and any metabolites, should be systemically inactive and nontoxic.[190]

It should be obvious that a local anesthetic with ideal properties for all clinical uses does not exist. Thus, the choice of local anesthetic must be individualized to each specific situation, and compromises, in terms of the ideal goal, are often necessary.

CHOICE OF LOCAL ANESTHETIC

Choice of a local anesthetic must take into consideration the duration of surgery, regional anesthetic technique employed, surgical requirements, the anesthesiologist's skills, the potential for local or systemic toxicity, and any metabolic constraints (Table 14-4).

Usually, a local anesthetic is chosen that will, at least minimally, outlast the duration of surgery. For operations of brief duration, a short-acting local anesthetic will usually suffice. For prolonged operations, either a long-acting local anesthetic or a continuous anesthetic technique is chosen. Long-acting aminoamide local anesthetics, such as bupivacaine or etidocaine, have safety margins as good as, if not better than, short-acting drugs, such as lidocaine and mepivacaine, when injected properly, because they have slower systemic absorption and they are more potent and can be injected in lower dosages.[178, 182] Continuous techniques using a short-acting local anesthetic have many advantages, including the ability to closely match the duration of anesthesia and surgery. However, this technique results in greater systemic accumulation of local anesthetic or metabolites than occurs with long-acting aminoamide local anesthetics, and may predispose to the development of tachyphylaxis.[182, 199, 319, 320]

The concentration of local anesthetic necessary to provide neural blockade varies among block techniques. Larger nerves are more difficult to anesthetize, and require higher concentrations of local anesthetic than smaller nerve fibers.[174] Thus, a higher concentration of local anesthetic is necessary for central neural blockade (e.g., epidural) than for peripheral blockade (e.g., posterior tibial nerve) (Table 14-4). Even lower concentrations are necessary for subcutaneous infiltration. Similarly, when higher concentrations are used for a given technique, such as using 0.75% rather than 0.5% bupivacaine for epidural anesthesia, the intensity, duration, and speed of onset of neural blockade may be increased.[173]

The quality of sensory and motor blockade, produced by the various anesthetics, differs considerably. For example, intrathecal administration of tetracaine appears to provide greater motor blockade than does bupivacaine, while bupivacaine provides a longer duration of sensory analgesia.[321] Similarly, mepivacaine provides a greater degree of motor blockade than lidocaine for brachial plexus blockade, yet also provides a longer duration of sensory anesthesia.[166] When profound muscle relaxation is needed during surgery,

mepivacaine and etidocaine may be the agents of choice for peripheral and epidural blockade (although high concentrations of bupivacaine provide excellent muscle relaxation), while tetracaine (or possibly lidocaine) may be preferred for spinal anesthesia.[322, 323]

The potential for systemic toxicity should also be considered when choosing a local anesthetic. Rapid clearance of ester-type local anesthetics should greatly reduce the potential for systemic toxicity, and provide a distinct advantage.[190] Indeed, chloroprocaine is so rapidly hydrolyzed that the risk of systemic toxicity is very low. However, its short duration of action limits its clinical utility. Tetracaine has a longer duration of action; however, it diffuses and spreads poorly through body tissues, and is surprisingly toxic when administered intravenously.[7] Prilocaine has an extremely high clearance, which helps to minimize C_{max} after a given dose, and, thus, increases the margin of safety compared to the other aminoamide local anesthetics.[175, 197]

REGIONAL ANESTHESIA

Bupivacaine and lidocaine can be used for all regional blocks, and are currently the most widely utilized local anesthetics. Mepivacaine is used extensively for peridural anesthesia and peripheral nerve blockade, but not for spinal anesthesia. Etidocaine is relatively comparable to bupivacaine, except that it produces more profound motor block. Consequently, its use

TABLE 14-8.   Preparations of Local Anesthetics Intended for Topical Anesthesia

ANESTHETIC	CONCENTRATION (%)	PHARMACEUTICAL APPLICATION FORM	INTENDED AREA OF USE
Benzocaine	1–5	Cream	Skin and mucous membrane
	20	Ointment	Skin and mucous membrane
	20	Aerosol	Skin and mucous membrane
Cocaine	4	Solution	Ear, nose, throat
Cyclonine	0.5–1	Solution	Skin, oropharynx, tracheobronchial tree, urethra, rectum
Dibucaine	0.25–1	Cream	Skin
	0.25–1	Ointment	Skin
	0.25–1	Aerosol	Skin
	0.25	Solution	Ear
	2.5	Suppositories	Rectum
Lidocaine	2–4	Solution	Oropharynx, tracheobronchial tree, nose
	2	Jelly	Urethra
	2.5–5	Ointment	Skin, mucous membrane, rectum
	2	Viscous	Oropharynx
	10	Suppositories	Rectum
	10	Aerosol	Gingival mucosa
Tetracaine	0.5–1	Ointment	Skin, mucous membrane, rectum
	0.5–1	Cream	Skin, mucous membrane, rectum
	0.25–1	Solution	Nose, tracheobronchial tree

(Covino BG, Vassallo HG: Local Anesthetics: Mechanism of Action and Clinical Use, p 93. New York, Grune & Stratton 1976, with permission.)

is limited to surgical anesthesia. Prilocaine is rarely used because of its propensity to produce methemoglobinemia. Procaine is largely used for local infiltration. Tetracaine, cocaine, and benzocaine are useful for topical anesthesia, and tetracaine is widely used for spinal anesthesia. Chloroprocaine produces peridural blockade of short duration that is particularly useful for cesarean section because of the low potential for toxicity to mother and fetus.

TOPICAL ANESTHESIA

Local anesthetics may be applied topically to provide anesthesia to such diverse sites as the eye, skin, tympanic membrane, oral mucosa, tracheobronchial tree, and rectum. To be effective topically, however, relatively high concentrations of local anesthetics are required (Table 14-8). Although increasing the concentration increases penetration of the tissues, the onset of anesthesia usually occurs in 5–10 min when applied to mucous membranes, and in 30–60 min when applied to the skin. Systemic absorption is also greater from mucous membranes, as is the risk of toxicity, if large volumes of local anesthetic are used.

MAXIMUM DOSE

Maximum doses of local anesthetic are frequently quoted for the safe administration of local anesthesia (i.e., avoidance of toxicity) (Table 14-3). Unfortunately, these recommendations are general in nature, and do not consider known pharmacokinetic variables. For example, different peak blood levels will result from the injection of the same dose of local anesthetic into different sites, yet maximum doses are quoted without consideration of the site of injection (Fig. 14-16). Furthermore, the maximum recommended dose of local anesthetic may not be rational in terms of known systemic blood levels. For example, the maximum recommended dose of bupivacaine is often quoted as 200 mg. However, when intercostal nerve blocks were performed with 400 mg of bupivacaine, only one in ten patients had a peak blood level that approached the seizure threshold.[324] Because intercostal injection produces the highest local anesthetic blood level of any regional technique, other techniques should produce even lower blood levels, and provide a greater margin of safety.[190] This data implies that the maximum recommended dose of bupivacaine is quite conservative. Finally, maximum doses are frequently quoted in terms of $mg \cdot kg^{-1}$, yet there is no evidence that weight significantly affects the peak blood level (Fig. 14-18). The maximum doses given in Table 14-3 are expressed in milligrams. Simple arithmetic indicates that a 1% solution of local anesthetic equals $10 \ mg \cdot ml^{-1}$.

A final consideration for determining the safe dose of local anesthetic is the skill of the anesthesiologist. Although proper injection of 200 mg of bupivacaine into the epidural space is very safe, as little as 50 mg injected intravenously, or 2.5 mg injected intraarterially, may be extremely toxic.[213, 278] Thus, the skill of the anesthesiologist may be *the* major factor determining the toxic dose of a local anesthetic.

ANTIARRHYTHMIC EFFECTS

Lidocaine has an antiarrhythmic effect that develops rapidly after intravenous infusion and dissipates quickly when the infusion is discontinued. Thus, it is easily titratable and extremely useful in situations where rapid control of ventricular

arrhythmias is necessary. Bupivacaine, etidocaine, and mepivacaine have also been found to be effective antiarrhythmics.[276, 277]

BLUNTING THE RESPONSE TO TRACHEAL STIMULATION

Lidocaine, injected intravenously or topically applied to the larynx and trachea, is variably effective at blunting the hemodynamic response to intubation.[325–328] Intravenous lidocaine may also prevent the rise in intraocular pressure seen with tracheal intubation, and the rise in intracranial pressure associated with tracheal suctioning.[329, 330] Intravenous lidocaine also has been shown to suppress coughing and prevent reflex bronchoconstriction.[331, 332]

OTHER THERAPEUTIC EFFECTS

Local anesthetics are anticonvulsants in low dosages, and, surprisingly, have been promoted as effective treatment for status epilepticus.[333, 334] Lidocaine blood levels of $1-2 \ \mu g \cdot ml^{-1}$ provide systemic analgesia, reduce MAC for inhalational anesthetics, and have been used to treat both acute and chronic pain.[335, 336] Lidocaine rapidly reduces raised intracranial pressure.[337] Intravenous infusions of local anesthetics can augment neuromuscular blockade.[338] Finally, infusions of local anesthetics can be used for general anesthesia.

ADJUVANTS AND COMBINATIONS

EPINEPHRINE

Epinephrine has been reported to produce beneficial effects when added to virtually every available local anesthetic for nearly every regional anesthetic technique. These beneficial effects include the ability to: 1) prolong the duration of anesthesia; 2) minimize the peak level of local anesthetic in the blood; 3) increase the intensity of the blockade; 4) reduce surgical bleeding; and 5) as a component of the test dose for regional anesthesia.

Prolonging the Duration of Anesthesia

In the concentrations typically used for regional anesthesia, local anesthetics universally cause local vasodilation. Epinephrine is added in an attempt to counteract this vasodilation, reduce absorption, and, therefore, prolong duration.[183] The ability of epinephrine to prolong duration is determined by the type of regional block, concentration of epinephrine, and type and concentration of local anesthetic utilized (Table 14-4).[175, 339, 340]

The addition of epinephrine to tetracaine consistently prolongs the duration of spinal anesthesia.[323] When added to bupivacaine or lidocaine, the results are less certain; some authors find a prolonged duration of spinal anesthesia, while others are unable to detect any significant effect.[321, 341–343] Epinephrine also prolongs the duration of most other regional anesthetic techniques (Table 14-4). However, epinephrine is less effective when added to bupivacaine and etidocaine, probably because the long duration of action of bupivacaine and etidocaine does not appear to be a function of local blood flow.

Minimizing Peak Blood Levels of Local Anesthetic

Peak blood levels of local anesthetics can approach the toxic range when used for regional blockade, especially for intercostal and peridural techniques.[177] Epinephrine can decrease peak blood levels, presumably by producing local vasoconstriction and decreasing the rate of local anesthetic absorption. However, epinephrine is less effective in reducing peak blood levels when administered with bupivacaine and etidocaine (Table 14-4).

Increasing the Intensity of Neural Blockade

Epinephrine has been considered for years to increase the intensity and quality of neural blockade. Hypalgesia or analgesia has been reported after the injection of epinephrine alone into the subarachnoid or epidural space.[344, 345] Similarly, the intensity of motor and sensory blockade has been reported to be improved for spinal analgesia, and for epidural anesthesia for labor and delivery.[339, 346, 347]

The increased intensity of analgesia may result from direct action of epinephrine on antinociceptive receptors in the spinal cord.[348] Epinephrine, and other alpha-adrenergic agonists, augment the ability of local anesthetics to block transmission of noxious stimuli in the spinal cord. Furthermore, the intensity and duration of these effects appear to depend on the dose of epinephrine.

Reducing Surgical Blood Loss

Subcutaneous, local infiltration of epinephrine-containing solutions can facilitate surgery by decreasing bleeding. The optimum concentration of epinephrine remains controversial. Definite conclusions are difficult to make because the site of injection, the concentration of local anesthetic, and the concentration of epinephrine all seem to be important. However, most clinical evidence suggests that near-maximal vasoconstriction occurs at epinephrine concentrations of 5 $\mu g \cdot ml^{-1}$ (1:200,000).

Optimal Concentration of Epinephrine

The optimal concentration of epinephrine for regional blockade is controversial. Since the degree of vasodilation is affected by the choice of local anesthetic, its concentration, and the site of injection, it is unlikely that one concentration of epinephrine is optimal for all regional techniques.[181, 295] However, most authors agree that 5 $\mu g \cdot ml^{-1}$ of epinephrine is optimal. Lower concentrations are ineffective, and higher concentrations are more likely to produce toxicity from the absorbed epinephrine.[175, 201, 349] The maximum dose of epinephrine probably should not exceed 200–250 μg.[350] Reduced quantities should be used in patients who may be placed at risk if they develop hypertension or tachycardia; such as those with coronary artery disease.

Component of a Test Dose

A test dose is frequently used for peridural anesthetic techniques in an attempt to minimize the chance of accidental subarachnoid or intravascular injection. Subarachnoid injection is detected by the rapid onset of spinal anesthesia. Intravascular injection is more difficult, but just as important to detect. If the test dose contains 15 μg of epinephrine, intravascular injection can be detected by an increase in the heart rate that begins in approximately 25 s, increases by at least 20%, and remains elevated for about 30 s.[351] These heart rate responses do not occur reliably in patients receiving beta-adrenergic blocking therapy.

Use in Obstetrics

The alpha-adrenergic effects of epinephrine may be dangerous to the fetus by decreasing uterine artery blood flow, and the beta-adrenergic effects may slow labor and increase the need for oxytocic supplementation.[352, 353] Although some clinical studies have found epinephrine to be safe, and free of these potential adverse effects, considerable controversy and uncertainty remain.[354-357] Some experts recommend the use of epinephrine in obstetrics, and others suggest that it should never be used.[358, 359]

Systemic Effects

Administration of epinephrine with local anesthetics results in significantly higher systemic levels of epinephrine than when epinephrine is injected alone.[360] The absorbed epinephrine produces predominantly beta-adrenergic effects, with little evidence of alpha-adrenergic effects at doses up to 400 μg.[349] Thus, heart rate, contractility, and cardiac output are all increased, while peripheral vascular resistance and blood pressure usually decrease. Systemic absorption, or accidental intravascular injection, of epinephrine may produce a variety of undesirable side effects, including tachycardia, arrhythmias, tremor, hypertension, and, possibly, decreased uterine blood flow. In contrast to all other regional techniques, injection of epinephrine into the subarachnoid space does not appear to produce systemic effects.

Potential Contraindications to the Use of Epinephrine

Epinephrine should not be used in situations where its undesirable side effects would be particularly dangerous, such as patients with: 1) severe or unstable angina; 2) malignant arrhythmias; 3) uncontrolled hypertension; or 4) uteroplacental insufficiency or fetal distress. Similarly, epinephrine should be avoided in patients with hyperthyroidism, and patients on medications that modify the effects of catecholamines (e.g., tricyclic antidepressants or monoamine-oxidase inhibitors). Finally, epinephrine should not be added to local anesthetics for peripheral nerve blocks in areas where there is not adequate collateral blood flow (e.g., digits, penis, wrist, ankle), or when performing intravenous regional anesthesia.

PHENYLEPHRINE

Phenylephrine is an alpha-adrenergic sympathomimetic that is effective for prolonging the duration of spinal and epidural anesthesia. However, phenylephrine does not appear to reduce peak blood levels of local anesthetic that result after epidural anesthesia, even when administered in doses that have vasoconstrictor effects equipotent with epinephrine.[234] Phenylephrine does not produce systemic effects when injected into the subarachnoid space, yet prominent alpha-adrenergic effects result when it is used for other regional techniques. The usual dose of phenylephrine used for prolongation of spinal anesthesia is 2–5 mg.

VASOPRESSIN ANALOGUES

Felypressin (octapressin) and Ornipressin are synthetic drugs, similar in structure to vasopressin, but without the antidiuretic or coronary vasoconstrictor effects. These drugs increase the intensity and duration of local anesthesia, decrease systemic absorption, and decrease bleeding, while producing minimal cardiovascular side-effects.[361-364] Octapressin and other catecholamines appear to have synergistic vasoconstrictor effects.[365] Finally, intravascular injection of octapressin-containing local anesthetic solutions appears to be less toxic than solutions that contain epinephrine.[363] Although these drugs enjoy considerable popularity in other countries, they are not currently available for use in the United States.

CARBONATED LOCAL ANESTHETICS

Carbonation of local anesthetics was first reported to hasten the onset and increase the intensity of local anesthesia over 20 years ago.[366] To this day, the clinical significance of this effect remains controversial, and commercially prepared solutions are not available in the United States for routine clinical use. The proponents of carbonated solutions speculate that the increased rate of onset of neural blockade results from more rapid intraneural diffusion, and more rapid penetration of connective tissue sheaths around the nerve trunk.[38-40, 367] The increased intensity of neural blockade is thought to result from the diffusion of carbon dioxide into the nerve, which reduces intraneural pH. This decrease in pH promotes iontrapping of the local anesthetic, increasing the intraneural concentration. Furthermore, carbon dioxide may have a direct anesthetic effect on the nerve membrane.[366] Several clinical studies report that carbonated local anesthetic solutions have advantages over typical solutions (prepared as the hydrochloride salt).[366-368]

In contrast, several studies report no clinical advantage of carbonated solutions.[369, 370] Furthermore, carbonated solutions may have some disadvantages. For example, peak blood levels of local anesthetics are higher after regional blockade with carbonated local anesthetic solutions.[371] Similarly, a faster rate of onset of epidural blockade could result in a greater magnitude, and rate, of decline of blood pressure.[372] This effect could be especially detrimental in obstetrical patients.

SODIUM BICARBONATE

Addition of sodium bicarbonate to local anesthetic solutions will raise the pH and increase the concentration of non-ionized free base. For example, increasing the pH of a solution of lidocaine from 6 to 7 increases the percent of non-ionized free base from less than 1% to 11% (Table 14-2). The increased percent of free base will theoretically increase the rate of diffusion and speed the onset of neural blockade.

Clinically, the addition of 1 mEq of sodium bicarbonate to each 10 ml of commercially prepared 1.5% lidocaine solution raises the pH to 7.15, and produces significantly faster onset of anesthesia and more rapid spread of sensory blockade.[37] Systemic blood levels were higher, but not statistically different. Similar to carbonated solutions, the faster onset of these solutions may contribute to a greater magnitude, and rate, of decline in blood pressure.[372]

DEXTRAN

The addition of dextran to local anesthetic solutions has been found to increase the duration of anesthesia.[373] Dextran also slows the rate of absorption of epinephrine, when used, so that the peak blood levels of epinephrine are decreased.[360]

However, the effect in individual patients is unpredictable, and dextran can provoke anaphylaxis.[374] Consequently, dextran is rarely added to local anesthetics for regional anesthesia.

HYALURONIDASE

Hyaluronic acid is a viscous polysaccharide that inhibits diffusion of foreign substances within interstitial spaces of tissues. Hyaluronidase hydrolyzes hyaluronic acid, facilitating the spread of local anesthetics. Proponents of hyaluronidase suggest that it improves the success rate of some regional techniques and prevents hematoma formation if an artery is punctured.[375] However, the addition of hyaluronidase can increase C_{max}, may provoke allergic reactions, may shorten the duration of anesthesia, and is technically awkward, since it cannot be heat sterilized (it is a protein).[375] Finally, most modern local anesthetic drugs diffuse rapidly; thus, the benefits of adding hyaluronidase are limited.

REFERENCES

1. Bean BP, Cohen CJ, Tsien RW: Lidocaine block of cardiac sodium channels. J Gen Physiol 81:613, 1983
2. Gintant GA, Hoffman BF: The role of local anesthetic effects in the actions of antiarrhythmic drugs. In Strichartz GR (ed): Local Anesthetics p 213. Berlin, Springer-Verlag, 1987
3. Covino BG: Cardiovascular effects of regional anesthesia. In Covino BG, Fozzard HA, Rehder K et al (eds): Effects of Anesthesia, p 207. Bethesda, MD; American Physiological Society, 1985
4. Steinback AB: Alteration of xylocaine (lidocaine) and its derivatives of the time course of the end plate potential. J Gen Physiol 52:144, 1986
5. Sine SM, Taylor P: Local anesthetics and histrionicotoxin are allosteric inhibitors of the acetylcholine receptor. J Biol Chem 257:8106, 1982
6. Garfield GM, Guigino L: Central effects of local anesthetic agents. In Strichartz GR (ed): Local Anesthetics, p 253. Berlin, Springer-Verlag, 1987
7. Liu PL, Feldman HS, Giasi R et al: Comparative CNS toxicity of lidocaine, etidocaine, bupivacaine, and tetracaine in awake dogs following rapid IV administration. Anesth Analg 62:375, 1983
8. Zipf HF, Dittman ECH: General pharmacological effects of local anesthetics. In Lechat P (ed): Local Anesthetics, p 191. Oxford, Pergamon Press, 1971
9. Strichartz G: Use-dependent conduction block produced by volatile general anesthetic agents. Acta Anaesthesiol Scand 24:402, 1980
10. Haydon DA, Urban BW: The action of alcohols and other nonionic surface active substances on the sodium current of the squid giant axon. J Physiol 341:411, 1983
11. Sangarlangkarn S, Klaewtanong V, Jonglerttrakool P et al: Meperidine as a spinal anesthetic agent: A comparison with lidocaine-glucose. Anesth Analg 66:235, 1987
12. Kendig JJ: Barbiturates: Active form and site of action at node of Ranvier sodium channels. J Pharmacol Exp Ther 218:175, 1981
13. Seeman P: The membrane actions of anesthetics and tranquilizers. Pharmacol Rev 24:583, 1972
14. Catterall WA: Neurotoxins that act on voltage-sensitive sodium channels in excitable membranes. Ann Rev Pharmacol Toxicol 20:15, 1980
15. Fink BR: History of local anesthesia. In Cousins MJ, Bridenbaugh PO (eds): Neural Blockade in Clinical Anesthesia and Management of Pain, p 3. Philadelphia, JB Lippincott, 1980
16. Covino B: One hundred years plus two of regional anesthesia. Reg Anesth 11:105, 1986

17. Fink BR: Leaves and needles: The introduction of surgical local anesthesia. Anesthesiology 63:77, 1985

18. Lee JA: Some foundations on which we have built. Reg Anesth 10:99, 1985

19. Vandam LD: Some aspects of the history of local anesthesia. In Strichartz BR (ed): Local Anesthetics, p 1. Berlin, Springer-Verlag, 1987

20. Liljestrand G: The historical development of local anesthesia. In Lechat P (ed): International Encyclopedia of Pharmacology and Therapeutics, p 1. Oxford, Pergamon Press, 1971

21. Moore DC: Regional block: Its history in the United States since World War II. In Rupreht J, van Lieburg M, Lee JA et al (eds): Anaesthesia—Essays on its History, p 128. Berlin, Springer-Verlag, 1985

22. Narahashi T, Frazier DT, Yamada M: The site of action and active form of local anesthetics. I. Theory and pH experiments with tertiary compounds. J Pharm Exp Ther 171:32, 1970

23. Ritchie JM, Ritchie B, Greengard P: The effect of the nerve sheath on the action of local anesthetics. J Pharm Exp Ther 150:160, 1965

24. Frazier DT, Narahashi T, Yamada M: The site of action and active form of local anesthetics. II. Experiments with quaternary compounds. J Pharm Exp Ther 171:45, 1970

25. Hille B: The pH-dependent rate of action of local anesthetics on the node of Ranvier. J Gen Physiol 69:475, 1977

26. Hille B: Local anesthetics: Hydrophilic and hydrophobic pathways for the drug-receptor reaction. J Gen Physiol 69:497, 1977

27. Hille B, Courtney K, Dum R: Rate and site of action of local anesthetics in myelinated nerve fibers. In Fink BR (ed): Molecular Mechanisms of Anesthesia. Progress in Anesthesiology, vol 1, p 13. New York, Raven Press, 1975

28. Ritchie JM: Mechanism of action of local anaesthetic agents and biotoxins. Br J Anaesth 47:191, 1975

29. Strichartz G: Interactions of local anesthetics with neuronal sodium channels. In Covino BG, Fozzard HA, Rehder K et al (eds): Effects of Anesthesia, p 39. Bethesda, American Physiological Society, 1985

30. de Jong RH: Local Anesthetics, p 41. Springfield, Charles C Thomas, 1977

31. Eckenstam BA: The effect of the structural variation on the local analgetic properties of the most commonly used groups of substances. Acta Anaesthesiol Scand 25(Suppl):10, 1966

32. Buchi J, Perlia X: Structure-activity relations and physicochemical properties of local anesthetics. In Lechat P (ed): Local Anesthetics, p 39. Oxford, Pergamon Press, 1971

33. Courtney KR, Strichartz GR: Structural elements which determine local anesthetic activity. In Strichartz GR (ed): Local Anesthetics, p 53. Berlin, Springer-Verlag, 1987

34. Setnikar I: Ionization of bases with limited solubility. Investigation of substances with local anesthetic activity. J Pharm Sci 55:1190, 1966

35. Moore DC: The pH of local anesthetic solutions. Anesth Anal 60:833, 1981

36. Hilgier M: Alkalinization of bupivacaine for brachial plexus block. Reg Anesth 8:59, 1985

37. Di Fazio CA, Carron HO, Grosslight KR et al: Comparison of pH adjusted lidocaine solutions for epidural anesthesia. Anesth Analg 65:760, 1986

38. Catchlove RFH: The influence of CO_2 and pH on local anesthetic action. J Pharmacol Exp Ther 181A:298, 1972

39. Park WY, Hagins FM: Comparison of lidocaine hydrocarbonate with lidocaine hydrochloride for epidural anesthesia. Reg Anesth 11:128, 1986

40. Bokesch PM, Raymond SA, Strichartz GR: Dependence of lidocaine potency on pH and P_{CO_2}. Anesth Analg 66:9, 1987

41. Weiner N: Norepinephrine, epinephrine, and the sympathomimetic amines. In Gilman AG, Goodman LS, Rall TW et al (eds): Goodman and Gilman's The Pharmacological Basis of Therapeutics, p 158. New York, Macmillan, 1985

42. Parnass SM, Baughman VL, Miletich DJ et al: The effects of pH on the oxidation rate of epinephrine. Anesthesiology 67:A280, 1987

43. Bonhomme L, Benhamou D, Martre BS et al: Chemical stability of bupivacaine epinephrine in pH-adjusted solutions. Anesthesiology 67:A279, 1987

44. Aldrete AJ, Johnson DA: Allergy to local anesthetics. JAMA 207:356, 1969

45. Nagel JE, Fuscaldo JT, Fireman P: Paraben allergy. JAMA 237:1594, 1977

46. Bray GM, Rasminsky M, Aguayo AJ: Interactions between axons and their sheath cells. Ann Rev Neurosci 4:127, 1981

47. Coggeshall RE: A fine structured analysis of the myelin sheath in rat spinal roots. Anat Rec 194:201, 1979

48. Landon N, Williams PL: Ultrastructure of the node of Ranvier. Nature 199:575, 1963

49. Langley OK, London DN: A light and electron histochemical approach to the nodes of Ranvier and myelin of peripheral nerve fibers. J Histochem Cytochem 15:722, 1967

50. London DN, Langley OK: The local chemical environment of nodes of Ranvier: A study of cation binding. J Anat 108:419, 1971

51. Langley OK: Local anesthetics and nodal polyanions in peripheral nerve. Histochem J 5:79, 1973

52. Gissen AJ, Covino BC, Gregus J: Differential sensitivity of fast and slow fibers in mammalian nerve: II. Margin of safety for nerve transmission. Anesth Analg 61:561, 1982

53. Angevine JB: The nervous tissue. In Fawcett DW (ed): A Textbook of Histology, p 311. Philadelphia, WB Saunders, 1986

54. Feng TP, Liu YM: The connective tissue sheath of the nerve as effective diffusion barrier. J Cell Comp Physiol 34:1, 1949

55. Stevens CF: The neuron. Sci Am 241:55, 1979

56. Singer SJ, Nicolson GL: The fluid mosaic model of the structure of cell membranes. Science 175:720, 1972

57. Pfenninger KH: Organization of neuronal membranes. Ann Rev Neurosci 1:445, 1978

58. Hille B: Ionic basis of resting and action potentials. In Handbook of the Nervous System. Handbook of Physiology, p 99. Baltimore, Williams & Wilkins, 1976

59. Hille B: Ionic channels in nerve membranes. Prog Biophys Mol Biol 21:1, 1970

60. Armstrong CM: Sodium channels and gating currents. Physiol Rev 61:644, 1981

61. Latorre R, Coronado R, Vergara C: K^+ channels gated by voltage and ions. Ann Rev Physiol 46:485, 1984

62. Schwarz W, Passow H: CA^{2+}-activated K^+ channels in erythrocytes and excitable cells. Ann Rev Physiol 45:359, 1983

63. Tsien RW: Calcium channels in excitable cell membranes. Ann Rev Physiol 45:341, 1983

64. DiPolo R, Beauge L: The calcium pump and sodium-calcium exchange in squid axons. Ann Rev Physiol 45:313, 1983

65. Catterall WA: The molecular basis of neuronal excitability. Science 223:653, 1984

66. Keynes RD: Ion channels in the nerve-cell membrane. Sci Am 240:126, 1979

67. Sigworth FJ: Sodium channels in nerve apparently have two conductance states. Nature 270:265, 1977

68. Aldrich RW, Corey DP, Stevens CF: A reinterpretation of mammalian sodium channel gating based on single channel recording. Nature 306:436, 1983

69. Goldman L, Schauf CL: Inactivation of the sodium current in myxicola giant axons. J Gen Physiol 59:659, 1972

70. Bezanilla F, Armstrong CM: Inactivation of the sodium channel: I. Sodium current experiments. J Gen Physiol 70:549, 1977

71. Aldrich RW, Corey DP, Stevens CF: A reinterpretation of mam-

malian sodium channel gating based on single recording. Nature 306:436, 1983

72. Agnew WS: Voltage-regulated sodium channel molecules. Ann Rev Physiol 46:517, 1984

73. Fozzard HA: Conduction of the action potential. In Berne RM *et al* (eds): Handbook of Physiology, sect 2, vol 1, p 335. Baltimore, Williams & Wilkins, 1979

74. Rall W: Core conductor theory and cable properties of neurons. In Brookhart JM, Mountcastle VB (eds): Handbook of Physiology, sect 1, vol 1, p 39. Baltimore, Williams & Wilkins, 1977

75. Ritchie JM: Mechanism of action of local anaesthetic agents and biotoxins. Br J Anaesth 47:191, 1975

76. Taylor RE: Effect of procaine on electrical properties of squid axon membrane. Am J Physiol 196:1071, 1959

77. Hille B: The common mode of action of three agents that decrease the transient change in sodium permeability in nerves. Nature 210:1220, 1966

78. Strichartz GR, Ritchie JM: The action of local anesthetics on ion channels of excitable tissues. In Strichartz GR (ed): Local Anesthetics. Handbook of Experimental Pharmacology, p 21. Berlin, Springer-Verlag, 1987

79. Strichartz G: Interactions of local anesthetics with neuronal sodium channels. In Covino BG, Fozzard HA, Rehder K *et al* (eds): Effects of Anesthetics, p 39. Bethesda, American Physiological Society, 1985

80. Strichartz GR, Ritchie JM: The action of local anesthetics on ion channels of excitable tissues. In Strichartz GR (ed): Local Anesthetics, p 21. Berlin, Springer-Verlag, 1987

81. Blaustein MP, Goldman DE: Competitive action of calcium and procaine on lobster axon. J Gen Physiol 49:1043, 1966

82. Arhem P, Frankenhaeuser B: Local anesthetics: Effects on permeability properties of nodal membrane in myelinated nerve fibres from xenopus. Potential clamp experiments. Acta Physiol Scand 91:11, 1974

83. Strichartz G: Molecular mechanisms of nerve block by local anesthetics. Anesthesiology 45:421, 1976

84. Shanes AM: Electrochemical aspects of physiological and pharmacological action in excitable cells. Part II: The action potential and excitation. Pharmacol 10:165, 1958

85. Johnson SM, Miller K: Antagonism of pressure and anaesthesia. Nature 228:75, 1970

86. Seeman P: The membrane expansion theory of anesthesia. In Fink BR (ed): Molecular Mechanisms of Anesthesia. Progress in Anesthesiology, vol 1, p 243. New York: Raven Press, 1975

87. Seeman P: The membrane actions of anesthetics and tranquilizers. Pharmacol Rev 24:583, 1972

88. Boulanger Y, Schreier S, Smith ICP: Molecular details of anesthetic-lipid interaction as seen by deuterium and phosphorus-31 nuclear magnetic resonance. Biochemistry 20:6824, 1981

89. Trudell JR, Cohen EN: Anesthetic-induced nerve membrane fluidity as a mechanism of anesthesia. In Fink BR (ed): Molecular Mechanisms of Anesthesia. Progress in Anesthesiology, vol 1, p 315. New York, Raven Press, 1975

90. Kelusky EC, Smith ICP: The influence of local anesthetics on molecular organization in phosphatidylethanolamine membranes. Molecular Pharmacology 26:314, 1984

91. Smith ICP, Butler KW: Location and dynamics of anesthetics in membranes: A magnetic resonance view. In Covino BG, Fozzard HA, Rehder K *et al* (eds): Effects of Anesthesia, p 1. Bethesda, American Physiological Society, 1985

92. Kendig JJ, Cohen EN: Pressure antagonism to nerve conduction block by anesthetic agents. Anesthesiology 47:6, 1977

93. Seeman P: Anesthetics and pressure reversal of anesthesia (editorial). Anesthesiology 47:1, 1977

94. Mrose HE, Ritchie JM: Local anesthetics: Do benzocaine and lidocaine act at the same single site? J Gen Physiol 71:223, 1978

95. Hille B: Charges and potentials at the nerve surface, divalent ions and pH. J Gen Physiol 51:221, 1968

96. McLaughlin S, Harary H: Phospholipid flip-flop and the distribution of surface charges in excitable membranes. Biophys J 14:200, 1974

97. Wei LY: Role of surface dipoles on axon membrane. Science 163:280, 1969

98. Blaustein MP, Goldman DE: Action of anionic and cationic nerve-blocking agents: experiment and interpretation. Science 153:429, 1966

99. McLaughlin S: Local anesthetics and the electrical properties of phospholipid bilayer membranes. In Fink BR (ed): Molecular Mechanisms of Anesthesia. Progress in Anesthesiology, vol 1, p 193. New York, Raven Press, 1975

100. Singer M: Effects of local anesthetics on phospholipid bilayer membranes. In Fink BR (ed): Molecular Mechanisms of Anesthesia. Progress in Anesthesiology, vol 1, p 223. New York, Raven Press, 1975

101. Aceves J, Machne X: The action of calcium and of local anesthetics on nerve cells, and their interaction during excitation. J Pharmacol Exp Ther 140:138, 1963

102. Strichartz GR: The inhibition of sodium currents in myelinated nerve by quaternary derivatives of lidocaine. J Gen Physiol 62:37, 1973

103. Hille B: Theories of anesthesia: general perturbations versus specific receptors. In Fink BR (ed): Molecular Mechanisms of Anesthesia. Progress in Anesthesiology, vol 2, p 1. New York, Raven Press, 1980

104. Hille B: Ionic channels in nerve membranes. Prog Biophys Mol Biol 21:1, 1970

105. Hille B: The permeability of the sodium channel to metal cations in myelinated nerve. J Gen Physiol 59:637, 1972

106. Ritchie JM: A pharmacological approach to the structure of sodium channels in myelinated axons. Ann Rev Neurosci 2:341, 1979

107. Strichartz GR, Ritchie JM: The action of local anesthetics on ion channels of excitable tissues. In Strichartz GR (ed): Local Anesthetics, Handbook of Experimental Pharmacology, p 21. Berlin, Springer-Verlag, 1987

108. Courtney KR: Mechanism of frequency-dependent inhibition of sodium currents in frog myelinated nerve by the lidocaine derivative GEA 968. J Pharmacol Exp Ther 195:225, 1975

109. Cahalan M, Shapiro BI, Almers W: Relationship between inactivation of sodium channels and block by quaternary derivatives of local anesthetics and other compounds. In Fink BR (ed): Molecular Mechanisms of Anesthesia. Progress in Anesthesiology, vol 2, p 17. New York, Raven Press, 1980

110. Hille B: Local Anesthetics: Hydrophilic and Hydrophobic Pathways for the Drug-receptor Interaction. J Gen Physiol 69:497, 1977

111. Schwartz W, Palade PT, Hille B: Local anesthetics: Effect of pH on use-dependent block of sodium channels in frog muscle. Biophys J 20:343, 1977

112. Hondeghem LM, Katzung BG: Time- and voltage-dependent interactions of antiarrhythmic drugs with cardiac sodium channels. Biochimica et Biophysica Acta 472:373, 1977

113. Courtney KR: Structure-activity relations for frequency-dependent sodium channel block in nerve by local anesthetics. J Pharmacol Exp Ther 213:114, 1980

114. Bean BP, Cohen CJ, Tsien RW: Lidocaine block of cardiac sodium channels. J Gen Physiol 81:613, 1983

115. Hondeghem LM, Katzung BG: Antiarrhythmic agents: The modulated receptor mechanism of action of sodium and calcium channel-blocking drugs. Ann Rev Pharmacol Toxicol 24:387, 1984

116. Khodorov B, Shishkova L, Peganov E *et al*: Inhibition of sodium currents in frog Ranvier node treated with local anesthetics: Role

of slow sodium inactivation. Biochimica et Biophysica Acta 433:409, 1976

117. Yeh JZ: Blockage of sodium channels by stereoisomers of local anesthetics. In Fink BR (ed): Molecular Mechanisms of Anesthesia, Progress in Anesthesiology, vol 2, p 35. New York, Raven Press, 1980

118. Ritchie JM, Rogart RB: The binding of saxitoxin and tetrodotoxin to excitable tissue. Rev Physiol Biochem Pharmacol 79:1, 1977

119. Cohen CJ, Bean BP, Colatsky TJ et al: Tetrodotoxin block of sodium channels in rabbit Purkinje fibers. Interactions between toxin binding and channel gating. J Gen Physiol 78:383, 1981

120. de Jong RH: Clinical physiology of local anesthetic action. In Cousins MJ, Bridenbaugh PO (eds): Neural Blockade in Clinical Anesthesia and Management of Pain, p 27. Philadelphia, JB Lippincott, 1980

121. de Jong RH: Local Anesthesia, p 51. Springfield, IL, Charles C Thomas, 1977

122. Franz DN, Perry RS: Mechanisms for differential block among single myelinated and non-myelinated axons by procaine. J Physiol (Lond) 236:193, 1973

123. Rosenberg PH, Heavner JE: Temperature-dependent nerve-blocking action of lidocaine and halothane. Acta Anaesthesiol Scand 24:324, 1980

124. Bromage PR: Epidural Anesthesia, p 525. Philadelphia, WB Saunders, 1978

125. Datta S, Lambert DH, Gregus J et al: Differential sensitivities of mammalian nerve fibers during pregnancy. Anesth Analg 62:1070, 1983

126. Flanagan HL, Datta S, Lambert DH et al: Effect of pregnancy on bupivacaine-induced conduction blockade in the isolated rabbit vagus nerve. Anesth Analg 66:123, 1987

127. Gasser HS, Erlanger J: The role played by the sizes of the constituent fibers of a nerve trunk in determining the form of its action potential wave. AM J Physiol 80:522, 1927

128. Gasser HS, Erlanger J: The role of fiber size in the establishment of a nerve block by pressure or cocaine. Am J Physiol 88:581, 1929

129. de Jong R: Local Anesthetics, 2nd edition, p 56. Springfield, IL, Charles C Thomas, 1977

130. Raymond SA, Gissen AJ: Mechanisms of differential nerve block. In Strichartz GR (ed): Local Anesthetics, p 95. Berlin, Springer-Verlag, 1987

131. Everett GM, Goodsell JS: The greater resistance to procaine of slow fiber groups in some peripheral nerves. J Pharmacol Exp Ther 106:385, 1952

132. Everett GM, Toman JEP: Procaine block of fiber groups in various nerves. Fed Proc 13:352, 1954

133. Franz DN, Perry RS: Mechanisms for differential block among single myelinated and non-myelinated axons by procaine. J Physiol (Lond) 236:193, 1974

134. Ford DJ, Raj PP, Singh P et al: Differential peripheral nerve block by local anesthetics in the cat. Anesthesiology 60:28, 1984

135. Heavner JE, de Jong RH: Lidocaine blocking concentrations for B- and C-nerve fibers. Anesthesiology 40:228, 1974

136. Scurlock JE, Heavner JE, de Jong RH: Differential B and C fibre block by an amide- and an ester-linked local anaesthetic. Br J Anaesth 47:1135, 1975

137. Rosenberg PH, Heinonen E: Differential sensitivity of A and C nerve fibres to long-acting amide local anaesthetics. Br J Anaesth 55:163, 1983

138. Rosenberg PH, Heinonen E, Jansson SE et al: Differential nerve block by bupivacaine and 2-chloroprocaine. Br J Anaesth 52:1183, 1980

139. Gissen AJ, Covino BG, Gregus J: Differential sensitivities of mammalian nerve fibers to local anesthetic agents. Anesthesiology 53:467, 1980

140. Wildsmith JAW, Gissen AJ, Gregus J et al: Differential nerve

141. Wildsmith JAW, Gissen AJ, Takman B et al: Differential nerve blockade: Ester v. amides and the influence of pKa. Br J Anaesth 59:379, 1987

142. Tasaki I: Conduction of the nerve impulse. In Magoun HW (ed): Handbook of Physiology, vol 1, Neurophysiology, p 108. Washington, American Physiological Society, 1959

143. Stampfli R: Overview of studies on the physiology of conduction in myelinated nerve fibers. In Waxman SG, Ritchie JM (eds): Demyelinating Diseases: Basic and Clinical Electrophysiology, p 11. New York, Raven Press, 1981

144. Tasaki I: Nervous Transmission, p 164. Springfield, IL, Charles C Thomas, 1953

145. Hiscoe NB: Distribution of nodes and incisures in normal and regenerated nerve fibers. Anat Rec 99:447, 1947

146. Nathan PW, Sears TA: Some factors concerned in differential nerve block by local anaesthetics. J Physiol (Lond) 157:565, 1961

147. Nathan PW, Sears TA: Differential nerve block by sodium-free and sodium-deficient solutions. J Physiol (Lond) 164:375, 1962

148. Gissen AJ, Covino BG, Gregus J: Differential sensitivity of fast and slow fibers in mammalian nerve: II. Margin of safety for nerve transmission. Anesth Analg 61:561, 1982

149. Gissen AJ, Covino BG, Gregus J: Differential sensitivity of fast and slow fibers in mammalian nerve: VI. Effect of pH on blocking action of local anesthetics. Reg Anesth 11:132, 1986

150. Grossman Y, Parnas I, Spira ME: Differential conduction block in branches of a bifurcating axon. J Physiol (Lond) 295:282, 1979

151. Raymond SA: Effects of nerve impulses on threshold of frog sciatic nerve fibres. J Physiol (Lond) 290:273, 1979

152. Raymond SA, Roscoe RF: After-effects of nerve impulses on threshold of frog sciatic fibers depends upon pH (pCO₂). Soc Neurosci Abstracts 9:513, 1983

153. Malenka RC et al: Modulation of parallel fiber excitability by postsynaptically mediated changes in extracellular potassium. Science 214:339, 1981

154. Gissen AJ, Covino BG, Gregus J: Differential sensitivity of fast and slow fibers in mammalian nerve: III. Effect of etidocaine and bupivacaine on fast/slow fibers. Anesth Analg 61:570, 1982

155. Fink BR, Cairns AM: Differential peripheral axon block with lidocaine: Unit studies in the cervical vagus nerve. Anesthesiology 59:182, 1983

156. Fink BR, Cairns AM: Differential slowing and block of conduction by lidocaine in individual afferent myelinated and unmyelinated axons. Anesthesiology 60:111, 1984

157. Fink BR, Cairns AM: Diffusional delay in local anesthetic block in vitro. Anesthesiology 61:555, 1984

158. Fink BR, Cairns AM: Differential margin of safety of conduction in individual peripheral axons. Anesthesiology 63:65, 1985

159. Fink BR, Cairns AM: Differential effect of nerve fiber structure on block by local anesthetic. Anesthesiology 63:157, 1985

160. Fink BR: Mechanisms of differential epidural block. Anesth Analg 65:325, 1986

161. Fink BR, Cairns AM: Lack of size-related differential sensitivity to equilibrium conduction block among mammalian myelinated axons exposed to lidocaine. Anesth Analg 66:948, 1987

162. Strichartz GR: The inhibition of sodium currents in myelinated nerve by quaternary derivatives of lidocaine. J Gen Physiol 62:37, 1973

163. Courtney KR, Kendig JJ, Cohen EN: Frequency-dependent conduction block: The role of nerve impulse pattern in local anesthetic potency. Anesthesiology 48:111, 1978

164. Scurlock JE, Meymaris E, Gregus J: The clinical character of local anesthetics: A function of frequency-dependent conduction block. Acta Anaesth Scand 22:601, 1978

165. Courtney KR: Structure-activity relations for frequency-depend-

ent sodium channel block in nerve by local anesthetics. J Pharm Exp Ther 213:114, 1980

166. Winnie AP, LaVallee DA, DeSosa B et al: Clinical pharmacokinetics of local anaesthetics. Canad Anaesth Soc J 24:252, 1977

167. Wildsmith JAW: Peripheral nerve and local anaesthetic drugs. Br J Anaesth 58:692, 1986

168. Selander D, Brattsand R, Lundborg G et al: Local anesthetics: Importance of mode of application, concentration and adrenaline for the appearance of nerve lesions. Acta Anaesthesiol Scand 23:127, 1979

169. Bromage PR: Spread of analgesic solutions in the epidural space and their site of action: a statistical study. Br J Anaesth 34:161, 1962

170. Burn JM, Guyer PB, Langdon L: The spread of solutions injected into the epidural space. Br J Anaesth 45:338, 1973

171. Erdemir HA, Soper LE, Sweet RB: Studies of factors affecting peridural anesthesia. Anesth Analg 44:400, 1965

172. Bromage PR: Mechanism of action of extradural analgesia. Br J Anaesth 47(Suppl):199, 1975

173. Scott DB, McClure JH, Giasi RM et al: Effects of concentration of local anaesthetic drugs in extradural block. Br J Anaesth 52:1033, 1980

174. Galindo A, Hernandez J, Benavides O et al: Quality of spinal extradural anaesthesia: The influence of spinal nerve root diameter. Br J Anaesth 47:41, 1975

175. Scott DB, Jebson PJ, Braid DP et al: Factors affecting plasma levels of lignocaine and prilocaine. Br J Anaesth 44:1040, 1972

176. Braid DP, Scott DB: Dosage of lignocaine in epidural block in relation to toxicity. Br J Anaesth 38:596, 1966

177. Tucker GT, Moore DC, Bridenbaugh PO et al: Systemic absorption of mepivacaine in commonly used regional block procedures. Anesthesiology 37:277, 1972

178. Tucker GT, Mather LE: Clinical pharmacokinetics of local anaesthetics. Clin Pharmacokin 4:241, 1979

179. Rosenberg PH, Heinonen J, Takasaki M: Lidocaine concentration in blood after topical anaesthesia of the upper respiratory tract. Acta Anaesthesiol Scand 24:125, 1980

180. Giasi RM, D'Agostino E, Covino BG: Absorption of lidocaine following subarachnoid and epidural administration. Anesth Analg 58:360, 1979

181. Blair MR: Cardiovascular pharmacology of local anaesthetics. Br J Anaesth 47S:247, 1975

182. Reynolds F: A comparison of the potential toxicity of bupivacaine, lignocaine and mepivacaine during epidural blockade for surgery. Br J Anaesth 43:567, 1971

183. Fink BR, Aasheim GM, Levy BA: Neural pharmacokinetics of epinephrine. Anesthesiology 48:263, 1978

184. Morikawa K-I, Bonica JJ, Tucker GT et al: Effect of acute hypovolaemia on lignocaine absorption and cardiovascular response following epidural block in dogs. Br J Anaesth 46:631, 1974

185. Bromage PR, Gertel M: Brachial plexus anesthesia in chronic renal failure. Anesthesiology 36:488, 1972

186. Mather LE, Tucker GT, Murphy TM et al: Hemodynamic drug interaction: Peridural lidocaine and intravenous ephedrine. Acta Anaesthesiol Scand 20:207, 1976

187. Bowdle TA, Freund PR, Slattery JT: Age-dependent lidocaine pharmacokinetics during lumbar peridural anesthesia with lidocaine hydrocarbonate or lidocaine hydrochloride. Regional Anesth 11:123, 1986

188. Veering BTH, Burm AG, van Kleef JW et al: Epidural anesthesia with bupivacaine: Effects of age on neural blockade and pharmacokinetics. Anesth Analg 66:589, 1987

189. Freund PR, Bowdle TA, Slattery JT et al: Caudal anesthesia with lidocaine or bupivacaine: Plasma local anesthetic concentration and extent of sensory spread in old and young patients. Anesth Analg 63:1017, 1984

190. Tucker GT: Pharmacokinetics of local anaesthetics. Br J Anaesth 58:717, 1986

191. Benowitz N, Forsyth RP, Melmon KL et al: Lidocaine disposition kinetics in monkey and man. I. Prediction by a perfusion model. Clin Pharmacol Ther 16:87, 1974

192. Tucker GT, Boyes RN, Bridenbaugh PO et al: Binding of anilidetype local anesthetics in human plasma: I. Relationships between binding, physicochemical properties, and anesthetic activity. Anesthesiology 33:287, 1970

193. Routledge PA, Stargel WW, Barchowsky A et al: Control of lidocaine therapy: New perspectives. Ther Drug Monit 4:265, 1982

194. Mather LE, Long GJ, Thomas J: The binding of bupivacaine to maternal and foetal plasma proteins. J Pharm Pharmacol 23:359, 1971

195. Kennedy RL, Miller RP, Bell JU et al: Uptake and distribution of bupivacaine in fetal lambs. Anesthesiology 65:247, 1986

196. Thomas J, Long G, Moore G et al: Plasma protein binding and placental transfer of bupivacaine. Clin Pharmacol Ther 19:426, 1976

197. Arthur GR, Scott DH, Boyes RN et al: Pharmacokinetic and clinical pharmacological studies with mepivacaine and prilocaine. Br J Anaesth 51:481, 1979

198. Mather LE, Runciman WB, Carapetis RJ et al: Hepatic and renal clearances of lidocaine in conscious and anesthetized sheep. Anesth Analg 65:943, 1986

199. Tucker GT: Plasma binding and disposition of local anesthetics. Int Anesthesiol Clin 13:33, 1975

200. Van Zundert A, Burm A, Van Kleef J et al: Plasma concentrations of epidural bupivacaine in mother and newborn. Anesth Analg 66:435, 1987

201. Kuhnert BR, Kuhnert PM, Philipson EH et al: The half-life of 2-chloroprocaine. Anesth Analg 65:273, 1986

202. Smith AR, Hur D, Resano F: Grand mal seizures after 2-chloroprocaine epidural anesthesia in a patient with plasma cholinesterase deficiency. Anesth Analg 66:677, 1987

203. Halkin H, Meffin P, Melmon KL et al: Influence of congestive heart failure on blood levels of lidocaine and its active monodeethylated metabolite. Clin Pharmacol Ther 17:669, 1975

204. Lescanic ML, Miller ED, DiFazio CA: The effects of lidocaine on the whole body distribution of radioactively labeled microspheres in the conscious rat. Anesthesiology 55:269, 1981

205. Sivarajan M, Amory DW, Lindbloom LE: Systemic and regional blood flow during epidural anesthesia without epinephrine in the rhesus monkey. Anesthesiology 45:300, 1976

206. Klein SW, Sutherland RI, Morch JE: Hemodynamic effects of intravenous lidocaine in man. Can Med Assoc J 99:472,1968

207. Wiklund L: Human hepatic blood flow and its relation to systemic circulation during intravenous infusion of bupivacaine or etidocaine. Acta Anaesthesiol Scand 21:189, 1977

208. Sivarajan M, Amory DW, Lindbloom LE et al: Systemic and regional blood-flow changes during spinal anesthesia in the rhesus monkey. Anesthesiology 43:78, 1975

209. Bonica JJ, Berges PU, Morikawa K-I: Circulatory effects of peridural block: I. Effects of level of analgesia and dose of lidocaine. Anesthesiology 33:619, 1970

210. Kennedy WF, Everett GB, Cobb LA et al: Simultaneous systemic and hepatic hemodynamic measurements during high peridural anesthesia in normal man. Anesth Analg 50:1069, 1971

211. Greiss FC, Still JG, Anderson SG: Effects of local anesthetic agents on the uterine vasculatures and myometrium. Am J Obstet Gynecol 124:889, 1976

212. Gibbs CP, Noel SC: Response of arterial segments from gravid human uterus to multiple concentrations of lignocaine. Br J Anaesth 49:409, 1977

213. Prescott LF, Adjepon-Yamoah KK, Talbot RG: Impaired ligno-

caine metabolism in patients with myocardial infarction and cardiac failure. Br Med J 1:939, 1976

214. Thomson PD, Melmon KL, Richardson JA et al: Lidocaine pharmacokinetics in advanced heart failure, liver disease, and renal failure in humans. Ann Intern Med 78:499, 1973

215. Roth RA, Rubin RJ: Role of blood flow in carbon monoxide- and hypoxic hypoxia-induced alterations in hexobarbital metabolism in rats. Drug Metab Dis 4:460, 1976

216. Branch RA, Shand DG, Wilkinson GR et al: The reduction of lidocaine clearance by dl-propranolol: An example of hemodynamic drug interaction. J Pharmacol Exp Ther 184:515, 1973

217. Adjepon-Yamoah KK, Nimmo J, Prescott LF: Gross impairment of hepatic drug metabolism in a patient with chronic liver disease. Br Med J 4:387, 1974

218. Collinsworth KA, Strong JM, Atkinson AJ et al: Pharmacokinetics and metabolism of lidocaine in patients with renal failure. Clin Pharmacol Ther 18:59, 1975

219. Reidenberg MM, James M, Dring LG: The rate of procaine hydrolysis in serum of normal subjects and diseased patients. Clin Pharmacol Ther 13:279, 1971

220. Finucane BT, Hammonds WD, Welch MB: Influence of age on vascular absorption of lidocaine from the epidural space. Anesth Analg 66:843, 1987

221. Moore RG, Thomas J, Triggs EJ et al: The pharmacokinetics and metabolism of the anilide local anaesthetics in neonates. III: Mepivacaine. Eur J Clin Pharmacol 14:203, 1978

222. Mihaly GW, Moore RG, Thomas J et al: The pharmacokinetics of the anilide local anesthetics in neonates. I: Lignocaine. Eur J Clin Pharmacol 13:143, 1978

223. Ecoffey C, Desparmet J, Maury M et al: Bupivacaine in children: pharmacokinetics following caudal anesthesia. Anesthesiology 63:447, 1985

224. Finholt DA, Stirt JA, DiFazio CA et al: Lidocaine pharmacokinetics in children during general anesthesia. Anesth Analg 65:279, 1986

225. Kennedy RL, Erenberg A, Robillard JE et al: Effects of changes in maternal-fetal pH on the transplacental equilibrium of bupivacaine. Anesthesiology 51:50, 1979

226. Friesen C, Yarnell R, Bachman C et al: The effect of lidocaine on regional blood flows and cardiac output in the non-stressed and the stressed foetal lamb. Can Anaesth Soc J 33:130, 1986

227. Denson D, Coyle D, Thompson G et al: Alpha₁-acid glycoprotein and albumin in human serum bupivacaine binding. Clin Pharmacol Ther 35:409, 1984

228. Bearn AG, Billing B, Sherlock S: The effect of adrenaline and noradrenaline on hepatic blood flow and splanchnic carbohydrate metabolism in man. J Physiol 115:430, 1951

229. Bowdle TA, Freund PR, Slattery JT: Propranolol reduces bupivacaine clearance. Anesthesiology 66:36, 1987

230. Burney RG, DiFazio CA: Hepatic clearance of lidocaine during N₂O anesthesia in dogs. Anesth Analg 55:322, 1976

231. Giasi RM, D'Agostino E, Covino BG: Interaction of diazepam and epidurally administered local anesthetic agents. Reg Anesth 5:8, 1980

232. Denson DD, Myers JA, Thompson GA et al: The influence of diazepam on the serum protein binding of bupivacaine at normal and acidic pH. Anesth Analg 63:980, 1984

233. Bonica JJ, Akamatsu TJ, Berges PU et al: Circulatory effects of peridural block. II. Effects of epinephrine. Anesthesiology 34:514, 1971

234. Stanton-Hicks M, Berges PU, Bonica JJ: Circulatory effects of peridural block: IV. Comparison of the effects of epinephrine and phenylephrine. Anesthesiology 39:308, 1973

235. Benowitz N, Forsyth RP, Melmon KL et al: Lidocaine disposition kinetics in monkey and man. II. Effects of hemorrhage and sympathomimetic drug administration. Clin Pharmacol Ther 16:99, 1974

236. Moore DC, Bridenbaugh LD, Bridenbaugh PO et al: Does compounding of local anesthetic agents increase their toxicity in humans? Anesth Analg 51:579, 1972

237. Cunningham NL, Major MC, Kaplan JA et al: A rapid-onset, long-acting regional anesthetic technique. Anesthesiology 41:509, 1974

238. Lalka D, Vicuna N, Burrow SR et al: Bupivacaine and other amide local anesthetics inhibit the hydrolysis of chloroprocaine by human serum. Anesth Analg 57:534, 1978

239. Raj PP, Ohlweiler D, Hitt BA et al: Kinetics of local anesthetic esters and the effects of adjuvant drugs on 2-chloroprocaine hydrolysis. Anesthesiology 53:307, 1980

240. de Jong RH, Bonin JD: Mixtures of local anesthetics are no more toxic than the parent drugs. Anesthesiology 54:177, 1981

241. Cohen SE, Thurlow A: Comparison of a chloroprocaine-bupivacaine mixture with chloroprocaine and bupivacaine used individually for obstetric epidural analgesia. Anesthesiology 51:288, 1979

242. Galindo A, Witcher T: Mixtures of local anesthetics: Bupivacaine-chloroprocaine. Anesth Analg 59:683, 1980

243. Corke BC, Carlson CG, Dettbarn W-D: The influence of 2-chloroprocaine on the subsequent analgesic potency of bupivacaine. Anesthesiology 60:25, 1984

244. Adriani J: Reactions to local anesthetics. JAMA 196:119, 1966

245. Aldrete JA, Johnson DA: Evaluation of intracutaneous testing for investigation of allergy to local anesthetic agents. Anesth Analg 49:173, 1970

246. Incaudo G, Schatz M, Patterson R et al: Administration of local anesthetics to patients with a history of prior adverse reaction. J Allergy Clin Immunol 61:339, 1978

247. Brown DT, Beamish D, Wildsmith JAW: Allergic reaction to an amide local anaesthetic. Br J Anaesth 53:435, 1981

248. De Shazo RD, Nelson HS: An approach to the patient with a history of local anaesthetic hypersensitivity: Experience with 90 patients. J Allergy Clin Immunol 63:387, 1979

249. Fisher M McD: Intradermal testing in the diagnosis of acute anaphylaxis during anaesthesia—Results of five years experience. Anaesth Intensive Care 7:58, 1979

250. Adriani T: Etiology and management of adverse reactions to local anesthetics. Int Anesthesiol Clin 10:127, 1972

251. Reisner LS, Hochman BN, Plumer MH: Persistent neurologic deficit and adhesive arachnoiditis following intrathecal 2-chloroprocaine injection. Anesth Analg 59:452, 1980

252. Ravindran RS, Bond VK, Tasch MD et al: Prolonged neural blockade following regional analgesia with 2-chloroprocaine. Anesth Analg 59:447, 1980

253. Gibbons RB: Chemical meningitis following spinal anesthesia. JAMA 3:900, 1969

254. Ready LB, Plumer MH, Haschke RH et al: Neurotoxicity of intrathecal local anesthetics in rabbits. Anesthesiology 63:364, 1985

255. Kane RE: Neurologic deficits following epidural or spinal anesthesia. Anesth Analg 60:150, 1981

256. Gissen AJ, Datta S, Lambert D: The chloroprocaine controversy. II. Is chloroprocaine neurotoxic? Reg Anesth 9:135, 1984

257. Wang BC, Hillman DE, Spielholz NI et al: Chronic neurological deficits and nesacaine-CE—An effect of the anesthetic, 2-chloroprocaine, or the antioxidant, sodium bisulfite? Anesth Analg 63:445, 1984

258. Ravindran RS, Turner MS, Muller J: Neurologic effects of subarachnoid administration of 2-chloroprocaine-CE, bupivacaine, and low pH normal saline in dogs. Anesth Analg 61:279, 1982

259. Ford DJ, Raj PP: Peripheral neurotoxicity of 2-chloroprocaine and bisulfite in the cat. Anesth Analg 66:719, 1987

260. Wagman IH, de Jong RH, Prince DA: Effects of lidocaine on the central nervous system. Anesthesiology 28:155, 1967

261. de Jong RH, Robles R, Corbin RW: Central actions of lidocaine-synaptic transmission. Anesthesiology 30:19, 1969

262. de Jong RH, Walts LF: Lidocaine-induced psychomotor seizures in man. Acta Anaesthesiol Scand 23:598, 1966

263. Munson ES, Tucker WK, Ausinsch B et al: Etidocaine, bupivacaine, and lidocaine seizure thresholds in monkeys. Anesthesiology 42:471, 1975

264. de Jong RH, Wagman IH, Prince DA: Effect of carbon dioxide on the cortical seizure threshold to lidocaine. Exp Neurol 17:221, 1967

265. Alexander CH, Berko RS, Gross JB et al: The effect of changes in arterial CO_2 tension on plasma lidocaine concentration. Can J Anaesth 34:343, 1987

266. Englesson S: The influence of acid-base changes on central nervous system toxicity of local anaesthetic agents. Acta Anaesthesiol Scand 18:79, 1974

267. Kim KC, Tasch MD: Effects of cimetidine and ranitidine on local anesthetic central nervous system toxicity in mice. Anesth Analg 65:840, 1986

268. Scott DB: Evaluation of the toxicity of local anaesthetic agents in man. Br J Anaesth 47:56, 1975

269. Ausinsch B, Malagodi MH, Munson ES: Diazepam in the prophylaxis of lignocaine seizures. Br J Anaesth 48:309, 1976

270. de Jong RH, Heavner JE: Local anesthetic seizure prevention: Diazepam vs. pentobarbital. Anesthesiology 36:449, 1972

271. Feinstein MB, Lenard W, Mathias J: The antagonism of local anesthetic induced convulsions by the benzodiazepine derivative diazepam. Arch Int Pharmacodyn 187:144, 1970

272. de Jong RH, Heavner JE, de Oliveira LF: Effects of nitrous oxide on the lidocaine seizure threshold and diazepam protection. Anesthesiology 37:299, 1972

273. Adams HJ, Kronberg GH, Takman BH: Local anesthetic activity and acute toxicity. (±)-2-(ethylpropylamino)-2', 6'-butyroxylidide: a new long-acting agent. J Pharm Sci 61:1820, 1972

274. Kozody R, Ready LB, Barsa JE et al: Dose requirements of local anaesthetic to produce grand mal seizure during stellate ganglion block. Can Anaesth Soc J 29:489, 1982

275. Aldrete JA, Romo-Salas F, Arora S et al: Reverse arterial blood flow as a pathway for central nervous system toxic responses following injection of local anesthetics. Anesth Analg 57:428, 1978

276. Dunbar RW, Boettner RB, Gatz RN et al: The effect of mepivacaine, bupivacaine, and lidocaine on digitalis-induced ventricular arrhythmias. Anesth Analg 49:761, 1970

277. Chapin JC, Kushins LG, Munson ES et al: Lidocaine, bupivacaine, etidocaine, and epinephrine-induced arrhythmias during halothane anesthesia in dogs. Anesthesiology 52:23, 1980

278. Albright GA: Cardiac arrest following regional anesthesia with etidocaine or bupivacaine. Anesthesiology 51:285, 1979

279. Block A, Covino B: Effect of local agents on cardiac conduction and contractility. Reg Anesth 6:55, 1981

280. de Jong RH, Ronfeld RA, DeRosa R: Cardiovascular effects of convulsant and supraconvulsant doses of amide local anesthetics. Anesth Analg 61:3, 1982

281. Kotelko DM, Shnider SM, Dailey PA et al: Bupivacaine-induced cardiac arrhythmias in sheep. Anesthesiology 60:10, 1984

282. Clarkson CW, Hondeghem LM: Mechanism for bupivacaine depression of cardiac conduction: Fast block of sodium channels during the action potential with slow recovery from block during diastole. Anesthesiology 62:396, 1985

283. Nath S, Haggmark S, Johansson G et al: Differential depressant and electrophysiologic cardiotoxicity of local anesthetics: An experimental study with special reference to lidocaine and bupivacaine. Anesth Analg 65:1263, 1986

284. Lynch C: Depression of myocardial contractility in vitro by bupivacaine, etidocaine, and lidocaine. Anesth Analg 65:551, 1986

285. Thomas RD, Behbehani MM, Coyle DE et al: Cardiovascular toxicity of local anesthetics: An alternative hypothesis. Anesth Analg 65:444, 1986

286. Heavner JE: Cardiac dysrhythmias induced by infusion of local anesthetics into the lateral cerebral ventricle of cats. Anesth Analg 65:133, 1986

287. Kasten GW: Amide local anesthetic alterations of effective refractory period temporal dispersion: Relationship to ventricular arrhythmias. Anesthesiology 65:61, 1986

288. Edouard A, Berdeaux A, Langloys J el al: Effects of lidocaine on myocardial contractility and baroreflex control of heart rate in conscious dogs. Anesthesiology 64:316, 1986

289. Bosnjak ZJ, Stowe DF, Kampine JP: Comparison of lidocaine and bupivacaine depression of sinoatrial nodal activity during hypoxia and acidosis in adult and neonatal guinea pigs. Anesth Analg 65:911, 1986

290. Morishima HO, Covino BG: Toxicity and distribution of lidocaine in nonasphyxiated and asphyxiated baboon fetuses. Anesthesiology 54:182, 1981

291. Morishima HO, Pedersen H, Finster M et al: Bupivacaine toxicity in pregnant and nonpregnant ewes. Anesthesiology 63:134, 1985

292. Rosen MA, Thigpen JW, Shnider SM et al: Bupivacaine-induced cardiotoxicity in hypoxic and acidotic sheep. Anesth Analg 64:1089, 1985

293. Komai H, Rusy BF: Effects of bupivacaine and lidocaine on AV conduction in the isolated rat heart: Modification by hyperkalemia. Anesthesiology 55:281, 1981

294. Avery P, Redon D, Schaenzer G et al: The influence of serum potassium on the cerebral and cardiac toxicity of bupivacaine and lidocaine. Anesthesiology 61:134, 1984

295. Johns RA, DiFazio CA, Longnecker DE: Lidocaine constricts or dilates rat arterioles in a dose-dependent manner. Anesthesiology 62:141, 1985

296. Johns RA, Seyde WC, DiFazio CA et al: Dose-dependent effects of bupivacaine on rat muscle arterioles. Anesthesiology 65:186, 1986

297. Fleisch JH, Titus E: Effect of local anesthetics on pharmacologic receptor systems of smooth muscle. J Pharmacol Exp Ther 186:44, 1973

298. Moore DC, Crawford RD, Scurlock JE: Severe hypoxia and acidosis following local anesthetic-induced convulsions. Anesthesiology 53:259, 1980

299. Moore DC, Bridenbaugh LD: Oxygen: The antidote for systemic toxic reactions from local anesthetic drugs. JAMA 174:842, 1960

300. Posner JB, Plum F, Van Poznak A: Cerebral metabolism during electrically induced seizures in man. Arch Neurol 20:388, 1969

301. Tommasino C, Maekawa T, Shapiro HM: Local cerebral blood flow during lidocaine-induced seizures in rats. Anesthesiology 64:771, 1986

302. Munson ES, Wagman IH: Diazepam treatment of local anesthetic-induced seizures. Anesthesiology 37:523, 1972

303. Moore DC, Balfour RI, Fitzgibbons D: Convulsive arterial plasma levels of bupivacaine and the response to diazepam therapy. Anesthesiology 50:454, 1979

304. Richards RK, Smith NT, Katz J: The effects of interaction between lidocaine and pentobarbital on toxicity in mice and guinea pig atria. Anesthesiology 29:493, 1968

305. Davis NL, de Jong RH: Successful resuscitation following massive bupivacaine overdose. Anesth Analg 61:62, 1982

306. Mallampati SR, Liu PL, Knapp RM: Convulsions and ventricular tachycardia from bupivacaine with epinephrine: Successful resuscitation. AnesthAnalg 63:856, 1984

307. Kendig JJ: Clinical implications of the modulated receptor hypothesis: Local anesthetics and the heart. Anesthesiology 62:382, 1985

308. Kasten GW, Martin ST: Bupivacaine cardiovascular toxicity: Comparison of treatment with bretylium and lidocaine. Anesth Analg 64:911, 1985

309. Kasten GW, Martin ST: Comparison of resuscitation of sheep and dogs after bupivacaine-induced cardiovascular collapse. Anesth Analg 65:1029, 1986

310. Kasten GW, Martin ST: Successful cardiovascular resuscitation after massive intravenous bupivacaine overdosage in anesthetized dogs. Anesth Analg 64:491, 1985

311. Chadwick HS: Toxicity and resuscitation in lidocaine- or bupivacaine-infused cats. Anesthesiology 63:385, 1985

312. Cregler LL, Mark H: Medical complications of cocaine abuse. N Engl J Med 315:1495, 1986

313. Wetli CV, Wright RK: Death caused by recreational cocaine use. JAMA 241:2519, 1979

314. Isner JM, Estes M, Thompson PD et al: Acute cardiac events temporally related to cocaine abuse. New Engl J Med 315:1438, 1986

315. Van Dyke C, Byck R: Cocaine. Sci Am March:128, 1982

316. Climie CR, McLean S, Starmer GA et al: Methaemoglobinaemia in mother and foetus during continuous epidural analgesia with prilocaine. Br J Anaesth 39:155, 1967

317. Lund PC, Cwik JC: Propitocaine (Citanest) and methemoglobinemia. Anesthesiology 26:569, 1965

318. Arens JF, Carrera AE: Methemoglobin levels following peridural anesthesia with prilocaine for vaginal deliveries. Anesth Analg 49:219, 1970

319. Inoue R, Suganuma T, Echizen H et al: Plasma concentrations of lidocaine and its principal metabolites during intermittent epidural anesthesia. Anesthesiology 63:304, 1985

320. Bromage PR, Pettigrew RT, Crowell DE: Tachyphylaxis in epidural analgesia: I. Augmentation and decay of local anesthesia. J Clin Pharmacol 9:30, 1969

321. Moore DC: Spinal anesthesia: Bupivacaine compared with tetracaine. Anesth Analg 59:743, 1980

322. Stanton-Hicks M, Murphy TM, Bonica JJ et al: Effects of extradural block: Comparison of the properties, circulatory effects and pharmacokinetics of etidocaine and bupivacaine. Br J Anaesth 48:575, 1976

323. Carpenter RL: How to optimize the success rate of spinal anesthesia. In Kirby RR, Brown DL (eds): Problems in Anesthesia, p 539. Philadelphia, JB Lippincott, 1987

324. Moore DC, Mather LE, Bridenbaugh PO et al: Arterial and venous plasma levels of bupivacaine following epidural and intercostal nerve blocks. Anesthesiology 45:39, 1976

325. Stoelting RK: Circulatory changes during direct laryngoscopy and tracheal intubation. Anesthesiology 47:381, 1977

326. Stoelting RK: Blood pressure and heart rate changes during short-duration laryngoscopy for tracheal intubation: Influence of viscous or intravenous lidocaine. Anesth Analg 57:197, 1978

327. Chraemmer-Jorgensen B, Hoilund-Carlsen PF, Marving J et al: Lack of effect of intravenous lidocaine on hemodynamic responses to rapid sequence induction of general anesthesia: A double-blind controlled clinical trial. Anesth Analg 65:1037, 1986

328. Laurito CE, Baughman VL, Polek WV et al: Aerosolized and intravenous lidocaine are no more effective than placebo for the control of hemodynamic responses to intubation. Anesthesiology 67:A29, 1987

329. Drenger B, Pe'er J, BenEzra D et al: The effect of intravenous lidocaine on the increase in intraocular pressure induced by tracheal intubation. Anesth Analg 64:1211, 1985

330. Yano M, Nishiyama H, Yokota H et al: Effect of lidocaine on ICP response to endotracheal suctioning. Anesthesiology 64:651, 1986

331. Yukioka H, Yoshimoto N, Nishimura K et al: Intravenous lidocaine as a suppressant of coughing during tracheal intubation. Anesth Analg 64:1189, 1985

332. Downes H, Gerber N, Hirshman CA: I.V. Lignocaine in reflex and allergic bronchoconstriction. Br J Anaesth 52:873, 1980

333. Berry CA, Sanner JH, Keasling HH: A comparison of the anticonvulsant activity of mepivacaine and lidocaine. J Pharmacol Exp Ther 133:357, 1961

334. Bernhard CG, Bohm E, Hojeberg S: A new treatment of status epilepticus. Arch Neurol Psychiatr 74:208, 1955

335. Cassuto J, Wallin G, Hogstrom S et al: Inhibition of postoperative pain by continuous low-dose intravenous infusion of lidocaine. Anesth Analg 64:971, 1985

336. Fenning WR: The use of local anesthetics for "beneficial" systemic effects. In Kirby RR, Brown DL (eds): Problems in Anesthesia, p 539. Philadelphia, JB Lippincott, 1987

337. Bedford RF, Persing JA, Pobereskin L et al: Lidocaine or thiopental for rapid control of intracranial hypertension? Anesth Analg 59:435, 1980

338. Carpenter RL, Mulroy MF: Edrophonium antagonizes combined lidocaine-pancuronium and verapamil-pancuronium neuromuscular blockade in cats. Anesthesiology 65:506, 1986

339. Littlewood DG, Buckley P, Covino BG et al: Comparative study of various local anaesthetic solutions in extradural block in labor. Br J Anaesth 51:47S, 1979

340. Tucker GT, Mather LE: Absorption and Disposition of Local Anesthetics. Pharmacokinetics, Neural Blockade in Clinical Anesthesia and Management of Pain, p 61. Philadelphia, JB Lippincott, 1980

341. Leicht CH, Carlson SA: Prolongation of lidocaine spinal anesthesia with epinephrine and phenylephrine. Anesth Analg 65:365, 1986

342. Chambers WA, Littlewood DG, Scott DB: Spinal anesthesia with hyperbaric bupivacaine. Effect of added vasoconstrictors. Anesth Analg 61:49, 1982

343. Chambers WA, Littlewood DG, Logan MR et al: Effect of added epinephrine on spinal anesthesia with lidocaine. Anesth Analg 60:417, 1981

344. Priddle HD, Andros GJ: Primary spinal anesthetic effects of epinephrine. Current Researches in Anesthesia and Analgesia 29:156, 1950

345. Bromage PR, Camporesi EM, Durant PA et al: Influence of epinephrine as an adjuvant to epidural morphine. Anesthesiology 58:257, 1983

346. Smith HS, Carpenter RL, Bridenbaugh LD: Failure rate of tetracaine spinal anesthesia with and without epinephrine. Anesthesiology 65:A193, 1986

347. Abouleish EI: Epinephrine improves the quality of spinal hyperbaric bupivacaine for cesarean section. Anesth Analg 66:395, 1987

348. Collins JG, Kitahata LM, Matsumoto M et al: Spinally administered epinephrine suppresses noxiously evoked activity of WDR neurons in the dorsal horn of the spinal cord. Anesthesiology 60:269, 1984

349. Kennedy WF Jr, Bonica JJ, Ward RJ et al: Cardiorespiratory effects of epinephrine when used in regional anesthesia. Acta Anaesthesiol Scand (Suppl) 22:320, 1966

350. Katz RL, Epstein RA: The interaction of anesthetic agents and adrenergic drugs to produce cardiac arrhythmias. Anesthesiology 29:763, 1968

351. Moore DC, Batra MS: The components of an effective test dose prior to epidural block. Anesthesiology 55:693, 1981

352. Hood DD, Dewan DM, Rose JC et al: Maternal and fetal effects of intravenous epinephrine containing solutions in gravid ewes. Anesthesiology 59:A393, 1983

353. Gunther RE, Bellville JW: Obstetrical caudal anesthesia: II. A randomized study comparing 1 per cent mepivacaine with 1 per cent mepivacaine plus epinephrine. Anesthesiology 37:288, 1972

354. Abboud TK, Sheik-ol-Eslam A, Yanagi T et al: Safety and efficacy of epinephrine added to bupivacaine for lumbar epidural analgesia in obstetrics. Anesth Analg 64:585, 1985

355. Jouppila R, Jouppila P, Hollmen A *et al:* Effect of segmental extradural analgesia on placental blood flow during normal labor. Br J Anaesth 50:563, 1978
356. Albright GA, Jouppila R, Hollmen A *et al:* Epinephrine does not alter human intervillous blood flow during epidural anesthesia. Anesthesiology 54:131, 1981
357. Jouppila R, Jouppila P, Kuikka J *et al:* Placental blood flow during caesarean section under lumbar extradural analgesia. Br J Anaesth 50:275, 1978
358. Albright GA: Epinephrine should be used with the therapeutic dose of bupivacaine in obstetrics. Anesthesiology 61:217, 1984
359. Marx GF: In reply to Ref. 358. Anesthesiology 61:218, 1984
360. Ueda W, Hirakawa M, Mori K: Acceleration of epinephrine absorption by lidocaine. Anesthesiology 63:717, 1985
361. Klingstrom P, Nylen B, Westermark L: A clinical comparison between adrenaline and octapressin as vasoconstrictors in local anesthesia. Acta Anaesthesiol Scand 11:35, 1967
362. Katz RL: Epinephrine and PLV-2: Cardiac rhythm and local vasoconstrictors effects. Anesthesiology 26:619, 1965
363. Akerman B: Effects of felypressin (Octopressin) on the acute toxicity of local anaesthetics. Acta Pharmacol Toxicol 27:318, 1969
364. Prokopiou AA, Pateromichelakis S, Rood JP: The effects of ornipressin and adrenaline on lignocaine nerve blocks. Acta Anaesthesiol Scand 30:647, 1986
365. Gerke DC, Frewin DB, Frost BR: The synergistic vasoconstrictor effect of octapressin and catecholamines on the isolated rabbit ear artery. Aust J Exp Biol Med Sci 55:737, 1977
366. Bromage PR, Burfoot MF, Crowell DE *et al:* Quality of epidural blockade. III. Carbonated local anaesthetic solutions. J Anaesth 39:197, 1967
367. Sukhani R, Winnie AP: Clinical pharmacokinetics of carbonated local anesthetics. I. Subclavian perivascular brachial block model. Anesth Analg 66:739, 1987
368. McClure JH, Scott DB: Comparison of bupivacaine hydrochloride and carbonated bupivacaine in brachial plexus block by the interscalene technique. Br J Anaesth 53:523, 1981
369. Martin R, Lamarche Y, Tetreault L: Comparison of the clinical effectiveness of lidocaine hydrocarbonate and lidocaine hydrochloride with and without epinephrine in epidural anaesthesia. Can Anaesth Soc J 28:217, 1981
370. Brown DT, Morison DH, Covino BG *et al:* Comparison of carbonated bupivacaine and bupivacaine hydrochloride for extradural anaesthesia. Br J Anaesth 52:419, 1980
371. Martin R, Lamarche Y, Tetreault L: Effects of carbon dioxide and epinephrine on serum levels of lidocaine after epidural anaesthesia. Can Anaesth Soc J 28:224, 1981
372. Parnass SM, Curran MA, Becker GL: Comparative hypotensive responses of the carbonated and hydrochloride salts of lidocaine in epidural blocks. Anesth Analg 66:S134, 1987
373. Navaratnarajah M, Davenport HT: The prolongation of local anaesthetic action with dextran. Anaesthesia 40:259, 1985
374. Bridenbaugh LD: Does the addition of low molecular weight dextran prolong the duration of action of bupivacaine? Reg Anesth 3:6, 1978
375. Moore DC: The use of hyaluronidase in local and nerve block analgesia other than spinal block: 1520 cases. Anesthesiology 12:611, 1951

Part III

Preparing for Anesthesia

Chapter 15

Leroy D. Vandam
Sukumar P. Desai

Evaluation of the Patient and Preoperative Preparation

Aside from the treatment of pain or application of life support measures, clinical anesthesia is not a therapeutic modality. The practice exists so that surgical and diagnostic procedures can be performed safely and without pain or other discomfort for the patients concerned. Anesthetics are among the most potent and rapidly acting drugs known, used not only to suspend consciousness but also to induce muscle relaxation and respiratory paralysis, occasionally to lower blood pressure to marginal levels, or to reduce skeletal body temperature to what might be considered nonsurvival limits in the waking state. No other specialty of medicine takes such liberties with the physiologic systems of humans.

Although the anesthetics available today are better understood and far safer than the older drugs, few, if any, are without some effect on the normal physiology of the vital systems—central nervous, circulatory, respiratory, hepatic, and renal—and more subtle influences on endocrine and intermediary metabolism. These effects are usually well tolerated in healthy people, but less so in those with pathophysiologic or physical abnormalities, and those at the extremes of age (*i.e.*, neonates or elderly). To avoid or minimize the attendant morbidity and mortality, one must be assured that a patient about to undergo operation, either elective or emergency, is at his or her best possible condition beforehand, both mentally and physically. A crude analogy might be the preparation of an athlete for a championship event involving severe physical strain.

The only way anesthesiologists may achieve the stated optimal conditions is to care for patients on a personal basis, that is, to become acquainted with patients, to examine them be-

forehand, direct the preparation for anesthesia, and to follow this course during and after operation. This is perhaps the only kind of activity that imparts true professional status to the specialty. Even though anesthesia and operation comprise a team effort involving referring physicians, surgeons, and nurses, only the anesthesiologist is knowledgeable in matters pertaining to anesthesia. It is not always possible for anesthesiologists to function appropriately. This might be so if every patient were to be referred to the anesthesiologist on a consultant basis by the other physicians concerned, as is often done in obstetric clinics, in preanesthetic clinics, or if the patient has been in the hospital for several days. Usually, however, anesthesiologists learn of their assignments late on an afternoon when the operating schedule is first posted. Although most patients will already have had a history, physical examination and essential laboratory tests performed and, for the most part, are admitted on time; now and then an important item is missing so that retrieval causes problems. Furthermore, except for ambulatory surgery, a host of professionals, including residents, attending physicians, nurses, and laboratory technicians (and medical students), will converge upon the patient to accomplish their duties. Thus, anesthesiologists must seek the right moment to carry out their missions.

In this chapter, we explain how the preoperative assessment and preparation for patients might be accomplished. In connection with each clinical problem, we shall discuss the philosophy of ordering and interpreting laboratory data, the concept of physical status, the risk involved in undergoing anesthesia and operation where facts are available, and the indications for consultation or delay of operation.

LOGISTICS OF THE PREANESTHETIC VISIT

Preferably, every patient who is to be anesthetized should be visited beforehand by the designated anesthesiologist, under any kind of arrangement, that is, inpatient status, morning admission, or ambulatory surgery, including emergency surgery. There is no substitute for seeing patients in order to learn about them, their concerns, their physical make-up, and pertinent laboratory data. In the process, a subtle bond will be established, as the patient senses the sympathy and professional qualities of the anesthesiologist. Several studies have shown that this kind of relationship results in a diminished need for sedative and analgesic medication before, probably during, and after anesthesia.[1, 2]

HOSPITAL RECORDS

Study of past and current hospital records saves time in questioning later on, because age, height, and body weight; body temperature; blood pressure; and the diagnosis will have been recorded on admission. Furthermore, a history and physical examination may already have been written both by the referring physician when a medical problem exists and by the surgeon. An earlier hospital record, particularly if anesthesia had been given for an operation, may reveal essential information either forgotten, misunderstood, or unknown to the patient in relation to problems and attendant complications. This is one of the main reasons why a conscientiously kept anesthetic record is so valuable for subsequent anesthetic administration and from the medicolegal standpoint. Every anesthetic given represents a clinical experiment. Was the preanesthetic medication adequate, which of the agents and techniques were used, and what were the results? Were there technical difficulties in relation to tracheal intubation or administration of a regional anesthetic, spinal, epidural or otherwise? The kinds of information gained are vital, as illustrated by the initial experience with halothane, where a single administration or multiple halogenated anesthetics were followed, in the rare instance (1:10,000), by development of fatal hepatic necrosis.[3] In some cases, the only clue to the ultimate complication was the onset of unexplained fever after the first anesthetic, an elusive symptom at best. Nevertheless, anesthesiologists have been faulted for not taking that clue into consideration before giving a halogenated anesthetic for subsequent anesthesia. On the other hand, a not uncommon problem is the inability to obtain from the same hospital a record dating back many years.

THE INTERVIEW

This should be accomplished in a professional manner, unhurried, and with regard to the impression created in the patient's mind, not being neglectful of attire, because a clean white coat helps to dispel the disconcerting effect of an operating room scrub suit. Since this is a private encounter, visitors and relatives might be asked to wait outside the room unless their help in answering questions is required, as in the case of children, for psychological reasons in adults or, in those with mental impediments of various kinds. An interpreter is required if a language barrier exists. The anesthesiologist might return later if the patient is eating, being examined by another physician, or undergoing special treatment. Confidentiality is important, as in the example of a young, unmarried woman who might not wish to divulge the use of contraceptives in the presence of her parents, others who may be unwilling to reveal drug abuse problems, still others who may not wish to reveal the fact that they have a socially unacceptable disease.

MENTAL ATTITUDES

At the start, even without questioning, one can discern elements of the patient's emotional constitution and relevant background from the point of view of comprehension. The conversation might begin by reference to the reading material that a patient has brought along for the hospital stay. The interviewer must not be prejudiced by a seemingly objectionable attitude while keeping in mind the effect of the physician's demeanor upon the patient. Some patients might appear to be too inquisitive or demanding, overly concerned, uncooperative, manipulative, or simply noncommunicative. Groves[4] has categorized "hateful patients" as not particularly those with whom the physician has an occasional personality clash, but those whom most physicians dread. The insatiable dependency of "hateful patients" leads to behaviors that group them into four stereotypes: dependent clingers, entitled demanders, manipulative help-rejectors, and self-destructive deniers. The physician's negative reactions constitute important clinical data that should facilitate better understanding and appropriate psychological management for each kind of patient. These manifestations may relate to anxiety, colored by a patient's ethnic and educational background, or simply the level of intelligence—attitudes that can be mollified or overcome by sympathetic understanding, patience, and gentle persistence in asking and answering questions. In another section, we shall discuss the assessment of patients with psychiatric problems, those with possible suicidal tendencies, and the special problems of the elderly. Rarely, it may be necessary to defer operation so that psychiatric consultation and appropriate care can be provided.

HISTORY TAKING

As long as the essential items are covered, it does not matter in which order the questioning proceeds; however, a routine plan is best (Table 15-1). For this purpose, anesthesiologists

TABLE 15-1.   The Order of the History Taking

Generalities
Previous anesthetics
Familial health and anesthetic experience
Current drug usage
Allergy (blood transfusion)
Drug abuse and addiction
Menstrual and obstetric experience
System review
Circulation
Respiration
Liver
Kidneys and urinary tract
Nervous system: central, peripheral
Musculoskeletal
Endocrine
Hematology
Dental and oral problems
Gastrointestinal

tend to use check lists or to fill in the spaces on the reverse of the anesthesia record. However, remarks written by the anesthesiologist on the patient's progress notes serve to call the attention of others to any anesthesia problems that might arise.

GENERALITIES

What is the state of the patient's well-being, physical activity and exercise tolerance, recent weight gain or loss, diet, and occupation? The latter is relevant to toxic exposures such as asbestosis in the shipfitter, chronic smoke inhalation in the firefighter, or exposure to cholinesterase inhibitors in the insecticides used by the farmer. Is the patient fully aware of the nature of the operation to be performed, and is the reaction appropriate to the occasion? Although an anesthesiologist must be fully cognizant of the details of the operation, it is best to refer leading questions to the surgeon and not to engage in discussion on the capability of the surgeon or the need for the procedure planned. Patients, out of anxiety, rarely have enough information to satisfy their concerns.

PREVIOUS ANESTHETICS

The patient should be asked to give details regarding any untoward reaction to previous anesthetics. Most people will not recall the details, such as for a tonsillectomy or myringotomy performed in infancy or childhood, but will simply recall how unpleasant the ether was. But the recollections can be vivid. An adult with a childhood history of ether convulsions, usually attributed to fever and acidosis, may have had an abortive, malignant hyperthermia (MH) incident. Despite the current association with halothane and succinylcholine, Denborough's original description of MH concerned a series of familial deaths where ether had been the sole anesthetic used.[5] The majority of women can relate their experiences with anesthesia during childbirth—having none at all, being put to sleep, development of post-lumbar puncture headache after spinal anesthesia, or an epidural anesthetic that was inadequate. For other anesthetics, there may have been prolonged awakening, awareness during operation, protracted postoperative nausea and vomiting, a neurologic complication of regional anesthesia, postoperative fever, jaundice and liver failure, or more serious matters such as intensive care admission, post-cardiac arrest or respiratory insufficiency. Few patients will have been fully informed or can recall or understand what might have happened to them. Even the MedicAlert bracelet may warn only of a serious drug reaction or a chronic disease that requires continuous attention and therapy, such as diabetes mellitus, epilepsy, hemophilia, adrenal insufficiency, or sickle cell disease. If the anesthetic record and postanesthetic notes are adequate, these facts may be found. However, as previously noted, it may not be possible to retrieve the record in that same hospital if the operation was performed many years ago with the records now in dead storage. If the anesthetic had been given elsewhere and the information is necessary for the patient's survival, a telephone call to an understanding anesthesiologist at the other hospital might enable the retrieval of the facts. If all attempts are to no avail, the anesthesiologist, in electing an anesthetic method, must proceed with a choice based on the odds of not encountering a major problem, for example, MH or an anaphylactoid reaction.

FAMILIAL HEALTH AND ANESTHETIC EXPERIENCES

In regard to anesthetic choice, hereditary diseases and familial anesthetic complications are highly relevant matters. What is the significance of a close relative's death on the operating table or admission to an intensive care unit in relation to inheritable disease, such as MH, cholinesterase abnormalities, glucose-6-phosphate deficiency; or was it a surgical or anesthetic catastrophe? Complications of this nature should be preventable, but a familial history of coronary artery disease, myocardial infarction, hypertension, or diabetes mellitus must also be taken into account because of the possibility of associated diffuse vascular disease.

CURRENT DRUG USAGE

Problems concerning the ancillary actions of therapeutic drugs and their interaction relate to modern improvements in pharmacotherapy with potent and highly specific agents and a heightened understanding of their dynamics and kinetics. In the early days of introduction of the corticosteroids for treatment of a variety of diseases and of reserpine for hypertension, anesthesiologists tended to adopt strict rules concerning discontinuance of these drugs before operation because of the possibility of adverse interactions with anesthetics. However, as experience accumulated, the problems proved to be not as serious as originally thought. In relation to reserpine, for example, comparative studies showed that untreated hypertensive patients have just as wide fluctuations of intraoperative blood pressure as those patients prepared with reserpine. Since then, circulatory active drugs, that is, those used in the treatment of hypertension, angina, congestive heart failure, and the complex of dysrhythmias, have actually been found to be advantageous from the anesthesia standpoint. Nevertheless, one must know how these drugs act, how compliant the patient has been with therapy, whether it is better to continue their use, and how to treat any kind of drug interaction. Only rarely does a specific drug need to be discontinued before anesthesia, and the possible consequences of that action for the patient's well-being must be taken into account. Specific drug interactions will be cited in a later section of this chapter in relation to the diseases concerned, but suffice it to say that those of most concern are used in the treatment of heart disease and hypertension, the immunosuppressive agents, including the corticosteroids, psychotherapeutic drugs, anticoagulants, and various endocrine replacement substances.

ALLERGY

A considerable proportion of the population will at some time have experienced an allergic reaction, usually of the atopic kind, many still undergoing therapy for hay fever, asthma, allergic rhinitis, or dermatitis. A few will have had more serious reactions of the anaphylactoid type: generalized hives, angioneurotic edema, erythema multiforme, anaphylaxis relating to hymenopteran sting or anesthetic drugs such as thiopental and althesin. The importance of a positive, allergic history is that such patients are more likely to develop sensitivity reactions during anesthesia.

If a reaction to a drug has been well documented—not always a simple matter—that drug should not be repeated unless deemed necessary. Such deviation from safe practice might involve a patient who has suffered a mild anaphylactoid reaction (urticaria) to an iodinated contrast medium during a radiodiagnostic study. Preparation for a second procedure usually involves pretreatment with an antihistamine and corticosteroid, with resuscitative equipment on hand, and an intravenous (iv) catheter in place. Those patients are labeled as being sensitive to iodine and should not undergo preoperative skin preparation with an iodinated antiseptic. Patients must always be informed of such reactions so that they can inform others who may be treating them. Specific query should always be made about prior blood transfusion and any reaction thereto.

DRUG ABUSE AND ADDICTION

Some confusion exists in the definition of drug abuse and addiction and the resulting pathophysiologic states. Alcohol, medical drugs, and nonmedical drugs may be used to excess, eventually giving rise to their compulsive use and dependence because of the altered mood and feelings engendered. *Addiction* is an extension of this kind of behavior, defined by the World Health Organization as a behavioral pattern of substance use characterized by overwhelming involvement with the use of a drug, the securing of its supply, and a high tendency to relapse into this state after withdrawal. With chronic usage, tolerance develops, in that an increasing amount of the substance is required for its effect. Coincidentally, physical dependence may develop wherein an altered physiologic state requires continuous use of the drug so that the withdrawal or abstinence syndrome will not develop. The implications of substance abuse are many for anesthesia and the agents include tobacco smoking; alcohol use (both discussed in the following sections); depressants such as the barbiturates; anxiolytics as typified by the benzodiazepines, opioids, and stimulants, including the hallucinogens, psychedelics, and cocaine. Many of these compounds are hepatic enzyme inducers.

Tobacco Smoking

Under the weight of public health efforts, the incidence of cigarette smoking has declined somewhat. However, a fair percentage of the population will present for anesthesia with a history of chronic smoking. The risk of development of health problems relates to amount and the age at which smoking first began, plus its continuance to the present time. The nicotine in tobacco is a strong adrenergic stimulus with resultant increases in heart rate, arterial blood pressure, and peripheral vascular resistance. Furthermore, studies on heavy smokers show that about 15% of the oxygen-binding sites on hemoglobin may be occupied by carbon monoxide, thus reducing the oxygen supply available to tissues. Considerable amounts of carbon monoxide may accumulate in anesthetic rebreathing systems. It has been said that smoking, particularly with certain additive factors (*e.g.*, obesity), causes approximately one half of the excess mortality resulting from cardiovascular disease and doubles the risk for development of myocardial infarction or death from coronary artery disease. Currently, there is little difference in this regard between men and women. Elevated blood pressure and hypercholesterolemia are independent risk factors additive to that of smoking.

A second serious effect is the development of airway disease, including emphysema and chronic bronchitis, leading to a marked increase in postoperative respiratory complications, additive to those of anesthesia and operation *per se*. More subtle effects include inhibition of the immune response, hepatic microsomal induction, the development of gastric hyperacidity, peptic ulcer, and reflux, so that aspiration of gastric contents is more lethal. Finally, smoking leads to a higher incidence of cancer of the lung, larynx, oral cavity, esophagus, stomach, and urinary bladder. A summary of the increased risks of tobacco smoking appears in Table 15-2.

According to this narrative, a patient would be well advised to stop smoking before a complicated operation, but a minimum of about 6 weeks of abstinence would be necessary to have an impact on morbidity. In that interval, deficiencies in the immune response should have recovered, along with improvement in bronchitis and reversible small airway disease. However, in the inveterate smoker facing the anxieties of a major operation, it may be too much to expect cessation of smoking. A prime candidate for development of a postoperative pulmonary complication, whether it be atelectasis or bronchopneumonia, is the male, long-term heavy smoker who must endure the pain and chest splinting associated with a thoracic or upper abdominal incision. Preoperative instruction in the techniques of pulmonary physiotherapy is believed to be beneficial in the prevention of these sequelae.

Alcohol Abuse

It is usually difficult to elicit an accurate history of alcohol dependency. In the aggressive business executive, the reply to the question might be that a drink or two is taken at lunch time, then several drinks with dinner and afterward, but not associated with inebriation. Nevertheless, this is the kind of person who might have a withdrawal seizure postoperatively or, in conjunction with the use of sedatives, might manifest confusion bordering upon delirium tremens. Although phenytoin is sometimes prescribed preoperatively to prevent a seizure, the efficacy is not established, and hydantoin is a well-known hepatic enzyme inducer. An alternative approach is to administer alcohol (iv) as part of fluid replacement. Intra-

TABLE 15-2.   Increased Risks for Cigarette Smokers

Cardiovascular Disease
Coronary artery disease
Peripheral vascular disease
Aortic aneurysm
Stroke (at younger ages)

Cancer
Lung
Larynx, oral cavity, esophagus
Bladder, kidney
Pancreas, stomach

Lung Disorders
Cancer (as noted above)
Chronic bronchitis with airflow obstruction
Emphysema

Complications of Pregnancy
Infants—small for gestational age, higher perinatal mortality
Maternal complications—placenta previa, abruptio placenta

Gastrointestinal Complications
Peptic ulcer
Esophageal reflux

(Reproduced with permission from Burns DM: Tobacco and health. In Wyngaarden JB, Smith LH Jr [eds]: Cecil Textbook of Medicine, 17th ed, p 47. Philadelphia, WB Saunders, 1985.)

venous alcohol is also an excellent sedative. It is believed that many housewives may surreptitiously consume considerable quantities of liquor during the course of the day. Many will admit the fact, and some will have obtained help from Alcoholics Anonymous. At any rate, the approximate amounts and kinds of alcohol consumed are of importance in the evaluation for anesthesia; even wine and beer consumption may be equivalent to lesser amounts of hard liquor. During social drinking, the blood alcohol level lies in the $50 \text{ mg} \cdot \text{dl}^{-1}$ range, while symptoms of excitement develop in the 70 to 100 $\text{mg} \cdot \text{dl}^{-1}$ range.

A list of alcohol-related illnesses is shown in Table 15-3. The heavy drinker may have fatty infiltration of the liver, abnormal liver function tests, elevation of transaminase in plasma, hepatitis, or cirrhosis. Although moderate alcohol consumption is said to lessen the risk of development of myocardial infarction, alcohol-induced myocarditis is an established entity. Tolerance to the ethyl radical may have developed on the basis of increased hepatic metabolism, thus larger amounts of general or iv anesthetics may be required. On the other hand, in the acute phase of alcohol intoxication, these drugs may cause additive depression. Clues to heavy alcohol consumption may be found in tremors of the hands, and telangiectasia and cyanosis of the nose and cheeks. During the physical examination, reflexes may be hyperactive and tenderness elicited over the liver.

Opioids, Marihuana, and Cocaine

OPIOIDS. Drugs in this group of substances can be taken by any of several routes, although oral ingestion is not usually used because of the lesser effect relating to first-pass metabolism in liver. These drugs are consumed because of the euphoria produced, and in no other instance are the phenomena of tolerance, physical dependence, and withdrawal effects so evident. The iv route of administration is beset with the possibility of skin infection, phlebitis, pulmonary embolism, lung infarction and abscess, bacterial endocarditis, and contraction of such diseases as hepatitis, acquired immunodeficiency syndrome (AIDS), tetanus, and even malaria when contaminated syringes and needles are used. The withdrawal symptoms produced by acute cessation of the drug, or unsuspecting use by a physician of an opioid antagonist or an agonist–antagonist, bear all the stigmata of catecholamine stimulation, both centrally and peripherally, often life threatening. Of late, the drug clonidine, used in the treatment of hypertension, has proved useful in treating those symptoms, probably because it is a centrally acting sympathetic nervous system inhibitor, apparently replacing opioid-mediated inhibition that is absent during withdrawal. In the alcohol withdrawal syndrome, clonidine has been shown to relieve the tremor, sweating, and tachycardia. The benzodiazepines and beta-adrenergic blockers have been used for similar reasons.

The simplest anesthetic approach to the opioid addict is to maintain drug usage at the accustomed level, or to substitute with methadone, and avoid use of the agonist–antagonists such as butorphanol, buprenorphine, nalbuphine, and the pure antagonists, naloxone and naltrexone. An increased requirement for anesthetics may be noticed during balanced techniques or opioid-supplemented general anesthesia.

MARIHUANA. The active ingredient of marihuana, widely smoked as a tranquilizer, is cannabis, which results in a state of well-being, relaxation, and disinhibition. Apparently there is no marked development of tolerance and physical dependence. Cannabis has been advocated as an antiemetic in persons undergoing cancer chemotherapy, as a mild bronchodilator in the asthmatic, and to reduce intraocular pressure in glaucoma. The pathophysiologic effects of cannabis may be more serious than currently believed, however, particularly in relation to the circulation (tachycardia and systolic hypertension) and in the psychotomimetic symptoms produced. This is

TABLE 15-3.   Alcohol-related Illnesses due to Toxic and Nutritional Effects of Ethanol

ORGAN	SYNDROMES DUE TO TOXIC EFFECTS	SYNDROMES DUE TO NUTRITIONAL EFFECTS
Brain	Alcoholic dementia (cortical atrophy)	Wernicke-Korsakoff syndrome Cerebellar degeneration Central pontine myelinosis (secondary to electrolyte changes during therapy)
Nerves		Peripheral polyneuropathy (thiamine deficiency)
Heart	Alcoholic cardiomyopathy	Beriberi heart disease (thiamine deficiency)
Blood	Leukopenia, anemia, thrombocytopenia	Macrocytic hyperchromic anemia (folic acid deficiency)
Gastrointestinal tract	Acute and chronic gastritis Acute and chronic pancreatitis Carcinoma of the head and neck and of the esophagus	Malabsorption syndrome (folic acid deficiency)
Liver	Fatty degeneration Acute hepatitis Laennec's cirrhosis	Laennec's cirrhosis
Metabolic	Hyperlipidemia Hyperuricemia (exacerbation of gout)	

(Reproduced with permission from Kissin B: Alcohol abuse and alcohol-related illness. In Wyngaarden JB, Smith LH Jr [eds]: Cecil Textbook of Medicine, 17th ed, p 55. Philadelphia, WB Saunders, 1985.)

the reason the drug is now listed as a Schedule I compound in the Controlled Substance Regulations.

COCAINE. Cocaine is now recognized as one of the most dangerous drugs of abuse, perhaps even more so than heroin.[6] The relative ease of acquisition, self-administration, and the short half-life lead to compulsive usage, and an increasing number of drug-related cardiovascular accidents have occurred, particularly in young male adults.

Known since precivilized times, cocaine is an alkaloid of Erythroxylon coca, made into an aqueous soluble hydrochloric acid salt for use as a local anesthetic. However, the free base is readily absorbed across mucous membranes, thus accounting for sniffing of preparations such as "rock" and inhalation of preparations such as "crack." The euphorogenic and toxic properties of cocaine apparently relate to the effect on the sympathetic nervous system, where presynaptic uptake of norepinephrine into sympathetic nerve endings is inhibited. Thus, an excess of catecholamines probably acts in the manner of some of the antidepressant, psychotherapeutic drugs or has an effect on dopaminergic transmission, which would also explain the vasoconstrictive effects on mucous membranes, the development of nasal fistula when inhaled, and the cardiovascular stimulative and arrhythmogenic effects. Euphorogenic and addictive properties may relate specifically to stimulation of dopaminergic neuronal complexes. In addition to the vasoconstriction, an acute rise in arterial blood pressure, tachycardia, ventricular arrhythmias, mydriasis, hyperglycemia, and hyperthermia are indicative of the catecholamine effect.

In cocaine intoxication, agitation, dysphoria, paranoia, hallucinations, and assaultive behavior may be present in addition to the cardiovascular manifestations. The long-term complications are similar to those seen in relation to systemic drug injection. Because of rapid hydrolysis in the circulation, the acute effects are short-lived, the treatment generally symptomatic, and the stimulatory effects diminished by use of the benzodiazepines.

MENSTRUAL AND OBSTETRIC HISTORY

For women in their childbearing years, the date of the last normal menstrual period should be learned to avoid the possibility of administering anesthesia during the first trimester of pregnancy. Information regarding possible adverse anesthetic effects on the fetus is not well documented; probably the stress of surgery is more of an influence. Insofar as spontaneous abortion is concerned, endocrine imbalance and a defective ovum may be the more responsible factors. Nevertheless, it is believed that nitrous oxide given to the mother might possibly be toxic to the fetus. Aside from these considerations, the degree of bleeding with menstruation may have resulted in chronic anemia, which must be considered in the context of the operation planned. The use of oral contraceptives predisposes to the development of thromboembolism.

The obstetric history, apart from the question of a current pregnancy, must be known, in that a patient may have had eclampsia followed by persistent hypertension, other problems such as placenta previa where bleeding occurred, requiring transfusions, or where disseminated intravascular coagulation (DIC) developed following amniotic fluid embolism. The kinds of anesthesia that were given for delivery and any problems that arose are essential factors in the selection of subsequent agents and techniques.

Having presented these general questions, it is apparent that in the average healthy patient, the answers to most, if not all, of these questions will be negative. Nonetheless, the details as given here are the thoughts that come to mind during history taking and planning the anesthetic.

SYSTEM REVIEW

In connection with each system reviewed, we shall list the questions to be asked. However, some of the major diseases are discussed in greater detail toward the end of this chapter.

The Circulatory System

Queries should focus on cardiac problems. Does the patient have heart disease, a murmur, palpitations, tightness in the chest, chest pain on exertion, high blood pressure? In connection with any of these symptoms or diseases, is medication required? Several of these problems such as the sick sinus syndrome, mitral valve prolapse, and idiopathic hypertrophic subaortic stenosis (IHSS) are discussed in the cardiovascular section of this chapter.

Respiratory System

As noted previously, we are concerned here with problems of cigarette smoking and obstructive airway disease, including asthma and emphysema. Chronic bronchitis is typified by long-standing productive cough. A history of tuberculosis or recent exposure, a past history of pneumonias, and recurrent lung infections are worthy of note.

Liver

Has the patient ever had jaundice, and was this related to gall stones or viral infection such as Type A or Type B hepatitis? If the latter is true, has infection persisted, and is the patient under therapy with corticosteroids? More serious ailments such as Laennec's or biliary cirrhosis will be readily evident during the history taking, as will the rarer diseases such as hemochromatosis.

Kidneys and Urinary Tract

Have there been problems with the kidneys or bladder, such as recurrent infection in the form of pyelonephritis, cystitis, calculi, symptoms of prostatism in the male, or incontinence in either sex. Polyuria might suggest the presence of diabetes mellitus—more rarely, diabetes insipidus. Any severe degree of renal failure will have been known to the patient and would be treated with dialysis. However, occasionally, a patient, particularly a male with long-standing, untreated prostatism or others with congenital malformations of the ureters, may be on the verge of renal failure. A uremic odor to the breath or unusual somnolence suggest this possibility. From an anesthetic standpoint, fluid and electrolyte disorders are the major concerns in renal failure.

Practically all patients in chronic renal failure are maintained on dialysis, usually hemodialysis performed in a renal failure facility or at home, a few others undergoing continuous, ambulatory peritoneal dialysis. These patients are kept in a reasonable state of fluid and electrolyte balance, particularly to avoid serious degrees of hyperkalemia, but the blood urea nitrogen (BUN) and creatinine remain abnormal. Anemia is usually present, with hematocrits remaining in the upper 20s or low 30s, because of the lack of erythropoietin, a hormone mainly synthesized in the normal kidney, which stimulates erythrocyte production in bone marrow. The anemia is accentuated by blood loss during hemodialysis and diminished survival of transfused red blood cells. Although repeated transfusions are necessary and probably lessen the immunogenic rejection of transplanted kidneys, chronic hepatitis B infection (and possibly AIDS) is common in dialysis units.

In choosing an anesthetic technique, one must remember that the patient with chronic renal failure is prone to infection, particularly if he or she is already being treated with immunosuppressive drugs. The anesthetic agents chosen should be those that do not depend upon elimination by the kidney for termination of their action. Thus, regional anesthesia is a good choice provided that large amounts of the amide-type local anesthetics are not given, as in continuous epidural anesthesia. Insofar as the general anesthetics are concerned, one might choose to avoid halothane because of difficulty in the differential diagnosis if hepatitis develops postoperatively, and not to use enflurane because its metabolic degradation results in production of fluoride ion, a known nephrogenic toxin. The longer-acting barbiturates (e.g., phenobarbital) and some of the neuromuscular blockers (e.g., tubocurarine and pancuronium in large doses, especially gallamine) are dependent upon the kidneys for elimination. Also, the effects of opioids may persist because of delayed renal excretion.

Central Nervous System

A history of seizures and their treatment with drugs is essential information for the anesthesiologist, and compliance with therapy must be ascertained, for example, by determination that plasma anticonvulsant levels are in the therapeutic range before induction of anesthesia. Other major diseases involving the brain and spinal cord will be apparent, including cerebrovascular occlusion with paralysis; transient ischemic attacks, or "little strokes"; unusual problems such as treated hydrocephalus or prior operation for brain tumor; and head trauma followed by loss of consciousness. Some patients will present with peripheral neuropathy—idiopathic or related to renal failure or diabetes. It is advantageous to know that the somatic component of the neuropathy is usually associated with autonomic neuropathy, so that one might expect to encounter inadequate neurocirculatory reflexes. As with the remainder of the findings in the history, each abnormality is significant from the standpoint of choice of anesthesia and management. Patients with paralysis or coma are particularly prone to develop hyperkalemia upon injection of succinylcholine (SCh).

The gamut of diseases encountered is extensive; multiple sclerosis, myasthenia gravis, parkinsonism, and Alzheimer's disease are not uncommon. One must not overlook the central nervous system (CNS) consequences of alcoholism, with metabolic encephalopathy and seizure tendencies.

Musculoskeletal System

The common problems in this category are rheumatoid arthritis and, to a lesser extent, osteoarthritis. Patients with severe rheumatoid disease will be taking a variety of analgesic drugs or drugs that affect the pathophysiology of the disease. Aspirin and the nonsteroidal anti-inflammatory drugs (NSAIDS) are commonly used, less frequently corticosteroids or methotrexate that affect the immunologic component, or gold injection in still others. In severe rheumatoid arthritis, there may be restrictive lung disease, spondylitis, pleural effusion, and myocarditis. Structural changes affecting the airway include cervical vertebral lordosis, inability to open the mouth because of temporomandibular ankylosis and laryngeal stenosis caused by cricoarytenoid joint involvement. Ankylosis and deformity of the joints lead to problems in intravenous therapy and positioning of the patient for operation, and difficult access in performing regional nerve blocks.

Endocrine System

DIABETES MELLITUS. The most common disease in this category is diabetes mellitus; more than 10 million people in the United States have the disease. The well-controlled diabetic patient does not pose major problems for anesthesia other than the need for perioperative management of glucose metabolism. Because of underlying pathophysiologic alterations, these mainly involve the cardiovascular system. The goal of therapy is to avoid the wide swings in metabolic control—hypoglycemia on the one hand, and ketoacidosis on the other hand. Along with a detailed description of glucose metabolism, the commonly prescribed perioperative diabetic regimens are presented later in this chapter and in Chapter 44.

ADRENAL CORTICAL DISEASES. Diseases involving the adrenal cortex involve either a hyperproduction or deficiency of a variety of corticosteroids, either on the basis of cortical abnormalities *per se* or alteration in the hypothalamic-pituitary-adrenal cortical axis.

Diseases of hypersecretion include Cushing's disease, with an overproduction of glucocorticoids (cortisol), or primary hyperaldosteronism, with excess secretion of the mineralocorticoid, aldosterone. Secretion of cortisol is controlled by a negative feedback system involving the hypothalamus (corticotropin-releasing factor), anterior pituitary gland (ACTH or corticotropin), and the adrenal cortex. Consequently, diagnostic tests are directed toward elements of this system. Cushing's syndrome and the effects of cortisol (plus androgens in the female) are marked by hypertension, diabetes, osteoporosis, hypokalemic alkalosis, muscle weakness, psychological problems and, in women, hirsutism and menstrual irregularities. A characteristic facies develops (bloated, plethoric appearance), with a "buffalo" distribution of body fat with abdominal and gluteal striae.

Hyperaldosteronism is also a cause of hypertension, but the major alterations involve salt and water retention and potassium loss. Although aldosterone secretion is partly under the influence of the anterior pituitary, the renin-angiotensin system has a more direct action on the cortex and secretion of the mineralocorticoid, aldosterone.

Adrenocortical insufficiency may be primary or idiopathic (Addison's disease, at one time caused by tuberculosis) or secondary to imbalance of the hypothalamic-pituitary-cortical axis (where aldosterone secretion may not be affected). The addisonian patient will show hyperpigmentation of skin and mucous membranes, hypotension, weight loss, hyperkalemia, muscle weakness, and salt-craving.

The preoperative assessment of any of these syndromes is complex, involving assays of the various hormones concerned, electrolyte determinations in plasma and urine, and both provocative and suppressive tests. (See Chapter 44.) Obviously, the Addisonian patient must have perioperative replacement therapy, with both glucocorticoids and mineralocorticoids. In the hypersecretory syndromes, replacement therapy is begun, coincident with adrenalectomy. Preoperatively, an effort is made to return fluid and electrolyte balance toward normal, in both hypo- and hyperadrenocorticism.

THYROID DISORDERS. A second, common endocrine disease pertains to the thyroid, whether hypo- or hyperactive, and a consideration of the drugs involved in therapy is warranted. Hypothyroidism is marked by an unusual susceptibility to effects of depressant drugs, a tendency to develop hypothermia, alveolar hypoventilation, hyponatremia, and hypoglycemia. As a rule, operation should not be undertaken unless the patient is in a euthyroid state. Oral thyroxine is the drug usually used, and it should be resumed postoperatively.

Hyperthyroidism rarely requires thyroidectomy today because of effective thyroinhibitory drugs. Nevertheless, for any type of operation, one must anticipate the possible development of thyroid storm, which is an acute, hypermetabolic state precipitated by a variety of stresses and managed with beta-adrenergic blocking drugs and agents that antagonize thyroid hormone already present in the circulation, such as propylthiouracil and sodium iodide. Glucocorticoids are also recommended because of the possibility of co-existing adrenal insufficiency; morphine is given for sedation; external body cooling is recommended to combat hyperthermia; and adequate fluid and electrolyte replacement is suggested.

In the patient with Graves' disease and exophthalmos, the eyes must be protected against damage during anesthesia. Further, the vocal cords should be examined pre- and postoperatively for signs of recurrent laryngeal nerve injury or paralysis.

PHEOCHROMOCYTOMA. Although pheochromocytoma is an endocrine disease, we shall discuss it under the heading of hypertension.

A final category of endocrine illness concerns the parathyroids and calcium regulation with resultant states of hyper- and hypocalcemia. (See Chapter 44.)

Hematologic Problems

The primary concern is with hemostasis and elements in the clotting process that are abnormal. Testing might reveal qualitative problems with blood platelets; thrombocytopenia; effects of the anticoagulants, heparin and dicoumarin derivatives; hemostatic deficiency resulting from hepatic failure; and, occasionally, von Willebrand's disease. Hemoglobinopathies such as sickle cell trait and disease and thalassemias have important implications for the preoperative period. Then there are the unusual syndromes, the hereditary porphyrias, the so-called myeloproliferative disorders that result in polycythemia or the leukemias, all associated with increased risk during the operative period.

Finally, the most common problem of all relates to the anemias, which require preoperative evaluation; perhaps replacement therapy prior to, during, and following operation, with attendant risks of blood transfusion or the more commonly used blood components. The most simple anemia is of the chronic blood loss variety as might occur with menometrorrhagia in women. Many patients with this disorder receive oral iron therapy. Another common cause of anemia is occult blood loss from the bowel, as might occur with high doses of aspirin or NSAIDS used to treat the arthritides. The discovery of significant anemia preoperatively in middle-aged men might suggest the presence of colon carcinoma, and, if the operation currently planned is elective (e.g., herniorrhaphy), the necessary colectomy might take precedence.

Considerable judgment is necessary in approaching the problem of anemia preoperatively. On the one hand, the oxygen-carrying capacity of blood should be improved in a patient with coronary artery disease, prior infarction, or angina. Conversely, for a young woman with anemia resulting from menorrhagia who is about to undergo a diagnostic dilatation and curettage (D&C) of the uterus, it makes little sense to submit that patient to the risk of transfusion therapy. If she were subsequently to require a hysterectomy, transfusion might be necessary.

The patient with renal failure has a severe degree of anemia because of deficient production of erythropoietin, which is formed in the normal kidney. Although transfusion of erythrocytes improves the oxygen-carrying capacity and in renal transplantation helps to minimize the rejection process, the transfused erythrocytes have a short survival time.

It is most important, however, to realize that in chronic anemia, there may be an expanded plasma volume brought about by those neurohumoral regulatory processes that maintain the plasma volume constant. In the acute phase of hypovolemia, as occurs in hemorrhage, massive burns, or gastrointestinal fluid losses, the sympathetic nervous system, by release of catecholamines, causes contraction of the vascular space, and antidiuretic hormone release results in oliguria. Subsequently, in hemorrhage, erythrocyte production in bone marrow replenishes red blood cell volume, while antidiuresis persists and aldosterone secretion is augmented by the renin-angiotensin pathway. This results in salt and water retention so that plasma and extracellular volume are restored, assisted by synthesis and release of protein from the liver. All these phenomena can be recognized by clinical observation and laboratory tests. Anemia, *per se*, therefore does not equate with hypovolemia, and the mistake should not be made of overzealous fluid replacement. The result might be development of pulmonary edema, often seen under these circumstances.

Dental and Oral Problems

From the anesthetic standpoint, the following derangements are considered important: 1) the presence of caries and periodontal disease with precariously loosened teeth and infection, the latter raising the possibility of bacteremia during oral manipulation, airway placement or tracheal intubation, and development of bacterial endocarditis in patients with valvular heart disease or valve prostheses; 2) the presence of dental appliances, which must either be removed or protected during the course of anesthesia; 3) the edentulous patient who poses problems with facial mask fit during induction of general anesthesia or risks injury to the gingiva and bony ridges during tracheal intubation so that dentures might not fit well later on; 4) temporomandibular joint syndrome accompanied by chronic pain or repeated dislocation of the jaw; and 5) salivary gland disease.

Gastrointestinal System

Major derangements of the gastrointestinal system are usually the reason for the proposed operation. Routinely, one is concerned with the following: gastrointestinal bleeding, overt or occult, with the prospect of anemia or pulmonary aspiration; peptic ulcer disease with hyperacidity, the threat of aspiration, and exacerbation of ulcer as a result of the stress of anesthesia and operation; and diaphragmatic hernia or gastric reflux, again with attendant problems of aspiration.

Many patients requiring gastrointestinal operations will have been started on nasogastric (NG) tube drainage, particularly if some form of obstruction is present. The purpose is to prevent gastric dilation owing to secretions and swallowing of air, but also to take care of gastroduodenal reflux. However, one should not depend upon a NG tube to ensure an empty stomach, since reflux may occur during the process of tracheal intubation when a neuromuscular blocker is used or during intubation with topical anesthesia. Therefore, the NG tube should remain on suction before, during, and after anesthesia. In the absence of obstruction, it is often better to insert the NG tube after induction of anesthesia and tracheal intubation, thereby avoiding problems with poor anesthesia mask fit. Retention of a NG tube postoperatively beyond 1 or 2 days usually causes sore throat and difficulty in coughing. Therefore, in the patient at risk for pulmonary complications, particularly the elderly, a surgeon may choose to establish temporary gastrostomy drainage to avoid intestinal distention and the threat to intestinal anastomotic suture lines.

Generally, anesthesiologists are on the alert to treat hyperacidity, whether in the obese patient or in the patient with a full stomach, where tracheal intubation is required, before induction of general anesthesia. In order to raise gastric pH and reduce the volume of gastric secretions, H_2 histamine-receptor antagonists may be given by mouth the night before operation or iv about 30 minutes before induction. There is controversy, however, concerning the effectiveness of either cimetidine (Tagamet) or ranitidine (Zantac) in these respects; both drugs have undesirable side-effects. Therefore, anesthesiologists might prefer to give a nonparticulate liquid antacid by mouth 30 minutes before induction of anesthesia. Sodium citrate solution (Bicitra), 30 ml, is the agent commonly used. In order to promote gastric emptying time and to prevent gastric reflux, metoclopramide (Reglan) may also be given, but here, too, the effectiveness is questionable in the context of the anesthetized patient.

PHYSICAL EXAMINATION

In general, those elements of the physical examination should be performed that relate to the possibility of occurrence of anesthetic complications. Auscultation of the heart and lungs should be performed in all patients, and blood pressure should be taken in both arms, or the legs when indicated. Peripheral pulses are palpated for their quality, particularly if arterial cannulation is to be done for monitoring of blood pressure. Similarly, the veins should be examined for ease of access in fluid administration, monitoring, or use of iv regional anesthesia. For regional anesthesia, the sites of needle insertion should be inspected for feasibility of success, and, if spinal, lumbar epidural, or caudal anesthesia is chosen, the bony landmarks should be identified and palpated and the skin condition checked. Body position of the patient as required for operation may be tried to determine whether the patient can tolerate the same position intraoperatively or whether physiologic embarrassment occurs. The lithotomy position may be intolerable for a patient with arthritis of the hips; the lateral decubitus position with the operating table "broken" or the prone position may prove harmful for obese patients or those with circulatory or respiratory insufficiency.

The best position for administration of spinal, epidural, or brachial blockade can also be ascertained beforehand. In these instances, a brief neurologic examination is recorded. Sensory and motor reflexes are evaluated to confirm that there is no antecedent neurologic disease that might be interpreted as an anesthetic complication postoperatively.

The operative site might also be examined if this does not involve invasion of a patient's privacy. Examination of an inguinal or ventral hernia or the site and dimensions of a superficial tumor enable one to determine the needs for anesthesia and to select the most satisfactory position of the patient both for surgery and anesthesia. There is no objection, indeed benefit may result, if the anesthesiologist confirms the surgical diagnosis. We have witnessed a misdiagnosis of cholecystitis when lower lobe pneumonia was responsible for the presenting physical signs, which included right upper quadrant abdominal pain, tenderness, and splinting of the muscles.

During the history and physical examination, the astute clinician uses all his or her senses, vision, hearing, smell, and touch, to help in the diagnosis of disease (Table 15-4). Obesity is always obvious, and from the standpoint of anesthesia management, it is not so much the weight but how it is distributed. Tissue wasting will also be apparent. The odor of the breath may suggest the presence of uremia, ketoacidosis, or recent alcohol consumption. One should be able to tell at a glance if a patient has Cushingoid, acromegalic, hyper- or hypothyroid features or the stigmata of other diseases, either congenital or acquired, such as parkinsonism or adrenal insufficiency (skin and mucous membrane pigmentation, asthenia).

In the arthritic patient, a high-pitched voice suggests the possibility of laryngeal stenosis; a hoarse voice is indicative of tobacco smoking, alcoholism, and, rarely, a laryngeal carcinoma. A halting speech suggests pulmonary insufficiency; intermittent productive cough suggests underlying bronchitis. The color of the skin tells much, although in the heavily pigmented person, it is difficult to detect cyanosis as a sign of hypoxemia. Cyanosis and clubbing of the digits (pulmonary osteoarthropathy) may be evident in congenital heart disease, advanced lung disease, and heart failure. Jaundice and telangiectasia accompany advanced degrees of liver failure. Plethora of the face, suffusion of the nose, and dilated cyanotic veins, plus tremor of the extremities, are strongly suggestive of chronic alcoholism. The eyes tell a great deal: exophthalmos, arcus senilis, scleral jaundice, pupillary size and reactivity or strabismus, the latter recalling the possibility of development of MH.

MOUTH AND AIRWAY

Examination of the mouth and airway is one of the more important aspects of the physical examination. Can the neck be flexed and the head extended to attain the "sniffing" position best suited for tracheal intubation? How much can the mouth be opened? Are there temporomandibular joint symptoms, pain, clicking, crepitus, or chronic dislocation? On opening the mouth, is the tongue found to be excessively

TABLE 15-4. Clues to Disease

Nutrition: Distribution of body fat tissue, wasting
Skin: Cyanosis, plethora, pigmentation, telangiectasia
Voice: Arthritis, tobacco smoking, alcoholism, laryngeal carcinoma
Speech: Pulmonary insufficiency, cerebrovascular accident
Cough: Chronic bronchitis, COPD
Breath: Uremia, ketoacidosis, alcoholism
Endocrine stigmata: Cushing's syndrome, acromegaly, hyper- and hypothyroidism, pituitary insufficiency, Addison's disease, Parkinson's disease
Eyes: Exophthalmos, Horner's syndrome, arcus senilis, jaundice, strabismus
Extremities: Pulmonary osteoarthropathy, nicotine stains, arthritis, nail-biting, intravenous (iv) drug use, tremor, edema
Posture and gait: Lordosis, kyphosis, scoliosis, arthritis, parkinsonism, poliomyelitis
Congenital syndromes

large? Is it coated or pink in color? How far can it be obtruded? Does it deviate to the side? Can the faucal pillars and uvula be seen on examination of the pharynx? These anatomic features determine whether tracheal intubation will be easy or difficult. Is there a postnasal discharge? Is there pharyngeal or tonsillar inflammation? Finally, the teeth are examined for loss of structure, periodontal disease, evidence of caries, and the presence of loose teeth, or fixed or removable prostheses. If there are any abnormalities in the dentition, they should be documented in the medical chart. The patient should be advised of the potential risks regarding subsequent dental damage. The teeth must be protected against damage and dentures removed before anesthesia unless their retention will offer a better mask fit for induction of general anesthesia.

LABORATORY TESTS

The routine tests to be performed and their putative value are subjects discussed and debated in every textbook of medicine.[7] For several decades after the transformation of medicine into a scientific discipline in the 1950s, routine tests included a hematocrit or hemoglobin, a white blood cell count and differential cell count, urinalysis, examination of the stool for occult blood, a chest x-ray, and the electrocardiogram (ECG) in the adult. These tests were meant to discover clues to disease not apparent on history taking and physical examination.

Of late, however, as a result of elucidation of complex disease processes, the practice has been to order a conglomeration of about 12 to 18 chemical and enzymatic analyses of blood and urine, accomplished by means of automated analyzers (e.g., the SMA 12), which reduce the cost below that of the individually, manually performed analyses. Initially, with the use of automated analysis, twice as many abnormalities were discovered (many in relation to plasma glucose and uric acid). However, the additional yield was neither impressive nor clinically significant. Many clinicians are now beginning to focus on fewer tests of the traditional variety, which, in addition to the stool guaiac and blood pressure measurement, offer the major protection in health maintenance examinations. Furthermore, the discovery of test results outside of the normal statistical range added to the cost of the hospital stay when the tests had to be repeated. Hidden in the supposed range of normality are such intangibles as the specificity, sensitivity, and repeatability of the tests performed and compounding factors such as diet, drug therapy, and gender of the individual.

Because the requirements for good anesthetic practice are not that demanding in relation to laboratory testing and for the reasons just cited, we do not intend to supply a table of normal laboratory values (these are extensive and can be found in any comprehensive textbook of medicine). Rather, we shall point out the vagaries and the cost–benefit ratios of some laboratory tests. We repeat: for the unusual test to be performed, there must be a sound clinical reason, and the interpretation of such tests should be carried out diligently by the clinician.

CHEST X-RAY

Both the philosophy and data relating to routine hospital admission chest x-ray examinations have been placed in context by Hubbell et al.[8] In 1983, the National Center for Devices and Radiological Health reported that for the year 1980, 52 million chest x-rays were taken in U.S. hospitals, thus, the most frequently performed radiologic procedure in this country. A previous study had shown that about 30 million such films had routinely been ordered on hospital admission (i.e., about 60% of the total). At an average cost of $50.00 per x-ray, about 1.5 billion dollars were spent annually for routine screening purposes. This practice had arisen when pulmonary tuberculosis was prevalent and because twice as many cases were discovered on hospital admission than were found on mass screening of the population. When the incidence of tuberculosis declined, the emphasis shifted to early discovery of lung cancer. However, at that time, comprehensive studies showed that no significant difference in mortality rate existed between patients in whom lung cancer was detected by chest x-ray and those in whom the disease was otherwise initially suspected. Thus, the American Cancer Society does not recommend the chest x-ray as a routine screening method. Furthermore, since the most common findings on routine examination include cardiomegaly, pulmonary interstitial changes, and chronic obstructive lung disease, many physicians now believe that routine examination is not necessary in patients younger than 20 years of age, in otherwise healthy patients preoperatively, in pregnant patients, and patients admitted to psychiatric facilities.

Hubbell et al[8] conducted a prospective study on the relevance of routine chest x-rays for patients admitted to the internal medicine wards of a Veterans Administration Hospital, where the population is known to have a high prevalence of cardiopulmonary disease. Of 491 patients studied, 294 (60%) had routine chest x-rays taken, and, of these, abnormalities were present in 106 (26%). Nevertheless, the findings were new in only 20 patients; the others represented known chronic cardiopulmonary disease. Of the 20 patients with new findings, treatment was altered in only 12 (4%), and in only one patient would appropriate treatment have been withheld because of the absence of x-ray.

According to the surveys, routine hospital admission chest x-rays are rarely cost-effective, and the radiologic examination is best directed toward the higher risk groups, where the patient's history and physical examination suggest the possibility of treatable chest disease.

ELECTROCARDIOGRAM

There is little question whether there is a need to record a baseline ECG before anesthesia in patients older than 40 years of age or whether the tracing is essential for the safe conduct of anesthesia. This recommendation is modified if an ECG has already been recorded within a reasonable period of time and if there is little clinical reason to expect change. The 12-lead ECG is of better diagnostic value than the limited number of leads used during anesthetic monitoring. Aside from these generalities, an ECG is essential if a patient has known heart disease, particularly of the ischemic type; heart block in any of its various forms; unusual entities such as Wolff-Parkinson-White syndrome, sick sinus syndrome, or symptomatic, prolapsed mitral valve; heart disease under treatment with drugs (for heart failure, arrhythmias, either atrial or ventricular, and hypertension); or major alterations in electrolytes, potassium, calcium, and magnesium. The ECG is then available for comparison with any change encountered during anesthesia. A compromise with this rule might be acceptable if the anesthesiologist is certain to carefully analyze the tracing on a monitor and to make a recording of it before induction of anesthesia.

On routine preoperative ECG screening, the findings should justify the expense and have a perceptible effect on reduction in morbidity and mortality. Few data are available to answer these questions—the best of them relating to patients with ischemic heart disease, as discussed subsequently. To reiterate, in a normal population, the reasons to request an ECG should be based on the results of the history and physical examination. Some physicians believe that the ECG should be recorded in all persons older than 40 years and that it should be repeated at 2-year intervals because of changes that may occur as people age, a recommendation based on the findings of Rabkin and Horne for the periodic health examination.[9]

Often, just before operation or on the evening prior to operation, an anesthesiologist may decide that an essential laboratory datum is missing and must be obtained, or that a consultation is necessary before proceeding with anesthesia. Acting with the best intentions and perhaps with medicolegal considerations in mind, this course of action may be warranted. However, considerable judgment must be brought to bear upon this decision before the operation is delayed or cancelled with the consequent disappointment, annoyance, and inconvenience for the patient, family, and surgeon. An extreme example of this kind of contretemps has been described by Mold and Stein as the "cascade effect in the clinical care of patients."[10]

A 59-year-old man was scheduled for elective inguinal herniorrhaphy. In addition to mild, chronic obstructive pulmonary disease and reflux esophagitis he gave a history of coronary artery disease with mild, stable angina. Coronary arteriography nine years before showed mild to moderate disease and the physician taking care of him now found the condition to be stable. Nevertheless, a cardiologist–consultant recommended that an exercise test be performed. After a delay of six hours, the patient became anxious and angry, with vague chest discomfort. The exercise test was cancelled and the patient was transferred to the telemetry unit where he became further agitated and nonspecific ECG changes developed. This resulted in transfer to the coronary care unit where treatment with nitroglycerine and a calcium channel blocker was instituted. However, repeat coronary arteriography at this time revealed that there was, in fact, improvement over the condition nine years ago. By this time, it was not possible to reschedule the herniorrhaphy until two weeks later. It remained for the family physician to try to reassure the patient that nothing of a serious nature had occurred.

Perhaps this course of action was justified, but the consultant possibly could not accept the small risk inherent in a situation in which the patient's condition had been stable. Perhaps this is an extreme example of the "cascade" effect, but one should not subject every patient of this type to such aggressive testing.

CHOOSING THE ANESTHETIC

OBTAINING A PATIENT'S CONSENT

Choice of anesthesia is a tripartite decision involving the anesthesiologist, surgeon, and patient and is based on the patient's physiologic status and the operation planned. With the varieties of anesthetics and techniques available today, it is difficult to conceive of only one choice of anesthetic for any procedure. One course might seem better than another, but rarely are the supporting data at hand to prove the point. For example, in anesthesia for uncomplicated coronary artery bypass surgery, mortality figures are so low that different groups of anesthesiologists can claim equal success with several kinds of anesthetic regimens, mainly because the preparation of patients, surgical techniques, and perioperative care have been perfected and standardized. One study has shown that transurethral resection of the prostate gland has an equally good outcome whether spinal or general anesthesia is given, and the same can be said for inguinal herniorrhaphy. Further, anesthesiologists perform best when they use methods with which they are most experienced, rather than choose a theoretically better regimen, particularly in cases in which there is a seriously ill patient.

In order to choose the appropriate method, anesthesiologists must thoroughly understand the nature of the operation proposed and how the surgeon might perform under different anesthetic situations. Surgeons deserve the best possible anesthetic conditions in order to perform the operation as easily and as expeditiously as possible without jeopardizing the patient. Furthermore, patients will have their own opinions about choice of anesthesia, even after having been explicitly informed as to what might be best for them. Rarely should there be argument, coercion, or resentment engendered over the choice of anesthesia. In the unusual situation in which it is apparent that the patient's preference is hardly the safest or most appropriate, the surgeon or referring physician might be asked to adjudicate the matter. What constitutes a truly informed consent on the part of the patient is a matter of conjecture, a subject more fully explored in Chapter 2. Nevertheless, the anesthesiologist should answer all questions posed by a patient without evasion and also volunteer information of importance. For example, when spinal anesthesia is suggested, the patient might be told that there is the possibility of development of post-lumbar puncture headache, but should also be informed that if such a headache occurs, there is a proven treatment with application of an epidural blood patch. The patient should also be told that residual paralysis is a distinctly rare event with the techniques used today. If the patient has a fear of being too much aware of what is happening during operation, he or she should be informed that sedation will be given according to need.

In the chapters devoted to the specialties, as in cardiothoracic anesthesia, neuroanesthesia, and obstetrics, choice of anesthesia will be more fully elucidated.

Once the history, physical examination, and interpretation of laboratory tests have been accomplished and a seemingly happy patient–physician relation has been established, a consultation note must be written, and the preanesthetic medication ordered. We have observed that many anesthesiologists will merely have filled in the blanks on an anesthesia check sheet, or the reverse of the anesthesia record. Rarely, unless a major complication occurs, are these notes read by other members of the professional staff of a hospital. Thus, we believe that a note should appear somewhere in the progress notes of the patient's record and be signed by the anesthesiologist so that all personnel involved will recognize this as a consultant's opinion and be informed thereby. This note should summarize the findings and indicate choice of anesthesia as mutually agreed upon by the patient and anesthesiologist. In the United States, the Joint Committee on Accreditation of Hospitals (JCAH) recommends that such a note be written.

THE CONCEPT OF PHYSICAL STATUS *VERSUS* RISK

Wilson and Crouch[11] have defined risk assessment "as a way of examining risks so that they be better avoided, reduced or otherwise managed. Risk implies uncertainty so that risk is largely concerned with uncertainty and hence with a concept of probability that is hard to grasp."

Every kind of human endeavor involves a risk of misadventure, whether it be mental or physical; certainly this pertains to anesthesia, with all the potential for harm. In the epidemiologic context, risk is usually evaluated in terms of the host (the patient), the agent (the anesthetic and the anesthesiologist), and the environment (hospital and operating room). Automobile and air traffic accidents can be analyzed according to this schema, but the term *risk* is not quite appropriate for an impending anesthetic and operation because of the large number of variables at play—human and otherwise. It is true that data are available to define mortality, not only according to a patient's disease and surgical procedure, but the percentage figures so derived from large population studies are not necessarily current or applicable to the individual.

A better way to categorize the patient–candidate for anesthesia is to use an estimate of the physical status, that is, the state of well-being in a pathophysiologic sense. This approach was first used by the New York Heart Association to prognosticate on the outcome of heart disease. There were four categories ranging from no disability to severe disability, so that some idea of risk or mortality might be gained. These designations were then applied to patients undergoing anesthesia, however, on the broader scale of physical status, in the American Society of Anesthesiologists' classification initially published in the 1940s. Thus, as may be seen in Table 15-5 in a revised classification of physical status,[12] a patient in physical status 1 would have no complicating ailment (nor would the surgical disease add to the disability). However, a patient in physical status 4 would have severely limiting disease so that the mortality might be expected to be high—all other factors considered. Further, the physical status 5 category implies that a patient is moribund—where operation is performed on the off-chance that a life might be saved. Finally, a patient who requires an anesthetic for an emergency operation, regardless of the category he or she is in, is deemed to be in a less satisfactory physical condition and is designated by the letter E.

A more detailed description of the physical status categories, as offered by Dripps *et al*[13] follows:

Class 1: The patient has no organic, physiologic, biochemical, or psychiatric disturbance. The pathologic process for which operation is to be performed is localized and does not entail a systemic disturbance.

Examples: A fit patient with inguinal hernia; fibroid uterus in an otherwise healthy woman.

Class 2: Mild to moderate systemic disturbance caused either by the condition to be treated surgically or by other pathophysiologic processes.

Examples: Nonorganic or only slightly limiting organic heart disease, mild diabetes, essential hypertension, or anemia. Some might choose to list the extremes of age here, either the neonate or the octogenarian, even though no discernible systemic disease is present. Extreme obesity and chronic bronchitis may be included in this category.

Class 3: Severe, systemic disturbance or disease from whatever cause, even though it may not be possible to define the degree of disability with finality.

Examples: Severely limiting organic heart disease; severe diabetes with vascular complications; moderate to severe degrees of pulmonary insufficiency; angina pectoris or healed myocardial infarction.

Class 4: Severe systemic disorders that are already life threatening, not always correctable by operation.

Examples: Patients with organic heart disease showing marked signs of cardiac insufficiency, persistent anginal syndrome, or active myocarditis; advanced degrees of pulmonary, hepatic, renal, or endocrine insufficiency.

Class 5: The moribund patient who has little chance of survival but is submitted to operation in desperation.

Examples: The burst, abdominal aneurysm with profound shock; major cerebral trauma with rapidly increasing intracranial pressure; massive pulmonary embolus. Most of these patients require operation as a resuscitative measure with little if any anesthesia.

Emergency Operation (E): Any patient in one of the classes listed previously who is operated on as an emergency is considered to be in poorer physical condition. The letter E is placed beside the numerical classification. Thus, the patient with a hitherto uncomplicated hernia now incarcerated and associated with nausea and vomiting is classified as 1E. By definition, status 5 would always constitute an emergency.

A physical status category should be assigned to every patient before anesthesia is administered. Often, whether it be a conscious or subconscious act on the part of the anesthesiologist, a poorer physical status is assigned to a patient only after a complication or a death has occurred. However, the use of this system permits one anesthesiologist to compare anesthetic outcomes with those of other anesthesiologists on the same basis—the physical status. All studies relating to anesthetic morbidity and mortality have shown a close correlation with the physical status designation (Table 15-6). On the whole, there is fairly close agreement among anesthesiologists concerning the physical status category assigned, but there are, nevertheless, differences in interpretation and misconceptions about the meaning of the classification.

PREANESTHETIC ORDERS

A patient should have been told what to expect in the way of preparation and will have been warned against eating and drinking at least during the 8-hour period preceding anesthesia. The reasons for the latter dictum should be made explicit, in that the stomach will be empty and the risk of aspiration of gastric contents is minimized. Whether the patient will require a sedative for sleep is a mutually determined decision.

TABLE 15-5.   Classification of Physical Status

1. A normal healthy patient.
2. A patient with mild systemic disease.
3. A patient with a severe systemic disease that limits activity but is not incapacitating.
4. A patient with an incapacitating systemic disease that is a constant threat to life.
5. A moribund patient not expected to survive 24 hours with or without operation.

In the event of emergency operation, precede the number with an E.

TABLE 15-6. Anesthesia Mortality (Primary and Contributory) and Physical Status

AUTHORS	TOTAL ANESTHETIC DEATHS	PERCENTAGE OF ALL ANESTHETIC DEATHS BY PHYSICAL STATUS CLASS					INCIDENCE BY PHYSICAL STATUS CLASS				
		1	2	3	4	5	1	2	3	4	5
Beecher and Todd	384	56			44		1:2,426			1:599	
Edwards et al*	586	17	21	46		16					
Dripps et al	80	0	15	34	41	10	0	1:1,013	1:151	1:22	1:11
Boba and Landmesser*	44 (cardiac arrests)		32		68						
Clifton and Hotten*	52		33		67						
Memery*	64	5	19	44	23	9					

(Reprinted with permission from Goldstein A Jr, Keats AS: The risk of anesthesia. Anesthesiology 33:130, 1970.)
*Breakdown of total population at risk not available.

At one time, the barbiturates were used for this purpose; now they are used less frequently because of their many disadvantages, including allergy, cross-tolerance with other hydrocarbon compounds, possibilities for abuse leading to suicide, and "hangover" effects. Today, one of the benzodiazepines might be given to induce sleep, other choices being hydroxyzine (Vistaril) or chloral hydrate, which is particularly useful in the elderly.

Other preanesthetic drugs that are prescribed are essentially part of the anesthetic plan. Further details on premedication are considered in subsequent chapters concerned with the specialties of anesthesia. One of the benzodiazepines might be given for sedation and relief of anxiety. If a patient is in pain and already requiring an opioid for relief and, where use of regional anesthesia might not otherwise be well accepted, an opioid is a good choice beforehand, bearing in mind the disadvantages of that category of drugs. If the general anesthetic plan calls largely for iv agents, the opioids are an essential component. These drugs can also be given iv in incremental doses as the need arises. Finally, the need for a vagolytic drug must be considered. At one time, atropine or scopolamine was given routinely to diminish excessive salivary and respiratory tract secretions resulting from the irritant, inhalation agents then available. The general anesthetics used today are far less irritating to the respiratory tract than diethyl ether, while the vagolytic drugs usually leave a patient with an uncomfortably dry mouth before operation. Currently, the vagolytic drugs are used selectively; for example, atropine is given to the child who is to undergo operation for strabismus or who is to receive an iv injection of SCh—in both circumstances where vagal response in the way of bradycardia is prominent; atropine is given in the presence of partial or complete heart block in order to avoid progression to complete blockade and ventricular standstill. Scopolamine offers the valuable attributes not only of being a better "drying" agent, dose for dose, compared with atropine, but also of producing bradycardia rather than tachycardia and a state of amnesia useful in avoiding the problem of awareness during general anesthesia. The commonly induced scopolamine disorientation can be reversed with injection of physostigmine (Antilirium). Under special circumstances, the vagolytic drug is given iv as the need arises.

Orders for preanesthetic medication should always be written for a given time, so that the patient will benefit according to the bioavailability of the drugs and the purposes for which they are intended.

Examples of Preanesthetic Notes

Physical Status #1

This 29-year-old white man and office worker with a long-standing right inguinal hernia is scheduled for herniorrhaphy at 8 A.M. tomorrow. The history and physical examination are entirely normal. He takes no medicines or drugs and has no allergies. He has not had an anesthetic or operation before this time, nor has he had a blood transfusion. He does not smoke tobacco and consumes alcohol purely on a social basis. There are no familial anesthetic problems.

On physical examination, he has a good airway and the lungs and heart are normal to percussion and auscultation. Blood pressure is 120/80, the pulse is 76 while supine. He has an easily reducible inguinal hernia on the right side. The hematocrit is 46, and urinalysis is negative.

He accepts the idea of spinal anesthesia after discussion, which included the possibility of development of post-lumbar puncture headache and the unlikely event of residual paralysis, but he would like to have sedation during the procedure. He also understands that general anesthesia may be required if adequate pain relief is not obtained with the spinal anesthetic. His back is normal and so is the neurologic examination. Plan for spinal anesthesia, with sedation. Weight 160 lb., height 5 ft. 10 in. Physical Status 1.

Signed _____

Physical Status 2E

Under different circumstances, the very same patient might enter the hospital, now with an irreducible, incarcerated painful hernia. He last drank a full glass of water about 3 hours ago; he is apprehensive but has not vomited. The blood pressure is now 160/80, the pulse rate is 96, and the hematocrit is 46. The urine is quite concentrated. Physical status might now be listed as 2E, because of the possibility of a full stomach, the apprehension, some degree of dehydration, and the emergency nature of the operation, which must be done as soon as possible. Probably this patient would be less willing to accept spinal anesthesia because of his apprehension. Many anesthesiologists might prefer primarily to give general, endotracheal anesthesia to protect the lungs against aspiration.

Physical Status 3E

This 69-year old black man with a history of myocardial infarction many years ago had onset of nausea, vomiting, and colicky abdominal pain 24 hours before entry. He had an uneventful spinal anesthetic for appendectomy at age 40 years, and the family history is noncontributory. There was no allergy and no recollection of blood transfusion. Alcohol consumption is confined to beer on weekends, but he has smoked two to three packs of cigarettes daily since youth. Exercise tolerance is fair, but he has occasional cough that is productive of yellow sputum. He takes one tablet daily of digitalis by mouth and recently started taking hydrochlorothiazide for mild elevation of blood pressure. There is some difficulty with the urinary stream. He has worked as a construction supervisor for many years.

On physical examination, he seems to be slightly obtunded—body weight is 160 lb, height 5 ft. 6 in., body temperature 100.2°F, blood pressure 160/100 in both arms. A NG tube is in place, draining feculent material, while an infusion of 5% dextrose in Ringer's lactated solution is running into an arm vein. A urinary bladder catheter drains dark colored urine. His teeth are in fair condition. He opens his mouth widely, and the neck is supple. The heart is not enlarged to percussion, but the sounds are distant, as are the lung sounds where a few coarse rales can be heard at the bases. The abdomen is typical for intestinal obstruction, with occasional high-pitched peristalsis.

Laboratory data: Hematocrit, 48, WBC, 10,000 with normal differential; urine specific gravity, 1.030; serum sodium, 146; chloride, 104; potassium, 3.2; creatinine, 2.0. ECG: LVH pattern, nonspecific T wave changes, possibly old myocardial infarction (MI). Chest x-ray: LV hypertrophy with increased lung markings and hyperluminescence. Abdomen: dilated small intestinal loops with fluid levels.

Plan: General, endotracheal anesthesia with rapid intubation and full monitoring as for any patient with an old MI and this combination of circumstances. Patient seems to understand and accepts this plan. Physical Status 3E.

Signed _____

IMMEDIATE PREPARATIONS FOR ANESTHESIA

Under the best of circumstances, the anesthesiologist who interviewed the patient and performed the physical examination and then wrote the preanesthetic orders should give the anesthetic or supervise a resident physician or nurse anesthetist in the procedure. Planning entails a reasonable understanding of the operation contemplated. For specialized anesthetic techniques or the management of unusual complications, detailed protocols may be followed: for example, deliberate hypotension for intracranial aneurysm. One may have to deal with such possible complications as malignant hyperthermia, anaphylactic shock, and cardiac arrest.

In some anesthesia departments where the nature of the operating schedule permits, briefing sessions can be held beforehand to determine the best plan for anesthetic management. The theme of this chapter has been that anesthesia can be given safely only if preparations have been thorough. An analogy might be made of the routine checks and human evaluations that must be made before an airplane flight so that a catastrophe should not occur. In anesthesia, where the human element is much more obvious and the apparatus used is less reliable from the standpoint of internal controls than in aviation, the chances for error are greater, even though only one life might be at stake in contrast to hundreds of lives in an aircraft.

There must be a plan for the procedure with enough latitude to change course if the patient does not respond as predicted or if the operation differs from that planned. Regardless of the situation, whether it be elective or emergency, sufficient time must be allowed to take care of the many details that constitute anesthetization. Usually the anesthesiologist will have tested the apparatus in the operating room before meeting the patient in a holding area. Additions, variations, or deletions regarding this plan will be required, depending upon the particular institution or the kinds of apparatus used.

TRANSPORT OF THE PATIENT TO THE OPERATING ROOM AND PRELIMINARY DETAILS

Transport to the operating room is no inconsequential matter, particularly for the extremely ill patient, and is usually carried out under nursing supervision with the aid of an orderly. A patient may not be able to tolerate the supine position without respiratory or circulatory embarrassment, and those medical devices, such as pacemakers, infusion pumps, dialysis–access sites, an insulin pump, traction apparatus, and iv alimentation lines, must be protected. The anesthesiologist may choose to personally supervise the transfer process in such cases. Last of all, a patient should be brought to the holding area in ample time so that eventual induction of anesthesia is neither hurried nor delayed.

In order not to delay the start of operation, certain tasks may be accomplished in the holding area (or in the operating room) under strict aseptic precautions and with the appropriate privacy; monitoring devices, such as intraarterial, central venous, or pulmonary artery catheters, may be placed. An epidural catheter may be inserted without injecting the entire volume of local anesthetic required for operation, or certain kinds of regional nerve blocks can be done, such as axillary, brachial plexus block, ankle block, intercostal nerve block, or femoral and sciatic nerve block, all accomplished with monitoring and resuscitative devices on hand.

Before any of these procedures are carried out, the patient must be interviewed to be sure that there has been no change in medical condition and that food and drink have not been ingested during the prescribed period of time. Vital signs, including body temperature, blood pressure, pulse rate, receipt of preanesthetic medication, as well as therapeutic drugs, should be checked. Results of laboratory tests that were previously not recorded and the floor nurse's notes should be read. A conscientious nurse is the patient's guardian against harm, up to and including the time of transport to the operating room. Sometimes the unexpected is encountered in the way of an abnormal laboratory finding, a change in the ECG, or discovery of a lung lesion on chest x-ray. If any one of these events is of major significance and if time permits, the test in question might be repeated or a missing item located. However, the anesthesiologist must be certain of the importance of the decision to delay operation because of the anticipated unhappy response of the patient and surgeon. Nevertheless, when the participants are taken into confidence and the evidence is convincing, few will disagree on the need for delay or even cancellation of operation. One should try to avoid the "cascade effect" in delaying operation, as previously described.

Finally, when all is in order, the patient is assisted in the move to the operating table, with all precautions as in transfer to the holding area. The patient should be covered with a warm cotton blanket, and there should be a lifting sheet beneath his or her back and a security strap gently applied above the knees. The extremities must be protected against neurologic injury and soft tissue compression. Slight flexion of the operating table may eliminate back strain and subsequent backache. Electrocautery grounding plates are carefully placed to avoid burns, electric shock, and interference with heart pacemaker function. The patient usually wears an operating room cap to contain the hair as a step toward antisepsis but, paradoxically, not a face mask unless a transmissible disease is present (viral hepatitis, AIDS, Jakob-Creutzfeldt disease). In such situations, the anesthetist may elect to use reverse precautions by wearing gloves, goggles, and an operating room gown. Once placed on an operating table, a patient should not be left unattended. If, after induction of anesthesia, positioning of the patient promises to be difficult, as in the very obese patient or in arthritic patients for D&C, the legs can be placed in stirrups beforehand, with the patient cooperating. Usually, shaving and preparation of the skin for operation are accomplished after induction of anesthesia.

Stethoscope and blood pressure cuff are applied to the arm, a precordial stethoscope is attached to the chest, ECG leads as well as other monitoring devices are affixed, including a pulse oximeter. Baseline data on the vital signs are recorded on the anesthesia record. Insofar as other technical matters are concerned, an iv infusion will have been begun to permit induction of anesthesia as well as access for resuscitative drugs. Rarely, if suitable venous access cannot be established beforehand, mask induction with general anesthesia usually results in venous dilation so that venipuncture should be easier. However, in seriously ill patients, preliminary venous cutdown may be necessary. All these matters are handled with the patient's safety and comfort foremost in mind. Little doubt exists as to the essentialness of alertness, technical skill, organization, and "applied brains" in the induction and maintenance of anesthesia. Anesthesiologists should try to be on time in order to help set the standards for operating room performance on the part of all concerned.

COMMON DISEASES/CONDITIONS

This section deals with anesthetic considerations in patients with commonly encountered major diseases. Owing to dissemination of medical information by the media, better diagnostic and therapeutic techniques and an aging population, anesthesiologists frequently encounter patients with severe systemic illness. Many of these patients undergo major operations in which invasive monitoring and intensive care nursing may be necessary. However, when these patients are scheduled for minor procedures, the anesthesiologist is often faced with a difficult choice. Usually, decisions regarding extent of monitoring techniques are based on severity of cardiorespiratory dysfunction. When such patients undergo minor operations, regional anesthesia might be favored, even though there are no convincing data that mortality is lower than when general anesthesia is used. Thus, anesthesiologists must know not only the consequences of anesthetic methods but also the pathophysiology of disease and the demands of the operation proposed.

CARDIOVASCULAR DISEASE

Although it is not possible to adequately discuss all cardiovascular diseases, or even to examine any particular disease in depth, an attempt is made here to provide the anesthesiologist with a general background on how to approach patients who have the more common cardiovascular diseases. The purpose of preoperative evaluation is to assess the risk of complications and to identify conditions that can be corrected beforehand. These considerations allow the rational recommendation of specific anesthetic methods and the character of monitoring required.

Ischemic Heart Disease

Ischemic heart disease constitutes an entity of diverse etiology, the common factor being an imbalance between myocardial oxygen supply and demand. This usually results from an absolute reduction in coronary artery blood flow or an inability to increase flow in order to match demand. Although atherosclerosis accounts for the majority of patients in this category, lesser causes include coronary insufficiency resulting from embolism, ostial stenosis, coronary artery spasm, and even coronary arteritis. Myocardial ischemia can also occur when myocardial work is greatly increased by the afterload associated with aortic stenosis or severe arterial hypertension. Still another cause of ischemia may be reduced oxygen-carrying capacity of blood as is present in anemia or hypoxemia.

Coronary atherosclerosis begins early in life, as documented by the frequent finding of significant lesions in young men killed in war or by accident. The recent interest in periodic heart evaluations, including stress testing, has resulted in another subset of persons—asymptomatic patients with documented ECG abnormalities during exercise. Symptomatic patients may have angina or a history of MI. Other evidence of coronary insufficiency may be found in congestive heart failure (CHF), ventricular ectopic activity, ECG evidence of ischemia, conduction defects, and so on.

The mortality rate in symptomatic patients averages about 4% per year. Subsets within this group have rates that may differ by a factor of 4. Normotensive patients with a normal resting ECG have a mortality of 2% per year, whereas in hypertensive patients with abnormal, resting ECGs, the mortality approaches 8% per year.[14] The most accurate prognostic factors appear to be the adequacy of left ventricular (LV) function and severity of coronary obstruction. In patients with left main coronary artery disease, the annual mortality rate averages 15%. In any subgroup, patients with elevated (LV) end-diastolic pressures are at greater risk. Thus, preoperative evaluation of the cardiovascular system should include not only a history and physical examination but also laboratory tests to enable evaluation of the degree of ischemia and LV function. Specific inquiry should be made about the presence of dyspnea, chest pain, fatigability, syncope, palpitation, and the precipitating conditions. Physical examination should include blood pressure measurement, quality of peripheral pulses, presence or absence of carotid bruits, and jugular venous distention or pedal edema, basal heart rates, S_3 gallop, and any irregularities in cardiac rhythm. Laboratory data are designed to confirm the clinical findings. In addition to the blood count, urinalysis, chest x-ray, and ECG, an assessment should be made of hepatic and renal function, serum electrolytes, and hemostasis. In patients with established coronary disease, current and old medical records should be evaluated for comparison of ECG, echocardiographic, x-ray, and angiographic findings. In addition, information on stress tests, 24-hour Holter monitoring, and noninvasive carotid blood flow studies should be sought. The anesthesiologist should also note the medications prescribed and whether they are to be discontinued preoperatively. It is also essential to know the patient's compliance with such therapy and whether it is effective in controlling blood pressure, heart rate, arrhythmias, and CHF.

The recent attitude has been to continue most, if not all, cardiac medications.

The overall risk of MI after general anesthesia is shown in Tables 15-7 and 15-8 and is between 0.1 and 0.7% in the population at large.[15, 16] In patients known to have had MI in the remote past (more than 6 months), the risk of perioperative reinfarction rises to about 6%. If MI occurred 3 to 6 months previously, risk of reinfarction is 15%, and within 3 months, the rate is 30%. If reinfarction occurs, the mortality rate is approximately 50%. Some of the important factors that have been independently related by Goldman et al[19] to perioperative cardiac complications include a history of recent MI (less than 6 months), S$_3$ gallop or jugular venous distention, and an abnormal ECG (Table 15-9). Of importance is the fact that more than half the "points" associated with cardiac risk are correctable. Using the Goldman classification, Figure 15-1 shows the relationship between severity of preoperative risk and the occurrence of cardiac complications. Currently, the belief is that if intraoperative cardiovascular function is monitored and if deviations from normal (evidence of ischemia, ventricular filling pressures, and afterload) are promptly corrected, including postoperative stay in the intensive care unit (ICU), the outcome should be improved. Recent data, shown in Tables 15-7 and 15-8, suggest that with this approach, reinfarction rates in the 3- to 6-month and 0- to 3-month groups may be reduced from 15 to 3.4%, and 30 to 7.8%, respectively.[20] Patients who have survived coronary bypass operations and subsequently undergo noncardiac surgery exhibit a lower risk of reinfarction.[21] The aim of preoperative assessment is to critically evaluate each patient for evidence of coronary insufficiency, factors which predispose to angina, the presence of left

TABLE 15-7.   The Risk of Myocardial Reinfarction after Surgery Related to the Presence of Previous Myocardial Infarction

AGE OF PREVIOUS INFARCTION	REINFARCTION RATE (%)	MORTALITY (%)
No previous infarction	0.13	64–73
>6 months	5	54
3–6 months	16	54
<3 months	37	54

(Reproduced with permission from Tarhan S, Moffitt EA, Taylor WF et al: Myocardial infarction after general anesthesia. JAMA 220:1451, 1972.)

TABLE 15-8.   The Risk of Myocardial Reinfarction after Surgery When Aggressive Hemodynamic Monitoring and Interventions and Postoperative ICU Admission are Used

AGE OF PREVIOUS INFARCTION (months)	REINFARCTION RATE (%)
7–12	1.0
3–6	2.3
0–3	5.8

(Reproduced with permission from Rao TLK, Jacobs KH, El Etr AA: Reinfarction following anesthesia in patients with myocardial infarction. Anesthesiology 59:499, 1983.)

TABLE 15-9.   Clinical Factors Independently Related to Perioperative Cardiac Complications

CRITERIA	POINTS
S$_3$ gallop or jugular venous distention on preoperative physical examination	11
Transmural or subendocardial myocardial infarction in the previous 6 months	10
Premature ventricular beats, more than 5/min documented at any time	7
Rhythm other than sinus or presence of premature atrial contractions on last preoperative ECG	7
Age over 70 years	5
Emergency operations	4
Intrathoracic, intraperitoneal, or aortic site of surgery	3
Evidence for important valvular aortic stenosis	3
Poor general medical condition*	3

*As evidenced by electrolyte abnormalities, renal insufficiency, abnormal blood gases, abnormal liver status, or any condition that has caused the patient to become chronically bedridden. (Reprinted by permission from Goldman L, Caldera DC, Nussbaum SR et al: Multifactorial index of cardiac risk in noncardiac surgical procedures. N Engl J Med 297:845–850, 1977.)

ventricular failure, and the presence of ECG evidence of myocardial ischemia, rhythm disturbance, or conduction defects. In some patients, information derived from echocardiography, angiography, stress tests, and hemodynamic evaluation may also be available. Recently, it has become possible to identify portions of the myocardium that are "at risk" by using thallium scanning in the presence of a vasodilator drug (dipyridamole).[22]

It is necessary to individualize the anesthetic plan to best meet the patient's and surgeon's needs. If the medical workup is complete and the patient's condition both optimal and stable, minor procedures might be performed under regional or even general anesthesia without extensive monitoring. At the other end of the spectrum, however, there is the patient who presents anew for elective surgery with a history suggestive of myocardial ischemia. If that patient also has untreated hypertension and other cardiac abnormalities, a complete cardiac workup is recommended. After mature consideration, this may dictate cancellation of operation until a stress test, echocardiogram and angiogram are done and medical therapy brings the patient into optimal condition. When such patients are encountered on morning admission or for ambulatory surgery, one must resist the pressure to proceed with administration of anesthesia.

Valvular Heart Disease

In the adult, valvular heart disease presents many diagnostic and therapeutic challenges. There is a large range in types of lesions and in the extent of valvular involvement, causes, and associated conditions. Thus, only generalizations will be made about anesthetic considerations in such patients.

The basic lesion might be stenosis or incompetence or both. In adults, aortic and mitral valve lesions are more common than those involving the tricuspid or pulmonic valve. Despite decreasing incidence, rheumatic heart disease is still the most common cause of adult valvular disease. Degenerative (sclerosis, fibrosis) disorders and congenital diseases are less common causes. With stenosis, the chamber proximal to the obstruction must increase the work of maintaining stroke

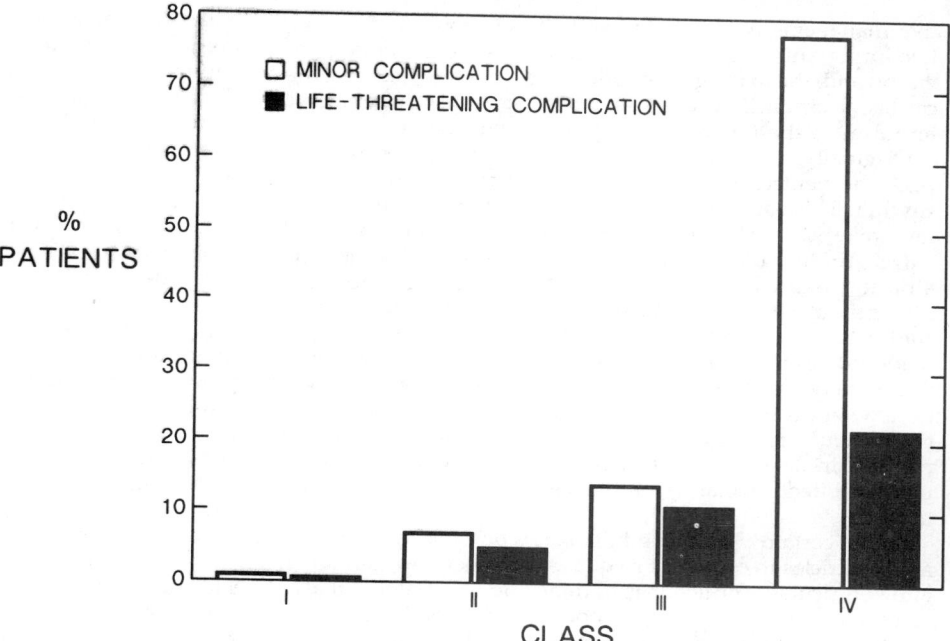

FIG. 15-1. Relationship between the multifactorial cardiac risk index class (Table 15-8) and postoperative cardiac complications. In Class IV patients (Cardiac Risk Index equal to or greater than 26 points), there is a significantly larger number of minor and life-threatening complications. Class IV also sustained the highest percentage of cardiac deaths in the series. Life-threatening complication includes documented intraoperative or postoperative myocardial infarction, pulmonary edema, or ventricular tachycardia without progression to cardiac death. (Reproduced with permission from Goldman L, Caldera DC, Nussbaum SR *et al:* Multifactorial index of cardiac risk in noncardiac surgical procedures. N Engl J Med 297:845, 1977.)

volume, eventually resulting in hypertrophy. Normal valves can episodically accommodate up to seven times the normal cardiac output, as in severe physical exercise in the normally active patient. Valvular stenosis is usually chronic and severe before cardiac output decreases. In valvular incompetence, the chambers both proximal and distal to the lesion are involved, because regurgitant flow during one phase of the cardiac cycle is added to forward flow during subsequent systole. Since lesions are almost never entirely unitary, in stenosis some regurgitation is common and *vice versa.* The resulting clinical classification describes valvular lesions as predominantly stenotic, predominantly regurgitational, or mixed stenosis and regurgitation.

Although detailed discussions on anesthetic management for patients with valvular heart disease are given elsewhere in this text, several fundamental issues are emphasized here. Since stenosis interferes with adequate diastolic filling of the distal chamber, any increase in heart rate would further limit diastolic filling, and stroke volume can fall precipitously. On the other hand, regardless of whether regurgitant flow occurs during systole or diastole, tachycardia may decrease regurgitant flow during the shortened systolic or diastolic phase, thus tending to balance the forces. Furthermore, regurgitant flow increases when pressure in the distal chamber is high; therefore, decreasing the pressure distally would lower regurgitant flow. For these reasons, patients with aortic or mitral stenosis do best with a slow pulse, whereas patients with aortic or mitral valvular insufficiency are better off with a higher heart rate and diminished afterload. Severe aortic stenosis poses the additional problems of a large increase in left ventricular systolic pressure. This results in concentric hypertrophy of the left ventricle, decreased ventricular compliance, and increased oxygen consumption, all predisposing to myocardial ischemia. Patients in the terminal phase of aortic stenosis are prone to sudden death and fare poorly during external cardiac resuscitation. Valvular lesions and prosthetic valves predis-

pose to development of bacterial endocarditis; thus, routine prophylactic use of antibiotics is common.

Mitral Valve Prolapse

A condition now frequently recognized is the syndrome of mitral valve prolapse (MVP),[23] features of which include atypical chest pain, palpitations, anxiety, breathlessness, dysrhythmias, conduction defects, abnormal T-wave patterns on the ECG, cerebral embolic events, mitral regurgitation, endocarditis, and sudden death. Auscultatory findings include a late apical systolic murmur and a nonejection systolic click. Valve motion abnormalities can be seen on echocardiography. Recognition of this syndrome has become common, occurring in at least 5% of the population, and in up to 17% in young women. An enlarged, diastolic ventricular dimension appears to be the best echocardiographic predictor of the subsequent but rare need for mitral valve replacement. In patients with MVP, a redundant mitral valve leaflet appears to be associated with a 10-fold greater risk of sudden death, infective endocarditis, or cerebral embolization. Nonetheless, the overall mortality in patients with MVP does not appear to be significantly different from age- and sex-matched controls. Patients at greatest risk appear to be those with abnormal resting ECGs, prolonged P–T intervals, a family history of sudden death, complex ventricular ectopy, evidence of a redundant mitral valve leaflet, or increased end-diastolic ventricular dimensions. Most patients with MVP are maintained on prophylactic antibiotic therapy.

Pacemakers

More then 300,000 patients in the United States have permanently implanted pacemakers. Anesthesiologists must be aware of the different types of pacemakers, the indications for insertion, evaluation of pacemaker function, and perioperative management of patients with these problems.[24, 25] The two important components of pacemakers are the pulse generator and the pacing electrode. The generator senses the cardiac electric activity and can, if necessary, discharge electric impulses to the myocardium by the pacing electrodes.

Originally, pacemakers were simple devices designed to pace the ventricles at a fixed rate, irrespective of intrinsic rhythm. This could result in ventricular fibrillation if the pacing spike were delivered during the intrinsically generated wave. Another disadvantage of any pacemaker in which the atria and ventricles are not paced synchronously is a decrease in ventricular filling owing to absence of coordinated atrial contraction. A second generation of pacemakers was designed to identify intrinsic cardiac activity, and the ventricular-inhibited variety would discharge only if the intrinsic rate were low, whereas the ventricular-triggered version fired during the absolute refractory period. The unnecessary discharge resulted in decreased battery life, a reason why the ventricular-inhibited "demand" pacemaker is now most frequently used.

Under certain clinical conditions, it is possible to allow atria and ventricles to contract in a quasi-normal cycle when nodal and ventricular conduction is normal, and an atrial pacemaker can act as a sinus node. When nodal conduction is abnormal, an atrial, synchronous pacemaker can detect atrial activity and stimulate the ventricle by means of a ventricular electrode. Finally, atrioventricular sequential units are available that stimulate the atrium and, after a fixed interval, activate the ventricle. These several devices are most likely to be encountered in patients undergoing open heart surgery.

Indications for insertion of a permanent pacemaker generally include conditions in which bradycardia or dysrhythmias result in symptoms suggestive of a low cardiac output, such as lightheadedness, syncope, or heart failure. Occasionally, such patients require temporary ventricular pacing on an emergency basis. Both temporary and permanent pacemakers are usually inserted transvenously, although, in patients undergoing open heart surgery, epicardial electrodes are frequently used. Another option that is available is the pacing-pulmonary artery catheter. In addition to components for the pulmonary artery, right atrium, balloon and infusion channels, these catheters also offer proximal and distal pacing leads. Recently, the use of transthoracic pacing (e.g., from a special skin electrode) has proved to be efficacious.

Anesthesiologists must sometimes decide whether a transvenous, temporary pacing wire should be inserted preoperatively. Persistent bradycardia not responding to iv atropine or exercise is one indication. Bifascicular block in a patient with a history of syncope suggests underlying, unrecognized complete heart block. Such patients, too, can benefit from the availability of transvenous pacing. Although asymptomatic patients with a history of complete heart block do not require routine, pacing wire insertion, these patients must be carefully observed, and a large-gauge venous cannula must be inserted in case pacemaker insertion is urgent. Patients with chronic, bundle branch block occasionally develop right bundle branch block during pulmonary arterial catheter insertion. Ordinarily, this does not present a major problem; however, in the patient with chronic left bundle branch block, complete heart block might develop. Usually, catheter removal effectively reverses complete heart block, but occasionally, temporary pacing is necessary. Interestingly, the converse is true about patients with chronic right bundle branch block who are undergoing left heart catheterization. Here, too, if complete heart block persists, temporary pacing may be necessary.

Preoperative evaluation of a patient with a permanent pacemaker is not as simple as may appear. Too often, anesthesiologists merely note the presence of a permanent pacemaker, whereas pacemakers can mask toxicity of antiarrhythmic drugs, electrolyte disorders, myocardial ischemia, and irritability. In general, the ECG should be examined for pacemaker malfunction, as evidenced by unexpected pauses. In addition, some clinicians evaluate the effects of the Valsalva maneuver to note how effectively the pacemaker functions when intrinsic rate is suppressed. The chest x-ray should provide information on electrode placement, the presence of electrode fracture, and even battery depletion.

During operation in patients with temporary pacemakers, care should be taken to cover the pacemaker generator with a nonconductive surface such as a rubber glove in order to prevent inadvertent conduction of static charge to the myocardium and the resultant microshock. In patients with permanent pacemakers, electromagnetic interference from the surgically employed cautery can cause bradycardia, and continuous use of the cautery converts most demand pacemakers to the fixed mode. In any given patient, if the pacemaker remains inhibited by cautery current, a magnet can be placed over the pacemaker generator to convert it to the fixed mode. Electric grounding pads must be placed away from the generator to decrease interference. During this time, monitoring of cardiac function should be continued by auscultation, pulse oximetry, and palpation of the pulse. Other sources of electric interference with the pacemaker generator are muscle potentials, particularly if severe, as in shivering, seizure activity, or following electroconvulsive therapy. The magnet may be used to revert the generator to the fixed mode. Other unusual situations requiring special attention include cardioversion where lower power settings may suffice and where paddles should not be placed directly over the generator. External cardiac compression during resuscitation may damage pacing electrodes; thus, pacemaker function should be re-evaluated after resuscitation. Many anesthesiologists hesitate to insert a pulmonary artery catheter in patients with permanent pacemakers. Unless pacing wire insertion has been done recently, reactive fibrosis should serve to secure the electrode firmly, and pulmonary catheterization should not be contraindicated.

The Athlete's Heart

A resurgence of interest in physical fitness and training has resulted in the need to consider those patients with "athlete's heart," a condition viewed as a normal, physiologic response to repetitive exercise.[26] With a knowledge of changes brought about by physical conditioning, one is better able to evaluate the relevant laboratory data and to reassure the athlete and other members of the operating room team in this regard. On examination, the pulse rate is slow, mid-systolic murmurs and mid-diastolic filling sounds are common, as are third and fourth heart sounds. The chest x-ray may reveal cardiomegaly; occasionally, it may show an increase in pulmonary vascularity. On the ECG, the frequency of sinus bradycardia, sinus dysrhythmias, first-degree block, Wenckebach's block, and junctional rhythm is higher than that found in age-matched controls. Increase in electric amplitude is found, and the heightened QRS axis is shifted to a more vertical position, while left and right ventricular hypertrophy patterns are common. Incomplete right bundle branch block and U waves may be seen. ST segment and T-wave changes are common, including ST-segment elevation or depression, peaked T waves, depressed J-point, or lateral T-wave inversion. In isotonic (dynamic) exercise, the size of both ventricular cavities increases, although the ejection fraction and myocardial contractility remain unchanged. Most of the morphologic, ECG, and echocardiographic changes appear soon after physical conditioning commences, then progress with additional training and resolve soon upon cessation of activity.

The Pericardium

Although pericardial disease is infrequently encountered in anesthetic practice, pathophysiologic changes presenting as cardiac tamponade and constrictive pericarditis are formidable. With rapid accumulation of pericardial fluid, pericardial pressures increase and affect determinants of ventricular filling. *Pari passu*, ventricular pressures increase until pressures equalize across the four cardiac chambers. Then, as ventricular filling declines, stroke volume and, therefore, cardiac output fall. Although filling pressures are thereby heightened, transmural pressures are low. Compensatory responses include endogenous adrenergic stimulation, resulting arteriolar constriction, and enhanced inotropy. The compensatory tachycardia is helpful in that stroke volume remains low and fixed because of impaired ventricular filling. Therefore, the anesthetic agents and techniques used should support, not counteract, these adaptive responses. Also, in constrictive pericarditis, the primary derangement is limited ventricular filling; the restriction is absent early in diastole, while right ventricular pressure increases abruptly during late diastole. As the thickened constrictive pericardium does not permit transmission of intrapleural pressure, filling pressures remain unaffected by respiration. Cardiac output is relatively well maintained by similar adrenergic compensatory mechanisms, and the anesthetic method should include adequate plasma volume maintenance and avoidance of bradycardia, vasodilation, or myocardial depression, if possible.

Idiopathic Hypertrophic Subaortic Stenosis

Idiopathic hypertrophic subaortic stenosis (IHSS) is an idiopathic disorder that includes nonuniform ventricular hypertrophy, obstruction to the left ventricular outflow tract, and, occasionally, mitral insufficiency.[27, 28] Thickening of the superior and anterior portions of the ventricular septum overlaps hypertrophy that is present in the posterior wall. Left ventricular contractility is greater than normal, as is the ejection fraction. This heightened contractility contributes to obliteration of the cavity during systole. Other features include poor ventricular filling related to impaired diastolic relaxation, late systolic subvalvular obstruction, and mitral insufficiency that develops late in systole. The ECG often reveals left ventricular hypertrophy (LVH), strain patterns, atrial and ventricular arrhythmias, with sudden death not uncommon. During anesthesia, attempts should be made to minimize close apposition of ventricular wall and aortic valve. Maneuvers that preserve stroke volume include a reduction in contractility, enhanced filling pressures, and moderate augmentation of afterload. Detrimental factors include increased positive inotropy, decreased filling pressures, and lowered mean arterial pressures. One should realize that arrhythmias are common and that they frequently contribute to sudden death. Thus, antiarrhythmic drugs and equipment for cardioversion and defibrillation should be available.

Sick Sinus Syndrome

The term *sick sinus syndrome (SSS)* is loosely applied to any form of sinus node depression characterized by marked sinus bradycardia, prolonged sinus pauses, sinus arrest, or sin-

oatrial block.[29] The term is most often applied to the "tachycardia–bradycardia syndrome," in which bouts of ectopic, atrial tachyarrhythmias alternate with periods of sinus and atrioventricular node depression. Isolated atrial fibrillation or a shifting atrial pacer are common early manifestations, especially in young patients. In these patients, heart rate does not increase appropriately with exercise, stress, or fever. The syndrome may be the cause of sudden death in young athletes.

This progressively disabling disease can be the result of ischemic, rheumatic, inflammatory, degenerative, or neoplastic disease. Transient sinus node depression can occur in vagotonic states such as subarachnoid hemorrhage, thyrotoxicosis, hyperkalemia, digitalis sensitivity, or upon the use of nicotine, beta blockers, or quinidine. Approximately 50% of patients with acute, inferior MI develop sinus bradycardia and remain prone to development of bradycardia. Diagnosis of SSS can be made by Holter monitoring and by evaluation of responses to iv atropine or isoproterenol. These patients also exhibit a prolonged, sinus node recovery time after rapid atrial pacing. Although most patients with SSS undergo permanent pacemaker placement, the anesthesiologist would do well to maintain vigilance in patients who develop signs suggestive of SSS. Young, healthy adults frequently have marked sinus bradycardia and sinus pauses exceeding 1.75 seconds. One should be assured that sinoatrial dysfunction appears to be a benign malady that does not significantly alter survival rates.

Toxic Cardiomyopathy

Many medicinal and environmental agents are known to cause myocardial toxicity, which is usually dose dependent. Chronic alcohol abuse has been associated with occurrence of congestive heart failure, arrhythmias, and coronary atherosclerosis. Cobalt, used in the past as a foaming agent in brewed liquors, has also been implicated in "beer drinker's cardiomyopathy."

Chemotherapeutic agents can also induce serious cardiotoxicity. Cyclophosphamide can produce myocardial necrosis and hemorrhagic myocarditis; the resulting heart failure and pulmonary edema may be resistant to treatment. Serum enzyme levels indicative of necrosis are found, and ECG reveals decreased voltage, QT prolongation, and ST–T-wave changes. Daunorubicin (Cerubidine) appears to cause cardiotoxic effects by binding to DNA in nuclei and mitochondria. Cumulative inhibition of protein synthesis causes slow onset but progressive myocardial damage, pump failure, and death. Toxic effects of doxorubicin (Adriamycin) are more widely recognized. In fact, cardiac toxicity is the major factor limiting its usefulness. The drug binds to DNA and inhibits nucleic acid synthesis. Myocardial interstitial fibrosis and mural thrombi are common. Frequently, heart failure appears 3 to 6 months after cessation of therapy. Depression of ventricular function is dose dependent, but heart failure is uncommon in patients receiving less than a total dose of 550 mg·m^{-2} of doxorubicin.[30] Echocardiography, systolic time intervals, and radionuclide ejection fraction studies are useful in evaluating the extent of toxicity. In addition, radiotherapy potentiates the toxic effects of doxorubicin. Heart failure is often resistant to therapy and commonly requires inotropic agents, vasodilators, and diuretics.

The anesthesiologist should aggressively monitor cardiac function when patients with cardiomyopathy undergo major operations. Rational intervention may be made only after determining cardiac output, filling pressures, and vascular resistance.

426   PREPARING FOR ANESTHESIA

Abnormal Serum Potassium

Potassium concentration in the intracellular and extracellular compartments is an important determinant of resting membrane potential and cardiac cell excitability. Anesthesiologists have recognized for a long time that potassium imbalance can predispose to cardiac dysrhythmias during operation. Respiratory alkalosis, administration of catecholamines, insulin, corticosteroids, and digoxin, gastrointestinal losses, hypothermia, and diuretics can all lower serum potassium. Hyperkalemia commonly accompanies renal failure, hypoaldosteronism, use of "potassium-sparing" diuretics, extensive tissue damage, and acidosis. Fasciculations and the minimal skeletal muscle injury that are observed with SCh administration also result in a small increase (average 0.5 mEq·l^{-1}) in serum potassium. Severe hyperkalemia associated with SCh administration is seen in patients with major burns or CNS disease of both recent and indeterminate duration. In these patients, the use of SCh is contraindicated, and muscle relaxation should be achieved with the use of noncompetitive blockers.

Recently it is has been recognized that attempts at *rapid* correction of chronic potassium imbalance are hazardous. This is particularly true when long-standing hypokalemia is aggressively treated with iv potassium; one of 200 such patients suffers life-threatening or fatal hyperkalemia.[31] It is also known that it is the ratio of intracellular to extracellular potassium that determines resting membrane potential and excitability. In mild to moderate chronic hypokalemia, it is believed that the ratio is not disturbed, and, therefore, cardiac dysrhythmias are uncommon. During anesthesia of various kinds, Vitez et al[32] showed that the incidence of cardiac dysrhythmias was the same in both normal and chronically hypokalemic patients (serum potassium 2.6 to 3.4 mEq·l^{-1}). The current belief is that in patients at low risk of cardiac complications, a modest reduction in serum potassium (3.0 to 3.5 mEq·l^{-1}) should not result in dysrhythmias and, therefore, does not require potassium therapy. In acute hypokalemia or severe chronic hypokalemia, postponement of operation is prudent. Chronic hyperkalemia is also well tolerated by patients undergoing dialysis. Here, too, unless serum potassium exceeds 6 mEq·l^{-1}, elective operations should not be postponed. In both severe, chronic hyperkalemia and acute hyperkalemia, appropriate therapy should be instituted before proceeding with anesthesia.

Hypertension

Hypertension is the most common circulatory derangement to affect humans. Patients with high blood pressure are subject not only to the usual surgical operations, but they also undergo procedures to correct the underlying cause of the elevated pressure. Anesthesiologists view these patients with more than usual concern, because the statistics show that life expectancy relates inversely to elevations both in systolic and diastolic pressure (Table 15-10 and Fig. 15-2).[33] Chief among the causes of death are cerebrovascular accidents, MI congestive heart failure, and renovascular sclerosis terminating in renal failure. Therefore, anesthesiologists are involved not only with maintenance of the patient's usual blood pressure but also with adequate tissue perfusion and oxygenation in the presence of probable vascular disease. In addition to the several kinds of circulatory derangement that may be present, one must take into account the variety of drugs used in treatment, the majority of which depress sympathetic nervous activity and therefore interact with anesthetic agents.

TABLE 15-10.   Etiology of Hypertension

I. Essential or primary hypertension
II. Primary renal disease: nephritis, renal arterial stenosis, congenital abnormalities
III. Toxemia of pregnancy
IV. Endocrinopathy
  A. Adrenal cortical hyperfunction
    1. Hyperaldosteronism
    2. Cushing's syndrome
    3. Adrenogenital syndrome (hypertensive form)
  B. Chromaffinomata
    1. Pheochromocytoma
    2. Paraganglionoma (especially organs of Zuckerkandl)
  C. Hyperthyroidism, acromegaly, hyperparathyroidism
V. Hemodynamic alterations
    1. Coarctation of the aorta
    2. Reduced elasticity of vascular system
    3. Decreased peripheral resistance
VI. Neurogenic hypertension
  A. Rapidly elevated intracranial pressure
  B. Seizures: grand mal, autonomic
  C. Denervation of the carotid sinus
  D. Polyneuritis, porphyria, bulbar poliomyelitis, tetanus

(Reproduced with permission from Hickler R, Vandam LD: Hypertension: Anesthesiology 33:219, 1970.)

FIG. 15-2. Mortality ratio (per cent) of actual to expected mortality rates for given levels of systolic and diastolic blood pressure in males ages 15-69 years. (Reproduced with permission from Hickler RB, Vandam LD: Hypertension. Anesthesiology 33:214, 1970.)

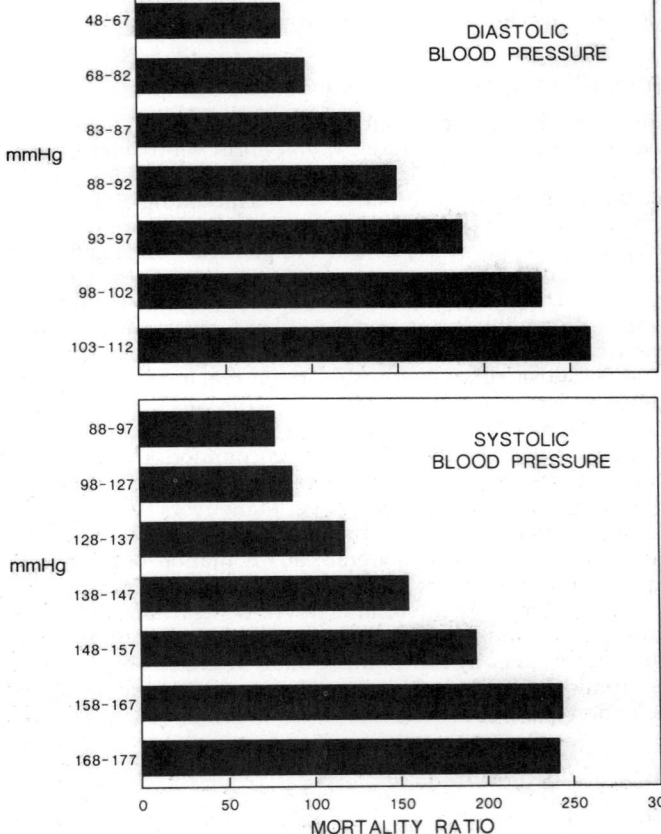

PREANESTHETIC CONSIDERATIONS. Men are more apt to have hypertension than are women, which may account in part for the higher overall male surgical mortality rate. Blacks have a higher incidence of hypertension than do whites, with a greater chance for development of malignant hypertension. Obesity is a common denominator among hypertensives. Chiang et al[34] found a genuine association between elevated blood pressure and increased body weight, independent of the large arm circumference that might affect blood pressure measurement. Not only was blood pressure higher in obese patients, but a significant portion of the hypertensive population was overweight. Obesity also causes problems in anesthetic management, as it is a well-known contributor to circulatory and respiratory complications. Surprisingly, despite the reputed relation between tobacco smoking and development of cardiovascular disease, no association has been found in relation to development of hypertension.

MEASUREMENT OF BLOOD PRESSURE. Little agreement exists as to what constitutes a normal blood pressure range, some extremists defining the limits as 120/80 mm Hg, a few accepting 180/110 mm Hg. Pressures are often falsely elevated when taken on admission to the hospital, and measurement is affected by the girth of the arm, width of the cuff, and presence or absence of vasoconstriction. These surgical patients can be identified at the preanesthetic visit. Although they have normal blood pressure *following* admission, their blood pressure is significantly elevated at the time of admission. Bedford and Feinstein[35] reported that 20–25% of hypertensive patients will develop severe postintubation hypertension.

TYPES OF HYPERTENSION. Sooner or later, every anesthesiologist will be confronted by a patient requiring anesthesia who has a background of one of the diseases listed in Table 15-10. With the exception of primary or essential hypertension, the other categories often call for surgical correction.

PRIMARY HYPERTENSION. The cause or causes of this type of hypertension are still undetermined, whereas the circulatory alterations differ according to the life history of the disease. Blood pressure may be elevated owing to an increase in cardiac output or a rise in peripheral vascular resistance or both. The genetic factors concerned in the development of a hyperdynamic heart and a hyperactive peripheral vascular bed suggest either a polygenic defect or single gene abnormality as inferred from a bimodal distribution of blood pressure in large population studies.[37] Some studies of hypertension have implicated altered sympathetic nervous system activity as evidenced by increased urinary excretion of norepinephrine[38] or alterations in its metabolism, although there is no real evidence that heightened sympathetic activity accounts for the increase in peripheral vascular resistance. Similarly, high sodium intake is not a primary factor, even though a low sodium diet and the use of diuretics may lower blood pressure. With the identification of angiotensin and elucidation of the renin-angiotensin-aldosterone complex, the belief was that this system might be involved in the elevated blood pressure of primary hypertension. However, except for malignant hypertension, where renin secretion plus secondary hyperaldosteronism are markedly enhanced, there is a lack of evidence that hyperaldosteronism is a primary factor. Nevertheless, several currently used antihypertensive drugs are designed to interfere with this endocrine pathway.

ENDOCRINE FORMS OF HYPERTENSION. This category constitutes approximately 5–10% of all cases of hypertension, all potentially curable by surgical means.

Pheochromocytoma. Fewer than 0.5% of hypertensive patients have a pheochromocytoma, a physiologic type of malignancy. On the whole, this is a relatively easily diagnosed and treated disease, but when left untreated, may lead to malignant hypertension and death. Pheochromocytoma may be a component of one of the familial, multiple endocrine syndromes in association with medullary carcinoma of the thyroid and parathyroid adenomas. In patients with untreated pheochromocytoma who are undergoing routine surgical procedures, the mortality rate may approach 10%. Thus, in taking a history from any patient, one must be alert to detect the characteristic symptoms. Because there are false-positive and false-negative findings, the diagnostic tests for pheochromocytoma must be carefully timed to coincide with hypertensive paroxysms.[39] Provocative methods may be used, including the cold pressor test or iv injection of glucagon (1 to 2 mg). The tumor or multiple tumors that are often present may be located with x-ray, computerized tomography, or selective venous sampling for catecholamines from the vena cava. The tumor, which develops from chromaffin tissues in the adrenal medulla or at other sites in the body, secretes excessive amounts of the catecholamines, epinephrine, and norepinephrine, which spill over into the circulation and give rise to the characteristic clinical syndrome. Although the latter is classically characterized by paroxysms of hypertension, headache, tachycardia, tremor, nervousness, ventricular arrhythmias and sweating, in many patients the elevated blood pressure is sustained at a low level, with episodic elevations. The diagnosis is confirmed by analysis of urine or plasma for free catecholamines and their metabolites, including epinephrine, norepinephrine, metanephrine, normetanephrine, and vanillylmandelic acid.

Because surgical removal of the tumor is the accepted treatment, meticulous preparation of the patient is essential. An attempt is made to return blood pressure to normal through the action of phenoxybenzamine (Dibenzyline), a short-acting alpha-blocker taken by mouth, 10 to 20 mg three to four times daily. Prazosin (Minipress), an alpha-adrenergic blocker, 2 to 5 mg bid, has a longer duration of action. However, its persistent hypotensive effect can conceal the blood pressure rise, which may help the surgeon to locate the tumor during surgical exploration. Because of the contracted vascular bed in the chronically hypertensive patient, therapy results in vasodilation, hemodilution, a decline in hematocrit, and a tendency toward postural hypotension. Thus, supplemental saline infusions, or whole blood or packed red cell transfusion, if the hematocrit is deemed too low before operation, may be necessary. Since tachycardia and ventricular arrhythmias may persist, these are controlled with propranolol (Inderal), a beta-adrenergic blocker, or labetalol (Normodyne), a combined alpha- and beta-blocker, in the perioperative period. Management of pheochromocytoma is discussed in detail in Chapter 44.

Cushing's Syndrome and Hyperadrenocorticism. Excess production of hydrocortisone, either as a result of adrenal hyperplasia, neoplasm, or a pituitary adenoma (classical Cushing's disease), results in hypertension in the majority of cases. Although the cause of the hypertension is still not clear, administration of excessive doses of corticosteroids to animals results in hypertension; furthermore, the vasopressor response to norepinephrine is potentiated while sodium and water are retained, thus increasing intravascular and extravascular volume. In some instances, hyperaldosteronism is an associated factor. Anesthesia is not so much complicated by the hypertension, which must be handled in the usual manner, but by altered sodium, potassium, and fluid balance and the need for steroid replacement therapy when the adrenals are removed.

Primary Hyperaldosteronism. Hypersecretion of aldosterone by the adrenal cortex as a result of benign or malignant cortical tumors, or hyperplasia, results in increased sodium reabsorption and potassium release in the renal tubules. The clinical manifestations of hyperaldosteronism derive from these biochemical alterations, hypertension and hypokalemia being the most prominent. Cardiac output is normal, peripheral vascular resistance is increased, and blood volume is expanded. Because the hypertension is usually mild except for the rare instance of progress into the malignant phase, problems in anesthesia concern alterations in the essential electrolytes and replacement therapy with steroids upon surgical removal of the adrenals.

RENOVASCULAR HYPERTENSION. Renal arterial stenosis results in the most common form of potentially curable hypertension. This type of hypertension is caused by an increase in renin secretion from the juxtaglomerular apparatus owing to diminished renal blood flow, as well as alterations of sodium content in the macula densa of the distal renal tubule. Increased renin output is followed by elaboration of the potent pressor substance, angiotensin. Then, because of action by angiotensin on the glomerulosa layer of the adrenal cortex, hyperaldosteronism occurs to a modest degree in some cases, more so in the malignant phase of renovascular disease. Anesthetically, the problems are similar to those encountered in other forms of endocrine hypertension, often with the additional factor of generalized arteriosclerosis.[40] In a cooperative study on renovascular hypertension in 570 patients who underwent operative treatment of renal artery stenosis, the mortality was 5.9%, a high rate wherein age, complicating disease, anesthesia, and operation must have been contributory.[40]

ANESTHESIA AND ANTIHYPERTENSIVE DRUGS. It is a rare hypertensive patient who is not treated by drugs today (Table 15-11). In general, the substances used affect the central and peripheral components of the sympathetic nervous system by altering synthesis, release, biotransformation, or action at end-organs, of norepinephrine (Fig. 15-3). Because the circulatory depressant effects of general anesthetics may be additive, the combination of antihypertensive drugs and anesthetics has caused concern.

When treatment of hypertension first began in the 1950s, anesthesiologists sought to discontinue these drugs prior to operation in order to preserve a functionally intact autonomic nervous system during anesthesia. This attitude arose when hypertensive patients given reserpine developed circulatory collapse, some resulting in cardiac arrest. Subsequent analysis of these complications, however, showed that hypertensive patients, without drug treatment, had considerable fluctuations in blood pressure during anesthesia, and, in treated patients, the percentage fall in pressure during anesthesia differed little from that in other patients.[41]

Recently, controversy has arisen over the preanesthetic use of beta-adrenergic blockers.[42, 43] These drugs were first used as antiarrhythmics, then for treatment of angina, now as adju-

TABLE 15-11.   Drugs Used in the Treatment of Hypertension

DRUGS	FREQUENT ADVERSE EFFECTS
DIURETICS	
Thiazide-type Chlorothiazide (Diuril), Others	Hypokalemia, hyperuricemia, hyperglycemia, hypomagnesemia, allergy
Loop diuretics Furosemide (Lasix)	Above, plus dehydration
Potassium-retaining Spironolactone (Aldactone), Others	Hyperkalemia, hyponatremia
PERIPHERAL SYMPATHOLYTICS	
Bradycardia, fatigue, sedation, increased airway resistance, CHF, beware of sudden withdrawal	Beta-adrenergic blockers Propranolol (Inderal) Prazosin (Minipress) Neserpine (Serpasil) Others
CENTRAL SYMPATHOLYTICS	
Clonidine (Catapres) Methyldopa (Aldomet)	Major rebound hypertension, headache, sedation, dry mouth
ARTERIOLAR DILATORS	
Hydralazine (Apresoline)	Tachycardia, postural hypertension
ANGIOTENSIN-CONVERTING (ACE) ENZYME INHIBITION	
Captopril (Capoten) Enalapril (Vasotec)	Hypotension, particularly with diuretics, hyperkalemia, renal and bone marrow effects
CALCIUM ENTRY BLOCKERS	
Nifedipine (Procardia) Verapamil (Isoptin) Others	Vasodilation, possible postural hypotension, reflex tachycardia

Note: In the initial treatment of mild hypertension, one drug may be used (*e.g.,* a thiazide diuretic). If blood pressure is not controlled, combinations of drugs are used. In addition to the adverse reactions listed, many other adverse effects can occur. The potential for interaction with anesthetics is apparent.

(Modified from: Some oral antihypertensive drugs. The Medical Letter 29:1, 1987.)

vants or the sole drugs used in the treatment of hypertension. Propranolol (Inderal), the first of the compounds introduced, has a negative inotropic and chronotropic effect on the heart, little influence on peripheral vascular resistance, and a tendency to induce bronchospasm. Thus, anesthesiologists were concerned with the possibility of additive effects with general anesthetics. It would have been necessary to discontinue the drug at least 8 to 12 hours preoperatively, because the half-life is approximately 4 to 6 hours after chronic use, and complete dissipation of effect requires about 48 hours. When this plan was adopted, however, some patients with angina who continued with their customary degree of daily activity developed myocardial ischemia and MI. Thus, adrenergic blockade is now considered essential during the perioperative period.[44] Accordingly, anesthesiologists regard the medically treated patient as a better candidate for anesthesia, a philosophy confirmed by quantitative studies on the circulation in hypertensives. During anesthesia, the aim is to maintain anesthesia and a level of blood pressure consistent with that tolerated during everyday activities.

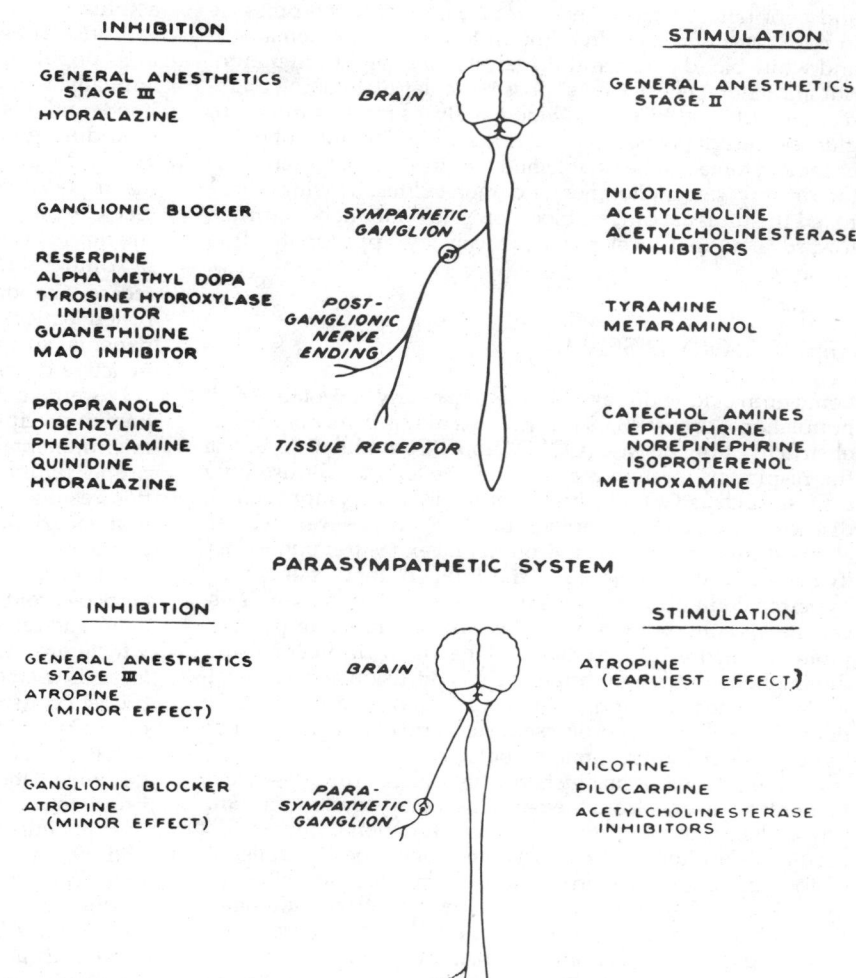

SYMPATHETIC SYSTEM

INHIBITION		STIMULATION
GENERAL ANESTHETICS STAGE III	*BRAIN*	GENERAL ANESTHETICS STAGE II
HYDRALAZINE		
GANGLIONIC BLOCKER	*SYMPATHETIC GANGLION*	NICOTINE ACETYLCHOLINE ACETYLCHOLINESTERASE INHIBITORS
RESERPINE ALPHA METHYL DOPA TYROSINE HYDROXYLASE INHIBITOR GUANETHIDINE MAO INHIBITOR	*POST-GANGLIONIC NERVE ENDING*	TYRAMINE METARAMINOL
PROPRANOLOL DIBENZYLINE PHENTOLAMINE QUINIDINE HYDRALAZINE	*TISSUE RECEPTOR*	CATECHOL AMINES EPINEPHRINE NOREPINEPHRINE ISOPROTERENOL METHOXAMINE

PARASYMPATHETIC SYSTEM

INHIBITION		STIMULATION
GENERAL ANESTHETICS STAGE III ATROPINE (MINOR EFFECT)	*BRAIN*	ATROPINE (EARLIEST EFFECT)
GANGLIONIC BLOCKER ATROPINE (MINOR EFFECT)	*PARA-SYMPATHETIC GANGLION*	NICOTINE PILOCARPINE ACETYLCHOLINESTERASE INHIBITORS
ATROPINE (MAJOR SITE OF EFFECT)	*END ORGAN*	PILOCARPINE (MAJOR SITE OF EFFECT) ACETYLCHOLINESTERASE INHIBITORS

FIG. 15-3. Action of antihypertensive drugs at various sites in the central and peripheral nervous systems. (Reproduced with permission from Hickler RB, Vandam LD: Hypertension. Anesthesiology 33:214, 1970.)

MORTALITY. Aside from anesthetic management of pheochromocytoma, there are few data pertaining to anesthetic morbidity and mortality in other hypertensive syndromes. Goldman and Caldera[45] found little correlation between preoperative blood pressure levels and development of cardiovascular complications. Patients with asymptomatic hypertension and diastolic blood pressures below 115 mm Hg were not at increased risk for cardiac complications regardless of whether blood pressure was adequately or inadequately treated. Moreover, although hypertension is usually associated with other cardiovascular abnormalities, when controlling for these conditions, mild to moderate hypertension *per se* was not a predictor of postoperative cardiac complications.

In essential hypertension, the associated vascular disease is a major factor in operative morbidity and mortality. The longer the duration of hypertension and the older the patient, the more prominent the arteriosclerosis. Baker *et al,*[46] in an analysis of autopsy material of patients 30 years of age or older in which they examined the circle of Willis for severity and extent of arteriosclerosis, found significant increases in the presence of hypertension. The changes were most pronounced when clinical criteria for the diagnosis of hypertension were used, but also when the weight of the heart was taken into account. In a prospective epidemiologic study of 5,127 men and women over a period of 14 years, Kannel *et al*[47] found a well-established association between hypertension and coronary heart disease (CHD). The incidence of all manifestations of CHD, including angina, coronary insufficiency, MI, and sudden death was significantly related to antecedent elevated levels of systolic and diastolic pressure. Further, Frank *et al*[48] found that the presence of hypertension prior to initial MI was associated with an increased mortality rate.

DISCOVERY OF HYPERTENSION BEFORE ELECTIVE OPERATION. Mild hypertension without symptoms, signs, or evidence of cardiovascular disease poses few problems, but the initial discovery of major hypertension shortly before operation calls for delay not only to find an unusual cause (pheochromocytoma) but also for more thorough assessment of the circulation. Physical examination should include examination of the blood vessels in the eye grounds, extracranial vessels, and peripheral arteries, and measurement of blood pressure in both arms and legs. In addition to the routine hematocrit and white blood count and urinalysis, one might order anterior and lateral chest x-rays, possibly a flat plate of the abdomen, a multilead ECG, and blood analyses for urea nitrogen, glucose, serum potassium, and uric acid. A diagnosis of pheochromocytoma can be established within 12 hours by analysis for urinary catecholamines and metabolites. Having eliminated the unusual causes, blood pressure should be returned toward a normal level preoperatively by appropriate drug therapy.

RESPIRATORY DISEASE

Some form of lung disease is present in nearly 25% of the adult population. Almost 40,000 Americans die each year of chronic obstructive lung disease (COPD) alone. Common disorders of the respiratory system are classified as follows: diffuse lung disease such as COPD (chronic bronchitis and emphysema); disease caused by immunologic mechanisms, as seen in bronchial asthma or noxious environmental exposure; pulmonary infection; vascular disease of the lung (primary pulmonary hypertension and thromboembolism); and tumors and miscellaneous conditions. Any of these disorders can impair respiratory function by one or more of the following mechanisms: diminished ventilation, impaired gas diffusion across the alveolar membrane, and altered ventilation–perfusion relations. Such abnormal processes are ultimately manifested by hypoxemia or hypercapnia, or both.

Although anesthesiologists readily learn of the presence of respiratory disease from the patient's history, symptoms, and physical examination, quantitation of functional impairment requires laboratory testing. Advanced age, obesity, a history of tobacco smoking, and associated cardiac, neurologic or thoracic cage disorders can add to the severity of pulmonary dysfunction. Reduced exercise tolerance, an altered sensorium, dyspnea, and abnormal respiratory signs (rate, pattern, and auscultatory findings) suggest the presence of respiratory impairment. Laboratory evaluation of respiratory function commonly includes chest x-ray, pulmonary function testing, ECG, and arterial blood gas analysis. Additional information can be obtained by means of ventilation and perfusion scanning, divided lung function testing, bronchoscopy, bronchography, and calculation of pulmonary vascular resistance when pulmonary artery pressures and flow are measured in the lesser circulation. However, laboratory testing can be misleading because the abnormalities may be nonspecific; they may not bear an exact chronologic relation to acute events, and they sometimes depend considerably upon the patient's cooperation and effort. Furthermore, few tests offer a means to accurately predict the likelihood of perioperative respiratory complications. In contrast to the patient with cardiovascular dysfunction, in many patients it is not easy to improve pulmonary function by therapeutic intervention. Beneficial effects can more often be achieved in patients with reversible bronchoconstriction, infection, and poorly drained secretions.

Bronchial Asthma

A disorder characterized by reversible airway narrowing, bronchial asthma is usually characterized by airway hyperreactivity.[49] Eosinophilia is a common accompaniment, confirming hypersensitivity as the cause in many patients. Other forms of asthma include exercise-induced asthma, infectious asthma, occupational asthma, and drug-induced (aspirin) asthma.

Bronchial asthma develops in approximately 2.5% of the U.S. population and accounts for several thousand deaths annually. Most patients first develop their symptoms in childhood, and it is unusual for asthma to be detected for the first time during anesthesia. Obstruction to gas flow occurs primarily during expiration, as confirmed by diminished maximal mid-expiratory flow rate and timed, forced vital capacity. (See Chapters 32 and 33.) Arterial blood gas values may be in the normal range, even in moderately severe disease because of compensatory hyperventilation; later, Pa_{O_2} and Pa_{CO_2} decrease. Carbon dioxide retention occurs only in severely afflicted patients. Because of the immunologic basis in most patients, eosinophilic counts are often greater than $300/mm^3$ in active disease.

Preventive therapy is directed toward avoiding contact with known precipitating factors, whether they are medications or environmental agents. In some patients, maintenance of proper hydration and prompt treatment of pulmonary infection results in reversal of the early bronchoconstrictive phenomena. Because asthma is an episodic illness, most patients do not require chronic drug therapy. Commonly used medications include beta$_2$-adrenergic agonists, aminophylline, and corticosteroids. Some patients benefit from mast cell stabilizers such as inhaled, nebulized cromolyn (Intal). Cromolyn, which prevents mast cell degranulation and is ineffective in treating bronchoconstriction, is used only for prophylaxis. Although anticholinergic drugs may increase bronchial caliber and respiratory dead space, they may result in airway obstruction owing to inspissated secretions. Of the beta-adrenergic agonists, epinephrine and isoproterenol are highly effective, but, because of their cardiovascular effects, their use is limited to patients with refractory and severe bronchoconstriction. Beta$_2$ specificity is progressively improved with isoetharine (Bronkosol), metaproterenol (Alupent), albuterol (Proventil), and terbutaline (Brethine). All these drugs can be administered by nebulizer (even in an anesthesia breathing circuit) or iv. Aminophylline, a phosphodiesterase inhibitor that enhances synthesis of cyclic AMP, is also effective in treating mild to moderate bronchoconstriction. Patients who have not previously received aminophylline can be given an iv loading dose of 5 to 7 $mg \cdot kg^{-1}$ over 15 to 20 minutes. Therapeutic blood levels lie between 10 and 20 $\mu g \cdot ml^{-1}$, and hepatic clearance of aminophylline is decreased during general anesthesia owing to decreased visceral blood flow; thus, toxic signs, including tachycardia, hypotension, ventricular irritability, and seizures, may develop. Corticosteroids are used in acute asthma as well as part of a chronic, maintenance regimen. Systemic effects can be diminished by administration in an aerosol such as beclomethasone (Beclovent).

Proper anesthetic management of asthmatic patients requires an appreciation of the pathophysiology and pharmacologic aspects of the disease process.[49, 50] Absence of wheezing and a normal eosinophil count suggest inactive disease. Where indicated, chest physiotherapy, hydration, and antibiotic therapy are useful preoperatively. There is little evidence that preoperative opioids or anticholinergic drugs have a significant effect on bronchomotor tone. Although rectal suppositories of aminophylline are an alternative to oral medication, the limited data available suggest that adequate plasma concentrations are not achieved without increasing dosage. When general anesthesia is elected, an attempt should be made to depress airway reflexes by the judicious use of opioids, proper depth of anesthesia, and local anesthetics such as lidocaine (topical or iv). Although several of the opioids (morphine, meperidine) do not appear to have deleterious effects, some of the competitive neuromuscular blockers such as curare and atracurium can cause bronchoconstriction by histamine release in susceptible patients. The inhalation agents—halothane, enflurane, and isoflurane—can provide the necessary depth of anesthesia and a degree of bronchodilation. Beta-adrenergic agents and aminophylline can cause dysrhythmias when given in the presence of anesthetics that sensitize the myocardium to catecholamines (*e.g.*, halothane). Enflurane and isoflurane are therefore acceptable alternatives to the traditionally used halothane. In spite of proper preoperative selection of anesthetic techniques, if bronchoconstriction develops intraoperatively, it may be necessary to use beta-adrenergic agonists, aminophylline, or corticosteroids.

Chronic Obstructive Pulmonary Disease

This disorder embraces the clinical gamut ranging from the progressive destruction of alveoli as seen in emphysema, to the excessive bronchoconstriction and mucous secretion of chronic bronchitis.[51] Cigarette smoking and other environmental factors are major causative factors. The loss of elastic recoil (emphysema) and excessive mucous secretions (chronic bronchitis) result in airway narrowing and obstruction. When emphysema predominates, the lungs are hyperinflated and radiolucent, and the diaphragm flattened.

The risk of postoperative pulmonary complications increases when obstruction to gas flow is severe enough to decrease FEV_1 below 50%; the same is true when respiratory insufficiency results in carbon dioxide retention. Long-standing COPD can result in pulmonary artery hypertension, chronic cor pulmonale, and, eventually, right heart failure. Although positive inotropic agents and diuretics appear to be useful, effective therapy should improve arterial oxygenation to relieve pulmonary vasoconstriction. As in bronchial asthma, adequate hydration and chest physiotherapy should help to mobilize secretions. Cessation of smoking for 4 to 8 weeks preoperatively, if feasible, will permit return toward normal of both pulmonary mechanics and mucociliary activity. Bronchodilators may be helpful in relieving the reversible component of bronchospasm.

Although, intuitively, regional anesthesia appears to be an attractive option, a word of caution is in order. In moderately severe COPD, the accessory muscles of respiration are recruited to combat expiratory obstruction and facilitate exhalation. In spinal anesthesia, when motor blockade extends to the upper thoracic segments, respiratory insufficiency may be precipitated. During general anesthesia, normal oxygenation of arterial blood is the goal. This might limit the usefulness of balanced anesthesia with nitrous oxide. Another disadvantage of high concentrations of nitrous oxide would be diffusion into emphysematous bullae or into the gas-containing gastrointestinal tract in patients already at a mechanical disadvantage owing to the flattened diaphragm. The inhalation agents suppress hypoxic pulmonary vasoconstriction and increase right-to-left intrapulmonary shunting, thus the need for increased, inspired oxygen concentrations.

The pattern of mechanical ventilation should be such that sufficient time is allowed for expiration. Failure to do so can result in gas trapping and ventilation mismatch. Clinical experience, too, would favor the use of large tidal volume (10 to 15 $ml \cdot kg^{-1}$) and a slow respiratory rate (6 to 8 breaths/min). Patients with severe COPD (FEV_1 less than 50%) who undergo upper adbominal operations often require mechanical, ventilatory support postoperatively.

The anesthesiologist can contribute in many ways to the limitation of development of pulmonary complications. In addition to therapist training of patients in the techniques of voluntary deep breathing, incentive spirometry and intermittent positive pressure breathing (IPPB) compliance with such maneuvers can be enhanced by several approaches to postoperative analgesia. Local anesthetic intercostal nerve block, intrathecal or epidural placement of an opioid, and local anesthetic infiltration of the surgical wound by the surgeon with a long-acting local anesthetic will all result in prolonged analgesia and improve the ability of such patients to perform the necessary respiratory exercises.

DIABETES MELLITUS

Literally, the term *diabetes* connotes a state of polyuria known as diabetes mellitus when the diuresis is caused by glucose, and diabetes insipidus when a deficiency of pituitary, antidiuretic hormone is present. Diabetes is the most common metabolic derangement in humans, often underdiagnosed and estimated to occur in about 2–4% of the population. The condition results from a deficiency in insulin availability or its action in relation to glucose metabolism, with resulting hyperglycemia that is superficially manifested by glycosuria. Untreated, the osmotic diuresis of glycosuria leads to fluid and electrolyte loss, dehydration, weight loss, and hyperphagia. Moreover, as part of a complex hormonal derangement, free fatty acids ordinarily mobilized from fatty stores for gluconeogenesis fail to undergo transformation in the liver, and ketone bodies are formed instead. The ketoacidosis, which can result in coma, is the most serious complication of untreated diabetes (Table 15-12). Another kind of coma may result from excessively high blood glucose levels, so-called hyperosmolar, nonketotic coma, which need not be accompanied by acidosis and is often related to ill-advised administration of glucose during fluid therapy, as in the treatment of body burns (Table 15-13). At the other end of the spectrum, when insulin is given to aid in metabolic utilization of glucose, hypoglycemia and attendant problems, especially coma, are not infrequent sequelae. Few severely diabetic patients have not experienced an insulin reaction at one time or another in the course of their treatment.

The autoregulatory processes relating to glucose homeostasis are primarily directed toward maintenance of sufficient substrate for cerebral aerobic metabolism, as the brain is an obligate glucose consumer, with ketones a secondary source of energy in the emergency[52] and mobilization of glucose from tissue stores by way of glycogenolysis, while glucose utilization in tissues is inhibited. In contradistinction, other tissues such as the myocardium and skeletal muscle can utilize free fatty acids (FFA), pyruvate, the amino acid alanine and possibly glycerol as energy sources. The dependence of the CNS on glucose substrate is clearly evident when the plasma levels begin to decline below $60 \ mg \cdot dl^{-1}$. At first, mental confusion occurs, then coma, followed by structural brain damage and death if hypoglycemia persists. Not only is the mental status indicative of hypoglycemia, but so are the other symptoms that relate to reactive epinephrine secretion, such as anxiety, sweating, palpitations and headache. Epinephrine acting by means of $beta_2$ adrenergic receptors is thus an emergency hormone that is active in glucose homeostasis so that cerebral metabolic and structural integrity may be preserved.

Insulin derived from pancreatic B cells is the major hormone concerned with glucose utilization. The signal for its release is an increase in blood sugar, with the result that glucose is

TABLE 15-12.   Clues to Complications in Diabetic Ketoacidosis

COMPLICATION	CLUES
Acute gastric dilatation or erosive gastritis	Vomiting of blood or coffee-ground material
Cerebral edema	Obtundation or coma with or without neurologic signs, especially if occurring after initial improvement
Hyperkalemia	Cardiac arrest
Hypoglycemia	Adrenergic or neurologic signs; rebound ketosis
Hypokalemia	Cardiac arrhythmias
Infection	Fever
Insulin resistance	Unremitting acidosis after 4–6 h of adequate therapy
Myocardial infarction	Chest pain, appearance of heart failure; appearance of hypotension despite adequate fluids
Mucormycosis	Facial pain, bloody nasal discharge, blackened nasal turbinates, blurred vision, proptosis
Respiratory distress syndrome	Hypoxemia in the absence of pneumonia, chronic pulmonary disease, or heart failure
Vascular thrombosis	Stroke-like picture or signs of ischemia in non-nervous tissue

(Reproduced with permission from Foster DW: Diabetes mellitus. In Braunwald E et al [eds]: Harrison's Principles of Internal Medicine, 11th ed, p 1790. New York, McGraw-Hill, 1987.)

TABLE 15-13.   Initial Laboratory Findings in Hyperosmolar Coma

SERIES	BROOKLYN*	WASHINGTON†
Age (years)	60	57
Glucose, $mg \cdot dl^{-1}$	1166	976
Sodium, $mEq \cdot l^{-1}$	144	142
Potassium, $mEq \cdot l^{-1}$	5	5
Chloride, $mEq \cdot l^{-1}$	99	98
Bicarbonate, $mEq \cdot l^{-1}$	17	22
BUN, $mg \cdot dl^{-1}$	87	65
Creatinine, $mg \cdot dl^{-1}$	5.5	—
Free fatty acids, $mM \cdot l^{-1}$	0.73	0.96
Osmolarity, $mOsm \cdot l^{-1}$	384	374

*Mean data from 33 episodes of hyperosmolar coma (AA Arieff, HJ Carroll: Medicine 51:73, 1972).

†Mean data from 20 episodes of hyperosmolar coma (JE Gerich et al: Diabetes 20:228, 1971).

(Reproduced with permission from Foster DW: Diabetes mellitus. In Braunwald E et al [eds]: Harrison's Principles of Internal Medicine, 11th ed, p 1791. New York, McGraw-Hill, 1987.)

phosphorylated and taken up by the body cells, while the remainder is taken up in liver and muscle. It is stored there as glycogen and is available as glucose by way of glycogenolysis. As in any homeostatic system with feedback controls, insulin is not unopposed in its action, as there is a compensating hormone, glucagon, derived from pancreatic A cells. The signal for glucagon release is a decline in the blood sugar level; its chief action is that of glycogenolysis.

Thus, three hormones are the major regulators of glucose metabolism: insulin, glucagon, and epinephrine. Several other hormones, not of the immediate regulatory kind, can also elevate the blood sugar, as both cortisol and growth hormone are known to antagonize the action of insulin. Anesthesia and operation also combine to induce a diabetic state not only by the stress response, which results in catecholamine and cortisol secretion, but also by an action of general anesthetics that interferes with phosphorylation and membrane transport of glucose. Episodes of hypoxemia, hypercarbia, and hypotension aggravate the surgical diabetic condition.

We have discussed the immediate consequences of hyper- and hypoglycemia. Anesthesiologists should also know that chronic diabetes, with the fluctuations in blood glucose levels that occur even during insulin therapy, results in macro- and microvascular disease, diabetic retinopathy, cataract formation, renal failure on a vascular basis, susceptibility to infection, and development of both somatic and autonomic neuropathy. These complications, which relate to the severity and duration of the diabetes, account for the excess mortality in diabetics with or without the complicating effects of anesthesia and operation.

It is well known that diabetes is not of unitary origin but, rather, is related to a variety of causes and is generally designated as Type 1, juvenile-onset or insulin-dependent diabetes mellitus (IDDM), or Type II, adult onset, which involves more of a chemical disturbance, usually controlled by diet alone or orally effective hypoglycemic agents. The two types of diabetes and their characteristic features are shown in Table 15-14.

On entry to the hospital, most patients will know of their diabetic state and insulin requirements as prescribed by a physician and with varying degrees of compliance. In others, diabetes may be discovered on entry because of suggestive symptoms and a familial history of the disease. The presence of glycosuria is a gross screening test, particularly if ketone bodies are found; however, the renal threshold for glucose excretion lies in the 60 to 150 $mg \cdot dl^{-1}$ range, and fasting blood sugars lie somewhere between 60 and 110 mg. Lower glucose levels may occasionally be discovered in children and in young women and after 2 to 3 days of fasting. As the goal of diabetic management is to maintain blood glucose and its utilization in the normal range, particularly in the face of surgical stress, we believe that it may be necessary that the IDDM patient be admitted to the hospital at least 24 hours in advance of operation in order that the degree of control and the presence of complicating disease be assessed, particularly in those patients who have experienced hypoglycemic or ketoacidotic episodes in the past. This precaution allows for consultation and control of the diabetic state or postponement of operation when diabetes is newly discovered. Even if IDDM is mild and well controlled, we do not believe it to be safe practice in the ambulatory care setting, whereby the patient would be asked to take nothing by mouth and to delay the morning dose of insulin until arrival at the hospital, where an iv infusion of glucose in water is first instituted. Ambulatory anesthesia and surgery can be done safely in the chemically dependent diabetic if the medical condition is acceptable.

Insofar as choice of anesthesia is concerned, that method which least disturbs glucose homeostasis is preferable. Thus, local or regional anesthesia seems to fulfill the requirements. Nevertheless, one might think twice about electing spinal anesthesia for inguinal herniorrhaphy or a rectal procedure either in young or elderly patients, in whom urinary retention is a common problem that requires bladder catheterization in

TABLE 15-14. Some Features Distinguishing Between Insulin-Dependent and Noninsulin-Dependent Diabetes

	IDDM	NIDDM
Synonym	Type I	Type II
Age of onset	Usually <30	Usually >40
Ketosis	Common	Rare
Body weight	Nonobese	Obese (80%)
Prevalence	0.2–0.3%	2–4%
Genetics		
HLA association	Yes	No
Monozygotic twin studies	40–50% concordance rate	Concordance rate near 100%
Circulating islet cell antibodies	Yes	No
Associated with other autoimmune phenomena	Occasional	No
Treatment with insulin	Always necessary	Usually not required
Complications	Frequent	Frequent
Insulin secretion	Severe deficiency	Variable: moderate deficiency to hyperinsulinemia
Insulin resistance	Occasional: with poor control or excessive insulin antibodies	Usual: due to receptor and postreceptor defects

(Reproduced with permission from Olefsky JM: Diabetes mellitus. In Wyngaarden JB, Smith LH Jr [eds]: Cecil Textbook of Medicine, 7th ed, p 1322. Philadelphia, WB Saunders, 1985.)

persons readily susceptible to urinary tract infections. Also, such a simple procedure as regional nerve blockade about the ankle is best avoided in those with evidence of peripheral vascular disease.

There are more than a few regimens, all incorporating the same general principles, for management of the diabetic patient perioperatively. In all these plans, one must know the kinds of insulin required and the dosage used by the patient (Table 15-15). One such plan of management is that advocated by Smith et al[53] and outlined in Tables 15-16 and 15-17. The overall rationale is as follows: (1) Glucose is infused iv at all times as the energy-yielding substrate; (2) insulin is given to ensure glucose utilization by tissues and to prevent tissue catabolism; and (3) the customary, morning insulin dose is reduced to avoid episodes of hypoglycemia. As a rule, diabetic control is best achieved if the patient is operated on early in the morning, according to the plan presented. For those patients whose diabetes is controlled by diet alone or by an oral hypo-

TABLE 15-15. Properties of Various Insulin Preparations

CLASS	TYPE	PEAK EFFECT	DURATION OF ACTION (hr)
Rapid	Regular crystalline insulin (CZI)	2–4	6–8
Intermediate	Semilente	2–6	10–12
	Neutral protamine (NPH)	6–12	18–24
	Lente	6–12	18–24
Long-acting	Protamine zinc, (PZI)	14–24	36
	Ultralente	18–24	36

(Reproduced with permission from Olefsky JB: Diabetes mellitus. In Wyngaarden JB, Smith LH Jr [eds]: Cecil Textbook of Medicine, 7th ed, p 1330. Philadelphia, WB Saunders, 1985.)

TABLE 15-16. Insulin Management During the Preoperative Period

BLOOD GLUCOSE (mg·dl⁻¹)	INSULIN-DEPENDENT DIABETIC	INSULIN-INDEPENDENT DIABETIC
<150	Decrease intermediate insulin (10–20%)	Discontinue oral agent
150–250	No change	No change
>250	Increase intermediate insulin (10–20%)	Discontinue oral agent and begin intermediate insulin (10–20 U)
>350	Increase intermediate insulin (10–20%) and add regular insulin (10–20% of intermediate dose)	

(Reproduced with permission from Smith RJ, Dluhy RG, Williams GH: Endocrinology. In Vandam LD [ed]: To Make the Patient Ready for Anesthesia, 2nd ed, pp 120, 121. Stoneham, Massachusetts, Butterworth Publishers, 1984.)

TABLE 15-17.   Insulin Management on the Day of Surgery

1. One-half usual intermediate (NPH or lente) insulin dose subcutaneously (SC) 1 hr preoperatively
2. IV D5W at 100 ml/hr starting 1 hr preoperatively
3. Determine blood glucose in recovery room and give one-half usual intermediate insulin dose SC
4. Follow blood glucose every 4–6 hr until next morning
5. Administer *regular* insulin SC every 4–6 hr according to the following schedule:

BLOOD GLUCOSE (mg · dl^{-1})	REGULAR INSULIN (SC)
>400	25% of usual A.M. dose
300–400	20% of usual A.M. dose
200–300	Observe; no insulin

(Reproduced with permission from Smith RJ, Dluhy RG, Williams GH: Endocrinology. In Vandam LD [ed]: To Make the Patient Ready for Anesthesia, 2nd ed, pp 120, 121. Stoneham, Massachusetts, Butterworth Publishers, 1984.)

glycemic agent, insulin is not given, but an infusion of glucose in water is administered at the rate shown. Blood glucose is measured immediately postoperatively, and, if it is above 250 mg · dl^{-1}, regular insulin is given, followed by glucose testing every 4 to 6 hours. Diet is resumed as soon as practicable. Smith *et al* also believe that use of urine glucose levels on the "sliding scale" as a guide to insulin therapy is not justified, since glycosuria is discovered only after the fact. Furthermore, the elderly diabetic, as a concomitant of the disease, may already have altered renal and bladder function, plus an elevated threshold for glucose clearance. Thus, what might seem to be mild glycosuria, may not reflect a considerable degree of hyperglycemia.

The poorly controlled diabetic, verging either upon hypoglycemia or, more importantly, ketoacidosis, will require appropriate treatment with fluids and insulin under expert guidance before operation is contemplated, even if several hours must be allowed to elapse before an emergency operation. (See also Chapter 44 for further information.)

OBESITY

Anesthetization of the obese patient poses many problems, as documented by the increased postoperative morbidity and mortality. In recent years, surgeons have attempted to cure morbid obesity by a variety of operations, even though the condition is obviously a medical problem. We have noted that in anesthesia, it is not so much the total body weight in the obese patient, but the distribution of the excess that causes difficulties. Thus, it is cogent to define the term *obesity*, particularly of the morbid kind. Usually, obesity is diagnosed when the body weight exceeds normal body weight by 20%; morbid obesity is diagnosed when the patient weighs twice the ideal weight. A better understanding is attained when body habitus is taken into account as defined by R. D. Levine.

1. In the male: height (cm) − 100 = ideal weight (kg)
2. In the female: height (cm) − 105 = ideal weight (kg)
3. Using the body mass index (BMI), obesity is said to exist when the ratio, body weight, kg/height, m, exceeds 30.

Markedly obese patients have both social and psychological problems to be considered at the outset in planning for anes-

thesia. One should keep in mind the actuarial data that suggest that a 30–40% increase in body weight carries approximately a 90% higher mortality rate than in age-matched persons of normal weight. For these social and medical reasons, surgical treatment has been advocated for morbidly obese patients. Those persons selected for operation are patients who have unsuccessfully tried to lose weight but are in fair general health, except for the often associated hypertension and chemical diabetes, and in the approximate age range, from 40 to 60 years.[54]

Although obese patients may require operation for all the usual reasons, the therapeutic obesity operation clearly illustrates the pathophysiologic problems. Aside from the relatively simple medical therapies, such as dieting, use of anorectics, thyroid hormone administration (a dangerous remedy), even wiring of the jaws, surgical procedures are designed to promote a sense of satiety, to decrease gastric capacity, to slow the emptying time, or to bypass absorptive segments of small bowel. Anesthesiologists may encounter patients already surgically treated, so it is well to know that the long-range efficacy of these procedures has not been established. Further, in addition to weight loss, there have been postoperative complications, including diarrhea, severe nutritional defects, thiamine deficiency, hyperuricemia, exacerbation of damage in the fatty liver, and arthritis, which may relate to the abnormalities listed.

Some of the specific problems of the obese in relation to anesthetic management during the perioperative period are discussed in the following sections.[55] (See also Chapter 41.)

Circulation

Obese persons develop hypertension, the diagnosis confounded by difficulty in measuring blood pressure because of the extra girth of the arm. The regular pressure cuff is too narrow in relation to circumference; thus, a higher cuff pressure is required to interrupt arterial circulation, using the Riva–Rocci method. Consequently, a thigh cuff may be necessary for both the physical examination and monitoring during anesthesia. In addition to the other hypertension-related complications and use of antihypertensive medications, some or all of the usual hypertension-related complications may be present, including left ventricular hypertrophy, along with coronary, cerebral, renal, and peripheral vascular disease. A cardiac myopathy of the obese has been described in addition to ventricular hypertrophy, fatty infiltration, and increase in pericardial fat.[56] Peripheral edema is often present, perhaps on a cardiac basis or owing to gravity effects. Thus, analysis of circulatory function by chest x-ray, ECG, and noninvasive cardiac tests provides essential information for anesthetic management.

Respiration

Because of the excessive weight of the fatty deposits about the chest, compounded by the weight of the breasts and the high diaphragms caused by the enlarged volume of abdominal viscera, thoracic compliance is reduced. Not only is the work of breathing augmented, but breathing becomes shallow, with decreased tidal volumes and increased rate. The diminution in expiratory reserve volume leads to small airway closure, a tendency toward miliary atelectasis, ventilation–perfusion mismatch and shunting. The possibilities for development of hypoxemia and hypercarbia are thus apparent, in turn affecting central control of respiration and adding to myocardial workload by means of pulmonary artery vasoconstriction and development of cor pulmonale; right heart failure and compensatory polycythemia are common features. The classic picture of the morbidly obese person is typified by Joe, the fat boy in Dickens' *Pickwick Papers* (*The Pickwickian Syndrome*), in whom lethargy, somnolence, periodic respiration, and apnea were highly suggestive of carbon dioxide retention and hypoxemia. Consequently, in anesthesia, maintenance of adequate alveolar ventilation is the goal, along with minimal use of respiratory depressant drugs, appropriate respiratory and circulatory monitoring, and documentation, beforehand, of the degree of pulmonary dysfunction.

Gastrointestinal and Metabolic Problems

Diaphragmatic herniation may compound the pulmonary deficiencies just listed, whereas increased gastric acidity and volume of secretion, plus esophageal reflux, pose the threat of pulmonary aspiration. Metabolically, chemical diabetes is common, exaggerated by a diminished sensitivity to insulin. Relatedly, there may be fatty infiltration of the liver not unlike that of chronic alcoholism. The implications for laboratory testing are apparent.

Physical Accompaniments

Under the section involving routine history taking and physical examination, we referred to obesity and the problems posed in airway management, positioning for operation, and circulatory access for fluids, and monitoring. In summary, in massively obese patients, and considering the magnitude of some of the operations performed to correct the obesity, the degree of circulatory and respiratory monitoring required is comparable to that used during major cardiovascular anesthesia.

ANXIETY/DEPRESSION/PSYCHIATRIC PROBLEMS

At the beginning of this chapter, we remarked that there is relatively little time for anesthesiologists to establish firm and satisfactory relations with patients just prior to operation. Since the patient's reactions may seem odd, anesthesiologists must understand the circumstances and not become antagonistic, all the while being aware of the influence of their own personalities and attitudes on the patient's behavior.

Anxiety is a normal response when a patient faces operation. It is important therefore, to determine whether the degree of apprehension is appropriate to the occasion, which is easier said than done. Underlying depression is always a possibility, perhaps enhanced by grief, as in the recent death of a loved one or a concurrent, serious illness in a family member. Other elements of the history may shed some light on the patient's mental state, in respect to habits such as tobacco smoking, alcohol intake, drug use, or recent onset of insomnia and weight loss. In other words, is the depression of a situational or delusionary nature? It is natural for a woman facing diagnostic breast biopsy for question of cancer to be concerned about the outcome, especially if there is a familial history of the disease.

Commonly, patients express fears about not awakening from general anesthesia or waking up too soon, others seek oblivion for the entire procedure, and still others express a death wish. If these attitudes seem extraordinary and implacable, psychiatric consultation should be sought, particularly if a state of panic exists. Usually, however, patience, explanation, and reassurance help to settle these matters while the appro-

priate amount of tranquilizing medicine adds to the solution. Additional visits to the patient, again in the evening, followed by another in the morning, both on the part of the anesthesiologist and the surgeon, help to mitigate the patient's fears and anxiety.[57] We have known patients to deliberately defy orders so that operation would be canceled (*e.g.*, consuming food and drink in spite of being warned against it, or signing out of the hospital against advice).

Depression as a manifestation of anxiety may relate to longstanding personal conflicts. There may be psychosomatic symptoms and complaints; the patient may already have been under therapy and taking medicines in that regard. Although antidepressant medications may interact with anesthetics, particularly in relation to sympathetic nervous activity, the combination is usually not harmful. Nevertheless, it is essential to know the medications taken and to continue their use, with the possible exception of the monoaminooxidase inhibitors, which have a long half-life and must be discontinued several weeks in advance. There is disagreement on this score, as the techniques of anesthesia can be adjusted to the situation, with specific anesthetics avoided. Psychotherapeutic drugs used in clinical practice have significant cardiorespiratory and CNS side-effects.

When a psychiatric problem seems severe and not amenable to resolution by simple means, operation should be postponed, because the perioperative period does not afford the time for adequate therapy. A suicidal tendency may be evident, but rarely is the intention carried out, as it is often merely an expression of the anxiety–depressive state. Kelly and Reich[57] state that suicide in the hospital is a rare event, perhaps more common in manic depressive and schizophrenic states. More often, suicide occurs in relation to an organic confusional state, in association with drug or alcohol withdrawal, and in the setting of postoperative psychosis, as might happen in the elderly. Treatment of these more complex mental problems are beyond the comprehension and abilities of the average anesthesiologist, so psychiatric evaluation is necessary. It is also well known that some nonpsychotherapeutic drugs can induce mental symptoms.

When a patient gives a history of having had a psychiatric problem that is now stable, drug therapy should be continued to maintain that state of relative well-being. One might expect that the patient's personal physician or psychiatrist would have advised on the situation; if not, psychiatric opinion should be sought.

ALLERGY

An anaphylactoid reaction is among the more injurious and potentially lethal events that can occur during the course of anesthesia. In daily existence, the prototypical example of this is the collapse and rapid death caused by a wasp sting. Persons susceptible to these kinds of accidents often give a history of allergy of the atopic kind, for example, allergic rhinitis, dermatitis, specific food intolerance, or asthma. Common iatrogenic offenders in atopy and the anaphylactoid response include the penicillins, codeine, radiodiagnostic contrast media, or chymopapain, once used to dissolve protruding intervertebral discs. During history taking, anesthesiologists may learn that morphine, meperidine, thiopental, Althesin, tubocurarine, or alcuronium, or preservatives such as methylparaben or the vehicle cremophor-L, may have produced an allergic reaction in the past.

In taking the patient's history, it is not easy to determine whether an allergic reaction to a drug has indeed occurred.

Testing by means of intradermal injection, of the substance in question while observing for a wheal and flare reaction yields both positive and negative results.[58] Diagnostically, one might rely on the nature of the allergic reaction that occurred. For example, in true anaphylaxis, there is often an aura of impending doom or uneasiness, followed by generalized itching, urticaria, dyspnea, respiratory obstruction owing to bronchospasm, and, finally, circulatory collapse. Any or all of these symptoms may have been present.

One of the reasons for problems in diagnosis and variation in symptomatology is the mechanism of the reaction. For example, the term *anaphylaxis*, rather than anaphylactoid, is used by some clinicians in cases in which immunoglobulin IgE is a factor. The antigen or allergen, as exemplified by a drug, forms a macromolecule with a protein, polysaccharide, or hapten to promote synthesis and release of IgE from plasma cells, in turn derived from B-lymphocytes. The IgE attaches to receptors on mast cells and basophils, and, when re-challenged with antigen, a conglomeration of potent mediators are released that affect smooth muscle and capillaries throughout the body, such as histamine, eosinophilic and neutrophilic chemotactic substances, kinins, possibly serotonin, newly synthesized prostaglandins, the leukotrienes and slow-reacting substance of anaphylaxis (SRSA). However, a similar anaphylactoid reaction, may be induced by means of the complement pathway, through drug action resulting in degranulation of mast cells, or by the cyclo-oxygenase pathway, where leukotrienes are formed from arachidonic acid. Further discussion regarding the allergic patient is found in Chapter 51.

GERIATRIC PATIENT

Certain features of aging explain the increased morbidity and mortality found in the elderly surgical population.[59] In a group of patients older than 80 years of age, a 1-month hospital mortality rate was 6.2%. Twenty-five percent of Physical Status 4 patients died.[60] For the most part, the problems that arise relate to a gradual deterioration in their physiologic performance, estimated to be in the range of 0.8–0.9% per year of the functional abilities present at age 30 years. There is a close resemblance between these changes and those that result from physical inactivity.[61] In the geriatric population, the rate and expectation of dying relate directly to age, and the percentage of the elderly in the population is slowly on the increase, now approaching 15% in the United States. In the context of anesthesia, the operations performed on older people are usually major, involving the heart and circulation, genitourinary system, orthopedics, the gastrointestinal tract, and malignancies of various types. Because of their seriousness, the operations tend to last longer; multistage procedures and reoperations are common because of complications.

The Aging Process

Some of the apparent features of old age are shown in Table 15-18.

Central Nervous System

Under the broad designation of senility, such changes occur as diminution in cognition, confusion, memory loss, emotional instability, and psychiatric syndromes, including delusion and infantile behavior. Often, the drugs prescribed to mini-

TABLE 15-18.　Characteristics of Old Age

High pain threshold	Dementia
Altered response to stress	Malnutrition
Arteriosclerosis	Anemia—low blood volume
Diminished autonomic tone	Diabetes
Edentia	Poor renal function
Emphysema	

(Reproduced with permission from Dripps RD, Eckenhoff JE, Vandam LD: Introduction to Anesthesia, 7th ed, p 357. Philadelphia, WB Saunders, 1988.)

mize these symptoms create additional problems; however, in anesthesia, one should not overlook the possibility that the original symptoms may relate to organic disease and that the use of opioids, sedatives, and tranquilizers must be sharply curtailed. This admonition is particularly appropriate in that many old people will complain of difficulty in sleeping or altered sleep patterns. Actually, studies have shown that sleeping time in the elderly is not greatly reduced, but that falling asleep takes longer, awakening is frequent, and the time devoted to the REM phase is lessened.

Neurophysiology

All phases of neural transmission are reduced with aging, probably relating to a reduction in neuronal density, reduced formation of neurotransmitters, and fewer receptors for their action. The result of these changes is an increased susceptibility to general anesthetics, so that the minimum alveolar concentration (MAC) declines. The pain threshold is elevated, perhaps as a result of the degenerative changes just noted. An example of this might be the declining incidence of post-lumbar puncture headache beyond the 7th decade. Bellville *et al* long ago demonstrated an increased effectiveness of opioids for pain relief. Thus, lesser amounts of the latter are needed; this is fortunate because of their depressant effects on respiration and circulation. Likewise, senescence affects the autonomic nervous system, which is mainly evident in sluggish baroreceptor reflexes.

Drug-Pharmacokinetics and Dynamics

An example of the altered geriatric response to drugs is apparent in the response to atropine, where tachycardia is less evident, atrioventricular dissociation is not uncommon in the ECG, and pupillary, mydriatic effects are diminished. In the anesthetic context, the usual doses of diazepam produce more profound and prolonged sedation. The so-called sleep dose of thiopental given for induction of anesthesia is reduced, while the metabolism of many drugs (*e.g.*, antipyrene and phenylbutazone) is slowed as shown by prolongation of their half-lives. Altered distribution in the body compartments is also a factor.

Circulation and Respiration

In the brain, as Kety first demonstrated during measurements of cerebral blood flow (CBF), a progressive, overall diminution in CBF and cerebral oxygen consumption occurs in the final decades of life. Cardiac output and cardiac index likewise decline while, during exercise in the aged, the ventricular ejection fraction falls, even as there is increase in peripheral vascular resistance, the result of "hardening of the arteries."[62]

In old age, as may be observed in postanesthetic recovery rooms, abnormal breathing patterns and periodic respiration are not unusual. Such phenomena and the tendency to develop apnea or hypoventilation are accentuated by the use of opioids. Just as there is a diminution in circulatory reflexes, so are the protective respiratory reactions diminished, as in coughing. With regard to the background of senescent pulmonary changes, emphysema, and bronchial obstruction, it is readily apparent why aspiration of gastric contents occurs with increased frequency and corresponding dire consequences.

The physical changes of advanced age are evident during history taking and physical examination: In the eye, there is arcus senilis, cataract formation, hyporeactive pupils, and frequent presence of glaucoma; in relation to iv therapy, one observes generalized loss of elastic tissue, tortuous and fragile blood vessels, and easy bruisability (as following application of a tourniquet or a failed iv needle insertion). We have spoken of the oral problems, edentia and prostheses, as they relate to anesthesia mask fit and tracheal intubation.

In preparation for and choice of anesthesia, all these pathophysiologic and physical factors play a role in the aged population.[63]

PERIOPERATIVE NAUSEA AND VOMITING

More than a few patients who are queried about their reactions to anesthetics will cite repeated episodes of nausea and vomiting. Nausea and vomiting may occur for a variety of reasons: 1) in regional or spinal anesthesia as a result of the cerebral ischemia during hypotensive episodes; 2) following the use of opioids that affect the medullary vomiting center's chemoreceptor and reflex components; 3) gastric dilation and increased volume caused by swallowing of blood and secretions or reflux from the small intestine; and 4) as reflex responses to a variety of surgical stimuli in the presence of inadequate afferent sensory blockade or a light plane of general anesthesia. There is also some evidence that the use of nitrous oxide increases the incidence of vomiting postoperatively.

A higher incidence of nausea and vomiting is noted in women than in men; this is probably estrogen related, as suggested by emesis gravidarum early in pregnancy and its occurrence during certain phases of the menstrual cycle. Thus, nausea and vomiting are frequent following gynecologic and breast surgery.

Often, this experience is not only distressing to patients, but it may actually produce complications such as wound dehiscence, prolonged hospital stay, or intraocular or conjunctival hemorrhage, so that a foolproof anesthetic technique might be sought. Since this is seldom ensured, a preventive approach is advised. Although theoretically expected to be effective, the parasympatholytic drugs, atropine and glycopyrrolate, are not useful, and the doses required to be effective would be excessive. Other drugs that exert a depressive effect on the vomiting centers, the barbiturates and phenothiazines, have the disadvantages of extrasedation and circulatory depression. However, droperidol (Inapsine) in low dosage iv, 2.5 to 5 mg, although also sedative, is a useful antiemetic, particularly when given postoperatively in smaller dosage, 1.25 to 2.5 mg. Gastric suction is useful in maintaining an empty stomach, whereas metoclopramide (Reglan), a dopaminergic antagonist, may facilitate gastric emptying and reduce the occurrence of reflux.

REFERENCES

1. Egbert LD, Battit GE, Turndorf H et al: The value of the preoperative visit by an anesthetist. JAMA 185:553, 1963
2. Leigh JM, Walker J, Janaganathan P: Effect of preanaesthetic visit on anxiety. Br Med J 2:987, 1977
3. Bunker JP, Forrest WH, Mosteller F et al (eds): The National Halothane Study. A study of the possible association between halothane anesthesia and postoperative hepatic necrosis. Bethesda, Maryland, U.S. Government Printing Office, 1969
4. Groves JE: Taking care of the hateful patient. N Engl J Med 298:883, 1978
5. Denborough MA, Forster JFA, Lovell RRH et al: Anaesthetic deaths in a family. Br J Anaesth 34:395, 1962
6. Cregler LL, Mark H: Medical complications of cocaine abuse. N Engl J Med 315:1495, 1986
7. Griner PF, Mayewski RJ, Mushlin AI et al: Selection and interpretation of diagnostic tests and procedures: Principles and applications. Ann Intern Med 1981 94:557, 1981
8. Hubbell FA, Greenfield S, Tyler JL et al: The impact of routine admission chest x-ray films on patient care. N Engl J Med 312:209, 1985
9. Rabkin SW, Horne JM: Preoperative electrocardiography: Effect of new abnormalities on clinical decisions. Can Med Assoc J 128:146,1983
10. Mold JW, Stein HF: The cascade effect in the clinical care of patients. N Engl J Med 314:512, 1986
11. Wilson R, Crouch EAC: Risk assessment and comparison: An introduction. Science 236:267, 1987
12. New Classification of Physical Status. Anesthesiology 24:111, 1963
13. Dripps RD, Eckenhoff JE, Vandam LD: Introduction to Anesthesia, 7th ed. Philadelphia, W.B. Saunders, 1988
14. Braunwald E, Cohn PF, Ross RS: Ischemic heart disease. In Isselbacher KJ, Adams RA, Braunwald E et al (eds): Harrison's Principles of Internal Medicine, p 1116. New York, McGraw-Hill, 1980
15. Knapp RB, Topkins MJ, Artusio JF: The cerebrovascular accident and coronary occlusion in anesthesia. JAMA 182:332, 1962
16. Topkins MJ, Artusio JF: Myocardial infarction and surgery: A five year study. Anesth Analg 43:716, 1964
17. Tarhan S, Moffitt EA, Taylor WF et al: Myocardial infarction after general anesthesia. JAMA 220:1451, 1972
18. Steen PA, Tinker JH, Tarhan S: Myocardial reinfarction after anesthesia and surgery. JAMA 239:2566, 1978
19. Goldman L, Caldera DC, Nussbaum SR et al: Multifactorial index of cardiac risk in noncardiac surgical procedures. N Engl J Med 297:845, 1977
20. Rao TLK, Jacobs, KH, EL Etr AA: Reinfarction following anesthesia in patients with myocardial infarction. Anesthesiology 59:499, 1983
21. Mahar LJ, Steen PA, Tinker JH et al: Perioperative myocardial infarction in patients with coronary artery disease with and without aorto-coronary bypass grafts. J Thorac Cardiovasc Surg 76:533, 1978
22. Engle KA, Singer DE, Brewster DC et al: Dipyramidole-thallium scanning in patients undergoing vascular surgery. JAMA 257:2185, 1987
23. Barlow JB, Pocock WA: The mitral valve prolapse enigma—two decades later. Mod Concepts Cardiovasc Dis 53:13, 1984
24. O'Neill MJ, David D: Pacemakers in noncardiac surgery. Surg Clin North Am 63:1103, 1983
25. Frye RL, Collins JJ, De Sanctis RW et al: Guidelines for permanent cardiac pacemaker implantation. J Am Coll Cardiol 4:434, 1984
26. Huston TP, Puffer JC, MacMillan RW: The athletic heart syndrome. N Engl J Med 313:24, 1985

27. Thompson RC, Liberthson RR, Lowenstein E: Perioperative anesthetic risk of non cardiac surgery in hypertrophic obstructive cardiomyopathy. JAMA 254:2419, 1985

28. Maron BJ, Bonow RO, Cannon RO, 3rd *et al:* Hypertrophic cardiomyopathy. Interrelations of clinical manifestations, pathophysiology, and therapy (I, II). N Engl J Med 316:780–789, 844–852, 1987

29. Belic N, Talano JV: Current concepts in sick sinus syndrome. II. ECG manifestation and diagnostic and therapeutic approaches. Arch Intern Med 145:722, 1985

30. Alexander J, Dainiak N, Berger HJ *et al:* Serial assessment of doxorubicin cardiotoxicity with quantitative radionuclide angiocardiography. N Engl J Med 300:278, 1979

31. Kassirer JP, Harrington JT: Diuretics and potassium metabolism: A reassessment of the need, effectiveness and safety of potassium therapy. Kidney Int 11:505, 1977

32. Vitez TS, Soper LE, Wong KC *et al:* Chronic hypokalemia and intraoperative dysrhythmias. Anesthesiology 63:130, 1985

33. Hickler RB, Vandam LD: Hypertension. Anesthesiology 33:214, 1970

34. Chiang BN, Perlman LV, Epstein FH: Overweight and hypertension. A review. Circulation 39:403, 1969

35. Bedford RF, Feinstein B: Hospital admission blood pressure: A predictor for hypertension following endotracheal intubation. Anesth Analg 59:367, 1980

36. Martin DE, Kammerer WS: The hypertensive surgical patient. Surg Clin North Am 63:1017, 1983

37. Platt R: Heredity in hypertension. Lancet 1:899, 1963

38. Von Euler US, Hellner S, Purkhold A: Excretion of noradrenaline in urine in hypertension. Scand J Clin Lab Invest 6:54, 1954

39. Bravo EL, Gifford RW Jr: Pheochromocytoma: Diagnosis, localization and management. N Engl J Med 311:1298, 1984

40. Franklin SS, Young JD, Maxwell MH *et al:* Operative morbidity and mortality in renovascular disease. JAMA 231:1148, 1975

41. Ominsky AJ, Wollman H: Hazards of general anesthesia in the reserpinized patient. Anesthesiology 30:443, 1969

42. Prys-Roberts C, Meloch R, Foëx P: Studies of anaesthesia in relation to hypertension. I: Cardiovascular responses of treated and untreated patients. Br J Anaesth 43:122, 1971

43. Low JM, Harvey JT, Prys-Roberts C *et al:* Studies of anesthesia in relation to hypertension. VII: Adrenergic responses to laryngoscopy. Br J Anaesth 58:471, 1986

44. Kopriva CJ, Brown ACD, Pappas G: Hemodynamics during general anesthesia in patients receiving propranolol. Anesthesiology 48:28, 1978

45. Goldman L, Caldera DL: Risks of general anesthesia and elective operation in the hypertensive patient. Anesthesiology 50:285, 1979

46. Baker AB, Resch JA, Loewenson RB: Hypertension and cerebral atherosclerosis. Circulation 39:701, 1969

47. Kannel WB, Schwartz MJ, McNamara PM: Blood pressure and risk of coronary heart disease. The Framingham Study. Dis Chest 56:43, 1969

48. Frank CW, Weinblatt E, Shapiro S *et al:* Prognosis of men with coronary heart disease as related to blood pressure. Circulation 38:432, 1968

49. Reynolds HY: Immunologic lung diseases (part 1). Chest 81:626, 1982

50. Benetar SR: Fatal asthma. N Engl J Med 314:423, 1986

51. Hudson LD: Management of COPD. State of the art. Chest 85:765, 1984

52. Cryer PE: Gerich JE: Glucose counterregulation, hypoglycemia, and intensive insulin therapy in diabetes mellitus. N Engl J Med 313:232, 1985

53. Smith RJ, Dluhy RG, Williams GH: Endocrinology, Chapter 5. In Vandam LD (ed): To Make the Patient Ready for Anesthesia, 2nd ed, pp 120, 121. Stoneham, Massachusetts, Butterworth Publishers, 1984

54. Gastric operations for obesity. The Medical Letter 26:113, 1984

55. Buckley FF, Robinson NB, Simonowitz DA *et al:* Anaesthesia in the morbidly obese. Anaesthesia 38:840, 1983

56. Messerli FH: Cardiomyopathy of the obese—a not so Victorian disease. N Engl J Med 314:378, 1986

57. Kelly MJ, Reich R: Psychiatric conditions, Chapter 9. In Vandam LD (ed): To Make the Patient Ready for Anesthesia, 2nd ed, pp 224–241. Stoneham, Massachusetts, Butterworth Publishers, 1984

58. Fisher M: Intradermal testing after anaphylactoid reaction to anesthetic drugs: Practical aspects of performance and interpretation. Anaesth Intensive Care 12:115, 1984

59. Kohn RR: Cause of death in very old people. JAMA 247:2793, 1982

60. Djokovic JL, Hedley-Whyte J: Prediction of outcome of surgery and anesthesia in patients over 80. JAMA 242:2301, 1979

61. Schneider EL, Brody JA: Aging, natural death and the compression of morbidity: Another view. N Engl J Med 309:854, 1983

62. Fleg J: Alterations in cardiovascular structure and function with advancing age. Am J Cardiol 57:33c, 1986

63. Williams WE: Clinical implications of aging physiology. Am J Med 76:1049, 1984

Chapter 16

Stephen F. Dierdorf

Rare Co-existing Diseases

Knowledge of the pathophysiologic characteristics of co-existing disease and an understanding of the implications of concomitant drug therapy are essential for the optimal management of anesthesia for an individual patient. In many instances, the nature of the co-existing disease has more impact on anesthesia than does the actual surgical procedure. A variety of rare disorders may influence the selection and management of anesthesia (Table 16-1).

MUSCULOSKELETAL DISEASES

MUSCULAR DYSTROPHY

There are several types of muscular dystrophy. Duchenne muscular dystrophy, also known as pseudohypertrophic muscular dystrophy, is the most severe form. Duchenne muscular dystrophy is characterized by painless degeneration and atrophy of skeletal muscle. This disorder is a sex-linked recessive trait that is clinically evident only in male patients. Typically progressive skeletal muscle weakness develops that produces symptoms when patients are between the ages of 2 and 5 yr. Progressive limitation of movement occurs, and these patients usually are confined to a wheelchair by the time they are 12 yr of age. Skeletal muscle imbalance generally produces kyphoscoliosis. Death occurs when patients are from 15 to 25 yr old, and it is usually secondary to congestive heart failure or pneumonia. Serum creatine kinase levels reflect the progression of skeletal muscle degeneration. Early in the patient's life the creatine kinase level is elevated. Later, however, as significant amounts of skeletal muscle have degenerated, the creatine kinase level decreases.

Cardiac muscle also degenerates in patients with this disease, as reflected by a progressive decrease in R wave amplitude on serial electrocardiograms (ECGs). Myocardial degeneration produces decreased myocardial contractility and in some cases mitral regurgitation secondary to papillary muscle dysfunction.[1] Interestingly, myocardial abnormalities are usually confined to the lateral and posterobasal walls of the left ventricle.[2] Obstruction of the right ventricular outflow tract can produce an insidious right heart failure, however.[3] Degeneration of respiratory muscles is evidenced by the restrictive pattern of pulmonary function tests. Diminished skeletal muscle strength produces an ineffective cough and subsequent retention of secretions, which lead to pneumonia and, ultimately, death.

Other forms of muscular dystrophy include fascioscapulo-humeral dystrophy and limb-girdle dystrophy. These types of dystrophies have clinical onset in adulthood and are not nearly as severe as Duchenne muscular dystrophy.

Management of Anesthesia

Myocardial dysfunction in the patient with Duchenne muscular dystrophy makes these patients potentially more sensitive to the myocardial depressant effects of potent inhaled anesthetics. There are several reports of cardiac arrest occurring during induction of anesthesia.[4] Consequently, cardiac function must be monitored carefully during induction of anesthesia. Succinylcholine should not be used because massive rhabdomyolysis, hyperkalemia, and cardiac arrest can occur.[5, 6] Some patients with Duchenne muscular dystrophy are also susceptible to malignant hyperthermia, but this susceptibility is unpredictable.[7, 8]

TABLE 16-1. Co-Existing Diseases That Influence Anesthesia Management

MUSCULOSKELETAL	CENTRAL NERVOUS SYSTEM	ANEMIAS	COLLAGEN VASCULAR	SKIN
Muscular dystrophy	Multiple sclerosis	Nutritional deficiency	Rheumatoid arthritis	Epidermolysis bullosa
Myotonic dystrophy	Epilepsy	Hemolytic	Lupus erythematosus	Pemphigus
Myasthenia gravis	Parkinson's disease	Hemoglobinopathies	Scleroderma	
Eaton-Lambert syndrome	Huntington's chorea	Thalassemias	Polymyositis	
Familial periodic paralysis	Alzheimer's disease			
Guillain-Barré syndrome	Amyotrophic lateral sclerosis			
	Creutzfeldt-Jakob disease			

Smooth muscle involvement results in hypomotility of the intestinal tract and delayed gastric emptying. The potential for aspiration of gastric contents is further enhanced by impaired swallowing mechanisms.[9] Precautions should be taken to prevent aspiration.

After operation the patient with Duchenne muscular dystrophy must be monitored closely for evidence of pulmonary dysfunction and retention of pulmonary secretions. Vigorous respiratory therapy and ventilatory support may be necessary.

MYOTONIC DYSTROPHY (MYOTONIA DYSTROPHICA, STEINERT DISEASE)

Myotonic dystrophy is the most common form of a group of diseases known as the myotonias. Other forms of myotonia include congenital myotonia (Thomsen disease) and paramyotonia. Myotonic dystrophy is an autosomal dominant trait with symptoms occurring when patients are in the second or third decades of life. The hallmark of myotonic dystrophy is persistent contracture of skeletal muscle after stimulation. Myotonic contraction of affected muscle is not relieved by regional anesthesia, nondepolarizing muscle relaxants, or deep anesthesia. Relaxation may be induced by infiltration of the affected muscle with a local anesthetic. The administration of quinine, tocainide, or mexiletine may also alleviate myotonic muscle contracture. These drugs depress rapid sodium influx into muscle cells and delay return of membrane excitability.[10, 11] There is progressive involvement and deterioration of function in skeletal, cardiac, and smooth muscle. Although myocardial contractile tissue degenerates, the cardiac conduction system, and in particular the His-Purkinje system, deteriorates more rapidly. Myocardial failure is rare but cardiac dysrhythmias and atrioventricular block are common.[12] First-degree atrioventricular block may actually precede the onset of clinical symptoms. Sudden death may be caused by the abrupt onset of third-degree atrioventricular block. Although mitral valve prolapse occurs in 20% of patients with myotonic dystrophy, the prolapse is secondary to geometric changes of the heart caused by thorax deformation. Systemic complications from mitral valve prolapse generally do not occur in patients with myotonic dystrophy.[13]

Pulmonary function studies demonstrate restrictive lung disease, mild arterial hypoxemia, and diminished ventilatory responses to hypoxia and hypercapnia.[14] Weakness of respiratory muscles diminishes the effectiveness of cough and may lead to pneumonia. Alteration of smooth muscle function produces gastric atony and intestinal hypomotility. Pharyngeal skeletal muscle weakness in conjunction with delayed gastric emptying increase the risk for aspiration of gastric contents. Endocrine dysfunction also occurs in patients with myotonic dystrophy and produces diabetes mellitus, thyroid dysfunction, adrenal insufficiency, and gonadal atrophy. Other clinical features include cataract formation, frontal baldness, and mental deterioration.

Pregnancy often produces exacerbations of myotonic dystrophy. It has been suggested that the increased progesterone levels of pregnancy contribute to increased symptoms. Cesarean section must often be performed because of uterine smooth muscle dysfunction.[15]

Congenital myotonia (Thomsen disease) develops during infancy or early childhood and usually manifests as swallowing dysfunction because of an inability to relax the oropharyngeal muscles. The condition generally improves with age and does not affect a patient's life expectancy. Paramyotonia is the third and most rare of the myotonic syndromes. Myotonic contracture develops when the patient's environment is cold. Warming will relax the contracted muscle.

Management of Anesthesia

Considerations for anesthesia in the patient with myotonic dystrophy include the presence of cardiac and respiratory muscle disease and the abnormal response to drugs used during anesthesia. Succinylcholine produces an exaggerated contracture and its use should be avoided (Fig. 16-1). Succinylcholine-induced myotonia can make ventilation of the lungs and tracheal intubation difficult or impossible.[16] The patient's response to nondepolarizing muscle relaxants appears normal. Neostigmine, however, may precipitate myotonia when administered for reversal of neuromuscular blockade.[17] Consequently, when one selects a neuromuscular blocking drug, a shorter-acting one such as atracurium or vecuronium would be useful.[18–20] Patients with myotonia are quite sensitive to the respiratory depressant effects of opioids, barbiturates, benzodiazepines, and inhaled anesthetics. Depression of ventilation increases as the disease progresses and seems to result from depression of the central respiratory center and a peripheral muscle effect.[21] Because patients with myotonia have mitral valve prolapse and cardiac conduction abnormalities, cardiac dysrhythmias may occur. The ECG taken before operation should be examined carefully for signs of atrioventricular conduction delay. Use of anesthetics known to delay conduction in the His-Purkinje system, specifically halothane, may be avoided for this reason.

Smooth muscle function is also affected by myotonia. Gastrointestinal motility is decreased and gastric emptying delayed. Precautions should be used to prevent pulmonary inspiration.[22]

Skeletal muscle weakness and myotonia are exacerbated during pregnancy. Labor is typically prolonged, and there is an increased incidence of postpartum hemorrhage from pla-

Succinylcholine (mg/kg)

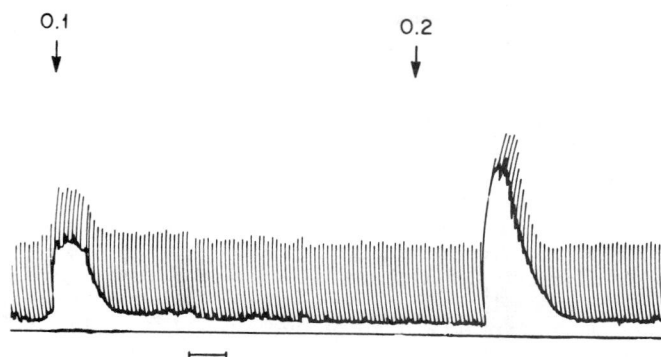

FIG. 16-1. Administration of small doses of succinylcholine to a patient with myotonic dystrophy produces an exaggerated contraction of skeletal muscle. (Reprinted with permission. Mitchell MM, Ali HH, Savarese JJ: Myotonia and neuromuscular blocking agents. Anesthesiology 49:44, 1978.)

centa accreta.[23] Anesthesia for cesarean section has been successful with general, spinal, or epidural anesthesia.[15, 25]

MYASTHENIA GRAVIS

Myasthenia gravis is a disease of the neuromuscular junction caused by a decrease in the population of acetylcholine receptors. The incidence is one in 20,000, and female patients are affected twice as often as male patients. Myasthenia gravis is considered an autoimmune disease because circulating antibodies destroy or inactivate acetylcholine receptors. Ninety per cent of myasthenic patients have antiacetylcholine receptor antibodies. The antigenic stimulus for antibody production may come from damaged muscle end-plate fragments or myoid cells within the thymus.[25] Damage to the muscle end-plate by acetylcholine receptor antibodies may initiate the production of antimuscle antibodies. Although the origin of the antibodies is unknown, the thymus gland undoubtedly occupies a central role. Indeed, 15–20% of patients with myasthenia gravis have thymomas. Thymomas are more likely to occur in patients older than 30 yr of age, whereas thymic hyperplasia frequently occurs in younger patients. Remission of the disease is common after thymectomy is performed. Many myasthenic patients also have antinuclear, antithyroid, and antimuscle autoantibodies.[26]

The clinical hallmark of myasthenia gravis is skeletal muscle weakness. Typically there are periods of exacerbations alternating with remissions.

There are several types of myasthenia gravis. The classification is based on the skeletal muscle groups that are affected. Types of myasthenia gravis include generalized, ocular, bulbar, and shoulder girdle. The course of the disease is frequently affected by environmental, physical, and emotional changes. Viral illness, pregnancy, and surgery may affect the patient with myasthenia gravis, but not predictably.[27] Patients with myasthenia gravis, especially those with thymoma, may have myasthenia gravis–related heart disease. Focal myocarditis is observed on examination of cardiac muscle. Clinically this myocarditis produces cardiac dysrhythmias, particularly atrial fibrillation and atrioventricular block.[28]

Pregnancy may produce either exacerbation or remission of

the disease. Forty per cent of pregnant women do have increased symptoms during gestation. Postpartum respiratory failure and death can occur. Fifteen to 20% of neonates born to myasthenic women have transient myasthenia resulting from the passive transfer of antiacetylcholine receptor antibodies. Neonatal myasthenia begins 12–48 h after birth and may persist for several weeks. Neonatal skeletal muscle strength must be monitored carefully during the early neonatal period.[29]

Treatment modalities for myasthenia gravis may include the use of the following: cholinesterase inhibitors, thymectomy, corticosteroids, and immunosuppressive therapy. Pyridostigmine is the most frequently used cholinesterase inhibitor. Consistent control of myasthenia with cholinesterase inhibitors can be quite challenging. Underdosage will result in increased skeletal muscle weakness, but an overdose will produce a "cholinergic crisis." Excessive doses of cholinesterase inhibitors will produce abdominal cramping, diarrhea, vomiting, and skeletal muscle weakness that mimics the weakness of myasthenia.

Management of Anesthesia

The primary concern for anesthesia for the patient with myasthenia gravis is the potential interaction between the disease, treatment of the disease, and neuromuscular blocking drugs. The myasthenic patient is exquisitely sensitive to nondepolarizing muscle relaxants. Even small defasciculating doses of nondepolarizing muscle relaxants can produce significant respiratory muscle paralysis. Vecuronium and atracurium, because of their relatively rapid elimination, are useful nondepolarizing drugs for patients with myasthenia.[30–33] The response to succinylcholine is unpredictable. The untreated myasthenic patient demonstrates a resistance to succinylcholine. The myasthenic patient treated with cholinesterase inhibitors may exhibit a prolonged response to succinylcholine, although this occurrence is poorly documented. Because of the patient's unpredictable response to succinylcholine, a nondepolarizing muscle relaxant is often preferred. Regardless of the muscle relaxant that is used, careful monitoring with a peripheral nerve stimulator is highly recommended. Patients with myasthenia gravis are clinically more sensitive to the ventilatory depressant effects of barbiturates, inhaled anesthetics, and opioids.

Ventilatory function must be monitored carefully in the myasthenic patient in the postoperative period. The unpredictable interactions of the disease, treatment drugs, and anesthetic drugs can make postoperative mechanical ventilation of the lungs necessary. The need for postoperative mechanical ventilation is substantially increased when transsternal thymectomy is used as opposed to transcervical thymectomy.[34–36] The patient with myasthenia gravis requiring mechanical ventilation can be one of the most challenging to wean from ventilatory support. Skeletal muscle strength can vary significantly in a short period of time. It is imperative that sustained respiratory muscle strength be confirmed before extubation of the trachea and resumption of spontaneous ventilation.

Exacerbation of myasthenia gravis may occur in the pregnant patient during late pregnancy and the early postpartum period. Consequently, skeletal muscle relaxation produced by regional anesthesia in conjunction with inherent muscle weakness may lead to hypoventilation. Regional analgesia and anesthesia have been used successfully in myasthenic patients, but careful monitoring is necessary. Because 15 to 20% of infants born to myasthenic mothers may exhibit transient neonatal myasthenia within 1–21 days of birth, anti-cholinesterase therapy and mechanical ventilation of the lungs may be necessary.

MYASTHENIC SYNDROME (EATON-LAMBERT SYNDROME)

The myasthenic syndrome is a disorder of neuromuscular transmission associated with carcinomas, particularly small cell carcinoma of the lung. This disorder is sometimes diagnosed inaccurately as myasthenia gravis. Typically the patient is a 50 to 70-yr-old man complaining of proximal extremity muscle weakness. Unlike myasthenia gravis, the patient with myasthenic syndrome generally has increasing skeletal muscle strength with exercise and has no improvement after anticholinesterase drugs are administered. It is believed that the basic lesion is a presynaptic abnormality that results in a decreased release of acetylcholine by nerve stimulation.[37] 4-aminopyridine, which acts in the presynaptic region, reverses skeletal muscle weakness in patients with myasthenic syndrome.[38]

Patients with myasthenic syndrome are sensitive to the effects of both depolarizing and nondepolarizing muscle relaxants. Consequently, the doses of these drugs should be reduced, and neuromuscular function should be monitored carefully. Because this syndrome is difficult to diagnose, a high index of suspicion must be maintained in patients who have diagnostic procedures such as bronchoscopic or mediastinoscopic examination or exploratory thoracotomy for suspected carcinoma of the lung.

FAMILIAL PERIODIC PARALYSIS

Familial periodic paralysis is characterized by intermittent but acute episodes of skeletal muscle weakness or paralysis. At-tacks begin when patients are in early childhood and may persist throughout their lives, although the frequency of episodes declines during middle age. There are three recognized forms of familial periodic paralysis: hypokalemic, normokalemic, and hyperkalemic (Table 16-2). It is believed that the defect involves abnormalities in the membrane transport of potassium and sodium.[39] The subsequent alterations in muscle membrane potentials may render the skeletal muscle inexcitable.

In the hypokalemic form, paralysis may be produced in the patient by his or her ingestion of carbohydrate loads, strenuous exercise, and infusion of glucose and insulin. Paralysis is generally incomplete and affects the limb and trunk muscles but spares the diaphragm. The low serum levels of potassium during acute episodes often produce cardiac dysrhythmias. Treatment consists of potassium infusion and administration of acetazolamide or dichlorophenamide (carbonic anhydrase inhibitors).[40] Permanent skeletal muscle weakness can occur in some patients with hypokalemic familial periodic paralysis.[41] There are several anesthetic considerations. If possible, any potassium abnormalities should be corrected before operation. During periods of hypokalemia these patients may be sensitive to nondepolarizing muscle relaxants. Because they have unpredictable responses to neuromuscular blocking drugs, doses should be reduced and the response monitored with a peripheral nerve stimulator. Metabolic changes (alkalosis) or medications (glucose and insulin, diuretics) that reduce serum potassium may initiate an episode of paralysis.[42] It would be desirable to measure serum potassium levels during prolonged use of anesthetics. The ECG should be monitored continuously during use of anesthesia for evidence of cardiac dysrhythmias secondary to hypokalemia. After surgery, adequate skeletal muscle strength must be ascertained before mechanical ventilation of the lungs is discontinued. Other recommendations include the avoidance of large carbohydrate loads and hypothermia. It should be remembered that any cause of severe potassium depletion, such as renal

TABLE 16-2. Clinical Features of Familial Periodic Paralysis

TYPE	SERUM POTASSIUM CONCENTRATION DURING ATTACK	PRECIPITATING FACTORS	OTHER FEATURES
Hypokalemic	<3 mEq·l^{-1}	Large meals Rest after strenuous exercise Glucose and insulin infusion	Changes of hypokalemia on electrocardiogram Cardiac dysrhythmias Sensitivity to nondepolarizing muscle relaxants
Normokalemic	3–5.5 mEq·l^{-1}	Alcohol Exercise Emotional stress	Muscle weakness persisting for as long as 14 days
Hyperkalemic	>5.5 mEq·l^{-1}	Exercise Potassium infusion Exposure to cold	Muscle weakness often localized to tongue and eyelids Sensitivity to succinylcholine

(Gibbs PS, Kim KC: Skin and musculoskeletal diseases. In Stoelting RK, Dierdorf SF [eds]: Anesthesia and Co-Existing Disease. New York, Churchill Livingstone, 1988. Reproduced with permission of the authors and publisher.)

tubular acidosis and chronic diarrhea, can also produce skeletal muscle weakness.[43, 44]

Hyperkalemic periodic paralysis is also characterized by episodic skeletal muscle weakness that develops in association with increased serum levels of potassium. Attacks may be initiated by fasting, cold, rest after exercise, or potassium administration. Acute episodes of paralysis generally are treated with acetazolamide or diuretics. Epinephrine and metaproterenol are also effective.[39] This disorder may be confused with paramyotonia because cold may trigger skeletal muscle weakness in patients with either disease. The use of succinylcholine is best avoided because it may enhance potassium loss from muscle cells and further increase serum potassium levels. Because of the potential for cardiac dysrhythmias, continuous ECG monitoring is recommended. If fasting is required, an intravenous infusion of glucose should be administered. Normothermia also must be maintained during anesthesia.

Normokalemic periodic paralysis can be triggered by a variety of stimuli, including alcohol ingestion, exercise, and emotional stress. Duration of skeletal muscle paralysis is quite variable but may exceed 14 days. Recorded anesthesia experience with this form of periodic paralysis is extremely limited. Cardiac tachydysrhythmias are common during attacks. Anesthetic considerations are similar to those for the hypokalemic form.[45]

GUILLAIN-BARRÉ SYNDROME (POLYRADICULONEURITIS)

Guillain-Barré syndrome (polyradiculoneuritis, acute idiopathic polyneuritis) is characterized by the acute or subacute onset of skeletal muscle weakness or paralysis in the legs. Sensory disturbances such as paresthesias often precede the paralysis. Typically, the paralysis progresses cephalad within a few days to include the muscles of the trunk and arms. Difficulty in swallowing and impaired ventilation resulting from intercostal muscle paralysis often occur. A variety of etiologic agents have been implicated, such as viruses (cytomegalovirus, para-influenza 2, herpes, measles, infectious mononucleosis), vaccinations, and prior surgical procedures. Nerve demyelination that occurs is felt to be immunologically mediated with a virus serving as an antigen.

Fifty per cent of patients with Guillain-Barré syndrome have a history of respiratory or gastrointestinal illness within 4 weeks of the onset of the neuropathy.[46] Although 85% of patients with this syndrome obtain a good or full recovery, chronic or recurrent neuropathy occurs in 3–5%. Treatment is primarily supportive particularly of the respiratory and cardiovascular systems. Controversial therapeutic modalities include the use of corticosteroids and plasmapheresis.

The most serious immediate problem is ventilatory insufficiency. The vital capacity should be monitored frequently. If the vital capacity decreases to 15 or 20 ml·kg^{-1}, then mechanical ventilation of the lungs is indicated.[47] The more rapid the onset of quadriplegia, the more likely the need for prolonged ventilatory support.[48]

Autonomic nervous system dysfunction occurs in many patients with Guillain-Barré syndrome. This dysfunction can produce wide fluctuations in blood pressure, tachycardia, cardiac dysrhythmias, and cardiac arrest.[49] Physical stimulation of the patient often precipitates hypertension, tachycardia, and cardiac dysrhythmias. Alpha- and beta-adrenergic blockade may be required for those patients.[50]

Management of Anesthesia

Autonomic nervous system dysfunction indicates that compensatory cardiovascular responses may be absent, resulting in significant hypotension secondary to postural changes, blood loss, or positive airway pressure. On the other hand, noxious stimuli such as laryngoscopic examination may produce exaggerated increases in heart rate and blood pressure. Direct acting vasopressors or vasodilators may be required to control the blood pressure. The cardiovascular system must be carefully monitored.

Use of succinylcholine may be avoided because of the danger of drug-induced potassium release and hyperkalemia. A nondepolarizing muscle relaxant with minimal cardiovascular effects, such as vecuronium, would be a useful choice for muscle relaxation. It is likely that mechanical ventilatory support will be required during the immediate postoperative period. Patients with Guillain-Barré syndrome who have pronounced sensory disturbances may benefit from the use of epidural opioids.[51]

It should be remembered that it can be very difficult to differentiate Guillain-Barré syndrome from anterior spinal artery syndrome in critically ill patients.[52]

CENTRAL NERVOUS SYSTEM DISEASES

MULTIPLE SCLEROSIS

Multiple sclerosis is an acquired disease of the central nervous system characterized by multiple sites of demyelination in the brain and spinal cord. Plaques of demyelination are found most often in areas along spinal fluid pathways. The optic tracts and periventricular regions have a particular predilection for plaque formation.[53] Multiple sclerosis is primarily a disease of young adults, with the onset of symptoms occurring when patients are between the ages of 15 and 40 yr.

The cause of multiple sclerosis appears to be multifactorial. The current theory is that multiple sclerosis is caused by a virus that either persists in the central nervous system or induces an autoimmunity.[54] The geographic correlation relative to susceptibility is impressive. The high-risk areas include the United States, Great Britain, Scandinavia, Europe, and New Zealand.

The symptoms of multiple sclerosis depend on the sites of demyelination in the brain and spinal cord. Demyelination of the optic nerves results in visual disturbances, whereas demyelination of oculomotor pathways usually produces nystagmus. Lesions of the spinal cord cause limb weakness and paresthesias. The legs are affected more frequently than the arms. Bowel retention and urinary incontinence are frequent complaints. Involvement of the brain stem can produce diplopia, trigeminal neuralgia, and, rarely, alterations in ventilation.[55] The course of multiple sclerosis is characterized by exacerbations of symptoms at unpredictable intervals over a period of several years. Residual symptoms eventually persist during remission and may lead to severe disability. In some patients the course is relatively benign, with infrequent periods of demyelination followed by prolonged remission. Pregnancy is generally associated with an improvement in multiple sclerosis, but the postpartum period is often associated with a high incidence of the appearance of new symptoms.[56]

The diagnosis of multiple sclerosis is made primarily on clinical determinations, although certain laboratory findings support the clinical diagnosis. Seventy per cent of patients with multiple sclerosis have elevated levels of immunoglobulin G in the cerebrospinal fluid. Magnetic resonance imaging

(MRI) is very sensitive in detecting the lesions of multiple sclerosis and indicating the severity of clinical disease.[57]

There is no known cure for multiple sclerosis. Corticosteroids or adrenocorticotrophic hormone (ACTH) are frequently used to promote remission. Immunosuppressive therapy with azathioprine and cyclophosphamide has also been used but with varying results.[58] Plasmapheresis has been employed with some benefit. Drugs used to treat skeletal muscle spasticity associated with multiple sclerosis include diazepam, dantrolene, and baclofen. Painful dysesthesias, tonic seizures, dysarthria, and ataxia are often treated with carbamazepine. Nonspecific therapeutic measures include the avoidance of excessive fatigue, emotional stress, and hyperthermia. Demyelinated fibers are extremely sensitive to increases in temperature. A temperature increase of as little as 0.5°C may block conduction in demyelinated fibers.[59]

Management of Anesthesia

The effect of surgery and anesthesia on the course of multiple sclerosis is controversial. Some reports indicate that symptoms of multiple sclerosis are exacerbated by anesthesia, particularly regional anesthesia.[60, 61] However, other studies report that anesthesia does not affect the course of multiple sclerosis.[55, 62] An unacceptably high number of patients with multiple sclerosis who receive spinal anesthesia do have an exacerbation of symptoms develop.[63] It could be speculated that demyelinated fibers might be more sensitive to the effects of local anesthetics. This increased sensitivity could explain exacerbations after anesthesia. Intrathecal morphine in conjunction with a combined spinal and general anesthetic has been used successfully in a patient with multiple sclerosis.[64] Certainly pyrexia and, most likely, metabolic changes induced by surgery and anesthesia can produce exacerbations of symptoms independent of the type of anesthesia. Despite the seeming confusion in the medical literature, certain conclusions seem warranted. Before operation the patient with multiple sclerosis should be advised that surgery and anesthesia could produce exacerbations of their disease despite a well-managed anesthetic. The patient should have a thorough neurologic examination before operation to document co-existing neurologic deficits. After surgery the neurologic examination can be repeated so that findings can be compared. In view of the fact that spinal anesthesia can cause unpredictable exacerbations, use of this type of anesthesia should be reserved for special situations. The patient's temperature should be monitored closely during anesthesia, and even slight temperature elevations must be treated actively.

Selection of agents for general anesthesia should take into consideration potential interactions with medications the patient is receiving. For example, patients receiving corticosteroids may need corticosteroid supplementation during the perioperative period. Theoretically succinylcholine could produce an exaggerated release of potassium, although this has not been reported in patients with multiple sclerosis. Anticonvulsants such as carbamazepine and phenytoin can produce resistance to nondepolarizing muscle relaxants.[65]

Autonomic dysfunction caused by multiple sclerosis may produce exaggerated hypotensive effects of volatile anesthetics. Consequently, careful monitoring of cardiovascular function is indicated.

EPILEPSY

A seizure disorder is a common manifestation of many types of central nervous system diseases. A seizure results from the excessive discharge of large numbers of neurons that become depolarized in a synchronous fashion. Idiopathic seizures generally begin when patients are children. The sudden onset of seizures in an adult should arouse suspicion of focal brain disease, particularly a tumor.

There are several types of seizures.

Grand Mal Seizure

A grand mal seizure is characterized by generalized tonic-clonic activity. All respiratory activity is arrested, and a period of arterial hypoxemia ensues. The tonic phase lasts for 20–40 s and is followed by the clonic phase. In the postictal phase the patient is lethargic and confused. Initial treatment is directed toward maintaining arterial oxygenation and stopping the seizure activity. Diazepam or thiopental are effective drugs for the treatment of acute seizures. Antiseizure drugs effective for control and prevention are phenytoin, valproate, and carbamazepine.

Focal Cortical Seizure

Focal cortical seizures, also known as Jacksonian epilepsy, may be sensory or motor, depending on the site of neuronal discharge. Usually there is no loss of consciousness, although the seizure activity may spread to produce a grand mal seizure.

Petit Mal Seizure

Petit mal seizures are characterized by a brief loss of awareness lasting about 30 s. Additional manifestations include staring, blinking, and rolling the eyes. Drugs used for treatment of petit mal seizures include valproate and ethosuximide.

Akinetic Seizure

Akinetic seizures are characterized by a sudden, brief loss of consciousness and loss of postural tone.

Myoclonic Seizure

Myoclonic seizures occur as isolated clonic jerks in response to a sensory stimulus. In most cases a single group of skeletal muscles is involved. Myoclonic seizures are often associated with degenerative and metabolic brain diseases.

Psychomotor Seizure

Psychomotor seizures are seen as an impairment of consciousness, inappropriate motor acts, hallucinations, amnesia, and unusual visceral symptoms. This type of seizure is usually preceded by an aura.

Status Epilepticus

Status epilepticus is a seizure disorder in which the seizure activity occurs unabated for 30 min or longer. Status epilepticus can include all types of seizure activity. Grand mal status epilepticus is of the greatest concern because mortality can be as high as 20%. Typically grand mal status epilepticus lasts for 48 h, with a seizure frequency of four to five per hour. As the seizures progress, skeletal muscle activity diminishes and seizure activity may only be evident on the electroencephalogram (EEG). Respiratory effects of status epilepticus include inhibition of respiratory centers, uncoordinated skeletal muscle activity that impairs ventilation, and abnormal autonomic activity that produces bronchoconstriction. In addition to the danger of arterial hypoxemia from inadequate airway control, there is a high likelihood of permanent neuronal damage by continued seizures.[66] Diazepam is considered the drug of choice for the treatment of status epilepticus. Because the effect of diazepam is transient, a longer acting anticonvulsant also must be administered. Thiopental is also quite effective for the initial treatment of status epilepticus, but the effect is transient. Muscle relaxants may be required for tracheal intubation if a secured airway is necessary. Although muscle relaxants will terminate the skeletal muscle manifestations of a seizure, there will be no effect on seizure activity in the brain. On rare occasions general anesthesia with halothane or isoflurane may be required for the treatment of status epilepticus.

Management of Anesthesia

Patients receiving anticonvulsant medications should be maintained on their normal medication regimen until the time of surgery. After operation, medications should be given parenterally until oral intake can be resumed. In management of anesthesia for the patient with a seizure disorder, the potential influence of anticonvulsant drugs on the response to anesthesia must be considered (Table 16-3). Conversely, an anesthetic technique must be used that will not increase the likelihood of seizure activity. Because anticonvulsant drugs affect the liver and neuromuscular systems, the potential for significant drug interaction certainly exists. Stimulation of hepatic microsomal enzymes by phenobarbital may accelerate and increase the magnitude of biotransformation of anesthetic drugs. Increased biotransformation of the volatile halogenated anesthetics may increase the risk of organ toxicity. Other known side effects of anticonvulsants include leukopenia, anemia, and hepatitis from phenytoin; pancreatitis and hepatic failure from valproate; and aplastic anemia and cardiotoxicity from carbamazepine.

Although most inhaled anesthetics, including nitrous oxide, have been reported to produce seizure activity, seizure activity during administration of halothane or isoflurane anesthesia is extremely rare. Enflurane predictably produces spike and wave activity on the EEG, particularly when hypocarbia exists. Children seem to be particularly susceptible to enflurane-induced seizure activity.[67] It would seem that halothane or isoflurane would be preferable to enflurane for anesthesia for patients with seizure disorders.

The use of ketamine is controversial. Ketamine has been shown to produce seizure activity in patients with known seizure disorders. However, there are also data indicating that ketamine is safe to use for patients with seizure disorders. It would seem reasonable to avoid the use of ketamine for patients with seizure disorders because alternative induction drugs such as barbiturates and benzodiazepines are available.[68]

Seizure-like activity has been reported to occur after the administration of fentanyl and sufentanil; however, other studies have found no seizure activity after use of fentanyl or sufentanil.[69-74] The reported seizure-like activity may represent myoclonic activity or a form of opioid-induced skeletal muscle rigidity. In relatively high doses fentanyl and sufentanil may produce seizures.[75, 76] High-dose fentanyl (200–400 $\mu g \cdot kg^{-1}$) or sufentanil (40–160 $\mu g \cdot kg^{-1}$) should be used with caution in patients with seizure disorders.

Methohexital has also been reported to produce seizures in children.[77] Certainly methohexital has been used for many patients with seizure disorders without adverse effects. Although methohexital may not be contraindicated in patients with seizures, thiopental would be a useful alternative.

Another potential drug interaction in patients receiving phenytoin and carbamazepine is their resistance to nondepolarizing muscle relaxants.[65, 78] The mechanism for this resistance appears to be pharmacodynamic rather than pharmacokinetic.

The patient with a seizure disorder should receive his or her normal therapeutic drug regimen up to and including the morning of surgery. After operation this regimen should be reinstituted as quickly as possible. A decline in blood levels of anticonvulsant drugs will only increase the likelihood of perioperative seizures.

PARKINSON'S DISEASE (PARALYSIS AGITANS)

Parkinson's disease is a degenerative disease of the central nervous system caused by loss of dopaminergic fibers in the basal ganglia of the brain. Subsequently dopamine is depleted in the basal ganglia. Recent discoveries have shown that Parkinson's disease is clearly secondary to dopamine deficiency.[79] Dopamine depletion produces diminished inhibition of the extrapyramidal motor system and unopposed action of acetylcholine. Parkinson's disease is one of the more common disabling neurologic diseases and affects 2.5% of the population older than 65 yr.

The typical features of Parkinson's disease include decreases in spontaneous movements, cogwheel rigidity of the extremities, facial immobility, and a rhythmic tremor at rest. These features are all secondary to diminished inhibition of

TABLE 16-3.   Anticonvulsant Drugs

DRUG	TYPE OF SEIZURE	THERAPEUTIC BLOOD LEVEL ($\mu g \cdot ml^{-1}$)	SIDE-EFFECTS
Phenobarbital	Generalized	15–35	Sedation, increased drug metabolism
Valproate	Generalized; petit mal	50–100	Pancreatitis, hepatic dysfunction
Phenytoin	Generalized; partial	10–20	Gingival hyperplasia, dermatitis, resistance to nondepolarizers
Carbamazepine	Generalized; partial	6–12	Cardiotoxic, hepatitis, resistance to nondepolarizers
Ethosuximide	Petit mal	40–100	Leukopenia, erythema multiforme
Primidone	Generalized; partial	6–12	Nausea, ataxia
Clonazepam	Petit mal	0.01–0.07	Ataxia

(Modified from The Medical Letter 28:91, 1986)

the extrapyramidal motor system as a result of depletion of dopamine from the basal ganglia. Other features that occur commonly in patients with Parkinson's disease include seborrhea, pupillary abnormalities, diaphragmatic spasm, and oculogyric crises. Mental depression can be severe enough to necessitate the use of antidepressant medications.

Parkinson's disease may be caused by a variety of disorders, including metabolic disorders; chemical agents; intracranial tumors; and arteriosclerotic changes. Other than in sporadic episodes of postencephalitic Parkinson's disease, there is no evidence that Parkinson's disease is caused by a virus.[80]

The treatment of Parkinson's disease is directed toward increasing dopamine levels in the brain and preventing adverse peripheral effects of dopamine. Consequently treatment protocols involve combinations of drugs used to achieve those goals. This approach does increase the likelihood of undesirable drug interactions, however. Levodopa, the immediate precursor of dopamine, is clearly the drug of choice for the treatment of Parkinson's disease. Unlike dopamine, levodopa can cross the blood–brain barrier and is converted to dopamine. Because the decarboxylating enzyme responsible for converting levodopa to dopamine is also present outside the brain, the dose of levodopa must be increased to compensate for systemic degradation. The addition of a peripheral decarboxylase inhibitor such as carbidopa or benserazide reduces the levodopa requirement. Currently, the combination of levodopa and carbidopa is the most effective drug available for the treatment of Parkinson's disease.[81] Patients receiving prolonged levodopa therapy may become less sensitive to levodopa and require increased doses. Side effects of levodopa administration include depletion of myocardial norepinephrine stores, peripheral vasoconstriction, and decreased intravascular fluid volume with resultant orthostatic hypotension. Bromocriptine, pergolide, and lisuride are dopaminergic agents that can relieve the tremor and rigidity of Parkinson's disease. Side effects of bromocriptine administration include hallucinations, nausea, orthostatic hypotension, angina pectoris, Raynaud-like digital vascular spasms, and cardiac dysrhythmias. Domperidone, a dopamine receptor antagonist, also prevents the peripheral side effects of dopamine agonists. Domperidone does not cross the blood–brain barrier or interfere with the effective treatment of Parkinson's disease. Because decreased dopamine activity in the basal ganglia enhances the excitatory effects of acetylcholine, anticholinergic drugs such as trihexyphenidyl, benztropine, and diphenhydramine are often administered to patients with Parkinson's disease. Amantadine is an antiviral drug that also increases the release of dopamine in the brain. The effects of amantadine are usually short lived.

Deprenyl (not yet approved in the United States) is a selective monoamine oxidase-B inhibitor that prevents degradation of dopamine in the brain. Consequently, the central action of levodopa is enhanced. Because of the synergism between deprenyl and levodopa, this combination reduces the incidence of levodopa side effects. Deprenyl is metabolized to methamphetamine and amphetamine, however, and can produce sympathomimetic activity. Deprenyl does not produce hypertensive crises when administered with levodopa.[82]

Management of Anesthesia

Management of anesthesia is generally determined by potential interaction between anesthesia drugs and anti-Parkinson medications. The patient's therapeutic regimen should be administered the morning of surgery. The half-life of levodopa is

short, and interruption of therapy for more than 6–12 h can result in severe skeletal muscle rigidity that interferes with ventilation. Phenothiazines and butyrophenones (droperidol) should be avoided because these drugs antagonize the effects of dopamine in the basal ganglia. The use of ketamine is controversial. Ketamine could potentially produce an exaggerated sympathetic nervous system response with resultant tachycardia and hypertension. Despite this concern, ketamine has been used without difficulty in patients treated with levodopa.[83] Theoretically halothane could cause cardiac dysrhythmias in patients receiving levodopa, but this has not been documented. The choice of muscle relaxant does not seem to be influenced by the presence of Parkinson's disease. However, there is a report of one patient in whom hyperkalemia developed after the administration of succinylcholine.[84] The significance of this isolated occurrence is not known.

The potential hazards of drug interactions in patients taking monoamine oxidase inhibitors are well known to anesthesiologists. The preliminary success with the use of deprenyl, a MAO-B inhibitor, for the treatment of Parkinson's disease increases the likelihood of having to anesthetize a patient who is receiving MAO inhibitors. There are no reported experiences of patients receiving deprenyl and anesthesia. B-type MAO enzyme acts on phenylethylamine, benzylamine, tyramine, and dopamine, with little effect on epinephrine and norepinephrine.[85] Conceivably there might be less risk of massive sympathetic discharge in patients receiving selective MAO-B inhibitors. Until this is substantiated, however, one should observe the usual precautions for patients receiving MAO inhibitors.

HUNTINGTON'S CHOREA

Huntington's chorea is a premature degenerative disease of the central nervous system characterized by marked atrophy of the basal ganglia. Neurochemical analysis of the brain reveals reductions in gamma-aminobutyric acid (GABA) and acetylcholine.[86] This disease is transmitted as an autosomal dominant trait, but its delayed appearance until a patient is 35–40 yr of age interferes with effective counseling and early diagnosis. It is hoped that recent genetic discoveries may lead to more effective genetic screening.

Disordered movement is the clinical hallmark of Huntington's chorea. In addition to the choreoathetosis, progressive dementia occurs. The disease progresses for several years, and accompanying mental depression makes suicide a frequent occurrence. Death usually results from malnutrition and aspiration pneumonitis. The duration of Huntington's chorea averages 17 yr from onset of symptoms to death.

There is no specific therapy for Huntington's chorea. Pharmacotherapy is directed toward relief of mental depression and movement disorders. The most useful therapy for control of involuntary movements is with drugs that interfere with the neurotransmitter effects of dopamine. Consequently the butyrophenones and phenothiazines may be helpful.

Management of Anesthesia

As the disease progresses and the pharyngeal muscles become more involved, the risk of aspiration pneumonitis increases. Consequently, appropriate antiaspiration maneuvers must be employed. If preoperative and postoperative sedation are necessary, the butyrophenones or phenothiazines are logical choices. Reported anesthetic experience with patients with Huntington's chorea is too limited to allow the proposal of specific anesthetic techniques. There are no specific contraindications to the use of intravenous or inhaled anesthetics. Delayed awakening and generalized tonic spasms have been observed after the administration of thiopental to one patient.[87] The significance of this observation is not clear. Decreased plasma cholinesterase activity, with a prolonged response to succinylcholine, has also been reported.[88] It has also been suggested that these patients may be sensitive to the effects of nondepolarizing muscle relaxants.[89]

ALZHEIMER'S DISEASE

Alzheimer's disease is the major cause of dementia in the United States. More than 2 million persons in the United States are afflicted with Alzheimer's disease, and it is the major reason patients are admitted to nursing homes. As life expectancy for men and women increases, a larger proportion of the population will be susceptible to this disease. Although dementia can be caused by more than 60 disorders, Alzheimer's disease causes 50–60% of the cases. Dementia is characterized by intellectual and cognitive deterioration that impairs social function. The clinical diagnosis of Alzheimer's disease can be made if a patient exhibits loss of memory and deficits in two or more areas of cognition. A mental status examination is central to the diagnosis of Alzheimer's disease. Any systemic causes of dementia, such as cerebral vascular disease, must be eliminated before the diagnosis of Alzheimer's disease is made. A cerebral computed tomography (CT) scan and EEG are helpful in diagnosis. Pathologic findings in the brain include a characteristic cortical atrophy and the presence of neurofibrillary tangles and neuritic plaques. Functionally there is a decrease in choline acetyltransferase and a subsequent cholinergic deficit. Interestingly, some studies have demonstrated an improvement in memory after the administration of physostigmine.[90] Unfortunately this effect is short lived. Aluminum and aluminum silicate are found in the neurofibrillary tangles, but the significance of this finding is not clear. Many patients with Alzheimer's disease also have a history of significant head trauma (loss of consciousness).[91] A small proportion of patients with Alzheimer's disease have a familial history for the disease.

Because there is no specific therapy for Alzheimer's disease, symptoms are treated. Medications may be used to treat the symptoms of mental depression or agitation.

Management of Anesthesia

No specific complications have been reported with anesthesia for patients with Alzheimer's disease. A few speculations and suggestions do seem warranted. Because of dementia these patients may be disoriented and uncooperative. Sedative drugs, as might be used for preoperative medication, should be administered rarely, because further mental confusion could result. There are no specific contraindications to use of intravenous anesthesia, although an inhaled anesthetic would permit a more predictable return to the patient's preoperative level of mental function. If an anticholinergic drug is required, glycopyrrolate, which does not cross the blood–brain barrier, would be preferable to scopolamine or atropine. Theoretically an anticholinergic drug that enters the brain could exacerbate the dementia. Finally, the patient's preoperative medication

list should be reviewed for the possibility of interaction with anesthetics.

AMYOTROPHIC LATERAL SCLEROSIS

Amyotrophic lateral sclerosis (ALS) is a degenerative disease of motor cells throughout the central nervous system and spinal cord. Progression of the disease is relentless, and death generally follows within 3 years of diagnosis. Upper and lower motor neurons are involved almost exclusively. The cause of ALS is unknown, but proposed causes include a slow viral infection, toxins, immune dysfunction, impaired DNA repair, altered axonal transport, and trauma.[92]

The signs and symptoms reflect the upper and lower motor neuron dysfunction. Frequently reported initial manifestations are atrophy, weakness, and fasciculation of skeletal muscles, often beginning in the intrinsic muscles of the hand. As the disease progresses, the atrophy and weakness involve most skeletal muscles, including those of the tongue, pharynx, larynx, and chest. Early symptoms of bulbar involvement include tongue fasciculations and dysphagia with pulmonary aspiration. Extraocular muscles usually are not involved. Respiratory failure eventually results, and mechanical ventilation of the lungs is necessary.

Many therapeutic agents have been tried with little success. Preliminary studies with the administration of thyrotropin-releasing hormone have produced transient improvements in some patients with ALS.[93]

Management of Anesthesia

Patients with lower motor neuron diseases such as amyotrophic lateral sclerosis are vulnerable to hyperkalemia after administration of succinylcholine. Patients with ALS also may have a prolonged response to nondepolarizing muscle relaxants. Bulbar involvement with dysfunction of pharyngeal muscles may predispose these patients to pulmonary aspiration. Use of postoperative ventilatory support is highly likely for the patient with ALS. There is no evidence that a specific anesthetic drug or combination of drugs is best for patients with ALS.

CREUTZFELDT-JAKOB DISEASE

Creutzfeldt-Jakob disease is one of three diseases that constitute the class of diseases known as the human spongiform encephalopathies. The other two diseases in this group are kuru and Gerstmann-Staussler syndrome. These disorders are most likely caused by an infectious agent, probably an atypical virus. These diseases are somewhat unique infectious diseases in that the incubation time is long (years) and there is an absence of fever and inflammation. Creutzfeldt-Jakob disease is much less common than multiple sclerosis, but, like multiple sclerosis, Creutzfeldt-Jakob disease is noted for its diverse presentations and varied neurologic signs.[94]

The typical clinical characteristics include subacute dementia, myoclonus, and electroencephalographic changes. The EEG pattern is relatively characteristic, with diffuse slow activity and periodic complexes. Because of the dementia and wide array of presenting symptoms, patients with Creutzfeldt-Jakob disease are often misdiagnosed as having psychiatric disorders. There is no specific therapeutic drug for Creutzfeldt-Jakob disease. Several antiviral drugs such as amantadine, idoxuridine, interferon, and vidarabine have been employed but with little success.

Management of Anesthesia

Creutzfeldt-Jakob disease should be regarded as transmissible. There are reports of cases developing after accidental inoculation and after surgery.[95-98] Consequently, appropriate precautions should be taken to protect other patients and medical staff persons. Three to 10% formalin and 70% alcohol do not inactivate the Creutzfeldt-Jakob virus. Sodium hypochlorite 0.5% and sterilization with steam and ethylene oxide will destroy the virus.[99]

Although reported anesthetic experience with Creutzfeldt-Jakob disease is limited, certain speculations and recommendations seem warranted. Patients with degenerative neurologic diseases are prone to aspirate gastric contents because they have impaired swallowing and decreased laryngeal reflexes. Therefore, appropriate antiaspiration maneuvers are indicated during anesthesia. Because lower motor neuron dysfunction also occurs in patients with Creutzfeldt-Jakob disease, use of succinylcholine should be avoided. The autonomic nervous system may also be involved.[100] This may produce abnormal cardiovascular responses to anesthesia and vasoactive drugs.

ANEMIAS

The causes of anemia are numerous (Table 16-4). Anemias can be conveniently classified as nutritional deficiency anemias, hemolytic anemias, hemoglobinopathies, and hemoglobin deficiency syndromes (thalassemia).

Irrespective of the cause of the anemia, compensatory physiologic mechanisms develop to offset the decreased oxygen-carrying capacity. Typically, an otherwise healthy person will not have symptoms develop from anemia until his or her hemoglobin level decreases below 7 g·dl^{-1}. Symptoms are highly variable and depend on other concurrent disease processes. Physiologic compensation includes increased plasma volume, increased cardiac output, and increased levels of red blood cell 2,3-diphosphoglycerate (2,3-DPG) (Table 16-5). Maximum levels of red blood cell 2,3-DPG will increase oxygen delivery by 30%.[101] Because elderly patients with chronic anemia have an increased plasma volume, transfusion of whole blood to these patients may result in congestive heart failure. Similarly, the myocardial depressant effects of anesthetics may be exaggerated in patients with increased cardiac output at rest as compensation for anemia.

TABLE 16-5.   Compensatory Mechanisms to Increase Oxygen Delivery with Chronic Anemia

Increased cardiac output
Increased red blood cell 2,3-diphosphoglycerate levels
Increased P_{50}
Increased plasma volume
Decreased blood viscosity

NUTRITIONAL DEFICIENCY ANEMIAS

The three primary causes of nutritional deficiency anemias are iron deficiency, vitamin B_{12} deficiency, and folic acid deficiency.

Iron deficiency anemia produces the typical microcytic hypochromic red blood cell. Iron deficiency may be an absolute deficiency secondary to decreased oral intake or a relative deficiency caused by rapid turnover of red blood cells (e.g., hemolysis).

Absorption of vitamin B_{12} by the gastrointestinal tract depends on production of intrinsic factor. Intrinsic factor is a glycoprotein produced by gastric parietal cells. Atrophy of the gastric mucosa will cause a vitamin B_{12} deficiency and a megaloblastic anemia. Vitamin B_{12} deficiency also causes a peripheral neuropathy because of degeneration of the lateral and posterior columns of the spinal cord. The neuropathy is manifest by symmetric paresthesias with loss of proprioception and vibratory sensation, especially in the lower extremities. Parenteral vitamin B_{12} will reverse both the hematologic and neurologic changes. The neurologic abnormalities must be considered when regional anesthesia or peripheral nerve blocks might be used. Nitrous oxide inactivates the vitamin B_{12} component of methionine synthetase. Prolonged exposure of a patient to nitrous oxide results in megaloblastic anemia and neurologic changes similar to those of pernicious anemia.[102] Use of nitrous oxide is best avoided in patients with vitamin B_{12} deficiency.[103]

Folic acid deficiency also produces a megaloblastic anemia. Although peripheral neuropathy may occur, it is not as common as with vitamin B_{12} deficiency. Causes of folic acid deficiency include alcoholism, pregnancy, and malabsorption syndromes. Methotrexate, phenytoin, and ethanol are among the drugs known to interfere with folic acid absorption.

HEMOLYTIC ANEMIAS

Causes of hemolytic anemia include structural erythrocyte abnormalities, enzyme deficiencies, and immune hemolytic anemias.

TABLE 16-4.   Types of Anemias

NUTRITIONAL	HEMOLYTIC	HEMOGLOBINOPATHIES	THALASSEMIAS
Iron deficiency	Spherocytosis	Hemoglobin S	Thalassemia major
B$_{12}$ deficiency	Pyruvate kinase deficiency		Thalassemia minor
Folic acid deficiency	Glucose-6-phosphate dehydrogenase deficiency		
Drug-induced ABO incompatibility			

Hereditary Spherocytosis

Hereditary spherocytosis is a disorder of red blood cell morphologic characteristics in which the red blood cell is rounded, more fragile, and more susceptible to hemolysis than is the normal biconcave red blood cell. As a result of the increased fragility, the spleen destroys the abnormal red blood cells and a chronic anemia ensues. Although the exact cause of the osmotic fragility is not known, the red blood cell membrane does permit a greater influx of sodium into the cell.[104] Cholelithiasis from chronic hemolysis and elevation of the serum bilirubin concentration occurs frequently in patients with hereditary spherocytosis. Patients with hereditary spherocytosis may have hemolytic crises develop with marked anemia, vomiting, and abdominal pain. These crises may be triggered by infection or folic acid deficiency.[105]

This disorder is treated by splenectomy, which is generally delayed until the patient is 6 yr or older. Splenectomy before that age is associated with a high incidence of bacterial infections, especially those secondary to pneumococcus. Before splenectomy most patients require a folic acid supplement because there is excessive utilization of folic acid for blood cell production. Transfusion is rarely necessary for patients with hereditary spherocytosis.

There are no special considerations during anesthesia for patients with hereditary spherocytosis. Preoperative transfusion is generally not necessary because adequate compensatory mechanisms have developed in these patients for their chronic anemia.

Glucose 6-Phosphate Dehydrogenase Deficiency

Glucose 6-phosphate dehydrogenase deficiency (G6PD) is the most common of the inherited erythrocyte enzyme deficiencies. One per cent of the black male population in the United States is afflicted by this disorder. Oriental and Mediterranean populations are also susceptible to G6PD deficiency. Glucose 6-phosphate dehydrogenase initiates the hexose monophosphate shunt. This shunt produces NADPH, the major reducing compound of the red blood cell. Without NADPH the red blood cell is susceptible to damage by oxidation. Oxidation produces denaturation of globin chains and causes premature erythrocyte destruction. There are a number of drugs that accentuate the oxidative destruction of erythrocytes (Table 16-6), which include analgesics, antibiotics, sulfonamides, and antimalarials. These persons are unable to reduce methemoglobin produced by sodium nitrate, and therefore sodium nitroprusside and prilocaine should not be administered.

TABLE 16-6. Drugs That Produce Hemolysis in Patients with Glucose-6-phosphate Dehydrogenase Deficiency

Phenacetin
Aspirin (large doses)
Penicillin
Streptomycin
Chloramphenicol
Isoniazid
Primaquine
Quinine
Quinidine
Parenteral vitamin K
Methylene blue

Characteristically, the crisis begins 2–5 days following drug administration. Bacterial infections can also trigger hemolytic episodes. Presumably, oxidant compounds produced by active white blood cells may hemolyze susceptible red blood cells.

Anesthetic drugs have not been implicated as hemolytic agents, however, early postoperative evidence of hemolysis might indicate a G6PD syndrome.

Pyruvate Kinase Deficiency

Pyruvate kinase is a glycolytic enzyme of the Embden-Meyerhof pathway. Clinically these patients exhibit anemia, premature cholelithiasis, and splenomegaly. The clinical features resemble those of patients with spherocytosis. There are no special considerations for anesthesia other than those for any patient with chronic anemia.

Immune Hemolytic Anemias

Immune hemolytic anemias are characterized by immunologic alteration of the red blood cell membrane. Immune hemolytic anemias are caused by drugs, diseases, or erythrocyte sensitization.

By attaching to the erythrocyte membrane, drugs may form an immunogenic complex that produces an antibody response. Levodopa, alpha-methyldopa, and penicillin can produce an immune hemolytic anemia. Collagen vascular diseases, neoplasms, and infections have also been known to trigger an autoimmune hemolytic anemia. The classic example of erythrocyte sensitization is hemolytic disease of the newborn produced by Rh sensitization. An Rh-negative mother with Rh antibodies may produce hemolysis in an Rh-positive fetus. Differences in fetal and maternal ABO groups may also produce hemolysis. This is unusual because A and B antibodies are of the IgM class and do not readily cross the placenta.

HEMOGLOBINOPATHIES

There are more than 300 different hemoglobinopathies described in the literature. Fortunately, most are quite rare and may never be encountered by an anesthesiologist during his or her career. Of the hemoglobinopathies, the most common in the United States are the sickle cell diseases. Eight to 10% of black persons in the United States have the sickle cell trait, and 1 in 400 black persons in the United States has sickle cell anemia.

Sickle Cell Disease

Hemoglobin S is a variant hemoglobin produced by substitution of valine for glutamic acid in the sixth position of the beta chain. When the hemoglobin deoxygenates, a gel structure is formed that produces structural changes in the red blood cell. Low oxygen tension and acidosis exaggerate sickle cell formation. Consequently, any condition that causes a decrease in oxygen tension, such as arterial hypoxemia, or decreased blood flow may produce sickling of red blood cells. Sickling begins at an oxygen tension less than 50 mmHg and becomes most pronounced when the arterial oxygen tension decreases to 20 mmHg. Local factors can also influence sickling. Systemic oxygenation may be adequate, but vascular occlusion may produce stasis with localized hypoxemia and initiate

TABLE 16-7. Hemoglobin S Variants

	HEMOGLOBIN SS	HEMOGLOBIN SC	HEMOGLOBIN SA
Hemoglobin level (g·dl^{-1})	7–8	9–12	13–15
Life expectancy (years)	30	Slightly reduced	Normal
Propensity for sickling	+ + + +	+ +	+
Clinical features	Vasoocclusive crises	Vasoocclusive crises	Few under physiologic
	Pneumonia	Retinal thrombosis	conditions
	Papillary necrosis	Femoral head necrosis	
	Splenic infarction		
	Hepatomegaly		
	Skin ulceration		

sickling. Similarly, if sickling occurs, increasing systemic oxygenation may not reverse the sickling if arteries supplying the area are occluded. It is better to prevent sickling rather than to treat it. The likelihood of sickling is directly related to the amount of S hemoglobin present in the blood.

The definitive diagnosis of sickle disease is made with hemoglobin electrophoresis. This test will not only detect hemoglobin S, but will also reveal any other type of hemoglobin present. Although there are several variants of sickle cell disease, the most common are SS (sickle cell anemia), SA (sickle cell trait), SC, and S-thalassemia. In sickle cell anemia, 70–98% of the hemoglobin is S and the remainder is hemoglobin F (fetal). In patients with sickle cell trait (SA), 10–40% of the hemoglobin is hemoglobin S. Cells with hemoglobin S and C are less likely to sickle than SS but more likely to sickle than SA cells. The clinical severity of the disorder is also related directly to the amount of hemoglobin S (Table 16-7).

CLINICAL MANIFESTATIONS. The patient with sickle cell trait (SA) generally has a normal life expectancy and few complications from the hemoglobinopathy. Hemoglobin levels are usually normal. Sickling occurs only under extreme physiologic alterations; however, anesthesia and surgery may produce such alterations. Although the risk of anesthesia for patients with sickle cell trait is considered small, there have been some reports of death from general anesthesia. Of the 514 patients with sickle cell trait and general anesthesia reported in the literature, there have been five deaths.[106, 107] Not all of the deaths could be attributed totally to the sickle cell trait, however.

Patients with sickle cell anemia (SS) are the most severely affected of those with sickle hemoglobinopathies. Clinical manifestations include chronic anemia and chronic hemolysis. Infarction of multiple organs is produced by occlusion of vessels with deformed erythrocytes. Pulmonary dysfunction may lead to cor pulmonale and an increased alveolar-to-arterial oxygen difference. Because of slow blood flow and decreased local oxygen tension, the renal medulla is particularly vulnerable to infarction and necrosis. Ultimately there will be an inability to concentrate urine. By the time the patient is about 6 yr of age, the spleen is virtually nonexistent because of repeated infarctions. The absence of splenic function increases the patient's vulnerability to bacterial infection. Chronic hemolysis of erythrocytes produces an elevated serum bilirubin level and results in a high incidence of cholelithiasis in patients with sickle cell anemia. Repeated cerebral infarction and hemorrhage can produce neurologic dysfunction. Priapism also occurs with increased frequency in patients with sickle cell disease. Most patients with sickle cell anemia die by 30 yr of age.

The clinical manifestations of SC disease represent an intermediate severity between SA and SS hemoglobinopathies.

Anemia is generally mild, with hemoglobin concentrations of 10–11 g·dl^{-1}. Sickle cell crises are less common in patients with SC disease than in those with SS. Pulmonary dysfunction secondary to upper respiratory tract infections, pneumonia, and pulmonary embolization are relatively common in patients with SC.[108] There are at least 40 other variants of the S hemoglobinopathy, some of which are quite rare. Hemoglobin SA, SS, and SC are the three most frequently encountered variants.

TREATMENT. Although the exact molecular nature of S hemoglobin has been known for nearly 40 yr, no definitive treatment is available. The best treatment is prevention of sickling. Maintenance of good systemic oxygenation and hydration to maintain good tissue perfusion are essential. In some instances transfusion with normal adult hemoglobin (AA) to dilute the hemoglobin S erythrocytes and decrease blood viscosity is indicated. A variety of techniques aimed at reversing the sickling process, such as alkalinization, carbamylation, and acetylation, have been attempted but with limited success. Because reversal of the sickling process is difficult, prevention becomes essential.

MANAGEMENT OF ANESTHESIA. Because arterial hypoxemia and vascular stasis are powerful stimuli for sickling, it is imperative that the risk of these be minimized during anesthesia. Preoperative sedation should not depress ventilation. During surgery and the postoperative period, the inspired oxygen concentration should be increased to maintain or increase the arterial oxygen tension. Monitoring arterial hemoglobin saturation with a pulse oximeter is a useful noninvasive monitor for patients with sickle cell disorders. Although regional anesthesia is often used for these patients, supplemental oxygen still may be indicated. Regional anesthesia may produce compensatory vasoconstriction and decreased oxygen tension in nonblocked areas, making red blood cells in those areas vulnerable to sickling. Circulatory stasis can be prevented with adequate hydration and anticipation of intraoperative volume loss to avoid acute hypovolemia. The use of extremity tourniquets is controversial. There are no studies documenting the safety or danger of tourniquet use. Some authors recommend that a tourniquet not be used for patients with hemoglobin S because of the potential dangers.[106] Other authors suggest that a tourniquet can be used if the tourniquet is critical to the success of the operation.[109] The environmental temperature should be controlled to maintain normothermia. Fever increases the rate of gel formation by S hemoglobin. Although hypothermia retards gel formation, the decreased temperature also produces peripheral vasoconstriction. Consequently, normothermia is desirable.

Although inhaled anesthetics accelerate precipitation of hemoglobin S in vitro, the clinical significance of this finding is not known. Maintenance of perfusion and oxygenation are more critical than the type of anesthesia. Because of low peripheral blood flow, hypothermia, and acidosis, cardiopulmonary bypass is especially dangerous for patients with sickle cell disease.[110]

One should continue carefully observing the patient and monitoring oxygenation into the postoperative period. Postoperative pain, analgesics, and transient pulmonary dysfunction will decrease arterial oxygen tension. Consequently, supplemental oxygen should be used after operation.

Although patients with sickle cell trait (SA) are at less risk than patients with hemoglobin SS, the same precautions applied to patients with SS should be used for those with SA. The patient with SC hemoglobin is also at risk during anesthesia and should be treated accordingly.[111]

Thalassemia

Thalassemia represents a number of inherited disorders that result in production of abnormal globin chains of hemoglobin. There are alpha- and beta-thalassemias, depending on which globin chain is affected. Beta-thalassemia major, or Cooley's anemia, is the most severe of the thalassemias. Untreated Cooley's anemia usually results in death. Transfusion therapy is essential but often produces iron toxicity. Splenectomy reduces transfusion requirements in some cases. Beta-thalassemia minor produces a mild hemolytic anemia and iron deficiency. Beta-thalassemia intermedia is an intermediate form of thalassemia but generally does not necessitate transfusion. Alpha-thalassemia produces a mild hemolytic anemia in most patients. Transfusion and splenectomy may be necessary in some patients with alpha-thalassemia.

Anesthetic considerations depend on the severity of the anemia. If the patient is transfusion dependent, then careful preoperative evaluation of hepatic and cardiac function are warranted because of iron toxicity. When an anesthetic is selected, the likelihood of cardiomyopathy and hepatic dysfunction must be considered, in addition to chronic anemia. Extramedullary hematopoiesis can produce hyperplasia of the facial bones and make direct laryngoscopic examination difficult.[112]

COLLAGEN VASCULAR DISEASES

There are a number of diseases that are classified as the collagen vascular diseases (Table 16-8). The four most common disorders of this group are rheumatoid arthritis, systemic lupus erythematosus, scleroderma, and polymyositis. The origin of these diseases is unknown, but current theories implicate the immune system and its effect on the vascular bed. Although all these diseases have localized features involving joints, each of the disorders also has diffuse systemic effects. Both the localized and systemic alterations in these patients are significant in the management of anesthesia.

RHEUMATOID ARTHRITIS

Rheumatoid arthritis is a chronic inflammatory disease characterized by a symmetric polyarthropathy and significant systemic involvement. Although genetics, immune responses, and inflammation are involved in the pathogenesis of rheumatoid arthritis, the cause is unknown. There are also infectious agents that produce rheumatoid arthritis-like diseases in animals.[113] Irrespective of the etiologic agent, the synovial membrane undergoes change beginning with cellular hyperplasia. The synovium is then invaded by lymphocytes, plasma cells, and fibroblasts. Ultimately, joint cartilage and bone are destroyed.

The hands and wrists are involved first, particularly the metacarpophalangeal and proximal interphalangeal joints. In the lower extremity the knee is involved most frequently. Compression of lower extremity nerves by the deformed knee can produce paresis and sensory loss over the lower leg. The cervical spine is generally involved, and altantoaxial subluxation can result. The odontoid process may impinge on the spinal cord and cause a cervical myelopathy. Synovitis of the temporomandibular joint may decrease jaw mobility. Cricoarytenoid arthritis is common and is evidenced by hoarseness, dysphagia, and stridor.

Extraarticular and systemic manifestations of rheumatoid arthritis are diverse (Table 16-9).[114] Pericardial thickening and/or effusion may lead to cardiac tamponade. Ventricular dysfunction may occur because of myocarditis and coronary arteritis. Formation of rheumatoid nodules in the cardiac conduction system can produce dysrhythmias. Aortitis with dilation of the aortic root can result in aortic insufficiency. Pleural effusions from pleural irritation frequently occur. Rheumatoid nodule deposition in the lung parenchyma in conjunction with costochondral arthritis produces restrictive pulmonary disease. Neurologic complications include peripheral nerve

---

TABLE 16-8. Collagen Vascular Diseases

Rheumatoid arthritis
Lupus
    Systemic lupus erythematosus
    Drug-induced lupus
    Discoid lupus
Scleroderma
    Progressive systemic sclerosis
    CREST syndrome (calcinosis, Raynaud, esophageal dysfunction, sclerodactyly, telangiectasias)
    Focal scleroderma
Polymyositis
    Dermatomyositis

TABLE 16-9. Extraarticular Manifestations of Rheumatoid Arthritis

Skin	Peripheral nervous system
Raynaud's phenomenon	Compression syndromes
Digital necrosis	Mononeuritis
Eye	Central nervous system
Scleritis	Dural nodules
Corneal ulceration	Necrotizing vasculitis
Lung	Liver
Pleural effusion	Hepatitis
Pulmonary fibrosis	
Heart	Blood
Pericarditis	Anemia
Tamponade	
Coronary arteritis	
Aortic insufficiency	
Kidney	
Interstitial fibrosis	
Glomerulonephritis	
Amyloid deposition	

compression (carpal tunnel syndrome) and cervical nerve root compression. Mononeuritis multiplex is presumed to be caused by deposition of immune complexes in blood vessels supplying the affected nerves. Cerebral necrotizing vasculitis can also occur. Mild anemia is almost always present. Rheumatoid arthritis with leukopenia (less than $2,000 \cdot mm^3$) and hepatosplenomegaly is Felty's syndrome.

Pharmacologic treatment of rheumatoid arthritis is directed at relief of pain and remission of the disease process.[115] Nonsteroidal antiinflammatory drugs include aspirin, phenylbutazone, indomethacin, ibuprofen, sulindac, and tolmetin. Aspirin is the standard against which all other drugs are compared. Unfortunately, significant side effects occur with chronic use of any of these drugs. Corticosteroids definitely reduce rheumatoid inflammation, but their deleterious side effects are well known.

Remission-inducing drugs include gold salts, antimalarial drugs, penicillamine, and azathioprine. Many of these drugs cause anemia, thrombocytopenia, and hepatitis. Synovectomy, tenolysis, and joint replacement are performed to relieve pain and restore function.

Management of Anesthesia

Arthritic involvement of the temporomandibular joints, cricoarytenoid joints, and cervical spine can make tracheal intubation extremely difficult. The patient's mobility of these joints must be evaluated before operation so that the anesthesiologist can select an intubation technique. Fiberoptic laryngoscopic examination may be necessary. Atlantoaxial instability is relatively common when the rheumatoid process involves the cervical spine. Flexion of the head in the presence of atlantoaxial instability could compress the spinal cord.[116] Neck pain with radiation to the occiput may be the first sign of cervical spine involvement.[117] Preoperative cervical radiographs may be necessary if the degree of cervical involvement is not known. Cricoarytenoid arthritis may be recognized by erythema and edema of the vocal cords. Involvement of the cricoarytenoid joints will reduce the size of the glottic inlet and necessitate the use of a smaller than predicted tracheal tube. Exaggerated postextubation edema and stridor also may occur.

The degree of cardiopulmonary involvement by the rheumatoid process will certainly influence the selection of the type of anesthesia. Functional evaluation of the lungs and heart are necessary if the clinical history suggests dysfunction. The need for postoperative ventilatory support should be anticipated if severe restrictive lung disease is present.

Medications the patient is receiving will influence the management of anesthesia (Table 16-10). Corticosteroid supplementation may be necessary during the operation, depending on the magnitude of the surgery. Aspirin will interfere with platelet function, and clotting may be abnormal. Many antirheumatoid drugs, including gold, suppress red blood cell function, and anemia is common. The antiinflammatory drugs also may alter hepatic function, which can influence the choice of anesthesia.

Restriction of joint mobility necessitates careful positioning during operation. The extremities should be positioned so as to minimize the risk of neurovascular compression and additional joint injury. Preoperative evaluation of joint motion helps determine how extremities should be positioned.

There are many systemic effects of rheumatoid arthritis. The degree and type of systemic involvement must be considered when an anesthetic is selected for the patient with rheumatoid arthritis.[118]

TABLE 16-10.   Adverse Effects of Drugs Used to Treat Collagen Vascular Diseases

DRUG	EFFECTS
Corticosteroids	Hypertension Osteoporosis Fluid retention Infection
Aspirin	Platelet dysfunction Peptic ulcer Hepatic dysfunction Hypersensitivity
Indomethacin	Peptic ulcer Hypertension Hyperglycemia Leukopenia
Gold	Aplastic anemia Dermatitis Nephritis
Antimalarials	Myopathy Retinopathy
Penicillamine	Glomerulonephritis Aplastic anemia Myasthenia
Azathioprine	Leukopenia Biliary stasis
Cyclophosphamide	Leukopenia Hemorrhagic cystitis

SYSTEMIC LUPUS ERYTHEMATOSUS

Lupus is a multisystem inflammatory disease of unknown origin. It is believed to be an autoimmune disease, and anti-DNA antibodies have been implicated. There are a number of potential mechanisms by which anti-DNA antibodies could produce clinical disease. The specific mechanism for systemic lupus has not been discovered, however.[119] There are a number of drugs—including hydralazine, procainamide, alpha-methyldopa, phenytoin, carbamazepine, and isoniazid—that can produce characteristics of systemic lupus.

Although the clinical features of lupus are diverse, there are several areas of involvement common to most patients. Arthritis occurs in most patients, which affects both large and small joints. Cutaneous manifestations include the characteristic erythematous butterfly rash over the nose and malar area, alopecia, and Raynaud's phenomenon. Renal disease from lupus is a significant cause of complications and death. Proteinuria, hypertension, and renal insufficiency invariably occur. During active phases of the disease, anemia, leukopenia, and thrombocytopenia are common.[120] Of special interest to anesthesiologists is the effect of systemic lupus on the central nervous system and the cardiopulmonary systems. The central nervous system manifestations of lupus include seizures, neuropathies, paralysis, and cerebrovascular accidents.[121]

Systemic lupus produces a serositis that manifests as pleuritis and pericarditis in the cardiopulmonary systems. In addition to pleural effusions, pneumonitis and pulmonary hemorrhage also may occur. The pneumonitis may be primary involvement or secondary to bacteria or uremia. Pericarditis is the most common cardiovascular manifestation of lupus. Despite the fact that more than 60% of patients with lupus have pericardial effusion, tamponade is a relatively uncommon condition.[122] Cardiomyopathy may be secondary to direct involvement of cardiac muscle or may be secondary to hypertension, anemia, uremia, or coronary artery disease. A noninfectious endocarditis (Libman-Sacks endocarditis) often affects the mitral valve and can produce mitral insufficiency. The leading causes of death in patients with systemic lupus erythematosus are renal failure and infection.

There is no specific therapeutic agent for lupus. Nonsteroidal antiinflammatory drugs are useful for treating arthritis. Glucocorticoids represent the main therapy because they are drugs with both antiinflammatory and immunosuppressive effects. Immunosuppressant drugs such as cyclophosphamide and azathioprine have also been used. Interestingly, antimalarial drugs seem to have beneficial effects for patients with lupus.

Management of Anesthesia

Because lupus is a multisystem disease with diverse clinical presentations, careful preoperative evaluation is necessary. Anesthesia management will be influenced by the drugs used to treat lupus and by the degree of dysfunction of organs affected by the disease.

Arthritic involvement of the cervical spine is unusual in patients with systemic lupus. Consequently, tracheal intubation is generally not difficult.

A preoperative echocardiogram may detect the presence and significance of a pericardial effusion. Certainly cardiac dysfunction will influence the choice of drugs for anesthesia. Because renal dysfunction is so common in patients with lupus, renal function should be quantified before operation. Pulmonary function testing generally will reveal a restrictive type of disease. Although minor abnormalities in liver function are present in many patients with lupus, these generally are not clinically significant. However, a lupoid hepatitis characterized by prolonged jaundice, hyperglobulinemia, and hepatomegaly develops in some patients. This form of hepatitis is usually fatal.[123]

Because most patients with systemic lupus receive corticosteroids, supplementation with steroids during the perioperative period generally is indicated. An initial dose of 1 mg·kg^{-1} of cortisol should be adequate.

There are no specific contraindications to any particular type of anesthesia. The ultimate selection will depend on the organ systems involved and the extent of involvement.

SCLERODERMA

Scleroderma (progressive systemic sclerosis) is a disorder characterized by deposition of fibrous connective tissue in many organs. It has been suggested that scleroderma is a disease of vascular control that permits direct transmission of arterial pressure to more distal, fragile blood vessels. This produces tissue edema, obstruction of lymphatics, and, ultimately, fibrosis.[124] This theory would explain the diffuse nature of the disease.

The manifestations of scleroderma are observed most readily in the skin, which becomes thickened and swollen. Eventually the skin becomes atrophic, hair and sweat glands are lost, and small arteries become sclerotic. Raynaud's phenomenon occurs in 95% of patients with scleroderma and is often the initial manifestation of the disease. As the disease progresses, the skin becomes taut and produces immobility of underlying structures. Joint mobility may become severely restricted.

Renal involvement is extremely common. Destruction of renal vessels leads to hypertension, anemia, and progressive renal failure. Chronic proteinuria is a common finding.

In the lung, scleroderma produces interstitial fibrosis and thickening of alveolar septa that impair oxygen diffusion. Sclerosis of the chest wall and diaphragm in conjunction with pleural fibrosis produces a severe restrictive defect. Pulmonary hypertension can be caused by compression of pulmonary arterioles or the formation of arteriovenous shunts. Ultimately cor pulmonale can ensue.

Myocardial fibrosis occurs in 60% of patients with scleroderma, although left ventricular function generally is preserved. A decreased resting ejection fraction is present in less than 20% of patients.[125] Fibrous atrophy of the cardiac conduction system may explain the high incidence of delayed atrioventricular conduction and supraventricular dysrhythmias. Pericardial effusion is also a common finding.

In most patients with scleroderma, the esophagus is involved, which permits gastroesophageal reflux. Small intestinal motility is also decreased.

Many of the treatment modalities are directed at relieving the symptoms of scleroderma. Although the exact mechanism of the disease is not known, it is felt to be a disease of the immune system. Consequently, immunosuppressive drugs, such as corticosteroids, and antimetabolites, such as 6-thioguanine and azathioprine, have been used. D-penicillamine, which reduces the number of immune responses, has been used somewhat successfully to treat scleroderma.

Management of Anesthesia

Much like systemic lupus, scleroderma is a multiorgan disease with diverse manifestations. Consequently, the affected organ systems must be evaluated thoroughly so that a logical plan for anesthesia can be selected. There are no specific contraindications to the use of any type of anesthetic, although the selection will be guided by the degree of organ dysfunction.

Tracheal intubation can be quite difficult. Lack of temporomandibular joint mobility may necessitate fiberoptic laryngoscopic examination with topical anesthesia. Orotracheal intubation may be preferable to nasotracheal intubation because of the fragility of the nasal mucosa and propensity for nasal hemorrhage. Tracheostomy may be necessary in severely affected patients.[126]

The patient with scleroderma is at risk for aspiration pneumonitis during the induction of anesthesia because of the high incidence of gastroesophageal reflux. Appropriate measures to prevent acid aspiration, such as the use of histamine-2 blocking agents and oral antacids, may be indicated.

Chronic arterial hypoxemia may be present because of restriction of lung expansion and impaired oxygen diffusion. Consequently, controlled mechanical ventilation of the lungs with an increased inspired oxygen concentration is generally necessary. Compromised myocardial function often necessitates the use of invasive cardiovascular monitoring. Venous access may be difficult to obtain. A venous cutdown or central venous catheterization may be necessary.

The anesthesiologist is often consulted as to the efficacy of sympathetic blockade for the treatment of vasospasm secondary to Raynaud's phenomenon.

POLYMYOSITIS

Polymyositis is an inflammatory myopathy affecting skeletal muscle. The diagnostic term dermatomyositis is used when characteristic skin lesions are associated with the myositis. Common presenting clinical features are proximal skeletal muscle weakness and the typical skin rash consisting of a violaceous eruption over the patient's eyelids with an erythematous rash over his or her face, neck, and upper chest. Ten percent of patients with polymyositis have an occult neoplasm. The origin is unknown, but, as with all of the collagen vascular diseases, altered cellular immunity has been suspected as a cause. Examination of skeletal muscle biopsy specimens reveals perivascular infiltrates, muscle degeneration, and interstitial infiltrates. Electromyography (EMG) demonstrates short polyphasic motor units and muscle fibrillation.[127]

Thirty to 40% of patients with polymyositis have ECG abnormalities that are secondary to myocardial fibrosis or atrophy of the cardiac conduction system. The magnitude of cardiac disease is an important prognostic factor.

Aspiration pneumonitis is the most common pulmonary complication of polymyositis.[128] Pulmonary interstitial fibrosis with restrictive lung disease occurs in nearly 70% of patients.

Most patients with polymyositis improve with corticosteroid therapy. Azathioprine, methotrexate, or cyclophosphamide have also been used.

Management of Anesthesia

Although mobility of the temporomandibular joint is not as severely affected by polymyositis as by scleroderma, some patients with dermatomyositis present a real challenge for tracheal intubation. Adequate mandibular and cervical mobility must be ascertained before induction of anesthesia.

Although the typical EMG findings suggest the potential for hyperkalemia after succinylcholine administration, this has not been documented clinically. Atypical cholinesterase activity has also been reported in patients with dermatomyositis, but the significance of this finding is unclear.[129] Sensitivity to nondepolarizing muscle relaxants is also likely.[130] Adequate monitoring of neuromuscular function during anesthesia is certainly indicated.

Dysphagia usually occurs, and there is an increased likelihood of aspiration pneumonitis. Appropriate antiaspiration maneuvers should be used during anesthesia induction.

The degree of cardiopulmonary dysfunction will influence the choice of anesthetic and selection of intraoperative monitors. Preoperative pulmonary and cardiac function studies will provide useful information in some patients with polymyositis. Because of skeletal muscle weakness, postoperative ventilatory support of the lungs may be necessary.

SKIN DISORDERS

EPIDERMOLYSIS BULLOSA

Epidermolysis bullosa is a rare hereditary skin disorder. The basic defect is felt to be increased collagenase production, which destroys intercellular bridges and causes skin layers to separate.[131] The separation of skin layers results in fluid accumulation and bullae formation. Even minor trauma produces skin blisters. Lateral shearing forces applied to the skin are particularly damaging because of skin separation. Pressure applied perpendicular to the axis of the skin surface is not as hazardous.

There are three types of epidermolysis: epidermolysis bullosa simplex, epidermolysis bullosa dystrophica, and junctional epidermolysis bullosa. The simplex form is characterized by a benign course and normal development. In contrast, patients with the junctional form rarely survive beyond early childhood, usually dying from sepsis. The dystrophic form produces severe scarring of the fingers and toes, with pseudosyndactyly formation, esophageal stricture, and malnutrition (Fig. 16-2). Anemia and hypoalbuminemia are common and result from chronic infection and malnutrition. Most patients do not survive after the second decade of life. Diseases associated with epidermolysis bullosa include porphyria cutanea tarda, amyloidosis, multiple myeloma, diabetes mellitus, and hypercoagulable states. Secondary bacterial infection of the bullae with *staphylococcus aureus* or beta-hemolytic streptococci is common.

Currently, specific treatment includes the use of phenytoin and retinoids, which appear to inhibit collagenase synthesis. More clinical trials with these drugs are necessary, however,

FIG. 16-2. Epidermolysis bullosa. (*A*) Bullous lesion on the finger of a neonate with epidermolysis. (*B*) Hands of an older child with epidermolysis showing progression of the disease to produce severe scarring and pseudosyndactyly. (Courtesy of James E. Bennett, M.D., Division of Plastic Surgery, Indiana University School of Medicine.)

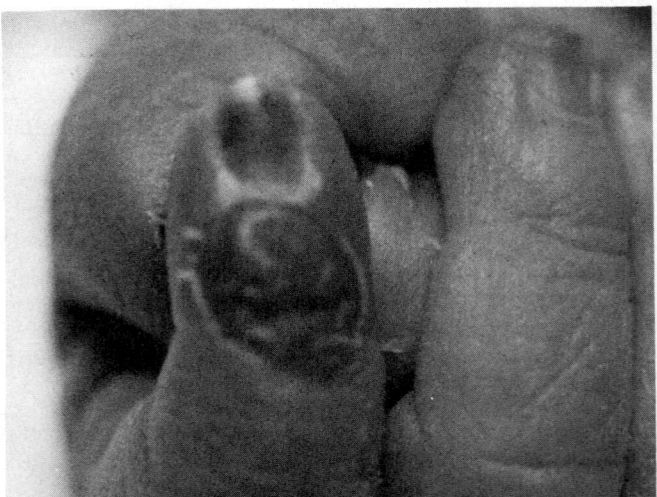

A

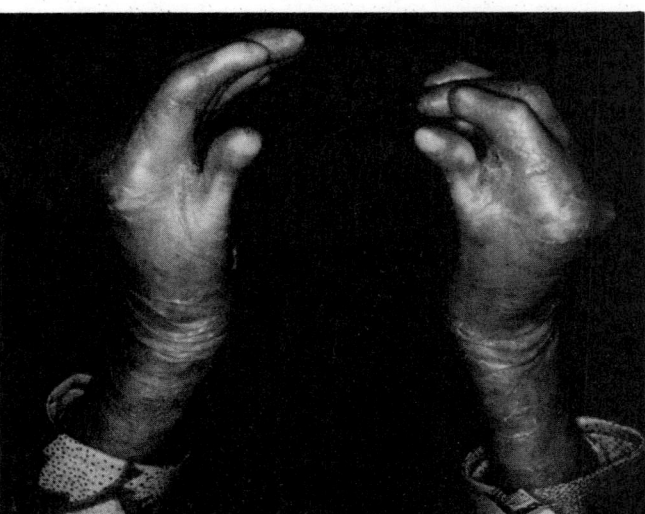

B

before conclusions can be made. Corticosteroids also have been used but are probably not effective.

Management of Anesthesia

It is critical that trauma to the skin and mucous membranes be avoided or minimized. Trauma from tape, blood pressure cuffs, tourniquets, and adhesive ECG electrodes may cause bulla formation. The blood pressure cuff should be padded with a loose cotton dressing. Intravenous and intraarterial catheters should be sutured or held in place with a gauze wrap rather than taped in place. Trauma from an anesthetic face mask must be reduced by gentle application against the skin. Lubrication of the patient's face and the mask with cortisol ointment can be helpful. Use of upper airway instruments should be kept to a minimum because the squamous epithelium that lines the oropharynx and esophagus is more susceptible to trauma than is the columnar epithelium of the trachea. Frictional trauma to the oropharynx, as produced by an oral airway, may result in large intraoral bullae formation and extensive hemorrhage from denuded mucosa.[132] A nasal airway is equally hazardous. Use of esophageal stethoscopes also should be avoided because it may lead to formation of intraoral or esophageal bullae. Hemorrhage from ruptured oral bullae has been treated successfully by application of epinephrine-soaked gauze to the bullae.[133] Despite theoretic hazards, intubation of the trachea has not been associated with laryngeal or tracheal complications, and its more routine use in these patients has been recommended.[134] Laryngeal involvement with the disease is rare, and tracheal bullae have not been reported. Lubrication of the laryngoscope blade and tracheal tube is recommended. Scarring of the oral cavity can result in a narrow oral aperture and immobility of the tongue. Esophageal scarring often produces esophageal stricture. Safety of tracheal intubation is unproven in children with junctional epidermolysis bullosa that involves all mucosa including the respiratory epithelium.[135]

Although porphyria occurs with increased incidence in patients with epidermolysis bullosa, it is porphyria cutanea tarda that does not have the same implications for anesthesia as acute intermittent porphyria[136] (see Chapter 17).

Ketamine is a useful anesthetic for procedures that do not require skeletal muscle relaxation or intraabdominal manipulation. Because patients with epidermolysis often require surgical procedures on the fingers and toes, use of ketamine is ideal. There are no known contraindications to the use of inhaled anesthetic drugs in these patients.

PEMPHIGUS

Pemphigus is a vesiculobullous disease that may involve extensive areas of the skin and mucous membranes. Pemphigus is an autoimmune disease in which there is a loss of cellular adhesiveness that leads to separation of skin and mucous membrane epithelium. The autoantibodies are highly specific and result in the excessive production of proteolytic enzymes that disrupt cell adhesion.

There are two types of pemphigus. Pemphigus vulgaris is the more common and severe form. It is characterized by bullae formation on the trunk and intertriginous areas. More than 60% of patients with pemphigus have oral lesions. Because extensive oropharyngeal involvement makes eating painful, patients may reduce oral intake to the extent that severe malnutrition develops. Skin denudation and bullae

formation can result in significant fluid and protein loss. The risk of secondary bacterial infection is great. As with epidermolysis bullosa, lateral shearing forces are more likely to produce bullae than pressure exerted perpendicular to the skin surface. Pemphigus foliaceus is a less severe form in which acantholysis occurs high in the epidermis. Mucous membrane involvement does not occur in pemphigus foliaceus.

Treatment with systemic corticosteroids has reduced mortality from 70 to 40%. The addition of immunosuppressants such as azathioprine, cyclophosphamide, and methotrexate has reduced mortality to less than 20%.

Management of Anesthesia

Preoperative drug therapy and the extreme fragility of mucous membranes are of primary consideration for anesthesia management. Management of the upper airway and intubation of the trachea should be performed as described for patients with epidermolysis bullosa. Ketamine has been used successfully in patients with pemphigus.[137] Regional anesthesia also has been used.[138]

There are no contraindications to use of any inhaled or intravenous anesthetics; however, potential side effects of treatment drugs and interactions with anesthetics must be considered. For example, perioperative supplementation with corticosteroids may be necessary. Methotrexate produces hepatorenal dysfunction and bone marrow suppression. Cyclophosphamide may prolong the effect of succinylcholine by inhibiting plasma cholinesterase activity.

REFERENCES

1. Sanyal SK, Johnson WW, Dische WR et al: Dystrophic degeneration of papillary muscle and ventricular myocardium. Circulation 62:430, 1980
2. Perloff JK, Henze E, Schelbert HR: Alterations in regional myocardial metabolism, perfusion, and wall motion in Duchenne muscular dystrophy studied by radionuclide imaging. Circulation 69:33, 1984
3. Ellis FR: Inherited muscle disease. Br J Anaesth 52:153, 1980
4. Seay AR, Ziter FA, Thompson JA: Cardiac arrest during induction of anesthesia in Duchenne muscular dystrophy. J. Pediatr 93:88, 1978
5. McKishnie JD, Muir JM, Girvan DP: Anaesthesia induced rhabdomyolysis—a case report. Can Anaesth Soc J 30:295, 1983
6. Rosenberg H: Neuromuscular blockade in the patient with neuromuscular disorders. Semin Anes 4:9, 1985
7. Wang JM, Stanley TH: Duchenne muscular dystrophy and malignant hyperthermia—two case reports. Can Anaesth Soc J 33:492, 1986
8. Brownell AKW, Paasuke RT, Elash A et al: Malignant hyperthermia in Duchenne muscular dystrophy. Anesthesiology 58:180, 1983
9. Smith CL, Bush GH: Anaesthesia and progressive muscular dystrophy. Br J Anaesth 57:1113, 1985
10. Hook R, Anderson EF, Noto P: Anesthetic management of a parturient with myotonia atrophica. Anesthesiology 43:689, 1975
11. Streib EW: Successful treatment with tocainide of recessive generalized congenital myotonia. Ann Neurol 19:501, 1986
12. Perloff JK, Stevenson WG, Roberts NK et al: Cardiac involvement in myotonic muscular dystrophy (Steinert's disease): A prospective study of 25 patients. Am J Cardiol 54:1074, 1984
13. Streib EW, Meyers DG, Sun SF: Mitral valve prolapse in myotonic dystrophy. Muscle Nerve 8:650, 1985

14. Jammes Y, Pouget J, Grimaud C et al: Pulmonary function and electromyographic study of respiratory muscles in myotonic dystrophy. Muscle Nerve 8:586, 1985

15. Cope DK, Miller JN: Local and spinal anesthesia for cesarean section in a patient with myotonic dystrophy. Anesth Analg 65:687, 1986

16. Mitchell MM, Ali HH, Savarese JJ: Myotonia and neuromuscular blocking agents. Anesthesiology 49:44, 1978

17. Buzello W, Kreig N, Schlickewei A: Hazards of neostigmine in patients with neuromuscular disorders. Br J Anaesth 54:529, 1982

18. Nightengale P, Healy TEJ, McGuinness K: Dystrophica myotonia and atracurium. Br J. Anaesth 57:1131, 1985

19. Stirt JA, Stone DJ, Weinberg G et al: Atracurium in a child with myotonic dystrophy. Anesth Analg 64:369, 1985

20. Boheimer N, Harris JW, Ward S: Neuromuscular blockade in dystrophia myotonica with atracurium besylate. Anaesthesia 40:872, 1985

21. Aldridge LM: Anaesthetic problems in myotonic dystrophy. Br J Anaesth 57:1119, 1985

22. Ishizawa Y, Yamaguchi H, Dohi S et al: A serious complication due to gastrointestinal malfunction in a patient with myotonic dystrophy. Anesth Analg 65:1066, 1986

23. Jaffe R, Mock M, Abramowicz J et al: Myotonic dystrophy and pregnancy: A review. Obstet Gynecol Surv 41:272, 1986

24. Paterson RA, Tousignant M, Skene SD: Cesarean section for twins in a patient with myotonic dystrophy. Can Anaesth Soc J 32:418, 1985

25. Fulpius BW: Antiacetylcholine receptor antibodies and myasthenia gravis. Int Rev Neurobiol 24:1, 1983

26. Penn AS, Schotland DL, Lamme S: Antimuscle and antiacetylcholine receptor antibodies in myasthenia gravis. Muscle Nerve 9:407, 1986

27. Seybold ME: Myasthenia gravis. A clinical and basic science review. JAMA 250:2516, 1983

28. Hofstad H, Ohm O, Mork SJ et al: Heart disease in myasthenia gravis. Acta Neurol Scand 70:176, 1984

29. Plauché WC: Myasthenia gravis. Clin Obstet Gynecol 26:592, 1983

30. Baraka A, Dajani A: Atracurium in myasthenics undergoing thymectomy. Anesth Analg 64:1127, 1984

31. Ramsey FM, Smith GD: Clinical use of atracurium in myasthenia gravis: A case report. Can Anaesth Soc J 32:642, 1985

32. Bell CF, Florence AM, Hunter JM et al: Atracurium in the myasthenic patient. Anaesthesia 39:961, 1984

33. Hunter JM, Bell CF, Florence AM et al: Vecuronium in the myasthenic patient. Anaesthesia 40:848, 1985

34. Sivak ED, Mehta A, Hanson M et al: Postoperative ventilatory dependence following thymectomy for myasthenia gravis. Cleve Clin Q 51:585, 1984

35. Leventhal SR, Orkin FK, Hirsch RA: Prediction of the need for postoperative mechanical ventilation in myasthenia gravis. Anesthesiology 53:26, 1980

36. Eisenkraft JB, Papatestas AE, Kahn CH et al: Predicting the need for postoperative mechanical ventilation in myasthenia gravis. Anesthesiology 65:79, 1986

37. Azar I: The response of patients with neuromuscular disorders to muscle relaxants: A review. Anesthesiology 61:173, 1984

38. Agoston S, VanWeerden T, Westra P et al: Effects of 4-aminopyridine in Eaton-Lambert syndrome. Br J Anaesth 50:383, 1978

39. Bendheim PE, Reale EO, Berg BO: β-adrenergic treatment of hyperkalemic periodic paralysis. Neurology 35:746, 1985

40. Dalakas MC, Engel WK: Treatment of "permanent" muscle weakness in familial hypokalemic periodic paralysis. Muscle Nerve 6:182, 1983

41. Buruma OJS, Bots GTAM, Went LN: Familial hypokalemic periodic paralysis. Arch Neurol 42:28, 1985

42. Rollman JE, Dickson CM: Anesthetic management of a patient with hypokalemic familial periodic paralysis for coronary artery bypass surgery. Anesthesiology 63:526, 1985

43. Christensen KS: Hypokalemic periodic paralysis secondary to renal tubular acidosis. Eur Neurol 24:303, 1985

44. Manary MJ, Keating JP, Hirshberg GE: Quadriparesis due to potassium depletion. Crit Care Med 14:750, 1986

45. Duncan PG: Neuromuscular diseases. In Katz J, Steward DJ (eds): Anesthesia and Uncommon Pediatric Diseases, p 509. Philadelphia, WB Saunders, 1987

46. Koski CL: Guillain-Barré syndrome. Neurol Clin 2:355, 1984

47. Newton-John H: Prevention of pulmonary complications in severe Guillain-Barré syndrome by early assisted ventilation. Med J Aust 142:444, 1985

48. Ropper AH: Severe acute Guillain-Barré syndrome. Neurology 36:429, 1986

49. Krone A, Reuther P, Fuhrmeister U: Autonomic dysfunction in polyneuropathies: A report of 106 cases. J Neurol 230:111, 1983

50. Moore P, James O: Guillain-Barré syndrome: Incidence, management, and outcome of major complications. Crit Care Med 9:549, 1981

51. Rosenfeld B, Borel C, Hanley D: Epidural morphine treatment of pain in Guillain-Barré syndrome. Arch Neurol 43:1194, 1986

52. Covert CR, Brodie SB, Zimmerman JE: Weaning failure due to acute neuromuscular disease. Crit Care Med 14:307, 1986

53. Powell HC, Lampert PW: Pathology of multiple sclerosis. Neurol Clin 1:631, 1983

54. Ellison GW, Visscher BR, Graves MC et al: Multiple sclerosis. Ann Intern Med 101:514, 1984

55. Reder AT, Antel JP: Clinical spectrum of multiple sclerosis. Neurol Clin 1:573, 1983

56. Birk K, Rudick R: Pregnancy and multiple sclerosis. Arch Neurol 43:719, 1986

57. Stevens JC, Farlow MR, Edwards MK et al: Magnetic resonance imaging. Clinical correlation in 64 patients with multiple sclerosis. Arch Neurol 43:1145, 1986

58. Schapiro RT, van den Noort S, Scheinberg L: The current management of multiple sclerosis. Ann NY Acad Sci 436:425, 1984

59. Eisen A: Neurophysiology in multiple sclerosis. Neurol Clin 1:615, 1983

60. Siemkowicz E: Multiple sclerosis and surgery. Anaesthesia 31:1211, 1976

61. Baskett PJF, Armstrong R: Anaesthetic problems in multiple sclerosis. Anaesthesia 25:397, 1970

62. Kytta J, Rosenberg PH: Anaesthesia for patients with multiple sclerosis. Ann Chir Gynaecol 73:299, 1984

63. Jones RM, Healy TEJ: Anaesthesia and demyelinating disease. Anaesthesia 35:879, 1980

64. Berger JM, Ontell R: Intrathecal morphine in conjunction with a combined spinal and general anesthetic in a patient with multiple sclerosis. Anesthesiology 66:400, 1987

65. Roth S, Ebrahim ZY: Resistance to pancuronium in patients receiving carbamazepine. Anesthesiology 66:691, 1987

66. Rawal K, D'Souza BJ: Status epilepticus. Critical Care Clinics 1:339, 1985

67. Steen PA, Michenfelder JD: Neurotoxicity of anesthetics. Anesthesiology 50:437, 1979

68. Defalque RJ, Musunuru VS: Diseases of the nervous system. In Stoelting RK, Dierdorf SF (eds): Anesthesia and Co-Existing Disease, p 239. New York, Churchill Livingstone, 1983

69. Safwat AM, Daniel D: Grand mal seizure after fentanyl administration (letter). Anesthesiology 59:78, 1983

70. Hoien AO: Another case of grand mal seizure after fentanyl administration (letter). Anesthesiology 60:387, 1984

71. Molbegott LP, Flashburg MH, Karasic HL *et al:* Probable seizures after sufentanil. Anesth Analg 66:91, 1987
72. Scott JC, Sarnquist FH: Seizure-like movements during a fentanyl infusion with absence of seizure activity in a simultaneous EEG recording. Anesthesiology 62:812, 1985
73. Sebel PS, Bovill JG, Wauquier A *et al:* Effects of high-dose fentanyl anesthesia on the electroencephalogram. Anesthesiology 55:203, 1981
74. Bovill JG, Sevel PS, Wauquier A *et al:* Electroencephalographic effects of sufentanil anaesthesia in man. Br J. Anaesth 54:45, 1982
75. Carlsson C, Smith DS, Keykhah MM, *et al:* The effects of high-dose fentanyl on cerebral circulation and metabolism in rats. Anesthesiology 57:375, 1982
76. Young ML, Smith DS, Greenberg J *et al:* Effects of sufentanil on regional cerebral glucose utilization in rats. Anesthesiology 61:564, 1984
77. Rockoff MA, Goudsouzian NG: Seizures induced by methohexital. Anesthesiology 54:333, 1981
78. Ornstein E, Matteo RS, Young WL *et al:* Resistance to metocurine-induced neuromuscular blockade in patients receiving phenytoin. Anesthesiology 63:294, 1985
79. Duvoisin RC: Etiology of Parkinson's disease: Current concepts. Clin Neuropharmacol 9 (suppl 1):S3, 1986
80. Lang AE, Blair RDG: Parkinson's disease in 1984: An update. Can Med Assoc J 131:1031, 1984
81. Medical Letter. Drugs for parkinsonism. 28:62, 1986
82. DaPrada M, Keller HH, Pieri L *et al:* The pharmacology of Parkinson's disease: Basic aspects and recent advances. Experientia 40:1165, 1984
83. Hetherington A, Rosenblatt RM: Letter: Ketamine and paralysis agitans. Anesthesiology 52:527, 1980
84. Gravlee GP: Succinylcholine-induced hyperkalemia in a patient with Parkinson's disease. Anesth Analg 59:444, 1980
85. McDaniel KD: Clinical pharmacology of monoamine oxidase inhibitors. Clin Neuropharmacol 9:207, 1986
86. Shoulson I: Huntington's disease. Neurology Clinics 2:515, 1984
87. Davies DD: Abnormal response to anaesthesia in a case of Huntington's chorea. Br J Anaesth 38:490, 1966
88. Propert DN: Pseudocholinesterase activity and phenotypes in mentally ill patients. Br J Psychiatry 134:477, 1979
89. Lamont AMS: Brief report: Anaesthesia and Huntington's chorea. Anesth Intens Care 7:189, 1979
90. Katzman R: Alzheimer's disease. N Engl J Med 314:964, 1986
91. Whitehouse PJ: Understanding the etiology of Alzheimer's disease. Neurology Clinics 4:427, 1986
92. Tandan R, Bradley WG: Amyotrophic lateral sclerosis: Part 2. Etiopathogenesis. Ann Neurol 18:419, 1985
93. Tandan R, Bradley WG: Amyotrophic lateral sclerosis: Part 1. Clinical features, pathology, and ethical issues in management. Ann Neurol 18:271, 1985
94. Bendheim PE: The human spongiform encephalopathies. Neurology Clinics 2:281, 1984
95. Duffy P, Wolf J, Collins G *et al:* Possible person-to-person transmission of Creutzfeldt-Jakob disease. N Engl J Med 290:692, 1974
96. Bernoulli C, Siegfried J, Baumgartner G: Danger of accidental person-to-person transmission of Creutzfeldt-Jacob disease by surgery. Lancet 1:478, 1977
97. Gajdusek MD, Gibbs CJ, Asher DM *et al:* Precautions in medical care of, and in handling material from, patients with transmissible virus dementia (Creutzfeldt-Jakob disease). N Engl J Med 297:1253, 1977
98. Brown P: An epidemiological critique of Creutzfeldt-Jakob disease. Epidemiol Rev 2:113, 1980
99. duMoulin GC, Hedley-Whyte J: Hospital-associated viral infection and the anesthesiologist. Anesthesiology 59:51, 1983
100. MacMurdo SD, Jakymec AJ, Bleyaert AL: Precautions in the anesthetic management of a patient with Creutzfeldt-Jakob disease. Anesthesiology 60:590, 1984
101. Keith AS: Introduction to the anemias. In Wyngaarden JB, Smith LH (eds): Cecil's Textbook of Medicine, 17th ed, p 870. Philadelphia, WB Saunders, 1985
102. Nunn JF, Chanarin J: Nitrous oxide inactivates methionine synthetase. In Eger EI (ed): Nitrous Oxide/N_2O, p 211. New York, Elsevier-Dutton, 1985
103. Schilling RF: Is nitrous oxide a dangerous anesthetic for vitamin B_{12}-deficient subjects? JAMA 255:1605, 1986
104. Chang H, Miller DR: Hemolytic anemias: Membrane defects. In Miller DR (ed): Blood Diseases of Infancy and Childhood, 5th ed, p 262. St Louis, CV Mosby, 1984
105. Hain WR: Diseases of blood. In Katz J, Steward DJ (eds): Anesthesia and Uncommon Pediatric Diseases, p 489. Philadelphia, WB Saunders, 1987
106. Luban NLC, Epstein BS, Watson SP: Sickle cell disease and anesthesia. Advances in Anesthesiology 1:289, 1984
107. The Anaesthesia Advisory Committee to the Chief Coroner of Ontario: Intraoperative death during cesarean section in a patient with sickle-cell trait. Can J Anaesth 34:67, 1987
108. Kin HC: Variants of sickle cell disease. In Schwartz E (ed): Hemoglobinopathies in Children, p 215. Littleton, PSG Publishing, 1980
109. Stein RE, Urbaniak J: Use of the tourniquet during surgery in patients with sickle cell hemoglobinopathies. Clin Orthop 151:231, 1980
110. Rockoff AS, Christy D, Zeldis N *et al:* Myocardial necrosis following general anesthesia in hemoglobin SC disease. Pediatrics 61:73, 1978
111. Heiner M, Teasdale SJ, David T *et al:* Aortocoronary bypass in a patient with sickle cell trait. Can Anaesth Soc J 26:428, 1979
112. Gibson JR: Anesthesia for sickle cell diseases and other hemoglobinopathies. Seminars in Anesthesiology 6:27, 1987
113. Phillips PE: Infectious agents in the pathogenesis of rheumatoid arthritis. Semin Arthritis Rheum 16:1, 1986
114. Krane SM, Simon LS: Rheumatoid arthritis: Clinical features and pathogenetic mechanisms. Med Clin North Am 70:263, 1986
115. Katz WA: Modern management of rheumatoid arthritis. Am J Med 79 (suppl 4C):24, 1985
116. Keenan MA, Stiles CM, Kaufman RL: Acquired laryngeal deviation associated with cervical spine disease in erosive polyarticular arthritis. Anesthesiology 58:441, 1983
117. White RH: Preoperative evaluation of patients with rheumatoid arthritis. Semin Arthritis Rheum 14:287, 1985
118. Reginster JY, Damas P, Franchimont P: Anaesthetic risks in osteoarticular disorders. Clin Rheumatol 4:30, 1985
119. Emlen W, Pisetsky DS, Taylor RP: Antibodies to DNA. Arthritis Rheum 29:1417, 1986
120. Pisetsky DS: Systemic lupus erythematosus. Med Clin North Am 70:337, 1986
121. Tsokos GC, Tsokos M, leRiche NGH *et al:* A clinical and pathologic study of cerebrovascular disease in patients with systemic lupus erythematosus. Semin Arthritis Rheum 16:70, 1986
122. Doherty NE, Siegel RJ: Cardiovascular manifestations of systemic lupus erythematosus. Am Heart J 110:1257, 1985
123. Mackay IR: Lupoid hepatitis and primary biliary cirrhosis: Autoimmune disease of the liver? Bull Rheum Dis 18:487, 1968
124. Rocco VK, Hurd ER: Scleroderma and scleroderma-like disorders. Semin Arthritis Rheum 16:22, 1986
125. Owens GR, Follansbee WP: Cardiopulmonary manifestations of systemic sclerosis. Chest 91:118, 1987
126. Thompson J, Conklin KA: Anesthetic management of a pregnant patient with scleroderma. Anesthesiology 59:69, 1983
127. Hochberg MC, Feldman D, Stevens MB: Adult onset polymyositis/dermatomyositis: An analysis of clinical and laboratory

features and survival in 76 patients with a review of the literature. Semin Arthritis Rheum 15:168, 1986

128. Dickey BF, Myers AR: Pulmonary disease in polymyositis/dermatomyositis. Semin Arthritis Rheum 14:60, 1984

129. Eielsen O, Stovner J: Dermatomyositis, suxamethonium action and atypical plasmacholinesterase. Can Anaesth Soc J 25:63, 1978

130. Eisele JH: Connective tissue diseases. In Katz J, Benumof J, Kadis LB (eds): Anesthesia and Uncommon Diseases, 2nd ed, p 508. Philadelphia, WB Saunders, 1981

131. Fine JD: Epidermolysis bullosa. Int J Dermatol 25:143, 1986

132. Broster T, Placek R, Eggers GWN: Epidermolysis bullosa: Anesthetic management for cesarean section. Anesth Analg 66:341, 1987

133. Pratilas V, Biezunski A: Epidermolysis bullosa manifested and treated during anesthesia. Anesthesiology 43:581, 1975

134. James I, Wark H: Airway management during anesthesia in patients with epidermolysis bullosa dystrophica. Anesthesiology 56:323, 1982

135. Holzman RS, Worthen HM, Johnson K: Anaesthesia for children with junctional epidermolysis bullosa (letalis). Can J Anaesth 34:395, 1987

136. Smith MF: Skin and connective tissues diseases. In Katz J, Steward DJ (eds): Anesthesia and Uncommon Pediatric Diseases, p 378. Philadelphia, WB Saunders, 1987

137. Vatashsky E, Aronson HB: Pemphigus vulgaris: Anaesthesia in the traumatised patient. Anaesthesia 37:1195, 1982

138. Jeyaram C, Torda TA: Anesthetic management of cholecystectomy in a patient with buccal pemphigus. Anesthesiology 40:600, 1974

Chapter 17

Henry Rosenberg
David Seitman

Pharmacogenetics

Due to physiologic, metabolic, or anatomic changes, many inherited disorders have significant implications for anesthetic management. In this chapter we discuss the inherited disorders whose manifestations are enhanced or instigated by drugs usually used by anesthesiologists. In some cases, such as with the porphyrias, the manifestations may be induced by agents other than anesthetics. In contrast, in other enzymatic disorders, *e.g.*, pseudocholinesterase deficiency, it would be extremely unlikely that a patient would have any problems until he or she were exposed to the depolarizing neuromuscular blocking agent succinylcholine. Malignant hyperthermia (MH) or malignant hyperpyrexia is perhaps the most significant inherited disorder that is triggered by exposure to anesthetic drugs.

MALIGNANT HYPERTHERMIA

Malignant hyperthermia was first formally described in 1960 in *Lancet* by Denborough and Lovell and subsequently in *The British Journal of Anesthesia*.[1, 2] That first case report laid the foundation for much of our understanding of the clinical presentations of MH. The patient was a young man who claimed that several of his relatives had died without apparent cause during anesthesia. He was anesthetized with halothane, and tachycardia, hot sweaty skin, peripheral mottling, and cyanosis developed. Early recognition and symptomatic treatment saved the patient. It therefore became apparent that this new syndrome had the following elements: patients were otherwise healthy unless exposed to an anesthetic agent; temperature elevation was a hallmark of the syndrome; a heritable or genetic component was present; and high mortality rate was associated. In addition, early recognition and treatment could abort the malignant effects of the syndrome.

In the 1960s other cases of MH were reported in increasing numbers, and a gene pool for MH was established in certain parts of the world. In addition, the association between porcine stress syndrome (PSS) or "pale soft exudative pork syndrome" and MH was described, thus providing an animal model for MH.[3] Porcine breeds such as the Landrace, Poland China, and Pietrain show the classic presentations of MH on induction of anesthesia with potent inhalation agents and succinylcholine.

In 1971 the first international symposium on MH was held in Toronto. During the 1970s many more clinical presentations of MH were reported. The development of the *in vitro* diagnostic test was suggested by Kalow *et al*, based on exposure of a skeletal muscle biopsy specimen to caffeine and then halothane.[4] In 1975, at the Second International Symposium on MH, Harrison's report showing that dantrolene could be effective in treating and preventing MH in pigs was brought to the attention of those interested in MH.[5] By 1979 a sufficient number of cases were described showing that intravenous dantrolene could successfully reverse the human form of MH, and it was approved for use by the Food and Drug Administration. During this decade studies of the pathophysiology of MH were also performed. By the late 1970s it was apparent that MH most likely resulted from metabolic alterations in skeletal muscle. By the 1980s regular workshops on MH were held every 2–4 yr, with an increasing number of investigators becoming interested in this unusual syndrome. In the 1980s lay organizations in the United States, Canada, and Great

Britain were formed to disseminate information to patients affected by MH as well as to enhance the awareness of the syndrome among physicians. Additional studies of the manifestations of MH and its association to other muscle disorders and the consolidation of our understanding and applicability of the muscle biopsy diagnostic halothane/caffeine contraction test have taken place in the 1980s. In addition, a variety of other tests for diagnosing MH were introduced, many of which subsequently were found to be of little or no validity.

A major step forward occurred in 1985, when the Lopez group demonstrated an increased intracellular concentration of calcium ion in muscle from MH–susceptible pigs and humans.[6] The intracellular calcium concentration dramatically increased during an MH crisis and was reversed by the administration of dantrolene. More widespread appreciation of MH, its clinical manifestations, and greater preparedness for treating this potentially fatal but curable disorder occurred in this decade.

The 1990s undoubtedly will bring about yet a greater awareness of MH, a further reduction in the mortality from this syndrome, and a better understanding of its pathophysiologic characteristics, which we hope will lead to a less invasive diagnostic test than present.

MALIGNANT HYPERTHERMIA: CLINICAL PRESENTATIONS

As our knowledge and understanding of MH has grown, the definition of MH has changed. At first MH was thought in all cases to be a heritable syndrome consisting of extremely elevated body temperature, skeletal muscle rigidity, acidosis, and associated with a high mortality rate. However, we have now begun to concentrate on the definition of MH in terms of its underlying pathophysiologic characteristics. MH is a hypermetabolic disorder of skeletal muscle with varied presentations, depending on species, breed, and triggering agents. An important pathophysiologic process is intracellular hypercalcemia. Intracellular hypercalcemia activates metabolic pathways that result, if untreated, in adenosine triphosphate (ATP) depletion, acidosis, membrane destruction, and cell death. Although a heritable component is present in many cases, it is not invariably apparent from patient family history. In addition, disorders that may have symptoms and signs similar to MH, such as neuroleptic malignant syndrome, may not have an inherited basis at all.

CLASSIC MALIGNANT HYPERTHERMIA

Malignant hyperthermia may present in several ways. Most commonly, the first manifestations of the syndrome occur in the operating room. However, MH may occur in the recovery room, or even on return to the ward, as well. In the classic case, the initial signs of tachycardia and tachypnea result from sympathetic nervous system stimulation secondary to underlying hypermetabolism and hypercarbia. Because most patients who receive general anesthesia are paralyzed, tachypnea usually is not recognized. Shortly after the increase in heart rate, an increase in blood pressure is manifest, often associated with ventricular arrhythmias induced by sympathetic nervous system stimulation from hypercarbia or due to hyperkalemia or catecholamine release. Thereafter, muscle rigidity or increase in muscle tone may become apparent. Desaturation of the blood in the operative field and then increase in body temperature, climbing at a rate of $1-2°C$ every 5 min, follows. With the increase in metabolism, the patient may "break through" the neuromuscular blockade. At the same time the carbon dioxide absorbant becomes activated and warm to the touch (because the reaction with carbon dioxide is exothermic). The patient will display peripheral mottling and, on occasion, sweating and cyanosis. Blood gas analysis usually reveals hypercarbia and respiratory and metabolic acidosis without marked oxygen desaturation. A mixed venous sample will show even more dramatic evidence of carbon dioxide retention and metabolic acidosis.[7] Hyperkalemia, hypercalcemia, and myoglobinuria are characteristic. Creatinine phosphokinase (CK) increase will be dramatic, often exceeding 20,000 units in the first $12-24$ h. Death will result unless the syndrome is promptly treated. Even with treatment and survival the patient is at risk for life-threatening myoglobinuric renal failure and disseminated intravascular coagulation. Another significant clinical problem is recrudescence of the syndrome within the first $24-36$ h.[8]

If succinylcholine is used during induction of anesthesia, an acceleration of the manifestations of MH may occur such that tachycardia, hypertension, marked temperature elevation, and arrhythmias are seen over the course of $5-10$ min. However, it is important to note that a completely normal response to succinylcholine may be present in some MH-susceptible patients. A potent inhalation agent apparently is necessary to trigger the syndrome in these cases.

Review of case reports of MH suggests that the syndrome becomes apparent most frequently shortly after induction, particularly when succinylcholine is used, and at the end of the procedure as the patient is emerging from anesthesia. Manifestations of MH are indeed rare several hours after the conclusion of surgery and anesthesia.

MASSETER MUSCLE RIGIDITY

Rigidity of the jaw muscles after administration of succinylcholine is referred to as masseter muscle rigidity (MMR). The association of this phenomenon with MH was underlined by Donlon et al when they reported several cases of MH occurring after episodes of MMR.[9] Others have also stated that MMR is often premonitory to MH.[10] Although MMR probably occurs in patients of all ages, it is distinctly most common in children and young adults. Several studies have shown a peak age incidence at $8-12$ yr of age.[11] Characteristically, anesthesia is induced by inhalation with halothane, after which succinylcholine is administered. Snapping of the jaw or rigidity upon opening of the jaw is seen. However, this rigidity can be overcome with effort and will usually abate within $2-3$ min. A peripheral nerve stimulator usually will reveal flaccid paralysis. However, increased tone of other muscles also may be noted. Repeat doses of succinylcholine will not relieve the problem. Tachycardia and arrhythmias are not infrequent. Only in rare cases will frank MH supervene immediately after MMR. More commonly (if the anesthetic is continued with a triggering agent), in $10-20$ min, the initial signs of MH will appear. If the anesthetic is discontinued, the patient usually will recover uneventfully. However, within $4-12$ h, myoglobinuria will occur and CK elevation will be detected.

Although MMR is seen with all types of surgical procedures, one recent report found a six times higher incidence in patients who have strabismus surgery. Muscle biopsy testing by caffeine/halothane contracture test has shown that approximately 50% of patients who experience MMR will also be MH susceptible.[12] Therefore, most authorities recommend that anesthesia (if elective in nature) be discontinued and surgery postponed after an episode of MMR. With the introduction of end-tidal carbon dioxide monitoring and the availability of dantrolene, and enhanced understanding of MH, some have questioned the advice that all anesthetics must be discontinued after MMR. Instead they recommend continuation with nontriggering anesthetics and the use of end-tidal carbon dioxide monitoring. If such a course is followed, it is nevertheless incumbent upon the anesthesiologist to discuss with the patient further diagnostic tests such as muscle biopsy for MH and to alert him or her to the possibility that MH may follow in subsequent procedures. The issue of whether to give dantrolene after an episode of MMR is also unsettled. It is our clinical impression that administration of dantrolene after MMR will prevent the characteristic myoglobinuria and marked elevation of CK.

The differential diagnosis of MMR consists of the following: 1) amytonic myotonia syndrome, 2) temporomandibular joint (TMJ) dysfunction, 3) underdosing, or 4) not allowing sufficient time for succinylcholine to act before intubation. Signs of TMJ dysfunction as well as myotonia should be sought in the postoperative period. Otherwise, patients need to be counseled regarding the need for a muscle biopsy and other diagnostic tests for MH.

If MMR were a rare phenomenon, it would be troublesome enough. However, based on two recent studies, this sign may occur in as many as 1 in 100 children anesthetized with halothane and given succinylcholine.[13] A third study based on the information supplied to the Danish Malignant Hyperthermia Registry showed that the incidence of MMR was 1 in 12,000 (including adults and children).[14] The discordance between the incidence of MH, which is felt to be in the range of 1 to 10,000 to 50,000 anesthetics, and the higher incidence of MMR in children may relate to the following: 1) the retrospective nature of the studies, 2) a greater susceptibility to MH in the younger age groups, 3) a peculiarity of the innervation or muscle structure of children, 4) a peculiarity of the masseter muscle itself.[15]

As perplexing as is the relationship between MMR and the susceptibility to MH, little or no information is available regarding patients who have experienced MMR along with myoglobinuria and who have normal results on biopsy testing for MH.

Our advice regarding MMR is as follows: 1) the anesthesiologist should, if at all possible, discontinue the anesthetic and postpone surgery. If end-tidal carbon dioxide monitoring and dantrolene are available and the anesthesiologist is experienced in managing MH, he or she may elect to continue with a nontriggering anesthetic. 2) After episodes of MMR, the patient should be observed carefully for a period of 12–24 h. One to 2 mg·kg^{-1} of dantrolene should be administered intravenously. 3) The family should be informed of the episode of MMR and its implications. 4) CK should be drawn at 6, 12, and 24 h after the episode. If the CK level is still grossly elevated at 12 h, additional CKs should be drawn until the CK is returning toward normal. Our recent studies have shown that if CK is greater than 20,000 IU in the perioperative period and there is not a concomitant myopathy present, then the diagnosis of MH can be made with virtual certainty.[16] 5) If muscle biopsy testing results are within normal limits after an episode of MMR, we currently do not recommend that other family members undergo testing but that use of succinylcholine be avoided in future anesthetics.

To date, MMR has been documented only in association with succinylcholine, although it may occur after induction with any anesthetic agent, intravenous or inhalation, before succinylcholine administration. As such, many pediatric anesthesiologists are avoiding the use of succinylcholine except on indication.

OTHER PRESENTATIONS OF MALIGNANT HYPERTHERMIA

Not only may MH occur in the operating room, but it may also become manifest in the early postoperative period, usually within the first few hours of recovery from anesthesia. The characteristic tachycardia, tachypnea, hypertension, and arrhythmias indicate that an episode of MH may be about to follow. Isolated myoglobinuria in the postoperative period should also alert the anesthesiologist that a problem has occurred. Succinylcholine may cause rhabdomyolysis in patients who have other muscle disorders that may not be clinically obvious on cursory examination.[17] Presence of myoglobinuria mandates that the patient be referred to a neurologist for further investigation.

NEUROLEPTIC MALIGNANT SYNDROME AND OTHER DISORDERS ASSOCIATED WITH MALIGNANT HYPERTHERMIA

The symptoms and signs of the neuroleptic malignant syndrome (NMS) include fever, rhabdomyolysis, tachycardia, hypertension, agitation, muscle rigidity, and acidosis.[18] The mortality is more than 20%. The observation that biopsied muscle from most patients with NMS will display enhanced contractures to halothane and caffeine suggests a common link between the two syndromes.[19] Also, dantrolene is an effective therapeutic modality in many cases of NMS. Therefore, it is not unusual for an anesthesiologist to be consulted in the management of patients with NMS.

Although the resemblance of NMS to MH is striking, there are significant differences between the two. MH is acute; NMS occurs after longer-term drug exposure. Phenothiazines and haloperidol alone or in combination are usually triggering agents for NMS. Sudden withdrawal of drugs used to treat Parkinson's disease may also trigger NMS. Electroconvulsive therapy (ECT) with succinylcholine usually does *not* trigger the syndrome.[20] Also, NMS does not seem to be inherited, and there are no case reports of NMS in family members who have had an episode of MH.

Many believe that the changes in NMS are a reflection of dopamine depletion in the central nervous system by psychoactive agents. In support of this theory, therapy with bromocriptine, a dopamine agonist, is often useful in treatment of NMS.[21] Therefore, although there appear to be similarities between MH and NMS, the common basis is not readily apparent. From an anesthesiologist's viewpoint, it is best to treat patients with NMS as though they were susceptible to MH until additional information is obtained and to conduct ECT therapy *without* the use of succinylcholine or other triggering agents of MH.

Duchenne muscular dystrophy (DMD) and other muscular dystrophies have also been linked to MH. Some patients with DMD anesthetized with MH-triggering agents will experience sudden cardiac arrest during operation or in the very early postoperative period. Hyperkalemia, acidosis, and temperature elevation are usually seen.[22] In others, significant rhabdomyolysis occurs in the early postoperative period, which leads to muscle weakness and early death.[23] In a series of 10 muscle biopsy specimens from patients with DMD and patients with a similar disorder, Becker's dystrophy, approximately 50% have shown the typical halothane contractures *in vitro* that are observed in MH-susceptible patients.[24] Therefore, MH-triggering agents should not be used in patients with DMD and related dystrophies. Dantrolene pretreatment must be considered before surgery in patients with myopathic disorders, although the muscle weakness that may follow dantrolene administration is of concern. In addition to avoiding the use of succinylcholine, cardiopulmonary and body temperature measurements must be monitored carefully in the perioperative period.

Central core disease is an unusual myopathy characterized by muscle weakness. It is probably inherited in a recessive manner. Many cases of MH have been reported in patients with central core disease. Therefore, precautions regarding MH must be taken for all patients with central core disease.[25]

Another myopathy associated with MH is myotonia congenita. Only a few cases of MH have been reported in patients with myotonia congenita, far fewer than would be expected if there were a high coincidence of susceptibility to MH in such patients.

King or King-Denborough syndrome is a rare myopathy characterized by cryptorchidism, markedly slanted eyes, low set ears, pectus deformity, scoliosis, small stature, and hypotonia. Several patients with this disorder have been diagnosed as MH susceptible both clinically and by muscle biopsy.[26] Schwartz-Jampal syndrome, a myotonic-like condition, is also associated with MH.

One of the few metabolic disorders associated with MH is osteogenesis imperfecta (OI).[27] Here again the association is sporadic. Despite a few well-documented cases of MH in patients with OI, we have not confirmed MH susceptibility in three cases of OI tested with the halothane/caffeine contracture test but have found typical contractures in one other biopsy.

Denborough *et al* have recently speculated that patients with MH are more likely to have offspring at risk for sudden infant death syndrome.[28] This observation needs further confirmation and investigation.

Pheochromocytoma may be mistaken for MH because of its presentation by tachycardia, hypertension, and fever during anesthesia. The link between the two disorders is not at all clear.

MALIGNANT HYPERTHERMIA OUTSIDE THE OPERATING ROOM

The concern that MH may occur outside the operating room without mediation of drugs in humans has been expressed repeatedly. This concern arrives from the oft-repeated observation that an MH-like syndrome can occur in certain pig breeds in response to stressful situations. However, documented cases of fulminant MH occurring without drug intervention in humans have not been convincing. Gronert *et al* have described a patient who had episodic fevers and had muscle biopsies positive for MH.[29] The fevers were controlled by dantrolene. Recently, Fishbein *et al* have reported on two young patients who had apparent heat stroke and were also MH susceptible.[30]

Some also believe that MH-susceptible patients are likely to die suddenly.[31] We are not convinced. Detailed information usually is not available regarding the medical history of young people who die suddenly and unexpectedly. Was there evidence of a recent infection? What were the results of previous medical examinations, drug levels, and other tests? Studies of sudden death in young people have found that infection and cardiac disease account for more than half the causes of such sudden death. Many times the symptoms of such problems are either mild and not recognized or are ignored. About 10% of sudden unexpected deaths in healthy young adults result from a cerebral bleed, 25% from asthma and epilepsy, and about 15% from undetermined causes. Neuspiel and Kuller state "both clinicians and coroners or medical examiners may have biased perceptions about sudden death in this age group."[32] A great deal of debate and very little data characterize the discussions regarding sudden death and MH. A more widespread easier-to-use diagnostic test and a better understanding of the pathophysiologic characteristics of MH are necessary to resolve this issue.

DRUGS THAT TRIGGER MALIGNANT HYPERTHERMIA

It is clearly established that the potent inhalation agents, including methoxyflurane, cyclopropane, and ether, may trigger MH. Succinylcholine and decamethonium are also triggers. The status of many other drugs is less clear. Table 17-1 indicates the drugs we believe to be safe *versus* those that are unsafe.

Local Anesthetics

The greatest controversy in regard to agents that trigger MH revolves around the local anesthetics. Based on studies indicating that neither amide or ester local anesthetics trigger MH in susceptible swine nor that amide local anesthetics trigger MH in susceptible humans, it seems clear that all local anesthetics are safe for MH-susceptible patients.[33, 34] Studies of local anesthetics during an MH crisis (*e.g.*, for arrhythmia control) are lacking. Therefore, most experts still recommend use of procaine or procainamide to manage arrhythmias during a crisis.

Ketamine

In our estimation, until additional data are available, it is best to avoid the use of ketamine in patients with suspected MH because elevated blood pressure, tachycardia, and temperature elevation are common in patients receiving ketamine.

TABLE 17-1.   Safe *versus* Unsafe Drugs in Malignant Hyperthermia

Unsafe Drugs	Safe Drugs
All inhalation agents (except nitrous oxide)	Barbiturates
Succinylcholine	Narcotics
Decamethonium	Antipyretics
Potassium salts	Antihistamines
	Antibiotics
	Local anesthetics
Insufficient Data/Controversial	Althesin
Curare	Pancuronium
Metocurarine	Atracurium
Calcium salts	Vecuronium
Ketamine	Propranolol
Catecholamines	Droperidol
Phenothiazines	Vasoactive drugs

Catecholamines

Although plasma catecholamine concentration increases during an MH crisis, such an elevation is usually secondary to metabolic and cardiovascular changes. Sympathetic denervation by spinal anesthesia does not delay the onset of halothane-induced MH in susceptible pigs.[35] Other data also support the contention that vasopressors and other catecholamines are not involved in triggering MH.[36] Therefore, these drugs should be used as necessary but only with simultaneous treatment of the MH crisis.

Nondepolarizing Relaxants

Although curare is a suspected trigger, vecuronium, atracurium, and pancuronium are considered safe to use in patients with MH.[37]

Anticholinesterases

Clinical studies have shown that anticholinesterase–anticholinergic combinations are safe for reversal of nondepolarizing relaxants in MH-susceptible patients.[38]

Phenothiazines

Phenothiazines increase intracellular calcium ion concentration and may cause contractures in vitro in muscle from MH-susceptible patients.[39] Phenothiazines also induce the related neuroleptic malignant syndrome. Therefore, although there have been several reports that phenothiazines are effective in managing temperature fluctuations during recovery from MH, in MH-susceptible patients these compounds should be used cautiously if at all.

Other Drugs

Digoxin, quinidine, and calcium salts do not induce MH in the swine caudal preparation.[40] Therefore, it is reasonable to assume that they are safe to use in clinical situations. However, potassium salts can trigger MH. This results from a depolarization of the muscle membrane, leading to muscle contracture.

Droperidol seems to be safe, based on clinical experience and in vitro studies.[41]

INCIDENCE AND EPIDEMIOLOGY

Although the incidence of reported episodes of MH has increased, the mortality rate from MH has declined. In part these two trends reflect a greater awareness of the syndrome, earlier diagnosis, and better therapy. The incidence of MH varies from country to country, based on differences in gene pools. In the upper midwest of the United States, for example, there are many families with a high incidence of MH. In contrast, other areas of the country and parts of the world have rarely reported MH. The overall incidence is said to be 1 in 50,000 anesthetics in adults and 1 in 15,000 anesthetics in children.[15] Results of large-scale studies of operative mortality are in general agreement with this figure. For example, a recent study in Great Britain revealed three cases of MH in 100,000 anesthetics. One of the better studies concerning the epidemiologic characteristics of MH is that of Ording.[14] Her study, based on information supplied to the Danish Malignant Hyperthermia Registry, comprising the reported incidence of MH in the approximately 5,000,000 population in Denmark,

revealed fulminant MH in approximately 1 in 250,000 anesthetics. However, if the definition of MH is expanded to include abortive cases of MH and is further refined to include only cases in which inhalation anesthetics and succinylcholine were used, then the incidence was as high as 1 in 4,000 anesthetic administrations!

Currently, the consensus is that the mortality from MH is approximately 10%. Indeed the Malignant Hyperthermia Association of the United States (MHAUS) is notified of eight to 10 deaths from MH during the course of the year. However, the epidemiologic characteristics of MH are very difficult to define for the following reasons:

1. Widespread diagnostic testing for MH is difficult to apply.
2. The clinical diagnosis of MH is often questionable.
3. Triggering of MH even in susceptible patients may not occur upon an individual anesthetic exposure. In some cases susceptible patients have received triggering agents for up to 13 anesthetics without any problems only to have MH triggered on the subsequent anesthetic.
4. There is no central reporting agency for MH.
5. Triggering agent use varies between countries. Organizations such as the Malignant Hyperthermia Association (of Canada) (MHA) as well as MHAUS are in the process of creating central registries for the reporting of MH cases.

A better diagnostic test and better reporting of MH will certainly enhance our knowledge of the incidence of this syndrome.

INHERITANCE OF MALIGNANT HYPERTHERMIA

Many of the reasons that limit our understanding of the epidemiologic characteristics of MH also limit our accurate assessment of its inheritance. It seems that studies of the animal model would clarify the issue of inheritance, but this has not been the case. In certain reports the inheritance appears to be autosomal dominant, whereas in others it is clearly autosomal recessive.[44, 45] This difference may result from differences in breeds. In at least four breeds of swine MH is quite common. Even in pigs the breeding experiments may fail to clarify inheritance because the diagnosis of MH in swine is often based on the animal's exposure to 3% halothane by mask and observation of a clinical response. However, this test does not detect all those that are susceptible.[46] Variabilities in clinical presentation, and the fact that MH is not regularly apparent on exposure to triggering agents even in those that are susceptible causes great difficulty in assessing the inheritance of MH in humans. The inheritance of MH in humans has been described as autosomal dominant, multifactorial, autosomal dominant with variable penetrance, as well as multigenetic.

Our studies, as well as anecdotal reports from other diagnostic centers, have supported the concept of autosomal dominant inheritance by a single gene with variable penetrance. Representative examples of such clinical documentation of autosomal dominance are as follows:

1. A 34-yr-old man died of the classic MH syndrome. Although his father had a family history of ptosis, he had MH-negative results on biopsy. His mother was too ill for biopsy. A maternal cousin was MH susceptible on contracture test, as was his maternal uncle.

2. A 4-yr-old child had masseter rigidity develop, with a postepisode level CK 8,000/IU. Her two siblings had negative biopsy results; however, her mother had MH-positive results. None of the children had anesthesia previously.
3. An 8-yr-old boy had masseter rigidity develop, with CK elevation after receiving succinylcholine. His father stated that his own father had died of hyperthermia during surgery years previously. The father was MH susceptible on contracture testing.

Studies of large families have also documented an autosomal dominant pattern. McPherson and Taylor studied 93 families in whom MH occurred.[47] Although MH was often diagnosed by inference, based on CK elevations as well as clinical histories and in some cases contracture testing, various patterns of inheritance did emerge (Table 17-2).[47]

We therefore advise patients that 50% of siblings and 50% of children of the MH-susceptible patients are potentially at risk. Although baseline CK determinations may be of no value in screening for MH, McPherson and Taylor reported that relatives of MH-susceptible patients with an elevated CK level (without recent trauma or muscle disorder) have a greater than 70% chance of being susceptible. However, relatives with a normal CK level may also be susceptible.

In cases of MH associated with a myopathy such as DMD, it is not clear whether MH is a manifestation of the underlying myopathy—and therefore those in a family who do not have evidence of a myopathy are not susceptible to MH—or whether the MH susceptibility is inherited apart from the myopathy—and therefore other family members may be at risk for MH.

DIAGNOSTIC TESTS FOR MALIGNANT HYPERTHERMIA

In 1970, Kalow et al demonstrated that isolated muscle from MH-susceptible patients behaved abnormally in response to caffeine when tested in vitro.[4] Shortly thereafter, investigators demonstrated that muscle from MH-susceptible patients responded in an abnormal fashion to halothane. Although others have shown that potassium chloride, thymol, other inhalation anesthetic agents, and succinylcholine can induce greater contractures in muscle from MH-susceptible patients than in those who are nonsusceptible, treatment of muscle biopsy specimens with halothane, caffeine, and/or the combination has come to be the standard test for diagnosing MH susceptibility.[48]

Other tests have been proposed to differentiate patients with MH from those who are normal. Some tests use skeletal muscle biopsy specimens, such as the test that measures ATP

TABLE 17-2.   Inheritance of Malignant Hyperthermia in 93 Families

Clearly autosomal dominant, 38%
Possibly autosomal dominant, 14%
Associated with dominant myopathies, 3%
Isolated, 17%
Questionable recessive (isolated), 21%
Insufficient information, 7%

(Based on data from McPherson EW, Taylor CA: The genetics of malignant hyperthermia: Evidence for heterogeneity. Am J Med Genet 11:273, 1982.)

concentration in isolated muscle after incubation with 4% halothane, whereas others employ blood elements such as platelets or white blood cells to determine susceptibility. Other less invasive tests also have been suggested to differentiate the MH-susceptible population, such as the twitch response to stimulation of the ulnar nerve during a period of tourniquet-induced ischemia and, more recently, measurements of the ratio of inorganic phosphate to phosphocreatine by nuclear magnetic resonance (NMR) techniques.

Tests That Have No Real Value in Diagnosis of Malignant Hyperthermia

BLOOD TESTS. Hypotonic red blood cell lysis may help differentiate MH-susceptible swine from nonsusceptible swine. However, this is not valid in humans.[49] Studies performed with red blood cells incubated with or without drugs have not shown any difference in hypotonic lysis between susceptible and nonsusceptible patients.

CREATININE PHOSPHOKINASE TESTS. Creatinine phosphokinase determinations may be valuable in differentiating MH-susceptible swine populations.[50] However, this is not the case in humans. CK is only useful in relatives of patients known to be susceptible; in that instance an elevated CK level predicts MH susceptibility with an approximate 70–80% accuracy. A normal CK level is not predictive.[47]

PLATELET NUCLEOTIDE DEPLETION TESTS. Platelets from patients susceptible to MH were reported to have a greatly reduced energy concentration ratio (ATP + APD/hypoxanthine + AMP) as compared with those from normal patients.[51] Several studies have failed to validate this test.[52]

TESTS USING SKELETAL MUSCLE BIOPSY SPECIMENS. Assay of the enzyme adenylate kinase was suggested as a possible marker for MH susceptibility. This has not been substantiated. Similarly, it was reported that myophosphorylase concentrations are elevated in susceptible patients, but this was not confirmed.[52a]

CALCIUM UPTAKE AND CALCIUM ATPase IN FROZEN MUSCLE. The advantage of this test was that samples could be frozen in liquid nitrogen and shipped to a laboratory that could perform this assay.[53] However, recent studies have found that calcium uptake, as well as calcium ATPase, in frozen thin muscle sections, does not differentiate MH-susceptible from nonsusceptible patients.[54] A double-blind study of 29 patients in whom the diagnosis of MH by halothane-contracture compared with calcium uptake was tested showed a large number of false-positive results by the uptake test.

SKINNED FIBER TESTS. In this test isolated muscle cells are dissected, the membrane is disrupted either mechanically or chemically, and the response to caffeine and or halothane is assessed in single fibers.[55] The advantage of the test is that muscle can be stored and shipped for analysis. However, the test is tedious and there are technical difficulties. Also, its results can only be considered supportive of the diagnosis by the standard halothane caffeine contracture test.

PROTEINS IN MALIGNANT HYPERTHERMIA. An abnormal protein in MH muscle was reported by one group.[56] However, subsequent studies have failed to confirm this finding.[57]

LESS INVASIVE TESTS. Enhanced response of the thenar muscles on stimulation of the ulnar nerve during a period of tourniquet ischemia was suggested to be a valid way of differentiating MH-susceptible from nonsusceptible patients. This finding also has not been substantiated by other investigators.[58]

New Tests for Malignant Hyperthermia

Klip *et al* have recently reported that isolated monocytes from blood from MH-susceptible patients will demonstrate an enhanced intracellular calcium release on exposure to halothane.[59] In this test the isolated cells are incubated with a calcium marker, Quin-2, whose light absorption varies, depending on calcium concentration.

We have recently reported that the ratio of inorganic phosphate to phosphocreatine is enhanced in MH-susceptible patients. Intracellular ratios of inorganic phosphate to phosphocreatine are measured easily by nuclear magnetic resonance of spectrometry.[6]

Although Lopez *et al* have elegantly demonstrated that intracellular calcium concentration is elevated in muscle from MH-susceptible swine and further enhanced by exposure to halothane, this observation has not reached a practical level for introduction for use as a diagnostic test.

Halothane–Caffeine Contracture Tests

This test is simple in concept and uncomplicated in operation (Table 17-3).[62] Skeletal muscle is usually obtained from the vastus lateralis muscle by biopsy. Strips of muscle weighing approximately 100 mg and measuring 1–2 cm in length by 2–5 mm in width by 1–4 mm in thickness are cut and mounted in standard muscle bath apparatus (Fig. 17-1). The tissue bath usually contains a modified Krebs solution at 37°C bubbled with oxygen and carbon dioxide (95%/5%), and the resting tension is adjusted to 2 g. The bundles are stimulated supramaximally with pulses of a frequency of 0.2 hz for 2–10 ms. After a 30-min equilibration CO_2 /O_2, halothane is added to mixture and the concentration is checked chromatographically.

Other strips are exposed to caffeine (see below). In our laboratory patients are judged MH susceptible when a contracture in one of the eight strips tested is greater than or equal to 0.7 g within a 5-min exposure to 3% halothane (Figs. 17-2A and 17-3) or greater than 0.5 g after exposure to 1–2% halothane. The European Malignant Hyperthermia Group has modified this halothane contracture test somewhat.[63] In one of the tests used by those investigators the muscle is allowed to rest at a fixed tension for several minutes and is then stretched at a rate of 4 ml·min^{-1} for 1.5 min. The preparation is held at this length for 1 min before the tension is decreased at the same rate. After three control cycles, halothane 0.5% is added for 3 min and another cycle completed. The halothane concentration is increased with each subsequent cycle. Contractures greater than 0.2 g are considered abnormal.

THE CAFFEINE CONTRACTURE TEST. The muscle strips are mounted as already described. After a 30-min equilibration, strips are exposed to incremental concentration of caffeine (0.125–16 mM) at twofold intervals. Two diagnostic criteria have been used in assessing the response to caffeine. The most common is the caffeine-specific concentration, in which the concentration that causes a 1-g contracture in the absence of halothane is estimated, based on a plot of the contracture response to incremental doses of caffeine. The second criterion is a contracture greater than or equal to 0.3 g to 2 mM caffeine (Fig. 17-2B).

HALOTHANE PLUS CAFFEINE CONTRACTURE TESTS. This test is similar to the caffeine contracture test but is done in the presence of 1% halothane. MH susceptibility is diagnosed by a caffeine-specific concentration less than 4 mM or a halothane caffeine-specific concentration less than 1 mM.[64]

In our laboratory almost all MH-susceptible patients will have significant contractures develop to halothane exposure alone. Far fewer respond to caffeine alone. Indeed false-negative results with a caffeine test only can be as high as 75%.[62] Nevertheless, some patients will display an abnormality on caffeine exposure with a normal response to halothane. Therefore, both tests should be used. The test combining halothane and caffeine has generated a great deal of controversy. Patients whose muscle responds in a normal fashion to halothane and caffeine but in an enhanced fashion to the combination of halothane and caffeine have been termed as having "K" phenotypes. It has been hypothesized that patients with a K phenotype may respond to MH-triggering agents in a fashion similar to MH-susceptible patients but with a slower response. Through selective breeding, Nelson *et al* have identified pigs whose muscle responds in a manner that would correspond to a K phenotype. On exposure to halothane and after repeated doses of succinylcholine, serum lactate levels will increase, *p*H levels will decrease, and carbon dioxide excretion levels will increase in these animals.[65] However, gross fulminant MH is not observed. Studies using human tissue have shown that the contracture response of the K type

TABLE 17-3. Contracture Responses to Halothane (3%) and Caffeine

CONTRACTURE TEST	MH NEGATIVE	MH POSITIVE	SIGNIFICANCE (*t* test)
CONTRACTURE IN g—$\overline{X} \pm$ SEM(N)			
Maximum halothane	0.32 ± 0.03 (39)	1.69 ± 0.17 (36)	$P < 0.001$
Average halothane	0.16 ± 0.01 (39)	0.95 ± 0.10 (36)	$P < 0.001$
Caffeine 2 mM	0.02 ± 0.00 (39)	0.10 ± 0.04 (35)	$P < 0.05$
CONCENTRATION IN mM—$\overline{X} \pm$ SEM(N)			
CSC	7.87 ± 0.48 (39)	6.23 ± 0.40 (35)	$P < 0.05$
HCSC	2.22 ± 0.27 (37)	1.62 ± .27 (34)	NS

CSC = caffeine-specific concentration; HCSC = caffeine-specific concentration in the presence of 1% halothane; ( ) = number of strips tested.
There is no significant difference between MH-positive and MH-negative results for the MHCSC test.

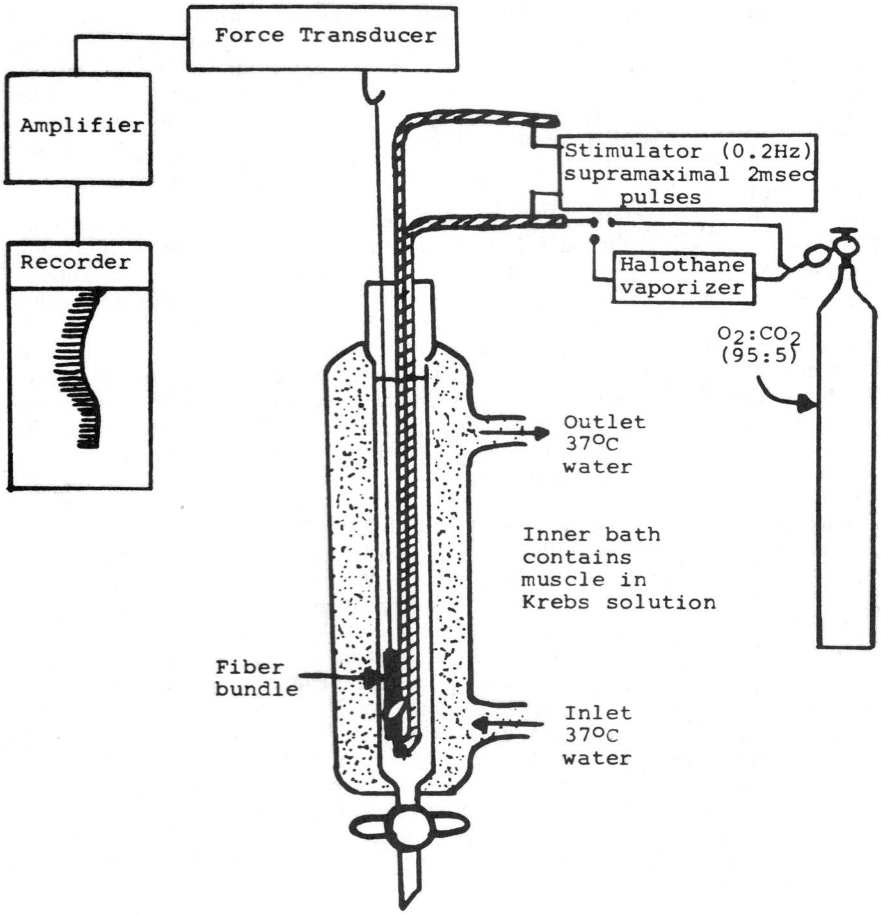

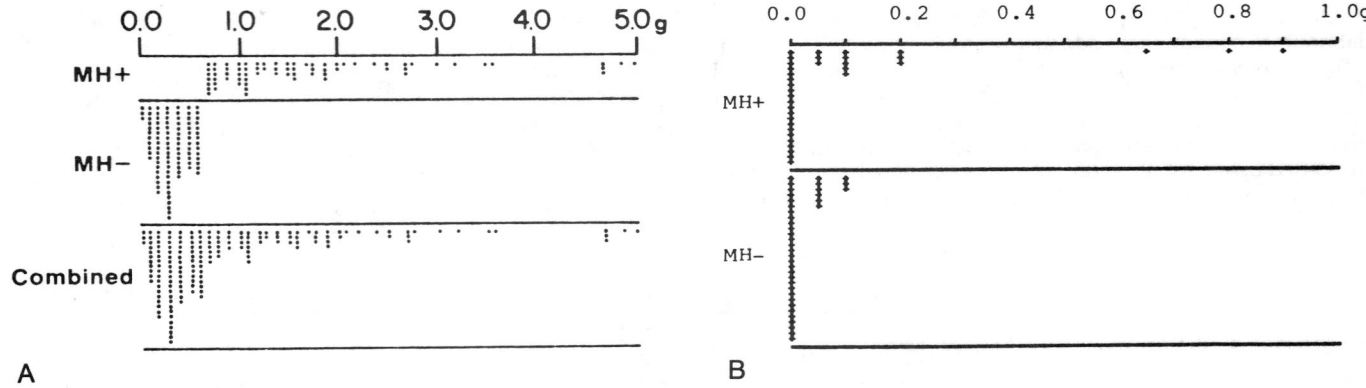

FIG. 17-1. Diagram of the muscle bath apparatus used for contracture testing for diagnosing malignant hyperthermia susceptibility.

FIG. 17-2. (*A*) Contracture response on exposure to 3% halothane in those susceptible and nonsusceptible to malignant hyperthermia. (*B*) The average contracture response to 2 mM caffeine in those susceptible and nonsusceptible to malignant hyperthermia.

can be found in up to 20% of the control population. Clearly this test variant will falsely diagnose many as MH susceptible.

PITFALLS IN THE CONTRACTURE TEST. Although at the present time more than 20 centers employ the caffeine–halothane contracture test for diagnosing MH, the criteria for differentiating susceptible from nonsusceptible patients are not always uniform between centers.

Incubation time, bath size, stimulation characteristics, and methods of introduction of halothane and caffeine are slightly different between centers. Most importantly, each laboratory needs to derive specimens from patients who are clearly and

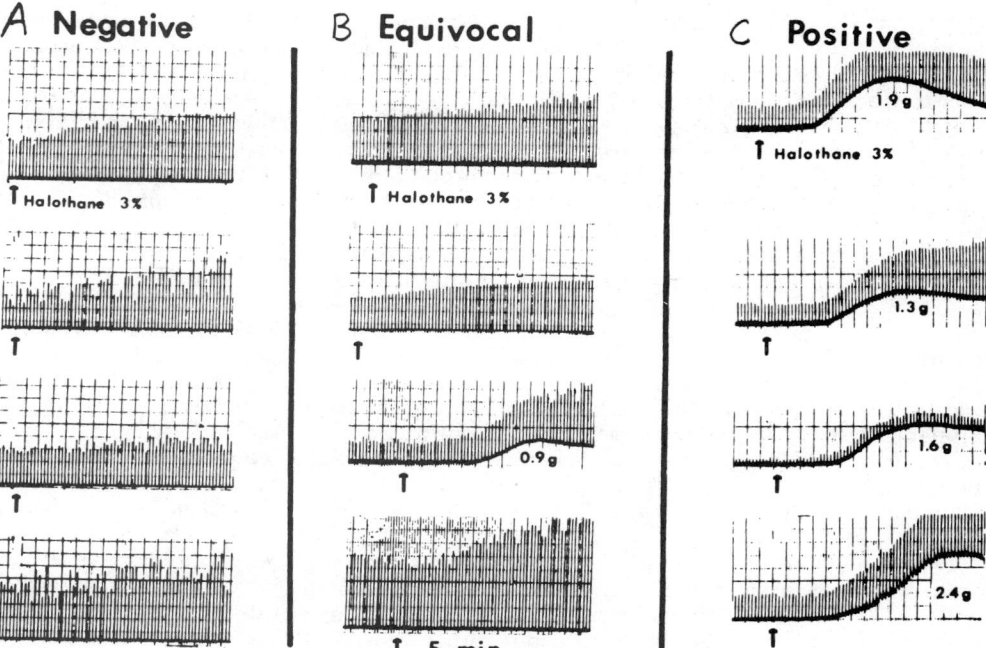

FIG. 17-3. Response to 3% halothane from representative biopsy specimens. (*A*) The normal response to 3% halothane. (*B*) Demonstration of a typical contracture indicative of malignant hyperthermia susceptibility in only one of four strips tested from a patient, who would be deemed malignant hyperthermia susceptible for clinical purposes. (*C*) A clear response in a susceptible patient.

unequivocally normal and those that are clearly and unequivocally MH susceptible. Unfortunately, it is not always possible to have complete agreement on the MH status of a patient. If an investigator determines the criteria for susceptibility in cases that are not unequivocally MH, a significant percentage of false-positive results can be reported. Although there has been some standardization of the caffeine–halothane contracture test in North America, further definition of standards and classifications of patients according to susceptibility is necessary. Investigators in Europe have agreed upon a standard protocol and testing for MH and employ similar equipment and similar techniques. This has facilitated the interchange of information and the creation of a larger pool of data for use in differentiating MH-susceptible from nonsusceptible patients.

One of the main problems in MH testing is that, rather than two separate groups being discernable on halothane–caffeine testing, there is instead a continuum of responses.[66] Susceptibility is determined by a response above or below a certain threshold. In addition, there may be variability between individual strips from the same biopsy specimen. A recent estimate from our laboratory showed that only 52% of fiber bundles from patients diagnosed as MH susceptible exhibited a positive response to halothane, whereas less than 25% of the strips tested positive for caffeine in biopsy specimens from 11 of 39 MH-susceptible patients. Therefore, to prevent sampling errors, it is best to test six to eight strips for each patient. On the positive side, however, contracture response of 1 g to halothane alone is uniformly recognized as indicating MH susceptibility in all laboratories. Furthermore, there is no reported incidence of a patient who has been diagnosed as MH negative by contracture testing who has subsequently experienced clinical episodes of MH. Anecdotal information indicates that several dozen patients who have been diagnosed as MH negative by contracture testing have indeed been exposed to halothane and succinylcholine without incident.

Until such time as the basic biochemical defect of MH is uncovered, the halothane–caffeine contracture test will al-

ways be subject to differences in interpretation. However, the halothane–caffeine contracture test is currently the only diagnostic test for MH that has been confirmed in any manner by multiple centers throughout the world. We recommend that laboratories continue to do the halothane–caffeine contracture test but that they test with 3% halothane alone, along with testing with caffeine alone. It is also necessary for each laboratory to establish its own controls and definitions of susceptibility, based on correlations with clinical events as well as standards of other laboratories.

MALIGNANT HYPERTHERMIA TREATMENT

Malignant hyperthermia is a treatable disorder. If it is diagnosed early and treated promptly with proper continued observation, mortality rate should be close to zero. All institutions in which anesthetic agents are administered should have dantrolene available (36 ampules is recommended, *i.e.,* 720 mg) and have a plan of management.

The Acute Episode

The following steps should be taken immediately when MH is diagnosed: 1) Administration of all inhalation agents and succinylcholine should be discontinued. 2) Hyperventilation with 100% oxygen should be instituted at high flow rates and assistance should be secured. (It is usually helpful to have a cart available containing the therapeutic agents for treatment of MH.) 3) Assistance should be obtained in mixing dantrolene. The present preparation of dantrolene is poorly soluble. Each ampule containing 20 mg should be mixed with 50 ml sterile distilled water (not saline solutions). Initial intravenous therapy should be started with a minimum dose of 2.5 $mg \cdot kg^{-1}$, with repeated doses as needed.[67] Although it is often recommended that the maximum dose of dantrolene is 10 $mg \cdot kg^{-1}$, more should be given as dictated by clinical circumstances. 4) Titration of dantrolene and bicarbonate to heart rate, body temperature, and Pa_{CO_2} are the best clinical guidelines of therapy. 5) In fulminant cases in which significant metabolic acidosis is present, 2–4 mEq·kg^{-1} bicarbonate should be given. 6) If not already available, a capnometer should be obtained so that carbon dioxide excretion can be followed. 7) If at all possible, the anesthesia circuit and carbon dioxide absorbent should be changed, because residual inhalation anesthetics may contaminate the anesthesia circuit. If not, very high flows of oxygen should be used. 8) Arrhythmia control will usually follow hyperventilation, dantrolene therapy, and correction of acidosis. On theoretic grounds, procaine or procainamide are the best choices for arrhythmia control. 9) Body temperature elevation should be managed by packing the patient with external icepacks and by use of gastric, wound, and rectal lavage. Gastric lavage is the quickest, most practical means for rapid temperature control. Some have recommended peritoneal dialysis and, others, cardiopulmonary bypass. Cooling should be stopped when body temperature reaches approximately 38°C to avoid hypothermia.

10) Although arterial blood gases are useful for assessing acidosis, central mixed venous blood gas determinations (or, if not available, femoral venous blood gases) will serve as a better guideline for therapy. Mixed venous carbon dioxide tension will be elevated and is a more appropriate measure of hypermetabolism. 11) Hyperkalemia should be managed in the usual fashion. The use of calcium for acute treatment of hyperkalemia has not been investigated. During therapy of MH, hypokalemia frequently results. However, potassium replacement should be undertaken very cautiously, if at all, because potassium may retrigger an MH episode.

Calcium channel blockers should not be used in the acute treatment of MH, particularly when dantrolene is administered.[68] Several studies have shown that verapamil may interact with dantrolene to produce hyperkalemia and a myocardial depression.

Management after the Acute Episode

After the acute episode, the clinician should be concerned about three complications of MH:

1. *Recrudescence of malignant hyperthermia.* Although most cases of MH resolve promptly with therapy, some cases are difficult to control. Temperature fluctuations may occur for several days and acute recrudescence may occur within hours of the first episode.[69]
2. *Disseminated intravascular coagulation.*[70] Disseminated intravascular coagulation (DIC) has often been described in cases of MH, probably resulting from release of thromboplastins secondary to shock and/or release of cellular contents upon membrane destruction. The usual regimen for DIC should be followed.
3. *Myoglobinuric renal failure.* Creatinine phosphokinase elevations may not occur for 6–12 h after an MH episode and should be followed as a rough guide for therapy. However, myoglobinuria classically occurs within 4–8 h of the episode; therefore, bladder catheterization is recommended. The guidelines for the dose and duration of dantrolene therapy after resolution of acute MH are empiric. It would seem prudent to continue dantrolene, 1–2 mg·kg^{-1} every 4 h intravenously, for at least 24 h. Some recommend conversion of dantrolene therapy from intravenous to oral form (4 mg·kg^{-1} per day or more) with continuation for several days.

Significant muscle weakness may follow MH, resulting from muscle destruction along with dantrolene administration; this should be managed symptomatically.

A variety of other electrolyte changes may occur, such as hypocalcemia and hyperphosphatemia. Sodium and chloride changes may occur secondary to fluid shifts during the acute episode. All these changes usually will respond to control of the acute episode.

DANTROLENE

In 1979 intravenous dantrolene was approved by the Food and Drug Administration for treatment of MH. Until that time, dantrolene primarily was used orally to manage spasticity. Dantrolene is a unique muscle relaxant. Unlike neuromuscular blocking agents, whose site of action is at the nicotinic receptor of the neuromuscular junction, or the nonspecific relaxants, which modulate spinal cord synaptic reflexes, dantrolene operates within the muscle cell itself by reducing intracellular levels of calcium. Most likely this results from a reduction of sarcoplasmic reticulum (SR) calcium release or inhibition of excitation contracture coupling at the transverse tubular level. It has now been demonstrated that during an MH episode dantrolene reduces intracellular calcium levels. Therefore, dantrolene is a specific and effective agent in the treatment of MH. In usual clinical doses dantrolene has little effect on myocardial contractility.[71]

Studies have also indicated that doses of neuromuscular blocking agents need not be changed significantly after dantrolene administration. However, the drug should be used cautiously in patients with neuromuscular diseases.[72]

The serum level of dantrolene required for prophylaxis against MH is about 2.5 μg·ml^{-1}. The half life of intravenous dantrolene, which is the only form recommended, is approximately 12 h. However, the therapeutic level of dantrolene usually persists for 4–6 h after a usual intravenous dose of 2.5 mg·kg^{-1}.[72] Therefore, dantrolene should be supplemented approximately every 4 h after a clinical episode. Some muscle weakness may persist for 24 h after dantrolene therapy is discontinued. Nausea and phlebitis are other complications of dantrolene administration. Hepatotoxicity has been demonstrated only with long-term use of oral dantrolene. Prophylaxis for MH should be conducted with intravenous rather than oral dantrolene.

MANAGEMENT OF THE MALIGNANT HYPERTHERMIA–SUSCEPTIBLE PATIENT

Because of an increasing awareness of MH and more widespread use of diagnostic tests, it is not unusual for an anesthesiologist to be confronted with an MH-susceptible patient or a patient who has a family history of MH. The management of such patients should be carefully planned.

In the preoperative interview the anesthesiologist should try to obtain sufficient information regarding previous episodes of MH and their documentation. The anesthesiologist should allow adequate time to reassure the patient and his or her family that he or she is familiar with MH and its implications and that appropriate prophylaxis and therapy will be instituted as necessary. It may be worth mentioning that there have been no deaths from MH in a previously diagnosed MH-susceptible patient when the anesthesia team was aware of the problem. Some believe that anxiety may predispose a patient to MH and therefore they recommend anxiolytic agents in the premedication. Standard premedicant drugs such as narcotics, benzodiazepines, ataractics, barbiturates, and antihistamines do not cause problems in MH-susceptible patients when administered in appropriate doses; however, we do not recommend phenothiazines for premedication. Anticholinesterases are also used routinely.

Where there is a high likelihood of MH susceptibility, dantrolene sodium, 2.5 mg·kg^{-1}, should be administered intravenously over a period of 15–30 min shortly before surgery. Oral dantrolene is no longer recommended to prevent signs of MH because of variable blood levels and clinical descriptions of failure of prophylaxis in at least two patients. Although dantrolene may cause nausea and vomiting and, in some cases, complaints of pain at the injection site, with the usual dose patients should have no significant discomfort.

The anesthesia machine is prepared according to empiric guidelines. Some operating rooms have a "clean" anesthesia machine available for MH-susceptible patients. However, if one uses a disposable circuit, removes or drains and disconnects vaporizers, changes carbon dioxide absorbant, and flows oxygen through the machine at 3–5 l·min^{-1} for several hours, we believe that the anesthesia machine can be used safely. Obviously, iced solutions and adequate supplies of dantrolene must be available in the vicinity of the operating room when MH-susceptible patients are anesthetized.

Exhaled carbon dioxide should be monitored because the earliest sign of MH is an increase in carbon dioxide production and excretion.[73] In the absence of capnography, arterial blood gas monitoring is recommended. Arterial and central venous monitoring is recommended for MH-susceptible patients, as dictated by the surgical procedure. Body temperature should be monitored by nasopharyngeal, rectal, or esophageal routes in all patients for all surgical procedures. Studies comparing skin temperature with core temperature during an MH crisis are lacking, but other studies have shown that forehead temperature may lag significantly behind core temperature.[74] Therefore, the value of peripheral temperature monitoring in detecting MH is not certain.

If possible, a regional, local, or major conduction anesthetic should be used with either amide or ester local anesthetics. If not possible, a barbiturate or narcotic induction followed by nitrous oxide, oxygen, pancuronium, narcotic technique is recommended. Other induction agents that have not been implicated in MH are midazolam, diazepam, droperidol, and althesin (alphaxalone and alphadolone).

Neuromuscular blocking agents such as pancuronium, vecuronium, and atracurium are safe, according to animal and human studies. We routinely reverse nondepolarizing relaxants with anticholinesterase and anticholinergic agents.

At the worst, nitrous oxide is a weak triggering agent. Many hundreds of safe anesthetics have been administered with nitrous oxide in MH-susceptible patients. Two cases have been reported in which early signs of MH have been documented despite the use of a safe anesthetic technique.[75] Therefore, even under the most controlled circumstances, the anesthesiologist should be alert to the early signs of MH.

We do not continue dantrolene after operation when there are no signs of MH. However, the patient must be observed closely for 4–6 h. MH has not occurred after surgery when dantrolene pretreatment and safe anesthetic techniques were used.

The same precautions should be taken for the obstetric patient as for the routine surgical patient. We are not convinced that the stress of labor may precipitate MH, and we recommend well-conducted epidural anesthesia for labor and delivery without dantrolene pretreatment but with careful monitoring of vital signs. If an emergency cesarean section with general anesthesia is necessary, dantrolene should be given intravenously along with nontriggering agents. In the very acute situation, anesthesia should be induced and dantrolene administered thereafter. The maternal/fetal partition ratio for dantrolene is probably 0.4.[76] Dantrolene has not been reported to produce significant problems for the fetus or newborn, but data are very scanty.

MALIGNANT HYPERTHERMIA IN SPECIES OTHER THAN PIGS AND PEOPLE

Malignant hyperthermia has been reported sporadically in many species. Clinical episodes have been documented in cats, dogs (especially greyhound species), and horses. Capture myopathy is a syndrome characterized by temperature elevation, rhabdomyolysis, acidosis, and death in wild animals (e.g., zebra, elk) after prolonged chase.[77] This also has been suggested to be an MH variant.

MEDICOLEGAL ASPECTS

In this litigious age it is not surprising that MH cases have been the subject of malpractice action. Because MH may be considered an inborn genetic problem that may be unrecognized before a patient's exposure to triggering agents and associated with an irreducible mortality, MH may be used as a "cover" for other problems.

Fever, opisthotonic posturing, and neurologic abnormalities may accompany hypoxic brain injury, and because of their similarity to MH, MH may be falsely implicated in the differential diagnosis. Furthermore, after cardiac arrest from any cause, CK and potassium levels may be significantly elevated. Mazzia and Simon have estimated that about 1% of MH cases have legal consequences, but this statistic is at least 10 yr old.[78] The incidence of lawsuits of true episodes of MH is probably much less. However, the incidence in regard to MH cases in which the patient died is undoubtedly much higher.

Although some have stated that with the advent of dantrolene there should be no deaths from MH, this is probably unrealistic because in some cases the syndrome may be truly explosive and impossible to control with current therapy. Also, we are not completely familiar with all factors that lead to MH, including drugs that may trigger MH, and the proper dose of dantrolene to employ in order to prevent recrudescence, and such. Nevertheless, certain common themes underlie the basis for litigation in MH:

1. Failure to obtain a thorough personal history in regard to anesthetic problems and a family history of unexplained perioperative problems.
2. Failure to monitor temperature continuously with an electronic temperature monitoring device. Several jury trial cases have been lost by the defense solely because the patient's temperature was not monitored. Intraoperative temperature monitoring is now considered a "standard of care" in the United States by the legal profession despite failure of the American Society of Anesthesiologists to recommend routine temperature monitoring during administration of all anesthetics.
3. Failure to have adequate supplies of dantrolene on hand with a plan of MH management.
4. Failure to investigate unexplained increases in body temperature and increased skeletal muscle tone (especially after succinylcholine administration) when associated with increased heart rate and arrhythmias.

Several examples of medicolegal cases in which these principles were not followed are described:

Increased heart rate developed in a 35-yr-old man who had a bowel resection for regional enteritis. His oral temperature by mercury thermometer was 37°C. The oral thermometer was left in place and the anesthetic continued with halothane and nitrous oxide. Toward the end of the procedure there was a rapid increase in heart rate followed by an increase in body temperature. Despite cooling and procainamide (this episode occurred in the predantrolene era) and other appropriate medical therapy, disseminated intravascular coagulopathy (DIC) eventually developed and the patient died. The plaintiff won the case when it was tried by jury primarily because continuous electronic temperature monitoring was available and was not used.

Another case involved a young male patient who had shoulder surgery with halothane–nitrous oxide–oxygen. Again, temperature was not monitored continuously. Intraoperative tachycardia to about 150 beats·min⁻¹ was treated with propranolol. At the end of the procedure, as the drapes were being removed, the patient felt warm. A temperature probe now revealed a reading of nearly 40°C. Shortly thereafter a cardiac arrest occurred, despite dantrolene administration, and the patient died. The case was settled out of court.

A man in his mid-thirties had a dental procedure in a dental operatory (not in the hospital). Halothane anesthesia was administered by an anesthesiologist. Despite increasing heart rate and temperature elevation, the anesthetic was continued until the patient had a cardiac arrest. This case was further aggravated because dantrolene was not available. Access to the operatory was limited, and the patient was dead on arrival at a nearby hospital. The case was settled out of court for an undisclosed sum. (Millions of anesthetics using MH-triggering agents are administered each year in dental operatories, outpatient surgical facilities, and, increasingly, physicians' offices. Standards and reviews applicable to hospitals are not applied to these locales.)

Symptoms of bowel obstruction developed in a middle-aged man. He was taken to a local hospital, and anesthesia was administered with nitrous oxide–oxygen–halothane and succinylcholine. His temperature was not monitored, but an unexplained tachycardia (140–160 beats·min⁻¹) was present throughout the 2-hr procedure. On arrival in the intensive care unit after operation, the patient was slightly hypotensive. Invasive monitoring was placed. Despite marked metabolic and respiratory acidosis, a P_{CO_2} of 100, and a recorded temperature of nearly 42°C, MH was not diagnosed. A cooling blanket and antibiotics failed to arrest the decrease in the patient's blood pressure, which eventually led to cardiac arrest. This case is in litigation.

PATIENT SUPPORT SERVICES

To answer the needs of patients and families who wished to learn more about MH and of those families whose relatives have died from MH, two support groups were founded—the Malignant Hyperthermia Association (of Canada) (MHA) and the Malignant Hyperthermia Association of the United States (MHAUS). Both groups serve as a repository of information about MH, provide names of physicians knowledgeable about MH and the location of MH diagnostic centers, and simply lend an ear to those with MH who have questions. Both organizations have an advisory committee of physicians but are run by volunteers who usually have a personal connection with MH. MHAUS and MHA organize annual meetings for physicians and nonphysicians. MHAUS publishes a quarterly newsletter, The Communicator, with excerpts from the medical literature, explanatory articles, questions and answers, and related information. In addition, a "hotline" has been organized so that a physician with an urgent question about MH can be placed in contact with a knowledgeable physician. Approximately 30–40 calls/month are handled by this hotline.

Besides the valuable function of providing patient advice, these associations gather information about MH, such as regarding variation in presentation and regional incidence.

The address of MHAUS is MHAUS, P.O. Box 3231, Darien, Connecticut 06820.

The hotline number is as follows: 209-634-4917. Ask for Index Zero.

The address of MHA of Canada is as follows: Room 314, Elizabeth Wing, Toronto General Hospital, 101 College Street, Toronto, Ontario M5G1L7.

The hotline number for MHA is as follows: 416-595-3000.

Physicians who want to provide patient services for MH must prepare for lengthy discussions about the disorder, because patients usually have only very limited information about MH.

PATHOPHYSIOLOGY AND ETIOLOGY OF MALIGNANT HYPERTHERMIA

Introduction

With the clinical implication of MH as a background, the pathophysiology and etiology can be more easily appreciated. Three major developments have contributed to the understanding of MH. The first was the recognition that the syndrome is genetically transmitted.[2] This finding is significant from a mechanistic standpoint, because it suggests that a single inheritable anomaly might explain the abnormal response to anesthetics. A second finding was identification of a greater sensitivity of skeletal muscle from MH-susceptible patients to halothane and/or caffeine.[4, 62] This was the basis for an in vitro system for patient diagnosis and study of the mechanisms underlying MH. The third was the recognition of similarities between human MH and PSS.[3] In addition to stress, the PSS could be triggered by halothane and succinylcholine, the two agents most often implicated in MH. Thus, an ideal animal model became available for studies of MH.

In Vivo and In Situ Studies

TRIGGERING AGENTS. PSS-susceptible pigs have been used to investigate agents that could potentially trigger an MH episode. As observed in human MH, PSS can be triggered by halothane or succinylcholine.[79] It seems unusual that two structurally unrelated agents with different presumed mechanisms of action can both trigger MH. Although halothane and succinylcholine are the agents most often implicated, most of the other halogenated volatile anesthetic agents are also associated with MH. Succinylcholine is the only neuromuscular blocking agent suggested to cause MH. Curare was once implicated in human MH; however, curare does not trigger MH in pigs.[80]

PHENOTYPES. Three to five PSS phenotypes have been reported as a result of outbreeding of pigs with PSS. One study has classified three phenotypes by contracture tests and in vivo halothane and succinylcholine challenge.[65] Phenotype H is unequivocally MH susceptible based on the *in vitro* contracture response to halothane 3%. Also, the contracture threshold to caffeine is lower in the presence of halothane for phenotype H than observed for normals. These pigs exhibit MH when challenged with halothane *in vivo*. The second phenotype (K) does not exhibit an abnormal contracture response to halothane 3% but does have a low contracture threshold to caffeine in the presence of halothane and is, therefore, considered an equivocal category. These pigs do not show signs of MH when challenged *in vivo* with halothane unless succinylcholine is also administered. Even when challenged with halothane and succinylcholine, these pigs do not demonstrate all the signs of an MH episode, despite repeated challenges or continuation of anesthesia for a prolonged time. The third phenotype (N) is the normal pig. These pigs have no contracture response to halothane 3% *in vitro*, they have a higher contracture threshold to caffeine in the presence of halothane than either the H or K phenotypes, and they do not exhibit signs of MH when challenged *in vivo* with halothane or succinylcholine, alone or in combination.

The existence of multiple phenotypes in humans is less clear. However, some investigators have reported a spectrum of contracture responses of muscle from MH-susceptible patients, which suggests that several phenotypes or different pathophysiologic mechanisms are possibly involved in MH.[81] Approximately 20% of normal patients would be classified as phenotype K, as determined by the contracture threshold to caffeine with halothane present.[82]

ROLE OF CATECHOLAMINES. Serum catecholamine levels are considerably elevated in both the MH syndrome and PSS and have been proposed to play an important role in the initiation of these syndromes.[83] A major *in situ* finding in the pig was the generation of MH signs in the absence of any sympathetic nervous system influence.[35] Therefore, it seems unlikely that catecholamine release alone initiates MH. However, this finding does not negate at least some role for catecholamines in the development of the full syndrome.

ROLE OF SKELETAL MUSCLE IN THERMOGENESIS. Most investigators believe that the hyperthermia characterizing an MH episode is not an effect of triggering agents on the thermoregulatory centers in the central nervous system, but rather is a direct effect of halothane and succinylcholine on skeletal muscle.[84] In support of this proposal, muscle from those that are MH susceptible exhibits a contracture to halothane when challenged *in vitro*.[6] Also, because the signs characteristic of halothane-induced MH are observed in the presence of curare or total spinal anesthesia, the central, peripheral, and autonomic nervous systems do not appear to be directly involved in the initiation of the syndrome.

In Vitro Contracture Studies

ANTAGONISTS OF CONTRACTURES. *In vitro* contracture studies have been used to study mechanisms underlying halothane and caffeine contracture induction and MH. Dantrolene is not only a very effective clinical antagonist of MH syndrome but is also the most potent inhibitor of halothane-induced contracture.[85] Phospholipase A2 inhibitors, local anesthetic agents, and calcium channel antagonists antagonize halothane-induced contractures but are not as potent as dantrolene in this regard.[86-88] Indeed, some local anesthetics, such as lidocaine, increase contractures to halothane. The results obtained with calcium antagonists have been interpreted as indicating a role for Ca^{++} influx across the sarcolemma in MH. Calcium is necessary both to initiate (*i.e.*, calcium-induced calcium release), as well as to sustain contractures (see below).

INTERACTION BETWEEN HALOTHANE AND SUCCINYLCHOLINE. Halothane and succinylcholine are the two agents most often implicated in triggering the MH syndrome. Clinically a synergism has been observed between halothane and succinylcholine in regard to incidence of MMR, increases in serum CK activity, core temperature elevation, and myoglobinemia.[62, 90] A similar *in vitro* synergism in contracture induction by halothane and succinylcholine also has been reported. As observed *in vivo* in regard to MH, the *in vitro* contractures induced by succinylcholine, but not those induced by halothane, are antagonized by curare.[91]

Succinylcholine is known to stimulate phospholipase A2 activity in skeletal muscle.[92] Agents known to inhibit phospholipase A2 have been shown to antagonize contractures synergistically induced by the combination of halothane and succinylcholine.[86] These findings suggest a role for phospholipase A2 activity in contractures synergistically induced by halothane and succinylcholine.

Biochemical and Electrophysiologic Studies

GENERAL. Biochemical and electrophysiologic studies have been aimed at understanding functional alterations occurring in various organelles and changes in the structure or concentration of various structural and regulatory molecules in muscle from MH-susceptible humans or PSS-susceptible swine. Often the results of one laboratory are in conflict with those of another. In many cases the conflicting data can be attributed to a questionable diagnosis of MH, different experimental conditions, poorly characterized or uncharacterized membrane fractions, or the use of postmortem instead of biopsy samples.

ROLE OF CALCIUM. The enhanced metabolism in MH is generally believed to result from abnormally high myoplasmic Ca^{++} concentrations.[6] Using electron microscopy and microprobe analysis, Stadhouders *et al* observed a large accumulation of mitochondrial Ca^{++} in muscle from pigs undergoing PSS, suggesting a greater increase than normal in myoplasmic Ca^{++} concentration.[94] Recently, it has been suggested that elevated resting myoplasmic Ca^{++} levels exist in MH-susceptible humans when calcium-selective microelectrodes were used. The elevated myoplasmic Ca^{++} levels are decreased by dantrolene.[6]

POSSIBLE CAUSES OF ELEVATED MYOPLASMIC CALCIUM LEVELS. Myoplasmic calcium levels could be drastically increased by the following: Ca^{++} release from the sarcoplasmic reticulum; Ca^{++} influx across the sarcolemma; Ca^{++} release from the mitochondria; and mechanisms blocking Ca^{++} extrusion or sequestration, including $(Ca^{++} + Mg^{++})$-ATPase, Na–Ca exchange, and mitochondrial oxidative and ATP-stimulated Ca^{++} accumulation. Most likely more than one of these processes eventually become altered in an episode of MH.

SOURCE OF HEAT PRODUCTION. The heat produced in skeletal muscle during an MH episode is believed to be derived from processes stimulated directly or indirectly by the Ca^{++} overload. These processes include aerobic and anaerobic metabolism, hydrolysis of ATP required for ion transport mechanisms (*e.g.* $[Na^{++} + Ca^{++}]$-ATPase and $[Ca^{++} + Mg^{++}]$-ATPase), and neutralization of H^- production.[94]

SARCOPLASMIC RETICULUM. Early studies of sarcoplasmic reticulum function in MH-susceptible humans and PSS-susceptible pigs examined Ca^{++} uptake into and release from the sarcoplasmic reticulum in the presence or absence of various drugs. In general, Ca^{++} uptake and the Ca^{++} capacity of the sarcoplasmic reticulum in humans appear to be decreased to some extent; however, these slight differences probably do not account for the MH syndrome.[95] These studies are adequately reviewed elsewhere.[96]

The Ca^{++}-induced Ca^{++} release process of the sarcoplasmic reticulum appears to be overly sensitive in skeletal muscle from MH-susceptible patients.[97] However, it is unlikely that this is the primary cause of MH, because dantrolene does not appear to alter Ca^{++}-induced Ca^{++} release from the sarcoplasmic reticulum.

Ohnishi *et al* have demonstrated a halothane-induced Ca^{++} release process in sarcoplasmic reticulum vesicles.[98] The main difference between MH-susceptible and normal patients is the amount of Ca^{++} preload necessary for the halothane effect. Dantrolene does inhibit halothane-induced Ca^{++} release from the sarcoplasmic reticulum.

Cheah and Cheah hypothesized that the Ca^{++} release from the sarcoplasmic reticulum results from increased production of unsaturated fatty acids.[99] Cheah and Cheah further demonstrated that this fatty acid–induced release of Ca^{++} from the sarcoplasmic reticulum is related to the degree of unsaturation of the fatty acids. More recent studies of halothane action on membranes have suggested that, not only can free fatty acids directly increase membrane permeability, but they can potentiate increases in membrane permeability induced by halothane. This interaction of halothane and free fatty acids is antagonized by dantrolene in red blood cells.[100]

MITOCHONDRIA. Several groups have reported alterations in the mitochondria of humans or animals that are MH or PSS susceptible. Morphologically, the mitochondria from PSS-susceptible pigs and humans appear swollen after an episode of PSS or MH. Studies of mitochondrial defects that might cause MH or PSS have yielded conflicting results. Although uncoupling of oxidative phosphorylation was postulated to possibly cause heat generation, much of the evidence does not support this possibility.[101]

Of particular interest is the observation that phospholipase A2 activity is increased in the mitochondria from PSS-susceptible pigs.[102] The elevated phospholipase A2 activity is believed to be responsible for a shift in the transition temperature of Ca^{++}-stimulated, but not ADP-stimulated, mitochondrial succinate oxidation. Cheah and Cheah have demonstrated that the free fatty acids generated by the mitochondria can cause Ca^{++} release from the sarcoplasmic reticulum and uncoupling of mitochondrial oxidative phosphorylation.[101]

SARCOLEMMA. Freeze-fracture analysis of the sarcolemma after an episode of MH has suggested a disintegration of the lipid–protein system. Although the resting membrane potential of muscle from PSS-susceptible pigs is normal, halothane induces a depolarization in PSS muscle that is not observed in normal muscle.[103] The depolarization of muscle and a different response of MH and normal muscle to external K^+ have been interpreted by this group as suggesting a sarcolemmal defect associated with MH. Also, using electron microscopy and microprobe analysis, Stadhouser *et al* calculated that the myoplasmic Ca^{++} overload could not be explained solely by release of Ca^{++} from the sarcoplasmic reticulum.[93] Defects have been reported in the ATP-dependent Ca^{++} transport system of isolated sarcolemma from PSS-susceptible swine.[104] Dantrolene was previously regarded as a specific inhibitor of calcium release from the sarcoplasmic reticulum by an action at the excitation–contracture coupling process, which brought into question the role of sarcolemmal involvement in MH. However, recent studies have demonstrated that dantrolene antagonizes halothane-induced increases in plasma membrane permeability, further supporting the possibility of a role for the sarcolemma in MH.[100]

ABNORMAL PROTEINS. Calmodulin concentrations have been reported to be increased in skeletal muscle from PSS-susceptible pigs.[105] These higher levels of calmodulin were postulated to be responsible for the increased activity of calmodulin-dependent phospholipase A2 activity observed previously. However, others have been unable to determine a role for calmodulin in PSS.[106]

A defect in contractile proteins resulting in an oversensitivity to Ca^{++} could account for MH. There is little evidence to support a role for differences in binding properties of contractile proteins in MH. This topic is reviewed by Ellis and Heffron.[96]

FIBER TYPE. The response to halothane has also been shown to correlate with type I fiber predominance when the contracture responses of different muscle groups are compared.[107] Most human striated muscles are of a heterogeneous nature, including the vastus lateralis, which is commonly used for MH diagnosis. It is possible that a predominance of type I fibers may exist in muscle from MH-susceptible patients. However, this seems an unlikely possibility because no correlation was observed between fiber type and strength of contracture when muscle strips of widely varying fiber type were examined from vastus lateralis.[108]

Summary

Malignant hyperthermia results from a genetic defect that appears to affect all membranes in skeletal muscle once the syndrome is triggered. The halothane challenge results in grossly elevated Ca^{++} levels in the myoplasm. It is possible that the release of free unsaturated fatty acids from the mitochondria, which is greater in MH-susceptible patients, can directly release Ca^{++} from the sarcoplasmic reticulum. In addition to this direct effect, the free fatty acids potentiate membrane permeability increases caused by halothane. Therefore, in the susceptible patient excessive Ca^{++} in the myoplasm may first be derived from the sarcoplasmic reticulum stores because of the extreme sensitivity of this organelle to halothane. However, halothane does increase the permeability of plasma membranes in synergy with free unsaturated fatty acids, suggesting the sarcolemmal barrier to Ca^{++} may also break down. It remains a mystery as to how succinylcholine triggers MH on its own, but this most likely involves stimulation of lipolytic activity in addition to some other process.

The exact mechanism by which dantrolene antagonizes the MH syndrome also remains unknown. Dantrolene appears to block halothane-induced Ca^{++} release from the sarcoplasmic reticulum and the sarcolemma.

OTHER INHERITED DISORDERS

Inherited diseases affect every body organ and every physiologic and biochemical process. Some are mild and allow a relatively normal life span, others are incompatible with extrauterine existence even for a few days. Adding to the complexity is a natural variability of penetrance and expressivity even in a single family. All of these disorders have as a common feature: an abnormality in one or more genes that affects the function of one or more enzymes. The metabolic basis of inherited diseases is the subject of several well-known monographs,[109, 110] which may be consulted for an in-depth appreciation of our state of knowledge of many of these disorders (see also Chapter 16).

DISORDERS OF PLASMA CHOLINESTERASE

Plasma cholinesterase, pseudocholinesterase, or nonspecific cholinesterase is an enzyme with a molecular weight of 320,000 and a tetrahedral structure. It is found in plasma and most tissue but not in red blood cells. Pseudocholinesterase degrades acetylcholine released at the neuromuscular junction.

The half-life of pseudocholinesterase has been estimated to be 8–16 h. It is very stable in serum samples and can be stored for long periods of time at $-20°C$ with little or no activity loss. Cholinesterase is manufactured in the liver. Therefore, decreased plasma cholinesterase activity occurs in advanced cases of hepatocellular dysfunction.

Inherited variants of pseudocholinesterase are of interest to the anesthesiologist because the duration of action of succinylcholine and, in some cases, ester-linked local anesthetics, is a function of the activity of this enzyme system. Prolonged apnea after succinylcholine administration occurs in patients who have very low absolute activity of pseudocholinesterase or have enzyme variants.[111, 112] These patients otherwise have no symptoms.

There are many physiologic, pharmacologic, and pathologic factors that can either increase or decrease the activity of this enzyme to a significant extent. However, it is only when there is a greater than approximately 75% decrease in the levels of the normal pseudocholinesterase that there is clinically evident prolongation of succinylcholine activity (see below). Table 17-4 lists some of the causes for variation in plasma cholinesterase activity.

Succinylcholine-Related Apnea

Succinylcholine is hydrolyzed by a two-step process: first to succinylmonocholine and then to succinic acid. It has been estimated that only about 5% of the injected drug reaches the end-plate region because of a combination of both hydrolysis and diffusion from the plasma. Urinary excretion and protein binding play an unimportant role in the disposition of the drug. The rate of metabolism determines the duration of action of succinylcholine.

There are a variety of assay procedures for pseudocholinesterase activity. However, most involve the reaction of a thiocholine (e.g., butyrylthiocholine) with serum or plasma containing cholinesterase. The reaction product is coupled to 5,5'-dithiobis-(2-nitrobenzoic acid) (DTNB) and forms a colored product that can be followed spectrophotometrically.

Kalow et al were the first to show that qualitative as well as quantitative differences in the pseudocholinesterase enzyme determine the duration of succinylcholine apnea.[113] Kalow found that in certain persons displaying succinylcholine sensitivity, the local anesthetic dibucaine (Nupercaine) inhibited the hydrolysis of a benzoylcholine substrate less than it inhibited the reaction in those displaying a normal response to succinylcholine. The percentage inhibition of the reaction was termed the dibucaine number (DN). It was found to be constant for a person and did not depend on the concentration

TABLE 17-4. Some Causes of Changes in Cholinesterase Activity[149-151]

Inherited
    Cholinesterase variants that may lead to decreased or increased activity (e.g., silent gene or C5 variant)
Physiologic
    Decreases in last trimester of pregnancy
    Reduced activity of the newborn
Acquired decreases
    Liver diseases
    Carcinoma
    Debilitating diseases
    Collagen diseases
    Uremia
    Malnutrition
    Myxedema
Acquired increases
    Obesity
    Alcoholism
    Thyrotoxicosis
    Nephrosis
    Psoriasis
    Electroshock therapy (EST)[161]
Drugs related to diseases
    Echothiophate iodide
    Neostigmine
    Pyridostigmine
    Chlorpromazine
    Cyclophosphamide
    MAO inhibitors
    Pancuronium
    Propanidid
    Contraceptives
    Organophosphorus insecticides
    Hexaflurenium
Other causes for decreased activity
    Plasmapheresis
    Extracorporeal circulation
    Tetanus
    X-ray therapy
    Burns

The significance of these factors will depend on the severity of disease, drug dosage, and individual variation.

(Adapted from Whittaker M: Plasma cholinesterase variants and the anesthetist. Anaesthesia 35:174, 1980.)

of the enzyme. A recent report by Ravindran et al suggests that, in patients with less than 10% of the normal pseudocholinesterase activity, the measurement of the DN (and the fluoride number) may be misleadingly low.[114]

A discontinuous distribution of DNs suggested an inheritance pattern based on alteration at a single gene locus (Table 17-5). Those with DNs in the range of 80 would be homozygote normal with a normal response to succinylcholine, those with DNs of 20 would be homozygous atypical with a marked prolongation of succinylcholine activity, and those with DNs in the 60 range would be heterozygotes and, in general, have a normal response to succinylcholine. This theory was substantiated by other workers.

Over the years two other major allelic variants were discovered. In one case, the silent gene, the enzyme is not produced completely. In the other (fluoride sensitive), there is a differential inhibition of cholinesterase activity.[115] In those with prolonged duration of succinylcholine activity with this genotype, fluoride ion inhibits the in vitro hydrolysis of substrate by the enzyme less than it does in normals. A fluoride number, similar to a dibucaine number, is so created. Other variants may exist.

TABLE 17-5. Biochemical Characteristics of Some Cholinesterase Variants[111]

GENOTYPE	CHOLINESTERASE ACTIVITY (u/10)	DIBUCAINE NUMBER	FLUORIDE NUMBER	CHLORIDE NUMBER	SUCCINYLCHOLINE NUMBER
E^uE^u	677–1,860	78–86	55–65	1–12	89–98
E^aE^a	140–525	18–26	16–32	46–58	4–19
E^uE^a	285–1,008	51–70	38–55	15–34	51–78
E^uE^f	579–900	74–80	47–48	14–30	87–91
E^fE^a	475–661	49–59	25–33	31–36	56–59
E^fE^s	351	63	26	25	81

E^u = normal enzyme gene; E^a = atypical enzyme gene; E^f = fluoride sensitive gene; E^s = silent gene.

TABLE 17-6. Hereditary Variants of Pseudocholinesterase Resulting from Four Allelic Genes[150]

GENOTYPE	FREQUENCY IN A BRITISH POPULATION	RESPONSE TO SUCCINYLCHOLINE	TYPICAL DIBUCAINE NUMBER	TYPICAL FLUORIDE NUMBER
N-N	96% normal	Normal	80	60
D-D	1 in 2,000	Greatly prolonged	20	20
F-F	1 in 154,000	Moderately prolonged	70	30
S-S	1 in 100,000	Greatly prolonged		
N-D	1 in 25	Slightly prolonged	60	45
N-F	1 in 200	Slightly prolonged	75	50
N-S	1 in 190	Slightly prolonged	80	60
D-F	1 in 20,000	Greatly prolonged	45	35
D-S	1 in 29,000	Greatly prolonged	20	20
F-S	1 in 150,000	Moderately prolonged	65	35

N = gene for normal pseudocholinesterase; D = gene for dibucaine-sensitive variant; F = gene for fluoride-sensitive variant; S = gene for absence of enzyme activity (silent gene).

(Adaped from Lehmann H, Lidell J: Human cholinesterase [pseudocholinesterase]: Genetic variants and their recognition. Br J Anaesth 41:243, 1969.)

When there is question of succinylcholine sensitivity, the absolute activity of the pseudocholinesterase should be determined as well as the DNs and fluoride numbers. In some cases, because of biologic variability or unusual combinations of genotype (*e.g.*, combination of atypical and fluoride genes), it is helpful to use other inhibitors of the cholinesterase reaction in genotyping the patient. Bromide, urea, NaCl, and succinylcholine have been used to distinguish the various genotypes (Table 17-5).

The frequencies of occurrence of the various genes vary to some extent with ethnic background. For example, Eskimo populations have the silent gene much more frequently, patients with Huntington's Chorea are more likely to have an E^f gene than are normal controls, and Israelis have a higher chance of having an atypical genotype than Americans. In European studies, the approximate percentage in the population of the genotypes are as follows: E^uE^u (96%), E^uE^a (2.5%), E^uE^f or E^uE^s (0.3%), E^aE^f (0.005%), E^aE^a (0.05%), and E^fE^f or E^fE^s (0.006%).[116]

Patients homozygous for atypical, fluoride, or silent genes as well as those with the combination of atypical with fluoride, atypical with silent genes, or fluoride with silent genes should wear Medic-Alert bracelets indicating that succinylcholine administration will lead to prolonged apnea. Relatives should be tested as well. There are only a few cholinesterase research units that investigate families and interpret results: Whittaker's in Great Britain, Hanel and Viby-Mogensen's in Denmark, and Rosenberg's in the United States.

Clinical Implications of Pseudocholinesterase Abnormalities

Important questions for the anesthesiologist are, of course: Which patients are at risk for development of an abnormal response to succinylcholine? What are the clinical characteristics of this response and treatment options?

Significant prolongation of succinylcholine's effects occurs in the following genotypes: E^aE^a, E^fE^f, E^aE^s, E^fE^a, and EsEs* (Table 17-6). The more common situations in which homozygote normals and heterozygotes are at risk are as follows: patients have been receiving echothiophate eye drops (up to 2 weeks after therapy is discontinued); patients undergoing plasmapheresis; patients have severe liver disease; patients

* The abbreviations are defined as follows: E^u—normal enzyme gene; E^a—atypical enzyme gene; E^f—fluoride sensitive gene; E^s—silent gene.

(particularly heterozygotes) received succinylcholine after reversal of nondepolarizing blockade with neostigmine.[117, 118]

Viby-Morgensen has studied the question of plasma cholinesterase apnea in detail. His cholinesterase unit found that 6.2% of patients who displayed apnea for 50–250 min after a "usual" dose of succinylcholine had an acquired deficiency of plasma cholinesterase.[111] He then studied 70 patients who were genotypically normal and administered 1 mg·kg^{-1} of succinylcholine during a 50% nitrous oxide–oxygen–1% halothane anesthetic and followed the depression and return of thumb twitch. He found that there was indeed a relation between the duration of apnea, the return of full twitch response, and plasmacholinesterase activity (Fig. 17-4).[119] However, only moderate prolongation of apnea was found when cholinesterase was depressed by as much as 70%. Apnea is only significantly prolonged with extreme depression of cholinesterase activity.

In a second study with a similar protocol he found that heterozygotes having one normal gene (e.g., E^{u}E^a; E^{u}E^f) had a normal response to succinylcholine, including typical fasciculations and a depolarizing type of block with train-of-four stimulations.[120] However, heterozygotes without the usual gene (e.g., E^{a}E^f) had a prolonged response to succinylcholine, with apnea lasting as long as 24 min. Most showed typical fasciculations. Fade with train-of-four stimulations was the rule. It should be noted that others have found that heterozygotes with one normal gene will display prolonged response to succinylcholine under certain conditions. About one in 500 heterozygotes are prone to such a response.

Apnea will develop in homozygote-atypical patients (E^{a}E^a) when they are given succinylcholine and will last from 120 to more than 300 min.[112] The onset of block is similar to that in normals; however, there is fade in response to train-of-four stimulation. Contrary to Baraka's report, fasciculations do occur with succinylcholine in these patients.[121]

The other class of patients who regularly display prolonged apnea after succinylcholine administration are patients homozygous for the silent gene.

Treatment of Succinylcholine Apnea

The safest course of treatment after the patient fails to breathe within 10–15 min after succinylcholine administration is to provide mechanical ventilation until adequate muscle tone has returned. Cholase, a protein preparation from human plasma (available in Europe), can be used to reverse the prolonged apnea in homozygote-atypical patients. One ampule corresponds to the amount of plasma cholinesterase in about 500 ml of human plasma. Ninety to 270 mg of Cholase given after 30 min of apnea can restore twitch response to normal. However, there is a risk of hepatitis transmission.

The use of cholinesterase inhibitors in treating succinylcholine apnea is controversial. When given along with Cholase the improvement is rapid and lasting. If it is administered without Cholase before there is evidence of fade with train-of-four, there may be a transient improvement followed by intensification of the neuromuscular block. The best chance for reversal of succinylcholine-related apnea in these situations occurs when no more than 0.03 mg·kg^{-1} of neostigmine is given 90–120 min after succinylcholine when a curare type of blockade is present.

C5 Variant

An isoenzyme of pseudocholinesterase has been demonstrated whereby the hydrolysis of succinylcholine is increased and, therefore, the duration of apnea decreased after succinylcholine administration. The gene does not appear to be an allele of the E^u and E^a gene and is found infrequently in the population.[122]

Plasma Cholinesterase Abnormalities and the Metabolism of Local Anesthetics

Although the ester-linked local anesthetics (e.g., procaine, tetracaine, 2-chloroprocaine) are metabolized by pseudocholinesterase, prolongation of block and/or clinical toxicity

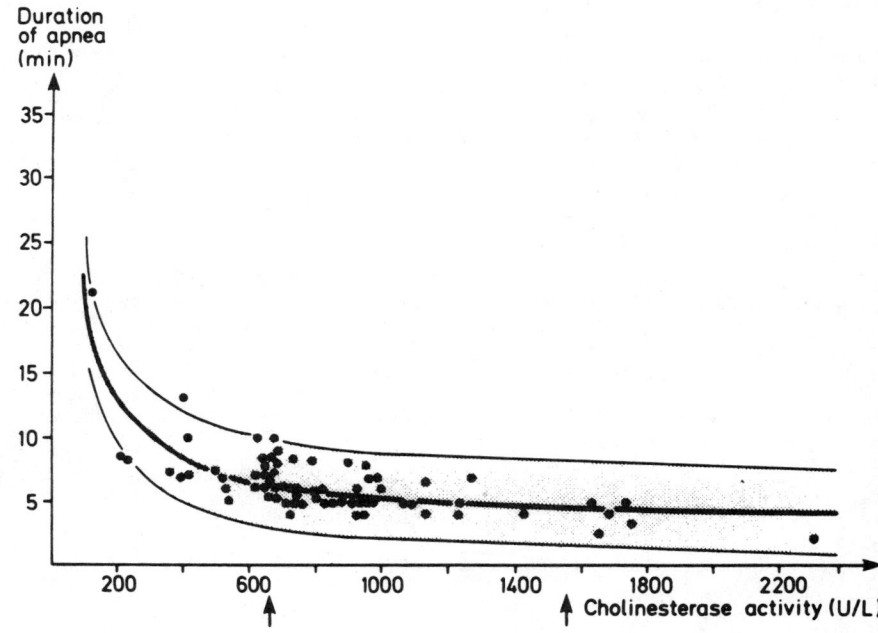

FIG. 17-4. Relationship between enzymatic activity and apnea after intravenous administration of succinylcholine, 1 mg·kg^{-1}, to 70 patients with the normal plasma cholinesterase genotype. The fitted regression line and 95% prediction region are given. *Arrows* indicate the normal range of plasma cholinesterase activity. (Reprinted with permission from Viby-Mogensen JV: Correlation of succinylcholine duration of action with plasma cholinesterase activity in subjects with normal enzyme. Anesthesiology 53:517, 1980.)

of these local anesthetics in homozygote atypicals has rarely been documented.

Brodsky et al[123] have reported a normal caudal epidural anesthetic with the use of chloroprocaine in a patient with low plasma cholinesterase activity secondary to chronic echothiophate iodide therapy.[123]

Raj et al reported that there were no clinical difficulties from prolonged elevation of the plasma concentration of chloroprocaine after epidural and brachial plexus block in homozygote atypicals.[124] On the other hand, Kuhnert et al have reported excessive somnolence and a prolonged chloroprocaine epidural block in a postpartum patient.[125] This patient also manifested sensitivity to succinylcholine during a postpartum anesthetic (prepregnancy response to succinylcholine was normal) and was believed to have either an E^aE^a or an E^aE^s genotype. Jatlow et al have shown delayed hydrolysis of cocaine in vitro with plasma from homozygote atypicals.[126] They theorized that such persons may be at risk to toxic reaction from normal doses of cocaine.

THE PORPHYRIAS

The porphyrias all involve a defect in heme synthesis. The heme pigments are tetrapyrroles that are the essential elements in hemoglobin, myoglobin, and the cytochromes, i.e., compounds that are involved in the transport of oxygen, activation of oxygen, and electron transport chain. Cytochrome P-450 is a hemoprotein intimately involved in the conversion of lipid-soluble nonpolar drugs to soluble polar compounds that may be excreted in the urine.

A complete deficiency of enzymes that are involved in heme synthesis is incompatible with life. However, a partial deficiency may lead to the accumulation of one or more of the molecular intermediates in heme production. Such an accumulation of precursors is responsible for the clinical manifestations of the porphyrias (in as yet an unexplained manner).

The rate-limiting step in heme synthesis is the conjugation of succinyl-CoA with glycine to form delta amino levulinic acid (the enzyme is ALA synthetase). In the porphyrias there is a partial deficiency of enzymes subsequent to this initial step, which results in a stimulation of this reaction to form ALA. The result is overproduction of intermediate products before the deficient step (Fig. 17-5).

The porphyrias generally become manifest after puberty. The inheritance is through an autosomal dominant pattern, but congenital erythropoietic porphyria is inherited as an autosomal recessive pattern.

A functional classification for the anesthesiologist is based on a division of the porphyrias into inducible and noninducible forms. The inducible porphyrias are those in which the acute symptoms are precipitated upon drug exposure (Table 17-7).

These forms are acute intermittent porphyria, variegate porphyria, and hereditary coproporphyria. These porphyrias have an acute neurologic syndrome and are therefore of interest to the anesthesiologist. Cutaneous manifestations, with particular sensitivity to ultraviolet light, which is exhibited by skin fragility and bleeding, are the chief features of the other porphyrias. About 80% of patients with variegate porphyria are photosensitive. Some patients with hereditary coproporphyria also may have skin lesions. The porphyrias are very difficult to diagnose in the latent phase of the disorder. A variety of tests (e.g., the Watson-Schwartz test) may be used in the acute state to measure the elevated levels of the heme intermediates. Variegate porphyria is common in South Africa, and acute intermittent porphyria is found with increased frequency in Sweden. The inducible porphyrias are seen as a neurologic syndrome with a variety of presentations (Table 17-8).

The central, peripheral, and autonomic nervous system

TABLE 17-7. Drugs Known to Precipitate Porphyria

Sedatives
  Barbiturates
  Hypnotics such as chlordiazepoxide, glutethimide, diazepam
Analgesics
  Pentazocine, antipyrine, aminopyridine
Local anesthetics
  Lidocaine
Anticonvulsants
  Phenytoin, methsuximide
Antibiotics
  Sulfonamides, chloramphenicol
Steroids
  Estrogens, progesterones
Hypoglycemic sulfonylureas
  Tolbutamide, chlorpropramide
Toxins
  Lead, ethanol
Miscellaneous
  Ergot preparations
  Amphetamines
  Methyldopa

FIG. 17-5. Biosynthesis of heme and sites of defects in certain porphyrias. (Reprinted with permission. Mees DL, Frederickson EL: Anesthesia and the porphyrias. South Med J 68:29, 1975.) Abbreviations: *ALA* = aminolevulinic acid; *PBG* = porphobilinogen; *URO* = uroporphyrinogen; *COPRO* = coproporphyrinogen; *PROTO* = protoporphyrinogen; *PRO* = protoporphyrin. In intermittent acute porphyria there is a partial deficiency of the enzyme at site 1. In hereditary coproporphyria there is an enzyme deficiency at site 2. In variegate porphyria the enzyme problem is at site 3. In porphyria cutanea tarda there is deficiency at site 4.

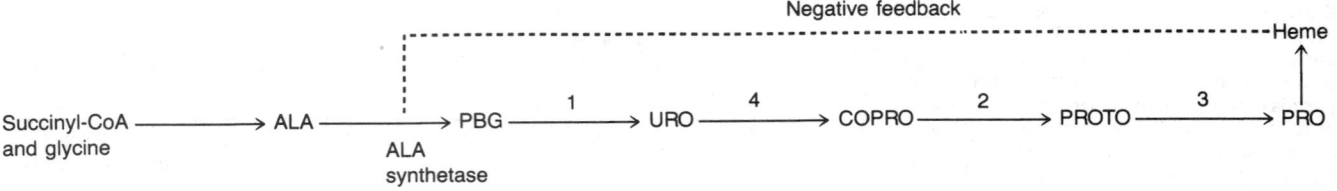

TABLE 17-8. Symptoms by Frequency
in Variegate Porphyria

Abdominal pain
Vomiting
Tachycardia
Hypertension
Neuropathy
Pyrexia
Pain in limbs
Confusion
Abnormal behavior
Seizures
Stupor

may be involved in porphyrias. A frequent manifestation is colicky abdominal pain, often with nausea and vomiting, which may suggest the diagnosis of acute abdomen, leading to exploratory laparotomy. Other symptoms are psychiatric disturbance, quadriplegia, hemiplegia, alterations of consciousness, and pain. Hyponatremia and hypokalemia may result from vomiting during the acute attack or may be related to hypothalamic disturbance. Death may result from paralysis of the respiratory muscles. The cause of these changes is unknown; they may be related to metabolites of the intermediates or result from deficiency of the heme pigment in the nerve cell itself.

In the anesthetic management of patients with porphyria, the chief concern is to avoid the administration of drugs that can induce a crisis; the drugs that induce cytochrome enzyme production can trigger the syndrome. Chief among those are the barbiturates; therefore, all barbiturates are contraindicated in porphyria. Ethyl alcohol, nonbarbiturate sedatives, hydantoin anticonvulsants, as well as a variety of other drugs, also can induce a crisis (Table 17-4). Endogenous factors, such as fasting, infection, and estrogens, may also precipitate porphyria. Diagnosis can be especially difficult because attacks may occur at a variable time period after drug administration or they may not occur at all despite administration of inducing drugs.

Because the porphyrias are unusual disorders, there is limited experience with the clinical use of many anesthetic drugs. *In vitro* studies suggest that certain anesthetics or anesthetic adjuvants may be contraindicated, but sufficient clinical experience is lacking (see below).

Management of Patients with Porphyria

It is important to recognize porphyria in patients. It may become apparent through a careful family history and personal history related to anesthesia. A careful history in the porphyric patient should concentrate on neurologic history and examination. Laboratory work should include electrolytes and blood urea nitrogen. Examination includes inspection of cutaneous lesions over the body. Most experts advise that regional techniques be avoided to prevent confusion should neurologic signs develop after operation. Glucose infusion should be started because starvation may induce an attack. Nitrous oxide, muscle relaxants, and narcotics are unequivocally safe drugs. Experience with other inhalation agents and reversal agents has been favorable, but *in vitro* studies suggest that they might exacerbate a crisis.[129] Blistered or fragile skin areas should be padded and given special attention.

The acute attack should be treated with glucose infusion, and hyponatremia, hypokalemia, and hypomagnesemia should be treated. Pyridoxine and hematin also have been valuable in some cases. Supportive therapy for respiratory insufficiency and treatment of pain is also suggested.

GLYCOGEN STORAGE DISEASES

The metabolic pathways involving glucose degradation to lactate, glucose conversion to glycogen, and the breakdown of glycogen to glucose are important to the whole body biochemistry as well as to cellular physiology in general. The enzymatic steps involved in glucose metabolism have been studied intensively since the earliest days of modern biochemistry. The glycogen storage diseases are inherited and are characterized by dysfunction of one of the many enzymes involved in glucose metabolism. To date, seven different glycogen storage disorders, each based on the deficiency of an enzyme involved in glucose metabolism, have been identified. Some of the glycogen storage diseases are incompatible with life past infancy, whereas others are not. Anesthetic experience with these diseases is limited, but several particular problems have been identified[130]:

Hypoglycemia. This results from failure to metabolize stored glycogen to glucose; there is a constant risk in these patients.
Acidosis. This is related to fat and protein metabolism because glycogen stores are not metabolically available.
Cardiac and hepatic dysfunction. This is secondary to destruction and displacement of normal tissue by the stored glycogen pools that accumulate.

Detailed descriptions of glucose metabolism are described elsewhere. Figure 17-6 outlines the glycogen–glucose–lactate pathway. There are, of course, multiple enzymatic steps to reach each of the end points.

FIG. 17-6. The glycogen–glucose–lactate pathway.

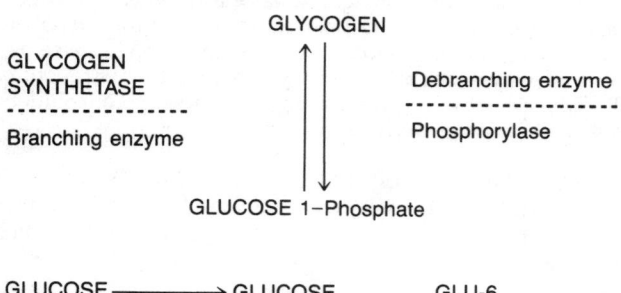

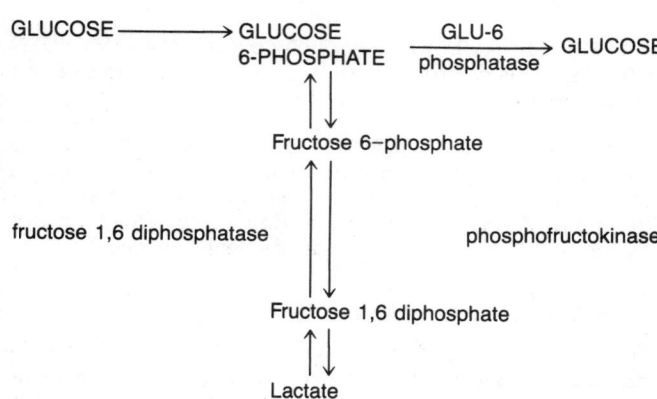

Defects in Glucose Metabolism

TYPE I (VON GIERKE'S DISEASE; GLUCOSE 6-PHOSPHATE DEFICIENCY). This is an autosomal recessive inheritance. The prognosis is moderately good, with many patients surviving into adulthood. Short stature and liver enlargement are characteristic.

The patients tolerate fasting very poorly. Hypoglycemia, acidosis, and convulsions may be a problem. Prolonged bleeding has been described. Often, preoperative hyperalimentation is used to reduce liver glycogen stores. Portocaval shunt has been performed with limited success in these patients. [131, 132]

TYPE II (POMPE'S DISEASE). Inheritance of this disease is considered to be autosomal recessive. This is a devastating disease with a very poor prognosis. Death usually occurs in childhood. There is a deficiency of lysosomal acid maltase with an accumulation of glycogen in the lysosomes, especially in the heart, liver, muscle, and central nervous system. Cardiac compromise resulting from outflow obstruction of hypertrophied muscle occurs, as does CHF secondary to myocardial disruption by glycogen stores. A case report has been described in which halothane was used without incident. [133] In another case, halothane led to prompt hypotension and intractable cardiac failure. [134] A late onset form with better prognosis has been described as well.

TYPE III (FORBE'S DISEASE; DEBRANCHING ENZYME DEFICIENCY). Inheritance of this is autosomal recessive.

TYPE IV (ANDERSEN'S DISEASE; BRANCHING ENZYME DEFICIENCY). This is a very rare disorder, characterized by a defect in the synthesis of normal glycogen. Cirrhosis of the liver and death before a patient reaches the age of 2 yr is characteristic.

TYPE V (McARDLE'S DISEASE; MUSCLE PHOSPHORYLASE DEFICIENCY). An autosomal recessive inheritance pattern and cramping with exercise are characteristic of this disorder. There is an inability of skeletal muscle to mobilize glycogen stores with exercise, the usual fuel in muscle for sustained exercise. Myoglobinuria occurs with overexertion in these patients and may occur after succinylcholine administration as well. Muscle atrophy occurs in adulthood. Tourniquets should not be used in these patients.

TYPE VI (HERS' DISEASE; REDUCED HEPATIC PHOSPHORYLASE). A decreased ability to mobilize hepatic glycogen occurs in this disorder with normal muscle and cardiac physiology.

TYPE VII (MUSCLE PHOSPHOFRUCTOKINASE DEFICIENCY). This disorder is similar to McArdle's disease and is characterized by muscle cramping.

TYPE VIII (DEFICIENT HEPATIC PHOSPHORYLASE KINASE). This results from a deficiency in the regulatory enzyme controlling the phosphorylase enzyme. A case report describing fever, and acidosis during succinylcholine, halothane, and ketamine anesthesia has been described. [135]

Defects of Fructose Metabolism

Fructose-6-phosphate is converted to fructose 1,6-diphosphate during glucose breakdown to lactate. Conversely, fructose 1,6-diphosphate is converted to fructose-6-phosphate by the enzyme fructose 1,6-diphosphatase during gluconeogenesis.

In fructose 1,6-diphosphatase deficiency there is an inability to produce glycogen from lactate. Hypoglycemia may result. Acidosis has been reported because lactate is formed preferentially. In errors of fructose metabolism, like those of glucose metabolism, hypoglycemia and acidosis pose the greatest threat to the patient. [136]

THE MUCOPOLYSACCHARIDOSES

The mucopolysaccharides are polysaccharides that yield mixtures of monosaccharides and derived products after hydrolysis. The mucopolysaccharides contain N-acetylated hexosamine in a characteristic repeating unit. For example, chondroitin sulfate A is a monosaccharide of d-glucuronic acid and N-acetyl d-galactosamine 4-sulfate. Monopolysaccharides are found in all cells.

The mucopolysaccharidoses are genetically determined diseases in which mucopolysaccharides are stored in tissues in abnormal quantities and excreted in large amounts in the urine. The disorders result from a deficiency of a specific lysosomal enzyme that is required to break down these compounds. As a result, mucopolysaccharides accumulate in tissues, producing specific clinical manifestations. There are seven basic forms of mucopolysaccharidoses and several subgroups. Most of the mucopolysaccharidoses are inherited as autosomal recessives. All the mucopolysaccharidoses are progressive and characteristically are marked by coarse facial features (gargoylism); associated skeletal abnormalities such as lumbar lordosis, stiff joints, chest deformity, dwarfing, and hypoplasia of the odontoid process (Morquio syndrome); corneal opacities; limitation of joint motion; and heart, liver, and spleen enlargement resulting from mucopoly saccharide accumulation. Mental deterioration also occurs frequently.

The Hunter and Hurler syndromes are best known variants of the mucopolysaccharidoses. The Hunter syndrome is an X-linked recessive disease. Respiratory infection and heart disease, both valvular and ischemic, often lead to death when patients are young. The patients may present for repair of inguinal hernia or orthopedic procedures. The thick soft tissues and the copious thick secretions make airway management a particular problem. In Leroy's and Crocker's series minor difficulties occurred with anesthesia in patients in more than one-third of 60 operations. [137] Postoperative respiratory obstruction was noted in several cases. Because of the underlying heart disease, these patients should have ECG and echocardiography tests performed before surgery.

Mucopolysaccharidosis IV (Morquio syndrome) is associated with perhaps the most significant skeletal deformities. In addition to cardiovascular disorders and respiratory insufficiency from marked chest wall deformity, acute, subacute, or chronic myelopathy is extremely common. This is secondary to severe hypoplasia or absence of the odontoid process of the second cervical vertebra. In anesthesia care the head should be positioned carefully and precautions, such as avoidance of succinylcholine, should be taken with patients with cord compromise.

When these patients die, it is usually of respiratory infection, or cardiac failure resulting from valvular lesions or cardiomyopathy. Patients come for surgical correction of orthopedic problems, corneal opacities, and carpal tunnel syndrome.

Other adverse reactions to anesthesia have been summarized recently. [138]

OTHER INHERITED DISORDERS

OSTEOGENESIS IMPERFECTA

Osteogenesis imperfecta is seen in approximately 1 of 50,000 births. Most cases are autosomal dominant; some are autosomal recessive. The pathophysiologic characteristics include decreased collagen synthesis, which leads to osteoporosis; joint laxity; and tendon weakness. The manifestations of osteogenesis imperfecta are small bowed limbs, large head, short neck, blue sclerae, otosclerosis, joint laxity, brittle teeth, and a tendency to fractures. One also sees an increased bleeding tendency resulting from abnormal platelet function, and aortic and mitral valve dysfunction resulting from dilation of the valve ring.

The patient should be handled carefully because minor trauma may lead to fractures. Airway management may also be difficult because of cervical spine involvement with this disorder. Patients with this disorder have short necks, and mandibular fractures frequently occur. The patient's cardiovascular status should be evaluated, especially mitral and aortic valve function. Kyphoscoliosis may also occur, with pulmonary compromise. Care should be taken to pad the pressure areas, particularly for long procedures. One should be prepared to obtain platelet transfusions. The patient's temperature should be monitored because hyperthermia (possibly resulting from central nervous system dysfunction) has been reported.[139] MH has also been associated with osteogenesis imperfecta.

NEUROFIBROMATOSIS (VON RECKLINGHAUSEN'S DISEASE)

Neurofibromatosis occurs in approximately one of 3,000 births.[140-142] The inheritance pattern is autosomal dominant, but there is a varied expression. The pathophysiologic characteristics include localized fibromas of skin and nerve. Manifestations include café au lait spots and neuromas located along peripheral nerves inside and outside the central nervous system. Meningiomas, gliomas, and acoustic neuromas are not uncommon and are seen in two-thirds of the cases. Laryngeal neurofibromas can lead to airway obstruction and dysphagia. Pheochromocytoma occurs in a small percentage of patients. Ten per cent of patients with pheochromocytoma have neurofibromatosis. Scoliosis and kyphoscoliosis can also occur.

There are numerous anesthetic considerations for the patient with neurofibromatosis. These include potential hypertensive crises resulting from pheochromocytomas or renal artery stenosis and hypersensitivity to nondepolarizing and depolarizing muscle relaxants. It is important to evaluate the airway because of the possibility of laryngeal tumors. Regional anesthesia may also be a problem in patients with fibroma involving the epidural space or peripheral nerves.

MARFAN'S SYNDROME

Marfan's syndrome is caused by abnormal collagen production.[143] Its inheritance follows an autosomal dominant pattern. The classical clinical features of Marfan's syndrome include aortic regurgitation, joint laxity, spindly extremities, ectopia lentis, and weakened arterial walls. Death often occurs by the time the patient reaches the mid-30s. Aortic dissection is the most feared complication in the perioperative period. Consequently, hypertension should be aggressively controlled.

EHLERS-DANLOS SYNDROME

Ehlers-Danlos syndrome is inherited through an autosomal dominant pattern.[144] However, there are both X-linked recessive and X-linked dominant patterns of inheritance. The clinical features include hypermobile joints, bleeding tendency, hernias, and vascular dissection. The major problem relates to the bleeding tendency. The treatment plan for patients with Ehlers-Danlos syndrome is to evaluate their coagulation profile and have large amounts of blood typed and crossed.

PHENYLKETONURIA

The inheritance of phenylketonuria follows an autosomal recessive pattern.[145] The inability to convert phenylalanine to tyrosine is the underlying defect. The clinical features include mental retardation and behavior abnormalities. These patients are prone to convulsions. Depression of the sympathoadrenal axis has also been seen. Hypoglycemia is common.

When anesthesia is administered, care should be taken to prevent hypoglycemia associated with preoperative fasting. The anesthesiologist should also remember that these patients can convulse. The precautions and appropriate plan for administering anesthesia include careful monitoring of blood glucose, avoidance of hypocarbia, avoidance of epileptogenic drugs, and continuation of all anticonvulsant therapy through the time of surgery.

PRADER-WILLI SYNDROME

The inheritance pattern of Prader-Willi syndrome is unknown.[146] Its clinical features include hypotonia, obesity, diabetes, hypogonadism, mental deficiency, and dental caries. The problems related to anesthesia are those that are secondary to the patient's hypoglycemia, obesity, and hypotonia. There are possible problems related to the neuromuscular blockade. The airway must be protected during surgery with an endotracheal tube, and during operation one should monitor the blood glucose level. Careful attention must also be paid to maintaining airway patency during operation, and after operation, airway obstruction has been seen.

RILEY-DAY (FAMILIAL DYSAUTONOMIA)

A deficiency of dopamine beta hydroxylase that leads to decreased noradrenaline at the nerve endings is thought to be the cause of Riley-Day syndrome.[147] This syndrome is inherited through an autosomal recessive fashion. Patients with Riley-Day exhibit copious pulmonary secretions, denervation supersensitivity, no sensitivity to pain, no response to histamine, and impairment of temperature control. The impairment of temperature control leads to intermittent fevers. There are numerous problems related to anesthesia. These include corneal abrasions, excess secretions, pneumonia, labile blood pressure, possible decreased response to hypoxia and hypercarbia, increased potential for aspiration because of swallowing problems, postural hypotension, and sensitivity to vasopressors. Anesthetic management should include temperature monitoring and careful blood pressure monitoring. Fresh gases should be humidified. Vasopressors need to be titrated carefully because of the hypersensitivity response. Secretions can be managed after operation with chest percussion therapy. One must also monitor for postoperative apnea. Chlorpromazine may be useful in managing emotional lability and cyclic fever.[148]

REFERENCES

1. Denborough MA, Lovell RRH: Anaesthetic deaths in a family. Lancet 2:45, 1960
2. Denborough MA, Forster JFA, Lovell RH et al: Anaesthesia deaths in a family. Br J Anaesth 34:395, 1962
3. Nelson TE: Porcine stress syndromes. In Gordon RA, Britt BA, Kalow W (eds): International Symposium on Malignant Hyperthermia, p 191. Springfield, Charles C Thomas, 1973
4. Kalow W, Britt BA, Terreau ME et al: Metabolic error of muscle metabolism after recovery from malignant hyperthermia. Lancet 2:895, 1970
5. Aldrete JA, Britt BA (eds): Second International Symposium on Malignant Hyperthermia. New York, Grune and Stratton, 1978
6. Lopez JR, Alamo L, Caputo C et al: Intracellular ionized calcium concentration in muscles from humans with malignant hyperthermia. Muscle Nerve 8:355, 1985
7. Gronert GA, Ahern CP, Milde JH: Treatment of porcine malignant hyperthermia: Lactate gradient from muscle to blood. Can Anaesth Soc J 33:729, 1986
8. Mathieu A, Bogosian AJ, Ryan JF et al: Recrudescence after survival of an initial episode of malignant hyperthermia. Anesthesiology 51:454, 1979
9. Donlon JV, Newfield P, Sreter I et al: Implications of masseter spasm after succinylcholine. Anesthesiology 49:298, 1978
10. Relton JES, Creighton RE, Conn AW et al: Generalized muscular hypertonicity associated with general anaesthesia. A suggested anaesthetic management. Can Anaesth Soc J 14:22, 1967
11. Carroll JB: Increased incidence of masseter spasm in children with strabismus anesthetized with halothane and succinylcholine. Anesthesiology (in press)
12. Ellis FR, Halsall PJ: Suxamethonium spasm. A differential diagnostic conundrum. Br J Anaesth 56:381, 1984
13. Schwartz L, Rockoff MA, Koka BV: Masseter spasm with anesthesia: Incidence and implications. Anesthesiology 61:772, 1984
14. Ording H: Incidence of malignant hyperthermia in Denmark. Anesth Analg 64:700, 1985
15. Britt BA, Kalow W: Malignant hyperthermia: A statistical review. Can Anaesth Soc J 17:293, 1970
16. Rosenberg H, Fletcher JE: Masseter muscle rigidity and malignant hyperthermia susceptibility. Anesth Analg 65:161, 1986
17. Miller ED, Sanders DB, Rowlingson JC et al: Anesthesia-induced rhabdomyolysis in a patient with Duchenne's muscular dystrophy. Anesthesiology 48:146, 1978
18. Caroff SN: The neuroleptic malignant syndrome. J Clin Psychiatry 41:679, 1980
19. Caroff SN, Rosenberg H, Fletcher JE et al: Malignant hyperthermia susceptibility in neuroleptic malignant hyperthermia syndrome. Anesthesiology 67:20, 1987
20. Addonizio G, Susman VL: ECT as a treatment alternative for patients with symptoms of neuroleptic malignant syndrome. J Clin Psychiatry 48:102, 1987
21. Granato JR, Stern BJ, Ringel A et al: Neuroleptic malignant syndrome: Successful treatment with dantrolene and bromocriptine. Ann Neurol 14:89, 1983
22. Kelfer H, Singer WN, Reynolds RN: Malignant hyperthermia in a child with Duchenne muscular dystrophy. Pediatrics 71:118, 1983
23. Smith CL, Bush GH: Anaesthesia and progressive muscular dystrophy. Br J Anaesth 57:1113, 1985
24. Heiman-Pattersohn TH, Natter H, Rosenberg H et al: Malignant hyperthermia susceptibility in X linked muscle dystrophies. Pediatric Neurology 2:356, 1986
25. Frank JP, Harate Y, Butler JS et al: Central core disease and malignant hyperthermia syndrome. Ann Neurol 7:11, 1980
26. McPherson EW, Taylor CA: The King syndrome: Malignant hypethermia, myopathy and multiple anomalies. Am J Med Genet 8:159, 1981
27. Rampton AJ, Kelly DA, Shanahan EC et al: Occurrence of malignant hyperpyrexia in a patient with osteogenesis imperfecta. Br J Anaesth 56:1443, 1984
28. Denborough MA, Galloway GJ, Hopkinson: Malignant hyperthermia and sudden infant death syndrome. Lancet 2:1068, 1982
29. Gronert GA, Thompson RL, Onofrio BM: Human malignant hyperthermia: Awake episodes and correction by dantrolene. Anesth Analg 59:377, 1980
30. Fishbein WN, Muldoon SM, Deuster PA et al: Myoadenylate deaminase deficiency and malignant hyperthermia susceptibility: Is there a relationship? Biochem Med 34:344, 1985
31. Wingard DW: Malignant hyperthermia: A human stress syndrome? Lancet 4:1450, 1974
32. Neuspiel DR, Kuller DH: Sudden and unexpected death in childhood and adolescence. JAMA 264:1321, 1985
33. Wingard DW, Bobko S: Failure of lidocaine to trigger porcine malignant hyperthermia. Anesth Analg 58:855, 1979
34. Berkowitz A, Rosenberg H: Femoral block with mepivacaine for muscle biopsy in malignant hyperthermia patients. Anesthesiology 62:651, 1985
35. Gronert GA, Milde JH, Theye RA: Role of sympathetic activity in porcine malignant hyperthermia. Anesthesiology 47:411, 1977
36. Gronert GA, Milde JH, Taylor SR: Porcine muscle responses to carbacol, alpha and beta adrenoreceptor agonist, halothane or hyperthermia. J Physiol 307:319, 1980
37. Britt BA, Webb GE, LeDuc C: Malignant hyperthermia induced by curare. Can Anaesth Soc J 21:371, 1974
38. Ording H, Nielsen VG: Atracurium and its antagonism by neostigmine (plus glycopyrrolate) in patients susceptible to malignant hyperthermia. Br J Anaesth 58:1001, 1986
39. Andersson K: Effects of chlorpromazine, imipramine and quinidine on the mechanical activity of single skeletal muscle fibers of the frogs. Acta Physiol Scand 85:532, 1982
40. Gronert GA, Ahern CP, Milde J et al: Malignant hyperthermia not produced by CO_2, calcium or digoxin in porcine cardial or skeletal muscle: Triggering effects of potassium in skeletal muscle. Anesthesiology 64:24, 1986
41. Fletcher JE, Rosenberg H: In vitro studies of droperidol for use in human malignant hyperthermia. Anesthesiology 63:A302, 1985
42. Lunn JN, Farrow SC, Fowkes FGR et al: Epidemiology in anaesthesia. Br J Anaesth 59:803, 1982
43. Lavad DG, Rice CP, Robinson R et al: Malignant hyperthermia: A study of an affected family. Br J Anaesth 44:93, 1972
44. Williams CH, Lasley JH: The mode of inheritance of the fulminant hyperthermia stress syndrome in swine. In Henschel EO (ed): Malignant Hyperthermia, Current Concepts, p 141. New York, Appleton-Century-Crofts, 1977
45. Eikelenboom G, Minkema D, Van Eldik P et al: Inheritance of the malignant hyperthermia syndrome in Dutch Landrace swine. In Aldrete JA, Britt BA (eds): Second International Symposium on Malignant Hyperthermia, p 141. New York, Grune and Stratton, 1977
46. Gallant EM, Rempel WE: Porcine malignant hyperthermia false negative in the halothane test. Am J Vet Res 48:488, 1987
47. McPherson EW, Taylor CA: The genetics of malignant hyperthermia: Evidence for heterogeneity. Am J Med Genet 11:273, 1982

48. Denborough MA: The pathopharmacology of malignant hyperpyrexia. Pharmacol Ther 9:357, 1980

49. Tolpin EI, Fletcher JE, Rosenberg H: Effects of anaesthetic agents on erythrocyte fragility: Comparison of normal and malignant hyperthermia susceptible patients. Can J Anaesth 34:366, 1987

50. Paasake RT, Brownell AKW: Serum creatine kinase level as a screening test for susceptibility to malignant hyperthermia. JAMA 255:769, 1986

51. Solomons CC, Masson NC: Platelet model for halothane-induced effects on nucleotide metabolism applied to malignant hyperthermia. Acta Anaesthesiol Scand 28:185, 1984

52. Lee MB, Adragna MHG, Edwards L: The use of a platelet nucleotide assay as a possible diagnostic test for malignant hyperthermia. Anesthesiology 63:311, 1985

52a. Traynor CA, Van Dyke EA, Gronent GA: Phosphorylase ratio and susceptibility to malignant hyperthermia. Anesth Analg 62:324, 1983

53. Allen PD, Ryan JF, Jones DE et al: Correspondence: Sarcoplasmic reticulum calcium uptake in cryostat sections of skeletal muscle from malignant hyperthermia patients and controls. Muscle Nerve 9:474, 1986

54. Nagarajan K, Fishbein WN, Muldoon S: Calcium uptake in frozen muscle biopsy sections compared with other predictions of malignant hyperthermia susceptibility. Anesthesiology 66:680, 1987

55. Britt BA, Frodis W, Scott E et al: Comparison of the caffeine skinned fibre tension (CSFT) test with the caffeine-halothane contracture (CHC) test in the diagnosis of malignant hyperthermia. Can Anaesth Soc J 29:550, 1982

56. Blanck TJJ, Fisher YI, Thompson M et al: Low molecular weight proteins in human malignant hyperthermia muscle. Anesthesiology 61:589, 1984

57. Walsh MP, Brownell AKW, Littmann V et al: Electrophoresis of muscle proteins is not a method for diagnosis of malignant hyperthermia susceptibility. Anesthesiology 64:473, 1986

58. Britt BA, Scott EA, Kleiman A et al: Failure of the tourniquet-twitch test as a diagnostic or screening test for malignant hyperthermia. Anesth Analg 66:1047, 1986

59. Klip A, Elliott ME, Frodis W et al: Anaesthetic induced increase in ionized calcium in blood mononuclear cells from malignant hyperthermia patients. Lancet 1:463, 1987

60. Olgin J, Argov Z, Rosenberg H et al: Noninvasive evaluation of malignant hyperthermia susceptibility with phosphorous nuclear magnetic resonance spectroscopy. Anesthesiology 68:507, 1988

61. Fletcher JE, Rosenberg H: In vitro muscle contractures induced by halothane and suxamethonium. 2. Human skeletal muscle from normal and malignant hyperthermia susceptible patients. Br J Anaesth 58:1433, 1986

62. Rosenberg H, Reed S: In vitro contracture tests for susceptibility to malignant hyperthermia. Anesth Analg 62:415, 1983

63. Ellis FR, Halsall JP, Ording H et al: A protocol for the investigation of malignant hyperpyrexia (MH) susceptibility. Br J Anaesth 56:1267, 1984

64. Britt BA, Endrenyi L, Frodis W et al: Comparison of effects of several inhalation anaesthetics on caffeine-induced contractures of normal and malignant hyperthermic skeletal muscle. Can Anaesth Soc J 27:12, 1980

65. Nelson TE, Flewellen EH, Gloyna DF: Spectrum of susceptibility to malignant hyperthermia—Diagnostic dilemma. Anesth Analg 62:545, 1983

66. Fletcher JE, Rosenberg H: Laboratory methods for malignant hyperthermia. In Williams CH (ed): Experimental Malignant Hyperthermia, pp 121–140. New York, Springer-Verlag, 1988

67. Kolb ME, Horne ML, Martz R: Dantrolene in human malignant hyperthermia. Anesthesiology 56:254, 1982

68. Rubin AS, Zablocki AD: Hyperkalemia, verapamil and dantrolene. Anesthesiology 66:246, 1987

69. Fletcher R, Blennow G, Olsson AK et al: Malignant hyperthermia in a myopathic child. Prolonged postoperative course requiring dantrolene. Acta Anaesth Scand 26:431, 1982

70. Jensen AG, Bach V, Werner M et al: A fatal case of malignant hyperthermia following isoflurane anaesthesia. Acta Anaesth Scand 30:293, 1986

71. Britt BA: Dantrolene. Can Anaesth Soc J 31:61, 1984

72. Watson CB, Reierson N, Norfleet EA: Clinically significant muscle weakness induced by oral dantrolene. Sodium prophylaxis for malignant hyperthermia. Anesthesiology 65:312, 1986

73. Neubauer K, Kaufman RD: Another use for mass spectroscopy: Detection and monitoring of malignant hyperthermia. Anesth Analg 64:837, 1985

74. Vaughan MS, Cork RC, Vaughan RW: Inaccuracy of liquid crystal thermometry to identify cone temperature trends in postoperative adults. Anesth Analg 61:284, 1982

75. Ruhland G, Hinkle A: Malignant hyperthermia after oral and intravenous pretreatment with dantrolene in a patient susceptible to malignant hyperthermia. Anesthesiology 60:159, 1984

76. Morison DH: Correspondence: Placental transfer of dantrolene. Anesthesiology 59:265, 1983

77. Harthorn AM, Young E: A relationship between acid base balance and capture myopathy in zebra (Equus burchelli) and apparent therapy. Vet Rec 95:337, 1974

78. Mazzia VDB, Simon A: Medicolegal implications of malignant hyperthermia. In Aldrete JA, Britt BA (eds): Malignant Hyperthermia, p 545. New York, Grune and Stratton, 1977

79. Gronert GA, Milde JH, Theye RA: Porcine malignant hyperthermia induced by halothane and succinylcholine: Failure of treatment with procaine and procainamide. Anesthesiology 44:124, 1976

80. Williams CH, Roberts JT, Hoech GP et al: The fulminant hyperthermia-stress syndrome: Total neuromuscular blockade with dimethyl curare prevents the development of the syndrome in susceptible pigs. J Thermal Biol 3:104, 1978

81. Kalow W, Britt BA, Richter A: The caffeine test of isolated human muscle in relation to malignant hyperthermia. Can Anaesth Soc J 678, 1977

82. Rosenberg H: International workshop on malignant hyperpyrexia. Anesthesiology 54:530, 1981

83. Williams CH: Some observations on the etiology of the fulminant hyperthermia-stress syndrome. Perspect Biol Med 20:120, 1976

84. Verburg MP, Oerlemansft JJJ, Van Bennekom CA et al: In vivo induced malignant hyperthermia in pigs: I. Physiological and biochemical changes and the influence of dantrolene sodium. Acta Anaesth Scand 28:1, 1984

85. Austin KL, Denborough MA: Drug treatment of malignant hyperpyrexia. Anaesth Intensive Care 5:207, 1977

86. Fletcher JE, Rosenberg H: In vitro muscle contractures induced by halothane and succinylcholine: I. The rat diaphragm. Br J Anaesth 58:1427, 1986

87. Moulds RFW, Denborough MA: Procaine in malignant hyperpyrexia. Br Med J 4:526, 1972

88. Ilias WK, Williams CH, Fulfer RT et al: Diltiazem inhibits halothane-induced contractions in malignant hyperthermia-susceptible muscles in vitro. Br J Anaesth 57:994

89. Fletcher JE, Lizzo FH: Contracture induction by snake venom cardiotoxin in skeletal muscle from humans and rats. Toxicon (in press)

90. Harrington JF, Ford DJ, Striker TW: Myoglobinemia after succinylcholine in children undergoing halothane and nonhalothane anesthesia. Anesthesiology 61:A431, 1984

91. Fletcher JE, Rosenberg H: In vitro interaction between halothane and succinylcholine in human skeletal muscle: Implications for

malignant hyperthermia and masseter muscle rigidity. Anesthesiology 190, 1985

92. Olthoff D, Kunze D, Kries H: Acyltransferase- and phospholipase activity in skeletal muscle homogenate with addition of muscle relaxants. Acta Biol Med Ger 31:317, 1973

93. Stadhouders AM, Viering WAL, Verburg MP et al: In vivo induced malignant hyperthermia in pigs. III. Localization of calcium in skeletal muscle mitochondria by means of electromicroscopy and microprobe analysis. Acta Anaesth Scand 28:14, 1984

94. Berman MC, Harrison GG, Bull AB et al: Changes underlying halothane-induced malignant hyperpyrexia in Landrace pigs. Nature (London) 225:653, 1970

95. Nelson TE, Flewellen EH, Belt M et al: Comparison of Ca^{2+} uptake and spontaneous Ca^{2+} release from sarcoplasmic reticulum vesicles isolated from muscle of malignant hyperthermia diagnostic patients. J Pharmacol Exp Ther 240:785, 1987

96. Ellis FR, Heffron JJA: Clinical and biochemical aspects of malignant hyperpyrexia. In Atkinson RS, Adams AP (eds): Recent Advances in Anaesthesia and Analgesia, p 173. Edinburgh, Churchill Livingstone, 1985

97. Endo M, Yagi S, Ishizuka T et al: Changes in the Ca-induced Ca release mechanism in the sarcoplasmic reticulum of the muscle from a patient with malignant hyperthermia. Biomed Res 4:83, 1983

98. Ohnishi ST, Taylor S, Gronert GA: Calcium-induced Ca^{2+} release from sarcoplasmic reticulum of pigs susceptible to malignant hyperthermia: The effects of halothane and dantrolene. FEBS Lett 161:103, 1983

99. Cheah KS, Cheah AM: Skeletal muscle mitochondrial phospholipase A2 and the interaction of mitochondria and sarcoplasmic reticulum in porcine malignant hyperthermia. Biochem Biophys Acta 638:40, 1981

100. Fletcher JE, Kistler P, Rosenberg H et al: Dantrolene and mepacrine antagonize the hemolysis of human red blood cells by halothane and bee venom phospholipase A2. Toxicol Appl Pharmacol 90:410, 1987

101. Cheah KS, Cheah AM: Malignant hyperthermia: Molecular defects in membrane permeability. Experientia 41:656, 1985

102. Cheah KS, Cheah AM: Mitochondrial calcium transport and calcium-activated phospholipase in porcine malignant hyperthermia. Biochem Biophys Acta 634:70, 1981

103. Gallant EM, Gronert GA, Taylor SR: Cellular membrane potentials and contractile threshold in mammalian skeletal muscle susceptible to malignant hyperthermia. Neurosci Lett 28:181, 1982

104. Mickelson JR, Ross JA, Hyslop RJ et al: Skeletal muscle sarcolemma in malignant hyperthermia: Evidence for a defect in calcium regulation. Biochem Biophys Acta 897:364, 1987

105. Cheah KS, Cheah AM, Waring JC: Phospholipase A2 activity, calmodulin, Ca^{2+} and meat quality in young and adult halothane-sensitive and halothane-insensitive British Landrace pigs. Meat Science 17:37, 1986

106. Marjanen LA, Collins SP, Denborough MA: Calmodulin and malignant hyperpyrexia. Biochem Med 32:283, 1984

107. Deuster PA, Brockman EL, Muldoon SM: In vitro responses of cat skeletal muscle to halothane and caffeine. J Appl Physiol 58:521, 1985

108. Heiman-Patterson T, Fletcher JE, Rosenberg H et al: No relationship between fiber type and halothane contracture test results in malignant hyperthermia. Anesthesiology 67:182, 1987

109. Nyhan WL, Sakata NO: Genetic and Malformation Syndromes in Clinical Medicine. Chicago, Year Book Medical Publishers, 1976

110. Stanbury JB, Wyngaarden JB, Frederickson DS: The Metabolic Basis of Inherited Disease. New York, McGraw-Hill, 1978

111. Viby-Mogensen J, Hanel HK: A Danish cholinesterase unit. Acta Anaesth Scand 21:405, 1977

112. Viby-Mogensen J: Succinylcholine neuromuscular blockade in subjects homozygous for atypical plasma cholinesterase. Anesthesiology 55:429, 1981

113. Kalow W, Genest K: A method for the detection of atypical forms of human serum cholinesterase. Determination of dibucaine numbers. Can J Biochem 35:339, 1957

114. Ravindran RS, Cummins DF, Pantazis KL et al: Unusual aspects of low levels of pseudocholinesterase in a pregnant patient. Anesth Analg 61:953, 1982

115. Harris H, Whittaker M: Differential inhibition of serum cholinesterase with fluoride. Recognition of two new phenotypes. Nature (London) 191:496, 1961

116. Hanel HK, Viby-Mogensen J, Schaffalitzky de Muckadell OB: Serum cholinesterase variants in the Danish population. Acta Anaesthesiol Scand 22:505, 1978

117. Packman P, Meyer DA, Verdun RM: Hazards of succinylcholine administration during electrotherapy. Arch Gen Psychiatry 35:1137, 1978

118. Patterson JL, Walsh ES, Hall GM: Progressive depletion of plasma cholinesterase during daily plasma exchange. Br Med J 2:580, 1979

119. Viby-Mogensen J: Correlation of succinylcholine duration of action with plasma cholinesterase activity in subjects with normal enzyme. Anesthesiology 53:517, 1980

120. Viby-Mogensen J: Succinylcholine neuromuscular blockade in subjects heterozygous for abnormal plasma cholinesterase. Anesthesiology 55:231, 1981

121. Baraka A: Absence of suxamethonium fasciculations in patients with atypical plasma cholinesterase. Br J Anaesth 47:419, 1975

122. Harris H, Hopkinson DA, Robson EB et al: Genetic studies on a new variant of serum cholinesterase detected by electrophoresis. Ann Hum Genet 26:359, 1963

123. Brodsky JB, Campos FA: Chloroprocaine analgesia in a patient receiving echothiophate iodide eye drops. Anesthesiology 48:288, 1978

124. Raj PP, Rosenblatt R, Miller J et al: Dynamics of local anesthetic compounds in regional anesthesia. Anesth Analg 56:110, 1977

125. Kuhnert BR, Philipson EA et al: A prolonged chloroprocaine epidural block in a postpartum patient with abnormal pseudocholinesterase. Anesthesiology 56:477, 1982

126. Jatlow P, Barash PG, Van Dyke C et al: Cocaine and succinylcholine sensitivity: A new caution. Anesth Analg 58:235, 1979

127. Murphy PC: Acute intermittent porphyria: The anaesthetic problem and its background. Br J Anaesth 36:801, 1964

128. Mustajoki P, Heinonen J: General anesthesia in "inducible" porphyrias. Anesthesiology 53:12, 1980

129. Parikh RK, Moore MR: Effect of certain anaesthetic agents on the activity of rat hepatic delta amino-levulinate synthetase. Br J Anaesth 50:1099, 1978

130. Cox JM: Anesthesia and glycogen storage disease. Anesthesiology 29:1221, 1963

131. Casson H: Anesthesia for portacaval bypass in patients with metabolic diseases. Br J Anaesth 47:969, 1975

132. Starzl TE, Putnam C et al: Portal diversion for the treatment of glycogen storage disease in humans. Ann Surg 178:525, 1973

133. Kaplan R: Pompe's disease presenting for anesthesia. Anesthesia Reviews 7:21, 1980

134. Ellis FR: Inherited muscle disease. Br J Anaesth 52:153, 1980

135. Edelstein G, Hirshman CA: Hyperthermia and ketoacidosis during anesthesia in a child with glycogen-storage disease. Anesthesiology 52:90, 1980

136. Hashimoto Y, Watanabe H, Satou M: Anesthetic management of a patient with hereditary fructose 1,6 diphosphate deficiency. Anesth Analg 57:503, 1978

137. Leroy JG, Crocker AC: Clinical definition of the Hurler-Hunter phenotypes. Am J Dis Child 112:518, 1966

138. Sjogren P, Pedersen T, Steinmetz H: Mucopolysaccharidoses and anaesthetic risk. Acta Anaesth Scand 31:214, 1987
139. Oliverio RM: Anesthetic management of intramedullary nailing in osteogenesis imperfecta: Report of a case. Anesth Analg 52:232, 1973
140. Fisher MM: Anaesthetic difficulties in neurofibromatosis. Anaesthesia 30:648, 1975
141. Magbagbeola JA: Abnormal responses to muscle relaxants in patients with von Recklinghausen's disease. Br J Anaesth 42:710, 1970
142. Yamashita M, Matsuki A, Oyama T: Anaesthetic considerations on von Recklinghausen's disease (multiple neurofibromatosis). Anaesthetist 26:317, 1977
143. Pyevitz RE, McKusick VA: The Marfan syndrome: Diagnosis and management. N Engl J Med 300:172, 1979
144. Donlan P, Sisko F, Riley E: Anesthetic considerations for Ehlers-Danlos syndrome. Anesthesiology 52:266, 1980
145. Jackson SH: Inborn errors of metabolism. In Katz J, Benumof J, Kadis LB (eds): Anesthesia and Uncommon Diseases, 2nd ed, p 1. Philadelphia, WB Saunders, 1981
146. Palmer SK, Atlee JL: Anesthetic management of the Prader Willi syndrome. Anesthesiology 44:161, 1976
147. Brown BR, Watson PD, Taussig LM: Congenital metabolic diseases of pediatric patients. Anesthesiology 43:197, 1975
148. Meridy HW, Creighton RE: General anaesthesia in eight patients with familial dysautonomia. Can Anaesth Soc J 18:563, 1971
149. Mirakhur RK, Lvery TD, Briggs, et al: Effects of neostigmine and pyridostigmine on serum cholinesterase activity. Can Anaesth Soc J 29:55, 1982
150. Whittaker M: Plasma cholinesterase variants and the anaesthetist. Anaesthesia 35:174, 1980
151. Sunew KY, Hicks RG: Effects of neostigmine and pyridostigmine on duration of succinylcholine action and pseudocholinesterase activity. Anesthesiology 49:188, 1978
152. Spurgeon MJ: Apparent resistance to succinylcholine. Anesth Analg 58:57, 1979
153. Mees DL, Frederickson EL: Anesthesia and the porphyrias. South Med J 68:29, 1975

Preoperative Medication

Anesthetic management for patients begins with the preoperative psychologic preparation and, if necessary, preoperative medication. Specific pharmacologic actions should be kept in mind when these drugs are administered before operation and they should be tailored to the needs of each patient. The anesthesiologist should assess the patient's mental and physical condition during the preoperative visit. Because it is part of and the beginning of the anesthetic, choice of preoperative medication is based on the same considerations as the choice of anesthesia, for example, the patient's medical problems, requirements of the surgery, and anesthesiologist's skills. Satisfactory preoperative preparation and medication facilitates an uneventful perioperative course. Poor preparation may begin a series of problems and misadventures.

No consensus on the choice of preoperative medications exists. Their use has been dominated in the past by tradition, which has been modified somewhat by the change in anesthetic agents and techniques over the years. Beecher stated that "empirical procedures firmly established in the habits of good doctors have a life, not to say, immortality of their own."[1] Similarly, "the emotional attachment of an anesthetist to his own regimen is often more obvious than his objective assessment of its effects."[2] Another reason for lack of consensus may be that several different drugs or combinations of drugs can accomplish the same goals. However, there is general agreement that most patients should enter the operating room after anxiety has been relieved and other specific goals have been met through preoperative preparation and medication. This should be accomplished without undue sedation interfering with patient safety.

PSYCHOLOGIC PREPARATION

Psychologic preparation of the patient involves the preoperative visit and interview with the patient and family members. The anesthesiologist should explain anticipated events and the proposed anesthetic management in an effort to reduce anxiety and allay apprehension. Patients may perceive the day of surgery as the biggest day in their lives. In the operating room they do not wish to be treated impersonally, as packages in a post office.[3] Preoperative visits must be conducted efficiently but must be informative and reassuring and answer all questions. Most of the anesthesiologist's time is spent with an unconscious or sedated patient. The anesthesiologist must take time before the operation to earn the trust and confidence of that patient.

Most patients are anxious before operation. Studies show, depending on the intensity of inquiry, that from 40 to 85% of patients are apprehensive before surgery.[4, 5] The preoperative anxiety states are at a high level, and patients expect apprehension to be relieved before arrival in the operating room, in the preoperative period.[6, 7] A study by Egbert et al showed an average of 57.2% patients were anxious before operation.[5] The highest levels of anxiety were noted in patients scheduled for major genitourologic surgery (79%) and for cancer surgery (85.7%). They found neither age nor sex differences in levels of apprehension among the study population. In a study of 500 adult patients scheduled for surgery, Norris and Baird found that female patients were more likely than male patients to be anxious before operation.[4] Also, they found an increased incidence of anxiety in female patients weighing more than 70 kg

485

and in patients previously or currently taking sedative drugs. They found a trend toward greater levels of anxiety in more ill patients. There was no difference with regard to anxiety in age, social status, nature of the operation, or previous hospital experience.

An informative and comforting preoperative visit may replace many milligrams of depressant medication. The study by Egbert *et al* showed that more patients were adequately prepared for surgery after a preoperative interview than after 2 mg·kg^{-1} of pentobarbital given intramuscularly 1 h before surgery (Table 18-1).[5] During ward rounds on the afternoon before surgery, the patients in their preoperative interview group were visited by the anesthesiologist, who discussed the patient's condition, the time of the operation, and the anesthetic. The patient was informed about perioperative events and asked about previous anesthetic experiences. The patients in this study who received pentobarbitol for preoperative medication but had no interview appeared and felt drowsy but were not calm. Leigh *et al* investigated adult patients, using objective tests of anxiety.[6] They found that the anesthesiologist's 10-min preoperative visit produced lower anxiety levels before operation than no visit at all. Furthermore, they found that the preoperative visit was more effective than a booklet given to the patients the day before surgery, which was specifically designed to reassure the patients about anesthesia. The booklet was not a substitute for a proper preoperative visit and interview.

Psychologic preparation cannot do everything. It will not relieve all anxiety. There are other goals of preoperative medication. Pain, amnesia, or sedation also will not be consistently achieved at satisfactory levels by the preoperative visit alone. In emergent situations there may be little or no time for a preoperative interview. Conversely, more ill or elderly patients may not tolerate the physiologic effects of sedative medications. One must always remember that the substitution of preoperative depressant drugs for a comforting and tactful preoperative visit may encroach on patient safety.

PHARMACOLOGIC PREPARATION

The ideal drug or combination of drugs for preoperative pharmacologic preparation is as elusive as the ideal anesthetic technique. Routine administration of the same drugs to all patients has fallen into disfavor as a selective approach has emerged. In selecting the appropriate drugs for preoperative medication, the patient's psychologic condition and physical status must be considered. The patient's age is important. Is the patient in the pediatric or the geriatric age group? The surgical procedure and its duration are important factors. Is

this an outpatient procedure? Is it elective surgery or emergency surgery? The anesthesiologist must know the patient's weight; prior response to depressant drugs, including unwanted side-effects; and allergies. Finally, the anesthesiologist's experience and familiarity with certain preoperative medications more than others are determinants.

The goals to be achieved for each patient with preoperative medication are intimately involved in the selection process (Table 18-2). The desired goals may be multiple and should be tailored to the needs of each patient. Some of the goals are traditional, with little modern indication, whereas others, such as relief of anxiety and production of sedation, apply to almost every patient. Prophylaxis against allergic reactions would apply in only a few instances. Prevention of autonomic reflexes mediated through the vagus or an antiemetic effect may be better attempted immediately before the anticipated need rather than achieved at the time of preoperative medication. However, administration of clonidine with diazepam 90–120 min before the induction of anesthesia blunts heart rate responses to laryngoscopic examination and reduces anesthetic requirements for inhaled and injected drugs.[8, 9] Conversely, most preoperative medication regimens do not produce sufficient obtundation to be significant clinically in reducing anesthetic requirement. Preoperative medication prevents preoperative elevations of plasma concentrations of beta-endorphins that normally accompany the stress response (Fig. 18-1).[10]

Some patients should not receive depressant drugs before surgery. Patients with little physiologic reserve, at the extremes of age, or with a head injury or the hypovolemic patient would probably be harmed more than they would be helped by many of the medications normally used before operation. In contrast, the conditions of others demand that pharmacologic attempts be made to reduce anxiety, increase gastric fluid *p*H, reduce gastric fluid volume, provide analgesia, or dry secretions in the airway to produce a safer perioperative course. For elective surgery, in most instances the anesthesiologist will want the patient to enter the operating room free of anxiety, sedated, but easily arousable and cooperative. The patient should not be overly obtunded or display other unwanted side effects of the preoperative drugs. The patient who asked to be "asleep" before leaving the hospital room should be told that apprehension and sedation may be reduced but it would be unsafe to produce a comatose state. The time and route of administration of the preoperative medications are important. As a general rule, oral medications should be given to the patient in the hospital room 60–90 min before

TABLE 18-1.   Comparison of Preoperative Visit and Pentobarbital (2 mg·kg^{-1} im) (Percentage of Patients)

	FELT DROWSY	FELT NERVOUS	ADEQUATE PREPARATION
Control group	18	58	35
Pentobarbitol only	30	61	48
Preoperative visit	26	40	65
Preoperative visit and pentobarbitol	38	38	71

(Data from Egbert LD, Battit GE, Turndorf H *et al*: The value of the preoperative visit by an anesthetist. JAMA 185:553, 1963.)

TABLE 18-2.   Various Goals for Preoperative Medication

1. Relief of anxiety
2. Sedation
3. Amnesia
4. Analgesia
5. Drying of airway secretions
6. Prevention of autonomic reflex responses
7. Reduction of gastric fluid volume and increased *p*H
8. Antiemetic effects
9. Reduction of anesthetic requirements
10. Facilitation of smooth induction of anesthesia
11. Prophylaxis against allergic reactions

(Modified from Stoelting RK: Psychological preparation and preoperative medication. In Miller RD [ed]: Anesthesia. New York, Churchill Livingstone, 1981.)

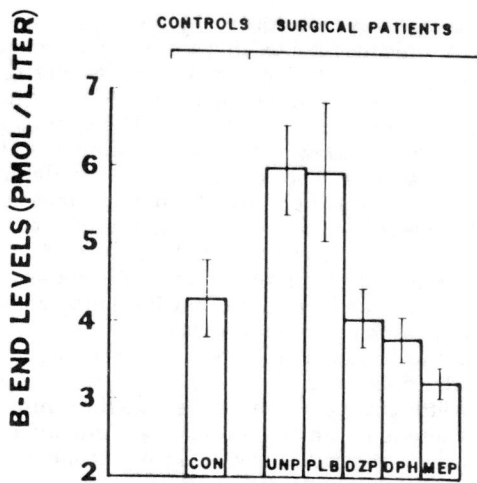

FIG. 18-1. Plasma beta-endorphin (B-END) concentrations as measured in control (CON) patients or in presurgical patients receiving no premedication (UNP), intramuscular saline (PLB), oral diazepam 10 mg (DZP), intramuscular diphenhydramine 1 mg · kg^{-1} (DPH), or intramuscular meperidine 1 mg · kg^{-1} (MEP). Measurements were made 1 h after treatment. Mean ± SEM. (Reprinted with permission. Walsh J, Puig MM, Lovitz MA *et al:* Premedication abolishes the increase in plasma beta-endorphin observed in the immediate preoperative period. Anesthesiology 66:402, 1987.)

TABLE 18-3.   Common Preoperative Medications, Doses, and Administration Routes

MEDICATION	ADMINISTRATION ROUTE	DOSE
Diazepam	Oral	5–20 mg
Lorazepam	Oral, im	1–4 mg
Midazolam	im	3–7 mg
	iv	Titration of 1–2.5-mg doses
Secobarbital	Oral, im	50–200 mg
Pentobarbital	Oral, im	50–200 mg
Morphine	im	5–15 mg
Meperidine	im	50–150 mg
Cimetidine	Oral, im, iv	150–300 mg
Ranitidine	Oral	50–200
Metoclopramide	Oral, im, iv	5–20 mg
Atropine	im, iv	0.3–0.6 mg
Glycopyrrolate	im, iv	0.1–0.3 mg
Scopolamine	im, iv	0.3–0.6 mg

im = intramuscular; iv = intravenous.
(Modified from Stoelting RK, Miller RD [ed]: Basics of Anesthesia. New York, Churchill Livingstone, 1984.)

the psychologic preoperative preparation has not been standardized.

SEDATIVE HYPNOTICS AND TRANQUILIZERS

Benzodiazepines

Benzodiazepines are among the most popular drugs used for preoperative medication (Table 18-4). They are used to produce anxiolysis, amnesia, and sedation. The anticonvulsant and muscle relaxant effects of the benzodiazepines are not usually important when preoperative medication is considered. Because the site of action of benzodiazepines is on specific receptors in the central nervous system, there is relatively little depression of ventilation or the cardiovascular system with premedicant doses. Benzodiazepines have a wide therapeutic index and a low incidence of toxicity. Other than central nervous system depression, there are few side-effects of this group of drugs. Specifically, nausea and vomiting are not usually associated with administration of benzodiazepines for preoperative medication. These drugs are often used before operation to reduce unpleasant dreams and delirium that may occur after ketamine administration.[11]

There are some hazards and unwanted side-effects of the

his or her arrival in the operating room. For full effect, intramuscular medications should be given at least 20 min and preferably 30–60 min before his or her arrival in the operating room. Every attempt should be made to have the preoperative medications achieve their full effect before the patient's arrival in the operating room rather than after induction of anesthesia. The drug(s), doses, route of administration, and effects should be recorded on the anesthetic record. A list of common preoperative medications is presented in Table 18-3.

Finally, the choice of premedicant drugs is not based on a large body of scientific data that are either definitive or persuasive. The subject is difficult to study. Often the investigations only involve one dose of drug or one dose of a number of drugs given in combination. In some studies drugs are given parenterally, whereas in others medications are administered orally or even rectally. Different investigations may study the effect of the drugs at different times after administration. The patients' responses and the investigators' observations of those responses are subjective and difficult to quantify. Also, the studies may involve heterogenous groups of patients, where

TABLE 18-4.   Comparison of Pharmacologic Variables of Benzodiazepines

	DIAZEPAM	LORAZEPAM	MIDAZOLAM
Dose equivalency (mg)	10	1–2	3–5
Time to peak effect after oral dose (hr)	1–1.5	2–4	0.5–1
Elimination half-time (hr)	20–40	10–20	1–4
Clearance (ml · kg^{-1} · min^{-1})	0.2–0.5	0.7–1.0	6.4–11.1
Volume of distribution (l · kg^{-1})	0.7–1.7	0.8–1.3	1.1–1.7

(Adapted from Reves JG, Fragen RJ, Vinick HR *et al:* Midazolam: Pharmacology and uses. Anesthesiology 62:310, 1985, and Stoelting RK: Pharmacology and Physiology in Anesthetic Practice. Philadelphia, JB Lippincott, 1987.)

benzodiazepines. Sometimes the central nervous system depression they cause is long and excessive, especially with lorazepam. There may be pain at the intramuscular or intravenous injection site with diazepam, as well as the likelihood of phlebitis.[11] These drugs are not analgetic agents. Benzodiazepines may not always produce a calming effect but may result in agitation, as evidenced by restlessness and delirium involving patients during labor and delivery.[12] However, in another study of patients during labor, a combination with an opioid produced satisfactory results.[13]

The proposed mechanisms of action of the benzodiazepines describe specific receptors and actions within the central nervous system (Fig. 18-2).[14, 15] The sedative action is said to result from a facilitation or enhancement of inhibitory neurotransmission mediated by GABA (gamma aminobutyric acid). The antianxiety effect comes from the action of glycine-mediated inhibition of neuronal pathways in the brain stem and in the brain. The site of action of the benzodiazepines in producing amnesia is unknown.

DIAZEPAM. The calming, amnesic, and sedative effects of diazepam make it a very popular choice for premedication. It is the standard to which other benzodiazepines are usually compared. Because diazepam is insoluble in water and must be dissolved in organic solvents, pain may occur on intramuscular or intravenous injection. Phlebitis is often a sequela of intravenous injection. More than 90% of an oral dose of diazepam is rapidly absorbed. Peak effect after oral administration occurs within ½ to 1 h and within 15–30 min in children (Fig. 18-3).[16] Diazepam does cross the placenta. Because the drug is highly protein bound, patients with low serum albumin levels, such as those with cirrhosis of the liver or chronic renal failure, may exhibit an increased effect of the drug.[17] Diazepam is metabolized by the hepatic microsomal enzymes to some metabolites that are active. Prolonged sedation resulting from active metabolites is usually seen after chronic use of diazepam rather than the use of a single dose of diazepam in the preoperative setting. The elimination half-time of diazepam is 21–37 h in healthy volunteers. It may be prolonged in patients with cirrhosis or in elderly patients.[19] Because absorption is unpredictable after intramuscular injection and because of pain with parenteral administration, many prefer to administer diazepam orally (Fig. 18-3).[16, 20, 21] Diazepam also may be given rectally.[22, 23] It is not as reliable in preventing recall as lorazepam, but the antegrade amnesia effect may be enhanced by scopolamine.[24] There is no evidence for the production of retrograde amnesia after diazepam administration.[25]

There is little effect of diazepam outside the central nervous system. There is minimal depression of ventilation, circulation, or hepatic or renal function. Soroker *et al* demonstrated little or no effect on ventilation after diazepam administration.[26] Detectable Pa_{CO_2} increases were demonstrable only after intravenous administration of $0.2 \ mg \cdot kg^{-1}$ of diazepam in another study.[27] The increase in carbon dioxide results from a decrease in tidal volume. In another investigation, after intravenous doses of $0.4 \ mg \cdot kg^{-1}$ the slope of the carbon dioxide response curve decreased but it was not shifted to the right.[28] Despite the safety of relatively large intravenous doses of diazepam, respiratory arrest has been reported with as little as 2.5 mg.[29-31] Furthermore, ventilatory depression may be compounded with other depressant drugs, especially the opioids. There is little cardiovascular depression seen after the doses of diazepam used for preoperative medication. Indeed, larger intravenous doses produce little circulatory depression.[27, 32] There is not much clinical effect on the neuromuscular junc-

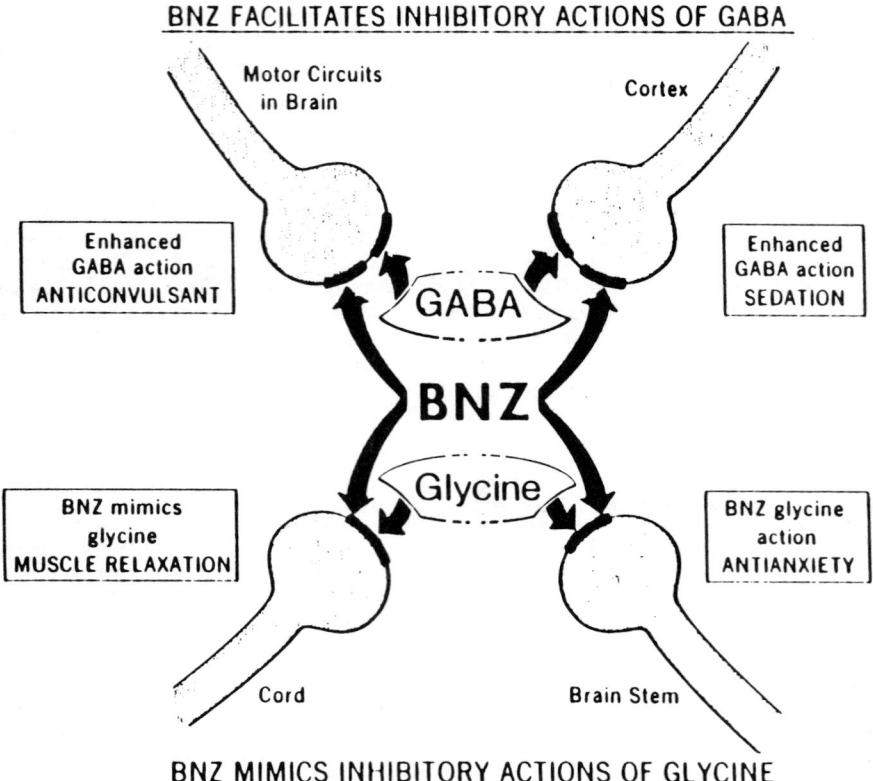

FIG. 18-2. Schematic diagram of possible mechanisms for pharmacologic effects of benzodiazepines (BNZ). (Reprinted with permission. Richter JJ: Current theories about the mechanisms of benzodiazepines and neuroleptic drugs. Anesthesiology 54:66, 1981.)

tion after diazepam has been given for preoperative medication. There have been attempts to reduce myalgias and fasciculations produced by succinylcholine with diazepam.[33, 34] The effect on fasciculations has been variable, but myalgias were reduced in one study.[33] Premedication with diazepam does not reliably prevent an increase in intraocular pressure after intubation of the trachea.[34–37] In animals diazepam has reduced the seizure threshold for lidocaine, but this effect has not been proven in humans.[38]

Some controversy exists with regard to interaction of diazepam with other drugs. Cimetidine will delay the hepatic clearance of diazepam.[39] The proposed mechanism is the inhibition of microsomal enzymes by cimetidine. There is some question as to whether this is clinically significant when diazepam is used as a single dose before operation. Diazepam $0.2 \text{ mg} \cdot \text{kg}^{-1}$ has been shown to decrease the MAC for halothane.[40] The magnitude in reduction of anesthetic requirement from premedicant doses may or may not be important to the anesthesiologist.

LORAZEPAM. Lorazepam resembles oxazepam and is five to 10 times as potent as diazepam. Lorazepam can produce profound amnesia, relief of anxiety, and sedation (Fig. 18-4).[41–52] When lorazepam is compared with diazepam, their effects are very similar. However, unlike with diazepam, pain on injection or phlebitis are not expected after lorazepam

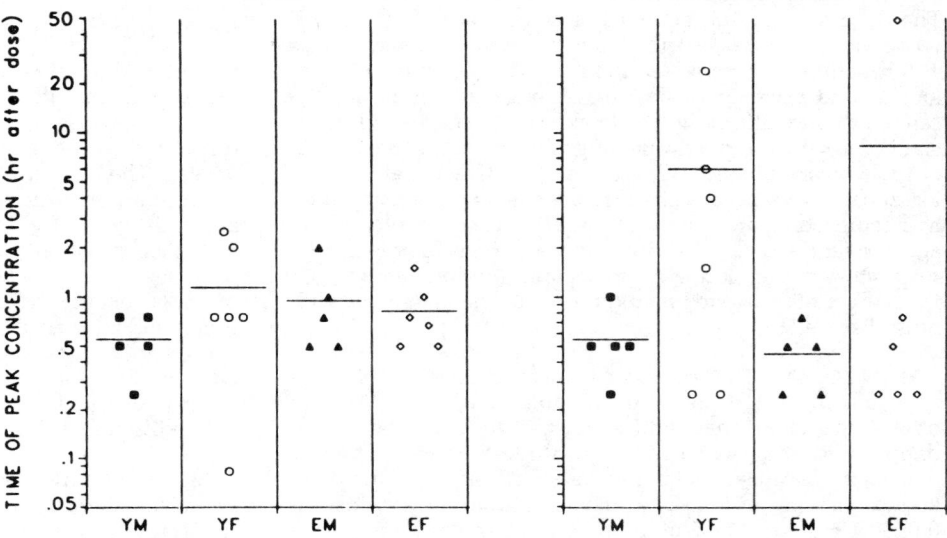

FIG. 18-3. Individual and mean (*horizontal bar*) times of peak plasma concentrations after oral or intramuscular (deltoid) administration of diazepam, 5 mg, to adult patients (20–78 yr old) categorized as young male (YM), young female (YF), elderly male (EM), and elderly female (EF) patients. (Reprinted with permission. Dwoll M, Greenblatt DJ, Ochs HR *et al:* Absolute bioavailability of oral and intramuscular diazepam: Effects of age and sex. Anesth Analg 62:1, 1983.)

FIG. 18-4. Percentage of patients in each group failing to recall specific events of the operative day. Medications were administered intramuscularly. (Reprinted with permission. Fragen RJ, Caldwell N: Lorazepam premedication: Lack of recall and relief of anxiety. Anesth Analg 55:792, 1976.)

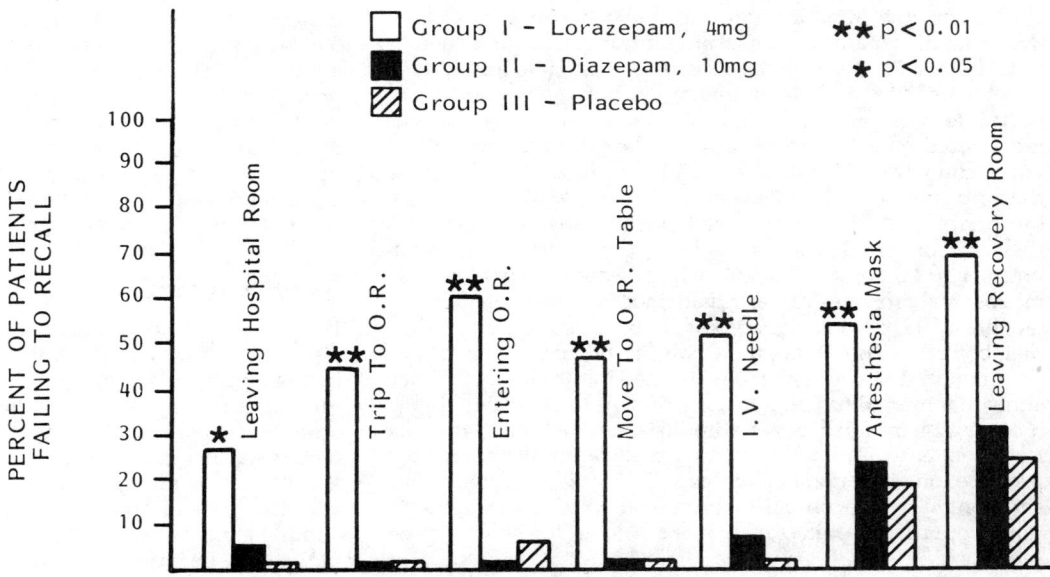

administration. Prolonged sedation is more likely after lorazepam administration. Even though the elimination half-life of diazepam is longer than that of lorazepam (20–40 h vs. 10–15 h), the effect of diazepam may be shorter because it more rapidly dissociates from the benzodiazepine receptor.[48]

Lorazepam is reliably absorbed both orally and intramuscularly. Maximal effect occurs 30–40 min after intravenous injection.[41] Bradshaw et al demonstrated clinical effects 30–60 min after oral administration of lorazepam.[49] A study by Blitt et al demonstrated that lack of recall was not produced until 2 h after intramuscular injection.[50] Peak plasma concentrations may not occur until 2–4 h after oral administration. Therefore, lorazepam must be ordered well before surgery so that the drug has time to be effective before the patient arrives in the operating room. Lorazepam also may be given sublingually.[51] As stated previously, the elimination of half-life is 10–20 h. The usual dose is about 25–50 $\mu g \cdot kg^{-1}$. The dose for an adult should not exceed 4 mg.[41, 42, 52] With recommended doses, amnesia may be produced for as long as 4–6 h without excessive sedation. Larger doses lead to prolonged and excessive sedation without more amnesia. Because of its length of action, lorazepam is not useful in instances in which rapid awakening is necessary, such as with outpatient anesthesia.[53] There are no active metabolites of lorazepam, and, because its metabolism is not dependent on microsomal enzymes, there is less influence on its effect from age or liver disease.[54] As with diazepam, there is little cardiorespiratory depression with lorazepam.[55–60] However, there is the danger of unwanted respiratory depression in those with lung disease.[61]

MIDAZOLAM. The physicochemical properties of midazolam allow water solubility and rapid metabolism. As with other benzodiazepines, midazolam produces anxiolysis, sedation, and amnesia. It is two to three times as potent as diazepam because of its increased affinity for the benzodiazepine receptor. The usual intramuscular dose is 0.05–0.1 $mg \cdot kg^{-1}$ and titration of 1–2.5 mg at a time intravenously. There is no irritation or phlebitis with injection of midazolam. The incidence of side-effects after administration is low, although depression of ventilation and sedation may be greater than expected, especially in elderly patients or when the drug is combined with other central nervous system depressants.[62] There is more rapid onset of action and predictable absorption after intramuscular injection of midazolam than after diazepam. The onset after intramuscular injection is 5–10 min, with peak effect occurring after 30–60 min. The onset after intravenous administration of 5 mg would be expected to occur after 1–2 min. In addition to quicker onset, more rapid recovery occurs after midazolam administration when compared with diazepam. This probably results from the lipid solubility of midazolam and the rapid distribution in the peripheral tissues and metabolic biotransformation. For these reasons, midazolam usually should be given within an hour of induction.[63] Midazolam is metabolized by hepatic microsomal enzymes to essentially inactive hydroxylated metabolites.[63] H_2 receptor antagonists do not interfere with its metabolism.[64] The elimination half-life of midazolam is approximately 1–4 h and may be extended in the elderly.[65] Tests show that mental function usually returns to normal within 4 h of administration.[63] After administration of 5 mg, amnesia lasts from 20 to 32 min.[66, 67] Intramuscular administration may produce longer periods of amnesia. The lack of recall may be augmented by concomitant administration of scopolamine.[68] The properties of midazolam make it ideal for shorter procedures.

OTHER BENZODIAZEPINES. Oxazepam is another benzodiazepine that has been used for preoperative medication.[69, 70] It is one of the pharmacologically active metabolites of diazepam. It is administered orally and is absorbed slowly after administration. Temazepam has been given in oral doses of 20–30 mg before surgery.[71–73] It must be given well before surgery because peak plasma levels do not occur until approximately 2½ h after administration. Triazolam is a short-acting benzodiazepine.[74, 75] The adult oral dose of the drug is 0.25–0.5 mg. Peak plasma concentrations occur in about 1 h. Elimination half-life of the drug is 1.7–5.2 h. However, a study by Pinnock et al did not show the short duration of triazolam to be a feature when compared with diazepam for premedication for minor gynecologic surgery.[75] Finally, the use of chlordiazepoxide for preoperative medication has largely been replaced by the other benzodiazepines.[76]

Barbiturates

Use of barbiturates for preoperative medication is a time-tested practice with a long record of safety. These drugs are used primarily for their sedative effects. There is little cardiorespiratory depression associated with the usual preoperative doses.[77] The barbiturates may be given orally as well as parenterally, and the drugs are relatively inexpensive. Barbiturates are unlikely to produce sedation in the presence of pain. In fact, disorientation may result. Small doses of barbiturates have been said to be antianalgetic. The agents lack specificity of action on the central nervous system and have a lower therapeutic index than the benzodiazepines. Barbiturates should not be used in patients with certain kinds of porphyria. Barbiturate administration for pharmacologic preparation before surgery has been replaced in many instances by the use of benzodiazepines.

SECOBARBITAL. Secobarbital usually is administered to adults in oral doses of 50–200 mg when used for preoperative medication. Onset usually occurs 60–90 min after administration, and sedative effects last 4 h or longer. Indeed, even though secobarbital traditionally has been considered a "short-acting" barbiturate, it may impair performance for as long as 10–22 h.[78]

PENTOBARBITAL. Pentobarbital may be administered orally or parenterally. The oral dose used for adults is usually 50–200 mg. Pentobarbital has a biotransformation half-life of about 50 h. Therefore, its use is not often suitable for shorter procedures. In an investigation by Dundee et al, 100 mg of pentobarbital given orally before surgery did not relieve anxiety or differ in effect from placebo.[79] These investigators postulated that larger doses may be necessary. In contrast, another study found pentobarbital equal to diazepam for the relief of preoperative anxiety.[80]

Butyrophenones

Intravenous or intramuscular doses of 2.5–7.5 mg of droperidol will produce the appearance of sedation in patients before operation. Calmness and tranquility may be observed, but patients often state that they feel dysphoric and restless and even experience fear of death.[81] The patient's dysphoric feeling has lead to refusal of surgery.[82, 83] Because droperidol is a dopamine antagonist, extrapyramidal signs may appear after its administration.[84, 85] This has been reported to occur in about 1% of patients. The butyrophenones also cause mild alpha-blocking effects. Another butyrophenone, haloperidol, is a long-acting antipsychotic drug that has been used infrequently for preoperative medication.

Currently, droperidol is usually administered for its antiemetic effect rather than its sedative properties (see the section on "Antiemetics"). Small clinical doses (up to 2.5 mg) of droperidol have been used before operation or just before emergence to prevent nausea and vomiting in the recovery room.

As a dopaminergic receptor blocker, droperidol counters the inhibitory effect of dopamine on the carotid body and the ventilatory response to hypoxia. Consequently, it preserves the carotid body response to hypoxia. For these reasons, it is said that droperidol may be a good premedicant for patients dependent on the hypoxic ventilatory drug (Fig. 18-5).[86]

Other Sedative Drugs

HYDROXYZINE. Hydroxyzine is a nonphenothiazine tranquilizer. It is often given for its proposed additive effects to opioids without an increase in side-effects.[87] Hydroxyzine has sedative action, anxiolytic properties, and limited analgetic properties. Hydroxyzine does not produce amnesia.[44, 88, 89] It is an antihistamine and an antiemetic.[90]

DIPHENHYDRAMINE. Diphenhydramine is a histamine receptor antagonist with sedative and anticholinergic activity. It

FIG. 18-5. Hypoxic sensitivity (change in ventilation for each 1% decrease in oxygen saturation) is increased after intravenous administration of droperidol, 2.5 mg. Solid symbols represent repeated experiments on the same subjects as those represented by the open symbols. (Reprinted with permission. Ward DS: Stimulation of hypoxic ventilatory drive by droperidol. Anesth Analg 63:106, 1984.)

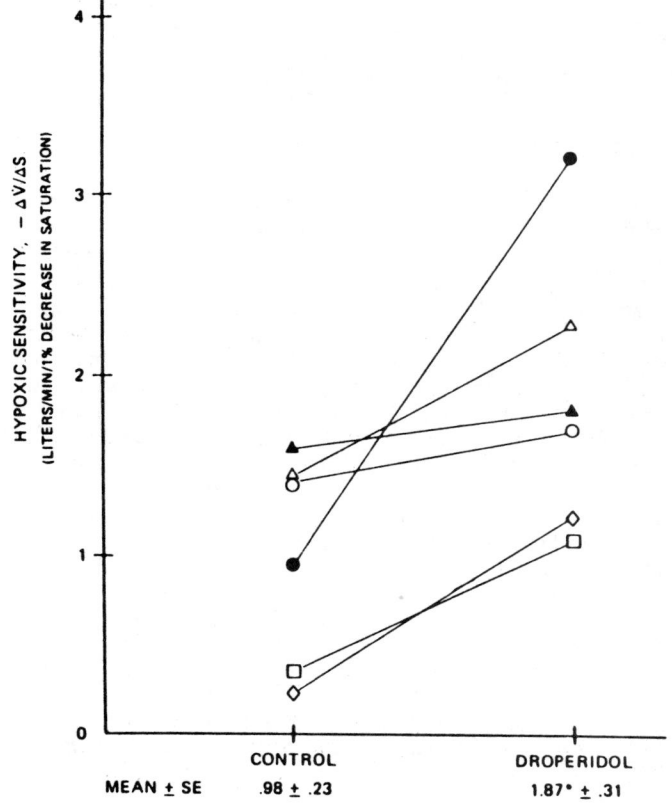

is also an antiemetic. A dose of 50 mg will last 3–6 h in an adult. Diphenhydramine has been used recently in combination with cimetidine, steroids, and other drugs for prophylaxis in patients with chronic atopy and for prophylaxis before chemonucleolysis and dye studies.[94] Diphenhydramine blocks the histamine receptor to prevent effects of histamine peripherally.

PHENOTHIAZINES. Promethazine, promazine, and perphenazine are often used in combination with opioids.[92, 93] Phenothiazines have sedative, anticholinergic, and antiemetic properties. These effects added to the analgetic effects of the opioids have been used for preoperative medication.

CHLORAL HYDRATE. Because of anxiolytic and amnestic qualities, chloral hydrate was used in the past as a premedicant, often in the elderly. Because of the advent of the benzodiazepines, chloral hydrate has a much smaller role in preoperative medications.

OPIOIDS

Morphine and meperidine are the most frequently used opioids for intramuscular preoperative medication. Recently the use of intranvenous fentanyl just before surgery has become popular. Opioids are used when analgesia is needed before operation. It has been stated in the strict sense that "unless there is pain, there is no need for narcotic in preanesthetic medication."[94] For the patient experiencing pain before operation, the opioids can produce good analgesia and even euphoria. Opioids have been ordered for patients before operation to ameliorate the discomfort that may occur during regional anesthesia or the insertion of invasive monitoring catheters or large intravenous lines. The dose of opioid may need to be reduced in the debilitated or the elderly patient.[95] The elderly patient often exhibits a reduced sensitivity to pain. Furthermore, elderly patients can have an increased analgetic response to opioids. Opioids also have been used before operation in the opioid-dependent patient.

Preoperative administration of opioids in other settings has been controversial. They have been given on the ward before surgery at the beginning of a nitrous-opioid anesthetic. This is done in attempt to have a basal state of anesthesia on board when the patient arrives in the operating room and to get a preview of the patient's response to opioids. Opioids have been given to patients before operation to provide analgesia upon their awakening in the recovery room. The other approach is to titrate the opioid intravenously during emergence or upon the patient's arrival in the recovery room. Preoperative administration of opioids can lower anesthetic requirements.[96, 97] This may or may not be clinically significant for a specific patient receiving a particular anesthetic technique. Some anesthesiologists use opioids in combination with other drugs before operation to facilitate anesthetic induction by mask. This is popular especially in those instances in which intravenous or rectal routes for induction agents cannot be used. It must be remembered that opioids will decrease ventilation during spontaneous breathing and therefore decrease uptake of inhalation drugs. If necessary, the anesthesiologist may want to use assisted or controlled ventilation of the lungs to overcome the respiratory depressant effects of the opioids. Finally, opioids are not the best drugs to relieve apprehension, produce sedation, or prevent recall.[98, 99]

Administration of opioids has the potential for several side-effects. They usually exhibit no direct myocardial effects except in the case of very large doses of meperidine. However, opioids do interfere with the compensatory constriction of smooth muscles of the peripheral vasculature. This may lead to orthostatic hypotension. Histamine release after injection of morphine may compound these circulatory effects. As with most preoperative medication, it is probably safest to have the patient remain at bedrest after opioid premedication. The analgetic properties and respiratory depressant effects of opioids go hand in hand.[77] The decrease in the carbon dioxide drive at the medulary respiratory center may be prolonged. Furthermore, there is a decrease in the responsiveness to hypoxia at the carotid body after injection of only small doses of opioids.[100] In general, the opioid agonist–antagonists produce less respiratory depression, but they also produce less analgesia. Rather than euphoria, the opioids may produce dysphoria. When this side-effect does occur, it is most commonly seen in a patient who does not have pain before operation and has received the opioid premedicant. Nausea and vomiting may result from opioid administration. Apomorphine is a profound emetic. The effect of opioids on the vestibular apparatus leading to motion sickness and/or stimulation of the medullary chemoreceptor trigger zone are postulated reasons for nausea and vomiting. Choledochoduodenal sphincter (sphincter of Oddi) spasm has been reported subsequent to injection of opioids.[101–103] The opioid produces smooth muscle constriction, which leads to right upper quadrant pain. Pain relief may be achieved with naloxone or possibly glucagon.[104] Occasionally the pain from biliary tract spasm is difficult to discern from the pain of angina pectoris. The administration of nitroglycerin should relieve angina pectoris and pain resulting from biliary tract spasm; an opioid antagonist should relieve only pain resulting from biliary tract spasm. Some question the use of opioid premedication in patients with biliary tract disease. All opioids have the potential to induce choledochoduodenal sphincter spasm. Meperidine is less likely than morphine to produce this side effect. Opioids may produce pruritis. Morphine, possibly through histamine release, often produces itching, especially around the nose. Opioids also may cause flushing, dizziness, and miosis.

Other drugs are often combined with opioids for their additive effects or to overcome the disadvantages of opioid side-effects. The sedative–hypnotics and scopolamine are often used with opioids to produce sedation, anxiolysis, and amnesia in addition to analgesia. Anesthesiologists often use the combination of morphine, a benzodiazepine, and/or scopolamine for pharmacologic preoperative preparation.

Morphine

Morphine is well absorbed after intramuscular injection. The onset of effect should occur within 15–30 min. The peak effect occurs in 45–90 min and lasts as long as 4 h. After intravenous administration the peak effect usually occurs within 20 min. Morphine is not reliably absorbed after oral administration. As with the other opioids, depression of ventilation and orthostatic hypotension may occur after injection of morphine. The effect of morphine on the chemoreceptive trigger zone may produce nausea and vomiting. Nausea and vomiting may also occur due to a vestibular component. This has been postulated because the supine patient is less likely to complain of nausea and vomiting. After morphine administration, motility of the gastrointestinal tract is decreased. Also, gastrointestinal secretions may be increased. Inclusion of morphine in the preoperative medication reduces the likelihood that unde-

sirable increases in heart rate will accompany surgical stimulation in the presence of volatile anesthetics.[105]

Meperidine

Meperidine is about one-tenth as potent as morphine. It may be given orally or parenterally. A single dose of meperidine usually lasts 2–4 h. The onset after intramuscular injection is unpredictable, and a great deal of variability in time to peak effect exists.[106] Meperidine is primarily metabolized in the liver. An increase in heart rate may be seen after meperidine administration, as well as orthostatic hypotension.

Other Opioids

Codeine has been used orally in doses of 50–60 mg for adults for preoperative medication. An intramuscular dose of 120 mg is equal to about 10 mg of morphine. Codeine can be administered intravenously, but histamine release is very likely. There is an advantage with methadone in that it can be given orally as well as intramuscularly. It is a long-acting opioid whose elimination half-life is approximately 35 h.[107] Hydromorphone is another opioid that may be given orally as well as intramuscularly.

Opioid Agonist–Antagonists

Opioid agonist–antagonists have been chosen for preoperative medication in an attempt to reduce the ventilatory side-effects of pure opioid agonists.[108–112] However, there is a ceiling on the analgesia that can be produced by agonist–antagonist drugs. They are similar to the pure opioids with regard to side-effects. In addition, dysphoria may be even more likely after their administration. Another issue to remember is that the agonist–antagonist drug can reduce the effectiveness of a pure opioid agonist needed to control postoperative pain. The most commonly used opioid agonist–antagonists are pentazocine, butorphanol, and nalbuphine.

GASTRIC FLUID pH AND VOLUME

Many patients who come to the operating room are at risk for aspiration pneumonitis. The classic example is the patient with a "full stomach" who must have emergency surgery. The pregnant patient, the obese patient, and the patient with hiatus hernia or gastroesophageal reflux may all be at risk for aspiration of gastric contents and subsequent chemical pneumonitis (Fig. 18-6).[113] Although it is not certain, it is believed that in adults aspiration of a volume of gastric fluid greater than 25 ml with a pH lower than 2.5 will cause pulmonary sequelae. Using these guidelines, it has been estimated that 40–80% of patients scheduled for elective surgery may be at risk.[114–116] This raises the question of the necessity of prophylaxis for aspiration pneumonitis during induction of anesthesia and emergence and extubation of the trachea and during long mask cases in which silent regurgitation and aspiration may occur. In addition, it has been shown that many outpatients exhibit an increase in gastric fluid volume (Fig. 18-7).[114]

The necessity of prolonged fasting (i.e., NPO after midnight) prior to induction of anesthesia for elective surgery has been challenged. Indeed, gastric fluid volume immediately after induction of anesthesia is not increased by ingestion of 150 ml of water, coffee, or orange juice 2 hours to 3 hours

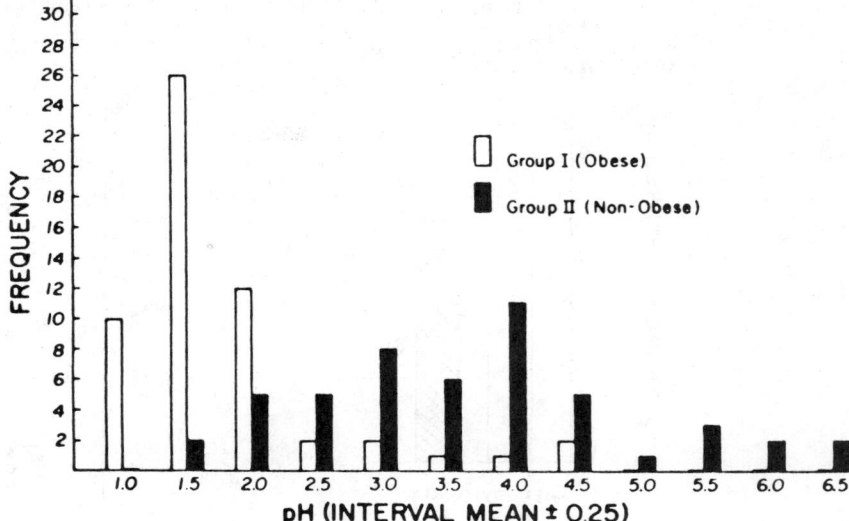

FIG. 18-6. Frequency distribution of gastric fluid pHs in obese (45 kg more than predicted ideal weight) and nonobese patients. (Reprinted with permission. Vaughan RW, Bauer S, Wise L: Volume and pH of gastric juice in obese patients. Anesthesiology 43:686, 1975.)

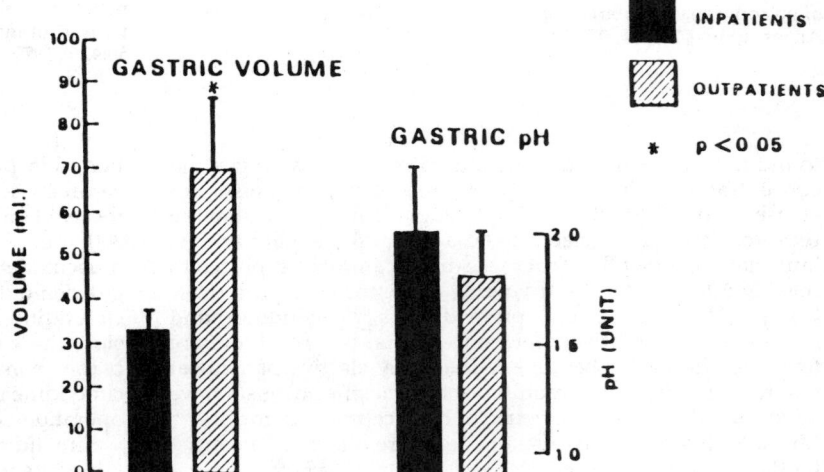

FIG. 18-7. Gastric fluid volume and pH as measured for inpatients and outpatients. Mean ± SD. (Reprinted with permission. Ong BY, Palahniuk RJ, Cumming M: Gastric volume and pH in outpatients. Can Anaesth Soc J 25:36, 1978.)

earlier.[117] Therefore, fears that ingestion of oral fluid on the morning of surgery will invariably result in a predictable increase in gastric fluid volume are unfounded. It must be appreciated, however, that these data are from healthy, nonpregnant patients in the absence of opioid preoperative medication and apply only to ingestion of liquids.

Many different kinds of drugs have been used to alter gastric fluid volume and increase the pH of gastric fluid. Anticholinergics, H_2 receptor antagonists, antacids, and gastrokinetic agents have all been employed to reduce the possibility for aspiration pneumonitis.

Anticholinergics

Neither atropine nor glycopyrrolate has been shown to be very effective in increasing gastric fluid pH or producing gastric fluid volume. A study by Stoelting demonstrated that, when given intramuscularly 1–1½ h before operation, neither atropine (0.4 mg) nor glycopyrrolate (0.2 mg) was successful in altering the gastric fluid pH or volume.[115] A similar study reported that glycopyrrolate (4–5 $\mu g \cdot kg^{-1}$), given before operation, did not reduce the percentage of patients at risk for aspiration pneumonitis.[116] That is, in a significant number of patients the gastric fluid pH remained below 2.5 and the gastric fluid volume was greater than 0.4 ml·kg^{-1}. Giving larger doses of glycopyrrolate (0.3 mg) is not more effective. Furthermore, intravenous doses of anticholinergics may cause relaxation of the gastroesophageal junction (Fig. 18-8).[118] Theoretically, this may also occur after neuromuscular doses. Therefore, the risk of aspiration pneumonitis may be increased, but this specific effect of intramuscular administration of anticholinergics for preoperative use has not been proven.

Histamine Receptor Antagonists

The H_2-receptor antagonists, cimetidine and ranitidine, reduce gastric acid secretion. They block the ability of histamine

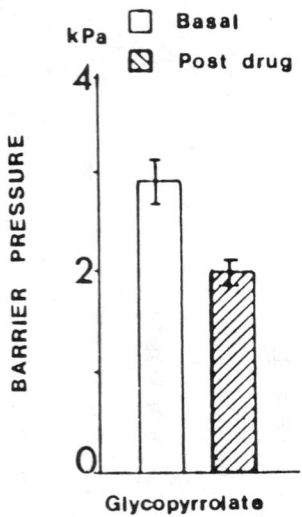

FIG. 18-8. Barrier pressure (esophageal sphincter pressure minus gastric pressure) before and after intramuscular administration of glycopyrrolate, 0.3 mg, to adult patients. Mean ± SE. (Reprinted with permission. Brock-Utne JG, Welman RS, Moshal MG, *et al:* The effect of glycopyrrolate (Robinul) on the lower oesophageal sphincter. Can Anaesth Soc J 25:144, 1978.)

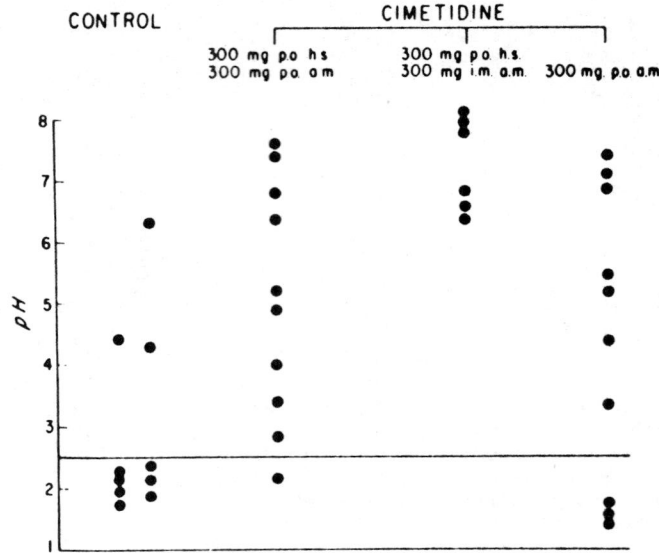

FIG. 18-9. Distribution of gastric fluid *p*Hs in control and cimetidine-treated adult patients. (Reprinted with permission. Weber L, Hirshman CA: Cimetidine for prophylaxis of aspiration pneumonitis: Comparison of intramuscular and oral dosage schedules. Anesth Analg 58:426, 1979.)

to induce secretion of gastric fluid with a high hydrogen ion concentration. Therefore, the H_2-receptor antagonists increase gastric fluid *p*H.[119] Their antagonism of the histamine receptor occurs in a selective and a competitive manner. It is important to remember that these drugs cannot be expected to reliably affect gastric fluid volume or gastric-emptying time. Compared with other premedicants, cimetidine and ranitidine have relatively few side-effects. Because there are few side-effects and because of the many elective patients at risk for aspiration pneumonitis, some anesthesiologists have advocated the preoperative use of H_2-receptor antagonists.[120] Multiple-dose regimens usually are more effective in consistently increasing gastric *p*H than a single dose before operation on the day of surgery (Fig. 18-9).[121] A multiple-dose regimen usually incorporates an oral dose of the H_2-receptor antagonist the night before surgery, followed by an intramuscular injection before operation on the day of surgery. As with most other drugs, parenteral administration produces a more rapid onset than the oral route. Cimetidine or ranitidine also may be used for the allergic patient or in preparation of a patient for exposure to a trigger of the allergic response, such as chymopapain or dye.

CIMETIDINE. Cimetidine usually is administered in 150–300-mg doses orally or parenterally.[121–125] Administration of 300 mg of cimetidine orally 1–1½ h before surgery has been shown to increase the gastric fluid *p*H above 2.5 in 80% of patients.[122] There was no effect on gastric fluid volume. However, a study by Maliniak *et al* reported that cimetidine (300 mg) given intravenously 2 h before operation increased gastric fluid *p*H and decreased gastric fluid volume. Cimetidine can be given intravenously for those unable to take oral medications. It may be necessary to increase the dose for the very obese patient. Cimetidine can cross the placenta, but adverse fetal effects are unproven.[126, 127] In one multicenter investiga-

tion, 126 patients were studied who were to have elective cesarean section with general anesthesia.[126] These patients received either 30 ml of an antacid 1–3 h before operation or 300 mg of cimetidine orally at bedtime and again intramuscularly 1–3 h before operation. There was an increase in gastric fluid *p*H and a reduction in gastric fluid volume in the cimetidine-treated group. Most importantly for this discussion, there were no differences in the neurobehavioral scores of the neonates between the two groups. The gastric effects of cimetidine last as long as 3 or 4 h and therefore are suitable for operations of that duration.[128]

Cimetidine has few side-effects, but there are some of note. It inhibits the hepatic mixed function oxidase enzyme system, therefore, it can prolong the half-life of many drugs, including diazepam, chlordiazepoxide, theophylline, propranolol, and lidocaine. The clinical significance of this after one or two preoperative doses of cimetidine is uncertain. There is also some question of hepatic blood flow reduction by cimetidine and a prolonged effect of the drug in patients with renal failure. Life-threatening cardiac dysrhythmias, hypotension, cardiac arrest, and central nervous system depression have been reported after cimetidine administration.[129, 130] These side-effects may be especially likely in critically ill patients after rapid intravenous administration. It has been postulated that airway resistance may increase in asthmatic patients because cimetidine could produce unopposed H_2 receptor-mediated bronchial constriction. As discussed previously, cimetidine will not affect gastric fluid already present.

RANITIDINE. Ranitidine is more potent, specific, and longer acting than cimetidine. The usual oral dose is 50–200 mg. Ranitidine, 50–100 mg, given parenterally will decrease gastric fluid *p*H within 1 h.[131, 132] It is as effective in reducing the number of patients at risk for gastric aspiration as cimetidine and produces fewer cardiovascular, or central nervous system side-effects.[133, 134] The effects of ranitidine last up to 9 h. Thus, it may be superior to cimetidine at the conclusion of lengthy procedures in reducing the risk of aspiration pneumonitis during emergence from anesthesia and extubation of the trachea.[123]

Antacids

Antacids are used to neutralize the acid in gastric contents. A single dose of antacid given 15–30 min before induction of anesthesia is almost 100% effective in increasing gastric fluid pH above 2.5.[115, 135–137] The nonparticulate antacid, 0.3 M sodium citrate, is commonly given before operation when an increase in gastric fluid pH is desired. The nonparticulate antacids do not produce pulmonary damage themselves if aspiration of gastric fluid should occur with these antacids in it.[138] Colloid antacid suspension may be more effective than the nonparticulate antacids in increasing gastric fluid pH.[139] However, aspiration of gastric fluid containing particulate antacids may cause significant and persistent pulmonary damage, despite the increase in gastric fluid pH.[140–143] The serious pulmonary sequelae have been manifested in the form of pulmonary edema and arterial hypoxemia.

Antacids work at the time given. There is no "lag time," as with the histamine receptor blockers. Antacids are effective on the fluid already present in the stomach. This makes them especially attractive in emergency situations for those patients able to take medications orally.

However, antacids do increase gastric fluid volume, unlike H_2-receptor blockers.[122, 144–145] The risk of aspiration depends on both the pH and the volume of gastric content. The increase in gastric fluid volume from antacid administration may become readily apparent after repeated doses, such as during labor, during which opioid administration may also contribute to delayed gastric emptying.[146] Withholding antacids because of concern of increasing gastric volume is not warranted, considering animal evidence documenting increased mortality after aspiration of low volumes of acidic gastric fluid (0.3 $ml \cdot kg^{-1}$, pH 1) compared with aspiration of large volumes of buffered gastric fluid (1–2 $ml \cdot kg^{-1}$, $pH \geq 1.8$).[147] Antacids may slow gastric emptying, and complete mixing with all gastric contents may be questionable in the immobile patient. The effect of antacids on food particles within the stomach is unknown.

Gastrokinetic Agents

Gastrokinetic agents are useful because of their effectiveness in reducing gastric fluid volume. Metoclopramide is an example of a gastrokinetic agent that may be administered before operation.

METOCLOPRAMIDE. Metoclopramide is a dopamine antagonist that stimulates upper gastrointestinal motility, increases gastroesophageal sphincter tone, and relaxes the pylorus and duodenum.[148, 149] It also has antiemetic properties. Metoclopramide speeds gastric emptying but has no known effect on acid secretion and gastric fluid pH. Metoclopramide may be administered orally or parenterally. A parenteral dose of 5–20 mg is usually given 15–30 min before induction. When the drug is administered intravenously over 3–5 min, it usually will prevent the abdominal cramping that can occur from more rapid administration. An oral dose of 10 mg will achieve onset within 30–60 min. The elimination half-life of metoclopramide is approximately 2–4 h.

The clinical usefulness of the gastrokinetic agents is found in those patients who are likely to have large gastric fluid volumes, such as parturients, patients scheduled for emergency surgery who have just eaten, obese patients, patients with trauma, outpatients, and those with gastroparesis secondary to diabetes mellitus.

However, the administration of metoclopramide does not guarantee gastric emptying. Significant gastric fluid volume may still be present despite its administration.[120] The effect of metoclopramide on the upper gastrointestinal tract may be offset by concomitant atropine administration[149] or prior injection of opioids.[150] It will not further reduce gastric volume in patients for elective surgery with already small gastric volumes.[151] It may not be effective after administration of sodium citrate.[152] In contrast, metoclopramide may be especially effective in reducing the risk of aspiration pneumonitis when combined with an H_2-receptor antagonist (for example, ranitidine) before elective surgery.[153–155]

As mentioned previously, the drugs used to alter gastric fluid pH and volume are relatively free of side-effects. The risk–benefit ratio for these drugs in reducing the risk of pulmonary sequelae from aspiration is often very favorable. Indeed, the drugs do decrease the number of patients at risk. However, none of the drugs or combination of drugs is absolutely reliable in preventing the risk of aspiration pneumonitis in all patients all of the time. Therefore, they do not eliminate the need for careful anesthetic techniques to protect the airway during induction, maintenance, and emergence from anesthesia.

ANTIEMETICS

There are several groups of patients in whom the antiemetic effects of drugs may be helpful in reducing nausea and vomiting. These are patients scheduled for opthalmologic surgery, patients with a prior history of nausea and vomiting, patients scheduled for gynecologic procedures, and patients who are obese. Many anesthesiologists prefer not to administer antiemetics as part of a preoperative regimen but believe that antiemetics should be administered intravenously just before they are needed at the conclusion of surgery.

Droperidol

Droperidol has been administered, usually intravenously, in small clinical doses to prevent postoperative nausea and vomiting.[156–164] An investigation by Korttila et al showed that 1.25 mg of droperidol given intravenously 5 min before the conclusion of surgery reduced the incidence of nausea and vomiting after operation.[156] They found the antiemetic effect of droperidol to be better than that of either metoclopramide or domperidone. Another study by Santos and Datta demonstrated the effectiveness of droperidol as an antiemetic for patients having cesarean section with spinal anesthesia (Fig. 18-10).[157] However, small doses of droperidol may not always be effective in preventing nausea and vomiting.[158] Larger doses at the end of surgery may lead to excessive sedation in the recovery room.

Metoclopramide

As mentioned in the previous section on gastrokinetic agents, metoclopramide does have antiemetic properties.[165–168] The effect is controversial and inconsistent, as demonstrated and

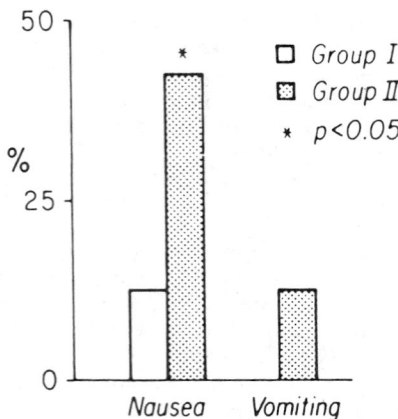

FIG. 18-10. Incidence of nausea and vomiting after elective cesarean section after intravenous administration of droperidol, 2.5 mg (Group 1), or saline (Group 2). (Reprinted with permission. Santos A, Datta S: Prophylactic use of droperidol for control of nausea and vomiting during spinal anesthesia for cesarean section. Anesth Analg 63:85, 1984.)

discussed in the study by Cohen *et al.*[158] This may partially result from brief duration of action of metoclopramide.

Other Antiemetics

Some of the phenothiazines, especially prochlorperazine, have antiemetic action. Hydroxyzine and diphenidol are two other drugs with antiemetic value.[90, 164] Although it has antiemetic properties, domperidone has not been proven effective in reducing postoperative nausea and vomiting.[156]

ANTICHOLINERGICS

Previously, anticholinergic drugs were widely used when inhalation anesthetics produced copious respiratory tract secretions and intraoperative bradycardia was a frequent danger.[169] The advent of newer inhalation agents has almost completely dispelled the routine use of anticholinergic drugs for preoperative medication. Their routine use has been questioned by several authors, who believe that the same care in selection of anticholinergics should be exhibited as with the choice of other drugs.[170-177] Specific indications for an anticholinergic before surgery are 1) antisialogogue effect, and 2) sedation and amnesia (Table 18-5). Uses that are less firmly established and not universally agreed upon include the preoperative prescription of anticholinergics for their vagolytic action or use in an attempt to decrease gastric acid secretion.

Antisialogogue Effect

Anticholinergics have been prescribed in a selective fashion when drying of the upper airway is desirable. For example, when endotracheal intubation is contemplated, an anesthesiologist may want to reduce secretions. In the study by Falick and Smiler, conditions were more often rated as satisfactory after endotracheal intubation when an anticholinergic drug had been administered.[178] The antisialogogue effect may be important for intraoral operations and instrumentations of the airway such as bronchoscopic examination. Administration of anticholinergics may be desirable before the use of topical anesthesia for the airway to prevent a dilutional effect of secretions and to allow contact of the local anesthetic with the mucosa.

Scopolamine is a more potent drying agent than atropine. It is less likely to increase heart rate and more likely to produce sedation and amnesia. Glycopyrrolate is a more potent and longer-acting antisialogogue than atropine, with less likelihood of increasing heart rate.[179-181] Because glycopyrrolate is a quaternary amine, it does not easily cross the blood–brain barrier and does not produce sedation. Anticholinergics are not the only drugs that can dry secretions. As demonstrated by the study of Forest *et al*, several other drugs and placebo (presumably a reflection of apprehension) can cause a patient to have a dry mouth before operation (Table 18-6).

Sedation and Amnesia

When sedation and amnesia are desired before operation, scopolamine is frequently the anticholinergic chosen, especially in combination with morphine. Scopolamine and atropine both cross the blood–brain barrier. Scopolamine is a much more potent sedative and amnestic drug than atropine. In a study of patient acceptance of preoperative medication, the combination of morphine and scopolamine was superior to morphine and atropine.[183] Scopolamine will not produce amnesia in all patients. It may not be as effective as lorazepam or diazepam in preventing recall. Scopolamine has an additive amnestic effect when combined with benzodiazepines. The study by Frumin *et al* showed that the combination of diazepam and scopolamine produced amnesia more often than did diazepam alone.[24]

Vagolytic Action

Vagolytic action of the anticholinergic drugs is produced through the blockade of effects of acetylcholine on the sinoatrial node. Atropine given intravenously is more potent than glycopyrrolate and scopolamine in increasing heart rate. The vagolytic action of the anticholinergic drugs is useful in the prevention of reflex bradycardia occurring during surgery. Bradycardia may result from traction on extraocular muscles

TABLE 18-5. Comparison of Some of the Effects of Anticholinergic Drugs

	ATROPINE	GLYCOPYRROLATE	SCOPOLAMINE
Increased heart rate	+++	++	+
Antisialogogue	+	++	+++
Sedation	+	0	+++

0 = no effect; + = small effect; ++ = moderate effect; +++ = large effect.
(Adapted from Stoelting RK: Pharmacology and Physiology in Anesthetic Practice. Philadelphia, JB Lippincott, 1987.)

TABLE 18-6. Incidence of Side-Effects One Hour After Preoperative Medication (percentage of patients)

MEDICATION	DRY MOUTH	SLURRED SPEECH	DIZZY	NAUSEATED	RELAXED
Pentobarbital (50–150 mg)	29	27	10	7	2
Secobarbital (50–150 mg)	41	32	8	9	4
Diazepam (5–15 mg)	35	20	10	3	12
Hydroxyzine (50–150 mg)	45	31	6	2	9
Morphine (5–10 mg)	80	33	15	7	20
Meperidine (50–100 mg)	85	45	20	12	25
Placebo	34	21	7	12	4

(Modified from Forrest WH, Brown CR, Brown BW et al: Subjective responses to six common preoperative medications. Anesthesiology 47:241, 1977.)

or abdominal viscera, from carotid sinus stimulation, or after the administration of repeated doses of intravenous succinylcholine. The prevention of reflex bradycardia with intramuscular doses of the anticholinergics is unreliable, given the drug dosages and timing usually involved with preoperative medication administered on the ward. Many anesthesiologists prefer to give atropine or glycopyrrolate intravenously just before surgery and the anticipated bradycardic stimulus.[184] Atropine and glycopyrrolate given intravenously immediately before surgery have been equally effective in preventing bradycardia resulting from repeated doses of succinylcholine.[185]

Elevation of Gastric Fluid pH Level

Large doses of anticholinergics often are needed to alter gastric fluid pH. Even then, when given in the preoperative setting anticholinergics cannot be relied upon consistently to decrease gastric hydrogen ion secretion.[115, 116] This function has largely been replaced by the use of histamine receptor antagonists. (See the section Gastric Fluid pH and Volume.)

Side-Effects in Anticholinergic Drugs

Scopolamine and atropine may cause central nervous system toxicity, the so-called "central anticholinergic syndrome."[186] This is most likely to occur after the administration of scopolamine but can be seen after large doses of atropine. The symptoms of central nervous system toxicity resulting from anticholinergic drugs include delirium, restlessness, confusion, and obtundation. Elderly patients and patients with pain appear to be particularly susceptible.[187] The central nervous system toxic effect of anticholinergics has been reported to be potentiated by inhalation anesthetics.[188] Some clinicians have successfully treated the syndrome after it occurs with 1–2 mg of physostigmine intravenously.[188, 189]

The anticholinergics relax the lower esophageal sphincter.[118] Theoretically, after parenteral administration of an anticholinergic drug, the risk of pulmonary aspiration of gastric contents is increased. This has yet to be proven as an important clinical issue.

Mydriasis and cycloplegia from anticholinergic drugs could be unwanted in patients with glaucoma because of increased intraocular pressure. This seems unlikely with the doses used for preoperative medication. Atropine and glycopyrrolate are less likely candidates than scopolamine.[190] In patients with glaucoma, most anesthesiologists feel safe in continuing medications for glaucoma up until the time of surgery and using atropine or glycopyrrolate when necessary (see Chapter 37).

Because anticholinergic drugs block vagal activity, relaxation of bronchial smooth muscle occurs and respiratory deadspace increases.[191] The magnitude of the increase in deadspace depends on prior bronchomotor tone; but increases as large as 25–33% have been reported. Anticholinergic drugs cause secretions to dry and thicken. Theoretically, a dose of anticholinergic drug given before operation could lead to inspissation of secretions and an increase in airway resistance. This may develop into more than a theoretic issue when patients with diseases such as cystic fibrosis are being considered.

Sweat glands of the body are innervated by the sympathetic nervous system and employ cholinergic transmission. Therefore, administration of anticholinergic agents interferes with the sweating mechanism, which may cause body temperature to increase. This side-effect of anticholinergic medication must be considered carefully in a child with a fever.

Atropine is more likely than glycopyrrolate or scopolamine to cause an increase in heart rate.[172] Unwanted increases in heart rate are much more likely after intravenous administration than intramuscular administration. In fact, heart rate may transiently decrease after intramuscular administration. This may result from a peripheral agonist effect of the anticholinergic agent.

DIFFERENCES IN PREOPERATIVE MEDICATION BETWEEN PEDIATRIC AND ADULT PATIENTS[192, 193]

Differences between children and adults with regard to preoperative medication include aspects of psychologic preparation, the emphasis on oral medications when pharmacologic preparation is desired, and more frequent use of anticholinergics for their vagolytic activity. What remains the same is the need to assess the needs of each child individually and tailor the psychologic preparation and preoperative medication accordingly.

PSYCHOLOGIC FACTORS IN PEDIATRIC PATIENTS

Hospital admission and major surgery can produce long-lasting psychologic effects in some children.[194, 195] The hospital stay is stressful and full of apprehension over the short term for almost all children. Psychologic stress and anxiety are less likely with minor procedures and brief hospitalizations.[196, 197] Contrary to what one might believe, repeated hospitalizations have not been shown to increase the number of pediatric patients manifesting long-lasting psychologic trauma.[195, 198] The demeanor and effort of the anesthesiologist can make a difference to the child who is getting ready for a trip to the operating room, anesthesia, and surgery.

Age is probably the most important aspect when psychologic preparation of the pediatric patient is considered.[193] A baby younger than 6 months of age is not emotionally upset when separated from his or her mother. Others in the health care team can substitute very easily. Preoperative preparation in this age group is often directed toward other goals, for example, obtundation of vagal reflex responses. However, preschool children are upset when separated from their mothers and fear the operating room. This is a time when hospitalization may be the most upsetting.[195, 199, 200] It is difficult to explain the forthcoming events to children in this age group. It is easier to communicate with patients from age 5 years to adolescence. The anesthesiologist can explain and offer reassurance about such issues as separation from parents and the home, operating room events, and any of the patient's perceived threats of surgery and anesthesia. The adolescent patient may already be anxious and apprehensive. They may also be worried about loss of consciousness, have a fear of death, or be apprehensive about what they will do or say after preoperative sedation or during anesthesia. The more fearful child may be difficult to identify.[193, 201] This is usually the child who does not talk much during the preoperative interview and appears nonchalant or even detached. If these patients can be identified before operation, they are often candidates for heavy pharmacologic preparation.

Other important psychologic aspects in preoperative preparation include the attitude and behavior of the parents, the socioeconomic status of the family, the magnitude of the planned surgery, and the hospital environment.[202, 203]

PSYCHOLOGIC PREPARATION

For the above reasons a good preoperative visit and proper psychologic preparation may be even more important in children than adults.[204-206] This is an art that is acquired by the anesthesiologist. The preoperative visit is a time of reassurance and explanation. It is an opportunity to gain the child's trust. Most anesthesiologists will want to involve the parents when possible. The child can then see the parents' acceptance of the anesthesiologist. Some hospitals have found motion pictures and slide shows to be helpful in preparing pediatric patients for the operating room.[202-208] The child may want to bring a personal belonging, such as a stuffed animal or blanket, to the operating room for security. Some children wish to take an active role by doing such things as holding the face mask during inhalation induction of anesthesia. It may be helpful to have the parents accompany the child to the operating room suite. In some hospitals parents may go into the operating room and stay until induction is complete.

DIFFERENCES IN PHARMACOLOGIC PREPARATION

The discussion of pharmacologic preparation for the pediatric patient presumes proper psychologic preparation, a satisfactory operating room environment, and preparation for an efficient and timely induction of anesthesia.

Sedative–hypnotics

As in adults, the sedative–hypnotic medications are used to reduce apprehension and produce sedation and amnesia. They are also used to facilitate smooth induction of anesthesia when an inhalation method is to be used. The use of preoperative medication is controversial in pediatric patients. It has not been proven to reduce unwanted psychologic outcome after surgery in anesthesia. It has been shown that the uneventful induction of anesthesia is less likely to produce long-lasting psychologic problems in children.[196, 199] After 6 months to 1 year of age, the child scheduled for a surgical procedure may benefit from a sedative hypnotic drug before surgery. There is some emphasis on avoiding intramuscular injections in children. The oral route is often used for preoperative medication in the older child, whereas in preschool children drugs may also be given rectally. Many sedative–hypnotic drugs have been prescribed for children before operation. Benzodiazepines and barbiturates have been chosen often, specifically diazepam and pentobarbital orally, which seem to be quite popular. Midazolam can be given intramuscularly. Perhaps unique to the pharmacologic preparation of children is the rectal administration of methohexital (Fig. 18-11).[209] Methohexital ($20-30$ mg·kg^{-1}) may be given immediately before operation, while the child is still in the parent's arms. The intramuscular route is also possible.

Opioids

There is the occasional need for opioid premedication in children. Methadone has the advantage of oral administration, usually prescribed in the $0.1-0.2$ mg·kg^{-1} dose range. Intramuscular morphine and meperidine are used, often in combination with other premedicant drugs. Intramuscular morphine is often seen as part of the pharmacologic preparation for the child with congenital heart disease.[210, 211] In many hospitals opioids have been combined with sedative–hypnotic and anticholinergic drugs to make a "cocktail" that may be given orally for preoperative medication.

Anticholinergics

Easily induced vagal reflexes make anticholinergics especially important in children.[193, 211-213] Bradycardia may result from airway manipulation, surgical manipulation, or anesthetic drugs such as halothane or succinylcholine. Also, the child's cardiac output depends more on heart rate than the adults. If no contraindication exists, most pediatric patients will receive atropine intravenously immediately after induction of anesthesia and an intravenous catheter has been placed. If the intramuscular route has been used for atropine, it will often be administered immediately after the patient becomes unconscious during induction of anesthesia. Glycopyrrolate also has been used in children in this setting. Scopolamine has a place

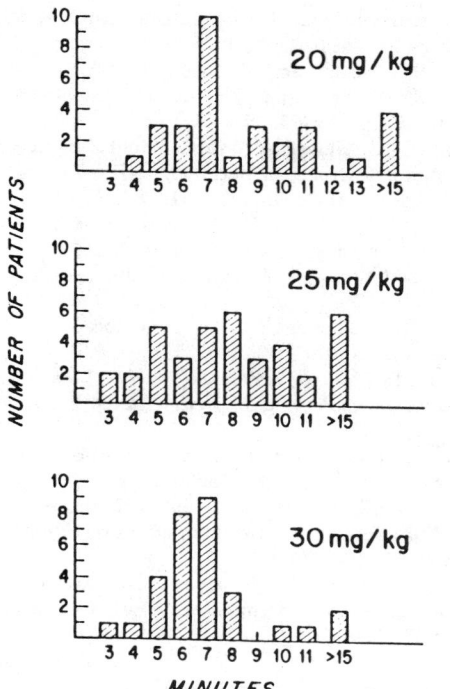

FIG. 18-11. Frequency distribution of sleep induction times after rectal instillation of methohexital. Patients averaged 3.3 yr in age and body weight, 15 kg. (Reprinted with permission. Liu LMP, Goudsouzian NG, Liu PL: Rectal methohexital premedication in children, a dose-comparison study. Anesthesiology 53:343, 1980.)

in premedication of the pediatric patient to produce sedation, amnesia, and drying of the airways. One must be aware of the hazards of administering an anticholinergic to a child with a fever or when inspissation of secretions is not wanted. Finally, it has been reported that patients with Down's syndrome appear to be sensitive to atropine.[215] This is especially evident with the effect on heart rate and mydriasis.

PREOPERATIVE MEDICATION FOR OUTPATIENTS

As with many aspects of preoperative medication, the pharmacologic preparation for outpatients is controversial.[48] Some anesthesiologists say it should be avoided. The patients are closer to their family and friends than inpatients, usually more minor surgery is scheduled, and postoperative obtundation and delayed discharge should be avoided.[216] Others believe a place exists for preoperative pharmacologic preparation for outpatients. In a study by Clark and Hurtig done in outpatients, intramuscular meperidine ($1.0\ mg \cdot kg^{-1}$) and atropine ($0.01\ mg \cdot kg^{-1}$) did not prolong recovery.[217] A retrospective analysis of 1,553 patients by Meridy showed that preoperative medication with diazepam or hydroxyzine did not delay discharge after surgery in outpatients.[218] Oral diazepam 0.25 $mg \cdot kg^{-1}$ has been used successfully in adults to reduce anxiety before outpatient surgery.[219] Horrigan et al reported that intravenous fentanyl ($1-2\ \mu g \cdot kg^{-1}$) did not prolong recovery time in the outpatient setting in their study.[220] Some investigators have found a place for preoperative medication when

pediatric patients were scheduled for outpatient procedures.[221, 222]

In some instances antiemetic drugs may be desirable before operation for outpatients, for example, patients scheduled for strabismus surgery, laparoscopic examination, and therapeutic abortions.[48] Small doses of droperidol have been used, with the consideration that larger doses can prolong recovery. Metoclopramide, hydroxyzine, and phenothiazines are other drugs that have been given before or during anesthesia to decrease the incidence of nausea and vomiting in the recovery room after outpatient surgery. One study has shown an increased gastric volume in outpatients.[114] Because of this and other factors, some authors recommend an H_2 receptor-antagonist (cimetidine or ranitidine) combined with metoclopramide in selected outpatients.[223]

REFERENCES

1. Beecher HK: Preanesthetic medication. JAMA 157:242, 1955
2. Lyons SM, Clarke RSJ, Vulgaraki K: The premedication of cardiac surgical patients. Anaesthesia 30:459, 1975
3. Nicholson MJ: Preanesthetic preparation and premedication. In Hale DE (ed): Anesthesiology, p 202. Philadelphia, FA Davis, 1954
4. Norris W, Baird WLM: Pre-operative anxiety: A study of the incidence and aetiology. Br J Anaesth 39:503, 1967
5. Egbert LD, Battit GE, Turndorf H et al: The value of the preoperative visit by the anesthetist. JAMA 185:553, 1963
6. Leigh JM, Walker J, Janaganathan P: Effect of preoperative anesthetic visit on anxiety. Br Med J 2:987, 1977
7. Korttila K, Aromaa U, Tammisto T: Patient's expectations and acceptance of the effects of the drugs given before anaesthesia: Comparison of light and amnesic premedication. Acta Anaesth Scand 25:381, 1981
8. Ghignone M, Calvillo O, Quintin L: Anesthesia and hypertension. The effect of clonidine on perioperative hemodynamics and isoflurane requirements. Anesthesiology 67:3, 1987
9. Flacke JW, Bloor BC, Flacke WE et al: Reduced narcotic requirement by clonidine with improved hemodynamic and adrenergic stability in patients undergoing coronary bypass surgery. Anesthesiology 67:11, 1987
10. Walsh J, Puig MM, Lovitz MA et al: Premedication abolishes the increase in plasma beta-endorphin observed in the immediate preoperative period. Anesthesiology 66:402, 1987
11. Ong BY, Pickering BG, Palahniuk RJ et al: Lorazepam and diazepam as adjuncts to epidural anesthesia for cesarean section. Can Anaesth Soc J 29:31, 1982
12. Houghton DJ: Use of lorazepam as a premedicant for caesarean section. Br J Anaesth 55:767, 1983
13. McAuley DM, O'Neill MP, Moore J et al: Lorazepam premedication for labour. Br J Obstet Gynecol 89:149, 1982
14. Richter JJ: Current theories about the mechanisms of benzodiazepines and neurolytic drugs. Anesthesiology 54:66, 1981
15. Study RE, Barker JL: Cellular mechanisms of benzodiazepine action. JAMA 247:2147, 1982
16. Divoll M, Greenblatt DJ, Ochs HR et al: Absolute bioavailability of oral and intramuscular diazepam: Effect of age and sex. Anesth Analg 62:1, 1983
17. Greenblatt DJ, Koch-Weser J: Clinical toxicity of chlordiazepoxide and diazepam in relation to serum albumin concentration: A report from the Boston Collaborative Drug Surveillance Program. Eur J Clin Pharmacol 7:259, 1974
18. Kaplan SA, Jack ML, Alexander RJ et al: Pharmacokinetic profile of diazepam in man following single intravenous and chronic oral administration. J Pharm Sci 62:1289, 1973

19. Klotz I, Avant GR, Hoyumpa A et al: The effects of age and liver disease on the disposition and elimination of diazepam in adult man. J Clin Invest 55:347, 1975

20. Hillestad L, Hansen T, Melson H et al: Diazepam metabolism in normal man. Serum concentrations and clinical effects after intravenous intramuscular and oral administration. Clin Pharmacol Ther 16:479, 1974

21. Assaf RAD, Dundee JW, Gamble JAS: The influence of the route of administration on the clinical action of diazepam. Anaesthesia 30:152, 1975

22. Lundgren S: Comparison of rectal diazepam and subcutaneous morphine-scopolamine administration for outpatient sedation in minor oral surgery. Acta Anaesthesiol Scand 29:674, 1985

23. Ravnborg M, Hasselstrom L, Ostergard D: Premedication with oral and rectal diazepam. Acta Anaesthesiol Scand 30:132, 1986

24. Frumin MJ, Herekar VR, Jarvik ME: Amnesic actions of diazepam and scopolamine in man. Anesthesiology 45:406, 1976

25. Liu S, Miller N, Waye JD: Retrograde amnesia effects of intravenous diazepam in endoscopy patients. Gastrointest Endosc 30:340, 1984

26. Soroker D, Barzilay E, Konichezky S et al: Respiratory function following premedication with droperidol or diazepam. Anesth Analg 57:695, 1978

27. Rao S, Sherbaniuk RW, Prasad K et al: Cardiopulmonary effects of diazepam. Clin Pharmacol 14:182, 1973

28. Gross JB, Smith L, Smith TC: Time course of ventilatory response to carbon dioxide after intravenous diazepam. Anesthesiology 57:18, 1982

29. Braunstein MC: Apnea with maintenance of consciousness following intravenous diazepam. Anesth Analg 58:52, 1979

30. Wingard DW: Physostigmine reversal of diazepam-induced depression. Anesth Analg 56:348, 1977

31. Dalen JE, Evans GL, Banas JS et al: The hemodynamic and respiratory effects of diazepam (Valium). Anesthesiology 30:259, 1969

32. McCammon RL, Hilgenberg JC, Stoelting RK: Hemodynamic effects of diazepam and diazepam-nitrous oxide in patients with coronary artery disease. Anesth Analg 59:438, 1980

33. Davies AO: Oral diazepam premedication reduces the incidence of postsuccinylcholine muscle pains. Can Anaesth Soc J 30:603, 1983

34. Verma RS: Diazepam and suxamethonium muscle pain (a dose response study). Anaesthesia 37:688, 1982

35. Feneck RD, Cook JH: Failure of diazepam to prevent suxamethonium-induced rise in intra-ocular pressure. Anaesthesia 38:120, 1983

36. Kruger AE, Roelofse JA: Precautions against intra-ocular pressure changes during endotracheal intubation—A comparison of pretreatment with intravenous lignocaine and diazepam. S Afr Med J 63:887, 1983

37. Fjeldborg P, Hecht PS, Busted N et al: The effect of diazepam pretreatment on the succinylcholine-induced rise in intraocular pressure. Acta Anaesthesiol Scand 29:415, 1985

38. Moore DC, Balfour RI, Fitzgibbons D: Convulsive arterial plasma levels of bupivacaine and the response to diazepam therapy. Anesthesiology 50:454, 1979

39. Greenblatt DJ, Abernathy DR, Morse DS et al: Clinical importance of the interaction of diazepam and cimetidine. N Engl J Med 310:1639, 1984

40. Perisho JA, Buechel DR, Miller RD: The effect of diazepam (Valium) in minimum alveolar anesthetic requirement (MAC) in man. Can Anaesth Soc J 18:536, 1971

41. Dundee JW, Lilburn JR, Nair SG et al: Studies of drugs given before anaesthesia. XXVI. Lorazepam. Br J Anaesth 49:1047, 1977

42. Heisterkamp DV, Cohen PT: The effect of intravenous premedication with lorazepam (Ativan), pentobarbital and diazepam on recall. Br J Anaesth 47:79, 1975

43. Pandit SK, Heisterkamp DV, Cohen PJ: Further studies of the antirecall effect of lorazepam: A dose-time-effect relationship. Anesthesiology 45:495, 1976

44. Wallace G, Mindlin LJ: A controlled double-blind comparison of intramuscular lorazepam and hydroxyzine as surgical premedicants. Anesth Analg 63:571, 1984

45. Aleniewski MI, Bulas BJ, Maderazo L et al: Intramuscular lorazepam versus pentobarbital premedication: A comparison of patient sedation, anxiolysis and recall. Anesth Analg 56:489, 1977

46. Russell WJ: Lorazepam as a premedicant for regional anaesthesia. Anaesthesia 38:1062, 1983

47. Pagano RR, Conner JT, Bellville JW et al: Lorazepam, hyoscine and atropine as IV surgical premedicants. Br J Anaesth 50:471, 1978

48. White PF: Pharmacologic and clinical apsects of preoperative medication. Anesth Analg 65:963, 1986

49. Bradshaw EG, Ali AA, Mulley BA et al: Plasma concentrations and clinical effects of lorazepam after oral administration. Br J Anaesth 53:517, 1981

50. Blitt CD, Petty WC, Wright WA et al: Clinical evaluation of injectable lorazepam as a premedicant: The effect on recall. Anesth Analg 55:522, 1976

51. Gale GD, Galloon S, Porter WR: Sublingual lorazepam: A better premedication? Br J Anaesth 55:761, 1983

52. Fragen RJ, Caldwell N: Lorazepam premedication: Lack of recall and relief of anxiety. Anesth Analg 55:792, 1976

53. George KA, Dundee JW: Relative amnesia actions of diazepam, flunitrazepam and lorazepam in man. Br J Clin Pharmacol 4:45, 1977

54. Kraus JW, Desmond PV, Marshall JP et al: Effects of aging and liver disease on disposition of lorazepam. Clin Pharmacol Ther 24:44, 1978

55. Gasser JC, Kaufman RD, Bellville JW: Respiratory effects of lorazepam, pentobarbital and pentazocine. Clin Pharmacol Ther 18:170, 1975

56. Comer WH, Elliott HW, Nomof W et al: Pharmacology of parenterally administered lorazepam in man. J Int Med Res 1:216, 1973

57. Conner JT, Katz RL, Bellville JW et al: Diazepam and lorazepam for intravenous surgical premedication. J Clin Pharmacol 18:285, 1978

58. Knapp RB, Fierro L: Evaluation of cardiopulmonary safety and effects of lorazepam as a premedicant. Anaesth Analg 53:122, 1974

59. Cormack RS, Milledge JS, Hanning CD: Respiration and amnesia after lorazepam or morphine premedication. Br J Anaesth 48:813, 1976

60. Dundee JW, Johnston HML, Gray RC: Lorazepam as a sedative—Amnesia in an intensive care unit. Curr Med Res Opin 4:290, 1976

61. Denaut M, Yernault JC, DeCoster A: Double blind comparison of the respiratory effects of parenteral lorazepam and diazepam in patients with chronic obstructive lung disease. Curr Med Res Opin 2:611, 1975

62. Mohler H, Okada T: Benzodiazepine receptor: Demonstration in the central nervous system. Science 198:849, 1977

63. Reves JG, Fragen RJ, Vinick HR et al: Midazolam: Pharmacology and uses. Anesthesiology 62:310, 1985

64. Greenblatt DJ, Locniskar A, Scavone JM et al: Absence of interaction of cimetidine and ranitidine with intravenous and oral midazolam. Anesth Analg 65:176, 1986

65. Greenblatt DJ, Abernathy DR, Locniskar A et al: Effect of age, gender and obesity on midazolam kinetics. Anesthesiology 61:27, 1984

66. Dundee JW, Wilson DB: Amnesic action of midazolam. Anaesthesia 35:459, 1980
67. Connor JT, Katz RL, Pagano RR et al: R021-3981 for intravenous surgical premedication and induction of anesthesia. Anesth Analg 59:1, 1978
68. Fragen RJ, Funk DI, Avram MJ et al: Midazolam versus hydroxyzine as intramuscular premedicants. Can Anaesth Soc J 30:136, 1983
69. Barrett RF, James PD, McLeod KCA: Oxazepam premedication in neurosurgical patients. Anaesthesia 39:429, 1984
70. Greenwood BK, Bradshaw EG: Preoperative medication for day care surgery. A comparison between oxazepam and temazepam. Br J Anaesth 55:933, 1983
71. Amarasekera K: Temazepam as a premedicant in minor surgery. Anaesthesia 35:771, 1980
72. Beechy APG, Etringham RJ, Studd C: Temazepam as premedication in day surgery. Anaesthesia 36:10, 1981
73. Clark G, Ervin D, Yate P et al: Temazepam as premedication in elderly patients. Anaesthesia 37:421, 1982
74. Thomas D, Tipping T, Halifax R et al: Triazolam premedication. Anaesthesia 41:692, 1986
75. Pinnock CA, Fell D, Hunt PCW et al: A comparison of triazolam and diazepam as premedication for minor gynaecologic surgery. Anaesthesia 40:324, 1985
76. Greenblatt DJ, Shader RI: Benzodiazepines. N Engl J Med 291:1239, 1974
77. Smith TC, Stephen GW, Zeiger L et al: Effects of premedicant drugs on respiration and gas exchange in man. Anesthesiology 28:883, 1967
78. Koch-Weser J, Greenblatt DJ: The archaic barbiturate hypnotics. N Engl J Med 291:790, 1974
79. Dundee JW, Nair SG, Assof RAE et al: Pentobarbital premedication for anesthetic. Anaesthesia 31:1025, 1976
80. Hovi-Viander M, Kangas L, Kanto J: A comparative study of the clinical effects of pentobarbital and diazepam given orally as preoperative medication. J Oral Surg 38:188, 1980
81. Herr GP, Conner JT, Katz RL et al: Diazepam and droperidol as IV premedicants. Br J Anaesth 51:537, 1979
82. Lee CM, Yeakel AE: Patients refusal of surgery following Innovar premedication. Anesth Analg 54:224, 1975
83. Briggs RM, Ogg MJ: Patient's refusal of surgery following Innovar premedication. Plast Reconstr Surg 54:224, 1975
84. Rivera VM, Keichian AH, Oliver RE: Persistent parkinsonism following neurolept analgesia. Anesthesiology 42:635, 1975
85. Patton CM: Rapid induction of acute dyskinesis by droperidol. Anesthesiology 43:126, 1975
86. Ward DS: Stimulation of the hypoxic ventilatory drive by droperidol. Anesth Analg 63:106, 1984
87. Hupert C, Yacoub M, Turgeon LR: Effect of hydroxyzine on morphine analgesia for the treatment of postoperative pain. Anesth Analg 59:690, 1980
88. Wender RH, Conner JT, Bellville JW et al: Comparison of IV diazepam and hydroxyzine as surgical premedicants. Br J Anaesth 49:907, 1977
89. Belleville JW, Dorey F, Capparell D et al: Analgesic effects of hydroxyzine compared to morphine in man. J Clin Pharmacol 19:290, 1979
90. McKenzie R, Wadhewa RK, Uy NTL et al: Antiemetic effectiveness of intramuscular hydroxyzine compared with intramuscular droperidol. Anaesth Analg 60:783, 1981
91. Beaven MA: Anaphylactoid reactions to anesthetic drugs. Anesthesiology 55:3, 1981
92. Keats AS, Telford J, Kurosu Y: "Potentiation" of meperidine by promethazine. Anesthesiology 22:34, 1961
93. Conner JT, Bellville JW, Wender R et al: Morphine and promethazine as intravenous premedicants. Anesth Analg 56:801, 1977
94. Cohen EN, Beecher HK: Narcotics in preanesthetic medication—A controlled study. JAMA 147:1664, 1951
95. Belleville JA, Forrest WH, Miller E et al: Influence of age on pain relief from analgesics. JAMA 217:1835, 1971
96. Saidman LJ, Eger EI II: Effect of nitrous oxide and of narcotic premedication on the alveolar concentration of halothane required for anesthesia. Anesthesiology 25:302, 1964
97. Tsunoda Y, Hattori Y, Takatsuko E et al: Effects of hydroxyzine, diazepam and pentazocine on halothane minimum alveolar anesthetic concentration. Anesth Analg 52:390, 1973
98. Conner JT, Bellville JW, Katz RL: Meperidine and morphine as intravenous surgical premedicants. Can Anaesth Soc J 24:559, 1977
99. Cormack RS, Milledge JS, Hanning CD: Respiratory effects and amnesia after premedication with morphine or lorazepam. Br J Anaesth 49:351, 1977
100. Weil JV, McCullough RE, Kline JS: Diminished ventilatory response to hypoxia and hypercapnia after morphine in man. N Engl J Med 292:1103, 1975
101. Economou G, Ward-McQuaid JN: A cross-over comparison of the effect of morphine, pethidine and pentazine on biliary pressure. Gut 12:218, 1971
102. Greenstein AJ, Kaynan A, Singer A et al: A comparative study of pentazocine and meperidine on the biliary passage pressure. Am J Gastroenterol 58:417, 1972
103. Radnay PA, Brochman E, Mankikar D et al: The effect of equianalgesic doses of fentanyl, morphine, meperidine, and pentazocine on common bile duct pressure. Anesthetist 29:26, 1980
104. Jones RM, Fiddian-Green R, Knight PR: Narcotic-induced choledochoduodenal sphincter spasm by glucagon. Anesth Analg 59:946, 1980
105. Cahalan MK, Lurz FW, Eger EI II et al: Narcotics decrease heart rate during inhalational anesthesia. Anesth Analg 66:166, 1987
106. Austin KL, Stapleton JV, Mather LE: Multiple intramuscular injections—A major source of variability in analgesic response to meperidine. Pain 8:47, 1980
107. Gourlay GK, Wilson PR, Glynn CJ: Pharmacodynamics and pharmacokinetics of methadone during the perioperative period. Anesthesiology 57:458, 1982
108. Laffey DA, Kay NH: Premedication with butorphanol: A comparison with morphine. Br J Anaesth 56:363, 1984
109. VanDam LD: Butorphanol. N Engl J Med 302:381, 1980
110. Hofmann RF, Weiler HH: Lorazepam and nalbuphine as local anesthetic ophthalmic surgery premedications. Ann Ophthalmol 15:64, 1983
111. Lake CL, Duckworth EN, DiFazio CA et al: Cardiorespiratory effects of nalbuphine and morphine premedication in adult cardiac surgical patients. Acta Anaesthesiol Scand 28:305, 1984
112. Pinnock CA, Bell A, Smith G: A comparison of nalbuphine and morphine as premedication agents for union gynaecological surgery. Anaesthesia 40:1078, 1985
113. Vaughn RW, Bauer S, Wise L: Volume and pH of gastric juice in obese patients. Anesthesiology 43:686, 1975
114. Ong BY, Palahniuk RJ, Cumming M: Gastric volume and pH in outpatients. Can Anaesth Soc J 25:36, 1978
115. Stoelting RK: Responses to atropine, glycopyrrolate and Riopan on gastric fluid pH and volume in adult patients. Anesthesiology 48:367, 1978
116. Manchikanti L, Roush JR: The effect of preanesthetic glycopyrrolate and cimetidine in gastric fluid pH and volume in outpatients. Anesth Analg 63:40, 1984
117. Hutchinson A, Maltby JR, Reid CRG: Gastric fluid volume and pH in elective inpatients. Part I: Coffee or orange juice versus overnight fast. Can J Anaesth 35:12–5, 1988
118. Brock-Utne JG, Rubin J, Welman S et al: The effect of glycopyrro-

late (Robinul) on the lower esophageal sphincter. Can Anaesth Soc J 25:144, 1978

119. Black JW, Duncan WAM, Durant CJ et al: Definition and antagonism of histamine H$_2$-receptors. Nature 236:385, 1972

120. Coombs DW: Aspiration pneumonia prophylaxis. Anesth Analg 62:1055, 1983

121. Weber L, Hirshman CA: Cimetidine for prophylaxis of aspiration pneumonitis: Comparison of intramuscular and oral dose schedules. Anesth Analg 58:426, 1979

122. Stoelting RK: Gastric fluid pH in patients receiving cimetidine. Anesth Analg 57:675, 1978

123. Coombs DW, Hooper D, Colton T: Acid aspiration prophylaxis by use of preoperative oral administration of cimetidine. Anesthesiology 51:352, 1979

124. Manchikanti L, Kraus JW, Edds SP: Cimetidine and related drugs in anesthesia. Anesth Analg 61:595, 1982

125. Maliniak K, Vakil AH: Pre-anesthetic cimetidine and gastric pH. Anesth Analg 58:309, 1979

126. Hodgkinson R, Glassenberg R, Joyce TH et al: Comparison of cimetidine (Tagamet) with antacid for safety and effectiveness in reducing gastric acidity before elective cesarean section. Anesthesiology 59:86, 1983

127. Johnston JR, Moore J, McCaughey W et al: Use of cimetidine as an oral antacid obstetric anesthesia. Anesth Analg 62:720, 1983

128. Coombs DW, Hooper DW: Cimetidine as a prophylactic against acid aspiration at tracheal extubation. Can Anaesth Soc J 28:33, 1981

129. Cohen J, Weetman AP, Dargie HJ et al: Life threatening arrhythmias and intravenous injection of cimetidine. Br Med J 2:768, 1979

130. Shaw RG, Mashford ML, Desmond PV: Cardiac arrest after intravenous injection of cimetidine. Med J Aust 2:629, 1980

131. Durrant JM, Strunin L: Comparative trial of the effect of ranitidine and cimetidine on gastric secretion in fasting patients at induction of anesthesia. Can Anaesth Soc J 29:446, 1982

132. Harris PW, Morison DH, Dunn GL et al: Intramuscular cimetidine and ranitidine as prophylaxis against gastric aspiration syndrome. Can Anaesth Soc J 31:599, 1984

133. Zeldis JE, Friedman LS, Iselbacher KJ: Ranitidine: A new N$_2$-receptor antagonist. N Engl J Med 309:1368, 1983

134. Gillett GB, Watson JD, Langford RM: Ranitidine and single dose antacid therapy as prophylaxis against acid aspiration syndrome in obstetric practice. Anaesthesia 39:638, 1984

135. Viegas OJ, Ravindran RS, Shumacker CA: Gastric fluid pH in patients receiving sodium citrate. Anesth Analg 60:521, 1981

136. Gibbs CP, Spohr L, Schmidt D: The effectiveness of sodium citrate as an antacid. Anesthesiology 57:44, 1982

137. Manchikanti L, Grow JB, Collvier JA et al: Sodium citrate and metoclopramide in outpatient anesthesia for prophylaxis against aspiration pneumonitis. Anesthesiology 63:378, 1985

138. Gibbs CP, Hempling RE, Wynne JW et al: Antacid pulmonary aspiration. Anesthesiology 51:S290, 1979

139. Frank M, Evans M, Flynn P et al: Comparison of the prophylactic use of magnesium trisilicate, sodium citrate or cimetidine in obstetrics. Br J Anaesth 56:355, 1984

140. Bond VK, Stoelting RK, Gupta CD: Pulmonary aspiration syndrome after inhalation of gastric fluid containing antacids. Anesthesiology 51:452, 1979

141. Gibbs CP, Schwartz DJ, Wynne JR et al: Antacid pulmonary aspiration in the dog. Anesthesiology 51:380, 1979

142. Heany GAH, Jones HD: Correspondence: Aspiration syndrome in pregnancy. Br J Anaesth 51:266, 1979

143. Schwartz J, Wynne JW, Gibbs CP et al: Pulmonary consequences of aspiration of gastric contents at pH values greater than 2.5. Am Rev Resp Dis 121:119, 1980

144. Foulkes E, Jenkins LC: A comparative evaluation of cimetidine and sodium citrate to decrease gastric acidity: Effectiveness at time of induction of anesthesia. Can Anaesth Soc J 23:29, 1981

145. Schmidt JF, Schierup L, Banning AM: The effect of sodium citrate on the pH and amount of gastric contents before general anesthesia. Acta Anaesthesiol Scand 28:263, 1984

146. O'Sullivan GM, Bullingham RE: Noninvasive assessment by radiotelemetry of antacid effect during labor. Anesth Analg 64:95, 1985

147. James CF, Modell JH, Gibbs CP et al: Pulmonary aspiration—Effects of volume and pH in the rat. Anesth Analg 63:665, 1984

148. Murphy DF, Nally B, Gardiner J et al: Effect of metoclopramide on gastric emptying before elective and emergency caesarean section. Br J Anaesth 56:1113, 1984

149. Wyner J, Cohen SE: Gastric volume in early pregnancy: Effect of metoclopramide. Anesthesiology 57:209, 1982

150. Nimmo WS: Drugs, diseases and altered gastric emptying. Clin Pharmacokinet 1:189, 1976

151. Cohen SE, Jasson J, Talafre M-L et al: Does metoclopramide decrease the volume of gastric contents in patients undergoing cesarean section? Anesthesiology 61:604, 1984

152. Schmidt JF, Jorgensen BC: The effect of metoclopramide on gastric contents after preoperative ingestion of sodium citrate. Anesth Analg 63:841, 1984

153. Manchikanti L, Marrero TC, Roush JR: Preanesthetic cimetidine and metoclopramide for acid aspiration prophylaxis in elective surgery. Anesthesiology 61:48, 1984

154. Manchikanti L, Colliver JA, Marrero TC et al: Ranitidine and metoclopramide for prophylaxis of aspiration pneumonitis in elective surgery. Anesth Analg 63:903, 1984

155. O'Sullivan G, Sear JW, Bullingham RES et al: The effect of magnesium trisilicate, metoclopramide and ranitidine on gastric pH, volume and serum gastrin. Anaesthesia 40:246, 1985

156. Korttila K, Kauste A, Auvinen J: Comparison of domperidone, droperidol and metoclopramide in the prevention and treatment of nausea and vomiting after balanced general anesthesia. Anesth Analg 58:396, 1979

157. Santos A, Datta S: Prophylactic use of droperidol for control of nausea and vomiting during spinal anesthesia for cesarean section. Anesth Analg 63:85, 1984

158. Cohen SE, Woods WA, Wyner J: Antiemetic efficacy of droperidol and metoclopramide. Anesthesiology 60:67, 1984

159. Tornetta FJ: A comparison of droperidol, diazepam and hydroxyzine hydrochloride as premedication. Anesth Analg 56:496, 1977

160. Patton CM, Moon MR, Dannemiller JT: The prophylactic antiemetic effect of droperidol. Anesth Analg 53:361, 1974

161. Iwamoto K, Schwartz H: Antiemetic effect of droperidol after ophthalmic surgery. Arch Ophthalmol 96:1378, 1978

162. Mortensen PT: Droperidol (Dehydrobenzperiodol): Postoperative antiemetic effect when given intravenously to gynaecologic patients. Acta Anaesth Scand 26:48, 1982

163. Karhunen U, Orko R: Nausea and vomiting after local anesthesia for cataract extraction in elderly female patients. Effect of droperidol premedication. Ophthalmic Surg 12:810, 1981

164. Winning TJ, Brock-Utne JG, Downing JW: Nausea and vomiting after anesthesia and minor surgery. Anesth Analg 56:674, 1977

165. Clark MM, Stores JA: The prevention of postoperative vomiting after abortion. Metoclopramide. Br J Anesth 41:890, 1969

166. Shah ZP, Wilson J: An evaluation of metoclopramide (Maxolon) as an antiemetic in anesthesia. Br J Anesth 44:865, 1972

167. Ellis FR, Spence AA: Clinical trials of metoclopramide (Maxolon) as an antiemetic in anaesthesia. Anaesthesia 25:368, 1970

168. Tornetta FJ: Clinical studies with the new antiemetic, metoclopramide. Anesth Analg 48:198, 1969

169. Greenblatt DJ, Shader RI: Anticholinergics. N Engl J Med 288:1215, 1973

170. Clarke RSJ, Dundee JW, Moore J: Studies of drugs given before anesthesia. 4. Atropine and hyoscine. Br J Anaesth 36:648, 1964

171. Eger EI II: Atropine, scopolamine and related compounds. Anesthesiology 33:365, 1962

172. Mirakhur RK: Anticholinergic drugs. Br J Anaesth 51:671, 1979

173. Shutt LE, Bowes JB: Atropine and hyoscine. Anaesthesia 34:476, 1979

174. Holt AI: Premedication with atropine should not be routine. Lancet 2:984, 1961

175. Middleton JJ, Zitzer JM, Urbach KF: Is atropine always necessary before general anesthesia? Anesth Analg 46:51, 1967

176. Kessel J: Atropine premedication. Anaesth Intensive Care 2:77, 1974

177. Mirakhur RA, Clarke RSJ, Dundee JW et al: Anticholinergic drugs in anaesthesia. A survey of their present position. Anaesthesia 33:133, 1978

178. Falick YS, Smiler BG: Is anticholinergic premedication necessary? Anesthesiology 43:472, 1975

179. Wyant GM, Kao E: Glycopyrrolate methobromide. Effect on salivary secretion. Can Anaesth Soc J 21:230, 1974

180. Russell-Taylor WJ, Llewellyn-Thomas E, Seller EA: A comparative evaluation of intramuscular atropine, dicyclomine and glycopyrrolate using healthy medical students as volunteer subjects. Int J Clin Pharmacol 4:358, 1970

181. McCubbin TD, Brown JH, Dewar KMS et al: Glycopyrrolate as premedicant: Comparison with atropine. Br J Anaesth 51:885, 1979

182. Forrest WH, Brown CR, Brown BW: Subjective responses to six common preoperative medications. Anesthesiology 47:241, 1977

183. Conner JT, Bellville JW, Wender R et al: Morphine, scopolamine and atropine as intravenous surgical premedicants. Anesth Analg 56:606, 1977

184. Meyers EF, Tomeldan SA: Glycopyrrolate compared with atropine in prevention of the ocularcardiac reflex during eye-muscle surgery. Anesthesiology 51:350, 1979

185. Sorensen O, Eriksen S, Hommegaard P et al: Thiopental-nitrous oxide-halothane anesthesia and repeated succinylcholine: Comparison of preoperative glycopyrrolate and atropine administration. Anesth Analg 59:686, 1980

186. Longo VG: Behavioral and electroencephalographic effects of atropine and related compounds. Pharmacol Rev 18:965, 1966

187. Smith DS, Orkin FK, Gardner SM et al: Prolonged sedation in the elderly after intraoperative atropine administration. Anesthesiology 51:348, 1979

188. Holzgrafe RE, Vondrell JJ, Mintz SM: Reversal of postoperative reactions to scopolamine with physostigmine. Anesth Analg 52:921, 1973

189. Duvoisin RC, Katz RL: Reversal of central anticholinergic syndrome in man by physostigmine. JAMA 206:1963, 1968

190. Garde JF, Aston R, Endler GC et al: Racial mydriatic response to belladonna premedication. Anaesth Analg 57:572, 1978

191. Severinghaus JW, Stupfel M: Respiratory dead space increase following atropine in man, and atropine, vagal or ganglionic blockade and hypothermia in dogs. J Appl Physiol 8:81, 1955

192. Korsch BM: The child and the operating room. Anesthesiology 43:251, 1975

193. Steward DJ: Psychological preparation and premedication. In Gregory GA (ed): Pediatric Anesthesia, p 423. New York, Churchill Livingstone, 1983

194. Chapman AH, Loeb DG, Gibbons MJ: Psychiatric aspects of hospitalizing children. Arch Ped 73:77, 1956

195. Vernon DTA, Schulman JL, Foley JM: Changes in children's behavior after hospitalization. Am J Dis Child 111:581, 1966

196. Davenport HT, Werry JS: The effect of general anesthesia, surgery and hospitalization on the behavior of children. Am J Orthopsychiatry 40:806, 1970

197. Steward DJ: Experiences with an out-patient anesthesia service for children. Anesthesiology 52:877, 1973

198. Jessner L, Blom GE, Waldfogel S: Emotional implications of tonsillectomy and adenoidectomy on children. Psychoanal Study Child 7:126, 1952

199. Eckenhoff JE: Relationship of anesthesia to post-operative personality changes in children. Am J Dis Child 86:587, 1953

200. Beeby DG, Hughes JOM: Behaviour of unsedated children in the anaesthetic room. Br J Anaesth 52:279, 1980

201. Bothe A, Galdston R: A child's loss of consciousness: A psychiatric view of pediatric anesthesia. Pediatrics 50:252, 1972

202. Rothman PE: A note on hospitalism. Pediatrics 30:995, 1962

203. Tisza VB, Angoff K: A play program for hospitalized children: The role of the playroom teacher. Pediatrics 28:841, 1961

204. Booker PD, Chapman DH: Premedication in children undergoing day-care surgery. Br J Anaesth 51:1083, 1979

205. Jackson K: Psychological preparation as a method of reducing the emotional trauma of anesthesia in children. Anesthesiology 12:293, 1981

206. Visintainer MA, Wolfer JA: Psychological preparation for surgical pediatric patients: The effect on children's and parents' stress responses and adjustment. Pediatrics 56:187, 1975

207. Vernon DTA, Bailey WC: The use of motion pictures in the psychological preparation of children for induction of anesthesia. Anesthesiology 40:68, 1974

208. Melamed BG, Siegel LJ: Reduction of anxiety in children facing hospitalization and surgery by use of filmed modeling. J Consult Clin Psychol 43:511, 1975

209. Liu LMP, Goudsouzian NG, Liu PL: Rectal methohexital in children, a dose-comparison study. Anesthesiology 53:343, 1980

210. McQuiston WO: Anesthetic problems in cardiac surgery in children. Anesthesiology 10:590, 1947

211. Moffitt EA, McGoon DC, Ritter DG: The diagnosis and correction of congenital cardiac defects. Anesthesiology 33:144, 1970

212. Gravenstein JS, Anton AH: Premedication and drug interaction. Clinical Anesthesia 3:199, 1969

213. Rackow H, Salanitre E: Modern concepts in pediatric anesthesiology. Anesthesiology 30:208, 1969

214. Kessel J: Atropine premedication. Anaesth Intensive Care 2:77, 1974

215. Harris WS, Goodman RH: Hyper-reactivity to atropine in Down's syndrome. N Engl J Med 279:407, 1968

216. Kortilla K, Linnoila M: Psychomotor skills related to driving after intramuscular administration of diazepam and meperidine. Anesthesiology 42:685, 1975

217. Clark AJM, Hurtig JB: Premedication with merperidine and atropine does not prolong recovery to the street fitness after outpatient surgery. Can Anaesth Soc J 28:390, 1981

218. Meridy HW: Criteria for selection of ambulatory surgical patients and guidelines for anesthetic management—A retrospective study of 1553 cases. Anesth Analg 61:921, 1982

219. Jakobsen H, Hertz JB, Johansen JR et al: Premedication before day surgery. Br J Anaesth 57:300, 1985

220. Horrigan RW, Moyers JR, Johnson BH et al: Etomidate vs. thiopental with and without fentanyl—A comparative study of awakening in man. Anesthesiology 52:362, 1980

221. Brustowicz RM, Nelson DA, Betts EK et al: Efficacy of oral premedication in pediatric outpatient surgery. Anesthesiology 60:475, 1984

222. Desjardins R, Ansara S, Charest J: Preanesthetic medication for paediatric day care surgery. Can Anaesth Soc J 28:141, 1981

223. Rao TLK, Suseela M, El-Etr AA: Metoclopramide and cimetidine to reduce gastric pH and volume. Anesth Analg 63:264, 1984

Anesthesia Systems

An anesthesia system consists of various components that may communicate with each other during the administration of inhalation anesthesia. The components include the anesthesia machine, the vaporizers, the ventilator, and the anesthetic circuit. A thorough understanding of these parts is essential to the safe practice of anesthesia. This chapter discusses the normal operation, function, and integration of major system components. More importantly, it illustrates some problems and hazards associated with each and describes appropriate preoperative checks.

ANESTHESIA MACHINES

Machine technology and emphasis on patient safety have increased over the years. The American National Standards Institute (ANSI) published the Z79.8 Machine Standard in 1979.[1] This document was a landmark for the advancement of machine technology and patient safety because it specifies the minimum performance, design characteristics, and safety requirements for anesthesia machines. It resulted from years of cooperative efforts of anesthesiologists, manufacturers, and engineers. Most machines produced in the United States today meet the ANSI Z79.8 Standard. The Ohmeda Modulus II (Fig. 19-1) and Drager Narkomed 3 (Fig. 19-2) are examples of machines that far exceed the standard.

GENERIC ANESTHESIA MACHINE

A standard two-gas anesthesia machine is shown in Figure 19-3. Both oxygen and nitrous oxide have two supply sources. They consist of a cylinder supply source and a pipeline supply source. The oxygen cylinder source is regulated from 2,200 pounds per square inch gauge (PSIG) to approximately 45 PSIG, and the nitrous oxide cylinder source is regulated from 750 to approximately 45 PSIG. The cylinders serve as back-up if the pipeline fails, and they should be turned off if a pipeline source is available. The pipeline source is normally 50 PSIG, the nominal working pressure of most machines.[2, 3]

Some machines have a second-stage oxygen regulator located downstream from the oxygen supply source. It is adjusted to a precise pressure level, such as 15 PSIG. This regulator supplies a constant pressure to the oxygen flow control valve, regardless of fluctuating oxygen pipeline pressures. For example, the output from the oxygen flow control valve will be constant if the oxygen supply pressure is greater than 15 PSIG. The oxygen flow control valve allows the operator to precisely control the oxygen flow rate, which is indicated on the oxygen flowmeter. The oxygen flow joins the flow from the nitrous oxide flowmeter in a common manifold and is directed to a calibrated variable-bypass vaporizer. Varying amounts of inhalation agent can be added to the mixture, depending on the vaporizer setting. The mixture flows toward the common gas outlet. Some machines may have a machine outlet check valve to protect the vaporizers from back pressure exerted during positive-pressure ventilation (see Vaporizers, Intermittent Back Pressure). The presence or absence of a check valve profoundly influences the preoperative machine check (see Checking Anesthesia Machines). The oxygen flush connection joins the mixed-gas pipeline between the one-way check valve and the machine outlet. Thus, the oxygen flush, when activated, has a "straight shot" to the common outlet.[2, 3]

Located downstream from the nitrous oxide supply source is a safety device traditionally referred to as the "fail-safe" system. It serves as an interface between the oxygen and

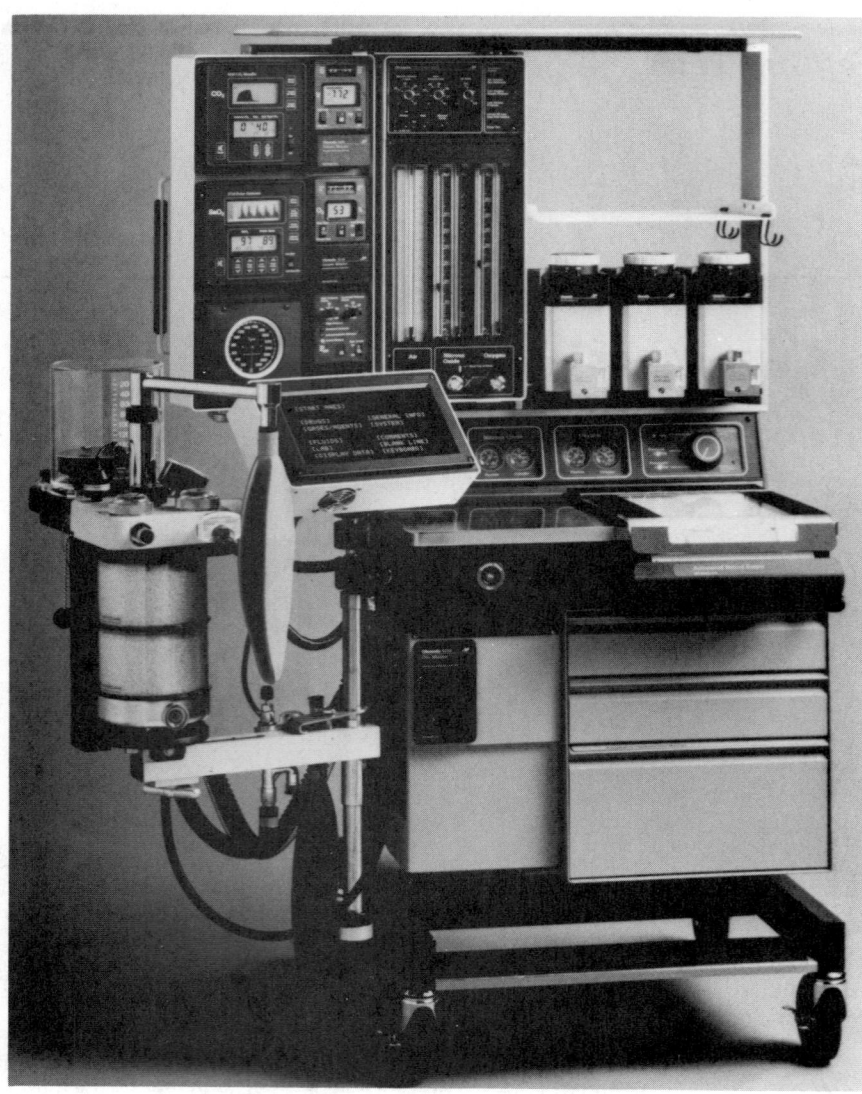

FIG. 19-1. Modulus II Anesthesia System. (Courtesy of Ohmeda, The BOC Group, Madison, WI.)

nitrous oxide supply sources. This device shuts off or proportionally decreases the supply of nitrous oxide (and other gases) if the oxygen supply pressure decreases. Finally, many machines have an alarm device to monitor the oxygen supply pressure. An alarm sounds at a predetermined oxygen pressure such as 30 PSIG.[2–4]

OXYGEN SUPPLY PRESSURE FAILURE SAFETY DEVICES

Oxygen and nitrous oxide supply sources existed as independent entities in older anesthesia machine models, and they were not interfaced. Therefore, abrupt or insidious oxygen pressure failure had the potential to lead to the delivery of a hypoxic mixture. Contemporary anesthesia machines have a number of safety devices that act together in a cascade manner to minimize the risk of hypoxia as oxygen pressure decreases. Several of these devices are described below.

Pneumatic and Electronic Alarm Devices

Ohmeda machines have been equipped with a pneumatic alarm called the oxygen supply failure alarm system. A decrease in oxygen supply pressure to a predetermined threshold value, such as 30 PSIG, sounds a warning for at least 7 s.[3, 5–7] Drager uses an electronic alarm, the oxygen supply pressure alarm, which is also activated at an oxygen supply pressure of 30 PSIG. Both visual and audible alarms alert the operator of oxygen pressures below this level.[4, 8, 9]

Fail-Safe Systems

A fail-safe valve is present in the gas line supplying each of the flowmeters (except oxygen) according to the Z79.8 Machine Standard. The valve is controlled by oxygen pressure. It shuts off or proportionally decreases the supply of gases other than oxygen (nitrous oxide, air, carbon dioxide, helium, nitrogen) as the oxygen supply pressure decreases. Unfortunately, the

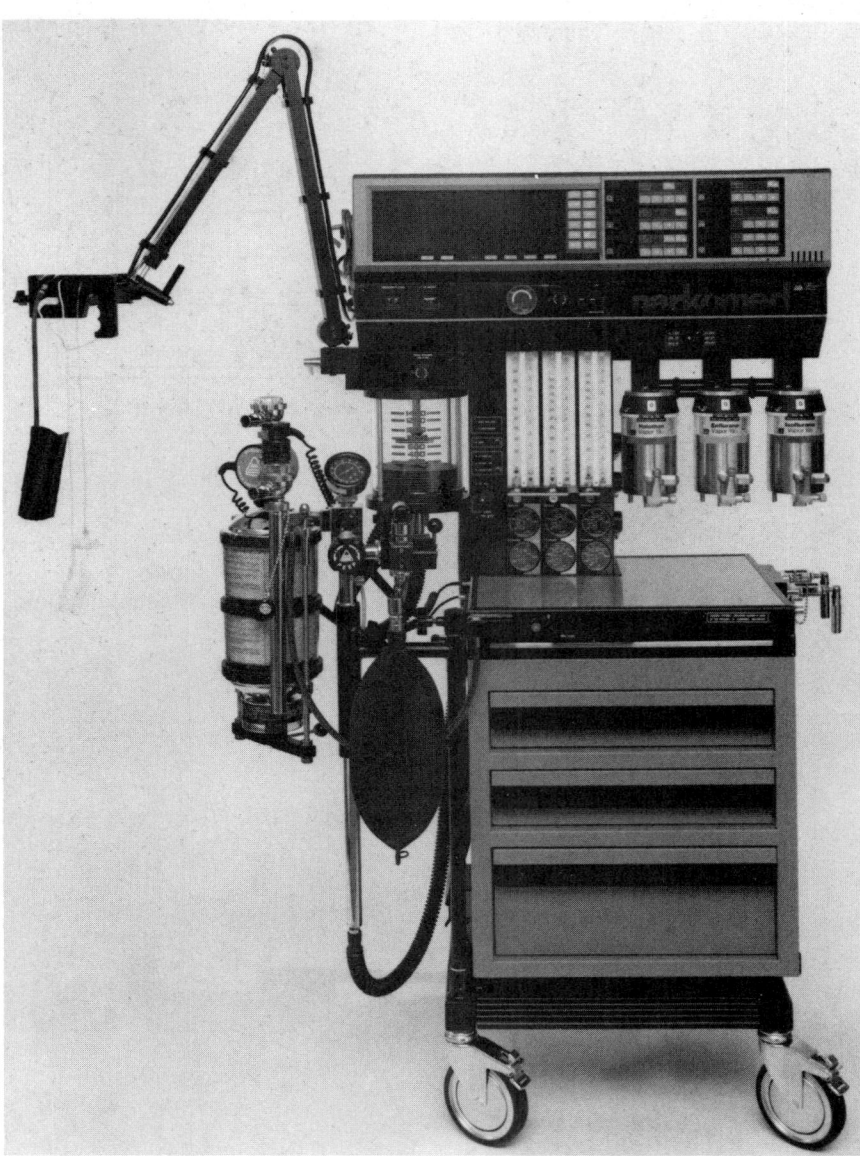

FIG. 19-2. Narkomed 3 Anesthesia System. (Courtesy of North American Drager, Telford, PA.)

misnomer of fail-safe has led to the misconception that the device prevents administration of a hypoxic mixture. This is not the case. Machines that are not equipped with a proportioning system (see Proportioning Systems) can deliver a hypoxic mixture under normal working conditions. The oxygen flow control valve can be closed intentionally or accidentally. Normal oxygen pressure will maintain other gas lines open so that a hypoxic mixture can result.[2, 3]

Ohmeda machines are equipped with a fail-safe valve known as the pressure-sensor shutoff valve. It is threshold in nature and is either open or closed. Figure 19-4 shows a nitrous oxide pressure-sensor shutoff valve with a threshold pressure of 20 PSIG. An oxygen pressure greater than the threshold value is exerted upon the mobile diaphragm in Figure 19-4A. This moves the piston, pin, and valve off the valve seat. Nitrous oxide flow passes freely to the nitrous oxide flow control valve. The oxygen supply pressure in Fig-

ure 19-4B is less than 20 PSIG, and the force of the valve return spring completely closes the valve.

Drager uses a fail-safe valve known as the Oxygen Failure Protection Device (OFPD), which interfaces the oxygen pressure with that of other gases, such as nitrous oxide, air, carbon dioxide, helium, and nitrogen. It differs from Ohmeda's oxygen pressure sensor shutoff valve because the OFPD is based on a proportioning principle rather than a threshold principle. The pressure of all gases controlled by the OFPD will decrease proportionally with the oxygen pressure. The OFPD consists of a seat/nozzle assembly, which is connected to a spring-loaded piston (Fig. 19-5). The oxygen supply pressure in the left illustration is 50 PSIG. This pressure pushes the piston upward, forcing the nozzle away from the valve seat. Nitrous oxide (or other gases) advances toward the flow control valve at 50 PSIG. The oxygen pressure in the right illustration is 0 PSIG. The spring is expanded and forces the nozzle against

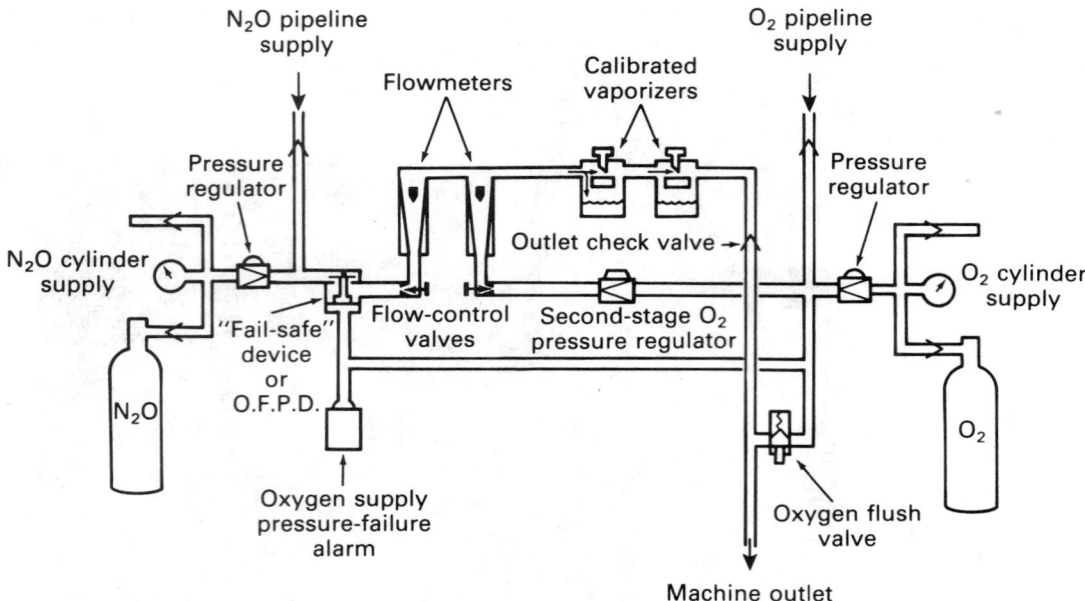

FIG. 19-3. Diagram of a generic two-gas anesthesia machine.

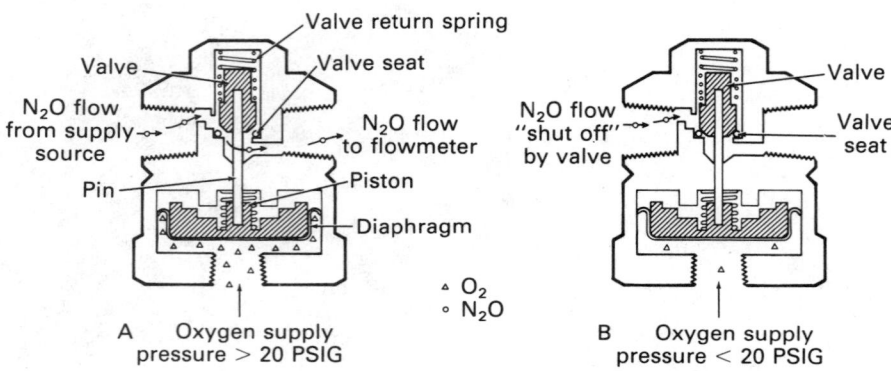

FIG. 19-4. Pressure sensor shutoff valve. The valve is open in (*A*) because the oxygen supply pressure is greater than the threshold value of 20 PSIG. The valve is closed in (*B*) because of inadequate oxygen pressure. (Redrawn with permission. Bowie E, Huffman LM: The Anesthesia Machine: Essentials for Understanding. Madison, WI, Ohmeda, The BOC Group, 1985.)

the seat, preventing flow through the device. Finally, the center illustration shows an intermediate oxygen pressure of 25 PSIG. The spring force partially closes the valve. The nitrous oxide pressure delivered to the flow control valve is 25 PSIG. There is a vast continuum of intermediate configurations between the extremes (0–50 PSIG) of oxygen supply pressure. These intermediate configurations are responsible for the proportional nature of the OFPD.[4]

Second-stage Oxygen Pressure Regulator

Most contemporary Ohmeda machines have a second-stage oxygen regulator set from 12 to 16 PSIG. Oxygen flowmeter output is constant when the oxygen supply pressure exceeds the set value. Ohmeda pressure sensor shutoff valves are set at a higher threshold value (20–30 PSIG). This ensures that oxygen is the last gas flow to decrease if oxygen pressure fails.[5–7, 10]

Oxygen Ratio Monitor Controller

The Oxygen Ratio Monitor Controller (ORMC) is a complex safety device used on contemporary Drager machines and is located downstream from the OFPD. Both devices work together in a cascade manner when the oxygen supply pressure decreases. First, the OFPD proportionally decreases the pressure of the other gases such as nitrous oxide.[4] Then, the spring-loaded ORMC shuts off the nitrous oxide slave control valve when the oxygen pressure decreases below 10 PSIG. Thus, oxygen flow is the last to cease. This action represents only one function of the ORMC, which also serves as a proportioning device and an alarm system. The ORMC will be discussed in detail in Proportioning Systems.

Integration of Oxygen Pressure Failure Safety Devices

Different brands and models of anesthesia machines respond differently to an insidious decline in oxygen supply pres-

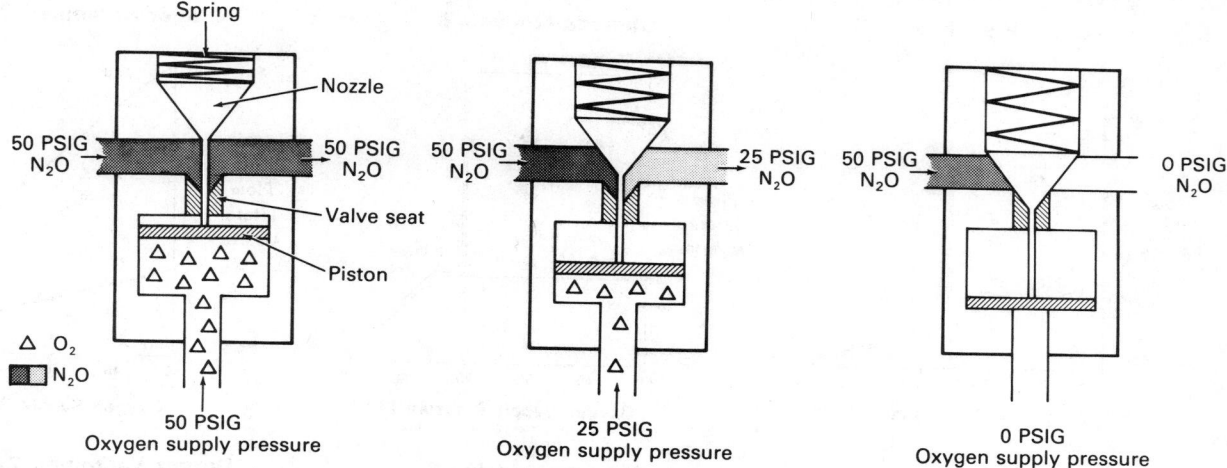

FIG. 19-5. Oxygen failure protection device—OFPD. The OFPD responds proportionally to changes in oxygen supply pressure. See text for details. (Redrawn with permission. Narkomed 2A Anesthesia System. Technical Service Manual. Telford, PA, North American Drager, June 1985.)

sure.[11] Careful evaluation of a machine's response to a decline in oxygen supply pressure serves as a noninvasive "fingerprint" of the design of the internal anesthesia machine. Examples of such fingerprints are shown in Fig. 19-6. They were generated in the following manner. All machine "E" cylinders were turned off, and a constant 50-PSIG nitrous oxide source was connected to the nitrous oxide pipeline inlet. With an initial oxygen pressure of 50 PSIG, the nitrous oxide and oxygen flow control valves were set to deliver 7 l·min⁻¹ nitrous oxide and 3 l·min⁻¹ oxygen. Total gas flow was calculated by adding the individual gas flows. An oxygen analyzer at the common outlet was used to determine the fresh gas oxygen concentration. The oxygen supply pressure was decreased in 5-PSIG decrements without the settings of the flow control valve being changed. Gas flow and oxygen concentration were remeasured at each decrement and the results were graphed.

Figure 19-6A represents the fingerprint of an older anesthesia machine that does not have a second-stage oxygen regulator. However, it does have a threshold pressure sensor shutoff valve set at 25 PSIG. A linear decline in oxygen flow occurs as the oxygen pressure decreases because of the absence of the second-stage regulator. Because the nitrous oxide supply pressure is adequate, the nitrous oxide flow remains constant at 7 l·min⁻¹ until the 25-PSIG oxygen pressure threshold is reached. A vulnerable oxygen pressure zone exists from 50 to 26 PSIG because the fresh gas oxygen concentration and total flow decrease. The oxygen concentration increases to 100% below 25 PSIG oxygen pressure because the nitrous oxide is shut off by the oxygen pressure sensor shutoff valve.

Figure 19-6B is the fingerprint of an Ohmeda Modulus II. It has a pneumatic low oxygen supply pressure alarm set at 30 PSIG, a pressure-sensor shutoff valve set at 20 PSIG, and a second-stage oxygen regulator set at 14 PSIG.[6, 10] The oxygen flow remains constant as long as the oxygen pressure is greater than 14 PSIG. This is unlike older machines without the second-stage oxygen regulator. As the oxygen supply pressure decreases from 50 to 21 PSIG, the flow of oxygen and nitrous oxide remain constant at 3 l·min⁻¹ and 7 l·min⁻¹,

respectively. A pneumatic low-oxygen pressure alarm sounds at 30 PSIG to alert the operator of a problem. It is important to note that when the alarm sounds, the oxygen concentration and the flows are identical to those noted at 50 PSIG. The nitrous oxide is shut off when the oxygen supply pressure decreases to 20 PSIG, which is the threshold pressure for the oxygen pressure sensor shutoff valve. The oxygen concentration at that point increases to 100%. Oxygen flow remains constant at 3 l·min⁻¹ from 20 to 15 PSIG because the second-stage oxygen regulator is set at 14 PSIG. Finally, there is a linear decrease in oxygen flow with decreasing oxygen supply pressure below 14 PSIG.

The Ohmeda Modulus II response to loss of oxygen supply pressure has several advantages over older machines. The oxygen concentration remains constant or increases, and the operator is alerted to a problem before flows decrease. Oxygen flow remains constant because the value of the second-stage oxygen regulator is set at a low pressure until the oxygen supply pressure is almost depleted.

The Drager Narkomed 2A ORMC response to decreasing oxygen supply pressure is unique (Fig. 19-6C). Several safety devices are recruited as the oxygen supply pressure decreases. These include the OFPD, the electronic low oxygen pressure alarm set at 30 PSIG, and the ORMC. First, the OFPD proportionally decreases nitrous oxide pressure in response to reduced oxygen pressure.[4] Flow reductions are proportional and the oxygen concentration of the fresh gas mixture remains constant at 30% from 50 PSIG to approximately 10 PSIG. The spring-loaded ORMC shuts off nitrous oxide flow entirely when the oxygen pressure is below 10 PSIG. The fresh gas oxygen concentration then increases to 100%.

An attractive feature of the Narkomed 2A response to decreasing oxygen pressure is that the oxygen concentration is maintained or increased. A vulnerable oxygen supply pressure zone theoretically exists from 50 to 31 PSIG, because flows can decrease as much as 30% before the operator is alerted to an oxygen pressure problem. Clinically, however, this is probably insignificant because oxygen supply failure is usually complete and abrupt instead of gradual.

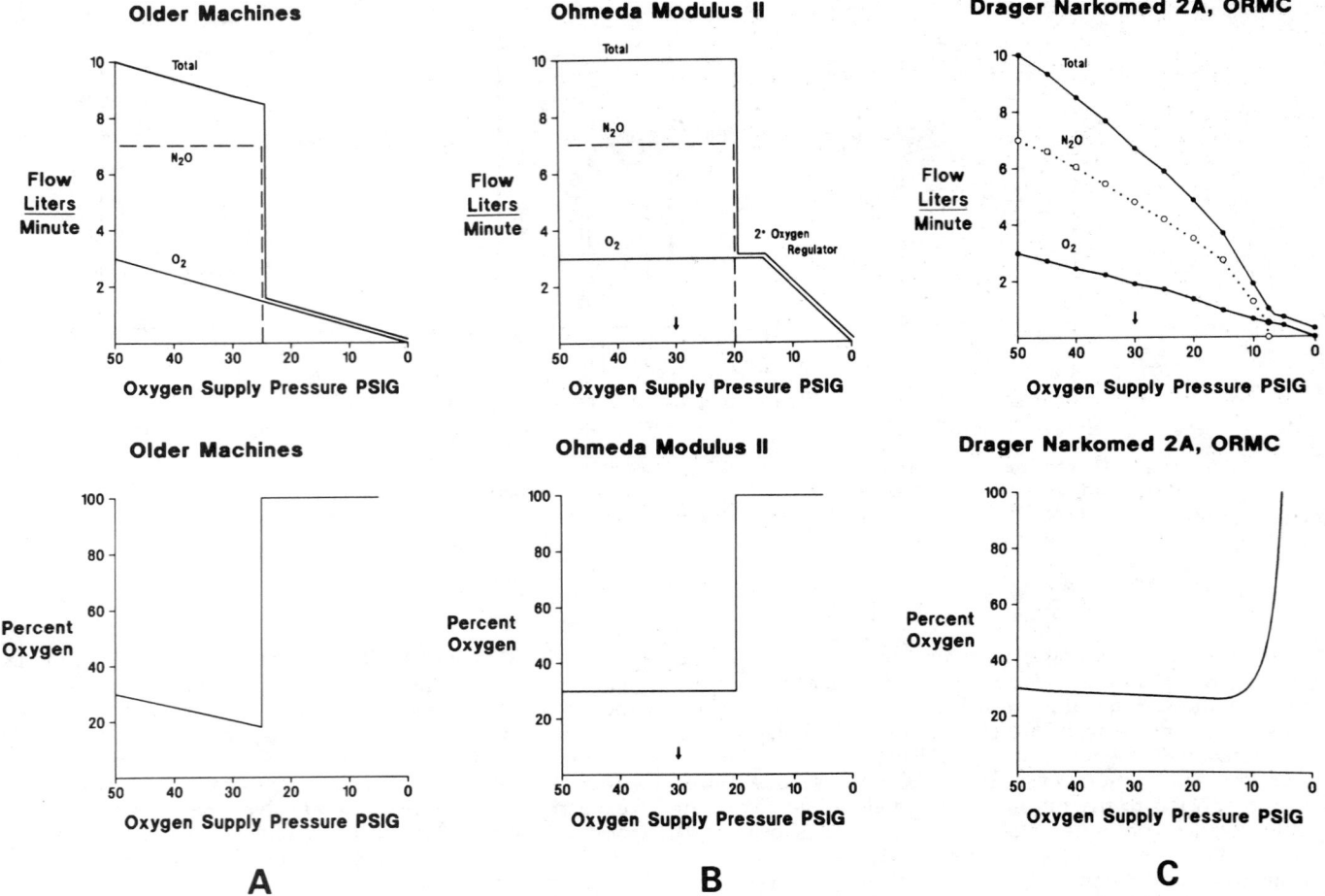

FIG. 19-6. Response of three anesthesia machines to a gradual decline in oxygen supply pressure. The responses of an older machine, an Ohmeda Modulus II, and a Drager Narkomed 2A are shown in *A, B,* and *C,* respectively. *Vertical arrows* represent the oxygen supply pressure at which the low oxygen pressure alarm sounds. See text for details.

FLOWMETER ASSEMBLY

The flowmeter assembly (Fig. 19-7) precisely controls and measures gas flow to the common gas outlet. The flow control valve regulates the amount of flow that enters a tapered, transparent flowtube known as a Thorpe tube. A mobile indicator float inside the flowtube indicates the amount of flow passing through the flow control valve. The quantity of flow is indicated on a scale associated with the flowtube.[2, 3]

Physical Principles of Flowmeters

Opening the flow control valve allows gas to travel through the space between the float and the flowtube. This space is known as the annular space (Fig. 19-8). The indicator float hovers freely in an equilibrium position in which the upward force resulting from gas flow equals the downward force on the float resulting from gravity at a given flow rate. The float moves to a new equilibrium position in the tube when flow is changed. These flowmeters are commonly referred to as constant pressure flowmeters because the pressure decrease across the float remains constant for all positions in the tube.[2, 12, 13]

Flowtubes are tapered, with the smallest diameter at the bottom of the tube and the largest diameter at the top. The term variable orifice designates this type of unit because the annular space between the float and the inner wall of the flowtube varies with the position of the float. The constriction created by the float can be tubular or orificial, depending upon the flow rate (Fig. 19-9). The gas characteristics that influence its flow rate through a given constriction are 1) its density, and 2) its viscosity. The annular space is tubular at low flow rates. Poiseuille's Law applies in this situation, and viscosity becomes dominant in determining gas flow rate. The annular space simulates an orifice at high flow rates, and gas flow rate then depends predominantly upon the density of the gas.[2, 12]

Components of Flowmeter Assembly

FLOW CONTROL VALVE ASSEMBLY. The flow control valve assembly is composed of a flow control knob, a needle valve, a valve seat, and a pair of valve stops.[2] The assembly can receive

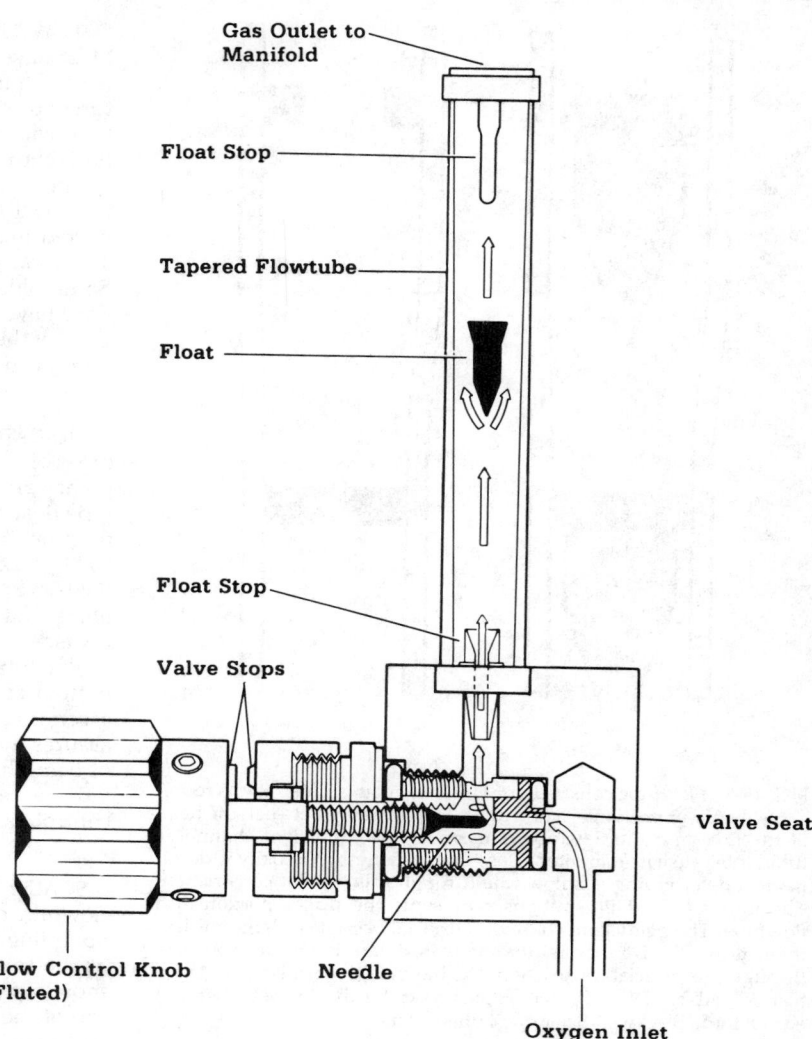

FIG. 19-7. Oxygen flowmeter assembly. The oxygen flowmeter assembly is composed of the flow control valve assembly plus the flowmeter subassembly. (Reprinted with permission. Bowie E, Huffman LM: The Anesthesia Machine: Essentials for Understanding. Madison, WI, Ohmeda, The BOC Group, 1985.)

its pneumatic input either directly from the pipeline source (50 PSIG) or from a second-stage pressure regulator.[3] The flow control valves are supplied by 50 PSIG on contemporary Drager machines such as the Narkomed 2A, 2B, and 3.[4, 9] In contrast, the Ohmeda Modulus II oxygen and nitrous oxide flow control valves are supplied by 14 PSIG and approximately 26 PSIG, respectively.[10]

The location of the needle valve in the valve seat changes to establish different orifices when the flow control valve is adjusted. Gas flow increases when the flow control valve is turned counterclockwise, and it decreases when the valve is turned clockwise. Extreme clockwise rotation damages the needle valve seat. Therefore, flow control valves are equipped with valve "stops" to prevent this occurrence.[3] The stops come into contact with each other at zero flow on most flow control valves. However, the oxygen flow control valve stops of the Ohmeda Modulus I, Modulus II, and Ohmeda 8000 are set at an oxygen flow rate of approximately 200 ml·min^{-1}.[5-7] Thus, on contemporary Ohmeda machines, minimum oxygen flow results from incomplete closure of the oxygen flow control valve. On contemporary Drager machines, the oxygen

FIG. 19-8. The annular space. The clearance between the head of the float and the flow tube is known as the annular space. It can be considered an equivalent to a circular channel of the same cross-sectioned area. (Redrawn with permission. Macintosh R, Mushin WW, Epstein HG: Physics for the Anaesthetist, 3rd ed. Oxford, Blackwell Scientific Publications, 1963.)

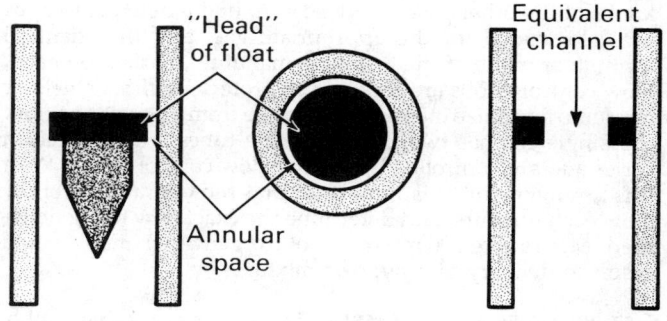

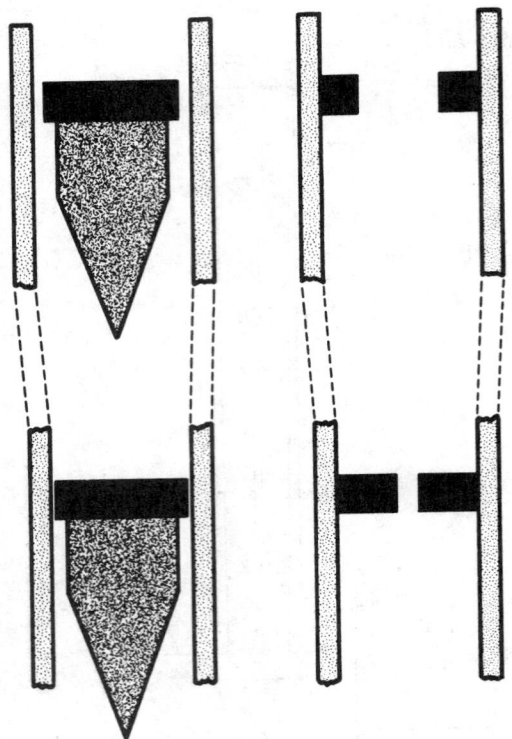

FIG. 19-9. Flowtube constriction. The lower pair of illustrations represents the lower portion of a flowtube. The clearance between the head of the float and the flowtube is narrow. The equivalent channel is tubular because its diameter is less than its length. Viscosity is dominant in determining gas flow rate through this tubular constriction. The upper pair of illustrations represents the upper portion of a flowtube. The equivalent channel is orificial because its length is less than its width. Density is dominant in determining gas flow rate through this orificial constriction. (Redrawn with permission. Macintosh R, Mushin WW, Epstein HG: Physics for the Anaesthetist, 3rd ed. Oxford, Blackwell Scientific Publications, 1963.)

flow control valve does close completely. Minimum oxygen flow enters the oxygen flow tube just downstream from the flow control valve.[4, 8, 9]

SAFETY FEATURES. Contemporary flow control valve assemblies have numerous safety features. The oxygen flow control knob is physically distinguishable from other gas knobs. It is distinctively fluted, projects beyond the control knobs of the other gases, and is larger in diameter. All knobs are color coded for the appropriate gas, and the chemical formula or name of the gas is permanently marked on each. Flow control knobs are recessed or protected with a shield or barrier to minimize inadvertent change from a preset position. If a single gas has two flowtubes, the tubes are arranged in series and are controlled by a single flow control valve.[1] With this arrangement, it is important that the operator carefully view each flowtube and determine the exact flow being delivered. Misreading 200 ml $\cdot$ min^{-1} of oxygen as 2 l $\cdot$ min^{-1} could result in delivery of a hypoxic mixture.

FLOWMETER SUBASSEMBLY. The flowmeter subassembly consists of the flowtube, the indicator float with float stops, and the indicator scale.[2]

FLOWTUBES. Contemporary flowtubes are made of glass. Most have a single taper in which the inner diameter of the flowtube increases uniformly from bottom to top. Manufacturers provide double flowtubes for oxygen and nitrous oxide to provide better visual discrimination at low flow rates. A fine flowtube indicates flow from approximately 200 ml $\cdot$ min^{-1} to 1 l $\cdot$ min^{-1}, and a course flowtube indicates flow from approximately 1 l $\cdot$ min^{-1} to 10–12 l $\cdot$ min^{-1}. The two tubes are connected in series and supplied by a single flow control valve. The total gas flow is that shown on the higher flowmeter. Some older machines manufactured before the Z79.8 Standard have two flow tubes for a single gas arranged in parallel. Each of the tubes has a flow control valve. The total flow is the sum of the individual flows.[2]

INDICATOR FLOATS AND FLOAT STOPS. Several different types of bobbins or floats are used to indicate flow on contemporary anesthesia machines. Ohmeda employs a plumb-bob type float on the Modulus I and Modulus II, a rotating skirted float on the Excel Series, and a ball float on the Ohmeda 8000.[5–7] Drager machines are equipped with sapphire ball floats.[4, 8, 9] Flow is read at the top of plumb-bob and skirted floats, but it is read at the center of the ball on the ball-type floats.[2]

Flowtubes are equipped with float stops at the top and bottom of the tube. The upper stop prevents the float from ascending to the top of the tube and plugging the outlet. It also assures that the float will be visible at maximum flows instead of being hidden in the manifold. The bottom float stop provides a central foundation for the indicator when the flow control valve is turned off.[2, 3]

SCALE. The flowmeter scale can be marked directly on the flowtube or located to the right of the tube.[1] Gradations corresponding to equal increments in flow rate are closer together at the top of the scale because the annular space increases more rapidly than does the internal diameter from bottom to top of the tube. Rib guides are used in some flowtubes with ball-type indicators to minimize this compression effect. They are tapered glass ridges that run the length of the tube. There are usually three rib guides that are equally spaced around the inner circumference of the tube. In the presence of rib guides, the annular space from the bottom to the top of the tube increases almost proportionally with the internal diameter. This results in a nearly linear scale.[2] Rib guides are employed on Drager flowtubes.

SAFETY FEATURES. The flowmeter subassembly for each gas on the Ohmeda Modulus I and Modulus II is housed in an independent, color-coded, pin-specific module. The flowtubes are adjacent to a gas-specific, color-coded backing. The flow scale and the chemical formula or name of the gas are permanently etched on the backing to the right of the flowtube.[5, 6] Flowmeter scales are individually hand calibrated by use of the specific float to provide a high degree of accuracy. The tube, float, and scale make an inseparable unit. The entire set must be replaced if any component is damaged.[3, 5, 6, 10]

Drager does not use a modular system for the flowmeter subassembly. The flow scale, chemical symbol, and the gas-specific color coding are etched directly onto the flowtube.[4, 8, 9] The scale in use is obvious when two flowtubes for the same gas are used.

Arrangement of Flowmeters

In 1963 Eger *et al* demonstrated that, in the presence of a flowmeter leak, a hypoxic mixture is less likely to occur if the oxygen flowmeter is located downstream from all other flowmeters.[14] Figure 19-10 is a contemporary version of that depicted in Eger's original publication. The unused air flowtube has a substantial leak. Nitrous oxide and oxygen flow rates are set at a ratio of 3 : 1.

A potentially dangerous arrangement is shown in Figures 19-10A and B because the nitrous oxide flowmeter is located in the downstream position. A hypoxic mixture can result because a substantial portion of oxygen flow passes through the leak and all nitrous oxide is directed to the common gas outlet. A safer configuration that complies with the Z79.8 Machine Standard is shown in Figures 19-10C and D. The oxygen flowmeter is located in the downstream position. A portion of the nitrous oxide flow escapes through the leak, and the remainder goes toward the common gas outlet. A hypoxic mixture is less likely because all the oxygen flow is advanced by the nitrous oxide.[14] Drager flowmeters are arranged as in Figure 19-10C, and Ohmeda flowmeters, Figure 19-10D. A broken oxygen flowtube, despite these "fail safe" arrangements, still can produce a hypoxic mixture.[15]

Problems with Flowmeters

LEAKS. Flowmeters are a common source of leaks. They can occur at the junction between the glass flowtube and the metal manifold because of problems associated with O-rings and gaskets. Glass flowtubes are the most fragile pneumatic component of the anesthesia machine. Gross damage is usually apparent, but subtle cracks and chips may be overlooked, resulting in errors of delivered flows.[15] As mentioned above, an oxygen flowmeter leak can produce a hypoxic mixture, regardless of flowmeter arrangement.

Flowmeter leaks are a substantial hazard because they are downstream from all machine safety devices except the oxygen analyzer. A broken oxygen flowtube of a contemporary anesthesia machine is shown in Figure 19-11. This leak was readily identified because the oxygen analyzer read much lower than expected. An appropriate preoperative leak test must be performed before each case. Drager recommends a positive-pressure leak test, and Ohmeda recommends a negative-pressure leak test (see Checking Anesthesia Machines).

INACCURACY. Flow error can occur even when flowmeters are assembled properly with appropriate components. Dirt or static electricity can cause a float to stick, and the actual flow may be higher or lower than that indicated. Sticking is more common in the low flow range because the annular space is smaller. A damaged float can cause inaccurate readings because of the precise relationship between the float and the flowtube. Back pressure from the breathing circuit can cause a float to drop so that it reads less than the actual flow. Finally, if flowmeters are not aligned properly in vertical position, readings can be inaccurate because tilting distorts the annular space.[2, 15, 17]

AMBIGUOUS SCALE. Before the standardization of flowmeter scales and the widespread use of oxygen analyzers, at least two deaths resulted from confusion created by ambiguous scales.[15, 17, 18] The operator read the float position beside an adjacent but erroneous scale in both cases. Today this is less likely to occur because contemporary flowmeter scales are marked either directly onto or to the right of the appropriate flowtube.[1] Confusion is minimized when the scale is etched directly onto the tube.

PROPORTIONING SYSTEMS

Manufacturers have equipped newer machines with proportioning systems in an attempt to prevent delivery of a hypoxic mixture. Nitrous oxide and oxygen are interfaced either mechanically or pneumatically so that the minimum oxygen concentration at the common outlet is 25%.

Ohmeda Link-25 Proportion Limiting Control System

Ohmeda uses the Link-25 System on the Ohmeda Modulus I and Modulus II, the Ohmeda 8000, and the Ohmeda Excel Series. The heart of the system is the mechanical integration of the nitrous oxide and oxygen flow control valves. It allows independent adjustment of either valve yet automatically intercedes to maintain a minimum 25% oxygen concentration with a maximum nitrous oxide/oxygen flow ratio of 3:1. An increased nitrous oxide flow beyond this maximum ratio results in a proportional 3:1 increase in oxygen flow.[5-7, 10]

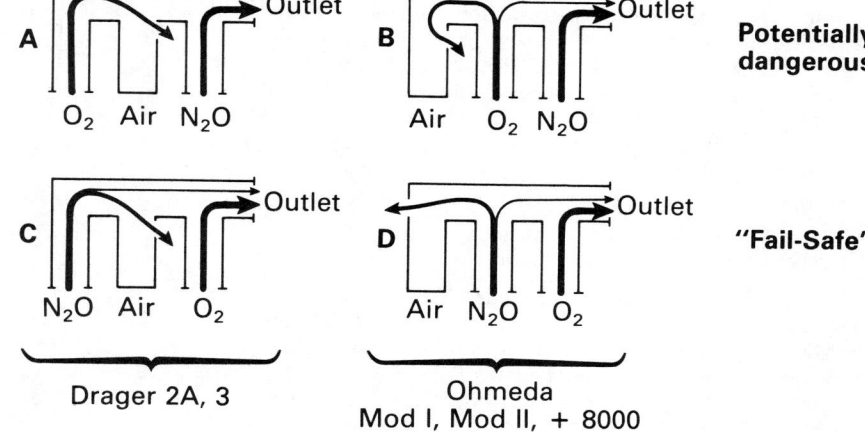

FIG. 19-10. Flowmeter sequence—a cause of hypoxia. In the event of a flowmeter leak, a potentially dangerous arrangement exists when nitrous oxide is located in the downstream position (A and B). The safest configuration exists when oxygen is located in the downstream position (C and D). See text for details. (Redrawn with permission. Eger EI, Hylton RR, Irwin RH *et al*: Anesthetic flow meter sequence—A cause for hypoxia. Anesthesiology 24:396, 1963.)

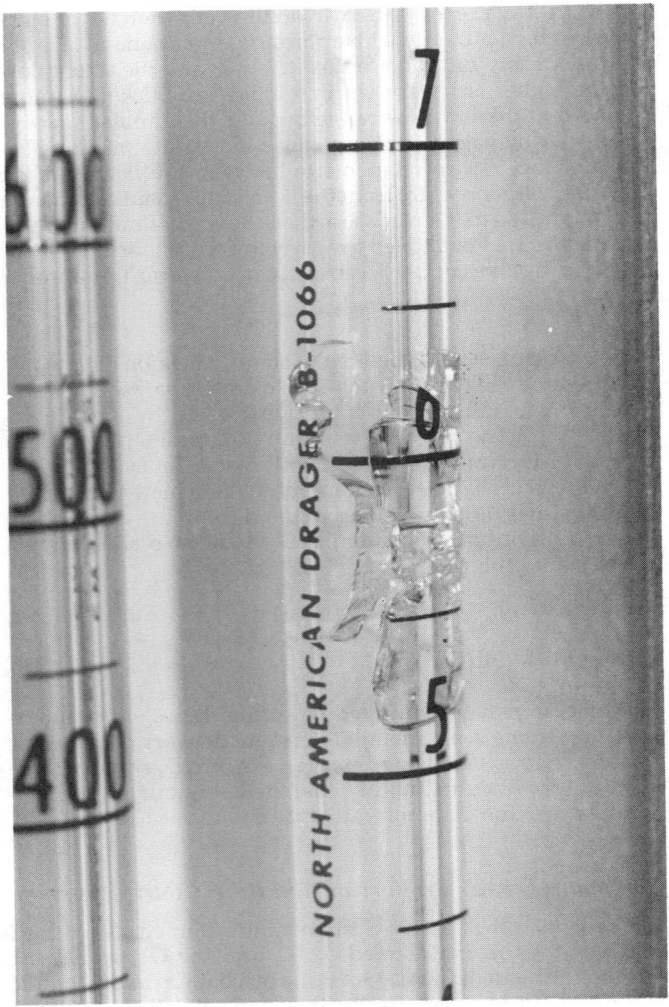

FIG. 19-11. Broken oxygen flowtube.

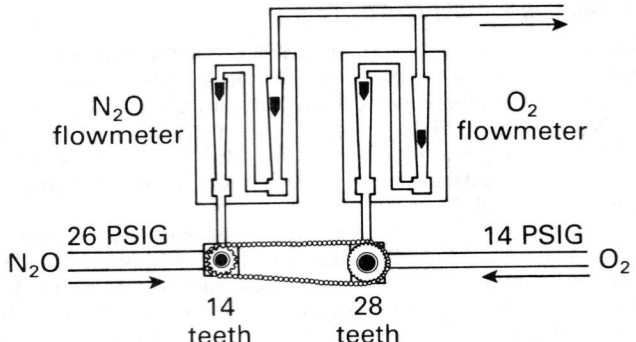

FIG. 19-12. Ohmeda Link-25 Proportion Limiting Control System. See text for details.

l·min^{-1} (Fig. 19-13). The ORMC limits nitrous oxide flow to prevent delivery of a hypoxic mixture.[4, 8, 9] This is unlike the Ohmeda Link-25, which actively increases oxygen flow.

A schematic of the ORMC is shown in Figure 19-14. It is composed of an oxygen chamber, a nitrous oxide chamber, and a nitrous oxide slave control valve; all are interconnected by a mobile horizontal shaft. The pneumatic input into the device is from the oxygen and the nitrous oxide flowmeters. These flowmeters are unique because they have specific resistors located downstream from the flow control valves. These resistors create back pressures that are directed to the oxygen and nitrous oxide chambers. The relative value of these resistors ultimately dictates the value of the controlled fresh gas oxygen concentration. The back pressure in the oxygen and nitrous oxide chamber pushes against rubber diaphragms that are attached to the mobile horizontal shaft. Movement of the shaft regulates the nitrous oxide slave control valve, which feeds the nitrous oxide flow control valve.[8, 16]

If the oxygen pressure is proportionally higher than the nitrous oxide pressure, the nitrous oxide slave control valve opens to a larger degree, allowing more nitrous oxide to flow.

Figure 19-12 Shows the Ohmeda Modulus II Link-25 System. The nitrous oxide and oxygen flow control valves are identical. A 14-tooth sprocket is attached to the nitrous oxide flow control valve, and a 28-tooth sprocket is attached to the oxygen flow control valve. A chain physically links the sprockets. When the nitrous oxide flow control valve is turned two revolutions, or 28 teeth, the oxygen flow control valve will revolve once because of the 2:1 gear ratio. The final 3:1 flow ratio results because the nitrous oxide flow control valve is supplied by approximately 26 PSIG, whereas the oxygen flow control valve is supplied by 14 PSIG. Thus, the combination of the mechanical and pneumatic aspects of the system yields the final oxygen concentration.[6, 10]

Drager Oxygen Ratio Monitor Controller

Drager's proportioning system, the ORMC, is employed on the Drager Narkomed 2A, 2B, and 3. It is a pneumatic oxygen/nitrous oxide interlock system designed to maintain a fresh gas oxygen concentration of at least 25 ± 3%. The device controls the fresh gas oxygen concentration to levels substantially higher than 25% at oxygen flow rates of less than 1

FIG. 19-13. Oxygen concentration control curve for the Drager Narkomed 2A. (Redrawn with permission. Narkomed 2A Anesthesia System. Technical Service Manual. Telford, PA, North American Drager, June 1985.)

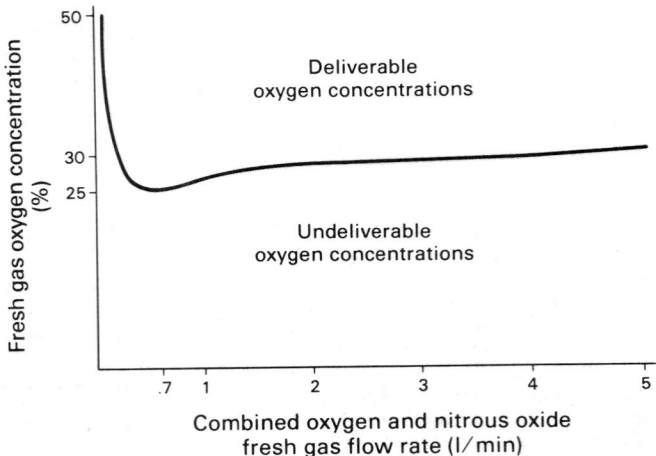

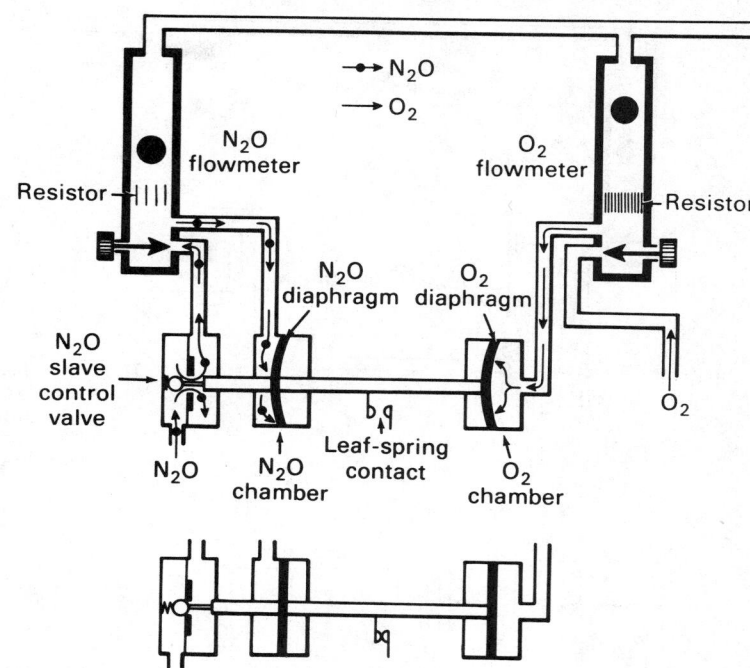

FIG. 19-14. Drager Oxygen Ratio Monitor Controller. See text for details. (Redrawn with permission. Schreiber P: Safety guidelines for anesthesia systems. Telford, North American Drager, 1985.)

As the nitrous oxide flow is increased manually, the nitrous oxide pressure forces the shaft toward the oxygen chamber. The valve opening becomes more restrictive and limits the nitrous oxide flow to the flowmeter. Figure 19-14 illustrates the action of a single ORMC under different sets of circumstances. The back pressure exerted on the oxygen diaphragm, in the upper configuration, is greater than that exerted on the nitrous oxide diaphragm. This causes the horizontal shaft to move to the left, opening the nitrous oxide slave control valve. Nitrous oxide can then proceed to its flow control valve and out through the flowmeter. In the bottom configuration, the nitrous oxide slave control valve is closed because of inadequate oxygen back pressure.[8, 16]

The ORMC has a dual role. It serves as a proportioning device and a monitor. An electrical contact attached to the mobile horizontal shaft activates an alarm when the ORMC is limiting the nitrous oxide flow to prevent a hypoxic fresh gas mixture. The alarm is functional only in the "O₂/N₂O" mode and not in the "All Gases" mode. However, the ORMC continues to control the oxygen–nitrous oxide ratio, regardless of the alarm status.[4, 8, 9]

Limitations

Proportioning systems are not fool-proof. Machines equipped with proportioning systems still can deliver a hypoxic mixture under the following conditions.

WRONG SUPPLY GAS. Both the Link-25 and the ORMC will be fooled if a gas other than oxygen is present in the oxygen pipeline. In the Link-25 System, the nitrous oxide and oxygen flow control valves will continue to be mechanically linked, and a hypoxic mixture will proceed to the common outlet. The oxygen rubber diaphragm of the ORMC will recognize adequate "oxygen" pressure, and flow of both the wrong gas plus nitrous oxide will result. The oxygen analyzer is the only

machine monitor that will detect this condition in both systems.

DEFECTIVE PNEUMATICS OR MECHANICS. Normal operation of the Ohmeda Link-25 and the Drager ORMC is contingent upon pneumatic and mechanical integrity. Pneumatic integrity in the Ohmeda System depends upon properly functioning second-stage regulators. A nitrous oxide–oxygen ratio other than 3:1 will result if the regulators are not precise. The chain connecting the two sprockets must be intact. A 97% nitrous oxide concentration can result if the chain is cut or broken.[19] In the Drager System, a functional Oxygen Failure Protection Device (OFPD) is necessary to supply appropriate pressure to the ORMC. The mechanical aspects of the ORMC, such as the rubber diaphragms, flowtube resistors, and nitrous oxide, must likewise be intact.

LEAKS DOWNSTREAM. The ORMC and the Link-25 function at the level of the flow control valves. A leak downstream from these devices (Figs. 19-15 and 19-16), such as a broken oxygen flowtube, can result in the delivery of a hypoxic mixture. Oxygen escapes through the leak, and the predominant gas delivered at the common outlet is nitrous oxide. The oxygen analyzer is the only machine safety device that can detect the problem.[16] Drager recommends a preoperative positive-pressure leak test to detect such a leak.[4, 8, 9] Ohmeda recommends a preoperative negative-pressure leak test because of the check valve located at the common outlet[5, 6, 20, 21] (see Checking Anesthesia Machines).

INERT GAS ADMINISTRATION. Administration of a third inert gas, such as helium, nitrogen, or carbon dioxide, can result in a hypoxic mixture because present-day proportioning systems link only nitrous oxide and oxygen.[5–9] The use of an oxygen analyzer is mandatory if the operator uses a third inert gas.

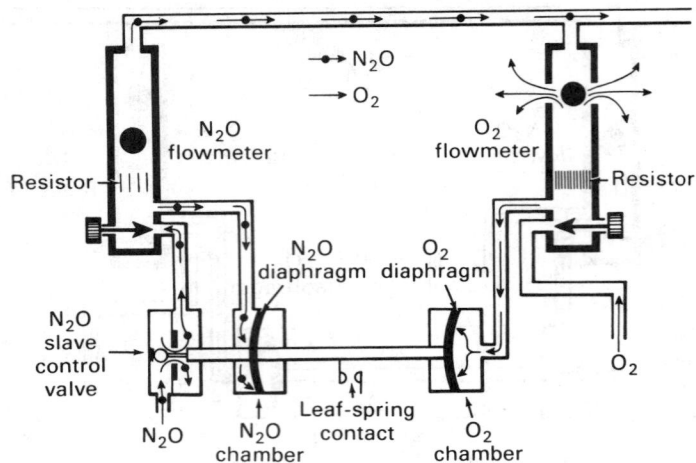

FIG. 19-15. Leak downstream from the Oxygen Ratio Monitor Controller (ORMC). A leak downstream from the ORMC, such as a broken oxygen flowtube, can result in the delivery of a hypoxic mixture. Drager recommends a preoperative positive pressure leak check to detect a leak of this type.

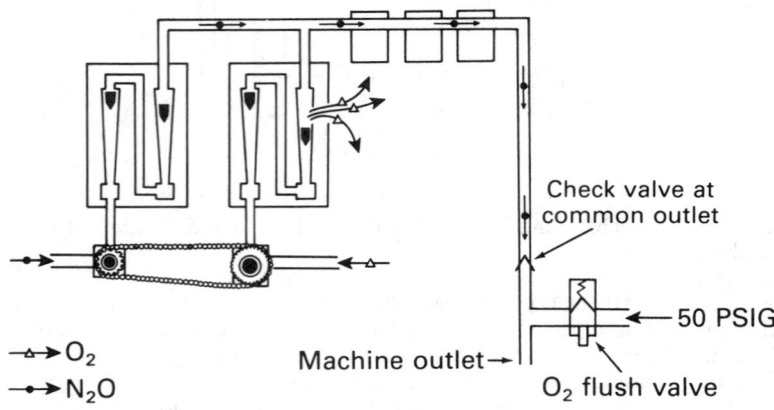

FIG. 19-16. Leak downstream from the Link-25. Proportion Limiting Control System. A leak downstream from the Link-25, such as a broken oxygen flowtube, can result in delivery of a hypoxic mixture. Ohmeda recommends a preoperative negative pressure leak test to detect a leak of this type.

VAPORIZERS

Through the years, vaporizers have evolved from rudimetary ether inhalers to the present sophisticated variable-bypass, temperature-compensated vaporizers. Bubble-through copper kettle vaporizers are no longer manufactured. Therefore, this section will be limited to newer variable-bypass vaporizers. Certain physical principles are reviewed briefly before the discussion so that the design, construction, and operation of these vaporizers can be understood.

PHYSICS

Vapor Pressure

Contemporary halogenated inhalation agents exist in the liquid state at room temperature. When a volatile liquid is in a closed container, molecules escape from the liquid phase to the vapor phase until the number of molecules in the vapor phase is constant. These molecules bombard the wall of the container and create a pressure known as the saturated vapor pressure. More molecules enter the vapor phase, and the vapor pressure increases as the temperature increases. Vapor pressure is independent of atmospheric pressure and is contingent only on the physical characteristics of the liquid and

the temperature. The boiling point of a liquid is that temperature at which the vapor pressure equals atmospheric pressure.[22-24]

Latent Heat of Vaporization

Energy must be expended to convert a molecule from the liquid to gaseous state because the molecules of a liquid tend to cohere. The latent heat of vaporization is defined as the number of calories required to change 1 g of liquid into vapor without a temperature change. The energy for vaporization must come from the liquid itself or an outside source. The temperature of the liquid decreases during vaporization in the absence of an outside energy source. Energy loss can lead to significant decreases in temperature of the remaining liquid. This temperature decrease will greatly decrease vaporization.[22, 24, 25]

Specific Heat

The specific heat of a substance is the number of calories required to increase the temperature of 1 g of a substance by 1° C.[22, 24, 26] The substance can be solid, liquid, or gas. The concept of specific heat is important to the design, operation, and construction of vaporizers because it is applicable in two ways: 1) the specific heat value for an inhalation agent is important because it indicates how much heat must be supplied to the liquid to maintain a constant temperature when heat is lost during vaporization; 2) manufacturers select vaporizer metals that have a high specific heat to minimize temperature changes associated with vaporization.

Thermal Conductivity

Thermal conductivity is a measure of the speed with which heat flows through a substance. The higher the thermal conductivity, the better the substance conducts heat.[22] Vaporizers are constructed of metals that have relatively high thermal conductivity, which helps maintain a uniform temperature.

VAPORIZER CLASSIFICATION

The Ohmeda Tec 4 and the Drager Vapor 19.1 are classified as variable-bypass, flow-over, temperature-compensated, agent-specific, out-of-circuit vaporizers. Variable-bypass refers to the method for regulating output concentration. After the total gas flow enters the vaporizer's inlet, the concentration control dial adjusts the amount of gas that goes to the bypass chamber and the vaporizing chamber. The gas channeled to the vaporizing chamber flows over the liquid agent and becomes saturated. Thus, flow-over refers to the vaporization method. The Tec 4 and the Vapor 19.1 are classified as temperature compensated because they are equipped with an automatic temperature-compensating device that helps maintain a constant vaporizer output over a wide range of temperatures. These vaporizers are classified as agent specific and out-of-circuit because they are designed to accommodate a single agent and to be located outside the breathing circuit. Conversely, copper kettle vaporizers are classified as measured-flow, bubble-through, non–temperature-compensated, multiple-agent, out-of-circuit vaporizers.[22]

BASIC DESIGN PRINCIPLES

The total gas flow in a variable-bypass vaporizer enters the vaporizer's inlet and splits into two portions, as shown in Figure 19-17. The first portion, which represents less than 20% of the total gas flow, passes through the vaporizing chamber, where it is enriched or saturated with vapor of the liquid anesthetic agent. The second portion, which represents more than 80% of the total gas flow, goes directly through the bypass chamber. Finally, both partial gas flows rejoin at the vaporizer outlet. The ratio of the two partial gas flows depends on the ratio of resistances in the two paths, that is, the resistance in the bypass chamber compared with the resistance in the vaporizing chamber. The concentration control dial can be located in the bypass chamber or in the vaporizing chamber outlet. A change in the dial setting causes a change in resistance, which alters the gas flow ratio.[27]

FACTORS THAT INFLUENCE VAPORIZER OUTPUT

The output of an ideal vaporizer should be constant at varying conditions such as flow rates, temperatures, back pressures, and carrier gases. Designing such a vaporizer is difficult because, as ambient conditions change, the physical properties of gases and of vaporizers themselves can change.[27] Contemporary vaporizers approach being ideal but still have some limitations. Several factors are listed below that can influence vaporizer output.

Flow Rate

Variable-bypass vaporizer output varies with the rate of gas flowing through it. This is particularly notable at extremes of flow rates. The output of all variable-bypass vaporizers is less than the dial setting at low flow rates (less than $250\ ml \cdot min^{-1}$).

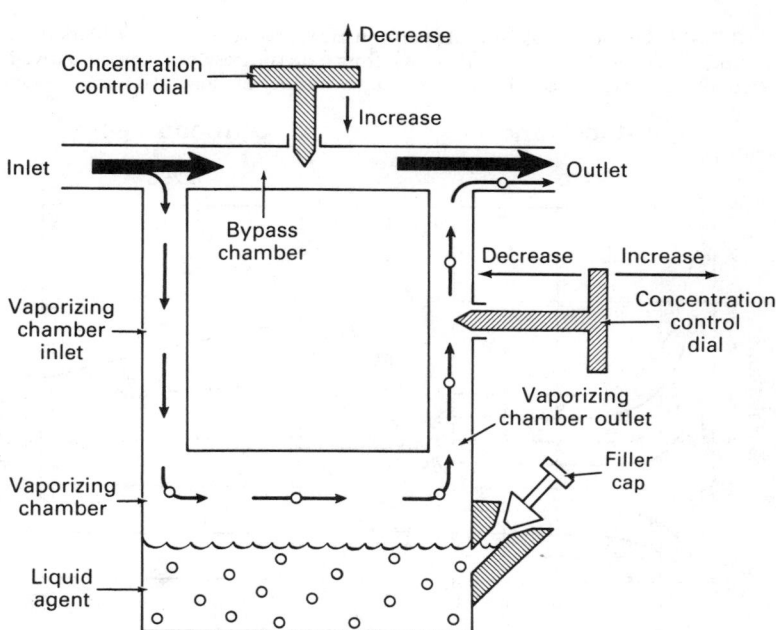

FIG. 19-17. Generic variable bypass vaporizer. See text for details.

This results from the relatively high specific gravity of volatile anesthetic agents. Insufficient pressure is generated at low flow rates in the vaporizing chamber to upwardly advance the molecules. At extremely high flow rates such as 15 l·min⁻¹, the output of most variable-bypass vaporizers is less than the dial setting. This is attributed to incomplete mixing and saturation in the vaporizing chamber. Also, the resistance characteristics of the bypass chamber and the vaporizing chamber can vary as flow increases. This can result in decreased output concentration.[27]

Figure 19-18 shows vaporizer output *versus* flow rate performance curves of three halothane vaporizers. These are the Fluotec Mark II, Ohmeda Tech 4, and Drager Vapor 19.1. In contrast to the older Fluotec Mark II, the output of contemporary vaporizers is near linear over a wide range of flow rates because of design improvements. An extensive wick and baffling system is employed in the Tec 4 and Vapor 19.1, which increases the effective surface area of the vaporizing chamber.[3, 28, 29] Also, both vaporizers have constant resistance characteristics over clinically useful flow rates.

Temperature

The output of older non-temperature-compensated vaporizers varies considerably with changes in temperature. This occurs because vapor pressure is a function of temperature. The output of contemporary temperature-compensated vaporizers, however, is almost linear over a wide range of temperatures. Several improvements in design are responsible for this linearity. Manufacturers have incorporated an automatic temperature-compensating mechanism in the bypass chamber to help maintain a constant vaporizer output with varying temperatures.[3, 28, 29] The valve can be a bimetallic strip or an expansion element. In either case, gas flow is apportioned in favor of the bypass chamber as temperature increases.[27] Wicks are placed in direct contact with the metal wall of the vaporizer to help replace heat that is used for vaporization. To minimize heat loss, vaporizers are constructed with metals with relatively high specific heat and high thermal conductivity.

Figure 19-19 shows vaporizer output *versus* temperature performance curves for the Ohmeda Tec 4. Within the temperature range of 20 to 35°C, there is only a slight increase in vaporizer output associated with an increase in temperature.[29] Accuracy cannot be assured at temperatures outside this range because vapor pressure varies nonlinearly with temperature whereas compensation varies linearly.

Intermittent Back Pressure

Intermittent back pressure associated with positive-pressure ventilation or oxygen flush can result in higher vaporizer output concentration than the dialed setting. This phenomenon is known as the pumping effect.[22, 27, 30–32] It is more pronounced at low flow rates, low dial settings, and low levels of liquid anesthetic in the vaporizing chamber. Additionally, the ventilator settings themselves are important because the pumping effect is exacerbated at rapid respiratory rates, high peak pressure, and at rapid decreases in pressure during expiration.[28–32] The Ohmeda Tec 4 and Drager Vapor 19.1 are relatively immune from the pumping effect, however, it is clinically important with older variable-bypass vaporizers such as the Fluotec Mark II.[28–30]

One proposed mechanism for the pumping effect is described as follows. Pressure is transmitted in a retrograde manner from the patient circuit to the vaporizer during the inspiratory phase of positive-pressure ventilation. This produces a no-flow state within the vaporizer. Gas molecules are compressed in both the bypass chamber and the vaporizing chamber. Then the back pressure is suddenly released during the expiratory phase of positive-pressure ventilation. Vapor exits the vaporizing chamber by two routes. One portion leaves in the conventional manner through the vaporizing chamber outlet. However, another portion exits in a retrograde manner through the vaporizing chamber inlet and joins

FIG. 19-18. Output *versus* flow rate performance curves of the Fluotec Mark II, the Ohmeda Tec 4, and the Drager Vapor 19.1. (Redrawn from data courtesy of Ohmeda, a division of the BOC Group, Madison, Wisconsin, and from data courtesy of North American Drager, Telford, PA.

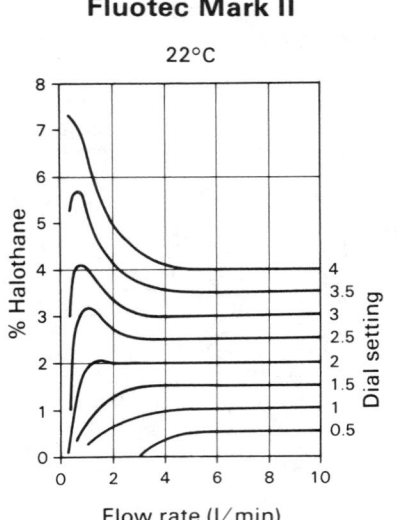

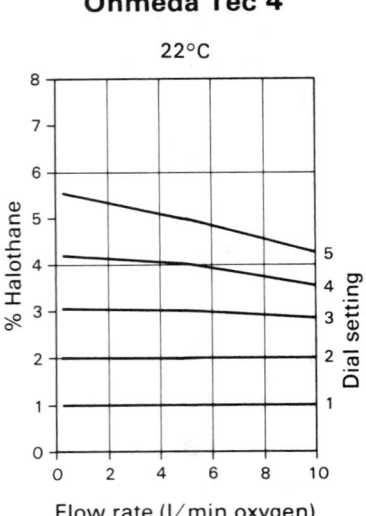

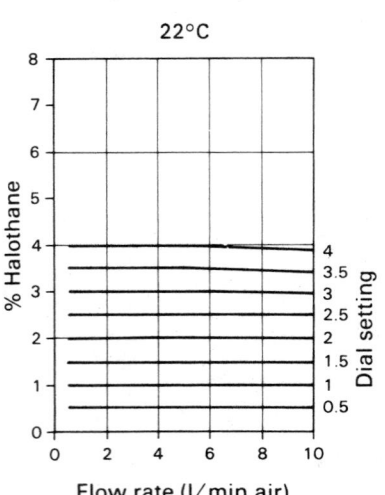

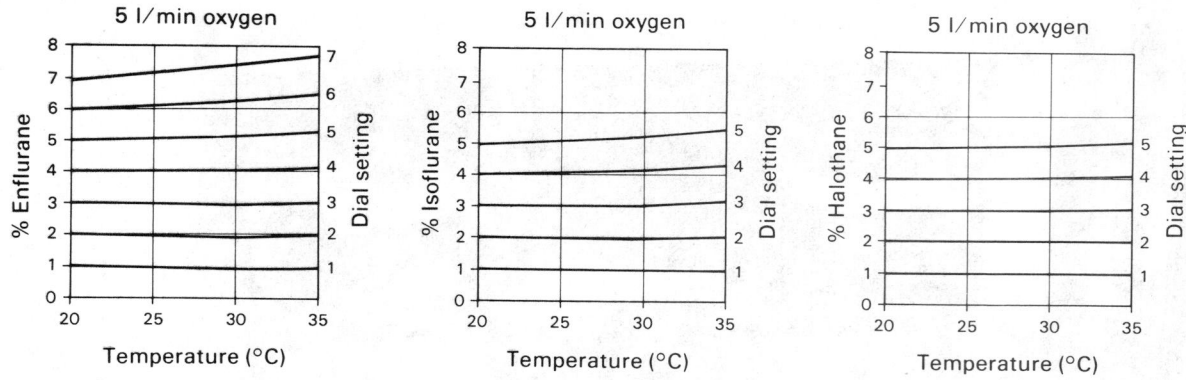

FIG. 19-19. Output *versus* temperature performance curves of Ohmeda Tec 4 Vaporizers. (Redrawn with permission. Tec 4 Continuous Flow Vaporizer Operator's Manual. Steeton, Ohmeda, The BOC Group, 1986.)

the bypass flow. This occurs because the output resistance of the bypass chamber is lower than that of the vaporizing chamber, particularly at low dial settings. The enhanced output concentration results from the increment of vapor that travels in the retrograde direction.[27, 30-32]

Ohmeda and Drager have addressed the pumping effect in the following manner. The vaporizing chambers of the Tec 4 and the Vapor 19.1 are smaller than those of older variable-bypass vaporizers such as the Fluotec Mark II (750 ml).[28, 29, 31] Therefore, no substantial volumes of vapor can be discharged from the vaporizing chamber into the bypass chamber during the expiratory phase. The Drager 19.1 has a patented, long spiral tube that serves as the inlet to the vaporizing chamber.[28, 31] When the pressure in the vaporizing chamber is released, some of the vapor enters this tube in a retrograde manner. The vapor does not enter the bypass chamber, however, because of tube length.[31] The Tec 4 has an extensive baffle system in the vaporizing chamber, and a one-way check valve has been inserted at the common outlet to minimize the pumping effect. This check valve may attenuate the pressure increase but does not prevent it, because gas still flows from the flowmeters during inspiration.[22, 33]

Carrier Gas Composition

The carrier gas composition influences the output of contemporary variable-bypass vaporizers.[34-40] Vaporizer output is approximately 10% less than the dial setting when the carrier gas is 100% nitrous oxide *versus* 100% oxygen.[39] A biphasic response occurs when the carrier gas is switched quickly from 100% oxygen to 100% nitrous oxide. First, there is a rapid initial 20–25% decrease in vaporizer output, which lasts less than 1 min. Then, during the next few minutes there is a gradual increase in vaporizer output until a new steady-state concentration is established. This concentration is approximately 10% less than the dial setting when 100% oxygen was the carrier gas.[39, 40] The rapid initial decrease in vaporizer output is attributed to the fact that nitrous oxide is more soluble than oxygen in halogenated liquid.[39] The steady-state response is ascribed to the difference in viscosity of the two gases, which presumably causes a different flow distribution within the vaporizer. When nitrous oxide is the carrier gas compared with oxygen, relatively more nitrous oxide flows through the bypass chamber. This results in a lower output

concentration.[36, 40] At routine flow rates and concentrations, this phenomenon probably is clinically insignificant.

SPECIFIC VAPORIZERS

Ohmeda Tec 4

The Ohmeda Tec 4 vaporizer system is used on all contemporary Ohmeda anesthesia machines, including the Modulus II, the Ohmeda 8000, and the Excel Series. As many as three vaporizers are attached to the Selectatec manifold, which provides a physical foundation for the system. A safety interlock mechanism ensures that only one vaporizer can be turned on when two or more adjacent Tec 4s are used. Turning on one vaporizer automatically activates an extension rod interlock mechanism that locks off the remaining vaporizer(s). In the "off" position, the vaporizers are automatically isolated from all circuits. This prevents delivery of more than one agent to the machine outlet. The same "on" action also automatically opens the inlet and outlet manifold port valves, which places the vaporizer in line. A locking lever located behind the concentration control dial ensures that the vaporizer inlet and outlet ports seal correctly. The Tec 4 can be turned on only when this lever is located in the "lock" position.[29]

Each vaporizer has a single control dial with a concentration scale calibrated in percentage of anesthetic vapor per total volume. Turning on a vaporizer requires two simultaneous actions. The operator must depress the control dial release button, located to the left of the concentration control dial, and rotate the control dial in a counterclockwise direction. This prevents accidental displacement of the control dial from the "off" to "on" position. Two filling mechanisms are available, including the screw cap filler and the agent-specific keyed filler. The low location of the filler port minimizes overfilling in either case. The liquid capacity of the Tec 4 is 125 ml, and the amount retained by the wick system is 35 ml.[29]

A vaporizer can be removed easily from the manifold if the control dial is in the "off" position and if the locking lever is in the "unlock" position. The manifold port valves continue to assure airtight seals. However, if the center vaporizer is removed, the extension rod interlock mechanism will not function, and two inhalation agents can be administered simultaneously (see Fig. 19-20). Thus, if the center vaporizer is

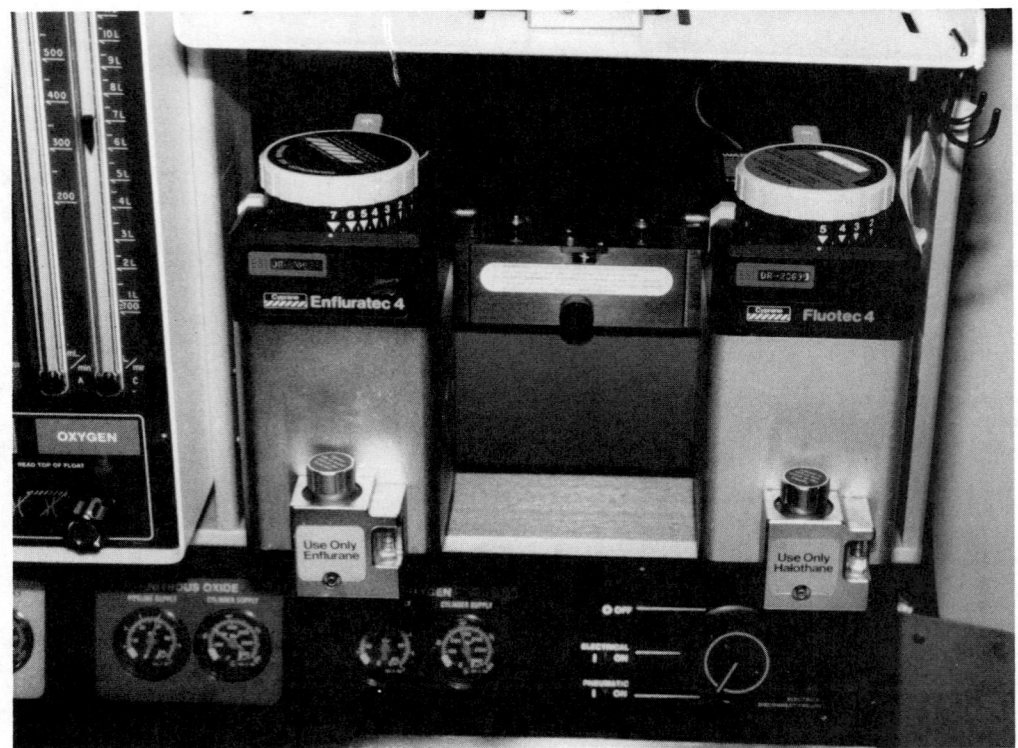

FIG. 19-20. Ohmeda Modulus II with center vaporizer removed. Simultaneous administration of inhalation agents is possible in this configuration. The dial settings of the enflurane and halothane vaporizers were intentionally set at 7% and 5%, respectively, for this illustration. Up to 12% inhalation agent can be delivered. The warning label between the two vaporizers reads, "If this label is visible, interlock is disabled. If only two vaporizers are used, one shall cover this label."

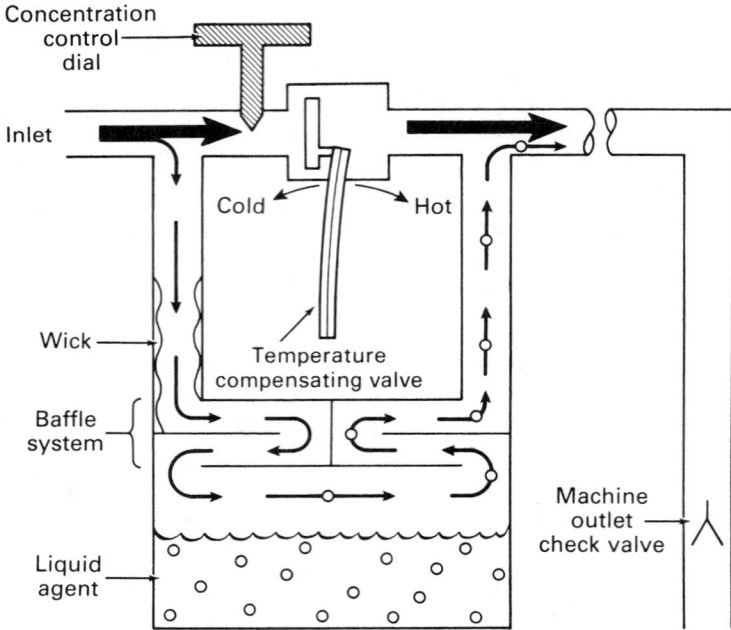

FIG. 19-21. Simplified schematic of the Ohmeda Tec 4 Vaporizer. See text for details.

removed, either the left or right vaporizer should be moved to the center position, as indicated by the manifold label. The extension rod interlock system will then be functional because the two remaining vaporizers are adjacent.[6]

A simplified diagram of the Ohmeda Tec 4 is shown in Figure 19-21. The total fresh gas flow enters the vaporizer's inlet and splits into two portions. The smaller first portion goes to the vaporizing chamber, which employs a wick and baffle system. The carrier gas becomes saturated with an agent and rejoins the larger bypass flow at the vaporizer outlet. The concentration control valve determines the relative flows through the vaporizing and bypass chambers. Temperature compensation is automatically accomplished by the bimetallic strip, which influences flow through the bypass chamber. A one-way check valve is incorporated at the common outlet to minimize the pumping effect.[3]

Drager Vapor 19.1

The Drager Vapor Exclusion System is used on the Narkomed 2A and Narkomed 3. As many as three vaporizers are attached semipermanently to the vaporizer mounting bracket, which is located to the right of the flowmeter bank (Fig. 19-22). A cam and lever interlock system is incorporated into the vaporizer bank, which prevents more than one vaporizer from being activated. All unused vaporizers are locked in the zero position. This external interlock system is different than the system employed by Ohmeda, in which the exclusion rods are an internal component of each vaporizer.[28]

When the control dial is set in the "O" position (off), fresh gas from the flowmeter passes with almost no resistance through a bypass inside the vaporizer directly to the common outlet. Thus, the actual vaporizing portion of the 19.1 is completely separated from the fresh gas flow. Also, in the "O" position, the inlet and the outlet of the vaporizing chamber are interconnected and vented through a hole. This ensures that no pressure builds in the vaporizing chamber. The anesthetic loss caused by venting in the "off" position is less than 0.5 ml/24 h at an ambient temperature of 22°C.[28]

Figure 19-23 shows a simplified schematic of the Drager Vapor 19.1 in the "on" position. Flow through the 19.1 is similar to that through the Tec 4, but back pressure and temperature compensation are different. The Vapor 19.1 uses a patented, long spiral tube as the inlet to the vaporizing chamber, which acts as a buffer against the pumping effect. Some inhalation agent gas molecules do travel in a retrograde manner up this tube during the expiratory phase of the pumping effect. However, they do not reach the bypass chamber because of the tube length. Drager does not employ a check valve at the common outlet because of this internal pressure compensation. Temperature compensation is achieved by an expansion element, which alters flow through the bypass chamber. The Vapor 19.1 has a wick and baffle system similar to that of the Tec 4.[28, 29]

The output of the 19.1 is regulated by a single concentration

dial calibrated in percentage and located on top of the vaporizer. It is turned on by simultaneously depressing the white "O" button while turning the dial in a counter-clockwise direction. Two types of filling mechanisms are available, which are the screw cap filler or the safety, agent-specific keyed filler. The liquid capacity of the 19.1 is 200 ml with a dry wick or 140 ml when the wick is wet.[28]

Removal of the Vapor 19.1 requires a service technician

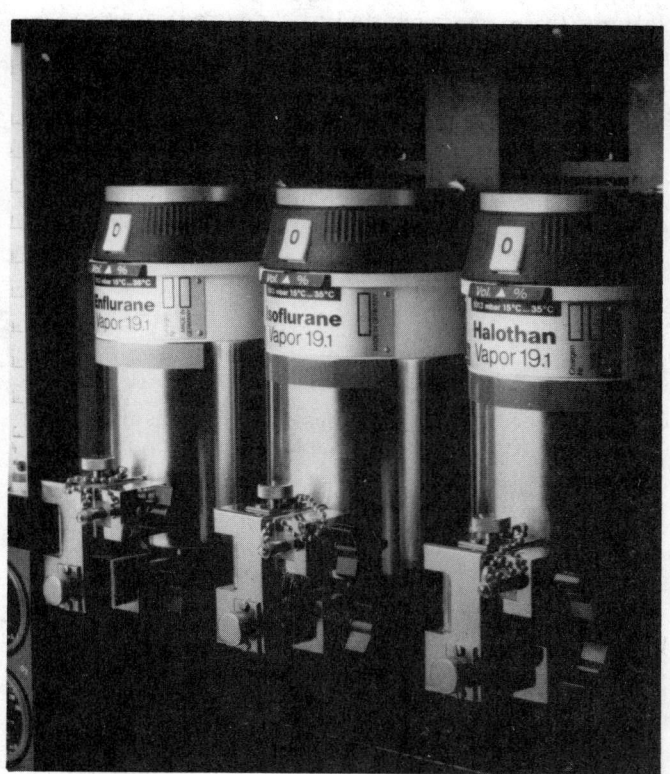

FIG. 19-22. Drager Vapor 19.1 Vaporizers with keyed filling devices. (Courtesy of North American Drager, Telford, PA.)

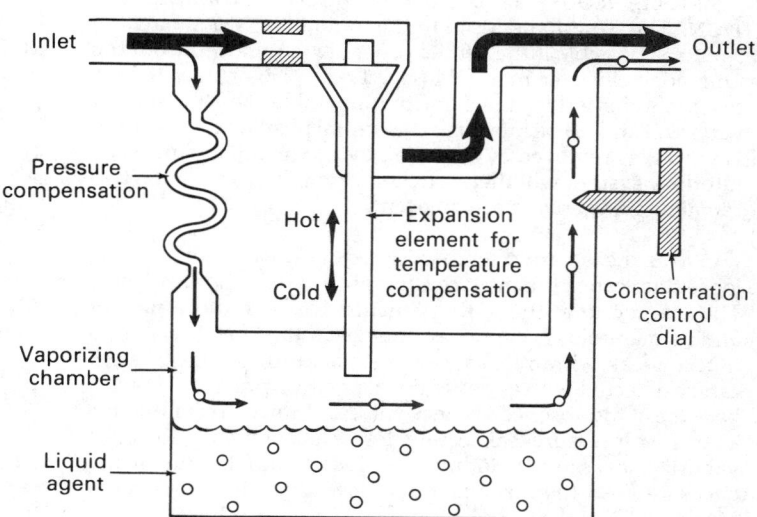

FIG. 19-23. Simplified schematic of the Drager 19.1 Vaporizer. See text for details.

because it is semipermanently affixed to its mounting bracket by two Allen screws. The interlock system continues to function when any of the three vaporizers are removed. However, a short-circuit block must be installed in place of the vaporizer, or a leak will occur.

SAFETY FEATURES

The Drager 19.1 and the Ohmeda Tec 4 have numerous safety features that have minimized or eliminated many hazards once associated with variable-bypass vaporizers. Agent-specific keyed filling devices help prevent a vaporizer from being filled with the wrong agent. Overfilling of these vaporizers is minimized because the filler port is located at the maximum safe liquid level. Today's vaporizers are soundly secured to the vaporizer manifold, and there is little need to move them. Thus, problems associated with tipping are minimized. Contemporary interlock systems prevent administration of more than one agent.[28, 29]

HAZARDS

Contemporary Variable-Bypass Vaporizers

Despite numerous safety features, some hazards are still associated with contemporary variable-bypass vaporizers.

INCORRECT AGENT. Many anesthesiologists prefer the screw-cap filler for convenience, although agent-specific keyed fillers are available. A vaporizer can be filled with the wrong agent when the former is employed.

TIPPING. Tipping can occur when vaporizers are incorrectly "switched out" or moved. However, tipping is unlikely when a vaporizer is attached to a manifold in the upright position. Excessive tipping can cause the liquid agent to enter the bypass chamber and can result in a high output concentration. The Tec 4 is slightly more immune to tipping than the Vapor 19.1 because of the extensive baffle system of the former. However, if either vaporizer is tipped, it should not be used until it has been flushed for 20–30 min at high flow rates with the vaporizer set at a low concentration.[2]

SIMULTANEOUS INHALATION AGENT ADMINISTRATION. The simultaneous administration of two inhalation agents is possible if the center vaporizer is removed from the Ohmeda Selectatec manifold (Fig. 19-20). This makes the extension rod interlock mechanism inoperable. The left or right vaporizer should be moved to the central position if the central vaporizer is removed as indicated by the manifold label. The interlock system will then function properly because the two remaining vaporizers are adjacent.

LEAKS. Leaks are often associated with vaporizers.[22, 41] A loose filler cap is the most common source of vaporizer leaks. They can occur at the O-ring junction between the vaporizer and its manifold. A vaporizer must be in the "on" position to detect a leak within it. Vaporizer leaks in the Drager System can be detected with a conventional positive-pressure leak test because of the absence of check valves. Ohmeda recommends a negative-pressure leak testing device (suction bulb) to detect vaporizer leaks in the Modulus I and Modulus II because of the check valve at the machine outlet (see Checking Anesthesia Machines).[5, 6]

Freestanding (add-on) Vaporizers

Freestanding, variable-bypass vaporizers have been "added on" to many anesthesia machines between the common outlet and the patient circuit. This practice is fraught with hazards. Tipping is a substantial possibility because the vaporizer is not permanently affixed to the machine. Furthermore, multiple agents can be administered because at least one agent from the machine plus the agent from the freestanding vaporizer can be delivered. Oxygen flushing ($35-75 \, l \cdot min^{-1}$) can deliver excess anesthetic agent from the freestanding vaporizer to the patient. Even though the inlet and outlet of freestanding vaporizers have different diameters, they can be connected in a reverse manner. Vaporizer output can be two times that which is indicated on the dial in this configuration.[42]

Many freestanding vaporizers have a check valve in the vaporizer outlet to minimize the pumping effect and to indicate reverse hook-up. This valve prevents leak detection in the low-pressure circuit when a traditional positive-pressure leak test is performed. Also, an intraoperative disconnect can go unnoticed if positive-pressure ventilation is employed. The pressure from the breathing circuit closes the check valve during inspiration, and the disconnection is not detectable by conventional means.[43]

VAPORIZER MAINTENANCE

Ohmeda recommends that Tec 4 vaporizers should be serviced annually at an authorized Ohmeda service center. The service includes complete disassembly of components, cleaning, inspection for damage and wear, and renewal of wicks, seals, and damaged items. Additionally, vaporizer output is checked at varying conditions.[29] North American Drager recommends in-house verification of vaporizer performance every 6 months by use of a Riken anesthetic gas analyzer.

ANESTHESIA VENTILATORS

CLASSIFICATION

The following section briefly reviews ventilator classification and terminology before the discussion of individual anesthesia machine ventilators. For additional details, refer to texts such as *Mechanical Ventilation*, by R. R. Kirby, R. A. Smith, and D. A. Desautels, and *Respiratory Therapy Equipment*, by S. P. McPherson.[44, 45]

Power Source

The power source required to operate a mechanical ventilator is provided by either compressed gas, electricity, or both. Older pneumatic ventilators such as the Ohio anesthesia ventilator, the Ohio V5, and the Ohio V5A require only a pneumatic power source to function properly.[46-50] Contemporary electronic ventilators such as the Ohmeda 7000 and the Drager AV-E require both an electronic and a pneumatic power source.[4, 8, 9, 51, 52]

Drive Mechanism

Anesthesia machine ventilators are classified as double-circuit, pneumatically driven ventilators. In a double-circuit system, a driving force compresses a bag or bellows, which in turn delivers gas to the patient. Compressed gases provide the actual driving force. Thus, the ventilators are pneumatically driven. In the Ohmeda 7000, the driving gas is composed of 100% oxygen.[51, 52] In the Drager AV-E, it is a mixture of oxygen and air because a Venturi is employed.[4, 8, 9]

An anesthesia machine ventilator may simplistically be viewed as a breathing bag (bellows) located within a clear plastic box. The bellows physically separates the driving gas circuit from the patient gas circuit. The driving gas circuit is located outside the bellows, and the patient gas circuit is inside the bellows. During the inspiratory phase, the driving gas exerts force upon the bellows, causing the anesthetic gas inside the bellows to be delivered to the patient. This compression action is analogous to the hand of the anesthesiologist squeezing the breathing bag. During the expiratory phase, the driving gas is vented to the atmosphere through the driving gas relief valve. Then anesthetic gas within the patient circuit fills the bellows. After the bellows is completely full, excess anesthetic gas is vented through the ventilator relief valve. This valve is analogous to the adjustable pressure-limiting (pop-off) valve of the circle system. The ventilator relief valve vents excess gas only during exhalation. Therefore, it is not good practice to activate the oxygen flush during inspiration because excess pressure can develop in the breathing circuit.

Bellows Classification

The bellows classification is determined by the direction of bellows movement during exhalation. Older, pneumatic ventilators employ weighted descending bellows, whereas most contemporary electronic ventilators have ascending bellows. Of the two configurations, the ascending bellows is substantially safer. If a breathing circuit disconnect occurs, an ascending bellows will not fill and the problem should be quickly recognized. However, a weighted descending bellows will continue its normal upward and downward movement despite a disconnection. This is caused by gravity acting upon the bellows. Room air is entrained to the system during the downward movement of the bellows, and it is discharged from the system during the upward movement. The gas flow during the upward movement may generate sufficient pressure to "fool" a pressure alarm. It is therefore extremely important to set the disconnect alarm point immediately below the peak inspiratory pressure when a descending bellows is used.[16]

Cycling Mechanism

Anesthesia machine ventilators are time cycled and provide ventilatory support in the control mode. Initiation of inspiration is accomplished by a timing device. Older pneumatic ventilators employ a fluidic timing device. Contemporary electronic ventilators use a solid-state timing device and are thus classified as time cycled and electronically controlled.

PNEUMATIC VENTILATORS

Pneumatic ventilators were most frequently used for mechanical ventilation in the operating room until recent years. Although they have become less popular, many are still being used today. Examples of pneumatic ventilators include the Ohio Anesthesia Ventilator, the Ohio V5, the Ohio V5A, and the Drager AV. They are classified as pneumatically powered, double-circuit, pneumatically driven, descending bellows, time-cycled, fluidically controlled, tidal volume preset ventilators that are generally used in the control mode. All use a

Venturi drive gas system. The entrained room air provides additional flow to the bellows chamber without substantially decreasing the oxygen supply pressure within the anesthesia machine.[46-50]

Pneumatic ventilators have several advantages. They require only a pneumatic power source. Therefore, they can be used effectively during an electrical power failure or in remote areas without electricity. The functional design of pneumatic ventilators is simple, and they are easy to operate. Most are mobile freestanding units that can readily be moved from room to room. The fluidic control components have no moving parts and depend solely on gas flow and pressure to function. Maintenance is minimal, and electrical knowledge is not necessary for servicing the ventilators.

Disadvantages of pneumatic ventilators, however, outweigh the advantages. The major disadvantage results from the descending bellows configuration coupled with a relatively low, factory-present, disconnect alarm threshold value (such as 8 cm H_2O pressure). As mentioned previously, disconnections can go unnoticed because the pressure generated by the weighted descending bellows can exceed the alarm threshold.[16] Most pneumatic ventilators have only one alarm: the disconnect alarm. This is in marked contrast to newer electronic ventilators, which may have as many as seven alarms.[51, 52] Finally, pneumatic ventilators lack flexibility. They have a limited number of controls and lack versatility.

ELECTRONIC VENTILATORS

Contemporary electronic anesthesia machine ventilators such as the Drager AV-E (Anesthesia Ventilator—Electronic) and the Ohmeda 7000 are an integral part of the global anesthesia system. Each will be discussed below.

Drager AV-E

The Drager AV-E is classified as a pneumatically and electronically powered, double-circuit, pneumatically driven, ascending bellows, time-cycled, electronically controlled, tidal volume preset controller. The AV-E is standard equipment on the Narkomed 2A, Narkomed 2B, and Narkomed 3, and it is not available as a freestanding ventilator. It consists of two major components: the control assembly and the bellows assembly. The control assembly contains the electronic and pneumatic components of the ventilator. It is located above the flowmeters and vaporizers, and it serves as a permanent shelf. Most of the ventilator control knobs are located on the face of the control assembly. The ascending bellows assembly is located to the left of the flowmeters. The ventilator relief valve is located behind the bellows chamber. The operator can observe the action of this valve because its dome is constructed of clear plastic.[4, 8, 9] This is in contrast to the ventilator relief valve of the Ohmeda 7000, which is located inside the bellows.[51, 52]

The AV-E has five controls. The ventilator power switch provides both pneumatic and electrical power to the ventilator. When turned to the "on" position, it automatically enables the apnea pressure alarm and the volume-related alarms of the respiratory volume monitor. The frequency control is used to adjust the respiratory rate from 1 to 99, using a two-digit thumb wheel. The I:E ratio control allows the operator to vary the inspiratory to expiratory phase time ratio in calibrated steps from 1:1 through 1:4.5. The inspiratory flow control regulates the flow rate of driving gas into the bellows chamber. A continuum of flow rates ranging from low to high can be selected. The flow setting should be adjusted so that the bellows is fully compressed at the end of the inspiratory phase. Finally, the last control is the tidal volume adjustment knob, which is located above the bellows assembly. The tidal volume scale ranges from 200 to 1,400 ml, and it increases from bottom to top.[4, 8, 9]

Two ventilator monitors are available on the Narkomed 2B and Narkomed 3. The breathing pressure monitor, or Baromed, is standard equipment. Pressure measurement from the patient circuit can be either at the absorber or the Y-piece. The operator sets a high-pressure alarm limit and a threshold pressure alarm limit. Alarms are provided for high pressure, pressure below the threshold for 15 and 30 s (apnea), continuing pressure above the set threshold for 15 s, and subatmospheric (≤ -10 cm H_2O) pressure. The respiratory volume monitor, or Spiromed, is an optional monitor. The tidal volume sensor is located between the expiratory valve and the CO_2 absorber. Alarms are provided for low tidal volume (< 70 ml), high respiratory rate (> 99 breaths $\cdot$ min^{-1}), and reverse flow through the sensor (> 20 ml).[4, 8, 9]

The operating principle of the AV-E is illustrated in Figures 19-24 and 19-25. Oxygen at 50 PSIG provides the pneumatic input to the driving gas circuit. Flow through this circuit is regulated by a solenoid valve, which serves as an interface between the pneumatic and electronic circuits of the ventilator. The electronic timing of the solenoid is determined by the settings of the frequency and I:E ratio controls. It is open during the inspiratory phase and closed during the expiratory phase.[4]

Inspiratory phase gas flows are illustrated in Figure 19-24. Oxygen at 50 PSIG passes through the solenoid valve and opens the control valve. This allows the preset gas flow from the flow regulator to proceed through the control valve to the Venturi. Back pressure from the Venturi is directed to the power relief valve and closes it. Then oxygen from the flow regulator passes through the Venturi, and a substantial volume of room air is entrained through the muffler. In fact, more than 80% of the driving gas flow is entrained room air, and the final oxygen concentration of the driving gas is approximately 35%. The flow of the driving gas increases considerably without depleting the oxygen pressure within the anesthesia machine because a Venturi device is used.[4]

The driving gas is forced into the bellows chamber, causing the pressure within it to increase. The pressure increase causes two events. First, the ventilator relief valve closes. This prevents anesthetic gas from escaping into the scavenging system. Second, the bellows is compressed downward, and

FIG. 19-24. Inspiratory phase gas flows of the Drager AV-E. See text for details.

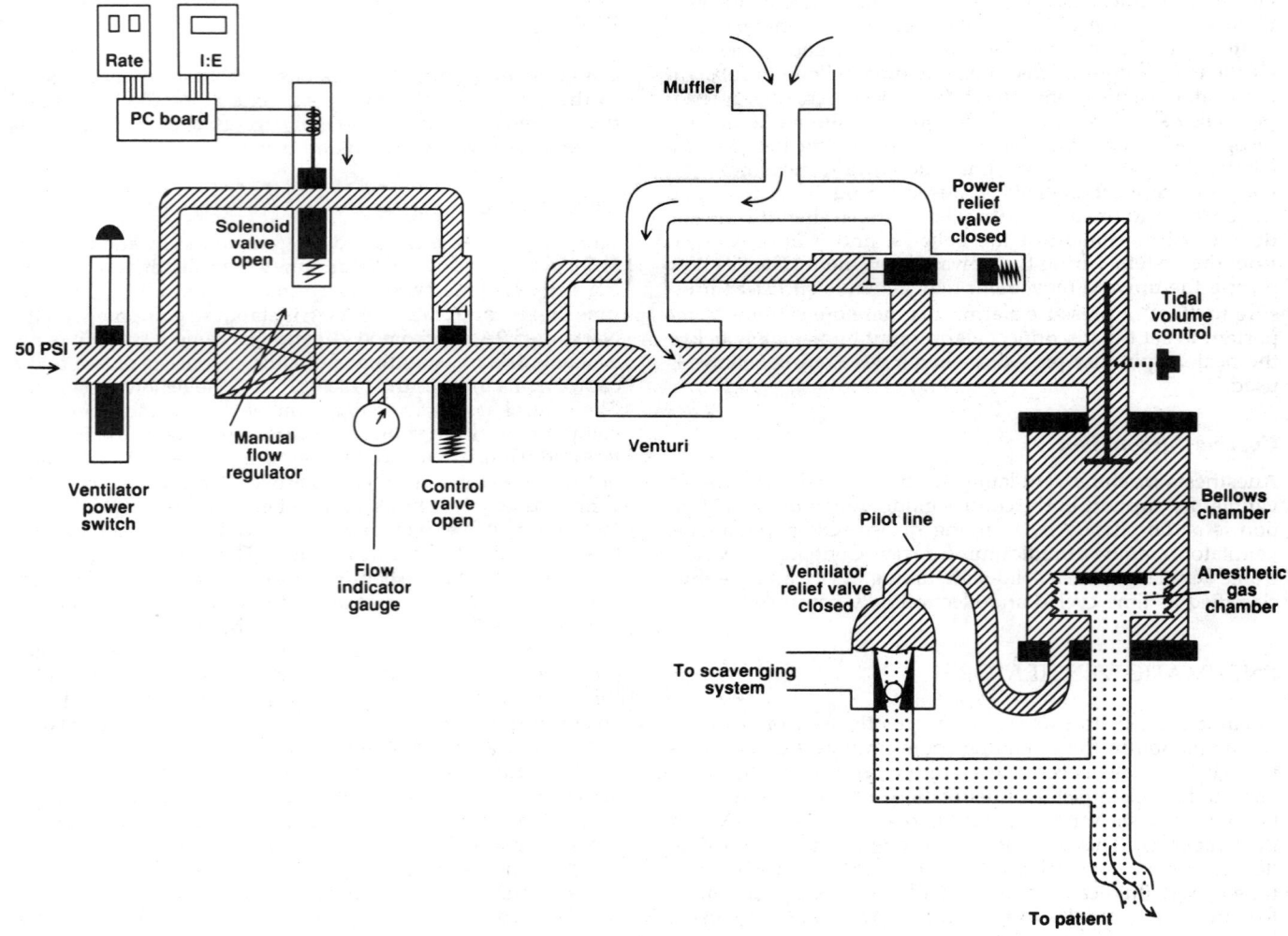

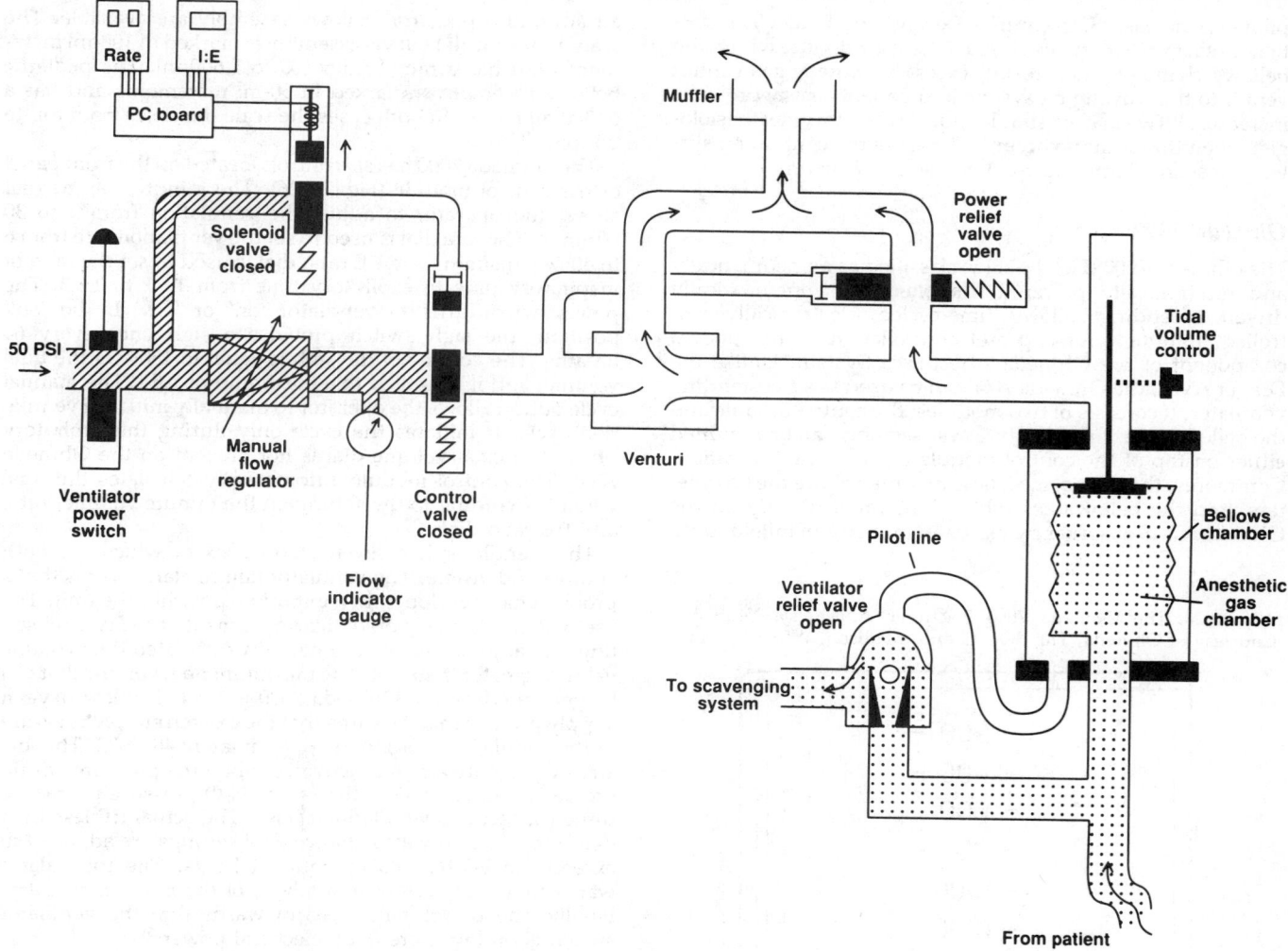

FIG. 19-25. Expiratory phase gas flows of the Drager AV-E. See text for details.

the anesthetic gas within the bellows is delivered to the patient's lungs. The ventilator relief valve remains closed as long as the bellows chamber contains pressure. The inspiratory pause time starts when the bellows is completely compressed, and it lasts until the bellows begins to ascend. The pressure in the bellows chamber, as preset by the flow regulator, cannot increase further. All excess pressure is released through the Venturi entrainment port, and the Venturi simultaneously ceases to entrain room air.[4] The volume of driving gas that circulates through the bellows chamber during the inspiratory phase may be substantially greater than the tidal volume delivered. This is particularly true at slow rates and prolonged inspiratory times. In contrast, the Ohmeda 7000 delivers a driving gas volume equal to the tidal volume.[51, 52]

The expiratory phase gas flows of the Drager AV-E are shown in Figure 19-25. The expiratory phase begins when the electric signal to the solenoid terminates. As soon as the electric signal stops, the solenoid valve closes. This closure terminates the 50-PSIG gas supply to the control valve, which also closes. The preset gas flow from the flow regulator is interrupted by the control valve. This causes an immediate pressure decrease at the Venturi, and no back pressure is supplied

to the power relief valve, which opens. Then the driving gas within the bellows chamber can exit through the power relief valve and through the entrainment port of the Venturi.[4] Regardless of the route taken, all driving gas is discharged through the ventilator muffler.

The pressure within the bellows chamber and in the pilot line declines to zero, causing the mushroom portion of the ventilator relief valve to open. To prevent premature outflow of anesthetic gas into the scavenging system, a weighted ball similar to those used in ball-type PEEP valves is incorporated into the base of the ventilator relief valve. The ball produces 2 cm H_2O back pressure. Thus, the bellows extends fully, and 2 cm H_2O pressure develops within the bellows chamber before anesthetic gas enters the scavenging system.[4] All ascending bellows ventilators have a minimum of 2 cm of PEEP because of this arrangement.

Global examination of the inspiratory and expiratory gas flows of the Drager AV-E reveals the importance of a clean, functional muffler. Most of the driving gas is entrained through the muffler during the inspiratory phase. All the driving gas exits through the muffler during the expiratory phase. Pressure within the bellows chamber and within the pilot line increases if the muffler becomes occluded. The ventilator relief valve remains closed if there is pressure within the bellows chamber. As a result, excess anesthetic gas cannot vent into the scavenging system and patient airway pressure increases.[53] Two alarms should quickly alert the anesthesiologist when this scenario occurs. These are the continuing system pressure alarm and the high-pressure alarm.

Ohmeda 7000

The Ohmeda 7000 (Fig. 19-26) is classified as a pneumatically and electronically powered, double-circuit, pneumatically driven, ascending bellows, time-cycled, electronically controlled, minute volume preset controller. It is an optional component of the Ohmeda Anesthesia System. Unlike the Drager AV-E, the Ohmeda 7000 can be used as a freestanding ventilator. It consists of two modules: the control module and the bellows assembly. The bellows assembly can be mounted either on top of the control module or in a remote location. Commonly, the control module is mounted above the flowmeters, and the bellows assembly is mounted directly on the Ohmeda GMS absorber by use of an interface manifold. Both

FIG. 19-26. The Ohmeda 7000 Electronic Anesthesia Ventilator. (Courtesy of Ohmeda, The BOC Group, Madison, WI.)

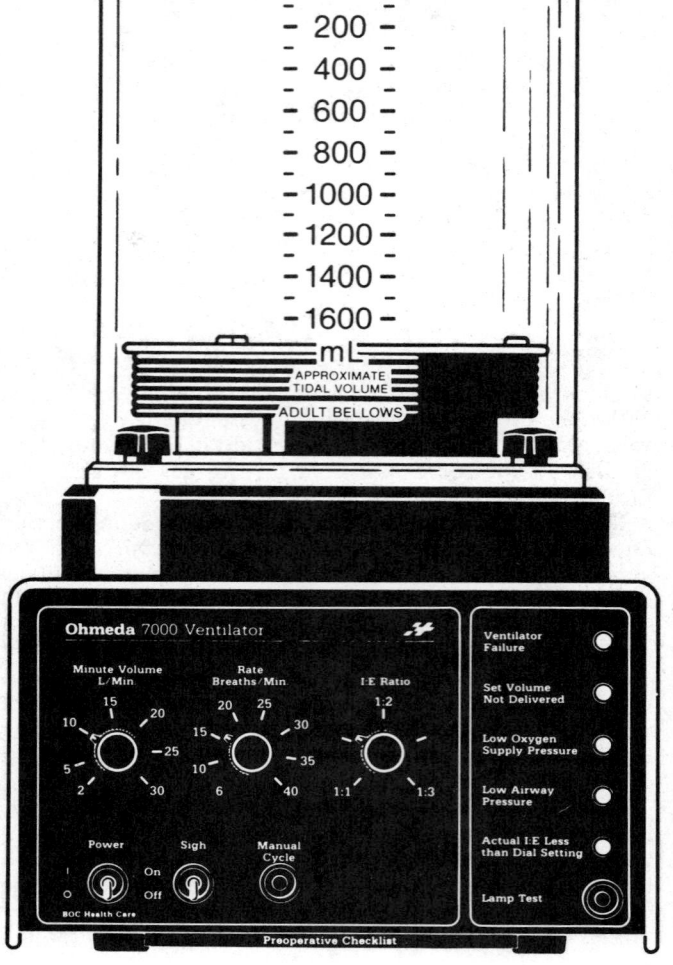

an adult and pediatric bellows assembly are available. The scale on the adult bellows assembly is marked in 100-ml increments and has a range from 100 to 1,600 ml. The pediatric bellows assembly is marked in 50-ml increments and has a 0–300 ml range. In both cases the scale increases from top to bottom.[51, 52]

The Ohmeda 7000 has six controls located on the front panel of the control module (Fig. 19-26). The minute volume dial allows the operator to adjust the ventilation from 2 to 30 $l \cdot min^{-1}$. The rate dial is used to set the ventilation rate from 6 to 40 breaths/min. The I:E ratio dial is used to set the ratio of inspiratory time to expiratory time from 1 : 1 to 1 : 3. The power switch turns the ventilator "on" or "off." In the "on" position, the sigh switch provides a sigh once every 64 breaths. The volume of the sigh is equal to 150% of the tidal volume, and it is limited to a maximum of 1.5 l. The manual cycle button allows the operator to manually initiate a ventilation cycle. It initiates the cycle only during the expiratory phase.[51] A tidal volume dial is not present on the Ohmeda 7000. The control module automatically calculates the tidal volume according to the setting on the minute volume, rate, and I:E ratio dials.

This ventilator has seven alarms, six of which are both audible and visible. The ventilator failure alarm warns that a problem has developed in a critical area within the unit. The "set volume not delivered" alarm warns that the control settings are adjusted to an automatically calculated tidal volume value of greater than 1.5l. The maximum tidal volume that can be generated by the Ohmeda 7000 is 1.6 l. The low oxygen supply pressure alarm warns that the oxygen supply pressure in the ventilator is less than approximately 40 PSIG. The low airway pressure alarm is activated when the pressure within the patient circuit is less than 6 cm H_2O pressure for two or three consecutive ventilation cycles. The actual I:E less than dial setting alarm warns that control settings are adjusted to exceed the ventilator's operational limits. The total alarm warns that there has been a failure of the internal circuitry. Finally, the power failure alarm warns that the ventilator switch is on but there is no electrical power.[51]

The operating principle of the Ohmeda 7000 is similar to that of the AV-E. Figure 19-27 is a schematic of the pneumatic circuitry of the Ohmeda 7000. The driving gas supply is 100% oxygen at 50 PSIG. A precision regulator reduces this pressure to 38 PSIG ± 0.5 PSIG. The regulated gas supply connects directly to a manifold of five solenoid valves. The control box electronically regulates the solenoid valves during the inspiratory time. Gas flow is directed through tuned orifices, which are calibrated for flows of 2, 4, 6, 8, 16, and 32 $l \cdot min^{-1}$. The range of flow selection is in 2-$l \cdot min^{-1}$ increments from 4 $l \cdot min^{-1}$ to 60 $l \cdot min^{-1}$. A precise volume of driving gas equal to the tidal volume is delivered to the bellows chamber at a specific rate, depending on the ventilator settings.[52]

During the inspiratory phase (Fig. 19-28, *top*), the control module delivers its computed driving gas flow into the bellows chamber. The bellows is compressed as the driving gas volume and pressure increase within the housing. Anesthetic gas is forced out of the bellows, through the patient circuit, and into the patient's lungs. Flow stops when the full volume of driving gas has been delivered into the bellows chamber. A relief valve located within the control module opens and vents excess driving gas into the atmosphere if high pressure occurs during the inspiratory phase. The threshold for this relief valve is 65 cm H_2O pressure.[51, 52]

Anesthetic gas enters the bellows chamber from the patient circuit during the expiratory phase (Fig. 19-28, *bottom*). The ventilator relief valve, located inside the bellows chamber, has

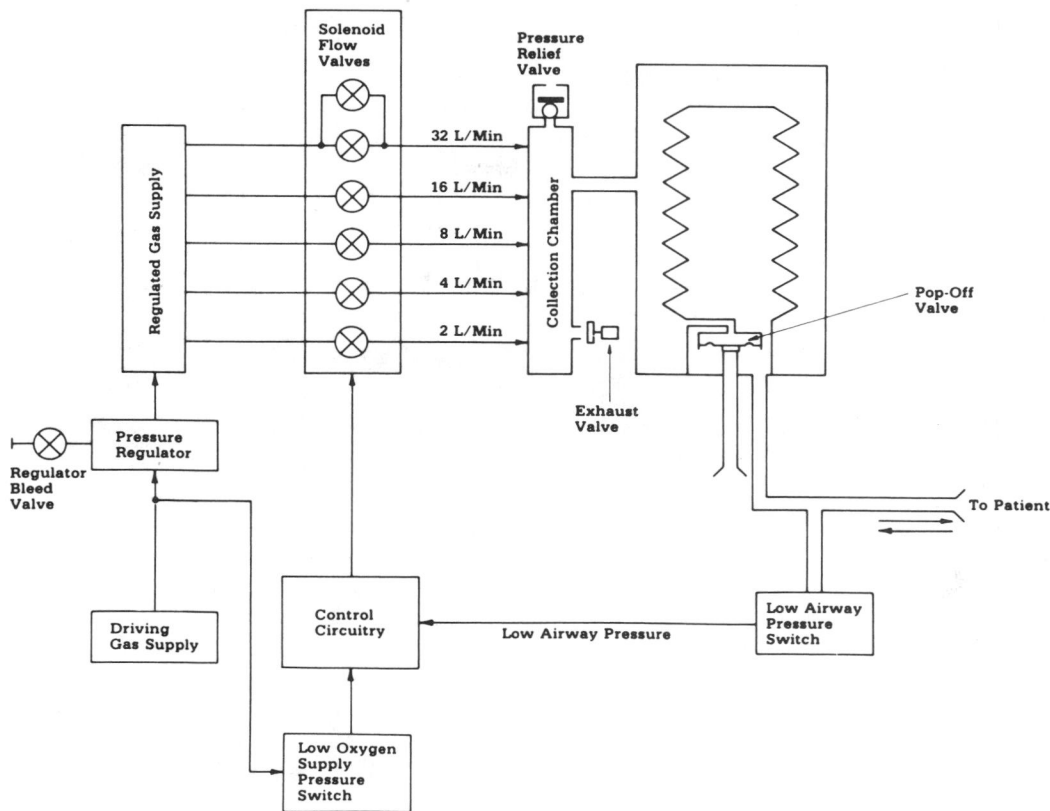

FIG. 19-27. Diagram of the Ohmeda 7000 Electronic Anesthesia Ventilator. See text for details. (Courtesy of Ohmeda, The BOC Group, Madison, WI.)

a threshold value of 2.5 cm H_2O pressure. Therefore, it opens only when the bellows is fully extended and the pressure within the bellows exceeds 2.5 cm H_2O. Then, excess patient gas is popped-off into the scavenging system.[51, 52]

Although the operating principles of the Ohmeda 7000 and the Drager AV-E are similar, there are several differences. The Ohmeda 7000 uses five solenoids to regulate driving gas flow, whereas the AV-E uses one. A Venturi device is not used on the Ohmeda 7000. Therefore, the driving gas of the Ohmeda 7000 is composed of 100% oxygen. In the AV-E, it is an air–oxygen mixture. The Ohmeda 7000 delivers a driving gas volume that is equal to the tidal volume. This is unlike the AV-E, which circulates a driving gas volume through the bellows chamber that is substantially larger than the tidal volume. Because of this difference, the tidal volume scale of the Ohmeda 7000 increases from top to bottom. On the AV-E it increases from bottom to top. Finally, the ventilator relief valve is located inside the bellows of the Ohmeda 7000. It is located outside the bellows of the AV-E in clear view.[4, 8, 9, 51, 52]

PROBLEMS AND HAZARDS OF ANESTHESIA VENTILATORS

Numerous problems are associated with anesthesia ventilators. They include breathing circuit failures, problems with the bellows assembly, and problems with the control assembly.[16, 53, 54]

Breathing Circuit Failure

Breathing circuit disconnection is a leading cause of critical incidents in anesthesia.[55] As mentioned previously, ventilators with ascending bellows are substantially safer than those with descending bellows (see Bellows Classification). Ascending bellows used in conjunction with contemporary pressure and volume monitors help minimize unrecognized disconnection.[16] Leaks within the breathing circuit can occur during mechanical ventilation. Failure to close the absorber pop-off valve accounts for most leaks. The bag/ventilator switch on contemporary absorbers minimizes this problem. Misconnections of the breathing system are common. Anesthesia machines, breathing systems, ventilators, and scavenging systems incorporate a multitude of hose terminals. Hoses can be connected easily to inappropriate terminals. Additionally, they may be improperly attached to a variety of cylindrically shaped protrusions on anesthesia machines. Committees writing standards on breathing systems, ventilators, and scavenging systems have attempted to increase safety by assigning different diameters to various terminals. Finally, incorrect insertion of unidirectional accessory devices such as PEEP valves and cascade humidifiers into the breathing system can result in a no-flow state.[16]

Bellows Assembly Problems

Leaks can occur in the bellows assembly. Improper seating of the plastic bellows housing can result in inadequate ventila-

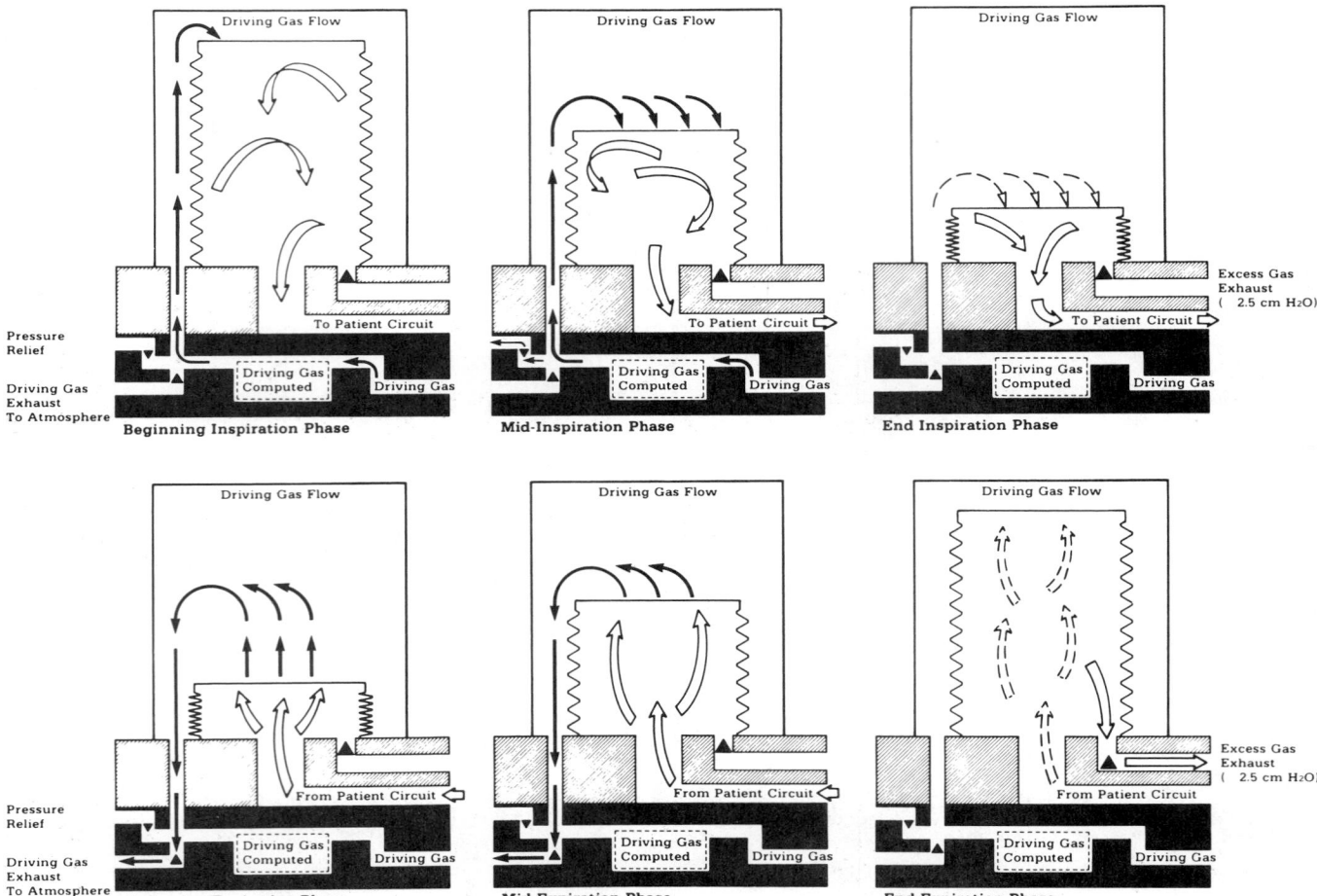

FIG. 19-28. Inspiratory and expiratory phase gas flows of the Ohmeda 7000 Electronic Anesthesia Ventilator. See text for details. (Courtesy of Ohmeda, The BOC Group, Madison, WI.)

tion because a portion of the driving gas is vented. A hole in the bellows can lead to alveolar hyperventilation and possibly barotrauma as the ventilator driving gas is forced into the anesthetic circuit. When this occurs the value on the oxygen analyzer may increase when the driving gas is 100% oxygen or it may decrease if the driving gas is composed of an air–oxygen mixture.[54]

The ventilator relief valve can cause problems. All ascending bellows produce a minimum of 2 cm H_2O pressure or PEEP in the breathing circuit. The upward movement of the bellows requires an above atmospheric pressure within the system.[16] The outflow resistance is necessary to assure complete filling of the bellows before scavenging of anesthetic gases. Oxygen flushing during the inspiratory phase of mechanical ventilation can result in barotrauma. The ventilator relief valve is closed during inspiration. Therefore, excess volume in the breathing circuit during oxygen flushing cannot be vented. The mushroom portion of the ventilator relief valve can rupture, which can result in inadequate ventilation during inspiration because anesthetic gas is delivered to the scavenging system instead of to the patient. Finally, excess suction from the scavenging system can cause the ventilator relief valve to malfunction. Subatmospheric pressure in the scavenging system can draw the diaphragm of the ventilator relief valve to its seat and close the valve. This can result in barotrauma.[16]

Control Assembly Problems

The control assembly can be the source of both electrical and mechanical problems. Electrical failure can be total or partial, with the former being more obvious. Some mechanical problems include leaks within the system, faulty regulators, and faulty valves. As mentioned previously, an occluded muffler can result in barotrauma (see Drager AV-E). Obstruction of driving gas outflow closes the ventilator relief valve, and excess patient gas cannot be vented.[53]

CHECKING ANESTHESIA MACHINES

A complete anesthesia apparatus checkout procedure should be performed each day before the first case. An abbreviated version should be performed before each subsequent case. Several checkout procedures exist, but the most popular one is the August 1986 Food and Drug Administration (FDA) Anesthesia Apparatus Checkout Recommendations, which is reproduced in Appendix A.[56–59] The FDA checkout is only a generic guideline because the designs of different machines vary considerably. Also, many machines have been modified in the field. Therefore, specific checks must be performed on specific machines. The user must refer to the operator's manual for special procedures or precautions. The best example of the importance of performing the appropriate preoperative check is the low-pressure leak test (#16 FDA). Several mishaps have resulted from application of the wrong leak test to the wrong machine.[17, 41, 60]

LOW-PRESSURE LEAK TEST

The low-pressure leak test checks the integrity of the anesthesia machine from the flow control valves to the common outlet. It is the most important preoperative check because it evaluates that portion of the machine that is downstream from all safety devices except the oxygen analyzer. The components located within this area are precisely the ones that are most subject to breakage and leaks. Flowtubes are the most delicate pneumatic component of the machine, and they can crack or break. Leaks can occur at the interface between the glass flowtube and the manifold because of problems associated with O-rings and gaskets. In fact, a typical three-gas anesthesia machine has 16 O-rings in the low-pressure circuit. Loose filler caps on vaporizers are a common source of leaks. Leaks can occur at the O-ring junction between the vaporizer and its manifold. Therefore, it is mandatory to perform the appropriate low-pressure leak test before every case. Most anesthesia machines have check valves located in the low-pressure circuit. The presence or absence of these check valves profoundly influences the type of leak test that should be employed. Each is discussed as follows.

Machines without Check Valves

A "traditional" positive-pressure leak test using the circle system can be performed on machines that do not have check valves in the low-pressure circuitry (see Table 19-1). The pop-off valve is closed, and the system is pressurized by use of the oxygen flush and flow from the oxygen flow control valve. The exact details of the test are outlined in Appendix A, #16. An uninterrupted pipe is present from the flow control valves to the circle airway pressure gauge. Therefore, a leak in the low-pressure circuit will be reflected by a decline in the value on the airway pressure gauge. This traditional test has two major advantages. First, it does not require accessory test devices. Second, it can be performed quickly. The main disadvantage of the traditional test is its lack of sensitivity when compared with leak tests using special devices (see below). This lack of sensitivity occurs because the traditional test is volume dependent. The pressurized volume in the breathing bag can mask leaks up to 250 ml/min.

Drager recommends a more sensitive positive-pressure leak test for the Narkomed 2A and Narkomed 3. It is not volume dependent because a positive-pressure leak test device (Fig. 19-29, *left*) is substituted for the breathing bag. The pop-off valve is closed, and the inspiratory and expiratory valves are interconnected by a single breathing hose. The system is pressurized to 50 cm H_2O by use of a squeeze bulb. The pressure decrease from 50 to 30 cm H_2O should take 30 s or longer.

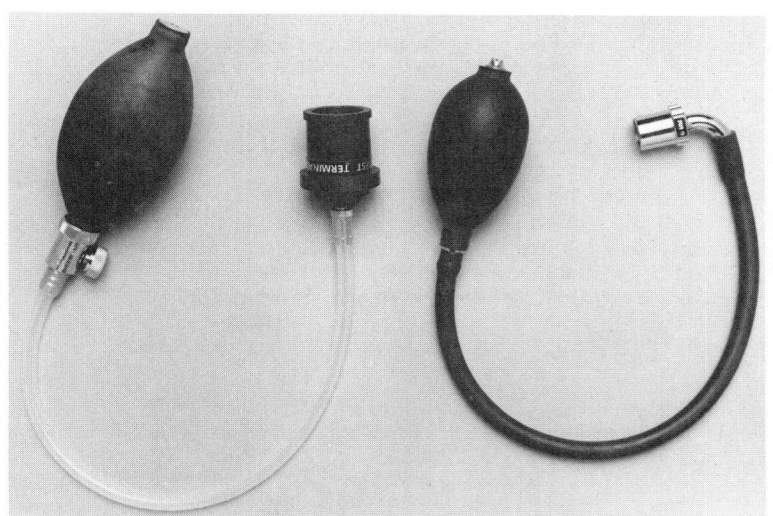

FIG. 19-29. Leak-testing devices. The Drager leak testing device is shown on the left, and the Ohmeda leak testing device is shown on the right. Although the devices are similar in appearance, their function is totally different. The Drager device is attached to the breathing bag mount, and it generates positive pressure. The Ohmeda device is attached to the common gas outlet, and it creates negative pressure. See text for details.

TABLE 19-1. Check Valves and Recommended Leak Test[5, 6, 8, 9, 20, 21]

ANESTHESIA MACHINE	MACHINE OUTLET CHECK VALVE	VAPORIZER OUTLET CHECK VALVE	RECOMMENDED LEAK TEST	
			Positive Pressure	Negative Pressure (Suction Bulb)
Drager Narkomed 2A	No	No	X	
Drager Narkomed 3	No	No	X	
Ohmeda Unitrol	Yes	Variable		X
Ohmeda 30/70	Yes	Variable		X
Ohmeda Modulus I	Yes	Variable		X
Ohmeda Modulus II	Yes	No		X

Machines with Check Valves

Most Ohmeda machines have a machine outlet check valve (Table 19-1) to minimize the pumping effect. These include the Unitrol, the 30/70, the Modulus I, and the Modulus II.[5, 6, 20, 21] The check valve is located downstream from the vaporizers and upstream from the oxygen flush. It is open (Fig. 19-30, *left*) in the absence of back pressure. Gas flow from the manifold moves the rubber flapper valve off its seat and allows gas to proceed freely to the common outlet. The valve closes (Fig. 19-30, *right*) when back pressure is exerted upon it. Intermittent positive pressure and oxygen flushing close the valve.

Ohmeda recommends the use of a negative-pressure leak test on the machines mentioned above. It is performed with the negative-pressure leak-testing device shown in Figure 19-29 (*right*). This is a suction bulb device, and it is included with all Ohmeda machines requiring it. A no-flow state is established. (The flow control valves are turned *off* when the Unitrol is tested. The master switch is turned *off* on the Modulus I and Modulus II, but the flow control valves are fully *open*.) The leak-testing device is attached to the common outlet. The bulb is compressed repeatedly until it remains collapsed. This action creates a vacuum in the low-pressure circuitry and opens the check valve. The machine is leak free if the hand bulb remains collapsed after 30 s, but a leak is present if the bulb reinflates during that interval. The leak test must be repeated with each vaporizer in the "on" position to detect vaporizer leaks.

Ohmeda's rationale for the negative-pressure leak test is as follows. First, the check valve separates the machine from the patient circuit. Pressuring the circle system will only reveal leaks downstream from the check valve.[61] Second, the test is extremely sensitive because it is not volume dependent. It can detect leaks as small as 30 ml·min^{-1}. Third, on the Modulus I and Modulus II, some components located upstream from the flow control valves are tested for leaks. These components include the oxygen flush, the pressure sensing system, and the pneumatics of the master on/off switch.

Application of a traditional positive-pressure leak test to a machine equipped with a check valve can lead to a false sense of security despite the presence of a huge leak.[17, 41, 60] Positive-pressure from the patient circuit closes the check valve, and the value on the airway pressure gauge does not decline. The

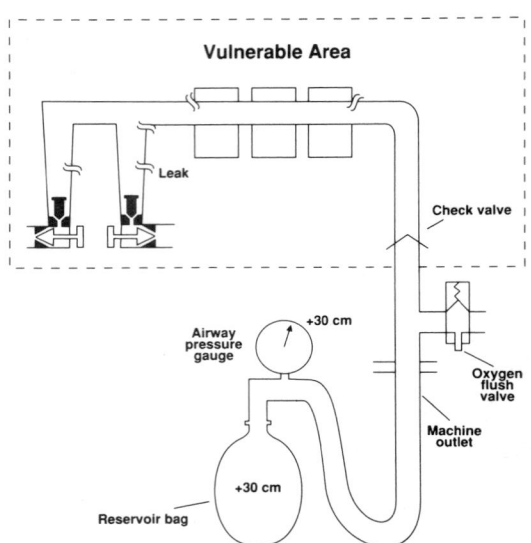

FIG. 19-31. Diagram of an anesthesia machine with a machine outlet check valve. The area within the rectangle is not checked by a traditional positive-pressure leak test. The components located within this area are precisely the ones that are most subject to breakage and leaks.

system appears to be tight, but, in actuality, only the circuitry distal to the check valve is leak free.[61] Thus, a vulnerable area (Fig. 19-31) exists from the check valve back to the flow control valves because this area is not tested by the traditional positive-pressure leak test. Addition of a freestanding vaporizer distal to the common outlet creates an even larger vulnerable area.

ANESTHETIC CIRCUITS

Anesthetic gases pass through a complex arrangement of tubing interposed between the anesthesia machine and the patient. The function of these conduits is to deliver anesthetic gases and oxygen and also to eliminate carbon dioxide. Carbon dioxide can be removed either by wash out with adequate fresh gas inflow or by soda lime absorption. These conduits are called anesthetic circuits. This discussion is limited to semiclosed rebreathing circuits and the Circle system.

MAPLESON SYSTEMS

Mapleson described and analyzed five different arrangements of fresh gas flow, tubing, mask, reservoir bag, and the expiratory valve to administer anesthetic gases.[62] They are now classically referred to as the Mapleson Systems, designated from A to E. Willis, Pender, and Mapleson added the F System to these original five.[63] The Mapleson circuits are shown in Figure 19-32. The amount of rebreathing associated with each type is highly dependent upon fresh gas flow rate. The performance of these circuits is best understood by studying the exhalation phase of the respiratory cycle.

Mapleson A

The Mapleson A is also known as Magill's Circuit. It has been extensively studied and consists of corrugated tubing, a reser-

FIG. 19-30. Machine outlet check valve. See text for details. (Reproduced with permission. Bowie E, Huffman LM: The anesthesia machine essentials for understanding. Madison, WI, Ohmeda, The BOC Group, 1985.)

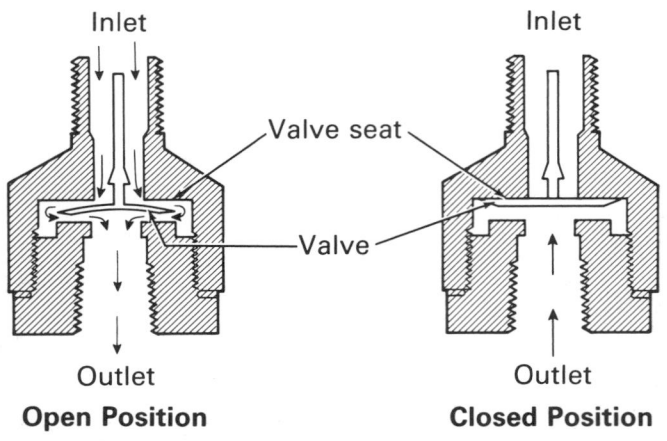

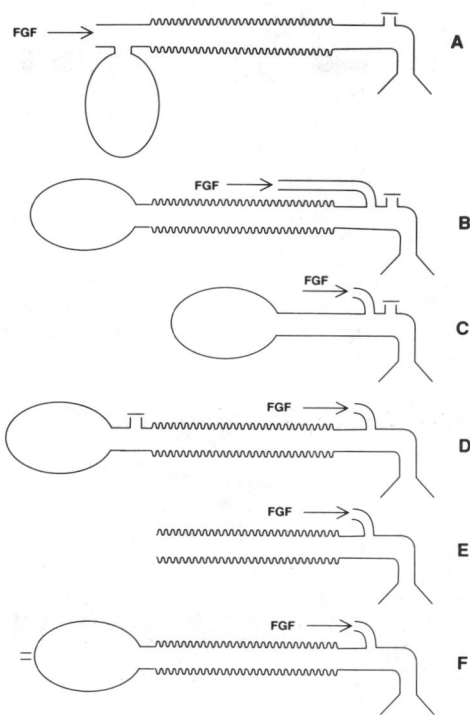

FIG. 19-32. (A–F) Mapleson breathing systems. (Redrawn with permission. Willis BA, Pender JW, Mapleson WW: Rebreathing in a T-piece: Volunteer and theoretical studies of the Jackson-Rees modification of Ayre's T piece during spontaneous respiration. Br J Anaesth 47:1239, 1975.)

voir bag, and fresh gas inflow at the machine end and a spring-loaded expiratory valve near the patient end (Fig. 19-32). Rebreathing during spontaneous ventilation in this circuit can be prevented with relatively low fresh gas flows. Upon exhalation, the patient end of the tubing is filled with dead space gas followed by the alveolar gas. This stream travels up the tubing and meets the fresh gas flowing into the circuit (Fig. 19-33, *left*). The pressure in the circuit increases and forces the expiratory valve to open, allowing the alveolar gas to escape. Most of the dead space gas is washed out if the fresh gas flow is adequate. During the inhalation phase, the fresh gas flushes the dead space gas down the tubing toward the patient. Rebreathing of dead space gas poses no problem because it does not contain carbon dioxide. Several studies have confirmed Mapleson's original finding that rebreathing of alveolar gas can be prevented if the fresh gas flow is equal to or exceeds the patient's minute ventilation.[64, 65] Rebreathing does not occur until the fresh gas flow is below 70% of the patient's minute ventilation.

The Mapleson A circuit is inefficient during controlled ventilation.[66] Expiratory valve pressure must be increased to ventilate the patient. Venting the gas in the circuit now occurs during the inspiratory phase, and the alveolar gases are retained in the tubing during the exhalation phase (Fig. 19-33, *right*). Thus, alveolar gas is rebreathed with the ensuing breath before the pressure in the system increases enough to force the expiratory valve open. This can cause an increase in arterial carbon dioxide tension. Adequate carbon dioxide elimination using controlled ventilation with a Mapleson A System requires a fresh gas flow of greater than $20 \, l \cdot min^{-1}$. In

practice, controlled ventilation should be avoided with this system.

Mapleson B

The Mapleson B System features the fresh gas inlet near the patient end just distal to the expiratory valve (Fig. 19-32). This circuit functions similarly during spontaneous and controlled ventilation, unlike the Mapleson A System. Location of the fresh gas inlet allows fresh gas to accumulate along with exhaled gases in the tubing (Fig. 19-33). The expiratory valve opens when pressure in the circuit increases, and a mixture of alveolar gas and fresh gas is discharged. During the next inspiration, the patient receives fresh gas flow from the machine and a mixture of retained fresh gas and alveolar gas from the tubing (Fig. 19-33). Composition of this inhaled mixture depends on fresh gas flow rate. Rebreathing can be prevented if the fresh gas flow rate is greater than twice the minute ventilation for both spontaneous and controlled ventilation.[66, 67]

Mapleson C

The Mapleson C System is also known as the Water's Circuit without an absorber. Arrangement of its component is similar to that of the Mapleson B, but the large-bore tubing is shorter (Fig. 19-32). This effectively reduces the reservoir volume and allows good mixing of fresh and exhaled gases. The inspired mixture contains more alveolar gas compared with the Mapleson B System. A fresh gas flow of twice the minute ventilation is required to prevent rebreathing.[67] Carbon dioxide will build up although at a slower rate than with Mapleson B Circuit, if rebreathing is allowed to occur.

Mapleson D

The Mapleson D Circuit can be described as a T-piece with an expiratory limb. The fresh gas inlet is located near the patient end, but the expiratory valve is toward the machine end close to the reservoir bag (Fig. 19-32). During spontaneous ventilation the dead space gas, alveolar gas, and fresh gas enter the tubing in the exhalation phase. The expiratory valve opens as pressure increases in the circuit and a portion of this mixture is expelled. The patient receives a combination of fresh gas and mixed gas from the tubing during the next inspiration. The content of this inspired mixture is determined by the rate of fresh gas flow, patient's tidal volume, and duration of the expiratory pause. A long expiratory pause (slow respiratory rate) allows the fresh gas to move down the tubing and flush the alveolar gas. A short expiratory pause (fast respiratory rate) provides inadequate time to flush the alveolar gas and allows rebreathing to occur. The amount of alveolar gas entering the tubing will increase if large tidal volumes are used. In this situation rebreathing can be prevented by high fresh gas flows and a long expiratory pause. Mapleson determined that a fresh gas flow greater than two times the minute ventilation was enough to prevent rebreathing. Recently, it has been shown that normocapnia can be maintained during spontaneous ventilation if the fresh gas flow is $100 \, ml \cdot kg^{-1} \cdot min^{-1}$, despite rebreathing.[68] Soliman and Laberge found that a flow rate of $206 \, ml \cdot kg^{-1} \cdot min^{-1}$ resulted in normocapnia in pediatric patients ages 1–5 yr.[69]

Dead space and alveolar gas enter the tubing in exhalation during controlled ventilation. Fresh gas is delivered to the patient on the next inspiration. Therefore, this system causes less rebreathing than the Mapleson B or C Systems. Bain and

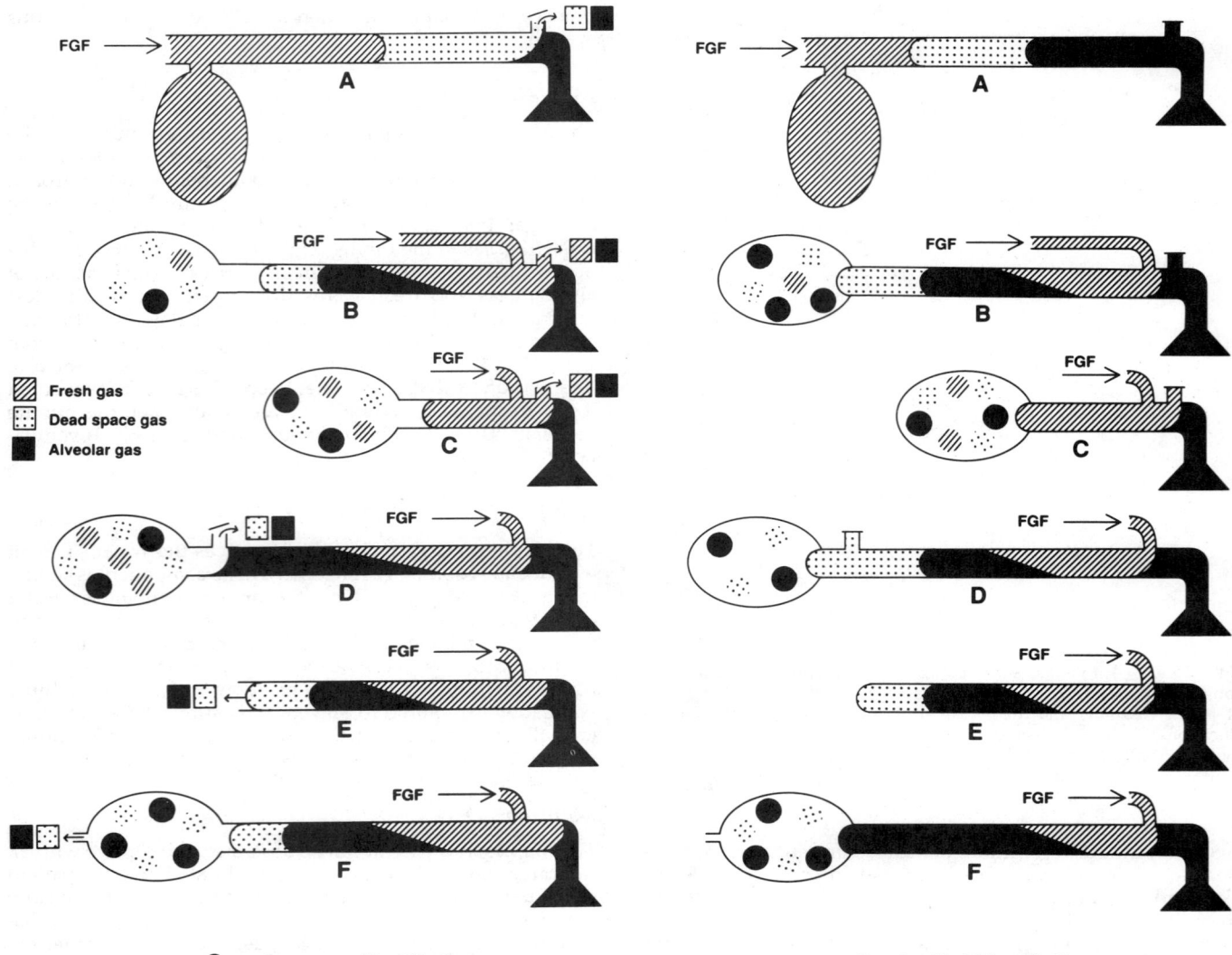

Spontaneous Ventilation   **Controlled Ventilation**

FIG. 19-33. Gas disposition at end-expiration during spontaneous (*left*) and controlled (*right*) ventilation in circuits *A–F*. (Modified with permission. Sykes MK: Rebreathing circuits: A review. Br J Anaesth 40:666, 1968.)

Spoerel have recommended the following fresh gas flow rates during controlled ventilation with the Mapleson D System[68]: $2 \, l \cdot min^{-1}$ for infants weighing less than 10 kg; $3.5 \, l \cdot min^{-1}$ for patients weighing from 10 to 50 kg; $70 \, ml \cdot kg^{-1} \cdot min^{-1}$ for patients weighing more than 60 kg. In each of these cases, the recommended tidal volume is $10 \, ml \cdot kg^{-1}$ and the respiratory rate, $12–16 \, breaths \cdot min^{-1}$.

Bain Circuit

The Bain Circuit is a modification of the Mapleson D System. It is a coaxial circuit in which fresh gas flows through a narrow inner tube within the outer corrugated tubing.[70] The central tube originates near the reservoir bag, but the fresh gas actually enters the circuit at the patient end (Fig. 19-34). Exhaled gases enter the corrugated tubing and are vented through the expiratory valve near the reservoir bag. The Bain Circuit may

be used for both spontaneous and controlled ventilation. The fresh gas flows necessary to prevent rebreathing are similar to those of the Mapleson D System. Normocarbia during spontaneous ventilation requires a fresh gas flow of 200–300, but a flow of only $70 \, ml \cdot kg^{-1}$ will produce normocarbia during controlled ventilation.[68, 71, 72]

There are many advantages of this circuit. It is lightweight, convenient, easily sterilized, and reusable. Scavenging of the gases from the expiratory valve is facilitated because it is located away from the patient. Exhaled gases in the outer reservoir tubing add warmth and humidity to inspired fresh gases. The hazards of the Bain Circuit include unrecognized disconnection or kinking of the inner fresh gas hose. These problems can cause hypercarbia from inadequate gas flow or increased respiratory resistance.

The outer tube should be transparent to allow inspection of the inner tube. The integrity of the inner tube can be assessed

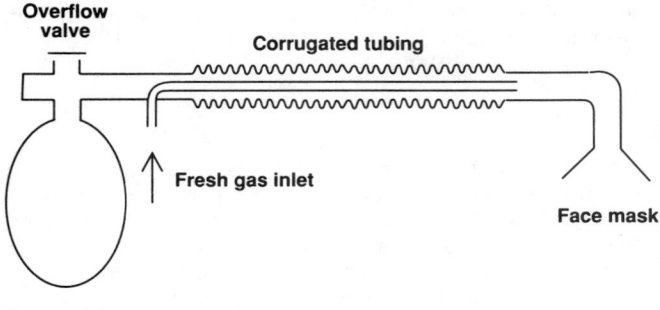

FIG. 19-34. The Bain circuit. (Redrawn with permission. Bain JA, Spoerel WE: A streamlined anaesthetic system. Can Anaesth Soc J 19:426, 1972.)

as described by Pethick.[73] High-flow oxygen is fed into the circuit while the patient end is occluded until the reservoir bag is filled. The patient end is opened, and oxygen is flushed into the circuit. If the inner tube is intact, the Venturi effect occurs at the patient end. This causes a decrease in pressure within the circuit, and the reservoir bag deflates. Conversely, a leak in the inner tube allows the fresh gas to escape into the expiratory limb, and the reservoir bag will remain inflated. This test is recommended as a part of the preanesthesia check if a Bain Circuit is used.

Mapleson E

The Mapleson E is a modification of Ayre's T-piece, which was developed in 1937 by Phillip Ayre for use in pediatric patients undergoing cleft palate repair or intracranial surgery.[74] It consists of a fresh gas inlet at the patient end and long corrugated tubing (Fig. 19-32). It has minimal dead space, no valves, and very little resistance.[75]

The expiratory limb is the reservoir. Volume of the expiratory limb greater than the patient's tidal volume prevents entrainment of room air and thereby prevents dilution of anesthetic gases and oxygen. A fresh gas flow greater than three times the minute ventilation prevents rebreathing.

During spontaneous ventilation, the fresh gas and exhaled gas flow down the expiratory limb (Fig. 19-33, left). Peak expiratory flow occurs early in exhalation. Therefore, the proportion of fresh gas added to the exhaled gases increases. The fresh gas accumulates at the patient end. During the next breath, fresh gas is drawn both from the fresh gas inlet and the expiratory limb or the reservoir. Controlled ventilation can be accomplished by intermittently occluding the end of the expiratory limb.

Mapleson F

The most commonly used T-piece system is the Jackson-Rees modification of Mapleson D.[76] This is a T-piece arrangement with a reservoir bag and incorporates a relief mechanism for venting exhaled gases. The relief mechanism is either an adjustable valve at the distal end of the reservoir bag or simply a hole in the side of the bag. During spontaneous ventilation when the patient exhales, the gases pass down the expiratory limb and mix with the fresh gas (Fig. 19-33, left). The expiratory pause allows fresh gas to push the exhaled gases down

the expiratory limb. With the next inspiration, the inhaled gas mixture comes from the fresh gas flow and the expiratory limb, including the reservoir bag. Considerations for fresh gas flow rates are similar to those for the Bain Circuit. Flow rates equivalent to three times the minute ventilation are recommended to prevent rebreathing.

The Jackson-Rees Circuit is commonly used for controlled ventilation during an anesthetic procedure and for transportation of intubated patients. Fresh gas flow rates are similar to those of the Bain Circuit. The degree of rebreathing is affected by venting and ventilation management.

The Jackson-Rees System is popular for pediatric anesthesia—especially for head and neck surgery—because it is lightweight and can be positioned easily. It is simply constructed and inexpensive and offers minimal resistance because there are no moving parts except the adjustable valve. Observation of the reservoir bag allows one to inspect respiratory excursions and judge the depth of anesthesia. Controlled ventilation can be instituted easily by squeezing the bag. Scavenging can be done either by enclosing the reservoir bag in a plastic chamber from which the waste gases are suctioned or by attaching various devices to the relief valves in the bag.

A disadvantage of this system is lack of humidification. However, this problem can be overcome by allowing the fresh gas to pass through an in-line heated humidifier. Incorporation of a water trap downstream from the humidifier accumulates condensed moisture from the fresh gas inlet tube. This prevents overhydration of the pediatric patient. Another disadvantage of the Jackson-Rees System is the need for high fresh gas flows. Finally, occlusion of the relief valve can rapidly increase the airway pressure, producing barotrauma.

CIRCLE SYSTEM

The circle system is the most popular breathing system in the United States. It is so named because its components are arranged in a circular manner. This system prevents rebreathing of carbon dioxide by soda lime absorption but allows partial rebreathing of other exhaled gases. The extent of rebreathing of the other exhaled gases depends upon component arrangement and the inflow rate.

A circle system can be semiopen, semiclosed, or closed, depending on the amount of fresh gas inflow.[77] A semiopen system has no rebreathing and requires a very high flow of fresh gas. A semiclosed system is associated with rebreathing of gases and is the most commonly used system in the United States. A closed system is one in which the inflow gas exactly matches that being taken up, or consumed, by the patient. There is complete rebreathing of exhaled gases after absorption of carbon dioxide, and the overflow (pop-off) valve is closed.

The circle system (Fig. 19-35) consists of seven components, including the following: 1) a fresh gas inflow source; 2) inspiratory and expiratory unidirectional valves; 3) inspiratory and expiratory corrugated tubes; 4) a Y-piece connector; 5) an overflow or pop-off valve; 6) a reservoir bag; and 7) a canister containing a carbon dioxide absorbent. The unidirectional valves are placed in the system so that the gases flow in only one direction and pass through the carbon dioxide absorber each time around. The fresh gas inflow enters the circle by a connection from the common gas outlet of the anesthesia machine.

Numerous variations of circle arrangement are possible, depending upon the relative positions of the unidirectional

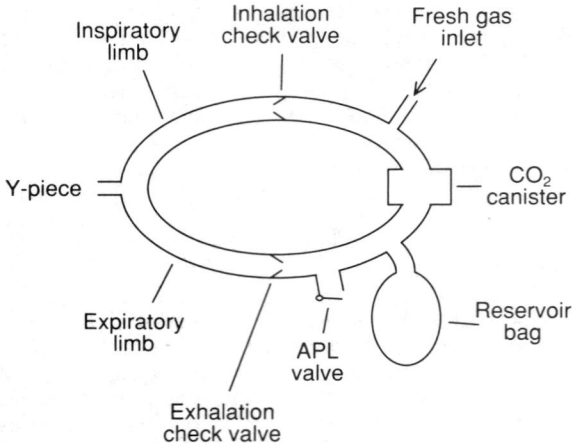

FIG. 19-35. Components of the circle system.

valves, the pop-off valve, the reservoir bag, the carbon dioxide absorber, and the site of fresh gas entry. However, to prevent rebreathing of carbon dioxide, three rules must be followed: 1) a unidirectional valve must be located between the patient and the reservoir bag on both the inspiratory and expiratory limbs of the circuit; 2) the fresh gas inflow cannot enter the circuit between the expiratory valve and the patient; and 3) the overflow (pop-off) valve cannot be located between the patient and the inspiratory valve. If these rules are followed, any arrangement of the other components will prevent rebreathing of carbon dioxide.[78]

The most efficient circle system arrangement that allows the highest conservation of fresh gases is one with the unidirectional valves near the patient and the pop-off valve just downstream from the expiratory valve. This arrangement conserves dead space gas and preferentially eliminates alveolar gas. A more practical but less efficient arrangement is the one used on all contemporary anesthesia machines (Fig. 19-35). It is less efficient because it allows alveolar and dead space gas to mix before venting.[78, 79]

The advantages of the circle system include a relative constancy of inspired concentration, conservation of respiratory moisture and heat, conservation of anesthetic gases, and minimization of operating room pollution. Additionally, it can be used for closed-system anesthesia or with low oxygen flows. The major disadvantage of the circle system stems from its complex design. The circuit has approximately 10 connections, all of which can disconnect and leak. Malfunctioning valves can cause serious problems. Rebreathing can occur if the valves stick in the open position. Total occlusion of the circuit can occur if they are stuck closed. Finally, the bulk of the circle offers less convenience and portability than the Mapleson Systems.

CARBON DIOXIDE ABSORPTION

Different anesthesia systems eliminate carbon dioxide with varying degrees of efficiency. This section will primarily be concerned with the closed or semiclosed circle system, which requires carbon dioxide absorption in order to make rebreathing possible. Desirable features in the carbon dioxide absorption mechanism are lack of toxicity with common anesthetics, low resistance to air flow, low cost, ease of handling, and relative efficiency.

HISTORY

In the early 1900s European scientists were experimenting with the carbon dioxide absorptive properties of lime water and caustic sodas. However, the real impetus to develop efficient carbon dioxide absorptive techniques came from submarine and chemical warfare applications during World War I.[80] In 1915 Wilson patented a new process to make soda lime, which greatly increased its efficiency.[81] Rebreathing techniques with carbon dioxide absorption were slow to gain popularity until cyclopropane was introduced.[80] Cyclopropane was an expensive and explosive anesthetic agent. Many additions and refinements in soda lime have occurred since its invention, but the essential ingredients have remained unchanged.

CHEMISTRY

Two formulations for carbon dioxide absorption are commonly used today. These are soda lime and baralyme. Soda lime consists of 94% calcium hydroxide, 5% sodium hydroxide, and 1% potassium hydroxide as an activator. Small amounts of silica are added to produce calcium and sodium silicate. This addition produces a hard compound and reduces dust formation. The efficiency of the soda lime absorption varies inversely with the hardness; therefore, little silicate is used in contemporary soda lime. Sodium hydroxide is the catalyst for the carbon dioxide absorptive properties of soda lime.[80, 82]

Baralyme is composed of 80% calcium hydroxide and 20% barium hydroxide. Baralyme is more stable than soda lime and does not require a silica binder. Barium hydroxide is the catalyst. Baralyme is more dense than soda lime and is approximately 15% less efficient, based on weight in absorbing carbon dioxide. Water is required for both formulations, but baralyme contains water as the barium hydroxide octohydrate salt. Therefore, it may perform better in a dry climate.[80, 82]

The soda lime used in the early days of carbon dioxide absorption was noted to regenerate its efficiency to absorb carbon dioxide after being exhausted.[83] The explanation for this regeneration is complex, but it is of little concern today. Regeneration is rarely seen today because of improved soda lime with less silica and the addition of potassium hydroxide. Baralyme has no regeneration capability.[80, 82]

The size of the absorptive granules has been determined by trial and error, which represents a compromise between resistance to air flow and absorptive efficiency.[84] The smaller the granules, the more surface area is available for absorption. However, air flow resistance increases. The granular size of soda lime and baralyme in anesthesia practice is between 4 and 8 mesh. Resistance to air flow at this size is negligible. Mesh refers to the number of openings per linear inch in a sieve through which the granular particles can pass. A 4-mesh screen means that there are four quarter-inch openings per linear inch. An 8-mesh screen has eight eighth-inch openings per linear inch.[80]

The absorption of carbon dioxide by soda lime is a chemical and not a physical process.[83] Carbon dioxide combines with water to form carbonic acid. Carbonic acid reacts with the hydroxides to form sodium (or potassium) carbonate and water. Calcium hydroxide accepts the carbonate to form calcium carbonate and sodium (or potassium) hydroxide. The equations are as follows:

1. $CO_2 + H_2O \rightleftharpoons H_2CO_3$
2. $H_2CO_3 + 2NaOH (KOH) \rightleftharpoons Na_2CO_3 (K_2CO_3) + 2H_2O + Heat$
3. $Na_2CO_3 (K_2CO_3) + Ca(OH)_2 \rightleftharpoons CaCO_3 + 2NaOH (KOH)$

Some carbon dioxide may react directly with $Ca(OH)_2$, but this reaction is much slower.

The reaction with baralyme differs because more water is liberated by a direct reaction of barium hydroxide and carbon dioxide.

1. $Ba(OH)_2 + 8H_2O + CO_2 \rightleftharpoons BaCO_3 + 9H_2O + Heat$
2. $9H_2O + 9CO_2 \rightleftharpoons 9H_2CO_3$
   Then by direct reactions and by KOH and NaOH
3. $9H_2CO_3 + 9Ca(OH)_2 \rightleftharpoons CaCO_3 + 18H_2O + Heat$

ABSORPTIVE CAPACITY AND INDICATORS

The maximum amount of carbon dioxide that can be absorbed with the above equations is 26 l of carbon dioxide per 100 g of absorbent. However, channeling of gas through granules may substantially decrease this efficiency and allow only 10–20 l of carbon dioxide to actually be absorbed.[85]

Several indicators are packaged with the absorbent to indicate exhaustion. These are acids or bases that change color when the hydrogen ion concentration changes. Common indicators and their respective colors are as follows: phenolphthalein (white → pink), ethyl violet (white → purple), clayton yellow (red → yellow), ethyl orange (orange → yellow), mimosa z (red → white).[86]

INCOMPATIBILITIES

As stated earlier, it is important and desirable to have carbon dioxide absorbents that are not intrinsically toxic and that are not toxic when exposed to common anesthetics. Soda lime fits this description, but it is important to note that when using an uncommon anesthetic, trichloroethylene, toxicity may result. In the presence of alkali and heat, trichloroethylene degrades into the cranial neurotoxin dichloroacetylene. Phosgene, a potent pulmonary irritant, is also produced. The resulting toxicities are manifested by cranial nerve lesions, encephalitis, and adult respiratory distress syndrome (ARDS).[87] A newer anesthetic, sevoflurane, is somewhat unstable in soda lime, but this apparently does not produce any toxic effects.[88]

HUMIDIFICATION

Historically the lung has been recognized as an organ that is highly vulnerable to disease. The benefits of using heated mist to treat airway disease have been recognized since the time of Hippocrates. A more modern recognition of these benefits is perhaps symbolized by the ubiquitous sick room croup kettle used by mothers to care for their children.

PHYSIOLOGIC CONSIDERATIONS

Mucus Blanket

The mucociliary blanket in the tracheobronchial tree provides a defense mechanism by which foreign particles and infectious debris are trapped and removed (Fig. 19-36). Warm, humidified air is needed for this defense to function properly.[89] The respiratory tract is an air conditioning system of remarkable efficiency. The upper airways warm and humidify the inspired air to 37°C and 95% humidity, despite wide variations in the external temperatures, ranging from 0 to 25°C, and humidities of less than 45–55%. Air reaching the laryngeal opening varies only a degree centigrade under a wide range of conditions.[90] The large surface area and high vascularity of the mouth and nose warm and humidify 10,000 l of air every 24 h. Nasal secretions amount to about 1 l per day. Seventy-five per cent of this moisture is used to humidify the inspired air. Most of this moisture is recaptured, limiting insensible water loss to only 25%, or 250 ml per day. However, fever, hyperventilation, endotracheal intubation, and inhalation of dry gases during an anesthetic procedure can dramatically increase this insensible loss in a patient.

Pseudostratified, ciliated, columnar epithelial cells of the respiratory tract keep the mucus blanket in a constant streaming motion toward the larynx.[91] Hence, the mucus blanket is also known as the "mucus escalator."[90] The production and transport of the mucus, as well as the ciliary movement, is affected by various physical and biochemical factors. Ciliary activity is optimal between the pHs of 6.8 and 7.2 and at a temperature of 28–33°C. Sodium chloride in 0.9% and 2% solution does not affect the ciliary activity. Opiates and nicotine directly depress the ciliary activity, but atropine inhibits it by increasing the viscosity of the mucus blanket. Inhalation anesthetics depress ciliary activity in concentrations required to produce general anesthesia.[89]

Precise administration of gases through the modern anesthesia machines depends upon clean and dry anesthetic gases. These are supplied as anhydrous gases free of particu-

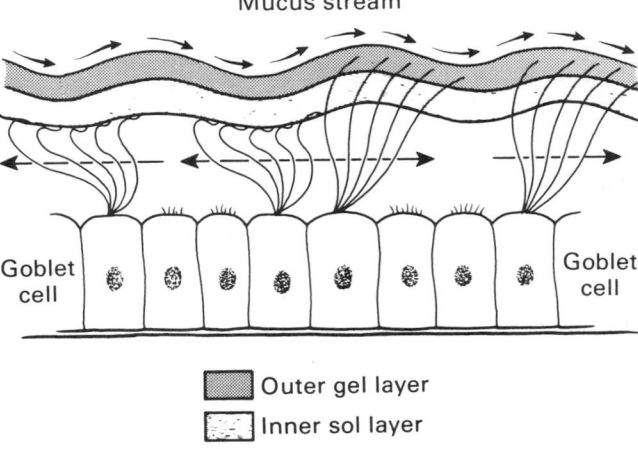

Mucus stream

☐ Outer gel layer
☐ Inner sol layer

FIG. 19-36. The mucociliary blanket. The gradient of water content of the mucus layer of the respiratory tree has led to the arbitrary classification of the blanket into two distinct layers: the inner sol layer and the outer gel layer, which is dryer and more viscous. The mucus blanket is kept in a constant streaming motion toward the pharynx by the ciliated epithelium.

late matter because the presence of moisture can cause the valves to malfunction, orifices to distort, and flowmeters to stray.[92] Inhalation of dry gases at room temperature or below imposes on the lower respiratory passages to humidify these gases.[93] In addition, endotracheal intubation bypasses nasopharyngeal air conditioning and compels the mucosa of the lower respiratory tract to perform the function of the nasopharynx.[90] Therefore, the water and heat losses from the respiratory tract become clinically significant in patients receiving unhumidified gases during a general anesthetic for any but the shortest surgical procedure. Breathing dry air can lead to dessication of mucus, impairment of ciliary function and mucus escalator activity, retention of secretions, atelectasis, bacterial colonization, and pneumonia (Table 19-2). Hence, in order to minimize postoperative pulmonary complications, warmth and humidity must either be added from external sources to these dry gases as they enter the patient's airway or conserved by using rebreathing techniques and low fresh gas flows.

HUMIDITY

Vaporization is the conversion of a liquid into a gas. Humidity is not true gaseous water because atmospheric temperature exists below the critical temperature of water (374°C or 705°F).[91] The amount of water vapor a volume of gas can potentially contain depends upon the temperature. The higher the temperature, the greater amount of water vapor a volume of gas can contain. The maximum amount of water that air can hold in the vapor state is called the saturated water content.[90] Figure 19-37 and Table 19-3 demonstrate that both the maximum water content of a gas and water vapor pressure increase exponentially with temperature.

Three terms are used to express water content of a gas: 1) Absolute humidity is the actual mass of water contained in a given volume of gas at a given temperature. Traditionally, this is measured as milligrams of water vapor per liter of gas ($mg \cdot l^{-1}$). 2) Maximum humidity is the maximum mass of water vapor that a given volume of gas can hold at a given temperature (saturated water content). 3) Relative humidity is a percentage expression of the actual water vapor content of a gas compared with its capacity to carry water at a given temperature.

The relative humidity can be computed if the temperature of the gas is known and either 1) the absolute humidity of the gas is known, or 2) the partial pressure of water vapor of the gas is known.[91] By referring to Table 19-3, the percentage relative humidity (% RH) can be calculated by substituting values into any of the simple formulas listed below.

$$\% \text{ RH} = \frac{\text{absolute humidity}}{\text{maximum humidity}} \times 100$$

TABLE 19-2.   Hazards of Breathing Dry Air

1. Ciliary paralysis and interference with mucociliary transport
2. Increase in viscosity of mucus leading to inspissation, encrustation, and atelectasis
3. Inflammation
4. Metaplasia
5. Increased incidence of postoperative pulmonary complication
6. Decrease in body temperature

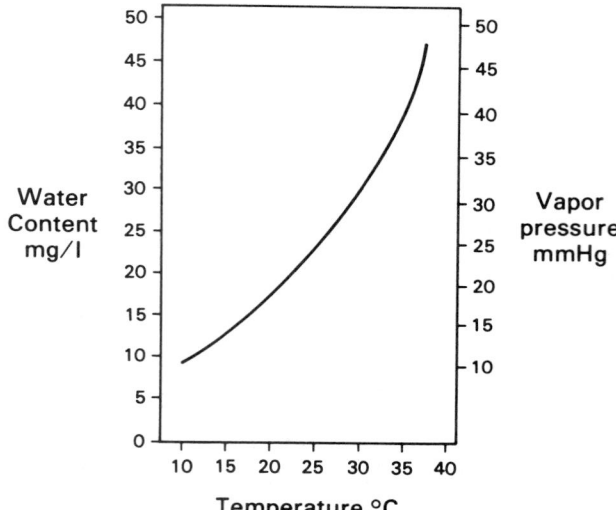

FIG. 19-37. Maximum water content and water vapor pressure curve of a fully saturated gas. Both the maximum water content and the water vapor pressure increase exponentially with an increase in temperature.

TABLE 19-3.   Maximum Water Content and Water Vapor Pressure

TEMPERATURE (°C)	MAXIMUM WATER CONTENT (mg/l)	WATER VAPOR PRESSURE (mm Hg)
0	4.85	4.58
5	6.80	6.54
10	9.41	9.21
15	12.83	12.79
20	17.30	17.54
21*	18.35	18.70
25	23.04	23.76
30	30.35	31.82
35	39.60	42.18
37	43.90	47.07

*Standard room air conditions are defined as 21° C and 50% humidity. Water content at these conditions is approximately $9 \, mg \cdot l^{-1}$.

$$\% \text{ RH} = \frac{\text{actual water content}}{\text{maximum water content}} \times 100$$

$$\% \text{ RH} = \frac{\text{actual water vapor pressure}}{\text{saturated water vapor pressure}} \times 100$$

EXAMPLE 1:

Given: Temperature = 21° C

Actual water content 9.2 $mg \cdot l^{-1}$

$$\% \text{ RH} = \frac{\text{actual water content}}{\text{maximum water content}} \times 100$$

$$= \frac{9.2}{18.35} = 50\%$$

(Saturated room air conditions have been defined as 21° C and 50% humidity. The actual water content at these conditions is 9 mg·l^{-1}. However, it is 18 mg·l^{-1} when fully saturated.)

EXAMPLE 2:

Given: Temperature = 37° C

water vapor pressure = 18.8 mm Hg

$$\% \text{ RH} = \frac{\text{actual water vapor pressure}}{\text{saturated water vapor pressure}} \times 100$$

$$= \frac{18.8 \text{ mm Hg}}{47 \text{ mm Hg}} \times 100 = 40\%$$

Humidity deficit is the lack of sufficient water vapor for saturation. Room air is rarely saturated, so additional moisture must be added when air enters the respiratory tree. A primary humidity deficit exists when inspired room air is less than saturated at a given temperature. A secondary humidity deficit occurs when inhaled air is warmed from room temperature to body temperature. This is because the capacity of air to carry moisture increases when the inspired air is warmed.[91-93] Under normal conditions, the nasal mucosa and the upper airways pay this deficit by giving up heat and water.

The water content to correct the humidity deficit at standard room air conditions can be calculated. Inspired air at 21°C and 50% humidity contains only 9 mg·l^{-1} of water. Once inhaled, the water content must increase to 44 mg·l^{-1} at 37°C and the humidity deficit is 35 mg·l^{-1}.

Humidity deficit (mg·l^{-1}) = maximum humidity
(37°C) − absolute humidity (21°C)

Compressed oxygen is 100% dry even at room temperature. Table 19-3 shows that 44 mg of water vapor must be added to each liter of oxygen to achieve maximum humidity at 37°C. The relative humidity is zero in this instance. The humidity deficit is 44 mg·l^{-1} because the difference between maximum water content (44 mg·l^{-1}) and absolute water content (0 mg·l^{-1}) is 44 mg·l^{-1}.

The loss of respiratory water can be calculated by the following formula:

Respiratory water loss g·hr^{-1} = 60 V_E (44 − A_t)

Water loss is the product of the minute ventilation (V_E) and the gradient of the inspired and exhaled water content. V_E can be measured or estimated from a nomogram. The water content of fully saturated exhaled air is 44 mg·l^{-1} at 37°C (Table 19-3). The absolute water content of the inspired air at a given temperature is expressed as A_t. The hourly water loss for a 70-kg adult breathing a standard room air mixture ($A_t = 9$ mg·l^{-1}) approximates 13 g·hr^{-1}. This value is near the estimated insensible daily respiratory water loss of 250 ml·day^{-1}. Total body water loss through this mechanism would increase only to 16 g/h if 100% anhydrous oxygen were administered. Thus, respiratory water loss resulting from humidity deficits has a negligible effect on body water balance and is replaced easily even in children. The importance of humidification of inspired gases is best understood in terms of the local preservation of the protective mucus blanket and thermal regulation.[94-97] Gases delivered at 37°C and those that are 50%−75% saturated will maintain the integrity of the mucus blanket.

HEAT LOSS

Humidity deficits require energy in two ways: The first way is the simple necessity of warming the inspired gases to body temperature. The heat loss for this activity depends upon the V_E, the temperature gradient between exhaled and inhaled gas, and the specific heat of the gas. It is expressed as follows:

Humidity heat loss/min = V_E (37 − t) (specific heat)

The caloric requirements for this activity are estimated to be 40 cal·min^{-1} for modern breathing systems in which the gases are delivered at room temperature.[91] The cooler the gases, the higher the delivered energy cost will be.

The most significant loss of heat and caloric debt results from the cost of vaporizing water to cover the humidity deficit. Heat is expended to vaporize enough water to saturate the inspired air at body temperature. The caloric expenditure for this activity has been estimated to be about 550 cal·g^{-1} of water vaporized. Because anhydrous oxygen administration will require 16 g·hr^{-1} of water vapor, three times as many calories are expended per hour to humidify inhaled air. A depression of thermal regulation during general anesthesia compounds the heat loss and can produce a significant threat to anesthetized patients, particularly children. The administration of anesthetic gases at 37°C and 100% humidity can maintain body temperature in anesthetized patients and can even be used in some situations to rewarm patients who have been deliberately cooled. Warming by inhalation of heated and rehumidified air or oxygen by the mask or endotracheal tube is an effective method of increasing the patient's core temperature. The temperature of inspired gases at the mouth or endotracheal tube, as well as the humidifier's temperature, should be monitored. Temperatures in excess of 40°C at the endotracheal tube can produce hemorrhagic, bronchospastic tracheobronchitis. Temperatures of 40°C or less at the endotracheal tube connection are safe for rewarming and allow a margin of safety in temperature regulation.

HUMIDIFIERS

The rate of humidification (vaporization) is influenced by three factors: 1) the surface area for gas/water contact, 2) the duration of exposure, and 3) the temperature.[90]

There are two basic types of humidifying devices: vaporizers and nebulizers. Nebulizers deliver water in droplet form as an aerosol. Heated nebulizers can produce 100% humidity at body temperature. Despite their efficiency, they present certain hazards (Table 19-4). Nebulizers can transmit bacteria in the water droplets, but vaporizers cannot because there is no particulate matter.[98] Nebulizers also present the hazard of producing overhydration, water intoxication, and increased respiratory resistance, especially in children.[90, 91] Vaporizers rarely add enough water to produce problems with water balance. The predominant humidifiers used on anesthesia machines are the vaporizer type because they are efficient and have a wider margin of safety than nebulizers.

TABLE 19-4. Hazards of Nebulized Humidification

1. Overheating
2. Overhydration, pulmonary edema, water intoxication (especially in children)
3. Infection
4. Increased airway resistance
5. Bronchopneumonia

ANESTHESIA CIRCUITS AND HUMIDITY

The minimum recommended humidity for anesthesia is 60% of 12 mg·l^{-1}. Optimum values are between 14 and 30 mg·l^{-1} of water vapor. Simple moistening of the insides of corrugated hoses and the reservoir bag has significantly increased the humidity in the circle system.[99] This achieves a water content of about 22 mg·l^{-1}. The humidity declines with time as evaporation within the circuit produces cooling. The adult or pediatric closed circle system can achieve a water content as high as 29 mg·l^{-1} when the gases are passed through a soda lime canister.[94, 100, 101] The relative humidity approaches 100% because of water production by neutralization during the process of carbon dioxide absorption by soda lime. Some of the water vapor also comes from the exhaled air. A closed circuit provides ideal inspired humidity. Humidification probably is not necessary in units designed for total rebreathing (closed system) because water loss is of a small magnitude. Humidification is required for systems that are open or semiopen and in which high gas flows are used for protracted periods of time. Table 19-5 lists the humidity achieved with some older anesthesia circuit systems. The to-and-fro system was particularly efficient in preserving water and heat because the soda lime canister was near the patient's mouth. Temperature within the canister rose as high as 45°C, and there was little time for cooling the gases *en route* to the patient.

Nonrebreathing circuits ordinarily deliver unhumidified gases. The Bain circuit is an exception. It is a modification of the Mapleson D System (see Anesthetic Circuits) and is conducive to the humidification of inspired gases.[91, 102] The Bain circuit is a coaxial circuit, and the inspiratory line is insulated by the warm exhaled gases in the outer expiratory tubing. This design minimizes temperature and humidity decreases once the system is heated. An absolute humidity between 21–25 mg·l^{-1} can be achieved within 30 min of use. Relative humidity will increase to 100% in approximately 80 min.

Humidity does not affect oxygen analyzers unless excess condensation accumulates on the sensors.[103] This problem is

TABLE 19-5. Relative Humidity of Gases in the Various Anesthetic Systems

ANESTHETIC SYSTEM	RELATIVE HUMIDITY OF GASES
Nonbreathing valve	0
T-piece	0
To-and-fro	40–100
Closed circle*	40–100
Bain modification	65–100
HUMAN NOSE	65

* Higher relative humidity is achieved by the low-flow, closed technique with a carbon dioxide absorber. Humidity is in the lower range with semiopen high-flow techniques.

minimized by the water-repelling membrane over the polymeric membrane. Condensation will cause an erroneously low reading if it occurs. The analyzer will therefore err in the patient's favor, should it occur. Condensation in the low-pressure alarm of anesthesia ventilators is a rare occurrence. Most condensation rains out in the large anesthesia circuits before reaching the low-pressure line. Condensation in the low-pressure alarm line will cause the alarm to sound. Condensation does not make the alarm inoperative but rather gives it a false disconnect response. Finally, condensation can occlude gas sampling lines for mass spectrometers and carbon dioxide analyzers.

HUMIDIFIERS–VAPORIZERS

Vaporizers, in contrast to nebulizers, are derived from two basic prototypes: 1) simple vaporizers, and 2) heated vaporizers.[91] Simple vaporizers do not employ heat and are designed to add only enough humidity to make the gas more comfortable. This type of humidifier is generally used only by mask or in an incubator. It allows the nasopharynx to provide the balance of humidification not provided by the humidifier. Although these devices may provide 100% humidity at room air temperature, they will supply about a third of the humidity required for the lower respiratory tract at 37°C. Two types of simple vaporizers have been used. These are the following: 1) the pass-over or blow-by humidifiers, and 2) the bubble humidifier. Two other humidifiers have been classified as simple vaporizers but are actually nebulizers that do not use heat. These are called the jet and underwater jet humidifiers.

Three major types of heated vaporizers are commonly used: 1) the Hopkins, or pass-over, vaporizer, 2) the bubbler, and 3) the heated cascade humidifier. The Hopkins, or pass-over, vaporizer is the simplest of the heated vaporizers. This type of humidifier is merely the heated version of the simple vaporizer. The large reservoir of the pass-over vaporizer is heated by an external hot plate element. It provides humidity by passing air over a relatively large surface area. This is the vaporizer used on the Emerson ventilator.[91]

Bubblers add vapor by streaming bubbles through a jar of water. A disadvantage of the bubbler is that the water in the jar is cooled as it evaporates. This lowers the temperature of the carrying gas and reduces its moisture-carrying capacity. The bubbler can only provide 20% relative humidity at body temperature unless it is heated. The deficit must be made up by the respiratory passages, and this may be poorly tolerated by a patient who already has lost mucociliary function. The addition of heat increases the performance of the bubbler, which is commonly used with nasal cannulas and oxygen masks.

Heated cascade humidifiers technically are bubblers. These devices deliver 100% humidity at body temperature. They break inspired gas into tiny bubbles and pass them through heated water. These are the mainstream humidifiers used with anesthesia systems and are the most effective of all the evaporative humidifiers. These vaporizers are typified by the Bennett cascade vaporizer. A potential hazard associated with the Bennett is misconnection. It has a one-way check valve, which retards the drift of humidity retrograde to the anesthesia machine.[91] Even though the inlet and outlet are labeled, they have the same diameter. Reverse hook-up results in a no-flow state.

The rationale for using heated humidity in anesthesia and respiratory therapy is to make the inspired gases comfortable for the patient, preserve the mucus blanket, heat inspired gases to provide 100% relative humidity, and counter the thermal loss resulting from water vaporization in the respiratory tree.

REFERENCES

1. Minimum Performance and Safety Requirements for Components and Systems of Continuous-Flow Anesthesia Machines for Human Use (ANSI Z79.8-1979). New York, American National Standards Institute, February 1979
2. Dorsch JA, Dorsch SE: The anesthesia machine. In Dorsch JA, Dorsch SE (eds): Understanding Anesthesia Equipment, 2nd ed, p 38. Baltimore, Williams & Wilkins, 1984
3. Bowie E, Huffman LM: The Anesthesia Machine: Essentials for Understanding. Madison, Ohmeda, The BOC Group, 1985
4. Narkomed 2A Anesthesia System. Technical Service Manual. Telford, North American Drager, June 1985
5. Modulus Anesthesia Gas Machine. Operation Maintenance. Madison, Ohio Medical Products, The BOC Group, 1981
6. Modulus II Anesthesia System. Operation and Maintenance Manual. Madison, Ohmeda, The BOC Group, 1985
7. Ohmeda 8000 Anesthesia Machine. Operation and Maintenance Manual. Madison, Ohmeda, The BOC Group, 1985
8. Narkomed 2A Anesthesia System. Instruction Manual. Telford, North American Drager, July 1985
9. Narkomed 3 Anesthesia System. Operator's Instruction Manual. Telford, North American Drager, 1986
10. Modulus II Anesthesia System. Service Manual. Madison, Ohmeda, The BOC Group, 1985
11. Loeb RG, Ross WT, Lawson D: How modern anesthesia machines respond to a decrease in oxygen line pressure. Anesth Analg 66:S1, 1987
12. Macintosh R, Mushin WW, Epstein HG: Flowmeters. In Macintosh R, Mushin WW, Epstein HG (eds): Physics for the Anaesthetist, 3rd ed, p 196. Oxford, Blackwell Scientific Publications, 1963
13. Andriani J: Clinical application of physical principles concerning gases and vapors to anesthesiology. In Adriani J (ed): The Chemistry and Physics of Anesthesia, 2nd ed, p 58. Springfield, Charles C Thomas, 1962
14. Eger EI, Hylton RR, Irwin RH et al: Anesthetic flow meter sequence—A cause for hypoxia. Anesthesiology 24:396, 1963
15. Eger EI, Epstein RM: Hazards of anesthetic equipment. Anesthesiology 24:490, 1964
16. Schreiber P: Safety Guidelines for Anesthesia Systems. Telford, North American Drager, 1985
17. Rendell-Baker L: Problems with anesthetic and respiratory therapy equipment. Int Anesthesiol Clin 20:1, 1982
18. Mazze RI: Therapeutic misadventures with oxygen delivery systems: The need for continuous in-line oxygen monitors. Anesth Analg 51:787, 1972
19. Abraham ZA, Basagoitia B: A potentially lethal anesthesia machine failure. Anesthesiology 66:589, 1987
20. Ohmeda Unitrol Anesthesia System. Operation and Maintenance Manual. Madison, Ohmeda, The BOC Group, 1985
21. 30/70 Proportionate Anesthesia machine (Canadian version). Madison, Ohio Medical Products, 1982
22. Dorsch JA, Dorsch SE: Vaporizers. In Dorsch JA, Dorsch SE (eds): Understanding Anesthesia Equipment, 2nd ed, p 77. Baltimore, Williams & Wilkins, 1984
23. Macintosh R, Mushin WW, Epstein HG: Vapor pressure. In Macintosh R, Mushin WW, Epstein HG (eds): Physics for the Anaesthetist, 3rd ed, p 68. Oxford, Blackwell Scientific Publications, 1963
24. Adriani J: Principles of physics and chemistry of solids and fluids applicable to anesthesiology. In Adriani J (ed): The Chemistry and Physics of Anesthesia, 2nd ed, p 7. Springfield, Charles C Thomas, 1962
25. Macintosh R, Mushin WW, Esptein HG: Vaporization. In Macintosh R, Mushin WW, Epstein HG (eds): Physics for the Anaesthetist, 3rd ed, p 26. Oxford, Blackwell Scientific Publications, 1963
26. Macintosh R, Mushin WW, Epstein HG: Specific heat. In Macintosh R, Mushin WW, Epstein HG (eds): Physics for the Anaesthetist, 3rd ed, p 17. Oxford, Blackwell Scientific Publications, 1963
27. Schreiber P: Anaesthetic equipment: Performance, classification, and safety. New York, Springer-Verlag, 1972
28. Vapor 19.1 Operating Manual. Lubeck, Federal Republic of Germany, Dragerwerk, 1985
29. Tec 4 Continuous Flow Vaporizer. Operator's Manual. Steeton, England, Ohmeda, The BOC Group, 1986
30. Hill DW, Lowe HJ: Comparison of concentration of halothane in closed and semi-closed circuits during controlled ventilation. Anesthesiology 23:291, 1962
31. Hill DW: The design and calibration of vaporizers for volatile anaesthetic agents. In Scurr C, Feldman S (eds): Scientific Foundations of Anaesthesia, 3rd ed, p 544. London, William Heineman Medical Books, 1982
32. Hill DW: The design and calibration of vaporizers for volatile anaesthetic agents. Br J Anaesth 40:648, 1968
33. Morris LE: Problems in the performance of anesthesia vaporizers. Int Anesthesiol Clin 12:199, 1974
34. Stoelting RK: The effects of nitrous oxide on halothane output from Fluotec Mark 2 vaporizers. Anesthesiology 35:215, 1971
35. Diaz PD: The influence of carrier gas on the output of automatic vaporizers. Br J Anaesth 48:387, 1976
36. Nawaf K, Stoelting RK: Nitrous oxide increases enflurane concentrations delivered by ethrane vaporizers. Anesth Analg 58:30, 1979
37. Prins L, Strupat J, Clement J et al: An evaluation of gas density dependence of anaesthetic vaporizers. Can Anaesth Soc J 27:106, 1980
38. Lin CY: Assessment of vaporizer performance in low-flow and closed-circuit anesthesia. Anesth Analg 59:359, 1980
39. Gould DB, Lampert BA, MacKrell TN: Effect of nitrous oxide solubility on vaporizer aberrance. Anesth Analg 61:938, 1982
40. Palayiwa E, Sanderson MH, Hahn CEW: Effects of carrier gas composition on the output of six anaesthetic vaporizers. Br J Anaesth 55:1025, 1983
41. Peters KR, Wingard DW: Anesthesia machine leakage due to misaligned vaporizers. Anesth Rev 14:36, 1987
42. Marks WE Jr, Bullard JR: Another hazard of free-standing vaporizers, increased anesthetic concentration with reversed flow of vaporizing gas. Anesthesiology 45:445, 1976
43. Capan L, Ramanathan S, Chalon J et al: A possible hazard with use of the Ohio Ethrane Vaporizer. Anesth Analg 59:65, 1980
44. Spearman CB, Sanders HG: Physical principles and functional designs of ventilators. In Kirby RR, Smith RA, Desautels DA (eds): Mechanical Ventilation, p 59. New York, Churchill Livingstone, 1985
45. McPherson SP, Spearman CB: Introduction to ventilators. In McPherson SP, Spearman CB (eds): Respiratory Therapy Equipment, p 230. St. Louis, CV Mosby, 1985
46. Ohio Anesthesia Ventilator. Operation Maintenance. Madison, Ohio Medical Products, The BOC Group, 1982
47. Anesthesia Ventilator. Service Manual. Madison, Ohio Medical Products, The BOC Group, 1983
48. Ohio V5 Anesthesia Ventilator. Operation and Maintenance Manual. Madison, Ohmeda, The BOC Group, 1983
49. V5A Anesthesia Ventilator. Operation and Maintenance Manual. Madison, Ohmeda, The BOC Group, 1986

50. V5/V5A Anesthesia Ventilator. Service Manual. Madison, Ohio Medical Products, The BOC Group, 1983

51. 7000 Electronic Anesthesia Ventilator: Operation Maintenance. Madison, Ohmeda, The BOC Group, 1985

52. 7000 Electronic Anesthesia Ventilator. Service Manual. Madison, Ohmeda, The BOC Group, 1985

53. Roth S, Tweedie E, Sommer RM: Excessive airway pressure due to a malfunctioning anesthesia ventilator. Anesthesiology 65:532, 1986

54. Feeley TW, Bancroft ML: Problems with mechanical ventilators. Int Anesthesiol Clin 20:83, 1982

55. Cooper JB, Newbower RS, Kitz RJ: An analysis of major errors and equipment failures in anesthesia management. Considerations for prevention and detection. Anesthesiology 60:34, 1984

56. Cooper JB: Toward prevention of anesthetic mishaps. Int Anesthesiol Clin 22:167, 1984

57. Spooner RB, Kirby RR: Equipment related anesthetic incidents. Int Anesthesiol Clin 22:133, 1984

58. Emergency Care Research Institute: Avoiding anesthetic mishaps through pre-use checks. Health Devices 11:201, 1982

59. Anesthesia Apparatus Checkout Recommendations, FDA. Rockville, Food and Drug Administration, August 1986

60. Comm G, Rendell-Baker L: Back pressure check valves a hazard. Anesthesiology 56:327, 1982

61. Dorsch JA, Dorsch SE: Equipment checking and maintenance. In Dorsch JA, Dorsch SE (eds): Understanding Anesthesia Equipment, 2nd ed, pp 401–414. Baltimore, Williams and Wilkins, 1984

62. Mapleson WW: The elimination of rebreathing in various semiclosed anaesthetic systems. Br J Anaesth 26:323, 1954

63. Willis BA, Pender JW, Mapleson WW: Rebreathing in a T-piece: Volunteer and theoretical studies of the Jackson-Rees modification of Ayre's T-piece during spontaneous respiration. Br J Anaesth 47:1239, 1975

64. Norman J, Adams AP, Sykes MK: Rebreathing with the Magill attachment. Anaesthesia 31:247, 1959

65. Kain ML, Nunn JF: Fresh gas economics of the Magill circuit. Anesthesiology 29:964, 1968

66. Sykes MK: Rebreathing during controlled respiration with the Magill attachment. Anaesthesia 31:247, 1959

67. Sykes MK: Rebreathing circuits: A review. Br J Anaesth 40:666, 1968

68. Bain JA, Spoerel WE: Flow requirements for a modified Mapleson D system during controlled ventilation. Can Anaesth Soc J 20:629, 1973

69. Soliman MG, Laberge R: The use of the Bain circuit in spontaneously breathing paediatric patients. Can Anaesth Soc J 25:276, 1978

70. Bain JA, Spoerel WE: A streamlined anaesthetic system. Can Anaesth Soc J 19:426, 1972

71. Ungerer MJ: A comparison between the Bain and Magill anesthetic systems during spontaneous breathing. Can Anaesth Soc J 25:122, 1978

72. Spoerel WE: Rebreathing and end tidal CO_2 during spontaneous breathing with the Bain circuit. Can Anaesth Soc J 30:148, 1983

73. Pethick SL: Letter to the Editor. Can Anaesth Soc J 22:115, 1975

74. Ayre P: Endotracheal anesthesia for babies with special reference to hare-lip and cleft-palate operations. Anesth Analg 16:331, 1937

75. Ayre P: The T-piece technique. Br J Anaesth 28:520, 1956

76. Jackson-Rees G: Anaesthesia in the newborn. Br Med J 2:1419, 1950

77. Moyers J: A nomenclature for methods of inhalation anesthesia. Anesthesiology 14:609, 1953

78. Eger EI II: Anesthetic systems: Construction and function. In Eger EI (ed): Anesthetic Uptake and Action, pp 206–227. Baltimore, Williams and Wilkins, 1974

79. Eger EI II, Ethans CT: The effects of inflow, overflow and valve placement on economy of the circle system. Anesthesiology 29:93, 1968

80. Adriani J: Carbon dioxide absorption. In The Chemistry and Physics of Anesthesia, p 151. Springfield, Charles C Thomas, 1962

81. Wilson RE: Soda lime an absorbent for industrial purposes. J Ind Eng Chem 12:1000, 1920

82. Dewey & Almy Chemical Division: The Sodasorb Manual of CO_2 Absorption, LOC #62-14923. New York, WR Grace and Company, 1962

83. Foregger R: The regeneration of soda lime following absorption of CO_2. Anesthesiology 9:15, 1948

84. Hunt HE: Resistance in respiratory valves and canisters. Anesthesiology 16:190, 1955

85. Brown ES: Performance of absorbents: Continuous flow. Anesthesiology 20:41, 1959

86. Adriani J: Soda lime indicators. Anesthesiology 5:45, 1944

87. Case History 39: Accidental use of trichloroethylene (trilene, trimar) in a closed system. Anesth Analg 43:740, 1964

88. Strum D, Eger EI, Johnson BH, et al: Toxicity of sevoflurane in rats. Anesth Analg 66:769, 1987

89. Burton JDK: Effects of dry anesthetic gases on the respiratory mucous membrane. Lancet 1:235, 1962

90. Shapiro BA, Harrison RA, Kacmarek RM et al: Humidity and aerosol therapy. In Shapiro BA, Harrison RA, Kacmarek RM et al (eds): Clinical Application of Respiratory Therapy, p 90. Chicago, Year Book Medical Publishers, 1985

91. McPherson SP, Spearman CB: Humidifiers and nebulizers. In McPherson SP, Spearman CB (eds): Respiratory Therapy Equipment, p 119. St. Louis, CV Mosby, 1985

92. Petty C: Anesthesia circuits. In Petty C (ed): The Anesthesia Machine, p 81. New York, Churchill Livingstone, 1987

93. Forbes AR: Humidification and mucus flow in the intubated trachea. Br J Anaesth 45:874, 1973

94. Chalon J, Ali M, Turndorf H et al: Humidification of Anesthetic Gases. Springfield, Charles C Thomas, 1981

95. Tausk HC, Miller R, Roberts RB: Maintenance of body temperature by heated humidification. Anesth Analg 55:719, 1976

96. Elder PT: Accidental hypothermia. In Shoemaker WC, Thompson WL, Holbrook PR (eds): Textbook of Critical Care, p 85. Philadelphia, WB Saunders, 1984

97. Bernard JM, Pinaud M, Souron R: Perioperative hypothermia prevention. Acta Anaesthesiol Scand 31:521, 1987

98. Spaepen MS, Bodman HA, Kundsin RB et al: Prevalence and survival of microbe contaminants in heated nebulizers. Anesth Analg 57:191, 1978

99. Chase HF, Trotta R, Kilmore MA: Simple methods for humidifying non-rebreathing anesthesia gas systems. Anesth Analg 41:249, 1962

100. Chalon J, Simon RS, Ramanathan S et al: A high-humidity circle system for infants and children. Anesthesiology 49:205, 1978

101. Weeks DB: Humidification of anesthetic gases using heat-and-moisture exchangers. Anesth Rev 12:22, 1985

102. Ramanathan S, Chalon J, Capan L et al: Rebreathing characteristics of the Bain anesthesia circuit. Anesth Analg 56:822, 1977

103. Westenskow DR, Jordan WS, Jordan R et al: Evaluation of oxygen monitors for use during anesthesia. Anesth Analg 60:53, 1981

APPENDIX A: ANESTHESIA APPARATUS CHECKOUT RECOMMENDATIONS

This checkout, or a reasonable equivalent, should be conducted before anesthesia administration. This is a guideline that users are encouraged to modify to accommodate differences in equipment design and variations in local clinical practice. Such local modifications should have appropriate peer review. Users should refer to the operators manual for special procedures or precautions.

*1. Inspect anesthesia machine for:
Machine identification number
Valid inspection sticker
Undamaged flowmeters, vaporizers, gauges, supply hoses
Complete, undamaged breathing system with adequate carbon dioxide (CO_2) absorbent
Correct mounting of cylinders in yokes
Presence of cylinder wrench

*2. Inspect and turn on:
Electrical equipment requiring warm-up (electrocardiogram/pressure monitor, oxygen monitor, etc.)

*3. Connect waste gas scavenging system:
Adjust vacuum as required

*4. Check that:
Flow-control valves are off
Vaporizers are off
Vaporizers are filled (not overfilled)
Filler caps are sealed tightly
CO_2 absorber bypass (if any) is off

*5. Check oxygen (O_2) cylinder supplies:
   a. Disconnect pipeline supply (if connected) and return cylinder and pipeline pressure gauges to zero with O_2 flush valve.
   b. Open O_2 cylinder; check pressure; close cylinder and observe gauge for evidence of high pressure leak.
   c. With the O_2 flush valve, flush to empty piping.
   d. Repeat as in b. and c. above for second O_2 cylinder, if present.
   e. Replace any cylinder less than about 600 PSIG. At least one should be nearly full.
   f. Open less full cylinder.

*6. Turn on master switch (if present).

*7. Check nitrous oxide (N_2O) and other gas cylinder supplies:
Use same procedure as described in 5a. and b. above, but open and close flow-control valve to empty piping. Note: N_2O pressure below 745 PSIG indicates that the cylinder is less than one-quarter full.

*8. Test flowmeters:
   a. Check that float is at bottom of tube with flow-control valves closed (or at minimum O_2 flow if so equipped).
   b. Adjust flow of all gases through their full range and check for erratic movements of floats.

*9. Test ratio protection/warning system (if present):
Attempt to create hypoxic O_2/N_2O mixture, and verify correct change in gas flows and/or alarm.

*10. Test O_2 pressure failure system:
   a. Set O_2 and other gas flows to midrange.
   b. Close O_2 cylinder and flush to release O_2 pressure.
   c. Verify that all flows fall to zero. Open O_2 cylinder.
   d. Close all other cylinders and bleed piping pressures.
   e. Close O_2 cylinder and bleed piping pressure.
   f. *Close flow control valves.*

*11. Test central pipeline gas supplies:
   a. Inspect supply hoses (should not be cracked or worn).
   b. Connect supply hoses, verifying correct color coding.
   c. Adjust all flows to at least midrange.
   d. Verify that supply pressues hold (45–55 PSIG).
   e. Shut off flow control valves.

*12. Add any accessory equipment to the breathing system: Add PEEP valve, humidifer, etc., if they might be used (if necessary remove after step 18 until needed).

13. Calibrate O_2 monitor:
   *a. Calibrate O_2 monitor to read 21% in room air.
   *b. Test low alarm.
   c. Occlude breathing system at patient end; fill and empty system several times with 100% O_2.
   d. Check that monitor reading is nearly 100%.

14. Sniff inspiratory gas:
There should be no odor.

*15. Check unidirectional valves:
   a. Inhale and exhale through a surgical mask into the breathing system (each limb individually, if possible).
   b. Verify unidirectional flow in each limb.
   c. Reconnect tubing firmly.

†16. Test for leaks in machine and breathing system:
   a. Close APL (pop off) valve and occlude system at patient end.
   b. Fill system *via* O_2 flush until bag just full, but negligible pressure in system. Set O_2 flow to 5 l/min.
   c. Slowly decrease O_2 flow until pressure *no longer rises* above about 20 cm H_2O. This approximates total leak rate, which should be no greater than a few hundred milliliters/minute (less for closed circuit techniques). Caution: Check valves in some machines make it imperative to measure flow in step c. above when pressure *just stops rising*.
   d. Squeeze bag to pressure of about 50 cm H_2O and verify that system is tight.

17. Exhaust valve and scavenger system:
   a. Open APL valve and observe release of pressure.
   b. Occlude breathing system at patient end and verify that negligible positive or negative pressure appears with either zero or 5 l/min flow and exhaust relief valve (if present) opens with flush flow.

18. Test ventilator:
   a. If switching valve is present, test function in both bag and ventilator mode.
   b. Close APL valve if necessary and occlude system at patient end.
   c. Test for leaks and pressure relief by appropriate cycling (exact procedure will vary with type of ventilator).
   d. Attach reservoir bag at mask fitting, fill system and cycle ventilator. Assure filling/emptying of bag.

19. Check for appropriate level of patient suction.

20. Check, connect, and calibrate other electronic monitors.

21. Check final position of all controls.

22. Turn on and set other appropriate alarms for equipment to be used.
(Perform next two steps as soon as is practical)

23. Set O_2 monitor alarm limits.

24. Set airway pressure and/or volume monitor alarm limits (if adjustable).

* If an anesthetist uses the same machine in successive cases, the steps marked with an asterisk (*) need not be repeated or may be abbreviated after the initial checkout.

† A vaporizer leak can only be detected if the vaporizer is turned on during this test. Even then, a relatively small but clinically significant leak may still be obscured.

(Reprinted with permission. Anesthesia Apparatus Checkout Recommendations, FDA. Rockville, Food and Drug Administration, August 1986.)

Chapter 20

Linda C. Stehling

Management of the Airway

Airway management involves more than proficiency with tracheal intubation techniques. The anesthesiologist must understand the physiologic consequences and complications of endotracheal intubation and have knowlege of the anatomy, innervation and pathologic conditions of the airway, and methods of assessment. He or she must be able to recognize patients in whom airway management may be difficult and be able to formulate and implement alternative plans in various clinical situations.

THE LARYNX

ANATOMY

Located at the level of the fourth to sixth cervical vertebrae in the adult, the larynx is composed of cartilage, ligaments, and muscle. It is lined by mucous membrane, which is continuous with that of the pharynx and trachea. The laryngeal cavity extends from the laryngeal inlet to the caudal border of the cricoid cartilage. The larynx is bounded anteriorly by the epiglottis, posteriorly by the mucous membrane that extends between the arytenoid cartilages, and laterally by the aryepiglottic folds. The vocal folds (vocal cords, true cords) extend from the thyroid cartilage to the arytenoid cartilages. The rima glottidis is the triangular opening between the vocal cords. The portion of the laryngeal cavity above the vocal cords is the vestibule that contains the ventricular folds (false vocal cords) (Fig. 20-1). In the adult, the area between the vocal cords is the narrowest part of the laryngeal cavity.

The infant's larynx differs from that of the adult in more than absolute size (Fig. 20-2). It is positioned relatively more cephalad and is slanted downward and anteriorly. The vocal cords are angled, whereas those of the adult are more perpendicular to the axis of the trachea. The epiglottis is less rigid, longer, and narrower. The angle between the glottis and epiglottis is more acute, and the aryepiglottic folds are redundant or closer to the midline. The infant's airway is narrowest at the cricoid.[1]

INNERVATION

The sensory and motor innervation of the larynx is provided by the vagus nerves. The internal branch of the superior laryngeal nerve is responsible for sensation down to the vocal cords and the recurrent laryngeal nerves for the area below the vocal cords. The cricothyroid muscle is innervated by the external branch of the superior laryngeal nerve, and the other laryngeal muscles are innervated by the recurrent laryngeal nerves.

FUNCTION

The larynx primarily protects the lower airway by preventing foreign matter from entering. Phonation is an important, but secondary, function.

AIRWAY ASSESSMENT

Although the same principles apply to patients examined outside the operating room, where decisions regarding emergency airway management must be based on less extensive evaluation, primary emphasis will be placed on management

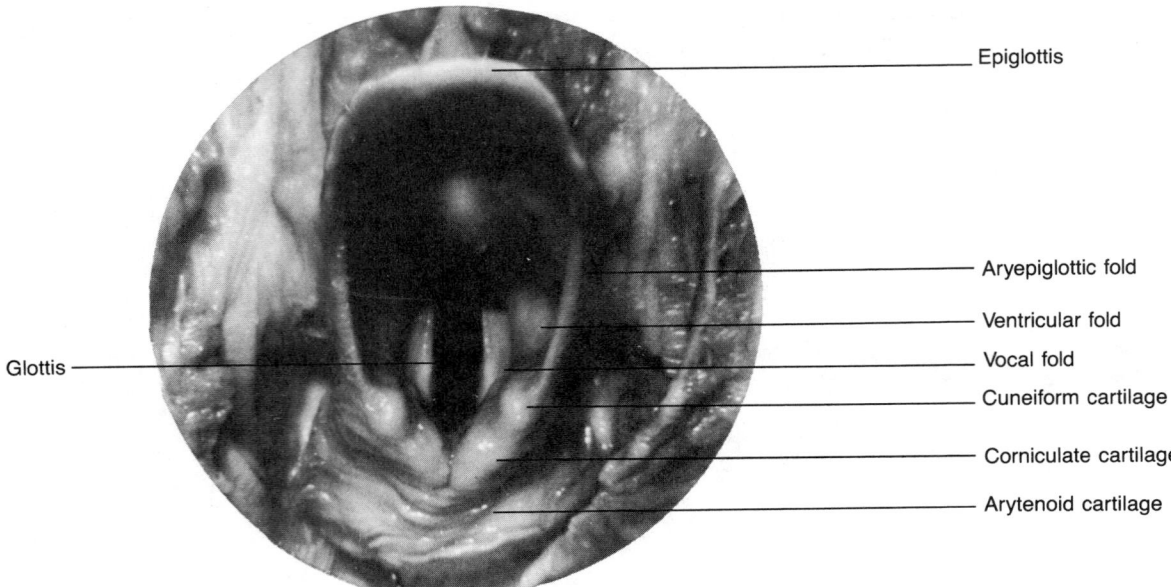

Epiglottis

Aryepiglottic fold

Ventricular fold

Vocal fold

Cuneiform cartilage

Corniculate cartilage

Arytenoid cartilage

Glottis

FIG. 20-1. Anatomic specimen of adult human larynx.

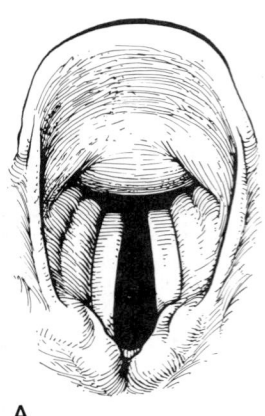

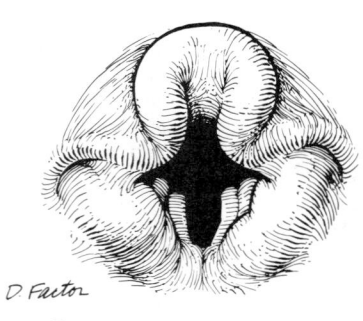

D. Factor

A   B

FIG. 20-2. (A) Adult larynx. (B) Infant larynx. The infant's epiglottis is relatively long, stiff, and "U" shaped.

of patients having surgery. The patient's diagnosis and the proposed surgical procedure are often the first clue to potential difficulties with airway management, as well as to the airway equipment required. A thorough preoperative history and physical examination are essential.

HISTORY

The patient should be questioned about signs and symptoms suggestive of airway abnormalities, such as hoarseness or shortness of breath, as well as information regarding prior surgery and trauma or neoplasia involving the airway. The history should include questions relating to prior anesthetic experiences. This is crucial if there is evidence suggesting that airway management may be difficult. Whenever possible, previous anesthesia records should be reviewed.

PHYSICAL EXAMINATION

The patient's head should be viewed in profile so that micrognathia can be detected, which is the most frequently encountered congenital feature associated with difficult endotracheal intubation. If the patient is seen only in the frontal plane, the degree of mandibular hypoplasia is frequently underestimated.

A cleft or long, high-arched palate, often associated with difficult tracheal intubation, may be an isolated finding or a component of a malformation syndrome. The tracheae of patients with certain congenital syndromes, such as Treacher-Collins, Goldenhar, Beckwith-Weideman, Weaver, Cruzon, and mucopolysaccharidoses, may be difficult or impossible to intubate.[1] The anesthetic implications of less common syndromes may not be as apparent, necessitating reference to texts dealing specifically with congenital anomalies.[2-4]

The presence of protruding or "buck" teeth, also best appreciated from the lateral aspect, may complicate endotracheal intubation. Conversely, it is very difficult to secure a tight seal with a face mask in edentulous patients. Loose, capped, and prosthetic teeth should be carefully noted. Occasionally it is preferable to extract loose teeth before airway manipulation to prevent them from being dislodged and possibly aspirated or swallowed. Nonfixed dental prostheses should be removed before anesthesia induction.

Temporomandibular joint mobility is assessed by asking the patient to open the mouth. Joint function can be further evaluated if the anesthesiologist places his or her middle finger of each hand just inferior and posterior to the patient's earlobes and the index fingers anterior to the tragus of the ears. When the patient opens the mouth maximally, the examiner should feel both rotation and forward gliding of the condylar heads bilaterally. If only the first phase of opening is palpated, limited opening of the mouth is to be expected.[5] Occasionally, forward pressure on the angles of the mandible or grasping the mandible anteriorly and pulling it forward allows wider opening.[6]

Ankylosis of the temporomandibular joints is seen most frequently in patients with rheumatoid arthritis. In patients who have sustained trauma or have an infection involving the mouth or neck, mobility may be restricted by pain rather than deformity. The cause of the joint dysfunction must be determined because voluntary limitation of motion will disappear once anesthesia is induced and a muscle relaxant is administered. However, the use of general anesthesia and muscle relaxants may be contraindicated in patients with decreased temporomandibular joint mobility until an endotracheal tube has been positioned or a tracheostomy performed.

The patient's cervical spine mobility must be evaluated because endotracheal intubation usually involves extension of the neck. The normal range of flexion–extension of the neck varies from 165 to 90 degrees, with the range decreasing approximately 20% by the time the patient is 75 yr old.[7] The patient with rheumatoid arthritis or ankylosing spondylitis may have virtually no neck mobility.[8, 9] Although radiographic evidence of cervical spine involvement is present in 25–90% of patients with rheumatoid arthritis, approximately half have no symptoms.[10] Any type of movement that produces paresthesias or sensory or motor deficits must be noted and avoided during intubation of the trachea. It is best to have the patient sitting or standing during this examination because the degree of restricted movement will be obscured if the patient's head is on a pillow.

The likely ease of tracheal intubation also can be assessed by measurement of the distance, normally 6.5 cm or more in adults, between the lower border of the mandible and the thyroid notch with the patient's neck fully extended. If the measurement is less than 6 cm, it will be impossible to visualize the larynx. If the distance is 6.5 cm and the patient has prominent teeth, a thick neck, or decreased neck mobility, one should anticipate difficulty in visualizing the larynx.[11] This can be measured with a ruler or an intubation gauge (Fig. 20-3). The anesthesiologist can also use his or her fingers to assess the distance, but, obviously, this measurement varies with the examiner.

The ease of tracheal intubation can also be predicted by having the seated patient open his or her mouth, and protrude the tongue maximally. When the faucial pillars, soft palate, and uvula are easily visualized, direct laryngoscopic examination should be easy. Laryngoscopic examination may be easy or difficult if only the faucial pillars and soft palate are visible

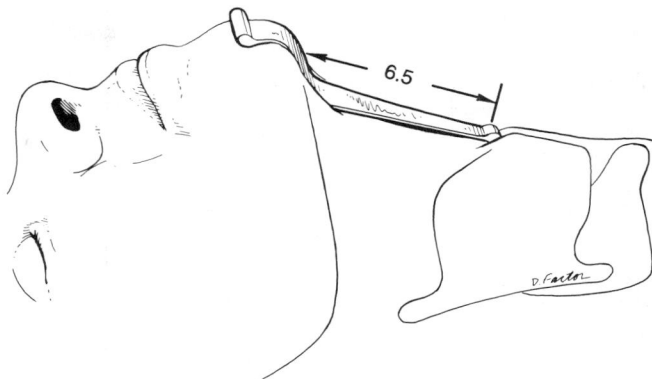

FIG. 20-3. An intubation gauge can be used to estimate the degree of difficulty with endotracheal intubation. The distance between the lower border of the mandible and the thyroid notch is normally greater than 6.5 cm in the adult.

but the uvula is obscured by the tongue. When only the soft palate is visualized, exposure of the glottis is almost invariably difficult.[12, 13]

The neck should be palpated so that masses and tracheal deviation can be detected. If the patient has a tracheostomy scar, the reason for the surgery must be determined. In patients with a tracheostomy *in situ*, it may be necessary to change the tube or use an adapter because some tubes are not compatible with anesthesia circuits.

RADIOGRAPHIC STUDIES

Standard anteroposterior and lateral x-rays of the neck and chest may be indicated to evaluate the cervical spine and ascertain the diameter and position of the trachea in patients with known or suspected airway abnormalities. Although not applicable in most clinical situations, radiographic measurements of the mandible are said to have predictive value in determining the ease of endotracheal intubation. Increased posterior depth of the mandible (the distance between the alveolus immediately posterior to the third molars and the lower border of the mandible) may hinder displacement of the soft tissues by the laryngoscope blade.[14] Computerized tomography can be invaluable in localizing and quantitating both intrinsic and extrinsic airway abnormalities.

LARYNGOSCOPY

A flexible fiberoptic nasopharyngoscope can be used by the anesthesiologist or otorhinolaryngologist to evaluate the pharynx and larynx. This examination can be performed with minimal discomfort in the awake patient and is especially useful in those with neoplasia involving the airway. However, visualization of the vocal cords, even if the laryngeal inlet appears adequate, does not guarantee that direct laryngoscopic examination and endotracheal intubation will be possible. A less reliable method of evaluating the glottis in the awake patient is indirect laryngoscopic examination with a laryngeal mirror.

AIRWAY EQUIPMENT

Certain items of equipment such as masks, airways, laryngoscopes, and endotracheal tubes are essential for management of any patient, regardless of the anesthetic technique employed. The nature of the patient's pathologic condition or the surgical procedure may dictate that additional equipment, such as a fiberoptic endoscope, also be available.

MASKS

The Connell anatomic mask (Fig. 20-4) is used most frequently for adults. It is available in a variety of sizes, and the malleable body allows it to be shaped to fit the patient's face. Rendell-Baker-Soucek masks (Fig. 20-4) are designed especially for children. Endoscopic masks (Fig. 20-4) may be employed during fiberoptic intubation of the trachea. Because flammable anesthetics are rarely used, it is no longer necessary to use carbon-containing black masks. Clear masks permit visualization of the mouth for secretions, emesis, and pinched lips.

AIRWAYS

Most oropharyngeal airways, available in several sizes and types, are made of plastic. Some are metal, including one specially designed for use during fiberoptic endotracheal intubation (Fig. 20-5). Nasopharyngeal airways are available in plastic and rubber. The binasal airway (Fig. 20-6) has an adapter for connection to the anesthesia circuit.

LARYNGOSCOPES

Laryngoscopes are composed of a handle and blade. Handles for fiberoptic blades are not interchangeable with those for blades with replaceable bulbs. Both are battery powered, but the area of contact between the handle and blade differs because the light source for the fiberoptic bundle is housed in the handle. Short handles are especially useful when patients who are obese or have short necks are intubated. One mod-

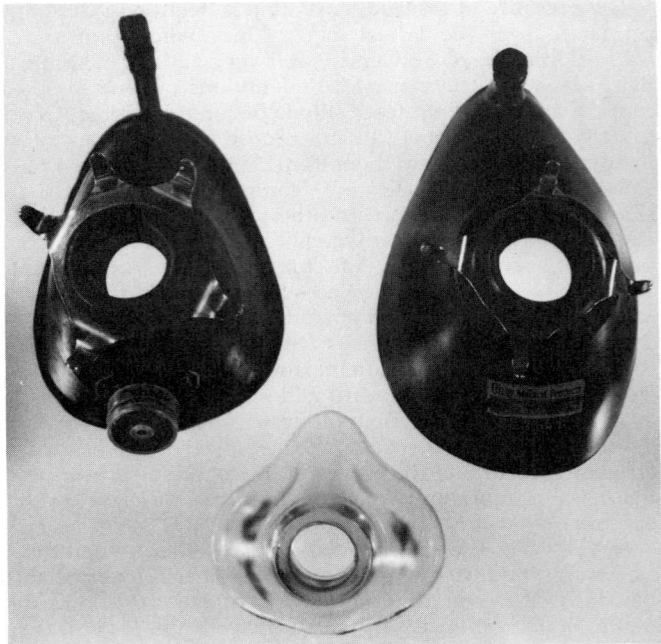

FIG. 20-4. The Connell anatomical mask (*right*) is most often used for adults, whereas the Rendell-Baker-Soucek mask (*center*) is designed specifically for children. The Patil-Syracuse endoscopic mask (*left*) (Anesthesia Associates, San Marcos, California) has an endoscopic port for insertion of a fiberoptic endoscope and endotracheal tube.

ification has a blade lock that allows the blade to be positioned at 180, 135, 90, or 45 degrees to the handle (Fig. 20-7).[15]

Curved and straight blades are the two general types available. The most commonly used are the Macintosh and Miller blades, which are manufactured in several sizes (Fig. 20-8). The tip of the curved blade is placed in the vallecula, superior to the epiglottis, whereas the tip of the straight blade is placed under the epiglottis to elevate it. Personal preference primarily

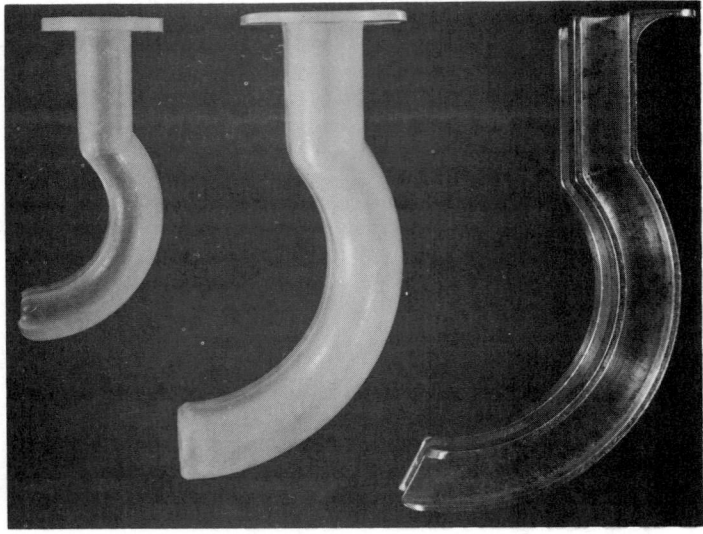

FIG. 20-5. Oropharyngeal airways are available in sizes suitable for children (*left*) and adults (*center*). The Patil-Syracuse endoscopic airway (*right*) (Anesthesia Associates, San Marcos, California) has a central groove to keep the insertion tube of a fiberoptic endoscope in the midline and a slit at the distal end to direct the instrument into the larynx. Lateral channels are provided for suctioning.

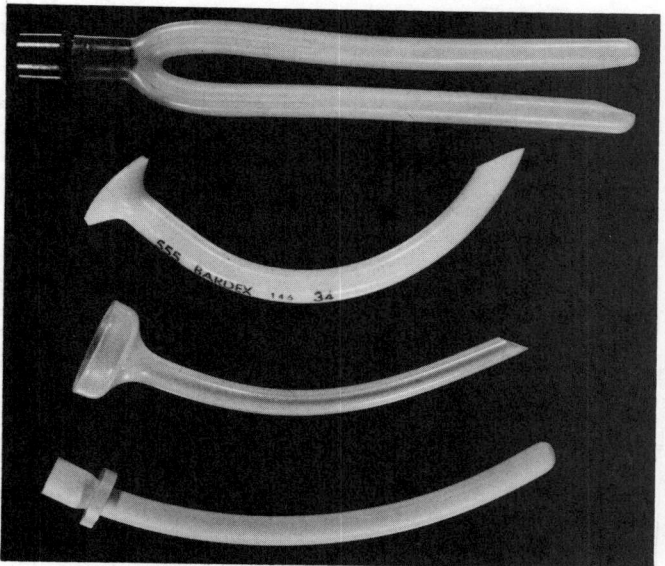

FIG. 20-6. Nasal airways are shown.

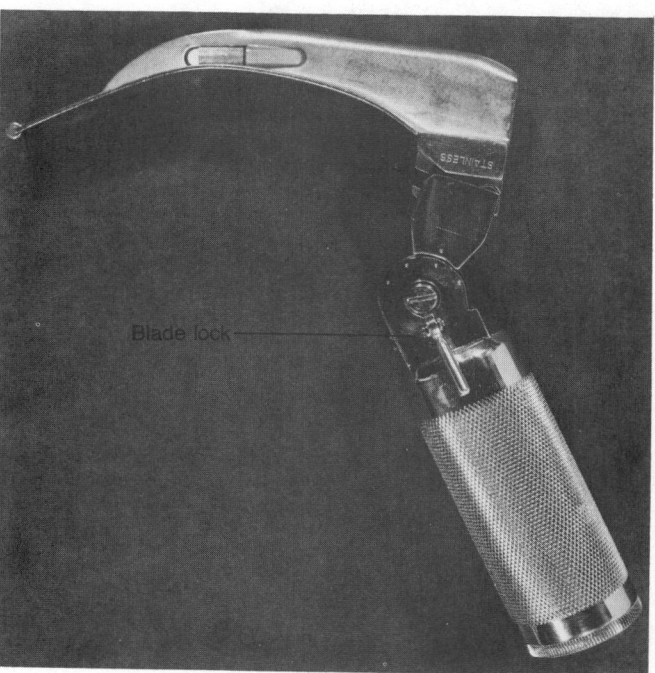

Blade lock

FIG. 20-7. Short, adjustable laryngoscope handle (Anesthesia Associates, San Marcos, California) with blade lock to allow the blade to be positioned at different angles.

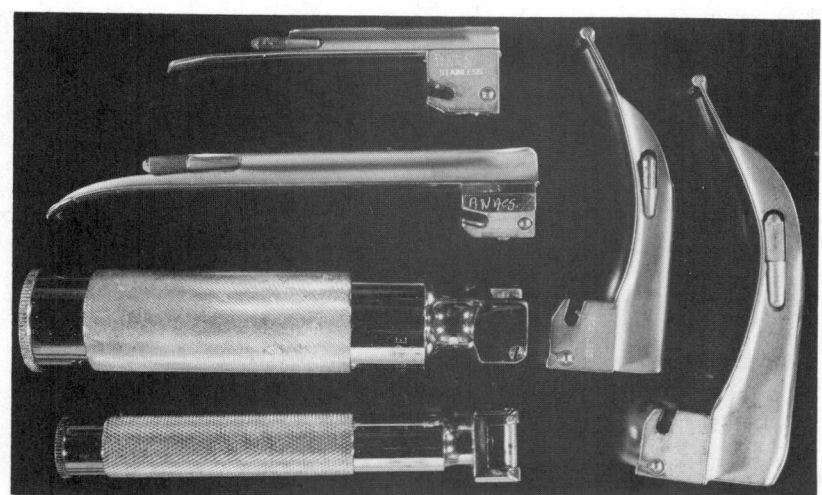

FIG. 20-8. Laryngoscope handles and Miller (*above*) and Macintosh (*right*) blades.

determines the type blade used for intubating adults. Alleged advantages of the curved blade include less potential for damage to the teeth and more space availability in the oropharynx for the endotracheal tube. Although inexperienced endoscopists tend to lever on the upper teeth when using a straight blade, the glottic exposure is often better, facilitating observation of the tube as it passes through the vocal cords. Straight blades are usually used for children because it is easier to lift the base of the tongue and fix the epiglottis, thereby facilitating visualization of the glottis.

Proponents of the Macintosh blade claim that the incidence

of laryngospasm and the magnitude of alterations in cardiac rate and rhythm are reduced because it does not contact the inferior surface of the epiglottis, which is innervated by the superior laryngeal nerve, a branch of the vagus. Rather, it is placed in the vallecula, which is innervated by the glossopharyngeal nerve. However, when studied, the incidence of changes in heart rate and rhythm was comparable with both curved and straight blades.[16] Because most patients receive a muscle relaxant before laryngosopic examination, the theoretic advantage of decreased laryngospasm with a curved blade has assumed less significance.

ENDOTRACHEAL TUBES

Endotracheal tubes are numbered according to the internal diameter (ID). The approximate size and length of the tube is determined by the patient's age and size (Table 20-1). In general, a 7.0–8.5-mm ID tube is appropriate for women and an 8.0–10.0-mm ID tube for men. In women, the length from the alveolar ridge to the tip of the tube should be approximately 21 cm and in men, 23 cm.[17] Although some anesthesiologists select an endotracheal tube for children that is approximately the same size as the child's little finger, others rely on formulae based on age. A useful guideline for children older than 1 yr is as follows:

$$\text{Endotracheal tube size (mm)} = 4 + \frac{\text{age (yr)}}{4}$$

$$\text{or}$$

$$= \frac{\text{age (yr)} + 16}{4}$$

The length of the tube can also be calculated:

$$\text{Length (cm)} = 12 + \frac{\text{age (yr)}}{2}$$

TABLE 20-1. Average Endotracheal Tube Sizes (internal diameter [ID]) and Lengths for Orotracheal Intubation

AGE	ID (mm)	LENGTH (cm)
Premature	2.5	10
Neonate	3.0–3.5	10–11
6–12 months	3.5–4	11–12
2 yr	4.5	13
4 yr	5	14
6 yr	5.5	15
8 yr	6.0	16
10 yr	6.5	17
12 yr	7.0	18

Nasotracheal tubes should be approximately 3 cm longer than orotracheal tubes.

Endotracheal tube resistance varies inversely with the tube size. Each millimeter decrease in tube size is associated with an increase in resistance of 25–100%. The work of breathing parallels changes in resistance. A 1-mm decrease in tube size increases the work of breathing 34–154%, depending upon the ventilatory pattern.[18]

Most endotracheal tubes are made of semirigid plastic and are disposable. The label IT (implant tested) or Z-79 (for the Z-79 Committee on Anesthesia Equipment of the American National Standards Institute [ANSI]) signifies that the tube material is nontoxic to tissue.

Tubes used in older children and adults have cuffs that are inflated to seal the airway. Uncuffed tubes are usually employed in children younger than 8–10 yr of age to decrease the risk of subglottic edema. In addition, the narrow subglottic area in young children provides an anatomic seal. When a cuffed tube is used, the size of the tube must be smaller to compensate for the added bulk of the cuff. Most endotracheal tubes have a radiopaque marker to facilitate radiologic verification of the tube position.

Anode or armored tubes (Fig. 20-9), designed to minimize kinking, have a wire coil embedded in the wall. Tubes molded with angles suitable for intraoral or intranasal use (Fig. 20-10) are available, or a flexible connector (Fig. 20-11) can be used to facilitate positioning of the anesthetic circuit away from the operative site during head and neck surgery. The Carden tube (Fig. 20-12) is placed below the vocal cords for surgery of the larynx or subglottic area. Double-lumen endobronchial or "split" tubes (Fig. 20-13) permit one or both lungs to be ventilated and are used primarily during thoracic surgery.

ANCILLARY EQUIPMENT

Malleable metal or firm rubber stylets are used to maintain the desired curve of the endotracheal tube during intubation. Although most are coated with a nonfriction covering to facilitate easy removal, they should be lubricated before insertion into endotracheal tubes.

Soft plastic or rubber tooth protectors (Fig. 20-14) can lessen

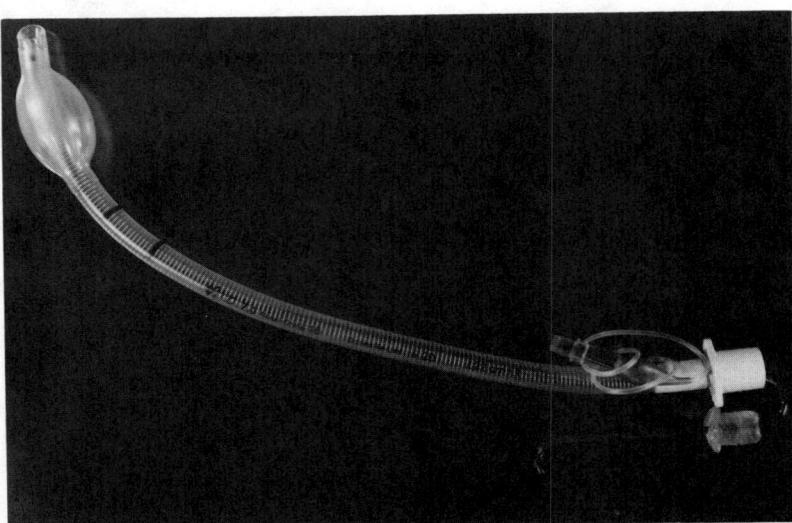

FIG. 20-9. A flexible armored (anode) tube. A metal stylet is inserted into the tube to facilitate placement.

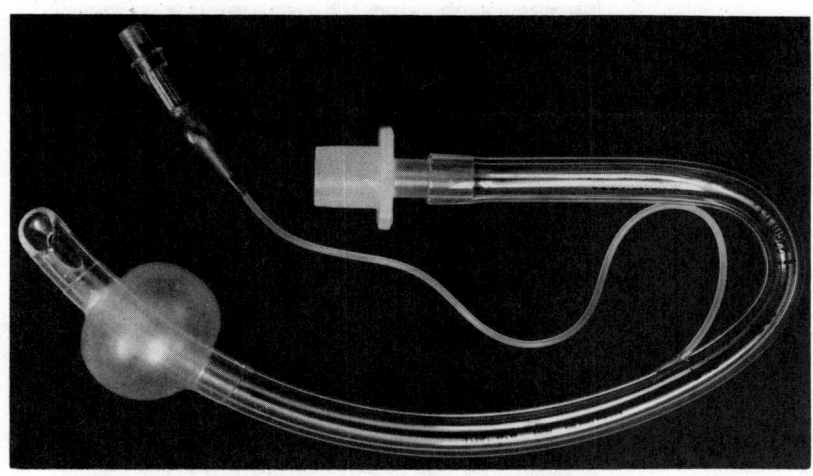

FIG. 20-10. Preformed RAE tube for orotracheal intubation.

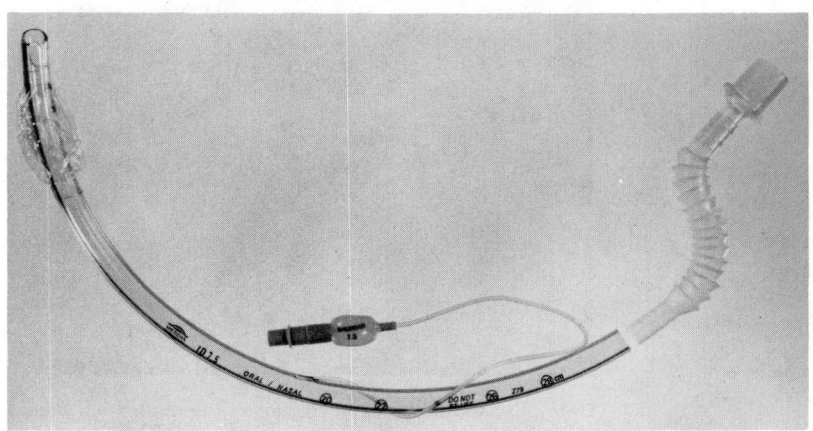

FIG. 20-11. A flexible connector.

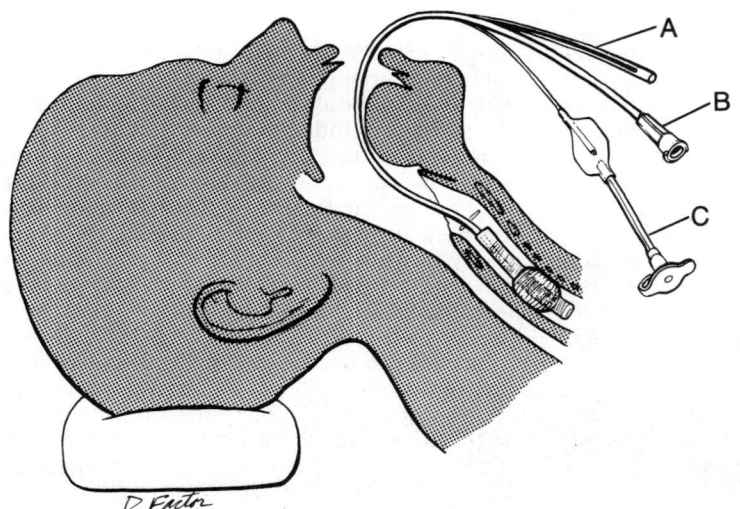

FIG. 20-12. The Carden tube is positioned below the vocal cords for surgical procedures involving the larynx. It has a stylet (A) to facilitate placement, an adapter (B) for attachment to a jet ventilator, and a pilot tube (C) for cuff inflation.

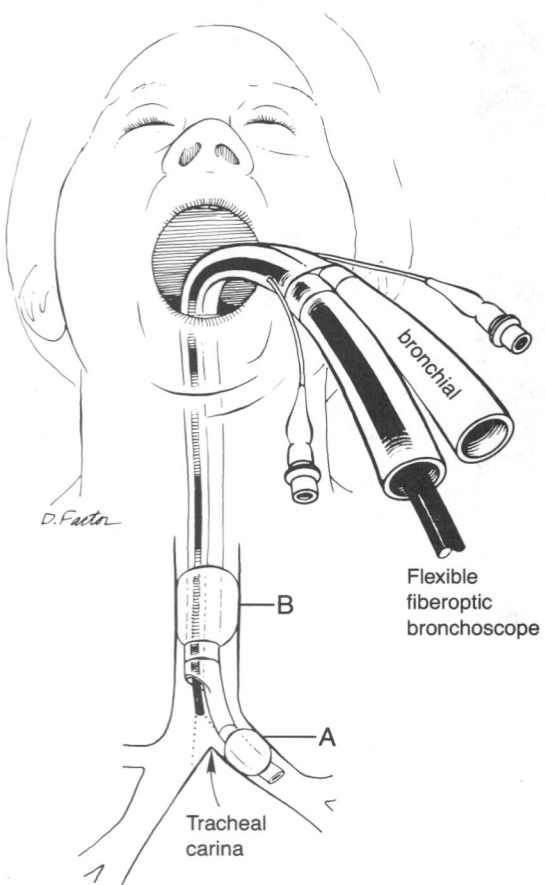

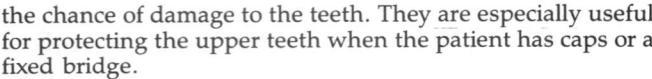

FIG. 20-13. Double-lumen endobronchial tubes permit one or both lungs to be ventilated. The left endobronchial tube is positioned with the distal cuff (*A*) in the left bronchus and the proximal cuff (*B*) in the trachea. A fiberoptic bronchoscope can be used to confirm proper tube placement.

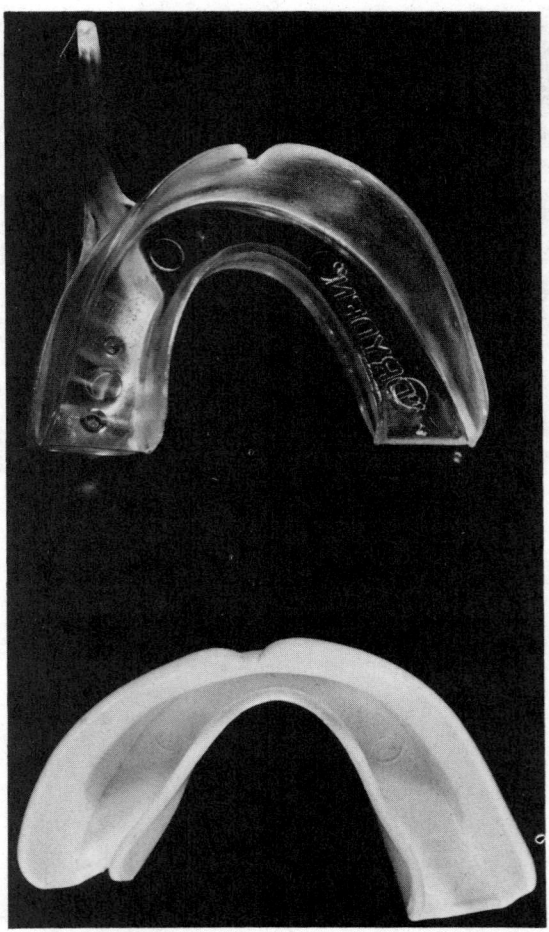

FIG. 20-14. Dental guards used to protect the teeth from damage during laryngoscopic examination.

the chance of damage to the teeth. They are especially useful for protecting the upper teeth when the patient has caps or a fixed bridge.

AIRWAY OBSTRUCTION

During anesthesia, the anesthesiologist assumes responsibility for establishment and maintenance of adequate ventilation of the lungs. An essential element in this process is prevention of airway obstruction. No anesthetic technique or device will guarantee a patent airway. The anesthesiologist's constant vigilance and technical skill are mandatory.

When the patient is breathing spontaneously, signs of airway obstruction include stridor, "noisy" breathing, decreased breath sounds, retraction of the trachea, flaring of the nostrils, and retraction of the thoracic cage. Unfortunately, chest and abdominal movement with airway obstruction can be misinterpreted as "breathing." Actual air movement must be verified by listening, feeling the warm exhaled air, or using a ventimeter or the rebreathing bag to measure the volume of air moved.

The most frequent site for airway obstruction is the oropharynx. With induction of anesthesia, there is relaxation of

the jaw and tongue such that the base of the tongue falls back in contact with the posterior pharynx. To relieve this obstruction, the anesthesiologist should place his or her hands behind the angle of the patient's mandible and move it forward. Care must be taken to avoid putting pressure on the anterior structures of the neck, which can accentuate the obstruction. Other measures useful in opening the upper airway include slight extension of the neck, turning the head to the side, application of positive airway pressure to "distend" the soft tissue, and insertion of an oral or nasal airway. The oropharynx also should be checked to ensure that the obstruction is not from a foreign body.

Airway obstruction can also be caused by reflex closure of the vocal cords, a condition known as laryngospasm. This typically occurs during "light" levels of anesthesia, when the larynx is irritated by contact with secretions, or when the patient experiences a painful stimulus. Partial laryngospasm is characterized by high-pitched phonation, or "crowing." Total occlusion is characterized by no sounds and the signs of airway obstruction mentioned above.

The incidence of laryngospasm can be reduced by keeping the airway clear of foreign material, avoiding abrupt inhalation of high concentrations of volatile anesthetics, and establishing a "deep" level of surgical anesthesia before instrumentation of the airway or allowing surgery to proceed. If laryngospasm occurs, it is usually brief and easily treated. Depending on the cause, treatment should include suctioning foreign material from the oropharynx, decreasing the inspired concentration of anesthetic, removing any painful stimulus, administering 100% oxygen, applying positive pressure to the airway, and placing of the fingers behind the angle of the mandible to thrust the jaw forward. If these measures do not resolve the laryngospasm quickly, a rapid-acting muscle relaxant should be administered.

ENDOTRACHEAL INTUBATION

General anesthesia is not, of itself, an indication for endotracheal intubation. In many cases it is unnecessary, and occasionally it is contraindicated. Similarly, endotracheal intubation is not always required to treat airway obstruction. However, once it is determined that endotracheal intubation is necessary, the anesthesiologist must decide whether nasotracheal or orotracheal intubation is most appropriate, choose the type and size of laryngoscope and tube to use, decide whether the patient is to be intubated while awake or after induction of anesthesia, and decide whether a muscle relaxant can be used safely.

INDICATIONS FOR ENDOTRACHEAL INTUBATION

Placement of an endotracheal tube before or immediately after induction of general anesthesia is indicated in the patient with a full stomach to minimize the possibility of aspiration of gastric contents. Endotracheal intubation is also necessary during operative procedures involving the head and neck, where a face mask would encroach upon the surgical field. Patient position during surgery may dictate placement of an endotracheal tube: it is essential for patients receiving general anesthesia in the prone and sitting positions and is usually necessary for those positioned laterally. Provision of a patent airway in patients with airway abnormalities and the need for prolonged positive-pressure ventilation are additional indications for endotracheal intubation. Intracranial, intrathoracic, and most intraabdominal operations mandate endotracheal intubation.

NASOTRACHEAL VERSUS OROTRACHEAL INTUBATION

Orotracheal intubation is performed much more frequently than nasotracheal intubation. Indications for the latter include intraoral operative procedures, during which the endotracheal tube could easily be displaced or obscure the operative site, and inability to open the patient's mouth. Nasotracheal intubation is contraindicated in the presence of intranasal abnormalities, extensive facial fractures, and systemic coagulopathy. Bleeding is not unusual after nasotracheal intubation and can produce significant complications in patients with disorders of hemostasis. When nasotracheal intubation is planned, the patient should be asked if it is easier to breathe better through one nostril than the other. If there is a difference, the nasotracheal tube should be passed through the presumably larger nasal passage after a topical vasoconstrictor such as phenylephrine or cocaine is applied. Placement of a soft, well-lubricated nasal airway before passage of the nasotracheal tube is useful in assessing the patency of the nostril and dilating the nasal passage. Endotracheal tubes used for nasotracheal intubation are usually smaller than those used for orotracheal intubation.

ANESTHESIA FOR INTUBATION OF THE TRACHEA

Although most patients' tracheae are intubated after thiopental and succinylcholine administration, other anesthetic agents and muscle relaxants also can be administered before intubation. However, the use of "fixed" agents such as thiopental, ketamine, opioids, sedatives, and muscle relaxants, which cannot be retrieved once given, must be viewed with caution. They may be contraindicated in patients with airway compromise or in those in whom it is anticipated that endotracheal intubation may be difficult. Muscle relaxants are particularly hazardous because they remove the patient's ability to protect the airway, and the loss of spontaneous ventilation precludes the anesthesiologist from guiding the endotracheal tube into the larynx by listening to breath sounds. If the anesthesiologist cannot *guarantee* that the patient's lung can be ventilated by mask, administration of neuromuscular blocking agents is contraindicated.

RAPID-SEQUENCE INDUCTION

A rapid-sequence or so-called "crash" induction, the most common method of securing the airway in the patient with a full stomach, minimizes the chances of regurgitation and aspiration. Strict adherence to all details of the technique and the availability of an assistant are mandatory. All equipment, including the suction apparatus with Yankauer or "tonsil" tip, must be checked before induction of anesthesia. Arguments can be advanced to justify placing the operating table in a head-up, head-down, or neutral (flat) position.[19] It is this author's opinion that a 40° head-up tilt is preferable, since gravity will minimize the risk of passive regurgitation of gastric contents. Although many anesthesiologists remove an indwelling nasogastric tube because it might increase the risk of aspiration by making the esophageal sphincter less competent or interfere with obliteration of the esophagus during application of cricoid pressure, studies indicate that it is safe to leave the tube *in situ*.[20]

The patient is usually preoxygenated for 3–5 min, however, 2–3 min is adequate if the mask fits tightly.[21] Four maximally deep breaths within 30 s or three vital capacity breaths of 100% oxygen also effectively increase arterial oxygenation.[22, 23] Respiration is not assisted until the airway is isolated to prevent air being forced into the stomach. A nondepolarizing muscle relaxant is administered before induction of anesthesia to minimize any increase in intragastric pressure from succinylcholine-induced muscle fasciculations. An assistant administers medications and applies cricoid pressure (Sellick's maneuver).[24] As soon as the drugs are injected, the assistant must apply cricoid pressure by placing his or her thumb and index finger on the cricoid cartilage and exerting pressure in an anteroposterior direction, occluding the esophagus (Fig. 20-15). The patient's trachea is intubated once spontaneous respiration ceases, and the cuff of the endotracheal tube is inflated by the assistant. Cricoid pressure is maintained until proper placement of the endotracheal tube is assured.

AWAKE INTUBATION OF THE TRACHEA

There are no absolute guidelines regarding indications for awake intubation of the trachea. It is necessary in some patients with congenital or acquired airway lesions, a full stomach, intestinal obstruction, upper gastrointestinal bleeding, cervical spine abnormalities, and facial trauma. Topical anesthesia can be applied to the patient's tongue to decrease gagging during orotracheal intubation. Although contraindicated in patients at risk of aspiration of gastric contents, superior laryngeal nerve blocks and translaryngeal injection of a local anesthetic significantly decrease the discomfort associated with awake intubation of the trachea.

LOCAL ANESTHESIA

Local anesthetic agents may be applied topically, infiltrated, or instilled. It must be remembered that local anesthetics are absorbed rapidly from mucous membranes and recommended doses must not be exceeded.[25]

Topical anesthesia of the lips, tongue, and oropharynx can be provided by direct application of pledgets soaked with a local anesthetic. In edentulous patients, the anesthetic also should be applied to the gums. After the tip of the tongue has been anesthetized, it is grasped with a gauze sponge and pulled forward to facilitate access to the oral cavity. The tongue can be held by the patient or an assistant, so that the anesthesiologist has both hands available to continue application of the anesthetic. This is best achieved with cotton pledgets soaked with the local anesthetic (usually cocaine), held with curved Krause forceps (Fig. 20-16). The superior surface of the tongue is anesthetized as the forceps are slowly advanced posteriorly. The pledgets then should be held in the piriform fossae for at least 2 min to anesthetize the internal laryngeal nerves.

Aerosolization of lidocaine is an effective, simple, and inexpensive method of topical anesthesia.[26] It can be employed alone or as an adjunct to other local anesthetic techniques. Ideally the patient is placed in a sitting position. A disposable nebulizer and face mask are used with an oxygen flow of approximately $8 \, l \cdot min^{-1}$. Phenylephrine (1 ml of 1% solution) can be added to the lidocaine (4 ml of 4% solution) as a vasoconstrictor. During the 5–7 min the patient breathes the mixture, the smaller nebulized particles are dispersed as far distally as the terminal bronchioles while the larger particles remain in contact with the nasal and pharyngeal mucosa. The technique is more effective if an antisialogogue is adminis-

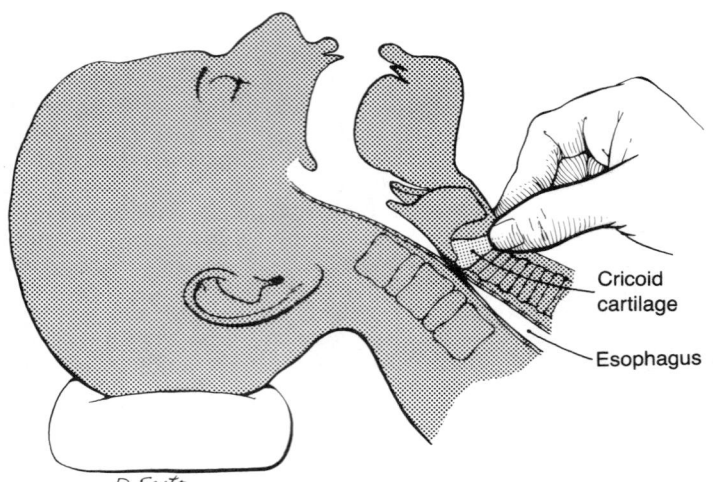

FIG. 20-15. Cricoid pressure (Sellick's maneuver) is applied to occlude the esophagus and prevent aspiration of gastric contents.

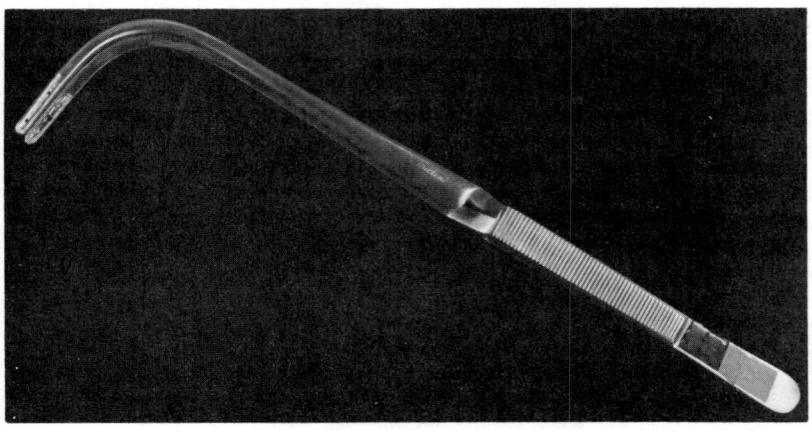

FIG. 20-16. Krause forceps for grasping cotton swabs used to anesthetize the tongue and pharynx. The design facilitates application of local anesthetic to the piriform fossae.

tered approximately an hour previously, because secretions may impair local anesthetic contact with the mucosa.

Bilateral superior laryngeal nerve blocks can be performed to anesthetize the internal laryngeal nerves (Fig. 20-17). The nerves pierce the thyrohyoid membrane just inferior to the greater cornu of the hyoid bone. Application of pressure to the opposite greater cornu displaces the laryngeal structures to the side to be blocked and facilitates identification of anatomic landmarks. After the skin is cleansed, the local anesthetic (3 ml of 2% lidocaine) is injected at the level of the thyrohyoid membrane with a 25-G needle. If air is aspirated, indicating that the pharynx has been entered, the needle is withdrawn slightly before the anesthetic is injected. Bilateral nerve blocks produce anesthesia of the inferior aspect of the epiglottis and the laryngeal outlet down to the vocal cords. The block should not be performed when there is local infection or tumor or when patients are at risk of aspiration of gastric contents.

Translaryngeal (often erroneously referred to as transtracheal) instillation of a local anesthetic provides anesthesia below the vocal cords. With the patient's neck fully extended, the cricothyroid membrane is palpated in the midline as a slight depression between the inferior border of the thyroid cartilage and the superior edge of the cricoid cartilage. The skin is cleansed and a 22-G needle introduced perpendicular to the skin (Fig. 20-17). After air is aspirated, the local anesthetic (3–5 ml of 2–4% lidocaine) is injected. The needle should be removed immediately because the patient will cough vigorously. Alternatively, a small-gauge intravenous catheter can be inserted and, when air is aspirated, the inner stylet withdrawn. Local anesthetic can then be injected through the soft catheter without the risk of tracheal injury when the patient coughs. Neither technique should be employed in the presence of local infection or tumor, when coughing is contraindicated, or if the patient is at risk of aspiration of gastric contents.

When nasotracheal intubation is to be performed, the nasal passage should be anesthetized. Use of cocaine is preferable because it is a potent vasocontrictor as well as topical anesthetic. Although the drug can be sprayed into the nose, best results are achieved when pledgets or cotton-tipped applicators soaked with the local anesthetic are placed in the nostrils and remain for 3–5 min.

Although not widely employed and somewhat technically difficult, maxillary nerve blocks can be used to provide analgesia and vasoconstriction before nasotracheal intubation. After topical application of a local anesthetic, a 27-G needle is inserted into the foramen of the greater palatine canal. The foramen is located between the second and third maxillary molars approximately 1 cm medial to the palatal gingival margin. After aspiration to ascertain that the sphenopalatine artery has not been entered, 2 ml of local anesthetic (2% lidocaine with 1 : 100,000 epinephrine) is injected. In addition to the nose, the maxillary teeth, alveolar bone, hard palate and part of the soft palate, upper lip, cheek, and lower eyelid are also anesthetized on the ipislateral side.

OROTRACHEAL INTUBATION

The operating table should be positioned so that the patient's head is approximately at the level of the anesthesiologist's xiphoid. In the adult, a pillow or pad is usually placed under the occiput to elevate the patient's head approximately 10 cm and thereby align the oral, pharyngeal, and laryngeal structures. Although this "sniffing" position should provide the most direct line of vision, some anesthesiologists find it easier to intubate when the patient's head is not elevated. Because children have relatively large heads, it is not necessary to use a pillow. Axial alignment is completed by extension of the atlantooccipital joint, and the patient's mouth is opened as widely as possible. The laryngoscope blade is inserted in the right side of the mouth and the tongue moved toward the left as the blade is advanced. When a curved blade is used, the tip is advanced into the vallecula, the space between the base of the tongue and the pharyngeal surface of the epiglottis (Fig. 20-18). The epiglottis is elevated and the glottis exposed as the handle of the laryngoscope is lifted forward and upward. In contrast, the tip of a straight blade is advanced beneath the laryngeal surface of the epiglottis to expose the glottic opening (Fig. 20-19). The most common errors made by the novice are levering on the upper incisors and trapping the lips between the laryngoscope blade and the teeth. The endotracheal tube should be observed until it passes through the vocal cords so that one can ascertain that it enters the larynx and gauge the

A

B

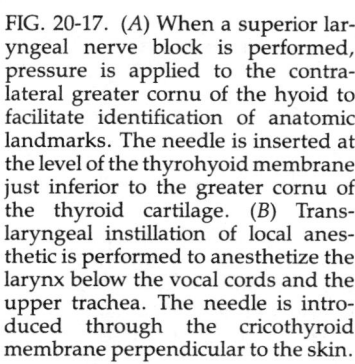

FIG. 20-17. (A) When a superior laryngeal nerve block is performed, pressure is applied to the contralateral greater cornu of the hyoid to facilitate identification of anatomic landmarks. The needle is inserted at the level of the thyrohyoid membrane just inferior to the greater cornu of the thyroid cartilage. (B) Translaryngeal instillation of local anesthetic is performed to anesthetize the larynx below the vocal cords and the upper trachea. The needle is introduced through the cricothyroid membrane perpendicular to the skin.

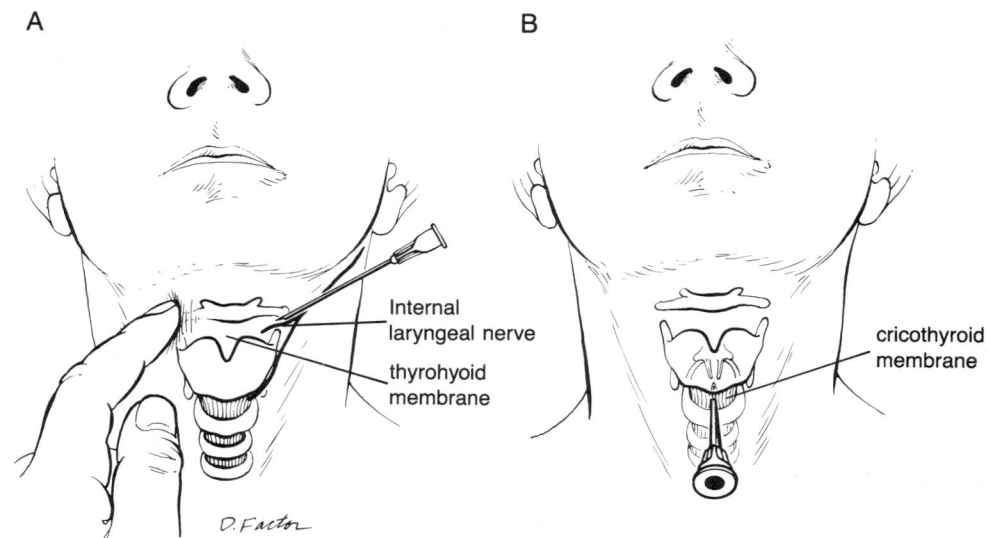

Internal laryngeal nerve
thyrohyoid membrane

cricothyroid membrane

D. Factor

A   B

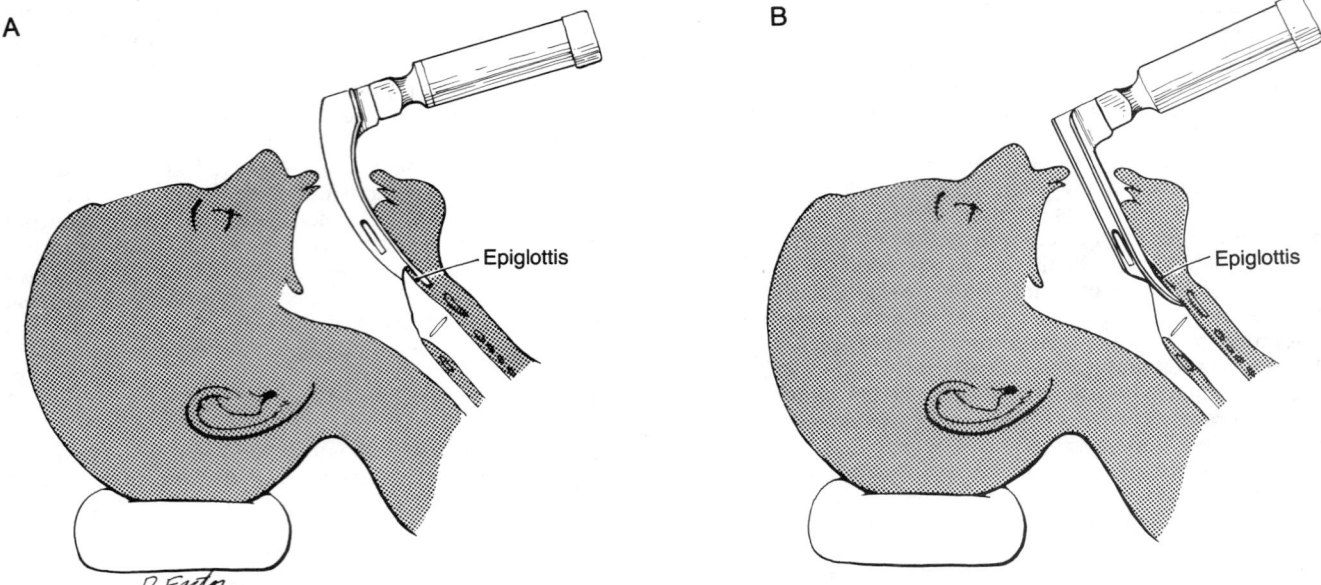

FIG. 20-18. (*A*) When a curved laryngoscope blade is used, the tip of the blade is placed in the vallecula, the space between the base of the tongue and the pharyngeal surface of the epiglottis. (*B*) The tip of a straight blade is advanced beneath the epiglottis.

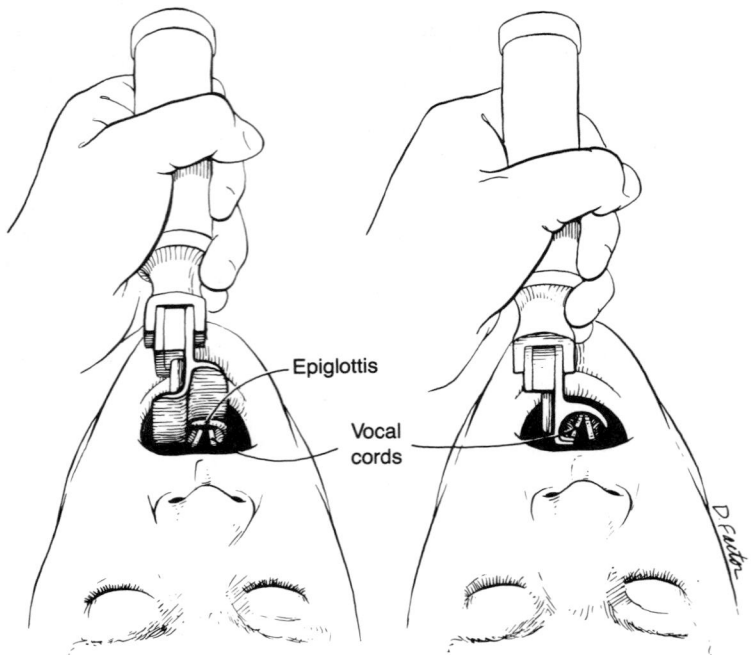

FIG. 20-19. (*A*) The curved laryngoscope blade is placed in the vallecula, and the vocal cords are exposed as the handle is lifted upward and forward. (*B*) A straight blade is advanced beneath the laryngeal surface and the epiglottis to expose the glottic opening.

depth of insertion. An assistant can apply external pressure to the thyroid cartilage to facilitate intubation of the trachea in the patient with an "anterior" larynx. In neonates and small children, the anesthesiologist can use the little finger of the left hand to apply pressure to the anterior neck.

Correct endotracheal tube placement usually can be ascertained by auscultation of the chest. The absence of air entry into the stomach, as determined by auscultation of the epi-

gastrium, is further assurance of proper tube placement. However, the detection of expired carbon dioxide with a capnograph or mass spectrometer provides the most reliable evidence of tracheal, rather than esophageal, intubation.[27]

If the tube is too long, endobronchial intubation will occur. It is an accepted fact that right endobronchial intubation is far more likely to occur in adults because of the relative angles of the right and left bronchi. The situation is more controversial in children. It has been reported that the right and left tracheobronchial angles are approximately equal in children younger than 3 yr of age, making intubation of either bronchus equally likely.[28] Recent studies refute this statement and confirm that even in premature infants, accidental right endobronchial intubation is more probable than left endobronchial intubation.[29, 30]

Once accurate tracheal placement is verified, the tube must be anchored securely to prevent later displacement into a bronchus or accidental extubation of the trachea. In patients with moist skin, tincture of benzoin should be applied before the tube is taped. In hirsute patients, cloth ties ("umbilical" or "hernia" tape) or Velcro straps should be used instead of adhesive tape. When these are not available, a surgical mask can be placed beneath the patient's head and the ties of the mask used to secure the tube.

NASOTRACHEAL INTUBATION

Nasotracheal intubation can be performed with direct vision, or a "blind" technique can be employed. If the patient states that it is easier to breathe through one nostril, that side should be used. A topical vasoconstrictor such as phenylephrine or cocaine should be applied. A soft nasal airway should be inserted first to determine the patency of the naris and to dilate the nasal passage.

When a general anesthetic is administered for intubation of the trachea, the nasal airway can be placed after the patient is anesthetized. Unless contraindicated, general anesthesia and a muscle relaxant are administered before laryngoscopic examination. The endotracheal tube is inserted into the nose until the tip is in the pharynx. Direct laryngoscopic examination is performed, the tip of the tube is visualized, and it is guided into the glottis. If necessary, forceps are used to grasp and direct the tip of the tube (Fig. 20-20). To avoid damage to the cuff, the tube should not be grasped by the cuff. The

direction of the tube is altered by rotating it to the right or left, as necessary. Occasionally, it is useful to rotate the patient's head (rather than the tube), especially in the patient with a deviated septum. Flexion of the neck is necessary when the tip of the tube impinges on the anterior commisure of the glottis. Extension of the neck may facilitate intubation when the tube persistently enters the esophagus.

When "blind" nasotracheal intubation is employed, direct laryngoscopic examination is not performed. The technique is similar whether the patient is anesthetized or awake. Breath sounds are used to guide the tube into the glottis in the spontaneously breathing patient. The anesthesiologist keeps an ear close to the tube to detect increased breath sounds as the tube nears the glottis. Alternatively, a whistle or amplifier can be placed in the tube to magnify the sounds.[31] Carbon dioxide inhalation or doxapram injection has been used to increase the depth of respiration, but these are rarely indicated. When the endotracheal tube enters the glottis, breath sounds are audible in the tube and there is movement of the breathing bag when the tube is connected to the anesthesia circuit.

PHYSIOLOGIC RESPONSES TO ENDOTRACHEAL INTUBATION

Hypertension, tachycardia, and increases in intracranial and intraocular pressure can occur in response to laryngoscopic examination and intubation.

CARDIOVASCULAR RESPONSES

The magnitude of the hypertensive response to laryngoscopic examination and intubation of the trachea appears to correlate with the blood pressure changes associated with stressful events such as hospital admission.[32] Hypertension and tachycardia may be inconsequential in healthy patients but detrimental to those with ischemic heart disease or increased intracranial pressure. Therefore, the patient's history determines the necessity for administering drugs to attenuate the response to laryngoscopic examination and intubation of the trachea. Among the methods used to decrease the circulatory responses are administration of deep inhalation anesthesia, intravenous opioids, topical or intravenous lidocaine, and intravenous adrenergic blocking agents.[33] Although 25–75 $\mu g \cdot kg^{-1}$ of fentanyl has been shown to block the response, smaller doses also offer some protection.[34-36] The rapid intravenous infusion of 1–2 $\mu g \cdot kg^{-1}$ of sodium nitroprusside is also effective.[37] The use of beta blockade alone is not recommended.[38] The effectiveness of inhalation of aerosolized lidocaine, gargling with viscous lidocaine, or translaryngeal instillation or intravenous administration of lidocaine may depends upon the duration of laryngoscopic examination.[39-41] Laryngoscopic examination with or without endotracheal intubation, provokes the cardiovascular and sympathoadrenal responses.[42] When the reports of the cardiovascular responses to intubation of the trachea are evaluated, it is apparent that the study conditions differ markedly in relation to premedication and anesthetic techniques employed. In addition, small numbers of patients are included in several studies. It seems reasonable to conclude that laryngoscopic examination and intubation of the trachea may induce cardiovascular changes that can jeopardize some patients. The best means of attenuating these responses depends upon the overall clinical situation. For example, the approach to the patient with a full

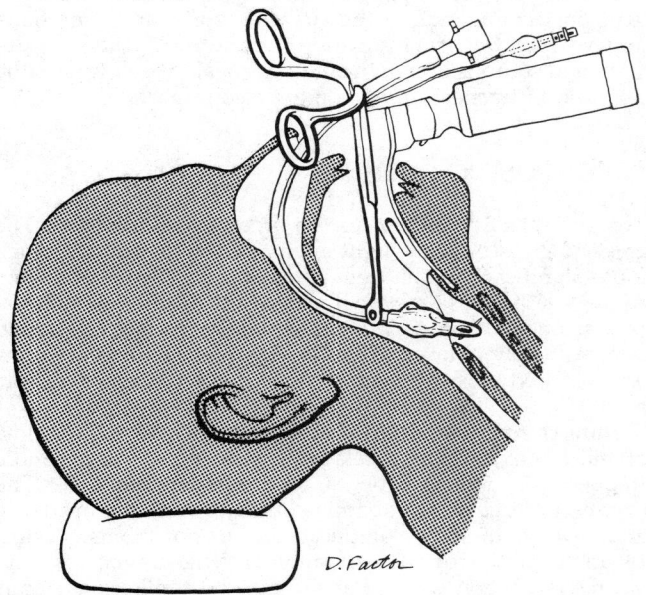

FIG. 20-20. McGill forceps are used to grasp and direct the endotracheal tube during nasotracheal intubation.

stomach, coronary artery disease, or known airway abnormalities may differ from that of the healthy patient scheduled for elective surgery. A combination of techniques may be employed, which include achieving an adequate depth of anesthesia before laryngoscopic examination, administration of fentanyl (6–8 μg·kg^{-1}), and intravenous administration of lidocaine (1.5 mg·kg^{-1} approximately 60–90 s before laryngoscopic examination). Translaryngeal administration of lidocaine is inferior to intravenous administration in blunting both cardiovascular responses and increases in intracranial pressure.[43]

INTRACRANIAL PRESSURE ALTERATION

Although transient increases in intracranial pressure associated with laryngoscopic examination and intubation of the trachea are of no consequence in patients without intracranial abnormalities, they may be significant in patients with increased intracranial pressure. Studies in both animals and humans have demonstrated an increase in intracranial pressure when administration of succinylcholine precedes intubation of the trachea.[44–46] Although the exact mechanism for the increase is uncertain, possible explanations include light anesthesia, hypercarbia, inadequate relaxation during intubation, a direct cerebral vasodilating effect of the succinylcholine, skeletal muscle fasciculations, and cerebral stimulation caused by afferent muscle spindle activity during depolarization.[47] Induction of adequate anesthesia, plus use of techniques normally used to control increased intracranial pressure, such as thiopental administration and hyperventilation before intubation of the trachea, will minimize this adverse effect of laryngoscopic examination and intubation.

EXTUBATION OF THE TRACHEA

Tracheae can be extubated while patients are deeply anesthetized or awake. Patients lightly anesthetized have active laryngeal reflexes and are prone to development of laryngospasm upon extubation of the trachea. Patients at risk of aspiration of gastric contents and those in whom reintubation would be difficult are best extubated while awake. Small children are usually extubated while awake because of the high incidence of laryngospasm associated with extubation of the anesthetized child.

Coughing or "bucking" on the endotracheal tube is associated with increases in intracranial and intraocular pressure, hypertension, and tachycardia. In addition, undue tension on sutures can lead to bleeding or wound dehiscence. The cardiovascular changes and coughing can be attenuated by intravenous injection of lidocaine (1 mg·kg^{-1}) approximately 2 min before extubation of the trachea.[48]

The pharynx is suctioned before extubation to remove secretions that can drain into the trachea or irritate the vocal cords and produce laryngospasm after the tube is withdrawn. Pressure on the breathing bag during tube removal may induce coughing and expulsion of any aspirated material.

COMPLICATIONS OF ENDOTRACHEAL INTUBATION

Complications can occur during intubation of the trachea or while the tube is *in situ* (Table 20-2). Some are evident when they occur; others are recognized during extubation of the

TABLE 20-2.   Complications of Endotracheal Intubation

During Intubation
  Laryngospasm
  Laceration, bruising of lips, tongue, and pharynx
  Fracture, chipping, dislodgment of teeth or dental appliances
  Perforation of trachea or esophagus
  Retropharyngeal dissection
  Fracture or dislocation of cervical spine
  Trauma to eyes
  Hemorrhage
  Aspiration of gastric contents or foreign bodies
  Endobronchial or esophageal intubation
  Dislocation of arytenoid cartilages or mandible
  Hypoxemia, hypercarbia
  Bradycardia, tachycardia
  Hypertension
  Increased intracranial or intraocular pressure

With Tube In Situ
  Accidental extubation
  Endobronchial intubation
  Obstruction or kinking
  Bronchospasm
  Ignition of tube by laser device
  Aspiration
  Excoriation of nose or mouth

Evident after Extubation
  Laryngospasm
  Aspiration of secretions, gastric contents, blood, or foreign
    bodies
  Glottic, subglottic, or uvular edema
  Dysphonia, aphonia
  Paralysis of vocal cords or hypoglossal, lingual nerves
  Sore throat
  Noncardiogenic pulmonary edema
  Laryngeal incompetence
  Sore, dislocated jaw
  Tracheal collapse
  Sinusitis
  Glottic, subglottic, or tracheal stenosis
  Vocal cord granulomata or synechiae

trachea or in the days to weeks after the endotracheal tube is removed. The incidence of complications varies with the patient population, skill of the laryngoscopist, and conditions under which tracheal intubation is performed. The size, design, and composition of the endotracheal tube as well as the duration of tracheal intubation are also important.

PREDISPOSING FACTORS

The patient's age influences the type of complications. The consequences of even slight edema of the airway are much more significant in children. In the infant, 1 mm of edema decreases the cross-sectional area of the glottic opening approximately 70% and increases flow resistance at the cricoid approximately 16 times. The same degree of laryngeal edema is associated with no symptoms or mild hoarseness in the adult.

Some complications vary with the patient's sex. Granuloma of the larynx, although relatively rare, occurs much more frequently in female patients, as does sore throat.[49, 50] The duration of tracheal intubation correlates with the incidence and severity of some complications but not others. Postextubation glottic edema, aspiration, laryngeal stenosis, and vocal dysfunction are well-documented complications occurring in patients intubated for a week or longer. However, the duration of translaryngeal intubation does not correlate with the incidence of granuloma formation.[51]

The type of endotracheal tube influences the incidence of both minor and major complications. Sore throat is a common complaint in patients whose tracheae have been intubated. The reported incidence varies markedly and is as high as 90%. Of interest, approximately 15% of patients who receive general anesthesia by mask also complain of sore throat.[52] Lubrication of the tube does not appear to decrease and may actually increase the incidence of sore throat.[52, 53] The incidence of sore throat and hoarseness is reduced by using smaller endotracheal tubes.[54] Although low-volume cuffs appear to be associated with a lower incidence of sore throat, the consequence of prolonged contact of these cuffs with tracheal mucosa indicates that high-volume, low-pressure cuffs should be used for all but brief tracheal intubations.[50, 55, 56]

The inhalation anesthetic agent employed is also important. Nitrous oxide diffuses into the endotracheal tube cuff and increases the volume and pressure of the cuff.[57, 58] These changes can be eliminated by inflation of the cuff with the same gas as that inspired, or with saline, or by periodic deflation of the cuff. Measurement of cuff pressures also has been recommended during prolonged operative procedures.[56]

PREVENTION OF COMPLICATIONS

Endotracheal intubation obviously has hazards. Tubes should be placed only when indicated. Attention to detail during intubation of the trachea is essential and can prevent most minor complications. Adequate fixation prevents migration of the tube into a bronchus, accidental extubation of the trachea, and unnecessary tube motion, which may increase the incidence of airway irritation. When prolonged intubation of the trachea is indicated, the risks must be weighed against those of tracheostomy. For periods of a week or less, translaryngeal intubation generally is preferred to tracheostomy. However, the relative merits of endotracheal intubation and tracheostomy are less clear when an artificial airway is required for a longer period of time.[51] Laryngoscopic examination immediately after extubation of the trachea is useful in evaluating the airway for abnormalities.

FIBEROPTIC ENDOSCOPY

The optimal method of managing the patient in whom airway difficulty is anticipated depends upon the patient's abnormalities, the anesthesiologist's skill, and the available equipment and personnel. Fiberoptic endoscopic examination is often appropriate.

UNANTICIPATED AIRWAY DIFFICULTY

It is not always possible to anticipate when endotracheal intubation will be difficult. However, when the larynx cannot be visualized and an endotracheal tube cannot be placed, the anesthesiologist must consider the alternatives, discuss them with the surgeon, and formulate a plan based on the origin of the difficulty and the urgency of surgery. If the procedure is elective, multiple tracheal intubation attempts have resulted in trauma, and there is no skilled fiberoptic endoscopist available, the procedure is best postponed. If the difficulty is recognized before airway trauma is produced, the patient is stable,

and an experienced fiberoptic endoscopist and appropriate equipment are available, it is reasonable to continue. An antisialagogue should be administered as soon as the decision is made to proceed with fiberoptic endoscopic examination. General anesthesia usually can be maintained with a potent inhalation agent. No additional muscle relaxants are administered. It may be necessary to reverse a nondepolarizing relaxant to allow resumption of spontaneous ventilation. If the esophagus was intubated or positive-pressure ventilation resulted in stomach distention, a nasogastric tube should be inserted and the stomach decompressed.

When the procedure is emergent and the patient's condition unstable, general anesthesia should be abandoned and the patient allowed to awaken. The patient whose condition is deteriorating because of cardiovascular instability or respiratory obstruction is almost never a candidate for fiberoptic endoscopic examination. Only if equipment is immediately available and a skilled endoscopist is in attendance should it even be considered. Cricothyrotomy, rigid bronchoscopic examination, or tracheostomy is usually preferable. If fiberoptic endoscopic examination is attempted in a patient with a full stomach, topical anesthesia and sedatives must be used with caution, if at all. The safest and most conservative approach is to avoid use of all local anesthetics because it is impossible to ensure that topical anesthesia will be confined to the area above the vocal cords. Translaryngeal and superior laryngeal nerve blocks are contraindicated in the patient at risk of aspiration of gastric contents.

ELECTIVE FIBEROPTIC LARYNGOSCOPY

Although the experienced endoscopist makes the procedure appear simple, fiberoptic laryngoscopic examination requires considerable skill and practice.[11] Practice with a fiberoptic device on an intubation mannequin is recommended. The model is immobile, does not fog the lens, is free of secretions and blood, and requires no monitoring or anesthesia. After gaining facility with the instrument, the anesthesiologist can then use it in normal patients in whom endotracheal intubation is indicated. Only after the anesthesiologist has successfully intubated the tracheae of several patients with normal airway anatomy should he or she use the instrument in less than optimal circumstances.

Fiberoptic endoscopic examination requires more time than conventional laryngoscopic examination, even when performed by an expert. The patient, surgeon, and operating room personnel must understand the indications for the procedure and the additional time required. It is imperative that the anesthetic technique be planned in advance, allowing sufficient time for induction of general anesthesia or for topical anesthesia and intravenous sedation to become effective. An assistant is useful when the procedure is performed with local anesthesia and mandatory if general anesthesia is administered. One person cannot monitor the patient, administer general anesthesia, and perform fiberoptic endoscopic examination.

Use of an endoscopic mask with a port through which the insertion tube of the endoscope is passed permits uninterrupted anesthesia and ventilation during the procedure (Fig. 20-21). As an alternative, adequate anesthesia and ventilation of the lungs can be maintained in most patients with a binasal airway attached to the anesthetic circuit. In order to maintain the midline position of the insertion tube as it is advanced through the pharynx into the trachea, an endoscopic airway is useful.

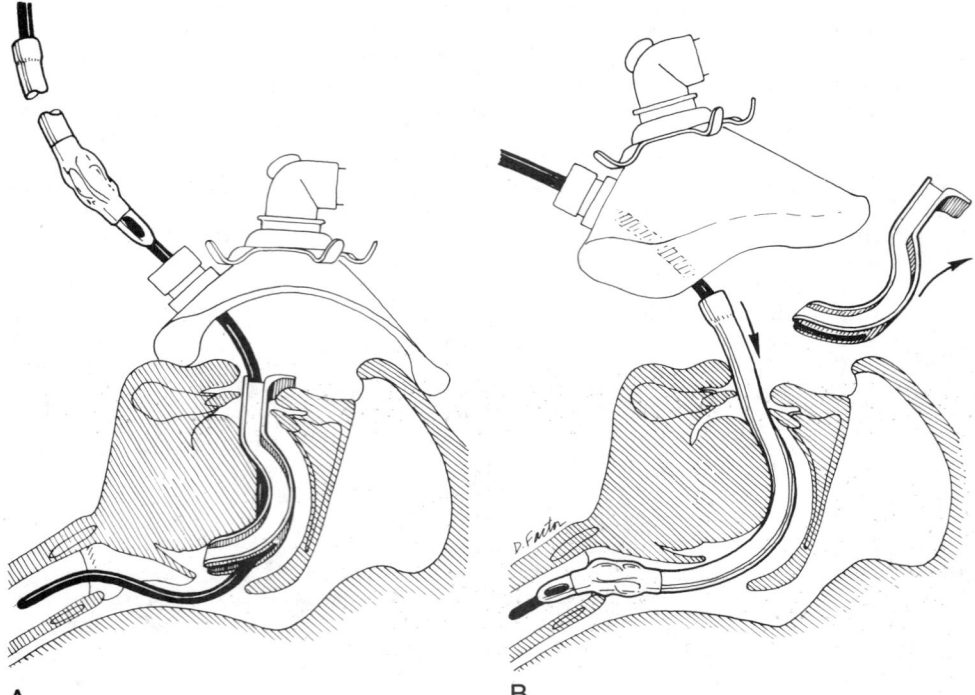

A   B

FIG. 20-21. (*A*) The insertion tube of the fiberoptic endoscope and the endotracheal tube are introduced through the port of the endoscopic mask. (*B*) The endoscopic airway is removed and the endotracheal tube advanced into the trachea.

The largest endoscope that will fit easily into the endotracheal tube should be used because it is more difficult to thread a large endotracheal tube over a small, flexible endoscope. Orotracheal intubation permits use of a larger endotracheal tube and is associated with less tissue trauma and bleeding. However, it may be difficult to thread the endotracheal tube once the endoscope is positioned in the trachea because of the acute angle formed between the oropharynx and trachea. Retraction of the tongue and anterior displacement of the mandible usually effectively overcome this problem. Nasotracheal intubation is often easier to perform because the natural curve of the nasopharynx guides the tube into the larynx (Fig. 20-22).

A step-by-step procedure should always be followed when fiberoptic endoscopic examination is performed. The endoscopist initially must determine that the working elements of the endoscope and light source are functional. It is essential that an antifog agent be applied to the lens. The sheath of the insertion tube must be lubricated thoroughly with a water-soluble jelly, beginning at the distal end and moving proximally to avoid the lens. Products containing oil or petroleum jelly should not be used. The lens of the instrument should be focused before use, not after the instrument is inserted. Visibility is enhanced if a constant oxygen flow is maintained through the operating channel of the instrument. In addition to providing a higher inspired oxygen concentration, the oxygen forces mucus, blood, and secretions away from the lens. Incorporation of a three-way stopcock in the suction tube allows alternating suction and oxygen flow.

The control section of the instrument is held in one hand, with the thumb positioned on the angle control and the index finger on the suction port. The insertion tube is held fully extended with the other hand, and the angle knob is manipulated to ensure that the end of the tube moves up and down, rather than sideways. When orotracheal intubation is performed in the adult, the insertion tube is advanced 8–10 cm into the pharynx. If the insertion tube is in the midline and has been advanced the proper distance, the vocal cords will come

into view as the tip of the scope is flexed upward. A local anesthetic agent can be instilled through the suction port directly onto the vocal cords if laryngeal anesthesia is inadequate. Slight rotation of the insertion tube may be necessary to bring the tip into the midline. The first view after the insertion tube is advanced through the vocal cords will be the thyroid cartilage, not the tracheal cartilages. The tip of the endoscope is straightened or returned to the neutral position and advanced until the tracheal cartilages and finally the carina are seen. The insertion tube is held firmly, the endotracheal tube threaded into the trachea, and the endoscope removed.

The primary reasons for technique failure are inexperience and insufficient planning. All too often the technique is considered only after multiple unsuccessful tracheal intubation attempts have resulted in tissue trauma, edema, and bleeding. In such circumstances anatomic landmarks are obscured

FIG. 20-22. Model demonstrating use of endoscopic mask and airway during fiberoptic nasotracheal intubation.

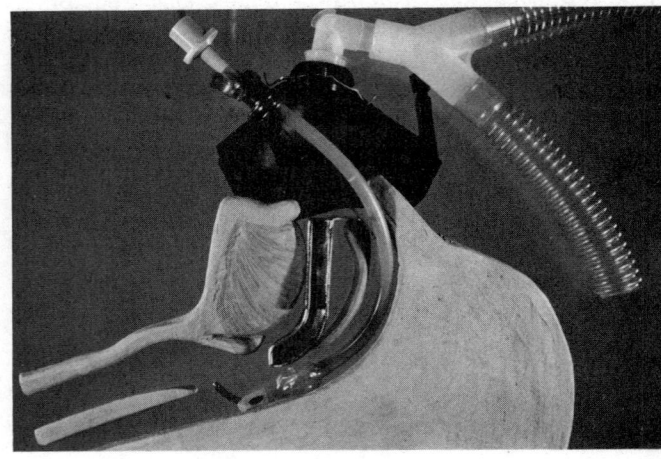

and there is little chance of success. If there is insufficient light or if the instrument is not properly focused, the image will be blurred or hazy. The lens becomes fogged after several minutes of use. If suctioning or flowing oxygen through the channel does not improve vision, the instrument must be withdrawn, cleaned, and defogged. The most frequent complaint of the beginning endoscopist is that everything appears pink. His or her first reaction is to withdraw the insertion tube on the presumption that the esophagus was intubated. If the endoscope easily advances more than 10 or 12 cm beyond the pharynx and no definable structures are evident, it can be assumed that this has occurred. However, the most common explanation is that the insertion tube is not in the midline and the tip is facing the piriform or tonsillar fossae or the oropharynx. In this case the endoscope should be withdrawn and reinserted to a depth of 8–10 cm.

The primary indication for fiberoptic laryngoscopic examination is endotracheal intubation. However, fiberoptic endoscopic examination also has diagnostic and therapeutic applications. The endotracheal, endobronchial (Fig. 20-22), and tracheostomy tube positions can be verified and the airway examined for abnormalities.[59] The fiberoptic bronchoscope is also useful for placing segmental bronchial blockers, changing endotracheal tubes and performing tracheobronchial toilet.[60]

OTHER SPECIALIZED TECHNIQUES OF AIRWAY MANAGEMENT

Altering the position of the patient's head and using a smaller endotracheal tube or a different laryngoscope blade is all that is necessary in some cases of difficult airway management. However, specialized equipment and techniques are useful when these maneuvers fail.

LIGHTWAND TECHNIQUE

Orotracheal intubation can be facilitated by use of a lighted stylet in the endotracheal tube.[61, 62] Although general anesthesia can be employed, topical anesthesia and sedation are recommended when the technique is used in the patient with known or suspected airway difficulty. The operating room lights are dimmed, the patient's tongue is grasped with a gauze sponge and pulled gently forward, and the endotracheal tube containing the lighted stylet is inserted into the oropharynx and advanced. When the tip is correctly positioned in the midline just superior to the larynx, a glow will be evident in the anterior neck. The tube is then slid off the lightwand and advanced into the trachea. If the tip of the stylet enters the esophagus, the light will be diminished. This technique compares favorably with both direct laryngoscopic and orotracheal intubation and blind nasotracheal intubation.[61, 62]

FLUOROSCOPIC TECHNIQUES

A flexible steerable catheter with an attached control handle (Medi-tech Inc., Watertown, MA) can be placed in the lumen of a nasotracheal tube and advanced with fluoroscopic control. Once the catheter has entered the trachea, the endotracheal tube is advanced over it and the catheter removed.[63]

Intubation of the trachea can sometimes be accomplished by threading a plastic catheter into a needle placed through the cricothyroid membrane and directing the catheter cephalad (retrograde) into the pharynx. The endotracheal tube is then threaded over the catheter and advanced through the larynx and into the trachea.[64, 65] Although fluoroscopic examination is not essential to the technique, it facilitates localization of the catheter, especially when it cannot be directed easily into the pharynx.

CRICOTHYROIDOTOMY

An intravenous needle and catheter (*e.g.*, 14-G for adults) is passed through the cricothyroid membrane. Once air is aspirated, the cannula is advanced caudally and the needle withdrawn. A 3-mm endotracheal tube adapter can be used for connection to the anesthesia circuit (Fig. 20-23). Alternatively, the barrel of a 3-ml syringe (from which the plunger has been removed) can be connected to the catheter and a 7-mm endotracheal tube adapter placed into the barrel of the syringe and the connection made to the anesthesia circuit.[66] There are a variety of other techniques which have been recommended, including placement of an endotracheal tube in the syringe, putting side holes in the tracheal cannula, and use of oxygen

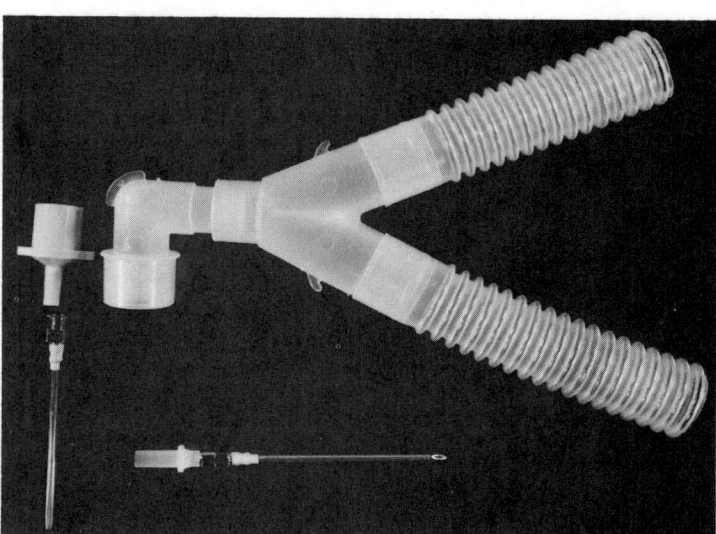

FIG. 20-23. An intravenous catheter (A) can be used for cricothyroidotomy. Insertion of a 3-mm endotracheal tube adapter (B) into the hub of the catheter permits attachment of the anesthesia circuit (C).

at high driving pressures.[67, 68] High-frequency jet ventilation by the transtracheal catheter has also been reported.[69, 70]

SURGICAL INTERVENTION

A rigid bronchoscope often can be passed when direct laryngoscopic examination and endotracheal intubation are impossible. When bronchoscopic examination is necessary, the anesthesiologist must determine that the appropriate bronchoscope and light sources are available and functional. Most bronchoscopes have a ventilating sidearm with a 15-mm adapter to connect to the anesthesia circuit. The anesthesiologist must be certain that the fittings are compatible before anesthesia induction. The Storz pediatric bronchoscopes and Hopkins telescopes provide optical detail not available with conventional bronchoscopes. However, air flow resistance is increased significantly, precluding spontaneous ventilation.[71] The problem of inadequate gas exchange is not eliminated by controlled ventilation, necessitating periodic removal of the telescope and inflation of the lungs with oxygen.

Although performed much less frequently for airway management since the introduction of fiberoptic endoscopy, tracheostomy is still indicated in some patients. It is better to perform a tracheostomy under controlled conditions than to resort to the technique once other measures have failed and the patient is *in extremis*.

SUMMARY

It is essential that every anesthesiologist formulate alternatives for airway management to be used when conventional methods fail.[72-75] Equipment necessary for management of the patient with a difficult airway should be assembled in one readily accessible area in the operating suite. The most efficient method is to have the equipment stored on a cart that can be moved quickly into the room when needed.

REFERENCES

1. Eckenhoff JE: Some anatomic considerations of the infant larynx influencing endotracheal intubation. Anesthesiology 12:401, 1951
2. Katz J, Benumof J, Kadis LB: Anesthesia and uncommon diseases. In Pathophysiologic and Clinical Correlations, 2nd ed. Philadelphia, WB Saunders, 1981
3. Katz J, Steward DJ: Anesthesia in Uncommon Pediatric Diseases. Philadelphia, WB Saunders, 1987
4. Smith DW: Recognizable Patterns of Human Malformation, 3rd ed. Philadelphia, WB Saunders, 1982
5. Block C, Brechner VL: Unusual problems in airway management. II. The influence of the temporomandibular joint, the mandible and associated structures on endotracheal intubation. Anesth Analg 50:114, 1971
6. Redick LF: The tempromandibular joint and tracheal intubation. Anesth Analg 66:675, 1987
7. Brechner VL: Unusual problems in the management of airways. I. Flexion-extension mobility of the cervical vertebrae. Anesth Analg 47:362, 1986
8. Jenkins CL, McGraw RW: Anaesthetic management of the patient with rheumatoid arthritis. Can Anaesth Soc J 16:407, 1969
9. Sinclair JR, Mason RA: Ankylosing spondylitis. The case for awake intubation. Anaesthesia 39:3, 1984
10. Pellicci PM, Ranawat CS, Tsairis P et al: A prospective study of the progression of rheumatoid arthritis of the cervical spine. J Bone Joint Surg 63:342, 1981
11. Patil VU, Stehling L, Zauder HL: Fiberoptic Endoscopy in Anesthesiology. Chicago, Year Book Medical Publishers, 1983
12. Mallampati SR, Gatt SP, Gugino LD et al: A clinical sign to predict difficult tracheal intubation: A prospective study. Can Anaesth Soc J 32:429, 1985
13. Sampson GLT, Young JRB: Difficult tracheal intubation. Anaesthesia 42:487, 1987
14. White A, Kander PL: Anatomical factors in difficult direct laryngoscopy. Br J Anaesth 47:468, 1975
15. Patil VU, Stehling LC, Zauder HL: An adjustable laryngoscope handle for difficult intubations. Anesthesiology 60:609, 1984
16. Cozanitis DA, Nuuttila K, Merrett JD et al: Influence of laryngoscope design on heart rate and rhythm changes during intubation. Can Anaesth Soc J 31:155, 1984
17. Owen RL, Cheney FW: Endobronchial intubation: A preventable complication. Anesthesiology 67:255, 1987
18. Bolder PM, Healy TEJ, Bolder AR: The extra work of breathing through adult endotracheal tubes. Anesth Analg 65:853, 1986
19. Salem MR: Anesthetic management of patients with "a full stomach." A critical review. Anesth Analg 49:47, 1970
20. Salem MR, Joseph NJ, Heyman HJ et al: Cricoid pressure is effective in obliterating the esophageal lumen in the presence of a nasogastric tube. Anesthesiology 63:443, 1985
21. Bertholid M, Read DH, Norman J: Preoxygenation—How long? Anaesthesia 38:96, 1983
22. Gold MI, Muravchick S: Arterial oxygenation during larygnoscopy and intubation. Anesth Analg 60:316, 1981
23. Drummond GB, Park GR: Arterial oxygen saturation before intubation of the trachea. Br J Anaesth 56:987, 1984
24. Sellick BA: Cricoid pressure to control regurgitation of stomach contents during induction of anaesthesia. Lancet 2:404, 1961
25. Sutherland AD, William SRT: Cardiovascular responses and lidocaine absorption in fiberoptic-assisted awake intubation. Anesth Analg 65:389, 1986
26. Bourke DL, Katz J, Tonneson A: Nebulized anesthesia for awake endotracheal intubation. Anesthesiology 63:690, 1985
27. Birmingham PK, Cheney FW, Ward RJ: Esophageal intubation: A review of detection techniques. Anesth Analg 65:886, 1986
28. Adriani J, Griggs TS: An improved endotracheal tube for pediatric use. Anesthesiology 15:466, 1954
29. Kubota Y, Toyoda Y, Nagata N et al: Tracheo-bronchial angles in infants and children. Anesthesiology 64:374, 1986
30. Tsuneto S, Yamashita M, Miyamoto Y: Tracheo-bronchial angles in neonates. Anesthesiology 67:151, 1987
31. Patil VU, Stehling L, Zauder HL: An aid to blind endotracheal intubation. Anesth Analg 63:882, 1984
32. Bedford RF, Feinstein B: Hospital admission blood pressure: A predictor for hypertension following endotracheal intubation. Anesth Analg 59:367, 1980
33. King BD, Harris LC Jr, Greifenstein FE et al: Reflex circulatory responses to direct laryngoscopy and tracheal intubation performed during general anesthesia. Anesthesiology 12:556, 1951
34. Lunn JK, Stanley TH, Eisele J et al: High dose fentanyl anesthesia for coronary artery surgery: Plasma fentanyl concentrations and influence of nitrous oxide on cardiovascular responses. Anesth Analg 58:390, 1979
35. Kautto UM: Attenuation of the circulatory response to laryngoscopy and intubation by fentanyl. Acta Anaesth Scand 26:217, 1982
36. Martin DE, Rosenberg H, Aukburg SJ et al: Low dose fentanyl blunts circulatory responses to tracheal intubation. Anesth Analg 61:680, 1982
37. Stoelting RK: Attenuation of blood pressure response to laryngoscopy and tracheal intubation with sodium nitroprusside. Anesth Analg 58:116, 1979
38. Derbyshire DR, Chmielewski A, Fell D et al: Plasma cate-

cholamine responses to tracheal intubation. Br J Anaesth 55:855, 1983

39. Kautto UM, Heinonen J: Attenuation of circulatory response to laryngoscopy and tracheal intubation: A comparison of two methods of topical anaesthesia. Acta Anaesth Scand 26:599, 1982

40. Stoelting RK: Circulatory changes during direct laryngoscopy and tracheal intubation: Influence of duration of laryngoscopy with or without prior lidocaine. Anesthesiology 47:381, 1977

41. Stoelting RK: Blood pressure and heart rate changes during short-duration laryngoscopy for tracheal intubation: Influence of viscous or intravenous lidocaine. Anesth Analg 57:197, 1978

42. Shribman AJ, Smith G, Achola KJ: Cardiovascular and catecholamine responses to laryngoscopy with and without tracheal intubation. Br J Anaesth 59:295, 1987

43. Hamill JF, Bedford RF, Weaver DC et al: Lidocaine before endotracheal intubation: Intravenous or laryngotracheal? Anesthesiology 55:578, 1981

44. Cottrell JE, Hartung J, Giffin JP et al: Intracranial and hemodynamic changes after succinylcholine administration in cats. Anesth Analg 62:1006, 1983

45. McLeskey CH, Cullen BF, Kennedy RD et al: Control of cerebral perfusion pressure during induction of anesthesia in high-risk neurosurgical patients. Anesth Analg 53:985, 1974

46. Burney RG, Winn R: Increased cerebrospinal fluid pressure during laryngoscopy and intubation for induction of anesthesia. Anesth Analg 54:687, 1975

47. Lanier WL, Milde JH, Michenfelder JD: Cerebral stimulation following succinylcholine in dogs. Anesthesiology 64:551, 1986

48. Bidwai AV, Bidwai VA, Rogers CR et al: Blood pressure and pulse-rate responses to endotracheal extubation with and without prior injection of lidocaine. Anesthesiology 51:171, 1979

49. Snow JC, Harano M, Balogh K: Postintubation granuloma of the larynx. Anesth Analg 45:425, 1966

50. Jensen PJ, Hommelgaard P, Sondergaard P et al: Sore throat after operation: Influence of tracheal intubation, intracuff pressure and type of cuff. Br J Anaesth 54:453, 1982

51. Bishop MJ, Weymuller EA, Fink BR: Laryngeal effects of prolonged intubation. Anesth Analg 63:335, 1984

52. Loeser EA, Stanley TH, Jordan W et al: Postoperative sore throat: Influence of tracheal tube lubrication versus cuff design. Can Anaesth Soc J 27:156, 1980

53. Stock MC, Downs JB: Lubrication of tracheal tubes to prevent sore throat from intubation. Anesthesiology 57:418, 1982

54. Stout DM, Bishop MJ, Dwersteg JF et al: Correlation of endotracheal tube size with sore throat and hoarseness following general anesthesia. Anesthesiology 67:419, 1987

55. Loeser EA, Orr DL, Bennett BM et al: Endotracheal tube cuff design and postoperative sore throat. Anesthesiology 45:684, 1976

56. Latto IP: The cuff. In Latto IP, Rosen M (eds): Difficulties in Tracheal Intubation. London, Bailliere Tindall, 1985

57. Stanley TH: Effects of anesthetic gases on endotracheal tube cuff gas volumes. Anesth Analg 53:480, 1974

58. Stanley TH: Nitrous oxide and pressures and volumes of high- and low-pressure endotracheal tube cuffs in intubated patients. Anesthesiology 42:637, 1975

59. Patil VU, Stehling LC, Zauder HL: Another use for the fiberoptic bronchoscope. Anesthesiology 55:484, 1981

60. Rosenbaum SH, Rosenbaum LM, Cole RP et al: Use of the flexible fiberoptic bronchoscope to change endotracheal tubes in critically ill patients. Anesthesiology 54:169, 1981

61. Ellis DG, Jakymec A, Kaplan RM et al: Guided orotracheal intubation in the operating room using a lighted stylet: A comparison with direct laryngoscopic technique. Anesthesiology 64:823, 1986

62. Fox DJ, Castro T, Rastrelli AJ: Comparison of intubation techniques in the awake patient: The Flexi-lum surgical light (light-wand) versus blind nasal approach. Anesthesiology 66:69, 1987

63. Davidson AJ, Reynolds AC, Stewart ET: Use of a flexible radiopaque directable catheter for difficult tracheal intubations. Anesthesiology 55:605, 1981

64. Powell WF, Ozdil T: A translaryngeal guide for tracheal intubation. Anesth Analg 46:231, 1967

65. Bouake D, Levesque PR: Modification of retrograde guide for endotracheal intubation. Anesth Analg 53:1013, 1974

66. Stinson TW III: A simple connector for transtracheal ventilation. Anesthesiology 47:232, 1977

67. Gildar JS: A simple system for transtracheal ventilation. Anesthesiology 58:106, 1983

68. Yealy DM, Stewart RD: Translaryngeal cannula ventilation: Continuing misconceptions. Anesthesiology 67:445, 1987

69. Ravussin P, Freeman J: A new transtracheal catheter for ventilation and resuscitation. Can Anaesth Soc J 32:60, 1985

70. Boucek CD, Gunnerson HB, Tullock WC: Percutaneous transtracheal high-frequency jet ventilation as an aid to fiberoptic intubation. Anesthesiology 67:247, 1987

71. Widlund B, Walczak S, Motoyama E: Flow-pressure characteristics of pediatric Storz-Hopkins bronchoscopes. Anesthesiology 47:A417, 1982

72. McIntyre JWR: The difficult tracheal intubation. Can J Anaesth 34:204, 1987

73. Tunstall ME: Failed intubation drill. Anaesthesia 31:850, 1976

74. Rosen M: Difficult and failed intubation in obstetrics. In Latto IP, Rosen M (eds): Difficulties in Tracheal Intubation, p 152. London, Bailliere Tindall, 1985

75. Latto IP: Management of difficult intubation. In Latto IP, Rosen M (eds): Difficulties in Tracheal Intubation, p 99. London, Bailliere Tindall, 1985

Chapter 21

Casey D. Blitt

Monitoring the Anesthetized Patient

Monitoring provides information that improves the administration of anesthesia with regard to safety, effectiveness of drugs and techniques, and recognition of adverse effects. Timely therapeutic intervention may therefore avoid or prevent disastrous consequences. Monitoring is also required to assess the effects of intervention or changes that have been made.

Monitoring is basically data collection, that is, providing input to the anesthesiologist who uses that information to develop output to the patient. The data must be processed by the anesthesiologist in order to be of real value. Data may be collected *manually*, such as by pulse palpation, or manual blood pressure determination; *by the senses*, such as by visual observation of reservoir bag movement; or *automatically*, such as by ECG, automatic blood pressure measurement, or pulse oximetry. All of these methods are useful, but it is becoming increasingly clear that automatic methods provide continual input and free the anesthesiologist from the tedious task of repetitive motions, thereby allowing more time for decision making. Automatic data collection is not without annoyances such as false alarms, incorrect data display, and occasional suboptimal performance in the electrically hostile operating room environment. Nevertheless, the practice of anesthesia has reached the stage where some automatic data collection devices are essential to safe clinical practice.

PATIENT SAFETY

Monitoring can substantially improve early recognition of many disasters such as esophageal intubation, anesthetic circuit disconnects, errors in gas supply/flow, and anesthetic overdosage. Monitoring should permit early intervention to help avoid a less than optimal outcome.

Multiple monitoring modalities with back-up are desirable. The more systems you have to tell you if your patient is hypoxemic, the greater chance you have to receive adequate input even if one system fails.

WHAT TO MONITOR

Two broad areas in anesthesia that should be monitored are easily identifiable: 1) the anesthetic delivery system (machine, gas flows, ventilator, vaporizer); and 2) the effect of anesthetic management on the patient. Monitoring the anesthetic delivery system includes monitoring of various pressures and concentrations of gaseous constituents of the system. There is clearly overlap of both of these areas because some monitoring of the anesthetic delivery system also monitors the anesthetic management of the patient (*i.e.*, halogenated anesthetics, carbon dioxide). Monitoring the anesthetic delivery system is discussed in an earlier chapter (Chapter 19) and will not be dealt with in depth in this chapter.

The effects of anesthesia on the patient may be categorized by organ system or by individual monitoring modalities. Some monitoring modalities monitor more than one organ system, and most organ systems have more than one monitoring modality available to them. I will discuss monitoring primarily by systems, with the exception of some modalities that affect so many systems that they must be discussed as separate entities.

INVASIVENESS *VERSUS* NONINVASIVENESS

Monitors can be categorized arbitrarily as invasive or noninvasive. Noninvasive monitors may be defined as any modality that does not require penetration of skin or mucous membrane, whereas invasive monitors do require such penetration. A noninvasive monitor may unintentionally become an invasive monitor in certain circumstances, such as when a nasopharyngeal temperature probe enters the brain or a tympanic membrane temperature sensor perforates the eardrum. Does a noninvasive modality, like computerized tomography (CT), become invasive when contrast (to enhance the image) is injected intravenously? Does nuclear cardiology fall into the invasive category when an injection of radiopharmaceutical is required? This author believes that categorizing monitoring modalities in terms of invasiveness *versus* noninvasiveness serves little useful purpose. All monitoring modalities are on a continuum of invasiveness to noninvasiveness, and categorization is always relative to other monitoring modalities.

ORGAN SYSTEMS

CENTRAL NERVOUS SYSTEM

Electroencephalogram

The electroencephalogram (EEG) is a monitor of cerebral function that is relatively noninvasive. Many physiologic variables as well as pharmacologic variables impact on the EEG. Theoretically, any factor that interferes with proper cerebral function, such as hypoxia, hypercarbia, or ischemia, should result in a change in the EEG. Opioids, barbiturates, and virtually all drugs used for induction or maintenance of anesthesia substantially affect the EEG.[1] Changes in carbon dioxide, oxygen, body temperature, sensory stimulation, and blood pressure also influence the EEG.[1]

The major use of EEG monitoring today is to ascertain adequacy of cerebral perfusion, such as during carotid endarterectomy. There are conflicting data regarding relevance of changes in the EEG to eventual neurologic outcome.[1] Major EEG changes lasting longer than 10 min appear to be significantly correlated with neurologic deficit.[1] The EEG has been advocated to monitor depth of anesthesia and has also been used to ascertain adequacy of brain perfusion during cardiopulmonary bypass and open heart surgery.

Because of the many factors that influence the EEG, because there have been continued difficulties in obtaining the EEG in the electrically hostile operating-room environment, and because few anesthesiologists have been trained or are experienced in interpreting EEG data, use of this modality has not been widespread.

Computer-assisted analysis of EEG data, designed to compress data and make them easier for the clinician to interpret, may improve the acceptability of EEG monitoring in the future. The cerebral function monitor (CFM), power spectrum analysis (PSA), the density-modulated spectral array (DSA), and the spectral edge frequency (SEF), all represent improved computer-based technology designed to aid the clinician in collecting and interpreting EEG data.[1] I do not feel that this instrumentation has yet reached a point where it is sufficiently cost effective, reliable, and simple for the average clinician to interpret and for it to be useful on a widespread basis. More information regarding the EEG is available in Chapter 30.

Evoked Potentials

A sensory-evoked potential is the electrophysiologic response to a stimulus. The stimulus may be somatosensory (pain), visual (light), or auditory (sound). The response is recorded by monitoring electrical activity in the central nervous system at the level of the spinal cord, brain stem, or cerebral cortex. Because the signals are of low amplitude and cannot be differentiated from normal electrical activity by the naked eye, computer processing of the electrical activity is required. When the signal response to a stimulus has been isolated, it is customary to measure the amplitude of the wave and the latency, or time required for the nerve impulse to travel from the point of the stimulus to the point where it is being recorded. The primary application of sensory-evoked potential monitoring is to assess continually the function and integrity of a neural pathway (such as the spinal cord or cranial nerve VIII).[2,3]

Evoked potential monitoring may be useful intraoperatively when four conditions are met. First, a structure amenable to monitoring is at risk. Second, equipment and personnel are available to record and interpret the wave forms. Third, appropriate sites are available for stimulation and recording. Finally, if the monitoring is to be significant, there should be some possibility of intervention to improve function in the event that deteriorating transmission of impulses is detected.[2] Neurosurgical procedures and operations, where neural pathways are at risk, comprise the majority of the cases in which this modality is used. Examples include operations for resection of spinal cord tumors, corrective surgery of the spine, and cranial tumor resection. Figure 21-1 shows the change in auditory evoked potential with traction on the eighth cranial nerve. Since anesthetics may substantially alter the electrophysiologic activity of the brain and spinal cord, a high level of communication among the anesthesiologist, the surgeon, and the neurophysiologist is extremely important. Drugs that substantially affect evoked potentials, such as the halogenated inhaled anesthetics, should be used in minimal concentrations.[2] Body temperature, arterial blood pressure, and arterial blood gas tensions may also influence evoked potentials and are somewhat under the control of the anesthesiologist.

The equipment for evoked-potential monitoring starts at about $25,000; a state-of-the-art system costs $125,000 or more. Complications of evoked potential monitoring are minimal except for inappropriate therapeutic intervention based on erroneous data interpretation. The modality is clearly worth the cost in operations where spinal cord function may be compromised.[2] Its worth in other areas is unclear. This modality will continue to mature and improve and as new developments are reported the modality will take its appropriate place in our monitoring armamentarium. This modality is more fully discussed in Chapter 30.

Intracranial Pressure

Intracranial pressure (ICP) is determined by the volume of the three "compartments" in the cranium: cerebral blood volume, cerebrospinal fluid volume, and brain tissue volume. Monitoring of ICP is important because an abnormal increase in ICP may cause a reduction in cerebral perfusion pressure (the difference between systolic blood pressure and ICP), cerebral ischemia, or herniation of brain tissue into the foramen magnum.

Intracranial pressure may be monitored by an intraventricular catheter, a subarachnoid screw, or by various epidural

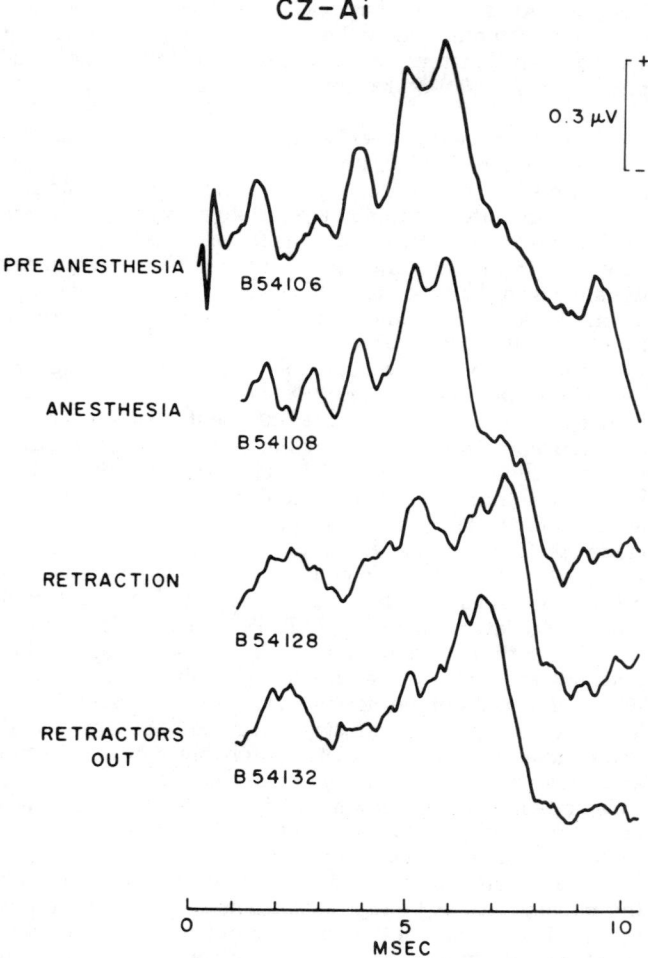

CZ-Ai

0.3 μV

+

−

PRE ANESTHESIA   B54106

ANESTHESIA   B54108

RETRACTION   B54128

RETRACTORS OUT   B54132

0   5   10
MSEC

FIG. 21-1. Brain stem auditory-evoked potential changes associated with retraction of the eighth cranial nerve and cerebellum. (Reprinted with permission. Grundy BL: Intraoperative monitoring of sensory-evoked potentials. Anesthesiology 58:72, 1983.)

transducers.[4] ICP measurement is clearly more useful when the cranial vault is closed than it is intraoperatively when the cranium may be open. The evolution and improvement in CT scanners seem to have resulted in a decrease in the use of intracranial pressure monitoring. ICP monitoring is most useful in evaluating therapy when patients are at risk for high ICP. Such patients might include those with a brain tumor, Reye's syndrome, or a head injury.

System leaks, transducer problems, and infections are the primary complications of this modality.[4] Ventriculitis from an intraventricular catheter is a particularly serious complication. This modality is additionally discussed in Chapters 30 and 31.

Anesthetic Depth

There is no uniformly applicable or consistently reliable measure of anesthetic depth. Anesthesiologists use their senses and powers of observation to determine adequate anesthetic depth in most circumstances. The presence or absence of movement in response to surgical stimulation in the patient who has not received muscle relaxants is frequently the most reliable sign of depth of anesthesia. The current pharmacologic armamentarium does not permit the reliable use of eye signs for determining depth of anesthesia. We have developed the habit of using the autonomic nervous system as a "mirror" of anesthetic depth. That is, we use the heart rate and blood pressure as a reflection of what is happening in the brain. Hypotension and bradycardia suggest "deep" anesthesia, whereas hypertension and tachycardia suggest "light" anesthesia. Unfortunately, a multitude of other factors can also affect these signs. Respiratory depression is an excellent hallmark of depth of anesthesia, but it is useful only if ventilation is spontaneous. Ventilation is also affected by surgical stimulation. The EEG is not an adequate measure of anesthetic depth. Subcortical awareness may persist even at "deep" levels of anesthesia.[5]

Inspired and end-tidal anesthetic concentration monitoring can allow us to use the ED_{50} (MAC) and ED_{95} and try to achieve what we estimate to be an adequate anesthetic depth. This still does not address individual variability in dose–response curves. The primary reason for monitoring anesthetic depth is to prevent overdosage and recall during anesthesia. Clearly, monitoring of anesthetic depth is more difficult with the injectable anesthetics than with the inhaled anesthetics. Assessment of anesthetic depth has traditionally relied on monitoring of physical signs. Technologic advances that have modernized cardiovascular monitoring have not made significant inroads in monitoring anesthetic depth.

The value of measuring lower esophageal contractility as a guide to the depth or adequacy of anesthesia has recently been investigated. The technique involves the detection and measurement of both spontaneous and provoked esophageal contractions in the lower one-third of the esophagus.[6] The smooth muscles of the lower esophagus remain active despite the use of muscle relaxants. This modality is currently in clinical testing stages, and the ultimate usefulness of lower esophageal contractility monitoring as a measure of anesthetic depth remains to be determined.

Computerized Tomography and Magnetic Resonance Imaging

CT and magnetic resonance imaging (MRI) are used primarily for their diagnostic value and not for routine patient monitoring. MRI spectroscopy has the potential for monitoring metabolism on a global nonspecific basis,[7] which may be of most value in the critical care setting. Neither MRI nor CT is likely to be used in the operating room simply because of logistic difficulties. For example, the magnet required in MRI or spectroscopy simply cannot coexist in the operating room environment. The major impact of CT and MRI involves selection of appropriate monitors when anesthetizing patients who are undergoing diagnostic studies using these modalities. Logistical difficulties (being far away from the patient)[8] and the need to eliminate ferrous metals from the room pose substantial challenges.

CARDIOVASCULAR SYSTEM

Senses

Although mechanical devices are appealing to many anesthesiologists, the senses of touch, hearing, and vision are extremely useful in monitoring the cardiovascular system. Pulse palpation, capillary refill, color of blood, and heart sounds may all be examined using the senses or the senses combined with simple instruments such as a precordial or esophageal stethoscope. These monitoring modalities are quite subjective (qualitative) and virtually impossible to quantitate except for heart rate. Furthermore, in critical situations they may be of value only to determine the presence or absence of pulse or heart sounds. Nevertheless, in an era of mechanization, with frequent appearance of artifacts, these sensory modalities are most useful as adjuncts or back-up systems for the more sophisticated and quantitative monitoring devices. Precordial or esophageal stethoscopes should not be discarded. Pulse oximetry and capnography may be important monitoring standards, but they like all other mechanical devices can fail or give erroneous information. Vigilance by machines should not totally replace vigilance by the anesthesiologist.

Blood Pressure

Blood pressure may be measured noninvasively by palpation, auscultation, or using the oscillometric method. The palpation method derives systolic blood pressure only. The auscultatory method makes use of the Korotkoff sounds and has come to be known as the Riva-Rocci method.[9] The oscillometric method is utilized in most automatic blood pressure devices.[10] Two commercially available devices that automatically determine systolic, diastolic, and mean arterial blood pressure using the oscillometric method are the Dinamap (Critikon, Tampa, FL) and the Accutorr (Datascope, Paramus, NJ). The obvious advantage of automatic determination of blood pressure is that it allows for measurements to be taken no matter what other tasks the anesthesiologist is performing. Many people recommend that an automatic blood pressure device should be available at every anesthetizing location.

Normal blood pressure varies and is lowest in the newborn and highest in the adult. Normal systolic blood pressure for a 3 kg newborn is 60 mm Hg. Normal systolic blood pressure for children 0–9 yr of age is 90–95 mm Hg and for adolescents 10-19 yr of age is 105–110 mm Hg. It is of paramount importance to match the size of the blood pressure cuff to the size of the patient's arm. If the cuff is too small, the blood pressure reading will be too high. A loosely wrapped cuff will also produce an erroneously high reading. The best width of a blood pressure cuff is 40% of the circumference of the arm.[9]

The location of the blood pressure determination is probably unimportant. The thigh, calf, arm, or forearm are all acceptable locations, particularly for oscillometric blood pressure determination. The significance of the blood pressure varies with the individual patient. Patients with long-standing cerebral vascular disease or coronary artery disease may require different blood pressure management than a healthy young teenager.

The addition of a recorder to an automatic blood pressure device to produce a written record is an important consideration. The written record allows the information to be transferred at a later time to the anesthesia record or it may be included as part of the permanent anesthetic record if desired. How to utilize the print-out obtained from the automatic blood pressure device must be decided on an individual basis. The written blood pressure record is invaluable as it represents "what actually happened,"[11] serves as a learning and teaching tool, and serves as an "inflight recorder" should a disaster occur. A further refinement is "computerization" of the anesthetic record so that all monitored information is recorded and stored automatically. Complications resulting from noninvasive blood pressure measurement are minimal. Nerve damage

has been reported secondary to continuous or rather frequent inflations of the automatic blood pressure cuff.[12] Petechiae secondary to pinching of the skin by the automatic blood pressure cuff also occur commonly but appear to be of no significance.

Noninvasive, beat-to-beat blood pressure measurement can also be determined utilizing a finger cuff (FINAP).[13] The finger blood pressure has been shown to reflect systemic arterial pressure accurately but there are certain instances where the modality is not effective.[13] Various factors affecting the measurement from this continuous finger cuff include hemodynamic disturbances, vasoactive drugs, sympathetic stimulation, hypovolemia, and the presence of an intraarterial cannula in the same hand.[13] Despite these drawbacks, the future for noninvasive continuous blood pressure measurement from the finger is very promising.

Invasive blood pressure measurement requires arterial catheterization. Indications are numerous and the procedure is used frequently. The radial artery at the wrist is the best vessel to cannulate in most circumstances. When the radial artery is unavailable other reasonable choices (in adults) include the dorsalis pedis, ulnar, femoral, and axillary arteries. Although a surgical cut-down is sometimes required, arterial cannulation can usually be achieved percutaneously. A test for adequate collateral circulation (Allen's test), while being emotionally soothing and possibly of some medicolegal value, does not appear to be of any predictive value in ascertaining who will or will not develop vascular problems secondary to arterial cannulation.[14, 15] Most vascular complications secondary to radial artery cannulation are probably embolic in nature and thus would not be predicted using a test for adequate collateral circulation. Because of this, many clinicians have abandoned performing tests for adequate collateral circulation prior to radial artery cannulation.

There are probably as many techniques for cannulation of the radial artery as there are clinicians performing the procedure. Dorsiflexion of the wrist, immobilization with adhesive tape, and identification of the course of the vessel with palpating fingers seem to be common recommendations for radial artery cannulation.[14, 16] These measures are necessary because the radial artery is rather tortuous as it passes over the wrist joint. The radial artery in fact is more easily cannulated slightly proximal to the wrist joint where it is straighter, although at this point its greater depth may make it somewhat more difficult to palpate. After the wrist has been stabilized the skin should be prepared with an antiseptic solution, and if the patient is awake, infiltration with local anesthetic should be performed. Radial artery catheterization is commonly performed with a small-gauge (20-gauge in adults and 22- or 24-gauge in pediatric patients) over-the-needle Teflon catheter apparatus. Two of the most commonly used techniques may be referred to as *front-entry* and *through-and-through techniques*. The front-entry technique is performed by inserting the catheter along the course of the radial artery at a 30–40° angle to the surface of the skin (Fig. 21-2). The return of arterial blood indicates that the needle has entered the artery. The cannula is then advanced into the lumen of the artery. While advancing the catheter into the artery, free blood flow must be continuously seen at the hub of the needle. If free blood flow is not seen, it must be assumed that either the catheter or the needle have migrated outside the lumen of the vessel.

There is no evidence that either the front-entry or the through-and-through method (transfixing of the radial artery) has an advantage over the other.[14] The single biggest technique problem in insertion of a radial artery catheter is the "no-thread" phenomenon. Experience in placing the leading

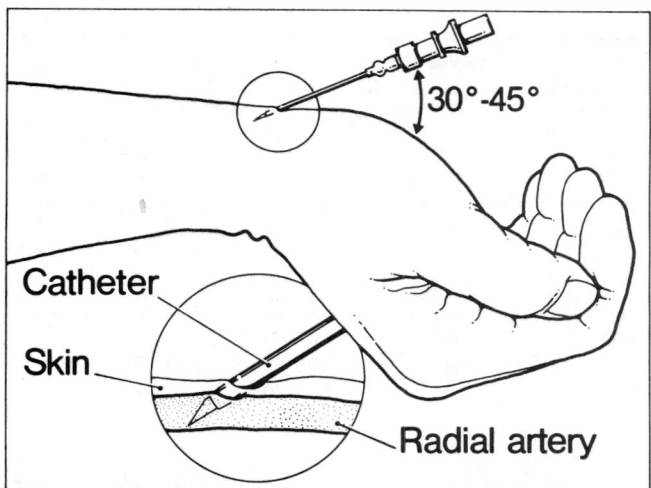

FIG. 21-2. Diagram of the appropriate angle for percutaneous radial artery cannulation. Note that it is important that both the needle bevel and the leading edge of the catheter be placed in the lumen of the artery. (Reprinted with permission. Brown BR, Blitt CD, Vaughn RW: St Louis, CV Mosby, 1985)

edge of the over-the-needle catheter as well as the bevel of the needle in the artery is helpful. The no-thread phenomenon is usually the result of the catheter impinging on the lateral or deep wall of the artery while only part of the tip of the needle is in the arterial lumen. Meticulous identification of the vessel, stabilization of the extremity, and finesse while introducing the catheter–needle assembly, all seem to minimize this problem. Using a straight angiographic wire catheter guide may also help. Once the catheter is inserted it should be firmly secured. All arterial catheters should be connected to a continuous flush system that contains heparin. One to two units of heparin per ml of flush solution is most commonly employed. The continuous flush is important in minimizing distal embolization and in minimizing nosocomial infections.

Vascular insufficiency and infection are the two most common complications associated with arterial cannulation. Because both catheter size and duration of cannulation have been implicated in the production of vascular occlusion,[14, 16] it would appear prudent to use as small a catheter as is feasible and to limit the duration of cannulation to that which is clinically necessary. As a general rule one might consider cannulating the radial artery of the nondominant hand both to facilitate patient mobility and to minimize the risk of causing severe disability in the unlikely event that distal vascular ischemia should occur. Since most vascular injuries related to arterial cannulation appear to be embolic in nature, it would also appear prudent to apply syringe suction to arterial cannulas at the time of decannulation to withdraw clots or other debris with the catheter. Observation of poor blood flow to the hand or fingers following radial artery cannulation indicates the need for decannulation. If signs of ischemia persist after decannulation, institution of sympathetic blockade in the affected extremity may be beneficial.

Because the hazards of arterial cannulation are minimal relative to the technical ease of performing arterial cannulation; and because the value of the information obtained is great, it is not surprising that radial artery cannulation has achieved widespread acceptance. Arterial cannulation should be performed unhesitatingly whenever clinical judgment dictates.

Central Venous Pressure

Central venous pressure (CVP) is an important determinant of both cardiac output and venous return. Multiple complex factors influence the CVP, cardiac output, and venous return. CVP measurement alone will not always allow correct clinical decisions. When CVP measurement is combined with other clinical observations and other influencing factors are considered, it can be an important adjunct to clinical management.[17] Improved techniques leading to increased safety and success in central venous system cannulation have enlarged the indications for placing catheters in the central circulation. Common indications include 1) measurement of central venous pressure; 2) rapid administration of fluids and blood; 3) insertion of a pulmonary artery catheter; 4) insertion of a transvenous pacemaker; 5) parenteral alimentation; 6) temporary hemodialysis; 7) long-term chemotherapy; 8) inability to cannulate peripheral veins for venous access; 9) operations in which venous air embolism is possible; 10) administration of drugs that cause sclerosis of peripheral veins; 11) frequent blood sampling; and 12) frequent therapeutic plasmapheresis.

Regardless of site of insertion, techniques for introducing a catheter into the central circulation can be categorized as one of three basic types: catheter over the needle; catheter through the needle; and catheter over a guide wire.[16, 17] Seldinger originally described inserting a needle into an artery and passing an angiographic wire catheter guide through the needle. The needle was then removed and a catheter passed over the wire.[18] The first application of this technique in the venous side of the circulation was reported in 1974.[19] The original technique was modified through use of a flexible angiographic wire catheter guide with the J configuration (J wire), which has made it easier to cannulate the external jugular vein and other tortuous vessels.

Central venous catheters are made of a variety of materials because no single material is ideal for all uses. The most common materials are polyvinyl chloride (PVC), polypropylene, polyethylene, polyurethane, tetrafluorethylene (Teflon), and silastic. Catheters vary in chemical inertness, thrombogenicity, and flexibility (Table 21-1).

Choice of a catheter must be made on an individual basis taking into consideration the primary purpose of the catheter. Long-term intravenous alimentation or chemotherapy probably warrants the most flexible and least reactive material available. Consequently silastic catheters would seem to be the best choice with siliconized polypropylene as an alternative. When rapid central venous cannulation is desired for administration of blood or fluid, polyethylene or polyurethane may be desirable. Polyurethane catheters seem to provide a good alternative between Teflon and silastic catheters. For short-term use all the materials have proven suitable. Catheters with side holes at the distal end are extremely valuable because they virtually eliminate aspiration difficulties.

Multiple-lumen central vascular access catheters are available with two, three, and as many as five lumens. These catheters have proven valuable for critically ill patients requiring multiple incompatible drug infusions. One must realize that incorporating multiple lumens into one catheter sacrifices internal diameter, and thus flow properties, unless the outer diameter of the catheter is increased. In order to maintain the flow properties, the outer diameter of some multiple-lumen catheters reach gargantuan proportions (i.e., 11–13 French). Infection is the most common complication of central

TABLE 21-1.   Comparison of Central Venous Catheter Materials

TYPE OF MATERIAL	CHEMICAL INERTNESS	THROMBOGENICITY	FLEXIBILITY	TRANSPARENT
Polyvinylchloride (PVC)	− − −	+ + +	+ +	Yes
Siliconized PVC	−	+ +	+ +	Yes
Polyethylene	− −	+ + +	+ +	Yes
Polypropylene	− −	+ + +	+ +	Yes
Siliconized polypropylene	0	+	+ +	Yes or no
Teflon	−	+	+	No
Silastic	0	0	+ + + +	No
Polyurethane	− −	+	+ + +	No

0 = none; + = minimal; + + = moderate; + + + and + + + + = large; − = less; − − = much less; − − − = markedly less.
(Reprinted with permission. Otto CW: Central venous pressure monitoring. In Blitt CD (ed): Monitoring and Anesthesia Critical Care Medicine. New York, Churchill Livingstone, 1985)

venous cannulation. Infection-free catheters can be maintained for prolonged periods only with strict adherence to aseptic protocols.[17] Prevention of infection begins with an aseptic insertion technique. A number of manufacturers now provide prepackaged central venous cannulation kits that include all the materials needed for sterile insertion. Securing a catheter so that it does not move is an important step in preventing future infection. Catheter fixation is best accomplished by suture. A monofilament suture such as Prolene or nylon is very nonreactive and does not collect blood or other debris. A sterile dressing should be applied to central vascular catheter sites. The introduction of water-vapor-permeable transparent adhesive plastic membranes has been a significant advance in decreasing infection in central venous access catheters.

Air embolism must be avoided when inserting central venous access catheters. The danger of air embolism during insertion can be minimized by proper patient positioning such that pressure in the vein is increased. Any time a needle or cannula is in a vein and the hub is open to the atmosphere there is a danger of air aspiration. These times should be kept to a minimum by keeping the hub occluded by a syringe or gloved finger. Particularly dangerous are the times when a guide wire is being inserted because air may pass around the guide wire. This manipulation should be accomplished expeditiously and the introducing needle or cannula removed from the vein as soon as possible. When a patient is breathing spontaneously, intrathoracic pressure decreases during inspiration. Consequently, air embolism is more likely if the patient takes a deep breath or sighs. A less obvious time of danger for air embolism is at the time of removal of a central venous catheter. If the catheter has been in place for several days, a tract may form around the catheter that is not immediately sealed when the line is removed. All central lines should be removed with the patient in the recumbent position and firm pressure should be applied over the insertion site to prevent aspiration of air. If there is any question of whether the insertion site has sealed itself, a temporary air-tight pressure dressing should be applied.

A number of techniques for central venous cannulation, when the vein cannot be seen, involve the use of a small locator needle prior to cannulation with a larger needle. This is widely recommended for internal jugular cannulation to minimize the incidence of carotid artery punctures with a large-bore catheter.

The ideal location of the tip of a central vascular catheter will depend to some extent on its purpose. If the catheter is needed for rapid administration of fluids or blood, a location freely within any large vein is adequate. If a highly accurate measurement of right ventricular filling pressure is needed, then a position in the right atrium may be indicated. The ideal location for a catheter to be used to aspirate potential air emboli during certain surgical procedures is at the superior vena cava–right-atrial junction or slightly higher.

Extravascular migration of central venous catheters is a serious, potentially fatal complication.[17] Factors related to extravascular migration include debility of the patient, stiffness and sharpness of the catheter, anatomic location of the catheter tip, and movement of the catheter tip resulting from the patient's movements (especially of the head and neck). A factor that contributes to vascular catheter erosion is positioning of the catheter tip perpendicular to a vessel wall. This problem is more commonly encountered with catheters inserted via left neck approaches. Care should be taken to ensure that catheters inserted via left neck approaches are long enough to pass into the superior vena cava. Too short a catheter is likely to lie transversely in the left innominate vein with its tip impinging on the wall. Extravascular migration can occur with any type catheter and with any insertion site. The most commonly used method of determining location of a central vascular access catheter tip is chest x-ray. Central vascular access catheter location should usually be confirmed by chest x-ray within a short time after insertion of the catheter. This will identify a pneumothorax as well as an aberrant catheter location. The chest x-ray subsequent to placement of the catheter may not, however, be a reliable indicator of potential for subsequent extravascular migration.

A number of routes and techniques have been described for central venous cannulation for central venous vascular access, making appropriate selection for the individual patient difficult.[16, 17] The primary considerations include the experience of the person inserting the catheter; the reason for cannulation; availability of equipment; condition of the patient and ability to withstand the positioning necessary for insertion; and success rate and complications of the technique. For many techniques success rate and complications are directly related to the expertise of the operator.

Figure 21-3 is a diagrammatic representation of the relationships of the major venous structures in the neck and thorax. Figure 21-4 emphasizes the major surface landmarks used in central venous cannulation. There are five major approaches to the central venous circulation: the basilic vein in the arm, the external jugular vein, the internal jugular vein, the subclavian vein, and the femoral vein. Table 21-2 describes how each site would rate relative to the others for several important considerations in central venous cannulation. The three most

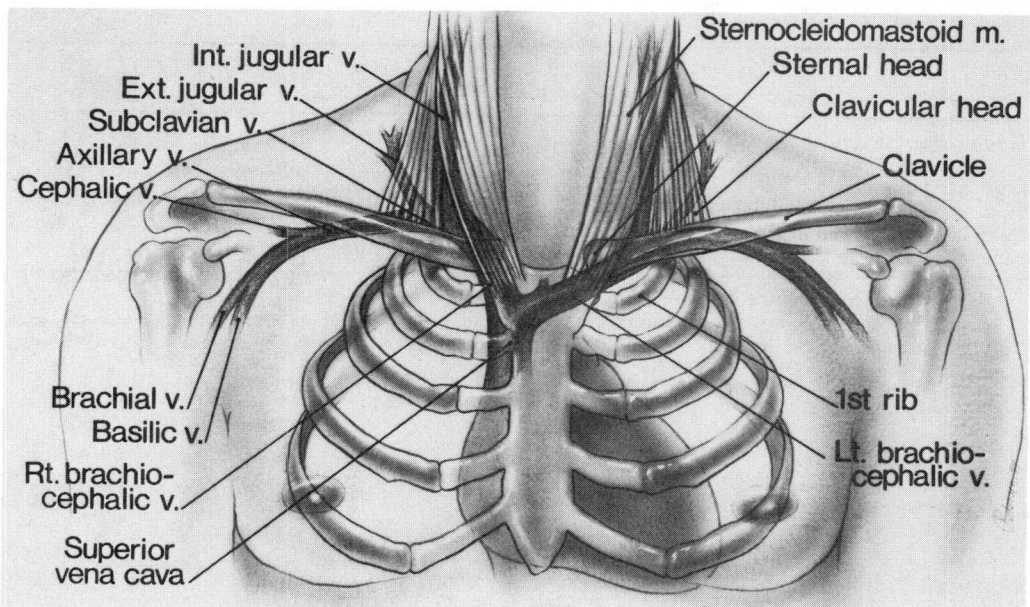

FIG. 21-3. The major venous structures of the neck and thorax. (Reprinted with permission. Otto CW: Central venous pressure monitoring. In Blitt CD (ed): Monitoring and Anesthesia Critical Care Medicine, p 121. New York, Churchill Livingstone, 1985)

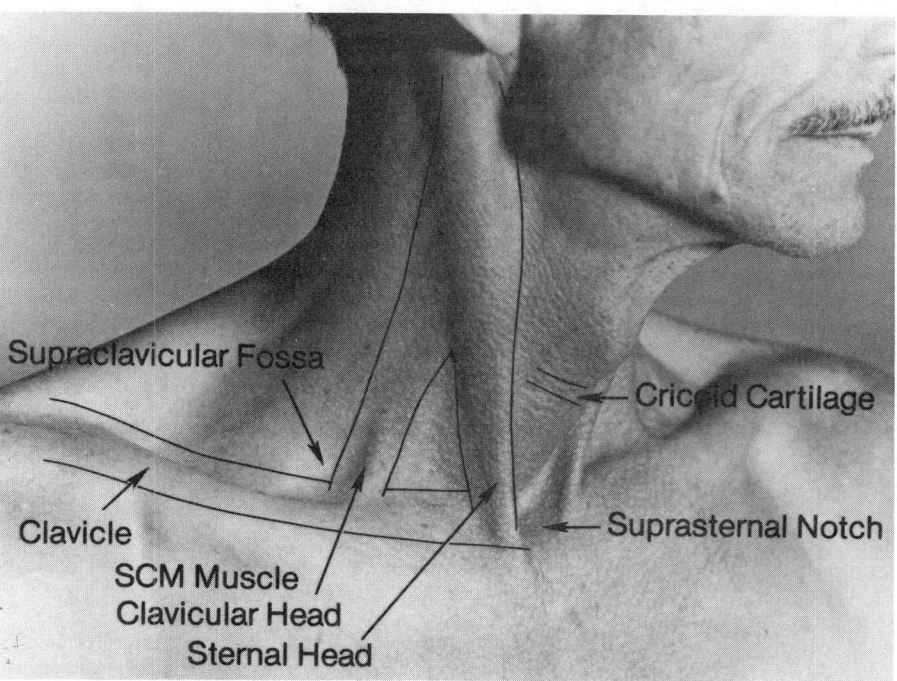

FIG. 21-4. Major surface landmarks used in central venous cannulation. SCM = Sterno-cleidomastoid. (Reprinted with permission. Otto CW: Central venous pressure monitoring. In Blitt CD (ed): Monitoring and Anesthesia Critical Care Medicine, p 121. New York, Churchill Livingstone, 1985)

commonly used access sites in anesthesia are the internal jugular, external jugular, and subclavian veins.

EXTERNAL JUGULAR VEIN CANNULATION. Although the position of the external jugular vein is quite constant, cannulation is recommended only if it is easily visible or palpable. The vessel is thin walled and movable in the subcutaneous tissues,

making cannulation slightly more difficult than for most arm veins. Cannulation is accomplished by placing the patient in the Trendelenburg position with the head turned away from the site of venipuncture. Either the right or left external jugular vein may be used. Venipuncture is performed slightly distal to the midpoint of the vein where it is easily seen. (Fig. 21-5). Venipuncture is made with a 6.25 cm over-the-needle

TABLE 21-2.   Relative Rating of Central Venous Access Techniques*

	BASILIC (ARM VEINS)	EXTERNAL JUGULAR	INTERNAL JUGULAR	SUBCLAVIAN	FEMORAL†
Ease of insertion and safety for the inexperienced	1	2	4	5	3
Long-term use	4	3	2	1	5
Success rate	5	4	1	3	2
Complications (technique related)	1	2	3	4	5
Ease of PA catheter insertion	5	2	1	4	3

*In each category 1 = best; 5 = worst.
†Because of the high incidence of complications, the femoral route should be used only as a last resort.
(Reprinted with permission. Otto CW: Central venous pressure monitoring. In Blitt CD (ed): Monitoring and Anesthesia Critical Care Medicine. New York, Churchill Livingstone, 1985)

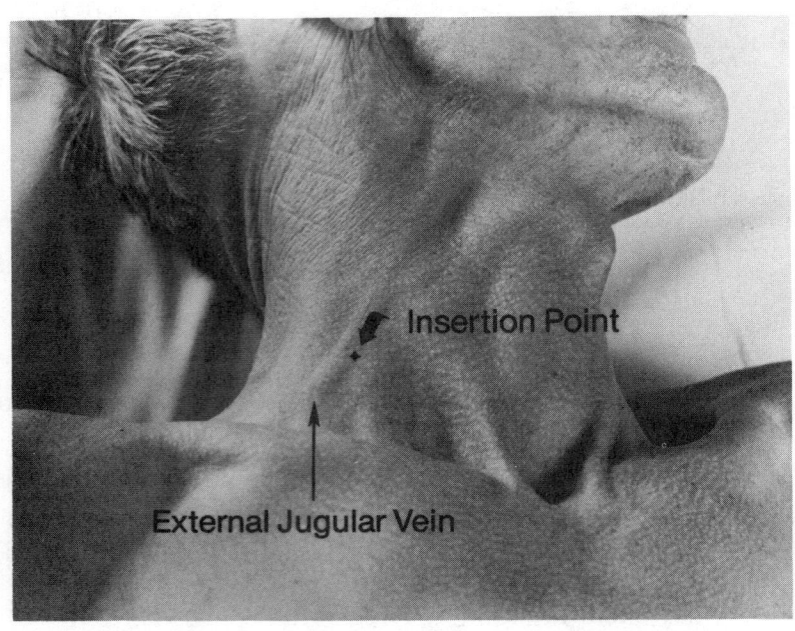

FIG. 21-5. Insertion point for external jugular venipuncture. (Reprinted with permission. Blitt CD (ed): Monitoring and Anesthesia Critical Care Medicine. New York, Churchill Livingstone, 1985.)

cannula attached to a syringe. A 16- or 18-gauge cannula is usually used in adults and an 18- or 20-gauge cannula is used in children. When free flow of blood is obtained, the cannula is advanced off the needle into the vein. The needle is removed and the syringe is reattached to the cannula and aspirated to verify free flow of blood. If free blood return is not obtained, the cannula is slowly withdrawn with intermittent gentle aspiration until free flow returns and the cannula is then fixed in that position. Following this initial cannulation, a J-wire with a 3-mm radius of curvature appropriate to the size of the cannula being used; and at least twice as long as the definitive catheter, is inserted through the catheter and advanced into the central circulation. To ease introduction of the wire into the hub of the cannula, a plastic sheath is slipped over the tip of the J to straighten it. When the J-wire is advanced it occasionally meets an obstruction and may need to be manipulated. Most success will be found by rotating the wire between the thumb and index finger while simultaneously moving the wire in and out 1–2 cm. This method of manipulation is more effective than rotating the wire while maintaining constant inward pressure against the obstruction. If an obstruction cannot be passed after multiple attempts, a smaller diameter

wire should be tried. Internal rotation of the ipsilateral arm with upward pressure on the scapula may also be of help in difficult wire passages as the maneuver raises the clavicle, allowing the wire to pass under. Care should be taken not to advance the wire too far because it will easily enter the right ventricle and cause arrhythmias. Once the guide wire is advanced into the chest, the short cannula is removed and the definitive catheter threaded over the wire using it as a guide. Depending on the size and type of catheter, there may be some resistance to passage through the skin and subcutaneous tissues. A #11 scalpel blade can be used carefully to widen the venipuncture site around the wire. A vessel dilator may also be used to widen the puncture site. Care should be taken to never lose control of the wire during catheter insertion or the wire may be advanced with the catheter, resulting in a wire embolism. After the catheter is inserted the wire is removed and a syringe is attached to verify free flow of blood from the catheter. An intravenous infusion is attached and the catheter is secured in place. The major complications associated with external jugular vein cannulation are those associated with all central venous access catheters regardless of site of insertion, that is, perforation of a vessel wall and infection.

The external jugular approach has much to recommend it under many circumstances. Although the technique is more complicated than the basilic vein approach, it shares many of the same advantages, has a higher success rate, and is usually accessible to the anesthesiologist during an operative procedure. Because the venipuncture is superficial and the vein directly visualized, it can be used safely by an inexperienced operator. It is a safe technique for the patient with a bleeding diathesis or who is receiving anticoagulants. The external jugular vein can be utilized for pulmonary artery catherization, although the large introducers necessary to accept a pulmonary artery catheter occasionally cannot be successfully passed under the clavicle by this route, or acute angulation of the introducer as it enters the subclavian vein causes it to kink so that the pulmonary artery catheter will not pass. The disadvantages of the external jugular approach are relative to other approaches. Catheters inserted through the neck are more difficult to fix and dress than some other sites and have a tendency to kink when the head is turned. For long-term catheterization the subclavian vein is the best choice. In the hands of experienced operators, success rates are slightly higher with internal jugular and subclavian vein approaches. Successful placement of a large introducer sheath for pulmonary artery catheter insertion is more likely with the internal jugular vein technique.

INTERNAL JUGULAR VEIN CANNULATION. The internal jugular vein has become a favorite site for central venous cannulation by anesthesiologists because of its ready accessibility, high success rate, and low incidence of complications.[17] Many approaches to the internal jugular vein have been described.[20] The most widely practiced is a central approach along the axis of the vein with venipuncture occurring several cm above the clavicle to minimize the risk of puncturing the pleura. The patient is placed in the Trendelenburg position with the head turned away from the site of venipuncture. Either the right or left internal jugular vein may be used, although the right is preferred because of the straight access to the superior vena cava, the presence of the thoracic duct on the left, and the fact that performance of the technique on the right is easier for right-handed operators. A wide area of the neck is prepped and draped. Local anesthesia is used if the patient is conscious.

An important landmark is the triangle formed by the sternal and clavicular heads of the sternocleidomastoid muscle and the clavicle. (Fig. 21-6) This landmark can be readily identified in nearly all people by placing a finger in the sternal notch and then moving laterally over the sternal head until a depression in the muscle is felt. Tensing the muscle by having the patient raise the head against resistance may help identification. The course of the vein and, therefore, the axis of needle insertion is determined by drawing a line connecting the mastoid process and the medial insertion of the sternocleidomastoid muscle on the clavicle. This latter point is also the lateral border of the aforementioned triangle. If the triangle cannot be reliably identified, this point can be found at the junction of the medial and middle thirds of the clavicle. Venipuncture is performed along this line with the needle following its course. Since the line so drawn represents the course of the vein, venipuncture could be performed at any point along the line; however, very high in the neck the carotid artery lies in front of the vein and the cupola of the lung lies low in the neck. Therefore, most operators prefer a puncture site approximately in the middle portion of the neck.

Occasionally, the triangle is small, with the apex occurring very low in the neck, or it is difficult to identify. In such cases the skin puncture site is determined by drawing a second line perpendicular to the first (which intersects with the cricoid cartilage) and venipuncture is performed through the sternocleidomastoid muscle. The carotid artery should be palpated prior to venipuncture to assure that it is medial to the intended puncture site. Prior to venipuncture with a larger needle the

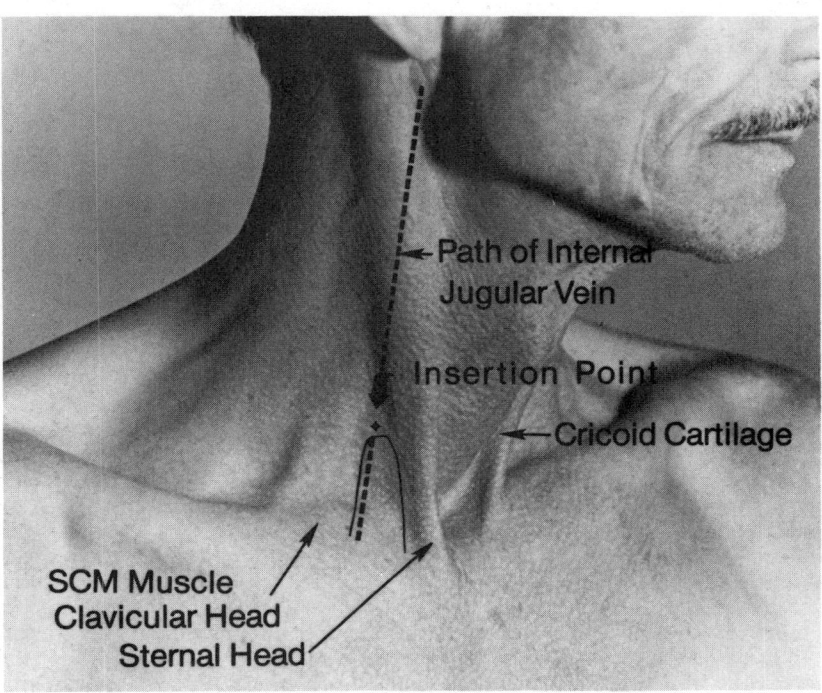

FIG. 21-6. Insertion site for internal jugular venipuncture. See text for details. SCM = sternocleidomastoid. (Reprinted with permission. Blitt CD (ed): Monitoring and Anesthesia Critical Care Medicine. New York, Churchill Livingstone, 1985.)

internal jugular vein should be located with a 22-gauge 3.75 cm needle attached to a syringe. A 23- or 25-gauge needle may be used in children. The needle is inserted from the previously identified entrance point at a 45° angle to the skin, caudad, and along the axis of the line from the mastoid to the clavicle. This direction is roughly toward the ipsilateral nipple. The angle of insertion should not be too narrow with the skin or the vein will not be encountered until the needle has passed very low in the neck. Continuous or intermittent gentle aspiration should be applied to the syringe so entry into the vein is identified immediately.

The use of the locator needle is important to minimize trauma to adjacent structures should the vein be missed. Puncture of the carotid artery can usually be identified by the color of the blood and rapidity of blood return when the syringe is removed (although pulsatile flow should not be expected through such a small needle). The vein should be encountered at a depth of 1.25–3.75 cm. If blood return is not encountered during insertion, gentle aspiration should be continued during slow needle withdrawal because the needle may have passed completely through the vein. If the vein is not found, changing the direction of the needle slightly lateral or medial should result in success. Once the vein has been located, the syringe is removed from the locator needle and the needle left in place as a guide for insertion of a large cannula. Some operators prefer to remove the locator needle immediately after determining the direction and depth of the vein. The locator needle does represent a potential port for air embolism but this is minimal in the head-down position. When the vein has been located, a 17- or 18-gauge thin-wall needle is inserted immediately adjacent to the locator needle in the same direction into the internal jugular vein. When free flow of blood is obtained the locator needle is removed and discarded. A flexible angiographic wire catheter guide of the appropriate size is passed through the thin wall needle. Either a straight wire or a J-wire can be used. After the wire has been inserted, the needle is removed and the definitive catheter is passed over the wire. Depending on the type and size of the catheter, there may be some resistance to passage through the skin and subcutaneous tissues. A #11 scalpel blade or a vessel dilator can be used carefully to widen the puncture site around the wire. After the catheter is inserted the wire is removed and a syringe attached to verify free blood flow from the catheter. An intravenous infusion is attached, and the catheter secured in place.

In experienced hands the complications associated with internal jugular vein cannulation are infrequent. Carotid artery puncture, the most frequent complication, occurs approximately 2% of the time in most series and rarely leads to significant sequelae.[17] Should the carotid artery be unintentionally punctured with a very large cannula, such as a sheath for a pulmonary artery catheter, surgical exploration and repair are advisable.[17] If doubt ever exists as to arterial placement of a locator needle, initial cannula, or Seldinger needle, connection to a transducer will permit one to determine whether the wave form is venous or arterial. Although internal jugular vein cannulation is not a technique recommended for the inexperienced, it is relatively easy to learn. It has a high success rate and a low incidence of complications. It is a useful technique for the anesthesiologist because of the accessibility of the neck during most operations. The internal jugular is probably the vein of choice for pulmonary artery catheterization. The site can be used for long-term catheterization but catheters inserted through the neck are more difficult to stabilize and dress than some other sites and have a tendency to kink when the head is turned.

SUBCLAVIAN VEIN CANNULATION. The subclavian vein is best approached by the infraclavicular route. The needle passes between the clavicle and the first rib. This is the most popular approach because it is safer than other approaches and because there is greater stability of the catheter on the anterior chest wall.[17] The patient is placed in the Trendelenburg position, arms at the sides, with the head turned away from the site of venipuncture. Either the right or left subclavian vein may be used. Placing a folded sheet, towel, or small pillow under the center of the back (between the shoulder blades) can help open the space between the clavicle and the first rib and let the shoulders fall back so that the head of the humerus is out of the way. A wide area of the neck and chest is prepped and draped. Local anesthetic is used if the patient is conscious. The skin puncture site in adults is approximately 1 cm below the midpoint of the clavicle. A 17- or 18-gauge thin-wall needle is used. The needle is placed at the insertion site and the index finger of the free hand is placed in the suprasternal notch. The needle is aimed toward the finger in the suprasternal notch and is advanced posterior to the clavicle, keeping close to the bone, with the syringe and needle parallel to the coronal plane (i.e., parallel to the bed). Apply continuous, gentle negative pressure to the syringe as the needle is advanced in order to identify the vein as soon as it is entered. In adults the vein should be reached at a depth of 3–5 cm. When free flow of blood is obtained, remove the syringe and insert a flexible angiographic wire catheter guide. The needle is then removed and the definitive catheter advanced over the wire. A vessel dilator is helpful in enlarging the path from the skin to the vein and facilitates easier definitive catheter passage.

The complications of most concern during subclavian catheterization are associated with lacerating adjoining structures during venipuncture. The incidence of pneumothorax ranges from 0–3% with the infraclavicular approach. The overall incidence of pneumothorax appears to be approximately 1%, which is high enough to recommend that bilateral attempts at subclavian cannulation not be made without an intervening chest radiograph in order to avoid bilateral pneumothorax.[17]

The major advantage of the infraclavicular subclavian approach is the ability to secure the catheter to the anterior chest wall. In this position the catheter has minimum movement with changes in body position, dressings stay secure, and the entrance site is away from potential neck wounds, such as tracheostomies, etc. These considerations have dictated that the approach be the site of choice for long-term parenteral alimentation catheters. The fact that surrounding tissue connections tend to keep the subclavian vein from collapsing has also made it a favorite for cannulation in the hypovolemic patient.

The supraclavicular route to the subclavian vein has little to recommend it. Since the insertion site is in the neck, it has none of the catheter stability advantages of the infraclavicular approach. It also has a higher complication rate than the internal jugular approach.

It becomes clear that complications related to central vascular access can be divided into two categories: those that are related to the insertion technique itself and those that are related to the presence of the catheter in the central circulation. The overall list of complications that may occur with central vascular access include air embolism, bleeding, cardiac tamponade, catheter erosion through skin, catheter embolism, catheter occlusion, catheter-related sepsis, endocarditis, exit-site infection, exit-site necrosis, extravasation, fibrin sheath formation at the tip of the catheter, hematoma, hemothorax, hydrothorax, chylothorax, nerve damage, laceration, perforation (extravascular migration), pneumothorax, thromboembolism, thrombophlebitis, venous thrombosis, and ventricular arrhythmia. Complications are rare, and central vascular access when indicated has clearly been shown to be a beneficial modality.

Pulmonary Artery Catheters

The development of a balloon-tipped catheter by Swan and Ganz[21] which could be "floated" into the pulmonary artery without use of radiography was a significant advance in critical care and intraoperative monitoring. The pulmonary artery catheter permitted measurement of three fundamental types of hemodynamic information:[21, 22] right- and left-sided intracardiac pressures; cardiac output by the thermodilution method; and mixed venous blood for gas and chemical analysis. In addition new catheters facilitate the diagnosis of complex cardiac arrhythmias and allow cardiac pacing as well as beat-to-beat determination of mixed venous oxygen saturation. The ability to obtain rapid, accurate measurements of cardiac output in critically ill patients and to repeat them as often as desired is one of the principal advantages of a pulmonary artery catheter. Thermodilution cardiac output is a variant of the dye indicator dilution technique, with "cold" as the trace indicator.

As originally reported, the primary indication for pulmonary artery catherization was hemodynamic assessment in complicated myocardial infarction.[21, 22] The benefits of the information obtained with the pulmonary artery catheter soon became apparent and led to its use in a variety of other situations. All of the numerous perioperative indications for a pulmonary artery catheter can be grouped into three categories. These are related to 1) the patient's physical status, especially cardiac reserve; 2) the extent of surgery (procedures associated with large blood loss or fluid shifts; or 3) a combination of the first two. In addition, high-risk obstetric patients and elderly patients are two other subgroups in whom the pulmonary artery catheter is being used with increased frequency to manage such problems as preeclampsia and acute respiratory failure, respectively. Patients undergoing aortic cross-clamping usually have some degree of coronary artery disease. In addition they are subject to significant variations in blood pressure, temperature changes, massive blood loss, and fluid shifts. Optimizing filling pressures can enable this patient group to adapt to the myocardial depression that accompanies aortic cross-clamping.

Shock of any variety is another indication for a pulmonary artery catheter. Information obtained facilitates decision-making in fluid replacement, correcting deficits of hemodynamic function, and changing respiratory parameters. Patients with severe pulmonary disease can benefit from a pulmonary artery catheter. Absolute pulmonary criteria for a pulmonary artery catheter are arbitrary. The more severe the impairment, particularly of oxygenation, the more likely the patient is to benefit. This is especially true in the presence of coexisting cardiac disease. Other subsets in which a pulmonary artery catheter is valuable include patients undergoing sitting craniotomies (early detection of air emboli), patients in barbiturate coma, and patients for whom questions exist regarding the adequacy of intravascular volume. The management of procedures associated with potentially large fluid deficits, those associated with a high mortality, or those performed in high-risk patients (ASA 4 or 5) is aided by the use of a pulmonary artery catheter. There is usually a high incidence of pulmonary artery catheterization in patients undergoing cardiac surgery. Indications for catheter insertion are summarized in Table 21-3.

TABLE 21-3. Indications for Pulmonary Artery Catheterization

In Patients Undergoing Cardiac Surgery
1. Poor ventricular function
   (EF < 0.4, LVEDP > 16 mm Hg
   CI < 2 l·min^{-1}·m^{-2})*
2. Noncompliant ventricle
3. Left main coronary lesion (or equivalent)
4. Aortic stenosis/aortic insufficiency
5. Mitral stenosis/mitral insufficiency
6. Acute ventricular septal defect
7. Acute papillary muscle dysfunction
8. Combined lesions (coronary + valvular)
9. Recent infarct (<6 mo)
10. Propranolol > 100 mg q.i.d.
11. Intraaortic balloon counter pulsation
12. Hemodynamic instability

In Patients Undergoing Noncardiac Surgery
1. Cardiac disease
   Coronary artery disease
   Valvular disease
   Cardiomyopathies
2. Pulmonary disease
   Severe COPD
   ARDS
   Other pulmonary diseases interfering with oxygenation
3. Shock
   Hemorrhage
   Sepsis
4. Induced hypotension
5. Complicated surgery
   High-risk patients (ASA IV or V)
   High mortality
   Large volume replacement
6. Assessment of intravascular volume
7. Miscellaneous
   Sitting craniotomies
   Aotic cross-clamping
   Bleomycin treated patients

*EF = Ejection fraction; LVEDP = left ventricular diastolic pressure; CI = cardiac index.
(Reprinted with permission. Keefer RJ, Barash PG: Pulmonary artery catheterization. In Blitt CD (ed): Monitoring in Anesthesia and Critical Care Medicine. New York, Churchill Livingstone, 1985)

Despite the multiplicity of indications, a fundamental question remains unanswered: Has the widespread use of pulmonary artery catheterization been rewarded by any decrease in patient morbidity or mortality?[23] Research to date has only hinted at the answer. No controlled prospective studies exist documenting patient benefits from pulmonary artery catheterization. One study showed that patients who have good cardiac function could safely undergo cardiac surgery with CVP monitoring at less cost and that patients who appear to require a pulmonary artery catheter were not benefited in mortality, morbidity, or cost by the addition of mixed venous oxygen saturation capability to the catheter.[24] In view of the cost of the catheter and the not insubstantial risk of complications, it is essential that the benefit of a pulmonary artery catheter, if it exists, be demonstrated.

Insertion of a pulmonary artery catheter is a simple, rapid, effective technique. Familiarity with the equipment as well as with the various wave forms likely to be encountered is essential for minimizing complications and ensuring successful passage of the catheter. Successful pulmonary artery catheterization starts with preparation for venipuncture and appropriate balancing and calibration of pressure monitoring equipment. It has been found to be efficient and cost effective to use prepackaged trays containing the appropriate items for venous cannulation and subsequent introduction of an 8.5 French sheath using the Seldinger technique. A pulmonary artery catheter sheath with a hemostasis valve (to prevent air embolism) is usually placed in the right internal jugular vein utilizing a sterile technique described in the section on Central Venous Pressure. Although a number of venous entry sites may be employed for pulmonary artery catheterization, the appropriate site should be easily accessible, a short distance from the right atrium, and should be associated with minimal complications. Based on these goals, most anesthesiologists inserting a pulmonary artery catheter choose the internal jugular vein approach.

Insertion of a pulmonary artery catheter requires constant display of pressure on an oscilloscope and recognition of characteristic wave forms (Fig. 21-7). Once the introducer sheath with hemostasis valve is in place, the pulmonary artery catheter is inserted carefully and advanced until the tip lies in a central vein. Approximate distances from various insertion sites are listed in Table 21-4. Intracardiac knotting is a consequence of inserting the catheter too far without the appropriate pressure trace being displayed on a monitor. Location of the tip of the catheter in a central vein can be confirmed by pressure changes related to respiration or coughing. With the catheter in the superior vena cava, the balloon is inflated with 1.5 ml of air (never more) and the catheter slowly advanced. When the right atrium is encountered typical venous A, C, and V waves will be noted. Normal right atrial pressure is 0–8 mm Hg. Further advancement of the catheter will produce a dramatic change in the pressure tracing as the tip of the catheter enters the right ventricle. Within one cardiac cycle pressures will change from those characteristic of the atrium to a phasic pressure in the range of 25/0 mm Hg typical of the right ventricle. The catheter is advanced quickly through the right ventricle until it enters the main pulmonary artery. This can be recognized by an increase in the diastolic pressure. Normal pulmonary artery pressure is in the range of 25/12. Usually there is no change in the systolic pressure. The catheter is advanced still further until it wedges (pulmonary capillary wedge pressure [PCWP]) in a branch of the pulmonary artery. The wedge trace will usually have the appearance of an atrial pressure pattern with A, C, and V wave components transmitted retrograde from the left atrium (normal PCWP = 8–12 mm Hg). Pulmonary capillary wedge position is verified by 1) a characteristic waveform and 2) a mean pressure lower than the mean pulmonary artery pressure. If an electronic mean is obtained on the oscilloscope, the pressure (in a normal patient) will be 1–4 mm Hg less than the pulmonary artery end-diastolic pressure. After achieving a wedge position, the balloon is deflated. This should produce a typical pulmonary artery pressure tracing. Reinflation of the balloon should reproduce the wedge tracing with 1.5 ml of air. If less than 1 ml of air results in a wedge trace, the catheter should be withdrawn to the point where 1–1.5 ml balloon inflation is associated with a PCWP. At no time should more air be injected into the balloon than is necessary to obtain PCWP. Once the catheter tip is satisfactorily located, a commercially available sterile sleeve can be secured over the catheter to allow for sterile repositioning of the catheter.

Diseases most commonly associated with difficult catheter insertions are low cardiac output states, pulmonary hypertension, and congenital cardiac defects. Table 21-5 outlines guidelines for the safe use of pulmonary artery catheters. A continuous flush device like that used for arterial catheterization is required for a pulmonary artery catheter.

The pulmonary artery thermodilution catheter by virtue of permitting measurement of cardiac output and left-sided heart pressures, has enabled extensive hemodynamic assessment to be made in the operating room or critical care unit. Various circulatory disease states can now be defined in terms of pump failure, hypovolemia, and high/low resistance states. With the emergence of new drugs, anesthesiologists have the opportunity to employ more precise therapy for a given type of circulatory failure. For the most prompt and effective therapy to be implemented, however, one needs not only the physiologic variables obtained *via* direct monitoring, that is, the pulse rate, the blood pressure, and the pulmonary artery pressure, but also those calculated from the original variables, *e.g.*, stroke work index and vascular resistances. Some of the more commonly made hemodynamic calculations are seen in Table 21-6.

A ventricular function curve defines the relationship between ventricular filling pressure and ventricular stroke work and is a unifying concept to explain the performance characteristics of a given ventricle. Although more sophisticated indices of cardiac performance have been advocated, the ven-

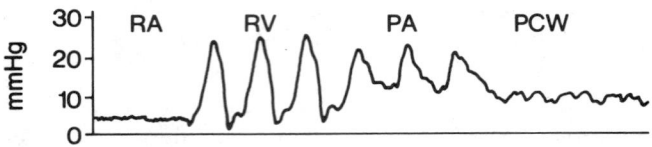

FIG. 21-7. Typical pressure tracings obtained during passage of a pulmonary artery catheter. RA = right atrium; RV = right ventricle; PA = pulmonary artery; PCW = pulmonary capillary wedge. (Reprinted with permission. Brown BR, Blitt CD, Vaughn RW: Clinical Anesthesiology, p 139. St Louis, CV Mosby, 1985)

TABLE 21-4. Distance (cm) to Right Atrium, Right Ventricle, and Pulmonary Artery

		RIGHT ATRIUM	RIGHT VENTRICLE	PULMONARY ARTERY
Internal jugular vein	Right	20	30	45
	Left	25	35	50
Antecubital vein	Right	50	65	80
	Left	55	70	85
Femoral vein		40	50	65
Subclavian vein		10	25	40

(Reprinted with permission. Keefer RJ, Barash PG: Pulmonary artery catheterization. In Blitt CD (ed): Monitoring in Anesthesia and Critical Care Medicine. New York, Churchill Livingstone, 1985)

tricular function curve is probably one of the better clinical means of physiologically describing the performance of the intact heart. This is because both the ordinate (left ventricular stroke work index) and the abscissa (LVEDP, LAP, PCWP) are related qualitatively to the two major symptom complexes of

TABLE 21-5.   Guidelines for Safe Use of Pulmonary Artery Flow Guided Catheters

1. Balance risk *versus* benefit
2. Slowly inflate balloon while continuously monitoring the pulmonary artery (PA) waveform
3. Upon transition from the pulmonary artery to the PCWP trace, immediately stop inflation
4. If an *overwedge pattern* is observed, the balloon should be immediately withdrawn 1–2 cm. The balloon is slowly reinflated and a normal wedge pressure waveform is noted.
5. Minimize duration of PCWP measurements
6. If balloon inflates with less than 1.5 ml of gas, the catheter should be withdrawn at least 1 to 2 cm
7. Spontaneous tip migration may occur: therefore continuously monitor the PA trace for "spontaneous wedging." If this occurs withdraw the catheter 1 to 2 cm or until a normal PA tracing reappears.
8. Minimize number of PCWP measurements in patients who are elderly, anticoagulated, or have pulmonary hypertension
9. If pulmonary artery diastolic pressure is less than 18 mm Hg, use pulmonary artery diastolic pressure rather than PCWP as an index of left ventricular filling pressure.

(Reprinted with permission. Keefer RJ, Barash PG: Pulmonary artery catheterization. In Blitt CD (ed): Monitoring in Anesthesia and Critical Care Medicine. New York, Churchill Livingstone, 1985)

patients with heart disease. In general an upward shift to the left is interpreted as an improvement in ventricular performance and a shift downward and to the right is considered to be deteriorating ventricular performance. In addition to changes in contractility, many interventions including alterations in preload, afterload, heart rate, and ventricular compliance can produce shifts in ventricular function curves. A ventricular function curve with three zones of ventricular function is depicted in Fig. 21-8.

The combination of pulmonary artery catheters with fiberoptic oximetry capability has further expanded the use of the pulmonary artery catheter.[25] Measurement of true mixed venous oxygen saturation, which is dependent on the balance between tissue oxygen demand and delivery, is now possible. Because delivery is more likely to change than demand (particularly in the anesthetized patient) minute-to minute-changes in mixed venous oxygen saturation can be used to track cardiac output. These catheters utilize the principle of reflectance spectrophotometry and employ a microprocessor to calculate mixed venous oxygen saturation. A decrease in mixed venous oxygen saturation can be due to decreased oxygen transfer at the lung, decreased oxygen transport to the tissue, or increased tissue utilization of oxygen. An increasing mixed venous oxygen saturation indicates improvement in pulmonary oxygen uptake, improvement in cardiac output, or decreased peripheral oxygen utilization. Episodes of low mixed venous oxygen saturation (less than 60% for more than 5 min) have been shown to be associated with major changes in a patient's clinical course in the perioperative period.[26] Although measuring mixed venous oxygen saturation has been advocated as an early warning indicator of hemodynamic instability, technical problems have been encountered with

TABLE 21-6.   Hemodynamic Calculations

Cardiac output (CO) $l \cdot min^{-1}$ = heart rate × stroke volume
Cardiac index (CI) $l \cdot min^{-1} \cdot m^{-2}$ is calculated as follows:

$$CI = \frac{CO}{Body\ Surface\ Area\ (BSA)\ in\ m^2}$$

Stroke volume (SV) or stroke volume index (SVI) overcomes some of the difficulties inherent in the use of CO or CI

$$SV = ml/stroke = \frac{CO}{Heart\ Rate}\ or\ SVI = \frac{CI}{Heart\ Rate}$$
$$SV = End\text{-}diastolic\ volume - end\text{-}systolic\ volume$$

Systemic vascular resistance (SVR) and systemic vascular resistance index are defined as

$$SVR\ (RU) = \frac{Mean\ Arterial\ Pressure\ (MAP) - Right\ Atrial\ Pressure\ (RAP)}{CO}$$
$$SVRI\ (RU \cdot m^{-2}) = \frac{MAP - RAP}{CI}$$

Left ventricular stroke-work index (LVSWI) is defined as

$$LVSWI = (MAP - \overline{PCWP}) \times SVI \times 0.0136$$

Pulmonary vascular resistance (PVR) and pulmonary vascular resistance index are defined as

$$PVR\ (RU) = \frac{PAP - PCWP}{CO}$$
$$PVRI\ (RU \cdot m^{-2}) = \frac{PAP - PCWP}{CI}$$

(Reprinted with permission. Keefer RJ, Barash PG: Pulmonary artery catheterization. In Blitt CD (ed): Monitoring in Anesthesia and Critical Care Medicine. New York, Churchill Livingstone, 1985)

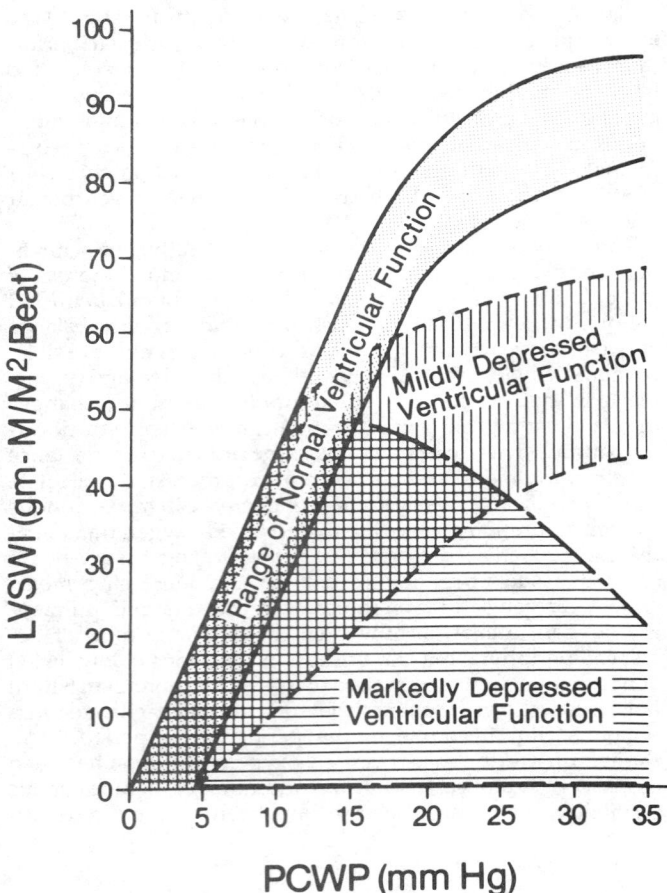

FIG. 21-8. Ventricular function curve plotting left ventricular stroke work index and pulmonary capillary wedge pressure. (Modified with permission. Barash PG, Chen Y, Kitahata LM *et al:* Hemodynamic tracking system. A method for data management and guide for cardiovascular therapy. Anesth Analg 59: 169, 1980)

TABLE 21-7.   Complications Associated with Pulmonary Artery (PA) Catheters

Venous Cannulation
  Air embolization
  Arterial puncture
  Bernard-Horner syndrome
  Hematoma
  Nerve injury
  Phrenic nerve blockade
  Pneumothorax

Catheter Passage
  Knotting
  Knotting on papillary muscle
  Pneumoperitoneum
  Separation of introducer from hub

Catheter In Situ
  Aberrant waveform due to balloon rupture
  Bradycardia secondary to thermodilution cardiac output
    measurement
  Cardiac valve injury
  Catheter fracture
  Deep venous thrombosis
  Endocarditis
  False positive lung imaging
  False positive echocardiography
  Hematuria
  Intraoperative transection of a catheter
  Migration of pediatric PA catheters
  PA perforation
  Pulmonary infarction
  Sepsis
  Suturing PA catheter to the heart
  Systolic clicks
  Thrombocytopenia
  Thrombosis caused by starch on PA catheters
  Vertebral arteriovenous fistula

the pulmonary artery oximeter catheters that include insertion problems, calibration problems, and faulty equipment.[25] Whether changes in mixed venous oxygen saturation accurately reflect changes in cardiac output is unclear because there have been conflicting reports.[27]

Complications associated with the use of pulmonary artery catheters include all those previously mentioned associated with central venous cannulation. Additionally, complications related to catheter passage and *in situ* have been described and are listed in Table 21-7.

Unquestionably, the most catastrophic complication occurring during maintenance of the catheter is pulmonary artery perforation and hemorrhage. Several significant risk factors have been identified.[22] Advanced age, hypothermia, and pulmonary hypertension place the patient at greater risk. Women have a higher risk of perforation. The presenting sign in most cases is the sudden appearance of hemoptysis. Characteristically, the blood is bright red and may vary in amount from less than 5 ml to massive bleeding. Usually the episode of bleeding is related to balloon inflation or catheter manipulation. Treatment is largely supportive in nature. If bleeding is massive, the patient's trachea should be intubated. If a double-lumen endotracheal tube is not available, an ordinary single-lumen endotracheal tube should be advanced into the main stem bronchus of the noninvolved lung, usually the left. If the patient has received heparin, it should be reversed if possible. Massive blood and fluid replacement may be necessary as may operative intervention. Positive end-expiratory pressure (PEEP) has been used in an attempt to compress the bleeding site. The common feature of this complication in most patients is distal location of the tip of the pulmonary artery catheter, although it has been reported with a more central catheter location as well.[22] When the tip is located too far distally, balloon inflation can distend the vessel wall, subjecting it to large transmural pressures. Mechanisms of pulmonary artery perforation other than overinflation of the balloon include tip perforation, tip propelled by an eccentric balloon, and balloon perforation.[22]

It is important to minimize the number of balloon inflations. In view of the fact that pulmonary artery diastolic pressure agrees very well with PCWP in the absence of pulmonary hypertension, it is recommended that the pulmonary artery diastolic pressure be used whenever possible as an indirect measurement of left atrial pressure. If this is done, the tip of the catheter can be left in a very proximal position, 4–5 cm beyond the pulmonic valve. If a true PCWP is required, the catheter can be floated into position through a sterile, protective external sheath enclosing the catheter.

Infection associated with pulmonary artery catheters can be minimized by adherence to the following recommendations: 1) insertion of the catheter should be performed with aseptic technique, including extensive skin preparation; 2) the catheter site should be covered with a sterile bioocclusive dressing; 3) performance of thermodilution cardiac output and changing of infusion sets should be performed as aseptically as possible and only when necessary; and 4) pulmonary artery catheters should be removed as soon as they are no longer necessary.

Pulmonary artery catheterization remains a valuable monitoring modality if used appropriately.

Transesophageal Echocardiography

Ultrasound is generated by applying voltage to a piezoelectric crystal and the reflected wave is then received by this same crystal.[7] Arrangement of these crystals on a gastroscope body and positioning the probe behind the heart (in the esophagus) results in a two-dimensional view of the heart. Transesophageal echocardiography (TEE) permits observation of heart wall motion, particularly ventricular wall motion, as well as providing a qualitative estimate of end-diastolic and end-systolic volumes, thereby giving a qualitative appreciation of ejection fractions.[28, 29] Wall motion abnormalities depicted by TEE have been shown to correlate with myocardial ischemia.[28, 29] TEE can also detect very small quantities of intravascular air. Cardiac surgery and certain neurosurgical procedures are associated with the entry of air into the circulation and this air can be rapidly detected and localized using TEE.[28] At this time the equipment required for data processing and display is rather expensive and has limited the widespread use of this modality. The complications seen with TEE have to do with the stiffness of the esophageal probe and include temporary vocal cord paralysis. Two-dimensional TEE has also been used to supplement inadequate echocardiography examinations in awake patients using local anesthesia in the hypopharynx. Pulsed Doppler velocity measurements utilizing Doppler flow probes mounted on a gastroscope body (just like TEE) can measure the velocity through the aorta (if positioned properly), and these devices calculate cardiac output by integrating flow velocity and heart rate.[7] Again, the basic modality is an application of ultrasound. Clinicians have not employed Doppler flow on a widespread basis at this point in time.

Transesophageal Doppler color flow mapping (TEDCFM) has recently been developed as an ultrasound modality.[30] It is reported to provide a convenient and relatively noninvasive way to image cardiac anatomy and intracardiac blood flow that may be used intraoperatively.[30] This modality was able to provide specific information about the presence, site, and severity of mitral regurgitation, aortic regurgitation, and interatrial shunting. The eventual fate of this modality is somewhat questionable, but if the cost of the signal processing is decreased substantially, there is no doubt that transesophageal cardiac imaging will be a useful modality in the operating room.

Nuclear Cardiology

The two basic nuclear cardiology modalities, ventriculography and scanning for coronary artery disease, do not appear to be useful intraoperative modalities at this point in time.[7, 29] They are useful primarily as diagnostic modalities. The applications of nuclear cardiology are broadly classified into 1) studies to predict the presence or absence of angiographically important coronary artery disease and 2) studies to quantitate the anatomic extent or functional importance of coronary artery disease.[31] The intravenous administration of thallium enables demonstration of abnormal myocardial perfusion. Administration of technetium and subsequent gated blood pool imaging allows assessment of abnormal left ventricular contraction.

Impedance Measurements

Instrumentation has been introduced that measures cardiac output (and other variables) using impedance technology.[7] The impedance measurements require the placement of multiple sensing electrodes on the thorax and elsewhere. (One instrument currently requires eight electrodes.) This modality clearly has limited use in the operating room simply because of difficulty in achieving proper electrode placement. The device (NCCOM 3, Medex Inc., Hilliard, OH) displays cardiac output, heart rate, stroke volume, thoracic fluid index, ventricular ejection time, and an index of cardiac contractility (ejection velocity index). The ultimate utilization of this modality for intraoperative care is uncertain at this point in time.

Oscilloscopic Electrocardiogram

Monitoring the heart's electrical activity is routine anesthetic practice and certainly constitutes one of the standards of monitoring care. The cost is moderate, operation of equipment is not complicated, and the risk to patients is small.

Use of the ECG is primarily for recognition of cardiac dysrhythmias, alterations in myocardial oxygen supply/demand balance, and changes caused by electrolyte abnormalities. Standard leads I or II are best for dysrhythmia determination and a modified V_5 lead configuration is best for ischemia determination.[32] Equipping instruments for monitoring ECG activity with recording devices so that a written record of the tracing can be obtained is recommended. This is very important for documentation as well as for recognition of complex arrhythmias or other abnormalities in the electrocardiogram. Chapter 22 discusses this modality in greater detail.

PULMONARY SYSTEM AND AIRWAY

Monitoring the adequacy of gas exchange in anesthetized patients is absolutely critical if hypoxia or hypercarbia is to be avoided.

The Senses

Hearing, vision, and touch, all can be used to monitor the respiratory system and airway. Auscultation of breath sounds, visual inspection of chest excursion, visual observation of reservoir bag movement (spontaneous ventilation), the feel of the reservoir bag, and observation of blood color can all be examined using the senses or senses combined with a stethoscope. Similar to the cardiovascular system, these modalities are very subjective and difficult to quantitate. A possible exception concerns auscultation of both lung fields in the midaxillary line as well as auscultation over the stomach to confirm tracheal placement of an endotracheal tube and lack of main stem bronchus intubation.[33] Even auscultation, however, may fail to detect esophageal intubation or main stem bronchus placement.[34] The use of the senses as respiratory monitors either alone or in combination with a stethoscope are most effective as corroborative modalities or back-up systems to more sophisticated and quantitative monitors.

Blood Gases

Analysis of arterial oxygen tension (partial pressure, mm Hg), carbon dioxide tension, and pH allows direct assessment of the adequacy of gas transfer at the lungs and adequacy of acid–base balance. Blood gas determination requires a sample of arterial blood. Continuous arterial blood gas analysis *via* the radial artery or other arterial catheter has been in developmental stages for a number of years and may be available soon. A more complete discussion of blood gas analysis is found in Chapter 25.

Respiratory and Anesthetic Gases

Monitoring of all the constituents of the anesthetic circuit represents the state of the art in indirect pulmonary and airway monitoring. The information may be obtained *via* a multiplexed mass spectrometer system or individual "stand alone" discrete gas-analysis instruments.[35, 36] Ideally, we should monitor all constituents of the anesthetic circuit including the life gases, oxygen, carbon dioxide, and nitrogen as well as the anesthetics, including nitrous oxide and the volatile halogenated anesthetics.

The mass spectrometer is capable of sensing the individual masses of elements or molecules in a mixture of unknown composition and reporting the makeup of that mixture broken down into its individual parts.[35, 36] Typically gases are sampled from a side port on an elbow inserted between the endotracheal tube or mask and the Y piece of a circle system. The gases ionize in an electric beam that accelerates the gas ions in a high-voltage field through a slit that creates a narrow ion beam. This beam passes through a magnetic field that deflects the heavier ions least, creating a spectrum of ions according to molecular weight. Each gas species is collected on a metal plate from which the current is amplified as a measure of concentration of that gas. Several gases commonly measured in anesthetized patients overlap in their mass to charge ratios. For example, nitrous oxide and carbon dioxide both have an atomic mass of 44. Because these two gases are always present during anesthesia with nitrous oxide, manufacturers measure the fragmentation products of ionization for nitrous oxide and carbon dioxide rather than the primary molecules. The halogenated anesthetics all generate "light" fragments that interfere with the accurate detection of other molecules. Complex corrections for "light" fragments are required when one is dealing with the halogenated hydrocarbon anesthetics. Analysis problems, vacuum leaks, and maintenance are the major drawbacks of a mass spectrometry system. Currently reliable and stable devices are available that have overcome these problems in a practical manner.

Discrete or stand-alone gas analyzers operate on the principle of nondispersive infrared absorption.[35, 36] Instruments are currently available to measure and display carbon dioxide, nitrous oxide, oxygen, and the halogenated anesthetic vapors. The current stand-alone gas analysis systems are unable, however, to measure nitrogen.

The value of measuring the constituents of the anesthetic circuit, gas by gas, with the exception of carbon dioxide, which will be handled separately, may be summarized as follows:[35, 36]

Oxygen: Verify fractional inspired oxygen concentrations from flow meters, track end-tidal oxygen values during closed circuit anesthesia, and help evaluate oxygen uptake

Nitrogen: Verify leak free anesthesia delivery system, monitor nitrogen washout during induction, and aid in detection of air emboli

Nitrous oxide: Verify inspired concentrations from flow meters, help evaluate uptake of nitrous oxide during anesthesia, and monitor washout during emergence and recovery

Halogenated anesthetics: Verify inspired concentration of anesthetic being used, ascertain appropriate calibration of vaporizers, evaluate anesthetic washout during recovery, evaluate uptake (end-tidal concentration) during anesthesia

In one cost analysis it was determined that discrete gas analyzers were less expensive than a multiplexed system when the number of locations to monitor was fewer than six.[36] The same evaluation stated that when there were more than eight locations to be monitored, the shared mass spectrometry system was less expensive, with an average cost between $2–3.00 per case in 1985.[36]

Irrespective of anesthetic and respiratory gas monitoring, it is mandatory to monitor oxygen delivery by the anesthetic delivery apparatus. Gaseous oxygen may be analyzed by either paramagnetic analyzers or polarographic oxygen electrodes.[35] These devices have a relatively slow response time and function to indicate mean concentrations. Almost all of the monitors now used on anesthesia machines use polarographic electrodes. The problems with the oxygen electrodes are relatively minor. The electrodes contain a liquid electrolyte that must be replaced periodically. The electrode itself may require replacement and the batteries periodically need replacement. Further discussion regarding monitoring of the anesthesia delivery system is found in Chapter 19.

Airway Pressures

Airway pressures should be measured with a pressure gauge, preferably incorporated into the anesthetic machine breathing circuit.[33] Alarms should sound when too high or too low pressures are encountered. Low circuit pressure alarms are mandatory if mechanical ventilation is employed to allow early detection of anesthetic circuit disconnections. High pressure alarms help to detect endotracheal tube obstruction and prevent barotrauma to the lungs. Further information on measurement of airway pressures is found in Chapter 19.

Ventimeter

The ability to measure the volume of gas moving out of the patient's lungs with each breath is critical to the safe conduct of anesthesia. Devices that are currently available are primarily flow sensors.[33] They are available only with circle systems. In general, the gas flow turns a vane or rotor on a spindle that is connected through a geared system to a point on a calibrated dial. Although problems include inertia and friction, collection of moisture and foreign material, and momentum (overshoot during high flow), ventimeters are invaluable and should be mandatorily incorporated in all anesthetic circuits. Ventimeters allow tidal volume as well as minute volume measurements.

Carbon Dioxide

End-exhalation or end-tidal carbon dioxide is an excellent indirect method to assess alveolar ventilation for patients with normal circulation and lung function. It approximates arterial carbon dioxide with only a small arterial to alveolar gradient.[33]

End-tidal carbon dioxide tension may be measured by an infrared analyzer or a mass spectrometer system. Some of the important uses of monitoring end-tidal carbon dioxide include helping to determine optimal minute ventilation; monitoring conditions of *no breathing* that may be related to ventilator malfunction, circuit disconnect, or airway obstruction; helping to detect inspired carbon dioxide concentrations that may be due to exhausted soda lime; and identifying esophageal intubation. End-tidal CO_2 is virtually infallible in detecting esophageal intubation when endotracheal tube placement is in doubt.[33, 34]

Measurement of carbon dioxide, known as *capnography*, is capable of providing a large amount of information. It is important that the operator be able to recognize and identify the various components of a normal capnogram. Although instruments that provide high and low carbon dioxide values in a breathing cycle, with a bar graph or digital readout are acceptable, instruments which display the CO_2 wave form provide far more information.[33, 36] The carbon dioxide wave form can be analyzed for five basic characteristics: height, frequency, rhythm, base line, and shape.[37] The height depends on the end-tidal carbon dioxide value. The frequency depends on the respiratory rate. The rhythm depends on the state of the respiratory center or on the function of the ventilator. The base line should be at 0. There is only one normal shape (Fig. 21-9).

Certain basic rules regarding capnography are easily identified. A sudden drop in carbon dioxide to 0 or to a very low level indicates a technical disturbance or defect such as a kinked endotracheal tube, defective carbon dioxide analyzer, circuit disconnection, or a defective mechanical ventilator.

A sudden change in baseline that may or may not be combined with changes in the plateau level usually indicates a calibration error, an exhausted carbon dioxide absorber, a faulty valve in the anesthesia circuit, or water condensation in the carbon dioxide analyzer. A sudden decrease in carbon dioxide value (but not to 0 with either spontaneous or mechanical ventilation indicates a leakage in the respiratory system (low airway pressure), or obstruction (high airway pressure). An exponential decrease in carbon dioxide (washout curve) within 1 or 2 min indicates a sudden disturbance in pulmonary blood flow or ventilation that may occur with circulatory arrest, pulmonary embolism, sudden hypotension, or sudden hyperventilation.

FIG. 21-9. The normal capnogram. A represents beginning of exhalation; AB represents anatomic dead space gas being exhaled; BC represents the ascending limb representing increasing concentration of carbon dioxide from increasingly distal airways; CD represents alveolar plateau containing mixed alveolar gases; D represents end-tidal carbon dioxide; DE represents the descending limb and the inspiratory phase of respiration showing rapidly decreasing carbon dioxide concentration as fresh gas is inhaled. (Reprinted with permission. Swedlow DB: Mass spectrometers and respiratory gas monitoring. In Barash PG (ed): American Society of Anesthesiologists Annual Refresher Courses, Philadelphia, JB Lippincott, 1985)

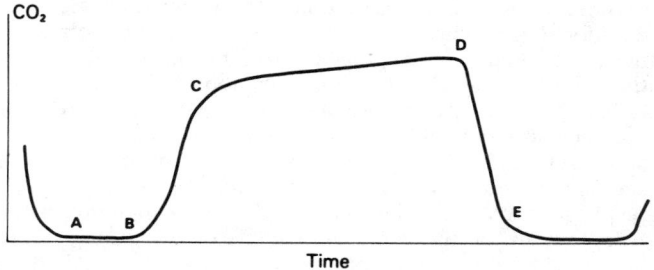

A gradual increase in carbon dioxide during either spontaneous or mechanical ventilation indicates hypoventilation, absorption of carbon dioxide from an external source such as the peritoneal cavity during laparoscopy, or rapidly rising body temperature such as may occur in malignant hyperthermia. A sudden increase in carbon dioxide during either spontaneous or mechanical ventilation may be due to the injection of sodium bicarbonate, the sudden release of a vascular occlusion tourniquet, or a sudden increase in pulmonary blood flow. A gradual upshift of the carbon dioxide baseline and top line usually indicates defective carbon dioxide absorption, a calibration or technical error in the carbon dioxide analyzer, or increasing dead space resulting in rebreathing. Gradual lowering of the end-tidal carbon dioxide (in which the curve retains its normal shape but the height of the plateau gradually drops) usually occurs in a mechanically ventilated patient and is caused by gradual hyperventilation, decreasing body temperature, or decreasing body or lung perfusion.

Thus, we see that capnography is capable of defining problems relating to gas supply to the patient as well as respiratory, circulatory, and central nervous system effects on the respiratory system as well. Three of the more common abnormalities in capnogram waveforms and their causes are seen in Figure 21-10.

Transcutaneous Gas Measurement

Measurement of arterial oxygen and carbon dioxide tensions can be accomplished with electrodes that are placed on the skin.[35] The electrodes are similar to those used for standard blood gas analysis. They are heated, which, in turn, causes an increase in blood flow in the skin beneath the electrode. Oxygen and carbon dioxide diffuse through the hyperemic skin to the electrodes. Unlike a pulse oximeter, which only measures hemoglobin saturation, transcutaneous electrodes measure P_{O_2} and P_{CO_2}. Because the sensors measure the gas tensions in the skin, the values reported will not only reflect changes in arterial gas tensions, but also changes in blood flow. Thus, a fall in transcutaneous P_{O_2} could signify either a decrease in arterial blood P_{O_2} or a decrease in blood flow to the skin, as might be seen with hypovolemia.

The primary use of transcutaneous electrodes is for monitoring adequacy of oxygenation and ventilation. This may especially be true when the trachea is not intubated and ventilation is uncertain. Such situations occur most often in children. The instruments require substantial set up and calibration and for this reason have not had wide appeal for intraoperative use. In addition, because the transcutaneous oxygen tension is dependent both on arterial oxygen tension and blood flow, interpretation of observations is somewhat difficult.[35] Carbon dioxide electrodes require calibration with a compressed gas and often drift on skin even when stable in calibration because of water movement in or out of the electrolyte layer. Because of the requirement for heating of the sensors (electrodes), these instruments have the potential to produce burns on the skin and changes in gas tensions are not detected as rapidly as they are with devices such as a pulse oximeter. Transcutaneous oxygen measurement is superior to pulse oximetry in situations of carbon monoxide poisoning.

RENAL MONITORING

The primary variables monitored intraoperatively to assess renal function are urine output (volume), urine specific gravity, and the presence or absence of substances in the urine

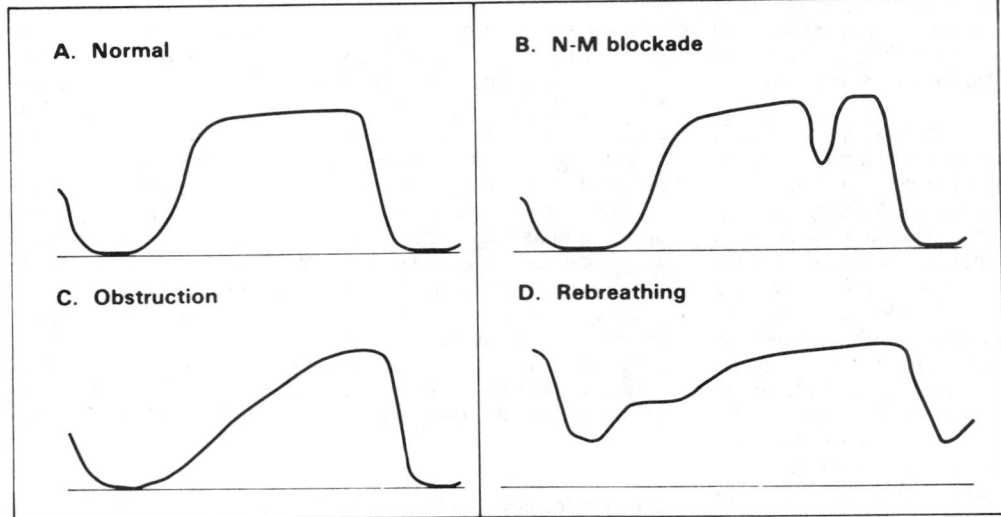

A. Normal

B. N-M blockade

C. Obstruction

D. Rebreathing

FIG. 21-10. *A* shows normal capnogram. In *B*, partial neuromuscular blockade with spontaneous diaphragmatic movement results in a cleft due to the inrush of carbon dioxide free gas as the diaphragm contracts. It may be the first clinical sign that neuromuscular function is returning. *C* shows prolonged exhalation secondary to a partially kinked endotracheal tube or small airway obstruction. The alveolar plateau is absent. This indicates that the lung units do not drain their carbon-dioxide-rich gas in a time-coordinated manner. *D* represents rebreathing that can occur in various circumstances such as faulty valves, exhausted carbon dioxide absorber, or inadequate fresh gas flow in a Mapleson D-type circuit. (Reprinted with permission. Swedlow DB: Mass spectrometers and respiratory gas monitoring. In Barash PG (ed): American Society of Anesthesiologists Annual Refresher Courses, Philadelphia, JB Lippincott, 1985)

such as sugar, hemoglobin, etc. Monitoring of the kidney is accomplished by use of an indwelling urinary catheter.

The primary reason for monitoring renal function is to monitor extracellular fluid volume and composition and adequacy of perfusion.[38] A second reason for monitoring kidney function is to prevent acute renal parenchymal failure. Additional reasons for monitoring renal function are the detection of several systemic disease states, including hemolysis, rhabdomyolysis, and ketoacidosis. A urinary catheter should be used whenever fluid and volume status is subject to substantial changes and whenever the combination of anesthesia and surgery suggests the potential development of renal failure. A more thorough discussion is found in Chapter 39.

MONITORING THE NEUROMUSCULAR JUNCTION

Monitoring the neuromuscular junction with a nerve stimulator has proven to be useful during anesthesia involving the use of neuromuscular blocking drugs.[39] These devices permit administration of muscle relaxants such that optimal surgical relaxation is achieved while permitting timely drug reversal either spontaneously or with antagonists. Muscle relaxant dosage can be titrated against the patient's response to nerve stimulation. This is particularly important because of the tremendous variability in patient response to muscle relaxants.

Prior to the development of nerve stimulators, anesthesiologists used other clinical indices of skeletal muscle strength. These include the ability to open the eyes or mouth widely, tongue protrusion, grip strength, head lift for 5 s, vital capacity, tidal volume, and inspiratory force.[39] Most of these clinical indices require a cooperative patient and are inappropriate while surgery is in progress.

The most satisfactory and reliable method for monitoring neuromuscular function, especially during surgery, is the stimulation of an appropriate nerve and observation of the evoked response in the skeletal muscles supplied by the nerve. This is accomplished by monitoring the mechanical force generated by the muscle or by its electrical response, the electromyogram.[39] The ulnar nerve–adductor pollicis muscle system of the thumb is most commonly used for mechanical force measurement, although the facial nerve may serve as an alternative site. The adductor pollicis muscle of the thumb is innervated solely by the ulnar nerve. Electrodes or subcutaneous needles are placed over the ulnar nerve at the wrist or elbow. A supramaximal electrical stimulus is delivered from the peripheral nerve stimulator and movement of the fingers observed.

There are four commonly used patterns of stimulation for monitoring neuromuscular blockade: single twitch, train-of-four, tetanus, and posttetanic stimulation. In clinical situations, these responses are evaluated visually or by touch. With appropriate equipment, these responses can be recorded and quantitated (Fig. 21-11).[39] The single twitch is a commonly observed response. The depth of neuromuscular blockade is defined as a per cent inhibition of twitch response and duration of blockade as the time for twitch response to recover to a per cent of control height. Train-of-four (four twitches at 2 Hz every 0.5 s) utilizes the concept that acetylcholine is depleted by successive stimulations. Only four twitches are necessary because additional stimulation fails to further alter release of additional acetylcholine. In the presence of nondepolarizing neuromuscular blockade, the height of the fourth twitch is less than the first twitch, allowing calculation of a train-of-four ratio (Fig. 21-12).[40] Recovery of the train-of-four ratio to 0.7 or greater correlates with complete return of single twitch response (Table 21-8). This confirms that train-of-four is a more sensitive monitor of neuromuscular blockade than is twitch response, which may be normal when 70% or more of the receptors are occupied by muscle relaxants. During depolarizing neuromuscular blockade, the train-of-four ratio does

succinylcholine (mg/kg)

0.3

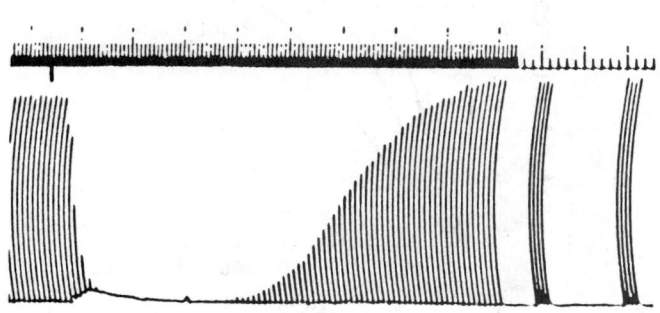

FIG. 21-11. Examples of evoked mechanical twitch recording. (Reprinted with permission. Crowley MP, Savarese JJ, Ali HH: Monitoring the neuromuscular junction. In Blitt CD [ed]: Monitoring in Anesthesia and Critical Care Medicine, p 523. New York, Churchill Livingstone, 1985)

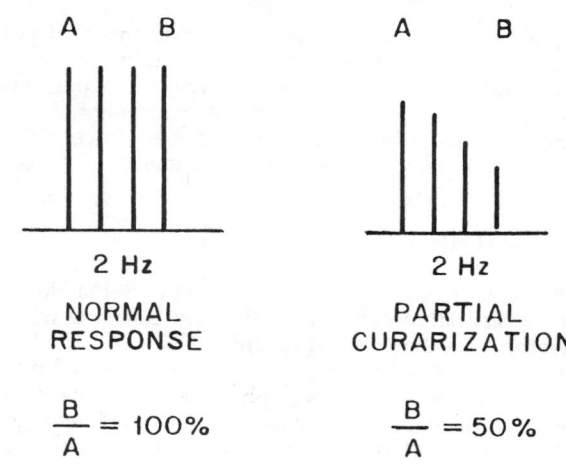

FIG. 21-12. Schematic depiction of responses to train-of-four stimulation. The ratio of the fourth twitch (B) to the first twitch (A) is calculated. (Reprinted with permission. Ali HH, Savarese JJ: Monitoring of neuromuscular junction. Anesthesiology 45:216, 1976)

TABLE 21-8.   Correlation of Evoked Responses with Clinical Signs

TWITCH HEIGHT (% of control)	CLINICAL RELAXATION	VENTILATION
100	None (train-of-four 70%, tetanus sustained at 50 Hz)	Normal
75	Poor, but head fit inadequate	Slight to moderate decrease in vital capacity
50	Fair	Moderate to marked decrease in vital capacity, tidal volume may be adequate
25	Good with volatile anesthetics	Diminished tidal volume
10	Good with injected anesthetics	Inadequate tidal volume
5	Very good, adequate for tracheal intubation	Some diaphragm motion possible
0	Excellent, good for tracheal intubation	Apnea

(Adapted with permission. Crowley MP, Savarese JJ, Ali HH: Monitoring the neuromuscular junction. In Blitt CD [ed]: Monitoring in Anesthesia and Critical Care Medicine, p 523. New York, Churchill Livingstone, 1985)

not change greatly as the height of all four twitches decreases simultaneously. A train-of-four ratio less than 0.3 in the presence of depolarizing neuromuscular blockade reflects a phase II blockade that may be susceptible to reversal with anticholinesterase drugs. Train-of-four stimulation should be repeated no more frequently than every 12 s. Continuous electrical stimulation for 5 s at 50 Hz (tetanus) is an intense stimulus to the neuromuscular junction for continued release of acetylcholine. In the presence of nondepolarizing neuromuscular blockade the initial response is not sustained (fades), while in the presence of depolarizing neuromuscular blockade the response is greatly reduced but does not fade. A sustained response to continuous stimulation for 5 s is present when the train-of-four ratio is 0.7 or greater. Following the end of a continuous stimulation, there is an increase in the immediately available store of acetylcholine such that subsequent twitch responses are transiently enhanced (postetanic potentiation). Although use of a nerve stimulator to assess the adequacy of reversal of neuromuscular blockade is efficacious,

determinants of skeletal muscle function by clinical tests should also be undertaken at the end of an anesthetic.

Does a peripheral nerve stimulator need to be used on every anesthetized patient who receives muscle relaxants? This question is not easily answerable, although the introduction of shorter-acting nondepolarizing muscle relaxants has made the peripheral nerve stimulator appear somewhat superfluous at times. There is considerable variation in patient response to muscle relaxants. Furthermore, the response to muscle relaxants can be unpredictable due to factors such as drugs, body temperature, acid–base balance, and co-existing neuromuscular diseases (see Chapter 16).

OXYGENATION

Adequate oxygenation of the anesthetized patient depends on a complex interaction of both pulmonary and cardiovascular systems. The ability to measure arterial oxygenation is critical to prevention of disasters such as hypoxic encephalopathy. Assessment of oxygenation can be accomplished by direct measurement of arterial blood gases, transcutaneous oxygen measurement, and pulse oximetry. Measurement of arterial and transcutaneous blood gases is discussed above. This discussion will therefore focus on pulse oximetry.

PULSE OXIMETRY

The oxygen saturation of hemoglobin in arterial blood can be fairly accurately determined by light reflected from, or passed through, the skin and subcutaneous vessels.[35] Arterial oxygen saturation of hemoglobin can be determined directly and continuously using spectrophotoelectric oximetric techniques. The wave length dependence of reduced hemoglobin *versus* oxyhemoglobin is evident from the prominent color differences in spectral light absorbance.[41] The light absorbance differences between reduced hemoglobin and oxyhemoglobin may be described quantitatively by the molecular extinction coefficients in Beer's law. Pulse oximetry functions by positioning any pulsating arterial vascular bed between a two-wave-length light source and a detector. The pulsating vascular bed expands and relaxes, thereby creating a change in the light path that modifies the amount of light detected. The amplitude of the detected light depends on the size of the arterial pulse change, the wave length of light used and the oxygen saturation of the arterial hemoglobin. The detected pulse or waveform is produced solely from arterial blood, and beat-to-beat continuous calculation of arterial hemoglobin saturation without interference from surrounding tissues, bone, or venous blood is accomplished. The technology utilizes a light source generated by two light-emitting diodes with wave lengths at approximately 660 and 940 nm. A photo diode is mounted in a receptacle that is placed somewhere on the body, usually an extremity such as a finger or toe. No heating or other arterialization techniques are required. Circuit control, saturation calculation, and display are managed by a computer. Calibration is not required. Pulse oximetry has been shown to be accurate linearly and to be precise between 8 and 100% saturation,[41] however, a study in volunteers demonstrated inaccuracies during transient episodes of profound hypoxia.[42] Because the technique uses light absorbance changes produced by arterial pulsations, any event that significantly reduces vascular pulsations will reduce the ability of the instrument to obtain and process the signal and thereby calculate arterial oxygen saturation. Thus, hypothermia, hypotension, and infusion of vasoconstrictor drugs can limit the usefulness of this monitoring modality.

Abnormal hemoglobin species such as carboxyhemoglobin, sulfhemoglobin, and methemoglobin will cause errors in measurement.[41, 43] Errors in measurement will also occur in patients receiving intravascular administration of certain dyes, such as indocyanine green, methylene blue, and indigo carmine.[43] This interference occurs because of overlapping of the absorbance spectra of the dyes and the wave lengths of light that are sensed by the pulse oximeter. Instrumentation that involves the production of wave lengths of light similar to those produced by the pulse oximeter will also interfere with determination of oxygen saturation. The most common clinical entity in this regard is the use of infrared heating lamps.[44] Motion and electrocautery also can interfere with the proper functioning of the instrument, although improvements are being made to minimize these effects. When employing pulse oximetry it is important to remember the relationship of hemoglobin oxygen saturation to arterial oxygen tension.[45]

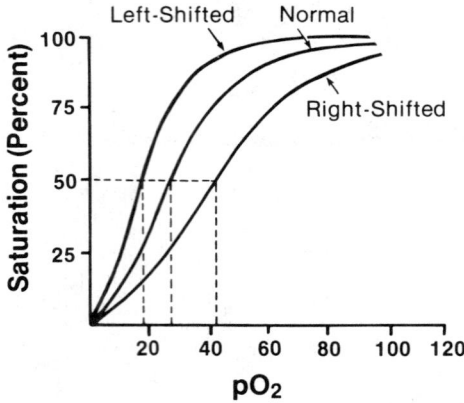

FIG. 21-13. Oxyhemoglobin dissociation curve with right and left shifts. (Reprinted with permission. Geha DG: Blood gas monitoring. In Blitt CD (ed): Monitoring in Anesthesia and Critical Care Medicine. New York, Churchill Livingstone, 1985)

This is graphically described with the oxyhemoglobin dissociation curve (Fig. 21-13). Pulse oximetry is also discussed in Chapter 5.

Since its introduction in 1983, pulse oximetry has proven to be quite valuable and has achieved widespread acceptance. Pulse oximetry is valuable in one-lung anesthesia, pulmonary artery banding, pigmented patients, as a home apnea monitor, and for assessment of adequacy of vascular reconstruction. Pulse oximetry is also valuable in the recovery room and in the critical care unit to assess adequacy of oxygenation. The device can substitute for multiple arterial blood gas determinations (for oxygen only) once a correlation between arterial oxygenation and arterial saturation is made for an individual patient. Pulse oximetry cannot replace an arterial catheter for beat-to-beat blood pressure determination. The major benefits of pulse oximetry are: it is noninvasive, it is easy to use, and nonanesthetic personnel may easily use the modality. Pulse oximetry enables early detection of incipient unsuspected arterial hypoxemia in the anesthetized patient so that therapeutic intervention may be instituted and disastrous consequences avoided.

TEMPERATURE MONITORING

Because abnormal temperature can adversely impact numerous organ systems, the anesthesiologist should monitor temperature and strive to maintain it within normal values. Heat production occurs by means of cellular metabolism that is affected by basal metabolic rate, muscular activity, sympathetic arousal, hormonal activity, and exogenously administered heat. Heat loss occurs by four specific physical phenomena: radiation, conduction, convection, and evaporation[46] (Fig. 21-14). Much of the heat loss from a patient (greater than 60%) occurs by radiation. Conduction accounts for a small fraction of heat loss, and convection also accounts for a relatively small amount of heat loss (approximately 12% in the operating room). Evaporation particularly from the skin surface and from the lungs (often referred to as insensible water loss) accounts for approximately 25% of heat loss. The physics of heat loss is discussed in detail in Chapter 5.

Infants represent a special situation regarding temperature control because of differences from the adult in the way heat is produced and lost.[46] The newborn does not shiver unless

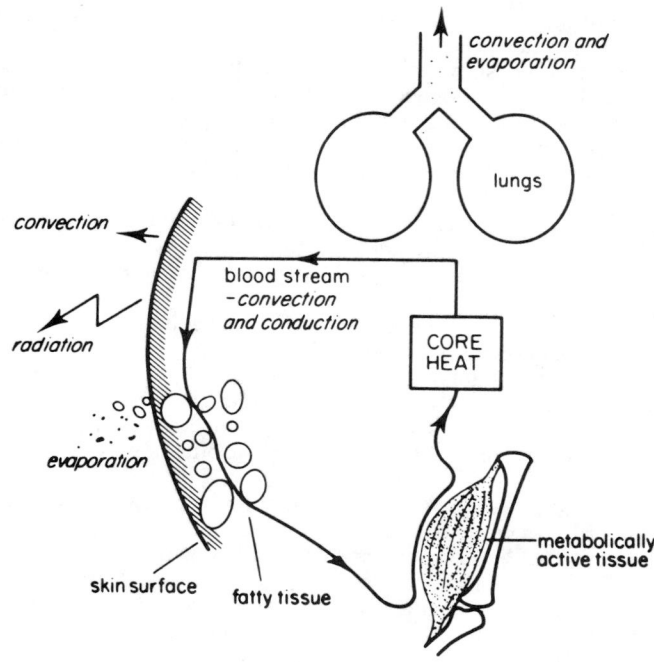

FIG. 21-14. Summary of heat production and heat loss. (Reprinted with permission. Holdcroft: Body Temperature Control in Anesthesia. In Surgery and Intensive Care. London, Balliére Tindall, 1980.)

5. Anesthesia reduces body metabolism (*i.e.*, heat production).
6. Anesthesia causes vasodilatation (*i.e.*, increased heat loss).
7. Anesthesia interferes with thermoregulatory mechanisms in the hypothalamus.

There are numerous physiologic consequences that result from hypothermia, and additional postoperative danger exists in the patient's own attempt at rewarming. Hypothermia reduces anesthetic requirements. Drugs that rely on liver metabolism for conjugation and excretion, such as morphine, have significantly prolonged half lives. Decreased glomerular filtration rate and renal blood flow increase the half lives of drugs that depend on the kidney for clearance. Blood viscosity increases during hypothermia, raising the risk of decreased perfusion.[46]

Shivering and increased metabolism are used by the awakening patient to restore normothermia. Shivering increases tissue oxygen consumption as much as 400–500%.[46] This requires an increased minute ventilation to provide the additional oxygen and an increased cardiac output to assure delivery of oxygen to the tissues. These demands occur at the same time when depressant effects of anesthetic drugs may still remain. As the patient's temperature returns toward normal, the peripheral vasoconstriction secondary to hypothermia becomes less marked and rewarming shock may result. The capacitance of the circulatory system increases during rewarming, and volume administration may be necessary to prevent hypotension.

Because the response to hypothermia and rewarming can be hazardous, prevention of hypothermia is preferred. Radiant heat lamps, warm blankets, heated humidification, warmer operating rooms, heated intravenous blood and fluids, and heat-retaining drapes and coverings provide us the means to help maintain normothermia. The use of low-flow (fresh gas) anesthesia is also an effective means of maintaining the patient's body heat.[46]

Causes of intraoperative hyperthermia include infection, hyperthyroidism, excessive external warming, and malignant hyperthermia. Clearly, malignant hyperthermia is the life-threatening disease entity that may be diagnosed (albeit somewhat late) by temperature monitoring. Malignant hyperthermia is discussed in detail in Chapter 17.

The most commonly used devices for measuring temperature are the thermistor and the thermocouple.[46] The major difference between the two devices is that the thermocouple is disposable while the thermistor is reusable. Numerous monitoring sites for measuring temperature have been described.[46] The most commonly used are rectal, nasopharyngeal, esophageal, and tympanic membrane locations. Although there are studies that support the tympanic membrane site as the best index of core temperature, a significant objection to the use of the tympanic membrane probe is tympanic membrane perforation.[46] Other monitoring sites that have been employed are the forehead and axilla. Rectal, bladder, esophageal, and nasopharyngeal temperatures most closely correlate with tympanic membrane and core temperature.[46] These sites are recommended rather than risking trauma to the tympanic membrane. Liquid crystal thermometers, in the form of a liquid crystal adhesive strip, can be affixed to the patient's skin and the temperature is read as the color of the liquid crystal changes with temperature. These devices have been found to correlate very poorly with other temperature monitors but they can be used as a trend indicator.

exposed to very low temperature. Newborns and infants use a method of heat production called *nonshivering thermogenesis*. Newborns and infants have a special tissue called *brown fat* located between the scapulae and around large blood vessels.[46] When an infant is exposed to cold temperature, a sympathetic discharge causes this brown fat to heat up and cardiac output becomes diverted to the brown fat so that this heat is distributed to the rest of the body.[46] Because infants have less insulation and proportionately more surface area, they are more apt to lose heat by radiation, conduction, and convection.

Hypothermia is the most common temperature disorder resulting from anesthesia and surgery. Approximately 60% of patients have temperatures of less than 36°C on admission to the recovery room.[46] Older patients become colder after anesthesia and surgery and remain colder for a longer period of time than do younger patients.[46] Thus, there is something that happens in the operating room that makes patients cool down. Factors that contribute to decrease patients' temperatures during anesthesia and surgery include the following:

1. The room is cold. Most operating rooms are kept at 18–21°C for the comfort of the sterile, heavily gowned operating team. It has been observed that patients lose heat in the operating room when the temperature is less than 21°C.[46]
2. The patient often receives nonwarmed intravenous fluids.
3. Heat is required to humidify the inspired anesthetic gases.
4. The patient's body core is often exposed to the environment during the surgical procedure and body cavities are frequently exposed to cold irrigating solutions on repeated occasions.

Should temperature monitoring be routine or should the *availability* of temperature monitoring be the standard of care? The ability to measure temperature should be available at every anesthetizing location and should be used whenever the anesthesiologist's clinical judgment deems it necessary. Although tympanic membrane perforation and burns from temperature probes have been reported,[46] the overall risk to the patient of temperature monitoring is extremely small compared with the information obtained.

STANDARDS FOR MONITORING

Which monitors should be used routinely, and which should be used selectively? These are difficult questions to answer. Medical judgment, good medical practice, and personal preference, all come into play. Even if there are little data to prove conclusively that monitors are beneficial, it is clear that certain minimum monitoring standards must be set, especially with regard to preplanned anesthetics given in designated anesthetizing locations. Monitoring in the labor and delivery suite should be the same as in the operating room. Monitoring for chronic pain management, predelivery labor, or sedation/amnesia or analgesia for various diagnostic and therapeutic procedures should be based on institutional guidelines. If minimum standards cannot be met, then appropriate documentation (in writing) as to why the standards cannot be complied with must be made. An example of such a circumstance might be monitoring for anesthesia given for MRI. Because of the powerful magnet, all ferrous-containing metals must be avoided in the MRI suite. Thus an automatic blood pressure cuff, telemetric ECG, and a plastic stethoscope may be all that are permitted.

Several groups have adopted minimum monitoring standards[47, 48] (See Chapter 2, Table 2-1). All require the physical presence of qualified anesthesia personnel in the room where the anesthetic is being administered. The interpretation of such a statement requiring the presence of the anesthesiologist is interesting. It implies that all of the modern, mechanical monitoring devices cannot take the place of a vigilant anesthesiologist. It also reflects the fact that monitors are only of great value if there is somebody present to observe the information that is obtained by the monitors.

Before starting an anesthetic, the anesthesiologist should undertake a thorough "preflight check" of anesthesia apparatus, such as that endorsed by the American Society of Anesthesiologists.[49] This check-out procedure is a guideline that users should be encouraged to use and modify to accommodate differences in equipment design and variations in local clinical practice.

The use of pulse oximetry and end-tidal carbon dioxide monitoring is gaining increasing favor and is strongly encouraged. Capnography is particularly useful for ascertaining proper placement of the endotracheal tube in instances where tracheal placement is in doubt.

COMPUTERS IN MONITORING

Computers are used now for signal processing, data manipulation, and display in many monitoring devices such as automatic blood pressure devices, pulse oximeters, evoked-potential monitors, and TEE. Computers can be valuable resources in data analysis, particularly for establishing a data base. Once a data base is established, computers can help with peer review, risk management, and educational conferences.[50]

Computers can be used to monitor equity of scheduling and equity of case assignments.

Computers show great promise for producing a fully automated anesthetic record.[50] Preliminary systems are now in place to perform this task. The following problems need to be addressed before the automated anesthesia record is a reality for the majority of practicing anesthesiologists.

1. There must be voice activation or minimal data entry requirement by anesthesiologists.
2. There must be a capability for adding comments in real time.
3. A variety of devices must be interfaced.
4. Data entry must be artifact free.
5. Anesthesiologists and lawyers must understand that artifacts can occur and that if brief episodes of hypotension are shown, even if real, that these do not necessarily contribute to poor patient outcome.

A study has shown a significant difference when the written record was compared with automated data collection.[11] This means that handwritten anesthetic records do not accurately reflect the totality of events that occur during anesthesia. Significant discrepancies that have been discovered between the anesthesia record and automatic data collection devices are somewhat unsettling. If in fact an accurate record is desired, particularly documentation of vital signs, then a computer-generated record is desirable. In addition, the anesthesiologists are freed from time-consuming record keeping so they can concentrate completely on patient care. This is particularly true during induction and emergence periods when physicians' concentration and efforts are and should be directed totally toward patient care.

SUMMARY

With the development of solid state electronics and miniature devices, a plethora of monitors has appeared in recent years. Physiologic variables are now being monitored that were considered impossible several years ago. Progress has been made, but there needs to be continual growth in the monitoring field. Interfacing of various pieces of monitoring equipment (even by the same manufacturer) has become frustrating at best and needs to be addressed—espcially by industry. We need to look forward to a complete centralized monitoring array without a spaghetti-like gaggle of wires, hoses, and power cords. Alarms need to be readily identifiable as to their source. The anesthetic work place needs to be improved and standardized (like an airplane cockpit) so as to minimize the occurrence of human error. Anesthesiologists must work with industry to accomplish these goals.

Regardless of biases, training, or age, we must realize that monitors and complex devices are here to stay and we must work with them, not against them. Monitoring is a means to achieve an end; that end is to make anesthesia as safe as possible.

REFERENCES

1. Donegan JH: The electroencephalogram. In Blitt CD (ed): Monitoring in Anesthesia and Critical Care Medicine, p 323. New York, Churchill Livingstone, 1985
2. Grundy BL: Evoked potential monitoring. In Blitt CD (ed): Mon-

itoring in Anesthesia and Critical Care Medicine, p 345. New York, Churchill Livingstone, 1985
3. Grundy BL: Intraoperative monitoring of sensory-evoked potentials. Anesthesiology 58:72, 1983
4. Sokoll MD: Monitoring intracranial pressure. In Blitt CD (ed): Monitoring in Anesthesia and Critical Care Medicine, p 413. New York, Churchill Livingstone, 1985
5. Grantham CD, Hameroff SR: Monitoring anesthetic depth. In Blitt CD (ed): Monitoring in Anesthesia and Critical Care Medicine, p 427. New York, Churchill Livingstone, 1985
6. Evans JM, Davies WL, Wise CC: Lower oesophageal contractility: A new monitor of anaesthesia. Lancet 1:1151, 1984
7. Stiff JL, Rogers MC: Monitoring modalities of the future. In Blitt CD (ed): Monitoring in Anesthesia and Critical Care Medicine, p 691. New York, Churchill Livingstone, 1985
8. Bashein G, Russell AH, Momii ST: Anesthesia and remote monitoring for intraoperative radiation therapy. Anesthesiology 64:804, 1986
9. Maier WR: Noninvasive blood pressure monitoring. In Blitt CD (ed): Monitoring in Anesthesia and Critical Care Medicine, p 29. New York, Churchill Livingstone, 1985
10. Geddes LA, Voel ZM, Combs C et al: Characterization of the oscillometric method for measuring indirect blood pressure. Ann Biomed Engl 10:271, 1982
11. Logas WG, McCarthy RJ, Narbone RF et al: Analysis of the accuracy of the anesthetic record. Anesth Analg 66:S107, 1987
12. Sy WP: Ulnar nerve palsy related to use of automatically cycled blood pressure cuff. Anesth Analg 60:687, 1981
13. Smith NT, Wesseling KH, DeWit B: Evaluation of two prototype devices producing noninvasive, pulsatile, calibrated blood pressure measurement from a finger. J Clin Monit 1:17, 1985
14. Bedford RF: Invasive blood pressure monitoring. In Blitt CD (ed): Monitoring in Anesthesia and Critical Care Medicine, p 41. New York, Churchill Livingstone, 1985
15. Slogoff S, Keats AS, Arlund C: On the safety of radial artery cannulation. Anesthesiology 59:42, 1983
16. Blitt CD: Catheterization techniques for invasive cardiovascular monitoring, p 33. Springfield, Charles C Thomas, 1981
17. Otto CW: Central venous pressure monitoring. In Blitt CD (ed): Monitoring and Anesthesia Critical Care Medicine, p 121. New York, Churchill Livingstone, 1985
18. Seldinger SI: Catheter replacement of the needle in percutaneous arteriography. Acta Radiol 39:368, 1953
19. Blitt CD, Wright WA, Petty WC et al: Central venous catheterization via the external jugular vein: A technique employing the J wire. JAMA 229:817, 1974
20. DeFalque RJ: Percutaneous catheterization of the internal jugular vein. Anesth Analg 53:116, 1974
21. Swan HJC, Ganz W, Forrester JS et al: Catheterizaton of the heart in man with use of a flow-directed-balloon-tipped catheter. N Engl J Med 283:447, 1970
22. Keefer RJ, Barash PG: Pulmonary artery catheterization. In Blitt CD (ed): Monitoring in Anesthesia and Critical Care Medicine, p 177. New York, Churchill Livingstone, 1985
23. Pace NL: A critique of flow-directed pulmonary artery catheterization. Anesthesiology 47:455, 1977
24. Pearson KS, Gomez MN, Carter JG et al: A cost/benefit analysis of randomized invasive monitoring in cardiac surgery. Anesth Analg 66:S138, 1987
25. Baele PL, McMichen JC, Marsh HM et al: Continuous monitoring of mixed venous oxygen saturation in critically ill patients. Anesth Analg 61:513, 1982
26. Schmidt CR, Frank LP, Estafenous FG: Continuous pulmonary artery oximetry: Early warning monitor in cardiac surgery patients. Anesthesiology 59:A139, 1983
27. Kyff JV, Vaughn S, Yang A et al: Significance of continuous monitoring of SV_{O_2} during acute myocardial infarction. Anesthesiology 65:A106, 1986
28. Clements FM, de Bruijn NP: Perioperative evaluation of regional wall motion by transesophageal two dimensional echocardiography. Anesth Analg 66:249, 1987
29. Cahalan MK, Litt L, Botvinick EH et al: Advances in noninvasive cardiovascular imaging: Implications for the anesthesiologist. Anesthesiology 66:356, 1987
30. de Bruijn NP, Clements FM, Kisslo JA: Intraoperative transesophageal color flow mapping: Initial experience. Anesth Analg 66:386, 1987
31. Gerson MC: Nuclear cardiology in the investigation of chronic coronary artery disease. JAMA 250:2037, 1983
32. Stevenson RL, Rogers MC: Electrocardiographic monitoring. In Blitt CD (ed): Monitoring in Anesthesia and Critical Care Medicine, p 87. New York, Churchill Livingstone, 1985
33. Fairley HB: Respiratory monitoring. In Blitt CD (ed): Monitoring in Anesthesia and Critical Care Medicine, p 229. New York, Churchill Livingstone, 1985
34. Birmingham PK, Cheney FW, Ward RW: Esophageal intubation: A review of detection techniques. Anesth Analg 65:886, 1986
35. Severinghaus JW: Monitoring anesthetic and respiratory gases. In Blitt CD (ed): Monitoring in Anesthesia and Critical Care Medicine, p 265. New York, Churchill Livingstone, 1985
36. Swedlow DB: Mass spectrometers and respiratory gas monitoring. In Barash PG (ed): American Society of Anesthesiologists Annual Refresher Courses, p 205. Philadelphia, JB Lippincott, 1985
37. Smalhout B: A quick guide to capnography and its use in differential diagnosis. Andover, MA, Hewlett-Packard, 1986
38. Tonnesen AS: Monitoring the kidney and urine. In Blitt CD (ed): Monitoring in Anesthesia and Critical Care Medicine, p 459. New York, Churchill Livingstone, 1985
39. Crowley MP, Savarese JJ, Ali HH: Monitoring the neuromuscular junction. In Blitt CD (ed): Monitoring in Anesthesia and Critical Care Medicine, p 523. New York, Churchill Livingstone, 1985
40. Ali HH, Savarese JJ: Monitoring of neuromuscular function. Anesthesiology 45:216, 1976
41. Yelderman M, New W: Evaluation of pulse oximetry. Anesthesiology 59:349, 1983
42. Severinghaus JW, Naifeh KH: Accuracy of response of six pulse oximeters to profound hypoxia. Anesthesiology 67:551, 1987
43. Scheller MS, Unger RJ, Kelner MJ: Effects of intravenously administered dyes on pulse oximetry readings. Anesthesiology 65:550, 1986
44. Brooks TD, Paulus DA, Winkle WE: Infrared heat lamps interfere with pulse oximeters. Anesthesiology 61:630, 1984
45. Geha DG: Blood gas monitoring. In Blitt CD (ed): Monitoring in Anesthesia and Critical Care Medicine, p 291. New York, Churchill Livingstone, 1985
46. Cork RC: Temperature monitoring. In Blitt CD (ed): Monitoring in Anesthesia and Critical Care Medicine, p 441. New York, Churchill Livingstone, 1985
47. Eichorn JH, Cooper JB, Cullen DJ et al: Standards for patient monitoring during anesthesia at Harvard Medical School. JAMA 256:1017, 1986
48. Standards for basic intraoperative monitoring. American Society of Anesthesiologists Newsletter. Chicago, American Society of Anesthesiologists, December 1986
49. Anesthesia apparatus checkout recommendations. Chicago, American Society of Anesthesiologists, October 1986
50. Saunders RJ: The computer in anesthesia. In Blitt CD (ed): Monitoring in Anesthesia and Critical Care Medicine, p 541. New York, Churchill Livingstone, 1985

Chapter 22   *James R. Zaidan*

Electrocardiography

Cardiac dysrhythmias occur at any time in the perioperative period. Although Levy and Lewis reported the development of dysrhythmias and sudden death during chloroform administration as early as 1911,[1, 2] it was not until 1968 that Vanik and Davis reported the incidence of perioperative dysrhythmias in a large series of patients:[3] 34% of the patients with heart disease in their study developed dysrhythmias. Interestingly, dysrhythmias occurred in 16.3% of the otherwise healthy patients. Administering regional anesthesia did not improve the incidence of dysrhythmias in the healthy patients. Kuner *et al*, in a study of Holter monitoring of 154 operative patients, reported that 62% of the patients had dysrhythmias.[4] As in the Vanik and Davis study, Kuner *et al* suggested that regional anesthesia did not reduce the incidence of perioperative dysrhythmias.

One must compare these perioperative studies to the occurrence of cardiac arrhythmias in the normal population. In 92 healthy children aged 7–11 years, heart rate varied between 37 and 197 beats·min^{-1}.[5] Junctional rhythms appeared in 45% of the children. Premature atrial and ventricular contractions occurred in 21%. Another study of healthy medical students revealed heart rates ranging from 37 to 180 beats·min^{-1}.[6] Minimal sleeping heart rates ranged from 33 to 55 beats·min^{-1}. Twenty-eight per cent had sinus arrests persisting greater than 1.75 s. Premature ventricular contractions occurred in 50% of the subjects, and 6% developed Wenkebach second-degree atrioventricular (AV) block. With these studies of unanesthetized subjects in mind, dysrhythmias occurring during anesthesia do not appear quite so ominous.

The decision to treat perioperative dysrhythmias depends on the overall cardiac status of the patient. For instance, a healthy patient undergoing uncomplicated surgery should not necessarily receive treatment for a junctional rhythm that does not significantly change blood pressure and clinical signs of perfusion. Conversely, this same dysrhythmia occurring in a patient with tight aortic stenosis might cause profound hemodynamic changes that require rapid treatment to prevent cardiovascular collapse.

This chapter aims to acquaint the reader with the electrocardiographic monitoring required to facilitate rapid diagnosing of intraoperative dysrhythmias. It will include lead placement and the surface electrocardiogram (ECG), methods of obtaining intracavitary ECGs, vector analysis, electrophysiology, and mechanisms of arrhythmias. Discussions of specific dysrhythmias will encompass supraventricular, nodal, and ventricular arrhythmias, bundle branch and AV nodal blocks, ischemic patterns, drug and electrolyte effects, and pacemakers.

Throughout the figures in this chapter, the top tracing is lead II and the bottom tracing is lead V_5 unless otherwise stated.

THE NORMAL ELECTROCARDIOGRAM

The electrocardiographic deflections separate into waves, complexes, intervals, and segments. Multiple waves form complexes, while intervals include waves and segments. Table 22-1 describes each of these deflections and their electrophysiologic significance. Sinoatrial (SA) nodal activity and atrial repolarization are invisible on the surface ECG.

Figure 22-1 reveals a normal surface ECG. Note that the P

587

TABLE 22-1.   Electrophysiologic Significance
of ECG Deflections

DEFLECTION	SIGNIFICANCE
P wave	Impulse spreads through atrium and AV node
PR interval	1. Conduction from AV node to Purkinje fibers 2. Atrial repolarization
QRS complex • Q wave • R wave • S wave	Ventricular activation • Any negative wave occurring before the R wave • Any positive wave • Any negative wave occurring after the R wave
ST segment	Occurs when the majority of myocardial cells are in phase 2 (plateau phase) Elevation or depression indicate ischemia
QT interval	Indicator of total ventricular depolarization and repolarization time; inversely proportional to heart rate
T wave	Represents ventricular repolarization
U wave	Related to ventricular repolarization

wave and T wave are upright in every lead except AVR and that the ST segment is isoelectric with the PR segment. With a standard paper speed of 25 mm·s^{-1}, each mm represents 0.04 s. Figure 22-1 therefore represents a PR interval of 0.152 s (normal range 0.12–0.20), a QRS duration of 0.088 s (normal <0.10 s), and a rate-corrected QT interval of 0.421 s. Figures 22-2–5 show different types of intraoperative interference that the anesthesiologist can encounter.

Figure 22-6 reveals the importance of calibrating and appropriately filtering the electrocardiographic signal. The first line, an ECG that was incorrectly calibrated, has almost 9 mm of ST-segment elevation. Correctly calibrated to 1 mV·cm^{-1} in the second line, the same patient had only 1.5 mm ST-segment elevation. Changes in low-frequency filtering create the difference in ST-segment elevation noted between the second and third tracings in Figure 22-6. The middle trace is filtered between 0.5 and 50 Hz, and the bottom trace is filtered from 0.05 to 100 Hz. Greater filtering of the ECG signal at the lower end of the signal (0.5 Hz $vs.$ 0.05 Hz) distorts the ST-segment change associated with ischemia. Generally accepted electrical filtering extends from 0.05 Hz high pass and 100 Hz low pass. Therefore, the third trace in Figure 22-6 is correctly filtered and reveals that the patient had a 4-mm ST-segment change. Although intraoperative lead placement tends to be haphazard, in fact, standardized placement helps interpret the ECG. Table 22-2 describes correct lead placement.

Impulses detected by the surface electrodes combine to cause deflections on the recorder in such a way that positive deflections have forces directed toward the electrode and negative deflections have forces directed away from the electrode. Electrical forces traveling perpendicular to the electrode do not cause a deflection on the ECG recorder and are therefore "invisible."

Three standard electrodes (right arm, left arm, and left leg) form a triangle, first described by Einthoven, in which the R-wave voltage in lead II should normally equal the combined voltages of leads I plus III. In the standard bipolar limb leads I, II, and III, each electrode equally influences the recorded ECG from locations on the extremities distant from the heart. Placing an exploring electrode close to the heart on the precordium and an indifferent electrode distant from the heart on an extremity lessens the influence of the indifferent electrode on the final ECG pattern. The "C" leads perform this task. The C

FIG. 22-1.   Normal ECG with sinus bradycardia.

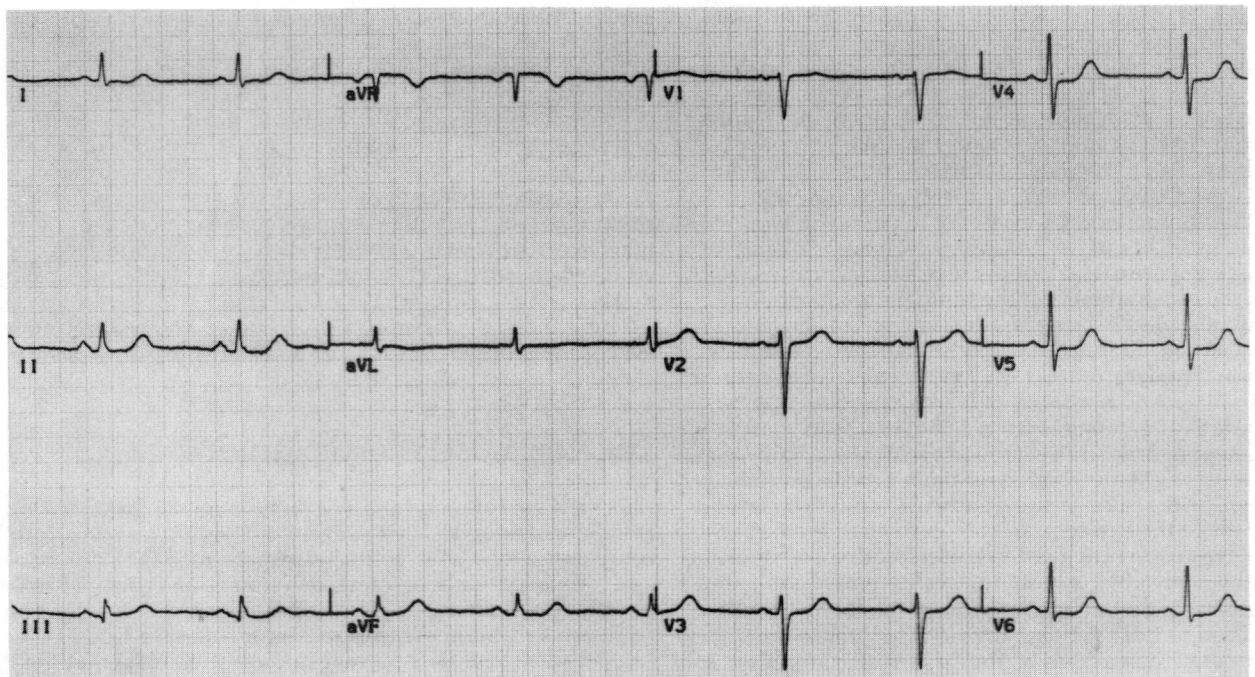

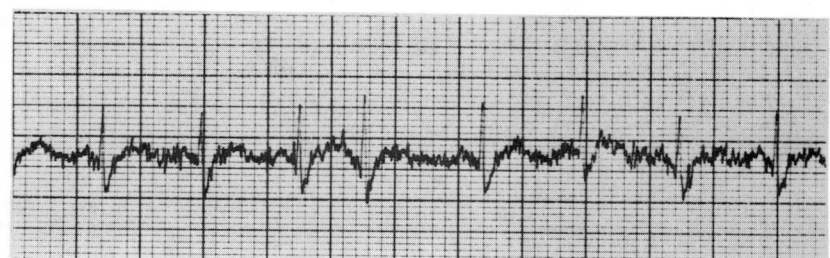

FIG. 22-2. Muscle artifact in the baseline makes it impossible to differentiate a premature atrial contraction from a junctional escape. Note the fourth R wave.

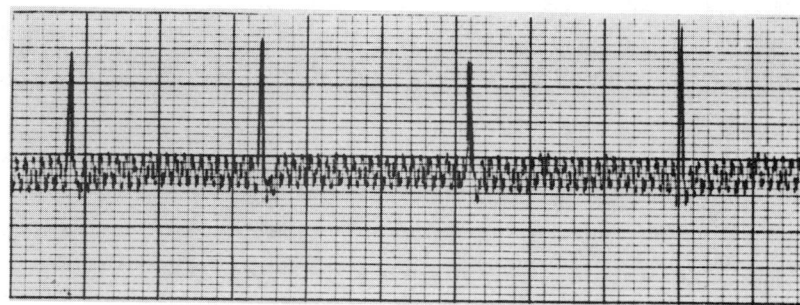

FIG. 22-3. 60-cycle interference affects the baseline.

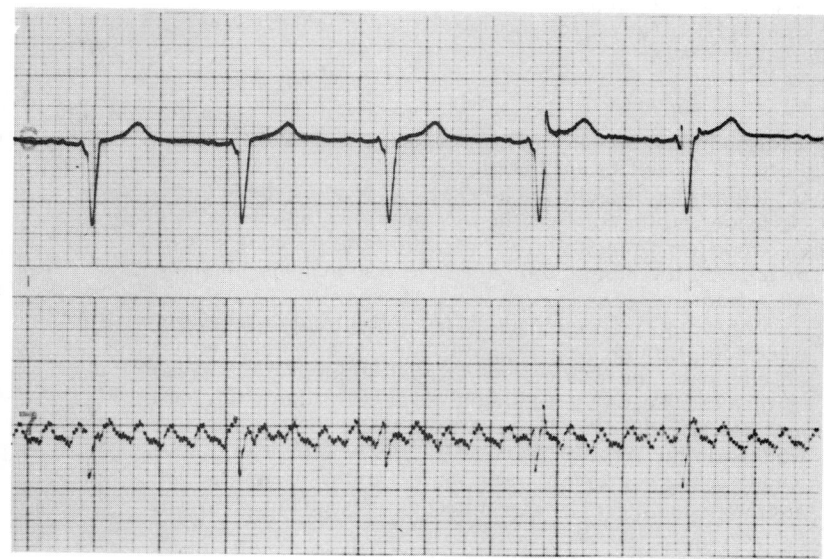

FIG. 22-4. The arterial pump head in the cardiopulmonary bypass machine distorts the ECG so that it appears like atrial flutter. This problem is created by the motor revolving within the column of blood in the arterial tubing. The top trace is lead II and the bottom trace is lead V_5.

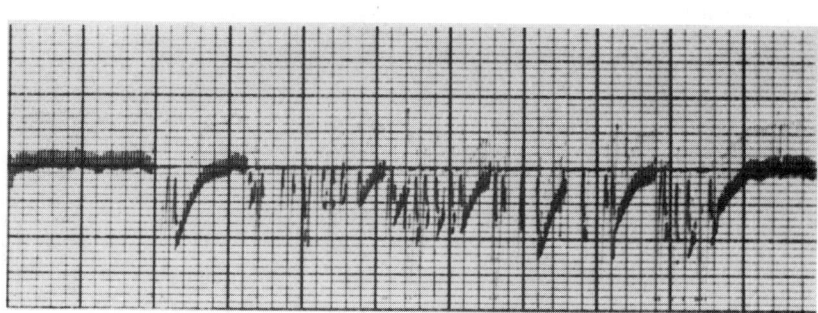

FIG. 22-5. The electrocautery totally distorts the electrogram.

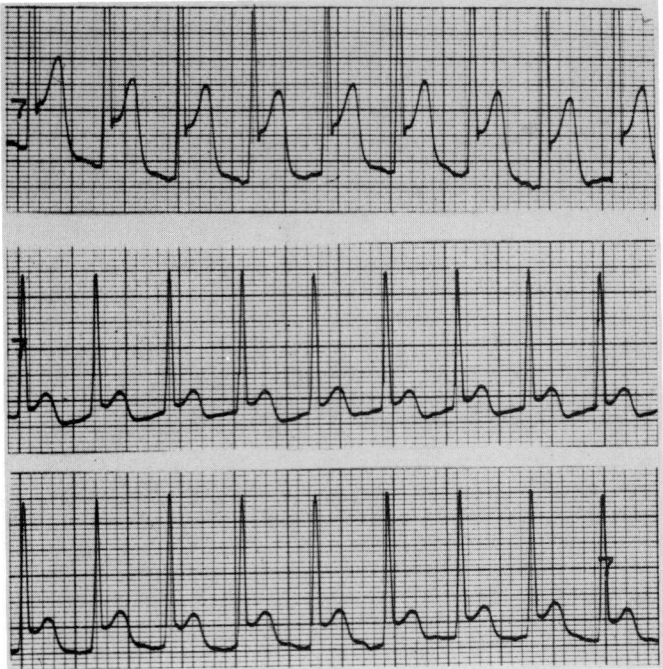

FIG. 22-6. A noncalibrated ECG (*top*) artifactually depicts 9-mm ST-segment elevation. The calibrated *middle* and *bottom* traces are filtered from 0.5–50 Hz and 0.05–100 Hz, respectively. The *bottom* trace is correctly filtered for ECG diagnosis of ST-segment change and reveals a 4-mm elevation.

leads are named according to the location of their indifferent electrode: C_F, left leg indifferent; C_R, right arm indifferent; and C_L, left arm indifferent. As an example, locating the left arm electrode (indifferent) over the left upper chest and the left leg electrode (exploring) over the V_1 position and selecting lead III on the ECG monitor modifies the C_L lead so that it is called the MC_{L1} lead.[7]

Connecting the combined left leg, left arm, and right arm electrodes through 5000 ohm resistances to a common terminal eliminates the indifferent electrode's influence on the precordial lead. Leads V_1–V_8, therefore, are considered unipolar and describe the impulse occurring under the surface electrode. Another type of unipolar lead is the limb lead. These leads are the commonly used V_R, V_L, and V_F leads that are augmented in height by disconnecting the right arm (V_R), left

arm (V_L), or left leg (V_F) electrodes from the common terminal. Augmentation performed by the ECG machine renames these leads aV_R, aV_L, and aV_F, respectively.

One can record impulses also from inside the heart if the monitor is appropriately electrically isolated. These intracavitary ECGs, which are called the *atrial electrogram (AEG)* and the *ventricular electrogram (VEG)* help to characterize complex atrial dysrhythmias. Figure 22-7 shows a typical AEG, and Figure 22-8 describes the intracavitary electrograms associated with placing an electrode into the ventricle. It is best when diagnosing an arrhythmia simultaneously to record the AEG and a surface lead II ECG. The VEG is not as clinically useful as the AEG. An esophageal ECG also can help to diagnose arrhythmias.[8] The esophageal probe, which contains large-surface-area electrodes, records impulses from the atrium or the ventricle.[9–11]

A special type of intracavitary electrogram, called the His bundle recording, requires multiple electrodes, special filtering, and fluoroscopy. After the impulse travels through the AV node, it enters the bundle of His. As shown in Figure 22-9, the very small His bundle deflection is located approximately midway between the atrial and ventricular deflections. Measuring the time between the P-wave or R-wave and His deflection estimates the time required for an impulse to travel from the atrium, through the AV node and bundle of His, to the ventricular conducting system. Normal conduction time intervals in the His bundle electrogram have wide variations. To ensure an accurate His bundle recording, the AEG and VEG recordings must be approximately equal in height (mv). Also, pacing from the electrode that is recording the His bundle deflection must produce a QRS complex identical to the surface lead's QRS complex. Once the catheter achieves good position, one can measure the PA (10–50 ms), SA (60–125 ms), and HV (35–55 ms) intervals.[12–16] The PA interval, measuring the time from the beginning of the surface P wave to the beginning of the intraatrial recording, estimates atrial activa-

FIG. 22-7. The AEG (*top*) clearly reveals atrial depolarizations compared to the V_5 lead (*bottom*). The *arrows* point out P waves on the AEG.

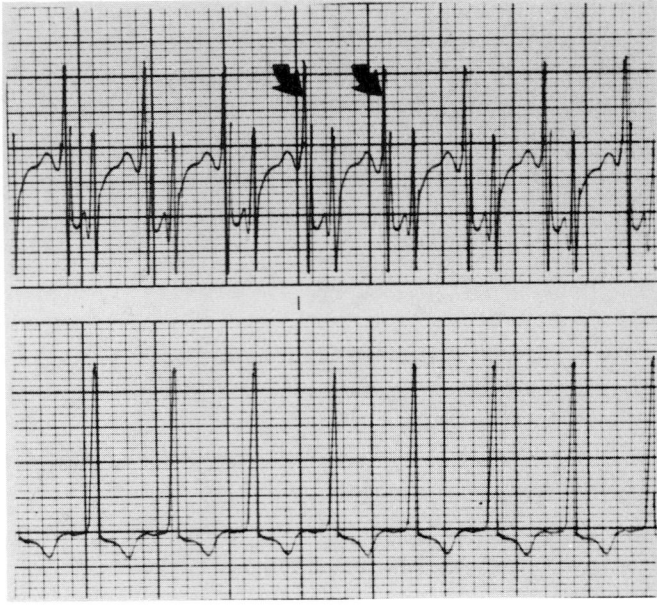

TABLE 22-2.   Correct ECG Lead Placement

LEAD	LOCATION
R_A	Right wrist
R_L	Right ankle
L_A	Left wrist
L_L	Left ankle
V_1	4th intercostal space, right of sternum
V_2	4th intercostal space, left of sternum
V_3	Between V2 and V4
V_4	5th intercostal space, left midclavicular line
V_5	5th intercostal space, left anterior axillary line
V_6	5th intercostal space, left midaxillary line

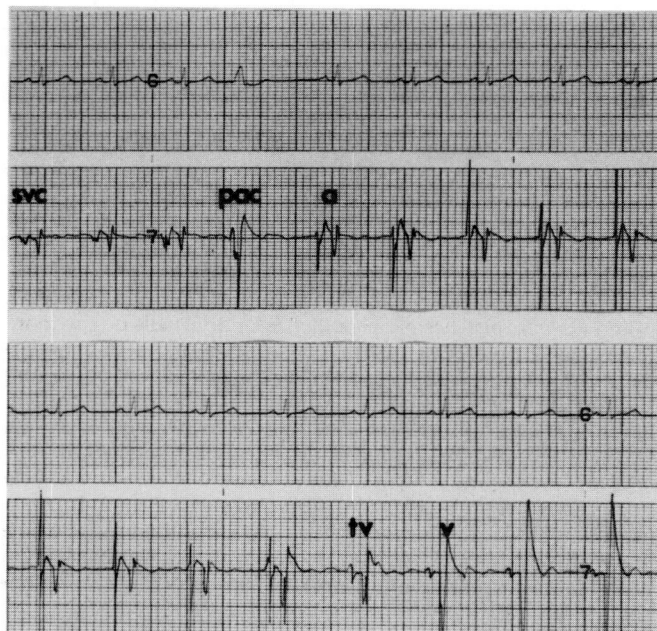

FIG. 22-8. Determine the exact location of an intracardiac electrode by observing the electrogram. In this example, the electrogram clearly shows the electrode as it enters the superior vena cava (SVC), atrium (A), tricuspid valve (TV), and ventricle (V). One premature atrial contraction (PAC) occurs.

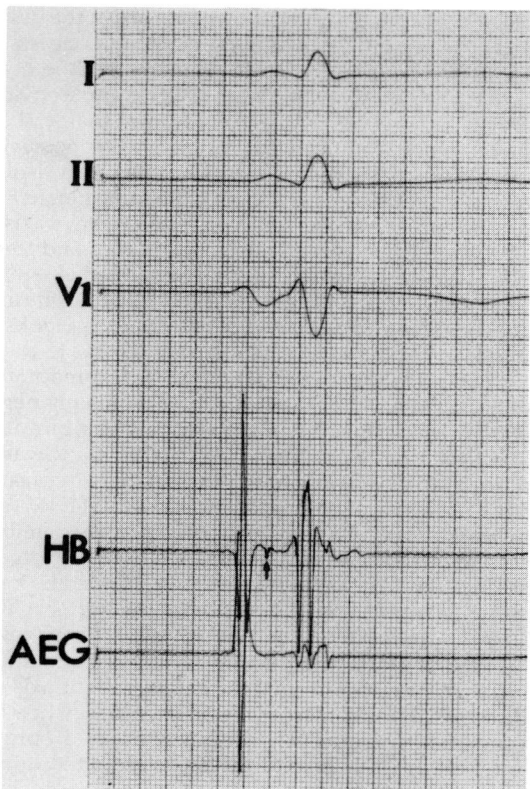

FIG. 22-9. The His bundle recording requires special catheters and electrical filtering. I, II, and V_1 are surface ECG leads. HB is the His recording showing the His deflection at the *arrow*. The atrial and ventricular depolarization are approximately equal in height compared to the atrial electrogram (AEG). (Courtesy of Paul Walter, M.D.)

tion time. The AH interval indicates the time for the impulse to proceed through the AV node, while the HV interval records the time necessary for the impulse to conduct through the His–Purkinje system. These intervals can be used to determine the effects of anesthetic drugs on conduction.[17]

Three methods exist for determining heart rate. The first method notes the number of 0.04 s units (1 mm) between R waves, multiplies 0.04 s times this number of units, and divides this number into 60. The second method quickly estimates heart rate. If two R waves have 5 mm between them (0.2 s), then the heart rate is 300. Each 0.2-s increase in the R–R interval indicates a decrease in the heart rate to 150, 100, 75, 60, 50, 43, 37, 35, and finally 30 beats · min^{-1} if there were 10 0.2-s units between R waves. The third method of determining heart rate involves knowing the number of seconds in the sweep speed of the ECG monitor. If the ECG monitor's sweep speed is 5 s, then the heart rate is 12 times the number of R waves in one sweep.

VECTORS AND ELECTRICAL AXIS

The sum of all of the impulses describes the electrical axis of the heart. One can determine an axis for the QRS complex, the P wave, and the T wave, and deviations from each normal axis have clinical significance. To determine an axis, one must first know the hexaxial reference system shown in Figure 22-10. Note that the standard limb leads are at 60° angles to each other, and that the augmented limb leads are oriented at 120° angles. Lead I, located at 0°, points directly to the right and aV$_F$ points directly downward. The directions of the other leads are easily placed by remembering the 60°/120° rule. The heart is theoretically placed on the hexaxial reference system so that

FIG. 22-10. The hexaxial reference system shows that leads I, II, and III are at 60° angles to each other, and leads aVR, aVL, and aVF are at 120° angles.

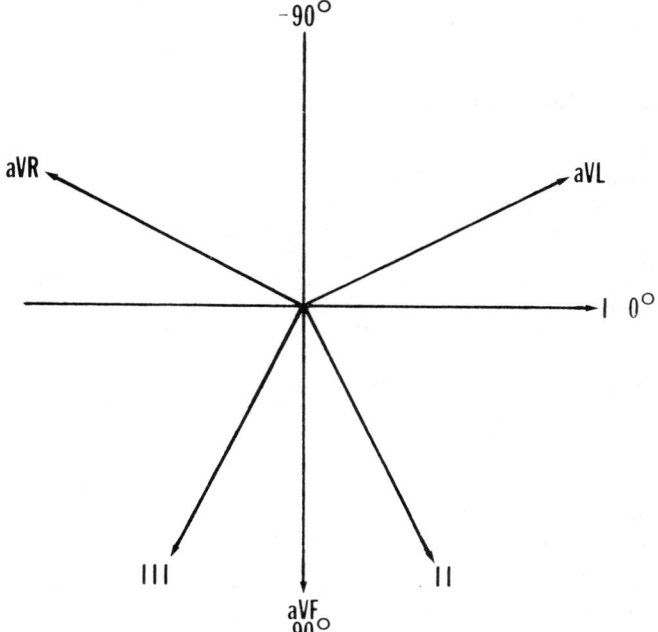

the septum lies on lead I, the left ventricle lies in the quadrant described by lead I and $-90°$, and the right ventricle lies in the quadrant between lead I and $+90°$. The first method of determining the QRS axis looks at the QRS complex with the highest voltage. The axis would point toward that lead on the hexaxial reference system if the voltage were positive and away from that lead if the voltage were negative. In Figure 22-1, leads I and II have approximately the same height R wave (6 mm). This configuration would place the R-wave axis equidistant between leads I and II. Since lead I is $0°$ and lead II is $+60°$, the estimated R-wave axis by this method is $+30°$. The second system first finds the ECG lead with equiphasic voltage (equal positive and negative voltage) and then looks at the voltage in lead II. The axis will be perpendicular to the equiphasic lead and toward lead II if lead II is predominately positive but away from lead II if II is predominately negative. Using Figure 22-1, lead III is slightly positive but approximately equiphasic. A positive lead II places the R-wave axis perpendicular to lead III and toward lead II, or in the vicinity of $+40-50°$. The final system of determining the QRS axis specifically measures the voltage in two of the standard limb leads and plots them on the hexaxial system. This last method, although simple in concept and can be performed by hand, is usually calculated by computer systems. The normal QRS axis is $-30+90°$. Minus $30°$ to $+90°$ indicates a left axis deviation and $+90-180°$ indicates a right-axis deviation. Left- and right-axis deviations can be normal variations. Right-axis deviations, however, should alert one to left posterior hemiblock, right ventricular hypertrophy, emphysema, and pulmonary embolus. Left anterior hemiblock and abdominal tumors or fluid that rotate the heart to the left are possibilities for left-axis deviation.[18] One may use the same methods to determine P-wave and T-wave axes. The T-wave axis generally points in the same direction as the QRS axis and should be within $50°$ of the QRS axis. The P-wave axis should point between leads I and II, but slightly closer toward lead II. Because the sum of all electrical forces in the atria point toward lead II, monitor this lead to see the most easily discernible P wave. A leftward shift of the P-wave axis indicates left atrial enlargement, and a rightward shift indicates right atrial enlargement. A right P-wave axis deviation greater than $+60°$ is strong evidence of chronic lung disease.[19]

ELECTROPHYSIOLOGY

A rapid influx of sodium ions through the cellular membrane creates phase 0 of the action potential and determines its maximal amplitude, overshoot, and rate of rise (V_{max}).[20] Hodgkin and Huxley later found that although sodium influx depolarizes, potassium extrusion repolarizes the membrane.[21] Hagiwara and Nakajina described two inward currents in cardiac conduction tissue.[22] One current, the fast channel responsible for phase 0 of the action potential, was due to the infux of sodium ions, and a second, slower current found later in the action potential was due to the influx of calcium ions.

The action potential encompasses five different phases (Figure 22-11A). Phase 0 occurs when an impulse of sufficient amplitude opens an activation "gate" or channel located in the external surface of the membrane that initiates entrance of sodium ions. Almost at the same instant, inactivation gates located in the internal surface of the membrane begin closing to impede the inward flow of sodium ions. The inactivation gates close slightly slower than the activation gates open. This slight delay is the period in which sodium enters the cell. Phase 1, extending from the peak of phase 0 to the beginning of the plateau phase, is thought to occur secondary to the beginning of an outward potassium current and an inward chloride current.[23, 24] During phase 2 the slow calcium channel that opened during phase 0 remains open because of its prolonged inactivation time constant of up to 500 ms. Calcium entrance counterbalances potassium extrusion, so that for up to 200 ms the transmembrane potential does not change. Phase 2, therefore, is called the plateau phase of the action potential. Phase 3 occurs when the slow inward flow of calcium ions diminishes and the outward potassium current continues.[25] The flow of potassium ions increases as the transmembrane voltage becomes more negative.

After reaching the maximal negative membrane potential, called the *maximal diastolic potential*, SA nodal cells begin spontaneously depolarizing during phase 4. Spontaneous depolarization in SA nodal cells is caused by the movement of calcium ions into the cell. When the SA nodal cell reaches the threshold potential, sodium quickly flows into the cell to create another phase 0. Automaticity in Purkinje fibers, unlike SA cells, is not secondary to calcium influx, but either to a slow decrease in an outward potassium current[26] or to an increasing diastolic inward sodium current.[27] Ventricular muscle normally does not have a phase 4 or a maximal depolarization potential, but rather has a constant resting membrane potential.

Figure 22-11B describes the appearance of action potentials in different areas of the heart. One notable fact is the lengthening of the action-potential duration in the distal Purkinje system and its shortening in ventricular muscle.[28] This lengthening of the action-potential duration in distal conducting fibers compared with ventricular muscle protects the ventricular muscle from receiving impulses in their relative refractory period.[29] Impulses entering ventricular muscle during the repolarizing phase could potentially fibrillate the heart.

ACTION POTENTIALS AND THE ECG

The relationship between multiple action potentials and the ECG is easy to visualize when one remembers that myocardial cells depolarize in sequence over a period of time.[30] It is this time delay in the onset of Phase 0 of the first action potential to the onset of phase 0 of the last action potential that inscribes the electrocardiographic pattern. The peak of the R wave occurs when the membrane potentials among the myocardial cells beneath the electrode are at their greatest differences. Phase 2, occurring simultaneously in most cells, creates a short period of time in which there are minimal voltage differences among the action potentials. Because the ECG electrode records no voltage difference, the ECG pattern becomes isoelectric and forms the ST segment. Phase 3 action potential delays create the T wave.

MECHANISMS OF ARRHYTHMIAS

Several cellular mechanisms create arrhythmias. These mechanisms either spontaneously initiate an impulse or require ongoing impulse formation with a circuit.

AUTOMATIC MECHANISMS

Changes in Normal Automaticity:

Cells in various areas of the heart display automaticity. These areas include the SA and distal AV nodes, bundle of His, bundle branches, Purkinje cells, and even cells in tricuspid

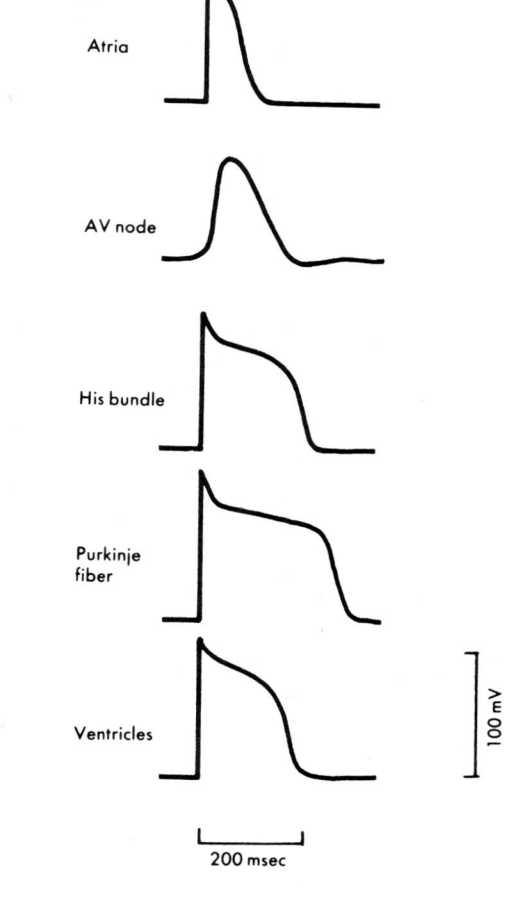

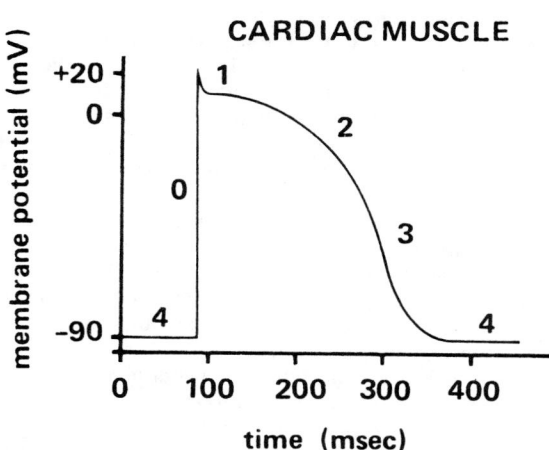

CARDIAC MUSCLE

FIG. 22-11. (A) Five phases (phase 0–4) comprise the cardiac action potential. These phases are described in the text. (B) Relationships of typical action potentials throughout the conduction system. Note the progressive lengthening of phase 2 from the atrium to the Purkinje fiber and then shortening of phase 2 in ventricular muscle. (Reproduced with permission. Marriott HJL, Conover MHB: Advanced Concepts in Arrhythmias. St Louis, CV Mosby, 1983.)

and mitral valves.[31–33] Normally, only SA nodal cells display sufficiently rapid automaticity and a less negative maximal diastolic potential to reach threshold before the other potential pacemaker cells.[34, 35] Changes in automaticity imply that slow depolarization during phase 4 of the action potential reaches threshold at a rate different than normal and is simply an enhancement of normal physiology. The slope of phase 4 could increase or decrease, causing an increase or decrease in heart rate or the ectopic rate.

Abnormal Automaticity:

Normal atrial and ventricular myocardial cells do not display phase 4 depolarization. Changing the resting membrane potential to −60 mV, however, creates abnormal automaticity through slow-response action potentials.[36–38] A less negative transmembrane potential not only initiates spontaneous depolarization in cells that normally do not have this type of activity[39, 40] but also permits spontaneously depolarizing cells to reach threshold before a pacemaker cell with a more negative transmembrane potential. In this instance, even ventricular or atrial muscle can initiate ectopic beats or tachycardias. Table 22-3 lists the effects of changes in maximal diastolic potential, threshold potential, and slope of phase 4 on heart rate.

TABLE 22-3.   Effect of Changes in Action Potential on Heart Rate

CHANGE	EFFECT
Increase slope of phase 4	Higher heart rate if in SA nodal cell Escape beats or ectopic focus
Decrease slope of phase 4	Slower heart rate if in SA nodal cell Less chance of escape beats or irritable focus
Less negative threshold	Slower heart rate if in SA nodal cell Less chance of escape beats or ectopic focus
More negative threshold	Faster heart rate if in SA nodal cell Escape beats or irritable focus
Less negative MDP	Higher heart rate if in SA nodal cell Escape beats or ectopic focus
More negative MDP	Slower heart rate if in SA nodal cell Less chance of escape beats or irritable focus

OSCILLATORY CURRENTS

Spontaneous oscillations can occur in transmembrane potentials. These oscillations in resting transmembrane potentials do not require a previous action potential to initiate them, and are thought by some to cause spontaneous impulses.[41] According to Lin et al, oscillatory currents that develop in response to repolarization are caused by calcium-initiated release of intracellular calcium that triggers a Na–Ca exchange.[42]

TRIGGERED ACTIVITY

Another mechanism responsible for cardiac dysrhythmias is the presence of early and delayed after-depolarizations.[43] Described by Bozler in atrial muscle[44] and by Cranefield and Aronson in Purkinje fibers,[45] delayed after-depolarizations occur after the cell has fully repolarized. Early after-depolarizations occur before completion of membrane repolarization. Both types of after-depolarizations can trigger another action potential of sufficient magnitude to reach the threshold potential. The dysrhythmias thereby created are called *triggered dysrhythmias.*

It is unclear how oscillatory currents described above relate to early after-depolarizations. They may represent the same phenomenon,[46] although Lin et al state that oscillatory currents are self initiating,[42] while after-depolarizations require a preceding depolarization.

The molecular mechanism responsible for creating after-depolarization remains unclear. Because cardiac glycosides are known to cause these depolarizations, the mechanism of after-depolarization is likely related to calcium.[46] The magnitude of after-depolarizations is increased by catecholamines and high levels of extracellular calcium.[47]

REENTRY

Reentry, another arrhythmogenic mechanism, can be ordered or random.

Ordered Reentry:

Schmitt and Erlanger described the requirements for reentry in 1929.[48] These requirements are a complete circuit by which an impulse can return to the beginning of the pathway, unequal conduction velocities in each limb of the circuit, and a unidirectional block.[46] Reentrant circuits that follow definite anatomic pathways are called *ordered reentry.* Reentrant circuits can be found in loops of Purkinje fibers;[49] unbranched collections of Purkinje fibers;[50] in the AV node;[51] at the junction of the atrium with the SA or at AV nodes;[52, 53] and at the junction of the Purkinje fibers with myocardial cells.[54] They give rise to many types of supraventricular dysrhythmias. Wolff-Parkinson-White (WPW) syndrome and AV nodal reentrant tachycardia are examples of ordered reentry.

Random Reentry:

In 1940, Wiggers noted that rapid rates of pacing fibrillated dog hearts.[55] Fibrillation requires a certain volume of myocardial cells for its initiation and persistence and represents fragmented wavefronts that are randomly conducted and blocked throughout the atrium or ventricle. The fragmented impulses block whenever they meet refractory tissue and retrogradely conduct to reactivate other limbs of the small circuits. Individual cells not receiving impulses in an orderly fashion respond by randomly contracting whenever they receive an impulse. Allessie et al suggest that the block does not necessarily require anatomically defined areas such as ischemia or infarction.[56] The blocks, however, can be the propagating impulse itself, creating a functionally inactive area of tissue. Atrial fibrillation is one example of random reentry.

Reflection:

It is possible for a quite small section of tissue, such as a group of myocardial cells, to have depressed conduction. Part of this section of tissue also could have total unidirectional blockade, while the remainder could continue transmitting impulses (Fig. 22-12). The transmitted impulse can reverse its direction, retrogradely proceed through the unidirectionally blocked area, and reenter the proximal segment. This type of reentry is called *reflection.* Reflection develops in longitudinally conducting fibers when a zone of depressed conduction separates two segments of normally conducting tissue.[57] Rozanski et al subdivided reflection into two types.[58] In their experiments, Rozanski et al characterized the action potentials of proximal (P) and distal (D) segments of ventricular muscle fibers separated by a nonelectrolytic sucrose gap (G) that represented the zone of depressed conduction. Normally conducting tissue would not retrogradely conduct to the proximal segment. A secondary depolarization that prolonged the action-potential duration in the proximal segment of the ventricular fiber characterized type I reflection (Fig. 22-13). Type II reflection (Fig. 22-14) occurs when the impulse returns to the segment proximal to the block after the proximal segment has fully repolarized. In type II reflection, the proximal segment actually develops two action potentials, the second of which can reenter normal areas. Reflection potentially causes premature beats.

PARASYSTOLE

Parasystole is the simultaneous existence of two totally independent pacemaker sites. As an example, one site could be in the sinus node that conducts normally, with a second site located in the distal Purkinje fibers. The second pacemaker site is protected from overdrive suppression by entrance block. If exit block does not exist, the secondary pacemaker continues discharging into the myocardium and causes an ectopic ventricular beat. This mechanism causes ventricular bigeminy, trigeminy, and so forth, depending on the discharge rate of the parasystolic site. It is very much like a patient having an asynchronous pacemaker that does not sense intrinsic electrical activity. This patient's ECG would reveal at least three different QRS morphologies: the sinus beat, the parasystolic ventricular beat, and fusion beats or a combination of the sinus and parasystolic beats.

ANTIDYSRHYTHMIC DRUG CLASSIFICATION

Anesthesiologists use many antidysrhythmic drugs. It is important to know the pharmacologic properties of these drugs to avoid their potentially serious side effects. Antidysrhythmic drugs are classified according to the drug's effect on a single myocardial cell's action potentials (Table 22-4 and 22-5).[59]

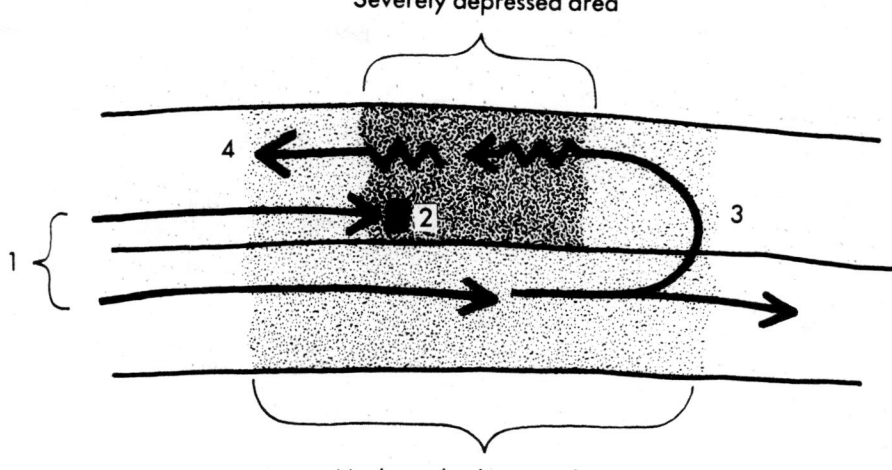

Severely depressed area

Moderately depressed area

FIG. 22-12. Illustration of reflection, in which the impulse (1) blocks in an ischemic area (2). The original impulse reflects at (3) and returns through the severely depressed area to its origin (4). (Reproduced with permission. Marriott HJL, Conover MHB: Advanced Concepts in Arrhythmias. St Louis, CV Mosby, 1983.)

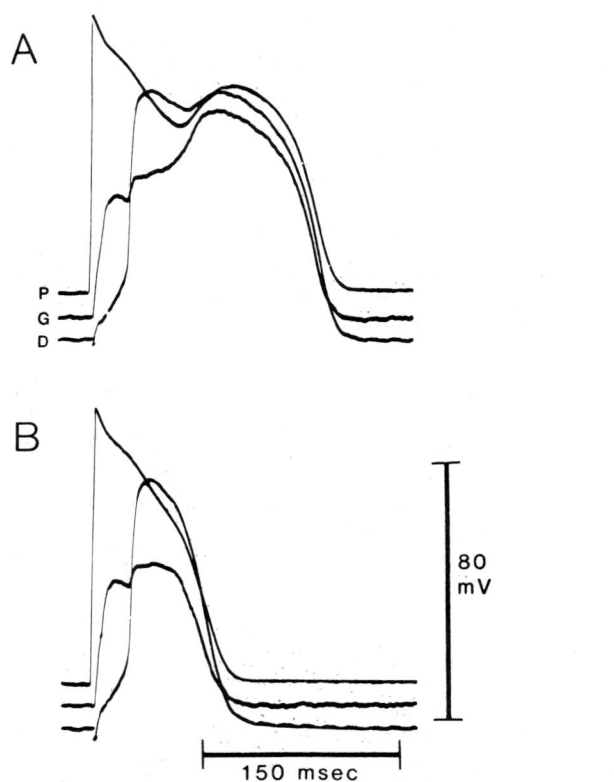

FIG. 22-13. (A) Type I reflection appears as a prolongation of phase 2 of depolarization in a proximal segment of a small section of ventricular muscle that was electrically divided into proximal (P) and distal (D) segments by a sucrose bath (G). (B) Conduction in the three segments when reflection does not occur. (Rozanski GJ, Jalife J, Moe GK: Reflected reentry in nonhomogeneous ventricular muscle as a mechanism of cardiac arrhythmias. Circulation 69:163, 1984. Reprinted by permission of the American Heart Association, Inc.)

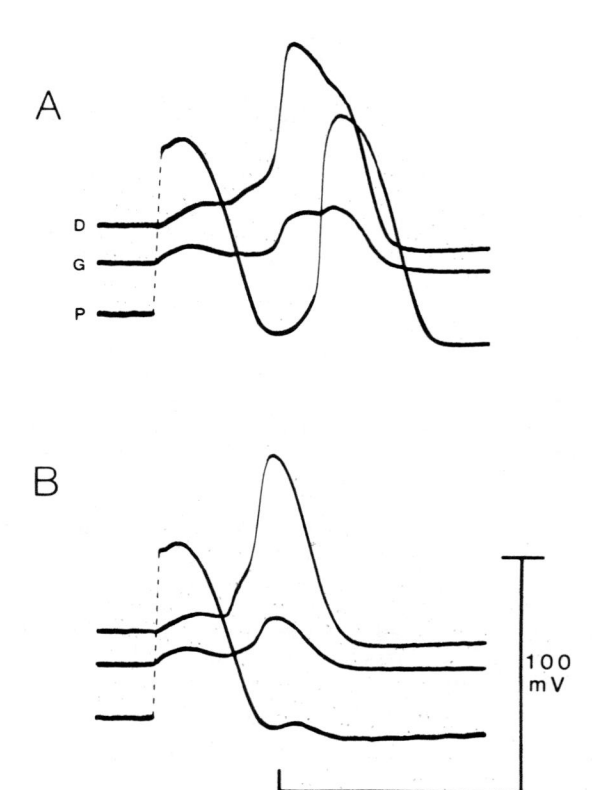

FIG. 22-14. (A) Type II reflection appears as a second action potential occurring in the proximal segment of a small section of ventricular muscle that was electrically divided by a sucrose gap. P = proximal segment; D = distal segment; G = sucrose gap. (B) Conduction in the three segments when reflection does not occur. (Rozanski GJ, Jalife J, Moe GK: Reflected reentry in nonhomogeneous ventricular muscle as a mechanism of cardiac arrhythmias. Circulation 69:163, 1984. Reprinted by permission of the American Heart Association, Inc.)

TABLE 22-4.   Classification of Antidysrhythmic Drugs

CLASS	ELECTROPHYSIOLOGIC ACTION	DRUGS
I. Membrane-stabilizing agents		
A	Depress phase 0 (dV/dt) Slow conduction moderately Prolong repolarization	Quinidine Procainamide Disopyramide
B	Minimal effect of phase 0 of the action potential Shorten repolarization	Lidocaine Mexiletine Tocainide Phenytoin
C	Markedly depress phase 0 of the action potential Marked slowing of conduction Minimal effect on repolarization	Encainide Flecainide Lorcainide
II. β-Adrenergic blocking agents		Propranolol Atenolol Metoprolol
III. Prolong repolarization	No effect on phase 0 of the action potential	Amiodarone Bretylium
IV. Calcium channel blockers		Verapamil Diltiazem

(Reprinted with permission. Platia EV: Management of Cardiac Arrhythmias, p 134. Philadelphia, JB Lippincott, 1987.)

CLASS I:

These membrane-stabilizing drugs block rapid sodium channels. Because of this effect, they reduce conduction velocity (reduce slope of phase 0 and decrease overshoot) and prolong the effective refractory period. Their ability to change conduction velocity and the refractory period make them useful in treating reentrant dysrhythmias. Automatic arrhythmias are terminated because class I drugs also slow phase 4 of depolarization. Investigators have further subdivided the class I drugs according to the degree of effect on the cell's action potential. Class IA drugs moderately reduce the slope of phase 0 and prolong the action-potential duration. Class IB agents have little effect of phase 0, but they increase the potassium repolarization current and therefore decrease the refractory period. Class IC drugs markedly slow phase 0 and conduction, but only minimally affect repolarization.

CLASS II:

These agents, the β-blocking drugs, terminate dysrhythmias solely by their action on the β-1 and β-2 receptors.[60]

CLASS III:

Drugs in the third category of antidysrhythmics prolong the action-potential duration and therefore lengthen the refractory period. Bretylium, which initially releases norepinephrine then later inhibits its release, extends the refractory period in His–Purkinje fibers and ventricular muscle cells.[61] By lengthening the refractory period in the His–Purkinje and ventricular cells, and therefore decreasing the dispersion of refractoriness, bretylium decreases the chance of microreentry. A totally different drug, amiodarone, functions similarly to bretylium, but is not limited to Purkinje and ventricular muscle cells.[62]

CLASS IV:

These drugs exert their influence primarily in the AV and SA nodes by blocking calcium channels. They have little if any effect on the fast sodium channels. Despite the fact that nifedipine is a calcium channel-blocking agent, it is not considered an antidysrhythmic drug, but rather a coronary vasodilator.

CLASS V:

This group, the cardiac glycosides, exerts its antidysrhythmic effect through the parasympathetic system.[63] It creates supraventricular and ventricular dysrhythmias by initiating triggered activity and increasing the slope of phase 4 of depolarization. Treatment of digitalis-induced dysrhythmias includes withholding the drug, administering potassium if the serum concentration is low, and possibly administering phenytoin, a drug known to terminate triggered activity.

SUPRAVENTRICULAR TACHYCARDIAS

Any tachycardia originating above the bundle of His is considered a supraventricular tachycardia. Included in this group of dysrhythmias are sinus arrhythmia and sinus tachycardia, atrial fibrillation and flutter, reentrant dysrhythmias, atrial

TABLE 22-5.   Pharmacologic Profile of Antidysrhythmic Drugs

CLASS	DRUG	COMMONLY USED DOSAGE	ELIMINATION HALF-LIFE	THERAPEUTIC PLASMA LEVEL ($\mu g \cdot ml^{-1}$)	SIDE-EFFECTS
IA	Quinidine	Oral: 200–600 mg q 6–8 hr IV: 6–10 mg $\cdot$ kg^{-1} over 30 min followed by 2–3 mg $\cdot$ min^{-1}	6 h	2–6	Quinidine syncope, conduction disturbances, nausea, vomiting, diarrhea, thrombocytopenia, hypotension
	Procainamide	Oral: 250–1000 mg q 4 h (q 6 for sustained-release form) IV: 10–20 mg $\cdot$ kg^{-1} over 20–40 min followed by 2–6 mg $\cdot$ min^{-1}	2–4 h	4–12 (8–15, N-acetyl procainamide)	Conduction disturbances, nausea, diarrhea, fever, lupus syndrome, hypotension
	Disopyramide	Oral: 150–300 mg q 6–8 h IV: 2 mg $\cdot$ kg^{-1} over 3–5 min	6–8 h	5–7	Cardiac depression, conduction disturbances, anticholinergic symptoms
IB	Lidocaine	IV: 1–2 mg $\cdot$ kg^{-1} bolus followed by 20–40 μg $\cdot$ kg^{-1} $\cdot$ min^{-1}	1–2 h	2–5	Drowsiness, hallucination, seizures, paranoid ideation
	Tocainide	Oral: 400–600 mg q 8 h	13–15 h	4–10	Tremor, dizziness, ataxia, paresthesia, rash, hepatitis, nausea, vomiting
	Mexiletine	Oral: 150–300 mg q 6–8 h	10–20 h	0.75–2.0	Tremor, convulsion, dizziness, photosensitivy, dermatitis, hypotension, nausea, vomiting
	Phenytoin	Oral: 200–400 mg once daily IV: 50–100 mg every 5 min to maximum 1 g	24 h	10–18	Hypotension, vertigo, lethargy, dysarthria, gingivitis, macrocytic anemia, lupus, pulmonary infiltrates
	Moricizine (ethmozine)	Oral: 75–200 mg q 8 h	4–10 h		Dizziness, headache, pruritus
IC	Encainide	Oral: 25–75 mg q 6–8 h IV: 0.5–1 mg $\cdot$ kg^{-1} over 15 min	3–4 h	0.01–0.02	Conduction disturbances, blurred vision, nystagmus, dizziness, ataxia, vertigo, paresthesia, nausea, proarrhythmic
	Flecainide	Oral: 100–200 mg q 12 h IV: 2 mg $\cdot$ kg^{-1} over 10 min	18–20 h	0.2–1.0	Blurred vision, headache, lightheadedness, ataxia, proarrhythmic
	Lorcainide	Oral: 100–200 mg q 12 h IV: 1–2 mg $\cdot$ kg^{-1} over 30 min	7–13 h (norlorcainide, 24 h)	0.05–0.3 0.08–0.3	Sleep disturbances, nightmares, tremor, hyponatremia, nausea, diarrhea
UNCLASSIFIED					
	Propafenone	Oral: 100–300 mg q 8 h IV: 2 mg $\cdot$ kg^{-1} over 15 min	4–8 h	0.5–2.0	Dizziness, metallic taste, conduction disturbances, nausea
II	Propranolol (β_1/β_2)	Oral: 20–80 mg q 6 h IV: 0.5–1 mg q 2 min to maximum 6–10 mg	3–6 h	0.05–0.1	Depression, fatigue, AV block, bradycardia, myocardial depression
	Acebutolol (β_1/β_2)	Oral: 600–1200 mg once daily	24 h		As above
	Atenolol (β_1)	Oral: 50–200 mg once daily	24 h		As above
	Nadolol (β_1/β_2)	Oral: 40–240 mg once daily	24 h		As above
	Timolol (β_1/β_2)	Oral: 20–60 mg	15 h		As above

(Continued)

TABLE 22-5. *(Continued)*

CLASS	DRUG	COMMONLY USED DOSAGE	ELIMINATION HALF-LIFE	THERAPEUTIC PLASMA LEVEL ($\mu g \cdot ml^{-1}$)	SIDE-EFFECTS
UNCLASSIFIED					
III	Amiodarone	Oral: 800–1600 mg · day^{-1} for 2 weeks then 200–600 mg · day^{-1} maintenance IV: 5–10 mg · kg^{-1} bolus over 5–15 min; then 800–1600 mg · day^{-1} as a continuous infusion or in divided doses	13–60 days		Corneal deposit, gastrointestinal disturbances, altered thyroid function, interstitial pulmonary disease, peripheral neuropathy, bradycardia, conduction block, hepatic dysfunction
	Bretylium	IV: 5–10 mg · kg^{-1} bolus over 10–30 min, then 1–4 mg · min^{-1}	6–8 h	0.8–2.0	Transient hypertension, sinus tachycardia, postural hypotension, proarrhythmic
IV	Verapamil	Oral: 80–160 mg q 6–8 h IV: 5–10 mg bolus, repeated after 10 min to a maximum of 20 mg Continuous infusion: 1–5 $\mu g \cdot kg^{-1} \cdot min^{-1}$	4–8 h	0.1	Cardiac depression, hypotension, AV block, asystole, edema, headache, constipation
	Diltiazem	Oral: 60–90 mg q 6 h	3–5 h		Edema, postural hypotension
OTHER AGENTS					
	Digoxin	Oral: 1–1.5 mg in divided doses over 24 h for digitalization; 0.125–0.25 mg once daily for maintenance IV: 0.75–1 mg in divided doses over 24 h for digitalization	1.5 days	1–2	Anorexia, nausea, vomiting, diarrhea, malaise, fatigue, confusion, headache, colored vision, arrhythmias, aggravation of heart failure

β_1/β_2, noncardioselective β-blockers; β_1, cardioselective β-blockers.
(Reprinted with permission. Platia EV: Management of Cardiac Arrhythmias, p 135. Philadelphia, JB Lippincott, 1987.)

tachycardia, multifocal atrial tachycardia, and AV junctional tachycardia. This section presents a brief discussion of each category of supraventricular tachycardia.

SINUS ARRHYTHMIA

Sinus arrhythmia is a normally occurring variation in heart rate that occurs with respiration. In older patients, however, the phenomenon can be symptomatic in the presence of hypothyroidism, digitalis, and calcium channel-blocking drugs (Fig. 22-15).

SINUS TACHYCARDIA

One of the most common dysrhythmias observed by the anesthesiologist is sinus tachycardia (Fig. 22-16). Causes include arterial hypoxemia, hypoventilation, light anesthesia, hypovolemia, hyperthermia, and antimuscarinic drugs. Treatment, directed toward correcting the underlying cause, includes evaluation of oxygenation and ventilation, deepening anesthesia, appropriate volume replacement, and possibly administration of β-blocking drugs. Pacing and cardioversion do not assume a role in controlling sinus tachycardia.

AV block generally does not occur in the presence of sinus tachycardia. Because impulses conduct through the AV node with gradual slowing, however, it is possible for AV nodal block to occur at a rate of 180–200 beats · min^{-1}. AV nodal block rarely occurs in hearts free of disease, but can potentially occur at lower rates in patients with coronary artery or valvular heart disease. If tachycardia-induced AV block occurs in patients with heart disease, then consider a β_1 blocking agent such as metoprolol in intravenous doses of 0.5 mg titrated to effect with a maximum dose of 5 mg. As atrial rate slows, 1:1 AV nodal conduction should resume.

ATRIAL FIBRILLATION

Atrial fibrillation produces an irregularly irregular QRS pattern and a fibrillatory baseline (Fig. 22-17). If the diagnosis is not obvious, then recording the AEG will confirm the presence of the fibrillatory baseline (Fig. 22-18).

Atrial fibrillation is associated with higher mortality in some patients.[64] Patients with chronic atrial fibrillation without associated cardiovascular disease have a higher mortality rate than patients in sinus rhythm. Patients with paroxysmal atrial fibrillation suffered a higher mortality rate only in the presence of cardiac disease such as mitral stenosis and coronary artery disease. The Framingham study shed light on antecedent factors for developing atrial fibrillation.[65, 66] There is a 2% risk of developing atrial fibrillation over a 20-yr period. This risk increases in the presence of congestive heart failure, rheumatic heart disease, and hypertensive cardiovascular disease. The average time to death after developing atrial fibrillation was 6 years. Investigators have demonstrated an increased risk of developing atrial fibrillation with increasing left atrial size, especially if the left atrial size is greater than 4.5 cm.[67]

Patients with atrial fibrillation persisting longer than ap-

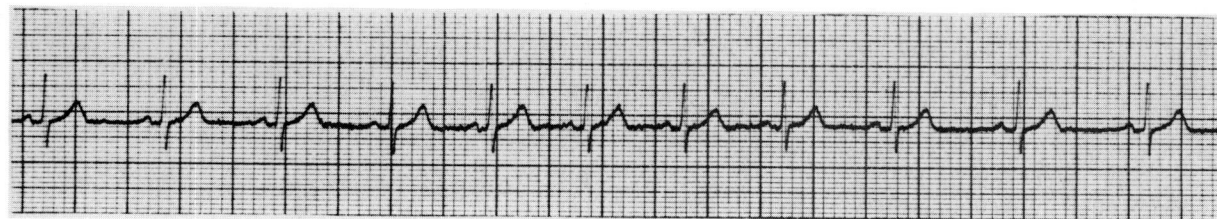

FIG. 22-15. Sinus arrhythmia.

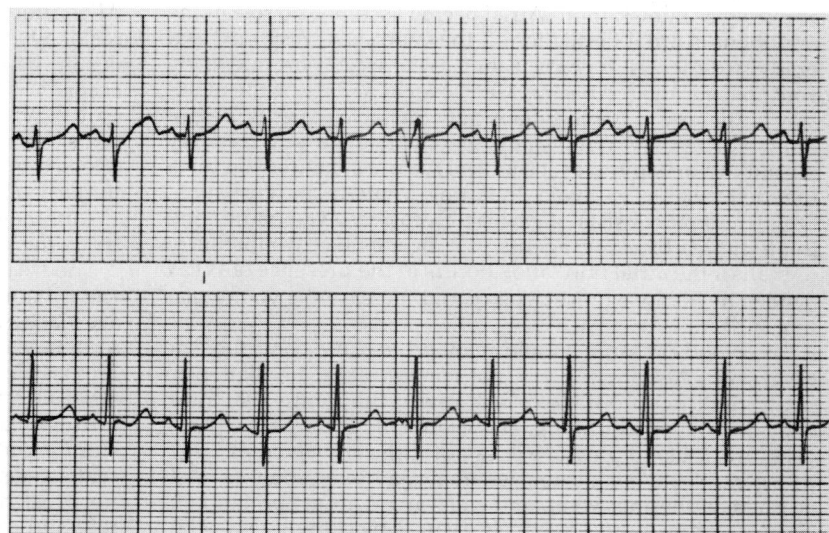

FIG. 22-16. At a rate of 125 beats · min^{-1}, and P waves occurring on a 1:1 basis with the R waves, this ECG shows sinus tachycardia. The top trace is lead II and the bottom is lead V$_5$.

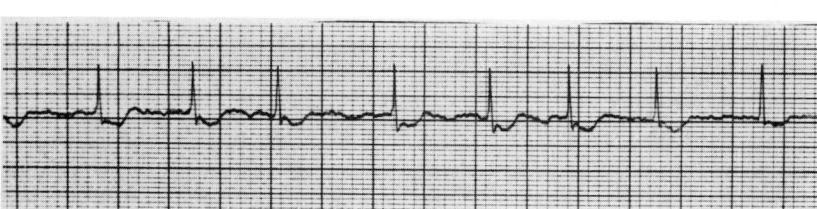

FIG. 22-17. This ECG demonstrates atrial fibrillation. It has a fibrillatory baseline and irregularly irregular R waves.

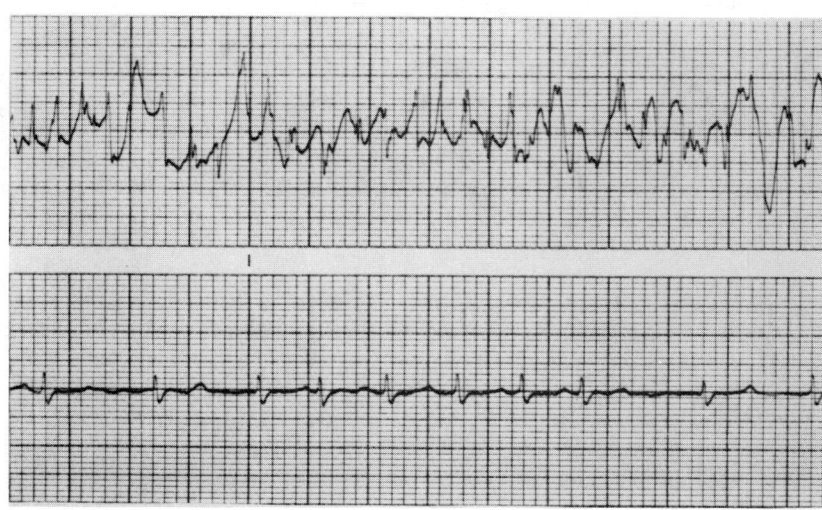

FIG. 22-18. The atrial electrogram (*top*) clearly reveals a fibrillatory pattern and is consistent with atrial fibrillation. The simultaneous surface ECG is shown in the *bottom* tracing.

proximately 1 week can develop an atrial thrombus and, eventually, an arterial embolus. Many patients experiencing chronic atrial fibrillation therefore take warfarin.

Patients with chronic atrial fibrillation without other significant cardiac disease generally are hemodynamically stable without major beat-to-beat changes in blood pressure if the ventricular response is 70–100 beats·min^{-1} (Fig. 22-19). Acute onset of atrial fibrillation, however, can create extreme hemodynamic instability. Initially, the very high ventricular rate substantially reduces ventricular filling. The end result is a high rate and low cardiac output and blood pressure.

Treatment focuses on controlling heart rate by cardioversion and drug administration. Atrial pacing assumes no role in the treatment of atrial fibrillation. If the ventricular response is at bradycardic levels, therapy is then to increase heart rate using ventricular inhibited pacing. Cardioversion remains the mainstay of therapy in hemodynamically unstable patients. Beginning with 50 watt/s (joules), incrementally increase the energy output to a maximum of 300 joules. Assure synchronization of the defibrillator to avoid initiating ventricular fibrillation. Drug therapy consists of cardiac glycosides, verapamil, and β-adrenergic blocking agents.[68–71] Do not use verapamil or digitalis if the atrial fibrillation occurs in the presence of WPW syndrome because these drugs could increase the ventricular rate.[72, 73]

The blood pressure should respond to acute control of the heart rate. Although it will not convert atrial fibrillation to sinus rhythm, propranolol will lower the ventricular rate, allow for ventricular filling, and eventually increase the blood pressure. If blood pressure does not sufficiently increase after rate control, then consider using an α-adrenergic agent such as phenylepherine. Verapamil will convert atrial fibrillation to sinus rhythm more effectively than β-blocking agents. Because acute hypokalemia could cause atrial fibrillation, judicious potassium replacement through a central intravenous catheter potentially can revert fibrillation to sinus rhythm without other therapy.

ATRIAL FLUTTER

Atrial flutter occurs less commonly than atrial fibrillation. One diagnoses this dysrhythmia by noting a saw-toothed base line with inverted P waves on the surface ECG (Fig. 22-20). The AEG unquestionably diagnoses atrial flutter (Fig. 22-21). Occasionally, the AEG will show a combination of fibrillation and flutter, as noted in Figure 22-22. Two types of atrial flutter occur.[74, 75] Type I flutter has an atrial rate of 250–350 beats·min^{-1}, while type II flutter has higher atrial rates of 340–430 beats·min^{-1}. Because of failure of AV conduction at high atrial rates, the ventricular response to type I and type II atrial flutter is approximately 150 beats·min^{-1}.

Automaticity and reentry cause atrial flutter; however, reentry is the more common cause.[76, 77]

The treatment of atrial flutter includes rapid atrial pacing, vagal maneuvers, cardioversion, and drug administration. Exact placement of an electrical impulse within the atrial cycle terminates reentrant type I atrial flutter. Clinically, it is almost impossible to place a stimulus in the precise location in the atrial electrical cycle to block the circuit and terminate the arrhythmia. Rapid atrial pacing, which delivers up to 800 stimuli per min, performs this task. Waldo *et al* have shown that atrial pacing at the flutter rate will entrain the atrium but not break the reentry.[78] One must pace higher than the flutter rate and create a morphologic change in the flutter wave in

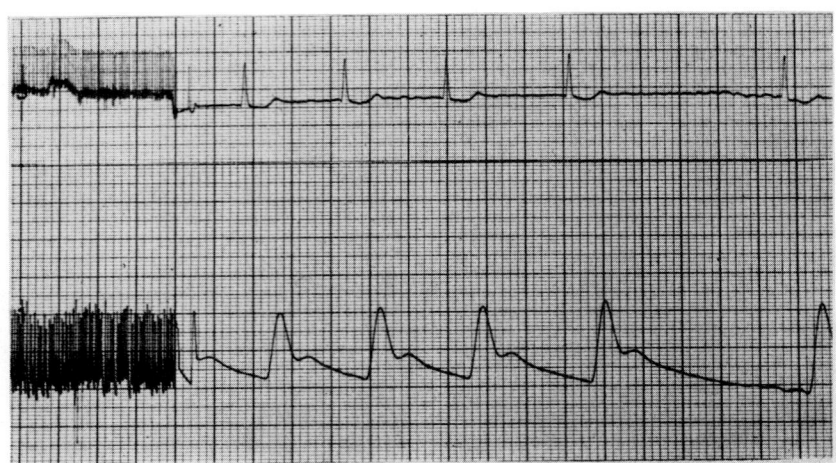

FIG. 22-19. Atrial fibrillation has a characteristic tracing in the arterial pressure line. Like the ECG, the pressure tracing is irregularly irregular occasionally with long pauses, but if the heart rate remains between 70 and 100 beats·min^{-1}, the blood pressure should remain stable.

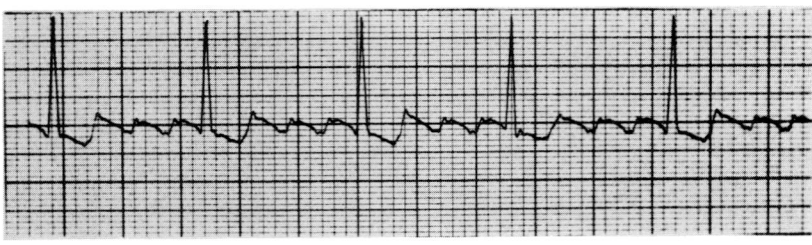

FIG. 22-20. A saw-toothed base line comprised of inverted P waves helps to diagnose atrial flutter. In this ECG, the atrial rate is 250, characteristic of type I flutter, and the ventricular rate is 57.

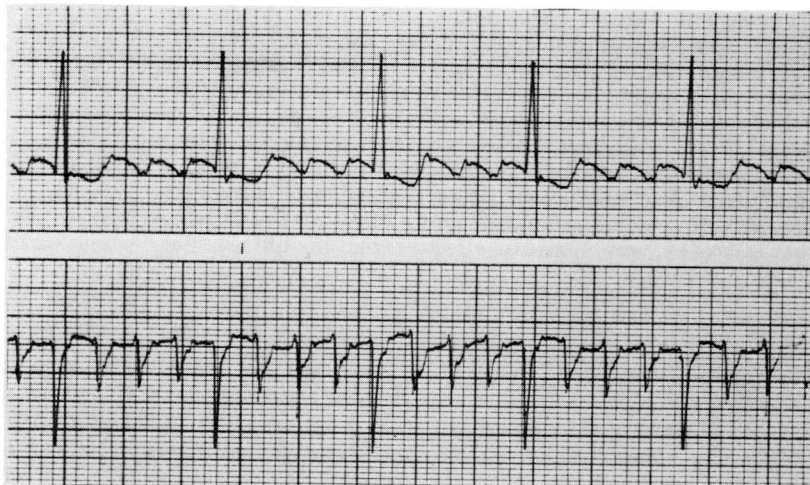

FIG. 22-21. The atrial electrogram (*bottom*) clearly reveals atrial flutter waves. The *top* trace is lead II.

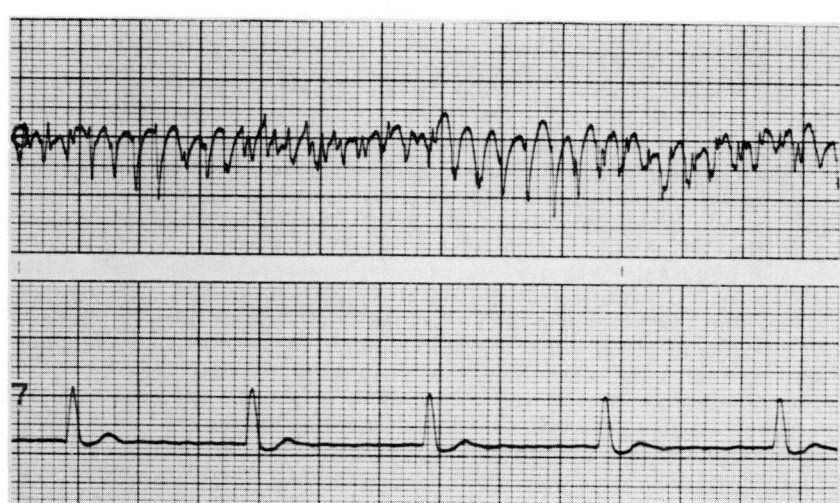

FIG. 22-22. The atrial electrogram (*top*) is a fibrillation–flutter pattern reminiscent of ventricular Torsade de Pointes. The *bottom* tracing is lead V₅.

order to terminate this arrhythmia. Type II atrial flutter generally will not terminate with rapid atrial pacing techniques.

Vagal maneuvers, such as carotid massage, do not always convert atrial flutter to sinus rhythm. Conversion occurs with increased vagal tone only if the reentrant circuit includes the AV node. If the reentrant circuit is located entirely within atrial tissue and does not include the AV node, then carotid massage could slow the ventricular response. Slowing the ventricular response might reveal previously undiagnosed atrial flutter waves.

Cardioversion is another form of treatment. Atrial flutter responds to energy levels as low as 25 joules.[79]

As in atrial fibrillation, the goal of drug therapy is control of ventricular rate. AV nodal blocking drugs such as verapamil, glycosides, and β-adrenergic blockers, represent primary drug therapy. Class IA antidysrhythmics may convert atrial flutter to sinus rhythm. By slowing the atrial flutter rate, thereby decreasing concealed conduction, and by their vagolytic action, class IA agents can increase the ventricular rate.[80] Class IA agents commonly are used in conjunction with β-adrenergic blocking drugs to control the ventricular rate.

ATRIOVENTRICULAR NODAL REENTRANT TACHYCARDIA

Another supraventricular tachycardia involves reentry in the AV node. The AV node is a highly complex structure that can dissociate into two conducting pathways that join proximally and distally into common pathways.[81–83] The AV node, therefore, represents a location for a reentrant dysrhythmia. In fact, it is possible to have two forms of AV nodal reentrant tachycardia.[84] The more common form (slow-fast) conducts slowly through the antegrade limb and rapidly through the retrograde limb, while the less common form (fast-slow) conducts rapidly through the antegrade limb and slowly through the retrograde limb. The slow-fast type of this dysrhythmia begins with a premature atrial beat and has its inverted P wave inscribed within the QRS complex because retrograde conduction is very rapid. The fast-slow form of this dysrhythmia begins with either a ventricular or atrial premature complex, or sinus tachycardia. The P wave occurs after the QRS complex because atrial activation takes place by way of the slow retrograde pathway.

Treatment focuses on vagal maneuvers, cardioversions, rapid atrial pacing, and drugs. Because the reentrant circuit includes the AV node, stimulating the parasympathetic system with a Valsalva maneuver or very careful carotid artery massage should terminate this arrhythmia. Rapid atrial pacing and DC cardioversion starting with 25 joules also should readily convert the arrhythmia to sinus rhythm. Verapamil is the drug of choice;[85] however, glycosides, β-adrenergic blockers, and edrophonium can also terminate the arrhythmia. Class IA agents are less effective than the other antiarrhythmic drugs.

ATRIOVENTRICULAR RECIPROCATING TACHYCARDIA

This supraventricular tachycardia commonly receives the name *preexcitation syndrome* or *Wolff-Parkinson-White syndrome* (Fig. 22-23). Patients with WPW syndrome have two AV nodal conducting pathways: one pathway is the normal AV node, bundle of His, and Purkinje system; and the second pathway is the anomalous AV nodal bypass tract or Kent bundle. The atrial impulse normally conducts over both of these pathways, leading to a short PR interval (<0.12 s) and a widened QRS complex with a delta wave or initial slurring of the PR interval into the QRS complex.[86] The reentrant circuit in WPW syndrome includes an atrium and a ventricle, the normal AV conducting pathway, and the anomalous tract.

WPW syndrome includes two subgroups, depending on the direction of the major deflection within the V_1 QRS complex. The QRS complex in type A has an R wave visible in V_1, while the QRS complex in type B contains an S wave in V_1. An R wave in V_1 indicates that the impulse arrives in the left ventricle and travels toward the V_1 electrode, and an S wave in V_1 describes an impulse that begins in the right ventricle and spreads toward the left ventricle away from the V_1 electrode. The QRS duration depends on several factors.[87] If the impulse traveling through the accessory pathway arrives at the ventricle many ms before the impulse traveling through the AV node, then the QRS complex will be very wide and bizarre. If, however, the two impulses arrive at approximately the same time, the QRS complex will be of normal duration. Abnormal repolarization leads to ST–T-wave abnormalities.

Concealed WPW syndrome occurs when the accessory pathway conducts only in a retrograde direction. Absence of anterograde conduction in the accessory pathways masks all of the electrocardiographic findings of WPW syndrome (short PR, delta wave, widened QRS), but these patients still develop supraventricular tachycardias.[88]

Patients with WPW syndrome can develop atrial fibrillation, atrial flutter, or the reciprocating tachycardia. Treatment focuses on controlling ventricular rate. Vagal maneuvers are a reasonable first-line therapy. Intraoperative onset of a supraventricular tachycardia could require cardioversion if hypotension occurs. Since digoxin decreases refractoriness in the accessory pathway, avoid its use. The class IA antidysrhythmics, quinidine, procainamide, and disopyramide, increase refractoriness in the accessory pathway and should help to maintain sinus rhythm.

SINOATRIAL REENTRANT TACHYCARDIA

Occasionally, the SA node forms part of a reentrant circuit that includes the atrium.[89] Premature atrial beats are an initiating event of this arrhythmia. During the tachycardia, the P waves appear similar to the normal P wave. This dysrhythmia masquerades as sinus tachycardia, but unlike sinus tachycardia, terminates with rapid atrial pacing.

ACCELERATED ATRIOVENTRICULAR JUNCTIONAL TACHYCARDIA

AV nodal cells normally have a phase 4 of depolarization that permits a rate of 40–60 beats·min^{-1} (Figs. 22-24 and 22-25). Although it is normally suppressed by SA nodal activity, the AV node occasionally increases its rate through enhanced automaticity. The factors causing enhanced automaticity in the AV node include hypokalemia, digitalis intoxication, and ischemia.[90] When the junctional rate increases to 70–100 beats·min^{-1}, the arrhythmia is called an accelerated AV junctional rhythm (Fig. 22-26). An accelerated junctional tachycardia occurs when the heart rate surpasses 100 beats·min^{-1}. The hemodynamic effect of a junctional rhythm reflects independent atrial and ventricular contractions with atrial cannon waves and hypotension alternating with a normal central

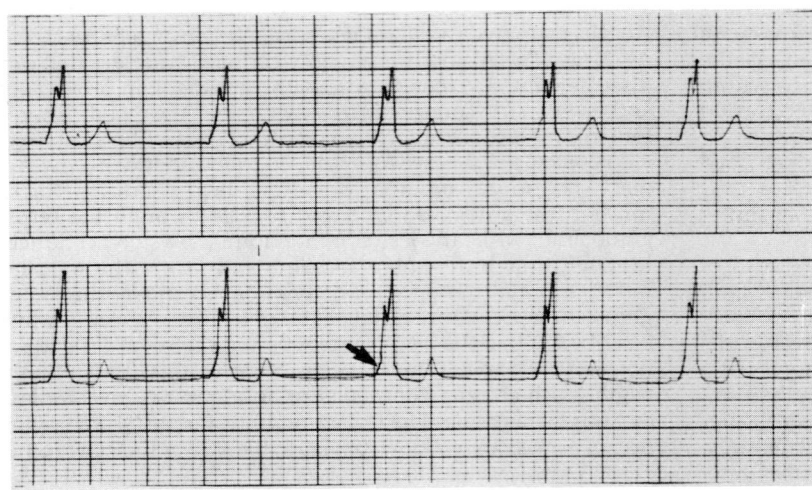

FIG. 22-23. Wolff-Parkinson-White syndrome includes a short PR interval (approximately 0.08 s), a delta wave (*arrow*), and an intraventricular conduction delay. The *top* trace is lead II, and the *bottom* trace is lead V_5.

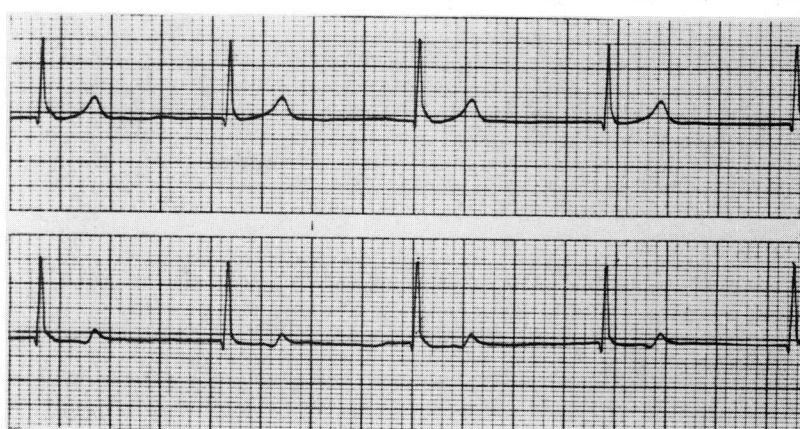

FIG. 22-24. Idiojunctional rhythms (rate = 40 beats·min⁻¹) commonly have visible P waves in the QRS complex. The P waves are noted here in the terminal phase of the R wave and cause the slurring effect. The *top* trace is lead II, and the *bottom* trace is lead V₅.

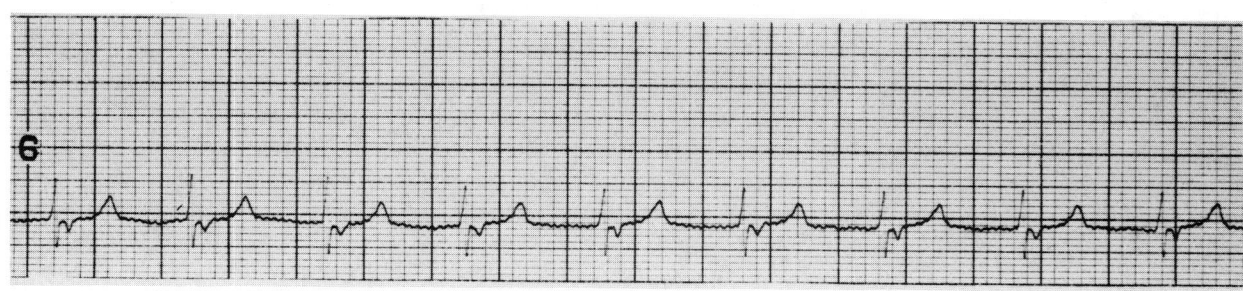

FIG. 22-25. This ECG demonstrates retrogradely conducted, and therefore inverted, P waves.

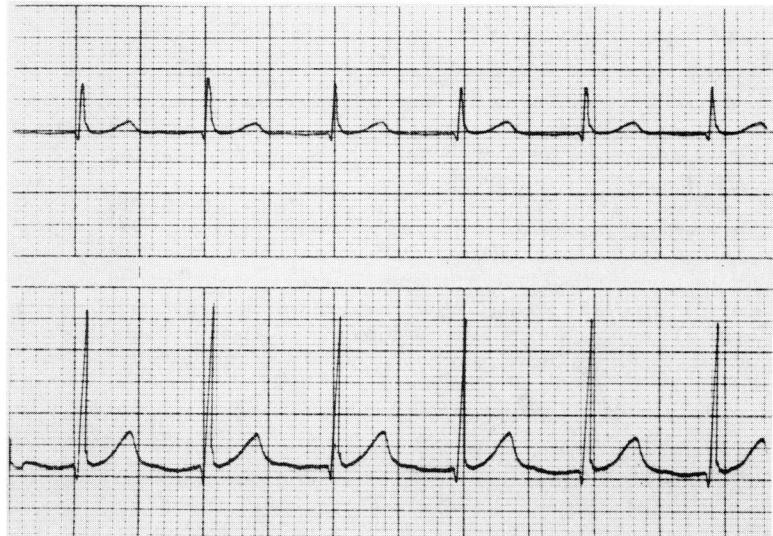

FIG. 22-26. An accelerated idiojunctional rhythm occurs when the junctional escape mechanism increases to greater than 70 beats·min⁻¹. In this case, the rate is 77 beats·min⁻¹, and the P waves slur the terminal phase of the R waves. The *top* trace is lead II, and the *bottom* trace is lead V₅.

venous pressure (CVP) tracing and normal blood pressure (Fig. 22-27).

These dysrhythmias are secondary to enhanced automaticity; therefore, rapid atrial pacing is not a therapeutic option. In the presence of intact AV conduction, atrial pacing restores atrial kick. Consider using AV sequential pacing if the patient has AV nodal block with the junctional rhythm.

ATRIAL TACHYCARDIA

The final group of supraventricular tachydysrhythmias is the atrial tachycardias. These dysrhythmias, entirely contained within the atrium, have reentry and enhanced normal or abnormal automaticity as their pathophysiologic mechanism. Because the reentrant atrial tachycardias do not include the

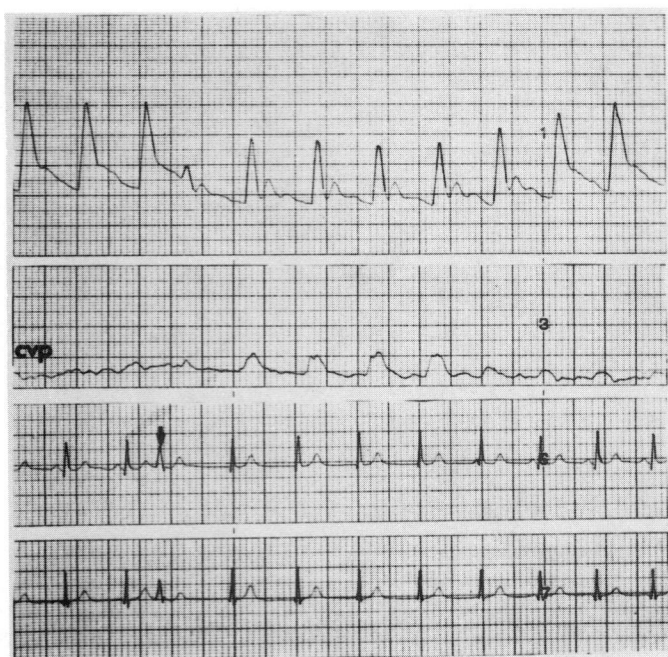

FIG. 22-27. The sudden onset of an idiojunctional rhythm occurs with an aberrantly conducted junctional beat (*arrow*). The loss of atrial kick causes a loss of blood pressure (*top*) and the appearance of cannon waves on the CVP (*second* trace). The reappearance of the sinus mechanism restores arterial pressure and the atrial cannon waves disappear. The *third* trace is lead II, and the *fourth* trace is lead V₅.

SA or AV nodes in their circuit, vagal maneuvers will not terminate the arrhythmia. Class IA drugs can successfully convert atrial tachycardia to sinus rhythm. Chronic lung disease and digitalis intoxication are common antecedents. It is nearly impossible to differentiate between an automatic atrial tachycardia and a reentrant atrial tachycardia without using specialized electrophysiologic testing.

Multifocal atrial tachycardia occurs in patients with chronic lung disease, coronary artery disease, and hypokalemia. This type of atrial tachycardia has varying P–P, P–R, and R–R intervals and at least three different P-wave morphologies.[91] Cardiac glycosides do not convert multifocal atrial tachycardia to sinus rhythm. Restoring potassium and magnesium levels, or administering procainamide or quinidine, however, can

stop the dysrhythmia.[92, 93] Unfortunately, this dysrhythmia commonly recurs.

VENTRICULAR ARRHYTHMIAS

Ventricular irritability presents as unifocal and multifocal premature contractions, ventricular tachycardia, and ventricular fibrillation (Figs. 22-28–30). The differential diagnosis of ventricular irritability during anesthesia should include myocardial ischemia with all of its possible antecedent factors; hypercarbia; direct stimulation from surgery and central monitoring catheters; reflex enhancement of parasympathetic tone; and drug interactions. Ventricular premature contractions associated with increased pulmonary artery pressures are caused by hypoventilation and arterial hypoxemia until proven otherwise.

Ventricular irritability occurring during myocardial ischemia likely originates through a reentrant mechanism because programmed stimulation initiates and terminates ventricular tachycardia.[94] More recently, clinical studies in patients with ventricular aneurysms and ventricular dysrhythmias revealed that resection of areas of the ventricle that had continuous electrical activity during diastole resulted in ablation of the arrhythmia.[95–97] Animal studies in infarcted dog heart models revealed that electrical activity occurring in the normally quiet diastolic period was related to ingrowth of scar tissue into myocardial tissue. This ingrowth of scar separated and disoriented myocardial muscle cells so that activation of this area was prolonged.[98] Investigators believe also that ventricular dysrhythmias occur due to triggered activity.[43, 99]

The clinical impression is that for a premature ventricular contraction to cause ventricular tachycardia, the premature ventricular contraction must fall on the T wave.[100] In fact, a premature ventricular beat located any place in the cardiac cycle can initiate ventricular tachycardia.[101–103] A depolarization traversing any repolarizing area can initiate reentry and ventricular tachycardia. The surface ECG reflects the electrical events not in one cell, but rather in all of the myocardial cells. For this reason, small areas of myocardium repolarize at various times around the T wave, not just during peak of the T wave; therefore, a premature ventricular contraction occurring late in the ST segment or after the T wave could cause ventricular tachycardia.

Hypercarbia with its associated hypertension and tachycardia potentially causes ventricular irritability. Also, reflex bradycardia secondary to surgical manipulation or laryngoscopy can result in idioventricular escape complexes. More direct

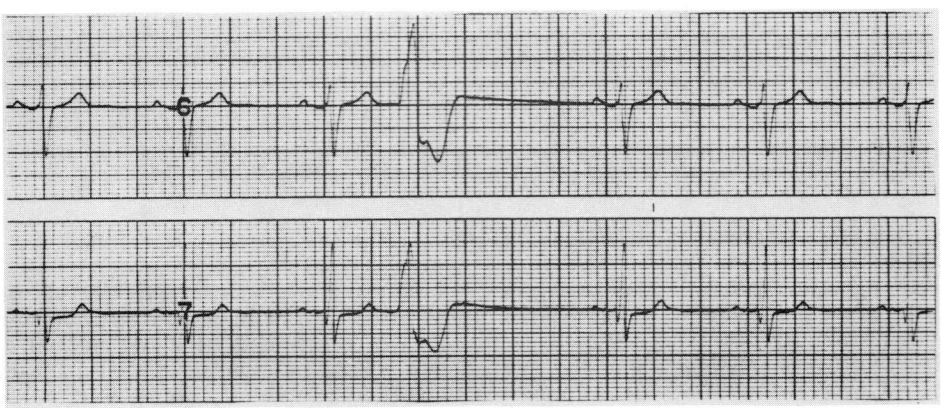

FIG. 22-28. It is difficult to distinguish an aberrantly conducted beat from a premature ventricular contraction (PVC), which is itself aberrantly conducted. This ECG likely reveals a PVC because it is unrelated to atrial activity, is fully compensated (see text), and has an increased QRS duration. The normal P wave occurs in the T wave of the PVC. The *top* trace is lead II, and the *bottom* trace is lead V₅.

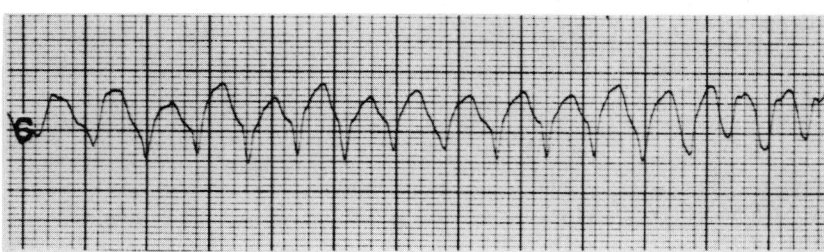

FIG. 22-29. Ventricular tachycardia.

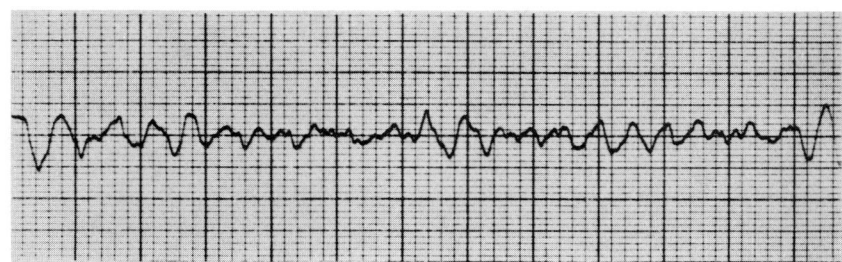

FIG. 22-30. Ventricular fibrillation.

causes of ventricular irritability include direct manipulation from pulmonary and esophageal surgical procedures and right ventricular stimulation from a pulmonary artery catheter.

Combinations of drugs may also cause ventricular dysrhythmias. Chronic administration of imipramine followed by pancuronium and halothane is associated with increased serum norepinephrine levels and ventricular arrhythmias.[104] Aminophylline plus halothane but not enflurane creates ventricular irritability if the serum concentration of aminophylline is greater than the therapeutic range.[105]

Epinephrine combines with the volatile anesthetics to cause ventricular irritability.[106–108] The irritability appears to occur through the α receptor;[109, 110] however, the β_1 and β_2 effects at lower doses could decrease diastolic pressure and increase heart rate and secondarily cause ventricular irritability in patients with coronary artery disease. Johnson et al determined in dogs that enflurane required the greatest dose of epinephrine, 10.9 $\mu g \cdot kg^{-1}$, to produce ventricular irritability. Isoflurane required 6.7 $\mu g \cdot kg^{-1}$ and halothane, the most sensitizing volatile anesthetic, required only 2.1 $\mu g \cdot kg^{-1}$.

Treatment of ventricular irritability focuses on terminating the premature beats as quickly as possible while determining and correcting the cause. Assure oxygenation and ventilation, remove the surgical stimulus that may have caused parasympathetic effects, and quickly treat hypertension and tachycardia. Consider the possibility that a pulmonary artery catheter might be coiled within the ventricle. It is seldom necessary to insert a pulmonary artery catheter further than 25% of the patient's height in cm. Bradycardia may result in ventricular escape beats. If the bradycardia has a sinus or an idiojunctional mechanism, then increase heart rate by administering an antimuscarinic or by atrial pacing if atrial electrodes are available. Drug therapy consists of lidocaine, 1 $mg \cdot kg^{-1}$, followed by an infusion at a rate of 2–4 $mg \cdot min^{-1}$. Also useful is bretylium, 5 $mg \cdot kg^{-1}$, with a 1–4 $mg \cdot min^{-1}$ infusion. Procainamide is occasionally useful. Administer 30 $mg \cdot kg^{-1}$ of procainamide up to a maximal dose of 1 g until the arrhythmia terminates, then maintain the serum level with an infusion of 1–4 $mg \cdot min^{-1}$. Stop the infusion of procainamide if the QRS complex widens by 50%.

It is important but very difficult to distinguish ventricular complexes from aberrant supraventricular complexes.[111] Unfortunately, lead II, the most commonly used ECG lead, cannot adequately distinguish ventricular contractions from aberrantly conducted beats (Figs. 22-31–33). Problems arise because ventricular tachycardias and bundle branch blocks have deep Q waves (QS pattern) in lead II. Another problem is that dissociated atrial activity, usually thought to imply ventricular tachycardia, occurs also during junctional tachycardia. If retrograde AV conduction remains intact, then ventricular tachycardia can create retrograde P waves.[112] Finally, although we think of a fusion beat as a supraventricular complex combining with a ventricular complex, it is possible, as shown by Kistin, that a supraventricular complex and an aberrantly conducted junctional complex can join to form a fusion beat.[113] Despite all of the pitfalls in differentiating supraventricular from ventricular complexes, clinicians generally accept the following criteria as indicative of ventricular activity:

1. QRS>0.12 s
2. Full compensation (two normal R–R intervals equals the R–R interval circumscribing the premature beat)
3. Dissociated from atrial activity
4. Premature in relation to the sinus beats

Wellens et al characterized the criterial for diagnosing ventricular ectopy.[114] When in doubt, treat a wide QRS complex as though it were ventricular in origin.

TORSADE DE POINTES

An unusual variety of ventricular tachycardia, torsade de pointes (Fig. 22-34), occurs in patients with prolonged QT intervals. The various causes of the QT interval prolongation include congenital prolongation; antidysrhythmic drugs such as procainamide, quinidine, and disopyramide; subarachnoid hemorrhage; and electrolyte disturbances.[115–118] It commonly occurs just after aortic unclamping during cardiac surgery. It is associated with variant angina and occurs in the presence of

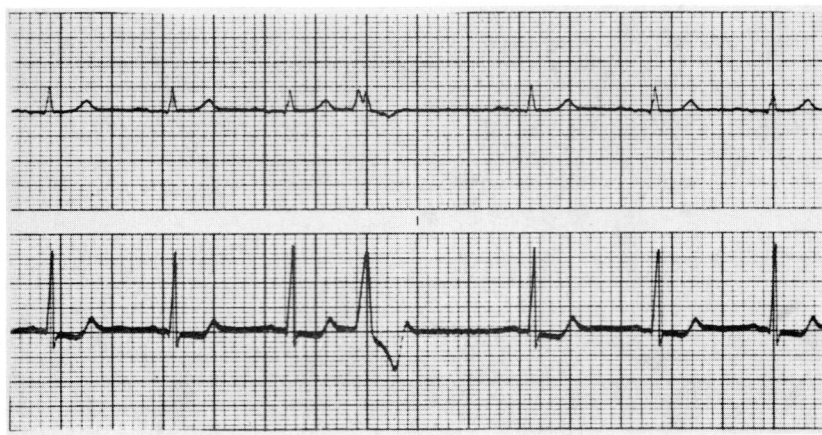

FIG. 22-31. Full compensation indicates a ventricular origin; however, QRS duration (0.14 s) and similar initial forces (upward) imply aberrant conduction. The *top* trace is lead II, and the *bottom* trace is lead V₅.

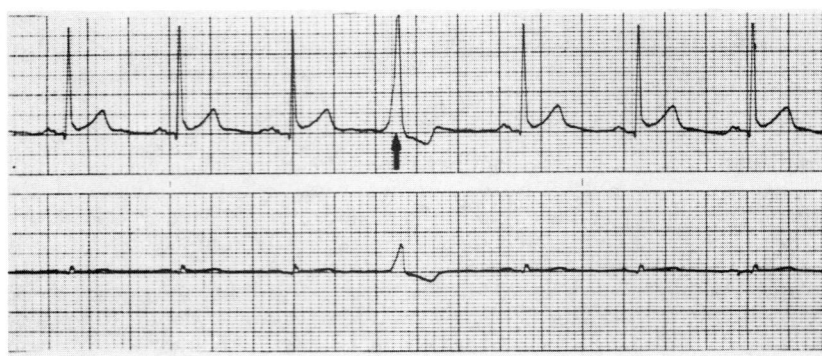

FIG. 22-32. This QRS complex (*arrow*) is likely a premature junctional with aberrant conduction. The *top* trace is lead II, and the *bottom* trace is lead V₅.

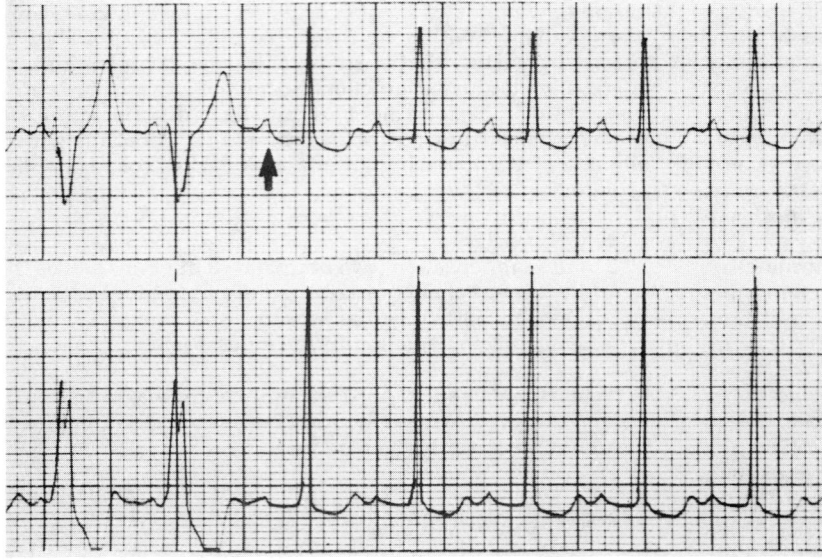

FIG. 22-33. A short PR interval finds the bundle branches somewhat refractory, leading to bundle branch block (first two QRS complexes). An increased time for the impulse to conduct through the AV node (first-degree block starting at *arrow*) finds the bundle branches fully repolarized and capable of normally conducting the impulse. The first two QRS complexes, therefore, represent abberant conduction and not ventricular contractions. The *top* trace is lead II, and the *bottom* trace is lead V₅.

bradycardia.[119] The electrocardiographic pattern is one of ventricular tachycardia twisting around a central axis.

The importance of torsade de pointes is that one must avoid administering the usual antiarrhythmic drugs. Treatment includes correcting the underlying electrolyte problem, pacing for bradycardia, and cardioversion.

BUNDLE BRANCH BLOCK

Ventricular activation proceeds in parallel, not in series. If one of the bundle branches slows or blocks conduction, then the impulses quickly travel to the normal ventricle. The impulse then slowly conducts through the intraventricular septum and

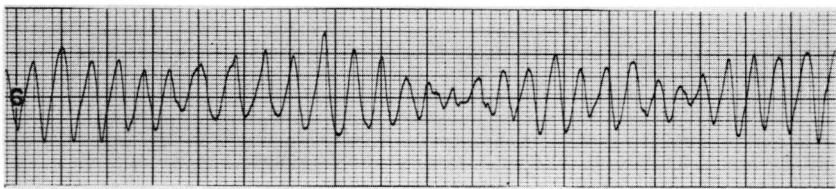

FIG. 22-34. A Torsade de Pointe pattern of ventricular tachycardia occurs when the depolarization waves twist around a central axis. Altered concentrations of myocardial potassium, calcium, or magnesium and prolonged QT interval syndrome, either drug induced or congenital, accompany this ECG pattern.

blocked ventricle. The electrocardiographic pattern reflects this concept.

RIGHT BUNDLE BRANCH BLOCK

The septum depolarizes from left to right, as is normal, before the left ventricular muscle mass depolarizes from the septum toward the free wall (right to left). Finally, the right ventricular electrical forces depolarize from the septum toward the right ventricular free wall (left to right). Overall, the ECG in V_1 initially shows an upward deflection (septal activation toward V_1); second, a downward deflection (left ventricular activation away from V_1); and third, another upward deflection (unopposed right ventricular forces toward V_1) (Fig. 22-35). This pattern in V_1 is an rSR' deflection.

LEFT BUNDLE BRANCH BLOCK

Abnormal right to left septal activation simultaneously occurs with right ventricular activation. The septal forces overwhelm the right ventricular forces. The left ventricle activates from the septum toward the free wall. Overall, the ECG in V_6 contains an initial upward deflection (right ventricular and septal forces combined), followed by a minimal downward deflection (septal activation finishing), quickly followed by another upward deflection (left ventricular activation). The pattern in V_6, therefore, is an R wave with a notch at the peak (Fig. 22-36). Leads I and aV_L can have the same general ECG patterns as V_6. Figure 22-37 compares leads I, V_1, and V_6 in right and left bundle branch block.

One would expect abnormal repolarization in the presence of abnormal depolarization. T waves should travel secondarily in a direction opposite to the terminal forces of the QRS complex. It is abnormal for T waves to move in the same direction as the terminal force of the QRS complex.[120]

Bundle branch blocks occasionally associate with abnormal left or right axis deviation. Combined complete left bundle branch block and left axis deviation is associated with a higher mortality rate.[121, 122] Bundle branch patterns can occur either as a single complex or runs of complexes related to heart rate. Premature atrial beats that are very early in the cardiac cycle can meet a refractory bundle branch that has not fully repolarized. Also, a very late premature atrial beat could meet a bundle branch that has already slightly depolarized during phase 4. In this instance, conduction could be slow enough to create an ECG picture of bundle branch block. In some patients with heart disease, a bundle branch block can occur during episodes of tachycardia.

THE HEMIBLOCKS

It is possible for the left bundle branch to have a block distal to its division into the anterior and posterior fascicles. A block occurring in one of the fascicles is called a *hemiblock*. It is difficult to relate a specific anatomic lesion in the left bundle branch to the electrocardiographic patterns associated with the hemiblocks.[123, 124] In posterior hemiblock (Fig. 22-38), look for a right axis deviation and sometimes a Q wave in II, III, and aV_F, and in anterior hemiblock (Fig. 22-39), look for a left axis deviation.[125]

Problems arise when trying to determine which patient with a bifascicular block would require perioperative temporary pacing. In a study of 544 patients with chronic bifascicular block and trifascicular disease, McAnulty *et al* reported that only 19 patients suffered from heart block. Of 160 deaths, 42% were attributable to tachycardia and acute myocardial infarction rather than bradycardia associated with heart block.[126]

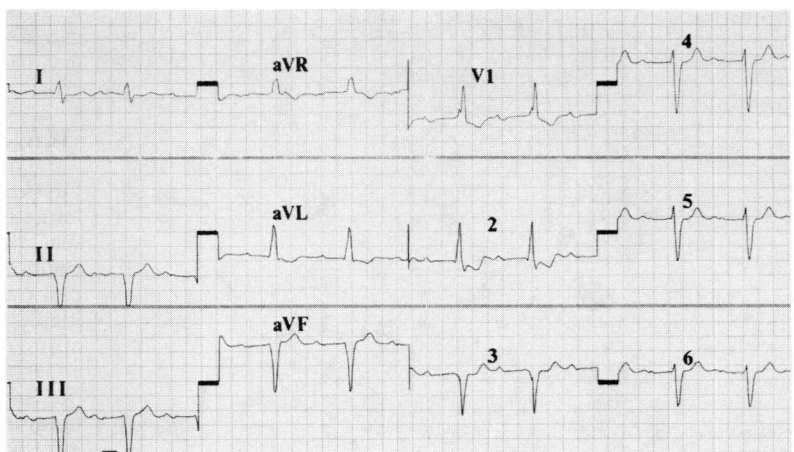

FIG. 22-35. Diagnose right bundle branch block by noting the QRS configuration in lead V_1. This patient also had a first-degree AV block. (Reprinted with permission. Zaidan JR, Curling PE: Cardiac dysrhythmias: Recognition and management. In Stoelting RK, Barash PG, Gallagher TH [eds]: Advances in Anesthesia, vol 2, p 232. Chicago, Year Book Medical Publishers, 1985.)

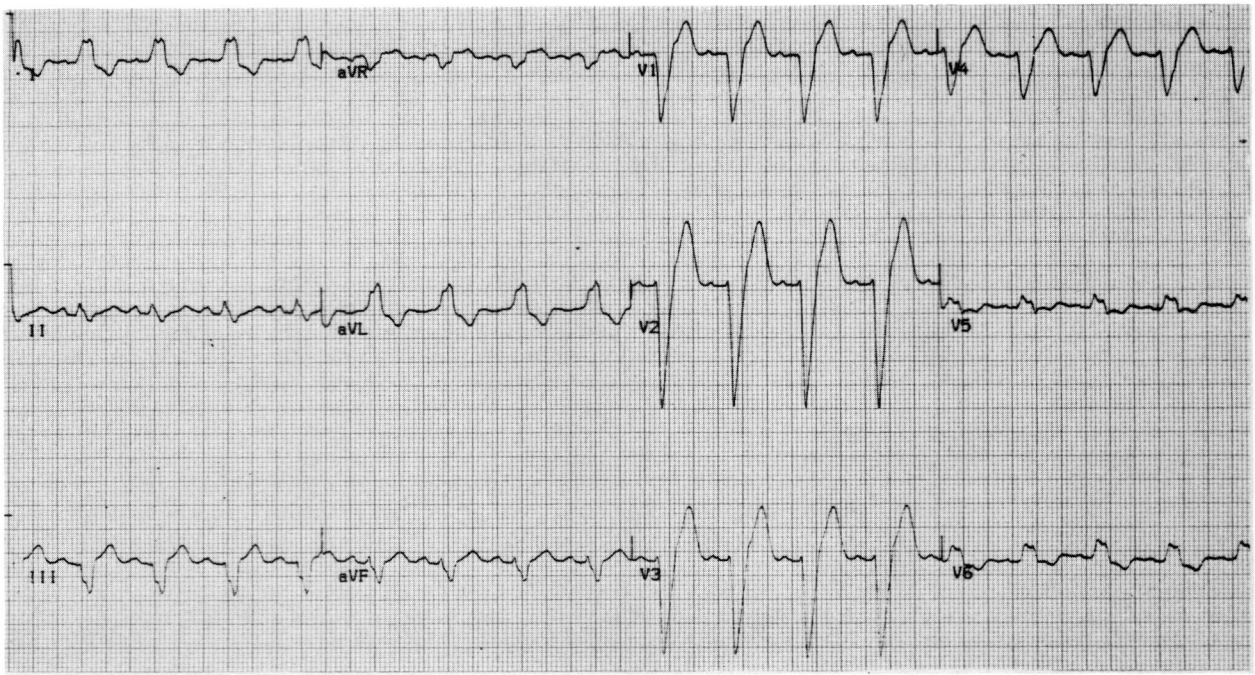

FIG. 22-36. The pattern in lead V₆ is consistent with left bundle branch block.

FIG. 22-37. Comparison of left (A) and right (B) bundle branch blocks in leads I, V₁, and V₆. (Reprinted with permission. Marriott HJL: Practical Electrocardiography, 7th ed, p 64. Baltimore, Williams and Wilkins, 1983.)

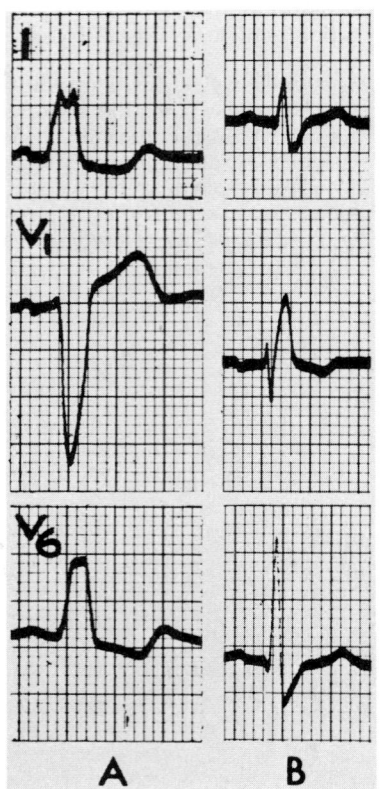

Predictors of sudden death were coronary artery disease and increasing age. Denes *et al* investigated sudden cardiac deaths in 30 patients of 277 who had chronic bifascicular block. Death was associated with coronary artery disease and ventricular arrhythmias rather than heart block.[127] Two Framingham studies of newly acquired right and left bundle branch block also imply that sudden death is related to cardiovascular abnormalities other than complete heart block.[128, 129] Investigations of anesthetized patients reveal the almost nonexistent chance of developing a perioperative complete heart block from bifascicular block.[130, 131] What the studies in anesthetized subjects do not address is the incidence of developing a third-degree block when the patient has either chronic bifascicular block plus first-degree block or evidence of trifascicular disease. In these latter two situations, if the patient is scheduled for major surgery associated with rapid fluid and electrolyte shifts and potentially major blood loss, then one should at least have pacing capabilities immediately available. Pacing can take the form of a typical ventricular electrode, a pulmonary artery catheter, or a transcutaneous system.[132]

HEART BLOCK

First-degree block occurs when the impulse requires a prolonged period to traverse the AV node. All of the impulses reaching the AV node from the atrium successfully cross the node and enter the ventricle. The ECG reflects first-degree block as a PR interval longer than 0.21 s (Fig. 22-40). The incidence of first-degree block in the normal population is approximately 1%.[133]

Second-degree block, indicating that some, but not all, of the impulses cross the AV node, occurs in two forms. One diagnoses type I second-degree block by noting a progressively lengthening PR interval until a P wave is not fol-

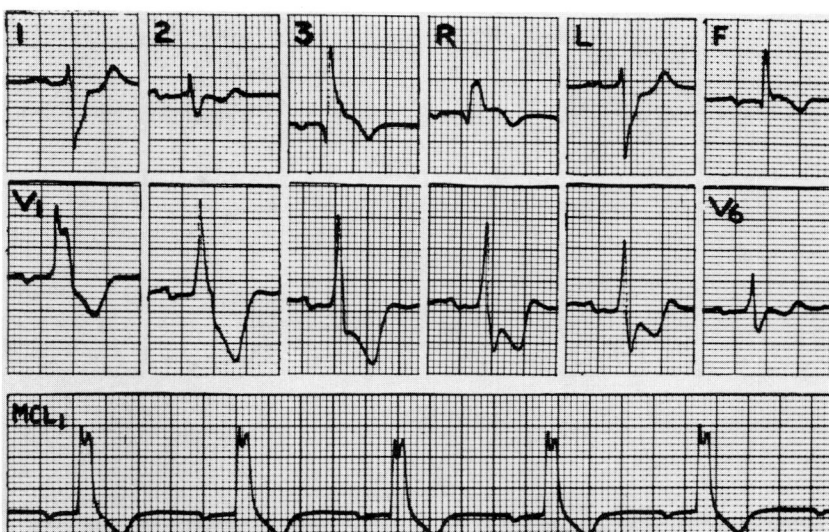

FIG. 22-38. Right axis deviation indicating left posterior hemiblock is diagnosed in this case by noting an R-wave axis of approximately 120°. (Reprinted with permission. Marriott HJL: Practical Electrocardiography, 7th ed, p 91. Baltimore, Williams and Wilkins, 1983.)

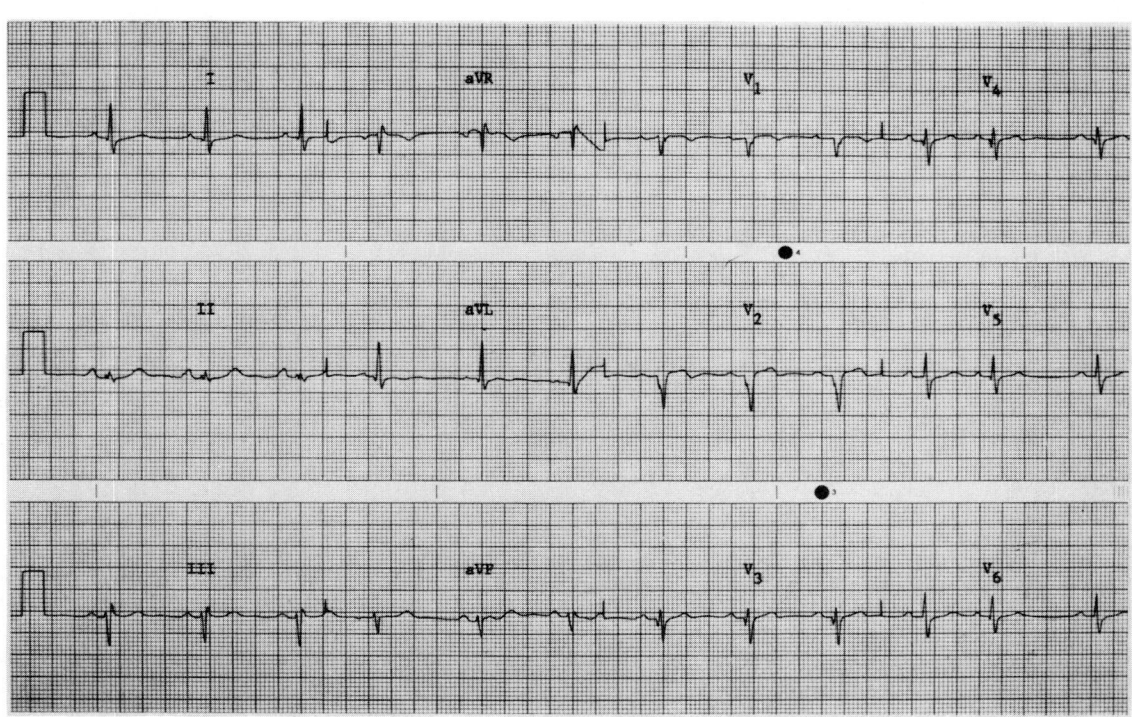

FIG. 22-39. Noting the R- and S-wave deflections in leads I, II, and III will indicate the R-wave axis. As a rough estimate, note the lead in which the R and S waves add to zero (lead II). The R-wave axis will be perpendicular to lead II. Since lead III is negative, the axis points away from lead III and would be in the quadrant between 0° and −90°. The exact axis is −30°, a left axis deviation consistent with left anterior hemiblock.

lowed by a QRS complex (Fig. 22-41). The problem is progressive slowing of conduction within the AV node.[134] Although type I second-degree block can be associated with cardiac disease such as ischemic heart disease, aortic valve disease, mitral valve prolapse, and atrial septal defects, it is also found in athletes who have no cardiac symptoms.[135, 136] Twenty-three per cent of the 35 athletes experienced second-degree

block compared with only 6% of the control group. As the P–R interval progressively lengthens, the R–P interval must progressively shorten. If type I second-degree block occurs after an acute inferior myocardial infarction, it generally does not proceed to a third-degree block.[137]

Type II second-degree block, the more serious of the two types of second-degree block, occurs in the bundle branches.

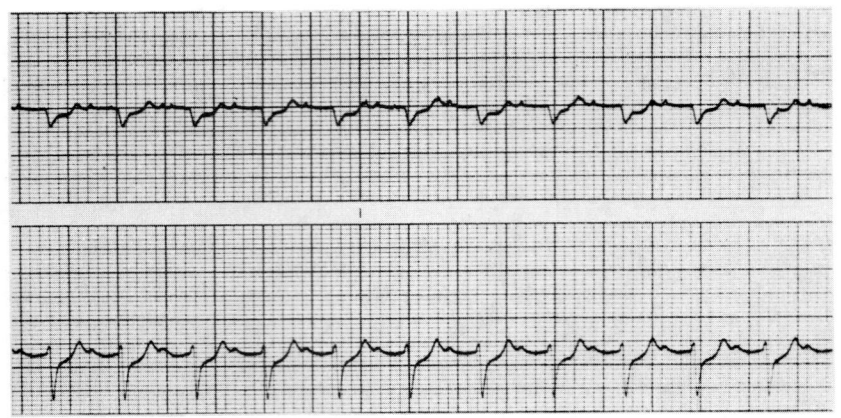

FIG. 22-40. First-degree block carries a prolonged PR interval >0.21 s. All of the impulses proceed through the AV node. This ECG also contains ST-segment depression. The *top* trace is lead II, and the *bottom* trace is lead V₅.

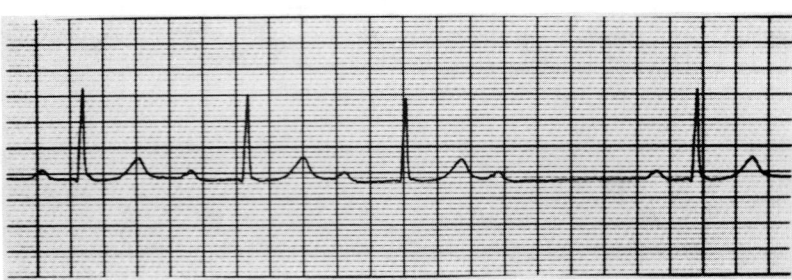

FIG. 22-41. Diagnose type I second-degree AV block by noting progressively lengthening PR intervals until complete block occurs. This cycle repeats with identical PR intervals. (Reprinted with permission. Zaidan JR, Curling PE: Cardiac dysrhythmias: Recognition and management. In Stoelting RK, Barash PG, Gallagher TH [eds]: Advances in Anesthesia, vol 2, p 235. Chicago, Year Book Medical Publishers, 1985.)

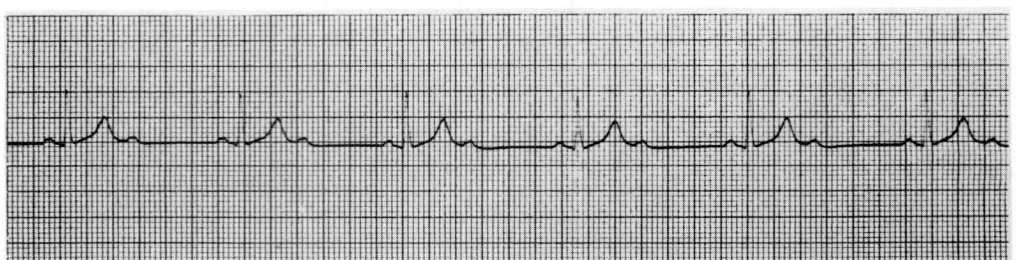

FIG. 22-42. Diagnose type II second-degree AV block by noting identical PR intervals in the conducted beats. In this case, the block is 2:1, indicating two P waves for each QRS complex.

For this reason, bundle branch block frequently accompanies type II block. To diagnose this dysrhythmia, one must see unvarying P–R intervals in the conducted beats, and if two consecutive P waves conduct, the consecutive P–R intervals must be equal (Fig. 22-42 and 22-43).

Third-degree or complete AV block occurs when no impulses cross the AV node. The ventricles will respond either by developing asystole or an idioventricular or idiojunctional rhythm (Fig. 22-44).[135] The atrial and ventricular rates dissociate. Idioventricular control will be associated with a wide bundle branch block pattern and idiojunctional control will have more narrow complexes. The block generally is located in the bundle branches rather than the AV node.[138–140] Ischemic heart disease, Lev's disease, and Lenegre's disease are common causes of trifascicular block.[141, 142]

The different types of heart block must be related to heart rate to determine if disease is actually present. A normal heart generally shows signs of fatigue of AV nodal conduction at approximately 180–200 beats · min⁻¹. If this person were atrially paced at 250 beats · min⁻¹, then probably a second-degree AV block would occur, even if the AV node were perfectly normal. This person does not actually have a second-degree block, but is experiencing a normal phenomenon. A patient with ischemic heart disease, however, might have normal AV conduction until atrial pacing increases the heart rate to 90 beats · min⁻¹. At this rate, second-degree heart block might develop. Both subjects have second-degree heart block by electrocardiographic criteria, but only one has clinically important disease.

BRADYCARDIA

Sinus rates below 60 beats · min⁻¹ classically fall into the category of sinus bradycardia (Fig. 22-45). Both well-trained athletes and critically ill patients with heart disease experience sinus bradycardia. Table 22-6 outlines several of the causes of sinus bradycardia during anesthesia. One must always assume that bradycardia is secondary to hypoxia until proven otherwise.

It is not necessary for bradycardia to have a sinus mechanism. Causes of nonsinus bradycardia include premature

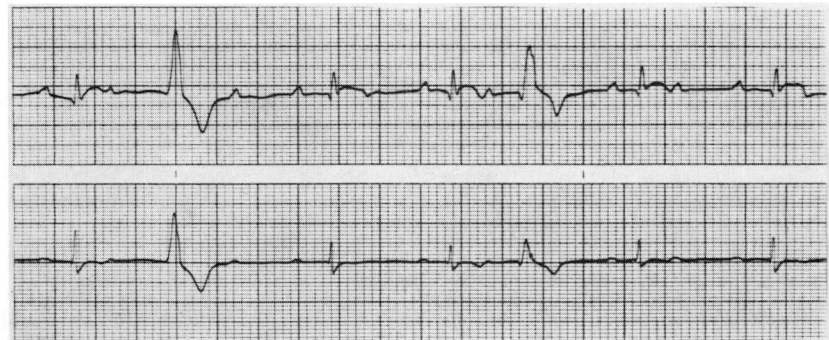

FIG. 22-43. Type II 2:1 second-degree block with either premature junctional or ventricular contractions. The *top* trace is lead II, and the *bottom* trace is lead V₅.

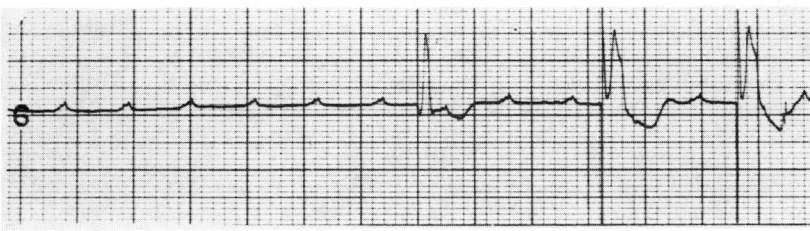

FIG. 22-44. Third-degree block with one junctional escape beat and initiation of ventricular pacing occurred in this patient. Occurrence of P waves without some escape beats is correctly called asystole.

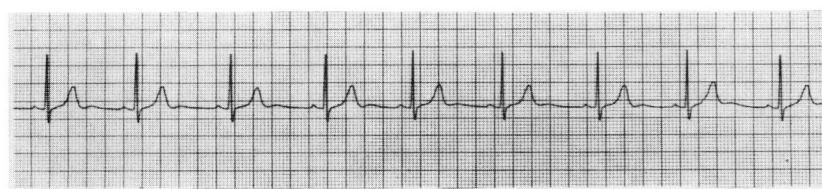

FIG. 22-45. Sinus bradycardia is defined as a heart rate below 60 beats·min⁻¹.

TABLE 22-6. Causes of Bradycardia

Vagal reflexes
Hypoxia
Intracranial hypertension
Anticholinesterase drugs
Beta-blocking drugs
Digitalis preparations

TABLE 22-7. Treatment of Bradycardia

Assure oxygenation
Sinus, no escape beats, otherwise healthy:
  No treatment, unless hypotensive
Sinus or idiojunctional, vagally induced, with hypotension and possibly escape beats:
  Removal vagal influence
  Atropine 0.4 mg iv repeated
  Ephedrine 5 mg iv repeated, if necessary
  Possible atrial pacing
Sinus, with hypertension:
  Treat hypertension
  Do not increase rate until hypertension is controlled
Third-degree block:
  Treat ischemia
  Sequential pacing if atrial activity intact
Chronic atrial fibrillation:
  Stop digoxin if serum concentration is high
  Ventricular pacing to physiologic rate
  Cardioversion might not be successful
Beta blockade:
  Stop drug
  Atropine 0.4 mg iv repeated
  Isoproterenol (4–8 μg·ml⁻¹) 0.5–2 μg·min⁻¹
  Atrial or sequential pacing
Anticholinesterase induced (muscle relaxant reversal):
  Atropine 0.4 mg iv repeated
Increased intracranial pressure:
  Hyperventilation, diuretics
  Surgery to relieve pressure

atrial complexes with nonconducted premature P waves, SA nodal block, third-degree block associated with an idioventricular rhythm, and atrial fibrillation or flutter.

Treatment of bradycardia (outlined in Table 22-7) depends on the hemodynamic and electrocardiographic responses. Maintenance of the sinus mechanism without ventricular or junctional escape beats and no loss of blood pressure in an otherwise healthy patient dictates vigilance with no specific treatment. In fact, uncontrolled treatment of bradycardia sometimes creates more problems. A patient with a "tight" left main coronary artery lesion can be asymptomatic at a heart rate of 40 beats·min⁻¹. Increasing the patient's rate to 90 beats·min⁻¹ likely will cause myocardial ischemia. Before treating bradycardia, consider the possibility that a tachycardia is potentially worse than bradycardia. Do not administer an antimuscarinic to a patient who has a reflex sinus bradycardia secondary to hypertension. Treating the hypertension will return the heart rate to more physiologic levels. Atrial pacing, when available, allows precise control of heart rate.

MYOCARDIAL ISCHEMIA AND INFARCTION

One of the initial electrocardiographic events in the presence of decreased oxygen delivery to the myocardium is T-wave inversion. If coronary flow does not return, the ST segment elevates and takes with it the inverted T wave. At this point, reestablishment of coronary flow will allow the ST–T wave changes to revert to normal. Continued insufficient oxygen delivery, however, eventually changes the QRS complex into a persistent QS complex or Q wave (Figures 22-46–52). This pattern of necrosis develops because the impulse no longer enters the area of the necrotic tissue. The electrical forces that formerly approached the ECG electrode do not exist; therefore, the electrode records activity directed toward the opposite side of the heart and away from the electrode. The overall ECG picture is a negative deflection recorded in the area of the necrosis and an unopposed, enhanced, positive deflection recorded from the other side of the heart.

An infarct has an area of necrosis associated with Q waves, an area of injury associated with ST segment changes, and a larger area of ischemia that creates T-wave changes. Electrodes placed directly on the heart can record each of these separate areas. An electrode located on the body's surface, however, simultaneously records all three of these areas. The result is possibly T-wave changes, ST-segment elevation, and Q waves recorded from one surface electrode. Characteristically, the Q wave must be 0.03 s in duration, the ST segments are convex upward (dome-shaped), and the T wave is pointed with two equal limbs.

Locating the exact position of an infarct is not well defined.[143] We can predict the general area of the heart affected by the infarct by observing specific ECG leads. Table 22-8 indicates these areas. If limb and precordial leads reveal persistent ST–T-wave changes, then the patient experienced a subendocardial infarct.[144]

Other subtle electrocardiographic changes suggest, but are not diagnostic of, myocardial ischemia. These changes include a perfectly horizontal ST segment that abruptly converts into the T wave, inverted U waves, and postextrasystolic T-wave changes.[145-147]

An atrial infarct is more difficult to diagnose than a ventricular infarct. Suspect an atrial infarct when a patient experiencing a ventricular infarct develops an atrial dysrhythmia.[148] Electrocardiographic signs of an atrial infarct include a change

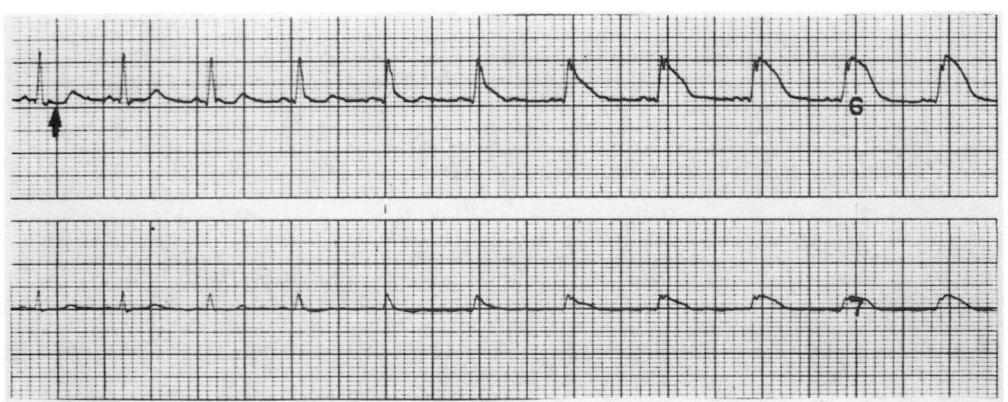

FIG. 22-46. Aortic cross-clamping (*arrow*) after initiation of cardiopulmonary bypass resulted in an intraventricular conduction delay and ST-segment change within three beats. The *top* trace is lead II, and the *bottom* trace is lead V₅.

FIG. 22-47. ST-segment depression is evident in lead II and V₅ (*left*). This patient had chest pain. Metoprolol decreased the heart rate from 96 to 80 beats·min⁻¹ (*middle*) with an obvious improvement in the ST-segment changes. Pain resolved within a few minutes after decreasing the heart rate, and the ST segments became isoelectric. The *top* tracing is lead II, and the *bottom* tracing is lead V₅.

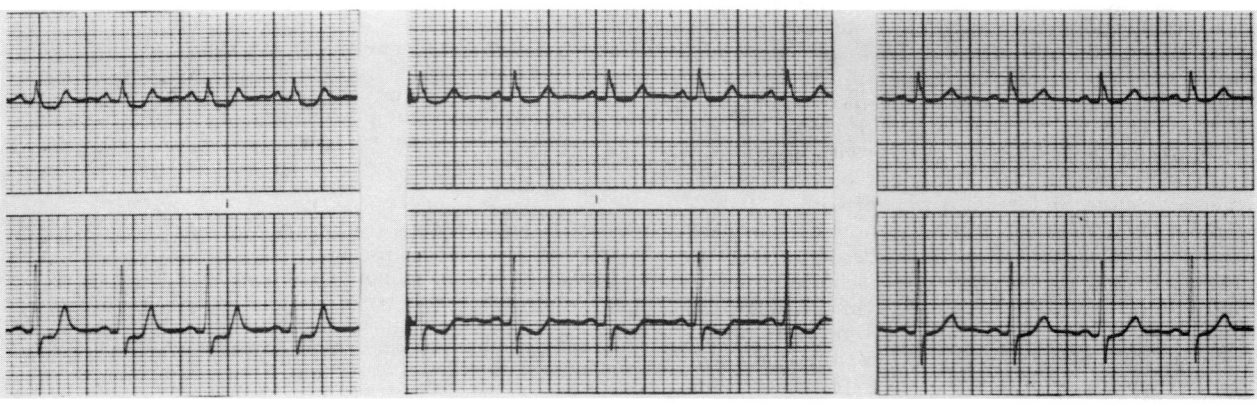

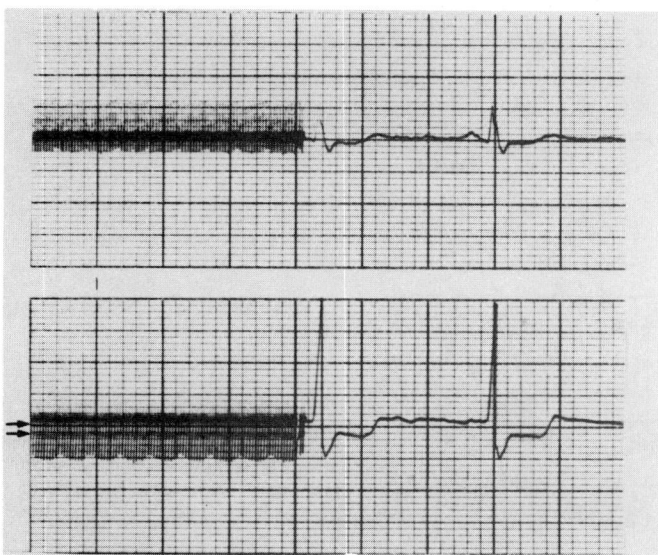

FIG. 22-48. The ECG recorder can reveal ST-segment depression even at very slow speeds. Note the lighter colored ink between the arrows and this area's corresponding location when the recorder was increased to 25 mm·s^{-1}. This lighter colored area would disappear when the ST segments returned to the base line. The *top* trace is lead II, and the *bottom* trace is V$_5$.

in the contour of the P wave and significant PR-interval elevation in lead I associated with PR-interval depression in lead III.[149]

The ST-segment change during exercise is significant if it undergoes 1–2 mm of depression 0.08 s after the J point regardless of the direction of the ST segment.[150–152] If stress produces ST-segment elevation, then one must consider severe ischemia, decreased ventricular function, wall motion abnormalities, and variant angina.[153–157]

Electrocardiographic changes indicative of myocardial ischemia occurring at rest portend infarction. If the patient experienced cardiovascular changes that led to the myocardial ischemia, then the anesthesiologist should promptly treat these undesirable changes. A common mistake is to avoid adequately anesthetizing the patient with coronary artery disease. In fact, it is the light anesthesia that causes hypertension and tachycardia. A lightly anesthetized patient must receive supplemental anesthetic drugs. Occasionally, the anesthesiologist will find it necessary to use β-adrenergic blocking drugs such as propranolol or metoprolol, α-adrenergic blocking drugs such as phentolamine, the α-β blocking drug labetalol, and directly acting vasodilators such as nitroprusside and nitroglycerin to control hypertension and tachycardia. Hypotension presents more difficult therapeutic problems. Although one might think that a hypotensive patient should not receive a vasodilator, reducing preload with nitroglycerin can restore the myocardial oxygen balance, increase contractility and secondarily increase cardiac output and blood pressure; therefore, if high filling pressures accompany the hypotension, then consider using nitroglycerin as a firstline drug, followed by a β$_1$ agonist such as dobutamine. "I" indicates that if low filling pressures led to the hypotension, then, as would be expected, volume replacement becomes the choice therapy. Patients experiencing ST-segment elevation during anesthesia can receive a nitroglycerin infusion at infusion rates of 0.25–0.5 μg·kg^{-1}·min^{-1} or 10 mg of sublingual nifedipine. Volatile anesthetic agents plus nifedipine can cause hypotension.

ELECTROCARDIOGRAMS ASSOCIATED WITH PACEMAKERS

Increased usage and sophistication of pacemakers create the possibility of misinterpretation of their ECG. The location of the electrodes and the type of generator determine the ECG's appearance. The generator can stimulate the atrium, ventricle, or both chambers sequentially. Electrodes located in the atrium will create P waves, and ventricular electrodes will cause a left bundle branch block if they are on the right ventricle or a right bundle branch block if they are on the left ventricle.

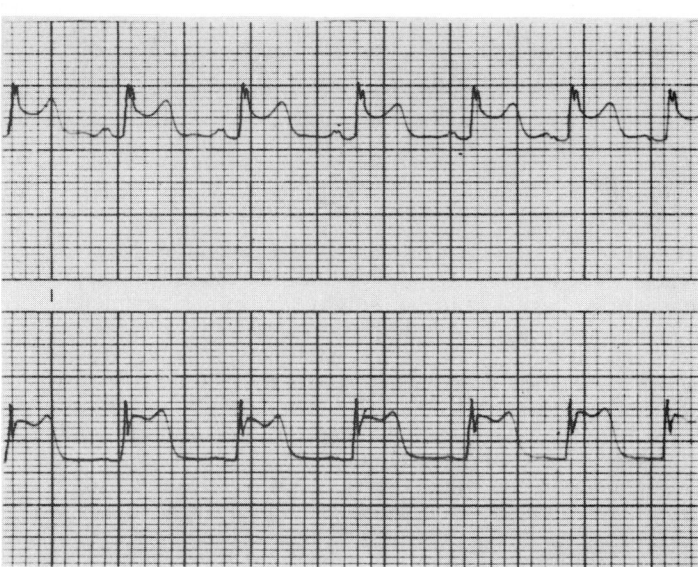

FIG. 22-49. Obvious in this figure is a 3-mm ST-segment elevation in lead II and a 6-mm elevation in V$_5$. The *top* trace is lead II, and the *bottom* trace is lead V$_5$.

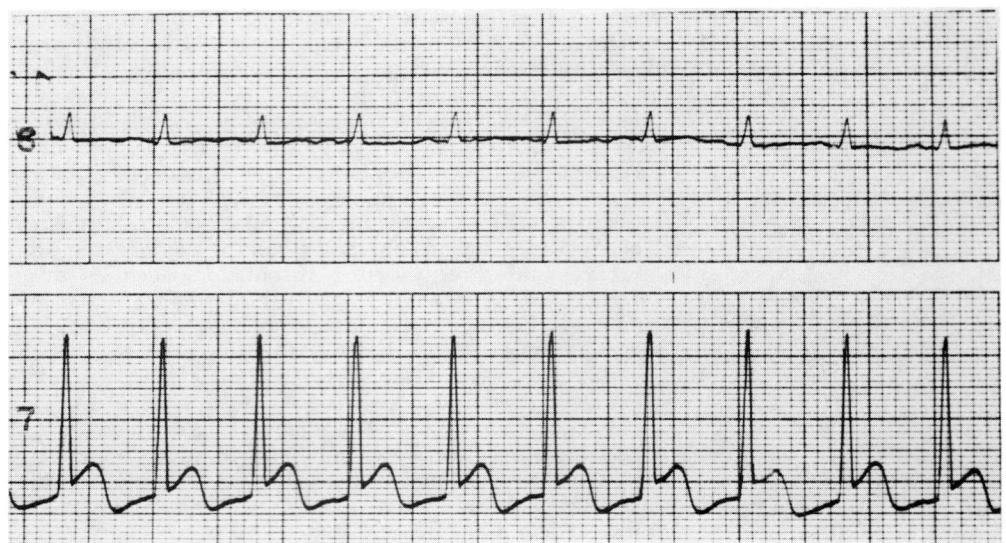

FIG. 22-50. Lead II does not always reveal ST-segment changes simultaneously with lead V₅. The *top* trace is lead II, and the *bottom* trace is lead V₅.

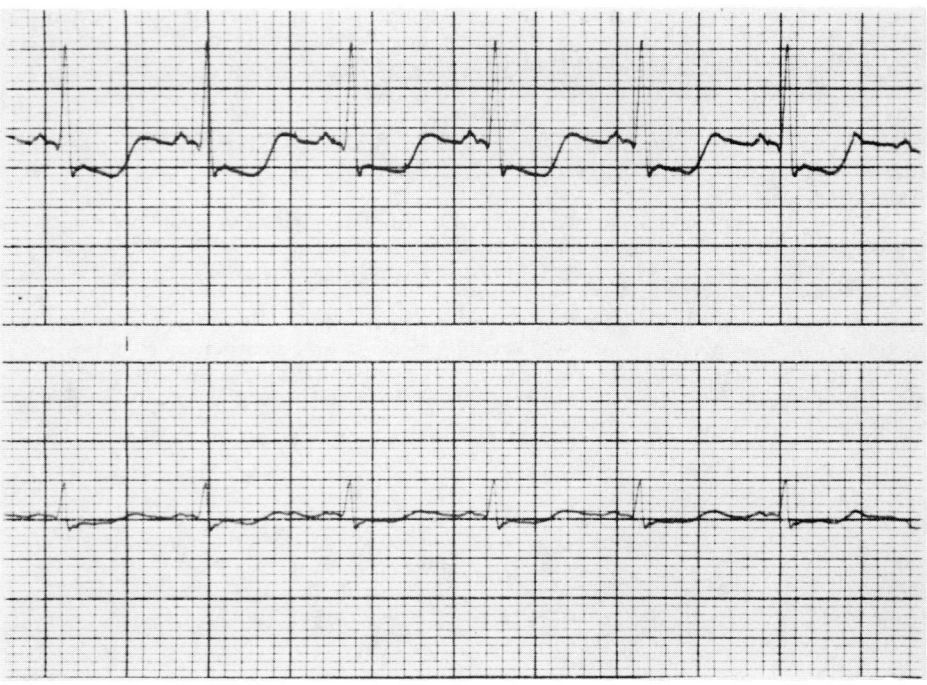

FIG. 22-51. In this example, lead II had signs of ischemia not evident in V₅. This patient had right coronary artery disease. The *top* trace is lead II, and the *bottom* trace is lead V₅.

At this time, almost all implanted pacemakers are programmable. Programmability implies that one can easily change the rate, voltage output, sensitivity, and other parameters. Two common generators have the three-letter designation, VVI and DDD. VVI indicates that stimulation (first letter) and sensing (second letter) take place in the ventricle (V). "I" indicates that if the pacemaker's sensing circuit detects sufficient R-wave voltage (usually about ±2 mV), the generator turns off (the sensing circuit inhibits the pacing circuit). With a VVI generator, one would expect to see ventricular pacing or no pacing, depending on the patient's intrinsic heart rate. A DDD pacemaker stimulates the atrium and ventrical (dual) and senses P waves from the atrium and R waves from the ventricle (dual). If it senses a P wave, the generator waits the

programmed period of time (the PR interval) then either triggers an impulse into the ventricle if an R wave does not occur, or continues pacing in the inhibited mode if the R wave does occur. The "fully automatic" DDD pacemaker can have four levels of pacing that depend on the patient's heart rate and PR interval: 1) total AV sequential pacing; 2) atrial pacing without ventricular pacing; 3) ventricular pacing without atrial pacing; and 4) no pacing.

Pacemakers must receive at least a simple evaluation before the patient can proceed to surgery. If the generator is less than 2 years old, does not produce pacing impulses when the patient's heart rate is above 72 beats · min⁻¹, and does produce pacing impulses associated with a peripheral pulse when the heart rate slows, then very likely the pacemaker system is

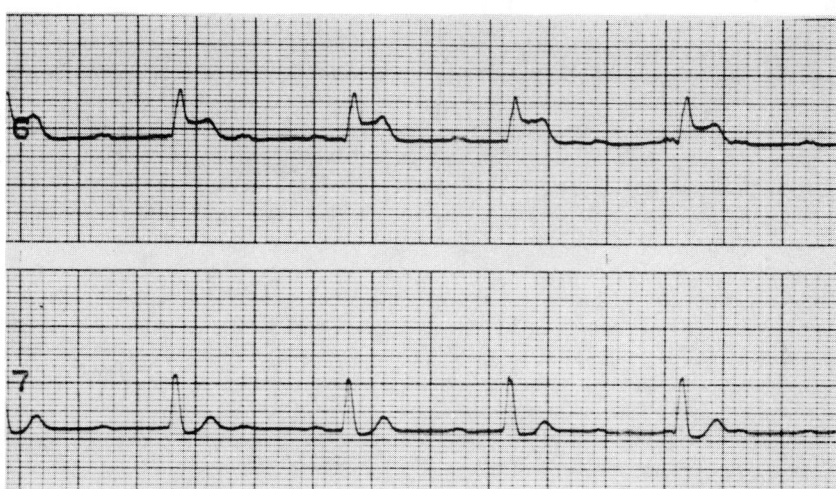

FIG. 22-52. ST-segment elevation, seen here in lead II, implies variant angina. The patient had AV dissociation and likely also had third-degree AV block. The top trace is lead II, and the bottom trace is lead V_5.

TABLE 22-8.   Locating the Myocardial Infarct

AREA OF INFARCT	AFFECTED ECG LEADS
Anterior	I, aV_L, V_3, V_4
Inferior	II, III, aV_F
Lateral	I, aV_L, V_5, V_6
Posterior	Reciprocal changes in V_1, V_2
Anterolateral[167]	V_{1-6}
Anteroseptal[168]	V_{1-4}
Inferolateral[169]	Inferior + V_5, V_6
Right Ventricle[170, 171]	V_{4R}–V_{6R}

properly functioning. The pacemaker should continue to function throughout the operative period unless one of several events occurs. Table 22-9 outlines the events that can cause intraoperative failure.

The remainder of this section presents commonly used normally and abnormally functioning pacemakers (Figs. 22-53 through 22-61).

OTHER CONDITIONS AFFECTING THE ELECTROCARDIOGRAM

Several other conditions that acutely affect the ECG could involve a patient scheduled for emergency surgery.

ACUTE PERICARDITIS

The ST stage develops first in acute pericarditis. It is characterized by elevated ST segments in many leads. The PR segment commonly undergoes depression.[158, 159]

TABLE 22-9.   Causes and Treatment of Pacemaker Failure

CHANGE	CAUSES	RESULT	CONSIDERATIONS
Acute K^+ Changes			
Extracellular K^+ decrease	Hyperventilation Acute diuretic therapy	Pacing loss	Increase output external generator
Extracellular K^+ increase	Myocardial ischemia Depolarizing muscle relaxants Rapid K^+ replacement	Pacing-related ventricular fibrillation	Treat ischemia Lidocaine $CaCl_2$
Electromagnetic interference	Electrocautery	Pacing loss Reprogramming	The pacemaker generator must not be between the ground plate and the active electrode of the electrocautery; do not place the magnet on the programmable generator
Myocardial infarction	Increase in size of electrode (dead tissue) and therefore decreased charge at the electrode–tissue interface	Pacing loss	Increase output of external generator; possible CPR

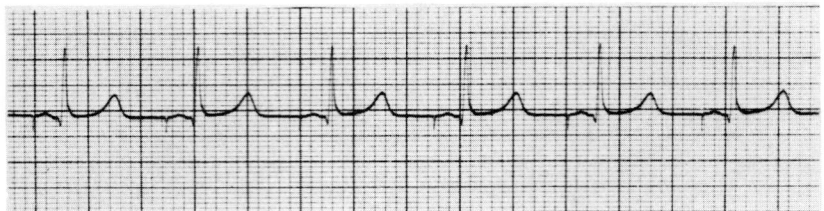

FIG. 22-53. Normal atrial pacing. A P wave follows each pacing impulse, and each P wave travels to the ventricle.

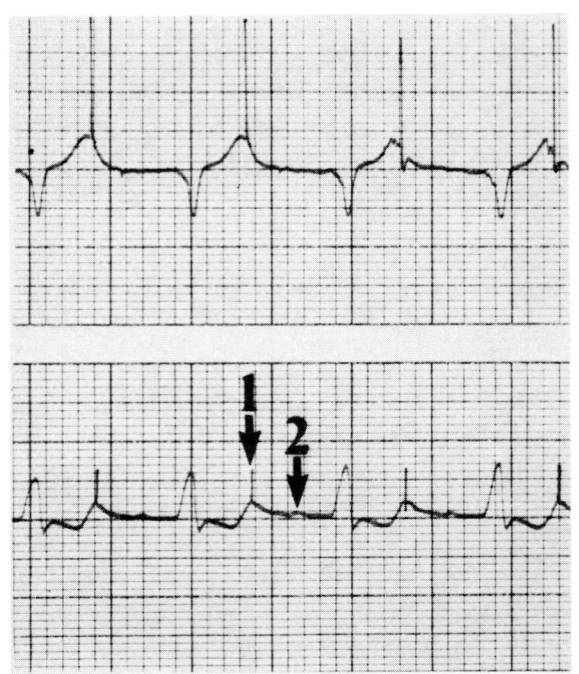

FIG. 22-54. This patient had a long delay between the atrial pacing impulse (*arrow 1*) and the P wave (*arrow 2*). This situation can occur after cardiopulmonary bypass and cardioplegia. The *top* trace is lead II, and the *bottom* trace is lead V₅.

The T-wave stage comprising the second phase of acute pericarditis persists for 10 days to 2 weeks. Widespread T-wave inversion is the characteristic finding.

PERICARDIAL EFFUSION

Electrocardiographic findings characteristic of pericardial effusion include low QRS voltage, ST-segment elevation, and electrical alternans. A patient experiencing electrical alternans of the P waves as well as the QRS complexes likely will have a malignant pericardial effusion.[160-162]

INTRACRANIAL HEMORRHAGE

Intracranial hemorrhage produces bradycardia and wide inverted T waves many times, coupled with an inverted U wave.[163, 164] Patients suffering subendocardial infarction can occasionally change their inverted T waves to the upright position and thereby mask the infarction.[165]

HYPOTHERMIA

Moderate hypothermia above approximately 32° C does not change the ECG. Below 30° C, bradycardia and an elevation of the J point develop (Fig. 22-62). Atrial fibrillation occurs below 29° C.[166]

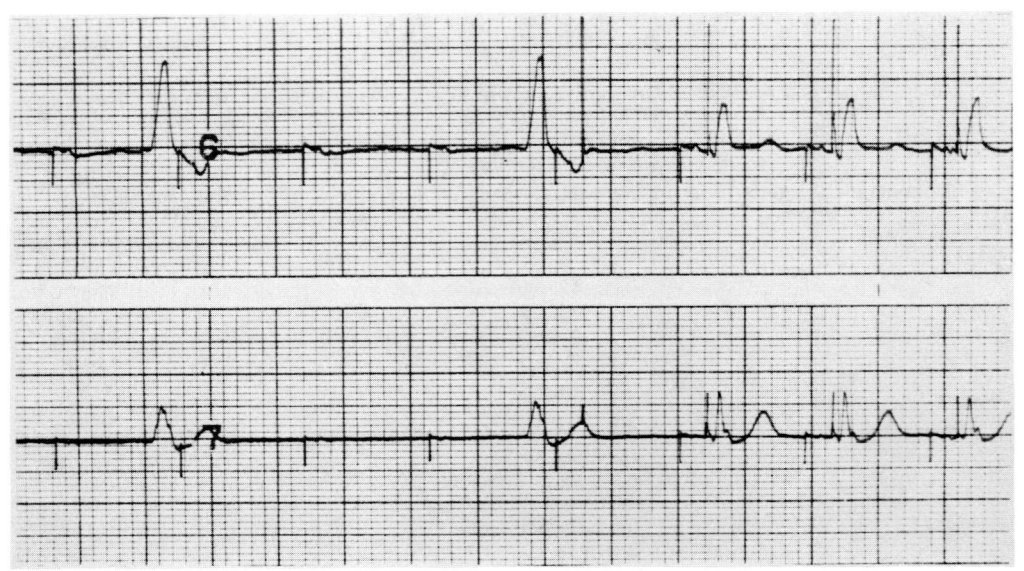

FIG. 22-55. Atrial pacing created an atrial depolarization that was not conducted to the ventricle. The first two QRS complexes are ventricular escapes, while the last three are associated with sequential pacing. The *top* trace is lead II, and the *bottom* trace is lead V₅.

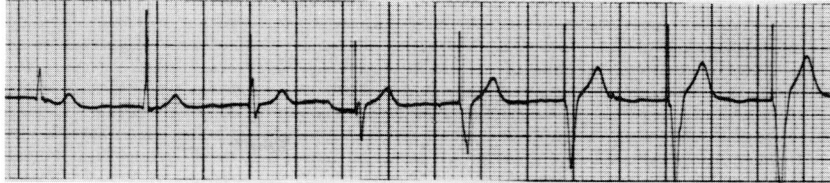

FIG. 22-56. Normal ventricular inhibited pacing showing, in sequence, a junctional escape, two pseudofusion beats, three fusion beats, and two ventricularly paced beats.

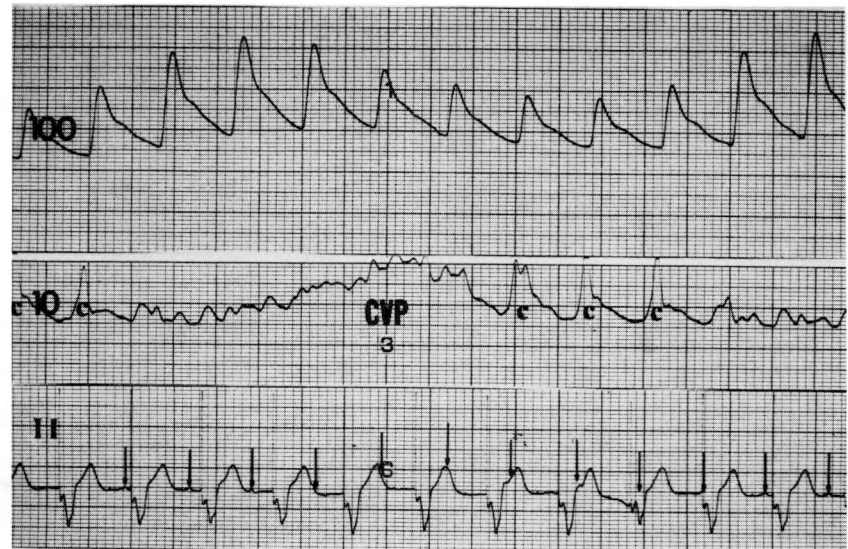

FIG. 22-57. Ventricular pacing with continued atrial activity (*arrows*) results in hemodynamic effects much like a junctional rhythm. The arterial blood pressure (*top* trace) decreases, and cannon waves (c) appear on the CVP tracing (*middle* trace). The third trace is lead II, and the fourth trace is lead V$_5$. (100 = 100 mm Hg; 10 = 10 mm Hg)

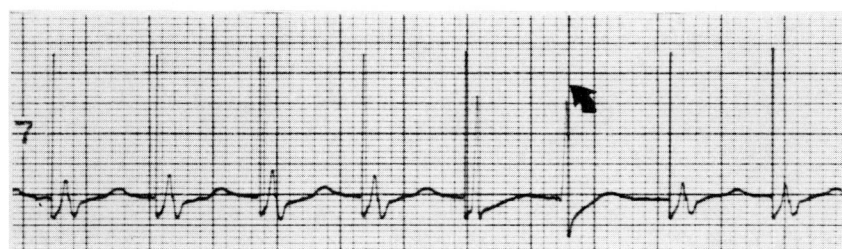

FIG. 22-58. The pacing spike at the *arrow* occurs after the peak of the R wave, showing abnormal sensing. The fifth complex is a fusion beat.

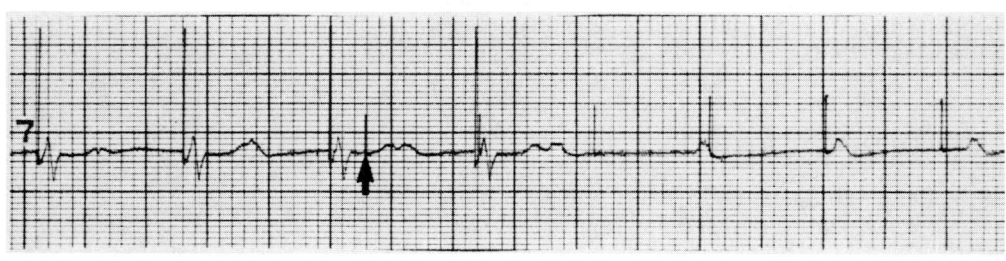

FIG. 22-59. A second, temporary pacemaker, turned on at the *arrow*, inhibited the patient's implanted pacemaker. The temporary pacemaker was not functioning and did not take over ventricular pacing. Only unrelated P waves occur.

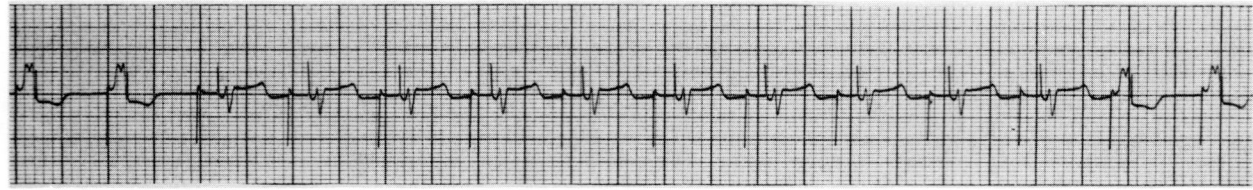

FIG. 22-60. AV sequential pacing reversed accidently when the atrial pacing electrode touched the ventricle (first three and last two QRS complexes). Ventricular pacing occurred with the atrial impulse, and the ventricular impulse therefore found a refractory ventricle. Had the PR interval been set to approximately 300 ms, the ventricular impulse could have initiated ventricular tachycardia or fibrillation by stimulating the ventricle in the repolarization period.

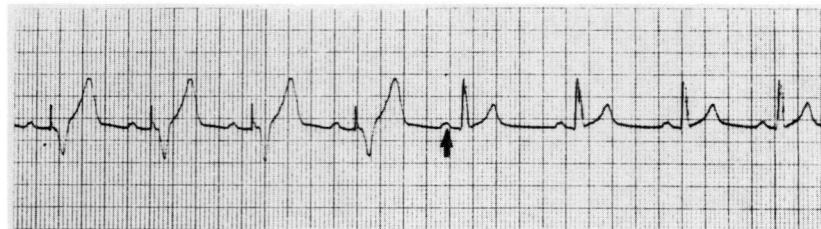

FIG. 22-61. Illustration of one aspect of totally automatic, or DDD pacing. P-wave sensing occurs (no impulse found before the P wave). The P wave took longer than the pacemaker's PR interval to cross the AV node; therefore, the ventricular circuit activated, and ventricular pacing occurred (first four complexes). The P wave crossed the AV node in a sufficiently short time period to inhibit the ventricular circuit at the *arrow*. An intraventricular conduction delay is evident.

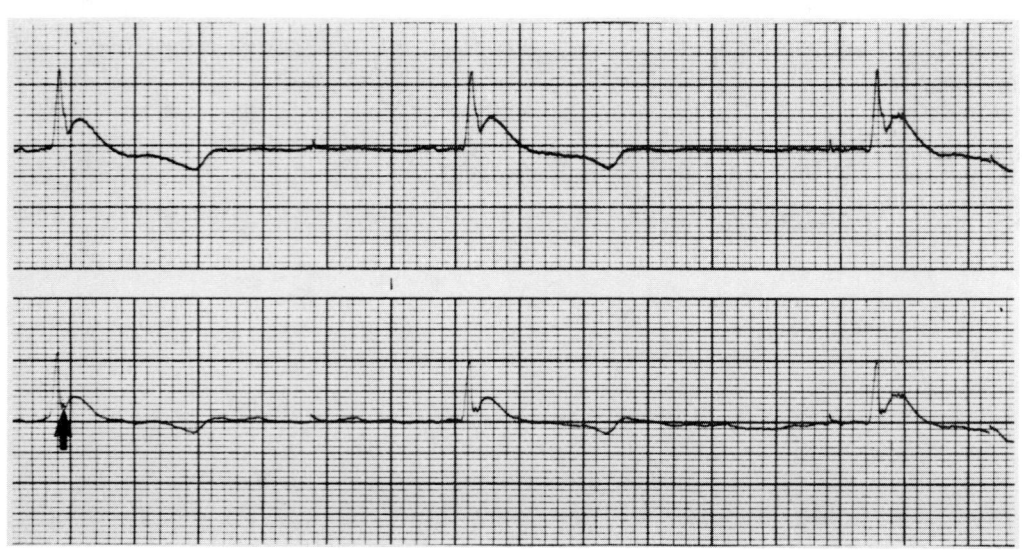

FIG. 22-62. Osborne waves (*arrow*) occur during hypothermia. Note that the Osborne wave is not an elevation of the ST segment. The *top* trace is lead II, and the *bottom* trace is lead V5.

ELECTROLYTES

Electrocardiographic changes associated with electrolyte abnormalities are listed in Table 22-10 (Fig. 22-63 and 22-64). These electrocardiographic changes may exist in the presence of normal serum electrolytes. Conversely, the ECG can be normal in the presence of abnormal serum electrolytes. Myocardial concentrations and transmembrane gradients, not serum electrolyte concentrations, create the ECG changes.

MONITORING CATHETERS

Atrial and ventricular arrhythmias and right bundle branch block can occur when a pulmonary arterial catheter floats through the heart and into the pulmonary artery (Fig. 22-65).

TABLE 22-10.   ECG Associated with Electrolyte Abnormalities

ELECTROLYTE CHANGE	ECG RESPONSE
Hypokalemia	ST-segment depression T wave flattening and inversion Tall U wave
Hyperkalemia	Tall T wave P–R interval prolongation ST-segment depression QRS widening Ventricular fibrillation
Hypocalcemia	Prolonged QT interval
Hypercalcemia	Short QT interval ST segment may disappear

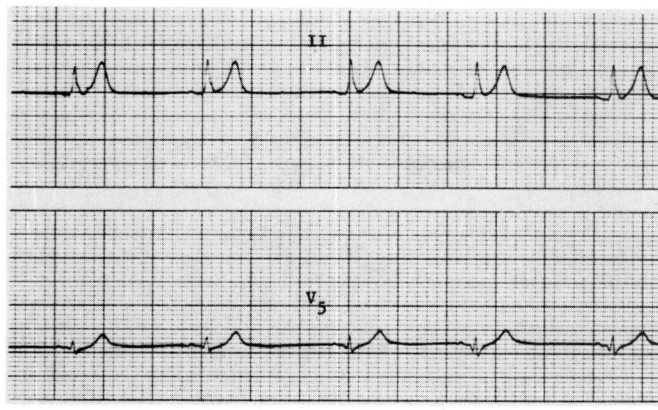

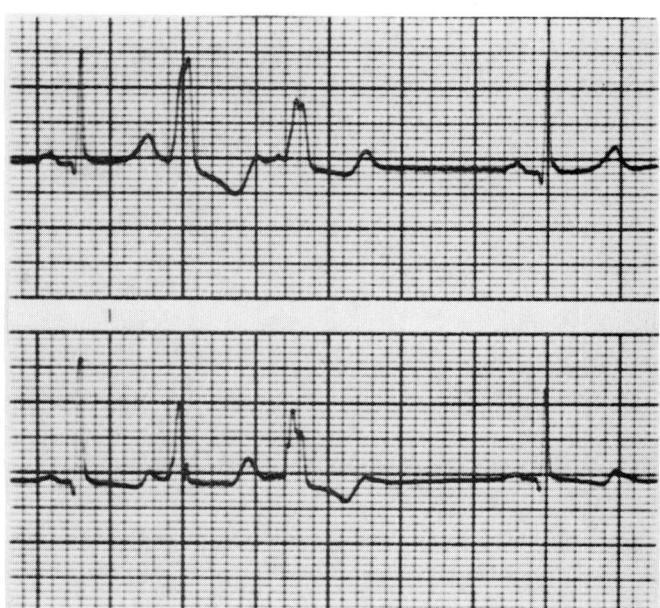

FIG. 22-65. The pulmonary arterial catheter created these ECG changes as it floated through the right ventricular outflow tract. It is difficult to distinguish between atrial and ventricular catheter-related dysrhythmias; however, these changes are likely ventricular in origin. The *top* trace is lead II, and the *bottom* trace is lead V₅.

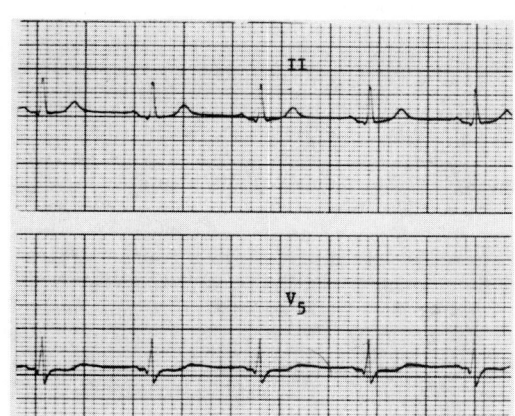

FIG. 22-63. Elevated myocardial potassium creates peaked T waves in relation to the R wave (*top* tracings). The *bottom* tracings show the ECG a short while after the patient received glucose and insulin.

Advancing a pulmonary artery catheter introduced through the right internal jugular vein no more than 25% of the patient's height in cm measured from the skin entry point should avoid arrhythmias due to coiling within the atrium or ventricle.

HEART TRANSPLANTATION

Heart transplantation creates an unusual ECG with P waves originating from the donor's heart and from the recipient's SA node and remaining atrial tissue. The donor's P wave will remain associated with the QRS complexes, and the recipient's atrial activity will dissociate from the QRS complexes (Fig. 22-66).

FIG. 22-64. Transient T-wave enhancement and R-wave changes were evident after the patient received 2 mEq of potassium through a central catheter. The *broad arrows* follow the T-wave changes, while the *narrow arrows* trace the R-wave changes. The heart rate also decreased. One can diagnose these changes even when the recorder speed is slow (25 mm·min⁻¹).

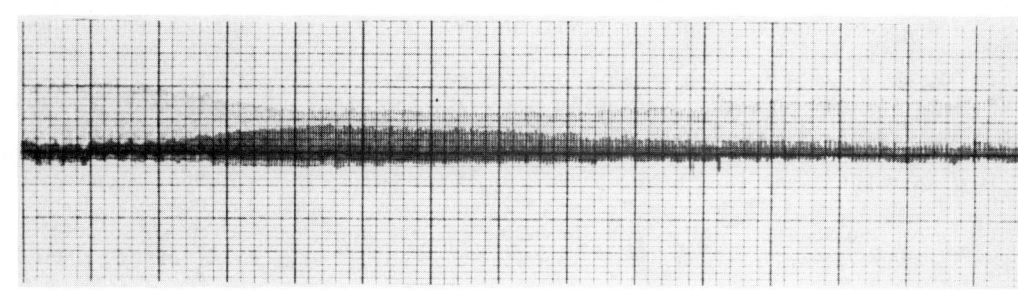

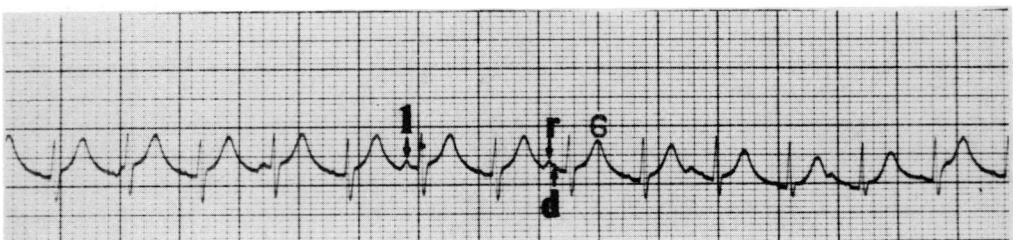

FIG. 22-66. The heart transplant patient will have recipient P waves (*arrow* r) and donor P waves (*arrow* d). They occasionally superimpose (*arrow* 1).

REFERENCES

1. Levy AG, Lewis T: Heart irregularities resulting from the inhalation of low percentages of chloroform vapor and their relationship to ventricular fibrillation. Heart 3:99, 1911
2. Levy AG: Sudden death under light chloroform anesthesia. J Physiol 42:3, 1911
3. Vanik PE, Davis HS: Cardiac arrhythmias during halothane anesthesia. Anesth Analg 47:299, 1968
4. Kuner J, Enescu V, Utsu F et al: Cardiac arrhythmias during anesthesia. Dis Chest 52:580, 1967
5. Southall DP, Johnston F, Shinebourne EA et al: A 24-hour electrocardiographic study of heart rate and rhythm patterns in populations of healthy children. Br Heart J 45:281, 1981
6. Brodsky M, Wu D, Denes P et al: Arrhythmias documented by 24 hour continuous electrocardiographic monitoring in 50 male medical students without apparent heart disease. Am J Cardiol 39:390, 1977
7. Marriott HJL, Fogg E: Constant monitoring for cardiac dysrhythmias and blocks. Mod Concepts Cardiovasc Dis 39:103, 1970
8. Kates RA, Zaidan JR, Kaplan JA: Esophageal lead for intraoperative electrocardiographic monitoring. Anesth Analg 61:781, 1982
9. Copeland GD: Clinical evaluation of a new esophageal electrode, with particular reference to the bipolar esophageal electrocardiogram. Am Heart J 57:862, 1959
10. Enselberg CD: The esophageal electrocardiogram in the study of atrial activity and cardiac arrhythmias. Am Heart J 41:382, 1951
11. Prystowsky EN, Pritchett EL, Gallagher JJ: Origin of the atrial electrogram recorded from the esophagus. Circulation 61:1017, 1980
12. Narula OS, Scherlag BJ, Samet P et al: Atrioventricular block: Localization and classification by His bundle recordings. Am J Med 50:146, 1971
13. Damato A, Schnitzler RN, Lay SH: Recent advances in the bundle of His electrograms. In Yu PN, Goodwin JF (eds): Progress in Cardiology, p 181. Philadelphia, Lea & Febiger, 1973
14. Gallagher JJ, Damato AN: Technique of recording His bundle activity in man. In Grossman W (ed): Cardiac Catheterization and Angiography, p 213. Philadelphia, Lea & Febiger, 1974
15. Castellanos A Jr, Castillo C, Agha A: Contribution of His bundle recording to the understanding of clinical arrhythmias. Am J Cardiol 28:499, 1971
16. Rosen KM: Evaluation of cardiac conduction in the cardiac catheterization laboratory. Am J Cardiol 30:701, 1972
17. Atlee JL, Brownlee SW, Burstrom RE: Conscious-state comparisons of the effects of inhalation anesthetics on specialized atrioventricular conduction times in dogs. Anesthesiology 64:703, 1986
18. Marriott HJL: Electrical axis. In Marriott HJL (ed): Practical Electrocardiography, p 32. Baltimore, Williams & Wilkins, 1983
19. Fowler NO, Daniels C, Scott RC et al: The electrocardiogram in cor pulmonale with and without emphysema. Am J Cardiol 16:500, 1965
20. Hodgkin AL, Katz B: Ionic currents underlying activity in the giant axon of the squid. J Physiol 108:37, 1949
21. Hodgkin AL, Huxley AF: A quantitative description of membrane current and its application to conduction and excitation in nerve. J Physiol 117:500, 1952
22. Hagiwara S, Nakajina S: Differences in Na and Ca spikes as examined by application of tetrodotoxin, procaine, and manganese ions. J Gen Physiol 49:793, 1966
23. Katz AM: Cardiac action potential. In Physiology of the Heart, p 229. New York, Raven Press, 1977
24. Kenyon JL, Gibbons WR: Effects of low-chloride solutions on action potentials of sheep cardiac Purkinje fibers. J Gen Physiol 70:63, 1977
25. Trautwein W: Membrane currents in cardiac muscle fibers. Physiol Rev 59:973, 1973
26. Bigger JT: Mechanisms and diagnosis of arrhythmias. In Braurswald E (ed): Heart Disease: A Textbook of Cardiovascular Medicine, p 630. Philadelphia, WB Saunders, 1980
27. DiFrancesco D: A new interpretation of the pacemaker current in calf Purkinje fibers. J Physiol 314:359, 1981
28. Myerburg RJ, Stewart JW, Hoffman BF: Electrophysiological properties of the canine peripheral AV conducting system. Circ Red 26:361, 1970
29. Myerburg RJ: The gating mechanism in the distal AV conducting system. Circulation 43:955, 1971
30. Surawicz B, Saito S: Exercise testing for detection of myocardial ischemia in patients with abnormal electrocardiograms at rest. Am J Cardiol 41:943, 1978
31. Wit AL, Fenoglio JJ, Wagner BM et al: Electrophysiological properties of cardiac muscle in the anterior mitral valve leaflet and the adjacent atrium in dog. Possible implications for the genesis of atrial dysrhythmias. Circ Res 32:731, 1973
32. Bassett AL, Wit AL: Ectopic impulses originating in the tricuspid valve and contiguous atrium. Fed Proc 33:445, 1974
33. Fenoglio JJ: Canine mitral complex, ultrastructure and electromechanical properties. Circ Res 31:417, 1972
34. Hoffman BF, Cranefield PF: Electrophysiology of the Heart, New York, McGraw Hill, 1960
35. Norma A, Irisawa H: A time and voltage-dependent potassium current in the rabbit sinoatrial node cell. Pfluegers Arch 366:251, 1976
36. Katzing B: Effects of extracellular calcium and sodium on depolarization-induced automaticity in guinea pig papillary muscle. Circ Res 37:118, 1975
37. Brown HF, Noble ST: Membrane currents underlying delayed rectification and pacemaker activity in frog atrial muscle. J Physiol (London) 204:717, 1969
38. Imaniski S, Surawicz B: Automatic activity in depolarized guinea pig ventricular myocardium: Characteristics and mechanisms. Circ Res 39:751, 1976
39. Lazzara R, El-Sherif M. Sherlag BJ: Electrophysiological properties of canine Purkinje cells in one day old myocardial infarction. Circ Res 33:722, 1973

40. Hordof AJ, Edie R, Malm JR et al: Electrophysiological properties and response to pharmacologic agents of fibers from diseased human atria. Circulation 54:774, 1976

41. DeHaan RL, DeFelice LJ: Electrical noise and rhythmic properties of embryonic heart cell aggregates. Fed Proc 37:2132, 1978

42. Lin CI, Kotake H, Vassalle M: On the mechanism underlying the oscillatory current in cardiac Purkinje fibers. J Cardiovasc Pharm 8:906, 1986

43. Cranefield PF: Action potentials, afterpotentials, and arrhythmias. Circ Res 41:415, 1977

44. Bozler E: The initiation of impulses in cardiac muscle. Am J Physiol 138:273, 1943

45. Cranefield PF, Aronson RS: Initiation of sustained rhythmic activity by single propagated action potentials in canine Purkinje fibers exposed to sodium-free solution or to ouabain. Circ Res 34:477, 1974

46. Hoffman BF, Rosen MR: Cellular mechanisms for cardiac arrythmias. Circ Res 49:1, 1981

47. Ferrier GR: Digitalis arrhythmias: Role of oscillatory afterpotentials. Prog Cardiovasc Dis 19:459, 1977

48. Schmitt FO, Erlanger J: Directional differences in the conduction of the impulse through heart muscle and their possible relation to extrasystolic and fibrillary contractions. Am J Physiol 87:326, 1929

49. Wit AL, Cranefield PF, Hoffman BF: Slow conduction and reentry in the ventricular conducting system. II. Single and sustained circuit movement in networks of canine and bovine Purkinje fibers. Circ Res 30:11, 1972

50. Wit AL, Hoffman BF, Cranefield PF: Slow conduction and reentry in the ventricular conducting system. I. Return extrasystole in canine Purkinje fibers. Circ Res 30:1, 1972

51. Mendez C, Moe GK: Demonstration of a dual AV nodal conduction system in the isolated rabbit heart. Circ Res 23:378, 1966

52. Han J, Malozzi AM: Sinoatrial reciprocation in the isolated rabbit heart. Circ Res 22:355, 1965

53. Bigger JT Jr, Goldreyer BN: The mechanism of paroxysmal supraventricular tachycardia in man. Circulation 42:673, 1970

54. Sasyniuk BI, Mendez C: A mechanism for reentry in canine ventricular tissue. Circ Res 28:3, 1971

55. Wiggers CS: The mechanism and nature of ventricular fibrillation. Am Heart J 20:399, 1940

56. Allessie MA, Bouke FIM, Schopman FJG: Circus movements in rabbit atrial muscle as a mechanism of tachycardia. III. The "leading circle" concept: A new model of circus movement in cardiac tissue without the involvement of an anatomical obstacle. Circ Res 41:8, 1977

57. Antzelevitch C, Moe GK: Electronically mediated delayed conduction and reentry in relation to "slow responses" in mammalian ventricular conducting tissue. Circ Res 49:1129, 1981

58. Rozanski GJ, Jalife J, Moe GK: Reflected reentry in nonhomogeneous ventricular muscle as a mechanism of cardiac arrhythmias. Circulation 69:163, 1984

59. Harrison DC: Antiarrhythmic drug classification: New science and practical application. Am J Cardiol 56:185, 1985

60. Single BN, Jewitt DE: Beta-adrenergic receptor blocking drugs in cardiac arrhythmias. Drugs 7:426, 1974

61. Heissenbuttel RH, Bigger JT: Bretylium tosylate: A newly available antiarrhythmic drug for ventricular arrhythmias. Ann Intern Med 91:229, 1979

62. Singh BN, Nademanee K, Josephson MA et al: The electrophysiology and pharmacology of verapamil, flecainide, and amiodarone: Correlations with clinical effects and antiarrhythmic actions. Ann NY Acad Sci 432:210, 1984

63. Gillis RA, Onset JA: The role of the nervous system in the cardiovascular effects of digitalis. Pharmacol Rev 31:19, 1980

64. Gajowski J, Singer RB: Mortality in an insured population with atrial fibrillation. JAMA 245:1540, 1981

65. Kannel WB, Abbott RD, Savage DD et al: Epidemiologic features of chronic atrial fibrillation: The Framingham study. N Engl J Med 306:1018, 1982

66. Kannel WB, Abbott RD, Savage DD et al: Coronary heart disease and atrial fibrillation: The Framingham study. Am Heart J 106:389, 1983

67. Henry WL, Morganroth J, Pearlman AS et al: Relation between echocardiography determined left atrial size and atrial fibrillation. Circulation 53:273, 1976

68. Hartel G, Louhija A, Konttinen A et al: Value of quinidine in maintenance of sinus rhythm after electric conversion of atrial fibrillation. Br Heart J 32:57, 1970

69. Hartel G, Louhija A, Konttinen A: Disopyramide in the prevention of recurrence of atrial fibrillation after electroconversion. Clin Pharmacol Ther 15:551, 1974

70. Waxman HL, Myerburg RJ, Appel R et al: Verapamil for control of ventricular rate in paroxysmal supraventricular tachycardia and atrial fibrillation or flutter. Ann Intern Med 94:1, 1981

71. Weiner P, Bassan MM, Jarchovsky J et al: Clinical course of acute atrial fibrillation treated with rapid digitalization. Am Heart J 105:223, 1983

72. Sellers TD, Bashmore TM, Gallagher JJ: Digitalis in the preexcitation syndrome: Analysis during atrial fibrillation. Circulation 56:260, 1977

73. Gulamhusein S, Ko P, Carruthers SG et al: Acceleration of the ventricular response during atrial fibrillation in the Wolff-Parkinson-White syndrome after verapamil. Circulation 65:348, 1982

74. Waldo AL, MacLean WAH: Diagnosis and Treatment of Cardiac Arrhythmias Following Open Heart Surgery, p 115. Mt Kisco, NY: Futura, 1980

75. Wells JL, MacLean WAH, James TN et al: Characterization of atrial flutter. Studies in man after open heart surgery using fixed atrial electrodes. Circulation 60:66, 1979

76. Boineau JP: Atrial flutter: A synthesis of concepts. Circulation 72:249, 1985

77. Guiney TE, Lown B: Electrical conversion of atrial flutter to atrial fibrillation: Flutter mechanism in man. Br Heart J 34:1215, 1972

78. Waldo AL, MacLean WAH, Karp RB et al: Entrainment and interruption of atrial flutter with atrial pacing: Studies in man following open heart surgery. Circulation 56:737, 1977

79. Treatment of cardiac arrhythmias. Med Lett Drugs Thera 25:21, 1983

80. Sung RJ, Myerburg RJ, Castellanos A: Electrophysiological demonstration of concealed conduction in the human atrium. Circulation 58:940, 1978

81. Anderson RH, Becker AE, Brechenmacker C et al: Ventricular preexcitation: A proposed nomenclature for its substrates. Eur J Cardiol 3:27, 1975

82. Mendez C, Moe GK: Demonstration of a dual AV nodal conduction system in the isolated rabbit heart. Circ Res 19:378, 1966

83. Moe GR, Preston JB, Burlington H: Physiological evidence for a dual AV transmission system. Circ Res 4:357, 1956

84. Sung RJ, Styperek JL, Myerburg RJ et al: Initiation of two distinct forms of atrioventricular nodal reentrant tachycardia during programmed ventricular stimulation in man. Am J Cardiol 42:404, 1978

85. Waxman HL, Myerburg RJ, Appel R et al: Verapamil for control of ventricular rate in paroxysmal supraventricular tachycardia and atrial fibrillation or flutter: A doubleblind randomized cross-over study. Ann Intern Med 94:1, 1981

86. Wolff L, Parkinson J, White PD: Bundle branch block with short PR interval in healthy young people prone to paroxysmal tachyarrhythmia. Am Heart J 5:685, 1930

87. Wellens HJJ: The Wolff-Parkinson-White syndrome. In Mandel

WJ (ed): Cardiac Arrhythmias: Their Mechanisms, Diagnosis, and Management, p 342. Philadelphia, JB Lippincott, 1980

88. Gillette PC: Concealed anomalous cardiac conduction pathways: A frequent cause of supraventricular tachycardia. Am J Cardiol 40:848, 1977

89. Narula OS: Sinus node reentry: A mechanism for supraventricular tachycardia. Circulation 50:1114, 1974

90. Sung RJ, Change MS, Chiang BN: Clinical electrophysiology of supraventricular tachycardia. Cardiol Clin 1:225, 1983

91. Shine KI, Kastor J, Yurchak PM: Multifocal atrial tachycardia: Clincal and electrocardiographic features in 32 patients. N Engl J Med 279:344, 1968

92. Iseri LT, Fairshter RD, Hardemann JL et al: Magnesium and potassium therapy in multifocal atrial tachycardia. Am Heart J 110:789, 1985

93. Levine JH, Michael JR, Guarnieri T: Treatment of multifocal atrial tachycardia with verapamil. N Engl J Med 312:21, 1985

94. Wellens HJJ, Duren D, Lie KI: Observations on mechanisms of ventricular tachycardia in man. Circulation 54:237, 1976

95. Josephson ME, Horowitz LN, Farshidi A: Continuous local electrical activity: A mechanism of recurrent ventricular tachycardia. Circulation 57:659, 1978

96. Marcus NH, Falcone RA, Harken AH et al: Body surface late potentials: Effects of endocardial resection in patients with ventricular tachycardia. Circulation 70:632, 1984

97. Wiener I, Mindich B, Pitchon R: Fragmented endocardial electrical activity in patients with ventricular tachycardia: A new guide to surgical therapy. Am Heart J 107:86, 1984

98. Gardner PI, Ursell PK, Fenoglio JJ et al: Electrophysiologic and anatomic basis for fractionated electrograms recorded from healed myocardial infarcts. Circulation 72:596, 1985

99. Kieval RS, Johnson NJ, Rosen MR: Triggered activity as a cause of bigeminy. J Am Coll Cardiol 8:644, 1986

100. Lown B, Temte JV, Arter WJ: Ventricular tachyarrhythmias: Clinical aspects. Circulation 47:1364, 1973

101. Thanavaro S, Kleiger RE, Miller JP et al: Coupling interval and types of ventricular ectopic activity associated with ventricular runs. Am Heart J 106:484, 1983

102. Bleifer SB, Karpman HL, Sheppard JJ et al: Relation between premature ventricular complexes and development of ventricular tachycardia. Am J Cardiol 31:400, 1973

103. Chou TC, Wenzke F: The importance of R on T phenomenon. Am Heart J 96:191, 1978

104. Edwards RP, Miller RD, Roizen MF et al: Cardiac response to imipramine and pancuronium during anesthesia with halothane of enflurane. Anesthesiology 50:421, 1979

105. Stirt JA, Berger JM, Riker SM et al: Arrhythmogenic effects of aminophylline during halothane anesthesia in experimental animals. Anesth Analg 59:410, 1980

106. Joas TA, Stevens WC: Comparison of the arrhythmogenic doses of epinephrine during Forane, halothane, and fluroxene anesthesia in dogs. Anesthesiology 35:48, 1971

107. Zahed B, Miletick DJ, Ivankovich AD et al: Arrhythmic doses of epinephrine and dopamine during halothane, enflurane, methoxyflurane, and fluroxene in goats. Anesth Analg 56:207, 1977

108. Sumikawa K, Ishizaka N, Suzaki M: Arrhythmogenic plasma levels of epinephrine during halothane, enflurane, and pentobarbital anesthesia in the dog. Anesthesiology 58:322, 1983

109. Maze M, Smith CM: Identification of receptor mechanism mediating epinephrine-induced arrhythmias during halothane anesthesia in the dog. Anesthesiology 59:322, 1983

110. Spiss CK, Maxe M, Smith CM: Alpha-adrenergic responsiveness correlates with epinephrine dose for arrhythmias during halothane anesthesia in dogs. Anesth Analg 63:297, 1984

111. Marriott HJL: Aberrant ventricular conduction and the diagnosis of tachycardia. In Marriott HJL (ed): Practical Electrocardiography, p 211. Baltimore, Williams & Wilkins, 1983

112. Marriott HJL: Differential diagnosis of supraventricular and ventricular tachycardia. Geriatrics 25:9, 1970

113. Kistin AD: Problems in the differentiation of ventricular arrhythmia with abnormal QRS. Prog Cardiovasc Dis 8:1, 1966

114. Wellens HJJ, Bar FW, Lie KI: The value of the electrocardiogram in the differential diagnosis of a tachycardia with a widened QRS complex. Am J Med 64:27, 1978

115. Strasberg B, Sclarovsky S, Endberg A et al: Procainamide-induced polymorphous ventricular tachycardia. Am J Cardiol 47:1309, 1981

116. Reynolds EW, Vanderark CR: Quinidine syncope and the delayed repolarization syndromes. Mod Concepts Cardiovasc Dis 45:117, 1976

117. Nicholson WJ, Martin CE, Gracey JG et al: Disopyramide-induced ventricular fibrillation. Am J Cardiol 43:1053, 1979

118. Carruth JE, Silverman ME: Torsade de Pointes: Atypical ventricular tachycardia complicating subarachnoid hemorrhage. Chest 78:886, 1980

119. Krikler DM, Curry PVL: Torsade de pointes, an atypical ventricular tachycardia. Br Heart J 38:117, 1976

120. Henry EI: Significance of the relation of QRS and T-waves in bundle branch block: A useful electrocardiographic sign. Am Heart J 54:407, 1957

121. Dhingra RC, Amat-Y-Leon F, Wyndham C et al: Significance of left axis deviation in patients with chronic left bundle branch block. Am J Cardiol 42:551, 1978

122. Rabkin SW, Mathewson FA, Tate RB: Natural history of left bundle branch block. Br Heart J 43:164, 1980

123. Rizzon P, Rossi L, Baissus C et al: Left posterior hemiblock in acute myocardial infarction. Br Heart J 35:711, 1975

124. Rossi L: Histopathology of conducting system in left anterior hemiblock. Br Heart J 38:1304, 1976

125. Marriott HJL: The hemiblocks and trifascicular block. In Marriott HJL (ed): Practical Electrocardiography, p 84. Baltimore, Williams & Wilkins, 1983

126. McAnulty JH, Rahimtoola SH, Murphy E et al: Natural history of "high-risk" bundle-branch block: Final report of a prospective study. N Engl J Med 307:137, 1982

127. Denes P, Dhingra RC, Wu D et al: Sudden death in patients with chronic bifascicular block. Arch Intern Med 137:1005, 1977

128. Schneider JF, Thomas E, Kreger BE et al: Newly acquired right bundle-branch block. Ann Intern Med 92:37, 1980

129. Schneider JF, Thomas E, Kreger BE: Newly acquired left bundle-branch block: The Framingham study. Ann Intern Med 90:303, 1979

130. Pastore JO, Yurchak PM, Janis KM et al: The risk of advanced heart block in surgical patients with right bundle branch block and left axis deviation. Circulation 57:677, 1978

131. Rooney SM, Goldiner PL, Muss E: Relationship of right bundle-branch block and marked left axis deviation to complete heart block during general anesthesia. Anesthesiology 44:64, 1976

132. Zoll PM, Zoll RH, Falk RH et al: External noninvasive temporary cardiac pacing: Clinical trials. Circulation 71:937, 1985

133. Johnson RL: Electrocardiographic findings in 67,375 asymptomatic individuals. VII. A-V block. Am J Cardiol 6:153, 1960

134. Narula OS: Wenckebach type I and type II atrioventricular block (revisited). Cardiovasc Clin 6:138, 1974

135. Marriott HJL: Atrioventricular block: Conventional approach. In Marriott HJL (ed): Practical Electrocardiography, p 322. Baltimore, Williams & Wilkins, 1983

136. Viitasalo MT, Kala R, Eisalo A: Ambulatory electrocardiographic recording in endurance athletes. Br Heart J 47:213, 1982

137. Lown B, Losowsky BD: Artificial cardiac pacemakers. II. N Engl J Med 283:971, 1970

138. Lepeschkin E: The electrocardiographic diagnosis of bilateral bundle branch block in relation to heart block. Prog Cardiovas Dis 6:445, 1964

139. Steiner C, Lau SH, Stein E et al: Electrophysiological documentation of trifascicular block as the common cause of complete heart block. Am J Cardiol 28:436, 1971

140. Rosenbaum MB, Elizari MV, Kretz A et al: Anatomical basis of A-V conduction disturbances. Geriatrics 25:132, 1970

141. Lev M: Anatomic basis for atrioventricular block. Am J Med 37:742, 1964

142. Lenegre J: Etiology and pathology of bilateral bundle branch block in relation to complete heart block. Prog Cardiovasc Dis 6:409, 1964

143. Roberts WC, Cardin JM: Locations of myocardial infarcts: A confusion of terms and definitions. Am J Cardiol 42:868, 1978

144. Yu PNG, Stewart JM: Subendocardial myocardial infarction with special reference to the electrocardiographic change. Am Heart J 39: 862, 1950

145. Evans W, McRae C: The lesser electrocardiographic signs of cardiac pain. Br Heart J 14:429, 1952

146. Gerson MC, Phillips JF, Morris SN et al: Exercise-induced U wave inversion as a marker of stenosis of the left anterior descending coronary artery. Circulation 60:1014, 1979

147. Mann RH, Burchell HB: The sign of T wave inversion in sinus beats following ventricular extrasystoles. Am Heart J 47:504, 1954

148. Marriott HJL: Myocardial infarction. In Marriott HJL (ed): Practical Electrocardiography, p. 373. Baltimore, Williams & Wilkins, 1983

149. Liu CK: Atrial infarction of the heart. Circulation 23:331, 1961

150. Kurita A, Chaitman BR, Bourassa MG: Significance of exercise-induced junction S-T depression in evaluation of coronary artery disease. Am J Cardiol 40:492, 1977

151. Rijneke RD, Ascoop CA, Talmon JL: Clinical significance of upsloping ST segments in exercise electrocardiography. Circulation 61:671, 1980

152. Stuart RJ, Ellestad MH: Upsloping S-T segments in exercise stress testing. Am J Cardiol 37:19, 1976

153. Yasui H: Comparison of coronary arteriography findings during angina pectoris associated with ST elevation or depression. Am J Cardiol 47:539, 1981

154. Stiles GL, Rosati RA, Wallace AG: Clinical relevance of exercise-induced ST segment elevation. Am J Cardiol 46:931, 1980

155. Sriwattanakomen S, Ticzon AR, Zubritsky SA et al: ST segment elevation during exercise: Electrocardiographic and arteriographic correlation in 38 patients. Am J Cardiol 45:762, 1980

156. Specchia G, deServi S, Falcone C et al: Coronary arterial spasm as a cause of exercise-induced ST segment elevation in patients with variant angina. Circulation 59:948, 1979

157. Specchia G, deServi S, Falcone C et al: Significance of exercise-induced ST segment elevation in patients without myocardial infarction. Circulation 63:46, 1981

158. Bruce MA, Spodick DH: Atypical electrocardiogram in acute pericarditis: Characteristics and prevalence. J Electrocardiol 13:61, 1980

159. Spodick DH: Electrocardiogram in acute pericarditis. Distributions of morphologic and axial changes by stages. Am J Cardiol 33:470, 1974

160. Bashour FA, Cochran PW: The association of electrical alternans with pericardial effusion. Dis Chest 44:146, 1963

161. McGregor M, Baskind E: Electrical alternans in pericardial effusion. Circulation 11:837, 1955

162. Nizet PM, Marriott HJL: The electrocardiogram and pericardial effusion. JAMA 198:169, 1966

163. Hersh C: Electrocardiographic changes in subarachnoid hemorrhage, meningitis, and intracranial space occupying lesions. Br Heart J 26:785, 1964

164. Surawicz B: Electrocardiographic pattern of cerebrovascular accident. JAMA 197:913, 1966

165. Gould L, Reddy RC, Kollali M et al: Electrocardiographic normalization after cerebral vascular accident. J Electrocardiol 14:191, 1981

166. Emslie-Smith D: The significance of changes in the electrocardiogram in hypothermia. Br Heart J 21:343, 1959

167. Myers GB: Correlation of electrocardiographic and pathologic function in large anterolateral infarcts. Am Heart J 36:838, 1948

168. Myers GB: Correlation of electrocardiographic and pathologic findings in anteroseptal infarction. Am Heart J 36:535, 1948

169. Myers GB: Correlation of electrocardiographic and pathologic findings in posterolateral infarction. Am Heart J 38:837, 1949

170. Erhardt LR, Sjögren A, Wahlberg I: Single right-sided precordial lead in the diagnosis of right ventricular involvement in myocardial infarction. Am Heart J 91:571, 1976

171. Croft CH, Nicod P, Corbett JR et al: Detection of acute right ventricular infarction by right precordial electrocardiography. Am J Cardiol 50:421, 1982

Electrical Safety

The myriad of electrical and electronic devices in the modern operating room greatly improves patient care and safety. However, these devices also subject both the patient and operating room personnel to increased risks. To combat this problem, these electrical systems are designed with specific safety features that reduce the risk of electrical shock. It is incumbent upon the anesthesiologist to have a thorough understanding of the basic principles of electricity and an appreciation of the concepts of electrical safety as they apply to the operating room environment.

PRINCIPLES OF ELECTRICITY

A basic principle of electricity is known as Ohm's law and is represented by the equation:

$$E = I \times R$$
$$E = \text{electromotive force (volts)}$$
$$I = \text{current (amperes)}$$
$$R = \text{resistance (ohms)}$$

Ohm's law has been used as the basis for the physiologic equation where the blood pressure is equal to the cardiac output times the total peripheral resistance ($BP = CO \times TPR$). In this case, the blood pressure of the vascular system is analogous to voltage, the cardiac output to current, and peripheral resistance to the forces opposing the flow of electrons. Electrical power is measured in units called *watts*. A watt is equal to the product of the voltage and the amperage and is defined by the formula:

$$W = E \times I.$$

The amount of electrical work done is measured in watts per unit of time. The watt-second (a joule) is a common designation for electrical energy expended in doing work. The energy produced by a defibrillator is measured in watt-seconds (or joules), and the kilowatt-hour is frequently used to measure very large quantities of electrical energy. Wattage not only can be thought of as measure of work done but can also be thought of as heat produced in any electrical circuit. Substituting Ohm's law in the formula

$$W = EI$$
$$W = IR \times I$$
$$W = I^2 R$$

Thus, wattage is equal to the square of the amperage times the resistance. Using these formulas, it is possible to calculate the number of amps and the resistance of a given device if the wattage and the voltage is known. For example, a 60-watt light bulb operating on a household 120-volt circuit would require 0.5 amperes of current for operation. Rearranging the formula so that

$$I = W/E$$
$$I = \frac{60 \text{ watts}}{120 \text{ volts}}$$
$$I = 0.5 \text{ amps}$$

Using this in Ohm's Law,

$$R = E/I$$

the resistance can be calculated to be 240 ohms.

$$R = \frac{120 \text{ volts}}{0.5 \text{ amps}}$$
$$R = 240 \text{ ohms}$$

It is obvious from the previous discussion that 1 volt of electromotive force flowing through a 1-ohm resistance will generate 1 amp of current. Similarly, 1 amp of current induced by 1 volt of EMF (electromotive force) will generate 1 watt of power.

DIRECT AND ALTERNATING CURRENTS

Any substance that permits the flow of electrons is defined as a conductor. Current is characterized by electrons flowing through a conductor. If the electron flow is always in the same direction, it is referred to as direct current (DC). However, if the electron flow changes direction (and goes in the opposite direction) at a regular interval, it is termed alternating current (AC). Either of these types of current can be pulsed or continuous in nature.[1]

The previous discussion of Ohm's law is accurate when applied to DC circuits. However, when dealing with AC circuits, the situation is more complex, because the current is opposed in its flow by more than resistance. This more complicated form of resistance to current flow is termed *impedance*.

IMPEDANCE

Impedance is defined as the sum of the forces that oppose electron movement in AC circuits and is designated by the letter Z. Impedance consists of resistance (ohms) but also takes into account capacitance as well as inductance. In actuality, when referring to AC circuits, Ohm's law is defined as:

$$E = I \times Z$$

An insulator is defined as a substance that opposes the flow of electrons and hence has a high impedance to flow, whereas a conductor is a material with a low impedance to electron flow.

In AC circuits, the capacitance and inductance can be important factors in determining the total impedance. Both capacitance and inductance are influenced by the frequency (cycles per second or Hertz, Hz) when the AC current reverses direction. The impedance is directly proportional to the inductance times the frequency ($Z \propto f \times IND$), and the impedance is inversely proportional to the product of the capacitance and the frequency:

$$Z / \propto \left(\frac{1}{f \times CAP} \right).$$

As the AC current frequency increases, both capacitance and inductance will increase. However, since impedance and capacitance are inversely related, total impedance will decrease as capacitance increases. Thus, as frequency increases, capacitance will rise, impedance will fall, and more current will be allowed to pass.[2]

CAPACITANCE

A capacitor consists of any two parallel conductors that are separated by an insulator (Fig. 23-1). A capacitor has the ability to store charge. Capacitance is the measure of that substance's ability to store charge. In a DC circuit, the capacitor plates are charged by a voltage source (*i.e.*, a battery), and

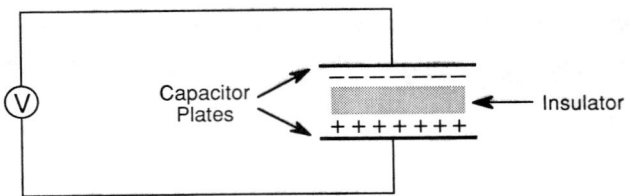

FIG. 23-1. A capacitor consists of two parallel conductors separated by an insulator. The capacitor is capable of storing charge supplied by a voltage source.

there is only a momentary current flow. The circuit is not completed, and there can be no further current flow unless a resistance is connected between the two plates and the capacitor is discharged.[3]

In contrast to DC circuits, a capacitor in AC circuits permits current flow, even when there is no completed circuit. This is due to the nature of AC circuits, whereby the current flow is constantly reversing itself. Since current flow results from the movement of electrons, every reversal of the AC current direction results in the capacitor plates being alternately charged positive and then negative. The consequence of this is an effective current flow as far as the remainder of the circuit is concerned, even though the circuit is not completed.[4]

Since capacitance varies directly with the AC frequency (Hz), the greater the AC frequency, the faster the electrons move back and forth. This results in a greater capacitance and a greater current flow. Therefore, high-frequency currents will have a high capacitance, and, since impedance and capacitance are inversely related, a marked decrease in impedance. As an example, a 20 million–ohm impedance in a 60-Hz AC circuit will be reduced to only a few hundred–ohm impedance when the frequency is increased to 1 million Hz.[5]

Electrical devices use capacitors for various beneficial purposes. There is, however, a phenomenon known as *stray capacitance*, which is defined as capacitance that was not designed into the system but is incidental to the construction of the equipment.[6] All AC-operated equipment produces stray capacitance. As an example, an ordinary power cord that consists of two insulated wires running next to each other will generate significant capacitance simply by being plugged into a 120-volt circuit, even though the piece of equipment is not turned on. Another example of stray capacitance is found in electric motors. The circuit wiring in electric motors generates stray capacitance to the metal housing of the motor.[7] The clinical importance of capacitance will be emphasized later in the chapter.

INDUCTANCE

Whenever electrons flow in a wire, a magnetic field is induced around the wire. If the wire is coiled repeatedly around an iron core, such as in a transformer, the magnetic field can be very strong. Inductance is a property of AC circuits in which an opposing electromotive force (EMF) can be electromagnetically induced in the circuit. The net effect of inductance is to increase impedance. Since inductance is also dependent upon AC frequency, as frequency is increased, inductance and thereby total impedance will also increase. Therefore, the total impedance of a coil will be much greater than its simple resistance.[4]

SHOCK HAZARDS

ALTERNATING AND DIRECT CURRENTS

Whenever an individual comes in contact with an external source of electricity, there is a potential for an electrical shock. Since an electrical current can cause stimulation of skeletal muscle cells, this can be used therapeutically in devices such as pacemakers or defibrillators. However, casual contact with an electrical current can also lead to an injury or death. Contact with either direct or alternating currents can be lethal. Although it takes approximately three times as much direct current as alternating current to cause ventricular fibrillation,[3] this by no means renders DC current harmless. Devices such as an automobile battery or a DC defibrillator can be sources of direct current shocks.

In the United States, utility companies supply electrical energy in the form of alternating currents of 120 volts at a frequency of 60 Hz.* The 60 Hz refers to the number of times in 1 second that the current changes its direction of flow.[8] The pattern that both the voltage and current waveforms assume is sinusoidal (Fig. 23-2).

In order to complete a circuit and have current flow, a closed loop must exist, and there must be a voltage source that drives the current through the impedance. If current is to flow in the electrical circuit, there has to be a voltage differential or a drop in the driving pressure across the impedance. According to Ohm's law, if the resistance is held constant, then the greater the current flow the larger the voltage drop must be.[9]

The power company labors to keep the line voltage constant at 120 volts. Therefore, by Ohm's law, the current flow is inversely proportional to the impedance. A typical power cord consists of two conductors. One is designated the "hot" and carries the current to the resistance; the other is the neutral, which returns the current to the source. The potential between the two is effectively 120 volts (Fig. 23-3). The amount of current that a given device uses is frequently referred to as the *load*. The load of the circuit is dependent upon the impedance. A very high impedance circuit will allow only a small current flow, and, thus, the load will be small. A very low impedance circuit will draw a large current and is said to be a large load. A *short circuit* is an example of an essentially zero impedance load with a very high current flow.[10]

In order to practice electrical safety, it is important for the anesthesiologist to have a thorough understanding of the basic principles of electricity as well as a thorough knowledge and understanding of how electrical accidents can occur. Electrical accidents or shocks occur because a person becomes part of or completes an electrical circuit. In order to receive a shock, the person must contact the electrical circuit at two points, and there must be a voltage source to drive the current (Fig. 23-4).

When an individual comes in contact with a source of electricity, there are two potential sources of damage. First, the electrical current can disrupt the normal electrical function of cells. Depending upon the magnitude of the current, it can cause contraction of muscles, alteration of brain function,

---

*The 120 volts of EMF and 1 amp of current are the effective voltage and amperage in an AC circuit. This is also referred to as *RMS*, which stands for Root–mean–square. In fact, it takes 1.414 amperes (amps) of peak amperage in the sinusoidal curve to give an effective amperage of 1 amp. Similarly, it takes 170 volts (120 × 1.414) at the peak of the AC curve to get an effective voltage of 120 volts.[8]

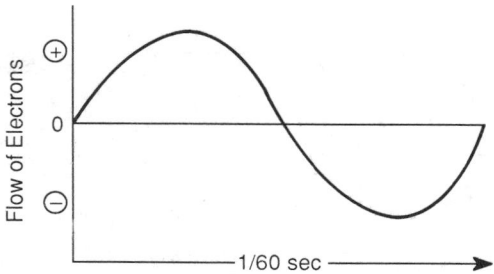

FIG. 23-2. Sine wave flow of electrons in a 60-Hz alternating current.

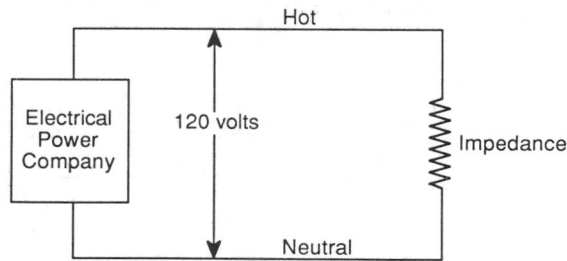

FIG. 23-3. A typical AC circuit where 120 volts potential difference exists between the hot and neutral side of the circuit. The current flows through a resistance, which in AC circuits is more accurately referred to as *impedance*, and then returns to the electrical power company.

paralysis of respiration, or disruption of the normal functioning of the heart, leading to ventricular fibrillation. The second mechanism involves the dissipation of electrical energy throughout the tissues of the body. Electrical current passing through any resistance raises the temperature. If enough energy is released, the temperature rises to the point at which a burn will occur. In accidents involving household currents, usually the burns are not severe, whereas in accidents involving very high voltages (*i.e.*, power transmission lines), severe burns are quite common.

Since current is the flow of electrical charges per unit of time, it is the amount of current (number of amps) that an individual comes in contact with that determines the severity of a shock. For the purposes of this discussion, electrical shocks are divided into two categories. *Macroshock* refers to gross amounts of current encountered by a human that can cause harm or death. *Microshock* applies only to the electrically susceptible patient who has an external conduit that is in direct contact with the heart. This can be a pacing wire or a saline-filled catheter such as central venous or pulmonary artery catheter. In the case of the electrically susceptible patient, minute amounts of current may cause ventricular fibrillation. Table 23-1 shows the typical effects that various currents will produce following a 1-sec contact with a 60-Hz current. When an individual comes in contact with a 120-volt household current, the severity of the shock will depend upon his skin resistance, the duration of the contact with the electrical source, and the current density. Skin resistance can vary from a few thousand ohms to over a million ohms. If a person with a skin resistance of 1000 ohms comes in contact

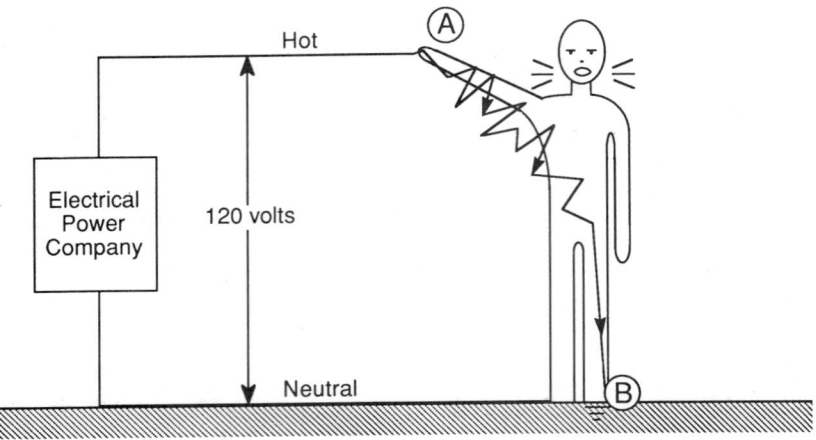

FIG. 23-4. An individual can complete an electric circuit and receive a shock by coming in contact with the hot side of the circuit (point A). This is because he or she is standing on the ground (point B), and the contact point A and the ground point B provide the two contact points necessary for a completed circuit. The severity of the shock that the individual receives, is dependent upon his or her skin resistance.

TABLE 23-1. Effects of 60-Hz Current on an Average Human for a 1-Second Contact[6]

CURRENT	EFFECT
MACROSHOCK	
1 mA (0.001A)	Threshold of perception
5 mA (0.005A)	Accepted as maximal harmless current intensity
10–20 mA (0.01–0.02A)	"Let-go" current before sustained muscle contraction
50 mA (0.05A)	Pain, possible fainting, mechanical injury; heart and respiratory functions continue
100–300 mA (0.1–0.3A)	Ventricular fibrillation will start, but respiratory center remains intact
6000 mA (6A)	Sustained myocardial contraction, followed by normal heart rhythm; temporary respiratory paralysis; burns if current density is high
MICROSHOCK	
100 μA (0.1 mA)	Ventricular fibrillation
10 μA (0.01 mA)	Recommended maximal 60-Hz leakage current

A = amperes; mA = milliamperes; μA = microamperes

with a 120-volt circuit, he or she would receive 120 mA of current, which would, in all probability, be a lethal shock. However, if that same person's skin resistance was 100,000 ohms, the current flow would be 1.2 mA, which would be barely perceptible.

$$I = \frac{E}{R} = \frac{120 \text{ volts}}{1000 \text{ ohms}} = 120 \text{ mA} \qquad \frac{120 \text{ volts}}{100,000 \text{ ohms}} = 1.2 \text{ mA}$$

The longer that an individual is in contact with the electrical source, the more dire the consequences, since more energy will be released and more tissue damage will result. Also, the longer the contact with the current, the greater will be the chance of ventricular fibrillation from excitation of the heart during the vulnerable period of the ECG cycle.

Current density is merely a way of expressing the amount of current that is applied per area of tissue. The current tends to diffuse in all directions in the body. The higher the current or the smaller the area to which it is applied, the higher the current density. In relation to the heart, a current of 100 mA (100,000 μA) is generally required to produce ventricular fibrillation when applied to the surface of the body. However, only 100 μA (0.1 mA) is required to produce ventricular fibrillation when that minute current is applied directly to the myocardium through a very small area such as a pacing wire electrode. In this case, the current density is 1000-fold higher when applied directly to the heart and, therefore, requires 1000-fold less energy to cause ventricular fibrillation. Therefore, the electrically susceptible patient can be electrocuted with currents that are well below the human threshold of perception which is 1 mA.

The frequency at which the current reverses itself is also an important factor in determining the amount of current that an individual can safely contact. Utility companies in the United States produce electricity at a frequency of 60 Hz. The "let-go" current is defined as that current above which sustained muscular contraction occurs and at which an individual would be unable to let go of an energized wire. The let-go current for 60-Hz AC power is 10 to 20 mA,[10–12] whereas at a frequency of 1 million Hz, up to 3 amp (3000 mA) is generally regarded as safe.[3] It should be noted that very high–frequency currents do not excite contractile tissue; consequently, they do not cause cardiac dysrhythmias.

Therefore, it can be seen that Ohm's Law governs the flow of electricity. For a completed circuit to exist, there must be a closed loop with a driving pressure to force a current through a resistance. Just as in the cardiovascular system there must be a blood pressure to drive the cardiac output through the peripheral resistance. Figure 23-5 illustrates that a hot wire carrying a 120-volt pressure through the resistance of a 60-watt light bulb produces a current flow of 0.5 amps. The voltage in the neutral wire is approximately 0 volts, whereas the current in the neutral wire remains at 0.5 amps. This correlates with our cardiovascular model, where a mean blood pressure drop of 80 mm Hg from the aortic root to the right atrium forces a cardiac output of 6 l/min through a peripheral resistance of 13.3 peripheral resistance units. However, the flow (in this case, the cardiac output or, in the case of the electrical model, the current) is still the same everywhere in the circuit, that is, the cardiac output on the arterial side is the same as the cardiac output on the venous side.

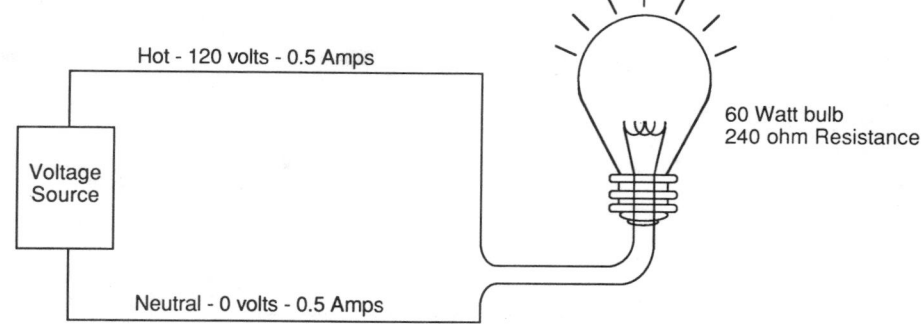

FIG. 23-5. A 60-watt light bulb has an internal resistance of 240 ohms and draws 0.5 amps of current. The voltage drop in the circuit is from 120 in the hot wire to 0 in the neutral wire, but the current is 0.5 amps in both the hot and neutral wires.

GROUNDING

In order to fully understand electrical shock hazards and their prevention, it is necessary to have a thorough knowledge of the concepts of grounding. These concepts of grounding are probably the single largest source of confusion in any discussion of electrical safety. This is because the same term is used to describe several different principles. In electrical terminology, grounding is applied to two separate concepts. The first is the grounding of electrical power, and the second is the grounding of electrical equipment. Thus, the concepts that power 1) can be grounded *or* ungrounded, and 2) may supply electrical devices that are themselves grounded or ungrounded are not mutually exclusive. It is vital to understand this point as the basis of electrical safety (Table 23-2). Electrical power in the home is grounded, whereas that in the operating room is ungrounded. Electrical equipment in the home may be grounded or ungrounded, but, in the operating room, it should always be grounded.

Electrical Power—Grounded

Electrical utilities universally provide power that is grounded. (By convention, the earth ground potential is zero, and all voltages represent a difference between potentials.) That is, one of the wires supplying the power to a home is intentionally connected to the earth. The utility companies do this as a safety measure to prevent electrical charges from building up in their wiring during electrical storms and to prevent the very high voltages used in transmitting power by the utility from entering the home in the event of an equipment failure in their high-voltage system.[3]

The power enters the typical home in the form of two wires. These two wires are attached to the main fuse or circuit breaker box at the service entrance. The "hot" wire supplies power to the "hot" distribution strip. The neutral is connected to the neutral distribution strip and to a service entrance ground (*i.e.*, a pipe buried in the earth) (Fig. 23-6).

TABLE 23-2.   Differences Between Power and Equipment Grounding in the Home and the Operating Room

	POWER	EQUIPMENT
Home	+	±
Operating room	−	+

+ = grounded; − = ungrounded; ± = may or may not be grounded.

From the fuse box, three wires leave to supply the electrical outlets in the house. The "hot" wire is color-coded black and carries a voltage 120 volts above ground potential. The second wire is the neutral or white wire; the third wire is the ground wire, which is the green or bare wire. The ground and the neutral wire are attached together at the same point in the circuit breaker box and then further connected to a cold water pipe (Figs. 23-7 and 23-8). Thus, this grounded power system is also referred to as a neutral grounded power system. The black wire is not connected to ground, as this would create a short circuit. The black wire is attached to the "hot" (*i.e.*, 120 volts above ground) distribution strip upon which the circuit breakers or fuses are located. From here, numerous branch circuits supply electrical power to the house. Each branch circuit is protected by a circuit breaker or fuse, which limits current to a specific maximal amperage. Most electrical circuits in the house are 15- or 20-amp circuits. These typically supply power for the electrical outlets and lights in the house. A number of higher amperage circuits are also provided for devices such as an electric stove or an electric clothes dryer, which can draw from 30 to 50 amps of current. The circuit breaker will interrupt the flow of current on the hot side of the line in the event of a short circuit or if too high a demand is placed on that circuit. For example, a 15-amp branch circuit will be capable of supporting 1800 watts of power.

$$W = EI$$
$$W = 120 \text{ volts} \times 15 \text{ amps}$$
$$W = 1800 \text{ watts}$$

Therefore, if two 1500-watt hair dryers were simultaneously plugged into one outlet, the load would be too great for a 15-amp circuit, and the circuit breaker would open or the fuse would melt. This is done to prevent the supply wires from melting and starting a fire. The wattage of the circuit breaker on the branch circuit is determined by the thickness of the wire that it supplies. If a 20-amp breaker is used with wire rated for only 15 amps, the wire could melt and start a fire before the circuit breaker would trip. It is important to note that a 15-amp circuit breaker provides no protection from lethal shocks to an individual. The 15 amps of current that will open the circuit breaker are far in excess of the 100 to 200 mA that can produce ventricular fibrillation.

The wires that leave the circuit breaker then supply the electrical outlets and lighting for the rest of the house. In older homes, the electrical cable consists of two wires, a hot and a neutral, which supply power to the electrical outlets (Fig. 23-9). In newer homes, a third wire has been added to the electrical cable (Fig. 23-10). This third wire is green or bare

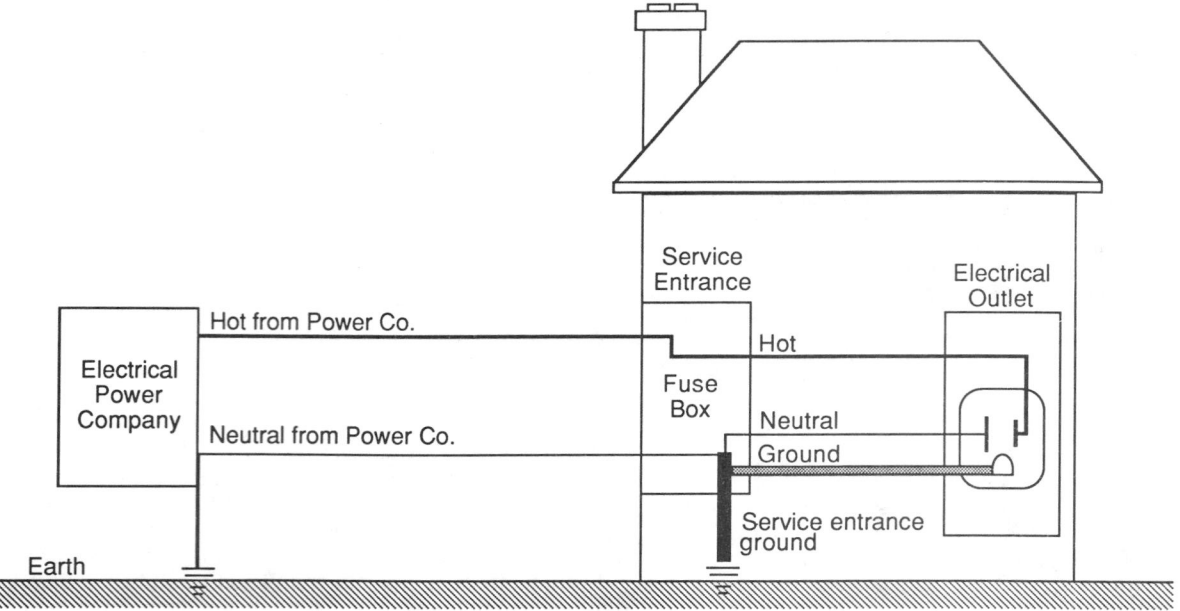

FIG. 23-6. In a neutral grounded power system, the electric company supplies two lines to the typical home. The neutral is connected to ground by the power company and is again connected to a service entrance ground when it enters the fuse box. Both the neutral and ground wires are connected together in the fuse box at the neutral bus bar, which is also attached to the service entrance ground.

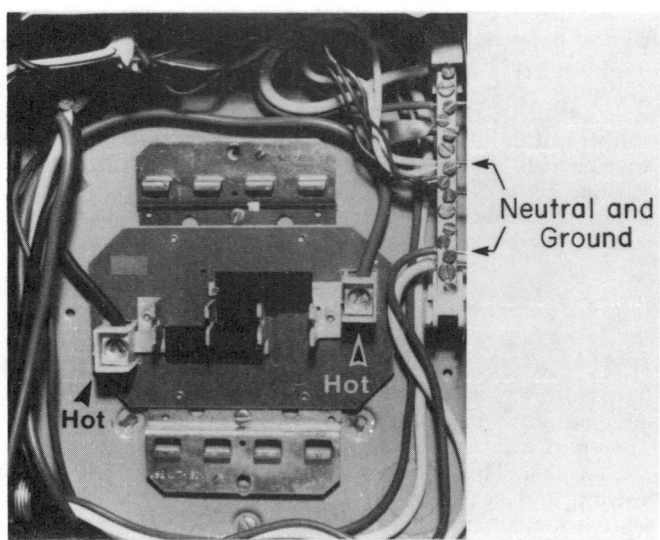

FIG. 23-7. Inside a fuse box with the circuit breakers removed. *Arrowheads* indicate the hot wires energizing the strips where the circuit breakers are located. The *arrows* point to the neutral bus bar where the neutral and ground wires are connected.

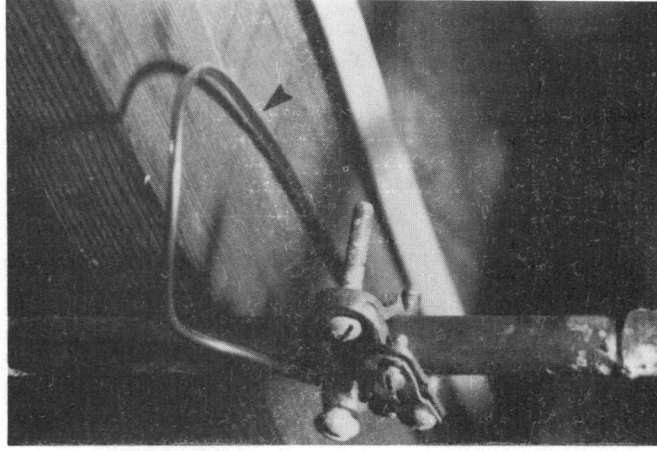

FIG. 23-8. The *arrow* indicates the ground wire from the fuse box attached to a cold water pipe.

and serves as a ground wire for the power receptacle (Fig. 23-11). On one end, the ground wire is attached to the electrical outlet (Fig. 23-12); on the other end, it is connected to the neutral distribution strip in the circuit breaker box where the white or neutral wires are also attached (Fig. 23-13).

It should be realized that in both the old and new situ-

ations, the power is still grounded, that is, a 120-volt potential exists between the black wire and the white wire and between the black wire and ground. In this case, ground is the earth (Fig. 23-14). In modern home construction, there is still a 120-volt potential difference between the black and the white wire as well as a 120-volt difference between the equipment ground wire, which is the third wire and 120-volt potential between the black wire and earth (Fig. 23-15).

A 60-watt light bulb can be used as an example to further demonstrate this point. Normally, the black and white wires are connected to the two wires of the light bulb socket, and,

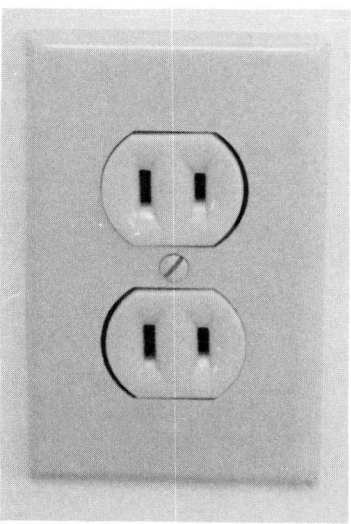

FIG. 23-9. An older style electrical outlet consisting of only two wires (a hot and a neutral). There is no ground wire.

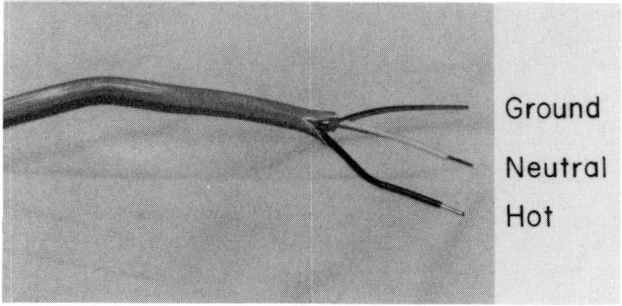

FIG. 23-10. Modern electrical cable in which a third or ground wire has been added.

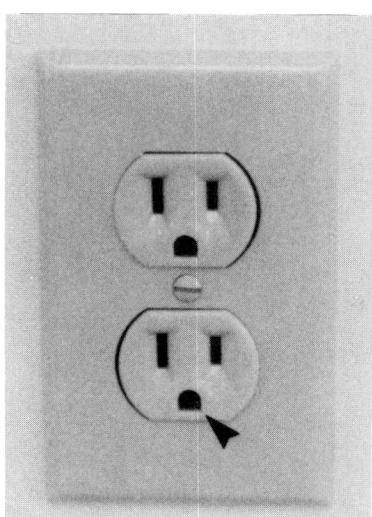

FIG. 23-11. Modern electrical outlet in which the ground wire is present. The *arrow* points to the part of the receptacle where the ground wire connects.

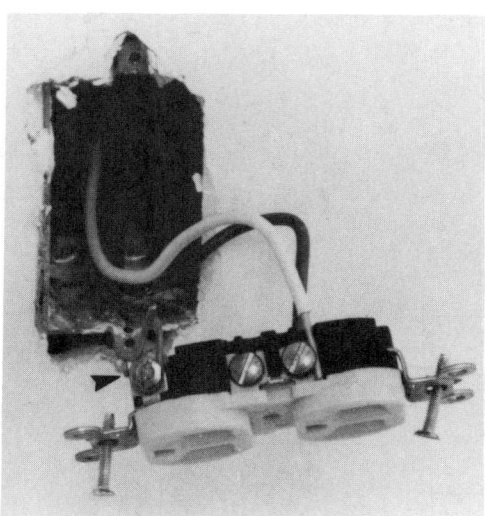

FIG. 23-12. Detail of a modern electrical power receptacle. The *arrow* points to the ground wire, which is attached to the grounding screw on the power receptacle.

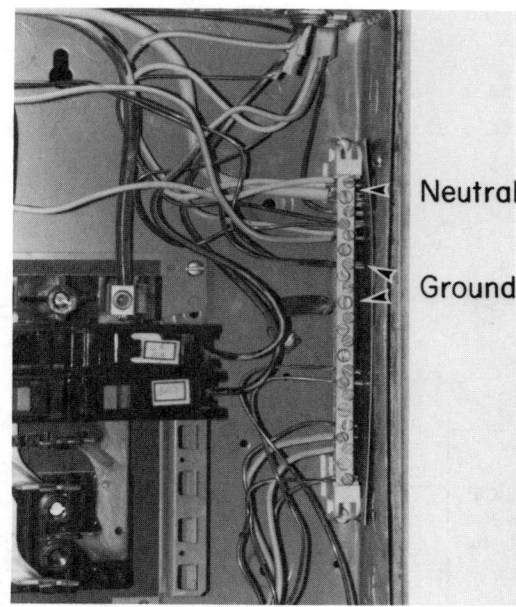

FIG. 23-13. The ground wires from the power outlet are run to the neutral bus bar, where they are connected with the neutral wires (*arrowheads*).

when the switch is thrown, the bulb will illuminate (Fig. 23-16). Similarly, if the black wire is connected to one side of the bulb socket and the other wire from the light bulb is connected to the equipment ground wire, the bulb will still illuminate. If the equipment ground wire is not present, the bulb will still light if the second wire is connected to any metallic grounded object such as a water pipe or a faucet. This illustrates that the 120-volt potential difference exists not only between the hot and the neutral wire but also between the hot wire and any object referenced to ground. Thus, in a

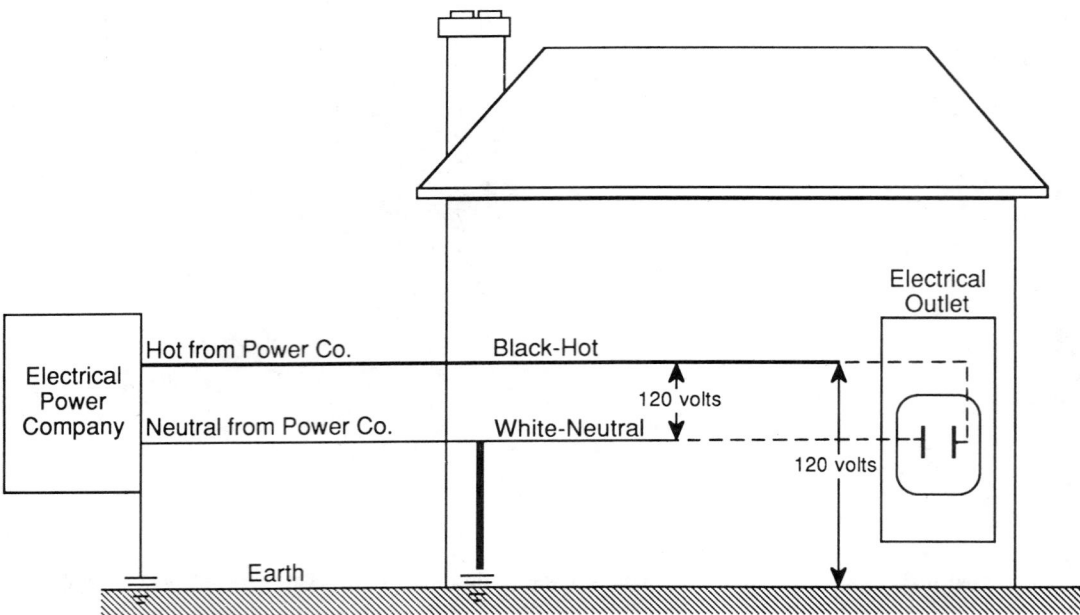

FIG. 23-14. Diagram of a house with older style wiring that does not contain a ground wire. A 120-volt potential difference exists between the hot and the neutral wire as well as between the hot wire and earth.

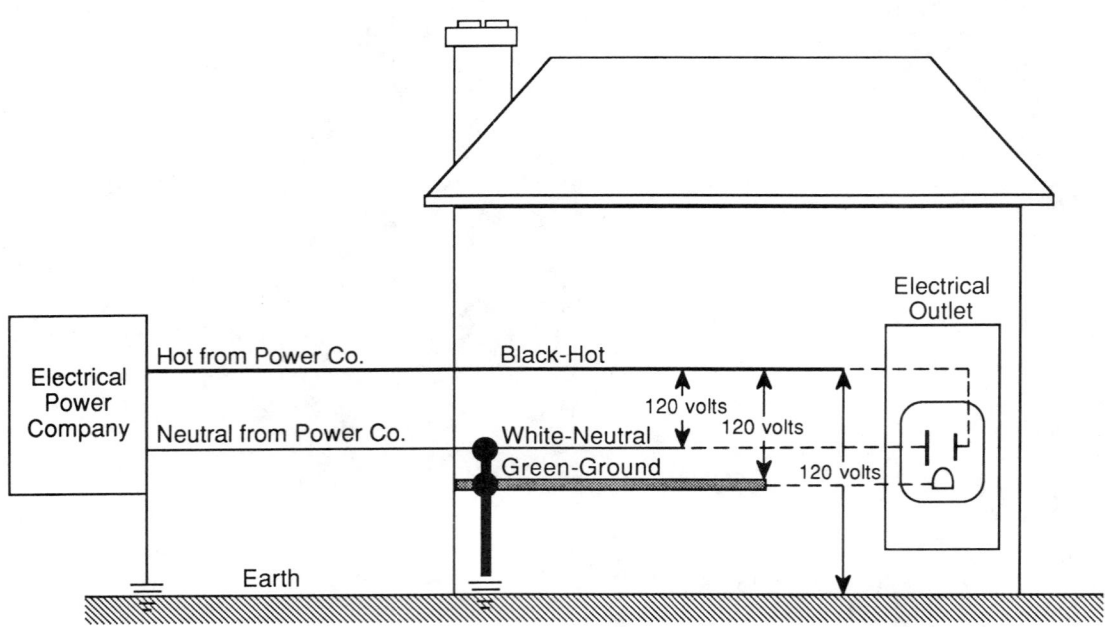

FIG. 23-15. Diagram of a house with modern wiring in which the third or ground wire has been added. The 120-volt potential difference exists between the hot and neutral wires, the hot and the ground wires, and the hot wire and earth.

grounded power system, the current will flow between the black wire and any conductor with an earth ground.

In order for current to flow, there must be a closed loop with a voltage source. For an individual to get an electric shock, he or she must contact the loop at two points. Since we may be standing on ground or be in contact with an object that is referenced to ground, only *one* additional contact point is necessary to complete the circuit and thus receive an elec-

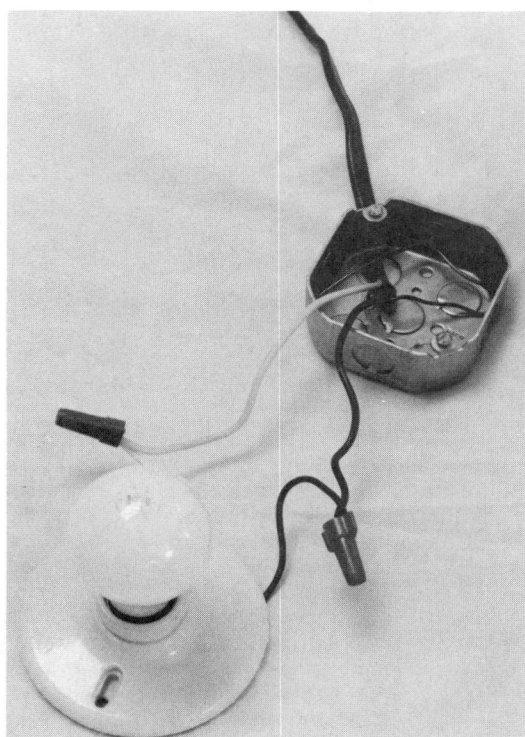

FIG. 23-16. A simple light bulb circuit in which the hot and neutral wires are connected with the corresponding wires from the light bulb fixture.

trical shock. This is an unfortunate and inherently dangerous consequence of grounded power systems. In the example of the modern wiring system, the third wire or the equipment ground wire has been added as a safety measure to reduce the severity of a potential electrical shock by providing an alternate, low-resistance pathway through which the current can flow.

Over time, the insulation on wires may deteriorate. It is then possible for a bare, hot wire to come in contact with the metal case or frame of an electrical device. This case would then become energized and present a shock hazard to someone coming in contact with it. Figure 23-17 illustrates a typical short circuit, where the individual has come in contact with the hot case of an instrument. This illustrates the type of wiring found in older homes: No equipment ground wire is present, or the electrical apparatus is not equipped with a ground wire. Here, the individual will complete the circuit and receive a severe shock. Figure 23-18 illustrates a similar example, but this time the equipment ground wire is supplied to an electrical distribution system that contains the equipment ground wire. In this example, the equipment ground wire provides a low-impedance pathway through which the current can travel. Therefore, the majority of the current would travel through the ground wire, and, although the person may get a shock, it would unlikely be a fatal one.

Electrical power supplied to homes is always grounded. A 120-volt potential always exists between the hot conductor and ground or earth. Modern electrical wiring systems use a third or equipment ground wire, which does not normally carry current. In the event of a short circuit, an electrical device that has a three-prong plug with a ground wire connected to the case will conduct the short circuited current or fault current through the ground wire and provide a significant safety benefit to someone accidentally contacting the defective device. If a large enough fault current exists, the ground wire will also provide a means to complete the short circuit back to the circuit breaker or fuse, and this will cause the fuse to melt or the circuit breaker to trip. Thus, in the grounded power system supplied to the house, it is possible to have equipment that is either grounded or ungrounded, depending upon the age of the electrical wiring and whether or not the electrical device is equipped with a three-prong plug containing a ground wire. Obviously, attempts to by-

FIG. 23-17. When a faulty piece of equipment without an equipment ground wire is plugged into an electrical outlet (not containing a ground wire), the case of the instrument will become hot. If an individual touches the hot case (point A), he will receive a shock, because he is standing on the earth (point B) and completes the circuit. The current (*dotted line*) will flow from the instrument through the individual touching the hot case.

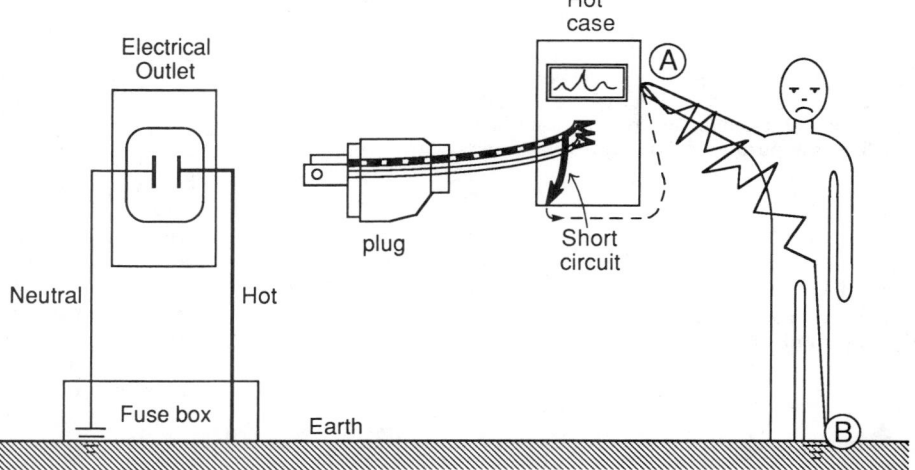

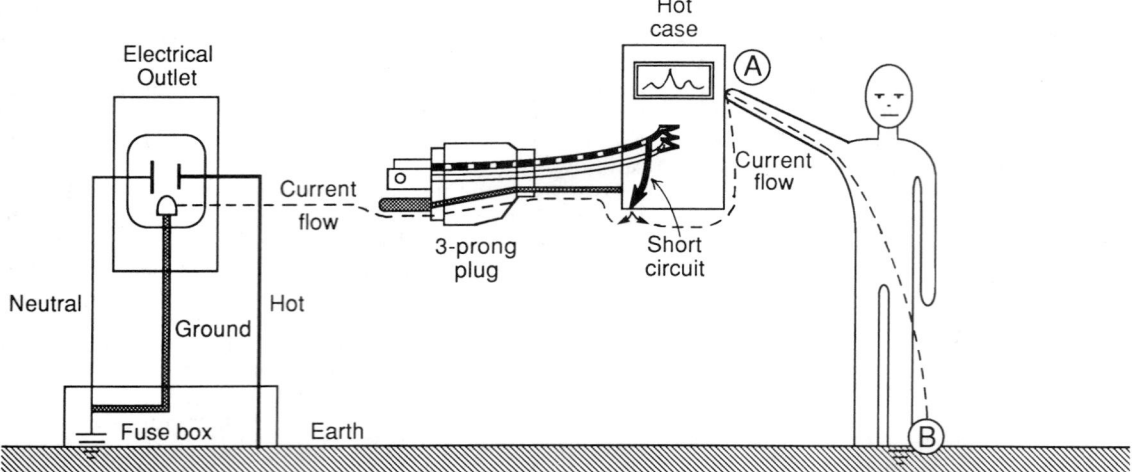

FIG. 23-18. When a faulty piece of equipment containing an equipment ground wire is properly connected to an electrical outlet with a grounding connection, the current (*dotted line*) will preferentially flow down the low-resistance ground wire. An individual touching the case (point A) standing on the ground (point B) will still complete the circuit; however, only a small part of the current will go through the individual.

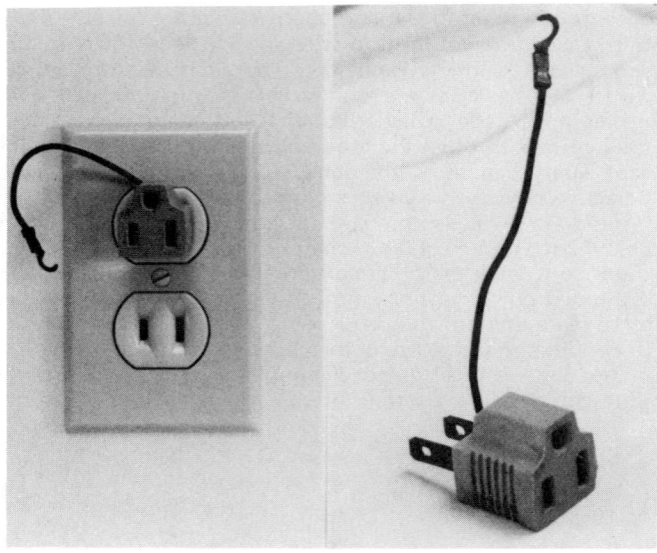

FIG. 23-19. The right side of the figure illustrates a "cheater plug" that converts a three-prong power cord to a two-prong cord. The left side of the picture illustrates that the wire attached to the cheater plug is rarely connected to the screw in the middle of the outlet. This totally defeats the purpose of the equipment ground wire.

pass the safety system of the equipment ground should be avoided. Devices such as a "cheater plug" (Fig. 23-19) should never be used, because they defeat the safety feature of the equipment ground wire.

Electrical Power—Ungrounded

Numerous electronic devices, power cords that run along the floor, and puddles of saline solutions tend to make the operating room an electrically hazardous environment for both patients and operating room personnel. Bruner and colleagues[13] found that 40% of electrical accidents that occur in hospitals took place in the operating room. The complexity of electronic equipment in the modern operating room demands that electrical safety be a factor of paramount importance. In order to provide an extra measure of safety from gross electrical shock (macroshock), the power supplied to most operating rooms is ungrounded. In this ungrounded power system, the current is isolated from ground potential. The 120-volt potential exists only between the two wires of the isolated power system, but no circuit exists between either of the isolated power lines and ground.

Supplying ungrounded power to the operating room requires the use of an isolation transformer (Fig. 23-20). This is a device that uses electromagnetic induction to induce a current in the ungrounded or secondary winding of the transformer using energy supplied to the primary winding. There is no direct electrical connection between the power supplied by the utility company on the primary side and the power induced by the transformer on the ungrounded or secondary side. Thus, the power supplied to the operating room is isolated from ground (Fig. 23-21). Since the 120-volt potential exists only between the two wires of the isolated circuit and not between ground, neither of the wires is hot or neutral with reference to ground. In this case, they are simply referred to as line 1 and line 2 (Fig. 23-22). Using the example of the light bulb, if we connect both wires of the light bulb socket to the two wires of the isolated power system, the light will illuminate. However, if we connect one wire of the light socket to one side of the isolated power and the other wire to ground, the light will not illuminate. If both wires of the isolated power system are shorted together, it will open the circuit breaker. In comparing the two systems, the standard grounded power has a direct connection to ground, whereas the isolated system imposes a very high impedance to any current flow to ground. The safety feature of this system can be seen in Figure 23-23. In this case, a person has come in contact with one side of the isolated power system (point A).

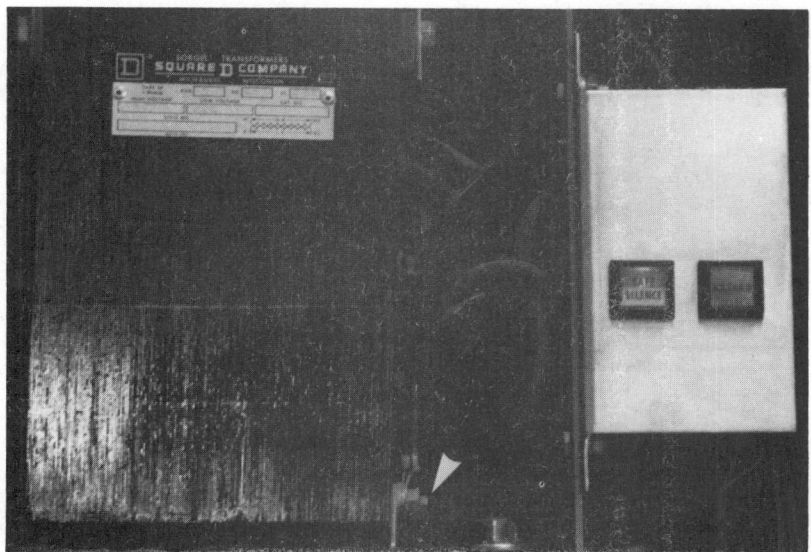

FIG. 23-20. Detail of an isolation transformer with the attached warning lights. The *arrowhead* points to ground wire connection on the primary side of the transformer. Note that no similar connection exists on the secondary side of the transformer.

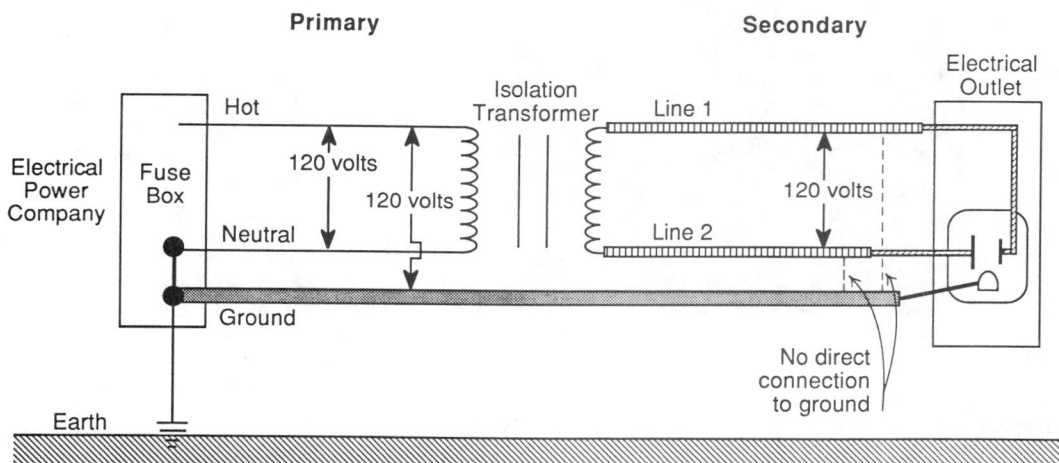

FIG. 23-21. In the operating room, the isolation transformer converts the grounded power on the primary side to an ungrounded power system on the secondary side of the transformer. A 120-volt potential difference exists between line 1 and line 2. There is no direct connection from the power on the secondary side to ground. The equipment ground wire, however, is still present.

Since standing on ground (point B) does not constitute a part of the isolated circuit, the person does not complete the loop and will not receive a shock. This is because the ground is part of the primary circuit (*solid lines*), and he is contacting only one part of the isolated secondary circuit (*striped lines*). He does not complete either circuit (*i.e.*, have two contact points); therefore, no electrical shock hazard exists. Of course, if he contacts both lines of the isolated power system (an unlikely event), he will receive a shock.

If an individual plugs a faulty electrical appliance into the standard household outlet and the appliance has an intact equipment ground wire and the home wiring has a properly connected ground wire, the amount of electrical current that will flow through the individual is considerably less than that which will flow through the low-resistance ground wire. In this case, the individual would be fairly well protected from a serious shock. However, if that ground wire was broken, the individual may receive a lethal shock. If the same faulty piece of equipment was plugged into the isolated power system, the individual would not receive a shock, even if the equipment ground wire was broken. Thus, the isolated power system provides a significant amount of protection from macroshock. Another feature of the isolated power system is that the faulty piece of equipment, even though it may be short-circuited, will not activate the circuit breaker. This is an important feature, since the faulty piece of equipment may be an important part of a life support system for a patient. It is important to note that even though the power is isolated from ground, the case or frame of all electrical equipment is still connected to an equipment ground. The third wire (equipment ground wire) is a necessary part of a total electrical safety program.

Figure 23-24 illustrates a faulty piece of equipment connected to the isolated power system. It does not present a hazard but merely converts the isolated power back to a grounded power system as is present outside the operating room. In fact, it takes a *second* fault before a hazard exists.

The previous discussion assumes that the isolated power system is perfectly isolated from ground. In fact, it is impossible to achieve perfect isolation. All AC-operated power systems and electrical devices exhibit some degree of capaci-

tance. As was previously discussed, electrical power cords, wires, and electric motors exhibit capacitive coupling to the ground wire and metal conduits and "leak" small amounts of current to ground (Fig. 23-25). This so-called leakage current partially ungrounds the isolated power system. The total amount of leakage current normally present in an operating room is in the range of a few milliamperes. So an individual contacting one side of the isolated power system would receive a very small shock in the range of 1 to 2 mA. This amount of current would be perceptible but not dangerous.

THE LINE ISOLATION MONITOR

The line isolation monitor (LIM) is a device that continuously monitors the integrity of the isolated power system. If a faulty piece of equipment is connected to the isolated power system, it will, in effect, change the system back to a conventional grounded system. The faulty piece of equipment will continue to function normally. Therefore, it is essential that there be a warning system in place that will alert the personnel that the power is no longer ungrounded. The LIM continuously monitors the isolated power to ensure that it is indeed isolated from ground. The LIM also has a meter that displays a continuous indication of the integrity of the system (Fig. 23-26). As previously discussed, if the isolation was perfect, the impedance would be infinitely high and there would be no current flow in the event of a first fault situation ($Z = E/I$ if $I = 0$, then $Z = $ infinity). Since all AC wiring and all AC-operated electrical devices have some capacitance, there will be small "leakage currents" that partially degrade the system. The meter of the LIM will indicate (in mA) the total amount of leakage in the system as a result of the capacitance, the electrical wiring, and any devices plugged into the isolated power system. The reading on the LIM meter is *not* an indication that current is actually flowing but merely indicates how much current would flow in the event of a first fault. The LIM is set to alarm at 2 or 5 mA, depending upon the age and make of the system. Once this preset limit is exceeded, a visual and audible alarm will be sounded (Fig. 23-27). This is an indication that the isolation from ground has been degraded beyond a predetermined limit. This does not indicate that there is a hazardous situation, but rather that the system is no longer totally isolated from ground. It would in fact require a second fault in order to create a dangerous situation.

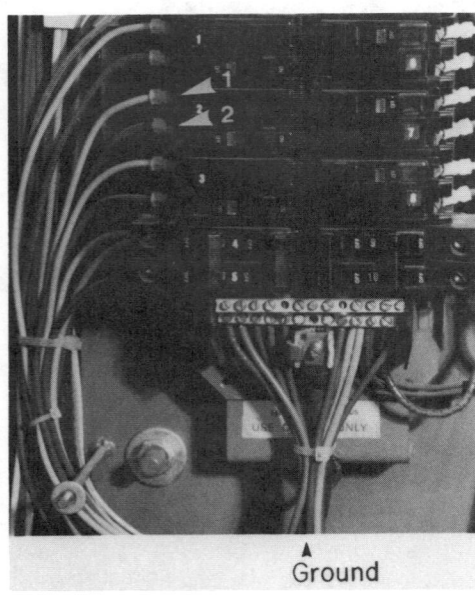

FIG. 23-22. Detail of the inside of a circuit breaker box in an isolated power system. The *black arrowhead* points to ground wires meeting at the common ground terminal. The *white arrowheads* indicate line 1 and line 2 from the isolated power circuit breaker. Neither line 1 nor line 2 is connected to the same terminals as the ground wires. This is in marked contrast to Figure 23-13, where the neutral and ground wires are attached at the same point.

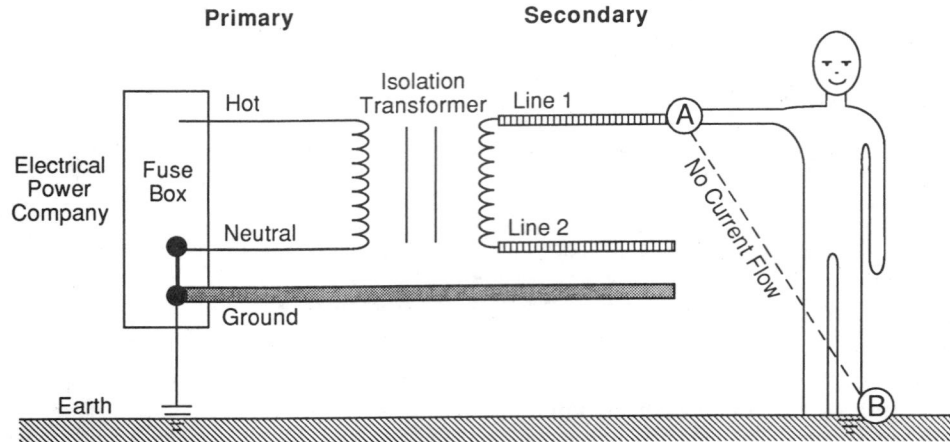

FIG. 23-23. This diagram illustrates a safety feature of the isolated power system. An individual contacting one side of the isolated power system (point A) and standing on the ground (point B) will not receive a shock. In this instance, the individual is not contacting the circuit at two points and thus not completing the circuit. Point A (*cross-hatched lines*) is part of the isolated power system, and point B is part of the primary or grounded side of the circuit (*solid lines*).

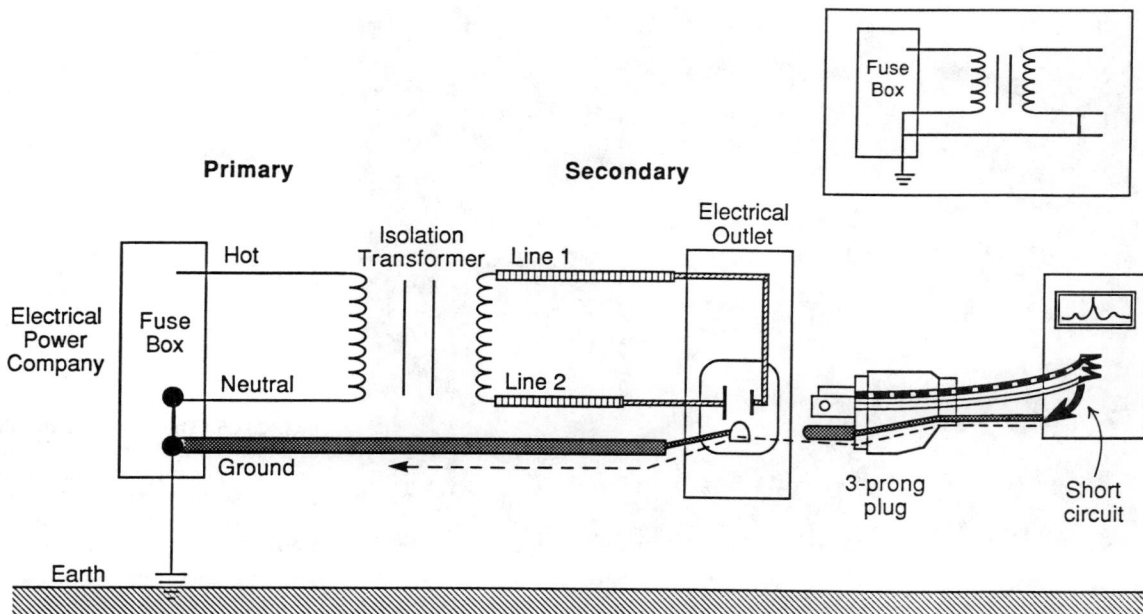

FIG. 23-24. A faulty piece of equipment plugged into the isolated power system does not present a shock hazard. It merely converts the isolated power system into a grounded power system. The figure insert illustrates that the isolated power system is now identical to the grounded power system. The dotted line indicates current flow in the ground wire.

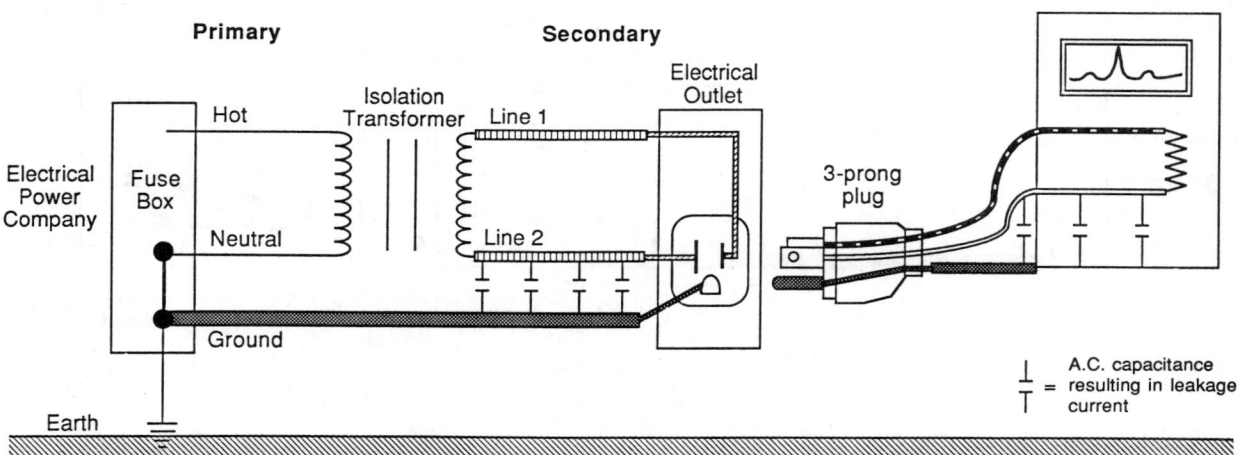

FIG. 23-25. The capacitance that exists in AC power lines and AC-operated equipment results in small "leakage currents" that partially degrade the isolated power system.

As an example, if the LIM was set to alarm at 2 mA, using Ohm's law either side of the isolated power would have an impedance of 60,000 ohms.

$$Z = \frac{E}{I}$$
$$Z = \frac{120 \text{ volts}}{0.002 \text{ amps}}$$
$$Z = 60,000 \text{ ohms}$$

Therefore, if either side of the isolated power system had less than 60,000 ohms impedance to ground, the LIM would alarm. There are two situations in which this might occur. In the event of a true fault to ground where there was a short circuit with essentially zero impedance from one line to ground, the system would be converted to the equivalent of a grounded power system. This would indicate that a faulty piece of equipment had been plugged into the power system and should be removed and serviced as soon as possible. This

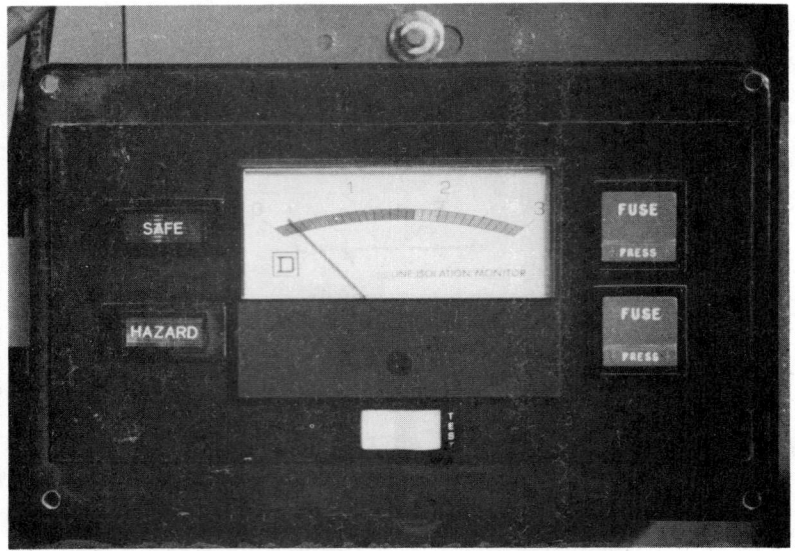

FIG. 23-26. The meter of the line isolation monitor is calibrated in milliamperes. If the isolation of the power system is degraded such that more than 2 mA of current could flow, the hazard light will illuminate and a warning buzzer will sound. Note the button for testing the hazard warning system.

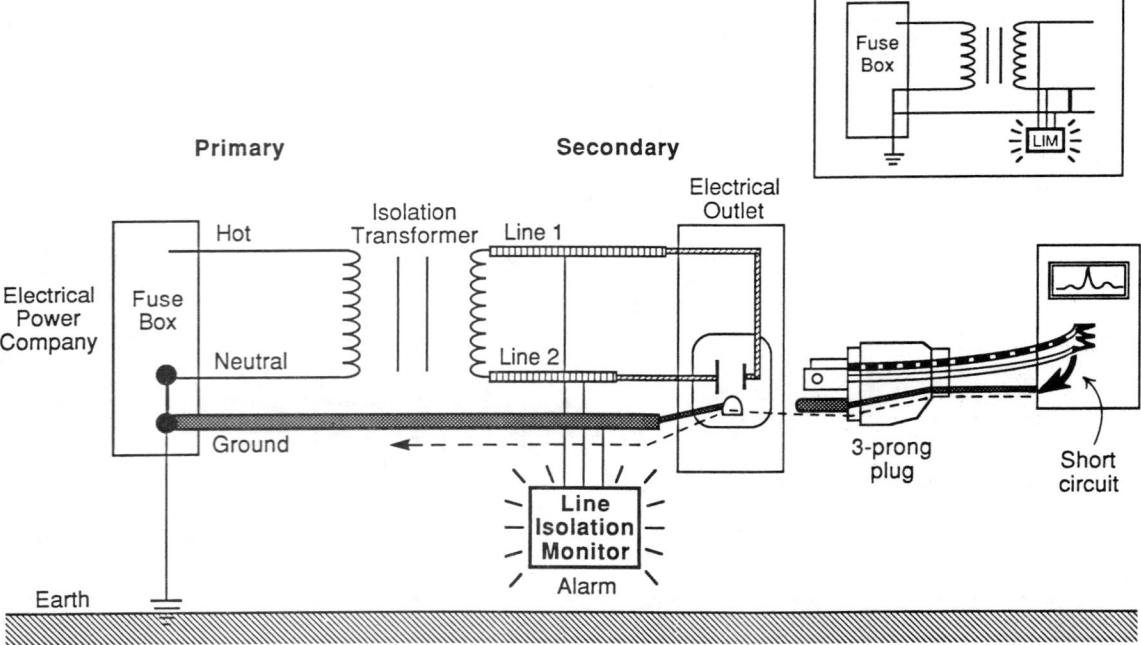

FIG. 23-27. When a faulty piece of equipment is plugged into the isolated power system, it will markedly decrease the impedance from line 1 or line 2 to ground. This will be detected by the line isolation monitor, which will sound an alarm.

would also create a true potential hazard, because a second faulty piece of equipment would now represent a serious electrical shock hazard. The second situation involves connecting a large number of perfectly normal pieces of equipment to the isolated power system. Each piece of equipment has a very small amount of leakage current; however, if the total leakage exceeds 2 mA, the LIM will then alarm. Let's assume that 30 electrical devices, each having 100 µA of leak-

age current, are simultaneously plugged in in the same operating room. The total leakage current (30 × 100 µA) would be 3 mA. The impedance to ground of the system would still be 40,000 ohms (120/0.003). The LIM would alarm, since the 2-mA set point was violated. However, the system is still very safe and represents a significantly different situation than in the first situation.

The equipment ground wire is again a very important part

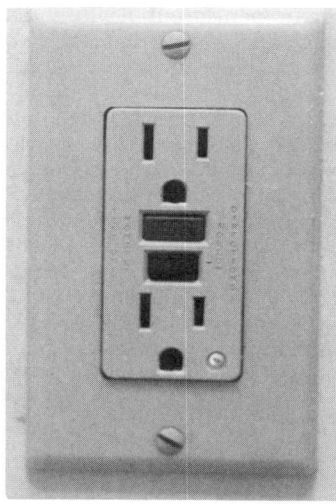

FIG. 23-28. A ground fault interrupter (GFI) electrical outlet with intergraded test and reset buttons.

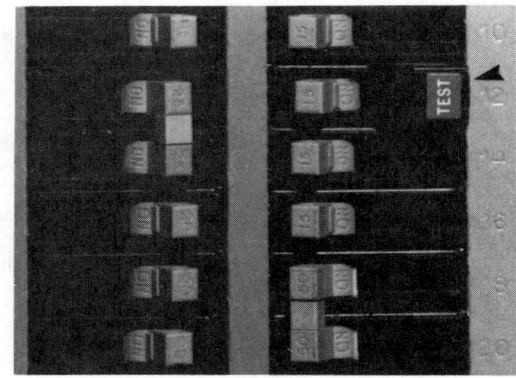

FIG. 23-29. Special GFI circuit breaker. The *arrowhead* points to the distinguishing red test button.

power system, the line isolation monitor would alarm, but the equipment could still continue to be used.

of the safety system. If the equipment ground wire is broken, when the faulty piece of equipment is plugged in, it would operate normally, but the LIM would not alarm. Therefore, the dangerous situation of a second fault could cause a shock, and the LIM would never have alarmed. Also, in the event of a second fault, the equipment ground wire provides a low resistance path to ground for the majority of the fault current (see Fig. 23-24). The LIM will only be able to register leakage currents from those pieces of equipment that are connected to the isolated power system and have intact ground wires.

GROUND FAULT INTERRUPTER

The ground fault interrupter (GFI) is another popular device used to protect individuals from receiving an electrical shock in a grounded power system. Electrical codes in most new construction require a GFI circuit to be present in potentially hazardous areas such as bathrooms or outdoor electrical outlets. The GFI may be installed as an individual power outlet (Fig. 23-28) or may be a special circuit breaker to which all the individual outlets are connected at a single point. The special GFI circuit breaker is located in the main fuse box and can be distinguished by its red test button (Fig. 23-29). Figure 23-5 demonstrates that the current flowing in both the hot and neutral wires is normally equal. The GFI monitors both sides of the circuit for equality of current flow, and, if it detects a difference, the power is immediately interrupted. If an individual should contact a faulty piece of apparatus where current was flowing through the individual, this would create an imbalance in the two sides of the circuit, which would be detected by the GFI. Very small amounts of current difference in the range of 5 mA can be detected and the GFI will open the circuit in a few milliseconds—the principle being that the GFI interrupts the current flow before the individual would receive a significant shock. Thus, the GFI provides a high level of protection at a very modest cost. The problem with using a GFI in the operating room is that it interrupts the flow of power. If the defective piece of equipment were of a life support nature, it could no longer be used. Whereas, if the same faulty piece of equipment was plugged into an isolated

MICROSHOCK

The previous discussion of electrical shock hazards dealt with the concept of macroshock. In macroshock, relatively large amounts of current are applied to the surface of the body. The current is conducted through all the tissues in proportion to their conductivity and area in a plane perpendicular to the current. Consequently, the "density" of the current (amperes per meter squared) that the heart sees is considerably less than what is applied to the body surface. However, an electrically susceptible patient who has a direct connection to the heart may be at risk from very small currents called *microshock*.[14] The catheter orifice or electrical wire with a very small surface area in contact with the heart produces a current density at the heart that is relatively large.[15] Stated another way, very small amounts of current applied directly to the myocardium will cause ventricular fibrillation. Microshock is a particularly difficult problem because of the insidious nature of the hazard.

Ventricular fibrillation can be produced in the electrically susceptible patient by a current that is below the threshold of human perception. The exact amount of current needed to produce ventricular fibrillation in the electrically susceptible patient is unknown. Whalen and colleagues[16] were able to produce fibrillation with 20 μA of current applied directly to the myocardium of dogs. Raftery et al[17] produced fibrillation with 80 μA of current in some patients. Hull[18] used data obtained by Watson et al[19] to show that 50% of patients would fibrillate at currents of 200 μA. Since 1000 μA (1 mA) is generally regarded as the threshold of human perception with 60-Hz AC current, the electrically susceptible patient can be electrocuted with currents that are one tenth of that which is normally perceptible. This is not only an academic but also a practical consideration, as many cases of ventricular fibrillation from microshock have been reported.[20–25]

The stray capacitance that is part of any AC-operated electrical instrument may result in significant amounts of charge build-up on the case of the instrument. An individual who simultaneously touches the case of an instrument where significant charge has built up and the electrically susceptible patient may unknowingly cause a discharge to the patient, resulting in ventricular fibrillation. Once again, the equipment ground wire provides the major source of protection against microshock for the electrically susceptible patient. In this case, the equipment ground wire provides a low-resistance path by which most of the leakage current is dissipated instead of stored as a charge. Figure 23-30 illustrates an example of a patient with a saline-filled catheter in the heart with a resistance of approximately 500 ohms. The ground wire with a resistance of 1 ohm is connected to the instrument case. A leakage current of 100 µA will divide according to the relative resistances of the two paths. In this case, 99.8 µA will flow through the equipment ground wire, and only 0.2 µA will flow through the fluid-filled catheter. This extremely small current does not present a hazard to the patient. In the

event that the equipment ground wire is broken, the electrically susceptible patient is at great risk. Now, all 100 µA of leakage current could flow through the catheter and cause ventricular fibrillation (Fig. 23-31).

Modern patient monitors incorporate another mechanism to reduce the risk of microshock to the electrically susceptible patient. This mechanism involves electronically isolating all direct patient inputs from the power supply of the monitor by placing a very high impedance between the patient and any device. This limits the internal leakage through the patient connection to a very small value. The standard currently is less than 10 µA. For instance, the output of the power supply of an ECG monitor is electrically isolated from the patient by placing a very high impedance between the monitor and the

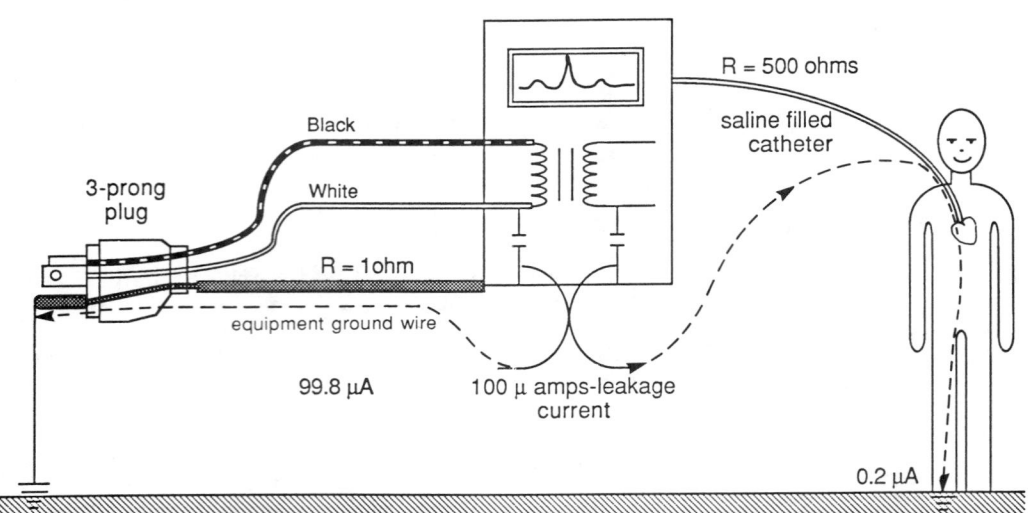

FIG. 23-30. The electrically susceptible patient is protected from microshock by the presence of an intact equipment ground wire. The equipment ground wire provides a low-impedance path in which the majority of the leakage current (*dotted lines*) can flow.

FIG. 23-31. A broken equipment ground wire results in a significant hazard to the electrically susceptible patient. In this case, the entire leakage current can be conducted to the heart and may result in ventricular fibrillation.

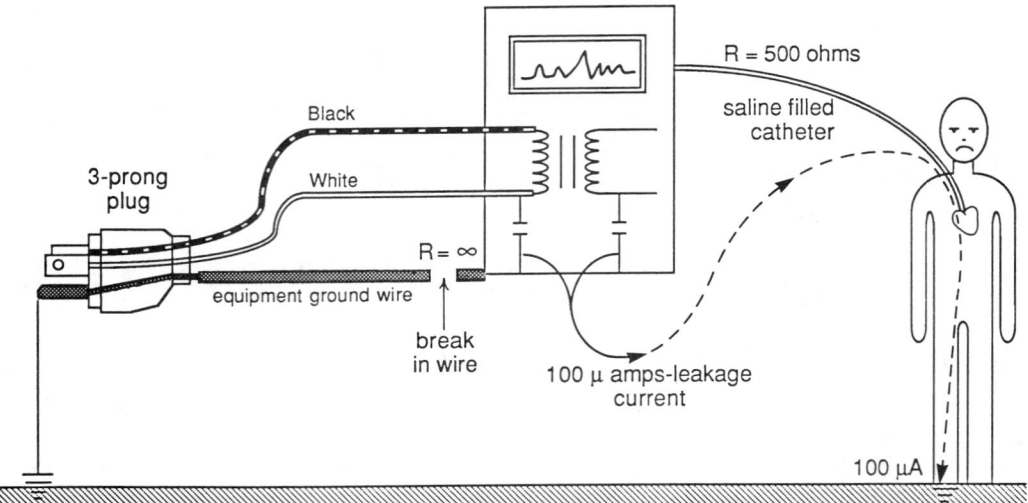

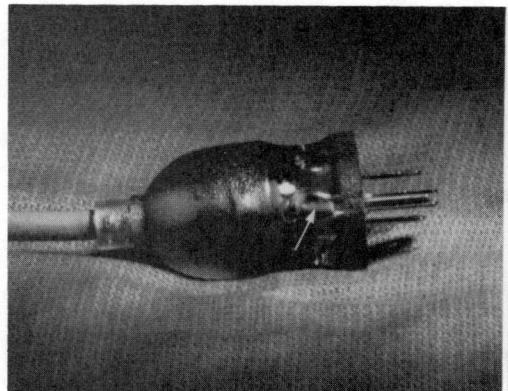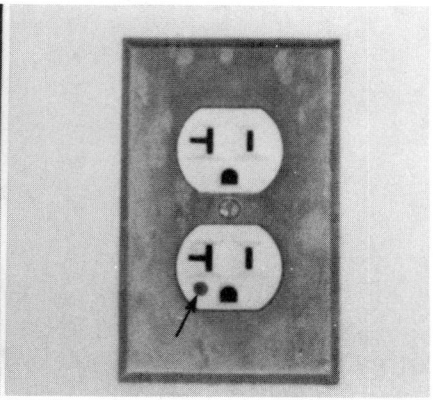

FIG. 23-32. (A) A hospital-grade plug that can be visually inspected. The *arrow* points to equipment ground wire whose integrity can be readily verified. (B) The *arrow* points to the green dot denoting a hospital-grade power outlet.

patient's ECG leads.[6, 26] Isolation techniques effectively inhibit hazardous electrical pathways between the patient and the monitor, yet allow the passage of the physiologic signal.

It must be remembered that the line isolation monitor is not designed to, nor does it, provide any protection against microshock. The microampere currents involved in microshock are far below the threshold of protection of the LIM. In addition, the LIM does not provide any information about the leakage of individual monitors. Rather, it provides a picture of the status of the total system. The reading on the LIM displays the amount of leakage current resulting from the total capacitance of the system. This is the amount of current that would flow to ground in the event of a first fault situation.

The essence of electrical safety is a thorough understanding of all the principles of grounding. As John Bruner states, "Grounding is neither safe nor unsafe. Its significance is dependent on what is grounded and in what context."[9] The object of electrical safety is to make it difficult for electrical current to pass through people. To that extent, both the patient and the anesthesiologist should be isolated from ground as much as possible. That is, they should have as high a resistance to current flow as is technologically possible. Because the operating room is inherently an unsafe electrical environment, several measures may be taken to help ensure the individual from contacting hazardous current flows. First, the grounded power that the utility company provides to the hospital is transformed to ungrounded power by means of an isolation transformer. The status of this isolation from ground is continuously checked by the LIM. The monitor will alarm and warn that the isolation of the power (from ground) has been lost in the event a defective piece of equipment is plugged into the electrical system. In addition, the shock that an individual could receive from a faulty piece of equipment is determined by the capacitance of the system and is limited to a few milliamperes. Second, all equipment plugged into the isolated power system is equipped with an equipment ground wire that is attached to the case of the instrument. This equipment ground wire provides an alternative low-resistance pathway for potentially dangerous currents to flow to earth ground. Thus, the patient and the anesthesiologist should be as insulated from ground as possible and all electronic equipment should be grounded.

The equipment ground wire serves three functions. First, it provides a low-resistance path for fault currents to reduce the risk of macroshock. Second, it dissipates leakage currents that are potentially harmful to the electrically susceptible patient. And, finally, it provides information to the LIM on the status of the ungrounded power system. If the equipment ground wire is broken, a significant factor in the prevention of electrical shock is lost. Additionally, the isolated power system will appear safer than it actually is because the LIM has no means to detect broken equipment ground wires.

Since power cord plugs and receptacles are subjected to higher degrees of abuse in the hospital than in the home, the Underwriters Laboratory has issued a strict specification for special "hospital-grade" plugs and receptacles (Fig. 23-32). The plugs and receptacles that conform to this specification are marked by a green dot.[27] The hospital-grade plug is one that can be visually inspected or easily disassembled to ensure the integrity of the ground wire connection. Molded opaque plugs are definitely not acceptable. Edwards[28] reported that 1800 of 3000 (60%) nonhospital-grade receptacles installed in a new hospital building were defective after 3 years. When 2000 of the nonhospital-grade receptacles were replaced with hospital-grade receptacles, there were no failures after 18 months of use.

ELECTROSURGERY

Ever since that fateful day in October 1926 when Dr. Harvey W. Cushing first used an electrosurgical machine invented by Professor William T. Bovie to resect a brain tumor, the course of modern surgery and anesthesia has been altered.[29] The ubiquitous use of electrosurgery in current times attests to the success of Professor Bovie's invention. However, the adoption of this technology has come at a cost. The widespread use of electrocautery has, at the least, hastened the elimination of explosive anesthetic agents from the operating room. In addition, as every anesthesiologist is aware, there are few things in the operating room that cannot be interfered with by the "Bovie." The high-frequency electrical energy that the electrosurgery unit generates can interfere with everything from the ECG signal to cardiac output computers, pulse oximeters, and even implanted cardiac pacemakers.[30]

The electrosurgical unit (ESU) operates by generating very high–frequency currents (radio frequency range) of anywhere from 500,000 to more than 1 million Hz. Whenever a current passes through a resistance, heat is generated. The amount of heat generated will be proportional to the square of the current and inversely proportional to the area that the current passes through ($H = I^2/A$).[31] By concentrating the energy at the tip of the "Bovie pencil," the surgeon is able to

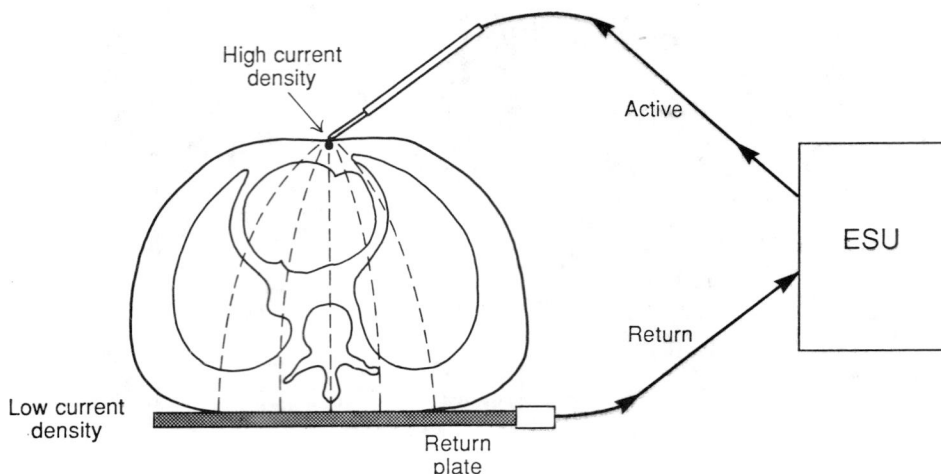

FIG. 23-33. A properly applied ESU return plate. The current density at the return plate is low, resulting in no danger to the patient.

produce a cut or a coagulation at any given spot. This very high–frequency current behaves much differently than standard 60-Hz AC current. The current generated by the ESU can pass directly across the precordium without causing ventricular fibrillation,[31] since high-frequency currents have a low-tissue penetration and do not excite contractile cells.

This large amount of energy generated by the ESU can pose other problems to the operator and the patient. Dr. Cushing became aware of one such problem. He wrote, "once the operator received a shock which passed through a metal retractor to his arm and out by a wire from his headlight, which was unpleasant to say the least."[32] The safe operation of the ESU is dependent upon the proper routing of the energy from the ESU through the patient and back to the unit. Ideally, the current generated by the active electrode is concentrated at the ESU tip, which consists of a very small surface area. This energy has a high current density and is able to create enough heat to produce a therapeutic cut or coagulation. The energy then passes through the patient to a dispersive electrode of large surface area that returns the energy safely to the ESU (Fig. 23-33).

One unfortunate quirk in terminology relates to the return (dispersive) plate of the ESU. This plate is often mistakenly referred to as a "ground plate." Operating room personnel may frequently ask "is the patient grounded?" As previously stated, the aim of electrical safety is to isolate the patient from ground. The use of ground when referring to the electrosurgical return plate is not only a misnomer but also leads to confusion. The ESU return plate is in reality a dispersive electrode of large surface area that safely returns the generated energy to the ESU via a low current density pathway. Because the current density is low at the area of the return plate, no harmful heat is generated and no tissue destruction occurs. Therefore, in a properly functioning system, the only tissue effect is at the site of the active electrode that is held by the surgeon.

Problems can arise if the electrosurgical return plate is not properly applied to the patient or if the cord from the return plate to the ESU is damaged or broken. In these instances, the high-frequency current generated by the ESU will seek an alternate return pathway. Anything connected to the patient such as ECG leads or a temperature probe can provide this alternate return pathway. Since the surface area of an ECG pad is considerably less than the area of the ESU return plate,

the current density at this site will be considerably higher than normal. In this case, a serious burn may occur at this alternate return site. Similarly, a burn may occur at the site of the ESU return plate if it is not properly applied to the patient or if it becomes partially dislodged during the course of the operation (Fig. 23-34). The numerous case reports involving patients who have received ESU burns attest to the fact that this is more than a theoretical possibility.[33-38]

The original ESUs were manufactured with the power supply connected directly to ground via the equipment ground wire. With these devices, it was extremely easy for ESU current to return by alternate pathways. In fact, the ESU would continue to operate normally even if the return plate was completely omitted. In order to help protect the patient from burns, most modern ESUs have the power supply isolated from ground. It was hoped that by isolating the return pathway from ground, the only route for current flow would be by the return electrode. This would in theory eliminate alternate return pathways and greatly reduce the incidence of burns.[5] Mitchell[39] found two incidences where the current could return via alternate pathways, even with the isolated ESU circuit. If the return plate was left on top of an uninsulated ESU cabinet or if the return plate was left in contact with the bottom of the operating room table, the ESU could operate in a reasonably normal manner and the current would return via alternate pathways. It will be recalled that the impedance is inversely proportional to the capacitance times the current frequency. Since the ESU operates at 500,000 to more than 1 million Hz, this leads to a large amount of capacitive coupling and a marked reduction in impedance. Therefore, even with isolated ESUs, the high degree of capacitance allows for current to return to the ESU by alternate pathways. Additionally, the isolated ESU does not protect the patient from burns if the return electrode is making poor contact with the patient. Although the isolated ESU does provide additional patient safety, it is by no means foolproof protection against patient burns.

The prevention of patient burns from the ESU is the responsibility of all professional staff in the operating room. Not only the circulating nurse, but also the surgeon and the anesthesiologist, must be aware of proper techniques and vigilant to potential problems. The most important factor is the proper application of the return plate. It is essential that the return plate have the appropriate amount of electrolyte

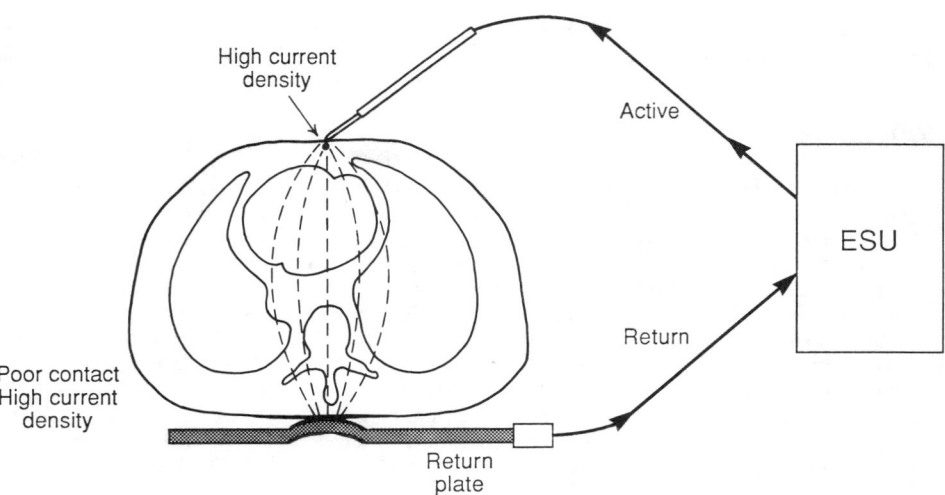

High current
density

Active

ESU

Poor contact
High current
density

Return

Return
plate

FIG. 23-34. An improperly applied ESU return plate. Poor contact with the return plate results in a high current density and a possible burn to the patient.

gel and an intact return wire. Reusable return plates must be properly cleaned between uses, and disposable plates must be checked to ensure that the electrolyte has not dried out during storage. In addition, it is prudent to place the return plate as close as possible to the site of the operation. Electrocardiographic pads should be placed as far away from the site of the operation as is feasible. Operating room personnel must be alert to the fact that pools of flammable prep solutions such as ether and acetone can be ignited when using the ESU. If the ESU must be used on the patient with a demand pacemaker, the return electrode should be located below the thorax, and preparations for treating potential dysrhythmias should be available, including a magnet to convert the pacemaker to a fixed rate, a defibrillator, and an external pacemaker. If the surgeon requests higher than normal power settings on the ESU, this should alert both the circulating nurse and the anesthesiologist of a potential problem. The return plate and cable needs immediate inspection to ensure that it is functioning and positioned properly. If this does not correct the problem, the return plate should be replaced. If the problem still remains, the entire ESU unit should be taken out of service. Finally, if the ESU is dropped or in any way damaged, it must be immediately removed from the operating room and thoroughly tested by a qualified biomedical engineer. If these simple safety steps are followed, most of the accidental patient burns from the ESU can be eliminated.

The previous discussion concerned unipolar ESUs. There is a second type of ESU, in which the current passes only between the two blades of a pair of forceps. This type of device is referred to as a bipolar ESU. Because the active and return electrodes are the two blades of the forceps, there is no need for another dispersive electrode to be attached to the patient unless a unipolar ESU is also being used. The power generated by the bipolar ESU is considerably less than that by the unipolar ESU, and they are mainly used for ophthalmic and neurologic surgery.[2]

Electrical safety in the operating room is a matter of applying common sense to some basic principles. Once operating room personnel understand the importance of safe electrical practice, they are able to develop a heightened awareness to potential problems. All electrical equipment must have routine periodic maintenance and be inspected to ensure conformity to designated electrical safety standards. These tests must be documented and records maintained for future inspection. This is because human error can easily compound electrical hazards. Starmer et al[40] site an incidence of a newly constructed laboratory where the ground wire was not attached to the receptacle. In another study, Albisser et al[41] found a 14% (198/1424) incidence of improperly or incorrectly wired outlets. Furthermore, potentially hazardous situations should be recognized and corrected before they become a problem. For instance, electrical power cords are frequently placed on the floor where they could be run over by various carts or the anesthesia machine. Often these cords could be located overhead or placed in an area of low traffic flow. Multiple plug extension boxes should not be left on the floor where they can come in contact with electrolyte solutions when they could easily be mounted on a cart or the anesthesia machine. Pieces of equipment that have been damaged or have obvious defects in the power cord must not be used until they have been properly repaired. If everyone is aware of potential problems, it takes only minor amounts of effort to prevent hazardous situations.

A final area of concern to the anesthesiologist is in the design of new operating room facilities. Frequently, an anesthesiologist is asked to consult with hospital administrators and architects in planning the design of new operating rooms. In the past, a very strict electrical code was enforced because of the use of flammable anesthetic agents. This included a requirement for isolated power systems and LIMs. In recent years, the National Fire Protection Association has revised its standard for health care facilities (NFPA 99–1984). These new standards state that in nonflammable anesthetizing locations, isolated power systems and LIMs are no longer required.[42, 43] Although NFPA standards are voluntary, they are usually adopted by local authorities when they revise their electrical codes.

It is possible that hospital administrators may want to eliminate isolated power systems in new operating room construction as a cost-saving measure. It is this author's opinion that this is a short-sighted and foolhardy measure. Although not perfect, the isolated power system and LIM do provide a significant amount of protection to the patient and operating room personnel in an electrically hazardous environment. Anesthesiologists need to be aware of this change and insist that new operating rooms are constructed with isolated power systems. The relatively small cost savings does not justify the elimination of an extremely useful safety system, and the alternative of using GFIs is not practical in the operating room environment.

REFERENCES

1. Bruner JMR: Hazards of electrical apparatus. Anesthesiology 28:396, 1967
2. Hull CJ: Electrical hazards in monitoring. Int Anesthesiol Clin 19(1):177, 1981
3. Leonard PF, Gould AB: Dynamics of electrical hazards of particular concern to operating-room personnel. Surg Clin North Am 45:817, 1965
4. Miller F: College Physics, 2nd ed, p 457. New York, Harcourt Brace and World, 1967
5. Uyttendaele K, Grobstein S, Svetz P: Monitoring instrumentation—Isolated inputs, electrosurgery filtering, burns protection: What does it mean? Acta Anaesthesiol Belg 29(3):317, 1978
6. Leonard PF: Characteristics of electrical hazards. Anesth Analg 51:797, 1972
7. Taylor KW, Desmond J: Electrical hazards in the operating room, with special reference to electrosurgery. Can J Surg 13:362, 1970
8. Leonard PF: Apparatus and appliances current thinking. III. Alternating current, the isolation transformer, and the differential-transformer pressure transducer. Anesth Analg 45:814,1966
9. Bruner JMR: Fundamental concepts of electrical safety. In Hershey SG (ed): ASA Refresher Courses in Anesthesiology, p 11. Philadelphia, JB Lippincott, 1974
10. Harpell TR: Electrical shock hazards in the hospital environment. Their causes and cures. Can Hosp 47:48, 1970
11. Wald A: Electrical safety in medicine. In Skalak R, Chien S (eds): Handbook of Bioengineering, p 341. New York, McGraw-Hill, 1987
12. Dalziel CF, Massoglia FP: Let-go currents and voltages. AIEE Trans 75(2):49, 1956
13. Bruner JMR, Aronow S, Cavicchi RV: Electrical incidents in a large hospital: A 42 month register. JAAMI 6:222, 1972
14. Weinberg DI, Artley JL, Whalen RE et al: Electric shock hazards in cardiac catheterization. Circ Res 11:1104, 1962
15. Starmer CF, Whalen RE: Current density and electrically induced ventricular fibrillation. Med Instrum 7:158, 1973
16. Whalen RE, Starmer CF, McIntosh HD: Electrical hazards associated with cardiac pacemaking. Ann NY Acad Sci III:922, 1964
17. Raftery EB, Green HL, Yacoub MH: Disturbances of heart rhythm produced by 50-Hz leakage currents in human subjects. Cardiovasc Res 9:263, 1975
18. Hull CJ: Electrocution hazards in the operating theatre. Br J Anaesth 50:647, 1978
19. Watson AB, Wright JS, Loughman J: Electrical thresholds for ventricular fibrillation in man. Med J Aust 1:1179, 1973
20. Furman S, Schwedel JB, Robinson G et al: Use of an intracardiac pacemaker in the control of heart block. Surgery 49:98, 1961
21. Noordijk JA, Oey FJI, Tebra W: Myocardial electrodes and the danger of ventricular fibrillation. Lancet 1:975, 1961
22. Pengelly LD, Klassen GA: Myocardial electrodes and the danger of ventricular fibrillation. Lancet 1:1234, 1961
23. Rowe GG, Zarnstorff WC: Ventricular fibrillation during selective angiocardiography. JAMA 192:947, 1965
24. Hopps JA, Roy OS: Electrical hazards in cardiac diagnosis and treatment. Med Electr Biol Eng 1:133, 1963
25. Mody SM, Richings M: Ventricular fibrillation resulting from electrocution during cardiac catheterization. Lancet 2:698, 1962
26. Leeming MN: Protection of the electrically susceptible patient: A discussion of systems and methods. Anesthesiology 38:370, 1973
27. Cromwell L, Weibell FJ, Pfeiffer EA: Biomedical instrumentation and measurements, 2nd ed, p 430. Englewood Cliffs, New Jersey, Prentice-Hall, 1980
28. Edwards NK: Specialized electrical grounding needs. Clin Perinatol 3(2):367, 1976
29. Goldwyn RM: Bovie: The man and the machine. Ann Plast Surg 2:135, 1979
30. Lichter I, Borrie J, Miller WM: Radio-frequency hazards with cardiac pacemakers. Br Med J 1:1513, 1965
31. Dornette WHL: An electrically safe surgical environment. Arch Surg 107:567, 1973
32. Cushing H: Electro-surgery as an aid to the removal of intracranial tumors. With a preliminary note on a new surgical-current generator by W.T. Bovie. Surg Gynecol Obstet 47:751, 1928
33. Meathe EA: Electrical safety for patients and anesthetists. In Saidman LJ, Smith NT (eds): Monitoring in Anesthesia, 2nd ed, p 497. Boston, Butterworths, 1984
34. Rolly G: Two cases of burns caused by misuse of coagulation unit and monitoring. Acta Anaesthesiol Belg 29:313, 1978
35. Parker EO: Electrosurgical burn at the site of an esophageal temperature probe. Anesthesiology 61:93, 1984
36. Schneider AJL, Apple HP, Braun RT: Electrosurgical burns at skin temperature probes. Anesthesiology 47:72, 1977
37. Bloch EC, Burton LW: Electrosurgical burn while using a battery-operated Doppler monitor. Anesth Analg 58:339, 1979
38. Becker CM, Malhotra IV, Hedley-Whyte J: The distribution of radiofrequency current and burns. Anesthesiology 38:106, 1973
39. Mitchell JP: The isolated circuit diathermy. Ann R Coll Surg Engl 61:287, 1979
40. Starmer CF, McIntosh HD, Whalen RE: Electrical hazards and cardiovascular function. N Engl J Med 284:181, 1971
41. Albisser AM, Parson ID, Pask BA: A survey of the grounding systems in several large hospitals. Med Instrum 7:297, 1973
42. Kermit E, Staewen WS: Isolated power systems: Historical perspective and update on regulations. Biomed Tech Today 1(3):86, 1986
43. NFPA: National electric code (ANSI/NFPA 70–1984). Quincy, Massachusetts, National Fire Protection Association, 1984

Chapter 24   *John T. Martin*

Patient Positioning

Positioning a patient for a surgical procedure is frequently a compromise between what the anesthetized patient can tolerate and the needs of the operating team for access to the surgical target. Physiologic instability resulting from disease or injury may sometimes be magnified by rapidly moving a seriously ill patient from bed to transport cart, through corridors and elevators, and onto the operating table. Induction of anesthesia and positioning may need to be delayed until the patient is hemodynamically stable, or establishment of the intended surgical posture may need to be modified to match the patient's tolerance. This chapter emphasizes the physiologic significance of various positions in which a patient may be placed during an operation and discusses the potential complications of positioning.[1]

Careful attention should be paid to accurate terminology in discussing positioning. *Decubitus* is a loosely defined term[2] that will be used in this chapter to indicate the part of the patient that is in contact with the supporting surface of the operating table. Thus, the term *left lateral decubitus position* describes a patient whose left shoulder and hip rest on the operating table and whose right side is accessible to the surgeon. The alternate term, *right chest position*, is sometimes used, but it is ambiguous and should be avoided; it could lead to making an incision on the wrong side.

DORSAL DECUBITUS POSITIONS

PHYSIOLOGY

Circulation

In the horizontal supine position (Fig. 24-1), the influence of gravity on the vascular system is minimal and intravascular pressures from head to foot vary little from mean pressures at the level of the heart; therefore, almost no perfusion gradient exists in the arterial tree between the heart and either the cerebral or lower extremity vessels. Similarly, in the venous circuits, gradients from the periphery to the right atrium consist principally of the cyclic intrathoracic pressure changes that occur with respiration.

If the patient in the dorsal decubitus position is tilted head high or head low, the effects of gravity on blood flow in the head or the feet can become quite significant as the gradient to or from the heart increases. Pressures have been shown to change by 2 mm Hg for each 2.5 cm that a given point varies in vertical height above or below the reference point at the heart.[3]

When the lower extremities are lower than the level of the heart, blood pools in the distensible dependent vessels, causing a reduction in effective circulating volume, cardiac output, and systemic perfusion. If the head is high and blood pressure measured at the level of the heart is low, the blood pressure in the brain is further decreased according to the magnitude of the head elevation.

The cardiovascular response to head-up tilt of 75° maintained for 3 min can be a useful indicator of the magnitude of acute blood loss.[4] If sustained tilt causes an increase in heart rate of more than 25 beats $\cdot$ min^{-1} but does not produce hypotension or syncope, the blood volume deficit is 9–14 ml $\cdot$ kg^{-1}. If syncope occurs on tilting, the deficit is likely to be as much as 20 ml $\cdot$ kg^{-1}. Hypotension without tilting indicates a deficit in excess of 20 ml $\cdot$ kg^{-1}.

If the head is tilted down (Fig. 24-2), pressure in the cerebral veins increases in proportion to the gradient upward to the heart. Many alert patients so positioned will complain of a rapidly occurring, pounding vascular headache. In the presence of intracranial pathology, such as with head injury, or stroke, elevations of cerebral venous pressure may provoke or intensify cerebral edema and dangerously raise intracranial

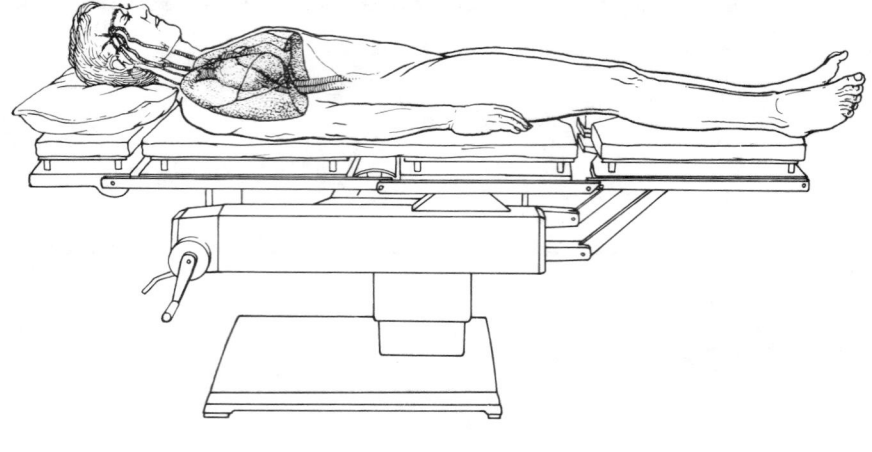

FIG. 24-1. Supine adult with minimal gradients in the horizontal vascular axis. Pulmonary vascular volume is congested dorsally and is relatively sparse substernally. Viscera displace dorsal diaphragm cephalad. Cerebral circulation is approximately at heart level.

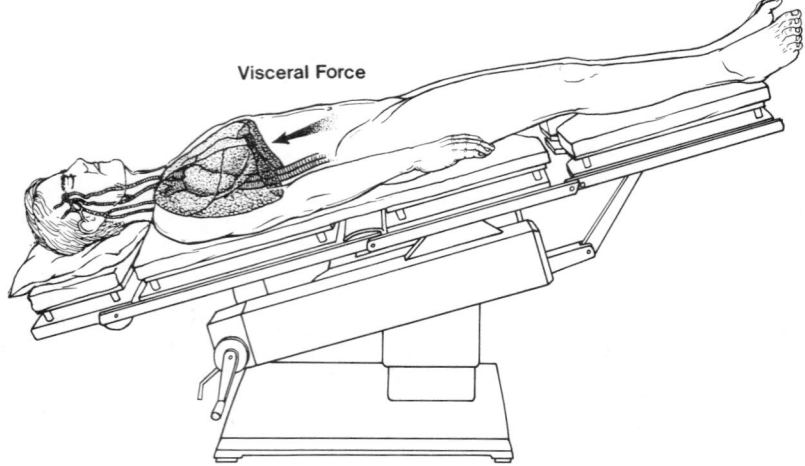

Visceral Force

FIG. 24-2. Head-down tilt promotes blood return from lower extremities but encourages reflex vasodilation, congests the pulmonary circuit in the poorly ventilated lung apices, and increases intracranial blood volume.

pressure. Head-down tilt also increases cerebrospinal fluid (CSF) pressure within the cranial vault, adding its effect to the total intracranial pressure elevation.

Kubal et al[5] have shown that myocardial oxygen consumption can increase in awake patients scheduled for coronary artery bypass grafting when they are placed in mild degrees of head-down tilt as a means of distending jugular vessels and facilitating the percutaneous introduction of pulmonary artery catheters. Measurements suggested an acute volume loading of the heart had occurred with the onset of the head-down tilt. Angina recurred in some patients, and one developed electrocardiographic changes indicative of myocardial ischemia.

Using the head-down tilt to treat hypotension, a well-entrenched practice that was based on the suggestions of physiologist Walter Cannon in World War I,[6] has been shown to be counterproductive.[7] While it does increase central blood volume by recovering pooled blood from caudad portions of the body, and while cardiac output is increased transiently, the enlarged central blood mass activates baroreceptors on the aortic arch and at the carotid bifurcation.[8] The result is rapid peripheral vasodilation, unchanged or reduced cardiac output, and decreased organ perfusion. In a study of patients in intensive care units, it was found that head-down tilt caused

an unpredictable further decrease in mean arterial pressure in some hypotensive patients.[7]

In the microcirculation, natural and spontaneous fluctuations in the flow exist to serve the nutritive requirements of the tissues.[9] When an awake human is supine and motionless, the spontaneous fluctuations weaken progressively until they disappear in approximately 1 hr. The subject then becomes uncomfortable and tissue blood flow continues to decrease if immobility is enforced.[10] A normal flow pattern returns if the subject becomes restless and moves about.

In the absence of hypocarbia, hypovolemia, or hypothermia, a similar impairment of changes in microcirculatory distribution of blood flow occurs after the induction of anesthesia, despite early augmentation of tissue flow due to the vasodilative properties of the anesthetic agents. Normal tissue perfusion is reestablished by awakening movements at the end of anesthesia.[10]

West et al[11] have identified three separate perfusion zones in the pulmonary circulation, based on the interrelationship between pressures in the alveoli, arterioles, and venules.

In Zone 1, alveolar pressure exceeds either arterial or venous pressure and perfusion of the lung unit is prevented. Although rarely present in a normal lung, Zone 1 can be produced by pulmonary hypotension, excessive positive end-expiratory pressure, or overdistension of alveolar units from large tidal volumes during intermittent positive pressure ventilation (IPPV).

In Zone 2, arterial pressure exceeds alveolar pressure while alveolar pressure remains higher than venous pressure. This relationship is found in nondependent portions of the lung, and perfusion is the result of a fluctuating balance between arterial and alveolar pressures.

In Zone 3, hydrostatic forces in the dependent portion of the lung have produced venous congestion, and perfusion is determined by the difference between arterial pressure and venous pressure.

In the dorsal recumbent positions, the pulmonary circulation tends to be most congested along the dorsal body wall and least substernally. When the patient is tilted head-high, Zone 3 moves toward the lung bases and optimum ventilatory mechanics. When the patient is tilted head-down, Zone 3 shifts cephalad into the poorly ventilated apices and can be expected to intensify abnormal ventilation/perfusion ratios.

Respiration

In the supine position, mobile abdominal viscera gravitate toward the dorsal body wall and move the dorsal parts of the diaphragm cephalad. The displacement lengthens muscle fibers in that portion of the diaphragm and increases the strength and effectiveness of its contractions during spontaneous ventilation. The benefit is improved ventilation of the congested, compacted, and less compliant lung bases. With head-up tilt (Fig. 24-3), the visceral weight shifts away from the diaphragm and ventilation is enhanced. In the head-down position, the visceral mass, its weight potentially increased by the presence of abdominal fat, fluid, tumors, *etc.*, can cause significant respiratory embarrassment by impeding caudad excursions of the contracting diaphragm and preventing adequate expansion of the lung bases.

In the supine position, gravity-induced vascular congestion forces the dorsal portions of the lung to function as a Zone 3.[11]

FIG. 24-3. Elevation of the head allows abdominal viscera to fall away from the diaphragm and improves ventilation of the lung bases. A gradient above the heart reduces pressure in cerebral arteries and may allow subatmospheric pressure in veins of the head and neck.

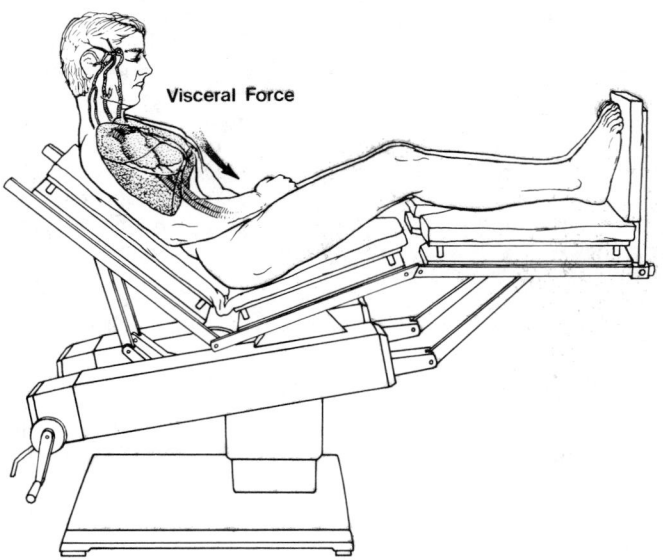
Visceral Force

Consequently, the compliance of the area is reduced and passive ventilation will tend to distribute gas preferentially to substernal units where pulmonary blood volume is less. To prevent development of clinically significant ventilation/perfusion imbalance during use of controlled ventilation, tidal volumes must be used that are greater than the average amount that is sufficient during spontaneous breathing.[12]

VARIATIONS OF THE DORSAL DECUBITUS POSITION

Supine

HORIZONTAL. In the horizontal supine position the patient lies on the back with a small pillow beneath the head. The arms are either comfortably padded and restrained alongside the trunk or abducted on padded arm boards. Either or both arms may be extended ventrally and secured to an elevated frame in such a way that perfusion of the hand is not compromised, that no skin-to-metal contact permits electrical burns if cautery is used, and that the axillary neurovascular bundle is not compromised at the axilla. The lumbar spine may need support to prevent backache. Bony contact points at the occiput, elbows, and heels should be padded.

While the horizontal supine posture (called by some the *crucifix position*) is traditional and widely used, it does not place hip and knee joints in neutral positions and is poorly tolerated for any length of time by an immobile, awake patient.

CONTOURED. A contoured supine posture (Fig. 24-4) has been termed the *lawn chair position*.[13] It is established by arranging the surface of the operating table so that the trunk–thigh hinge is angulated about 15° and the thigh–knee hinge is angulated a similar amount in the opposite direction. The patient then lies with hips and knees each flexed gently in an approximately neutral position. Quite often a patient who has been required to lie motionless on a rigid horizontal table and then is changed to the contoured supine position will offer an almost involuntary expression of relief and appreciation.

As with the horizontal supine position, the patient should have a pad or pillow beneath the occiput, and bony pressure points at elbows and heels should be padded. Arms can be accommodated as described for the horizontal supine posture.

Lithotomy

STANDARD. In the standard lithotomy position (Fig. 24-5), the patient lies supine with arms crossed on the abdomen or extended laterally on arm boards. Both legs are flexed at the hip and knee and simultaneously elevated so that the perineum becomes accessible to the surgeon.

Numerous devices are available to hold legs elevated during delivery or an operation. Each should be fitted to the stature of the individual patient.

When the legs are to be lowered to the original supine position at the end of the procedure, they should be first brought together in the sagittal plane and then lowered slowly. This minimizes torsion stress on the lumbar spine that would occur if each leg were lowered independently. It also slows the process of adding the vascular volume of the legs to the circulatory capacitance, thereby allowing vasocompensation to adjust perfusion and avoid sudden hypotension.[14]

For most urologic procedures, and for procedures that require simultaneous access to the abdomen and perineum, the

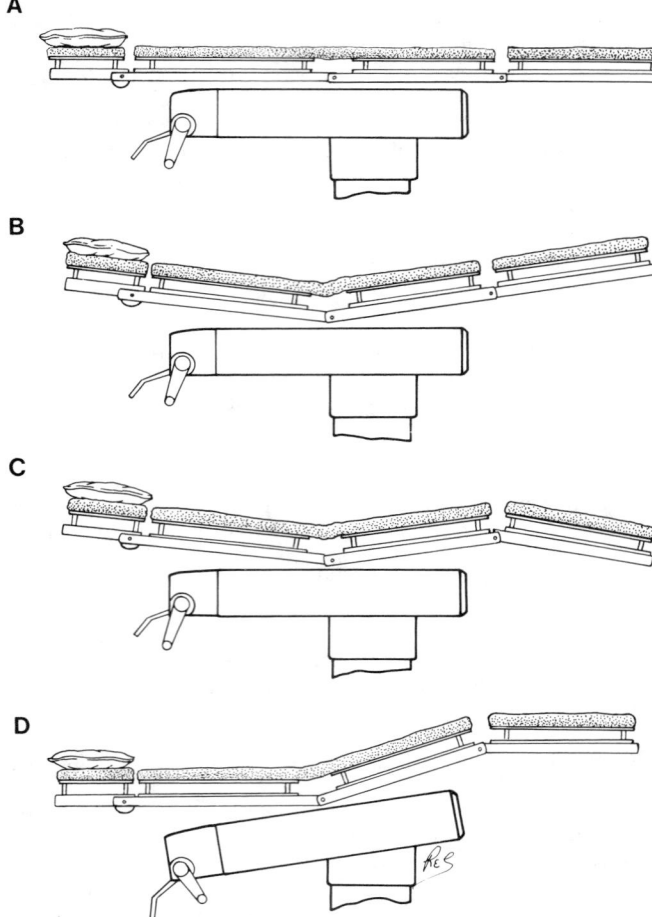

FIG. 24-4. Establishment of the contoured supine (*lawn-chair*) position. (*A*) Traditional flat supine table top. (*B*) Thighs flexed on trunk. (*C*) Knees gently flexed. (*D*) Trunk section leveled to stabilize floor-supported arm board. (Reprinted with permission. Martin JT: Positioning in Anesthesia and Surgery. Philadelphia, WB Saunders, 1987.)

degree of thigh elevation desired is only about 45°, with enough knee flexion to permit the lower leg to be nearly parallel to the floor (Fig. 24-6*A*). For gynecologic procedures, however, the degree of thigh elevation may be almost 90° (Fig. 24-6*B*).

EXAGGERATED. Some surgical procedures on the perineum require that the thighs be almost forcibly flexed on the abdomen and the lower legs be aimed skyward to be out of the way (Fig. 24-7). This exaggerated lithotomy position stresses the lumbar spine, produces a significant uphill gradient for perfusion of the feet, and may restrict ventilation because of abdominal compression by the thighs. It can be tolerated under anesthesia, but can rarely be assumed by an awake patient. Control of the patient's ventilation is usually necessary. If painful lumbar spine pathology exists, an alternate surgical position may need to be chosen in order to avoid severely accentuating the lumbar distress postoperatively.

Lithotomy Plus Trendelenburg

Frequently, some degree of head-down tilt is added to the exaggerated lithotomy position so that the retropubic area is more readily accessible from a perineal approach; however, the posture combines the worst features of both the Trendelenburg and the extreme lithotomy positions. It is often necessary to add shoulder braces to the table to retain the patient in the desired position despite the head-down tilt.

The tilt adds the weight of abdominal viscera to whatever compression of the abdomen is produced by the flexed thighs. Consequently, the work of spontaneous ventilation is increased for an anesthetized patient in a posture that already worsens the ventilation/perfusion relationship because of increased pulmonary blood volume in the poorly ventilated lung apices. Some increase also occurs in the perfusion gradient to the elevated feet, and reductions in mean arterial pressure may cause relative ischemia of the raised lower extremities.

Intracranial vascular congestion and increased intracranial pressure can be expected. The position should be used in patients with intracranial pathology only in the rare instances in which a surgically useful alternate posture cannot be found; the operation should then be as brief as possible, and postoperative neurologic intensive care may be required.

Trendelenburg

Friedrich Trendelenburg, a renowned Leipzig surgeon of the late 1800s, received widespread recognition for tilting a patient 30–45° head-down (Fig. 24-8) during an operation as a means of having abdominal viscera gravitate cephalad out of the pelvis and improve exposure of pathology that involved the urinary bladder, rectum, and vagina. His technique originated about 1870 and was publicized in an article by his pupil, Dr. Willy Meyer,[15] more than a decade later.

During World War I, Walter Cannon, the eminent physiologist, espoused the notion that the Trendelenburg position was advantageous in the treatment of shock. He believed that it improved circulatory return from the lower extremities and improved cerebral circulation.[6] As a result, the head-down position was used to treat shock until just recently. Reports of Cole in 1952,[16] Weil in 1957,[17] Guntheroth et al in 1964,[18] Taylor and Weil in 1976,[19] and Sibbald's group in 1979[7] have carefully detailed the disadvantages of the Trendelenburg position as a means of treating shock, but the tenacious persistence of the practice, particularly among older physicians, has been astonishing.

The classic Trendelenburg position employs 30–45° of head-down tilt and requires some means of preventing the patient from sliding cephalad out of position. Hewer developed a contoured mattress with raised areas that supported the Achilles tendons, lumbar spine, and neck.[20] This English device has not been widely used in the United States. Wristlets affixed to the table edge have been used, but they have the potential of stretching the brachial plexuses as the weight of the patient hangs from the fixed wrists. Ischemia of the hands is possible if the wristlets are too tight.

Shoulder braces are useful if placed over the acromioclavicular joints, but care must be taken to see that the brachial neurovascular bundle is not compressed between the clavicle and the first rib. If the braces are placed medially against the root of the neck, they may easily compress neurovascular structures that emerge from the area of the lateral edge of the scalene musculature.

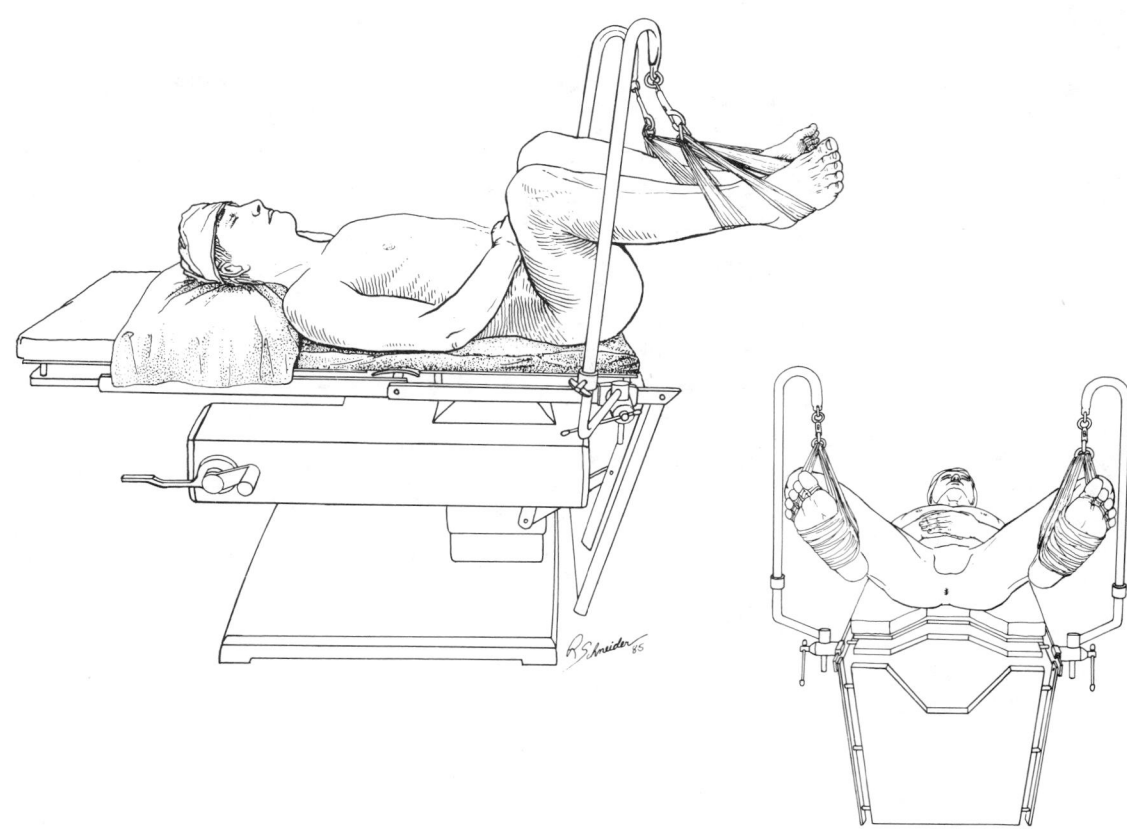

FIG. 24-5. Standard lithotomy position. (Reprinted with permission. Martin JT: Positioning in Anesthesia and Surgery. Philadelphia, WB Saunders, 1987.)

Anklets and bent knees are a satisfactory method of retaining the tilted patient in position if the anklets are not excessively tight and if the flexed knee joint is placed sufficiently caudad of the leg–thigh hinge of the table top so that the adjacent edge of the depressed leg section is not digging into the patient's proximal calf. If it does so, compressive ischemia and phlebitis are likely.

Scultetus

The usual amount of head-down tilt now employed in most surgical suites is probably about 10–15° (Fig. 24-8). This corresponds to a posture referred to as the Scultetus position,[2, 21] possibly associated with the German surgeon, Johann Schultes (1595–1645), who was known as Scultetus, and for whom the bandage is named. While the minimal angulation used does not threaten to dislodge the patient, it has been shown to increase myocardial oxygen consumption in spontaneously ventilating patients.[5] In principle, even this small amount of head-down tilt is poorly tolerated by many patients with impaired myocardial perfusion. It should be avoided in the presence of increased intracranial pressure.

An alternate position that is effective for treating patients with moderate hypovolemia, such as that associated with blood loss or spinal anesthesia, is elevation of the legs with the rest of the body flat. The blood in the legs is "autotransfused" into the central circulation, yet there is no compromise of ventilation or dangerous increase in cerebral venous pressure.

COMPLICATIONS OF THE DORSAL DECUBITUS POSITIONS

Postural Hypotension

Depending on the resilience of the patient's vasocompensatory mechanisms, postural hypotension may be seen when a head-elevated position is established. On a statistical basis, it is probably the most frequent complication of a head-elevated posture. If mean arterial pressure at the circle of Willis remains above 60 mmHg in a patient who is not hypertensive, little treatment may be needed other than appropriately decreasing the concentration of anesthetic drugs to protect compensatory reflexes as much as possible. If the degree of hypotension encountered is more severe, further head elevation should be delayed until decreasing the level of anesthetic plus judicious use of fluids and vasopressors can reestablish effective perfusion.

Postural hypotension may also appear in the presence of inadequately replaced blood loss and a functionally increased intravascular space when either the legs are lowered to horizontal at the termination of the lithotomy position or when a head-down tilt is returned to horizontal. Volume repletion is the indicated therapy.

Pressure Alopecia

Prolonged compression of hair follicles can produce hair loss. Abel and Lewis[22] described patients who had pain, swelling,

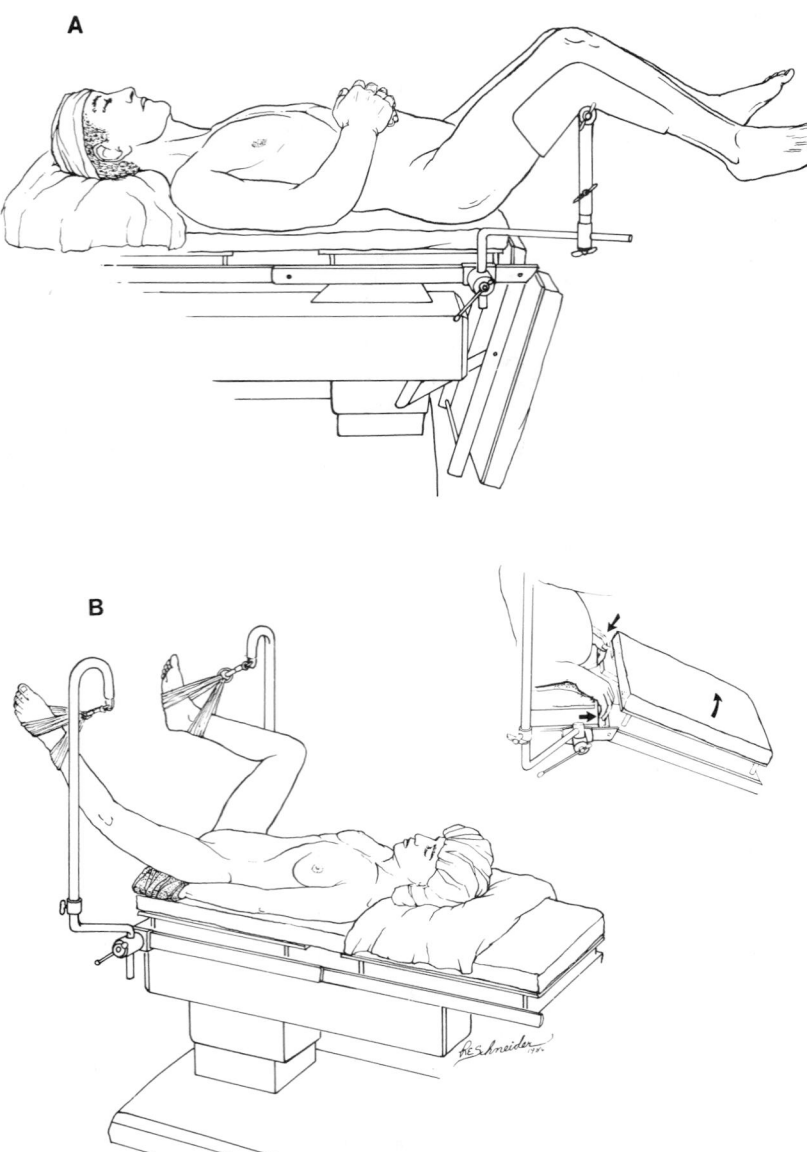

FIG. 24-6. (*A*) Usual lithotomy position for urologic procedures such as transurethral prostatic resection. (*B*) Usual gynecologic lithotomy position. Note the possibility for scissoring injury to fingers as the leg section of the table top is returned to horizontal; towel-wrapping the hands keeps digits out of the hinge. (Reprinted with permission. Martin JT: Positioning in Anesthesia and Surgery. Philadelphia, WB Saunders, 1987.)

and exudation where the occiput had been supporting the weight of the head for long periods in the Trendelenburg position. Alopecia occurred between the 3rd and 28th postoperative day; regrowth was complete within 3 months. Use of tight headstraps to hold anesthetic face masks has also been associated with compression alopecia.[23] Prolonged hypotension and hypothermia may also predispose to pressure alopecia.[24] Recommendations for minimizing the risk of this complication include frequent turning of the head during lengthy operations and the use of padded, soft head supports.

Pressure Point Reactions

Weight-bearing bony prominences can develop ischemic necrosis of overlying tissue unless proper padding is applied. Hypothermia and vasoconstrictive hypotension may enhance the process. Heels, elbows, and the sacrum are particularly vulnerable and should be carefully padded as a prophylactic routine. This is especially important when patients are thin or the operation will last several hours.

Brachial Plexus Injuries

ROOT INJURIES. Shoulder braces placed tight against the base of the neck can compress and injure the roots of the brachial plexus. The braces are less harmful when placed laterally over the acromioclavicular joint.

The dorsal decubitus positions do not usually threaten structures within the patient's neck unless considerable lateral displacement of the head occurs. In that position the roots of the brachial plexus on the side of the obtuse head–shoulder angle can be stretched and damaged. If the upper extremity is fixed at the wrist, the stretch injury of the plexus can be accentuated as the head moves laterally away from the an-

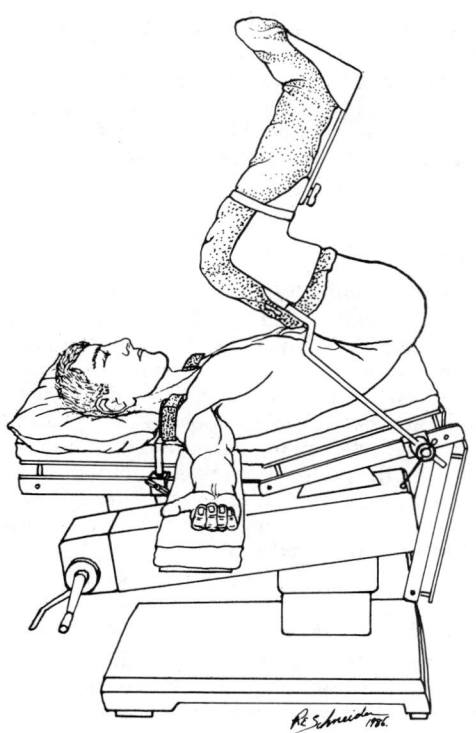

FIG. 24-7. The exaggerated lithotomy position of Young. Shoulder braces are placed over the acromioclavicular area to minimize compression of the brachial plexus and adjacent vessels. (Reprinted with permission. Martin JT: Positioning in Anesthesia and Surgery. Philadelphia, WB Saunders, 1987.)

choring point of the wrist. Similarly, exaggerated rotation of the head away from an extended arm can be associated with brachial plexus injury.

COMPRESSION BETWEEN CLAVICLE AND FIRST RIB. If the shoulder is allowed to move dorsally or the supine patient shifts cephalad while the upper extremity is immobilized at the wrist, the clavicle can be pressed forcibly against the underlying first rib. In the process, the subclavian neurovascular bundle can be compressed and its structures injured. Occasionally a dampened pulse at the wrist will identify this situation in the sitting position and will require support under the elbow to lift the shoulder and relieve the obstruction.

LONG THORACIC NERVE INJURY. Several lawsuits have centered about postoperative serratus anterior dysfunction and winging of the scapula alleged to be the result of positioning injuries to the long thoracic nerve of Bell, which arises from nerve roots C5, C6, and C7. Emergence of the nerve from the lateral portion of the middle scalene muscle supports the premise that its neuropathy is traumatic in origin.[25] Johnson and Kendall[26] described the widely variable etiology of serratus anterior paralysis in a review of 111 cases and found only 7% occurring after a surgical procedure. Foo and Swann[27] thought that most occurred as the result of a viral infection. Because the nerve is not routinely involved in a stretch injury of the brachial plexus, the relationship between postoperative long thoracic nerve dysfunction and patient positioning maneuvers remains speculative.

AXILLARY TRAUMA FROM THE HUMERAL HEAD. Excessive abduction of an arm on an arm board may thrust the head of the humerus into the axillary neurovascular bundle. The bundle is stretched at that point and neural structures may be damaged. In the same manner, vessels can be compressed or occluded and perfusion of the extremity can be jeopardized.

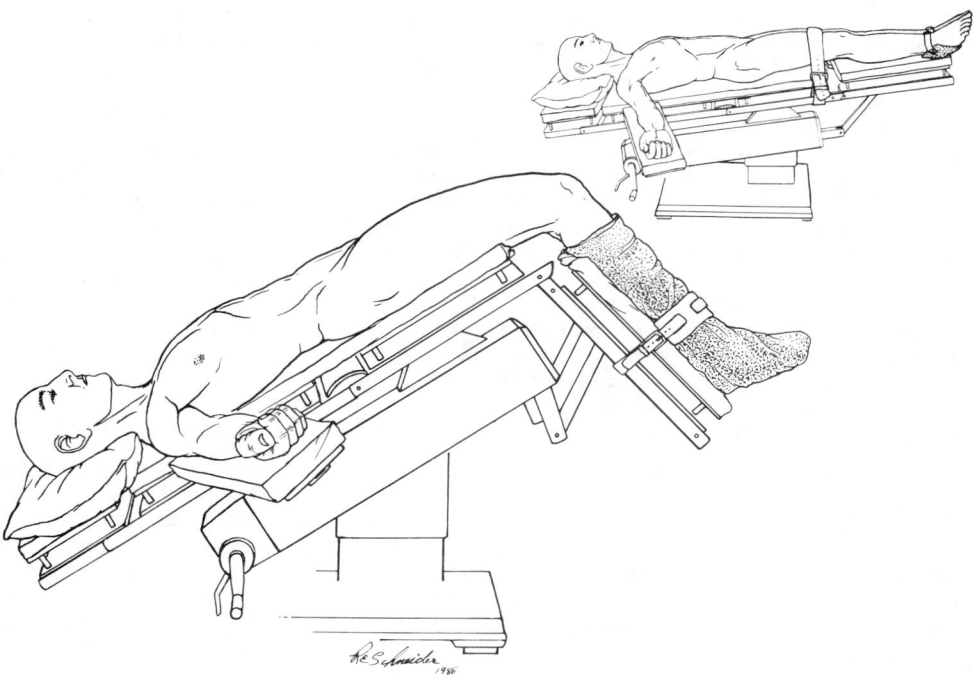

FIG. 24-8. *Foreground* shows traditional steep (30–45°) tilt described by Trendelenburg. Leg restraints and knee flexion stabilize the patient, avoiding the need for wristlets or shoulder braces that threaten the brachial plexus. *Upper* shows 10–15° of head-down tilt (Scultetus' position) more common in modern surgical procedures. (Reprinted with permission. Martin JT: Positioning in Anesthesia and Surgery. Philadelphia, WB Saunders, 1987.)

RADIAL NERVE COMPRESSION. The radial (musculospiral) nerve, arising from roots C6–8 and T1, passes dorsally and laterally around the middle and lower portion of the humerus in the musculospiral groove. At a point on the lateral aspect of the arm about three fingerbreadths proximal to the lateral epicondyle of the humerus, the nerve can be compressed against the underlying bone and injured. Clinical manifestations of a radial nerve lesion include wrist drop, weakness of abduction of the thumb, inability to extend the metacarpophalangeal joints, and loss of sensation in the web space between the thumb and index finger.[28] Its function can be rapidly assessed by noting the patient's ability to extend actively the distal phalanx of the thumb.[29] The vertical bar of an "ether screen," or a similar device, can be the offending source of pressure against the lateral arm and radial nerve.[30]

ULNAR NERVE AT THE ELBOW. Direct trauma to the ulnar nerve, arising from roots C8 and T1, as it passes behind the medial epicondyle of the humerus is not uncommon. It can occur during sleep or anesthesia if the thin arm of a supine person rests on the flexed elbow with the forearm across the trunk. The nerve can also be traumatized in some patients as the arm lies abducted on an arm board with the hand pronated and the contents of the groove between the medial epicondyle and the olecranon compressed between bones and board. Clinical manifestations of ulnar nerve dysfunction vary with the location and extent of the lesion,[31] but rapid assessment can identify an acute injury if a pin prick cannot be felt in the fifth finger.[29] Supination of the hand on an arm board (shifting the weight of the elbow to the olecranon process), and carefully padding the medial aspect of the elbow regardless of arm position, are preventative measures that help to minimize the opportunities for ulnar nerve compression during anesthesia and surgery.

Arm Complications

An arm board that is hyperabducted, whether intentionally or by inadvertent pressure from the hip of a surgical assistant, is dangerous. It can force the head of the humerus into the axillary neurovascular bundle and damage nerves and vessels to the arm. Abduction of the arm to more than 90° from the trunk is not recommended.

The attachment of an arm board to the operating room table must be very secure to prevent accidental release. Occasionally surgeons will seek comfort for their tired lumbar spine by placing one foot on the base of the operating table. If their knee fits comfortably beneath the arm board in that position, and if they exercise the calf muscle by extending the foot, the arm board may be dislodged from the table edge and damage the patient's shoulder, axillary contents, or humerus.

An arm that is not properly secured can slip over the edge of the table or arm board and result in injury to the capsule of the shoulder joint by excessive dorsal extension of the humerus, fracture of the neck of an osteoporotic humerus, or injury to the ulnar nerve at the elbow.

Backache

Lumbar backache can be made worse by the ligamentous relaxation that occurs with either general or spinal anesthesia. Loss of normal lumbar curvature in the supine position is apparently the issue. Several folded towels placed under the lumbar spine before the induction of anesthesia may retain lordosis and make a patient with known lumbar distress more comfortable.

When the lithotomy position is contemplated, elevation of the legs can worsen the pain of a herniated nucleus pulposus. Gently attempting to assume the posture before anesthesia is induced may be helpful in determining whether the position can be tolerated.

Perineal Crush Injury

The supine patient who is placed on a fracture table to repair a fractured femur usually has the pelvis retained in place by a perineal pole (Fig. 24-9), while the foot of the injured extremity is fixed to a mobile rest. A worm gear on the rest lengthens the distance between the foot and the pelvis to distract and realign the bone fragments. Unless the pole is well padded, severe pressure can be exerted on the pelvis and damage can occur to the genitalia and the pudendal nerves. Complete loss of penile sensation following use of the fracture table has been reported.[32, 33] The correct position for the pole is between the genitalia and the uninjured limb.[32]

Compartment Syndrome

If, for whatever reason, perfusion is inadequate to a lower extremity, a compartment syndrome may develop. Characterized by ischemia, hypoxic edema, elevated tissue pressure within fascial compartments of the leg, and extensive rhabdomyolysis, the syndrome produces extensive damage to nerves within the area. Ferrihemate, resulting from myoglobin destruction, exerts a direct toxic effect on renal tubular epithelium, and renal failure is likely.[34]

Causes of a compartment syndrome while a patient is in any of the dorsal decubitus positions include systemic hypotension, vascular obstruction of major leg vessels by intrapelvic retractors, compression of the elevated extremity by straps that are too tight or by the arm of a surgeon, and obstruction to distal perfusion by excessive flexion of knees or hips. Fasciotomies are the only means of terminating the cycle of ischemia and compartment edema. Alkalinizing the urine and promoting diuresis may reduce the degree of renal damage.

Finger Injury

In 1968 Courington and Little[35] described the amputation of a young woman's fingers that were caught in the hinge between the leg and thigh sections of the operating table as the leg section was returned to horizontal at the termination of an operation in the lithotomy position. Welborn[36] has advocated putting a boxing glove-like wrap on the hands to preclude such a tragic misadventure (Fig. 24-6B), but withdrawal of the hands from the risky position prior to raising the foot of the table is both less troublesome and safer.

Other Complications

Placing the supine patient in a head-down tilt position (Trendelenburg or Scultetus position) causes blood to pool in the central and cerebral veins. This acute increase in volume has been associated with myocardial ischemia[5] and an increase in intracranial pressure. When treating hypovolemic hypotension, elevation of the legs, while keeping the rest of the body flat, is preferable to tilting the entire patient in a head-down position.[17–19]

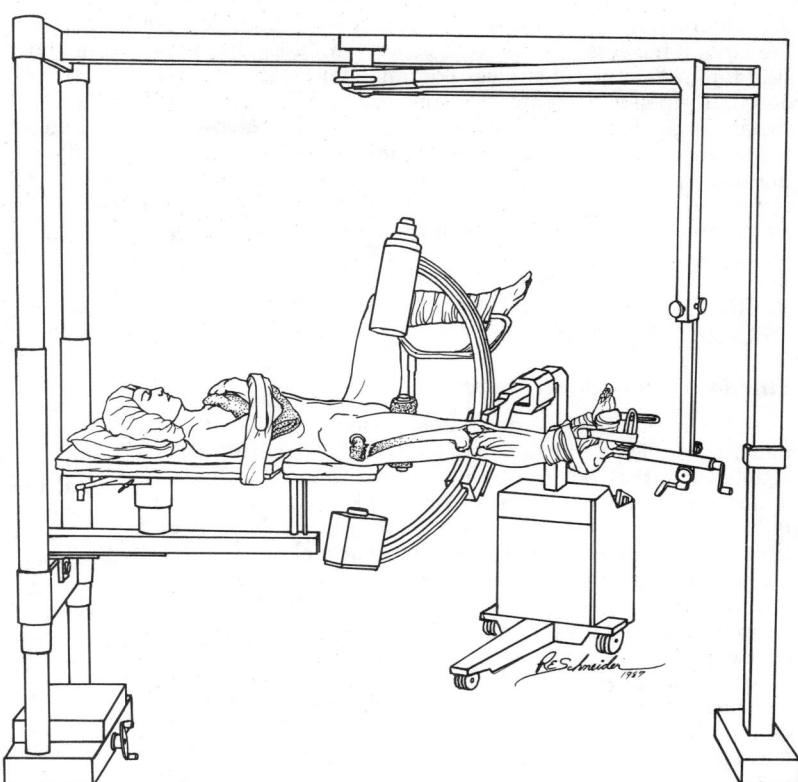

FIG. 24-9. Traction table with perineal post stabilizing patient while leg is elongated to reposition bone ends. (Reprinted with permission. Martin JT: Positioning in Anesthesia and Surgery. Philadelphia, WB Saunders, 1987.)

LATERAL DECUBITUS POSITIONS

PHYSIOLOGY

Circulatory

In the lateral decubitus position the patient is turned onto one side of the trunk and stabilized to prevent accidental rolling toward either the supine or the prone positions. If the legs are maintained in the long axis of the body, almost no pressure gradients exist along the great vessels from head to foot. Small hydrostatic differences will be detected between the values recorded by blood pressure cuffs placed on the two arms. If the legs are flexed laterally at the hips and allowed to remain below the level of the heart, blood will pool in the dangling lower extremities because of dependent increases in venous pressure and resultant venous stasis. Wrapping the legs and thighs in compressive bandages is the usual means of combatting dependent venous pooling. Lateral flexion of the lower extremities can also partially or completely obstruct venous return to the inferior vena cava. A small support should be placed just caudad of the down-side axilla to lift the thorax enough to relieve pressure on the axillary neurovascular bundle and prevent reduced blood flow to the hand.

In the low-pressure pulmonary circuit, hydrostatic gradients occur between the two hemithoraces. Although the degree of gravity-induced lateral displacement of the heart is different in the two lateral decubitus positions, it is generally true that most of the down-side lung lies below the level of the atrium and that the up-side lung lies above it. Vascular congestion of the down-side lung resembles a Zone 3 of West,[11] while the relative hypoperfusion of the up-side lung resembles a

Zone 2. Kaneko *et al*[37] found that the transition between Zone 3 and Zone 2 occurred at approximately 18 cm above the most dependent part of the lung.

If the cervical spine of the patient who is placed in a lateral decubitus position is carefully maintained in alignment with the thoracolumbar spine, almost no gradient will occur between pressures in the mediastinum and those in the head. If the head is improperly supported and sufficient lateral angulation of the neck occurs in either direction, obstruction of jugular flow may be produced and intracranial vascular dynamics can be disturbed.

Respiratory

With a supple chest the lateral decubitus position can decrease the volume of the down-side hemithorax. The weight of the chest may force the rib cage into a less expanded conformation. Gravity-induced shifts of mediastinal structures toward the down-side chest wall tend to further reduce the volume of the dependent lung. Viscera force the down-side diaphragm cephalad if the long axis of the trunk is horizontal or head-down.

While spontaneous ventilation can partially compensate for the diaphragmatic stretching in the down hemithorax, because the contractile efficiency of the elongated muscle fibers is increased, the compacted lung base and Zone 3 vascular congestion decrease compliance and interfere with the distribution of gas during IPPV. An elevated kidney rest that is either placed against the down-side rib margin or flank, or that migrates into that position as the patient shifts on it, further interferes with passive ventilation of the dependent lung.

The up-side hemithorax is much less compressed than is the

dependent side and, because the lung lies above the level of the atria, it has less vascular congestion than does the down-side lung. As a result, unless contralateral flexion has rendered the up-side flank muscles quite taut and imprisoned the costal margin, ventilation is easier and preferential to the more compliant up-side lung. The result is often hyperventilation of the underperfused up-side lung and hypoventilation of the congested down-side lung. The potential for a clinically significant ventilation/perfusion mismatch is obvious.

VARIATIONS OF THE LATERAL DECUBITUS POSITIONS

Standard (Horizontal) Lateral Position

In the horizontal lateral decubitus position (Fig. 24-10), the patient is rolled onto one side on a flat table surface and stabilized in that posture by flexing the down-side thigh to almost 90° on the trunk. The down-side knee is bent to retain the leg on the table. The peroneal nerve of that side is padded to minimize compression damage from the weight of the legs. The up-side thigh and leg are extended comfortably and pillows are placed between the lower extremities. The head is supported so that the cervical and thoracic spines are properly aligned.

Arms may be extended ventrally and retained on a single arm board with suitable padding between them, or they may be individually retained on a padded two-level arm support that can help also to stabilize the thorax (Fig. 24-11A).

An additional method is to flex each elbow and place the arms on suitable padding on the table in front of the patient's face (Fig. 24-11B). A small pad, thick enough to raise the thorax and prevent excessive compression of the shoulder, is placed just caudad to the down-side axilla. It should assure adequate perfusion of the down-side hand and minimize circumduction of the dependent shoulder that might stretch the suprascapular nerve.

The patient is stabilized in the lateral position by the use of one or more retaining tapes stretched across the hip and fixed to the underside of the table top. Care must be taken to see

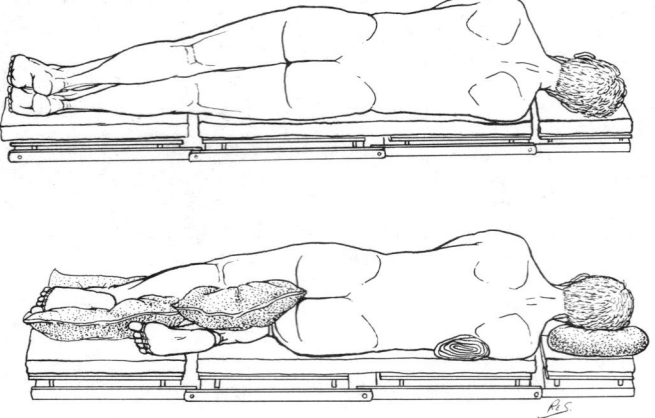

FIG. 24-10. Standard lateral decubitus position. Proper padding and head support are shown in lower figure. Flexed down-side leg stabilizes torso. Retaining straps not shown. (Reprinted with permission. Martin JT: Positioning in Anesthesia and Surgery. Philadelphia, WB Saunders, 1987.)

that the hip tapes lie safely between the iliac crest and the head of the femur rather than over the head of the femur in a compressive manner that could eventuate in its aseptic necrosis (Fig. 24-11B). An additional restraining tape may be used across the thorax just caudad to the axilla if necessary, but it should never be placed across the costal margins where it could restrict ventilation.

Semisupine and Semiprone

The semilateral postures are designed to reach anterolateral (semisupine) or posterolateral (semiprone) structures of the trunk. The semiprone position is commonly used in the postoperative management of patients who have had surgical procedures within the upper airway and in the recovery-room care of children.

In the semisupine position the up-side arm must be carefully supported so that it is not hyperextended and so that no traction or compression is applied to the brachial and axillary neurovascular bundles (Fig. 24-12). Padding should be placed under the dorsal torso and hip to prevent the patient from rolling supine.

In the semiprone position the down-side arm is usually placed behind the patient to avoid stress on the shoulder (Fig. 24-13). The down-side lower extremity is straight, while the up-side lower extremity is flexed at hip and knee in order to maintain the posture.

Sims

In 1857 the prominent New York City gynecologist, J. Marion Sims, began to use a modification of the lateral position for operations on the perineum, rectum, vagina, and bladder (Fig. 24-14). Subsequently, it became widely used as a birthing position. It resembles the semiprone position in that the down-side lower extremity is extended, the up-side is flexed at hip and knee to expose the perineum, and the patient rolls slightly ventrad.

Flexed Lateral Positions

LATERAL JACKKNIFE. The lateral jackknife position places the down-side iliac crest over the hinge between the back and thigh sections of the table (Fig. 24-15). The table top is angulated at that point to flex laterally the thighs on the trunk. After the patient has been suitably positioned and restrained, the chassis of the table is then tipped so that the uppermost surface of the flank and thorax is essentially horizontal. As a result, the feet are below the level of the atria and significant amounts of blood may pool in distensible vessels in each leg.

The lateral jackknife position is usually intended to stretch the up-side flank and widen intercostal spaces as an asset to a thoracotomy incision. Its physiologic price is high, however, and it is no longer needed once the rib-spreading retractor is placed in the incision.[38]

KIDNEY. The kidney position (Fig. 24-16) resembles the lateral jackknife position, but it adds the use of an elevated rest under the down-side iliac crest that increases the amount of lateral flexion and improves access to the up-side kidney under the overhanging costal margin. Unlike the lateral jackknife position, the kidney position does not have a useful alternative for a flank approach to the kidney. Thus, the physiologic insults associated with the position, such as venous pooling and ventilation/perfusion mismatch, need to be carefully combatted by vigilant anesthesia and rapid surgery. Strict stabiliz-

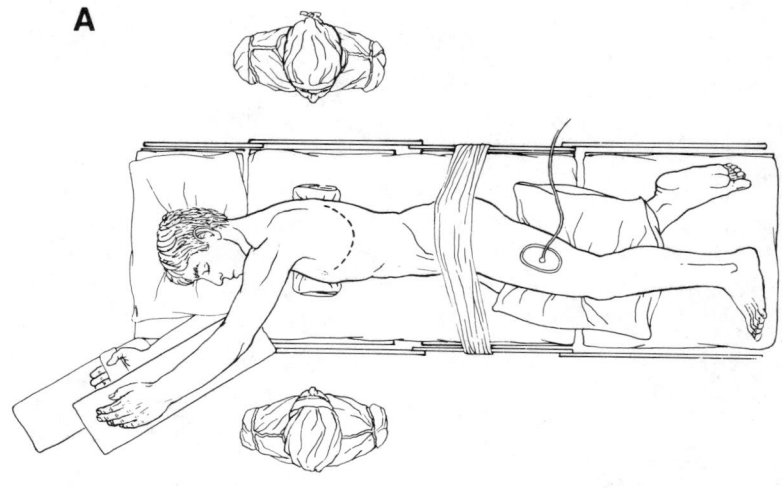

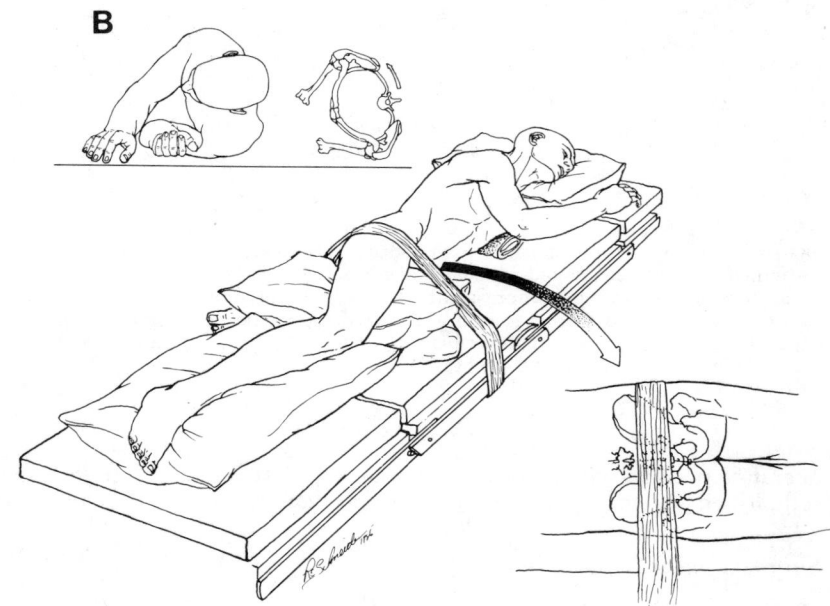

FIG. 24-11. Lateral position with arms arranged on two-tiered arm supports (*A*) or positioned on pillows on the table surface (*B*) in front of the patient's head. Note the location of the stabilizing strap(s) between the iliac crest and the head of the up-side femur (*B, lower right*) rather than on the head of the femur. Potential ventral displacement of the torso can threaten the down-side axillary neurovascular bundle (*B, upper left*). (Reprinted with permission. Martin JT: Positioning in Anesthesia and Surgery. Philadelphia, WB Saunders, 1987.)

ing precautions should be taken to prevent the patient from shifting on the table so that the elevated rest ("kidney rest") relocates into the down-side flank and becomes a severe impediment to ventilation of the dependent lung.

COMPLICATIONS OF THE LATERAL DECUBITUS POSITION

Eyes and Ears

Injuries to the dependent eye are unlikely if the head is properly supported during and after the turn from supine to the lateral position. If the face turns toward the mattress, however, and the lids are not closed, preventable abrasions of the surface of the eye can occur.

In the lateral position, the down-side ear can be pressed by the weight of the head against a rough or uneven supporting surface. Careful padding with a pillow or a foam sponge is usually sufficient protection against contusion of the ear.

Neck

Lateral flexion of the neck is possible when the head of a patient in the lateral position is inadequately supported. If the cervical spine is arthritic, postoperative neck pain can be troublesome. Pain from a symptomatic protrusion of a cervical disc can be intensified unless the head is carefully positioned so that flexion, extension, or rotation are avoided. Lee *et al*[39] reported a technique in which patients with unstable cervical spines can be intubated awake and turned gently into the

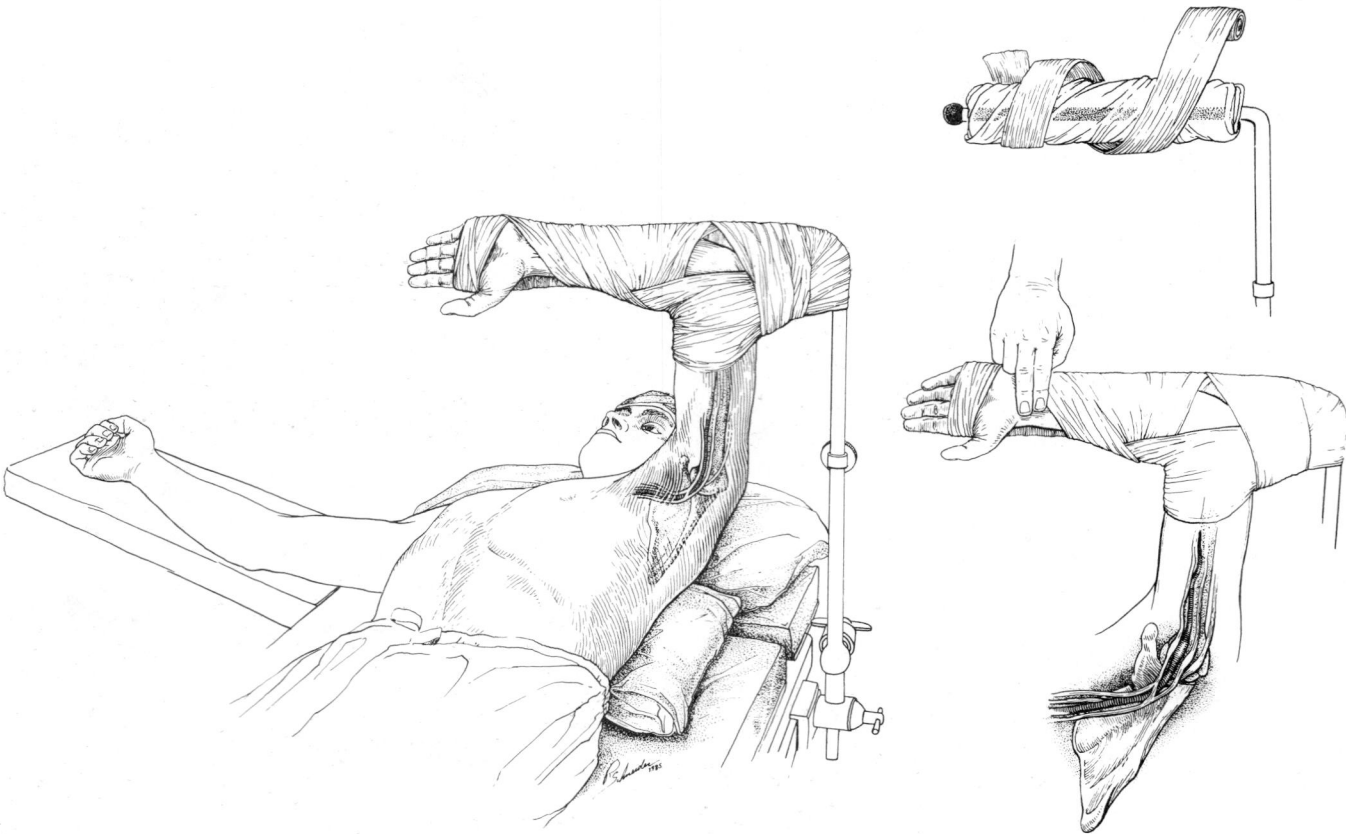

FIG. 24-12. The semisupine position with dorsal pads supporting the torso and the relaxed arm restrained on a well-cushioned adjustable overhead bar. Axillary contents (*lower inset*) are not under tension and are not compressed by the head of the humerus; the radial pulse is not compromised. The position is safe only if arm does not become a hanging mechanism to support the torso. (Reprinted with permission. Collins VJ [ed]: Principles of Anesthesiology, 3rd ed. Philadelphia, Lea & Febiger, in press.)

operative position while repeated neurologic checks are accomplished to detect the development of a positioning injury.

Suprascapular Nerve Injury

Ventral circumduction of the dependent shoulder can rotate the suprascapular notch away from the root of the neck (Fig. 24-17). Since the suprascapular nerve is fixed both at the neck and at the notch, circumduction can stretch the nerve and produce troublesome diffuse, dull shoulder pain. This problem has been the source of litigation.* The diagnosis is established by blocking the nerve at the notch and producing pain relief. Treatment may require resecting the ligament over the notch to decompress the nerve. A supporting pad placed under the thorax just caudad to the axilla, and thick enough to raise the chest off of the shoulder, should prevent the circumduction injury to the nerve.

Unstable Thorax

When the rib cage is unstable following an injury, turning the patient onto the injured side should be avoided if there is a

*Schweiss JF: Personal Communication, 1986

useful alternate position. Sharp ends of fractured ribs can be displaced by the weight of the thorax to puncture the down-side lung. A tension pneumothorax that develops during a surgical procedure on the opposite chest or at a distant site can be chaotic and life threatening before it is accurately diagnosed.

Atelectasis

Atelectasis of an imprisoned and poorly expanding dependent lung can occur in the lateral decubitus positions, particularly the flexed lateral position, if the flexion point is in the flank or on the costal margin instead of at the down-side iliac crest. Careful positioning and adequate passive IPPV should reduce the risk.

Aseptic Necrosis of Up-side Femoral Head

Compression of the head of the femur into the acetabulum by pressure from a misplaced restraining tape in the lateral decubitus position can result in aseptic necrosis of the hip. Obstruction of the nutrient artery to the femoral head is the assumed cause and the incidence of the complication is not known. Nevertheless, the tapes that stabilize the patient

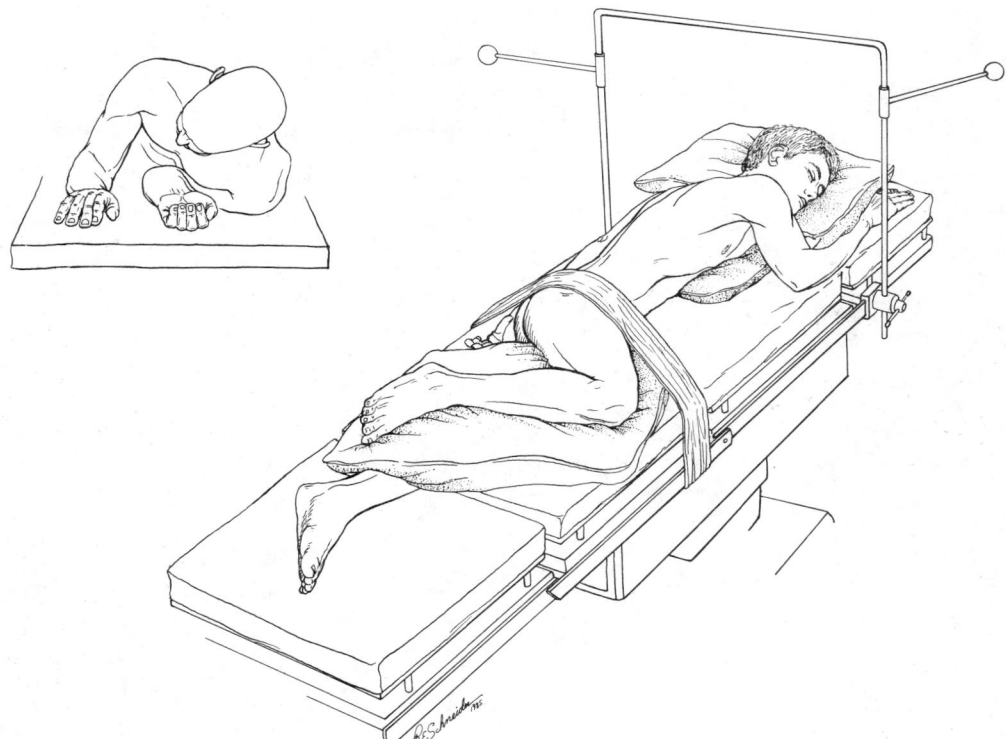

FIG. 24-13. The semiprone position with down-side leg extended and up-side leg flexed at the knee, permitting ventral rotation of the trunk. The down-side arm should be just behind the trunk to prevent axillary compression, as shown in the inset. (Reprinted with permission. Martin JT: Positioning in Anesthesia and Surgery. Philadelphia, WB Saunders, 1987.)

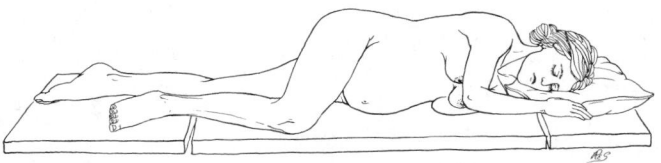

FIG. 24-14. The Sims position, used as a means of access to the structures of the perineum. (Reprinted with permission. Martin JT: Positioning in Anesthesia and Surgery. Philadelphia, WB Saunders, 1987.)

should be placed across the up-side hip on the soft tissue in the space between the head of the femur and the crest of the ilium in order to avoid causing ischemia of the femoral head (Fig. 24-15). Apparently, aseptic necrosis of the head of the down-side femur is unlikely.

Unstable Spine

Turning a patient with an unstable vertebral column into the lateral position requires careful teamwork and a sufficient number of personnel to assure gentle handling. Bivalved frames such as the Foster or the Stryker are rarely used. If the trachea is intubated while the patient is awake, a neurologic evaluation can be accomplished after the patient is finally positioned. Use of somatosensory-evoked potential (SSEP) recordings before and after the turn may also be helpful. Having the responsible surgeon present and involved in establishing the desired position is prudent.

Peroneal Nerve Injury

Pressure from weight of the down-side knee against the mattress may compress the common peroneal nerve as it passes laterally around the neck of the fibula. Inability to dorsiflex the foot and loss of sensation over the dorsum of the foot indicate dysfunction of the nerve.[40] Padding the area of the head of the fibula is usually a sufficient precautionary measure.

VENTRAL DECUBITUS POSITIONS

PHYSIOLOGY

Circulatory

In the prone position, the circulatory dynamics vary according to the postural modification in use. If the legs remain essentially horizontal, pressure gradients in the vessels are minimal. If the patient is kneeling, or if the table chassis is rotated head high, significant venous pooling of blood is likely in distensible dependent vessels.

With the patient lying on the soft ventral abdominal wall, pressure of compressed viscera is transmitted to the dorsal surface of the abdominal cavity. Mesenteric and paravertebral vessels are compressed, causing engorgement of veins within the spinal canal. Obstruction of the inferior vena cava can produce immediate, visible distention of vertebral veins.[41] Because bleeding from incised vessels about the spine is increased under these circumstances, numerous modifications of the prone position have been created to free the abdomen from pressure, reduce the congestion of intraspinal veins, and facilitate surgical hemostasis.[42, 43]

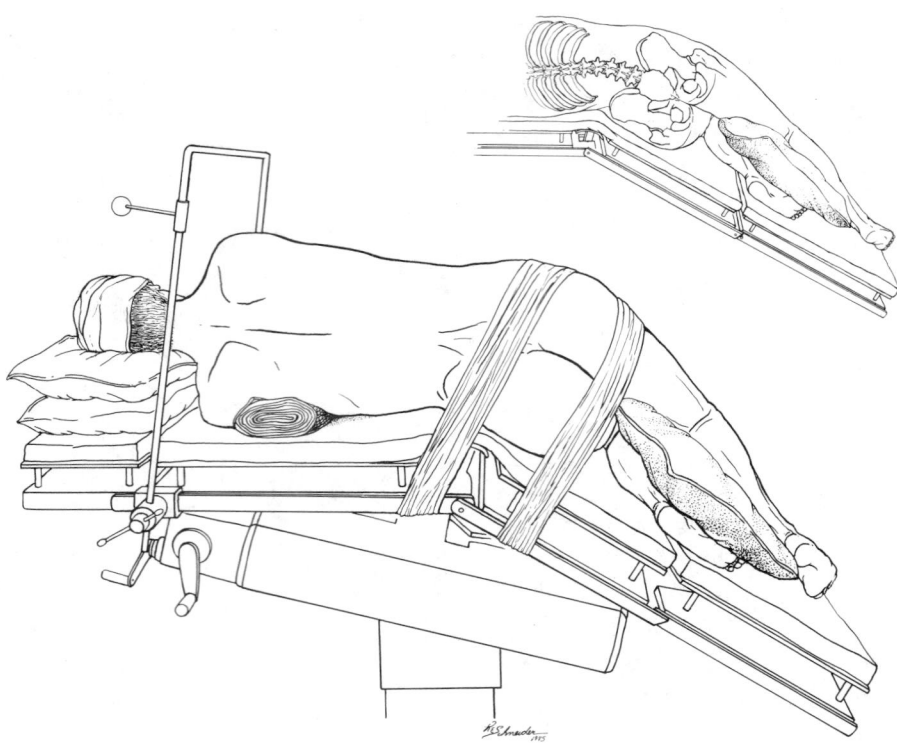

FIG. 24-15. The lateral jackknife position, intended to open intercostal spaces. Note the properly placed restraining tapes intended to retain the iliac crest at the flexion point of the table and prevent caudad slippage that compresses the down-side flank (*inset*). (Reprinted with permission. Martin JT: Positioning in Anesthesia and Surgery. Philadelphia, WB Saunders, 1987.)

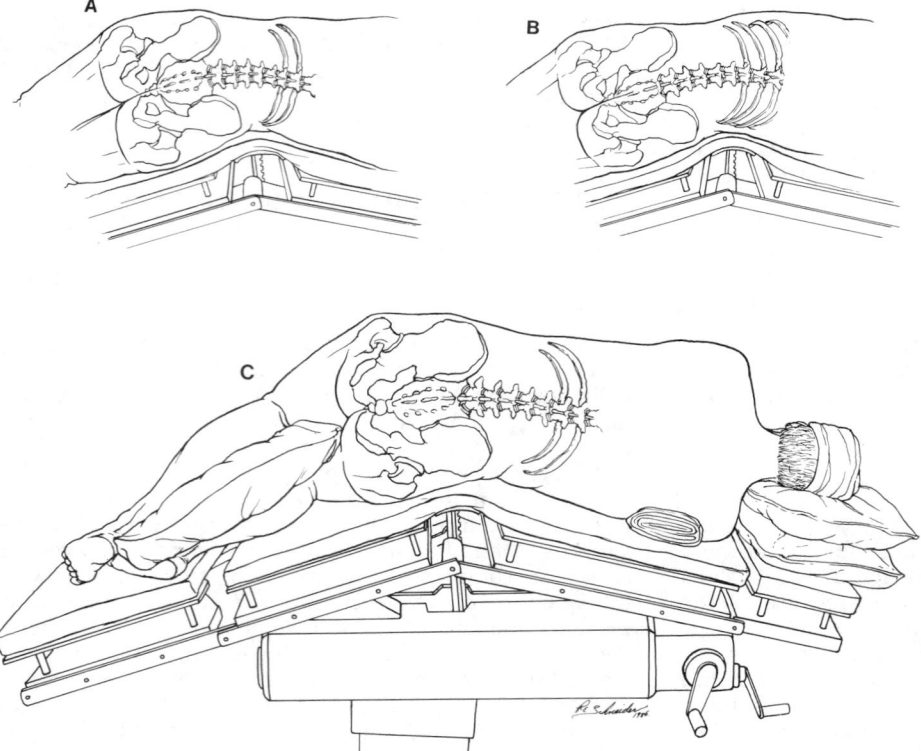

FIG. 24-16. The flexed lateral (kidney) position. (*A and B*) Improper location of the flexion point of the table in the flank or at the lower costal margin impeding ventilation of the down-side lung. (*C*) The iliac crest is shown as the flexion point with best possible expansion of the down-side lung resulting. Restraining tapes deleted for clarity. (Reprinted with permission. Martin JT: Positioning in Anesthesia and Surgery. Philadelphia, WB Saunders, 1987.)

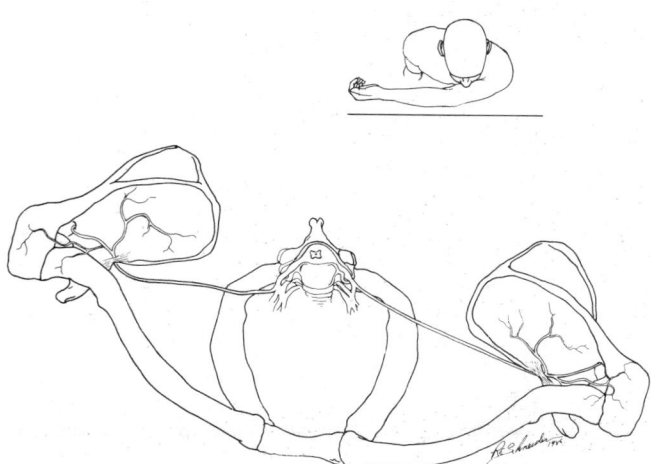

FIG. 24-17. Circumduction of the arm displacing the scapula and stretching the suprascapular nerve between its anchoring points at the cervical spine and the suprascapular notch. (Reprinted with permission. Martin JT: Positioning in Anesthesia and Surgery. Philadelphia, WB Saunders, 1987.)

If the head of a prone patient is below the level of the heart, venous congestion of the face and neck becomes evident. Turning the head can alter arterial perfusion and venous drainage in both extracranial and intracranial vessels. Conjunctival edema, most abundant in the down-side eye, is usual and reflects the influence of gravity on accumulation of extravascular fluid. If the head is above the level of the heart, mean vascular pressures are decreased, air entrainment in open veins is possible, and conjunctival edema will be less evident or absent.

Kaneko et al[37] described the perfusion of the entire lung of prone subjects in terms that would subsequently fit the Zone 3 of West.[11] Backofen and Schauble,[44] monitoring patients with systemic arterial and pulmonary artery thermodilution catheters before and after pronation, found that even the carefully established and supported prone position caused a significant fall in stroke volume and cardiac index, despite the development of increased vascular resistance in both the systemic and pulmonary circuits, while no changes were detected in mean arterial pressure, right atrial pressure, or pulmonary artery occlusion pressure.

On the basis of these results, it is recommended that patients with a precarious cardiovascular status have invasive hemodynamic monitors introduced prior to pronation in order to detect otherwise unrecognizable deterioration of cardiac function due to positioning.[44]

Respiratory

If the thorax is supple and compliant, the body weight of an anesthetized prone patient will compress the anteroposterior diameter of the chest to a degree that is real but poorly defined. If visceral pressure is sufficient to force the diaphragm cephalad, the lung is shortened along its long axis. With both the dorsoventral and cephalocaudad dimensions of the lung decreased, and in the presence of the relative vascular congestion of a Zone 3 of West,[11] the compliance of the compacted prone lung can be anticipated to decrease.

The result of decreased pulmonary compliance in a poorly positioned prone, anesthetized patient is either an increased work of spontaneous ventilation or the need for higher inflation pressures during IPPV. If the latter is the case, the potential exists for the development of pulmonary barotrauma and its possible sequelae, including pulmonary interstitial edema, a pneumothorax, mediastinal emphysema, subcutaneous emphysema, or a pneumomesentery.

Proper positioning can retain more nearly normal pulmonary compliance by minimizing the cephalad shift of the diaphragm caused by compressed abdominal viscera. If the patient is arranged so that the abdomen hangs free, the loss of functional residual capacity (FRC) is less in the prone position than in either the supine or the lateral positions.[45] Rehder et al.[46] noted that the weight of the freed abdominal contents had an "inspiratory effect on the diaphragm" when the pronated patient was properly supported by pads under the shoulder girdle and pelvis.

VARIATIONS OF THE VENTRAL DECUBITUS POSITION

Full (Horizontal) Prone

In the so-called "full" or "horizontal" prone position, (Fig. 24-18), the requirement to elevate the trunk and free the ventral abdominal wall from compression almost always results in the head and lower extremities being lower than the level of the spine. If the table top is angulated at the trunk–thigh hinge in order to remove lumbar lordosis and separate the spinous processes, and if the chassis is then rotated head-up enough to level the patient's back, a significant perfusion gradient may develop between the legs and the heart. Wrapping the legs will minimize pooling of blood in distensible vessels and support venous return.

Various ventral supports, including parallel sheet rolls, reusable soft pads, padded and adjustable metal frames, and four-pillar frames have been devised to free the abdomen from compression.[42, 43] Each has merit, and none is unquestionably superior to the others. The choice is based on local custom and the physique of the patient.

Patients with limited mobility of the neck should have their heads retained in a sagittal plane, either with a skull-pin head clamp or with a device similar to the rocker-based head rest developed by Ray.[43] If neck mobility is satisfactory, the head can be supported on one of several soft sponge devices that prevents pressure on the down-side eye and ear.[43, 47] Forced head rotation should be carefully avoided.[47]

When a patient is scheduled to be pronated after induction of anesthesia, the preanesthetic interview should obtain information about any limitations that may exist in his or her ability to raise the arms overhead during work or sleep.[43] If dysesthesias have been experienced when the arms were elevated, the upper extremities should be retained alongside of the trunk in the prone position. If the arms are to be flexed at the shoulder and elbow and abducted onto arm boards, the musculature about the shoulders should be under no tension, neither humeral head should distend its axillary neurovascular bundle, ulnar nerves at the elbows should be padded, and the pulses at the wrists should remain full.

Prone Jackknife

The prone jackknife posture is used to provide access to the sacral, perianal, and perineal areas as well as to the lower alimentary canal (Fig. 24-19). The thighs are flexed on the trunk more than is usual in the full prone position, and man-

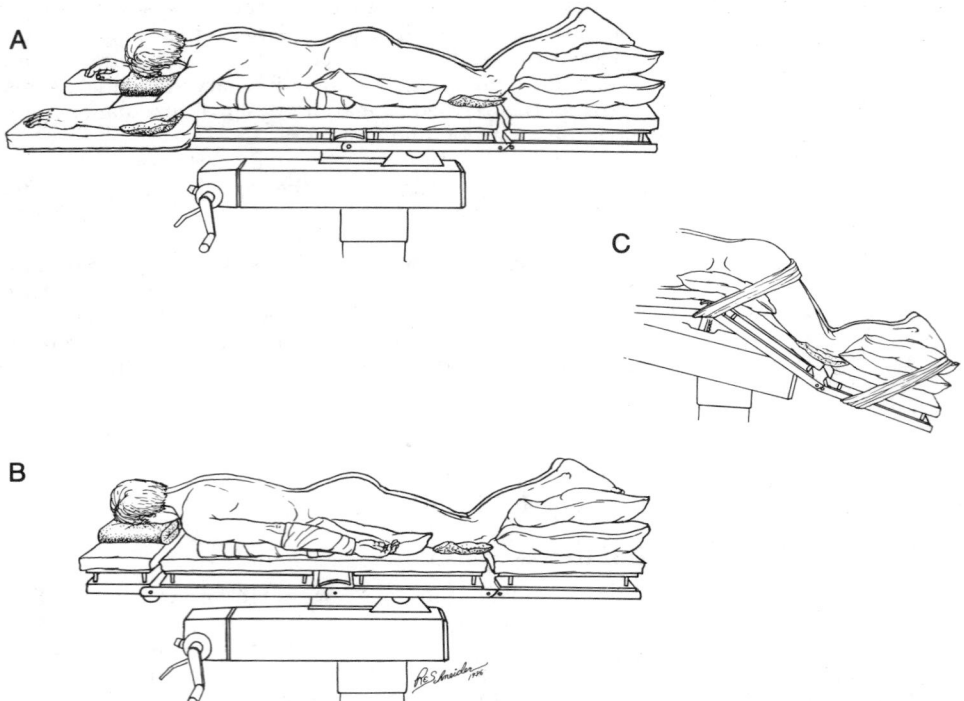

FIG. 24-18. The classic prone position. (*A*) Flat table with relaxed arms extended alongside head. Parallel chest rolls extend from clavicle to just beyond inguinal area with pillow over pelvic end. Elbows and knees are padded and legs are bent at the knees. Head is turned onto a C-shaped foam sponge that frees the down-side eye and ear from compression. (*B*) Same posture with arms snugly retained alongside torso. (*C*) Table flexed to reduce lumbar lordosis and gluteal straps placed to thrust cephalad and prevent caudad slippage as legs are lowered. (Reprinted with permission. Martin JT: Positioning in Anesthesia and Surgery. Philadelphia, WB Saunders, 1987.)

FIG. 24-19. The prone jackknife positions. (*A*) Low jackknife position with trunk–thigh hinge of table used as flexion point and augmented by a pillow under the pelvis. (*B*) Full jackknife position with the thigh–leg hinge of the table used as the flexion point to achieve more acute angulation of the hips on the torso. (Reprinted with permission. Martin JT: Positioning in Anesthesia and Surgery. Philadelphia, WB Saunders, 1987.)

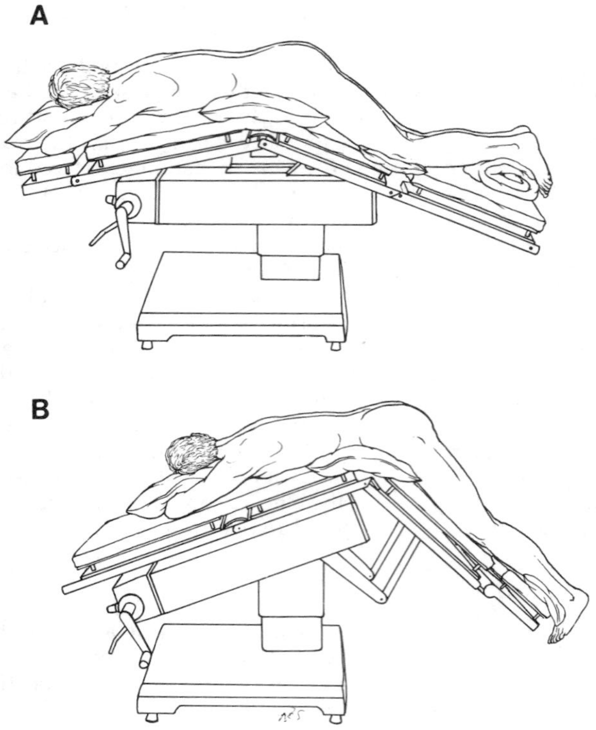

agement of the table surface hinges determines the degree of flexion available.[43]

Kneeling

Kneeling positions have been used to improve operative conditions in the lumbar and cervico-occipital areas (Fig. 24-20). Numerous frames have been constructed to support the weight of a kneeling patient, and their usefulness again depends on local custom and the physique of the patient. Kneeling frames are not as useful as longitudinal supports if the vertebral column is unstable because they tend to apply shearing forces to the fracture site that could damage the contents of the spinal canal. In massively obese patients who must be operated on in the prone position, the kneeling frames tend to prevent pressure on the abdomen more successfully than do longitudinal frames.

COMPLICATIONS OF THE VENTRAL DECUBITUS POSITIONS

Eyes and Ears

The eyes and ears are at risk in the prone position even when the head is turned to one side. The eyes should be lubricated and covered in some manner so that the lids cannot be accidentally separated and the cornea scratched. The eyes should also be protected against the head turning medially after positioning and pressure being exerted on the globe. The anterior chamber and crystalline lens can be injured. If intraocular pressure exceeds retinal artery pressure, blindness can result. Monitoring wires and tubing should be checked after positioning to see that none has migrated underneath the head. If the head is retained in the sagittal plane, the eyes

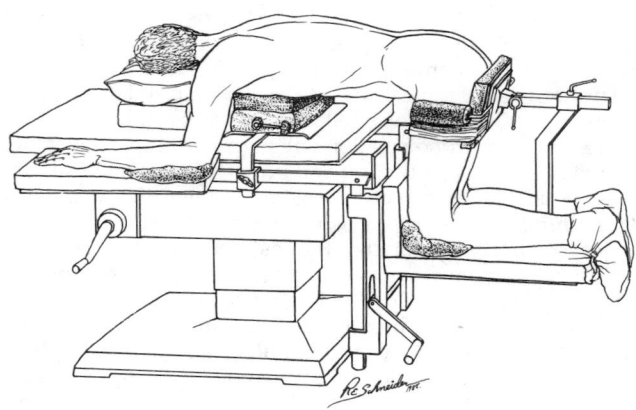

FIG. 24-20. The Andrews kneeling frame with Wiltse thoracic jack in use. (Reprinted with permission. Martin JT: Positioning in Anesthesia and Surgery. Philadelphia, WB Saunders, 1987.)

should be checked after positioning to assure that they are safe from pressure.

Conjunctival edema usually occurs in the eyes of the pronated patient if the head is at or below the level of the heart. It is generally transient, inconsequential, and requires only reestablishment of the normal tissue pressure gradients of the supine position, or of a low Fowler's position, to be redistributed.

The down-side ear should not be bent or distorted lest cartilagenous injury occur. Soft foam padding is usually sufficient protection.

Neck Problems

Anesthesia impairs reflex muscle spasm that protects the skeleton against motion that would be painful in an alert patient.

Lateral rotation of the head and neck of an anesthetized, pronated patient, particularly one with an arthritic cervical spine, can stretch relaxed skeletal muscles and ligaments and injure cervical articulations. Neck pain and limitation of motion can result. The arthritic neck is usually best managed by keeping it in the sagittal plane when the patient is prone.

Extremes of head and neck rotation can also interfere with flow in either ipsilateral or contralateral vessels to and from the head. Excessive head rotation can reduce flow in both the carotid[48] and vertebral[49] systems. Impaired cerebral perfusion can result.

Brachial Plexus Injuries

Stretch injuries to roots of the brachial plexus (Fig. 24-21) on the side contralateral to the turned face are possible if the contralateral shoulder is held firmly caudad. If an arm is placed on an arm board alongside the head, care must be taken to see that the head of the humerus is not stretching and compressing the axillary neurovascular bundle.

When the arm is placed on an arm board alongside the head, the forearm naturally pronates. As a result the ulnar nerve is vulnerable to pressure at the elbow, in the groove between the olecranon process and the medial epicondyle of the humerus. As a result, when an arm is to be placed alongside the head of a patient who is in the prone position, the medial aspect of the elbow must be well padded and its weight borne principally on the medial epicondyle of the humerus.

Thoracic Outlet Syndrome

Some patients complain of pain and paresthesias in their arms after working with items on an overhead shelf, changing an overhead light bulb, or sleeping with one or both arms elevated alongside the head. The most likely explanation for the distress is the presence of a thoracic outlet syndrome with

FIG. 24-21. Sources of potential injury to the brachial plexus and its peripheral components when the patient is in the prone position. A: Neck rotation stretching roots of the plexus. B: Compression of the plexus and vessels between the clavicle and first rib. C: Injury to the axillary neurovascular bundle from the head of the humerus. D: Compression of the ulnar nerve above, below, and within the cubital tunnel. E: Area of vulnerability of the radial nerve to lateral compression above the elbow. (Reprinted with permission. Martin JT: Positioning in Anesthesia and Surgery. Philadelphia, WB Saunders, 1987.)

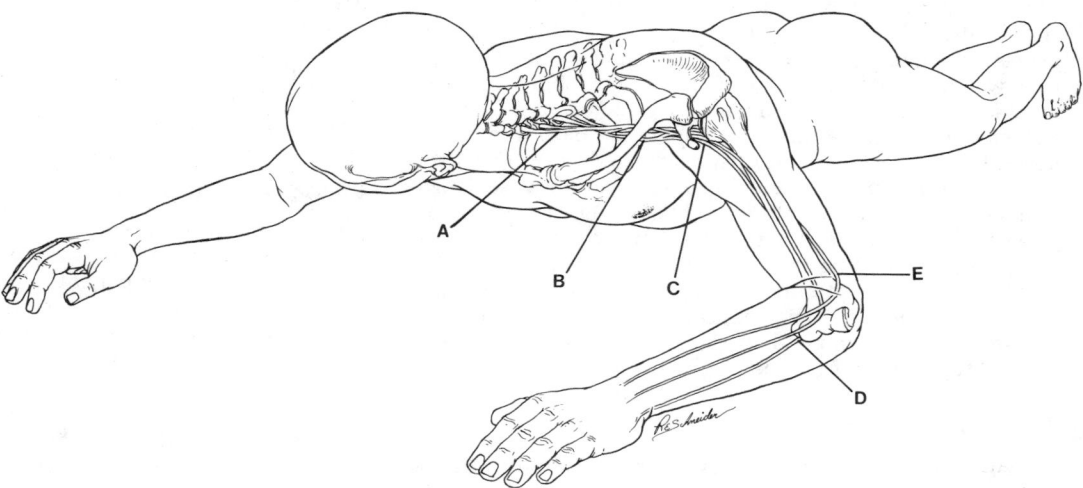

compression of the brachial plexus and subclavian vessels near the first rib. The preanesthetic interview should inquire about this possibility whenever a patient is scheduled to be placed in a prone position. When present, the condition requires that the patient's arms be retained alongside of the trunk. Debilitating postoperative arm and hand pain may result if the arms are alongside of the head during a lengthy operation.[43]

Unstable Chest Wall

Patients with an unstable chest wall are apt to displace jagged rib fragments into underlying lung tissue when they are pronated and the weight of the thorax rests on the sternum and rib cage. In most instances alternate operative postures are possible and should be chosen despite the surgical inconvenience produced. If the prone position must be used following a destabilizing injury to the thorax, serious consideration should be given to prophylactic introduction of chest tubes.

Breast Injuries

Female breasts of average size can be stretched and injured if forced laterally when the patient is prone. Medial and cephalad displacement seems better tolerated. Massive breasts of a very large patient, if forced laterally, may not cause distress to the patient; however, they may force the arms far enough laterally to cause the surgical team difficulty in reaching the depths of an incision in the dorsal midline.

Direct pressure on breasts containing enhancement prostheses can rupture the prosthesis. Tense skin grafts over mastectomy sites require considerable soft padding to prevent pressure necrosis and loss of the graft. Male breasts with gynecomastia are usually enlarged and firm but are apparently nontender; however, prudence would indicate that they be appropriately padded before pronation.

Coronary Artery Grafts

Mediastinal contents shift somewhat ventrad when a patient assumes the prone position. Apparently, the degree to which the ventrodorsal dimension of a stable chest is compressed by the prone position can vary with the patient and the type of ventral supporting system used. Weinlander et al[50] have reported an occurrence with a patient who had received a coronary artery bypass graft 8 years previously and who had, in the interim, been successfully anesthetized for a lumbar laminectomy that was done in the prone position on longitudinal chest rolls. Subsequently needing a repeat laminectomy, he was anesthetized and placed on a kneeling frame. The sternum was elevated by a pad to relieve venous congestion of the head and neck. Electrocardiographic evidence of myocardial ischemia followed placement of the sternal pad, was not relieved by drug therapy, and necessitated intraaortic balloon pump support for emergency coronary artery revascularization following the laminectomy. While a number of questions remain unanswerable, Weinlander's group felt that sternal compression resulting from the pad adversely affected the previously functional coronary artery grafts and probably caused the ischemia.[50] The implication that a sternal pad compresses the chest more than does a longitudinal frame is interesting, but the issue needs further proof.

The Unstable Spine

Pronating the patient whose spine is unstable requires skillful teamwork. Enough people are required to control the weight of the patient without sudden shifts of posture. Participation of the principle surgeon should be a requirement if stabilizing traction must be removed during positioning.

Through use of topical anesthesia and mild sedation, awake intubation of the trachea followed by a careful turn of the patient into the prone position will permit multiple neurologic checks after final positioning and prior to induction of surgical anesthesia.[39] Detection of neurologic changes that occur during turning permits rapid correction of the faulty posture.

Use of bivalved nursing frames, such as the Foster or Stryker, allows anesthesia and intubation to be accomplished with the patient on the dorsal shell of the frame while traction is unchanged. Depending on the position of the neck in traction and the mobility of the mandible, fiberoptic or "blind" techniques may be needed for intubation of the trachea. Addition of the ventral shell to the frame provides firm fixation of the patient during pronation. Removal of the dorsal shell after the turn permits the operation to be carried out on the remaining ventral shell without further risk from positioning torsion and without removing the corrective traction.

Abdominal Compression

Compression of the abdomen by the weight of the trunk of the prone patient can cause the diaphragm to be forced cephalad enough to impair ventilation. If intraabdominal pressure approaches or exceeds venous pressure, return of blood from the pelvis and lower extremities is obstructed. Because the vertebral venous plexuses communicate directly with abdominal veins, increased intraabdominal pressure is transmitted to the surgical field in the form of venous distension and increased bleeding. All of the various supportive pads and frames are designed to remove pressure from the abdomen and avoid these problems.[42, 43]

Injuries to Viscerocutaneous Stomata

Stomata that drain viscera into containers affixed to the abdominal wall are at risk in the prone position if they lie against a part of the ventral supporting frame or pad. Compressive ischemia of the stomal orifice can cause it to slough subsequently.

Knee Injuries

Extremely heavy patients, or those whose knees are pathologic, can injure knee joints in the kneeling position if the ledges that support them are not heavily padded. Often there is no suitable alternate position for these patients, and the possibility of postoperative knee problems due to the kneeling prone position should be carefully discussed in the preanesthetic interview.

Thermal Instability

Because many of the operations that require the prone position are lengthy, and because ventral supporting frames prevent contact between patients and heating blankets, heat loss in the prone position is problematic. Use of heated humidifiers added to the airway, and low flow rates delivered from the anesthesia machine to the rebreathing system, are satisfactory methods of maintaining normothermia. If significant hyperthermia is encountered, vigorous cooling methods, including intragastric cooling and packing available body surfaces with ice, must be used while the surgical procedure is terminated as rapidly as possible.

HEAD-ELEVATED POSITIONS

PHYSIOLOGY

Circulatory

Coonan and Hope have reviewed circulatory changes that occur in alert humans with the change from the supine to the erect position.[51] As the head is raised above the level of the heart, pressure gradients develop and increase with the degree of elevation. Blood shifts from the upper body toward the feet. Atrial filling pressures decrease, sympathetic tone increases, parasympathetic tone decreases, the renin–angiotensin–aldosterone system is activated, and fluid and electrolytes are retained by the kidneys.[52, 53] Intrathoracic blood volume decreases as much as 500 ml, pulmonary vascular resistance can double, and left atrial pressure falls more than does the right.[54] Cardiac output decreases 20%–40% and stroke volume decreases by as much as 50%. Heart rate accelerates by as much as 30%. The arterial tree constricts, and systemic vascular resistance increases 30%–60% to maintain a steady or increased mean arterial pressure, but the venous capacitance system is essentially unaffected.[55, 56] Oxygen consumption by the tissues is unchanged, so the reduced oxygen supply (reduced cardiac output) causes an increased arteriovenous oxygen content difference.[57]

Cerebral blood flow decreases by approximately 20% with high head elevation.[55] Renal blood flow decreases as much as 30% (in massively obese patients in the sitting position, as much as 76%), glomerular filtration decreases, and reduced secretion of antidiuretic hormone and aldosterone result in retention of water and sodium.[58]

Albin et al[59, 60] and Dalrymple[61] noted similar alterations in cardiovascular parameters when the head-elevated position was established after patients were anesthetized. While significant changes were not encountered with less than 60° of head-up tilt, the magnitude of changes was often greater than the awake values presented above, and the alterations increased progressively for more than 1 hr after the posture was finalized. The question arose as to whether an impaired circulatory system could or should adjust to these stresses.

One can infer that the presence of intracranial pathology may exacerbate potentially harmful reductions in cerebral blood flow associated with head elevation.[62] Mean arterial pressure should be measured at the level of the circle of Willis, since that site is more reliable as an indicator of cerebral blood flow and perfusion pressure in the anesthetized, seated patient than is measurement at the level of the arm or wrist.[51]

Respiratory

As the patient becomes more upright in the head-elevated dorsal decubitus position, the inspiratory stroke of the diaphragm becomes less impeded by the bulk of abdominal viscera. Spontaneous chest wall motion requires less effort, and less inspiratory pressure is needed to inflate the lungs during IPPV. FRC increases in the head-elevated positions.[63] Age-related increases in shunting are less in the head-elevated position than in the supine.[63] Gurtner[64] found that the diffusing capacity for oxygen was reduced in the sitting position as a result of the gravity-related decreases in perfusion of the upper portions of the lungs. Slutsky et al, however, found no difference between the supine and the sitting positions when measuring the ventilatory responses to hypoxia in volunteers.[65]

VARIATIONS

Sitting

The full sitting position, characterized by the patient sitting upright in a chair, is uncommon in current practice. It was used frequently for installation of air prior to pneumoencephalography but was uncommon as a surgical position.

The classic sitting position for surgery has the patient in a semireclining posture on an operating table, with the legs elevated to about the level of the heart and the head flexed ventrally on the neck (Fig. 24-22). Compressive wraps about the legs reduce pooling of blood in the lower extremities. The head is held in place by some type of face rest or a three-pin skull fixation frame.

Supine, Head-elevated

A dorsal recumbent position with the head of the table elevated somewhat is used for many operations about the ventral and lateral aspects of the head and neck (Fig. 24-23). Its purpose is to improve access to the surgical target for the operating team as well as to drain blood and irrigation solutions away from the wound. The entire table may be rotated head-high or the back section alone can be elevated as needed. While the degree of tilt involved is not great, small pressure gradients are created along the vascular axis that can pool blood in the lower extremities or entrain air in patulous vessels that are incised above the level of the heart.

Vidabek has described a position (Fig. 24-24) that uses a small degree of head elevation along with a carefully arched thoracolumbar spine to improve access to the organs of the upper abdomen.[66] In a small series, he noted its usefulness to the surgeon and its difficulties for patients with precarious cardiovascular systems.

For operations about the shoulder joint, the patient is often placed in a head-elevated supine position, with the upper torso moved across the lateral edge of the operating table so that head and hips are supported but the surgical shoulder is beyond the edge. A pad under the thorax slightly rotates the trunk to elevate the shoulder above the table surface and further improve access. The posture has been called the *barber chair position*.[67]

Lateral, Head-elevated

The lateral recumbent position with the head somewhat elevated, apparently created at the Montreal Neurological Institute as a means of access to occipitocervical pathology, has also been referred to as the *park bench position*.[68] All of the stabilizing requirements needed for the usual lateral decubitus position apply. The head is held firmly in a three-pin skull fixation holder, which can be readjusted as needed during surgery. While the degree of head elevation used is mild, the position does not completely remove the threat of air embolization. The anesthesiologist has good access to the patient's face and ventral thorax for purposes of monitoring, manipulation, and resuscitation.

Prone, Head-elevated

The ventral decubitus posture with the table rotated head-high (Fig. 24-25) has become a widely used replacement for the sitting position as a means of access to dorsal structures within the head and neck. In many instances, the avowed advantage of the position is the avoidance of air embolization.

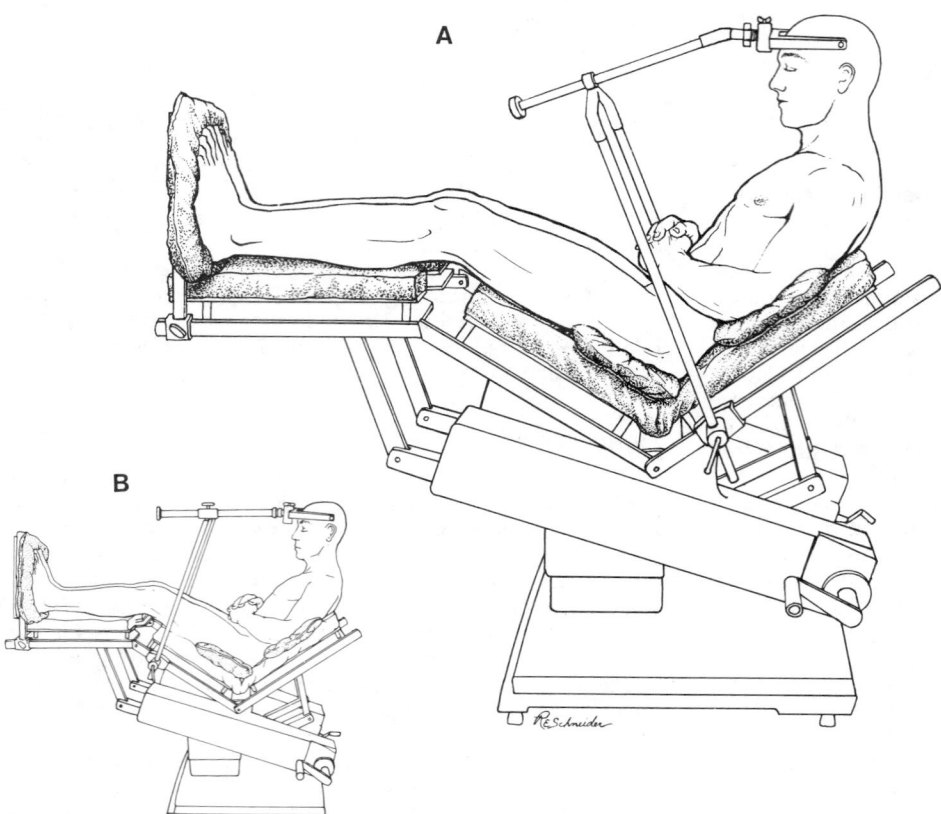

FIG. 24-22. Conventional neurosurgical sitting position, with legs approximately at the level of the heart. (A) The frame of the head-holder is properly clamped to the side rails of the trunk section of the table so that the patient's torso can be leveled in the event of a venous air embolus at the cervico–occipital operative site. (B) The frame is clamped to the side rails of the thigh section of the table, making it difficult or impossible to level the back section in an emergency. (Reprinted with permission. Martin JT: Positioning in Anesthesia and Surgery. Philadelphia, WB Saunders, 1987.)

However, as the result of the positive-pressure inflation cycle of passive ventilation, a bothersome recurrent flux of CSF in and out of the exposed wound may be encountered and hemostasis may be complicated. The position also severely restricts resuscitative access to the ventral thorax.

COMPLICATIONS

Postural Hypotension

In the anesthetized patient, establishment of any of the head-elevated positions is frequently accompanied by some degree of reduction in systemic blood pressure. The normal protective reflexes are inhibited by anesthesia. Measuring mean arterial pressures at the level of the circle of Willis is recommended to assess cerebral perfusion pressures more accurately. Treatment of hypotension consists of temporarily delaying the elevation of the head as the patient is positioned; reducing the concentrations of anesthetic drugs; infusing crystalloids or colloids to increase effective circulating volume; and using appropriately small amounts of a vasopressor as a temporary expedient.

Air Embolus

Air embolization is potentially lethal. If air gets into the circulation, it foams with blood in the heart into a compressible mass that destroys the propulsive efficiency of ventricular contractions and irritates the conduction system. As air moves into the pulmonary vasculature, the bubbles obstruct small vessels and compromise gas exchange.

Opportunities for venous air embolization *via* an incised vein in a surgical wound located above the heart increase with the degree of elevation of the operative site. While the occurrence of air emboli is a relatively frequent phenomenon in head-elevated positions, most of the emboli are small in volume, clinically silent, and recognizable only by sophisticated detection techniques. Nevertheless, the potential for continuing and dangerous accumulations of entrained air requires its immediate detection and prompt treatment. Prudence indicates the need for careful precautions against air entrainment in incised veins as well as persistent monitoring of those situations in which a significant potential for embolization exists. Air embolism may be diagnosed by the presence of one or several of the following: a cardiac murmur; arrhythmias; hypotension; air hunger; a decrease in expired carbon dioxide; and a change in heart sounds noted by a Doppler probe placed over the sternum. For a more detailed consideration of venous air embolization, the reader is referred to Chapter 31 on neurosurgical anesthesia.

Approximately 20%–35% of the population[69] has a residual foramen ovale that is functionally closed as long as pressure in the left atrium exceeds that in the right. However, in the sitting position, right atrial pressure can be higher than left. That gradient, augmented by the presence of air in the right heart, IPPV, and positive end-expiratory pressure, may be sufficient to reopen an existing, but functionally closed, foramen ovale. Air in the right atrium thereby gains paradoxical access to the coronary, cerebral, and systemic circulations.[70] In anesthetized and newly positioned patients, Perkins-Pearson *et al*[71] suggest that if pulmonary artery occlusion pressures are lower than right atrial pressures, it is an indication that the head-

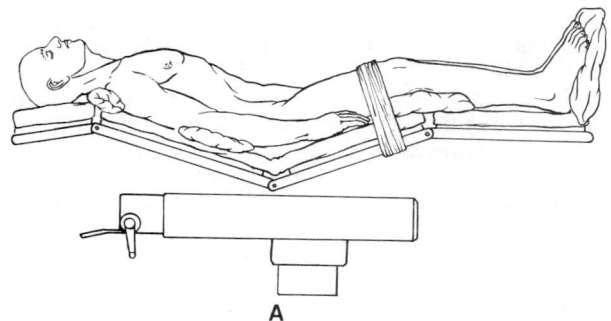

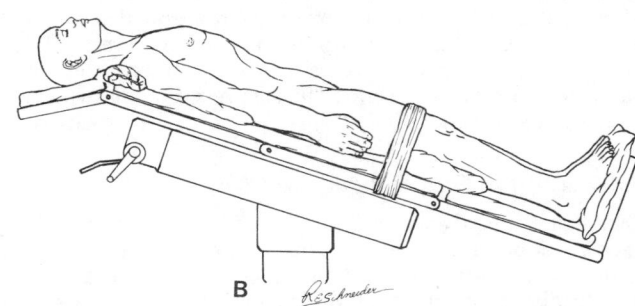

FIG. 24-23. Head-elevated positions often used for operations about the ventral and ventrolateral aspects of the head, face, neck, and cervical spine. (A) The legs are at approximately heart level and the gradient into the head is appreciable but slight. (B) The flat table and foot rest are useful when a thyroidectomy is planned under regional anesthesia. (Reprinted with permission. Martin JT: Positioning in Anesthesia and Surgery. Philadelphia, WB Saunders, 1987.)

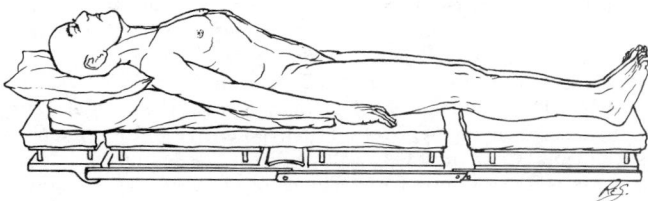

FIG. 24-24. The xyphoid-high posture of Vidabek used to gain access to the upper abdomen. (Reprinted with permission. Martin JT: Positioning in Anesthesia and Surgery. Philadelphia, WB Saunders, 1987.)

elevated posture should be abandoned in favor of a position in which the head is level with the heart. Cucchiara et al[72] have injected agitated saline through a right atrial catheter and used transesophageal echocardiography to detect paradoxical passage of the fluid across the atrial septum. Positive airway pressure aided in determining paradoxical flow in 3 of their 20 patients.

Pneumocephalus

In the usual craniotomy, most of the brain lies subjacent to the incision. After the dura is incised, CSF is removed to improve working conditions and the surgical field is open to the air. During the subsequent closure of the craniotomy, most of the air escapes and the residual pneumocephalus is of little consequence. When an incision is made through the dura in the posterior fossa or cervical spine of a seated patient, however, the bulk of the brain lies above the incision. CSF drains downward out of the wound, and tissue retraction can allow air to bubble up over the surfaces of the brain and to become trapped in the upper reaches of the cranium.[73] When brain mass is decreased by ventricular drainage, steroids, and diuresis, the space available to a pneumocephalus is enlarged. Diffusion of nitrous oxide into the accumulated air or warming of the trapped gas can produce a tension pneumocephalus with signs of increased intracranial pressure and delayed awakening from anesthesia. Twist drill holes over the air mass can be used to vent the gas and decompress the brain.

Toung et al[74] found postoperative pneumocephalus in all of

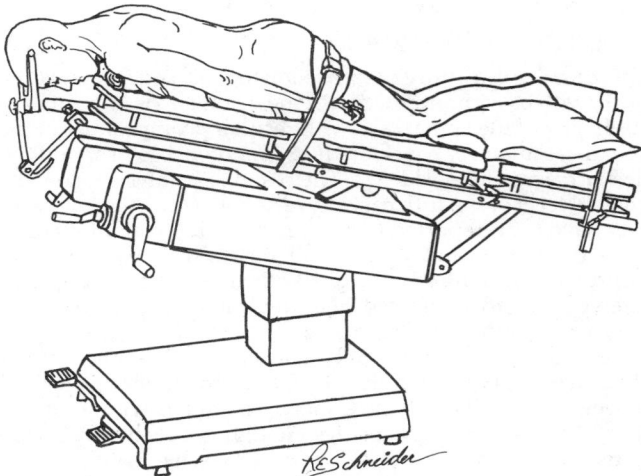

FIG. 24-25. The skull-pin head rest used to stabilize a patient in the head-elevated prone position. Note the chest rolls used to free the abdomen from compression and the gluteal strap to minimize caudad slippage after head-up tilt. (Reprinted with permission. Martin JT: Positioning in Anesthesia and Surgery. Philadelphia, WB Saunders, 1987.)

a group of seated patients, and in most of those who had been prone or in the park bench position. Intraventricular air was present in most of the seated patients and was rare in the other positions. None of their group of 100 patients had neurologic changes attributable to the trapped intracranial air. Standefer et al[75] reported a 3% incidence of symptomatic (tension) pneumocephalus in seated, anesthetized patients whose dura was opened.

Ocular Compression

Pressure on the eyes of a patient who has been placed in a head-elevated position can dislocate a crystalline lens or render the globe ischemic. Unilateral blindness has been reported as a result.[76] In earlier years, the padded head rests that were in general use were difficult to secure firmly to the head and face; sometimes they allowed heads to shift during surgery.

Eye trauma was a constant threat.[76] Modern skull-pin head clamps that grip firmly when properly applied have made ocular compression in the sitting position now a rarity. In the head-elevated lateral decubitus or prone positions, the threats to the eyes are those described in the preceding discussions of nonelevated positions.

Edema of the Face, Tongue, and Neck

McAllister[77] has encountered severe postoperative macroglossia, apparently due to venous and lymphatic obstruction caused by prolonged, marked neck flexion. The patient's chin was firmly against the chest and an oral airway was in place to protect the endotracheal tube. Ellis et al[78] reported a similar patient who needed a tracheostomy because of massive swelling of the tongue, lips, pharynx, and epiglottis that occurred within several hours of extubation following lengthy hypotensive anesthesia in the sitting position. Extremes of neck flexion, with or without head rotation, have been widely used to gain access to structures in the posterior fossa and cervical spine, but their potential for damage should be understood.

Midcervical Tetraplegia

This devastating injury occurs following marked flexion of the neck, with or without rotation of the head, and is attributed to stretching of the spinal cord with resultant compromise of the spinal vasculature. An element of spondylosis or a spondylotic bar may be involved.[79, 80] The result is paralysis below the general level of the fifth cervical vertebra. While the few cases that have been reported (less than 40 in the world literature) have most often followed use of the sitting position, I am aware of an infant who awoke with midcervical tetraplegia after prolonged nonforced head flexion for intracranial surgery in the supine position.

Reversible changes in SSEPs elicited by stimulation of the median nerve have been shown to occur after neck flexion;[81, 82] however, Cottrell et al[83] have shown in studies with monkeys that SSEPs may not be sensitive enough to detect midcervical tetraplegia, and Levy et al[84] have suggested using motor-evoked potentials for this purpose.

Sciatic Nerve Injury

Stretch injuries of the sciatic nerve can occur in some patients if the hips are markedly flexed without bending the knees. Prolonged compression of the sciatic nerve as it emerges from the pelvis is possible in a thin, seated patient unless the buttocks are suitably padded. Foot drop may be the result of injuries to either the sciatic nerve or the common peroneal nerve and can be bilateral.

Thermal Instability

A seated patient may have much of the ventral surface of the torso exposed for the purposes of monitoring. The ability of a wet exposed head to lose body heat is well known to water safety experts. In a cold operating room, despite the use of an antishock garment about the abdomen and lower extremities of the patient, accidental hypothermia can be a vexing problem. Often body weight plus the angulations of the surface of the operating table combine to defeat flow of fluid through the channels of a thermal mattress. Heat losses can be minimized, and often thermal recovery promoted, by using carefully warmed and humidified respiratory gases. An additional method is to suspend a safety-certified electrician's trouble light alongside of the uncovered torso of the patient. In doing so, care should be taken to avoid overheating either the airway or the exposed skin.

Elevations of body temperature are uncommon during operations involving head-elevated patients. If significant or accelerating hyperthermia does occur, vigorous cooling methods and suitable drug therapy should be instituted at once. The surgical procedure should be terminated as promptly as possible.

REFERENCES

1. Martin JT: Positioning in Anesthesia and Surgery. Philadelphia, WB Saunders, 1987
2. Dorland's Illustrated Medical Dictionary. Philadelphia, WB Saunders, 1965
3. Enderby GEH: Postural ischemia and blood pressure. Lancet 1:185, 1954
4. Green DM, Metheny D: Estimation of acute blood loss by tilt test. Surg Gynecol Obstet 84:1045, 1947
5. Kubal K, Komatsu T, Sanchala V et al: Trendelenburg position used during venous cannulation increases myocardial oxygen demands. Anesth Analg 63:239, 1984
6. Porter WT: Shock at the Front. Boston Med Surg J 175:874, 1916
7. Sibbald WJ, Patterson NAM, Holliday RL et al: The Trendelenburg position: Hemodynamic effects in hypotensive and normotensive patients. Crit Care Med 7:218, 1979
8. Dripps RD, Comroe JH Jr: Circulatory physiology: The adjustments to blood loss and postural changes. Surg Clin North Am 26:1368, 1946
9. Burch GE: Method for recording simultaneously the time course of digital rate and of digital volume of inflow and outflow during a single pulse cycle in man. J Appl Physiol 7:99, 1954
10. Coonan TJ, Hope CE: Cardiorespiratory effects of changes of body position. Can Anaesth Soc J 30:424, 1983
11. West JB, Dollery CT, Naimark A: Distribution of blood flow in isolated lung: Relations to vascular and alveolar pressures. J Appl Physiol 19:713, 1964
12. Froese AB, Bryan AC: Effects of anesthesia and paralysis on diaphragmatic mechanics in man. Anesthesiology 41:242, 1974
13. Martin JT: The lawn chair (contoured supine) position. In Martin JT (ed: Positioning in Anesthesia and Surgery, p 37. Philadelphia, WB Saunders, 1987
14. Little DM: Posture and anesthesia. Can Anaesth Soc J 7:2, 1960
15. Meyer W: Ueber die Nachbehandlung des hohen Steinschnittes sowie ueber Verwendbarkeit desselben zur Operation von Blasenscheidenfisteln. Archiv Klinische Chirurgie 31:494, 1885
16. Cole F: Head lowering in the treatment of hypotension. JAMA 150:273, 1952
17. Weil MH: Current concepts in the management of shock. Circulation 16:1097, 1957
18. Guntheroth WG, Abel FL, Mullins GL: The effect of Trendelenburg's position on blood pressure and carotid flow. Surg Gynecol Obstet 119:354, 1964
19. Taylor J, Weil MH: Failure of the Trendelenburg position to improve circulation during clinical shock. Surg Gynecol Obstet 124:1004, 1976
20. Hewer CL: Latest pattern of non-slip mattress. Anaesthesia 8:198, 1953
21. Collins VJ: Principles of Anesthesiology, p 163. Philadelphia, Lea and Febinger, 1976
22. Abel RR, Lewis GM: Postoperative alopecia. Arch Dermatol 81:72, 1960
23. Gormley T. Sokoll MD: Permanent alopecia from pressure of a headstrap. JAMA 199:157, 1967

24. Lawson NW, Mills NL, Ochsner JL: Occipital alopecia following cardiopulmonary bypass. J Thorac Cardiovasc Surg 71:342, 1976
25. Gregg JR, Labosky D, Harty M et al: Serratus anterior paralysis in the young athlete. J Bone Joint Surg (Am) 61A:825, 1979
26. Johnson JTH, Kendall HO: Isolated paralysis of the serratus anterior muscle. J Bone Joint Surg 37A:567, 1955
27. Foo CL, Swann M: Isolated paralysis of the serratus anterior. J Bone Joint Surg 65B:552, 1983
28. Chusid JG: Correlative Neuroanatomy and Functional Neurology, p 145. Los Altos, Lange Medical Publications, 1985
29. McAlpine FS, Seckel BR: Peripheral nervous system complications. In Martin JT (ed): Positioning in Anesthesia and Surgery, p 303. Philadelphia, WB Saunders, 1987
30. Britt BA, Gordon RA: Peripheral nerve injuries associated with anesthesia. Can Anaesth Soc J 11:514, 1964
31. Chusid JG: Correlative Neuroanatomy and Functional Neurology, p 149. Los Altos, Lange Medical Publications, 1985
32. Hofmann A, Jones RE, Schoenvogel R: Pudendal nerve neuropraxia as a result of traction on the fracture table. J Bone Joint Surg 64A:136, 1982
33. Lindenbaum SD, Fleming LL, Smith DW: Pudendal nerve palsies associated with closed intramedullary femoral fixation. J Bone Joint Surg 64A:934, 1982
34. Matsen FA III: Compartmental syndrome. A unified concept. Clin Orthop 113:8, 1975
35. Courington FW, Little DM Jr: The role of posture in anesthesia. Clin Anesth 3:24, 1968
36. Welborn SG: The lithotomy position: Anesthesiologic considerations. In Martin JT (ed): Positioning in Anesthesia and Surgery, p 57. Philadelphia, WB Saunders, 1987
37. Kaneko K, Milic-Emily J, Dolovich MB et al: Regional distribution of ventilation and perfusion as a function of body position. J Appl Physiol 21:767, 1966
38. Lawson NW: The lateral decubitus position: Anesthesiologic considerations. In Martin JT (ed): Positioning in Anesthesia and Surgery, p 156. Philadelphia, WB Saunders, 1987
39. Lee C, Blarneys A, Nagel EL: Neuroleptanalgesia for awake pronation of surgical patients. Anesth Analg 56:276, 1977
40. Chusid JG: Correlative Neuroanatomy and Functional Neurology, p 157. Los Altos, Lange Medical Publications, 1985
41. Smith RH: The prone position. In Martin JT (ed): Positioning in Anesthesia and Surgery, p 79. Philadelphia, WB Saunders, 1978
42. Singh I: The prone position: Surgical aspects. In Martin JT (ed): Positioning in Anesthesia and Surgery, p 181. Philadelphia, WB Saunders, 1987
43. Martin JT: The prone position: Anesthesiologic considerations. In Martin JT (ed): Positioning in Anesthesia and Surgery, P 191. Philadelphia, WB Saunders, 1987
44. Backofen JE, Schauble JF: Hemodynamic changes with prone position during general anesthesia. Anesth Analg 64:194, 1985
45. Douglas WW, Rehder K, Beynen FM et al: Improved oxygenation in patients with acute respiratory failure: The prone position. Am Rev Resp Disp 115:559, 1977
46. Rehder K, Knopp TJ, Sessler AD: Regional intrapulmonary gas distribution in awake and anesthetized-paralysed prone man. J Appl Physiol 45:528, 1978
47. Gravenstein N, Grundy BL, Reid SA: Complications of positioning: The central nervous system. In Martin JT (ed): Positioning in Anesthesia and Surgery, p 291. Philadelphia, WB Saunders, 1987
48. Sherman DD, Hart RG, Easton JD: Abrupt change in head position and cerebral infarction. Stroke 12:2, 1981
49. Toole JF: Effects of change of head, limb and body position on cephalic circulation. N Engl J Med 297:307, 1968
50. Weinlander CM, Coombs DW, Plume SK: Myocardial ischemia due to obstruction of an aortocoronary bypass graft by intraoperative positioning. Anesth Analg 64:933, 1985
51. Coonan TJ, Hope CE: Cardio-respiratory effects of change of body position. Can Anaesth Soc J 30:424, 1983
52. Sonkodi S, Agabiti-Rosei E, Fraser R et al: Response of the renin–angiotensin–aldosterone system to upright tilting and to intravenous furosemide: Effect of prior metoprolol and propranolol. Br J Clin Pharmacol 13:341, 1982
53. Williams GH, Cain JP, Dluly RG et al: Studies on the control of plasma aldosterone concentration in normal man. I. Response to posture, acute and chronic volume depletion and sodium loading. J Clin Invest 51:1731, 1972
54. Fournier P, Mensch-Dechene J, Ranson-Bitker B et al: Effect of sitting up on pulmonary blood pressure, flow and volume in man. J Appl Physiol 46:36, 1979
55. Gauer OH, Thron HL: Postural changes in the circulation. In Hamilton WF, Dow P (eds): Handbook of Physiology, vol 3, p 2409. Washington DC, American Physiological Society, 1965
56. Ward RJ, Danziger F, Bonica JJ et al: Cardiovascular effects of change of posture. Aerospace Med 37:257, 1966
57. Bevegard S, Holmgren A, Jonsson B: The effect of body position on the circulation at rest and during exercise, with special reference to the influence on the stroke volume. Acta Physiol Scand 49:279, 1960
58. Rhodes JM, Graham-Brown RAC, Sarkany I: Reversible renal failure in an obese patient: Hazard of sitting with feet continuously elevated. Lancet 2:96, 1979
59. Albin MS, Janetta PJ, Maroon JC et al: Anaesthesia in the sitting position. In Recent Progress in Anesthesiology and Resuscitation. Amsterdam, Excerpta Medica International Congress Series No. 347, 1974
60. Albin MS, Babinski M, Wolf S: Cardiovascular response to the sitting position. Br J Anaesth 52:961, 1980
61. Dalrymple DG: Cardiorespiratory effects of the sitting position in neurosurgery. Br J Anaesth 51:1079, 1979
62. Shenkin HA, Scheuerman EB, Spitz EB et al: Effect of change of posture upon cerebral circulation of man. J Appl Physiol 2:317, 1949
63. Don HF: The measurement of trapped gas in the lungs at functional residual capacity and the effects of posture. Anesthesiology 35:582, 1971
64. Gurtner GH: Interrelationships of factors affecting pulmonary diffusing capacity. J Appl Physiol 30:619, 1979
65. Slutsky AS, Goldstein RG, Rebuck AS: The effect of posture on ventilatory response to hypoxia. Can Anaesth Soc J 27:445, 1980
66. Vidabek F. Posture with elevated and extended thorax. Acta Anaesthiol Scand 24:458, 1980
67. Day LJ: Unusual positions: Orthopedics: Surgical aspects. In Martin JT (ed): Positioning in Anesthesia and Surgery, p 223. Philadelphia, WB Saunders, 1987
68. Gilbert RGB, Brindle F, Galindo A: Anesthesia for Neurosurgery. Boston, Little, Brown, 1966
69. Hagen PT, Scholz DG, Edwards WD: Incidence and size of patient foramen ovale during the first ten decades: A necropsy study of 965 normal hearts. Mayo Clinic Proc 59:17, 1984
70. Gronert GA, Messick JM, Cucchiara RF et al: Paradoxical air embolism from a patent foramen ovale. Anesthesiology 50:548, 1979
71. Perkins-Pearson NAK, Marshall WK, Bedford RF: Atrial pressures in the seated position: implications for paradoxical air embolism. Anesthesiology 57:493, 1982
72. Cucchiara RF, Seward JB, Nishimura RA et al: Identification of patent foramen ovale during sitting position craniotomy by transesophageal echocardiography with positive airway pressure. Anesthesiology 63:107, 1985
73. Kitahata LM, Katz JD: Tension pneumocephalus after posterior fossa craniotomy, a complication of the sitting position. Anesthesiology 44:448, 1976
74. Toung TKJ, McPherson RW, Ahn H: Pneumocephalus: Effects of

patient position on incidence of aerocele after posterior fossa and upper cervical cord surgery. Anesth Analg 65:65, 1986

75. Standefer M, Bay JW, Trusso R: The sitting position in neurosurgery: A retrospective analysis of 488 cases. Neurosurgery 14:649, 1984

76. Hollenhorst RW, Svein HJ, Benoit CF: Unilateral blindness occurring during anesthesia for neurosurgical operations. Arch Ophthalmol 52:819, 1954

77. McAllister RG: Macroglossia—A positional complication. Anesthesiology 40:199, 1974

78. Ellis SC, Bryan-Brown CW, Hyderally H: Massive swelling of the head and neck. Anesthesiology 42:102, 1975

79. Hitselberger WE, House WF: A warning regarding the sitting position for acoustic tumor surgery. Arch Otolaryngol 106:69, 1980

80. Wilder BL: Hypothesis: The etiology of midcervical quadriplegia after operation with the patient in the sitting position. Neurosurgery 11:530, 1982

81. McCallum JE, Bennett MH: Electrophysiologic monitoring of spinal cord function during intraspinal surgery. Surg Forum 26:469, 1975

82. McPherson RW, Szymanski J, Rogers MC: Somatosensory evoked potential changes in position-related brain stem ischemia. Anesthesiology 61:88, 1984

83. Cottrell JE, Hassan NF, Hartung J et al: Hyperflexion and quadriplegia in the seated position. Anesthesiol Rev 5:34, 1985

84. Levy WJ, York OH, McCaffrey M et al: Motor evoked potentials from transcranial stimulation of the motor cortex in humans. Neurosurgery 15:287, 1984

Chapter 25

Edwin A. Bowe
E. F. Klein, Jr.

Acid Base, Blood Gas, Electrolytes

Although ubiquitous in modern medical practice, accurate determinations of gas tensions and pH are a relatively recent development. Thirty years ago, electrodes were not available for the measurement of the partial pressures (tensions) of oxygen or carbon dioxide in blood. Measurement of pH, although possible using electrodes initially developed in 1933, were not widely available. Without the ability to measure these parameters, evaluation was based primarily on inferences drawn from history, physical examination, and other laboratory tests. The years between 1955 and 1960 saw the development of the Sanz electrode for measuring pH,[1] the Severinghaus modification[2] of the electrode initially proposed by Stowe[3] for measuring the partial pressure of carbon dioxide (P_{CO_2}), and the Clark electrode[4] for measuring the partial pressure of oxygen (P_{O_2}). It took several years following the development of the new electrodes before they became available in university hospitals and several more years before their availability extended to community settings. As a consequence of their relatively recent advent on the clinical scene, most physicians trained prior to the 1970s had little or no exposure to blood gases and acid–base physiology. In modern clinical practice, blood–gas machines are commonly available not only in the pathology laboratory or respiratory therapy department but also in the operating room, recovery room, and intensive care units.

CARBON DIOXIDE

Carbon dioxide (CO_2) is produced primarily in the mitochondria as a major end-product of metabolism.[5] It then diffuses from the mitochondria, through the cytoplasm of the cell, and into the blood where it is transported in several different forms to the lungs for elimination in the form of gaseous CO_2.[6] The partial pressure of CO_2 in arterial blood (Pa_{CO_2}) is determined by the balance between the production and elimination of CO_2.

$$Pa_{CO_2} \propto \frac{CO_2 \text{ production}}{CO_2 \text{ elimination}} \qquad (25\text{-}1)$$

Arterial P_{CO_2} is an indication of the ventilatory response to metabolism, that is, CO_2 production.[7] Since in most operating room and intensive care unit settings, CO_2 production is relatively constant, Pa_{CO_2} is most commonly used only to evaluate the ventilatory function of the lungs.[8–11] This is possible because of the absence of CO_2 from the inspired gas mixture. If inadequate fresh gas flows are administered in the absence of a functional carbon dioxide absorber or if unidirectional valves do not function properly, significant inspired CO_2 concentrations may occur. The presence of CO_2 in the inspired gas mixture substantially complicates the evaluation of pulmonary status on the basis of the Pa_{CO_2}.[5] Additionally, Pa_{CO_2} plays a vital role in the interpretation of acid–base disorders.

CARBON DIOXIDE PRODUCTION

Carbon dioxide production ($\dot{V}_{CO_2}$) is largely ignored when evaluating Pa_{CO_2}.[8, 9] Failure to recognize the role of $\dot{V}_{CO_2}$ in determining Pa_{CO_2} may lead to inaccurate diagnosis and inappropriate management in some clinical settings. Increased Pa_{CO_2} will occur if CO_2 production exceeds CO_2 elimination. Conversely, an isolated decrease in CO_2 production will produce a fall in Pa_{CO_2}. Patients suffering from thermal injuries receiving parenteral nutrition[12, 13] are classic examples of a population with massively increased $\dot{V}_{CO_2}$.

Carbon dioxide production is determined by metabolic rate and respiratory quotient (R). Metabolic rate is influenced by the following factors: physical activity, temperature, thyroid hormone, other endocrine factors, and respiratory quotient.

Physical Activity

Exercise is the factor that most commonly causes acute changes in metabolic rate.[14] While it is true that patients in the operating room or intensive care unit rarely experience the increase in $\dot{V}_{CO_2}$ associated with jogging or other forms of exercise, seizures and shivering[15] are other examples of physical activity that increase CO_2 production. Similarly, decreases in $\dot{V}_{CO_2}$ are associated with the lack of physical activity occurring during sleep or general anesthesia.

Temperature

Reductions in body temperature produce a generalized decrease in metabolic rate of approximately 7%–9% for each 1°C decrease. Both oxygen consumption and CO_2 production demonstrate similar changes.[16, 17] These changes in CO_2 production are valid only as long as there is no response in the form of shivering to the decrease in body temperature. Increases in CO_2 production, however, result from the increased muscular activity associated with attempts to restore body temperature by shivering. Decreases in body temperature may be induced intentionally (as is common during cardiopulmonary bypass) or may result from exposure to a cold environment (such as an operating room).[18, 19] Accidental hypothermia is a significant consideration for some intensive care unit and emergency room patients.[20–22]

Conversely, $\dot{V}_{CO_2}$ is increased by the rise in metabolic rate associated with increased body temperature. Perhaps the most dramatic example of this phenomenon is the increase in $\dot{V}_{CO_2}$ associated with malignant hyperthermia.[23, 24]

Thyroid Hormone

Changes in $\dot{V}_{CO_2}$ are associated with thyroxine-induced changes in almost all chemical reactions throughout the body. Although most hyperthyroid patients manifest a 40%–60% increase in metabolic rate, fulminant hyperthyroidism (such as thyroid storm) may be associated with a 100% increase in metabolic rate.[14] The complete absence of thyroid hormone secretion may be associated with a metabolic rate 40%–50% of normal.[14, 15]

Other Endocrine Factors

Sympathetic stimulation and catecholamine release, as occur with trauma or inadequate (light) anesthesia, produce a generalized increase in cellular activity and, therefore, increase $\dot{V}_{CO_2}$. Catecholamines have been implicated as the factor mediating the increased metabolic rate following burn injuries.[14, 26] Male sex hormone and growth hormone are also associated with increases in metabolic rate.[14]

Respiratory Quotient

Carbon dioxide production is also determined in part by the respiratory quotient (R)

$$R = \frac{\text{carbon dioxide production}}{\text{oxygen utilization}} \qquad (25\text{-}2)$$

In turn, the respiratory quotient is effected by the substrates being consumed, varying from 0.7 with lipid oxidation to 1.0 during carbohydrate utilization.[27, 28] Under normal circumstances, R averages approximately 0.8 (i.e., 20% less CO_2 is produced than O_2 is consumed). If carbohydrates are the predominant form of metabolic substrate being utilized, an increase in $\dot{V}_{CO_2}$ may occur as the result of an increase in R to 1.0. (i.e., the amount of CO_2 produced is the same as the amount of O_2 consumed). This situation is not uncommon in the surgical patient relying solely on intravenous (iv) glucose as a source of exogenous calories.

The nutritional state of the patient is also capable of altering R. During starvation, CO_2 production decreases as R declines to 0.7, reflecting almost complete reliance on fat for metabolic substrate.[27] Conversely, conversion of carbohydrates to fat during parenteral nutrition with high glucose loads may be associated with values for R as high as 8.0 (e.g., 8 moles of CO_2 produced for each mole of O_2 consumed).[29] The ventilatory state of the patient has also been associated with alterations in R, with values approximating 1.0 being reported if hyperventilation is present.

In the past, only gross disturbances in $\dot{V}_{CO_2}$ owing to changing values of R were detectable. With the advent of indirect calorimetry and other devices capable of accurately determining R, the significance of this factor in determining Pa_{CO_2} can be more accurately assessed.[30]

CARBON DIOXIDE IN BLOOD

Carbon dioxide is carried in blood in four different forms: 1) in physical solution, 2) hydrated to carbonic acid, 3) dissociated to bicarbonate ion, and 4) as carbamino compounds (Fig. 25-1).

Carbon Dioxide in Physical Solution

Carbon dioxide in physical solution constitutes only approximately 5%–7% of CO_2 carriage in whole blood.[31, 32] Despite its relatively insignificant contribution to total carbon dioxide content, the importance of CO_2 in physical solution is enhanced for several reasons. First, most cell membranes are freely permeable to this form of CO_2. Although most membranes (especially those of the central nervous system) are relatively impermeable to HCO_3^- and H^+, molecular CO_2 easily penetrates these barriers and may thereby alter intracellular pH.[5, 32] Second, it is in this form that most CO_2 enters and leaves the blood. Rapid hydration to carbonic acid with subsequent dissociation to bicarbonate requires the presence of carbonic anhydrase, which is present in the red blood cell. Similarly, bicarbonate and carbamino-CO_2 must be converted back to CO_2 in physical solution before pulmonary elimination is possible.[33] Third, this is the only form that is routinely and directly measured without interference from other forms of CO_2.[34] Being a gas, dissolved CO_2, like dissolved O_2, is measured in terms of its partial pressure.

PARTIAL PRESSURE. Earth's atmosphere consists of a layer of gas that exerts a pressure that can be quantitated either in terms of weight (millimeters of mercury, mm Hg; pounds per square inch, psi) or pure pressure (torr; kiloPascal, kPa). In blood, the partial pressure of a gas is determined by the number of molecules in solution. In any gas mixture, each gas exerts its own pressure (partial pressure) independently of all other gases. Additionally, the total gas pressure is the simple sum of partial pressures of all gases present.

A TOTAL CO₂ CONTENT

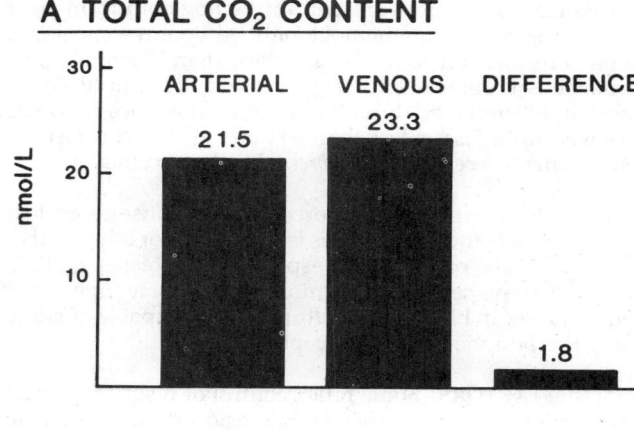

B PERCENT CO₂

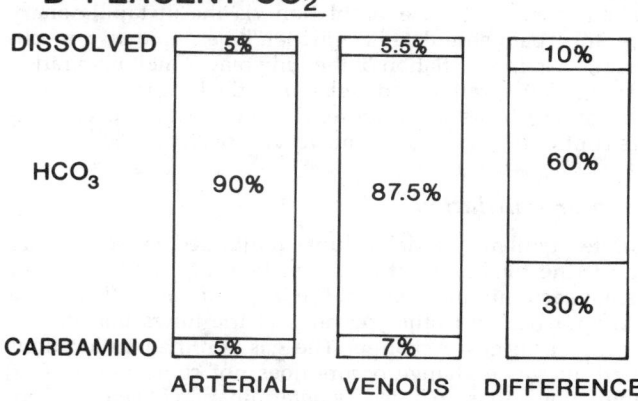

FIG. 25-1. Carbon dioxide (CO₂) content of blood. (*A*) Quantity of CO₂ in arterial blood, venous blood, and the difference between the two. (Modified from West JB: Respiratory Physiology—The Essentials, 3rd ed, p 74. Baltimore, Williams & Wilkins, 1985. (*B*) Forms of CO₂ in arterial and venous blood. Composition of the venous-arterial CO₂ difference is also presented. See text for description of forms and their significance.

Carbonic Acid

Hydration of CO₂ produces carbonic acid by Equation 25-3.

$$CO_2 + H_2O \rightleftharpoons H_2CO_3 \qquad (25\text{-}3)$$

This reaction is very slow, requiring minutes to achieve equilibrium.[1] The presence of a catalytic enzyme, carbonic anhydrase, in erythrocytes and renal tubular cells substantially accelerates this reaction. The presence of carbonic anhydrase not withstanding, less than 1% of total CO₂ content of blood is in the form of carbonic acid.[5] Both CO₂ in physical solution and carbonic acid are sometimes referred to as H_2CO_3. More correctly, H_2CO_3 refers only to carbonic acid.

Bicarbonate Ion

The majority of CO₂ in blood is carried in plasma as bicarbonate ion (HCO_3^-). Bicarbonate is formed as the result of dissociation of carbonic acid, as shown in Equation 25-4.

$$H_2CO_3 \rightleftharpoons H^+ + HCO_3^- \qquad (25\text{-}4)$$

Under physiologic conditions, approximately 96% of H_2CO_3 is dissociated to H^+ and HCO_3^-. This occurs as a result of diffusion, hydration, and dissociation as illustrated in Figure 25-2. Although classic teaching is that all HCO_3^- exists in its dissociated state, more recent work has documented the presence of sodium and potassium bicarbonate ($NaHCO_3$ and $KHCO_3$, respectively) under physiologic conditions.[35]

Carbamino Compounds

Carbon dioxide may combine with terminal amino groups of each protein and with side-chain amino groups of arginine and lysine.[5]

$$R\text{-}NH_2 + CO_2 \rightleftharpoons R\text{-}NH\text{-}COOH \qquad (25\text{-}5)$$

Hydration of CO₂ is not necessary for this reaction to occur. Although plasma proteins provide little carbamino carriage, hemoglobin may carry a significant amount of CO₂. Reduced hemoglobin carries approximately 3.5 times as much CO₂ as does oxyhemoglobin. This increased capacity of reduced hemoglobin to carry CO₂ in the form of carbamino compounds produces, at the same P_{CO_2}, a higher total CO₂ content in the presence of reduced hemoglobin. This phenomenon, termed the Haldane effect, is responsible for the fact that 30% of the CO₂ diffusing from the cell into the blood is carried in the form of carbamino compounds, whereas only 5% of total arterial CO₂ content is present in this form (Fig. 25-1).[5, 31]

CARBON DIOXIDE ELIMINATION

Once CO₂ is transported to the lungs, it must gain entrance to functional lung units in order to be eliminated by ventilation. All CO₂ must be converted to its gaseous form for ventilatory elimination to occur.[36] This requirement necessi-

FIG. 25-2. Transport of CO₂ in blood. Following diffusion from cells into the blood, the majority of CO₂ diffuses into the red blood cell (RBC) where it is either bound to hemoglobin and carried as carbaminohemoglobin or hydrated to H_2CO_3 by carbonic anhydrase. Most H_2CO_3 dissociates to produce HCO_3^-, which diffuses down a concentration gradient from the RBC into the plasma. (Modified from Nunn JF: Applied Respiratory Physiology, 3rd ed, p 215. London, Butterworths, 1987.)

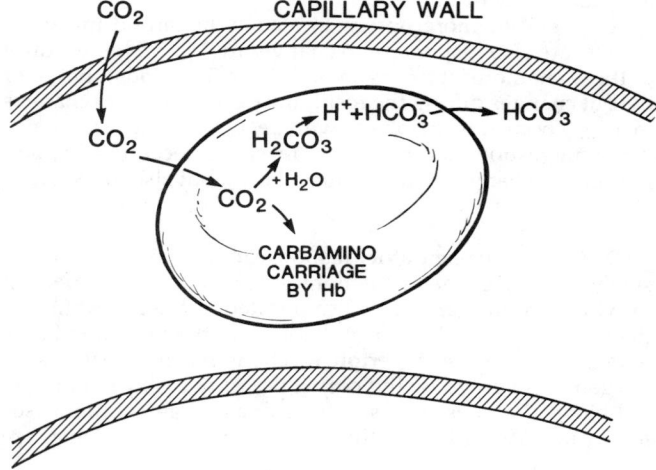

tates the diffusion of HCO_3^- back into the red blood cell where it combines with H^+ to form H_2CO_3. The action of carbonic anhydrase on carbonic acid produces CO_2. Likewise, CO_2 carried as carbamino-hemoglobin must be released, a process facilitated by the oxygenation of hemoglobin.[36] Carbon dioxide in the red blood cell (i.e., that carried either as HCO_3^- or carbamino hemoglobin) must then diffuse across the red blood cell membrane, through the plasma, and across the capillary endothelium, interstitial space, and alveolar epithelium before entering the alveolus.[37] The high solubility of CO_2 ensures that, under normal circumstances, there is no limitation to diffusion and that the partial pressures of CO_2 in alveolar gas and end-capillary blood are identical.[38]

Carbon dioxide elimination is determined by the interactions of tidal volume (V_T), respiratory rate, and dead space (V_d), which determine alveolar ventilation (V_A). Tidal volume and respiratory rate are regulated by neural mechanisms that control respiration. The normal value for the partial pressure of CO_2 in arterial blood is 40 mm Hg. Long-standing chronic obstructive pulmonary disease (COPD) may produce a resetting of ventilatory drive based on a chronically elevated Pa_{CO_2}.[39] Although 40 mm Hg may no longer be a "normal" value for these patients, the presence of an increased Pa_{CO_2} still indicates pulmonary pathology.

Control of Ventilation

CHEMICAL CONTROL. Although arterial hypoxemia and acidosis can stimulate ventilation, the single most important regulator of ventilation under normal circumstances is the Pa_{CO_2}. The control mechanism is sensitive enough that under normal circumstances, Pa_{CO_2} is held almost completely constant, varying by as little as 3 mm Hg even during exercise.[40] Increases in CO_2 production should increase alveolar ventilation to maintain a constant Pa_{CO_2}. Similarly, decreases in CO_2 production should stimulate a decrease in alveolar ventilation.

CARBON DIOXIDE. Central chemoreceptors located on the surface of the medulla provide approximately 80% of the respiratory response to CO_2.[41] Cerebrospinal fluid (CSF) pH is the most important factor stimulating the central chemoreceptors. Acutely, Pa_{CO_2} is the single most significant determinant of CSF pH. This occurs because the vascular membrane, which is freely permeable to molecular CO_2, is relatively impermeable to HCO_3^-. Changes in Pa_{CO_2} rapidly alter CSF pH, whereas changes in blood HCO_3^- concentrations are only gradually evident in the CSF.[32]

Peripheral chemoreceptors, located in the carotid and aortic bodies, are also responsive to changes in Pa_{CO_2}. The response of these chemoreceptors is so rapid (1 to 3 seconds) that their output changes during the respiratory cycle owing to changes in Pa_{CO_2} occurring in phase with respiration. There is also some suggestion that the peripheral chemoreceptors respond not only to changes in the value of Pa_{CO_2}, but also to its rate of rise.[41]

OXYGEN. The respiratory response to hypoxemia is located solely in the peripheral chemoreceptors, the most important of which are the carotid bodies (located at the bifurcation of the common carotid arteries). Because of the high blood flow in relation to their size, peripheral chemoreceptor response to oxygen is governed by the partial pressure of oxygen in arterial blood (Pa_{O_2}) as opposed to arterial oxygen content (see following). Accordingly, the peripheral chemoreceptors are

not affected by anemia or aberrant hemoglobin forms (carboxyhemoglobin or methemoglobin). Although some stimulation of respiration occurs if Pa_{O_2} is less than 500 mm Hg, the response is nonlinear and largely insignificant until Pa_{O_2} is less than 100 mm Hg.[41] Prominent stimulation does not occur, however, until Pa_{O_2} is less than 60 mm Hg.[42] In contrast, the central chemoreceptors are depressed by hypoxemia.

ACIDOSIS. Peripheral chemoreceptor response to acidosis is the same whether the acidosis is due to CO_2 or other acids.[43] Only 15%–20% of the total response to increases in Pa_{CO_2} is located in the peripheral chemoreceptors.[41] Hypoperfusion and increases in blood temperature are also capable of stimulating the peripheral chemoreceptors.[41]

OTHER FACTORS. Some reflex control of respiration exists under certain circumstances: Hypotension stimulates a baroreceptor-induced increase in ventilation, pulmonary capillary distention may increase ventilation via the juxtapulmonary receptors, pain stimulates ventilation by an unknown mechanism, sustained inflation of the lung may inhibit inspiration via the inflation reflex, and deflation of the lung may augment inspiration via the deflation reflex. The most important factors controlling respiration, however, are chemical.[40]

Alveolar Ventilation

Minute ventilation (tidal volume multiplied by respiratory rate) is the total amount of gas moved into the respiratory system each minute. Some of the inspired gas is distributed to the trachea and other portions of the lungs that do not participate in gas exchange. The gas confined to locations where no gas exchange occurs does not contribute to CO_2 elimination and is excluded by determination of alveolar ventilation (Eqn. 25-6).

$$V_A = \text{Respiratory rate} \times (V_T - V_D) \qquad (25\text{-}6)$$

DEAD SPACE. Dead space (V_d) is that portion of the minute ventilation (V) or tidal volume (V_T) that does not participate in gas exchange. Dead space may be categorized as anatomic, alveolar, physiologic, or apparatus.

Anatomic dead space (Fig. 25-3) is the volume of air in the conducting airways (e.g., trachea, bronchi). Patient size is the single most important determinant of anatomic dead space,[44] which is reasonably approximated as $0.5 \text{ ml} \cdot \text{kg}^{-1}$.[45] In addition to body size, anatomic dead space during normal spontaneous ventilation is determined by posture (decreased in the supine position),[46] age (increased with increasing age),[47] and head position (increased with neck extension and forward thrust of mandible, decreased by neck flexion).[48] Other factors that increase anatomic dead space include positive pressure ventilation, bronchodilators (including atropine),[49] ganglionic blocking drugs,[50] and general anesthesia.[51] Conversely, reductions in anatomic dead space occur during spontaneous ventilation with small tidal volumes.[52]

Alveolar dead space (Fig. 25-4) is that volume of gas that enters nonperfused lung units, thereby failing to participate in gas exchange.[53] Alveolar dead space occurs because of the absence of blood flow (perfusion) to the affected lung unit (ventilation present, perfusion = 0, V/Q = ∞).[54] In the upright position, alveolar dead space occurs as a normal phenomenon because pulmonary artery pressure is inadequate to perfuse the most superior lung units.[55] West's zone I of the lung, where alveolar pressure (P_A) exceeds pulmonary artery pres-

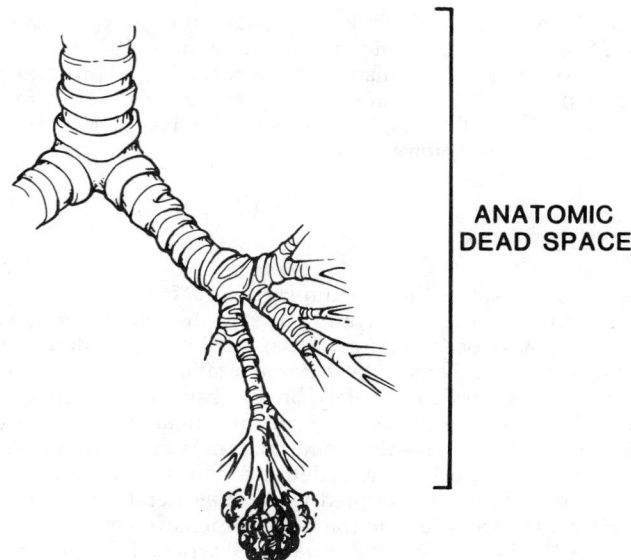

ANATOMIC
DEAD SPACE

FIG. 25-3. Subglottic conducting airways. A portion of each inspiratory volume comes to rest in the conducting passages of the respiratory system. Because no gas exchange occurs in these locations, the volume constitutes anatomic dead space. Not shown, but also contributing to the volume of anatomic dead space, are the nasopharynx and oropharynx.

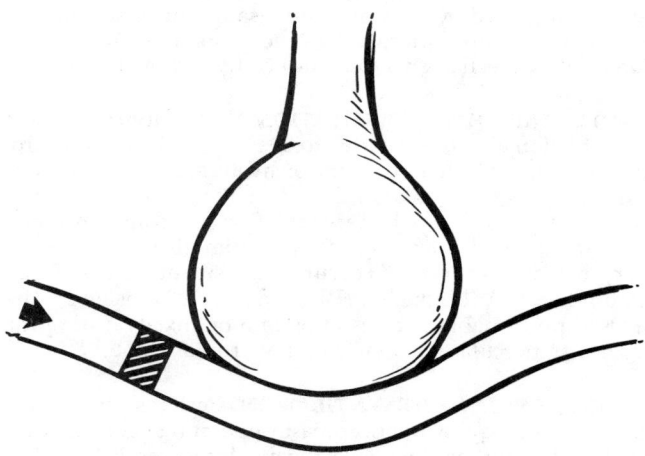

FIG. 25-4. Alveolar dead space. Obstruction to blood flow in the pulmonary vascular bed produces dead space when ventilation, V, continues despite the absence of perfusion, Q, (V/Q = ∞).

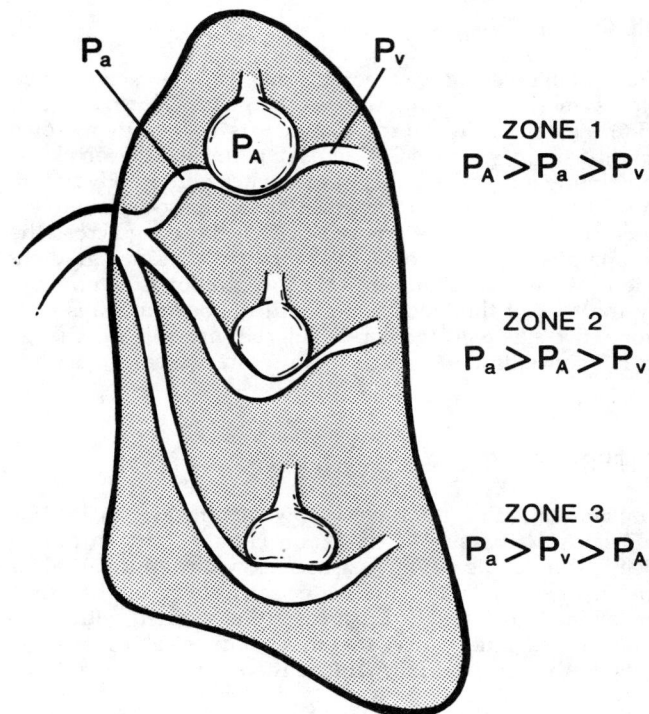

P_a P_v

P_A

ZONE 1
$P_A > P_a > P_v$

ZONE 2
$P_a > P_A > P_v$

ZONE 3
$P_a > P_v > P_A$

FIG. 25-5. West's zones of the lung. (Zone 1) Alveolar pressure (P_A) in excess of pulmonary artery pressure (P_a) compresses the vasculature and prevents perfusion, thereby creating dead space. (Zone 2) Perfusion is determined by the difference between P_a and P_A. Increases in alveolar pressure (as may occur with mechanical ventilation or application of expiratory distending pressure) or decreases in pulmonary artery pressure (as may occur with hypovolemia or vasodilator infusion) may convert lung units in Zone 2 to a Zone 1 relationship. (Zone 3) Perfusion is determined by the difference between pulmonary artery and pulmonary venous pressures.

sure (P_a), describes the conditions present in alveolar dead space (Fig. 25-5).[56] From this relationship, it is evident that alveolar dead space will be increased by factors that decrease P_a (vasodilator-induced deliberate hypotension, severe hypovolemia). Additionally, increases in P_A (most notably mechanical ventilation and/or expiratory distending pressure, i.e., positive end-expiratory pressure [PEEP], or continuous positive airway pressure [CPAP]) increase alveolar dead space. Other factors increasing alveolar dead space include upright posture,[53] pulmonary emboli (occlusion of pulmonary capillaries by thrombi,[57] air,[58] or fat[59]), general anesthesia,[53, 58] and ventilation of nonvascular air spaces (destruction of alveolar septa and pulmonary capillaries produced by chronic lung disease).[53, 60]

Physiologic dead space is the sum of anatomic and alveolar dead space. Dead space to tidal volume ratio (V_D/V_T) is the most commonly used method for quantitating physiologic dead space.[61] Normal values for V_D/V_T range from 0.2 to 0.4 during spontaneous ventilation. During conventional mechanical ventilation, V_D/V_T is routinely increased to 0.4 to 0.6.[61] This occurs ultimately because during mechanical ventilation, blood flow is distributed preferentially to dependent lung units,[62] while ventilation is preferentially distributed to nondependent lung units.[63]

Apparatus dead space is another type of dead space that becomes a consideration with the addition of an anesthestic circuit or a mechanical ventilator. In addition to that generated by anesthesia masks, anesthetic circuits provide a variable amount of apparatus dead space.[5] With most currently available anesthesia and ventilator circuits, apparatus dead space is not a significant consideration, provided that the circuits are correctly configured and fresh gas flow rates are adequate (see Chapter 19).

MEASUREMENT

The partial pressure of carbon dioxide (P_{CO_2}) in a blood sample is measured using the Severinghaus electrode (Fig. 25-6).[5,7,9,11] The P_{CO_2} in the sample acts as the driving force for diffusion of gaseous CO_2 across a permeable silicon elastic membrane into an aqueous bicarbonate solution. Hydration of the CO_2 produces carbonic acid, which dissociates into H^+ and HCO_3^-. Since the amount of CO_2 diffusing across the membrane is proportional to the partial pressure gradient (Henry's law), the change in H^+ concentration is determined by the P_{CO_2} of the blood sample. In the Severinghaus electrode, two silver-silver chloride half cells measure the change in H^+ concentration, which is an indirect measurement of P_{CO_2}.[5,7,9,11]

INTERPRETATION

The normal value for the Pa_{CO_2} is 40 mm Hg. In healthy subjects, increases of 45 to 47 mm Hg are common during sleep.[5] Certain disorders are associated with abnormal values for Pa_{CO_2} as a result of normal compensatory mechanisms. Metabolic acid–base disturbances are associated with alterations in respiratory drive that may produce values for Pa_{CO_2} outside the range of normal (see the section entitled Acid–

FIG. 25-6. Carbon dioxide electrode. CO_2 diffuses across the gas-permeable silicon membrane into a thin layer of electrolyte solution containing HCO_3^-. A nylon spacer separates the electrolyte solution from a pH electrode. Diffusion of CO_2 into the $NaHCO_3$ produces a change in pH proportional to the difference in CO_2 concentrations between the sample and the electrolyte solution. The voltage produced by the change in H^+ concentration is electronically transformed to report PCO_2. (Modified from Shapiro BA, Harrison RA, Walton JR: Clinical Application of Blood Gases, 3rd ed, p 33. Chicago, Year Book Medical Publishers, 1982.)

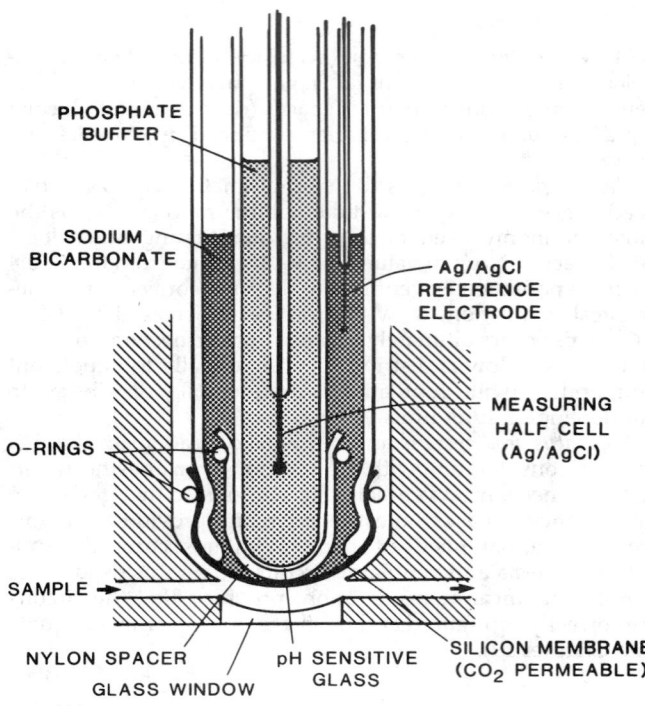

PHOSPHATE BUFFER

SODIUM BICARBONATE

Ag/AgCl REFERENCE ELECTRODE

O-RINGS

MEASURING HALF CELL (Ag/AgCl)

SAMPLE

NYLON SPACER

GLASS WINDOW

pH SENSITIVE GLASS

SILICON MEMBRANE (CO_2 PERMEABLE)

Base Physiology). Similarly, patients with long-standing COPD may routinely maintain $Pa_{CO_2} > 40$ mm Hg as a result of a "resetting" of ventilatory drive based on a chronically elevated Pa_{CO_2}.[64] In either of these circumstances, the presence of a "normal" Pa_{CO_2} (i.e., 40 mm Hg) may be indicative of additional pathology.

HYPOCAPNIA

Values of Pa_{CO_2} less than 35 mm Hg are generally considered to constitute hypocapnia and, in the absence of primary metabolic acid–base derangements, would be considered by most authors to constitute hyperventilation. Some authors define hyperventilation solely on the basis of a decreased Pa_{CO_2}.[13,67,68] In the presence of primary metabolic acid–base disorders, others consider the normal respiratory compensation that should occur and redefine a "normal" Pa_{CO_2}.[65]

This disagreement, coupled with other literature defining hyperventilation solely on the basis of increased minute ventilation,[66,67] has produced a situation in which the same term may have three different interpretations. For the purposes of clarity, it is probably best to describe hyperventilation as being associated with $Pa_{CO_2} < 40$ mm Hg, an elevated arterial pH, or a high minute ventilation.

Etiology

Hypocapnia occurs when alveolar ventilation is excessive compared with CO_2 production.[5] It may be voluntary, iatrogenic, or induced by normal compensatory mechanisms mediated by chemoreceptors or baroreceptors. In certain conditions, reflex mechanisms may induce hypocapnia.

VOLUNTARY HYPERVENTILATION. The voluntary aspect of ventilation allows the cortex to override brain stem control to some degree. Anxiety, pain, or hysteria may also induce "voluntary hyperventilation."[5,68] In either of these circumstances, all criteria for hyperventilation are commonly met (minute volume is increased, Pa_{CO_2} is diminished, and a primary increase in arterial pH occurs as a result of increased CO_2 elimination.) Additionally, Pa_{CO_2} may be transiently depressed presumably as a result of pain or anxiety during the process of percutaneous sampling of arterial blood.[5,69]

IATROGENIC HYPERVENTILATION. Perhaps the most common etiology of hypocapnia in operating room and intensive care unit settings is iatrogenic hyperventilation. Despite the fact that it is not benign, intentional hyperventilation has long been advocated as a means of suppressing spontaneous inspiratory efforts during controlled mechanical ventilation.[70,71] Additionally, hypocapnia is commonly associated with assist mode mechanical ventilation.[72]

There are at least two additional potential etiologies of iatrogenic hyperventilation. Some **pharmacologic agents** (nicotine, doxapram, acetylcholine) stimulate ventilation by means of peripheral chemoreceptors.[41] Other agents such as salicylates, xanthines (aminophylline), and progesterone appear to act centrally.[73]

Under conditions of fixed ventilation (i.e., during mechanical ventilation), **decreases in CO_2 production** may be associated with hypocapnia. Ventilator settings that produced a normal Pa_{CO_2} at the beginning of an anesthetic may produce hypocapnia as VCO_2 decreases owing to a lower metabolic rate and a fall in temperature.

HYPOXEMIA. A low Pa_{O_2}, especially below 60 mm Hg, stimulates respiration via the carotid bodies.[41] Any etiology of low Pa_{O_2} (e.g., cyanotic congenital heart disease, high altitude) may be the stimulus for this response. Hypocapnia occurring as a result of this hypoxemia-induced peripheral chemoreceptor stimulation will tend to diminish respiratory drive via CSF alkalosis (the so-called braking effect). Over a period of 48 to 72 hours, pH of the CSF and blood will be adjusted toward normal (the former by the egress of HCO_3^- from the CSF, the latter by renal excretion of HCO_3^-). With restoration of pH, hypoxemia once again becomes effective in increasing ventilation. Ultimately, a balance will occur between the hypoxia-induced peripheral stimulation and the hypocapnia-induced respiratory depression.[74]

HYPOTENSION. Decreased blood pressure may induce a baroreceptor-stimulated increase in ventilation.[41] Ventilation may also be stimulated by a decreased rate of perfusion of peripheral chemoreceptors.[41, 45]

ACIDOSIS. Both central and peripheral chemoreceptors respond to acidosis by stimulating ventilation.[41] Hypocapnia may be induced by an increase in H^+ concentration of arterial blood, which acutely stimulates respiration, primarily by the peripheral chemoreceptors.

Central chemoreceptors are responsive to changes in pH of the brain extracellular fluid, which may be induced by alterations in local blood flow or metabolism and by changes in CSF composition. Local factors that produce an acidosis of the CSF or decrease cerebral blood flow are believed to be responsible for the hypocapnia that commonly accompanies central nervous system (CNS) lesions.[41, 75, 76]

DISTORTED PULMONARY ARCHITECTURE. Certain pulmonary anatomic abnormalities have been documented to stimulate respiration. Vagal afferents are commonly involved in the increased ventilation associated with abnormal architecture of the lung.[5, 41] Most lesions that induce mechanical abnormalities (pneumonia, adult respiratory distress syndrome [ARDS], pulmonary edema) also produce hypoxemia and may induce hypocapnia by this mechanism as well. However, in some conditions (e.g., asthma, pulmonary fibrosis), anatomic abnormalities are believed to play a significant role in the production of hypocapnia.[5, 41]

MISCELLANEOUS. During exercise, ventilation is increased with the initiation of physical activity. It is believed that the motor cortex, in addition to producing skeletal muscle contraction, stimulates the respiratory center by collateral impulses. Additionally, proprioceptors at the joints are also capable of stimulating the respiratory center. Although increases in ventilation proportionate to increases in CO_2 production normally maintain a constant Pa_{CO_2}, hypocapnia may result from excessive respiratory stimulation during exercise.[77]

Similarly, increased body temperature stimulates respiration not only as a result of increases in metabolic rate and CO_2 production but also as a direct effect on the respiratory center. Under these conditions, disproportionate increases in ventilation may produce hypocapnia despite increased CO_2 production.[77]

Effects

The method of hyperventilation (spontaneous vs mechanical) used to induce hypocapnia may play a role in determining the ultimate physiologic response. For example, mechanical ventilation is associated with increased intrathoracic pressure, which decreases venous return, whereas the negative intrathoracic pressure generated by spontaneous ventilation is associated with an augmentation of venous return. Accordingly, the method used to generate hypocapnia must be ascertained before the results and their implications can be fully and accurately interpreted.

CARDIOVASCULAR. Heart rate, cardiac rhythm,[78] and myocardial contractility[79, 80] are basically unaffected by decreases in Pa_{CO_2}. Peripheral blood vessels tend to vasoconstrict as a result of the direct effect of hypocapnia. This is at least partially offset by decreased sympathetic activity (and therefore vasodilatation) occurring as a result of the central effects of hypocapnia.[78] Although cardiac output may be increased when hypocapnia is due to spontaneous ventilation,[81] mechanical hyperventilation produces a reduction in cardiac output.[82] This decrease, combined with an increase in O_2 consumption,[83] produces reductions in mixed venous P_{O_2}. Postulated mechanisms for the reduction in cardiac output include decreased preload (owing to increased intrathoracic pressure)[82] and increased afterload (owing to systemic vasoconstriction).[78]

Decreased myocardial blood flow[84] resulting from hyperventilation-induced increases in coronary vascular resistance has been documented in dogs.[85] Hypocapnia has been demonstrated to provoke coronary artery spasm in some patients with Prinzmetal's variant angina[86, 87] or coronary artery disease with typical angina.[88]

PULMONARY. Pulmonary vasodilation occurs as a consequence of decreases in Pa_{CO_2}. Dilatation of pulmonary vasculature is commonly accompanied by increased intrapulmonary shunting.[89, 90] In addition, decreased cardiac output and increased oxygen consumption combine to produce a decrease in Pa_{O_2}.[78, 89]

Increased airway resistance[90] (bronchoconstriction) commonly accompanies hypocapnia. Functional residual capacity[91] and lung compliance[90] are also decreased.

CENTRAL NERVOUS SYSTEM. Decreases in Pa_{CO_2} produce vasoconstriction of cerebral blood vessels.[92, 93] Cerebral blood flow and cerebral blood volume are reduced as a consequence of the vasoconstriction.[92, 93] Although efficacious in lowering intracranial pressure,[94, 95] excessive hyperventilation may produce decreases in cerebral oxygen tension[92, 93] and alterations in brain metabolism.[92, 96, 97] Electroencephalographic (EEG) changes similar to those seen with cerebral hypoxia may be demonstrated during these episodes.[98, 99]

Central nervous system manifestations of hypocapnia include generalized depression, confusion, and euphoria.[100, 101] Loss of consciousness may occasionally occur.

MISCELLANEOUS. Decreases in Pa_{CO_2} produce increases in pH, which ultimately decrease serum ionized calcium concentrations.[102, 103] Although clinical manifestations of decreases in ionized calcium are rare in mechanically hyperventilated patients, spontaneous hyperventilation is commonly accompanied by some manifestations resembling classic hypocalcemic tetany. The most frequently occurring presentation is carpal spasm. Chvostek's and Trousseau's signs rarely accompany hyperventilation, even when carpal spasm is present.[78]

Serum potassium concentrations decrease an average of 0.5 $mEq \cdot l^{-1}$ for each 10 mm Hg decrease in Pa_{CO_2}.[78] Decreases in serum sodium[78] and phosphorous[102, 103] concentrations also occur.

Hemoglobin and hematocrit as well as erythrocyte, platelet, and leukocyte counts have been reported to increase during spontaneous hyperventilation.[104]

HYPERCAPNIA

Values of Pa_{CO_2} in excess of 45 mm Hg are considered pathologic in most circumstances. As described for hyperventilation, however, some paradoxes occur if Pa_{CO_2} is the sole criterion used to define hypoventilation. (Increased Pa_{CO_2} may exist in the presence of increased, decreased, or normal minute ventilation, for example.) Failure to consider pH of arterial blood (and/or CSF), alveolar ventilation, and CO_2 production as well as Pa_{CO_2} when defining hypoventilation is likely to produce confusion in some circumstances.

Etiology

Hypercapnia occurs when alveolar ventilation is inadequate compared with CO_2 production. Diminished respiratory drive, pulmonary pathology, musculoskeletal or neuromuscular disease, or metabolic disturbances may all produce hypercapnia.

RESPIRATORY DEPRESSION. Opioids and general anesthetics are obvious examples of pharmacologic agents that depress the respiratory center response to CO_2. Numerous other drugs, including barbiturates, benzodiazepines,[105] ethyl alcohol,[106] and local anesthetics,[107] are less obvious respiratory depressants. Some drugs (e.g., monoamine oxidase inhibitors,[108] chlorpromazine[109]) that have little or no intrinsic respiratory depressant effects themselves are capable of interacting with other drugs to produce significant respiratory depression.

Respiratory drive may also be altered by any of the factors regulating respiration. It should be noted, however, that although mild hypoxemia stimulates respiration, hypoxia has a direct depressant effect on CNS neurons[110] and may actually result in respiratory depression.[111] Similarly, extreme hypercapnia can depress ventilation[41] by decreasing respiratory neuron excitability owing to hyperpolarization.[112]

Cerebrospinal fluid alkalosis deserves special mention in this context. For example, the relative impermeability of the blood–brain barrier to HCO_3^- initially blunts the respiratory response to increases in arterial pH. Eventually, however, CSF pH will be influenced by arterial pH, and alkalosis of the CSF may diminish respiratory drive.[113] Decreased alveolar ventilation produces an increase in alveolar P_{CO_2} and a reciprocal decrease in alveolar P_{O_2}. In patients breathing room air, the resultant decrease in Pa_{O_2} may stimulate respiration and limit the increase in Pa_{CO_2}. This phenomenon may account for the relatively infrequent reports of hypercapnia accompanying metabolic alkalosis.[114, 115] Administration of supplemental O_2 may attenuate this response and produce a further increase in Pa_{CO_2}.[116]

INCREASED DEAD SPACE. By wasting more of each tidal volume breath, increased dead space may decrease CO_2 elimination, thereby producing an increase in Pa_{CO_2}. With most pulmonary pathology, minute ventilation may be increased sufficiently to compensate for increases in dead space.[53] During anesthesia or mechanical ventilation, consideration must be given to potential problems with anesthetic

system circuitry, which could produce increased apparatus dead space. Incompetent[117, 118] or absent[119] valves on circle systems, defective inner tubing on Bain systems,[120, 121] and inadequate fresh gas flows on Mapleson Systems[118, 122, 123] are examples of circuitry problems that are capable of producing increased apparatus dead space.

INADEQUATE TIDAL VOLUME OR RESPIRATORY RATE. Neuromuscular disease or residual effects of muscle relaxants may compromise the patient's ability to respond to a normal respiratory drive.[124, 125] Similarly, pulmonary pathology (e.g., bronchospasm) may limit tidal volume or respiratory rate.[125] Rarely, neurologic disorders (e.g., phrenic nerve damage,[126, 127] Ondine's curse,[128] medullary infarction[129]) may cause increased Pa_{CO_2}.

Although mechanical ventilation is generally instituted to ensure adequate ventilation, the simple process of attaching an endotracheal tube to a ventilator circuit does not guarantee that this objective is met. Reliance on assist mode ventilation (with which a breath is delivered only when a predetermined negative airway pressure is generated by the patient) or low rate intermittent mandatory ventilation may result in inadequate respiratory rates in the presence of sedation or paralysis. Ventilator rate may be confirmed by the simple process of counting machine-delivered breaths, however.

Assessment of tidal volume is more sophisticated. Administration of a mechanical tidal volume equal to a normal spontaneous tidal volume is generally inadequate for mechanically ventilated patients. Most authors advocate administration of a mechanical tidal volume of at least 10 ml·kg^{-1}.[130] This is necessitated in part by the increase in physiologic dead space resulting from the rise in alveolar pressure induced by positive pressure ventilation. Additionally, some of the preset tidal volume is unavailable to the patient with each mechanical breath, because it remains in the circuit as a result of expansion of ventilator tubing and humidification devices. This "compression volume," which may exceed 4 ml·cmH_2O^{-1} peak inspiratory pressure, is significant if small tidal volumes are delivered to patients requiring high peak inspiratory pressures. Because the gas exits from the ventilator circuit during the expiratory phase, it will be measured as part of the exhaled volume, and its magnitude cannot be ascertained by this determination.

Calculation of the compliance of a ventilator circuit is a relatively easy task and is the only way to accurately estimate compression volume. (With the patient end of the ventilator circuit occluded, a large tidal volume breath is delivered into the circuit. Observation of the peak inspiratory pressure coupled with measurement of the exhaled volume allows calculation of the compliance of the circuit. The value derived in this manner may be used in conjunction with the peak inspiratory pressure generated during mechanical ventilation of the patient to estimate compression volume.)

INCREASED CO_2 PRODUCTION. Carbon dioxide production is proportional to metabolic rate, and CO_2 elimination is proportional to alveolar ventilation. Accordingly, for Pa_{CO_2} to remain constant, increases in metabolic rate should stimulate increases in CO_2 elimination. If alveolar ventilation is fixed, as occurs with control mode mechanical ventilation, Pa_{CO_2} will increase as metabolic rate increases. Additionally, pulmonary pathology may prohibit adequate increases in alveolar ventilation during spontaneous ventilation. Finally, even in the absence of pulmonary pathology, massive increases in CO_2 production (e.g., with malignant hyperthermia) may exceed the ability of the respiratory system to compensate.

Effects

Physiologic consequences of hypercapnia occur not only as a consequence of the direct effects of increased CO_2 concentrations but also through the resulting decreases in pH. Separation of those effects owing to increased Pa_{CO_2} from those owing to acidosis is not possible. Furthermore, in most organ systems, the observed effects of hypercapnia are the result of the balance between the direct effects of CO_2 itself and the indirect effects mediated by the autonomic nervous system or some other control mechanism. Finally, species differences are such that it is often not appropriate to extrapolate results from one species to another.[131] Accordingly, reports of the consequences of hypercapnia must be critically evaluated with regard to the acid–base status present during hypercapnia, status of the autonomic nervous system, and species studied.

CARDIOVASCULAR. The direct effects of CO_2 on the cardiovascular system are vasodilatation and a decrease in myocardial contractility[132] (mediated by acidosis).[133] In conscious patients, the excitatory effects of mild hypercapnia (Pa_{CO_2} to 50 mm Hg) on the sympathetic nervous system result in increases in heart rate, myocardial contractility, stroke volume, and cardiac output.[134] Reductions in cardiac output are likely to occur at very high levels of Pa_{CO_2}.[135] Under anesthesia, the ultimate presentation may be further altered by anesthesia-induced changes in the status of the autonomic nervous system.[136–140]

Cardiac dysrhythmias are uncommon in conscious humans below Pa_{CO_2} of 80 mm Hg. Even at higher levels, the most common cardiac dysrhythmia is an atrioventricular (AV) junctional rhythm.[131] Under anesthesia, however, the increased sympathetic activity associated with hypercarbia[141] is capable of combining with the direct effects of CO_2 on the myocardium[142] to produce significant cardiac dysrhythmias.[143]

There is some suggestion that hypercapnia may be associated with coronary vasodilatation resulting in a disproportionate increase in coronary blood flow compared with left ventricular work.[131]

CENTRAL NERVOUS SYSTEM. Carbon dioxide may be considered to be a generalized depressant of the CNS. Hypercarbia, induced by the administration of exogenous CO_2, has been used to produce anesthesia in humans.[144] Its use, in concentrations required for anesthesia, has been complicated by the occurrence of seizures.[145] The opioid effects of CO_2 are apparently due to the alteration of neuronal intracellular pH.[144, 146]

Pa_{CO_2} is the single most important, easily measured factor regulating cerebral blood flow (CBF). Both CBF and intracranial pressure are directly proportional to Pa_{CO_2}.

Hypercapnia is associated with stimulation of the autonomic nervous system. Increases in plasma epinephrine and norepinephrine levels have been documented with moderate increases in Pa_{CO_2}.[147, 148] In many of the target organs, sympathic stimulation reverses the direct depressant effects of CO_2 itself.[131, 135] Additionally, acidosis is commonly associated with decreased sensitivity to circulating catecholamines.[149]

MISCELLANEOUS. Hypercapnia produces a loss of K^+ from the intracellular compartment, resulting in an increased serum K^+ level.[144] Pharmacokinetics and pharmacodynamics for drugs in general may be altered by changes in organ perfusion and by acidosis, which may alter ionization, solubility, and protein binding of pharmacologic agents.

OXYGEN

Evaluating the partial pressure of O_2 in arterial blood (Pa_{O_2}) should involve two specific considerations: 1) appraising the adequacy of arterial O_2 content (Ca_{O_2}), and 2) assessing lung function as it relates to oxygenation. Although the adequacy of arterial O_2 content will be determined primarily by hemoglobin concentration, in some circumstances, Pa_{O_2} may become a significant factor. Assessing oxygenation function of the lung involves some form of comparison between Pa_{O_2} and alveolar P_{O_2} (PA_{O_2}).

Role in the Body

Approximately 90% of total O_2 consumption occurs in the mitochondria during the process of generating high-energy compounds (e.g., adenosine triphosphate, ATP), which are utilized for the short-term storage of energy throughout the body.[150] The presence of adequate O_2 concentrations allows the aerobic oxidation of glucose, which produces CO_2, water, and 38 moles of ATP from each mole of glucose. Inadequate O_2 concentrations necessitate anaerobic metabolism, which generates 2 moles of lactic acid and 2 moles of ATP from each mole of glucose.[151] Whereas aerobic oxidation of one mole of glucose stores 456,000 calories of energy (representing 66% efficiency of energy transfer) in the form of ATP, only 24,000 calories (approximately 3% efficiency) of energy can be stored from metabolism of the same amount of glucose under anaerobic conditions.[152] In addition to impaired efficiency, anaerobic metabolism is associated with the production of an additional quantity of "metabolic acid," which must be cleared from the body.

Oxygen is necessary for the generation of energy from fats and proteins, since no significant anaerobic metabolism of these compounds occurs.[14] Finally, O_2 is also necessary for incorporation into mixed function oxidases (including cytochrome P-450, which is involved with biotransformation of drugs) and oxygenases.[151]

Partial Pressure Gradients

Before reaching the mitochondria, its primary site of utilization, O_2 must move from the atmosphere, through the lungs, and into the cell by way of arterial and capillary blood (Fig. 25-7). Each step along the way is associated with a further reduction in the P_{O_2}. Other than in blood, where O_2 is bound to hemoglobin and therefore actively distributed to the tissues by cardiac output, entry to each subsequent step is achieved by diffusion.

According to Fick's law, rate of diffusion is directly proportional to surface area, partial pressure difference, temperature, and solubility and inversely proportional to molecular weight and tissue thickness.[38, 153] Since all other factors are essentially constant, the partial pressure difference may be viewed as the driving force for O_2 diffusion, and the magnitude of the gradient becomes a significant factor in determining the rate of diffusion.[154]

MEASUREMENT

Determining the P_{O_2} in blood is done polarographically by the Clark electrode (Fig. 25-8). Upon injection into the blood-gas machine, blood comes in contact with a thin polypropylene membrane, which is permeable to O_2. Oxygen diffuses through the membrane into a dilute solution of potassium

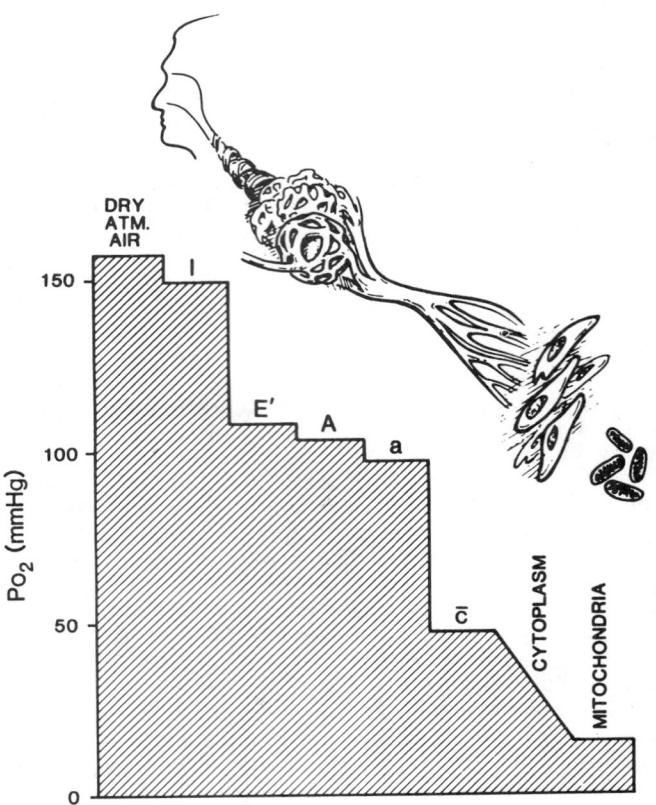

FIG. 25-7. Concentration gradient for oxygen. Oxygen diffuses down a concentration gradient from dry atmospheric air to humidified inspired gas (I), end-expiratory gas (E'), alveolar gas (A), arterial (a) and capillary (c̄) blood, cytoplasm, and eventually to mitochondria. (Modified from Nunn JF: Applied Respiratory Physiology, 3rd ed, p 243. London, Butterworths, 1987.)

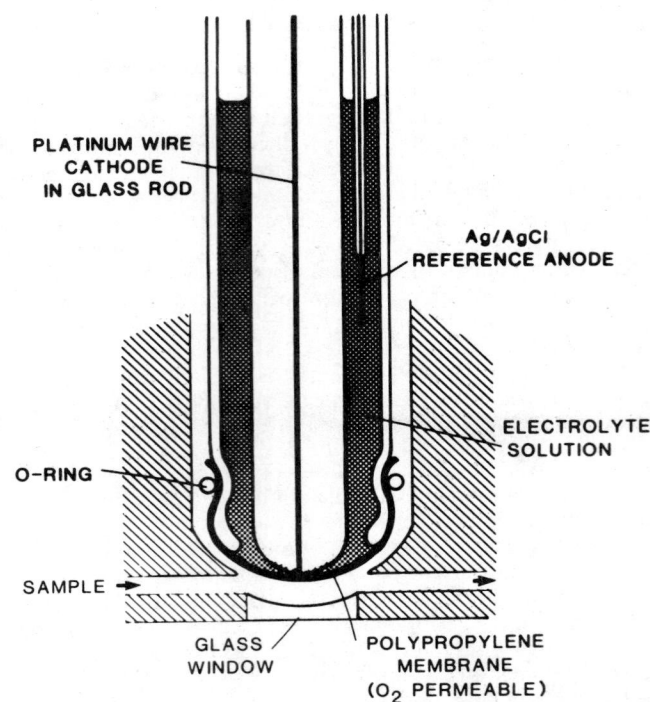

FIG. 25-8. Oxygen electrode. A thin polypropylene membrane separates the blood sample from an electrolyte solution consisting of KCl and phosphate buffer saturated with AgCl. This solution is in contact with a reference electrode and a polarized platinum cathode. Oxygen diffuses into the electrode solution and reacts with the platinum cathode to produce current flow that is measured and reported as P_{O_2}. (Modified from Ledingham IM, Macdonald AM, Douglas IHS: Monitoring of ventilation. In Shoemaker WC, Thompson WL, Holbrook PR (eds): Textbook of Critical Care, p 123. Philadelphia, WB Saunders, 1984.)

chloride, which is in contact with a silver anode and a platinum cathode. A current, which is directly proportional to the P_{O_2}, is observed as a result of diffusion of O_2 from the blood through the membrane to the cathode, where it is reduced.[155]

Errors in determination may occur owing to addition or loss of O_2 from the sample as a result of exposure of the blood to air, most commonly in the form of a bubble in the sampling syringe. Under these circumstances, O_2 moves from a higher to a lower concentration by simple diffusion. If Pa_{O_2} exceeds the P_{O_2} in the bubble (as may occur in patients receiving supplemental O_2), a falsely low value will occur as a result of O_2 diffusion from the blood into the bubble. More commonly, however, the P_{O_2} in the bubble will exceed the Pa_{O_2}, and O_2 will move from the bubble into the blood and produce a spuriously high Pa_{O_2}.[156] Assuming appropriate maintenance and calibration of the blood gas machine, the second most common cause of erroneous P_{O_2} values results from delays in measurement.[151] Although red blood cells lack mitochondria and accordingly do not utilize O_2, the same cannot be said for white blood cells and platelets.[157, 158] (The markedly increased numbers of white blood cells present in patients with leukemic crises may be responsible for a clinically relevant decrease in Pa_{O_2} occurring, even with normal sampling to measurement intervals.)[158] Despite the fact that graphs have been developed to estimate O_2 consumption based on the duration

of time between obtaining a sample and determining P_{O_2},[159] it is more prudent to endeavor to reduce the rate of O_2 consumption by storing the sample in ice and performing the determination with minimal delays.[160]

Oxygen Content of Blood

Oxygen is present in arterial blood in two forms: 1) bound to hemoglobin, and 2) dissolved in plasma. Just as calculation of alveolar P_{O_2} is essential when using Pa_{O_2} to evaluate lung function, calculation of arterial oxygen content (Ca_{O_2}) is necessary when evaluating the adequacy of O_2 delivery to the tissues. Although there is some disagreement among physiologists regarding the exact value of the constants to be used when determining the amount of O_2 that may be bound to hemoglobin or dissolved in plasma,[32, 151] Equation 25-7 is clinically useful in determining Ca_{O_2}.[32]

$$Ca_{O_2} = (1.34)(Hgb)(\% \text{ Sat}) + (0.003)(Pa_{O_2}) \quad (25\text{-}7)$$

Using Equation 25-7, it is evident that, by far, the greater amount of O_2 is carried bound to hemoglobin. In fact, in "normal" arterial blood ($Pa_{O_2} = 100$, $Hgb = 15 \text{ g·dl}^{-1}$), only about 1.5% of the total Ca_{O_2} is dissolved in plasma. Despite its relatively insignificant contribution to Ca_{O_2}, dissolved O_2 is important because it is this dissolved O_2 that determines the magnitude of the partial pressure gradient down which O_2 must diffuse before it reaches the tissues. Furthermore, it is the dissolved O_2 that is measured when arterial blood gases (ABG) are determined.

Based on an arterial P_{O_2} of 673 mm Hg (the maximum that can be attained if barometric pressure (P_B) = 760 mm Hg and Pa_{CO_2} = 40 mm Hg), the maximal amount of O_2 that can be dissolved in 100 ml of blood is 2.0 ml. It should be noted that in order to accomplish this, the patient must be breathing 100% O_2, and Pa_{O_2} must equal PA_{O_2}, the latter being highly unlikely. If Pa_{O_2} is maintained equal to or greater than 60 mm Hg (90% Sa_{O_2}), increasing hemoglobin by 1 g·dl^{-1} will increase Ca_{O_2} by 1.2 ml in every 100 ml of blood. Accordingly, the most efficient way to increase Ca_{O_2} is to increase the patient's hemoglobin.

Oxyhemoglobin Dissociation Curve

Under normal circumstances, the majority of arterial oxygen is reversibly bound to the heme portion of hemoglobin.[151] The amount of O_2 bound to hemoglobin is determined by the partial pressure of O_2 in blood and is described under normal conditions (*p*H = 7.40, temperature = 37° C, Pa_{CO_2} = 40 mm Hg) by the curve shown in Figure 25-9. From this curve, it can be determined that, under normal conditions, hemoglobin is 90% saturated when Pa_{O_2} is 60 mm Hg. It is also evident that Pa_{O_2}s less than 60 mm Hg are associated with substantial reductions in hemoglobin saturation, whereas Pa_{O_2}s greater than 60 mm Hg produce only modest increases in the percentage of hemoglobin saturated with O_2. An increase of 40 mm Hg from Pa_{O_2} of 60 mm Hg to Pa_{O_2} of 100 mm Hg is associated with only a 7%–8% increase in hemoglobin saturation, whereas a 30 mm Hg decrease from Pa_{O_2} of 60 mm Hg

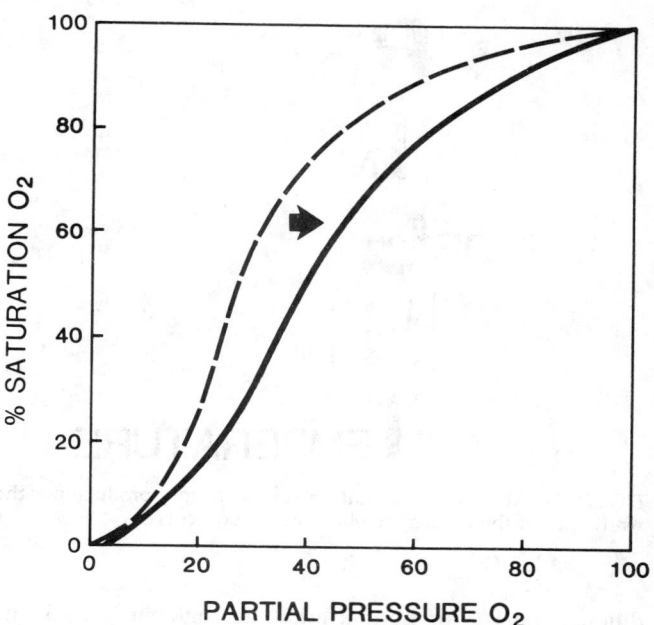

FIG. 25-10. Shift to the right of the oxyhemoglobin dissociation curve is associated with lower saturations at equivalent values for P_{O_2}.

to Pa_{O_2} of 30 mm Hg is associated with a 30% decrease in hemoglobin saturation. A "normal" Pa_{O_2} (100 mm Hg) represents 97% saturation, whereas a "normal" $P\bar{v}_{O_2}$ (40 mm Hg) represents approximately 75% saturation.

Changes in temperature, *p*H, P_{CO_2}, or 2,3 DPG levels are associated with shifts in the oxyhemoglobin dissociation curve[31, 151] as shown in Figure 25-10. Aberrant forms of hemoglobin may also produce alterations in the curve.[151] The most common hemoglobin variation is normal fetal hemoglobin, which is associated with a leftward shift of the oxyhemoglobin dissociation curve.[161] More than 40 other stable variations of hemoglobin with a high affinity for O_2 have been described.[162] Other hemoglobin variants, including sickle hemoglobin, are associated with decreased affinity for O_2.[151]

Shifts of the oxyhemoglobin dissociation curve to the left are associated with an increased affinity of hemoglobin for O_2. This is advantageous during fetal existence by facilitating O_2 uptake on the fetal side of the placenta[163] and allowing increased arterial O_2 content. (Hemoglobin saturation averages only 65% in the fetal ascending aorta.[164]) Although a leftward shift may seem advantageous even after birth, during extrauterine existence, increased affinity is associated with only minimal increases in CaO_2. (A "normal" Pa_{O_2} of 100 mm Hg is already at least 97% saturated. Even if Pa_{O_2} decreases to 60 mm Hg, hemoglobin remains 90% saturated.) The same leftward shift in the oxyhemoglobin dissociation curve produces a reduction in O_2 unloading at the tissue level, which may result in reduced tissue O_2 levels.[151] By contrast, a rightward shift of the oxyhemoglobin dissociation curve, which is associated with minimal decreases in arterial O_2 saturation at "normal" values for Pa_{O_2}, facilitates O_2 unloading at the tissue level.[151] Figure 25-11 presents a mnemonic for recalling some of the more common factors producing a shift of the oxyhemoglobin dissociation curve.

Evaluating changes in the oxyhemoglobin dissociation curve is most commonly performed by comparing the O_2 partial pressures at 50% saturation (P_{50}). Under standard con-

FIG. 25-9. Oxyhemoglobin dissociation curve for normal adult hemoglobin. Point A represents normal mixed venous blood (P_{O_2} = 40 mm Hg corresponds to approximately 75% saturation). Hemoglobin is approximately 90% saturated when P_{O_2} = 60 mm Hg (Point B). The P_{O_2} at which hemoglobin is 50% saturated (P_{50}) serves as a method of comparing different oxyhemoglobin dissociation curves.

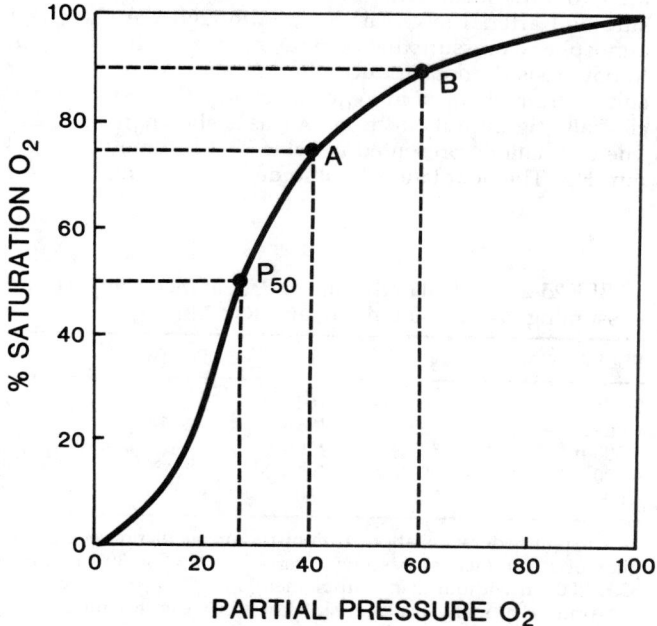

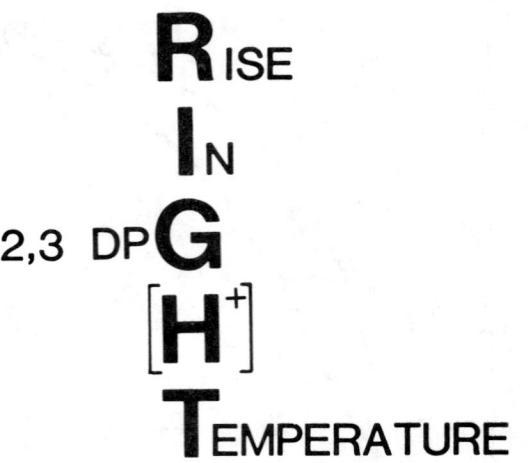

RISE

IN

2,3 DP**G**

[**H**+]

TEMPERATURE

FIG. 25-11. Mnemonic illustrating several factors producing rightward shift of the oxyhemoglobin dissociation curve.

ditions, the P_{50} for normal adult hemoglobin is 26.3 mm Hg.[165] Left-shifted curves, which represent increased affinity, are associated with lower values for P_{50}. (The P_{50} for fetal hemoglobin is approximately 20 mm Hg.)[163] Decreases in affinity, which produce right-shifted curves, are associated with higher values for P_{50}.

ASSESSMENT OF LUNG FUNCTION

Alveolar P_{O_2}

In evaluating lung function, isolated knowledge of the Pa_{O_2} may be almost meaningless. Since O_2 enters blood by diffusing down a concentration gradient from the alveolus, the PA_{O_2} represents the highest possible value for the Pa_{O_2}. Accurate assessment of lung function based on Pa_{O_2} necessitates quantification of PA_{O_2}, which may be calculated with some precision using the "alveolar air equation" (Eqn 25-8).[53]

$$PA_{O_2} = (P_B - P_{H_2O})\, F_{I_{O_2}} - Pa_{CO_2} \times F \qquad (25\text{-}8)$$

P_B = barometric pressure
P_{H_2O} = saturated water vapor pressure
    (47 mm Hg at 1 atmosphere at 37° C)
$F_{I_{O_2}}$ = fractional concentration of inspired O_2
PA_{CO_2} = alveolar partial pressure of CO_2
    F = correction factor determined by both
        the respiratory quotient and the $F_{I_{O_2}}$.

By convention, Pa_{CO_2} is assumed equal to PA_{CO_2}. For the purposes of this calculation, this assumption is valid, since, under most clinical circumstances, it is rare to achieve a $Pa_{CO_2} - PA_{CO_2}$ gradient as high as 2 mm Hg.[5] The value of the correction factor, F, in the above formula may be determined by Equation 25-9.

$$F = F_{I_{O_2}} + \frac{1 - F_{I_{O_2}}}{R} \qquad (25\text{-}9)$$

    F = correction factor for alveolar air from
        Equation 25-8
$F_{I_{O_2}}$ = fractional concentration of inspired O_2
    R = respiratory quotient

Use of the correction factor is necessary because of the

TABLE 25-1. Comparison of Calculated PA_{O_2} Using True Alveolar Air Equation and Modified Alveolar Air Equation (Assuming $Pa_{CO_2} = 40$ and $R = 0.8$)

$F_{I_{O_2}}$	$P_{I_{O_2}}$	F	PA_{O_2} (with F)	PA_{O_2} (w/o F)
1.0	713	1.00	673	673
0.8	570	1.05	528	530
0.6	428	1.10	384	388
0.4	285	1.15	239	245
0.3	214	1.18	167	174
0.25	178	1.19	130	138

inequality between the rate of O_2 uptake and the rate of CO_2 production. Since normally the volume of CO_2 diffusing into the alveolus is 80% of the volume of O_2 leaving the alveolus, a "hole" is created in the alveolar volume that must be filled by inspired gas. If R were 1.0, the amount of CO_2 entering the alveolus would equal the amount of O_2 leaving the alveolus, and no "hole" would be created. The value of F would be 1. If R is less than 1.0, failure to utilize the correction factor may artificially raise the calculated value of PA_{O_2} by assuming that all the gas that fills the "hole" is O_2. If $F_{I_{O_2}} = 1.0$, all gas filling the "hole" would in fact be O_2 and the value of F would again be 1. Clinically, for patients breathing 50% O_2 or more (and probably even for those breathing 30% O_2 or more), the correction factor may be ignored and PA_{O_2} may be calculated by the modified alveolar air equation (Eqn 25-10).

$$PA_{O_2} = (P_B - 47)\, F_{I_{O_2}} - Pa_{CO_2} \qquad (25\text{-}10)$$

Deletion of the correction factor results in a clinically useful approximation of PA_{O_2} under these circumstances, because the value of the correction factor decreases with increasing inspired O_2 concentrations, while the number from which it is subtracted increases. As a result, as $F_{I_{O_2}}$ increases, the correction factor has a reduced effect on PA_{O_2}. (Table 25-1)

Examining the modified alveolar air equation (Eqn 25-10) reveals that, in addition to inspired O_2 concentrations, there are two other factors that influence PA_{O_2}: atmospheric pressure and arterial (alveolar) P_{CO_2}. Although the changes in atmospheric pressure that occur at a given location on a day-to-day basis do not produce relevant alterations in PA_{O_2} resulting from changes in P_B, changes in altitude may have a clinically significant effect on PA_{O_2} as is shown in Table 25-2. The calculations presented in Table 25-2 assume Pa_{CO_2} of 40 mm Hg. The adaptation to altitude involves an increase in

TABLE 25-2. Calculated Value of PA_{O_2} at Increasing Altitude (Assuming $Pa_{CO_2} = 40$ mm Hg and $R = 0.8$)

ELEVATION	P_B	$P_{I_{O_2}}$	$P_{I_{O_2}}$ (wet)	PA_{O_2}
Sea Level	760	160	150	102
Denver	635	133	124	76
3,300 m*	523	110	100	52
4,000 m†	483	101	91	43
6,000 m	380	80	70	22

*Current Federal Aviation Administration regulations permit the pilot of a commercial passenger carrier to fly for 30 minutes at 3300–4000 m without using supplemental O_2.[166]

†Altitude of many peaks at ski slopes in western United States.

ventilation that lowers Pa_{CO_2} and thereby increases PA_{O_2}. Even if alveolar ventilation was doubled (a difficult achievement to sustain), Pa_{O_2} would be increased at most 24 mm Hg. Similarly, PA_{O_2} may be significantly increased by exposure to hyperbaric conditions.

While clinically relevant changes in P_B rarely occur provided that altitude is constant, significant alterations in Pa_{CO_2} do occur. Increases in PA_{CO_2} commonly accompany sleep and may be responsible for a significant reduction in PA_{O_2} at that time. Spontaneous ventilation under general anesthesia, in the absence of surgical stimulation, is associated with even greater increases in Pa_{CO_2}. Hypercarbia (*e.g.*, resulting from drug overdose) may cause a substantial increase in Pa_{CO_2}, which in itself may produce arterial hypoxemia (Table 25-3).

Normal Pa_{O_2}

Although a Pa_{O_2} of 75 to 80 mm Hg may be normal when the PA_{O_2} is 100 mm Hg, the same value is grossly abnormal when the PA_{O_2} is 500 mm Hg. Defining a minimal normal Pa_{O_2} as 80 to 100 mm Hg[166–168] involves several unstated assumptions ($P_B = 760$ mm Hg, $Pa_{CO_2} = 40$ mm Hg, $Fi_{O_2} = 0.21$).

It is impossible to achieve a "normal" Pa_{O_2} on room air at 3,300 m elevation (See Table 25-2). Similarly, it is evident that these "normal" values cannot be achieved at Denver (where PA_{O_2} is only 76 mm Hg) without increasing alveolar ventilation (and thereby decreasing Pa_{CO_2} or increasing Fi_{O_2}). Additionally, as demonstrated in Table 25-3, hypercarbia may make it impossible to achieve a "normal" Pa_{O_2} without enhancing inspired O_2 concentrations.

Despite these limitations, most discussions of blood gases customarily include some formula or table describing "normal" Pa_{O_2}. Any such guidelines must consider the deterioration in oxygenation that accompanies increasing age. For those who prefer this approach, Equation 25-11 provides a reasonable approximation of the predicted Pa_{O_2} for patients with a normal Pa_{CO_2} breathing room air at sea level.

$$\text{"Normal" } Pa_{O_2} = 102 - \frac{\text{age (in years)}}{3} \quad (25\text{-}11)$$

The value derived from Equation 25-9 represents the mean Pa_{O_2}. Variations of 10 mm Hg either side of this calculated value represent 5% confidence intervals (± 2 standard deviations).[169] This formula may be applied only as long as the predicted Pa_{O_2} is at least 70 mm Hg. Most authors recognize 70–75 mm Hg as a minimal acceptable Pa_{O_2} regardless of age.

A–a D_{O_2}

Since the majority of blood gases obtained in the operating room and intensive care unit are on patients receiving more than 21% O_2, some way of objectively evaluating and comparing Pa_{O_2} under these circumstances is desirable. The most commonly used system for evaluation of Pa_{O_2} in patients on supplemental O_2 is the calculation of the difference between alveolar and arterial P_{O_2}s (often termed the A–a gradient.)[170–174]

$$D(A\text{-}a)_{O_2} = PA_{O_2} - Pa_{O_2} \quad (25\text{-}12)$$

This system takes into account the effect on PA_{O_2} of all three previously mentioned factors (P_B, Pa_{CO_2}, and Fi_{O_2}).

The major drawback in using $D(A\text{-}a)_{O_2}$ to evaluate lung function is the absence of a single acceptable value. The magnitude of the normal $D(A\text{-}a)_{O_2}$ is altered by factors that influence PA_{O_2}, foremost of which are Fi_{O_2} and P_B. A normal $D(A\text{-}a)_{O_2}$ under standard conditions ($P_B = 760$ mm Hg, $Pa_{CO_2} = 40$, $Fi_{O_2} = 0.21$) is 5 to 10 mm Hg,[151, 175, 176] but gradients less than 20 to 25 mm Hg are generally considered acceptable.[151, 176] With $Fi_{O_2} = 1.0$ ($P_B = 760$ mm Hg, $Pa_{CO_2} = 40$), normal $D(A\text{-}a)_{O_2}$ is less than 100 mm Hg. Because the magnitude of the gradient is not *linearly* related to either Fi_{O_2} or PA_{O_2},[151, 177] a different acceptable $D(A\text{-}a)_{O_2}$ must be learned or a table must be consulted for PA_{O_2}. The A–a gradient system, as a result of these shortcomings and the lack of data on normal gradients with Fi_{O_2} between 0.21 and 1.0, has been described as "difficult" to interpret.[178]

a/A Ratio

Although not as widely used as the A–a gradient, calculation of the a/A ratio (Eqn. 25-13) offers many advantages.

$$\text{a/A ratio} = Pa_{O_2}/PA_{O_2} \quad (25\text{-}13)$$

To utilize the a/A ratio, PA_{O_2} must be calculated; therefore, all factors effecting PA_{O_2} are taken into account. The major advantage of the a/A ratio is its ease of interpretation. A normal a/A ratio is 0.75 or greater no matter what the PA_{O_2} or Fi_{O_2}. Under general anesthesia, a/A ratios in excess of 0.5 may be considered normal. Lung oxygenation function may be easily compared between two samples obtained on different Fi_{O_2}s simply by calculating and comparing the different a/A ratios—the higher the a/A ratio, the better the lung is functioning as an organ of O_2 exchange.

Pa_{O_2}/Fi_{O_2}

The Pa_{O_2}/Fi_{O_2} ratio is another method designed to permit evaluation of Pa_{O_2} in patients receiving various amounts of supplemental O_2. In its simplest form, Pa_{O_2} is divided by Fi_{O_2}. The result should equal or exceed 400 to 500 mm Hg (corresponding to a Pa_{O_2} of 80 to 100 mm Hg on room air).[166] Values less than 400 mm Hg would be anticipated to be associated with hypoxemia on room air.

Although simple, this system, like others designed to estimate normal Pa_{O_2}, suffers from failure to include consideration of barometric pressure or PA_{CO_2} in its calculations. Although it is true that decreases in Pa_{O_2}/Fi_{O_2} ratio owing to hypercarbia would predict room air hypoxemia, the therapeutic implications are different for hypercarbia-induced hypoxemia.

One variation of this approach involves the determination of the minimal acceptable Pa_{O_2} at any Fi_{O_2}. Pa_{O_2} should meet or exceed five times the inspired O_2 percentage (Eqn. 25-14). Failure to achieve this level predicts arterial hypoxemia on room air.

$$\text{Minimal } Pa_{O_2} = \text{Inspired } O_2 \text{ per cent} \times 5 \quad (25\text{-}14)$$

TABLE 25-3. Calculated Value of PA_{O_2} at Increasing Carbon Dioxide Levels (Assuming R = 0.8 and $PA_{CO_2} = Pa_{CO_2}$)

Fi_{O_2}	Pa_{CO_2} (mm Hg)	PA_{O_2} (mm Hg)
0.21	40	102
0.21	50	90
0.21	60	78
0.21	80	54

Comparison of Evaluation Systems

In addition to estimating the magnitude of lung oxygenation defects present at any one time, evaluation systems should ideally permit the clinician to compare lung function at different times under conditions of a changing FI_{O_2} and Pa_{CO_2}. Consider the following scenario. A patient with a drug overdose is admitted to the emergency room, where his trachea is intubated and the lungs are mechanically ventilated with 100% O_2. ABGs under these conditions are $Pa_{O_2} = 550$ mm Hg, $Pa_{CO_2} = 40$ mm Hg. FI_{O_2} is decreased to 0.3, and repeat ABGs reveal $Pa_{O_2} = 100$ mm Hg and $Pa_{CO_2} = 40$ mm Hg. The following day, with $FI_{O_2} = 0.40$, ventilatory support is reduced. ABGs are again obtained, and $Pa_{O_2} = 118$ mm Hg and $Pa_{CO_2} = 60$ mm Hg. In all circumstances, Pa_{O_2} meets or exceeds the textbook normal. The question to be answered is whether any of these ABGs reflect the presence of significant lung function defects. This assessment becomes more difficult in the face of changing values for FI_{O_2} and Pa_{CO_2}. Table 25-4 summarizes the results of the various evaluation methods when applied to these ABGs.

Determination of the a/A ratios for these ABGs reveal that lung oxygenation function is best at time C and clearly acceptable at time A. ABGs obtained at time B, however, are associated with a defect in lung oxygenation function (a/A = 0.53) according to this evaluation system. Interpretation of the derived information involves only a simple comparison with a single normal value.

The calculated values for $D(A-a)_{O_2}$ range from 123 mm Hg with $FI_{O_2} = 1.0$ to 74 mm Hg with $FI_{O_2} = 0.3$. Although this calculation compensates for all factors that effect PA_{O_2}, the interpretation of the resulting information is not simple. It is not immediately evident that there is any significant difference in these values in Table 25-4, given the changes in FI_{O_2}. In fact, in the conditions previously presented, the worst lung oxygenation function is associated with the lowest $D(A-a)_{O_2}$.

Calculation of Pa_{O_2}/FI_{O_2} reveals that ABGs B and C reflect the presence of lung oxygenation defects. Although this agrees with the a/A ratio in condition B, ABGs at time C are associated with the highest a/A ratio but the lowest value for Pa_{O_2}/FI_{O_2}. The failure of Pa_{O_2}/FI_{O_2} to compensate for aberrant values of Pa_{CO_2} makes this evaluation system subject to error when attempting to quantitate lung oxygenation function in the presence of abnormal Pa_{CO_2}s. While it is true that hypoxemia would likely occur on room air in both conditions B and C, the etiology of this problem at time C is related to hypercarbia and not to any intrinsic lung dysfunction. The best therapeutic intervention in this circumstance is mechanical ventilation of the lungs rather than the administration of supplemental oxygen.

One additional advantage offered by the a/A ratio system

is the ability to use the calculated value in making changes in FI_{O_2}. Since a/A ratio remains relatively constant despite changes in FI_{O_2}, it may be used to predict the Pa_{O_2} that will occur at a new FI_{O_2}. On the most basic level, if $Pa_{O_2} = 250$ mm Hg and $PA_{O_2} = 500$ mm Hg, a change in FI_{O_2} that produces $PA_{O_2} = 300$ mm Hg would be expected to produce $Pa_{O_2} = 150$ mm Hg. In a more sophisticated utilization, the a/A ratio may be used to predict the FI_{O_2} necessary to achieve a desired value for Pa_{O_2}. If the current a/A ratio is determined, the formula for a/A ratio may be used to estimate the PA_{O_2}, which should produce a given Pa_{O_2}, that is, if a/A = 0.5, to achieve $Pa_{O_2} = 100$ mm Hg, $PA_{O_2} = 200$ mm Hg should be provided. Using the value for PA_{O_2} derived in this manner, the necessary FI_{O_2} may also be calculated, that is, with $P_B = 760$ mm Hg and $Pa_{CO_2} = 40$ mm Hg, $FI_{O_2} = 0.35$ should produce $PA_{O_2} = 200$ mm Hg (713 mm Hg × 0.35 to 40 mm Hg = 248 mm Hg − 40 mm Hg = 208 mm Hg). A nomogram has been developed to simplify this process.[180]

EVALUATION OF HYPOXEMIA

There is a tendency to attribute any decrease in Pa_{O_2} to lung dysfunction. This is not necessarily valid, as there are other potential causes for a low Pa_{O_2}. A differential diagnosis should be developed, and each potential factor should be evaluated. The following factors should be considered in determining the etiology of arterial hypoxemia.

Low PA_{O_2}

The most important first step in evaluating a low Pa_{O_2} is to calculate PA_{O_2} (Eqns. 25-8, 25-10). A low Pa_{O_2} may be the result of alveolar hypoxia. The simple calculation of PA_{O_2} will determine not only the presence but also the magnitude of a problem. (No lung function problem exists if $Pa_{O_2} = 60$ mm Hg in a patient breathing room air in Denver, but a major defect is present with the same Pa_{O_2} in a patient breathing 100% O_2 at sea level).

Potential etiologies of alveolar hypoxia include hypercarbia (which should be evident on the blood gas), low barometric pressure, or low FI_{O_2}. Although the latter condition is less likely with modern ventilators and anesthesia machines, older models lacked O_2 monitors and the protective mechanisms that prevented the administration of hypoxic gas mixtures. Administration of 100% N_2O was possible when tank O_2 was depleted in the absence of an oxygen fail-safe mechanism. Hypoxic gas mixtures could also be administered by simply failing to provide adequate O_2 flows. Low Pa_{O_2}s are clearly to be expected in these circumstances and do not reflect lung dysfunction. It is prudent to recheck FI_{O_2} with each blood gas determination and especially important if the sample demonstrates a low Pa_{O_2}.

Treatment of Pa_{O_2} secondary to low PA_{O_2} simply involves restoring PA_{O_2} to normal values. This is most commonly accomplished by correcting hypercarbia or ensuring an adequate FI_{O_2}. In those rare circumstances in which alveolar hypoxia is due to low barometric pressure, efforts should be directed toward achieving a normal P_B (by descending the mountain, decreasing aircraft elevation, or pressurizing the aircraft cabin.)

Absolute Shunt

If venous blood enters the arterial circulation without benefit of exposure to functional lung units, Pa_{O_2} will be decreased.

TABLE 25-4.   Comparison of $D(A-a)_{O_2}$, a/A ratio, and Pa_{O_2}/FI_{O_2} in Evaluating Oxygenation Function of the Lung

	A	B	C
FI_{O_2}	1.0	0.3	0.4
Pa_{CO_2} (mm Hg)	40	40	60
PA_{O_2} (mm Hg)	673	174	225
Pa_{O_2} (mm Hg)	550	100	118
$D_{(A-a)O_2}$ (mm Hg)	123	74	80
a/A	0.82	0.57	0.94
Pa_{O_2}/FI_{O_2}	550	333	295

The ventilation/perfusion ratio (V/Q) is used to describe abnormalities in the pulmonary distribution of gas (ventilation) and blood flow (perfusion). Ventilation of an unperfused lung unit (V = finite, Q = 0, V/Q = ∞) constitutes dead space (Fig. 25-4). Absolute shunt (Fig. 25-12) occurs when blood perfuses atelectatic or otherwise nonfunctional lung units (V = O, Q = finite, V/Q = 0).[181, 182] The most obvious situation in which this occurs is the presence of a right-to-left intracardiac shunt, such as an uncorrected transposition of the great vessels, where the bulk of the blood in the systemic arterial circulation has gone directly from the systemic venous circulation into the aorta. Absolute shunt exists in normal persons in the form of the blood draining from the bronchial veins (some of which empty venous blood into the pulmonary vein)[183] and the Thebesian veins[184] (some of which direct venous blood into the left side of the heart).[185]

Pulmonary pathologic processes may also produce an absolute shunt. The presence of an unrecognized right mainstem intubation of the trachea, for example, will eventually produce alveoli in the left lung with values for $P_{A_{O_2}}$ and $P_{A_{CO_2}}$ identical to those of venous blood. Continued perfusion of these lung units will constitute an absolute shunt.[53] Vascular lung tumors, intrapulmonary fistulae,[186] and bronchial obstruction[53] are other pulmonary pathologic processes that may produce an absolute shunt.[187]

Correction of the reduced $P_{a_{O_2}}$ owing to absolute shunt necessitates correction of the pathologic process (reinflation of atelectatic lung units, closure of anatomic right-to-left shunts). Decreases in $P_{a_{O_2}}$ produced by this phenomenon are refractory to O_2 administration.[181] Because the shunted blood does not perfuse functioning lung units, it is never exposed to the increased $P_{A_{O_2}}$ produced by supplemental O_2. Although additional O_2 will be present in blood perfusing other lung units, this will be carried primarily in the form of dis-

solved O_2. Little additional O_2 will be added to hemoglobin, since blood perfusing normal lung units is nearly fully saturated on room air.[187]

Relative Shunt

Lung units with a V/Q ratio greater than 0 but less than 1 are said to constitute relative shunt.[182, 188] In patients breathing room air, this results in blood perfusing these lung units having a lower O_2 content than blood perfusing normal lung units (Fig. 25-13). Unlike absolute shunt, some gas exchange does occur in the presence of relative shunt. Decreases in $P_{a_{O_2}}$ result because the bulk O_2 flow into these lung units is inadequate to achieve an O_2 content or partial pressure equal to that of blood perfusing normal lung units. Although some O_2 has been added to the mixed venous blood, it is inadequate to achieve the O_2 content of blood perfusing normal lung units.[189] Relative shunt may occur as a result of either inadequate ventilation or excessive perfusion.[190]

Relative shunts, sometimes termed venous admixture,[181] shunt effect,[181] physiologic shunt,[53] low V/Q units,[53, 191] or (nonspecifically) V/Q inequality,[69, 167, 186] are the most common cause of decreased $P_{a_{O_2}}$.[64, 167] (Description of relative shunts as "V/Q mismatch" may lead to confusion, since deadspace and absolute shunts may also be accurately described as constituting "V/Q mismatch," Fig. 25-14.) All patients manifest some degree of relative shunting as a result of normal V/Q scatter.[53, 69, 187] (Ventilation of dependent lung units is generally reduced compared with perfusion of those units.)[53, 69] Pathologic processes that may create areas of relative shunt by decreased ventilation of affected lung units include pulmonary edema, interstitial lung disease, neonatal respiratory distress syndrome (hyaline membrane disease), and ARDS.[53] Pulmonary embolism is an example of a patho-

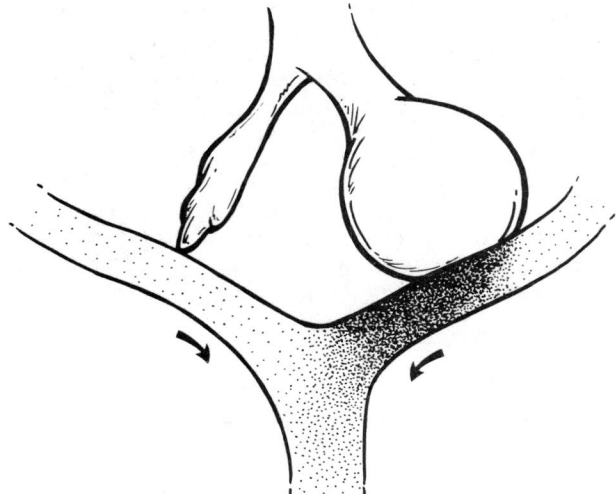

FIG. 25-12. Absolute shunt. Continued perfusion of nonventilated lung units constitutes absolute shunt. Oxygen in blood is schematically represented as stipling. Venous blood returns to the lungs with a low O_2 content. Although normal amounts of O_2 are added to blood perfusing functional lung units, reductions in O_2 content occur when shunted blood is added. Because no ventilation is present in lung units that constitute absolute shunt, the associated hypoxemia is resistant to the administration of supplemental O_2. See text for further details.

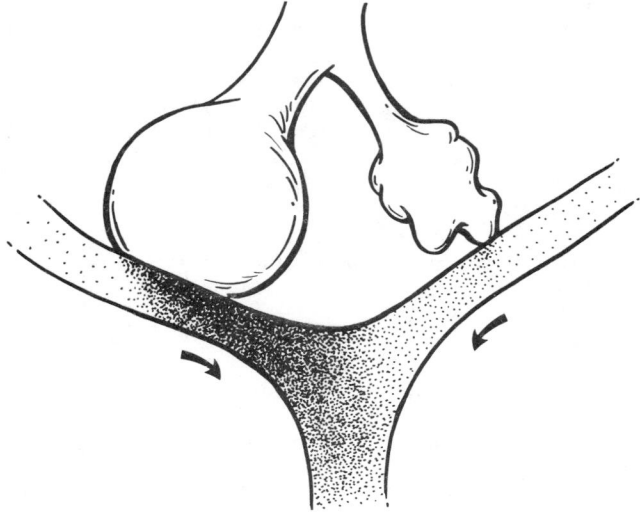

FIG. 25-13. Relative shunt. Perfusion in excess of ventilation constitutes relative shunt. Oxygen in blood is schematically represented by stipling. Although some O_2 is added to venous blood in relative shunt, the O_2 content in this blood is reduced. Arterial blood resulting from the combination of normal and relative shunt blood flow has a reduced O_2 content. Administration of supplemental O_2 may permit the addition of sufficient O_2 to achieve a "normal" O_2 content despite the existence of the relative shunt. See text for further details.

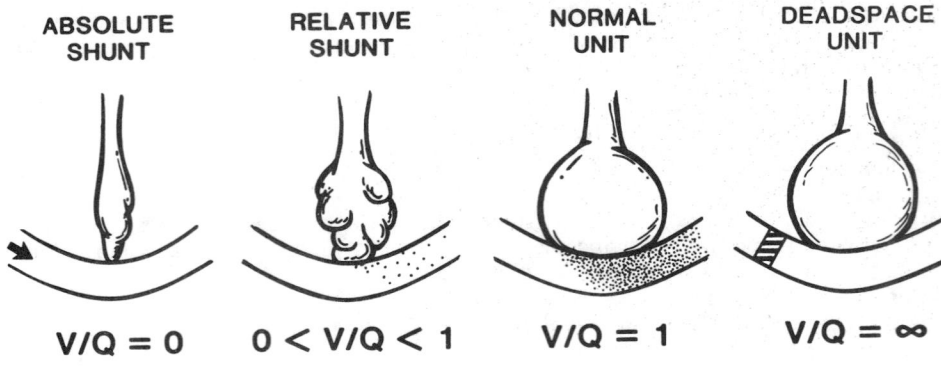

FIG. 25-14. Ventilation/perfusion relationships. The functional status of a lung unit may be represented by its V/Q ratio. Under normal circumstances, ventilation and perfusion are matched (V/Q = 1). Perfusion in excess of ventilation (most commonly produced by reductions in ventilation) constitutes relative shunt (0 < V/Q < 1). Perfusion in the absence of ventilation creates absolute shunt (V/Q = 0). Dead space occurs when ventilation occurs in the absence of perfusion.

logic process that may increase relative shunt by increasing perfusion of lung units.[53, 192] (If a major portion of the pulmonary circulation is occluded by the embolus, all blood must flow through the remaining portion of the pulmonary vascular bed. Unless ventilation of these lung units is also increased, a relative shunt may develop.)

The fact that lung units that generate relative shunt continue to receive some ventilation makes the decrease in Pa_{O_2} caused by this process amenable to O_2 therapy.[181] Although the pathologic process itself remains unchanged, its effects on Pa_{O_2} are minimized by the higher PA_{O_2} in the affected lung units. It should be noted, however, that treatment with high inspired O_2 concentrations may accelerate the conversion of areas with low but finite V/Q ratios from relative to absolute shunt by the process of absorption atelectasis.[181, 193–195] This response to supplemental O_2 may be used to differentiate cyanotic congenital heart disease from respiratory dysfunction in hypoxemic neonates. (The absolute shunting associated with cyanotic congenital heart disease produces little increase in Pa_{O_2} when 100% O_2 is administered. In contrast, a significant increase in Pa_{O_2} is almost always seen following the administration of 100% O_2 to neonates with the relative shunting associated with lung disease.)[196]

ESTIMATION OF SHUNT. Calculation of venous admixture or physiologic shunt by Equation 25-15 allows a means of quantitating the magnitude of combined relative and absolute shunt.[53] If the calculations are performed using numbers obtained with the patient breathing 100% O_2, the value obtained primarily reflects the amount of absolute shunt present.[197] (With $F_{I_{O_2}} = 1.0$, areas of relative shunt should be either masked by the high PA_{O_2} or converted to absolute shunt by absorption atelectasis.) Breathing less than 100% O_2, however, the equation combines the effects of relative and absolute shunt to generate a value for the physiologic shunt (Q_{sp}/Q_t). Essentially, the equation considers the blood from all lung units as having a P_{O_2} equal to either mixed venous P_{O_2} ($P\bar{v}_{O_2}$) or PA_{O_2}.[53, 167] Although entirely artificial (combining, as it does, absolute and relative shunt), the calculated shunt fraction is still a useful method of quantitating lung dysfunction and following response to therapeutic interventions.[53]

$$\frac{Q_{sp}}{Q_t} = \frac{Cc'_{O_2} - Ca_{O_2}}{Cc'_{O_2} - C\bar{v}_{O_2}} \qquad (25\text{-}15)$$

Q_{sp} = physiologic shunt flow
Q_t = cardiac output
Q_{sp}/Q_t = shunt fraction
Cc'_{O_2} = O_2 content of idealized pulmonary capillary ($Pc'_{O_2} = PA_{O_2}$)
Ca_{O_2} = arterial O_2 content
$C\bar{v}_{O_2}$ = mixed venous O_2 content

(Oxygen contents are calculated using Eqn. 25-7; mixed venous and idealized pulmonary capillary values are calculated using the respective values for S_{O_2} and P_{O_2}.)

Decreased Mixed Venous P_{O_2}

If all lung units functioned perfectly and no shunt (either relative or absolute) existed, mixed venous P_{O_2} ($P\bar{v}_{O_2}$) would not affect Pa_{O_2}. Since this is not true and some degree of shunting is present in all patients, decreases in $P\bar{v}_{O_2}$ may also produce a decrease in Pa_{O_2}.[198] Consider a patient in whom 50% of pulmonary blood flow occurs through an absolute shunt, with the remaining pulmonary blood flow perfusing "perfect" lung units and achieving a P_{O_2} equal to alveolar P_{O_2}. A reduction in $P\bar{v}_{O_2}$ will have a significant effect on Pa_{O_2}, as demonstrated in (Fig. 25-15). By utilizing a 50% shunt fraction, this example admittedly accentuates the effect of a decrease in $P\bar{v}_{O_2}$ on Pa_{O_2}. It should be evident from the example, however, that 1) changes in $P\bar{v}_{O_2}$ may influence Pa_{O_2}, and 2) the magnitude of the effect on Pa_{O_2} is determined by the magnitude of the shunt fraction.

$P\bar{v}_{O_2}$ is determined by the balance between O_2 supply and O_2 demand. Reductions in $P\bar{v}_{O_2}$ may occur as a result of either increases in demand (owing to fever, hyperthyroidism, seizures, or shivering) or decreases in supply. Since O_2 supply is determined by arterial O_2 content and cardiac output,[199] this mechanism of decreased Pa_{O_2} permits an isolated reduction in cardiac output to produce a decrease in Pa_{O_2} without any change in lung function.[53] (It should be noted, however, that many studies have documented a decrease in shunt fraction occurring apparently as a consequence of reduced cardiac output.[200, 201] It has been proposed that the decrease in shunt is due to pulmonary vasoconstriction stimulated by the decreased $P\bar{v}_{O_2}$.[202] Ultimately, the changes in Pa_{O_2} induced by decreases in cardiac output may be minimized by simultaneous reductions in shunt fraction.)[53]

Treatment of decreased Pa_{O_2} produced by decreased $P\bar{v}_{O_2}$ is best addressed by providing an adequate O_2 supply to meet O_2 demands. In practice, this involves normalizing O_2 demands (by treating fever, seizures, or hyperthyroidism) or increasing O_2 supply (by increasing cardiac output or hemoglobin in an anemic patient).

Diffusion Block

Impaired diffusion of O_2 from the alveolus into pulmonary capillary blood (diffusion block, alveolar capillary block) has classically been considered another potential etiology of reduced Pa_{O_2}.[186, 203] Diseases that are associated with an increased distance between alveolar gas and red blood cell (and therefore have been considered to produce hypoxemia by

FIG. 25-15. Mechanisms of hypoxemia. Calculations assume Hb=15 g·dl^{-1}, normal Pv̄$_{O_2}$=40 mm Hg (approximately 75% saturation producing mixed venous O_2 content, Cv̄$_{O_2}$, of 15 ml O_2·dl^{-1}. (A) Qs/Qt=50%, normal cardiac output. Equal volumes of blood flow through each route. Blood perfusing normal lung units achieves C$_{O_2}$=20 ml·dl^{-1}. No O_2 is added to blood constituting shunt (C$_{O_2}$ remains 15 ml·dl^{-1}). Combining equal amounts of blood with each O_2 content produces Ca$_{O_2}$=17.5 ml·dl^{-1}. (B) Qs/Qt=50%, cardiac output reduced. In the absence of decreases in O_2 demand, reductions in cardiac output produce a decrease in Cv̄$_{O_2}$, here depicted as 10 ml·dl^{-1}. Qs/Qt remains 50%, unchanged from A. Blood perfusing normal lung units still achieves C$_{O_2}$=20 ml·dl^{-1}. As in A, no O_2 is added to shunt blood, that is, C$_{O_2}$ remains 10 ml·dl^{-1}. Combining equal amounts of blood with each C$_{O_2}$ produces Ca$_{O_2}$=15 ml·dl^{-1}. Although *lung* function has remained unchanged (Qs/Qt is still 50%), C$_{O_2}$ has been reduced solely by a decrease in Cv̄$_{O_2}$. (C) Qs/Qt=25%, cardiac output normal. Decreases in Qs/Qt produce increase in Ca$_{O_2}$. As in A, Cv̄$_{O_2}$=15 ml·dl^{-1}, but a decrease in Qs/Qt from 50% to 25% produces a higher Ca$_{O_2}$.

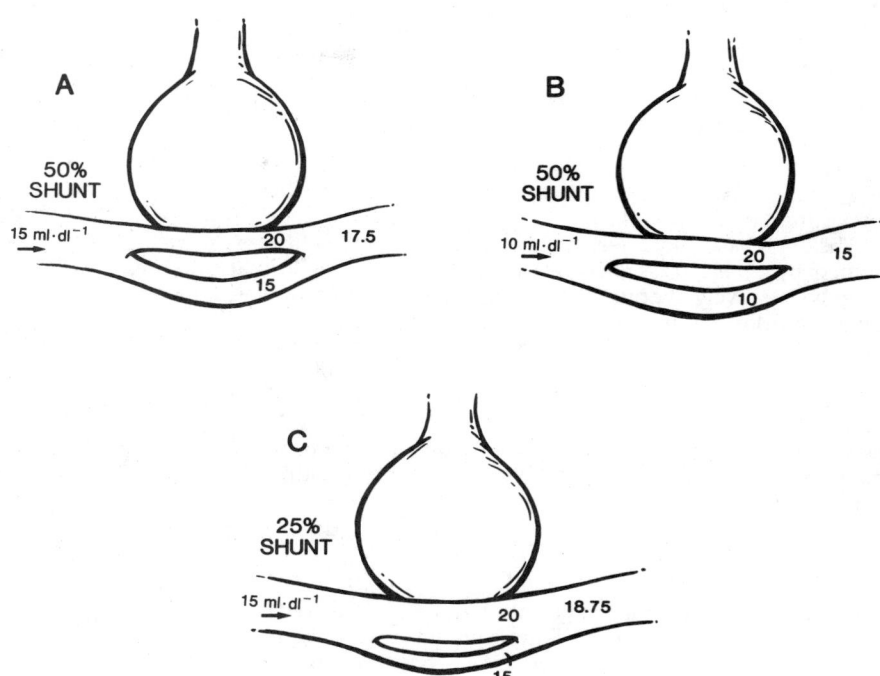

diffusion block) include alveolar cell carcinoma, collagen diseases with pulmonary involvement, diffuse interstitial fibrosis, asbestosis, and sarcoidosis.[69] The concept is appealing and appears intuitively valid. Nonetheless, the distorted pulmonary architecture probably prevents normal ventilation and blood flow in the affected areas. Use of the multiple inert gas technique to evaluate V/Q relationships has determined that all of the hypoxemia present under these circumstances may be attributed to uneven ventilation and blood flow.[167] Although diffusion block continues to be mentioned as an etiology of hypoxemia in some textbooks, most authors now consider that the majority of circumstances formerly attributed to diffusion block (sarcoidosis, pulmonary fibrosis) are in reality manifestations of shunts, either relative or absolute.[69, 154]

The potential role of diffusion in the development of arterial hypoxemia is increased in the presence of low PA$_{O_2}$ (as occur with low barometric pressures or the administration of hypoxic gas mixtures).[53] Additionally, under conditions of exercise, when cardiac output and the rate of pulmonary blood flow are increased, blood is exposed to lung units for shorter periods of time and diffusion has a greater potential to become a limiting factor in the bulk flow of O_2 from the alveolus into the pulmonary capillary blood.[53, 69]

Since rate of diffusion is a function of the P$_{O_2}$ gradient from alveolus to pulmonary capillary, administration of even low concentrations of supplemental O_2 increase the P$_{O_2}$ gradient from alveolus to pulmonary capillary blood so drastically that any component of diffusion block that existed on room air should be completely corrected by supplemental O_2.[69, 186]

TEMPERATURE CORRECTION

In the past, it was recommended that blood gases and pH should be corrected for temperature if the temperature of the measuring electrode (usually 37° Celsius) differed from the patient's body temperature. This recommendation is based on the knowledge that the solubility of O_2 and CO_2 in the blood are temperature-dependent. Therefore, placing blood from patients with body temperatures less than 37° Celsius into electrodes maintained at 37° Celsius means that more molecules enter the gas phase to be sensed as partial pressure than would be present *in vivo* at the lower body temperature of the patient. Nomograms are available to correct blood gases and pH measurements for temperature. The need, however, to correct P$_{CO_2}$ and pH measurements for body temperature is questionable.[204] It is argued that a normal P$_{CO_2}$ and pH measured at an electrode temperature of 37° Celsius reflects an unperturbed acid–based status of the patient regardless of the body temperature that existed at the time the sample was drawn. This argument is based on the concept that maintenance of electrochemical neutrality (pH = pOH) requires the pH to rise with reductions in body temperature. Conversely, with increases in body temperature, the neutral point falls, and maintenance of electrochemical neutrality requires a decrease in pH. If this concept is accepted, it is unnecessary to correct P$_{CO_2}$ and pH for variations in body temperature from the temperature of the electrodes that are usually maintained at 37° Celsius. Temperature correction of the P$_{O_2}$ remains important, however, to assess oxygenation.

ACID–BASE

Acid–base balance has been conceptually difficult for many physicians. This confusion is understandable given that 1) the measurement system (based as it is on negative logarithms) is unique in clinical medicine, and 2) the concentrations of hydrogen ion (H$^+$) are 1/1,000,000th the concentration of most other commonly measured ions in the body.

Definition

The concept of acids and bases is more easily grasped if the Brönsted–Lowry definitions of the two terms are accepted.

Using this nomenclature, acids are H^+ donors and bases are H^+ recipients.

$$HA \rightleftharpoons H^+ + A^- \qquad (25\text{-}16)$$

In Equation 25-16, HA is an acid, since it is capable of donating one H^+. Similarly, A^- is a base, since it is capable of accepting one H^+.

The acid–base characteristics of a substance are *not* determined by its electrical charge. Table 25-5 shows acids that may be positively charged, negatively charged, or neutral. A single substance (NH_3 in Table 25-5) may constitute either an acid (when it releases H^+ to form NH_2^-) or a base (when it accepts H^+ to form NH_4^+). The behavior of such substances is determined by the H^+ concentration of the solution. When the H^+ concentration is very high, NH_3 will likely act as a base by accepting H^+ to form NH_4^+. When the H^+ concentration is very low, NH_3 will likely act as an acid by donating H^+ and forming NH_2^-.

pH System

Although most other ion concentrations are measured and expressed in terms of equivalents or moles, by convention, H^+ concentrations are expressed as *pH*. This system greatly impedes comprehension. First, the system is logarithmic rather than linear (an increase from $pH = 6.0$ to $pH = 7.0$ reflects a tenfold change in H^+ concentration). Second, the system is negative rather than positive (an *increase* from $pH = 7.0$ to $pH = 7.4$ reflects a *decrease* in H^+ concentration). Both concepts are alien to all other conventional clinical measurements. Conceptual understanding of H^+ concentration might be improved by utilizing nanoequivalents (nEq) instead of *pH* as measurement units.[205, 206] However, the *pH* system is so ingrained in physiology, pharmacology, and, for that matter, clinical medicine that physicians are compelled to conform to its eccentricities.

From Table 25-6, the logarithmic nature of the measuring scale should be evident. By definition, a 1.0 unit change in *pH* is associated with a tenfold change in H^+ concentration ($pH\ 6.0 = H^+\ 1000\ nEq \cdot l^{-1}$, $pH\ 7.0 = H^+\ 100\ nEq \cdot l^{-1}$, $pH\ 8.0 = H^+\ 10\ nEq \cdot l^{-1}$). A change in *pH* from 7.4 to 7.0 represents a $60\ nEq \cdot l^{-1}$ change in H^+ concentration, but the same magnitude change in *pH* when going from 7.4 to 7.8 represents only a $24\ nEq \cdot l^{-1}$ change in H^+ concentration.

The strength of an acid is determined by the magnitude of dissociation in solution and by the resultant concentration of H^+. The *pH* at which the substance is 50% dissociated (equal amounts of A^- and HA are present) is termed the pKa of that substance. The lower the pKa of a substance, the stronger the acid. Lactic acid (pKa = 3.86) is said to be a stronger acid than carbonic acid (pKa = 6.1), because at any given *pH*, lactic acid will be more dissociated and release more H^+ than carbonic acid.

TABLE 25-5.   Examples of Acids and Bases

ACID		BASE
NH_4^+	$\rightleftharpoons$	$H^+ + NH_3$
NH_3	$\rightleftharpoons$	$H^+ + NH_2^-$
$H_2PO_4^-$	$\rightleftharpoons$	$H^+ + HPO_4^=$

TABLE 25-6.   Comparison of H^+ Concentration in $nEq \cdot l^{-1}$ and *pH*

H^+ ($nEq \cdot l^{-1}$)	*pH*
1000	6.0
160	6.8
125	6.9
100	7.0
80	7.1
63	7.2
50	7.3
40	7.4
35	7.5
25	7.6
20	7.7
16	7.8
10	8.0

ROLE OF HYDROGEN ION

Water may be considered an acid, dissociating as it does to form hydroxyl (OH^-) and hydrogen ions (Eqn. 25-17).

$$H_2O \rightleftharpoons H^+ + OH^- \qquad (25\text{-}17)$$

Pure water dissociates into equal amounts of H^+ and OH^- the concentration of each being 0.000000.01 (or 1×10^{-7} $mEq \cdot l^{-1}$) at 25° Celsius. Since the concentration of H^+ is 1×10^{-7}, the *pH* (negative logarithm of H^+ concentration) of water is 7.0. An *increase* in H^+ concentration is manifested by a *decrease* in *pH*. For example, the addition to water of a strong acid (such as HCl) will result in an increase in H^+ concentration. If HCl is added until H^+ concentration is 0.0000001 (or $10 \times 10^{-7} = 1 \times 10^{-6}$) $mEq \cdot l^{-1}$, the new *pH* will be 6.0. A tenfold increase in H^+ concentration is associated with a 1.0 unit decrease in *pH*. Similarly, *pH* will increase by addition of a base (which decreases H^+ concentration).

Despite its low concentration relative to other ions, H^+ still plays a significant role in altering body functions. Changes in H^+ concentration have been described as altering the electrochemical behavior of water itself,[205] thereby affecting the distribution of other ions. One of the best examples of this principle is the alkalinization of serum produced by hyperventilation or the administration of sodium bicarbonate ($NaHCO_3$) in the acute therapy of hyperkalemic-induced cardiac dysrhythmias. The increase in *pH* produced by either intervention causes extracellular K^+ to move into the cells. A 0.10 unit increase in *pH* produces a 0.5 to 1.5 $mEq \cdot l^{-1}$ decrease in serum K^+.[207] Although total body potassium remains unchanged, the alteration in distribution normalizes the ratio between intracellular and extracellular potassium concentrations, thus ameliorating the cardiac dysrhythmias.[208]

Changes in H^+ concentration also alter protein configuration. Perhaps the most relevant example is the ease with which hemoglobin binds and releases O_2 in the face of changes in *pH*.[151, 209] Alteration in H^+ concentration tends to change the stereochemistry of hemoglobin, which ultimately changes the ability of hemoglobin to bind O_2[151] (as indicated by the shift in the oxyhemoglobin dissociation curve in Fig. 25-10). Alterations in protein configuration may also produce changes in biodegradation, detoxification, energy metabolism, and biosynthesis.[205]

ACID PRODUCTION

Essentially all acids normally present in the body occur as a result of metabolism. Carbon dioxide, which becomes an H^+ donor following its hydration to carbonic acid (Eqn. 25-18), constitutes the majority of the daily acid load with which the body must cope.

$$H_2O + CO_2 \rightleftharpoons H_2CO_2 \rightleftharpoons H^+ + HCO_3^- \qquad (25\text{-}18)$$

The production of 200 ml $\cdot$ min^{-1} of CO_2 is associated with a daily production of 12,960 mEq of acid in the form of CO_2.[210] Because of its unique ability to be eliminated by the lungs, CO_2 is termed a "volatile" or "respiratory" acid.[211-213] Acid–base disturbances owing to abnormalities of CO_2 production or elimination are therefore described as "respiratory" disorders.[64, 211, 214-216]

All remaining acids produced in the body are described as "fixed,"[212, 213] "nonvolatile,"[206, 213] or metabolic acids[216]; acid–base disturbances resulting from abnormalities of their production or elimination are termed *metabolic* disorders.[65, 211, 213-216] The majority of these metabolic acids (pyruvic acid,[152] lactic acid,[217] acetoacetic acid,[152] and beta-hydroxybutyric acid[217]) are capable of undergoing further metabolic degradation, eventually being reduced to CO_2 and H_2O. In this manner, many metabolic acids are converted to respiratory acids and eliminated by way of the lungs. The kidneys are the major avenue for the excretion of inorganic acids (*e.g.*, phosphoric acid, sulfuric acid, uric acid) and those fixed acids that are not converted to CO_2 and H_2O.[206] Under normal circumstances, renal excretion of H^+ is approximately 1 mEq $\cdot$ kg^{-1} daily.[206, 210, 213, 216]

MEASUREMENT

When assessing acid–base status in the clinical laboratory, three different measurements are commonly obtained: pH, P_{CO_2}, and bicarbonate ion (HCO_3^-).[205, 216] The Henderson–Hasselbalch equation can be modified to relate all three of these components.[205, 216]

$$pH = pKa + \log \frac{HCO_3^-}{H_2CO_3}$$

pKa = dissociation constant for carbonic acid/bicarbonate
HCO_3^- = bicarbonate concentration (mEq $\cdot$ l^{-1})
H_2CO_3 = CO_2 in physical solution in plasma (including H_2CO_3)   (25-19)

By using the solubility coefficient for CO_2 in plasma and the pKa of carbonic acid, the equation can be reconstructed:[205, 210, 216, 218, 219]

$$pH = 6.1 + \log \frac{HCO_3^-}{0.03P_{CO_2}}$$

6.1 = pKa of H_2CO_3 system
0.03 = solubility coefficient of CO_2
P_{CO_2} = partial pressure of CO_2 (25-20)

The Henderson–Hasselbalch equation has at least three redeeming qualities. First, the equation separates the "marker" used to evaluate metabolic disorders (HCO_3^-) from the marker used to evaluate respiratory disorders (CO_2). Although neither marker is affected solely by one specific type of disturbance (*i.e.*, alterations in Pa_{CO_2} owing to respiratory

disorders will have a direct influence on HCO_3^- concentrations, the metabolic marker), the concept is clinically useful and reflects the characterizations of most disturbances as primarily a result of either respiratory or metabolic disturbances.

Second, the equation emphasizes the fact that pH is not determined by the absolute amounts of either HCO_3^- or CO_2, but rather by the ratio between the two (*i.e.*, pH will remain normal despite an increased Pa_{CO_2} if HCO_3^- is increased proportionally). It is this fact that provides the basis for normal compensatory mechanisms. (The pH change induced by respiratory depression, which produces a primary increase in Pa_{CO_2}, is minimized by renal mechanisms that increase HCO_3^- concentration. In this manner, changes in the ratio of HCO_3^- and CO_2 in the blood are minimized.)

Third, using the Henderson–Hasselbalch equation allows any one of the three components to be determined from measurements of the other two.[210, 213, 219] Under normal circumstances, HCO_3^- is approximately 24 mEq $\cdot$ l^{-1} and Pa_{CO_2} is 40 mm Hg. Since Pa_{CO_2} must be multiplied by 0.03 to determine the CO_2 in physical solution (Eqn. 25-20), the ratio is 24/1.2 or 20. Normal arterial pH equals 6.1 plus log 20. Since log 20 is 1.3, normal arterial pH = 6.1 + 1.3 = 7.4. An increase in the ratio (owing to either an increase in HCO_3^- or a decrease in Pa_{CO_2}) produces an increased pH (alkalosis). Decreases in the ratio (owing to a decrease in HCO_3^- or an increase in Pa_{CO_2}) produce a decrease in pH (acidosis).

pH

Determination of the pH of a blood sample relies on the unique properties of special "pH-sensitive glass." If two samples of different pH are separated by a membrane of pH-sensitive glass, a measurable voltage will develop across the glass. The modern electrode uses a measuring electrode composed of silver–silver chloride embedded in a buffer solution of known pH. The reference electrode of mercury–mercurous chloride is connected by a potassium chloride solution to the measuring electrode. A voltmeter is used to measure the electrical potential difference that occurs when substances of two different H^+ concentrations, the blood sample and the buffer solution with pH = 6.840, are separated by the pH-sensitive glass.[220]

The modern Sanz electrode (Fig. 25-16) incorporates these elements in a design that maintains a constant temperature by encasing the measuring electrode and the sample chamber in a water bath.[220] Configuration of the pH-sensitive glass as a fine capillary tube allows pH determinations on samples as small as 25 μl.[1]

pH, like P_{CO_2} and P_{O_2}, is most commonly determined on an arterial blood sample. Also like P_{CO_2} and P_{O_2}, pH should be determined as quickly as possible after the sample is obtained in order to minimize changes in H^+ concentration owing either to the formation of lactic acid by the metabolism of glucose or to the loss of CO_2.[219, 221] Anaerobic techniques are necessary during sampling, transportation, storage, and measurement in order to minimize changes in pH owing to loss of CO_2 from the sample.[219, 222]

Bicarbonate Ion Concentration

Serum bicarbonate concentration cannot be measured directly.[219, 223] Because all forms of CO_2 (CO_2 in physical solution, H_2CO_3, HCO_3^-, and carbamino compounds) are in equilibrium, the process of titration measures the total content of all forms of CO_2 in the sample (ctCO_2). The value of

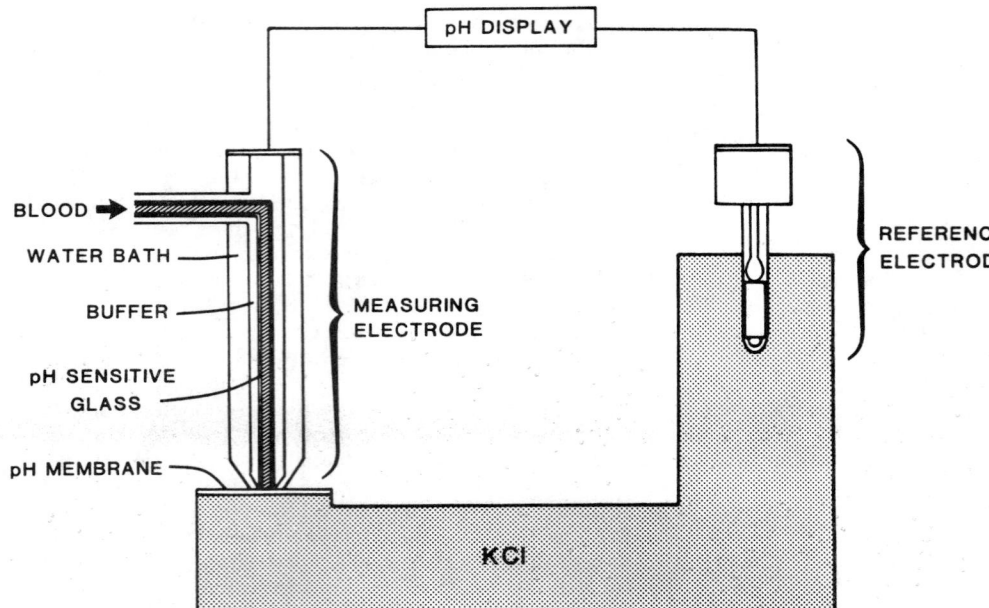

FIG. 25-16. pH electrode. When two solutions with different H^+ concentrations are separated by a special pH-sensitive glass, a measurable voltage occurs. The modern electrode consists of two half cells (measuring and reference electrodes) connected by a KCl salt bridge. Blood is injected into a capillary tube composed of pH-sensitive glass and surrounded by a buffer solution with pH = 6.84. The measuring electrode is encased in a constant temperature water bath. The blood gas machine converts the voltage created by the difference in pH between the blood sample and the buffer solution into pH. (Modified from Shapiro BA, Harrison RA, Walton JR. Clinical Application of Blood Gases, 3rd ed, p 32. Chicago, Year Book Medical Publishers, 1982.)

"bicarbonate" reported from chemistry laboratories is actually a measure of the total CO_2 content of the sample.[219, 221, 222]

Once again, comprehension is obfuscated by imprecise terminology. Confusion is enhanced by referring to the value derived for total CO_2 as either "CO_2" (which may be confused with P_{CO_2}) or "bicarbonate" (which may be confused with true HCO_3^- concentrations). Because most such determinations are performed on serum or plasma, the carbamino compounds contribute little, and the value reported is influenced largely by the concentrations of HCO_3^- and H_2CO_3 as well as P_{CO_2}. (Measurement of total CO_2 content in whole blood would result in a higher value, primarily because of the additional quantity of CO_2 present in the form of carbamino compounds.)[219, 222]

Accurately interpreting total CO_2 content involves recognizing the components being measured. Changes in the quantity of CO_2 present in any of the three forms may produce changes in total CO_2 content. Further, reciprocal changes in the quantity of one form of CO_2 may minimize or completely obscure a change in the quantity of another form (e.g., total CO_2 may be normal despite a decreased HCO_3^- concentration if Pa_{CO_2} is sufficiently increased). Fortunately, normal compensatory mechanisms prevent the common occurrence of this problem. As dictated by the Henderson–Hasselbalch equation, compensation for decreased HCO_3^- concentrations produces a *decrease* in Pa_{CO_2}. Since decreases in the quantity of either HCO_3^- or Pa_{CO_2} will produce a reduction in total CO_2 content, the simultaneous occurrence of these changes will magnify the deviation of total CO_2 content from normal. Only under the rare circumstances of combined defects of the same type (i.e., simultaneous metabolic and respiratory acidosis) may total CO_2 content be normal in the presence of a significant acid–base disturbance. The fact remains, however, that total CO_2 content is more affected by changes in Pa_{CO_2} and other nonbicarbonate forms of CO_2 in the blood than the serum HCO_3^- concentration calculated by the Henderson–Hasselbalch equation. This has led some authors to compare interpreting total CO_2 content without

knowing the pH to interpreting white blood cell count without a differential cell count.[219, 224, 225]

While the value for "bicarbonate" reported by chemistry laboratories is actually total CO_2 content, blood gas laboratories routinely report a value for HCO_3^- concentration that is calculated from the Henderson–Hasselbalch equation using the measured values of pH and P_{CO_2}. Although questions have been raised regarding the validity of calculated values for HCO_3^- derived from the Henderson–Hasselbalch equation,[226] these questions have centered on the stability of the value used for pKa[227, 228] and/or the existence of equilibrium at the time that the sample was obtained.[227, 229] At this time, the preponderance of evidence seems to indicate that pKa is a stable value, at least within the range of clinically encountered conditions.[230-233] Even those who voice concern agree that the values derived from the Henderson–Hasselbalch equation are sufficiently accurate for use in the clinical setting.[226, 230] Despite disparaging remarks regarding the "calculated" nature of this value, assuming that the values for pH and P_{CO_2} are correct, it more accurately represents serum HCO_3^- concentration than the "measured" determination of total CO_2 content.[230] Although the reported value of total CO_2 content reflects all forms of CO_2 in the sample, according to the Henderson–Hasselbalch equation, there is only one possible value for HCO_3^- for each pair of pH and P_{CO_2} values.[210]

DEFENSE MECHANISMS

Classic teaching is that H^+ concentration is very carefully controlled in the body.[213, 216] It is true that changes of 60 $nEq \cdot l^{-1}$ in sodium concentrations would go undetected, whereas the same change in H^+ concentrations produce significant changes in pH. On the other hand, it should be recognized that the range of pH that is acutely compatible with life represents a seven- to tenfold increase in H^+ concentration from the lowest concentration to the highest concentration.[213, 214] Imagine serum sodium or potassium varying by such percentages! No other ions in the body are allowed this magnitude of variation in concentration.

Under most circumstances, however, arterial pH is maintained between 7.35 and 7.44 (corresponding to H^+ concentrations of approximately 35 to 45 $nEq \cdot l^{-1}$).[213, 214] Two separate defense mechanisms, compensation and buffering, minimize the change in pH resulting from normal metabolism and disturbances in acid production and/or elimination.

Compensation

Acid–base abnormalities can result from increased loss or excessive production of acids or bases. The body responds to such problems by minimizing both the magnitude and duration of the abnormality. The development of a primary acid–base problem, reflected in an alteration of arterial pH, stimulates compensatory mechanisms as well as responses intended ultimately to correct the primary problem.

The magnitude of pH change resulting from the addition (or loss) of a given amount of acid (or base) is minimized by compensatory mechanisms that restore the bicarbonate/carbonic acid ratio (HCO_3^-/CO_2) toward normal.[213] Primary changes in the concentration of one variable produce compensatory alteration in the other. Metabolic derangements, which alter pH by changes in HCO_3^- concentration, stimulate ventilatory compensation. (P_{CO_2} is altered to minimize changes in HCO_3^-/CO_2. If HCO_3^- concentration decreases, decreases in P_{CO_2} will minimize the change in pH by reducing the derangement of HCO_3^-/CO_2).[213, 214, 216] Primary alterations in P_{CO_2} stimulate metabolic compensation in the form of alterations in HCO_3^- concentration. (The effect on pH produced by increases in P_{CO_2} will be minimized by increasing HCO_3^- concentration, thus restoring HCO_3^-/P_{CO_2}.)[64, 213, 216]

Respiratory compensation for metabolic acid–base derangements is limited to alterations in the excretion of CO_2. Decreases in HCO_3^- concentration stimulate an increase in alveolar ventilation, which restores HCO_3^-/CO_2 toward normal by decreasing Pa_{CO_2}.[213, 214, 216] Increases in HCO_3^- concentration invoke a decrease in CO_2 elimination by reducing alveolar ventilation. Decreased ventilation produces not only an increase in Pa_{CO_2}, but also a reduction in Pa_{O_2}. In the absence of supplemental O_2 administration, respiratory compensation for primary increases in HCO_3^- concentration may be limited by the respiratory stimulation from the carotid body in response to arterial hypoxemia.

Renal compensation for acid–base disorders may be possible not only in response to a primary respiratory disturbance but also in response to a metabolic derangement. Normal renal function permits increased H^+ excretion and/or increased HCO_3^- reabsorption in disease states such as diabetic ketoacidosis or lactic acidosis.[206] These mechanisms are obviously unavailable in metabolic acidosis owing to renal failure. In response to decreases in Pa_{CO_2}, HCO_3^- concentration may be reduced by renal dumping of HCO_3^- or by decreased elimination of H^+.[206, 213]

Although restoration of pH to normal by compensation would be optimal, a completely normal pH removes the stimulus for compensation, and the primary problem becomes manifest again.[213] Complete compensation for a primary problem (i.e., restoration of a normal pH) almost never results from compensatory mechanisms alone.

Buffers

Ultimately, acids must be physically removed from the body to prevent an undesirable decrease in pH. As indicated previously, this is accomplished with the elimination of CO_2 by the lungs and of metabolic acids by the kidneys. The presence of a system of chemical compounds known as buffers minimizes the variations in pH occurring before and after acids are eliminated. Without buffering systems, venous pH would be substantially lower than arterial pH because of added CO_2 and metabolic acids.

The typical buffer system of the body consists of a weak acid (HBuffer), which is capable of dissociating as shown in Equation 25-21, and its salt (NaBuffer), Equation 25-22.

$$HBuffer \rightleftharpoons H^+ + Buffer^- \qquad (25\text{-}21)$$

$$NaBuffer \rightleftharpoons Na^+ + Buffer^- \qquad (25\text{-}22)$$

The buffer pair is capable of combining with H^+ produced by addition of stronger acids (Eqn. 25-23) or OH^- produced by adding stronger bases (Eqn. 25-24) to minimize the change in H^+ concentration induced by the addition of one of these compounds.

$$HCl + NaBuffer \rightleftharpoons H^+ + Cl^- + Na^+ + Buffer^-$$
$$\rightleftharpoons HBuffer + NaCl \qquad (25\text{-}23)$$

$$NaOH + HBuffer \rightleftharpoons Na^+ + OH^- + H^+ + Buffer^-$$
$$\rightleftharpoons NaBuffer + H_2O \qquad (25\text{-}24)$$

Equation 25-23 demonstrates the buffering of an acid. HCl, a strong acid (i.e., largely dissociated), is added to a system containing the salt of a weak acid (NaBuffer). The H^+ released by HCl combines with the dissociated Buffer$^-$ to form the weak acid HBuffer. Because HBuffer is a weak acid, it is less dissociated than HCl. Accordingly, less free H^+ exists, and the pH decreases less than if HCl were added to the system without a buffer.

A similar circumstance is portrayed in Equation 25-24. In the absence of a buffer, the free OH^- released from NaOH, a strong base, combines with most free H^+, reducing H^+ concentration and thereby substantially raising pH. In Equation 25-24, H^+ released from HBuffer combines with the OH^- to produce H_2O and NaBuffer. The presence of the buffer has converted some of the strong base NaOH to the weaker base NaBuffer. The H^+ concentration is maintained closer to the initial value because NaBuffer is less dissociated than NaOH.

The efficacy of a buffer is determined by comparing the pKa of the components to the starting pH of the solution to be buffered (the closer pKa is to the initial pH, the more effective the buffer) and to the concentration of the buffer substances (the greater the concentration, the more H^+ that can be buffered).[213] There are three major buffer systems in the body: 1) carbonic acid–bicarbonate, 2) phosphate, and 3) protein.

CARBONIC ACID–BICARBONATE. Producing carbonic acid by dissolving CO_2 in water was demonstrated in Equation 25-18. In the presence of HCO_3^-, usually in the form of (extracellular) $NaHCO_3$ or (intracellular) $KHCO_3$, the reaction shown in Equation 25-25 will occur when a strong acid is added to the system.

$$HCl + NaHCO_3 \rightleftharpoons H^+ + Cl^- + Na^+ + HCO_3^- \rightleftharpoons NaCl$$
$$+ H_2CO_3 \rightleftharpoons NaCl + H_2O + CO_2 \qquad (25\text{-}25)$$

Ventilation eliminates the CO_2 produced from carbonic acid, thus effectively removing the acid introduced initially in the form of HCl. Because of its ability to convert a strong acid to CO_2, a volatile acid that can be eliminated by the lungs, bicarbonate is unique among the buffering systems of the body.[206, 210] Obviously, however, the bicarbonate system cannot buffer respiratory acid, CO_2.

A strong base, such as NaOH, is buffered by carbonic acid, as shown in Equation 25-26.

$$NaOH + H_2CO_3 \rightleftharpoons Na^+ + OH^- + H^+ \\ + HCO_3^- \rightleftharpoons NaHCO_3 + H_2O \qquad (25\text{-}26)$$

The continuous production of CO_2 by metabolism ensures that adequate quantities are available to rapidly buffer any strong base and convert it to HCO_3^-.[206]

Based on the pKa (6.1) of the system and the concentration of its components, the bicarbonate buffering system would be anticipated to be minimally significant in modulating pH changes.[213] Notwithstanding these inadequacies, the efficacy of bicarbonate as a buffer of metabolic acids probably equals all the others in the body.[210, 211, 213] The reason for this disproportionate significance is that both components of the system, CO_2 and HCO_3^-, can be regulated independently.[210, 213]

PHOSPHATE. The phosphate buffer system is of greatest significance intracellularly.[206, 213] The system, which is similar to bicarbonate, is illustrated in Equations 25-27 and 25-28.

$$HCl + Na_2HPO_4 \rightleftharpoons H^+ + Cl^- + Na^+ \\ + NaHPO_4 \rightleftharpoons NaCl + NaH_2PO_4 \qquad (25\text{-}27)$$

$$NaOH + NaH_2PO_4 \rightleftharpoons Na^+ + OH^- + H^+ \\ + NaHPO_4 \rightleftharpoons Na_2HPO_4 + H_2O \qquad (25\text{-}28)$$

Equation 25-27 demonstrates the conversion of the strong acid HCl into the weak acid NaH_2PO_4. Although the NaH_2PO_4 formed during the buffering of HCl is capable of dissociating into $NaHPO_4^-$ and H^+, because it is a weak acid (*i.e.*, poorly dissociated), less H^+ is produced than if the buffer were not present.

Since the pKa of the phosphate buffer system is 6.8, the system operates near its maximal efficiency in arterial blood.[213] The efficacy of this system in plasma is substantially reduced, however, by the low concentration of its components in extracellular fluid.[206] The concentration of the phosphate buffer components in the extracellular fluid is less than 10% of that of the components of the bicarbonate systems.[206] The small amount of Na_2HPO_4 present in plasma is capable of buffering very few hydrogen ions. Its contribution is increased in intracellular fluids because of its higher concentrations there.[206] Additionally, normal mean intracellular pH, which has been estimated as 6.9[234] is almost exactly the same as the pKa of this buffer system. Renal tubular cells, where phosphate concentrations are even higher, are the site of maximal phosphate buffering activity in the body.[213]

PROTEIN BUFFERS. Proteins account for the majority of intracellular buffering potential.[206, 213] Although protein buffering capacity is greatest in the cells, it is also effective for buffering extracellular fluid. In spite of the fact that protein concentrations in extracellular fluids are relatively low, the ability of CO_2 to easily pass cell membranes, combined with the ability (albeit limited) of H^+ and HCO_3^- to also diffuse across this barrier, allows the intracellular buffer systems to participate in the buffering of extracellular fluids as well.[213] It has been estimated that 75% of the body's chemical buffering power is intracellular.[213]

Some amino acids have the ability to neutralize H^+ by lib-

erating OH^- from free basic radicals, most often in the form of $-NH_3OH$ (Eqn. 25-29).

$$-NH_3OH + H^+ \rightleftharpoons -NH_3^+ + H_2O \qquad (25\text{-}29)$$

Similarly, free acidic radicals, most often in the form of $-COOH$, have the ability to liberate H^+ and thereby neutralize excessive base (Eqn. 25-30).

$$-COOH + OH^- \rightleftharpoons COO^- + H_2O \qquad (25\text{-}30)$$

Protein buffering is important because of the large quantities of protein that are distributed throughout the body and because the pKa of several proteins approximates 7.4.[213]

The hemoglobin buffering system is a special example of the protein buffers. Although the protein involved (hemoglobin) is still intracellular, it assumes added significance because it is located within the blood, thereby facilitating transport of the buffered respiratory acid to the lungs for elimination. Figure 25-2 illustrates this process. After CO_2 diffuses from the cells into the plasma, it enters the red blood cell (RBC). Carbonic anhydrase in the RBC facilitates the conversion of CO_2 into H_2CO_3, which immediately dissociates into H^+ and HCO_3^-. These intracellular ions react with potassium (K^+) and reduced hemoglobin (Hb^-), as shown in Equations 25-31 and 25-32.

$$K^+ + HCO_3^- \rightleftharpoons KHCO_3 \qquad (25\text{-}31)$$

$$H^+ + Hb^- \rightleftharpoons HHb \qquad (25\text{-}32)$$

By this process, HCO_3^- accumulates within the RBCs. When intracellular concentration exceeds plasma concentration, HCO_3^- diffuses out of the RBCs and into the plasma. Chloride (Cl^-) enters the cell, replacing HCO_3^-, to maintain electrical neutrality.[5, 213]

When blood reaches the lungs, the reduced hemoglobin becomes oxygenated, and the H^+ is released to react with $KHCO_3$.

$$HHb + O_2 + KHCO_3 \rightleftharpoons HHbO_2 \\ + KHCO_3 \rightleftharpoons KHbO_2 + H_2CO_3 \qquad (25\text{-}32)$$

With the formation of carbonic acid, a gradient is established favoring the diffusion of HCO_3^- back into the RBCs, and Cl^- diffuses out. The H_2CO_3 is converted by carbonic anhydrase to CO_2, which diffuses from the RBCs, through the plasma, and into the alveolus for elimination from the body.[5, 213]

BUFFERING CAPACITY. The efficiency of the body in buffering acids was most graphically demonstrated when a dog was given a dose of HCl equal to 14,000,000 nEq $H^+ \cdot l^{-1}$ total body water.[235] In response to this acid load, arterial pH decreased from its initial value of 7.44 ($H^+ = 36$ nEq $\cdot l^{-1}$) to 7.14 ($H^+ = 72$ nEq $\cdot l^{-1}$). Only 36 nEq $\cdot l^{-1}$ remained as free H^+. The remaining 13,999,964 nEq $H^+ \cdot l^{-1}$ had been bound to buffers in the body.[211]

In addition to demonstrating the buffering capacity of the body, this study also demonstrates the futility of attempting to quantitate the magnitude of an acidosis directly from an isolated measurement of arterial pH.[211] Accurate assessment of the problem would require measurement of the change in buffer anion concentrations.

Fortunately, if multiple buffer systems are in equilibrium in a homogeneous solution (such as plasma), the changes of components in any one buffer system will reflect alterations in all the other systems.[210, 211, 213] In clinical medicine, the bicarbonate–carbonic acid buffer pair is the system most readily assessed.[210, 211]

EVALUATION SYSTEMS

Despite the presence of buffering systems and compensatory mechanisms, acid–base disturbances may occur that produce either an increase in H^+ concentration causing pH to fall or a decrease in H^+ concentration causing pH to rise. Either aberration may be produced primarily by abnormalities in CO_2 (primary respiratory problems) or by nonrespiratory ("metabolic") abnormalities. All four primary disturbances (metabolic acidosis, metabolic alkalosis, respiratory acidosis, respiratory alkalosis) induce some degree of compensation. Accurate and thorough analysis of an acid–base problem requires knowledge of pH, HCO_3^-, and Pa_{CO_2}. Based on these three values, the primary disturbance may be categorized into one of the four disturbances just mentioned, and the degree of compensation may be evaluated. Accurate characterization is essential to determine etiology and guide not only supportive but also definitive therapy.

Several systems[236–239] have been developed in an effort to simplify the process of characterization and quantification (primarily of *metabolic* acid–base disorders). As with most shortcuts, each system has flaws that may lead to incorrect diagnoses.[211] Prior to the 1950s, when accurate electrodes became available for the determination of blood pH,[1] analysis of acid–base disturbances was limited solely to measurement of total CO_2 content ($ctCO_2$) by sample acidification, as described previously. Any decrease in $ctCO_2$ was equated with metabolic acidosis, and any increase in $ctCO_2$ was attributed to a metabolic alkalosis. Unfortunately, this approach does not always lead to an accurate diagnosis.

As previously indicated, changes in acid–base status are not confined to the intravascular compartment. Appreciation of this fact explains the evolution and shortcomings of systems designed to diagnose and quantitate metabolic acid–base disturbances. Initial determinations were performed on plasma,[236] thereby excluding not only the buffering potential of the extravascular fluids but also the significant contribution of hemoglobin to intravascular buffering. Although subsequent determinations were performed on whole blood,[237] they, too, evaluated only the bicarbonate–carbonic acid buffer pair. The magnitude of contribution by the other buffer systems could not be readily discerned from this information. With the development of the concepts of whole blood buffer base[238] and base excess/deficit,[239] attempts were made to consider all intravascular buffer systems. *In vivo* titration curves have subsequently been performed[240–243] and allow consideration of the extravascular acid–base status. Despite the shortcomings of the base excess/deficit system, it currently remains the one most widely used.

CO₂ Combining Power (Alkali Reserve)

With the ability to measure pH and P_{CO_2}, respiratory disorders could be more easily quantitated and separated from metabolic disturbances. The problems associated with relying solely on $ctCO_2$ measurements became more readily apparent. Prior to the development of pH and CO_2 electrodes, in an endeavor to eliminate the contribution of respiratory disturbances, plasma from sample blood was equilibrated with the laboratory technician's alveolar gas, where, presumably, $P_{CO_2} = 40$ mm Hg.[219, 236] It was believed that this technique corrected for any respiratory problems by establishing P_{CO_2} at (presumably) a normal value. Measurement of $ctCO_2$ (termed *combining power* or *alkali reserve*) under these circumstances was believed to accurately reflect metabolic acid–base status.[219] Measured HCO_3^- combined with knowledge of P_{CO_2} (fixed at 40 mm Hg) allowed determination of pH, by use of either a specifically constructed graph or the Henderson–Hasselbalch equation.

By using serum or plasma instead of whole blood, this system failed to account for the buffering capacity of hemoglobin (Hb). The inaccuracies imposed by this system have resulted in its exclusion from modern medical practice.

ASTRUP METHOD. The Astrup apparatus permits determination of a value for Pa_{CO_2} without use of a CO_2 electrode. After initial pH measurements, the sample is equilibrated against two different known CO_2 concentrations, with the pH being determined after each period of equilibration. These two pairs of values can be used to construct a straight line plot of pH versus the logarithm of P_{CO_2}, which describes all possible pH and P_{CO_2} values for that sample. Initial P_{CO_2} value can then be determined from the pH-log P_{CO_2} line by use of the initial value.[239, 244] Additionally, values for actual bicarbonate, standard bicarbonate, total CO_2 content, buffer base, and base excess concentration may be derived using the Astrup method.[244]

Standard Bicarbonate

The standard bicarbonate method, essentially a modification of the alkali reserve method just described, measures CO_2 concentration in whole blood equilibrated against gas with P_{CO_2} fixed at 40 mm Hg.[237] Additional accuracy is achieved by ensuring that hemoglobin is fully oxygenated and by performing the analysis at 38° Celsius rather than room temperature (as was done for alkali reserve).[240]

Normal standard bicarbonate is 24 (22–26) $mEq \cdot l^{-1}$. Although the results achieved with standard bicarbonate calculations are more accurate than the alkali reserve determination, like all *in vitro* titrations, this method does not account for buffering systems outside the blood or for the movement of HCO_3^- from blood into interstitial and intracellular fluids. Furthermore, like all current systems that rely solely on bicarbonate determinations, it evaluates the status of only the bicarbonate/CO_2 system, which accounts for approximately 75% of the buffering action of the blood.[239]

In the absence of an acid–base disturbance, standard HCO_3^- and actual HCO_3^- are equal, since both determinations are performed at $P_{CO_2} = 40$ mm Hg. In the presence of a respiratory acidosis, actual HCO_3^- exceeds standard HCO_3^-. In the presence of a respiratory alkalosis, CO_2 is absorbed into the blood sample when it is exposed to the higher P_{CO_2} (40 mm Hg) during the determination of the standard HCO_3^-. The increase in P_{CO_2} produces an increase in HCO_3^-, and standard HCO_3^- exceeds actual HCO_3^-.[240]

Buffer Base and Base Excess

These systems attempt to evaluate all intravascular buffering capacity rather than just that associated with the bicarbonate/CO_2 system. In addition, they also attempt to quantitate (exactly) the excess or deficit of base in the blood. Both systems have been described as unnecessary and difficult to comprehend.[245] Despite objections to attempts to quantitate any buffer other than bicarbonate, the base excess system remains widely used in clinical medicine.[215, 216, 240]

Both systems rely on the Siggaard–Andersen nomogram, Figure 25-17, which relates pH, P_{CO_2} and HCO_3^-. Based on the actual measurement of pH and P_{CO_2} in conjunction with the calculation of HCO_3^- concentration, the amount of available buffering capacity (including plasma and intracellular bicarbonate and phosphates, plasma proteins, and hemoglobin) in the blood sample may be determined.[239, 240]

In vitro titration curves have been performed, which, based on actual measurements of pH and Pa_{CO_2} (and calculation of HCO_3^- concentration), permit quantitation of the amount of buffering capacity available in whole blood.[239] *In vitro* titrations, however, fail to consider movement of HCO_3^- into the interstitial space.[241, 246] This shortcoming is of greatest significance in the presence of a pure respiratory acidosis. In the presence of an elevated Pa_{CO_2} when *in vivo* values of HCO_3^- are compared to levels predicted by *in vitro* titrations, an apparent metabolic acidosis will exist.[246, 247] Although *in vitro* HCO_3^- is confined to the test tube, *in vivo* HCO_3^- diffuses into the interstitial space. This diffusion of HCO_3^- into the

interstitial space produces a lower than predicted level of HCO_3^- in the patient's blood. This, in turn, leads to the erroneous diagnosis of a metabolic acidosis.

Buffer base simply defines the amount of buffering capacity in whole blood (normal = 45 to 50 $mEq \cdot l^{-1}$). Conceptually, buffer base was initially defined as the content of buffer anions (expressed in $mEq \cdot l^{-1}$) in whole blood.[238, 240] Added H^+ must either appear as free H^+ (in which case pH is changed) or be bound to a buffer (in which case the remaining buffering capacity is reduced). Accordingly, determination of pH and all the available buffers should provide a better indication of the added acids than determination of pH and $ctCO_2$. Increases in Pa_{CO_2}, while generating H^+, which consume some of the buffering capacity, also produce increases in HCO_3^- according to Equation 25-33.

$$CO_2 + H_2O \rightleftharpoons H_2CO_3 \rightleftharpoons H^+ + HCO_3^- \qquad (25\text{-}33)$$

Since the amount of HCO_3^- and H^+ produced are equal,

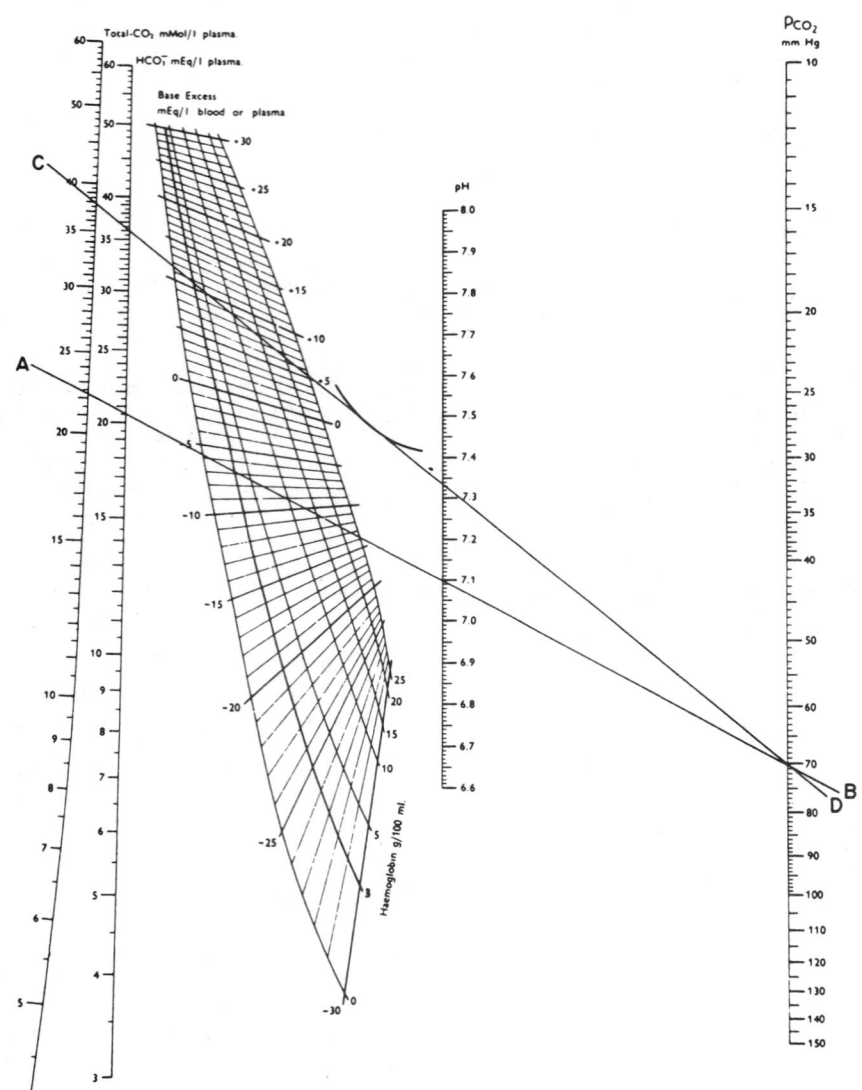

FIG. 25-17. Siggaard–Andersen nomogram. Plotting any two measured parameters (pH, Pa_{CO_2}, ct_{CO_2}) allows determination of base excess, actual HCO_3^- concentration, and the third measurable parameter. (Reproduced with permission. Siggaard-Andersen O: Blood acid-base alignment nomogram. Scand J Clin Invest 15:211, 1963.)

changes in buffer base are relatively unaffected by respiratory disorders and are considered to reflect only metabolic disturbances.[213, 240]

Base excess (BE) compares the buffering capacity in the patient's blood to normal.[239, 240, 248] Instead of reporting the buffer base value of the sample, normal buffer base is subtracted from the calculated value (*i.e.*, if the calculated buffer base of the sample is 35 mEq $\cdot$ l^{-1} and normal buffer base is 45 mEq $\cdot$ l^{-1}, base excess = −10 mEq $\cdot$ l^{-1}, or base deficit = 10 mEq $\cdot$ l^{-1}).

Increased buffering capacity (base excess or buffer base greater than 50 mEq $\cdot$ l^{-1} may occur as a result of decreased metabolic acids or increased buffering content (hemoglobin, protein, phosphates). Reductions in buffering capacity (buffer base < 45 mEq $\cdot$ l^{-1}, base deficit or negative base excess) may likewise be associated with either reductions in buffer content or increased metabolic acids.

Part of the appeal of the base excess system is its simplicity[211, 213, 240, 248]—normal base excess = 0 (range = +2.5 to −2.5 in mEq $\cdot$ l^{-1}); metabolic alkalosis is associated with a positive base excess, and metabolic acidosis is associated with a negative base excess (or a base deficit).

Although convenient, shortcomings still exist with the buffer base and base excess systems. It must be recognized that, in addition to the aforementioned problems with HCO$_3^-$ as a metabolic marker in respiratory acidosis, the base excess system does not consider the contribution of the intracellular and interstitial compartments in the body's response to acid–base disturbances. Although *p*H changes in the interstitial fluid (ISF) tend to parallel changes in the intravascular compartment, the total buffering capacity of the ISF is much reduced compared with that of blood. This decrease in buffering capability is due primarily to the absence of hemoglobin and the lower protein concentration in the ISF. Utilization of the base excess system to quantitate acid–base changes in the entire extracellular fluid (ECF) volume will overestimate the magnitude of the acidosis. Consideration of the intracellular fluid (ICF) compartment complicates the picture even further. Whereas P$_{CO_2}$-induced changes in ECF *p*H are paralleled in the ICF, the same is not always true of metabolic disturbances. On some occasions, ICF *p*H moves in the opposite direction compared with ECF *p*H.[249–252] Under these circumstances, it is clearly not possible to predict with any accuracy the magnitude of total body metabolic acid–base disturbance on the basis of the calculated base excess.

Despite the imposition of a great deal of complexity (if understanding is to be achieved), the systems offer no advantage over those systems using *p*H, P$_{CO_2}$ and HCO$_3^-$ and a knowledge of *in vivo* titrations.

As with any system designed to simplify a complex process, exceptions and errors exist. In the base excess system, these range from incorrectly diagnosing a combined metabolic and respiratory acidosis when a pure respiratory disturbance is present to fallacious assumptions regarding the precision of the calculated value.

Finally, the base excess system is designed to evaluate only acute disorders. Normal renal compensation for a primary increase in carbonic acid (Pa$_{CO_2}$) will appear as a metabolic alkalosis complicating a respiratory acidosis. Similarly, a patient with normal renal compensation for a chronic respiratory alkalosis will, using the base excess system, present with a metabolic acidosis. The practitioner must then attempt to estimate the magnitude of the normal "metabolic acidosis" present with a pure respiratory alkalosis. Since data are not provided by the base excess system for the magnitude of normal compensation, it is not possible to quantitate the magnitude of abnormal metabolic disorders under these conditions. This inadequacy has been described as self-defeating. The primary virtue of the base excess system, the ability to quantitatively evaluate the metabolic component of any acid–base disturbance, is absent.[253] These problems have led some authors to describe the base excess system as worthless.[247] Most other detractors simply describe the system as difficult to understand and needlessly complex.[211, 253]

In Vivo Titrations

Evaluation of respiratory disturbances is based on changes in Pa$_{CO_2}$. Unfortunately, the only "marker" commonly available for the evaluation of metabolic disturbances is HCO$_3^-$ concentration. Although it can be calculated from the Henderson–Hasselbalch equation, HCO$_3^-$ cannot be measured directly without including all forms of CO$_2$. Additionally, changes in Pa$_{CO_2}$ (*i.e.*, respiratory disturbances) also affect HCO$_3^-$ concentrations. The base excess system, which some clinicians believe to be the best way to resolve the apparent contradictions, is flawed, as previously described. These problems were anticipated[253] and subsequently documented in animals[240] and humans.[241]

Undoubtedly, the most accurate method of evaluating acid–base disturbances utilizes information obtained from *in vivo* titration curves.[210, 211, 247, 253] The objective of these studies was to determine normal HCO$_3^-$ levels in the presence of isolated respiratory acid–base disorders. On the basis of human experimental data with laboratory evaluation of *p*H, Pa$_{CO_2}$, and HCO$_3^-$, the normal response to acute and chronic respiratory disorders can be predicted. The actual values in a given patient can then be compared with the anticipated values, and deviations from the predicted responses can be analyzed and quantitated.[65, 210, 211, 253, 254]

Increases in Pa$_{CO_2}$ are associated with increased formation of carbonic acid, thereby producing increases in the concentrations of H$^+$ and HCO$_3^-$. In the *acute* setting, each 10 mm Hg increase in Pa$_{CO_2}$ is associated with an increase of 0.8 mEq $\cdot$ l^{-1} in HCO$_3^-$ concentration and an increase of 8 nEq $\cdot$ l^{-1} in H$^+$ concentration (Table 25-7).[241] Although the relationship between Pa$_{CO_2}$ and H$^+$ concentration is linear, this is obscured to some degree by the logarithmic nature of the *p*H scale. In order to avoid the need to convert *p*H to H$^+$ concentration, attempts have been made to generalize regarding the effect of acute increases in Pa$_{CO_2}$ on *p*H. Under these conditions, each 10 mm Hg increase in Pa$_{CO_2}$ is predicted to produce a *p*H decrease of 0.07.[210, 254] Although this association is useful and sufficiently accurate for Pa$_{CO_2}$ between 30 and 60 mm Hg, as would be anticipated based on the logarithmic nature of the *p*H scale, the greater the devi-

TABLE 25-7. Respiratory Acidosis—Changes Predicted by *in vivo* Titration Curves

10-mm Hg increase in Pa$_{CO_2}$
Acute
HCO$_3^-$ increased 0.8 mEq $\cdot$ l^{-1}
H$^+$ increased 8 nEq $\cdot$ l^{-1}
*p*H decreased 0.07
Chronic
HCO$_3^-$ increased 4 mEq $\cdot$ l^{-1}
H$^+$ increased 3.2 nEq $\cdot$ l^{-1}
*p*H decreased 0.03

ation from a normal Pa_{CO_2}, the less accurate the generalization becomes.

Renal compensation (H^+ excretion and HCO_3^- reabsorption), which requires 3 to 5 days to become maximal, attenuates changes in pH but cannot restore the value to normal. On the basis of this compensation, the values for pH and HCO_3^- present during *chronic* hypercapnia differ from the initial acute values. Under these conditions, each 10-mm Hg increase in Pa_{CO_2} is associated with an HCO_3^- increase of approximately 4 $mEq \cdot l^{-1}$ and an increase in H^+ concentration of 3.2 $nEq \cdot l^{-1}$.[242, 243] This H^+ concentration change has been generalized to a pH decrease of 0.03 for each chronic 10-mm Hg increase in Pa_{CO_2}.[210]

When levels of Pa_{CO_2} are decreased, carbonic acid formation is reduced, and concentration of HCO_3^- and H^+ fall. Acute hypocapnia produces a decrease in HCO_3^- of 2 $mEq \cdot l^{-1}$ for each 10 mm Hg decrease in Pa_{CO_2}. Changes in H^+ concentration are equal in magnitude but opposite in direction compared with those of acute hypercapnia (*i.e.*, each 10 mm Hg decrease in Pa_{CO_2} is associated with an 8 $nEq \cdot l^{-1}$ decrease in H^+ concentration). Recognizing that the accuracy diminishes with greater deviations from normal, the increase in pH associated with each acute 10 mm Hg decrease in Pa_{CO_2} is approximately 0.08 (Table 25-8).[210, 254]

With chronic primary hypocapnia, renal compensation in the form of decreased renal tubular reabsorption of HCO_3^- and decreased H^+ excretion occur. With this compensation comes not only a restoration of pH toward a more normal value, but also a change in HCO_3^- concentration. *In vivo* titration curves demonstrate that for each sustained 10 mm Hg decrease in Pa_{CO_2} below 40 mm Hg, HCO_3^- decreases approximately 6 $mEq \cdot l^{-1}$,[255] H^+ decreases 1.7 $nEq \cdot l^{-1}$,[210, 255] and pH increases approximately 0.03 (Table 25-8).[210]

Decreases in pH induced by nonrespiratory acids (*i.e.*, metabolic acidosis) induce an almost immediate respiratory response (increased alveolar ventilation), which decreases Pa_{CO_2}, restoring pH toward normal.[210, 213] It has been stated that the respiratory system is ordinarily capable of compensating for only 50%–75% of a metabolic acidosis (*i.e.*, respiratory compensation for a metabolic acidosis, which, if uncorrected, would produce a pH of 7.0, normally increases pH only to 7.2 or 7.3).[213] Observations indicate that each 1 $mEq \cdot l^{-1}$ decrease in HCO_3^- concentration normally produces a 1.1-mm Hg reduction in Pa_{CO_2}.[256] Alternatively, normal Pa_{CO_2} with a pure metabolic acidosis may be predicted by Equation 25-34.[65]

$$\text{Predicted } Pa_{CO_2} = 1.5(HCO_3^-) + 8 \ (\pm 2) \qquad (25\text{-}34)$$

In the setting of a pure metabolic acidosis, a 4 $mEq \cdot l^{-1}$ decrease in HCO_3^- concentration produces approximately a decrease in pH of 0.08. As with respiratory disturbances, the logarithmic nature of the pH scale is responsible for this generalization becoming progressively less accurate the greater the deviation in HCO_3^- concentration from normal (Table 25-9).

In primary metabolic alkalosis, HCO_3^- concentration increases. The Henderson–Hasselbalch equation predicts that consequent changes in pH would be minimized by concomitant increases in Pa_{CO_2}. Reductions in alveolar ventilation, which increase Pa_{CO_2}, would be the anticipated respiratory compensation for a primary metabolic alkalosis.[113, 213, 214, 257] It will be recalled from earlier discussions, however, that increases in Pa_{CO_2} are associated with reductions in Pa_{O_2}. Significant hypercarbia in response to metabolic alkalosis is not always seen in patients breathing room air[114, 115, 257–259] because the mild hypoxemia induced by increased Pa_{CO_2} stimulates respiratory drive. Administration of supplemental O_2 may ameliorate or prevent hypoxemia and permit greater respiratory compensation.[116] The lack of a consistent respiratory response under normal circumstances has prompted some authors to state that the body prefers alkalosis to hypoxemia.[210] Although metabolic alkalosis has been described as "the most poorly compensated acid–base disorder,"[205] respiratory compensation in the form of hypercapnia can occur in patients with[260] or without[116] pre-existing pulmonary disease. Equation 25-35 may be used to predict the normal Pa_{CO_2} in the presence of a metabolic alkalosis.[65, 261]

$$\text{Predicted } Pa_{CO_2} = 0.7(HCO_3^-) + 20 \ (\pm 2) \qquad (25\text{-}35)$$

Deviations in Pa_{CO_2} from this predicted value may be considered an indication of a coexistent respiratory acid–base disturbance.[65]

UTILIZING IN VIVO TITRATION CURVES. There are three basic steps to utilization of *in vivo* titration curves for the diagnosis of acid–base disorders.

1. *Evaluate the arterial pH.* Acidemia is defined as arterial pH = 7.35 or less. Alkalemia is defined as arterial pH = 7.45 or greater. Since normal compensatory mechanisms do not fully restore arterial pH to normal,[206, 213] a pH between 7.35 and 7.45 generally indicates the absence of acid–base pathology. A normal pH does not guarantee the absence of any acid–base disorders, however. Rarely, two disorders of equal magnitude but opposite direction (*i.e.*, alkalosis and acidosis) may exist simultaneously and produce a normal arterial pH despite the presence of pathology.
2. *Evaluate the markers to determine the nature of the primary disorder.* Carbon dioxide is used to evaluate respiratory disorders, and HCO_3^- is used for metabolic derangements. The inability of the compensatory responses to achieve a normal pH means that the pH will be changed

---

TABLE 25-8.   Respiratory Alkalosis—Changes Predicted by *in vivo* Titration Curves

10-mm Hg decrease in Pa_{CO_2}
Acute
HCO_3^- decreased 2 $mEq \cdot l^{-1}$
H^+ decreased 8 $nEq \cdot l^{-1}$
pH increased 0.08
Chronic
HCO_3^- decreased 6 $mEq \cdot l^{-1}$
H^+ decreased 1.7 $nEq \cdot l^{-1}$
pH increased 0.03

TABLE 25-9.   Metabolic Acidosis—Changes Predicted by *in vivo* Titration Curves

4 $mEq \cdot l^{-1}$ decrease of HCO_3^-
Produces
4.5-mm Hg decrease in Pa_{CO_2}
pH decreases 0.08
Alternatively, $Pa_{CO_2} = 1.5 \ (HCO_3^-) \times 8$

in the direction of the primary disorder. (Example: Consider a patient with $pH = 7.22$, $Pa_{CO_2} = 24$ mm Hg, $HCO_3^- = 10$ mEq $\cdot$ l^{-1}. An acidemia is evident from arterial pH; low Pa_{CO_2} indicates a respiratory alkalosis; low HCO_3^- indicates a metabolic acidosis. Based on the low arterial pH, the primary disorder is a metabolic acidosis. A compensatory respiratory alkalosis may also be diagnosed, based on the low Pa_{CO_2}).

3. *Compare the observed compensation with that which is predicted.* In the aforementioned example, HCO_3^- is decreased by 14 mEq $\cdot$ l^{-1}. The anticipated respiratory response (a 1.1-mm Hg decrease in Pa_{CO_2} for each 1 mEq $\cdot$ l^{-1} decrease in HCO_3^-) should produce a 15-mm Hg decrease in Pa_{CO_2}, that is, predicted $Pa_{CO_2} = 25$ mm Hg. An appropriate respiratory compensation is present in this example.

Quantitation of Disturbance

Studies have attempted to quantitate the magnitude of the excess or deficit of metabolic acids in the body based on the difference between the reported and predicted values for HCO_3^-. No system, whether based on standard bicarbonate, base excess, or *in vivo* titration curves, can quantitate this value with any degree of accuracy. Not even the *direction* of change in intracellular pH can be accurately predicted based on measurements of values in blood. It seems highly unlikely, therefore, that a valid system of quantitating the magnitude of acid–base changes in the total body will be possible in the near future.

One of the reasons that many clinicians prefer the base excess system is its ease of use in guiding therapeutic interventions. Various formulae exist for using the calculated base excess to estimate the dose of $NaHCO_3$ in treating metabolic acidosis (Eqn. 25-36).

$$\text{total base excess} = \text{BE} \times \frac{\text{BW(kg)}}{3} \qquad (25\text{-}36)$$

Example: 70 kg pt with BE $= -10$ mEq $\cdot$ l^{-1}
extracellular water $= 70$ kg/(3 l $\cdot$ kg^{-1}) $= 23$ l
Total BE $= (-10$ mEq $\cdot$ l^{-1})(23 l) $= -230$ mEq.

Based on this calculation, most authors recommend treating with half the calculated deficit which, in this case, is 115 mEq $NaHCO_3$ (approximately 2 ampules).

PRIMARY DISTURBANCES

There are four possible primary disturbances in acid–base physiology: 1) respiratory acidosis occurs when the primary derangement is retention of CO_2; 2) respiratory alkalosis occurs when the primary derangement is a reduction in Pa_{CO_2}; 3) metabolic acidosis occurs when the primary derangement is either an excess accumulation of metabolic acids or a decrease in HCO_3^- concentration from some nonrespiratory cause; and 4) metabolic alkalosis occurs when the primary derangement is either an excess nonrespiratory loss of H$^+$ or an increased HCO_3^-.

Respiratory Acidosis

PATHOPHYSIOLOGY. The initiating abnormality is an inability to adequately eliminate the CO_2 being produced. Because CO_2 is capable of producing H$^+$ (Eqn. 25-18), H$^+$ concentration increases and pH decreases.

ETIOLOGY. Retention of CO_2 may occur because of decreased elimination or increased production. The etiologies of hypercarbia have been discussed in the section concerning CO_2.

COMPENSATION. Given the fact that the primary problem is an inability to adequately eliminate CO_2, renal compensation is the only mechanism (other than the buffering systems) available to minimize the decrease in pH induced by primary respiratory acidosis. In addition to retaining HCO_3^-, renal compensation increases excretion of H$^+$, primarily in the form of ammonium ions (NH_4^+) and other buffer anions, predominantly a dihydrogen phosphate salt (NaH_2PO_4). Unfortunately, renal compensation is slow, requiring several days to complete. This results in differing degrees of compensation, depending upon the duration of the respiratory acidosis (acute or chronic).

LABORATORY EVALUATION. Whether acute or chronic, respiratory acidosis presents with a decreased pH and an increased Pa_{CO_2}. In acute conditions, the actual (calculated) HCO_3^- and measured CO_2 content are also increased. Standard bicarbonate should remain normal. Although base excess should remain zero, this is not always true. When renal compensation has occurred (*i.e.*, chronic respiratory acidosis), pH increases toward normal. Renal retention of HCO_3^- leads to an increase in actual HCO_3^-, standard bicarbonate, CO_2 content, and base excess. If compensation were complete (*i.e.*, $pH = 7.40$), it would be difficult if not impossible to distinguish a primary respiratory acidosis with renal compensation from a primary metabolic alkalosis with respiratory compensation (Table 25-10).

TREATMENT. It is important to differentiate respiratory from metabolic acidosis. As will be discussed, alkali therapy (most commonly in the form of $NaHCO_3$) is the cornerstone of therapy for metabolic acidosis requiring treatment. Use of $NaHCO_3$ in respiratory acidosis is generally not prudent, as it produces even more CO_2 for eventual elimination. Acute bronchospasm is one setting in which $NaHCO_3$ therapy may be warranted in the presence of an uncomplicated respiratory acidosis.[261] Since the acidosis itself decreases the responsiveness of airway smooth muscle to bronchodilators,

TABLE 25-10.   Respiratory Acidosis—Laboratory Manifestations

UNCOMPENSATED
Pa_{CO_2} increased
pH decreased (0.07 per 10 mm Hg increase in Pa_{CO_2})
HCO_3^- increased (0.8 mEq $\cdot$ l^{-1} per 10 mm Hg increase in Pa_{CO_2})
ctCO_2 increased
Standard HCO_3^- normal
Base excess normal
Actual HCO_3^- exceeds standard HCO_3^-

COMPENSATED
Pa_{CO_2} increased
pH decreased (0.03 per 10 mm Hg increase in Pa_{CO_2})
HCO_3^- increased (4 mEq $\cdot$ l^{-1} per 10 mm Hg increase in Pa_{CO_2})
ctCO_2 increased
Standard HCO_3^- increased
Base excess positive
Actual HCO_3^- exceeds standard HCO_3^-

NaHCO$_3$ administration, with its resultant increase in pH, may facilitate the action of pharmacologic bronchodilators, thereby enhancing the primary therapeutic intervention.

ACUTE. Augmentation of alveolar ventilation is generally indicated in the therapy of acute, uncomplicated, primary respiratory acidosis. Although mechanical ventilation is the most common therapeutic intervention used to achieve this goal, other modalities may also be efficacious in some settings (*e.g.*, naloxone administration in opioid overdose). Occasionally, consideration must also be given to decreasing CO$_2$ production (*e.g.*, with malignant hyperthermia).

Respiratory Alkalosis

PATHOPHYSIOLOGY. Primary respiratory alkalosis has been described as the least common of the four primary acid–base disturbances.[262] In respiratory alkalosis, elimination of CO$_2$ is excessive compared with production. Diminished levels of Pa$_{CO_2}$ produce an increase in both HCO$_3$$^-$/CO$_2$ and pH.

ETIOLOGY. Some potential etiologies of primary respiratory alkalosis are listed in Table 25-11.

COMPENSATION. The only mechanism of compensation, other than the buffer systems, is renal. Under normal circumstances, the kidneys excrete an acid urine as a result of excretion of H$^+$ and NH$_4$$^+$ as well as conservation of HCO$_3$$^-$. In the presence of a respiratory alkalosis, these acidification processes are reduced or terminated. Hydrogen ion concentration of the serum is also increased by a shift of K$^+$ into the cells, accompanied by movement of H$^+$ and Na$^+$ into the extracellular fluid. Serum HCO$_3$$^-$ is decreased by a combination of increased HCO$_3$$^-$ excretion and increased H$^+$ retention.[206]

LABORATORY EVALUATION. The primary disturbance is a decrease in Pa$_{CO_2}$. In uncompensated respiratory alkalosis, the decrease in Pa$_{CO_2}$ increases the HCO$_3$$^-$/CO$_2$ ratio, which results in an increased pH.[206] Even in the absence of renal compensation, the measured HCO$_3$$^-$ is decreased, since reduced amounts of CO$_2$ are available to produce HCO$_3$$^-$. Stan-

dard bicarbonate, however, is normal (indicating the presence of a respiratory derangement), and base excess should be zero[262] (Table 25-12).

Renal compensation will further decrease HCO$_3$$^-$, which will tend to restore the HCO$_3$$^-$/CO$_2$ ratio and thereby decrease pH. Renal compensation is indicated by a decrease in standard bicarbonate, the presence of a negative base excess, and an HCO$_3$$^-$ lower than that calculated using the generalizations based on *in vivo* titrations (Table 25-12).

TREATMENT. Hypocarbia induced by spontaneous hyperventilation is a common finding in patients with intracranial hypertension. In these circumstances, restoration of a "normal" Pa$_{CO_2}$, by whatever means, may be associated with a further increase in intracranial pressure. Increasing Pa$_{CO_2}$ by the use of paralysis and/or pharmacologic suppression of respiratory drive in conjunction with mechanical ventilation may produce a detrimental effect on the CNS. Addition of deadspace or the presence of CO$_2$ in the inspired gas mixture in spontaneously breathing patients will simply further increase alveolar ventilation and maintenance of the pre-existing respiratory alkalosis. Only when alveolar ventilation can no longer be increased will a catastrophic increase in Pa$_{CO_2}$ occur.

Metabolic Acidosis

PATHOPHYSIOLOGY. Metabolic acidosis occurs as the result of either an excess accumulation of acids other than CO$_2$ or a loss of base. In either circumstance, HCO$_3$$^-$ concentrations are reduced, leading to a decrease in HCO$_3$$^-$/CO$_2$ and pH.

ETIOLOGY. Metabolic acidosis may result from the generation of excessive amounts of normal metabolic acids, from impaired elimination of usual amounts of metabolic acids, from excess intake (either dietary or parenteral) of metabolic acids, or from loss of normal base (chiefly HCO$_3$$^-$). Unlike respiratory acidosis, which results from excess production or decreased elimination of only one acid (CO$_2$), in metabolic acidosis, the acids whose production may be increased or

TABLE 25-11.   Etiologies of Respiratory Alkalosis

Hyperventilation syndrome
Interstitial pulmonary disease
Chronic liver disease
Endotoxemia
Carbon monoxide poisoning
Hypotension
Salicylate intoxication
Progesterone (pregnancy or pharmacologic agents)
Central nervous system lesions (tumor, increased intracranial pressure)
Hypoxemia
Iatrogenic mechanical hyperventilation
Fever
Paraldehyde intoxication
Disulfiram plus alcohol
Intraabdominal pathology (ascites, metastatic neoplasms, peritonitis)
Respiratory stimulants Nicotine Doxapram Acetylcholine

TABLE 25-12.   Respiratory Alkalosis—Laboratory Manifestations

UNCOMPENSATED
Pa$_{CO_2}$ decreased
pH increased (0.08 per 10 mm Hg decrease in Pa$_{CO_2}$)
HCO$_3$$^-$ decreased (2 mEq·l^{-1} per 10 mm Hg decrease in Pa$_{CO_2}$)
ctCO$_2$ decreased
Standard HCO$_3$$^-$ normal
Base excess normal
Actual HCO$_3$$^-$ less than standard HCO$_3$$^-$

COMPENSATED
Pa$_{CO_2}$ decreased
pH increased (0.03 per 10-mm Hg decrease in Pa$_{CO_2}$)
HCO$_3$$^-$ decreased (6 mEq·l^{-1} per 10 mm Hg decrease in Pa$_{CO_2}$)
ctCO$_2$ decreased
Standard HCO$_3$$^-$ decreased
Base excess negative (*i.e.*, base deficit present)
Actual HCO$_3$$^-$ less than standard HCO$_3$$^-$

TABLE 25-13.   Etiologies of Metabolic Acidosis

Ketoacidosis
    diabetic, starvation, alcoholic
Lactic acidosis
    hypoperfusion, malignancy, hepatic failure, drugs
    (phenformin, fructose)
Renal dysfunction
    renal tubular acidosis, renal failure (acute or chronic)
Endocrine disorders
    thyrotoxicosis, hypoaldosteronism, diabetic
    ketoacidosis, hyperparathyroidism
Excessive gastrointestinal losses
    diarrhea, small bowel drainage, ureterosigmoidostomy
Pharmacologic agents
    HCl, NH₄Cl, carbonic anhydrase inhibitors, cholestyramine,
    sulfamylon, K⁺-sparing diuretics, intravenous hyper-
    alimentation
Toxic ingestion
    salicylate, methyl alcohol, ethylene glycol, paraldehyde, boric
    acid, oxalic acid
Inherited diseases
    familial lactic acidosis, aminoacidurias, glycogen disorders

whose elimination may be impaired are much more numerous for the development of metabolic acidosis. Some of the etiologies of metabolic acidosis are listed in Table 25-13.

ANION GAP. The presence and magnitude of a metabolic acidosis are determined by measurements of pH, P_{CO_2}, and HCO_3^-. Once the diagnosis of metabolic acidosis is made, calculation of the "anion gap" is often advocated to facilitate determination of the etiology of the problem.[205, 210, 234, 263, 264] Table 25-14 classifies etiologies of metabolic acidosis based on the anion gap. The anion gap is calculated by Equation 25-37.

$$Anion\ gap = (Na^+ + K^+) - (HCO_3^- + Cl^-).\quad (25\text{-}37)$$

A normal anion gap is approximately 16 mEq·l⁻¹ or less. The concept of anion gap may be misleading. There is no actual "gap" between the total concentrations of positively and negatively charged ions as a "normal" gap of 16 mEq·l⁻¹ implies. The normal gap occurs because routinely screened electrolytes measure a greater percentage of positively charged ions (Na^+ and K^+) than those that are negatively charged (HCO_3^- and Cl^-). Electrical neutrality is actually maintained at all times.

If the calculated value exceeds 20 to 22 mEq·l⁻¹, the anion gap is increased ("abnormal" or "large"). As previously described, HCO_3^- will be decreased in any patient with a metabolic acidosis. The concept of anion gap may be used to determine the presence or absence of accompanying reciprocal elevation of Cl^-. Increased anion gap occurs in the absence of Cl^- elevations and is due to the presence of an unmeasured anion that replaces increases in Cl^- concentration.

COMPENSATION. Respiratory compensation consists of increased elimination of CO_2 in an attempt to restore HCO_3^-/CO_2 (and therefore pH) by decreasing CO_2 in the face of decreased HCO_3^-. In the absence of kidney disease, renal compensation, consisting primarily of increased H^+ excretion and HCO_3^- retention, may also be possible.

LABORATORY EVALUATION. In uncompensated primary metabolic acidosis, pH and HCO_3^- are low and Pa_{CO_2} is normal. The standard and actual HCO_3^- are the same (indicating the absence of a respiratory component), and the base excess is negative (Table 25-15).

Because respiratory compensation is relatively rapid (hours as opposed to days for renal compensation), it is uncommon to find an isolated metabolic acidosis without respiratory compensation. Increased elimination of CO_2 produces a decrease in Pa_{CO_2} and a partial restoration of pH owing to an increase in HCO_3^-/CO_2. Standard bicarbonate exceeds actual HCO_3^-, indicating the presence of a respiratory component of the acid–base disorder (in this case, a compensatory respiratory alkalosis). Base excess remains unchanged.

Depending upon the etiology of the metabolic acidosis, renal compensation may also occur. To the degree that renal compensation is successful, HCO_3^- (both actual and standard) concentration will increase, further increasing pH. The increase in HCO_3^- occurring with renal compensation will return the negative base excess (base deficit) toward zero.

TREATMENT. Successful treatment of metabolic acidosis requires correction of the etiologic factors and replacement

TABLE 25-14.   Classification of Metabolic Acidosis by Anion Gap

Increased Anion Gap
    Ketoacidosis
    Lactic acidosis
    Toxic ingestion
    Renal failure
    Glycogen disorders

Normal Anion Gap
    Renal tubular acidosis
    Hypoaldosteronism
    Potassium-sparing diuretics
    Excessive gastrointestinal losses
    Carbonic anhydrase inhibitors
    Acid administration
        (HCl, NH₄Cl, arginine HCl)
    Intravenous hyperalimentation
    Sulfamylon, cholestyramine

TABLE 25-15.   Metabolic Acidosis—Laboratory Manifestations

UNCOMPENSATED
HCO_3^- decreased
pH decreased (0.08 per 4 mm Hg decrease in HCO_3^-)
Pa_{CO_2} normal
ctCO₂ decreased
Standard HCO_3^- decreased
Base excess negative (*i.e.*, base deficit present)
Actual HCO_3^- equals standard HCO_3^-

COMPENSATED
HCO_3^- decreased
pH decreased
Pa_{CO_2} decreased (4.5 mm Hg per 4 mEq·l⁻¹ decrease in HCO_3^-)
ctCO₂ decreased
Standard HCO_3^- decreased/normal
Base excess negative (*i.e.*, base deficit present)
Actual HCO_3^- less than standard HCO_3^-

of any lost electrolytes. Although sodium bicarbonate ($NaHCO_3$) has long been advocated in the therapy of metabolic acidosis,[265-268] recent studies have highlighted the potential problems associated with its administration[269-276] (Table 25-16). Many authors now claim either that there is no role for $NaHCO_3$ in the therapy of metabolic acidosis[277] or that the role of $NaHCO_3$ needs to be re-evaluated.[269, 278-281] Authors who still favor the use of $NaHCO_3$ often recommend that it be withheld unless $pH < 7.20$[65] and/or that $NaHCO_3$ administration be directed toward achieving $pH = 7.20$.[269]

In the past, $NaHCO_3$ was most commonly administered based on a formula using the value derived for base excess (Eqn. 25-38).[213, 240]

$$mEq \ NaHCO_3 = 0.3 \times BD \times Wt$$
$$BD = base \ deficit$$
$$(negative \ base \ excess)$$
$$wt = body \ weight \ (in \ kg)$$
$$0.3 = correction \ factor \quad (25-38)$$

Although simple and widely accepted, based on the inaccuracies of the system, the wisdom of using this value to determine the dose of a drug has always seemed dubious. In light of the controversy surrounding the use of $NaHCO_3$, it is not surprising that, at this time, there is no widely accepted formula to calculate dosage. Indications for $NaHCO_3$ must be decided on a case-by-case basis. If the acidosis is severe and organ failure is threatened, pharmacologic therapy may still be indicated.

Metabolic Alkalosis

PATHOPHYSIOLOGY. Metabolic alkalosis occurs because of a loss of H^+ or an accumulation of excess base. The increase in HCO_3^- under conditions of a constant Pa_{CO_2} produces an increase in pH.

TABLE 25-16.   Reported Deleterious Effects of $NaHCO_3$

Cardiovascular
    Hypotension[276, 279]
    Myocardial depression[276, 289]
    Decreased peripheral resistance[274, 276]
    Volume overload (pulmonary edema)[279]
    Decreased ventricular fibrillation threshold[289]
    Increased threshold for ventricular defibrillation[289]
    Decreased liver and gut blood flow[275]
Respiratory
    Respiratory acidosis[269, 273, 274]
    Pulmonary edema[279]
Metabolic
    Impaired O_2 delivery to tissues[269]
    Increased CO_2 production[273, 274]
    Increased blood lactate[271, 275]
    Further decrease in intracellular pH[275]
    Metabolic alkalosis[269]
    Delayed clearance of ketone bodies[267]
      (diabetic ketoacidosis)
Central Nervous System
    Increased intracranial pressure[274]
    Decreased consciousness[279]
    CSF acidosis[269]
    Intracranial hemorrhage[290]
Blood
    Hypernatremia[269, 290]
    Hyperosmolarity[269, 290]
    Hypokalemia[269]
    Hypocalcemia[269]

ETIOLOGY. Metabolic alkalosis commonly occurs owing to the loss of HCl from the body during nasogastric suctioning. Normally, H^+ (formed by dissociation of H_2CO_3 produced from CO_2 and H_2O by the parietal cells of the stomach) enters the lumen of the stomach with Cl^- to form HCl. The HCO_3^- produced by this process diffuses back into the blood stream; subsequently, H^+ formed by cells of the small intestine pass back into the blood neutralizing the excess HCO_3^-. Loss of H^+ owing to vomiting or nasogastric suction leaves this HCO_3^- unneutralized and produces a metabolic alkalosis.

Loss of H^+ from the body can also be caused by hypokalemia. Low serum K^+ values are associated with loss of K^+ from the cells. In addition to Na^+, H^+ enters the cells to replace the lost K^+, thus effecting a loss of H^+ from the extracellular fluid. H^+ may also be lost by way of the kidneys. Normally, the distal tubule actively secretes about 10% of the filtered K^+ load in exchange for Na^+; in the presence of hypokalemia, urinary loss of H^+ occurs when H^+ replaces K^+ in the exchange process.[282]

Use of thiazide or loop diuretics may also produce an alkalosis. In addition to producing hypokalemia, these agents directly stimulate H^+ losses by the excretion of ammonium ions, NH_4^+. Although increased, Na^+ excretion is not adequate to keep pace with the diuretic-induced Cl^- excretion. Electrical neutrality is maintained in the urine by increased excretion of K^+ and NH_4^+.[283]

Sudden correction of chronic hypercapnia may produce a metabolic alkalosis. As discussed previously, renal compensation for respiratory acidosis includes HCO_3^- retention and increased H^+ excretion. A sudden decrease in Pa_{CO_2}, as may occur with injudicious mechanical ventilation of a patient with long-standing hypercapnia, may produce a metabolic alkalosis because of the increased serum HCO_3^- concentration.[283]

COMPENSATION. Compensation for metabolic alkalosis involves both renal and pulmonary mechanisms. Renal compensation is similar to that described for respiratory alkalosis, assuming that renal function permits compensation. As discussed previously, respiratory compensation for metabolic alkalosis may become more evident if the hypoxemia-induced limitation is alleviated by the administration of supplemental oxygen.

LABORATORY EVALUATION. In uncompensated, primary metabolic alkalosis, blood pH is elevated, P_{CO_2} is normal, and HCO_3^- is increased (Table 25-17). Base excess is positive, and standard bicarbonate is increased. Unless alkalosis is due to hypokalemia, when an acid urine is produced, urine is alkaline.

With respiratory compensation, Pa_{CO_2} increases and actual HCO_3^- exceeds standard HCO_3^-. The old doctrine that $Pa_{CO_2} > 55$ mm Hg cannot be due to compensation for metabolic alkalosis has been proved invalid.[116, 257]

TREATMENT. As with the therapy of metabolic acidosis, the most important therapeutic intervention is correction of the underlying disturbance. Appropriate fluid replacement should be provided for gastrointestinal losses; consideration should be given to the use of H_1 receptor antagonists (cimetidine, ranitidine) instead of, or in addition to, oral antacids for patients in whom they are necessary[284]; and hypokalemia should be treated appropriately. In most circumstances, treatment of the underlying disorder alone will be adequate.

Rarely, oral therapy with NH_4Cl or HCl may be necessary. Parenteral HCl is also available for use in extreme metabolic alkalosis unresponsive to other therapeutic interventions. If

TABLE 25-17.   Metabolic Alkalosis—Laboratory
Manifestations

UNCOMPENSATED

HCO_3^- increased
pH increased
Pa_{CO_2} normal
$ctCO_2$ increased
Standard HCO_3^- increased
Base excess positive
Actual HCO_3^- equals standard HCO_3^-

COMPENSATED

HCO_3^- increased
pH increased (0.08 per 10 mm Hg decrease in Pa_{CO_2})
Pa_{CO_2} decreased ($Pa_{CO_2} = 0.7(HCO_3^-) + 20$
$ctCO_2$ increased
Standard HCO_3^- increased
Base excess positive
Actual HCO_3^- exceeds standard HCO_3^-

$ctCO_2$ = total CO_2 content

parenteral HCl is necessary, most authors recommend the use of a 0.15 normal solution (150 ml of 1.0 normal HCl added to 850 ml sterile water) at infusion rates up to 125 ml·hr^{-1}.[283] The HCl solution must be administered from a glass container.[283] Although infusion into a central vein is generally recommended,[283–286] peripheral infusions have been used,[284, 287] provided that the HCl is buffered in an amino acid solution and administered with a fat emulsion.[287]

Other pharmacologic agents have been used in the therapy of metabolic alkalosis. Carbonic anhydrase inhibitors may decrease the alkalosis and restore renal response to diuretics in thiazide-induced metabolic alkalosis.[283] NH_4Cl produces additional H^+ to reduce the alkalosis, but it must be metabolized by the liver before entering the systemic circulation and is associated with potentially deleterious side-effects, especially in the presence of hepatic or renal dysfunction.[286] Arginine hydrochloride likewise requires hepatic metabolism and has been associated with hyperkalemia, thrombocytopenia, and allergic reactions.[286] L-lysine monohydrochloride has been used in the treatment of diuretic-induced metabolic alkalosis.[283] Although hemodialysis has been used in the treatment of transfusion-related metabolic alkalosis,[288] it has been described as "expensive and cumbersome" because of the need to establish vascular access and heparinize the patient.

MIXED DISORDERS

In addition to isolated respiratory or metabolic disorders, simultaneous primary disturbances may occur. In general, any etiology of one primary disturbance may combine with an etiology of the other primary disturbance to produce a mixed disorder. The two primary disorders may produce opposite or similar changes in pH. In the presence of two primary disorders producing opposite changes in pH, history and clinical course may be essential in diagnosing two independent disturbances as opposed to normal compensation. Simultaneous disturbances producing similar changes in pH are more severe and, fortunately, less common.

Since primary disorders affect both the metabolic and respiratory systems, little compensation is possible. Treatment is directed toward underlying etiologies.

TABLE 25-18.   Mixed Respiratory Alkalosis and Metabolic Acidosis—Laboratory Manifestations

Pa_{CO_2} decreased*
HCO_3^- decreased*
pH increased, decreased, or normal
$ctCO_2$ decreased
Standard HCO_3^- decreased
Base excess negative (base deficit present)
Actual HCO_3^- less than standard HCO_3^-

*Values are decreased beyond those predicted by *in vivo* titration curves based on actual levels of either HCO_3^- or Pa_{CO_2}.

Mixed Respiratory Alkalosis and Metabolic Acidosis

PATHOPHYSIOLOGY. Primary (*i.e.*, not compensatory) changes in both Pa_{CO_2} and HCO_3^- occur. Because the two etiologies have opposite effects on H^+ concentration, the change in pH is minimized. The primary decrease in Pa_{CO_2} tends to minimize the change in pH produced by the simultaneous decrease in HCO_3^-.

ETIOLOGY. Salicylate intoxication is an example of a single entity capable of producing both a primary respiratory alkalosis and a primary metabolic acidosis. One example of two different etiologies combining to produce this entity would be iatrogenic mechanical hyperventilation in the presence of lactic acidosis owing to hypoperfusion.

LABORATORY EVALUATION. If the magnitude of the disturbances is equal, pH may remain normal. If one disorder is more severe than the other, pH will change in the direction dictated by the more severe disturbance. Low values will be obtained for HCO_3^- and Pa_{CO_2}. Actual values for HCO_3^- and Pa_{CO_2} will not correspond to those predicted by *in vivo* titration curves. (HCO_3^- will be lower than predicted on the basis of Pa_{CO_2}, and Pa_{CO_2} will be lower than predicted based on HCO_3^- concentration); (Table 25-18).

Mixed Respiratory Acidosis and Metabolic Alkalosis

PATHOPHYSIOLOGY. Primary increases in Pa_{CO_2} minimize changes in pH induced by primary increases in HCO_3^-.

ETIOLOGY. Excessive administration of $NaHCO_3$ to a patient with limited alveolar ventilation (*i.e.*, controlled mechanical ventilation) is one combination of etiologies that may produce this disorder.

LABORATORY EVALUATION. Increased levels of Pa_{CO_2} and HCO_3^- are present. Depending upon the relative severity of the two conditions, pH may be increased, decreased, or normal. The values for Pa_{CO_2} and HCO_3^- are higher than those predicted by *in vivo* titration curves (Table 25-19).

TABLE 25-19.   Mixed Respiratory Acidosis and Metabolic Alkalosis—Laboratory Manifestations

Pa_{CO_2} increased*
HCO_3^- increased*
pH increased, decreased, or normal
$ctCO_2$ increased
Standard HCO_3^- increased
Base excess positive
Actual HCO_3^- exceeds standard HCO_3^-

*Values are increased beyond those predicted by *in vivo* titration curves based on actual levels of either HCO_3^- or Pa_{CO_2}.

TABLE 25-20.   Mixed Metabolic Acidosis and Respiratory Acidosis—Laboratory Manifestations

Pa_{CO_2} increased
HCO_3^- decreased
pH decreased
$ctCO_2$ decreased
Standard HCO_3^- decreased
Base excess negative (base deficit present)
Actual HCO_3^- exceeds standard HCO_3^-

TABLE 25-21.   Mixed Metabolic Alkalosis and Respiratory Alkalosis—Laboratory Manifestations

HCO_3^- increased
Pa_{CO_2} decreased
pH increased
$ctCO_2$ increased
Standard HCO_3^- increased
Base excess positive
Actual HCO_3^- less than standard HCO_3^-

Mixed Respiratory Acidosis and Metabolic Acidosis

PATHOPHYSIOLOGY. Increases in Pa_{CO_2} and decreases in HCO_3^- combine to produce an extreme decrease in pH.

ETIOLOGY. Although rare, one combination of etiologies that may produce this disturbance is respiratory depression in a patient with a pre-existing metabolic acidosis.

LABORATORY EVALUATION. The presence of two primary disorders producing pH change in similar directions cannot be confused with compensation. The primary manifestations are a low pH and HCO_3^- in addition to increased Pa_{CO_2} (Table 25-20).

Mixed Metabolic Alkalosis and Respiratory Alkalosis

PATHOPHYSIOLOGY. Primary increase in HCO_3^- combines with primary decrease in Pa_{CO_2} to produce a high pH.

ETIOLOGY. Simultaneous administration of $NaHCO_3$ and hyperventilation have been combined to produce this mixed disorder.

LABORATORY EVALUATION. An increase in pH is produced by a decrease in Pa_{CO_2} and an increase in HCO_3^-. Normal compensation for either disorder predicted by *in vivo* titration curves is absent (Table 25-21).

REFERENCES

1. Sanz MC: Ultramicro methods and standardization of equipment. Clin Chem 3:406, 1957
2. Severinghaus JW, Bradley AF: Electrodes for blood PO_2 and PCO_2 determinations. J Appl Physiol 12:65, 1958
3. Stowe RW, Baer RF, Randall BF: Rapid measurement of the tension of carbon dioxide in blood. Arch Phys Med Rehabil 38:646, 1957
4. Clark LC: Monitor and control of blood and tissue oxygen tensions. Trans Am Soc Artif Intern Organs 2:41, 1956
5. Nunn JF: Carbon dioxide. In Applied Respiratory Physiology, 3rd ed, p 207. London, Butterworths, 1987
6. Jobsis FF: Basic processes in cellular respiration. In Fenn WO, Rahn H (eds): Handbook of Physiology—Respiration I, p 63. Washington D.C., American Physiological Society, 1964
7. Severinghaus JW: Blood gas concentrations. In Fenn WO, Rahn H (eds): Handbook of Physiology—Respiration II, p 1475. Washington, D.C., American Physiological Society, 1965
8. West JB: Acid–base balance and regulation of H^+ excretion. In West JB (ed): Best and Taylor's Physiological Basis of Medical Practice, p 516. Baltimore, Williams & Wilkins, 1985
9. Gravenstein JS, Paulus DA: Monitoring ventilation and gases. In Clinical Monitoring Practice, 2nd ed, p 157. Philadelphia, JB Lippincott, 1987
10. Ledingham IM, Macdonald AM, Douglas IHS: Monitoring of ventilation. In Shoemaker WC, Thompson WL, Holbrook (eds): The Society of Critical Care Medicine Textbook of Critical Care, p 184. Philadelphia, JB Lippincott, 1987
11. West JB: Disorders of ventilation. In Braunwald E, Isselbacher KJ, Petersdorf RG et al (eds): Harrison's Principles of Internal Medicine, p 1049. New York, McGraw-Hill, 1987
12. Bartlett RH, Allyn PA, Medley T et al: Nutritional therapy based on positive caloric balance in burn patients. Arch Surg 112:974, 1977
13. Demling RH: Burn injury. Acute Care 178:138, 1985
14. Guyton GC: Energetics and metabolic rate. In Textbook of Medical Physiology, 7th ed, p 841. Philadelphia, WB Saunders, 1986
15. Bay J, Nunn JF, Prys–Roberts C: Factors influencing arterial PO_2 during recovery from anaesthesia. Br J Anaesth 40:398, 1968
16. Hegnauer AH, D'Amato HE: Oxygen consumption and cardiac output in the hypothermic dog. Am J Physiol 40:398, 1968
17. Michenfelder JD, Theye RA: Hypothermia: Effect on canine brain and whole body metabolism. Anesthesiology 29:1107, 1968
18. Searle JF: Incidental hypothermia during surgery for peripheral vascular disease. Br J Anaesth 43:1095, 1971
19. Shanks CA: Heat balance during surgery involving body cavities. Anaesth Intensive Care 3:114, 1975
20. Sekar TS, MacDonnell KF, Namsirikul P et al: Survival after prolonged submersion in cold water without neurologic sequelae. Report of two cases. Arch Intern Med 140:775, 1980
21. Southwick FS, Dalglish PH Jr: Recovery after prolonged asystolic cardiac arrest in profound hypothermia. A case report and literature review. JAMA 243:1250, 1980
22. Fitzgerald FT, Jessop C: Accidental hypothermia: A report of 22 cases and review of the literature. Adv Intern Med 27:127, 1982
23. Verburg MP, Oerlemans FTJ, Van Bennekom CA et al: In vivo induced malignant hyperthermia in pigs. I. Physiological and biochemical changes and the influence of dantrolene sodium. Acta Anaesthesiol Scand 28:1, 1984
24. Liebenschutz F, Mai C, Pickerodt VMA: Increased carbon dioxide production in two patients with malignant hyperpyrexia and its control by dantrolene. Br J Anaesth 51:899, 1979
25. Szepesi B, Freedland RA: Effect of thyroid hormones on metabolism. IV. Comparative aspects of enzyme responses. Am J Physiol 216:1054, 1969
26. Wilmore DW, Long JM, Mason AD et al: Catecholamines: Mediator of the hypermetabolic response to thermal injury. Ann Surg 180:653, 1974
27. Biebuyck JF (ed): Nutritional Aspects of Anesthesia. Philadelphia, WB Saunders, Clin Anesthesiol 3:707, 1983
28. Weissman C, Hyman AI: Nutritional care of the critically ill patient with respiratory failure. In Weissman C (ed): Nutritional Support. Philadelphia, WB Saunders, Crit Care Clin, 3(1):185, 1987
29. Mansell AL, Anderson JC, Muttart CR et al: Short-term pulmonary effects of total parenteral nutrition in children with cystic fibrosis. J Pediatr 104:700, 1984

30. Damask MC, Schwarz Y, Weissman C: Energy measurements and requirements of critically ill patients. In Weissman C (ed): Nutritional Support. Philadelphia, WB Saunders, Crit Care Clin, 3(1):71, 1987

31. West JB: Gas Transport to the periphery. In Respiratory Physiology—The Essentials, 3rd ed. p 67. Baltimore, Williams & Wilkins, 1985

32. Guyton GC: Transport of oxygen and carbon dioxide in the blood and body fluids. In Textbook of Medical Physiology, 7th ed, p 493. Philadelphia, WB Saunders, 1986

33. Jehle D, Harchelroad F: Bicarbonate. Emerg Med Clin North Am 4:145, 1986

34. Garfinkel HB, Gelfman NA: Bicarbonate, not "CO_2". Arch Intern Med 143:2063, 1983

35. Wimberley PD, Siggaard–Andersen O, Fogh–Anderson N et al: Are sodium bicarbonate and potassium bicarbonate fully dissociated under physiological conditions? Scan J Clin Lab Invest 45:7, 1985

36. Thews G: Pulmonary respiration. In Schmidt RF, Thews G (eds) (translated by Brederman–Thorsn MA): Human Physiology, p 456. Berlin, Springer-Verlag, 1983

37. Lenfant C: Gas transport and gas exchange. In Ruth TC, Patton HD, Scher AM (eds): Physiology and Biophysics. Circulation, Respiration and Fluid Balance, p 325. Philadelphia, WB Saunders, 1974

38. West JB. Diffusion. In Respiratory Physiology—The Essentials, 3rd ed, p 21. Baltimore, Williams & Wilkins, 1985

39. West JB: Obstructive diseases. In Pulmonary Pathophysiology—The Essentials, p 59. Baltimore, Williams & Wilkins, 1982

40. West JB: Control of ventilation. In Best and Taylor's Physiological Basis of Medical Practice, 11th ed, p 605. Baltimore, Williams & Wilkins, 1985

41. Nunn JF: Control of Breathing. In Applied Respiratory Physiology, 3rd ed, p 72. London, Butterworths, 1987

42. Guz A: Regulation of respiration in man. Ann Rev Physiol 37:303, 1975

43. Hornbein TF, Roos A: Specificity of H ion concentration as a carotid chemoreceptor stimulus. J Appl Physiol 18:580, 1963

44. Radford EP: Ventilation standards for use in artificial respiration. J Appl Physiol 7:451, 1955

45. West JB: Ventilation. In Respiratory Physiology—The Essentials, 3rd ed, p 11. Baltimore, Williams & Wilkins, 1985

46. Fowler WS: Lung function studies. IV. Postural changes in respiratory dead space and functional residual capacity. J Clin Invest 29:1937, 1950

47. Fowler WS: Lung function studies. V. Respiratory dead space in old age and pulmonary emphysema. J Clin Invest 29:1439, 1950

48. Nunn JF, Campbell EJM, Peckett BW: Anatomical subdivisions of the volume of respiratory dead space and effect of position of the jaw. J Appl Physiol 14:174, 1959

49. Nunn JF, Bergman NA: The effect of atropine on pulmonary gas exchange. Br J Anaesth 36:68, 1964

50. Severinghaus JW, Stupfel M: Respiratory dead space increase following atropine in man, and atropine, vagal or ganglionic blockade and hypothermia in dogs. J Appl Physiol 8:18, 1955

51. Loh L, Seed RF, Sykes MK: The cardiorespiratory effects of halothane, trichloraethylene, and nitrous oxide in the dog. Br J Anaesth 45:125, 1973

52. Shepard RH, Campbell EJM, Martin HB et al: Factors effecting pulmonary dead space as determined by single breath analysis. J Appl Physiol 11:24, 1957

53. Nunn JF: Distribution of pulmonary ventilation and perfusion. In Applied Respiratory Physiology, 3rd ed, p 140. London, Butterworths, 1987

54. West JB: Blood flow and metabolism. In Respiratory Physiology—The Essentials, 3rd ed, p 31. Baltimore, Williams & Wilkins, 1985

55. West JB: Regional differences in gas exchange in the lung of erect man. J Appl Physiol 17:893, 1962

56. West JB, Dollery CT, Naimark A: Distribution of blood flow in isolated lung. Relation to vascular and alveolar pressures. J Appl Physiol 19:713, 1964

57. Stein M, Forkner CE, Robin ED et al: Gas exchange after autologous pulmonary embolism in dogs. J Appl Physiol 16:961, 1961

58. Severinghaus JW, Shupfel M: Alveolar dead space as an index of distribution of blood flow in pulmonary capillaries. J Appl Physiol 10:335, 1957

59. Greenbaum R, Nunn JF, Prys–Roberts C et al: Cardio-pulmonary function after fat embolism. Br J Anaesth 37:554, 1965

60. Donald KW, Renzetti A, Riley RL et al: Analysis of factors affecting the concentrations of oxygen and carbon dioxide in gas and blood of lungs—results. J Appl Physiol 4:497, 1952

61. Shapiro BA, Harrison RA, Walton JR: Arterial carbon dioxide tension. In Clinical Application of Blood Gases, 2nd ed, p 69. Chicago, Year Book Medical Publishers, 1977

62. Hedenstierna G, McCarthy G: Mechanics of breathing, gas distribution, and functional residual capacity at different frequencies of respiration during spontaneous and artificial ventilation. Br J Anaesth 47:706, 1975

63. Bergman NA: Effect of varying respiratory waveforms on distribution of inspired gas during artificial ventilation. Am Rev Respir Dis 100:518, 1969

64. Shapiro BA, Harrison RA, Walton JR: Respiratory acid–base balance. In Clinical Application of Blood Gases, 2nd ed, p 111. Chicago, Year Book Medical Publishers, 1977

65. Bernards WC: Practical management of acid–base disorders: metabolic component. In 38th Annual Refresher Course Lectures and Clinical Update Program, p 124B(1). Chicago, American Society of Anesthesiologists, 1987

66. Rogers TA: Elementary Human Physiology, p 153. New York, John Wiley & Sons, 1961

67. Auchincloss JH: Ventilatory disturbances in disease. In Fenn WO, Rahn H (eds): Handbook of Physiology—Respiration II, p 155. Washington, D.C., American Physiological Society, 1965

68. Shapiro BA, Harrison RA, Walton JR: Clinical Application of Blood gases, 2nd ed, p 206. Chicago, Year Book Medical Publishers, 1977

69. West JB: Gas exchange. In Pulmonary Pathophysiology—The Essentials, 2nd ed, p 19. Baltimore, Williams & Wilkins, 1982

70. Douglas ME, Downs JB: Cardiopulmonary effects of intermittent mandatory ventilation. Int Anesthesiol Clin 18(2):81, 1980

71. Safar P, Berman B, Diamond E et al: Cuffed tracheotomy tube vs tank respirator for prolonged artificial ventilation. Arch Phys Med Rehabil 43:487, 1962

72. Downs JB, Douglas ME, Ruiz BC et al: Comparison of assisted and controlled mechanical ventilation in anesthetized swine. Crit Care Med 7:5, 1979

73. Lamberstein CJ: Effects of drugs and hormones on the respiratory response to carbon dioxide. In Fenn WO, Rahn H (eds): Handbook of Physiology—Respiration I, p 545. Washington, D.C., American Physiological Society, 1964

74. West JB: Respiratory physiology in unusual environments. In Respiratory Physiology—The Essentials, 3rd ed, p 129. Baltimore, Williams & Wilkins, 1985

75. West JB: Control of ventilation. In Respiratory Physiology—The Essentials, 3rd ed, p 113. Baltimore, Williams & Wilkins, 1985

76. Shapiro BA, Harrison RA, Walton JR: Common clinical causes of abnormal blood gases. In Clinical Application of Blood Gases, 2nd ed, p 207. Chicago, Year Book Medical Publishers, 1977

77. Guyton AC: Textbook of Medical Physiology, 7th ed, p 511. Philadelphia, WB Saunders, 1986

78. Utting JE: Hypocapnia. In Gray TC, Nunn JF, Utting JE (eds): General Anaesthesia, 4th ed, p 461. London, Butterworths, 1980

79. Foex P, Prys–Roberts C: Effect of CO_2 on myocardial contractility

and aortic input impedance during anaesthesia. Br J Anaesth 46:669, 1975

80. Foex P, Prys–Roberts C: Effects of changes in $PaCO_2$ on pulmonary input impedance. J Appl Physiol 38:156, 1975

81. Burnum JF, Hickman JB, McIntosh M: Effect of hypocapnia on arterial blood pressure. Circulation 9:89, 1954

82. Prys–Roberts C, Kelman GR, Greenbaum R et al: Circulatory influences of artificial ventilation during nitrous oxide anaesthesia in man. II. Results: The relative influence of mean intrathoracic pressure and arterial carbon dioxide tension. Br J Anaesth 39:533, 1967

83. Karetzky MS, Cain SM: Effect of carbon dioxide on oxygen uptake during hyperventilation in normal man. J Appl Physiol 28:8, 1970

84. Neill WA, Hattenhauer N: Impairment of myocardial oxygen supply due to hyperventilation. Circulation: 52:854, 1975

85. Marshall M, Williams WG, Creighton RE et al: A technique for measuring regional myocardial blood flow and its application in determining the effects of hyperventilation and halothane. Can Anaesth Soc J 23:244, 1976

86. Girotti LA, Crosaho JR, Messuti H et al: The hyperventilation test as a method for developing successful therapy in Prinzmetal's angina. Am J Cardiol 49:34, 1982

87. Yasue H, Nagao M, Omote S et al: Coronary arterial spasm and Prinzmetal's variant form of angina induced by hyperventilation and Tris-buffer infusion. Circulation 58:56, 1978

88. Rasmussen K, Bagger JP, Bottzauw J et al: Prevalence of vasospastic ischaemia induced by the cold pressor test or hyperventilation in patients with severe angina. Eur Heart J 5:354, 1984

89. Bindslev L, Jolin–Carlsson A, Santesson J et al: Hypoxic pulmonary vasoconstriction in man: Effects of hyperventilation. Acta Anaesthesiol Scand 29:547, 1985

90. Monkcom W, Patterson RW: Ventilation perfusion inequalities resulting from hypocapnic changes in lung mechanics. J Thorac Cardiovasc Surg 63:577, 1972

91. Hewlett AM, Hulands GH, Nunn JF et al: Functional residual capacity during anaesthesia III. Artificial ventilation. Br J Anaesth 46:495, 1974

92. Alexander SC, Smith TC, Strobel G et al: Cerebral carbohydrate metabolism of man during respiratory and metabolic alkalosis. J Appl Physiol 24:66, 1968

93. Wasserman AJ, Patterson JL: The cerebral vascular response to reduction in arterial carbon dioxide tension. J Clin Invest 40:1297, 1961

94. Kjallquist A, Siesjo BK, Zwetnow N: Effects of increased intracranial pressure in cerebral blood flow and on cerebral venous PO_2, PCO_2, pH, lactate and pyruvate in dogs. Acta Physiol Scand 75:267, 1969

95. Reivich M: Arterial PCO_2 and cerebral hemodynamics. J Appl Physiol 206:25, 1964

96. Granholm L, Siesjo BK: The effects of hypercapnia and hypocapnia upon the cerebrospinal fluid lactate and pyruvate concentrations and upon the lactate, pyruvate, ATP, ADP, phosphocreatine and creatine concentrations of cat brain tissue. Acta Physiol Scand 77:179, 1969

97. Granholm L, Lukjanova L, Siesjo BK: The effect of marked hyperventilation upon tissue levels of NADH, lactate, pyruvate, phosphocreatine and adenosine phosphates of rat brain. Acta Physiol Scand 75:257, 1969

98. Davis H, Wallace WM: Factors affecting changes produced in electroencephalogram by standardized hyperventilation. Arch Neurol Psychiatr 47:606, 1942

99. Morgan P, Ward B: Hyperventilation and changes in the electroencephalogram and electrocardiogram. Neurology 20:1009, 1970

100. Kety S, Schmidt CF: The effects of active and passive hyperventilation on cerebral blood flow, cerebral oxygen consumption, cardiac output and blood pressure of normal man. J Clin Invest 25:107, 1946

101. Robinson JS, Gray TC: Observations on the cerebral effects of passive hyperventilation. Br J Anaesth 33:62, 1961

102. Knochel JP: Hypophosphatemia. West J Med 134:15, 1981

103. Watchko D, Bifano EM, Bergstrom WH: Effect of hyperventilation on total calcium, ionized calcium, and serum phosphorus in neonates. Crit Care Med 12:1055, 1984

104. Stauble M, Stauble UP, Waber U et al: Hyperventilation—Induced changes of the blood picture. J Appl Physiol 54:1170, 1985

105. Bellville JW, Seed JC: The effect of drugs on the respiratory response to carbon dioxide. Anesthesiology 21:397, 1960

106. Ritchie JM: The aliphatic alcohols. In Gilman AG, Goodman LS, Rall TW, et al (eds): Goodman and Gilman's The Pharmacologic Basis of Therapeutics, p 372. New York, Macmillan, 1985

107. Telivuo L, Katz RL: The effects of modern intravenous local analgesics on respiration during partial neuromuscular block in man. Anaesthesia 25:30, 1970

108. Campbell GD: Dangers of monoamine oxidase inhibitors. Br Med J 1:750, 1963

109. Steen SN: The effects of psychotropic drugs on respiration. Pharmacol Ther 2:717, 1976

110. Edelman NH, Epstein PE, Lahin S et al: Ventilatory responses to transient hypoxia and hypercapnia in man. Respir Physiol 17:302, 1973

111. Cherniak NS, Longobardo GS: Abnormalities in respiratory rhythm. In Cherniak NS, Widdicombe JG (eds): Handbook of Physiology, The Respiratory System, Control of Breathing, Part 2, p 729. Bethesda, Maryland, American Physiological Society, 1986

112. Yamamoto WS: Computer simulation of ventilatory control by both neural and humoral CO_2 signals. Am J Physiol (Regulatory Integrative Comp Physiol) 7:R28, 1980

113. Stone DJ: Respiration in man during metabolic alkalosis. J Appl Physiol 17:33, 1962

114. Roberts KE, Poppell JW, Vanamee P et al: Evaluation of respiratory compensation in metabolic alkalosis. J Clin Invest 35:261, 1956

115. Mulhausen RO, Blumenthals AS: Metabolic alkalosis. Arch Intern Med 116:729, 1965

116. Tuller MA, Mehdi F: Compensatory hypoventilation and hypercapnia in primary metabolic alkalosis. Am J Med 50:281, 1971

117. Kerr JH, Evers JL: Carbon dioxide accumulation: Valve leaks and inadequate absorption. Can Anaesth Soc J 5:154, 1958

118. Eger EI, Epstein RM: Hazards of anesthetic equipment. Anesthesiology 25:490, 1964

119. Smith RH, Volpitto PP: Volume ventilation valve. Anesthesiology 20:885, 1959

120. Inglis MS: Torsion of the inner tube. Br J Anaesth 52:705, 1980

121. Wildsmith JAW, Grubb DJ: Defective and missing coaxial circuits. Anaesthesia 32:293, 1977

122. Dunn AJ: Empty tanks and Bain circuits. Can Anaesth Soc J 25:337, 1978

123. Nimocks JA, Modell JH, Perry PA: Carbon dioxide retention using a humidified "nonrebreathing" system. Anesth Analg 54:271, 1975

124. Roussos C, Macklem PT: Inspiratory muscle fatigue. In Macklem PT, Mead J (eds): Handbook of Physiology, p 511. Bethesda, Maryland, American Physiological Society, 1986

125. Pride NB, Macklem PT: Lung mechanisms in disease. In Macklem PT, Mead J (eds): Handbook of Physiology, p 659. Bethesda, Maryland, American Physiological Society, 1986

126. Riley EA: Idiopathic diaphragmatic paralysis. A report of eight cases. Am J Med 32:404, 1962

127. Markland ON, Moorthy SS, Mahomed Y et al: Postoperative

phrenic nerve palsy in patients with open-heart surgery. Ann Thorac Surg 39:68, 1985

128. Severinghaus JW, Mitchell RA: Ondine's curse—a failure of respiratory center automaticity while awake. Clin Respir 10:122, 1952

129. Devereaux MW, Keans JR, Davis RL: Automatic respiratory failure associated with infarction of the medulla: Report of two cases with pathologic study of one. Arch Neurol 29:46, 1973

130. Downs JB, Douglas ME: Intermittent mandatory ventilation and weaning. Int Anesthesiol Clin 18(2):81, 1980

131. Prys–Roberts C: Hypercapnia. In Gray TC, Nunn JF, Utting JE (eds): General Anaesthesia, 4th ed, p 435. London, Butterworths, 1980

132. Pannier JL, Brutsaert DL: Contractility of isolated cat papillary muscle and acid–base changes. Arch Int Pharmacodyn Ther 172:244, 1968

133. Foex P, Fordham RMM: Intrinsic myocardial recovery from the negative inotropic effects of acute hypercapnia. Cariovasc Res 6:257, 1972

134. Cullen DJ, Eger EI: Cardiovascular effects of carbon dioxide in man. Anesthesiology 41:345, 1974

135. Nunn JF: The effects of changes in carbon dioxide tension. In Applied Respiratory Physiology, 4th ed, p 460. London, Butterworths, 1987

136. Prys–Roberts C, Kelman GR, Greenbaum R et al: Hemodynamics and alveolar-arterial PO_2 differences at varying $PaCO_2$ in anesthetized man. J Appl Physiol 25:80, 1968

137. Cullen DJ, Eger EI, Gregory GA: The cardiovascular effects of carbon dioxide in man, conscious and during cyclopropane anesthesia. Anesthesiology 31:407, 1969

138. Cullen BF, Eger EI, Smith NT et al: The circulatory response to hypercapnia during fluroxene anesthesia in man. Anesthesiology 34:415, 1971

139. Fourcade HE, Stevens WC, Larson CP et al: The ventilatory effects of forane, a new inhaled anesthetic. Anesthesiology 35:26, 1971

140. Calverly RK, Smith NT, Jones CW et al: Ventilatory and cardiovascular effects of enflurane anesthesia during spontaneous ventilation in man. Anesth Analg 57:610, 1978

141. Katz RL, Epstein RA: The interaction of anesthetic agents and adrenergic drugs to produce cardiac arrhythmias. Anesthesiology 29:763, 1968

142. Price HL, Lurie AA, Jones RE et al: Role of catecholamines in the initiation of arrhythmic cardiac contraction by carbon dioxide inhalation in anesthetized man. J Pharmacol Exp Ther 122:63A, 1958

143. Black GW, Linde HW, Dripps RD et al: Circulatory changes accompanying respiratory acidosis during halothane (Fluothane) anaesthesia in man. Br J Anaesth 31:238, 1959

144. Clowes GHA, Hopkins AL, Simeone FA: A comparison of physiological effects of hypercapnia and hypoxia in the production of cardiac arrest. Ann Surg 142:446, 1955

145. Leake CD, Waters RM: The anesthetic properties of carbon dioxide. J Pharmacol Exp Ther 33:280, 1928

146. Woodbury DM, Karler R: The role of carbon dioxide in the nervous system. Anesthesiology 21:686, 1960

147. Nahas GC, Ligou JC, Mehlman B: Effects of pH changes on O_2 uptake and plasma catecholamine levels in the dog. J Appl Physiol 198:60, 1960

148. Millar RA: Plasma adrenaline and noradrenaline during diffusion respiration. J Physiol 150:79, 1960

149. Tenney SM: Sympatho-adrenal stimulation by carbon dioxide and the inhibitory effect of carbonic acid on epinephrine response. Am J Physiol 187:341, 1956

150. Cohen PJH: Oxygen and intracellular metabolism. Int Anesthesiol Clin 19:9, 1981

151. Nunn JF: Oxygen. In Applied Respiratory Physiology, 3rd ed, p 235. London, Butterworths, 1987

152. Guyton AC: Metabolism of carbohydrates and formation of adenosine triphosphate. In Textbook of Medical Physiology, 7th ed, p 808. Philadelphia, WB Saunders, 1986

153. Forster RE: Diffusion of gases. In Fenn WO, Rahn H (eds): Handbook of Physiology—Respiration II, p 839. Washington D.C. American Physiological Society, 1964

154. Nunn JF: Diffusion and alveolar/capillary permeability. In Applied Respiratory Physiology, 3rd ed, p 184. London, Butterworths, 1987

155. Siggaard–Andersen O: Electrochemistry. In Tietz NW (ed): Fundamentals of Clinical Chemistry, 3rd ed, p 87. Philadelphia, WB Saunders, 1987

156. Pruden EL, Siggaard–Andersen O, Tietz NW: Blood gases and pH. In Tietz NW (ed): Fundamentals of Clinical Chemistry, 3rd ed, p 625. Philadelphia, WB Saunders, 1987

157. Kennedy SK, Wilson RS: Oxygen measurement. Int Anesthesiol Clin 19:201, 1981

158. Lenfant C, Aucult C: Oxygen uptake and change in carbon dioxide tension in human blood stored at 37° C. J Appl Physiol 20:503, 1965

159. Kelman GR, Nunn JF: Nomograms for the correction of blood PO_2, PCO_2, pH and base excess for time and temperature. J Appl Physiol 21:1484, 1966

160. Gravenstein JS, Paulus DA: Clinical Monitoring Practice, 2nd ed, p 316. London, JB Lippincott, 1987

161. Delivoria–Papadopoulos M, Ronceric NP, Oski FA: Postnatal changes in oxygen transport of term premature and sick infants. The role of 2,3 diphosphoglycerate and adult hemoglobin. Pediatr Res 5:235, 1971

162. Bunn HF: Disorders of hemoglobin. In Braunwald E, Isselbacher KJ, Petersdorf RG et al (eds): Harrison's Principles of Internal Medicine, p 1518. New York, McGraw-Hill, 1987

163. Auld PAM: Concepts in pulmonary physiology. In Scarpelli EM, Auld PAM (eds): Pulmonary Physiology of the Fetus, Newborn and Child, p 1. Phildelphia, Lea & Febiger, 1975

164. Rudolph AM: The fetal circulation. In Congenital Diseases of the Heart, p 1. Chicago, Year Book Medical Publishers, 1974

165. Morse M, Cassels DE, Holder M: The position of the oxygen dissociation curve of blood in normal children and adults. J Clin Invest 29:1091, 1950

166. Shapiro BA, Harrison RA, Walton JR: Guidelines for interpretation. In Clinical Application of Blood Gases, 2nd ed, p 129. Chicago, Year Book Medical Publishers, 1977

167. Hug CC: Monitoring. In Anesthesia, 2nd ed; page 411, Miller RD ed. New York, Churchill Livingstone, 1986

168. Severinghaus JW: Blood gas concentrations. In Fenn WO, Rahn H (eds): Handbook of Physiology—Respiration II, p 1475. Washington D.C., American Physiological Society, 1965

169. Marshall BE, Wyche MQ: Hypoxemia during and after anesthesia. Anesthesiology 37:178, 1972

170. West JB: Disturbances of respiratory function. In Braunwald E, Isselbacher KJ, Petersdorf RG et al (eds): Harrison's Principles of Internal Medicine, 11th ed, p 1049. New York, McGraw-Hill, 1987

171. Ingram RH: Adult respiratory distress syndrome. In Braunwald E, Isselbacher KJ, Petersdorf RG et al (eds): Harrison's Principles of Internal Medicine, 11th ed, p 1134. New York, McGraw-Hill, 1987

172. Said SI, Bannerjee CM: Venous admixture to the pulmonary circulation in human subjects breathing 100 percent oxygen. J Clin Invest 42:507, 1963

173. Bergman NA: Components of the alveolar—arterial oxygen tension difference in anesthetized man. Anesthesiology 28:517, 1967

174. Raine JM, Bishop JM: A–a difference in O₂ tension and physiological dead space in normal man. J Appl Physiol 18:284, 1963

175. Murray JF: Exercise. In The Normal Lung: The Basis for Diagnosis and Treatment of Pulmonary Disease, 2nd ed, p 183. Philadelphia, WB Saunders, 1986

176. Harris EA, Kenyon AM, Nisbet HD et al: The normal alveolar-arterial oxygen tension gradient in man. Clin Sci 46:89, 1974

177. Lemaire F, Harf A, Teisseire BP: Oxygen exchange across the acutely injured lung. In Zapol WM, Falke KJ (eds): Acute Respiratory Failure, p 521. New York, Marcel Dekker, 1985

178. Klocke RA: Intrapulmonary distribution of air and blood. In Fishman AP (ed): Pulmonary Diseases and Disorders, p 373. New York, McGraw-Hill, 1980

179. Gilbert R, Keighley JF: The arterial/alveolar oxygen tension ratio: Index of gas exchange applicable to varying inspired oxygen concentration. Am Rev Respir Dis 109:142, 1974

180. Gross R, Israel RH: A graphic approach for prediction of arterial oxygen tension at different concentrations of inspired oxygen. Chest 79:311, 1981

181. Shapiro BA, Harrison RA, Walton JR: Arterial oxygenation. In Clinical Application of Blood Gases, 2nd ed, p 79. Chicago, Year Book Medical Publishers, 1977

182. Bowe EA, Klein EF: Postoperative respiratory care. Int Anesthesiol Clin 21:77, 1983

183. Gray H: The respiratory system. In Epstein RM, Malm JR, Goss CM (eds): Anatomy of the Human Body, 28th ed, p 1159. Philadelphia, Lea & Febiger, 1966

184. Ravin MB et al: Contribution of thebesian veins to the physiologic shunt in anaesthetized man. J Appl Physiol 20:1148, 1965

185. Gray H: The veins. In Epstein RM, Malm JR, Goss CM (eds): Anatomy of the Human Body, 28th ed, p 686. Phildelphia Lea & Febiger, 1966

186. Shapiro BA, Harrison RA, Walton JR: Shunt and deadspace disease. In Clinical Application of Blood Gases, 2nd ed, p 185. Chicago, Year Book Medical Publishers, 1977

187. West JB: Ventilation-perfusion relationships. In Respiratory Physiology—The Essentials, 3rd ed, p 49. Baltimore, Williams & Wilkins, 1985

188. Smith RA: Oxygen delivery systems. In Kirby RR, Taylor RW (eds): Respiratory Failure, p 515. Chicago, Year Book Medical Publishers, 1986

189. Riley RL, Pernell S: Venous admixture component of the A–aDO₂ gradient. J Appl Physiol 35:430, 1973

190. Riley RL, Cournand A: Analysis of factors affecting partial pressure of oxygen and carbon dioxide in gas and blood of lungs: Theory. J Appl Physiol 4:77, 1951

191. Rahn H, Farhi LE: Ventilation, perfusion, and gas exchange—the V$_A$/Q concept. In Fenn WO, Rahn H (eds): Handbook of Physiology—Respiration I, p 735. Washington DC. American Physiological Society, 1964

192. Dantzker DR, Wagner PD, Tornabene VW et al: Gas exchange after pulmonary thromboembolization in dogs. Circ Res 42:92, 1978

193. Nunn JF: Pulmonary collapse and atelectasis. In Applied Respiratory Physiology, 3rd ed, p 440. London, Butterworths, 1987

194. West JB: Oxygen therapy. In Pulmonary Pathophysiology—The Essentials, 2nd ed, p 171. Baltimore, Williams & Wilkins, 1982

195. Webb SJS, Nunn JF: A comparison between the effects of nitrous oxide and nitrogen on arterial PO₂. Anaesthesia 22:69, 1967

196. Klaus MH, Fanaroff AA: Care of the High-Risk Neonate, p 242. Philadelphia, WB Saunders, 1973

197. Goudsouzian N, Karamanian A: Ventilation-perfusion relationships. In Physiology for the Anesthesiologist, 2nd ed, p 195. Norwalk, Connecticut, Appleton-Century-Crofts, 1984

198. Cheney FW, Colley PS: The effect of cardiac output on arterial blood oxygenation. Anesthesiology 52:496, 1980

199. Gravenstein JS, Paulus DA: Clinical Monitoring Practice, 2nd ed, p 144. Philadelphia, JB Lippincott, 1987

200. Dantzker DR, Lynch JP, Weg JG: Depression of cardiac output is a mechanism of shunt reduction in the therapy of acute respiratory failure. Chest 77:636, 1980

201. Lynch JP, Mhyre JG, Dantzker DR: Influence of cardiac output on intrapulmonary shunt. J Appl Physiol 46:315, 1979

202. Marshall BE, Marshall C: Anesthesia and pulmonary circulation. In Covino BG, Fozzard HA, Rehderk SG (eds): Effects of Anesthesia, p 121. Bethesda, Maryland, American Physiological Society, 1985

203. Cohen R, Overfield E: The diffusion component of arterial hypoxemia. Am Rev Respir Dis 105:532, 1972

204. Ream AK, Reitz BA, Silverberg G: Temperature correction of P$_{CO_2}$ and pH in estimating acid–base status: An example of the emperor's new clothes? Anesthesiology 56:41, 1982

205. Robin ED: Respiratory medicine. In Rubenstein E, Federman DD (eds): Scientific American Medicine, p I-1. New York, Scientific American, 1987

206. Goldberger E: The principles of acid–base chemistry and physiology. In A Primer of Water, Electrolyte and Acid–Base Syndromes, 7th ed, p 119. Philadelphia, Lea & Febiger, 1986

207. Davis RF: Etiology and treatment of perioperative cardiac dysrhythmias. In Kaplan JA (ed): Cardiac Anesthesia, 2nd ed, p 411. Orlando, Florida, Grune & Stratton, 1987

208. Levinsky NG: Fluids and electrolytes. In Braunwald E, Isselbacher KJ, Petersdorf RG et al (eds): Harrison's Principles of Internal Medicine, 11th ed, p 198. New York, McGraw-Hill, 1987

209. Roughton FJW: Transport of oxygen and carbon dioxide. In Fenn WO, Rahn H (eds): Handbook of Physiology—Respiration I, Vol I, p 767. Washington DC, American Physiological Society, 1964

210. Bear RA, Gribik M: Asssessing acid–base imbalances through laboratory parameters. Hosp Pract 9:157, 1974

211. Bernards WC: Interpretation of clinical acid–base data. In (eds): ASA Refresher Courses in Anesthesiology, vol 1, p17. Philadelphia, J.B. Lippincott

212. Smith TC: Practical management of acid–base disorders. Pulmonary component. In 38th Annual Refresher Course Lectures and Clinical Update Program, p 124. Chicago, American Society of Anesthesiologists, 1987

213. Guyton AC: Regulation of acid–base balance. In Textbook of Medical Physiology, 7th ed, p 438. Philadelphia, WB Saunders, 1986

214. Shapiro BA, Harrison RA, Walton JR: Metabolic acid–base balance. In Clinical Application of Blood Gases, 2nd ed, p 95. Chicago, Year Book Medical Publishers, 1977

215. Goldberger E: Acidosis and alkalosis. In A Primer of Water, Electrolyte and Acid–Base Disturbances, 7th ed, p 131. Philadelphia, Lea & Febiger, 1986

216. Grogono AW: Acid–base balance. In Racz (ed): Problems and Advances in Respiratory Therapy. Boston, Little, Brown and Co, 1986

217. Guyton AC: Lipid metabolism. In Textbook of Medical Physiology, 7th ed, p 818. Philadelphia, Lea & Febiger, 1986

218. Shapiro BA, Harrison RA, Walton JR: Chemistry of acid–base balance. In Clinical Application of Blood Gases, 2nd ed, p 11. Chicago, Year Book Medical Publishers, 1977

219. Goldberger E: Clinical measurement of acid–base balance. In A Primer of Water, Electrolyte and Acid–Base Syndromes, 7th ed, p 137. Philadelphia, Lea & Febiger, 1986

220. Shapiro BA, Harrison RA, Walton JR: Physics and chemistry of blood gas measurement. In Clinical Application of Blood Gases, 2nd ed, p 29. Chicago, Year Book Medical Publishers, 1977

221. Tietz NW: Electrolytes. In Tietz NW, Caraway WT, Freier EF et al (eds): Fundamentals of Clinical Chemistry, p 873. Philadelphia, WB Saunders, 1976

222. Tietz NW: Blood gases and electrolytes. In Tietz NW, Caraway WT, Freier EF et al (eds): Fundamentals of Clinical Chemistry, p 849. Philadelphia, WB Saunders, 1976

223. Garfinkel HB, Gelfman NA: Bicarbonate, not 'CO₂'. Arch Intern Med 143:2063, 1983

224. Gambino SR: The clinical value of routine determinations of venous plasma pH in acid–base problems. Am J Clin Pathol 32:301, 1959

225. Gambino SR: Comparison of pH in human arterial, venous, and capillary blood. Am NY Acad Sci 133:235, 1966

226. Hood I, Campbell EJM: Is pK' OK? N Engl J Med 306:864, 1982

227. Natelson S, Nobel D: Effect of the variation of pK' of the Henderson–Hasselbalch equation on values obtained for total CO₂ calculated from PCO₂ and pH values. Clin Chem 23:767, 1977

228. Tietz NW: Comparison of calculated and experimental PCO₂ values. Ann Clin Lab Sci 3:341, 1973

229. Trenchard D, Noble NIM, Guz A: Serum carbonic acid pK', abnormalities in patients with acid–base disturbances. Clin Sci 32:199, 1967

230. Halperin ML, Goldstein MB, Pickette C et al: Evaluation of the bicarbonate buffer system: Does the pK' really vary in the blood? Am J Nephrol 3:245, 1983

231. Gennar FJ: Is pK' OK? N Engl J Med 307:683, 1982

232. Ryan DH, Holt J: Is pK' OK? N Engl J Med 307:683, 1982

233. Austin WH, Ferrante V, Anderson C: Evaluation of whole blood pK' in the acutely ill patient. J Lab Clin Med 72:129, 1968

234. Levinsky NG: Acidosis and alkalosis. In Braunwald E, Isselbacher KJ, Petersdorf RG et al (eds): Harrison's Principles of Internal Medicine, 11th ed, p 208. New York, McGraw-Hill, 1987

235. Pitts RF: Mechanisms for stabilizing the alkaline reserves of the body. Harvey LE, Lect 48:172, 1952–1953

236. Van Dyke DD, Cullen GE: Studies of acidosis. I. The bicarbonate concentration of the blood plasma, its significance, and its determination as a measure of acidosis. J Biol Chem 30:289, 1917

237. Jorgensen K, Astrup P: Standard bicarbonate: Its clinical significance and a new method for its determination. Scand J Clin Lab Invest 2:122, 1957

238. Singer RB, Hastings AB: An improved clinical method for the estimation of disturbances of the acid–base balance of human blood. Medicine 27:223, 1948

239. Astrup P, Siggaard–Andersen O, Jorgensen K et al: Acid–base metabolism. New approach. Lancet 1:1035, 1960

240. Cohen JJ, Brackett NC, Schwartz WB: Carbon dioxide titration curve in the normal dog. J Clin Invest 43:777, 1964

241. Brackett NC, Cohen JJ, Schwartz WB: Carbon dioxide titration curve of normal man. The effect of increasing degrees of acute hypercapnia on acid–base equilibrium. N Engl J Med 272:6, 1965

242. Schwartz WB, Brackett NC, Cohen JJ: The response of extracellular hydrogen ion concentration to graded degrees of chronic hypercapnia: The physiologic limits of the defense of pH. J Clin Invest 4:291, 1965

243. Brackett NC, Wingo CF, Muren O et al: Acid–base response to chronic hypercapnia in man. N Engl J Med 280:124, 1969

244. Goldberger E: Clinical measurement of acid–base balance (continued): The Astrup method of determining acid–base disturbances. In A Primer of Water, Electrolyte and Acid–Base Disturbances, 7th ed, p 145. Philadelphia, Lea & Febiger, 1986

245. Nunn JF: Nomenclature and presentation of hydrogen ion regulation data. Modern Trends in Anesthesia 2: Hydrogen Ion Regulation and Biochemistry in Anesthesia. In Evans F, Gray T (eds): Washington DC, Butterworths, 1962

246. Roos A, Thomas LJ: The in vivo and in vitro carbon dioxide dissociation curves of true plasma. Anesthesiology 28:1048, 1967

247. Bunker JP: The great trans-Atlantic acid–base debate. Anesthesiology 26:591, 1965

248. Collier CR, Hackney JD, Mohler JG: Use of extracellular base excess in diagnosis of acid–base disorders. A conceptual approach. Chest 61:65, 1972

249. Holmdahl MH, Nahas GG, Hassam D et al: Acid–base changes in CSF following rapid changes in the bicarbonate/carbonic acid ratio in the blood. Ann NY Acad Sci 92:520, 1961

250. Robin ED, Wilson RJ, Bromberg PA: Intracellular acid–base relation and intracellular buffers. Ann NY Acad Sci 92:539, 1961

251. Tizianello A, De Ferrari G, Gurreri G et al: Effects of metabolic alkalosis, metabolic acidosis and uraemia on whole-body intracellular pH in man. Clin Sci 52:125, 1977

252. Graf H, Leach W, Arieff AI: Metabolic effects of sodium bicarbonate in hypoxic lactic acidosis in dogs. Am J Physiol 249 (Renal Fluid Electrolyte Physiol 18): F630, 1985

253. Schwartz WB, Relman AS: A critique of the parameters used in the evaluation of acid–base disorders. N Engl J Med 268:1382, 1963

254. Sladen A: Acid–base balance. In McIntyre KM, Lewis AJ (eds): Textbook of Advanced Cardiac Life Support, p 135. Dallas, Texas, American Heart Association, 1983

255. Gennari JF, Goldstein MB, Schwartz WB: The nature of the renal adaptation to chronic hypocapnia. J Clin Invest 51:1722, 1972

256. Lennon EJ, Lemann J: Defense of hydrogen concentration in chronic metabolic acidosis. Ann Intern Med 65:265, 1966

257. Goldberger E: Metabolic alkalosis syndromes. In A Primer of Water, Electrolyte, and Acid–Base Disorders, 7th ed, p 265. Philadelphia, Lea & Febiger, 1986

258. Roberts KE, Poppell JW, Vanamee P et al: Evaluation of respiratory compensation in metabolic alkalosis. J Clin Invest 35:261, 1956

259. Mulhausen RO, Blumenthals AS: Metabolic alkalosis. Arch Intern Med 116:729, 1965

260. Miller PD, Berns AS: Acute metabolic alkalosis perpetuating hypercarbia: A role for acetazolamide in chronic obstructive pulmonary disease. JAMA 238:2400, 1977

261. Javaheri S, Shove NS, Rose B et al: Compensatory hypoventilation in metabolic alkalosis. Chest 81:296, 1982

262. Goldberger E: Respiratory alkalosis. In A Primer of Water, Electrolyte and Acid–Base Syndromes, 7th ed, p 260. Philadelphia, Lea & Febiger, 1986

263. Emmett M, Narins RG: Clinical use of the anion gap. Medicine 56:38, 1977

264. Goldberger E: The body water. In A Primer of Water, Electrolyte and Acid–Base Syndromes, 7th ed, p 3. Philadelphia, Lea & Febiger, 1986

265. Foster DW: Lactic acidosis. In Petersdorf RG, Adams RA, Braunwald P et al (eds): Harrison's Principles of Internal Medicine, 10th ed, p 679. New York, McGraw-Hill, 1983

266. Andreoli TE: Disorders of fluid balance, electrolyte and acid–base balance. In Wyngaarden JB, Smith LH (eds): Cecil Textbook of Medicine, 17th ed, p 515. Philadelphia, WB Saunders, 1985

267. Alberti KGMM, Naltrass M: Lactic acidosis. Lancet 2:25, 1977

268. Sapir DG, Walker WG: Acid–base disturbances. In Harvey AM, Johns RJ, McKusick VA et al (eds): The Principles and Practices of Medicine, 21st ed, p 70. Norwalk, Connecticut, Appleton-Century-Crofts, 1984

269. Hazard PB, Griffin JP: Sodium bicarbonate in the management of systemic acidosis. South Med J 73:1339, 1980

270. Lever E, Jaspon JB: Sodium bicarbonate therapy in severe diabetic ketoacidosis. Am J Med 75:263, 1983

271. Arieff AI, Leach W, Park R et al: Systemic effects of NaHCO₃ in experimental lactic acidosis in dogs. Am J Physiol 242:F586, 1982

272. Ostrea EM, Odell GB: The influence of bicarbonate administration on blood pH in a "closed system": Clinical implications. J Pediatr 80:671, 1972

273. Bishop RL, Weisfeldt ML: Sodium bicarbonate administration during cardiac arrest. JAMA 235:506, 1976

274. Huseby JS, Gumprecht DG: Hemodynamic effects of rapid bolus hypertonic sodium bicarbonate. Chest 79:552, 1981

275. Graf H, Leach W, Arieff AI: Metabolic effects of sodium bicarbonate in hypoxic lactic acidosis in dogs. Am J Physiol 249:F630, 1985

276. Dumont L, Stanley P, Chartrand C: The cardiovascular effects of hypertonic sodium bicarbonate in conscious dogs: Underlying mechanisms of action. Can J Physiol Pharmacol 62:314, 1984

277. Weil MH, Trevino RP, Rackow EC: Sodium bicarbonate during CPR. Does it help or hinder? Chest 88:487, 1985

278. White RD: Cardiovascular pharmacology—part I. In McIntyre KM, Lewis AJ (eds): Textbook of Advanced Cardiac Life Support, p 99 Dallas, Texas, American Heart Association, 1983

279. Ryder RE: Lactic acidosis: High-dose or low-dose bicarbonate therapy? Diabetes Care 7:99, 1984

280. Stacpoole PW: Lactic acidosis. The case against bicarbonate therapy. Ann Intern Med 105:276, 1986

281. Hale PJ, Crase J, Nattrass M: Metabolic effects of bicarbonate in the treatment of diabetic ketoacidosis. Br Med J 289:1635, 1984

282. Goldberger E: Metabolic alkalosis syndromes: Hypokalemia. In A Primer of Water, Electrolyte and Acid–Base Syndromes, 7th ed, p 277. Philadelphia, Lea & Febiger, 1986

283. Goldberger E: Metabolic alkalosis syndromes. In A Primer of Water, Electrolyte and Acid–Base Syndromes, 7th ed, p 265. Philadelphia, Lea & Febiger, 1986

284. Wagner CW, Nesbit RR, Mansberger AR: The use of intravenous hydrochloric acid in the treatment of thirty-four patients with metabolic alkalosis. Am Surg 46:140, 1980

285. Worthley LIG: The rational use of IV hydrochloric acid in the treatment of metabolic acidosis. Br J Anaesth 49:811, 1977

286. Wagner CW, Nesbitt RR, Mansberger AR: Treatment of metabolic alkalosis with intravenous hydrochloric acid. South Med J 72:1241, 1979

287. Knutsen OH: New method for administration of hydrochloric acid in metabolic alkalosis. Lancet 1:953, 1983

288. Barcenas CG, Fuller TJ, Knochel JP: Metabolic alkalosis after massive blood transfusion. JAMA 236:953, 1976

289. Niemann JT, Rosborough JP: Effects of acidemia and sodium bicarbonate therapy in advanced cardiac life support. Ann Emerg Med 13:9, 1984

290. Simmons MA, Adcock EW, Bard H et al: Hypernatremia and intracranial hemorrhage in infants. N Engl J Med 291:5, 1974

Chapter 26   *Norig Ellison*

Hemostasis and Hemotherapy

Bleeding as a result of a defect in hemostasis may have numerous etiologies ranging from congenital deficiencies of coagulation factors, through trauma, to iatrogenic causes such as thrombocytopenia secondary to cancer chemotherapy or surgery. In the last instance some bleeding is to be expected and is not necessarily a cause for concern; however, blood loss in excess of that which would be expected at any stage in the procedure should be investigated. Furthermore, although the body's ability to seal off leaks in the circulatory system with a platelet plug or clot is essential, that ability to respond with rapid, localized hemostasis in a fluid medium is not without risk.

While imbalance in one direction, such as deficiency in platelet number or Factor X concentration, leads to excessive bleeding, imbalance in the other direction leads to thrombosis. The problem of imbalance in the direction of excessive thrombosis formation has become more widely recognized in the past two decades. For example, while bleeding disorders associated with specific clinical entities such as dead fetus or hemolytic transfusion reaction have long been recognized, the recognition of a common denominator and use of the terms *disseminated intravascular coagulation* (DIC) are recent developments. It was not until 1972 that DIC first appeared as a separate heading in *Index Medicus*. While DIC may be considered as a "disease of medical progress" in that it is now being diagnosed more frequently because more critically ill patients are surviving for longer periods of time, a more likely explanation is that the entity is now well accepted and, thus, just being recognized more readily and earlier.[1]

HEMOSTASIS

NORMAL PHYSIOLOGY

When a leak in the circulatory system develops, a primary hemostatic plug will form within 5 min of injury, requiring only interaction between the injured vessel and platelets (Fig. 26-1). The coagulation mechanism is not involved in the formation of the primary hemostatic plug. As a platelet plug forms, vasoactive substances, which are released from the platelets, produce vasoconstriction, a salutory effect in that decreasing the orifice that must be plugged will also decrease the leak. The formation of the definitive or secondary hemostatic plug, which will require an additional 1–2 hr, involves two more steps. First, a loose fibrin clot will be formed by the conversion of fibrinogen to fibrin through activation of the coagulation mechanism. Second, Factor XIII activation induces cross-polymerization of the loose fibrin to produce a firm, insoluble clot that in turn retracts into a firm, definitive hemostatic plug under the influence of platelets. Finally, fibrinolysis, a physiologic process, is activated to localize the clot and to remodel the area of injury as the endothelium regenerates.

The Blood Vessel

In the absence of such injury, the endothelium, which functions as a permeable barrier that prevents loss of colloid from the circulation, exerts multiple antithrombotic properties.

707

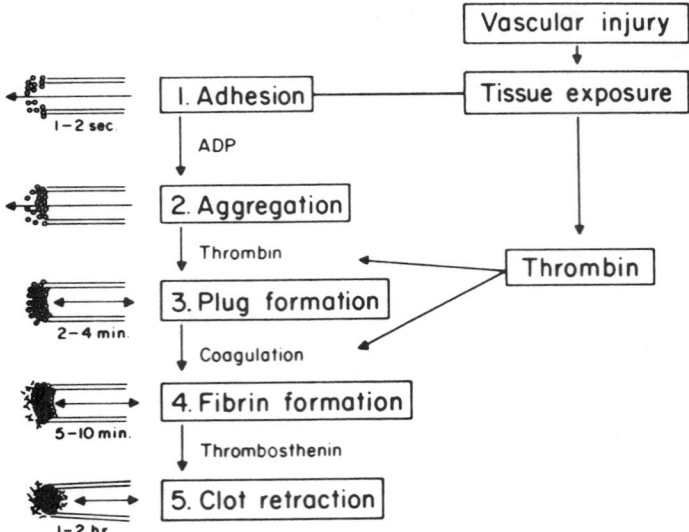

FIG. 26-1. Formation of the primary and secondary (definitive) hemostatic plugs. (Reprinted with permission. Herker LA: Hemostasis Manual, p 4. Seattle, University of Washington Press, 1970.)

First, there is contained on the luminal surface heparan sulfate, which can weakly stimulate antithrombin III (AT-III) and provide an ideal localized surface for AT-III to act. Second, the vascular endothelial cell produces prostacyclin (PGI2), which is both a potent vasodilator and an inhibitor of the hemostatic function of platelets. Third, the vascular endothelial membrane also contains a receptor, thrombomodulin, which forms a complex with thrombin to alter its activity radically.[2] Instead of forming a complex with Factor VIII to activate Factor Xa, or converting fibrinogen to fibrin, the thrombin–thrombomodulin complex converts protein C, a vitamin K-dependent physiologic anticoagulant, to its activated form. Active protein C inactivates Factor V and Factor VIII and regulates the release of tissue plasminogen activator (TPA). Once a definitive hemostatic plug has been formed, the vascular endothelial cells will play a role in fibrinolysis by synthesizing TPA, which appears to bind to fibrin and facilitates the action of fibrin-bound plasminogen, leading to clot lysis and healing.

Surgery cannot be performed without routinely creating multiple blood vessel defects. While the spontaneous arrest of bleeding from ruptured vessels conveying blood under pressure involves autonomic mechanisms that are extremely complex in detail, the mechanical principles governing the laws of blood flow through such a defect are quite simple. Blood loss will continue as long as pressure within the vessel exceeds the pressure outside the vessel. Blood vessel mechanisms to arrest blood loss include 1) vasoconstriction to decrease the size of the defect; 2) anastomotic dilatation to shunt blood away from the defects; 3) bleeding into tissues to increase the extravascular pressure and decrease the intravascular-extravascular gradient; 4) increased permeability of the microcirculation to promote further increase in extravascular pressure as edema fluid escapes from the blood vessels; 5) hemoconcentration, resulting from diminished plasma volume as fluid leaves the vascular compartment due to the increased permeability, to slow circulation and further reduce intravascular pressure; and 6) continual blood loss without replacement to produce sufficient hypotension to minimize or halt blood loss.[3] Finally, surgical ligation of the bleeding vessel will restore vascular integrity more quickly and completely in instances where these mechanisms would not suffice until irreparable harm had occurred.

Coagulation Mechanism

Because most blood vessels are less than 1 mm in diameter, and in vessels of this caliber platelets and coagulation factors play the major role in hemostasis, an efficient coagulation mechanism is essential to prevent bleeding. Figure 26-2 out-

FIG. 26-2. Schematic representation of the coagulation mechanism as measured *in vitro*. Factors involved in the prothrombin time, partial thromboplastin time (PTT), and the thrombin time are noted. (Adapted with permission. Morrison FS: Hemorrhagic complications in surgery. In Artz, Hardy [eds]: Management of Surgical Complications. Philadelphia, WB Saunders.)

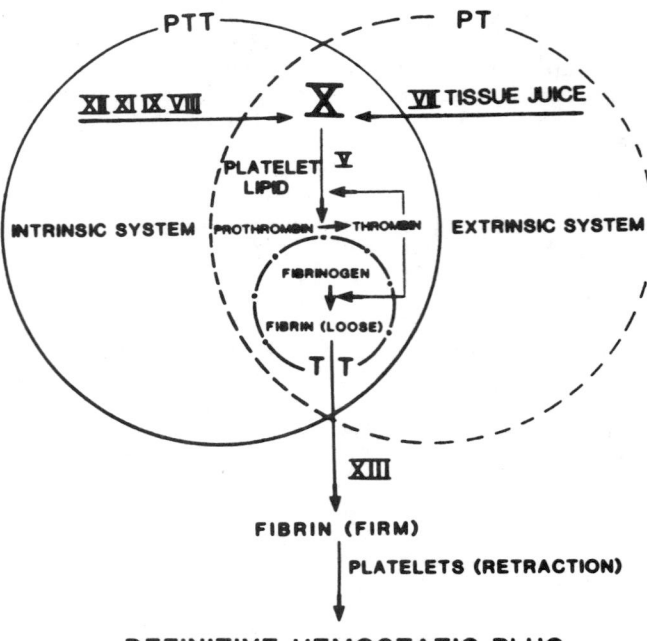

lines the currently accepted theory of the coagulation scheme, and Table 26-1 lists the coagulation factors with some of their synonyms. By common consent, the suffix "a" is used to designate the activated form, and the numeral VI has not been assigned to another factor. Three factors (I, V, VIII) do not exist in an enzymatically active form. With the exception of Factors III and IV, all of the factors are plasma proteins.

Primary hemostasis, the formation of the platelet plug, is accompanied by activation of the coagulation mechanism or cascade, the end result of which is formation of the definitive hemostatic plug. In the final common pathway, Factor X is activated by the end-product of either the intrinsic or extrinsic system. The complex sequence of events that leads up to activation of Factor X serves as a biologic amplifier, so that only a small stimulus is needed to initiate fibrin formation from fibrinogen. With a molecular weight of 340,000, fibrinogen conversion proceeds with thrombin splitting off two fibrinopeptides, A and B, which constitute about 3% of the fibrinogen molecule. Spontaneous polymerization of fibrin monomers into a loose fibrin net ensues and then, under the stimulus of Factor XIIIa, conversion of the loose fibrin net by covalent bonds into a more stable clot occurs. Finally, platelets induce retraction of the clot to form the definitive hemostatic plug.[4]

The concept of a rigid division of the coagulation cascade into an intrinsic and extrinsic system is no longer valid. In fact, not only can Factor VIIa activate Factor IX as indicated in Figure 26-3, Factors IXa, Xa, thrombin, and XIIa can probably activate Factor VII. Clearly, both systems are necessary for effective hemostasis because patients with isolated deficiencies in either system do present with clinical bleeding syndromes. Activation of coagulation factors is surface oriented, with platelet surfaces providing a protective environment that allows such activation to proceed unimpeded by the physiologic anticoagulants such as plasma AT-III.

Factor VIII is a complex consisting of von Willebrand factor (Factor VIII:vWF) and Factor VIII:C. The latter is that property of normal plasma missing in patients with hemophilia, measured in the standard coagulation assays, and, due to the presence of a procoagulant glycoprotein, that can be identified by immunoassay. Factor VIII:vWF is a large polymeric glycoprotein that mediates platelet adhesion to a foreign surface such as collagen during formation of the primary hemostatic plug. It is also necessary for formation of the definitive hemostatic plug because Factor VIII:vWF regulates the production or release of Factor VIII:C. While these two are noncovalently bound and closely associated in plasma, they are the products of different genes and have different immunologic properties.[5]

Platelets

Platelets have been called the keystone to the hemostatic arch because of their involvement in all phases of hemostasis. Not only are they the first nonvascular direct response of the body to bleeding, they are involved in activating the coagulation mechanism as well as initiating clot retraction. The initial event in platelet activation is exposure of the platelet to an appropriate stimulus, which produces a shape change in the platelet from its natural disc form to a "spiny sphere." After completing the shape change, platelet adhesion and platelet aggregation appear to develop simultaneously. Platelet adhesion is the affinity of platelets for nonplatelet surfaces, and platelet aggregation is an affinity of platelets for each other.

This phase of platelet activation culminates with the release reaction during which the contents of cytoplasmic granules are released extracellularly. The released substances include adenosine diphosphate (ADP), serotonin, platelet factor 4 (PF-4), catecholamines, and factors that modify vascular permeability and integrity. ADP is a potent aggregating agent, and its escape from platelets undergoing a release reaction causes more platelets to become activated. The released vasoactive substances stimulate contraction of the injured blood vessel. Platelets also actively participate in several steps of the

TABLE 26-1. List of Coagulation Factors With Some of Their Eponyms

FACTOR	SYNONYM	CLINICAL SYNDROME CAUSED BY DEFICIENCY
I	Fibrinogen	Yes
II	Prothrombin, prethrombin	Yes
III	Tissue factor, tissue thromboplastin	No
IV	Calcium	No
V	Labile factor, proaccelerin, plasma accelerator globulin (ac-G)	Yes
VI	No factor assigned to this numeral	
VII	Stable factor, proconvertin, autoprothrombin I, serum prothrombin conversion acceleration (SPCA)	Yes
VIII	Antihemophilia globulin (AHG), antihemophilic factor (AHF), thromboplastinogen, platelet cofactor I, antihemophilic Factor A	Yes
IX	Plasma thromboplastin component (PTC), Christmas factor, autothrombin II, antihemophilic Factor B, platelet cofactor II	Yes
X	Stuart-Prower factor, autoprothrombin C (or III)	Yes
XI	Plasma thromboplastin antecedent (PTA), Rosenthal syndrome, antihemophilic Factor C	mild
XII	Hageman factor, glass factor	No
XIII	Fibrin stabilizing factor (FSF), Laki-Lorand factor, fibrinase serum factor, urea-insolubility factor	Yes

(Reprinted with permission. Ellison N: Coagulation evaluation and management. *In* Ream AK, Fogdall RP [eds]: Acute Cardiovascular Management, p 773. Philadelphia, JB Lippincott, 1982.)

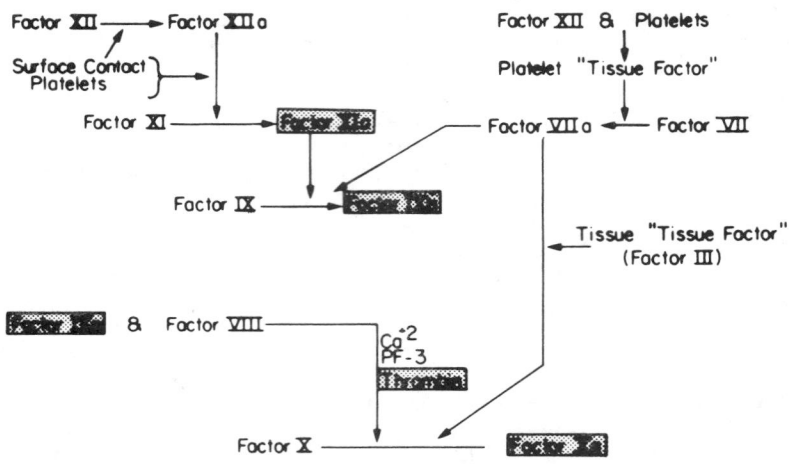

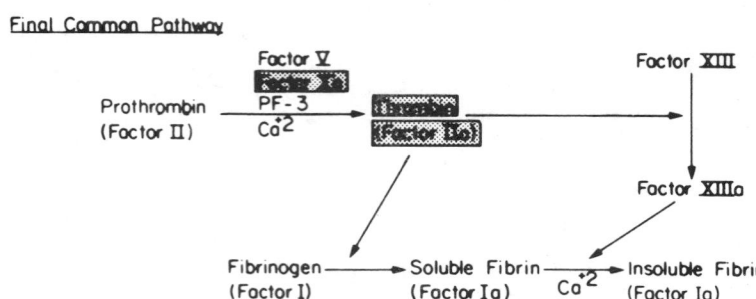

Final Common Pathway

FIG. 26-3. Coagulation cascade and its interrelationships. The four factors that comprise the prothrombin complex and are sensitive to coumarin administration, II (prothrombin), VII, IX, and X, are enclosed in boxes. The four activated factors that are inhibited by heparin, IIa (thrombin), IXa, Xa, and XIa, are shaded. This cascade demonstrates the interrelationships between extrinsic and intrinsic pathways in the first stage of coagulation. The concept of separate pathways is no longer valid.[14] PF-3 = platelet factor 3. (Reprinted with permission. Ellison N et al: Implications of anticoagulant therapy. Int Anesthesiol Clin 20:121–136, 1982.)

coagulation cascade as indicated in Figure 26-3. PF-3 is a property of lipoproteins within, and inseparable from, the platelet membrane. In contrast, PF-4, which neutralizes heparin, can be recovered from plasma after platelet aggregation and is a protein present in the granular fraction of platelet homogenates. The activated platelet membrane acts as a surface upon which the macromolecular complexes of blood coagulants (IXa, VIII, X, CA^{++}, and Xa, V, CA^{++}) are assembled.[6]

Platelets have also been reported to play a role in the activation of Factor XII in the presence of ADP, and possibly to provide an alternative route bypassing Factor XIIa by collagen-induced activation of Factor XI. This may explain why patients who are deficient in Factor XII and have markedly abnormal coagulation profiles do not bleed excessively. The final step in the sequence, clot retraction, is due to another platelet protein, thrombosthenin.

Fibrinolysis

There are several natural built-in checks to keep thrombus formation localized and to prevent the process from continuing to the point of complete intravascular thrombosis. These built-in checks include 1) rapid blood blow, producing dilution of coagulation factors below threshold levels; 2) clearance of activated coagulation factors by the liver and reticular endothelial system (RES); 3) blocking action of naturally occurring inhibitory plasma proteins such as AT-III on the action of thrombin. When the insult is overwhelming, the fibrinolytic system may be activated.

The fibrinolytic system digests fibrin to remodel the area of injury and prevent or reopen thrombotic occlusion of the

vessel. A classic example of the ability of the fibrinolytic system to recanalize occluded vessels is presented in the study of Bedford and Wollman, who reported 100% recanalization of radial arteries in 20 patients following demonstrated total occlusion after radial artery catheters were removed.[7] Both the plasminogen and coagulation systems contain inactive profactors, activators, and inhibitors. The primary activator of the plasminogen system is TPA, which selectively binds to fibrin and activates fibrin-bound plasminogen to plasmin, an event that tends to limit the extent of the fibrin formation. Plasmin is a serine protease that digests many substrates, including fibrinogen and Factors V and VIII. Ordinarily, upon escape from the fibrin surface, plasmin is rapidly activated by an extremely efficient inhibitor, α_2 antiplasmin.

The physiologic function of fibrinolysis is to localize fibrin deposition to the area of injury as well as to remove the secondary hemostatic plug during the course of healing. Recognized physiologic activators include vigorous exercise, anoxia, and stress in addition to the coagulation mechanism where both Factor XIIa and thrombin can activate plasminogen to plasmin. The activation of the fibrinolytic system in response to the intravascular deposition of fibrin is, therefore, a normal defense mechanism.

The pathologic form of fibrinolysis represents a response to increased thrombogenesis and occurs in the setting of disseminated intravascular coagulation (DIC). Rarely, pathologic fibrinolysis may occur in the absence of any obvious thrombogenic stimulus. In both types plasmin circulates intravascularly and digests not only fibrin but also fibrinogen and Factors V and VIII. Ordinarily, in vivo plasmin acts primarily on fibrin, breaking it down into successively smaller fragments known as fibrin split products (FSP), which possess anticoagulant properties of their own by inhibiting polymerization of fibrin monomers.

TESTS OF HEMOSTASIS

General Principles

The best means of detecting a hemorrhagic diathesis is a properly taken history. Especially important is information about the hemostatic response to a prior surgical procedure. Specific questions concerning dental extractions, for example, may suggest the need for further tests. Equally important is a detailed history of drug ingestion. Patients will usually volunteer the information if they were taking anticoagulants when interviewed, but perhaps not if they have been taking aspirin, which has a profound effect in small doses on platelet function.

The first step in the laboratory analysis of hemostasis is obtaining a blood specimen, which must be done with the same attention to detail as performing the test. Although the use of silicon needles and syringes has been advocated, disposable needles and plastic syringes are satisfactory. The venipuncture should be accurate and atraumatic to avoid introducing tissue fluid. One way to insure this is to use a two-syringe technique in which the first syringe is discarded after collection of 2 ml, and a second syringe is attached to the indwelling needle to collect the sample. The second syringe size and additives will vary, depending on what tests are to be performed.

An alternate approach to obtaining a blood specimen is the use of indwelling arterial or central venous cannulas. These lines may contain herapin flush solutions, and the frequent contamination of samples with heparin has prompted many laboratories to proscribe samples for coagulation tests being obtained from such lines. This proscription is not necessary if samples are collected with the same attention to detail as with venipuncture collection. Withdrawing an adequate aliquot prior to collecting a sample is particularly important. Withdrawing twice the dead space from the line prior to collecting the sample will eliminate the chance of herapin contamination. Additionally, the use of indwelling catheters around which hemostasis has been secured will obviate the need for venipuncture, which should ideally be avoided in patients with a hemorrhagic diathesis who are already bleeding from previous venipuncture sites.[8]

An increasing number of mechanical devices are available to perform coagulation tests, with the end-point being measured by electrical, magnetic, mechanical, or optical means. While all these machines have the advantage of reducing human variability in a given test, they are more expensive except in large-volume laboratories where their use has resulted in more efficient processing of many samples and usually more rapidly available results.

One of the limiting factors on the value of any test is how fast the results will be available. For this reason, tests that can be performed in the operating room appeal to many. Table 26-2 lists the criteria that are desirable for a hemostasis testing device designed for use in the operating room.[9] An alternative approach to evaluation of hemostasis directly by the anesthetist is the use of laboratory technicians in the operating room vicinity. With the increasing availability of clinical laboratories adjacent to or within the confines of operating suites to provide rapid arterial blood gas, pH and electrolyte analysis, incorporation of basic tests of hemostasis into such clinical

TABLE 26-2.   Characteristics of the Ideal Device for Testing Hemostasis in the Operating Room

Simple test procedures yield reproducible results
Equipment is compact, inexpensive, and operates quietly
Result is available quickly, even with abnormally prolonged time
Test is performed on whole blood rather than plasma
Test reagents are stable indefinitely
Test must not require prolonged attention away from operator's usual duties
Heparin concentration is linearly related to the test results (for open heart surgery)

(Adapted with permission. Ellison N, Jobes DR, Schwartz AJ: Implications of anticoagulant therapy. Int Anesthesiol Clin 20:121, 1982.)

laboratories may be desirable. No one test or pair of tests is sufficient to make the diagnosis of a bleeding disorder.

Tests of Coagulation Mechanisms

The activated coagulation time (ACT), a modification of the whole blood coagulation time in which celite is added to promote maximal activation of Factor XII, is a test of the intrinsic system and the final common pathway. The automated ACT is widely used to monitor heparin therapy, especially in the operating room.[9] Normal values for the automated variation of the ACT as provided by the manufacturer are usually in the range of 90–120 s.

The partial thromboplastin time (PTT) evaluates the intrinsic system and final common pathway, but eliminates the platelet variable by adding cephalin as a substitute for the PF-3. The original test, when modified by the addition of kaolin to produce maximal contact activation, is called the activated PTT (aPTT). Normal values are less than 35 s. This test will detect deficiencies of coagulation factors below 25% of normal levels except for Factors VII and XIII.

The prothrombin time (PT), one of the oldest and most commonly performed tests of coagulation today, is used to monitor coumarin anticoagulation. The PT tests the extrinsic system in the same way that the aPTT tests the intrinsic system. Both the PT and aPTT, of course, test the final common pathway. One of the principal determinants of the PT will be the strength of the thromboplastin suspension, which may vary greatly. For this reason, the use of control plasma and reporting both values is recommended in lieu of "per cent activity."[10] Prolongation of the PT or aPTT may be due to a coagulation factor deficiency or to a circulating anticoagulant. To differentiate these, the tests are repeated, with equal volumes of control plasma and patient plasma being compared with a 9:1 patient:control plasma. Continued prolongation in the former suggests the presence of an inhibitor, whereas shortening with the latter suggests a coagulation factor deficiency in the patient is more likely.

The thrombin time (TT) bypasses all but the final stage of fibrin formation. Thrombin solution is prepared and diluted until the TT of the controlled oxalated plasma usually falls into the range of 20–35 s. By diluting the thrombin suspension, this test can be made even more sensitive. Prolonged TT is due to a fibrinogen level less than $90 \text{ mg} \cdot \text{dl}^{-1}$, heparin or heparin-like anticoagulants that inhibit thrombin, or an abnormal fibrinogen. As with the PT, mixture of a patient's plasma with control plasma will confirm or disprove the presence of an anticoagulant.

Tests of Platelet Function

All platelet tests suffer from the same potential pitfall inherent in handling platelets, which tend to clump, fragment, and adhere to the sides of the collecting implements. To reduce the influence of this inherent platelet characteristic on test results, tissue damage and blood manipulation during collection must be minimized. Because most bleeding attributed to platelet problems is secondary to a reduction in platelet numbers, a platelet count should be the first test performed. The platelet count is a quantitative test only and does not measure platelet function. Counts can be performed with either light or phase microscopy, but electronic counters seem to offer greater accuracy. Bleeding rarely occurs unless the platelet count decreases to less than 50,000–70,000 mm^3.

The Ivy bleeding time, the most widely accepted clinical test of platelet function, measures both quality and quantity. Inability to control the many variables has made the Duke earlobe method obsolete. These variables include the length and depth of incision, the venous pressure, and patient cooperation. For that matter, in children or uncooperative adults who may not keep their arms still, the Ivy bleeding time may be invalidated. The introduction of a disposable template, which produces an incision of standard depth and width, has also improved the reproducibility of the Ivy bleeding time.[11] A normal bleeding time is 3–8 min.

The platelet aggregometer is designed to measure this function spectrophotometrically. The aggregometer has provided much information about the physiology of platelets. Platelet-rich plasma (PRP) and platelet-poor plasma (PPP) are prepared from citrated plasma and used to standardize an aggregometer, with PRP representing 0% light transmission and PPP 100% transmission. Aliquots of 0.5 ml PRP are tested with various reagents. The amount of a given reagent required to produce the release reaction is a measure of how sensitive the platelets are.

Clot retraction is another function of platelets that can be grossly measured. When maintained at 37° C, a clot should begin to retract within 2–4 hr. Efforts to quantitate the degree of retraction have not been successful and the test remains a qualitative test, with the presence of any clot retraction being considered positive.

Tests of Fibrinolysis

A clot should not lyse while maintained at 37° C for up to 48 hr. Lysis may occur in less than 1 hr in the presence of fibrinolysis. Care must be taken, however, not to mistake the fragmentation of the weak, friable clot of hypofibrinogenemia for fibrinolysis. A fibrinogen level obviously helps in distinguishing these two possibilities. A confirmatory test of fibrinolysis is performed by mixing a clot from normal plasma with an equal volume of test plasma or serum. If a normal clot lyses within 24 hr in the test plasma, increased fibrinolytic activity is present.

Plasminogen activator, plasminogen, plasmin, and fibrinogen are all euglobulins and can be separated from water-soluble inhibitors by precipitation when diluted with water. Sampling is extremely important in this test because prolonged venostasis (e.g., tourniquet on too long) and trauma (e.g., excessive alcohol rub of the skin) stimulate the release of plasminogen activator. Platelets will prolong the ELT because of their antiplasmin activity, so PPP should be used in this test. A normal euglobulin lysis time (ELT) is greater than 2 hr.

Fibrin(ogen) split products formed from the breakdown of either fibrin or fibrinogen cause coagulase positive Staphylococcus aureus to become adherent to one another and to produce visible clumping in contrast to the smooth suspension usually seen when no clumping has occurred. Serial dilutions of fibrinogen standards and patient serum are prepared and mixed with the bacterial suspension to measure the lowest dilution where clumping is easily visualized as an end-point. The comparison to standard fibrinogen dilution end-points gives the final answer, which is expressed in $\mu g \cdot ml^{-1}$ fibrinogen equivalents with values greater than 12 $\mu g \cdot ml^{-1}$, indicating active fibrinolysis.

Routine Evaluation

Again, a properly taken history is the best means of detecting a hemorrhagic diathesis, and together with a complete physical examination is the first and most important step in evaluating the hemostatic status of any patient. In patients who are poor historians or who have acquired a hemostatic defect since their last surgical experience, a history obtained regarding the hemostatic response to prior surgery is of little value. Rappaport has proposed performing screening tests of various levels depending on the magnitude of the surgery contemplated.[12] Conversely the concept that preoperative hemostasis tests should not be arbitrarily ordered has been advanced.[13] Nevertheless, a screening coagulation profile on any patient scheduled for major surgery as well as those whose history suggests a hemorrhagic diathesis is recommended. A useful profile includes a PT, aPTT, platelet count, fibrinogen level, and bleeding time. In the operating room, a baseline automated ACT is usually performed. While the yield from such a profile may be low, the advantage of not having to include a preexisting defect in the differential diagnosis of a bleeding disorder that occurs intraoperatively justifies the effort. With a negative history and a normal screening coagulation profile, this is a valid assumption. In addition, baseline values are available for comparison.

Figure 26-3 illustrates why no one test or pair of tests is sufficient to make an accurate diagnosis of a coagulopathy. While the aPTT and PT test both the intrinsic and extrinsic systems as well as the final common pathway, more refined mixing tests using plasma known to be deficient in Factor VIII, for example, are necessary before a definitive diagnosis of hemophilia A can be made. For that reason, a history of excessive bleeding must be given serious consideration and quantitative assays of at least the three hemophilia factors (VIII, IX, and XI) should be performed in such a patient to be certain that there is no preexisting hemorrhagic diathesis.

PATHOLOGY

Congenital Defects

The relative frequency of congenital hemostatic deficiencies varies greatly, with estimates of von Willebrand's disease as high as 1% of the population compared with less than 100 cases of familial afibrinogenemia having been reported. Some of the latter are believed to have represented DIC because they were associated with a low platelet count.[1] The relative frequencies of the three hemophilias are 85% for Factor VIII, 14% for Factor IX, and 1% for Factor XI, with the incidence of classic hemophilia A, Factor VIII deficiency, reported to be as high as 1 per 10,000–25,000 live births. The remainder of the congenital defects are extremely rare.[14]

Factor VIII, for which the kinetics have best been worked out, will be discussed to illustrate the eight variables that

TABLE 26-3.   Minimum Levels of Coagulation Factors and Platelets Necessary for Effective Hemostasis; Distribution and Fate of Clotting Factors After Transfusion Therapy; and Treatment Schedules

	MINIMAL LEVEL FOR SURGICAL HEMOSTASIS (% of normal)	GENETIC PATTERN IN CONGENITAL DEFICIENCIES	*IN VIVO* HALF-LIFE (hr)	THERAPEUTIC AGENT	DOSE (per kg body weight)	
					Initial	*Maintenance*
FACTORS						
I (Fibrinogen)	50–100	Autosomal recessive	72–144	Cryoprecipitate	Ppt from 100 ml	Ppt from 14–20 ml, once daily
II	20–40	Autosomal recessive	72–120	Plasma	10–15 ml	5–10 ml, once daily
V	5–20	Autosomal recessive	12–36	Fresh or frozen plasma	10–15 ml	10 ml, once daily
VII	10–20	Autosomal recessive	4–6	Plasma	5–10 ml	5 ml, once daily
VIII	30	Males affected Females carriers	10–18	Cryoprecipitate	Ppt from 70 ml	Ppt from 35 ml, twice daily
von Willebrand's	30	Autosomal dominant Variable penetrance		Plasma	10 ml	10 ml every 2–3 days
IX	20–25	Males affected Females carriers	18–36	Plasma or II, VII, IX, X concentrate	60 ml Variable	7 ml once daily
X	10–20	Autosomal recessive	24–60	Plasma	15 ml	10 ml, once daily
XI	20–30	Autosomal recessive	40–80	Plasma	10 ml	5 ml, once daily
XII	0	Autosomal recessive	?50–70	Plasma	5 ml	5 ml, once daily
XIII	1–3	Autosomal recessive ? Some sex link	?72–120	Plasma	2–3 ml	None
PLATELETS	50,000– 100,000 mm³			Platelet concentrate	1–2 units per desired 10,000 increment in count	

(Adapted with permission. Ellison N: Coagulation evaluation and management. *In* Ream AK, Fogdall RP [eds]: Acute Cardiovascular Management, p 733. Philadelphia, JB Lippincott, 1982.)

determine the dose. *Patient size, initial level of the deficient factor,* and *potency of the preparation* are three obvious determinants. *Hemostatic level* of each factor varies greatly. Table 26-3 lists the coagulation factors and the minimum level (% of normal) of each necessary for surgical hemostasis. Even this is not complete, as evidenced by Table 26-4, which equates the recommended levels of Factor VIII with surgical procedures. From this it can been seen that during the preoperative and convalescent period Factor VIII level should be maintained above 30% at all times. The *magnitude of the operation* influences the treatment mainly with respect to the duration of treatment—24-hr treatment or just one dose may be given in cases of minor dental surgery, whereas sustained levels above 30% are necessary in major orthopedic reconstruction for several weeks. The *half life* of coagulation factors varies greatly with Factor VIII levels at 10–12 hr, necessitating treatment at 8–12-hr intervals in contrast to von Willebrand's where treatment at 3-day intervals may suffice. *Redistribution* occurs out of the vascular space following the administration of all coagulation factors. The administration of any blood component results in a characteristic double exponential decay curve with the early rapid decrease due to redistribution. Again, for Factor VIII the extravascular distribution is twice the intravascular distribution, whereas for Factor VII extravascular distribution is one half the intravascular distribution. The *metabolic rate* will affect the dose in that an increase of metabolism with a fever, for example, will decrease the half-life of the products.

Deficiencies of hemophilia A and von Willebrand's disease and their treatment will be discussed as examples of a complete approach to these patients.

HEMOPHILIA A. Factor VIII deficiency, hemophilia A, is transmitted as a sex-linked recessive trait, but in 25%–30% of patients no family history of hemophilia can be obtained. There have been three dramatic breakthroughs in the management of patients with hemophilia.[2] The first was the isolation by Pool in 1964 in 3% of the original plasma volume of 30%–60% of the Factor VIII originally present. Prior to this isolation, fresh frozen plasma (FFP) was the only blood component available to treat hemophilia. This new component, cryoprecipitate, eliminated the volume constraints that previously plagued physicians and patients alike. The second breakthrough was the recognition that patients or their families could treat the patient at home at the first suggestion of a hemorrhage or on a regular schedule, a development that was

TABLE 26-4.   Recommended Factor VIII Levels and Duration of Treatment for Certain Operations or Bleeding Conditions

	FACTOR VIII LEVEL (Unit · ml⁻¹)	TREATMENT	
		Frequency (hr)	*Duration* (day)
Hemarthrosis	0.3	every 12	1
Dental (minor)	0.3	every 12	1
Dental (extraction)	0.3	every 8	1–2
All surgery	0.5	every 8	2–10

made possible after the introduction of lyophylized plasma concentrates eliminated the need for storing frozen cryoprecipitate. In particular the mangement of hemarthrosis and limb hematomas are very effectively managed on a home treatment program. The two major advantages of home programs are rapid treatment, which minimizes the crippling effects of hemorrhage, and economy of time and money by avoiding multiple trips to the clinic or hospitalizations, as well as the need for repeated infusions which early treatment may obviate. Home treatment also effectively eliminated the chain that kept patients with hemophilia in close proximity to their treatment centers.

The third breakthrough was the development of regional hemophilia centers to provide total care. These centers contain hematologists with special interest in the treatment of hemophilia, general and orthopedic surgeons who are well versed in the care of these patients, as are the dentists, oral surgeons, and social workers. The intraoperative care of these patients is also greatly facilitated by anesthesiologists who have a similar special knowledge. Usually these patients, who have lived with this disease all their life, are extremely knowledgeable and can educate physicians and nurses caring for them. Each program needs a coordinator who serves as the focal point for provision of care. The average patient with hemophilia will receive approximately 40,000–50,000 units of Factor VIII annually at a mean cost of $4000–5000. Today, in most states the financial burden has been eased greatly through the development of programs supported by the National Hemophilia Foundation or a state agency.

One unit of Factor VIII:C clotting activity is defined as the amount present in 1 ml of fresh normal, pooled plasma. A concentrate of one unit of Factor VIII:C activity per ml (i.e., 100 units·dl^{-1} is expressed as 100% with the normal range being 60%–140%. The practical way to plan treatment is based on the plasma volume, as follows:[2]

The initial dose before surgery = 1 PV

where PV = 1 unit of Factor VIII for each ml of plasma

Maintenance dose = ½ PV every 8 hr × Postoperative day 1
= ½ PV every 12 hr × for 7–10 days
= ¼ PV every 12 hr × for 5–7 days

In theory, Factor VIII requirements could be reduced while maintaining desired levels if the concentrate were given by continuous infusion. Treatment routinely should start 1½ hr before surgery and adequate plasma factor level goals should be confirmed before surgery. In recent years some patients have been discharged from the hospital to continue home treatment during further convalescence.

As in many disease states, treatment often carries complications. Because of the large number of donors to whom patients are exposed, acute and chronic hepatitis have long been recognized as complications of treatment. This is probably true whether the patient receives the cryoprecipitate, where each bag comes from one donor, or the commercial lyophilized products prepared from plasma pools of 10,000 donors. However, some centers treat hemophiliacs who are only mildly deficient in Factor VIII or IX, and all children less than 5 yr with cryoprecipitate or FFP in an attempt to decrease the incidence of hepatitis. Donors for commercial concentrates are all checked for hepatitis B surface antigen, but the tests lack sufficient sensitivity to detect 100%. Thus, small amounts of surface antigen can contaminate an entire plasma pool. For that reason, hepatitis B vaccine should be administered to all patients with hemophilia. The risk of acquired immuno deficiency syndrome (AIDS) transmission is discussed below.

The development of antibodies or inhibitors, which is seen in 7%–10% of patients, usually occurs in patients with severe hemophilia. In the case of "nonresponding inhibitors" that do not increase in titer when challenged by infusion of the antigen, merely increasing the level of Factor VIII will suffice to achieve hemostasis. In the case of a "responding inhibitor," the titer will increase 4–6 days after infusion and will remain elevated for months or even years. Attempts to treat these patients with porcine Factor VIII or plasmapheresis have not met with universal success. As improved fractionation has led to Factor IX concentrates that contain less activated factors, larger doses of Factor IX concentrate are required. For that reason today activated Factor IX concentrates that have Factor VIII inhibitor bypassing activity (FIBA) are used. These products presumably work by bypassing the Factor VIII step in the coagulation cascade. A future alternative therapy may be porcine Factor VIII.

Recent reports of decreased Factor VIII infusion requirements in patients who are maintained on danazol, an anabolic steroid, are conflicting. The promising early reports, which suggested that hemophilia therapy may be radically altered, have not been confirmed subsequently.[2]

VON WILLEBRAND'S DISEASE. Von Willebrand's disease, a milder bleeding disorder than hemophilia A, is characterized by mucosal rather than visceral bleeding and is unique in that it involves both primary and secondary hemostasis. The disease is inherited as either an autosomal dominant (types 1 and 2) or, rarely, as an autosomal recessive trait (type 3). Type 1 involves a quantitative abnormality of Factor VIII:vWF and type 2 involves a qualitative abnormality. The former also have low levels of Factor VIII:C, whereas the latter may have normal levels. Type 3 involves markedly defective synthesis of Factor VIII and an autosomal recessive inheritance pattern resulting in a bleeding pattern similar to that seen in severe hemophilia. Recognition that Factor VIII is a complex consisting of two portions, Factor VIII:vWF and Factor VIII:C, has permitted a better understanding of the relationships between these two diseases. Whereas in hemophilia A only Factor VIII:C production is deficient in amount and quality, in von Willebrand's disease there is a decrement in both Factor VIII:C and Factor VIII:vWF. Infusion of Factor VIII concentrate in hemophilia will result in levels that peak at the conclusion of the infusion and demonstrate a half-life of 10–18 hr as they decrease. In contrast, infusion of plasma or cryoprecipitate in von Willebrand's disease produces peak levels of Factor VIII:C 48 hr after the conclusion of the infusion that are sustained for 72 hr. This response has prompted the recommendation to infuse plasma or cryoprecipitate the evening before surgery to permit the delayed response to occur. However, correction of the bleeding time, a manifestation of the primary hemostatic defect, will last only 2–6 hr. To achieve both the increase in Factor VIII levels and the decrease in bleeding time, treatment with plasma or cryoprecipitate both the evening before and immediately before surgery is recommended. Repeat infusion of cryoprecipitate need be administered only at 24–48 hr intervals because of the sustained response.

In type 2 von Willebrand's disease, in which Factor VIII:C levels are normal, often only a single treatment given in the immediate preoperative period may be required. Cryoprecipitate is the blood product of choice to be used to treat von Willebrand's disease because Factor VIII concentrate lacks Factor VIII:vWF. Factor VIII concentrates are also not used to raise Factor VIII:C levels because supplemental plasma infusion will still be required to provide Factor VIII:vWF. 1-Deamino, 8-d-arginine vasopression (DDAVP) will increase Factor VIII:C levels in normal individuals, in patients with hemophilia who are mildly deficient in Factor VIII, and especially in patients with von Willebrand's disease, type 1. Intravenous administration is more effective than the intranasal route. Although not a form of treatment, it should be emphasized that aspirin ingestion by patients with von Willebrand's disease may markedly increase the hemostatic defects.

Acquired Defects

Defects in vascular integrity, deficiencies in coagulation factor levels, and quantitative or qualitative deficiencies in platelets comprise the possible etiologies of acquired defects of hemostasis. Within the framework of that classification the following causes of defective hemostasis will be discussed: 1) anticoagulants; 2) liver failure; 3) massive transfusion; 4) DIC; and 5) thrombocytopenia.

ANTICOAGULANTS. Coumarin-like drugs inhibit production of prothrombin (Factor II) and Factors VII, IX, and X, which together are known as the prothrombin complex or vitamin K-dependent factors, while heparin inhibits the action of thrombin (Factor IIa), IXa, Xa, and XIa. Small doses of coumarin inhibit Factor IX, resulting in prolongation of the PT while the aPTT remains normal. Larger doses of coumarin produce depression of prothrombin and Factors VII, IX, and X in addition, resulting in prolongation of both PT and aPTT. Small doses of heparin inhibit Factor IXa initially, resulting in a prolonged aPTT and a normal PT. Larger doses affect thrombin, Factors Xa and XIa, also resulting in a prolongation of both PT and aPTT. The presence of heparin in the patient's blood can be confirmed by adding protamine to the patient's citrated plasma and assessing whether this improves the aPTT. Coumarin can also be measured in the patient's plasma, a technique especially valuable in suspected cases of surreptitious ingestion or "coumarin malingerers."

A rebound hypercoagulable state resulting in exacerbation of the original condition for which the anticoagulant was originally prescribed has been suggested as a theoretical hazard of anticoagulant neutralization. There are no reliable data on which this theory is based and, furthermore, in an emergency situation such gradual tapering is impossible. Cessation of anticoagulant therapy because of hemorrhage carries no greater risk of recurrent embolism than does elective discontinuation, nor does the manner of termination (gradual or abrupt) affect the incidence of thromboembolism.[10]

Although protamine is the only commercial antidote available for neutralizing heparin, protamine requirements remain a confused and controversial area. *In vitro*, protamine will retard clot formation and has been shown to impair platelet aggregation in response to ADP. This may explain the bleeding problem seen following excessive doses of protamine.[15] Recent reports of adverse responses (allergic reactions, pulmonary hypertension) on administration of protamine have alerted clinicians to the possibility of severe and potentially lethal complications.[16]

Bleeding following neutralization of heparin and not due to obvious inadequate surgical hemostasis may be due to heparin rebound, which is defined as the recurrence of heparin effect in blood following laboratory-demonstrated adequate neutralization with protamine. Heparin rebound has been described as occurring up to 24 hr following heparin neutralization, and is most likely to occur in the first 4–6 hr after neutralization. While the occurrence of heparin rebound is probably a relatively rare event in the usual clinical setting, the diagnosis is easily made by means of an ACT and a protamine titration, and specific, simple treatment with protamine is readily available.

Transfusion of blood or plasma or the administration of vitamin K are the two methods available to neutralize coumarin. Vitamin K is the specific antidote for coumarin, but will take at least 3–6 hr for an effect in patients with normal liver function. Vitamin K in doses of 2.5–50 mg should be given orally or parenterally depending on severity. Response to therapy should be monitored with serial prothrombin times to insure a satisfactory response. Because the action of coumarin may last 4–5 days, it is advisable to follow the PT daily for that period. In the emergency situation, transfusion is required. While transfusion produces immediate results, there is no formula available to predict the volume of blood or plasma required because the degree of depression of the patient's coagulation factors for a given PT and the level of coagulation factors present in each unit of blood or plasma are extremely variable. Because the four vitamin K-dependent factors (II, VII, IX, and X) are all present in banked blood, administration of fresh whole blood or FFP is not necessary. Concentrates of the prothrombin complex are no longer recommended as an antidote for coumarin because as a pooled product, they have a high risk of hepatitis and also contain thrombogenic material or activated clotting factors that may initiate DIC.

LIVER FAILURE. In advanced cases of liver failure, bleeding may be due to portal hypertension and mechanical factors such as esophageal varices or thrombocytopenia secondary to hypersplenism, to excessive fibrinolysis, or to decreased production of clotting factors. Thus, isolated or combined defects in vascular integrity or decreased levels of platelets or coagulation factors are all possible in these patients. The synthesis of clotting factors in the liver decreases in proportion to the loss of liver cells. For this reason the PT is a good prognostic indicator in patients with liver failure. Treatment of bleeding episodes associated with liver failure depends on an accurate diagnosis whenever possible and will vary from vitamin K administration or platelet transfusion to surgical decompression of the portal vein.

Factors I, V, and XI are produced in the liver as well as the four vitamin K-dependent factors (II, VII, IX, and X); therefore, vitamin K alone, even in massive doses, will not correct the deficiency seen in liver failure. Slight improvement following parenteral vitamin K may be seen because of malabsorption of vitamin K due to lack of bile salts. More often, clinically significant depression of fibrinogen is a feature of advanced liver disease or of increased fibrinolysis and DIC more than the result of decreased synthesis of coagulation factors.

One iatrogenic cause of bleeding due to decreased production that may be seen in critically ill patients is the intestinal sterilization syndrome. The intestinal flora are a major source of vitamin K in humans. Patients who have their gastrointestinal tracts sterilized with large doses of antibiotic preoperatively lose this source of vitamin K. If they are maintained on intravenous fluids or receive a restricted diet without vitamin K-containing foods, their vitamin K stores will be depleted in approximately 1 week. This syndrome is easily diagnosed on the basis of history, the finding of an isolated prolonged PT, and the prompt response to vitamin K administration.

MASSIVE TRANSFUSION. Ideally, therapy should be designed to treat a pathologic condition without producing another one. The need to correct an acute hypovolemic state with large volumes of blood, however, may produce a hemostatic defect inherent in bank blood. Factor VIII levels decrease by 50% after 2 days, but Factor V levels do not decrease to 50% for over 2 weeks. However, the remaining levels are well above the minimal hemostatic level for Factor V and usually for Factor VIII. Thus, deficiencies of these two factors are rarely a primary cause of bleeding.

In contrast, the hemostatic effectiveness of stored platelets rapidly decays over 48–72 hr. In what amounted to a bioassay that clearly demonstrated this, Miller et al[17] infused 500–1000 ml of FFP (which contains Factors V and VIII but no platelets) into combat casualties who were bleeding after receiving more than 20 units of blood. They demonstrated return to normal of the aPPT and PTs without correction of the bleeding disorders. Subsequent administration of fresh whole blood resulted in correction of these bleeding disorders.[17] Nevertheless, the potential production of a qualitative or quantitative defect in platelets does not justify routine administration of platelets in massive transfusion.[18] It is not clear whether mild deficiencies of Factor V and VIII, which are insufficient to produce bleeding on their own, may possibly aggravate the bleeding seen in patients with thrombocytopenia.

DISSEMINATED INTRAVASCULAR COAGULATION. DIC is a pathologic syndrome in which formation of fibrin thrombi, consumption of Factors V and VIII, loss of platelets, and activation of the fibrinolytic system suggest the presence of thrombin in the systemic circulation. The clinical findings of DIC may vary, with patients manifesting thrombotic, hemorrhagic, or mixed signs and symptoms. Furthermore, some patients with no clinical manifestations may have classic laboratory findings of DIC. Table 26-5 lists the potential causes of DIC.

The hemorrhagic component of the DIC spectrum is readily appreciated and has been characterized as a paradox in that bleeding and thrombosis are occurring simultaneously, and are further complicated by another paradox in that one of the recommended forms of treatment of the hemorrhage is the administration of an anticoagulant, heparin.[19] The thrombotic component of the DIC spectrum, although obviously a necessary precursor to the hemorrhagic component, is less readily appreciated.

There is no one pathognomonic laboratory test for DIC. Colman and Robboy have established the following criteria.[20]

TABLE 26-5. Potential Causes of Disseminated Intravascular Coagulation (DIC) Divided Into Three Basic Mechanisms*

1. Cellular damage releasing into the blood stream phospholipids, which are necessary for both the extrinsic and intrinsic systems of coagulation to function
    Examples: hemolytic transfusion reaction, malaria, trauma, extracorporeal circulation, near drowning
2. Endothelial damage resulting in activation of the intrinsic clotting system through exposure of blood to collagen
    Examples: viremia, heat stroke, meningococcemia, trauma, aortic aneurysm, shock, glomerulonephritis
3. Introduction of tissue factor into the blood stream resulting in activation of the extrinsic clotting system
    Examples: neoplasms, leukemia, trauma and tissue injury, obstetrical defibrination syndromes, extracorporeal circulation, burns, transplant rejection

* The difficulty in dividing cases of DIC into different categories is illustrated by the listing of trauma in all three categories. Trauma can damage cells, injure blood vessels and expose collagen, and introduce tissue factor into the blood stream.

In the absence of hepatic disease or blood transfusion, they use a screening triad of PT greater than 15 s, fibrinogen level less than 160 $mg \cdot dl^{-1}$, and platelet count less than 150,000 mm^3. Abnormalities of all three indicate DIC. If results of two of these three tests are abnormal, then either the TT time or FSP must be abnormal to confirm the laboratory diagnosis of DIC.[20] While these criteria may sound straightforward, patients have frequently received at least a blood transfusion before the diagnosis is entertained. In that case, a high index of suspicion permits the diagnosis to be made on clinical grounds. Perhaps the *sine qua non* from the lab tests to support a diagnosis of DIC is a decrease in the platelet count. As a practical matter in a patient who presents with a typical clinical setting, and both the platelet count and fibrinogen level are decreased, Hattersley has suggested that the diagnosis can be presumed until proven otherwise.[21]

The differential diagnosis of primary *versus* secondary fibrinolysis must be considered, although the validity of differentiating primary and secondary fibrinolysis is now being questioned.[22] The conversion of plasminogen to plasmin as a defense mechanism (secondary fibrinolysis) to the intravascular deposition of fibrin, would destroy fibrin or fibrinogen and Factors V and VIII. Both the consumption of platelets and coagulation factors and the presence of FSPs, which result from the plasmin degradation of fibrin or fibrinogen and which possess anticoagulant properties of their own, will further aggravate the bleeding disorder. If differentiation of primary from secondary fibrinolysis is vital, a normal platelet count most likely suggests primary fibrinolysis. Certain disease states such as cirrhosis or prostatic surgery are also commonly associated with primary fibrinolysis.

DIC is never a primary disease state, nor will every patient who receives, for example, an incompatible blood transfusion develop DIC because of the natural defense mechanisms that will facilitate elimination of thrombin within the vascular tree. Thus, in most cases of incompatible blood transfusion for example, the combination of rapid blood flow–dilution, hepatic–RES clearance, and naturally occurring inhibitors will prevent DIC; however, in cases of stagnant blood flow such as shock, hepatic–RES impairment such as hypoxemia, or where the insult is so overwhelming such as massive transfusion of ABO incompatible blood, DIC may develop.

The initial treatment of DIC is not heparin. The first goal of treatment should be correction of the primary disorder. This may be all that is necessary and DIC will be self limited. In some patients with primary disorders such as septic shock or neoplasia, however, correction of the primary disorder may not be readily accomplished. Heparin therapy in these patients is designed to stop clot formation, and thus to inhibit the continued consumption of coagulation factors and platelets so that they can reach normal levels. Heparin doses of 40–80 $units \cdot kg^{-1}$ are administered every 4–6 h, the object being to prolong the whole blood coagulation time (WBCT) to two to three times normal. Ideally, this should produce sufficient anticoagulation to prevent clot formation but not produce bleeding. Monitoring heparin therapy with a WBCT is recommended instead of the aPTT because the latter is more sensitive to depleted coagulation factors and the anticoagulant effects of FSPs and cannot distinguish between them and the effect of heparin.[20]

Heparin therapy is by no means universally accepted in the treatment of DIC, and the decision to employ heparin is not to be taken lightly. There is some disagreement that heparin therapy at best merely replaces one cause of bleeding with another and that theoretical grounds are not sufficient to justify the use of such a dangerous drug. We have been

extremely reluctant to use heparin therapy in surgical patients, especially in patients with severe fibrinogenemia (less
than 50 mg·dl^{-1}), an accompanying vasculitis, or local defect
in vasculature.[1]

The most recent addition to the therapeutic regimen for DIC
is cryoprecipitate. While this blood product was originally
developed for the treatment of hemophilia, a unit of
cryoprecipitate contains one third of the fibrinogen in the
plasma from which it is derived. There is less risk of hepatitis
with cryoprecipitate than with fibrinogen, which is a pooled
product that contains no Factor VIII. The use of cryoprecipitate
will therefore increase levels of fibrinogen and Factor VIII,
both of which are depressed in DIC. FFP and platelet concentrates may be required also to treat other deficiencies.

THROMBOCYTOPENIA. Thrombocytopenia can occur in
massive transfusion, liver failure, or DIC. Thrombocytopenia
may also develop independently of these conditions due to
decreased production as in cases of aplastic anemia or in
oncologic patients who are receiving chemotherapy or due to
increased destruction as in idiopathic thrombocytopenic purpura, which could well be called "immune" thrombocytopenic purpura.

In a review article we stated that the cut-off below which
elective surgery should not be performed in patients with
thrombocytopenia ranged from 50,000–100,000 per mm^3.[4]
More recently, Tomasullo and Lenes have stated that if the
bleeding time is less than twice the upper limit of normal and
the platelet count is greater than 50,000 per mm^3, a patient
may undergo surgery without prophylactic transfusion.[23]
They base this recommendation in part on the fact that bleeding due to thrombocytopenia is not rapid. Where blood loss is
rapid in the patient with thrombocytopenia, a significant
bleeding lesion should be sought, and the repair of such lesion
requires more attention than increasing the platelet count. In
fact, since transfused platelets would just be lost during the
period of rapid blood loss, transfusion should always be delayed until a modicum of surgical hemostasis has been
achieved.

HEMOTHERAPY

RED BLOOD CELL *VERSUS* WHOLE BLOOD ADMINISTRATION

To increase oxygen-carrying capacity, red blood cells (RBC)
only are required. Ideally, therefore, only RBCs, formally referred to as "packed red blood cells" or PRBC should be
administered. Certainly that is the case in treating anemia
where the administration of RBC produces almost a twofold
greater increase in the hemoglobin level than a similar volume
of whole blood. In the surgical patient, however, especially
one who is bleeding massively and losing plasma as well as
RBCs, the use of whole blood seems logical.

The pressing need to provide Factor VIII concentrate to treat
patients with hemophilia and platelet concentrates to treat
oncology patients has led many blood banks to fraction increasing amounts of blood. Figure 26-4 illustrates our local
practice in which a 1200% increase in RBCs transfused has
been associated with a 77% decrease in whole blood transfused in the past decade. Mollison has questioned whether
the current practice of fractionating approximately 80% of
units will leave sufficient units of whole blood to satisfy the
needs in cases of massive transfusion.[24] Schmidt has outlined
his practice as follows: preoperative orders to cross-match four

or more units of blood are filled with whole blood; for three or
fewer units, RBCs are prepared and supplemented as necessary by crystalloid solutions.[25] Recently it has been recommended that patients who lose more than 25% of their blood
volume and are continuing to bleed should receive whole
blood.[26]

What are the objections to using RBCs in surgical patients?
Slow flow rate, inadequate volume replacement, and deficiency of coagulation factors are frequently mentioned. The
major objection seems to be that because of the increased
viscosity, the RBCs flow more slowly, especially through a
microfilter. This objection can easily be overcome, however, by
reconstitution with saline. In cases where rapid replacement
of blood loss is required, some form of pressurized system is
usually employed and this will also markedly improve flow
rate. The issue of volume replacement is also answered by
reconstitution. The third major objection to the use of RBCs is
that the level of plasma coagulation factors and platelets may
decrease to the point that a hemorrhagic diathesis is produced, further complicating the bleeding. Because blood
stored over 24 hr contains few viable platelets, the need for
platelet concentrates to treat dilutional thrombocytopenia is
not lessened by using whole blood in lieu of RBCs unless fresh
whole blood is used. Logistically, a requirement for fresh
whole blood cannot be met by most blood banks. FFP may be
required to correct a coagulation factor deficiency; however,
Counts *et al* responded to the need for Factor VIII and platelets
while providing blood products for the trauma patient by
collecting blood in a triple-bag system from which 85% of the
platelets, 60% of Factor VIII, and 25% of fibrinogen are removed. The supernatant plasma remaining after cryoprecipitate removal is then returned to the RBCs to provide modified
whole blood.[27]

FRESH FROZEN PLASMA

In cases of liver failure, the administration of FFP, which
contains all the clotting factors generally produced by the liver
and is often prescribed in massive doses, has recently been
questioned. During the past decade there has been a tenfold
increase in the use of FFP in the United States. It has been
suggested that "FFP is used most commonly as a volume
replacement solution," although it is not specifically required
for this purpose.[28] This same review concluded that the role of
FFP in the management of coagulopathy in patients receiving
large volumes of stored blood is not well defined despite
widespread advocacy for FFP in these situations. A Consensus Development Conference held at the National Institutes of Health in September 1984 reached the same conclusions.[29] Two large-scale prospective studies of massively
transfused patients have failed to indicate that either the PT or
aPTT possess sufficient specificity to justify FFP administration. Therefore, rigid use of the outlined screening tests to
determine when FFP is to be administered cannot be recommended. Again, laboratory tests must be correlated with the
clinical picture to guide appropriate therapy. Clearly the need
for FFP in nonbleeding patients on a prophylactic basis is not
likely to be beneficial, nor has the value of any preestablished
FFP regimen (*e.g.*, 1 unit FFP for every 3ˆ6 units of RBCs) been
proven effective. In summary, while FFP may be the most
widely overprescribed blood product, the guidelines for the
use of FFP based on current literature are necessarily vague. In
view of the potential hazards of infection and severe pulmonary complications, the use of these products should be minimized.

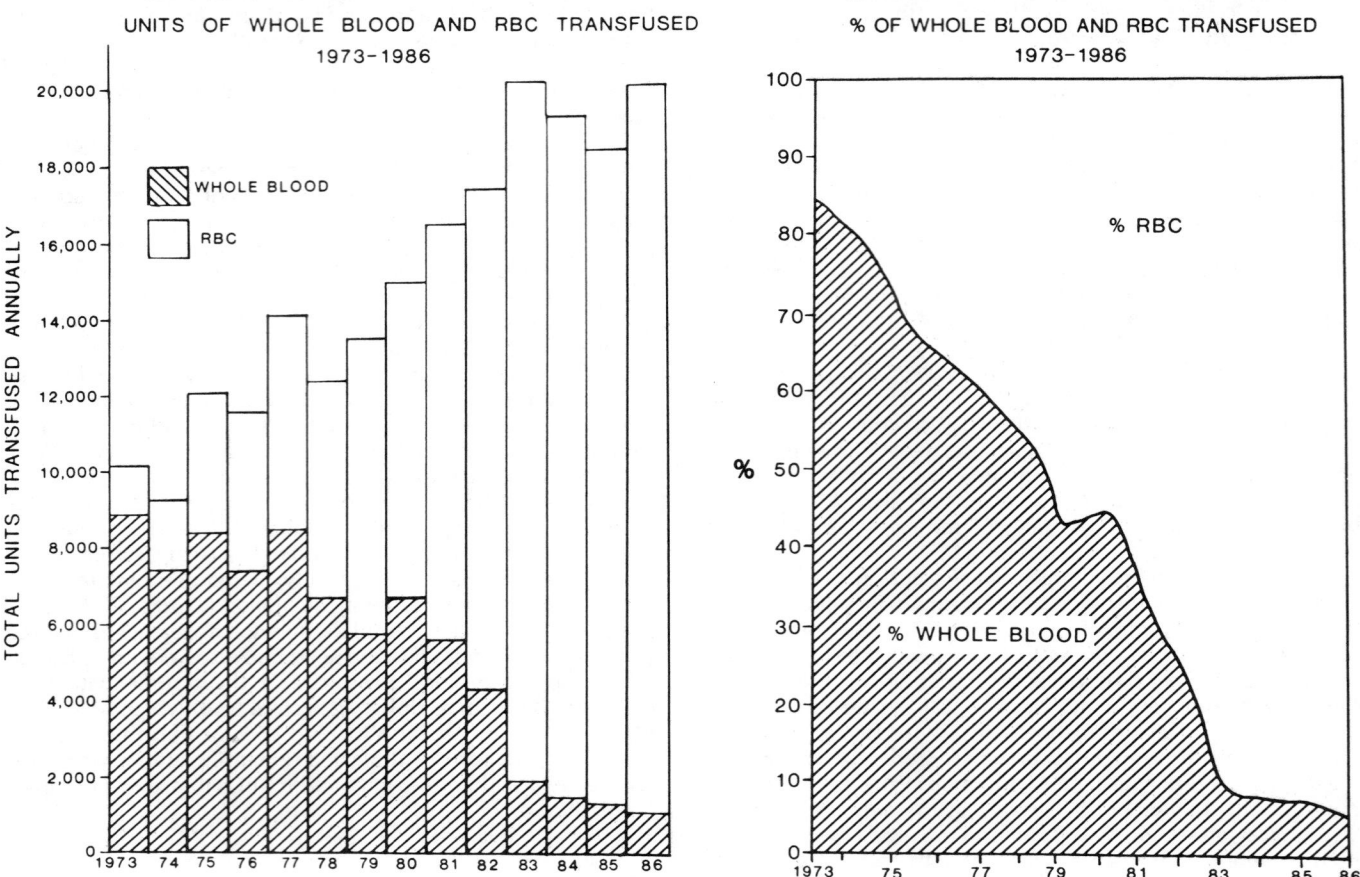

FIG. 26-4. Blood component therapy at the Hospital of the University of Pennsylvania, 1973–1986. (*A*) While the total units of whole blood (WB) and red blood cells (RBC) infused has more than doubled (9823 to 20,079) in the past decade, the increase represents a 1200% increase in RBC and a concomitant 77% decrease in WB usage. (*B*) This translates into a change from 14.7% RBC/85.3% WB in 1973 to 94.7% RBC/5.6% WB in 1986. (Adapted with permission. Ellison N, Silberstein LE: Hemostasis in the perioperative period. Advances in Anesthesia 3:67, 1986.)

PLATELETS

For the surgical patient who has not previously received platelet transfusions, administration of ABO-nonidentical platelets is acceptable. If the patient has received platelets previously and the desired increase in platelet count and decrease in bleeding time is not achieved with a platelet transfusion, alloimmunization to HLA antigens may be responsible. If HLA-matched platelets produce the desired results, one can definitely assume this to be the case. In women of child-bearing potential who are Rh negative, platelets from Rh positive donors should be avoided whenever possible. Alternatively, Rh immune globulin should be administered after the transfusion to reduce the risk of Rh sensitization.

One unit contains 5.5 x 10¹¹ platelets and 1 unit · 10 kg^{w1} has been suggested as a dose that should raise the platelet count to effective hemostatic levels.[23] Platelets should be ad-

ministered as rapidly as the patient's cardiovascular system will permit because the peak posttransfusion increment is probably related to the effectiveness of the transfusion. Slow infusions of platelets are inappropriate. In the past decade the American Red Cross has increased its annual platelet processing almost tenfold. Much of this increase can be attributed to the demonstrable effectiveness of such transfusions in patients who are receiving chemotherapy for hematologic malignancy. More recently there has been an increased use of platelets in patients who are having open heart surgery. Studies to document the effectiveness of platelet transfusion in these patients are lacking.[30] What documentation should be sought? Ideally an increase in the platelet count at 1 hr and 24 hr and a decrease in the bleeding time should be documented. However, these measures are frequently not practical during the intraoperative period. Patients should receive platelet therapy only if they have excessive bleeding as a result of thrombocytopenia or thrombocytopathia.

COMPLICATIONS OF TRANSFUSION

The most severe complication of blood transfusion is an acute hemolytic transfusion reaction (AHTR), something that can be avoided with a properly performed crossmatch and meticulous clerical attention to detail to insure that the correct unit of blood is administered to the correct patient. In addition, the chances of an AHTR are extremely small if ABO- and Rh-type specific blood is administered. Fever, nausea, shaking chills, and flank pain may herald the onset of an AHTR in the awake patient. Recognition of an acute AHTR in an anesthetized patient may be difficult. The onset of red urine due to free plasma hemoglobin in a patient whose bladder is catheterized or because of uncontrollable bleeding due to DIC may be the first sign. Support of blood pressure as necessary to maintain renal blood flow and fluid and diuretic therapy to maintain urine flow are the mainstays of treatment. If a shut-down occurs, hemodialysis may be necessary.

Other potential causes of acute hemolysis during transfusion include faulty blood warmers, concurrent infusion of nonisotonic solutions with osmotic lysis of RBCs, infusion under pressure especially through a small needle, unrecognized paroxysmal nocturnal hemoglobinuria, glucose-6-phosphate dehydrogenase (G6PD) deficiency, or sepsis on the patient or with contaminated blood.[31]

Febrile reactions, the most common type of reaction, are defined as a temperature elevation of more than 1ºC occurring in association with a transfusion and they can be effectively prevented by the use of white blood cell-poor saline washed blood, RBCs, or microaggregate filtration.[32] While febrile reactions are relatively benign, differentiating them from an AHTR or sepsis at the time of presentation are reasons for stopping the transfusion.

Allergic reactions are the second most common reaction and are usually easily treated with an antihistamine. Under general anesthesia the appearance of hives in a patient receiving blood transfusion may be the only manifestation. Rarely, after the infusion of a few ml of blood, patients may develop respiratory distress, cyanosis, and shock. This usually occurs in IgA-deficient patients who have developed IgA antibodies. In addition to discontinuing the transfusion, treatment with epinephrine is required.

Delayed hemolytic transfusion reactions occur in patients who have a compatible cross-match, but over a 4–21 day period the transfused RBCs are destroyed. The reactions are usually subclinical and only diagnosed when a positive Coombs' test and an antibody not present on a previous cross-match is subsequently detected.

Infection due to virus, bacteria, or spirochetes may be transmitted via blood transfusion. Hepatitis and AIDS are the two most feared diseases of this type. Hepatitis transfusion has been markedly decreased by the elimination of paid blood donors and perfection of third-generation testing for HBsAg. Nevertheless, with the near elimination of hepatitis B the prevalence of non-A, non-B hepatitis has apparently increased. Reported incidence of posttransfusion hepatitis depends on the intensity of follow-up because the incubation and clinical courses may be highly variable. Of note is the fact that 33 of the 133 deaths related to blood transfusion reported to the FDA were due to hepatitis.[33]

Transmission of AIDS is the most feared complication, and while that fear has developed a healthy conservative approach to blood transfusion, the hysteria that has accompanied the recognition of transfusion-associated AIDS is regrettable. Recipients of blood products constitute 2% of AIDS cases.[34] Since the human immunodeficiency virus (HIV) is heat sensitive,

lyophylized concentrates of Factors VIII and IX can now be prepared using techniques that greatly decrease AIDS transmission. The development for tests for HIV antibody are another positive development. Unfortunately there is a "window" between infection and seropositivity that makes the test less than perfect.

Another complication is microaggregate infusion. Microaggregates consisting of platelets and leukocytes form during storage of whole blood, and accumulation of these microaggregates becomes significant after 3–5 days of storage. Infusion of whole blood containing microaggregates has been implicated as a cause of posttransfusion pulmonary dysfunction. As a result, micropore filters have been developed to remove particles with diameters in the 10–40 mm range. Nevertheless, use of micropore filters has not been conclusively documented to be useful.[35] Regardless of the attitude about micropore filters, it must be appreciated that blood should always be administered through 170 mm filters.

BLOOD SUBSTITUTES

Autologous blood is technically not a substitute for blood, but when blood is needed, predeposited autologous blood is absolutely the best substitute for homologous blood. Units may be collected weeks, or if frozen, months in advance for elective surgical procedures. Most patients are able to donate 3 units of blood up to 72 hr before surgery, assuming the preoperative hematocrit is greater than 30%. Alternatively, acute isovolemic hemodilution and collection of 1–2 units of blood immediately before surgery can provide fresh whole blood for use toward the end of the operation. Intraoperative scavenging, washing, and subsequent infusion of blood collected intraoperatively is a third method of autologous blood transfusion.

Use of type and screen permits more efficient utilization of stored blood and is cost effective. Type and screen denotes blood that has been typed for A, B, and Rh antigens and screened for antibodies. A type and cross-match, in contrast to a type and screen, makes that blood unavailable to other patients, resulting in the possible loss of storage time if that blood is not used. Type and screen is used when the scheduled surgical procedure is unlikely to require transfusion of blood, but is one for which blood should be available.

Crystalloid infusion to maintain normovolemia in a patient who is losing blood is a standard practice, and usually 2–4 ml of crystalloid must be infused for each ml of blood loss due to crystalloid's extravascular distribution. Crystalloid is administered until a predetermined hemoglobin level is achieved. While a hemoglobin level of 10 mg·dl^{-1} is frequently used, there is a move to lower that level now to further decrease the need for homologous blood transfusion.[36]

Colloid may be used in lieu of crystalloid to replace blood loss and has the advantage that colloid may be used in a 1:1 ratio, but the disadvantage of being more expensive. In addition, some of these products contain vasoactive substances which may produce hypotension.[37] Plasma protein fraction (PPF) and 5% and 25% albumin are blood products that have been heated to 60ºC for 10 hr, which removes the risk of disease transmission. Hydroxyethyl starch and dextran are other colloids that stay largely within the vascular compartment.

A long-standing controversy in fluid management is the need for colloid administration. Does colloid administration increase survival or decrease morbidity in surgical patients? The number of studies on this subject is impressive and the preponderance of evidence suggests that if sufficient crystalloid is administered, there are no important differences in the two groups. In particular, lung water accumulation and pulmonary edema are usually not increased when crystalloid is used.[38] In cases of hypoproteinemia where the body stores of protein are depleted, there may be a greater need for colloid administration.[39]

Artificial blood development would be a tremendous breakthrough. The current precarious balance between supply and demand would be obviated and the complications associated with homologous blood products avoided. Unfortunately, the current perfluro compound under limited investigation, Fluosol-DA is not likely to gain widespread acceptance clinically because of its limited oxygen-carrying capacity. Furthermore, reports of pulmonary complications analogous to those seen following the administration of other perfluorocarbons provide additional justification for restraint in using this product.[40]

SUMMARY

Effective hemostasis in the perioperative period rests on a triad of vascular integrity, platelets, and coagulation factors. A working knowledge of the normal hemostatic process, of the tests for hemostasis, and of the available blood products for treating deficiencies are essential. A high index of suspicion will permit the development of a hemostatic defect to be detected early and treatment started promptly. In this way the effects of hemostatic defects will be minimized and outcome improved. In appropriate cases, the administration of blood, especially large volumes of blood, can be life saving. Alternatively, injudicious administration of blood is wasteful of a precious national resource and can even have fatal consequences. Intelligent individualization is necessary for each unit of blood or blood product administered to each patient.

REFERENCES

1. Ellison N: Diagnosis and management of bleeding disorders. Anesthesiology 47:171, 1977
2. Ellison N, Silberstein LE: Hemostasis in the perioperative period. In Stoelting RK, Barash PG, Gallagher TJ (eds): Advances in Anesthesia, vol. 3, p 67. Chicago, Year Book Medical Publishers, 1986.
3. McFarlane RG: Symposium No. 27. Zoological Society of London. The Hemostatic Mechanism in Man and Other Animals. London, Academic Press, 1970
4. Barrer MJ, Ellison N: Platelet function. Anesthesiology 46:202, 1977
5. Ware AJ: Desmopression acetate in hemorrhagic conditions. In Ellison N, Jobes DR (eds): Effective Hemostasis in Cardiac Surgery, Orlando, Grune & Stratton, (in press)
6. Triplett DA: Overview of hemostasis. In Menitove JE, McCarthy LJ (eds): Hemostatic Disorders and the Blood Bank, p 1. Arlington, VA, American Association of Blood Banks, 1984
7. Bedford RF, Wollman H: Complications of percutaneous radial artery cannulation. Anesthesiology 38:228, 1973
8. Palermo LM, Andrews RA, Ellison N: Avoidance of heparin contamination in coagulation studies drawn from indwelling lines. Anesth Analg 59:222, 1980
9. Jobes DR, Schwartz AJ, Ellison N et al: Monitoring heparin anticoagulation and its neutralization. Ann Thorac Surg 31:161, 1981
10. Ellison N, Jobes DR, Schwartz AJ: Implications of anticoagulant therapy. Int Anesthesiol Clin 20:121, 1982
11. Mielke CH, Dodds J, Johnson G et al: Measurement of the bleeding time. Thromb Hemostas 52:210, 1984
12. Rappaport SI: Preoperative hemostatic evaluation: Which tests, if any? Blood 61:229, 1983
13. Barber A, Green D, Galluzzo T et al: The bleeding time as a preoperative screening test. Am J Med 78:761, 1985
14. Greenwalt TJ: General Principles of Blood Transfusion. Chicago, American Medical Association, 1977
15. Ellison N, Edmunds LH Jr, Colman RW: Platelet aggregation following heparin and protamine administration. Anesthesiology 48:65, 1978
16. Morel DR, Zapol WM, Thomas SJ et al: C5A and thromboxane generation associated with pulmonary vaso- and broncho-constriction during protamine reversal of heparin. Anesthesiology, 66:597, 1987
17. Miller RD, Robbins TO, Tong MJ et al: Coagulation defects associated with massive blood transfusion. Ann Surg 174:794, 1971
18. Harrigan C, Lucas CE, Ledgerwood AM: Serial changes in primary hemostasis after massive transfusion. Surgery 98:836, 1985
19. Miller RD: Problems in massive transfusion. Anesthesiology 39:82, 1973
20. Colman RW, Robboy SS: Postoperative disseminated intravascular coagulation. Urol Clin North Am 3:107, 1974
21. Hattersley PG, Kunkel M: Cryoprecipitates as a source of fibrinogen in treatment of disseminated intravascular coagulation. Transfusion 16:641, 1976
22. Marengo-Rowe AJ: Experts opine. Survey of Anesthesia 37:377, 1986
23. Tomasullo BA, Lenes BA: Platelet transfusion therapy. In Menitove JE, McCarthy LJ (eds): Hemostatic Disorders in the Blood Bank, p 63. Arlington, VA, American Association of Blood Banks, 1984
24. Mollison PL: Summary of reports presented at the XVI Congress of the International Society of Blood Transfusion. Vox Sang 40:289, 1981
25. Schmidt PJ: Whole blood transfusion. Transfusion 24:368, 1984
26. Grindon AJ, Tomasulo PS, Bergin JJ et al: The hospital transfusion committee: Guidelines for improving practice. JAMA 253:540, 1985
27. Counts RB, Haisch C, Simon TL: Hemostasis in massively transfused patients. Ann Surg 190:91, 1979
28. Braunstein AH, Oberman HA: Transfusion of plasma components. Transfusion 24:281, 1984
29. Tullis JL, Alvin B, Bove JR et al: Fresh frozen plasma. JAMA 253:251, 1985
30. Aster RH, Bartolucci AA, Collins JA et al: Platelet transfusion therapy. JAMA 257:1777, 1987
31. Peschel MB: Adverse effects of blood transfusion. In Reynolds AW, Steckler D (eds): Practical Aspects of Blood Administration, p 95, Arlington, VA, American Association of Blood Banks, 1986
32. Meryman H, McCullough J: The preparation of red cells depleted of leukocytes: Review and evaluation. Transfusion 26:101, 1986
33. Myhre BA: Fatalities from blood transfusion. JAMA 244:1333, 1980
34. Kunkel SE, Warner MA: Human T-cell lymphotropic virus type III (HTLV-III) infection: How it can effect you, your patients, and your anesthesia practice. Anesthesiology 66:195, 1987
35. Snyder EL, Hazzey A, Barash PG et al: Microaggregate blood filtration in patients with compromised pulmonary function. Transfusion 22:21, 1982
36. Stehling LC, Ellison N, Faust RJ et al: A survey of transfusion practices among anesthesiologists. Vox Sang 52:60, 1987
37. Ellison N, Behar M, MacVaugh HA III et al: Bradykinin, plasma protein fraction, and hypotension. Ann Thorac Surg 29:15, 1980
38. Gallagher JD, Moore RA, Kerns D et al: Effects of colloid or crystalloid administration on pulmonary extravascular water in the postoperative period after coronary artery bypass grafting. Anesth Analg 64:753, 1985
39. Rackow EC, Weil MH, MacNeil AR et al: Effects of crystalloid and colloid fluids on extravascular lung water in hypoproteinemic dogs. J Appl Physiol 62:2421, 1987
40. Police AM, Waxman K, Tominage G: Pulmonary complications after fluosol administration to patients with life-threatening blood loss. Crit Care Med 13:96, 1985

Chapter 27

B. Skeie
J. Askanazi
H. Khambatta

Nutrition, Fluid, and Electrolytes

Nutritional and electrolyte disturbances in surgical and intensive care patients correlate with increased morbidity and mortality rates. Recent advances in understanding these disturbances coupled with introduction of new nutrient regimens and refinements in delivery methods have resulted in nutritional and metabolic support developing as a major form of therapy. For optimal metabolic support for the acutely ill or the surgical patient, a basic understanding of the changes in body composition and metabolic responses to starvation, surgical trauma, and stress is necessary. The goals for treatment include maintaining body tissue stores, prevention and correction of specific deficiencies, and use of synthetic nutrients to optimize organ function. Currently, a new generation of synthetic nutrients are available or being developed as solutions with modified amino acid composition (high branched-chain amino acids), altered fatty acid profile (medium chain triglycerides, polyunsaturated fatty acids), and small molecular-weight substrates such as ketones and ketoacids. These nutrient mixtures may lead to more specific metabolic support for specific diseases in the coming years.

The basic knowledge of the changes in body composition and metabolism in response to malnutrition, surgical stress, and injury is important for the understanding and proper treatment of nutritional and electrolyte disturbances in surgical and intensive care patients and will therefore be outlined first.

BODY COMPOSITION

DEFINITIONS

The body is composed of fat and lean body mass (LBM). The latter is subdivided into extracellular fluid (ECF), body cell mass (BCM), and extracellular supportive structures such as skeleton, cartilage, and tendons. The sum of the LBM and adipose tissue is equal to total body weight (TBW).

The fat functions as the energy storage area. It is a relatively anhydrous mass, with water representing only about 20% by weight, whereas in skeletal muscle total water content is 80% by weight. If total caloric intake and energy expenditure are equal, there is no reduction or gain of fat mass. Since fat provides $9.5 \text{ cal} \cdot \text{g}^{-1}$ and fat tissue is only 20% water, this is a very compact storage area. Metabolic use of fat results in only one-eighth the amount of weight loss as compared with skeletal muscle, i.e., 2000 calories of fat or protein would be equal to the loss of 275 g of adipose tissue or 2500 g of skeletal muscle.

Extracellular mass consists of plasma, interstitial water, transcellular water (cerebral spinal fluid, pericardial fluid, and the fluid that is in the joint spaces), and the supporting structures such as skeleton, tendons, and cartilage.

BCM is the metabolically active portion of the LBM. It consists of skeletal muscle (60%), viscera (30%), and the cells of the supporting structure of the extracellular mass such as red blood cells and the cellular component of adipose tissue.

The standard 70-kg man contains 20 kg of fat and 50 kg of LBM that is equally divided by weight as ECF and BCM. These parameters vary with sex, body build, and age. Women tend to have decreased LBM and increased adipose tissue. The ratio of LBM to TBW also decreases with age. Very muscular individuals will have a LBM : TBW ratio that is greater than normal.

These relationships remain constant as long as caloric intake equals expenditures. With excess caloric intake, there will be an increase in the adipose tissue unless a vigorous exercise program is undertaken, in which circumstances an increase in skeletal muscle mass will occur if adequate protein is supplied. Excess energy is stored as fat; there are no storage deposits of protein as glycogen cannot be stored in any significant amounts.

BODY COMPOSITION MEASUREMENTS

There are two major approaches to measuring body composition: 1) balance measurements, which only measure changes in amount of body constituents; and 2) direct body composition measurements, which measure the total amount of any constituent.[1]

Measurements of balance have been used most extensively for nitrogen, although sodium, potassium, calcium, phosphorus, energy, fat, and carbohydrate have been studied as well. As previously noted, balance studies measure only changes in constituents and cannot assess absolute body content. Methodologic problems in measurements of balances stem from estimation of both intake and output. Use of a defined enteral or parenteral diet greatly simplifies the problems of analysis of individual foods for nitrogen. Output of each constituent must be determined in urine, stool, vomitus, and all drainages. The common practice of measuring 24-hr urinary urea nitrogen and adding a constant for other losses is sometimes useful for clinical evaluation of patients, but is inadequate for research purposes.[2] Total nitrogen and all other elements under study, such as sodium, potassium, and phosphorus, should be analyzed in all samples.

Early methods used to perform direct measurement of body composition include underwater weighing to determine density and thereby estimate the LBM:fat ratio, and indicator dilution methods to compartmentalize the various water compartments. The latter methods make use of a compound not normally present in the body that penetrates a known body water compartment. By dividing the amount administered by the concentration in plasma, the volume or space or distribution of the indicator can be determined. The dye, T-1825, which binds to albumin, was introduced to measure plasma volume; sodium thiocyanate has been used to measure extracellular space; and antipyrine is used for TBW. The introduction of a variety of radioisotopes after World War II greatly extended the use of the indicator dilution method; plasma volume of the extracellular mass can now be measured by radioactive albumin; red blood cell mass can be measured by using radioactive chromium-tagged red blood cells; tritium can be used to measure total body water; radioactive bromine can be used to measure the total extracellular water. Recently, potentially useful methods have been introduced; these include neutron activation analysis, which provides simultaneous measurements of whole body calcium, chloride, sodium, potassium, phosphorus, and nitrogen, and electrical conductance, which measures the size of fat and LBM components.

Most of the methods for measuring changes in body composition are not available in the usual clinical setting. Although they are important as research tools, these methods have not yet been shown to be important in the management of the critically ill patient. The clinical evaluation, based on history taking and physical examination, is probably almost as effective as objective measurement for body composition. Of particular importance are indications of weight loss, edema, anorexia, vomiting, diarrhea, and decreased food intake. Frequent measurements of body weight are probably the most important nutritional parameter clinically available. Large day-to-day changes in weight usually represent changes in the ECF, whereas long-term changes represent changes in BCM as well as fat and consequently are more difficult to interpret. Additional useful clinical measurements are 24-hr values for urinary excretion of sodium, potassium, urea, and creatinine. These, together with accurate estimates of intake,

can be used to calculate daily balance and serve as an approximation of the changes in ECF (sodium) and BCM (potassium and nitrogen). Measurement of daily creatinine excretion serves as a quality control measure on the completeness of urine collection; creatinine excretion is quite constant from day to day, even in sick patients. Large daily variations should alert the investigator to inadequate specimen collection. In addition, daily urine creatinine output permits calculation of the creatinine height index, which serves as an index of prior loss of BCM.[3]

BODY COMPOSITION CHANGES IN ACUTE ILLNESS

The alterations in body composition during illness and malnutrition can be classified in three fundamental categories. Starvation in unstressed patients causes a decrease in BCM and fat; the ECF also decreases, but to a lesser extent, hence the ratio of ECF to BCM increases. When carbohydrate is administered as the sole nutrient (as in the common practice of infusing 5% dextrose/0.45 normal saline), there is both a relative and absolute expansion of the ECF. Finally, injury or sepsis also causes increases in the ECF independent of nutrient administration.

Starvation

Complete starvation in the unstressed patient results in a loss of fat and LBM. With partial starvation the amount and proportion of the two compartments lost will depend on both the amount and the composition of nutrients ingested. The rates of loss differ greatly for the three components of LBM: ECF, BCM, and extracellular structural components.

With nutrient intakes that are just below energy expenditure, losses of LBM and fat occur approximately in the proportion of 0.5:1.[4] During complete starvation the ratio approximates 2.6:1 (Table 27-1).[5] Further, the composition of weight loss changes with duration even on a fixed nutrient intake. In the first few days, water losses are high when compared with fat and protein loss, and include the loss of water associated with glycogen depletion and a preferential loss of ECF.[6] This occurs because initially there is a diuresis and naturesis secondary to an anti-antidiuretic hormone and antialdosterone effect because of the increased glucagon levels. However,

TABLE 27-1.   Tissue Composition of Weight Loss in Different Conditions

CONDITION	BCM (kg) Ratio Fat (kg)	REFERENCE
Normal subjects		
Marginal intake	0.35–0.51	Calloway[4]
Fasting	2.6	Benedict[5]
Postoperative		
Men	2.6	Kinney et al[6]
Women	1.7	Kinney et al[6]
Major injury	4.5	Kinney et al[6]

BCM = body cell mass.
(Reprinted with permission. Insel J, Elwyn DH: Body composition. In Askanazi J, Starker PM, Weissman C [eds]: Fluid and Electrolyte Management in Critical Care, p 1. Boston, Butterworths 1986.)

losses of protein, fat, and water diminish with time, the rate of water loss declines more rapidly, and the rate of fat loss declines less rapidly than that for protein, indicating conservation of LBM and a relative expansion of ECF with respect to BCM.[7] Although weight loss is more rapid during fasting than with balanced hypocaloric diets, the pattern of compartmental changes is very similar. As starvation progresses, adipose tissue and BCM continue to erode and ECF continues to increase relative to BCM. Thus, weight loss may only be about 16%, but adipose tissue and BCM may have decreased by 37% and 40%.[8] For this reason it is obvious that body weight does not adequately reflect the extent of BCM loss during malnutrition.

The relative expansion of ECF and blood volume that is seen during uncomplicated starvation or fasting is not due to renal failure or to decreases in plasma total protein or albumin levels, which are maintained at relatively normal levels during starvation and balanced hypocaloric diets. The relative ECF expansion stems from the failure of the ECF to contract during weight loss.[1] It has been hypothesized[7] that because there is no decrease in the size of the blood vessels in parallel with BCM during nutritional depletion, there should be no decrease in blood volume. If the processes that regulate the volume of the extravascular ECF in relation to blood volume continue to operate normally, these two compartments will remain at the usual size despite shrinkage of BCM and fat. If starvation is complicated by infection, hypoproteinemia, kidney failure, or other conditions, additional factors contribute independently to the relative and absolute expansion of ECF.

Effects of Carbohydrate Administration

When carbohydrate is administered alone in the complete absence of protein, there is an absolute and relative increase in the ECF. Kwashiorkor, a form of malnutrition, results from intake of little or no protein, with fairly adequate caloric levels derived mainly from carbohydrate. In this condition there is a marked expansion of ECF with pitting edema, ascites, and anasarca. One week of carbohydrate feeding can produce the fully developed kwashiorkor syndrome in an already undernourished child.[9]

In hospitalized patients it is routine to administer 2 l of 5% dextrose as nutritional support. This regimen provides only $100 \text{ g} \cdot \text{day}^{-1}$ of glucose and results in a kwashiorkor-like syndrome in hospitalized patients if used for prolonged duration. Ingestion of $100 \text{ g} \cdot \text{day}^{-1}$ of glucose has been reported to result in marked retention of sodium when given to volunteers during a 6-day fasting period.[10] There was little effect on potassium losses; i.e., carbohydrate administration exacerbates the increased ECF/BMC that occurs during starvation. Combined glucose (100 g) and sodium chloride (4.5 g) ingestion (equivalent to 2 l of 50% dextrose, 0.45 normal saline solution) have been found to abolish completely the sodium loss, while potassium loss exceeds that of a complete fast. Thus the use of 5% dextrose in saline results in a greater ECF/BCM ratio than total starvation.

Carbohydrate can increase the ECF when given in great excess even if protein is present. Volunteers receiving normal diets with an excess of carbohydrate equal to $1500 \text{ kcal} \cdot \text{day}^{-1}$ above energy requirements had an average weight gain in 7 days of 5.1 kg, much of which must been an expanded ECF.[11] Thus, glucose may increase ECF by providing calories in the complete absence of protein, apparently resulting in cellular dysfunction, or it may have direct renal effects. Increased plasma glucose levels necessitate an increased ECF volume if isotonicity is to be maintained. Carbohydrate may also inhibit glucocorticoid production and thereby potentiate the effect of antidiuretic hormone on water and sodium retention.

Effects of Injury and Sepsis

At any given nutrient intake, injury increases the rate of loss of LBM; after elective operations weight loss occurs in the ratio of LBM:fat of 2:1. With severe injury the ratio rises to 4:1 (Table 27-1).[6] Both surgical and accidental trauma have been shown to cause acute increases in the ECF compartment.[12, 13] These increases in ECF often necessitate the intravenous administration of large quantities of fluids during resuscitation and the perioperative period. Such fluids are not retained when administered to normal subjects but are retained when given to stressed patients. Several days following the injury, there is usually a diuresis of both sodium and water and the excess ECF is lost. Failure to diurese suggests an underlying complication such as sepsis.

After initial resuscitation following injury, sepsis has been shown to be associated with a further increase in ECF volume and a decrease in serum sodium concentration. Several authors have reported that patients with sepsis are generally hyponatremic with an expanded ECF; as the sepsis resolves, they diurese and their serum sodium concentration increases. The more severe the infectious process, the more exaggerated are the changes in the ECF. This phenomenon has been attributed to numerous factors, including expansion and dilution of ECF volume, fluid therapy, inappropriate ADH secretion, and salt losses resulting from sweating, vomiting, and diarrhea.[1] It seems clear that nutritional therapy cannot reverse the increased ECF volume in septic patients unless the sepsis is controlled.

CLINICAL IMPLICATIONS OF BODY COMPOSITION IN CRITICALLY ILL PATIENTS

Body composition changes in acutely ill patients can result from various combinations of starvation, carbohydrate administration, and injury or sepsis, and other factors that may be less well defined. Typically, patients who have lost weight experience an increase in ECF and a decrease in BCM. If absolute increase in ECF is found, it suggests that the starvation has been of the kwashiorkor form or complicated by trauma or sepsis. In the critically ill patient prior loss of BCM as a result of protein–calorie insufficiencies will affect therapy. Recent weight losses of less than 10% of normal body weight may not require urgent nutritional treatment. Losses of 10–30% represent a serious complication, and failure to provide nutritional therapy will almost certainly interfere with recovery despite treatment that is optimum in other respects. Losses greater than 30% are life threatening and can cause permanent damage to the musculoskeletal system. Nutritional therapy must be administered immediately, but with caution, because overfeeding in these conditions can cause life-threatening complications.[7]

An expanded ECF volume is generally considered undesirable. As outlined below, it is correlated with postoperative complications and undesirable effects on pulmonary and cerebral function.[14] Adequate nutrition will result in a relative decrease of the ECF when the water retention has occurred for nutritional reasons alone. If the expanded ECF results from trauma or sepsis, however, nutritional support alone may not be sufficient.

NUTRITION

GENERAL PRINCIPLES

Metabolism

ENERGY GENERATION. By metabolism of carbohydrate, lipid, and protein, energy is released for mechanical work, synthesis, membrane transport, and thermogenesis. Glucose, amino acids, fatty acids, triglycerides, lactate, and ketones all, under different circumstances, play a role in energy generation. Glucose metabolism generally occurs along the glycolysis and the oxidative phosphorylation pathways. Glycolysis produces a small amount of adenosine triphosphate (ATP) as compared with oxidative phosphorylation because it can proceed anaerobically; however, it becomes important during anoxic and hypoxic conditions. Fatty acids and amino acids are metabolized aerobically and use slightly more oxygen per kcal of energy generated than does glucose; this is true even during aerobic glucose metabolism.

FUEL STORES. To maintain adequate metabolism during periods with enhanced energy needs or reduced dietary intake, expenditure of endogenous tissue stores is required. The energy available from circulating substrates is negligible. Carbohydrate is stored as glycogen in liver and muscle. The average healthy adult stores 200–300 g of carbohydrate, which gives a total energy available of approximately 900 kcal. This can only fulfill energy requirements for 8–10 hr and thus the glycogen stores become depleted within 24 hr during starvation. Fat contributes to about 15–30% of the body weight. The average 70-kg adult man has 15–20 kg adipose tissue, making the total available caloric storage from fat to be about 140,000 kcal. This constitutes 85% of the total body energy stores and is the major energy source during periods of prolonged starvation. Fat is stored as triglyceride.

Protein is present in lean body tissue, the major part in skeletal muscle and visceral organs. Fourteen to twenty per cent of the body weight is protein, giving a total amount available of approximately 24,000 kcal. There is no protein whose sole function is energy storage, but during poor dietary intake protein can be oxidized for energy. Some degree of functional loss always accompanies the use of LBM for energy generation.

An individual's total caloric storage could potentially sustain life for about 4–5 months; however, functionally most persons would be at the point of death on burning about 140,000 kcal, or about 75% of the fat and 50% of the protein. This occurs in approximately 60 days during a complete fast.

METABOLIC RESPONSES TO FASTING AND STARVATION. After the first day of starvation the carbohydrate stores are exhausted and fat and protein are expended to meet whole body energy needs. A wide variety of metabolic adaptations takes place if the starvation state continues. The metabolic changes in response to starvation are aimed primarily at conservation of fuel stores and reduction of the body's dependence on glucose.

Complete starvation of 1 week's duration without any intervening stress causes a progressive decrease in urinary nitrogen loss. The decrease is due to ketoadaptation; the liver starts to synthesize ketones from incoming fatty acids that are used for energy. In the absence of any significant carbohydrate intake, gluconeogenesis is the main source of glucose resulting in protein breakdown as amino acids are converted to glucose. Most amino acids are glucogenic and can be converted to Krebs cycle intermediates, which may then be converted to glucose *via* gluconeogenesis. In addition, as much as 20 g·day^{-1} of glucose can be synthesized from the glycerol that is released by hydrolysis of adipose tissue triglyceride. Other adaptive mechanisms include reduction in the rate of glucose utilization by tissues capable of using fat and changes in the insulin release affecting protein catabolism and gluconeogenesis. A decrease in resting energy expenditure (REE) occurs during a fast; this decrease appears to be an adaptive mechanism designed to minimize tissue losses.

Most tissues can oxidize fat as the primary fuel for energy requirements. Free fatty acids do not cross the blood–brain barrier and are not available to the brain as metabolic substrate. In the complete absence of glucose intake, the central nervous system (CNS) progressively increases its use of ketones produced by the liver as an energy substrate.[15] In the absence of ketones, 100–150 g·day^{-1} of glucose is required, mainly derived through gluconeogenesis from amino acids provided by protein breakdown. Thus, use of ketones for fuel lowers the cerebral glucose requirements and spares protein breakdown that would otherwise be expended for gluconeogenesis and is regarded as being crucial to the development of a protein-sparing state.

Under normal steady-state conditions, nitrogen excretion equals dietary nitrogen intake (10–30 g·day^{-1}). Starvation of 1 week causes a progressive decrease in urinary nitrogen to 6–8 g·day^{-1}, which represents a loss of about one half pound of lean tissue a day. Administration of 100 g of carbohydrates reduces the nitrogen losses to about 3–4 g·day^{-1}.[16] A protein-free diet with adequate carbohydrate can cut protein losses; however, this nitrogen-sparing effect of carbohydrate may not be entirely beneficial because it seems to result in a diffuse whole body expansion of the ECF compartment.

The healthy subject will adapt over 5–10 days by excreting less nitrogen during fasting. In the critically ill patient, however, the compensations do not occur readily. In addition there are the increased nitrogen requirements associated with tissue repair, synthesis of immune proteins, and the acute-phase reactants. These patients may also often have extrarenal nitrogen losses from gastrointestinal tract or direct tissue injury after trauma or from hemorrhage. Metabolic requirements during this condition are increased rather than decreased, as during a fast. The hyperglycemia seen in critically ill patients prevents the development of the ketotic, nitrogen-sparing state observed in starvation.

The respiratory quotient (RQ) is calculated from the carbon dioxide production divided by the oxygen consumption. The RQ of carbohydrate is 1.00, fat 0.71, and protein 0.82. Lipogenesis, the synthesis of fat from glucose, is associated with an RQ of approximately 8.0. A whole body RQ greater than 1.0 would imply net lipogenesis. Prolonged starvation is associated with a whole body RQ approaching 0.7 as fat and fat-derived fuels provide substrates for the major portion of the organism's energy needs. During refeeding, the RQ reflects the composition of the fuel being administered. If a hypertonic solution of glucose and amino acids is given, the RQ will rise from 0.7 to 1.0 or higher as glucose becomes the major fuel substrate and excess glucose is converted to fat (lipogenesis).

METABOLIC RESPONSES TO TRAUMA AND SURGICAL STRESS. Cuthbertson divided the response to injury into three stages.[17] The shock phase is associated with an early period of weight gain due to fluid sequestration. The metabolic rate is depressed, body temperature is lowered, and the circulating blood volume reduced. It is followed after a day or two by the catabolic phase (flow stage) with increased metabolic activity. In this stage body energy stores are mobilized to meet increased needs. Weight is lost as the retained fluid is mobilized; this is combined with a mobilization of fat and LBM. Maximal nitrogen loss generally occurs between the 4th and 8th day after injury. The nitrogen excretion is increased as a function of the severity of the trauma.[18] Kinney et al[19] found that multiple fractures resulted in a 10–20% increase in REE for 1–3 weeks, while infection produced increases of 15–50%. Extensive burns resulted in increases from 40% to 100% that lasted for several weeks. Uncomplicated elective operations did not increase REE (Fig. 27-1). The catabolic phase is followed by the anabolic or recovery phase.

The degree of the catabolic response depends on the severity and duration of the trauma or stress. After an uncomplicated surgical procedure in an otherwise healthy patient, the catabolic response persists for about 1 week with a net nitrogen loss. These mild nitrogen losses are well tolerated and readily replaced by subsequent oral feeding. By contrast the fasting patient recovering from severe trauma or stress catabolizes considerable amounts of lean body tissue and fat.

The catabolic response can be viewed as a mobilization of body protein, fat, and carbohydrate stores to ensure adequate circulatory levels of substrate (glucose, fatty acids, and amino acids) when dietary intake is limited. The increased available amino acid pool occurs predominantly at the expense of skeletal muscle. These amino acids may be oxidized directly for fuel

FIG. 27-1. The effects of injury, sepsis, and nutritional depletion on resting energy expenditure. (Reprinted with permission. Kinney JM: The application of indirect calorimetry to clinical studies. In Kinney JM [ed]: Assessment of Energy Metabolism in Health and Disease, p 42. Columbus, Ross Laboratories, 1980.)

Resting Energy Expenditure

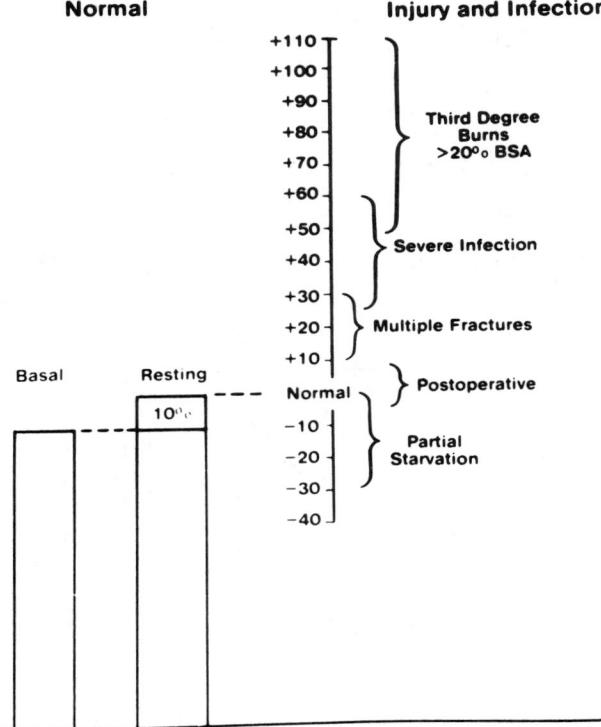

or used for gluconeogenesis; this process also makes more precursors available for synthesis of visceral protein and the proteins of tissue repair.

In response to injury gluconeogenesis is increased in the presence of high levels of glucose.[20] This hyperglycemia, referred to as the *diabetes of injury*, reflects the urgent nature of glucose requirements that the healing tissues require.[21] Fat is mobilized to obtain high circulating levels and is used for the energy needs of cardiac, skeletal, and respiratory muscles; this allows glucose to be spared for tissues that specifically require it, such as the CNS, the cellular immune system, and the healing wound. There is an increased body metabolism in response to trauma that is characterized by fever and enhanced oxygen consumption. The hormonal changes include an increased adrenal glucocorticoid, glucagon, and catecholamine release.

Nutritional Requirements

Maintenance of the BCM and organ function requires a supply of water, energy, and all the 36 essential nutrients. The recommended enteral intake of these nutrients is presented in several sources[22] and suggested allowances for intravenous intake are also presented. In this section the basic rules for estimating the normal requirements will be outlined. In patients the requirements may vary greatly depending on the type of disease and on organs involved. Specific nutritional support during metabolic stress and failure of vital organs (heart, lung, liver, brain, kidney) will be discussed in a separate section.

WATER. Normal individuals require about 1 ml of water for each ingested calorie, or about 2000–3000 ml·day^{-1} for adult subjects. When intake and output records are measured, water requirements are usually estimated as following: 500 ml (insensible loss) + urine output (ml) + nonurinary losses (ml) (*e.g.*, enteral drainage, *etc.*).

ELECTROLYTES, MINERALS, AND TRACE ELEMENTS. Electrolytes need to be tailored to the individual patient's need. For example, the patient with a metabolic alkalosis due to gastrointestinal losses may require more chloride and less acetate, and the patient with a chronic metabolic acidosis may require addition of lactate to the system. Similarly, calcium, potassium, magnesium, and trace element requirements may vary with the clinical setting. Guidelines for maintenance dose of electrolytes and trace elements are listed in Table 27-2. An outline of electrolyte balance and disturbances and their treatment are described in the section "Fluid and Electrolytes."

ENERGY. Caloric requirements should be predicted to prevent insufficient caloric intake as well as overfeeding. The basal caloric requirements can be calculated from the Harris-Benedict equation.[23] The equation is based on the patient's sex, age (A), height (H), and weight (W):

$$\text{Female: } 655 + 9.6(W) + 1.8(H) - 4.7(A) = \text{kcal·day}^{-1}$$
$$\text{Male: } 66 + 13.7(W) + 5(H) - 6.8(A) = \text{kcal·day}^{-1}$$

In clinical practice the caloric requirements usually are estimated on the patients weight: 25–30 kcal·kg^{-1}·day^{-1}.

Depending on the clinical condition of the patient, the energy intake may be increased. If the patient has fever, the energy expenditure will increase by approximately 17% for each degree Celsius of body temperature above normal. Major surgery, sepsis, and burns increase energy expenditure (Fig.

TABLE 27-2.   Recommended Daily Basic Requirements per Kg Body Weight During Intravenous Nutrition

ELEMENT	AMOUNT mMol
Sodium	1–1.4
Potassium	0.7–0.9
Calcium	0.11
Phosphorus	0.15
Magnesium	0.04
Iron	0.25–1.0
Manganese	0.1
Zinc	0.7
Chloride	1.3–1.9
Fluoride	0.7
Iodide	0.015
Chromium	0.015
Molybdenum	0.003
Selenium	0.006

(Adapted with permission from Shenkin A, Wretlind A: Parenteral nutrition. World Rev Nutr Diet 28:1, 1978.)

27-2). Intake must be adjusted upward if urinary and fecal calorie losses are increased. On the other hand, semistarvation, which is often seen in surgical patients, may reduce energy expenditure by as much as 30%. In a nutritionally depleted patient a greater intake than calculated expenditure is necessary for deposition of new tissue. For nutritional repletion energy intake should exceed REE by 50%. For maintenance, only 20% above REE is necessary. In the previously malnourished individual with more than 10% weight loss one should aim for repletion, while the previously healthy individual who is acutely ill requires maintenance only. Overfeeding, particularly with glucose, may lead to hypermetabolism, hepatic steatosis, and elevated carbon dioxide production.

NON-PROTEIN ENERGY. Normally, carbohydrates contribute 40–60%, protein 10–15%, and fat 30–40% of the total energy intake. The amount of the protein intake used for energy varies because parts of the amino acids are used for protein synthesis. The body is more sensitive to protein intake than to total energy provision. Optimal nutritional support therefore first optimizes protein intake and then adds sufficient calories. The non-protein calories can be provided by carbohydrates or fat. A minimum of approximately 500 kcal · day^{-1} should be administered as glucose to supply carbohydrate for the brain, bone marrow, and injured tissue. On the other hand at least 10% of the energy should be given as fat to provide sufficient essential fatty acids (linoleic and linolenic acid). The essential fatty acid deficiency syndrome has been reported in patients who received fat-free intravenous nutrition.

Once the minimal intake for glucose and fat is met, the additional nonprotein calories may be provided as either of these substrates. Total parenteral nutrition (TPN) systems have been described that provide nonprotein calories from 83% lipid/17% glucose to the traditional 100% glucose. The optimum balance of fat and glucose is not yet determined. TPN systems with 50% of nonprotein calories delivered as fat are as effective in maintaining nitrogen balance as those with 100% glucose and seem to minimize complications.

PROTEIN. In healthy humans the normal ingestion is about 1 g of protein · kg^{-1} · day^{-1}. Losses of protein (nitrogen) occur through urine and stool. The adult human usually remains in zero nitrogen balance. With a daily protein intake of 70 g, the urinary nitrogen losses will be about 9 g and fecal nitrogen about 1–2 g.

To calculate the nitrogen balance, the nitrogen intake and nitrogen output must be determined. The nitrogen intake in g is determined from the equation protein intake (g) = 6.25 × N(g). The total urinary nitrogen is 70 to 80% urea nitrogen under normal conditions and because the latter is easily measured, the nitrogen output (g · day^{-1}) can be estimated as urea (g · day^{-1}) + 4 g. The equation for nitrogen balance will be:

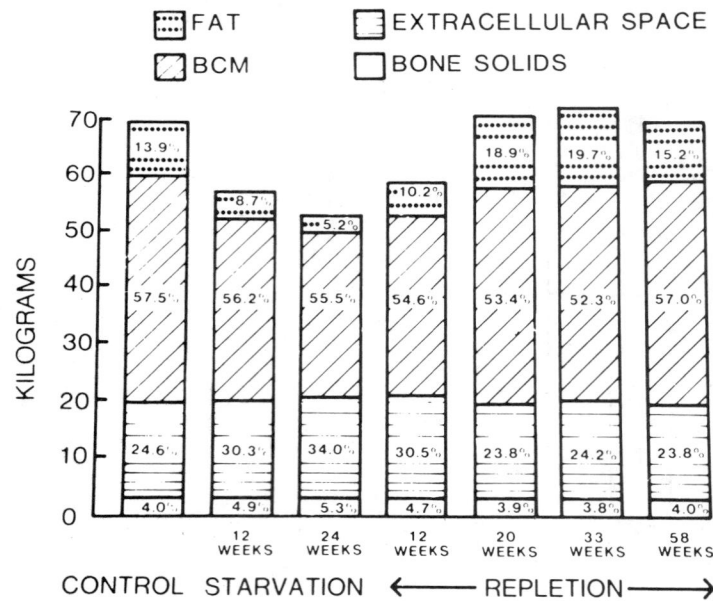

FIG. 27-2. Effects of 24 weeks of starvation followed by 58 weeks of repletion on body composition of active young men. Control energy requirements were estimated at 3490 Kcal · day^{-1}. Energy intake during starvation averaged 1570 Kcal · day^{-1}, 45% of the control level. Energy intake was restricted to an average of 2900 Kcal · day^{-1} for the first 12 weeks of repletion; subsequently, the subjects had free access to food. (Adapted with permission. Keys A, Brozek J, Henschel H et al: The Biology of Human Starvation. Minneapolis, University of Minnesota Press, 1950.)

$$N \text{ balance } (g \cdot day^{-1}) = N \text{ intake } (g \cdot day^{-1})$$
$$- N \text{ output } (g \cdot day^{-1})$$

where:

$$N \text{ Intake } = \text{ Protein intake}:6.25 \ (g \cdot day^{-1})$$
$$N \text{ output } = \text{ urea in urine } + 4 \ (g \cdot day^{-1})$$

Negative nitrogen balance is associated with resorption and positive nitrogen balance with deposition of cellular protoplasm. In healthy adults a nitrogen equilibrium is established when daily protein intake is about $0.6-1 \ g \cdot kg^{-1} \cdot day^{-1}$. Surgical stress and possible postoperative complications increase nitrogen requirements, and protein intake has to be increased accordingly to prevent loss of cellular protoplasmic mass. As a simple guide to make up for the increased protein needs after major surgery and postoperative complications, protein must be increased in proportion to energy (calorie/nitrogen ratio) to about $100 \ kcal \cdot g^{-1}$ of nitrogen. For example if energy expenditure is estimated at $2000 \ kcal \cdot day^{-1}$, the nitrogen intake would be $2000/100 = 20 \ g$ N per day $\times 6.25 = 130 \ g$ protein. Renal or hepatic failure will increase this ratio. Patients with malabsorption have an increased protein demand varying from $2-8 \ g \cdot kg^{-1} \cdot day^{-1}$ depending on the severity of the disease. When a nutritional program is aimed at repleting LBM, protein intake must be increased above maintenance protein requirements.

VITAMINS. The vitamins are important to normal metabolic functions. They are essential nutrients and therefore have to be supplied to the nutritional support regimen (Table 27-3).

Nutritional Failure

MALNUTRITION. Nutritional failure is associated either with protein depletion in the presence of adequate calories or with combined protein–calorie deficiency. In protein–caloric deficiency the food has adequate proportions of proteins but the total caloric intake is inadequate. In their respective end-stage forms protein deficiency corresponds to kwashiorkor and combined protein–calorie deficiency corresponds to marasmus.

Protein depletion will affect the protein content of all organs. The liver and gut are rapidly depleted while the brain is affected less than other organs. In severe protein depletion the gut may be unable to tolerate or digest food presumably because protein is needed to produce digestive enzymes. The

skeletal muscle is most affected and may lose as much as 70% of its protein.

Protein–calorie depletion is a frequent finding in surgical patients as well as in the critically ill. Nutritional deficits are often unsuspected and remain unnoticed. Patients with malnutrition have been shown to be at an increased risk for infections and mechanical complications in the postoperative period, as outlined below. TPN can be used to correct the nutritional abnormalities and thus decrease the risk of perioperative morbidity and mortality with a shortening of the hospital stay.

DIAGNOSIS OF MALNUTRITION. An evaluation of the nutritional status is an important means of identifying the patient who needs nutritional intervention as well as assessing the efficacy of the nutritional support. The lack of a specific test for protein–calorie malnutrition makes the diagnosis difficult in many cases.

Nutritional assessment begins with a medical history and physical examination, including recording of height and weight. During the start of TPN weight should be measured daily. Acute changes in weight reflect changes in water and sodium. In the chronically malnourished patient with underlying disease, extracellular volume is expanded, with a relatively increased total body water and exchangeable sodium and a decreased exchangeable potassium.[13] The body weight thus may underestimate the degree of malnutrition. On the other hand nutritional repletion may be associated with a diuresis and contraction of the ECF compartment so that early weight loss may occur even though BCM is increasing. Nevertheless, the best single index of malnutrition is evidence of weight loss from the patient's normal level of weight.

Practical clinical tools of anthropometric measurement of body composition include the triceps skinfold thickness and midarm circumference. The former is an indicator of body fat, and the latter is an indicator of muscle and, thereby, of LBM. These are simple tests that can be quickly performed. Both measurements however, have a wide range of normal values and are rather insensitive to early changes in nutritional status. Further, the tests are limited in that it is difficult to differentiate kwashiorkor from marasmus.

Dynamic nutritional assessment is performed using energy and nitrogen balance. Energy balance measurements, however, require calorimetry. Nitrogen balance requires careful collection of all drainage and excreta. In the clinical setting, nitrogen loss is usually estimated by measuring 24-hr urinary urea nitrogen excretion and adding correction factors for non-urea urinary nitrogen. The nitrogen balance provides an estimate of net protein degradation or synthesis. Creatinine excretion is directly related to muscle mass, and expected creatinine excretion can be calculated based on sex and height.[24] The creatinine/height index is a useful indicator of muscle mass.

Analysis of the visceral proteins synthesized in the liver includes measurement of serum albumin, transferrin, retinol-binding protein, and prealbumin. There are limitations to the use of albumin as an index of nutritional status; other causes of low albumin other than malnutrition must be considered. Albumin is distributed throughout the extra-cellular compartment so that changes in total body water will influence the level of albumin independent of changes in nutritional status. There also exists a large exchangeable pool of albumin; the albumin half time is approximately 17 days and this limits its usefulness as a short-term indicator of efficacy of nutritional support. Serum albumin appears to be most useful in the initial assessment of chronic malnutrition. Transferrin has a

TABLE 27-3.   Maintenance Dose of Vitamins

VITAMIN	DOSE
Vitamin A	3300 IU
Vitamin D	200 IU
Vitamin E	10 IU
Vitamin C	100 mg
Thiamine	3 mg
Riboflavin	3.6 mg
Niacin	40 mg
Pyridoxine	4 mg
Biotin	60 mg
Folate	400 mg
B_{12}	5 mg

shorter half-life (approximately 8 days); however, it is also an acute-phase reactant and is affected by the status of iron stores. This lack of specificity limits the clinical usefulness of transferrin. Retinol-binding protein and prealbumin turn over more rapidly, with half-lives of 12 and 36 hr, respectively. They may be potentially more sensitive and specific indicators of nutritional status, but their clinical usefulness has not yet been established. Decreased humoral and cellular immunity is a serious consequence of protein–calorie malnutrition. Total lymphocyte count and cutaneous reactivity are commonly used in the clinical setting. Sepsis and carcinoma, however, also cause anergy independent of nutritional status. This lack of specificity limits their use in the clinical setting.

There is today no single best indicator of nutritional status or the efficacy of nutritional support. The prognostic nutritional index[25] and the protein–energy malnutrition scale[26] attempt to develop more objective measures to predict outcome based on a combination of parameters; however, clinical judgment has been reported to be as good as any of the objective measurements in predicting morbidity and mortality.[27]

Nutritional Treatment

Nutritional therapy has three main goals. The first is to maintain body tissue. It is a prophylactic support to give TPN to prevent the development of malnutrition (e.g., postoperatively). The second is to replete body tissues in the already malnourished patient. The third goal is the prevention and correction of specific micronutrient deficiencies (vitamins, trace elements, etc.).

The first step in planning any nutritional regimen is to identify the need for intervention; the next step is to determine the route of delivery. The last step is to prescribe the amounts of macronutrients and micronutrients based on the clinical setting and nutritional assessment of the patient.

INDICATIONS. Critically ill patients are often in a hypercatabolic state and are at high risk of rapidly developing malnutrition, even though their premorbid nutritional status was adequate. The goal is to meet their increased nutritional requirements to minimize the loss of LBM and function during the catabolic phase. Patients with severe injury, major burns, or sepsis fall into this group. Patients with chronic diseases with or without gastrointestinal tract involvement often require intravenous nutrition. Patients with short gut syndrome, gastrointestinal fistula, severe malabsorption, or inflammatory bowel disease may require intravenous nutrition. Often, nutritional debilitation is seen in chronic diseases even though the gastrointestinal tract is not directly involved, for example, in patients with chronic renal failure. Malnutrition is common in patients with cancer. In the patient with malignancy who is about to undergo a surgical procedure, the risk of TPN, the risk of delaying the operation, and the benefit in terms of morbidity and mortality must be considered in each patient. There is evidence that TPN may improve patient tolerance to chemotherapy and radiation.[28, 29] No significant long-term benefit, however, has been demonstrated to date.

For hepatic encephalopathy, renal failure, and hypercatabolic stress states, specific amino acid formulations have been developed in order to affect the specific metabolic derangements of each of these conditions. Their clinical use will be outlined later in this chapter. Intravenous fat emulsions have also been proposed to alter the inflammatory profile of the lung via alterations in prostaglandin (PG) synthesis.[30] When nutritional support is used for these indications to achieve specific metabolic and pharmacologic effects, it may be considered as a drug.

Perioperative nutritional support is outlined in a separate section (see below)

ENTERAL ROUTE OF ADMINISTRATION. Patients can be fed by either the enteral or the parenteral route or by a combination of the two. Intravenous feeding is an alternative to oral feeding and should be used only when the gastrointestinal tract is unavailable. When ad libitum food intake is negligible (less than 500 kcal · day^{-1}), enteral solutions are used to supply the total daily requirements. The solutions can be sipped or administered through a nasogastric feeding tube with a thin lumen.

Enteral solutions vary in composition, palatability, and cost. The formula ingredients are either premixed by the manufacturer or added together shortly before use. The two major groups of fixed-composition formulas are elemental and polymeric; the formulas prepared de novo are termed modular.

Elemental solutions consist of an easily digested and absorbed nitrogen source, a carbohydrate source requiring little amylase activity, and a small amount of fat in the form of medium chain triglycerides (MCTs) or essential fatty acids. They provide all essential nutrients and most of them contain about 1 kcal · ml^{-1} of fluid.[31] Elemental formulas are generally used in patients who have maldigestion and malabsorption. The disadvantages of these formulas are that they are unpalatable and require tube feeding; they are hyperosmolar (500–900 mOsm · kg^{-1}), which may result in cramping and osmotic diarrhea if infused too rapidly; they are relatively high in carbohydrates, which in turn increases carbon dioxide production and ventilation; and they are expensive relative to polymeric solutions.

Polymeric solution are indicated in patients with normal or near-normal gastrointestinal function. Their protein, carbohydrate, and fat are provided in high-molecular-weight forms. Many of the polymeric formulas are palatable and can be tolerated without tube feeding. They are less expensive and generally lower in osmolality than elemental solutions.

A modular formula is prepared by combining two or more ingredients to form the mixture. The type and amount of protein, carbohydrate, and fat, and the mineral and vitamin content can be adjusted to meet the needs of each patient. Modular solutions are thus prepared from available sources of protein, carbohydrate, fat, minerals, and proteins.[32] Alternatively, any one of the individual modules can be added to one of the complete formulas, which serves as a base solution. Modular formulas offer specific advantages in patients with cardiac failure, decreased pulmonary function, malabsorption, diabetes and renal insufficiency.

The nutrition-depleted patient does not tolerate an adequate diet instantly; diarrhea almost always occurs. The first goal, therefore, is to provide volume, and then slowly increase concentration until adequate nutrition is achieved without diarrhea. If an isotonic enteral formula used, however, the initial infusion in most situations can be started at full strength if an appropriate slow speed is selected. The infusion rate is then advanced as tolerated.

PARENTERAL NUTRITION. It is possible to supply all nutrients by the intravenous route. Intravenous nutrition may be given alone as TPN or as a supplement in some patients if oral or tube feeding may be possible but insufficient.

HISTORY. In 1913, Henriques and Anderson provided a major stepping stone in the history of intravenous nutrition with the intravenous administration of a protein hydrolysate in a goat.[33] They were able to keep the goat in a positive N balance for 14 days. In the ensuing decades the effort was devoted to the development of intravenous protein and energy sources as well as to methods of administration. There also were a growing understanding and clinical awareness of the influence of nutritional status on the outcome following injury or surgery.[33-36] The major obstacle to total intravenous nutritional support remained the inability to deliver adequate non-protein calories. Two major advancements, however, opened the door to the clinical application of TPN. In 1960 Wretlind and Haakansson in Sweden developed a fat emulsion that was without complication when given to animals and to patients.[37, 38] This fat emulsion, Intralipid, was made from soybean oil, with purified egg phosphatides as the emulsifier. In the United States in 1968, Wilmore and Dudrick reported their experience with central venous catheterization for the delivery of hypertonic dextrose solution.[39] They demonstrated that administration of intravenous nutrients exclusively could not only support life, but also promote growth and development.

The last two decades have seen advancements in the understanding of the metabolic response to starvation and stress and refinements in methodology. A current interest in nutritional support is the attempt to differentiate various nutritional support solutions for different disease states.

ROUTES OF PARENTERAL ADMINISTRATION. Parenteral nutrition can be delivered by central or peripheral vein. The subclavian or internal jugular vein may be cannulated percutaneously and the central catheter placed with the tip in the superior vena cava. The Hickman or Broviac type of Silastic catheter with Dacron cuff placed *via* venotomy with subcutaneous tunneling may also be used. They may be inserted by venotomy *via* the cephalic, basilic, or external jugular vein.[40-43] A peel-away introducer has been developed that allows percutaneous placement into the subclavian or internal jugular vein. A subcutaneous tunnel is used to increase the distance between the exit site and the vein to reduce infection. The major disadvantages of the percutaneous subclavian catheter is that it is associated with a 5–7% incidence of significant mechanical complications such as pneumothorax and subclavian artery puncture.[44]

Short-term intravenous nutrition can be administered by peripheral vein. Lipids are then used as a substantial proportion of the non-protein calories to reduce the toxicity of the solution. An example of such a mixture would be 500 ml of a 20% fat emulsion, 1000 ml of 8.5% amino acid solution, and 1000 ml of 10% dextrose. This provides nearly 1800 kcal·day^{-1} when infused at 100 ml·hr^{-1}. The final concentration of dextrose is less than 5%, hence the phlebitis rate is quite low and comparable with that observed with 5% dextrose and saline solution. The vein puncture site should be rotated every 2–3 days. The use of an arteriovenous shunt or fistulas for TPN has been attempted but is not in general use.[42]

NUTRITIONAL PROGRAM COMPONENTS. In Table 27-4 we have outlined a nutritional program based on a glucose–lipid system for an average 70-kg man who has lost weight to 60 kg due to stress and illness. Formulas for nutrition for specific disease states are discussed below.

Nitrogen balance is sensitive to protein intake as well as to total energy (calories) consumed; for comparative calories the effect of protein exceeds that of nonprotein calories. Optimal nutritional support first maximizes protein intake and only then adds sufficient calories in the form of glucose and fat.[45] A positive nitrogen balance cannot be achieved by giving amino acids alone, with no other calories. Nonprotein calories can reduce the nitrogen excretion, but only to a minimum level in the absence of protein intake.[46] Thus, both protein and nonprotein energy are required. The effects of nitrogen and en-

TABLE 27-4. Nutrient Regimen for the Standard 70-kg Man Following Weight Loss Aiming for Nutritional Repletion

REGIMEN	CONTENT
NUTRIENT MIXTURE:	
Protein	110 g
Nonprotein calories	1000–2000
Distribution	50% glucose and 50% fat
PARENTERAL SOLUTIONS:*	
1000 ml	11% amino acids
1000 ml	20% glucose
500 ml	20% fat emulsion

*The parenteral solutions can be mixed in one bag and infused over 24 hr at 100 ml·hr^{-1}. Electrolytes, trace elements, and vitamins are added to the TPN mixture.

ergy intake on nitrogen balance, however, are not independent of one another; their interaction is complex. If nitrogen intake is adequate, zero nitrogen balance is achieved when caloric intake meets caloric expenditure. Similarly, increasing caloric intake above requirements increases nitrogen retention and results in net positive nitrogen balance.[47] Changes in body composition that occur with hyperalimentation have been found to consist of approximately two parts fat to one part LBM,[4, 48] but will depend on kind of nutritional composition. During nutritional repletion, as during starvation, there are no appreciable changes in ECF. In the study of Keys et al,[7] fat was restored more rapidly than LBM (Fig. 27-2). By 20 weeks excess fat has been deposited; this fat is gradually lost between weeks 33 and 58. Restoration of BCM is not completed until the 58th week, and it is only by this time that body compartments are returned to their control pattern.[7] During nutritional repletion there is a greater positive nitrogen balance in the beginning that declines as the BCM returns more to its prestarvation levels.

The large nitrogen loss that occurs during the first 6 days of fasting can be halved by daily ingestion of only 100 g of glucose.[10] The nitrogen-sparing effect of a relatively small (400 kcal·g^{-1}) caloric load occurs with carbohydrate only because fat does not produce the same suppression of nitrogen excretion during fasting.[49] On the other hand, restriction of either fat or carbohydrate in the diet increases nitrogen output, although nitrogen loss is greater with carbohydrate restriction,[50] while adding either back improves nitrogen retention.[51] The ability of fat as compared with glucose to spare nitrogen has been studied extensively. At low dosages, glucose is clearly superior to fat. When carbohydrate is administered in amounts of more than 600 kcal·day^{-1}, the nitrogen-sparing effects of fat and carbohydrate are equal,[51] while fat has only a small nitrogen-sparing effect in the absence of 600 kcal·day^{-1} of carbohydrates;[52, 53] however, no differences in N balances have been detected in studies comparing groups receiving the nonprotein calories in form of glucose with those whose nonprotein calories were supplied as one-half fat and one-half glucose[54, 55] (Fig. 27-3). When the lipid-based system is administered, a lesser calorigenic response and a decreased norepinephrine excretion have been found compared to the "glucose system."[56] A reduction in carbon dioxide production has also been observed in patients receiving "the lipid system."[57] Liver function tests have shown fewer abnormalities when lipid was used to replace one-third of the glucose calories.[58] These studies provide evidence of the efficacy of 20% fat emulsion as a concentrated nutrient source that allows provision of calories without overhydration and hemodilution.

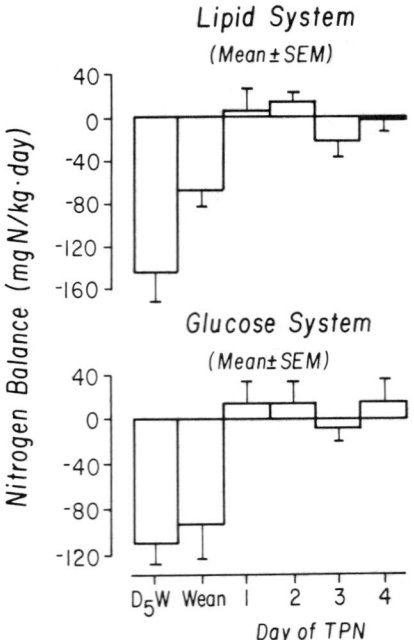

Lipid System
(Mean ± SEM)

Glucose System
(Mean ± SEM)

FIG. 27-3. Nitrogen balance in subjects given two forms of nutritional support systems: a lipid-based system *vs.* a glucose-based system. During administration of parenteral nutrition, nitrogen balance with both systems is equivalent. (Reprinted with permission. Nordenstrøm J, Askanazi J, Elwyn DH *et al:* Nitrogen balance during total parenteral nutrition: Glucose *versus* fat. Ann Surg 197:27, 1983.)

General usage of fat as a calorie source in TPN in the United States has only gradually developed even though fat emulsions represent a logical alternative to glucose loading, especially in patients with an exaggerated caloric requirement and a diminished ability to clear exogenous glucose (*e.g.,* in metabolic stress), as well as in those with hepatic or pulmonary dysfunction.

DELIVERY OF NUTRIENTS. The most common mode of delivery of nutrients is continuous administration *via* the central route. Cyclic administration of nutrients has been suggested, alternating dextrose-containing with dextrose-free solutions. This method has the theoretical advantage of avoiding prolonged hyperinsulinemia and allowing release of endogenous fatty acids from adipose tissue and may also optimize visceral protein preservation and avoid alterations in hepatic function.[59]

Mixing of all the components for TPN in one mix ("three-in-one" system) before administration simplifies procedures for the nursing personnel and may also reduce the risk of infection. Until now the most common mode of delivery has been to give separate infusion of amino acids, fat and carbohydrate and add vitamins and trace elements into the solutions before infusion ("bottle system"). The nursing personnel has to mix the components, monitor infusion rate of more solutions given at the same time, and change bottles several times during the day. In addition to the work for the nursing staff, the mixing of solutions on the floor may not be satisfactory from a hygienic point with the often required manipulations with infusion sets and connections.

COMPLICATIONS. Complications of parenteral nutrition arise as the result of placement or maintenance of the intravenous catheter required for the infusion or from excessive or insufficient provision of one or more nutrients. Virtually every component of TPN has been associated with metabolic complications, usually from deficient or excess administration. The most common metabolic complication is hyperglycemia and glucosuria. This is dependent on the rate of infusion and carbohydrate source. Frequent monitoring of glucose in urine and serum is required during TPN. If glucose in serum is more than 250 mg·dl^{-1}, insulin is usually added to the TPN solution. Hyperglycemic hyperosmolar coma has been reported from infusion of the TPN solution. Hypoglycemia and shock have been reported after TPN infusion has been suddenly discontinued. A frequent metabolic complication is hyperchloremic acidosis, which can be prevented by decreasing the ratio of chloride to acetate in the TPN.[60] Rapid infusion of amino acid solutions have been associated with nausea, headache, and a warm sensation. When the patient begins to become anabolic, large amounts of potassium and phosphate shift into the intracellular space; to avoid a deficit of these, supplementation will be needed. Hepatic dysfunction has been reported. Replacement of part of the TPN glucose calories with fat, however, leads to better glucose tolerance and fewer hepatic complications.[58]

The mechanical catheter-related complications are outlined in Table 27-5. Of these complications sepsis deserves special mention. The venous catheters are often in place for long periods, and the fluids used are ideal for supporting growth of microorganisms. In one large, multi-hospital study, an infection rate of 7% was reported.[61] Strict antiseptic conditions should prevail during catheter placement, and the catheter should be used only for the infusion of TPN. The frequency of the induction of sepsis is increased with the use of multilumen catheters for TPN. In one large study the frequency of sepsis was 14.6% for multilumen catheters compared with 3.2% for single-lumen catheters.[60]

PATIENT MONITORING. Table 27-6 gives guidelines for monitoring the patient for the development of infection or metabolic complications. When the patient is stable and tolerating a

TABLE 27-5.   Mechanical Complications of TPN

Central Venous Catheter Placement
  Malposition
  Catheter embolism
  Air embolism
  Thrombosis and thromboembolism
  Sepsis
  Cardiac dysrhythmias
  Myocardial perforation

Subclavian or Internal Jugular Venipuncture
  Arterial puncture
  Pneumothorax, hemothorax, chylothorax
  Brachial plexus injury
  Mediastinal hematoma

Peripheral Venipuncture
  Pain
  Hematoma
  Thrombosis
  Phlebitis
  Extravasation

TABLE 27-6. Suggested Monitoring Schedule During TPN

PARAMETER	Early	After Stable
Volume in (iv and oral)	Daily	Daily
Volume out (urine and drainage)	Daily	Daily
Body temperature	Daily	Daily
Urine S&A	4 Times daily	Twice daily
Electrolytes	Daily	Biweekly
BUN/creatinine	Biweekly	Biweekly
Ca^{++}, PO_4^{--}, Mg^{++}	Biweekly	Weekly
CBC, platelets	Weekly	Weekly
Glucose	Daily	Biweekly
PT, PTT	Weekly	Weekly
Triglycerides, cholesterol	Weekly	Weekly
Liver profile	Biweekly	Weekly
ABGs, urine electrolytes, drainage analysis, blood cultures, serum insulin, ketones, plasma amino acids, plasma fatty acids	Weekly	Weekly
Weight	Biweekly	Biweekly

iv = intravenous; S&A = sugar and acetone; BUN = blood urea nitrogen; CBC = complete blood count; PT = prothrombin time; PTT = partial thromboplastin time; ABGs = arterial blood gases. (Reprinted with permission. Robin AR, Greig PD: Basic principles of intravenous nutritional support. Clin Chest Med 7:29, 1986.)

particular regimen, most of those determinations can be performed less frequently.

Weight should be measured daily; acute changes reflect changes in water and sodium. Body weight changes may underestimate the degree of malnutrition because ECF does not change during malnutrition, and nutritional repletion may be associated with a diuresis and contraction of the extracellular (ECV) compartment, so that early weight loss may occur, even though BCM is increasing.

If the patient becomes hyperglycemic (blood glucose > 250 $mg \cdot dl^{-1}$), the infusion rate of glucose should be reduced[62] and insulin may be administered. The requirement for insulin often decreases rapidly when the patient's stress resolves and the patient shifts from the catabolic to the anabolic state. The need for insulin should be reevaluated daily by close monitoring of blood and urinary sugars. The discontinuing of glucose–insulin mixtures should be done with caution to avoid hypoglycemia. As the effect of the insulin lasts longer than that of glucose, the tendency toward hyperosmolarity can be prevented if the plasma osmolarity, sodium, blood urea nitrogen, acid–base balance, and blood sugar levels are carefully monitored.

When the patient begins to become anabolic, additional supplementation of potassium and phosphate will be needed as these shift into the intracellular space. Hypophosphatemia may reduce cardiac and muscle contraction, as well as CNS, red blood cell, and leucocyte function.[63]

SPECIFIC NUTRIENT SUPPORT IN DISEASE STATES

Liver Disease

Protein–calorie malnutrition is common in the patient with liver disease; therefore, nutritional support is an important part of the therapy. The protein component of the nutrition, however, presents a problem to the patient with hepatic insufficiency who is intolerant to protein, and who may develop hepatic encephalopathy.

There are a number of metabolic alterations in liver disease that affect design of a nutritional support regimen. Diminished degradation of circulating hormones and portal–systemic shunting may result in a persistent elevation of glucagon and insulin.[64, 65] The increase in glucagon may be greater than insulin,[66] resulting in a decreased insulin:glucagon ratio and a catabolic state.[67] In addition to the tendency toward catabolism, there may also exist an energy deficit in liver failure due to impaired utilization of carbohydrates and lipids.[66, 68] The cirrhotic liver fails to store glucose as glycogen. The chronic hyperglucagonemia presumably results in depletion of glycogen. Increased lipolysis also lessens the requirement for glucose. Lipolysis liberates glycerol, which contributes to gluconeogenesis, and fatty acids, which are used directly or oxidized to ketones (although this latter pathway may be impaired). The increased lipolysis combined with a decreased metabolism of fatty acids leads to high blood levels of nonesterified fatty acids.[69] The tendency toward gluconeogenesis from amino acids from muscle breakdown requires an equal capacity for ureagenesis in order to prevent hyperammonemia. In addition to hyperammonemia caused by diminished ureagenic capacity, there is a shunting of ammonia of gut origin resulting in persistent elevation of plasma ammonia concentrations.

A specific amino acid pattern is seen in hepatic failure. Amino acids dependent on hepatic metabolism show increases. The aromatic amino acids (e.g., tyrosine, tryptophan) levels are elevated.[70] Conversely, the branched-chain amino acids that are catabolized in the periphery (e.g., skeletal muscle) are decreased due to the increased peripheral demand and utilization.[70, 71]

The increased level of aromatic amino acids and a decreased level of branched-chain amino acids in plasma has been correlated with the presence of encephalopathy.[72] Members of the neutral amino acid group compete at the blood–brain barrier (BBB) for a single transport system (termed the L-system) that mediates their entry across the BBB.[73, 74] In hepatic encephalopathy there may be a derangement of the BBB,[75] which results in a selective increase in transport of the neutral amino acids. Within this group it is hypothesized that the transport of the aromatic amino acids is preferentially increased due to their elevated plasma levels as well as the decreased competition for the transport system due to decreased plasma branch-chain amino acids.[71, 76] According to this theory, which is by no means generally accepted,[77] a decrease in the branched-chain/aromatic amino acid plasma ratio would be responsible for an imbalance of central aminergic neurotransmitters. The aromatic amino acids (phenylalanine, tyrosine, tryptophan) are precursors of neurotransmitters, and there has been found an increase in brain concentrations of serotonin and false neurotransmitters in hepatic encephalopathy.[72] The false neurotransmitters are produced locally in the brain and may replace the physiologic transmitters (dopamine, noradrenaline) at the synapse. It has become clear, however, that one cannot predict the brain or cerebrospinal fluid amino acid content from plasma amino acid levels alone.[78] Although controversy continues, it seems that the ratio of branched-chain to aromatic amino acids is a good predictor of hepatic function but not encephalopathy.[79] According to this hypothesis, ammonia does not exert a direct toxic effect, but rather appears to contribute to the pathogenesis of hepatic encephalopathy indirectly through the brain metabolite glutamine, which may accelerate transport of aromatic amino acids across the BBB.[80, 81]

The administration of branched-chain amino acid-enriched solutions was originally advocated for patients with liver failure. The standard balanced amino acids used in nutrition contain 19–25% of their amino acids as branched-chain, while the branched-chain amino acid-enriched solutions have about 45% of the amino acids as branched-chain. The branched-chain amino acids are unique in their partial utilization as an energy source by tissues (primarily muscle), other than the liver. At the same time NH_2 groups are formed from the branched-chain amino acids for the synthesis of alanine and glutamine. Alanine is released from muscle and used as substrate for gluconeogenesis by the liver (alanine–glucose cycle).[82] Glutamine is mainly used as an energy source by the intestine and the kidneys. In addition to their use as an energy source, the branched-chain amino acids also have been found to play a role in the regulation of protein turnover; the branched-chain amino acids may decrease muscle breakdown[83] and promote protein synthesis in muscle[84] as well as in the liver.[85] The ketoacid analogs of the branched-chain amino acids seem to be more efficacious in this regard than the amino acids themselves.[86]

The branched-chain amino acid-enriched solutions offer a theoretically attractive solution in hepatic failure by their properties to provide usable calories that can be utilized by peripheral conversion to arrest protein catabolism and promote protein synthesis, and to normalize the branched-chain/aromatic amino acid plasma levels.[87] Promising reports of studies in dogs and monkeys clearly indicated that a branched-chain amino acid-enriched solution was superior over commercially available amino acid mixture in achieving positive nitrogen balance and normalizing of neurologic symptoms.[78, 88, 89] Encouraged by these reports, numerous anecdotal studies were published in which branched-chain amino acid infusions were found to be useful in patients with liver disease.[90, 91, 95] Subsequently at least seven controlled, randomized studies have been published.[92–98] These studies have given conflicting results. It seems apparent that the branched-chain amino acids are of some value in treatment of hepatic encephalopathy. Patients in hepatic coma awoke as quickly in response to administration of branched-chain amino acids and hypertonic dextrose solution as they did in response to the conventional treatment with starvation and neomycin/lactulose therapy, and both regimens worked much more quickly than placebo. The exceptions to this trend, which used fat as the principal energy source,[92, 95, 98] failed to show efficacy of branched-chain amino acid-enriched solutions as preferable to standard amino acid solutions in hepatic encephalopathy. In the opinion of certain authors, the high lipid intake would not constitute a source of calories and could possibly worsen the encephalopathy.[97]

Of the controlled studies, only the U.S. multi-center trials[97] have achieved nitrogen equilibrium. A study indicates that patients with cirrhosis may be able to tolerate protein administered in a branched-chain amino acid-enriched form better than conventional protein.[99] Two of the controlled studies have suggested improved survival in patients with liver disease when treated with branched-chain amino acid-enriched solutions.[96, 97] However, patients treated with conventional amino acids also have improved survival,[98] which indicates that the nutritional support in itself seem to be associated with increased survival.

As a conclusion, branched-chain amino acid-enriched solutions seem indicated in hepatic failure with encephalopathy to reduce the cerebral symptoms and to provide usable calories. It is still not clear, however, whether the *in vitro* effects on protein turnover and possible promotion of hepatic protein synthesis are of clinical importance.

Metabolic Stress

The response to injury and infection can be described as a mobilization of body protein, fat, and carbohydrate stores to provide normal or above-normal circulating levels of substrate (glucose, free fatty acids, and amino acids) in the absence of dietary intake. Injury increases the rate of loss of LBM at any given nutrient intake; after elective operations weight loss occurs in the ratio of 2:1 (LBM:fat);[6] with severe injury the ratio rises to 4:1 (Table 27-1). The persistence of gluconeogenesis, despite high serum concentrations of glucose, demonstrates the urgent nature of the need for glucose. Fat is mobilized to meet the energy needs of cardiac and skeletal muscle; this spares glucose for the tissues that specifically oxidize it, such as the CNS and the cellular immune system. This pattern, unlike that observed in fasting normal humans, does not respond easily to nutritional manipulation. As a result, hypertonic glucose dosages are usually ineffective in these patients and may add additional stress by precipitating increases in oxygen consumption, carbon dioxide production, and noradrenaline excretion, and by inducing hepatic complications. These findings do not indicate that glucose infusion is contraindicated in stressed patients; a certain amount of carbohydrate intake is essential to meet obligatory glucose requirements. The importance of glucose has been underscored by data associating the administration of amino acids alone (without supplementary glucose) with reduced cellular energy levels in injured patients.[100] A nutritional regimen appropriate for a patient under metabolic stress would therefore consist of a relatively modest amount of glucose administered with amino acids and other essential nutrients. Fat emulsions represent the logical alternative to glucose loading in patients with an exaggerated caloric requirement. The fat emulsion allows provision of calories without overhydration and hemodilution. It seems, therefore, that a regimen supplying nonprotein calories in the form of both glucose and fat may be particularly appropriate for the stressed patient.

The amino acid requirement is increased by sepsis or trauma. A plasma amino acid pattern resembling that seen in hepatic failure has been noted in patients with systemic sepsis. These findings led to investigations of the utility of branched-chain amino acid-enriched solutions for critically ill patients. In addition branched-chain amino acids can serve as fuel energy substrates, to promote the synthesis of muscle and visceral protein, and to reduce the breakdown of muscle protein.[101–105] All these effects may be beneficial in states with metabolic stress to decrease catabolism.

Several animal and human studies have indicated beneficial effects of the use of branched-chain amino acid solutions to patients with metabolic stress.[106–110] Other studies, however, have not found any difference in nitrogen retention in normal (25%) and high (45%) branched-chain amino acid groups.[111–113] The overall conclusions from the controlled human studies are clouded by the variability of stress and the number of septic patients included. The studies showing promotion of nitrogen balance with enriched branched-chain amino acid solutions have not used a balanced substrate for nonprotein caloric support. Several investigators have shown that a balanced TPN regimen where the nonprotein calories have been given as carbohydrates and lipids can lead to a positive nitrogen balance.[55, 114] In one study no significant difference was found in nitrogen balance promotion when a 44.6% branched-chain amino acid solution was compared with a standard TPN regimen (19% branched-chain amino acid, carbohydrate:lipid ratio 7:3.[112] The lack of difference may be due to an effective utilization of lipids as fuel source by both the groups.[115]

The *in vitro* studies that have suggested a beneficial effect of the branched-chain amino acids in decreasing protein degradation have investigated muscle tissue from nonseptic animals. Preliminary results, however, suggest that the controls of muscle degradation may be different in septic animals than in normal[116] and this may explain the marginal effects demonstrated with the branched-chain amino acids in septic patients. It has also been proposed that the most important property of the branched-chain amino acids in sepsis may be the apparent effect of the branched-chain amino acids on hepatic protein synthesis, with indirect synthesis of proteins involved in host defense.[117]

As a conclusion, the role of branched-chain amino acids in the support of the critically ill stressed patient remains unclear. Further studies of the control of protein synthesis in the stressed state and the effect of a balanced TPN on N balance have to be undertaken.

Respiratory Disease

The effects of nutrition on respiration involve respiratory drive, respiratory muscle function, and pulmonary parenchyma as well as metabolic demand. In general nutritional support increases the respiratory work load by increasing metabolic demand and ventilatory drive, but it seems that improvements in respiratory muscle and lung function also occur if nutrition is given over a longer period.

When hypertonic glucose is used as the sole source of nonprotein calories in TPN, a marked rise in carbon dioxide production occurs.[118, 119] As substrates shift from fat oxidation to glucose oxidation, an increase in RQ occurs; if sufficient glucose is given, lipogenesis occurs with a further rise in the level of carbon dioxide production.[120] This increase in carbon dioxide production, with its increase in ventilatory demand, can lead to respiratory distress in patients with impaired lung function. Substitution of fat emulsions for nonprotein calories lowers the RQ and reduces minute ventilation and ventilatory demand.[57] Thus, administration of the nonprotein calories as a mixture of fat and carbohydrate is important in patients with pulmonary disease.

A series of studies has demonstrated that amino acids stimulate ventilation.[121-123] Solutions that are high in the branched-chain amino acids seem to have a greater stimulatory effect than the standard amino acid solutions.[123] This would suggest that part of this phenomenon is an effect of amino acids on neurotransmission as precursors for neurotransmitter production.

Malnutrition is followed by a deterioration of the respiratory muscles. It is becoming increasingly evident that nutritional support can result in an improvement of the respiratory muscles as positive nitrogen balance occurs.[124] These improvements require time to have a discernible effect (from 2 to 3 weeks). Malnutrition also has important effects on the pulmonary parenchyma by causing emphysema-like changes and indirectly by impairment of the immune function. It is not yet clear whether and to what extent these malnutrition-induced lesions on the pulmonary parenchyma can be reversed.[125] Surfactant production also seems to be impaired in depletion with improvement during refeeding.

Cardiac Disease

The effect of nutrition on the myocardium is a two-fold phenomenon. Nutrition has an acute effect on the myocardium.

The extent to which different fuels are used has important implications in myocardial function and the myocardial tissue damage that occurs under stressed states. A second important effect of nutrition on the myocardium involves protein synthesis and degradation; the myocardium is not spared in starvation and stress conditions, and during catabolic states there is protein loss by the myocardium as well as protein loss by skeletal muscle throughout the body. The loss of protein occurring from the myocardium during starvation is restored during refeeding. The effect of nutrition on myocardial protein synthesis and degradation is important in the preoperative and postoperative periods; whereas in the intraoperative and immediate postoperative period the effects of nutrients to alter substrate supply (glucose, fat, lactate, *etc.*) become more significant.

ACUTE NUTRITIONAL EFFECTS ON THE MYOCARDIUM. Cardiac muscle is capable of using a wide variety of substrates as sources of energy.[126-128] Glucose and plasma free fatty acids are the primary fuels but lactate, pyruvate, ketone bodies, triglycerides, and to a lesser extent amino acids, can all serve as sources of energy under varying conditions. Utilization of these substrates by the heart is a function of their plasma concentrations, availability of alternate competing substrates, mechanical activity of the heart, supply of oxygen, and plasma levels of certain hormones. Under normal circumstances, oxidative phosphorylation accounts for almost all of the ATP produced. In a well-oxygenated heart all substrates are completely oxidized in the citric acid cycle. The importance of fatty acids in myocardial metabolism is well known. Their oxidation normally accounts for 60-70% of oxidative metabolism, but may under some conditions account for as much as 100%.[129, 130] Under most conditions free fatty acids are utilized in preference to carbohydrate. This is particularly true at high levels of cardiac work where fatty acids are the main substrate utilized.[131, 132] Although fatty acids appear to be the preferred fuel under most circumstances, glucose represents an important fuel for respiration in hypoxic hearts. Its metabolism through glycolysis is a major source of ATP in hypoxic tissue. The acceleration and alterations of substrate utilization under various conditions involve a complicated system of regulatory interactions in various metabolic pathways, the glucose fatty acid cycle.[126] This cycle controls the substrate utilization and adjusts rates to match substrate supply with energy needs.

Physiologic studies over a 50-year period suggest that glucose, insulin, and potassium (GIK) are beneficial to myocardial performance; GIK, therefore, has been the preferred choice for substrate support of the myocardium in the perioperative period and under conditions of acute myocardial ischemia. In 1926, it was reported that insulin has positive inotropic effects on the isolated, beating turtle heart,[133] and diphtheritic myocarditis was reported to respond positively to dextrose and insulin administration in 1930.[134] Anoxia has been found to increase the glucose uptake and anoxia plus insulin further accelerates glucose uptake.[135] Elevations in cardiac glycogen have resulted in increased glycolytic reserve and improved resistance to hypoxia by enhancing glycolytic and anaerobic ATP production.[136] On the other side, experimental and clinical observations of infusion of free fatty acids during ischemia have demonstrated a depression of the contractile myocardial function, an increase in the frequency of serious rhythm disturbances[137-139] and an increase in oxygen consumption.[140]

The list of potential beneficial sites of GIK on the ischemic myocardium includes favorable action on metabolic pathways, increased availability of glucose, decreased availability of FFAs, stabilization of the membranes, and favorable influence on prostaglandin synthesis.[141]

Experimental data have demonstrated a preservation of function and structure of hypoxic myocardium with increased perfusion of glucose.[142, 143] In early infusion of GIK during experimental acute coronary occlusion, the predicted size of the myocardial infarction was reduced.[144] In human studies GIK solutions have been found to stabilize ischemic myocardium;[145] to improve ventricular function;[146] to reduce the infarction size;[147] and to reduce hospital mortality in acute myocardial infarction.[148]

NUTRITION IN CARDIAC CACHEXIA. The heart has often been considered to be protected from chronic protein–energy starvation. Undernutrition, however, also affects the myocardium, and nutritional support can prevent or partially reverse the heart disease associated with undernutrition. The undernourished state characteristic of severe heart disease is usually called *cardiac cachexia*.[149] There are two types of cardiac cachexia: the "classic" type, which occurs in patients suffering from severe heart failure; and the "nosocomial" type, which develops in the postoperative state when complications develop, preventing a resumption of normal eating after surgery. One-third of patients with class III or IV heart disease have been found to suffer from cardiac cachexia.[150] A study has estimated that 1 out of every 15 patients in the surgical intensive care unit are suffering from nosocomial cardiac cachexia.[151] In hospitalized patients suffering from both types of cardiac cachexia, approximately one-half of the cardiac patients have been found to have some degree of undernutrition diagnosed by serum albumin and anthropometric measurements.[152]

Patients with classic cardiac cachexia frequently complain of poor appetite, which is compounded by the prescription of unappealing diets. There may be drug-induced vitamin and mineral losses and often some degree of malabsorption. The body weight is frequently normal, but physical and biochemical examinations indicate chronic undernutrition. In nosocomial cardiac cachexia the preoperative nutritional status usually is adequate. The cachexia develops in days or weeks postoperatively because of complications; the intake is sharply reduced and nutrient losses are excessive. The cachexia often is clinically deceptive because many patients will appear to be normally nourished according to standard assessment techniques, despite severe depletion of lean body tissue. If large amounts of carbohydrates but little or none of the other essential nutrients are infused, the glucose-induced insulin response prevents breakdown of adipose tissue without completely stopping lean tissue breakdown. Nutritional support is indicated when the underlying surgical complication cannot be corrected in 3–5 days.

It is clear that malnutrition results in a loss of cardiac mass and that nutritional repletion can restore cardiac tissue; however, the clinical implications and appropriate use of nutritional support in the preoperative and postoperative patient have been poorly studied. A profound difference in mortality and morbidity rates has been found between patients with cardiac disease who suffered from preoperative malnutrition compared with patients of good nutritional status.[153] It has been suggested that preoperative nutritional care could reduce myocardial complications following surgery[154] and result in improved myocardial function.[155]

Although some studies conclude that the undernutrition of cardiac cachexia can be at least partially corrected, the available reports about the beneficial effects of nutritional support on cardiac performance are incomplete and further controlled studies are needed to resolve these questions. There are now specifically formulated enteral and parenteral feeding solutions available for treating cardiac cachexia. Minimal recommended therapy in the classic form of cardiac cachexia is vitamin and mineral replacement; some patients may benefit from complete nutritional supplements. When the undernourished cardiac patient is scheduled for surgery, some workers recommend a 2-week preoperative course of hyperalimentation.[152] Postoperative complications following cardiac surgery often lead to rapid depletion of LBM and therefore nutritional therapy using nutrient solutions infused enterally, peripherally, or centrally is indicated.

Brain Injury

Development of irreversible brain tissue damage in brain ischemia is not always proportional to the degree of tissue oxygen deficiency. This paradox suggests that factors other than the severity of tissue hypoxia may influence postischemic recovery.

In experimental animal studies, raising the blood glucose level before a global ischemic insult increases brain damage.[156–158] This suggests that pre-ischemic hyperglycemia may have contributed to the neurologic injury. Findings similar to those in animals have been described in patients with ischemic stroke.[159] In a retrospective study, blood glucose level on admission was significantly related to neurologic recovery after cardiac arrest, with a high blood glucose level on admission being associated with poor neurologic recovery.[160] The mechanism for glucose-mediated injury may be related to enhanced tissue lactic production, or the glucose may exert the effect by acting as an osmotic agent.[161] The results may have important clinical implications and suggest that hyperglycemia be avoided in patients at risk for significant cerebral ischemia (cardiopulmonary bypass, induced hypotension, cerebral vascular surgery, and head injury).

There is considerable controversy regarding glucose administration during intracranial surgery. The administration of $100–150 \text{ g} \cdot \text{day}^{-1}$ of glucose produces protein sparing in starving individuals, decreases fat and protein mobilization during a short fast, and provides free water; it has, therefore, been advocated for patients undergoing general surgery.[162] Glucose administration during neurosurgery has also been advocated for the same reasons. Intraoperative ischemia, however, can occur in patients undergoing neurosurgical procedures. In view of the risk of intraoperative ischemia and the experimental and clinical findings noted above, it may be prudent to avoid giving excessive amounts of glucose intraoperatively, thus possibly avoiding the potential risk that glucose may aggravate intraoperative ischemic insults.[163] The same considerations apply for glucose infusion to patients with head injury. Sieber *et al*[164] found that intraoperative glucose infusion ($11–15 \text{ g} \cdot \text{hr}^{-1}$) produces glucose levels greater than 200 $\text{mg} \cdot \text{dl}^{-1}$, which are the levels that have been associated with potentiation of ischemic neurologic damage. Patients receiving saline had much lower glucose levels. Because there did not appear to be any metabolic compromise in those not receiving glucose, the results suggest that glucose should be avoided during intracranial and cerebrovascular surgical procedures. Similarly, the intensive care management of patients with head trauma should include avoidance of hyperglycemia.

Acute Renal Failure

Most patients with acute renal failure (ARF) have some degree of net protein breakdown and disordered fluid, electrolyte, or acid–base status. There is often excess total body water, azotemia, hyperkalemia, hyperphosphatemia, hypocalcemia, hyperuricemia, and a large anion-gap metabolic acidosis. The net protein degradation in ARF can be massive.[165] Patients are more likely to be catabolic when the ARF is caused by shock or sepsis. It is likely that the profound catabolic response of many patients with ARF may increase the risk of infection and delayed wound healing, prolong convalescence, and increase mortality. The net protein catabolism may accelerate the rate of rise in the plasma levels of potassium, phosphorus, nitrogenous metabolites, and acids.[166] The mechanisms for the catabolic effects of ARF are not well defined. The uremia *per se* may have potential catabolic effects, but other causes for wasting and malnutrition in ARF (*e.g.*, anorexia and vomiting, underlying medical disorders, loss of nutrients during dialysis) clearly also contribute. The aim of nutritional therapy in ARF is to counter the increased protein breakdown and to maintain protein stores. This goal should be accomplished without an increase in the production of uremic toxins, *e.g.*, without worsening azotemia. Ultimately, improved nutritional status in ARF patients should improve recovery, renal function, and survival.

Clinical studies performed in the 1960s suggested that amino acid therapy hastened recovery and lessened mortality in ARF.[167, 168] Patients with ARF who received an essential amino acid solution and hypertonic glucose had an improved recovery of renal function but no significant improvement in overall hospital survival.[168] In a more recent study three treatment regimens were compared: hypertonic dextrose alone; dextrose in combination with essential amino acids; and dextrose in combination with essential and nonessential amino acids.[165] They found no improvement in the recovery of renal function or in patient survival among the three groups, and the patients in the amino acid groups did not show an improvement in nitrogen balance. Increasing the nitrogen intake of patients with ARF does not seem to improve nitrogen balance.[169] It has been suggested that a different formulation of amino acids might be required for patients with ARF. Solutions with enhanced branched-chain amino acid content have been reported to reduce net protein catabolism in nonuremic patients. Further studies are needed to assess the high branched-chain amino acid solutions in ARF. However, in experimental ARF, amino acid solutions have been reported to increase the rapidity and severity of ARF and to increase the severity of postischemic ARF.[170, 171] Lysine has recently been suggested to have nephrotoxic effects,[172] but it is unknown whether the lysine in standard amino acid solutions exerts a nephrotoxic effect in humans.

Another important factor in the nutritional therapy is the calorie intake. Adequate calorie intake in nonuremic patients is correlated with positive nitrogen balance and better outcome. Because the provisions of adequate calories in many patients requires an infusion of 1–1.5 l of fluid daily, an increased frequency of dialysis may be needed. Those patients undergoing dialysis usually tolerate standard amino acid solutions, but special attention should be given to monitoring fluid and electrolyte balance. Those who are not undergoing dialysis tolerate standard amino acid formulations poorly, and administration of an essential amino acid formulation with adequate amounts of carbohydrate may result in better utilization of endogenous urea by conversion to nonessential amino acids.[173]

PERIOPERATIVE NUTRITIONAL SUPPORT

Preoperative Nutritional Support

There is a well-established relationship between the nutritional status of patients undergoing surgical procedures and the risk of perioperative morbidity and mortality.[3, 6–8] This relationship has led investigators to explore whether preoperative nutritional support can decrease morbidity and mortality. Several studies have reported a decreased incidence of complications (sepsis, wound infections, pneumonia, and mortality) after preoperative nutritional support.[3, 174–176] The impact on mortality and morbidity is unclear,[175, 177–182] however, and the optimal duration of nutritional support and criteria for the use of preoperative TPN remain poorly defined. Some data indicate that TPN should not be given for a fixed time interval; rather, the patient's response to TPN in terms of weight, albumin, and so forth should be the indicator of when to proceed with an elective operation.[175] Patients who lost weight and showed a rise in serum albumin levels during 1 week of TPN were at a reduced risk for postoperative complications. Patients who respond to TPN with decreased serum albumin values and increased weight remain at a high risk for postoperative complication and should be considered candidates for prolonged preoperative nutritional support.

Patients who are well nourished and require intravenous fluids for less than 5 days should receive conventional hypocaloric fluid therapy postoperatively. If the patient is depleted, TPN should be considered even if a return to an oral diet is anticipated within a few days. TPN should always be considered if the postoperative semistarvation is likely to be greater than 4 or 5 days. In general, one should begin TPN early, based on this estimation, rather than waiting in anticipation of a return to gastrointestinal function.

Interactions Among Nutrition, Body Composition, and Perioperative Mortality and Morbidity

With nutritional depletion, the ECF compartment increases in relation to total body water.[13, 183–184] It is clear that the regulation of albumin synthesis is sensitive to the patient's nutritional status[185, 186] but the relationship between serum albumin, protein synthesis, and body composition has not been well defined.

With nutritional repletion, as defined by positive nitrogen balance, it has been observed that the expected increases in albumin concentrations are not consistently seen. The relation between serum albumin and nutritional status appears to be more dependent on changes in body composition than on protein synthesis.

Patients with anorexia nervosa are markedly protein–calorie depleted, but since this occurs on a balanced nutritional regimen (including protein), there is no absolute expansion of the ECF compartment. Under these conditions serum albumin tends to remain normal. In the healthy adult who is injured or has an acute septic episode, a marked degree of fluid resuscitation is required. This is accompanied by a fall in serum albumin even though whole body protein status is fairly intact. Nitrogen balance is negative, but there is no significant depletion of body protein at this time that might explain the fall in serum albumin levels. This indicates that expanding ECF, rather than negative nitrogen balance, is the cause of the reduction in serum albumin. When parenteral nutrition is administered and albumin synthesis is increased, an expanded ECF prevents an increase in serum albumin concentration; the albumin simply diffuses through an enlarged fluid space.

Consequently, when the ECF is expanded due to capillary leak syndromes, an increase in albumin synthesis in response to nutritional support results in an increased whole body albumin pool. The albumin pool may increase by means of further expansion of the ECF rather than an increase in concentration. When the stress response and capillary leak phenomenon diminish, however, the ECF compartment contracts; this contraction is associated with a return of serum albumin to normal levels.

Starker et al[187, 188] used nitrogen balance to document the nutritional status of hospitalized patients during refeeding. Measurements of sodium balance were used to show alterations in the ECF. By examining concurrent changes in plasma levels of albumin, body weight, and sodium balance, the relation of albumin to the status of the ECF compartment, rather than to nitrogen balance, was established.[187] Patients were categorized as being either stressed or nonstressed; the stressed group consisted mostly of patients with active underlying infection. Figure 27-4 demonstrates that there was no significant difference in nitrogen balance between the stressed and the unstressed group. Figure 27-5 shows the changes in sodium balance and serum sodium concentrations. During nutritional depletion, sodium balance was positive. It appears that weight loss under hospital conditions does not necessarily reflect the loss of body tissue, since an expanded ECF compartment tends to mask the loss of body protein. During repletion, the nonstressed group displayed a negative sodium balance, whereas in the stressed group sodium balance was markedly positive. Thus there was a contraction of the ECF compartment during repletion in the nonstressed group.

Serum albumin levels are shown in Figure 27-6. They seem to have a closer correlation with the alterations in ECF than with nitrogen balance. There is a rise in serum albumin in the nonstressed group, while it falls during the first 2 weeks of repletion in the stressed group of patients. The response observed among the stressed group probably reflect an altered response of the fluid compartment to nutritional therapy. Many of the patients in this group had underlying infection or tumor. It is likely that one of these stresses played a part in the failure of this group to diurese and normalize the ECF. The expanded ECF compartment presumably diluted the albumin pool, which prevented a rise in serum concentration of albumin.

It should be emphasized that these patients were in positive

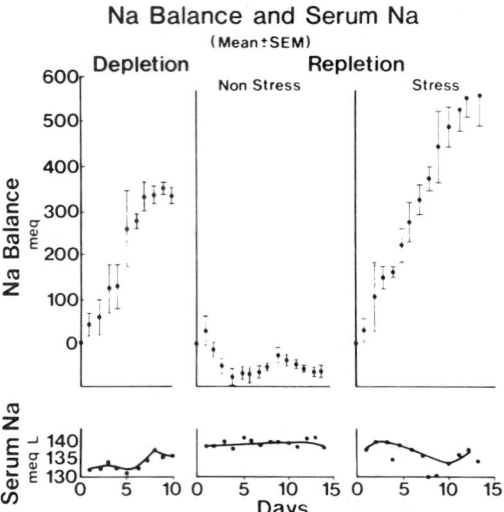

FIG. 27-5. Alterations in sodium balance are shown. The stressed patients retain sodium, while the unstressed patients contract their ECF, as evidenced by a negative Na balance. (Reprinted with permission. Starker PM, Gump FE, Askanazi J et al: Serum albumin levels as an index of nutritional support. Surgery 91:194, 1982.)

nitrogen balance, and hence were in the anabolic state. Under these conditions, we would have expected albumin synthesis to increase.[186] In a study of patients who were in a poor nutritional state postoperatively, Shizgal[189] noted that one patient, who developed an intraabdominal abscess, had a markedly greater ECF expansion than the other patients, indicating that nutritional depletion can exacerbate the expansion of the ECF seen in sepsis. Furthermore, ongoing sepsis can prevent normalization of the ECF despite nutritional support.

FIG. 27-4. Changes in nitrogen (N) balance in stressed and unstressed patients. Both groups were in positive N balance. (Reprinted with permission. Starker PM, Gump FE, Askanazi J et al: Serum albumin levels as an index of nutritional support. Surgery 91:194, 1982.)

FIG. 27-6. Serum albumin levels increase in relation to negative sodium balance and not in relation to nitrogen balance. (Reprinted with permission. Starker PM, Gump FE, Askanazi J et al: Serum albumin levels as an index of nutritional support. Surgery 91:194, 1982.)

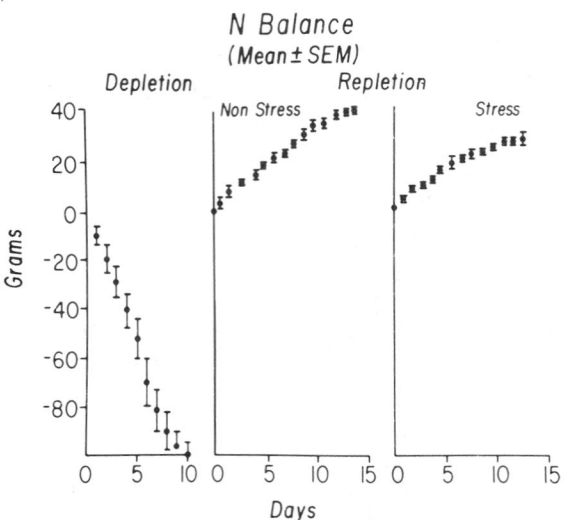

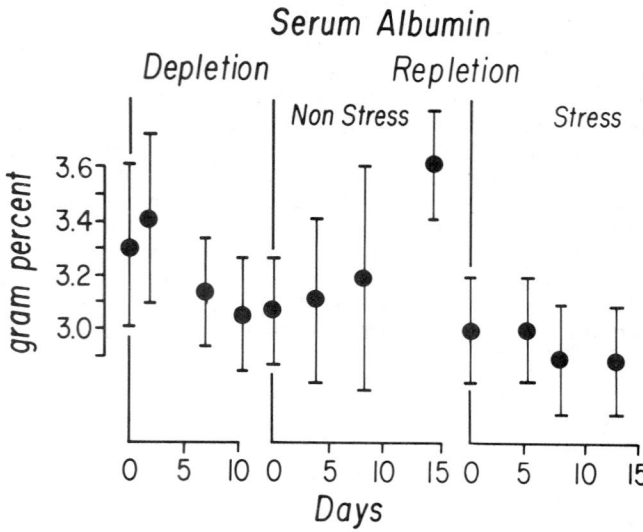

This may have profound implications for patients, particularly those with respiratory and neurologic dysfunction. Larca *et al*,[190] studying patients who received nutritional support while on mechanical ventilation, demonstrated that patients who had a rise in plasma protein in response to nutritional therapy could be weaned from a mechanical ventilator, while those whose plasma protein fell during TPN could not. Bryan-Brown *et al*[191] reported three cases in which cerebral edema, although unresponsive to conventional therapy, improved as a result of adequate nutritional support. Body composition changes in these patients demonstrate that the ECF returned to normal with adequate nutrition.

Starker *et al*[188] correlated changes in skeletal muscle composition with whole body electrolyte and nitrogen balance, to establish the contribution made by skeletal muscle to changes in whole body fluid and electrolyte composition during nutritional repletion. In this study, TPN was administered to 10 patients for up to 25 days. Metabolic rate and balances of nitrogen, sodium, and potassium were measured daily. Muscle biopsies were taken prior to the administration of TPN, in the middle, and at the end of the nutritional regimen. Prior to the institution of parenteral nutrition, muscle concentrations of water, sodium, and chloride were greater than normal. With the administration of exogenous nutrients, all three declined. The calculated loss in muscle water, however, accounted for only about one-half of the whole body changes. It would appear then, that nutritional support results in a restoration of cell mass and a contraction of the ECF compartment (Fig. 27-7). The restoration of cell mass may occur primarily in muscle, but the contraction of the ECF must occur in other

tissues. The contraction of the ECF is believed to occur in such tissues as the brain and the lung, thus resulting in the improvements in pulmonary and cerebral status observed in patients receiving nutritional support.

For patients who need parenteral nutrition before undergoing operation, the expansion of the ECF represents a serious risk factor. A study has correlated the postoperative course with the preoperative response to nutritional support.[174] Nutritionally depleted patients received an average of 1 week of TPN prior to major abdominal operation. Of the 16 patients who exhibited the characteristic response to early nutritional support, diuresis of the expanded ECF with a resultant loss of weight and rise in serum albumin, only one developed a complication in the postoperative period. The other 16 patients did not exhibit this response to TPN. They retained additional fluid, gained weight, and showed a decrease in serum albumin levels. Eight of these patients developed a total of 15 postoperative complications (Table 27-7). In a follow-up study, Starker *et al*[175] demonstrated that patients who do not diurese and show a rise in serum albumin after 1 week can do so if TPN is maintained for 4–6 weeks, with a consequent reduction in the rate of mortality and morbidity (Group III in Table 27-7).

Postoperative Nutritional Support

A study by Askanazi *et al*[176] reviewed the effect of nutritional support on duration of hospitalization in patients undergoing radical cystectomy. Thirty-five patients were randomly assigned to either 5% dextrose solution plus electrolytes or TPN following operation. The assigned nutritional regimen was continued for 1 week after operation until oral intake resumed. The group receiving immediate postoperative TPN had a median duration of hospital stay of 17 days, while median hospital stay for the group receiving 5% dextrose solution was 24 days (Fig. 27-8). All other patient characteristics such as age,

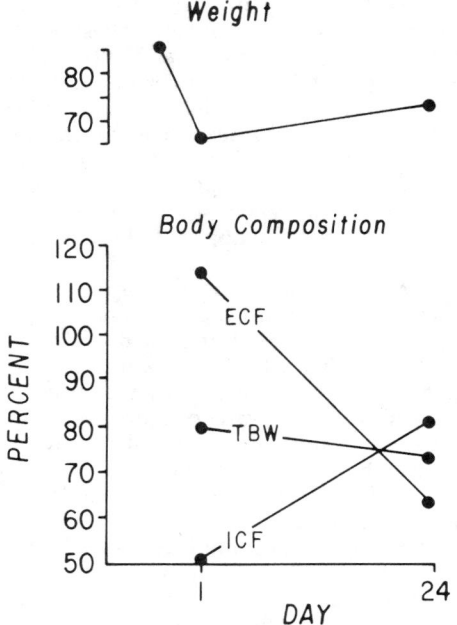

FIG. 27-7. Changes in body weight (kg) and body composition (% of predicted) during nutritional repletion in a patient with neurologic damage. The study demonstrates a reduction in ECF after the institution of nutritional support, which corresponds to an improvement in clinical condition. (Reprinted with permission. Bryan-Brown CW, Savitz MH, Elwyn DH *et al*: Cerebral edema unresponsive to conventional therapy in neurosurgical patients with unsuspected nutritional failure. Crit Care Med 1:125, 1973.)

TABLE 27-7.   Postoperative Complications Related to Response to TPN

COMPLICATIONS	GROUP I (n = 16)	GROUP II (n = 16)	GROUP III (n = 16)
Mechanical			
Prolonged ventilatory support	0	4	0
Fistula	0	0	1
Wound dehiscence	0	1	0
Anastomotic leak	0	1	0
Total	0	6	1
Infections			
Sepsis	0	2	0
Pneumonia	1	3	0
Wound infection	0	3	1
Abscess	0	1	0
Total	1	9	1
Death (nutritionally related)	0	2	0
Total complications	1	15	2
Total number of patients developing complications*	1	9	2
Per cent of patients developing complications	4.3	45	12.5

* $P < 0.01$ (Group I/Group II); $P < 0.05$ (Group II/Group III).
Source: References 174 and 175.

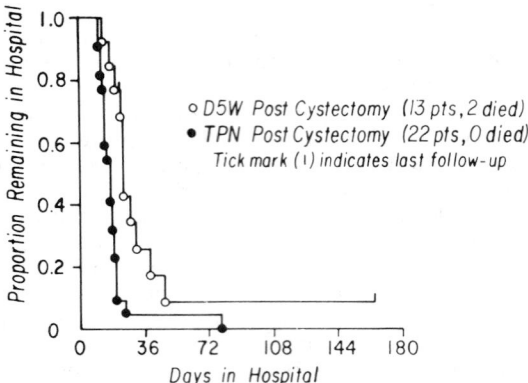

FIG. 27-8. Length of hospital stay following radical cystectomy. In the group receiving immediate postoperative parenteral nutrition, median duration of hospitalization is reduced by 7 days. (Reprinted with permission. Askanazi J, Hensle TW, Starker PM *et al:* Effect of immediate postoperative nutritional support on length of hospitalization. Ann Surg 203:236, 1986.)

sex, stage/grade of tumor, and extent of preoperative radiotherapy were similar. These results demonstrated that immediate postoperative institution of nutritional support reduced hospitalization time following radical cystectomy and indicated that the routine use of 5% dextrose as postoperative nutrition should be reevaluated.

FLUID AND ELECTROLYTES

FLUID AND ELECTROLYTE BALANCE

Water Balance

In the 70-kg man, 60% of TBW is water (42 l). Forty per cent of TBW (28 l) is intracellular fluid (ICF) and 20% (14 l) is ECF. The ECF is divided into 11 l of interstitial fluid and 3 l of plasma volume. The hydration of LBM is quite constant in the healthy individual. Because adipose tissue contains little water, water constitutes a larger proportion of body weight in lean individuals and infants and a smaller proportion in obese individuals and women, who have proportionally larger amounts of adipose tissue than men. LBM decreases with age, with fat representing relatively more body weight. Thus, the ratio of body water to TBW decreases with age.

There is a higher concentration of protein in plasma than in interstitial fluid, while the electrolyte compositions of plasma and interstitial fluid are virtually equivalent. Sodium and chloride are the primary electrolyte components of ECF. Magnesium, phosphorus, and potassium are present in relatively low concentrations. All the cells of the body maintain a low intracellular concentration of sodium despite a high concentration in the fluid surrounding them.

The osmolality of all body fluid compartments is considered equal because the cell membrane is completely permeable to water. Sodium constitutes 90% of the osmotically active cations in the ECF and plays a unique role in the regulation of the ECF compartment. When the osmolality of ECF changes secondary to gain of water or sodium, however, the redistribution of water between the ICF and ECF compartments is minimized by ADH and aldosterone release. Studies of total exchangeable potassium reveal that less than 2% of total body potassium stores are in the ECF; therefore, potassium gains do not significantly affect ECF osmolality. Both different ionic composition of ICF and ECF and the osmotic balance are maintained by selective cell membrane permeability and active, energy-requiring transport of sodium ions up the electrochemical gradient.

OSMOLALITY AND OSMOTIC PRESSURE. The concentration of solutes in water is expressed in osmoles. One osmole (osm) is equivalent to the molecular weight of the solute divided by the number of particles liberated when it is dissolved. Thus, sodium chloride, with a molecular weight of 58, dissociates into two particles in very dilute solutions and contributes 1 osm for every 29 g dissolved in water. Osmolal concentration is commonly measured by freezing point depression or vapor pressure. For each osm dissolved in 1 kg of water, the freezing point is depressed by 1.86° C.

OSMOTIC PRESSURE. Osmolality plays a critical role in the movement of water across semipermeable membranes. The movement of water across membranes impermeable to electrolytes can create a pressure equivalent to 7.3 atm at an osmolality of 290 mOsm.

Water moves from areas of high thermodynamic activity to areas of low activity. Pure water has a thermodynamic activity of 1 (aH₂O). The more solute dissolved in water, the lower the thermodynamic activity of the remaining water.

The flux of water from an area of high to an area of low thermodynamic activity is directly proportional to the product of osmotic pressure and the difference in aH₂O between the two regions.

CONTROL OF WATER BALANCE. The control of the volume and composition of the intracellular and extracellular spaces is complex. Figure 27-9 outlines the factors affecting water intake and output. The water balance is intimately related to the regulation of solute balance.

The supraoptic and paraventricular nuclei of the hypothalamus function as the integrating regions for regulation of water, receiving inputs from many areas and controlling water intake and output by affecting thirst and release of ADH. Because the regulation system is influenced by multiple factors, priorities have been established that best serve the needs of the body. Normally, water intake and output are controlled in response to the osmolality of the ECF. Osmolal regulation is, however, subordinate to the maintenance of ECF volume and, in particular, the intravascular compartment of the ECF volume. This, in turn, is subordinate to some correlate of perfusion or delivery of essential elements to tissues. Thus, hypotension stimulates a response by the system even though osmolality and ECF volume appear to be normal.[192]

WATER INTAKE. Thirst appears to be stimulated by the same mechanisms that control the release of ADH. The release of ADH, however, has a lower threshold than does stimulation of thirst.[193] Thus, thirst acts as a back-up mechanism in osmolal regulation and is activated only when renal conservation of water fails to match water output to water intake. This osmotic thirst is thought to be stimulated by the sodium concentration in the cerebrospinal fluid. In addition to osmotic regulation, a reduction in ECF volume, and particularly a reduction in effective circulating blood volume, stimulates thirst. Thirst is not satisfied until osmolality has fallen to a value significantly below the threshold at which thirst is initiated. Drinking causes a temporary inhibition of thirst before absorption of the ingested water changes osmolality. This

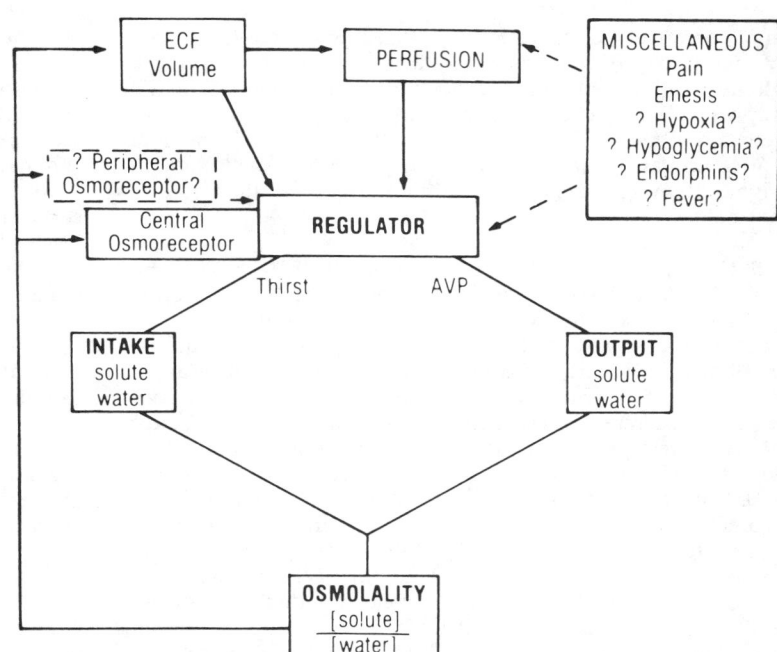

FIG. 27-9. Water balance: factors affecting water intake and output. *Question marks* and *dashed lines* indicate areas of uncertain understanding. ECF = extracellular fluid; AVP = arginine–vasopressin. (Reprinted with permission. Tonnesen AS: Water balance and control of osmolality. In Askanazi J, Starker PM, Weissman C [eds]: Fluid and Electrolyte Management in Critical Care, p 93. Boston, Butterworths, 1986.)

temporary inhibition of thirst appears to arise from oropharyngeal and gastroduodenal regions.[194]

ANTIDIURETIC HORMONE. Arginine–vasopressin (AVP) is the ADH in all mammals except swine. AVP is produced in the supraoptic and paraventricular nuclei of the hypothalamus. The pituitary gland serves as a reservoir of the hormone. The release of AVP is primarily in response to changes in osmolality, circulating blood volume, and perfusion pressure. In addition, hypoxia and hypoglycemia are capable of stimulating AVP release. Many other stimuli such as pain, emesis, emotions, fever, drugs, and possibly endorphins contribute indirectly to the regulation of AVP release.

Osmolality is the normal factor responsible for changes in AVP secretion. Increases in plasma osmolality of as little as 2% can cause major changes in the rate of AVP secretion. In general, the threshold for AVP release in normovolemic, recumbent humans is between 276 and 290 mOsm·l^{-1}.[195] The response to volume changes is mediated *via* stretch receptors in the left and right atrium that send afferent signals *via* the vagus nerve to the medulla,[196] and the medulla sends projections to the supraoptic nucleus neurons. Reductions in blood pressure elevate the threshold for AVP release. This response is apparently mediated *via* the baroreceptor mechanism, of which the afferent limb includes the glossopharyngeal nerve.

The induction of anesthesia in humans with a variety of drugs causes little or no increase in AVP levels.[197, 198] In general, even where increases occur, continuation of anesthesia is associated with a gradual decline in AVP levels. In contrast to the induction of general anesthesia, surgical procedures on humans under anesthesia are consistently associated with marked increases in AVP levels. The skin incision typically causes a dramatic rise in AVP.[197, 198] A rough correlation between the magnitude of surgery and AVF levels has been observed,[199] but the roles of the anesthesia level, blood pressure, osmolality, blood volume, and fluid replacement have

not been clarified. AVP levels tend to remain increased, although to a lesser degree, for about 2 days postoperatively.[200]

Prolonged mechanical ventilation of the lungs has been associated with water retention in about 20% of patients.[201] The addition of positive end-expiratory pressure (PEEP) to mechanical ventilation decreases urine output and free water clearance, whereas urine osmolality increases. Continuous positive-pressure breathing probably increases AVP levels by activating volume receptors.[202] The effects of ventilation and PEEP on AVP, however, will require more study to separate the effects of blood gas changes, cardiac output, and changes in volume status and pressure.

The two most important effects of AVP are antidiuresis and vasoconstriction. The antidiuretic effect is caused by AVP's ability to increase the permeability of the cortical collecting tube. In addition to AVP, the production of maximally concentrated or maximally dilute urine involves adjustments in renal blood flow, glomerular filtration rate, and proximal tubular electrolyte reabsorption, as well as an intact loop of Henle and distal tubule, and a variable permeability to water in the collecting tube.[203] Maximal antidiuresis and urine osmolality (1200–1400 mOsm·l^{-1}) occur at an AVP plasma level of 5–6 pg·ml^{-1}. Maximal diuresis is associated with barely detectable plasma levels of AVP and urine osmolalities of between 50 and 100 mOsm·l^{-1}. The ability of AVP to develop a highly concentrated urine is enhanced by its action on the renal vessels. AVP produces a redistribution of blood flow, with increased inner renal flow and decreased cortical flow without changing the total flow.[204] This shift in blood flow would shift glomerular filtration to juxtamedullary nephrons with longer loops of Henle. In addition, high plasma levels of AVF constrict the renal vasculature to a degree that will reduce the glomerular filtration rate, and this effect complements the fluid-reabsorbing effect of AVP.

Excessive and deficient AVP secretion typically are presented as hyponatremia and polyuria, respectively. There are, however, physiologic limits to this reduction in urine output and, conversely, a deficiency of AVP is but one possible cause of polyuria. Urine output is the difference between the glomerular filtration rate and total fluid reabsorption along the nephron. A reduction in urine output may be the result of reduced filtration or increased absorption. Even with maximal AVP stimulation, however, urine output levels usually remain higher than 50 ml·hr^{-1} if the glomerular filtration rate is normal.[205]

SYNDROME OF INAPPROPRIATE ANTIDIURETIC HORMONE SECRETION. In the syndrome of inappropriate ADH secretion (SIADH), there exists a decreased ability to dilute the urine because the secretion of AVP is inappropriate. It should be emphasized that the secretion of AVP is only inappropriate in relation to ECF osmolality. Although osmolality usually controls AVP secretion, it is the lowest in the hierarchy, and states of inadequate perfusion and hypovolemia will stimulate AVP secretion physiologically regardless of osmolality.[205]

SIADH has been reported in intracranial disease, intrathoracic disease, endocrine disease, malignancy, and in response to drugs.[206] The excessive AVP release may result from hypothalamic or pituitary regions, ectopic AVP production, or potentiation of AVP effects on the collecting ducts. As excess water is retained, the osmolality of the body fluids is diluted and the ECF volume expands. The latter leads to reduced renal sodium reabsorption with a secondary natriuresis and sodium depletion.

The diagnosis of SIADH is one of exclusion. The criteria for the diagnosis are listed in Table 27-8. In the critically ill patient, it is often difficult to rule out hypovolemia and edema-forming states. In addition the renal function is often changing, diuretics are commonly used, and the function of adrenal glands may be difficult to assess. Thus, the diagnosis should be made only after appropriate measurements have eliminated alternate diagnoses. Direct measurements of AVP in patients with the clinical SIADH have reported unpredictable results.[207]

The signs and symptoms associated with SIADH reflect such CNS dysfunctions as nausea, anorexia, emesis, lethargy, confusion, seizures, and somnolence.[207]

The therapy of SIADH ideally should include elimination of the underlying disease. The symptomatic treatments include water restriction, sodium administration (with or without diuretics), and administration of drugs that block AVP release or interfere with its renal actions. The goal in fluid restriction is to match fluid intake to the limited water output. However, it is often difficult to achieve water restriction in critically ill patients and the response to fluid restriction is slow. If sodium depletion is present, correction of hyponatremia by water restriction is accompanied by reduced ECF and plasma volume. This stimulates an appropriate release of AVP, and sodium supplementation will then be required. The infusion of sodium chloride alone is not effective therapy for SIADH. A hypertonic sodium chloride infusion should be used immediately to raise the plasma sodium level when the patient develops symptoms or when plasma sodium levels decrease below 120–125 mMol·1^{-1},[205] but sodium replacement must be accompanied by other measures to reduce total body water. When a combination of sodium supplementation and diuretics is administered, the excess water is excreted, whereas sodium balance is corrected by overreplacing urinary sodium losses. In addition, renal medullary washout reduces urinary osmolality despite high AVP levels. In some instances the release of AVP may be blocked by phenytoin or opioid antagonists. The action of AVP on the collecting duct can be inhibited by demeclocycline or lithium, and the ability of the kidney to generate a hypertonic interstitium can be impaired by furosemide, mannitol, or urea.[207]

DIABETES INSIPIDUS. Diabetes insipidus may be nephrogenic (AVP resistant) or caused by low AVP levels. It is an important metabolic problem in neurosurgical patients, particularly those undergoing pituitary procedures.[208] Following hypophysectomy, diabetes insipidus occurs within the first week and may then remit, only to occur again several days later.[209] Diabetes insipidus may be partial or transient.

The clinical hallmark of diabetes insipidus is polyuria, and diabetes insipidus is one of the differential diagnoses of polyuria (Table 27-9). The diagnosis is confirmed by the kidney's inability to concentrate the urine, despite water deprivation. An increased urine osmolality in response to exogenous AVP distinguishes central diabetes insipidus from the nephrogenic form, which does not respond to AVP therapy.

In critically ill patients, the use of aqueous vasopressin by the intramuscular or subcutaneous route in doses of 5–10 units leads to a prompt antidiuresis that lasts for 4–6 hr. For long-term management of central diabetes insipidus the drug of choice is desmopressin (DDAVP), which is administered intranasally every 12–24 hr. Agonist therapy necessitates frequent monitoring of plasma electrolyte levels and osmolality with appropriate adjustments in fluid intake and doses of agonist. Chlorpropamide potentiates AVP action on the kidney and is useful in long-term therapy of diabetes insipidus.

TABLE 27-8. Criteria for the Diagnosis of SIADH

Hyponatremia
Low serum osmolality
Osmolality of the urine greater than appropriate for plasma
  osmolality
Excessive renal excretion of Na
Normal ECF and plasma volume
Normal renal, adrenal, and thyroid function
Absence of edema-forming states
Absence of diuretic use

TABLE 27-9. Causes of Polyuria

Nephrogenic (AVP resistance)
  Hereditary
  Primary renal dysfunction
  Renal dysfunction secondary to systemic disease
  Drug induced
Hypoosmolality (AVP suppression)
  Polydipsia
    Psychogenic
    Central nervous system damage
  Iatrogenic fluid administration
  Central diabetes insipidus (AVP deficiency)
    Defective regulation
    Deficient production
      Hereditary
      Surgical damage
      Trauma
      Idiopathic

AVP = arginine–vasopressin.
(Reprinted with permission. Tonnesen AS: Water balance and control of osmolality. In Askanazi J, Starker PM, Weissman C [eds]: Fluid and Electrolyte Management in Critical Care, p 93. Boston, Butterworths 1986.)

Because nephrogenic diabetes insipidus does not respond to AVP therapy, fluid replacement is of key importance. The only useful treatment currently available is solute depletion and fluid replacement. Diuretic therapy has met with some success in nephrogenic diabetes insipidus by causing volume contraction, which in turn enhances proximal fluid reabsorption.

Sodium Balance

Sodium is the principal cation in the ECF of the human body and virtually determines the state of ECF. As a result, sodium, measured by its plasma concentration or by sodium balance, is used to assess the extracellular compartment. The ECF includes blood, lymph, transcellular fluid, and interstitial fluid. The ECF is composed of a heterogeneous group of fluids and the ion concentration is not exactly the same for each of the spaces. For the purposes of this discussion, however, the sodium concentration and ECF will be referred to as a single space. The osmotic and electrical effects, as well as other factors, result in an intracellular sodium concentration of 10 $mMol \cdot 1^{-1}$ and an extracellular concentration of 145 $mMol \cdot 1^{-1}$. Sodium, together with the associated osmotically active anions chloride and bicarbonate, are responsible for more than 90% of the solute load of the ECF. As a result, sodium and its accompanying anions are the major determinant of the ECF.

Following a decrease in extracellular sodium, the osmolality of the ECF will decrease. Water will diffuse across the membranes from the ECF into cells, increasing the intracellular volume with an associated decrease in the ECF. The result is a decreased osmolality, which will be reflected in both the ECF and intracellular volume. The consequence of the loss of water from the ECF is a decreased circulating volume. With an increase in extracellular sodium, there is a shift of fluid from the intracellular volume, with an associated increase in the ECF. Such changes will then activate various physiologic systems to correct the alterations.

There exist two closely related systems that control the body sodium and thereby the ECF. The first system is the afferent or sensing system, and the second system is the efferent or effector system. The sensing system detects changes in the ECF, while the effector system responds to changes in the ECF by altering either the input or output of sodium in the ECF.[210]

The sensing system is affected by changes in the ECF volume primarily through changes in the pressure. Current data support both a low-pressure and a high-pressure system of detection.[210] A direct correlation has been demonstrated between the renal excretion of sodium and left atrial pressure in animal models.[211] The atrial receptors appear to contribute to ECF regulation by exerting nonosmotic control over AVP secretion and thereby renal water excretion. An example of the high-pressure receptors is the renal afferent arteriolar baroreceptors. Decreased arterial pressures and renal blood flow release renin from the juxtaglomerular cells. Renin splits angiotensin I from angiotensinogen. Angiotensin I is converted to angiotensin II, which controls the rate of aldosterone secretion. In turn, it is the vasoconstrictor effect of angiotensin II and the sodium-retaining effect of aldosterone that act to restore the effective circulating volume. Systemic baroreceptors located near the carotid artery and aorta also cause renin release when blood pressure falls. Aldosterone has been documented as the major agent altering sodium balance. In addition, a kind of autoregulation seems to exist in the kidney in which the reabsorption of the glomerular filtrate responds to changes in the filtered load of sodium.[212] Other factors that appear to affect sodium excretion are renal hemodynamics, the sympathetic nervous system, the "third factor," prostaglandins, and others.[210]

Potassium Balance

In contrast to sodium and chloride, which are predominantly in the ECF and regulated by the kidneys, potassium is predominantly in the intracellular volume. The plasma potassium concentration is not closely related to the total body potassium because 98% of the potassium is intracellular.[213] Fluctuations in the plasma potassium level are more closely related to changes in pH, nutritional status, and other neural and hormonal factors affecting the distribution of intracellular and extracellular potassium than to total body potassium. Because of the effects at the level of the cell membrane, however, even small fluctuations in the plasma potassium level can be clinically significant.

In general, acidosis leads to hyperkalemia, whereas alkalosis leads to hypokalemia; furthermore, metabolic states have a more pronounced effect on plasma potassium levels than do respiratory states. A rapid increase in plasma osmolality results in mild elevation in the plasma potassium, apparently because of the rapid movement of ICF to the ECF. As this shift occurs, potassium is drawn out of the cell.[214] Increases in plasma potassium have been shown experimentally to be in the range of 0.1 to 0.6 $mMol \cdot 1^{-1}$ per 10 mOsm increase in osmolality.[215]

Potassium moves in relation to glucose and other substrates of energy metabolism. Both the endogenous and the exogenous administration of insulin are associated with decreases in plasma potassium that are due to the movement of potassium into liver and skeletal muscle cells. This movement of potassium depends partially on the active transport of glucose. This mechanism is so rapid and effective that insulin secretion serves as one of the body's first responses to hyperkalemia.

Adrenergic activity also plays a role in potassium flux. Experimental evidence shows that α-adrenergic activity results in hyperkalemia, whereas β-adrenergic activity produces hypokalemia.[216, 217] Exogenous administration of catecholamines has similar effects on potassium flux. Infusion of α agents such as noradrenaline produces a hyperkalemic effect, while administering a β agonist such as isoproterenol produces a hypokalemic effect. Adrenaline, which is a mixed adrenergic agent, has two effects on potassium flux: the rapid infusion results primarily in hyperkalemia, whereas a continuous infusion of adrenaline produces hypokalemia.

The mineralocorticoids, particularly aldosterone, are important modulators of body potassium. Increases in plasma potassium stimulates the adrenal gland to increase secretion of mineralocorticoids, which leads to increased renal potassium excretion. No definite evidence exists that the mineralocorticoids induce movement of potassium from the plasma to the intracellular space. Thus, the role of mineralocorticoids seems to be related to renal excretion of potassium.

Chronic wasting diseases, prolonged catabolism, cachexia, muscle wasting, and generalized debility reduce total body potassium stores. The potassium shifts are associated with protein breakdown, and each 1 g loss of total body nitrogen is accompanied by approximately 4 mMol loss of potassium. This effect is reversible with anabolism. The gradual erosion of the body cells is reflected with a reduction in intracellular water and exchangeable potassium and a relatively expanded ECF. Hypotonicity is seen in all body compartments.

Plasma potassium levels increase shortly after the onset of

trauma with a peak in about 8 hr, and return to normal over the subsequent 24–48-hr period. Severe trauma may be accompanied by late hypokalemia. Trauma increases potassium losses, causing a net negative potassium balance that is maximal in the first 24 hr and persists for 2 or 3 days. When the patient begins adequate oral intake, the potassium balance rapidly becomes positive. When the patient without complications is given the standard nutritional requirements after a moderately stressful cholecystectomy, an average of 60 mMol of potassium is lost on the day of operation, an average of 35 mMol on the first postoperative day, and about 20 mMol · day^{-1} for 4 days. Total potassium loss is 175 mMol, approximately 5% of the total body potassium.[218]

Magnesium Balance

Magnesium ranks next to potassium as the chief intracellular cation. The body distribution of magnesium is similar to that of potassium, except that 50% is in the bone where it comprises a magnesium reserve that can be readily mobilized. The plasma concentration of magnesium is 1.5–2.5 mEq · l^{-1}; similar to calcium, magnesium is bound to plasma proteins, predominantly albumin, and in fact competes with calcium for binding sites.

Magnesium metabolism and the homeostatic mechanisms regulating magnesium concentration in the ECF are not well understood. Serum magnesium levels may not accurately reflect body magnesium stores because intracellular and extracellular concentrations can vary independently. The dietary requirements of magnesium are estimated to be about 40 mEq · day^{-1}. About 40% of ingested magnesium is normally absorbed and excreted in the urine. The net absorption of magnesium generally varies in a linear fashion with the dietary supply.

Magnesium is important in the function of many enzymes, including adenylate cyclase, creatinine phosphokinase, and alkaline phosphatase. It is essential for protein synthesis, neurochemical transmission, and muscular excitability. At the neuromuscular junction, magnesium decreases the sensitivity of the motor end-plate to acetylcholine and impairs acetylcholine release. Although the factors regulating the magnesium concentration in cells and plasma are unclear, they appear to be correlated with aldosterone secretion in a manner not unlike that of K. Further, the movements of magnesium in relation to pH changes are similar to those of K, with a net movement of magnesium from the intracellular volume to the extracellular volume during acidosis, while magnesium moves into the cells in alkalosis.

Calcium Balance

Calcium is an essential inorganic element that helps to regulate many cellular functions, including the maintenance of membrane integrity, neuromuscular activity, blood coagulation, enzyme activation, and transport and secretory functions of the cell. Most of the calcium is in the skeleton. The serum calcium level is 4.5–5.3 mEq · l^{-1} (9 to 10.5 mg · dl^{-1}) and consists of two approximately equal fractions: ionizable calcium, which is diffusible and physiologically active, and nonionizable calcium. Most non-ionizable calcium is bound to protein; a small portion is chelated to anions such as citrate and gluconate. Hospital laboratories routinely determine the total serum calcium concentration, which includes both bound calcium and free calcium. Direct determination of the free calcium level requires a calcium-specific electrode and is not routinely available. Under most circumstances, however,

ionized calcium can be estimated to be approximately one-half the total measured serum calcium. There are circumstances, however, under which this approximation may not be accurate. In acidosis, calcium binds less well to albumin, giving rise to a disproportionately high free level. Conversely, in alkalosis, calcium binds more avidly to albumin, giving rise to disproportionately low free calcium level relative to the total value. The second situation in which free calcium cannot simply be estimated as 50% of total calcium occurs when the serum albumin level is low. Hypoalbuminemia gives rise to a low total serum calcium concentration, although the free calcium level is normal and symptoms of hypocalcemia do not develop. An estimate of the apparent total serum calcium concentration can be made by increasing the measured calcium level by 0.8 mg · dl^{-1} for every 1 g · dl^{-1} decrease in serum albumin. Citrated blood transfusions may also lower ionized calcium levels. For most patients receiving transfusion this effect is not important, but if transfusions are required at a rate of 1–2 ml · kg^{-1} · min^{-1} over a sustained period, calcium supplementation is indicated.[219]

Calcium levels are regulated by two hormones. Parathormone is a single-chain polypeptide produced by the parathyroid gland; it maintains serum ionizable calcium by increasing reabsorption of bone calcium. This hormone also reduces renal phosphate reabsorption and increases calcium absorption by the intestine. Elevation of plasma phosphorus lowers ionizable calcium, thereby stimulating parathormone secretion. Parathormone secretion is thus regulated in part by a feedback mechanism; a decrease in ionizable calcium stimulates parathormone secretion, and a calcium increase inhibits this hormone.

Calcitonin is the second calcium-regulating hormone. This polypeptide, coming from the thyroid C cells, inhibits calcium resorption in bone; this effect is opposite to that of parathormone. It acts faster than parathormone and regulates plasma calcium levels more precisely.

Phosphate Balance

Phosphate shares with calcium a role as a major constituent of bone mineral. It is found in all tissues and, in one of its several derivatives, is involved in virtually all energy-requiring metabolic processes. Phosphate also is an essential component of nucleic acids, proteins, and intermediary metabolites. Phosphate constitutes about 1% of the TBW, and about 70–80% is in the skeleton. The normal phosphorous level in the blood is 1–2 mEq · l^{-1} (3–4.5 mg · dl^{-1}). The serum phosphorus level is under less tight control than the serum calcium level and may undergo daily variations of as much as 1 mg · dl^{-1}.

The plasma phosphates are filtered by the glomerulus and 90% are reabsorbed by the proximal tubule. If plasma levels fall below 3 mg · dl^{-1}, virtually all phosphate will be reabsorbed. Parathormone reduces phosphate reabsorption by the proximal tubule; this increases the urinary phosphate level and decreases the serum phosphate concentration. There may also be an independent effect of vitamin D on the renal handling of phosphate.

FREQUENT WATER AND ELECTROLYTE ABNORMALITIES

Overhydration

Signs of water intoxication include drowsiness, restlessness, muscular weakness, cardiac arrhythmia, fever, convulsions, and coma. Migration of water into the brain tissue from the hypoosmolar plasma produces cerebral edema. The hematocrit and plasma sodium levels are low.

Overhydration is produced by overadministration of non-electrolyte fluids, increased endogenous vasopressin secretion secondary to stress, renal insufficiency with oliguria, nephritis, or overadministration of vasopressin in the treatment of diabetes insipidus. Overhydration is a common postoperative problem because large volumes of intravenously administered sodium-poor or nonelectrolyte fluids decrease serum sodium, especially when renal function is impaired. Elderly patients with debility and malnutrition are often mistakenly considered to be dehydrated and are therefore given several liters of nonelectrolyte solutions with a concomitant water intoxication. The patient with large volumes of gastric aspirate is another candidate for overhydration when gastric aspirate is replaced by a nonelectrolyte solution.

Cessation of fluid administration may reverse mild cases of water intoxication. Advanced cases may require diuretics and hypertonic solutions. Hypertonic solutions reduce cerebral edema and can be given as 50–100 ml doses of 3% saline, 50% glucose, or 20% mannitol.

Dehydration

Fever, exposure of the peritoneum during surgical procedures, inhalation of dry gases, and burns all increase evaporative water losses. The accumulation of fluid associated with ascites and pleural effusion or fluid sequestration in the bowel lumen during intestinal obstruction are other forms of more insidious development of water losses. Patients with ileus usually lose 2–4 l of fluid by vomiting and may have accumulated 4–6 l in the lumen of the gastrointestinal tract.

A patient who is dehydrated requires replacement of the losses in addition to daily needs. In general about 50% of the losses should be rapidly replaced over 4–8 hr, and the remainder within 16–20 hr. The fluid lost may be replaced with a physiologic saline solution or with a 5% solution of glucose in Ringer's lactate. Since fluid losses are only roughly estimated, physiologic criteria must be used to warn of overhydration when large fluid volumes are given rapidly. Oliguria, low peripheral temperature, hypotension, and tachycardia indicate the need for more rapid fluid replacement, while central venous pressure measurements higher than 15 cmH$_2$O indicate that fluids are being infused too rapidly. In mild to moderate dehydration the fluid losses are approximately 3–6% of body weight, while severe dehydration correlates with approximately 10% fluid loss.

Hyponatremia

The main causes of hyponatremia can be divided into three groups: reduced ECF volume (sodium deficit, water deficit); nonedematous ECF volume expansion; and edematous ECF volume expansion (Table 27-10). Hyponatremia is frequently observed after surgical and traumatic injury. Plasma sodium concentration decreases, paradoxically, during the postinjury phase of maximal sodium retention and normalizes when renal sodium excretion returns to normal. Increased levels of AVP following injury lead to retention of water in excess of sodium, dilutional hyponatremia, and expansion of the ECF. Catabolic release of cell water may also contribute to posttraumatic hyponatremia.[220] Iatrogenic hyponatremia occurs when lost isotonic fluid (e.g., third-space loss) is replaced with hypotonic sodium solutions or following overhydration with nonelectrolyte fluids. Despite the fact that serum sodium is low in dilutional hyponatremia, the patient has both too much

TABLE 27-10. Causes of Hyponatremia

Reduced ECF volume (Na deficit; H$_2$O deficit)
Renal loss
Diuretic therapy
Hypoaldosteronism
Salt-losing nephritis
Renal tubular acidosis
Nonrenal loss
Gastrointestinal loss
Burns
Sweating
Peritonitis
Nonedematous ECF volume expansion
Endocrine
SIADH
Hypothyroidism
Glucocorticoid deficiency
Edematous ECF volume expansion
Renal
Renal failure
Nephrotic syndrome
Cardiac failure
Cirrhosis

(Reprinted with permission. Schrier RW, Szatalowics VL: Disorders of water metabolism. Contrib Nephrol 21: 48, 1980.)

sodium and too much water; therefore, the treatment of choice is fluid and sodium restriction with or without diuretics.

Hyponatremia and hypotonicity are common also in starvation, malnutrition, and other depleted states. In the latter situations failure or inadequacy of the sodium pump due to depletion of energy stores probably leads to accumulation of intracellular sodium and water.[218] According to this, correction of plasma sodium levels depends primarily on replenishment of energy stores, as well as excretion of excess water.

Hypernatremia

An elevated serum sodium paradoxically usually means a depleted total body sodium with an ECF deficit. This usually occurs secondarily to marked dehydration or desalting water loss. Loss of hypotonic body fluids, such as gastric juice, results in ECF depletion and hypernatremia. If these lost fluids are replaced with hypertonic sodium solution, hypernatremia will persist. Hypovolemic hypernatremia may also result from diuretic administration, glucosuria, and inappropriate replacement of evaporative loss from skin and lungs, which may be greatly increased by hyperventilation and fever.[221] Normally functioning kidneys, however, will in most cases compensate for errors in fluid management. The treatment is repletion of the ECF space. Guidelines for fluid replacement are outlined in the "Dehydration" section. The electrolyte concentration is calculated on the basis of fluid lost.

Hypokalemia

Marked differences in the behavior and distribution of sodium versus potassium are apparent in the clinical syndromes produced by their deficiencies or excesses. In general, plasma potassium concentrations move in the opposite direction to plasma sodium.

Hypokalemia may be defined as plasma potassium concentrations less than 3.5 mMol·l^{-1}; however, because only 2% of body potassium is in the ECF and about 0.5% in the plasma volume, these small potassium compartments are not representative of total body potassium; normal plasma potassium values are frequently associated with intracellular and total body potassium depletion. The minimum daily potassium requirement is assumed to be 30–50 mMol of potassium. A normal varied diet contains an excess of potassium. A potassium deficiency therefore usually occurs when normal intake is reduced during malnutrition and starvation as well as in chronic wasting diseases, sepsis, carcinomatosis, prolonged complicated postoperative states, and multiple organ failure.

Hypokalemia is frequently seen in patients with prolonged vomiting. With severe vomiting and prolonged nasogastric suction, a loss of both H^+ and potassium occurs, leading to a hypokalemic alkalosis; the hypokalemia makes the alkalosis worse and alkalosis makes the hypokalemia worse. This combination may be particularly hazardous because the loss of plasma volume associated with vomiting stimulates aldosterone secretion and the adrenal stress response. Aldosterone aggravates the hypokalemia. Ordinarily, the loss of H^+ by vomiting would be compensated by the loss of OH^- in the urine, resulting in an alkaline urine. However, the aldosterone response initiated by the hypovolemia leads to resorption of sodium and HCO_3^- by the kidneys with increased urinary potassium. This paradoxical aciduria tends to aggravate the alkalosis, which in turn further worsens the hypokalemia.

Hypokalemia is seen with acute or chronic diarrhea and in the chronic overuse of laxatives or diuretics. Hyperfunction of the adrenal cortex (Cushing's disease) or overadministration of steroids depletes total body potassium. Initially, potassium is released from the cells into the ECF, but this increased potassium is promptly excreted in the urine because of the low renal threshold for potassium. In severe diabetes, both acidosis and the breakdown of intracellular constituents reduce cellular potassium. Most of this potassium is excreted into the urine, especially when there is polyuria, leaving a net loss of body potassium. Insulin treatment will drive potassium into the cells along with glucose, resulting in hypokalemia. Hypokalemia is treated with enteral or intravenous potassium supplements. If alkalosis is present, this also requires correction. The rate of intravenous potassium infusion should not exceed 5–10 mMol·hr^{-1}, i.e., 120–240 mMol·day^{-1}. This is usually adequate and safe for several days if urine output is satisfactory and potassium levels are monitored. If more rapid infusions are thought to be required, the patient should receive electrocardiographic monitoring during the infusion. The goal of rapid intravenous infusion is to fill the small extracellular potassium space. It is important to recognize that intravenously administered potassium may take 8–48 hr before it is incorporated intracellularly.[222] Hypokalemia, alkalosis, and dehydration must all be corrected. It is necessary to begin correction of the hypokalemia before attempting to correct dehydration by massive saline infusions because the volume load will further dilute already low plasma potassium levels and may precipitate arrythmias or convulsions. Patients with hypokalemic alkalosis are particularly vulnerable to the additional stress of surgery, which aggravates the hypokalemia and thereby intensifies the aldosterone response. Moreover, iatrogenic hyperventilation during anesthesia causes a respiratory alkalosis that exacerbates hypokalemia.

Hyperkalemia

Moderate stresses usually cause a transient hyperkalemia that peaks within 8 hr of the stressful stimulus. This hyperkalemia is due to redistribution of potassium from the cells into the ECF and there is no increase in total body potassium. If renal function is not severely impaired, the increased plasma potassium is quickly excreted by the kidney. Transient hyperkalemia may be followed by hypokalemia if total body potassium losses and substrates for energy are not replaced.

Hyperkalemia may occur in a variety of clinical settings, including renal failure, diabetic ketoacidosis, adrenocorticoid insufficiency, rapid administration of potassium, and massive transfusions of stored blood. Hyperkalemia is usually associated with hyponatremia and hypocalcemia. Poor perfusion and metabolic acidosis result in hyperkalemia. There is loss of bicarbonate with a decrease in the carbon dioxide combining power. Correction of the etiology of the poor perfusion will usually correct the acidosis and hyperkalemia.

Treatment in less severe cases of hyperkalemia consists of administration of hypertonic glucose solutions, insulin, diuretics, and iv fluids and correction of the hypocalcemia and acidosis. The hypertonic glucose tends to drive potassium back into the cells, correct dehydration, and improve plasma volume. The acidosis can be corrected by sodium bicarbonate infusions. Glucose and sodium bicarbonate usually produce transient effects that are only of temporary benefit in chronic renal failure. Oral administration of ion exchange resin and nasogastric suction will remove both potassium and H^+. In hyperkalemia above 6 mMol·l^{-1}, peritoneal dialysis or hemodialysis is indicated to reduce plasma potassium levels.

Hypomagnesemia

Hypomagnesemia occurs most often during late-stage cirrhosis or after a prolonged magnesium-free diet. It is also found in patients receiving diuretic therapy, and in patients with metabolic alkalosis, severe burns, acute pancreatitis, or hyperparathyroidism.[218] Hypomagnesemia is often seen with other electrolyte abnormalities and the symptoms are ill defined. It may produce muscular fasciculations, hyperirritability, hyperreflexia, tremors, convulsions, depression, and psychiatric disturbances.

Severe hypomagnesemia responds dramatically to magnesium administration. Those patients who tolerate oral feeding should be given a magnesium hydroxide mixture. Those patients with severe hypomagnesemia and those for whom oral medication is inappropriate may be given 2–4 ml intramuscular injections of a 50% magnesium sulfate solution at 6-hr intervals. Intramuscular injections of magnesium sulfate are painful, but most of the magnesium is retained; with the intravenous route, the bulk of the magnesium will be cleared rapidly by the kidney.

With no oral intake there is an obligatory urinary magnesium loss of about 0.5–1 mEq·day^{-1}. Surgical stress transiently decreases urinary magnesium excretion. This decrease is followed by a rapid return toward normal excretion rates beginning on the first postoperative day.[223] In patients with impaired renal function serum levels of magnesium should be measured frequently to titrate magnesiumtherapy.

Hypermagnesemia

Although hypermagnesemia is rare, it may be fatal, so the signs of high magnesium plasma levels are important to recognize. Loss of deep tendon reflexes is seen at serum concentrations of 7 mEq·l^{-1} and greater. Weakness and, finally, paralysis of all muscles may occur at higher levels. The action of muscle relaxants such as d-tubocurarine is potentiated.[224] Above 10 mEq·l^{-1} the respiratory center is progressively depressed, causing shallow respirations and, eventually, prolonged apnea.[225] The presence of deep tendon reflexes can usually be relied on to indicate that life-threatening hypermagnesemia is not present.[226]

Hypermagnesemia may be associated with overdoses of magnesium sulfate in the treatment of preeclampsia. It may also be seen after overdoses of magnesium salts in patients with chronic constipation. Finally, it may be produced by diabetic acidosis with dehydration or renal failure. The therapy of hypermagnesemia is cessation of magnesium combined with iv administration of calcium. Usually, normal plasma levels gradually return; however, patients with renal failure may require dialysis.

Hypocalcemia

The usual differential diagnosis of hypocalcemia considered in the noncritically ill, ambulatory patient is different from that to be considered in the acutely ill individual. For example, hypoparathyroidism is unlikely to be found in the acutely ill hypocalcemic patient, unless that patient had this disorder as a chronic preexisting condition. The diagnosis then is self evident. A very common cause of apparent hypocalcemia in the acutely ill patient, namely low serum albumin level, is rare in the ambulatory setting, however. Causes of hypocalcemia are listed in Table 27-11.

The gravely ill patient may have a decreased total calcium plasma concentration because of hypoalbuminemia. The patient is asymptomatic, and the ionized calcium level is normal. The total calcium level should be adjusted to the serum albumin level as indicated earlier. The acid–base status is also an important consideration in assessing the hypocalcemic state. An alkalotic patient will be more symptomatic of hypocalcemia, reflecting a decreased amount of ionized calcium for a given level of total calcium. For every 0.1 unit increase in the pH, the ionized calcium level will decrease by $0.1 \text{ mg} \cdot \text{dl}^{-1}$ because of greater calcium binding to albumin when the pH is above normal.

One group of disorders associated with a decrease in both total and ionized calcium is characterized by a deficiency of the active metabolite of vitamin D. The deficiency may be due to an impairment of renal conversion of 25-hydroxyvitamin D to 1,25-dihydroxyvitamin D. Hepatic failure also can lead to a failure of production of 25-hydroxyvitamin D from the parent vitamin. An altered hepatic vitamin D metabolism is also associated with the long-term administration of anticonvulsants such as phenytoin and phenobarbital. The hypocalcemia that occurs in association with acute pancreatitis probably is due to a variety of factors, including deposition of calcium soaps in areas of fat necrosis. Rarely, hypocalcemia is associated with osteoblastic metastases of bone or prostatic carcinoma. Affected patients may develop hypocalcemia from calcium influx into osteoblastic lesions.

A very important cause of hypocalcemia is hypomagnesemia. Hypocalcemia develops because of impaired parathyroid hormone secretion at very low magnesium levels and also because of impaired responsiveness of target tissues to parathyroid hormone when magnesium levels are low. Associated with hypomagnesemia is often marked hypokalemia resulting from renal potassium wasting.

The symptoms of hypocalcemia vary from paresthesias to acute tetany. Decreased ionizable calcium levels increase neuromuscular excitability, which may be reflected in classic signs of the disorder: Chvostek's or Trousseau's sign, or spontaneous carpal–pedal spasm. When the condition is severe, bronchospasm and seizures may develop.

Hypocalcemia should be treated if total calcium concentrations are less than $7.5 \text{ mg} \cdot \text{dl}^{-1}$, especially if symptoms are present. Acutely ill patients with serious symptoms should receive calcium intravenously until the acute problem is relieved. An ampul of calcium gluconate is injected over 5–10 min. If the hypocalcemia is not life threatening, it is preferable to administer a more dilute calcium-containing solution in dextrose over a longer period. In general, $15 \text{ mg} \cdot \text{kg}^{-1}$ of calcium given over 4–6 hr will raise the serum calcium level by approximately $2–3 \text{ mg} \cdot \text{dl}^{-1}$. A special consideration pertains to the patient with hypomagnesemia who is hypocalcemic. The proper approach in this case is the administration of magnesium, either intramuscularly or intravenously.

Hypercalcemia

Hypercalcemia is a relatively common metabolic disturbance. The cause of the particular hypercalcemic state should always be considered concurrently with therapy, because, in addition to those measures useful in all hypercalcemic patients, certain selective approaches are based on the underlying cause of the condition. The causes of hypercalcemia are listed in Table 27-12. Of greatest concern are those situations associated with symptomatic hypercalcemia in which the serum calcium level is usually well above the upper limits of normal (i.e., well above $10.5 \text{ mg} \cdot \text{dl}^{-1}$).

Malignancy and primary hyperparathyroidism are the most common causes of hypercalcemia in the hospitalized patient. Much less common, hypercalcemia may occur as a manifestation of vitamin D toxicity or during the recovery from ARF.

Hypercalcemic crises are a rare complication. The clinical features are vomiting, diarrhea, mental confusion, disorientation, and shock. If hypercalcemic crisis is untreated, renal failure may develop. If the serum calcium level is moderately elevated, between 12 and $14 \text{ mg} \cdot \text{dl}^{-1}$, the patient may or may not have symptoms. Low serum albumin levels and acidosis will tend to increase the ionized calcium with an increase in signs and symptoms of hypercalcemia. When the level is greater than $14 \text{ mg} \cdot \text{dl}^{-1}$, treatment should be instituted, not only because patients are invariably symptomatic in this range, but also because they are at significant risk for developing damage to the cardiovascular and renal systems.[227]

The general principles of management of hypercalcemia are

TABLE 27-11.   Causes of Hypocalcemia

Impaired production of 1,25-dihydroxyvitamin D
  Malabsorption*
  Severe hepatic failure*
  Anticonvulsant therapy*
  Renal failure*
Pancreatitis*
Hypomagnesemia
  Nutritional (alcoholism)*
  Gentamicin
  Cis-platinum
Alkalosis*
Decreased serum albumin level*
Hypoparathyroidism
  Idiopathic
  Postsurgical*
  Pseudohypoparathyroidism
Osteoblastic metastases

*Causes most commonly occurring in the acutely ill individual.
(Reprinted with permission. Shane EJ, Bilezikian JP: Disorders of calcium, phosphate, and magnesium metabolism. In Askanazi J, Starker PM, Weissman C [eds]: Fluid and Electrolyte Management in Critical Care, p. 337. Boston, Butterworths 1986.)

TABLE 27-12.   Causes of Hypercalcemia

Most common
  Neoplasms*
    Multiple myeloma
    Malignancies with evident metastases in bone
    Humoral hypercalcemia of malignancy (without detactable
      bone metastases)
  Primary hyperparathyroidism*
Uncommon
  Hyperthyroidism
  Thiazide diuretic administration
  Hypervitaminosis D*
  Sarcoidosis
  Lithium administration
  Immobilization (in children and in Paget's disease of bone)
  Recovery phase of acute renal failure*
Rare
  Other granulomatous diseases (tuberculosis, histoplasmosis)
  Hypervitaminosis A*
  Adrenal insufficiency
  Hypophosphatasia
  Familial hypocalciuric hypercalcemia
  Milk–alkali syndrome

*Causes most commonly occurring in the acutely ill individual.
(Reprinted with permission. Shane EJ, Bilezikian JP: Disorders of
calcium, phosphate, and magnesium metabolism. In Askanazi J,
Starker PM, Weissman C [eds]: Fluid and Electrolyte Management in
Critical Care, p 337. Boston, Butterworths 1986.)

to lower the serum calcium levels by increasing urinary calcium excretion. These therapeutic maneuvers include rehydration with intravenous fluids, saline administration, diuretics, and mobilization. When hypercalcemia is associated
with renal failure, dialysis should be considered. If hyperparathyroidism is present, phosphates and sulfates are added
to the intravenous fluids. Steroids may be useful, particularly
in vitamin D intoxication and metastatic carcinoma. Calcitonin
has been reported to be effective in situations with vitamin D
toxicity and hyperthyroidism, but with less impressive effects
in the more common causes of hypercalcemia such as hyperparathyroidism and malignancy. Mithramycin is used in the
short-term therapy of severe hypercalcemia. It acts to prevent
the resorption of calcium from bone. Unfortunately, mithramycin has serious adverse effects, including thrombocytopenia, hepatic dysfunction, and nephrotoxicity. If the serum
calcium level is markedly elevated and associated with life
threatening signs or symptoms, however, mithramycin
should be used without hesitation.[227]

Hypophosphatemia

In acutely ill patients a moderate hypophosphatemia occurs
commonly in a wide variety of situations: after injection of
saline, sodium bicarbonate, glucose, and lactate, as well as
following administration of insulin, epinephrine, diuretics,
and corticosteroids. In addition, low phosphate levels may be
seen during hemodialysis, salicylate intoxication, sepsis, and
in electrolyte disturbances such as hypokalemia and hypomagnesemia. The degree of hypophosphatemia in these situations is usually moderate (i.e., phosphate levels between 1.5
and 2.5 $mg \cdot dl^{-1}$) and is rarely associated with specific symptoms related to the phosphate level. The hypophosphatemia
frequently corrects spontaneously when the underlying problem is treated and does not require specific therapy.[227]

In contrast, when the serum phosphate level declines to
below 1.5 $mg \cdot dl^{-1}$, several important problems may arise as a
direct consequence. The scarcity of extracellular phosphate
lowers the intracellular ATP levels and affects the hematologic
and neuromuscular systems, which are critically dependent
on ATP and on normal oxygen delivery to the tissues. Consequently, low serum phosphate levels can be responsible for
profound muscle weakness and even cellular breakdown, i.e.,
rhabdomyolysis.[228] With severe hypophosphatemia there also
is an impairment in red blood cell, leukocyte, and platelet
function.[63] Low phosphate levels have also been suggested to
cause hepatic dysfunction.

In an acutely ill patient where multiple abnormalities of
organ function may coexist, low phosphate serum levels can
jeopardize what would under different circumstances be effective therapy. For example, poor respiratory muscle function
associated with hypophosphatemia could jeopardize recovery
from a pulmonary event, and leukocyte dysfunction caused
by hypophosphatemia could compromise the effectiveness of
antibiotic administration.

Intravenous phosphate therapy is instituted when the serum phosphate level is below 1.5 $mg \cdot dl^{-1}$. Lesser degrees of
hypophosphatemia are often not treated because it is believed
that these values cause cell dysfunction only rarely. If total
body phosphate stores are not likely to be very low or if the
hypophosphatemia is of short duration, an initial dose of 0.08
$mMol \cdot kg^{-1}$ of body weight (2.5 $mg \cdot kg^{-1}$) should be administered. If more marked total body phosphate depletion is suspected, 0.16 $mMol \cdot kg^{-1}$ of body weight (5 $mg \cdot kg^{-1}$) is used.
The phosphate solution is infused over 6 hr and the serum
phosphate concentration should be obtained soon after the
infusion to estimate the size of subsequent doses.[227]

REFERENCES

1. Insel J, Elwyn DH: Body Composition. In Askanazi J, Starker P,
   Weissman C (eds): Fluid and Electrolyte Management in Critical
   Care, p 3. Boston, Butterworths, 1986
2. Shaw SN, Elwyn DH, Askanazi J et al: Effects of increasing
   nitrogen intake on nitrogen balance and energy expenditure in
   nutritionally depleted adult patients receiving parenteral nutrition. Am J Clin Nutr 37:930, 1983
3. Blackburn GL, Bistrian BR, Miani BS et al: Nutritional and metabolic assessment of the hospitalized patient. JPEN 1:11, 1977
4. Calloway DH: Nitrogen balance of men with marginal intakes of
   protein and energy. J Nutr 105:914, 1975
5. Benedict FG: A study of prolonged fasting. Washington, DC,
   Carnegie Institute, 1915
6. Kinney JM, Long CL, Gump FE et al: Tissue composition of
   weight loss in surgical patients. Ann Surg 168:459, 1968
7. Keys A, Brozek J, Henschel H et al: The biology of human starvation. Minneapolis, University of Minnesota Press, 1950
8. Shizgal HM: Body composition and nutritional support. Surg
   Clin North Am 61:727, 1981
9. Viteri F, Behar M, Arroyave G et al: Clinical aspects of protein
   malnutrition. In Munro HN, Allison JB (eds): Mammalian Protein Metabolism, vol 2, p 235. New York, Academic Press, 1964
10. Gamble JL: Physiological information gained from studies on the
    life raft ration. Harvey Lect 42:247, 1946–1947
11. Schutz Y, Acheson K, Bessard T et al: Effects of a 7-day carbohy-
    drate hyperalimentation on energy metabolism in healthy indi-
    viduals: JPEN 6:351, 1982
12. Ariel IM, Kremen AJ: Compartmental distribution of sodium
    chloride in surgical patients pre- and post-operatively. Ann
    Surg 132:1009, 1950
13. Elwyn DH, Bryan-Brown CW, Shoemaker WC: Nutritional as-

pects of body water dislocations in postoperative and depleted patients. Ann Surg 182:76, 1975

14. Abrams JS, Deane RS, Davis HJ: Adverse effects of salt and water retention on pulmonary functions in patients with multiple trauma. J Trauma 13:788, 1973

15. Owen OE, Morgan AP, Kemp HG et al: Brain metabolism during fasting. J Clin Invest 46:1589, 1967

16. Aoki TT, Muller WA, Brennan MF et al: Metabolic effects of glucose in brief and prolonged fasted man. Am J Clin Nutr 28:507, 1975

17. Cuthbertson DP: Post-shock metabolic response. Lancet 1:433, 1942

18. Cuthbertson DP, Tilstone WJ: Metabolism during the post injury period. Adv Clin Chem 12:1, 1969

19. Kinney JM, Duke JH Jr, Long CL et al: Tissue fuel and weight loss after injury. J Clin Pathol (Suppl 23) 4:65, 1970

20. Long CL, Spencer JL, Kinney JM et al: Carbohydrate metabolism in man: Effect of elective operations and major surgery. J Appl Physiol 31:110, 1971

21. Chen RW, Postlethwart RW: The biochemistry of wound healing. Monogr Surg Sci 1:215, 1964

22. Recommended Dietary Allowances, 9th ed. Washington, DC, Nutritional Academy of Sciences, 1980

23. Blackburn GL, Bistrian BR, Miani BS et al: Nutritional and metabolic assessment of the hospitalized patient. JPEN 1:11, 1977

24. Kudsk KA, Sheldon GF: Nutritional assessment. In Fisher JE (ed): Surgical Nutrition, p 407. Boston, Little, Brown, 1983

25. Mullen JL, Buzby GP, Waldman MT et al: Prediction of greater morbidity and mortality by preoperative nutritional assessment. Surg Forum 30:80, 1979

26. Linn BS: A protein energy malnutrition scale (PEMS). Ann Surg 200:747, 1984

27. Baker JP, Detsky AS, Wesson DE et al: Nutritional assessment: A comparison of clinical judgment and objective measurements. N Engl J Med 306:969, 1982

28. Copeland EM, MacFayden BV, Lanzotti VF: Intravenous hyperalimentation as an adjunct to cancer therapy. Am J Surg 129:167, 1975

29. Dematteis R, Herman RE: Supplementary parenteral nutrition in patients with malignant disease. Cleve Clin Q 40:139, 1973

30. Skeie B, Askanazi J, Rothkopf MM et al: Intravenous fat emulsions and lung function. Crit Care Med 16:183, 1987

31. Heymsfield SB, Erbland M, Casper BS et al: Enteral nutritional support. Clin Chest Med 7:41–67, 1986

32. Smith JL, Heymsfield SB: Enteral nutritional support: Formula preparation from modular ingredients. JPEN 7:280, 1982

33. Henriques V, Anderson AC: Über parenteral Ernahring durch intravenous Injection. J Physiol Chem 23:31, 1977

34. Brunschwig AD, Clark DE, Corbin N: Symposium on abdominal surgery: Postoperative nitrogen loss and studies on parenteral nitrogen nutrition by means of casein digestion. Ann Surg 115:1091, 1942

35. Cuthbertson DP: Further observations on the disturbance of metabolism caused by injury, with particular reference to the dietary requirements of fracture cases. Br J Surg 23:505, 1936

36. Rhoads JE, Alexander CE: Nutritional problems of surgical patients. Ann NY Acad Sci 63:268, 1955

37. Schuberth O, Wretlind A: Intravenous infusion of fat emulsions, phosphatides and emulsifying agents. Clinical and experimental studies. Acta Chir Scand (Suppl) 278:1021, 1961

38. Wretlind A: Development of fat emulsions. JPEN 5:230, 1981

39. Wilmore DW, Dudrick SJ: Growth and development of an infant receiving all nutrients exclusively by vein. JAMA 203:860, 1968

40. Starker PM, LaSala PA, Askanazi J: Placement of Broviac catheters for total parenteral nutrition. Surg Gynecol Obstet 156:229, 1983

41. Heimbach DM, Ivey TD: Technique for placement of a permanent home hyperalimentation catheter. Surg Gynecol Obstet 143:635, 1976

42. Broviac JW, Cole JJ, Scribner BH: A silicone rubber atrial catheter for prolonged parenteral alimentation. Surg Gynecol Obstet 136:602, 1973

43. Hickman RO, Buckner D, Chift RA et al: A modified right atrial catheter for access to the venous system in marrow transplant recipients. Surg Gynecol Obstet 148:871, 1979

44. Bernhard RW, Stahl WM: Subclavian vein catheterizations: A prospective study. I. Noninfectious complications. Ann Surg 173:184, 1971

45. Calloway DH, Spector H: Nitrogen balance as related to calorie and protein intake in active young men. Am J Clin Nutr 2:405, 1954

46. Wolfe BM, Culebras JM, Sim AJ et al: Substrate interaction in intravenous feeding: Comparative effects of carbohydrate and fat on amino acid utilization in fasting man. Ann Surg 186:518, 1977

47. Cuthbertson DP, McCutcheon A, Munro HN: A study of the effect of overfeeding on the protein metabolism of man. Biochem J 31:681, 1937

48. Keys A, Anderson JT, Brozek J: Weight gain from single overeating. Character of tissue gained. Metabolism 4:427, 1955

49. Cathcart ED: The influence of carbohydrates and fats on protein metabolism. J Physiol (Lond) 39:311, 1909

50. Werner SC, Habif DV, Randall HT et al: Postoperative nitrogen loss: Comparison of effects of trauma and of caloric readjustment. Ann Surg 130:668, 1949

51. Munro HN: General aspects of the regulation of protein metabolism by diet and by hormones. In Munro HN, Allison JB (eds): Mammalian Protein Metabolism, vol. 1, p 381. New York, Academic Press, 1964

52. Brennan MF, Fitzpatrick GF, Cohen KH et al: Glycerol: Major contributor to the short term protein sparing effect of fat emulsions in normal man. Ann Surg 182:386, 1975

53. Long JM III, Wilmore DW, Mason AD Jr et al: Effect of carbohydrate and fat intake on nitrogen excretion during total intravenous feeding. Ann Surg 185:417, 1977

54. Nordenstrøm J, Askanazi J, Elwyn DH et al: Nitrogen balance during total parenteral nutrition: Glucose versus fat. Ann Surg 197:27, 1983

55. MacFie J, Smith RC, Hill GL: Glucose or fat as a nonprotein energy source. Gastroenterol 80:103, 1981

56. Nordenstrøm J, Jeevanandam M, Elwyn DH et al: Increasing glucose intake during total parenteral nutrition increases norepinephrine excretion in trauma and sepsis. Clin Physiol 1:525, 1981

57. Askanazi J, Nordenstrøm J, Rosenbaum SH et al: Nutrition for the patient with respiratory failure: Glucose versus fat. Anesthesiology 54:373, 1981

58. Meguid MM, Akahoshi M, Jeffers S et al: Amelioration of metabolic complications of conventional TPN: A prospective randomized study. Arch Surg 119:1294, 1984

59. Miani B, Blackburn GL, Bistrian BR et al: Cyclic hyperalimentation: An optimal technique for preservation of visceral protein. J Surg Res 20:515, 1976

60. Wolfe BM, Ryder MA, Nishikawa RA et al: Complications of parenteral nutrition. Am J Surg 152:93, 1986

61. Maki DG, Goldman DA, Rhame FS: Infection control in intravenous therapy. Ann Intern Med 79:867, 1973

62. Parsa MH, Habif DV, Ferrer JM et al: Intravenous hyperalimentation: Indications, technique and complications. Bull NY Acad Med 48:920, 1972

63. Knochel JP: Hypophosphatemia. West J Med 125:15, 1981

64. Sherwin R, Joshi P, Hendler R et al: Hyperglucagonemia in

Laennec's cirrhosis. The role of portal-systemic shunting. N Engl J Med 290:239, 1974

65. Striebel JP, Holm E, Lutz H et al: Parenteral nutrition and coma therapy with amino acids in hepatic failure. JPEN 3:240, 1979

66. Soeters PB, Fisher JE: Insulin, glucagon, amino acid imbalance, and hepatic encephalopathy. Lancet 2:880, 1976

67. Unger RH: Glucagon and the insulin: Glucagon ratio in diabetes and other catabolic illnesses. Diabetes 20:834, 1971

68. Bower RH, Fisher JE: Nutritional management of hepatic encephalopathy. In Draper HH (ed): Advances in Nutritional Research, vol. 5, p 1. New York, Plenum Publishing, 1983

69. Fischer JE: Currents concepts of pathogenesis of hepatic encephalopathy. In Preisig R, Bircher J (eds): The Liver, p 374. Bern, Edito Cantor Aulendorf, 1979

70. James JH, Freund H, Fischer JE: Amino acids in hepatic encephalopathy. Gastroenterology 77:421, 1979

71. Rosen HM, Yoshimura N, Hodgman JM et al: Plasma amino acid patterns in hepatic encephalopathy of differing etiology. Gastroenterology, 72:483, 1977

72. Fischer JE, Rosen HM, Ebeid AM et al: The effect of normalization of plasma amino acids on hepatic encephalopathy in man. Surgery 80:77, 1976

73. Christensen HN, Liang M: An amino acid transport system of unassigned function in the Ehrlich ascites tumor cell. J Biol Chem 240:3601, 1965

74. James JH, Fischer JE: Transport of neutral amino acids at the blood brain barrier. Pharmacology 22:1, 1981

75. Cangiano C, Cascino A, Fiaccadori F et al: Is the blood-brain barrier really intact in portal-systemic encephalopathy? Lancet 1:1367, 1981

76. James JH, Escourrou J, Fischer JE: Blood-brain neutral amino acid transport activity is increased after portacaval anastomosis. Science 200:1395, 1978

77. Shaw W, Lieber CS: Plasma amino acid abnormalities in the alcoholic: Respective role of alcohol, nutrition, and liver injury. Gastroenterology 74:677, 1978

78. Smith AR, Rossi-Fanelli F, Ziparo V et al: Alternations in plasma and CSF amino acids, amines and metabolites in hepatic coma. Ann Surg 187:343, 1978

79. McCullough AJ, Czaja AJ, Jones JD et al: The nature and prognostic significance of serial amino acid determinations in severe chronic active liver disease. Gastroenterology 81:645, 1981

80. Fischer JE, Baldessarini RJ: False neurotransmitters and hepatic failure. Lancet 2:75, 1971

81. James JH, Cangiano C, Cardelli-Cangiano P et al: Glutamine linked hyperammonemia and neurotransmitter derangements in portal systemic shunting. Gastroenterology 78:1308, 1980

82. Felig P, Wahren J: Protein turnover and amino acid metabolism in the regulation of gluconeogenesis. Fed Proc 33:1092, 1974

83. Buse MG, Reid SS: Leucine: A possible regulator of protein turnover in muscle. J Clin Invest 56:1250, 1975

84. Chua B, Seihl DL, Morgan HE: Effect of leucine and metabolites of branched chain amino acids on protein turnover in heart. J Biol Chem 254:8358, 1979

85. Freund HR, James JH, Fischer JE: Nitrogen-sparing mechanisms of singly administered branched chain amino acids in the injured rat. Surgery 90:237, 1981

86. Sapir DG, Owen OE, Pozefsky T et al: Nitrogen-sparing induced by ketoanalogues of essential amino acids. J Clin Invest 53:70a, 1974

87. Cardelli-Cangiano P, Cangiano C, James JH et al: Uptake of amino acids by brain microvessels isolated from rats after portocaval anastomosis. J Neurochem 36:627, 1981

88. Fischer JE, Funovics JM, Aguirre A et al: The role of plasma amino acids in hepatic encephalopathy. Surgery 78:276, 1975

89. Smith AR, Rossi-Fanelli F, Freund H et al: Sulfur-containing amino acids in experimental hepatic coma in the dog and the monkey. Surgery 85:677, 1979

90. Freund H, Dienstag J, Lehrich J et al: Infusion of branched-chain enriched amino acid solution in patients with hepatic encephalopathy. Ann Surg 196:209, 1982

91. Okada A, Kamata S, Kim CW et al: Treatment of hepatic encephalopathy with BCAA-rich amino acid mixture. In Walser M, Williamson R (eds): Metabolism and Clinical Implications of Branched-Chain Amino and Ketoacids, p 447. New York, Elsevier/North Holland, 1987

92. Michel H, Pomier-Layrargues G, Duhamel O et al: Intravenous infusion of ordinary and modified amino acid solutions in the management of hepatic encephalopathy (controlled study of 30 patients). Gastroenterology 79:1038, 1979

93. Rossi-Fanelli F, Riggio O, Cangiano C et al: Branched-chain amino acids versus lactulose in the treatment of hepatic coma. A controlled study. Dig Dis Sci 27:929, 1982

94. Gluud C, Dejgaard A, Hardt F et al: Preliminary treatment results with balanced amino acid infusion to patients with hepatic encephalopathy. Scand J Gastroenterol 18 (suppl 86): 19, 1983

95. Wahren JJ, Denis J, Desurmont P et al: Is intravenous administration of branched chain amino acids effective in treatment of hepatic encephalopathy? A multicenter study. Hepatology 3:475, 1983

96. Fiaccadori F, Ghinelli F, Pedretti G et al: Branched chain amino acid enriched solutions in the treatment of encephalopathy: A controlled study. In Capocaccia L, Fischer JE, Rossi-Fanelli F (eds): Hepatic Encephalopathy in Chronic Liver Failure, p 311. New York, Plenum Press, 1984

97. Cerra FB, Cheung NK, Fischer JE et al: Disease-specific amino acid infusion (FO80) in hepatic encephalopathy: A prospective, randomized, double-blind, controlled trial. JPEN 9:288, 1985

98. Michel H, Bories P, Aubin JP et al: Treatment of acute hepatic encephalopathy in cirrhotics with a branched-chain amino acids enriched versus a conventional amino acids mixture. Liver 5:282, 1985

99. Marchesini G, Zoli M, Dondi C et al: Anticatabolic effect of branched-chain amino acid-enriched solutions in patients with liver cirrhosis. Hepatology 2:420, 1982

100. Liaw KY, Askanazi J, Michelson CB et al: Effect of postoperative nutrition on muscle high energy phosphates. Ann Surg 195:12, 1982

101. Sakamato A, Moldawer LL, Usui S et al: In vivo evidence for the unique nitrogen-sparing mechanism of branched-chain amino acid administration. Surg Forum 30:67, 1979

102. Odessey RK, Khairallah EA, Goldberg AL: Origin and possible significance of alanine production by skeletal muscle. J Biol Chem 249:7623, 1974

103. Blackburn GL, Moldawer LL, Usui S et al: Branched chain amino acid concentrations and metabolism during starvation, injury, and infection. Surgery 86:307, 1979

104. Freund HR, Yoshimura N, Fischer JE: The effect of branched chain amino acids and hypertonic glucose infusions on post injury catabolism in the rat. Surgery 87:401, 1980

105. Blackburn GL, Desai SP, Keenan RA et al: Clinical use of branched chain amino-acid enriched solutions in the stressed and injured patient. in Walser M, Williamson JR (eds): Metabolism and Clinical Implications of Branched Chain Amino and Ketoacids, p 521. New York, Elsevier/North Holland, 1981

106. Gimmon Z, Freund HR, Fischer JE: The optimal branched-chain to total amino acid ration in the injury-adapted amino acid formulation. JPEN 9:133, 1985

107. Cerra FB, Upson D, Angelico R et al: Branched chains support postoperative protein synthesis. Surgery 92:192, 1982

108. Cerra FB, Mazuski J, Teasley K et al: Nitrogen retention in critically ill patients is proportional to the branched chain amino acid load. Crit Care Med 11:775, 1983
109. Desai SP, Bistrian BR, Moldawer LL et al: Plasma amino acid concentrations during branched-chain amino acid infusions in stressed patients. J Trauma 22:747, 1982
110. Echenique MM, Bistrian BR, Moldawer LL et al: Improvement in amino acid use in the critically ill patient with parenteral formulas enriched with branched chain amino acids. Surg Gynecol Obstet 159:223, 1984
111. Van Way CW, Moore EE, Allo M et al: Comparison of total parenteral nutrition with 25 percent and 45 percent branched chain amino acids in stressed patients. Ann Surg 51:609, 1985
112. Wounde PV, Morgan RE, Kosta JM: Addition of branched-chain amino acids to parenteral nutrition of stressed critically ill patients. Crit Care Med 14:685, 1986
113. Daly JM, Mihranian MH, Vehoe JE et al: Effects of postoperative infusion of branched chain amino acids on nitrogen balance and forearm muscle substrate flux. Surgery 94:151, 1983
114. Kirkpatrick JR, Dahn M, Lewis L: Selective versus standard hyperalimentation. A randomized prospective study. Am J Surg 141:116, 1981
115. Nanni G, Siegel JH, Coleman B et al: Increased lipid fuel dependence in the critically ill septic patient. J Trauma 24:14, 1984
116. Sax HC, Talamini MA, Fischer JE: Clinical use of branched chain amino acids in liver disease, sepsis, trauma and burns. Arch Surg 121:358, 1986
117. Bower RM, Muggia-Sullham M, Vallgren S et al: Branched chain amino acid-enriched solutions in the septic patient. Ann Surg 1:13, 1986
118. Askanazi J, Carpentier YA, Elwyn DH et al: Influence of total parenteral nutrition on fuel utilization in injury and sepsis. Ann Surg 194:40, 1980
119. Askanazi J, Rosenbaum SH, Hyman AL et al: Respiratory changes induced by the large glucose loads of total parenteral nutrition. JAMA 243:1444, 1980
120. Askanazi J, Elwyn DH, Silverberg PA et al: Respiratory distress secondary to a high carbohydrate load: A case report. Surgery 87:596, 1980
121. Weissman C, Askanazi J, Rosenbaum SH et al: Amino acids and respiration. Ann Intern Med 98:41, 1983
122. Askanazi J, Weissman C, LaSala P et al: Effect of protein on ventilatory drive. Anesthesiology 60:106, 1984
123. Takala J, Askanazi J, Weissman C et al: Branched chain amino acids and respiration. Anesthesiology 63:A277, 1985
124. Goldstein S, Thomashow B, Askanazi J: Functional changes during nutritional repletion in patients with COPD. Clin Chest Med 7:141, 1986
125. Sahebjami H: Nutrition and the pulmonary parenchyma. Clin Chest Med 7:111, 1986
126. Newsholme EA, Leech AR: Biochemistry for the Medical Sciences. New York, John Wiley, 1983
127. McGinty DA: Blood lactic acid and coronary circulation. Proc Soc Exper Biol Med 28:451, 1931
128. Bing RJ: Myocardial metabolism. Circulation 12:635, 1956
129. Miller HI, Yum KY, Durham BX: Myocardial free fatty acid in unanesthetized dogs at rest and during exercise. Am J Physiol 220:589, 1971
130. Most AS, Brachfeld N, Gorlin R et al: Free fatty acid metabolism of the human heart at rest. J Clin Invest 48:1177, 1969
131. Neely JR, Bowman RH, Morgan HE: Effects of ventricular pressure development and palmitate on glucose transport. Am J Physiol 216:804, 1969
132. Crass MF III, McCaskill ES, Shipp JC: Effect of pressure develop-
ment on glucose and palmitate metabolism in perfused heart. Am J Physiol 216:1569, 1969
133. Visscher MB, Muller EA: The influence of insulin upon the mammalian heart. J Physiol 62:341, 1926
134. Schwenther FF, Noel WW: Circulatory failure of diphtheria: Carbohydrate metabolism in diphtheria intoxication. Bull Johns Hopkins Hosp 46:259, 1930
135. Morgan HE, Henderson MJ, Regen DM et al: Regulation of glucose uptake in heart muscle from normal and alloxan-diabetic rats: The effects of insulin, growth hormone, cortisone and anoxia. Ann NY Acad Sci 82:387, 1959
136. Scheuer J, Stezoski SW: Protective role of increased myocardial glycogen stores in cardiac anoxia in the rat. Circ Res 27:835, 1970
137. Henderson AH, Most AS, Parmley WW et al: Depression of myocardial contractility in rats by free fatty acids during hypoxic periods. Circ Res 26:439, 1970
138. Kjekshus JK, Mjos OD: Effect of free fatty acids on myocardial function and metabolism in the ischemic dog heart. J Clin Invest 51:1767, 1972
139. Oliver MF, Kurien VA, Greenwood TW: Relation between serum free-fatty-acids and arrhythmias and death after acute myocardial infarction. Lancet 1:710, 1968
140. Oram JF, Bennetch SL, Neely JR: Regulation of fatty acid utilization in isolated rat hearts. J Biol Chem 248:5299, 1973
141. Rogers WJ, Russell RO Jr, McDaniel HG et al: Acute effects of glucose–insulin–potassium infusion on myocardial substrates, coronary blood flow and oxygen consumption in man. Am J Cardiol 40:421, 1977
142. Weissler AM, Kurger FA, Bab N et al: Role of anaerobic metabolism in the preservation of functional capacity and structure of anoxic myocardium. J Clin Invest 47:403, 1968
143. Ahmed SS, Lee CH, Oldwurtel AH et al: Sustained effect of glucose–insulin–potassium on myocardial performance during regional ischemia. J Clin Invest 61:1123, 1978
144. Opie LH, Bruyneel K, Owen P: Effects of glucose, insulin and potassium infusion on tissue metabolic changes within first hour of myocardial infarction in the baboon. Circulation 52:49, 1975
145. Rackley CE, Russell RO Jr, Rogers WJ et al: Morcardial metabolism in coronary artery disease. In Rackley CI, Russell RO Jr (eds): Coronary Artery Disease: Recognition and Management, p 261. Mt Kisco, NY, Futura, 1979
146. Gwata T, Edwards IR: Glucose, insulin, potassium (GIK) in the treatment of congestive cardiomyopathy. Cent Afr J Med 26:249, 1980
147. Whitlow PL, Rogers WJ, Smith LR et al: Enhancement of left ventricular function by glucose–insulin–potassium infusion in acute myocardial infarction. Am J Cardiol 49:811, 1982
148. Rogers WJ, Stanley AW, Breinig JB et al: Reduction of hospital mortality rate of acute myocardial infarction with glucose–insulin–potassium infusion. J Am Heart 92:441, 1976
149. Pittman JG, Cohen P: The pathogenesis of cardiac cachexia. N Engl J Med 271:403, 1964
150. Heymsfield SB, Bleier J, Wenger N: Detection of protein–calorie undernutrition in advanced heart disease. Circulation (Suppl III) 56:102, 1977
151. Abel RM: Parenteral nutrition for patients with severe cardiac illness. In Greep JM, Soeters PB, Wesdorp RIC et al (eds): Current Concepts in Parenteral Nutrition, p 147. The Hague, Martinus Hijnoff Medical Division, 1977
152. Blackburn GL, Gibbons GW, Bothe A et al: Nutritional support in cardiac cachexia. J Thorac Cardiovasc Surg 73:480, 1977
153. Abel RM, Fischer JE, Buckley MJ et al: Malnutrition in cardiac surgical patients: Result of a prospective randomized evaluation of early postoperative total parenteral nutrition (TPN). Arch Surg 111:45, 1976

154. Lolley DM, Myers WO, Roy JR III et al: Clinical experience with preoperative myocardial nutrition management. J Cardiovasc Surg 26:236, 1985

155. Heymsfield SB, Bethel RA, Ansley JD et al: Cardiac abnormalities in cachectic patients before and during nutritional repletion. Am Heart J 95:584, 1978

156. Siemkowicz E, Gjedde A: Post-ischemic coma in rat: Effect of different preischemic blood glucose levels on cerebral metabolic recovery after ischemia. Acta Physiol Scand 110:225, 1980

157. Myers RE: Anoxic brain pathology and blood glucose. Neurology 26:345, 1976

158. Ginsberg MD, Welsh FA, Budd WW: Deleterious effect of glucose pretreatment on recovery from diffuse cerebral ischemia in the cat. I. Local cerebral blood flow and glucose utilization. Stroke 11:347, 1980

159. Pulsinelli WA, Levy DE, Sigsbee B et al: Increased damage after ischemic stroke in patients with hyperglycemia with or without established diabetes mellitus. Am J Med 74:540, 1983

160. Longstreth WT Jr, Inui TS: High blood glucose level on hospital admission and poor neurological recovery after cardiac arrest. Ann Neurol 15:59, 1984

161. Welsh FA, Ginsberg MD, Rider W et al: Deleterious effect of glucose pretreatment on recovery from diffuse cerebral ischemia in the cat. II. Regional metabolite levels. Stroke 11:355, 1980

162. Elwyn DH: Nutritional requirements of adult surgical patients. Crit Care Med 8:9, 1980

163. Seiber FE, Smith DS, Traystman RJ et al: Glucose: A revaluation of intraoperative use. Anesthesiology 67:72, 1987

164. Sieber F, Smith DS, Kupferberg J et al: Effects of intraoperative glucose on protein catabolism and plasma glucose levels in patients with supratentorial tumors. Anesthesiology 64:453, 1986

165. Feinstein EI, Blumenkrantz MJ, Healy H et al: Clinical and metabolic responses to parenteral nutrition in acute renal failure: A controlled double-blind study. Medicine 60:124, 1981

166. Kopple JD: Altered metabolic and nutritional status in acute renal failure. American Society for Parenteral and Enteral Nutrition, 11th Clinical Congress, New Orleans, p 27, 1987

167. Abel RM, Beck CH Jr, Abbott WM et al: Improved survival from acute renal failure after treatment with intravenous essential amino acids and glucose: Results of a prospective double-blind study. New Engl J Med 288:685, 1973

168. Toback FG: Amino acid enhancement of renal regeneration after acute tubular necrosis. Kidney Int 12:193, 1977

169. Feinstein EI, Kopple J, Silberman H et al: Total parenteral nutrition with high or low nitrogen intakes in patients with acute renal failure. Kidney Int 24:S–319, 1983

170. Solez K, Stout R, Bendush B et al: Adverse effect of amino acid solutions in amino glycoside-induced renal failure in rabbits and rats. In Eliahou H (ed): Acute Renal Failure, p 241. London, Libbey and Co, 1982

171. Zager RA, Venkatachalam MA: Potentiation of ischemic renal injury by amino acid infusion. Kidney Int 24:620, 1983

172. Racusen LC, Whelton A, Solez K: Effects of lysine and other amino acids on kidney structure and function in the rat. Am J Pathol 120:436, 1985

173. Abel RM, Shih VE, Abbott WM et al: Amino acid metabolism in acute renal failure. Ann Surg 180:350, 1974

174. Starker PM, LaSala PA, Askanazi J et al: The response to TPN: A form of nutritional assessment. Ann Surg 198:720, 1983

175. Starker PM, LaSala PA, Askanazi J et al: The influence of preoperative TPN on morbidity and mortality. Surg Gynecol Obstet 162:569, 1986

176. Askanazi J, Hensle TW, Starker PM et al: Effect of immediate postoperative nutritional support on length of hospitalization. Ann Surg 203:236, 1986

177. Hadfield JIH: Preoperative and postoperative intravenous fat therapy. Br J Surg 52:291, 1965

178. Heatley RV, Williams RHP, Lewis MH: Preoperative intravenous feeding: Controlled trial. Postgrad Med J 55:541, 1979

179. Muller JM, Brewer V, Dienst C et al: Preoperative parenteral feeding in patients with gastrointestinal carcinoma. Lancet 1:68, 1982

180. Holter AR, Fischer JE: The effects of perioperative hyperalimentation on complications in patients with carcinoma and weight loss. J Surg Res 23:31, 1977

181. Mullen JL, Buzby GP, Matthews DC et al: Reduction of operative morbidity and mortality by combined preoperative and postoperative nutritional support. Ann Surg 192:604, 1980

182. Mullen JL: Consequences of malnutrition in the surgical patient. Surg Clin North Am 61:465, 1981

183. Barac-Nieto M, Spurr GB, Lotero H et al: Body composition during nutritional repletion of severely undernourished men. Am J Clin Nutr 32:981, 1979

184. Deo MG, Bhan AK, Ramalingaswami V: Metabolism of albumin and body fluid compartments in protein deficiency: An experimental study in the rhesus monkey. J Nutr 104:858, 1974

185. Morgan EH, Peters T Jr: The biosynthesis of rat serum albumin. V. Effect of protein depletion and refeeding on albumin and transferrin synthesis. J Biol Chem 246:3500, 1971

186. Skillman JJ, Rosenoer VM, Smith PC et al: Improved albumin synthesis in postoperative patients by amino acid infusion. N Engl J Med 295:1037, 1976

187. Starker PM, Gump FE, Askanazi J et al: Serum albumin levels as an index of nutritional support. Surgery 91:194, 1982

188. Starker PM, Askanazi J, LaSala PA et al: The effect of parenteral nutritional repletion on muscle water and electrolytes: Implications for body composition. Surg Gynecol Obstet 152:22, 1981

189. Shizgal HM: The effect of malnutrition on body composition. Surg Gynecol Obstet 152:22, 1981

190. Larca L, Greenbaum DM: Effectiveness of intensive nutritional regimes in patients who fail to wean from mechanical ventilation. Crit Care Med 10:297, 1982

191. Bryan-Brown CW, Savitz MH, Elwyn DH et al: Cerebral edema unresponsive to conventional therapy in neurosurgical patients with unsuspected nutritional failure. Crit Care Med 1:125, 1973

192. Johnson JA, Zehr JE, Moore WW: Effects of separate and concurrent osmotic and volume stimuli on plasma ADH in sheep. Am J Physiol 218:1273, 1970

193. Anderson B, Rundgren MR: Thirst and its disorders. Ann Rev Med 33:231, 1982

194. Thrasher TN, Nistal-Herrera JF: Satiety and inhibition of vasopressin secretion after drinking in dehydrated dogs. Am J Physiol 240:E394, 1981

195. Robertson GL, Shelton RL: The osmoregulation of vasopressin. Kidney Int 10:25, 1976

196. Gauer OH, Henry JP: Cardiac receptors and fluid volume control. Prog Cardiovasc Dis 4:1, 1961

197. Oyama T, Sato K: Plasma levels of antidiuretic hormone in man during halothane anesthesia and surgery. Can Anaesth Soc J 18:614, 1971

198. Cochrane JP, Forsling ML: Arginine vasopressin release following surgical operations. Br J Surg 68:209, 1981

199. Ukai M, Moran WH Jr: The role of visceral afferent pathways on vasopressin secretion and urinary excretory patterns during surgical stress. Ann Surg 168:16, 1968

200. Soliman MG, Brindle GF: Plasma levels of anti-diuretic hormone during and after heart surgery with extracorporeal circulation. Can Anaesth Soc J 21:195, 1974

201. Sladen A, Laver MB, Pontoppidan H: Pulmonary complications

and water retention in prolonged mechanical ventilation. N Engl J Med 279:448, 1968

202. Moran WH Jr: CPPB and vasopressin secretion. Anesthesiology 34:501, 1971
203. Jamison RL, Oliver RE: Disorders of urinary concentration and dilution. Am J Med 72:308, 1982
204. Azzawi SA-O, Shirley DG: The effect of vasopressin on renal blood flow and its redistribution in the rat. Am J Physiol 232:F111, 1977
205. Tonnesen AS: Water balance and control of osmolality. In Askanazi J, Starker PM, Weissman C (eds): Fluid and Electrolyte Management in Critical Care, p 93. Boston, Butterworths, 1986
206. Abramow M, Cogan E: Clinical aspects and pathophysiology of diuretic-induced hyponatremia. Adv Nephrol 13:1, 1984
207. Zerbe R, Tropes L: Vasopressin function in the syndrome of inappropriate antidiuresis. Ann Rev Med 31:315, 1980
208. Balestrieri FJ, Chernow B, Rainey TG: Post-craniotomy diabetes insipidus: Who's at risk? Crit Care Med 10:108, 1982
209. Moses AM, Notman DD: Diabetes insipidus and syndrome of inappropriate antidiuretic hormone secretion (SIADH). Adv Intern Med 27:73, 1982
210. Forse RA: Sodium regulation. In Askanazi J, Starker PM, Weissman C (eds): Fluid and Electrolyte Management in Critical Care, p 39. Boston, Butterworths, 1986
211. Gillespie DJ, Sandberg RL, Koike TI: Dual effect of left atrial receptors on excretion of sodium and water in the dog. Am J Physiol 225:706, 1973
212. Lindheimer MD, Lalone RC, Levinsky NG: Evidence that an acute increase in glomerular filtration rate has little effect on sodium excretion in the dog unless extracellular volume is expanded. J Clin Invest 46:256, 1967
213. Forbes GB, Lewis AM: Total sodium, potassium and chloride in adult man. J Clin Invest 35:596, 1956
214. Makoff DL, DaSilva JA, Rosenbaum BJ et al: Hypertonic expansion: Acid-base and electrolyte changes. Am J Physiol 218:1201, 1970
215. Cox M: Potassium homeostasis. Med Clin North Am 65:363, 1981
216. Williams ME, Gervino EV, Rosa RM et al: Catecholamine modulation of rapid potassium shifts during exercise. N Engl J Med 312:823, 1985
217. Brown MJ, Brown DC, Murphy MB: Hypokalemia from beta$_2$-receptor stimulation by circulating epinephrine. N Engl J Med 309:1414, 1983
218. Shoemaker WC: Fluids and electrolytes in the acutely ill adult. In Shoemaker WC, Thompson WL, Holbrook PR (eds): Textbook of Critical Care, p 614. Philadelphia, WB Saunders, 1984
219. Mathews D, Cirella V, Rosenbaum SH: Serum electrolytes and the heart. In Askanazi J, Starker PM, Weissman C (eds): Fluid and Electrolyte Management in Critical Care, p 217. Boston, Butterworths, 1986
220. Moore FD: Metabolic Care of the Surgical Patient, p 266. Philadelphia, WB Saunders, 1959
221. Gump FE, Kinney JM, Long CL et al: Measurement of water balance: A guide to surgical care. Surgery 64:154, 1968
222. O'Meara MP, Birkenfeld LW, Gotch FA et al: The equilibration of radiosodium, radiopotassium, and denterium oxide in hydropic human subjects. J Clin Invest 36:784, 1957
223. Davidson I, Gelin LE, Hedman L et al: Hemodilution and recovery from experimental intestinal shock in rats: A comparison of the efficacy of three colloids and one electrolyte solution. Crit Care Med 9:42, 1981
224. Ghoneim MM, Long JP: The interaction between magnesium and other neuromuscular blocking agents. Anesthesiology 42:545, 1975
225. Young BK, Weinstein HM: Effects of magnesium sulfate on toxemic patients in labor. Obstet Gynecol 49:681, 1977
226. Weissman C: Signs and symptoms of electrolyte disturbances. In Askanazi J, Starker PM, Weissman C (eds): Fluid and Electrolyte Management in Critical Care, p 135. Boston, Butterworths, 1986
227. Shane EJ, Bilezikian JP: Disorders of calcium, phosphate, and magnesium metabolism. In Askanazi J, Starker PM, Weissman C (eds): Fluid and Electrolyte Management in Critical Care, p 337. Boston, Butterworths, 1986
228. Knochel JP: The pathophysiology and clinical characteristics of severe hypophosphatemia. Arch Intern Med 137:203, 1977

Part IV

Management of Anesthesia

Chapter 28

Benjamin G. Covino
Donald H. Lambert

Epidural and Spinal Anesthesia

The introduction of regional anesthesia into clinical practice is attributed to Carl Koller,[1] a young Viennese ophthalmologist, who employed cocaine in 1884 for topical anesthesia of the cornea in patients scheduled for eye surgery. In 1885, Corning[2] accidentally performed the first spinal anesthetic while performing experiments on the action of cocaine on the spinal nerves of dogs. Corning coined the term *spinal anesthesia* in 1888. In 1898, Sicard described the toxic effects of subarachnoid cocaine.[3] August Bier is considered the father of spinal anesthesia. In 1899, he reported that he and his assistant had performed spinal anesthesia on each other, and then employed this technique to provide anesthesia for surgical procedures.[4] In 1899, Tait and Caglieri[5] performed the first spinal anesthetic for surgery in the United States. However, Matas[6] provided the first description of spinal anesthesia in the USA.

Cathelin,[7] in France, is believed to have performed the first caudal epidural anesthetic in surgical patients in 1901. In 1921, Pages[8] described the lumbar approach to the epidural space for surgical patients. However, Dogliotti[9] is usually given credit for describing a more practical approach to the lumbar epidural space and for popularizing the use of segmental epidural analgesia for surgery. Epidural and spinal anesthesia continue to be two of the most popular regional anesthetic procedures employed for surgery, obstetrics, and postoperative analgesia. Today, spinal anesthesia is probably the most widely employed regional anesthetic technique for surgical patients. The introduction of continuous epidural techniques has helped to popularize the use of this procedure, particularly for analgesia during labor and for postoperative analgesia.

RATIONALE FOR THE USE OF EPIDURAL AND SPINAL ANESTHESIA

Anesthesia can clearly influence the physiological state of patients during the intraoperative and postoperative periods. In some patients, regional anesthesia may be preferable to general anesthesia for certain surgical procedures in which either form of anesthesia may be employed. Prospective studies have elucidated the influence of various anesthetic techniques on the endocrine-metabolic responses to surgery, perioperative blood loss, frequency of thromboembolic complications, cardiopulmonary complications, postoperative recovery phase, and morbidity and mortality.[10]

METABOLIC AND ENDOCRINE ALTERATIONS

Regional anesthesia itself appears to have little influence on endocrine function and metabolic activity. A decrease in plasma epinephrine and norepinephrine levels has been reported following epidural and spinal anesthesia that extend to the upper thoracic dermatomes.[11]

With regard to metabolic products, epidural anesthesia extending to the midthoracic level does not produce any significant changes in blood glucose, lactate, alanine, free fatty acids, glycerol, or ketones.[12, 13] Spinal anesthesia extending to upper thoracic dermatomal levels will inhibit the release of insulin, which usually occurs in response to hyperglycemia.[12]

Surgical stimulation results in an increase in plasma concentrations of cortisol, aldosterone, renin, vasopressin, growth hormone, epinephrine, norepinephrine, glucose, and lactate.

TABLE 28-1. Effect of Epidural Anesthesia on Surgically Induced Endocrine Functions

ENDOCRINE PARAMETERS	SURGERY	EPIDURAL BLOCKADE
PITUITARY HORMONES		
Prolactin	Increase	Inhibit
Growth hormone	Increase	Inhibit
ACTH	Increase	Inhibit
ADH	Increase	Inhibit
ADRENAL AND RENAL HORMONES		
Cortisol	Increase	Inhibit
Aldosterone	Increase	Inhibit
Renin	Increase	Inhibit
Epinephrine	Increase	Inhibit
Norepinephrine	Increase	Inhibit
PANCREATIC HORMONES		
Insulin	No effect	Decrease
Glucagon	No effect	No effect
THYROID HORMONES		
Thyroxine	No effect	No effect
Triiodothyronine	Decrease	No effect

Most of these surgically induced endocrine and metabolic changes can be inhibited by adequate afferent blockade (Tables 28-1, 28-2).

Epidural anesthesia can block the increase in plasma prolactin, growth hormone, ACTH, and antidiuretic hormone associated with surgery. Epidural anesthesia will also inhibit the surgically induced increase in plasma cortisol, aldosterone, renin, epinephrine, and norepinephrine.[14] The extent of the epidural blockade and the site of surgery will influence the degree of inhibition of these various hormones.

A decrease in plasma insulin levels has been observed following surgery performed under epidural anesthesia, whereas there was little or no change in plasma glucagon.[12, 15] Glucose tolerance is much less affected by surgery if epidural rather than general anesthesia is employed.[16] Epidural anesthesia does not appear to exert a significant influence on changes in plasma thyroxine or plasma triiodothyronine levels during surgery.[17]

Increases in plasma glucose, lactate, and 3-hydroxybutyrate, which usually occur following the start of surgery, can be effectively inhibited by epidural anesthesia.[13, 15] Surgical procedures involving the lower abdomen performed under epidural anesthesia are associated with decreased levels of plasma glycerol and free fatty acids.[13] Upper abdominal surgi-

TABLE 28-2. Effect of Epidural Anesthesia on Surgically Induced Changes in Metabolic Functions

METABOLIC PARAMETERS	SURGERY	EPIDURAL BLOCKADE
Glucose	Increase	Inhibit
Lactate	Increase	Inhibit
3-Hydroxybuterate	Increase	Inhibit
Glycerol	Increase	Inhibit
Free fatty acids	Increase	Inhibit
Alanine	Decrease	No effect
Cyclic AMP	Increase	Inhibit

cal procedures or analgesia extending to lower thoracic dermatomes only have not been associated with similar changes in free fatty acids.[18]

The ability of epidural or spinal anesthesia to inhibit the release of pituitary hormones is probably due to the blockade of afferent nociceptive pathways. On the other hand, the inhibition of the release of adrenal cortical hormones, such as cortisol, may result from an inhibition of efferent pathways or, more likely, from the inhibition of the release of ACTH from the pituitary gland during afferent blockade. Inhibition of the release of catecholamines from the adrenal medulla is probably related to the blockade of efferent autonomic pathways. Similarly, the decrease in the release of insulin from the pancreas is probably due to the blockade of efferent sympathetic fibers to the pancreas.

The inability of epidural and spinal anesthesia to block the endocrine-metabolic stress response for upper abdominal surgical procedures may be due to a failure to block afferent pathways conducted through the vagus nerve. However, vagus nerve blockade by local infiltration failed to inhibit the increase in cortisol blood levels observed during surgery in the upper abdominal area carried out under epidural anesthesia. The stress associated with an upper abdominal surgical procedure may be sufficiently great that it is difficult for an epidurally or intrathecally administered local anesthetic to inhibit completely all nociceptive afferent pathways.

BLOOD LOSS

A number of studies have evaluated intraoperative blood loss during various surgical procedures performed under either general or regional anesthesia. The average intraoperative blood loss was 22–50% lower during total hip replacements performed under epidural or spinal anesthesia, as compared to similar procedures performed under general anesthesia.[19, 20] Blood loss was reduced by 37% during retropubic prostatectomy and 18% during transurethral prostatectomy performed under regional anesthesia as compared to general anesthesia.[22] Spinal anesthesia has been associated with a reduction in intraoperative blood loss of 45% during abdominal hysterectomies.[23] However, other studies involving abdominal surgery failed to demonstrate any difference in blood loss between general and regional anesthesia.[24, 25]

The diminished bleeding during regional anesthesia may be related to the hypotension caused by the sympathetic block. Hypotensive anesthesia with halothane and nitroprusside also results in a similar reduction in intraoperative blood loss during hip replacement. Some studies have shown that the decreased blood loss during epidural blockade was not associated with a significant reduction in blood pressure. It has been postulated that epidural or spinal anesthesia may lead to a redistribution of blood flow away from the operative site, resulting in a reduced blood loss.[21]

THROMBOEMBOLIC COMPLICATIONS

Thromboembolic complications have been reported to be reduced 50–60% when hip surgery is performed under lumbar epidural anesthesia.[20, 21, 26] A similar reduction was observed during prostatectomy.[22] Epidural anesthesia did not significantly reduce thromboembolic complications following abdominal surgical procedures.[25, 27]

The mechanism responsible for the reduction in thromboembolism is probably an increased blood flow to the lower extremities following sympathetic blockade by regional anesthesia. An additional factor may be an increase in fibrinolytic activity during regional anesthesia.[28, 29]

CARDIOPULMONARY COMPLICATIONS

Continuous epidural analgesia for postoperative pain relief may ameliorate the usual postoperative deterioration of pulmonary function. A comparison of either intramuscular morphine, continuous intravenous morphine, or continuous epidural bupivacaine for postoperative pain relief following cholecystectomy revealed that patients given epidural analgesia had better analgesia than patients receiving morphine, and had significantly higher arterial oxygen tensions during the first three postoperative days, and had a lower incidence of pulmonary complications and chest infections.[30] In a review of multiple studies in which regional or general anesthesia had been employed for various surgical procedures, 25 of 198 patients (13%) who received regional anesthesia developed postoperative pulmonary complications, in contrast to 43 of 203 patients (21%) in the general anesthesia group.[14] This suggests that regional anesthesia may alter the rate of postoperative pulmonary complications.

The cardiovascular effects of general or regional anesthesia in healthy patients do not differ markedly. Both general anesthesia and epidural or spinal anesthesia may cause a decrease in blood pressure. The hypotension related to general anesthesia is usually due to a decrease in cardiac output, while spinal or epidural blockade decreases systemic vascular resistance secondary to sympathetic blockade. However, a comparison of neuroleptic anesthesia and epidural anesthesia combined with light general anesthesia in patients with a recent history of myocardial infarction scheduled for major abdominal surgery revealed significant differences in the two groups with regard to various hemodynamic parameters.[31] A mean pulmonary artery occlusion pressure of greater than 18 mm Hg was observed in 75% of the neuroleptic anesthesia patients, compared to 17% in the epidural group. A decrease in coronary vascular resistance of greater than 25% occurred in 57% of the neuroleptic anesthesia patients, compared to 13% of the epidural patients. All of the neuroleptic anesthesia patients demonstrated an increase in myocardial oxygen consumption of greater than 25%, compared to only one patient in the epidural group. Fifty percent of the neuroleptic anesthesia patients showed ST–T segment depression of greater than 1 mm, compared to 13% in the epidural group. Finally, ventricular arrhythmias developed intraoperatively in 36% of the neuroleptic anesthesia patients, while only 8% of the epidural patients showed signs of ventricular arrhythmias. No difference in the frequency of perioperative myocardial infarction or 1-month postoperative mortality existed between the two groups. Two patients in the neuroleptic anesthesia group and one patient in the epidural group suffered an intraoperative myocardial infarction. In addition, three patients in the neuroleptic anesthesia group developed a myocardial infarction during the first postoperative week. Two patients in the neuroleptic anesthesia group and one patient in the epidural group died within the first postoperative month. The results of this study suggest that patients with diagnosed cardiac disease who undergo major non-cardiac surgery may develop more serious alterations in coronary hemodynamics, and may be at greater risk in terms of myocardial ischemia and ventricular arrhythmias, when a general anesthetic, rather than a regional anesthetic technique, is employed.

MORBIDITY AND MORTALITY

Little difference in perioperative mortality exists between various anesthetic techniques in relatively healthy patients scheduled for elective surgery. In elderly patients admitted for emergency repair of hip fractures, contradictory results have been reported.[32, 33] A lower mortality within the 1-month postoperative period was observed in several studies in patients in whom spinal anesthesia had been employed compared to the use of general anesthesia. However, no difference in the number of deaths during a 1–2-yr postoperative period was observed in patients in whom an emergency repair of a hip fracture was carried out under either spinal or general anesthesia.[33, 34] Therefore, emergency surgery performed under spinal anesthesia in elderly patients who presumably have a certain degree of cardiac disease may be associated with a lower morbidity and mortality, but only during the immediate, i.e., 1–2 weeks, postoperative period. A recent study has also demonstrated that epidural anesthesia and postoperative analgesia may improve the outcome in high-risk patients in whom major surgical procedures are performed.[35]

ANATOMY

BONY STRUCTURES

The spinal canal extends from the foramen magnum to the sacral hiatus. The bony arches of the vertebra posterior to the vertebral bodies form a continuum which makes up the spinal canal (Fig. 28-1). The spaces between the vertebra are occupied by the spinal ligaments. The vertebral column consists of seven cervical, 12 thoracic, and five lumbar vertebrae. The sacrum and coccyx are caudad extensions of the vertebral column. The shape and size of the vertebrae differ in the cervical, thoracic, and lumbar areas (Fig. 28-2). The vertebrae increase in size from the cervical to the lumbar areas, which are related to the function of the vertebrae in the various locations. Cervical vertebrae are smallest and have the least weight-bearing function. The lumbar vertebrae are largest in size and support the greatest amount of weight.

The vertebrae consist of a vertebral body behind which is a bony arch. The arch consists of two pedicles anteriorly and two laminae posteriorly. The transverse processes are formed by the junction of the pedicles and laminae, while the spinal process is formed from the union of opposing laminae.

The spinal processes vary in their angulation in the cervical, thoracic, and lumbar regions. The degree of angulation will influence the direction of a needle to be placed in the epidural or subarachnoid space. In the cervical, lower thoracic, and lumbar regions, the spinal processes are almost horizontal, and the needle may be directed at right angles to the sagittal plane. However, in the mid-thoracic region, the spinal processes have a marked caudad angulation that is maximal between the T3 and T7 vertebrae. Thus, an epidural or spinal needle must be inserted at varying degrees from the horizontal plane to enter the epidural or subarachnoid space. The sacrum is formed by the fusion of the five sacral vertebrae, and the coccyx is attached to the caudad end of the sacrum.

LIGAMENTS

The vertebrae are joined together posteriorly by a series of short ligaments. The laminae of the vertebrae are connected by the ligamentum flavum, while the posterior spinous proc-

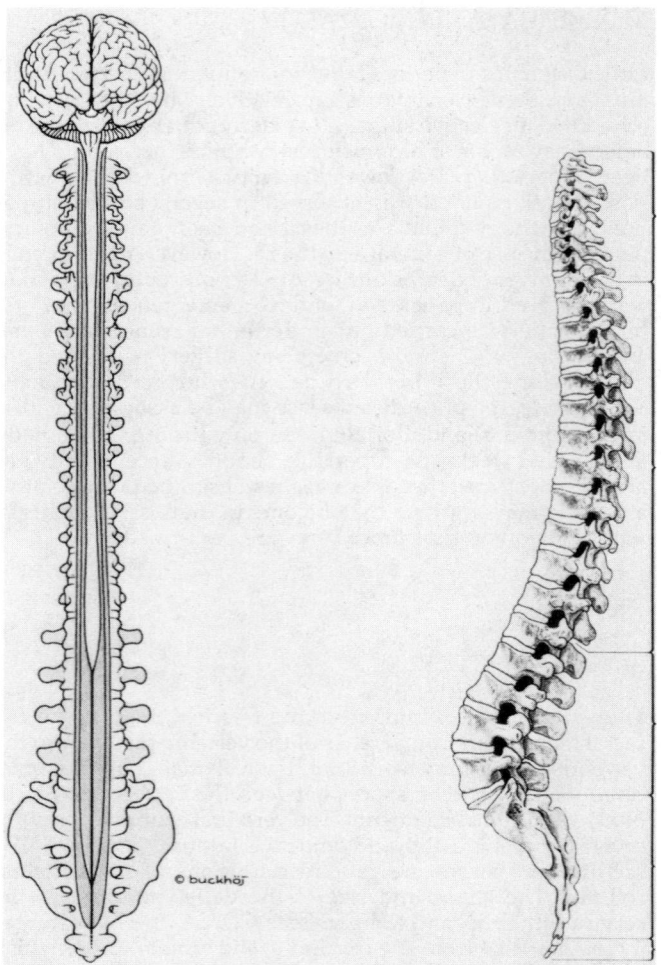

FIG. 28-1. (*Left*) The spinal canal runs from the foramen magnum to the sacral hiatus. (*Right*) The vertebral column is composed of 7 cervical, 12 thoracic, and 5 lumbar vertebrae, with the sacrum and coccyx inferiorly. The vertebrae vary in size and shape according to their position and function. (Reproduced with permission: Covino BG, Scott DB: Handbook of Epidural Anaesthesia and Analgesia, p 10. Orlando, Grune & Stratton, 1985.)

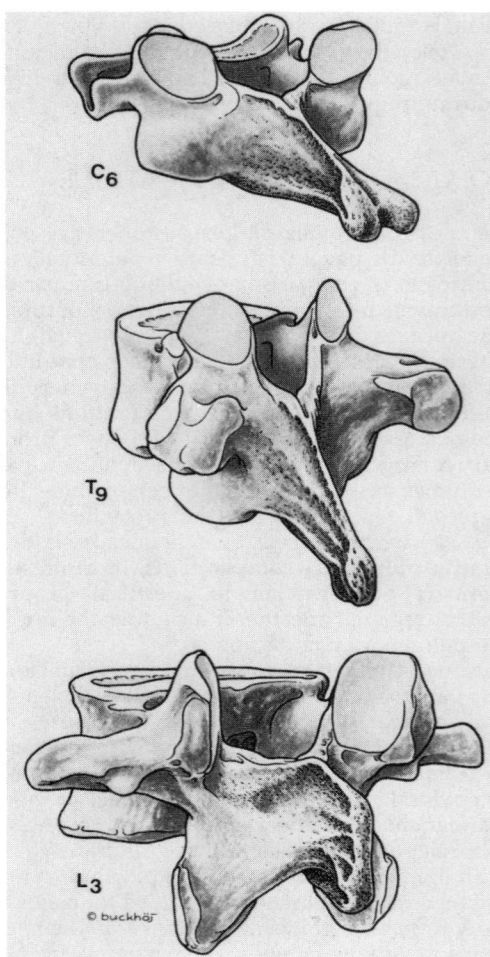

FIG. 28-2. Oblique views of a cervical, a thoracic, and a lumbar vertebra. (Reproduced with permission: Covino BG, Scott DB: Handbook of Epidural Anaesthesia and Analgesia, p 11. Orlando, Grune & Stratton, 1985.)

esses are connected by the interspinous ligaments. The supraspinous ligaments run superficial to the tips of the spinal processes. The vertebral bodies are separated anteriorly by the intervertebral discs, and the anterior longitudinal ligament runs from the base of the skull to the sacrum with an attachment to the discs and the adjacent margins of the vertebral bodies. The posterior longitudinal ligament connects the posterior surface of the vertebral bodies and forms the anterior wall of the vertebral canal. The intervertebral foramina exist as openings between the vertebral pedicles, through which the spinal nerves pass.

EPIDURAL SPACE

The spinal canal contains the spinal cord and its coverings, the pia mater, arachnoid mater, and dura mater. The epidural space (Fig. 28-3) is located between the dura mater and the connective tissue covering the vertebrae and the ligamentum flavum. The epidural space has been described as a potential

space, since, normally, it is completely filled with a loose type of connective tissue, fatty tissue, and blood vessels. It is particularly rich in venous plexuses. No free fluid exists in the epidural space. However, solutions injected into the epidural space will spread in all directions between the loose tissue structures that occupy this area.

The subdural space is the area between the arachnoid mater and the dura mater. The subdural space is also a potential space, since it contains lymph. The pia mater is closely attached to the spinal cord and the spinal nerves. The area between the arachnoid mater and the pia mater is the subarachnoid space, which contains cerebrospinal fluid (Fig. 28-3).

The space within the spinal canal is primarily occupied by the spinal cord that extends from the foramen magnum to the first or second lumbar vertebra. The spinal cord has a longitudinal cylindrical shape that is somewhat flattened, anteroposteriorly, particularly in the lumbar region. The cord is characterized by cervical and lumbar enlargements. Below the lumbar area, the cord tapers into the conus medullaris, from which the filum terminale continues down to attach to the coccyx.

The anterior and posterior (dorsal) spinal nerve roots exit

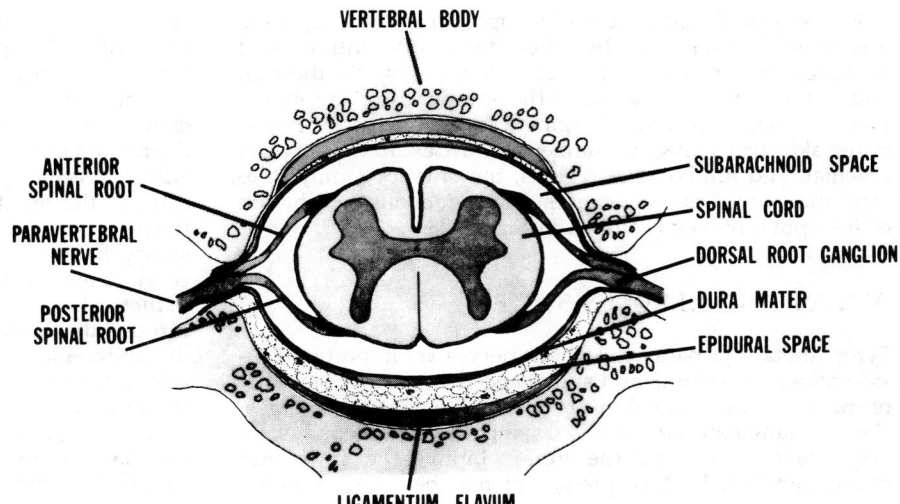

FIG. 28-3. Cross-sectional diagram of the vertebral column and spinal cord. (Reproduced with permission: Covino BG, Vassallo HG: Local Anesthetics: Mechanism of Action and Clinical Use, p 76. New York, Grune & Stratton, 1976.)

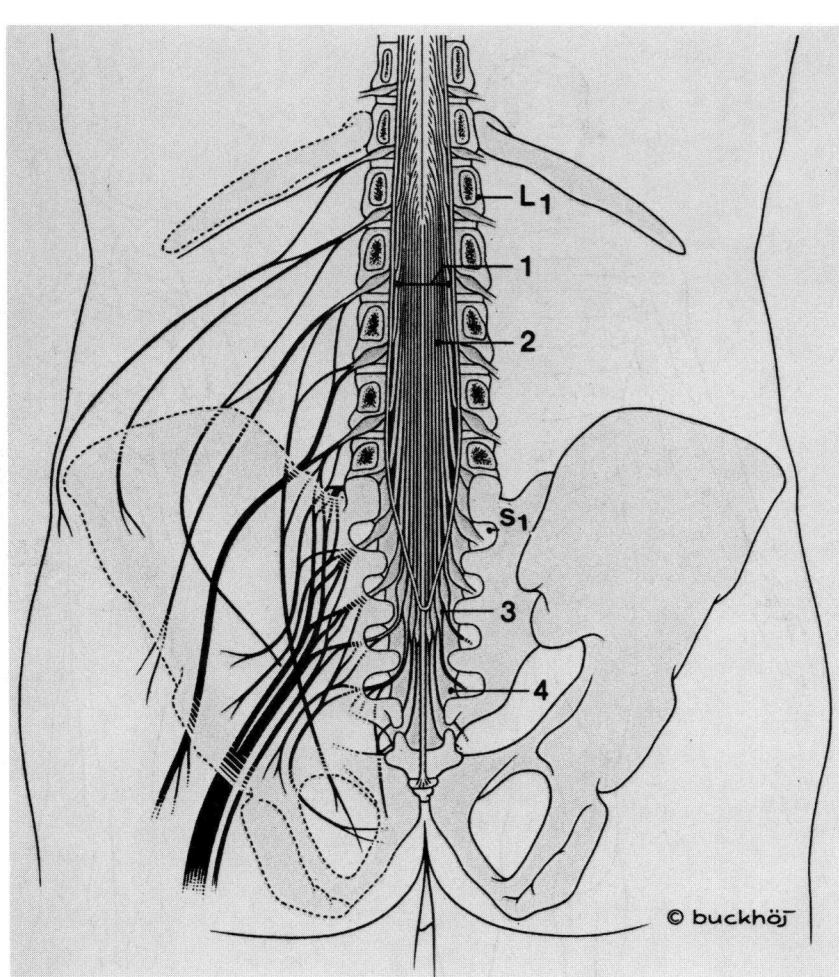

FIG. 28-4. Schematic diagram of the cauda equina and the formation of the lumbosacral plexus. (1) Cauda equina. (2) Subarachnoid space. (3) Dorsal root ganglion. (4) Sacral epidural space. (Reproduced with permission: Covino BG, Scott DB: Handbook of Epidural Anaesthesia and Analgesia, p 24. Orlando, Grune & Stratton, 1985.)

from the spinal cord and then join to form the spinal nerves at each intervertebral space. The spinal nerves leave the spinal canal *via* the intervertebral foramina (Fig. 28-3). The dorsal root ganglia are located on the dorsal spinal roots just prior to the junction at which the ventral and dorsal roots unite. In the cervical and thoracic regions, the spinal nerves immediately

leave the spinal canal by way of intervertebral foramina shortly after their formation. However, because the spinal cord ends at the level of L1-2, the lower lumbar and sacral nerve roots extend for some distance within the spinal canal as the cauda equina before leaving the spinal canal to enter the sacral epidural space (Fig. 28-4).

As the spinal nerves leave the spinal canal through the intervertebral foramina, they then divide into anterior and posterior primary rami. The posterior rami supply the skin and muscles of the back, while the anterior rami supply the rest of the body. Each spinal segment supplies a specific region of the skin and a specific number of muscles. In the cervical, brachial, and lumbosacral regions, the anterior rami join to form the various nerve plexuses. The cutaneous distribution of the spinal nerves is shown in Figure 28-5.

AUTONOMIC NERVOUS SYSTEM

Sympathetic and parasympathetic nerves are important considerations in epidural and spinal anesthesia, since blockade of these nerves can lead to profound physiological changes. The pre-ganglionic nerves of the sympathetic nervous system originate in nerve cells in the lateral column of the gray matter of the spinal cord. These pre-ganglionic fibers pass from the spinal cord through the spinal nerves from the T1 to the L2 level. After the spinal nerves exit through the intervertebral foraminae, the pre-ganglionic sympathetic nerve fibers leave the spinal nerves to become part of the white rami communicantes which run to the sympathetic chain. The pre-ganglionic fibers then run up or down the sympathetic chain to synapse within specific sympathetic ganglia. The sympathetic chain extends the length of the spinal column along the antero-lateral aspect of the vertebral bodies. In the cervical region, the sympathetic ganglia make up the superior cervical, middle cervical, and stellate ganglia. In the thoracic region, the sympathetic chain gives rise to the splanchnic nerves, which pass through the diaphragm and terminate in the coeliac plexus. In the abdominal area, these nerves connect with the coeliac, aortic, and hypogastric plexuses. The sympathetic chain ends in the pelvis on the anterior surface of the sacrum.

Post-ganglionic sympathetic nerves originate in the various ganglia and are widely distributed to various organs. Post-ganglionic sympathetic nerves play an important role in con-

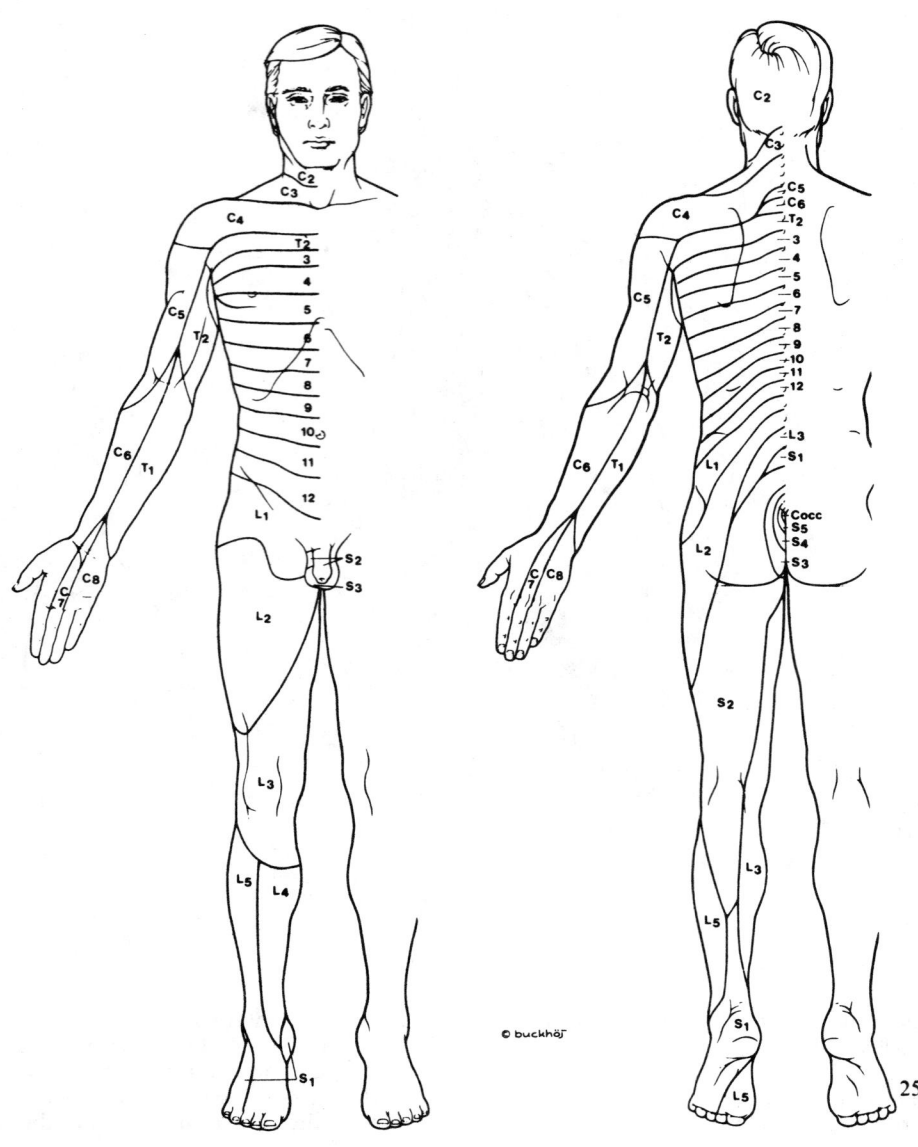

FIG. 28-5. Cutaneous distribution of the spinal nerves. (Reproduced with permission: Covino BG, Scott DB: Handbook of Epidural Anaesthesia and Analgesia, p 25. Orlando, Grune & Stratton, 1985.)

trolling cardiac function, vascular tone, gastro-intestinal tone, and motility.

Pre-ganglionic parasympathetic nerve fibers are contained within the cranial nerves, or in the second, third, or fourth sacral nerves. The pre-ganglionic parasympathetic fibers extend to the various organs that they innervate, and synapse within the walls of these organs with the short post-ganglionic parasympathetic fibers. The parasympathetic nervous system is also of importance in terms of regulating cardiovascular and gastrointestinal function.

BLOOD SUPPLY OF THE SPINAL CANAL

The anterior spinal artery and posterior spinal arteries and their branches supply blood to the spinal cord, spinal roots, and meninges (Fig. 28-6). The anterior spinal artery is formed by the union of two branches of the terminal portion of the vertebral artery at the level of the foramen magnum. The anterior spinal artery then descends along the median sulcus on the anterior surface of the cord to the conus medullaris, and then terminates as an arteriole on the filum terminale. The anterior spinal artery supplies the anterior two-thirds of the spinal cord. Two posterior spinal arteries are located on each side of the posterior surface of the cord. They arise from the posterior inferior cerebellar arteries and descend on the dorsal surface of the cord medial to the dorsal nerve roots. The posterior spinal arteries supply the posterior one-third of the spinal cord.

Branches of the vertebral, deep cervical, intercostal, and lumbar arteries enter the vertebral canal through the intervertebral foraminae. These spinal branches divide into anterior and posterior radicular arteries that travel along the nerve roots to reach the cord where they anastomose with the anterior and posterior spinal arteries. One of the radicular arteries is considerably larger than the rest, and represents the major blood supply to the lower two-thirds of the cord. This particular branch is known as the arteria radicularis magna, or the

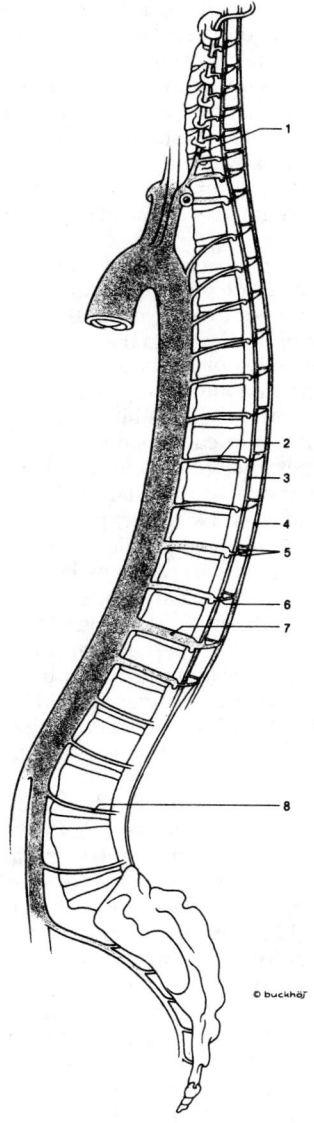

1. Vertebral artery
2. Intercostal artery
3. Anterior spinal artery
4. Posterior spinal artery
5. Anterior and posterior radicular arteries
6. Spinal branch of intercostal artery
7. Artery of Adamkiewicz
8. Lumbar artery

FIG. 28-6. Blood supply of the spinal cord. Radicular arteries, which run in the anterior and posterior nerve roots to the cord, are derived from the vertebral artery in the neck, the intercostal arteries in the thorax, and the lumbar arteries in the abdomen. The artery of Adamkiewicz is the main supply of the lower two-thirds of the cord. (Reproduced with permission: Covino BG, Scott DB: Handbook of Epidural Anaesthesia and Analgesia, p 21. Orlando, Grune & Stratton, 1985.)

artery of Adamkiewiez. It is located in the lower thoracic or upper lumbar area, and is more common on the left side.

Blood from the contents of the spinal canal drains into a tortuous venous plexus in the pia mater which contain six longitudinal veins. These connect with the internal vertebral plexus in the epidural space from which blood flows by way of the intervertebral veins into the azygos and hemiazygos systems.

PATIENT EVALUATION AND PREPARATION FOR EPIDURAL AND SPINAL ANESTHESIA

The preanesthetic evaluation and examination of patients scheduled for epidural or spinal anesthesia should be no less vigorous than for patients scheduled for general anesthesia. The anesthesiologist should explain to patients the reasons for suggesting an epidural or spinal anesthetic technique and the potential advantages of these techniques. Patients should be made aware of what they might hear or see in an operating room if the decision is made to have the patient awake during a surgical procedure. Although a complete medical history should be obtained on any patient scheduled for surgery, a careful evaluation of the patient's cardiovascular and neurological status should be made if epidural or spinal anesthesia is selected. A pre-surgical physical examination should have been performed by the surgical staff and reviewed by the anesthesiologist. The patient's drug history should be taken, since many agents that affect the cardiovascular system, such as adrenergic blocking agents or anti-hypertensive agents, may influence the patient's physiological response to epidural or spinal blockade.

Physical examination of the patient's back should be made to determine the appropriate site of entry of the epidural or spinal needle. Any spinal deformities or excessive calcification should be noted that may make epidural or spinal anesthesia difficult, or, in fact, impossible. Any history of back problems or trauma to the spinal canal should be elicited from the patient, which, again, may determine the feasibility of performing a central neural block in a particular patient.

Laboratory data required preoperatively for patients scheduled for epidural or spinal anesthesia are similar to those required for general anesthetic patients. However, particular attention should be paid to the coagulation profile to determine the possibility of any coagulation defects and any laboratory data that might be indicative of abnormal bleeding tendency. Coagulation profiles and, possibly, bleeding times should be obtained on any patient who has been on anticoagulants preoperatively, even if the anticoagulants have been discontinued prior to surgery. Similar studies should be available on patients who have been taking medications that are known to influence platelet adhesiveness that may result in prolonged bleeding times.

The technique of epidural or spinal anesthesia should be described to the patient. The advantages relative to general anesthesia and the possible complications of epidural or spinal anesthesia intraoperatively and postoperatively should also be explained. Patient concerns regarding remaining in an awake state intraoperatively should not be an automatic contraindication to the use of an epidural or spinal anesthetic technique. Various forms of sedation may be employed intraoperatively. The use of earphones for listening to music or other forms of entertainment can provide a distraction for patients intraoperatively. Alternatively, general anesthetic agents in sufficiently low concentrations to allow patients to sleep, but not be fully anesthetized, may also be utilized. If a combined general and regional anesthetic technique is suggested for a particular patient, the primary anesthetic procedure is the epidural or spinal, and the general anesthetic should be merely sufficient to allow a state of somnolence, rather than a state of full general anesthesia. Patients in whom a combined general and regional anesthetic procedure is anticipated may or may not require intubation of the trachea. The choice of intubation of the trachea will depend on the ability to maintain a patent airway with a mask and the position of the patient intraoperatively.

Preoperative medication for patients scheduled for epidural or spinal anesthesia is dependent on the level of anxiety of the patient, the ability of the anesthesiologist to allay fear and anxiety, and the ability of the patient to tolerate some pain associated with insertion of the epidural or spinal needle. Anticholinergic agents are probably not indicated in patients scheduled for regional anesthesia.

INDICATIONS AND CONTRAINDICATIONS FOR EPIDURAL AND SPINAL ANESTHESIA

Table 28-3 includes a list of those surgical procedures that can be performed under epidural or spinal anesthesia. Surgical procedures in the upper abdomen have been performed under high spinal anesthesia, but, today, lumbar or thoracic epidural techniques are usually employed. There are relatively few absolute contraindications to epidural and spinal anesthesia. These include localized infection at the puncture site, patients who refuse regional anesthesia, severe uncorrected hypovolemia, uncorrected coagulation defects, or pathological situations resulting in excessive bleeding times and anatomic abnormalities that make epidural or spinal techniques difficult or impossible. Relative contraindications include generalized infection, such as bacteremia, neurologic disorders, such as multiple sclerosis, and minidose heparin

TABLE 28-3. Surgical Procedures Often Performed Under Spinal or Epidural Anesthesia

1. Any intraabdominal procedure
2. Gynecological procedures
   A. Hysterectomy
   B. Cone biopsy
   C. D & C
   D. Ovarian cystectomy
3. Obstetrical procedures
   A. Cesarean section
   B. Circlage
   C. Vaginal delivery
4. Herniorraphies
5. Lower limb procedures
   A. Orthopedic
   B. Vascular
   C. Amputations
6. Urological procedures
   A. Transurethral resections
   B. Cystoscopy
   C. Open prostatectomies
   D. Penile implant
   E. Orchiectomy
7. Perineal and rectal surgery
   A. Bartholin cyst
   B. Rectal fissures
   C. Hemorrhoids
8. Others

therapy. In these cases, the benefits of employing epidural or spinal anesthesia may sometimes outweigh the risks.

TECHNICAL ASPECTS

The most important landmarks for performance of a lumbar epidural or spinal block are the vertebral spinal processes and the iliac crests (Fig. 28-7). The spinous processes clearly define the midline. A line drawn between the iliac crests crosses the fourth lumbar vertebra. Thus, the interspace above this line represents the L3–L4 interspace, and the space below the line is the L4–L5 interspace. These spaces are usually chosen for insertion of the epidural or spinal needle, since the spinal cord ends at the L1–L2 level. For thoracic epidural blocks, a line passing between the inferior angle of the scapulae crosses the seventh thoracic vertebra. The T7–T8 interspace is usually the site of needle entry for a mid-thoracic epidural block.

EPIDURAL BLOCKADE

The epidural space is most easily entered in the lumbar region, since the spinous processes are not angulated in relation to the vertebral body, and the space between adjacent laminae, covered by the ligamentum flavum, is wide. The patient should be positioned with the lumbar spine in maximal flexion so that the intervertebral spaces are maximally opened. This can be done in the lateral or the sitting position. In the lateral position, the patient's knees are flexed as high as possible in front of the abdomen, and the head is bent onto the chest. In the sitting position, the patient should be flexed with the elbows resting on the knees or on a table, and head bent with the chin on the chest.

Numerous prepackaged and sterile kits are available for epidural blocks. A 17- or 18-gauge Tuohy needle is most commonly employed. The curved Huber point is designed to decrease the possibility of accidental dural puncture and facilitate the passage of a plastic catheter into the epidural space. Various types of epidural needles are available, such as the Crawford needle, which has a short blunt bevel, and the Weiss

needle, with wings attached to the needle hub. The latter is particularly useful if a hanging-drop technique is employed.

Epidural blocks should only be attempted in a location where complete anesthetic equipment is readily available, including an anesthetic machine and resuscitative equipment and drugs. An intravenous infusion should be initiated prior to the performance of an epidural block. In addition, blood pressure, heart rate, and the electrocardiogram should be recorded prior to and during the epidural procedure.

Epidural anesthesia must be performed utilizing an aseptic technique. The patient's back should be sterilized with an antiseptic solution. The decision to employ sterile drapes is at the discretion of the anesthesiologist, but it is useful to ensure a sterile field. The anesthesiologist should wear a mask and sterile surgical gloves.

The iliac crest is observed or palpated, and the L3–L4 interspace identified. The L2–L3 and L4–L5 spaces should also be identified, and the space that appears to offer the easiest access to the epidural space is chosen for needle insertion (Fig. 28-7). An intradermal wheal is raised with a local anesthetic over the chosen interspace. Subcutaneous infiltration may also be employed to decrease the pain associated with insertion of the epidural needle and to identify the appropriate direction for the epidural needle. A 16- or 18-gauge needle is used to perforate the skin to facilitate penetration with the epidural needle. The skin should be held firmly over the spinous process above the chosen interspace with the index and middle finger of one hand, while the epidural needle is inserted in the middle of the chosen interspace at right angles to the skin with the opposite hand.

The most common method to identify the epidural space is the loss-of-resistance technique. There are many variations of this technique. Usually, a syringe containing saline or air is attached to the needle lying in the interspinous ligament (Fig. 28-8). If the needle is properly positioned, it will be difficult to inject at this point. At this time, the direction of the tip of the needle should be slightly cephalad.

The dorsum of the non-injecting hand is placed on the patient's back, and the thumb and index or middle finger is used to grasp the hub of the needle. This hand is used to advance the needle. The opposite hand is placed on the

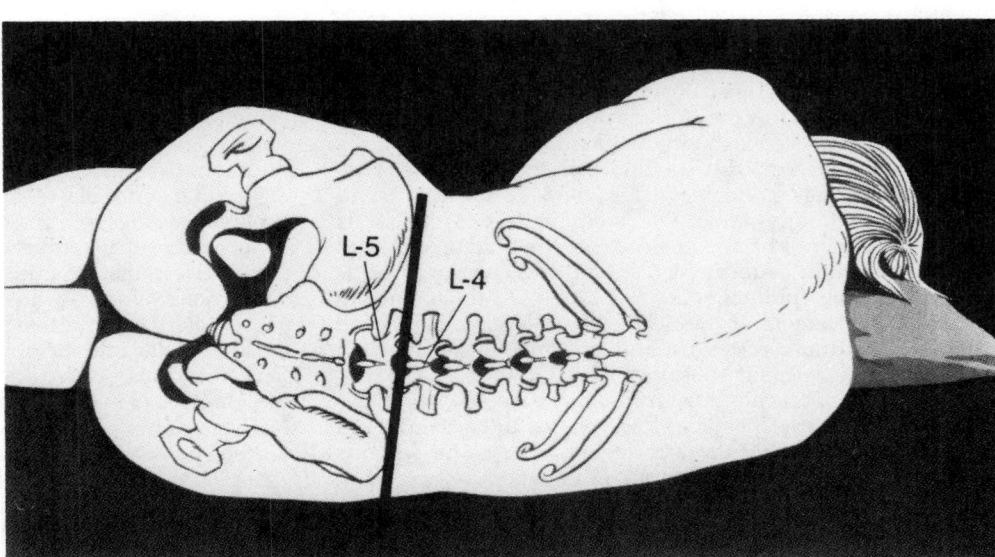

FIG. 28-7. Patient position for epidural and/or spinal anesthesia. Anatomical landmarks are illustrated.

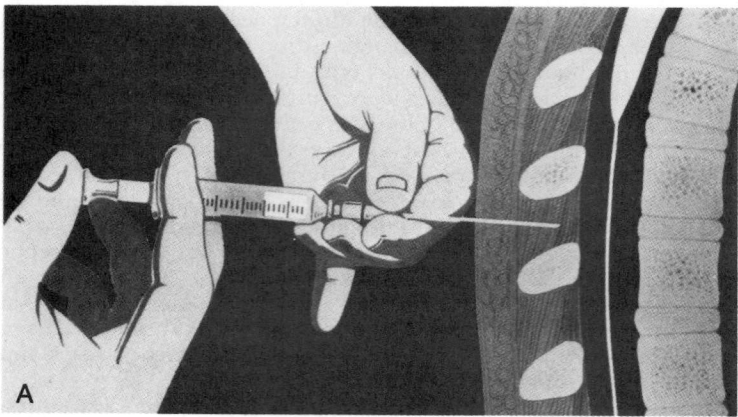

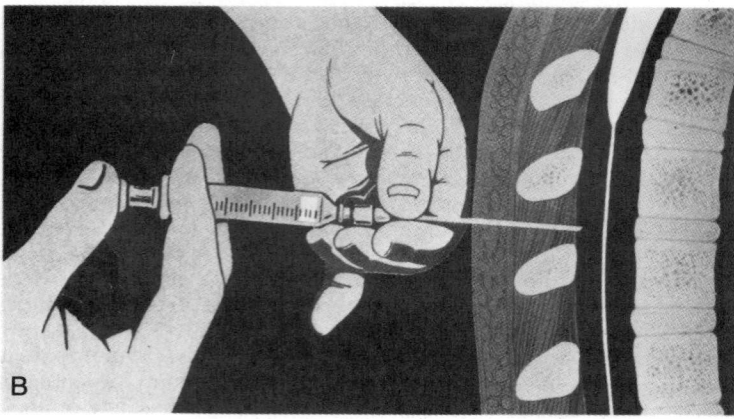

FIG. 28-8. Correct hand positions for the "loss of resistance" method of identifying the epidural space. The needle should be advanced slowly and firmly (*A*), until loss of resistance is encountered, signifying entry of the needle into the epidural space (*B*).

plunger of the syringe, and gentle but continuous pressure is applied. Resistance to advancement of the plunger is noted as the needle is advanced toward the ligamentum flavum. As the needle passes through the ligamentum flavum and enters the epidural space, a sudden loss of resistance will occur. The saline or air can be injected with ease into the epidural space. The advancement of the needle should cease once the epidural space has been identified.

The hanging-drop technique is based on the presence of negative pressure in the epidural space. A winged, Weiss-type epidural needle is usually employed. The needle is inserted percutaneously in the same fashion as described above. Once the needle is engaged in the interspinous ligament, the stylet is removed and a drop of fluid is placed in the hub of the needle. The wings of the needle are held with the thumb and index finger of both hands. The lateral surface of the hands rest on the patient's back. The needle is slowly advanced until the ligamentum flavum is pierced and the hanging drop is sucked into the epidural space (Fig. 28-9). At this point, no further advancement of the needle should occur. Identification of the epidural space is usually confirmed by the injection of saline or air without resistance.

A midline approach is most commonly employed for insertion of the epidural needle. However, for thoracic epidural anesthesia in the mid-thoracic region, where the spinous processes are markedly angulated, or in patients who cannot flex their spine adequately or where there is excessive vertebral calcification, a paramedian or lateral approach to the epidural space may prove useful. The needle is inserted 1–1.5 cm lateral to the midline on a level with the upper border of the spinous process below the selected interspace. Following cutaneous penetration, the needle is directed in a cephalad and mediad direction in order to perforate the ligamentum flavum and enter the epidural space in the midline. Identification of the epidural space is accomplished by a loss of resistance or hanging drop technique.

Catheter Placement

Although single-shot epidural techniques, in which local anesthetic solution is injected through the needle and the needle withdrawn, are employed for surgical procedures of limited duration, the primary advantage of epidural blockade is the ability to insert a plastic catheter into the epidural space and provide anesthesia or analgesia of indefinite duration. A variety of commercial epidural catheters are available. Some have a single terminal opening, while others may have several lateral holes with or without a terminal opening. Most, but not all, catheters are supplied with a stylet to allow easier passage of the catheter into the epidural space. The catheters usually have markings spaced 1 cm apart at their distal end. The catheter is held in one hand, and the distal end of the catheter is advanced through the needle into the epidural space. As the catheter passes through the tip of the needle into the epidural space, a slight resistance is usually encountered. The first marking on the catheter denotes the distance from the tip of the needle to the hub. The catheter should be advanced 2–3 markings beyond the hub of the needle, which will ensure that

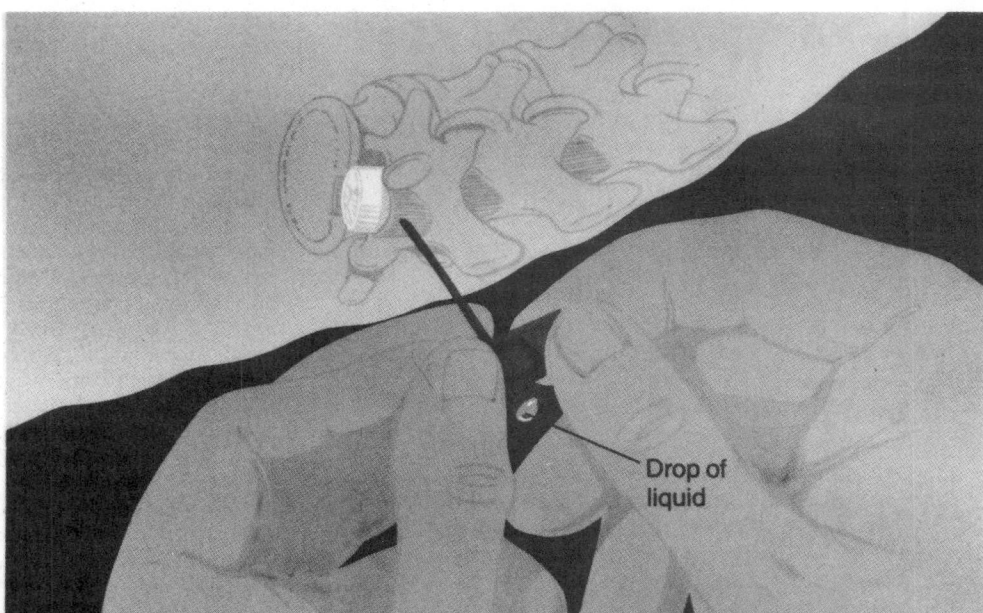

FIG. 28-9. Correct hand position for using the hanging drop method of locating the epidural space. The needle should be moved slowly until the drop is sucked into the needle, signifying entry of the needle tip into the epidural space.

Drop of liquid

2–3 cm of catheter have entered the epidural space. One should not attempt to insert an extensive length of the catheter into the epidural space, since this may result in the tip of the catheter entering an intervertebral foramen, resulting in an inadequate epidural blockade. The tip of the epidural needle is usually directed in a cephalad or caudad direction in hopes of advancing the catheter in a cephalad or caudad direction. However, radiological studies indicate that the direction of the needle tip does not guarantee the direction of the catheter in the epidural space.

Once the catheter has been inserted into the epidural space, the needle is then slowly withdrawn. The needle should be withdrawn over the catheter with one hand, while the other hand applies gentle inward pressure on the catheter to ensure that the catheter is not withdrawn with the needle (Fig. 28-10). No attempt should ever be made to withdraw a catheter back through the needle, since this may result in shearing of a portion of the catheter in the epidural space.

Once the needle and stylet have been withdrawn, the catheter is taped to the patient's back, usually with a loop formed as the catheter exits from the back to prevent kinking of the catheter. The catheter is taped to the back from the point of cutaneous exit to the shoulder of the patient, so that injections can be made at the head of the patient. A syringe adapter is fastened to the proximal end of the catheter, to which a syringe may then be attached. A bacterial filter may also be employed between the catheter and the syringe.

Test Dose

A local anesthetic test dose is recommended to detect an accidental intravascular or subarachnoid placement of the needle or catheter. Three to four milliliters of a local anesthetic solution with epinephrine, *e.g.*, 3–4 ml of 1.5% lidocaine with 1:200,000 epinephrine, should be used as a test dose. Heart rate and blood pressure should be monitored. An intravascular injection will usually be detected due to the increase in heart rate and blood pressure that will occur following the

intravascular injection of epinephrine. The failure to elicit an increase in heart rate or blood pressure is often, but not always, indicative of a non-intravascular injection. For example, patients on chronic β-adrenergic receptor blockers will not demonstrate an increase in rate following the intravenous injection of epinephrine.[36]

Following the administration of the test dose, sensory and motor function in the lower limbs should be assessed in order to detect the possibility of an accidental subarachnoid injection. If any signs of an intravascular injection are noted, no further injections should be made, the epidural needle or catheter should be withdrawn, and the entire placement procedure should be reinstituted at another interspace. If signs of an intrathecal injection are observed, spinal anesthesia may be considered as an alternative to epidural anesthesia.

Due to the relatively rapid absorption of drugs from the epidural space and the relatively large doses required for epidural blockade, the main portion of injectate should be made slowly and, preferably, in a fractionated dose regimen. In the latter instance, volumes of 3–5 ml of anesthetic solution are administered intermittently at 3–4-min intervals. The patient should be continually evaluated for signs of an accidental intravascular or intrathecal injection. The total dose of drug administered will be dependent on the physical status of the patient and the location of the surgical procedure. The dermatomal analgesic level can be evaluated by pin-prick or use of an alcohol swab at approximately 1-min intervals during and following the intermittent injection of the anesthetic solution.

SPINAL ANESTHESIA

Spinal anesthesia is usually induced with the patient in the lateral decubitus or the sitting position. The lateral decubitus position has the advantage that it is more comfortable for the patient and the patient is not as likely to experience a faint. The disadvantage is that it is often difficult to communicate the posture that the anesthesiologist would like the patient to

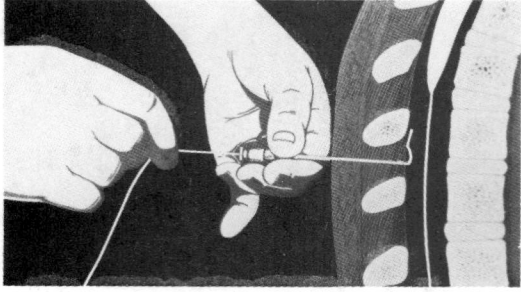

A

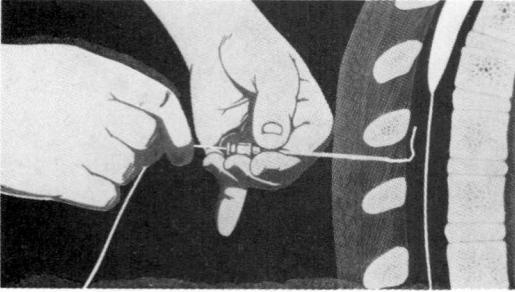

B

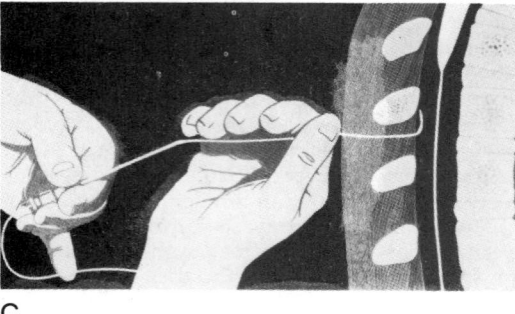

C

FIG. 28-10. Removing the needle following insertion of the catheter. With one hand holding the catheter, the other hand should pull the needle (*A*) until both hands meet (*B*). When the needle is free, it should be removed by holding the catheter and gently easing the needle off with the other hand (*C*).

assume. Furthermore, it is easy for patients to make their back lordotic at the precise moment when an arched out back is more desirable. Lastly, if the patient is obese, it is more difficult to locate the midline with the patient in the lateral decubitus position.

The advantage of the sitting position is that the proper curvature of the back for lumbar puncture is easier to obtain. The correct posture is easily communicated to the patient by asking him/her to merely lean forward. Another advantage is that it is more difficult for the patient to "move away from the needle" when in this position. The sitting position is also valuable for patients with certain injuries. For example, it is often less painful for patients with hip fractures to achieve a sitting position than to lay on either side. The major disadvantage to this position is the increased incidence of fainting.

Preparation of the patient's back for spinal anesthesia is the same as previously described for epidural anesthesia.

Midline Approach

The L4–5 interspace is the site most commonly used for spinal anesthesia. The spinal cord ends at the L1–2 interspace in adults (it ends at L2 in small children). However, even at this level, the spinal cord has tapered, becoming the filum terminalis, and the possibility of damaging the cord with the spinal needle is remote. Therefore, lumbar puncture performed at L2 and below is virtually free of risk of injuring the spinal cord itself. Nerve injury involving the cauda equina is, on the other hand, possible, although extremely rare, since these structures are free to move away from the advancing needle.

The anesthesiologist should choose the interspace below L2, which appears to afford the easiest access to the subarachnoid space. A skin wheal is raised with local anesthetic in the midline of the chosen interspace. The spinal needle, with the bevel parallel to the dural fibers, is inserted through the skin wheal in the midline and parallel to the spinous processes. Some prefer a two-handed method of advancing the needle. However, advancement of the needle with thumb and index finger of one hand while identifying the appropriate space with the fingers of the opposite hand appears to afford greater opportunity for successful lumbar puncture. The needle is angled slightly cephalad, and is advanced slowly and gently until it lodges in the supraspinous ligament. Once lodged in the supraspinous ligament, the direction which the tip of the needle will take is "fixed by the ligament," and is no longer under the control of the anesthesiologist. Any attempts to guide or change the direction of the needle tip by bending the shaft of the needle remaining outside of the patient will not be successful. The needle is slowly advanced without bending it, through the ligaments toward the dura. One often notices a "firming up" as the needle enters the ligamentum flavum, and a distinct "pop or click" as it leaves this ligament and enters the dura. If cerebrospinal fluid is not obtained, or if blood, paresthesia, or bone are encountered, the needle is withdrawn to the subcutaneous tissue and redirected, and the process of advancing the needle is repeated. If, after one or two attempts, cerebrospinal fluid is not obtained, it is best to move to another interspace. Usually, unless there is some anatomical problem, lumbar puncture is successful after one or two attempts. Time should not be wasted at an interspace that is causing problems.

Some anesthesiologists prefer to use an introducer to guide the spinal needle in the proper direction. If an introducer needle is to be used, it is inserted in the center of the skin wheal and directed along the intended path of the spinal needle, stopping short of the ligamentum flavum. The spinal needle is then inserted *via* the introducer through the ligamentum flavum and the dura, and into the subarachnoid space. If resistance is encountered, the introducer and the needle are withdrawn to the subcutaneous plane and redirected.

The incidence of post-dural puncture headache is related to needle gauge and patient age.[37, 38] A 25- or 26-gauge needle should be employed in young patients. However, 22-gauge needles may be used in elderly patients. Skill with lumbar puncture can be improved by using larger (22-gauge) needles in patients 60 yr of age and older. These larger needles facilitate lumbar puncture and help to build confidence with the technique without increasing the incidence of post-lumbar puncture headache in this age group. Once the spinal needle has entered the subarachnoid space and flow has been achieved, it is not necessary to rotate it. The volar surface of the nondominant hand is placed on the patient's back, and the hub of the needle grasped between the thumb and index finger. The syringe containing the spinal anesthetic solution is securely attached to the needle, a small amount of cerebrospinal fluid is gently aspirated to verify that the needle has not been dislodged, and the spinal anesthetic solution injected. Once the solution has been injected, the needle is removed and the patient positioned for surgery.

Paramedian or Lateral Approach

This technique is performed at a distance of 1.5–2.0 cm lateral to the midline opposite the center of the selected interspace. The needle is directed medially at an angle of approximately 25° with the midline and at right angles to the vertebral column. If bone is encountered, the needle is withdrawn slightly and then readvanced in a slightly cephalad or caudad direction. Often, the needle can be "walked" off the bone into the ligamentum flavum and, thence, into the subarachnoid space. Minimal resistance is encountered as the needle is advanced until the ligamentum flavum is reached, because the path of the needle is lateral to the supra- and interspinous ligaments. Free flow of cerebrospinal fluid indicates proper placement of the spinal needle.

The advantages of this approach are that calcified ligaments and osteophytes, often encountered in the midline in the aged patient, are avoided. Furthermore, the opening between the vertebrae through which the spinal needle passes en route to the cerebrospinal fluid is larger when approached from this direction, as compared to the midline approach. This is especially true, and may be particularly advantageous, in patients who have difficulty assuming the flexed position for lumbar puncture, e.g., pregnant patients, patients with rheumatoid arthritis, and patients in the prone position.

Taylor Approach

The lowest prominence of the posterior superior iliac spine is located and a skin wheal raised 1.0 cm medial and 1.0 cm caudad to this point. The spinal needle is directed through the skin wheal, medially and cephalad, in such a manner as to enter the spinal canal in the midline at the lumbosacral (L5–S1) interspace. As with the lateral or paramedian approach, if the needle contacts the bony sacrum, it may be "walked off" into the lumbosacral foramen.

The advantages of this technique are the same as for the lateral or paramedian approach. In addition, the Taylor approach employs the largest interspace in the vertebral column and, therefore, should be the easiest place to perform lumbar puncture. This technique has been employed to ensure low segmental levels of spinal anesthesia for urologic and rectal surgery in geriatric patients.

MECHANISM OF SPINAL AND EPIDURAL ANESTHESIA

SPINAL BLOCKADE

Nerve fibers are classified on the basis of size and degree of myelination. Size and degree of myelination, in turn, determine the conduction velocity. Fiber size is also related to function and sensitivity to local anesthetics. Table 28-4 shows the sensitivity of the various fiber types to the subarachnoid injection of procaine. The table shows the classical concept relating local anesthetic blockade to fiber size as described by Gasser and Erlanger in 1929.[39]

Recent studies in isolated nerves have suggested that the classical concept may be incorrect.[40] These studies have shown that the large myelinated fibers are more sensitive to local

TABLE 28-4. Classification of Nerve Fibers on the Basis of Fiber Size, Relating Size to Fiber Function and Sensitivity to Local Anesthetics

FIBER GROUP	DIAMETER (μm)	CONDUCTION VELOCITY (m · s⁻¹)	MODALITY SUBSERVED	SENSITIVITY TO LOCAL ANESTHETICS (Subarachnoid Procaine-%)
A (Myelinated)				
Alpha	20	100	Large motor Proprioception	1
Beta	↑	↑	Small motor Touch Pressure	1
Gamma	│	│	Muscle Spindle	1
Delta	4	5	Temperature Sharp pain	0.5
B (Myelinated)	3	3–14	Preganglionic Autonomic	0.25
C (Unmyelinated)	0.5–1	1.2	Dull pain Temperature Touch	0.5

(Reproduced with permission from Winnie AP: Differential diagnosis of pain mechanisms. In Hershey SG (ed): ASA Refresher Courses in Anesthesiology. 6:171, 1978. Copyright, 1978, The American Society of Anesthesiologists.)

anesthetic blockade than the smaller unmyelinated fibers. However, *in vivo* diffusion of local anesthetics to the membrane receptor site and interaction with those receptors are both involved in determining the apparent sensitivity of the various nerve fibers to local anesthetic blockade. Thus, in spinal anesthesia, the anatomy of the dorsal roots brings small-diameter nerve fibers close to the nerve root surface, thereby shortening the diffusion path of a drug instilled into the spinal subarachnoid space. The diffusion path to the large-diameter fibers, which are situated deep to the nerve bundle, is longer. This makes it appear that the small-diameter fibers are more susceptible to drug action than are the large-diameter fibers.

The amount of local anesthetic employed during spinal anesthesia represents an overdosage in relation to the minimum concentration required to block the various nerve fiber types. Furthermore, the distribution of the local anesthetic in the spinal subarachnoid space results in a relatively rapid blockade of all fiber types during clinical spinal anesthesia.

Spinal anesthesia is induced with the express purpose of interrupting the nociceptive A delta and C fiber afferents (dorsal roots) that subserve the pain modality. At the same time, the proprioceptive and sympathetic afferent fibers (dorsal root) and motor and sympathetic (both ventral root) nerve fibers are also blocked. Blockade of motor and proprioceptive fibers is also desirable because such blockade improves the surgical operative conditions and patient comfort. Nociceptive viscero-sensory afferent sympathetic fiber impulses traveling *via* the sympathetic trunk must also be interrupted in order that the patient remain comfortable during the surgical procedure. Since these fibers enter the spinal cord *via* the dorsal root, they are blocked along with the other fibers in this structure.

EPIDURAL BLOCKADE

The dorsal and the ventral spinal roots appear to be the primary sites of action of epidurally administered local anesthetic agents due to the unique anatomy of the membranous structures around the spinal roots. In this area, the dura mater is relatively thin and arachnoid granulations are believed to be present, which increase the surface area available for diffusion of anesthetic agents from the epidural space into the subarachnoid space.[41] Local anesthetics administered epidurally are concentrated to a greater extent in spinal roots than either the dorsal root ganglion or the spinal cord itself.[42] Additional evidence favoring the spinal roots as the initial site of action of epidurally administered local anesthetics is obtained from clinical studies evaluating the onset pattern of epidural blockade. A significant delay in onset of anesthesia at the S1 and S2 dermatomal levels is usually observed following the epidural administration of various local anesthetics.[43] In some cases, little or no anesthesia is present at the S1 and S2 levels, although adequate anesthesia is obtained above and below those dermatomes. This delay of, or failure to achieve, anesthesia in the S1–S2 region is believed related to the large size of the nerve roots in this area. The increased fiber size of the nerve roots, which is due to a greater density of connective tissue, impedes the rate of diffusion of local anesthetic agents to the nerve membrane receptor sites. The spinal cord may also represent a site of action of epidurally injected local anesthetic drugs. Tissue distribution studies following the epidural administration of labelled local anesthetics have shown that these agents can cross the dura and penetrate the spinal cord. However, the concentration of local anesthetics in the spinal

cord following epidural administration was less than that found in the spinal roots.[42] During the recovery phase from epidural blockade, analgesia regresses from the highest to the lower dermatomes in a caudad direction, similar to the regression observed following subarachnoid blockade. This suggests that spinal cord blockade does occur following epidural administration of local anesthetic agents, but the initial onset of anesthesia is probably related to inhibition of conduction in spinal roots.

PHYSIOLOGICAL EFFECTS OF SPINAL AND EPIDURAL BLOCKADE

SPINAL BLOCKADE

Spinal anesthesia profoundly affects the cardiovascular system and, to a lesser degree, the pulmonary, hepatic, renal and endocrine systems. Sympathetic nerve fiber blockade is unavoidable during spinal anesthesia. The preganglionic sympathetic nerve fibers originate in the lateral horn of the spinal cord and exit *via* the ventral roots. Because of the distribution of local anesthetic solution during the conduct of spinal anesthesia, these fibers are blocked along with the other fibers in the ventral roots.

The degree of sympathetic efferent denervation is often unpredictable, and may be quite extensive during spinal anesthesia. Since the sympathetic B fibers are among the smallest in the body, it is generally assumed that the level of sympathetic blockade during spinal anesthesia exceeds the level of sensory anesthesia level because the B fibers are more sensitive to the action of local anesthetics. Recently, Gissen *et al*[40] have shown that B fibers are blocked at intermediate concentrations and that C fibers are the most resistant to block. As mentioned above, the sympathetic fibers may be blocked to a greater extent than somatic sensory fibers because they are more peripherally located in the nerve roots than the sensory fibers.

An alternative explanation lies in the anatomy of the distribution of the sympathetic nerve fibers. Sympathetic preganglionic fibers leaving the spinal cord travel up or down segments before entering the sympathetic ganglia. Therefore, sensory blockade, for example, to the 4th thoracic dermatome may be associated with interruption of sympathetic activity as high as the first thoracic level. It has, in general, been assumed that sympathetic blockade exceeds somatic blockade by two dermatomes.[44] However, Chamberlain and Chamberlain[45] utilizing thermographic measurements of skin temperature during lidocaine or tetracaine spinal anesthesia have recently shown that skin temperature increases (assumed to represent sympathetic blockade) occurred as much as six dermatomal levels higher than the somatic sensory block. These findings may explain the profound hypotension sometimes associated with relatively low sensory levels of spinal anesthesia.

The Cardiovascular System

Numerous studies have been conducted concerning the cardiovascular effects of spinal anesthesia. For example, Ward *et al* reported that a level of spinal anesthesia to T_5 resulted in an increase in pulse rate of 3.7%.[46] Generally, spinal anesthesia is associated with a slowing of the pulse rate depending on the level of block, premedication, the patient's age, and the patient's position. Bradycardia is due to blockade of the cardio-accelerator fibers and to diminished venous return. The cardio-accelerator fibers arise from the T1–T4 dermatomes.

Levels of spinal anesthesia that include these dermatomes not only inhibit the cardiac accelerator nerves, but also result in total preganglionic sympathetic blockade that produces venodilatation and decreased venous return. The decreased venous return activates great vein and right atrial cardiac receptors that reflexly slow the heart.[47]

Ward et al also showed a decrease in mean arterial blood pressure of 21.3%, while the decline in total peripheral resistance was only 5.0%. The hypotension seen with spinal anesthesia is clearly the result of a decrease in cardiac output (17.7%). The decline in cardiac output results from venodilatation and decreased stroke volume (25.4%). It should be appreciated that all of these cardiovascular effects associated with spinal anesthesia are the direct result of preganglionic sympathetic blockade by the local anesthetic.

The Respiratory System

Many studies have shown that even high levels of spinal anesthesia have little, if any, effect on resting ventilatory mechanics.[48] Furthermore, it has also been shown that blood gas tensions are only slightly affected under these conditions.[49] On the other hand, intercostal muscle paralysis resulting from high levels of spinal anesthesia does interfere with the ability to cough and clear secretions.[50]

The Renal System

The preganglionic sympathetic innervation of the kidney arises from the T_{11}–L_1 dermatomes. Despite levels of spinal anesthesia above these dermatomes, autoregulation maintains renal blood flow as long as the mean arterial blood pressure remains greater than 80 mm Hg. Spinal anesthesia resulting in hypotension, sufficient to cause renal hypoperfusion, is accompanied by transient decreases in glomerular filtration and urinary output. Restoration of the blood pressure results in recovery of renal function.[51]

The Gastrointestinal System

The effect of spinal anesthesia on hepatic blood flow and function are minimal. Hepatic blood flow is diminished in direct proportion to any reduction in arterial blood pressure. There are no major changes in hepatic function following spinal anesthesia, even in situations where there are dramatic decreases in blood pressure, such as in cases where deliberate hypotension has been produced to minimize surgical blood loss.[52, 53]

The innervation of the bowel is both sympathetic and parasympathetic. The parasympathetic innervation arises from the vagus nerve and the hypogastric nerves (S2–S4). The sympathetic innervation comes from the T5–L1 dermatomes. Spinal anesthesia is capable of blocking all of the sympathetic fibers innervating the bowel and the hypogastric nerves. The vagus nerve, of course, will remain unblocked. The result of spinal anesthesia to the T5 dermatome is to contract the intestines, increase peristalsis and secretion, and relax sphincters. The contracted state of the bowel during spinal anesthesia may improve the surgical field.

The etiology of nausea during spinal anesthesia is poorly understood. Possible causes include the unopposed vagal activity, increased peristalsis, hypotension, cerebral hypoxia, and adjuvant medications used for sedation. If nausea is persistent, the operative conditions will obviously be poor. The combination of nausea and a high spinal blockade may in-crease the risk of aspiration, because the ability to clear secretions and protect the larynx is diminished with high spinal anesthesia.[50]

EPIDURAL BLOCKADE

Administration of local anesthetics in sufficient dosage into the epidural space will inhibit conduction of sensory, motor, and autonomic fibers. The small unmyelinated sensory fibers are usually affected initially following epidural injection due to the lack of diffusion barriers. The larger, heavily myelinated motor fibers of the A type are usually much more resistant to blockade due to the thick myelin sheath surrounding them, which serves as a barrier to the diffusion of local anesthetics. The rate of blockade of preganglionic autonomic B fibers varies according to the dosage of local anesthetic and the specific drug administered into the epidural space. Sympathetic blockade sufficient to cause systemic hypotension rarely occurs before sensory anesthesia is well established. Thus, sensory analgesia is usually the first indication of successful epidural blockade.

Hemodynamic Effects

Interruption of sympathetic impulses can lead to cardiovascular alterations following the establishment of epidural anesthesia. In most patients, cardiovascular changes are not very marked. On the other hand, profound hypotension may be observed in some patients following the onset of epidural anesthesia. The changes in blood pressure, heart rate, and cardiac output are related to the level of blockade, the amount of drug administered, the specific local anesthetic employed, the inclusion of a vasoconstrictor in the anesthetic solution, and the cardiovascular status of the patient (Fig. 28-11).

The dermatomal level of sympathetic blockade will determine the degree of hypotension following the epidural administration of local anesthetics. Blocks below T5 are seldom associated with marked hypotension due to compensatory vasoconstriction in unblocked segments. Higher blocks will not only prevent compensatory vasoconstriction, but also affect the cardiac sympathetic nerves which arise in the T1–4 segments. At these dermatomal levels of block, a fall in heart rate and cardiac output may occur. The blockade of sympathetic fibers to the heart and the failure to block the vagus nerves can cause vasovagal attacks, which are associated with profound bradycardia and, in some patients, with transient cardiac arrest. This may represent the most common cause of profound hypotension following high levels of epidural anesthesia. The venous capacitance vessels will also be affected by the sympathetic blockade. Pooling can occur if the venous return is obstructed by gravity or a pregnant uterus. Thus, patients are very susceptible to the head-up posture, which causes expansion of the capacitance vessels and can lead to a marked decrease in venous return and cardiac output.

Relatively large amounts of local anesthetic drugs are required to achieve a satisfactory degree of epidural blockade. The local anesthetic agents are absorbed rather rapidly, and may produce systemic effects involving the cardiovascular system. Most local anesthetic agents produce a biphasic effect on the cardiovascular system. For example, it has been shown that blood levels of lidocaine of less than 4 $\mu g \cdot ml^{-1}$ following epidural blockade resulted in a slight increase in blood pressure owing mainly to an increase in cardiac output. Doses of epidural lidocaine that produce blood levels in excess of 4 $\mu g \cdot ml^{-1}$ caused hypotension owing in part to the negative

% Change

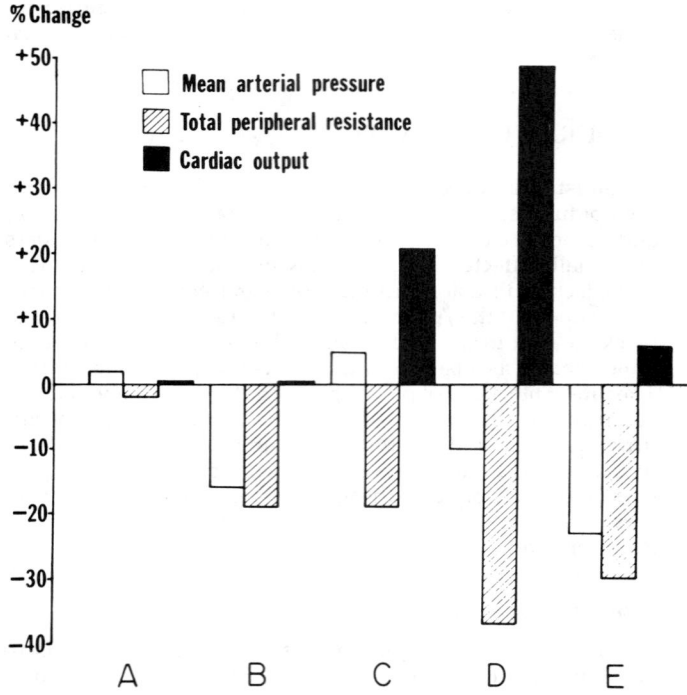

FIG. 28-11. Cardiovascular effects of epidural anesthesia as influenced by analgesic dermatomal level, epinephrine, and presence of hypovolemia. The sensory level of anesthesia was T5 at A, D, and E; T1 at B; and T2-3 at C. Epinephrine was present at D and E. Hypovolemia was present at E. (Modified and reproduced with permission: Covino BG, Vassallo HG: Local Anesthetics: Mechanism of Action and Clinical Use, p 137. New York, Grune & Stratton, 1976.)

inotropic action of lidocaine and the peripheral vasodilator effect of this agent.[54]

Differences in the onset of epidural anesthesia occur as a function of the specific agent employed. The more rapidly acting agents, such as chloroprocaine and etidocaine, tend to produce a more profound degree of hypotension due to the more rapid blockade of sympathetic fibers. In addition, certain agents, such as etidocaine, can penetrate myelinated fibers more readily and, again, may be associated with a more profound degree of sympathetic blockade and hypotension.

A more profound degree of hypotension may occur following the use of epinephrine-containing local anesthetics for epidural blockade. The absorbed epinephrine is believed to stimulate B_2-adrenergic receptors in peripheral vascular beds, leading to an enhanced state of vasodilation and a fall in diastolic pressure.[55] The B_1-adrenergic receptor stimulating effect of epinephrine results in an increase in heart rate and cardiac output that will counteract the peripheral vasodilator state to some extent. Although absorbed epinephrine may be responsible for the early cardiovascular changes observed following epidural block, the more prolonged hypotension seen with local anesthetics containing epinephrine is probably related to the achievement of a more profound degree of sympathetic blockade.

Cardiovascular depression is more severe and more dangerous following the production of epidural anesthesia in hypovolemic subjects.[56] Epidural anesthesia in mildly hypovolemic volunteers was associated with profound hypotension and bradycardia. Hypovolemia is usually accompanied by compensatory vasoconstriction, which will be abolished by the block, and cardiovascular collapse may ensue. The addition of epinephrine to the anesthetic solution may result in a less profound degree of hypotension in hypovolemic subjects. However, even the positive inotropic and chronotropic action of absorbed epinephrine cannot completely counteract the

hypotensive effect of epidural blockade owing to the reduced circulating blood volume in these patients.

Effects on Regional Blood Flow

The sympathetic nervous system plays an important part in regulating regional blood flow. Blockade of sympathetic nerve fibers and resulting loss of vasomotor tone will, therefore, cause considerable changes in the distribution of cardiac output, and epidural anesthesia will produce significant changes in blood flow to various organs, depending on the level of blockade achieved. Investigations in monkeys have shown that a T10 dermatomal level of anesthesia resulted in an increase in lower limb blood flow, but no significant change in coronary, cerebral, renal, or hepatic blood flow.[57] High levels (T1) of epidural blockade caused a 55% decrease in coronary blood flow. This decrease in coronary blood flow occurred concomitantly with a 47% decrease in mean arterial blood pressure. The decrease in myocardial work was greater than the decrease in coronary flow. The low coronary flows may be related, in part, to extensive sympathetic blockade or to the peripheral vasodilator effect of lidocaine, both of which will cause systemic hypotension and decreased coronary perfusion.

A significant decrease in cerebral blood flow of approximately 35% was also observed following achievement of a T1 dermatomal level of epidural anesthesia. Normally, cerebral blood flow is maintained constant owing to autoregulation, but, below a critical arterial pressure, the blood flow decreases and is compensated for by increased oxygen extraction from the arterial blood.

Renal blood flow also decreased significantly following attainment of a T1 level of epidural anesthesia in the monkey studies. A 31–37% decrease in renal blood flow occurred at the time when mean arterial blood pressure and cardiac output were markedly reduced, suggesting that renal autoregulation may also be affected by hypotension.

Significant decreases in total hepatic blood flow of 20–40% were observed following achievement of a T1 level of anesthesia. These changes in hepatic blood flow followed a 14–47% decrease in mean arterial pressure.

Limited studies have been conducted in man with regard to regional blood flow during epidural anesthesia. A 14% decrease in renal blood flow was observed in volunteers when a T5 level of epidural blockade was produced.[58] This change in renal blood flow occurred despite the lack of a significant decrease in mean arterial pressure and cardiac output. On the other hand, hepatic blood flow changes during epidural anesthesia in man parallel changes in mean arterial pressure.

The effect of epidural blockade on blood flow in the lower limbs below the level of blockade is predictable. A marked increase in blood flow in the lower limbs below the level of block is accompanied by a compensatory decrease in blood flow in the upper limbs above the level of blockade.[59] As a result, blood pressure may not change very much with a low level of epidural anesthesia. However, high levels of epidural blockade will cause inhibition of sympathetic outflow to both upper and lower limbs, resulting in extensive vasodilation and a marked decrease in peripheral vascular resistance. Under these conditions, limb blood flow will be directly related to the patient's blood pressure.

PHARMACOLOGICAL CONSIDERATIONS

SPINAL ANESTHESIA

The selection of a specific local anesthetic for spinal anesthesia is related to a number of factors, such as:

1. The desired segmental level of sensory anesthesia.
2. The duration of the surgical procedure.
3. The intensity of the motor blockade desired.

Greene[60] has recently reviewed the factors which are believed to influence the distribution of local anesthetics in the cerebrospinal fluid (Table 28-5). The density of the local anesthetic solution, the shape of the spinal canal, and the position of the patient are probably the most important factors involved.[61]

Density, Specific Gravity, and Baricity

Local anesthetics used for spinal anesthesia are described as hypobaric, isobaric, or hyperbaric. Hypobaric solutions are less dense than cerebrospinal fluid, while isobaric and hyperbaric solutions are equally dense and more dense than cerebrospinal fluid, respectively.

Density is the weight in grams of 1 ml of a solution $(g \cdot ml^{-1})$ at a specific temperature.

Specific gravity is the ratio of the density of a solution at a specific temperature to the density of water at that same temperature.

Baricity is the ratio of the density of a (local anesthetic) solution at a specific temperature to the density of cerebrospinal fluid at that same temperature.[60] Some authors have used specific gravity to determine the baricity of local anesthetic solutions. Baricity, in this case, is the ratio of the specific gravity of a local anesthetic solution at a specific temperature to the specific gravity of cerebrospinal fluid at the same tem-

TABLE 28-5. Factors Influencing Distribution of Local Anesthetics in Cerebrospinal Fluid*

PATIENT CHARACTERISTICS
Age
Height
Weight
Gender
Intraabdominal pressure
Anatomic configuration of spinal column
Position

TECHNIQUE OF INJECTION
Site of injection
Direction of injection
  Direction of needle
  Direction of bevel
Turbulence
  Rate of injection
  Barbotage

DIFFUSION

CHARACTERISTICS OF SPINAL FLUID
Composition
Circulation
Volume
Pressure
Density

CHARACTERISTICS OF ANESTHETIC SOLUTION
Density
Hypobaric solutions
Isobaric solutions
Hyperbaric solutions
Amount of anesthetic
Concentration of anesthetic
Volume injected
  Isobaric solutions
  Hypobaric solutions
  Hyperbaric solutions
Vasoconstrictors

*Hypothetical or demonstrable.
(Reproduced with permission from Greene NM: Distribution of local anesthetic solutions within the spinal subarachnoid space. Anesth Analg 64:715, 1985.)

perature. This is less accurate than determining baricity from density.

An isobaric local anesthetic solution has a baricity of unity, while hypobaric and hyperbaric solutions have baricities less than and greater than unity, respectively. It is important to note that density varies inversely with temperature. Therefore, a local anesthetic that has the same density as cerebrospinal fluid at 37° C[62] will be more dense (hyperbaric) at room temperature than cerebrospinal fluid at 37° C. However, the clinically important density of local anesthetic solutions is that which is measured at 37° C because, during spinal anesthesia, local anesthetic solutions rapidly equilibrate with the temperature of cerebrospinal fluid.[63]

The density of normal human cerebrospinal fluid with 95% confidence limits at 37° C is 1.0001 to 1.0005. Therefore, local anesthetic solutions with baricity less than 0.9998 (99.9% confidence limits) at 37° C will be hypobaric in *all* patients. Similarly, local anesthetic solutions at 37° C with baricity greater than 1.0008 (99.9% confidence limits) will be reliably hyperbaric in *all* patients. Because of the normal variability in the density of cerebrospinal fluid, it is difficult to precisely know that a local anesthetic solution will, in fact, be isobaric in *all* patients. Nevertheless, local anesthetic solutions with densities between 0.9998 and 1.0008 behave functionally as if they have the same density as cerebrospinal fluid.[60]

The local anesthetics most commonly used for spinal anesthesia in the United States are lidocaine, bupivacaine, and tetracaine (Table 28-6). Procaine is also available for spinal anesthesia, but is not widely used.

Dibucaine is a popular spinal anesthesia agent outside of the USA. However, in the USA, it is no longer available.

Local anesthetic solutions used for spinal anesthesia are generally formulated with sodium chloride to make them isotonic. Solutions without added glucose are either isobaric (lidocaine, tetracaine, and dibucaine) or are very close to isobaric (bupivacaine is very slightly hypobaric). Procaine that is formulated as a 10% solution for spinal anesthesia is hyperbaric. Hyperbaric solutions of lidocaine, tetracaine, bupivacaine, and dibucaine are prepared by adding glucose in sufficient quantity to increase their density to greater than 1.0008. Other agents may be used to make a local anesthetic solution hyperbaric. For example, 1% tetracaine is sometimes made hyperbaric by mixing it in a 1:1 ratio with 10% procaine. Hypobaric solutions of procaine, tetracaine, and dibucaine are prepared by diluting them with distilled water to a density of less than 0.9998. Dilution of lidocaine with distilled water to make it hypobaric results in concentrations of lidocaine too low to provide adequate spinal anesthesia. The adequacy of spinal anesthesia with hypobaric solution of bupivacaine is not well documented at this time. Table 28-6 summarizes the density and baricity of the commonly used spinal anesthetic solutions.

Effect of Baricity and Patient Position on Spinal Anesthesia

Utilizing an *in vitro* model of the spinal canal and injecting local anesthetic solutions colored with methylene blue dye, one can observe the effect of baricity, gravity (patient position), shape of the spinal canal, etc., on the distribution of local anesthetics within the spinal subarachnoid space. Isobaric solutions remain in the vicinity of the injection site, hyperbaric solutions gravitate to dependent areas, and hypobaric solutions "float" to the least dependent areas. The shape of the average human spinal canal with the patient in the supine position is such that there is a lumbar lordosis (high point) at the L3–4 interspace and a thoracic kyphosis (low point) at the T5–6 interspace (Fig. 28-12). These curves will influence the distribution of hyperbaric and hypobaric solutions within the spinal subarachnoid space. The distribution of isobaric solutions are unaffected by the shape of the spinal canal.

For surgical procedures performed in other than the supine position, the baricity of the local anesthetic solution and gravity have been employed to "direct" the local anesthetic towards the spinal nerves innervating the surgical site. For example, hemorrhoidectomy with the patient in the lithotomy position is often performed under "saddle block" spinal anesthesia. This is accomplished by administering a hyperbaric local anesthetic solution with the patient in the sitting position and allowing the solution to gravitate to the sacral nerves. Alternatively, hemorrhoidectomy in the prone jackknife position and hip surgery in the lateral recumbent position are often performed under hypobaric spinal anesthesia. In these cases, the spinal anesthesia is performed with the patient positioned for the surgical procedure that results in the surgical site (and the spinal nerves to be anesthetized) being uppermost. After injection, the hypobaric solution "floats" up to the nerves innervating the surgical site. These relationships are illustrated in Figure 28-13. It is important to note that surgery performed on areas innervated by nerves below the L1 dermatomes may be easily performed with an isobaric solution. Since these solutions are unaffected by patient position, the spinal anesthesia can be induced in the most convenient position for the patient and the anesthesiologist. The patient can then be turned to the position dictated by the surgical procedure. Because spinal nerves L1 to S5 pass through the cerebrospinal fluid into which the isobaric solution is injected, anesthesia in all of these dermatomes will result (Fig. 28-14).

TABLE 28-6. Density and Baricity of Local Anesthetics Commonly Used for Spinal Anesthesia

AGENT	USUAL CONC (%)	GLUCOSE CONC (%)	DENSITY (37° C)	BARICITY (37° C)
CSF			1.0003	1.0000
Procaine	2.5	DW	0.9986	0.9983 (HO)
Procaine	10.0		1.0107	1.0104 (H)
Lidocaine	2.0	S	1.0007	1.0004 (I)
Lidocaine	5.0	7.5	1.0265	1.0262 (H)
Bupivacaine	0.5	S	0.9993	0.9990 (HO*)
Bupivacaine	0.75	8.25	1.0230 (CAL)	1.0227 (H)
Tetracaine	<0.33	DW	<0.9980	<0.9977 (HO)
Tetracaine	0.5	S	1.0000	0.9997 (HO*)
Tetracaine	0.5	5.0	1.0136	1.0133 (H)
Dibucaine	0.66	S	0.9967	0.9964 (HO)
Dibucaine	0.5	S	0.9992	0.9990 (HO*)
Dibucaine	0.25	5.0	1.0111	1.0108 (H)

CSF = cerebrospinal fluid; CSF density (37° C) 99.9% confidence limits = 0.9998–1.0008. Dibucaine is no longer manufactured. DW = distilled water; S = saline; HO = hypobaric; I = isobaric; H = hyperbaric; HO* = solution considered to be clinically isobaric; CAL = approximate value calculated from specific gravity.

(Reproduced with permission from Lambert DH, Covino BG: Hyperbaric, hypobaric and isobaric spinal anesthesia. Res Staff Phys 33:79, 1987.)

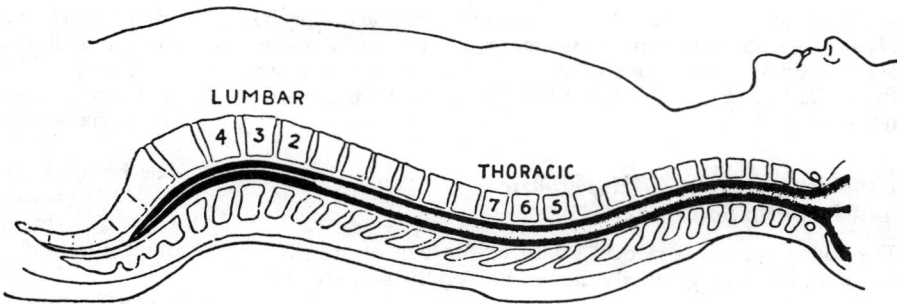

FIG. 28-12. The shape of the spinal canal with the patient in the supine horizontal position. The lumbar lordosis produces a high point at L3, while the thoracic kyphosis produces a low point at T6. (Reproduced with permission: Lee JA, Atkinson RS: Sir Robert MacIntosh's Lumbar Puncture and Spinal Analgesia: Intradural and Extradural, p 138. Edinburgh, Churchill Livingstone, 1978.)

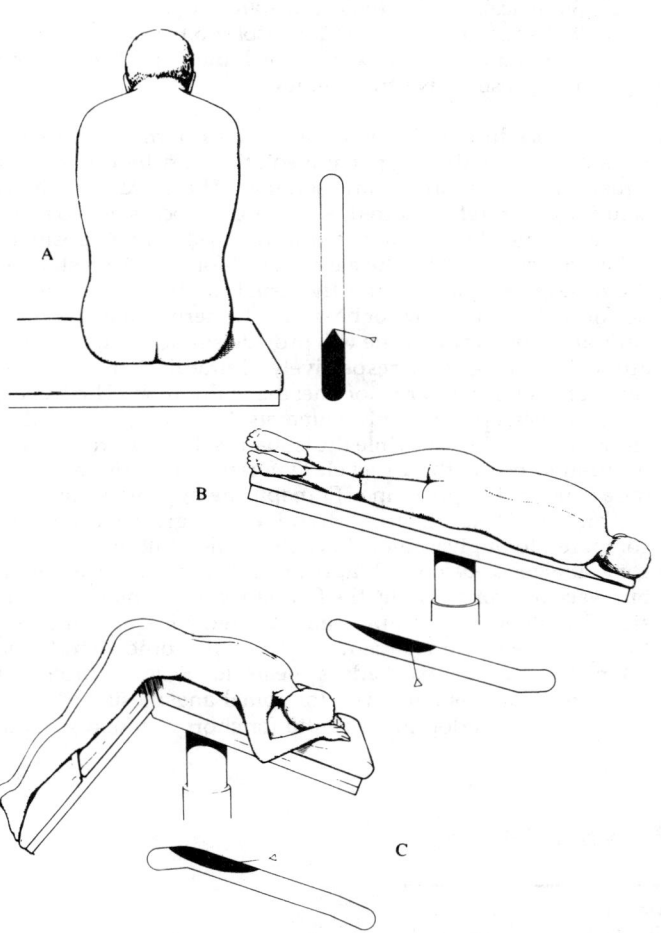

FIG. 28-13. The effect of position and baricity on the distribution of a local anesthetic in the spinal subarachnoid space. The tubular figures to the right are meant to represent the dural sac, which contains the cerebrospinal fluid. The darkened areas indicate the disposition of the local anesthetic solution. (A) The patient is in the seated position undergoing "saddle block." A hyperbaric solution, which gravitates to the most dependent area, is used. (B) The patient is in the right lateral recumbent position with head-down tilt for left hip surgery. A hypobaric solution that "floats" to the uppermost area is employed. (C) The patient is in the prone jackknife position for rectal surgery. Again, a hypobaric solution is used. All three procedures could be done equally well with an isobaric solution. Isobaric solutions are unaffected by position and remain localized to the site of injection. (Reproduced with permission: Lambert DH, Covino BG: Hyperbaric, hypobaric and isobaric spinal anesthesia. Res Staff Phys 33:79, 1987. Copyright, 1987 Romaine Pierson Publishers.)

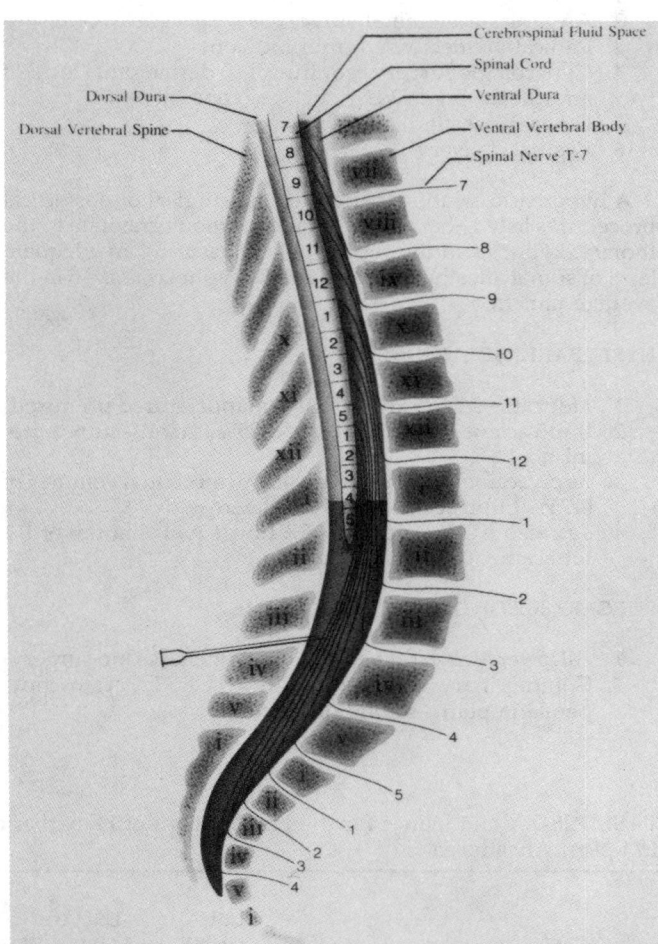

FIG. 28-14. Longitudinal section through the distal portion of the vertebral column and spinal cord. Notice that the spinal cord terminates at the L-1 vertebral body, and that the spinal nerves extend downward for considerable distances before exiting beneath their respective vertebral bodies. Isobaric local anesthetics injected into the spinal subarachnoid space at the L3-4 interspace clinically occupy the darkened area and block all spinal nerves distal to L-1. Furthermore, isobaric solutions tend to remain localized and are unaffected by patient position. (Reproduced with permission: Lambert DH, Covino BG: Hyperbaric, hypobaric and isobaric spinal anesthesia. Res Staff Phys 33:79, 1987. Copyright, 1987 Romaine Pierson Publishers.)

Hyperbaric solutions of lidocaine and tetracaine are probably the most common solutions employed for spinal anesthesia. Hyperbaric solutions achieved their popularity because of the belief that it is easier to control the spread of these solutions.

Guidelines for Use of Hyperbaric and Isobaric Solutions

The following is a practical guide to the use of anesthetic solutions of varying baricity, depending on the surgical site.[64]

SURGERY ABOVE THE L1 DERMATOME

1. Hernias
2. Any intra-abdominal surgery
3. Radical orchiectomy (groin incision)
4. Gynecologic surgery requiring T10 dermatomal level of anesthesia (e.g., D&C, circlage, cone biopsy)
5. Cesarean section
6. Vaginal delivery

A hyperbaric solution is used for the surgical or obstetrical procedures listed above. Hyperbaric solutions gravitate to the thoracic kyphosis in the supine patient assuring an adequate level of spinal anesthesia. The thoracic kyphosis is at T6 in the average patient.

HYPERBARIC SOLUTIONS

1. Lidocaine 5%, dextrose 7.5% (manufactured premixed)
2. Bupivacaine 0.75%, dextrose 8.25% (manufactured premixed)
3. Bupivacaine 0.375%, dextrose 5% (mix equal volumes of 0.75% bupivacaine and 10% dextrose)
4. Tetracaine 0.5%, dextrose 5% (mix equal volumes of 1% tetracaine and 10% dextrose)

SURGERY BELOW THE L1 DERMATOME

1. All lower limb orthopedic surgery (includes hip surgery)
2. Genitourinary surgery (TURP, TURBT, cystoscopy, penile implant, scrotal orchiectomy)

3. Perineal surgery (Bartholin cyst)
4. Lower limb vascular surgery (femoral-popliteal bypass graft)
5. Amputations of the lower limbs
6. Rectal surgery

For the surgical procedures listed above, an isobaric solution is ideal. As indicated above, these solutions tend to remain in the lower dermatomes, providing intense anesthesia of prolonged duration.

ISOBARIC SOLUTIONS

1. Lidocaine 2% (epidural solution)
2. Bupivacaine 0.5% (epidural solution)
3. Bupivacaine 0.75% (epidural solution)
4. Tetracaine 0.5% (mix equal volumes of 1% tetracaine and preservative free saline)

Any procedure performed below the L1 dermatome that is usually done with a hypobaric solution can be carried out equally well with an isobaric solution. Therefore, hypobaric solutions are rarely required, except for the occasional patient in whom anesthesia is induced in the "jack-knife" position. Table 28-7 summarizes the agents used for spinal anesthesia, the dosages employed, and the usual durations for surgery performed at sites above or below the L1 dermatomes. Hyperbaric and isobaric lidocaine will provide surgical anesthesia of approximately 1–2 h, respectively. Tetracaine and bupivacaine are similar in terms of anesthetic duration. The hyperbaric solutions provide approximately 2 h of surgical anesthesia above the L1 level, while the isobaric solutions provide 3–4 h duration below the L1 level. Differences do exist between tetracaine and bupivacaine. Epinephrine appears to prolong the anesthetic duration of tetracaine to a greater extent, as compared to bupivacaine, above the L1 dermatome.[65, 66] Sensory analgesia below L1 appears more pronounced with bupivacaine. For example, the frequency of tourniquet pain is significantly lower in bupivacaine-treated patients compared to tetracaine-treated patients.[67, 68] On the other hand, the intensity of motor blockade appears to be more profound when tetracaine is employed for spinal anesthesia.

In summary, lidocaine is useful for short-duration surgical

TABLE 28-7.   Guidelines for the Employment of Hyperbaric and Isobaric Solutions In Spinal Anesthesia

SURGICAL SITE	SOLUTION	CONC (%)	USUAL DOSE (mg)	USUAL VOLUME (ml)	USUAL DURATION NO EPI* (hours)	USUAL DURATION 0.2 mg EPI (hours)
ABOVE L1: HYPERBARIC	Bupivacaine	0.75	10–15	1.5–2	2	2
	Tetracaine	0.5	10–15	2–3	3	3
	Lidocaine	5.0	50–75	1–1.5	1	1
BELOW L1: ISOBARIC	Bupivacaine	0.5	15	3	3–4	4–6
	Tetracaine	0.5	15	3	3–4	4–6
	Lidocaine	2.0	60	3	1–2	2–4

* EPI = Epinephrine.
Isobaric solutions of bupivacaine and lidocaine are not yet approved by the FDA for spinal anesthesia. However, this use has been reported in numerous publications. Solutions intended for spinal anesthesia should NOT contain any preservatives or antioxidants, such as methylparaben, sodium bisulfite, or sodium metabisulfite.
(Reproduced with permission from Lambert DH, Covino BG: Hyperbaric, hypobaric and isobaric spinal anesthesia. Res Staff Phys 33:79, 1987.)

and obstetrical procedures, i.e., 30–90 min. Hyperbaric tetracaine is probably still the most useful solution for abdominal surgical procedures of 2–4 h duration. Isobaric bupivacaine is particularly valuable for lower limb vascular and orthopedic procedures of 2–5 h duration.

Vasoconstrictors

Epinephrine or phenylephrine are frequently added to local anesthetics to prolong the duration of spinal anesthesia. Vasoconstrictors are believed to prolong spinal anesthesia by constriction of blood vessels supplying the dura and the spinal cord, which results in decreased spinal cord and dural blood flow. This, in turn, leads to decreased vascular absorption of the local anesthetic and, therefore, more of the local anesthetic remains in contact with the neural tissue for a longer period, creating a more intense and prolonged neural blockade. The dose of epinephrine (1:1000) used to extend the duration of spinal anesthesia is usually 0.2–0.3 ml (200–300 µg). The recommended dosage for phenylephrine (1% solution) is 0.2–0.5 ml (2–5 mg).

The ability of vasoconstrictors to prolong the duration of spinal anesthesia may vary, depending on the specific local anesthetic employed. Epinephrine and phenylephrine have been shown to prolong the duration of spinal anesthesia induced with tetracaine.[65] It has been reported that epinephrine does not significantly prolong two- and four-segment (lower thoracic) regression of spinal anesthesia with lidocaine and bupivacaine.[66, 69] Nevertheless, the duration of anesthesia in the lumbar and sacral dermatomes was prolonged by the addition of epinephrine to lidocaine and bupivacaine. Other studies have demonstrated that vasoconstrictors can significantly prolong the duration of lidocaine- and bupivacaine-induced spinal anesthesia.[70–73]

Kozody et al[74–76] have shown that lidocaine and tetracaine increased, whereas bupivacaine decreased, spinal cord and dural blood flow in dogs. Tetracaine was responsible for the greatest increase in blood flow. Epinephrine was found to inhibit the increase in spinal cord and dural blood flow produced by lidocaine and tetracaine. These results suggest that epinephrine should markedly prolong the action of tetracaine and moderately increase the duration of lidocaine, but not alter the duration of bupivacaine.

Epinephrine and phenylephrine are believed to prolong spinal anesthesia primarily by vasoconstriction. However, a direct antinociceptive effect in the spinal cord may also be operative.[77] The most profound effect of adding a vasoconstrictor to the spinal anesthetic solution occurs in the lumbo-sacral region. This is most likely due to the fact that the concentration of the local anesthetic and the vasoconstrictor are greatest here simply because this is the customary site of injection.

In general, vasoconstrictors appear useful in prolonging the duration of spinal anesthesia below L1 with all local anesthetic agents. Thus, the duration of spinal anesthesia for orthopedic or vascular procedures in the lower extremities may be prolonged by the addition of a vasoconstrictor to lidocaine, bupivacaine, and tetracaine. However, for abdominal surgical procedures, vasoconstrictors added to lidocaine or bupivacaine may not be as efficacious as they are with tetracaine in terms of prolonging anesthetic duration.

EPIDURAL ANESTHESIA

Local anesthetic agents intended for epidural (Table 28-8) use may be classified as follows: 1) agents of low anesthetic potency and short duration of action (chloroprocaine); 2) agents of intermediate anesthetic potency and duration of action (lidocaine, mepivacaine, and prilocaine); and 3) agents of high anesthetic potency and prolonged duration of action (bupivacaine and etidocaine).[78] In terms of latency, chloroprocaine, lidocaine, mepivacaine, prilocaine, and etidocaine possess a relatively rapid onset of action. Bupivacaine has a relatively slow onset of anesthesia. Procaine and tetracaine are rarely used for epidural blockade because of their slow onset of action.

Chloroprocaine has enjoyed popularity as an epidural anesthetic agent for obstetrical use. This local anesthetic is characterized by a rapid onset time and a wide therapeutic ratio in terms of systemic toxicity for mother and fetus. The very short duration of chloroprocaine limits its usefulness for surgical epidural anesthesia, except for short ambulatory procedures or unless a catheter technique is employed.

Lidocaine, mepivacaine, and prilocaine are similar in terms of their anesthetic profile when used for epidural blockade. Lidocaine may possess a slightly shorter onset time, while mepivacaine and prilocaine produce a longer duration of anesthesia than lidocaine when these drugs are used without a vasoconstrictor. Prilocaine is systemically the least toxic of the various amide local anesthetics. Unfortunately, doses above 600 mg are associated with the formation of methemaglobinemia that has limited the use of this drug. Nevertheless, it is an excellent local anesthetic if such doses are not exceeded.

Bupivacaine and etidocaine are employed as epidural drugs of relatively long duration. They differ considerably in their anesthetic profile, although they are both potent, long-acting

TABLE 28-8.   Agents for Epidural Blockade

AGENT	USUAL CONCENTRATION (%)	USUAL ONSET (min)	USUAL DURATION OF SURGICAL ANESTHESIA	MAIN CLINICAL USE
Chloroprocaine	2–3	5–15	30–90	Obstetrics
Lidocaine	1–2	5–15	60–120	Obstetrics Surgery
Mepivacaine	1–2	5–15	60–150	Surgery
Prilocaine	1–3	5–15	60–150	Surgery
Bupivacaine	0.25–0.75	10–20	120–140	Obstetrics Surgery
Etidocaine	1–1.5	5–15	120–240	Surgery

local anesthetics. Bupivacaine is widely used for both surgical and obstetrical epidural anesthesia. It is of particular value for continuous epidural blockade during labor. When used as a 0.25% solution, it provides satisfactory sensory analgesia with minimal motor blockade. The 0.5% solution is also used during labor, but at the expense of greater motor blockade. Thus, the patient in labor can be rendered pain free and still be able to move her legs. In addition, bupivacaine usually provides 1–3 h of adequate analgesia, although this depends greatly on the dosage. The onset of anesthesia is relatively slow, frequently requiring 15–20 min for development of an adequate epidural blockade. For surgical procedures, the 0.75% concentration of bupivacaine appears more useful than the 0.25% or 0.5% solution. The latency is shortened, the depth of analgesia is more profound, and skeletal muscle relaxation is improved. However, 0.75% bupivacaine is no longer recommended for obstetrical anesthesia due to reports of severe cardiotoxic reactions.

Etidocaine is especially useful for surgical procedures. When used as a 1.5% solution, this drug provides the most rapid onset of any local anesthetic administered epidurally. Initial signs of analgesia appear in 3–5 min, and may be complete in 10 min. Etidocaine shows little sensory/motor discrimination. Thus, dosages of this drug that provide satisfactory analgesia invariably produce profound motor blockade. In surgical situations in which optimal skeletal muscle relaxation is desirable, etidocaine has proven to be a valuable local anesthetic for epidural use, since it combines a rapid onset, duration of 3–4 h, and a satisfactory quality of analgesia combined with profound skeletal muscle relaxation. However, this marked effect on motor function renders etidocaine of limited value for obstetrical analgesia.

The quality of epidural blockade will be influenced primarily by the local anesthetic employed. Other factors that may influence the adequacy of epidural blockade include: 1) dose, volume, and concentration of the local anesthetic agent; 2) addition of a vasoconstrictor to the local anesthetic solution; 3) site and speed of injection; 4) patient position; and 5) patient age, height, and clinical status.

Dose, Volume, and Concentration of the Local Anesthetic Agent

The volume of the anesthetic solution administered into the epidural space may influence the vertical spread of anesthesia. For example, 30 ml of 1% lidocaine produced a level of analgesia following lumbar epidural administration that was 4.3 dermatomes higher than that achieved by 10 ml of 3% lidocaine.[79] However, the relationship between spread and volume of local anesthetic solution is neither linear nor predictable. The essential qualities of epidural anesthesia, that is, onset, depth, and duration of sensory analgesia and motor blockade, are related to the mass of drug, rather than variations in volume or concentration of solution. For example, a comparison of 600 mg of prilocaine administered epidurally either as 30 ml of a 2% solution or 20 ml of a 3% solution failed to show any difference in onset, adequacy, or duration of anesthesia, and onset, depth, and duration of motor blockade.[80] An increase in the dosage of local anesthetic administered epidurally will tend to decrease the onset time, increase the frequency of satisfactory anesthesia, and significantly prolong the duration of anesthesia (Fig. 28-15). Studies with bupivacaine administered epidurally in obstetrics have shown that increasing the concentration from 0.125% to 0.5% while maintaining the same volume of injection shortened the latency time, improved the incidence of satisfactory analgesia, and increased the duration of sensory anesthesia. In addition, the degree and duration of motor blockade was also enhanced by an increase in the concentration and dosage of bupivacaine.[81]

Addition of a Vasoconstrictor

Epinephrine is frequently added to local anesthetic solutions intended for epidural administration in order to increase the depth of blockade and significantly prolong the duration of anesthesia. The effect of epinephrine is believed to be related primarily to its effects on the local vasculature, which causes a decrease in absorption of the local anesthetic. Thus, more of

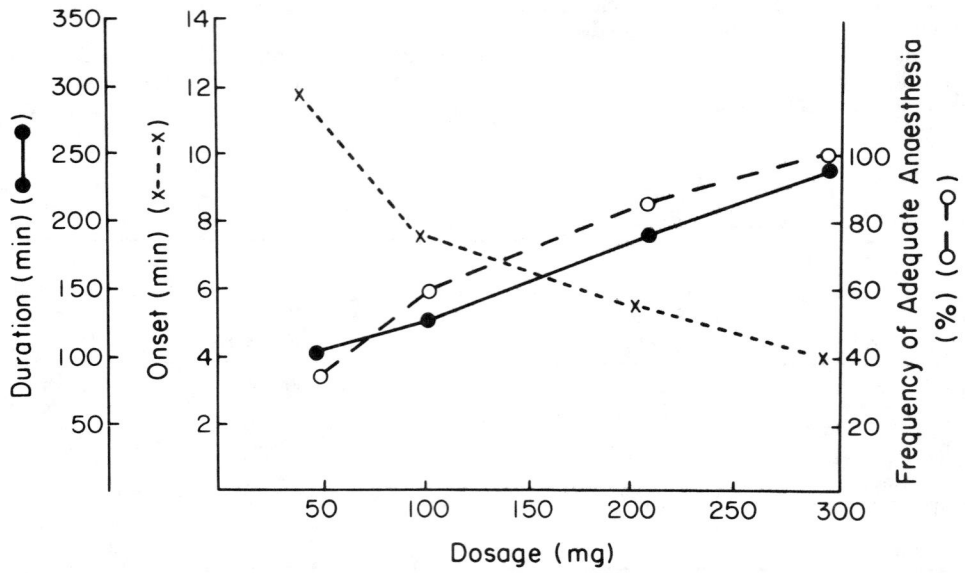

FIG. 28-15. Illustrating the effect of increasing dosage of local anesthetic agent on the onset, duration, and frequency of adequate anesthesia during epidural anesthesia. The figure shows that increasing the dose decreases the onset time, while increasing the duration and frequency of adequate anesthesia.

the drug remains in the epidural space and is available for diffusion to the spinal roots and cord to produce a more profound degree and longer duration of anesthesia. A 1:200,000 (5 $\mu g \cdot ml^{-1}$) concentration of epinephrine is usually employed when used in conjunction with a drug such as lidocaine. While other vasoconstrictor drugs, such as phenylephrine, have also been used as additives to solutions of local anesthetics intended for epidural anesthesia, the available evidence suggests that epinephrine is the most effective vasoconstrictor.[82]

Prilocaine, bupivacaine, and etidocaine administered epidurally do not appear to benefit as much as lidocaine or mepivacaine from the addition of epinephrine. In the case of bupivacaine, the effect of epinephrine on the frequency and duration of adequate anesthesia is dependent on the concentration of bupivacaine employed for epidural blockade. The frequency of adequate anesthesia and/or the duration of sensory analgesia is improved when epinephrine 1:200,000 is added to 0.125% and 0.25% bupivacaine for epidural blockade in obstetrical patients.[81] However, the addition of epinephrine to 0.5% and 0.75% bupivacaine intended for epidural use in either obstetrical or surgical patients is not associated with a significant improvement in the frequency of adequate anesthesia.[81, 83] The duration was prolonged in some studies, but not in others.[83, 84] Addition of epinephrine to either bupivacaine or etidocaine does appear to increase the profoundness of motor blockade.[83]

Site and Speed of Injection

Injection of local anesthetics into different epidural sites will produce marked differences in the spread of anesthesia. For example, injections of small volumes, i.e., 3–5 ml, into the relatively narrow midthoracic epidural space results in a discrete but wide segmental blockade. Lumbar epidural administration usually requires the use of volumes of 15–25 ml to achieve surgical anesthesia. Cephalad spread occurs more easily than caudad spread following lumbar epidural injections, due in part to the negative intrathoracic pressure and to the resistance afforded by the narrowing of the epidural space at the lumbosacral junction. A significant delay and/or absence of analgesia at the first and second sacral segments is frequently observed following lumbar epidural injections. This has been attributed in part to the narrowing of the epidural space at the lumbosacral junction, and also to the thickness of the spinal roots in this area.[43] Caudal anesthesia usually requires greater amounts of drug due to loss of solution through the anterior sacral foramina and the rapid vascular absorption from this site. Little cephalad spread beyond the lumbosacral junction occurs following caudal injections because of the peculiar anatomy of the epidural space in this region.

Rate of injection appears to have little effect on the profile of epidural anesthesia. Twenty milliliters of 2% lidocaine injected into the lumbar epidural space at a rate of $1 \, ml \cdot s^{-1}$ and $1 \, ml \cdot s^{-1}$ did not influence the duration of anesthesia or motor block or the level of anesthesia in a clinically significant manner.[79] Greater patient discomfort may be associated with the rapid injection of local anesthetics into the epidural space.

Patient Position

Posture was originally thought to influence the spread of epidural analgesia.[85] However, studies involving the use of radioisotopes administered into the epidural space failed to demonstrate any effect of posture on the spread of these materials in the epidural space.[86] Controversy exists concerning the onset of sensory anesthesia following the epidural administration of local anesthetics to patients in the sitting or lateral decubitus position. Some studies have suggested a greater spread in patients in the lateral decubitus position.[85] Other investigators have failed to confirm these findings.[87] In general, patient position per se does not appear to predictably influence the spread or duration of epidural anesthesia in a fashion similar to that following the administration of local anesthetics into the subarachnoid space.

Age, Height, and Pregnancy

Discrepancies exist between studies that evaluated the influence of age and height of patients on the spread of anesthetics in the epidural space.[87, 88] Originally, the level of epidural blockade was reported to be related to height and age. Other investigators have failed to demonstrate any correlation between age, height, and spread of epidurally administered local anesthetics. More recent studies comparing the spread of anesthetic solution in patients of varying age have shown little correlation between the maximal dermatomal analgesic level obtained and the age of patients up to the age of 40 yr.[89] Patients 40 yr and older did show a greater spread of epidural anesthesia compared to patients less than 40 yr of age when the volume and dose of local anesthetic solution was the same in both groups. However, the mean difference between the various age groups was only two to three segments.

Pregnancy is believed to affect the level of epidural anesthesia. For example, similar levels of anesthesia were obtained following the use of 6–10 ml of 2% lidocaine in obstetrical patients and 15–30 ml of 2% lidocaine in nonpregnant patients.[90] This difference is believed to be related to inferior vena caval compression in pregnancy, which results in a marked distention of the epidural venous plexi. Recent studies suggest that the greater sensitivity and spread of epidural anesthetics in pregnant patients may be related to hormonal, rather than mechanical, factors. The dose per segment requirements of epidurally administered local anesthetics was decreased in patients during their first trimester of pregnancy compared to a similar group of non-pregnant patients.[91] Since distention of venous plexi by inferior vena caval occlusion is not a factor at this early stage of pregnancy, the increased sensitivity to local anesthetics is believed related to hormonal influences. Moreover, isolated nerve studies have confirmed a more rapid onset of conduction blockade and a greater sensitivity to local anesthetics in nerves from pregnant rabbits compared to nerves from non-pregnant animals.[92, 93]

COMPLICATIONS OF SPINAL AND EPIDURAL ANESTHESIA

SPINAL BLOCKADE

Complications associated with spinal anesthesia may be classified as minor or major. Minor complications consist of limited, transient alterations in physiologic function. Hypotension, the high spinal with depression of ventilation, postdural puncture headache, and back pain fall in the minor complication category. The major complication category consists largely of neurologic injuries—isolated nerve injuries, meningitis, and cauda equina syndrome. Fortunately, the major complications of spinal anesthesia occur infrequently. Although the minor complications occur with greater frequency, they are, in general, easy to manage.

Hypotension

Hypotension during spinal anesthesia is the result of decreased cardiac output, which is, in turn, the result of decreased venous return. The amount of venous pooling and, therefore, decreased venous return is directly related to the degree of sympathectomy in turn related to the level of the spinal blockade. The degree of hypotension that can be tolerated depends on the age and physical status of the patient. Elderly patients with cardiac and cerebrovascular disease may be at risk, if the blood pressure is allowed to decline to low levels during spinal anesthesia. Although the absolute level of hypotension that can be tolerated by these patients is not known, it is probably best to not allow the mean blood pressure to decline more than 20% in these individuals.

In pregnancy, placental perfusion is dependent upon maternal blood pressure. Maintaining maternal mean blood pressure above 100 mm Hg will ensure placental perfusion and improve fetal outcome. On the other hand, young, healthy, nonpregnant individuals may experience greater falls in blood pressure without ill effects.

Attention to a few details will minimize the occurrence of hypotension. These include adequate hydration prior to the induction of spinal anesthesia, and proper positioning of the patient once spinal anesthesia is induced. Both of these maneuvers will improve venous return, cardiac output, and blood pressure. All patients should have fluid deficits replaced prior to spinal anesthesia. An additional 500 ml of balanced salt solution will usually mitigate the response to venodilatation due to sympathectomy. Patients with congestive failure should receive less fluid as their vascular system is already at or above capacity. Once the spinal anesthetic drug has been injected, positioning the patient so as to ensure adequate venous return is paramount. Usually the horizontal supine position is all that is required. If, however, after adequate fluid loading, and after the patient is in the supine horizontal position, the blood pressure cannot be maintained in the desired range, a slight head-down position, so that the right atrium is below the great veins, will often improve the situation. The head-down tilt need not be steep. A modest Trendelenburg position of 5–10° will improve venous return without greatly exaggerating the cephalad spread of the spinal anesthetic. Occasionally, despite both of these maneuvers, the blood pressure will need to be supported with vasoactive agents. Patients should not be placed in the head-up position to prevent an exaggerated cephalad spread of the local anesthetic, since this will tend to cause a more profound degree of hypotension.[94]

During spinal anesthesia, systemic vascular resistance (arteriolar dilatation) is only minimally decreased. The major decline in mean arterial pressure is due to decreased cardiac output resulting from decreased venous return. Therefore, vasopressors that constrict veins in preference to arterioles provide a more rational method for treating the hypotension that results from spinal anesthesia. Drugs commonly used are ephedrine, mephentermine, and phenylephrine. Ephedrine and mephentermine have mixed alpha and beta receptor activity, and are potent venoconstrictors, whereas phenylephrine is an alpha-receptor agonist and a more potent arteriolar constrictor. While improving venous return, ephedrine and mephentermine will also increase heart rate. Phenylephrine will increase blood pressure by arteriolar constriction, with little or no change in, or a decline in, heart rate.[95–97]

One approach to treating hypotension during spinal anesthesia is to administer boluses of ephedrine (5–10 mg) iv. Usually, one or two boluses are all that is required. Occasionally, however, it is necessary to administer a vasoconstrictor for more prolonged periods. Under these conditions, an intramuscular injection of ephedrine (25–50 mg) or an infusion of phenylephrine (10 mg in 250 ml of D_5W or balanced salt solution) is indicated because tachyphylaxis precludes the intravenous administration of ephedrine or mephentermine for prolonged intervals.[98]

Post-Dural Puncture Headache

Post-dural puncture headache is believed to be due to decreased cerebrospinal fluid pressure resulting from the leakage of cerebrospinal fluid through the opening in the dural sheath created by the lumbar puncture needle. Post-dural puncture headache is probably the most common complication of spinal anesthesia. The incidence of spinal headache is believed to be related to age, sex, pregnancy, size of the dural puncture needle, direction of the needle bevel, and the angle at which the needle penetrates the dura.[37, 38, 99, 100] The headache is classically described as frontal or occipital, is made worse by erect posture, is improved in the recumbent position, and may be accompanied by tinnitus and/or photophobia. A true post-dural puncture headache must have a postural component, i.e., be made worse by the sitting or standing position. It is important to remember that many patients may have a headache postoperatively that is not related to the dural puncture.

Table 28-9 shows the effect of sex, age, and needle size on the incidence of post-dural puncture headache. Women appear to be more prone to develop a post-dural puncture headache than men.[37] This may be related to the influence of hormones, e.g., progesterone and estrogen. Age is inversely related, and needle diameter is directly related, to the incidence of post-dural headache. Midline approaches to the subarachnoid space result in greater leakage of cerebrospinal fluid than paramedian approaches.[100] Midline approaches may, therefore, result in a higher incidence of post-dural puncture headache. Inserting the spinal needle with the bevel parallel to the orientation of the dural fibers, as opposed to cutting across them with the bevel inserted at right angles to the fibers, has been reported to decrease the incidence of post-dural puncture headache.[99] The incidence of post-dural puncture headache is higher in the pregnant patients than in nonpregnant females. At the Brigham and Women's Hospital, the incidence of post-spinal headache in obstetric patients averages approximately 7%, despite the use of 26-gauge needles. Once again, hormonal factors may be involved. However, an interesting observation and alternative explanation is the increased incidence of post-dural puncture headache associated with the concentration of glucose injected with the local anesthetic.[101] Figure 28-16 shows a direct relationship between the incidence of spinal headache and the amount of glucose contained in the local anesthetic solution.

Once the diagnosis of post-dural puncture headache is confirmed, three methods of therapy are available: 1) analgesics, bed rest, and hydration; 2) epidural blood patch; and 3) intravenous caffeine.

Nearly all post-dural puncture headaches will resolve without therapy in time. Bed rest, analgesics, and hydration are often satisfactory for the patient who has had extensive surgery and who is unlikely to be ambulatory postoperatively. Hydration in the form of "forcing fluids" is done with the intent of increasing the production of cerebrospinal fluid, so that cerebrospinal fluid production exceeds loss through the dural puncture site, thus restoring the cerebrospinal fluid pressure to normal. Some authors have recommended the use of pitressin to augment the process by preventing diuresis.[102]

If a post-dural puncture headache persists following 24 h of rest, fluid, and analgesic therapy, the patient should be of-

TABLE 28-9. Relation of Sex, Age, and Needle Gauge Used for Lumbar Puncture to Incidence of "Spinal" Headache

	NUMBER OF SPINAL ANESTHETICS	NUMBER OF "SPINAL" HEADACHES	PERCENT
SEX			
Male	4063	302	7
Female	5214	709	14
Vaginal delivery	938	220	22
Other procedures	4276	489	12
Totals	9277	1011	21
AGE (YEARS)			
10–19	537	51	10
20–29	1994	321	16
30–39	1833	261	14
40–49	1759	192	11
50–59	1736	133	8
60–69	1094	45	4
70–79	297	7	2
80–89	27	1	3
Totals	9277	1011	11
NEEDLE GAUGE			
16	839	151	18
19	154	16	10
20	2698	377	14
22	4952	430	9
24	634	37	6

(Reproduced with permission from Vandam LD, Dripps RD: Long-term follow up of patients who received 10,098 spinal anesthetics: III. Syndrome of decreased intracranial pressure [headache and occular and auditory difficulties]. JAMA 161:586, 1956. Copyright 1956, American Medical Association.)

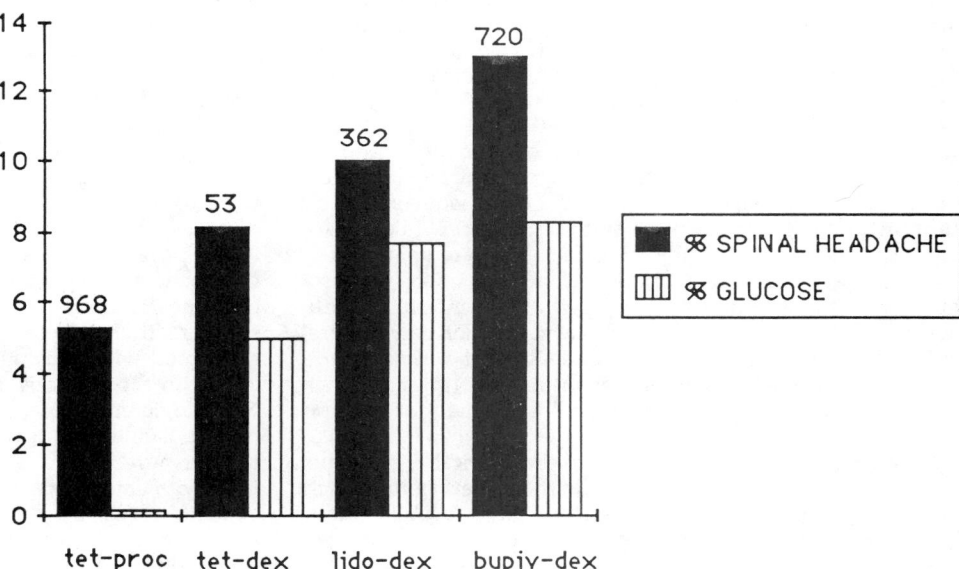

FIG. 28-16. The relationship between glucose concentration of the spinal anesthetic and the incidence of spinal headache. As the glucose concentration increases, the incidence of spinal headache also increases. Tet-proc = tetracaine 0.5%-procaine 5% (no dextrose); lido = lidocaine (5%); bupiv = bupivacaine (0.75%); and dex = dextrose (concentration as indicated by the open bars). The numbers above the solid bars indicate the number of spinal anesthetics. (Reproduced with permission of the author: Naulty JS: Unpublished.)

fered an epidural blood patch. This is accomplished by placing a needle in the epidural space in the vicinity of the dural puncture and injecting 10–20 ml of autologous blood aseptically. The optimum amount of blood injected has been determined to be 15 ml in the average patient.[103] This procedure is very effective. If relief of the headache is not observed, the procedure may be repeated. If two epidural blood patches are not effective in curing the headache, the diagnosis of post-dural puncture headache is suspect. Complications associated with epidural blood patch are minimal. Low back pain and nuchal discomfort are the most common complaints. These usually resolve in 24–48 h with analgesics. Epidural saline has been recommended for post-dural puncture headache,[104] but does not appear to be as efficacious as an epidural blood patch.[105]

Recently, the use of caffeine infusions for the treatment of post-dural puncture headache has been reinvestigated. The initial studies involving caffeine were conducted by Sechzer and Abel.[106, 107] The mechanism by which caffeine infusion reverses spinal headache is not clear, although it may be related to its vasoconstrictor action. Jarvis et al[108] have shown that 80% of patients with post-dural puncture headache, infused with D5-Ringer's lactate (1 liter) containing caffeine sodium benzoate (500 mg), followed by an additional infusion of 1000 ml of D5-Ringer's lactate resulted in significant improvement in symptoms.

Extensive Spread of Spinal Blockade

High spinal anesthesia with respiratory and vascular embarrassment can occur in any patient. However, the patients most susceptible to high spinal anesthesia are parturients. This may result from a number of factors—decreased cerebrospinal fluid volume, the use of hyperbaric solutions in the presence of an exaggerated lumbar lordosis, increased neuronal sensitivity to local anesthetics, ventilatory insufficiency due to the enlarged uterus, etc. High spinal anesthesia is most likely to occur shortly after the induction of spinal anesthesia. Nevertheless, late occurring respiratory distress has been reported. It is important, therefore, to closely monitor the patient during and following the induction of spinal anesthesia until the level of spinal anesthesia has significantly regressed.

Most patients will become agitated with a high spinal, and nausea and hypotension are frequent. These symptoms should alert the anesthesiologist to the possibility that the spinal is higher than desired. The diagnosis should be made as quickly as possible, and can be made in combination with the therapy. The patient should be given oxygen, preferably by mask attached to the anesthesia circuit. Ask the patient to take a deep breath and observe intercostal muscle function and the movement of the reservoir bag. Good intercostal muscle function and exchange of large volumes of oxygen from the reservoir bag are inconsistent with high spinal anesthesia. Agitation, nausea, and hypotension most likely represent exaggerated sympathectomy. Treatment consists of restoring the blood pressure with positioning, fluids and/or vasopressors, and reassurance. Lack of intercostal muscle function and minimal movement of the reservoir bag indicates very high spinal anesthesia. Again, the treatment consists of supporting the blood pressure and reassurance while assisting ventilation. Usually, the phrenic nerves are spared and diaphragmatic breathing will suffice. This may not be the case in the parturient, where the enlarged uterus interferes with diaphragmatic excursions. Inadequate ventilation may require induction of general anesthesia and assisted ventilation of the lungs following endotracheal intubation. Intubation of the trachea is especially indicated for the patient at risk for aspiration.

When spinal anesthetics spread to the cervical region, the concentration of the local anesthetic in the upper regions is not great. Therefore, the exaggerated spread is usually short lived, and respiratory function can be expected to return relatively quickly. It is usually advisable, however, to keep the patient unconscious until the surgical procedure is complete once intubation of the trachea has been accomplished.

Backache

Surprisingly, backache following spinal anesthesia is relatively infrequent. It may be related to the spinal anesthetic procedure itself. Small hematomas, ligamentous irritation, reflex skeletal muscle spasm, and positioning during surgery are also possibilities. Profound skeletal muscle relaxation occurs with spinal anesthesia. This, coupled, for example, with the lithotomy position, may result in ligament strain postoperatively. Backache does occur, however, and it sometimes takes on the same significance as the spinal headache. Serious neurological damage should be ruled out. Otherwise, reassurance, rest, heat, and analgesics will usually rectify the problem. Physical examination and the "laying on of hands" is often beneficial, and should be done if practical. Occasionally, paraspinous muscle spasm is the culprit, and skeletal muscle relaxant medication, e.g., diazepam, can help.

Nausea

Nausea during spinal anesthesia can be a vexing problem. Because nausea can be a symptom of cerebral ischemia, it is imperative that the anesthesiologist think first of providing oxygen and determining if severe hypotension is the cause when nausea appears. Treatment involves restoration of the arterial blood pressure, while providing oxygen therapy. Datta et al[109] have shown that immediate treatment of arterial hypotension in parturients minimizes the incidence of nausea during cesarean section.

Another cause of nausea during spinal anesthesia is an imbalance between the parasympathetic and sympathetic nervous systems resulting from chemical sympathectomy or from parasympathetic mediated traction reflexes from surgical manipulation. Atropine (0.4 mg) may help, but not invariably. Adjuvant medications, especially opioids, may cause nausea in some cases. In this instance, small amounts of droperidol (0.625 mg) may be beneficial.[110]

Major Neurologic Injuries

Major neurologic injuries are extremely rare following spinal anesthesia. This is due, in part, to the use of disposable spinal kits and the relative safety and small doses of the local anesthetics employed. The pre-packaged sterile spinal kits have virtually eliminated meningitis as a complication of spinal anesthesia. A review[111] of 11 spinal anesthetic studies involving approximately 65,000 patients with various agents lists 31 cases of neurologic sequelae (an incidence of 1:2000). Many of these 31 sequelae were exacerbations of previous neurologic diseases.[112]

The possible causes of neurologic injury include: 1) spinal cord ischemia; 2) needle trauma; 3) chemical contamination of local anesthetic solutions; and 4) toxicity of the local anesthetic solutions themselves. Spinal cord ischemia is believed to be associated with prolonged arterial hypotension in combination with a precarious anterior spinal arterial blood supply. Neurologic injury resulting from needle trauma is extremely rare. It usually results from multiple attempts during difficult lumbar puncture.[113] Contamination of local anesthetic solutions with detergents or other chemicals has been responsible, in some cases, for the production of neurological sequelae following spinal anesthesia. For example, cases of aseptic meningitis have been attributed to soaking syringes with disinfectants.[114] The use of disposable equipment has virtually eliminated this complication, as well as bacterial meningitis. The incidence of neurological complications due to spinal anesthesia has decreased since the 1940s, probably due to the use of disposable equipment and elimination of solutions containing such substances as alcohol, acacia, and strychnine.[115]

When a major neurologic complication occurs following spinal anesthesia, a neurologist should be consulted and every effort should be made to determine the etiology of the neurologic injury. Neurologic injury can be caused by an errantly placed needle or injection of the wrong substance into the subarachnoid space. However, nerve injury can also result from other causes, *e.g.*, pre-existing neurologic lesion, retractors, the birth process, or pressure on nerves due to faulty positioning during surgery.

Unfortunately, there is often little that can be done once neurologic injury has occurred. With the exception of evacuation of a hematoma or drainage of an abscess, treatment is usually symptomatic. The best therapy, however, is attention to details and avoidance of injury.

EPIDURAL ANESTHESIA

Toxicity Due to Local Anesthetics

Relatively large doses of local anesthetic agents are required in order to achieve adequate sensory anesthesia for surgery following epidural administration. In addition, the epidural space contains numerous venous plexus, which may be penetrated by an epidural needle or catheter leading to the accidental intravascular administration of local anesthetic agents. As a result, toxicity may occur due to either the administration of an excessive amount of drug extravascularly or accidental intravascular injection. The blood and tissue levels of local anesthetic agents associated with systemic toxic reactions are determined by the rate of absorption, tissue redistribution, metabolism, and excretion of the anesthetic compound.

The systemic absorption and potential toxicity of epidurally administered local anesthetics are related to the site of injection, dosage and addition of a vasoconstrictor, and the pharmacological profile of the local anesthetic itself. Little difference in the rate of absorption is seen following cervical, thoracic, or lumbar epidural injections.[116] However, with caudal injections, mean peak venous blood levels are significantly higher than those following lumbar epidural injections.[78] This may reflect the greater lateral spread of the injected solution, and exposure to a larger vascular surface area in the caudal canal.

Blood levels of local anesthetics are related to the total dose of drug administered. For most local anesthetics, a linear relationship exists between the amount of drug administered and the resultant peak blood level (Fig. 28-17). For example, the mean venous blood level of lidocaine increased from approximately 1.5 μg · ml^{-1} to 4 μg · ml^{-1}, as the total dose administered into the lumbar epidural space was increased from 200 to 600 mg.[78] For certain local anesthetics, such as bupivacaine and etidocaine, a nonlinear relationship has been observed between the total dose administered and the peak venous blood level. This may be due to the high lipid solubility of bupivacaine and etidocaine that results in sequestration of these drugs in epidural fat, such that the rate of systemic absorption is less when relatively small doses are used. However, when large doses are administered, lipid depots may be saturated so that more free drug is available for absorption. The peak blood level achieved following epidural blockade is a function of the dose in milligrams, and does not appear to be related to either the concentration or volume of the local anesthetic solution employed. No significant difference in the venous plasma levels of different local anesthetics has been observed following the lumbar epidural administration of these drugs at varying volumes and concentrations if the total dose was the same.[78]

Many local anesthetic solutions contain a vasoconstrictor agent, usually epinephrine in a concentration of 5 μg · ml^{-1}

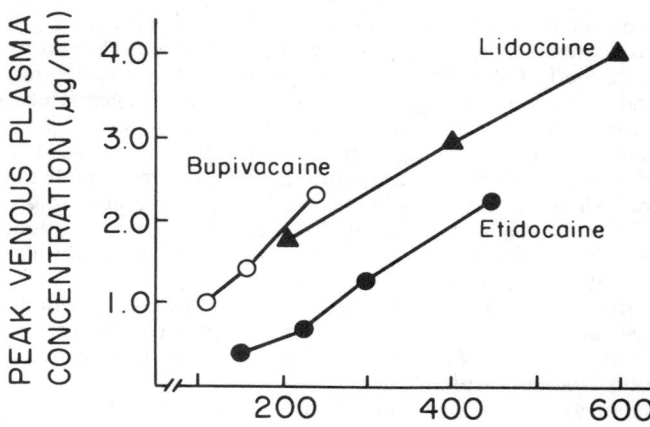

FIG. 28-17. Relationship between the amount of drug administered epidurally and the resultant peak blood levels. For lidocaine, a linear relationship is observed. Bupivacaine and etidocaine demonstrate a nonlinear relationship.

(1:200,000). A concentration of 5 μg · ml^{-1} of epinephrine appears to be optimal in terms of reducing the rate of absorption of local anesthetic agents, such as lidocaine and mepivacaine, from the lumbar epidural space.[117] The vascular uptake from the epidural space of local anesthetics such as prilocaine, bupivacaine, and etidocaine appears to be less influenced by the addition of a vasoconstrictor than are lidocaine and mepivacaine.[117–119]

Differences exist in the rate of absorption of various local anesthetics from the epidural space. For example, prilocaine blood levels are significantly lower than those of lidocaine following lumbar epidural administration of equal doses of both drugs. This difference may reflect the greater vasodilator activity of lidocaine, but more important is the larger distribution volume and the rapid rate of elimination of prilocaine.[120] Among the more potent drugs, etidocaine blood levels are significantly lower than those of bupivacaine if equal doses of both local anesthetics are administered epidurally.[118] This may be related, in part, to the greater lipid solubility, the larger distribution volume, and more rapid rate of elimination of etidocaine.[120] The lower blood level of etidocaine has practical clinical implications. Although 1.0–1.5% etidocaine is required to provide a similar degree of sensory analgesia as 0.5–0.75% bupivacaine, no difference in blood levels or potential toxicity exists between the two drugs following lumbar epidural administration.

Systemic Toxicity of Local Anesthetic Agents

When properly performed, epidural anesthesia does not usually result in blood levels of local anesthetics that are sufficient to cause systemic effects. However, accidental intravascular injection or the administration of an excessive amount of local anesthetic into the epidural space can result in blood and tissue levels that will cause profound systemic effects.

The central nervous system is particularly susceptible to the systemic actions of local anesthetics.[121] The signs and symptoms of central nervous system toxicity are as follows: initially, feelings of numbness of legs and tongue, lightheadedness, and dizziness are usually reported, followed frequently by visual and auditory disturbances, such as difficulty in focusing, and tinnitus. Other subjective central nervous system symptoms include disorientation and occasional feelings of drowsiness. Objective signs of an excitatory central nervous system effect include shivering, skeletal muscular twitching, and tremors, involving, at first, muscles of the face and distal parts of the extremities. This may progress to generalized convulsions of a tonic-clonic nature. If a sufficiently large dose of a local anesthetic agent is administered systemically, these initial signs of central nervous system excitation are rapidly followed by a state of generalized central nervous system depression. Seizure activity ceases and depression of ventilation and, ultimately, apnea occurs.

In general, the cardiovascular system appears to be more resistant to the effects of local anesthetics than the central nervous system. However, local anesthetics can cause profound cardiovascular toxicity.[121]

The sequence of cardiovascular events that usually occurs following the accidental intravascular administration of local anesthetics is as follows: at relatively non-toxic blood levels of these drugs, either no change in blood pressure or a slight increase in blood pressure may be observed. The slight increase in blood pressure may be related to an increase in cardiac output and heart rate that has been seen in some animal preparations and is believed to be due to an enhancement of sympathetic activity by these drugs. In addition, the direct vasoconstrictor action of local anesthetics on certain peripheral vascular beds at low concentrations may be responsible, in part, for a slight increase in systemic blood pressure. As the blood level of local anesthetic agents approaches toxic concentrations, a fall in blood pressure is usually the first sign of a systemic effect. The hypotension appears to be related to the negative inotropic action of these agents, which results in a decrease in cardiac output and stroke volume. The initial reduction in blood pressure is transient in nature, and is spontaneously reversible in most patients. However, if the amount of local anesthetic administered is excessive, a profound and irreversible state of cardiovascular depression occurs. This is due not only to the negative inotropic action of the local anesthetics, but also to massive peripheral vasodilation. Local anesthetic toxicity is best avoided by administering these agents slowly into the epidural space, or by the use of a fractionated dose technique, as described previously.

Treatment of central nervous system toxicity consists initially of maintaining a patent airway and assisting ventilation of the lungs with oxygen. Most convulsive reactions are of brief duration, and terminate spontaneously. If convulsive activity persists for more than 1–2 min, therapy should be instituted. Central nervous system depressants, such as iv thiopental or diazepam, are most frequently employed to terminate convulsive activity. Succinylcholine has also been advocated as a means of controlling the muscular activity associated with convulsions. In addition, succinylcholine will facilitate endotracheal intubation in a convulsing patient in whom ventilation of the lungs cannot be adequately supported.

Hypotension due to local anesthetic-induced toxicity is probably best treated with a drug like ephedrine that has positive inotropic activity and a peripheral vasoconstrictor action.

Local Tissue Toxicity

The potential of epidurally administered local anesthetics to cause localized nerve damage is very low. The accidental subarachnoid injection of large doses of local anesthetics may be of concern, since the spinal cord and spinal roots lack a connective tissue sheath. Most local anesthetics are free of local neural irritation in the concentrations employed for epidural anesthesia. Recently, some concern has existed with regard to the local irritant properties of chloroprocaine, due to reports of prolonged sensory/motor deficits in patients following the accidental subarachnoid injection of large amounts of this local anesthetic.[122, 123] Experimental studies have indicated that the combination of the low pH and sodium bisulfite in solutions of chloroprocaine may be responsible for the neurotoxic effects, rather than the chloroprocaine itself.[124] It is obvious that epidural blockade should be performed with great care to avoid the accidental intrathecal injection of large amounts of local anesthetics. Again, a fractionated dose technique should preclude the intrathecal administration of large amounts of local anesthetics.

Technique-related Complications

HYPOTENSION. This is the most common cardiovascular complication of epidural anesthesia, and results primarily from widespread sympathetic blockade. The hemodynamic effects of epidural blockade are similar to those previously described for spinal blockade. However, due to the slower onset of sympathetic blockade following epidurally administered local anesthetics, an excessive fall in arterial pressure is usually not seen in normovolemic patients. Epidural blockade to the T10 level seldom causes any decrease in arterial pressure. Blocks extending into the upper thoracic segments frequently result in a decrease in mean arterial pressure of no more than 10–20 mm Hg. The vasodilation below the level of sympathetic blockade is usually compensated by vasoconstriction above the level of blockade, such that the decrease in blood pressure is relatively mild. On the other hand, an extremely high level of sympathetic blockade resulting in a reduction in cardiac output can lead to a profound fall in blood pressure. In addition, in hypovolemic patients, or patients in whom inferior vena caval occlusion is present, epidural blockade can result in a severe degree of hypotension. As is the case with spinal blockade, patients should be kept supine or in a slightly head-down position in order to increase venous return and ensure an adequate cardiac output that will tend to prevent a marked fall in blood pressure.

The combined use of light general anesthesia with epidural blockade will generate a greater fall in blood pressure due to the peripheral vasodilation produced by the epidural blockade and the negative inotropic action of the general anesthetic. However, in healthy patients, the decrease in blood pressure is usually well tolerated, unless the depth of general anesthesia is excessive.

Treatment of hypotension due to sympathetic blockade is dependent on the degree of hypotension and the physical status of the patient. In most healthy patients, a fall of approximately 20 mm Hg in mean arterial pressure is usually well tolerated, and may be beneficial in terms of decreasing blood loss. If the fall in blood pressure is excessive, or occurs in patients with cardiovascular disease in whom it is important to maintain blood pressure, positioning of patients in a head-down position and administration of fluids is frequently adequate to reverse the hypotensive state. A marked fall in blood pressure due to extensive sympathetic blockade may require pharmacological intervention. If the extent of the sympathetic blockade is sufficiently great to cause a fall in heart rate, atropine should be administered to treat the bradycardia. In addition, the use of vasopressor agents may also be required to reverse the profound state of hypotension. An intravenous infusion of an alpha-adrenergic receptor stimulant, such as phenylephrine, may be employed. Drugs such as ephedrine or mephentermine, which possess both alpha- and beta-receptor stimulating activity, may be of value. Some authors have advocated the intramuscular use of ephedrine prophylactically in order to prevent a decrease in blood pressure following the induction of epidural anesthesia. However, this is rarely necessary in healthy patients or if the dose of epidurally administered local anesthetic is controlled in order to avoid an excessive level of sympathetic blockade.

VENTILATORY COMPLICATIONS. Epidural blockade rarely has any profound effect on ventilation. Even epidural blockade extending to the upper thoracic dermatome is usually not associated with a significant degree of ventilatory depression. Although high epidural blocks may result in paralysis of intercostal muscles, the diaphragm is usually able to function normally and achieve adequate ventilation of the lungs. In certain patients, such as the grossly obese, diaphragmatic activity may be inadequate, and assisted ventilation of the lungs will be required.

ACCIDENTAL SUBDURAL OR SUBARACHNOID INJECTIONS. Profound depression of ventilation following the performance of an epidural block is usually indicative of an accidental subdural or subarachnoid injection. The inadvertent administration of local anesthetics subdurally or intrathecally always represents a potential complication of epidural blockade. The hemodynamic and respiratory consequences of a high spinal blockade have been discussed previously. An accidental subdural injection would result in hemodynamic and ventilatory changes similar to those seen following an accidental high spinal blockade. However, the onset of hypotension and ventilatory depression following a subdural injection is usually slower than that observed following an accidental intrathecal injection. Treatment of hypotension or ventilatory depression due to high accidental spinal blockade is the same as that described previously. The accidental intrathecal or subdural administration of local anesthetics is best prevented by the use of a fractional dose technique when performing an epidural blockade. Early signs of motor weakness, extensive spread of sensory anesthesia, and hypotension following the administration of 3–4 ml of local anesthetic solution is usually indicative of an inadvertent subarachnoid injection.

DURAL PUNCTURE AND POST-SPINAL HEADACHE. Accidental puncture of the dura is always a potential risk when performing an epidural blockade. Spinal headache does not always occur following dural puncture with a 17- or 18-gauge epidural needle. In older patients in whom epidural anesthesia is performed, dural puncture is frequently not associated with the occurrence of a spinal headache. However, in younger patients and, in particular, pregnant patients, dural puncture during an attempted epidural block results in a high incidence of post-spinal headache. Some authorities have advocated the immediate use of an epidural blood patch in such patients in whom dural puncture has occurred during an attempted epidural blockade. However, since the extent to which the dura has been punctured is unknown, and since not all patients develop a classical spinal headache, it is probably prudent to wait 12–24 h postoperatively to determine if a spinal headache develops, and then offer the patient the option of an epidural blood patch.

NEURAL DAMAGE. Neurological deficits may occur following epidural blockade, although the incidence of this problem is low. A review of seven epidural studies involving approximately 45,000 patients listed 40 cases of neurological sequelae, 22 of which were simply identified as paresthesias.[111] Neurological deficits are usually due to trauma, anterior spinal artery syndrome, or space-occupying lesions, such as a hematoma. The etiology and management of these neural injuries are similar to those described previously for spinal anesthesia. The concurrent use of epidural anesthesia and anticoagulants is a concern with regard to the possible dangers associated with the puncture of an epidural vein and the development of an epidural hematoma.[125] Epidural anesthesia should not be attempted in a patient who is fully anticoagulated, or in patients in whom an abnormal coagulation profile or bleeding time is present. Anticoagulation of a patient following the placement of an epidural catheter does appear justified. Studies involving several thousand patients have been reported in which patients have been anticoagulated with heparin primarily for vascular surgical procedures following the placement of an epidural catheter without reports of epidural hematomas occurring.[126, 127] Concern is frequently expressed with regard to patients in whom an epidural vein is punctured during an attempted epidural block, and in whom heparinization is planned for the surgical procedure. Puncture of an epidural blood vessel should not be an automatic cause for cancellation of surgery or abandonment of the epidural technique. If heparinization is not accomplished until 30–60 min following the puncture of the epidural blood vessel, this should allow sufficient time for clot formation to occur at the site of the venous puncture. The use of mini-dose heparin or oral anticoagulants to prevent postoperative deep venous thrombosis may restrict the use of epidural anesthesia. However, reports exist in which epidural anesthesia has been employed in patients on oral anticoagulants without adverse complications.[126]

Nevertheless, the potential risk of an epidural hematoma should be fully explained to any patient in whom an epidural anesthetic is employed, and in whom anticoagulant therapy is anticipated. In addition, these patients should be carefully monitored preoperatively to evaluate their coagulation profile, and examined postoperatively to determine whether any signs of neurological deficits related to a space-occupying lesion are present.

CATHETER COMPLICATIONS. Insertion of plastic catheters into the epidural space is usually a simple and safe procedure. Complications related to catheter insertion may occur, although the incidence is very low. Catheters may be inserted directly into a blood vessel or, more rarely, may be placed into the subarachnoid space. Negative aspiration of blood is not a guarantee that a catheter has not been placed into an epidural vein. Thus, the use of an epidural test dose or a fractionated dose regimen is advocated in order to avoid the intravascular injection of an excessive dose of local anesthetic.

The most common concern associated with the use of an epidural catheter involves the breaking off of a segment of the catheter in the epidural space.[128] This usually occurs if an attempt is made to withdraw a catheter through the epidural needle. One must never withdraw a catheter backward through the epidural needle. If it is not possible to advance the catheter into the epidural space, then the needle and catheter should be withdrawn together, and the procedure repeated at another interspace. If an epidural catheter is sheared, most authorities believe that it is best to inform the patient of this occurrence, but indicate that no attempt should be made to retrieve the catheter segment. Catheter segments remaining in the epidural space are rarely associated with clinically significant problems. It has also been reported that epidural catheters can curl and turn on themselves in the epidural space, and can actually form a knot, such that it may be difficult to remove the catheter from the epidural space. This is an extremely rare occurrence, and is usually due to attempts to advance an excessive length of catheter into the epidural space.[128] For this reason, catheters should never be advanced more than 2–3 cm into the epidural space.

CAUDAL ANESTHESIA

Caudal anesthesia is produced by placement of local anesthetic solution in the epidural space via a needle or catheter introduced through the sacral hiatus into the sacral canal. The patient may be positioned in either the lateral or prone position, with the latter position preferred for palpating bony landmarks. The sacral hiatus and the adjacent sacral cornu are identified (usually about 5 cm from the tip of the coccyx in the midline), and an 18 gauge 7 cm needle is inserted at a 45° angle into the sacral hiatus between the two cornu. The needle is advanced through the sacrococcygeal membrane until the sacrum is contacted. At this point, the needle is withdrawn a small distance and the angle changed to 5° to 15° before advancing the needle in the sacral canal for a distance of about 2 cm. Further advancement of the needle increases the risk of dural puncture because the dural sac typically extends to the level of S2. Aspiration tests are necessary to confirm the absence of cerebrospinal fluid or blood. A test dose of local anesthetic solution containing epinephrine is then injected. Approximately twice the dose of local anesthetic solution (3 ml of drug par spinal segment) is needed for caudal, compared with lumbar epidural, anesthesia because of the relatively large sacral canal and free leakage of solution through sacral foramina. Although infection is rare, the nearness of this approach to the rectum requires strict aseptic technique. In adults, most anesthesiologists prefer lumbar rather than caudal (sacral) approach to the epidural space because the former is a more predictable and easier technique to use.

Caudal anesthesia is becoming a popular technique for provision of anesthesia and postoperative analgesia in pediatric patients.[129] In contrast to adults, the sacral hiatus is usually easy to locate in children (especially neonates), and local anesthetic dose requirements seem more predictable. The needle should not be advanced more than 1 cm into the sacral canal because the dural sac may extend more caudal in children compared with adults.

REFERENCES

1. Koller K: Über die Verwendung des Cocain zur Anasthesirung am Auge. Wien Med Blatter 7:1352, 1884
2. Corning JL: Spinal anesthesia and local medication of the cord. NY J Med 42:483, 1885
3. Sicard A: Essais d'injections microbiennes toxiques et therapeutiques, par voie cephalo-racidenne. CR Soc Biol (Paris) 50:472, 1898
4. Bier A: Versüche über Cocainisirung des Ruckensmarkes. Deutsch Z Chir 51:361, 1899
5. Tait D, Caglieri G: Experimental and clinical notes on the subarachnoid space. Trans Med Soc Calif 35:6, 1900
6. Matas R: Report of successful spinal anesthesia. Medical News. JAMA 33:1650, 1899
7. Cathelin MF: Une novelle voie d'injection rachidienne. Methode des injections epidurales par le procede du canal sacre. Applications a l'homme. CR Soc Biol (Paris) 53:452, 1901
8. Pages F: Anesthesia metamerica. Rev Sanid Mil Madr 11:351, 1921
9. Dogliotti AM: Anesthesia. Chicago, SB Dubour, 1939
10. Carron H, Covino BG: Influence of anaesthetic procedures on surgical sequelae. Reg Anesth 7(Suppl), 1982
11. Enqquist A, Brandt MR, Fernandes A et al: The blocking effect of epidural analgesia on the adrenocortical and hyperglycemic response to surgery. Acta Anaesthesiol Scand 21:330, 1977
12. Halter JB, Pflug AE: Relationship of impaired insulin secretion during surgical stress to anesthesia and catecholamine release. J Clin Endocrinol 51:1093, 1980
13. Kehlet H, Brandt MR, Prange Hanson A et al: Effect of epidural analgesia on metabolic profiles during and after surgery. Br J Surg 66:543, 1979
14. Kehlet H: Influence of regional anesthesia on postoperative morbidity. Ann Chir Gynaecol 73:171, 1984
15. Brandt MR, Kehlet H, Binder C et al: Effect of epidural analgesia on the glycoregulatory endocrine response to surgery. Clin Endocrinol 5:107, 1976
16. Brandt MR, Kehlet H, Faber O et al: C-peptide and insulin during blockade of the hyperglycemic response to surgery by epidural analgesia. Clin Endocrinol 6:167, 1977
17. Brandt MR, Kehlet H, Skovsted L et al: Rapid decrease in plasmatriiodothyronine during surgery and epidural analgesia independent of afferent neurogenic stimuli and of cortisol. Lancet ii:1333, 1976
18. Hallberg D, Oro L: Free fatty acids of plasma during spinal anaesthesia in man. Acta Med Scand 178:281, 1965
19. Keith I: Anaesthesia and blood loss in total hip replacement. Anaesthesia 32:444, 1977
20. Modig J, Hjelmstedt A, Sahlstedt B et al: Comparative influences of epidural and general anaesthesia on deep vein thrombosis and pulmonary embolism after total hip replacement. Acta Chir Scand 147:125, 1981
21. Modig J, Borg T, Karlstrom G et al: Thromboembolism after total hip replacement: Role of epidural and general anesthesia. Anesth Analg 62:174, 1983
22. Hendolin H, Mattila MAK, Poikolainen E: The effect of lumbar epidural analgesia on the development of deep vein thrombosis of the legs after open prostatectomy. Acta Chir Scand 147:425, 1981
23. McKenzie PJ, Wishart HY, Dewar MS et al: Comparison of the effects of spinal anaesthesia and general anaesthesia on postoperative oxygenation and perioperative mortality. Br J Anaesth 52:49, 1980
24. Hendolin H, Tuppurainen T, Lahtinen J: Thoracic epidural analgesia and deep vein thrombosis in cholecystectomized patients. Acta Chir Scand 148:405, 1982
25. Mellbring G, Dahlgren S, Reiz S et al: Thromboembolic complications after major abdominal surgery: Effect of thoracic epidural analgesia. Acta Chir Scand 149:263, 1983
26. Davis FM, Laurenson VG: Spinal anaesthesia or general anaesthesia for emergency hip surgery in elderly patients. Anaesth Intensive Care 9:352, 1981
27. Hjortso NC, Andersen T, Froosig F et al: A controlled study of the effect of epidural analgesia with local anaesthetics and morphine on morbidity after abdominal surgery. Acta Anaesthesiol Scand 29:790, 1985
28. Modig J, Borg T, Bagge L et al: Role of extradural and of general anaesthesia in fibrinolysis and coagulation after total hip replacement. Br J Anaesth 55:625, 1983
29. Simpson PJ, Radford SG, Forster SJ et al: The fibrinolytic effects of anaesthesia. Anaesthesia 37:3, 1982
30. Cuschieri RJ, Morran CG, Howie JC et al: Postoperative pain and pulmonary complications: Comparison of three analgesic regimens. Br J Surg 72:495, 1985

31. Reiz S, Balfors E, Sorenson MB et al: Coronary hemodynamic effects of general anesthesia and surgery: Modification by epidural analgesia in patients with ischemic heart disease. Reg Anesth 7(Suppl):S8, 1982
32. McLaren AD: Mortality studies. A review. Reg Anaesth 7(Suppl): S192, 1982
33. McKenzie PJ, Wishart HY, Dewer MS et al: Long-term outcome after repair of the fractured neck of the femur. Br J Anaesth 56:581, 1984
34. Valentin N, Lomholt B, Jensen JS et al: Spinal or general anaesthesia for surgery of the fractured hip? A prospective study of mortality in 578 patients. Br J Anaesth 58:284, 1986
35. Yeager MP, Glass DD, Neff RH et al: Epidural anesthesia and analgesia in high-risk surgical patients. Anesthesiology 66:729, 1987
36. Soni V, Peeters C, Covino B: Value and limitations of test dose prior to epidural anesthesia. Reg Anesth 6:23, 1981
37. Vandam LD, Dripps RD: Long term follow up of patients who received 10,098 spinal anesthetics: III. Syndrome of decreased intracranial pressure (headache and occular and auditory difficulties). JAMA 161:586, 1956
38. Bromage PR: Neurologic complications of regional anesthesia for obstetrics. In Shnider SM, Levinson G (eds): Anesthesia for Obstetrics, 2nd ed, p 317. Baltimore, Williams and Wilkins, 1987
39. Gasser HS, Erlanger J: The role of fiber size in establishment of a nerve block by pressure or cocaine. Am J Physiol 88:581, 1929
40. Gissen AJ, Covino BG, Gregus J: Differential sensitivities of mammalian nerve fibers to local anesthetic agents. Anesthesiology 53:467, 1980
41. Shantha TR, Evans JA: The relationship of epidural anesthesia to neural membranes and arachnoid villi. Anesthesiology 37:543, 1972
42. Bromage PR, Joyal AC, Binney JC: Local anesthetic drugs. Penetration from the spinal extradural space into the neuraxis. Science 140:392, 1963
43. Galindo A, Hernandez J, Benavides O et al: Quality of spinal extradural anesthesia: The influence of spinal nerve root diameter. Br J Anaesth 47:41, 1975
44. Greene NM: The area of differential block during spinal anesthesia with hyperbaric tetracaine. Anesthesiology 19:45, 1958
45. Chamberlain DP, Chamberlain BDL: Changes in skin temperature of the trunk and their relationship to sympathetic blockade during spinal anesthesia. Anesthesiology 65:139, 1986
46. Ward RJ, Bonica JJ, Freund FG et al: Epidural and subarachnoid anesthesia: Cardiovascular and respiratory effects: JAMA 191:275, 1965
47. Greene NM: Physiology of Spinal Anesthesia, 3rd ed, p 95. Baltimore, Williams and Wilkins, 1981
48. Askrog VF, Smith TC, Eckenhoff JE: Changes in pulmonary ventilation during spinal anesthesia. Surg Gynecol Obstet 119:563, 1964
49. DeJong RH: Arterial carbon dioxide and oxygen tensions during spinal block. JAMA 191:608, 1965
50. Egbert LD, Tamersoy K, Deas TC: Pulmonary function during spinal anesthesia: The mechanism of cough depression. Anesthesiology 22:882, 1961
51. Kennedy WF Jr, Sawyer TK, Gerbenshagen HJ et al: Simultaneous systemic cardiovascular and renal hemodynamic measurements during high spinal anesthesia in man. Acta Anaesthesiol Scand (Suppl) 37:163, 1970
52. Greene NM, Bunker JP, Kerr WS et al: Hypotensive spinal anesthesia: Respiratory, metabolic, hepatic, renal and cerebral effects. Ann Surg 140:641, 1954
53. Kennedy WF Jr, Everett GB, Cobb LA et al: Simultaneous systemic and hepatic hemodynamic measurements during high spinal anesthesia in normal man. Anesth Analg 49:1016, 1970
54. Bonica JJ, Berges PU, Morikawa K: Circulatory effects of peridural block: I. Effect of level of analgesia and dose of lidocaine. Anesthesiology 33:619, 1971
55. Bonica JJ, Akamatsu TJ, Berges PU et al: Circulatory effects of peridural block: II. Effect of epinephrine. Anesthesiology 34:514, 1972
56. Bonica JJ, Kennedy WF, Akamatsu TJ et al: Circulatory effects of peridural block: III. Effects of acute blood loss. Anesthesiology 36:219, 1972
57. Sivarajan M, Amory DW, Lindbloom LE: Systemic and regional blood flow during epidural anesthesia without epinephrine in the rhesus monkey. Anesthesiology 45:300, 1976
58. Kennedy WF, Sawyer TK, Gerbershagen HU et al: Systemic cardiovascular and renal hemodynamic alterations during peridural anesthesia in normal man. Anesthesiology 31:414, 1969
59. Stanton-Hicks M, Murphy TM, Bonica JJ et al: Effects of peridural block: V. Properties, circulatory effects, and blood levels of etidocaine and lidocaine. Anesthesiology 42:398, 1975
60. Green NM: Distribution of local anesthetic solutions within the subarachnoid space. Anesth Analg 64:715, 1985
61. Wildsmith JAW, McLure JH, Brown WT et al: Effects of posture on the spread of isobaric and hyperbaric amethocaine. Br J Anaesth 53:273, 1981
62. Levin E, Muravchick S, Gold MI: Density of normal human cerebrospinal fluid and tetracaine solutions. Anesth Analg 60:814, 1981
63. Ernst EA: In-vitro changes of osmolality and density of spinal anesthetic solutions. Anesthesiology 29:104, 1968
64. Lambert DH, Covino BG: Hyperbaric, hypobaric and isobaric spinal anesthesia. Res Staff Phys 33:79, 1987
65. Armstrong IR, Littlewood DG, Chambers WA: Spinal anesthesia with tetracaine—Effect of added vasoconstrictors. Anesth Analg 62:793, 1983
66. Chambers WA, Littlewood DG, Scott DB: Spinal anesthesia with hyperbaric bupivacaine: Effect of added vasoconstrictors. Anesth Analg 61:49, 1982
67. Concepcion M, Lambert DH, Welch KA et al: Tourniquet pain during spinal anesthesia: A comparison of plain solutions of tetracaine and bupivacaine. Anesth Analg 67: In press, 1988
68. Stewart A, Lambert DH, Concepcion M et al: Decreased incidence of tourniquet pain during spinal anesthesia with bupivacaine: A possible explanation. Anesth Analg 67: In press, 1988
69. Chambers WA, Littlewood DG, Logan MR et al: Effect of added epinephrine on spinal anesthesia with lidocaine. Anesth Analg 60:417, 1981
70. Lawrence VS, Rich CR, Magitsky L et al: Spinal anesthesia with isobaric lidocaine 2% and the effect of phenylephrine. Reg Anesth 9:17, 1984
71. Racle JP, Benkhadra A, Poy JY et al: Effect of increasing amounts of epinephrine during isobaric bupivacaine spinal anesthesia in elderly patients. Anesth Analg 66:882, 1987
72. Vaida GT, Moss P, Capan LM et al: Prolongation of lidocaine spinal anesthesia with phenylephrine. Anesth Analg 65:781, 1986
73. Moore DC, Chadwick HS, Ready LB: Epinephrine prolongs lidocaine spinal: Pain in the operative site the most accurate method of determining local anesthetic duration. Anesthesiology 67:416, 1987
74. Kozody R, Ong B, Palahniuk RJ et al: Subarachnoid bupivacaine decreases spinal cord blood flow in dogs. Can Anaesth Soc J 32:216, 1985
75. Kozody R, Palahniuk RJ, Biehl DR: Spinal cord blood flow following subarachnoid lidocaine. Can Anaesth Soc J 32:472, 1985
76. Kozody R, Palahniuk RJ, Cumming MO: Spinal cord blood flow following subarachnoid tetracaine. Can Anaesth Soc J 32:23, 1985
77. Collins JG, Kitahata LM, Matsumoto M et al: Spinally adminis-

tered epinephrine suppresses noxiously evoked activity of WDR neurons in the dorsal horn of the spinal cord. Anesthesiology 60:269, 1984

78. Covino BG, Scott DB: Handbook of Epidural Anaesthesia and Analgesia. p 70. Orlando, Grune and Stratton, 1985

79. Erdermir HA, Soper LE, Sweet RB: Studies of the factors affecting peridural anesthesia. Anesth Analg 44:400, 1965

80. Covino BG, Bush DF: Clinical evaluation of local anaesthetic agents. Br J Anaesth (Suppl) 47:289, 1975

81. Littlewood DG, Buckley P, Covino BG et al: Comparative study of various local anesthetic solutions in block in labour. Br J Anaesth 51:47S, 1979

82. Stanton-Hicks M, Berges PU, Bonica JJ: Circulatory effects of peridural block: IV. Comparison of the effects of epinephrine and phenylephrine. Anesthesiology 39:308, 1973

83. Sinclair CJ, Scott DB: Comparison of bupivacaine and etidocaine in extradural blockade. Br J Anaesth 56:147, 1984

84. Kier L: Continuous epidural analgesia in prostatectomy: Comparison of bupivacaine with and without epinephrine. Acta Anaesthesiol Scand 18:1, 1974

85. Bromage PR: Spread of analgesic solutions in the epidural space and their site of action: A statistical study. Br J Anaesth 34:161, 1962

86. Nishimura N, Kitahara T, Kusakafe T: The spread of lidocaine and I^{131} solution in the epidural space. Anesthesiology 20:785, 1959

87. Park MY, Hagins FM, Massengale MD et al: The sitting position and anesthetic spread in the epidural space. Anesth Analg 63:863, 1984

88. Bromage PR: Aging and epidural dose requirements. Br J Anaesth 41:1016, 1969

89. Park WY, Massengale M, Kim S-I et al: Age and the spread of local anesthetic solutions in the epidural space. Anesth Analg 59:768, 1980

90. Hehre FW, Moyes AZ, Senfield RM et al: Continuous lumbar peridural anesthesia in obstetrics, II: Use of minimal amounts of local anesthetics during labor. Anesth Analg 44:89, 1965

91. Fagraeus L, Urban BJ, Bromage PR: Spread of epidural analgesia in early pregnancy. Anesthesiology 58:184, 1983

92. Datta S, Lambert DH, Gregus J et al: Differential sensitivities of mammalian nerve fibers during pregnancy. Anesth Analg 62:1070, 1983

93. Flanagan HL, Datta S, Lambert DH et al: Effect of pregnancy on bupivacaine-induced conduction blockade in the isolated rabbit vagus nerve. Anesth Analg 66:123, 1987

94. Greene NM: Present concepts of spinal anesthesia. ASA Refresher Courses in Anesthesiology 7:131, 1979

95. Butterworth JF IV, Austin JC, Johnson MD et al: Effect of total spinal anesthesia on arterial and venous responses to dopamine and dobutamine. Anesth Analg 66:209, 1987

96. Butterworth JF IV, Piccione W, Berrizbeitia LD et al: Augmentation of venous return by adrenergic agonist during spinal anesthesia. Anesth Analg 65:612, 1986

97. Greene NM: (Abbott Lecture) Perspectives in spinal anesthesia. Reg Anesth 7:55, 1982

98. Gilman AG, Goodman LS, Gilman A: The Pharmacologic Basis of Therapeutics, 6th ed, p 163. New York, Macmillan, 1980

99. Mihic DN: Postspinal headache and relationship of needle bevel to longitudinal dural fibers. Reg Anesth 10:76, 1985

100. Ready LB, Woodland RV, Haschke RH: Spinal needle angle affects rate of fluid leak across human dura. Anesthesiology 65:A241, 1985

101. Naulty JS, Hertwig L, Datta S et al: Influence of local anesthetic solution on post dural puncture headache. Anesthesiology 63:A454, 1985

102. Zuspan FP: Treatment of postpartum post spinal headache. Obstet Gynecol 16:1, 1960

103. Szeinfeld M, Ihmeidan IH, Moser MM et al: Epidural blood patch: Evaluation of the volume and spread of blood injected into the epidural space. Anesthesiology 64:820, 1986

104. Crawford JS: Prevention of headache consequent on dural puncture. Br J Anaesth 44:598, 1972

105. Shnider SM, Levinson G: Anesthesia for cesarean section. In Shnider SM, Levinson G (eds): Anesthesia for Obstetrics, p 165. Baltimore, Williams & Wilkins, 1987

106. Sechzer PH, Abel L: Post-spinal anesthesia headache treated with caffeine. Evaluation with demand method. Part I. Curr Ther Res 24:307, 1978

107. Sechzer PH: Post-spinal anesthesia headache treated with caffeine. Part II: intracranial vascular distention, a key factor. Curr Ther Res 26:440, 1979

108. Jarvis AP, Greenawalt JW, Fagraeus L: Intravenous caffeine for post-dural puncture headache. Reg Anesth 11:42, 1986

109. Datta S, Alper MH, Ostheimer GO et al: Method of ephedrine administration and nausea and hypotension during spinal anesthesia for cesarean section. Anesthesiology 56:68, 1982

110. Santos A, Datta S: Prophylactic use of droperidol for control of nausea and vomiting during spinal anesthesia for cesarean section. Anesth Analg 63:85, 1984

111. Kane RE: Neurologic deficits following epidural or spinal anesthesia. Anesth Analg 60:150, 1981

112. Vandam LD, Dripps RD: Exacerbation of pre-existing neurologic disease after spinal anesthesia. N Engl J Med 255:843, 1956

113. Dripps RD, Vandam LD: Hazards of lumbar puncture. JAMA 147:1118, 1951

114. Garfield JM, Andriole GL, Vetto JT et al: Prolonged diabetes insipidus subsequent to an episode of chemical meningitis. Anesthesiology 64:253, 1986

115. Greene NM: Neurological sequelae of spinal anesthesia. Anesthesiology 22:682, 1961

116. Mayumi T, Dohi S, Takahashi T: Plasma concentrations of lidocaine associated with cervical, thoracic and lumbar epidural anesthesia. Anesth Analg 62:578, 1983

117. Braid DP, Scott DB: The systemic absorption of local analgesic drugs. Br J Anaesth 37:394, 1965

118. Lund PC, Bush DF, Covino BG: Determinants of etidocaine concentration in the blood. Anesthesiology 42:497, 1975

119. Abdel-Salam AR, Vonwiller JB, Scott DB: Evaluation of etidocaine in extradural block. Br J Anaesth 47:1081, 1975

120. Tucker GT, Mather LE: Clinical pharmacokinetics of local anaesthetics. Clin Pharmacokinet 4:241, 1979

121. Covino BG: Toxicity of local anesthetics. Adv Anesth 3:37, 1986

122. Ravindran RS, Bond VK, Tasch MD et al: Prolonged neural blockade following regional analgesia with 2-chloroprocaine. Anesth Analg 58:447, 1980

123. Reisner LS, Hochman BN, Plumer MH: Persistent neurological deficit and adhesive arachnoiditis following intrathecal 2-chloroprocaine injection. Anesth Analg 58:452, 1980

124. Gissen AJ, Datta S, Lambert D: The chloroprocaine controversy: II. Is chloroprocaine neurotoxic? Reg Anesth 9:135, 1984

125. Varkey GP, Brindle GF: Peridural anaesthesia and anticoagulant therapy. Can Anaesth Soc J 21:106, 1974

126. Odoom JA, Sih IL: Epidural analgesia and anticoagulation therapy. Experience with one thousand cases of continuous epidurals. Anaesthesia 38:254, 1983

127. Rao TLK, El-Etr AA: Anticoagulation following placement of epidural and subarachnoid catheters: An evaluation of neurologic sequelae. Anesthesiology 55:618, 1981

128. Bromage PR: Epidural Analgesia, p 664. Philadelphia, WB Saunders, 1978

129. Broadman LM. Regional anesthesia for the pediatric outpatient. Anes Cl North 5:53, 1987

Chapter 29   *Michael F. Mulroy*

Peripheral Nerve Blockade

GENERAL PRINCIPLES

Regional anesthesia of the extremities and of the trunk is a useful alternative to general anesthesia in many situations. Regional techniques have recently attracted greater interest because of awareness of their salutary role in reducing the stress response to anesthesia and surgery,[1] in reducing postoperative complication rates,[2] and for their potential in improving outpatient anesthesia recovery.[3] Regional techniques are also the most favored choice of anesthesia by anesthesiologists,[4] but their application is often limited by inconsistent teaching in our residency training programs.[5] They are not applicable for every patient or procedure, but familiarity with the techniques described in this chapter and in Chapter 28 will broaden the alternatives we have to offer patients. The specific advantages of regional techniques will be mentioned briefly as appropriate in this chapter but will be discussed in greater detail in chapters relating to specific surgical situations. Some aspects of the selection of drugs and equipment and the preparation, sedation, and monitoring of patients must be modified when dealing with regional anesthesia and will be discussed before the description of specific techniques.

LOCAL ANESTHETIC DRUG SELECTION AND DOSES. The pharmacology of local anesthetics is reviewed at length in Chapter 14. A few points deserve emphasis, particularly in regard to peripheral nerve blockade. Although high concentrations of drug are needed to produce anesthesia in the epidural space, lower concentrations (*e.g.*, 1% lidocaine, 0.25% or 0.5% bupivacaine) are more appropriate on peripheral nerves because of concerns about local and systemic toxicity. Local toxicity of these anesthetics appears to be concentration-dependent[6, 7] (unless injected directly intraneurally); thus, high concentrations are best avoided. Lower concentrations are also indicated because larger volumes are often required to anesthetize poorly localized peripheral nerves or to block a series of nerves (such as the intercostals). The use of a high-concentration solution presents the patient with a high total milligram dose of local anesthetic, which may produce toxic blood levels. In simplest terms, one can use twice as much 1% lidocaine as 2% lidocaine before reaching the same level of concern about toxicity.[8] For both of these reasons, high concentrations are best avoided in peripheral nerve blockade.

The absorption of drug and the duration of anesthesia will vary with the dose, drug, location injected, and presence of vasoconstrictors. The anesthesiologist must remain aware that the highest blood levels of local anesthetic occur after intercostal blockade, followed by epidural, caudal, and brachial plexus blockade. Similarly, the duration is dependent upon the blood supply of the area of injection. Equivalent doses of local anesthetic may produce only 3 to 4 hr of anesthesia in the epidural space, but 24 to 36 hours on the sciatic nerve. Care should be taken in choosing drugs of appropriate concentration, duration, and total dose. Specific comments are made in conjunction with each of the techniques described, but familiarity with the material and tables in Chapter 14 is needed for appropriate choices. In general, the addition of epinephrine 1:200,000 is advantageous in prolonging the duration of blockade and in reducing the systemic blood levels of local anesthetic. Its use is not appropriate in the vicinity of "terminal" blood vessels, such as in the digits or penis, or when using an intravenous regional technique, but, generally, all the recommended doses and drugs in this chapter include the addition of epinephrine to the solution.

NERVE LOCALIZATION. A few general principles apply to methods of nerve localization. The blockade techniques associated with reliable *proximity of nerves to bones or arteries* are the easiest technically to perform (*e.g.*, epidural, intercostal, axillary). Less-reliable landmarks, such as the psoas compartment or obturator foramen, require either large volumes of local anesthetic solution or the establishment of a distinct paresthesia of the desired nerve to provide adequate anesthesia. *Paresthesias* have been recommended as the ultimate sign of successful localization, and the older dictum of "no paresthesia, no anesthesia" has merit. Nevertheless, there are some potential problems associated with this technique. Of greatest concern is the potential for intraneural injection if paresthesias are obtained. This is usually signaled by a complaint from the patient of a "cramping" or "aching" pain during the initial injection. If this occurs, the needle should be immediately withdrawn a few millimeters and a small test injection repeated. Even without intraneural injection, residual neuropathy of peripheral nerves appears more likely if paresthesias are obtained. Selander et al[9] have reported a 2.8% incidence of residual ulnar neuropathy when paresthesias were used to locate nerves compared with a 0.8% incidence with other techniques of axillary blockade. Although careful technique and attention to needle design (see below) and drugs (see Chapter 14) may reduce this, caution should be taken when using paresthesias for nerve localization. A third problem with this technique is the inevitable discomfort associated with it; patient education and sedation must be handled appropriately (see below).

One alternative method for nerve localization is the use of a *nerve stimulator*. This is based on the observation that a low-current electrical impulse applied to a peripheral nerve will produce stimulation of the motor fibers and, thus, will identify the proximity of the nerve without actual needle contact or patient discomfort (or cooperation). This technique is particularly suited to the patient who is uncooperative as a result of inebriation or heavy sedation. Since the nerve stimulator does not actually have to contact the nerve to produce a motor response, its use may reduce the chance for nerve injury. Its use does not improve the success rate of regional anesthesia in a training program,[10] since a familiarity with the anatomy and the techniques are necessary to bring the needle into proximity to the nerve. Nevertheless, this is a promising adjunct to regional anesthesia, and some comments about appropriate use of these devices are warranted.

The ideal stimulator should have a variable amperage output.[11] This allows a high current to be delivered in the exploration phase, and then a progressively lower current to document proximity of the nerve. Whereas 10 mA can be used to produce the first motor twitch, actual injection of anesthetic should be delayed until stimulation is produced by as little as 0.1 mA. At that point, 2 to 3 ml of local anesthetic should be sufficient to abolish motor twitch and indicates that it is appropriate to inject the remainder of the proposed dose. The accuracy of the localization can be improved by the use of insulated needles. A plastic sheath along the shaft allows the current flow to be concentrated at the tip and is more likely to produce stimulation only when the tip is near the nerve fiber, rather than after the tip has moved past its target.[12] Current flow can also be improved by using the positive (red) pole of the stimulator as the ground (or reference) electrode and the negative (black) lead as the connection to the needle itself. Despite these steps, the stimulator is still only an adjunct to nerve localization and not a reliable substitute for good technique. Its potential advantages must be weighed against the small amount of extra time involved in its use and the usual require-ment for an assistant to operate the machine while the anesthesiologist performs the actual blockade.

EQUIPMENT. In addition to the nerve stimulator, some other items of regional blockade equipment deserve general comment. The most frequent discussion in this regard is the debate over disposable versus reusable *trays*. This is a matter of personal preference and of economy. If a large volume of regional anesthetics are performed in an institution, the cost of maintenance of trays (technician time and sterilization) will be less than the use of disposable equipment.[13] Reusable trays also allow the department to select high-quality needles and syringes to meet their specifications. Manufacturers usually do not produce disposable equipment to the same high tolerances that characterize reusable instruments. On the other hand, there are a large number of quality disposable kits available on the market today, and many of the major manufacturers will customize their packages at the request of large institutions willing to commit to purchasing a sufficient volume. The use of disposable trays also provides the advantage of placing the burden of sterilization on the manufacturer, although the liability for checking the sterility of contents always remains with the user. In the final analysis, cost is a major factor, but personal choice is usually the critical element.

For greater safety and efficacy, the *needles* used for regional techniques require some modifications from the standard injection needles (Fig. 29-1). First, for most cases of peripheral blockade, the "short bevel" or "B bevel" is used. This shorter angulation of the bevel (16 to 20 degrees vs conventional 12 to 13 degrees) was introduced by Selander et al[14] and has been shown to produce less injury to nerves, perhaps by pushing the nerve away rather than piercing it when contact is made. Other modifications, such as the "pencil point"–insulated needle have also been introduced in attempts to reduce nerve injury. Another feature of regional blockade needles is the

FIG. 29-1. Regional anesthesia needles. Characteristic features of needles used for peripheral nerve blockade include the "security bead" on the shaft just below its juncture with the hub and the shorter bevel angle compared with standard Quincke-type needle points. Further modifications to enhance the use of a nerve stimulator include the attachment prong for the electrode and the insulated shaft.

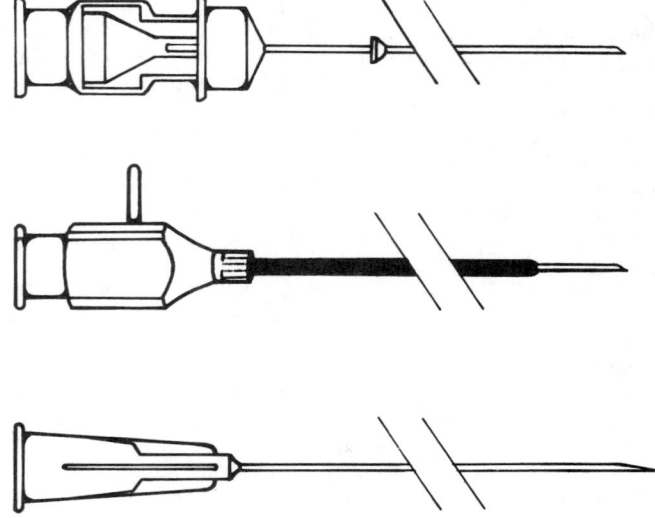

addition of a "security bead" to the shaft. This small bead is added approximately 6 mm from the juncture of the shaft and the hub and prevents the shaft of the needle from retracting below the skin in the event that it becomes separated from the hub. These two modifications are useful features for peripheral nerve blockade. In addition, the regional anesthesiologist should have an assortment of needle sizes and lengths available for various types of blockade.

Special *syringes* are also useful for performing peripheral nerve blockades. Although glass syringes are often preferred for epidural techniques, the loss of resistance is rarely needed in peripheral blockade. Plastic or glass may be equally useful. With respect to size, a 10-ml syringe is usually a good compromise. Large volumes are usually required for peripheral nerve blockade, so that 3 ml and 5 ml syringes are rarely adequate. Larger than 10-ml volume often presents such bulk and weight that fine control is hampered. If a larger syringe is used, it is usually advisable to have an assistant manipulate the syringe and have it attached to the needle by a short length of extension tubing. The use of finger rings (the "control syringe") is helpful in controlling injection and allowing the operator to refill the syringe with one hand (Fig. 29-2). Luer-Lok adaptors for the syringe–hub connection are also advantageous. Although friction fittings produce tight seals, the amount of force required for attaching or removing the syringe may displace a needle that has been meticulously maneuvered into the appropriate close contact with a nerve.

The selection of *antiseptic solutions* is usually a local preference. Organic iodine preparations are the current standard for skin asepsis. They are usually nonirritating to tissues and carry the added advantage of a distinct color. Colorless prep solutions are dangerous because of the possibility of confusion with (or contamination of) local anesthetic solutions. Colored alcohol solutions are acceptable skin cleansers for many of the simple infiltrations that do not require extensive preparation. For major deep blockade, a wide area of skin preparation is more desirable, and the borders of the clean area can be extended by draping on four sides with sterile towels. Regional anesthesia does not require the same degree of sterile preparation and gowning as indicated for surgery, but

FIG. 29-2. The three-ring ("control") syringe. Use of this adaptation to the plunger of a standard 10-ml syringe allows greater control of injection, easier aspiration, and the opportunity to refill the syringe with one hand. Plastic adapters are available for disposable syringes as demonstrated; glass syringes are supplied with a metal plunger and ring attached. (Reproduced with permission. From Mulroy M: Handbook of Regional Anesthesia. Boston, Little, Brown, 1988.)

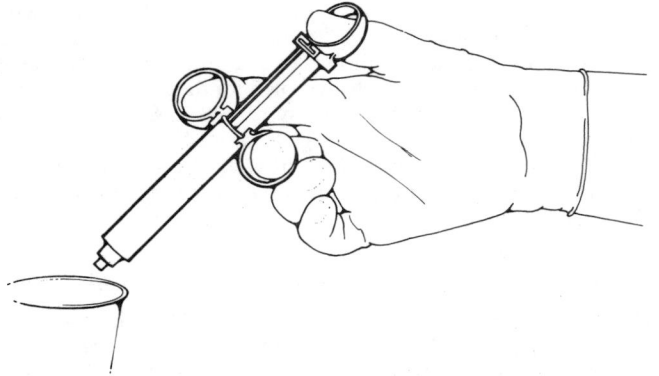

strict attention to asepsis is desirable to reduce the chance of infection.

COMMON COMPLICATIONS. Although specific complications of each of the individual techniques will be discussed in the following sections, there are a few recurrent common problems of peripheral nerve blockade that merit mention. *Systemic toxicity of local anesthetics* is the most serious concern. This syndrome, as well as the problems of allergy and other unique toxicities, is addressed in Chapter 14. Central nervous system excitation and myocardial depression are the two most common hazards associated with high blood levels of local anesthetics. No peripheral nerve blockade using significant quantities of local anesthetic should be performed without appropriate resuscitation equipment immediately available. This includes blockades using small quantities of anesthetic but near cerebral vessels, such as stellate ganglion or cervical plexus blockade. With peripheral nerve blockade, careful use of a test dose and small incremental injections are needed if intravascular injection is a risk. Although attention is usually focused on this possibility, toxicity can also occur owing to slow absorption of large doses. Patients should be observed carefully for 20 to 30 minutes following injection, since peak levels occur at this time.

Peripheral *neuropathy* usually results from intraneural local anesthetic injection or needle trauma, although it should be kept in mind that there are other causes.[15] Careful attention should be paid to positioning the patient with numb extremities. Postoperative follow-up is important in confirming that neurologic function has returned to normal. If a deficit is detected, early neurologic assessment is critical in determining whether a pre-existent neuropathy was involved.[16] Fortunately, most of these syndromes resolve uneventfully, but full recovery of some peripheral injuries requires several months as a result of slow regeneration of injured peripheral nerves. Sympathetic concern and involvement of the anesthesiologist in arranging physical therapy during recovery will help reduce patient dissatisfaction.

Other minor complications such as *pain at the site of injection* and local *hematoma* formation are not uncommon but are usually of short duration and respond to reassurance by the anesthesiologist. Hematoma around a peripheral nerve is not of the same significance as that in the epidural or subarachnoid space. Again, expressed concern and help with local therapy and analgesics will alleviate patient dissatisfaction.

PATIENT PREPARATION

PATIENT SELECTION. In general, all patients scheduled for extremity, thoracic, abdominal, or perineal surgery should be considered candidates for a regional anesthetic technique. This can be used as the only anesthetic, as a supplement to provide analgesia and muscle relaxation along with general anesthesia, or as the initial step for provision of prolonged postoperative analgesia such as with intercostal blockade or continuous epidural anesthesia. *Patient refusal* can often be an impediment to regional anesthesia, although this is frequently a "relative" refusal. Often the patient's real objections to "being awake" or "being aware" can be managed by the use of sedatives and amnestic drugs. True unwavering refusal of "any needles" is a contraindication to regional anesthesia, although gentle attempts at patient education should be offered. Other contraindications include local *infection* and perhaps systemic *coagulopathy*. The presence of pre-existing *neu-*

rologic disease is often discussed. Some data are available in the case of spinal anesthesia, but the use of peripheral nerve blockade in this situation is unclear. A classic example is whether an arm blockade should be used for a scheduled ulnar nerve transposition at the elbow. Although some physicians will avoid any procedure that may confuse the picture of postoperative neuropathy, others believe that if there is a clear difference in the potential injury and the pre-existent disease, regional techniques are appropriate. There are no clear answers in this regard, and full patient education and cooperation are most appropriate. Finally, the level of *patient anxiety* is an important consideration. Extreme apprehension regarding surgery will necessitate heavy sedation, and the advantages of regional anesthesia in providing rapid recovery, alertness, and protection of airway reflexes may be negated. The use of regional anesthesia in these situations is a matter of judgment and experience.

PREMEDICATION AND SEDATION. The best preparation for a regional technique is careful patient education. Calm gentle explanation of the technique as it is performed will reduce most patient anxiety to a manageable level. In most cases, though, supplemental medication is also useful. In addition to the general comments about premedication discussed in earlier chapters, regional anesthesia techniques have some special requirements. First, sedation must be adjusted to the required level of patient cooperation. If paresthesias are to be sought, medication must be light enough to allow patient identification and reporting of nerve contact. Although a mild dose of opioid (50 to 100 μg of fentanyl or equivalent) will help ease the discomfort of nerve localization, patient awareness must be maintained. This does not preclude the use of an amnestic agent, and midazolam in 1 mg to 3 mg doses may provide excellent amnesia at levels of consciousness that still allow cooperation. This is also an excellent supplement in the outpatient setting, where short duration of effect is desired. If paresthesias are not needed, as in intercostal blockade, heavy sedation may allow greater patient tolerance of the injections. In such situations, longer-acting opioids such as 8 to 12 mg of morphine and more sedative amnestics such as scopolamine may be useful. Although intramuscular premedication is common with hospitalized patients, careful titration of intravenous drugs at the time of the blockade is the most effective way to adjust the level of sedation to individual patient needs and sensitivities.

MONITORING. Along with the consideration of degree of sedation is the question of the appropriate degree of monitoring for patients receiving regional anesthetic techniques. Although current discussions of "monitoring" typically revolve around mechanical and electrical devices, repetitive assessment of the patient's *mental status* when receiving local anesthetics is of paramount importance. The anesthesiologist must maintain verbal contact with these patients on a frequent basis and ideally have an uninvolved assistant available to assess the level of consciousness at all times. There are no electrical or mechanical devices that detect rising blood levels of local anesthetic; close observation for peak levels owing to intravenous (within 2 min) and subcutaneous absorption (about 20 min) is essential. An *electrocardiogram* (ECG) is appropriate to detect the pulse rise seen with epinephrine when it is included in a test dose. It is also useful in case systemic toxicity occurs with bupivacaine, particularly whenever large doses of that drug are used. Other pulse counters such as mechanical meters and pulse oximeters are also useful when monitoring the pulse rate change with epinephrine. *Blood pressure* monitoring

should be performed as with any anesthetic. A baseline pressure should be obtained whenever any sympathetic blockade is performed and at frequent intervals thereafter. Other circumstances in which blood pressure measurement is important include following the injection of celiac plexus anesthesia or to detect intravascular epinephrine injection. Beyond these specific comments, the standards for monitoring and recordkeeping on any patient undergoing regional anesthesia are the same as for patients undergoing any general anesthetic. One must be particularly careful not to be lulled into a false sense of security because it is "just a regional anesthetic." Patients may still develop life-threatening cardiovascular or ventilatory depression owing to delayed absorption of local anesthetic or too liberal use of sedation.

DISCHARGE CRITERIA. Concern is occasionally expressed about discharging patients from Post-Anesthesia Care Units when an extremity is still anesthetized. If regional anesthesia is administered to provide prolonged analgesia, numbness may be expected to persist for 10 (with intercostal anesthesia) to 24 (sciatic blockade) hours after bupivacaine administration. It is clearly unreasonable to delay discharge in this situation, and patients have been successfully discharged to the wards as long as their mental alertness is adequate. Even outpatients may be discharged home with numb arms or legs as long as the patient is reliable and adequate instruction about care of the insensitive extremity is provided. The major problem arises with orthostatic hypotension following sympathetic blockade. Patients receiving celiac plexus blockade or spinal or epidural sympathectomies should be assessed for stable blood pressure and ambulated gradually before discharge from close supervision.

SPECIFIC TECHNIQUES

The remainder of this chapter is devoted to the details of the performance of specific types of blockade, arranged by sections of the body. There has not been an attempt to describe every regional technique practiced but to focus on those of clinical usefulness to the anesthesiologist. The common methods are described, recognizing that several alternative approaches have been advocated in each case.

HEAD AND NECK

Regional anesthesia of the head and neck has limited surgical application. Concern about control and maintenance of the airway makes many anesthesiologists uncomfortable with regional techniques when intraoperative airway intervention is awkward. Nevertheless, occasionally there are patients who may benefit from regional techniques in the head or neck. More commonly, the techniques of trigeminal nerve blockade and occipital nerve blockade are used for diagnostic or neurolytic blockade for chronic pain syndromes. Cervical plexus blockade is useful for some surgical procedures on the neck, and topical/regional airway anesthesia is effective in reducing the subjective discomfort and hemodynamic responses to intubation.

Trigeminal Nerve Blockade

Sensory and motor nerve function of the face is provided by the branches of the 5th cranial (trigeminal) nerve. The roots of this nerve arise from the base of the pons and send sensory branches to the large gasserian (or semilunar) ganglion, which lies on the superior margin of the petrous bone just inside the skull above the foramen ovale. A smaller motor fiber nucleus lies behind it and sends motor branches to one terminal nerve, the mandibular. The three major branches of the trigeminal each have a separate exit from the skull (Fig. 29-3). The uppermost ophthalmic branch passes through the sphenoidal fissure into the orbit. The main terminal fibers of this nerve, the frontal nerve, bifurcate into the supratrochlear and supraorbital nerves. These two branches traverse the orbit along the superior border and exit on the front of the face in the easily palpated supraorbital notch for the former, and along the medial border of the orbit for the latter.

The two major branches of the trigeminal are the middle (maxillary) and lower (mandibular). The maxillary nerve contains only sensory fibers and exits the skull through the foramen rotundum. It passes beneath the skull anteriorly through the sphenomaxillary fossa. At this point, it lies medial to the lateral pterygoid plate on each side. At the anterior end of this channel, it again moves superiorly to re-enter the skull in the infraorbital canal in the floor of the orbit. Within the sphenomaxillary fossa, it branches to form the sphenopalatine nerves and to give off the posterior dental branches. The anterior dental nerves arise from the main trunk as it passes through the infraorbital canal. The terminal infraorbital nerve emerges from the foramen of the same name just below the eye and lateral to the nose and gives off the terminal palpebral, nasal, and labial nerves. The mandibular nerve is the third and largest branch of the trigeminal, and the only one to receive motor fibers. It exits the skull posterior to the maxillary nerve through the foramen ovale. At this point, it is just posterior to the lateral pterygoid plate of the sphenoid bone. The motor nerves separate into an anterior branch immediately below the foramen ovale. The main branch continues as the inferior alveolar nerve medial to the ramus of the mandible. This nerve curves anteriorly to follow the mandible and exits as a terminal branch through the mental foramen. The mental nerve provides sensation to the lower lip and jaw.

GASSERIAN GANGLION BLOCKADE. Ideally, the simplest blockade of the trigeminal nerve is performed in the central ganglion, which includes all three branches, and is frequently recommended for treatment of disabling trigeminal neuralgia. In fact, this blockade is technically the most difficult and has the most undesirable potential for the complications of subarachnoid injection of anesthetic after neurolytic blockade. Residual numbness of the face is sometimes unpleasant, and a neuritis may be as unpleasant as the original condition. Protective corneal sensation may also be lost, and special care of the eye may be needed. Nevertheless, it is a technique useful in severe cases of trigeminal neuralgia that are unresponsive to more peripheral blockade. Alcohol injection has been performed in the past, although radio-frequency ablation by neurosurgeons has become more accepted recently. The procedure for blockade follows:

1. Three landmarks are needed to help locate the foramen ovale. First, a skin wheal is raised 3 cm lateral to the corner of the mouth on the involved side. A second mark is made on the skin 1 cm anterior to the midpoint of the zygoma (the midpoint lies just above the deepest part of the sigmoid notch of the mandible). The third landmark is the pupil of the eye itself on the ipsilateral side.
2. A 12.5 cm needle is introduced through the skin wheal on the cheek. The needle is advanced posteriorly in the sagittal plane formed by an imaginary line between the pupil and the point of insertion. As it moves posteriorly, it is angled superiorly toward the third point (anterior to the midpoint of the zygomatic arch). If advanced properly, the needle will pass through the muscles of the cheek without entering the oral cavity and will contact the base of the skull medial to the mandible and the zygoma. If it has remained in the plane of the pupil, it will be near the foramen ovale.
3. Once bone is contacted, the needle is withdrawn and reinserted to angle slightly more posteriorly until the foramen is entered. At this point, paresthesias of the maxillary branch are sought. The needle should not be advanced more than 1 cm beyond the opening of the foramen. If there is any question about localization, biplanar fluoroscopy is useful in confirming position.
4. After localization of the nerve, careful aspiration is performed to detect unwanted subarachnoid placement of the needle. Two milliliters of 1% lidocaine injected slowly will usually produce anesthesia of all three sensory branches. If alcohol is used, the anesthesia is preceded by a severe burning sensation; this can be reduced by prior injection of a few drops of local anesthetic.

FIG. 29-3. Lateral view of major branches of trigeminal nerve. Each major branch exits the skull by a separate foramen. The ophthalmic branch travels in the orbit. The maxillary and mandibular branches emerge from the skull medial to the lateral pterygoid plate, which serves as the landmark for their identification. (Reproduced with permission. From Mulroy M: Handbook of Regional Anesthesia. Boston, Little, Brown, 1988.)

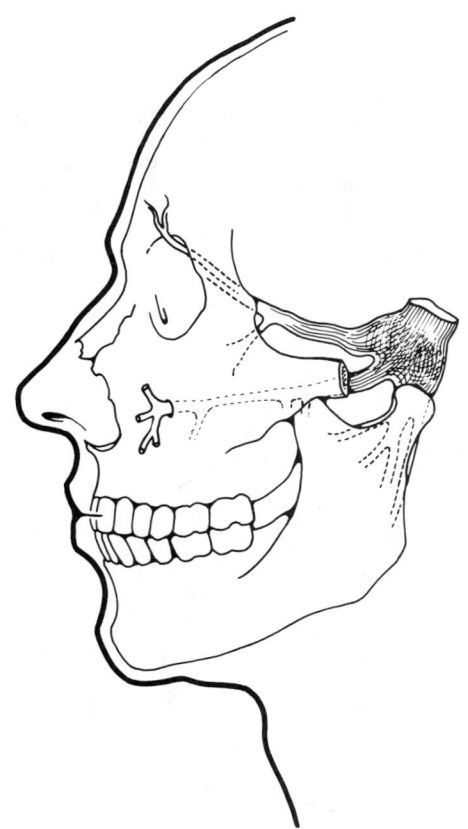

SUPERFICIAL TRIGEMINAL NERVE BRANCH BLOCK-ADE. Fortunately, most anesthetic applications of trigeminal blockade can be more easily performed by injection of the individual terminal superficial branches. This is relatively simple, since the three superficial branches and their associated foramen all lie in the same sagittal plane on each side of the face (Fig. 29-4). Each of these foramina are readily palpable, and these nerves can be easily blocked with superficial injections of small quantities of local anesthetic. Although the bony landmarks are usually sufficient themselves, paresthesias are desirable before alcohol injection. Each of these blocks can be performed with the patient in the supine position. The procedure for blockade follows:

1. The supraorbital notch is easily palpated along the medial superior rim of the orbit, usually 2.5 cm from the midline. Two to 3 ml of local anesthetic injected immediately in the vicinity of the notch will produce anesthesia of the ipsilateral forehead. Anesthesia of the supratrochlear nerve by superficial infiltration of the medial aspect of the orbital rim is needed if the band of anesthesia is to cross the midline.
2. The infraorbital foramen lies below the inferior orbital rim in the same plane at approximately the same dis-

tance from the midline as the supraorbital notch (usually 2.5 cm). If the foramen cannot be palpated directly, it can be sought by gently probing with a small-gauge needle. This needle should be introduced through a skin wheal approximately 0.5 cm below the expected opening, because the canal angles cephalad from this point toward the orbital floor. Again, injection of a small quantity of local anesthetic immediately in the vicinity of the foramen will produce anesthesia of the middle third of the ipsilateral face.

3. The mental nerve also emerges approximately 2.5 cm from the midline, usually midway between the upper and lower border of the mandible. The mental canal angles medially and inferiorly so that, in this case, needle insertion should start approximately 0.5 cm above and 0.5 cm lateral to the anticipated location of the orifice if it cannot be palpated directly. In older patients, resorption of the superior margin of the mandibular bone itself will make the foramen appear to lie more superiorly along the ramus. Again, 2 ml of local anesthesia injected into the canal will produce anesthesia of the mandibular area.

MAXILLARY NERVE BLOCKADE. If anesthesia in superior dental nerves is also required or if superficial infraorbital nerve blockade does not produce adequate anesthesia, proximal block of the maxillary nerve is required. This can be performed by a lateral approach to the sphenopalatine fossa (Fig. 29-5). The procedure for blockade follows:

1. The patient lies supine with a small towel under the occiput and the head turned slightly away from the side to be blocked. The zygomatic arch is marked along its course, and the patient is asked to open and close the mouth slowly so that the curved upper border of the

FIG. 29-4. Terminal branches of the trigeminal nerve. Each of the three terminal branches (the supraorbital, infraorbital, and mental) exits its respective bony canal in the same sagittal plane, approximately 2.5 cm from the midline. The infraorbital canal is angled slightly cephalad, while the mental canal can be entered if the needle is directed medial and slightly caudad. (Reproduced with permission. From Mulroy M: Handbook of Regional Anesthesia. Boston, Little, Brown, 1988.)

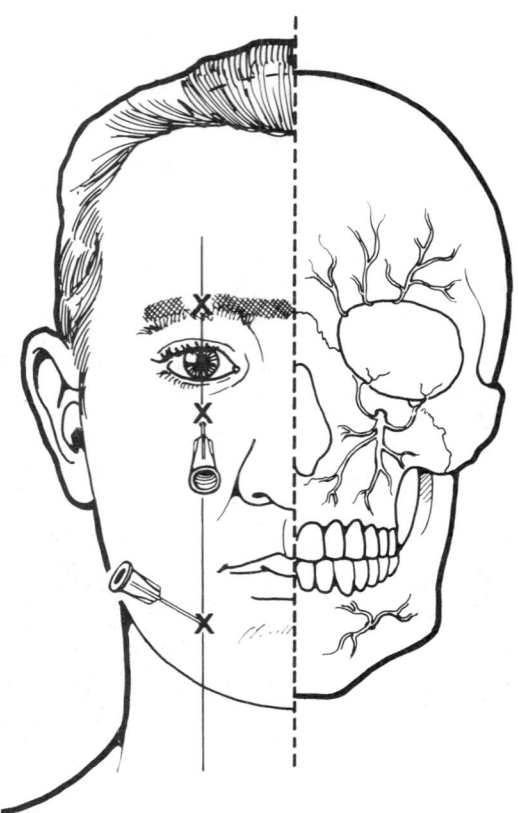

FIG. 29-5. Lateral approach to the maxillary nerve. The needle is introduced through the skin just over the notch of the mandible and directed anterior and cephalad to identify the pterygoid plate. As the needle is advanced anteriorly off the plate, the maxillary nerve is encountered before it re-enters the skull in the infraorbital canal in the base of the orbit. (Reproduced with permission. From Mulroy M: Handbook of Regional Anesthesia. Boston, Little, Brown, 1988.)

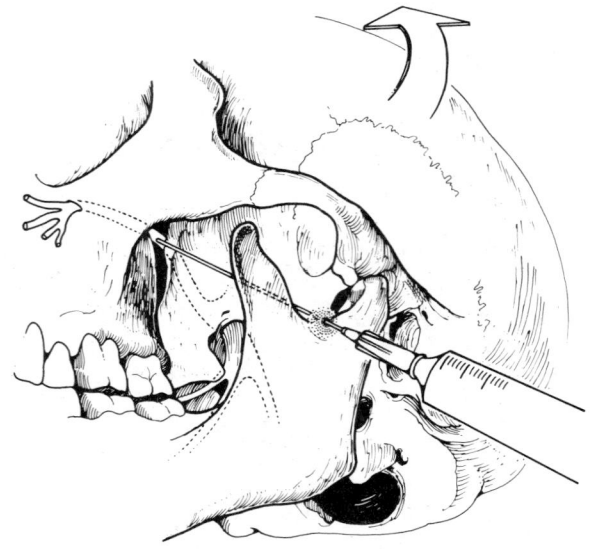

mandible can be identified. The lowest point of the mandibular notch is palpated, and an "X" marked at this spot, which is usually at the midpoint of the zygoma. A skin wheal is raised at the "X" after the appropriate skin preparations.

2. With the patient's jaw in the open position, a 7.5 cm needle is introduced through the "X" and directed 45 degrees cephalad and slightly anterior. This direction should be toward the imagined posterior border of the globe of the eye.
3. The needle should contact the pterygoid plate. It is then withdrawn and redirected slightly anterior until it succeeds in passing beyond the pterygoid plate. At this point, the nerve should lie approximately 1 cm deeper. A paresthesia in the nose or the upper teeth will confirm the nerve localization.
4. Anesthesia can be achieved by injecting 5 ml into the fossa, either on obtaining the paresthesia or blindly by advancing 1 cm beyond the plate.

The major complication of concern is spread of the anesthetic to adjacent structures, especially to the nerves in the orbit.

MANDIBULAR NERVE BLOCKADE. This nerve can also be blocked for inferior dental pain. It is the only branch where anesthesia carries the risk of loss of motor (mastication) function (Fig. 29-6). The procedure for blockade follows:

1. Head position and landmarks are the same as those described for the maxillary nerve blockade.

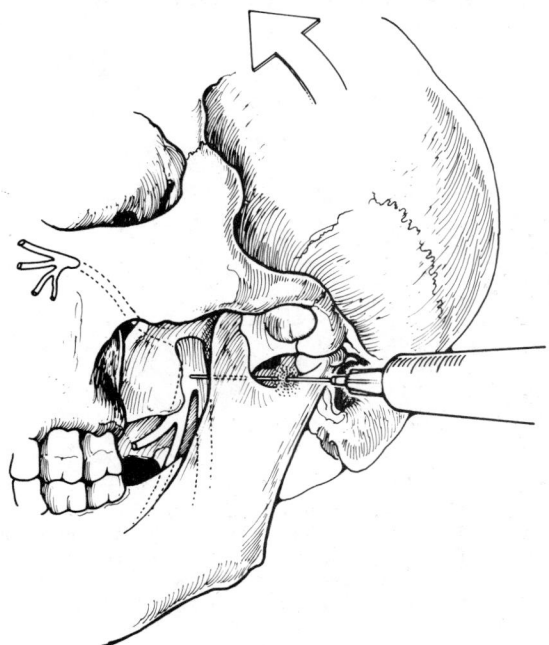

FIG. 29-6. Lateral approach to the mandibular nerve. The needle is introduced in the same manner as for the maxillary nerve block but directly posteriorly. After contacting the pterygoid plate, it is directed further posteriorly until it passes behind the plate, where it should encounter the nerve. (Reproduced with permission. From Mulroy M: Handbook of Regional Anesthesia. Boston, Little, Brown, 1988.)

2. A 2-inch needle is introduced through the skin wheal and directed medially but slightly posterior and without the cephalad angulation required for maxillary nerve anesthesia. This will leave the needle approximately perpendicular to the skin in all planes.
3. When the pterygoid plate is contacted, the needle is redirected posteriorly until it passes beyond the plate. It should contact the nerve 0.5 to 1 cm deep to this point.
4. Paresthesia of the jaw or cheek will confirm identification of the nerve. Five to 10 ml of solution injected incrementally at this point should produce anesthesia of the terminal branches. If paresthesias are essential, exploration should be carried gently cephalad and caudad from the initial point where the needle passes posterior to the plate. As with maxillary blockade, paresthesias can be painful to the patient, and the use of an assistant to secure the head is occasionally necessary.

Facial nerve anesthesia can occasionally be seen when large volumes are injected to block the mandibular nerve. This is of little consequence unless neurolytic agents are used. A more serious complication is the possibility of intravascular injection in this highly vascularized area. Injection should be performed incrementally with small quantities, with constant observation for signs of central toxicity.

Cervical Plexus Blockade

Sensory and motor fibers of the neck and posterior scalp arise from the nerve roots of the 2nd, 3rd, and 4th cervical nerves. This cervical plexus is unique in that the sensory fibers separate from the motor fibers early in their course and can be blocked separately. Classic plexus anesthesia along the tubercles of the vertebral body produces both motor and sensory blockade. The transverse processes of the cervical vertebrae form peculiar elongated troughs for the emergence of their nerve roots. These troughs lie immediately lateral to a medial opening for the cephalad passage of the vertebral artery. The trough at the terminal end of the transverse process divides into an anterior and posterior tubercle, which can often be easily palpated. These tubercles also serve as the attachments for the anterior and middle scalene muscles, which thus form a compartment for the cervical plexus as well as for the brachial plexus immediately below. The compartment at this level is less developed than the one formed around the brachial plexus. The motor branches (including the phrenic nerve) curl anteriorly around the lateral border of the anterior scalene and proceed caudad and medially toward the muscles of the neck. They give anterior branches to the sternocleidomastoid as they pass behind it. The sensory fibers, as mentioned, also emerge behind the anterior scalene muscle but separate from the motor branches and continue laterally to emerge superficially under the posterior border of the sternocleidomastoid. They provide sensory anesthesia to the anterior and posterior skin of the neck and shoulder.

Anesthesia of either the superficial cervical nerves or the cervical plexus itself can be used for operations on the lateral or anterior neck. Thyroidectomy and carotid endarterectomy fall into this category, although supplemental local infiltration of the thyroid gland may occasionally be necessary because of sensory innervation from cranial nerves. In carotid surgery, local infiltration of the carotid bifurcation may be necessary to block reflex hemodynamic changes associated with glossopharyngeal stimulation. Cervical plexus anesthesia alone is rarely adequate for shoulder surgery. It is preferable to perform interscalene anesthesia of the brachial plexus for these procedures, since the likelihood of adequate motor relaxation is greater and the cervical plexus is usually blocked incidentally. The procedure for cervical plexus blockade follows:

1. The patient is placed supine with a small towel under the head, with the head turned slightly to the side opposite the one to be blocked.
2. The mastoid process is identified and marked. The transverse processes can often be palpated. If not, the most prominent tubercle, that of the 6th cervical vertebra, is marked, and a line is drawn between it and the mastoid process (Fig. 29-7).
3. The cervical processes should be felt approximately 0.5 cm posterior to the line drawn between the mastoid and the 6th cervical tubercle. The 2nd vertebral process should lie approximately 1.5 cm below the mastoid itself. (There is no process for the first vertebra.)
4. The 3rd and 4th processes lie approximately 1.5 cm below their respective superior neighbors.
5. Skin wheals are raised at the three "X" marks that have been placed over the transverse processes.
6. A 3.75 cm needle is introduced perpendicular to the skin and directed posterior and slightly caudad at each "X" until it rests on the transverse process. It is important to maintain a caudad direction in order to avoid entry directly into the intervertebral foramina. The needle is walked caudad. It should slip off the bone if it is truly on the process rather than continuing to contact bone if it is on the vertebral body. It is important to contact the transverse process as far laterally as possible in order to avoid any contact of the needle with the vertebral artery (Fig. 29-8).
7. Paresthesias are usually not necessary. A syringe is connected directly to the needle, and 5 ml of local anesthetic solution is deposited along the transverse process itself. Anesthesia should follow within 5 minutes in the distribution of the nerve.

The major potential complication of this procedure is intravascular injection into the vertebral artery. Again, injection should be made in small increments, with frequent observation of the patient's mental status and frequent aspiration to detect intravascular placement. If the needle is advanced too far medially into the vertebral foramen, epidural or even subarachnoid anesthesia may be produced. This is more likely in the cervical region because of longer sleeves of dura that accompany these nerve branches. Again, frequent aspiration and careful lateral placement of the needle is important.

Phrenic nerve blockade occurs frequently with deep cervical plexus anesthesia. This blockade is not indicated in any patient who is dependent upon his or her diaphragm for tidal ventilation, nor is bilateral blockade desirable in most patients. Recurrent laryngeal nerve or vagal blockade can also occur because of diffusion of the local anesthetic. This is a troublesome but not serious complication. It may interfere with the ability to evaluate vocal cord function following thyroid surgery.

SUPERFICIAL CERVICAL PLEXUS BLOCKADE. This is performed in the same position, and results in anesthesia only of the sensory fibers of the plexus. The procedure for blockade follows:

1. An "X" is made along the posterior border of the sternocleidomastoid muscle at the level of the 4th cervical

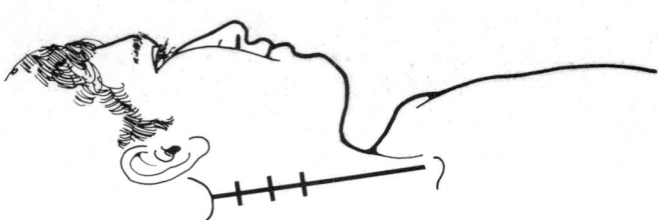

FIG. 29-7. Superficial landmarks for cervical plexus blockade. A line is drawn from the mastoid process to the prominent tubercle of the 6th cervical vertebra. The transverse processes of the 2nd, 3rd and 4th cervical vertebrae lie 0.5 cm posterior to this line and at 1.5-cm intervals below the mastoid. (Reproduced with permission. From Mulroy M: Handbook of Regional Anesthesia. Boston, Little, Brown, 1988.)

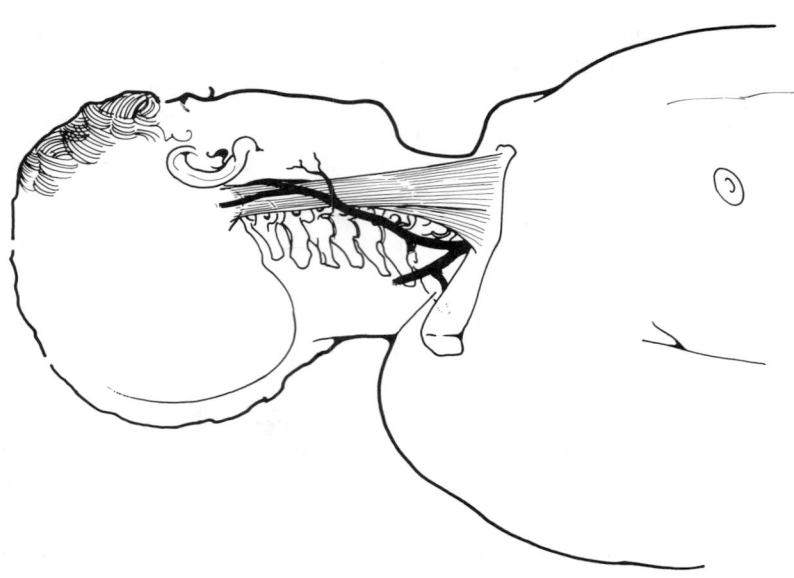

FIG. 29-8. Anatomy of deep cervical plexus blockade. The transverse processes lie under the lateral border of the sternocleidomastoid muscle, each with a distal trough or sulcus that defines the path of nerve exit. (Reproduced with permission. From Mulroy M: Handbook of Regional Anesthesia. Boston, Little, Brown, 1988.)

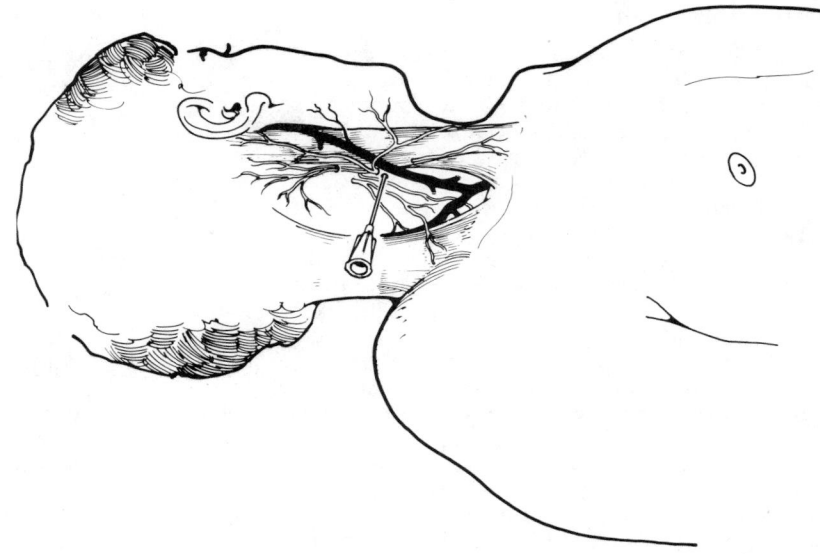

FIG. 29-9. Superficial cervical plexus blockade. The sensory fibers of the plexus all emerge from behind the lateral border of the sternocleidomastoid muscle. A needle inserted at its midpoint, usually where the external jugular vein crosses the muscle, can be directed superiorly and inferiorly to block all these terminal branches. (Reproduced with permission. From Mulroy M: Handbook of Regional Anesthesia. Boston, Little, Brown, 1988.)

vertebra. This usually corresponds with the junction of the external jugular vein as it crosses the posterior border of the muscle (Fig. 29-9).

2. A skin wheal is raised at this mark, and superficial local anesthetic infiltration is performed along the posterior border of the sternocleidomastoid muscle 4 cm above and below the level of the "X." Ten to 12 ml of local anesthetic solution will usually provide sensory anesthesia of the anterior neck and shoulder.

Occipital Nerve Blockade

The ophthalmic branch of the trigeminal nerve provides sensory innervation of the forehead and anterior scalp, but the remainder of the scalp is innervated by fibers of the greater and lesser occipital nerves, terminal branches of the cervical plexus. These nerves can be blocked by superficial injection at the point on the posterior skull where they emerge from below the muscles of the neck (Fig. 29-10). Anesthesia is rarely used for surgical procedures; it is more often applied as a diagnostic step in evaluating head and neck pain complaints. The procedure for blockade follows:

1. The block is perfomed in the sitting position, with the patient leaning the head forward to expose the prominent nuchal ridge of bone at the posterior base of the skull.

2. The external occipital protuberance is identified in the midline, and a mark is placed lateral to this prominence along the nuchal line at the lateral border of the insertion of the erector muscles of the neck, usually 2.5 cm from the midline. The branches of the greater occipital nerve usually pass laterally from behind the muscle to cross the nuchal line at this point.

3. After skin preparation, a small needle is introduced through the mark to the depth of the skull itself. A ridge of 14 ml of local anesthetic (1% lidocaine or equivalent) is then deposited across the path of the emerging nerves just above the level of the bone. Paresthesias are occasionally encountered but are not essential to obtaining simple skin anesthesia.

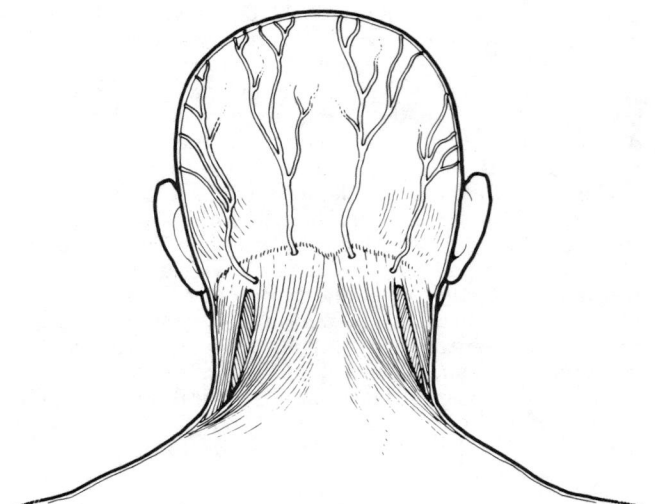

FIG. 29-10. Occipital nerve blockade. The greater and lesser branches of the occipital nerve emerge from under the muscles at the level of the nuchal ridge on the posterior scalp. They can be easily blocked by a subcutaneous ridge of anesthetic solution. (Reproduced with permission. From Mulroy M: Handbook of Regional Anesthesia. Boston, Little, Brown, 1988.)

4. If more anterior anesthesia of the scalp is required, the lesser occipital nerve branches are also blocked by advancing the needle subcutaneously from this point in an anterior direction toward the mastoid process. A band of anesthetic solution is deposited along the line between the skin entry and the mastoid. A larger volume (6 to 8 ml) will be required.

Complications of this technique are rare. Care must be taken not to advance the needle anteriorly under the skull itself, as the foramen magnum might be unintentionally entered with a long needle. Local hematoma may be produced with the superficial injection, but this is only a temporary problem.

Airway Anesthesia

Manipulation of the airway either during laryngoscopy or endotracheal intubation is often associated with laryngospasm, coughing, and cardiovascular reflexes that are undesirable. The anesthesiologist can abolish or blunt these reflexes by anesthetizing one or all of the sensory pathways involved. The nasal mucosa is innervated by fibers of the sphenopalatine ganglion, a branch of the middle division of the fifth cranial nerve. These branches lie on the lateral wall of the nasal passages on each side, under the mucosa just posterior to the middle turbinate (Fig. 29-11). The branches of these fibers continue caudad to provide sensory innervation to the superior portion of the pharynx, uvula, and tonsils. Anesthesia of the maxillary branch of the trigeminal is possible but not a practical solution for airway anesthesia. Transmucosal topical application of local anesthetic is more appropriate. Below the sphenopalatine fiber distribution, sensory innervation of the oral pharynx and supraglottic regions is provided by branches of the glossopharyngeal nerve. These nerves lie laterally on each side of the pharynx submucosally in the region of the posterior tonsillar pillar. Direct submucosal injection can be performed but carries the risk of unintentional intravascular injection into several blood vessels in this area. Topical anesthesia of the terminal branches in the mouth and throat is again an easier approach. The larynx itself is innervated by the superior laryngeal branch of the vagus nerve in the area above the vocal cords. This branch leaves the main vagal trunk in the carotid sheath and passes anteriorly. Its internal branch penetrates the thyrohyoid membrane and divides to provide the sensory fibers to the cords, epiglottis, and arytenoids.

The recurrent laryngeal nerve provides innervation to the areas below the vocal cords, including motor innervation for all but one of the intrinsic laryngeal muscles. The trachea itself is also innervated by the recurrent laryngeal nerve. Topical anesthesia is again the simplest approach to this nerve.

Airway anesthesia can be performed by anesthetizing one or all of these sensory distributions. Full anesthesia will facilitate procedures such as nasal intubation or fiberoptic laryngoscopy. Airway anesthesia below the vocal cords might best be avoided if there is concern about potential aspiration, as this may blunt the reflex cough reaction to the presence of foreign bodies in the trachea. Topical postpharyngeal anesthesia may also ablate protective laryngeal reflexes.

In the performance of airway anesthesia, the patient can be anesthetized in the supine position, although many patients will find it more comfortable to be semi-upright or sitting when topical anesthesia is sprayed into the posterior pharynx. These positions allow them greater ease in swallowing excess solutions and may reduce gagging. In whatever position chosen, there should be a firm support behind the head to reduce the possibility of involuntary withdrawal motions by the patient, which might dislocate needles being used for injections. The procedure for airway anesthetic administration follows:

1. For nasal mucosal anesthesia, cotton pledgets soaked with anesthetic solution are introduced through the nares and passed along the turbinates all the way to the posterior end of the nasal passage (Fig. 29-11). A second set of pledgets is introduced with a cephalad angulation to follow the middle turbinate back to the mucosa overlying the sphenoid bone. This pledget is the more critical one, since anesthesia in this mucosal area is most likely to anesthetize the branches of the sphenopalatine ganglia as they pass along the lateral wall of the airway. Bilateral anesthesia is preferable, even if a nasal tube is to be inserted only on one side; bilateral blockade of the sphenopalatine fibers will also produce posterior pharyngeal anesthesia caudad to this level. The pledgets should be allowed to remain in contact with the nasal mucosa for at least 2 to 3 minutes to allow adequate diffusion of local anesthetic.

   Cocaine in a 4% solution has been the traditional topical anesthetic for this application because of its unique vasoconstrictive properties. Cocaine produces shrinkage of the mucosa and reduces the chance of bleeding. Because of the toxicity of cocaine and a significant abuse problem in this country, alternate solutions have been recommended—primarily a mixture of 3 to 4% lidocaine and 0.25 to 0.5% phenylephrine.[17, 18]

2. Topical anesthesia to the posterior pharynx can be performed while the nasal applicators are in place. This can be done with a commercial spray or with an atomizer filled with a 4% solution of lidocaine. (A higher concentration of local anesthetic is required in order to pene-

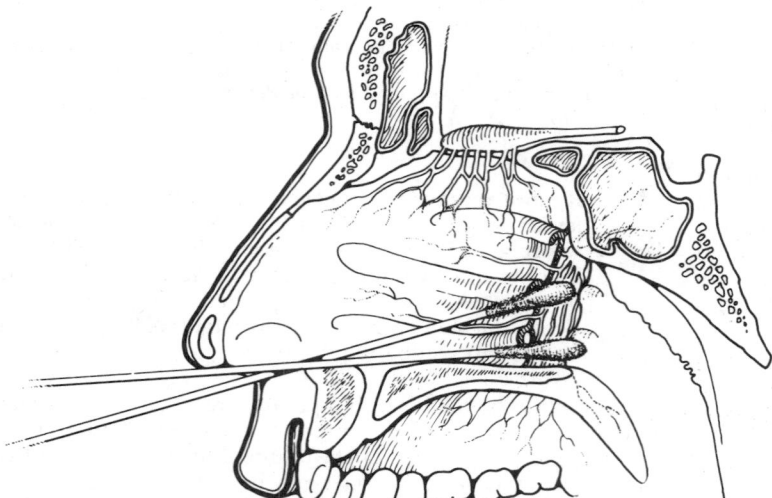

FIG. 29-11. Nasal airway anesthesia. Cotton pledgets soaked with anesthetic are inserted along the inferior and middle turbinates to produce anesthesia of the underlying sphenopalatine ganglion by transmembrane diffusion of the solution. Wide pledgets are needed to also provide maximal topical anesthesia and vasoconstriction of the nasal mucosa as well. (Reproduced with permission. From Mulroy M: Handbook of Regional Anesthesia. Boston, Little, Brown, 1988.)

trate mucosal membranes.) For effective anesthesia in the posterior pharyngeal wall, topical application is performed in two stages. First, the tongue itself is sprayed with a local anesthetic, and the patient is encouraged to gargle and swallow the residual liquid in the mouth. The numb tongue is then grasped with a gauze pad with one hand while the spray device is inserted into the mouth with the other. The patient is then encouraged to take rapid deep breaths ("pant like a puppy") while the spray is applied on inspiration. The inspiratory flow of gases should be enough to draw the lidocaine solution into the posterior pharynx and even to the vocal cords themselves. If superior laryngeal nerve blockade has been performed prior to this, it is likely that the aerosol will be carried on into the trachea itself. Again, a few minutes are needed for adequate onset of topical anesthesia in the pharynx. Topical anesthesia is less effective if there are copious secretions. Premedication with an anticholinergic is frequently beneficial.

3. Superior laryngeal nerve blockade can also be performed while the nasal pledgets are in place (Fig. 29-12). This nerve is blocked bilaterally by identifying the superior ala of the thyroid cartilage, which usually lies just inferior to the posterior position of the hyoid bone on each side. A 5-ml syringe with a 1% lidocaine solution with a 23-g 1.75-cm needle is used. The index finger of one hand retracts the skin of the neck caudad down over the thyroid cartilage; the needle is inserted until it rests on the superior margin of the cartilage. The tension on the skin is then released, and the needle is withdrawn slightly and allowed to walk superiorly off the cartilage. The needle is then reinserted and passed through the thyrohyoid membrane, which is perceived as a discernible resistance. After careful aspiration, 2.5 ml of solution is injected into the space below the membrane. This procedure is repeated on the opposite side. This blockade can be performed as part of total airway anesthesia,

or it can be used independently to provide increased acceptance of indwelling endotracheal tubes in the intensive care unit.[19]

4. Tracheal anesthesia can be performed by a direct transcrycoid ("transtracheal") injection. This is accomplished by raising a small skin wheal over the cricothyroid membrane. A 20-g intravenous catheter is then inserted gently through this skin wheal and through the membrane itself. Entry into the trachea can be confirmed by the ability to aspirate air through the catheter. The steel stylet is then removed, and the plastic catheter is left in the trachea. A syringe with 4 ml of 4% lidocaine is attached to the catheter, and the local anesthetic is sprayed into the trachea during inspiration. The flow of air will usually carry the local anesthetic distally; the resultant cough will continue to spread the anesthetic more proximally up to the underside of the vocal cords and the larynx. Not uncommonly, if the local anesthetic is injected while the patient forcibly exhales, it is possible to obtain adequate anesthesia of the trachea, larynx, and posterior pharynx, without the need for either steps 2 or 3.

5. After each of these steps has been completed, the pledgets can be removed from the nasal passages and nasal intubation performed. If tracheal or laryngeal anesthesia has been omitted because of concern of aspiration, there should be some pharmacologic intervention to reduce the cardiovascular response to the passage of the tube into the trachea. This can be facilitated by pretreatment with intravenous beta-adrenergic blocking drugs, by administration of sedation, or by administration of rapid-acting thiobarbiturates immediately after the airway is secured.

Complications of these techniques are rare. Systemic toxicity from the local anesthetics is a distinct possibility because of the large quantities of drug required to produce sufficient mucosal anesthesia. If all four stages of airway anesthesia are undertaken, the total milligram doses applied will usually exceed the maximal recommended dose for peripheral injection. Fortunately, the mucosal absorption is less than the peripheral absorption, but close attention to the patient's mental status and preparation for treatment of toxicity are necessary. As has been mentioned, aspiration of gastric contents is also a possibility when the protective reflexes of the airway are interrupted. Precautions should be taken in the form of the usual prophylaxis to reduce stomach acidity, as well as provision for suction and adequate oxygenation if emesis or regurgitation occurs.

UPPER EXTREMITY

The innervation of the upper extremity is conveniently derived from five closely approximated nerve roots, extending from the 5th cervical to the 1st thoracic segment of the spinal cord. These roots undergo a series of mergers and divisions that produce the terminal nerves of the arm and hand. The plexus branches are close enough to each other to allow reliable anesthesia to be achieved at several points associated with consistent bony or vascular landmarks.

In their proximal course, the nerve roots all lie in a well-demarcated fascial envelope formed by the anterior fascia of the middle scalene muscle and the posterior fascia of the anterior scalene. These muscles attach to the posterior and anterior tubercles of the transverse processes of the cervical

FIG. 29-12. Superior laryngeal nerve blockade. The needle is advanced superiorly off the lateral wing of the thyroid cartilage to drop through the thyrohyoid membrane. (Reproduced with permission. From Mulroy M: Handbook of Regional Anesthesia. Boston, Little, Brown, 1988.)

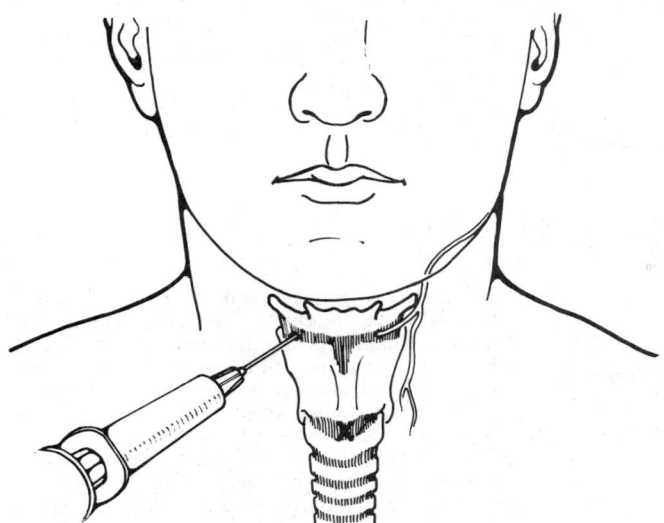

vertebrae from which the nerves emerge. The tubercle can be used as a faithful landmark to guide localization of the nerve, and the fascial planes serve to keep anesthetic solution injected between them in close proximity to the nerve bundle. The fascia extends outward for a variable distance from the lateral border of the muscles themselves to enclose the nerves in a "sheath," which can extend into the axilla. This enclosed bundle passes over the 1st rib just behind the midpoint of the clavicle (and just posterior to the insertion of the anterior scalene on the rib) where it is joined by the subclavian artery, which rises from the mediastinum to cross the rib and pass into the axilla. At the midpoint of the rib, the plexus has consolidated into only three trunks; these rapidly subdivide into the terminal branches. The musculocutaneous nerve is the first branch to leave the companionship of its partners as it passes into the body of the coracobrachialis muscle high in the axilla. As the individual nerves form, separate compartments in the sheath are formed by developing septae, and reliable blockade of all the nerves with a single injection is not practical distal to the axilla.

Although many techniques of approach to the brachial plexus have been described, there are basically three anatomic locations where anesthetics are placed: 1) the interscalene groove near the transverse processes; 2) the subclavian sheath at the first rib; and 3) the axillary sheath surrounding the artery in the axilla. Because of the specific configuration of the nerves at each of these levels, the anesthesia produced is significantly different with each approach and applicable to different situations.[20] Interscalene injection at the level of the 6th cervical transverse process produces extension of the blockade to the lower fibers of the cervical plexus and, thus, is ideally suited for shoulder operations and upper arm procedures. It frequently spares the lowest branches of the plexus, the C-8 and T-1 fibers, which innervate the caudad (ulnar) border of the forearm. Blockade at the level of the 1st rib is most reliable in producing anesthesia of all four terminal nerves of the forearm and hand. The axillary technique is simpler but carries the risk of missing the musculocutaneous nerve that departs the sheath high in the axilla and, thus, might produce inadequate anesthesia of the forearm. The choice of the appropriate approach depends not only upon the patient's anatomy but also on the site of surgery.

The terminal branches can also be anesthetized by local anesthetic injection along their peripheral courses as they cross the joint spaces, or by the injection of a dilute local anesthetic solution intravenously below a pneumatic tourniquet on the upper arm.

Interscalene Approach

This technique was first popularized by Winnie,[21] who stressed the advantages of the fascial sheath provided by the "envelope" of muscles that surround the origins of the brachial plexus in the neck. Localization of the nerves uses a combination of the muscular and bony landmarks surrounding the nerves. The procedure for blockade follows:

1. The patient is positioned supine, with the head turned to the side opposite that to be blocked. A small towel is placed under the occiput. The arm on the side to be blocked is held at the side, and the patient is asked to hold the shoulder down by pretending to reach for his hip or knee.
2. The lateral border of the sternocleidomastoid muscle (SCM) is identified and marked, and the patient is then asked to raise his head slightly into a "sniffing" position (Fig. 29-13). This tenses the scalene muscle behind the SCM, and the groove between the anterior and middle scalene is palpated by rolling the fingers posteriorly off the lateral border of the SCM. This groove is marked along its entire extent, as high up as possible. The patient then relaxes the muscles of the neck, and the level of the cricoid cartilage is marked. The index finger then gently palpates in the groove at the level of the cricoid. The prominent transverse process of the 6th cervical vertebra can often be felt directly.
3. After aseptic skin preparation, a skin wheal is raised in the groove at the level of the cricoid. A 22-g 3.75-cm needle is introduced through the wheal *perpendicular to the skin in all planes* so that it is directed medially, caudad, and slightly posterior. Resting one hand on the clavicle will allow better control of the syringe (Fig. 29-14).
4. The needle is advanced until the tubercle is contacted or a paresthesia is elicited (or a motor twitch obtained with a nerve stimulator) (Fig. 29-15). If bone is contacted before nerve, the needle is withdrawn and re-directed in

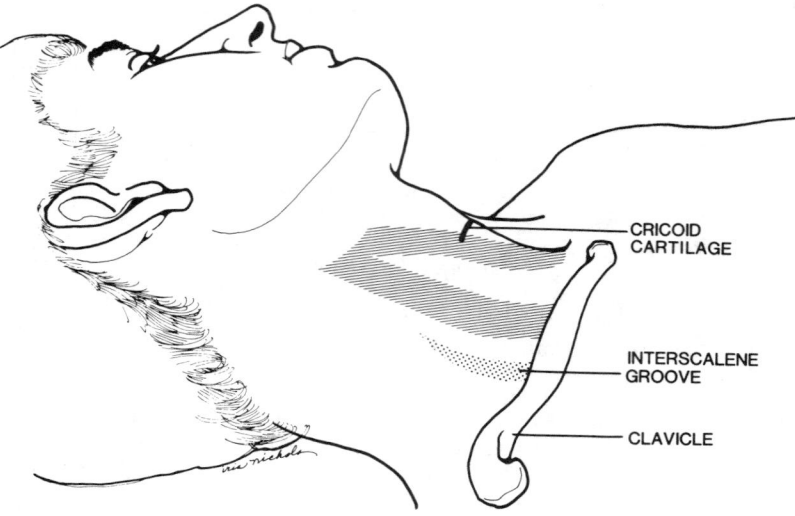

FIG. 29-13. Superficial landmarks for interscalene brachial plexus blockade. The sternocleidomastoid muscle is identified, and the anterior scalene muscle is found by moving the fingertips over the lateral border of the larger muscle while it is slightly tensed. The groove between the anterior and middle scalene muscle can usually be felt easily, along with the tubercle of the 6th cervical vertebra, which lies at the level of the cricoid cartilage. (Reproduced with permission. From Mulroy M: Handbook of Regional Anesthesia. Boston, Little, Brown, 1988.)

CRICOID CARTILAGE

INTERSCALENE GROOVE

CLAVICLE

small steps in an anteroposterior (AP) plane until the nerves are identified.

5. Once the nerve is located (usually a paresthesia to the thumb or upper arm), the needle is fixed in this position with one hand while 25 to 30 ml of local anesthetic solution is injected. Careful aspiration is performed

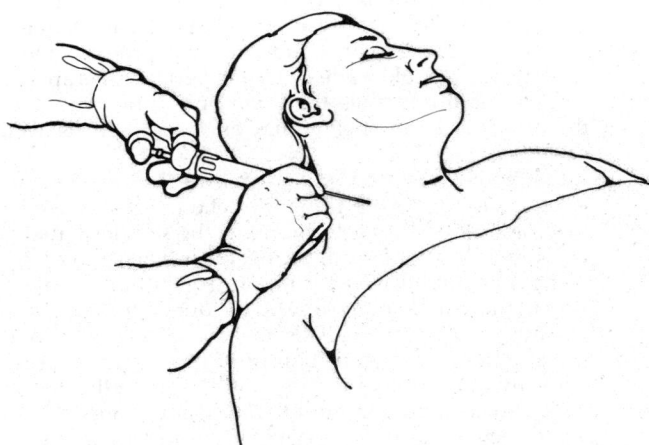

FIG. 29-14. Hand position for interscalene blockade. The needle is directed medially and caudad into the interscalene groove while one hand exerts constant control of the depth by resting on the clavicle. (Reproduced with permission. From Mulroy M: Handbook of Regional Anesthesia. Boston, Little, Brown, 1988.)

FIG. 29-15. Needle direction for interscalene blockade. The needle is always kept in a caudad direction; medial insertion will allow the point to pass into the intervertebral foramen and produce epidural, spinal, or intraarterial injection of anesthetic. Note the relation of the vertebral artery and the nerve roots to the transverse processes. (Reproduced with permission. From Mulroy M: Handbook of Regional Anesthesia. Boston, Little, Brown, 1988.)

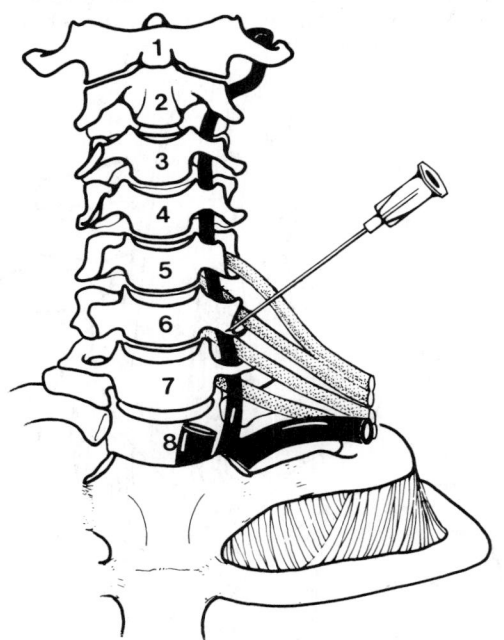

first, and the initial injection is performed in small increments to detect intraneural or intraarterial placement of the needle. A larger volume (30 to 40 ml) is required if greater spread is desired, such as to the cervical plexus or inferiorly to the C-8 to T-1 fibers.

6. If arm surgery requiring a tourniquet is planned, a subcutaneous ring of anesthetic across the axilla is usually required to block the superficial intercostobrachial fibers crossing from the chest wall into the axilla.

Complications from this approach are related to the structures located in the vicinity of the tubercle. The cupola of the lung is close and can be contacted if the needle is directed too far inferior. Pneumothorax should be considered if cough or chest pain is produced while exploring for the nerve. If the needle is allowed to pass directly medially, it may enter the intervertebral foramina, and injection of local anesthetic may produce spinal or epidural anesthesia. The vertebral artery passes posteriorly at the level of the 6th vertebra to lie in its canal in the transverse process; direct injection into this vessel can rapidly produce central nervous system toxicity and convulsions. Careful aspiration and incremental injections are helpful in avoiding both of these potential problems.

Even with appropriate injection, the local anesthetic solution will spread to contiguous nerves. This may produce cervical plexus blockade with high volumes, which may be desirable if shoulder surgery is contemplated. The involvement of the motor fibers of the cervical roots may also produce diaphragmatic paralysis, which may be a problem in patients with respiratory insufficiency. The phrenic nerve may be blocked by lower volumes because of diffusion to the anterior side of the anterior scalene or because of inappropriate injection anterior to the muscle.

Neuropathy of the C6 root is a potential problem, because the needle may unintentionally pin the nerve root against the tubercle and predispose to intraneural injection. The needle should be withdrawn slightly if the first injection produces the characteristic "crampy" pain sensation.

Inadequate anesthesia is most likely to occur in the ulnar distribution. As mentioned previously, this can be reduced by the use of higher volumes. Supplemental local anesthesia of the ulnar nerve may also be helpful.

Supraclavicular Approach

The description of the approach to the brachial plexus at this level is originally attributed to Kulenkampff, but the current recommended technique is based on the modifications recommended by Moore[22] and Winnie and Collins.[23] The current technique avoids the originally described medial direction of the needle, which may contact the pleura. It uses the same anatomic consideration, however, in that it attempts to intercept the nerve trunks at their closest approximation to one another as they pass over the first rib. The procedure for blockade follows:

1. The patient lies in the same position as for interscalene blockade, with the ipsilateral arm held at the side and pulled downward to exaggerate the landmarks of the clavicle and the neck muscles.
2. The outline of the clavicle is drawn on the skin, as well as the interscalene groove (as described previously). The midpoint of the clavicle is marked. An "X" is placed posterior to this midpoint in the interscalene groove, usually 1 cm behind the clavicle. The groove will ideally extend all the way to the first rib, where the muscles

insert, but palpation of the rib is usually difficult. On the thin patient, the pulsation of the subclavian artery can be appreciated in the groove or just anterior to it.

3. After aseptic preparation, a skin wheal is raised at the mark, and a 3.75-cm 22-g needle attached to a 10-ml syringe is introduced in the sagittal plane and advanced caudad until the first rib is contacted (Figs. 29-16 to 29-18). It is important that the direction of the needle

remains perpendicular to the rib, which usually requires that the syringe remain parallel to the axis of the head and neck. If the rib is not contacted, careful exploration should be carried out first laterally to the mark and, last of all, medially. The greatest danger of contacting the pleura occurs when probing medially.

4. If a paresthesia is produced during the course of exploration, the anesthetic solution is injected while the needle is fixed in position. Twenty-five to 40 ml of 1% lidocaine or 0.25% bupivacaine will produce adequate anesthesia; higher concentrations will produce more profound motor blockade. Multiple paresthesias are not usually required, since there are only three trunks at this level and the sheath that encloses them is well defined.

5. If a paresthesia is not obtained on insertion, exploration is continued until the rib is identified. A 5-cm needle may be needed to reach the rib in the heavier patient. Once the rib is contacted, the needle is walked in an AP plane until a paresthesia is found. Again, the needle is kept in the safe sagittal plane on the dorsal surface of the rib during exploration. If the needle advances beyond the anterior or posterior border of the rib as it curves medially at these two points, it is simply redirected in the opposite direction until the rib is found again. Medial direction is avoided. While exploring along the direction of the rib, the needle should be withdrawn almost to the skin before re-direction for each pass. If it is lifted only a few millimeters from the rib, it may simply push the nerve bundle ahead of it without making contact.

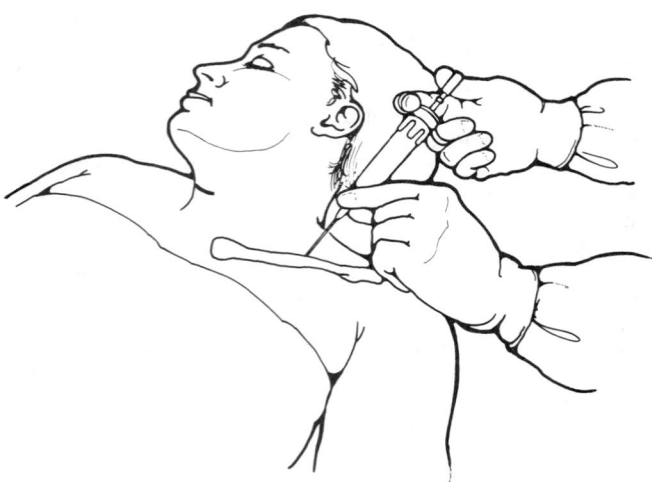

FIG. 29-16. Hand position for supraclavicular blockade. The needle is directed caudad behind the midpoint of the clavicle in the interscalene groove. Again, control of depth is maintained by the hand resting on the clavicle. The syringe is kept in the sagittal plane parallel to the patient's head to prevent medial angulation, which would increase the chance of pneumothorax. (Reproduced with permission. From Mulroy M: Handbook of Regional Anesthesia. Boston, Little, Brown, 1988.)

FIG. 29-17. Needle direction for supraclavicular blockade (AP view). The needle is directed downward onto the first rib, where it can be expected to contact the three trunks of the brachial plexus as they cross over the rib. The rib at this point lies along the AP plane of the body. (Reproduced with permission. From Mulroy M: Handbook of Regional Anesthesia. Boston, Little, Brown, 1988.)

FIG. 29-18. Needle direction for supraclavicular blockade (lateral view). The subclavian artery rises from the chest to join the three trunks of the brachial plexus in crossing over the first rib. The nerves usually lie posterior to the artery at this point, although they rapidly encircle it as it becomes the axillary artery. Note that once the needle contacts the rib, it should be withdrawn almost completely to the skin before redirection, since short steps along the bone may simply "push" the nerves ahead of the needle. (Reproduced with permission. From Mulroy M: Handbook of Regional Anesthesia. Boston, Little, Brown, 1988.)

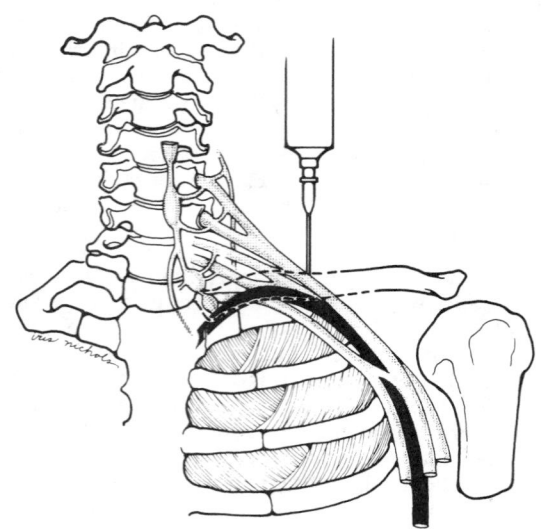

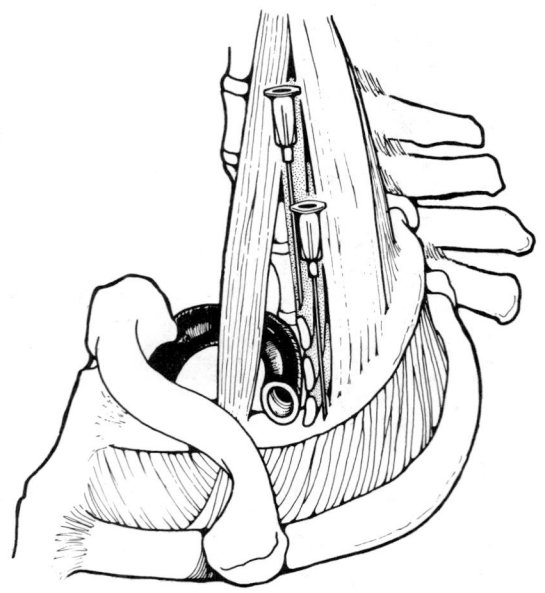

6. If no paresthesia is obtained, the artery can be used as a landmark. Once it is entered with the needle, a series of injections posterior to it can be used to produce a "wall" of 40 ml of anesthetic solution in this area.
7. If a tourniquet is to be used, a ring of subcutaneous anesthesia should be infiltrated along the axilla to block the sensory fibers from the chest wall that cross here to innervate the inner aspect of the upper arm.

Pneumothorax is the most serious complication of this technique. Although it is rare in experienced hands,[24] it does occur more frequently with this approach to the brachial plexus than with any other approach. This may limit the use of this technique, particularly in outpatients, in whom the insertion of a chest tube would then require hospitalization. The other complications of peripheral blockade do not occur with any greater frequency with this blockade than with other methods of blockade.

Axillary Technique

Of the central approaches, the axillary technique carries the least chance of pneumothorax and thus may be ideal for the outpatient. The nerves are anesthetized around the axillary artery, where they have regrouped into their terminal branches. The technique does generate some controversy because of the observation that at this point the single sheath may be broken up into separate compartments by fascial septae, which now surround the individual nerves. Although the septae do not limit diffusion of drug in every case,[25] Thompson and Rorie[26] have identified several patients in whom the development of these divisions has limited the spread of anesthetic to other nerves at this level. This has led to the recommendation that local anesthetic be injected at multiple sites with this technique, in contrast to the single injections possible with the other approaches. Another obstacle to single-injection technique at this level is the early departure of the musculocutaneous branch from the sheath high in the axilla. In light of these controversies, several variations of this technique are possible.

CLASSIC APPROACH, SEEKING PARESTHESIAS. This is probably the most common practice. The procedure for blockade follows:

1. The patient lies supine with the arm extended 90 degrees from the side and flexed at the elbow. Extension beyond 90 degrees will potentially compress the axillary artery because of the pressure from the head of the humerus and may make identification of the landmarks more difficult. A pillow under the forearm will also reduce rotation of the shoulder joint, which can also obscure the pulse.
2. The axillary artery is marked as high in its course in the axilla as is practical. It is usually felt in the intramuscular groove between the coracobrachialis and the triceps. It also passes between the insertions of the pectoralis major and the latissimus dorsi muscles on the humerus.
3. After aseptic preparation, a skin wheal is raised over the proximal portion of the artery. The index and middle finger of the nondominant hand straddle the artery just below this point, both localizing the pulsation and compressing the sheath below the intended site of injection (Fig. 29-19).
4. A three-ring syringe with a 2.5-cm short bevel needle is held in the other hand, and the needle is introduced alongside the artery seeking a paresthesia. Ideally, the

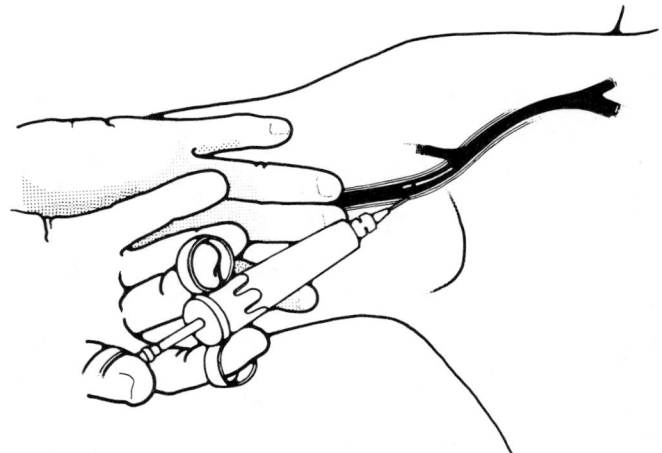

FIG. 29-19. Hand position for axillary blockade. Two fingers of equal length straddle the artery while the needle is introduced along its long axis with a central angulation. The palpating fingers serve not only to identify the vessel but also to compress the perivascular sheath and encourage the spread of anesthetic solution centrally. (Reproduced with permission. From Mulroy M: Handbook of Regional Anesthesia. Boston, Little, Brown, 1988.)

nerves serving the area of proposed surgery are sought first. The median and the musculocutaneous nerves lie on the superior aspect of the artery (as viewed by the operator), whereas the ulnar and radial nerves lie below and behind the vessel (Fig. 29-20).
5. When a paresthesia is obtained, the contents of the syringe are injected, taking precautions to avoid intraneural injection. Firm pressure is maintained on the distal sheath to encourage the solution to move centrally from the point of injection, hopefully to include the point of origin of the musculocutaneous nerve. At this point, the anesthesiologist may elect to fix the needle in position, refill the syringe, and inject a total dose of 25 to 40 ml of anesthetic solution near this single paresthesia. As an alternative, the larger bolus may be injected from a 50-ml syringe attached to the needle by an intravenous extension tube.
6. If other paresthesias are desired, they should be elicited within 5 minutes of the original injection. Beyond this time, spread of the solution may produce hypesthesia of the other nerves, which prevents their identification. A second paresthesia should be sought on the side of the artery opposite the original one. With this approach, 15 to 20 ml of solution is injected following elicitation of each paresthesia.
7. If separate supplementary anesthesia of the musculocutaneous nerve is sought, it can be obtained by injecting an additional 5 to 10 ml of anesthetic solution into the body of the coracobrachialis muscle. This muscle can be easily grasped between the thumb and forefinger, and the entry into its fascial compartment is readily identified. This step may be required even if 40 ml of solution is used in the perivascular injection, since the musculocutaneous nerve may be spared as often as 25% of the time even with this or larger volumes.[27]

ALTERNATE APPROACH OF MULTIPLE INJECTIONS WITHOUT PARESTHESIAS. As an alternative to the classic technique, anesthesia can be obtained without seeking par-

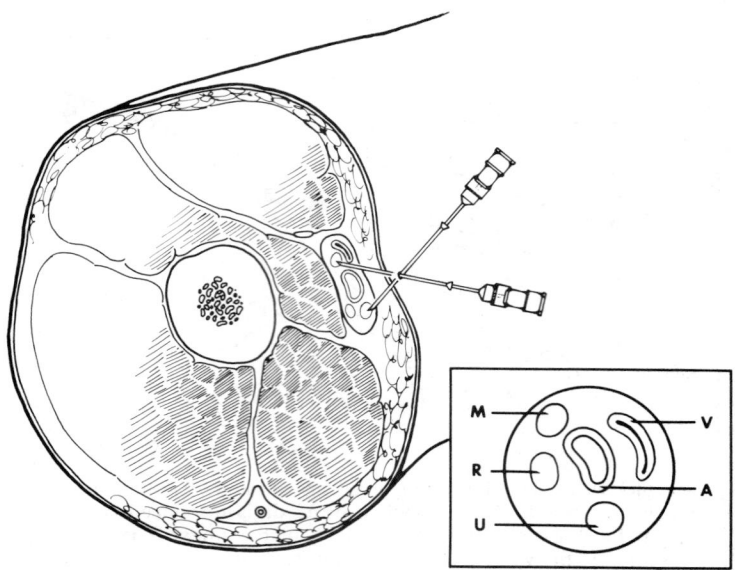

FIG. 29-20. Needle position for axillary injection. The median and musculocutaneous nerves lie on the superior side of the artery, although the latter may have already departed the axillary sheath at the level of injection. The ulnar lies inferior, and the radial is inferior and posterior.

esthesias. This approach may reduce nerve injury.[28] The technique is identical to that just described except that no paresthesias are elicited and the anesthetic solution is simply injected on each side of the artery in multiple small increments covering all the perivascular area and producing a "wall" of solution that intercepts the paths of each of the branches. This approach is potentially less reliable and requires meticulous attention to localization of the artery and the surrounding fascial compartment.

TRANSARTERIAL APPROACH. This is another alternative that seeks to avoid paresthesias. Again, the preparation and landmarks are identical to those of the classical approach. Here the artery is deliberately entered directly with the needle. The needle is advanced through the vessel until aspiration confirms that it has passed just posterior; at this point, half the anesthetic solution is injected incrementally with careful attention to avoid intravascular placement. The needle is then withdrawn back through the vessel until aspiration confirms that it is just anterior to the artery. The other half of the solution is injected.

This technique is simple and effective and should be kept in mind as an alternative while the classic approach is being used. If paresthesias cannot be obtained with the former or (more commonly) if the vessel is unintentionally entered during the search, the transarterial approach should be used.

The complications of all these approaches are minimal compared with those of the other central approaches. The problem of neuropathy is the foremost consideration. Hematoma can occur if the vessel is punctured, but this is rarely a problem. The use of small-gauge needles may reduce this possibility.

Distal Upper Extremity Blockade

As in the leg, the nerves to the hand can be blocked at the point where they cross the two major joints, the elbow and the wrist (Fig. 29-21). At these two levels, the overlying muscles are thinned and the bony landmarks are more prominent, allowing easier identification of the nerves. Peripheral blockade is usually not quite as dense as central blockade but may be useful in anesthetizing one branch that was missed with a

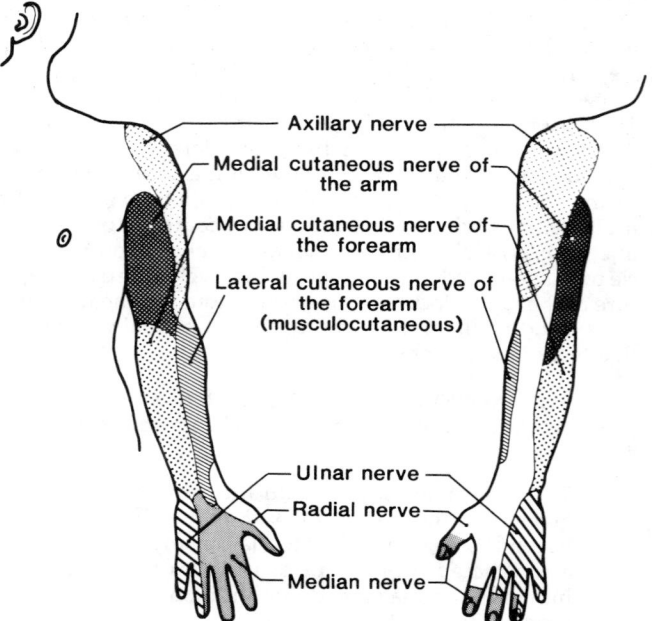

FIG. 29-21. Sensory dermatomes of the arm. Sensation is provided by the terminal nerves as identified. This pattern is different from the classic dermatomal distribution of the nerve roots. Different patterns of anesthesia will develop if the blockade is performed at the root level (interscalene blockade) or terminal nerve level (axillary blockade). (Reproduced with permission. From Mulroy M: Handbook of Regional Anesthesia. Boston, Little, Brown, 1988.)

central blockade or in providing very localized anesthesia on the hand. Since the sensory branches to the forearm from the musculocutaneous nerve and the internal cutaneous nerve have already branched so extensively that adequate anesthesia of the forearm is not easily obtained, blockade at the elbow really produces no greater anesthesia than blockade at the wrist.

BLOCKADE AT THE ELBOW. Two nerves to the hand cross this joint on the inner aspect, whereas the ulnar travels posteriorly in its well-known superficial groove. The procedure for blockade follows:

1. The ulnar nerve is blocked by injection of 1 ml to 4 ml local anesthetic in the groove formed by the medial condyle of the humerus and the olecranon. This is easily done with the joint flexed at about 30 degrees. Further flexion may cause the nerve to roll medially and anterior to the condyle. Paresthesias can usually be readily obtained, but direct injection on a paresthesia or directly into the groove under pressure is not advised because of the risk of damage to the nerve. If the injection is made deep to the fascia, anesthesia should commence within 5 minutes.
2. The median nerve crosses the joint in the company of the brachial artery. A line is drawn between the two condyles on the inner aspect of the joint, and a skin wheal is raised at the point where this line crosses the pulsation of the brachial artery, usually 1 cm to the ulnar side of the biceps tendon. A needle is introduced perpendicularly at this point, and paresthesias are sought immediately adjacent to the artery. Five milliliters of solution are sufficient to produce anesthesia, and, again, intraneural injection is carefully avoided.
3. The radial nerve is identified along the same intracondylar line, approximately 2 cm lateral to the biceps tendon. Another skin wheal is raised here, and, again, a needle is inserted to search for paresthesias in a fan-shaped pattern. If paresthesias are not obtained, a wall of anesthetic solution can be deposited here but with less chance of reliable anesthesia.

BLOCKADE AT THE WRIST. The nerves lie more superficially at this joint and are closely associated with easily identified landmarks (Fig. 29-22). For this reason, blockade at this level is usually preferred to other distal approaches. The procedure for blockade follows:

1. The ulnar nerve lies between the ulnar artery and the flexor carpi ulnaris. A skin wheal is raised at the level of the styloid process on the palmar side of the forearm between these two landmarks. A small-gauge needle is inserted, and 3 ml of solution is injected into the area, with or without paresthesias.
2. At the same level on the forearm, the median nerve lies between the tendons of the palmaris longus and the flexor carpi radialis. If only the palmaris longus can be felt, the nerve is just to the radial side of this tendon. A skin wheal is raised, and a needle is inserted until it pierces the deep fascia. Three milliliters of solution will produce anesthesia.
3. The radial nerve requires a broader injection, as it has already started to ramify as it crosses the wrist. The anatomic "snuff box" formed by the tendons of the extensor pollicis longus and extensor pollicis brevis tendons is located, and 3 ml of solution is injected here. A subcutaneous wheal is then raised from this point, extending over the dorsum of the wrist 3 to 4 cm onto the back of the hand.

Intravenous Regional Anesthesia

The simplest technique of arm anesthesia is the injection of local anesthetic into the venous system below an occluding

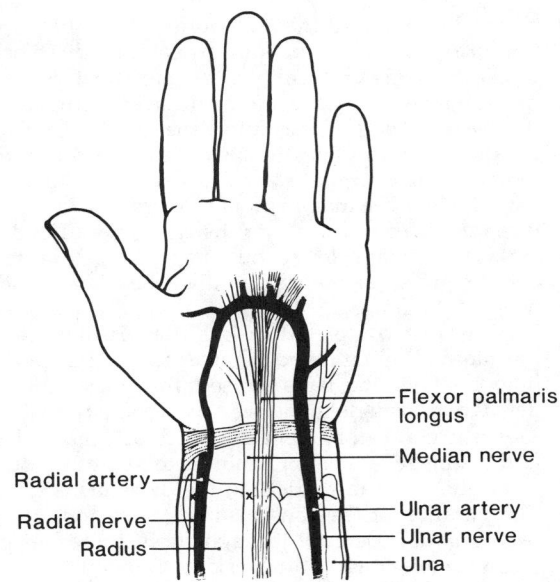

FIG. 29-22. Terminal nerves at the wrist. The median nerve lies just to the radial side of the flexor palmaris longus. The ulnar and radial nerves lie just "outside" their respective arteries. The radial nerve has already begun branching at this level and must be blocked by a wide subcutaneous ridge of anesthetic. (Reproduced with permission. From Mulroy M: Handbook of Regional Anesthesia. Boston, Little, Brown, 1988.)

tourniquet. This appears to produce anesthesia by direct diffusion of the anesthetic from the vessels into the nearby nerves. The technique is often referred to as a *Bier block*, in honor of August Bier who first described anesthesia produced in this manner. His technique required a cutdown and ligation of a vein; the modern adaptation is elegant in its simplicity. The procedure for blockade follows:

1. A small-gauge (20 or 22) intravenous plastic catheter is inserted in the arm to be blocked on the dorsum of the hand. It is taped firmly in place, and a heparin port or small syringe is attached and saline is injected to maintain patency. A pneumatic tourniquet is applied over the upper arm.
2. The arm is elevated to promote venous drainage. An elastic bandage may be applied to produce further exsanguination. After exsanguination, the tourniquet is inflated to 300 mm Hg or 2.5 times the systolic blood pressure and is tested carefully for adequate occlusion of the radial pulse.
3. The arm is returned to the horizontal position, a 50-ml syringe with 0.5% lidocaine or prilocaine (or 0.25% bupivacaine) is attached to the previously inserted cannula, and the contents are injected. The forearm will discolor, and the patient will perceive a transient "pins and needles" sensation as anesthesia ensues over the following 5 minutes. Epinephrine should *not* be added to the local anesthetic solution.
4. For short procedures, the cannula can be removed at this point. If surgery may extend beyond 1 hour, the cannula can be left in place and re-injected after 90 minutes.
5. Beyond 45 minutes of surgery, many patients will expe-

rience discomfort at the level of the tourniquet. Special "double-cuff" tourniquets are available for this blockade to alleviate this problem. The proximal cuff is inflated first, allowing anesthesia to be induced in the area under the distal cuff. If discomfort ensues, the distal cuff is inflated over the anesthetized area of skin, and the uncomfortable proximal cuff is released. This step is critical, since the major risk of this procedure is premature release of solution into the circulation. If a double cuff is used, both cuffs should be tested before starting and the proper sequence for inflation and deflation meticulously followed.

6. If surgery is completed in less than 20 minutes, the tourniquet is left inflated for at least that total period of time. If 40 minutes have elapsed, the tourniquet can be deflated as a single maneuver. Between 20 and 40 minutes, the cuff can be deflated, re-inflated immediately, and finally deflated after a minute to reduce the sudden absorption of anesthetic into the systemic circulation.

7. The duration of anesthesia is minimal beyond the time of tourniquet release. Although bupivacaine may give a slight prolongation of analgesia, the advantage is short.

The simplicity of this technique is offset by the significant risk of systemic local anesthetic toxicity if the tourniquet fails or is released prematurely. Careful testing of the tourniquet and slow injection of solution into a peripheral (not antecubital) vein will reduce the chance of leakage under the tourniquet.[29] Systemic blood levels are time-dependent,[30] and careful attention should be paid to the sequence of tourniquet release and patient monitoring during this period. A separate intravenous site for injection of resuscitation drugs is needed, as well as ready availability of all needed equipment. With careful attention to these details, this technique is one of the most effective and reliable available to the anesthesiologist.

TRUNK

Anesthesia of the abdomen and chest is most simply obtained with spinal and epidural injections of local anesthetics, as discussed in Chapter 28. In some situations, a narrower band of intercostal or paravertebral anesthesia is preferable, or epidural injection may be hazardous because of infection or coagulopathy. In many clinical situations, it may also be desirable to separate the anesthesia of the somatic and sympathetic fibers that inevitably occurs in combination when these axial blockades are performed. The sympathetic nerves separate from their somatic counterparts early in their course, which makes independent somatic and sympathetic blockade a practical consideration. Sympathetic blockade is most commonly performed at the major ganglia, particularly the stellate, celiac, and lumbar plexus. These blockades often require multiple injections and are technically more difficult than axial anesthesia, but they do offer advantages in certain clinical situations.

The somatic nerves of the chest emerge from their respective intervertebral foramina and pass through the narrow triangular-shaped paravertebral space. In this triangle, they give off the sympathetic branch and also a small dorsal branch, which provides sensation to the midline of the back. The main trunks then pass into the intercostal groove along the ventral caudad surface of each rib. An artery and vein travel along with each of these nerves in the groove under the protection of the overhanging external edge of the rib. The fascia of the internal and external intercostal muscles provide interior and external borders of this intercostal groove. As the nerves travel beyond the midaxillary line, they give off a lateral sensory branch while the main trunk continues on to the anterior abdominal wall to provide sensory and motor innervation for the trunk and abdomen down to the level of the pubis. The intercostal groove becomes much less well defined anterior to the midaxillary line, and the nerve begins to move away from its protected position. The lowermost intercostal nerve (the 12th) is much less closely applied to its accompanying rib and is less easy to identify and anesthetize using a classic intercostal blockade technique. The upper lumbar roots form the ilioinguinal nerves, which pass laterally within the muscles of the abdominal wall at the level of the iliac crest and eventually move anteriorly to provide innervation of the groin region as the ilioinguinal nerves.

The anatomic basis for separate sympathetic anesthesia is produced by the early separation of sympathetic fibers from their somatic roots in the form of the white rami communicantes, which separate from the somatic nerves shortly after their emergence from the intervertebral foramina and join the sympathetic ganglia, which lie anteriorly on each side of the vertebral bodies. These preganglionic fibers of the sympathetic system usually arise only from the 1st thoracic through the 2nd lumbar segments. The spinal ganglia formed by these fibers constitute the sympathetic trunks, which extend upward into the neck and caudad along the lumbar spine. They give terminal sympathetic branches to all the areas of the body. The sympathetic innervation of the head and the lower extremities is derived from fibers that originate from the spinal cord, join sympathetic trunks, and then pass cephalad or caudad along the chain of ganglia before reaching their target organs. Segmental sympathetic innervation of the body from the cervical to the sacral roots is provided by postganglionic nerves departing from the chains (the grey rami communicantes), which re-join the somatic nerves early in their course. In the head (where motor and sensory innervation is by cranial nerves), the sympathetic fibers reach their end organs by traveling with the arterial vascular supply. The sympathetic ganglia in the neck lie along the lateral border of the relatively flat vertebral bodies. In the chest, the vertebral bodies become more rounded, and the chain of ganglia lie more posteriorly on the lateral side of the vertebral body near the head of each rib. In the abdomen and pelvis, the sympathetic chains begin to move anteriorly and lie on the ventral surface of the vertebral bodies and thus are more widely separated from their respective somatic nerves.

Intercostal Nerve Blockade

Anesthesia of the intercostal nerves provides both motor and sensory anesthesia of the entire abdominal wall from the xiphoid to the pubis. The 6th to 11th ribs are usually easily identified, and their accompanying nerves are reliably blocked by injections along the easily palpated sharp posterior angulation of the ribs, which occurs between 5 and 7 cm from the midline in the back.[31] Ribs above the 5th are difficult to palpate because of the overlying scapula and paraspinous muscles and are thus most easily blocked using the paravertebral technique. Establishing five or six levels of intercostal nerve blockade is a useful anesthetic procedure for providing analgesia and motor relaxation for upper abdominal procedures such as cholecystectomy and gastric surgery. This form of anesthesia usually requires supplementation with light general anesthesia or an additional sympathetic blockade, since much of the intraperitoneal and subdiaphragmatic sensation is carried by other nerve trunks. This form of anesthesia for upper abdominal surgery offers the advantages of muscle relaxation without the necessity of an accompanying sympathetic blockade (unless celiac plexus blockade is chosen as an optional supplement). Intercostal blockade with long-acting amide local anesthetics will also provide postoperative analgesia for 8 to 12 hours, which may greatly facilitate patient satisfaction and immediate recovery.[32] Unilateral blockade of these nerves is a useful treatment for the pain of rib fracture and also serves to reduce postoperative analgesia requirements in patients with subcostal incisions. Several segments must be blocked in each of these applications because of the overlap of the intercostal nerves. This technique is also useful in reducing the pain associated with the insertion of chest tubes or percutaneous biliary drainage procedures. The procedure for blockade follows:

1. For the performance of intercostal blockade, the patient may be in the lateral, sitting, or prone position. For operative anesthesia, the prone position is most practical. A pillow is placed under the abdomen in order to provide slight flexion of the thoracic spine. The arms are draped over the edge of the stretcher or operating table so that the scapula falls away laterally from the midline. The anesthesiologist stands at the patient's side. Most anesthesiologists prefer to stand on the side that allows their dominant hand to hold the syringe (the caudad side of the patient).

2. The spinous processes in the midline from T-6 through T-12 are marked (Fig. 29-23). The ribs are then identified along the line of their most extreme posterior angulation. For the 12th rib, this is usually 7 cm from the midline. At the level of the 6th rib, this posterior angulation will be best appreciated somewhat more medially, usually 5 cm from the midline. These two ribs are marked first at their inferior borders, and a line is drawn between these two points. The rest of the ribs between them are identified, and a mark is placed on the inferior border of each rib along the angled parasagittal plane identified by the first line between the 6th and 12th ribs.

3. After aseptic preparation, light sedation is provided for the patient, and a skin wheal is raised at each mark.

4. The ribs are usually blocked starting with the lowermost and moving upward. The 12th rib is not closely associated with its intercostal nerve, and a reliable blockade is not usually possible. For upper abdominal procedures, blockade of this nerve can be omitted without jeopardizing the anesthesia.

5. Starting with the lowest rib on the side closest to the anesthesiologist, the index finger of the cephalad hand is placed on the skin above the identifying mark; this finger should lie immediately over the midpoint of the rib. The skin is then retracted in a cephalad direction, so that the previous mark now lies over the rib itself, somewhat toward the inferior side. The other hand inserts a 22-g 3.75-cm needle directly onto the rib. This needle is attached to a 10-ml syringe filled with local anesthetic. The syringe and needle are held in such a way that they maintain a constant 10-degree cephalad angulation.

6. Once the needle is safely "parked" on the dorsal surface of the rib, the cephalad hand releases the tension on the skin and takes control of the needle and syringe (Fig. 29-24). This is done by placing the ulnar border of the hand firmly against the skin and grasping the hub of the needle firmly between the thumb and index

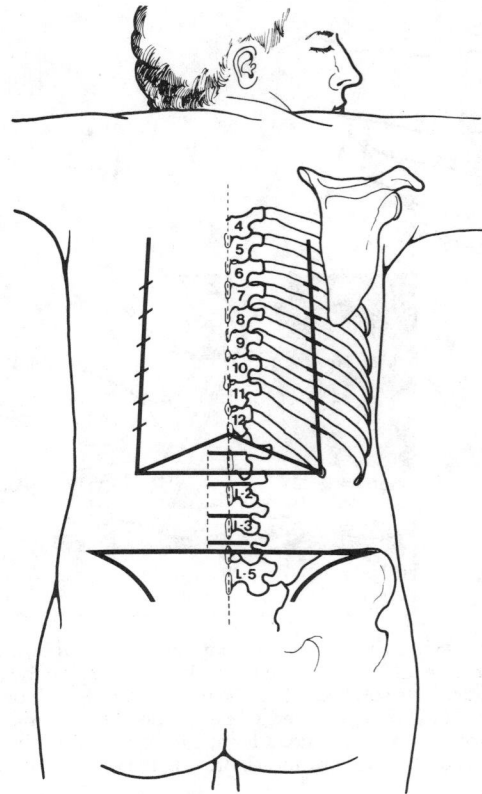

FIG. 29-23. Landmarks for intercostal blockade. The inferior borders of the ribs are identified at their most prominent point on the back. The marks then usually lie along a line that angles slightly medially from the 12th to the 6th rib. The triangle drawn between the 12th ribs and their spinous process is used for the celiac plexus blockade. (Reproduced with permission. From Mulroy M: Handbook of Regional Anesthesia. Boston, Little, Brown, 1988.)

finger. The middle finger of this hand rests along the shaft of the needle to provide guidance. Once the syringe is firmly gripped by the cephalad hand, the fingers of the caudad hand are placed in an "injection" position, either in the rings of a three-ring syringe or on the plunger of a straight syringe.

7. The needle and syringe are then raised slightly off the bone and "walked" in a caudad direction until they pass below the inferior border of the rib. The entire needle and syringe unit is kept at a 10-degree cephalad angle to the rib at all times. As it passes the inferior border, the needle is advanced 4 to 6 mm under the rib, with the needle actually pointing slightly cephalad into the intercostal groove.

8. Once in the groove, aspiration is performed, and 3 to 5 ml of local anesthetic solution is injected. Generally, 0.25% bupivacaine will produce good sensory anesthesia, whereas 0.5% bupivacaine is required for prolonged anesthesia with motor blockade. Aspiration is not reliable in preventing intravascular injection of the anesthetic; a slight "jiggling" motion of the needle during the injection will reduce this chance by ensuring that the needle is in a vessel only transiently if it does occur.

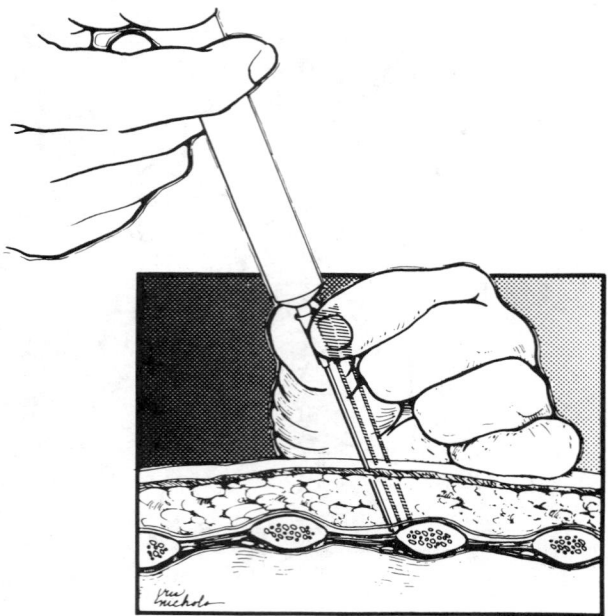

FIG. 29-24. Hand and needle position for intercostal blockade. The depth of the needle is controlled by the hand resting on the back. The other hand injects solution when the needle is under the rib, but that is the only function performed while the needle is near the pleura. (Reproduced with permission. From Mulroy M: Handbook of Regional Anesthesia. Boston, Little, Brown, 1988.)

9. As soon as the injection is complete, the needle is withdrawn from the groove and moved cephalad and parked again on the safe dorsal surface of the rib. The fingers of the caudad hand are then removed from the injection position and assume control of the syringe again. The cephalad hand now relinquishes control and is moved up to the next rib to repeat this cyclical process.

10. The six or seven designated ribs on each side are blocked in this process by progressively moving up the back, with control of the syringe alternating between the cephalad and caudad hands at the time of injection. The ribs on the opposite side are blocked in a similar manner. This can be done with the anesthesiologist standing on the same side and reaching across the back, or by moving to the opposite side of the patient. If the contralateral blockades are performed from the opposite side of the bed, an attempt should be made to "switch hands," so that the functions of cephalad and caudad hand remain the same even though the right and left hands have changed roles. It is sometimes more difficult for operators to control the syringe with their nondominant hand. It is worth the effort, since attempting to hold the syringe in the cephalad hand often makes maintenance of the proper cephalad angulation difficult. The syringe often ends up being rotated along its long axis as it is moved to the caudad edge of the rib, with the result that by the time the needle moves off the rib, it is pointed in a caudad rather than a cephalad direction. This will produce an injection of solution away from the nerve rather than into the groove.

11. If the intercostal nerve blockades are to be supple-

mented with a number of somatic paravertebral nerve blockades or sympathetic blockade of the celiac plexus, these are performed at the end of intercostal anesthesia. Care should be taken to adjust the total dosage of drug in such combinations of techniques so that the maximal recommended amounts are not exceeded.

Despite frequent concern about the incidence of pneumothorax with intercostal blockade, this complication is rare in experienced hands.[33] This depends primarily upon maintaining strict safety features of the described technique. Primarily, emphasis should be placed on absolute control of the syringe and needle at all times, particularly during the injection. This control requires that the cephalad hand, which is securely resting on the back, is the one that controls the depth of needle insertion. The needle rests on the safe dorsal side surface of the rib at all other times except for the brief moment of injection.

A common complication is related to the sedation required to perform this blockade in the prone position. The 12 to 14 needle insertions are uncomfortable, and patients usually require some narcotic and amnestic sedation. Overdosage can lead to airway obstruction and respiratory depression in the prone position. Ideally, the sedation should be administered by an assistant who will monitor the patient's airway and breathing closely while the anesthesiologist is performing the blockade. Care should be exercised in patients with reflux esophagitis to avoid regurgitation and aspiration during this procedure. Attention must also be paid to the patient's mental status, since this blockade produces the highest blood levels of local anesthetics when compared with any other regional anesthetic technique. Because this blockade is frequently supplemented by a light general anesthetic for surgery, systemic toxicity signs are rarely seen because of the overlying general anesthetic. When the blockade is performed for postoperative pain relief, the dosage should be reduced to 0.25% bupivacaine in order to minimize the chance for toxicity.

Although one of the advantages of this blockade is the avoidance of sympathetic blockade and its attendant cardiovascular changes, it is possible to produce partial spinal or epidural anesthesia if the injection is made close to the midline and the anesthetic tracks along a dural sleeve to the epidural or subarachnoid space.[34] This appears to be more likely if intrathoracic injection is performed intraoperatively by a surgeon. Hypotension may result in this situation. Hypotension has also been observed rarely when this blockade is used for postoperative pain relief in a patient who has received generous doses of opioids. Once the local anesthetic succeeds in relieving the pain, the patient's intrinsic sympathetic response is reduced, and the respiratory depressant effect of previously injected opioids is unmasked. Patients should be observed for at least 20 to 30 minutes following performance of intercostal blockade. Respiratory insufficiency can also be seen if the intercostal muscles are blocked in a patient dependent upon them for ventilation. Patients with chronic obstructive disease with ineffective diaphragm motion are not good candidates for this technique.[35]

Paravertebral Blockade

The upper five ribs are more difficult to palpate laterally, and blockade of their associated intercostal nerves is best performed with a paravertebral injection. This approach is technically more difficult and has slightly greater potential for complications because of the proximity of the lung and of the intervertebral foramina. Anatomically, the injection is made into the triangle formed by the intervertebral body, the pleura, and the plane of the transverse processes (Fig. 29-25). The intervertebral foramina at each level lie between the transverse processes and approximately 2 cm anterior to the plane formed by the transverse processes in their associated fascia. At this point, the sympathetic ganglia lie very close to the somatic nerves, and coincidental sympathetic blockade is usually attained. This is also related to the injection of larger volumes of local anesthetic that is required because location of the nerve is less reliable with this technique. Nevertheless, it is a useful technique for segmental anesthesia, particularly of the upper thoracic segments. It is also useful if a more proximal blockade is needed, such as to relieve the pain of herpes zoster or a proximal rib fracture.

The paravertebral approach varies somewhat depending upon the spinal level. In the upper thoracic spine, the transverse process is located lateral to the spinous process of the vertebral body above it. In the lower thoracic spine, the spinous processes are less steeply angled, so that the 11th and 12th spinous processes lie between the associated transverse processes. In the lumbar region, the spinous processes are straight, and the transverse processes lie opposite their own respective spinous process. Thus, paravertebral blockade in the upper thoracic region is performed at each level by identifying the spinous process of the vertebra *above* the level to be blocked; in the lumbar region, the spinous process of the level to be blocked is used to locate the transverse process. The procedure for blockade follows:

1. This blockade is also performed in the prone position, with a pillow under the abdomen to produce flexion of the thoracic and lumbar spine. The spinous processes in the region to be blocked are marked. These can be identified by counting upward from the 4th lumbar process (which usually lies just at or above the line joining the two iliac crests) or by counting down from the 7th cervical process (which is the most prominent in the cervical region).

2. Transverse lines are drawn across the cephalad border of the spinous processes and extended laterally to overlie the transverse process (approximately 1cm to 4 cm). In the lumbar region, the lines will overlie the transverse process of the associated vertebra. In the thoracic region, they will indicate the transverse process of the vertebral body immediately below the associated spinous process. Finally, a vertical line is drawn parallel to the spine 3 to 4 cm lateral to it joining the transverse lines from the spinous processes. For a diagnostic blockade, a single nerve may need to be anesthetized. For pain control, several levels must be identified. The injection of at least three segments (as in intercostal blockade) is required to produce reliable segmental blockade because of sensory overlap.

3. Following aseptic skin preparation, skin wheals are raised at the intersections of the vertical and transverse lines.

4. A 22-g needle is introduced through the skin wheal in the sagittal plane and directed slightly cephalad to contact the transverse process. A 7.5-cm needle is usually required in the average patient, and the transverse process will lie between 3 and 5 cm from the skin. Gentle cephalad or caudad exploration may be required to identify the bone. The depth of the transverse process is carefully noted on the needle shaft.

5. The needle is now withdrawn from the transverse process and "walked" inferiorly to pass below its caudad edge. This will usually require more perpendicular direction relative to the skin. The needle is advanced 2 cm below the transverse process and angled slightly medial to attempt to contact the vertebral body. Paresthesias are not sought unless a neurolytic injection is planned. When the needle has entered the paravertebral space, 5 to 10 ml of local anesthetic solution is injected after careful aspiration.

The complication of pneumothorax is more likely in the thoracic region with this technique than with intercostal blockade.[36] The needle should be directed medially as it passes below the transverse process and never more than 2 cm beyond the transverse process (see Fig. 29-25). If cough or chest pain occurs, a chest x-ray should be performed to rule out pneumothorax. Subarachnoid injection is also more likely in the thoracic area because of the extension of the dural sleeves to the level of the intervertebral foramina. Careful aspiration is important but may not prevent the unintentional injection of local anesthetic into a subdural pocket. Total spinal anesthesia can result with a 5 to 10-ml injection. Systemic toxicity is also a possibility because of the need for relatively large volumes of local anesthetic. Attention must be paid to the total milligram dosage injected. The volume required for each level obviously limits the concentrations that can be used and the total number of levels that can be blocked. If lumbar paravertebral injections are combined with intercostals, the concentration and total volume for both blockades may have to be reduced.

Sympathetic Blockade—Stellate

Separate blockade of the sympathetic fibers of the upper extremity and head can be achieved by a single injection of a local anesthetic on the stellate ganglion. The ganglion is the large fusion of the first thoracic sympathetic ganglion with the lower cervical ganglion on each side, and it lies on the generally flat

FIG. 29-25. Paravertebral blockade. As it exits the intervertebral foramen, the thoracic somatic nerve enters a small triangular space formed by the vertebral body, the plane of the transverse process, and the pleura. Medial direction of the needle is obviously important in reducing the chance of a pneumothorax.

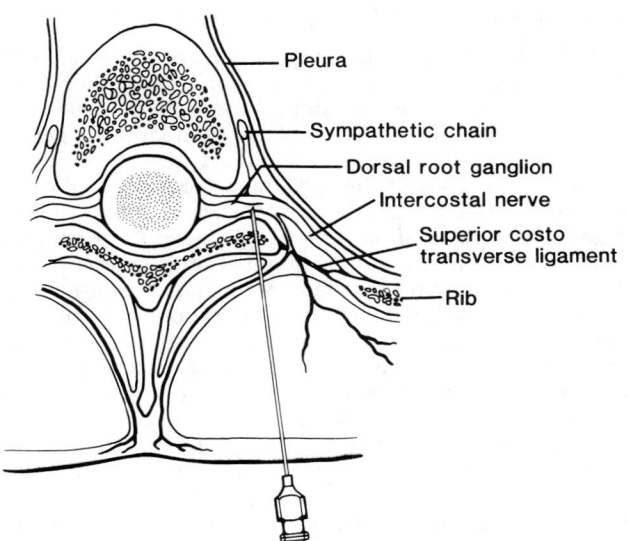

Pleura

Sympathetic chain

Dorsal root ganglion

Intercostal nerve

Superior costo transverse ligament

Rib

lateral border of the vertebral body of C-7. All the fibers to the middle and superior cervical ganglia pass through this lowermost collection and thus can be anesthetized with a single injection. Although technically simple, the location of this ganglia in close proximity to the carotid artery, the vertebral artery, and the pleura make this a challenging blockade. It is very useful in providing pain relief for sympathetic dystrophies of the upper arm. Stellate ganglion blockade may relieve the pain of acute herpes zoster infection of the head or neck region. It has also been advocated as a means of reducing postthoracotomy pain by blocking the sympathetic sensory fibers to the pleural cavity. The procedure for blockade follows:

1. The patient is placed in a supine position with a small towel or pillow under the neck, and the arms are held at the side.
2. The medial border of the SCM on the involved side is marked with a pen as well as the level of the cricoid cartilage. Gentle palpation approximately 2 cm lateral to the cartilage will often reveal the anterior tubercle of the transverse process of the 6th cervical vertebra (Chassaignac's tubercle). A circle is marked over this tubercle, and an "X" is placed 1.5 to 2 cm caudad to this mark at the same distance from the midline. This "X" should overlie the tubercle of the 7th cervical vertebra and should fall at the medial border of the SCM body and approximately two fingerbreadths above the clavicle itself.
3. A skin wheal is made at the "X" after aseptic skin preparation.
4. With the index and middle finger of one hand, the SCM and the carotid sheath are retracted laterally (Fig. 29-26). A 22- or 25-g 3.75-cm needle is introduced through the "X" and passed directly posterior until it rests on bone.

FIG. 29-26. Stellate ganglion blockade. The sternocleidomastoid muscle and the carotid sheath are retracted laterally with one hand while the needle is introduced directly onto the lateral border of the 7th vertebral body, just medial to the transverse process. The vertebral artery is passing posteriorly at this level to enter its canal in the transverse processes, but here lies near the level of intended injection. After contacting bone, the needle is withdrawn slightly and careful aspiration is performed before incremental injection. (Reproduced with permission from Mulroy M: Handbook of Regional Anesthesia. Boston, Little, Brown, 1988.)

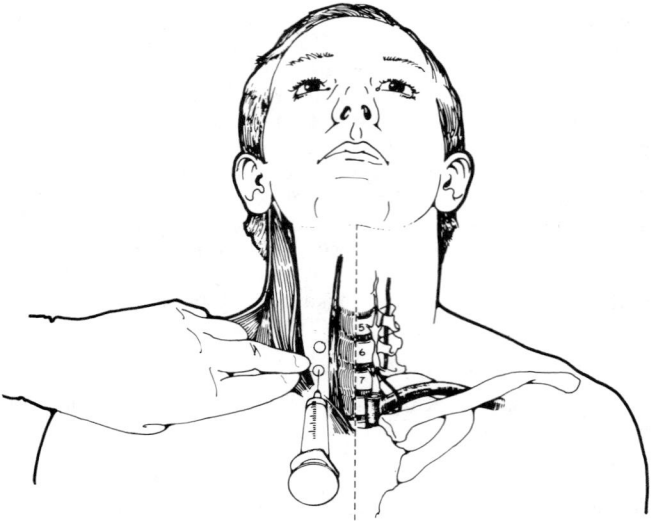

Paresthesia of the brachial plexus implies that the needle is too far laterally and has passed beyond the transverse process. It may have to be readjusted slightly more medially and perhaps more cephalad or caudad.

5. Once bone is contacted, the needle is withdrawn a few millimeters, and very careful aspiration is performed to rule out contact with the vertebral artery. A 2-ml test dose is injected to further evaluate an unrecognized intravascular position. The patient's mental status must be closely observed.
6. If no change occurs, a total of 10 ml of local anesthetic can be injected incrementally with frequent aspiration. One per cent lidocaine or 0.25% bupivacaine or their equivalents are more than adequate to produce anesthesia of the sympathetic nerves.
7. Onset of sympathectomy is usually indicated by the appearance of a Horner's syndrome on the ipsilateral side. Ptosis, miosis, and anhydrosis usually develop within 10 minutes as well as vasodilatation in the arm. Nasal congestion is another common sign usually associated with Horner's syndrome.

As implied, there are several potential complications of stellate ganglion blockade related to the surrounding anatomy. The pleura can be punctured with resulting pneumothorax. Intravascular injection is the most serious complication because of the close proximity of the vertebral artery to the site of injection.[37] Careful aspiration and incremental injections are essential. Only a few milligrams of local anesthetic are required to produce cerebral symptoms when injected directly into the vertebral circulation. Cardiovascular changes are possible with the loss of the cardiac accelerator fibers from the cervical sympathetic ganglia. This is particularly a problem if bilateral blockade is performed—a procedure rarely indicated. Hoarseness from recurrent laryngeal nerve paralysis is a minor but troublesome side-effect. Somatic anesthesia of the brachial plexus nerves can be produced by injection behind the level of the tubercle, and phrenic nerve paralysis has also been reported. Subarachnoid injection is also a possibility if the needle is misplaced. The close association of so many vital structures has discouraged the use of neurolytic agents in the region of the stellate ganglion.

Sympathetic Blockade—Celiac Plexus

The thoracic sympathetic ganglia send branches anteriorly that merge as greater and lesser splanchnic nerves to pass below the diaphragm and around the aorta to coalesce in a diffuse periaortic supplementary sympathetic ganglion known as the *celiac plexus*. This extensive network is generally located at the level of the 1st lumbar vertebra in the retroperitoneal space along the aorta at the level of the origin of the celiac artery. Fibers from this ganglion send postganglionic innervation to all the intraabdominal organs and appear to carry pain sensation from many of the intraperitoneal organs such as the pancreas and liver. Injection into this retroperitoneal space will allow anesthetic solution to diffuse around the ganglia and the splanchnic nerves to provide blockade of these fibers.[38] This blockade produces supplementary intraabdominal anesthesia when used in conjunction with intercostal blockade or general anesthesia. It is more commonly applied as a neurolytic sympathetic blockade for the relief of pain from malignancy of the pancreas, liver, or other upper abdominal organs.[39] The procedure for blockade follows:

1. As with intercostal blockade, the patient is placed in the prone position with the thoracic spine flexed by the use of a pillow under the abdomen.
2. The spinous process of the 12th thoracic and the 1st lumbar vertebral bodies are identified and marked along their entire extent. The 12th rib is likewise identified and marked 7 cm from the midline. A line is drawn between the 12th ribs on each side, usually crossing the midline at the level of the spinous process of the 1st lumbar vertebra. Lines are also drawn from the spinous process of the 12th thoracic vertebra to the points on these ribs on both sides. The net result is a shallow ipsilateral triangle, with the spinous process of the 12th vertebra at its apex.
3. Skin wheals are raised bilaterally at the marks along the ribs after aseptic skin preparation. Deeper infiltration of local anesthetic with a 22-g needle is often helpful in improving patient tolerance of this procedure.
4. On each side, a 12.5-cm 22- or 20-g needle is introduced through the skin wheals and advanced anteriorly and medially and cephalad along the two lines of the triangle that was previously drawn (Fig. 29-27). The needle should be passed at approximately a 45-degree angle anteriorly so that it will contact the lateral border of the vertebral body of L-1 at a depth of approximately 5 cm from the skin. (The 12th spinous process partially overlies the L-1 vertebral body.)
5. When contact with a vertebral body is made, the needle is withdrawn several centimeters, and the angle of insertion is steepened so that it advances more anteriorly with subsequent passage, hoping to "walk off" the anterior border of the vertebral body. The periosteum may be encountered several times during this attempt and should always be palpated gently because of the associated discomfort. Intravenous sedation may be required for tolerance of this blockade, although it must be kept to a minimum if evaluation of a diagnostic pain blockade is desired.
6. Once the anterior border of the vertebral body is reached, the needle is advanced 2 to 3 cm beyond this, and careful aspiration is performed. On the left side, advancement should be halted whenever aortic pulsation is appreciated. If the artery is unintentionally punctured, the needle should be withdrawn slightly and cleared immediately of blood. On the right side, the needle can often be advanced a centimeter or two further than the needle on the left side.
7. If radiologic confirmation is desired, it is obtained at this point, before injection of the anesthetic. The bony landmarks themselves are usually sufficient to identify the retroperitoneal space anterior to the first lumbar vertebral body. If neurolytic agents are to be used or if the anatomy is difficult, x-ray confirmation may be desirable. Although simple flat-plate radiographs are usually sufficient, the use of fluoroscopy may be indicated in difficult cases. The use of a computed tomography (CT) scan is not economically justified except in the most difficult of anatomic localizations.
8. Careful aspiration is performed, and a test dose is injected on each side to rule out subarachnoid or intravascular injection.
9. A large volume of local anesthetic solution is required. Twenty to 25 ml of 0.75% lidocaine or 0.25% bupivacaine are usually adequate, but a large volume is needed to diffuse in the retroperitoneal space to reach the ganglia.
10. The most reliable sign of successful anesthesia is the disappearance of pain in cancer patients or the appearance of hypotension in normal patients. Pain patients must remain supine for several hours and should have appropriate intravenous fluid supplementation to avoid orthostatic hypotension. Gradual ambulation is mandatory.

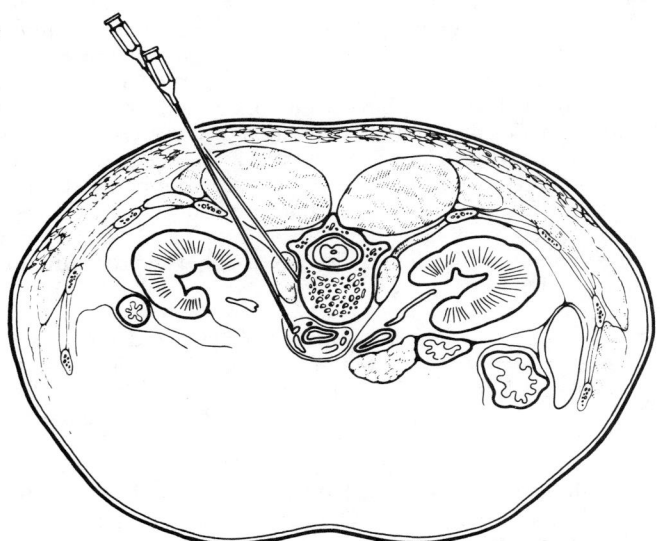

FIG. 29-27. Celiac plexus blockade. The surface landmarks are described in Figure 29-23. The needles are advanced medially and superiorly to contact the lateral aspect of the vertebral body. They are then advanced more anteriorly to pass beyond the vertebra to the prevertebral space where the greater and lesser splanchnic nerves and their subsequent celiac plexus lie. No attempt is made to advance the needles to the anterior aspect of the vessels. (Reproduced with permission from Mulroy M: Handbook of Regional Anesthesia. Boston, Little, Brown, 1988.)

Hypotension is the most common complication of celiac plexus blockade. As mentioned previously, it can be reduced by the administration of a liter of balanced salt solution before performing the blockade. The most serious complication is the development of paralysis from unrecognized subarachnoid injection of a neurolytic drug.[40] Radiographic confirmation of needle location is advisable before injection of any neurolytic drug. Even with correct placement of neurolytic drugs, back pain is common and may require intravenous opioids. This pain can be reduced by diluting the alcohol solution with an equal volume of local anesthetic, such that a total volume of 50 ml is injected, consisting of 25 ml of alcohol and 25 ml of anesthetic. Even with this approach, diaphragmatic irritation (manifested as shoulder pain) is not uncommon. The duration of pain relief in the chronic pain patient is unpredictable but is often sufficient for 2 to 6 months. The blockade appears to be repeatable as often as necessary, although a trial diagnostic blockade with a local anesthetic agent is indicated before each use of neurolytic drugs. One minor side effect of celiac plexus blockade is the increased peristalsis of the gut that is produced by the shift in the balance of the parasympathetic and sympathetic innervation. This may produce diarrhea within the first 12 hours after the blockade and may be a source of relief to patients on chronic opioid therapy for cancer pain.

Sympathetic Blockade—Lumbar

Lumbar sympathetic blockade combines some of the anatomic considerations for stellate ganglion blockade and paravertebral anesthesia. As with the sympathetic innervation of the head and arm, the sympathetic nerves to the lower extremities all exit the cord above the 2nd lumbar vertebra and all pass through a common "gateway" ganglia in the sympathetic chain at the L-2 level. Thus, as in the neck, sympathetic blockade of the lower extremity can be achieved by a single injection of one ganglion. The approach to this ganglion is very similar to paravertebral anesthesia as discussed previously except that in the lumbar region, the sympathetic chain lies much further anterior from the somatic nerves, and, thus, a clean separation of sympathetic blockade from somatic blockade can be more easily attained.

As in the upper extremity, lumbar sympathectomy can be used in the treatment of sympathetic dystrophies or herpes zoster in an early stage. It is also occasionally used in the lower extremities in the presence of severe vascular disease to give some indication of whether a patient would profit from permanent chemical or surgical sympathectomy. The procedure for blockade follows:

1. The patient position is similar as that for celiac plexus blockade. The patient lies prone with a pillow under the lumbar spine.
2. The spinous processes of the 2nd and 3rd lumbar vertebrae are identified and marked over their entire course. A horizontal line is drawn through the midpoint of the 2nd lumbar spinous process and extended 5 cm to either side of the midline. An "X" is placed at this point, which should overlie the space between the transverse process of the 2nd and 3rd vertebrae or the caudad edge of the second transverse process.
3. A skin wheal is raised after aseptic skin preparation at each "X."
4. A 10-cm needle is introduced on each side through the "X," angled 30 to 45 degrees cephalad, and advanced until it contacts the transverse process (Fig. 29–28).

FIG. 29-28. Lumbar sympathetic blockade. The needle is first placed on the transverse process of the 2nd lumbar vertebra and then advanced below it to pass 5 cm deeper. The needle can be angled slightly medially to contact the body of the vertebra; the sympathetic chain lies along the anterior margin of these bodies. (Reproduced with permission from Mulroy M: Handbook of Regional Anesthesia. Boston, Little, Brown, 1988.)

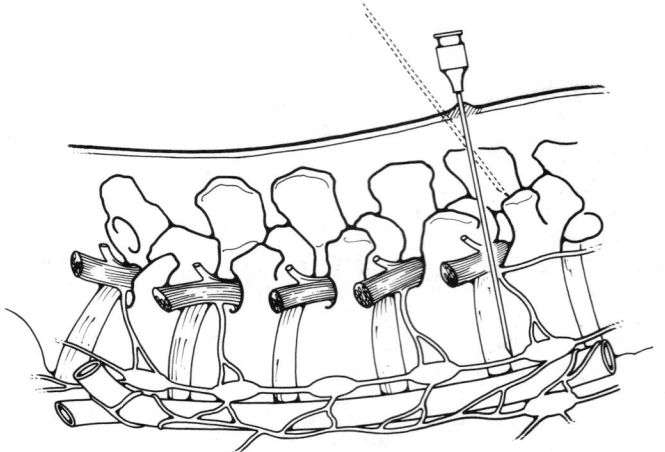

5. The depth of the needle insertion is marked, and the needle is then withdrawn slightly, angled caudad, and "walked" inferiorly off the transverse process (usually in a direction perpendicular to the skin). A slight medial angulation is used in the hope of contacting the vertebral body below the transverse process. The needle is advanced 5 cm below the depth of the transverse process. If it encounters a vertebral body, it is angled slightly more anteriorly to "walk off" that body at the desired depth.
6. Once the needle is in position, careful aspiration is performed, and a test dose is injected on both sides. Ten milliliters of local anesthetic solution injected on each side should produce sympathetic blockade. Again, 1% lidocaine, 0.25% bupivacaine, or an equivalent concentration is more than sufficient to produce sympathetic nerve blockade. If a neurolytic drug such as phenol is used, confirmation of needle position by radiography should be performed. A slightly more caudad site of injection may be more effective for neurolytic blockade[41]; injection of smaller quantities at several levels may be more appropriate for neurolytic drugs.
7. Care is taken not to inject anesthetic solution as the needle is withdrawn, because this may produce a somatic nerve blockade as the needle passes the course of the L-2 nerve root.
8. Vasodilatation and increase in skin temperature should be noted within the leg in 5 to 10 minutes. This can be quantitated objectively if a skin temperature probe is placed on the foot before the start of the blockade.

Complications with this technique are unusual, but, again, intravascular or subarachnoid injection can be a potential problem. The most troublesome and frequent complication is simultaneous blockade of the 2nd lumbar somatic nerve root. This will produce a band of anesthesia across the lateral and anterior thigh. This may confuse the evaluation of a diagnostic sympathetic blockade.

Ilioinguinal Blockade

The L-1 nerve root (occasionally joined by a branch of the T-12 root) provides sensory anesthesia to the lowermost portion of the abdominal wall and the groin by means of its superior iliohypogastric branch and its inferior ilioinguinal branch. These nerves travel in a path very similar to that of the intercostal nerves, but without the convenient bony landmark of a rib to identify them. Nevertheless, they can be anesthetized relatively easily in the groin because of their relationship to the anterosuperior iliac spine. Anesthesia of these two nerves is useful in providing lower abdominal wall anesthesia to supplement intercostal blockade. It is more commonly used to produce field anesthesia for hernia repair surgery. Anesthesia of these nerves alone is not sufficient for hernia repair, and subcutaneous infiltration is also necessary. The procedure for blockade follows:

1. The patient lies in a supine position, and the anterosuperior iliac spine is identified. An "X" is placed on the skin 2.5 cm medial to the spine and slightly cephalad.
2. After aseptic preparation, a skin wheal is raised at the "X."
3. A 2.5-cm 22-g needle is introduced through the "X" and directed perpendicular to the skin until it reaches the fascia of the external oblique muscle. A "wall" of local anesthetic solution is then laid down between this point

and the iliac spine, and also opposite the mark on an imaginary line extending toward the umbilicus. Injections are made at and below the level of the external oblique, with some solution injected at the level of the internal oblique. A total of 10 to 15 ml of anesthetic is usually required. A solution of 1% lidocaine, 0.25% bupivacaine, or an equivalent is adequate.

4. If field anesthesia for hernia repair is required, further subcutaneous infiltration of anesthetic is performed along the skin crease of the groin and along the imaginary line extending to the umbilicus. This will produce a triangular-shaped area of skin anesthesia. For hernia operations, further anesthesia of the spermatic cord is required. This is usually performed by local injections in the area of the cord and the internal ring. Although epinephrine is useful in the subcutaneous and ilioinguinal blockade, it should be avoided in solutions used to anesthetize the base of the penis or the spermatic cord.

Further anesthesia of the groin area and below can be obtained by blockade of the femoral and lateral femoral cutaneous nerves (see next section), but this may result in unwanted weakness of the leg musculature, which may prevent ambulation.

Complications of this procedure are extremely rare. Hematoma formation as well as unwanted motor blockade of the femoral nerve is possible. These complications are rare. More commonly, anesthesia produced by this technique is inadequate for hernia repair because the patient is still able to perceive the discomfort of peritoneal traction. Administration of local anesthesia by the surgeon or systemic opioids may be required.

Penile Blockade

If surgery is confined to the penis (circumcision, urethral procedures), the organ should be blocked with simple local infiltration. Two skin wheals are raised at the dorsal base of the penis, one on each side just below and medial to the pubic spine. A 22-g 3.75-cm needle is introduced on each side, and 5 ml of anesthetic is deposited superficially and deep along the lower border of the pubic ramus to anesthetize the dorsal nerve. An additional 5 ml is infiltrated in the subcutaneous tissue around the underside of the shaft to produce a complete ring of anesthetic. A larger needle or a second injection site may be needed to complete the ring. Twenty to 25 ml of 0.75% lidocaine or 0.25% bupivacaine will usually suffice. Epinephrine is strictly avoided.

LOWER EXTREMITY

The nerves to the lower extremity are most easily blocked by the spinal, caudal, or epidural techniques described in Chapter 28. There are occasions where anesthesia by these routes is contraindicated because of systemic sepsis or coagulopathy, or where selective anesthesia of one leg or foot is needed. Peripheral nerve blockade is possible because the motor and sensory fibers to the lower extremities are somewhat similar to those of the upper extremities in that they form a series of intertwined branching roots and divisions that are enclosed in a fascial sheath before they emerge as the terminal nerves to the extremity. They can also be successfully blocked by a single injection in one plane, although the anatomic landmarks identifying this fascial sheath are not as clearly defined as those in the upper extremity. Because of this, the majority

of lower extremity blockades are performed more distally, where the nerves have already separated into terminal branches. Thus, in addition to the fascial compartment approach (psoas blockade), there are peripheral approaches described at the hip, at the knee, and at the ankle.

The nerves to the legs emerge from the roots of the 2nd lumbar though the 3rd sacral spinal segments (Fig. 29-29). The upper nerve roots from the 2nd to the 4th lumbar vertebrae form the lumbar plexus, which then ramifies to eventually form the lateral femoral cutaneous, femoral, and obturator nerves. These primarily provide sensory–motor innervation of the upper leg, although a branch of the femoral nerve commonly extends along the medial side of the knee as far down as the big toe. A branch of this lumbar plexus, the lumbosacral trunk of L-4 and L-5, joins the sacral fibers to form the major trunks of the large nerve of the posterior thigh and lower leg, the sciatic. The sciatic nerve is made up of two main trunks, the tibial and the common peroneal, which divide just above the knee. As in the brachial plexus, the upper nerve roots emerge from their foramina into a compartment lined by the fascia of muscles anterior and posterior to it. In this case, the quadratus lumborum is posterior, while the posterior fascia of the psoas muscle provides the anterior border of the compartment. The sacral roots have a similar envelope except that the posterior border is the bone of the ilium, which prevents approach with a needle.

The lumbar plexus branches form their three terminal nerves early. Each of these pass anteriorly and laterally to circle around the pelvis and emerge anteriorly in the groin. The femoral nerve is the only one to continue in the fascial

FIG. 29-29. Psoas compartment anatomy. The roots of the lumbar plexus emerge from their foramina into a fascial plane between the quadratus lumborum muscle posteriorly and the psoas muscle anteriorly. The origin of the lumbosacral plexus is broader than the corresponding brachial plexus in the neck, and the lower sacral roots cannot be easily reached by a single injection. (Reproduced with permission from Mulroy M: Handbook of Regional Anesthesia. Boston, Little, Brown, 1988.)

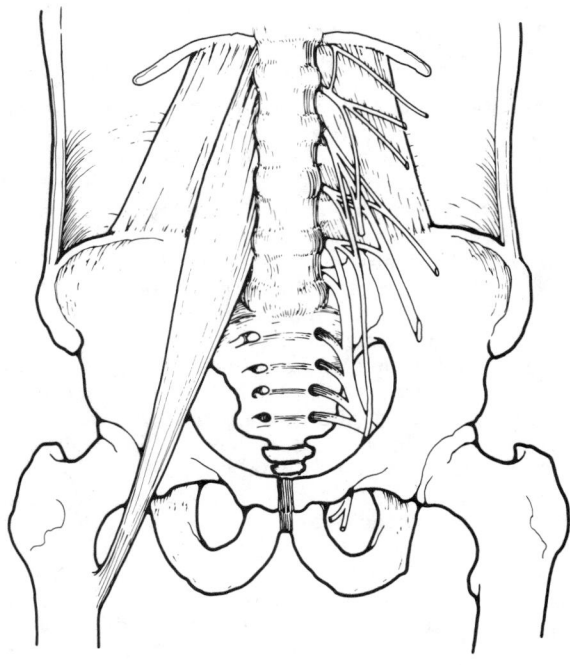

compartment formed by the psoas fascia as it passes into the groove between the psoas and the iliac muscle. The femoral nerve becomes associated with the femoral artery in the area of the groin and passes under the inguinal ligament just lateral to the artery. The lateral femoral cutaneous nerve migrates laterally early and passes under the inguinal ligament near the anterosuperior iliac spine. The third branch of the lumbar plexus, the obturator, remains somewhat medial and posterior in the pelvis and emerges under the superior ramus of the pubis through the obturator foramen to supply motor and sensory fibers to the medial thigh and medial border of the knee.

The branches of the sacral plexus also travel laterally within the pelvis before exiting posteriorly through the sciatic notch as the sciatic nerve. This largest nerve of the body is actually the conjunction of two trunks. The lateral trunk forms from the roots of L-4 through S-2 and eventually emerges as the common peroneal nerve. Other branches of L-4 through S-3 form the medial trunk, eventually to become the tibial nerve. These combined nerves exit through the sciatic notch and pass anteriorly to the piriformis muscle between the ischial tuberosity and the greater trochanter of the femur. They curve caudad and descend the posterior thigh immediately behind the femur. After their bifurcation high in the popliteal fossa, the peroneal nerve provides the motor and sensory fibers to the anterior calf and dorsum of the foot, while the tibial nerve remains posterior and provides sensation to the calf and sole of the foot. Thus, there are three major branches that cross the knee—the femoral, tibial, and peroneal. By the time that these nerves reach the ankle, there are five branches that cross this joint to provide innervation for the skin and muscles of the foot.

Psoas Compartment Blockade

As described previously, the roots of the lumbar plexus lie in an envelope similar to the interscalene fascial compartment in the neck (Fig. 29-29). Unfortunately, this fascial compartment is more difficult to identify in the lower than in the upper extremity and lies much deeper beneath the skin than its equivalent in the neck. Nevertheless, it is useful to attempt if single-injection anesthesia of the leg is desired. The procedure for blockade follows:

1. The patient is placed in the prone or in the lateral position. The spinous processes of the lumbar vertebrae are identified, and an "X" is placed on the skin 5 cm lateral to the spinous process of the 3rd lumbar vertebra. This is similar to the technique described for lumbar paravertebral blockade.
2. After aseptic preparation, a skin wheal is raised at the "X." A 10-cm needle is advanced perpendicular to the skin in all planes and passed through the muscles of the back. The nerve roots should lie at a depth of between 7 and 10 cm. Although in some patients the well-demarcated fascial planes can identify the entry into the perineural sheath, anesthesia is much more reliable if paresthesias are obtained. If they are not obtained at a 10-cm depth, probing with the needle in a fan-like manner should be performed in a cephalad caudad plane (which is perpendicular to the known paths of the emerging nerves).
3. When a paresthesia is obtained, the needle is fixed in position, and careful aspiration and administration of a test dose are used to rule out intravascular or subarachnoid placement. Forty milliliters of local anesthetic

solution is usually required to fill the sheath. 1.5% lidocaine or 0.5% bupivacaine are adequate to provide sensory and motor anesthesia. Lower concentrations will provide adequate sensory anesthesia with less profound motor blockade. Fifteen to 20 minutes may be required for spread of the anesthetic to all the roots of the lumbosacral plexus. It may take longer to produce anesthesia of the caudad branches (the lower sacral fibers that form the tibial nerve).

Complications of this technique are rare, although hematoma in the muscle sheath and neuropathy of the nerves are possible. Inadequate anesthesia of some of the branches may occur more frequently than these rare complications.

Anesthesia at the Level of the Hip

Many anesthesiologists feel more confident when administering regional anesthesia in the hip region when paresthesias are sought for each of the major nerves. This technique is cumbersome and usually requires the patient to assume at least two separate positions for the injections. The anesthesia will be more reliable but will also require a larger volume of anesthetic drug. Each of the four nerves may be blocked selectively on an individual basis. Anesthesia of the lateral femoral cutaneous nerve is occasionally used to provide sensory anesthesia for obtaining a skin graft from the lateral thigh. It can also be blocked as a diagnostic tool to identify cases of meralgia paresthetica. A sciatic nerve blockade alone will provide adequate anesthesia for the sole of the foot and lower leg. Procedures on the knee will require anesthesia of the femoral and the obturator nerve. Anesthesia of the lateral femoral cutaneous is also required if a tourniquet is to be placed on the thigh during foot surgery.

SCIATIC NERVE BLOCKADE, CLASSIC POSTERIOR APPROACH. This is the most commonly described approach to the sciatic nerve and requires that the patient be able to lie in the lateral position and flex the hip and the knee (Fig. 29-30). The procedure for blockade follows:

1. The patient lies with the side to be blocked uppermost and rolls slightly anterior, flexing the knee so that the ankle of the involved side rests on top of the knee of the opposite side. This position tends to rotate the femur so that the trochanter is more easily palpated and the muscles overlying the sciatic nerve become stretched.
2. The superior aspect of the greater trochanter of the hip is marked with a circle. A similar circle is placed on the posterosuperior iliac spine, and a line is drawn between these two points.
3. A perpendicular line is drawn from the midpoint of this original line and extended 5 cm in the caudad direction. An "X" is marked at this point. A third line drawn between the greater trochanter and the sacral hiatus should intersect this "X." In the taller patient, the original perpendicular may need to be extended caudad to provide and intersect with the third line, and the nerve may lie closer to the intersection of the second and third line than to the original "X."
4. A skin wheal is raised at the "X" after aseptic skin preparation.
5. A 10-cm needle is introduced perpendicular to the skin in all planes, and paresthesias of the lower leg and foot are sought. If they are not obtained at the full depth of the needle, the needle is withdrawn to the skin and

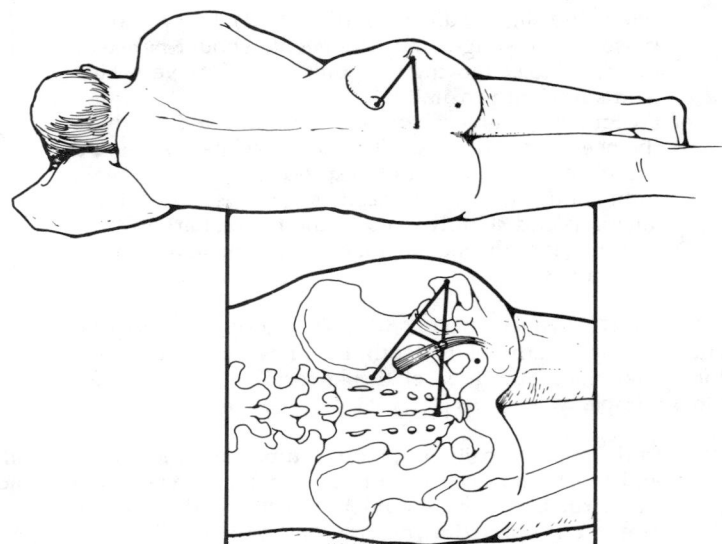

FIG. 29-30. Sciatic nerve blockade, classic posterior approach. With the patient in the lateral position and the hip and knee flexed, the muscles overlying the sciatic nerve are stretched to allow easier identification. The nerve lies beneath a point 5 cm caudad along the perpendicular line that bisects the line joining the posterosuperior iliac spine and the greater trochanter of the femur. This is also usually the intersection of that perpendicular line with another line joining the greater trochanter and the sacral hiatus. (Reproduced with permission from Mulroy M: Handbook of Regional Anesthesia. Boston, Little, Brown, 1988.)

reintroduced in a fanwise fashion in a path perpendicular to the imagined course of the nerve in the hip. This path can usually be visualized by following the muscular groove on the back of the thigh up and into the imagined position of the sciatic notch. The bony edges of the sciatic notch itself may be encountered. These should be noted, and the search continued. The nerve should lie at approximately this depth as it emerges from inside the pelvis. Paresthesias are critical in this blockade, since the blind infiltration of a large quantity of local anesthetic rarely produces adequate anesthesia because of multiple muscle planes in this area. If a paresthesia cannot be obtained in the first 10 minutes, the landmarks should be reassessed. Alternatively, the blockade can be performed with a nerve stimulator, which will also reduce patient discomfort.

6. When a paresthesia to the foot is obtained, the needle is held immobile, and 25 ml of local anesthetic is injected. Again, 1.5% lidocaine, 0.5% bupivacaine, or the equivalent are adequate. A lower concentration may be needed if several nerves are to be blocked, which would then require a large total volume of anesthetic in several locations.

SCIATIC NERVE BLOCKADE, SUPINE APPROACH (LITHOTOMY). If a patient is uncomfortable in the lateral position or cannot be turned to the side because of a fracture or pain, the nerve can be blocked with the patient in the supine position. An assistant is required to elevate the leg into a lithotomy-type position so that the posterior aspect can be reached. The procedure for blockade follows:

1. With the patient supine, the hip is flexed by an assistant so that the upper leg is at a 90-degree angle to the torso.
2. The greater trochanter is identified as well as the ischial tuberosity, and a line is drawn between these two. An "X" is marked on the midpoint of this line.
3. A skin wheal is raised at the "X" after aseptic skin preparation. A 10-cm needle is introduced, and paresthesias are sought in a direction along the length of this line (which is perpendicular to the course of the nerve).

4. When a paresthesia is obtained, 25 ml of local anesthetic is injected.

LATERAL FEMORAL CUTANEOUS NERVE BLOCKADE. The other three nerves of the leg can be blocked at the level of the hip with the patient in the supine position. If no paresthesias are sought, the patient can be sedated more heavily than was used for the sciatic nerve blockade. If the single-injection technique (see below) is used, paresthesias are needed and sedation should be lighter. The procedure for blockade follows:

1. In the supine position, the anterosuperior iliac spine is identified and marked. An "X" is placed on the skin 2.5 cm below and 2.5 cm medial to the spine.
2. A skin wheal is raised at the "X" after aseptic preparation.
3. A 3.75-cm 22-g needle is introduced through the wheal and directed laterally until a "pop" is felt as it pierces the fascia lata. Three to 5 ml of local anesthetic solution is injected as the needle is withdrawn slowly. The needle is then reinserted slightly medially, and the procedure is repeated until a "wall" of anesthesia has been spread over a 5-cm area above and below the fascia lata extending medially from the level of the anterosuperior spine. A total of 15 to 20 ml of local anesthetic may be required. No paresthesias are sought.

FEMORAL NERVE BLOCKADE. This blockade can be performed blindly without eliciting paresthesias, or paresthesias can be sought for a "three-in-one" blockade (see below). The procedure for blockade follows:

1. In the supine position, a line is drawn from the anterosuperior iliac spine to the pubic tubercle. The femoral artery is identified as it passes below this line, and an "X" is marked on the skin lateral to the artery 2.5 cm below the line.
2. After aseptic preparation, a skin wheal is raised at the mark.
3. A 5-cm 22-g needle is introduced through the "X" and passed perpendicular to the skin until it lies next to the

artery and slightly deep to it (Fig. 29-31). Entry into the vessel is not sought, but the needle should be easily perceived to be moving with pulsation of the vessel if it is in sufficient proximity.

4. Five milliliters of local anesthetic are injected slowly as the needle is withdrawn. The needle is then reinserted slightly more laterally, and the process is repeated again until another "wall" of anesthesia has been laid down lateral to and slightly deep to the femoral artery.

5. Anesthesia of the medial thigh should ensue within 5 to 10 minutes.

OBTURATOR NERVE BLOCKADE. This nerve is more difficult to locate because of its depth, but anesthesia is essential for operations in the area of the knee. The procedure for blockade follows:

1. In the supine position, the pubic tubercle is identified, and an "X" is placed 1.5 cm below and 1.5 cm lateral to this structure. This should lie medial to the femoral artery, and a line drawn between the three "X's" used for these three nerve blockades should be parallel to the line between the superior spine and the pubic tubercle.

FIG. 29-31. Blockade of the anterior lumbosacral branches in the groin. The lateral femoral cutaneous nerve emerges approximately 2.5 cm medial to the anterosuperior iliac spine and is best blocked 2.5 cm caudad to this point. The femoral nerve emerges alongside and slightly posterior to the femoral artery and is again easily approached approximately 2.5 cm below the inguinal ligament. On that same line, the obturator nerve emerges from the obturator canal but is deeper and less reliably located. (Reproduced with permission from Mulroy M: Handbook of Regional Anesthesia. Boston, Little, Brown, 1988.)

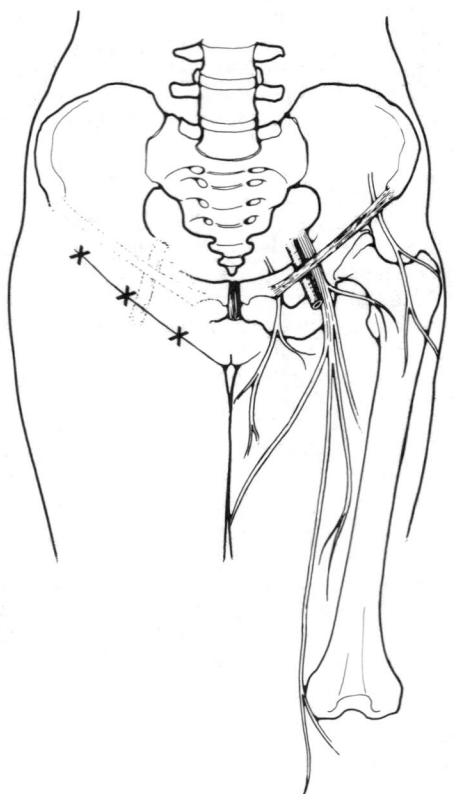

2. After aseptic skin preparation, a skin wheal is raised at the "X," and a 7.5-cm 22-g needle is introduced through the "X" perpendicular to the skin.

3. The needle is advanced until it contacts bone, which should be the inferior ramus of the pubis. The needle is withdrawn slightly and redirected laterally and slightly caudad to enter the obturator foramen. It is advanced another 2 to 3 cm, and 5 ml of anesthetic is injected as the needle is withdrawn through the presumed depth of the obturator foramen.

4. The needle is then reinserted slightly more laterally, and the process is repeated again until 20 ml of anesthetic solution has been injected to form another "wall" along the presumed path of the obturator nerve (see Fig. 29-31).

LUMBAR PLEXUS ("THREE-IN-ONE") BLOCKADE. Winnie et al[42] have popularized the concept of a single-injection blockade for the lumbar plexus, utilizing the fascial plane that the femoral nerve travels in as it crosses the pelvis. The object of this blockade is to inject a large quantity of local anesthetic solution in this plane so that it will spread upward into the pelvis and anesthetize the obturator and lateral femoral cutaneous nerves at the point where they still travel in conjunction with the femoral nerve. Because it is essential to have the needle exactly in the plane of the nerve, paresthesias are critical for this approach. Light sedation is therefore more appropriate than for the relatively "blind" traditional approaches to the three nerves of the groin. The procedure for blockade follows:

1. Preparation for femoral nerve blockade is made as described previously.

2. The needle is inserted in a cephalad manner rather than in a perpendicular angle recommended previously. It is advanced alongside the artery angled at about 45 degrees so that it passes under the inguinal ligament. A paresthesia is sought, recognizing that the nerve lies slightly posterior to and occasionally partially under the femoral artery. When the paresthesia is obtained, the needle is fixed and the fingers of an assistant are used to compress the femoral artery and the neural sheath below the inguinal ligament while the operator injects 40 ml of anesthetic solution. The injection is performed incrementally after careful aspiration.

Complications of these techniques are rare. Hematomas can occur in any of the areas of injection and are annoying but rarely serious. The problem of systemic toxicity is a major one because of the large volumes of anesthetic solution required. As mentioned previously, careful attention must be paid to the total milligram dose involved when these multiple injections are used. Neuropathy is a possibility. Interneural injection must be avoided by watching for signs of any discomfort at the time of actual injection.

Popliteal Fossa Blockade

The nerves of the lower leg can also be anesthetized by injections at the level of the knee.[43] The success of this technique depends upon locating the sciatic nerve near its bifurcation into the tibial and peroneal branches high in the popliteal fossa (Fig. 29-32). Supplemental anesthesia of the femoral nerve is needed in order to block its terminal saphenous branch, which serves the medial anterior calf and the dorsum of the foot. The procedure for blockade follows:

1. The patient is placed in a prone position. The triangular borders of the popliteal fossa are outlined by drawing the borders of the biceps femoris and the semitendinosus muscles. The base of the triangle is the skin crease behind the knee. The patient can help identify the muscles by slightly flexing the lower leg.

2. After the triangle is drawn, a perpendicular line is drawn from the midpoint of the base to the apex of the triangle. Five centimeters from the base, an "X" is drawn 1 cm lateral to this bisecting line.

3. After aseptic skin preparation, a skin wheal is raised at the "X."

4. A 7.5-cm or 10-cm needle is introduced through the "X" and directed 45 degrees cephalad along the middle of the triangle (Fig. 29-33). The nerves should be passing down the back of the leg parallel to the bisecting line of the triangle. A fanwise search is conducted perpendicular to this line until the nerve is contacted. If the femur is contacted by the needle, the depth is noted. The nerve should lie midway between the skin and the femur.

5. Once a paresthesia is obtained, the needle is fixed in position and 30 to 40 ml of local anesthetic solution is injected.

6. The femoral branches can be injected in the same position by raising a subcutaneous wheal of 5 to 10 ml of local anesthetic along the medial tibial head just below the knee.

Ankle Blockade

All the nerves of the foot can be blocked at the level of the ankle.[44] Although this approach is ideal in producing the least amount of immobility of the lower extremity, it is technically more difficult because at least five nerves must be anesthetized (Fig. 29-34). Several of these nerves can be blocked by simple infiltration of a "wall" of anesthesia, but increased reliability can be produced by seeking paresthesias of the major branches. If paresthesias are not sought, this blockade may actually be less time consuming than other techniques, even though five separate injections are required. The procedure for blockade follows:

1. The *posterior tibial nerve* is the major nerve to the sole of the foot. It can be approached with the patient either in the prone position or with the hip and knee flexed so that the foot rests on the bed. The medial malleolus is identified along with the pulsation of the posterior tibial artery behind it. A needle is introduced through the skin just behind the posterior tibial artery and directed 45 degrees anteriorly, seeking a paresthesia in the sole of the foot. Five milliliters of a local anesthetic will produce anesthesia if a paresthesia is identified. If not, a fan-shaped injection of 10 ml can be performed in the trian-

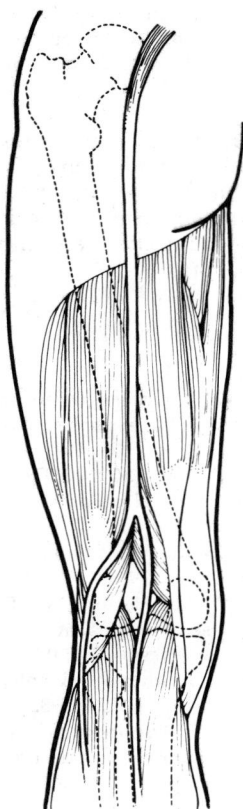

FIG. 29-32. Popliteal fossa blockade. The two major trunks of the sciatic bifurcate in the popliteal fossa 7 to 10 cm above the knee. A triangle is drawn using the heads of the biceps femoris and the semitendinosus muscles and the skin crease of the knee; a long needle is inserted 1 cm lateral to a point 5 cm cephalad on the line from the skin crease that bisects this triangle. (Reproduced with permission from Mulroy M: Handbook of Regional Anesthesia. Boston, Little, Brown, 1988.)

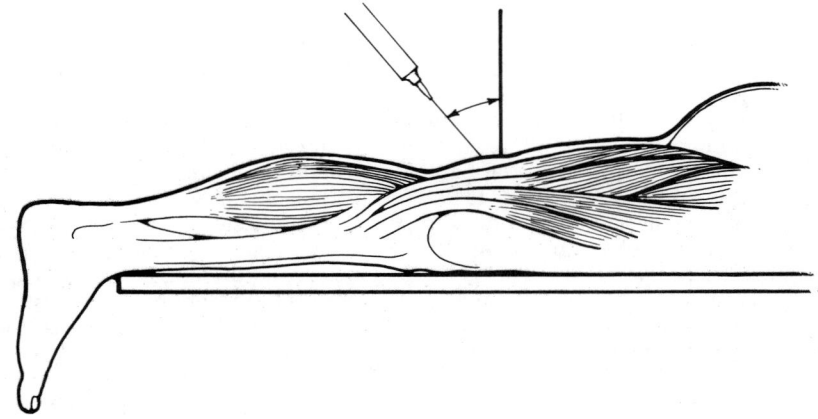

FIG. 29-33. Popliteal fossa blockade, needle direction. The needle is inserted at the point described in Figure 29-32 and angled 45 degrees cephalad. The nerves will usually be contacted halfway between the skin and the femur. (Reproduced with permission from Mulroy M: Handbook of Regional Anesthesia. Boston, Little, Brown, 1988.)

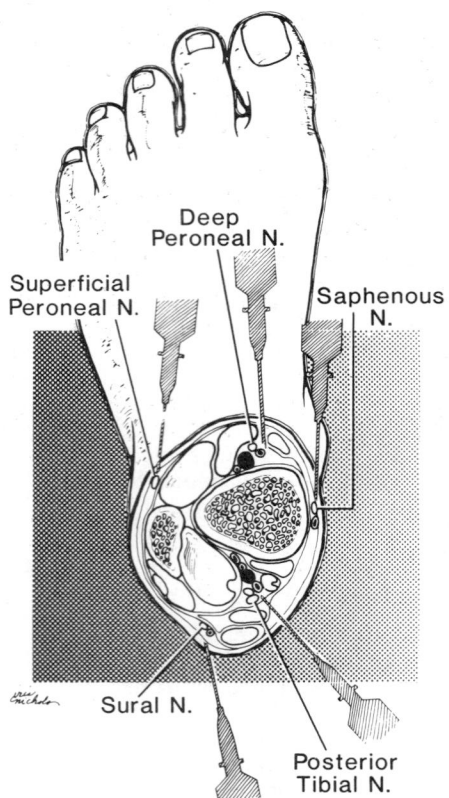

FIG. 29-34. Ankle blockade. Injections are made at five separate nerve locations. The superficial peroneal nerve, sural nerve, and saphenous are usually blocked simply by subcutaneous infiltration, since they may have already generated many superficial branches as they cross the ankle joint. Paresthesias can be sought in the posterior tibial nerve or the deep peroneal, but the bony landmarks will usually suffice to provide adequate localization for the deeper injections. (Reproduced with permission from Mulroy M: Handbook of Regional Anesthesia. Boston, Little, Brown, 1988.)

gle formed by the artery, the achilles tendon, and the tibia itself.

2. *Sural nerve.* With the foot in the same position, the other posterior nerve of the ankle can be blocked by injection on the lateral side. The subcutaneous injection of a ridge of anesthesia behind the lateral malleolus filling the groove between it and the calcaneus will produce anesthesia of the sural nerve. This will require another 5 ml of local anesthetic.

3. *Saphenous nerve.* The last three branches of the ankle lie anteriorly. The patient is either turned supine, or the leg can now be extended so that attention of the anesthesiologist is turned to the anterior surface. The saphenous nerve is anesthetized by infiltrating 5 ml of local anesthetic around the saphenous vein at the level where this vein passes anterior to the medial malleolus. A wall of anesthesia between the skin and the bone itself will suffice to block the nerve.

4. *Deep peroneal nerve.* This is the major nerve to the dorsum of the foot and lies in the deep plane of the anterior tibial artery. Pulsation of the artery is sought at the level of the skin crease on the anterior midline surface of the ankle. If it can be felt, 5 ml of local anesthetic is injected just lateral to this. If the artery is not palpable, the

tendon of the extensor hallucus longus can be identified by asking the patient to extend the big toe. Injection can be made into the deep planes below the fascia using either one of these landmarks.

5. *Superficial peroneal branches.* Finally, a subcutaneous ridge of anesthetic solution is laid along the skin crease between the anterior tibial artery and the lateral malleolus. This subcutaneous ridge will overlie the previous subfascial injection for the deep peroneal nerve. Another 5 to 10 ml of local anesthetic may be required to cover this area.

Anesthesia of the foot should ensue within 10 minutes after the performance of these five injections. Complications of this blockade are rare, although neuropathy can be produced. Care should be taken not to pin any of the deep nerves against the bone at the time of injection, and intraneural injection should be avoided as usual.

REFERENCES

1. Kehlet H: The modifying effect of general and regional anesthesia on the endocrine-metabolic response to surgery. Reg Anesth (Suppl) 7:S38, 1982
2. Yeager MP, Glass DD, Neff RK *et al:* Epidural anesthesia and analgesia in high-risk surgical patients. Anesthesiology 66:729, 1987
3. Wetchler BV: Anesthesia for Ambulatory Surgery, pp 225–269. Philadelphia, JB Lippincott, 1985
4. Buffington CW, Ready LB, Horton WG: Training and practice factors influence the use of regional anesthesia; implications for resident education. Reg Anesth 10:2, 1985
5. Bridenbaugh LD: Are anesthesia resident programs failing regional anesthesia? Reg Anesth 7:26, 1982
6. Selander D, Brattsand R, Lundborg G *et al:* Local anesthetics: Importance of mode of application, concentration, and adrenaline for the appearance of nerve lesions. Acta Anaesth Scand 23:127, 1979
7. Ready LB, Plummer MH, Haschke RH *et al:* Neurotoxicity of intrathecal local anesthetics in rabbits. Anesthesiology 63:364, 1985
8. Kelly DA, Henderson AM: Use of local anesthetic drugs in hospital practice. Br Med J 286:1784, 1983
9. Selander D, Edshage S, Wolff T: Paresthesiae or no paresthesiae? Acta Anaesthesiol Scand 23:27, 1979
10. Smith BL: Efficacy of a nerve stimulator in regional anesthesia; experience in a resident training programme. Anaesthesia 31:778, 1976
11. Pither CE, Raj PP, Ford DJ: The use of peripheral nerve stimulators for regional anesthesia. Reg Anesth 10:49, 1985
12. Bashein G, Haschke RH, Ready LB: Electrical nerve location: Numerical and electrophoretic comparison of insulated vs uninsulated needles. Anesth Analg 63:919, 1984
13. McMahon DJ: Managing regional anesthesia equipment. In Problems in Anesthesia, Vol 1, No 4, pp 592–596. Philadelphia, JB Lippincott, 1987
14. Selander D, Dhuner KG, Lundborg G: Peripheral nerve injury due to injection needles used for regional anesthesia. Acta Anaesthesiol Scand 21:182, 1977
15. Thompson GE: Perioperative nerve injuries. In Problems in Anesthesia, Vol 1, No 4, pp 580–587. Philadelphia, JB Lippincott, 1987
16. Marinacci AA, Rand CW: Electromyogram in peripheral nerve complications following general surgical procedures. West J Surg 67:199, 1959
17. Gross JB, Hartigan ML, Schaffer DW: A suitable substitute for 4%

cocaine before blind nasotracheal intubation: 3% lidocaine–0.25% phenylephrine nasal spray. Anesth Analg 63:915, 1984

18. Sessler CN, Vitaliti JC, Cooper KR et al: Comparison of 4% lidocaine/0.5% phenylephrine with 5% cocaine: Which dilates the nasal passages better? Anesthesiology 64:274, 1986

19. Gotta AW, Sullivan CA: Anesthesia of the upper airway using topical anesthesia and superior laryngeal nerve block. Br J Anaesth 53:1055, 1981

20. Lanz E, Theiss D, Jankovic D: The extent of blockade following various techniques of brachial plexus block. Anesth Analg 62:55, 1983

21. Winnie AP: Interscalene brachial plexus block. Anesth Analg 49:455, 1970

22. Moore DC: Regional Block. Springfield, Illinois, Charles C Thomas, 1954

23. Winnie AP, Collins VJ: The subclavian perivascular technique of brachial plexus anesthesia. Anesthesiology 25:353, 1964

24. Moore DC, Bridenbaugh LD: Pneumothorax: its incidence following brachial plexus block analgesia. Anesthesiology 15:475, 1954

25. Partridge BL, Katz J, Benirschke K: Functional anatomy of the brachial plexus sheath: Implications for anesthesia. Anesthesiology 66:743, 1987

26. Thompson GE, Rorie DK: Functional anatomy of the brachial plexus sheaths. Anesthesiology 59:117, 1983

27. Vester–Andersen T, Christiansen C, Sorensen M et al: Perivascular axillary block II: Influence of injected volume of local anesthetic on neural blockade. Acta Anaesthesiol Scand 27:95, 1983

28. Selander D: Axillary plexus block: Paresthetic or perivascular (editorial). Anesthesiology 66:726, 1987

29. Grice SC, Morell RC, Balestrieri FJ et al: Intravenous regional anesthesia: Evaluation and prevention of leakage under the tourniquet. Anesthesiology 65:316, 1986

30. Tucker GT, Boas RA: Pharmacokinetic aspects of intravenous regional anesthesia. Anesthesiology 34:538, 1971

31. Moore DC, Bush WH, Scurlock JE: Intercostal nerve block: A roentgenographic anatomic study of technique and absorption in humans. Anesth Analg 59:815, 1980

32. Bridenbaugh PO, DuPen SL, Moore DC et al: Postoperative intercostal nerve block analgesia versus narcotic analgesia. Anesth Analg 52:81, 1973

33. Moore DC, Bridenbaugh LD: Pneumothorax: Its incidence following intercostal nerve block. JAMA 182:1005, 1962

34. Sury MRJ, Bingham RM: Accidental spinal anesthesia following intrathoracic intercostal nerve blockade. Anaesthesia 41:401, 1986

35. Cory P, Mulroy MF: Postoperative respiratory failure following intercostal block. Anesthesiology 54:418, 1981

36. Eason MJ, Wyatt R: Paravertebral thoracic block—a reappraisal. Anaesthesia 34:638, 1979

37. Korevaar WC, Burney RG, Moore PA: Convulsions during stellate ganglion block: A case report. Anesth Analg 58:329, 1979

38. Moore DC, Bush WH, Burnett LL: Celiac plexus block: A roentgenographic, anatomic study of technique and spread of solution in patients and corpses. Anesth Analg 60:369, 1981

39. Brown DL, Bulley K, Quiel EL: Neurolytic block for pancreatic cancer pain. Anesth Analg 66:869, 1987

40. Cherry DA, Lamberty J: Paraplegia following coeliac plexus block. Anesth Intensive Care 12:59, 1984

41. Umeda S, Arai T, Hatano Y et al: Cadaver anatomic analysis of the best site for chemical lumbar sympathectomy. Anesth Analg 66:643, 1987

42. Winnie AP, Ramamurthy S, Durrani Z: The inguinal paravascular technique of lumbar plexus anesthesia. "The 3-in-1 block." Anesth Analg 52:989, 1973

43. Rorie DK, Byer DE, Nelson DO et al: Assessment of block of the sciatic nerve in the popliteal fossa. Anesth Analg 59:371, 1980

44. Schurman DJ: Ankle block anesthesia for foot surgery. Anesthesiology 44:342, 1976

Chapter 30

William E. Hoffman
Betty L. Grundy

Neuroanatomy and Neurophysiology

The purpose of this chapter is to review neuroanatomy and neurophysiology as related to anesthetic action, neurosurgical anesthesia, and acute care of patients with neurologic disorders. This chapter is divided into three sections. The first section addresses the physiology and anatomy of the central nervous system (CNS). In this section, the cerebrovascular effects and cerebral metabolic actions of anesthetic drugs are also considered; cerebrospinal fluid (CSF) production and blood-brain barrier (BBB) function during anesthesia and disease are also discussed. In the second section, we evaluate neurophysiological monitoring techniques, such as the electroencephalogram (EEG), evoked potentials (EP), and intracranial pressure (ICP). Changes in each of these parameters during anesthesia and in the presence of brain lesions are summarized. Finally, neuroradiology procedures for patient evaluation are discussed. Computerized tomography (CT), sonography, and magnetic resonance imaging (MRI) are presented, and these methods are compared with regard to diagnostic value in neurologic disease states and provision of anatomical definition for neurological surgery. Throughout, the direct and indirect actions of anesthetic drugs on neurophysiology and pathophysiology are indicated, and methods of monitoring the CNS are described.

ANESTHETIC ACTIONS ON CEREBRAL BLOOD FLOW AND METABOLISM

Under normal conditions, the functional metabolic activity of the brain is maintained by aerobic oxidation of glucose.[1] Because of limited stores of these substrates within the brain, particularly oxygen, minute-to-minute activity and viability of neurons are dependent upon adequate cerebrovascular perfusion with delivery of oxygen and glucose. Normally, the brain regulates its own perfusion according to the demand for energy substrates. The metabolic activity of the brain is heterogeneous, and cerebral perfusion is controlled at the microvascular level. Cerebral autoregulation maintains a constant cerebrovascular perfusion when mean arterial blood pressure ranges from about 70–160 mm Hg.[2, 3] The normal cerebral autoregulatory curve shifts to the right with chronic hypertension, and this shift may be reversed with antihypertensive drug treatment.[4] Blood flow to the brain increases if blood content of oxygen or glucose is decreased, as the brain attempts to maintain a constant supply of these substrates.[5, 6]

The cerebrovascular system is reactive to changes in Pa_{CO_2}, cerebral blood flow (CBF) being linearly correlated with Pa_{CO_2} between 20 and 80 mm Hg. Normal CO_2 response curves may be depressed by high-dose barbiturate therapy.[7] Experimental studies in the cat indicate that the cerebrovascular effects of CO_2 are mediated by the extracellular brain tissue pH and by CO_2 directly.[6] Other components contributing to brain extracellular fluid pH are local production of lactic acid and CSF bicarbonate ion concentrations. Blood lactic acid and bicarbonate concentrations have little effect on short-term changes in CBF.[7, 8] Adenosine, a potent vasodilator, may be important in local control of cerebrovascular resistance. Increased concentrations of adenosine in brain tissue have been shown during challenges of hypoxia or brain ischemia,[9] and adenosine antagonists attenuate the increase in CBF produced by hypoxia (Fig. 30-1).[10]

Under normal conditions, there is a coupling between local

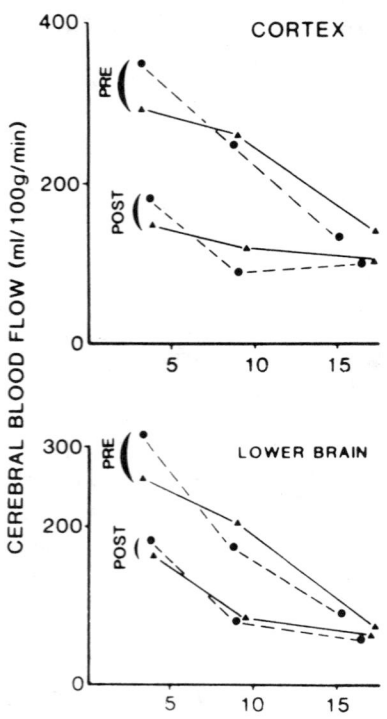

FIG. 30-1. Cortical and subcortical cerebral blood flow (CBF) changes during hypoxia in young (dashed line) and aged (solid line) rats before (pre) and after (post) intracerebrovascular infusion of theophylline, an adenosine antagonist. Aged rats showed an attenuated increase in CBF at severe hypoxic levels compared with the young rats. Theophylline decreased the difference in CBF between young and old rats during severe hypoxia. (Hoffman WE *et al:* The role of adenosine in CBF increases during hypoxia in young vs aged rats. Stroke 15:124, 1984. By permission from the American Heart Association.)

brain tissue perfusion (CBF) and metabolic demand.[1, 11] Anesthetic agents that depress brain metabolism also decrease CBF.

INHALED ANESTHETICS

In general, the volatile anesthetics—halothane, enflurane, and isoflurane—produce cerebral metabolic depression and cerebrovasodilation (Fig. 30-2).[12] The degree of change in each component depends on the particular drug used. The cerebral metabolic depression produced by volatile anesthetics is similar to that seen with many intravenous drugs. The concomitant cerebrovasodilation produced by volatile anesthetics, however, represents an uncoupling of the normal relationship between CBF and cerebral metabolism rate for oxygen ($CMRO_2$). Halothane, enflurane, and isoflurane seem to directly dilate the cerebrovasculature.[13]

Halothane

Early studies in dogs, baboons, and man showed that halothane produced significant increases in CBF and decreases in $CMRO_2$.[14-16] However, work in monkeys showed that halothane anesthesia may be associated with no change or a reduction in CBF when arterial blood pressure is decreased. Amory et al[17] reported that 0.8% and 1.2% end-expired halothane decreased CBF to 65% and 89% of unanesthetized control values, respectively, in monkeys. Arterial blood pressure was also decreased to 68 mm Hg (0.8% halothane) and 52 mm Hg (1.2% halothane), which suggests that CBF changes produced by halothane may be pressure-dependent. Lees et al[18] reported small increases in CBF with 0.5–0.7% halothane and decreases in flow with 1.5–2% halothane. Harp et al[19] observed similar biphasic CBF changes in rats during 0.6 and 2% halothane, which were closely related to blood pressure. These apparent inconsistencies in CBF changes during halothane were resolved by the work of Miletich et al,[20] who found that, in goats, 1 minimal alveolar concentration (MAC), but not 0.5 MAC, of halothane or enflurane abolished cerebral autoregulation, so that CBF was pressure-dependent and not regulated by oxygen demand (Fig. 30-3). The nonspecific cerebrovasodilation produced by halothane has been shown to

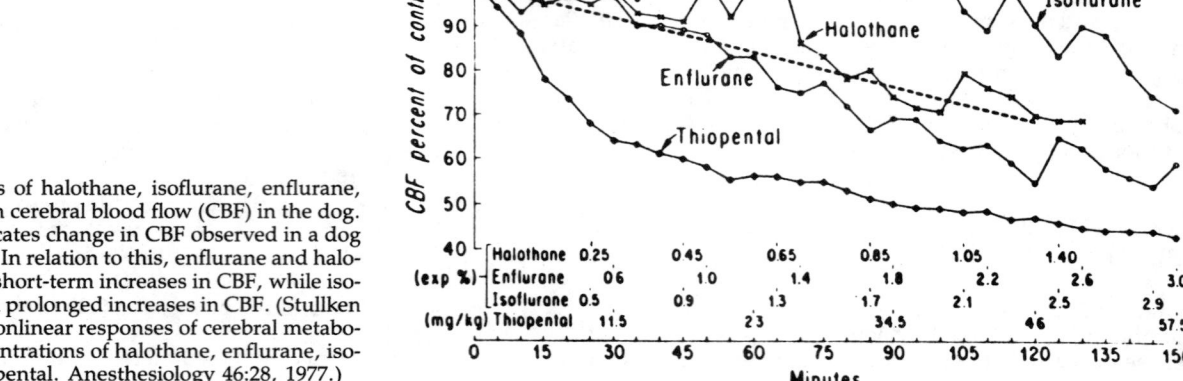

FIG. 30-2. Effects of halothane, isoflurane, enflurane, and thiopental on cerebral blood flow (CBF) in the dog. Dashed line indicates change in CBF observed in a dog model over time. In relation to this, enflurane and halothane produced short-term increases in CBF, while isoflurane produced prolonged increases in CBF. (Stullken EH Jr *et al:* The nonlinear responses of cerebral metabolism to low concentrations of halothane, enflurane, isoflurane and thiopental. Anesthesiology 46:28, 1977.)

TABLE 30-1.   Effects of Various Anesthetics on Cerebral Spinal Fluid (CSF)

ANESTHETIC	SPECIES	CSF PRODUCTION	RESISTANCE TO CSF REABSORPTION
Isoflurane	Dog	0	↓ 50%
Enflurane	Dog	↑ 50%	↑ 23%
Halothane	Dog	↓ 30%	↑ 10%
Nitrous oxide	Dog	0	
Pentobarbital	Cat	0	
Fentanyl	Dog	0	↓ 4%
Ketamine	Rat	0	↑ 200%

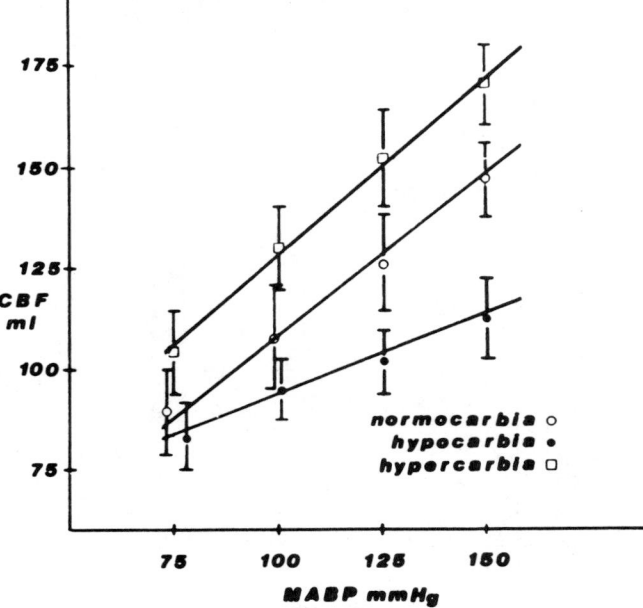

FIG. 30-3. Effects of systemic mean arterial blood pressure (MABP) on cerebral blood flow (CBF) during 1 minimal alveolar concentration (MAC) halothane anesthesia and hyper-, normo-, and hypocarbia. Under unanesthetized conditions, CBF autoregulated to show no change in flow over a MABP range of 75–100 mm Hg. Cerebral autoregulation is abolished by 1 MAC halothane at all Pa_{CO_2} levels. (Miletich DJ et al: Absence of autoregulation of cerebral blood flow during halothane and enflurane anesthesia. Anesth Analg 55:100, 1976.)

impair perfusion of ischemic regions of the brain. Vasodilation in non-ischemic zones "steals" flow from under-perfused tissue.[21] However, the cerebral vasculature remains responsive to changes in Pa_{CO_2} at halothane concentrations of 1 MAC and higher.[15, 22, 23]

The time course of CBF changes during halothane anesthesia is important in analyzing results of different studies. Albrecht et al[24] demonstrated that, during inspiration of 1% halothane, goats show a 100% increase in brain flow at 30 min, but that CBF returns to control levels by 150 min. This normalization of CBF during prolonged halothane anesthesia is neither pressure-dependent nor related to CSF pH changes.[25] In addition, blockade of alpha- or beta-adrenergic receptors does not alter the normalization response.[24] More recent work sug-

gests that normalization of cerebrovascular resistance over time occurs with other inhaled anesthetics as well.[26] The addition of nitrous oxide (N_2O) to halothane anesthesia appears to have little effect on CBF in man.[27, 28] Nitrous oxide may increase CBF during halothane anesthesia, but these effects appear to be related to changes in blood pressure. Manohar and Parks[29] and Tranquilli et al[30] reported higher arterial blood pressure and CBF in pigs during anesthesia with halothane and N_2O than with halothane alone. An increase in blood pressure when cerebral autoregulation is abolished by halothane would produce a passive increase in CBF that is unrelated to any direct central effects of N_2O.

Halothane decreases cerebral metabolism in man and animals, but the magnitudes of these changes vary. Studies in man indicate that 1% halothane reduces $CMRO_2$ by about 25%.[15, 31] Keaney et al[32] reported a 30% decrease in $CMRO_2$ from light to profound halothane anesthesia. In dogs, McDowall[16] observed a 12% decrease in $CMRO_2$ with 0.5% halothane and a 30% reduction with 2% halothane. Harp et al[19] indicated that 0.6% halothane produced a 20% decrease in $CMRO_2$ in rats, while 2% halothane decreased brain metabolism by 50%, which was comparable to the reduction in $CMRO_2$ produced by barbiturates. However, 2% halothane does not produce an isoelectric EEG, and halothane concentrations (4.5%) required to abolish cortical electrical activity in dogs produce a dose-related, possibly toxic effect on oxidative phosphorylation. This suggests that, while cerebral metabolism may be depressed 25–40% by nontoxic doses of halothane, maximum decreases are not comparable to those produced by barbiturates.

Enflurane

The effects of enflurane on CBF and $CMRO_2$ at low concentrations are similar to those produced by halothane. Stullken et al[12] showed, in dogs, that CBF increases during induction of enflurane anesthesia, but that overall changes in brain perfusion are modest during enflurane, and less than those produced by halothane. This is consistent with reports that enflurane produces moderate increases in CBF in humans, which are less than those produced by halothane.[33, 34] Others have reported no change or a decrease in CBF in dogs during enflurane anesthesia to a depth of 2 MAC,[12] while, simultaneously, cortical $CMRO_2$ decreased to 70% of control values. In man, Sakabe et al[34] reported that 1.2 MAC enflurane produced an EEG pattern of spiking and suppression and a 17% reduction in whole brain $CMRO_2$.

The association of enflurane anesthesia with EEG seizure patterns, particularly during hypocapnia, focused attention on cerebral metabolism during these seizures. In dogs, 2.2%

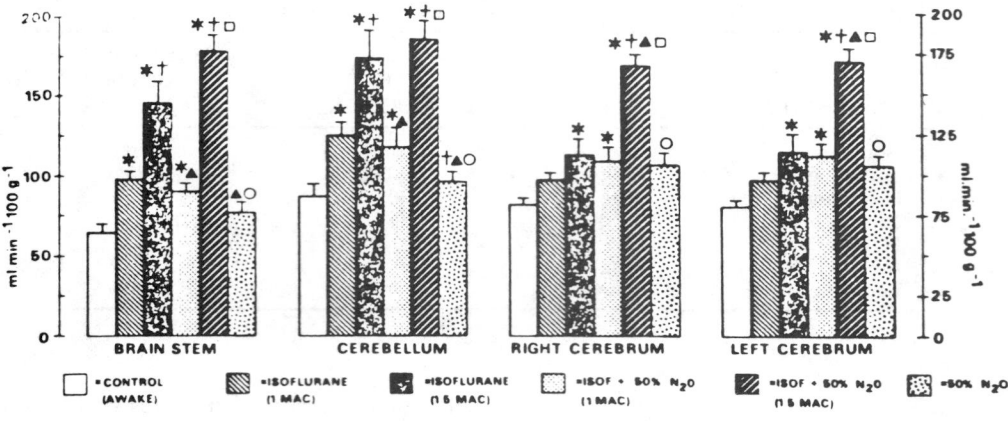

FIG. 30-4. Regional cerebral blood flow (CBF) during isoflurane anesthesia with and without N₂O in the dog. Isoflurane produced increases in CBF, which were potentiated by addition of N₂O. (Manohar M, Parks C: Regional distribution of brain and myocardial perfusion in swine while awake and during 1.0 and 1.5 MAC isoflurane anaesthesia produced without or with 50% nitrous oxide. Cardiovasc Res 18:344, 1984.)

end-tidal enflurane decreases CMRO₂ by 34%, but induction of seizures by hypocapnia and hand-clapping at 3.4% enflurane increases CMRO₂ by 48% from pre-seizure values.[35] Seo et al[36] measured the cerebral energy state in rats during deep enflurane anesthesia with and without hypocapnia. They found that spiking EEG activity was not associated with any change in brain energy charge or glycolytic metabolites. They concluded that there is no derangement in brain energy state or evidence of anaerobic metabolism during enflurane anesthesia.

Isoflurane

Initial studies evaluating the central effects of isoflurane show that this drug produces cerebrovasodilation and depresses CMRO₂ more than either halothane or enflurane. Cucchiara et al[37] showed, in dogs, that 2.4% end-expired isoflurane produced a 63% increase in CBF and a 30% decrease in CMRO₂. In a comparison of the cerebral effects of the three volatile anesthetics in dogs, Stullken et al[12] found that isoflurane produces greater, more prolonged increases in CBF than halothane or enflurane. Gelman et al[38] compared the regional vascular effects of 1 and 2 MAC halothane and isoflurane in dogs, and showed that both anesthetics produce comparable dose-related increases in CBF, compared with awake controls, despite decreases in blood pressure to 60–70 mm Hg with 2 MAC anesthesia. Manohar and Parks[39] reported significant increases in CBF in pigs during 1 and 1.5 MAC isoflurane. This effect was enhanced by the addition of 50% N₂O (Fig. 30-4). The blood pressure-related changes in CBF produced by the addition of N₂O or phenylephrine infusion suggest that autoregulation may be impaired with isoflurane concentrations greater than 1 MAC.[40]

Time-dependent changes in CBF have also been reported during prolonged isoflurane anesthesia. Turner et al[26] found that CBF was increased in dogs 2 h after induction of anesthesia with 0.8% isoflurane and 70% N₂O. CBF gradually decreased 40–50% from this level over the following 2.5 h to levels seen in normal, awake animals, even though blood pressure increased slightly. These results suggest that isoflurane, halothane, and enflurane act in a similar manner to increase CBF, which gradually returns to control levels during prolonged anesthesia.

In contrast to the above reports indicating that isoflurane may increase CBF, Todd and Drummond[41] demonstrated, in cats, that CBF increases with 0.5, 1.0, and 1.5 MAC halothane and N₂O, but not during isoflurane anesthesia (Fig. 30-5).

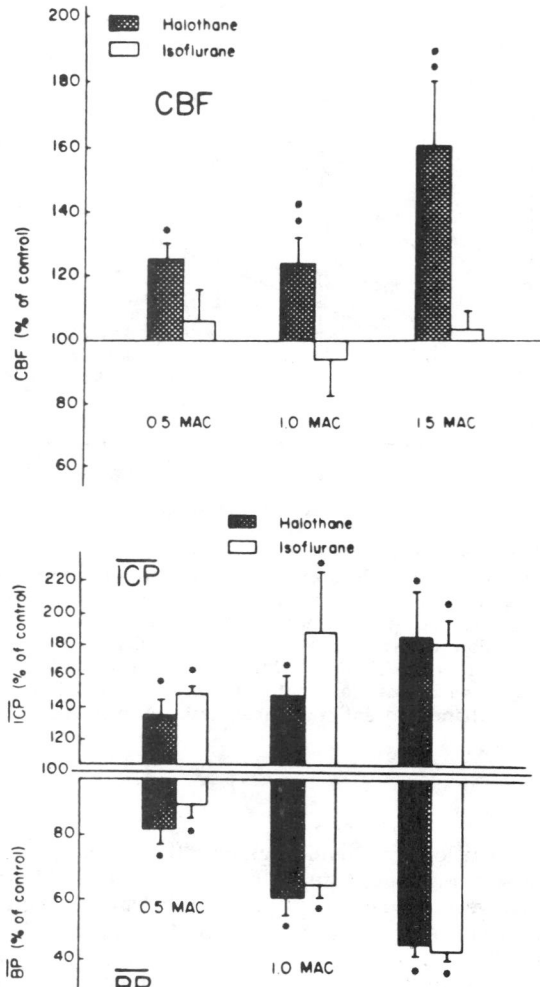

FIG. 30-5. Cerebral blood flow (CBF) and intracranial pressure (ICP) changes during halothane and isoflurane anesthesia. Despite similar decreases in blood pressure, halothane increased CBF and isoflurane produced no change. At the same time, ICP increased in a similar pattern with both anesthetics. (Todd MM, Drummond JC: A comparison of the cerebrovascular and metabolic effects of halothane and isoflurane in the cat. Anesthesiology 60:276, 1984.)

Comparable decreases in blood pressure are produced by both anesthetics. Cerebrovascular autoregulation is also intact during 1 MAC isoflurane, but not during 1 MAC halothane anesthesia, which suggests that cerebrovascular reactivity is better maintained with isoflurane. Additional reports from these investigators show that CBF may be controlled during isoflurane anesthesia by normal ventilation or by hyperventilation, but that flow increases during halothane anesthesia under similar conditions.[42, 43] This is consistent with reports that halothane increases CBF more than does isoflurane[33] (Fig. 30-6) in humans, and that ICP can be controlled more easily by using hyperventilation during isoflurane anesthesia than during halothane anesthesia.[44]

Reports also indicate that isoflurane decreases $CMRO_2$ to a greater degree than either halothane or enflurane. Todd and Drummond[41] found, in cats, that 1.5 MAC halothane decreased $CMRO_2$ to 70% of control, while 1.5 MAC isoflurane decreased brain metabolism by 50%, comparable to the depression that can be produced by high-dose barbiturates. Newberg et al[45] reported that maximum cerebral metabolic depression was produced in dogs with 3% end-expired isoflurane concentrations, coincident with complete EEG suppression. Greater increases in isoflurane dosage to 6% did not further depress brain metabolism or produce a decrement in brain energy states (Fig. 30-7).

In summary, isoflurane, halothane, and enflurane produce cerebrovasodilation and may increase CBF. However, CBF changes are pressure-dependent during halothane or enflurane anesthesia at concentrations of 1 MAC or greater because cerebral autoregulation is abolished. Recent work sug-

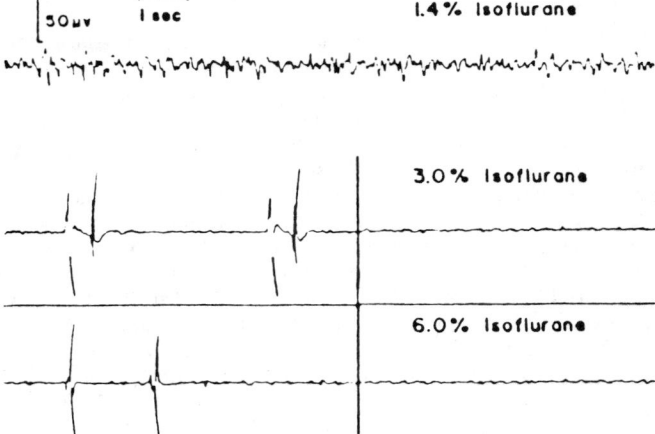

FIG. 30-7. Electroencephalogram in a dog with increasing isoflurane concentrations. An anesthetic pattern is seen at 1.4% isoflurane, which changed to rhythmic spikes separated by isoelectric silence at 3% and 6%. (Newberg LA et al: The cerebral metabolic effects of isoflurane at and above concentrations that suppress cortical electrical activity. Anesthesiology 59:23, 1983.)

gests that, with 1 MAC isoflurane, CBF is not increased and autoregulation is intact. Furthermore, the cerebrovasculature may be more reactive to decreases in Pa_{CO_2} with isoflurane than with halothane anesthesia. It is possible, however, that isoflurane concentrations above 1 MAC may produce cerebrovasodilation, increases in CBF, and loss of autoregulation. Isoflurane, in nontoxic doses, like barbiturates, can produce an isoelectric EEG and up to 50% decreases in $CMRO_2$. In contrast, high doses of halothane have been shown to be toxic, and high doses of enflurane combined with hypocapnia may produce seizures. At present, isoflurane is preferred for use during neurosurgical anesthesia because of its cerebrovascular and cerebral metabolic effects and its ability to decrease brain protrusion.[46]

Regional brain metabolism has been measured during isoflurane anesthesia. Ori et al[47] found, in rats, that 1.5% inspired isoflurane decreases glucose utilization in all cortical areas and in the primary sensory relay nuclei of visual and auditory pathways (superior and inferior colliculus and medial and lateral geniculate). Metabolism is also decreased in the extrapyramidal motor system (red nucleus, ventral thalamus, and cerebellum). Increases in glucose utilization were observed in regions associated with the limbic system (medial habenulo-interpeduncular system and the CA_3 field of the hippocampus). Similarly, Maekawa et al[48] reported that 0.5–2 MAC isoflurane produced dose-related depression of brain glucose utilization in cortical and subcortical regions associated with auditory, visual, and somatosensory input. Maximum (50–70%) depression of glucose metabolism was observed at 2 MAC isoflurane, associated with burst-suppression EEG activity. Two limbic structures (dentate gyrus and interpeduncular nucleus) showed no depression, even at the higher anesthetic concentrations. A similar pattern of alterations in local cerebral glucose utilization has been reported during halothane and enflurane anesthesia.[49, 50] The increased metabolism in the medial habenulo-interpeduncular system is apparently a common phenomenon seen with several intravenous and inhalational anesthetics.[49, 51, 52]

FIG. 30-6. Cerebral blood flow (CBF) changes in man during control (c), halothane (h), enflurane (e), and isoflurane (i) anesthesia. Both h and e produced increases in CBF from pretreatment control. (Eintrei C et al: Local application of ^{133}xenon for measurement of regional cerebral blood flow (rCBF) during halothane, enflurane and isoflurane anesthesia in humans. Anesthesiology 63:391, 1985.)

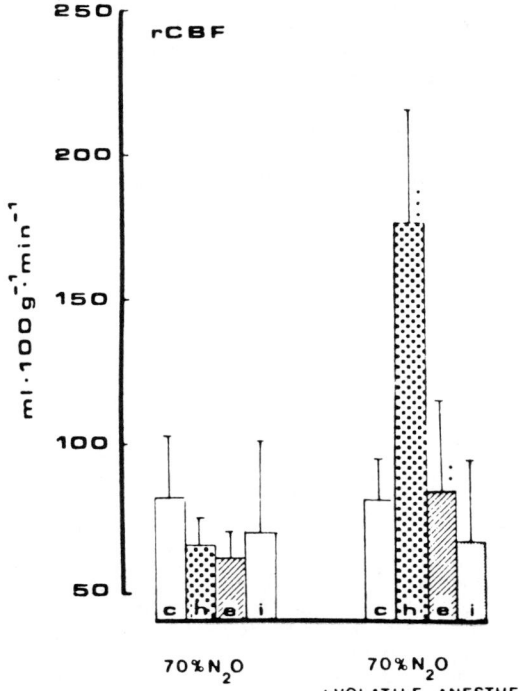

Nitrous Oxide

In clinical doses, N_2O does not produce cardiovascular depression but produces additive analgesic and sedative effects when given with other anesthetics.[53] For these reasons, N_2O is often used in combination with other anesthetic drugs. Cerebrovascular autoregulation and reactivity to changes in Pa_{CO_2} are intact during N_2O anesthesia. Sedation with N_2O is often used alone to produce a "control" level, which is suggested to represent the unanesthetized state during experiments in animals. This proposal is controversial. Studies in man indicate that N_2O produces either no change or a slight decrease in brain metabolism and CBF.[27, 28, 54] However, the effects of N_2O in these studies may have been modified by sedative or other anesthetic drugs. N_2O increases CBF and $CMRO_2$ in dogs and goats up to 200% from unanesthetized control levels, with most of the increase in blood flow observed in cerebral cortical regions (Fig. 30-8).[55–57] In rats, N_2O produces minimal changes in CBF and $CMRO_2$.[58] Regional cerebral glucose utilization is generally unchanged during N_2O in rats, but may be increased in the thalamus, caudate-putamen, and hippocampus.[59, 60] The possible cerebral stimulatory effects of N_2O are dramatically reduced by pretreatment with other anesthetics.[56] However, modest but significant cerebral metabolic stimulation by N_2O can be demonstrated in the presence of halothane, barbiturates, and midazolam.[56, 60, 61]

INTRAVENOUS ANESTHETICS

Barbiturates

Early studies of the cerebrovascular and cerebral metabolic effects of barbiturates showed that low, sedative doses of these drugs produce little change in brain metabolism and EEG activation.[62] Barbiturates produce dose-dependent depression of CBF and $CMRO_2$,[63, 64] and maximum doses of thiopental, pentobarbital, or phenobarbital produce a quiescent EEG and depression of CBF and $CMRO_2$ to 40–50% of normal.[65–68] Michenfelder[69] showed that massive doses of thiopental in dogs produce a maximum depression of brain metabolism to approximately 50% of control, which correlates with a quiescent EEG (Fig. 30-9). Further increases in thiopental dosage produce no greater depression of $CMRO_2$. Maximum thiopental doses depress electrical function of neurons but have little effect on basal neuronal metabolic functions. Kassell et al[70] confirmed these results with a similar study in dogs and found that maximum depression of $CMRO_2$ can be produced with thiopental doses that do not seriously depress the cardiovascular system. This indicates a separation of thiopental's cerebral metabolic and cardiovascular depressant effects. Phenobarbital also produces EEG suppression and maximum decreases in $CMRO_2$ with high doses in the rat (Fig. 30-10),[68] but aged rats show a greater depression of $CMRO_2$ with high doses.[71] This suggests that barbiturate anesthesia may depress neuronal metabolic function, as well as electrical function, in elderly patients.

It is uncertain whether barbiturates produce additional cerebrovascular effects besides those produced by cerebral metabolic depression and the coupling between CBF and $CMRO_2$. Marin et al[72] found that pentobarbital inhibits spontaneous

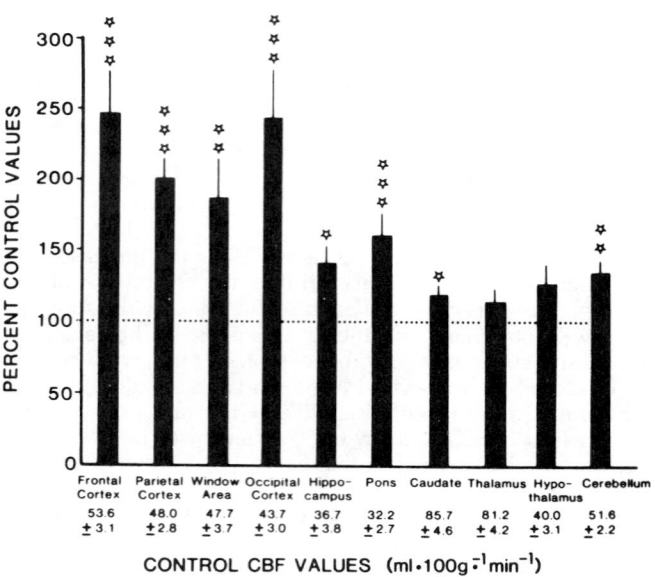

FIG. 30-8. Regional cerebral blood flow (CBF) changes during N_2O anesthesia in the goat. Note the global increases in CBF, although constant, Pa_{CO_2} was maintained. (Pelligrino DA et al: Nitrous oxide markedly increases cerebral cortical metabolic rate and blood flow in the goat. Anesthesiology 60:405, 1984.)

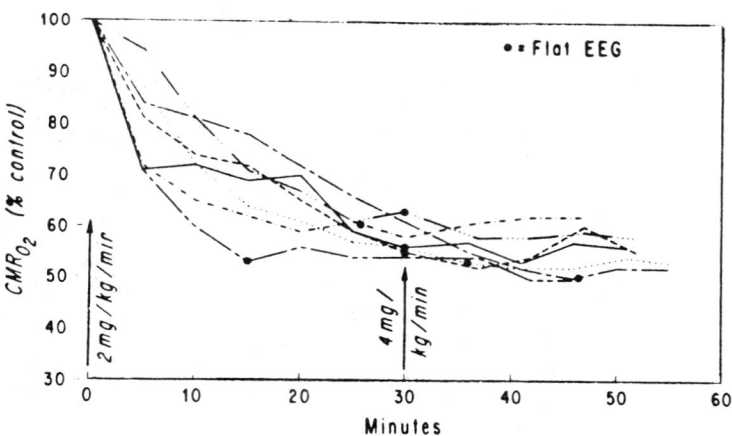

FIG. 30-9. Effect of thiopental infusion on maximum cerebral metabolic rate for oxygen ($CMRO_2$) in the dog. Thiopental produced $CMRO_2$ depression at doses that completely suppressed neuronal electrical activity. (Michenfelder JD: The interdependency of cerebral functional and metabolic effects following massive doses of thiopental in the dog. Anesthesiology 41:231, 1974.)

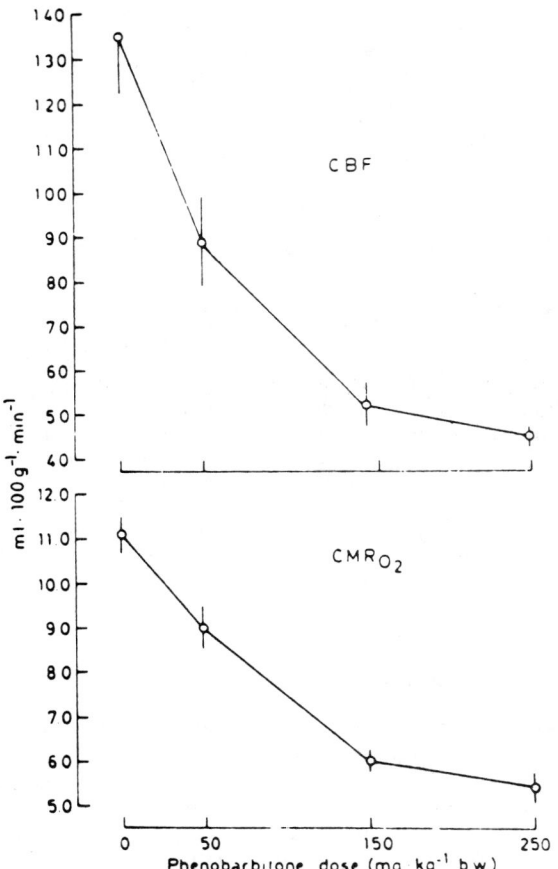

FIG. 30-10. Cerebral blood flow (CBF) and maximum cerebral metabolic rate for oxygen (CMRO₂) decreased in rats with increasing phenobarbitone doses, which produced maximum suppression of CBF and CMRO₂, as well as electroencephalogram burst suppression or silence. (Nilsson L, Siesjo BK: The effect of phenobarbitone anaesthesia on blood flow and oxygen consumption in the rat brain. Acta Anaesthesiol Scand 57(suppl):18, 1975.)

mechanical activity and produces relaxation of cortical branches of the middle cerebral artery *in vitro*. However, *in vivo* studies suggest that barbiturates produce vasoconstriction, in addition to what is necessary for normal coupling between CBF and CMRO₂, and that the magnitude of this vasoconstriction is age-related.[71]

The decrease in CBF produced by barbiturates may be regionally specific. Goldman and Sapirstein[73] reported that, in rats, pentobarbital anesthesia produces more depression of flow in high-flow than in low-flow regions. Thus, flow in all regions tends to equilibrate at a basal level. This is consistent with the results of Abdul-Rahman et al,[74] who found the greatest decreases in local CBF in cortex and other subcortical gray matter regions, and less CBF reduction in brain stem structures that have lower baseline flow rates. Laurent et al[75] observed a compartmental shift in Xenon-133 wash-out curves from the fast to the slow component. It has been suggested that the fast and slow components relate to perfusion of gray matter and white matter, respectively. A shift of blood flow from metabolically active brain regions to areas that are less metabolically active may be linked with the ability of barbiturates to provide brain protection and decrease ICP.

The regional brain metabolic effects of barbiturates have been studied by several investigators. Sokoloff et al[76] reported that, in rats, thiopental reduces the rate of glucose utilization in all cortical and subcortical brain regions measured. Herkenham[51] found similar brain depression in rats during pentobarbital anesthesia, but observed that metabolism of the limbic medial habenulo-interpeduncular system is not decreased. This specific sparing of metabolic activity with barbiturates is neurally mediated, since destruction of afferent input to the region abolishes the effect.

Opioids

Opioids such as morphine and fentanyl produce analgesia and anesthesia, with very little cardiovascular depression, by stimulation of central opioid receptors.[77] For this reason, opioids are often part of the anesthetic regimen for critically ill, unstable patients, in whom maintenance of blood pressure is a concern. The effect of morphine on cerebral hemodynamics has been studied by several investigators. Takeshita et al[78] reported, in dogs, that incremental doses of morphine up to 1.2 mg·kg⁻¹ produce dose-related decreases in CBF and CMRO₂ to 45% and 85% of control, respectively. These results were supported in a later study, which showed that 1 mg·kg⁻¹ of intravenous morphine reduces both CBF and spinal cord blood flow to 73% of control. In both studies, the depression of cerebral metabolism and blood flow produced by morphine could be reversed by the opioid antagonists, nalorphine and naloxone. Work in man suggests that morphine produces little effect on cerebral metabolism or cerebrovascular reactivity.[79, 80]

The cerebral effects of synthetic opioids have also been studied. Michenfelder and Theye[81] gave fentanyl (6 µg·kg⁻¹) to dogs sedated with N₂O. They saw a short-term decrease in CBF (45%) and CMRO₂ (18%), which reached a maximum in appoximately 16 min and returned to control by 40 min. This agrees with work in rats, which showed that intravenous fentanyl infusions in doses of 50–500 µg·kg⁻¹·h⁻¹ produce dose-related decreases in CBF and CMRO₂, with maximum decreases to 50% and 70% of control, respectively.[82] Experiments comparing the cerebral response to fentanyl in old and young animals showed that aged rats have less cerebrovascular and cerebral metabolic depression during fentanyl infusion than do young rats.[83]

Sufentanil, an opioid five to ten times more potent than fentanyl, produces dose-related decreases in CBF and CMRO₂, which reach a maximum of 47% and 60% of control, respectively, in rats (Fig. 30-11).[84] In high doses, both fentanyl and sufentanil produce seizure activity in rats.[82, 84, 85] This seizure activity is accompanied by global increases in CBF, with elevations persisting during the seizure episode and the post-seizure phase of EEG suppression. Evidence of seizure activity has also been reported in humans with sufentanil and fentanyl, but the seizure threshold has not been determined for either drug.[86–88]

The regional brain metabolic effects of sufentanil were studied by Young et al[89] in the rat. With sufentanil (160 µg·kg⁻¹), glucose utilization is decreased 20–45% in cortical regions and 40–55% in the caudate and ventral thalamic nuclei. Focal limbic areas in the hippocampus and amygdala show marked increases in glucose metabolism, which are associated with EEG seizure activity. These results support findings of moderate cerebral cortical metabolic depression during opioid anesthesia, and suggest that EEG seizure patterns may reflect subcortical limbic activation.

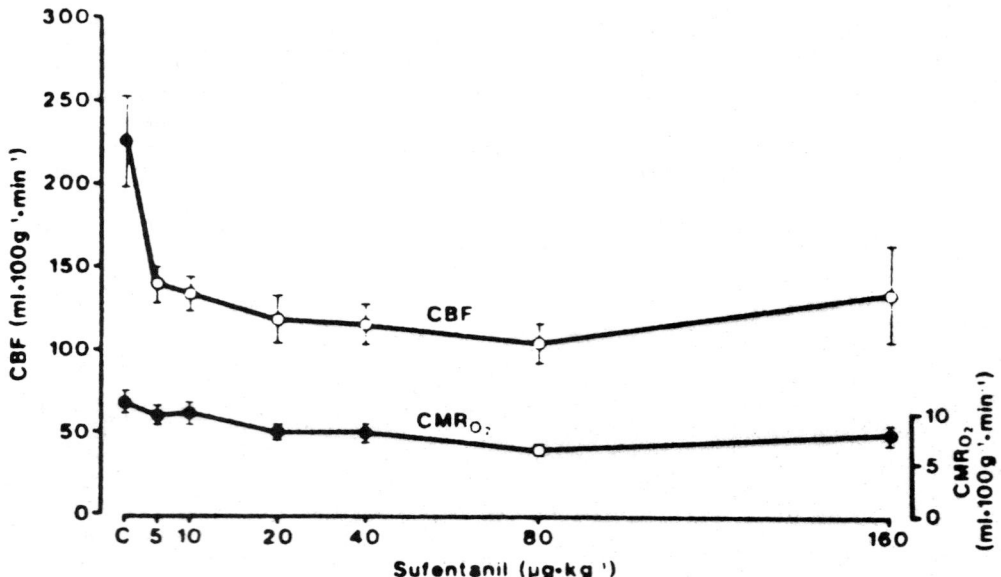

FIG. 30-11. Cerebral blood flow (CBF) and cerebral metabolic rate for oxygen ($CMRO_2$) changes seen with sufentanil infusion in the rat. Sufentanil produced decreases in CBF, and small but significant decreases in $CMRO_2$ with increasing doses. (Keykhah MM *et al:* Influence of sufentanil on cerebral metabolism and circulation in the rat. Anesthesiology 63:274, 1985.)

Benzodiazepines

Benzodiazepines produce sedation and amnesia by stimulation of brain receptors in the benzodiazepine/gamma aminobutyric acid (GABA) receptor complex.[90] These drugs decrease CBF and $CMRO_2$ by 21–30% in dogs.[92] Carlsson *et al*[93] found that 0.75 mg·kg^{-1} and 7.5 mg·kg^{-1} of diazepam increase CBF and $CMRO_2$ in the presence of N_2O. However, other investigators report that N_2O does not potentiate, and may attentuate, the cerebral metabolic depressant effects of benzodiazepines.[61, 94] When central benzodiazepine receptors are pharmacologically saturated, these drugs may decrease $CMRO_2$ as much as 40%, but they do not produce complete EEG suppression.[95]

The relatively new specific benzodiazepine antagonists have shown significant clinical potential. Work in animals[96] and humans[97] indicates that these drugs reverse the behavioral, EEG, CBF, and cerebral metabolic effects of midazolam. Although some of these benzodiazepine antagonists have agonistic cerebral-stimulating effects when used alone,[96] flumazenil appears to be a specific antagonist with very little agonistic action.[97]

Etomidate

Etomidate, a carboxylated imidazole derivative, was introduced in 1971 as an intravenous hypnotic.[98] The anesthetic action of etomidate is mediated by stimulation of brain GABA receptors and enhancement of their central inhibitory effects. Studies of the cerebral effects of etomidate in dogs have shown that this drug produces direct cerebrovasoconstriction and up to 50% decreases in $CMRO_2$, coincident with an isoelectric EEG (Fig. 30-12).[100] Analyses of cerebral metabolites indicate that etomidate alone does not alter the normal brain energy state and provides protection from the energy state depletion produced by hypotensive ischemia.[99, 100] The depression in CBF and $CMRO_2$ produced by etomidate in dogs is consistent with a report that a single injection of etomidate (15 mg) in humans produces a maximum 45% decrease in $CMRO_2$ and comparable changes in CBF.[101] These reports suggest that etomidate, like barbiturates and isoflurane, is capable of producing complete EEG suppression and maximum decreases in $CMRO_2$.

A study of the regional brain metabolic effects of etomidate in rats show that forebrain regions are generally depressed by this anesthetic.[102] Etomidate in doses of 1–12 mg·kg^{-1} produced 25–35% decreases in glucose utilization of cortical and diencephalic structures, with little change in hindbrain metabolic function. Forebrain limbic structures, such as the hippocampus and amygdala, were depressed, while metabolism in the mesencephalic interpeduncular nucleus was not changed by etomidate. These results support earlier findings that etomidate anesthesia may produce marked brain depression associated with an isoelectric EEG, while hindbrain regions that control blood pressure and other physiological variables are spared.

Ketamine

Ketamine is a cataleptoid anesthetic that produces both excitatory and depressant actions in the brain. Studies in dogs and rats have shown that ketamine anesthesia produces modest but significant stimulation of brain metabolism and an increase in CBF, while cerebral autoregulation remains intact.[103–105] In humans, ketamine produces regionally specific changes in cortical CBF, with marked increases occurring in the fronto-temporal and parieto-occipital regions.[106] These changes in CBF probably reflect drug-induced increases in local neuronal activity, rather than a direct cerebrovasodilator effect. A study of regional brain glucose utilization in rats showed that ketamine significantly increases activity in the hippocampus and decreases activity in the medial geniculate and inferior colliculus.[107] It is hypothesized that ketamine produces cataleptic phenomena by hippocampal excitation and anesthesia by depression of sensory input.

CENTRAL NEUROTRANSMITTERS IN ANESTHESIA

In addition to central opioid, benzodiazepine, and GABA receptors, other brain receptor mechanisms may be involved

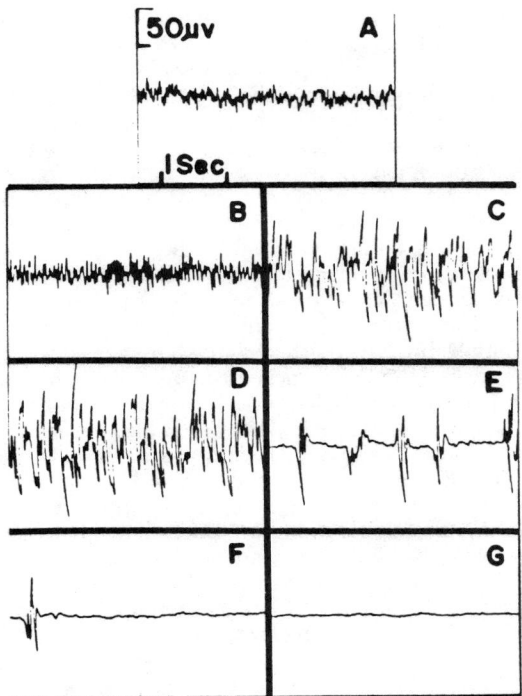

FIG. 30-12. Electroencephalogram (EEG) changes with etomidate infusion in the dog from control *(A)* to a state of maximum depression of cerebral metabolic rate for oxygen and EEG *(G)*. Note change in EEG from low-frequency fast activity to high-amplitude slow activity, then burst suppression. (Milde LN *et al*: Cerebral functional, metabolic, and hemodynamic effects of etomidate in dogs. Anesthesiology 63:371, 1985.)

in cerebral metabolic and vascular responses to drug treatment. Muscarinic cholinergic receptors, which appear to reflect pharmacological subtypes, have been identified in brain tissue.[108] These receptors may mediate the cerebral metabolic-stimulating effects of physostigmine.[109] Physostigmine, when given alone, produces cerebral metabolic and cerebrovascular stimulation. It may reverse the cerebral depressant and sedative effects of benzodiazepines (Fig. 30-13).[109–111] Histamine H_2 receptor subtypes have also been identified in brain tissue, closely associated with cerebrovascular tissue.[112] These receptors may be important in mediating histamine-induced cerebrovasodilation following treatment with histamine-releasing drugs, such as D-tubocurarine or morphine.[113–115] Circulating histamine produces cerebrovasodilation only if the amine is allowed to cross the BBB to obtain access to cerebral resistance vessels. This may be seen in association with head trauma or other cerebral injury when the BBB is disrupted. The cerebrovasodilatory effects of histamine, in these cases, can exacerbate the increased ICP that may be present with the original lesion.

Adrenergic receptors are also present in brain tissue, and may modulate cerebral metabolic activity under normal and pathological conditions. Stimulation of central beta-adrenergic receptors in humans and animals produces increases in CBF and $CMRO_2$, which can be blocked by pretreatment with propranolol.[116, 117] The cerebral metabolic activation produced by catecholamines is affected when these agents cross the BBB to stimulate adrenergic receptors in brain tissue.

Breakdown of the BBB may occur following hypertensive or hyperosmotic episodes,[113] or may be associated with head trauma or other brain injury. Clinically, the risk of brain ischemia is greater when brain metabolism is increased by catecholamines, while the BBB is compromised and local cerebral tissue perfusion is depressed by brain edema and/or elevated ICP. In support of this possibility, it has been shown that adrenalectomy significantly lowers the BBB response to hypoxic stress.[118] However, propranolol has not been found effective in the treatment of focal cerebral ischemia.[119]

BLOOD-BRAIN BARRIER

The BBB separates the brain interstitial space from blood, and is formed by brain capillary endothelial cells that are fused together by epithelial-like tight junctions. The BBB prevents free diffusion of circulating molecules and cells into brain interstitial space, and is present in virtually all vertebrates.[120] The physiochemical properties of solutes within the plasma determine their ability to move across the capillary endothelium and to enter the brain extracellular space. Solutes with a high affinity for membrane lipid, compared with water, can readily penetrate the BBB. This explains the fast onset of central action seen with most anesthetics. Membrane transport systems are also available to accelerate the movement of compounds with a high affinity for water, such as glucose, that are necessary for brain function. These transport systems are saturable and provide the brain with nutrients at a relatively constant rate in the face of the fluctuating plasma levels of these compounds.

FIG. 30-13. Effect of physostigmine $(0.4 \ mg \cdot kg^{-1})$ on cerebral blood flow (CBF) and cerebral metabolic rate for oxygen ($CMRO_2$) in the rat with increasing midazolam doses. Physostigmine, alone, increased CBF and $CMRO_2$, compared with placebo (controls), and reversed the depression of CBF and $CMRO_2$ produced by midazolam. (Hoffman WE *et al*: Cerebrovascular and cerebral metabolic effects of physostigmine, midazolam, and a benzodiazepine antagonist. Anesth Analg 65:639, 1986.)

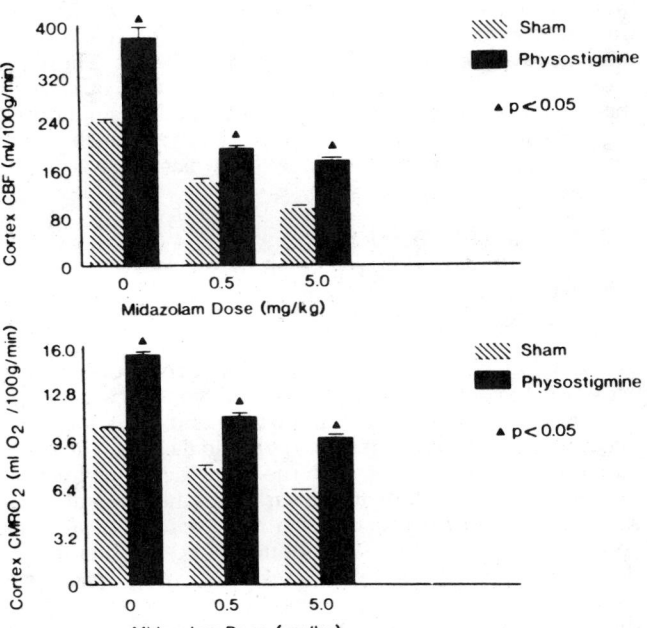

Several pathological states, including head trauma and cerebral ischemia,[121, 122] can compromise function of the BBB. This is of concern to the anesthesiologist, because an inadequate BBB can lead to enhanced solute and water movement into brain tissue and the production of cerebral edema and elevated ICP.[123] Compromised BBB function can thus decrease brain perfusion in already ischemic tissue or increase the region of focal ischemia. Conditions that may lead to BBB impairment during anesthesia include acute hypertensive crises that may occur during intubation of the trachea, seizures, microembolization of air or particulate matter, surgical manipulation and retraction of the brain, or hypoperfusion of brain tissue that may occur during hypotension or with cerebrovascular stenosis or occlusion. Ishikawa et al[124] demonstrated, in dogs, that nitroprusside-induced hypotension with cerebral perfusion pressure (CPP) of 30 mm Hg produces acute dysfunction of the BBB, which resolves within 3 days. This dysfunction may be related to the presence of cerebral ischemia or to nitroprusside-mediated cerebrovasodilation and disruption of endothelial tight junctions without ischemia. Similar BBB dysfunction can be produced when hypertension is combined with a cerebrovasodilating anesthetic, such as halothane.[125]

Therapeutic disruption of the BBB may be of benefit in treating CNS malignancies. Central tumors respond poorly to peripherally administered chemotherapeutic agents,[126] perhaps because the BBB excludes access of these drugs to the site of the malignancy. Osmotic BBB disruption with hypertonic solutions is effective and reversible.[127-129] This technique has been used in patients to facilitate delivery of chemotherapeutic agents to primary and metastatic CNS lesions.[130, 122] It is necessary to discontinue corticosteroids prior to BBB disruption because of their ability to stabilize the BBB and limit the effectiveness of osmotic therapy. A potential problem in patients with space-occupying intracranial lesions is the presence of elevated ICP. Studies in animals have shown a 1–1.5% increase in brain water after BBB disruption,[128] and studies in patients have revealed only small (<10 mm Hg), transient increases in ICP with osmotic disruption.[131] Likewise, any increase in neurological deficit produced by osmotic disruption of the BBB is transient, and resolves within 48–72 h.[122] The initial, successful results obtained with osmotic disruption of the BBB, combined with chemotherapy, suggest that this regimen may be used more extensively in the future. These procedures also offer the possibility of therapy with other drugs that do not easily cross the BBB. Unfortunately, osmotic opening of the BBB may increase neurotoxicity by enhancing delivery of anticancer drugs to normal brain tissue.[132]

BRAIN MONITORING

ANESTHESIA AND THE ELECTROENCEPHALOGRAM

The EEG, as recorded from the scalp, reflects the electrical activity of the cerebral cortex. The signals consist, primarily, of the graded summations of inhibitory and excitatory postsynaptic potentials (PSPs) in the pyramidal cells of the granular cortex. These neurons, with their long dendritic trees, are oriented perpendicularly to the surface of the cerebral cortex, so that PSPs create dipole fields with phase reversal at a mean cortical depth of about 900 μm and a zero isopotential at a depth of about 800 μm. Recordings from closely spaced electrodes on the cortical surface show activity in the tangential direction. The pyramidal cells are the only neurons at right angles to the cortex that receive similar synaptic inputs and have dendritic trees long enough to act as effective dipoles. A clear statistical relationship exists between unit action potentials of single pyramidal cells and surface EEG spindles.[133] The diagnostic EEG is normally recorded on paper as a plot of voltage against time. Most often, the voltage calibration is 50 microvolts (μV) and paper speed is 30 mm·s^{-1}. These values may vary, and calibration marks must be shown.

Clinically, the EEG is usually described in terms of rhythms and complexes that are nominally indicated according to frequency bands of specific patterns. Delta rhythm is 0–4 Hz, and may be seen with deep sleep, deep anesthesia, or pathologic conditions, such as brain tumors, in the underlying white matter that cuts off the normal transmission of controlling impulses from subcortical structures of the brain. Delta rhythm is also characteristic of hypoxic and other metabolic encephalopathies. Theta rhythms, 4–8 Hz, are seen during sleep and anesthesia in adults. They are common with hyperventilation in normal, awake children and young adults. Alpha rhythm, nominally 8–13 Hz, is the characteristic EEG pattern of the resting, alert adult, particularly when the eyes are closed. This rhythm is seen predominantly in occipital leads, and is usually abolished by opening the eyes or when startled. Beta activity, 13–30 Hz, is seen during mental concentration, as when the subject is performing arithmetic calculations, and during light stages of anesthesia. Fast frontal activity in the beta range is characteristically seen in patients who take barbiturates or benzodiazepines, and may persist as long as 2 weeks after the withdrawal of these drugs.

Under normal awake conditions, the dominant EEG frequency is alpha in 75–90% of cases; beta frequencies occur in 7%. Intermittent irregular delta and theta rhythms with high- or low-amplitude variants occur approximately 20% of the time. The normal amplitude of the EEG is 10–50 μV, but may be higher or lower. At ages greater than 65 yr, alpha activity slows, and the incidence of a slow variant of alpha (7–8 Hz) increases. Beta activity increases with aging, as does the incidence of irregular slowing of EEG frequency and focal abnormalities. The focal abnormalities observed with aging may reflect impairment of local cerebral perfusion and metabolism at a time when clinical manifestations are not present (Fig. 30-14).

Anesthetics produce systematic changes in the EEG, which are related to the level of anesthesia. The changes probably reflect the ability of anesthetic drugs to depress normal brain function, produce analgesia, and decrease awareness.

Increasing doses of most anesthetics produces anesthesia, which progresses from a euphoric state, possibly associated with agitation or excitation, to deeper levels of sleep, until a surgical level of anesthesia is reached. In most cases, induction of anesthesia initially produces a decrease in alpha and an increase in beta activity, coincident with the clinical state of excitation. This may be related to generalized cortical activation due to loss of normal inhibitory mechanisms.[134] As the depth of anesthesia increases, EEG frequency decreases until theta or delta activity is predominant. Further increasing the dose of anesthesia at this level can produce suppression of the EEG to a burst suppression pattern. This coincides with near-maximal depression of cerebral metabolic activity. An additional increase in anesthesia from this stage will produce complete cortical electrical silence and a quiescent EEG.

Because anesthesia usually produces the same general pattern of EEG changes, the EEG may be considered an indicator of the depth of anesthesia. However, not all anesthetics produce the same maximal state of cerebral depression. For example, high doses of anesthetics such as isoflurane or barbitu-

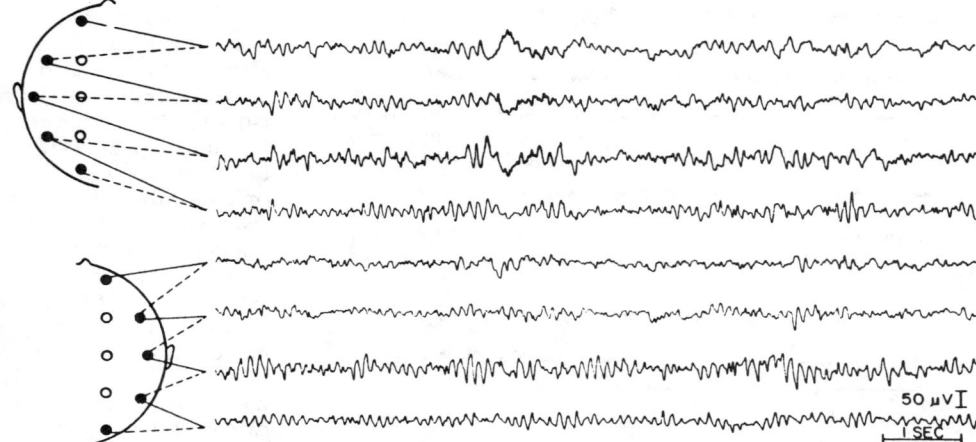

FIG. 30-14. Electroencephalogram record showing abnormal sporadic left temporal slow waves observed in a 61-yr-old subject without clinical manifestations. (Spehlman R: EEG primer, p 216. New York, Elsevier-North Holland Biomedical Press, 1981.)

rates can produce complete EEG suppression, while other anesthetic agents such as halothane and opioids will only produce marked slowing of EEG activity. Furthermore, anesthetics may produce other varying patterns of EEG activation and suppression.[135-137]

Inhaled Anesthetics

The pattern of the EEG change during halothane anesthesia is consistent with the general pattern described above. During induction of anesthesia, there is a shift from a dominant unanesthetized alpha pattern to increasing beta activity. The frequency then slows as anesthesia deepens until, at a surgical anesthetic level, high amplitude delta and theta activity are dominant.[135] Deep halothane anesthesia may depress the EEG to a burst suppression or quiescent pattern,[138] but this may represent a secondary toxic effect, rather than a direct anesthetic effect.[139]

The dominant EEG activity shifts from alpha to beta during induction of anesthesia with enflurane. Surgical anesthesia with enflurane is marked by high voltage delta and theta activity, as with halothane.[139, 140] With higher concentrations of enflurane, spiking activity may occur (Fig. 30-15).[141] This may be followed by a generalized seizure pattern with occasional tonic-clonic muscle activity. Seizures are most likely to occur when enflurane is the sole anesthetic and Pa_{CO_2} levels are decreased due to hyperventilation of the lungs.[35]

Isoflurane may provide greater cerebral metabolic depression and less cardiovascular depression than halothane.[41, 45] The effect of isoflurane on the EEG is similar to that of halothane during induction and at surgical levels of anesthesia. However, the ability of isoflurane to produce greater cerebral metabolic depression than halothane is coincident with the ability of this drug to suppress the EEG to burst suppression, then silence at high doses.[45]

Intravenous Anesthetics

Barbiturates, such as thiopental, produce anesthesia coincident with a general depression of brain metabolic activity. After intravenous injection, thiopental quickly moves across the BBB and rapidly equilibrates with brain tissue. The anesthetic effect of short-acting barbiturates, such as thiopental, is brief (7–8 min), because the drug is redistributed to less well-perfused tissues, such as muscle and fat. Other barbiturates

may have a longer anesthetic action due to differences in lipid solubility, dissociation, and plasma protein binding.

With slow intravenous injection of barbiturates, EEG changes are similar to those seen with other anesthetics.[143] An initial phase of low-voltage, fast EEG activity is seen, followed by an increase in amplitude in all frequency ranges. This changes to a dominant pattern of high-amplitude delta and theta activity as anesthesia deepens. The EEG may progress to burst suppression or to complete electrical silence if the barbiturate dose is further increased.[143, 144] These changes in EEG activity are closely linked with the cerebral metabolic depressant effects of barbiturates, as with inhalational agents. With fast intravenous injections of barbiturates, the initial phases of EEG change are passed through quickly, and high-amplitude delta and theta activity may be observed within 1–2 min. As the subject recovers from barbiturate anesthesia, the pattern of EEG suppression also reverses, with high-amplitude, slow-wave activity eventually being replaced by alpha and beta activity. This reversal may occur within 7–8 min following a single intravenous injection of thiopental.

In contrast to barbiturates, ketamine stimulates, rather than depresses, cerebral metabolic activity and is thought to produce anesthesia by a dissociative mechanism. Following intravenous or intramuscular injection, ketamine disrupts the normal EEG pattern. High-amplitude theta activity, together with secondary patterns of beta activity, may be seen coincident with surgical anesthesia. This pattern slowly reverses to normal over 20–40 min as the patient recovers from a single dose of the anesthetic. The theta EEG rhythm and cerebral metabolic activation seen with ketamine are thought to be due to inhibition of normal cortical antagonism and to secondary activation of subcortical rhinencephalic structures.[107]

Opioids also produce anesthesia without marked cerebral metabolic or cardiovascular depression, specifically acting on brain opioid receptors.[77] Recently available opioids, such as fentanyl, sufentanil, and alfentanil, have a rapid onset and brief duration of action, which enhances the potential use of these drugs in anesthetic procedures.

During induction with anesthetic doses of opioids, alpha activity slows and beta activity ceases in the EEG within 1–2 min (Fig. 30-16).[137] This is followed rapidly by diffuse theta and some delta activity. Within 5 min of induction, high-amplitude delta activity is dominant and is synchronized in a high percentage of patients. These changes slowly reverse 15–20 min after induction; delta activity becomes lower in

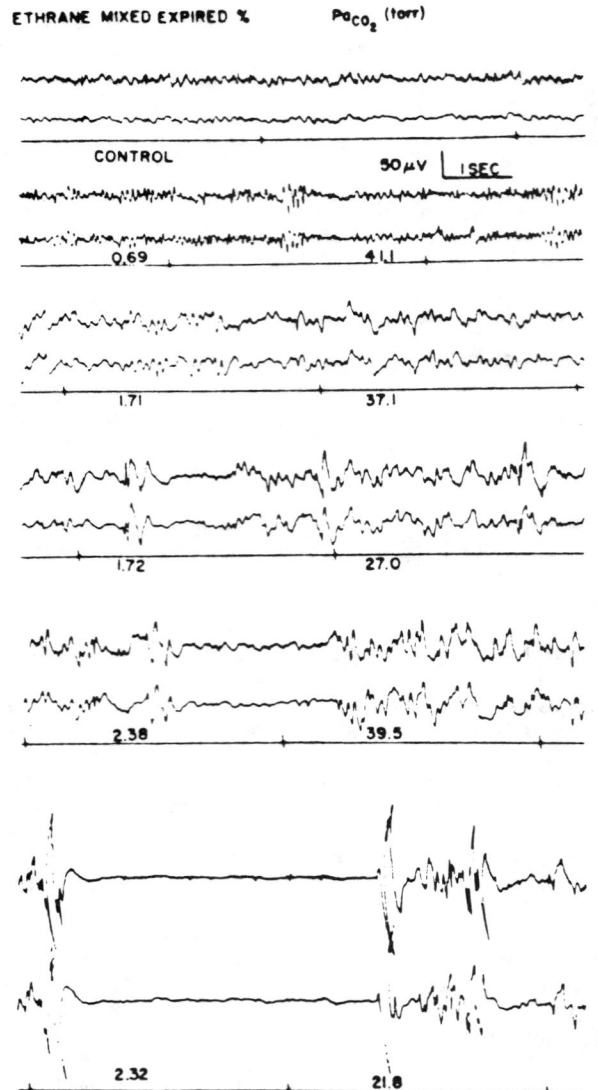

ETHRANE MIXED EXPIRED %   Pa$_{CO_2}$ (torr)

CONTROL   50μV | 1 SEC

0.69   4.1.1

1.71   37.1

1.72   27.0

2.38   39.5

2.32   21.8

FIG. 30-15. Effect of increasing depth of enflurane concentration and changes in Pa$_{CO_2}$ in man. Note spiking activity at high enflurane concentration and low Pa$_{CO_2}$. (Clark DL *et al:* Neurophysiological effects of different anesthetics in unconscious man. J Appl Physiol 31:884, 1971.)

amplitude and irregular, while theta activity increases. If additional doses of opioids are not given, alpha and beta activity slowly return. Sharp-wave and spiking EEG patterns have been observed with sufentanil and fentanyl,[82, 84–87] and supraclinical doses of these drugs produce seizure-like EEG activity in animals (Fig. 30-17).[84, 85] An inability to produce maximal brain metabolic or EEG suppression with high doses of opioids indicates that the mechanism of anesthesia is different than with other anesthetics.[82] It is likely that these agents do not depress overall neuronal activity, but act more specifically at limbic and other subcortical sites to disassociate afferent sensory activity from conscious cortical function.

Etomidate is an intravenous drug that produces anesthesia and depresses neuronal metabolic function, but provides little analgesia.[99] Etomidate is unusual in that it suppresses brain metabolism and EEG substantially, but has little effect on cardiovascular function. This is probably because the primary site of action of etomidate is at forebrain neuronal GABA receptor sites, which modulate brain metabolic and electrical functions. Following anesthetic induction with etomidate, electrical activity at all frequencies initially increases with transient neuronal excitation. This pattern quickly reverts to high-amplitude, slow-wave synchronous delta activity (Fig. 30-18).[147, 148] An overdose of etomidate manifests as further depression of EEG to burst suppression or quiescence.[99, 149] Reversal of anesthesia occurs quickly; the phases of anesthesia are passed through in reverse order and dominant alpha activity returns in 8–10 min. Some reports suggest that etomidate may activate epileptogenic cortical regions selectively, enhancing the production of seizure activity.[150] For this reason, the use of etomidate in epileptic patients should perhaps be limited to those occasions when epileptic foci are being identified for possible resection.

Epilepsy

Epilepsy may be defined as hyperactive or hypersynchronous neuronal discharges within the brain. The overactive state of neuronal function is thought to arise from an imbalance of excitatory and inhibitory mechanisms. Normal excitatory mechanisms relay information from lower centers to the cortex, producing arousal, while inhibitory mechanisms provide feedback inhibition and allow focusing of cortical function on specific sensory input. Feedback inhibitory interneurons that utilize GABA as a neurotransmitter have been identified in the brain.[151] Benzodiazepine receptors interact with the GABA receptor to increase chloride conductance and decrease neuro-

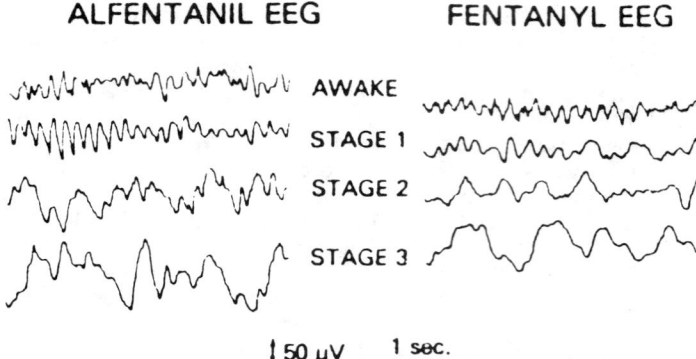

ALFENTANIL EEG   FENTANYL EEG

AWAKE

STAGE 1

STAGE 2

STAGE 3

| 50 μV   1 sec.

FIG. 30-16. Electroencephalogram stages for alfentanil and fentanyl. Activity changes from mixed alpha and beta activity in the awake state to high-amplitude delta activity at stage 3 with both anesthetics. (Scott JC *et al:* EEG quantitation of narcotic effect: The comparative pharmacodynamics of fentanyl and alfentanil. Anesthesiology 62:234, 1985.)

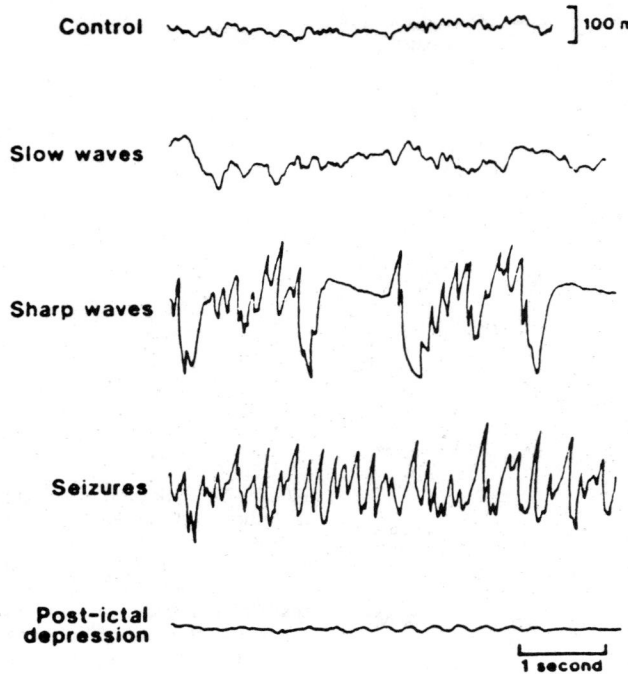

Control ⟩ 100 mV

Slow waves

Sharp waves

Seizures

Post-ictal depression

1 second

FIG. 30-17. Representative record of electroencephalogram (EEG) changes in rats with increasing sufentanil doses. Anesthetic EEG pattern changes to sharp waves and seizure activity with elevated doses of sufentanil. (Keykhah MM *et al:* Influence of sufentanil on cerebral metabolism and circulation in the rat. Anesthesiology 63:274, 1985.)

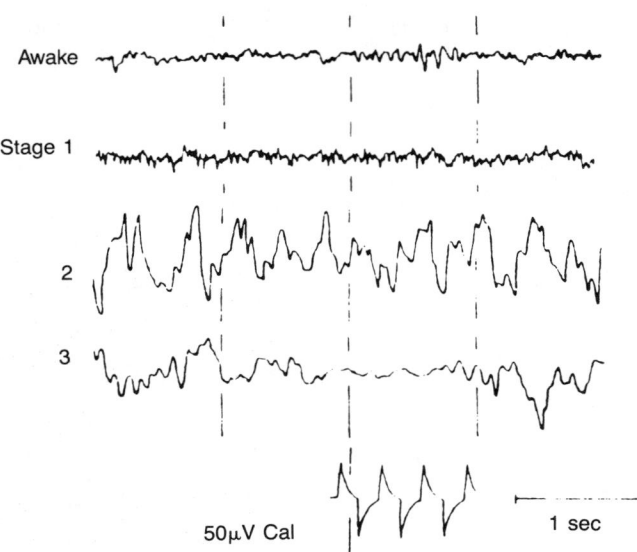

Awake

Stage 1

2

3

50μV Cal   1 sec

FIG. 30-18. Electroencephalogram progression with increasing etomidate dosage. Activation of beta activity is seen in stage 1, which reverts to high-amplitude, low-frequency waves and periods of quiescence at stage 3. (Arden JR *et al:* Increased sensitivity to etomidate in the elderly: Initial distribution versus altered brain response. Anesthesiology 65:19, 1986.)

nal excitability. Both GABA and benzodiazepine receptors have been identified in cortical and subcortical tissue, and have been proposed to be primarily involved in controlling neuronal excitability in the onset of epilepsy.[152]

Clinically, epilepsy may be characterized as being either cortical or subcortical in origin. Subcortical epilepsy reportedly originates from cortical-activation mechanisms located in the reticular formation and intralaminar nuclei of the thalamus.[153] This concept is supported by experiments showing that electrical or chemical stimulation of these areas produces cortical epileptic-like activity.[154] The EEG preceding a grand mal seizure in subcortical epilepsy shows low-voltage, fast beta activity. This is followed by high-voltage spikes of 8–12 Hz frequency, which coincide with the tonic phase of the seizure. The high voltage spikes quickly decay into short bursts of spike activity, separated by slow 1.5- to 3-Hz waves, which coincide with the clonic phase of grand mal seizure. Finally, the EEG becomes quiescent with slow delta activity while the patient becomes flaccid. This slow activity corresponds to clinical postictal depression, and may persist for several hours.

Petit mal seizures are also subcortical in origin.[154] They are seen in children, rather than in adults, and may be precipitated by alkalosis due to hypocapnia, or by hypoglycemia. The EEG pattern seen with petit mal consists of bilateral, generalized spike and wave activity occurring at a rate of 3–4 per second. Most attacks of petit mal are accompanied by slight myoclonic twitchings often restricted to the eyelids. Myoclonic epileptic attacks, also subcortical in origin, are accompanied by myoclonic jerks that are bilateral and symmetri-

cal.[155] The EEG pattern with these attacks resembles the spike and wave pattern of petit mal, but the spikes are usually multiple rather than single. Myoclonic attacks occur frequently in cases of subcortical epilepsy, and have been regarded as smaller episodes of grand mal.[156]

Localized or focal EEG seizure patterns are most likely of cortical origin. A variety of pathological processes can lead to hypersensitivity of cortical foci, which probably involves chronic dendritic polarization of pyramidal neurons (Fig. 30-19).[156, 157] Seizure activity within these cortical foci may then spread both locally and to other associated cortical regions by means of recruitment.[158] The interictal discharges of epileptogenic foci are accompanied by strong inhibitory patterns in surrounding cortical tissue, and it is this mechanism that maintains the focus of these seizures. The EEG pattern shows a transition from sporadic interseizure activity to rhythmical spikes or sharp waves, usually at a rate of 10–12 Hz. As the attack develops clinically, this rate may decrease to as low as 2 Hz. In psychomotor epilepsy, the epileptic focus is most often located in the temporal lobe. Often, the seizure activity spreads bilaterally to mirror foci in the opposite cortex by means of commissural connections. Additional bilateral recruitment of epileptic activity may also occur by association with subcortical generators, which makes the diagnosis of primary focal epilepsy more difficult.[158]

Tumors

Tumor tissue in the brain is not active in generating electrical activity. EEG abnormalities that occur as a result of a tumor are produced primarily because of the space-occupying effect of the tumor and the possible impedance of blood flow to surrounding tissue. Early reports described EEG slowing resulting from cerebral tumors, which may be used to locate the site of the tumor.[159] Slow activity that is bilaterally symmetrical,

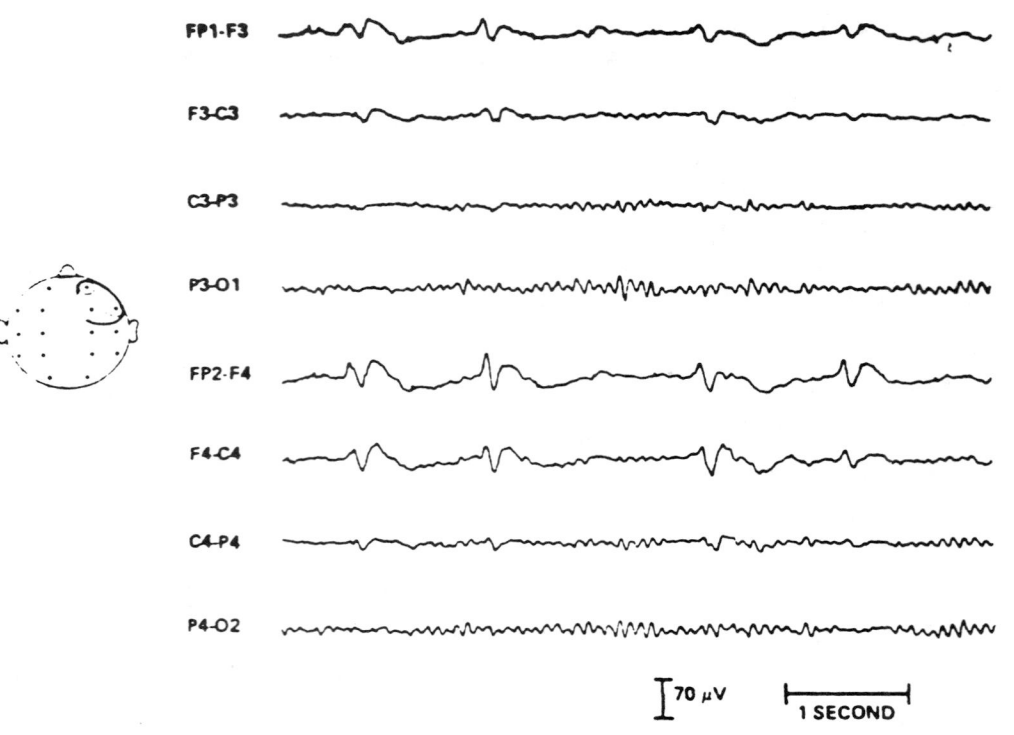

FP1-F3

F3-C3

C3-P3

P3-O1

FP2-F4

F4-C4

C4-P4

P4-O2

$\int 70\ \mu V$ 1 SECOND

FIG. 30-19. Spike and wave activity indicating focal seizure pattern in the right frontal cortex with spread of this activity to left and posterior regions. (Wyllie E *et al:* Ipsilateral forced head and eye turning at the end of the generalized tonic-clonic phase of versive seizures. Neurology 36:1212, 1986.)

synchronous, and rhythmic is often associated with infratentorial tumors, due to the displacement and distortion of subcortical centrencephalic structures.[160] ICP is often increased with these tumors due to obstruction of CSF flow, but this is not likely to be the source of EEG abnormalities. Supratentorial tumors involving subcortical structure may produce widespread EEG abnormalities due to the distortion of centrencephalic structures. Depending on the location of the tumor, this distortion may be unilateral or bilateral. Cortical tumors may produce focal delta activity or spikes as a result of direct pressure, induction of edema, or vascular insufficiency in local neurons. Delta activity may be due to a lack of input from subcortical sites. Cerebral abscesses and chronic subdural hematomas often produce similar EEG slowing due to their space-occupying effects. With a subdural hematoma, EEG amplitude is usually depressed due to compression of cortical neurons and increased distance between the cortex and the scalp electrodes.

Cerebral Trauma

Acute head injury may be associated with both short- and long-term changes in EEG, which are dependent on the severity of the injury and help to provide a prognosis for eventual recovery. Experimentally, head injury produces an immediate reduction in EEG amplitude.[161] This is followed by a generalized slowing of EEG to delta activity. The rapid recovery of the EEG from this state is dependent on the severity of the head injury and correlates roughly with the clinical picture. In mild head injury in man, there is a generalized slowing of EEG to theta or delta activity, which usually resolves to a normal EEG pattern within 10 min.[162] In severe head injury, the extent and persistence of EEG attenuation is dependent on the degree of injury, and marked attenuation is associated with coma and, most often, with eventual death. EEG amplitude

attenuation usually changes to a slowing of activity within 1–2 days. The extent of this slowing depends on the degree of head injury, and the prognosis for the patient is poor if the dominant EEG activity is 4 Hz or below.[163] From this state, the EEG eventually returns to a normal pattern if the patient recovers. This return may occur slowly over a period of several days to several months. Localized brain injury may also be associated with focal EEG attenuation and slowing, then posttraumatic epilepsy.[164] Epilepsy may be prefaced by high-amplitude spiking activity, and may occur several days to several weeks following the injury.

Cerebrovascular disease may produce ischemia and neuronal damage by infarction or brain hemorrhage. The extent and degree of ischemia produced by these lesions and the associated brain edema may produce widespread or localized changes in EEG, which depend on the neuronal mechanisms that are affected. Infarction of the brain stem may produce no observable changes in EEG unless portions of the mesencephalic tegmentum and the reticular activating system are damaged.[165] In these cases, normal EEG is replaced by bilaterally synchronous slow-wave activity.

Unilateral occlusion of the internal carotid artery may produce little change in EEG if clinical signs of cerebral ischemia are not apparent. This is due to the ability of the contralateral arterial system to produce adequate blood flow and oxygenation to the affected cortex through the circle of Willis. When carotid occlusion is accompanied by cerebral arterial disease or hypotension, a diffuse slowing of EEG and a decrease in amplitude may be observed throughout the ipsilateral cortex.[166] Focal slowing and decreases in amplitude are usually most apparent in the temporal or frontotemporal regions. When cerebrovascular accidents affect specific areas of the cortex, the slowing and diminution of EEG may be more localized. Focal delta activity may be apparent within a few hours of the infarction. Surrounding cortical tissue may also show a slowing to theta activity, which may be associated with perifocal edema. In some cases in which the lesion affects thalamic regions, the slowing of EEG and decrease in amplitude may be apparent over the entire cortex, with little localization. The extent to which EEG is affected throughout the cortex is related to the state of consciousness. If EEG changes are unilateral and particularly focal in nature, consciousness is often preserved. Resolution of EEG abnormalities usually occurs over a period of several weeks, particularly if the abnormalities are focal in nature. Long term, there is good correlation between the persistence of EEG slowing and decreased regional CBF.[167] Clinically, the correlation between recovery of function and resolution of EEG abnormalities is not precise. EEG may recover over a period of time with little improvement of clinical symptoms. On the other hand, as with head injury, the state of consciousness and clinical symptoms may improve rapidly following a cerebrovascular accident, while EEG slowing continues over a much longer period.

Computerized EEG Processing

Interpretation of the raw multi-channel EEG is difficult, particularly for the anesthesiologist who has not been trained in that area. Computerized analysis of the EEG now enables presentation of the raw EEG in a format that is simpler to understand and that can be quantitated.[168] By complex mathematical manipulation of the signal, the EEG can be presented in a three-dimensional graphic form where power (amplitude) is plotted on the y-axis, frequency on the x-axis, and time on the z-axis. There are several methods to process and display the EEG, such as the compressed spectral array (CSA),[169] the density-modulated spectral array (DSA),[170] an aperiodic analysis,[171] and the cerebral function monitor (CFM).[172] The usefulness of computerized EEG analysis has yet to be fully determined, since interpretation of the processed EEG, like the raw EEG, requires learning and experience. Nevertheless, reports have been published describing the use of the processed EEG for monitoring of anesthetic depth[173] and cerebral perfusion during carotid endarterectomy[174] and cardiopulmonary bypass.[175]

EVOKED POTENTIALS DURING ANESTHESIA

Analysis of the EEG is of value in evaluating anesthetic effects, as well as the presence of brain pathology. Another electrophysiologic technique for monitoring brain function is the evoked potential (EP). EPs can be obtained by using somatosensory, auditory, or visual stimulation. They reflect the functional integrity of neural pathways, as well as subcortical and cortical processing.

Several factors, such as body temperature, Pa_{CO_2}, and patient age, affect EPs. Therefore, these factors must be controlled in some way during any study evaluating the effects of anesthesia on EPs.

Somatosensory Evoked Potentials

Somatosensory evoked potentials (SEPs), such as those elicited by stimulation of the median nerve, produce well-defined reproducible wave forms with peaks and complexes that, for clinical purposes, are associated with different neural generators. Nomenclature of the characteristic peaks and complexes is not fully standardized, but designations according to polarity and nominal post-stimulus latency seem most appropriate. For example, a negative peak recorded about 20 msec after stimulation of the median nerve at the wrist is referred to as "N20." Emerson and Pedley[176] concluded that the Erb's point potential (P9) is the afferent volley in the brachial plexus at Erb's point. N13 is a postsynaptic potential generated near the cervicomedullary junction by dorsal gray matter of the rostral cervical spinal cord or the nucleus cuneatus. N20 is probably the first cortical response to median nerve stimulation; its source may be in the primary somatosensory cortex or in the thalamus or thalamocortical radiations. All observers agree that the P22, or initial cortical positivity, arises in the somatosensory cortex.

SEPs persist during administration of a large dose of thiopental, even after the EEG becomes isoelectric.[177] Drummond et al[178] concluded that, although large doses of thiopental increase the latency of the cortical primary specific complex and decrease its amplitude, the wave forms are compatible with effective monitoring. The smaller doses that are normally used produce smaller changes.[179] Very large doses of the drug are required to markedly attenuate the SEP.[177, 178] Low doses of morphine and fentanyl produce variable effects on SEP amplitude with little or no change in the latency of the response.[180, 181]

Several investigators have studied the effect of inhaled anesthetics on the SEP. Peterson et al[182] reported that enflurane, halothane, and isoflurane, in neurologically intact patients premedicated with morphine, each reduced the amplitude of the cortical SEP elicited by stimulation of the median nerve (Fig. 30-20). Post-stimulus latencies were increased. Reductions in SEP amplitude greater than 50% were observed with 1 MAC halothane, 0.5 MAC enflurane, and 0.5 MAC isoflurane, all given with 60% N_2O in oxygen. These authors concluded that halothane is least disruptive of the SEP, while enflurane is most disruptive, and that N_2O added to stable concentrations of volatile inhaled anesthetics attenuates the response.

Pathak et al[183] also reported that halothane, enflurane, and isoflurane given in 60% N_2O decreased the amplitude and increased the latency of the SEP. However, in contrast to the results of Peterson et al,[182] they found halothane the most disruptive, and enflurane the least disruptive, of the SEP. Taken together, both studies indicate that halothane, enflurane, and isoflurane produce marked attenuation of the SEP in 1 MAC concentrations, possibly with little difference among the three agents.

McPherson et al[184] studied the effects of uncontrolled concentrations of enflurane and isoflurane and 50% N_2O in clinical studies. They found that all three drugs decreased the SEP amplitude when one was administered after anesthesia was induced with fentanyl. Enflurane and isoflurane increased the latency of the responses while N_2O did not. Although these workers suggested that 50% N_2O alone depressed the SEP as much as isoflurane or enflurane alone, the design of their study and their data do not clearly support that conclusion. Several investigators[182, 183, 185] have observed reductions in SEPs when N_2O is combined with volatile anesthetics, but the well-controlled study by Peterson et al[182] suggests that N_2O alters SEPs less than equivalent MAC levels of halothane, enflurane, or isoflurane. Samra et al[186] found that, when isoflurane is given alone, SEPs can still be recorded in at least some patients with end-tidal isoflurane concentrations as high as 1.7 MAC.

Auditory Evoked Potentials

Brain stem auditory evoked potentials (BAEPs) consist of seven peaks. The purported neural generators of these peaks are: peak 1 = extracranial portion of the acoustic nerve; peak

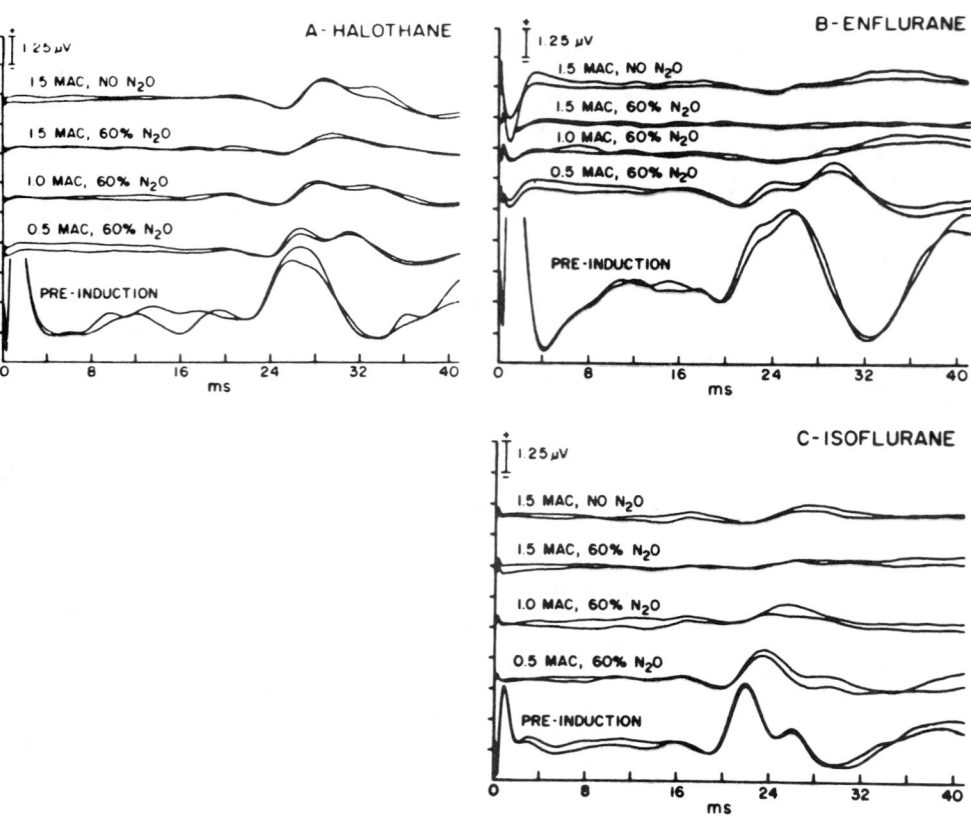

FIG. 30-20. Cortical somatosensory evoked responses at various minimal alveolar concentration (MAC) levels of halothane, enflurane, and isoflurane. Note marked alteration of evoked responses at 1 MAC and higher levels of inhaled agents and the modest improvement of the evoked response when N_2O was withdrawn. (Peterson DO *et al:* Effects of halothane, enflurane, isoflurane and nitrous oxide on somatosensory evoked potentials in humans. Anesthesiology 65:35, 1986.)

2 = intracranial portion of the acoustic cochlear nucleus; peak 3 = superior olive; peak 4 = lateral lemniscus; peak 5 = inferior colliculus; peak 6 = medial geniculate; and peak 7 = thalamocortical radiations.[187] The subcortical generators of BAEPs are generally more resistant to alteration by anesthesia than the later cortical waveforms; this is probably due to the greater effect of anesthetics on cortical metabolic and functional activity, and may be related to the number of synapses in the transmitting pathway.

The latencies of BAEP peaks are increased with increasing levels of isoflurane, but peak amplitudes show little change, even with 1.65% end-tidal concentrations.[185, 188] N_2O also produces little effect on BAEP latencies or amplitudes when given alone or added to isoflurane. Although isoflurane causes only small increases in BAEP latencies and amplitudes, the middle-latency cortical components of the auditory evoked potential (AEP) show dose-related decrements in amplitude.[189] The increases in BAEP latencies produced by isoflurane are similar to those reported for enflurane and halothane.[190] Intravenous anesthetics, such as etomidate and fentanyl, produced no change in the subcortical BAEP.[191, 192] Thornton *et al*[193] found that, although etomidate did not change the subcortical BAEP, the middle-latency cortical peaks were attenuated and prolonged by etomidate in a dose-related manner. Drummond *et al*[178] found small increases in latency in the subcortical BAEP with high doses of thiopental (77.5 mg · kg^{-1}). However, this drug dose was three times that required to produce an isoelectrical EEG, and the increases in latency occurred without a change in peak amplitudes. Overall, the above reports indicate that subcortical BAEPs are resistant to change during anesthesia, while the middle-latency cortical components of the AEP show dose-related depression and prolongation with

anesthetics.[190] This suggests that cortical responses to auditory stimulation may be useful in evaluating anesthetic depth.

Visual Evoked Potentials

The visual evoked potential (VEP) represents cortical electrical responses to visual stimulation, and anesthetic effects on the VEP are similar to those seen with the SEP. The VEP shows little change during neuroleptanalgesia with low doses of fentanyl, but N_2O and isoflurane produce dose-related decreases in VEP amplitudes.[194] Chi and Field[195] showed that increasing isoflurane concentrations in man increases VEP latencies and decreases VEP amplitudes until the response is abolished at end-tidal concentrations of 1.8%. These authors reported that increasing the concentrations of isoflurane from 0.5 MAC to 1 MAC produces greater changes in VEP latencies and amplitudes than does addition of 60% N_2O to 0.6% isoflurane. Uhl *et al*[196] found that end-tidal halothane concentrations of 0.75–1.1% produce a significant increase in VEP latency when compared with that recorded before anesthesia, but that no systematic change in the VEP amplitude occurs. This may indicate that the VEP, like the SEP,[182] is more resistant to change with halothane than with isoflurane anesthesia.

In summary, changes are more likely to occur in cortical than in subcortical EPs during anesthesia. Inhaled anesthetics, particularly the volatile agents, depress these responses more than intravenous agents. Subcortical components of the SEP and the BAEP remain intact, perhaps with small increases in latency, while cortical responses are depressed to undetectable levels with high doses of volatile anesthetics. On the other hand, intravenous agents such as morphine, fentanyl, and thiopental produce little change in either cortical or subcortical EPs, unless very large doses are used. With thiopental, early cortical EPs are altered, but can still be recorded beyond the level at which the EEG becomes isoelectric.Thus, the effects of anesthetics on EPs seem to depend on both the sources of electrophysiologic activity and the mechanisms of drug action. Volatile inhaled agents are more potent inhibitors of evoked cortical electrical activity than are the intravenous drugs, but none of these anesthetics produce marked attenuation of subcortical function except, perhaps, at extremely high concentrations.

INTRACRANIAL PRESSURE

The intracranial space, which is about 1500 ml in volume, is occupied by three compartments: brain tissue (about 85%), CSF (about 10%), and blood (about 5%). Changes in any of these may affect intracranial pressure (ICP). Enlargement of the tissue space may increase ICP in the presence of a brain tumor or with tissue edema following head injury. The CSF compartment compensates, within limits, for increases in other compartments by shifting fluid from the intracranial space to the spinal subarachnoid space (Fig. 30-21).[197, 198] The rate of CSF production, about 0.35 mg·min^{-1} in a normal adult, is relatively insensitive to changes in ICP.[199] In contrast, reabsorption of CSF increases as ICP rises to about 30 mm Hg.[200]

Intracranial blood volume is affected by alterations in cerebral arterial and venous pressures, vasoactive drugs or metabolites, and intracranial bleeding or other mass effects within the cranial vault. When intracranial capacitance has been depleted, further increases in volume lead to marked increases in ICP. Sustained increases in ICP are important because they may lead to brain herniation or to prolonged and critical decreases in cerebral perfusion pressure (CPP).

Mass lesions may block normal pathways of CSF flow and pressure transmission, with marked regional changes in pressure and even tissue herniation from one intracranial compartment to another. Normally, cerebral autoregulatory mechanisms allow the arterial vascular system to maintain relatively

constant cerebral perfusion until CPP decreases below 60–70 mm Hg. Below this level, CBF may be decreased and cerebral ischemia may result.

Anesthesia

Anesthetic management of the patient with elevated ICP involves a high degree of risk, because some anesthetic agents and procedures may further increase ICP while decreasing arterial blood pressure, which dangerously compromises CPP. Laryngoscopy and intubation of the trachea increase ICP, the greatest changes being observed in patients with decreased intracranial compliance.[201] Major determinants of the rise in ICP are transmission of the cough-induced increase in intrathoracic pressure to the cerebral venous system and the hypertension and tachycardia associated with instrumentation of the airway under light anesthesia. Both arterial and venous pressures may, thus, be markedly elevated, so that cerebral blood volume is transiently increased.

Intratracheal and, to some extent, intravenous lidocaine suppress ICP increases produced by endotracheal suctioning.[202, 203] Both techniques suppress coughing. Either endoscopy or intratracheal instillation of lidocaine through an endotracheal tube or tracheostomy may provoke hypertension or a cough, however. The combined use of general anesthetics, muscle relaxants, and topical anesthetics may, therefore, be most effective in preventing the increase in ICP produced by laryngoscopy.[203] On the other hand, Minton et al[204] have suggested that succinylcholine, rather than the cough reflex, may be primarily responsible for increases in ICP during these procedures (Fig. 30-22). Use of a nondepolarizing relaxant

FIG. 30-22. Intracranial pressure (ICP) increases following succinylcholine (SCH) injection and subsequent treatment with thiopental. Pa$_{CO_2}$ remained at 40 mm Hg after SCH injection. (Minton MD et al: Increases in intracranial pressure from succinylcholine: Prevention by prior nondepolarizing blockade. Anesthesiology 65:165, 1986.)

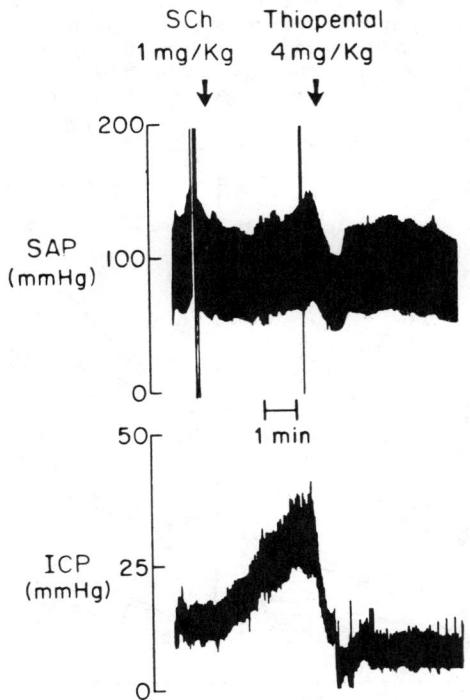

FIG. 30-21. Idealized intracranial pressure (ICP) relationship to increasing intracranial volume. Note shift to higher ICP with small increases in intracranial volume when intracranial compliance is reduced. (Gravenstein N et al: The central nervous system. In Martin JT [ed]: Positioning in Anesthesia and Surgery, 2nd ed, p 291. Philadelphia, WB Saunders, 1987.)

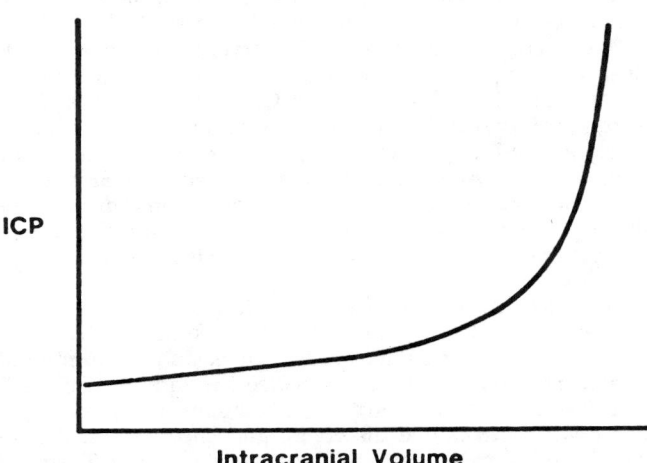

with minimal effect on the cardiovascular system, such as vecuronium, may be useful.

Changes in head position may elevate ICP by impeding cerebral venous return and increasing cerebral blood volume. This is most likely to produce marked increases in ICP when intracranial capacitance is depleted or when cerebrovasodilating drugs or anesthetics are used. Direct vasodilators, such as nitroglycerin, nitroprusside, hydralazine, and verapamil, may increase ICP, particularly in patients with decreased intracranial compliance (Fig. 30-23).[205-209] These changes are more closely related to increases in cerebral blood volume than to changes in CBF.[205] Aortic cross-clamping produces arterial hypertension, which may translate directly to increases in ICP when cerebrovasodilating anesthetics, such as enflurane, halothane, or isoflurane, are used. Intracranial hypertension may be reversed with a short-acting barbiturate that produces cerebrovasoconstriction.[210] Anesthetics that constrict cerebral blood vessels, such as barbiturates, benzodiazepines, and etomidate, are often effective in controlling elevated ICP (Fig. 30-24).[211-217] These drugs are thought to act by reducing intracranial blood volume, not only by constricting cerebral vessels, but also by stabilizing and/or lowering arterial blood pressure.

Ketamine is contraindicated in patients with decreased intracranial compliance because it produces stimulation and increases both CBF and ICP.[218] Diazepam or other benzodiazepines may attenuate the cerebral metabolic stimulation and intracranial hypertension normally produced by ketamine anesthesia.[219]

Fentanyl does not change the rate of CSF production in dogs,[220] but this agent decreases the resistance to CSF reabsorption.[221] Cerebral blood volume is decreased 7–10% for more than 3 h by fentanyl, but ICP is decreased for only the first 20 min.[222]

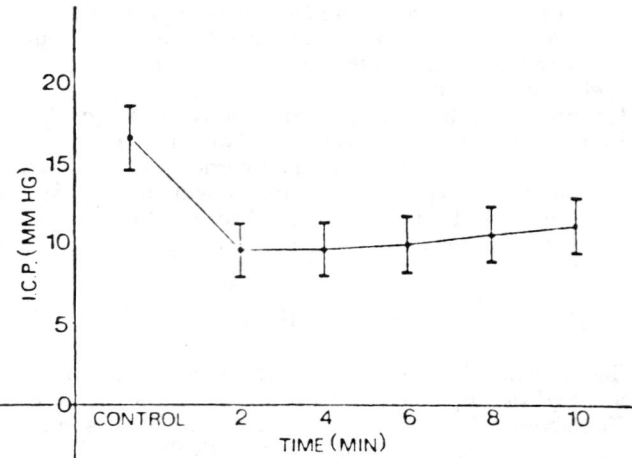

FIG. 30-24. Intracranial pressure (ICP) changes in patients before (control) and after administration of 0.2 mg·kg^{-1} etomidate. (Moss E et al: Effect of etomidate on intracranial pressure and cerebral perfusion pressure. Br J Anaesth 51:347, 1979.)

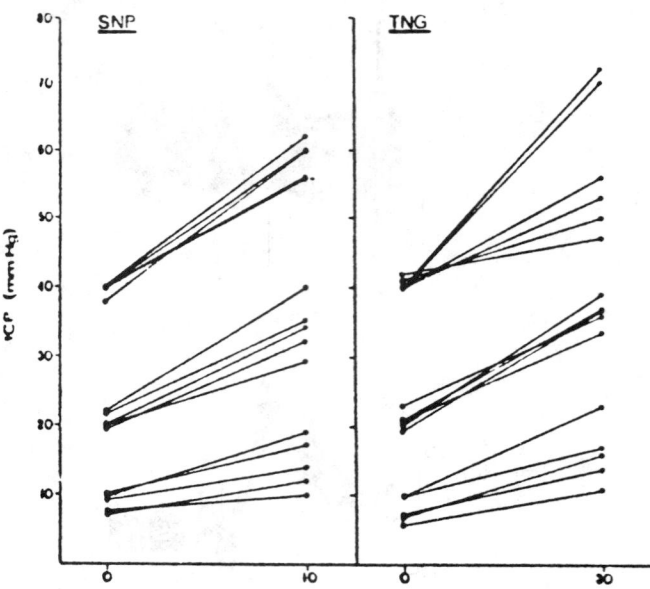

FIG. 30-23. Intracranial pressure (ICP) response to infusion of 10 μg·kg^{-1}·min^{-1} nitroprusside (SNP) and 30 μg·kg^{-1}·min^{-1} glyceryl trinitrate (TNG) in relation to pretreatment control ICP. Note the larger increases in ICP when it was elevated initially. (Morris PJ et al: Changes in canine intracranial pressure in response to infusions of sodium nitroprusside and trinitroglycerin. Br J Anaesth 54:991, 1982.)

Inhaled anesthetics, such as halothane and enflurane, increase ICP by direct cerebrovasodilation and increases in cerebral blood volume.[223] The increase in ICP produced by halothane is closely related to increases in cerebral blood volume, while enflurane produces prolonged increases in ICP that are greater than can be accounted for by changes in cerebral blood volume alone. Later elevations in ICP seen with enflurane may be due to the fact that enflurane increases both CSF production and resistance to CSF reabsorption.[224, 225] This observation is consistent with reports that, in patients with space-occupying intracranial lesions, hyperventilation minimizes the increases in ICP produced by halothane,[226] but not those produced by enflurane.[227] Halothane decreases production of CSF throughout more than 3 h of anesthesia,[220] but increases the resistance to its reabsorption.[221]

Of the volatile inhaled anesthetics, isoflurane is currently the most popular for neurosurgical anesthesia. In normal cats, 1 MAC isoflurane produces little change in CBF. Furthermore, this agent depresses cerebral metabolism more than does halothane, while impairing autoregulation of CBF less.[41] In patients with supratentorial tumors or hematomas, however, isoflurane increases CSF pressure in the presence of normocapnia.[228] This increase is not seen in the presence of hypocapnia, but isoflurane may increase CBF and ICP in patients with intracranial mass lesions if hyperventilation is not used. Even with hyperventilation, isoflurane increases ICP in patients with a large brain shift on CT scan.[229] In dogs, 1.4% isoflurane increases cerebral blood volume over 3.5 hr of anesthesia, while ICP is increased only for the first 20 min or so (Fig. 30-25).[222] Artru suggests that changes in CSF volume may compensate for increases in blood volume during isoflurane anesthesia. Isoflurane does not increase the rate of CSF production,[230] and it decreases the resistance to reabsorption of CSF.[231]

Nitrous oxide may also have a deleterious effect in patients with elevated ICP. Moss and McDowall[232] found that 50% N$_2$O in oxygen produces significant ICP increases in head-injured patients; this rise in ICP can be reversed by withdrawing N$_2$O. Henriksen and Jorgensen[233] reported similar results in patients with intracranial disorders, and showed that the increases in ICP can be reversed by hyperventilation. The most

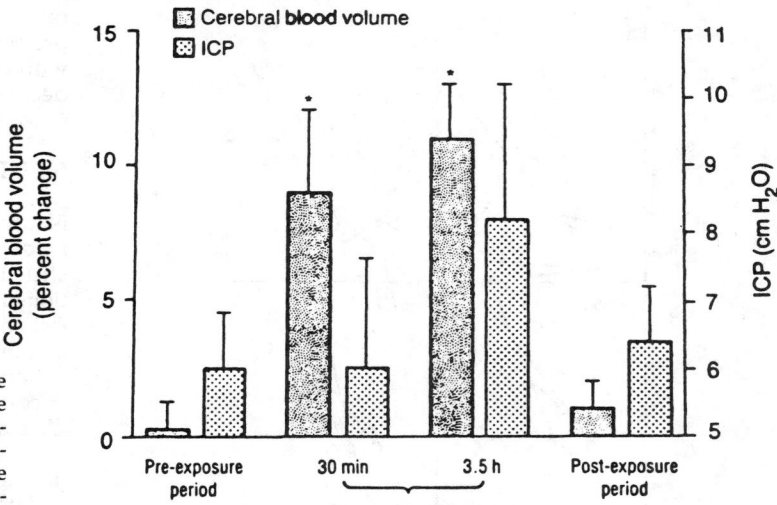

FIG. 30-25. Cerebral blood volume and intracranial pressure (ICP) changes to prolonged isoflurane anesthesia in dogs. Note increases in blood volume and marked but nonsignificant increases in ICP during isoflurane anesthesia. (Artru AA: Relationship between cerebral blood volume and CSF pressure during anesthesia with isoflurane or fentanyl in dogs. Anesthesiology 60:575, 1984.)

likely cause of this increase in ICP is cerebrovasodilation, which leads to increased cerebral blood volume. Other authors, however, have seen little or no change in ICP during N_2O administration.[234, 235] This discrepancy may be related to the initial ICP seen before N_2O is given. Patients showing an increase in ICP with N_2O typically have an elevated ICP before receiving N_2O. Hyperventilation and administration of thiopental prior to introduction of nitrous oxide reduce the risk of an increase in ICP with N_2O when intracranial compliance is reduced.

Another drug that may cause an increase in ICP is succinylcholine, a depolarizing muscle relaxant.[204, 236-238] A study in dogs indicated that the increases in ICP following succinylcholine are produced by cerebral metabolic stimulation and increases in CBF.[239] It is apparent that the depolarizing action of succinylcholine is responsible for the brain-stimulating effects and the increase in ICP, since these effects are attenuated by prior treatment with nondepolarizing agents.[204] Neuromuscular blockade with nondepolarizing agents may also affect ICP and CPP. The hypertension and tachycardia occasionally seen with pancuronium may increase ICP by increasing cerebral blood volume. Agents that release histamine, such as curare, metocurine, and atracurium, may cause vasodilation both systemically and intracranially, which simultaneously increases cerebral blood volume and decreases CPP. The clinical importance of cerebral stimulation by laudanosine, a compound produced by the degradation of atracurium, is probably negligible.

Mechanical ventilation plays a role in the physiologic management of patients with increased ICP. Although it may improve arterial oxygenation, positive end-expiratory pressure (PEEP) can reduce cardiac output and blood pressure while, at the same time, increasing central venous pressure, cerebral venous pressure, and ICP.[240] These changes are most apparent when brain compliance is reduced or ICP is elevated.[241] When the lungs are abnormal, consolidated, and noncompliant, however, airway pressures may not be fully transmitted to the CNS. High-frequency positive-pressure ventilation has been suggested as an alternative to low-frequency ventilation because of its ability to eliminate ventilator-linked fluctuations in blood pressure and ICP.[242]

Head Injury

The effects of head injury and increased ICP on CBF have been studied by several investigators. Under normal conditions in animals without brain injury, increasing ICP by artificial means, as by CSF infusion or balloon inflation, produces a normal autoregulatory response; CBF remains constant until CPP decreases below 60 mm Hg.[243] At this stage, arterial blood pressure may increase (Cushing response) and CSF lactate is increased, suggesting the presence of anaerobic metabolism.[244] Following acute head injury, there is often a diffuse derangement of cerebrovasomotor regulation, accompanied by increased ICP.[245] Initially, CBF may be normal or low,[245, 246] but marked reductions in CBF are not observed unless ICP increases above 30 mm Hg and perfusion pressure is reduced.[247] Vasomotor reactivity to changes in Pa_{CO_2} is reportedly lost during the first few days following severe head injury (Fig. 30-26).[248, 249] In contrast, cerebral autoregulation in the face of changes in arterial blood pressure may be intact. It has been questioned whether cerebral autoregulation is preserved following head injury, or whether it is the result of vasoparalysis and pseudo-autoregulation during intracranial hypertension.[250, 251] Some time after head injury, prolonged hyperemia may develop that is not responsive to hyperventilation.[246] The presence of hyperemia may be closely correlated with the presence of high ICP and decreased CBF during the initial phase of head injury. Focal hyperemic or ischemic patterns occur in severely injured brain areas,[248, 249] and extensive distribution of either pattern usually indicates a poor prognosis.[245, 246] CBF typically shows little correlation with $CMRO_2$ or brain function in the early stages of head injury.[252] Mannitol may help increase CBF in patients with brain edema even when CPP does not change.[253] This treatment, however, may not affect the prognosis for survival. Mannitol is effective in treating increased ICP, although the method of administration may be important in the efficacy of the drug.[254, 255] McGraw and Howard[255] reported that high cumulative doses of mannitol, given over 6 h, negatively influenced the response of ICP to mannitol, and led to a subsequent requirement for excessive doses of mannitol.

In summary, evaluation and control of ICP and CPP are

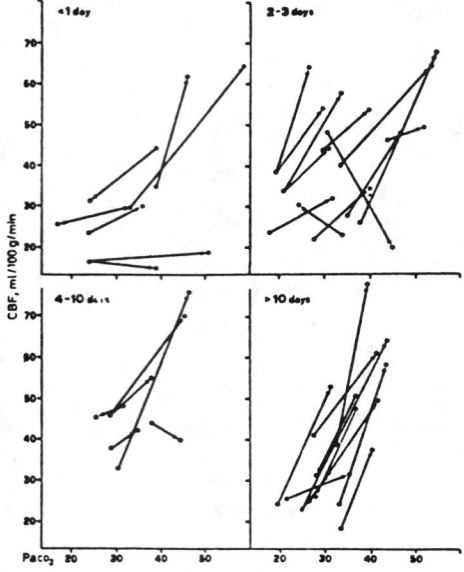

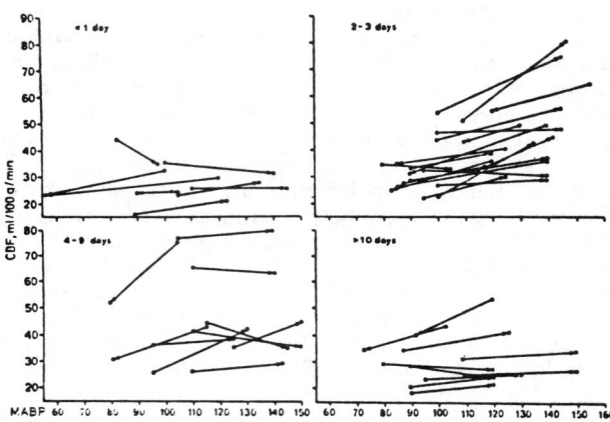

FIG. 30-26. Cerebrovascular reactivity to changes in Pa_{CO_2} *(top)* and mean arterial blood pressure (MABP) *(bottom)* at various intervals following head injury. Reactivity to Pa_{CO_2} is attenuated initially following head injury, while cerebral autoregulation is apparently intact. (Fieschi C *et al:* Regional cerebral blood flow and intraventricular pressure in acute head injuries. J Neurol Neurosurg Psychiatr 37:1378, 1974.)

critical during anesthetic management of patients with head injury or intracranial space-occupying lesions. Agents such as inhaled anesthetics and succinylcholine, which produce no untoward effects in the normal patient, can markedly increase ICP in the patient with reduced intracranial compliance. The blood volume compartment, the most labile of the intracranial compartments, may change dramatically during hypertensive episodes or during treatment with drugs that cause cerebrovasodilation. Means of controlling ICP during anesthesia include hyperventilation, administration of cerebral metabolic depressant and cerebrovasoconstrictor drugs (*e.g.*, barbitu-

rates, benzodiazepines, and etomidate, which produce a prominent decrease in cerebral blood volume), and treatment with diuretics, mannitol, or other hyperosmolar agents that decrease brain water content.

NEURORADIOLOGY

Neuroradiology and nuclear medicine are rapidly developing fields that offer exciting new methods for evaluating both structure and function of the nervous system. Clinical applications are invaluable in the diagnosis of neoplastic, vascular, ischemic, metabolic, and congenital brain disorders. Using CT, the extent of a lesion can be evaluated to characterize focal abnormalities and their anatomical relationships, the presence of brain edema, and the development of brain atrophy.[259] CT scans are used in longitudinal studies for the prognosis of malignant cerebral tumors. Levin *et al*[256] noted a direct relationship between the size of a tumor, as determined by CT, and its rate of progression over a year. Murovic *et al*[257] reported that, in patients with supratentorial malignant gliomas, the sustained disappearance of the lesion from CT after surgery, radiation therapy, and chemotherapy provided a good prognosis for survival. In cases of chiasmal glioma, Fletcher *et al*[258] reported that CT facilitates detection of hydrocephalus and monitoring of shunt function. The ability to distinguish tumor appearance with CT may also be of benefit in the diagnosis of chiasmal glioma, possibly obviating the need for craniotomy.

MRI is a relatively new diagnostic technique that provides excellent anatomical characterization of the brain.[260] This technology differs from CT in the method of acquiring images and in the kind of information that is obtained. Studies comparing MRI and CT have generally found the anatomical resolution to be superior with MRI. Brant-Zawadzki *et al*[261] detected focal brain abnormalities in 48 of 51 patients using a spin-echo multisection MRI technique. Thin-section CT techniques identified two intrasellar masses and one intracanalicular lesion not detected by MRI. However, CT failed to demonstrate focal lesions in 17 of the 48 patients whose lesions were observed with MRI. Thus, MRI appears to be more sensitive than CT in detecting most brain abnormalities.

In acute cerebral infarction, CT scanning can help to determine the extent of brain edema. This technique can demonstrate BBB disruption by showing the movement of contrast material from the vascular space into the brain. In an animal model of cerebral ischemia, however, Kuroiwa *et al*[262] found that CT did not detect the early presence of brain edema or BBB disruption that could be verified by other techniques. These results question the sensitivity of CT in the early diagnosis of brain infarction. Xenon-enhanced CT imaging for measurement of regional CBF, however, may be of clinical value for detecting poorly perfused brain regions that might be amenable to surgical treatment.

High-resolution sonography can be used to localize intracranial mass lesions.[263, 264] Smith *et al*[265] identified brain edema surrounding brain lesions by using regional ultrasound examination of the brain. The diffuse echogenic region encircling a mass lesion corresponds to an area of brain edema as identified by CT. The heterogenous nature of echogenicity in these regions, however, hampers accurate mapping of the extent of the brain lesion.

The low sensitivity of CT as a diagnostic tool for acute stroke and the lack of adequate anatomical definition with other techniques led to the proposal that MRI might be useful in the morphological evaluation of stroke.[266] Indeed, MRI appears to provide greater sensitivity and better specificity in the detection of acute stroke than traditional methods.[267]

Early prognosis is important following severe head injury. The factors that provide the greatest prognostic significance include the clinical neurological status of the patient and evaluation of intracranial pathology. The use of CT in head injury has shown that patients who will have prolonged coma do not have normal CT scans, and that normal scans in head injury usually lead to favorable outcome.[268] This is not always true, however, because brain damage due to impact or hypoxia may initially be unrecognized with CT.[269] Long-term follow-up CT scans show a higher incidence of brain atrophy in patients developing permanent disability than in those who make a good recovery.

Comparisons have been made between standard skull radiography, CT, MRI, and positron-emission tomography (PET) in the study of brain trauma. MRI is superior to radiography and CT for demonstrating extracerebral, as well as intracerebral, traumatic lesions.[270–272] Subdural hematomas

FIG. 30-27. Computerized tomography scans *(upper)* and magnetic resonance imaging (MRI) scans made in a patient with a frontal lesion *(arrow)* produced by a fall down a flight of stairs. Arrows on superior cuts of T1 weighted *(center)* and T2 weighted MRI *(lower)* show a fluid level between two portions of an intraparenchymal hematoma. (Langfitt TW et al: Computerized tomography, magnetic resonance imaging, and positron emission tomography in the study of brain trauma. J Neurosurg 64:760, 1986.)

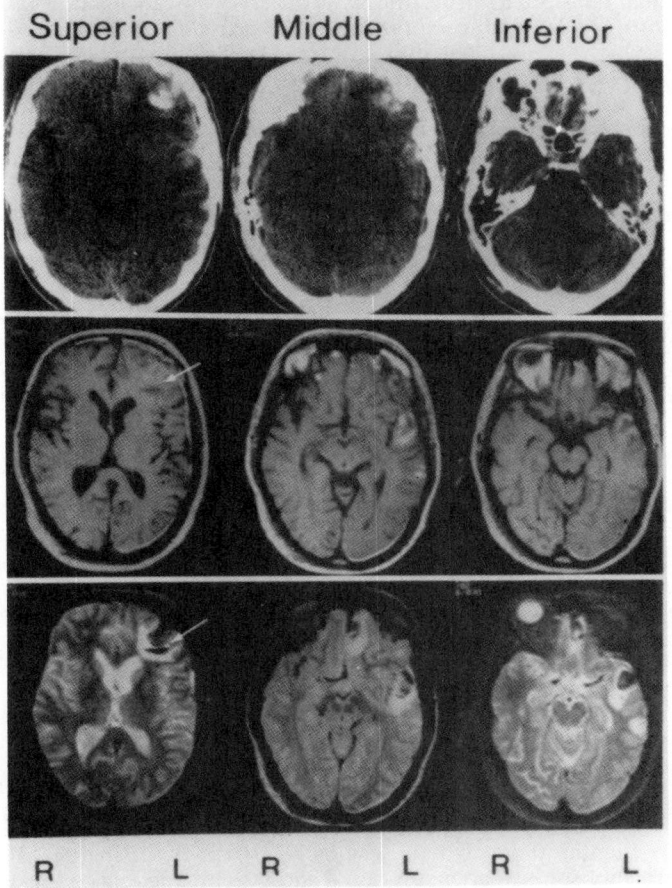

and nonhemorrhagic contusions, which present a diagnostic dilemma in CT, are clearly seen with MRI (Fig. 30-27). Neurophysiological assessment of brain function and memory during hospitalization showed a correlation with the size and location of frontal lesions, as determined by MRI, and follow-up exams disclosed a reduction in MRI lesion size that was related to improved cognition and memory. Comparison of PET to MRI and CT in head injury showed disturbances in glucose metabolism, which extended beyond the structural abnormalities identified by MRI and CT.[273] The clinical significance of metabolic abnormalities in this penumbra region is unknown at present. Neuropsychological testing confirmed the presence of frontal lesions identified by CT and MRI, but did not predict lesions identified in the anterior temporal lobes. These studies indicate that outcome following head injury is clearly related to the length and depth of coma and the extent of brain lesions identified by CT or MRI. MRI provides a more accurate description of the size and location of brain lesions, but CT is adequate for locating large lesions that require surgical treatment. MRI also provides a high correlation with neuropsychological evaluations and with improvement in follow-up studies.

The advent of CT, MRI, and ultrasound techniques for neuroanatomical definition has led to a resurgence of interest in stereotactic ablation or removal of deep intracranial lesions. Devices have been developed that provide stereotactic guidance to defined intracranial targets and lesions.[274] More recently, MRI has been integrated with modified stereotactic systems to provide better definition of neuroanatomical structures.[275] This has allowed the comparison of CT to MRI in stereotactic surgical procedures. Lunsford et al[276] described cases in which patients underwent stereotactic surgery for mass lesions identified by both CT and MRI scans. They concluded that MRI provides better contrast resolution and target determination than CT (Fig. 30-28). Superior resolution of tumor margins, as well as superior definition of adjacent histological features with MRI, allows better stereotactic surgical manipulation of the target structure. In addition, an ultrasound-guided stereotactic biopsy apparatus has been described that may simplify surgical procedures normally performed with CT guidance.[277] The ability of ultrasound-guided neurosurgery to expedite anesthetic and scanning procedures, however, is offset by a lack of anatomical resolution with this technique. Of the neuroradiological methods that have been reported, MRI provides the greatest potential for definition of anatomical structures and accurate stereotactic guidance for neurosurgical procedures.

PET may have even greater research potential than CT and MRI, since it allows examination of biochemical and physiological events in the brains of living human subjects. CBF and the metabolic rates for glucose and oxygen have been measured for several years by using PET, and recent developments allow the imaging of specific neurotransmitter receptors in living brains of animals and humans.[278] Similarly, *in vivo* imaging of neurotransmitter receptors can be accomplished by using a gamma-emitting isotope, a gamma camera, and single-photon emission-computed tomography (SPECT). PET techniques are far more sensitive than CT and MRI but, at present, they are limited by spatial resolution of 4 mm.

The choice of appropriate ligands for binding to the neurotransmitter receptors is critical. At present, ligands have been developed for visualization in humans of receptors for dopamine (D1 and D2), serotonin (5-hydroxytryptamine), gamma-aminobutyric acid (GABA-A, GABA-B, benzodiazepine), opioids, and acetylcholine (muscarinic).[279] Ligands for imag-

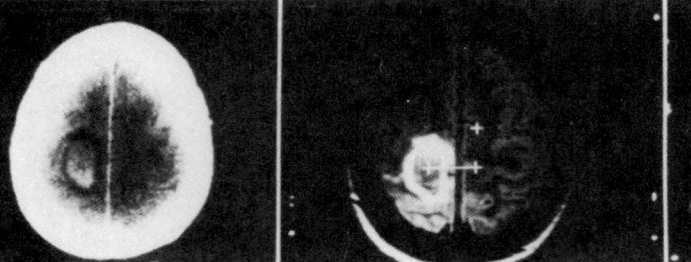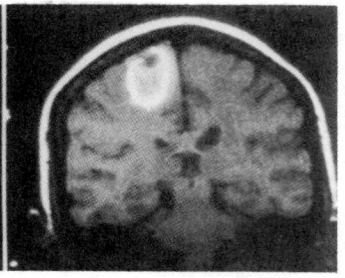

FIG. 30-28. *(Left)* Stereotactic computerized tomography scan disclosing a right parietal mass and surrounding low density. *(Center)* Stereotactic axial T₂ weighted magnetic resonance imaging (MRI) scan. *(Right)* T1 weighted scan of same mass. The MRI signals suggest "layering" of the lesion, later identified as a hematoma with surrounding edema. (Reprinted by permission of the publisher from Lunsford LD, Martinez AJ: Stereotactic exploration of the brain in the era of computed tomography. Surg Neurol 22:222, 1984. Copyright 1984 by Elsevier Science Publishing Co., Inc.)

ing other neurotransmitter receptors in humans, such as the adrenergic receptors, are currently being developed.[280, 281] These techniques are tremendously exciting for anesthesiologists, not only as a means of characterizing receptors in health and disease, but particularly as a means of directly imaging the effects of anesthetics on brain receptors. For example, 2-N-(11C) methylspiperone has a high affinity for dopamine receptors *in vitro,* and this compound concentrates in the basal ganglia, known to be rich in dopamine receptors, in living primates and normal persons.[282] It has now been determined that dopamine receptor levels fall significantly in persons between the ages of 19 and 73 yr, to a greater degree in men than in women. Furthermore, D2 receptor levels in the caudate nucleus and putamen are increased in patients with schizophrenia. Carfentanil, an ultrapotent synthetic opioid, binds mainly to mu receptors, which are involved in pain perception. Thirty to sixty minutes after injection in humans, 11C-labeled carfentanil can be seen on PET scanning, bound to receptors in the frontal and temporoparietal regions, the medial thalamus, and the caudate nucleus and putamen.[283] The highest concentrations of opiate receptors are found in the amygdala, and may be involved in the production of euphoria by opiates.[284] Dense bands of opioid receptors have also been demonstrated in the spinal cord. Binding of carfentanil is diminished in the thalamus during sexual arousal[285]; this observation supports the hypothesis that sexual arousal induces the secretion of endogenous opioids that then block accumulation of the tracer. PET has also been used to label monoamine oxidases A and B in human brain.[286]

Magnetic resonance spectroscopy (MRS) derives information from the RF signals emitted when paramagnetic nuclei are placed in a strong, uniform magnetic field and then stimulated at their resonance frequencies by RF pulses.[287] Magnets can be "tuned" to specific nuclei, such as 1-Hydrogen, 31-Phosphorus, 19-Fluorine, 13-Carbon, or 23-Sodium. The frequency and amplitude of the emitted signals are mathematically transformed to show frequency relationships, and the integrated intensity of the transformed signal is proportional to concentration of each nuclear species present. Brain metabolism can now be analyzed non-invasively in both animals and humans with a technique that, so far, shows no evidence of tissue damage.[288] With phosphate MRS, changes in adenosine triphosphate (ATP), phosphocreatinine (PCr), inorganic phosphate (Pi), and intracellular *p*H can be observed non-invasively. Proton MRS is used to analyze changes in

lactate and some amino acids. 19-Fluorine MRS has been used to examine the uptake and elimination of anesthetics.[289–292]

CONCLUSION

This chapter has described the effects of anesthetic drugs on cerebral function, and has introduced brain monitoring techniques to evaluate anesthetic and disease states. It is apparent that anesthetic drugs have a variety of actions on cerebrovascular and cerebral metabolic activity. Inhaled anesthetics, such as halothane, enflurane, and isoflurane, produce cerebral metabolic depression, but isoflurane may produce more depression of brain metabolism, less direct cerebrovasodilation, and better maintenance of cerebrovascular reactivity. Some intravenous anesthetics, such as barbiturates and etomidate, produce cerebral metabolic depression and concomitant cerebrovasoconstriction. Others, such as opioids and ketamine, produce regional increases and decreases in brain metabolic function. A common finding with regard to the regional metabolic action of anesthetics is the sparing of metabolic activity in the medial habenulo-interpeduncular nucleus regions. The significance of this observation is not yet clear.

Numerous techniques for monitoring the brain are now available. The EEG shows reproducible changes that may be useful for evaluating anesthetic depth. EPs also show changes that are related to the type and depth of anesthesia used. Inhaled anesthetics produce the greatest dose-related change in cortical evoked responses, while opioids produce little effect. Subcortical SEPs and BAEPs are more resistant to change with all anesthetic drugs than are cortical EPs. Both EEG and EP are used to monitor the functional integrity of the CNS in the operating room and critical care unit.

ICP monitoring may be of critical importance in the patient with head injury or space-occupying intracranial lesions. When intracranial compliance is reduced, increases in ICP may be produced by procedures such as endotracheal intubation or administration of inhaled anesthetics. In these cases, critical reductions in CPP may produce general or regional ischemia in brain tissue, particularly when cerebral autoregulation is impaired.

Identification of brain lesions and their neuroanatomical relationships with neuroradiological techniques is of great importance in evaluating patient status. Methods using CT,

MRI, and sonography are valuable in defining the course of anesthetic and neurosurgical treatment and for stereotactic brain surgery. Of these, MRI appears to provide the most promise, both for neuroanatomical resolution of the intracranial space and for diagnosis of brain lesions. In the future, on-line computer analysis of EEG, EP, and other physiological variables, combined with stereotactic neuroradiological methods, will provide better diagnosis and outcome in treatment of neurological lesions. New radiological techniques that allow imaging of neurotransmitter receptors and enzymes in the human brain hold great promise for increasing our understanding of the mechanisms of anesthetic action. MRS methods permit non-invasive observations of brain metabolism, as well as localization of drugs and their metabolites.

REFERENCES

1. Siesjo BK: Brain Energy Metabolism. New York, John Wiley & Sons, 1978
2. Lassen NA: Control of cerebral circulation in health and disease. Circ Res 34:749, 1974
3. Strandgaard S, MacKenzie ET, Sengupta D et al: Upper limit of autoregulation of cerebral flow in the baboon. Circ Res 34:435, 1974
4. Hoffman WE, Miletich DJ, Albrecht RF: Cerebrovascular response to hypotension in hypertensive rats: Effect of antihypertensive therapy. Anesthesiology 58:326, 1983
5. Duckrow DB, Beard DC, Brennan RW: Regional cerebral blood flow decreases during hyperglycemia. Ann Neurol 17:267, 1985
6. Kontos HA: Mechanisms of regulation of the cerebral microcirculation. Curr Conc Cereb Dis Stroke 10:7, 1975
7. Harper AM: The inter-relationship between Pa_{CO_2} and blood pressure in the regulation of blood flow through the cerebral cortex. Acta Neurol Scand 41(Suppl 14):94, 1965
8. Pannier JL, Demeester G, Leusen I: The influence of nonrespiratory alkalosis on cerebral blood flow in cats. Stroke 5:324, 1974
9. Winn HR, Rubio R, Berne RM: Brain adenosine concentration during hypoxia in rats. Am J Physiol 241:H235, 1981
10. Hoffman WE, Albrecht RF, Miletich DJ: The role of adenosine in CBF increases during hypoxia in young vs aged rats. Stroke 15:124, 1984
11. Lebrun-Grandie P, Baron J-C, Soussaline F: Coupling between regional blood flow and oxygen utilization in the normal human brain. A study with positron tomography and oxygen 15. Arch Neurol 40:230, 1983
12. Stullken EH Jr, Milde HJ, Michenfelder JD et al: The nonlinear responses of cerebral metabolism to low concentrations of halothane, enflurane, isoflurane and thiopental. Anesthesiology 46:28, 1977
13. Smith AL: The mechanism of cerebral vasodilation by halothane. Anesthesiology 39:581, 1973
14. Theye RA, Michenfelder JD: The effect of halothane on canine cerebral metabolism. Anesthesiology 29:1113, 1968
15. Christensen MS, Hoedt-Rasmussen K, Lassen NA: Cerebral vasodilatation by halothane anaesthesia in man and its potentiation by hypotension and hypercapnia. Br J Anaesth 39:927, 1967
16. McDowall DG: The effects of clinical concentrations of halothane on the blood flow and oxygen uptake of the cerebral cortex. Br J Anaesth 39:186, 1967
17. Amory DW, Steffenson JL, Forsyth RP: Systemic and regional blood flow changes during halothane anesthesia in the rhesus monkey. Anesthesiology 35:81, 1971
18. Lees MH, Hill J, Ochsner AJ et al: Regional blood flows of the rhesus monkey during halothane anesthesia. Anesth Analg 50:270, 1971
19. Harp JR, Nilsson L, Siesjo BK: The effect of halothane anaesthesia upon cerebral oxygen consumption in the rat. Acta Anaesthesiol Scand 20:83, 1976
20. Miletich DJ, Ivankovich AD, Albrecht RF: Absence of autoregulation of cerebral blood flow during halothane and enflurane anesthesia. Anesth Analg 55:100, 1976
21. deRood M, Capon A, Mouawad E: Effects of halothane on regional cerebral blood flow. Acta Anaesth Belgica 1:82, 1974
22. Albrecht RF, Miletich DJ, Rosenberg R et al: Cerebral blood flow and metabolic changes from induction to onset of anesthesia with halothane or pentobarbital. Anesthesiology 47:252, 1977
23. Alexander SC, Wollman H, Cohen PJ et al: Cerebrovascular response to Pa_{CO_2} during halothane anesthesia in man. J Appl Physiol 19:561, 1964
24. Albrecht RF, Miletich DJ, Madala LR: Normalization of cerebral blood flow during prolonged halothane anesthesia. Anesthesiology 58:26, 1983
25. Warner DS, Boarini DJ, Kassell NF: Cerebrovascular adaptation to prolonged halothane anesthesia is not related to cerebrospinal fluid pH. Anesthesiology 63:243, 1985
26. Turner DM, Kassell NF, Sasaki T et al: Time-dependent changes in cerebral and cardiovascular parameters in isoflurane-nitrous oxide-anesthetized dogs. Neurosurgery 14:135, 1984
27. Jobes DR, Kennel EM, Bush GL et al: Cerebral blood flow and metabolism during morphine nitrous oxide anesthesia in man. Anesthesiology 47:16, 1977
28. Wollman H, Alexander SC, Cohen PJ et al: Cerebral circulation during general anesthesia and hyperventilation in man. Thiopental induction to nitrous oxide and d-tubocurarine. Anesthesiology 26:329, 1965
29. Manohar M, Parks C: Porcine regional brain and myocardial blood flows during halothane-O_2 and halothane-nitrous oxide anesthesia: Comparisons with equipotent isoflurane anesthesia. Am J Vet Res 45:465, 1984
30. Tranquilli WJ, Manohar M, Parks CM et al: Systemic and regional blood flow distribution in unanesthetized swine and swine anesthetized with halothane + nitrous oxide, halothane, or enflurane. Anesthesiology 56:369, 1982
31. McHenry LC Jr, Slocum H, Bivens HE et al: Hyperventilation in awake and anesthetized man. Arch Neurol 12:270, 1965
32. Keaney NP, Pickerodt VW, McDowall DG et al: Cerebral circulatory and metabolic effects of hypotension produced by deep halothane anaesthesia. J Neurol Neurosurg Psychiatr 36:898, 1973
33. Eintrei C, Leszniewski W, Carlsson C: Local application of ^{133}xenon for measurement of regional cerebral blood flow (rCBF) during halothane, enflurane, and isoflurane anesthesia in humans. Anesthesiology 63:391, 1985
34. Sakabe T, Maekawa T, Fujii S et al: Cerebral circulation and metabolism during enflurane anesthesia in humans. Anesthesiology 59:532, 1983
35. Michenfelder JD, Cucchiara RF: Canine cerebral oxygen consumption during enflurane anesthesia and its modification during induced seizures. Anesthesiology 40:575, 1974
36. Seo K, Maekawa T, Takeshita H et al: Cerebral energy state and glycolytic metabolism during enflurane anesthesia in the rat. Acta Anaesthesiol Scand 28:215, 1984
37. Cucchiara RF, Theye RA, Michenfelder JD: The effects of isoflurane on canine cerebral metabolism and blood flow. Anesthesiology 40:571, 1974
38. Gelman S, Fowler KC, Smith LR: Regional blood flow during isoflurane and halothane anesthesia. Anesth Analg 63:557, 1984
39. Manohar M, Parks C: Regional distribution of brain and myocardial perfusion in swine while awake and during 1.0 and 1.5 MAC isoflurane anaesthesia produced without or with 50% nitrous oxide. Cardiovasc Res 18:344, 1984

40. Madsen JB, Cold GE, Hansen EF *et al:* The effect of isoflurane on cerebral blood flow and metabolism in humans during craniotomy for small supratentorial cerebral tumors. Anesthesiology 66:332, 1987

41. Todd MM, Drummond JC: A comparison of the cerebrovascular and metabolic effects of halothane and isoflurane in the cat. Anesthesiology 60:276, 1984

42. Drummond JC, Todd MM: The response of the feline cerebral circulation to Pa_{CO_2} during anesthesia with isoflurane and halothane and during sedation with nitrous oxide. Anesthesiology 62:268, 1985

43. Scheller MS, Todd MM, Drummond JC: Isoflurane, halothane and regional cerebral blood flow at various levels of Pa_{CO_2} in rabbits. Anesthesiology 64:598, 1986

44. Adams RW, Cucchiara RF, Gronert GA *et al:* Isoflurane and cerebrospinal fluid pressure in neurosurgical patients. Anesthesiology 54:97, 1981

45. Newburg LA, Milde JH, Michenfelder JD: The cerebral metabolic effects of isoflurane at and above concentrations that suppress cortical electrical activity. Anesthesiology 59:23, 1983

46. Drummond JC, Todd MM, Toutant SM *et al:* Brain surface protrusion during enflurane, halothane and isoflurane anesthesia in cats. Anesthesiology 59:288, 1983

47. Ori C, Dam M, Pizzolato G *et al:* Effects of isoflurane anesthesia on local cerebral glucose utilization in the rat. Anesthesiology 65:152, 1986

48. Maekawa T, Tommasino C, Shapiro HM *et al:* Local cerebral blood flow and glucose utilization during isoflurane anesthesia in the rat. Anesthesiology 65:144, 1986

49. Myers RR, Shapiro HM: Local cerebral metabolism during enflurane anesthesia: Identification of epileptogenic foci. Electroencephalgr Clin Neurophysiol 47:153, 1979

50. Kofke WA, Hawkins RA, Davis DW *et al:* Comparison of the effects of volatile anesthetics on brain glucose metabolism in rats. Anesthesiology 66:810, 1987

51. Herkenham M: Anesthetics and the habenulo-interpeduncular system: Selective sparing of metabolic activity. Brain Res 210:461, 1981

52. Duffy TE, Cavazzuti M, Cruz NF *et al:* Local cerebral glucose metabolism in newborn dogs: Effects of hypoxia and halothane anesthesia. Ann Neurol 11:233, 1982

53. Dahlgren N, Ingvar M, Yokoyama H *et al:* Influence of nitrous oxide on local cerebral blood flow in awake, minimally restrained rats. J Cereb Blood Flow Metab 1:211, 1981

54. Smith AL, Hoffman SC, Wollman H: Effect of general anesthesia on auto-regulation of cerebral blood flow in man. J Appl Physiol 29:665, 1970

55. Pelligrino DA, Miletich DJ, Hoffman WE *et al:* Nitrous oxide markedly increases cerebral cortical metabolic rate and blood flow in the goat. Anesthesiology 60:405, 1984

56. Oshita S, Ishikawa T, Totutsu Y: Cerebral circulatory and metabolic stimulation with nitrous oxide in the dog. Acta Anaesthesiol Scand 23:177, 1979

57. Theye RA, Michenfelder JD: The effect of nitrous oxide on canine cerebral metabolism. Anesthesiology 29:1119, 1968

58. Carlsson C, Hagerdal M, Siesjo BK: The effect of nitrous oxide on oxygen consumption and blood flow in the cerebral cortex of the rat. Acta Anaesthesiol Scand 20:91, 1976

59. Ingvar M, Abdul-Rahman A, Siesjo BK: Local cerebral glucose consumption in the artificially ventilated rat: Influence of nitrous oxide analgesia and of phenobarbital anesthesia. Acta Physiol Scand 109:177, 1980

60. Ingvar M, Siesjo BK: Effects of nitrous oxide on local cerebral glucose utilization in rats. J Cereb Blood Flow Metab 2:481, 1982

61. Hoffman WE, Miletich DJ, Albrecht RF: The effects of midazolam on cerebral blood flow and oxygen consumption and its interaction with nitrous oxide. Anesth Analg 65:729, 1986

62. Kety SS, Woodford RB, Harmetl MH *et al:* Cerebral blood flow and metabolism in schizophrenia. Effects of barbiturate seminarcosis, insulin coma and electro shock. Am J Psychiatr 104:765, 1947-1948

63. Wechsler RL, Dripps RD, Kety SS: Blood flow and oxygen consumption of the human brain during anesthesia produced by thiopental. Anesthesiology 12:308, 1951

64. McCall ML, Taylor HW: Effect of barbiturate sedation on the brain in toxemia of pregnancy. JAMA 149:51, 1952

65. Pierce ED, Lambertsen CJ, Deutsch S *et al:* Cerebral circulation and metabolism during thiopental anesthesia and hyperventilation in man. J Clin Invest 41:1644, 1962

66. Homburger E, Himwich WA, Etstein B *et al:* Effect of pentothal anesthesia on canine cerebral cortex. Am J Physiol 147:343, 1946

67. Messick JM, Theye RA: Effects of pentobarbital and meperidine on canine cerebral and total oxygen consumption rates. Can Anaesth Soc J 16:321, 1969

68. Nilsson L, Siesjo BK: The effect of phenobarbitone anaesthesia on blood flow and oxygen consumption in the rat brain. Acta Anaesthesiol Scand 57(suppl):18, 1975

69. Michenfelder JD: The interdependency of cerebral functional and metabolic effects following massive doses of thiopental in the dog. Anesthesiology 41:231, 1974

70. Kassell NF, Hitchon PW, Gerk MK *et al:* Alterations in cerebral blood flow, oxygen metabolism and electrical activity produced by high dose sodium thiopental. Neurosurgery 7:598, 1980

71. Baughman VL, Hoffman WE, Miletich DJ *et al:* Effects of phenobarbital on cerebral blood flow and metabolism in young and aged rats. Anesthesiology 65:500, 1986

72. Marin J, Lobato RD, Rico ML: Effect of pentobarbital on the reactivity of isolated human cerebral arteries. J Neurosurg 54:521, 1981

73. Goldman H, Sapirstein LA: Brain blood flow in the conscious and anesthetized rat. Am J Physiol 224:122, 1973

74. Abdul-Rahman A, Dahlgren N, Ingvar M *et al:* Local versus regional cerebral blood flow in the rat at high (hypoxia) and low (phenobarbital anesthesia) flow rates. Acta Physiol Scand 106:53, 1979

75. Laurent J, Lawner P, Simeone F *et al:* Pentobarbital changes compartmental contribution to cerebral blood flow. Neurosurgery 56:510, 1982

76. Sokoloff L, Reivich M, Kennedy C, *et al:* The [^{14}C]deoxyglucose method for the measurement of local cerebral glucose utilization: Theory, procedure, and normal values in the conscious and anesthetized albino rat[1]. Neurochemistry 28:897, 1977

77. Snyder SH: Drug and neurotransmitter receptors in the brain. Science 224:22, 1984

78. Takeshita H, Michenfelder JD, Theye RA: The effects of morphine and n-allylnormorphine on canine cerebral metabolism and circulation. Anesthesiology 37:605, 1972

79. Jobes DR, Kennel E, Bitner R *et al:* Effects of morphine-nitrous oxide anesthesia on cerebral autoregulation. Anesthesiology 42:30, 1975

80. Jobes DR, Kennell EM, Bush GL *et al:* Cerebral blood flow and metabolism during morphine-nitrous oxide anesthesia in man. Anesthesiology 47:16, 1977

81. Michenfelder JD, Theye RA: Effects of fentanyl, droperidol, and innovar on canine cerebral metabolism and blood flow. Br J Anaesth 43:630, 1971

82. Carlsson C, Smith DS, Keykhah MM *et al:* The effects of high dose fentanyl on cerebral circulation and metabolism in rats. Anesthesiology 57:375, 1982

83. Baughman VL, Hoffman WE, Albrecht RE *et al:* Cerebral vascu-

lar and metabolic effects of fentanyl and midazolam in young and aged rats. Anesthesiology 67:314, 1987

84. Keykhah MM, Smith DS, Carlsson C et al: Influence of sufentanil on cerebral metabolism and circulation in the rat. Anesthesiology 63:274, 1985

85. Maekawa T, Tommasino C, Shapiro HM: Local cerebral blood flow with fentanyl-induced seizures. J Cereb Blood Flow Metab 4:88, 1984

86. Sebel PS, Bovill JG, Wauquier A et al: Effects of high-dose fentanyl anesthesia on the electroencephalogram. Anesthesiology 55:203, 1981

87. Bovill JG, Sebel PS, Wauquier A et al: Electroencephalographic effects of sufentanil anaesthesia in man. Br J Anaesth 54:45, 1982

88. Rao TLK, Mummaneni N, El-Etr AA: Convulsion: An unusual response to intravenous fentanyl administration. Anesth Analg 61:1020, 1982

89. Young ML, Smith DS, Greenberg J et al: Effects of sufentanil on regional cerebral glucose utilization in rats. Anesthesiology 61:564, 1984

90. Rockoff MA, Naughton KVH, Shapiro HM et al: Cerebral circulatory and metabolic responses to intravenously administered lorazepam. Anesthesiology 53:215, 1980

91. Denson DD, Myers JA, Thompson GA et al: The influence of diazepam on the serum protein binding of bupivacaine at normal and acidic pH. Anesth Analg 63:980, 1984

92. Sari A, Fukuda Y: Effects of psychotropic drugs on canine cerebral metabolism and circulation related to EEG-diazepam, clomipramine, and chlorpromazine. J Neurol Neurosurg Psychiatr 38:838, 1975

93. Carlsson C, Hagerdal M, Kaasik AE et al: The effects of diazepam on cerebral blood flow and oxygen consumption in rats and its synergistic interaction with nitrous oxide. Anesthesiology 45:319, 1976

94. Nugent M, Artru AA, Michenfelder JD: Cerebral metabolic, vascular and protective effects of midazolam maleate. Comparison to diazepam. Anesthesiology 56:172, 1982

95. Newman LM, Hoffman WE, Miletich DJ et al: Regional blood flow and cerebral metabolic changes during alcohol withdrawal and following midazolam therapy. Anesthesiology 63:395 1985

96. Hoffman WE, Feld JM, Larscheid P et al: Cerebrovascular and cerebral metabolic effects of flurazepam and a benzodiazepine antagonist, 3-hydroxymethyl-beta-carboline. Eur J Pharmacol 106:585, 1985

97. Forster A, Juge O, Louis M et al: Effect of specific benzodiazepine antagonist (RO 15-1788) on cerebral blood flow. Anesth Analg 66:309, 1987

98. Janssen PAJ, Niemegeers CJE, Schellekens KHL et al: Etomidate (R-(+)-ethyl-l-(-methyl-benzyl) imidazole-5-carboxylate) (R 16659)—A potent, short acting and relatively atoxic intravenous hypnotic agent in rats. Arzneim Forsch 21:1234, 1971

99. Milde LN, Milde JH, Michenfelder JF: Cerebral functional, metabolic, and hemodynamic effects of etomidate in dogs. Anesthesiology 63:371, 1985

100. Milde LN, Milde JH: Preservation of cerebral metabolites by etomidate during incomplete cerebral ischemia in dogs. Anesthesiology 65:272, 1986

101. Renou AM, Vernhiet J, Macrez PT et al: Cerebral blood flow and metabolism during etomidate anaesthesia in man. Br J Anaesth 50:1047, 1978

102. David DW, Mans AM, Biebuyck JF et al: Regional brain glucose utilization in rats during anesthesia. Anesthesiology 64:751, 1986

103. Takeshita H, Okuda Y, Sari A: The effects of ketamine on cerebral circulation and metabolism in man. Anesthesiology 36:69, 1972

104. Dawson B, Michenfelder JD, Theye RA: Effects of ketamine on canine cerebral blood flow and metabolism: Modification by prior administration of thiopental. Anesth Analg 50:443, 1971

105. Hoffman WE, Miletich DJ, Albrecht RF: The influence of aging and hypertension on cerebral autoregulation. Brain Res 214:196, 1981

106. Hougaard K, Hansen A, Broderson P: The effect of ketamine on regional cerebral blood flow in man. Anesthesiology 41:562, 1974

107. Nelson SR, Howard RB, Cross RS et al: Ketamine-induced changes in regional glucose utilization in the rat brain. Anesthesiology 52:330, 1980

108. Garvey JM, Rossor M, Iversen LL: Evidence for multiple muscarinic receptor subtypes in human brain. J Neurochem 43:299, 1984

109. Hoffman WE, Albrecht RF, Miletich DJ et al: Cerebrovascular and cerebral metabolic effects of physostigmine, midazolam, and a benzodiazepine antagonist. Anesth Analg 65:639, 1986

110. Blitt CD, Petty WC: Reversal of lorazepam delirium by physostigmine. Anesth Analg 54:607, 1975

111. Caldwell CB, Gross JB: Physostigmine reversal of midazolam-induced sedation. Anesthesiology 57:125, 1982

112. Burkard WP: Histamine H_2-receptor binding with 3H-cimetidine in brain. Eur J Pharmacol 50:449, 1978

113. Vesely R, Hoffman WE, Gil KSL et al: The cerebrovascular effects of curare and histamine in the rat. Anesthesiology 66:519, 1987

114. Moss J, Rosow CE, Savarese JJ et al: Role of histamine in the hypotensive action of d-tubocurarine in humans. Anesthesiology 55:19, 1981

115. Kubota Y: Effects of tubocurarine on plasma histamine concentration in the rat. Br J Anaesth 58:1397, 1986

116. Berntman L, Dahlgren N, Siesjo BK: Influence of intravenously administered catecholamines on cerebral oxygen consumption and blood flow in the rat. Acta Physiol Scand 104:101, 1978

117. King BD, Sokoloff L, Wechsler RL: The effects of 1-epinephrine and 1-norepinephrine upon cerebral circulation and metabolism in man. J Clin Invest 31:273, 1952

118. MacKenzie ET, McCulloch J, O'Keane M et al: Cerebral circulation and norepinephrine: Relevance of the blood-brain barrier. Am J Physiol 231:483, 1976

119. Capraro JA, Reedy DP, Latchaw JP et al: Treatment of acute focal cerebral ischemia with propranolol. Stroke 15:486, 1984

120. Lane NJ: A comparison of the construction of intercellular junctions in the CNS of vertebrates and invertebrates. Trends Neurosci 7:95, 1984

121. O'Brien MD, Jordan MM, Waltz AG: Ischemic cerebral edema and the blood-brain barrier. Arch Neurol 30:461, 1974

122. Williams WT, Lowry RL, Eggers GWN Jr: Anesthetic management during therapeutic disruption of the blood-brain barrier. Anesth Analg 65:188, 1986

123. Klatzo I, Chui E, Fujiwara K et al: Resolution of vasogenic brain edema. Adv Neurol 28:359, 1980

124. Ishikawa T, Funatsu N, Okamoto K et al: Blood-brain barrier function following drug-induced hypotension in the dog. Anesthesiology 59:526, 1983

125. Forster A, Van Horn K, Marshall LF et al: Anesthetic effects on blood-brain barrier function during acute arterial hypertension. Anesthesiology 49:26, 1978

126. Benjamin RS, Wiernik PH, Bachur NR: Adriamycin chemotherapy—Efficacy, safety and pharmacologic basis of intermittent single high-dose schedule. Cancer 33:19, 1974

127. Neuwelt EA, Frenkel EP, Rapoport SI et al: Effect of osmotic blood brain barrier disruption on methotrexate pharmacokinetics in the dog. Neurosurgery 7:36, 1980

128. Rapoport SI, Matthews K, Thompson HK et al: Osmotic opening of blood brain barrier in rhesus monkey without measurable brain edema. Brain Res 136:23, 1977

129. Neuwelt EA, Maravilla KR, Frenkel E et al: The use of enhanced computerized tomography to evaluate osmotic blood brain barrier disruption. Neurosurgery 6:49, 1980

130. Neuwelt EA, Balaban E, Diehl J et al: Successful treatment of primary central nervous system lymphomas with chemotherapy after osmotic blood brain barrier opening. Neurosurgery 12:662, 1983

131. Neuwelt EA, Frenkel EP, Diehl J et al: Reversible osmotic blood brain barrier disruption in humans: Implication for the chemotherapy of malignant brain tumors. Neurosurgery 7:44, 1980

132. Inoue T, Fukui M, Nishio S et al: Hyperosmotic blood-brain barrier disruption in brains of rats with an intracerebrally transplanted RG-C6 tumor. J Neurosurg 66:256, 1987

133. Ball GJ, Gloor P, Thompson CJ: Computed unit-EEG correlations and laminar profiles of spindle waves in electroencephalogram of cats. Electroencephalogr Clin 43:330, 1977

134. Guedel AE: Signs of inhalation anesthesia. In Guedel AE (ed): Inhalation Anesthesia, A Fundamental Guide, p 10. New York, Macmillan, 1938

135. Oshima E, Shingu K, Mori K: EEG activity during halothane anaesthesia in man. Br J Anaesth 53:65, 1981

136. Stockard JJ, Bickford RG: The neurophysiology of anesthesiology. In Amsterdam GE: (ed). A Basis and Practice of Neuroanesthesia, 2nd ed. New York, Exerpta Medica, 1981

137. Scott JC, Ponaganis KV, Stanski DR: EEG quantitation of narcotic effect: The comparative pharmacodynamics of fentanyl and alfentanil. Anesthesiology 62:234, 1985

138. Gain EA, Paletz SG: An attempt to correlate the clinical signs of fluothane anaesthesia with the electroencephalographic levels. Can Anaesth Soc J 4:289, 1957

139. Bassell GM, Cullen BF, Fairchild MD et al: Electroencephalographic and behavioral effects of enflurane and halothane anaesthesia in the cat. Br J Anaesth 54:659, 1982

140. Levy WJ: Power spectrum correlates of changes in consciousness during anesthetic induction with enflurane. Anesthesiology 64:688, 1986

141. Clark DL, Hosick EC, Rosner BS: Neurophysiological effects of different anesthetics in unconscious man. J Appl Physiol 31:884, 1971

142. Moorthy SS, Reddy RV, Paradise RR et al: Reduction of enflurane-induced spike activity by scopolamine. Anesth Analg 59:417, 1980

143. Pichlmayr I, Lips U, Kunkel H: The electroencephalogram in anesthesia. Fundamentals, practical applications, examples. New York, Springer-Verlag, 1984

144. Quasha AL, Tinker JH, Sharbrough FW: Hypothermia plus thiopental: Prolonged electroencephalographic suppression. Anesthesiology 55:636, 1981

145. Todd MM, Drummond JC, Sang H: The hemodynamic consequences of high-dose methohexital anesthesia in humans. Anesthesiology 61:495, 1984

146. Smith NT, Dec-Silver H, Sanford TJ et al: EEGs during high-dose fentanyl-, sufentanil-, or morphine-oxygen anesthesia. Anesth Analg 63:386, 1984

147. Doenicke A, Loffler B, Kugler J et al: Plasma concentration and EEG after various regimens of etomidate. Br J Anaesth 54:393, 1982

148. Arden JR, Holley FO, Stanski DR: Increased sensitivity to etomidate in the elderly: Distribution versus altered brain response. Anesthesiology 65:19, 1986

149. Ghoneim MM, Yamada T: Etomidate: A clinical and electroencephalographic comparison with thiopental. Anesth Analg 56:479, 1977

150. Ebrahim ZY, DeBoer GE, Luders H et al: Effect of etomidate on the electroencephalogram of patients with epilepsy. Anesth Analg 65:1004, 1986

151. Kiloh LG, McComas AJ, Osselton JW: Clinical electroencephalography, 3rd ed. London, Butterworths, 1972

152. Penfield W, Jasper H: Highest level seizures. Res Publ Assoc Nerv Ment Dis 26:252, 1947

153. Gastaut H, Fischer-Williams M: Encephalographic study of syncope, its differentiation from epilepsy. Lancet II: 1018, 1957

154. Jasper H, Droogeleever-Fortuyn J: Experimental studies on the functional anatomy of petit mal epilepsy. Res Publ Assoc Nerv Ment Dis 26:272, 1947

155. Janeway R, Ravens RJ, Pearce LA et al: Progressive myoclonus epilepsy with Lafora inclusion bodies. Arch Neurol 16:565, 1967

156. Ward AA: The epileptic neurone. Epilepsia 2:70, 1961

157. Wyllie E, Luders H, Morris HH et al: Ipsilateral forced head and eye turning at the end of the generalized tonic-clonic phase of versive seizures. Neurology 36:1212, 1986

158. Ralston BL: Mechanisms of transition of interictal spiking foci into ictal seizure discharges. Electroencephalogr Clin Neurophysiol 10:217, 1958

159. Walter WG: The location of cerebral tumours by electroencephalography. Lancet II: 305, 1936

160. Bagchi BK, Kooi KA, Selving BT et al: Subtentorial tumours and other lesions: An electroencephalographic study of 121 cases. Electroencephalogr Clin Neurophysiol 13:180, 1961

161. Williams D, Denny-Brown D: Cerebral electrical changes in experimental concussion. Brain 64:223, 1941

162. Ulett GA: Clinical and experimental studies of mild head injuries. Electroencephalogr Clin Neurophysiol 7:496, 1955

163. Dawson RE, Webster JE, Gurdjiian ES: Serial electroencephalography in acute head injuries. J Neurosurg 8:613, 1951

164. Kaufman IC, Walker AE: The electroencephalogram after head injury. J Nerv Ment Dis 109:383, 1949

165. Titeca J: Contribution of EEG to the study of hemiplegias of vascular origin. J Belg Med Phys Rhum 11:89, 1965

166. Roger J, Naquet R, Gastaut H et al: Electroencephalographic and electrocardiographic manifestations provoked by carotid compression in cerebral circulatory insufficiencies. In Gastaut H, Meyer JS (eds): Cerebral Anoxia and the Electroencephalogram. Springfield, Charles C Thomas, 1961

167. Ingvar DH: The pathophysiology of occlusive cerebrovascular disorders. Acta Neurol Scand 43(Suppl 31):93, 1967

168. Levy WJ, Grundy BL, Smith NT: Monitoring the electroencephalogram and evoked potentials during anesthesia. In Saidman LJ, Smith NT (eds): Monitoring in Anesthesia, pp 238–245. Boston, Butterworths, 1984

169. Bickford RG, Billinger TW, Fleming NI et al: The compressed spectral array (CSA)—A pictorial EEG. Proc San Diego Biomed Symp 11:365, 1972

170. Fleming RA, Smith NT: Density modulation: A technique for the display of three-variable data in patient monitoring. Anesthesiology 50:543, 1979

171. Demetrescu M: The aperiodic character of the electroencephalogram (EEG): New approach to data analysis and condensation (abstr). Physiologist 18:189, 1975

172. Levy WJ, Shapiro HM, Maruchak G et al: Automated EEG processing for intraoperative monitoring: A comparison of techniques. Anesthesiology 53:223, 1980

173. Bart AH, Homi J, Linde HW: Changes in power spectra of electroencephalograms during anesthesia with fluroxene, methoxyflurane, and ethrane. Anesth Analg 50:53, 1971

174. Chiappa KH, Burke SR, Young RR: Results of electroencephalographic monitoring during 367 carotid endarterectomies: Use of a dedicated minicomputer. Stroke 10:381, 1979

175. Stockard JJ, Bickford RG, Myers RR et al: Hypotension-induced changes in cerebral function during cardiac surgery. Stroke 5:730, 1974

176. Emerson RG, Pedley TA: Generator sources of median somatosensory evoked potentials. J Clin Neurophysiol 1:203, 1984
177. Ganes T, Lundar T: The effect of thiopentone on somatosensory evoked responses and EEGs in comatose patient. J Neurol Psych 46:509, 1983
178. Drummond JC, Todd MM, Hoi Sang U: The effect of high dose sodium thiopental on brain stem auditory and median nerve somatosensory evoked responses in humans. Anesthesiology 64:249, 1985
179. Abrahamian HA, Allison T, Goff WR et al: Effects of thiopental on human cerebral evoked responses. Anesthesiology 24:650, 1963
180. Pathak KS, Brown RH, Cascorbi HF et al: Effect of fentanyl and morphine on intraoperative somatosensory cortical-evoked potentials. Anesth Analg 63:833, 1984
181. Grundy BL, Brown RH, Berilla JA: Fentanyl alters somatosensory cortical evoked potentials (abstr). Anesth Analg 59:544, 1980
182. Peterson DO, Drummond JC, Todd MM: Effects of halothane, enflurane, isoflurane and nitrous oxide on somatosensory evoked potentials in humans. Anesthesiology 65:35, 1986
183. Pathak KS, Ammadio M, Kalamchi A et al: Effects of halothane, enflurane, and isoflurane on somatosensory evoked potentials during nitrous oxide anesthesia. Anesthesiology 66:753, 1987
184. McPherson RW, Mahla M, Johnson R et al: Effects of enflurane, isoflurane, and nitrous oxide on somatosensory evoked potentials during fentanyl anesthesia. Anesthesiology 62:626, 1985
185. Sebel PS, Ingram DA, Flynn PJ et al: Evoked potentials during isoflurane anaesthesia. Br J Anaesth 58:580, 1986
186. Samra SK, Vanderzant CW, Domer PA et al: Differential effects of isoflurane on human median nerve somatosensory evoked potentials. Anesthesiology 66:29, 1987
187. Grundy BL, Jannetta PJ, Procopio PT et al: Intraoperative monitoring of brain-stem auditory evoked potentials. J Neurosurg 57:674, 1982
188. Manninen PH, Lam AM, Nicholas JF: The effects of isoflurane and isoflurane-nitrous oxide anesthesia on brainstem auditory evoked potentials in humans. Anesth Analg 64:43, 1985
189. Jones JG: The effects of isoflurane on the auditory evoked response in man. Br J Anaesth 57:352P, 1985
190. Heneghan CPH, James MFM, Jones JG: Effects of halothane or enflurane with controlled ventilation on auditory evoked potentials. Br J Anaesth 56:315, 1984
191. Navaratnarajah M, Thornton C, Heneghan CPH et al: Effect of etomidate on the auditory evoked response in man. Br J Anaesth 55:1157, 1983
192. Samra SK, Lilly DJ, Rush NL et al: Fentanyl anesthesia and human brain-stem auditory evoked potentials. Anesthesiology 61:261, 1984
193. Thornton C, Heneghen CPH, Navaratnarajah M et al: Effect of etomidate on the auditory evoked response in man. Br J Anaesth 57:554, 1985
194. Sebel PS, Flynn PJ, Ingram DA: Effect of nitrous oxide on visual, auditory and somatosensory evoked potentials. Br J Anaesth 56:1403, 1984
195. Chi OZ, Field C: Effects of isoflurane on visual evoked potentials in humans. Anesthesiology 65:328, 1986
196. Uhl RR, Squires KC, Bruce DL et al: Effect of halothane anesthesia on the human cortical visual evoked response. Anesthesiology 53:273, 1980
197. Langfitt TW, Tannanbaum HM, Kassell NF et al: Acute intracranial hypertension, cerebral blood flow and the EEG. Electroencephalogr Clin Neurophysiol 20:139, 1966
198. Gravenstein N, Grundy BL, Reid SA: The central nervous system. In Martin JT (ed): Positioning in Anesthesia and Surgery, 2nd ed, p 291. Philadelphia, WB Saunders, 1987
199. Cutler RWP, Page LK, Galicich J: Formation and absorption of cerebrospinal fluid in man. Brain 91:707, 1968
200. Rosenberg GA, Saland L, Kyner WT: Pathophysiology of periventricular tissue changes with raised CSF pressure in cats. J Neurosurg 59:606, 1983
201. Burney RG, Winn R: Increased cerebrospinal fluid pressure during laryngoscopy and intubation for induction of anesthesia. Anesth Analg 54:687, 1975
202. Yano M, Nishiyama H, Yokota H et al: Effect of lidocaine on ICP response to endotracheal suctioning. Anesthesiology 64:651, 1986
203. White PF, Schlobohm RM, Pitts LH et al: A randomized study of drugs for preventing increases in intracranial pressure during endotracheal suctioning. Anesthesiology 57:242, 1982
204. Minton MD, Grosslight K, Stirt JA et al: Increases in intracranial pressure from succinylcholine: Prevention by prior nondepolarizing blockade. Anesthesiology 65:165, 1986
205. Dohi S, Matsumoto M, Takahashi T: The effects of nitroglycerin on cerebrospinal fluid pressure in awake and anesthetized humans. Anesthesiology 54:511, 1981
206. Turner JM, Powell D, Gibson RM et al: Intracranial pressure changes in neurosurgical patients during hypotension induced with sodium nitroprusside or trimethaphan. Br J Anaesth 49:419, 1977
207. Cottrell JE, Gupta B, Rapaport H et al: Intracranial pressure during nitroglycerin-induced hypotension. J Neurosurg 53:309, 1980
208. Morris PJ, Todd M, Philbin D: Changes in canine intracranial pressure in response to infusions of sodium nitroprusside and trinitroglycerin. Br J Anaesth 54:991, 1982
209. Marsh ML, Aidinis SJ, Naughton KVH et al: The technique of nitroprusside administration modifies the intracranial pressure response. Anesthesiology 54:538, 1979
210. Hantler CB, Knight PR: Intracranial hypertension following cross-clamping of the thoracic aorta. Anesthesiology 56:146, 1982
211. Hayashi M, Kobayashi H, Kawano H et al: The effects of local intraparenchymal pentobarbital on intracranial hypertension following experimental subarachnoid hemorrhage. Anesthesiology 66:758, 1987
212. Shapiro HM, Galindo A, Wyte SR et al: Rapid intraoperative reduction on intracranial pressure with thiopentone. Br J Anaesth 45:1057, 1973
213. Giffin JP, Cottrell JE, Shwiry B et al: Intracranial pressure, mean arterial pressure, and heart rate following midazolam or thiopental in humans with brain tumors. Anesthesiology 60:491, 1984
214. Moss E, Powell D, Gibson RM et al: Effect of etomidate on intracranial pressure and cerebral perfusion pressure. Br J Anaesth 51:347, 1979
215. Dearden NM, McDowall DG: Comparison of etomidate and althesin in the reduction of increased intracranial pressure after head injury. Br J Anaesth 57:361, 1985
216. Woodcock J, Ropper AH, Kennedy SK: High dose barbiturates in non-traumatic brain swelling: ICP reduction and effect on outcome. Stroke 13:785, 1982
217. Rea GL, Rockswold GL: Barbiturate therapy in uncontrolled intracranial hypertension. Neurosurgery 12:401, 1983
218. Wyte SR, Shapiro HM, Turner P et al: Ketamine-induced intracranial hypertension. Anesthesiology 36:174, 1972
219. Thorsen T, Gran L: Ketamine/diazepam infusion anaesthesia with special attention to the effect on cerebrospinal fluid pressure and arterial blood pressure. Acta Anaesthesiol Scand 24:1, 1980
220. Artru AA: Effects of halothane and fentanyl on the rate of CSF production in dogs. Anesth Analg 62:581, 1983

221. Artru AA: Effects of halothane and fentanyl anesthesia on resistance to reabsorption of CSF. J Neurosurg 60:252, 1984

222. Artru AA: Relationship between cerebral blood volume and CSF pressure during anesthesia with isoflurane or fentanyl in dogs. Anesthesiology 60:575, 1984

223. Artru AA: A comparison of the effects of isoflurane, enflurane, halothane and fentanyl on cerebral blood volume and ICP (abstr). Anesthesiology 57:A374, 1982

224. Mann JD, Cookson SL, Mann ES: Differential effects of pentobarbital, ketamine hydrochloride, and enflurane anesthesia on CSF formation rate and outflow resistance in the rat. In Shulman K, Marmarous A, Miller JD et al (eds): Intracranial Pressure IV, p 466. Berlin, Springer-Verlag, 1980

225. Artru AA, Nugent M, Michenfelder JD: Enflurane causes a prolonged and reversible increase in the rate of CSF production in the dog. Anesthesiology 57:255, 1982

226. Adams RW, Gronert GA, Sundt TM Jr et al: Halothane, hypocapnia and cerebrospinal fluid pressure in neurosurgery. Anesthesiology 37:510, 1972

227. Zattoni J, Siani C, Rivano C: The effects of ethrane on intracranial pressure. Proceedings of the First European Symposium on Modern Anesthetic Agents. Anesthesiol Resus 84:272, 1975

228. Adams RW, Cucchiara RF, Gronert GA et al: Isoflurane and cerebrospinal fluid pressure in neurosurgical patients. Anesthesiology 54:97, 1981

229. Grosslight K, Foster R, Colohan AR et al: Isoflurane for neuroanesthesia: Risk factors for increases in intracranial pressure. Anesthesiology 63:533, 1985

230. Artru AA: Isoflurane does not increase the rate of CSF production in the dog. Anesthesiology 60:193, 1984

231. Artru AA: Effects of enflurane and isoflurane on resistance to reabsorption of cerebrospinal fluid in dogs. Anesthesiology 61:529, 1984

232. Moss E, McDowall DG: I.C.P. increases with 50% nitrous oxide in oxygen in severe head injuries during controlled ventilation. Br J Anaesth 51:757, 1979

233. Henriksen HT, Jorgensen PB: The effect of nitrous oxide on intracranial pressure in patients with intracranial disorders. Br J Anaesth 45:486, 1973

234. Misfeldt BB, Jorgensen PB, Rishoj M: The effect of nitrous oxide and halothane upon the intracranial pressure in hypocapnic patients with intracranial disorders. Br J Anaesth 46:853, 1974

235. Gordon E, Greitz T: The effect of nitrous oxide on the cerebrospinal fluid pressure during encephalography. Br J Anaesth 42:2, 1970

236. Cottrell JE, Hartung J, Giffin JP et al: Intracranial and hemodynamic changes after succinylcholine administration in cats. Anesth Analg 62:1006, 1983

237. McLeskey CH, Cullen BF, Kennedy RD et al: Control of cerebral perfusion pressure during induction of anesthesia in high-risk neurosurgical patients. Anesth Analg 53:985, 1974

238. Halldin M, Wahlin H: Effect of succinylcholine on intraspinal fluid pressure. Acta Anaesthesiol Scand 38:155, 1959

239. Lanier WL, Milde JH, Michenfelder JD: Cerebral stimulation following succinylcholine in dogs. Anesthesiology 64:551, 1986

240. Huseby JS, Pavlin EG, Butler J: Effect of positive end-expiratory pressure on intracranial pressure in dogs. J Appl Physiol 44:25, 1978

241. Aidinis SJ, Lafferty J, Shapiro HM: Intracranial responses to PEEP. Anesthesiology 45:275, 1976

242. Todd MM, Toutant SM, Shapiro HM: The effects of high-frequency positive-pressure ventilation on intracranial pressure and brain surface movement in cats. Anesthesiology 54:496, 1981

243. Haggendal E, Lofgren J, Nilsson JN et al: Effects of varied cerebrospinal fluid pressure on cerebral blood flow in dogs. Acta Physiol Scand 79:262, 1970

244. Zwetnow NN: Effects of increased cerebrospinal fluid pressure on the blood flow and on the energy metabolism of the brain. Acta Physiol Scand Suppl 339:1, 1970

245. Fieschi C, Beduschi A, Agnoli A et al: Regional cerebral blood flow and intraventricular pressure in acute brain injuries. Eur Neurol 8:192, 1972

246. Bruce DA, Langfitt TW, Miller JD et al: Regional cerebral blood flow, intracranial pressure, and brain metabolism in comatose patients. J Neurosurg 38:131, 1973

247. Overgaard J, Tweed WA: Cerebral circulation after head injury. Part 1: Cerebral blood flow and its regulation after closed head injury with emphasis on clinical correlations. J Neurosurg 41:531, 1974

248. Kety SS, Shenkin HA, Schmidt CF: The effects of increased intracranial pressure on cerebral circulatory functions in man. J Clin Invest 27:493, 1948

249. Enevoldsen EM, Cold G, Jensen FT et al: Dynamic changes in regional CBF, intraventricular pressure, CSF pH and lactate levels during the acute phase of head injury. J Neurosurg 44:191, 1976

250. Enevoldsen EM, Jensen FT: Autoregulation and CO_2 responses of cerebral blood flow in patients with acute severe head injury. J Neurosurg 48:689, 1978

251. Miller JD, Garibi J, North JB et al: Effects of increased arterial pressure on blood flow in the damaged brain. J Neurol Neurosurg Psychiatr 38:657, 1975

252. Fieschi C, Battistini N, Beduschi A et al: Regional cerebral blood flow and intraventricular pressure in acute head injuries. J Neurol Neurosurg Psychiatr 37:1378, 1974

253. Levin AB, Duff TA, Javid MJ: Treatment of increased intracranial pressure: A comparison of different hyperosmotic agents and the use of thiopental. Neurosurgery 5:570, 1979

254. Muizelaar JP, Lutz HA III, Becker DP: Effect of mannitol on ICP and CBF and correlation with pressure autoregulation in severely head-injured patients. J Neurosurg 61:700, 1984

255. McGraw CP, Howard G: Effect of mannitol on increased intracranial pressure. Neurosurgery 23:269, 1983

256. Levin VA, Hoffman WF, Heilbron DC: Prognostic significance of the pretreatment CT scan on time to progression for patients with malignant gliomas. J Neurosurg 52:642, 1980

257. Murovic J, Turowski K, Wilson CB et al: Computerized tomography in the prognosis of malignant cerebral gliomas. J Neurosurg 65:799, 1986

258. Fletcher WA, Imes RK, Hoyt WF: Chiasmal gliomas: Appearance and long-term changes demonstrated by computerized tomography. J Neurosurg 65:154, 1986

259. Moss AA, Gamsa G, Genant HK: Computed Tomography of the Body. Philadelphia, WB Saunders, 1983

260. Stark DD, Bradley WG: Magnetic Resonance Imaging. St. Louis, CV Mosby, 1988

261. Brant-Zawadzki M, Norman D, Newton TH et al: Magnetic resonance of the brain: The optimal screening technique. Radiology 152:71, 1984

262. Kuroiwa T, Seida M, Tomida S: Discrepancies among CT, histological, and blood-brain barrier findings in early cerebral ischemia. J Neurosurg 65:517, 1986

263. Gooding GAW, Edwards MSB, Rabkin AE et al: Intraoperative real-time ultrasound in the localization of intracranial neoplasms. Radiology 146:459, 1983

264. Rubin JM, Dohrmann GJ: Intraoperative neurosurgical ultrasound in the localization and characterization of intracranial masses. Radiology 148:519, 1983

265. Smith J, Vogelzang L, Marzano M: Brain edema: Ultrasound examination. Radiology 155:379, 1985

266. Hawkes RC, Holland GN, Moore WS et al: Nuclear magnetic resonance (NMR) tomography of the brain: A preliminary clini-

cal-assessment with demonstration of pathology. J Comput Assist Tomogr 4:577, 1980

267. Bryan RN, Willcott MR, Schnieders NJ *et al:* Nuclear magnetic resonance evaluation of stroke. A preliminary report. Radiology 149:189, 1983

268. Clifton GL, Grossman RG, Makela ME: Neurological course and correlated computerized tomography findings after severe closed head injury. J Neurosurg 52:611, 1980

269. Lobato RD, Sarabia R, Rivas JJ *et al:* Normal computerized tomography scans in severe head injury. J Neurosurg 65:784, 1986

270. Han JS, Kaufman B, Alfidi RF *et al:* Head trauma evaluated by magnetic resonance and computed tomography: A comparison. Radiology 150:71, 1984

271. Gandy SE, Snow RB, Zimmerman RD *et al:* Cranial nuclear magnetic resonance imaging in head trauma. Ann Neurol 16:254, 1984

272. Levin HS, Amparo E, Eisenberg HM *et al:* Magnetic resonance imaging and computerized tomography in relation to the neurobehavioral sequelae of mild and moderate head injuries. J Neurosurg 66:706, 1987

273. Langfitt TW, Obrist WD, Alavi A *et al:* Computerized tomography, magnetic resonance imaging, and positron emission tomography in the study of brain traumas. Preliminary observations. J Neurosurg 64:760, 1986

274. Lunsford LD, Martinez AJ: Stereotactic exploration of the brain in the era of computed tomography. Surg Neurol 22:222, 1984

275. Leksell L, Herner T, Leksell D: Visualisation of stereotactic radiolesions by nuclear magnetic resonance. J Neurol Neurosurg Psychiatr 48:19, 1985

276. Lunsford LD, Martinez AJ, Latchaw RE: Stereotaxic surgery with a magnetic resonance- and computerized tomography-compatible system. J Neurosurg 64:872, 1986

277. Berger MS: Ultrasound-guided stereotaxic biopsy using a new apparatus. J Neurosurg 65:550, 1986

278. Sedvall G, Farde L, Persson A *et al:* Imaging of neurotransmitter receptors in the living human brain. Arch Gen Psychiatr 43:995, 1986

279. Wagner HN: Chemical neurotransmission in man. Curr Concepts Diagnos Nucl Med, Winter, p 14, 1986

280. Thomas KD, Greer DM, Couch MW *et al:* Radiation dosimetry of I-123 HEAT, an alpha-1 receptor imaging agent. J Nucl Med 28:1745, 1987

281. Thornoor CM, Couch MW, Greer DM *et al:* In vivo binding in rat brain and radiopharmaceutical preparation of radioiodinated HEAT, an alpha-1 adrenoceptor ligand. J Nucl Med (in press)

282. Wagner HN, Burns HD, Dannals RF *et al:* Imaging dopamine receptors in the human brain by positron tomography. Science 4617:1264, 1983

283. Frost JJ, Wagner HN, Dannals RF *et al:* Imaging opiate receptors in the human brain by positron tomography. J Comput Assist Tomogr 9:231, 1985

284. Kuhar MJ, Pert CB, Snyder SH: Regional distribution of opiate receptor binding in monkey and human brain. Nature 245:447, 1973

285. Frost JJ, Mayberg HS, Berlin F: Alteration in brain opiate receptor binding in man following sexual arousal using C-11 carfentanil and positron emission tomography (abstr). J Nucl Med 27:1027, 1986

286. Fowler JS, MacGregor RR, Wolf AP *et al:* Mapping human brain monoamine oxidase A and B with ^{11}C-labeled suicide inactivators and PET. Science 235:481, 1987

287. Smith DS, Chance B: New techniques, new opportunities, old problems. Anesthesiology 67:157, 1987

288. Budinger TF, Cullander C: Health effects of *in vivo* nuclear magnetic resonance. In James TL, Margulis AR (eds): Biomedical Magnetic Resonance, p 7. San Francisco, Radiology Research and Education Foundation, 1984

289. Wyrwicz AM, Yao-En Li, Schofield JC *et al:* Multiple environments of fluorinated anesthetics in intact tissues observed with ^{19}F NMR spectroscopy. FEBS Lett 162:334, 1983

290. Wyrwicz AM, Pszenny MH, Schofield JC *et al:* Noninvasive observations of fluorinated anesthetics in rabbit brain by fluorine-19 nuclear magnetic resonance. Science 222:428, 1983

291. Litt L, Gonzalez-Mendez R, James TL *et al:* An in vivo study of halothane uptake and elimination in the rat brain with fluorine nuclear magnetic resonance spectroscopy. Anesthesiology 67:161, 1987

292. Mills P, Sessler DI, Mosely M *et al:* An in vivo ^{19}F nuclear magnetic resonance study of isoflurane elimination from the rabbit brain. Anesthesiology 67:169, 1987

Chapter 31

Roy F. Cucchiara
Susan Black
Jeffrey A. Steinkeler

Anesthesia for Intracranial Procedures

In neurosurgery, the anesthesiologist has a definite impact on making the surgical procedure possible, safe, and even easier. Although sometimes difficult, communication between anesthesiologist and neurosurgeon is essential to provide the very best operating conditions and the safest anesthetic care. This communication must be based on known facts tempered with experience. We are involved because we are interested in the patient's safety, provision of the best operating conditions, and provision of high quality anesthesia care. We must be knowledgeable about the physiology, pathology, and pharmacology of the brain to apply clinical principles effectively in the operating room.

BASIC PRINCIPLES OF NEUROANESTHESIA

CEREBRAL BLOOD FLOW AND METABOLISM

Autoregulation

In the normal brain, cerebral blood flow (CBF) is regulated to provide adequate oxygen and substrate supply to meet the metabolic needs of the tissue. Normal human CBF is 40 to 54 ml · 100 gm^{-1} · min^{-1}.[1-5] Cerebral blood flow is influenced by many physiologic and pathologic factors, including metabolic requirements, cerebral perfusion pressure, and arterial partial pressures of carbon dioxide (Pa_{CO_2}) and oxygen (Pa_{O_2}). In addition, drugs, cerebrovascular diseases, and pathologic processes resulting in loss of autoregulation or increased intracranial pressure affect CBF.[6]

Autoregulation is the maintenance of a constant CBF over a wide range of cerebral perfusion pressures (CPP). Cerebral perfusion pressure is equal to mean arterial pressure (MAP) minus intracranial pressure (ICP). Increases in ICP or decreases in MAP will both result in a decreased CPP. In patients without neurologic or vascular pathology, CBF is constant between the range of MAPs of 50 to 150 mm Hg. With increases in MAP, arteriolar vasoconstriction occurs, and, with reductions in MAP, vasodilation occurs to maintain CBF. Above and below the limits of autoregulation, the vasoconstrictive and vasodilatory capacity of the cerebral vasculature is exhausted, and flow follows pressure passively.[6, 7]

Autoregulation is affected by many factors. Chronic hypertension results in a shift of the autoregulatory curve to the right so that, with hypotension, CBF begins to decrease early, passively following decreases in pressure above a MAP of 50 mm Hg, but autoregulation is maintained during hypertension to a higher MAP than in normotensive patients.[8, 9] Chronic antihypertensive therapy with adequate blood pressure control results in a return of the autoregulatory range toward normal.[9] Cerebral autoregulation is impaired in regions of cerebral ischemia. CBF decreases passively as MAP decreases, indicating a failure of autoregulation during relative hypotension.[10] Hypertension results in no increase in CBF in regions of ischemia.[10, 11] This observation is explained by some as due to intact autoregulation to increasing perfusion pressures.[11] Others suggest that blood flow to the ischemic area (*via* collaterals) is already maximal, and cannot increase further with increases in pressure.[10] Impaired cerebral autoregulation might also be expected in areas of relative ischemia surrounding mass lesions, following grand mal seizures,[6] after head injury,[12] and during hypercarbia and hypoxemia.[6]

Many drugs used perioperatively affect cerebral autoregulation. Volatile anesthetic drugs narrow the pressure range over which CBF is autoregulated. This effect increases with increasing concentrations. At 1.0 MAC halothane or enflurane autoregulation is abolished, while, at 0.5 MAC, autoregulation is partially maintained.[13] Isoflurane impairs autoregulation less than halothane.[14] Intact cerebral autoregulation has been demonstrated in healthy volunteers anesthetized with morphine (2 mg·kg^{-1}) and 70% N_2O.[15] Fentanyl does not impair cerebral autoregulation.[16] In general, drugs that are cerebral vasodilators, such as the volatile anesthetics, impair cerebral autoregulation, and agents such as the opioids, that cause cerebral vasoconstriction, do not (Table 31-1).

CBF varies directly with Pa_{CO_2}. CBF is most sensitive to changes in Pa_{CO_2} over a range of Pa_{CO_2} values from 20 to 80 mm Hg.[3, 17] CBF increases linearly with increasing Pa_{CO_2}, increasing 1 ml·100 g^{-1}·min^{-1} for each 1 mm Hg increase in Pa_{CO_2} from 20 to 60 mm Hg.[18] Outside these values, there is a plateau in the CBF response to changes in Pa_{CO_2} such that further increases above a Pa_{CO_2} of 80 mm Hg or decreases below a Pa_{CO_2} of 20 mm Hg result in little further change in CBF.[17, 18] Several factors influence the normal CBF response to changing Pa_{CO_2}. Areas of regional cerebral ischemia in which maximal vasodilation has occurred in response to inadequate tissue perfusion have been demonstrated to have an altered responsiveness to changes in Pa_{CO_2}.[19, 20, 21] Following severe head injury, CBF responsiveness to changes in Pa_{CO_2} may be altered.[12] Aging also alters the responsiveness of CBF to changes in Pa_{CO_2}. With aging, both the vasoconstrictive response to hypocapnia[22] and the vasodilator response to hypercapnia are blunted.[23] This has been attributed to the "normal" mild degrees of atherosclerosis occurring with aging.[22, 23] In patients with risk factors for cerebrovascular disease, the response to hypercarbia is more affected than by normal aging, and is severely altered in patients with symptomatic cerebrovascular disease.[23]

Many agents used intraoperatively may alter the effect of changes in Pa_{CO_2} on CBF. CBF increases linearly with increases in Pa_{CO_2} between 30 and 56 mm Hg during isoflurane anesthesia at 1 MAC in dogs.[24] Likewise, the CBF response to changes in Pa_{CO_2} is linear between a Pa_{CO_2} of 20-60 mm Hg in dogs under halothane anesthesia.[25, 26] Because these drugs can cause an increase in CBF (halothane more than isoflurane), the combination of a volatile anesthetic and hypercarbia can result in higher levels of CBF than either alone. Intravenous drugs resulting in cerebral vasoconstriction, such as barbiturates, midazolam, fentanyl, and Innovar, also result in a preservation of a linear CBF responsiveness to alterations in Pa_{CO_2}. However, with these drugs, decreases in CBF in response to decreases in Pa_{CO_2} may be blunted.[16, 25, 27-29] Most commonly used volatile and intravenous anesthetic drugs result in a preservation of the CBF response to alterations in Pa_{CO_2} in the clinical situation (Table 31-1).

Changes in Pa_{O_2} have little effect on CBF at normal values. However, hypoxemia is a potent cerebral vasodilator and, at values of Pa_{O_2} below 50 mm Hg, CBF increases markedly. Near maximal vasodilation occurs. Flow follows perfusion pressure passively, and changes in Pa_{CO_2} have little, if any, effect on CBF. High levels of Pa_{O_2} achieved at 1 ATM result in minimal cerebral vasoconstriction.[6, 30]

Cerebral Ischemia

Cerebral ischemia can be categorized as complete or incomplete, and as global or focal. During complete cerebral ischemia, there is no blood flow to the brain, as in cardiac arrest. In this situation, cerebral electrical activity ceases within seconds, and irreversible cell damage occurs within 4-5 min. Following restoration of CBF after an episode of complete cerebral ischemia, a brief period of hyperemia is followed by a period of hypoperfusion lasting at least 6 h. This phenomenon may contribute significantly to tissue damage. During incomplete ischemia, some cerebral blood flow persists, although it is inadequate to meet metabolic demands. This is the situation during severe hypotension and when ischemic regions are supplied by collateral blood flow. In this situation, some electrical activity persists, and the degree of cell damage depends both on duration of ischemia and degree of reduction of blood flow. Global cerebral ischemia reflects inadequate blood flow to all regions of the brain. Focal ischemia involves only tissue in the distribution of a particular vessel. Tissue tolerance to focal cerebral ischemia depends on the degree to which flow is obstructed, availability of blood flow via collateral vessels, and duration of the ischemia.[31-33] Intraoperatively focal and incomplete ischemia are more commonly encountered than complete global ischemia.

Diagnosis of cerebral ischemia depends on the ability to assess function of the central nervous system. In an awake patient, alterations in mental status and changes in or new appearance of neurologic deficits occur with cerebral ischemia. Many methods have been devised in an attempt to detect cerebral ischemia intraoperatively. Monitoring the unprocessed EEG,[34] processed EEG,[35] and evoked potentials[36] allow intraoperative monitoring of neurologic function. All demonstrate characteristic progressive changes with worsening degrees of cerebral ischemia.

Other methods assess risk of developing cerebral ischemia. These include measurement of CBF and comparison of that value with "minimal" acceptable CBF.[37] "Critical" CBF is that flow below which EEG changes occur. The Kety-Schmidt technique and its modifications are utilized both in humans and experimental animals to measure CBF.[2] Tissue clearance techniques are also utilized in which a radioactive labelled substance (usually ^{133}Xe) is administered via inhalation or intra-

TABLE 31-1.

	AUTOREGULATION	CBF RESPONSE TO INCREASED Pa_{CO_2}	CBF RESPONSE TO DECREASED Pa_{CO_2}
Halothane	Impaired	Intact	Intact
Enflurane	Impaired	Intact	Intact
Isoflurane	Less impaired than with halothane	Intact	Intact
Thiopental	Intact	Intact	Blunted
Opioids	Intact	Intact	Blunted

arterially, and the washout of radioactivity is measured to determine CBF. Blood flow in the middle cerebral artery following internal carotid artery occlusion will determine the rate of radioactive decay, and the measured CBF will reflect the blood supply to the potentially ischemic brain.[37] In addition, stump pressures have been suggested to accurately reflect adequacy of collateral circulation during carotid artery cross clamping. However, this measure is felt by some not to accurately reflect CBF, agreeing with CBF measurement and EEG analysis in only 58% of cases, with a high rate of both false positives (28%) and false negatives (14%).[38] In anesthetized patients continuous monitoring of the EEG and determination of CBF have proved to reliably predict the occurrence of cerebral ischemia.[34, 38]

Effects of Anesthetic Agents on Cerebral Blood Flow and CMRO₂

INHALATION AGENTS. The volatile anesthetic agents are direct cerebral vasodilators that cause an increase in CBF[14, 24, 39-44] and also depress cerebral metabolism, decreasing cerebral metabolic rate for oxygen (CMRO₂) and glucose.[14, 24, 40, 43-45] As a result, they are said to "uncouple" the relationship between CBF and metabolism (Fig. 31-1). A number of studies in both animal models and man have indicated that halothane is the most potent cerebral vasodilator and isoflurane is the least potent cerebral vasodilator of the three commonly used volatile anesthetic drugs.[14, 39, 41-44, 46] Enflurane in higher concentrations (1.5 MAC) and in combination with hypocapnea has been documented to cause seizure activity that results in a marked increase in both CBF and CMRO₂.[43]

Increases in CBF due to volatile anesthetic-induced decreases in cerebrovascular resistance (CVR) lead to increases in cerebral blood volume (CBV) with resultant increases in ICP.[47] This effect is potentially deleterious in neurosurgical patients with altered intracranial compliance. Halothane-induced increases in CBF and resultant increase in ICP seen in some neurosurgical patients can be prevented by hyperventilation of the lungs prior to the addition of halothane to the inspired gas mixture. However, simultaneous institution of hyperventilation with administration of halothane will not blunt the increases in CBF and ICP caused by halothane.[48] In contrast, increases in CBF and ICP caused by isoflurane in neurosurgical patients are effectively blocked by simultaneous institution of hyperventilation.[49] The combination of isoflurane anesthesia and marked hyperventilation (Pa$_{CO_2}$ 20–25 mm Hg) has been demonstrated to cause a decrease in CBF.[50] This decrease in CBF, even during isoflurane-induced hypotension, did not result in adverse effects on the cerebral metabolic balance.[51]

Volatile anesthetics cause a dose-dependent decrease in CMRO₂. This response is nonlinear at concentrations below 1.0 MAC, with the greatest decrease in CMRO₂ occurring at the anesthetic concentrations causing a change in the EEG pattern from awake to anesthetized.[45] The degree of depression of cerebral metabolism varies among halothane, enflurane, and isoflurane. Both enflurane and halothane result in decreases in CMRO₂ of 16%–30%.[40, 42, 43] However, with enflurane-induced seizure activity, CMRO₂ increases by 48%.[43] Isoflurane causes the greatest decrease in CMRO₂. In clinically relevant concentrations, 2.0 MAC, isoflurane results in complete suppression of cerebral electrical activity and a decrease of CMRO₂ to approximately 50% of control values. This property of isoflurane is unique among the currently available volatile agents.[14, 24, 44, 52, 53]

It has been suggested that the net effect on CBF of a volatile anesthetic agent is a combination of the direct cerebral vasodilation to increase CBF and the indirect decrease in CBF "coupled" to the decrease in CMRO₂. Isoflurane causes the greatest degree of depression of cerebral metabolism opposing the direct vasodilator properties with a net result of little to no change in CBF. In animal studies with maximal depression of cerebral electrical activity by barbiturates prior to the administration of isoflurane and halothane, both agents resulted in equal increases in CBF and decreases in cerebral vascular resistance.[39] This supports the concept that isoflurane has as potent a direct vasodilator activity as halothane, and that the markedly different effects on CBF in most clinical situations are due to the more potent depressant effect on cerebral metabolism of isoflurane. Caution should be exercised in administering isoflurane to patients whose cerebral metabolism is

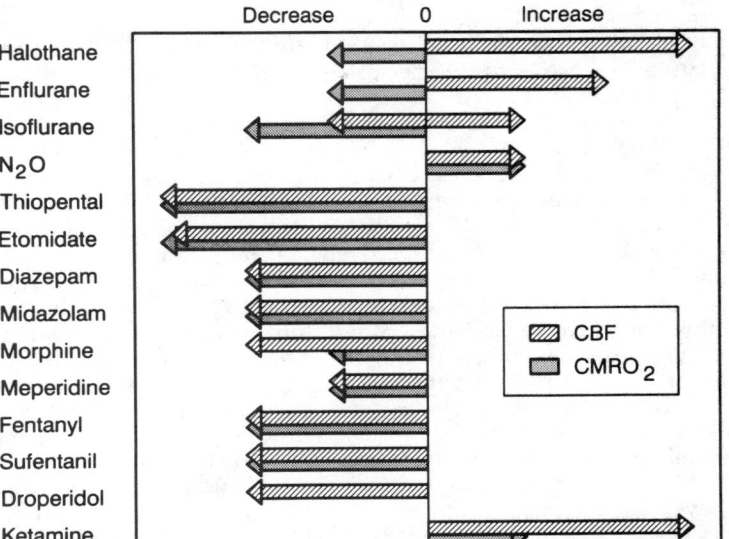

FIG. 31-1. The effects of anesthetic agents on cerebral blood flow and cerebral metabolism.

depressed either by other drugs, such as barbiturates, or by pathologic conditions causing decreases in cerebral function and metabolism, as these patients may exhibit a greater than expected increase in CBF with administration of isoflurane.

The effect of nitrous oxide (N_2O) on cerebral metabolism and blood flow is the subject of much controversy and conflicting reports. In several well-controlled studies using a rat model, N_2O was consistently found to have only minimal effects on both CBF and $CMRO_2$. In these studies, either no effect or clinically insignificant decreases in CBF or $CMRO_2$ were found.[54, 55] However, in other studies using several different animal models, including dogs, goats, and cats, and in humans, N_2O was found to result in small increases in $CMRO_2$ (11%–21%) and significant (35%–103%) increases in CBF.[56–61] One factor contributing to these conflicting results is the inability to deliver N_2O in concentrations equal to or above 1 MAC. The varying results could be due to the effects of either sympathetic stimulation under light anesthesia or the effects of the different drugs administered to supplement the N_2O anesthesia in different models. However, even while taking these factors into consideration and attempting to control for them, a species difference between rats and other animal models persists. In rats, N_2O has minimal effects on cerebral metabolism or blood flow, but, in the other animal models, N_2O causes mild increases in $CMRO_2$ and significant increases in CBF. Considering these results, in man, it is likely that N_2O causes significant cerebral vasodilation. However, these effects are easily modulated by other factors, including hyperventilation of the lungs[48, 49] and vasoconstrictive drugs, such as thiopental, diazepam, and morphine.[56, 62]

INTRAVENOUS DRUGS. Most intravenous drugs cause some degree of cerebral vasoconstriction, decrease in CBF, and a depression of $CMRO_2$, and do not "uncouple" the relationship of blood flow to metabolism (Fig. 31-1). Thiopental and other barbiturates result in a dose-dependent decrease in CBF and $CMRO_2$, with a maximal decrease in $CMRO_2$ of 50%–55% and in CBF of 40%–60%. This occurs at a dose adequate to completely suppress cerebral function and result in electrical silence.[27, 63, 4] Further doses of thiopental beyond that causing an isoelectric EEG result in no further decreases in $CMRO_2$ or CBF.[63] This suggests that the decrease in $CMRO_2$ requirements by thiopental is due to a decrease in cerebral function. Like the barbiturates, etomidate causes a dose-dependent decrease in CBF or $CMRO_2$, which is maximal at doses sufficient to cause electrical silence. Further increases in etomidate dose cause no further decreases in CBF or $CMRO_2$. $CMRO_2$ decreases by 45%–52%, and CBF by 34%–77%.[64, 65] Cases of etomidate-induced seizures have been reported, suggesting a potential for increased $CMRO_2$ and CBF in those patients. The benzodiazepines, diazepam and midazolam, both cause dose-dependent decreases in $CMRO_2$ and CBF. The decreases in CBF and $CMRO_2$ with diazepam are reported to be 15%–40% and 16%–40%, respectively,[66, 67] and, for midazolam, 33%–45% and 45%–55%, maintaining a favorable CBF to $CMRO_2$ ratio.[5, 29, 239] Opioids increase cerebrovascular resistance and decrease CBF and $CMRO_2$. Intravenous morphine causes a decrease in CBF of 27%–55% and a decrease in $CMRO_2$ of 15%–30%.[68, 69] Meperidine (2 mg·kg^{-1}) decreases CBF by only 10% and $CMRO_2$ by 13%.[70] Fentanyl at high doses decreases CBF by 40%–50% and $CMRO_2$ by 18%–40%.[25, 71, 72] Sufentanil results in similar decreases in CBF (53%) and $CMRO_2$ (53%).[73] Very high doses of both fentanyl and sufentanil have been demonstrated to result in seizure activity and increases in $CMRO_2$ in animal models.[71–73] It is likely that, in clinical doses, opioids cause relatively little decrease in CBF. Droperidol causes a decrease in CBF of 40% and no significant change in $CMRO_2$.[25] Ketamine differs from the other intravenous agents in that it results in an increase in CBF and $CMRO_2$. Ketamine increases CBF by 62%–80% with lesser increases in $CMRO_2$ (0–16%).[74–76]

The osmotic diuretic, mannitol, which is used relatively frequently in neurosurgical patients, results in an early transient increase in CBF during and immediately following mannitol infusion, with CBF returning to control values by 10 min following completion of the infusion in experimental animals.[77]

INTRACRANIAL PRESSURE (ICP)

The cranial contents of cerebral tissue (85%), cerebral blood (5%), and cerebrospinal fluid (10%) volumes can be altered with varying response rates. One compartment of the intracranial vault may change volume to accommodate a change in another compartment, allowing the intracranial pressure to remain unchanged. Acute increases in cerebral blood volume allow cerebrospinal fluid to shift caudally with sufficient ease to prevent any noticeable ICP change. Chronically developing mass lesions may shift CSF into the more distensible spinal subarachnoid space, increase CSF absorption, decrease cerebral venous volume, and compress brain tissue so as to become quite large with slow elevation of ICP and few symptoms.

ICP may be measured directly from the cerebral ventricles by ventriculostomy, from the cerebral subdural space by a catheter or hollow bolt, from the cerebral epidural space by an implanted transducer, or by inference from a needle or catheter in the lumbar subarachnoid space (Fig. 31-2). Each of these methods has its particular problems in providing accurate and reliable values. The zero reference point must be established to compensate for changes in pressure values with changes in patient position. Usually, either the heart level supine or the base of the skull is used.

Intracranial hypertension is defined as a sustained ICP at the head level exceeding 15 mm Hg. Symptoms may include headache and nausea progressing to a reduced level of consciousness. Signs may include papilledema, cranial nerve VI dysfunction, and progression to irregular respirations. The diagnosis is usually confirmed by a CT scan showing a midline shift of greater than 0.5 cm with a mass lesion, or obstruction of CSF pathways by tumor with resulting hydrocephalus.[78]

Intracranial compliance is the change in ICP related to a given change in volume (change volume/change ICP).[79] The greater the change in ICP with small changes in volume, the lower the compliance of the intracranial contents. Intracranial volume can increase moderately with no change in ICP (Fig. 31-3). It is difficult to know where on the curve a given patient fits, but this is most important on the seemingly safest part of the curve between points 1 and 2. If a patient has clinical or CT evidence of elevated ICP, precautions are needed to avoid further increases. If a patient has no clinical or CT signs of elevated ICP but has a mass lesion, we have no clinical method of accurately predicting intracranial compliance. For this reason, most of these patients are treated as though they are near the "elbow" of the curve at point 2. Their compliance markedly decreases, and small changes in volume produce large and clinically important increases in ICP. Correlation of clinical signs with ICP values is not exact.[80, 81]

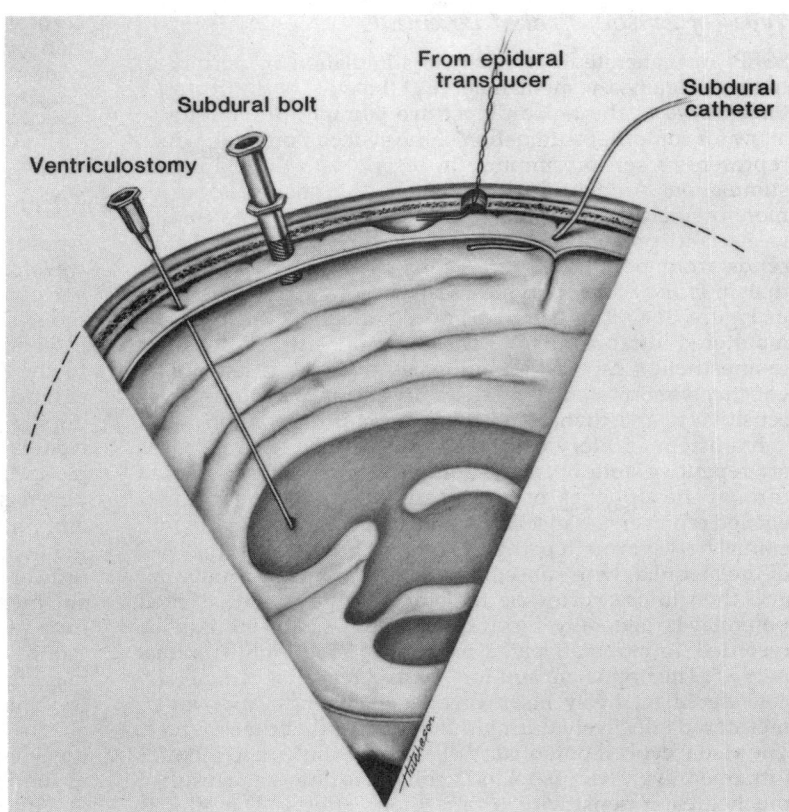

FIG. 31-2. Clinical methodology for measurement of ICP.

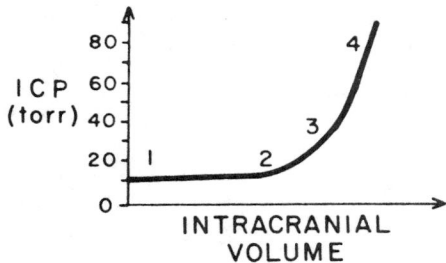

FIG. 31-3. A stylized intracranial volume-pressure curve describing intracranial compliance. (Modified from Langfitt TW: Increased intracranial pressure. Clin Neurosurg 14:436, 1968.)

ELECTROPHYSIOLOGIC NEUROLOGIC TECHNIQUES

EVOKED POTENTIALS

Intraoperative monitoring of sensory evoked potentials (SEP) allows for continuous assessment of neural pathways at a time when these pathways are at a risk of damage during operations on the spine and spinal cord, brainstem, and posterior fossa structures.[82, 83] An understanding of the origin of these potentials and the effects of anesthesia and operation is crucial to effective monitoring. It is a goal of monitoring SEP that alterations detected intraoperatively will reliably predict pos-

sible embarrassment of neural structures. Effective monitoring implies that equipment utilized is sensitive enough to record such changes, that trained observers can detect alterations in the potentials, and that therapeutic manipulations may subsequently alter outcome if changes are detected. Current experience with SEP monitoring indicates good reliability in predicting and preventing adverse postoperative outcome in most cases, but concerns over the sensitivity of isolated pathways predicting global dysfunction still exist.

Nature of Evoked Potentials

SEP represent pathways elicited by stimulation of sensory structures. Monitoring of SEP requires computer signal averaging of sensory stimulus-induced events that can be separated from the background EEG. The waves of the evoked potential are plotted as a voltage *versus* time response, and are felt to represent potentials from specific neural generators. The evoked potential is described in terms of the type of eliciting sensory stimulus (somatosensory, auditory, visual), post-stimulus latency, wave amplitude, and distance separating the neural generators and recording electrodes.

SEP can also be described in terms of monitoring location. For example, the generated somatosensory evoked potential (SSEP) can be monitored with surface electrodes at the level of the peripheral nerve, spinal cord, and cerebral cortex. In addition, the SSEP can be monitored *via* direct recording from the spine or epidural space. Knowledge of timing of specific events at the spinal and cortical level allows calculation of impulse conduction time through central neuronal pathways.

Types of Sensory Evoked Potentials

SSEP are generated *via* electrical stimulation of peripheral nerves, usually, the median nerve at the wrist or the posterior tibial nerve at the ankle. Repetitive stimuli are required to allow for computer summation of the evoked potential, which represents a sensory impulse in response to the peripheral stimulation. As described previously, the potentials can be monitored at various levels from peripheral nerve to cortical levels, and probably represent a sensory pathway that ascends from peripheral nerve to dorsal spinal columns to thalamus and cortex. A typical scalp–recorded SSEP is shown in Figure 31-4. The early cortical components are typically monitored intraoperatively. These components are sensitive to anesthetics, especially the inhaled drugs, but can still be effectively monitored. The later cortical components are very sensitive to anesthetics and more difficult to monitor.

Brainstem auditory evoked responses (BAER) are elicited *via* repetitive auditory click stimulation, which is achieved through headphones or ear inserts. The sensory pathway elicited represents transmission through the peripheral eighth cranial nerve through pathways into the brainstem at the level of the medulla, with subsequent relay to the pons, midbrain, and then to the cortex *via* thalamic pathways. The elicited potential is generally recorded over the scalp, but can be recorded intraoperatively directly from the eighth cranial nerve.[84] The brainstem auditory evoked response is generally considered relatively insensitive to anesthetics, and can be monitored effectively during different anesthetic techniques. The visual evoked potential (VEP) is more difficult to monitor intraoperatively because of its likelihood to be lost as a result of much greater sensitivity to anesthetic effects. The VEP is typically stimulated intraoperatively *via* flashes emitted by light-emitting diodes in eye goggles. Monitoring is at the cortical level, and the potentials are felt to represent transmission *via* optic pathways. These potentials have not found widespread intraoperative application due to sensitivity to anesthetics and overall difficulty in obtaining satisfactory intraoperative monitoring.

Effects of Anesthetic Agents

Anesthetic agents may produce alterations of evoked potential waveform latency and amplitude. In general, the sensitivity to waveform changes induced by anesthetic agents in decreasing order of sensitivity is VEP, SSEP, with BAER being the most insensitive. Studies on specific agents show that, with respect to the SSEP, induction doses of thiopental, fentanyl, and etomidate preserved monitoring of SSEP. Thiopental (4 mg·kg^{-1}) and fentanyl (25 µg·kg^{-1}) produced minor increases in latency and decreases in amplitude of the early cortical components, while 0.4 mg·kg^{-1} of etomidate produced slight increases in latency but dramatic increase in amplitude of the early cortical components.[85] High-dose thiopental has been noted to increase latency and decrease amplitude of the early cortical peaks of the median nerve SSEP, but still preserve ability to monitor, while the BAER showed some increased latency of early peaks with good preservation of monitoring ability.[86] Etomidate has been shown to have minimal effects on the early peaks of the BAER.[87] Fentanyl and morphine have been shown, in addition, to have minimal effects on early components of BAER,[88, 89] while producing dose-related latency increases with variable amplitude effects in the SSEP.[90]

With respect to the BAER, clinically applicable concentrations of the inhaled drugs halothane, enflurane, and isoflurane increased brainstem wave latencies, but preserved

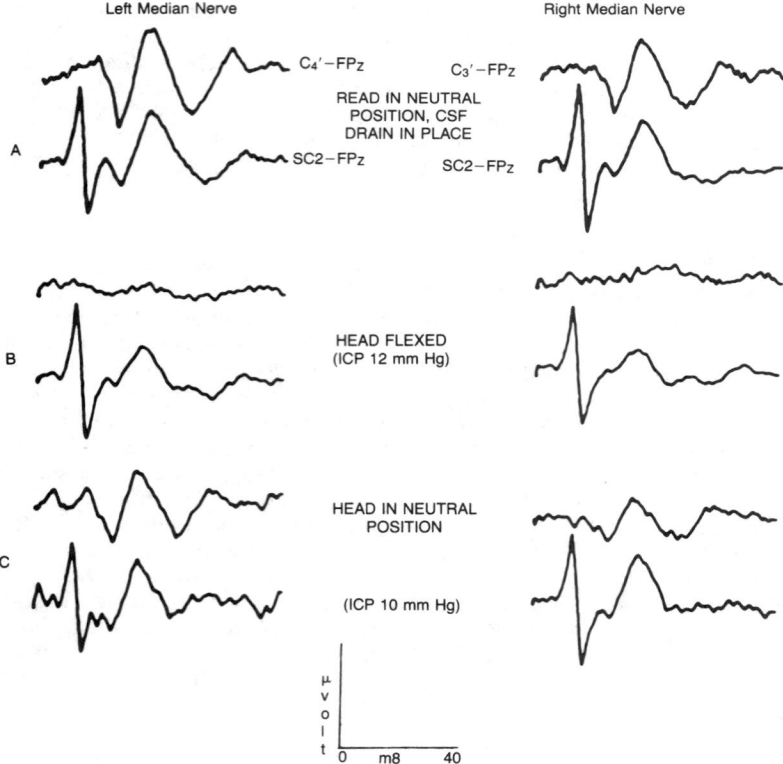

FIG. 31-4. Dramatic change in SSEP at the scalp, and not at the neck, with head flexion (*B*), returning to normal as head position is returned to neutral (*C*). Note that ICP is essentially unchanged. (From McPherson RW, Szymanski J, Rogers M: Somatosensory evoked potential changes in position-related brain stem ischemia. Anesthesiology 61:88, 1984.)

wave morphology, thus allowing for continued monitoring ability.[91-94] The SSEP demonstrates greater sensitivity to volatile drugs, with significant dose-related alterations in the recorded potentials. For example, increasing dose of isoflurane during isoflurane anesthesia to 2% end-tidal has been shown to produce significant decreases in the amplitude and latency increases of early cortical components,[95] while satisfactory traces could be obtained in all patients at end-tidal concentrations of 0.5% and 1%, with 1.5% being variable. The ability to obtain satisfactory monitoring waveforms after median nerve stimulation has been shown to be greater with halothane than with isoflurane or enflurane.[96] This study suggested that successful recording could be maintained with 60% N_2O plus 1.0 MAC halothane or 0.5 MAC isoflurane or enflurane. A quantitative difference was found in a study of halothane, enflurane, and isoflurane effects on SSEP generated by posterior tibial nerve stimulation.[97] These authors found that clinically useful monitoring could be maintained at levels up to 0.75 MAC plus 60% N_2O with all drugs, and at 1.0 MAC plus 60% N_2O with enflurane and isoflurane. It is important, however, to consider the effects of N_2O alone. N_2O has been shown to produce significant decreases in amplitude with minimal latency change in the cortical SSEP.[98-100] The VEP is also sensitive to the effects of N_2O and isoflurane with latency and amplitude changes.[100, 101]

Intraoperative Uses of Evoked Potentials

Monitoring of SEP has been utilized widely with hopes of preventing intraoperative neurologic impairment.[102] Typical applications include monitoring of SSEP during spinal surgery[103] and monitoring of BAER during operations in the cerebellopontine angle.[104] BAER have been utilized in cerebral posterior circulation vascular surgery as an indicator of brainstem injury.[105, 106] SSEP have been similarly monitored during intracranial aneurysm surgery.[107-110] SSEP monitoring has been utilized during carotid endarterectomy[111-113] and to assess potential spinal cord ischemia during aortic operations.[114, 115] VEP have been monitored during operations in the anterior visual pathways.[116]

Anesthetic management for operations in which evoked potentials are to be monitored should seek to obtain a steady state, so that waveform changes detected are presumed to reflect operative events. In addition, when monitoring SSEP during spinal surgery, consideration must be given to the possibility of performing a "wake-up test" for intraoperative assessment of motor function.[117] With these factors in mind, thiopental induction with N_2O and opioid infusion for anesthetic maintenance has been suggested for scoliosis surgery.[118] A technique utilizing volatile agents for maintenance would be appropriate if consideration is given to the fact that higher level of inhalation agents may greatly alter the SSEP waveform. Since the BAER is more resistant to anesthetic effects, a variety of anesthetic agents may be utilized with this technique, but it is still essential to strive for steady-state conditions. Other factors can alter SEP, such as hypotension, hypoxia,[119] and hypothermia,[120, 121] and must be considered if alterations in the SEP waveform occur. Alteration of cortical SEP has also been noted with accumulation of intracranial gas during operations in the sitting position.[122, 123]

Reliability of Evoked Potentials

As stated previously, evoked potential monitoring seeks to monitor neural pathways at risk and predict and prevent neural dysfunction. Monitoring of BAER in cerebello-pontine angle tumor patients has been shown to play a role in hearing

preservation,[124] but some authors feel that intraoperative BAER are routinely too sensitive, and that changes in operative conditions should be based only on gross changes of the BAER waveform.[125]

SEP monitoring has found wide application, especially to help preserve function during operations on the spinal cord. In general, reliability has been good with changes in SSEP predicting postoperative events,[126] but concern exists because the SSEP monitors dorsal column function, and not motor function, directly. In fact, postoperative neurologic deficits have occurred despite preserved intraoperative SSEP.[127, 128] In order to more specifically monitor motor function, evoked potentials obtained via direct motor tract stimulation are being investigated.[129, 130]

INTRAOPERATIVE ELECTROMYOGRAPHY

Electromyography (EMG) is a technique widely utilized in the diagnosis of neuromuscular disorders.[131] EMG recording electrodes measure motor unit potentials, which originate from the summated action potentials of the fibers of the motor unit. Adaptation of this monitoring technology, for intraoperative use to monitor and prevent potential nerve injury, is currently being accomplished.[132]

The widest application of intraoperative EMG has been monitoring and preservation of facial nerve function during acoustic neuroma resection.[133, 134] The technique of intraoperative EMG for facial nerve preservation involves preoperative placement of indwelling fine wire electrodes into the facial muscles (orbicularis oculi, orbicularis oris, mentalis, frontalis, masseter, or temporalis), which is verified by preanesthetic recording to verify location, followed by intraoperative recording to determine potential facial nerve damage during tumor resection. Spontaneous muscle action potentials are recorded continuously intraoperatively, and neurotonic discharges that indicate nerve irritation are a signal that surgical maneuvers are affecting the facial nerve. These maneuvers may then be altered to reduce potential nerve damage. In addition, to help localize the facial nerve during the resection, compound muscle action potentials may be recorded from the fine wire electrodes in response to direct electrical stimulation of the facial nerve by the surgeon via a hand-held stimulating electrode. These processes of measuring spontaneous EMG and elicited muscle action potentials are effective in preserving facial nerve function, especially with larger acoustic neuromas. The use of intraoperative EMG is currently being expanded to provide monitoring of cranial nerve function during surgery in proximity to the brainstem, and for monitoring during spinal surgery.

Anesthetic management of patients who are to undergo intraoperative EMG must be altered to allow its effective assessment. A major consideration is to avoid further use of muscle relaxants after the initial doses of relaxants necessary for endotracheal intubation. Because of this necessity, anesthesia techniques are chosen that will accomplish immobility as part of the technique. At the Mayo Clinic, anesthetic induction is generally accomplished with intravenous administration of thiopental and an intermediate-acting non-depolarizing muscle relaxant, the effects of which will have dissipated prior to the time of intraoperative EMG recording of facial nerve function. No further muscle relaxants are administered. Anesthetic maintenance utilizing a combination of potent inhaled drug and N_2O with small supplemental doses of an intravenous opioid is generally utilized. The patient with an acoustic neuroma or other cerebello-pontine angle tumor can thus provide considerable anesthetic challenge. Anesthetic management must be tailored to allow for effective electrophysiologic monitoring that will involve measurement of brainstem auditory evoked potentials and EMG, and must provide immobility without the use of muscle relaxants at a time when the surgeon is dissecting delicate structures under the operating microscope.

ANESTHETIC MANAGEMENT OF THE TUMOR PATIENT

SUPRATENTORIAL TUMORS

Choice of Anesthetic Agent

The factors in selection of the anesthetic drug are multiple. In neuroanesthesia, the effects of the agent on ICP, cerebral perfusion pressure (CPP), CBF, $CMRO_2$, and promptness of return to consciousness are major considerations. Secondary considerations include drug-related protection from ischemia or edema, blood pressure control, and compatibility with neurophysiologic monitoring techniques.

All of the volatile anesthetics can cause an increase in ICP at deeper levels of anesthesia and normocarbia. These circumstances are rarely used in neoplastic neurosurgery. Moderate hypocarbia with less than 1.0 MAC volatile agent represents the most common application of this anesthetic technique. In cerebrovascular surgery, light volatile anesthesia avoids blood pressure depression, and mild hypocarbia is a reasonable choice to avoid excessive cerebral vasoconstriction.

Halothane produces the greatest reduction in cerebral vascular resistance and the clearest increase in ICP. This can be blunted or even eliminated if hyperventilation of the lungs is established before beginning halothane administration.[48] Isoflurane produces a reduction in cerebral vascular resistance and an elevation of ICP at normocarbia. This response can be blocked by hyperventilation in tumor patients.[49] Other work suggests that patients with a midline shift on CT scan are more likely to show an elevation of ICP during isoflurane anesthesia.[135] On balance, human studies suggest that isoflurane is a safe anesthetic drug when used for intracranial tumor surgery.[136]

Intravenous drugs (e.g., thiopental, fentanyl) are useful in neuroanesthesia because they decrease CBF and $CMRO_2$ together. This allows a reduction in ICP to be accomplished by modification of the vascular compartment without producing cerebral ischemia. Thiopental safely produces a profound linked reduction of CBF and $CMRO_2$ to near half of awake values.[4] This is reflected in the dramatic reduction of ICP that can be achieved by utilizing thiopental with this goal in mind. For decades, thiopental has seen waxing and waning of enthusiasm for its use as a constant infusion in combination with N_2O to provide desirable operating conditions for neurosurgical neoplastic cases. The effectiveness of thiopental as a cerebral protective drug should probably be viewed as applicable to the experimental conditions at which that protection is most solidly demonstrated, i.e., cerebral ischemia by vascular occlusion techniques. Cerebral protection by barbiturates in brain tumor patients produced by lowering ICP is a distinctly different, although useful, concept.

Fentanyl decreases CBF slightly more than the decrease in $CMRO_2$.[25] Theoretically, this imbalance could predispose to cerebral ischemia, but such a consideration does not seem to be clinically important. The usefulness of fentanyl in neurosurgical anesthesia is based on its ability to lower ICP through decreased CBF, and on its control of heart rate and blood pressure during surgical stimulus.

Most craniotomy surgery in the United States today is probably performed following a thiopental induction of anesthesia with intubation of the trachea after a non-depolarizing relaxant, and maintenance with N_2O/isoflurane/fentanyl in various combinations during hypocarbia to Pa_{CO_2} levels of 28–33 mm HG.

Choice of Muscle Relaxants

Muscle relaxant use can probably affect the conduct of a neuroanesthetic as much as the primary agent. Succinylcholine as yet appears unequaled in achieving total rapid paralysis for the rapid sequence intubation of the trachea. There is still controversy regarding succinylcholine-induced increases in ICP.[137, 138] However, such increases are probably clinically insignificant, except, perhaps, in the most extreme cases of intracranial hypertension. Since complete flaccidity is required to avoid coughing and straining during intubation of the trachea and thus avoid ICP increases, it is reasonable to use a nerve stimulator during induction and intubation in these cases. The shorter acting non-depolarizing relaxants (vecuronium, atracurium) are well suited for intubation paralysis in cases of elevated ICP. They do not increase ICP, and have little or no effect on heart rate and blood pressure.[139, 140]

Hemiplegia from cerebral ischemia or from cerebral tumor is associated with differences in response to non-depolarizing muscle relaxants on the two sides of the body. The affected extremities are resistant to neuromuscular blockade by non-depolarizing relaxants.[141, 142] In most operating room arrangements, the face and endotracheal tube are turned toward the anesthetist so that the operative field is uppermost. This places the extremities contralateral to the tumor in a position that allows easy monitoring of neuromuscular transmission. But that arm, e.g., is likely to be more resistant to non-depolarizing relaxants than the rest of the body, thus leading us to use a relative overdose of drug. Perhaps this is fortunate, since it ensures that the patient will not move intraoperatively, because we are providing neuromuscular blockade of the most resistant muscles. Succinylcholine is also associated with a special consideration in the hemiplegic patient, that of hyperkalemia.[143] The time of sensitivity is not well defined, but cases are reported from 1 week to 6 months following onset of hemiplegia

Intraoperative Fluids

Choice of intraoperative intravenous fluids for tumor patients must take into account the patient's overall fluid and electrolyte status and specific electrolyte imbalances present preoperatively or likely to occur intraoperatively. For most patients, replacement of overnight fluid deficit does not seem necessary. However, angiographic dye used in cerebral studies is osmotically active, and substantial intravascular fluid volume can be lost in the urine following such a study. An important factor in fluid administration is the integrity of the blood-brain barrier. For practical purposes, the surgical effort necessary to remove cerebral tumors can always leave the area immediately surrounding the resection with a damaged blood-brain barrier from trauma of resection or retractor ischemia. It is generally felt that limiting fluid administration to what is necessary to maintain hemodynamic stability helps to prevent brain edema; perhaps the converse is more applicable, i.e., large volumes of fluid administered to the injured blood-brain barrier patient contribute to cerebral edema. It is clinically unwise to allow significant intravascular hypovolemia to occur for fear of exacerbation of cerebral edema.

The effect of these fluids on neural tissue that has been injured by trauma or ischemia has been an area of increasing interest. It has long been realized that the use of 5% dextrose in water can result in cerebral edema in the patient with a damaged blood-brain barrier. The mechanism appears to be the passage of sugar and water into the brain tissue, with subsequent metabolism of sugar leaving free water in excess. This phenomenon was actually used in years gone by to increase brain size to fill large intracranial spaces left after removal of subdural hematoma. It is now generally appreciated that isotonic electrolyte solutions provide the most physiologic replacement for neurosurgical patients. Elevated blood glucose has been demonstrated to worsen cerebral ischemic injury in a variety of animal models, including intact primates.[144] Patients admitted with stroke and elevated blood sugar (>120 mg·dl^{-1}) have increased neurologic damage.[145] Neurologic deficits are more common and more severe in postcardiac arrest patients with higher blood sugars.[146] Based on this body of work, it seems reasonable to delete glucose from intravenous fluid administration to patients in whom central neural ischemia is likely to occur. Patients undergoing brain tumor surgery would seem to fall into this category.

With current attention focused on the risk of blood transfusion, more dependence can be placed on colloid products to maintain blood volume intraoperatively. Albumin and hetastarch are reasonable choices. There is a theoretical possibility that these osmotically active agents could cross the damaged blood-brain barrier and remain there to cause cerebral edema. However, this has not been identified as a clinical problem, and the risk of colloid in these patients still seems less than the risk of blood transfusion. Hetastarch has been anecdotally linked with decreased blood coagulability in neurosurgical cases, possibly contributing to postoperative cerebral hematoma.[147]

Intraoperative Management of "Tight Brain"

Intracranial hypertension can result in the extrusion of brain tissue when craniotomy is performed. The first sign of difficulty is usually noted by the neurosurgeon as the craniotomy flap is removed and the dura is bulging and tense. The term "tight brain" gives no clue as to etiology or course of treatment. Some observations can help assess the severity and tractability of the situation. If the dura is tense and bulging only at the lower portion of the craniectomy, palpation may reveal that the brain tissue is easily displaced upward, and that the superior dura is tense only from being pushed out at the lower level. Surgical exposure may be slightly compromised in this situation, and some maneuvers may improve the situation. If the dura is tense at all edges of the craniectomy and palpation reveals fairly immobile brain beneath, surgical exposure may be severely compromised. Maneuvers may help the situation, but are unlikely to bring the brain profile to the bone edge. A large dural incision will result in brain extrusion with trapping at the edges and little room to achieve exposure. A small dural incision allows the surgeon some control of the brain as he seeks to obtain exposure. While the usual cause of such extreme tenseness of the dura is not amenable to anesthetic maneuvers, it is important to rule out correctable problems (Table 31-2). The usual cause is intracranial hypertension because of the tumor mass itself. As resection is performed, the dural opening can be enlarged and the offending mass will be removed, eventually leaving a cavity where, previously, there was bulging brain. An ominous cause of such swelling is occult acute bleeding into the tumor. Vital signs give a clue to this. Hypertension may de-

TABLE 31-2. Therapeutic Maneuvers to Improve "Tight Brain"

Position, venous return
P_{CO_2}, P_{O_2}
Anesthetic drug
Thiopental
Muscle relaxants
Diuretics
Spinal fluid drainage
Steroids
Pneumocephalus

velop without apparent cause, and appears unusually resistant to increasing anesthetic depth. Heart rate may initially rise, but then slows. This response is somewhat masked by the complexity of pharmacologic and surgical interventions superimposed during anesthesia. Timing is also important. If the brain begins to vigorously bulge where it was slack before, intracerebral hemorrhage must be strongly suspected. It is helpful to the surgeon to be informed of the subtle vital sign changes suggesting this etiology, because he will need to proceed more rapidly and boldly with decompression. Because of the relationship of cerebral perfusion pressure to ICP and blood pressure, it may be unwise to try to reduce blood pressure before decompression, despite the probability of bleeding.

With the use of the operating microscope, the surgeon may adjust the position of the table for best exposure without realizing that the patient is slowly being placed horizontal or head-down. Readjusting the operating room table to allow the head to be slightly elevated can dramatically improve the situation. Venous drainage may be compromised by extreme head positions and go unnoticed until the dura is exposed. Repositioning the alignment of head and chin to body may be necessary.

Because it is a powerful cerebral vasodilator, an increase in Pa_{CO_2} may cause a dramatic increase in ICP. Hypoxic cerebral vasodilation may produce the same effect. Reassurance that hypocarbia is achieved and hypoxia is absent can be obtained by arterial blood gas determinations supported by pulse oximetry and capnography.

Despite the overall evidence of safety of volatile anesthetics, it seems prudent to discontinue such drugs and utilize an opioid in the presence of "tight brain." There may be no causal connection between volatile drugs and brain size, but changing to an opioid anesthetic eliminates any such possibility. N_2O may increase CBF, but its effect is likely to be less pronounced and easily altered by thiopental or opioids. Acute administration of a sleep dose of thiopental can be expected to reduce ICP. Lack of any visible response of the brain to thiopental suggests a serious situation.

Patients receiving anti-seizure medications may have a shortened response to non-depolarizing muscle relaxants.[148] Return of abdominal and thoracic muscle tone during light anesthesia can raise central venous pressure and, thus, cerebral venous pressure. Thus, the origin of the anecdote that "curare relaxes the brain." Evaluation of the level of neuromuscular blockade is an important subtle step in seeking a cause for "tight brain."

Osmotic diuretics have long been shown to be effective at reducing brain size in normal brain tissue by drawing water from the interstitial tissue. In patients with intact autoregulation, mannitol results in no change in CBF and a decrease of ICP by 27% at 25 min. However, in patients with impaired autoregulation, the CBF increases by 5%, and there is less decrease in ICP (18%) at 25 min.[149] Furosemide in fairly large doses (*e.g.*, 80 mg) reduces ICP, but its mechanism of action is not entirely clear.[150]

Drainage of cerebrospinal fluid is a rapid and effective method of reducing intracranial bulk directly. Generally effective methods include subarachnoid needle and catheter techniques. Rarely, pneumocephalus may be present from some previous diagnostic test, and can increase with the use of N_2O.

Monitoring for Supratentorial Brain Tumor Surgery

General routine monitoring should be used as for any other case of this magnitude. The use of direct arterial pressure recording is usually appropriate. Specific considerations for additional monitoring and ancillary techniques can aid materially in the management of these patients. Hypocarbia is a part of all neuroanesthetic techniques for tumor resection, and capnography or mass spectrometry is useful for quantitating Pa_{CO_2} levels, especially when coupled with blood gas determinations. Meningiomas and metastatic tumors to the brain tend to bleed, suggesting monitoring that provides information on hemodynamic parameters. A lesion invading a major cerebral venous sinus may bleed profusely if venous sinus pressure is high, but may entrain air if venous sinus pressure is subatmospheric. Special monitoring for venous air embolism (VAE) is useful in early detection of air, and a right heart catheter may be lifesaving in a case of massive air embolism through an open cerebral venous sinus. Intracranial pressure monitoring is popular in some centers. Some authors find this particularly useful during induction of and emergence from anesthesia. To be helpful during induction, the ICP monitor must be placed in the awake patient. Induction drugs can then be titrated to produce the desired level of ICP.[151]

INFRATENTORIAL TUMOR SURGERY

Infratentorial tumors require a change in body and head position to provide surgical access to the posterior fossa. For some lesions, this can be achieved with the patient supine and with the head turned dramatically to the side. For others, the park-bench, prone, or sitting position provides the desired surgical exposure.

The sitting position is said to offer some surgical advantages (Table 31-3). Surgeons might weigh these advantages differently, but most would agree that ease of surgical exposure, the amount of blood pooling in the operative field, and the operative position of the surgeon are different among the sitting,

TABLE 31-3. Practical Reasons for Selective Use of Sitting Position

Better surgical exposure
Less tissue retraction and damage
Less bleeding
Less cranial nerve damage
More complete resection of the lesion
Ready access to airway, chest and extremities
Modern monitoring gives early warning of Venous air embolism Brain stem compromise
Serious problems due to venous air embolism are uncommon

lateral, supine, and prone positions. Some anesthesiologists feel that access to the endotracheal tube, the reduction of facial swelling, and the ability to observe facial nerve function are notable advantages of the sitting position in anesthetic management. The two most common procedures performed in the sitting position are cervical laminectomy and posterior fossa exploration. Hazards to the patient in the sitting position include VAE, hypotension, vital sign changes due to brain stem manipulation, specific cranial nerve stimulation, airway obstruction, and position–related brain stem ischemia. Our management should be directed at the prevention, early detection, and treatment of these problems.

There is much concern about the use of the sitting position, some even suggesting that it is malpractice to use this position for today's surgery. These intimidating statements have some basis in fact, but, in general, do not consider what has become a large body of information about the safety of the sitting position.

Safety

There are several large series of sitting cases that have a remarkably similar and favorable safety record.[152–155]

The practice at our institution reflects the practice in the United States in general. The sitting position is being used less, and more posterior fossa procedures are being performed in horizontal positions. The use of the sitting position is becoming a conscious selection, rather than automatic, for any posterior fossa lesion. There is risk and benefit in each position, and these must be weighed in the overall care of the patient.

A recent study puts the problem into perspective, and is consistent with other studies.[155] Five hundred and seventy-nine posterior fossa craniectomies (333 sitting and 246 horizontal) performed at the Mayo Clinic between 1981 through 1984 were reviewed retrospectively.

Intraoperatively, the incidence of hypotension was not different between groups either from induction of anesthesia to incision or from incision to closure. About 20% of the patients in both groups became hypotensive during each of these periods. All responded to vasopressors and/or fluids. The incidence of VAE in patients monitored with the Doppler was significantly greater in the sitting patients (45%) as compared to the horizontal patients (12%).

An important difference was found in the need for blood transfusion between the two groups, confirming the traditional surgical impression that upright patients "bleed less." More than two units of blood were required in 13% of the horizontal patients and in only 3% of the upright patients. Average blood volume transfused was also lower in the sitting patients.

Postoperatively, no differences were found in cardiac or respiratory complications. The perioperative myocardial infarction rate was less than 1% overall, and not different between groups. Respiratory complications were found in 2.5%, and were not different between groups, nor from other studies.[152]

Thus, the data does not support the general selection of either the sitting or down positions based on outcome. There are certain risks and advantages to each, and selection of position should be made with those in mind.

In our opinion, there are some conditions that seem prudent to consider as relative contraindications to the sitting position (Table 31-4). However, there is little objective data to support our approach. If a shunt tube is in place from the cerebral ventricular system to the right atrium, air may enter

TABLE 31-4.   Relative Contraindications to Operative
Sitting Position

Ventriculo-atrial shunt in place and open
Cerebral ischemia upright awake
Left atrial pressure < Right atrial pressure
Platypnea-orthodeoxia
Preoperative demonstration of patent foramen ovale or right-to-left shunt

? cardiac instability	chest compression and resuscitation
? age extremes	not really better in prone or lateral position

the end of the shunt as CSF drains out and be pulled into the heart. The non-collapsible tubing acts as a non-collapsible vein to allow air to pass unimpeded into the heart. This is not a potential problem with a ventriculo-peritoneal shunt, since the air would have no venous access. We recommend that a patient having a ventriculo-atrial shunt in place should have the shunt tied off before having an intracranial procedure performed in the sitting position. There are some patients who suffer cerebral ischemia whenever they assume the upright position. Their cardiovascular and cerebral vascular systems may both be implicated in this situation. These patients may present for an extracranial-intracranial bypass procedure for the posterior cerebral circulation. Some surgeons feel the sitting position gives the best exposure for this procedure. We feel that we cannot be sure that we will maintain cerebral circulation in this circumstance, since we must not only put the patient upright, but also give him an anesthetic. It seems a reasonable balance of risk/benefit ratio to place such a patient in a horizontal position.

There has been a suggestion that, if the left atrial pressure (as measured by pulmonary artery occlusion pressure, PAOP) is less than the right atrial pressure in the sitting position, the patient should be operated horizontally because of increased risk of paradoxical embolism.[156] This is based on two important assumptions. First, that the left atrial pressure will be greater than the right atrial pressure in the horizontal position. Second, that the atrial pressure gradient and its direction is a prognostic indicator of whether VAE will become paradoxical air embolism. We have some recent unpublished laboratory data to indicate that the atrial pressure gradients have little, if any, predictive value during air embolism. There are some patients who have a potential right-to-left shunt demonstrated preoperatively. There is an unusual cardiovascular illness in which the atrial gradients apparently reverse upon assuming the upright position.[157] In platypnea-orthodeoxia the patient is well oxygenated in the supine position, but becomes desaturated in the upright position because of unsaturated blood passing from right to left at the atrial level. There are other patients in whom a patent foramen ovale is demonstrated preoperatively during a cardiac work-up. Still others may have a known right-to-left shunt. It seems that these patients might be at greater risk for paradoxical air embolism should VAE occur, and, therefore, it seems prudent to avoid using the sitting position for them.

Some suggest that patients with cardiac instability or at extremes of age should not be placed in a sitting position based on a possible need to resuscitate intraoperatively. We feel that it is really no easier to provide chest compression in the prone or lateral position than in the sitting position; they are equally undesirable. The rare occurrence of the need to resuscitate probably does not justify giving up whatever surgical advantage is felt to be gained by using the sitting position. Thus, in

our opinion, these last considerations are not really relative contraindications.

Monitoring

In collating the data from many studies, the sitting position seems relatively safe, provided adequate monitoring is used.

CENTRAL NERVOUS SYSTEM. Central nervous system monitoring techniques for patients in the sitting position are directed not only at minimizing the hazards of the position, but also at providing positive information to the surgeon, particularly during posterior fossa exploration. The response of the vital signs to brain stem manipulation and the response of the cranial nerves to stimulation can provide pathophysiologic data that the surgeon can utilize in real time during his dissection (Table 31-5).

Blood pressure and pulse rate are monitors of several interrelated systems and factors. Some operations performed in the sitting position tend to be of a type that might result in sudden and extreme changes in heart rate and blood pressure, either because of the surgery or because of VAE. Intra-arterial blood pressure measurements will yield instantaneous information, particularly in regard to cerebral perfusion pressure. This is most easily accomplished when the strain gauge is zeroed to the base of the skull.

The electrocardiogram (ECG) is an effective monitor of brain stem compression. Spontaneous respiration has been advocated as a means of detecting transgression of the respiratory centers during posterior fossa exploration. However, large series indicate that monitoring of the ECG provides adequate warning of brain stem compromise during light anesthesia, while using mechanical ventilation to maintain reduced Pa_{CO_2} levels.[158] BAER and SSEP can provide an electrophysiologic monitor for detection of early brain stem compromise. Stimulation of the seventh cranial nerve results in a facial twitch that is visible in the seated patient. Electromyography over the distribution of VII can aid in detecting stimulation of the facial nerve when the face is not accessible to palpation or visual assessment.

Venous Air Embolism (VAE)

DIAGNOSIS. Monitoring for VAE can be approached from several aspects. Monitors include a precordial Doppler, a right-heart catheter, capnograph or mass spectrometer,

TABLE 31-5.   Cranial Nerve Stimulation During Posterior Fossa Surgery

CLASSIC ACTIVITY DESCRIPTION—PHYSICAL SIGNS	ELECTRONIC DEVICE
V—motor—jaw jerk	EMG
sensory—hypertension	arterial line
bradycardia	ECG
VII—facial twitch	EMG
X—hypotension	arterial line
bradycardia	ECG
XI—shoulder jerk	EMG
Pons, brainstem compression	BAER, SEP
ectopic cardiac foci	ECG
hyper/hypo tension	arterial line
tachy/brady cardia	ECG
gasp, irregular respirations	respirator "trigger"

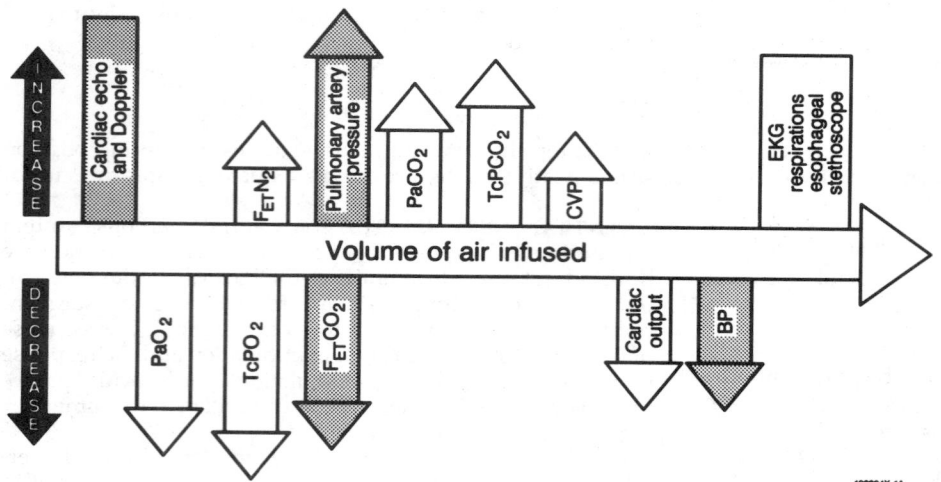

FIG. 31-5. Changes in detection parameters for venous air embolism with increasing air volume. Data are aggregated from human and animal studies under a wide variety of circumstances.

esophageal stethoscope, transcutaneous O_2, and transesophageal echocardiography (TEE). The most sensitive of these are the TEE and Doppler, followed by expired N_2 ($F_E N_2$), end-tidal CO_2, transcutaneous O_2, right heart catheter, and, least sensitive, the esophageal stethoscope. None of these monitors is totally reliable. We feel that it is generally necessary to use at least three of these to insure that VAE can be detected (Fig. 31-5).

The risk of VAE is not eliminated by putting the patient horizontal, but it is reduced. A 12% incidence of Doppler detected air occurs in supine infratentorial craniectomy cases.[155] Once VAE has occurred, about 20% of those patients will have hypotension, regardless of the position of the patient.

The precordial Doppler is advocated as the basic monitoring device for the reduction of hazards due to VAE. It is reasonably priced, relatively easy to use, non-invasive, and very sensitive; its position over the right heart can be verified by rapid injection of saline into the central venous circulation, and its sounds can be heard by both surgeon and anesthesiologist. Its sensitivity has led some to criticize its use as indicating "insignificant air" before hemodynamic consequences ensue. Protagonists argue that such sensitivity is precisely the early warning needed to identify the occurrence of VAE and stop its entry surgically.

The use of the right heart catheter has evolved and improved such that air can frequently be aspirated when detected on Doppler. But what are the real functions of the right heart catheter?[159] Rapid injection of saline through it can help confirm that the Doppler is properly placed over the right heart. The aspiration of air confirms or establishes the diagnosis of VAE. The role of the catheter in the treatment of VAE is more anecdotal and less solidly founded. The aspiration of air from the right atrium during VAE is occasionally lifesaving, but such occasions must be very rare situations of massive VAE. Whether the routine aspiration of smaller or medium quantities of air from the heart can prevent paradoxical air embolism or cardiopulmonary complications is not known. Right atrial multiorifice catheters allow a larger amount of air to be aspirated than single-orifice catheters. Proper placement of the right atrial catheter in the high right atrium by ECG control can increase its effectiveness by placing it where the air tends to "hang up" (Fig. 31-6).[160]

The right heart catheter may be positioned by ECG control, x-ray, or pressure recordings. It is likely that the ECG trace

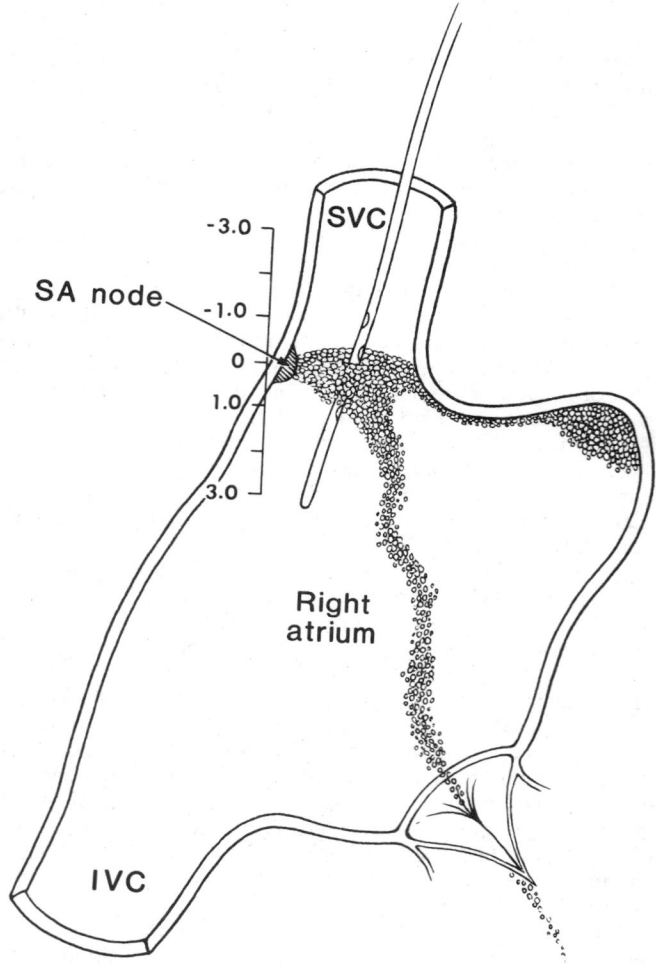

FIG. 31-6. The air tends to localize at the atrial-SVC junction, moving through the tricuspid valve or into upright portions of the atrium. The multiorifice catheter placement most likely to aspirate air is shown. The ECG tracing from the catheter in this position is described in Figure 31-7. Conceptualization of localization of air embolism in the upright heart based on a human cardiac model and human echocardiographic findings.

from a multiorifice catheter comes from the proximal hole, usually 2 cm from the tip.[161] Thus, the tracing sought is a little different with these catheters. The standard concept of a progressively more negative P wave as the catheter is advanced still applies, but the proximal orifice should be placed in the superior vena cava (SVC), allowing the portion of the catheter that has the holes to float at the SVC-high right atrial level (Fig. 31-6). The P wave should be large and negative, with no positive component (Fig. 31-7). This indicates that the proximal orifice is not in the atrium. In practice, one can usually obtain an increasingly negative P wave that finally develops a small positive deflection, and then withdraw slightly to an all-negative P wave. Care must be taken when the arm is returned to the side, because the catheter will likely migrate a little more centrally and may need to be withdrawn slightly.[162]

The use of the pulmonary artery catheter for the aspiration of VAE has generally been unsatisfactory, because of the small lumen size and slow speed of blood return. However, other information can be obtained from the pulmonary artery catheter. The entry of air into the pulmonary circulation causes the pulmonary artery (PA) pressures to rise. One can utilize this information to evaluate when VAE has cleared the pulmonary circulation. If PA pressure rises during VAE and the Doppler clears, a return of PA pressure to previous levels suggests that the air obstructing the pulmonary circulation has been moved more distally, and probably excreted through the lungs.[156]

Capnography and mass spectrometry demonstrate a decrease in end-tidal CO_2 during VAE with intermediate sensitivity. One can expect to see changes in end-tidal CO_2 after Doppler changes but before hemodynamic changes occur. When enough air is entrained to cause hemodynamic changes, the end-tidal CO_2 will usually drop within a few breaths of the Doppler change. Sensitive mass spectrometry can show increases in F_EN_2 as the VAE is excreted through the lung. Transcutaneous P_{O_2} is also of intermediate sensitivity, but has more practical and technical problems, making its use in the operating room somewhat less popular.[163]

Transesophageal echocardiography (TEE) is still a research tool, but holds considerable promise in the diagnosis of VAE.

FIG. 31-7. The intracardiac electrocardiogram from each position is shown. With a single orifice catheter, tracing 4 indicates mid-right atrial position. Since the ECG trace originates from the proximal orifice of a multiorifice catheter and since placement as shown in Figure 31-6 is desirable, tracing 2 should be sought. (From Cucchiara RF, Messick JM, Gronert GA *et al:* Time required and success rate of percutaneous right atrial catheterization: Description of a technique. Can Anaesth Soc J 27:572, 1980.)

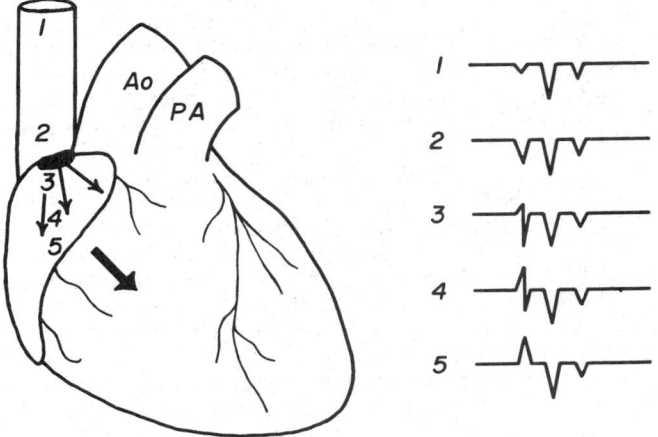

It is very sensitive, and allows us to visualize air in the cardiac chambers themselves. This gives us the unique opportunity to identify the occurrence of left heart air (Fig. 31-8).[164] The only other clinical way to identify paradoxical air embolism during sitting position surgery is for the surgeon to visualize air in the small arteries of the brain or spinal cord. This implies that it is already late, since the air is already in the vessels to the brain in large enough amounts to be readily seen.

TREATMENT OF VENOUS AIR EMBOLISM (VAE). The team approach is critical in achieving a reduction in complications from VAE. The anesthesiologist can make the diagnosis from the devices discussed above. The surgeon often makes the diagnosis at the same time, because he can see that the vein that he has opened is entraining air rather than bleeding back. The role of the anesthesiologist is to support the cardiovascular system so that ischemic injury can be avoided; the role of the surgeon is to stop the influx of air at the surgical site. We can help identify the problem area in the surgical field by several maneuvers. The surgeon can flood the field with saline to submerge the area of air entry. The application of jugular pressure at the anterior neck for about 15 seconds will frequently raise the venous pressure in the wound enough so that the vessel will back bleed. We would suggest two cautions in applying this pressure. One must attempt to feel the carotid pulsation so that it is not occluded as well. Prolonged occlusion of the jugular veins may raise cerebral venous pressure sufficiently to cause the brain to bulge from the wound. The discontinuation of N_2O will slow the increase in size of the aspirated bubbles and hasten their reabsorption. The use of vasopressors and volume for pre-load may increase cardiac output and thereby aid in moving the air through the heart to the peripheral pulmonary circulation.

The use of positive end-expiratory pressure (PEEP) in these circumstances is controversial. There is evidence to suggest that, although PEEP may raise the central venous pressure, it may also facilitate the passage of air through a patent foramen ovale. PEEP may raise right atrial pressures to levels which exceed PAOP in seated patients. In examining for patent foramen ovale, cardiologists have shown that a Valsalva maneuver can cause injectate to cross right-to-left at the atrial level on echocardiogram.[165] The application of PEEP in humans does not eliminate VAE. In dogs, PEEP was less effective in raising cerebral venous pressure than was a neck tourniquet. There are preliminary data that suggest that PEEP may not increase paradoxial air embolism, but, when PEEP is released, air tends to move paradoxically.

The mechanics of elevation of cerebral venous pressure are not as simple as was previously thought. It appears that cerebral venous flow is carried in both collapsible (jugular veins) and non-collapsible (vertebral venous sinuses) vessels. When venous sinus pressure is highly negative, cerebral venous drainage is carried primarily through non-collapsible vessels that are protected from the neck tourniquet. Neck compression is most effective when venous drainage is through the collapsible channels. That occurs when the venous sinus pressure is only slightly negative or positive. PEEP increased venous sinus pressure when it was very negative only if cardiac output was maintained.[166]

The use of PEEP thus remains controversial, but it is our opinion, based on current literature, that the potential risks of PEEP outweigh its potential benefits.

Anesthetic Considerations

There are several viable choices in agent selection for sitting position cases, and each has its advantages and disadvan-

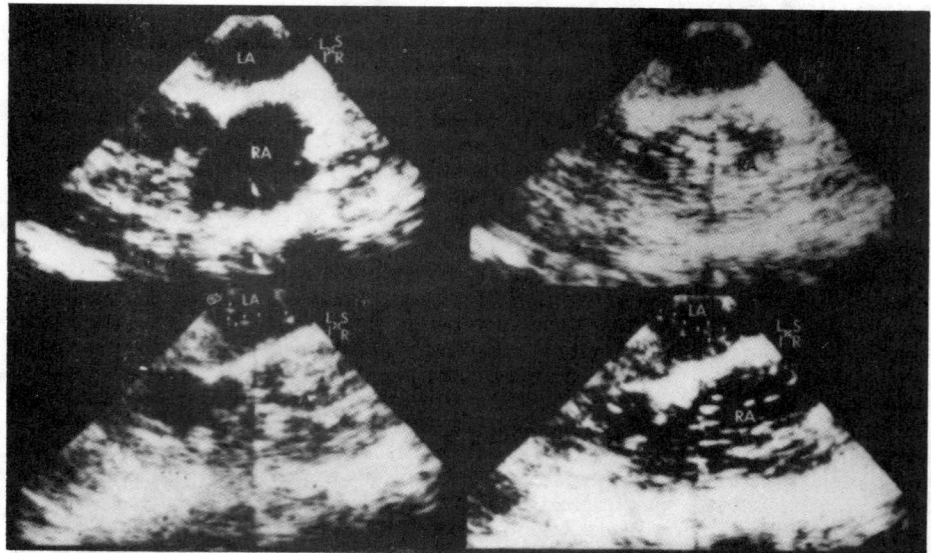

FIG. 31-8. Paradoxical air as noted by transesophageal echocardiography. (*top, left*) Normal: (*top, right*) air in right atrium; (*bottom, left*) air in left atrium, right atrium nearly opacified; (*bottom, right*) more air in left and right atrium. (From Cucchiara R, Nugent M, Seward J *et al*: Air embolism in upright neurosurgical patients: detection and localization by 2-D transesophageal echocardiography. Anesthesiology 60: 353, 1984.)

tages. Some of the disadvantages can be minimized by skillful administration. Volatile anesthetics are generally the mainstay for these types of cases at our institution. They provide smooth, easily controlled anesthetic depth; the anesthetic depth can be measured using mass spectrometry; little cardiovascular depression is encountered in the low concentrations required; and a predictable awakening can be accomplished at the end of the case. The supplemental use of N_2O is an area of controversy, particularly in these cases, because of the risk of VAE. When VAE occurs in the presence of N_2O, the bubbles will increase in size as the N_2O diffuses into the bubble faster than the nitrogen can diffuse out. Some have suggested that N_2O should be deleted in sitting cases because of this risk. Many feel that more volatile agents must be used when N_2O is deleted, and it is a little more difficult to end a sitting case without the added analgesia provided by N_2O. These cases can be done with a high-dose opioid technique, but, in general, it is difficult to have the patient actively responding at the end of surgery with this technique. The significance of apnea may be confusing, since it may be due to the surgery or to the opioid. Continued intubation of the trachea may be necessary to support ventilation of the lungs. We use an isoflurane/N_2O low-dose fentanyl technique to circumvent these problems and to allow the versatility required to use or withhold muscle relaxants. Most neurosurgeons want to see the patient awake at the end of the case in the operating room to assess their work and to be sure that a catastrophic event requiring reopening has not occurred. An anesthetic technique that permits this is desirable.

With the advent of SSEP and intraoperative EMG, our use of long-acting muscle relaxants is compromised. Muscle relaxants do not interfere with SSEP monitoring of a cervical laminectomy, for example, but, when cranial nerve motor function (VII, for example) is being tested, we are limited in practice to muscle relaxants for intubation of the trachea and closure only. This poses additional risks, because it is most undesirable to have an open craniotomy patient suddenly strain on the endotracheal tube or move. We have avoided that situation previously by using long-acting non-depolarizing muscle relaxants. As more motor monitoring comes into practice, our use of muscle relaxants will be more limited. This is not only true for

sitting cases. These same procedures done in the horizontal position will likely be monitored in the same way. The anesthetic plan must incorporate consideration of these aspects of the procedure. Thus, our overall anesthetic-muscle relaxant technique must be altered to assure, as best we can, that the patient will not move and that the monitoring can be used at critical times.

Postoperative Considerations

The most serious immediate postoperative complication following posterior fossa craniectomy is apnea. It is very important to be able to define anesthetic-related apnea at the end of the case, since apnea resulting from surgical complications, especially hematoma, may require immediate reoperation. For this reason, it is desirable to return the Pa_{CO_2} to near normal and to verify that only the smallest concentration of anesthetic drugs are present, that muscle relaxants are reversed, that temperature is near normal, and that any opioid effects are dissipated. The anesthetic technique should be managed with these goals in mind.

Posterior fossa craniectomy patients are subject to cranial nerve injuries that have implications for the anesthesiologist.[167] Whenever the lower cranial nerves are disturbed, traumatized, or even severed during the procedure, the anesthesiologist should be notified. If cranial nerve V is injured, sensation to the cornea will be impaired, and an eye patch should be used. The most dangerous cranial nerve injuries are to the sensory and motor nerves to the pharynx and larynx. If cranial nerves IX, X, or XI are injured, the patient is at increased risk of aspiration pneumonitis and hypoxia. The pathophysiology seems to involve inability to handle secretions either because the patient is not aware that these are in the pharynx and does not swallow them, or because motor coordination of the pharyngeal muscles is impaired so that swallowing is ineffective. Sometimes the cords are paretic and unable to effectively close the glottis to secretions. The process of aspiration of their own secretions is an insidious one in these patients. We have the clinical impression that they become hypoxic some hours after emerging from anesthesia. If the lower cranial nerves are significantly compromised, the patient's trachea is probably best left intubated overnight. We prefer to see the patient swallow on the endotracheal tube before extubation of the trachea to assure ourselves that at least pharyngeal sensation is present. Depending on the anesthetic technique used, this is not always possible, but observation of the event when it occurs can give one a little more confidence in removing the endotracheal tube.

Pneumocephalus occurs regularly in posterior fossa patients, but symptomatic tension pneumocephalus is uncommon. When it occurs, it requires immediate decompression. There is controversy surrounding the use of N_2O and its relationship to the frequency and severity of tension pneumocephalus.[168, 169]

TRANSSPHENOIDAL SURGERY

The pituitary gland is anatomically and functionally separated into the anterior pituitary (adenohypophysis) and posterior pituitary (neurohypophysis). Excision of adenomas of the anterior pituitary represent the vast majority of transsphenoidal operations performed, but understanding of total glandular function is necessary, as even selective removal of anterior pituitary microadenomas may often lead to posterior pituitary dysfunction. Normal anterior pituitary function is influenced both by hypothalamic releasing and inhibiting factors and by feedback from endocrine organ hormones. The posterior pituitary is responsible for storage and release of the hormones, antidiuretic hormone (ADH) and oxytocin, which are synthesized in the hypothalamus and transported to the posterior pituitary as granules in neurosecretory axons. The hormones released by the pituitary gland are listed in Table 31-6.

Clinical presentation of pituitary tumors is generally manifested as pressure effects secondary to tumor growth with impingement on adjacent intracranial structures or by altered endocrine function.[170, 171] Pressure effects may result in headaches, cranial nerve palsies, and visual disturbances secondary to optic tract involvement. In addition, pituitary endocrine deficiency may occur secondary to compression of normal gland. Functioning pituitary adenomas may cause hypersecretion of anterior pituitary hormones, resulting in a variety of clinical syndromes. The hormones most commonly involved are prolactin, growth hormone (GH), and adrenocorticotrophic hormone (ACTH), with adenomas secreting thyroid stimulating hormone (TSH), follicle stimulating hormone or luteinizing hormone being rare. Prolactinomas represent the most common hyperfunctioning adenoma, followed by GH and ACTH adenomas. Hyperprolactinemia may produce the amenorrhea-galactorrhea syndrome in females and impaired libido and potency in males. Hypersecretion of GH prepuberty may lead to gigantism, while, postpuberty, the result is acromegaly. ACTH adenomas result in the increased adrenal cortisol production of Cushing's disease. Endocrine hypofunction secondary to pressure effects on normal pituitary can be reflected as panhypopituitarism necessitating hormone replacement preoperatively. Hyposecretion of ADH, secondary to pressure effects on the posterior pituitary, may produce diabetes insipidus, which manifests as impairment of urinary concentrating ability and overall inability to maintain body water balance, especially in the face of hyperosmolarity and hypovolemia.

Anesthetic Considerations

Preoperative assessment of the patient scheduled for transsphenoidal surgery necessitates an evaluation with emphasis on physiologic changes related to endocrine dysfunction. Glucose tolerance may be disturbed secondary to endocrine dysfunction, and patients should be evaluated for possible hyperglycemia. Adequacy of ADH reserve of the posterior pituitary may be determined by measuring urinary concentrating ability following water deprivation.[171] Knowledge of baseline function is important, as operative manipulations may alter pituitary function, even if a small adenoma is microscopically removed. This necessitates perioperative provision of glucocorticoids and awareness of the potential postoperative development of diabetes insipidus.[172] In addition to the endocrine evaluation, the radiologic features of the tumor should be reviewed in order to ascertain whether pathology is limited to the sella turcica or involves suprasellar extension.

Special consideration must be given to the patient presenting with Cushing's disease or acromegaly. The patient with Cushing's disease is susceptible to hypertension, hyperglycemia, hyperkalemia, skeletal muscle weakness, and increased intravascular fluid volume.[173] The acromegalic may have hypertension, hyperglycemia, and skeletal muscle weakness, as well as skeletal, soft tissue, and connective tissue abnormalities that may manifest as neuropathies, organomegaly, and alterations in airway anatomy that may make tracheal intubation difficult and may predispose to sleep apnea.[174] Airway changes include prognathism, macroglossia, pharyngeal, tonsillar and epiglottic soft tissue hypertrophy, vocal cord fixation, and laryngeal stenosis.[175, 176] Careful preoperative assessment of the airway in the patient with acromegaly may help to anticipate difficult airway management. This may involve difficulty with obtaining good mask fit and ventilating the patient, visualizing the larynx, and advancing an endotracheal tube.[177] These authors suggest that patients with preoperatively ascertained glottic abnormalities or those with soft tissue abnormalities and glottic abnormalities should be considered for elective tracheostomy preoperatively. Other authors suggest that tracheostomy is rarely necessary in these patients, even with advanced acromegalic changes. Fiberoptic laryngoscopy and intubation of the trachea should be initially considered in acromegalic patients in whom airway management difficulties are anticipated.[178, 179]

The transsphenoidal approach for microsurgical excision of pituitary adenomas is generally performed under general anesthesia, and principles for management of patients with intracranial lesions should be observed if there is associated suprasellar extension and potential increased intracranial pressure. Patient monitoring routinely includes directly or indirectly measured arterial pressure, ECG, temperature, esophageal auscultation, and urine output. Right atrial/central venous pressure monitoring and precordial Doppler ultrasonic air detection have been suggested by some in order to diagnose and treat potential VAE in operations performed

TABLE 31-6. Pituitary Hormone Products

ANTERIOR PITUITARY	POSTERIOR PITUITARY
Growth hormone (GH)	Antidiuretic hormone (ADH)
Prolactin (PRL)	Oxytocin
Adrenocorticotrophic hormone (ACTH)	
Beta-lipotropin (B-LPH)	
Follicle-stimulating hormone (FSH)	
Luteinizing hormone (LH)	
Thyrotropin (TSH)	

with a 40° head up tilt,[180] while others suggest that the monitoring may be omitted if head up tilt is limited to less than 5 to 15 degrees.[181] Induction of general anesthesia can generally be accomplished with intravenous thiopental and a non-depolarizing muscle relaxant to facilitate endotracheal intubation. Succinylcholine may be utilized, especially if a shorter duration of relaxation is desired in cases when difficult airway management is anticipated. The acromegalic airway might be such a case. The transsphenoidal approach to the pituitary usually involves nasal septal and sublabial incisions, thus necessitating oral endotracheal intubation, with the endotracheal tube and esophageal stethoscope secured to the corner of the mouth opposite to the side where the surgeons are operating (Fig. 31-9). The mouth and posterior pharynx may be packed with moist cotton gauze to prevent bleeding into the esophagus and glottic regions and thus prevent postoperative vomiting of blood. Anesthetic maintenance can be achieved either with an opioid-N$_2$O or inhalation technique. Selection of anesthetic agents must consider the potential hypertensive and arrhythmogenic effects of epinephrine and cocaine used in submucosally injected local anesthetic mixtures by the surgeon[172] with halothane most likely to sensitize toward these effects.

When there is suprasellar extension of the tumor, subarachnoid air may be injected to allow the tumor outline to be visualized on intraoperative fluoroscopy. The elevation of ICP produced by the air may help to deliver the tumor downward into the surgeon's field. Inhaled N$_2$O will increase the volume of the injected air rapidly. There are several possible approaches to this ancillary technique, none of which has been shown to be clearly superior. One may continue the N$_2$O and inject smaller volumes of air (e.g., 5 ml), realizing that it will expand as it reaches the cranium. One may discontinue the N$_2$O and inject subarachnoid air (e.g., 10 ml), or one may draw the gas mixture from the inspired line and inject it. We do not utilize this third option if volatile drugs are in use. The air is injected through a lumbar subarachnoid needle or catheter. As long as CSF can be aspirated from the lumbar drainage system, one can help the surgeon by controlling the degree of downward push on the tumor (related to increased ICP) by removing CSF. Thus, if the air volume proves to be too large as seen from the surgeon's view of the tumor, removal of CSF can optimize the intracranial fluid dynamics. Occasionally, air will

be injected but not seen on head fluoroscopy. There may be two reasons for this: 1) the lumbar drain is not subarachnoid (this can be ruled out by withdrawing CSF before and after air injection); and 2) the drain is too caudad, and the air is passing caudad in the subarachnoid space rather than cephalad.

One must bear in mind the potential for operative complications. The sella turcica is bordered laterally by the cavernous sinus, which, in addition to venous structures, contains the intracavernous portion of the internal carotid artery and cranial nerves III, IV, V, and VI. Operative manipulation in the region of the cavernous sinus can thus result in: 1) hemorrhage from the carotid artery or arterial spasm secondary to arterial manipulation, 2) venous hemorrhage and potential entrainment of air into the venous system if head up tilt is excessive, and 3) cranial nerve weakness secondary to trauma or stretching.[182] Visual complications secondary to damage to the optic nerve or chiasm may occur, as well as hypothalamic damage and intracranial hemorrhage. Other complications include postoperative alterations in endocrine function, including the development of diabetes insipidus, which may manifest as a hypotonic polyuria and necessitates frequent reassessment of fluid status. If diabetes insipidus should develop, fluid replacement should include maintenance fluids plus an amount to cover urinary losses. In addition, exogenous vasopressin may need to be administered. This may be accomplished *via* intranasal administration of DDAVP once nasal packing is removed.

SURGERY FOR INTRACTABLE SEIZURES

Cortical resection for seizure control offers an alternative for certain patients with epilepsy who are refractory to medical therapy. Epilepsy is not a disease itself, but a symptom of altered brain function resulting in recurrent seizure activity secondary to epileptogenic cortical discharges. Despite the extensive ability of neurons to generate electrical activity and a widespread network of synaptic connections, the normal pathways for generation and for spread of electrical excitation within the brain are well regulated. In epileptogenic disorders, cortical discharges are felt to arise from a local subpopulation of abnormal neurons with altered membrane function leading to burst discharges, with spread *via* widespread

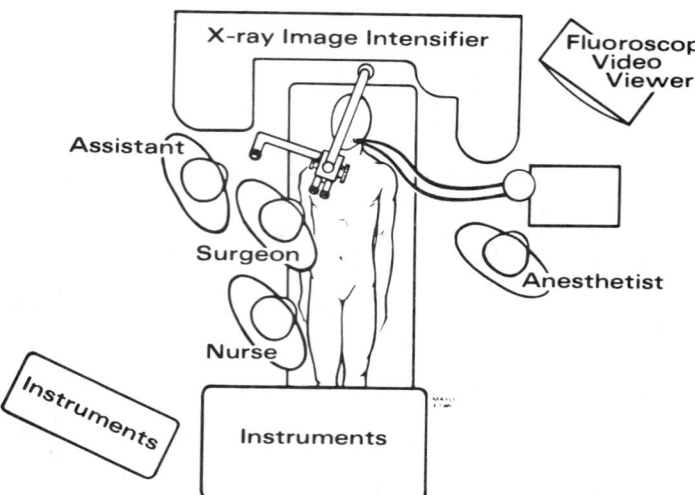

FIG. 31-9. A typical operating room arrangement for transsphenoidal pituitary surgery. (From Messick JM, Faust RJ, Cucchiara RF: Anesthesia for transsphenoidal microsurgery. In Laws ER, Randall RV, Kern EB *et al* [eds]: Management of Pituitary Adenomas and Related Lesions with Emphasis on Transsphenoidal Surgery, p. 253. New York; Appleton-Century-Crofts, 1982.)

excitatory synaptic connections after failure of normal local synaptic inhibition.[183] This widespread activation may lead to clinical seizures.

CLASSIFICATION

The epilepsies are generally classified clinically into generalized and partial categories (Table 31-7), and this classification is important in medical and surgical management. Generalized seizures are defined as those in which clinical signs and EEG changes indicate initial involvement of both hemispheres, while partial (focal) epilepsies indicate initial activities limited to a part of one or both hemispheres.[184] Partial seizures that result in impairment of consciousness are known as complex partial seizures. This classification is important, as the surgically manageable epilepsies are generally of partial origin, with psychomotor (temporal lobe) seizures being most amenable to surgical therapy. In addition, correct classification is important, as the different seizures respond to different medication. The classic generalized absence (petit mal) seizures traditionally respond to valproic acid or ethosuximide, while partial epilepsies, such as temporal lobe epilepsy, typically respond to carbamazepine, phenytoin, phenobarbital, or primidone.

SURGICAL MANAGEMENT

Craniotomy may be considered in patients who demonstrate sufficiently frequent seizures with life impairment and demonstrate medical refractoriness indicated by continued seizures, despite correct seizure classification and treatment with appropriate drugs used to their maximal effectiveness.[185] In addition, surgery may be considered in patients who demonstrate unacceptable toxicity to the anticonvulsant agents. The goals of surgical management are to obtain a reduction in seizure frequency on medications postoperatively, with eventual potential long-term tapering of anticonvulsants. Studies have generally indicated improved seizure control in 60%–90% of patients with temporal lobe epilepsy managed by surgery.[186]

The ideal surgical candidate, in addition to demonstrating medical refractoriness, must be of an age and intelligence to tolerate and cooperate with the extensive pre-surgical evaluation. This evaluation is undertaken to accurately define the area of epileptogenesis and to estimate and prevent impairment of cerebral language and memory function secondary to the planned surgical resection. Routine initial evaluation generally includes prolonged recording of the scalp EEG with videotape monitoring to record clinical seizures; radiographic studies, including CT or MRI, to delineate possible structural lesions; and neuropsychologic testing to assess intelligence, language, and memory function. Further evaluation includes cerebral angiography to assess possible vascular malformations and selective intracarotid injection of amobarbital. Intracarotid injection of amobarbital produces temporary unilateral cerebral anesthesia, and allows for determination of the language dominant hemisphere and the memory function of the hemisphere not involved in the planned surgical resection.[187] To further define the site of epileptogenesis, anticonvulsant medications may be tapered or withdrawn completely, and further scalp EEG recording may be performed. In some centers, further seizure presurgical evaluation involves invasive placement of intracranial electrodes.[188] This involves either stereotactic intracerebral placement of depth electrodes, or operative placement of epidural recording electrode assays.[189] Subsequent recording from these invasive electrodes during spontaneous seizures may help to localize the seizure focus prior to resection surgery.

Traditional surgical management for seizure resection involves performance of a craniotomy under local anesthesia with intraoperative electrocorticographic recording from cortical electrodes to localize seizure focus and mapping *via* stimulating electrodes of sensorimotor and language areas.[190] This requires that the patient be minimally sedated during mapping; full patient cooperation is needed. Resection of the identified seizure focus can then be performed using the information from the stimulation process to gauge the limits of the resection. Surgical resection of epileptic foci under general anesthesia has also been described.[191] This is accomplished *via* extraoperative recording by epidural electrode assays placed during initial craniotomy to localize the seizure focus, and cortical SSEP to localize the sensorimotor response. After 24–72 h of extraoperative recording, the patient undergoes repeat craniotomy for resection of the localized focus. Stereotactic seizure focus resection under general anesthesia with intraoperative depth recording has also been utilized.[192] Extent of surgical resection for temporal lobe epilepsy varies with the side of localized seizure focus. Foci in the non-dominant speech hemisphere may be resected with a more traditional temporal lobectomy, while foci in the dominant speech hemisphere may require a more limited resection of medial and anterior temporal lobe structures to avoid language areas in the posterolateral temporal lobe.

ANESTHETIC CONSIDERATIONS

Preanesthetic evaluation should include an assessment of: 1) type and frequency of seizures; 2) anticonvulsant medications utilized; 3) complications of anticonvulsant therapy; and 4) functional status and ability of the patient to cooperate with the planned procedure, especially if awake craniotomy is to be performed. Serious complications, including hematologic and hepatic dysfunction, have resulted from anticonvulsant therapy,[193] and blood counts and liver function tests should be measured preoperatively. A summary of potential drug toxicities is found in Table 31-8.

Intraoperative management of the patient undergoing awake craniotomy for seizure resection requires excellent patient cooperation, long-acting local anesthetic infiltration by the surgeon, judicious use of neuroleptic agents by the anesthesiologist, ability to rapidly treat overt seizures, and preparedness for rapid airway management, including possible induction of general anesthesia. A technique utilizing conscious-sedation analgesia with fentanyl and droperidol has been described.[194]

TABLE 31-7. Classification of Epilepsies

I. Primary Generalized Epilepsies
    Absence
    Myoclonic
    Clonic-tonic-clonic (grand mal)
    Tonic-clonic (grand mal)
II. Partial Epilepsies
    Simple partial
    Complex partial
III. Secondary Generalized Epilepsies

TABLE 31-8. Potential Toxicity of Drugs Used
to Treat Epilepsy

DRUG	
Valproic acid	Thrombocytopenia, hypofibrinogenemia, elevation of serum transaminases and possible severe hepatic dysfunction
Ethosuximide	Thrombocytopenia
Phenytoin	Gingival hyperplasia, teratogenicity, ataxia, Stevens-Johnson disorder
Carbamazepine	Leukopenia, anemia, bone marrow depression
Phenobarbital	Sedation, occasional drug sensitivity reaction
Primidone	Sedation

In some centers, and with certain patients unable to cooperate with awake craniotomy, general anesthesia is utilized. At the Mayo Clinic, where intraoperative electrocorticography is performed,[195] anesthesia is induced with a short-acting barbiturate and maintained with N_2O and fentanyl, with a volatile anesthetic often added. At the time of electrocorticography, it is sometimes necessary to reduce or discontinue the volatile drug to optimize recording of the seizure focus. Muscle relaxation is maintained throughout the procedure, as no intraoperative cortical stimulation and movement testing is performed. Higher and more frequent doses of muscle relaxants may be required, because resistance to blockade has been demonstrated in patients receiving anticonvulsant therapy.[148, 196, 197]

Etomidate may activate epileptogenic foci during electrocorticography,[198, 199] and ketamine causes EEG activation. The use of fentanyl and droperidol during seizure resection can be accomplished with minimal effects on epileptogenicity. Among the inhalation drugs, N_2O has minimal effects on epileptic foci, while enflurane in high concentrations and in association with hypocarbia can activate the EEG.[43] Halothane and isoflurane in lower doses should allow for adequate intraoperative recording, but might need to be withdrawn if adequate electrocorticography cannot be obtained.

After seizure resection, anticonvulsant therapy is resumed intravenously, as incidence of seizures may initially be increased. Postoperatively, it is important to be prepared to rapidly terminate seizure activity should it occur. Small doses of thiopental or diazepam may be efficacious initially, while intravenous phenytoin or phenobarbital may be required to prevent seizure recurrence.

CEREBROVASCULAR SURGERY

CEREBRAL ANEURYSMS

Principles of Management

Anesthetic management of patients with cerebral aneurysms requires consideration of two major sources of morbidity and mortality from cerebral aneurysms, aneurysm rupture, and vasospasm-induced cerebral ischemia. Rebleeding occurs most frequently during the first 10 days following subarachnoid hemorrhage (SAH), and 29% of aneurysm patients presenting with SAH have more than one episode of bleeding. Rebleeding is a major cause of morbidity and mortality in aneurysm patients with good neurologic function at the time of presentation. Aneurysmal rupture during induction of anesthesia or craniotomy (prior to dissection of the cerebral aneurysm or its feeding vessels) results in an extremely high incidence of morbidity and mortality. Factors influencing risk of bleeding include size of the aneurysm, strength of the aneurysmal wall, timing of prior episodes of bleeding, and the transmural pressure across the wall of the aneurysm.[200-203] Anesthetic management can alter the transmural pressure, but has little influence on the other factors. Transmural pressure is equal to the difference between the arterial pressure within the aneurysmal sac and the ICP. Flow within the aneurysm is pulsatile, and the systolic, diastolic, and mean arterial pressures inside the aneurysm are roughly equal to the pressures measured peripherally.[204] Any marked or sudden increase in systemic arterial pressure or decrease in ICP would cause an increase in the transmural pressure gradient and increase the risk of rupture of the aneurysm.

Vasospasm is a relatively frequent occurrence, developing in 40%–60% of aneurysm patients following subarachnoid hemorrhage. Cerebral vasospasm may be asymptomatic, detected only by angiography, or can result in symptomatic ischemia and development of new neurologic deficits that may prove to be reversible or irreversible. It occurs most frequently 5–14 days following SAH, but has been reported to occur from the first day to several weeks after SAH. Vasospasm may develop initially pre- or postoperatively, and has been suggested to occur more commonly in those patients with severe meningeal signs, worsened neurologic status, or larger volumes of subarachnoid blood (as determined by CT) and in patients noted intraoperatively to have a "red, angry, swollen" brain, considerable amounts of clotted blood around the feeding vessels, or impaired cerebral autoregulation.[205-207] Caution should be exercised in administering agents causing cerebral vasoconstriction in patients with documented or suspected cerebral vasospasm. However, no anesthetic technique has been demonstrated to either increase or decrease the risk of cerebral vasospasm. Given the multitude of factors present perioperatively, it is unlikely that any drug will ever be demonstrated to be the anesthetic technique of choice to prevent vasospasm.

Preoperative care should include a careful preoperative assessment and appropriate premedication. The pre-anesthetic evaluation should include history of prior aneurysmal bleeds and their timing, current neurologic status, evidence of vasospasm with or without cerebral ischemia, size and location of the aneurysm, and any focal neurologic abnormality due to compression by the aneurysm. Any medications the patient is receiving and concurrent acute or chronic medical problems should be noted. Premedication should be tailored to the individual patient. Those patients who are receiving sedation following SAH should have this continued. Premedication for other patients should balance the need to decrease anxiety and sympathetic tone in these patients with the risk of excessive sedation, and the deleterious effects of hypercarbia and hypoxia on cerebral hemodynamics. In many instances, a reassuring pre-anesthetic visit may be adequate.

Nimodipine, a calcium blocker, has been found in clinical trials to decrease the incidence of cerebral vasospasm following SAH, while causing few significant adverse effects.[208] It is likely that, in the future, many patients coming to surgery for aneurysm clipping following SAH will be on nimodipine therapy. Nimodipine results in cerebral vasodilation following cerebral ischemia,[209] but has no effect on CBF or $CMRO_2$ in normal brain,[210] and, therefore, is unlikely to cause dangerous increase in CBF, cerebral blood volume, or ICP. In patients receiving nimodipine preoperatively and undergoing aneurysm repair with an anesthetic technique of thiopental induction, halothane or enflurane for maintenance, and induced hypotension, there was no increase in the incidence of untoward events as compared to the same technique utilized in patients not receiving nimodipine. Hemodynamic parameters were similar, suggesting that patients receiving nimodipine are not at increased risk for intraoperative hemodynamic instability, and can be safely managed with current anesthetic regimens.[211]

The period of induction of anesthesia and intubation of the trachea is one of the most crucial points in the anesthetic management of these patients. During this time, wide fluctuations in MAP and ICP are possible, altering the transmural pressure gradient and the risk of aneurysmal rupture. A smooth, adequately monitored induction of anesthesia and intubation of the trachea are essential. In addition to the basic monitors of an ECG, blood pressure cuff, and a pulse oximeter established prior to induction of anesthesia, direct arterial pressure monitoring prior to the intubation of the trachea is important, allowing continuous monitoring of blood pressure and control of the systemic pressure, avoiding excessive increases in arterial and transmural pressure. Placement of a radial artery cannula under local anesthesia prior to induction of anesthesia allows direct arterial pressure to be monitored throughout induction. However, painful stimuli in an awake patient may result in sympathetic stimulation and increases in systemic pressure. For this reason, some prefer to place the arterial cannula following induction of anesthesia, but prior to intubation of the trachea.

Drugs utilized for induction of anesthesia should be chosen with consideration of the necessity of minimizing the transmural pressure gradient. Wide swings in arterial pressure and ICP should be avoided, especially hypertension and sudden decreases in ICP. A combination of thiopental induction followed by a non-depolarizing muscle relaxant with minimal cardiovascular effects, such as vecuronium or atracurium, and adequately controlled ventilation of the lungs without airway obstruction, hypoventilation, or marked hyperventilation can provide the desired smooth induction of anesthesia.[212] Prior to intubation of the trachea, adequate muscle relaxation should be achieved, and additional anesthesia to block the cardiovascular and ICP response to laryngoscopy and intubation should be given. This can be accomplished with additional thiopental, fentanyl, sufentanyl, or intravenous lidocaine.[212-215] Laryngotracheal lidocaine at the time of laryngoscopy is probably inadequate, as significant pressor responses occur with laryngoscopy alone.[213, 214] Consideration should also be given to blocking the effects of sympathetic stimulation with beta blockers such as propranolol, labetolol, or esmolol.[216, 217] Esmolol, with its ultrashort duration, may be superior to the long-acting agents propranolol or labetolol in this setting.[216]

Following the critical period of induction of anesthesia and intubation of the trachea, careful assessment of arterial pressure, depth of anesthesia, and anticipated stimulation should be continued. Positioning of the patient either for surgery or placement of a CSF drainage catheter or needle may result in an increase in sympathetic stimulation and cardiovascular instability. Prior to placement of the pinions, an adequate depth of general anesthesia must be obtained, and infiltration of the pinion sites with local anesthetics should also be utilized. Regardless of the agents or techniques chosen, achieving and maintaining an adequate depth of anesthesia for the expected stimulation, adequate skeletal muscle relaxation, and adequate ventilation of the lungs and oxygenation are crucial. More important than which specific drugs and techniques are utilized, it must be remembered that light anesthesia, airway obstruction, and "bucking on the tube" may have disastrous consequences.[212]

A variety of techniques for maintenance of anesthesia during cerebral aneurysm surgery including opioids, volatile drugs, and high-dose barbiturates as primary anesthetics have all been used with success.[211, 218-220] None has been proven to be superior, and any can be utilized safely if consideration is given to maintaining cardiovascular stability and adequate cerebral perfusion without significant increases in the transmural pressure gradient, and to providing an adequately "slack" brain to facilitate surgical exposure. Theoretically, high dose opioid techniques may be inadvisable in patients with evidence of cerebral vasospasm because of the vasoconstrictive properties of these agents. Systemic blood pressure should not exceed the pressure range tolerated by the patient preoperatively. Commonly, the arterial pressure is maintained at the lower end of the normal range for a patient prior to dissection of the aneurysm or its feeding vessels. Moderate hyperventilation of the lungs to a Pa_{CO_2} of 28–30 mm Hg is useful to blunt any anesthetic-induced increase on CBF and ICP, and to facilitate surgical exposure.[48, 49] Greater degrees of hyperventilation prior to opening the dura may result in an undesirable degree of decrease in ICP and increase of the transmural pressure gradient.

Several interventions by the anesthesiologist may be utilized to "shrink" the brain and facilitate dissection. The timing of these efforts should coincide with opening the dura in order to avoid marked increases in the transmural pressure gradient. Hyperventilation of the lungs, barbiturates, osmotic diuretics, and CSF drainage have been utilized.[200, 218, 220] Mannitol is the osmotic diuretic used most often and, given in doses of 0.5–1.0 $g \cdot kg^{-1}$ around the time of incision, will decrease brain mass maximally as the dura is opened.[149, 200, 221] CSF drainage may be accomplished by placing either a lumbar subarachnoid needle or catheter prior to positioning the patient for the operative procedure. It is important that only a minimal amount of CSF be lost at the time of placing the needle or catheter to avoid significant decreases in ICP. Removal of CSF can be done cautiously following opening of the dura with guidance by the surgeon.

The anesthetic technique should be modified to allow assessment of neurologic status as soon as possible following completion of the operative procedure. This is usually possible in the immediate postoperative period using both a volatile agent and a N_2O-opioid technique. With high-dose barbiturate anesthesia, such assessment is usually delayed for 3–4 h postoperatively.[218-221] Prompt diagnosis of complications, such as ischemia due to improper clip placement, movement of a clip, or hematoma formation, allows for rapid treatment and potential reversal of any resultant neurologic deficit. During emergence from anesthesia, hypertension should be avoided. It may be necessary to administer antihypertensive agents during this period of light anesthesia and continued stimulation. Hydralazine is a direct-acting vasodilator with an onset of action in 15–20 min and may be useful. Labetolol, a combined alpha and beta blocker with more rapid onset (approximately 5 min) or esmolol, the ultrashort-acting beta blocker, may be more suitable.[216] Nitroprusside infusion may be necessary.

Special Techniques

Hypothermia causes a depression of $CMRO_2$ that is proportional to the degree of temperature reduction below 37° C, with $CMRO_2$ decreasing approximately 50% for each 8° C decrease in body temperature. The depression of $CMRO_2$ by hypothermia results from a decrease in all cell functions, both those related to neuronal activity and those responsible for maintenance of cellular integrity. Unlike barbiturates, hypothermia decreases $CMRO_2$ in the absence of cerebral electrical activity.[222] The hypothermia-induced decrease in $CMRO_2$ provides cerebral protection, prolonging safely tolerated periods of cerebral ischemia.[223] Varying degrees of hypothermia have been utilized during cerebral aneurysm surgery to prolong ischemic tolerance in the event that temporary occlusion of cerebral vessels is necessary. Moderate hypothermia to 28–30° C can be produced with surface cooling, and does not require cardiopulmonary bypass. Unfortunately, the technique of surface cooling is cumbersome and time consuming. Moderate hypothermia is frequently complicated by cardiac dysrhythmias, including bradycardias and ventricular fibrillation, hypotension, acidosis, downward "drift" of temperature below the desired level, and rewarming shock. Profound hypothermia (12–28° C) makes possible circulatory arrest for up to 60 min, and can only be achieved with cardiopulmonary bypass. The technique requires systemic heparinization, two surgical teams, and much extra equipment. The major problems are coagulation defects causing difficulties in obtaining hemostasis at the operative site and a high incidence of reopenings for bleeding. After several years of use of hypothermia, and with the development of new operative and anesthetic techniques, institutions utilizing hypothermia compared their results following cerebral aneurysm surgery with and without hypothermia. The mortality from aneurysm surgery was the same, regardless of whether hypothermia was used. There was some morbidity associated with the hypothermic techniques, and as a result, deliberate hypothermia is no longer routinely utilized. Some suggest that it may be used rarely for giant cerebral aneurysms of the basilar system that would be inoperable without the aid of profound hypothermia and circulatory arrest.[32, 223]

The most common technique currently utilized to facilitate cerebral aneurysm surgery is induced hypotension. Systemic blood pressure is reduced during dissection of the aneurysm and its feeding vessels to reduce the risk of rupture during surgical manipulation. Hypotension may also facilitate application of clip by "softening" the aneurysmal sac. In the event of intraoperative rupture, hypotension may decrease bleeding and facilitate clip application. The "safe" level of hypotension is usually considered to be the lower limit of cerebral autoregulation, a MAP of 50 mm Hg in patients free of cardiovascular disease. Induced hypotension with a variety of agents in a number of animal models and in humans to a MAP of 50 mm Hg has been produced without evidence of cerebral ischemia.[51, 224–228]

Induced hypotension may be necessary in patients with cardiovascular disease, hypertension, and occlusive cerebrovascular disease, and in elderly patients. In these patients, hypotension should be produced cautiously with a MAP about 50 mm Hg as the limit of hypotension, because cerebral autoregulation may be impaired. It has been suggested that MAP may be decreased by 30% below a patient's usual MAP safely. Potential complications of induced hypotension include cerebral ischemia, myocardial ischemia, systemic acidosis, oliguria, thrombotic events, persistent hypotension, and potential for rebound hypertension and increased bleeding following discontinuation of the hypotensive drug.[229] Properly administered and monitored induced hypotension in selected patients can be a very valuable technique with low morbidity and mortality (<1%).[229]

A number of drugs and techniques have been utilized to induce and maintain hypotension. Accurate and reliable measurement of blood pressure, as provided by direct arterial cannulation, is needed. Many neurosurgical patients are fluid restricted preoperatively and, as a result, volume depleted. Induction of hypotension in volume-depleted patients may be complicated by precipitous drops in blood pressure. Ideally, the hypotensive drug chosen should provide easily controlled degrees of hypotension, have rapid onset and offset, be easily titratable, and be free from the development of tachyphylaxis or toxicity. Although this perfect drug has yet to be found, a number of techniques are successfully utilized clinically.

Sodium nitroprusside is one of the most commonly utilized hypotensive drugs. Nitroprusside is a direct-acting vasodilator with arteriolar dilating capacity exceeding its effect on the venous system. Some degree of reflex increase in heart rate is common, and may limit the degree of hypotension produced. Beta blockers may be necessary to blunt the sympathetically mediated tachycardia. Tachyphylaxis is uncommon.[228, 230–232] Rebound hypertension has been reported after discontinuing the nitroprusside infusion. Because nitroprusside is also a direct cerebral vasodilator, it can cause an increase in CBF and cerebral blood volume, resulting in increases in ICP, especially in patients with reduced intracranial compliance.[230, 233, 234] Systemic toxicity can occur with large doses of nitroprusside, and is due to the release of cyanide by the metabolism of nitroprusside. Doses in excess of 1 $mg \cdot kg^{-1}$ over several hours should be avoided. For longer use, the maximum recommended infusion rate is 5 $\mu g \cdot kg^{-1} \cdot min^{-1}$.[230]

Hypotension to a MAP of 50 mm Hg has been produced with nitroprusside without resulting in impairment of cerebral energy state or evidence of cerebral ischemia.[228] In spite of the potential problems of systemic toxicity, elevated CBF and ICP, and rebound hypertension, nitroprusside continues to be used safely and effectively for induced hypotension in neurosurgical patients.[232]

Nitroglycerin may also be used to induce hypotension during neurosurgical procedures. Like nitroprusside, it is a direct vasodilator and, as such, shares with nitroprusside the potential for increasing CBF and ICP. Nitroglycerin-induced hypotension to a MAP of 50 mm Hg results in no evidence of altered cerebral energy state or cerebral ischemia.[226, 231, 235] In patients with coronary artery disease, nitroglycerin has an important advantage over other hypotensive agents, such as nitroprusside and isoflurane, in that it improves distribution of coronary blood flow, increasing blood flow to regions of the myocardium that are ischemic or at risk for ischemia.[236]

Trimethaphan is a ganglionic blocking agent that has been used to produce induced hypotension. Evaluations in ICP have also been reported, but to a lesser degree than with nitroprusside. In addition, trimethaphan produces mydriasis and acycloplegia, which may complicate intraoperative and postoperative neurologic evaluation. In an animal model used to study cerebral metabolic effects of induced hypotension, evidence of cerebral ischemia and altered cerebral metabolic state was present during induced hypotension to a MAP of 55 mm Hg with trimethaphan, but not at similar levels of hypotension produced by nitroprusside, adenosine, isoflurane, or nitroglycerin.[224, 229, 233, 235] It is less commonly used now than some of the other hypotensive drugs.

Labetalol is a unique drug for producing controlled hypotension by virtue of selective alpha-1 and nonselective beta-1 and beta-2 blockade. Prompt reductions in blood pressure that follow intravenous administration of this drug reflect simultaneous decreases in cardiac output and peripheral vascular resistance. Bronchospasm is less likely to occur with labetalol than with other non-selective beta-adrenergic antagonists.

Both halothane and isoflurane have been used to induce hypotension. Halothane reduces blood pressure primarily by myocardial depression, decreasing cardiac output. The desired levels of hypotension can be readily produced and, at a MAP of 50 mm Hg, no evidence of cerebral metabolic disturbance develops.[46, 228] Isoflurane is the volatile drug used more commonly to induce hypotension. Isoflurane produces hypotension primarily by decreasing systemic vascular resistance, while causing a less marked decrease in cardiac output.[224, 237] Some evidence suggests, however, that isoflurane is a myocardial depressant, and that the cardiac output is likely maintained in the face of decreased contractility by the decrease in afterload.[238] The desired level of hypotension can be achieved within 5–6 min by increasing the inspired isoflurane concentrations to 4%, and, thereafter, can be maintained by adjusting the inspired concentration to between 2% and 3%. Rapid return of blood pressure to control levels within 7 min can be achieved following further decreases in inspired concentration (to 0.25%) without rebound hypertension.[237] Concentrations necessary to induce and maintain hypotension have been shown to be free of cerebral toxicity.[224] Like nitroprusside and nitroglycerin, hypotension to MAP of 50 mm Hg with isoflurane does not result in an altered cerebral metabolic state.[51, 224] Emergence from anesthesia is not delayed by this technique. Isoflurane is unique among the commonly used hypotensive agents in significantly decreasing $CMRO_2$ and providing some potential cerebral protection.[224, 225, 240]

Adenosine is a new hypotensive agent. Like many of the other hypotensive agents, adenosine does not result in an altered cerebral metabolic state at hypotensive levels of a MAP of 50 mm Hg. It has been studied extensively in animal models and used successfully to induce hypotension in neurosurgical patients. Adenosine produces prompt, easily controlled levels of hypotension, maintenance of cardiac output, rapid return of blood pressure to control levels without rebound hypertension, and no evidence of toxicity. Currently, this drug has not been approved for clinical use in the United States.[227, 241]

Selection of the best hypotensive agent or agents and the appropriate level of induced hypotension requires understanding of the pharmacology of the agents, the patient's condition and associated medical problems, and the surgical requirements. Consideration of these factors and attention to maintenance of adequate cerebral perfusion pressures, oxygenation, ventilation, and hemodynamic stability provide optimal management.

CEREBRAL ARTERIOVENOUS MALFORMATIONS

Anesthetic management of the patient with an arteriovenous malformation (AVM) for ligation of feeding vessels and removal of the AVM is similar to management of a cerebral aneurysm patient. AVM present more commonly in a younger age group than aneurysms,[202] and the most frequent presenting symptom is bleeding. However, 30% of these patients present with seizures.[242] AVM may present in several ways, and the anesthetic approach should concentrate on the presenting problem. The AVM that has recently bled a small amount is similar to a ruptured or leaking aneurysm. A large bleed with clot may present with elevated ICP and mass effect. The large intact AVM may have high flow and cause a "steal," so that cerebral ischemia develops in the remainder of the brain. Each of these presentations can be cared for by management that focuses on that problem, realizing that they are interrelated to various degrees in different patients. As in cerebral aneurysm patients, close attention must be paid to maintenance of systemic blood pressure within the patient's normal range and avoiding wide swings in blood pressure or wide swings in ICP. A smooth, adequately monitored induc-

tion of anesthesia as described for cerebral aneurysm patients is appropriate. Maintenance of anesthesia is also similar to that for aneurysm patients. A volatile drug or an opioid-based technique may be used if attention is given to maintaining hemodynamic stability and adequate cerebral perfusion. Moderate hyperventilation of the lungs is often useful. In addition, spinal cerebrospinal fluid drainage or mannitol may be necessary to further "shrink" the brain to facilitate surgical exposure. Induced hypotension is often used during the dissection and ligation of feeding vessels to improve surgical exposure and decrease bleeding. Prompt emergence from anesthesia following completion of the surgical procedure to allow for neurologic assessment is optimal. This technique results in relatively light anesthesia during completion of the closure and application of the head dressing that may cause hypertension. Excessive elevations in blood pressure may result in unacceptable amounts of bleeding into the bed of the AVM. It is advisable, in this setting, to control blood pressure as the anesthetic is lightened with antihypertensive agents such as labetolol, esmolol, hydralazine, or nitroprusside.

CEREBRAL BYPASS PROCEDURES

Extracranial to intracranial cerebral bypass procedures (EC-IC bypass), have been used in the treatment of occlusive cerebrovascular disease. Controversy continues to surround the efficacy of EC-IC bypass in preventing ischemic stroke and which subgroups of patients, if any, might benefit from the procedure.[243-248] Results from a multicenter randomized trial showed no decrease in stroke rate in patients treated with an EC-IC bypass *versus* those with medical management. Recently, this study has come under heavy criticism, leaving the issue unresolved.[246-248]

Anesthetic management of patients undergoing EC-IC bypass for occlusive cerebrovascular disease is similar to that for carotid endarterectomy patients (See Chapter 36).

CEREBRAL PROTECTION

The topic of cerebral protection has been the subject of a great deal of study in recent years. In considering cerebral protection, the distinction must be made between ischemic damage due to complete global ischemia and to focal or incomplete cerebral ischemia. Some agents found to be protective against one type of ischemia are not protective against the other. Initial work suggested the barbiturates might lessen the degree of neurologic damage resulting from complete cerebral ischemia.[249] However, further studies have repeatedly failed to demonstrate any degree of cerebral protection against complete global ischemia by barbiturates.[250, 251] Hypothermia does exert a protective effect during complete cerebral ischemia, increasing tolerance to ischemic insults.[222] The explanation of the different effects of hypothermia and barbiturate in complete cerebral ischemia, although both decrease $CMRO_2$, is found in the mechanism through which each agent decreases $CMRO_2$ (Fig. 31-10). Barbiturates decrease $CMRO_2$ by decreasing cerebral electrical activity and, in the absence of cerebral function, no decrease in $CMRO_2$ occurs with barbiturate administration. Hypothermia decreases the rate of all metabolic reactions in cerebral tissue, both those related to function and those related to the maintenance of cellular integrity. In the absence of cerebral function, decreases in temperature decrease $CMRO_2$. Since ischemic tolerance is prolonged by decreasing $CMRO_2$ and consumption of energy stores, a drug

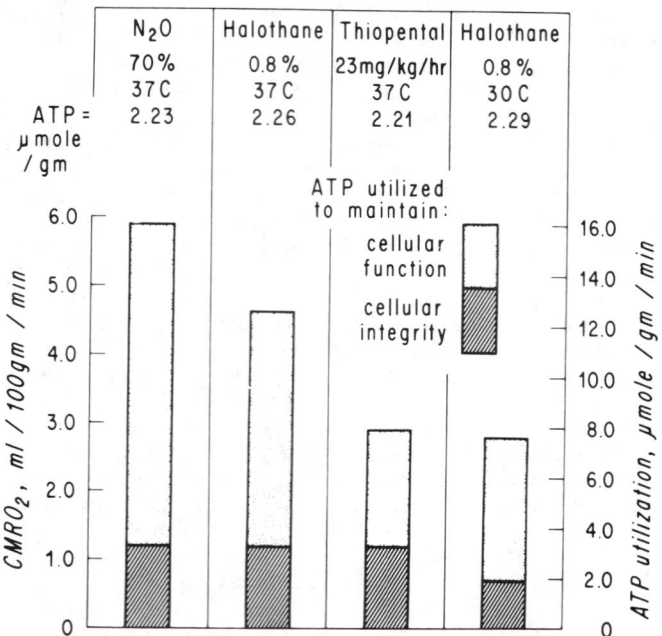

FIG. 31-10. Differences in metabolic rates between different anesthetics are accounted for only by differences in functional needs. Energy for maintenance of integrity is the same for all. By contrast, hypothermia slows the rates of all energy-consuming processes. It is coincidental that deep thiopental and moderate hypothermia (30° C) result in a similar total metabolic rate. (From Michenfelder JD: Brain hypoxia: Current status of experimental and clinical therapy. Seminars in Anesthesia 2:81, 1983.)

decreasing $CMRO_2$ would be expected to provide cerebral protection. With complete cerebral ischemia, electrical silence occurs within seconds. In this situation, barbiturates cause no further decrease in $CMRO_2$. On the other hand, hypothermia decreases $CMRO_2$ and, therefore, offers some degree of cerebral protection.[222] Recently, the calcium channel blocker, nimodipine, administered either before or following complete cerebral ischemia, has been found to decrease the degree of neurologic injury. Nimodipine has been shown to increase cerebral blood flow during the postischemic hypoperfusion period as compared to untreated animals. This effect on CBF has been suggested as a possible mechanism for the improvement in neurologic outcome with nimodipine treatment following complete ischemia.[209, 210, 252–254] Other calcium blockers have failed to demonstrate equal cerebral protective effects.[255, 256]

Episodes of complete cerebral ischemia are uncommon intraoperatively. The more common events are temporary episodes of incomplete or focal ischemia that might occur during very low levels of induced hypotension or temporary occlusion of major vessels. During incomplete or focal cerebral ischemia, electrical activity persists. In this situation, agents that decrease $CMRO_2$ by decreasing cerebral electrical activity should have some protective effects. Barbiturates and isoflurane in adequate doses cause complete electrical silence and decrease cerebral metabolic rate to approximately 40% of awake values.[44, 63] Indeed, in both animal models and human studies, there is evidence of cerebral protection by barbiturates and isoflurane during incomplete cerebral ischemia.[257–259] This degree of metabolic depression has not been

demonstrated with benzodiazepenes or, opioids. Midazolam and diazepam have been demonstrated to provide a degree of cerebral protection less than that by barbiturates.[260] There has been one study (occlusion of the MCA in monkeys during induced hypotension to a MAP of 45 mm Hg) in which isoflurane did not provide cerebral protection. The authors suggested that the failure of isoflurane to offer protection in this model might be due either to the inability of isoflurane to further decrease $CMRO_2$ in the area of focal ischemia or to the vasodilatory effects of isoflurane and unfavorable redistribution of CBF (steal phenomenon) in this model of combined vessel occlusion and induced hypotension.[261]

Some conclusions can be drawn from these studies. First, during complete global cerebral ischemia, the only class of drugs that has reproducably produced cerebral protection is the calcium channel blockers, with nimodipine being the most efficacious thus far. Profound hypothermia, as is utilized during complete circulatory arrest to facilitate complex repairs of congenital cardiac anomalies, prolongs ischemic tolerance. This technique has very limited applicability in neurosurgical patients.[223] Barbiturates are ineffective in improving outcome after complete cerebral ischemia.[250, 251] Fortunately, perioperative global ischemia is uncommon. Both barbiturates and isoflurane have been demonstrated to provide cerebral protection during incomplete cerebral ischemia.[257–259]

It is appropriate to discuss the role of a glucose in neurologic outcome following cerebral ischemia. Work in humans suggested than those patients with elevated blood glucose at hospital admission for ischemic stroke had a worse neurologic outcome than those with normal glucose levels, suggesting that hyperglycemia may be detrimental.[145] In a primate model of complete cerebral ischemia, those animals receiving a 5% glucose infusion fared worse neurologically than those not receiving glucose, although blood glucose levels in the animals receiving the glucose infusion were not significantly elevated at the time of the ischemic insult. It seems likely that elevated brain glucose results in increased neurologic damage following cerebral ischemia, possibly due to increased lactate production.[144]

There are several potential clinical applications of this information. Little is currently available to improve neurologic outcome following complete ischemia other than prompt and effective resuscitation as irreversible brain damage begins to develop by 4–5 min. Nimodipine may prove to be useful in this situation by increasing CBF after ischemia. The potential for incomplete cerebral ischemia exists intraoperatively during profound induced hypotension, especially in patients with cerebrovascular disease. It may be that isoflurane is the ideal agent in this situation. It produces easily controlled levels of hypotension, decreases cerebral metabolic rate, and results in better preservation of cerebral energy stores at a MAP of 40 mm Hg than other available hypotensive agents. In addition, cerebral protection during incomplete ischemia by isoflurane has been demonstrated in some animal models. Focal cerebral ischemia may also occur intraoperatively as a result of occlusion of major vessels during aneurysm clipping or during the EC-IC anastomosis. Administration of a ''sleep dose'' of thiopental (3–5 mg·kg⁻¹) adequate to provide near maximal suppression of $CMRO_2$ just prior to occlusion should result in a decreased $CMRO_2$ in the potentially ischemic area, prolonging the tolerance to cerebral ischemia. Additional doses of barbiturate during occlusion are less likely to be of benefit. If there is no blood flow to the ischemic area, barbiturate administered prior to occlusion should not ''wash out,'' and barbiturate given after occlusion will not reach the ischemic tissue. If, on the other hand, adequate collateral flow exists to deliver enough barbiturate to the ischemic area to depress cerebral function, the protection may not be necessary. It has been suggested that a moderate dose of barbiturate prior to occlusion, limited occlusion times, temporary restoration of flow when possible, and additional small doses of thiopental (1–2 mg · kg^{-1}) prior to reocclusion is a rational approach.[32] Finally, in patients at risk for cerebral ischemic insults, routine administration of glucose-containing solutions may be inadvisable. In addition, during these periods of stress, maintenance of adequate oxygenation and ventilation and hemodynamic stability is critical, and should not be overlooked during attempts to provide some degree of cerebral protection.

REFERENCES

1. Michenfelder JD, Messick JM, Theye RA: Simultaneous cerebral blood flow measured by direct and indirect methods. J Surg Res 8:475, 1968
2. Kety SS, Schmidt CF: The nitrous oxide method for quantitative determination of cerebral blood flow in man: Theory, procedure and normal values. J Clin Invest 27:476, 1948
3. Grubb RL, Raichle ME, Erchling JO et al: The effects of changes in Pa$_{CO_2}$ on cerebral blood volume, blood flow, and vascular mean transit time. Stroke 5:630, 1974
4. Cucchiara RF, Michenfelder JD: The effect of interruption of the reticular activating system on metabolism in canine cerebral hemispheres before and after thiopental. Anesthesiology 39:3, 1973
5. Forster A, Juge O, Morei D: Effects of midazolam on cerebral blood flow in human volunteers. Anesthesiology 56:453, 1982
6. Smith AL, Wollman H: Cerebral blood flow and metabolism: Effects of anesthetic drugs and techniques. Anesthesiology 36:378, 1972
7. Lassen NA: Cerebral blood flow and oxygen consumption in man. Physiol Rev 39:183, 1959
8. Kety SS, Hafkenschiel JH, Jeffers WA et al: The blood flow, vascular resistance and oxygen consumption of the brain in essential hypertension. J Clin Invest 27:511, 1948
9. Hoffman WE, Miletich DJ, Albrecht RF: The influence of antihypertensive therapy on cerebral autoregulation in aged hypertensive rats. Stroke 13:701, 1982
10. Waltz AG, Sundt TM: Influence of systemic blood pressure on blood flow and microcirculation of ischemic cerebral cortex: A failure of autoregulation. Prog Brain Res 30:107, 1968
11. Kogure K, Masgtoshi F, Scheinberg P et al: Effects of changes in carbon dioxide pressure and arterial pressure on blood flow in ischemic regions of the brain in dogs. Circ Res 24:557, 1969
12. Enevoldsen EM, Jensen FT: Autoregulation and CO$_2$ responses of cerebral blood flow in patients with acute severe head injury. J Neurosurg 48:689, 1978
13. Miletich DJ, Ivankovich AD, Albrecht RF et al: Absence of autoregulation of cerebral blood flow during halothane and enflurane anesthesia. Anesth Analg 55:100, 1976
14. Todd MM, Drummond JC: A comparison of the cerebrovascular and metabolic effects of halothane and isoflurane in the cat. Anesthesiology 60:276, 1984
15. Jobes DR, Kennell E, Bitner R et al: Effects of morphine-nitrous oxide anesthesia on cerebral autoregulation. Anesthesiology 42:30, 1975
16. McPherson RW, Traystman RJ: Fentanyl and cerebral vascular responsivity in dogs. Anesthesiology 60:180, 1984
17. Artru AA, Michenfelder JD: Effects of hypercarbia on canine cerebral metabolism and blood flow with simultaneous direct and indirect measurement of blood flow. Anesthesiology 52:466, 1980
18. Reivich M: Arterial P$_{CO_2}$ and cerebral hemodynamics. Am J Physiol 206:25, 1964
19. Boysen G, Ladogaard-Pedersen HJ, Henriksen H et al: The effects of Pa$_{CO_2}$ on regional cerebral blood flow and internal carotid artery pressure during carotid clamping. Anesthesiology 35:286, 1971
20. Pistolese GR, Citone G, Faraglia V et al: Effects of hypercapnia on cerebral blood flow during the clamping of carotid arteries in surgical management of cerebrovascular insufficiency. Neurology 21:95, 1971
21. Syman L: Regional cererbrovascular responses to acute ischaemia in normocapnia and hypercapnia. J Neurol Neurosurg Psychiatry 33:756, 1970
22. Yamaguchi F, Meyer JS, Fumihito S et al: Normal human aging and cerebral vasoconstrictive responses to hypocapnia. J Neurol Sci 44:87, 1979
23. Yamamoto M, Meyer JS, Sakai F et al: Aging and cerebral vasodilator responses to hypercarbia. Responses in normal aging and in persons with risk factors for stroke. Arch Neurol 37:489, 1980
24. Cucchiara RF, Theye RA, Michenfelder JD: The effects of isoflurane on canine cerebral metabolism and blood flow. Anesthesiology 40:571, 1974
25. Michenfelder JD, Theye RA: Effects of fentanyl, droperidol, and innovar on canine cerebral metabolism and blood flow. Br J Anaesth 43:630, 1971
26. Alexander SC, Wollman H, Cohen PJ et al: Cerebrovascular response to Pa$_{CO_2}$ during halothane anesthesia in man. J Appl Physiol, 19:561, 1964
27. Kassell NF, Hitchon PW, Gerk MK et al: Influence of changes in arterial P$_{CO_2}$ on cerebral blood flow and metabolism during high-dose barbiturate therapy in dogs. J Neurosurg 54:615, 1981
28. Pierce EC, Lambertsen CJ, Deutsch S et al: Cerebral circulation and metabolism during thiopental anesthesia and hyperventilation in man. J Clin Invest 41:1664, 1962
29. Forster A, Juge O, Morei D: Effects of midazolam on cerebral hemodynamics and cerebral vasomotor responsiveness to carbon dioxide. J Cereb Blood Flow Metab 3:246, 1983
30. Kety SS, Schmidt CF: The effects of altered arterial tensions of carbon dioxide and oxygen on cerebral blood flow and cerebral oxygen consumption of normal young men. J Clin Invest 27:484, 1948
31. Michenfelder JD: Brain hypoxia: Current status of experimental and clinical therapy. Seminars in Anesthesia II:81, 1983
32. Michenfelder JD: Cerebral preservation for intraoperative focal ischemia. Clin Neurosurg 32:105, 1985
33. Meyer FB, Sundt TM Jr, Yanagihara T et al: Focal cerebral ischemia: Pathophysiologic mechanisms and rationale for future avenues of treatment. Mayo Clin Proc 62:35, 1987
34. Sundt TM, Sharbrough FW, Anderson RE et al: Cerebral blood flow measurements and electroencephalograms during carotid endarterectomy. J Neurosurg 41:310, 1974
35. Spackman TN, Faust RJ, Cucchiara RF: A comparison of Lifescan EEG monitor with EEG and cerebral blood flow for detection of cerebral ischemia. Anesthesiology 63:A187, 1985
36. Carter LP, Raudzens PA, Gaines C et al: Somatosensory evoked potentials and cortical blood flow during craniotomy for vascular disease. Neurosurgery 15:22, 1984
37. McKay RD, Sundt TM, Michenfelder JD et al: Internal carotid artery stump pressure and cerebral blood flow during carotid endarterectomy: Modification by halothane, enflurane, innovar. Anesthesiology 45:390, 1976
38. Sundt TM, Sharbrough FW, Piepgras DG et al: Correlation of cerebral blood flow and electroencephalographic changes during carotid endarterectomy with results of surgery and hemodynamics of cerebral ischemia. Mayo Clinic Proc 56:533, 1981
39. Drummond JC, Todd MM, Scheller MS et al: A comparison of the

direct cerebral vasodilating potencies of halothane and iso-flurane in the New Zealand white rabbit. Anesthesiology 65:462, 1986

40. Sakabe T, Maekawa T, Fujii S et al: Cerebral circulation and metabolism during enflurane anesthesia in humans. Anesthesiology 59:532, 1983
41. Eintrei C, Leszniewski W, Carlsson C: Local application of ^{133}Xenon for measurement of regional cerebral blood flow (rCBF) during halothane, enflurane, and isoflurane anesthesia in humans. Anesthesiology 63:391, 1985
42. Theye RA, Michenfelder JD: The effect of halothane on canine cerebral metabolism. Anesthesiology 26:1113, 1968
43. Michenfelder JD, Cucchiara RF: Canine cerebral oxygen consumption during enflurane anesthesia and its modification during induced seizures. Anesthesiology 40:575, 1974
44. Newberg LA, Milde JH, Michenfelder JD: The cerebral metabolic effects of isoflurane at and above concentrations that suppress cortical electrical activity. Anesthesiology 59:23, 1983
45. Stullken EH, Milde JH, Michenfelder JD et al: The nonlinear responses of cerebral metabolism to low concentrations of halothane, enflurane, isoflurane, and thiopental. Anesthesiology 46:28, 1977
46. Boarini DJ, Kassell NF, Coester HC et al: Comparison of systemic and cerebrovascular effects of isoflurane and halothane. Neurosurgery 15:400, 1984
47. Artru AA: Relationship between cerebral blood volume and CSF pressure during anesthesia with halothane or enflurane in dogs. Anesthesiology 58:533, 1983
48. Adams RW, Gronert GA, Sundt TM et al: Halothane, hypocapnia, and cerebrospinal fluid pressure in neurosurgery. Anesthesiology 37:510, 1972
49. Adams RW, Cucchiara RF, Gronert GA et al: Isoflurane and cerebrospinal fluid pressure in neurosurgical patients. Anesthesiology 54:97, 1981
50. Scheller MS, Todd MM, Drummond JC: Isoflurane, halothane and regional cerebral blood flow at various levels of Pa_{CO_2} in rabbits. Anesthesiology 64:598, 1986
51. Artru AA: Cerebral metabolism and EEG during combination of hypocapnia and isoflurane-induced hypotension in dogs. Anesthesiology 65:602, 1986
52. Michenfelder JD, Theye RA: In vivo toxic effects of halothane on canine cerebral metabolic pathways. Am J Physiol 229:1050, 1975
53. Stockard JJ, Bickford R: The neurophysiology of anesthesia. In Gordon E (ed): A Basis and Practice of Neuroanaesthesia, p3. Amsterdam, Excerpta Medica, 1975
54. Carlsson C, Hagerdal M, Siesjo BK: The effect of nitrous oxide on oxygen consumption and blood flow in the cerebral cortex of the rat. Acta Anaesthesiol Scand 20:91, 1976
55. Dahlgren N, Ingvar M, Yokoyama H et al: Influence of nitrous oxide on local cerebral flow in awake, minimally restrained rats. J Cereb Blood Flow Metab 1:211, 1981
56. Dhirman JR, Shapiro HM: Modification of nitrous oxide-induced intracranial hypertension by prior induction of anesthesia. Anesthesiology 46:150, 1977
57. Pelligrino DA, Miletich DJ, Hoffman WE et al: Nitrous oxide markedly increases cerebral cortical metabolic rate and blood flow in the goat. Anesthesiology 60:405, 1984
58. Sakabe T, Kuramoto T, Inove S et al: Cerebral effects of nitrous oxide in the dog. Anesthesiology 48:195, 1978
59. Oshito S, Ishikawa T, Tokutsu Y et al: Cerebral circulatory and metabolic stimulation with nitrous oxide in the dog. Acta Anaesthesiol Scand 23:177, 1979
60. Manohar M, Parks CM: Porcine brain and myocardial perfusion during enflurane anesthesia without and with nitrous oxide. J Cardiovasc Pharmacol 6:1092, 1984
61. Theye RA, Michenfelder JD: The effects of nitrous oxide on canine cerebral metabolism. Anesthesiology 20:1119, 1964

62. Jobes DR, Kennell EM, Bush GL et al: Cerebral blood flow and metabolism during morphine-nitrous oxide anesthesia in man. Anesthesiology 47:16, 1977
63. Michenfelder JD: The interdependency of cerebral functional and metabolic effects following massive doses of thiopental in the dog. Anesthesiology 41:231, 1974
64. Milde LN, Milde JH, Michenfelder JD: Cerebral functional, metabolic, and hemodynamic effects of etomidate in dogs. Anesthesiology 63:371, 1985
65. Renou AM, Vernhiet J, Macrez P et al: Cerebral blood flow and metabolism during etomidate anesthesia in man. Br J Anaesth 50:1047, 1978
66. Carlsson C, Hagerdal M, Kaasik AE et al: The effects of diazepam on cerebral blood flow and oxygen consumption in rats and its synergistic interaction with nitrous oxide. Anesthesiology 45:319, 1976
67. Maekawa T, Sakabe T, Takeshita H: Diazepam blocks cerebral metabolic and circulatory responses to local anesthetic-induced seizures. Anesthesiology 41:389, 1974
68. Takeshita H, Michenfelder JD, Theye RA: The effects of morphine and N-allylnormorphine on canine cerebral metabolism and circulation. Anesthesiology 37:605, 1972
69. Matsumiya N, Dohi S: Effects of intravenous or subarachnoid morphine on cerebral and spinal cord hemodynamics and antagonism with naloxone in dogs. Anesthesiology 59:175, 1983
70. Messick JM Jr, Theye RA: Effects of pentobarbital and meperidine on canine cerebral and total oxygen consumption rate. Can Anaesth Soc J 16:321, 1969
71. Carlsson C, Keykhah M, Smith DS et al: Influence of high dose fentanyl on cerebral blood flow and metabolism. Acta Physiol Scand 113:271, 1981
72. Carlsson C, Smith DS, Keykhah MM et al: The effects of high-dose fentanyl on cerebral circulation and metabolism in rats. Anesthesiology 57:375, 1982
73. Keykhah MM, Smith DS, Carlsson C et al: Influence of sufentanil on cerebral metabolism and circulation in the rat. Anesthesiology 63:274, 1985
74. Dawson B, Michenfelder JD, Theye RA: Effects of ketamine on canine cerebral blood flow and metabolism: Modification by prior administration of thiopental. Anesth Analg 50:443, 1971
75. Hougaard K, Hansen A, Brodersen P: The effect of ketamine on regional cerebral blood flow in man. Anesthesiology 41:562, 1974
76. Takeshita H, Okuda Y, Sari A: The effects of ketamine on cerebral circulation and metabolism in man. Anesthesiology 36:69, 1972
77. Johnston JH, Harper AM: The effect of mannitol on cerebral blood flow. J Neurosurg 38:461, 1973
78. Tabaddor K, Danziger A, Whisoff H: Estimation of ICP by CT scan in closed head trauma. Surg Neurol 18:212, 1982
79. Marmarou A, Shulman K, LaMorgese J: Compartmental analysis of compliance and outflow resistance of the cerebrospinal fluid volume. Arch Neurol 28:265, 1973
80. Risberg J, Lundberg N, Ingvar D: Regional cerebral blood volume during acute transient rises of the intracranial pressure (plateau waves). J Neurosurg 31:303, 1969
81. Tans J, Poortvliet D: Intracranial volume-pressure relationship in man. J Neurosurg 59:810, 1983
82. Grundy B: Intraoperative monitoring of sensory-evoked potentials. Anesthesiology 58:72, 1983
83. Raudzens PA: Intraoperative monitoring of evoked potentials. Ann NY Acad Sci 388:308, 1982
84. Moller AR, Jannetta PJ: Monitoring auditory functions during cranial nerve microvascular decompression operations by direct recording from the eighth nerve. J Neurosurg 59:493, 1983
85. McPherson RW, Sell B, Traystman RJ: Effects of thiopental, fentanyl and etomidate on upper extremity somatosensory evoked potentials in humans. Anesthesiology 65:584, 1986
86. Drummond JC, Todd MM, U HS: The effect of high dose sodium

thiopental on brainstem auditory and median nerve somatosensory evoked responses in humans. Anesthesiology 63:249, 1985

87. Thornton C, Heneghan CPH, Navaratnarajah M et al: Effect of etomidate on the auditory evoked response in man. Br J Anaesth 57:554, 1985

88. Samra SK, Lilly DJ, Rush NL et al: Fentanyl anesthesia and human brainstem auditory evoked potentials. Anesthesiology 61:261, 1984

89. Samra SK, Krutak-Krol H, Pohorecki R et al: Scopolamine, morphine and brainstem auditory evoked potentials in awake monkeys. Anesthesiology 62:437, 1985

90. Pathak KS, Brown RH, Cascorbi HF et al: Effects of fentanyl and morphine on intraoperative somatosensory cortical-evoked potentials. Anesth Analg 63:833, 1984

91. Dubois MY, Sato S, Chassy T et al: Effects of enflurane on brainstem auditory evoked responses in humans. Anesth Analg 61:898, 1982

92. Manninen PH, Lam AM, Nicholas JP: The effects of isoflurane and isoflurane-nitrous oxide anesthesia on brainstem auditory evoked potentials in humans. Anesth Analg 64:43, 1985

93. Thornton C, Catley DM, Jordon C et al: Enflurane anaesthesia causes graded changes in the brainstem and early cortical auditory evoked response in man. Br J Anaesth 55:479, 1983

94. Thornton C, Heneghan CPH, James MFM et al: Effects of halothane or enflurane with controlled ventilation on auditory evoked potentials. Br J Anaesth 56:315, 1984

95. Samra SK, Vanderzant CW, Domer PA et al: Differential effects of isoflurane on human median nerve somatosensory evoked potentials. Anesthesiology 66:29, 1987

96. Peterson DO, Drummond JC, Todd MM: Effects of halothane, enflurane, isoflurane and nitrous oxide on somatosensory evoked potentials in humans. Anesthesiology 65:35, 1986

97. Pathak KS, Ammadio M, Kalamchi A et al: Effects of halothane, enflurane, and isoflurane on somatosensory evoked potentials during nitrous oxide anesthesia. Anesthesiology 66:753, 1987

98. McPherson RW, Mahla M, Johnson R et al: Effects of enflurane, isoflurane, and nitrous oxide on somatosensory evoked potentials during fentanyl anesthesia. Anesthesiology 62:626, 1985

99. Sloan TB, Koht A: Depression of cortical somatosensory evoked potentials by nitrous oxide. Br J Anaesth 57:849, 1985

100. Sebel PS, Flynn PJ, Ingram DA: Effect of nitrous oxide on visual, auditory and somatosensory evoked potentials. Br J Anaesth 56:1403, 1984

101. Chi OZ, Field C: Effects of isoflurane on visual evoked potentials in humans. Anesthesiology 65:328, 1986

102. Grundy BL: Monitoring of sensory evoked potentials during neurosurgical operations: Methods and applications. Neurosurgery 11:556, 1982

103. Grundy BL, Nash CL, Brown RH: Deliberate hypotension for spinal fusion: Prospective randomized study with evoked potential monitoring. Can Anaesth Soc J 29:452, 1982

104. Grundy BL, Jannetta PJ, Procopio PT et al: Intraoperative monitoring of brainstem auditory evoked potentials. J Neurosurg 57:674, 1982

105. Little JR, Lesser RP, Lueders H et al: Brainstem auditory evoked potentials in posterior circulation surgery. Neurosurgery 12:496, 1983

106. Lam AM, Keane JF, Manninen PH: Monitoring of brainstem auditory evoked potentials during basilar artery occlusion in man. Br J Anaesth 57:924, 1985

107. Carter LP, Raudzens PA, Gaines C et al: Somatosensory evoked potentials and cortical blood flow during craniotomy for vascular disease. Neurosurgery 15:22, 1984

108. Grundy BL, Nelson PB, Lina A et al: Monitoring of cortical somatosensory evoked potentials to determine the safety of sacrificing the anterior cerebral artery. Neurosurgery 11:647, 1982

109. Symon L, Wang AD, Costa E et al: Perioperative use of so-

matosensory evoked responses in aneurysm surgery. J Neurosurg 60:269-275, 1984

110. McPherson RW, Niedermeyer EF, Otenasek RJ et al: Correlation of transient neurological deficit and somatosensory evoked potentials after intracranial aneursym surgery. Case Report. J Neurosurgery 59:146, 1983

111. Markand ON, Dilley RS, Moorthy SS et al: Monitoring of somatosensory evoked responses during carotid endarterectomy. Arch Neurol 41:375, 1984

112. Moorthy SS, Markand ON, Dilley RS et al: Somatosensory evoked responses during carotid endarterectomy. Anesth Analg 61:879, 1982

113. Russ W, Fraedrich G, Hehrlein FW et al: Intraoperative somatosensory evoked potentials as a prognostic factor of neurologic state after carotid endarterectomy. Thorac Cardiovasc Surg 33:392, 1985

114. Kaplan BJ, Friedman WA, Alexander JA et al: Somatosensory evoked potential monitoring of spinal cord ischemia during aortic operations. Neurosurgery 19:82, 1986

115. Takaki O, Okumura F: Application and limitation of somatosensory evoked potential monitoring during thoracic aortic aneurysm surgery: A case report. Anesthesiology 63:700, 1985

116. Costa E, Silva I, Wang AD et al: The application of flash visual evoked potentials during operations on the anterior visual pathways. Neurol Res 7:11, 1985

117. Vaazelle C, Stagnara P, Jouvinroux P: Functional monitoring of spinal cord activity during spinal surgery. Clin Orthop 93:173, 1973

118. Pathak KS, Brown RH, Nash CL et al: Continuous opioid infusion for scoliosis fusion surgery. Anesth Analg 62:841, 1983

119. Grundy BL, Heros RC, Tung AS et al: Intraoperative hypoxia detected by evoked potential monitoring. Anesth Analg 60:437, 1981

120. Van Rheineck Leyssius AT, Kalkman CJ, Bovill JG: Influence of moderate hypothermia on posterior tibial nerve somatosensory potentials. Anesth Analg 65:475, 1986

121. Stockard JJ, Sharbrough FW, Tinker JA: Effects of hypothermia on the human brainstem auditory response. Ann Neurol 3:368, 1978

122. Schubert A, Zornow MH, Drummond JC et al: Loss of cortical evoked responses due to intracranial gas during posterior fossa craniectomy in the seated position. Anesth Analg 65:203, 1986

123. McPherson RW, Toung TJK, Johnson RM et al: Intracranial subdural gas: A cause of false-positive change of intraoperative somatosensory evoked potential. Anesthesiology 62:816, 1985

124. Jannetta PJ, Moller AR, Moller MB: Technique of hearing preservation in small acoustic neuromas. Ann Surg 200:513, 1984

125. Friedman WA, Kaplan BJ, Gravenstein D et al: Intraoperative brainstem auditory evoked potentials during posterior fossa microvascular decompression. J Neurosurg 62:552, 1985

126. Grundy BL, Nelson PB, Doyle E et al: Intraoperative loss of somatosensory evoked potentials predicts loss of spinal cord function. Anesthesiology 57:321, 1982

127. Ginsberg HH, Shetter AG, Raudzens PA: Postoperative paraplegia with preserved intraoperative somatosensory evoked potentials. J Neurosurg 63:296, 1985

128. Lesser RP, Raudzens P, Luders H et al: Postoperative neurological deficits may occur despite unchanged intraoperative somatosensory evoked potentials. Ann Neurol 19:22, 1986

129. Levy WJ: Spinal evoked potentials from the motor tracts. J Neurosurg 58:38, 1983

130. Levy WJ: Clinical experience with motor and cerebellar evoked potential monitoring. Neurosurgery 20:169, 1987

131. Buchthal F: Electromyography in the evaluation of muscle diseases. Neurol Clin 3:573, 1985

132. Harner SG, Daube JR, Ebersold MJ: Electrophysiologic monitoring of facial nerve during temporal bone surgery. Laryngoscope 96:65, 1986

133. Prass RL, Luders H: Acoustic (loudspeaker) facial electromyographic monitoring: Part 1. Neurosurgery 19:392, 1986

134. Harner SG, Daube JR, Ebersold MJ et al: Improved preservation of facial nerve function with use of electrical monitoring during removal of acoustic neuromas. Mayo Clin Proc 62:92, 1987

135. Grosslight K, Foster R, Colohan AR, et al: Isoflurane for neuroanesthesia: Risk factors for increases in intracranial pressure. Anesthesiology 63:533, 1985

136. Madsen JB, Cold GE, Hansen ES et al: The effect of isoflurane on cerebral blood flow and metabolism in humans during craniotomy for small supratentorial cerebral tumors. Anesthesiology 66:332, 1987

137. Marsh ML, Dunlop BJ, Shapiro HM et al: Succinylcholine—Intracranial pressure effects in neurosurgical patients. Anesth Analg 59:550, 1980

138. Minton MD, Stirt JA, Bedford RF: Increased intracranial pressure from succinylcholine: Modification by prior nondepolarizing blockade. Anesthesiology 63:A391, 1985

139. Minton MD, Stirt JA, Bedford RF et al: Intracranial pressure after atracurium in neurosurgical patients. Anesth Analg 64:1113, 1985

140. Unni VK, Gray WJ, Young MB: Effects of atracurium on intracranial pressure in man. Anaesthesia 41:1047, 1986

141. Graham D: Monitoring neuromuscular block may be unreliable in patients with upper motor neuron lesions. Anesthesiology 52:74, 1980

142. Brown JC, Charlton JE: Study of sensitivity to curare in certain neurological disorders using a regional technique. J Neurol Neurosurg Psychiatry 38:34, 1975

143. Cooperman LH, Strobel GE, Kennell EM: Massive hyperkalemia after administration of succinylcholine. Anesthesiology 32:161, 1970

144. Lanier WL, Stangland KJ, Scheithauer BW et al: The effects of dextrose infusion and head position on neurologic outcome after complete cerebral ischemia in primates: Examination of a model. Anesthesiology 66:39, 1987

145. Pulsinelli WA, Levy DE, Sigsbee B et al: Increased damage after ischemic stroke in patients with hyperglycemia with or without established diabetes mellitus. Am J Med 74:540, 1983

146. Longstreth WI, Inui TS: High blood glucose level on hospital admission and poor neurological recovery after cardiac arrest. Ann Neurol 15:59, 1984

147. Cully MD, Larson CP, Silverberg GD: Hetastarch coagulopathy in a neurosurgical patient. Anesthesiology 66:706, 1987

148. Messick JM, Maass L, Faust RJ et al: Duration of pancuronium neuromuscular blockade in patients taking anticonvulsant medication. Anesth Analg 61:203, 1982

149. Muizelaar JP, Lutz HA, Becker DP: Effect of mannitol on ICP and CBF and correlation with pressure autoregulation in severely head-injured patients. J Neurosurg 61:700, 1984

150. Samson D, Beyer CW: Furosemide in the intraoperative reduction of intracranial pressure in the patient with subarachnoid hemorrhage. Neurosurgery 10:167, 1982

151. Bedford R, Colley P: Intracranial tumors. In Matjasko J, Katz J (eds). Clinical Controversies in Neuroanesthesia and Neurosurgery, p 135. Orlando, Grune and Stratton, 1986

152. Standefer M, Bay JW, Trusso DO: The sitting position in neurosurgery: A retrospective analysis of 488 cases. Neurosurgery 14:649, 1984

153. Matjasko J, Petrozza P, Cohen M et al: Anesthesia and surgery in the seated position: Analysis of 554 cases. Neurosurgery 17:695, 1985

154. Young ML, Smith DS, Murtagh F et al: Comparison of surgical and anesthetic complications in neurosurgical patients experiencing venous air embolism in the sitting position. Neurosurgery 18:157, 1986

155. Oliver S, Cucchiara R: Comparison of outcome following posterior fossa craniectomy done in either a sitting or horizontal position. Anesthesiology 65:A305, 1986

156. Perkins-Pearson NAK, Marshall WK, Bedford RF: Atrial pressures in the seated position: Implication of paradoxical air embolism. Anesthesiology 57:493, 1982

157. Seward JB, Hayes DL, Smith HC et al: Platypnea-orthodeoxia: Clinical profile, diagnostic workup, management and report of seven cases. Mayo Clin Proc 59:221, 1984

158. Michenfelder JD, Gronert GA, Rehder K: Neuroanesthesia. Anesthesiology 30:65, 1969

159. Michenfelder JD: Central venous catheters in the management of air embolism: Whether as well as where. Anesthesiology 55:339, 1981

160. Bunegin L, Albin M, Helsel P et al: Positioning the right atrial catheter: A model for reappraisal. Anesthesiology 55:343, 1981

161. Cucchiara RF, Messick JM, Gronert GA et al: Time required and success rate of percutaneous right atrial catheterization: Description of a technique. Can Anaesth Soc J 27:572, 1980

162. Lee D, Kuhn J, Shaffer M et al: Migration of tips of central venous catheters in seated patients. Anesth Analg 63:949, 1984

163. Glenski JA, Cucchiara RF: Transcutaneous O_2 and CO_2 monitoring of neurosurgical patients: Detection of an embolism. Anesthesiology 64:546, 1986

164. Cucchiara RF, Nugent M, Seward JB et al: Air embolism in upright neurosurgical patients: Detection and localization by 2-D transesophageal echocardiography. Anesthesiology 60:353, 1984

165. Lynch JJ, Schuchard GH, Gross CM et al: Prevalence of right to left atrial shunting in a healthy population: Detection by Valsalva maneuver contrast echocardiography. Am J Cardiol 53:1478, 1984

166. Toung T, Ngeow YK, Long DL et al: Comparison of the effects of PEEP and jugular venous compression on canine cerebral venous pressure. Anesthesiology 61:169, 1984

167. Artru AA, Cucchiara RF, Messick JM: Cardiorespiratory and cranial nerve sequelae of surgical procedures involving the posterior fossa. Anesthesiology 52:83, 1980

168. Skahen S, Shapiro HM, Drummond JC et al: Nitrous oxide withdrawal reduces intracranial pressure in the presence of pneumocephalus. Anesthesiology 65:92, 1986

169. Artru AA: Breathing nitrous oxide during closure of the dura and cranium is not indicated. Anesthesiology 66:719, 1987

170. Randall RV: Clinical presentation of pituitary adenomas. In Laws ER, Randall RV, Kern EB et al (eds): Management of Pituitary Adenomas and Related Lesions with Emphasis on Transphenoidal Surgery, p 15. New York, Appleton-Century-Crofts, 1982

171. Tindall GF, McLanahan CS: Hyperfunctional pituitary tumors: pre- and postoperative management considerations. Clin Neurosurg 27:48, 1980

172. Messick JM, Laws ER, Abboud CF: Anesthesia for transphenoidal surgery of the hypophyseal region. Anesth Analg 57:206, 1978

173. Tasch MD: Endocrine diseases. In Stoelting RK, Dierdorf SF (eds): Anesthesia and Co-existing Disease, p 437. New York, Churchill Livingstone, 1983

174. Cadieux RJ, Kales A, Santen RJ et al: Endoscopic findings in sleep apnea associated with acromegaly. J Clin Endocrinol Metab 55:18, 1982

175. Hassan SZ, Matz GJ, Lawrence AM et al: Laryngeal stenosis in acromegaly: A possible cause of airway difficulties associated with anesthesia. Anesth Analg 55:57, 1976

176. Kitahata LM: Airway difficulties associated with anesthesia in acromegaly. Br J Anaesth 43:1187, 1971

177. Southwick JP, Katz J: Unusual airway difficulty in the acromegalic patient–Indications for tracheostomy. Anesthesiology 51:72, 1979
178. Ovassapian A, Doka JC, Romsa DE: Acromegaly–Use of a fiberoptic laryngoscopy to avoid tracheostomy. Anesthesiology 54:429, 1981
179. Messick JM, Cucchiara RF, Faust RJ: Airway management in patients with acromegaly. Anesthesiology 56:157, 1982
180. Newfield P, Albin MS, Chestnut JC et al: Air embolism during transsphenoidal pituitary operations. Neurosurgery 2:39, 1978
181. Messick JM, Faust RJ, Cucchiara RF: Anesthesia for transsphenoidal microsurgery. In Laws ER, Randall RV, Kern EB et al (eds): Management of Pituitary Adenomas and Related Lesions with Emphasis on Transsphenoidal Surgery, 253. New York, Appleton-Century-Crofts, 1982
182. Laws ER, Kern EB: Complications of transsphenoidal surgery. In Laws ER, Randall RV, Kern EB et al (eds): Management of Pituitary Adenomas and Related Lesions with Emphasis on Transsphenoidal Surgery, 329. New York, Appleton-Century-Crofts, 1982
183. Prince DA, Connors BW: Mechanisms of interictal epileptogenesis. Adv Neurol 44:275, 1986
184. Delgado-Escueta AV, Treiman DM, Walsh GO: The treatable epilepsies. N Engl J Med 308:1508, 1983
185. Spencer DD, Spencer SS: Surgery for epilesy. Neurologic Clinic 3:313, 1985
186. King DW, Flanigin HF, Gallagher BB et al: Temporal lobectomy for partial complex seizures: Evaluation, results and 1-year follow-up. Neurology 36:334, 1986
187. Wada J, Rasmussen T: Intracarotid injection of sodium amytal for the lateralization of cerebral speech dominance. J Neurosurg 17:266, 1960
188. Engel J Jr, Crandall PH: Intensive neurodiagnostic monitoring with intracranial electrodes. Adv Neurol 46:85, 1987
189. Goldring S, Gregorie EM: Surgical management of epilepsy using epidural recordings to localize the seizure focus. J Neurosurg 60:457, 1984
190. Ojemann GA: Mapping of neuropsychological language parameters at surgery. Int Anesthesiol Clin 24:115, 1986
191. Goldring S: A method for surgical management of focal epilepsy, especially as it relates to children. J Neurosurg 49:344, 1978
192. Kelly PJ, Scarbrough FW, Kall BA et al: Magnetic resonance imaging-based computer-assisted stereotactic resection of the hippocampus and amygdala in patients with temporal lobe epilepsy. Mayo Clin Proc 62:103, 1987
193. Delgado-Escueta AV, Treiman DM, Walsh GO: The treatable epilepsies. N Engl Med 308:1576, 1983
194. Trop D: Conscious-sedation analgesia during the neurosurgical treatment of epilepsies—Practice at the Montreal Neurological Institute. Int Anesthesiol Clin 24:175, 1986
195. Meyer FB, Marsh WR, Laws ER et al: Temporal lobectomy in children with epilepsy. J Neurosurg 64:371, 1986
196. Ornstein E, Matteo RS, Young WL et al: Resistance to metocurine-induced neuromuscular blockade in patients receiving phenytoin. Anesthesiology 63:294, 1985
197. Roth S, Ebrahim Z, Subichin S: Resistance to pancuronium in patients receiving carbamazepine. Anesthesiology 65:A286, 1986
198. Gancher S, Laxer KD, Krieger W: Activation of epileptogenic activity by etomidate. Anesthesiology 61:616, 1984
199. Ebrahim ZY, DeBoer GE, Luders H et al: Effect of etomidate on the electroencephalogram of patients with epilepsy. Anesth Analg 65:1004, 1986
200. Sundt TM, Kobayashi S, Fode NC et al: Results and complications of surgical management of 809 intracranial aneurysms in 722 cases. J Neurosurg 56:753, 1982
201. Whisnant JP, Philips LH, Sundt TM: Aneurysmal subarachnoid hemorrhage. Timing of surgery and mortality. Mayo Clin Proc 57:471, 1982
202. Locksley HP: Report on the cooperative study of intracranial aneurysms and subarachnoid hemorrhage. J Neurosurg 25:219, 1966a
203. Locksley HP: Report on the cooperative study of intracranial aneurysms and subarachnoid hemorrhage. J Neurosurg 25:321, 1966b
204. Ferguson GC: Direct measurement of mean and pulsatile blood pressure at operating in human intracranial saccular aneurysms. J Neurosurg 36:560, 1972
205. Chyatt D, Sundt TM: Cerebral vasospasm after subarachnoid hemorrhage. Mayo Clin Proc 59:498, 1984
206. Sundt TM: Management of ischemic complication after subarachnoid hemorrhage. J Neurosurg 43:418, 1975
207. Farrar JK, Gamache FW, Ferguson CG: Effects of profound hypotension on cerebral blood flow during surgery for intracranial aneurysms. J Neurosurg 58:857, 1981
208. Allen GS, Ahn HS, Preziosi TJ et al: Cerebral arterial spasm—A controlled trial of nimodipine in patients with subarachnoid hemorrhage. N Engl J Med 308:619, 1983
209. Steen PA, Newberg LA, Milde JH et al: Cerebral blood flow and neurologic outcome when nimodipine is given after complete cerebral ischemia in the dog. J Cereb Blood Flow Metab 4:82, 1984
210. Forsman M, Fleischer JE, Milde JH et al: The effects of nimodipine on cerebral blood flow and metabolism. J Cereb Blood Flow Metab 6:763, 1986
211. Stullken EH, Balestrieri FJ, Prough DS et al: The hemodynamic effects of nimodipine in patients anesthetized for cerebral aneurysm clipping. Anesthesiology 62:346, 1985
212. McLeshey CH, Cullen BF, Kennedy RD et al: Control of cerebral perfusion pressure during induction of anesthesia in high-risk neurosurgical patients. Anesth Analg 53:985, 1974
213. Hamill JF, Bedford RF, Weaver DC et al: Lidocaine before endotracheal intubation: Intravenous or laryngotracheal? Anesthesiology 55:578, 1981
214. Kiny BD, Harris LC, Greifenstein FE et al: Reflex circulatory responses to direct laryngoscopy and tracheal intubation performed during general anesthesia. Anesthesiology 12:556, 1951
215. de Lange S, Boscue MJ, Stanley TH et al: Comparison of sufentanil-O_2 and fentanyl-O_2 for coronary artery surgery. Anesthesiology 56:112, 1982
216. Cucchiara RF, Benefiel DJ, Matteo RS et al: Evaluation of esmolol in controlling increases in heart rate and blood pressure during endotracheal intubation in patients undergoing carotid endarterectomy. Anesthesiology 65:528, 1986
217. Sufwat AM, Reitan JA, Misle GR et al: Use of propranolol to control rate-pressure product during cardiac anesthesia. Anesth Analg 60:732, 1981
218. Sokoll MD, Kassell NF, Davies LR: Large dose thiopental anesthesia for intracranial aneurysm surgery. Neurosurg 10:555, 1982
219. Varkey GP, Thompson WR: Anesthetic considerations in the surgical repair of intracranial aneurysms: Anesthetic management. Int Anesthesiol Clin 20:159, 1982
220. Luben V, Easton J, Messick J et al: Anesthetic considerations in the surgical repair of intracranial aneurysms: The practice at some centers. Int Anesthesiol Clin 20:195, 1982
221. Sokoll MD, Kassell NF, Gergis SD: Hemodynamic effects of N_2O, O_2, barbiturate anesthesia and induced hypotension in early years versus aneurysm clipping. Neurosurgery 11:352, 1982
222. Steen PA, Newberg L, Milde JH et al: Hypothermia and barbiturates: Individual and combined effects on canine cerebral oxygen consumption. Anesthesiology 58:527, 1983
223. Michenfelder JD, Terry HR, Daw EF et al: Induced hypothermia: Physiologic effects, indications, and techniques. Surg Clin North Am 45:889, 1965

224. Newberg LA, Milde JH, Michenfelder JD: Systemic and cerebral effects of isoflurane-induced hypotension in dogs. Anesthesiology 60:541, 1984

225. Newman B, Gelb AW, Lam AM: The effect of isoflurane-induced hypotension on cerebral blood flow and cerebral metabolic rate for oxygen in humans. Anesthesiology 64:307, 1986

226. Chestnut JS, Albin MS, Gonzales-Abola E et al: Clinical evaluation of intravenous nitroglycerin for neurosurgery. J Neurosurg 48:704, 1978

227. Sollevi A, Lagerkranser M, Irestedt L et al: Controlled hypotension with adenosine in cerebral aneurysm surgery. Anesthesiology 61:400, 1984

228. Michenfelder JD, Theye RA: Canine systemic and cerebral effects of hypotension induced by hemorrhage, trimethaphan, halothane, nitroprusside. Anesthesiology 46:188, 1977

229. Larson AG: Deliberate hypotension. Anesthesiology 25:682, 1964

230. Tinker JH, Michenfelder JD: Sodium nitroprusside: Pharmacology, toxicology and therapeutics. Anesthesiology 45:340, 1976

231. Maktabi M, Warner D, Sokoll M et al: Comparison of nitroprusside, nitroglycerin, and deep isoflurane anesthesia for induced hypotension. Neurosurgery 19:350, 1986

232. Siegel P, Moraca PP, Greer JR: Sodium nitroprusside in the surgical treatment of cerebral aneurysms and arteriovenous malformations. Br J Anaesth 43:790, 1971

233. Turner JM, Powel D, Gibson RM et al: Intracranial pressure changes in neurosurgical patients during hypotension induced with sodium nitroprusside or trimethaphan. Br J Anaesth 49:417, 1977

234. Larson R, Teichmann J, Hilfiter O et al: Nitroprusside-hypotension: Cerebral blood flow and cerebral oxygen consumption in neurosurgical patients. Acta Anaesthesiol Scand 26:327, 1982

235. Artru AA, Wright K, Colley PS: Cerebral effects of hypocapnia plus nitroglycerin-induced hypotension in dogs. J Neurosurg 64:924, 1986

236. Kaplan JA: Nitrates. In Kaplan JA (ed): Cardiac Anesthesia, Volume 2: Cardiovascular Pharmacology, p 151. New York, Grune and Stratton, 1983

237. Lam AM, Gelb AW: Cardiovascular effects of isoflurane-induced hypotension for cerebral aneurysm surgery. Anesth Analg 62:742, 1983

238. Weinlander CM, Abel MD, Piehler JM et al: Isoflurane is a potent myocardial depressant in patients with ischemic heart disease. Anesthesiology 65:A4, 1986

239. Hoffman WE, Miletich DJ, Albrecht RF: The effects of midazolam on cerebral blood flow and oxygen consumption and its interaction with nitrous oxide. Anesth Analg 65:729, 1986

240. Newberg LA, Michenfelder JD: Cerebral protection by isoflurane during hypoxemia or ischemia. Anesthesiology 59:29, 1983

241. Newberg LA, Milde JH, Michenfelder JD: Cerebral and systemic effects of hypotension induced by adenosine or ATP in dogs. Anesthesiology 62:429, 1985

242. Frost EAM: Anesthesia for intracranial vascular malformations. Bull NY Acad Med, 60:759, 1984

243. The ECI JC Bypass Study Group: Failure of extracranial-intra-cranial arterial bypass to reduce the risk of ischemic stroke. N Engl J Med 313:1191, 1985

244. Whisnant JP, Sundt TM, Fode NC: Long-term mortality and stroke morbidity after superficial temporal artery-middle cerebral artery bypass operations. Mayo Clin Proc 60:241, 1985

245. Sundt TM, Whisnant JP, Fode NC et al: Results, complications, and follow-up of 415 bypass operations for occlusive disease of the carotid system. Mayo Clin Proc, 60:230, 1985

246. Sundt TM: Was the international randomized trial of extracranial-intracranial bypass representative of the population at risk? N Engl J Med 316:814, 1987

247. Goldring S, Zervas N, Langfitt T: The extracranial-intracranial bypass study. A report of the committee appointed by the American Association of Neurologic Surgeons to examine the study. N Engl J Med, 316:817, 1987

248. Barnett HJM, Sackett D, Taylor DW et al: Are results of the extracranial-intracranial bypass trial generalizable? N Engl J Med 316:820, 1987

249. Bleyaert AL, Nemoto EM, Safar P et al: Thiopental amelioration of brain damage after global ischemia in monkeys. Anesthesiology, 49:390, 1978

250. Steen PA, Milde JH, Michenfelder JD: No barbiturate protection in a dog model of complete cerebral ischemia. Ann Neurol 5:343, 1978

251. Michenfelder JD, Theye RA: Cerebral protection by thiopental during hypoxia. Anesthesiology 5:510, 1973

252. Steen PA, Newberg LA, Milde JH et al: Nimodipine improves cerebral blood flow and neurologic recovery after complete cerebral ischemia in the dog. J Cereb Blood Flow Metab 3:38, 1983

253. Milde LN, Milde JH, Michenfelder JD: Delayed treatment with nimodipine improves cerebral blood flow after complete cerebral ischemia in the dog. J Cereb Blood Flow Metab 6:332, 1986

254. Steen PA, Gisvold SE, Milde JH et al: Nimodipine improves outcome when given after complete cerebral ischemia in primates. Anesthesiology 62:406, 1985

255. Newberg LA, Steen PA, Milde JH et al: Failure of flunarizine to improve cerebral blood flow or neurologic recovery in a canine model of complete cerebral ischemia. Stroke 15:666, 1984

256. Fleischer JE, Lanier WL, Milde JH et al: Effect of lidoflazine on cerebral blood flow and neurologic outcome when administered after complete cerebral ischemia in dogs. Anesthesiology 66:304, 1987

257. Michenfelder JD, Milde JH, Sundt TM Jr: Cerebral protection by barbiturate anesthesia use after middle cerebral artery occlusion in Java monkeys. Arch Neurol 33:345, 1976

258. Newberg LA, Michenfelder JD: Cerebral protection by isoflurane during hypoxemia in ischemia. Anesthesiology 39:29, 1983

259. Nussmeier NA, Arlund C, Slogoff S: Neuropsychiatric complications after cardiopulmonary bypass: Cerebral protection by a barbiturate. Anesthesiology 64:165, 1986

260. Nugent M, Artru AA, Michenfelder JD: Cerebral metabolic, vascular and protective effects of midazolam maleate. Anesthesiology 56:172, 1982

261. Gelb AW, Boisnert DD, Tary C et al: A comparison in primates of the tolerance to focal cerebral ischemia during isoflurane or nitroprusside induced hypotension. Anesth Analg 66:S65, 1987

Chapter 32

Ronald A. Harrison

Respiratory Function and Anesthesia

In many respects, the lung is a truly unique organ system. It is the only system that essentially receives the entire cardiac output. Although its primary function, without question, is maintenance of adequate gas exchange and external respiration, its importance on many metabolic regulatory processes is also of major significance. The lung is a valveless mechanical system with bi-directional flow, which introduces additional complexities to functional analysis. The large number of compactly arranged air passages, blood, and lymph vessels require precise integration to form a cohesive unit. This network is designed to maintain appropriate respiratory function, in spite of dynamic changes in dimensions and internal forces associated with breathing and postural changes. Because of the complexity of the lung, the chapter is subdivided into the following major topics 1) Anatomy 2) Neurological Control Mechanisms, 3) Lung Mechanics, 4) Physiology of Gas Exchange, and 5) Tests of Pulmonary Function. This approach is intended to provide the clinician with a logical, integrated concept of lung function along with pertinent clinical applications.

ANATOMY OF THE LUNG

Precise delineation of structural lung tissue measurements on *in vitro* examination is subject to error. The tissues uniformly collapse, resulting in alterations in size and shape, upon removal from the intact organism. Also, the use of fixatives or reagents to prepare the lung for examination can cause variable amounts of shrinkage, thus introducing additional inaccuracies. Emphasis on improving techniques has resulted in better standardization in the methods for fixing, preserving, and sectioning lung tissues.[1–3] This has provided lung anatomists with a more reliable means of comparison and a better

appreciation of spatial relationships. The most reliable light microscopy studies demonstrating the three-dimensional characteristics of lungs have been performed on *in vivo* studies.[4] The most sophisticated and accurate studies of structural detail have been achieved using the electron microscope. Studies of lung anatomy in all mammals reveal general similarities, but significant variations in detailed structure within different species. Thus, it is not always possible to extrapolate anatomic findings from experimental animal studies to the human lung.

It is impractical to present a complete and fully detailed analysis of all the anatomical characteristics of the human lung. For the dedicated reader, there are numerous excellent textbooks and illustrated handbooks in basic anatomy that have already accomplished this task.[5,6] The emphasis in this chapter will be on functional lung anatomy describing structure in the context of its mechanical and physiologic function.

HUMAN THORAX

The human thorax, composed of 12 thoracic vertebral bodies, 12 pairs of ribs, and the sternum, must be sufficiently rigid to protect the organ systems contained within, but pliable enough to allow the lungs to act as a bellows. Thus, the ribs must be capable of movement and, therefore, cannot be rigidly attached to their points of articulation on the vertebral bodies. To facilitate both protection and movement, the rib structure is rounded in its dorsal portion, providing increased strength, but flattened laterally and anteriorly to facilitate muscle and cartilage attachments.[7] The thoracic cage is characterized geometrically as a truncated cone with a rather small superior opening and large inferior opening where the diaphragm is attached. The thoracic vertebral column is the major supporting vertical structure. It is designed so that flexion and extension movements are readily permitted, being limited only by the relative thickness or thinness of the thoracic intervertebral disks. Rotational movement around the long axis of the body is not severely limited, since the articular facets for rib attachments are ideally positioned, as though on the circumference of a large circle. This arrangement permits a greater degree of rotational and bending motion in the upper trunk than otherwise could be tolerated. The most important anterior supporting skeletal chest wall structure is the sternum, so named because of its "sword-like" appearance. Its individual components consist of a handle (the manubrium), a body (corpus sterni), and a tip (the xiphoid process). The upper border of the manubrium positioned between the two sternoclavicular joints is called the suprasternal notch. It is in the same horizontal plane as the mid-portion of the second thoracic vertebral body. Another important anatomical landmark is the junction between the manubrium and body, the sternal angle. This sternal angle is located in a horizontal plane passing through the lung, intersecting the vertebral column at a T4 or T5 level. Anteriorly, it is formed by the junction of the second rib with the sternum. One important characteristic is that it represents the plane of separation between the superior and inferior mediastinum. There are seven pairs of true ribs that have direct connections to the vertebral column and sternum. In addition, there are five pairs of false ribs indirectly joined to the sternum and two free-floating ribs. A typical rib has a head for articulation with a vertebra and a constricted portion, or neck, that contains the axis around which the rib rotates. This part of the rib has a crest for ligamentous attachments and a tubercle for articulation with the vertebral transverse process. The rib then continues ventrally, initially turning at its dorsal angle, and finally turning medially towards the sternum. With the exception of floating ribs, all pairs of ribs articulate with thoracic vertebral bodies so that their anterior portion and sternum can be raised and lowered with inspiration and expiration. In general, the ribs take a curved, oblique, downward course in passing from the dorsal or vertebral portion to their sternal attachment, when viewed from an upright position. Ultimately, freedom of chest cage motion with breathing is dependent on the movable synovial joints between each rib and corresponding vertebral articular facet. Mechanically, the greatest overall displacement of any rib is at a point of the greatest directed distance from the neck axis. Because of the differences in the angle of attachment of the ribs to vertebral bodies, the greatest radial distance is near the sternum in the upper lung region and positioned laterally in the lower lung fields.[8] Therefore, the predominant changes in respective lung diameters are in an anterior-posterior direction in the upper lung region, and in a lateral or transverse direction in the lower portion of the lungs.[9] The net effect is that inspiration results in an increase in both transverse and anterior-posterior dimensions of the thoracic cavity with converse movement during expiration.

MUSCLES OF RESPIRATION

At rest, the primary breathing muscle is the diaphragm, with some minor contributions by intercostal muscles. As respiratory effort is increased, abdominal muscles begin to play an important role assisting in rib depression and increasing intra-abdominal pressure to facilitate forced exhalation. With further increase in respiratory effort, cervical strap muscles become active, helping to elevate the sternum and upper costal portions of the chest. Finally, large back and intravertebral muscles of the shoulder girdle are called into play with development of maximum respiratory effort. In general, the muscles of respiration that raise the ribs can be functionally considered as inspiratory in nature, whereas muscles that lower the ribs are primarily important in expiration.

The amount of force (subatmospheric pressure) that can be generated by respiratory muscles is dependent upon their thickness or mass and respective properties of individual fibers. Muscle fiber type is determined by the number of motor units and their frequency of contraction.[10] There is ample experimental evidence for a positive correlation between type of muscle fiber, fatigability of a muscle fiber and its oxidative capacity.[11] Fatigue resistant fibers are characterized by their slow twitch response to electrical activity. They comprise approximately 50% of diaphragmatic fibers and, because of their oxidative capacity, function as endurance muscle units.[12] The other types of muscle fibers are termed fatigue susceptible and fatigue prone, both of which have rapid responses to electrical activity. These fibers facilitate a greater development in magnitude of force, but are limited in endurance.[13] Work capacity is dependent on the magnitude of generated force and the initial length of the muscle. Maximum shortening of skeletal muscle fibers, including respiratory muscles, is approximately 50% of its resting length.[14] The amount of energy required for muscle shortening is dependent on the type of muscle activity involved.[15] In *myometric* activity, the muscle tension increases and the muscle physically shortens, which requires maximum muscle energy expenditure. In *isometric* activity, the muscle develops increased tension, while its length remains unchanged; thus, there is less energy expenditure. Finally, in *pliometric* activity, an effect secondary to contraction of opposing muscles, the length of the contracting muscle actually increases, requiring minimum energy.

Energy—in essence, oxygen—is required to reverse the chemical reactions of muscle contraction. The innervation ratio; that is, the number of muscle fibers per motor unit, is the important factor affecting the degree of fine muscle movements and potential for fatigue. For most skeletal muscle, the ratio of muscle fibers per innervated motor unit is approximately 100. In the diaphragm, it varies between 15 and 30 muscle fibers per motor unit. This obviously permits a finer gradation of muscular control, but makes the diaphragm potentially more susceptible to fatigue. A muscle must be firmly anchored at both its origin and its insertion to effectively accomplish mechanical work. As a muscle, the diaphragm is unique, since its insertion is mobile, an untethered central tendon. It originates from fibers attached directly to vertebral bodies and costal portions of the lower ribs and sternum. Diaphragmatic muscle contraction results in descent of the diaphragmatic dome and expansion of the base of the thorax. This results in decreased intrathoracic pressure and a corresponding increase in abdominal pressure.

The electrical activity of the human diaphragm has been extensively studied by means of both surface and needle electrodes, and this gives additional insight into its function.[16] During resting inspiratory breathing, there is a gradual, progressive rise in electrical activity during the early portion of inspiration, which gradually fades to zero by mid- to end-expiration.[17] In forced exhalation or with expulsive efforts, such as coughing, electrical activity remains strong throughout expiration.[18] Considerable debate remains as to the importance of external and internal intercostals during inspiration. All external intercostal muscles and the inter-cartilage portion of internal intercostals are primarily active during inspiration. The remaining portion of internal intercostal muscles are associated with exhalation.[19] The abdominal wall muscles, the most powerful muscles of expiration, are essential to successful expulsive efforts.[20] The important muscles in this group are the external and internal obliques, transversus abdominus, and rectus abdominus. Their function is to increase intra-abdominal pressure by compressing the abdominal contents. This activity results in some flexion of the trunk and depression of the lower ribs. The cervical strap muscles in the neck are involved in elevation and fixation of the first two ribs. This activity is observed even during resting inspiratory and expiratory breathing patterns. The primary function of the sternocleidomastoid muscle is to elevate the sternum, thus increasing the dorsoventral diameter of the chest wall. Cervical strap muscles are the most important accessory inspiratory muscles. Their importance is enhanced when there is partial loss of diaphragmatic function, such as with a cervical spinal cord transection. Other large back muscles, such as the pectoralis major and minor, latissimus dorsi, and serratus anterior, are used to augment inspiration by enlarging the rib cage during very high levels of respiratory activity.

MEDIASTINUM

The area between the right and left mediastinal pleura is a space containing the thoracic components of cardiovascular and gastrointestinal systems, the great vessels, nerves, nerve plexuses, lymphatics, and connective tissue. This mediastinal space is divided into a superior and inferior compartment. The inferior compartment is further sub-divided into an anterior, middle, and posterior portion. The middle portion of the inferior mediastinum is the largest subcompartment, and contains the pericardial sac and its contents. Because of the thin layer of tissue separating the mediastinum from the pleural cavities, viscera contained within it are subject to changes in pressure transmitted from the intrapleural space.

LUNG PARENCHYMA

With an intact respiratory system, the expandable lung tissue completely fills the pleural cavity. Upon opening the thorax, healthy lung retracts, collapsing against the lower innermost surfaces of the mediastinum. Both the right and left lungs have oblique fissures, separating the upper from the lower lobes. In addition, the right lung has a horizontal fissure separating the middle and lower lobe. The major divisions of the right and left lungs into their respective lobes and bronchopulmonary segments are listed in Table 32-1. A working knowledge of bronchopulmonary segments is clinically important to localization of lung pathology, interpretation of lung radiographs, identification of lung regions during bronchoscopy, and for surgical lung resection. Each bronchopulmonary segment is separated from adjacent segments by well-defined connective tissue planes. Therefore, pulmonary disease initially tends to remain segmental in scope.

LUNG MORPHOMETRICS

The term *lung morphometrics* implies the study of dimensions of various structures within the lung. Many of these types of

TABLE 32-1.   Major Divisions of the Lung

	LOBES	BRONCHOPULMONARY SEGMENTS
RIGHT LUNG	Upper	Apical
		Anterior
		Posterior
	Middle	Medial
		Lateral
	Lower	Superior
		Medial basal
		Lateral basal
		Anterior basal
		Posterior basal
LEFT LUNG	Upper	Apical posterior
		Anterior
	Lingula	Superior
		Inferior
	Lower	Superior
		Posterior basal
		Anteromedial basal
		Lateral basal

studies have been published by Weibel et al.[21-23] Physical forces govern gas movement through airways, blood flow through vascular channels, and the exchange of oxygen and carbon dioxide between blood and air. An understanding of the effects of these forces on lung function in health and disease requires a knowledge of the design and geometric properties of the system. Based on these considerations, the pulmonary system can be functionally sub-divided into three basic areas (Table 32-2).

Direct measurements and calculations of size related to macro- and microstructure in various lung areas are essential to an understanding of physiologic function. Sophisticated methodologies involving random sampling techniques leading to systematic analysis are required to obtain unbiased measurements. In general, branching of sequential airway structures is such that each parent gives rise to two daughter branches, which, in turn, repeat the process. This dichotomy is somewhat imperfect in that some large airway branches manifest major variations in individual lengths and diame-

TABLE 32-2.   Functional Anatomic Lung Areas

ZONE	ANATOMIC STRUCTURES	CHARACTERISTIC GAS TRANSPORT FUNCTION
Conductive	Multiple branching airways (trachea to terminal bronchioles) and blood vessel branches: blood and gas movement to and from lung periphery.	Gas convection
Transition	Respiratory bronchioles, alveolar ducts, and pre- and post-capillary networks.	Convection and diffusion
Respiratory	Alveoli, alveolar sacs, and corresponding true capillary networks.	Gas exchange Diffusion Ventilation/ perfusion relationships

ters. Therefore the branches are not dichotomous in some of the very large airways, such as lobar bronchi and bronchopulmonary segments. Direct measurements of airway dimensions for the first 11 generations have been averaged and are an accurate reflection of lung structure. Estimation of structure size is based on theoretical calculations for all remaining smaller airways, pre- and post-capillaries, alveolar ducts, alveoli, and capillary segments, since they are too small to be reliably measured and counted. An example of this type of morphometric data, extrapolated in part, from work done by Weibel and others, is presented in Table 32-3.[24] A primary assumption of this model is that each subsequent airway branch is increased by a factor of two. Although not representative of some major airway divisions, such as the lobar and bronchopulmonary segmental bronchi, it is a reasonably accurate representation of the branching architecture of smaller airway divisions.

The sequential series and parallel arrangement of branching airways result in a progressive accumulation in total cross-sectional area as gas moves from the trachea toward alveoli. It is instructive to note that the diameter of the seventh generation airway has decreased to about 2 mm, and the cumulative cross-sectional area is more than 5.0 square cm. Conventionally, airways with diameters equal to or larger than 2 mm are considered large airways, and are the locus of 90% of total lower airway resistance. A major reason for this phenomena is the marked decrease in peripheral flow velocity resulting from the rapidly increasing cumulative cross-sectional area as gas is transported to the lung periphery.

Some important estimations of lung microstructure are briefly summarized. There are approximately 300 million alveoli in an adult. The number of alveoli progressively increases with age, starting out at approximately 24 million at birth, and reaching their adult number of 300 million by the age of 8–9 yr. These alveoli are associated with about 250 million pre-capillaries and 280 billion capillary segments. Each capillary segment is minimally in contact with two adjacent alveoli. This anatomic arrangement results in approximately 70 square meters of surface area for gas exchange. The air blood barrier, the alveolar capillary membrane, has been shown to vary in diameter between 0.4 and 2.5 microns (one micron = 1×10^{-4} cm). The alveolar capillary membrane is composed of capillary endothelial cells, a basement membrane, and alveolar epithelial cells. Histologic features of structures within the lung airways have an important role in regional and overall function of the lungs, and require more detailed discussion.

TRACHEA

The trachea is a fibromuscular tube, approximately 10–12 cm in length, with a diameter of approximately 20 mm. It is primarily supported by 20 U-shaped hyaline cartilages. It is tethered by the cricoid membrane to the cricoid cartilage at the level of the sixth cervical vertebral body. It enters the chest cavity through the superior mediastinum and bifurcates at the sternal angle at the lower border of the fourth thoracic vertebral body. The trachea is normally positioned so that one-half is intrathoracic and one-half extrathoracic. The intrathoracic portion of the trachea is subject to pressure changes within the chest cavity, and the extrathoracic portion is subject to atmospheric pressure. Therefore, with rapid and deep inspiration, the thoracic portion of the trachea becomes wider, whereas the cervical portion of the trachea is narrowed. Since the trachea is attached to movable structures at either end, the longitudinal dimensions of the trachea are subject to considerable lengthening either by elevation of the

TABLE 32-3.   Representative Model: Dimensions and Numbers of Lung Airways*

AIRWAY GENERATION	AIRWAY NAME	NUMBER OF AIRWAYS	DIAMETER (cm)	LENGTH (cm)	CUMULATIVE CROSS-SECTIONAL AREA (cm²)
0	Trachea	1	1.80	12.0	2.54
1	Mainstem bronchi	2	1.22	4.8	2.33
2	Lobar bronchi	4 (5)†	0.83	1.9	2.13
3	Segmental (bronchopulmonary) bronchi	8 (18)†	0.56	0.8	2.00
4	Sub-segmental bronchi (#1)	16	0.45	1.3	2.48
⋮					
7	Sub-segmental bronchi (#4)	128+	0.23	0.7	5.10
8	Sub-segmental bronchi (#5)	256+	0.18	0.6	6.95
⋮					
⋮					
16	Terminal bronchiole	131,000+	0.06	0.14	180.0
⋮					
17	Respiratory bronchiole (#1)	65,536+	0.05	0.11	300.0
⋮					
20	Alveolar duct (#1)	1,048,000+	0.045	0.08	1,600.0
⋮					
23	Alveolar sac	8,388,000+	0.041	0.05	11,800.0

*Model assumes dichotomous branching.
†Actual number of anatomic divisions.

larynx and/or diaphragmatic depression. Because of this, the anatomical position of the tracheal bifurcation can be moved upward as much as 5 cm from its normal resting position. At the trachea bifurcation, the carinal cartilage is responsible for maintaining consistency of the take-off angles of the right and left mainstem bronchus.

Certain cellular structures making up the tracheal wall are important in the removal of mucus from the lungs.[25] The tracheal epithelial layer is primarily composed of pseudo-stratified columnar ciliated epithelium. Interspersed between these cells are goblet cells and brush cells. Chronic exposure to irritants, such as tobacco smoke, influences the number and distribution of various cell types.[26] With chronic irritation, the number of mucus-producing goblet cells is increased, whereas the number of ciliated cells is diminished. This situation is obviously prone to result in an increased amount of secretions and limited capability of secretion removal. The cilia of all cells beat in an organized, coordinated manner, and are responsible for a wave-like propulsive movement of the serous mucous layer towards the mouth. The total functions of brush cells have not been completely delineated, but they appear to be a source of low viscosity fluid for the serous layer. The histologic structures in other, larger airways are similar to those in the trachea.

RIGHT AND LEFT MAINSTEM BRONCHI

The next generation of airways is composed of the right and left mainstem bronchi. The right main bronchus is approximately 2.5 cm long prior to its initial branching into lobar bronchi. Following its respective division into branches to the right upper and middle lobes, the bronchus continues on as the main channel to the right lower lobe bronchus. The left main bronchus is approximately 5 cm long prior to its initial branching point to the left upper lobe and lingula, and then continues on to the left lower lobe. The diameter of the right bronchus is generally greater than that of the left bronchus. At this level, the combined cross-sectional areas of both bronchi is approximately the same as that of the trachea. The take-off angle of the right bronchus from the long vertical axis of the trachea is approximately 25° in adults, whereas the angle for the left bronchus is approximately 45°. Thus, in the adult, inadvertent endobronchial intubation or aspiration of foreign material is likely to end up in the right lower lung field. In children less than 3 yr of age, the bifurcations of both the right and left bronchi are approximately equal, with take-off angles of about 55°.

BRONCHOPULMONARY SEGMENTS AND SMALLER BRONCHI

The anatomic positions, and their relation to gravity, of the next generation of airways, the 18 bronchopulmonary segments, are very important for normal clearance of secretions and postural drainage, a commonly employed therapeutic technique in bronchial hygiene. Depending on the lung segment, successive generations of bronchi, prior to the appearance of bronchioles, reportedly number between eight and 13. For each successive generation beyond the bronchopulmonary segments, there is a progressive, and rather significant, increase in total cross-sectional area (Table 32-3). The ciliated epithelial cells gradually change into an ever-greater number of cuboidal epithelial cells similar to those in primary bronchioles. By the seventh airway generation, the airway

diameter has decreased to approximately 2 mm, the transition point between large and small airways. The smallest bronchi, an airway containing some cartilage elements, is approximately 1 mm in diameter. In general, the larger bronchi have histologic structures identical to the trachea. At the level of the medium-sized bronchi, the eighth to tenth airway generations, the cartilage plates becomes less helical and well-developed, occurring more irregularly. The bronchial mucous glands and goblet cells start to diminish after the tracheal bifurcation, but persist to the level of the smallest bronchi, progressively becoming less frequent in number. These are associated with an equal decrease in number of mucus tubules and serous accini. The venous plexus surrounding the epithelial wall becomes more extensive in the peripheral bronchi. The fibromuscular cylindrical arrangement responsible for elastic recoil in the airways becomes more prominent in the peripherally placed bronchi. It is this muscular arrangement that facilitates changes in both length and caliber of the airways during normal inspiration and expiration.

BRONCHIOLES

The bronchioles, extremely small airways, have diameters of less than 1 mm. They are devoid of cartilaginous support and have the highest proportion of smooth muscle in the wall when compared to lumen diameter. There are approximately three to four generations, with the final element referred to as the terminal bronchiole. The terminal bronchiole is the last airway component of the tracheal-bronchiole tree that is not directly involved in gas exchange. Goblet cells are not found in bronchioles, and there is a continued gradual transition of ciliated epithelial cells to cuboidal epithelium.

GAS EXCHANGE AREA

The respiratory bronchiole following the terminal bronchiole is the first portion of the tracheal-bronchial tree where true gas exchange takes place. These airways are characterized by intermittent alveolar outpockets and a gradual change in the cuboidal epithelial layer to squamous cells. The respiratory bronchioles make up a small part of the total adult respiratory surface area. In adults, there are usually two to three divisions of respiratory bronchioles, which, in turn, lead to alveolar ducts. There are generally four to five generations of alveolar ducts, each with multiple openings leading to alveolar sacs. The closely spaced multiple openings in the walls of alveolar ducts are an integral part of lung parenchyma. During the respiratory cycle, they are subjected to traction forces that tend to distort their structure. The normal architecture is maintained by a framework consisting of elastic, collagenous reticular fibers and slender bundles of smooth muscle fibers. The final divisions of alveolar ducts terminate in alveolar sacs, which, in turn, open into clusters of alveoli. Intact alveolar diameters have been determined to range between 100 and 300 microns. The configuration of alveoli depends to some extent upon their location within the lung.[27] Those alveoli, positioned peripherally just underneath the parietal pleura or along bronchopulmonary segmental planes, are dome-shaped and open widely into the lumina of alveolar sacs. Deeper alveoli share straight flat walls with adjacent alveoli, and can exhibit four to six sides. The supporting lattice-work of the alveolar structures, the intraalveolar septum, is composed of elastic, collagenous, and reticular fibers.

The pulmonary capillaries are also incorporated into, and supported by, this fibrous lattice-work.

ALVEOLAR-PULMONARY CAPILLARY NETWORKS

The pulmonary capillary beds are the most dense of any found within the entire body. The calculated diameter for pulmonary capillaries is between 10 and 14 microns. This extensive vascular branching system starts with pulmonary arterioles in the region of respiratory bronchioles. Each alveolus is closely associated with approximately 1000 short capillary segments. The alveolar capillary membrane, an extremely sophisticated interface, is well-designed to facilitate gas exchange. At its thinnest portion, it is lined with flattened or squamous Type I alveolar cells. The electron microscope shows that, in cross-section, each cell consists of a thin capillary epithelial cell, a surfactant lining layer, a basement membrane, and a pulmonary capillary endothelial cell. The alveolar Type I cells cover approximately 80% of the alveolar surface. It has a flattened nucleus and extremely thin extensions of cytoplasm that provide the surface area for gas exchange. The volume of a Type I cell is twice that of a Type II alveolar cell, but its surface area is 50 times greater.[28] It is highly differentiated and, therefore, metabolically limited. These types of constraints make it highly susceptible to injury. When Type I cells are seriously damaged, there is some evidence that Type II cells become modified after serial replication to form new Type I cells.[29] Type II alveolar cells are interspersed between the Type 1 cells, primarily at the alveolar septa junctions, and are polygonal in shape. These cells have considerable metabolic and enzymatic activity, and have clearly been shown to be a source of a surfactant type material.[30] The enzymatic activity related to surfactant production is less than 50% of the total enzymatic activity present in the Type II alveolar cells.[31] The other enzymatic activity has been attributed to the production of substances affecting endothelial and lymphatic cell functions and the modulation of local electrolyte balance, although evidence for these functions is not as clearly well-defined as it is for surfactant metabolism.[32] Both Type I and II pneumocytes have tight intracellular junctions, thus providing a relatively impermeable barrier to fluids. The third type of alveolar cell, the alveolar macrophage, is considered an important element of lung defense mechanisms. It is migratory in nature, and its phagocytic activity has clearly been documented, as evidenced by ingestion of foreign materials within alveolar spaces.[33] The source of Type III alveolar cells remains controversial, although there is evidence to suggest that it is of mesodermal origin from intra-alveolar septi. The capillary endothelial cells have a greatly increased surface area because of numerous finger-like projections. This provides extremely close contact between each cell and circulating blood volume. This arrangement makes these cells ideally suited for anabolism and catabolism of circulating substances. Therefore, the alveolar capillary membrane has two primary functions: transport of oxygen and carbon dioxide, and metabolic activity associated with activation or deactivation of circulating substances such as hormones, enzymes, and other vasoactive substances.

MECHANISMS OF COLLATERAL VENTILATION

Airways less than or equal to 1 mm in diameter are readily subject to blockage. This results in loss of normal traction forces, accumulation of inflammatory and infectious fluids, or aspirated secretions. The pores of Kohn have long been appreciated and identified as a primary structure in collateral ventilation. These structures facilitate intra-alveolar communication and are located in the interspaces between the alveolar capillary networks.[34] Potentially more important sources of collateral ventilation are pathways directly communicating between small distal or terminal respiratory bronchioles and neighboring alveoli. Their existence has been difficult to prove, as they often appear on histologic sections as a fold in the bronchiolar lining or as an irregularity in an alveolar outline. Their theoretical advantages over the pores of Kohn relate to their size and anatomic location. They have larger diameters than the pores of Kohn, 30 microns versus 8–10 microns, and their anatomic position provides access to a greater number of alveoli.[35]

VASCULAR SYSTEMS

The two major circulatory systems within the lung consist of the pulmonary and bronchial vasculatures. The primary role of the pulmonary vascular system is to deliver aerated blood to the left atrium via the pulmonary veins. The veins are located independently along the intralobular connective tissue planes. The pulmonary capillary system is deemed adequate to provide for the metabolic needs of all lung parenchyma. However, the bronchial system is a primary source of metabolic substances that influence conducting airway and pulmonary vessel tissues. Anatomic connections between the bronchial and pulmonary circulation have been demonstrated and are a source of anatomic shunt. The branches of the pulmonary arteries have a specialized connective tissue arrangement capable of maintaining blood vessel patency in spite of changes in lung volume during breathing and/or with change in anatomic position.

MECHANISMS FOR CONTROL OF VENTILATION

The mechanisms controlling breathing are extremely complex, requiring integration with many areas of the central and peripheral nervous systems. The respiratory centers were first localized in the brainstem in 1812 by LeGallois, when it was demonstrated that breathing did not depend on an intact cerebrum, but on a small region of the medulla near the origin of the vagus nerves.[36] Countless studies over the past 2 centuries have greatly increased our knowledge and understanding of the numerous anatomic components involved in the control of breathing. However, since many of these studies have been done in experimental animals whose central nervous systems are not identical to humans', it has not been feasible to extrapolate much of this information to the human organism.

CONTROL OF RESPIRATION (VENTILATION)

A respiratory center, a term used to identify a central control mechanism, can be defined as a specific area in the brain whose functional characteristics are designed to integrate individual responses of the organism to produce the act of breathing. In actuality, there are several discrete areas or neuronal networks within the central nervous system that function as respiratory centers. These centers process afferent sensory impulses and appropriately modify the organism's response. In turn, the respiratory centers can be modified by other inputs from within and outside the central nervous system. Using terminology designed to characterize a functional approach to the control of breathing, the respiratory centers are designated as the control system.[37] In this context, they are referred to as integrators, oscillators or modulators that act on the entire respiratory system, including peripheral nerves, respiratory muscles, the vascular system, and lung parenchyma. This approach is useful in that it provides a model, a graphic explanation, of how the entire system functions, although all the individual components may not be completely identified.[38, 39] A simplified type of model for control of ventilation will be used to coalesce the important concepts at the conclusion of this section.

From the clinician's perspective, the respiratory centers are collections of neural structures capable of organizing and regulating the complex act of breathing. The respiratory centers are primarily located in the reticular formation of the pons and medulla oblongata as aggregates of richly interconnected neurons. One of the most important sensory inputs acting upon the centers are those receptors responsive to chemical changes in the blood milieu. However, frequently, the rhythmical breathing process is subservient to other important functions, such as temperature control, vomiting, deglutition, and vocalization for speech.

BREATHING PATTERNS

Certain types of breathing patterns merit further amplification to insure that their meanings are clearly understood, since they occur frequently. The term *eupnea* refers to the continuous rhythmical inspiratory and expiratory breathing movement without any undue interruption. In simple terms, this represents the integrated motor output of the intact respiratory centers and is the characteristic activity of normal breathing. *Apnea* is the cessation of respiration in the resting expiratory position where the patient's lung volume is at functional residual capacity. On the other hand, *apneusis* is a cessation of respiration with the patient's lung situated in the maximum inspiratory position or at volumes approaching total lung capacity.[40] *Apneustic respiration* is the pattern associated with alternating phases of apneusis and expiratory spasm.[41] Finally, *Biot's respiration* is characterized by a series of ventilatory gasps interposed between periods of apnea.[42]

IDENTIFICATION OF BRAINSTEM RESPIRATORY CENTERS

The majority of experimental work designed to anatomically localize respiratory centers has been done in rabbits, dogs, and especially, cats. Because of species differences some structures have no direct counterpart in human respiratory centers. Initial descriptions of brainstem respiratory center functions are based on classic ablation or electrical stimulation studies.[43-46] Another method for localization of respiratory centers consists of recording action potentials from different areas of the brainstem with microelectrodes. The assumption is that local brain activity in phase with specific observed respiratory activity is evidence that the area being studied has "respiratory neurons."[47] All the aforementioned techniques are subject to serious flaws for precisely localizing a discrete collection of brainstem neurons specifically responsible for a particular respiratory behavior pattern. It is even more complex because of the abundance of interconnecting neurons to the different respiratory centers. Many combinations of techniques involving ablation, action potential

recordings, and electrical stimulation have resulted in classic descriptions of several unique brainstem respiratory centers. A simplified schematic identifying the classic CNS respiratory centers and important peripheral inputs is illustrated in Figure 32-1.

Pneumotaxic Center

The pneumotaxic respiratory center is located in the rostral portion of the pons. In experimental studies, a simple transection through the brainstem isolating this portion of the pons from the rest of the brainstem results in some reduction in respiratory rate with increased tidal volume amplitude. If in addition, both vagus nerves are transected, the result is apneusis.[48] On this basis, the primary function of the pneumotaxic center is to limit the depth of inspiration. When maximally activated, it has a secondary effect, an increase in breathing frequency, since each new cycle of inspiraton starts at an earlier time. With minimal activity, the response is to simply decrease respiratory rate. The modulating function of the pneumotaxic center is entirely dependent upon inputs from other parts of the brainstem and peripheral nerve inputs, such as the vagus nerve, as it has no intrinsic rhythmicity. Functionally, it can be conceptualized as a negative feedback circuit to the brainstem with the role of terminating inspiration.

Apneustic Center

A second major respiratory center is the apneustic center located in the middle or lower portion of the pons. Electrical stimulation of this area results in inspiratory spasm.[49] With activation, this center sends impulses to inspiratory neurons in the medulla designed to sustain inspiration. More detailed studies of the middle to lower pons have revealed specific areas where inspiratory-expiratory and expiratory-inspiratory neurons, referred to as phase-spanning neurons, are located.[50] These neurons appear to play a role in the transition between phases of respiration, rather than exerting direct control over respiratory muscles. These elements are important in control of ventilation, since neurologic activity is frequently out of phase with the inspiratory/expiratory mechanical activity of the respiratory system.

Medullary Centers

The basic respiratory control areas in the brain are located in the medulla oblongata. Specific areas are primarily active either during inspiration or expiration with many neuronal inspiratory or expiratory interconnections between individual areas. The inspiratory centers are primarily located in the dorsal portion of the reticular formation, whereas the expiratory centers are located in the ventral portion of the reticular formation. The inspiratory center is the source of the elementary baseline respiratory rhythmicity.[51, 52] This rhythmical activity is still present when all incoming peripheral and interconnecting nerves to the area have been sectioned or completely blocked. In a sense, it functions as an indigenous rhythm or inspiratory "pacemaker" for the respiratory system.[53] This rhythmical pattern is usually ataxic, gasping in nature, and frequently associated with intermittent maximum inspiratory efforts involving all muscles of respiration. Some neuro-anatomic studies have suggested that the summation of discharge activity for all the inspiratory-expiratory neurons in the medulla is a constant. This would suggest that the total population of inspiratory-expiratory neurons is linked *via* a system of reciprocal innervation.[47] These studies

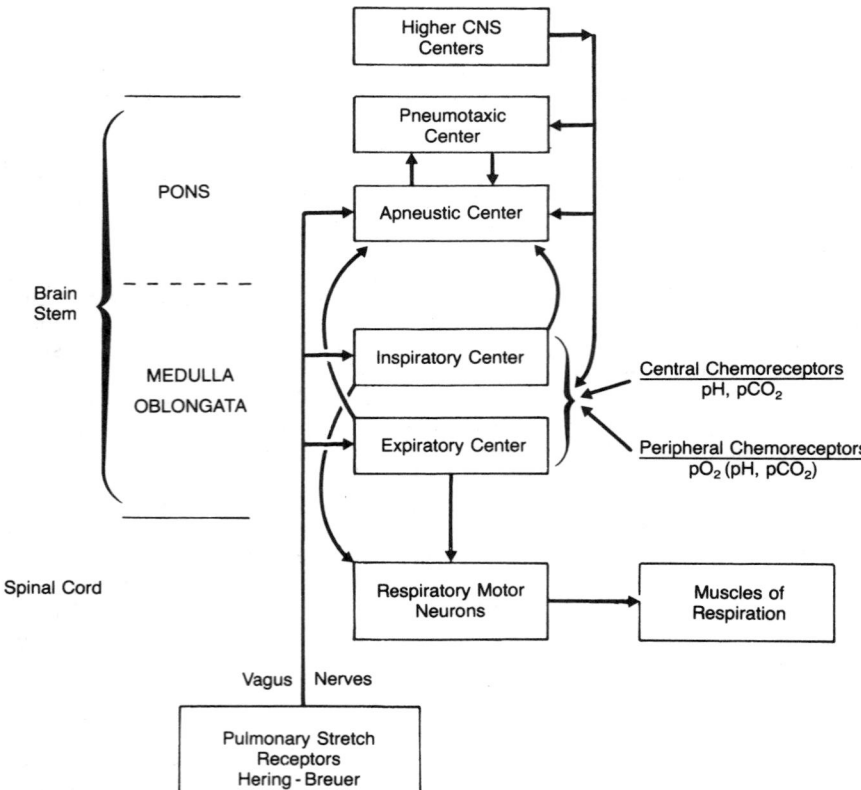

FIG. 32-1. Schematic diagram of classic CNS respiratory centers. Diagram illustrates major respiratory centers, neuro feedback circuits, primary neuro-humoral sensory inputs, and mechanical outputs.

provide strong evidence for a hypothesis that the generation of a normal breathing pattern (eupnea) is greatly dependent on input from both higher brain centers and other peripheral sensory inputs.

Many higher level brain structures clearly affect ventilatory control processes. In the mid-brain, stimulation of the reticular activating system (RAS) has been shown to increase the rate and amplitude of respiration.[54] The effects of the cerebral cortex on breathing are well documented, although the precise responsible neuronal pathways have not been clearly delineated.[55] In some circumstances, specific behavior patterns require the ventilatory control process to be subservient to other regulatory centers. The anterior and posterior hypothalamus are portions of the brain responsible for thermal regulation. The respiratory system is an important effector organ for body temperature control, as it provides a large surface area for heat loss. This is especially important in animals, where the process of panting is the only effective means of losing heat. This respiratory pattern is felt to be related to neural input *via* descending pathways from the hypothalamus to the pneumotaxic center in the upper pons. Several studies have suggested that cardiovascular vasomotor control and certain respiratory responses are closely linked together. Stimulation of the carotid sinus leads to both inhibition of respiration and decreased vasomotor tone. In certain circumstances, stimulation of the carotid body chemoreceptors results in an increase in both respiratory activity and vaso-motor tone. Specific relationships between vasomotor tone and respiratory activity have been attributed to neural inputs modulating the medullary respiratory centers.[56, 57] Deglutition, the act of swallowing, is related to activity of the glossopharyngeal (ninth cranial nerve) and vagus

(tenth) cranial nerve. The receptor areas for swallowing are in the anterior and posterior pillars of the posterior pharynx. With active swallowing, there is a momentary inhibition of inspiration, usually immediately followed by increased tidal volume and respiratory rate. The exact respiratory centers involved in coordinating breathing with deglutition have not been identified.[58] Finally, vomiting or emesis, a result of prolonged vigorous stimulation of the posterior pharynx, is an activity that requires significant modification of normal respiratory activity.[59] Vomiting is a complex activity that takes into consideration salivation, deglutition, gastrointestinal reflexes, rhythmical spasmodic respiratory movements, and, finally, significant muscle activity by the diaphragm and abdominal wall muscles. It is an obvious advantage to the whole organism to terminate inspiration during the act of vomiting.

CHEMICAL REGULATION OF RESPIRATION: PERIPHERAL CHEMORECEPTORS

The primary goal of respiration is to maintain appropriate amounts of oxygen, carbon dioxide, and hydrogen ions in the body. Hypoxia, a generalized decrease in oxygen in either the blood (hypoxemia), alveoli, or tissues, results in increased breathing activity. Lack of oxygen does not appear to have a significant direct stimulating effect on the brain respiratory centers. Its effect on controlling ventilation is secondary to stimulation of peripheral chemoreceptors located in carotid and aortic bodies.[60, 61] The carotid bodies are located bilaterally at the bifurcation of the common carotid arteries. The output of these receptors is transmitted to the respiratory centers *via* afferent fibers in the glossopharygeal nerves. The output of aortic bodies, located along the arch of the aorta, reaches the medullary centers *via* the vagus nerve. The receptors become strongly stimulated when arterial oxygen concentration falls below certain critical levels. This behavior is not an all-or-nothing phenomena or step function response dependent on a specific arterial P_{O_2}. Neural activity gradually increases above baseline starting at an arterial P_{O_2} 100 mm Hg with marked increase in activity as P_{O_2} falls to the range between 60–30 mm Hg. This phenomena is graphically shown in Figure 32-2. Blood flow through the carotid and aortic bodies is extremely high relative to their tissue mass, so that the normal oxygen extraction is less than one volume percent. Therefore, the tissue P_{O_2} is usually approximate to arterial P_{O_2} rather than venous P_{O_2}. When this delicate physiologic condition is perturbed, such as with low arterial P_{O_2} or with decreased cardiac output causing hypotension, especially with arterial pressures below 60 mm Hg, there is a significant increase in neural activity. This initiates reflexes that enhance respiratory activity and cause peripheral vasoconstriction.

Increased carbon dioxide tension or hydrogen ion concentration also activates the receptors, but their magnitude of response, compared to their corresponding effects on central chemoreceptors, is several orders of magnitude smaller. Thus, the peripheral chemoreceptors can be conceptualized as primarily sensitive to oxygen.

CHEMICAL REGULATION OF RESPIRATION: CENTRAL CHEMORECEPTORS

Acid base regulation involving carbon dioxide, hydrogen ions, and bicarbonate is primarily related to chemosensitive receptors located in the medulla positioned close to or in direct contact with cerebrospinal fluid. The studies almost uniformly support the hypothesis that these receptors are sensitive to changes in hydrogen ion concentration. However, the exact location of the chemosensitive area, whether in extracellular tissue fluid, intracellular fluid, or cerebrospinal fluid, is still debated.[62]

Carbon dioxide has little direct stimulating effect on these chemosensitive areas. It does have a potent indirect effect by reacting with water to form carbonic acid, which, in turn, dissociates into free hydrogen and bicarbonate ions.[63] Increased blood CO_2 is a more potent stimulator of respiration than increased blood hydrogen ions from a metabolic source, since only carbon dioxide passes readily through the blood-brain and blood-cerebrospinal fluid barriers. Under most circumstances, many of the hydrogen ions in blood, extracellular, and intracellular fluid are immediately neutralized by extremely effective buffering systems. In contrast, the cerebrospinal fluid (CSF) has minimal buffering capacity. Thus, for any given increase in CO_2, the number of free hydrogen ions in the CSF would be considerably greater than those found in blood or tissue fluids. In addition, the CSF is in intimate contact with the rich blood supply of the arachnoid plexus. If the CSF is the primary chemoreceptive area, this could readily explain the rapid respiratory response, a large increase in ventilation, to relatively small increases in blood CO_2. The respiratory effects of acutely increased blood P_{CO_2} peaks within a minute or two after the change. Then the effect of increased ventilation declines over a period of several hours, probably as a result of active transport of bicarbonate from the blood into the CSF through arachnoid villi.[64]

VENTILATORY RESPONSE TO BREATH-HOLDING

In general, total activity or input from peripheral and central chemoreceptors are integrated in the medullary respiratory centers. Their summation effect on respiratory center stimulation is dependent upon individual levels of oxygen, carbon

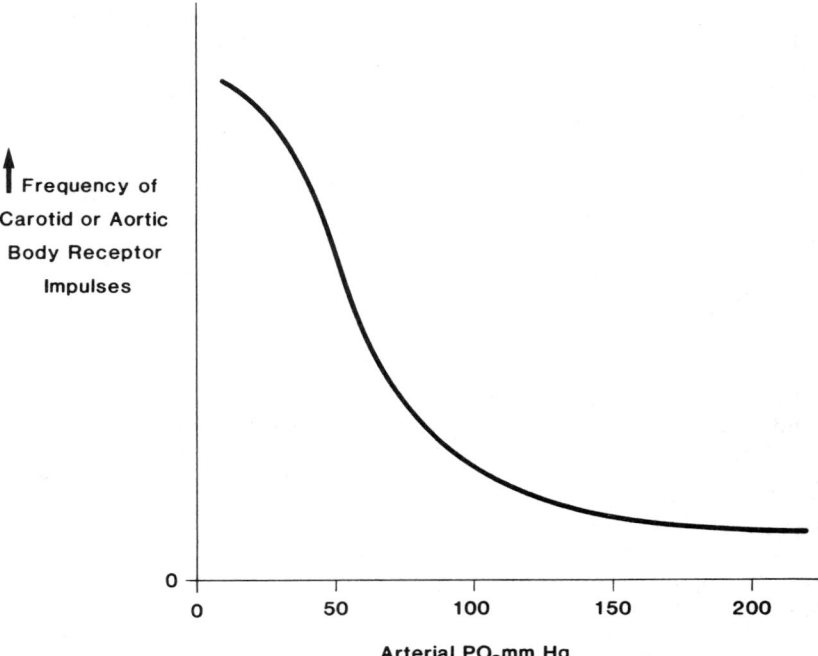

FIG. 32-2. Graphic representation of neural activity of aortic/carotid bodies in response to changes in arterial oxygen tension.

dioxide, and hydrogen ions in the blood and body. Because of its complexity, it is not feasible to specifically describe all the combined effects of manipulations in CO_2, O_2, and pH. A simplified way to grasp the interdependence and complexity of these parameters on control of ventilation is to record the response to prolonged breath-holding. When a volunteer with normal lungs and gas exchange function is asked to breath-hold without previous hyperventilation, the usual time limit is approximately 1 min. Under these circumstances, alveolar P_{O_2} decreases to 65–70 mm Hg, and there is a 10 mm Hg increase in alveolar P_{CO_2} to 50 mm Hg. If individuals are allowed to breathe 100% oxygen prior to this maneuver, they can lengthen their breath-holding time to 2–3 min. The major drive to start re-breathing is an increased P_{CO_2} (60 mm Hg). If a person breathing room air is instructed to hyperventilate prior to breath-holding (to reach an alveolar P_{CO_2} level of 20 mm Hg), he can frequently hold his breath for up to 3–4 minutes.[65] If a volunteer both hyperventilates and breathes 100% oxygen prior to breath-holding, he can breath-hold for periods as long as 6–10 min. Finally, if subjects are given gas mixtures containing decreased oxygen and increased carbon dioxide following an initial breath-holding maneuver, they are still capable of repeated prolonged breath-holding periods following short interspersed periods of breathing. This phenomenon occurs even when subsequent gas mixtures used had oxygen tensions below, and carbon dioxide tensions above, values recorded in the alveoli from the previous trial.[66] This strongly supports the hypothesis that other sensory inputs, such as pulmonary stretch receptors or inputs from higher brain centers, can independently stimulate or depress ventilatory drive. Spontaneous apnea, a process of breath-holding for even short time periods, following hyperventilation in unanesthetized man is rarely observed. In contrast with administration of extremely light anesthesia, the phenomena of spontaneous apnea is frequently observed following even mild hyperventilation.[67]

RESPIRATORY RECEPTOR ORGANS AND REFLEXES

Input to respiratory centers from respiratory reflex receptors is *via* afferents from both cranial and spinal cord nerves. There are several types of receptors that originate from the chest wall or lungs and airways, although the precise effects that some of them have on control of ventilation is still uncertain.

Sub-epithelial receptors are located in the trachea, especially along the posterior wall, and bronchial walls of the larger airways. These receptors are primarily responsible for the cough reflex.[68] Muscle spindle receptors, proprioceptors sensitive to pressure changes, are located within smooth muscle in all airways in the lungs.[69] Receptors resembling muscle spindles have also been identified in the perichondrial portion of larger bronchi. Tendon spindles (Golgi tendon organs) positioned in a series arrangement with respiratory muscles tend also to facilitate a proprioceptive control mechanism. The intercostal muscles are rich in tendon spindles, whereas the diaphragm has a limited number. This is correlated with a well-demonstrated stretch reflex in intercostal muscles, but such a reflex does not exist in the diaphragm.[70] This supports the hypothesis that the diaphragm is designed to perform routine inspiratory function, while the intercostals are activated only with additional workloads on the system. Encapsulated receptor endings have been identified in respiratory bronchioles, and unencapsulated receptor endings in alveolar ducts, atria, alveolar sacs, and alveoli. These receptor organs may have a role in modulation of both inspiration and expiration. Finally, there are several different types of receptors, diffusedly spread throughout the pulmonary vascular bed, whose function remains undefined. The variety and number of receptor end organs in the lungs provides anatomic justification for multiplicity of respiratory reflexes.

A few reflexes involved in ventilatory control have been extensively studied. The Hering-Breuer reflex, first reported in 1868, noted that a time period of sustained distension of the lungs in lightly anesthetized animals was followed by decreased to absent respiratory efforts.[71] The response was blocked with bilateral vagotomy. It is more prominent in lower order mammals, such as rabbits, but only weakly present in man. This response, termed the inflation reflex, has been associated with inspiratory muscle inhibition documented by marked reduction in electrical activity in both the phrenic nerve and diaphragmatic muscle itself. The second component of the Hering-Breuer reflex, the deflation reflex, is increased respiratory muscle activity associated with sustained lung collapse. This reflex has not been demonstrated to be of any significance in man. The pulmonary stretch receptors are the smooth muscle spindle receptors responsible for sensing mechanical changes associated with inflation and deflation of the lungs. These proprioceptive receptors slowly adapt to changes in pressure, and are subject to pressure thresholds. The stretch reflex can be demonstrated with distension of isolated airways, so that airway pressure, rather than volume distension *per se*, would appear to be the primary sensitive factor.[72] Thus, clinical conditions resulting in decreased lung compliance leading to increased traction on the airways would predictively be prone to produce this response. Clinical conditions in which pulmonary stretch receptors are sensitized are pulmonary vasculator congestion, atelectasis, and pulmonary edema, as well as many other infectious and inflammatory causes of acute lung injury. Certain drugs, such as acetylcholine, pilocarpine, or histamine, administered intravenously or in aerosol doses large enough to result in decreases in lung compliance, have also been shown to enhance the stretch reflex.[73] In contrast, the pulmonary stretch receptors are inhibited by inhalation of vaporized water, intravenous injection of antihistamines, and topically administered local anesthetics.

PHYSIOLOGIC ROLE OF RESPIRATORY REFLEXES

Although it is tempting to think of respiratory reflexes as being primary modifiers of respiratory activity, their function is more likely to be of a secondary nature. Some of the known effects of respiratory-related reflexes are:

1. Serving as modulators of timing in phasic respiratory activity.
2. Terminating inspiration with high discharge frequency and augmentation of early inspiration with slow discharge frequency of pulmonary stretch receptors.
3. Altering tonic baseline muscle activity of the diaphragm. Resultant nerve activity has been shown to enhance resting respiratory muscle tone at small lung volumes and depress it at large lung volumes.
4. Modifying the sensitivity of respiratory centers to other major input stimuli, such as changes in P_{CO_2}, pH, and/or P_{O_2}.
5. Producing secondary effects on cardiac function, related to increase in heart rate or development of sinus

arrhythmia, phenomena associated with the cyclic activity of inspiration and expiration.

ORGANIZATION OF THE VENTILATORY CONTROL SYSTEM

The control of breathing is a multifactorial process involving respiratory centers, afferent and efferent nerves, reflex feedback networks, skeletal and smooth muscle, and intrinsic mechanical and physiologic properties of a passive lung system. In spite of the extreme complexity, a practical understanding of system functions can be achieved by establishing a model depicting a logical sequential order of events. Since all the elements have not been clearly identified, the model would not be parametric, but, of necessity, would have constrained parameters. The respiratory system is ideally suited to such an analytical approach, and the technique has been effectively used and published in both biomedical engineering and physiology disciplines.[74,75] Such a simplified representative model identifying the important elements in the respiratory system is graphically illustrated in Figure 32-3.

The primary respiratory centers are anatomically located in the medulla oblongata and pons portion of the brainstem. These primary respiratory and higher level central nervous system centers make up the control system directing behavior and ultimate function of the respiratory system. In order for the controlling system to properly function, it must have negative feedback loops to minimize the effects of under-desired inputs. This function is performed by chemoreceptor reflexes and internal reflexes from a "passive respiratory system" plus external respiratory reflexes. The entire respiratory system, nerves, muscles, lung, and chest wall tissues, is the passive system, or structures being acted upon by the ventilatory controllers. Since breathing is cyclic in nature, the timing of events, whether inspiratory or expiratory, is important in characterization of function. Intrinsic properties of the system are correlated with variations in mechanical and fluid (gas) behavior and energy expenditure. The amount of work done, the pressure–volume product, is greatly dependent on the magnitude of pulmonary resistance and compliance. This impacts on energy expenditure as well as the organisms "ventilatory reserve," which itself is dependent upon respiratory muscle function. Because of real time lag in mechanical systems, there are phase differences between neural and muscle activity and the mechanics of gas flow or volume displacement in and out of the lung. In obstructive lung diseases (with prolonged system time constants), there can be considerable time delay between respiratory nerve activation, muscle contraction, and gas flow from the mouth down the airways. Therefore, a description of activity as inspiratory or expiratory in time is often greatly dependent upon the intrinsic mechanical properties of the passive respiratory system.

The undisputed output of the system is ventilation, reinforcing the notion that the lung is primarily a ventilator and not a respirator. The effectiveness of ventilation is dependent

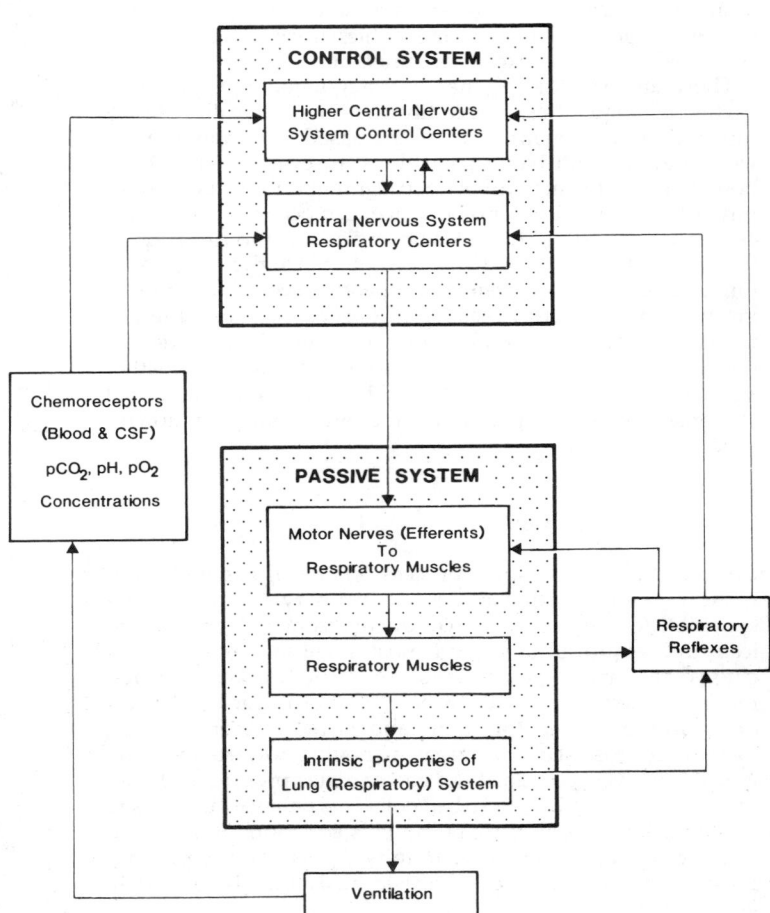

FIG. 32-3. Model of the respiratory system. The two major subdivisions are 1) the ventilation control system component, which acts on 2) the passive respiratory system component.

on lung mechanics and gas exchange function, which will be discussed in detail in the following section. In summary, this type of model provides a basic framework and is a valuable tool for delineating the effects of control and feedback mechanisms on physiologic and mechanical behavior of the respiratory system. As interest and knowledge in a particular area is increased, it is readily feasible to expand that portion of the model. This obviously includes specific effects of various agents and drugs used by anesthesia clinicians.

PHYSIOLOGY AND MECHANICS OF GAS TRANSPORT IN THE LUNG

The primary function of the lungs is transport of oxygen from the ambient environment into pulmonary capillaries, as well as removal of carbon dioxide from pulmonary capillaries by releasing it into the atmosphere. This gas exchange process, termed external respiration, is an equivalent counterpart to internal respiration, the gas exchange process between systemic capillary beds and body tissues. From the immediate surrounding atmosphere through the upper and lower airways into alveoli, gas transport is entirely dependent upon the mechanical properties of airways, lungs, and chest wall tissues. The bidirectional exchange of gases between alveolar spaces and pulmonary capillary beds is dependent on both lung mechanical properties and cardiac function. Therefore, it is equally important to evaluate cardiovascular function, including myocardial pump capability and distribution of blood flow (cardiac output), within the lungs. The presence of limited cardiovascular reserves and/or significant disparities in regional pulmonary mechanics invariably results in abnormalities in gas exchange function.

These abnormalities, generally categorized as ventilation/perfusion inequalities, are readily identified clinically, as they cause signs and symptoms of increased cardiopulmonary work and aberrant blood gas values. In order to appreciate how a severe mismatch between ventilation and perfusion, physiologic shunt and/or deadspace, can occur, it is first necessary to understand the roles of convection and diffusion in transporting gases to and from alveoli. Since the lung's anatomic architecture is a system of repeating sequential branching tubes with ever-increasing cross-sectional area, the potential for significant abnormal distribution of ventilation in the presence of lung disease may occur, even under anesthesia. Therefore, as shown in Table 32-4, gas exchange should be considered only the final component of total pulmonary lung gas transport.

GAS CONVECTION

Convection, the transport process where all gas molecules move in a given direction, is the primary mechanism responsible for gas flow in the conductive zone, which anatomically makes up all large and most small airways. This includes all airway generations from the trachea through medium-sized and small bronchi and bronchiolar airways down to the 14th or 15th generations. Because of the ever-increasing cross-sectional area in moving toward the lung periphery, average velocity of gas particles progressively decreases as they travel toward alveoli. This behavior in a closed system is characterized by Bernoulli's equation, and is often referred to as the Law of Continuity.[76] It is also the primary reason why the majority of airway resistance is located in larger airways.

TABLE 32-4.   Pulmonary Gas Transport

I. Convection [bulk flow]
II. Mixed—convection/diffusion
III. Gas exchange
    A. Diffusion
    B. Ventilation/perfusion relationships ($\dot{V}_{alv}/\dot{Q}_{cap}$)

GAS DIFFUSION

The second major gas transport process is diffusion, defined as random molecular motion leading to complete mixing of all gases. As gas moves further toward the lung periphery, starting with terminal bronchioles (16th airway generation), diffusion gradually becomes the predominant component of gas transport. This transition zone is exemplified by the terminal divisions of respiratory bronchioles and larger alveolar ducts. Finally, effective gas transport in small alveolar ducts, alveolar sacs, and alveoli, the gas exchange zone, is dependent upon both diffusion and regional ventilation/perfusion relationships. Historically, presumed defects in gas diffusion have often been presented as the reason for inadequate blood oxygen values (hypoxemia). Realistically, the most frequent cause of hypoxemia is physiologic shunt; anatomic right-to-left shunts or persistent capillary perfusion with inadequate or absent alveolar ventilation.[77]

There are several physical and physiologic relationships affecting gas diffusion, listed in Table 32-5, which are important factors in gas transport.[78]

Combining the physical properties of molecular weight and gas solubility as expressed by Graham's and Henry's law, respectively, results in the familiar 20 : 1 diffusibility ratio between carbon dioxide and oxygen. An important clinical point is that hypercarbia is the result of inadequate alveolar ventilation, and should never be attributed to a diffusion defect. The evaluation of diffusion requires a consideration of lung area available for diffusion. This is a common explanation for an apparent decrease in diffusing capacity in patients with significant chronic obstructive lung disease. It is actually the inequalities in ventilation/perfusion relationships, func-

TABLE 32-5.   Important Factors in Diffusion of Oxygen and Carbon Dioxide

1. Physical properties
  a) Graham's law (molecular weight of the gas)

$$\text{Diffusion gas} = D_{gas} = \frac{1}{\sqrt{MW_{gas}}}$$

  b) Henry's law (gas solubility)
    Dissolved gas = (S)* P_{gas}
    *S = Solubility coefficient (cc gas/cc blood/atmos P_{gas})

  c) Combined Effects of Graham's and Henry's Laws on Diffusion (D) of CO_2 and O_2

$$\frac{D_{CO_2}}{D_{O_2}} = \left[\frac{1/[MW\ CO_2]^{1/2}}{1/[MW\ O_2]^{1/2}}\right] \times \left[\frac{S_{CO_2}}{S_{O_2}}\right]$$

$$\frac{D_{CO_2}}{D_{O_2}} = \left[\frac{[1/44]^{1/2}}{[1/32]^{1/2}}\right] \times \left[\frac{0.592}{0.024}\right] = (0.85)(24.3) \cong \frac{20}{1}$$

2. Area for diffusion (~70 m² in adult man)
3. Histologic characteristics of alveolar-capillary membrane.
4. Average gas pressure difference across the Alv-pulmonary capillary membrane.

tionally resulting in less surface area, that decreases diffusing capacity.[79] The prototype abnormality of a diffusion defect, an alveolar capillary block, is secondary to alterations in histologic characteristics of the alveolar capillary membrane. Finally, average pressure difference for oxygen and carbon dioxide between alveoli and pulmonary capillaries is an important factor when quantitatively evaluating gas diffusion across the alveolar-capillary membrane. Because of a continuous variation in blood oxygen tension with time as it moves through the pulmonary capillary, oxygen cannot be used to directly assess diffusion capability. A gas mixture containing carbon monoxide (CO), which has essentially zero gas tension in blood because of its high affinity for hemoglobin, is the traditional diagnostic gas used to quantitatively evaluate lung diffusing capacity.[80]

BASIC CONCEPTS OF CONVECTION MECHANICS

In order for gas to enter or leave gas exchange areas, it must pass through the complex branching airway system. Thus, a knowledge of mechanical factors affecting convection or bulk gas movement is essential to overall understanding of pulmonary gas transport.[81, 82]

Several variables are necessary to adequately describe functional characteristics of gas transport in any cyclic mechanical system. These mechanical variables and their corresponding clinical parameters are presented in Table 32-6, and represent the functional determinants of any ventilator system. The relative importance of each is greatly dependent upon design or specific application of the system. The inertial effects of acceleration or deceleration of gas flow have no routinely specified clinical parameters, since they only play an important role when high frequency ventilation techniques are considered.[83]

Since ventilation is cyclic, time is the primary independent variable; tidal volume delivered to a patient, gas flow, and pressure developed within the system are all subject to time constraints. The concept of pressure as a "forcing function" is that pressure represents the force causing the entire system to behave in some prescribed manner. More specifically, during inspiration, whether spontaneous or secondary to positive pressure ventilation, and during forced exhalation, the pressure changes within the lungs are forcibly directed. The pressure changes during inspiration are, to a great extent, a reflection of respiratory muscle activity with spontaneous breathing, dependent upon a clinician's manipulation of an attached mechanical ventilator or a combination of both factors. In contrast, during passive exhalation, the changes in system pressures (airway, alveolar, intrapleural) with time are simply a passive reflection of all mechanical properties of the airways, lung parenchyma, and chest wall tissues. In this case, the pressure changes are referred to as a "free (unforced) response." One of the most important aspects of pressure is that it is the unifying variable reflecting superimposed respiratory muscle effort and/or the force of a mechanical ventilator and, finally, the magnitudes of all respective lung mechanical factors in the pulmonary system. This relationship facilitates the derivation of mathematical expressions that can be used to quantitatively characterize convective gas flow within the pulmonary system.[84]

SYSTEM PRESSURE: A FORCE BALANCE OF OPPOSING *VERSUS* GENERATED PRESSURES

Newton's third law of motion states that force applied to a body is met by an equal, opposing force developed by the body. This law provides the justification for application of a force balance equation to the pulmonary and any other mechanical ventilator support system used for lung ventilation.[85] The applied force is represented by positive pressure generated by a mechanical ventilator or subatmospheric pressure developed by a patient's respiratory muscles to facilitate tidal volume delivery. The opposing force or opposing pressure, in this case, reflects all the mechanical properties within a patient's lungs tending to inhibit tidal volume delivery. The magnitude of total opposing pressure or lung impedance is a reflection of the relative contributions of chest wall and lung tissue elastic forces and dynamic resistive forces of airways. Acceleration or deceleration of gas flow, the inertial forces, only contribute significantly to opposing pressure when ventilation frequency is greatly increased. Therefore, this factor only need be included when high frequency ventilation techniques are considered. Elastance or elastic recoil, a property of static lung mechanics, is frequently conceptualized as the difficulty in distending the pulmonary system. Since lung parenchyma and chest wall tissues are superimposed on top of each other, a series arrangement, their elastances are added directly:

Elastance (total) = elastance (lung) + elastance (chest wall)

Compliance, the reciprocal of elastance (C = 1/E), or lung distensibility characterizes the relationship between changes in lung volume and transpulmonary pressure, the pressure difference between the mouth and "intrapleural space." Intrapleural pressures are indirectly measured from a properly placed esophageal pressure transducer. Because of its reciprocal relationship to elastance, total compliance is always less than individual chest wall or lung compliance:

$$\frac{1}{C_{(Total)}} = \frac{1}{C_{(Lung)}} + \frac{1}{C_{(Chest\ wall)}}$$

The normal value for $C_T = 0.1$ l/cm H_2O, which is based on C_{Lung} and $C_{chest\ wall}$, each equalling 0.2 l/cm H_2O. Airway resistance and tissue resistance are the properties of dynamic lung mechanics. However, with normal breathing patterns the component of resistance due to tissue deformation can be ignored. Normal values for R_A, in the lower airway, are 1–2 cm $H_2O \cdot l^{-1} \cdot sec^{-1}$.[81]

TABLE 32-6.   Functional Determinants of Ventilator Systems

MECHANICAL VARIABLE	CLINICAL PARAMETER
Time	Frequency (respiratory rate)
	Inspiratory/expiratory time ratio
Volume	Average tidal volume
	Minute ventilation
Flow (volume/time)	Peak flow
	Average flow
Flow (volume/time^2) Acceleration/deceleration	*
Pressure (forcing function)	Intrathoracic pressure (tracheal, alveolar, intrapleural)

* Clinical parameter applicable only with the use of high frequency ventilator (HFV) techniques.

Since the pressure generated during inspiration must be adequate to meet the opposing or lung impedance pressure in order to deliver a tidal volume, this permits a solution to the force balance equation.

Opposing Pressure = Generated Pressure

$$\left\{\begin{array}{c} \text{Compliance} \\ \text{and} \\ \text{Resistance} \end{array}\right\} \quad \left\{\begin{array}{c} \text{Respiratory muscles and/or} \\ \text{Mechanical ventilation} \end{array}\right\}$$

When pressure generated over the specified inspiratory time is constant or time-dependent, it greatly simplifies the right-hand side of the equation and can be set equal to some representative pressure (Po). When using standard ventilation techniques or with most spontaneous breathing patterns, it is quite apparent that airway resistance, lung and chest wall compliance are the major factors governing the pressure required to deliver a given tidal volume. The delta symbol (δ) is used to signify a rate of change in volume or flow with time.

$$R\frac{\delta V}{\delta t} + \frac{1}{C}V = P_o$$

The left-hand side of the equation can be further simplified by letting $[\delta V/\delta t]$ be represented by flow (F) and then dividing both sides of the equation by resistance (R), which is also assumed to be constant:

$$F + \frac{1}{RC}V = \frac{P_o}{R}$$

Additional information on gas movement in the lung under passive conditions, a free or unforced system response, can be determined by excluding the constant pressure and resistance terms on the right-hand side of the equation. It represents characteristic gas flow in the lungs during passive exhalation. Mathematically, this is accomplished by assessing the change in flow with respect to time. Since both pressure and resistance have been defined as constant terms, which do not change with time, the right-hand side of the equation becomes zero.

$$\frac{\delta F}{\delta t} + \frac{1}{RC}F = 0$$

In this form, the equation permits a determination of the effects of resistance and compliance on changes in flow with time. The solution is represented by a first order equation with flow at time zero indicated as F(0) and flow at any time indicated as F(t).[84]

$$F(t) = F(0)\ e^{-t/RC}$$

The graph of this equation is an exponential decay curve as shown in Fig. 32-4. The exact character of the flow curve is dependent upon initial flow and individual values for airway resistance, lung and chest wall compliance. Establishing a convenient frame of reference facilitates comparison of different lung and mechanical ventilatory systems. The two most commonly used parameters are half-life ($t\frac{1}{2}$) and the time constant, tau (τ). For a more detailed discussion of these concepts, the interested reader is referred to a specific article on the mechanics and physics of patients' lungs and ventilator systems.[84]

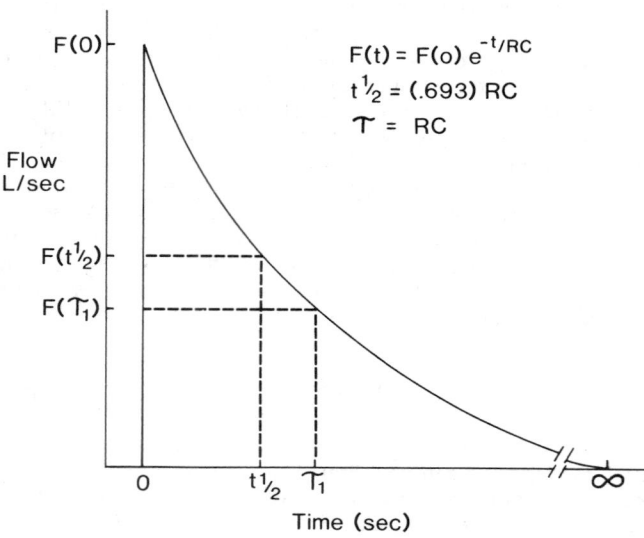

Exponential Decay Curve

$$F(t) = F(o)\ e^{-t/RC}$$
$$t\frac{1}{2} = (.693)\ RC$$
$$\tau = RC$$

FIG. 32-4. Characteristic flow profile observed with a passive exhalation, a free response. The initial flow F(o) represents the flow at the start of exhalation, zero time. Flow at any time F(t) can be calculated when values for resistance, compliance, and the initial flow are known.

THE TIME CONSTANT

The concept of half-life is familiar to most clinicians, since it is routinely used in assessing pharmacokinetic activity and radioactive decay behavior. Half-life represents the amount of time required for a reaction rate to equal one-half the initial rate, or radioactivity to be one-half its initial value. In addressing behavior of mechanical systems, the reference time is more frequently related to the number e (2.71828...), which simplifies the mathematics. This turnover time, or time constant, indicated by the Greek letter tau (τ), represents the amount of time required for flow to decrease to a value of 1/e of the initial flow:[84]

$$\tau\ (\text{time constant}) = RC,$$

where R = resistance and C = compliance. A comparison of both half-life and time constant reference times is shown in the exponential decay curve in Figure 32-4. The standard units for resistance and compliance are substituted into the equation to reinforce the concept that tau (τ) is a measure of real time:

$$\tau\ (\text{sec}) = R\left[\frac{\Delta P\ (\text{cm } H_2O)}{F\ (\text{l/sec})}\right] C\left[\frac{\Delta V\ (\text{l})}{\Delta P\ (\text{cm } H_2O)}\right] = \text{sec}$$

A practical use of time constants is that it provides sequential quantitative assessment of reduction in flow with time.[84] Thus, the decrease in flow, equal to 1/e for the first time constant T_1, is approximately 37% of initial flow. Continued reduction in flow at T_2, equal to (1/e) × (1/e), or (1/e²), is about 14% of the initial flow. The required time in seconds to reach each time constant is entirely dependent upon the specific values for resistance and compliance. The changes in flow and percent maximum volume associated with several time

TABLE 32-7. Reduction in Flow and Volume Accumulated and Removed Using a Constant Pressure Generator

NO TIME CONSTANTS	F(t)/F(o)	% INITIAL FLOW	% MAXIMUM VOLUME REMOVED OR ADDED
τ_0	$[1/e^0]$	100.0	0.0
τ_1	$[1/e]$	36.7	63.3
τ_2	$[1/e^2]$	13.5	86.5
τ_3	$[1/e^3]$	4.9	95.1
τ_4	$[1/e^4]$	1.8	98.2
τ_5	$[1/e^5]$	0.7	99.3
$\vdots$	$\vdots$	$\vdots$	$\vdots$
τ_∞	$[1/e^\infty]$	0.0	100.0

Two Compartment Lung Model

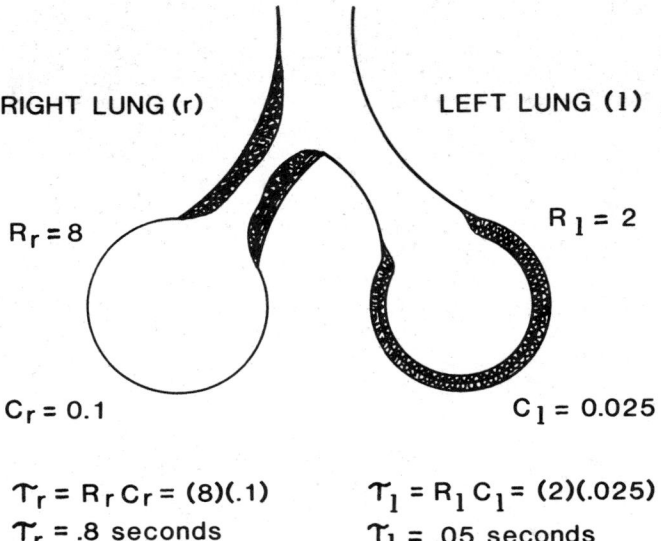

RIGHT LUNG (r)   LEFT LUNG (l)

$R_r = 8$ $R_l = 2$

$C_r = 0.1$ $C_l = 0.025$

$\tau_r = R_r C_r = (8)(.1)$ $\tau_l = R_l C_l = (2)(.025)$
$\tau_r = .8$ seconds $\tau_l = .05$ seconds

FIG. 32-5. Schematic representation of a two-compartment lung with normal compliance and increased airway resistance in the right unit and normal airway resistance and decreased compliance in the left unit. T_r and T_l are the first respective time constants for each component.

constants are listed in Table 32-7. In this simplified example, a constant generated pressure (Po) is applied throughout inspiration; it can be seen that a unique relation exists between percentage of maximum volume added or removed and decrease in flow from initial flow. Passive exhalation into the atmosphere, with the respiratory muscles totally at rest, represents a condition where back pressure tending to inhibit further flow is always atmospheric or zero, so that, in effect, the pressure generator is constant.

Several practical aspects of lung mechnical function can be derived from the time constant concept. Although flow theoretically continues to infinite time, when elapsed real time is equal to three time constants or three times the product of the patient's resistance and compliance, the flow has decreased to about 5% of initial flow. Volume delivered to the lung is approximately 95% of maximum volume for that specific constant generated pressure. This concept can also be a valuable guide to help the clinician determine the most appropriate mechanical ventilatory support during anesthesia or in the postoperative period in patients with significant lung pathology. It provides a theoretical basis to help the clinician appreciate what effect regional differences in pulmonary lung mechanics have on volume distribution within the lung.

CLINICAL APPLICATION OF TIME CONSTANTS

Gas transport through the multi-branching airway configuration leading to respiratory gas exchange areas is reasonably effective when the lungs are healthy. With development of lung pathology, the non-uniform effects of disease on individual airway resistances and variations in regional lung compliance will significantly interfere with gas transport and gas exchange, causing increased ventilation/perfusion inequalities.[86] This situation frequently poses the challenging problem for the anesthetist of how to structure a ventilatory pattern that will minimize gas exchange defects. The solution to the problem is more frequently realized when effects of pulmonary disease on gas transport are understood.

For purposes of illustration and simplicity, a two-compartment lung model is used (Fig. 32-5), and convenient values for right and left airway resistance and lung compliance are arbitrarily chosen. In addition, it will be assumed that a constant positive pressure generator (a standard ventilator) provides the force for inspiration, and exhalation is passive.

In this example, the increased airway resistance to the right lung field, coupled with decreased compliance in the left lung field, results in major maldistribution of ventilation to the respective lung areas. The first time constant (τ_{1r}), the time required to remove or add 63% of maximum volume in the right lung field, is prolonged to 0.8 s. This type of lung area is referred to as a "slow lung unit," because of the prolonged time necessary for filling and emptying. It would require 2.4 seconds, three times the time constant τ_{3r} for delivery of 95% of maximum volume to the right lung field. If, in addition, the regional compliance was increased, it would further increase time requirements. In general, this type of condition is primarily associated with lung areas that have significantly increased regional airway resistances.[87] If this situation was representative of both lung fields, for example, in a patient with generalized chronic obstructive lung disease, this information would be helpful in establishing a more appropriate ventilatory pattern. In summary, it would dictate a slow respiratory rate with large tidal volumes. Time for exhalation should be considerably prolonged over inspiration, since the differences between generated inspiratory (ventilator) pressure and alveoli are likely to be substantially greater than generated exhalatory pressure between alveoli and the atmosphere.

In contrast, the left lung field has a decreased first time constant (T_{1l}) of 0.05 s. This is primarily due to decreased regional compliance. These type of gas exchange units, called "fast lung units," fill and empty rapidly as alveolar pressure quickly rises to approach generated pressure. The time required to reach 95% of maximum volume, (T_{3l}) in this lung field is only 0.15 s. If this decrease in compliance was representative of the entire lung, for example, in a patient with pulmonary fibrosis, a reasonable ventilatory pattern would incorporate an increased frequency and small tidal volumes. The time allotted for exhalation could be quite close to that for inspiration without causing any adverse effects.

A more realistic and commonly encountered challenge is

ventilation of a patient with widespread disparities in local airway resistances and regional compliances. This example is represented by the simplified two-compartment lung model used for illustration. It should be emphasized that there are numerous combinations of regional differences in lung mechanical properties that can result in equally divergent gas transport to respective lung gas exchange areas. In this simplified example, the left lung field will have received 95% of its potential maximum volume in about 1/16th (0.15 s/2.4 s) of the time required for the right lung field. In all probability, towards the end of inspiration, the left lung field or "fast lung units" would be emptying into the "slow lung units" on the right side. This type of behavior, called penduluft, is likely to be exaggerated in lung disease, presumably plays a role in gas mixing and transport in HFV techniques, and probably even occurs, to a small extent, in normal healthy lungs. An important clinical goal in this situation is to establish a mechanical ventilatory pattern, which will promote a more uniform distribution of lung ventilation. The use of a slow rate, larger tidal volumes, prolonged time for exhalation with an "inspiratory hold" maneuver is a simple, practical way to obtain the desired result. The inspiratory hold, by keeping delivered volume within the lung, facilitates a more equitable, uniform distribution of tidal volume.[88] In essence, it uses penduluft to the patient's advantage, since it provides extra time to compensate for slow lung units, while still permitting fast lung units to effectively participate in gas transport and potentially improve gas exchange or ventilation/perfusion relationships.

GAS EXCHANGE (VENTILATION/PERFUSION RELATIONSHIPS)

The primary function of the lung is external respiration or gas exchange between the ambient environment and the pulmonary capillary bed. Gas diffusion and adequate amounts of alveolar ventilation and pulmonary capillary blood flow are necessary elements in this process. The effectiveness of gas exchange is greatly dependent on an appropriate matching of regional capillary perfusion ($\dot{Q}_{cap}$) and alveolar ventilation ($\dot{V}_{alv}$).

DISTRIBUTION OF BLOOD FLOW

Blood flow to the lungs in the upright position is mainly gravity-dependent. The lateral wall pressure in the pulmonary artery (Ppa) decreases by approximately $1.25 \, mm \cdot cm^{-1}$ of vertical distance up the lung. The amount of blood flow along the vertical axis depends upon the relationship between the Ppa, the alveolar pressure (P_A), and the pulmonary venous pressure (Ppv) (Fig. 32-6). Traditionally, the lung is divided into three zones as described by West. Zone 1 is the upper part of the lung above the level where Ppa is equal to P_A. Since P_A is equal to atmospheric pressure, the Ppa in zone 1 is subatmospheric ($P_A > Ppa > Ppv$). The P_A transmitted to the pulmonary capillaries would lead to their collapse ("collapse zone") with the consequence of zero blood flow to this lung region. Since no gas exchange is possible in this zone, it represents alveolar deadspace. Normally, zone 1 is of limited extent, but in conditions where Ppa decreases, such as in hypovolemic shock or with positive pressure ventilation which increases P_A, zone 1 may extend, causing a wide discrepancy between Pa_{CO2} and end-tidal CO_2 (PET_{CO2}).

Zone 2 extends from the lower limit of zone 1 (Ppa = P_A) vertically down as a consequence of and increase in Ppa, which becomes positive and exceeds P_A up to the point at which Ppv = P_A (Ppa > P_A > Ppv). The blood flow in this zone is determined by the pressure difference between Ppa and P_A, while the Ppv has no influence. This zone is referred to as a Starling resistor or the "waterfall zone" by analogy to waterfall over a dam. The rate of blood flow is determined by the difference between upstream arterial pressure (Ppa) and the magnitude of alveolar pressure (the dam) and is not affected by the downstream venous pressure (Ppv). It is important to keep in mind that the relationships among arterial, alveolar, and venous pressure vary during the respiratory and cardiac cycles, so that the amount of blood flow also varies accordingly.

Zone 3 is termed the "distention zone", where Ppa > Ppv > P_A, and blood flow is governed by the downstream Ppa–Ppv pressure difference. Because of the higher venous pressure in this zone, the pulmonary capillaries are maximally distended. Recruitment of previously unperfused capillaries from zone 1 into zone 2 can take place with an increase in Ppa. Similarly, underperfused capillaries can be recruited from zone 2 to zone 3. Thus, the limits of various zones are not fixed, but can vary according to physiologic or pathologic changes.

DISTRIBUTION OF VENTILATION

A healthy lung is a viscoelastic organ that will collapse inward upon itself without chest wall support. In essence, the viscoelastic tissues of the intact thoracic cage exert an outwardly directed force tending to keep the lung inflated. This results in a subatmospheric (negative) pressure in the potential space between the visceral and parietal pleura (intrapleural space). Due to gravity, there is a relatively greater subatmospheric pressure at the top of the upright lung compared with tissues at the bottom. The difference in intrapleural pressures between the top and the bottom of the lung is approximately 7.5 cm water (the lung is 30 cm in height with one-fourth the density of water; thus, 30 cm divided by 4 is 7.5 cm). Pleural pressure is therefore increased by 0.25 cm per centimeter of lung dependency. A greater subatmospheric pressure at the apical area of the lung in the presence of equal P_A increases alveolar or transpulmonary distending pressure (P[mouth] minus P[intrapleural]), resulting in more distended alveoli. The transpulmonary distending pressure is less at the base of the lung, where intrapleural pressure is relatively more positive. This results in less distended alveoli, since they are on a lower portion of their pressure volume curve.

VENTILATION-PERFUSION RATIO

In the upright position, most of the blood flow and the largest portion of tidal volume is distributed to the gravity-dependent part of the lung, resulting in reasonably good matching of ventilation ($\dot{V}$) and perfusion ($\dot{Q}$). However, ventilation and perfusion are not perfectly matched from the top to the bottom of the lung, creating different $\dot{V}/\dot{Q}$ ratios down the lung. A $\dot{V}/\dot{Q}$ ratio of 1.0 is believed to occur at the level of the third rib; above this, the ventilation is in excess of perfusion ($\dot{V}/\dot{Q} > 1$), while below the third rib, the ratio is less than 1.0 (Fig. 32-7).

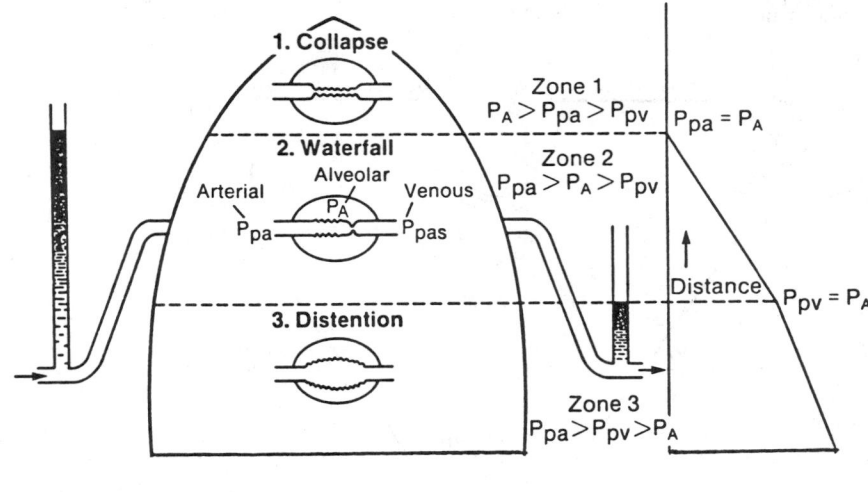

FIG. 32-6. The figure is a schematic that accounts for the distribution of blood flow in the isolated lung. In zone 1, alveolar pressure (P_A) exceeds pulmonary artery pressure (P_{pa}), and no flow occurs because the vessels are collapsed. In zone 2, arterial pressure exceeds alveolar pressure, but alveolar pressure exceeds pulmonary venous pressure (P_{pv}). Flow in zone 2 is determined by the arterial–alveolar pressure difference ($P_{pa} - P_A$), which steadily increases down the zone. In zone 3, pulmonary venous pressure now exceeds alveolar pressure, and flow is determined by the arterial–venous pressure difference ($P_{pa} - P_{pv}$), which is constant down this zone of the lung. However, the pressure across the walls of the vessels increases down the zone, so that their caliber increases, as does flow. (West JB, Dollery CT, Naimark A: Distribution of blood flow in isolated lung: Relation to vascular and alveolar pressures. J Appl Physiol 19:713, 1964. Reproduced by permission.)

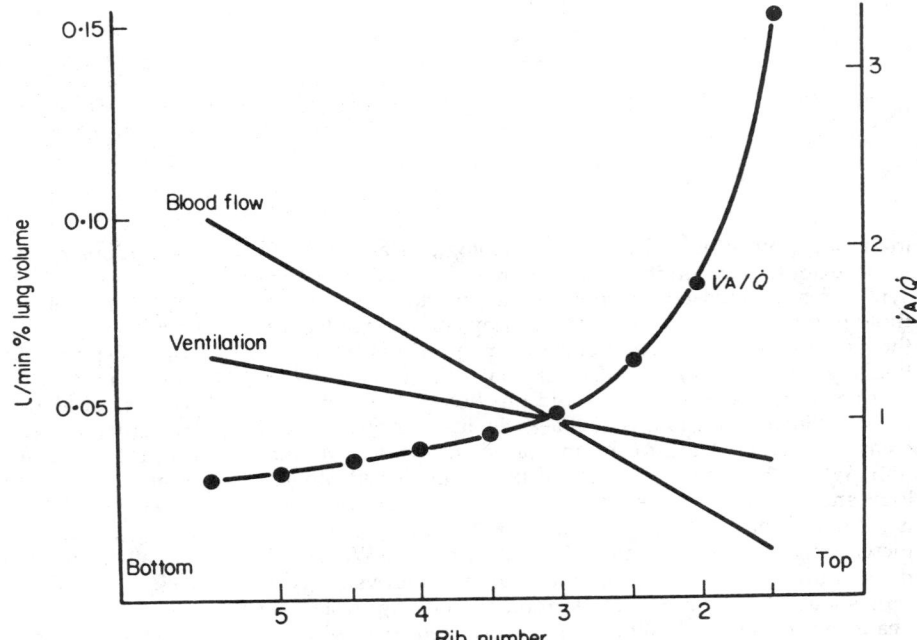

FIG. 32-7. Distribution of ventilation, blood flow, and ventilation-perfusion ratio in the normal upright lung. Straight lines have been drawn through the ventilation and blood flow data. Because blood flow falls more rapidly than ventilation with distance up the lung, ventilation-perfusion ratio rises; slowly at first, then rapidly. (West JB: Ventilation/Blood Flow and Gas Exchange. Oxford, Blackwell Publications, 1985. Reproduced by permission.)

The concept of a gas exchange unit, traditionally designated as a normal, deadspace, shunt, or silent unit, has been used to differentiate the various ventilation/perfusion relationship possibilities.[89] Interrelationships between various gas exchange unit types can be more clearly perceived by considering individual units as a continuum in the gas exchange process (Fig. 32-8).

In healthy lungs, the majority of alveolar-capillary units are, in essence, normal gas exchange units. At one end of the spectrum, the "absolute deadspace" unit represents clinical situations in which blood flow to a particular alveolar area is totally absent. The "deadspace effect" units are characterized by a progressive diminution of blood flow relative to ventilation in going from normal gas exchange to absolute deadspace. In contrast, the "absolute shunt" unit represents an alveolar-capillary unit with blood flow and total absence of

ventilation. The "shunt effect" units are associated with a progressive decrease in ventilation relative to blood flow in moving from normal gas exchange to absolute shunt. Since neither deadspace or shunt units facilitate effective gas exchange, it is logical to have physiologic mechanisms diminish ventilation and/or perfusion away from these lung areas. Pulmonary vaso-hypoxic constrictive reflexes present in the pulmonary circulation are activated for shunt units, and bronchiolar constrictive reflexes in the small bronchioles are activated for deadspace units to achieve this purpose.[90, 91] When this occurs, shunt and/or deadspace units are converted to silent units.

Pulmonary diseases causing pathophysiologic changes in the lung would generally result in both physiologic shunt and deadspace abnormalities. However, in the early developmental stages, most disease processes primarily cause either

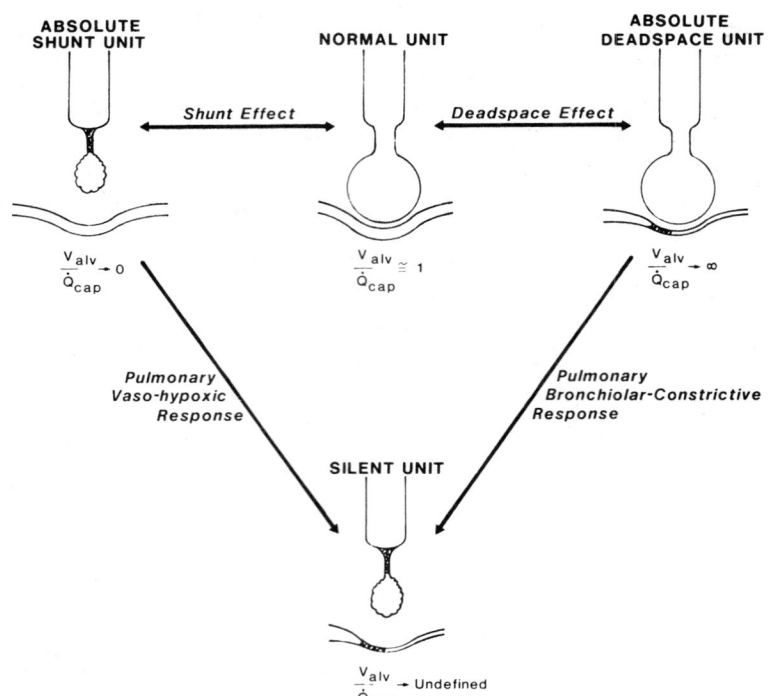

FIG. 32-8. Continuum of ventilation/perfusion relationships. Gas exchange is maximally effective in normal lung units and only partially effective in shunt and deadspace effect units. It is totally absent in silent units, absolute shunt, and deadspace units.

increased physiologic shunt or physiologic deadspace. To some extent, both entities will result in clinical signs and symptoms of increased cardiopulmonary work. When the pathology inherently causes increased physiologic deadspace, the patients' expected compensatory response is increased total mechanical ventilation. The arterial blood gas parameter that correlates best with increased physiologic deadspace is carbon dioxide tension. The Pa_{CO_2} is inappropriately decreased corresponding to the increased mechanical ventilation. When the disease process results in increased physiologic shunt, the patients appropriate compensatory response is increased cardiac output.[92] Whenever physiologic shunt is increased, arterial hypoxemia is invariably present. When initially evaluating the nature of pulmonary pathophysiology, it is reasonable to assume that the problem is either physiologic deadspace or shunt. It should be emphasized that, with extensive lung involvement or advanced disease, the artificial separation between physiologic shunt and deadspace is no longer practical, since they become clinically and physiologically indistinguishable.

PHYSIOLOGIC DEADSPACE

A practical way to functionally differentiate type of ventilation is to divide minute volume into alveolar ($\dot{V}_{alv}$) and physiologic deadspace ($\dot{V}_{D_{physio}}$) ventilation. Physiologic deadspace is further subdivided into anatomic ($\dot{V}_{D_{anat}}$) and alveolar ($\dot{V}_{D_{alv}}$) deadspace. In lung areas where deadspace effect is present, mathematically, it is analogous to assigning an appropriate portion to either the alveolar or physiologic deadspace component:

$$\text{Minute ventilation} = (RR)(V_T) = \dot{V}_{alv} + \dot{V}_{D_{physio}}$$

where

$$V_{D_{physio}} = V_{D_{anat}} + V_{D_{alv}}$$

Traditionally, arterial CO_2 is clinically used to evaluate the effectiveness of alveolar ventilation. Patients are determined to be hyperventilating or hypoventilating depending upon their Pa_{CO_2} status; whether it's below or above the normal range, respectively. Arterial P_{CO_2} is a reliable index, since it is a function of only two variables: the rate of CO_2 elimination, alveolar ventilation; and rate of CO_2 production, metabolic rate. Thus, a meaningful evaluation of arterial P_{CO_2} must always include assessment of metabolic function and alveolar ventilation. Teleologically, since physiologic deadspace is wasted ventilation, the appropriate response is to increase minute ventilation. The majority of physiologic deadspace normally consists of anatomic deadspace, approximately 2 $ml \cdot kg^{-1}$ ideal body weight.[93] It includes all anatomic airway structures from the oronasal pharynx, including terminal bronchioles, down to the respiratory bronchioles. Clinical conditions resulting in modification of anatomic deadspace include endotracheal intubation, tracheostomy, and positive airway pressure therapy. However, the primary concern is with clinical conditions resulting in a significant increase in alveolar deadspace.[94] Pulmonary embolism, irrespective of its source; blood clot, fat, air, or amniotic fluid, is the prototype example of an acute increase in alveolar deadspace. The most frequent cause of increased alveolar deadspace is secondary to conditions resulting in decreased cardiac output.[95] The use of positive pressure ventilation or PEEP therapy can potentially cause increased alveolar deadspace (increased zone 1) secondary to interference with venous return to the right heart and decreased cardiac output.[96]

ASSESSMENT OF PHYSIOLOGIC DEADSPACE

It is clinically useful to have a readily available means of assessing physiologic deadspace. A simple, straightforward approach is a direct comparison between minute ventilation and alveolar ventilation. More sophisticated assessment techniques include: 1) measurements of differences between end-tidal CO_2 and arterial CO_2, and 2) calculaton of total physiologic deadspace using the modified Bohr equation.

A disparity between mechanical ventilation and corresponding arterial P_{CO_2}, a reflection of alveolar ventilation, is present whenever physiologic deadspace and/or metabolic rate is increased above normal. The simple correlation of measured minute volume with arterial P_{CO_2} is, at best, a semiquantitative technique. Its validity, however, depends upon the precisely defined relation between metabolic rate, alveolar ventilation, and alveolar P_{CO_2}. Subtracting physiologic deadspace from tidal ventilation is equivalent to alveolar ventilation ($V_A = V_T - V_D$). This can also be re-stated for minute ventilation (MV). The volume of physiologic deadspace ventilated in 1 min ($\dot{V}_{D_{physio}}$) is subtracted from minute ventilation (MV) to yield minute alveolar ventilation ($\dot{V}_A$). Arterial P_{CO_2} represents a reasonably good approximation of alveolar P_{CO_2}. These relations are shown in the following equations:

$$\alpha\ \dot{V}_{CO_2} \text{ (metabolic rate)} = [Pa_{CO_2}][\dot{V}_{alv}]$$
$$= [Pa_{CO_2}][MV - \dot{V}_{D_{physio}}],$$

where α = a unit conversion constant and MV = minute ventilation. For increased clarity, the equation solved for Pa_{CO_2} is graphically illustrated in Figure 32-9 by a series of hyperbolic curves representing different metabolic rates. The graph also shows clearly that increased physiologic deadspace without appropriate increased minute ventilation will result in decreased alveolar ventilation. As an initial approximation, doubling normal baseline minute ventilation, assuming normal distribution between alveolar and deadspace ventilation and a stable metabolic rate, should result in a reduction in arterial P_{CO_2} to approximately one-half its baseline value.

When a disparity between mechanical ventilation and arterial P_{CO_2} is present, it is necessary to determine if the cause is increased alveolar or increased anatomic deadspace or a result of an atypical metabolic rate. If the patient has a reasonably "normal" ventilatory pattern, appropriate for body size, the anatomic deadspace component can be considered reasonably normal.[97] The patient's metabolic function, as reflected by minute carbon dioxide production, should also be within acceptable limits. Cardiovascular function must be adequate to maintain peripheral tissue perfusion to legitimately reflect the metabolism of the entire body. When these criteria are fulfilled, doubling baseline normal minute ventilation decreases baseline arterial P_{CO_2} from 40 to 30 mm Hg. Quadrupling minute ventilation results in a decrease in arterial P_{CO_2} to 20 mm Hg. If the arterial P_{CO_2} is not appropriately reduced in response to increased mechanical ventilation, this represents strong supportive evidence for an acute increase in alveolar deadspace. The practical advantage of this assessment technique is that required measurements are easily performed and, generally, part of a normal clinical evaluation routine.

A non-invasive and quite sensitive technique for assessing increased physiologic deadspace is evaluation of differences between end-tidal and arterial CO_2. In Figure 32-10, the distinctive profiles of carbon dioxide exhalation curves are illustrated. During phase I, the initial portion of exhaled volume, carbon dioxide is absent, since anatomic deadspace has the same concentration of CO_2 as inspired air. The rapid increase in CO_2, during phase II, the transition zone, marks the gradual change from airway to alveolar gas. The volume of gas exhaled at the mid-point of the transition zone (V_F) represents an average pathway length from the mouth to the gas exchange area. This exhaled volume from zero to this point is anatomic deadspace, and is frequently called Fowler's dead-

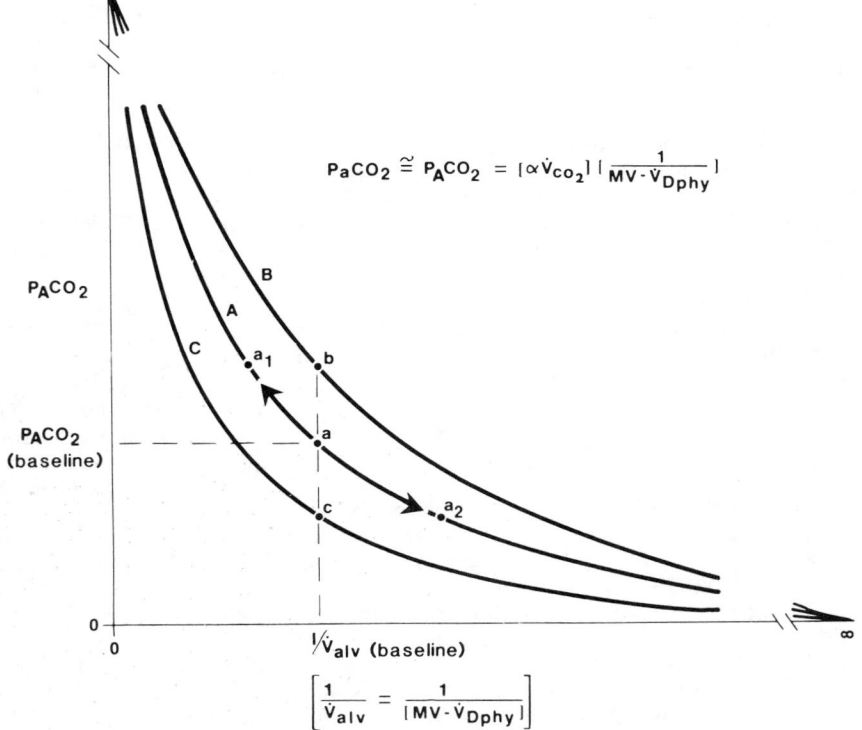

FIG. 32-9. Metabolic hyperbolas. Curve A represents normal state of metabolism; curve B, increased metabolism (*e.g.*, hyperthermia); and curve C, decreased metabolism (*e.g.*, hypothermia). With a stable "normal baseline" alveolar ventilation and metabolic rate, point *a* would represent eucapnia Pa_{CO_2} = 40 mm Hg), point *b* hypercapnia, and point *c* hypocapnia secondary to a respective increase and decrease in metabolic rate. Even with metabolic rate unchanged from baseline, decreased alveolar ventilation results in hypercapnia, point a_1, and increased alveolar ventilation results in hypocapnia, point a_2. Alveolar ventilation (V_{alv}) can be effectively changed by either specific changes in minute ventilation (MV) or changes in physiologic deadspace.

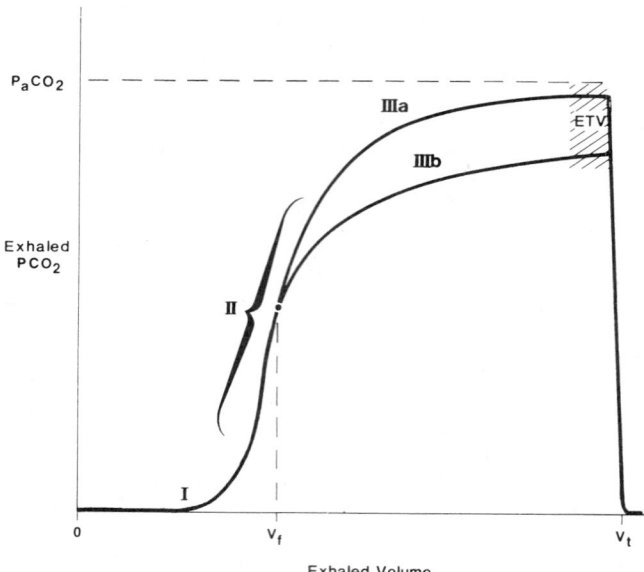

FIG. 32-10. Exhalation CO_2 curves. Phase I = anatomic deadspace. Phase II = transition zone from airways to alveoli; V_F is the midpoint or Fowler's anatomic deadspace volume. Phase III = Alveolar plateau non-uniform emptying of alveoli with the CO_2 value at end-tidal volume (ETV) close to arterial Pa_{CO_2} in normal lungs (IIIa), and considerably less than arterial Pa_{CO_2} with increased alveolar deadspace (IIIb), whether on an acute or chronic basis.

space. Phase III, often called the alveolar plateau, represents gas mixtures in lung alveoli. Generally, the last group of alveoli to empty are those from the gravity-dependent portion of the lung (zone 3) containing the highest percentage of carbon dioxide. In patients with normal lungs, the P_{CO_2} in end-tidal volume is usually only 2–3 mm Hg less than arterial P_{CO_2}. When blood flow to an alveolar portion of the lung is absent, there is a corresponding decrease in exhaled, end-tidal CO_2, as gas leaving that lung area no longer contains carbon dioxide. This is characterized by an increased difference between arterial and end-tidal CO_2. An increased difference between arterial and end-tidal P_{CO_2}, $[P(a–A)_{CO_2}]$, is the physiologic result of increased alveolar deadspace, as the configuration of the curve (III b) in Figure 32-10 illustrates. This assessment technique is extremely sensitive for ascertaining acute increases in alveolar deadspace, such as occurs with air embolus.

The most quantitative assessment technique used to measure physiologic (both anatomic and alveolar) deadspace utilizes the modified Bohr equation:

$$\frac{V_D}{V_T} = \frac{Pa_{CO_2} - P\overline{E}_{CO_2}}{Pa_{CO_2}}$$

The value for alveolar P_{CO_2} is replaced by arterial P_{CO_2} (Pa_{CO_2}), and an averaged P_{CO_2} value is obtained from an expired gas sample ($P\overline{E}_{CO_2}$). In spontaneous breathing patients, the normal V_D/V_T ratio is between 0.2 and 0.4. In patients receiving positive pressure ventilatory support using large tidal volumes or on PEEP therapy, the V_D/V_T ratio can normally be as high as 0.55. The major limitation to application of this measurement is the inability to obtain an accurate $P\overline{E}_{CO_2}$ from an exhaled gas sample in non-intubated patients.

Measurements of exhaled CO_2 can be easily contaminated with inspired air or supplemental oxygen. The measurement will also be inaccurate if the patient does not maintain a steady-state pattern of ventilation. Therefore, when this measurement is used as part of a physiologic and clinical evaluation, extreme care must be taken to insure that all measurements are accurately performed.

PHYSIOLOGIC SHUNT

Whereas physiologic deadspace applies to lung areas that are ventilated but inadequately perfused, physiologic shunt occurs in lung areas that are perfused but inadequately ventilated. Defective to absent gas exchange is the net effect of both abnormalities.[98]

In general terms, a shunt is simply a "bypass," but its meaning is more restricted in pulmonary physiology. Physiologic shunt can be operationally defined as that portion of total cardiac output ($\dot{Q}_t$) that is returned to the left heart and systemic circulation without participating in alveolar-pulmonary capillary gas exchange. Total cardiac output can be mathematically divided into two components, pulmonary capillary or effective cardiac output ($\dot{Q}_c$), and wasted or physiologic shunted cardiac output ($\dot{Q}_s$). When lung units are totally devoid of ventilation, this condition can be defined as an *absolute shunt*, a ventilation/perfusion inequality ($\dot{V}_{alv}/\dot{Q}_{cap}$) equal to zero. The term *shunt effect* or venous admixture is applied to lung units where alveolar ventilation is deficient compared to the amount of perfusion ($0 < [\dot{V}_{alv}/\dot{Q}_{cap}] \ll 1$).

Frequently, the concepts and terminology applied to physiologic shunt are misunderstood; thus, it is imperative to clearly define terms used in this discussion and establish a practical analytical approach, such as that illustrated in Figure 32-11. The initial division of physiologic shunt is based on the specific vascular pathway, anatomic or pulmonary capillary, the blood takes in going from the right to left ventricle. In this context, the term "anatomic" refers to a complete bypass of all pulmonary alveolar-capillary beds. Although some anatomic right-to-left shunts can cause significant clinical problems, pathologic conditions leading to capillary shunt are more frequently encountered. A second analytical level categorizes type of physiologic shunt based on an individual's response to supplemental oxygen therapy. Finally, a quantitative value for defects in pulmonary oxygen gas exchange can be determined using the physiologic shunt equation.

Anatomic Shunts

A small percentage of venous blood normally bypasses the right ventricle, emptying directly into the left atrium. This "universal" anatomic shunt is primarily secondary to venous return from pleural, bronchial, and Thebesian veins. It usually comprises 2%–5% of total cardiac output, and explains, in part, the discrepancy between the theoretical end pulmonary capillary oxygen tension and measured arterial oxygen tension. Anatomic shunts of greatest magnitude are usually associated with cyanotic heart disease, those congenital lesions responsible for right-to-left shunts. Intrapulmonary anatomic shunts, such as arterio-venous anastomoses or fistulas, can be a prominent cause of anatomic shunt. Occasionally, this phenomenon is observed in patients with advanced liver cirrhosis and associated systemic and pulmonary A-V anastomoses.

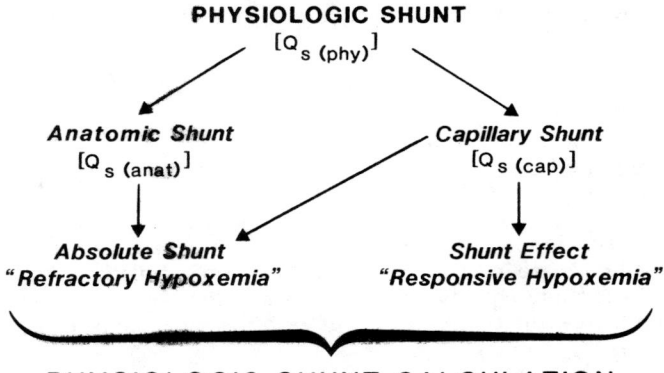

FIG. 32-11. Organization of physiologic shunt. Level (I) is based on the specific types of vascular pathways the blood takes in going from the right ventricle to the left ventricle. Level (II) is based on the patient's clinical response to supplemental oxygen. The physiologic shunt calculation is classically expressed as a ratio of shunted cardiac output to total cardiac output $[\dot{Q}_{sp}/\dot{Q}_t]$.

Capillary Shunts

Capillary shunt occurs in lung areas where gas exchange should normally take place. Clinical entities causing capillary shunt can be considered in the general context of alveolar collapse, atelectasis, or as a result of fluid-filled alveoli. Atelectasis or alveolar collapse due to gas absorption occurs because of airway obstruction secondary to retained secretions, foreign bodies, lung tumors, or even an inadvertent bronchial intubation. It can be the result of passive lung collapse due to accumulation of fluid, blood, or air in the intrapleural space. Fluid-filled alveoli are generally the result of inflammatory or infectious disease processes: pneumonia, cardiogenic pulmonary edema, or acute lung injury.

Hypoxemia and Physiologic Shunt

Since hypoxemia is invariably a clinical manifestation of physiologic shunt, its response to supplemental oxygen therapy can be used to help evaluate the underlying pathology (Fig. 32-11). When a disease process causes a large *absolute shunt* (major areas of the lung where ventilation is totally absent), minimal improvement is observed in arterial P_{O_2}. This refractory hypoxemia occurs irrespective of the concentration of administered oxygen. Acute lobar atelectasis, an extensive acute lung injury, massive pulmonary edema, or bilateral pneumonias are frequent causes of this pathophysiologic response. In contrast, *shunt effect* is characterized by a marked improvement in arterial P_{O_2}, a responsive or non-refractory hypoxemia, following supplemental oxygen. The majority of patients have clinical entities that act as shunt effect and, therefore, show dramatic improvement in arterial oxygen tension with supplemental oxygen. An "oxygen challenge" can be used to differentiate refractory from responsive hypoxemia. Conceptually, it depends on the magnitude of increase in arterial P_{O_2} associated with a precise increase in FI_{O_2}. This requires the use of an oxygen analyzer or administration of oxygen using a "high flow" consistent delivery system. One advantage to this therapeutic approach is that the clinician develops a frame of reference for changes in arterial P_{O_2} secondary to a known change in FI_{O_2} related to specific clinical entities.

PHYSIOLOGIC SHUNT CALCULATION

The physiologic shunt calculation is a ratio of shunted cardiac output over total cardiac output $(\dot{Q}_{sp}/\dot{Q}_t)$. In this form, a measurement of cardiac output is not required; however, a pulmonary artery blood sample (mixed venous blood) is necessary. A specific calculated value is, in essence, a measure of total oxygen gas exchange deficiencies within the lung.[8] For any given evaluation, it is not possible to distinguish the individual sub-components related to absolute shunt, shunt effect, or even that secondary to a diffusion defect. The calculated percentage of shunt represents a deviation from a theoretical ideal gas exchange state, a zero percent shunt value. Mathematically, the classic shunt equation compares a theoretical "end pulmonary capillary" oxygen content (Cc_{O_2}) with a measured arterial oxygen content (Ca_{O_2}) in the numerator and a measured mixed venous (pulmonary artery) oxygen content ($C\bar{v}_{O_2}$) in the denominator. The end pulmonary capillary oxygen content represents an idealized maximum value with end-pulmonary capillary oxygen tension set equal to alveolar oxygen tension (PA_{O_2}) obtained from the ideal alveolar gas equation.[99]

$$\frac{\dot{Q}_{sp}}{\dot{Q}_t} = \frac{[Cc_{O_2} - Ca_{O_2}]}{[Cc_{O_2} - C\bar{v}_{O_2}]}$$

The magnitude of the numerator directly reflects defects in pulmonary gas exchange. The denominator represents the difference between a theoretical maximum blood oxygen content and a minimum or residual oxygen content following tissue oxygen extraction. Changes in cardiac output and/or oxygen consumption can have major effects on mixed venous oxygen content, which, in turn, indirectly influences the calculated shunt value.[100]

THE FICK EQUATION

The relationship between mixed venous and arterial oxygen contents, cardiac output, and oxygen utilization is expressed by the Fick equation:[101]

$$\dot{V}_{O_2} = [\dot{Q}_T][Ca_{O_2} - C\bar{v}_{O_2}]$$

A primary objective of the human organism is to maintain adequate (consistent) tissue oxygen supply ($\dot{V}_{O_2}$), so that changes in cardiac output ($\dot{Q}_T$) and oxygen extraction $[Ca_{O_2} - C\bar{v}_{O_2}]$ are reciprocally related. Cardiac output is generally increased in the presence of decreased arterial oxygen tension and content secondary to increased physiologic shunt. Conversely, with decreased cardiac output secondary to myocardial disease, oxygen extraction is increased to maintain adequate tissue oxygenation. Solving for mixed venous oxygen content in the Fick equation can serve to show these effects:

$$C\bar{v}_{O_2} = Ca_{O_2} - \frac{\dot{V}_{O_2}}{\dot{Q}_T}$$

Decreased mixed venous oxygen content is frequently due to decreased arterial oxygen content secondary to increased physiologic shunt. However, an increase in the ratio of oxygen consumption to cardiac output can also cause a significant decrease in $C\bar{v}_{O_2}$.[102] An appropriate manipulation of the classic shunt equation clearly illustrates the potential effects on the calculated shunt ratio of each these physiologic variables:

$$\frac{\dot{Q}_{sp}}{\dot{Q}_t} = \frac{[Cc_{O_2} - Ca_{O_2}]}{[Ca_{O_2} - C\bar{v}_{O_2}] + [Cc_{O_2} - Ca_{O_2}]}$$

$$= \frac{[Cc_{O_2} - Ca_{O_2}]}{\dot{V}_{O_2}/\dot{Q}_T + [Cc_{O_2} - Ca_{O_2}]}$$

ALVEOLAR TO ARTERIAL OXYGEN TENSION DIFFERENCES

Various gas tension indices have traditionally been used to quantitate differences between ideal alveolar (maximum) oxygen and existing arterial oxygen values. The most commonly employed has been the alveolar-to-arterial oxygen tension differences $P(A-a)_{O_2}$. This approach was the only practical means of assessing pulmonary gas exchange deficiencies prior to development of the pulmonary artery balloon-tipped catheter. Without a Swan-Ganz catheter, pulmonary artery blood samples for mixed venous blood are now easily obtained.[103]

The $P(A-a)_{O_2}$ tension difference is a simplified extraction of alveolar and arterial oxygen tensions from the total oxygen content difference (oxyhemoglobin and dissolved oxygen) in the numerator of the shunt equation. There are two factors that frequently limit the use of this evaluation technique as a *quantitative* assessment. Its accuracy depends on a linear relationship for dissolved oxygen content applied to differences between alveolar and arterial oxygen tensions. Thus, the comparison is only quantitatively valid when arterial oxygen tensions are high enough to insure complete saturation of all arterial hemoglobin. When arterial P_{O_2} values are theoretically less than 150 mm Hg and certainly less than 100 mm Hg, the relationship between oxygen content and oxygen tension is non-linear as hemoglobin unloads oxygen. In other words, very small changes in oxygen tension are associated with large changes in oxygen content related to desaturation of hemoglobin. The second factor affecting the validity of the relationship presumes that no significant changes in cardiac output and/or oxygen consumption affecting mixed venous oxygen content have occurred, a condition infrequently observed in critically ill patients.

The evaluation of any abnormal arterial oxygen tension requires a multi-factorial analysis. It is essential that the clinician clearly understands the interactions between physiologic shunt and hypoxemia. As a general guideline, the presence of hypoxemia is almost always indicative of the existence of physiologic shunt. It is always important to precisely monitor the amount of oxygen administered (FI_{O_2}). In certain circumstances, variation in oxygen consumption above or below normal, due to alterations in metabolic rate, can affect arterial oxygen tension. The importance of hemoglobin con-

centration on oxygen content, at lower oxygen tensions, at the non-linear portion of the oxygen dissociation curve, is critical to this evaluation. The role of cardiovascular function, cardiac output, tissue perfusion, and the reciprocal relationship between cardiac output and oxygen extraction, are extremely important considerations when assessing the cause of inadequate arterial oxygen tension.

MECHANICAL TESTS OF PULMONARY FUNCTION

A complete assessment of pulmonary function necessitates evaluation of lung mechanics, pulmonary cardiovascular hemodynamics, diffusing capacity, arterial blood gases, and, finally, the distribution and matching of alveolar ventilation and pulmonary capillary perfusion. Anesthesiologists are frequently involved in intraoperative and postoperative care of patients with significant defects in pulmonary function. Risk factors predisposing patients for increased probability of pulmonary complications include type of operation, past smoking history, obesity, and elderly patients. When pulmonary function tests are abnormal, the incidence of postoperative pulmonary complications is greatly increased.[104, 105] It is, therefore, incumbent upon the anesthesia clinician to intelligently interpret the available mechanical tests of pulmonary function. (Additional applications of pulmonary function testing are found in Chapter 33.)

LUNG VOLUMES AND CAPACITIES

Specific reproducible lung gas volumes and capacities are well known, and provide a reliable basis for comparisons between normal and abnormal measurements.[106] Normal measurements obviously vary within the population, and are dependent upon age, sex, and body size. Although body surface area correlates best with body size, height can be used as a reliable index, and is generally the parameter used for most tables. By definition, lung capacities are comprised of two or more basic lung volumes. The four basic lung volumes and capacities are schematically illustrated in Figure 32-12.

Tidal volume (V_T), the gas volume moved in and out of the lungs during quiet breathing, is approximately 6–8 ml · kg^{-1}

FIG. 32-12. Lung volumes and capacities. The expressed percents for individual lung volumes comprising (TLC) are subject to considerable variation, and these values represent average values.

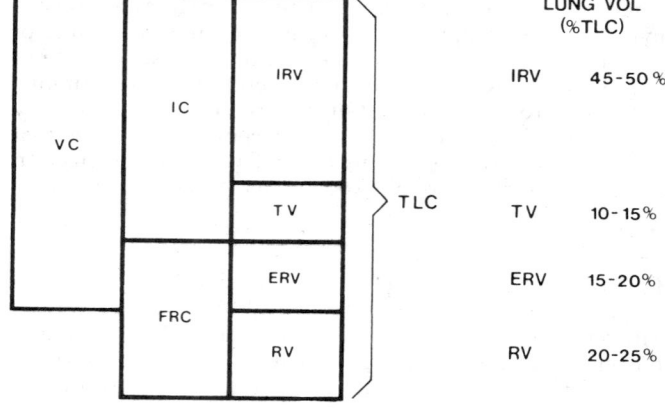

	LUNG VOL (%TLC)
IRV	45-50%
TV	10-15%
ERV	15-20%
RV	20-25%

of ideal body weight. Tidal volume invariably changes in pulmonary disease states. It decreases when lung and/or chest wall compliance is reduced or the patient has decreased respiratory muscle strength. Since inspiratory reserve volume (IRV) is approximately 50% of total lung capacity, it is the primary volume used for augmentation of tidal volume. Vital capacity (VC), the maximum volume of gas that can be exhaled following maximum inspiration, is composed of tidal volume and inspiratory and expiratory reserve volumes (V_T, IRV, ERV). For clinical purposes, normal vital capacity measurements for healthy subjects are established on the basis of height, age, and sex. Values generally range between 40 and 80 $ml \cdot kg^{-1}$ of ideal body weight. Vital capacity measurements correlate well with a patient's ventilatory reserve, capability for deep breathing, and effective coughing. Forced vital capacity (FVC) measurements less than 15 $ml \cdot kg^{-1}$ have clearly been associated with decreased ventilatory reserve and increased incidence of postoperative pulmonary complications.[105]

Functional residual capacity (FRC), the volume of gas remaining in the lungs following exhalation of a normal tidal volume, is composed of ERV and residual volume (RV). An accurate measurement of residual volume, the gas remaining in the lungs following a maximum exhalation, is entirely dependent on the subject's total cooperation. Its value is obtained indirectly by subtracting the measurement of ERV from FRC. With normal breathing at rest, exhalation is passive, continuing until FRC is reached, the point at which opposing elastic recoil forces of lung and chest wall tissues are in equilibrium. Diseases and pathological processes associated with a decrease in pulmonary compliance (lung and/or chest wall) result in decreased FRC. Common examples of pathological processes causing decreased FRC include acute lung injury, pulmonary edema, pneumonitis, and pulmonary interstitial fibrosis. Respiratory muscle weakness or paralysis, secondary to neuromuscular disease or muscle relaxants, is associated with decreased FRC because of lost chest wall and diaphragmatic muscle tone. In contrast, patients with chronic obstructive pulmonary disease or emphysema, entities associated with increased lung compliance, have an increased FRC.

Inspiratory capacity (IC), the maximum volume of gas that can be inspired when initiating an inspiratory breath from FRC, is composed of IRV and V_T. Inspiratory capacity is frequently decreased in the presence of significant extrathoracic airway obstruction. This measurement is one of the few simple tests sensitive enough to detect extrathoracic airway obstruction. Most routine pulmonary function tests only measure exhaled flows and volumes that may be relatively unaffected by extrathoracic airway obstruction until it is quite severe. Finally, total lung capacity (TLC), the maximum volume of gas that can be contained within the lungs, is indirectly obtained by combining measured volumes for inspiratory capacity and functional residual capacity.

SCREENING PULMONARY FUNCTION TESTS

Because of its anatomical complexity, it is impossible to identify a single test uniformly sensitive enough to detect significant pulmonary mechanical dysfunction. Therefore, several measurements are required to determine the type of abnormality caused by restrictive, obstructive, or mixed patterns of lung disease. Some of the measurements commonly utilized, referred to as screening pulmonary function tests, which are

TABLE 32-8.   Standard Screening Lung Function Tests

Slow vital capacity [SVC]
Timed vital capacity [FVC]
Peak flow [PF]
Forced expiratory vol. (1 s) [FEV_1]
Ratio of FEV_1/FVC [FEV_1 %]
Max. expiratory flow rate [$MEF_{200-1200}$]
Max. mid-expiratory flow rate [$MMF_{25-75\%}$]
Max. voluntary ventilation [MVV]

relatively inexpensive and easy to perform, are listed in Table 32-8.

These tests only accurately reflect pulmonary mechanics if equipment is properly calibrated and personnel are appropriately trained to correctly perform the testing procedures. An additional advantage to many screening tests is that the data can be graphically displayed to ascertain measurement reliability and provide a permanent record. A normal expiratory flow curve is graphically displayed, illustrating the important derived parameters in Figure 32-13. A TLC of 8 l is arbitrarily chosen to provide a set of real numbers for calculation of values.

Expiratory Flow Curve

One of the most frequently obtained screening tests is the timed or forced vital capacity (FVC). Starting from TLC, the subject exerts maximum voluntary effort so as to exhale the largest gas volume in the shortest time frame possible. Sequential volumes are measured at 1-s intervals. In normal subjects, measurements obtained by deliberately exhaling slowly, a slow vital capacity, or exhaling rapidly (FVC) are almost identical. However, in patients with significant obstructive lung disease, air trapping occurs during the forced maneuver, so that the vital capacity measurement is greater for a slow exhalation. It is important to recognize that severe pulmonary impairment can still be present with a relatively normal vital capacity measurement. When both vital capacity and the gas exhaled in 1 s (FEV_1) are measured, more definitive information about lung mechanics is obtained. Measurements of FEV_1 have been used as a needle predictor, differentiating patients who can or cannot tolerate major lung resections. The FEV_1 %, the ratio of gas volume exhaled in 1 s divided by the vital capacity, is an effective measurement to document significantly increased airway resistance. However, the FEV_1 % is primarily sensitive to increased resistance associated with large airways, those greater than 2 mm in diameter. These larger airways are responsible for approximately 90% of total lower airway resistance. Measurements such as peak flow and maximum expiratory flow rate [$MEF_{200-1200}$], a 1-liter measurement following exhalation of an initial 200 ml, are primarily dependent on voluntary effort, and, therefore, are not definitive with respect to cause of dysfunction. Decreased initial flow can be secondary to increased airway resistance in obstructive lung disease, suboptimal effort, generalized muscular weakness, or decreased pulmonary compliance secondary to restrictive lung diseases. Therefore, measurements of lung mechanics, early in the course of exhalation, are not definitive with respect to the precise cause of an abnormality.

Maximum mid-expiratory flow rate [$MMF_{25-75\%}$] measures the middle 50% of the exhaled volume during a forced vital capacity maneuver. When this volume is divided by the required time ($l \cdot s^{-1}$), it represents the average flow during

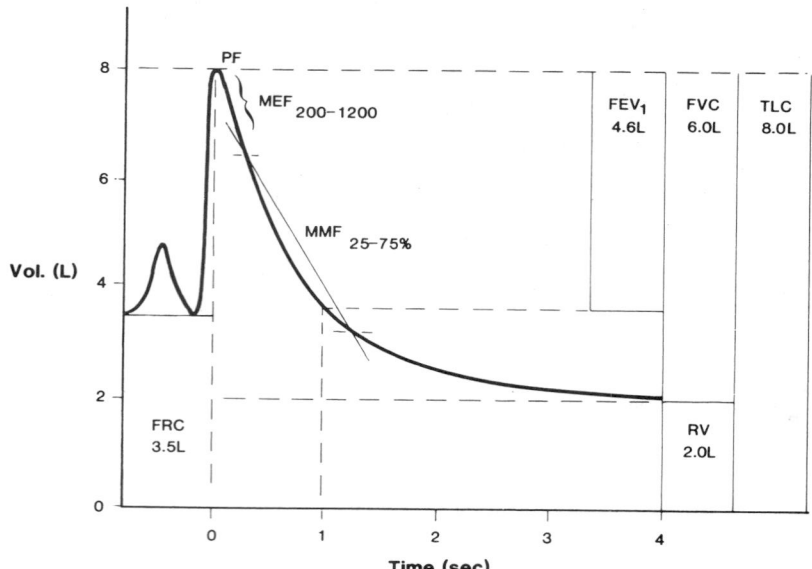

FIG. 32-13. Representative (normal) expiratory flow curve. The diagnostically important measurements include the FVC, FEV_1, $FEV_1\%$, and the MMF (25%–75%). Peak flow (PF) and maximum expiratory flow, MEF (200-1200), are not routinely used for preoperative diagnostic testing. The $FEV_1\% = FEV_1/FVC$ in this case is $[(4.6/6.0) \times 100]$, which equals 77%. The value for MMF (25%–75%) is routinely expressed in liters per second; in this case, approximately 3.7 l/sec.

mid-exhalation. This measurement is considered the most effort-independent of all pulmonary function screening tests. It more accurately reflects the physical properties of both large and small airways. Air flow in the small airways is primarily a function of alveolar pressure generated by respiratory muscles, elastic forces in lung tissue, and the geometric characteristics of non-rigid, potentially collapsible airways.

Maximum voluntary ventilation (MVV), sometimes referred to as maximum breathing capacity (MBC), is obtained by having the patient breathe as much air as possible for a defined time period, generally between 10 and 15 s. This test is frequently criticized as being non-specific. However, it is the only simple pulmonary function test that evaluates mechanical aspects of air movement in and out of the lungs.[79] When abnormally low values for maximum voluntary ventilation are obtained, in the presence of normal exhaled pulmonary function tests, it strongly supports the possibility of a significant extrathoracic airway obstruction or less than maximal voluntary effort. As a general guideline, the measured gas volume exhaled in 1 s (FEV_1) multiplied by 40 should approximate the value obtained for maximum voluntary ventilation. If MVV is less than the calculated value, the subject has either put forth suboptimal effort or, very likely, has an extrathoracic upper airway obstruction that requires more sophisticated testing procedures.

LABORATORY PULMONARY FUNCTION TESTS

Many pulmonary function tests require sophisticated instrumentation and personnel with expertise to obtain accurate measurements, so these tests are best performed in a specialized laboratory. Some of the more important specialized pulmonary function tests, outlined in Table 32-9, will be considered.

FRC Measurement

The determination of total lung capacity is dependent on an accurate measurement of functional residual capacity. Two basic methodologies can be used to obtain this measurement;

gas dilution techniques and body plethysmography. Gas dilutional techniques commonly employed are either helium dilution or nitrogen washout. The helium dilution technique uses a closed system that incorporates a spirometer with a known volume containing a mixture of air and 10% helium, an inert, insoluble gas.[108] Starting from FRC, the subject breathes into and out of a closed system until uniform mixing of air and helium in the spirometer and lung is completed. Carbon dioxide is removed from the system by a soda lime absorber, and oxygen is added to replace that required for tissue metabolism. With the subject's lung volume at FRC, the final concentration of helium in the entire system is decreased in proportion to the subject's FRC. Since spirometer volume is known and the initial (i) and final (f) concentrations of helium are measured, it is possible to calculate the subject's FRC:

$$[\text{Conc(He)}_i][V_{\text{spiro}}] = [\text{Conc(He)}_f][V_{\text{spiro}} + \text{FRC}]$$

$$\text{FRC} = \frac{[V_{\text{spiro}}][\text{Conc(He)}_i - \text{Conc(He)}_f]}{\text{Conc(He)}_f}$$

In the nitrogen washout technique, the patient breathes from a 100% oxygen reservoir, and all exhaled gas is collected. The accuracy of this measurement is based on the assumption that insignificant amounts of nitrogen diffuse from the body as a whole into the lungs, since it is a relatively insoluble gas. Required measurements are total exhaled gas volume and initial lung nitrogen concentration, and final nitrogen concentration in the exhaled volume. Since nitrogen concentration in the exhaled gas multiplied by exhaled volume equals functional residual capacity times the initial concentration of nitrogen in the lung, the FRC can be calculated.

TABLE 32-9.   Laboratory Lung Function Tests

Functional residual capacity [FRC]	
Lung compliance [C_L] ⎫	
Chest wall compliance [C_C] ⎬ ——— Total compliance [C_T]	
Airway resistance [R_A]	
Flow-volume loops [V–V]	

The determination of FRC with a body plethysmograph requires the subject to be seated in a closed chamber and inspire/expire against an obstructed airway.[109] Manometers are positioned to measure both mouth pressure, assumed equal to alveolar pressure, and body chamber pressure. The increase/decrease in lung volume and mouth pressure [ΔP_{mo}] is reflected by reciprocal changes in chamber pressure [ΔP_{pleth}] according to Boyle's law (constant gas temperature). Both alveolar and body chamber pressure start at atmospheric pressure, and changes in thoracic volumes are reflected by changes in pressure in the body plethysmograph:

$$(P_{atmos})(V_{FRC}) = (P_{atmos} + \Delta P_{mo})(V_{FRC} - \Delta P_{pleth})$$
$$V_{FRC} = (P_{atmos}) \frac{(\Delta P_{pleth})}{\Delta P_{mo}} + (\Delta P_{pleth})$$

Since changes in plethysmograph pressure are small relative to atmospheric pressure, the relationship can be further simplified to its general clinical expression:

$$FRC = [\text{pressure (atmosphere)}] \frac{\Delta P_{pleth}}{\Delta P_{mo}}$$

In patients with significant obstructive lung disease, many airways have prolonged time constants, resulting in poor gas exchange. The measurement of FRC using a body plethysmograph is independent of the mechanics of lung airways, and, therefore, more accurate. Inaccuracies using gas dilution techniques are prone to result in erroneously low values for FRC in patients with severe obstructive disease.

Measurements of Static and Dynamic Lung Mechanics

In the range of normal inspired and exhaled volumes in cooperative subjects, total compliance can be considered constant, so that a linear relationship exists between changes in tidal volume and static airway or pressure. However, this pressure volume relationship becomes non-linear at volumes approaching TLC and RV.

Resistance or interference with gas flow and lung tissue deformation represents the major component of dynamic lung mechanics with spontaneous ventilation or using traditional ventilatory support techniques. Total resistance is composed of pulmonary resistance (airways and lung tissue) plus chest wall tissue resistance. Airway resistance comprises more than 90% of pulmonary resistance. The upper respiratory tract can be a major contributor to total airway resistance, with as much as 50% attributed to the nasal passages when the patient is nose breathing. The oral and nasal pharynx, larynx, and extrathoracic trachea normally account for 20%–30% of total airway resistance during quiet breathing. The primary locus of lower airway resistance includes the large and medium-sized bronchi, including all airway branches from the trachea through the seventh airway generation, those airways with diameters greater than 2 mm. Since airway caliber changes with changing lung volumes, airway resistance also changes. Therefore, measurement of airway resistance is frequently indexed to a particular lung volume, and is referred to as "specific airway conductance."[110] This airway resistance measurement is usually determined when the subject's lung volume is at vital capacity mid-point. Airway resistance is theoretically determined from measurements of flow and the transairway pressure difference, the average pressure drop between the mouth and alveoli. Since it is impractical to directly measure transairway pressure, airway resistance volumes are extrapolated from measurements of transpulmonary pressure and pulmonary resistance.

Clinically useful measurements of airway resistance, lung compliance, and chest wall compliance are obtained when the subject is tested in a body plethysmograph (Table 32-10). Measurements are made both during the dynamic phase of gas movement and under static conditions. The important measured clinical indices are pulmonary (airway) resistance and both total and lung compliance. Chest wall compliance can be determined by simple subtraction of lung compliance from total compliance.

Assessment of Flow-volume Loops

Assessment of flow resistive properties in the airways are readily obtained by analyzing inspiratory and expiratory flow volume curves.[111] Measured parameters are displayed such that lung volume is on the horizontal axis, with expiratory flow on the positive portion and inspiratory flow on the negative portion of the vertical axis, as shown in Figure 32-14.

Since changes in flow are synchronized with changes in lung volume, a more detailed assessment of lung mechanical function is obtained. Since many pulmonary disease states have characteristic flow-volume loop patterns, this test can be used to help confirm the presence of specific pulmonary abnormalities.[112] The rate of exhaled flow is influenced by both intrinsic mechanical properties of the airways and voluntary muscular effort, especially at lung volumes greater than 75% of total lung capacity. At intermediate and low lung volumes, expiratory flow reaches a maximum level and is not further increased with either moderate or extreme increases in muscular effort. This is dramatically illustrated by analyzing serial expiratory flow curves in subjects who exert varying degrees of respiratory muscle effort.[113] The terminal portion of the exhalation curves, representing flows at smaller lung volumes, tends to be superimposed. The mechanical explanation proposed for this behavior is embodied in the concept of a movable equal pressure point in the airways.[114] During forced exhalation, intrapleural pressure greatly exceeds atmospheric pressure, causing a significant increase in both alveolar and extraluminal airway pressure, tending to constrict small airways. Total force affecting gas flow is the sum of tissue elastic recoil forces and transmitted pleural pressure. As gas leaves the alveoli intraluminal airway, pressure progressively falls due to airway resistance. Initially, intraluminal airway pressure in peripheral airways, close to the alveoli, is greater than extraluminal pressure. At some point

TABLE 32-10.   Measurements of Compliance and Resistance Using a Body Plethysmograph

PRESSURE DIFFERENCE	STATIC CONDITIONS	DYNAMIC CONDITIONS
Transairway P $P_{mo} - P_{alveolar}$		$R_{(airway)}$
Transpulmonary P $P_{mo} - P_{intrapleural}$	$C_{(lung)}$*	$R_{(pulmonary)}$†
Transthoracic P $P_{mo} - P_{plethysmograph}$	$C_{(total)}$*	$R_{(total)}$

* Calculation of C (chest wall):

$$\frac{1}{C \text{ (chest wall)}} = \frac{1}{C \text{ (total)}} - \frac{1}{C \text{ (lung)}}$$

† R (airway) $\cong$ R (pulmonary).

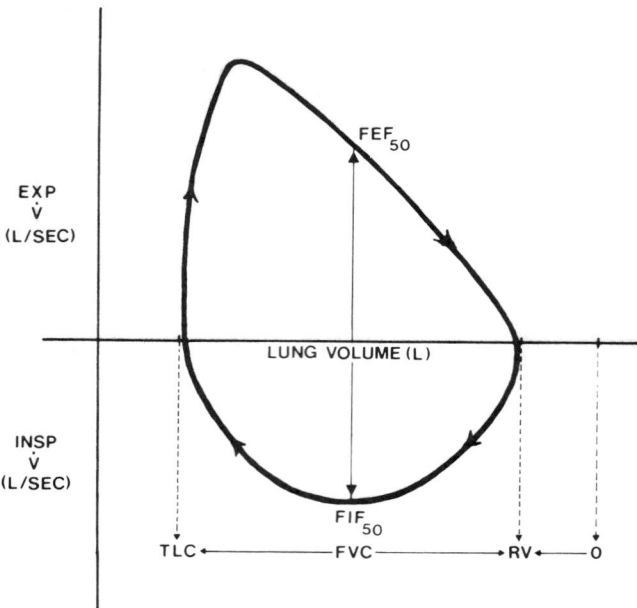

FIG. 32-14. Idealized flow-volume ($\dot{V}$–$\dot{V}$) loop. During forced expiration, the rate of airflow increases rapidly at volume close to TLC. As lung volume decreases, flow progressively falls in a near-linear fashion secondary to increasing airway resistance. With maximum inspiratory effort, flow normally peaks at a lung volume near the midportion of FVC. At mid-point lung volume, the forced inspiratory flow (FIF_{50}) and forced expiratory flow (FEF_{50}) should normally be equal. When the ratio (FIF_{50}/FEF_{50}) is less than unity, it suggests an extrathoracic obstruction, compromising inspiratory flow. If greater than one, it supports a diagnosis of intrathoracic airway obstruction.

in the airway, the intraluminal airway pressure has decreased and becomes equal to extraluminal airway pressure, the equal pressure point. From this point on, airway segments have interluminal pressures less than extraluminal pressure, and are subject to dynamic compression. Additional increases in muscular effort result in further positive increases in extraluminal pressure, leading to additional airway compression and collapse. The airway geometry has become the primary limiting factor determining gas flow. Under normal circumstances, in healthy lungs, this equal pressure point is located either at the glottis or in the intrathoracic but extraparenchymal large airways. Since these airways have rigid cartilage supporting structures, they do not undergo dynamic compression. When significant obstructive pulmonary disease is present, the phenomenon of airway compression is accentuated, and the equal pressure point moves peripherally to smaller airways, resulting in airtrapping and intermittent interruption of exhalation.

CLINICAL APPLICATION OF PULMONARY FUNCTION TESTS

With the large array of available pulmonary function tests, the anesthesiologist needs to know which tests are definitive and reliable for specific pulmonary pathological processes. This is especially important in preoperative evaluation of patients with suspect pulmonary function who are scheduled for major procedures (see Chapter 33). Pulmonary function tests should meet the following minimum goals.

1. Identify the patient at increased risk of morbidity: the patient with increased probability for postoperative complications. The tests must help the clinician determine the need for a) a more complete preoperative evaluation, b) relevant preoperative pulmonary and bronchial hygiene therapy, and c) a logical postoperative management plan of the patient's cardiopulmonary system.
2. Identify the patient at increased risk of mortality: for example, the patient scheduled for lung resection who has such limited pulmonary function that the proposed surgical procedure might be life-threatening.[115] The anesthesiologist must recognize the need for more specialized and definitive studies designed to define appropriate surgical limits.

Two pulmonary screening tests which have served the clinician well are 1) the forced vital capacity test and 2) the forced expiratory volume test (1 s) %. The results need to be evaluated, not only as a percentage of the predicted value, but also as absolute values. In addition, valuable information can be obtained from 3) the mid-expiratory flow rate (25–75), a measure of exhaled volume that is most effort-independent, and 4) maximum voluntary ventilation.[116] The major advantage to this last test is that both inspiratory and expiratory mechanics are evaluated. More sophisticated and detailed tests of pulmonary function are indicated when pulmonary functioning screening tests reveal significantly abnormal values. This is especially important if the patient is scheduled for an abdominal and/or thoracic surgical procedure or a lung resection, or has a well-documented history of pulmonary disease.

REFERENCES

1. Loosli CG, Krahl VE, Tobin CE et al: Report of committee on preparation of human lungs for macroscopic and microscopic study. Am Rev Respir Dis 80:114, 1959
2. Heard BE: Fixation of the lung with respect to lung volume and air space size. In Ruecke AVS, O'Connor M (eds): CIBA Foundation Symposium on Pulmonary Structure and Function, p 291. Boston, Little Brown and Company, 1962
3. Pratt PC, Klugh GA: A technique for the study of ventilatory capacity, compliance and residual volume of excised lungs and for fixation, drying and serial sectioning in the inflated state. Am Rev Respir Dis 83:690, 1961
4. De Alva WE, Rainer WG: A method of high speed in vivo pulmonary microcinematrography under physiologic conditions. Angiology 14:160, 1963
5. Gray H: Anatomy of the Human Body, 29th edition. In Goss CM (ed). Philadelphia, Lea & Febiger, 1966
6. Netter FH: CIBA Collection of Medical Illustrations, Vol 7. In Divertic MB, Brass A (ed): Respiratory System. CIBA, 1979
7. Luciani L: Human Physiology, Vol 2, p 408. Welby FA (trans). London, Macmillan, 1911
8. Berggren SM: The oxygen deficit of arterial blood caused by nonventilating parts of the lung. Acta Physiol Scand 4:9(Suppl 11), 1942
9. Wade OL: Movements of thoracic cage and diaphragm in respiration. J Physiol (Lond) 124:193, 1954
10. Bigland B, Lippold DO: Motor unit activity in the voluntary contraction of human muscle. J Physiol (Lond) 125:322, 1954
11. Burke RE, Levine DN, Zojas FE et al: Mammalian motor units: Physiologic histochemical correlation in these types of cat gastrocnemius. Science 174:709, 1971
12. Lieberman DA, Falkner JA, Craig AB Jr et al: Performance of

histochemical composition of guinea pig and human diaphragm. J Appl Physiol 34:233, 1973

13. Roussos C, Macklin PT: Diaphragmatic fatigue in man. J Appl Physiol 43:189, 1977
14. Fenn WO: A comparison of respiratory and skeletal muscles. In Cori CF, Foglia VG, Leloir LF et al (eds): Perspective in Biology, p 293. Amsterdam, Elsevier, 1963
15. Hubbard AW, Stetson RH: An experimental analysis of human locomotion. Am J Physio 124:300, 1938
16. Murphy AJ, Koepec GH, Smith EM et al: Sequence of action of diaphragm and intercostal muscles during respiration. II. Expiration. Arch Phys Med 40:337, 1959
17. Petit JM, Milic-Emili G, Delhez L: Role of the diaphragm in breathing in conscious normal man: An electromyographic study. J Appl Physiol 15:1101, 1960
18. Coryllos PN: Action of the diaphragm in cough. Experimental and clinical study on the human. Am J Med Sci 194:523, 1937
19. Campbell EJM: An electromyographic examination of the role of the intercostals muscles in breathing in man. J Physiol (Lond) 129:12, 1955
20. Campbell EJM, Green JH: The behaviour of the abdominal muscles and the intra-abdominal pressure during quiet breathing and increased pulmonary ventilation. A study in man. J Physiol (Lond) 127:423, 1955
21. Weibel ER: Morphometry of the Human Lung. Berlin, Springer-Verlag, 1963
22. Weibel ER, Gomez DM: A principle for counting tissue structures on random sections. J Appl Physiol 17:343, 1962
23. Weibel ER, Gomez DM: Architecture of the human being. Science 137:577, 1962
24. Weibel ER: Morphometrics of the lung. In Fenn WO, Rahn H (eds): Handbook of Physiology, Sec 3, Vol 1, p 285. Washington, DC, Am Physiol Soc, 1964
25. Rhodin JAG: An Atlas of Ultrastructure. Philadelphia, W.B. Saunders, 1963
26. Auerbach O, Stout AP, Hammond EC et al: Changes in bronchial epithelium in relation to cigarette smoking and in relation to lung cancer. N Engl J Med 265:253, 1961
27. Krahl VE: Microstructure of the lung. Arch Environmental Health 6:37, 1963
28. Gail DB, L'Enfant CJM: Cells of the lung. Biology and clinical implications. Am Rev Respir Dis 127:366, 1983
29. Bachoven M, Weibel ER: Basic pattern of tissue repair in human lungs following unspecific injury. Chest 65:145 1974
30. Kikkawa Y, Yoneda K, Smith F: The type II epithelial cells of the lung: Chemical composition and phospholipid synthesis. Lab Invest 32:295, 1975
31. Fishman AP: Non-respiratory function of lung. Chest 72:84, 1977
32. Mason RJ, Williams MC, Widdicombe JH: Secretion and fluid transport by alveolar type II epithelial cells. Chest (Suppl) 81:61, 1982
33. Hocking WG, Golden DW: The pulmonary-alveolar macrophage. N Engl J Med 301:580, 1979
34. Macklin CC: Alveolar pores and their significance in the human lung. Arch Pathol 21:202, 1936
35. Lambert MW: Accessory bronchio-alveolar channels. Anat Record 127:472, 1957
36. Legallois CJJ: Expériences sur le Principe de la Vie, p 325. Paris, D'Hautel, 1812
37. Brodie DA, Borison HL: Evidence for a medullary inspiratory pacemaker. Functional concept of central regulation of respiration. Am J Physiol 188:347, 1957
38. von Euler C, Herrero F, Wexler L: Control mechanisms determining rate and depth of respiratory movements. Respir Physiol 10:93, 1970
39. Grunstein MD, Youres M, Milic-Emili J: Control of tidal volume and respiratory frequency in anesthetized cats. J Appl Physiol 35:463, 1973
40. Lumsden TL: The regulation of respiration. Part I. J Physiol (Lond) 58:81, 1923
41. Hoff HE, Breckenridge CG: The medullary origin of respiratory periodicity in the dog. Am J Physiol 158:157, 1949
42. Hoff HE, Breckenridge CG: Intrinsic mechanisms in periodic breathing. AMA Arch Neurol Psychiatr 72:11, 1954
43. Comroe JH Jr: The effects of direct chemical and electrical stimulation of the respiratory center in the cat. Am J Physiol 139:490, 1943
44. Ngai SH, Wang SC: Organization of central respiratory mechanisms in the brainstem of the cats: Localization by stimulation and destruction. Am J Physiol 190:343, 1957
45. Pitts RF: The differentiation of respiratory centers. Am J Physiol 134:192, 1941
46. Pitts RF, Magoun HW, Ranson SW: Localization of the medullary respiratory centers in the cat. Am J Physiol 126:673, 1939
47. Salmoiraghi GC, Burns BD: Localization and patterns of discharge of respiratory neurons in the brainstem of a cat. J Neurophysiol 23:2, 1960
48. Stella G: On the mechanism of production and the physiologic significance of "apneusis." J Physiol (Lond) 93:10, 1938
49. Lumsden TL: Observations on the respiratory centers in the cat. J Physiol (Lond) 57:153, 1923
50. Cohen MI, Wang SC: Respiratory neuronal activity in pons of cat. J Neurophysiol 22:33, 1959
51. Cohen MI: Neurogenesis of respiratory rhythm in the mammal. Physiol Rev 51:1105, 1979
52. Guz A: Regulation of respiration in man. Ann Res Physiol 37:303, 1975
53. Pitts RF, Magoun HW, Ranson SW: The origin of respiratory rhythmicity. Am J Physiol 127:654, 1939
54. Kabat H: Electrical stimulation of points in the forebrain and mid-brain: The resultant alterations in respiration. J Comp Neurol 64:187, 1936
55. Kaada BR: Somato-motor, autonomic and electrocorticographic responses to electrical stimulation of "rhinencephalic" and other structures in primates, cat and dog. A study of responses from the limbic, subcallosal, orbito-insular, periform and temporal cortex, hippocampus-fornix and amygdala. Acta Physiol Scand 24(Suppl 83):1, 1951
56. Chai CY, Wang SC: Localization of central cardiovascular control mechanism in lower brainstem of the cat. Am J Physiol 202:25, 1962
57. Uvnas B: Central cardiovascular control. In Handbook of Physiology, Section I, Vol. II, Neurophysiology, p 1131. Washington, DC, Am Physiol Soc, 1960
58. Bosma JF: Deglutition: Pharyngeal stage. Physiol Rev 37:275, 1957
59. Wang SC, Borison HL: The vomiting center: A critical experimental analysis. AMA Arch Neurol Psychiatr 63:928, 1950
60. Biscoe TJ: Carotid body: Structure and function. Physiol Rev 58:604, 1978
61. Coleridge HM: Thoracic chemoreceptors in the dog: A histological and electrophysiologic study of the location, innervation and blood supply of the aortic bodies. Circ Res 26:235, 1970
62. Leusen I: Regulation of cerebrospinal fluid composition with reference to breathing. Physiol Rev 52:1, 1972
63. Cohen MI: Discharge patterns of brainstem respiratory neurons in relation to carbon dioxide tension. J Neurophysiol 31:142, 1968
64. Heinemann HO, Golaring RM: Bicarbonate and the regulation of ventilation. Am J Med 57:361, 1974
65. Engle GL, Ferris EB, Webb JP et al: Voluntary breathholding. II. The relation of the maximum time of breathholding to the oxygen tension of the inspired air. J Clin Invest 23:734, 1946

66. Fowler WS: Breaking point of breath-holding. J Appl Physiol 6:539, 1954

67. Fink BR: The stimulant effect of wakefulness on respiration: Clinical aspects. Br J Anaesth 33:97, 1961

68. Gaylor JB: The intrinsic nervous mechanisms of the human lung. Brain 57:143, 1934

69. von Euler C: On the role of proprioceptors in perception and execution of motor acts with special reference to breathing. In Pengelly LD, Rebuck AS, Campbell JBL (eds): Loaded Breathing, p 139. Longman, Don Mills, 1974

70. Jung-Caillot MC, Duron B: Number of neuromuscular spindles and electrical activity of the respiratory muscles. In Durm B (ed): Respiratory Centers and Afferent Systems, p 165. Paris, INSERM, 1976

71. Hering E, Breuer J: Die Sebsteuerung der Athmung durch den Nervus vagus. Stizber Akad Wiss Wien 57(II):672, 1868

72. Davis HL, Fowler WS, Lambert EH: Effect of volume and rate of inflation and deflation on transpulmonary pressure and response of pulmonary stretch receptors. Am J Physiol 187:558, 1956

73. Dawes GS, Comroe JH Jr: Chemoreflexes from the heart and lungs. Physiol Rev 34:167, 1954

74. Derenne JP: Methodes d'investigation clinique des mecanismes rigulateins de la ventilation. Bull Physiopathol Respir 13:681, 1977

75. Milhorn HJ Jr, Benten R, Ross R et al: A mathematical model of the human respiratory control system. Biophys J 5:27, 1965

76. Berlin JJ: Engineering Fluid Mechanics, p 146. Englewood Cliffs, Prentice-Hall, Inc, 1984

77. West JB: Ventilation/Blood Flow and Gas Exchange. 4th edition. Oxford, Blackwell Scientific Publications, 1985

78. Butler J, Caro CS, Alcala R: Physiologic factors in normal subjects and in patients with obstructive respiratory disease. J Clin Invest 39:584, 1960

79. Piiper J, Haab P, Rahn H: Unequal distribution of pulmonary diffusing capacity in the unanesthetized dog. J Appl Physiol 16:499, 1961

80. Apthorp GH, Marshall R: Pulmonary diffusing capacity: A comparison of breath-holding and steady-state methods using carbon monoxide. J Clin Invest 40:1775, 1961

81. Comroe JH Jr, Forster RE, DuBois AB et al: The Lung: Clinical Physiology and Pulmonary Function Tests. Chicago, Year Book Medical Publishers, 1962

82. Mead J: Mechanical properties of lungs. Physiol Rev 281, 1961

83. Fredberg JJ, Hoenig AE: Mechanical response of the lungs at high frequency. J Biomed Eng 100:57, 1978

84. Harrison RA: Mechanics and physics of patient-ventilator systems. In Shapiro B, Cane R (eds): Positive Airway Pressure Therapy: PPV and PEEP, Anesthesia Clinics of North America, p 1 (Appendix 19–21). Philadelphia, WB Saunders, 1987

85. Mead J, Milic-Emili T: Handbook of Physiology, Respiration, Vol 1, p 363. Washington, DC, American Physiologic Society, 1964

86. West JB: Gas exchange. In West JB (ed): Regional Differences in the Lung, p 202. New York, Academic Press, 1977

87. Otis AB, McKerrow CB, Bartlett RA: Mechanical factors in distribution of pulmonary ventilation. J Appl Physiol 8:427, 1956

88. Wilson TA, Fredberg JJ, Rodarte JR: Interdependence of regional expiratory flow. J Appl Physiol 59:1924, 1985

89. Bendixen HH, Egbert LD, Hedley-Whyte J et al: Respiratory Care. St Louis, CV Mosby, 1965

90. Benumof JL, Pirla AF, Johanson I et al: Interaction of P_vO_2 with Pa_{O_2} on hypoxia pulmonary vasoconstriction. J Appl Physiol 51:871, 1981

91. Swenson EW, Finley TN, Guzman SV: Unilateral hypoventilation in man during temporary occlusion of one pulmonary artery. J Clin Invest 40:828, 1961

92. Lynch JP, Mhyre JG, Dantzker DR: Influence of cardiac output on intrapulmonary shunt. J Appl Physiol 46:315, 1979

93. Fowler WS: Lung function studies, II. The respiratory deadspace. Am J Physiol 154:405, 1948

94. Fisher SR, Duranceau A, Floyd RD et al: Comparative changes in ventilatory deadspace following micro- and massive emboli. J Surg Res 20:195, 1976

95. Freeman J, Nunn JF: Ventilation-perfusion relationships after haemorrhage. Clin Sci 24:135, 1963

96. Bergman NA: Effect of varying respiratory waveforms on distribution of inspired gas during artificial ventilation. Am Rev Respir Dis 100:518, 1969

97. Brisco WA, Forster RE, Comroe JH Jr: Alveolar ventilation at very low tidal volumes. J Appl Physiol 7:27, 1954

98. West JB: State-of-the-art: Ventilation-perfusion relationships. Am Rev Respir Dis 116:919, 1977

99. Riley RL, Cournand A: Ideal alveolar air and the analysis of ventilation/perfusion relationships in the lungs. J Appl Physiol 1:825, 1949

100. Riley RL, Cournand A: Analysis of factors affecting partial presence of oxygen and carbon dioxide in gas and blood of lungs: Theory. J Appl Physiol 4:77, 1951

101. Fick A: Ueber die Messung des Blutquantums in dem herz-ventikelm Sitzungsb. Der phys med Ges Za Wurzburg 36, 1870

102. Prys-Robert S, Kelman GR, Greenbaum R: The influence of circulating factors on arterial oxygenation during anesthesia in man. Anaesthesia 22:257, 1967

103. Swan HJC, Ganz W, Forrester J et al: Catheterization of the heart in man with use of a flow limited balloon-tipped catheter. N Engl J Med 283:447, 1970

104. Block AJ, Olson GN: Preoperative pulmonary function testing. JAMA 235:257, 1976

105. Tisi GM: State-of-the-art; Preoperative evaluation of pulmonary function. Am Rev Respir Dis 119:293, 1979

106. Christie RV: Lung volume and its subdivisions. J Clin Invest 11:1099, 1932

107. Bendixen HH, Smith GM, Mead J: Pattern of ventilation in young adults. J Appl Physiol 19:195, 1964

108. Meneely GR, Kaltreider NL: Volume of the lung determined by helium dilution. J Clin Invest 28:129, 1949

109. Mead J: Volume displacement body plethysmograph for respiratory measurements in human subjects. J Appl Physiol 15:736, 1960

110. Brisco WA, DuBois AB: Relationship between airway resistance, airway conductance and lung volume in subjects of different age and body size. J Clin Invest 37:1279, 1958

111. Hyatt RE, Black LF: The flow volume curve; A current perspective. Am Rev Resp Dis 107:191, 1973

112. Golish JA, Muzaffar A, Yarnal JR: Practical application of the flow volume loop. Cleveland Clin Quart 47:39, 1980

113. Hyatt RE, Schilder DP, Fry DL: Relationship between maximum expiratory flow and degree of lung inflation. J Appl Physiol 13:331, 1958

114. Mead J, Turner JM, Macklem PT et al: Significance of the relationship between lung recoil and maximum expiratory flow. J Appl Physiol 22:95, 1967

115. Lockwood P: The principles of predicting risk of post-thoracotomy function related complications in bronchiogenic carcinoma. Respiration 30:329, 1973

116. Matheson HW, Spies SN, Gray JS et al: Ventilatory function tests. II. Factors affecting the voluntary ventilation capacity. J Clin Invest 29:682, 1950

Chapter 33

James B. Eisenkraft
Edmond Cohen
Joel A. Kaplan

Anesthesia for Thoracic Surgery

The number of noncardiac thoracic surgical operations has dramatically increased in recent years and is expected to increase further in the future. A recent report, using data from the National Center for Health Statistics in the USA, showed that, in 1979, approximately 53,000 procedures on the lung and bronchus were performed; this number had grown to 73,000 in 1983.[1] Mediastinoscopies increased from 33,000 in 1979 to 44,000 in 1983. The increase in this type of surgery has been associated with, and sometimes made possible by, advances in anesthesia care. Indeed, thoracic anesthesia is developing into a subspecialty in its own right, with a number of reference texts exclusively devoted to this subject.[2-4]

The physiologic, pharmacologic, and clinical considerations for the patient undergoing pulmonary surgery will be reviewed; followed by sections on anesthesia for diagnostic and therapeutic procedures, high-frequency ventilation, and special situations, including bronchopleural fistula and tracheal reconstruction. A discussion of myasthenia gravis is included because of the relationship between the thymus gland and myasthenia, and because thymectomy is one of the most commonly performed thoracic surgical procedures in these patients. The chapter concludes with a review of the postoperative management of the thoracic surgical patient.

PREOPERATIVE EVALUATION

The preoperative evaluation of the patient for thoracic surgery should, in addition to the routine assessment for major surgery, focus on the extent and severity of pulmonary disease and of cardiovascular involvement.

HISTORY

Dyspnea

Dyspnea occurs when the requirement for ventilation is greater than the patient's ability to respond appropriately. Dyspnea is quantitated as to the degree of physical activity required to produce it, the level of activity possible (*e.g.*, ability to walk on level ground, climb stairs, etc.), and management of daily activities. Severe exertional dyspnea usually implies a significantly diminished ventilatory reserve and an FEV_1 of less than 1500 ml, with possible need for postoperative ventilatory support.

Cough

Recurrent productive cough for 3 months of the year for two consecutive years is necessary to make the diagnosis of chronic bronchitis. Cough indirectly increases airway irritability. If the cough is productive, the volume, consistency, and color of the sputum should be assessed. Sputum should be cultured to rule out infection and to establish if there is a need for preoperative antibiotic therapy. Blood-stained sputum or episodes of gross hemoptysis should alert the anesthesiologist to the possibility of a tumor invading the respiratory tract, *e.g.*, mainstem bronchus, which might interfere with endobronchial intubation.

Cigarette Smoking

Cigarette smoking increases the risk of chronic lung disease and malignancy, as well as the incidence of postoperative pulmonary complications. The number of pack-years (packs smoked per day multiplied by the number of years) is directly related to measurable changes in air flow and closing capacity, making these patients prone to postoperative atelectasis and arterial hypoxemia.

PHYSICAL EXAMINATION

The physical examination of the patient should particularly address the following aspects.

Respiratory Pattern

The presence of cyanosis and clubbing, the breathing pattern, and the type of breath sounds should be noted.

CYANOSIS. The presence of peripheral cyanosis (fingers, toes, ears) should be distinguished from causes of poor circulation (acrocyanosis). The presence of central cyanosis (buccal mucosa) is usually secondary to arterial hypoxemia. If cyanosis is present, the arterial saturation is 80% or less (Pa_{O_2} less than 50–52 mm Hg), which indicates a limited margin of respiratory reserve.

CLUBBING. Clubbing is often seen in patients with chronic lung disease, malignancies, or congenital heart disease associated with right-to-left shunt.

RESPIRATORY RATE AND PATTERN. The inability to complete a normal sentence without pause for breath is an indication of severe dyspnea. Inspiratory paradox, the abdomen moving in while the chest moves out, suggests diaphragmatic fatigue and respiratory dysfunction. Paroxysmal retraction (Hoover's sign), limited diaphragmatic movement because of hyperinflation, asymmetry of chest movement secondary to phrenic nerve involvement, hemothorax, pleural effusion, and pneumothorax should be assessed. The pattern and rate of breathing have important roles in distinguishing between obstructive and restrictive lung disease. For a constant minute ventilation, the work done against elastic resistance decreases when breathing is slow and deep. Work done against air flow resistance decreases when breathing is rapid and shallow (pulmonary infarct, pulmonary fibrosis, etc.).

BREATH SOUNDS. Wet sounds (crackles) are usually due to excessive fluid in the airways and indicate sputum retention or edema. Dry sounds (wheezes) are produced by high-velocity air flow through bronchi, and are a sign of airway obstruction. Distant sounds are an indication of emphysema and, possibly, bullae. The trachea should be midline. Displacement of the trachea may be secondary to a number of causes, including mediastinal mass and should alert the anesthesiologist to a potentially difficult intubation of the trachea and/or airway obstruction on induction of anesthesia.

Evaluation of Cardiovascular System

One of the most important factors in the evaluation of patients scheduled for thoracic surgery is the presence of an increase in pulmonary vascular resistance (PVR) secondary to a fixed reduction in the cross-sectional area of the pulmonary vascular bed. The pulmonary circulation is a low-pressure high-compliance system that is capable of handling an increase in blood flow by recruitment of normally underperfused vessels. This acts as a compensatory mechanism, which normally pre-

vents an increase in pulmonary arterial pressure. In chronic obstructive pulmonary disease (COPD), there is distention of the pulmonary capillary bed with reduced ability to tolerate an increase in blood flow (reduced compliance). Such patients will demonstrate an increase in PVR when cardiac output (CO) increases because of a reduced ability to compensate for an increase in pulmonary blood flow. This results in pulmonary hypertension, signs of which include a split second heart sound, increased intensity of the pulmonary component of the second heart sound, and right ventricular and atrial hypertrophy.

An increase in PVR is of significance in the management of the patient during anesthesia, since several factors such as acidosis, sepsis, hypoxia, and application of PEEP will all further increase the PVR and increase the likelihood of right ventricular (RV) failure.

In patients with ischemic or valvular heart disease, the function of the left side of the heart should also be carefully evaluated. This is discussed elsewhere in this volume (Chapter 35).

LABORATORY STUDIES

Electrocardiogram

A patient with COPD may present with electrocardiographic (ECG) features of right atrial and ventricular hypertrophy and strain. These include a low voltage QRS complex due to lung hyperinflation and poor R-wave progression across the precordial leads. An enlarged P-wave ("P-pulmonale") is diagnostic of right atrial hypertrophy. The ECG changes of right ventricular hypertrophy are an R/S ratio of greater than 1.0 in lead V_1 (i.e., R-wave voltage exceeds S-wave voltage).

Chest X-ray

Hyperinflation and increased vascular markings are usually present with COPD. Prominent lung markings often occur in bronchitis while they are decreased in emphysema, particularly at the bases where, in severe cases, actual bullae may be present. Hyperinflation, with an increased antero-posterior chest diameter, may be present, together with an enlarged retrosternal air space of greater than 2 cm in diameter.

The location of the lung lesion should be assessed by PA and lateral projections on chest radiography. A mediastinal mass may indicate, in addition to tracheal or carinal shift, a difficult intubation, difficult and bloody dissection, inability to use a double-lumen tube (because of deviation of the mainstem bronchus), or a collapsed lobe due to bronchial obstruction with possible sepsis. Review of a computerized tomography study is also useful, often providing more information about tumor size and location than does the chest radiograph.

ARTERIAL BLOOD GAS (ABG). A common finding in ABG analysis of COPD patients is hypoventilation and CO_2 retention. The "blue bloaters" (chronic bronchitics) are cyanotic, hypercarbic, hypoxemic, and, usually, overweight. They are in a state of chronic respiratory failure and have a reduced ventilatory response to CO_2. In these patients, the high Pa_{CO_2} increases cerebrospinal fluid bicarbonate concentration, the medullary chemoreceptors become reset to a higher level of CO_2, and sensitivity to CO_2 is decreased. These patients will hypoventilate when given high oxygen concentrations because of a decreased hypoxic drive.

The "pink puffers" (patients with emphysema), typically

are thin, dyspneic, and pink, with essentially normal blood gas values. They present with an increase in minute ventilation to maintain their normal Pa_{CO_2}, which explains the increase in work of breathing and dyspnea.

PULMONARY FUNCTION TESTING AND EVALUATION FOR LUNG RESECTABILITY. There are three goals in performing pulmonary function tests (PFT) in patients scheduled for lung resection. The first is to identify those patients at risk of increased morbidity and mortality postoperatively. In thoracic surgery for lung cancer, the specific question is: How much lung tissue may be safely removed without creating a pulmonary cripple? This should be weighed against the 1-year mean survival of the surgically untreated lung carcinoma. The second is to identify those patients who will need short- or long-term ventilatory support postoperatively. The third is to evaluate the beneficial effect and reversibility of airway obstruction with the use of bronchodilators.

EFFECTS OF ANESTHESIA AND SURGERY ON LUNG VOLUMES. Anesthesia and postoperative medications can cause changes in lung volumes and ventilatory pattern (see Chapter 32). Total lung capacity (TLC) decreases after abdominal surgery but not after surgery on the extremities.[6] Vital capacity (VC) is reduced by 25–50% within 1–2 days following surgery, and generally returns to normal after 1–2 weeks. Residual volume (RV) increases by 13%, while expiratory reserve volume (ERV) decreases by 25% following lower abdominal surgery and 60% following upper abdominal and thoracic surgery. Tidal volume (V_T) decreases by 20% within 24 h following surgery, and gradually returns to normal after 2 weeks. Pulmonary compliance decreases by 33%, with similar reductions in functional residual capacity (FRC) secondary to small airway closure. Most of the patients who undergo lung resection are smokers with a certain degree of COPD, and will be prone to postoperative complications in direct relation to the amount of lung to be resected (lobectomy or pneumonectomy) and to the severity of the preoperative lung disease.

SPIROMETRY. Forced vital capacity (FVC), forced expiratory volume in 1 s (FEV_1), and peak expiratory flow rate (PEFR) can be measured at the patient's bedside using a spirometer. The measurement can be recorded as a volume-time trace or as a flow-volume loop.

A VC of at least three times the V_T is necessary for an effective cough.[7] A VC of less than 50% of predicted or less than 2 liters is an indicator of increased risk.[8] An abnormal preoperative VC can be identified in 30–40% of postoperative deaths. A patient with an abnormal VC has a 33% chance of complications and a 10% risk of postoperative mortality.

FEV_1 is a more direct indication of airway obstruction. An FEV_1 of less than 800 ml in a 70 kg male is probably incompatible with life, and is an absolute contraindication to lung resection. Mortality in patients with an FEV_1 greater than 2 liters is 10%, and in patients below 1 liter is between 20–45%.[9]

The ratio FEV_1/FVC is useful in differentiating between restrictive and obstructive disease. It is normal in restrictive disease, since both decrease, while, in obstructive disease, the ratio is generally low, since the FEV_1 is markedly reduced.

Maximum voluntary ventilation (MVV) is a non-specific test, and is an indicator of both restriction and obstruction. Although MVV has not been systematically evaluated as a predictor of morbidity, it is generally accepted that an MVV below 50% of predicted value is an indication of high risk.

A ratio of residual volume-to-total lung capacity (RV/TLC) of greater than 50% is generally indicative of a high-risk pa-

tient for pulmonary resection. Mittman[10] found that a RV/TLC ratio of greater than 40% was associated with a 30% mortality, compared to 7% when RV/TLC was less than 40%.

FLOW-VOLUME LOOPS. The flow-volume loop displays essentially the same information as a spirometer, but is more convenient for measurement of specific flow rates (Fig. 33-1). The shape and peak air flow rates during expiration at high lung volumes are effort-dependent, but indicate the patency of the larger airways. Effort-independent expiration occurs at low lung volumes, and usually reflects small airways resistance, best measured by maximum mid-expiratory flow rate between 25 and 75% of vital capacity (MMEFR $_{25-75}$).

In general, patients with obstructive airways disease (Fig. 33-2), such as asthma, bronchitis, and emphysema, have grossly reduced FEV_1/FVC ratios because of increased airways resistance and a reduction in FEV_1. Peak expiratory flow rate and MMV are usually reduced, while TLC increases secondary to increases in RV. In these patients, the effort-independent portion of the flow-volume curve is markedly depressed inward, with reduction of the flow rate at 25–75% of FVC.

In patients with restrictive disease (Fig. 33-2), such as pulmonary fibrosis and scoliosis, there is a reduction in FVC with a normal FEV_1. Since the airways resistance is normal, FEV_1/FVC is also normal. Total lung capacity is markedly reduced, while MMV and MMEFR$_{25-75}$ are usually normal. The flow-volume curves of these patients will be normal in shape, but there are lower lung volumes and peak flow rates (Fig. 33-2).

SIGNIFICANCE OF BRONCHODILATOR THERAPY. Pulmonary function tests (PFT) are usually performed before and

FIG. 33-1. Flow-volume loop in a normal subject $\dot{V}_{75}$, $\dot{V}_{50}$, and $\dot{V}_{25}$ represent flow at 75, 50, and 25% of vital capacity, respectively. RV = residual volume. (Goudsouzian N, Karamanian A: Physiology for the Anesthesiologist, 2nd ed. Norwalk, Appleton-Century-Crofts, 1984. Reproduced by permission.)

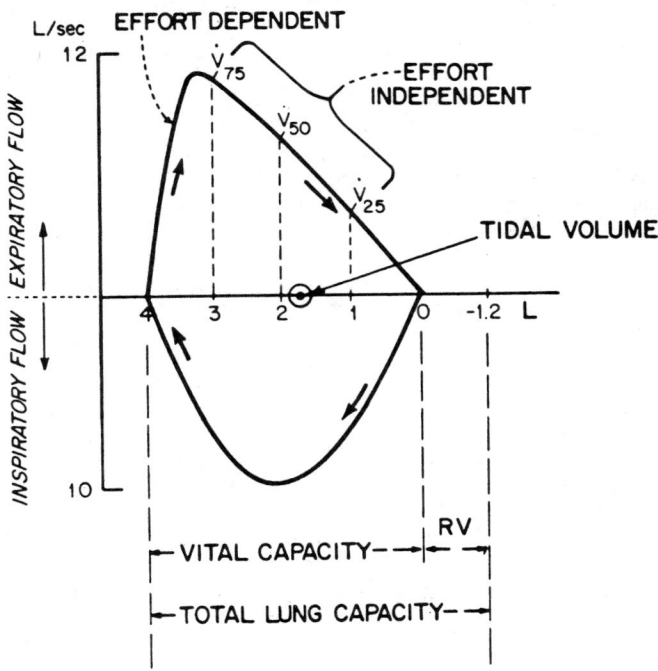

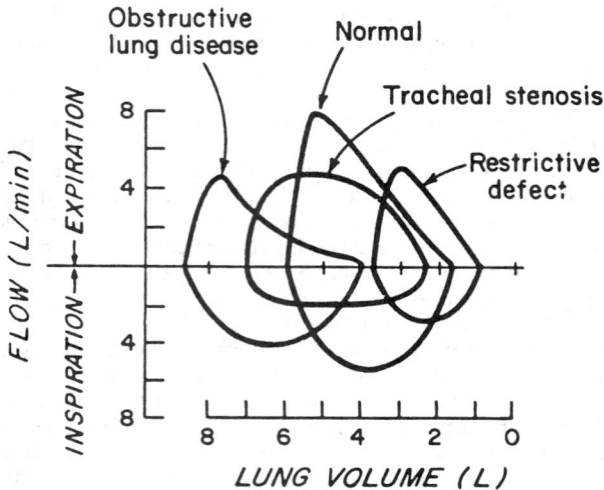

FIG. 33-2. Flow volume loops relative to lung volumes (1) in a normal subject, (2) in a patient with COPD, (3) in a patient with fixed obstruction (tracheal stenosis), and (4) in a patient with pulmonary fibrosis. Note the concave expiratory form in the patient with COPD and the flat inspiratory curve in the patient with a fixed obstruction. (Goudsouzian N, Karamanian A: Physiology for the Anesthesiologist: 2nd ed. Norwalk, Appleton-Century-Crofts, 1984. Reproduced by permission.)

after bronchodilator therapy to assess the reversibility of the airways obstruction.[11] This is useful in the assessment of the degree of airway obstruction and the patient's effort ability. Following treatment with bronchodilators, increases in PEFR compared to a baseline indicate reversibility of airway obstruction (often seen in asthmatic patients). A 15% improvement in PFTs may be considered as a positive response to bronchodilator therapy, and indicates that this therapy should be initiated preoperatively. The overall prognosis of COPD is better related to the level of spirometric function following bronchodilator therapy rather than to a baseline function.

SPLIT LUNG FUNCTION TESTS. Regional lung function studies serve to predict the functioning of the lung tissue that would remain post-lung resection. A whole (two) lung test may fail to estimate whether the amount of post-resection lung tissue will allow the patient to function at a reasonable level of activity, without disabling dyspnea or cor pulmonale.

REGIONAL PERFUSION TEST. This involves the iv injection of insoluble radioactive Xenon (Xe[133]). The peak radioactivity of each lung is proportional to the degree of perfusion of each lung.

REGIONAL VENTILATION TEST. Using an inhaled insoluble radioactive gas, the peak radioactivity over each lung is proportional to the degree of ventilation. Combining radiospirometry with whole lung testing (FEV_1, FVC, MBC) has resulted in a fair degree of correlation between predicted volumes and pulmonary function tests measured post-pneumonectomy. It is generally held that an FEV_1 of 0.8 liters is the minimum accepted volume for post-resection survivability.

REGIONAL BRONCHIAL BALLOON OCCLUSION TEST. This test basically simulates preoperatively the post-resection con-

dition by using balloon occlusion of the bronchus to the segment of the lung to be resected. Spirometry and ABGs with the remaining functioning lung are then performed.

PULMONARY ARTERY BALLOON OCCLUSION TEST. The postoperative stress on the right ventricle and remaining pulmonary vascular bed can be simulated by occluding the pulmonary artery of the lung to be resected using a balloon-tipped pulmonary artery catheter. This test may be done with or without exercise. If the mean pulmonary artery pressure increases above 40 mm Hg, Pa_{O_2} is less than 60 mm Hg, or Pa_{CO_2} is greater than 45 mm Hg, it is unlikely that the patient will be able to tolerate pneumonectomy without developing respiratory failure or cor pulmonale postoperatively.

The preoperative pulmonary evaluation of patients considered for lung resection is summarized as follows. First, a whole lung test with spirometry and ABGs should be done. If any of the following values, $Pa_{CO_2} > 40$ mmHg, $FEV_1 < 50\%$, FVC < 2 l, MBC < 50%, or RV/TLC > 50%, is found to be outside these limits, then a second level of split lung function testing should be done to estimate the exact contribution of the resected portion of the lung to either ventilation or perfusion. Conventional spirometry should yield a predicted post-resection FEV_1 greater than 800 ml. If these criteria cannot be met, surgery is usually contraindicated. A postoperative simulation of ventilation or perfusion by bronchial or PA occlusion can produce additional information, and risk-benefit ratio must be considered for each individual patient.

PREOPERATIVE PREPARATION

The wide spectrum of physiologic changes occurring during thoracic surgery puts patients at great risk of developing postoperative complications. The morbidity and mortality increase when these changes are superimposed on an acutely or chronically compromised patient. Several conditions show particular correlations with postoperative complications. Such conditions include infection, dehydration, electrolyte imbalance, wheezing, obesity, cigarette smoking, cor pulmonale, and malnutrition. Proper vigorous preoperative preparation can improve the patient's ability to face the surgery with a reduced risk of morbidity and mortality. Stein et al[12] found that postoperative pulmonary complications developed in 4 of 17 well-prepared patients, compared to 13 of 17 unprepared patients; therefore, it is important that conditions predisposing to postoperative complications be effectively treated preoperatively.

SMOKING

Approximately 33% of adult patients presenting for surgery are smokers, and there is now extensive evidence that they are at increased risk.[13, 14] Smoking increases airway irritability, decreases mucociliary transport, and increases secretions. Smoking also decreases FVC and MMEFR, thereby increasing the incidence of postoperative pulmonary complications.[15] On the other hand, cessation of smoking for a period of greater than 4–6 weeks prior to surgery is associated with a decreased incidence of postoperative complications.[14, 16, 17] Furthermore, cessation of smoking for 48 h prior to surgery has been shown to decrease the level of carboxyhemoglobin, to shift the oxyhemoglobin dissociation curve to the right, and to increase tissue oxygen availability. It should be emphasized that most of the beneficial effects of cessation of smoking, such as improvement in ciliary function, improvement in closing volume, increase in MMEFR, and reduction in sputum production, usually occur 2–3 months following the cessation of smoking.

INFECTION

Acute or chronic infection should be vigorously treated prior to surgery. Broad-spectrum antibiotics, such as ampicillin or tetracycline, are commonly used. Treatment of the acutely ill patient will depend upon the Gram stain of the sputum and on blood culture. In one prospective study, the incidence of mortality was lower (9%) in the group treated with prophylactic antibiotics compared with 17% of the untreated patients, and a lower incidence of postoperative pulmonary infection was shown as well.[18] Although not all surgeons administer antibiotics prophylactically to their patients, infection, when present preoperatively, should be vigorously treated.

HYDRATION AND REMOVAL OF BRONCHIAL SECRETIONS

Correction of hypovolemia and electrolyte imbalance should be accomplished prior to surgery, since hydrating the patient decreases the viscosity of the bronchial secretions and facilitates their removal from the bronchial tree. Humidification using a jet humidifier or ultrasonic mist system is extremely useful. The use of mucolytic drugs, such as acetylcysteine (Mucomyst) or oral expectorants (potassium iodide), can be of benefit to patients with viscous secretions.[19, 20] Commonly used methods for removing the secretions from the bronchial tree include postural drainage, vigorous coughing, chest percussion, deep breathing, and the use of an incentive spirometer. These often require patient cooperation and frequent verbal encouragement to maximize the beneficial effect.

WHEEZING AND BRONCHODILATATION

The presence of acute wheezing represents a medical emergency, and elective surgery should be postponed until effective proper treatment has been instituted. Chronic wheezing is often seen in patients with COPD, and is due to the presence of gas flow obstruction secondary to smooth muscle constriction, accumulation of secretions, and mucosal edema. Smooth muscle contraction may occur in small airways only (detectable by changes in FEF 25–75%), or may be widespread, with a large reduction of FEV_1 and FVC. The efficacy of bronchodilators in reversing the bronchospastic component is extremely important. A trial of bronchodilators and measurement of their effects on pulmonary function should be performed in any patient who shows evidence of airflow obstruction.[21] Several classes of bronchodilators are available.

Sympathomimetic Drugs

Sympathomimetic drugs increase the formation of 3, 5, cyclic AMP (cAMP). The balance between cAMP, which produces bronchodilatation, and cyclic GMP (cGMP), which produces bronchoconstriction, determines the state of contraction of the bronchial smooth muscle.[22] Thus, increasing cAMP production causes relaxation of the bronchial tree. Sympathomimetic drugs, such as epinephrine, isoproterenol, isoetharine, and

ephedrine, all have mixed β_1 and β_2 sympathetic agonist effects. The B_1 (cardiac effects) of these drugs are often undesirable in treating patients with COPD. Selective β_2 sympathomimetic drugs, such as albuterol, terbutaline (Brethine), and metaproterenol, given as inhaled aerosols, are the preferred drugs in the treatment of bronchospasm, particularly in patients with cardiac disease.

Phosphodiesterase Inhibitors

Phosphodiesterase inhibitors inhibit the breakdown of cAMP by cytoplasmic phosphodiesterase. The methylxanthines, such as aminophylline, increase the level of cAMP, resulting in bronchodilatation. In addition, aminophylline improves diaphragmatic contractility and increases the patient's resistance to fatigue.[23] Therapeutic blood levels of aminophylline are $5–20\ \mu g \cdot ml^{-1}$, and can be achieved by giving a loading dose of $5–7\ mg \cdot kg^{-1}$ infused over 20 min, followed by a continuous iv infusion of $0.5–0.7\ mg \cdot kg^{-1} \cdot h^{-1}$. Aminophylline may cause ventricular dysrhythmias, and this side effect should be borne in mind when treating patients who have myocardial ischemia.

Steroids

While not true bronchodilators, steroids are traditionally considered to decrease mucosal edema, and may prevent the release of bronchoconstricting substances. They are of questionable benefit in an acute bronchospastic situation. Steroids may be given orally, parenterally, or in aerosol form, such as beclomethasone by inhaler.

Cromolyn Sodium

Cromolyn sodium stabilizes mast cells and inhibits degranulation and histamine release. It is useful in the prevention of bronchospastic attacks, but is of little value in the treatment of the acute situation.

Parasympatholytics

Parasympatholytics include atropine and ipratropium. In the past, atropine has been avoided in patients with COPD and bronchitis due to the concern regarding increases in the viscosity of mucous. However, atropine blocks the formation of cGMP and, therefore, has a bronchodilator effect. Marini et al[24] found that inhaled atropine alone improved FEV_1 in 85% of patients with COPD. Given together with terbutaline, the FEV_1 improved in 93% of patients, while terbutaline alone improved FEV_1 in only 56% of patients. The antimuscarinic drugs, such as atropine, therefore, potentiate the bronchodilator effect of the sympathomimetic agents.

In conclusion, the preoperative preparation of the patient for thoracic surgery should focus on those conditions that are treatable prior to surgery so that the patient is in optimal condition at the time of surgery.

INTRAOPERATIVE MONITORING

All patients undergoing thoracic surgical procedures require monitoring with an electrocardiogram (lead II and/or V_5), chest and/or esophageal stethoscopes for heart and breath sound monitoring, and a temperature probe. In addition, a non-invasive blood pressure system can be used during surgery. The following invasive monitoring is also indicated, and has led to markedly improved patient care.

Direct Arterial Catheterization

Peripheral arterial cannulation has become an essential tool for the anesthesiologist in the management of patients undergoing major thoracic surgical procedures. It allows for continuous beat-to-beat measurement of blood pressure, as well as frequent sampling for the determination of arterial blood gases. The risk, when utilizing 20-gauge Teflon catheters in the radial artery, has been shown to be extremely low, and any risk can be further decreased by assuring patency of the ulnar artery. This can be done by the use of a modified Allen test, digital plethysmography, or Doppler ultrasound.[25]

Continuous blood pressure readings are critical during thoracic surgery, since surgical manipulations or intravascular volume shifts can cause sudden, major changes in the blood pressure. Immediate recognition of the change allows time for proper identification of the etiology and the institution of appropriate treatment.[26]

Serial blood gas determinations are essential in the management of patients undergoing one-lung anesthesia, or during cases in which part of the lung may be "packed away" for a period of time. Arterial hypoxemia is commonly seen due to increased pulmonary shunting and inadequate hypoxic pulmonary vasoconstriction. Significant changes in acid-base status, as well as hyper- or hypoventilation, can also be determined. The arterial blood samples can be used to confirm the readings obtained by pulse oximetry, as well as to aid in the interpretation of transcutaneous arterial oxygen tension values (i.e., respiratory versus cardiac abnormalities) and end-tidal CO_2 concentrations (i.e., inadequate ventilation versus shunting).

A radial arterial catheter can be placed in either extremity during thoracic surgery. For a mediastinoscopy, it is useful to place the catheter in the right arm and to use it to monitor compression of the innominate artery by the mediastinoscope.[27] This can help to avoid central nervous system complications resulting from inadequate cerebral blood flow through the right carotid artery (see the section on Mediastinoscopy). During thoracotomy, the radial arterial catheter is often placed in the dependent arm to aid in stabilizing the catheter. However, a roll must be placed under the axilla to avoid compression of the axillary artery and bradial plexus in this arm. In rare cases, the arterial catheter can be placed in the brachial, femoral, or dorsalis pedis artery if the ulnar collateral cirulation is thought to be inadequate.[28]

Central Venous Pressure Monitoring

The central venous pressure (CVP) is usually measured as an indication of right atrial and right ventricular pressures. It is a useful monitor if the factors affecting it are realized and its limitations understood. The CVP reflects the patient's blood volume, venous tone, and right ventricular performance; however, it is also affected by central venous obstructions and alterations of intrathoracic pressure (e.g., PEEP).[25] Serial measurements are more useful than an individual number, and the response of the CVP to a volume infusion is a useful test of right ventricular function. The CVP reflects *right* heart function, and not left ventricular performance (Fig. 33-3). The combination of the CVP to monitor right atrial pressure and the esophageal stethoscope to monitor left atrial pressure (i.e., rales, S_3) is still a useful monitoring technique in patients with good left ventricular function. A CVP catheter is often used in patients with good left ventricular function during thoracic surgical procedures for either monitoring or infusion/insertion applications. In monitoring: 1) large volume shifts, which may

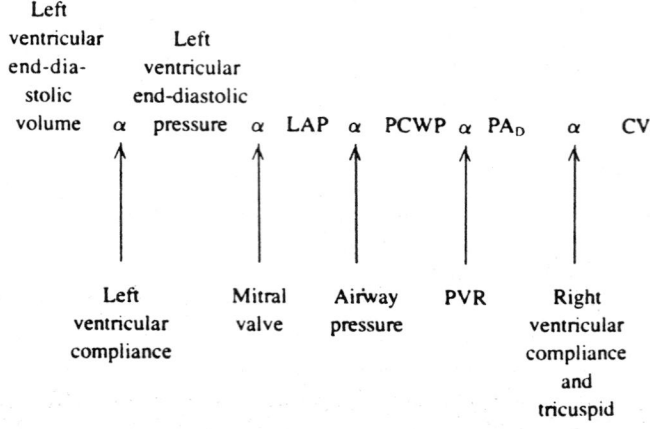

FIG. 33-3. Directional changes in central venous pressure (CVP) may reflect alterations in left ventricular performance. However, in the presence of severe pulmonary disease alteration in valve function or CVP is a poor monitor of LV function. (LAP = left atrial pressure; PCWP = pulmonary capillary wedge pressure; PA_D = pulmonary artery diastolic pressure. (From Kaplan JA [ed]: Cardiac Anesthesia, p 192. New York, Grune and Stratton, 1979, with permission.)

occur (e.g., pneumonectomy); 2) hypovolemia if suspected (e.g., hyperalimentation preoperatively); and 3) where trauma has produced acute hypovolemia. In infusion/insertion: 1) insertion of a transvenous pacemaker may be necessary; 2) vasoactive drugs may be indicated; and 3) a pulmonary arterial catheter may be subsequently required during surgery or in the postoperative period.

The CVP catheter can be placed centrally from either the external or internal jugular veins, from the subclavian veins, or from one of the arm veins. The success rate is highest using the right internal jugular vein, and a pacemaker or pulmonary arterial catheter can be inserted most easily from this vein.[29] The major disadvantage of the external jugular veins during thoracotomy is that the catheter often kinks when the patient is turned to the lateral decubitus position. The subclavian technique leads to a high incidence of pneumothorax that can be disastrous if it occurs in the dependent lung during one-lung ventilation.

Pulmonary Artery Catheterization

The use of the pulmonary artery catheter (PAC) allows measurements of left-sided filling pressures, the determination of cardiac output by thermodilution, calculation of derived hemodynamic and respiratory parameters (e.g., systemic vascular resistance and intrapulmonary shunt, respectively) and clinical use of Starling function curves. In addition, advanced versions of the basic catheter allow measurement of mixed venous oxygen saturation or right ventricular ejection fraction, as well as the application of atrial or ventricular pacing. The PAC is indicated during thoracic surgery in specific situations (Table 33-1).[26]

In the past, CVP catheters were used to monitor patients with left-sided heart disease or pulmonary disease; however, the CVP has been shown to have a poor correlation with the left atrial pressure in these types of patient. Many studies have shown the disparity between left- and right-sided pressures due to the many factors separating the CVP reading from the true left ventricular preload (Fig. 33-3).

TABLE 33-1. Indications for Pulmonary Artery Catheterization in Thoriac Surgery

1. Patients with known cardiovascular disease, with or without heart failure
2. Surgery in which cross-clamping of the thoracic aorta is anticipated
3. Patients with respiratory failure
4. Patients with suspected or diagnosed pulmonary emboli
5. Patients who have undergone previous cardiac surgery
6. When a pneumonectomy is anticipated
7. Significant shifts of intravascular volume are anticipated
8. The presence of sepsis
9. Patients who receive continuous infusions of inotropes or vasodilators
10. Patients with pulmonary hypertension or elevated pulmonary vascular resistance
11. In the presence of cor pulmonale
12. Bleomycin-treated patients

(Reproduced by permission from Kaplan JA [ed]: Thoracic Anesthesia. New York, Churchill-Livingstone, 1983.)

The PAC is most reliably inserted via the right internal jugular vein using a modified Seldinger technique that has been extensively described.[25] Insertion of the PAC through either external jugular vein or subclavian vein often leads to obstruction of the catheter when the patient is placed in the lateral decubitus position. Complications of PAC insertion and use can be divided into immediate and long-term.[30] Immediate complications include the development of supraventricular and ventricular dysrhythmias during insertion, onset of a right bundle branch block, and/or complete heart block in patients with a pre-existing left bundle branch block, as well as all the potential complications of inserting a needle into a central vein (*e.g.*, arterial puncture, pneumothorax, nerve damage, or thoracic duct injury).[31, 32] Long-term complications of the PAC include balloon rupture and gas embolization, pulmonary infarction, pulmonary artery rupture, knotting of the catheter in the right ventricle, infection, vascular obstruction, and erroneous diagnosis from misinterpretation of data.[33, 34]

Misinterpretation of data from a PAC is a real risk in a patient with cardiac and pulmonary disease undergoing thoracic surgery with one-lung ventilation. These errors can be produced by altered ventilatory modes, location of the PAC tip, ventricular compliance changes, or ventricular independence.[33, 34] A major limitation of the PAC is the assumption that the pulmonary capillary wedge pressure (PCWP) is a good approximation of left ventricular end-diastolic volume. The use of the PCWP to directly assess preload assumes a linear relationship between ventricular end-diastolic volume and ventricular end-diastolic pressure. However, alterations in ventricular compliance affect this pressure-volume relationship during surgery. Reductions in ventricular compliance can be seen with myocardial ischemia, shock, right ventricular overload, or pericardial effusion (Fig. 33-4). Numerous investigators have demonstrated a poor correlation between PCWP and left ventricular end-diastolic volume in acutely ill patients.[33-35] This correlation is worsened even further by the application of PEEP. Therefore, whenever the PCWP is used to estimate left ventricular preload, the number must be interpreted in light of the clinical situation. The interdependence of the right and left ventricles must also be remembered when interpreting PCWP.[36] Ventricular interdependence can be misleading when the interventricular septum encroaches on the left ventricular cavity, leading to elevated measurements of PCWP. An elevated PCWP associated with a decreased cardiac output can be interpreted as left ventricular failure, when, in fact, there may not be an increased left ventricular end-diastolic volume, but a decreased volume due to compression of the left ventricle by a distended right ventricle (Fig. 33-5). This situation can occur with acute respiratory failure and high levels of PEEP.[37] Techniques such as echocardiography, which directly measure ventricular dimensions, are necessary to resolve this complex situation.

Since the highest percentage of pulmonary blood flow is to the right lower lobe, the tip of a flow-directed PAC will usually be located in the right lower lobe. During a left thoracotomy with one-lung ventilation, the catheter tip would then be in the dependent lung and should produce accurate hemodynamic measurements. However, during a right thoracotomy with one-lung ventilation, the catheter tip should be in the non-dependent lung. Cohen *et al* reported that, during right thoracotomies with the tip of the PAC catheter in a West zone 1 or 2 region of the right lung, hemodynamic measurements may be inaccurate.[38] These authors found that cardiac output measurements were lower during right thoracotomies than left thoracotomies, and the derived parameters of stroke

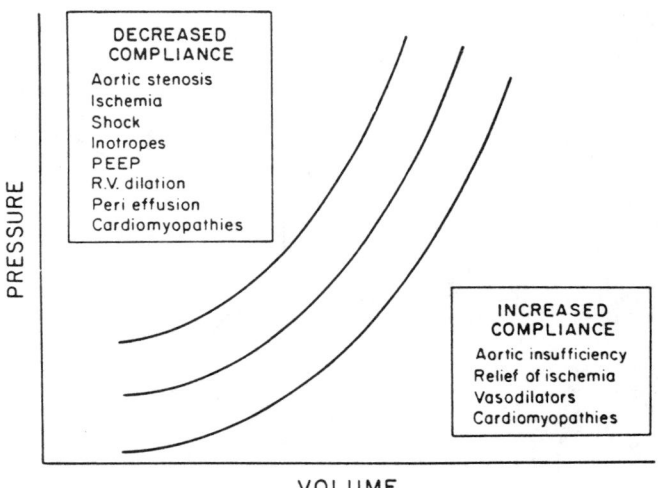

FIG. 33-4. The left ventricular compliance is the relationship between the LVEDP and the LVEDV. An increased compliance shifts the curve down and to the right, while a decreased compliance shifts it up and to the left. Examples of increased and decreased compliance are shown in the boxes. Peri effusion = pericardial effusion. (From Kaplan JA [ed]: Cardiac Anesthesia, 2nd Ed, p. 207. Orlando, Grune and Stratton, 1987, with permission.)

FIG. 33-5. Comparison of left ventricular failure and ventricular interdependence. (From Keefer JR, Barash PG: Pulmonary artery catheterization. In Blitt CD [ed]: Monitoring in Anesthesia and Critical Care Medicine. New York, Churchill Livingstone, 1985, with permission.)

	PCWP	Cardiac Output	LVEDV
LV failure	↑	↓	↑
Ventricular interdependence	↑	↓	↓

volume index and oxygen delivery were also inappropriately low (Fig. 33-6). It was thought that these results were due to the fact that the PAC tip located in the collapsed lung was affected by abnormalities in blood flow due to hypoxic pulmonary vasoconstriction. This hypothesis is supported by the concurrent finding that the mixed venous oxygen saturation also decreased during right thoracotomies as compared with left thoracotomies. This decrease in mixed venous oxygen saturation may have been caused by stagnant blood flow through the partially collapsed lung. Therefore, hemodynamic data derived from a PAC in the nondependent collapsed lung must be carefully evaluated.

FIG. 33-6. Oxygen delivery variables with left and right thoracotomies (see text for explanation). CO = cardiac output; $S\bar{v}O_2$ = mixed venous O_2 saturation; SVI = stroke volume index. (Cohen E, Eisenkraft JB, Thys DM et al: Hemodynamics and oxygenation during one lung anesthesia: Right versus left, p 126. Phoenix, Society of Cardiovascular Anesthesiologists Meeting, April 1985, with permission.)

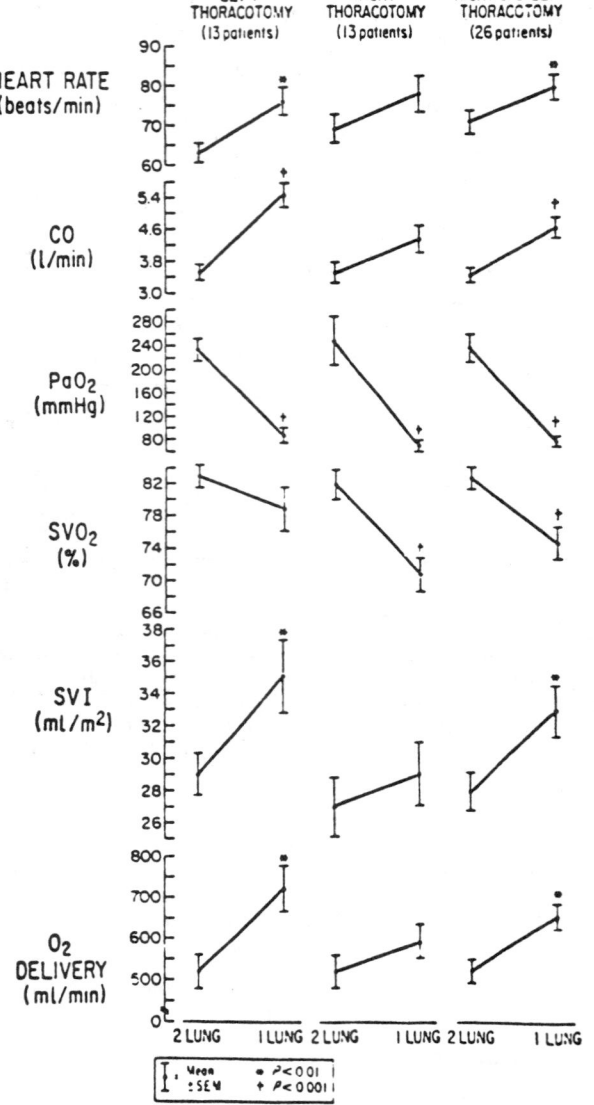

Assessment of right ventricular function is made difficult by the complex geometry and shape of the right ventricle. The thermodilution technique used to measure cardiac output with the PAC can also determine right ventricular ejection fraction (RVEF) if a fast-response thermistor is used. There are numerous situations during thoracic surgery when decreased right ventricular function precludes adequate right heart output to a normal left ventricle. Since the right ventricle is very sensitive to increases in afterload, right ventricular function can be evaluated by comparing RVEF with a measure of right ventricular afterload, such as pulmonary vascular resistance.[39] Right ventricular function curves may be even more useful than left ventricular function curves in patients with chronic pulmonary disease undergoing thoracic surgical procedures.

The multipurpose PAC, with five pacing electrodes, is now widely available. This catheter can be used for atrial, ventricular, or A-V sequential pacing in patients who require a PAC for hemodynamic monitoring.[40] Indications for the pacing PAC are: 1) intermittent third-degree heart block; 2) second-degree heart block; 3) left bundle branch block; 4) digitalis toxicity; and 5) severe bradycardia.

A major development in the area of PAC monitoring has been the addition of fiberoptic bundles for light transmission, allowing continuous measurement of oxygen saturation of the mixed venous blood ($S\bar{v}O_2$) by an oximeter. Four mechanisms can account for a decreased $S\bar{v}O_2$: 1) decreased Sa_{O_2}; 2) decreased cardiac output; 3) increased oxygen consumption; and 4) decreased hemoglobin concentration. $S\bar{v}O_2$ represents a measure of global tissue oxygen extraction and consumption, and is generally directly related to cardiac output via the Fick formula. The monitoring of $S\bar{v}O_2$ has been evaluated in patients undergoing one-lung anesthesia, and was found to show little change with changes in Pa_{O_2}.[41] This was probably due to an associated increase in cardiac output that resulted in no change or an increase in tissue oxygen delivery and, therefore, no change in $S\bar{v}O_2$. This type of monitoring may be of value, however, in the detection of patients who are unable to compensate for a decreased Pa_{O_2} by increasing cardiac output and, therefore, have a compromised oxygen delivery system. For example, Guffin et al showed that shivering after intrathoracic surgery led to a marked decrease in $S\bar{v}O_2$ due to an increased oxygen consumption, which could not be compensated for by changes in cardiac output (Fig. 33-7).[42] Utilizing this type of catheter, many oxygen delivery parameters can be calculated during and after thoracic surgery.

MONITORING OF OXYGENATION AND VENTILATION

Oxygenation

During all thoracic surgical anesthetics, the concentration of oxygen in the breathing system must be measured using an oxygen analyzer with a low oxygen concentration limit alarm. Such analyzers vary in sophistication from fuel cells, polarographic and paramagnetic analyzers, to mass spectrometers that can monitor all of the gases used during anesthesia. Adequacy of blood oxygenation must also be ensured, and adequate illumination and exposure of the patient is necessary to assess the color of shed blood, or the presence of cyanosis of the lips, nailbeds, or mucous membranes. Most patients undergoing thoracic surgical or diagnostic procedures will have an arterial catheter in place for continuous monitoring of blood

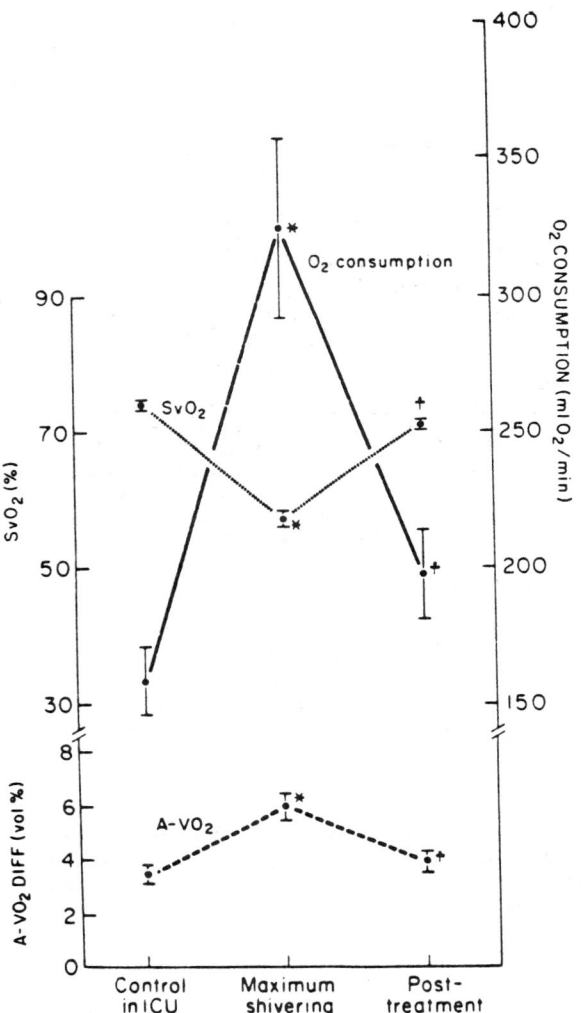

FIG. 33-7. Postoperative shivering in a group of patients after coronary artery bypass graft operation (CABG) produced a decrease in SvO_2 due to a doubling of total body O_2 consumption. This was corrected after treatment with meperidine or pancuronium. (From Guffin A, Girard D, Kaplan JA: Shivering following cardiac surgery: Hemodynamic changes and reversal. J Cardiothorac Anesth 1:24, 1987, with permission.)

pressure and sampling of arterial blood for ABG. In such cases, baseline ABG values should be obtained with an $FI_{O_2} = 0.21$ (room air), prior to starting the procedure, and repeated regularly and/or whenever indicated during surgery. Arterial blood is usually analyzed for oxygen tension (Pa_{O_2}), and saturation (Sa_{O_2}) is calculated from the oxygen-hemoglobin dissociation curve, correcting for temperature, pH and Pa_{CO_2}.

The oxygen content of arterial blood can be assessed using a bench co-oximeter, such as the IL282 (Instrumentation Laboratory, Lexington, MA), which uses spectrophotometric principles to measure the total hemoglobin ($g \cdot dl^{-1}$) and the percentages of oxyhemoglobin (HbO_2), methemoglobin (MetHb), and carboxyhemoglobin (COHb). Reduced hemoglobin (RHb) is the difference between 100% and the sum of COHb, MetHb, and HbO_2. The oxyhemoglobin percentage* (previously termed fractional concentration) is the more important index for assessing oxygen delivery. The oxygen saturation of available hemoglobin* (total amount of hemoglobin available to bind oxygen, or Sa_{O_2}, and previously known as functional saturation) will differ from HbO_2% depending upon the amount of dyshemoglobins (COHb, MetHb) present. Thus, if the hemoglobin concentration is $15\,g \cdot dl^{-1}$, and 1 gram of hemoglobin combines with 1.34 ml O_2 when fully saturated, the formula ($15 \times HbO_2\% \times 1.34$) provides the more accurate estimate of ml $O_2 \cdot dl^{-1}$ of blood than using ($15 \times Sa_{O_2} \times 1.34$) or using the calculated saturation from a saturation nomogram based upon Pa_{O_2}.

Pulse oximetry is now a commonly employed method for non-invasively obtaining a quantitative assessment of oxygenation. A sensor containing two light-emitting diodes (LEDs) and one photodetector is placed on a fingertip or earlobe. The LEDs emit light at 660 and 940 nm, and absorbance of light is measured by the photodetector. The ratio of the amplitude of the pulse-added absorptance signal at 660 to that at 940 nm is related, *via* an algorithm, to some previously empirically determined measure of oxygenation (Sa_{O_2} or HbO_2%) and is displayed as the pulse oximeter's estimate of oxygen saturation (Sp_{O_2}).[43] Subject to certain limitations (*i.e.*, presence of dyshemoglobins, dyes, hypothermia, low cardiac output states, heating lamps, use of diathermy), pulse oximeters are fairly accurate in estimating oxygenation over the range of 60–100%. Their value has also been demonstrated during one-lung ventilation, when rapid assessment of oxygenation is extremely important, and where blood gas analysis may involve some delay (Fig. 33-8).[44]

The monitoring of transcutaneous oxygen tension (P_{tcO_2}) has also been used during thoracic surgery and one-lung anesthesia. While these monitors are non-invasive and continuous, a warm-up time is required before use, and the skin underlying the sensor must be heated to 45° C to arterialize the blood. Generally, Ptc_{O_2} is approximately 80% of actual arterial oxygen tension (Pa_{O_2}), and is accurate only when the patient is hemodynamically stable with a cardiac index in excess of 2.2 $1 \cdot min^{-1} \cdot m^{-2}$. During periods of hypotension, Ptc_{O_2} does not follow Pa_{O_2}, but decreases. Thus, a low Ptc_{O_2} may be misleading in the presence of an adequate Pa_{O_2} and poor tissue perfusion.[45] For these reasons, pulse oximetry is usually preferred over transcutaneous oxygen monitoring during thoracic surgery.

The most recent advance in continuous monitoring of oxygenation is the "optode" (American Bentley, Irvine, CA), a fiberoptic probe for continuous intraarterial measurement of Pa_{O_2}. The device consists of a single optical fiber with a luminescent dye coating at the tip. It is heparin-coated, less than 0.5 mm in diameter, and passes easily through a 20-gauge arterial cannula. It does not appear to interfere with the arterial pressure waveform, and blood samples can be easily withdrawn from the cannula with the optode in place. A flash lamp emits light that excites the molecules of the luminescent dye. The excited electrons of the dye can either decay to a lower energy level by emitting light, or react with oxygen without light emission. Thus, the light emitted is inversely proportional to the amount of oxygen. This device has been evaluated, but further improvements in accuracy are required for use at a low Pa_{O_2}.[46] Nevertheless, once improved, this

*National Committee for Clinical Laboratory Standards, Villanova, Pennsylvania. Vol 2, No 10, p 342, 1982

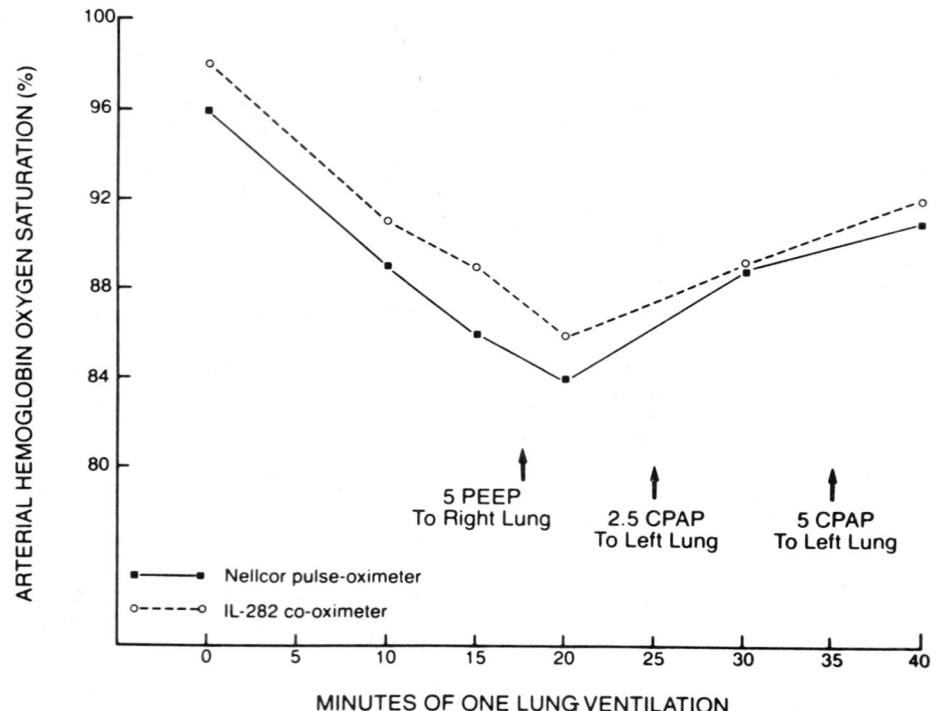

FIG. 33-8. Changes in hemoglobin oxygen saturation during one-lung ventilation. Early detection of hypoxemia with pulse oximetry facilitates prompt treatment with PEEP (5 cm H_2O) and incremental CPAP (2.5–5 cm H_2O) until arterial saturation is returned to an acceptable level. PEEP = positive end expiratory pressure; CPAP = continuous positive airway pressure. (Brodsky JB *et al*: Pulse oximetry during one-lung ventilation. Anesthesiology 65:213, 1985, with permission.)

device holds great promise for use in thoracic surgical patients, since it also permits simultaneous arterial pressure monitoring and blood sampling.

Ventilation

All patients must be continually monitored to ensure adequate ventilation. Monitoring includes such qualitative signs as chest excursion (visual observation of the lung when the chest is open), observation of the reservoir bag, and auscultation of breath sounds. An esophageal or precordial stethoscope should be used routinely. In addition, during one-lung ventilation, a stethoscope should be placed on the chest wall under the ventilated dependent lung. During controlled ventilation, a disconnect alarm with an audible signal must be utilized. The respiratory rate, V_T, minute volume, and inflation pressures should be observed.

Adequacy of ventilation should be confirmed by monitoring arterial blood gases, Pa_{CO_2} in particular. This may be estimated continuously and non-invasively by using a capnograph or mass spectrometry system. The end-tidal CO_2 concentration represents alveolar CO_2 (PA_{CO_2}), which approximates PA_{CO_2}. There is normally a small arterial-to-alveolar CO_2 gradient (4–6 mm Hg), depending on alveolar dead space. The capnogram waveform is also helpful in diagnosing airway obstruction, incomplete relaxation, and even malposition of the double-lumen tube.[47] In the latter application, a capnograph is coupled to each port of the double-lumen tube (one or two capnographs may be used) and the correct position of the double-lumen tube is identified by simultaneous and synchronous CO_2 readings on of the two analyzers. The waveforms from each lung are examined for shape, height, and rhythm, depending upon the correct postion of the tube, as well as on the ventilation-perfusion ratio for each lung.[47] A decrease in end-

tidal CO_2 in the gas from one lumen of the double-lumen tube suggests malposition of the tube. During one-lung ventilation, systemic hypoxemia is usually a greater problem than hypercarbia.[48] This is because CO_2 is some twenty times more diffusible than oxygen and Pa_{CO_2} is more dependent upon ventilation, as compared to Pa_{O_2}, which is perfusion weighted.

PHYSIOLOGY OF THE LATERAL DECUBITUS POSITION

Having considered ventilation and blood flow in the upright position (Chapter 32), these variables will now be considered as they pertain to the lateral decubitus position under the following five circumstances, which are encountered during thoracic surgery.[49]

Lateral, Awake, Breathing Spontaneously, Chest Closed

In the lateral decubitus position, the distribution of blood flow and ventilation is similar to that in the upright position, but turned by 90° (Fig. 33-9). Blood flow and ventilation to the dependent lung are significantly greater than to the nondependent lung. Good V/Q matching at the level of the dependent lung results in adequate oxygenation in the awake patient breathing spontaneously. There are two important concepts in this situation. First, since perfusion is gravity-dependent, the vertical hydrostatic gradient is smaller in the lateral, as compared to the upright, position; therefore, zone 1 is usually less extended. Second, in regard to ventilation, the dependent hemidiaphragm is pushed higher into the chest by the abdominal contents in the region of the dependent lung hemidiaphragm as compared with the non-dependent lung

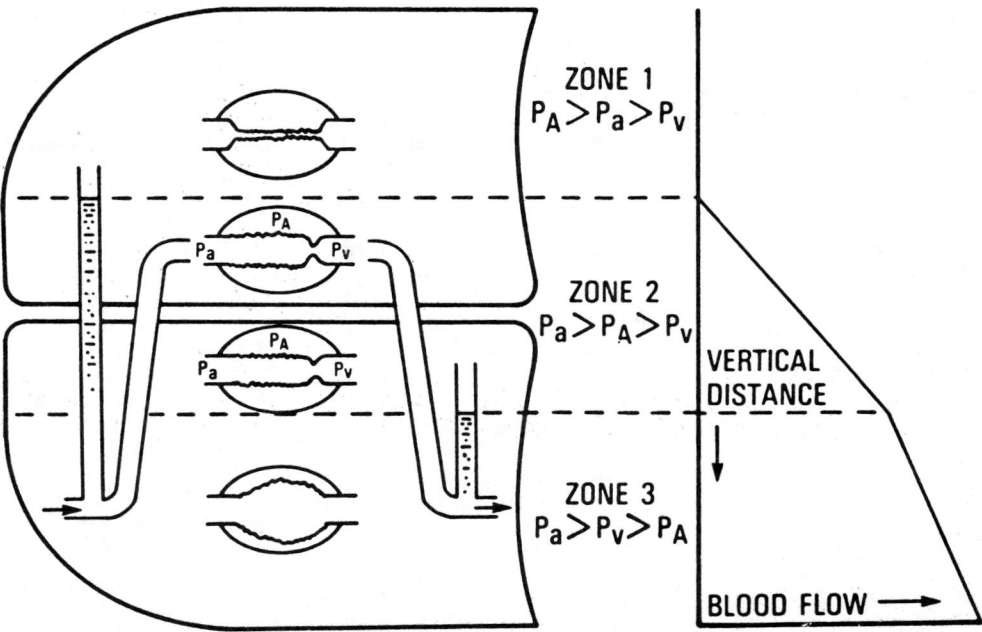

FIG. 33-9. Schematic representation of the effects of gravity on the distribution of pulmonary blood flow in the lateral decubitus position. Vertical gradients in the lateral decubitus position are similar to those in the upright position, and cause the creation of zones 1, 2, and 3. Consequently, pulmonary blood flow increases with lung dependency and is largest in the dependent lung and least in the non-dependent lung. (Benumof JL: Physiology of the open-chest and one lung ventilation. In Kaplan JA [ed]: Thoracic Anesthesia. New York, Churchill-Livingstone, 1983. Reproduced by permission.)

hemidiaphragm. During spontaneous ventilation, the conserved ability of the dependent diaphragm to contract will result in an adequate distribution of V_T to the dependent lung. Since most of the perfusion is also to the dependent lung, the $\dot{V}/\dot{Q}$ matching is good in this position and similar to that in the upright position.

Lateral, Awake, Breathing Spontaneously, Chest Open

Controlled positive pressure ventilation is the only way to provide adequate ventilation and ensure gas exchange in an open-chest situation. Frequently, thoracoscopy is performed using intercostal blocks with the patient breathing spontaneously in order to allow proper lung examination. The thoracoscope provides an adequate seal of the open chest to prevent a "free" open-chest situation. Two complications can arise from the patient breathing spontaneously with an open chest. The first is mediastinal shift, usually occurring during inspiration (Fig. 33-10). The negative pressure of the intact hemithorax compared with the relative positive pressure of the open hemithorax can cause the mediastinum to move vertically downward and push into the dependent hemithorax. The mediastinal shift can create circulatory and reflex changes that may result in a clinical picture similar to shock and respiratory distress. Sometimes, depending upon the severity of the distress, the patient will need to be immediately

FIG. 33-10. Schematic representation of mediastinal shift in the spontaneously breathing open-chested patient in the lateral decubitus position. During inspiration, negative pressure in the intact hemithorax causes the mediastinum to move downward. During expiration, relative positive pressure in the intact hemithorax causes the medastinum to move upward. (From Tarhan S, Moffitt EA: Principles of Thoracic Anesthesia. Surg Clin North Am 53:813, 1973. Reproduced by permission.)

EXPIRATION

Pneumothorax

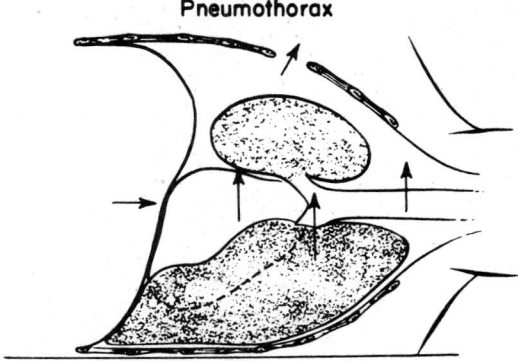

INSPIRATION

Pneumothorax

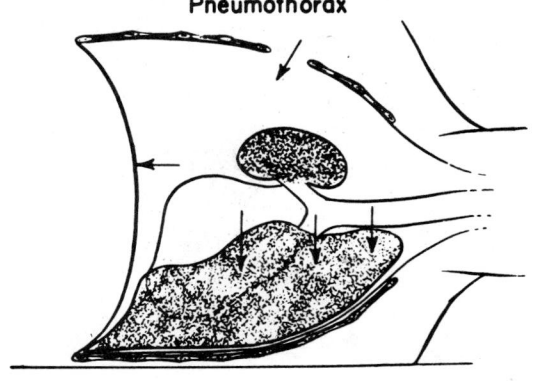

intubated, with initiation of positive pressure ventilation, and the anesthesiologist must be prepared to intubate the patient in this position without disturbing the surgical field. The second phenomenon is paradoxical breathing (Fig. 33-11). During inspiration, the relatively negative pressure in the intact hemithorax compared with atmospheric pressure in the open hemithorax can cause movement of air from the non-dependent into the dependent lung. The opposite occurs during expiration. This gas movement reversal from one lung to another represents wasted ventilation and can compromise the adequacy of gas exchange. Paradoxical breathing is increased by a large thoracotomy or by an increase in airway resistance in the dependent lung. Positive pressure ventilation or adequate sealing of the open chest will eliminate paradoxical breathing.

Lateral Position, Anesthetized, Chest Closed

The induction of general anesthesia does not cause signnificant change in the distribution of blood flow, but has an important impact on the distribution of ventilation. The majority of the V_T passes to the non-dependent lung, and this results in a significant $\dot{V}/\dot{Q}$ mismatch. Induction of general anesthesia causes a reduction in the volumes of both lungs secondary to a reduction in functional residual capacity (FRC). Any reduction in volume in the dependent lung is of a greater magnitude than in the non-dependent lung, for several reasons. First, the cephalad displacement of the dependent diaphragm by the abdominal contents is more pronounced, and will be increased by paralysis. Secondly, the mediastinal structures pressing on the dependent lung, and/or poor positioning of the dependent side on the operating table, will prevent the lung from expanding properly. The above mentioned factors will move both lungs to a lower volume on the S-shaped volume-pressure curve (Fig. 33-12). The non-dependent lung moves to a steeper position on the compliance curve and receives most of the V_T while the dependent lung will be on the flat non-compliant part of the curve.

Lateral Position, Anesthetized, Breathing Spontaneously, Chest Open

Opening the chest has little impact on the distribution of perfusion. However, the upper lung is now no longer restricted by the chest wall and will be free to expand, resulting in a further increase in $\dot{V}/\dot{Q}$ mismatch as the non-dependent lung is preferentially ventilated due to a now increased compliance.

Lateral Position, Anesthetized, Paralyzed, Chest Open

During paralysis and positive pressure ventilation, diaphragmatic displacement is maximal over the non-dependent lung, where there is the least amount of resistance to diaphragmatic movement caused by the abdominal contents (Fig. 33-13).

FIG. 33-11. Schematic representation of paradoxical respiration in the spontaneously breathing open-chested patient in the lateral decubitus position. During inspiration, movement of gas from the exposed lung into the intact lung and movement of air from the environment into the open hemithorax causes collapse of the exposed lung. During expiration, the reverse occurs, and the exposed lung expands. (From Tarhan S, Moffitt EA: Principles of thoracic anesthesia. Surg Clin North Am 53:813, 1973. Reproduced by permission.)

EXPIRATION
Pneumothorax

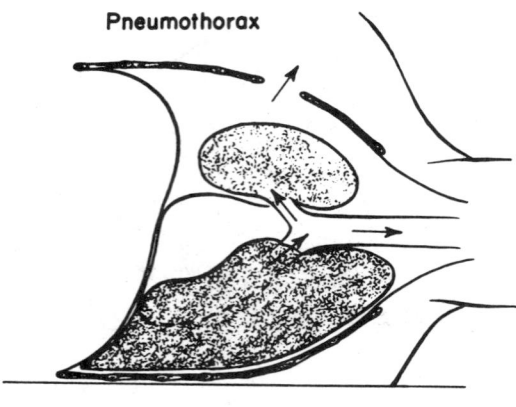

INSPIRATION
Pneumothorax

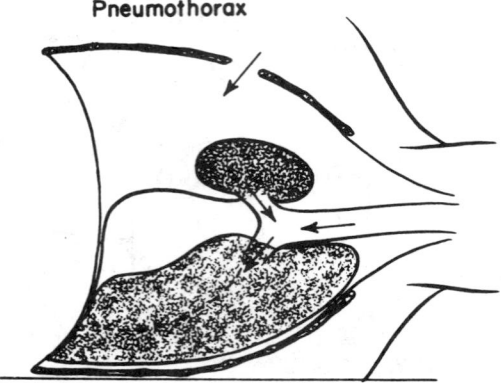

FIG. 33-12. The left-hand side of the schematic shows the distribution of ventilation in the awake patient (closed chest) in the lateral decubitus position, and the right-hand side shows the distribution of ventilation in the anesthetized patient (closed chest) in the lateral decubitus position. The induction of anesthesia has caused a loss in lung volume in both lungs, with the non-dependent (up) lung moving from a flat, noncompliant portion to a steep compliant portion of the pressure-volume curve, and the dependent (down) lung moving from a steep compliant part to a flat, noncompliant part of the pressure-volume curve. Thus, the anesthetized patient in the lateral decubitus position has the majority of the tidal ventilation in the non-dependent lung (where there is the least perfusion) and the minority of the tidal ventilation in the dependent lung (where there is the most perfusion.) (Benumof JL: Physiology of the open-chest and one lung ventilation. In Kaplan JA [ed]: Thoracic Anesthesia. New York, Churchill-Livingstone, 1983. Reproduced by permission.)

AWAKE   ANESTHETIZED

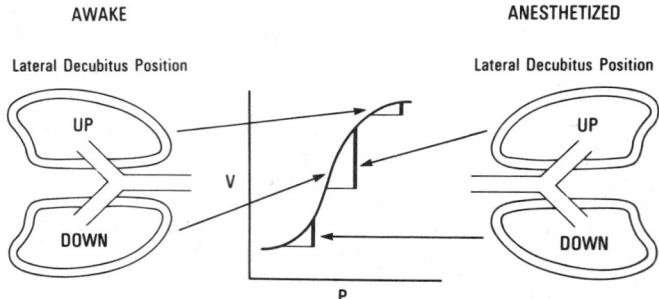

This will further compromise the ventilation to the dependent lung and increase the $\dot{V}/\dot{Q}$ mismatch.

One-lung Ventilation, Anesthetized, Paralyzed, Chest Open

During two-lung ventilation in the lateral position, the mean blood flow to the non-dependent lung is assumed to be 40% of cardiac output (CO), and 60% of CO goes to the dependent lung (Fig. 33-14). Normally, venous admixture (shunt) in the lateral position is 10% of CO, and is equally divided as 5% in each lung. Therefore, the average percentage of CO participating in gas exchange is 35% in the non-dependent lung and 55% in the dependent lung.

One-lung ventilation creates an obligatory right-to-left trans-pulmonary shunt through the non-ventilated non-dependent lung, since the $\dot{V}/\dot{Q}$ ratio of that lung is zero. In theory, an additional 35% should be added to the total shunt during one-lung ventilation. However, assuming normal hypoxic pulmonary vasoconstriction (HPV), blood flow to the non-dependent hypoxic lung will be reduced by 50%, and, therefore, will be $40-(35/2)=22.5\%$, all of which represents venous admixture (Fig. 33-14).[50] Together with the 5% shunt in the dependent lung, total shunt during one-lung ventilation is $22.5 + 5 = 27.5\%$. This will result in a Pa_{O_2} of approximately 150 mm Hg ($FI_{O_2} = 1.0$).

Since 72.5% of the perfusion is directed to the dependent lung during one-lung ventilation, the matching of ventilation in this lung is important for adequate gas exchange. The dependent lung is no longer on the steep, compliant portion of the volume-pressure curve because of reduced lung volume and FRC. There are several reasons for this reduction in FRC, including general anesthesia, paralysis, pressure of abdominal contents, compression by the weight of mediastinal structures, and suboptimal positioning on the operating table. Other considerations that impair optimal ventilation to the dependent lung include absorption atelectasis, accumulation of secretions, and the formation of a fluid transudate in the dependent lung. All of these will create a low $\dot{V}/\dot{Q}$ ratio and a large $P(A-a)_{O_2}$ gradient.

ONE-LUNG VENTILATION

ABSOLUTE INDICATIONS FOR ONE-LUNG VENTILATION

Separation of the lungs to prevent spillage of pus or blood from an infected or bleeding source is an absolute indication for OLV (Table 33-2). Life-threatening complications, such as massive atelectasis, sepsis, and pneumonia, can result from bilateral contamination. Bronchopleural and broncho-cutaneous fistulae both represent low-resistance pathways for the V_T delivered by positive pressure ventilation, and both prevent adequate alveolar ventilation. Giant cysts or unilateral bullae may rupture under positive pressure ventilation. This can be avoided by selective lung ventilation. Finally, during bronchopulmonary lavage, an effective separation of the lungs is mandatory to avoid accidental spillage of fluid from the lavaged lung to the non-dependent ventilated lung.

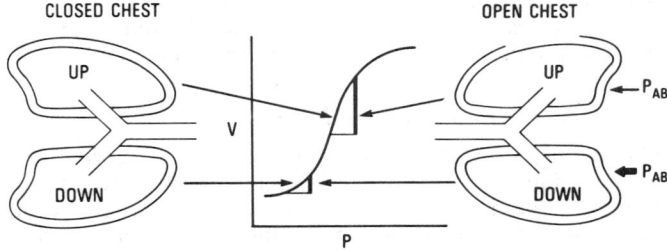

FIG. 33-13. This schematic of a patient in the lateral decubitus position compares the closed-chested anesthetized condition with the open-chested anesthetized and paralyzed condition. Opening the chest increases non-dependent lung compliance, and reinforces or maintains the larger part of the tidal ventilation going to the non-dependent lung. Paralysis also reinforces or maintains the larger part of tidal ventilation going to the non-dependent lung, because the pressure of the abdominal contents (P_{AB}) pressing against the upper diaphragm is minimal, and it is, therefore, easier for positive pressure ventilation to displace this lesser resisting dome of the diaphragm. (Benumof JL: Physiology of the open-chest and one lung ventilation. In Kaplan JA [ed]: Thoracic Anesthesia. New York, Churchill-Livingstone, 1983. Reproduced by permission.)

FIG 33-14. Schematic representation of two-lung ventilation *versus* one-lung ventilation. Typical values for fractional blood flow to the non-dependent and dependent lungs, as well as Pa_{O_2} and $\dot{Q}_s/\dot{Q}_t$ for the two conditions, are shown. The $\dot{Q}_s/\dot{Q}_t$ during two-lung ventilation is assumed to be distributed equally between the two lungs (5% to each lung.) The essential difference between two-lung and one-lung ventilation is that, during one-lung ventilation, the nonventilated lung has some blood flow and, therefore, an obligatory shunt, which is not present during two-lung ventilation. The 35% of total flow perfusing the non-dependent lung, which was not shunt flow, was assumed to be able to reduce its blood flow by 50% by hypoxic pulmonary vasconstriction. The increase in $\dot{Q}_s/\dot{Q}_t$ from two-lung to one-lung ventilation is assumed to be solely due to the increase in blood flow through the nonventilated non-dependent lung during one-lung ventilation. (Benumof JL: Anesthesia for Thoracic Surgery. Philadelphia, WB Saunders, 1987. Reproduced by permission.)

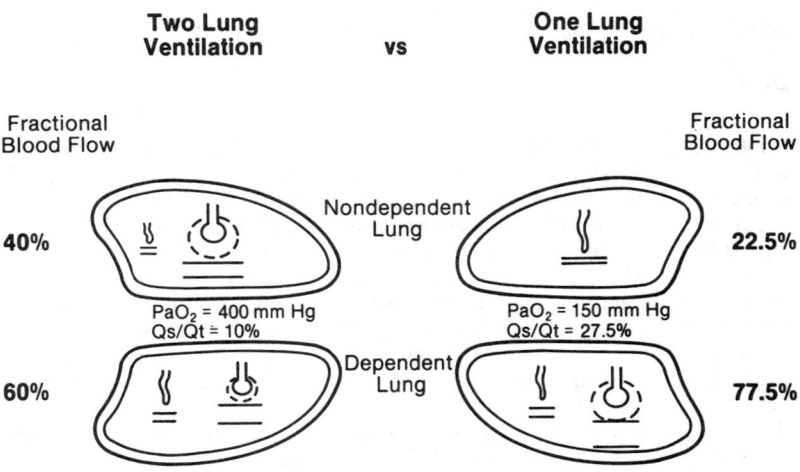

TABLE 33-2.   Indications for One-Lung Ventilation

Absolute
1. Isolation of each lung to prevent contamination of a healthy lung:
   a. Infection (abscess, infected cyst, etc.)
   b. Massive hemorrhage
2. Control of distribution of ventilation to only one lung
   a. Bronchopleural fistula
   b. Bronchopleural cutaneous fistula
   c. Unilateral cyst or bullae
   d. Major bronchial disruption or trauma
3. Unilateral lung lavage

Relative
1. Surgical exposure—high priority
   a. Thoracic aortic aneurysm
   b. Pneumonectomy
   c. Upper lobectomy
2. Surgical exposure—low priority
   a. Esophageal surgery
   b. Middle and lower lobectomy
   c. Thoracoscopy under general anesthesia

(Modified from Benumof JL: Physiology of the open chest and one-lung ventilation. In Kaplan JA [ed]: Thoracic Anesthesia, p 299. New York, Churchill Livingstone, 1983.)

RELATIVE INDICATIONS FOR ONE-LUNG VENTILATION

In clinical practice, a double-lumen tube is commonly used for a lobectomy or pneumonectomy; these represent relative indications for lung separation. Upper lobectomy, pneumonectomy, and thoracic aortic aneurysm repair are relatively high-priority indications. These procedures are technically difficult, and optimal surgical exposure and a quiet operative field are highly desirable. Lower or middle lobectomy and esophageal resection are of lower priority. Nevertheless, many surgeons are accustomed to operating with a collapsed lung, which minimizes lung trauma from retractors and manipulation, helps surgeons to better visualize lung anatomy, and facilitates identification and separation of anatomic structures and lung fissures. Thoracoscopy, if not performed with an intercostal block in the spontaneously breathing patient, is greatly facilitated by collapse of the lung under examination.

METHODS OF LUNG SEPARATION

Bronchial Blockers

BRONCHIAL BLOCKER. Lung separation can be achieved with a reusable bronchial blocker. Magill described an endobronchial blocker that is placed with the help of a bronchoscope and directed to the non-ventilated lung. Inflation of the cuff at the distal end of the blocker serves to block ventilation to that lung. The lumen of the blocker permits suctioning of the airway distal to the catheter tip. Depending on the clinical circumstance, oxygen can be insufflated through the catheter lumen. A conventional endotracheal tube is then placed in the trachea. This technique can be useful in achieving selective ventilation in children under 12 yr of age, since the smallest double-lumen tube presently available is 28 French. However, since the blocker balloon requires a high distending pressure, it easily slips out of the bronchus into the trachea, obstructing ventilation and losing the seal between the two lungs. This displacement can be secondary to changes in position or to surgical manipulation. The loss of lung separation can be a life-threatening situation if it is performed to prevent spillage of pus, blood, or fluid from bronchopulmonary lavage. For this reason, bronchial blockers are rarely used in present day practice.

ARTERIAL EMBOLECTOMY CATHETER. Selective airway occlusion can be produced by the use of Fogarty catheters designed for embolectomy procedures.[51] Placement of the embolectomy catheter is best performed under direct vision with the aid of a fiberoptic bronchoscope. A conventional endotracheal tube is then placed alongside the catheter after withdrawing the bronchoscope.

UNIVENT TUBE. Introduced in 1982 by Fuji Systems Corporation, Tokyo, Japan, this is a single-lumen endotracheal tube with a movable endobronchial blocker. In this tube, the bronchial blocker is housed in a small channel bored in the endotracheal tube wall. Following intubation of the trachea, the movable blocker is manipulated into the desired mainstem bronchus with the aid of a fiberoptic bronchoscope.[52, 53]

Single-lumen Endobronchial Tubes

Historically, a number of single-lumen tubes were designed for insertion into a mainstem bronchus in order to achieve lung separation.[2–4] However, these tubes are rarely, if ever, used today due to technical difficulties and less satisfactory performance.

Double-lumen Endobronchial Tubes

These are currently the most widely used means of achieving lung separation and one-lung ventilation. There are several different types of double-lumen tubes, but all are essentially similar in design in that two catheters are bonded together. One lumen is long enough to reach a mainstem bronchus, and the second lumen ends with an opening in the distal trachea. Lung separation is achieved by inflation of two cuffs, the proximal tracheal cuff and the distal bronchial cuff, located in the mainstem bronchus (see section on double-lumen tubes positioning). The endobronchial cuffs of the right-sided tubes are slotted or otherwise designed to allow ventilation of the right upper lobe, since the right mainstem bronchus is too short to accommodate both the right lumen tip and a right bronchial cuff.

CARLENS. A left-sided double-lumen tube with a carinal hook to aid in positioning and to minimize dislocation is shown in Figure 33-15. It is made of red rubber and each catheter has a D-shaped cross-sectional lumen. Although the carinal hook may help in the correct placement of the tube, it can increase difficulty during insertion, cause vocal cord trauma, and can sometimes be amputated and lost during the insertion and manipulation of the tube.

WHITE. This tube is essentially a right-sided Carlens tube (Fig. 33-16). It is used for right endobronchial intubations and left-sided surgical procedures. The distal endobronchial cuff is slotted to permit ventilation of the right upper lobe bronchus.

ROBERTSHAW. This is a double-lumen tube available in left- and right-sided forms without a carinal hook, which makes insertion easier (Fig. 33-17). This tube has the advantages of having D-shaped large diameter lumens that allow easy suctioning and offer low resistance to gas flow, and a fixed curvature to facilitate proper positioning and to reduce the possibility of kinking. The right-sided endobronchial tube is designed to minimize occlusion of the right upper lobe. The original red rubber tubes are available in three sizes: small, medium, and large. Clear, polyvinyl, disposable Robertshaw-design double-lumen tubes are also in wide use today. These tubes are available in a right or left design and in French sizes 35, 37, 39, and 41. The advantages of the disposable tubes include relative ease of insertion, proper positioning, easy recognition of the blue color of the endobronchial cuff when fiberoptic bronchoscopy is used, confirmation of position on a chest radiograph using the radio-opaque lines in the wall of

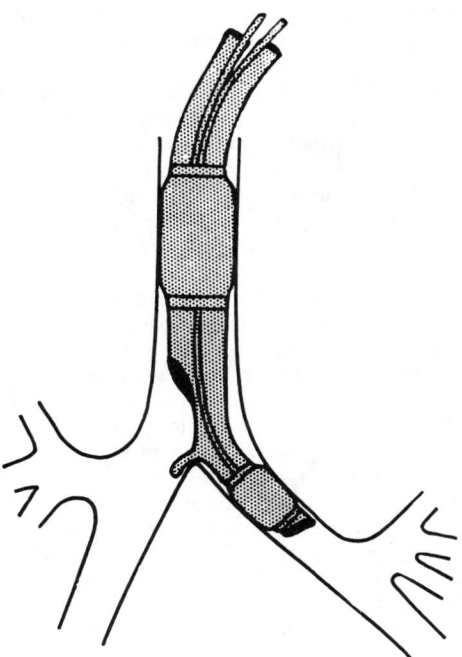

FIG. 33-15. Left mainstem endobronchial intubation using a Carlens tube. Note carinal "hook" used for correct positioning. (Hillard EK, Thompson PW: Instruments used in thoracic anaesthesia. In Mushin WW [ed]: Thoracic Anaesthesia, p 315. Oxford, Blackwell Scientific, 1963. Reproduced with permission.)

FIG. 33-16. Right mainstem endobronchial intubation with a White tube. Note the slot in the endobronchial cuff to facilitate ventilation of the right upper lobe. (Hillard EK, Thompson PW: Instruments used in thoracic anaesthesia. In Mushin WW [ed]: Thoracic Anaesthesia, p 309. Oxford, Blackwell Scientific, 1963. Reproduced with permission.)

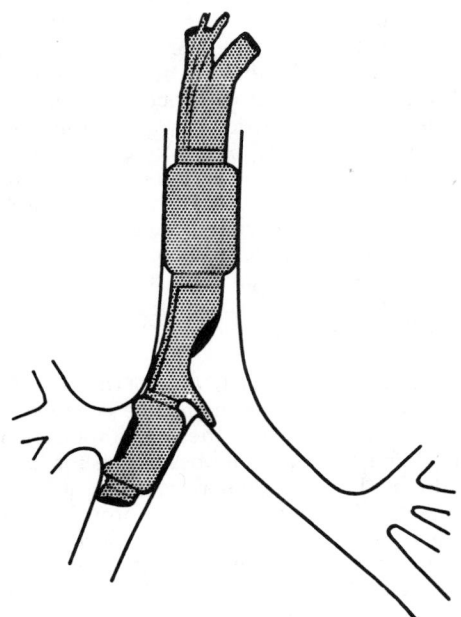

FIG. 33-17. Right- and left-sided Robertshaw tubes. (Wilson RS: Endobronchial Intubation. In Kaplan JA (ed): Thoracic Anesthesia. New York, Churchill-Livingstone, 1983. Reproduced by permission.)

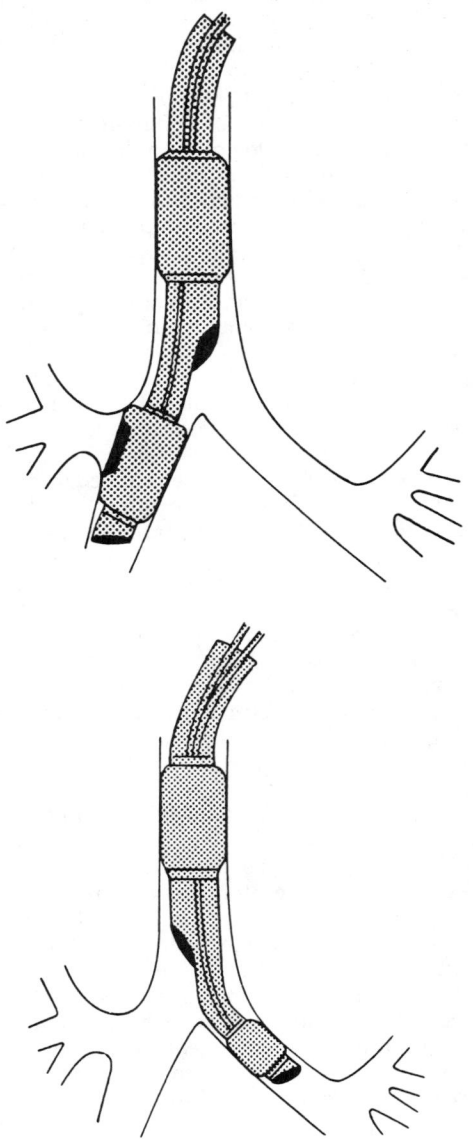

the tube, and continuous observation of tidal gas exchange and of respiratory moisture through the clear plastic. The right endobronchial cuff is doughnut-shaped and allows the right upper lobe ventilation slot to ride over the right upper lobe orifice. The tube is also suitable for use in long-term ventilation in the intensive care unit because it has a high-volume low-pressure cuff. These are now considered the tubes of choice for achieving lung separation and one-lung ventilation.

Despite the availability of disposable double-lumen tubes, many centers continue to use the red rubber Robertshaw tubes. There are several reasons for this. First, the cost of reusable tubes is significantly less than that of the disposable tubes. Second, some anesthesiologists believe that although the red rubber tubes may be more difficult to insert, they are less likely to dislocate during patient positioning and surgical manipulation. Third, during insertion of the double-lumen tube, the tracheal cuff often directly rubs against the patient's upper teeth. If the latter are prominent and sharp, the thin-walled tracheal cuffs of the disposable tubes are much more likely to tear, as compared to the thicker-walled cuffs of the red rubber tubes. Fourth, if the wrong size of disposable tube is selected and insertion attempted, the tube cannot be reused, since sterility is compromised. This does not apply to the red rubber tubes, which withstand repeated sterilizations.

POSITIONING DOUBLE-LUMEN TUBES. This section will concentrate on the insertion of Robertshaw-type double-lumen tubes (both disposable and non-disposable), since they are the most widely used. Prior to insertion, the double-lumen tube should be prepared and checked. The tracheal cuff (low pressure, high volume) can accommodate up to 20 ml of air, and the bronchial cuff should be checked using a 3 ml syringe. The tube should be coated liberally with lubricating ointment and the stylet should be withdrawn, lubricated, and gently placed back into the bronchial lumen without disturbing the tube's preformed curvature. The MacIntosh 3 blade is preferred for intubation of the trachea, since it provides the largest area through which to pass the tube. The insertion of the tube is performed with the distal concave curvature facing anteriorly. After the tip of the tube is past the vocal cords, the stylet is removed and the tube is then rotated through 90°. The left-sided tube is rotated 90° to the left and the right-sided tube is rotated to the right. Advancement of the tube ceases when moderate resistance to further passage is encountered, indicating that the tube tip has been firmly seated in the mainstem bronchus. It is important to remove the stylet before rotating and advancing the tube in order to avoid tracheal or bronchial lacerations. Rotation and advancement of the tube should be performed gently and under continuous laryngoscopy to prevent hypopharyngeal structures from interfering with proper positioning. Once the tube is thought to be in the proper position, a sequence of steps should be performed to check its location.

First, the tracheal cuff should be inflated and equal ventilation of both lungs established. If breath sounds are not equal, the tube is probably too far down and the tracheal lumen opening is in a mainstem bronchus or is lying at the carina. Withdrawal of the tube by 2–3 cm usually restores equal breath sounds. The second step is to clamp the right side (in the case of the left-sided tube) and remove the right cap from the connector. Then the bronchial cuff is slowly inflated to prevent an air leak from the bronchial lumen around the bronchial cuff into the right tracheal lumen. This ensures that no excessive pressure is applied to the bronchus, and helps avoid laceration. Inflation of the bronchial cuff rarely requires more than 2 ml of air. The third step is to remove the clamp

and check that both lungs are ventilated with both cuffs inflated. This will ensure that the bronchial cuff is not obstructing the contralateral hemithorax, either totally or partially. The final step is to selectively clamp each side and watch for absence of movement and breath sounds on the ipsilateral side, while the ventilated side should have clear breath sounds, chest movement that feels compliant, respiratory gas moisture with each tidal ventilation, and no air leak. If peak airway pressure during two-lung ventilation is 20 cm H_2O, it should not exceed 40 cm H_2O for the same tidal volume during one-lung ventilation.

Other common methods for ensuring the correct placement of a double-lumen tube include fluoroscopy, chest x-ray, selective capnography, and the use of an underwater seal. Determination of the presence of air leaks when positive pressure is applied to one lumen of double-lumen tube is easily done in the operating room. If the bronchial cuff is not inflated and positive pressure is applied to the bronchial lumen of the double-lumen tube, gas will leak past the bronchial cuff and return through the tracheal lumen. If the tracheal lumen is connected to an underwater seal system, gas will be seen to bubble up through the water. The bronchial cuff can then be gradually inflated until no gas bubbles are seen and the desired cuff seal pressure can be attained. This test is of extreme importance when absolute lung separation is needed, such as in bronchopulmonary lavage.

The most important advance in checking the proper position of a double-lumen tube is the introduction of the pediatric fiberoptic bronchoscope. Recently, Smith et al showed that, when the disposable double-lumen tube was thought to be in correct position by auscultation and physical examination, subsequent fiberoptic bronchoscopy showed that 48% of tubes were, in fact, malpositioned.[54] When using a left-sided double-lumen tube, the bronchoscope is usually first introduced through the tracheal lumen. The carina is visualized and no bronchial cuff herniation should be seen. The upper surface of the blue endobronchial cuff should be just below the tracheal carina. The bronchial cuff of the disposable double-lumen tube is very easily visualized because of its blue color. The bronchoscope should then be passed through the bronchial lumen and the left upper lobe orifice should be identified. When a right-sided double-lumen tube is used (Fig. 33-18), the carina should be visualized through the tracheal lumen; but, more importantly, the orifice of the right upper lobe bronchus should be identified when the bronchoscope is passed through the right upper lobe ventilating slot of the double-lumen tube. Pediatric fiberoptic bronchoscopes are available in several sizes: 5.6, 4.9, and 3.6 mm in external diameters. The 4.9 mm-diameter bronchoscope can be passed through double-lumen tube of French sizes 37 and larger. The 3.6 mm-diameter bronchoscope is easily passed through all sizes of double-lumen tube. In general, it is recommended that the largest size that can pass through the lumen of a double-lumen tube be used, since it provides better visualization and facilitates identification of the bronchial anatomy.

PROBLEMS OF MALPOSITION OF THE DOUBLE-LUMEN TUBE. The use of a double-lumen tube is associated with a number of potential problems, the most important of which is malposition. There are several possibilities for tube malposition. The double-lumen tube may be accidentally directed to the side opposite the desired mainstem bronchus. In this case, the lung opposite the side of the connector clamped will collapse. Generally inadequate separation, increased airway pressures, and instability of the double-lumen tube occur. In addition, due to the morphology of the double-lumen tube

Use of Fiberoptic Bronchoscope to Determine
Precise Right-Sided Double-Lumen Tube Position

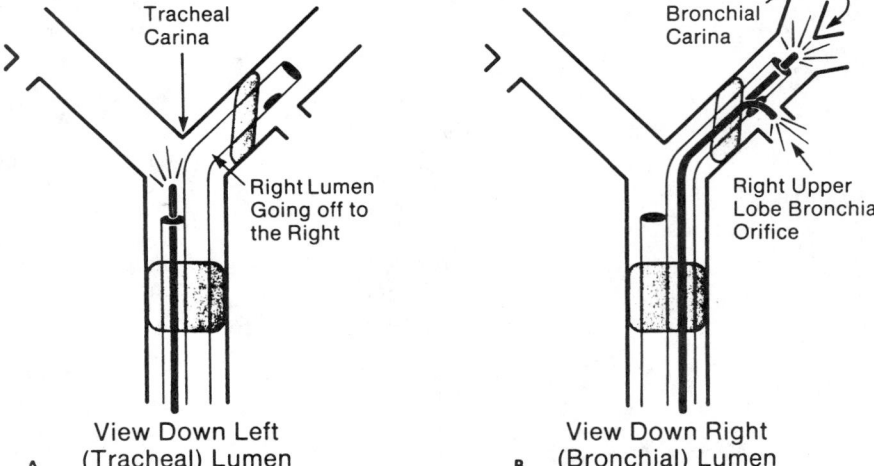

FIG. 33-18. Use of fiberoptic bronchoscope to determine the position of a right-sided double-lumen tube. (*A*) When passed down the left (tracheal) lumen, the endoscopist should see a clear view of the tracheal carina and right lumen going off into the right mainstem bronchus. (*B*) When the bronchoscope is passed *via* the right (bronchial) lumen, the endoscopist should see the bronchial carina off in the distance; when the bronchoscope is flexed cephalad and passed through the right upper lobe ventilation slot, the right upper lobe bronchial orifice should be visualized. (Benumof JL: Intraoperative considerations for all thoracic surgery. In Benumof JL: Anesthesia for Thoracic Surgery. Philadelphia, WB Saunders, 1987.)

Double-Lumen Tube Malpositions

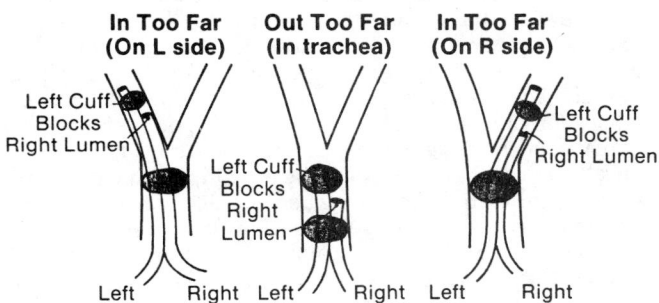

FIG. 33-19. Diagram showing the three major malpositions of a left-sided double-lumen endotracheal tube. The tube can be in too far on the left (*left*), out too far (*center*), or down the right mainstem bronchus (*right*). In each case, the left cuff, when fully inflated, can completely block the right lumen. (Benumof JL: Intraoperative considerations for all thoracic surgery. In Benumof JL: Anesthesia for Thoracic Surgery. Philadelphia, WB Saunders, 1987.)

curvatures, tracheal or bronchial lacerations may result. If a left-sided double-lumen tube is inserted into the right mainstem bronchus, it will obstruct the ventilation to the right upper lobe (Fig. 33-19, *right*). It is, therefore, essential to recognize and correct such a malposition as soon as possible.

Second, the double-lumen tube may have been passed too far down into either the right or left mainstem bronchus. In this case, breath sounds will be very diminished, or not audible at all, over the contralateral side. This situation is corrected when the tube is withdrawn until the opening of the tracheal lumen is above the carina.

Third, the double-lumen tube may not be inserted far enough with the bronchial lumen opening above the carina. In this position, good breath sounds will be heard bilaterally when ventilating through the bronchial lumen, but no breath sounds will be audible when ventilating through the tracheal lumen, since the inflated bronchial cuff obstructs gas flow arising from the tracheal lumen. The cuffs should be deflated and the double-lumen tube rotated and advanced into the desired mainstem bronchus.

Fourth, a right-sided double-lumen tube may occlude the right upper lobe orifice (Fig. 33-20). The mean distance from the carina to the right upper lobe orifice is 2.3 ± 0.7 cm in males, and 2.1 ± 0.7 cm in females.[55] With the right-sided double-lumen tubes, the ventilatory slot in the side of the bronchial catheter must overlie the right upper lobe orifice to permit ventilation of this lobe. The margin of safety, however, is extremely small, and varies from 1–8 mm.[55] It is, therefore, difficult to assure proper ventilation to the right upper lobe and to avoid dislocation of the double-lumen tube during surgical manipulation. Where right endobronchial intubation is required, a disposable right-sided double-lumen tube is perhaps the best choice because of the slanted doughnut shape of the bronchial cuff. The latter allows the ventilation slot to ride off the right upper lobe ventilation orifice, and increases the margin of safety.

Fifth, the left upper lobe orifice may be obstructed by a left-sided double-lumen tube. Traditionally, it was believed that the take-off of the left upper lobe bronchus was at a safe distance from the carina, and that it would not be obstructed by a left-sided double-lumen tube. However, the mean distance between the left upper lobe orifice and the carina is 5.4 ± 0.7 cm in males and 5.0 ± 0.7 cm in females.[55] The average distance between the right and left lumen openings on the left-sided disposable tubes is 6.9 cm.[4] Therefore, an obstruction of the left upper lobe is possible while the tracheal lumen is still above the carina. There is also a 20% variation in the location of the blue endobronchial cuff on the disposable tubes, since this cuff is attached by hand at the end of the manufacturing process.

Finally, bronchial cuff herniation may occur and obstruct the bronchial lumen, if excessive volumes are used to inflate the cuff. The bronchial cuff has also been known to herniate over the tracheal carina; and, in the case of a left-sided double-lumen tube, to obstruct ventilation to the right mainstem bronchus.

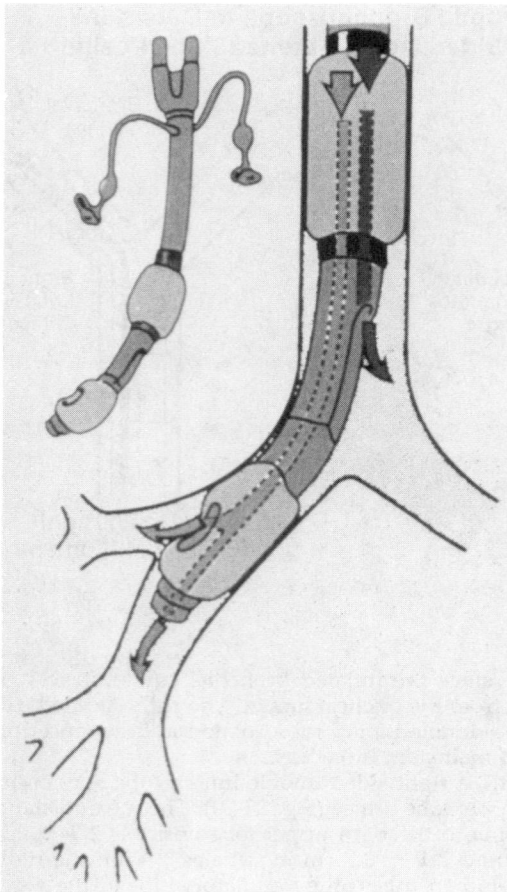

FIG. 33-20. A right-sided Robertshaw design double-lumen tube showing slotted endobronchial cuff overlying the origin of the right upper lobe bronchus. Malposition of the tube may cause the bronchial cuff to occlude the origin of the right upper lobe bronchus.

Another reported complication with double-lumen tubes is tracheal rupture. Guernelli *et al*[56] reported 5 of 2700 patients with tracheobronchial rupture caused by intubation with Carlens tubes. Most of these were thought to be secondary to the carinal hook or use of an inappropriately sized tube. Overinflation of the bronchial cuff, inappropriate positioning, and trauma due to intraoperative dislocation that resulted in bronchial rupture have also been described in association with the Robertshaw tube and the disposable double-lumen tube.[57] Therefore, the pressure in the bronchial cuff should be monitored and decreased if the cuff is found to be overinflated. If absolute separation of the lungs is not needed, the bronchial cuff should be deflated and then reinflated slowly to avoid excessive pressure on the bronchial walls. The bronchial cuff should also be deflated during any repositioning of the patient unless lung separation is absolutely required during this time.

CONTRAINDICATIONS TO USE OF THE DOUBLE-LUMEN TUBE. Use of a double-lumen tube to achieve lung separation is relatively contraindicated in situations where there is a lesion in the airway itself or a difficult upper airway that results in poor laryngeal visualization, and in some critically ill patients in whom short periods of apnea or hypoxemia, which

may occur during insertion of a double-lumen tube, may be life-threatening. In patients requiring rapid intubation (*i.e.* full stomach), a double-lumen tube is not necessarily contraindicated, since the disposable tubes with stylets are as easily inserted as a single-lumen tube in most cases.

MANAGEMENT OF ONE-LUNG VENTILATION

This section will discuss the management of one-lung ventilation in a paralyzed patient in the lateral decubitus position with an open chest. Inspired oxygen fraction (FI_{O_2}), V_T and respiratory rate, dependent lung PEEP, and non-dependent lung CPAP will be reviewed, and an approach to the management of one-lung ventilation will be presented.

INSPIRED OXYGEN FRACTION

Usually, an FI_{O_2} of 1.0 is used during one-lung ventilation. This high oxygen concentration serves to protect against hypoxemia during the procedure. In many studies, an FI_{O_2} of 1.0 has been used, and resulted in mean Pa_{O_2} values between 150 and 210 mm Hg during one-lung ventilation.[58-61] In addition to a higher margin of safety, high inspired oxygen fractions cause vasodilatation of the vessels in the dependent lung, which increases the capability of this lung to accept blood flow redistribution due to non-dependent lung HPV. A high FI_{O_2} may, however, cause absorption atelectasis and potentially further increase the degree of shunt because of the collapsed alveoli.[62] The risk can be reduced by using a lower FI_{O_2}, by the application of positive pressure ventilation, or by the use of a high V_T and positive end-expiratory pressure (PEEP). Theoretically, a high FI_{O_2} can also cause lung injury due to oxygen toxicity, although this complication is unlikely to occur in the time frame of a surgical operation. Lower oxygen concentrations have been used in the past[63, 64] and more recently,[65, 66] with resulting Pa_{O_2} values as shown in Table 33-3.

The use of an FI_{O_2} inhaled less than 1.0 during one-lung ventilation offers the benefits of reducing the risk of absorption atelectasis, and may permit use of lower concentrations of potent inhaled anesthetics, which, in higher concentrations, might be more depressant to the myocardium, particularly in high-risk patients. An FI_{O_2} of less than 1.0 may also be indicated in patients with bleomycin toxicity.[68] The combination of N_2O/O_2 with pulse oximetry monitoring represents an optimal solution in such cases. However, the risk/benefit for each patient should always be carefully considered.

TIDAL VOLUME AND RESPIRATORY RATE

During one-lung ventilation, the dependent lung should be ventilated with a V_T of 10–12 ml·kg^{-1}. Tidal volumes ranging between 8 and 15 ml·kg^{-1} produced no significant effect on transpulmonary shunt or Pa_{O_2}.[67] A V_T of less than 8 ml·kg^{-1} can result in a decrease in FRC and enhanced formation of atelectasis in the dependent lung. A V_T of greater than 15 ml·kg^{-1} can increase the PVR of the dependent lung (similar to the application of PEEP) and divert blood flow into the non-dependent lung. The value of 10–12 ml·kg^{-1} is a middle range between 8 and 15 ml·kg^{-1} and appears to have the least effect on Pa_{O_2} and percent shunt ($\dot{Q}_s/\dot{Q}_t$).[60]

The respiratory rate should be adjusted to maintain a Pa_{CO_2} 40 ± 3mm/Hg. Elimination of CO_2 is usually not a problem

TABLE 33-3.   Mean Pa_{O_2} during One-Lung Ventilation Using $F_{I_{O_2}} = 0.5$

INVESTIGATORS	REF NO.	NO. OF PATIENTS	$F_{I_{O_2}}$	TWO LUNG Pa_{O_2} (mm Hg)	ONE LUNG Pa_{O_2} (mm Hg)
Lunding and Fernandes	63	6	0.50	163	77
Lunding and Fernandes	63	15	0.25	98	67
Khanam and Branthwaite	170	28	0.40	NR	73
Torda *et al*	64	9	0.50	116	64
Torda *et al*	64	10	0.35	126	62
Jenkins *et al*	65	10	0.50	165	87
Cohen *et al*	66	20	0.50	248	80

NR = not reported.

during one-lung ventilation, if the double-lumen tube is positioned correctly. The shunt during one-lung ventilation has little influence on Pa_{CO_2} values, since the $P_{(A-\bar{v})CO_2}$ difference is normally only 6 mm/Hg. Furthermore, CO_2 is 20 times more diffusible than O_2. It is also important not to hyperventilate the patient's lungs, because hypocapnia will increase dependent lung PVR, inhibit non-dependent lung HPV, increase shunt, and decrease Pa_{O_2}. Finally, one-lung ventilation decreases the $(\dot{V}_D/\dot{V}_T)$ ratio and enhances CO_2 elimination.

PEEP TO THE DEPENDENT LUNG

The beneficial effect of selective PEEP 10 cm H_2O ($PEEP_{10}$) to the dependent lung is due to an increased lung volume at end-expiration (FRC), which improves the V/Q relationship in the dependent lung. The increase in FRC prevents airway and alveolar closure at end-expiration. Therefore, it is not surprising that attempts have been made to improve oxygenation during one-lung ventilation by the application of PEEP to the dependent lung. However, the results were somewhat disappointing (Table 33-4). Most of the studies showed either no change in Pa_{O_2}, a decrease, or a slight increase in Pa_{O_2},[61, 66-67, 69] probably due to the PEEP inducing an increase in lung volume that caused compression of the small interalveolar vessels and increased PVR. If this increase in resistance is limited to the dependent lung, blood flow can only be diverted to the non-dependent lung, increasing Q_s/Q_t and further decreasing Pa_{O_2}.

The studies of PEEP cited above used an $F_{I_{O_2}} = 1.0$ with a

mean Pa_{O_2} during one-lung ventilation of between 150 and 200 mm Hg, where further improvement in Pa_{O_2} is clinically unnecessary. The possibility that, in a diseased dependent lung (low lung volume and low V/Q ratio) with a low Pa_{O_2} (below 80 mm Hg) during one-lung ventilation, the application of PEEP can improve Pa_{O_2} has been addressed by Cohen et al.[70] Using an $F_{I_{O_2}} = 0.5$ in 18 patients, 11 patients had a Pa_{O_2} below 80 mm Hg during one-lung ventilation. The application of $PEEP_{10}$ significantly increased Pa_{O_2} in 10 out of 11 patients. In the other group of seven patients, who had Pa_{O_2} greater than 80 mm Hg with one-lung ventilation, the application of $PEEP_{10}$ did not improve mean Pa_{O_2}. It was concluded from this study that the application of $PEEP_{10}$ during one-lung ventilation in patients with a low Pa_{O_2} may increase FRC to normal values, resulting in a lower PVR and in improved V/Q ratio and Pa_{O_2}. Presumably, patients with a higher Pa_{O_2} had a dependent lung with an adequate FRC, and the application of PEEP had the negative effect of distributing blood flow away from the dependent ventilated lung (Fig. 33-21).

CONTINUOUS POSITIVE AIRWAY PRESSURE (CPAP) TO THE NON-DEPENDENT LUNG

The single most effective maneuver to increase Pa_{O_2} during one-lung ventilation is the application of CPAP to the non-dependent lung. This has been clearly demonstrated in several studies.[61, 66, 71] A lower level of CPAP (5–10 cm H_2O) maintains the patency of the non-dependent alveoli, allowing some oxygen uptake to occur in the distended alveoli. The

TABLE 33-4.   Effect of PEEP on Pa_{O_2} During One-Lung Ventilation in Man

INVESTIGATORS	REF NO.	NO. OF PATIENTS	$F_{I_{O_2}}$	PEEP cm H_2O	Pa_{O_2} (mm Hg) DURING ONE-LUNG VENTILATION WITH ZEEP	Pa_{O_2} (mm Hg) ONE-LUNG VENTILATION WITH PEEP
Tarhan and Lundborg	58	14	1.0	10	170	120
Aalto-Setala *et al*	171	11	1.0	5	160	153 (NS)
Capan *et al*	61	11	1.0	10	155	85
Katz *et al*	67	17	1.0	10 ($V_T = 7$ ml · kg^{-1})	184	157 (NS)
Katz *et al*	67	17	1.0	10 ($V_T = 7$ ml · kg^{-1})	210	162
Cohen *et al*	70	17	0.5	10	80	105 (NS)

ZEEP = zero end expiratory pressure.
NS = not statistically significant.

CPAP should be applied after delivering a V_T to the non-dependent lung to keep it slightly expanded. The CPAP, applied by insufflation of oxygen under positive pressure, will keep this lung "quiet" and prevent it from collapsing completely. Inflation of oxygen without maintaining a positive pressure failed to improve Pa_{O_2},[61, 71] although some improvement in Pa_{O_2} occurred after 45 min of one-lung ventilation (from 140 ± 107 to 206 ± 76 mm Hg) with oxygen insufflation only.[72] The beneficial effects of $CPAP_{10}$ are not due solely to the

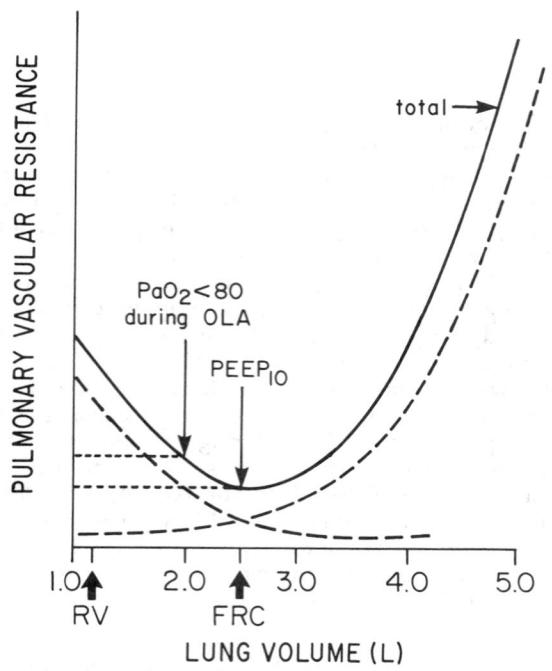

FIG. 33-21. Effect of $PEEP_{10}$ on FRC. It is postulated that, in patients having $Pa_{O_2} < 80$ mm Hg with ZEEP, FRC is low. $PEEP_{10}$ increases FRC and thereby increases Pa_{O_2}. PEEP = positive end expiratory pressure (10 cm H_2O); OLA = one-lung anesthesia; FRC = functional residual capacity; RV = residual volume; ZEEP = zero end expiratory pressure.

effect of positive pressure in causing blood flow diversion away from the collapsed lung, since Alfery *et al* showed, in dogs, that the hyperinflation of N_2 into the non-dependent lung under 10 cm H_2O failed to improve Pa_{O_2}.[71]

The application of high-level CPAP (15 cm H_2O) is not beneficial. At this pressure, the lung becomes over-distended and interferes with surgical exposure. Also, this level of CPAP might have hemodynamic consequences, while $CPAP_{10}$ has been shown to have no significant hemodynamic effects.[66, 73]

CPAP can be applied to the non-dependent lung using a number of simple systems.[74-77] All these systems have essentially the same features: an O_2 source, tubing to connect the oxygen source to the non-ventilated lung, a pressure relief valve, and a pressure gauge. The catheter to the non-dependent lung is usually insufflated with $5\ l \cdot min^{-1}$ of O_2 using a modified Ayre's T-piece pediatric circuit, and the valve on the expiratory limb is adjusted to the desired pressure as read on the attached gauge (Fig. 33-22). Instead of a pressure gauge or manometer inserted into the circuit, Brown *et al* described the use of a weighted pop-off valve, such as a ball or spring-loaded PEEP valve.[78]

High-frequency ventilation (HFV) with oxygen to the non-dependent lung and conventional ventilation to the dependent lung has also been used to improve Pa_{O_2} during one-lung ventilation (see section on HFV).

CLINICAL APPROACH TO MANAGEMENT OF ONE-LUNG VENTILATION

Once the patient is in the lateral position, the position of the double-lumen tube should be rechecked. Two-lung ventilation should be maintained for as long as possible, and, when one-lung ventilation needs to be instituted, it is recommended that an $FI_{O_2} = 1.0$ be used. The lungs should be ventilated using a V_T of 10–12 ml $\cdot$ kg^{-1} at a rate adjusted to maintain Pa_{CO_2} at 35 ± 3 mm Hg. This is usually monitored with the use of a mass spectrometer or capnograph.

Following the initiation of one-lung ventilation, Pa_{O_2} can continue to decrease for up to 45 min.[67] Close monitoring of arterial blood gases or use of a pulse oximeter should be available throughout the operative period. It is also essential to work closely with the surgeon. If there are any questions

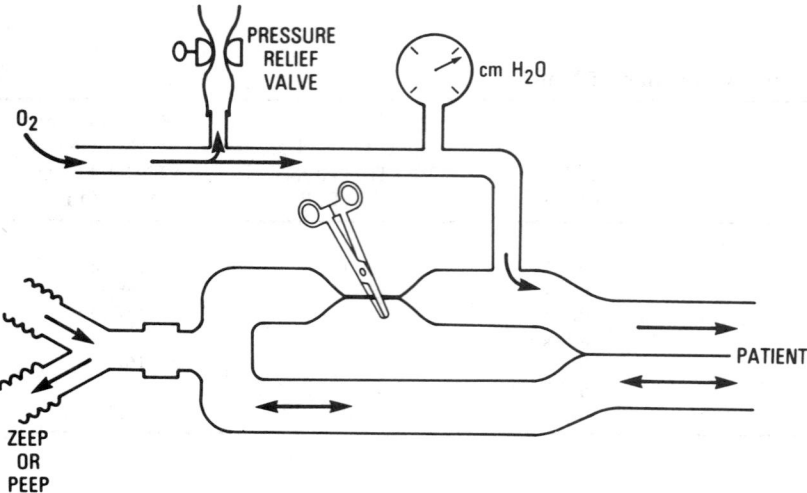

FIG. 33-22. Schematic of a simple, selective up-lung CPAP system. The fresh inflow of oxygen is restricted or limited by a pressure release valve and, therefore, a constant distending airway pressure to the nonventilated lung occurs. The dependent lung can be ventilated with positive end-expiratory pressure (PEEP) or zero end-expiratory pressure (ZEEP). (Benumof JL: Physiology of the open-chest and one lung ventilation. In Kaplan JA [ed]: Thoracic Anesthesia. New York, Churchill-Livingstone, 1983. Reproduced by permission.)

concerning the position of the double-lumen tube position and if fiberoptic bronchoscopy is not available, then the surgeon can palpate the tube and help to manipulate it into correct position with direct digital guidance.

If hypoxemia occurs during one-lung ventilation, the position of the double-lumen tube should be rechecked using a fiberoptic bronchoscope. If the dependent lung is not severely diseased, a satisfactory Pa_{O_2} on two-lung ventilation should not decrease to dangerously hypoxic levels on one-lung ventilation. If a left thoracotomy is being performed using a right-sided double-lumen tube, the ventilation to the right upper lobe should be assured. After the tube position has been confirmed as being correct, $CPAP_{10}$ should be applied to the non-dependent lung following a V_T that expands the lung. In most cases, the Pa_{O_2} will increase to a safe level. If a CPAP device is not readily available and the Pa_{O_2} is below 80 mm Hg, $PEEP_{10}$ can be applied to the dependent lung. The combination of $CPAP_{5-10}$ with $PEEP_{5-10}$ can be applied in different combinations in search of optimal oxygenation.

In the very rare case in which, despite all of these maneuvers, the Pa_{O_2} remains low, intermittent two-lung ventilation can be reinstituted with the surgeon's cooperation. Also, depending upon the stage of surgical dissection, if a pneumonectomy is being performed, ligation of the pulmonary artery will eliminate the shunt.

During one-lung ventilation, the peak airway pressure, the effective V_T delivered (measured by a spirometer), and the shape of the capnogram should be checked continuously. A sudden increase in peak airway pressure may be secondary to tube dislocation because of surgical manipulation, resulting in impaired ventilation. In addition, continuous auscultation by a stethoscope over the dependent lung is extremely important.

If any questions arise about the stability of the patient, or if the patient should become hypotensive, dusky, or tachycardic, two-lung ventilation should be resumed until the problem has been resolved. It should be remembered that the majority of thoracic surgical procedures represent only relative indications for one-lung ventilation. Because of pericardial manipulation (left thoracotomy, in particular) and pulling on the great vessels, cardiac dysrhythmias and hypotension are not uncommon. Cardiotonic drugs should be prepared and kept available for use during any thoracic surgical procedures.

CHOICE OF ANESTHESIA FOR THORACIC SURGERY

The choice of anesthetic technique for thoracic surgical procedures must take into account the patient's cardiovascular and respiratory status and the particular effects of anesthetic drugs on these and other organ systems.

Thoracic surgical patients are more likely than others to have increased airway reactivity and a propensity to develop bronchoconstriction. This is because many of these patients are cigarette smokers and have chronic bronchitis and/or COPD. In addition, surgical manipulation of the airways and bronchial tree by instruments, double-lumen tube, or surgeon make bronchoconstriction more likely to occur. The potent inhaled drugs halothane, enflurane, and isoflurane have all been shown to decrease airways reactivity and bronchoconstriction provoked by hypocapnia or inhaled or irritant aerosols. Their mechanism of action is probably a direct one on the airway musculature itself, and these agents are, therefore, the drugs of choice in patients with reactive airways. For an inhalation induction, halothane might be preferable, since it is

the least pungent of the three drugs, although, once the patient is asleep, isoflurane may be the preferred drug because it increases the cardiac dysrhythmia threshold and provides greater cardiovascular stability. Fentanyl does not appear to influence bronchomotor tone, but morphine may increase tone by a central vagotonic effect and by releasing histamine.

In most patients, anesthesia is safely induced with a barbiturate, thiopental or thiamylal. In patients with reactive airways, ketamine may be the drug of choice for induction of anesthesia because it has a bronchodilator effect and has been successfully used in the treatment of asthma. Thiopental has been associated with bronchospasm in asthmatic patients, although the reactivity in such cases may be related to inadequate levels of anesthesia prior to instrumentation of the airway.

The muscle relaxants of choice for thoracic procedures are those that lack a histamine-releasing or vagotonic effect and that have some sympathomimetic effect. In this respect, pancuronium and vecuronium probably represent the drugs of choice. Succinylcholine is useful to provide rapid profound relaxation for intubation of the trachea, and is not associated with an increase in airways reactivity.

Intravenous lidocaine ($1-2$ mg·kg^{-1}) can be used prior to manipulations of the airway to prevent reflex bronchospasm. It has also been given by infusion to depress airways reactivity in patients who have poor cardiovascular function and cannot tolerate normal doses of the potent inhaled drugs. Intravenous lidocaine has also been used to treat bronchospasm occurring during anesthesia. Lidocaine nebulized and administered via the airways has a similar salutary effect on bronchial tone.

Atropine may be used to block the antimuscarinic effects of acetylcholine and thereby protect against cholinergically induced bronchoconstriction. It may be administered iv or in nebulized form (see section on Bronchoscopy).

HYPOXIC PULMONARY VASOCONSTRICTION (HPV)

General anesthesia may impair pulmonary gas exchange, and arterial hypoxemia may occur as a result. In patients undergoing halothane-oxygen anesthesia with spontaneous two-lung ventilation, Nunn found a calculated shunt of 14% of pulmonary blood flow as compared to a calculated shunt of 1% in normal conscious supine patients measured using the same techniques.[79] He suggested that the large shunt observed was probably due to perfusion of totally unventilated parts of the lung. Marshall et al confirmed this, and concluded that postoperative hypoxemia may also be a result of the residual effects of the anesthetic on venous admixture.[80] With this background, many investigators have studied the regulation of the pulmonary circulation through a homeostatic mechanism called HPV, which normally diverts blood away from hypoxic regions of the lung and thereby optimizes the gas exchange function of the lung.

HPV was first described by Von Euler and Liljestrand in 1946.[81] They were studying changes in the pulmonary circulation of the cat in response to changes in inspired gas mixtures, and found that 10.5% inspired O_2 (in N_2) mixtures caused an increase in pulmonary arterial pressure. Breathing 100% O_2 caused a decrease in pulmonary arterial pressure. They concluded that the increased pressure during hypoxia was due to a direct effect on the pulmonary vessels. Whereas they delivered hypoxic gas mixtures to both lungs, others have studied the effects of the size of the hypoxic segment and the size of the hypoxic stimulus on perfusion pressure and on flow diversion. Thus, Marshall *et al* studied the effects of changing FI_{O_2} in lung segments of seven different sizes in a dog model.[82] In each test, the rest of the lung received oxygen, while HPV in the test segment was demonstrated by both increased perfusion pressure and diversion of blood flow away from the hypoxic test segment. Marshall *et al* found that pulmonary perfusion changes increased with the size of the hypoxic segment from zero (smallest hypoxic segment) to approximately 2.2 times baseline for the hypoxic whole lung. Flow diversion, as a percentage of flow to the test segment under normoxic conditions, decreased with increasing size of the hypoxic test segment from a maximum of 75% for very small segments to zero when the whole lung was made hypoxic. Flow diversion increased linearly as Pa_{O_2} was decreased over the range of 128 to 28 mm Hg. In both flow diversion and changes in perfusion pressure, the response to HPV was predictable, continuous, and maximal at a predicted Pa_{O_2} of 30 mm Hg (4% oxygen). Thus, HPV causes a rise in both perfusion (pulmonary arterial) pressure and flow diversion.

The choice of anesthetic technique for one-lung ventilation must take into consideration the effects on oxygenation and, therefore, on HPV. Normally, collapse of the non-ventilated, non-dependent lung results in activation of reflex HPV in this lung. This causes local increases in pulmonary vascular resistance and diversion of blood flow to other better-oxygenated parts of the pulmonary vascular bed (*i.e.*, the dependent oxygenated and ventilated lung). The stimulus to HPV appears to be a function of both Pa_{O_2} and $P\bar{v}_{O_2}$ in lungs ventilated with hypoxic mixtures, but, in the atelectatic lung, the stimulus is the $P\bar{v}_{O_2}$.[83] The response is believed to be accounted for by each smooth muscle cell in the pulmonary arterial wall responding to the oxygen tension in its vicinity. Because HPV causes flow diversion, Pa_{O_2} should be higher than if there were no HPV. The relationship between Pa_{O_2} and the size of the hypoxic segment (Fig. 33-23) shows that, when little of the lung is hypoxic, HPV has little effect on Pa_{O_2} because, in this

situation, shunt will be small. When most of the lung is hypoxic, there is no significant normoxic region to which the hypoxic region can divert flow, and then it does not matter, in terms of Pa_{O_2}, whether the hypoxic region has active HPV or not. When the amount of lung made hypoxic is 30–70%, such as occurs during one-lung ventilation, then there may be a large difference between the Pa_{O_2} to be expected with normal HPV as compared to that expected in its absence. HPV can raise Pa_{O_2} from potentially dangerous levels to higher and safer ones. Conversely, inhibition of HPV may cause or contribute to hypoxemia during anesthesia.

EFFECTS OF ANESTHETICS ON HPV

All of the inhaled and many of the intravenous drugs used in anesthesia have been studied for their effects on HPV. The results have not always been consistent. Benumof has classified the preparations used to study these effects as *in vitro*, *in vivo*, non-intact, *in vivo* intact, and human studies.[84] In the *in vitro* preparations, such as isolated rat lungs in which all variables could be controlled, it was found that HPV was depressed in a dose-related manner by all potent inhaled anesthetics,[85] but not by intravenous agents.[86] In the *in vivo*, non-intact preparation, such as the dog in which the left lower lobe had been isolated for ventilation purposes, the inhaled agents had variable effects on HPV,[87, 88] while intravenous agents had no effect.[89] In the *in vivo*, intact dog preparations, inhaled drugs have been shown to depress HPV,[90] while intravenous drugs had no effect.[91] Based upon the results of the above three types of preparation, it is generally believed that inhaled drugs inhibit HPV, whereas intravenous drugs do not have this effect.

Human studies are, perhaps, the most significant because of their applicability to the clinical situation. Bjertnaes used perfusion scans (scintigraphy) to assess the effect of anesthetics on human HPV.[92] In his patients, lung separation was

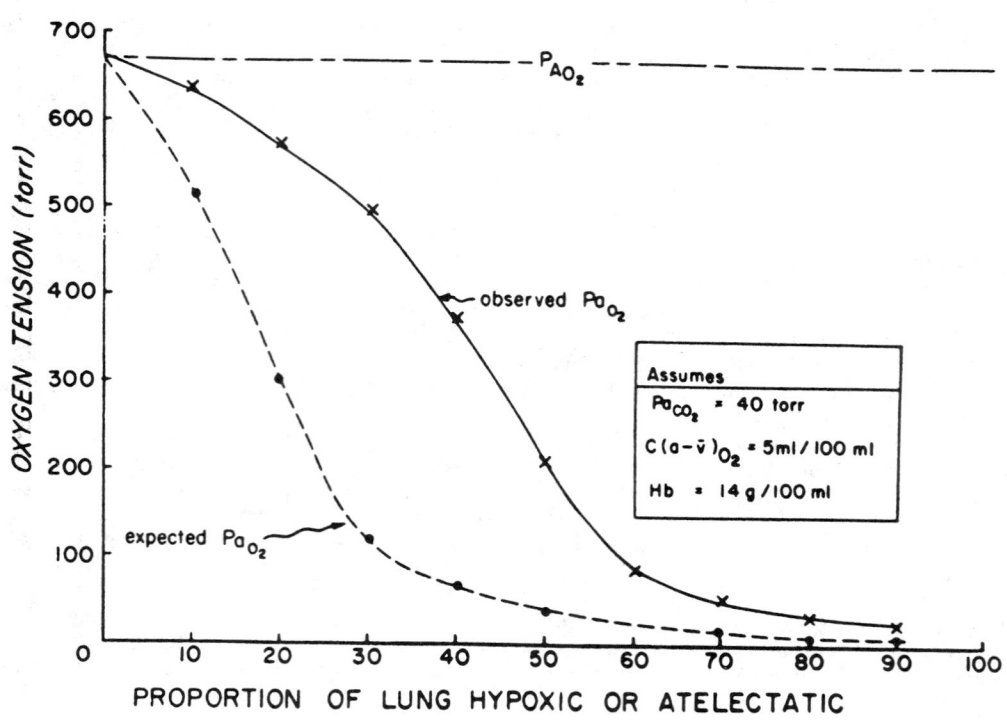

FIG. 33-23. Role of hypoxic vasoconstriction (HPV) in preserving Pa_{O_2} (in dogs). Assumptions are shown in insert. Lung is ventilated with $FI_{O_2} = 1.0$, while increasing portions of lung are subjected to hypoxia or atelectasis. In the absence of HPV, the expected Pa_{O_2} would follow the broken line, whereas, in the presence of an active HPV response, observed Pa_{O_2} is maintained close to the solid line. (Adapted from Marshall BE *et al*: HPV in dogs: Effects of lung segment size and oxygen tension. J Appl Physiology 51:1543, 1981. Reproduced by permission.)

achieved using a double-lumen tube. One lung could then be ventilated with 100% O_2 and the other with 100% N_2. HPV was assessed in the presence and absence of ether, halothane, and intravenous drugs (thiopental and fentanyl). Based upon his scintigraphic findings, Bjertnaes concluded that the inhalation agents, in clinically useful concentrations, inhibited HPV in humans.

Jolin Carlsson et al used separate lung ventilation and a triple gas washout technique to study HPV in eight patients.[93] They demonstrated the presence of HPV in response to 8% O_2 in 92% N_2 in the test lung, but found no further change with the addition of 1.0 or 1.5% end-tidal isoflurane, and blood gases remained essentially unaltered. Attempts to use higher concentrations caused unacceptable hypotension. These authors concluded that isoflurane might be indicated for anesthesia in the presence of lung disease or during one-lung ventilation, since arterial oxygenation might be better preserved than would be the case with an anesthetic that more effectively inhibited HPV. Thus, while it is possible that higher concentrations of isoflurane might have caused a clear change in the differential blood flow distribution, at clinically used concentrations, the effect of HPV in their subjects was all but unmeasurable.

Others have studied the effects on oxygenation of intravenous and inhaled anesthetic techniques during one-lung ventilation. Weinreich et al[94] used a ketamine infusion and found a lower incidence of hypoxemia (defined as $Pa_{O_2} < 70$ mm Hg) than other studies reporting the use of halothane for one-lung ventilation. Rees and Gaines[95] compared a ketamine-oxygen technique with an enflurane (1–3% inspired)-oxygen technique for one-lung ventilation, and found no differences between the groups in Pa_{O_2} or shunt. These findings suggested that ketamine afforded no advantage over enflurane during one-lung ventilation.

Rogers and Benumof[96] compared the effects of inhaled (isoflurane and halothane) with intravenous (methohexital and ketamine) anesthesia during one-lung ventilation, and concluded that the inhaled drugs at about 1-MAC concentrations do not significantly affect HPV in humans, as evidenced by a lack of significant differences in Pa_{O_2} between use of the two techniques.

In a subsequent study, Benumof et al investigated the changes in Pa_{O_2} and shunt that occurred following conversion from 1-MAC halothane or isoflurane anesthesia to intravenous anesthesia (fentanyl, diazepam, and sodium thiopental) during one-lung ventilation for thoracic surgery in 12 patients.[97] In this study, they found that, during one-lung atelectasis, 1-MAC halothane anesthesia slightly but significantly increased shunt and decreased Pa_{O_2} (compared to intravenous anesthesia), whereas 1-MAC isoflurane anesthesia very slightly but nonsignificantly increased shunt and decreased Pa_{O_2} (compared to intravenous anesthesia). Fundamental differences between the two studies[96, 97] were in the duration of the periods of one-lung ventilation with the potent inhalational drug, and in the MAC multiples of the drugs used. In the earlier study,[96] end-tidal concentrations of halothane and isoflurane were kept constant for approximately 20 min at 1.45 and 1.15 MAC, respectively. In the later study,[97] patients were maintained with one-lung anesthesia with the potent inhaled drug (1 MAC) for 40 min before final measurements under these conditions were taken.[97] The authors also concluded that halothane and isoflurane had only a small inhibitory effect on the one-lung HPV response.[97]

The contrast between the results of the in vitro and in vivo studies in sufficiently striking to suggest that other variables are obscuring the effects of inhibition of HPV in the in vivo studies. One such variable is CO, which is altered to a mark-edly different extent by different inhaled drugs. Studying this relationship, Marshall found that the effectiveness of HPV varied inversely with CO.[98] Thus, during the administration of halothane, a direct inhibition of HPV may be offset by the enhanced responsiveness accompanying decreased cardiac output, with the result that flow diversion and gas exchange (as assessed by Pa_{O_2}), and, by inference, HPV, may also appear to be unaffected. This may explain the findings in some of the human studies.

Thus, overall, the potent inhaled anesthetics are the drugs of choice during thoracic surgery. The technique chosen should, however, always be dictated by the needs of the particular patient, so that, in the presence of cardiovascular instability or poor oxygenation where depression of HPV is a possibility, a balanced technique may be preferable.

OTHER DETERMINANTS OF HPV

Aside from potent inhaled drugs, other drugs and maneuvers used during anesthesia may also have an inhibitory effect on regional or whole-lung HPV. Factors associated with an increase in pulmonary arterial pressure will antagonize the effect of increased resistance due to HPV, and will result in increased flow to the hypoxic region. Such indirect inhibitors of HPV include mitral stenosis, volume overload, thromboembolism, hypothermia, vasoconstrictor drugs, and a large hypoxic lung segment. Direct inhibitors of HPV include infection; vasodilator drugs, such as nitroglycerin and nitroprusside; hypocarbia; and metabolic alkalemia. All of these potential inhibitors should be considered when evaluating a patient for hypoxemia during thoracic surgery.

POTENTIATORS OF HPV

Whereas, in the past, most of the research effort has been directed to studying inhibition of HPV, more recent research has investigated substances that may potentiate HPV. Almitrine, a respiratory stimulant drug, has been found to improve Pa_{O_2} in patients with COPD and to have this effect in the absence of ventilatory stimulation. Indirect evidence suggested that it may potentiate HPV in intact dogs, although a subsequent and more extensive dog study concluded that almitrine caused non-specific pulmonary vasoconstriction that was greater in the 100% O_2-ventilated lung than in the hypoxic lung regions, thus causing a reduction of the HPV response.[99]

It has been suggested that prostaglandins have a role in HPV inhibition and, therefore, prostaglandin inhibitors have been investigated as potentiators of HPV. Ibuprofen, a cyclo-oxygenase inhibitor, has been found to potentiate HPV in hypoxic isolated rat lung preparation and to reverse the inhibition of HPV caused by halothane.[100] The value, if any, of such potentiators in humans undergoing one-lung anesthesia has not yet been reported.

ANESTHESIA FOR DIAGNOSTIC PROCEDURES

BRONCHOSCOPY

The translaryngeal approach to bronchoscopy was first described by Killian at the turn of the century, when he introduced an esophagoscope under topical anesthesia with cocaine to remove an aspirated pork bone from the right

TABLE 33-5.   Indications for Bronchoscopy

Diagnostic	Therapeutic
Cough	Foreign bodies
Hemoptysis	Accumulated secretions
Wheeze	Atelectasis
Atelectasis	Aspiration
Unresolved pneumonia	Lung abscess
Diffuse lung disease	Reposition endotracheal
Preoperative evaluation	tubes
Rule out metastases	Placement of
Abnormal chest x-ray	endobronchial tubes
Assess local disease recurrence	Laser surgery
Recurrent laryngeal nerve palsy	
Diaphragm paralysis	
Acute inhalation injury	
Exclude tracheo-esophageal	
fistula	
During mechanical ventilation	
Selective bronchography	

(Adapted from Landa JF: Indications for bronchoscopy. Chest 73 (suppl): 686, 1978, with permission of author and publisher.)

bronchus. Early bronchoscopes were of the rigid type, but, in 1966, the Machida and Olympus Companies introduced the first practical bronchofiberscopes. Since then, these have been improved dramatically, and have simplified many otherwise complicated bronchoscopies. The indications for bronchoscopy are shown in Table 33-5, and the instruments of choice in Table 33-6. Operator preferences and experience may play a major role in the choice of instrument.

Prior to bronchoscopy, the patient must be evaluated preoperatively for chronic lung disease, respiratory obstruction, bronchospasm, coughing, hemoptysis, and infectivity of secretions. Medications should be reviewed and the need for a more major procedure should always be anticipated. Thus, bronchoscopy may lead to thoracotomy or sternotomy. The planned technique for bronchoscopy should be discussed with the surgeon preoperatively, and all equipment and connectors should be checked for compatibility. Monitoring dur-

TABLE 33-6.   Instrument of Choice for Bronchoscopy

Rigid
Foreign bodies
Massive hemoptysis
Vascular tumors
Small children
Endobronchial resections

Fiberoptic/Flexible
Mechanical problems of neck
Upper lobe and peripheral lesions
Limited hemoptysis
During mechanical ventilation
Pneumonia, for selective cultures
Positioning of double-lumen tubes
Difficult intubation
Checking position of endotracheal tube
Bronchial blockade

Combination
Positive cytology with negative chest x-ray

(Adapted from Landa JF: Indications for bronchoscopy. Chest 73 (suppl): 686, 1978, with permission of author & publisher.)

ing bronchoscopy should include an ECG, a blood pressure cuff, a precordial stethoscope, and a pulse oximeter. If thoracotomy is planned, an arterial cannula should also be placed, as well as other monitors (*e.g.,* PA or CVP catheters) that may be indicated by the patient's condition. There are many anesthetic techniques that are useful for bronchoscopy.

Local Anesthesia

The patient should first be pretreated with a drying agent, such as atropine, glycopyrrolate, or scopolamine. The local anesthetics most commonly used are lidocaine and tetracaine. In all cases, the total dose of anesthetic must be considered and the potential for toxicity recognized. A nebulizer can be used to spray the oropharynx and base of the tongue, or the patient may gargle viscous lidocaine. The tongue is then held forward, and pledgets soaked in local anesthetic are held in each pyriform fossa using Krause's forceps to achieve block of the internal branch of the superior laryngeal nerve. Tracheal anesthesia is achieved either by a transtracheal injection of local anesthetic or by spraying the cords and trachea under direct vision, using a laryngoscope, or *via* the suction channel of the bronchofiberscope. Alternatively, a superior laryngeal nerve block can be performed by an external approach, and a glossopharyngeal block can be used to depress the gag reflex. These blocks cause depression of airway reflexes, so that patients must be kept NPO for several hours following the bronchoscopy. If a fiberoptic bronchoscopy is to be performed transnasally, the nasal mucosa should be pretreated topically with 4% cocaine, and/or viscous lidocaine may be administered through the nares. Local anesthesia for bronchoscopy has the advantage that the patient is awake, cooperative, and breathing spontaneously. Sedatives may be added to make the patient more comfortable. Disadvantages are poor tolerance of any bleeding and the occasional lack of patient cooperation.

General Anesthesia

General anesthesia for bronchoscopy is often combined with topical laryngeal anesthesia so that less general anesthesia is needed. A balanced technique uses N_2O/O_2, incremental doses of an intravenous drug such as thiopental, an opioid (*e.g.,* fentanyl), and a muscle relaxant (*e.g.,* succinylcholine, atracurium, vecuronium). A potent inhaled drug technique (*e.g.,* O_2/halothane or N_2O/O_2/halothane) is also satisfactory, although the use of N_2O may cause some optical distortion for the surgeon because of changes in the refractive index of the gas mixture. Additionally, the use of N_2O and potent inhaled drugs creates an operating room contamination problem for the waste anesthesia gases, but limited scavenging may be possible by placing a suction catheter into the patient's oropharynx. Unless there is some contraindication, ventilation of the lungs is generally controlled. In any patient undergoing a thoracic diagnostic procedure for a suspected malignancy, the possibility of the myasthenic syndrome with sensitivity to nondepolarizing muscle relaxants must always be considered. Muscle relaxant doses should be titrated to effect using a neuromuscular monitoring system.

Rigid Bronchoscopy

A modern rigid ventilating bronchoscope is essentially a hollow tube with a blunted, bevelled tip. Various sizes and designs are available, but, in all, a side arm is provided for connection to an anesthesia source. A number of techniques have been described for maintaining ventilation and oxygenation during rigid bronchoscopy.

Apneic Oxygenation

Following pre-oxygenation and induction of general anesthesia and skeletal muscle paralysis, oxygen is insufflated at $10–15 \, l \cdot min^{-1}$ *via* a small catheter placed above the carina. If the patient has been adequately denitrogenated, this technique can provide adequate oxygenation for more than 30 min.[101] The apneic period should not be allowed to extend beyond 5 min, however, since the technique is limited by buildup of CO_2 (at a rate of $3 \, mm \, Hg \cdot min^{-1}$), respiratory acidosis, and cardiac dysrhythmias. Fraoli *et al*[102] demonstrated that the FRC/body weight ratio is important in considering apneic oxygenation techniques, and recommended that only patients with predicted FRC/body weight ratios of 50 $ml \cdot kg^{-1}$ or more have apneic oxygenation for longer than 5 min.

Apnea and Intermittent Ventilation

Oxygen and anesthesia gases are delivered to the bronchoscope *via* the anesthesia circuit. Ventilation is only possible when the eye piece is in place, and this limits the period for instrumentation by the surgeon. Intermittent ventilation of the lungs is achieved by squeezing the reservoir bag. In this way, assuming a good bronchoscope fit in the airway, compliance is constantly monitored, the risk of barotrauma is reduced, and V_T may be estimated. The disadvantage of this technique is that, with prolonged bronchoscopies, poor blood gases, in particular hypercarbia, may result. This may lead to cardiac dysrhythmias.

SANDERS INJECTION SYSTEM

Sanders applied the venturi principle to provide ventilation of the lungs by attaching a jet ventilator to the bronchoscope.[103] Oxygen from a high-pressure source (50 psi) is delivered, *via* a controllable pressure-reducing valve and toggle switch, to a 2.5 to 3.5 cm 18- or 16-gauge needle inside and parallel to the long axis of the bronchoscope. When the toggle switch is depressed, the jet of oxygen entering the bronchoscope entrains air, and the air/O_2 mixture resulting at the distal tip of the bronchoscope emerges at a pressure to provide adequate ventilation and oxygenation. The intraluminal tracheal pressure is a function of the driving pressure from the reducing valve, the size of the needle jet, and the length, internal diameter, and design of the bronchoscope. Increasing the size of the needle jet increases the total gas flow for any given driving pressure. For each combination of gas driving pressure, jet orifice, and bronchoscope diameter, only one inflation pressure can be attained, regardless of the volume or compliance of the lung. As long as the proximal end of the bronchoscope is open, the system is strictly pressure-limited, and the pressure will not rise because of obstruction at the distal end. Pressure varies inversely with the cross-sectional area of the bronchoscope, so that insertion of a suction catheter or biopsy forceps into the lumen causes the intratracheal pressure to increase. Provided there is not a tight fit between the bronchoscope and the airway, the risk of barotrauma is unlikely. If the fit is tight, driving pressure should be reduced.

The advantages of the Sanders system are that, because continuous ventilation is possible (since the presence of an eye piece is not necessary for ventilation of the lungs), the dura-

tion of the bronchoscopy procedure is minimized, but the efficiency also permits extended bronchoscopy. A disadvantage is that entrainment of air by the O_2 jet results in a variable FI_{O_2} at the distal end of the bronchoscope, ventilation of the lungs may be inadequate if compliance is poor, and adequacy of ventilation may be difficult to assess. Giesecke *et al* have compared the intermittent ventilation and the Sanders techniques, and found that Pa_{O_2} was satisfactory with either method, but it was higher in the intermittent ventilation group.[104] Pa_{CO_2} was lower and arterial *p*H higher in the Sanders group, indicating superiority of this method, particularly for long procedures.

The basic Sanders technique has been modified to increase FI_{O_2} and to deliver N_2O and potent inhaled drugs. Carden[105] has replaced the 16-gauge O_2 jet with a longer jet (Carden side arm) that allows ventilation with 100% O_2 and the development of much higher pressures at the tracheal end of the bronchoscope, while using a driving pressure of 50 psi. The Sanders injector system may also be used with a ventilating bronchoscope whose side arm is connected to a supply of anesthesia gases, so that the injection jet will entrain the anesthesia gases.

Mechanical Ventilator

Ventilation of the lungs may be achieved by attaching a mechanical ventilator to an anesthesia circuit connected to the bronchoscope side arm.

High-frequency Positive-pressure Ventilation

HFPPV has been used in conjunction with rigid bronchoscopy and compared to the Sanders injector in patients with tracheobronchial stenosis. With HFPPV of up to 150 $breaths \cdot min^{-1}$, blood gases were identical with both techniques. At a frequency of 500 $breaths \cdot min^{-1}$, oxygenation deteriorated and CO_2 was not removed effectively. HFPPV has the advantage that the tracheobronchial wall remains perfectly immobile during ventilation.[106]

Other Techniques

Cuirass ventilation, external chest compression, and a ventilating catheter or endotracheal tube placed alongside the bronchoscope have also been used to provide ventilation during bronchoscopy.

Fiberoptic Bronchoscopy

The new generations of fiberscopes, with their improved optics and smaller diameter, have revolutionized bronchoscopy. Examination of the fifth order of bronchial branching is now possible, and the diagnostic potential of this instrument is thereby enhanced. The flexibility has also been applied in preoperative assessment of the airway, management of difficult tracheal intubations, endotracheal tube positioning and change, bronchial toilet, correct positioning of double-lumen tubes, bronchial blockade, and evaluation of the larynx and trachea.[3, 107]

Nasal fiberoptic bronchoscopy under topical anesthesia is well tolerated by most awake patients. A suction catheter in the mouth is useful to remove oral secretions. Oral insertion is also possible in both awake and asleep patients, and should be performed *via* a specially designed airway, which guides the fiberscope over the back of the tongue and prevents potential damage by the patient's teeth.

PHYSIOLOGIC CHANGES ASSOCIATED WITH FIBEROPTIC BRONCHOSCOPY. In all patients, insertion of the fiberoptic bronchoscope is associated with hypoxemia. The average decline in Pa_{O_2} is 20 mm Hg, and lasts for 1–4 h after the procedure. By 24 h, the blood gases are usually back to normal. It is, therefore, recommended that if the initial Pa_{O_2} is <70 mm Hg ($F_{I_{O_2}} = 0.21$), bronchoscopy should be performed only with the administration of supplemental O_2. This can be provided using mouth-held nasal prongs, using a special face mask with a diaphragm through which the fiberscope can be passed, or *via* an endotracheal tube with a T-piece diaphragm adapter.

During and after fiberoptic bronchoscopy, patients develop increased airway obstruction. Matsushima *et al*[108] studied alterations in pulmonary mechanics in 35 patients, and found that insertion of the bronchoscope was associated with an increase in FRC (17–30%) and decreases in Pa_{O_2}, VC, FEV_1, and forced inspiratory flow (FIF). All returned to baseline by 24 h. These changes are thought to be secondary to direct mechanical activation of irritative reflexes in the airway and, possibly, also to mucosal edema. They may be avoided if atropine, either intramuscular or aerosolized into the airway, is administered preoperatively. Isoproterenol has a similar salutary effect on lung function, but is associated with an increased incidence of cardiac dysrhythmias. Overall, atropine is recommended as premedication for fiberoptic bronchoscopy. Concern that atropine may have an overall undesirable effect by increasing viscosity of secretions in patients with COPD is unsubstantiated.

The standard adult fiberoptic bronchoscope has an external diameter of 5.7 mm and a 2 mm-diameter suction channel. If suction at 1 atmosphere is applied to the fiberscope, air is removed at a rate of 14 liters/minute. If the fiberscope is in the airway, this will cause decreases in $F_{I_{O_2}}$, PA_{O_2}, and FRC, leading to decreased Pa_{O_2}. Suctioning should, therefore, be kept brief. The adult fiberscope will pass through endotracheal tubes of 7.0 mm or greater internal diameter. Clearly, passage through an endotracheal tube decreases the cross-sectional area available for ventilating the patient, so that, if fiberscopy is planned, the largest possible diameter endotracheal tube should be used.

Insertion of the bronchoscope also causes a significant PEEP effect, which may result in barotrauma in ventilated patients. If the patient is already being ventilated with PEEP, the latter should be discontinued prior to the passage of the bronchoscope. A post-endoscopy chest x-ray is advisable to exclude mediastinal emphysema or pneumothorax. In patients whose tracheae are intubated with endotracheal tubes of less than 8.0 mm internal diameter, use of pediatric fiberscopes, with diameters as small as 3.5 mm, would be more appropriate.

The suction channel of the adult fiberoptic bronchoscope has been used to oxygenate and ventilate the lungs of patients. By attaching a jet ventilation system (similar to that used to drive the Sanders injector for rigid bronchoscopy) to the suction connection at the head of a fiberoptic bronchoscope, Satyanaryama *et al*[109] were successful in ventilating lungs of patients undergoing gynecological procedures. A driving pressure of 50 psi of O_2 was used with a ventilatory rate of 18–20 per minute. Tracheal pressures of 6–8 mm Hg, tracheal oxygen concentrations of 88–93%, and Pa_{O_2} values of 340–478 mm Hg were obtained. This technique will permit adequate ventilation of patients with normally compliant lungs and chest walls, but, to date, has not been attempted in patients with lung disease. Ventilation of the lungs should only be performed with the tip of the instrument in the trachea, as a more peripheral location may produce barotrauma.

Neodymium-yttrium-aluminum garnet (Nd-YAG) lasers have recently been used for the resection of obstructing and endobronchial lesions. This procedure is conducted under general anesthesia. The lasers may be introduced into the bronchial tree through a fiberoptic bundle passed *via* the suction port of the fiberoptic bronchoscope. During laser resection, $F_{I_{O_2}}$ should be kept to a minimum and titrated against oxygen saturation (as continuously monitored by pulse oximeter) in order to make endotracheal fire less likely.[110] Laser therapy of bronchial tumors is also possible using a rigid bronchoscope.[111] Vourc'h *et al* found that HFPPV *via* a rigid bronchoscope provided satisfactory operating conditions for laser resection of tracheal tumors, and had the advantage of producing airway immobility.[106]

Complications of Bronchoscopy

Complications of rigid bronchoscopy include mechanical trauma to the teeth, hemorrhage, bronchospasm, loss of sponge, bronchial or tracheal perforation, subglottic edema, and barotrauma. The incidence of complications is much less with fiberoptic bronchoscopy. Nevertheless, complications may arise due to overdosage with topical anesthetic drug, insertion trauma, local trauma, hemorrhage, upper airway obstruction related to passage of the instrument through an area of tracheal stenosis, hypoxemia, and bronchospasm. In most cases, it is best to intubate the trachea with an endotracheal tube in patients following bronchoscopy under general anesthesia. This permits avoidance or treatment of some of these problems, particularly the increased airway irritability. Intubation also facilitates effective suctioning of the trachea and bronchi, and allows the patient to recover more gradually from a general anesthesia. Overall, with careful evaluation of the patient and an understanding of the techniques employed, bronchoscopy is a relatively safe procedure.[112]

DIAGNOSTIC PROCEDURES FOR MEDIASTINAL MASSES

Patients with an anterior mediastinal mass present a special problem to the anesthesiologist. While such masses may cause superior vena cava (SVC) obstruction that is obvious, they may also cause obstruction of major airways and cardiac compression, which is less obvious and may become apparent only upon induction of anesthesia. Neuman *et al*[113] described three cases of anterior mediastinal mass, in two of which airway obstruction occurred following induction of anesthesia and onset of paralysis. In the first case, total occlusion of the trachea starting 2–3 cm above the carina and extending to both mainstem bronchi was observed, and a bronchoscope was passed through the obstruction. In the second case, extrinsic compression of the left mainstem bronchus occurred on inspiration during recovery from anesthesia. In the third case of anterior mediastinal mass, flow-volume studies were performed in the upright and supine positions, and demonstrated marked reductions in FEV_1 and PEFR in the latter position. These findings suggested potential obstruction with onset of anesthesia, and radiotherapy to the mediastinum was commenced, following which, the flow-volume studies showed improved function. The surgical procedure planned was then performed under local anesthesia.

Airway obstruction due to an anterior mediastinal mass has been attributed to changes in lung and chest wall mechanics associated with changes in position, or to onset of paralysis in muscles that were previously maintaining airway patency. Neuman *et al* have proposed a flow chart (Fig. 33-24) describing the preoperative evaluation of a patient with an anterior mediastinal mass in order to avoid life-threatening total airway obstruction.[113] It is important to determine in the history if there is dyspnea in the supine position, and to examine the CT scan to determine the extent of the tumor and its effect on surrounding structures. If such obstruction occurs, it may be relieved by passage of a rigid bronchoscope or anode tube past the obstruction, by direct laryngoscopy,[114] or by changing the position of the patient.

In a situation where the biopsy procedure cannot be performed under local anesthesia (Fig. 33-24) and there is concern that muscle paralysis may result in airway compression, an awake fiberoptic intubation followed by general anesthesia with spontaneous ventilation has been described for thoracotomy.[115] Thus, during spontaneous inspiration, the normal transpulmonary pressure gradient distends the airways and helps to maintain their patency, even in the presence of extrinsic compression.

MEDIASTINOSCOPY

Mediastinoscopy was introduced by Carlens[116] as a means of assessing spread of carcinoma of the bronchus. The lymphatics of the lung drain first to the subcarinal and para-

tracheal areas, and then to the sides of the trachea, the supraclavicular areas, and the thoracic duct. Examination of these nodes has provided a tissue diagnosis and greater selectivity of patients for thoracotomy. It is most useful in right-lung tumors, since left-lung cancers tend to spread to subaortic nodes that are more accessible by an anterior mediastinoscopy in the second or third interspace (Chamberlain procedure). Apart from diagnostic uses, mediastinoscopy has also been used to place electrodes for atrial-triggered pacing.[117] The transcervical approach to the thymus is another adaptation of this technique.

The anesthetic considerations for mediastinoscopy follow naturally from an understanding of the anatomy of this procedure and its potential complications. For cervical mediastinoscopy, the patient is placed in reverse Trendelenburg position, and the mediastinoscope is inserted into the superior mediastinum *via* a transverse incision just above the suprasternal notch. The instrument is advanced along the anterior aspect of the trachea and passes behind the innominate vessels and the aortic arch (Fig. 33-25). The left recurrent nerve is vulnerable as it loops around the aortic arch, and any of

FIG. 33-24. Flow chart describing the preoperative evaluation of the patient with an anterior mediastinal mass. + indicates positive finding; − indicates negative work-up. (Neuman GG *et al*: Anesthetic management of the patient with an anterior mediastinal mass. Anesthesiology 60:144, 1984. Reproduced by permission.)

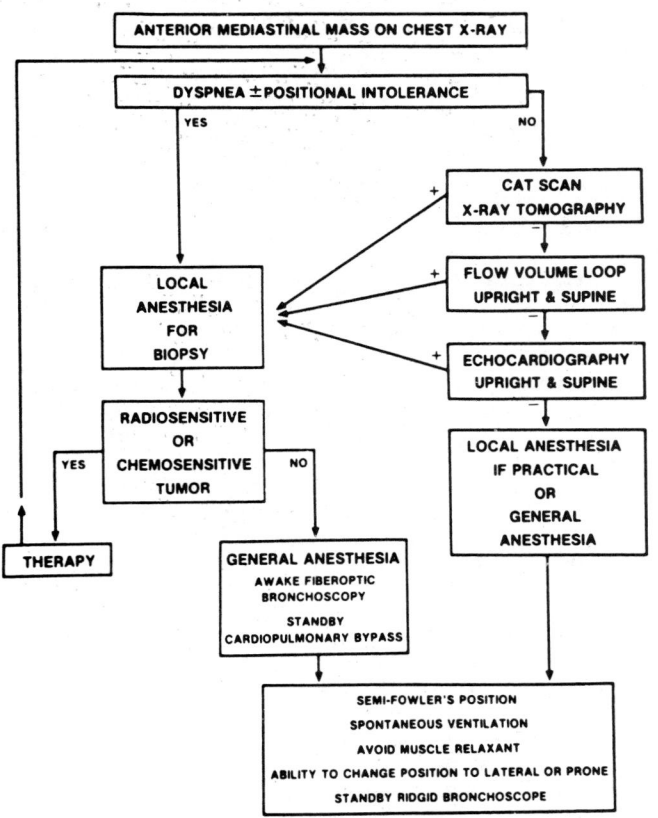

FIG. 33-25. Anatomic relationships during mediastinoscopy. Note the position of the mediastinoscope behind the right innominate artery and aortic arch and anterior the trachea. Reproduced with permission from Carlens E: Mediastinoscopy: A method for inspection and tissue biopsy in the superior mediastinum. Dis Chest 36:343, 1959.

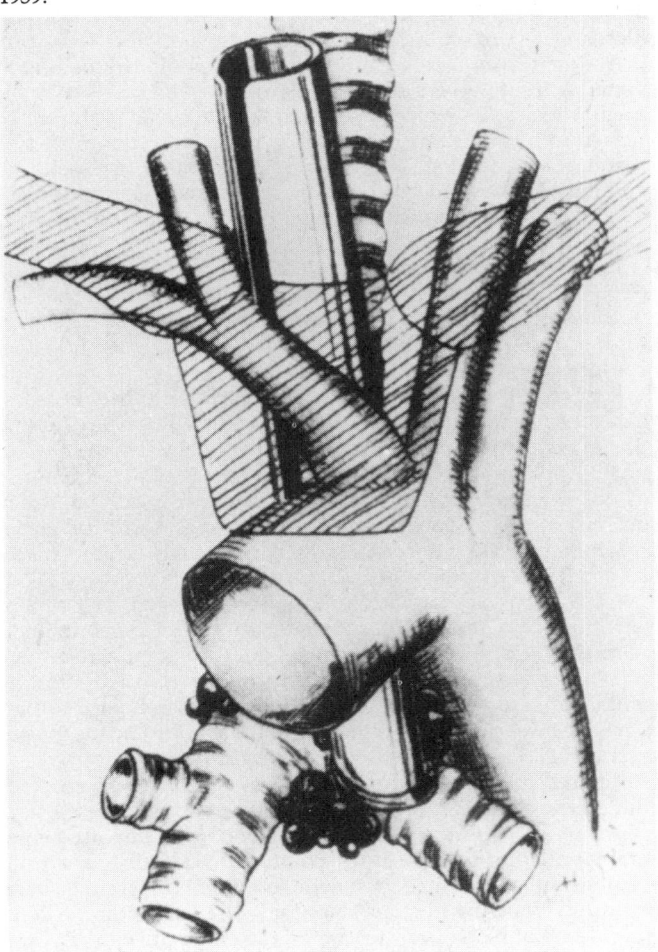

these structures may be traumatized. Because of scarring, previous mediastinoscopy is a contraindication to a repeat examination. Relative contraindications include superior vena caval obstruction, tracheal deviation, and aneurysm of the thoracic aorta.

Preoperative evaluation should include a search for airway obstruction or distortion. Review of a CT scan is very helpful in this regard. Evidence of an impaired cerebral circulation, history of stroke, or signs of the Eaton-Lambert syndrome due to oat cell carcinoma should be sought. Blood must be available for the procedure, because hemorrhage is a real risk and may be life-threatening.

Mediastinoscopy may be performed under local anesthesia, and this approach is claimed to offer greater simplicity and safety in patients with limited pulmonary reserve or in those with cerebrovascular disease.[118] However, most surgeons and anesthesiologists prefer general anesthesia using an endotracheal tube and continuous ventilation, as this offers a more controlled situation and greater flexibility in terms of surgical manipulations. The anesthetic technique should include a muscle relaxant to prevent the patient from coughing, since this may produce venous engorgement in the chest or trauma by the mediastinoscope to surrounding structures. The morbidity of mediastinoscopy has been reported as 1.5–3.0%, and mortality as 0.09%.[119] The most common complication is hemorrhage (0.73%) because of the proximity of major vessels and the vascularity of certain tumors. Tamponade may be the only recourse, and thoracotomy or median sternotomy may be required to achieve hemostasis. Needle aspiration of any structure is essential prior to any biopsy being taken. If severe bleeding occurs, induced arterial hypotension may be helpful in reducing the size of the tear in a vessel. If bleeding is venous, fluids given *via* an upper limb vein may enter the mediastinum, in which case a large-bore catheter should be placed in a lower limb vein.[120] A venous laceration may also result in air embolism, particularly if the patient is breathing spontaneously. Some authors, therefore, recommend the use of a precordial Doppler probe if the risk of air embolism is likely.

Pneumothorax is the second most common complication (0.66%). It is usually right-sided, often recognized at the time of the occurrence, and is treated according to size. A symptomatic pneumothorax should be treated by chest tube decompression.

Recurrent laryngeal nerve injury occurred in 0.34% of cases, and was permanent in 50% of these cases.[119] The nerve may be damaged by the mediastinoscope or be involved in tumor. It is not a problem unless both nerves are damaged, in which case upper airway obstruction may result. Autonomic reflexes may be initiated by manipulation of the trachea or of the aorta, which has pressor receptors located in the arch. Vagally mediated reflexes may be blocked by atropine.

"Apparent" cardiac arrest has been reported by Lee and Salvatore.[121] They monitored the right radial pulse using a plethysmograph, and the tracing suddenly disappeared in the presence of a normal ECG. A normal pulse returned after the mediastinoscope was removed, and the etiology of the apparent arrest was pressure on the innominate artery by the instrument (Fig. 33-25). Decreases in right arm blood pressure, as compared to left, were found by Petty in four of seven cases undergoing mediastinoscopy.[27] Duration was 15–360 s. This is of particular significance if there is a history of impaired cerebral circulation or transient ischemic attacks, or if a carotid bruit is present, since transient left hemiparesis has been reported following mediastinoscopy.[119] It is, therefore, recommended that blood pressure be monitored in the left arm and

that the right radial pulse be monitored continuously during mediastinoscopy. A decrease in the right radial pulse would be an indication for repositioning the mediastinoscope, especially in a patient with a history of cerebrovascular disease.

Other reported complications, which may require prompt intervention by the anesthesiologist, include acute tracheal collapse,[122] tension pneumomediastinum, mediastinitis, hemothorax, and chylothorax.[123] A chest radiograph taken in the immediate postoperative period is a useful precaution in all patients who have undergone mediastinoscopy.

THORACOSCOPY

Thoracoscopy involves the insertion of an endoscope into the thoracic cavity and pleural space. It is used for the diagnosis of pleural disease, effusions, and infectious disease (especially in immunosuppressed and AIDS patients), and for staging procedures, chemical pleurodesis, and lung biopsy. A small incision is made in the lateral chest wall and, with the insertion of the instrument, fluid and biopsies are easily obtained.

This procedure may be performed using local, regional, or general anesthesia, the choice depending upon the expected duration of the procedure and the physical status of the patient. The most common methods are local anesthetic infiltration or intercostal nerve blocks two spaces above and below the usual sixth intercostal space. Intercostal blocks also anesthetize the parietal pleura. The addition of a stellate ganglion block helps to suppress the cough reflex that is sometimes provoked during manipulation of the hilum of the lung.

When air enters the pleural cavity under inspection, a partial pneumothorax occurs, permitting good surgical visualization. Changes in Pa_{O_2}, Pa_{CO_2}, and ECG rhythm are usually minimal when the procedure is performed using local or regional anesthesia.[124] The physiology of this situation is discussed in an earlier section on lateral position, chest open, spontaneous ventilation.

With local anesthesia, the spontaneous pneumothorax is usually well-tolerated because the skin and chest wall form a seal around the thoracoscope and limit the degree of lung collapse. Occasionally, however, the procedure is poorly tolerated, and general anesthesia must be induced. The insertion of a double-lumen tube with the patient in the lateral position may be difficult, in which case the patient may be temporarily placed supine for the intubation.

If general anesthesia is required, either a single- or a double-lumen tube may be used. Positive pressure ventilation will interfere with visualization *via* the endoscope, however, and, therefore, a double-lumen tube is preferable. Additionally, if pleurodesis is being performed, general anesthesia *via* a double-lumen tube allows for complete re-expansion of the lung and avoids the pain associated with instillation of talc for recurrent pneumothorax. To overcome the pathophysiological effects of the pneumothorax, albeit small, a high FI_{O_2} is recommended for either local or general anesthesia. Blood gas monitoring may not be essential, but pulse oximetry during this procedure is extremely useful.

ANESTHESIA FOR SPECIAL SITUATIONS

Management of patients with bronchopleural fistula, empyema, cysts, and bullae, and for tracheal reconstruction are considered here. Many of these cases are appropriately managed using high-frequency ventilatory techniques; therefore, these techniques are described first.

HIGH-FREQUENCY VENTILATION

With conventional positive pressure ventilation, V_T and rates usually exceed or approach those in the normal spontaneously breathing patient. Gas transport to the alveoli occurs by convection in the larger airways, and then by convection and molecular diffusion in the more distal airways and alveoli. HFV differs from conventional positive pressure ventilation in that smaller V_T and more rapid rates are used, and gas transport may depend more upon molecular diffusion, high velocity flow, and coaxial gas flow in the airways, with gas in the center moving distally, and that on the periphery moving proximally.

There are three different types of HFV. HFPPV uses small V_T at rates of 60–120 breaths·min^{-1} (1–2 Hz). The ventilator used (e.g., Bronchovent) has a negligible internal compliance, so that the V_T generated, which usually approximates the dead space volume, equals the volume set on the ventilator and represents all fresh gas. The high instantaneous gas flows generated facilitate gas exchange and movement in the conducting airways.

HFPPV may be delivered via an open or a closed system. An example of the former would be the percutaneous placement of a transtracheal catheter or placement of a catheter via the nose or mouth with its distal end above the carina. Inflow is intraluminal, and outflow extraluminal. This technique has been used during bronchoscopy and tracheal resection and reconstructive surgery. When open systems are used, the gas outflow pathway is not established mechanically, and depends upon natural airway patency. It is, therefore, subject to compromise. Also, aspiration is a potential complication with open systems.

The closed system is superior, since it integrates both airway patency and outflow protection. A closed system is represented by a catheter placed within a short segment of an endotracheal tube for delivery of the HFPPV, while the remainder of the tube lumen represents the exit pathway for gas. A quadruple-lumen endotracheal tube has been designed specifically for delivery of HFPPV. One lumen is for the HFPPV delivery, one for gas outflow, one for cuff inflation, and one for measuring airway pressures at the distal end of the tube. The use of a closed system also permits application of PEEP, a situation not possible with an open arrangement.

High frequency jet ventilation (HFJV) uses a pulse of a small jet of fresh gas introduced from a high-pressure source (50 psi) into the airway via a small catheter or additional lumen in an endotracheal tube. Rates used are usually 100–400 breaths·min^{-1}. The fresh gas jet entrains gas from an injection cannula side port reservoir. This system is somewhat analogous to the Sanders injector system described in the bronchoscopy section, and FI_{O_2} is similarly variable. The jet and entrained gas flows cause forward motion of the mass of gas in the airways. HFJV can be used with an open system or with a closed arrangement, as described above. In the latter, PEEP may be added to enhance oxygenation. Also, using high fresh gas flows from an anesthesia circuit, inhaled drugs may be delivered as an entrained gas mixture.

High frequency oscillation ventilation (HFOV) employs a mechanism that oscillates gas at rates of 400–2400 breaths·min^{-1}. It has not been described in association with thoracic surgical procedures. In this system, V_T are small (50–80 ml), and gas exchange occurs via enhanced molecular diffusion and coaxial airway flow.

The potential advantages offered by HFOV during thoracic anesthesia are as follows: lower V_T and inspiratory pressures result in a "quiet" lung field for the surgeon with minimal movements of airway, lung tissue, and mediastinum. Thus, HFPPV has been used to ventilate both the non-dependent lung and the dependent lung during thoracic surgical procedures, with adequate ABG being obtained throughout.[125, 126] At high frequencies (>6 Hz), however, CO_2 retention may become a problem.

HFJV has been used to ventilate the non-dependent lung to improve Pa_{O_2} during one-lung anesthesia, while the dependent lung was ventilated with conventional IPPV.[127] In this study, the Pa_{O_2} increased compared with that obtained during simple collapse of the non-dependent lung. However, no study to date has compared HFV to the non-dependent lung with CPAP to this lung. Since similar increases in Pa_{O_2} may be obtained using selective CPAP to the non-dependent lung and while using much simpler equipment than that necessary to deliver HFV, the use of CPAP would seem preferable to HFV to increase Pa_{O_2} during most one-lung anesthesia situations. Also, during HFJV, a driving pressure of 25–35 psi is generally used to maintain normocapnia, but such pressures could lead to overdistention of the operated lung and poor surgical conditions. Wilks et al[127] showed that low driving pressures (15 psi) caused minimal distention to the non-dependent lung and improved Pa_{O_2}, while CO_2 removal was mainly a function of the dependent, conventionally ventilated lung. In certain situations, however, HFJV to the non-dependent lung may offer some advantage. Thus, Morgan et al[128] have described combined unilateral HFJV and contralateral IPPV in the management of a patient who required a right lower lobectomy for bronchial carcinoma associated with emphysema, pneumoconiosis, and a previous thoracoplasty for pulmonary tuberculosis. These authors and others recommended consideration of the use of this technique in any patient presenting for partial lung resection in the presence of severe pulmonary impairment.[129, 130]

The lower pressures and V_T associated with HFV result in a small leak via bronchopleural fistulae, and HFJV is now generally considered the conservative treatment of choice in this condition. Another advantage of HFV is that the rapid rate small V_T can be delivered via small tubes or catheters, so that, if an airway has to be divided, the passage of a small tube across the surgical field will permit ventilation of the distal airway and lung tissue. This use has been applied during sleeve resection of the lung, tracheal reconstruction, and surgery for tracheal stenosis. In all three situations, the surgeon is able to work easily around the small catheter used to provide the HFV.

Most recently, Jenkins et al[65] have compared conventional IPPV (650 ml × 14 breaths·min^{-1}) with HFJV (150–200 breaths·min^{-1}; minute volume 10–15 liters) to the dependent lung during one-lung ventilation, in ten patients, using $FI_{O_2} = 0.5$. There were no significant differences between the groups in Pa_{O_2}, Pa_{CO_2}, or hemodynamic indices, although shunt fraction was higher in the HFJV group. A significant PEEP effect was also noted in this group, but not in the IPPV group. The unintentional generation of PEEP during HFJV is well known, and is thought to be due to expiratory flow limitation. The PEEP to the dependent lung increases pulmonary vascular resistance (PVR) in this lung and causes diversion of blood flow to the non-dependent, non-ventilated lung, thereby increasing shunt fraction (32.9% vs. 42.4%). These authors concluded that the theoretical benefits of HFJV on the cardiovascular system are outweighed by the effects of mean airway pressure increasing shunt to the non-ventilated lung during one-lung anesthesia.[65] Although adequate gas exchange was maintained with HFJV during one-lung anesthesia with $FI_{O_2} = 0.5$, they found that it was more difficult to assess the adequacy of ventilation with HFJV and, therefore, recommend against its routine use during one-lung anesthesia.

BRONCHOPLEURAL FISTULA AND EMPYEMA

A bronchopleural fistula is an abnormal communication between the bronchial tree and the pleural cavity. Occasionally, there is an additional communication to the surface of the chest, a bronchopleural cutaneous fistula. A bronchopleural fistula occurs most commonly following pulmonary resection for carcinoma. Other causes include traumatic rupture of a bronchus or bulla (sometimes due to barotrauma or PEEP), penetrating chest wound, or spontaneous drainage into the bronchial tree of an empyema cavity or lung cyst. The incidence is higher following pneumonectomy than following other types of lung resection. The problems associated with bronchopleural fistula and empyema are that positive pressure ventilation may result in contamination of healthy lung, loss of air, decreased alveolar ventilation leading to CO_2 retention, and the development of a tension pneumothorax.

If an empyema is present, it should first be drained under local anesthesia prior to any surgery to close the bronchopleural fistula. Drainage is performed with the patient sitting up and leaning toward the affected side. It must be recognized that empyemas are often loculated and that complete drainage is not always possible. A drain to an underwater seal system is left in the cavity prior to administration of anesthesia for surgery to the bronchopleural fistula and, following the drainage of an empyema, a chest radiograph should be obtained to determine the efficacy.

The priorities in the anesthetic management of bronchopleural fistula are the isolation of the affected side in terms of contamination and ventilation. The ideal approach is an awake intubation of the trachea using a double-lumen tube with the patient breathing spontaneously. Supplemental oxygen should be administered, and the patient should be constantly reassured. Neuroleptanalgesia is satisfactory in providing a suitably cooperative patient, and the airway is then pretreated with topical anesthesia. The endobronchial tube selected should be such that the bronchial lumen is on the side opposite to the bronchopleural fistula. Selection of the largest possible tube provides a close fit in the trachea, which helps to stabilize the tube. Once the tube is adequately positioned in the trachea, there may be a considerable outpouring of pus from the tracheal lumen if an empyema is present, and so this lumen should be immediately suctioned using a large-bore suction catheter. The healthy and, possibly, the affected lung may then be ventilated, adequacy of oxygenation and ventilation being assessed by pulse oximetry or ABG analysis.

An alternative technique is to insert the double-lumen tube under general anesthesia, with the patient breathing spontaneously to avoid a tension pneumothorax. With either technique, the chest drainage tube must be left unclamped to avoid any bouts of coughing and to prevent the build-up of a tension pneumothorax if a predisposing valvular mechanism should exist. In patients who do not have an empyema, use of a single-lumen tube has been described and may be satisfactory if the bronchopleural fistula (and airleak) is small. A rapid-sequence induction with ketamine or thiopental followed by a relaxant has also been described, but is associated with considerable risk of contamination and tension pneumothorax.

Bronchopleural fistulae may also be treated conservatively using various ventilatory techniques. Thus, the bronchus of the normal lung may be intubated and ventilated, allowing the bronchopleural fistula to rest and heal. This approach may result in an intolerable shunt, however, and PEEP may be necessary to maintain Pa_{O_2}. Differential lung ventilation *via* a double-lumen tube has also been described, the healthy lung being ventilated with normal V_T, while the affected lung is exposed to smaller V_T[131] or to CPAP with O_2 at pressures just below the critical opening pressure of the fistula. The latter can be assessed by determining at what level of CPAP continuous bubbling appears *via* the underwater seal chest drain.

For large bronchopleural fistulae, HFJV may be the nonsurgical treatment of choice. The use of small V_T results in minimal gas loss through the fistula, which may heal more quickly. In addition, hemodynamic effects are usually minimal, and spontaneous efforts at ventilation are usually abolished, thereby decreasing the work of breathing and eliminating the need for relaxants or excessive sedation.

Bishop *et al*[132] have recently demonstrated that HFJV may not always be superior to conventional ventilation in the conservative management of bronchopleural fistula. They showed that HFJV is less effective in reducing the ventilatory leak through a bronchopleural fistula when the peripheral leak is combined with severe injury and decreased compliance in the remainder of the lung than when only an airway is disrupted. In the seven patients they reported, HFJV was compared with controlled ventilation of the lungs, and it was found that adequate gas exchange could not be achieved at comparable mean airway pressures with HFJV, although peak airway pressures decreased. Indeed, in some patients, flow through the bronchopleural fistula actually increased with HFJV. These authors concluded that HFJV should be used selectively in patients with bronchopleural fistula.[132]

LUNG CYSTS AND BULLAE

Air filled cysts of the lung are usually bronchogenic, postinfective, infantile, or emphysematous. They may be associated with COPD or be an isolated finding. A bulla is a thin-walled space filled with air that results from the destruction of alveolar tissue. The walls are, therefore, composed of visceral pleura, connective tissue septa, or compressed lung tissue. In general, bullae represent an area of end-stage emphysematous destruction of the lung.

Patients may be considered for surgical bullectomy when dyspnea is incapacitating, when the bullae are expanding, when there are repeated pneumothoraces due to rupture of bullae, or if the bullae compress a large area of normal lung. Most of these patients have severe COPD and CO_2 retention and little functional respiratory reserve. The first consideration in management is that a high $F_{I_{O_2}}$ should be maintained. If the bulla or cyst communicates with the bronchial tree, positive-pressure ventilation may cause it to expand if it is compliant, or even to rupture, producing a situation analogous to tension pneumothorax. If the bulla is very compliant, most of the applied V_T may be wasted in this additional dead space. N_2O should be avoided, since it causes expansion of any air spaces within the body, including bullae. Once the chest is open, even more of the V_T may enter the compliant bulla, which is no longer limited by chest wall integrity; and an increase in ventilation is needed until the bulla is controlled.

The anesthetic management of these patients is challenging, particularly if the disease is bilateral. The use of a pulse oximeter is very helpful in the continuous assessment of oxygenation. Ideally, a double-lumen tube is inserted with the patient awake or under general anesthesia, but breathing spontaneously. The avoidance of positive-pressure ventilation (where possible) helps to decrease the likelihood of the potential problems described above, although it must be recognized that oxygenation may be precarious with spontaneous ventilation. Once the endotracheal tube is in place, each lung may be controlled separately, and adequate ventilation can be applied to the healthy lung if bilateral disease is not present. Gentle positive-pressure ventilation with rapid, small V_T and pressures not to exceed 10 cm H_2O may be used during the induction and maintenance of anesthesia, especially if the bullae have been shown to have no, or only poor, bronchial communication by preoperative ventilation scanning. While the surgery is being performed, as each bulla is resected, the operated lung can be separately ventilated to check for air leaks and presence of additional bullae.

If positive-pressure ventilation is to be applied prior to opening of the chest, the possibility of a tension pneumothorax must be borne in mind, and treatment should be readily available. The diagnosis of pneumothorax may be made by a unilateral decrease in breath sounds (may be difficult to distinguish in a patient with bullous disease), increase in ventilatory pressure, progressive tracheal deviation, wheezing or cardiovascular changes. Treatment of a pneumothorax involves the rapid placement of a chest tube. An added risk of the latter is the creation of a bronchopleural-cutaneous fistula, which creates problems for ventilation. Alternatively, general anesthesia is induced only after the surgeon has prepared the operative field and draped the patient. In the event of sudden deterioration in the patient's condition during induction, the surgeon may make an immediate median sternotomy. In any event, the time from induction of anesthesia to sternotomy must be kept to a minimum.

In order to avoid these problems in a patient with known bullae, HFJV has been used in a patient with a large bulla undergoing CABG[133] and in another patient undergoing bilateral bullectomy.[134] If bilateral bullectomy is to be performed, a median sternotomy is generally used. Benumof[135] has described the use of sequential one-lung ventilation using a double-lumen tube in the management of a patient for bilateral bullectomy. The side with the largest bulla and least lung function, as assessed preoperatively by ventilation and perfusion scans, should be operated on first. In this way, the lung with the better function should support gas exchange first. If hypoxemia develops during this one-lung situation, application of CPAP to the non-ventilated lung during the deflation phase of a tidal breath should increase Pa_{O_2}.

In an extreme situation where no respiratory reserve exists, it may not be possible to maintain an adequate Pa_{O_2} on one-lung ventilation, and, in such a situation, the use of an extra-corporeal oxygenator and femoro-femoral bypass may be needed. Heparinization is an additional surgical problem in such cases. Such a severe situation may also be well-suited to surgery in a hyperbaric chamber. Oxygenation can be assured, and the cyst or bulla will diminish in size under hyperbaric conditions.

Unlike most cases of pulmonary resection, patients following bullectomy are left with a greater amount of functional lung tissue than was previously available to them, and the mechanics of respiration are improved. At the end of the case, the double-lumen tube is replaced by a standard tube, and the patients generally require several days to be weaned from the respirator. During this time, the positive airway pressure used should be minimized to avoid causing a pneumothorax due to rupture of suture or staple-lines or of residual bullae.

ANESTHESIA FOR RESECTION OF THE TRACHEA

Trachael resection and reconstruction are technically difficult for the surgeon and challenging for the anesthesiologist.[136] Indications for this type of procedure include congenital lesions (agenesis, stenosis), neoplasia (primary or secondary), injuries (direct, indirect), infections, and post-intubation injuries (due to endotracheal tube or tracheotomy). For the surgical team, the major problems are the maintenance of ventilation to the lungs while the airway is being operated on, and the integrity of the anastomoses postoperatively. In this respect, the presence of lung disease that is of sufficient severity to require postoperative ventilatory support is a relative contraindication to tracheal resection or reconstruction.

Monitoring of these patients should include an arterial cannula placed in the left radial artery to permit continuous measurement of blood pressure during periods of innominate artery compression. Steroids should be administered to help reduce any tracheal edema, and a high Fi_{O_2} should be used throughout the procedure to ensure an adequate oxygen reserve at all times in the FRC, so that temporary interruptions of ventilation are less likely to produce hypoxemia.

Numerous methods have been reported to provide oxygenation and ventilation of the lungs during these procedures. A small-bore anode tube may be pushed through and distal to an upper lesion, so that resection may occur around the tube. This technique is useful only in mild stenoses. Alternatively, an endotracheal tube may be passed *via* the glottis to above the stenosis, and a sterile endotracheal or bronchial tube may later be inserted into the trachea opened distal to the site of stenosis, with the sterile anesthesia tubing being led across the surgical field. Following resection of the lesion, the sterile and distally placed endotracheal tube is withdrawn, and the upper tube (originally passed through the glottis) is advanced across the anastomosis. With low tracheal or bronchial lesions, resection and reconstruction may be performed around an endobronchial or double-lumen tube. During these procedures, the patient is kept in a head-down position to minimize aspiration of blood and debris into the alveoli, and ventilation must be carefully monitored throughout.

Clearly, the presence of large-bore tubes in the airway may make these resections technically difficult, and the use of HFV techniques may improve surgical access. Thus, a small-diameter catheter or catheters may be placed across or through the stenotic lesion or transected airway(s), and ventilation to the distal airways and lungs maintained using HFPPV or HFJV. Potential disadvantages of these HFV techniques are that, by necessity, the system is "open" (see section on HFV), and egress of gas during exhalation may be compromised if the stenosis is tight. Also, the catheter may become occluded by blood and may become displaced, and distal aspiration of debris or blood may occur. With complex resections, two anesthesia teams with two circuits or sets of ventilating equipment may be necessary to ensure adequate ventilation of the two distal airway segments, although, during carinal resections, HFPPV to the left lung alone generally provides adequate oxygenation and ventilation.

In very difficult cases, cardiopulmonary bypass has been used to provide oxygenation and CO_2 removal during the period of resection, while, following resection, anesthesia can be maintained *via* a standard endotracheal tube. With the use of bypass comes an attendant risk of massive hemorrhage due to the necessary heparinization.

Following tracheal resection or reconstructive surgery, patients should be kept with their necks and heads flexed in order to reduce tension on the anastomotic suture lines. In some cases, this is maintained by using sutures between the chin and the anterior chest wall. Extubation of the trachea is performed as early as possible, so as to minimize tracheal trauma due to the endotracheal tube and cuff.

BRONCHOPULMONARY LAVAGE

This procedure involves irrigation of the lung and bronchial tree, and is used as a treatment for alveolar proteinosis, radioactive dust inhalation, cystic fibrosis, bronchiectasis, and asthmatic bronchitis. Lung lavage is performed under general anesthesia using a double-lumen tube, so that one lung may be ventilated while the other is being treated with lavage fluid.[137]

The preoperative assessment of these patients should include ventilation-perfusion scans, so that lavage can be performed first on the more severely affected lung (i.e., the one with the least ventilation). If involvement is equal, the left lung is generally lavaged first, since gas exchange should be better through the larger right lung. The patients are premedicated and supplied with supplemental O_2 en route to the operating room.

Anesthesia is induced with an intravenous drug and maintained with an inhaled drug in O_2 to maintain the highest FI_{O_2}. Muscle relaxation facilitates placement of the double-lumen tube, and the cuff seal should be checked to maintain perfect separation at a pressure of 50 cm H_2O to prevent leakage of lavage fluid around the cuff. A fiberoptic bronchoscope is useful to check the position of the bronchial cuff of the double-lumen tube. Other monitoring should include an arterial catheter, and oxygenation should be continuously monitored by pulse oximetry. A stethoscope should be placed over the ventilated lung to check for rales that may indicate leakage of lavage fluid into this lung.

The patient is maintained on an $FI_{O_2} = 1.0$ throughout the procedure, and, prior to lavage, this serves to denitrogenate the lungs, so that only O_2 and CO_2 remain. Instillation of fluid will then allow the latter gases to be absorbed, resulting in greater access by the fluid to the alveolar spaces than if more insoluble nitrogen bubbles remained.

Once the trachea is intubated, the patient is turned so that the side to be treated is lowermost, and the double-lumen tube position and seal are checked once again. With the patient in a head-up position, warmed heparinized isotonic saline is infused by gravity from a reservoir 30 cm above the mid-axillary line, into the catheter to the dependent lung, while the non-dependent lung is ventilated. When fluid ceases to flow in (usually after 700–1000 ml in the adult), the patient is placed in a head-down position and fluid is allowed to drain out. The lavage is continued until the effluent is clear (as opposed to the milky fluid that drains initially when lavage is being performed for alveolar proteinosis) when the lung is suctioned and ventilation is re-established with large V_T (and pressures), since the compliance will be decreased due to loss of surfactant. With each lavage, inflow and outflow volumes are monitored, so that the patient is not "drowned" in fluid and there is no excessive absorption or leakage to the ventilated side. At least 90% of the saline volume should be recovered with each lavage. Two-lung ventilation is re-established and, as compliance improves, an air-O_2 mixture (addition of N_2) may be introduced to help maintain alveolar patency. After a further period of ventilation, most patients' tracheae can be extubated

in the operating room. In the post-treatment period, patients are encouraged to cough and engage in breathing exercises to fully re-expand the treated lung. At 3 days to a week following lavage of the first lung, the patient may return to the operating room for lavage of the other lung.

Problems sometimes encountered with this procedure include spillage of lavage fluid from the treated to the ventilated lung. This must be managed by stopping the lavage and assuring functional separation of the lungs before continuing. Double-lumen tube positioning is critical. Spillage may cause profound decreases in oxygenation, which may necessitate terminating the procedure and maintaining two-lung ventilation with oxygen and PEEP.

During periods when lavage fluid is being instilled into the dependent lung, oxygenation usually improves, because the increased intraalveolar pressure due to the fluid causes diversion of the pulmonary blood flow to the non-dependent, ventilated lung (Fig. 33-26). Conversely, when the fluid is drained out of the dependent lung, hypoxemia may occur.[138] In some cases where severe hypoxemia was anticipated during right lung lavage, the risk has been reduced by passing a balloon-tipped catheter into the right main pulmonary artery (checked by x-ray) and inflating the balloon during periods of right lung drainage. In this way, blood flow to the dependent, right, non-ventilated lung would be minimized during periods of drainage. This technique is not without risk (e.g., pulmonary artery rupture) and is reserved for those patients considered to be at greatest risk for hypoxemia during lavage.

If the patient has recently had a diagnostic open lung biopsy, a bronchopleural fistula may be present. If this is a

FIG. 33-26. Changes in Pa_{O_2}, $S\bar{v}_{O_2}$, CO, and $\dot{Q}s/\dot{Q}_T$ during seven unilateral lung lavages. Instillation of fluid caused an increase in Pa_{O_2}, decreases in CO and in $\dot{Q}s/\dot{Q}_T$, and no change in $S\bar{v}_{O_2}$. ($S\bar{v}_{O_2}$ should be read as % on the ordinate scale.) Pa_{O_2} = arterial oxygen tension; $S\bar{v}_{O_2}$ = mixed venous oxygen saturation; CO = cardiac output; $\dot{Q}s/\dot{Q}_T$ = intrapulmonary shunt; OLA = one-lung anesthesia. (Reproduced with permission from Cohen E, Feinberg BI, Camunas JC: Unilateral lung lavage, p 112. Phoenix, Society of Cardiovascular Anesthesiologists Meeting, April 1985.)

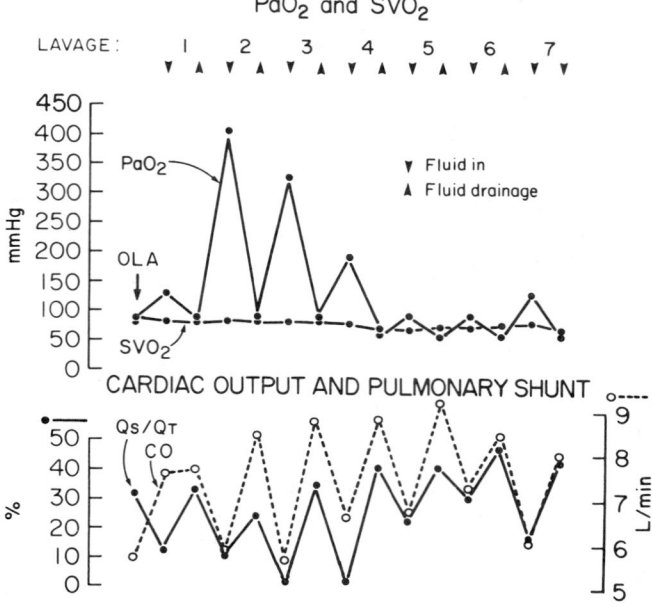

possibility, a chest tube should be inserted into the side of the bronchopleural fistula, and this side should be lavaged first. The chest drain is removed several days later.

Limitations in the sizes of available double-lumen tubes preclude their use for lavage in patients weighing less than 40 kg. In such cases, cardiopulmonary bypass may be required to provide oxygenation during lavage.

MYASTHENIA GRAVIS (MG)

The thoracic anesthesiologist will likely have to manage myasthenia gravis (MG) patients for thymectomy, which is now considered the treatment of choice in most cases of MG. MG is a disorder of the neuromuscular junction, the function of which is altered routinely in the modern practice of anesthesia. The worldwide prevalence is one per 20,000 to 30,000 of the population; it is more common in females than males in a 6:4 ratio. Any age may be affected, but peaks of incidence occur in the third decade for females and the fifth for males. MG is a chronic disorder characterized by weakness and fatigability of voluntary muscles with improvement following rest. Onset is frequently slow and insidious, any skeletal muscle or group of muscles may be affected, and the condition is associated with relapses and remissions. The most common onset is ocular, and, if the disease remains localized to the eyes for 2 yr, the likelihood of progression to generalized MG is low. In some cases, the disease is generalized, and may involve the bulbar musculature, causing problems with breathing and swallowing. Peripheral muscle involvement may cause weakness, clumsiness, and difficulty in holding up the head or in walking. The most commonly used clinical classification of MG is shown in Table 33-7.[139]

The basic abnormality in MG is a decrease in the number of postsynaptic acetylcholine receptors at the end-plates of affected muscles. This causes a decrease in the margin of safety of neuromuscular transmission. MG is an autoimmune disorder, and most affected patients have circulating antibodies to the acetylcholine receptors. These antibodies may cause complement-mediated lysis of the postsynaptic membrane, direct blockade of the receptors, or modulate the receptor turnover such that the degradation rate exceeds the resynthesis rate. Studies of the end-plate area show loss of synaptic folds and a widening of the synaptic cleft.[140]

The diagnosis is suspected from the history and confirmed by pharmacological, electrophysiological, and/or immunological testing. Patients cannot sustain or repeat muscular contraction. The electrical counterpart of this is a decrement in the muscle action potentials evoked by repetitive stimulation of a motor nerve. Mechanical and electrical (EMG) decrements improve with 2–10 mg of intravenous edrophonium (Tensilon test). Myasthenic patients are characteristically sensitive to D-tubocurarine. Where the routine EMG results are equivocal, a regional curare test may be performed using a tourniquet to isolate the limb and to limit the action of the drug. In the regional curare test, EMGs are performed before and after the administration of O.2 mg curare. In equivocal cases, a positive result of a test for anti-acetylcholine receptor antibodies is considered diagnostic.

MEDICAL THERAPY

Anticholinesterases are used to prolong the action of acetylcholine at the postsynaptic membrane, and may also exert their own agonist effect on the acetylcholine receptors. They are the most commonly used therapy in MG (Table 33-8). Myasthenic patients learn to regulate their medication and titrate dose against optimum effect. Overdosage causes the muscarinic effects of acetylcholine (Ach), and may cause a cholinergic crisis. Underdosage causes weakness or a myasthenic crisis. In a patient with weakness, distinction between the two types of crisis may be made by performing a Tensilon test or by examining pupillary size, which will be large (mydriatic) in a myasthenic, but small (miotic) in a cholinergic crisis. Muscarinic side effects are treatable with atropine.

The immunologic basis of MG has led to the use of immunosuppressive drugs, such as steroids, azathioprine, cyclophosphamide, and, most recently, cyclosporine, in MG. Steroids often produce initial deterioration before an improvement. The usual regime is prednisone $1 \text{ mg} \cdot \text{kg}^{-1}$ on alternate days. The other drugs mentioned represent third and fourth lines of treatment.

Plasma exchange or plasmapheresis may produce dramatic but transient improvements in muscle strength with decreases in anti-acetylcholine receptor antibody titers. Usually reserved for severe MG, it has been shown to improve respiratory function in both operated and non-operated MG patients. Plasmapheresis causes a decrease in plasma cholinesterase levels that may prolong the effect of drugs, such as suc-

TABLE 33-7.   Clinical Classification of Myasthenia Gravis (MG)[139]

I   Ocular Myasthenia—Involvement of ocular muscles only. Mild with ptosis and diplopia. Electrophysiologic (EMG) testing of other musculature is negative for MG.

IA   Ocular Myasthenia with peripheral muscles showing no clinical symptoms but showing a positive EMG for MG.

II   Generalized Myasthenia

IIA   Mild—Slow onset, usually ocular spreading to skeletal and bulbar muscles. No respiratory involvement. Good response to drug therapy. Low mortality rate.

IIB   Moderate—As IIA but progressing to more severe involvement of skeletal and bulbar muscles. Dysarthria, dysphagia, difficulty chewing. No respiratory involvement. Patient's activities limited. Fair response to drug therapy.

III   Acute Fulminating—Rapid onset of severe bulbar and skeletal weakness with involvement of muscles of respiration. Progression usually within 6 months. Poor response to therapy. Patient's activities limited. Low mortality rate.

IV   Late Severe—Severe MG developing at least 2 yr after onset of Group I or Group II symptoms. Progression of disease may be gradual or rapid. Poor response to therapy and poor prognosis.

TABLE 33-8.   Anticholinesterase Drugs Used to Treat Myasthenia Gravis

DRUG	DOSAGE mg			EFFICACY
	Oral	iv	im	
Pyridostigmine (Mestinon)	60	2.0	2.0–4.0	1
Neostigmine (Prostigmine)	15	0.5	0.7–1.0	1
Ambenonium (Mytelase)	6	not available		2.5

cinylcholine, which are normally broken down by this enzyme system.

Abnormalities are found in 75% of thymus glands removed from MG patients (85% show hyperplasia; 15% thymoma). Following thymectomy, some 75% of patients either go into remission or are improved. Thymectomy is now considered to be the treatment of choice in most patients with MG, exceptions being those in Osserman class I.[141] A retrospective controlled study of 80 MG patients treated medically matched (as regards age, sex, severity, and duration of MG) with 80 treated by thymectomy showed that the group treated surgically lived longer and showed more clinical improvement than the group treated medically.[142] Thymectomy may be performed either *via* a classical sternum-splitting approach, or transcervically using a technique similar to mediastinoscopy. Controversy exists over which is the best surgical approach to thymectomy. Although a more radical thymectomy can be performed by the transsternal route, the morbidity would appear to be greater than by the transcervical route. Furthermore, the results in terms of clinical improvement and remission rate following transcervical thymectomy are reported to be equally as good as those following transsternal thymectomy.[143]

Management of General Anesthesia

Where possible, MG patients should be admitted for elective surgery while in remission. Upon admission, the patient's physical and emotional states should be optimized. Other diseases occasionally associated with MG should be excluded (Table 33-9). Current drug therapy should be reviewed and possible drug interactions considered. Because the patients are less active while in the hospital, their anticholinesterase dosage may need to be decreased. If the patient has a history of respiratory disease or bulbar involvement, preoperative evaluation should include respiratory function studies. Breathing exercises and instruction in the use of incentive spirometers may be indicated. The patients should be told of the possible need for postoperative intubation of the trachea and ventilation of the lungs. Myasthenic patients should be scheduled to be the first case of the day in the operating room. Patients on steroid therapy should receive perioperative coverage.

TABLE 33-9.   Disorders Associated with Myasthenia Gravis

Thymoma
Thyroid disease
   hyperthyroidism
   hypothyroidism
   thyroiditis
Idiopathic thrombocytopenic purpura
Rheumatoid arthritis
Systemic lupus erythematosus
Anemias
   pernicious
   hemolytic
Multiple sclerosis
Ulcerative colitis
Leukemia
Lymphoma
Convulsive disorders
Extrathymic neoplasia
Polymyositis
Sjögren's syndrome
Scleroderma

Since the patient's trachea is to be intubated and the lungs ventilated for the planned procedure, anticholinesterase therapy should be withheld on the morning of surgery so that the patient is weak on arrival to the operating room. This avoids interactions with other drugs used in the operating room. Anticholinesterase therapy may be continued if the patient is physically or psychologically dependent on it. Premedication is satisfactorily achieved with a benzodiazepine or barbiturate. Opioids are generally avoided for fear of producing respiratory depression.

Monitoring should be as dictated by the patient's state and planned surgical procedure, but should include an assessment of neuromuscular transmission (mechanomyogram/twitch monitor or integrated EMG monitor) if agents affecting neuromuscular transmission are to be used.

Induction of anesthesia is readily achieved with a short-acting barbiturate. In elective cases intubation of the trachea, maintenance, and relaxation are readily achieved using potent inhaled drugs. Anesthesia may be deepened using halothane, enflurane, or isoflurane, and the trachea intubated under their effect. Myasthenic patients are more sensitive than normals to the neuromuscular depressant effects of the potent inhaled drugs. Thus, while concentrations of 3.5% enflurane are needed to produce twitch depression in normals, as little as 1% enflurane or 0.4% isoflurane may produce profound depression in MG patients.[144] Because these drugs are easily administered and withdrawn, they are the most commonly used anesthetic drugs for MG patients. At the end of the procedure, the drug is discontinued and recovery of neuromuscular function begins.

Non-depolarizing Relaxants

In some cases, the patients cannot tolerate the cardiovascular depressant effects of the potent drugs, in which case muscle relaxants may be employed, titrating dose against monitored effect. MG patients are sensitive to the non-depolarizing relaxants. A usual precurarizing dose in a normal patient may represent an ED in MG.[141] All of the non-depolarizing relaxants have been successfully and uneventfully used, with careful monitoring, in MG patients. They should be titrated in $\frac{1}{10}$ to $\frac{1}{20}$ of the usual dose. Atracurium is now probably the preferred agent because of its short elimination half-life (20 min), small volume of distribution, lack of cumulative effect, and high clearance. The Hofmann elimination pathway gives it very reproducible pharmacodynamics and kinetics, and most patients do not require reversal if monitored carefully. A recent review suggests that the average intubating dose of atracurium in MG patients is $0.1-0.2 \, mg \cdot kg^{-1}$.[138] Relaxation is readily maintained thereafter using an atracurium infusion, and recovery time is not prolonged with this drug. While the other non-depolarizers may be used, they do have cumulative effects, which may represent a potential disadvantage. If necessary, the non-depolarizers may be reversed by increments of anticholinesterases, while carefully monitoring neuromuscular transmission to obtain maximum antagonism yet avoid a cholinergic crisis. All anticholinesterases have been safely used. Edrophonium may be the drug of choice, since its onset of action is rapid and larger doses have a prolonged duration of action. Because of the risk of cholinergic crisis with anticholinesterase agents, the rapid, predictable, spontaneous recovery from atracurium may represent an additional advantage in that reversal may not be necessary.

The sensitivity of MG patients to non-depolarizers is very variable, depending upon the individual patient, severity of MG, and treatment. There are conflicting reports as to the sensitivity of MG patients who are "in remission." All such patients should be considered sensitive until proven otherwise.[141]

Depolarizing Relaxants

MG patients are resistant to succinylcholine. The ED_{95} is 2.6 times normal in these patients.[145] Clinically, however, its use has been without incident, with normal clinical doses producing adequate relaxation for endotracheal intubation and a normal recovery time, despite the occasionally reported early onset of phase II block. Doses of $0.2-1.0$ mg·kg^{-1} have been used in a number of MG patients, and most did not fasciculate before becoming paralyzed.[141] Fade in response to train-of-four stimulation was observed in some patients during recovery, but the latter was not delayed. It should be noted that the prior administration of an anticholinesterase may complicate the response to succinylcholine by delaying its metabolism. Where a rapid-sequence intubation of the trachea is required, rapid onset of muscle relaxation may be achieved with succinylcholine or with moderate doses of a non-depolarizer; in the latter case, with an associated prolongation of effect.

Medications with neuromuscular blocking properties should be used with caution in MG, particularly if relaxants are being used concurrently. Such drugs include antidysrhythmics (quinidine, procainamide, calcium channel blockers), diuretics (hypokalemia), nitrogen mustards, quinine, and aminoglycoside antibiotics. Dantrolene has been used safely in MG.[146]

Recovery from anesthesia must be carefully monitored. Extubation of the trachea should be performed when the patients are responsive and able to generate negative inspiratory pressures of greater than -20 cm H_2O. Following extubation of the trachea, the patients are carefully observed in the recovery area or the intensive care unit. As soon as possible, patients should resume their usual pyridostigmine regimen. Cases of mild respiratory depression may be treatable with parenteral anticholinesterase; more severe cases may require reintubation of the trachea and mechanical ventilation of the lungs. In the immediate postoperative period, post-thymectomy patients often show a marked improvement in their condition and a decreased need for anticholinesterase therapy.

Myasthenic patients are at increased risk of developing respiratory failure postoperatively.[147] There have been several attempts at predicting preoperatively which MG patients will require prolonged postoperative ventilation of the lungs.[148] For patients who underwent transsternal thymectomy, Leventhal et al[149] found that positive predictors were a duration of MG greater than 6 yr; history of chronic respiratory disease, other than directly due to MG; pyridostigmine dosage greater than 750 mg·day^{-1}; and preoperative VC of less than 2.9 l. This predictive system has not been found useful when applied in MG patients undergoing transsternal thymectomy at other centers, and of no value in MG patients undergoing other types of surgical procedure.[148] Each patient should, therefore, be treated on his or her own merits.

A more recent study of transsternal thymectomy patients suggested that the need for postoperative mechanical ventilation correlated best with preoperative maximum static *expiratory* pressure.[150] It was concluded that expiratory weakness, by reducing cough efficacy and ability to clear secretions, was the main predictive determinant. Adequate clearance of secretions is essential in these patients, and may occasionally necessitate bronchoscopy.

In general, the postoperative morbidity in terms of respiratory failure is less following transcervical than transsternal thymectomy.[143, 148] Techniques described which may be useful in reducing postoperative ventilatory failure include preoperative plasma exchange and high-dose steroid therapy perioperatively. If the anticipated duration of the surgical procedure is $1-2$ h, preoperative oral anticholinesterase therapy may be of value, since the peak effect of the drug will coincide with the conclusion of the surgical procedure and attempts at extubation.[141]

Postoperative Care

In the immediate postoperative period, pain relief is usually provided by opioid analgesics, such as meperidine, but in reduced dosages. The analgesic effect of morphine and other opioid analgesics has been reported as being increased by anticholinesterases, which has led to the recommendation that the dose of opiate analgesics be reduced by one-third in patients receiving anticholinesterase therapy.[151] The use of epidural or intrathecal opioids in myasthenic patients following thymectomy has not yet been reported.

MYASTHENIC SYNDROME (Eaton Lambert Syndrome, ELS)

The myasthenic syndrome is a very rare disorder of neuromuscular transmission, which is sometimes associated with small-cell carcinoma of the lung. Complaints of weakness may be mistaken for MG, but, in ELS symptoms do not respond to anticholinesterases or steroids, and activity *improves* strength. The defect in this condition is thought to be prejunctional, associated with diminished release of Ach from nerve terminals, and improved by agents, such as 4-aminopyridine, guanidine, and germine, that increase repetitive firing. Affected patients are particularly sensitive to the effects of all muscle relaxants, which should be used with great caution or avoided entirely. The possibility of ELS should be considered in all patients with known malignant disease and those patients undergoing diagnostic procedures for suspected carcinoma of the lung. Anesthesia considerations in these patients are essentially the same as in those with MG.

POSTOPERATIVE MANAGEMENT AND COMPLICATIONS

ATELECTASIS

Patients who require thoracotomy often have preexisting pulmonary disease which, when combined with the operative procedure, is likely to result in significant pulmonary dysfunction. Atelectasis, the most significant cause of postoperative morbidity, has been reported to occur in up to 100% of patients undergoing thoracotomy for pulmonary resection.[152] It occurs more frequently in the basal lobes than in the middle or upper lung regions, and is thought to be secondary to reduction of normal respiratory effort due to pain, intrathoracic blood and fluid accumulation, and decreased compliance, which leads to rapid shallow constant V_T. Such a respiratory pattern produces small airway closure and obstruction with inspissated secretions, resulting ultimately in alveolar air resorption and terminal airway collapse. The diagnosis of atelectasis can be made by clinical findings, chest x-ray, or ABGs. This problem is best resolved by increasing resting lung volume or functional residual capacity (FRC). FRC can be increased by an increase in transpulmonary pressure (difference between airway and intrapleural pressures: PL = [Paw - Ppl]) or lung compliance.

The tracheae of many patients can be extubated shortly after brief thoracic surgical procedures using standard extubation criteria. However, most patients with COPD undergoing extensive thoracic surgical procedures require postoperative ventilation to avoid atelectasis and other pulmonary complications.[153] Mechanical ventilation raises airway pressure and, to a lesser extent, intrapleural pressure; therefore, transpulmonary pressure increases. Most postoperative thoracotomy patients are ventilated using intermittent mandatory ventilation (IMV) and PEEP. Ventilation settings include: $V_T = 12$ $ml \cdot kg^{-1}$, rate 8 breaths $\cdot min^{-1}$, $FI_{O_2} = 0.5$, and PEEP 5–20 cm H_2O. The goal is to keep the Pa_{O_2} between 80–100 mm Hg and the Pa_{CO_2} and pH normal. The IMV rate is decreased as tolerated to two breaths per minute, and then the PEEP level is reduced to 5 cm H_2O. When ABGs are adequate at these settings and the VC is greater than 10 $ml \cdot kg^{-1}$, inspiratory force is greater than -20 cm H_2O, and the level of consciousness is adequate, the patient's trachea is ready for extubation.[154]

POSTOPERATIVE PAIN CONTROL

After extubation of the trachea, respiratory therapy and pain management become critical components of postoperative care. Adequate postoperative pain control is necessary to ensure a good respiratory effect. Administration of iv opioids has been the standard form of pain management for years. These drugs may improve pulmonary function slightly or allow respiratory therapy maneuvers; however, meperidine (50 mg) has been shown to be relatively ineffective at allowing patients to increase their ability to cough. Advantages of iv opioids are the ease of administration, relatively low toxicity, and the lack of a need for close medical supervision. The key disadvantage is the inadequate pain relief leading to postoperative atelectasis and great discomfort on the part of the patient. Patient-controlled analgesia allows for better pain relief for the patient and, possibly, will lead to some improvement in respiratory parameters. It has recently been shown to be very popular and safe in patients after major surgery.

Many clinicians have suggested the use of intercostal nerve blocks before, during, or after thoracic surgery to decrease pain and improve postoperative respiratory function. Studies have documented a decrease in requirements for postoperative opioids, improved respiratory function (Fig. 33-27), and some decrease in hospital stay.[155] The intercostal block can be performed externally before or after surgery using a standard technique. However, the easiest method during thoracic surgery is to have the surgeon perform the block under direct vision from inside the thorax with the chest open. Bupivacaine, 0.5%, in doses of 2–3 ml can be placed in the five intercostal spaces around the incision and in intercostal spaces where chest tubes will be placed. This provides for 6–24 h of moderate pain relief, but patients still complain of diaphragmatic shoulder discomfort due to the chest tubes. Larger volumes of local anesthetic (i.e., 5–10 ml) should not be used in the intercostal space due to the high absorption rate and attendant systemic toxicity that can be produced, as well as the possibility of pushing the drug centrally and producing a paravertebral sympathetic or epidural block with central sympatholysis and severe hypotension.[156]

A prolonged duration intercostal nerve block may be obtained by cryoanalgesia, a technique of freezing the nerve

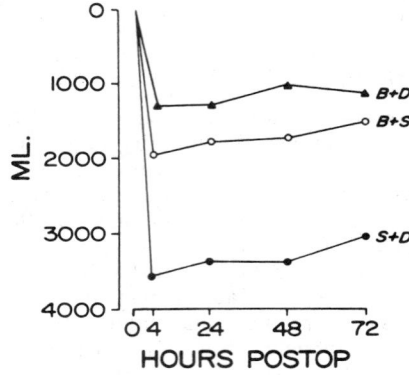

CHANGE IN VITAL CAPACITY FROM CONTROL

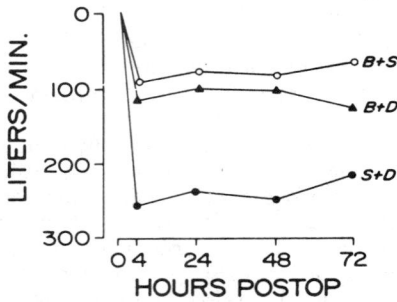

CHANGE IN FORCED EXPIRATORY FLOW RATES FROM CONTROL

FIG. 33-27. (*Top*) Mean decrease in vital capacity from control and after thoracotomy with intercostal nerve block; (*bottom*) mean decrease in forced expiratory flow rates from control and after thoracotomy with intercostal nerve block. Nerve block performed with the following solutions: bupivacaine-dextran (B + D); bupivacaine-saline (B + S); saline-dextran (S + D). (Kaplan JA, Miller ED, Gallagher EG: Postoperative analgesia for thoracotomy patients. Anes Analg 54:774, 1975, with permission.)

under direct vision at time of thoracotomy.[157] A cryoprobe is applied directly to the nerve to disrupt the axon but not the support structures. In this way, conduction is interrupted until the nerve regenerates over the next 3–4 months, by which time full structure and function are usually restored. During the postoperative period, the patients are numb in the segments thus treated. Ideally, any drains or chest tubes should be located within the area made analgesic with the cryoprobe so as to minimize immediate postoperative discomfort. Since cryoanalgesia is of prolonged duration, it is not used routinely following thoracotomy, but, rather, in cases where prolonged analgesia would be necessary, such as following surgery for chest trauma.

The newest approach to postoperative pain control after thoracic surgery is the use of epidural or intrathecal opioids. Epidural morphine has been shown to produce profound analgesia lasting from 16–24 h after thoracotomy and not to cause a sympathetic block or sensory or motor loss.[158] These are significant advantages over other methods of administering opioids or local anesthetics. The opioids have been successfully used by both the thoracic and lumbar epidural routes. Morphine, in a dose of 5–7 mg diluted in 15–20 ml of fluid, has been used in the lumbar epidural technique. This technique has led to a 30% increase in postoperative expiratory flow rates without significant side effects, even in patients with chronic lung disease.

Intrathecal morphine, in a dose of 10–15 $\mu g \cdot kg^{-1}$, has also been successfully used after thoracic surgery. With this technique, the drug acts directly on the spinal cord, and analgesia can be produced with a smaller dose than by the epidural or intravenous routes. Gray et al[159] showed the effectiveness of this technique in post-thoracotomy pain management. When the drug is given intrathecally prior to the induction of anesthesia, a reduction in the dose of anesthetic drugs required may occur. However, Wynands et al recently showed that intrathecal morphine (1.5 mg) did not reduce postoperative pain or improve respiratory parameters in a group of patients anesthetized with fentanyl undergoing intrathoracic surgery (Fig. 33-28).[160] The authors stated that this was due to the opioid receptors being saturated by the iv fentanyl. All previous studies showing the benefits of epidural or intrathecal opioids have been performed after anesthetic techniques that were not dependent on large doses of opioids.

All patients who have received intrathecal or epidural opioids must be closely observed for potential side effects. These include delayed respiratory depression, urinary retention, pruritus, nausea, and vomiting, and they appear to be dose-related. All of these effects may be reversed with naloxone.

FIG. 33-28. FVC, FEV₁, and PEFR measured preoperatively (Preop), and 1 and 24 h postextubation. $P < .05$ when compared with baseline values ITM = intrathecal morphine; ITS = intrathecal saline. (Wynands JE, Casey WF, Ralley FF et al: The role of intrathecal morphine in the anesthetic management of patients undergoing coronary artery bypass surgery. J Cardiothoracic Anesth, 1:510, 1988, with permission.)

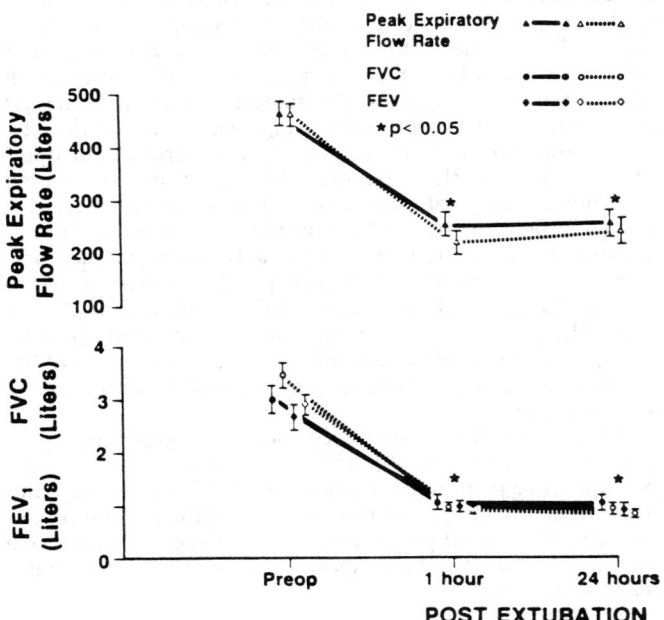

RESPIRATORY THERAPY TECHNIQUES

Physiotherapy is one of the oldest forms of therapy for the prevention and treatment of respiratory complications. Techniques include postural drainage, breathing exercises, vibration, deep breathing, coughing, and percussion. Many clinicians feel that chest physical therapy is useful despite the sparse data to support its physiologic benefits. Decades ago, it was also felt that forced exhalation against resistance would create increased airway pressures and inflation of the lungs. Thus, water-filled blow bottles were designed for postoperative use. However, studies subsequently showed that a forced exhalation decreases the expiratory transpulmonary pressure and lung volumes, and should be avoided in postoperative patients. Bartlett et al suggested that the blow bottles were only useful because of the large inspiration that preceded the forced exhalation.[161]

Intermittent positive-pressure breathing (IPPB) has also been used extensively in the postoperative period to prevent and treat respiratory insufficiency. However, most of the studies demonstrated little physiologic benefit. In fact, some authors showed that IPPB could be harmful after thoracotomy due to the hypoventilation that subsequently occurred after the forced hyperventilation.[162] The hyperventilation led to a decreased FRC and Pa$_{O_2}$ secondary to the decreased expiratory transpulmonary pressure.

Incentive spirometry is the most widely used postoperative respiratory care device. This device, producing a long, deep breath, has been shown to cause less complications and atelectasis than IPPB, blow bottles, or chest physiotherapy.[163] Patients with a decreased FRC and decreased Pa$_{O_2}$ experience a reduction of atelectasis on chest x-ray and improved arterial oxygenation. Bartlett showed that the technique produces an increase in inspiratory transpulmonary pressure, but not an increase in expiratory pressure.[161] Expiratory transpulmonary pressure can best be increased by the use of CPAP by mask. This technique was first described in the mid-1930s. Andersen et al compared mask CPAP to chest physical therapy, postural drainage, and endotracheal suction in the treatment of postoperative atelectasis.[163] They found that 15 cm H_2O CPAP applied once an hour for 25–35 breaths led to a clinically significant improvement within 12 h, while the other techniques produced little change. This technique appears to be very useful in the treatment of atelectasis in order to avoid reintubation of the trachea in patients after surgery. Gastric distention, regurgitation, and pulmonary aspiration are the potential dangers of mask CPAP.

OTHER COMPLICATIONS AFTER THORACIC SURGERY

The other major complications after thoracic surgery can be grouped into cardiovascular, pulmonary, and related problems (Table 33-10). The cardiovascular complications are often the most difficult to manage in patients with associated respiratory insufficiency. The low CO syndrome and postoperative cardiac dysrhythmias are the most common and life-threatening of these problems. In the postoperative period, advanced hemodynamic monitoring is used to make the differential diagnosis of left or right ventricular failure and the low output syndrome. The key monitor is the pulmonary arterial catheter that facilitates the construction of Starling function curves.[164] New diagnostic modalities, such as echocardiography, may be required to rule out the presence of pericardial effusions or

TABLE 33-10. Complications of Thoracic Surgery

I. Cardiovascular complications
   1. Hypotension
   2. Low-output syndrome
   3. Dysrhythmias
   4. Postoperative hypertension
   5. Myocardial ischemia and infarction
   6. Pacing problems
II. Pulmonary complications
   1. Pulmonary emboli
   2. Bronchopleural fistula
   3. Empyema and mediastinitis
   4. Pulmonary torsion
   5. Tracheostomy problems
   6. Diagnostic procedure complications
   7. Chest wall complications
   8. Pleural drainage
   9. Pulmonary hemorrhage
III. Related complications
   1. Monitoring equipment
   2. Neurologic—central and peripheral

tamponade after opening the pericardium during certain types of thoracic surgical procedure. The low CO syndrome must be differentiated from hypovolemia resulting from intrathoracic hemorrhage, tamponade, pulmonary emboli, or the effects of mechanical ventilation with PEEP. Therapeutic interventions for postoperative myocardial dysfunction include inotropic drugs, vasodilators, and combinations of these drugs, as needed, to improve ventricular function. The goal is to shift the Starling function curve up and to the left by reducing preload of either the left or right side of the heart and increasing cardiac output. Vasodilators are very effective at decreasing right ventricular afterload and improving right ventricular function, since this side of the heart is especially afterload-dependent.[165] Combinations of inotropes and vasodilators, such as isoproterenol and nitroglycerin, or combined drugs, such as amrinone, can be especially useful in the treatment of right heart failure.

Postoperative cardiac dysrhythmias are common after thoracic surgery. Patients undergoing pulmonary resection have postoperative supraventricular tachycardias with a frequency and severity proportional to both their age and the magnitude of the surgical procedure. Many factors contribute to these dysrhythmias, including underlying cardiac disease, degree of surgical trauma, effects of anesthetics and cardioactive drugs, and metabolic abnormalities.

Beck-Nielson reported on cardiac dysrythmias in a series of 300 thoracotomies for lung resection and found that atrial fibrillation occurred in 20% of patients with malignant disease but in only 3% with benign disease.[166] The prophylactic use of digitalis in thoracic surgical patients is controversial, particularly in patients with signs of congestive heart failure. Factors against its use include the potential toxic effects of the drug and the difficulty in assessing adequacy of digitalization in the absence of heart failure. A factor in favor of its use is the drug's efficacy in reducing the incidence of potentially fatal complications in older patients.[167] If digitalis is to be instituted, normokalemia should be ensured to reduce the likelihood of digitalis toxicity.

Supraventricular tachycardias can also be treated with either beta- or calcium channel-blocking drugs after ruling out

underlying reversible physiologic abnormalities, such as hypoxia. Verapamil has been the standard treatment for these problems until the recent introduction of the ultrashort-acting beta-blocker, esmolol. Esmolol has been shown to be equally effective in controlling the ventricular rate in patients with postoperative atrial fibrillation or flutter and in increasing the conversion rate to regular sinus rhythm from 8–34%.[168] Due to its short duration of action (beta-elimination half-life of 9 min, and beta$_1$-cardioselectivity, it is the drug of choice in the postoperative period to control these dysrhythmias. Doses of $50–200 \ \mu g \cdot kg^{-1} \cdot min^{-1}$ have been shown to be most effective in the control of supraventricular tachycardias.

Hemorrhage and pneumothorax are always major concerns after intrathoracic surgery. Due to these problems, intrapleural thoracostomy tubes with an underwater seal system are routinely used after thoracic surgery. Slippage of a suture on any major vessel or airway in the chest can lead to the slow or rapid development of hypovolemic shock or a tension pneumothorax. Drainage of greater than $200 \ ml \cdot hr^{-1}$ of blood is an indication for surgical reexploration for hemorrhage. Management of the pleural drainage system is fraught with confusion. The chest bottles must be kept below the level of the chest, and the tubes should not be clamped during patient transport. These tubes can be life-saving, but errors in technique can lead to serious complications.

Both central and peripheral neurologic injuries can occur during intrathoracic procedures. Such injuries often result in serious and disabling loss of function, and are very distressing to the patient. Peripheral nerves can be injured, either in the chest or in other parts of the body, by pressure or stretching.[169] It has been recognized for years that the majority of these postoperative neuropathies are due to malpositioning of the patient on the operating table, with subsequent stretching or compression of the nerves. The nerve injury may be apparent immediately after surgery, or may not become obvious until several days later. These patients often complain of a variety of unpleasant sensations, including paresthesias, coldness, pain, or anesthesia in the area supplied by the affected nerves. The brachial plexus is especially vulnerable to trauma during thoracic surgery due to its long superficial course in the axilla between two points of fixation, the vertebrae above and the axillary fascia below. Stretching is the chief cause of damage to the brachial plexus, with compression having only a secondary role.[169] Branches of the brachial plexus may also be injured lower in the arm by compression against objects such as an ether screen or other parts of the operating table. Intrathoracic nerves can be directly injured during a surgical procedure by being transected, crushed, stretched, or cauterized. The intercostal nerves are the ones most frequently injured during intrathoracic surgical procedures. The recurrent laryngeal nerve can become involved in lymph node tissue and injured at the time of a node biopsy, especially when the biopsy is performed through a mediastinoscope. This nerve can also be injured during tracheostomy or radical pulmonary dissections. The phrenic nerve is frequently injured during pericardiectomy, radical pulmonary hilar dissections, division of the diaphragm during esophageal surgery, or dissection of mediastinal tumors.

Prevention is the treatment of choice for all these intraoperative nerve injuries. Analgesics may be necessary to control postoperative pain in the distribution of the nerve injury and to aid in maintaining joint mobility during the healing phase. Subsequent surgical procedures may be necessary to move a swollen ulnar nerve at the elbow, or to stent a partially paralyzed vocal cord.

REFERENCES

1. Rutkow IM: Thoracic and cardiovascular operations in the United States, 1979 to 1984. J Thoracic Cardiovasc Surg 92:181, 1986
2. Kaplan JA (ed): Thoracic Anesthesia. New York, Churchill Livingstone, 1983
3. Marshall BE, Longnecker DE, Fairly HB: Anesthesia for Thoracic Procedures. Oxford, Blackwell Scientific, 1987
4. Benumof JL: Anesthesia for Thoracic Surgery. Philadelphia, WB Saunders, 1987
5. Beck GJ, Doyle CA, Schacter FN: Smoking and lung function. Am Rev Respir Dis 155:149, 1981
6. Tisi GN: Preoperative evaluation of pulmonary function: Validity, indications, and benefits. Am Rev Respir Dis 119:293, 1979
7. O'Donoghue WJ, Baker JP, Bell GM et al: Respiratory failure in neuromuscular disease: Management in respiratory intensive care unit. JAMA 235:733, 1976
8. Gass GD, Olsen GN: Clinical significance of pulmonary function tests. Preoperative pulmonary function testing to predict postoperative morbidity and mortality. Chest 89:127, 1986
9. Lockwood P: Lung function test results and the risk of postthoracotomy complications. Respiration 30:529, 1973
10. Mittman C: Assessment of operative risk in thoracic surgery. Am Rev Respir Dis 84:197, 1961
11. Traver GA, Chine MG, Burrows B: Predictors of mortality in chronic obstructive pulmonary disease—A 15-year follow-up study. Am Rev Respir Dis 119:895, 1979
12. Stein M, Koota GM, Simon M et al: Pulmonary evaluation of surgical patients. JAMA 181:765, 1962
13. Jones RM, Rosen M, Seymour L: Smoking and anaesthesia (editorial). Anaesthesia 42:1, 1987
14. Jones RM: Smoking before surgery: The case for stopping smoking. Br Med J 290:1763, 1985
15. Buist AS, Sexton GV, Nagy JM et al: The effects of smoking cessation and modification of lung function. Am Rev Resp Dis 123:149, 1981
16. Pearce AC, Jones RM: Smoking and anesthesia: Preoperative abstinence and preoperative morbidity. Anesthesiology 61:576, 1984
17. Warner MA, Tinker JH, Divertie MB: Preoperative cessation of smoking and pulmonary complications in pulmonary dysfunction. Anesthesiology 59:A 60, 1983
18. Cooper DKL: The incidence of postoperative infection and the role of antibiotic prophylaxis in pulmonary surgery: A review of 221 consecutive patients undergoing thoracotomy. Br J Dis Chest 75:154, 1981
19. Chopru SK, Tuplin GV, Simmons DH et al: Effects of hydration and physical therapy on tracheal transport velocity. Am Rev Respir Dis 115:1009, 1977
20. Scheffiner AC: The mucolytic activity and mechanism of action and metabolism of acetylcysteine. Pharmacol Ther 1:47, 1964
21. Lertzman MM, Chernich RM: Rehabilitation of patients with chronic obstructive disease. Chest 73 (suppl):927, 1978
22. Crabb-Johnson DC, Chir B, Andrew JL: Bronchodilator therapy. NEJM 297:476, 1977
23. Aubier M, DeTroyer A, Sampson M et al: Aminophylline improves diaphragmatic contractility. NEJM 249:305, 1981
24. Marini JJ, Lakshmimara Y, Kradyan WA: Atropine and terbutaline aerosols in chronic bronchitis. Chest 80:285, 1981
25. Kaplan JA: Hemodynamic Monitoring. In Kaplan JA (ed): Cardiac Anesthesia, 2nd ed, p 179 Orlando, Grune and Stratton, 1987
26. Nobak CR: Intraoperative monitoring. In Kaplan JA (ed): Thoracic Anesthesia, 197. New York, Churchill-Livingstone, 1983

27. Petty C: Right radial artery pressure during mediastinoscopy. Anesth Analg 58:428, 1979
28. Gurman GM, Kriemerman S: Cannulation of big arteries in critically ill patients. Crit Care Med 13:217, 1985
29. Verweis J, Kester A, Stroes W et al: Comparison of 3 methods for measuring central venous pressure. Crit Care Med 14:288, 1986
30. Sznajder JI, Zveibil FR, Bitterman H et al: Central vein catheterization: Failure and complication rates by 3 percutaneous approaches. Arch Intern Med 146:259, 1986
31. Shah KB, Rao TLK, Laughlin S et al: A review of pulmonary artery catheterization in 6245 patients. Anesthesiology 61:271, 1984
32. Patel C, Laboy V, Venus B et al: Acute complications of pulmonary artery catheter insertion in critically ill patients. Crit Care Med 14:195, 1986
33. Nadeau S, Noble WH: Misinterpretation of pressure measurements from the pulmonary artery catheter. Can Anaesth Soc J 33:352, 1986
34. Schmitt EA, Brannigan CO: Common artifacts of pulmonary artery pressures: Recognition and interpretation. J Clin Monit 2:4, 1986
35. Raper R, Sibbald WJ: Misled by the wedge. Chest 89:427, 1986
36. Kaul S: The interventricular septum in health and disease. Am Heart J 112:568, 1986
37. Jardin F, Farcot JC, Boisante L et al: Influence of PEEP on left ventricular performance. NEJM 304:387, 1981
38. Cohen E, Eisenkraft JB, Thys D et al: Hemodynamics and oxygenation during OLA. Right vs left. Anesthesiology 63:A 566, 1985
39. Hines R, Barash PG: Right ventricular failure. In Kaplan JA, (ed). Cardiac Anesthesia, 2nd ed, p 995. Orlando, Grune and Stratton, 1987
40. Zaidan J, Freniere S: Use of a pacing pulmonary artery catheter during cardiac surgery. Ann Thorac Surg 35:633, 1983
41. Cohen E, Eisenkraft JB, Thys JA: Continuous monitoring of $S\bar{v}_{O_2}$ during one-lung anesthesia. Anesthesiology 615:A512, 1984
42. Guffin A, Girard D, Kaplan JA: Shivering following cardiac surgery: Hemodynamic changes and reversal. J Cardiothorac Anesth 1:24, 1987
43. Eisenkraft JB: Pulse oximeter desaturation due to methemoglobinemia. Anesthesiology 68:279, 1988
44. Brodsky JB, Shulman MS, Swan M et al: Pulse oximetry during one-lung ventilation. Anesthesiology 63:212, 1985
45. Tremper KK, Konchigeri HN, Cullen BF et al: Transcutaneous monitoring of oxygen tension during one-lung anesthesia. J Thorac Cardiovasc Surg 88:22, 1984
46. Barker SJ, Tremper KK, Heitmann HA: Continuous fiberoptic arterial oxygen tension in dogs. Crit Care Med 15:403, 1987
47. Shafieha MA, Sit J, Kartha R et al: End-tidal CO_2 analyzers in proper positioning of double-lumen tubes. Anesthesiology 64:844, 1986
48. Riley RH, Marcy JH: Unsuspected endobronchial intubation—Detection by continuous mass spectrometry. Anesthesiology 63:203, 1985
49. West JB, Dollery CT, Naimark A: Distribution of blood flow in isolated lung. Relation to vascular and alveolar pressures. J Appl Physiol 19:713, 1964
50. Marshall BE, Marshall C, Benumof JL et al: Hypoxic pulmonary vasoconstriction in dogs: Effects of lung segment size and oxygen tension. J Appl Physiol 51:1543, 1981
51. Ginsberg RJ: New techniques for one lung anesthesia using an endobronchial blocker. J Thorac Cardiovasc Surg 32:542, 1981
52. Inoue H, Shohtsu A, Ogawa J et al: New device for one-lung anesthesia: Endotracheal tube with movable blocker. J Thorac Cardiovasc Surg 83:940, 1982

53. Hultgren BL, Krishna PR, Kamaya H: A new tube for one lung ventilation: Experience with the Univent tube. Anesthesiology 65:3A, A481, 1986

54. Smith G, Hirsch N, Ehrenwerth J: Sight and sound: Can double-lumen endotracheal tubes be placed accurately without fiberoptic bronchoscopy? Br J Anaesth 58:1317, 1987

55. Benumof JL, Partridge BL, Salvatierra C et al: Margin of safety in positioning modern double-lumen endotracheal tubes. Anesthesiology 67:729, 1987

56. Guernelli N, Bragaglia RB, Briccoli A et al: Tracheobronchial rupture due to cuffed Carlens tubes. Thorac Surg 28:66, 1979

57. Wagner DL, Gammage GW, Wong ML: Tracheal rupture following the insertion of a disposable double-lumen endotracheal tube. Anesthesiology 63:698, 1985

58. Tarhan S, Lundborg RO: Carlens endobronchial catheter versus regular endobronchial tube during thoracic surgery: A comparison of blood gas tensions and pulmonary shunting. Can Anaesth Soc J 18:594, 1971

59. Kerr JH, Crampton Smith A, Prys-Roberts C et al: Observations during endobronchial anesthesia II, Oxygenation. Br J Anaesth 46:84, 1974

60. Flacke JW, Thompson DS, Read RC: Influence of tidal volume and pulmonary artery occlusion on arterial oxygenation during endobronchial anesthesia. South Med J 69:619, 1976

61. Capan LM, Turndorf H, Patel K et al: Optimization of arterial oxygenation during one-lung anesthesia. Anesth Analg 59:847, 1980

62. Dantzker DR, Wagner PD, West JB: Instability of lung units with low V/Q ratio during O_2 breathing. J Appl Physiol 38:886, 1975

63. Lunding M, Fernandes A: Arterial oxygen tensions and acid-base status during thoracic anaesthesia. Acta Anaesthesiol Scand 11:43, 1967

64. Torda TA, McCulloch CH, O'Brinh HD et al: Pulmonary venous admixture during one-lung anaesthesia: Effect of inhaled oxygen tension and respiration rate. Anaesthesia 29:272, 1974

65. Jenkins J, Cameron EWJ, Milne AC et al: One-lung anaesthesia. Cardiovascular and respiratory function compared during conventional ventilation and HFJV. Anaesthesia 42:938, 1987

66. Cohen E, Eisenkraft JB, Thys DM et al: Oxygenation and hemodynamic changes during one-lung ventilation. J Cardiothoracic Anesthesia, 2:34–40, 1988

67. Katz JA, Larlane RG, Rairby HB et al: Pulmonary oxygen exchange during endobronchial anesthesia: Effect of tidal volume and PEEP. Anesthesiology 56:164, 1982

68. Goldiner PL, Carlon GC, Cvitkovic E et al: Factors influencing postoperative morbidity and mortality in patients treated with bleomycin. Br Med J 1:1664, 1978

69. Tarhan S, Lundborg RO: Effects of increased expiratory pressure on blood gas tensions and pulmonary shunting during thoracotomy with use of the Carlens catheter. Can Anaesth Soc J 17:4, 1970

70. Cohen E, Thys DM, Eisenkraft JB et al: PEEP during one lung anesthesia improves oxygenation in patients with low PaO_2. Anesth Analg 64:200, 1985

71. Alfery D, Benumof JL, Trousdale FR: Improving oxygenation during one lung ventilation: The effects of PEEP and blood flow restoration to the non-ventilated lung. Anesthesiology 55:381, 1981

72. Rees DI, Wansbrough SR: One-lung anesthesia and arterial oxygen tension during continuous insufflation of oxygen to the non-ventilated lung. Anesth Analg 61:501, 1982

73. Eisenkraft JB, Thys DM, Cohen E et al: CPAP and PEEP during one-lung ventilation with isoflurane. Anesthesiology 61:3A520, 1984

74. Hannenberg AA, Sotwicz PR, Pienes RS Jr et al: A device for applying CPAP to the non-ventilated upper lung during one-lung ventilation II. Anesthesiology 60:254, 1984

75. Thiagarajah S, Job C, Rao A: A device for applying CPAP to the non-ventilated upper lung during one-lung ventilation. Anesthesiology 60:253, 1984

76. Lyons TE: A simplified method of CPAP delivery to the non-ventilated lung during unilateral pulmonary ventilation. Anesthesiology 61:217, 1984

77. Arandia HY, Patel VU: PEEP and the Mapleson D circuit. Anesthesiology 62:846, 1985

78. Brown DR, Kafer ER, Robertson VO et al: Improved oxygenation during thoracotomy with selective PEEP to the dependent lung. Anesth Analg 56:26, 1977

79. Nunn JF: Factors influencing the arterial oxygen tension during halothane anesthesia with spontaneous respiration. Br J Anaesth 36:327, 1964

80. Marshall BE, Cohen PJ, Klingenmaier CH et al: Pulmonary venous admixture before, during and after halothane: Oxygen anesthesia in man. J Appl Physiol 27:653, 1967

81. Von Euler US, Liljestrand G: Observations on the pulmonary arterial blood pressure in the cat. Acta Physiol Scand 12:301, 1946

82. Marshall BE, Marshall C, Benumof JL et al: Hypoxic pulmonary vasoconstriction in dogs: Effects of lung segment size and alveolar oxygen tensions. J Appl Physiol 51:1543, 1981

83. Domino KB, Wetstein L, Glasser SA et al: Influence of mixed venous oxygen tension (PvO_2) on blood flow to atelectatic lung. Anesthesiology 59:428, 1983

84. Benumof JL: One-lung ventilation and hypoxic pulmonary vasoconstriction: Implications for anesthetic management, Anesth Analg 64:821, 1985

85. Marshall C, Lindgren L, Marshall BE: Effects of halothane and isoflurane in rat lungs in vitro. Anesthesiology 60:304, 1984

86. Bjertnaes LJ: Hypoxia-induced vasoconstriction in isolated perfused lungs exposed to injectable or inhalational anaesthetics. Acta Anaesthesiol Scand 21:133, 1977

87. Mathers J, Benumof JL, Wahrenbrock EA: General anesthetics and regional HPV. Anesthesiology 46:111, 1977

88. Saidman LJ, Trousdale FR: Isoflurane does not inhibit HPV. Anesthesiology 57:A472, 1982

89. Gibbs JM, Johnson H: Lack of effect of morphine and buprenorphine on HPV in the isolated perfused cat lung and the perfused lobe of the dog lung. Br J Anaesth 50:1197, 1978

90. Domino KB, Borowec L, Alexander CM et al: Influence of isoflurane on HPV in dogs. Anesthesiology 64:423, 1986

91. Lumb PD, Silvay G, Weinreich AI et al: A comparison of the effects of continuous ketamine infusion and halothane on oxygenation during OLV in dogs. Can Anaesth Soc J 26:394, 1979

92. Bjertnaes LJ: Hypoxia-induced pulmonary vasoconstriction in man: Inhibition due to diethyl ether and halothane anaesthesia. Acta Anaesthesiol Scand 22:578, 1978

93. Jolin Carlsson A, Bindslev L, Hedenstierna G: Hypoxia-induced pulmonary vasoconstriction in the human lung. The effect of isoflurane anesthesia. Anesthesiology 66:312, 1987

94. Weinreich AI, Silvay G, Lumb PD: Continuous ketamine infusion for one-lung ventilation. Can Anaesth Soc J 27:485, 1980

95. Rees DI, Gaines GY: One-lung anesthesia—A comparison of pulmonary gas exchange during anesthesia with ketamine or enflurane. Anesth Analg 63:521, 1984

96. Rogers SM, Benumof JL: Halothane and isoflurane do not decrease Pa_{O_2} during one-lung ventilation in intravenously anesthetized patients. Anesth Analg 64:946, 1985

97. Benumof JL, Augustine SD, Gibbons JA: Halothane and isoflurane only slightly impair arterial oxygenation during one-lung ventilation in patients undergoing thoracotomy. Anesthesiology 67:910, 1987

98. Marshall BE, Marshall C: Anesthesia and the pulmonary circulation. In Covino BJ, Fozzard HA, Rehder K et al (eds): Effects of Anesthesia, Clinical Physiology Series, p 121. Bethesda, American Physiological Society, 1985

99. Chen L, Miller FL, Malmkvist G et al: High-dose almitrine bimesylate inhibits hypoxic pulmonary vasoconstrictin in closed-chest dogs. Anesthesiology 67:534, 1987

100. Marshall C, Kim SD, Marshall BE: The actions of halothane, ibuprofen and BW 755C on hypoxic pulmonary vasconstriction. Anesthesiology 66:537, 1987

101. Frumin MJ, Epstein R, Cohen G: Apneic oxygenation in man. Anesthesiology 20:789, 1959

102. Fraoli RL, Sheffe LA, Steffanson JL: Pulmonary and cardiovascular effects of apneic oxygenation in man. Anesthesiology 39:588, 1973

103. Sanders RD: Two ventilating attachments for bronchoscopes. Delaware Med J 39:170, 1967

104. Giesecke AH, Gerbershagen H, Dortman C et al: Comparison of the ventilating and injection bronchoscopes. Anesthesiology 38:298, 1973

105. Carden E: Recent improvements in anesthetic techniques for use during bronchoscopy. Otol Rhinol Laryngol 83:777, 1974

106. Vour'h G, Fishler M, Michon F et al: Manual jet ventilation v high-frequency jet ventilation during laser resection of tracheobronchial stenosis. Br J Anaesth 55:973, 1983

107. Sackner MA. State of the art—Bronchofiberscopy. Am Rev Respir Dis 111:62, 1975

108. Matsushima Y, Jones RL, King EG et al: Alterations in pulmonary mechanics and gas exchange during routine fiberoptic bronchoscopy. Chest 86:184, 1984

109. Satyanarayana T, Capan L, Ramanathan S et al: Bronchofiberscopic jet ventilation. Anesth Analg 59:350, 1980

110. Warner ME, Warner M, Leonard P: Anesthesia for neodymium-YAG laser resection of major airway obstructing tumors. Anesthesiology 60:230, 1984

111. Duckett JE, McDonnell TJ, Unger M et al: General anesthesia for Nd:YAG laser resection of obstructing endo-bronchial tumors using the rigid bronchoscope. Can Anaesth Soc J 32:67, 1985

112. Watson CB: Fiberoptic bronchoscopy in thoracic anaesthesia. In Gotthard JW (ed): Thoracic Anaesthesia, p 33. Philadelphia, Bailliere Tindall, 1987

113. Neuman G, Weingarten AE, Abramowitz RM et al: The anesthetic management of the patient with an anterior mediastinal mass. Anesthesiology 60:144, 1984

114. DeSoto H: Direct laryngoscopy as an aid to relieve airway obstruction in a patient with a mediastinal mass. Anesthesiology 67:116, 1987

115. Sibert K, Biondi JW, Hirsch NP: Spontaneous respiration during thoracotomy in a patient with a mediastinal mass. Anesth Analg 66:904, 1987

116. Carlens E: Mediastinoscopy: A method for inspection and tissue biopsy in the superior mediastinum. Dis Chest 36:343, 1959

117. Carlens E, Ericsson M, Levander-Lindgren M et al: Detector electrode introduced by mediastinoscopy for atrial triggered cardiac pacing. Br Heart Journal 39:1265, 1977

118. Morton JR, Guinn GA: Mediastinoscopy using local anesthesia. Am J Surg 122:696, 1971

119. Ashbaugh DG: Mediastinoscopy. Arch Surg 100:568, 1970

120. Roberts JT, Gissen AJ: Management of complications encountered during anesthesia for mediastinoscopy. Anesthesiology Review 6:31, 1979

121. Lee J, Salvatore A: Innominate artery compression simulating cardiac arrest during mediastinoscopy. A case report. Anesth Analg 55:748, 1976

122. Barash PG, Tsai B, Kitahata LM: Acute tracheal collapse following mediastinoscopy. Anesthesiology 44:67, 1976

123. Vaughan RS: Anesthesia for mediastinoscopy. Anaesthesia 33:195, 1978

124. Faurschou P, Madsen G, Viskum K: Thoracoscopy: Influence of the procedure on some respiratory and cardiac values. Thorax 38:341, 1983

125. Malina JF, Nordstrom SG, Sjostrand UH et al: Clinical evaluation of high-frequency positive-pressure ventilation (HFPPV) in patients scheduled for open-chest surgery. Anesth Analg 60:324, 1981

126. Glenski JA, Crawford M, Rehder K: High-frequency small-volume ventilation during thoracic surgery. Anesthesiology 64:211, 1986

127. Wilks D, Schumann T, Riley R et al: Selective high-frequency jet ventilation of the operative lung improves oxygenation during thoracic surgery. Anesthesiology 63:A568, 1985

128. Morgan BA, Perks D, Conacher ID et al: Combined unilateral HFJV and contralateral IPPV. Anaesthesia 42:975, 1987

129. Capan LM, Miller S, Patel KP: Pro: Application of CPAP to the non-dependent lung is preferable to HFV for optimal oxygenation during pulmonary surgery. J Cardiothoracic Anesth 1:584, 1987

130. El-Baz N: Application of CPAP to the non-dependent lung is not preferable to HFV to optimize oxygenation during pulmonary surgery. J Cardiothoracic Anesth 1:587, 1987

131. Rafferty TD, Palma J, Motoyama et al: Management of a bronchopleural fistula with differential lung ventilation and PEEP. Resp Care 25:654, 1980

132. Bishop MJ, Benson MS, Sato P et al: Comparison of high-frequency jet ventilation with conventional ventilation for bronchopleural fistula. Anesth Analg 66:833, 1987

133. Normandale JP: Bullous cystic lung disease. Anaesthesia 40:1182, 1985

134. McCarthy G, Coppel DL, Gibbons JR et al: High-frequency jet ventilation for bilateral bullectomy. Anaesthesia 42:411, 1987

135. Benumof JL: Sequential one-lung ventilation for bilateral bullectomy. Anesthesiology 67:268, 1987

136. Grillo HC: Carinal reconstruction. Ann Thorac Surg 34:357, 1984

137. Lippman M, Mok MS: Anesthetic management of pulmonary lavage in adults. Anesth Analg 56:661, 1977

138. Smith JC, Millen JE, Safar P et al: Intrathoracic pressure, pulmonary vascular pressures and gas exchange during pulmonary lavage. Anesthesiology 33:401, 1978

139. Osserman KE, Genkins G: Studies in myasthenia gravis—Review of a 20-year-experience in over 1200 patients. Mount Sinai J Med 38:497, 1971

140. Engel AG: Myasthenia gravis and myasthenic syndromes. Ann Neurol 16:516, 1984

141. Eisenkraft JB: Myasthenia gravis and thymic surgery—Anaesthetic considerations. In Gotthard JWW (ed): Thoracic Anaesthesiology, p 133. London, Balliere Tindall, 1987

142. Buckingham JM, Howard FM, Bernatz PE: The value of thymectomy in myasthenia gravis. A computer-assisted matched study. Ann Surg 184:453, 1976

143. Papatestas AE, Genkins G, Kornfeld P et al: Effects of thymectomy in myasthenia gravis. Ann Surg 206:79, 1987

144. Eisenkraft JB, Papatestas AE, Sivak M: Neuromuscular effects of halogenated agents in patients with myasthenia gravis. Anesthesiology 61:3A, A307, 1984

145. Eisenkraft JB, Book WJ, Papatestas AE, Hubbard M: Resistance to succinylcholine in myasthenia gravis: A dose-response study. Anesthesiology (in press)

146. Mora CT, Eisenkraft JB, Papatestas AE: Intravenous dantrolene in a patient with myasthenia gravis. Anesthesiology 64:371, 1986

147. Gracey DR, Divertie MB, Howard FM: Mechanical ventilation for respiratory failure in myasthenia gravis. Mayo Clinic Proceedings 58:597, 1983
148. Eisenkraft JB, Papatestas AE, Kahn CH et al: Predicting the need for postoperative mechanical ventilation in myasthenia gravis. Anesthesiology 65:79, 1986
149. Leventhal R, Orkin FK, Hirsch RA: Prediction of the need for postoperative mechanical ventilation in myasthenia gravis. Anesthesiology 53:26, 1980
150. Younger DS, Brawn NMT, Jaretzski A: Myasthenia gravis: Determinants for independent ventilation after transsternal thymectomy. Neurology 34:336, 1984
151. Foldes FF, Nagashima H: Myasthenia gravis and anesthesia. In Oyama T (ed): Endocrinology and the Anaesthetist. Monographs in Anesthesiology, p 171. New York, Elsevier, 1983
152. Downs JB: Postoperative respiratory care. In Kaplan JA (ed): Thoracic Anesthesia, p 635. New York, Churchill-Livingstone, 1983
153. Hirschler-Schultz CJ, Hylkema BS, Beyer RW: Mechanical ventilation for acute postoperative respiratory failure after surgery for bronchial carcinoma. Thorax 40:387, 1985
154. Cane RD, Shapiro B: Mechanical ventilatory support. JAMA 254:87, 1985
155. Kaplan JA, Miller ED, Gallagher EG: Postoperative analgesia for thoracotomy patients. Anesth Analg 54:773, 1975
156. Gallo JA, Lebowitz PW, Battit GE et al: Comparison of intercostal nerve blocks performed under direct vision during thoracotomy. J Thorac Cardiovasc Surg 86:628, 1983
157. Glynn CJ, Lloyd JW, Barnard JD: Cryoanalgesia in the management of pain after thoracotomy. Thorax 34:325, 1980
158. Shulman M, Sandler AN, Bradley JW et al: Post-thoracotomy pain and pulmonary function following epidural and systemic morphine. Anesthesiology 61:564, 1984
159. Gray JR, Fromme GA, Nauss LA et al: Intrathoracic morphine for post-thoracotomy pain. Anesth Analg 65:873, 1986
160. Wynands JE, Casey WF, Ralley FE et al: The role of intrathecal morphine in the anesthetic management of patients undergoing coronary artery bypass surgery. J Cardiothorac Anesth 1:510, 1987
161. Bartlett RH, Gazzaniga AB, Geraghty TR: Respiratory maneuvers to prevent postoperative pulmonary complications. JAMA 224:1017, 1973
162. Iverson LI, Ecker RR, Fox HE et al: A comparison study of IPPB, the incentive spirometer and blow bottles: The prevention of atelectasis following cardiac surgery. Ann Thorac Surg 25:197, 1978
163. Andersen JB, Olesen KP, Eikard B et al: Periodic CPAP by mask in the treatment of atelectasis. Eur J Resp Dis 61:20, 1980
164. Altschule M: Reflections on Starling's Laws of the Heart. Chest 89:444, 1986
165. Prewitt R, Ghignone M: Treatment of right ventricular dysfunction in acute respiratory failure. Crit Care Med 5:346, 1983
166. Beck-Nielsen J, Sorenson HR, Astroup P: Atrial fibrillation following thoracotomy for non cardiac disease; in particular cancer of the lung. Acta Med Scand 193:425, 1973
167. Shields TW, Uyiki GT: Digitalization for prevention of arrhythmias following pulmonary surgery. Surg Gynecol Obstet 126:743, 1968
168. Morganroth J, Horowitz LN, Anderson J et al: Comparative efficacy and tolerance of esmolol to propranolol for control of supraventricular tachyarhythmias. Am J Cardiol 56:335, 1985
169. Seyfer AE, Grammer NY, Bogumill GP et al: Upper extremity neuropathies after cardiac surgery. J Hand Surg 10:16, 1985
170. Khanam T, Branthwaite MA: Arterial oxygenation during one-lung anesthesia (1): A study in man. Anaesthesia 28:132, 1973
171. Aalto-Setala M, Heinonen J, Salorinne Y: Cardiorespiratory function during thoracic anesthesia: Comparison of two-lung ventilation and one-lung ventilation with and without PEEP. Acta Anesthesiol Scand 19:287, 1975

Chapter 34

Carol L. Lake

Cardiovascular Anatomy and Physiology

A basic knowledge of the anatomy and physiology of the heart and vascular system is essential for the anesthesiologist caring for patients for either cardiac or non-cardiac surgery. This chapter focuses upon those aspects of cardiovascular anatomy and physiology important to perioperative management. It also details some of the pathophysiologic alterations associated with cardiovascular diseases.

ANATOMY

HEART

Right Atrium

Systemic veins drain into the right atrium *via* the superior vena cava (SVC), the inferior vena cava (IVC), and the coronary sinus. The right atrium consists of two parts: 1) a thin-walled trabeculated portion, often termed the right auricle, which is separated by a ridge of muscle, the crista terminalis, from 2) the smooth-walled portion, into which the SVC and IVC enter. On frontal chest x-ray, the right upper portion of the cardiac silhouette is the SVC (or ascending aorta in older patients) (Fig. 34-1). At the junction of the SVC with the right atrium is the sinoatrial node. The ostium of the inferior vena cava is guarded by the eustachian valve.[1] The third structure entering the right atrium is the coronary sinus with its ostium guarded by the thebesian valve.[2] The right and left atria are separated by the inter-atrial septum with its central ovoid portion, the fossa ovalis, the remnant of the fetal foramen ovale.

As blood leaves the right atrium, it passes through the tricuspid valve, which directs it anteriorly, inferiorly, and to the left toward the right ventricular outflow tract. As its name implies, the tricuspid valve consists of three leaflets, anterior, posterior, and medial, comprising an area of 8–11 cm² (Fig. 34-2). The anterior leaflet, the largest, is attached to the crista

supraventricularis (described below) and controlled by the anterior papillary muscle, which originates from a prominent intraventricular muscle, the moderator band, and the anterolateral ventricular wall. The septal leaflet attaches to the junction of the interatrial and interventricular septum.[3] The posterior leaflet originates from the diaphragmatic portion of the right ventricle. Connecting the papillary muscles to the valve leaflets are strong, fibrous structures known as the chordae tendineae. The small posterior and septal papillary muscles receive chordae from the posterior and medial tricuspid valve leaflets.

Right Ventricle

The right ventricle (RV) is a pocket wrapped around one-third of the left ventricle. Its muscle fibers are continuous with those of the left ventricle. Anatomically, it consists of inflow (sinus) and outflow (conal) portions divided by the crista supraventricularis. The crista supraventricularis also joins the interventricular septum and left ventricle to the right ventricular free wall. Because of these connections, the crista may be important in the integration of right and left ventricular function.[3] The heavily trabeculated inflow portion of the RV, containing the tricuspid valve, is posterior and inferior. Anterosuperiorly is the infundibulum or pulmonary outflow tract and pulmonic valve. Within the inflow portion are prominent muscle bands (moderator, septal, and parietal).

Pulmonary Artery and Peripheral Pulmonary Circulation

The pulmonic valve separates the right ventricular infundibulum from the main pulmonary artery. It is a trileaflet valve (right, left, and anterior cusps), normally about 4 cm² in area (Fig. 34-2). As it originates from the superior portion of the right ventricle, the pulmonary artery passes backward and upward under the aorta before it bifurcates into right and left pulmonary arteries. On the frontal chest x-ray, the superior portion of the left cardiac silhouette is the aorta, and just beneath is the main pulmonary artery (Fig. 34-1). The remnant of the fetal ductus arteriosus, the ligamentum arteriosum, connects the upper aspect of the bifurcation to the inferior aortic surface. The pulmonary arteries and veins of the lower lobes are normally larger and more prominent than those of the upper lobes. Pulmonary arteries branch into arterioles, and thence into capillaries, which spread over the alveolar surfaces between two alveolar endothelial layers.

The size of the peripheral pulmonary vessels indicates pulmonary blood volume and flow. With left-to-right cardiac shunts, the main pulmonary artery and hilar vessels are prominent. With pulmonary hypertension, however, dilation of the main pulmonary artery and abrupt tapering of the peripheral pulmonary vessels is noted.

Left Atrium

The left atrium (LA) is slightly larger than the right, and receives one or two pulmonary veins on its left and two or three on its right side. Enlargement of the left atrium appears on chest x-ray as a straightening of the left heart border, a double density near the right heart border, or displacement of the left mainstem bronchus (Fig. 34-1). Normally, the margins of the LA are the right main and intermediate bronchi and the left main and left lower lobe bronchi.

Leaving the LA, blood traverses the mitral valve. It consists of four cusps: 1) a large anterior (aortic) cusp; 2) the large posterior (mural) cusp; and 3) two small septal or commissural cusps. The surface area of the normal mitral valve is 6–8 cm² in adults.[4] Valves of less than 1 cm² are severely stenotic. As in the tricuspid valve, papillary muscles and chordae tendineae loosely anchor the leaflets or cusps to the left ventricular myocardium. The blood supply to the chordae and papillary muscles is often quite tenuous.[5, 6]

Left Ventricle

Normally, the left ventricle (LV) is thicker than the right, measuring about 8–15 mm. Its maximal cross-sectional dimension is also greater, about 4.5 cm compared to 3.5 cm for the RV.[7] Trabeculae are less coarse, but more dense, in the LV apex than in the RV. The interventricular septum with its membranous superior portion near the aortic valve and muscular inferior portion divides RV from LV. Separating the membranous and the muscular portion of the septum is the limbus marginalis.[8]

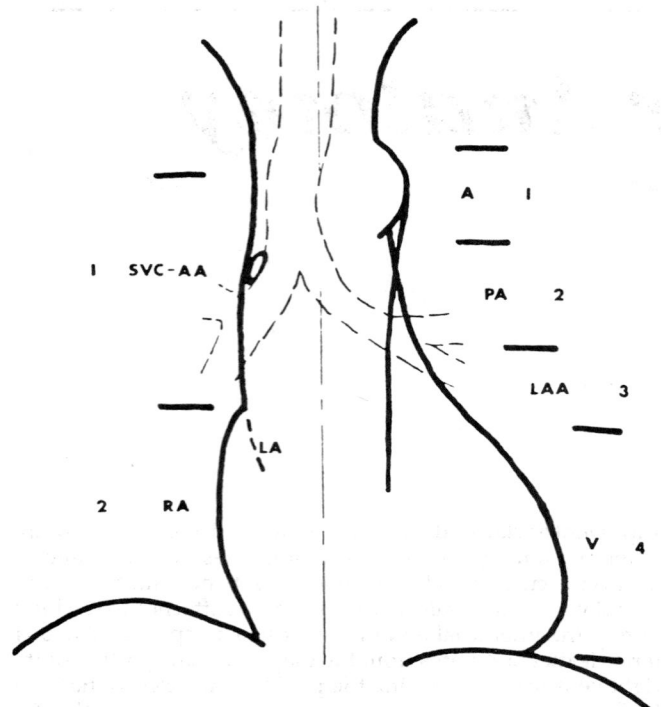

FIG. 34-1. The frontal chest radiograph in a diagrammatic view. *A* is the aortic arch, *PA* is the main pulmonary artery, *V* is the left ventricle, *LAA* is the left atrial appendage, *RA* is the right atrium, and *SVC-AA* is the superior vena cava or aortic segment. (New York Heart Association: Nomenclature and Criteria for Diagnosis of Disease of the Heart and Great Vessels, 8th Ed, Boston, Little, Brown and Company, 1973 with permission of the New York Heart Association and the publisher. Copyright 1973.)

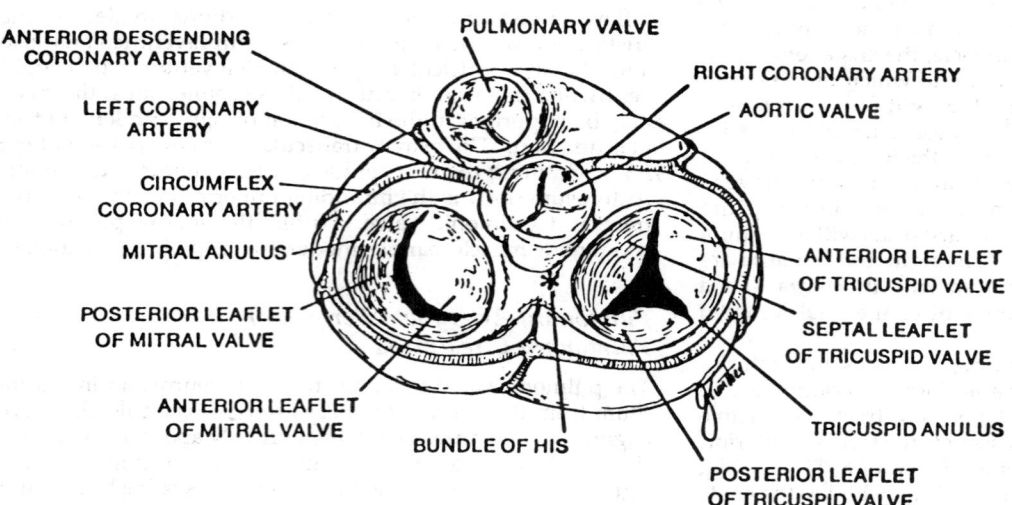

FIG. 34-2. A coronal section of the heart at the level of the valves. The close association between all four cardiac valves is easily recognized. The coronary arteries, arising from the coronary cusps of the aortic valve, pass between aorta and pulmonic valve. The left coronary artery divides into the anterior descending and circumflex branches. The mitral valve is composed of anterior and posterior leaflets, while the tricuspid valve has anterior, posterior, and septal leaflets. (Lowe DA: Abnormalities of the atrioventricular valves. In Lake CL (ed): Pediatric Cardiac Anesthesia. East Norwalk, Appleton and Lang, 1988.)

AORTA AND ITS BRANCHES

The aortic valve is adjacent to the mitral valve within the left ventricle, separated only by a fibrous tissue framework that comprises the annuli of both valves (Fig. 34-2). Three pocket-like structures of unequal size, the right and left (coronary) and posterior (noncoronary) cusps, form the aortic valve. A normal aortic valve is 3–4 cm^2 in area, but the area, weight, and volume of the cusps increase with age and heart weight.[4, 9] In the center of each cusp is a small nodule, the nodule of Arantius, while the free edge of the cusp is termed the lunula.[10] Coaptation of the nodules during ventricular diastole prevents regurgitation.[10] The aorta at the level of the valve dilates to form the sinuses of Valsalva, in which the coronary ostia are located.

The ascending aorta, just beyond the aortic valve, has no branches. Major branches of the aorta, the innominate, left carotid, and left subclavian arteries, arise from the aortic arch. The innominate subdivides into the right subclavian and right carotid arteries.

PERIPHERAL CIRCULATION

Arterial Circulation

The anatomy of many peripheral arteries is important to anesthesiologists, either for direct arterial cannulation or as a target to be avoided during venous cannulation (Fig. 34-3). Other portions of the peripheral circulation are important to the understanding of complications arising from certain surgical procedures. Among these are the carotid, cerebral, renal, bronchial, and spinal cord circulations.

CEREBRAL CIRCULATION. The cerebral circulation consists of the anterior communicating arteries, the internal carotid arteries, the posterior communicating arteries, the internal carotid arteries, the posterior communicating arteries, and the vertebral arteries. Together, these vessels form the circle of Willis (Fig. 34-4). The external carotid arteries supply the face and neck, but not the brain. During carotid artery surgery, a needle inserted in the internal carotid artery while the external and common carotid arteries are clamped allows measurement of the stump pressure, the arterial pressure occurring in the carotid as a result of blood flow via the circle of Willis (Fig. 34-4).

ARTERIES OF THE UPPER EXTREMITY. In the upper extremity, the subclavian artery gives rise to the axillary, brachial, radial, and ulnar arteries (Fig. 34-3). Because the basilic vein frequently overlies the brachial artery, the brachial artery may be punctured or cannulated when attempting vascular access in the antecubital fossa. Aberrant radial arteries often traverse the radial styloid process to enter the thenar webbed space. Attempted cannulation of veins over the anatomic "snuff box" may result in cannulation of an aberrant radial artery.

INTRA-ABDOMINAL AND LOWER EXTREMITY ARTERIES. The abdominal branches of the aorta include the superior mesenteric, inferior mesenteric, and celiac arteries, principally supplying the gastrointestinal tract (Fig. 34-3). The kidneys receive about 20% of the cardiac output via a single renal artery. The aorta bifurcates into right and left iliac arteries in the lower torso. At the level of the inguinal ligament, the iliacs have bifurcated into superficial and deep femoral arteries. The femoral artery can be easily cannulated just below the inguinal ligament. Distal to the knee, the femoral artery bifurcates into anterior and posterior tibial arteries. In the foot, the superficial arteries are the dorsalis pedis, located just lateral to the extensor hallucis longus tendon, and the posterior tibial, behind the medial malleolus.

SPINAL CORD. The blood supply to the spinal cord consists of the anterior spinal arteries, which traverse the length of the cord and arise from the vertebral arteries.[11] The anterior spinal arteries supply the majority (75%) of the cross-sectional area of the grey and white matter of the spinal cord. Only the posterior parts of the posterior columns and posterior horns are supplied by the posterior spinal artery (25%). Anastomoses between the anterior and posterior spinal arteries (circumflex arteries) are inconstant and insufficient to sustain adequate cord circulation. In addition, there are also radicular arteries that are branches of the intercostal and lumbar arteries, which anastomose with the anterior-posterior spinal artery system (Fig. 34-5). There are usually eight (the number varies from four to ten) radicular branches, at least one in the cervical, two in the thoracic, and one in the lumbar region. The largest of these is the arteria radicularis magna, or artery of Adamkiewicz, in the lower thoracic or upper lumbar region. When this vessel originates from the suprarenal aorta in the lower thoracic or upper lumbar region, it is generally the only significant radicular artery. However, if the origin of the arteria radicularis magna is infrarenal (lumbar segments 2 to 4), the segmental blood supply to the cord is usually good, and, thus, there is another major radicular vessel in the thoracic area.

Precise radiologic verification of the spinal cord blood supply is difficult and not routinely performed. Since either the radicular or the anterior-posterior spinal artery system predominates in most patients, ischemia can occur from decreased flow in either system.

BRONCHIAL CIRCULATION. Three bronchial arteries (two for the left lung and one for the right lung) originate from the thoracic aorta at T5 and T6 or intercostal arteries, and provide nutrients to the lung.[12] The bronchial circulation also permits heat and water exchange in the airways. Although normally small compared to the pulmonary circulation (it receives only 1% of the cardiac output), the bronchial circulation can enlarge in respone to injury, tumor growth, and inadequate pulmonary blood flow (as in cyanotic congenital heart disease), and can even perform gas exchange function.[12] Branches of the bronchial arteries accompany the bronchi down to the terminal bronchioles, where they form a plexus in the peribronchial space. They also anastomose with pulmonary alveolar microvessels, and coronary, thyroid, esophageal, thymic, internal mammary, thyrocervical, vertebral, and subclavian arteries.

HEPATIC AND PORTAL CIRCULATION. Surgery for hepatic transplantation or portal hypertension requires a knowledge of the blood supply to the liver. The liver is supplied by both the hepatic artery and the portal vein. Hepatic blood flow (hepatic artery and portal vein) is about 20% of the cardiac output, and averages 100 ml · min · 100 g^{-1} of tissue. This supplies about 65–80% of the hepatic blood flow, with the remainder coming from the portal system. The portal vein, which carries nutrients from the gut to the liver, arises from the superior mesenteric, splenic, and renal veins before entering the liver.

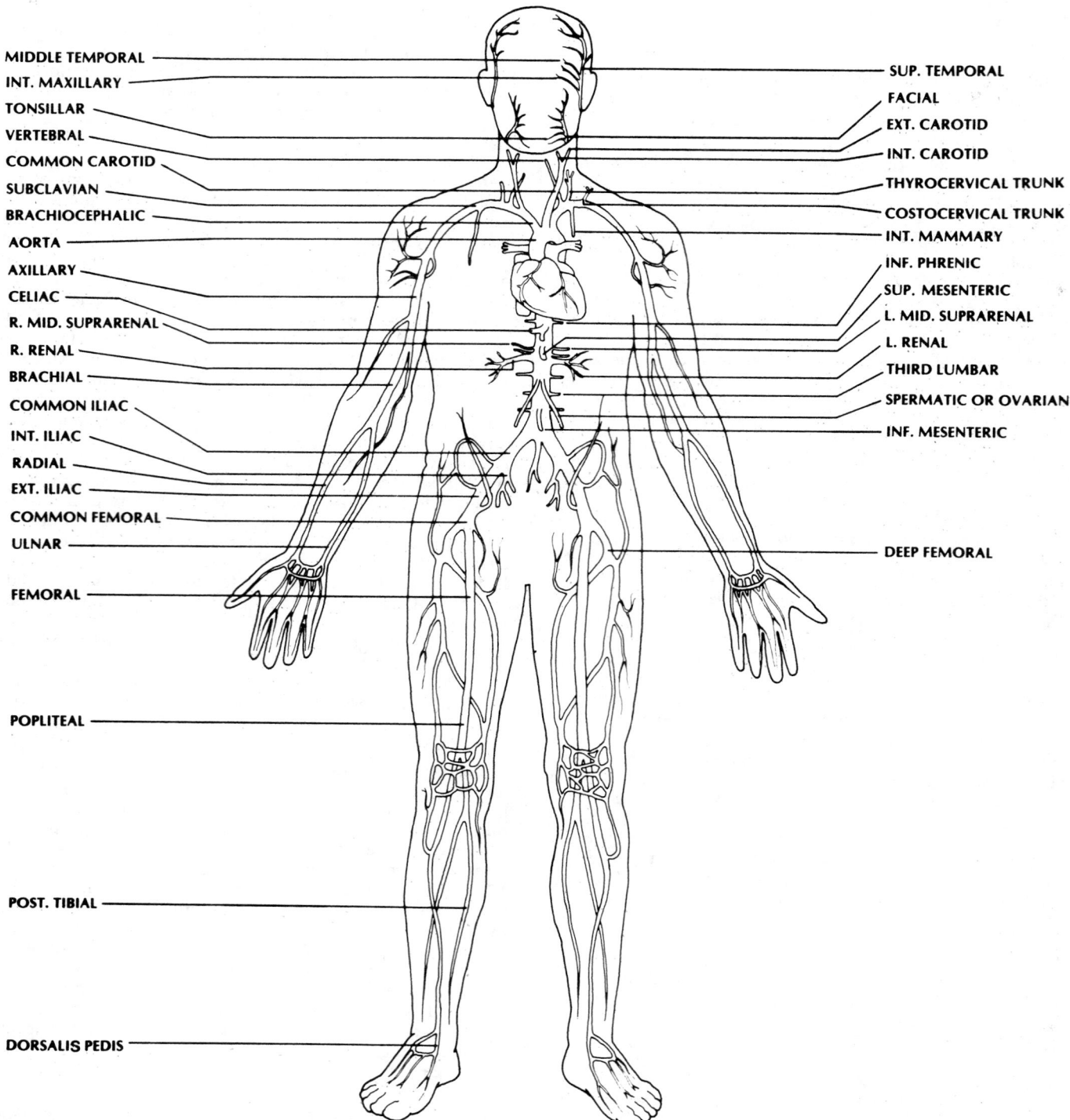

FIG. 34-3. The major arteries of the human body used by anesthesiologists to directly monitor arterial pressure include the radial, ulnar, femoral, brachial, axillary, dorsalis pedis, and superficial temporal.

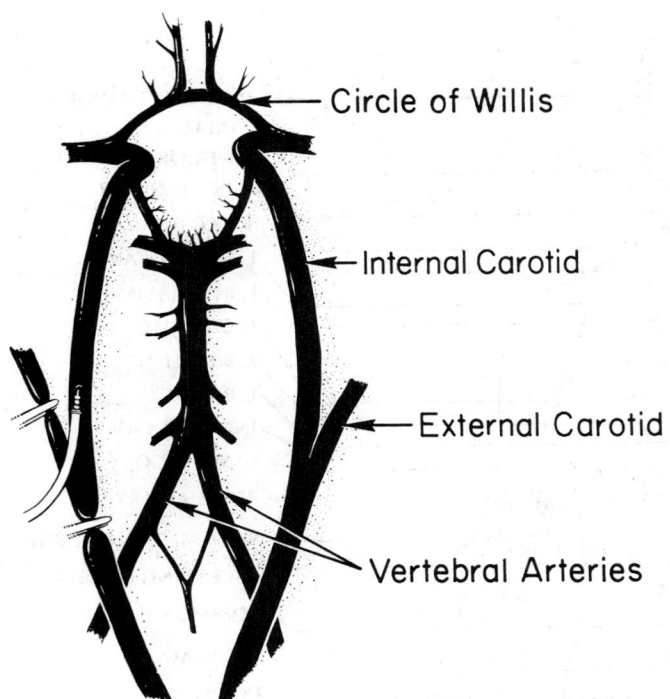

FIG. 34-4. The cerebral circulation includes the internal carotid and the vertebral arteries. Together with the anterior communicating and posterior communicating arteries, the carotid arteries from both sides join to form the Circle of Willis, which provides collateral circulation to the brain in the event of stenosis or occlusion of one carotid artery. The diagram also shows the position of a clamp on the carotid artery during measurement of "stump" pressure, the pressure present in the cerebral circulation during acute occlusion of the ipsilateral carotid artery. (Lake CL: Cardiovascular Anesthesia, p 411. New York, Springer Verlag, 1985, with permission of the publisher.)

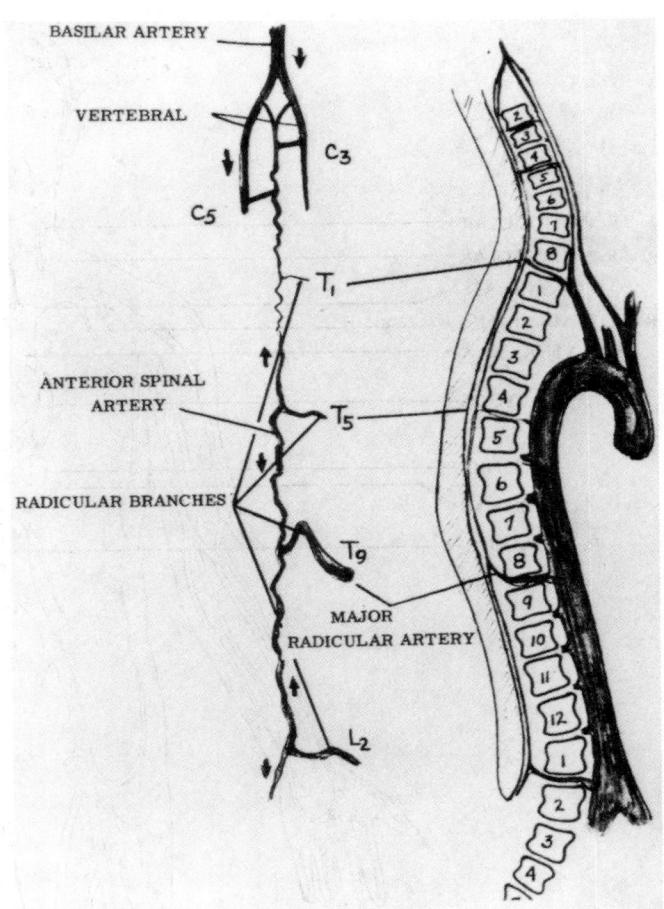

FIG. 34-5. The circulation to the spinal cord is often tenuous. It consists of anterior and posterior spinal arteries, which arise from the vertebral arteries, and radicular arteries, which originate from the intercostal and lumbar arteries. However, the radicular branches are quite variable, and ligation of a significant radicular branch causes spinal cord ischemia. (Brewer LA *et al:* Spinal cord complications following surgery for coarctation of the aorta. J Thorac Cardiovasc Surg 64:368, 1972 with permission of author and publisher.)

Peripheral Venous Circulation

Major veins follow a similar course to the arteries. From the head, the internal and external jugular veins join the subclavian veins of either side (Fig. 34-6). The course of the external jugular is often tortuous and variable, with two sets of valves, one at the entrance to the subclavian and the other about 4 cm superior to the clavicle. From the arms, the basilic (medial aspect) and cephalic veins join as the brachial vein. This vein becomes the axillary vein in the axilla, and thence the subclavian. Normally, subclavian veins from both sides unite to form the SVC.

In the legs, there are both superficial and deep veins. The greater and lesser saphenous veins are the principle superficial veins. The vein overlying the medial malleolus is the greater saphenous vein, which is frequently used as a conduit during aortocoronary bypass grafting. The lesser saphenous is located in the posterior aspect of the calf. The saphenous vein joins the femoral vein in the thigh to enter the pelvis as the iliac vein. Right and left iliac veins unite to form the inferior vena cava. Veins leaving the liver, the right, left, and middle hepatic veins, enter the inferior vena cava.

Bronchial veins from the extrapulmonary portions of the proximal tracheobronchial tree drain into the azygous and hemizygous veins (right heart). The azygous vein also drains perispinal areas and esophagus. Bronchial venous drainage from the intrapulmonary branches is to the pulmonary veins (left heart).

CARDIAC CONDUCTION SYSTEM

The system of electrical activation in the heart is termed the conduction system. It consists of the sinoatrial (SA) node, the atrioventricular (AV) node, the bundle of His, the right and left bundle branches, and the Purkinje system. The body of the SA node lies in the right atrial wall at the junction of the right atrium with the superior vena cava. In human hearts, the AV node is located in the floor of the right atrium, near the opening of the coronary sinus.[13] The SA and AV nodes are connected *via* the internodal conduction system, which consists of three tracts; the anterior, middle, and posterior internodal systems.[14–16] At the lower end of the AV node, the fibers form the common bundle of His, which passes along the superior edge of the membranous interventricular septum to the apex of the muscular portion of the septum (Fig.

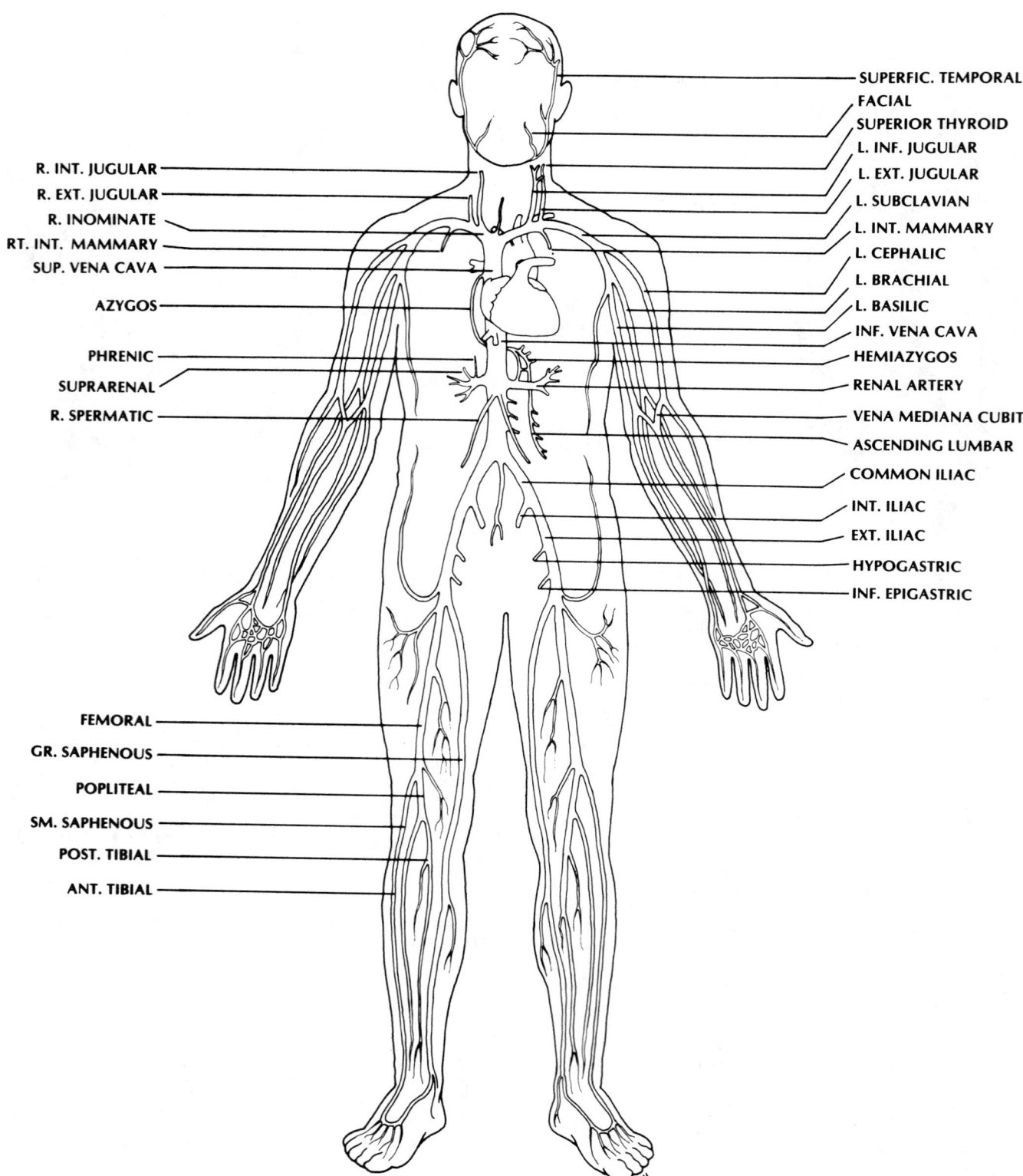

R. INT. JUGULAR

R. EXT. JUGULAR

R. INOMINATE

RT. INT. MAMMARY

SUP. VENA CAVA

AZYGOS

PHRENIC

SUPRARENAL

R. SPERMATIC

SUPERFIC. TEMPORAL

FACIAL

SUPERIOR THYROID

L. INF. JUGULAR

L. EXT. JUGULAR

L. SUBCLAVIAN

L. INT. MAMMARY

L. CEPHALIC

L. BRACHIAL

L. BASILIC

INF. VENA CAVA

HEMIAZYGOS

RENAL ARTERY

VENA MEDIANA CUBITI

ASCENDING LUMBAR

COMMON ILIAC

INT. ILIAC

EXT. ILIAC

HYPOGASTRIC

INF. EPIGASTRIC

FEMORAL

GR. SAPHENOUS

POPLITEAL

SM. SAPHENOUS

POST. TIBIAL

ANT. TIBIAL

FIG. 34-6. The major veins of the human body accessible for cannulation include the internal and external jugular, subclavian, femoral, basilic, cephalic, median cubital, and saphenous. The azygous and hemizygous systems assume importance if the inferior vena cava is occluded. It should also be noted that the veins follow the course of most of the major arteries. Therefore, during attempts at venous cannulation, accidental arterial cannulation is always possible.

34-2). Here, the bundle divides into right and left bundle branches, which extend subendocardially along the surfaces of both ventricles. The right bundle branch passes through the interventricular septum to emerge in the right ventricular endocardium near the moderator band at the base of the anterior papillary muscle. It usually extends for some distance without dividing, but one branch passes through the moderator band and the other passes over the right ventricular endocardial surface. Subdivision of the left bundle into anterior and posterior fascicles occurs shortly after its origin. There is also a small collection of short medial fascicles that originate from the left bundle just after the anterior fascicle, and activate the septal myocardium. The posterior fascicle terminates in the posterior papillary muscle.

Peripherally, the fascicles of both right and left bundle branches subdivide to form the Purkinje network. The left bundle branch fascicles make their initial functional contact with the left endocardial surface of the interventricular septum below the aortic valve. Right bundle branch fascicles contact ventricular subendocardium near the base of the anterior papillary muscle.

CARDIAC NERVES

Sympathetic System

Nerves to the heart and blood vessels originate from sympathetic neurons of the thoracolumbar region and parasympathetic nerves from the cervical region. Sympathetic fibers originate from the stellate ganglion and the caudal halves of the cervical sympathetic trunks below the level of the cricoid cartilage. There are three major sympathetic cardiopulmonary nerves from the stellate and middle cervical ganglia bilaterally: 1) stellate cardiopulmonary nerve; 2) dorsal cardiopulmonary nerves (three on the left side); and 3) dorsal lateral (right) and dorsal medial cardiopulmonary nerve (right).[17] The right dorsal medial and dorsal lateral cardiac nerves frequently unite to form one large nerve that follows the course of the left main coronary artery. It further separates into branches along the anterior descending and circumflex coronary arteries. Cholinergic fibers extend into the ventricular myocardium with considerable numbers in ventricular conducting tissue.[18] No sympathetic cardiac nerves arise from the superior cervical ganglia or the thoracic sympathetic trunks inferior to the stellate ganglia.[17] Transmission through the sympathetic ganglia occurs by release of acetylcholine, which interacts with the postsynaptic nicotinic cholinergic receptors on the postganglionic neuron. This stimulates norepinephrine release at the neuroeffector junction to activate beta$_1$ adrenergic receptors.

Parasympathetic System

Parasympathetic preganglionic neurons arise in the medulla oblongata in the dorsal vagal nucleus and the nucleus ambiguus. These fibers enter the thorax as branches from the recurrent laryngeal and thoracic vagus. The dorsal and ventral cardiopulmonary plexuses between the aortic arch and the tracheal bifurcation receive both sympathetic and parasympathetic branches. From the plexuses emerge three large cardiac nerves, the right and left coronary cardiac nerves and the left lateral cardiac nerve. Smaller cardiac nerves also arise from the plexuses and the thoracic vagi.[17] Ganglia occur within the heart, usually close to the structures innervated by the short postganglionic neurons. Postganglionic transmission occurs from stimulation of nicotinic cholinergic receptors at the postganglionic junction by acetylcholine. Release of acetylcholine at the neuroeffector junction activates muscarinic receptors in the heart.

Cerebral Vasomotor Center

Afferent nerves from the heart ascend via the tenth cranial nerve (vagus) and spinal cord to the nucleus tractus solitarius and the dorsal vagal nucleus of the medullary vasomotor center. The dorsal vagal nucleus plus the nucleus ambiguous comprise the parasympathetic motor efferent system. Although the vasomotor center independently regulates arterial pressure, blood flow distribution, and cardiac contractility influences from higher centers such as the cerebral cortex, hypothalamus, and pons are present.

Cardiac Receptors

Three types of vagal receptors, located in various cardiac chambers, are sensitive to changes in heart rate or chamber pressure. These include: 1) myelinated vagal afferents located at the venous-atrial junctions that indicate changes in atrial filling and heart rate; 2) unmyelinated vagal afferent nerves present in all cardiac chambers that indicate alterations of contractility, preload, and afterload; and 3) myelinated and nonmyelinated afferents that pass to the spinal cord, present in all chambers but of unknown significance.[19] These receptors may be important in coronary vasospasm, ischemia-induced arrhythmias, maintenance of cardiac volume, perception of cardiac pain, and responses to chemical stimuli, such as bradykinin or lactic acid.[19]

Vagal innervation principally affects the atrial musculature and SA and AV nodes, but also reaches the ventricular myocardium.[20, 21] The greatest concentrations of parasympathetic nerves are in the SA node, with lesser numbers in the AV node, right atrium, left atrium, and ventricles.[22] Parasympathetic alpha$_1$, but not alpha$_2$, receptors have been identified. Sympathetic fibers extend to all portions of the atria, ventricles, and conduction system. Both beta$_1$ and beta$_2$ subtypes of adrenergic receptors are present. Human right atrium contains about 74% beta$_1$ and 26% beta$_2$ receptors.[23] The proportions of beta receptors differ in the ventricle, which contains 86% beta$_1$ and 14% beta$_2$.

Neural Supply of the Peripheral Vasculature

Innervation of the peripheral circulation, with the exception of the cerebral and coronary vasculature, originates from the thoracolumbar sympathetic fibers. Vasodilation results from reduced alpha adrenergic tone or activation of vasodilatory (beta$_2$) receptors. Stimulation of alpha adrenergic fibers causes constriction in the arterial vascular beds of the skin, skeletal muscle, splanchnic, renal, and in systemic veins. Stimulation of beta$_2$ receptors dilates systemic veins and arteries of the muscle, splanchnic, and renal circulations.

BLOOD SUPPLY OF THE HEART

Arterial Circulation

Two coronary arteries, right and left, originating from the sinuses of Valsalva near the aortic valve, supply arterial blood to the myocardium. The left coronary artery usually has a short common or left main coronary artery before it bifurcates or trifurcates. The branches of the left coronary artery are the anterior descending, which courses downward over the anterior left ventricular wall and supplies the interventricular groove and the circumflex. The circumflex branch follows the atrioventricular groove, giving off the posterior interventricular branch and supplying all the posterior LV and part of the right ventricular wall[24] (Fig. 34-7; Table 34-1).

From the right coronary artery originates the sinus node artery and atrioventricular nodal artery. The right atrial myocardium is also supplied by the sinus node artery. The right coronary terminates on the diaphragmatic surface of the heart as the posterior descending artery[25] (Fig. 34-8). The blood supply to the AV node and common Bundle of His is the atrioventricular branch of the right coronary artery (90% of hearts) and septal perforating branches of the left anterior descending coronary artery (10% of hearts).[26, 27] Branches to the inter-atrial septum and posterior interventricular septum also arise from the AV nodal artery. The right bundle branch and the left anterior fascicle are supplied by branches of the left anterior descending artery, but can be supplied by the AV nodal artery.[26, 27] Both the left anterior and posterior descending coronary arteries supply the posterior fascicle.[27]

CORONARY DOMINANCE. Descriptions of the coronary circulation often refer to the dominance of one or the other coronary artery. Dominance is determined by which artery crosses the crux or junction between atria and ventricles to supply the posterior descending coronary branch. In about 50% of humans, the right coronary is dominant; in 20%, the left; and, in 30%, a balanced pattern exists. Areas of the myocardium affected by stenosis or occlusion of individual coronary arteries are shown in Table 34-1.

Venous Circulation

The principle cardiac veins are the great and middle cardiac veins and posterior left ventricular vein. These veins drain into the coronary sinus. The marginal vein drains into the great cardiac vein. Near the orifice of the great cardiac vein, the oblique vein of Marshall (vein of the LA) enters the coronary sinus. Anterior cardiac veins and the small cardiac vein may enter the right atrium independently of the coronary sinus. Thebesian veins, which traverse the myocardium, drain into various cardiac chambers.[28] Thebesian venous flow, coupled with bronchial and pleural venous flow, contributes the normal 1–3% arteriovenous shunt.

PERICARDIUM

The normal pericardium consists of thick fibrous and serous visceral layers. Although it is nonessential, it has certain anatomic and physiologic functions, among which are the isolation of the heart from other mediastinal structures, maintenance of the heart in optimal functional shape and position, minimization of cardiac dilatation, and prevention of adhesions.[29–31] The pericardium also contains vagal nerve branches, stimulation of which decreases heart rate and blood pressure. The pericardium also acts as a hydrostatic system to apply a compensating hydrostatic force to the heart under conditions of acceleration and other gravitational forces.[31, 32]

TABLE 34-1.   Coronary Artery Distribution

Left Coronary Artery
Anterior Descending Branch
  Right bundle branch
  Left bundle branch
  Anterior and posterior papillary muscle (mitral)
  Anterolateral left ventricle
Circumflex Branch
  Lateral left ventricle

Right Coronary Artery
SA and AV nodes
Right atrium and ventricle
Posterior interventricular septum
Posterior fascicle of left bundle branch
Inter-atrial septum

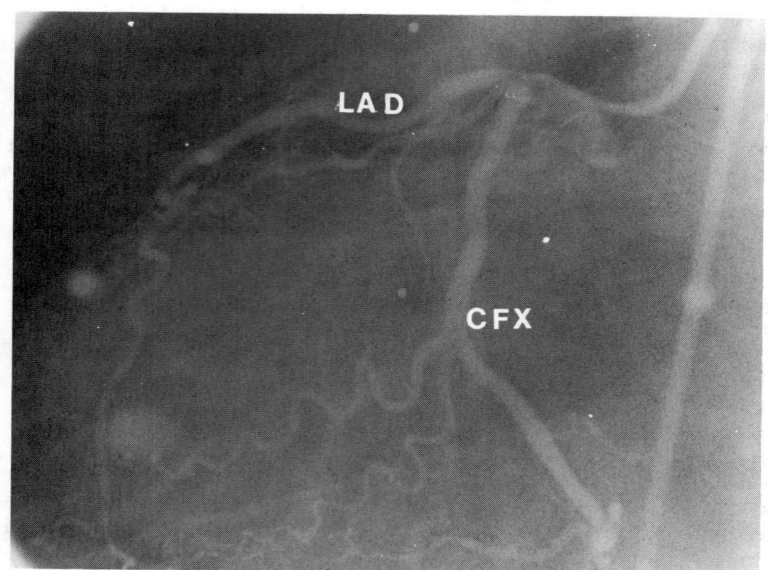

FIG. 34-7. The anatomy of the normal left coronary artery is seen in the coronary angiogram. It divides into the anterior descending (LAD) and circumflex (CFX) coronary arteries. (Lake CL: Cardiovascular Anesthesia, p 38. New York, Springer Verlag, 1985, with permission of the publisher.)

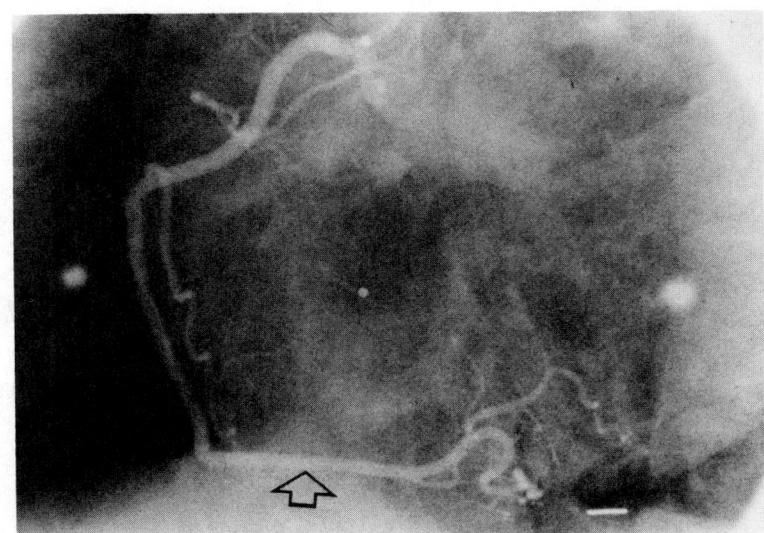

FIG. 34-8. The distribution of the right coronary artery as seen on coronary angiography. The right coronary artery usually gives off the arteries to the sinus and atrioventricular nodes before terminating on the inferior surface of the heart as the posterior descending artery (*arrow*). (Lake CL: Cardiovascular Anesthesia, p 38. New York, Springer Verlag, 1985, with permission of publisher.)

CARDIOVASCULAR CATHETERIZATION AND ANGIOGRAPHY

Abnormalities of both the anatomy and physiology of the cardiovascular system are diagnosed by invasive catheterization. However, noninvasive procedures, such as echocardiography, are increasingly being used to determine valvular lesions, ventricular function, and congenital defects.

CATHETERIZATION

General anesthesia is rarely required for cardiovascular catheterization, except in children, although intravenous sedation is often used. In all age groups, cardiac catheterization is usually performed *via* the femoral vessels. Occasionally, the brachial vessels are used in adults if the femoral vessels cannot be entered or catheters manipulated through the abdominal aorta.[33] Direct vascular cutdowns are rarely necessary, as the Seldinger technique, with various sizes of sheaths and introducers, provides adequate access in most patients.[34] The passage of catheters through either the venous or arterial systems is guided by fluoroscopic control. Pressure measurements are made in each cardiac chamber or great vessel, their pressure waveforms recorded, and vascular or ventricular angiography performed. Normal pressure values and oxygen saturations are shown in Table 34-2. Normal pressure waveforms are shown in Figure 34-9. Catheters can be specifically placed in virtually any major artery to demonstrate the presence of occlusion, dilatation (aneurysm), or congenital abnormalities, or to collect blood samples (such as renin from the renal arteries).

ANGIOGRAPHY

Either spot films or cineangiography are performed to quantitate ventricular contractility, to evaluate shunting between cardiac chambers, to demonstrate valvular regurgitation, or to delineate vascular outlines (pulmonary venous return, aortic dissection, pulmonary embolism, etc). Iodinated dyes, such as diatrizoate and ioxaglate, are injected to produce contrast. The total amount of injected contrast should not exceed 5 ml · kg^{-1} body weight, because contrast media are hyperosmolar substances that depress the myocardium, dilate the coronary arteries, decrease blood pH, increase serum osmolarity, and cause allergic reactions.[35] Adequate fluid replacement must be given after contrast angiography to prevent hypovolemia from the induced osmotic diuresis.

Angiography assesses the amount of valvular regurgitation by grading the amount of contrast re-entering the chamber preceding the valve. For instance, in the case of aortic regurgitation, 1+ regurgitation is a small amount of contrast entering the LV during diastole, but clearing with each systole. The LV is faintly opacified during diastole, and fails to clear with systole with 2+ regurgitation. In 3+ aortic regurgitation, the LV is progressively opacified during diastole and, eventually, completely opacified; while, in 4+ aortic regurgitation, the LV is completely opacified on the first diastole and remains opacified for several beats.[35]

CORONARY ARTERIOGRAPHY

Selective coronary angiography using either retrograde brachial technique of Sones or the percutaneous femoral approach of Amplatz or Judkins evaluates each coronary artery

TABLE 34-2. Normal Catheterization Data

SITE	PRESSURE (mm Hg)	OXYGEN SATURATION (%)
Inferior vena cava	0–8	80 ± 5
Superior vena cava	0–8	70 ± 5
Right atrium	0–8	75 ± 5
Right ventricle	15–30/0–8	75 ± 5
Pulmonary artery	15–30/4–12	75 ± 5
Pulmonary wedge	5–12 (mean	75 ± 5
Left atrium	12 (mean)	95 ± 1
Left ventricle	100–140/4–12	95 ± 1
Aorta	100–140/60–90	95 ± 1

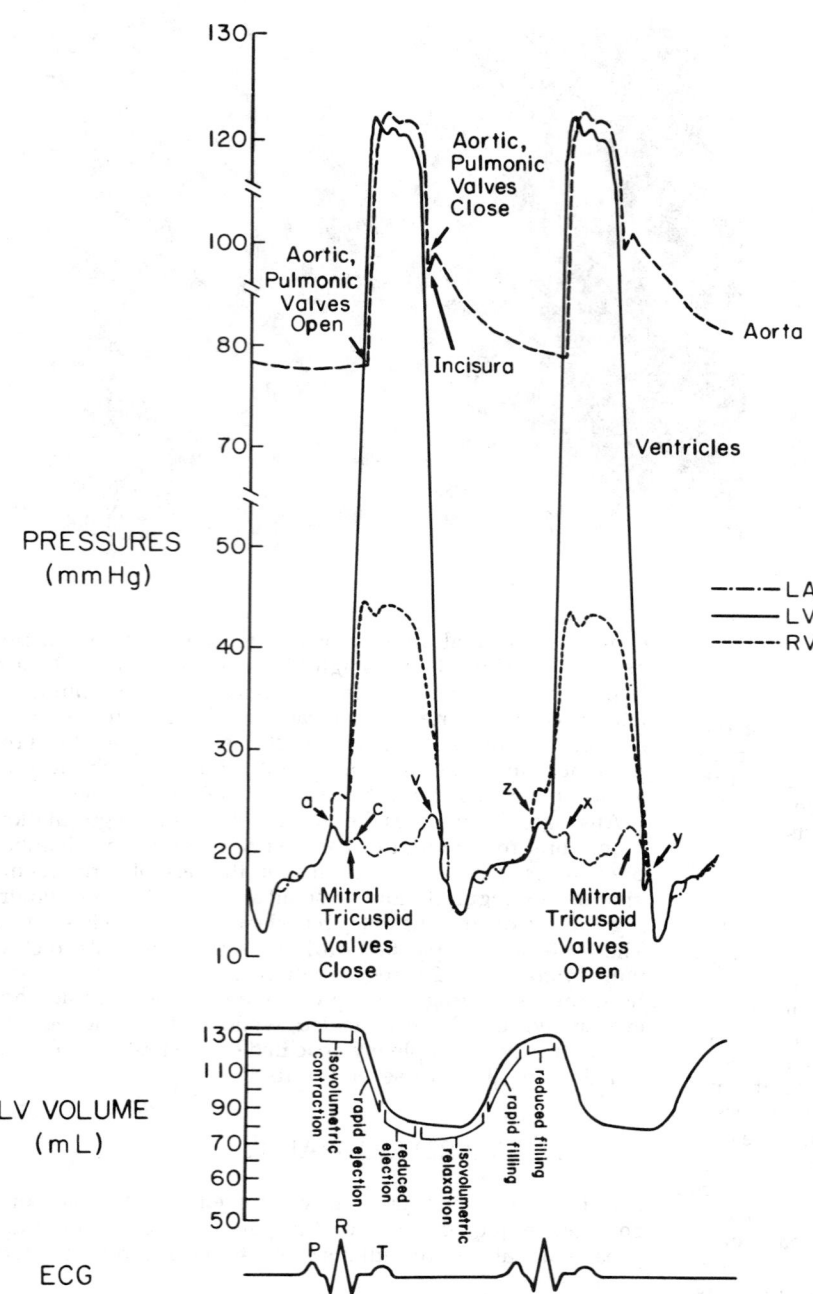

FIG. 34-9. The events of the cardiac cycle from filling of the atria to ventricular emptying are demonstrated using waveforms from the aorta, pulmonary artery, right and left ventricles, and central veins. The relationship between the electrocardiogram and the phases of the cardiac cycle shows that ventricular systole occurs immediately following the QRS complex. The changes in ventricular volume coincide with ventricular ejection and filling.

for the presence and extent of coronary occlusive disease, aneurysm formation, or congenital anomalies (Figs. 34-7, 34-8). Coronary arteriography occasionally causes ventricular ectopy, the vonBezold-Jarisch reflex, ventricular asystole, or fibrillation. More common are T-wave changes, bradycardia, and mild hypotension. Even in normal coronary arteries, injection of the right coronary produces T-wave inversion in lead II, and injection of the left artery produces T-wave peaking in lead II.[36] These changes revert to normal when the catheter is removed from the coronary ostia or the blood pressure is increased by having the patient cough.[37]

DETERMINATION OF CARDIAC OUTPUT

Cardiac output is determined by the Fick principle, dye dilution, thermodilution, or Doppler flow techniques. The Fick method requires the measurement or estimation of oxygen consumption, as well as collection of arterial and venous blood.

$$\text{Cardiac output } (l \cdot min^{-1}) = \dot{V}_{O_2}/Ca_{O_2} - Cv_{O_2} \times 100,$$

where $\dot{V}_{O_2}$ = oxygen consumption, Ca_{O_2} = arterial oxygen content, and Cv_{O_2} = venous oxygen content. The principle of the Fick measurement is that the size of a fluid stream is calculated by the amount of substance entering or leaving the stream and the concentration difference resulting from entry or removal of the substance. Arterial and mixed venous oxygen contents are calculated using the relationship:

$$C_{O_2} = \text{alpha } P_{O_2} + 1.34 \text{ hemoglobin concentration} \times \text{percent hemoglobin saturation,}$$

where alpha = the solubility of oxygen in whole blood (0.0031 $ml \cdot dl^{-1} \cdot mm\ Hg$). In the dye dilution method, the concentration of an indicator, usually indocyanine green, injected into the venous circulation, is measured by passing arterial blood through a densitometer. This method, which is based on the Fick principle, although requiring a cumbersome calculation of the area under the dye curve, can be used to measure outputs in the presence of, and to detect, intravascular shunts. Because recirculation of the dye occurs, some portion of the downslope of the curve must be extrapolated to near zero.

A normal dye dilution curve has an uninterrupted buildup slope, a steep disappearance slope with a short disappearance time, and a prominent recirculation peak. In right-to-left shunts, there is a deformity on the buildup slope by the abnormal early appearance of the dye in the arterial circulation. Left-to-right shunting causes a decreased peak dye concentration, absence of the recirculation peak, and a prolongation of the disappearance time.

Doppler echocardiography permits non-invasive assessment of cardiac output by measurement of the cross-sectional area of the aorta and the velocity of blood flow from the Doppler shift of the reflected sound waves. Although this method correlates well with thermodilution technique in experimental situations, clinical application has been less reliable.[38]

Thermodilution cardiac output determinations are presently the most widely used in clinical situations. The principle for thermodilution measurements is the indicator-dilution technique. A known quantity of room temperature or cooled dextrose is injected into the central venous circulation. A thermistor in the pulmonary artery detects the bolus of injectate and records the temperature change over time. The output of the right heart only is measured. Thermodilution outputs are subject to inaccuracies due to wandering baselines, improper volume or speed of injection, and too peripherally placed pulmonary catheters.

DETERMINATION OF SHUNTS

A shunt exists when arterial and venous blood mix at some site in the circulatory system, either an intracardiac or extracardiac location, usually due to a congenital cardiac malformation. The site of a shunt can be determined by measurement of oxygen saturations in various cardiac chambers or by calculation of pulmonary and systemic flow by the Fick principle. A 10% increase ("step-up") in oxygen saturation at the atrial level indicates left-to-right shunting into the right atrium. A 5% step-up at ventricular or aorticopulmonary level indicates shunting at the site.

The measurement of pulmonary and systemic flow is performed by direct measurement or by the Fick principle using estimated oxygen consumption and measured systemic and pulmonary oxygen contents. The pulmonary ($\dot{Q}_P$) to systemic flow ($\dot{Q}_s$) is equal in the absence of shunting, and the

flow ratio is 1. In a bidirectional shunt, the effective pulmonary flow ($\dot{Q}_{pe}$) is

$$\dot{V}_{O_2}/Pv_{O_2} - Mv_{O_2},$$

where Pv_{O_2} is the pulmonary venous oxygen content and Mv_{O_2} is the mixed venous oxygen content. Flow in left-to-right shunting is $\dot{Q}_P - \dot{Q}_{pe}$. Flow in right-to-left shunting is $\dot{Q}_s - \dot{Q}_{pe}$.

CALCULATON OF VALVE AREAS

Valve areas and flows can be calculated from the heart rate, cardiac output, and vascular pressure.[39] The aortic valve area is calculated by determining the systolic ejection period per beat (SEP) from the pressure waveforms. The systolic ejection period per minute is calculated by multiplying the SEP per beat by the heart rate. The pressure gradient across the aortic valve is the difference between left ventricular systolic mean pressure and aortic systolic mean pressure. The aortic valve flow (AVF) is cardiac output/SEP$_{minute}$. The aortic valve area is calculated using the following equation:

$$\text{Aortic valve area} = \frac{\text{aortic valve flow}}{1 \times 44.5 \times \sqrt{\text{systolic pressure gradient}}}$$

1 = the empiric constant for the aortic valve, which combines the coefficient of orifice contraction (a factor to compensate for the physical reduction of the stream to an area of less than the actual orifice area), the coefficient of velocity, the conversion factor of centimeters of water to millimeters of mercury, and other factors. Recent evidence suggests that this constant varies with the transvalvular pressure gradient.[40]

A similar calculation is made for mitral valve area, except that the diastolic filling period per beat, the gradient between left atrial and left ventricular pressure, and an empiric constant of 0.7 are used.[41] The diastolic filling period (DFP) per beat is determined from pressure waveforms. The diastolic fillling period per minute is calculated by multiplying the DFP per beat by the heart rate. The pressure gradient across the mitral valve is the difference between left atrial pressure and left ventricular diastolic pressure. The mitral valve flow is cardiac output (ml/min)/DFP$_{minute}$. The mitral valve area is calculated using the following equation:

$$\text{Mitral valve area} = \frac{\text{mitral valve flow}}{0.7 \times 44.5 \times \sqrt{\text{diastolic pressure gradient}}}$$

PHYSIOLOGY

CARDIAC CYCLE

The cardiac cycle begins with the filling of the right and left atria while the tricuspid and mitral valve are closed (Fig. 34-9). The V wave on the venous pressure waveform represents the gradual increase in atrial blood volume as blood returns from the periphery. Once the aortic valve has closed, but ventricular pressure still exceeds atrial pressure, the ventricle is in the phase of isovolumetric relaxation. About 0.02–0.04 s after closure of the aortic valve, atrial and ventricular pressure equalize and a small gradient develops across the atrioventricular valves as ventricular pressure decreases further. The atrioventricular valve cusps bulge into the ventricle and separate slightly. At 0.03–0.05 s after crossover of the atrial and ventricular pressure waves, the atrioventricular valves open completely over 0.02–0.04 s. The V wave of the atrial pressure waveform crests when the atriae are filled and the tricuspid and mitral valves open to initiate ventricular filling. The Y wave results from opening of the atrioventricular valves combined with ventricular relaxation. Effective atrial systole at resting heart rates contributes about 5–20% of the stroke volume.[22] Acute atrial fibrillation increases atrial pressures, reduces atrial compliance, increases atrial oxygen consumption, and eliminates the contribution of the atriae to ventricular filling.[42]

Initially, there is a rapid increase in ventricular volume, the rapid filling phase of about 0.06–0.10 s, during which time the ventricular pressure continues to decrease because ventricular expansion exceeds filling. Peak ventricular filling in early diastole occurs at 500–700 ml · s^{-1} as the ventricle "sucks" blood from the atria (diastolic suction). The elastic recoil of the heart and great vessels during diastole contributes to the accelerated filling phase of the ventricle, particularly during tachycardia. The third heart sound, S_3, occurs at the point of transition from rapid ventricular filling to reduced filling.

The previous ventricular contraction provides much of the energy for the subsequent diastolic expansion through the energy expenditure of the gross movement and deformation of the heart during systole.[43] The nadir of the ventricular pressure curve at the end of the rapid filling phase probably marks the end of ventricular relaxation and the beginning of elastic distention of the ventricle. A period of reduced ventricular filling follows the rapid filling phase. During this period, there is an upswing in the ventricular pressure that abolishes forward movement of blood and can force the atrioventricular valves into a semiclosed position unless venous return is great. Atrial systole, the A wave on the venous pressure waveform, which coincides with the P wave on the electrocardiogram (ECG), concludes ventricular filling. Measurement of the mean right atrial pressure provides a guide to right atrial and right ventricular function.

Although venous return is the most important factor contributing to ventricular filling, atrial contraction is often important to the heart with poorly functioning ventricles. In such hearts, a fourth heart sound, S_4, occurs 0.04 s after the P wave, resulting from vibrations of left ventricular muscle and mitral valve. The S_4 most likely represents vigorous atrial contraction. The adequacy of ventricular filling is determined by the distensibility (compliance) of the ventricles, the filling time, and the effective filling pressure. The effective filling pressure is the transmural ventricular pressure. Tachycardia also decreases the time available for ventricular filling, decreasing filling time from 400–500 msec at a heart rate of 60 bpm to 10 ms or less at 160 bpm. Mitral stenosis slows ventricular filling and alters the change in ventricular wall motion associated with filling. Hypertrophic cardiomyopathy slows the distention of the ventricle associated with filling. Reduced diastolic filling is also seen in patients with coronary artery disease, probably resulting from changes in compliance and regional wall motion during ischemia. The intraventricular pressure just prior to the beginning of ventricular contraction is end-diastolic pressure (Table 34-2). However, normal end-diastolic pressures do not imply normal ventricular function. Increased end-diastolic pressures occur with hypervolemia or changes in ventricular compliance, as well as decreased contractility.

The period just before the sudden increase in ventricular pressure is presystole, which includes atrial systole and the time just before isovolumetric ventricular contraction. The Z point on the venous pressure waveform immediately precedes ventricular systole. The isovolumetric phase of ventricular contraction is marked by the C wave on the venous waveform. Isovolumetric contraction is the period between closure of the atrioventricular valves and opening of the semilunar (aortic, pulmonic) valves. Intraventricular pressure increases, but there is no change in intraventricular volume. After this point, the atrioventricular valves close, atrial diastole begins, the ventricles begin to contract, and ventricular pressure soon exceeds atrial pressure. Ventricular systole occurs immediately after the QRS complex on the ECG, about 0.12–0.20 s after atrial contraction. Atrioventricular valve closure is facilitated by the increased ventricular pressure and the cessation of atrial systole. Closure of the atrioventricular valves is noted clinically by the first heart sound, S_1. However, some investigators suggest that S_1 results from reverberations of the left ventricular muscle, mitral valve, and left ventricular outflow tract in response to the accelerating and decelerating of blood during early systole.[44, 45] Since right and left ventricular contraction is normally slightly asynchronous, S_1 is usually split.

The aortic and pulmonic valves open at the summit of the C wave. The atrial pressure decreases, resulting in the X descent, because blood goes into the aorta and pulmonary artery. Once the ventricular pressure exceeds aortic pressure, the aortic and pulmonic valves open. The majority of ventricular ejection occurs during the rapid ejection phase. The pressure in the aorta is slightly lower, while ventricular pressure increases rapidly. Initially, the output into the aorta exceeds the runoff into the peripheral circulation. Peak aortic pressure occurs slightly after peak aortic blood flow.[46] As aortic runoff and ventricular output equilibrate, the period of reduced ventricular ejection occurs. Forward flow continues until the end of ventricular diastole, protodiastole, when a brief period of retrograde flow initiates aortic and pulmonic valve closure. On pressure waveforms, semilunar valve closure is marked by a notch, or incisura. The second heart sound, S_2, which also results from rapid deceleration of blood causing vibration of the outflow tracts and great vessels, as well as closure of the semilunar valves, is heard on auscultation.

CARDIAC ELECTROPHYSIOLOGY

Cellular Electrophysiology

Cardiac pacemaker and ventricular muscle cells have an intracellular ionic composition that differs from that found in the extracellular fluid. The most important ions are calcium, sodium, and potassium. An active transport system in the cell membrane, the sodium/potassium pump, maintains normal concentration gradients for sodium and potassium by pumping sodium out of, and potassium into, the cell. Ionic transfer is facilitated by the energy released from the hydrolysis of ATP. Extracellular ions cross the cell membrane in channels that are either fast sodium channels or slow calcium channels. The compound action potential (AP) in these cells results from local ionic transmembrane fluxes, or currents, through the channels[47] (Fig. 34-10). When the cell is excited, there is an increase in the permeability of the membrane that permits positively charged sodium ions to move across the cell membrane into the cell, resulting in depolarization. This sodium influx reverses the transmembrane potential from −80 mvolts to 20–30 mvolts, and initiates phase 0 of the AP in a ventricular muscle cell (Fig. 34-11). During phase 0, there

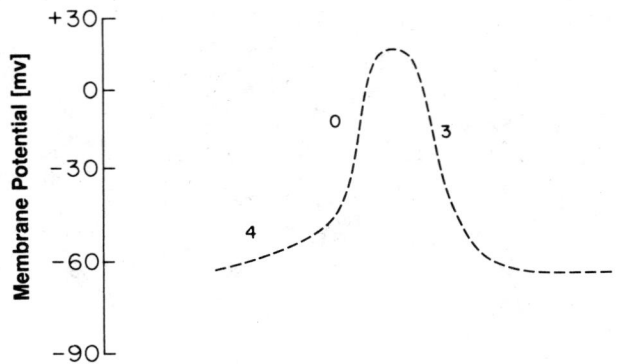

FIG. 34-10. The action potential of an automatic cell, such as the sinoatrial node, differs from that of the ventricular muscle cell in that the cell slowly depolarizes spontaneously during phase 4. Phase 0 is the depolarization phase that results from sodium ion influx through the fast channel and calcium ion influx through the slow channel. Phase 3 is the repolarization phase that results from potassium movement through the cell membrane. (Lake CL: Cardiovascular Anesthesia, p 250. New York, Springer Verlag, 1985, with permission of publisher.)

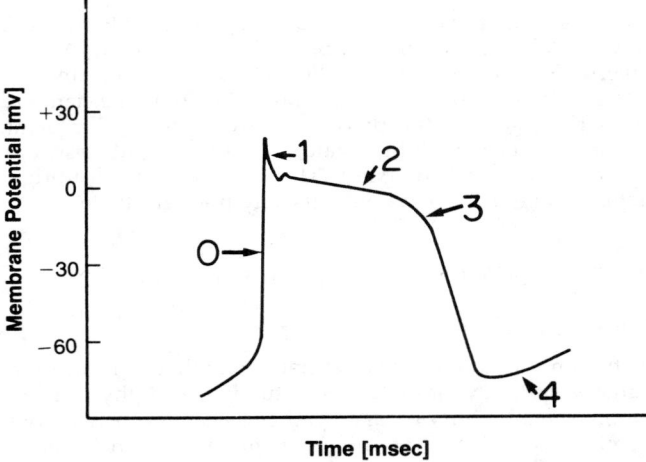

Time [msec]

FIG. 34-11. The action potential in a ventricular muscle cell. When the cell is stimulated, an action potential occurs due to a rapid influx of sodium ions into the cell (phase 0). Phase 1 is the beginning of the repolarization phase. Phase 2 is the plateau of the action potential resulting principally from calcium entry through the slow channel of the cell membrane. During Phase 3, repolarization of the cell occurs; while, during Phase 4, the sodium entering during Phase 0 is actively pumped out of the cell. (Lake CL (ed): Pediatric Cardiac Anesthesia. East Norwalk, Appleton and Lang, 1987, with permission of publisher.)

is also a decrease in permeability to potassium. At about -30 mvolts, inward calcium transfer begins through the slow channel.[48,49] Phase 0 corresponds to the QRS complex of the electrocardiogram (ECG). After excitation, the cell membrane undergoes an initial period of rapid repolarization (phase 1), followed by a period of variable duration in which the membrane potential remains close to 0. This is termed the plateau of the AP. The plateau is caused by slow inactivation of the

calcium current. The duration of the plateau is probably the result of complicated interactions between calcium influx and potassium efflux.[47] Phase 3, the repolarization phase that results from potassium ions moving from an intracellular to an extracellular site, corresponds to the T wave of the ECG. During phase 4, the resting membrane potential (RMP) is generated by active exchange of intracellular sodium for potassium. In the latter part of phase 4, the RMP is stable in ventricular muscle cells until the cell is excited again. In automatic cells such as the SA and AV nodes, slow, spontaneous depolarization occurs during phase 4 due to calcium transport through the slow channel.

During depolarization, the cell membrane is absolutely refractory to other stimuli. The end of the absolute refractory period is signalled by the earliest transient depolarization that can be elicited. The absolute refractory period ends at the beginning of the T wave of the ECG. Once repolarization reaches the threshold potential, the cell is relatively refractory, since an unusually strong stimulus can produce depolarization. This period is marked by the T wave of the ECG. The earliest propagated AP defines the end of the effective or functional refractory period.

The SA node is normally the dominant pacemaker because, in it, automaticity is most highly developed. It also initiates impulses at the fastest rate. The rate of phase 4 depolarization is faster in the SA node than in the terminal Purkinje fibers, causing less highly developed pacemakers to be depolarized by the propagated wave from above before they spontaneously depolarize.[50]

FACTORS AFFECTING CELLULAR CARDIAC ELECTROPHYSIOLOGY. Changes in the AP itself, or factors that affect the AP, alter the rate of firing of an automatic cell. For example, hypothermia decreases the slope of phase 4, while hyperthermia increases heart rate.[51] Hypoxia or ischemia increase the slope of phase 4 and reduce the maximum diastolic potential.[52] Acetylcholine has little effect on AP duration in Purkinje cells, but antagonizes the effect of isoproterenol and decreases AP duration.[53]

ACTION POTENTIAL ALTERATIONS. The rate of firing of an automatic cell depends upon the slope of phase 4 depolarization, the maximum diastolic potential (the maximum level of resting membrane potential achieved at the end of repolarization), and the threshold potential. If the difference between the threshold potential and the RMP is increased, a greater stimulus is needed for depolarization. A smaller stimulus is required if only a small difference exists between RMP and threshold. Other factors affecting rate include increases or decreases in the RMP, an increased or decreased rate of spontaneous phase 4 depolarization, and shifting of the threshold potential toward or away from the RMP.[54]

ELECTROLYTE EFFECTS. Hypokalemia increases the rate of phase 4 depolarization in the SA node.[54] Hyperkalemia reduces the rate of phase 4 depolarization and decreases the maximum diastolic potential of Purkinje, but not sinus node, fibers.[55] Diastolic depolarization is abolished in Purkinje fibers at very high potassium concentrations with the membrane stabilized at 20 mvolts.

Decreased sodium decreases the slope of phase 4 depolarization and the height of the action potential without a change of RMP in atrial, ventricular, or Purkinje fibers.[54] Neither hypocalcemia nor hypercalcemia alters the RMP or phase 4 in the SA node or Purkinje fibers. However, hypocalcemia makes the threshold potential more negative. Hypercalcemia shifts the threshold potential away from the maximum diastolic potential and toward 0, which makes it more difficult for the cell to reach threshold.[56] The changes caused by magnesium are similar to those of calcium.

ACID-BASE CHANGES. Hypercarbia and increased pH increase the slope of phase 4 and reduce maximum diastolic potential.[54] Slow channels are selectively blocked by metabolic acidosis. Spontaneous depolarization in Purkinje fibers is enhanced by decreased bicarbonate concentrations.[57]

Clinical Electrophysiology

The first wave of the normal ECG is the P wave, which is produced by atrial depolarization resulting from an AP in the SA node. Sinus node rate exhibits a circadian rhythm, decreasing nocturnally. Sinus node recovery time is also prolonged at night.[58] The P wave usually does not normally exceed 3 mm in height or 0.11 s in duration. It is usually upright, except in lead avR.

Transmission of an impulse elicited by an AP in the SA node to the AV node takes about 0.04 s. The electrical impulse travels from the SA node to the AV node *via* atrial tissue, specialized atrial conducting tissue, or the anterior, middle, and posterior tracts of the right atrium. Transmission is further delayed in the AV node because its conduction velocity is about $0.2 \text{ m} \cdot \text{s}^{-1}$. The effective refractory period of the AV node also demonstrates circadian rhythm and is increasingly refractory at night.[58] The PR interval (normally 0.2 msec or less), which occupies the time between atrial and ventricular depolarization, is nearly isoelectric, because atrial repolarization is not recordable. Significant interactions between the parasympathetic and sympathetic nervous system control the conduction through the AV node. Unlike the SA node, sympathetic activity predominates in AV nodal conduction.[59]

Ventricular depolarization begins about 0.12–0.20 s, in adults, and 0.15–0.18 s, in children, after depolarization of the SA node.[60] Ventricular depolarization produces the QRS complex on the ECG. The first negative wave seen in the QRS complex is the Q wave, which should be 0.04 s or less in duration and less than one-fourth of the subsequent R wave in amplitude. The first positive wave in the QRS is the R wave, and the second negative wave is the S wave. The entire QRS complex should be less than 0.10 s. The right and left branches of the Bundle of His connecting with the Purkinje fibers conduct the depolarizing impulse rapidly over the endocardial surface of the heart. Normally, in sinus rhythm, the earliest area of activation is the trabecular area on the anterior right ventricular surface about 18–25 msec after the surface QRS complex (Fig. 34-12). Activation then spreads toward the apex and base of the heart, with the latest activation at the cardiac base. Electrical activation also spreads from endocardium to epicardium.

Abnormal ventricular activation is recognized by an area exhibiting activation before the onset of the surface QRS complex. Mapping of the direct cardiac electrogram to determine such abnormal areas of activation is the basis of clinical electrophysiologic studies in patients with ventricular dysrhythmias.

On the ECG, the time from the end of ventricular depolarization to the beginning of repolarization, the S-T segment, is isoelectric. More than 1 mm of elevation in the standard leads or 2 mm of elevation in the precordial leads is abnormal in this segment. No more than 0.5 mm of depression should be seen in any lead. The J point, the junction between the QRS complex and the ST segment, is depressed or elevated with

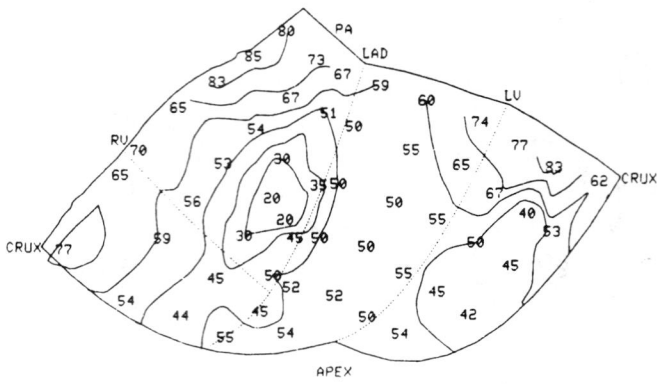

FIG. 34-12. In this representation, the heart has been cut along its posterior surface from the base to the apex and laid flat. The numbers indicate the time in milliseconds after the QRS complex is seen on the ECG until electrical activity is noted. The right ventricle is activated earliest, about 19 to 20 milliseconds after the QRS complex, while the latest activation occurs at the base of the heart at 75 to 80 milliseconds. (Gallagher JJ *et al*: Techniques of intraoperative electrophysiologic mapping. Am J Cardiol 49:224, 1982 with permission of author and publisher.)

the ST segment. Ventricular repolarization results in the T wave. T waves are normally upright in leads I, II, and V_3–V_6, inverted in lead aV_R, and variable in II, aV_L, aV_F, V_1, and V_2. The T wave should not exceed 5 mm in height in the standard leads or 10 mm in the precordial leads. The Q-T interval, varying inversely with heart rate, should be slightly less than one-half of the RR interval.[61] The U wave, a small upright deflection after the T wave, is usually not detectable.

PHYSIOLOGY OF THE CARDIAC NERVES

Neural Regulation

Although the dominance of either sympathetic or parasympathetic system varies with age, situation, and physical condition, the inhibitory parasympathetic system is usually predominant.[62, 63] However, neural regulation of the heart is complex. Stimulation of dorsal cardiac nerves increases or decreases heart rate and blood pressure in humans.[64] In some patients, the vagal influence may be excessive, causing vagotonia.[65] Parasympathetic stimulation, particularly of the right vagus, decreases heart rate. Intense vagal stimulation depresses both atrial and ventricular contractility by stimulation of cardiac muscarinic receptors, which alter the myocyte cyclic AMP level, inhibition of norepinephrine release from nearby sympathetic nerve terminals by acetylcholine, and inhibition of adrenergic receptor activation.[22] Vagal stimulation can suppress ventricular automaticity, which may facilitate termination of ventricular dysrhythmias. Stimulation of the stellate ganglion or other sympathetic cardiac fibers increases heart rate, contractility, and ejection fraction. The right stellate ganglion has a greater effect on heart rate, while the left has more effect on contractility.[22] Abnormalities of sympathetic cardiac nerve tone occur in long Q-T interval syndromes.[66] Only alpha$_1$ receptors have been conclusively demonstrated in cardiac tissue. However, both beta$_1$ and beta$_2$ receptors are present in the heart. Beta$_1$ postsynaptic receptors increase the rate, force of contraction, and conduction velocity of the heart by stimulation of adenylcyclase. Activation of beta$_2$ receptors in the heart increases rate and contractility.

Cardiac Receptors

There are two major types of nerve endings that interconnect in the heart. They are: 1) the nerve net; and 2) diffuse or compact unencapsulated endings.[67]

Atrial Receptors

The atria have three types of parasympathetic receptors; type A, type B, and receptors innervated by Group C fibers. Atrial receptors usually reflexly alter intravascular volume or heart rate. Atrial receptor types A and B are innervated by myelinated vagal afferent fibers. The primary location of types A and B are the cavoatrial junction, pulmonary venous-atrial junction, atrial appendage, and atrial body.[67] Type A receptors discharge at the time of the A wave of the atrial pressure waveform. They may actually respond to heart rate rather than atrial pressure, since they are unaffected by the amplitude of the A wave or the rate of atrial pressure increase.[67] Their rate of firing is maximal during normal cardiac cycles, with no change in firing frequency with hemorrhage or volume.

Type B receptors are stretch receptors that discharge during late systole, during the V wave of the atrial pressure waveform in conjunction with the upstroke of the aortic pressure. Their discharge is closely related to atrial volume, and varies with the rate of atrial pressure increase. Although type B receptors are inactive during normal atrial contraction, tachyarrhythmias, which increase atrial volume, increase their rate of discharge.[67]

Atrial receptors innervated by group C fibers are located through the atria. Such receptors discharge in the pattern of either Type A or Type B receptors. Usually, their rate of discharge is low, but they respond to stretch at a threshold pressure of 2–3 mm Hg. Generally, they respond less to changes in atrial pressures than types A and B.[67]

Ventricular Receptors

Stimulation of ventricular receptors causes either cardiovascular excitation or bradycardia and hypotension. Several types of ventricular receptors have been described. They include the pressure-sensitive coronary baroreceptors, coronary pressure receptors, mechanoreceptors (innervated by nonmyelinated vagal afferent fibers), and sympathetic mechanosensitive or chemosensitive receptors.[67]

The Bainbridge reflex, described below, is mediated by the parasympathetic receptors. Myocardial ischemia increases discharge of both vagal and sympathetic receptors. The sympathetic afferent fibers may transmit the pain sensation associated with coronary occlusion. Postcardiotomy hypertension results from a cardiogenic reflex transmitted through the sympathetic afferent fibers of the stellate ganglion.[67]

The tension- or pressure-sensitive ventricular receptors discharge at the onset of ventricular ejection, and their frequency response is related to the rate of pressure rise. Other ventricular receptors are unresponsive to ventricular distension, but respond to changes in mean coronary pressure. Another type, located in or near the coronary sinus, is affected by changes in coronary pressure and ventricular contraction.

Two types of unmyelinated ventricular vagal afferent fibers

are present in the heart. One type innervates chemosensitive receptors that are stimulated by capsaicin or veratridine, while the other innervates mechanoreceptors that respond to aortic constriction.[67] Unmyelinated sympathetic afferent fibers with either mechanosensitive or chemosensitive receptors are present throughout the heart, great vessels, and pericardium.[67]

CORONARY CIRCULATORY PHYSIOLOGY

About 5% of the cardiac output, or 250 ml·min^{-1}, perfuses the coronary arteries of a 70-kg human. Physiologically, the coronary circulation consists of large, low-resistance epicardial vessels and higher-resistance intramyocardial arteries and arterioles. Coronary blood flow is locally regulated by metabolic, mechanical, anatomic, and, possibly, myogenic factors.[8] The majority of left coronary artery flow occurs in diastole, because intramyocardial pressure is lowest at that time.[69] Right coronary artery flow occurs in both systole and diastole because intramyocardial pressure is lower in the thinner-walled right ventricle.

Coronary flow also decreases from epicardium to endocardium as a consequence of extravascular pressure. During systole, about 15–25% of the coronary flow distends and is stored in the extramural coronary arteries. Only a small amount actually perfuses the myocardium. During diastole, this stored blood perfuses the myocardium[70] (Fig. 34-13).

There is a minimum coronary pressure required to initiate flow, the zero flow pressure. Normally, zero flow pressure ranges from 12 to 50 mm Hg. The source of this pressure includes the collapse of intramyocardial coronary microvessels at tissue pressures exceeding intraluminal pressures and the magnitude of the intracavitary back pressure. Coronary flow ceases completely at 20 mm Hg, the critical closure, or critical flow, pressure.[71]

Myocardial oxygen consumption is high. Consequently, coronary venous blood is only 30% saturated, and its P_{O_2} of 18–20 mm Hg is the lowest of any organ in the body. Because oxygen extraction cannot be increased further, coronary flow must increase if the heart requires additional oxygen.

FIG. 34-13. This diagrammatic relationship between aortic pressure and coronary flow demonstrates that little coronary flow occurs during systole, while the majority occurs during diastole. This relationship is particularly true for the left coronary artery, which supplies the left ventricle. The right ventricle, being thinner and developing less pressure, produces less impediment to systolic coronary flow.

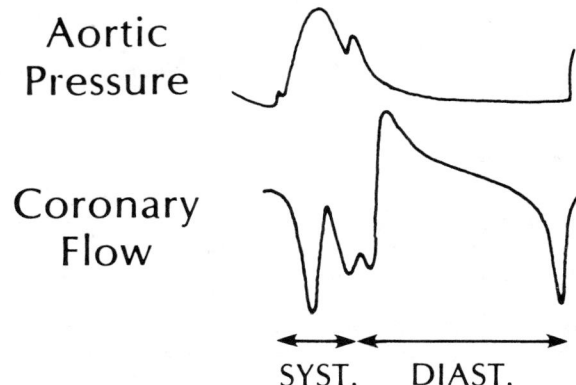

Coronary Autoregulation

Coronary perfusion is autoregulated to maintain a constant flow over a range of perfusion pressures (usually between 50 and 120 mm Hg) at any given myocardial oxygen demand.[72] Above and below these limits, coronary flow varies with perfusion pressure. The term autoregulation refers strictly to pressure-dependent changes in coronary resistance unrelated to changes in myocardial metabolism.[72] However, flow does not return to precisely its previous level after a change of perfusion pressure. Decreased heart rate attenuates autoregulation, while pharmacologic coronary constriction augments it.[73]

The autoregulatory mechanism may even extend into different myocardial layers.[70] Autoregulation is greater in the subepicardium than in the subendocardium, possibly due to the transmural gradient to which the subendocardial vessels are exposed.[72] Autoregulation in the right coronary artery may be less than in the left coronary artery. Pressure and flow-dependent changes in myocardial oxygen consumption in the right ventricle explain these differences.[72]

The most important regulators of coronary vascular tone are metabolic, with adenosine being the most likely local mediator to link blood flow to oxygen consumption. Other mediators, such as oxygen, potassium, carbon dioxide, prostaglandins, prostacyclin, histamine, and ATP, may affect coronary tone.[68] Prostaglandin E_1 dilates the coronary arteries, probably acting through adenosine as a mediator. Prostaglandin E_2, however, is a coronary vasoconstrictor.[74] Acting through the H_1 receptor, histamine contracts epicardial coronary arteries, provoking spasm, but the H_2 receptor mediates vasodilation.[75] Histamine also promotes production of prostaglandin in the heart.[75]

A metabolic mechanism for autoregulation appears most likely. Although it is difficult to separate myogenic and metabolic contributions to autoregulation, changes in myocardial oxygen demand alter autoregulation. The involved metabolite, therefore, is oxygen (specifically, myocardial oxygen tension—P_{O_2}) acting through mediators such as adenosine.[70] The threshold oxygen tension for autoregulation is 32 mm Hg.[73] Coronary autoregulation is also closely coupled to coronary venous P_{O_2}.[70,73]

Changes in myocardial oxygen demand and coronary resistance affect the epicardial vessels and the resistance coronary arteries to the same extent. Reperfusion flow, immediately after occlusion of a coronary artery, increases beyond pre-occlusion levels. This process is termed reactive hyperemia. In a related process, reactive dilatation, large coronary arteries dilate after relief of occlusion, but, unlike reactive hyperemia, the onset is delayed to 60 s and sustained for 150 s after relief of occlusion.[76] Coronary flow is determined by the duration of diastole and the difference between diastolic aortic pressure and left ventricular end diastolic pressure only after local autoregulation has produced maximum coronary vasodilation.[77]

Coronary Flow Reserve

Coronary flow also increases by maximal dilatation of the coronary arteries. The difference between resting and maximal coronary flow is the coronary flow reserve. Although coronary vasodilation occurs in response to ischemia or other endogenous stimuli, maximal flow, which is unavailable to the heart, may be achieved with pharmacologic agents. Exhaustion of autoregulatory vasodilator reserve does not necessarily mean that exhaustion of pharmacologic vasodilator reserve has occurred. Coronary flow reserve can be decreased by: 1) decreased maximal flow; and 2) increased regulated coronary flow.[78] Maximal coronary flow is decreased by tachycardia, increased blood viscosity, increased myocardial contractility, and myocardial hypertrophy.[70]

As epicardial coronary artery stenosis occurs, arteriolar vasodilation occurs to maintain flow at normal levels. Once the vasodilator reserve is exhausted (usually at stenoses of greater than 90%), however, an increase in the stenosis of the coronary artery will decrease flow. Administration of a vasodilator to a vascular bed served by a normal and a stenotic coronary artery connected by collaterals will dilate the normal arterioles, but produce little change in the arterioles served by the stenotic artery, since they are maximally dilated. The increased flow to the normal arterioles is termed "myocardial or coronary steal."

Endocardial/Epicardial Flow Ratio

The distribution of coronary flow is as important as total flow. The ratio of flow in the endocardium to that in the epicardium, the endo/epi ratio, is used to assess what subendocardial flow should be. Since subepicardial flow is usually adequate, if the endo/epi ratio remains constant, adequate subendocardial blood flow is inferred.[78] However, with maximal coronary vasodilation, the endo/epi ratio varies with the coronary perfusion pressure.[70] The ratio is minimally affected by changes in afterload, but increased preload reduces it. The latter results either from a disproportionate increase in subendocardial diastolic tissue pressure or an increase in coronary sinus pressure.[70] Transient subendocardial ischemia accompanies the onset of severe exercise. Although anemia increases coronary blood flow by autoregulation, severe anemia decreases the endo/epi ratio, indicating subendocardial ischemia.[70] Hypoxia, on the other hand, increases both coronary blood flow and the endo/epi ratio.

The onset of atrial fibrillation increases atrial blood flow. However, increased right ventricular preload decreases right ventricular blood flow without altering its intramyocardial distribution.[79] In ischemic hearts, atrial fibrillation or volume loading may impair myocardial oxygenation.

Neural Influences

Coronary arteries are also responsive to neural stimuli.[80] Parasympathetic and sympathetic nerves extend to the precapillary coronary vessels. Parasympathetic stimulation activates coronary muscarinic receptors, directly inducing dilation. Sympathetic stimulation causes coronary dilatation due to the metabolic dilation produced by increased myocardial oxygen requirements. Beta$_1$ adrenergic receptors predominate over alpha$_1$ receptors in canine circumflex coronary artery.[81]

Alpha$_2$ adrenoceptors and muscarinic receptors are present in the sympathetic nerve endings of coronary arteries. Activation of such receptors by norepinephrine and acetylcholine (via the vagus) reduces sympathetic neurotransmitter output, which would reduce the dilation of these vessels. Coronary artery spasm may result from unopposed alpha$_1$ adrenoceptor stimulation in the presence of beta adrenergic blockade, or when a pure alpha$_1$ agonist is given. Acute coronary occlusion attenuates the baroreflex responses of heart rate and systemic vascular resistance.[82]

CARDIAC OUTPUT

Cardiac output is the volume of blood pumped by the heart each minute. It is the product of the heart rate and the volume of each beat (stroke volume), but is determined by preload, afterload, heart rate, contractility, and ventricular compliance (Fig. 34-14). Cardiac output measurements are usually corrected for the size of the patient by dividing the output by the body surface area to give the cardiac index. A normal cardiac index is 2.5–3.5 $l \cdot min^{-1} \cdot m^{-2}$ (Table 34-3). Cardiac output increases with increased heart rate, preload, or contractility and decreased afterload. Decreases in cardiac output result from decreased heart rate, contractility, or preload and increased afterload.

Determinants

PRELOAD. Preload is defined as the end diastolic stress on the ventricle (end diastolic fiber length or end diastolic volume). The determinants of preload are blood volume, venous tone, ventricular compliance, ventricular afterload, and myocardial contractility. The distribution of the blood volume between intrathoracic and extrathoracic compartments also affects preload. Extrathoracic blood volume increases with standing, while the negative intrathoracic pressure during inspiration increases intrathoracic blood volume.

Stroke volume is determined by the volume of blood in the heart at the beginning of systole (end-diastolic volume—EDV) and the amount of blood remaining in the ventricle at closure of the aortic valve at the end of systole (end-systolic volume—ESV). The degree of stretch of the left ventricular fibers, determined by the amount of blood in the ventricle, determines the amount of work the ventricle can do.[83] An increase in preload increases end-diastolic volume and wall tension.

End-diastolic volume is not synonymous with end-diastolic pressure, nor are they linearly related. The ejection fraction, normally 0.6–0.7, is the ratio of the stroke volume to the end-diastolic volume. Severe impairment of left ventricular function is present when the LV ejection fraction is less than 0.4.

$$\text{Ejection fraction} = \frac{EDV - ESV}{EDV}$$

AFTERLOAD. Afterload is the wall stress or tension faced by the myocardium during ventricular ejection. It is the force opposing ventricular fiber shortening during ejection. Afterload is related to the shape, size, radius, and wall thickness of the ventricle, with the principle factors being the radius (related to preload and chamber volume) and aortic impedance (controlled by arterial compliance and systemic vascular resistance). Usually, the ejection phase stress is implied in discussions of afterload, although there are wall stresses during the isovolumetric contraction phase.

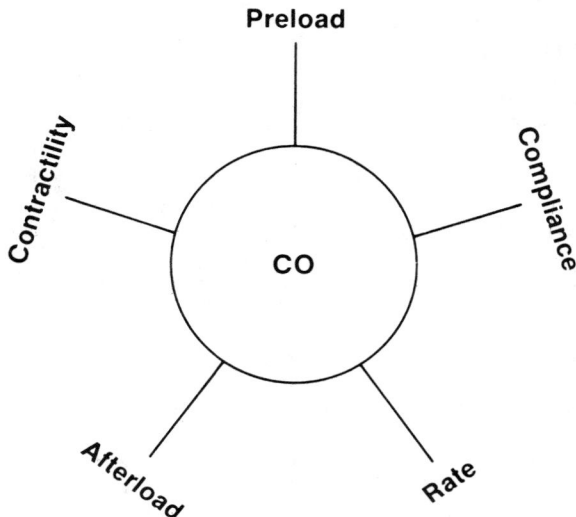

FIG. 34-14. The major determinants of cardiac output are preload, afterload, contractility, compliance, and heart rate. Alterations in any of these variables affect cardiac output, although the overall effect depends upon intrinsic cardiac function, compensatory mechanisms, and the magnitude of the change. Increased preload increases cardiac output to a point where subsequent increases cause heart failure (Starling's law). Increased afterload is more likely to reduce cardiac output in the failing heart than in the normal heart. The optimum heart rate for maximum cardiac output is approximately 120 beats · min^{-1} in the adult.

TABLE 34-3. Hemodynamic Variables: Calculations and Normal Values

VARIABLE	CALCULATION	NORMAL VALUES
Cardiac index (CI)	CO/BSA	2.5–4.0 $l \cdot min^{-1} \cdot m^{-2}$
Stroke volume (SV)	CO × 1000/HR	60–90 $ml \cdot beat^{-1}$
Stroke index (SI)	SV/BSA	40–60 $ml \cdot beat^{-1} \cdot m^{-2}$
Mean arterial pressure (MAP)	Diastolic pressure + ⅓ pulse pressure	80–120 mm Hg
Systemic vascular resistance (SVR)	$\dfrac{MAP - \overline{CVP}}{CO} \times 79.9$	1200–1500 dynes-cm-sec^{-5}
Pulmonary vascular resistance (PVR)	$\dfrac{\overline{PAP} - PWP}{CO} \times 79.9$	100–300 dynes-cm-sec^{-5}
Right ventricular stroke work index (RVSWI)	0.0136 ($\overline{PAP}$ − PWP) × SI	5–9 $g\text{-}m \cdot beat^{-1} \cdot m^{-2}$
Left ventricular stroke work index (LVSWI)	0.0136 (MAP − CVP) × SI	45–60 $g\text{-}m \cdot beat^{-1} \cdot m^{-2}$

$\overline{CVP}$ = mean central venous pressure; BSA = body surface area; CO = cardiac output; $\overline{PAP}$ = mean pulmonary artery pressure; PWP = pulmonary wedge pressure; MAP = mean arterial blood pressure; g-m = gram meter; sec^{-5} = seconds$^{-5.}$

Clinically, systemic vascular resistance (SVR) is frequently used as an estimate of afterload (Table 34-3). However, SVR reflects only peripheral arteriolar tone rather than left ventricular systolic wall tension. A true measure of left ventricular afterload, such as left ventricular end-systolic wall stress, which incorporates left ventricular chamber pressure, ventricular dimensions, wall thickness, and peripheral loading conditions, should be used to accurately assess afterload.[84] However, these measurements require direct intraventricular pressure determination and echocardiographic evaluation of wall thickness and ventricular dimensions. Compared to left ventricular end-systolic wall stress, systemic vascular resistance underestimates afterload when afterload is increased or decreased or contractility improved.[84]

When afterload is reduced, the ventricle shortens more rapidly and completely.[85] An increase in afterload decreases the extent and velocity of shortening, and increases active tension and the time to peak tension in cardiac muscle. Wall tension, ventricular radius, and end-diastolic volume are also increased to maintain stroke volume. In the poorly contractile heart, acute increases in afterload severely reduce stroke volume. For this reason, vasodilator therapy benefits patients with heart failure. Hearts facing chronically increased afterload adapt by hypertrophy, which returns wall stress and shortening characteristics toward normal.

HEART RATE. Heart rate is primarily determined by the automaticity of the sinus node. However, its intrinsic rate depends upon both neural and humoral influences. Neural influences are paramount, with sympathetic stimulation increasing, and parasympathetic or vagal stimulation decreasing, heart rate. An increase in heart rate increases cardiac output, even if the stroke volume remains constant, by increasing the extent and velocity of shortening and the developed tension. This effect is often prominent during anesthesia. Between 120 and 160 beats $\cdot$ min^{-1}, cardiac output increases, but not as greatly as at more optimal heart rates (Fig. 34-15). An increase in heart rate shortens the filling time between beats, reducing end-diastolic volume. Because most cardiac filling occurs during the first half-second of the rapid filling phase, cardiac output decreases at heart rates over 160 beats $\cdot$ min^{-1} because of inadequate filling time.

Cardiac output is also increased during the heartbeat after a ventricular extrasystole. This extrasystolic potentiation results from increased ejection fraction, decreased left ventricular end-diastolic volume, and enhanced diastolic filling. The mechanism is probably increased availability of calcium to the contractile mechanism.[86]

CONTRACTILITY. Contractility has been defined as the degree of inotropic state independent of changes in preload, afterload, or heart rate.

CARDIAC SYSTOLE. Myocardial contraction begins when an action potential, acting through the T system of the sarcoplasmic reticulum, results in calcium release into the sarcoplasm. A cyclic adenosine monophosphate (cAMP) dependent protein kinase in the heart stimulates calcium transport by the vesicles of the sarcoplasmic reticulum. Intracellular cAMP protein kinase is activated and transfers the terminal phosphate of adenosine triphosphate (ATP) to troponin I, phospholamban, or other intracellular proteins. Troponin has three components; troponin I, the inhibitory factor inhibiting the magnesium-stimulated ATPase of actomyosin; troponin C, which is the calcium-sensitive factor; and troponin A, which allows attachment of the troponin complex to actin and

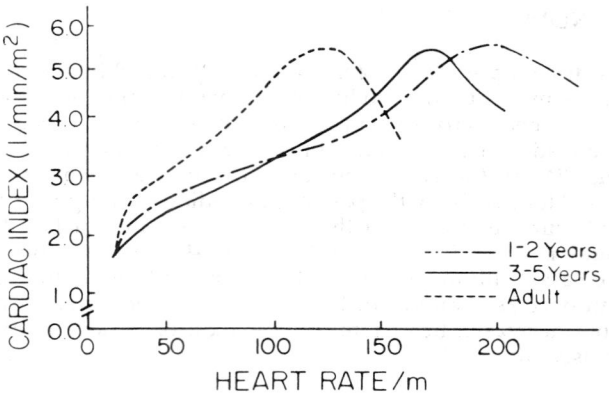

FIG. 34-15. The effect of heart rate on cardiac output varies with age. In children, an increase in heart rate increases cardiac output because the immature heart is relatively noncompliant and does not increase its stroke volume in response to increased demands. In the adult, however, an increase in heart rate beyond 120 beats/min does not increase cardiac index. (Wetsel RC: Critical Care State of the Art, 1981 with permission of author and publisher.)

tropomyosin. Phospholamban, a membrane-bound protein, which is a calcium-stimulated magnesium ATPase, permits increased calcium uptake and calcium release by the sarcoplasmic reticulum.[87] ATPase from the calcium pump, which couples hydrolysis of one molecule of ATP to the active transport of two calcium ions, is the channel through which the activator calcium is released to initiate systole. The increased free calcium is bound to troponin C, releasing the inhibition of actin-myosin interaction by the troponin-tropomyosin complex. Contraction of actin and myosin occurs. Both developed tension and relaxation depend upon the rate of calcium delivery to troponin, the quantity of available calcium, and the rate of calcium removal from troponin.[88]

DIASTOLE. Relaxation of the heart and its return to a precontractile configuration actually begins during late systole and continues during isovolumic relaxation and rapid ventricular filling. Myocardial relaxation occurs due to reuptake of or binding of calcium ion by the sarcoplasmic reticulum, a lusitropic or relaxing effect of cAMP.[89] Relaxation is a load-dependent process. In the relaxing heart, load is the premature lengthening of cardiac muscle. Myocardial relaxation depends upon internal restoring forces, such as cardiac fibers; hemodynamic loading, such as the impedance of the arterial system; and external restoring forces resulting from deformation of the wall of the intact heart.[90] During relaxation, load dependence indicates the dissipation of activation, and diastolic "suction" occurs as a consequence. During hypoxia, load dependence of relaxation is suppressed, probably from inhibition of the reuptake of calcium by the sarcoplasmic reticulum or impaired detachment of the force-generating site of actin and myosin.[90] These findings explain the relaxation abnormalities associated with ischemic disease.

ALTERATIONS IN CONTRACTILITY. Myocardial contractility is evaluated by the rate of ventricular pressure change with time (dP/dt), mean circumferential fiber shortening rate (during ejection phase), force-velocity curves, pressure-volume loops, or other derived parameters described later. The cardiac output can be increased by increasing load, either volume or pressure (heterometric autoregulation); the Anrep effect (homeometric autoregulation), in which ventricular performance improves several beats after the initial stretching of the myocardial fibers; and the treppe phenomenon. The Anrep effect, which results from abrupt elevation of aortic or left ventricular pressure, by increased contractility resulting from more rapid activation of the contractile process, increased developed force, and increased velocity of shortening, is operative for only a few minutes as the initially increased ventricular end-diastolic volume and circumference decrease with recovery of stroke work.[90] The treppe (staircase effect) or Bowditch phenomenon is a progressive increase in contractile force associated with a sudden increase in heart rate. A long pause between beats also increases the force of contraction, and is known as the reverse or negative staircase effect.[91] Increasing contractility increases the ejection fraction if end-systolic volume decreases while end-diastolic volume remains the same. Contractility is decreased by hypoxia, acidosis, cardiomyopathy, myocardial ischemia or infarction, and drugs such as calcium entry or beta blockers.

COMPLIANCE. Compliance is defined as the change in end-diastolic volume as related to the change in end-diastolic pressure. The relationship between ventricular volume and diastolic pressure is nonlinear. The rapidity of diastolic filling is a major determinant of cardiac output, which is reduced by decreased compliance. Although the contractility of the ventricle may be normal, reduced relaxation from coronary artery disease, hypertrophic cardiomyopathy, cardiac tamponade, and hypertensive heart disease impairs diastolic filling, which, in turn, limits cardiac output.

Myocardial Mechanics

The mechanical function of the heart is determined by evaluation of velocity of shortening, exerted force or tension, instantaneous length, and time after activation. Among the traditional indices of myocardial contractility are ventricular function (Starling) curves, ejection phase indices (force-velocity curves, ejection fraction, velocity of circumferential fiber shortening), isovolumic phase indices (rate of left ventricular pressure development [dP/dt], velocity of circumferential fiber shortening [V_{cf}], and maximal velocity of contractile element shortening [V_{max}]), and end-systolic indices (pressure/volume relationship at end-systole). Normal dP/dt is 800–1700 mm Hg · s^{-1}, but measurements are affected by intrapatient variation and complicated recording equipment. Complexity of measurement is also a problem with measurement of circumferential fiber shortening, and it is sensitive to acute changes in afterload. Measurements of V_{max} are research-oriented, since the range of normal is large, and includes some patients with cardiac disease. End-systolic indices are better methods of measuring contractility, less affected by either preload or afterload. End-systolic volume is independent of initial ventricular volume. However, the completeness of ventricular emptying depends upon both afterload and contractility.[92] Ejection fraction is affected by changes in loading conditions independent from changes in ventricular contractility.

STARLING (VENTRICULAR FUNCTION) CURVE. Myocardial contractility and function can be altered with or without changes in end-diastolic myocardial fiber length. If the cardiac muscle is stretched, it develops greater contractile tension. This observation is the basis of Starling's Law, which states that "the Law of the Heart is therefore the same as that of skeletal muscle, namely, that the mechanical energy set free

on passage from the resting the contracted state depends . . . on the length of the muscle fibers."[93] Atrial, as well as ventricular, muscle obeys Starling's Law. However, the Starling curve of the right ventricle is upward and to the left of the left ventricular function curve. Increased preload or initial fiber length increases resting tension, velocity of tension development, and peak tension. An increase in venous return will stretch the muscle fibers to increase contractility and improve cardiac output. However, this finding appears to occur only at subnormal filling pressures. In the upright position, ventricular filling pressures decrease to about 4 mm Hg, and the normal heart operates on the ascending limb of the ventricular function curve. Peak ventricular output occurs at normal filling pressures of about 10 mm Hg in normal humans.[94] Whether the heart can fall onto a descending limb of the length-stroke volume curve like skeletal muscle is unclear.[94] On the descending limb, the heart decompensates, and further increases in end-diastolic volume decrease stroke volume, but disengagement of actin and myosin does not occur. In all probability, the heart actually moves to a different curve.

Ventricular function curves are influenced by afterload, although they incorporate the effects of preload alterations (Fig. 34-16). To assure that a change in contractility has occurred when using Starling curves, preload, afterload, and heart rate must be controlled. Starling curves, as a measure of pump function, are used clinically during weaning from cardiopulmonary bypass, to assess the effects of anesthetic agents on the heart, and to guide fluid and cardiac therapy in the perioperative period.

PRESSURE-VOLUME LOOPS. Another index of contractility that is less affected by preload, afterload, or other conditions

FIG. 34-16. The ventricular function (Starling) curve of the normal left ventricle is demonstrated. The output of the normal heart (*solid line*) is affected much more by changes in preload (left ventricular end diastolic pressure) than it is by an increase in afterload (*dotted line*). The failing heart moves to a curve downward and to the right of the normal heart. Venodilator therapy decreases preload without increasing cardiac index (the heart moves to the left on the curve), while reduction of afterload increases cardiac index without a change in preload. Combined preload and afterload reduction decrease filling pressure and increase cardiac index.

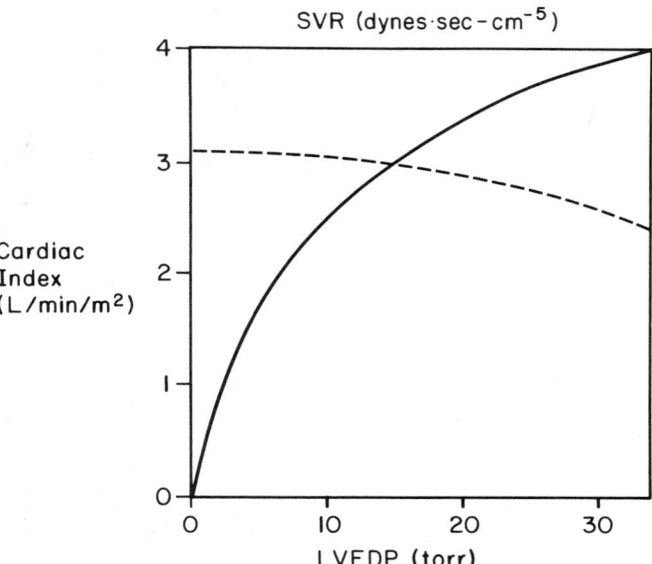

is the pressure-volume loop, an end-systolic index (Fig. 34-17). At end systole, ejection ceases and the aortic valve closes with the ventricle at minimum dimension and volume.

Although pressure-volume loops can be measured in humans using gated blood pool scintigraphy, two-dimensional echocardiography, or contrast angiocardiography and intravascular catheterization, performance is difficult and results not immediately available for patient care.[95]

In such loops, the height and width of the loop are determined by the ventricular systolic pressure and stroke volume. The area subtended by the systolic portion of the curve provides a measure of stroke work during ejection, while the area of the diastolic limb is a measure of diastolic work performed during ventricular filling and distention. The volume between the systolic and diastolic portions of the loop is the stroke volume. Cardiac work, the product of pressure and volume, is the area of the pressure/volume loop. In a given ventricle, all of the end-systolic points are positioned on the same line that represents the elastance of that ventricle (the change in end-systolic pressure/change in end-systolic volume).[96] Contractility is directly proportional to elastance with its slope becoming steeper with increased contractility and flatter with decreased contractility. The slope of the end-systolic pressure-volume relation correlates well with ejection fraction and is linear.[95, 97]

Pressure-volume loops also reveal information about ventricular compliance. The normal relationship between diastolic pressure and volume is curvilinear. There is a relatively gentle slope at low end-diastolic pressures (e.g., little change in pressure for large changes in volume). At end-diastolic pressures at the upper limits of normal (12 mm Hg or more), the curve becomes steeper and pressure is almost exponentially related to end-diastolic volume. Ventricular compliance decreases under such conditions. Thus, compliance actually changes during each contraction.

The ventricular end systolic pressure-volume relation is load independent, and can be used to assess left ventricular performance under various conditions (Fig. 34-17). However, one limitation of pressure-volume loops is that pressure may inaccurately reflect end-systolic afterload.[92] The ratio of pressure to volume at end-systole can also be used as an index of contractile function. However, this assumes that, at higher pressures, there are larger volumes at a given inotropic state.[92]

FORCE-VELOCITY CURVE. Myocardial contractility can also increase when the myocardial fibers increase their developed force or velocity of shortening without a change in fiber length. Force-velocity curves evaluate contractility (velocity of

FIG. 34-17. The relationship of ventricular pressure and volume over the entire cardiac cycle is the pressure-volume loop shown in A. The loop begins on the bottom with opening of the mitral valve and filling of the ventricle to end-diastolic volume. An extension of the bottom portion of the loop (without ventricular systole) would give a diastolic pressure-volume curve for the ventricle. Isovolumetric contraction begins at the lower right portion of the curve with closure of the mitral valve. The aortic valve opens at the upper right portion of the loop and ventricular ejection begins. At the upper left of the loop, the aortic valve closes (end systolic volume) and isovolumetric relaxation returns the loop to the starting point. Stroke volume is the difference between the volume at the end of diastole and the end of systole. The effects of afterload reduction on the pressure-volume loop are shown in B, while E shows the changes with increased afterload. C shows the changes in the pressure-volume loop in a patient with aortic stenosis with a high peak systolic pressure and steep diastolic slope representing reduced ventricular compliance. Venodilation and coronary vasodilation improve both contractility and compliance of the ischemic heart in E. In a normal heart (F), an increase in heart rate markedly reduces left ventricular volume.

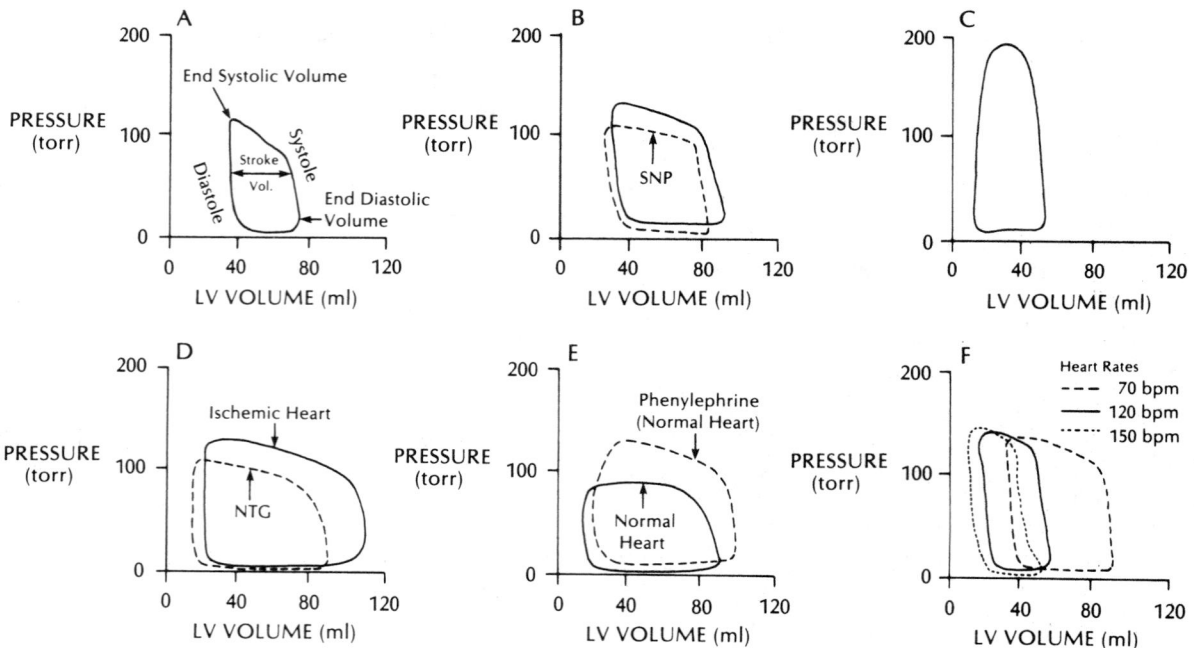

shortening) at constant fiber length in a passively stretched muscle (preloaded) that is stimulated to contract against either no load or an afterload. They are much more sensitive indicators of contractility than Starling curves, and are based upon the Hill model of isolated muscle.

As afterload is increased, the initial rate of shortening follows a hyperbolic relationship (Fig. 34-18). The force or tension developed during contraction is measured by dP/dt_{max}, the maximum rate of rise of intraventricular pressure during the isometric phase of ventricular contraction. The point of the curve where no shortening occurs, although the muscle develops maximal force, is termed Po. Extrapolation of the curve back to zero load where the maximal velocity of shortening occurs is termed V_{max}. Both preload and afterload affect dP/dt max. As preload increases, the maximum isometric tension that the muscle develops increases, but the maximal velocity of shortening is unchanged. An increase in myocardial contractility increases both the developed tension and the maximum velocity of shortening, shifting the force/velocity curve upward and to the right.

CARDIAC WORK. Because of the difficulties in obtaining the data for pressure-volume loops or force-velocity curves under clinical conditions, cardiac work is often measured as a substitute. Cardiac work describes pump function in terms of the load carried and the distance moved. The calculation of cardiac work and its indexing to body surface area (left and right ventricular stroke work indexes) is shown in Table 34-3. The advantages of using cardiac work instead of cardiac output or stroke volume to describe pump function are: 1) calculation includes heart rate, preload, and afterload, the major variables affecting cardiac function; 2) stroke work index defines the area of the pressure/volume loop; and 3) stroke work index measures both systolic and diastolic performance.[98]

FIG. 34-18. A force velocity curve of cardiac muscle shows the point of maximal shortening with no load or V_{max} (Point A). Point B is Po, where no shortening occurs, although tension development is maximal. Curve C is a force/velocity curve with increased preload. Curve D demonstrates increased myocardial contractility. On any curve, load (afterload) increases from left to right. (Lake CL: Cardiovascular Anesthesia, p 10. New York; Springer Verlag, 1985, with permission of the publisher.)

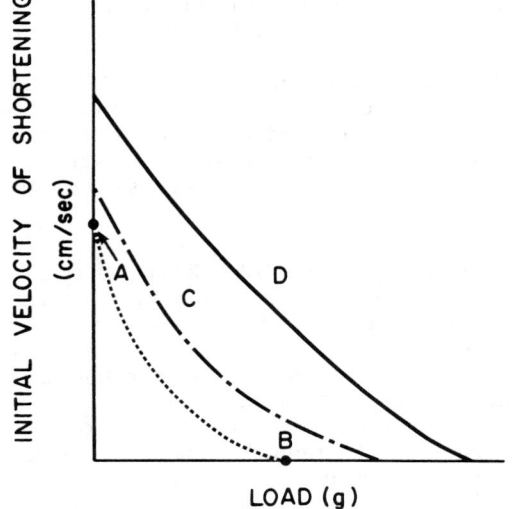

RIGHT VENTRICULAR FUNCTION. The functional significance of the right ventricle in normal circulatory homeostasis is minimal. After excitation, the wave of contraction spreads over the right ventricular free wall from the sinus to the conal (outflow) portion, with contraction of the conal portion lagging 25–50 milliseconds behind the inflow portion.[99] During ventricular systole, right ventricular free wall is pulled toward the interventricular septum by alignment of septal fibers and the greater left ventricular pressure, although its spiral muscles also contract.[100] Intraventricular pressure develops more gradually in the right ventricle and declines more slowly during diastole. Peak ejection occurs later than in the left ventricle. This difference in function results because the right ventricular free wall is flattened by the pull of the interventricular septum toward the left ventricle during systole, giving a bellows-like action for expulsion of blood.[101] Because of this mechanism, RV function is less likely to be impaired during right coronary arterial occlusion.

During systole, RV stroke volume is more sensitive to ejection pressure than the LV. Factors that oppose blood flow from the right ventricle include the resistance of the pulmonary vascular bed, pulmonary arterial compliance, the inertness of the ejected blood, and pulse wave reflection altering pulmonary artery pressure.[99]

In diastole, the right ventricle is twice as distensible (more compliant) as the left ventricle.[100, 102] Right ventricular pumping capability depends upon: 1) pressure against which it ejects; 2) filling volume; and 3) right ventricular contractility.[102] The right ventricle obeys Starling's Law except at higher end-diastolic pressures where its response is flatter than that of the left ventricle.[99] Increases in filling volume increase right ventricular stroke volume up to the limit imposed by the restraint of the pericardium (normally about a 20% acute increase in cardiac volume).[101] The contractility of the right ventricle depends upon sympathetic tone, myocardial structural integrity, and the chemical content of the coronary perfusate.[102]

Normally, right ventricular systolic pressures are only 30–40 mm Hg because the recruitable vasculature of the pulmonary circulation allows between 5 and 20 liters of blood to flow within it. RV ejection fraction is approximately 0.4. However, under conditions of pressure overload, such as increased pulmonary vascular resistance or left ventricular failure, it hypertrophies to generate systemic pressures. Although acute right ventricular failure is compatible with life, the symptoms caused by increased venous pressure suggest that right ventricular function is important for maintenance of normal venous pressures.[99, 101]

VENTRICULAR INTERDEPENDENCE. Because the ventricles are anatomically associated, alterations of volume and pressure in one ventricle can affect these parameters in the other.[103] During normal inspiration, right ventricular end-diastolic volume increases, left ventricular diastolic volume decreases, and left ventricular transmural pressure is unchanged.[104] Important factors in ventricular interdependence are septal position and deformability, ventricular distensibility, and the transeptal pressure gradient. Interdependence is somewhat dependent upon the presence of the pericardium, although an interaction can be demonstrated after pericardiotomy.

In vitro experimental animal models confirm that, when left ventricular pressure increases, both decreased diastolic compliance and depressed systolic ventricular function occur in the right ventricle and vice versa. The mechanisms are: 1) Frank Starling effect due to increased ventricular diastolic volume, and 2) decreased systolic ventricular function.[105] The etiology of the depressed systolic function is unclear.[105]

Increased distention of either ventricle alters the compliance and geometry of the opposite ventricle. Myocardial infarction that decreases left ventricular free wall compliance causes right ventricular pressure and volume displacement to be more responsive to changes in left ventricular volume.[103] Computer models confirm that hypertrophy from right ventricular pressure overload, which increases septal thickness and decreases septal compliance, decreases transfer of pressure and volume between the ventricles, limiting ventricular interdependence.

Myocardial Metabolism

An understanding of myocardial metabolism is essential to the preservation of the heart during conditions of stress, cardiac arrest, or elective asystole during cardiac surgery. Metabolism includes both substrate utilization and oxygen consumption.

SOURCES OF ENERGY. The energy supply of the heart is derived primarily from lactate and fatty acids delivered by the coronary blood. Free or nonesterified fatty acids (palmitic and oleic acids) are the preferred fuel.[106] Myocardial uptake of fatty acids is almost linear with the plasma concentration above the threshold of 345 μmol·l^{-1}.[107] Fatty acid uptake by the heart from either fatty acid-albumin complexes or lipoprotein triglyceride occurs by either passive diffusion or carrier-mediated transport. During fasting, free fatty acids are always used as fuel. The heart has a limited ability to synthesize fatty acids from acetyl coenzyme A except for the formation of structural lipids. The oxidation of fatty acids and ketone bodies inhibits uptake of glucose, pyruvate oxidation, and glycolysis while facilitating glycogen synthesis.[107] Oxidation of nonesterified fatty acids accounts for 90% of myocardial oxygen consumption.[10]

Fuel selection by the heart probably depends upon regulatory enzymes controlled by factors other than substrate availability and product removal. Myocardial lactate utilization is regulated by the arterial lactate concentrations and pyruvate oxidation in the Kreb's tricarboxylic acid cycle. Glucose, pyruvate, acetate, and triglycerides can also be used by the heart as energy sources. Utilization of glucose by the myocardium depends upon the arterial glucose and insulin concentration. Glucose is normally used postprandially. However, glucose use by the myocardium as the primary energy source occurs only with high glucose levels, insulin secretion, or hypoxia. Glucose is the only substrate used by the heart anaerobically. As long as the entry of acetyl coenzyme A into the Kreb's cycle is not inhibited, the heart will use as much pyruvate as it is given. Substrates such as fructose, glycogen, or proteins are used for energy only during special circumstances, such as starvation, diabetic ketoacidosis, or anoxia.[109]

MYOCARDIAL OXYGEN CONSUMPTION. The heart has one of the highest metabolic rates of any organ. At rest, it uses 8–10 ml of oxygen per 100 g of myocardium per minute. The subendocardium requires about 20% more oxygen than the epicardium. For this reason, the subendocardium is more vulnerable to ischemia. Myocardial oxygen consumption is determined by heart rate, wall tension, and myocardial contractility (Table 34-4). The relative importance of each of these factors is difficult to evaluate, since they are interrelated through wall tension.[110] Less important factors include the oxygen costs of shortening of muscle fibers, electrical acti-

TABLE 34-4. Factors Involved in Myocardial Oxygen Supply and Demand

Myocardial Oxygen Consumption
Heart rate
Contractile state
Myocardial wall tension
Arterial oxygen content
Basal oxygen requirements
Oxen cost of muscle fiber shortening
Oxygen cost of electrical activation
Myocardial Oxygen Supply
Aortic diastolic pressure
Left ventricular end-diastolic pressure
Coronary artery diameter
Arterial oxygen content

vation, and catecholamines, as well as the basal oxygen requirements and the level of arterial oxygenation. Tension development constitutes about 50% of myocardial oxygen consumption.

Myocardial wall tension is related to the tension-time index, left ventricular end-diastolic pressure, and ventricular size. Wall tension can be divided into its components: the rate of force development, the magnitude of force development, the interval during which force is generated and maintained for each contraction, and the frequency with which force is developed per unit time.[110] Wall tension is measured according to LaPlace's law:

$$T = Pr/2h,$$

where radius is cardiac radius, T is cardiac tension, P is interventricular pressure, and h is ventricular muscle thickness. Increases in ventricular chamber pressure or volume increase both the magnitude of force development and the force maintained during ejection.

Tachycardia is well tolerated in the normal heart, although myocardial oxygen consumption and blood flow must increase. There is little change in arteriovenous oxygen difference across the coronary bed with moderate increases in heart rate. At extremely rapid heart rates, the arteriovenous oxygen difference increases. Tachycardia shortens diastole more than systole, increases myocardial contractility, and decreases both stroke volume and ventricular volume to maintain aortic pressure.[78]

Variables such as the rate-pressure product (RPP), the product of systolic blood pressure or the triple index, the product of rate-pressure product, and wedge pressure have been used clinically to monitor myocardial oxygen consumption. However, they often fail to correlate significantly in the anesthetized patient.

MYOCARDIAL SUPPLY-DEMAND RATIO. A balance must always exist between oxygen consumption (demand) and myocardial oxygen supply if ischemia is to be avoided. Factors important to this relationship are shown in Table 34-4. Myocardial oxygen supply is dependent upon the diameter of the coronary arteries, left ventricular end-diastolic pressure, aortic diastolic pressure, and arterial oxygen content. Myocardial blood flow is determined by the blood pressure at the coronary ostia, arteriolar tone, intramyocardial pressure or extravascular resistance, coronary occlusive disease, heart rate, coronary collateral development, and blood viscosity. The epicardial coronary arteries contribute little to coronary vascular resistance, while the intramural coronary vessels are the principal determinants.

In the normal heart, the coronary perfusion pressure is the difference between the aortic diastolic pressure and the left ventricular end-diastolic pressure. Because the pressure distal to a coronary stenosis will be lower than aortic diastolic pressure, this relationship is not applicable in coronary occlusive disease. Myocardial blood flow is also reduced by a low aortic diastolic pressure, increased pulmonary wedge pressure (both of which increase subendocardial tissue pressure), and tachycardia, which shortens diastole, reducing the duration of blood flow. Increasing preload or intracavitary pressure increases wall tension and oxygen demand, while decreasing subendocardial perfusion.

Myocardial oxygen supply is also affected by the level of arterial oxygenation. Oxygen content, resulting from Pa_{O_2}, hemoglobin, 2,3 DPG, and pH, P_{CO_2}, or temperature effects on the oxyhemoglobin dissociation curve, can be an important factor in patients with obstructive lung disease or severe anemia. Normal oxygen extraction by the heart is 60–70%, and changes very little with increased cardiac work because coronary vascular resistance decreases. However, if the coronary vascular resistance response is limited, oxygen extraction can be increased over 90%.[110] An increase in oxygen extraction and coronary vasodilation constitute the metabolic reserve of the heart to increased demand.

Heart rate and diastolic ventricular volume are the two factors most likely to produce ischemia if either or both are increased. Myocardial contractility or increased afterload, by increasing arterial pressure and myocardial oxygen supply, offset their tendency to increase myocardial oxygen consumption.

DISTRIBUTION OF CARDIAC OUTPUT

The cardiac output is distributed to the organ systems as follows: brain 12%, coronary 4%, liver 24%, kidneys 20%, muscle 23%, skin 6%, and intestines 8%. The total tissue blood flow in a given vascular bed is a function of the effective perfusion pressure and vascular resistance. Effective perfusion pressure is the difference between arterial and venous pressure across the vascular bed. Organs that autoregulate to keep blood flow constant in the face of changes in perfusion pressure include the cerebral, renal, coronary (described earlier), hepatic arterial, intestinal, and muscle circulation.

FACTORS REGULATING CARDIAC OUTPUT

Cardiovascular Reflexes

CAROTID SINUS REFLEX. This reflex, also called the pressoreceptor or baroreceptor reflex, occurs when an increase in blood pressure stretches pressoreceptors in the carotid sinus or arch of the aorta to increase their frequency of discharge. The impulses are transmitted along the afferent nerve of Hering[111] to the glossopharyngeal (carotid receptors) or vagus (aortic receptors) to the cardiovascular centers in the medulla. The medullary cardiovascular center, in turn, inhibits sympathetic activity, resulting in decreased cardiac contractility, heart rate, and vasoconstrictor tone. Parasympathetic activity is increased, which decreases heart rate. When the arterial pressure decreases as a result of medullary input, there are

fewer afferent impulses to the cardiovascular center, sympathetic tone increases, and vagal tone decreases. The baroreceptor reflex reduces changes in arterial pressure to about one-third of expected. The threshold of the reflex is about 60 mm Hg, and its limits are pressures of 175–300 mm Hg.[112] Its gain is determined by the pulse pressure.[113]

VALSALVA MANEUVER. The response to the Valsalva maneuver is mediated by the pressoreceptor reflex. The Valsalva maneuver is accomplished by voluntarily closing the glottis while performing a forced expiration to increase intrathoracic pressure. Venous pressure in the head and extremities increases while venous return to the right ventricle decreases.[104] As a consequence, cardiac output and blood pressure decrease, resulting in a reflex increase in heart rate. With glottic opening, venous return to the right heart suddenly increases, causing forceful right, and, subsequently, left, ventricular contraction. The increase in blood pressure then elicits the pressoreceptor response to produce transient bradycardia.

MUELLER MANEUVER. The Mueller maneuver is an inspiratory effort against a closed airway. During this maneuver, right ventricular end-diastolic volume and left ventricular end-diastolic pressure increase, while left ventricular end-diastolic volume is unchanged or decreased.[104] Ejection fraction is unchanged. Pleural pressure decreases and the afterloading effects of decreased pleural pressure increase left ventricular volume. The net effect of these changes on left ventricular function depends upon ventricular interdependence, heart rate, and contractility (position of heart on diastolic pressure/volume curve).

In patients with coronary artery disease, regional wall akinesis may be seen during the Mueller maneuver. This is possibly due to increased wall stress increasing myocardial oxygen demand, or increased left ventricular transmural pressure decreasing motion in nonfunctional ventricular myocardium.

BEZOLD-JARISCH REFLEX. Noxious stimuli to the ventricular wall activate left ventricular mechanoreceptors, which reflexly cause hypotension, bradycardia, and parasympathetically induced coronary vasodilation.[114–116] The afferent pathway is nonmyelinated vagal c fibers.[115] Reperfusion of previously ischemic tissue also elicits the reflex.[117, 118]

CUSHING'S REFLEX. Increased cerebrospinal fluid pressure compresses cerebral arteries, causing cerebral ischemia. The response to cerebral ischemia is an increase in arterial pressure sufficient to reperfuse the brain. Intense sympathetic activity causes severe peripheral vasoconstriction as a result of this reflex.

ATRIAL REFLEXES. Bainbridge described a reflex increase in heart rate when vagal tone was high and the right atrium or central veins were distended. The response of heart to atrial distention depends upon the pre-existing heart rate. There is no effect with pre-existing tachycardia, but volume loading at slow heart rate causes progressive tachycardia.[67] Although the Bainbridge reflex is primarily mediated through vagal myelinated afferent fibers, activation of sympathetic afferent fibers may also occur.[67] Increased right atrial pressure directly stretches the SA node and enhances its automaticity, increasing the heart rate, making the existence of this reflex questionable. Experimental distention of the cavoatrial junctions or other small portions of the atriae increases heart rate, but clinical conditions, such as heart failure, usually do not produce such locally increased atrial pressure.[119] Global atrial distention to high pressures causes bradycardia, hypotension, and decreased systemic vascular resistance.[120]

CHEMORECEPTOR REFLEX. Peripheral chemoreceptors sensitive to decreasing oxygen tension or increased hydrogen ion concentrations in the blood are located in the carotid and aortic bodies. Nerve fibers from the chemoreceptors pass through the nerve of Hering and the vagus to the medullary vasomotor centers. Normally, the peripheral chemoreceptors are minimally active. However, occlusion of the carotid artery decreases their oxygen supply and activates the reflex to increase pulmonary ventilation and blood pressure while decreasing heart rate. Stimulation of the aortic bodies causes tachycardia.

OCULOCARDIAC REFLEX. Traction on the extraocular muscles or pressure on the globe causes bradycardia and hypotension as a consequence of this reflex. Traction on the medial rectus, rather than the lateral rectus, is likely to elicit the reflex. Afferent fibers run with the short or long ciliary nerves to the ciliary ganglion, and then with the ophthalmic division of the trigeminal nerve to the Gasserian ganglion. Between 30 and 90% of patients undergoing ophthalmic surgery will demonstrate the oculocardiac reflex, which can be attenuated by intravenous administration of atropine.

CELIAC REFLEX. Traction on the mesentery or gall bladder, stimulation of vagal nerve fibers in the respiratory tract, or rectal distention stimulate afferent vagal nerve endings to cause bradycardia, apnea, and hypotension (vagovagal reflex). Manipulation around the celiac plexus decreases systolic pressure, narrows pulse pressure, and slightly decreases heart rate.

PERIPHERAL CIRCULATORY PHYSIOLOGY

The peripheral circulation consists of resistance and capacitance vessels. The majority of the resistance is in the arterial circulation, which consists of the Windkessel vessels, the precapillary resistance vessels, and the capillary exchange vessels. Windkessel vessels, named for the air-filled compression chamber of 18th century fire engines, are distensible elastic arteries, such as the aorta, and large muscular arteries that damp the pulsatile output of the ventricle. The arterioles, the precapillary resistance vessels, are muscular vessels that provide more than 60% of the peripheral resistance. At the most distal portion of the terminal arterioles are precapillary sphincters, which regulate the flow of blood into specific capillary beds. The capillary exchange vessels contribute about one-fourth of the total peripheral resistance, although most capillaries consist of a single endothelial cell layer without any surrounding smooth muscle.[22] The venous system, discussed below, is the capacitance system.

Arterial Pulse

The arterial pulse is a wave of vascular distention resulting from the impact of the stroke volume of each beat being ejected into a closed system. The wave of distention begins at the base of the aorta and passes over the entire arterial system with each heartbeat. The pulse is not due to the passage of the blood itself. The pulse waveform is due to the combined effects of the forward-propagating pressure wave and its reflectance back toward the heart from various parts of the

vasculature. Wave reflection may occur in high resistance arterioles, branching points, or sites of changes in arterial distensibility, but the major source is the arteriole.[121] The velocity of the pulse wave depends on the elasticity of the vessel. The pulse wave velocity is most rapid in the least distensible arteries. In the aortic arch, the pulse wave travels $3-5\ m \cdot s^{-1}$, and the aortic pulse waveform precedes the brachial waveform by about 0.05 s. In large distensible arteries, such as the subclavian, the pulse wave travels $7-10\ m \cdot s^{-1}$; while, in the small nondistensible peripheral arteries, it travels $15-30\ m \cdot s^{-1}$. Such differences become important when timing the counterpulsation of an intra-aortic balloon.

The arterial pressure waveform changes as it moves peripherally (Fig. 34-19). Peripheral pulse waveforms have a greater amplitude, more pronounced diastolic wave, and lower mean pressure, and the foot of the wave is delayed.[121] Systolic pressure is higher and diastolic pressure lower in the periphery. Such changes are best explained by a tubular model of the vascular system. In such a system, the contour of the pressure wave depends upon the velocity of the pressure wave, the duration of the pulse, and the length of the tube.[121]

Pulse contour also changes with hemodynamic conditions. In children, wave reflection facilitates cardiac performance by a relative decrease in arterial pressure during systole and a relative increase during diastole. As aging occurs, wave reflection occurs earlier in the cardiac cycle, increasing systolic pressure and decreasing diastolic pressure. In shock, the pulse wave velocity is reduced by hypotension, increased heart rate reduces the duration of cardiac systole, and peripheral vasoconstriction increases the peripheral reflection coefficient. Pulse waveforms vary in atrial fibrillation with beats

FIG. 34-19. The change in the pulse waveform as it moves from the aortic root to the dorsalis pedis artery is dramatic. These changes result from both forward wave propagation and wave reflection at branch points in the circulation. The waveform has a greater amplitude, higher systolic pressure, lower diastolic pressure, and reduced mean pressure in the peripheral circulation. (Bedford RF: Invasive blood pressure monitoring. In Blitt CD (ed): Monitoring in Anesthesia and Critical Care Medicine, p 50. New York, Churchill Livingstone, 1985, with permission of author and publisher.)

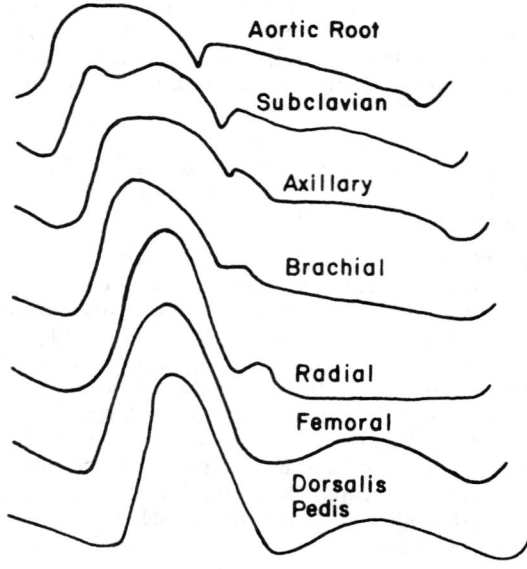

with short systolic duration demonstrating diastolic waves and those with long durations having accentuated systolic peaks. Patients with hypertrophic cardiomyopathy have double systolic pulse waveforms, because the initial systolic wave of ventricular ejection occurs during the first half of systole, and the reflected wave returns during the same systole.[121]

Blood Pressure

Arterial pressure is the lateral pressure exerted by the contained blood on the walls of the vessels. Mean arterial pressure is the product of the cardiac output and the systemic vascular resistance. If a normal arterial waveform is present, mean blood pressure is about one-third the difference between the systolic and diastolic pressures. MBP = (Diastolic Pressure) + ($\frac{1}{3}$ S − D). However, mean pressure remains constant, while pulse pressure and systolic pressure increase in the peripheral circulation.

Arterial pressure varies with the respiratory cycle. It normally decreases 6 mm Hg or less during inspiration, because pulmonary venous capacitance increases during inspiration to a greater extent than the increase in right heart venous return and output, thus causing a decrease in left ventricular stroke output and pressure. These changes are exaggerated in pericardial tamponade, causing pulsus paradoxus. Clinically, pulsus paradoxus is measured by auscultation of the blood pressure until the first heart sound is heard intermittently. Further deflation of the cuff to the pressure where all beats are heard yields the difference known as the paradoxical pulse.

FACTORS CONTROLLING BLOOD PRESSURE. Factors controlling blood pressure include central and autonomic nervous function, cardiac output, systemic vascular resistance, antidiuretic hormone, catecholamines, renin-angiotensin system, and atrial natriuretic factor. Arteriolar tone is regulated by intrinsic and extrinsic mechanisms. The intrinsic mechanism is the inherent myotonic activity of the vascular smooth muscle. Extrinsic factors include neural (sympathetic) and humoral factors. Sympathetic neural activity provides rapid alteration of tone in response to need for greater blood flow. Humoral factors are less important in overall circulatory regulation.

ANF. Atrial natriuretic factor (ANF) or atriopeptin is a peptide stored in the perinuclear granules of human atrial myocytes.[122] Secretion of ANF is limited to cells specialized for mechanical, rather than conductive, activity. More storage granules containing the prohormone, atriopeptigen (the primary storage form), are found in the right than in left atrium. During release from the granules, selective enzymatic cleavage occurs, to yield atriopeptin-28, the form circulating in the plasma.[123] The primary effects of ANF are direct peripheral vasodilation, suppression of antidiuretic hormone (ADH) release when elevated by hemorrhage or dehydration, inhibition of aldosterone release, and direct renal effects, such as increased glomerular filtration, natriuresis, and diuresis.[123] Kaliuresis does not occur. ANF affects not only blood pressure (by decreasing cardiac output and vascular resistance), but also water and electrolyte balance and blood volume. It has no direct inotropic or chronotropic properties. In animals, ANF causes profound renal vasodilation with lesser vasodilatory effects on the carotid, femoral, and coronary vascular beds.[124]

Release of ANF is caused by increased vascular volume, epinephrine, arginine vasopressin, acetylcholine, and increased myocardial (atrial) pressure.[122] Normal circulating plasma levels are 25–100 μg·ml^{-1}, but atrial tissue concentrations are unknown.[122, 125] Disease states such as congestive heart failure and atrial tachyarrhythmias increase circulating ANF levels.[122]

Therapeutic uses of ANF for diuresis and vasodilation appear particularly likely, since it has a circulating half-life of 3 min.[123] It may also be useful in renal failure by increasing glomerular filtration rate, and in congestive heart failure by promoting diuresis and inhibition of vasoconstriction. In normal volunteers, administration of ANF does not cause significant changes in renin, aldosterone, cortisol, norepinephrine, or ADH at doses which increase urinary output, decrease blood pressure, and reduce forearm vascular resistance.[126, 127]

RENIN-ANGIOTENSIN SYSTEM. Renin is a proteolytic enzyme produced in the granular juxtaglomerular cells of the kidney. Its release is governed by the macula densa, an intrarenal stretch-type receptor, circulating potassium angiotensin II, epinephrine, and ADH concentrations; and by the renal sympathetic nerves. Renin secretion is also inversely related to renal perfusion.[128] The half-life of renin is 4–15 min, during which it initiates the formation of angiotensin I from angiotensinogen, which is synthesized in the liver. Angiotensin I is biologically inactive until it is cleaved by angiotensin converting enzyme in lung and other tissues to angiotensin II.[129] Angiotensin II and angiotensin III, formed by hydrolysis of angiotensin II, stimulate the secretion of aldosterone and inhibit renin release through a negative feedback loop. The half-life of angiotensin II is about 30 s.

SYMPATHETIC NERVOUS SYSTEM. The receptors of the adrenergic nervous system are conveniently divided into alpha$_1$, alpha$_2$, beta$_1$, and beta$_2$ types (see Chapter 7). Presynaptic alpha$_2$ receptors inhibit the release of norepinephrine from the nerve terminal. However, they are also located on postsynaptic membranes of vascular smooth muscle. Post-synaptic alpha$_1$ receptors mediate smooth muscle vasoconstriction in the presence of agonist with norepinephrine, the more important agonist. Alpha receptor stimulation constricts arteries and veins.

Epinephrine is more potent as a beta receptor agonist than norepinephrine. Beta$_2$ receptors are located in both pre- and postsynaptic regions. Acting by stimulation of adenylcyclase, they dilate arteries.

Physiology of Specific Peripheral Circulations

PULMONARY CIRCULATION: FUNCTIONS. The pulmonary circulation has five principal functions: 1) metabolic transport of humoral substances and drugs;[130] 2) transport of blood through the lungs; 3) reservoir for the left ventricle; 4) filtration of venous drainage; and 5) transport of gas, fluid, and solutes across the walls of exchanging vessels. Normally, all circulating blood passes through the pulmonary circulation at least once each minute. Nevertheless, it is a low-pressure, high-flow system. The lung also has a large, metabolically active, endothelial surface.

METABOLIC TRANSPORT. The pulmonary vascular endothelium is important for removal, biosynthesis, and release of various vasoactive hormones, including biogenic amines, prostaglandins, leukotrienes, and peptides. Norepinephrine is removed by the lung by a carrier-mediated, temperature- and drug-sensitive transport process. Epinephrine, histamine, vasopressin, and dopamine, however, are unaltered by transpulmonary passage.[131] Almost complete removal of 5-hydroxytryptamine, adenosine triphosphate, and monophosphate occurs in the lungs. Acetylcholine is rapidly inactivated in the lung. Bradykinin is inactivated by the lungs, probably by an enzymatic process. Prostaglandins of the E and F series are also removed by either a carrier-mediated, energy-requiring process or by rapid degradation by 15-hydroxyprostaglandin-dehydrogenase. Prostacyclin (PGI₂) is not inactivated in the lung. ANF is rapidly removed from the blood by rabbit lung by an unknown mechanism,[132] and the lung is ideally situated to regulate the physiologic actions of right atrial ANF. Many drugs, such as propranolol, lidocaine, bupivacaine, captopril, and fentanyl, are removed during transpulmonary passage.[132, 133]

INTRAVASCULAR TRANSPORT. The passage of blood and its distribution to various segments of the lung depends upon pulmonary blood flow, pulmonary vascular resistance, or impedance and left atrial pressure. It also depends upon transmural distending pressure and the distensibility of the vessel walls. Blood flow to the lung apex is less than that to the base because of regional differences in pulmonary venous, alveolar, and pulmonary arterial pressures. However, the pulmonary circulation accommodates a large increase in flow with little change in pressure by a substantial decrease in resistance. Although there are some similarities between pulmonary and systemic impedance, there are also substantial differences. Among these are pulmonary resistance about one-fifth systemic, pulmonary impedance about one-half systemic, and stronger pulse wave reflections in the pulmonary beds due to similar reflecting sites (related to the smaller size of the vascular bed).[99]

Capillary endothelium, endothelial basement membrane, interstitial space, epithelial basement membrane, and alveolar epithelium form the alveolar-capillary membrane that separates the blood and gas phases in the lung. Abundant vascular smooth muscle is present in pulmonary vessels, distributed evenly between arteries and veins. Muscular arterioles are absent in the lung. The pulmonary veins perform primarily a reservoir function, preventing pulmonary edema in the event of reduced left ventricular compliance.[134]

Measurements of Pulmonary Tone. Drugs and maneuvers to dilate or constrict the pulmonary vasculature have clinical applications. However, measurements of pulmonary tone are essential to therapeutic investigations. Pulmonary artery pressures are clinically measured using flow-directed catheters. Wedging of the tip of these catheters in a small branch of the pulmonary artery measures the pulmonary artery wedge (PCWP) or occluded pressure (PA_o) (Table 34-2). From the tip of the catheter beyond the point of occlusion, the pressure in the pulmonary artery equilibrates with left atrial pressure. Normally, left atrial pressure is similar to left ventricular end-diastolic pressure (LVEDP) in the absence of mitral valvular stenosis. Other reasons for PWP greater than LVEDP are increased airway pressures or the presence of an intraatrial mass. Normally, the PCWP is 1–4 mm Hg lower than pulmonary end-diastolic pressure. However, with tachycardia or increased pulmonary resistance, the PCWP may be the same or slightly higher than pulmonary end-diastolic pressure.

Methods for the measurement of pulmonary resistance are either difficult or have limitations. The normal value for pulmonary resistance is listed in Table 34-3. Direct measurements of pulmonary blood flow using either isolated vessels *in vitro* or individual vessels *in situ* are affected by: 1) measurements made in a single artery that may differ in size or response from

other vessels; 2) technical factors related to vessel harvest and handling; and 3) isolated vessels unaffected by reflexes and other factors, such as airway pressure and cardiac output.[135]

Indirect estimations using the classic formula in the following equation have significant problems:

$$PVR = \frac{MPA - LAP}{\dot{Q}_{P \text{ or } CO}}$$

For example, pulmonary artery pressure is not linearly related to either flow or left atrial pressure. An increase in pulmonary flow or left atrial pressure is unaccompanied by a proportional increase in pulmonary arterial pressure. Therefore, calculated PVR decreases when either pulmonary flow or left atrial pressure increase. The nonlinearity results from distention or recruitment of vessels when flow or pressure increase. However, in zone 3 of the lung (where left atrial pressure is greater than airway pressure), pulmonary artery pressure is the most important factor determining pulmonary blood flow.[136] Therefore, regardless of the effect on the pulmonary vascular tone, agents or manipulations that change pulmonary flow or left atrial pressure will change calculated PVR. Only if a particular intervention does not change pulmonary flow or left atrial pressure or if the changes in pulmonary resistance can only be explained by active changes in pulmonary tone (*e.g.*, a decrease in pulmonary artery pressure accompanied by an increase in pulmonary blood flow) can PVR be accurate. However, even in these circumstances, reflex effects caused by the drug or maneuver cannot be eliminated.[137]

Another major factor affecting indirect measurements is airway pressures, since the degree of lung inflation and the ventilatory pressure directly influence pulmonary pressure/flow relationships. Either increases or decreases in lung volume beyond normal functional residual capacity increase pulmonary resistance due to compression of small intra-alveolar vessels. Baseline pulmonary tone, stimulation of pulmonary chemoreceptors, autonomic influences, and bronchospasm also directly affect the pulmonary vasculature or modify its response to drugs.

Effects of Drugs and Maneuvers on Pulmonary Tone. Various physiologic and nonphysiologic conditions alter pulmonary vascular resistance either actively or passively. These factors are summarized in Table 34-5. Alveoli in an area of lung that is poorly ventilated and contains hypoxic gas cause the precapillary arterial vessels supplying that area to constrict to divert blood away from that area. This process is termed hypoxic pulmonary vasoconstriction (HPV). Pulmonary hypertension does not occur because the hypoxia is localized. Drugs such as nitroprusside, nitroglycerin, and the inhalation anesthetics decrease HPV, resulting in worsening of venous admixture and arterial P_O₂.[138] If hypoxia is generalized, pulmonary hypertension ensues.[139] However, increased pulmonary artery pressure from one of several mechanisms inhibits hypoxic pulmonary vasoconstriction.

Pulmonary blood vessels can be dilated by acetylcholine or bradykinin, which act by release of endothelial-derived relaxing factor. Angiotensin converting enzyme in the lung, however, inactivates bradykinin. Hypoxia, which inactivates converting enzyme, may permit bradykinin to increase vascular permeability in the systemic circulation.[140] Serotonin increases pulmonary tone in animals, but not in man.[141] Vagal stimulation, by releasing acetylcholine from preganglionic cholinergic neurons, also dilates the pulmonary vasculature. Alpha adrenergic stimulation, also *via* the vagus, increases

TABLE 34-5. Alterations in Pulmonary Vascular Resistance

ACTIVE CHANGES		PASSIVE CHANGES	
Factors	Changes	Factors	Changes
Sympathetic stimulation	↑ or →	Pulmonary hypertension	↓
Parasympathetic stimulation	→	Left atrial hypertension	
Catecholamines	↑	Increased pulmonary interstitial pressure	↑
Angiotensin	↑	Increased blood viscosity	↑
Acetylcholine	↓	Increased pulmonary blood volume	↓
Histamine	→		
Bradykinin	↓		
Serotonin	↑		
Prostaglandin E₁	↓		
Prostaglandin F	↑		
Hypoxia	↑		
Hypercarbia	↑ →		
Acidemia	↑		

(Data from Murray JP: The Normal Lung, p. 128. Philadelphia, WB Saunders, 1976.)

pulmonary vascular resistance. When alpha-adrenergic blockers increase pulmonary vascular tone, agents such as norepinephrine, epinephrine, or adrenergic stimulation can actually decrease pulmonary tone (β effect).[142] However, the lung also has beta receptors, since isoproterenol decreases pulmonary tone.[142] Acidosis increases pulmonary resistance and decreases pulmonary blood flow.[139] Histamine is usually a pulmonary vasodilator, but is a vasoconstrictor if resting tone is low.[22] The leukotrienes are also powerful pulmonary vasoconstrictors.

TRANSVASCULAR TRANSPORT. The filtration of fluid across the alveolar-capillary membrane is described by the following equation, Starling's equation:

$$\text{Fluid filtration rate} = K_f\{(Pmv - Ppmv) - \sigma(\pi mv - \pi mv)\},$$

where Pmv is the pulmonary capillary hydrostatic pressure and $Ppmv$ is the interstitial fluid hydrostatic pressure (the hydrostatic pressures inside and outside of the pulmonary vessels), πmv is the colloid osmotic pressure inside and πpmv the interstitial colloid osmotic pressures outside the pulmonary vessels, K_f is the filtration coefficient of the pulmonary vessel (the capillary permeability), and σ is the reflection coefficient for proteins. The reflection and filtration coefficients describe the resistance of the pulmonary vessels to passage of fluid and protein. The filtration coefficient is the product of the effective capillary surface area in a given mass of tissue and the permeability per unit surface area of the capillary wall. Normally, the intravascular colloid osmotic pressure = 25 mm Hg keeps water within the capillaries while the pulmonary capillary hydrostatic pressure = 10 mm Hg attempts to force water across the endothelium into the interstitial space. Fluid filtered into the interstitial compartment is removed by the lymph. Transvascular fluid movement increases if there is a decrease in resistance of the vessel wall (increased permeability) or increased filtration pressure (either osmotic or hydrostatic). Pulmonary edema from left heart failure occurs because of an increase in Pmv, an increase in the amount of fluid filtered because of increased pulmonary venous and microvascular pressures, which overwhelms to capacity of the lymph removal system. Adult respiratory distress syndrome, on the other hand, results from increased vascular permeability, rather than a change in pressure.

BRONCHIAL CIRCULATION. Bronchial flow depends upon the cardiac output and blood pressure, ceasing at aortic pressures less than 40 mm Hg.[143] It is decreased by positive airway pressure and increased by hypoxia and hypercarbia.[12] Sympathetic stimulation or epinephrine decrease bronchial flow, while parasympathetic or vagal stimulation increase it.[143] Bronchial veins are more responsive to autonomic influences than bronchial arteries.[143] Histamine also increases bronchial flow, but prostaglandins decrease it.[12]

RENAL CIRCULATION. Renal blood flow is well in excess of the amount needed for renal perfusion. It is autoregulated so that glomerular filtration remains relatively constant, despite changes in arterial pressure between 70 and 180 mm Hg.[144, 145] Theories proposed to explain renal autoregulation include the juxtaglomerular theory (vasoactive hormonal release from the juxtaglomerular apparatus in response to the quantity or quality of filtrate reaching the macula densa) and the myogenic theory. Of these, the myogenic theory, in which changes in afferent arteriole tone provide the autoregulation, seems most likely.[146]

The main purpose of the excessive renal flow is to provide energy for active renal tubular reabsorption of sodium. Renal oxygen consumption is high, and the arteriovenous oxygen content difference is low. Of the blood delivered to the glomeruli, about 20% is filtered to form an ultrafiltrate of plasma. The main driving force is the glomerular hydrostatic pressure, which is essentially the systemic arterial pressure modified by the renal vasculature. Glomerular capillary pressure is, thus, about two-thirds of systemic pressure.[146] Glomerular capillary pressure is modified by afferent and efferent capillary tone. It is increased by dilatation of the afferent arteriole or constriction of the efferent arteriole. Arteriolar tone is also influenced by sympathetic stimulation, catecholamines, kinins, prostaglandins, and other vasoactive substances. Other factors affecting glomerular filtration include the total surface area available for filtration and the permeability of the glomerular membrane. The ultrafiltrate collects in Bowman's space before passing into the renal tubular system.

HEPATIC CIRCULATION. Hepatic arterial flow increases in response to decreased portal venous flow. The mechanisms for this alteration (the arterial "buffer response") include myogenic, metabolic, and neural controls, as well as the quality of the portal venous blood and the washout of some endogenous substance, probably adenosine, generated by hepatic tissue.[147]

Portal flow is controlled by preportal arterioles in the splanchnic organs from which the portal vein originates. Precapillary sphincters (presinusoidal) adjust portal flow to maintain an even distribution throughout the liver. The major site of resistance to portal flow is postsinusoidal, regulated by alpha sympathetic receptors affecting venous smooth muscle.[147] Normally, the liver contains about 15% of the blood volume. Sympathetic neural activation can mobilize one-half of the hepatic blood volume. Like the systemic vasculature, the hepatic arteriole is the major site of resistance.

PHYSIOLOGY OF THE VENOUS SYSTEM

Systemic veins have a conduit and a reservoir function. Since the smallest postcapillary venules lack muscular layers, while venules and small veins have only small amounts of muscle, the postcapillary resistance is usually small. However, it is important because the ratio of precapillary to postcapillary resistance determines the capillary filtration pressure.[22] The major capacitance vessels are medium and large veins, as well as the venae cavae. About 60% of the systemic blood volume is in small veins and venules of 20 μm to 2 mm in diameter.[148]

Venodilation to accommodate as much as 70–75% of the systemic blood volume buffers sudden increases in arterial blood pressure by allowing sequestration of blood in systemic veins. The compliance of the venous system is regulated by venomotor tone, which is controlled by cerebral autonomic impulses. Sympathetically mediated venoconstriction adds about 1 l of blood to the circulation, but passive constriction from a reduction in venous pressure contributes about two-thirds of the total volume mobilized. Individual organs contribute about 30–50% of their blood volume by sympathetically mediated venoconstriction.[22] The term vascular capacitance is used for the vascular pressure/volume relationship at a given level of venous tone. Venous tone is normally at 70% of maximum in the standing human.[22]

Venous return, the rate of flow of blood from the periphery to the heart, is a major determinant of cardiac preload. It is determined by the pressure gradient from the peripheral vascular beds to the right side of the heart and the resistance to venous return.[148] The upstream driving pressure from the peripheral tissue to the right atrium is the mean circulatory filling pressure (Pmcf). Pmcf is an equalization of pressures between the venous and arterial beds when flow is 0, and is usually about 10 mm Hg, similar to the mean systemic filling pressure. It is increased by catecholamines or increased sympathetic activity.[148] An increase in right atrial pressure decreases the pressure gradient and venous return. Cutaneous venous tone is determined by thermoregulatory mechanisms, rather than systemic pressure regulatory mechanisms.

Loss of venous tone, as in autonomic neuropathy or during anesthesia, limits the normal compensatory increases in venous tone to changes in posture, positive airway pressure, or decreased blood volume. If these factors are excessive, ventricular preload is adversely affected. Venoconstriction induced by hypovolemia, anxiety, or exercise augments intrathoracic blood volume and preload.

PHYSIOLOGY OF THE PERICARDIUM

In addition to the anatomic separation of the heart from the mediastinum, the pericardium also has physiologic functions. The pericardium may be important in the maintenance of normal ventricular compliance. The pericardium restrains the left ventricle and modifies its response to an increase in preload.[149] As dilatation of the left ventricle occurs, intrapericardial pressure limits right ventricular filling and reduces forward flow to the lungs, possibly preventing pulmonary edema. However, shifts of the left ventricular diastolic pressure-volume relationship are equal to changes in pericardial pressure and volume.[150] Mangano noted that neither left ventricular systolic function nor compliance are affected by the presence of the pericardium.[151] Thus, the role of the pericardium in the maintenance of normal ventricular systolic and diastolic function appears to be limited.

During pathologic conditions, the pericardium assumes more physiologic importance. Increased intrapericardial fluid (cardiac tamponade) causes hypotension, decreased cardiac output, myocardial ischemia, and tachycardia. However, a vagally mediated depressive reflex is also operative, contributing further to the decreased cardiac output resulting from the presence of pericardial fluid.[152] Intrapericardial pressure results in an underfilled ventricle, which operates on the ascending limb of Starling's curve.[153]

Lymph drainage of the myocardium occurs *via* the pericardium. Myocardial edema is particularly deleterious, since it reduces both systolic and diastolic ventricular performance. Normally, lymph flow rate adjusts rapidly to changes in myocardial interstitial fluid pressure. The relationship is defined as follows:

$$Jv = Lp \cdot A\,[(Pcap - Pint) - \sigma(\pi cap - \pi int)]$$

where Jv is the rate of fluid filtration, $Lp \cdot A$ is the filtration coefficient, $Pcap$ is capillary hydrostatic pressure, $Pint$ is interstitial hydrostatic pressure, πcap is capillary oncotic pressure, σ is the protein reflection coefficient, and πint is interstitial oncotic pressure.[154] Lymph, from interstitial myocardial lymphatics, collects on the epicardial surfaces and in the pericardial space before drainage into the lymphatic system *via* pericardial lymphatic vessels.[155]

REFERENCES

1. Powell EDU, Mullaney JM: The Chiari network and the valve of the inferior vena cava. Br Heart J 22:579, 1960
2. Hellerstein HK, Orbison JL: Anatomic variation of the orifice of the human coronary sinus. Circulation 3:514, 1951
3. James TN: Anatomy of the crista supraventricularis: Its importance for understanding right ventricular function, right ventricular infarction and related conditions. J Am Coll Cardiol 6:1083, 1985
4. Westaby S, Karp RB, Blackstone EH et al: Adult valve dimensions and their surgical significance. Am J Cardiol 53:552, 1984
5. Estes EH, Dalton FM, Entman ML et al: The anatomy and blood supply of the papillary muscles of the left ventricle. Am Heart J 71:356, 1966
6. Lam JHS, Ranganathan N, Wigle ED et al: Morphology of the human mitral valve. I. Chordae tendineae. Circulation 41:449, 1970
7. Byrd BF, Schiller NB, Botvinick EH et al: Normal cardiac dimensions by magnetic resonance imaging. Am J Cardiol 55:1440, 1985

8. Rosenquist GC, Sweeney LJ: The membranous ventricular septum in the normal heart. Johns Hopkins Med J 1345:9, 1974
9. Silver MA, Roberts WC: Detailed anatomy of the normally functioning aortic valve in hearts of normal or increased weight. Am J Cardiol 55:454, 1985
10. Zimmerman J: The functional and surgical anatomy of the aortic valve. Isr J Med Sci 5:862, 1969
11. Adams HD, Van Geertruyden HH: Neurologic complications of aortic surgery. Ann Surg 144:574, 1956
12. Deffebach ME, Charan NB, Lakshminarayan S et al: The bronchial circulation. Am Rev Respir Dis 135:463, 1987
13. James TN: Morphology of the human atrioventricular node, with remarks pertinent to its electrophysiology. Am Heart J 62:756, 1961
14. Bachmann G: The inter-auricular time interval. Am J Physiol 41:309, 1916
15. Thorec C: Über den Aufbau des Sinuskotens und seine Verbendung mit der Cava Superior und den Wenckebachschen Bundeln. Munch Med Wochenschr 57:183, 1910
16. Wenckebach KF: Beiträge zur Kenntnis der Menschlichenherztägtigkeit. Arch fur Physiol (Suppl BD) 3:53, 1908
17. Janes RD, Brandys JC, Hopkins DA et al: Anatomy of human extrinsic cardiac nerves and ganglia. Am J Cardiol 57:299, 1986
18. Rardon DP, Bailey JC: Parasympathetic effects on electrophysiologic properties of cardiac ventriocular tissue. J Am Coll Cardiol 2:1200, 1983
19. Shepherd JT: The heart as a sensory organ. J Am Coll Cardiol 5:83B, 1985
20. De Geest H, Levy MN, Zieske H et al: Depression of ventricular contractility by stimulation of the vagus nerves. Circ Res 17:222, 1965
21. Williams RS, Dukes DF, Lefkowitz RJ: Subtype specificity of alpha adrenergic receptors in rat heart. J Cardiovasc Pharmacol 3:522, 1981
22. Perloff WH: Physiology of the heart and circulation. In Swedlow DB, Raphaely RC (eds): Cardiovascular Problems in Pediatric Critical Care, p 1. New York, Churchill Livingstone, 1986
23. Stiles GL, Taylor S, Lefkowitz RJ: Human cardiac beta adrenergic receptors: Subtype heterogeneity delineated by direct radiological binding. Life Sci 33:467, 1983
24. James TN: Blood supply of the human interventricular septum. Circulation 17:391, 1958
25. Nerantzis CE, Toutouzas P, Avgoustakis D: The importance of the sinus node artery in the blood supply of the atrial myocardium. Acta Cardiol 38:35, 1983
26. Anderson KR, Murphy JG: The atrioventricular node artery in the human heart. Angiology 34:711, 1983
27. Scheinman MM, Gonzalez RP: Fascicular block and acute myocardial infarction. JAMA 244:2646, 1980
28. Wearn JT, Mettier SR, Klumpp TG et al: The nature of the vascular communications between the coronary arteries and the chambers of the heart. Am Heart J 9:143, 1933
29. Bartle SH, Herman HJ, Cavo JW et al: Effect of the pericardium on left ventricular volume and function in acute hypervolemia. Cardiovasc Res 2:284, 1968
30. Spodick DH: The normal and diseased pericardium: Current concepts of pericardial physiology, diagnosis and treatment. J Am Coll Cardiol 1:240, 1983
31. Spodick DH: The pericardium: Structure, function, and disease spectrum. Cardiovasc Clin 7:1, 1976
32. Banchero N, Rutishauser WJ, Tsakiris AG et al: Pericardial pressure during transverse acceleration in dogs without thoracotomy. Circ Res 20:65, 1967
33. Kennedy JW: Registry Committee of the Society for Cardiac Angiography: Complications associated with cardiac catheterization and angiography. Cathet Cardiovasc Diagn 8:5, 1982
34. Seldinger SI: Catheter replacement of the needle in percutaneous arteriography. Acta Radiol 39:368, 1953
35. Levin AR, Grossman H, Schubert ET et al: The effect of angiocardiography on fluid and electrolyte balance. Am J Roentgenol 105:777, 1969
36. Conti CR: Coronary arteriography. Circulation 55:227, 1977
37. Criley JM, Blaufuss AH, Kissel GL: Cough-induced cardiac compression: Self administered form of cardiopulmonary resuscitation. JAMA 236:1246, 1976
38. Rose JS, Nanna M, Rahimtoola SH et al: Accuracy of determination of changes in cardiac output by transcutaneous continuous-wave Doppler computer. Am J Cardiol 54:1099, 1984
39. Gorlin R, Gorlin G: Hydraulic formula for calculation of area of stenotic mitral valve, other cardiac valves, and central circulatory shunts. Am Heart J 41:1, 1951
40. Cannon SR, Richards KL, Crawford M: Hydraulic estimation of stenotic orifice area: A correction of the Gorlin formula. Circulation 71:1170, 1985
41. Cohen MV, Gorlin R: Modified orifice equation for the calculation of mitral valve area. Am Heart J 84:839, 1972
42. White CW, Holida MD, Marcus ML: Effects of acute atrial fibrillation on the vasodilator reserve of the canine atrium. Cardiovasc Res 20:683, 1986
43. Robinson TF, Factor SM, Sonnenblick EH: The heart as a suction pump. Sci Am 254:84, 1986
44. Abrams J: Current concepts of the genesis of heart sounds. I. First and second sounds. II. Third and fourth sounds. JAMA 239:2787, 1978
45. Luisada AA, MacCanon DM, Kumas S et al: Changing views of the mechanism of the first and second heart sounds. Am Heart J 88:503, 1974
46. Spencer MP, Greiss FC: Dynamics of ventricular ejection. Circ Res 10:274, 1962
47. Morad M, Maylie J: Calcium and cardiac electrophysiology. Some experimental considerations. Chest 78:16, 1980
48. New W, Trautwein W: The ionic nature of slow inward current and its relation to contraction. Pflug Arch 334:24, 1972
49. Noble D: The surprising heart: A review of recent progress in cardiac electrophysiology. J Physiol 353:1, 1984
50. Durrer D, Van Dam RT, Freud GE et al: Total excitation of the isolated human heart. Circulation 41:899, 1970
51. Coraboeuf E, Wiedman S: Temperature effects on the electrical activity of Purkinje fibers. Helv Physiol Pharmacol Acta 12:32, 1954
52. Kohlhardt M, Mnich Z, Maier G: Alteration of the excitation process of the sinoatrial pacemaker cell in the presence of anoxia and metabolic inhibitors. J Mol Cell Cardiol 9:477, 1977
53. Bailey JC, Watanabe AM, Besch HR et al: Acetylcholine antagonism of the electrophysiological effects of isoproterenol on canine cardiac Purkinje fibers. Circ Res 44:378, 1979
54. Russell PH: Electrophysiology of the heart. The key to understanding and management of electrocardiographic abnormalities. JAMA 27:181, 1972
55. Fisch C, Knoebel SB, Feigenbaum H et al: Potassium and the monophasic action potential, electrocardiogram, conduction, and arrhythmias. Prog Cardiovasc Dis 8:387, 1966
56. Trautwein W: Generation and conduction of impulses in the heart as affected by drugs. Pharmacol Rev 15:278, 1963
57. Von Bogaert PP, Vereecke J, Carmeliet E: Cardiac pacemaker currents and extracellular pH. Arch Intern Physiol Biochem 603, 1975
58. Cinca J, Morja A, Figueras J et al: Circadian variations in the electrical properties of the human heart assessed by sequential bedside electrophysiologic testing. Am Heart J 112:315, 1986
59. Urthaler F, Neely BH, Hageman GR et al: Differential

sympathetic-parasympathetic interactions in sinus node and AV junction. Am J Physiol 250:H43, 1986

60. Hoffman BF, Moore EN, Stuckey JH et al: Functional properties of the atrioventricular conduction system. Circ Res 13:308, 1963

61. Kovacs SJ: The duration of the QT interval as a function of heart rate: A derivation based on physical principles and comparison to measured values. Am Heart J 110:876, 1985

62. de Marneffe M, Jacobs P, Haardt R et al: Variations of normal sinus node function in relation to age: Role of autonomic influence. Eur Heart J 7:662, 1986

63. Musha H, Murayama M, Ito H et al: Estimation of autonomic nervous tone by evaluating minimal hourly heart rate. Respiration and Circulation 34:1003, 1986

64. Murphy DA, Johnstone DE, Armour JA: Preliminary observations on the effects of stimulation of cardiac nerves in man. Can J Physiol Pharmacol 63:649, 1985

65. Sapire DW, Casta A: Vagotonia in infants, children, adolescents, and young adults. Int J Cardiol 9:211, 1985

66. Medak R, Benumof JL: Perioperative management of prolonged Q-T interval syndrome. Br J Anaesth 55:361, 1983

67. Longhurst JC: Cardiac receptors: Their function in health and disease. Prog Cardiovasc Dis 27:201, 1984

68. Wilcken DEL: Local factors controlling coronary circulation. Am J Cardiol 52:8A, 1983

69. Steinhausen M, Tillmanns H, Thederan H: Microcirculation of the epimyocardial layer of the heart. Pflug Arch 378:9, 1978

70. Hoffman JIE: Determinants and prediction of transmural myocardial perfusion. Circulation 58:381, 1978

71. Rubio P, Berne RM: Regulation of coronary blood flow. Progr Cardiovasc Dis 43:105, 1975

72. Dole WP: Autoregulation of the coronary circulation. Prog Cardiovasc Dis 29:293, 1987

73. Dole WP, Nuno DW: Myocardial oxygen tension determines the degree and pressure range of coronary autoregulation. Circ Res 59:202, 1986

74. Karmazyn M, Dhalla NS: Physiological and pathophysiological aspects of cardiac prostaglandins. Can J Physiol Pharmacol 61:1207, 1983

75. Marone G, Triggiani M, Cirillo R et al: Chemical mediators and the human heart. Prog Biochem Pharmacol 20:38, 1985

76. Vatner SF: Regulation of coronary resistance vessels and large coronary arteries. Am J Cardiol 56:16E, 1985

77. Kirk ES, Sonnenblick EH: Newer concepts in the pathophysiology of ischemic heart disease. Am Heart J 103:756, 1982

78. Hoffman JIE: Transmural myocardial perfusion. Progr Cardiovasc Dis 29:429, 1987

79. Dyke CM, Brunsting LA, Salter DR et al: Preload dependence of right ventricular blood flow. I. The normal right ventricle. Ann Thorac Surg 43:478, 1987

80. Vatner SF: Alpha adrenergic regulation of the coronary circulation in the conscious dog. Am J Cardiol 52:15A, 1983

81. Shepherd JT, Vanhoutte PM: Mechanisms responsible for coronary vasospasm. J Am Coll Cardiol 8:50A, 1986

82. Trimarco B, Ricciardelli B, Cuocolo A et al: Effects of coronary occlusion on arterial baroreflex control of heart rate and vascular resistance. Am J Physiol 252:H749, 1987

83. Little RC, Little WC: Cardiac preload, afterload, and heart failure. Arch Intern Med 142:819, 1982

84. Lang RM, Borow KM, Neumann A et al: Systemic vascular resistance: An unreliable index of left ventricular afterload. Circulation 74:1114, 1986

85. Prewitt RM, Wood LDH: Effect of altered resistive load on left ventricular systolic mechanics in dogs. Anesthesiology 56:195, 1982

86. Wisenbaugh T, Nissen S, DeMaria A: Mechanics of postextra-

systolic potentiation in normal subjects and patients with valvular heart disease. Circulation 74:10, 1986

87. Katz AM: Regulation of myocardial contractility 1958–1983: An odyssey. J Am Coll Cardiol 1:42, 1983

88. Braunwald E, Sonnenblick EH, Ross J: Contraction of the normal heart. In Braunwald E (ed): Textbook of Cardiovascular Medicine, p 409. Philadelphia, WB Saunders, 1983

89. Katz AM: Cyclic adenosine monophosphate effects on the myocardium: A man who blows hot and cold with one breath. J Am Coll Cardiol 2:143, 1983

90. Brutsaert DL, Rademakers FE, Sys SU et al: Analysis of relaxation in the evaluation of ventricular function of the heart. Prog Cardiovasc Dis 28:143, 1985

91. Woodworth RS: Maximal contraction, "staircase" contraction, refractory period, and compensatory pause of the heart. Am J Physiol 8:213, 1902

92. Carabello BA, Spann JF: The uses and limitations of end-systolic indexes of left ventricular function. Circulation 69:1058, 1984

93. Starling EH: The Lineacre lecture on the law of the heart. In Chapman CB, Mitchell JH (eds): Starling on the Heart, p 119. London, Pall Mall, 1965

94. Parker JO, Case RB: Normal left ventricular function. Circulation 60:4, 1979

95. McKay RG, Aroesty JM, Heller GV et al: Left ventricular pressure-volume diagrams and end systolic pressure-volume relations in human beings. J Am Coll Cardiol 3:301, 1984

96. Thuys DM: Monitoring the left ventricle. Volume versus pressure. Mt Sinai J Med 52:526, 1985

97. Grossman W, Braunwald E, Mann T et al: Contractile state of the left ventricle in man as evaluated from end-systolic pressure volume relations. Circulation 56:845, 1977

98. Barash PG, Kopriva CJ: Cardiac pump function and how to monitor it. In Thomas SJ (ed): Manual of Cardiac Anesthesia, p 1. New York, Churchill Livingstone, 1984

99. Piene H: Pulmonary arterial impedance and right ventricular function. Physiol Rev 66:606, 1986

100. Hines R, Barash PG: Right ventricular function in the perioperative period. Mt Sinai J Med 52:529, 1985

101. Barnard D, Alpert JS: Right ventricular function in health and disease. Curr Probl Cardiol 12:423, 1987

102. Weber KT, Janicki JS, Shroff SG et al: The right ventricle: Physiologic and pathophysiologic considerations. Crit Care Med 11:323, 1983

103. Santamore WP, Shaffer T, Hughes D: A theoretical and experimental model of ventricular interdependence. Basic Res Cardiol 81:529, 1986

104. Santamore WP, Hickman JL, Bove AA: Right and left ventricular pressure-volume response to respiratory maneuvers. J Appl Physiol 57:1520, 1984

105. Maruyama Y, Nunokawa T, Koiwa T et al: Mechanical interdependence between the ventricles. Basic Res Cardiol 78:544, 1983

106. Opie LH: Metabolism of the heart in health and disease. Am Heart J 77:100, 1969

107. Berne RM, Rubio R: Coronary Circulation. In Berne RM (ed): Handbook of Physiology. The Cardiovascular System, p 873. Baltimore, Williams and Wilkins, 1979

108. Bing RJ: Cardiac metabolism. Physiol Rev 45:171, 1965

109. Merin RG: Inhalation anesthetics and myocardial metabolism. Anesthesiology 39:216, 1973

110. Weber KT, Janicki JS: The metabolic demand and oxygen supply of the heart: Physiologic and clinical considerations. Am J Cardiol 44:722, 1979

111. Hering HE: Der Karotisdruckversuch. Munch Med Wochenschr 70:1287, 1923

112. Aviado DM, Schmidt CF: Reflexes from stretch receptors on blood vessels, heart and lungs. Physiol Rev 35:247, 1955

113. Schmidt RM, Kumada M, Sagewa K: Cardiovascular responses to various pulsatile pressures in the carotid sinus. Am J Physiol 223:1, 1972

114. Von Bezold A, Hirt L: Über die physiologischen Wirkungen des essigsauren Veratrins. Physiol Lab Wuerzburg Untersuchungen 1:75, 1867

115. Mark AL: The Bezold Jarisch reflex revisited: Clinical implications of inhibitory reflexes originating in the heart. J Am Coll Cardiol 1:90, 1983

116. Jarisch A, Richter H: Die afferenten Bahnen des Veratrine Effektes in den Herznerven. Arch Exp Pathol Pharmacol 193: 355, 1939

117. Wei JY, Markis JE, Malagold M et al: Cardiovascular reflexes stimulated by reperfusion of ischemic myocardium in acute myocardial infarction. Circulation 67:796, 1983

118. Koren G, Weiss AT, Ben-David Y et al: Bradycardia and hypotension following reperfusion with streptokinase (Bezold-Jarisch reflex): A sign of coronary thrombolysis and myocardial salvage. Am Heart J 112:468, 1986

119. Ledsome JR, Linden RJ: A reflex increase in heart rate from distention of the pulmonary vein-atrial junction. J Physiol 170: 456, 1964

120. Lloyd TC Jr: Control of systemic vascular resistance by pulmonary and left heart baroreflexes. Am J Physiol 225:1511, 1972

121. O'Rourke MF, Yaginuma T: Wave reflections and the arterial pulse. Arch Intern Med 144:366, 1984

122. Rodeheffer RJ, Tanaka I, Imada T et al: Atrial pressure and secretion of atrial natriuretic factor into the human central circulation. J Am Coll Cardiol 8:18, 1986

123. Needleman P, Greenwald JE: Atriopeptin: A cardiac hormone intimately involved in fluid, electrolyte, and blood-pressure homeostasis. N Engl J Med 314:828, 1986

124. Baum T, Sybertz EJ, Watkins RW et al: Hemodynamic actions of a synthetic atrial natriuretic factor. J Cardiovasc Pharmacol 8:898, 1986

125. de Bold AJ: Atrial natriuretic factor. A hormone produced by the heart. Science 230:767, 1985

126. Richards AM, Nicholls MG, Ikram H et al: Renal, hemodynamic, and hormonal effects of human alpha atrial natriuretic peptide in healthy volunteers. Lancet 1:545, 1985

127. Bolli P, Muller FB, Linder L et al: The vasodilator potency of atrial natriuretic peptide in man. Circulation 75:221, 1987

128. Reid IA: The renin-angiotensin system and body function. Arch Intern Med 145:1475, 1985

129. Ryan J, Smith U, Niemeyer R: Angiotensin I: Metabolism by plasma membrane of lung. Science 176:64, 1972

130. Brigham KL, Newman JH: The pulmonary circulation. Basics of RD 8:1, 1979

131. Said SI: Metabolic functions of the pulmonary circulation. Circ Res 50:325, 1982

132. Gillis CN: Pharmacological aspects of metabolic processes in the pulmonary microcirculation. Ann Rev Pharmacol Toxicol 26: 183, 1986

133. Roerig D, Bunke S, Dawson CA et al: Inhibition of fentanyl uptake in the isolated perfused rat lung by propranolol. Fed Proc 44:1758, 1985

134. Goto M, Arakawa M, Suzuki T et al: A quantitative analysis of reservoir function of the human pulmonary "venous" system for the left ventricle. Jpn Circ J 50:222, 1986

135. Kulik TJ, Lock JE: The assessment of pulmonary vascular tone: A review of experimental methodologies. Pediatr Pharmacol 4: 73, 1984

136. Thorvaldson J, Ilebekk A, Loraand S et al: Determinants of pulmonary blood volume. Effects of acute changes in pulmonary vascular pressure and flow. Acta Physiol Scand 121:45, 1984

137. Rich S, Martinez J, Lam W et al: Reassessment of the effects of vasodilator drugs in primary pulmonary hypertension. Guidelines for determining a pulmonary vasodilator response. Am Heart J 105:119, 1983

138. Marshall BE, Marshall C: Anesthesia and the pulmonary circulation. In Covino BG, Fozzard HA, Strichartz G (eds): Effects of Anesthesia, p 121. Bethesda, American Physiological Society, 1985

139. Rudolph AM, Yuan S: Response of the pulmonary vasculature to hypoxia and H$^+$ ion concentration changes. J Clin Invest 45: 399, 1966

140. Stalcup A, Lipsit J, Waan J et al: Inhibition of angiotensin converting enzyme activity in cultured endothelial cells by hypoxia. J Clin Invest 63:966, 1979

141. Murray JP: Circulation. In Murray JP (ed): The Lung, p 113. Philadelphia, W.B. Saunders Co, 1976

142. Hyman AL, Lippton HL, Kadowitz PJ: Autonomic regulation of the pulmonary circulation. J Cardiovasc Pharmacol 7 (Suppl 3): S80, 1985

143. Baier H: Functional adaptations of the bronchial circulation. Lung 164:247, 1986

144. Navar LG: Renal autoregulation. Perspectives from whole kidney and single nephron studies. Am J Physiol 234:F357, 1978

145. Roberts CR, Deen WM, Troy JL et al: Dynamics of glomerular ultrafiltration in the rat. III. Hemodynamics and autoregulation. Am J Physiol 223:1191, 1972

146. Fried TA, Stein JH: Glomerular dynamics. Arch Intern Med 143: 787, 1983

147. Kang YG, Gelman S: Liver Transplantation. In Gelman S (ed): Organ Transplantation, p 142. Philadelphia, WB Saunders, 1987

148. Rothe CF: Physiology of venous return. Arch Intern Med 146: 977, 1986

149. Glantz SA, Misbach GA, Moores WY et al: The pericardium substantially affects the left ventricular diastolic pressure volume relationship in the dog. Circ Res 42:433, 1978

150. Refsum H, Junemann M, Lipton MJ et al: Ventricular diastolic pressure volume relation and the pericardium. Circulation 64: 997, 1981

151. Mangano DT, Van Dyke DC, Hickey RF et al: Significance of the pericardium in human subjects: Effects on left ventricular volume, pressure, and ejection. J Am Coll Cardiol 6:290, 1985

152. Friedman HS, Lajam F, Gomes JA et al: Demonstration of a depressor reflex in acute cardiac tamponade. J Thorac Cardiovasc Surg 73:278, 1977

153. Grose R, Greenberg M, Steingard R et al: Left ventricular volume and function during relief of cardiac tamponade in man. Circulation 66:149, 1982

154. Laine GA, Granger HJ: Microvascular, interstitial, and lymphatic interactions in normal heart. Am J Physiol 249:834, 1985

155. Miller AJ, Pick R, Johnson PJ: Lymphatic drainage of the heart. Am J Physiol 26:463, 1971

Chapter 35

Peter G. Andriakos
Cindy W. Hughes
Stephen J. Thomas

Anesthesia for Cardiac Surgery

Anesthetizing patients for open heart surgery is exciting, intellectually challenging, and emotionally rewarding. Competent and skillful clinical management requires a thorough understanding of normal and altered cardiac physiology; an intimate knowledge of the pharmacology of anesthetic, vasoactive and cardioactive drugs; and familiarity with the physiologic derangements associated with cardiopulmonary bypass (CPB) and the surgical procedures themselves. This chapter will present a brief overview of the subject in order to familiarize the reader with the critical physiologic and technical considerations when caring for cardiac surgical patients. The initial discussions concerning coronary artery and valvular heart disease lay the physiologic and some of the pharmacologic groundwork upon which anesthetic planning and therapeutic decisions are based. First, we will describe the balance of myocardial oxygen supply and demand with particular reference to the patient with coronary artery disease. Next, we will focus on those variables that regulate myocardial performance, specifically myocardial contractility, heart rate, and loading conditions (both preload and afterload). We will then discuss the bells, whistles, and mechanics of CPB. Following this, we will describe anesthetic considerations relevant to all adults undergoing open heart surgery, including preoperative evaluation, choice of monitoring techniques, selection of anesthetic drugs, and the actual conduct of the anesthetic pre-, during, and postbypass. The chapter concludes with some special topics as well as a brief introduction to the child with congenital heart disease. Some of the issues discussed are controversial, since the field is continuously evolving. We have tried whenever possible to sug-gest what is the consensus about these topics, but, inevitably, our own preferences will also be apparent.[1] For the sake of brevity, numerous tables are included in order to summarize data and to provide readily available guidelines for the various phases of the operative procedure. Many monographs are available for those who desire more detailed analysis of any aspect of cardiac anesthesia.[2-8]

CORONARY ARTERY DISEASE

The prevention or treatment of ischemia prior to CPB in patients undergoing coronary artery bypass graft (CABG) surgery reduces the incidence of perioperative myocardial infarction.[9-11] The hemodynamic profile during the prebypass period, how the anesthetic is managed, and who does the managing is also important, since the avoidance or treatment of factors known to increase myocardial oxygen demand (MVO_2) reduces the frequency of pre-CPB ischemic episodes.[9] In addition, not only is control of MVO_2 critical, but it is now apparent that many ischemic events occur with minimal or no changes in MVO_2, suggesting that a primary reduction in oxygen supply is also a major etiologic factor for intraoperative ischemia.[9, 10, 12, 13] Therefore, successful management of patients with coronary artery disease requires controlling the factors determining MVO_2 and, in so far as possible, optimizing oxygen delivery to the myocardium.[14] The determinants of myocardial oxygen supply and demand are listed in Table 35-1 and are also discussed in Chapter 34. A few points merit special attention.

TABLE 35-1. Myocardial Oxygen Balance

DEMAND	SUPPLY
Wall tension	Coronary blood flow
Ventricular radius	Driving pressure
Pressure generation	Diastolic time
Contractility	Arteriolar tone
Heart rate	Collaterals
	Arterial O_2 content
	Myocardial O_2 extraction

MYOCARDIAL OXYGEN DEMAND

Wall tension and contractility are the principal determinants of MVO_2.[15] LaPlace's law states that wall tension is directly proportional to *both* developed intracavitary pressure and ventricular radius and inversely proportional to wall thickness. Therefore, preventing or promptly treating ventricular distention is desirable in helping to control or reduce MVO_2. Since contractility is also of major importance, myocardial depression can be very beneficial as long as such depression does not result in ischemia-producing hypotension[16] or increases in wall tension.

MYOCARDIAL OXYGEN SUPPLY

Any increase in myocardial oxygen requirements can be met only by raising coronary blood flow (CBF). Blood oxygen content (hemoglobin concentration $\times$ O_2 saturation $\times$ 1.34) is obviously important, as is oxygen extraction by the myocardium, but these are infrequently the basis of intraoperative ischemia. Oxygenation and blood volume are usually well maintained during anesthesia. Coronary sinus P_{O_2} is about 27 mm Hg (50% saturation), and although extraction can be increased somewhat under conditions of stress, this is inadequate to meet the continuously changing levels of demand.[15]

Therefore, the principal mechanism for matching oxygen supply to alterations in MVO_2 is exquisite regulation and control of CBF.

CORONARY BLOOD FLOW. The critical factors that modify CBF are diastolic time available for perfusion (namely, heart rate), perfusion pressure, coronary vascular tone, and the presence and severity of intraluminal obstructions. We are most concerned with flow to the subendocardial region of the left ventricle, since this is the area most vulnerable to ischemia. As shown in Figure 35-1 and as will become more evident in the following discussion, the subendocardium is most at risk for the development of ischemia, because metabolic requirements are greater owing to greater shortening and because flow is restricted during systole.[17, 18]

Perfusion of the left ventricular subendocardium takes place almost entirely during diastole; the majority of right ventricular flow occurs during systole (Fig. 35-2). This temporal disparity is explained by the differences (in the absence of pulmonary hypertension) in intracavitary pressures during systole. Since left ventricular flow is diastolic, it is evident that not only is diastolic pressure important, but duration of diastole is also critical in determining the volume of left ventricular subendocardial flow. The time available for diastole decreases with increasing heart rate, with the greatest percentage reductions occurring at lower heart rates[19] (Fig. 35-3).

Coronary perfusion pressure for the left ventricle is often defined as aortic diastolic pressure (AoDP) minus left ventricular end diastolic pressure (LVEDP). This is an oversimplification, since there is no single AoDP. Rather, it is likely that there is a range of pressures that drive blood to the subendocardium. In the presence of intraluminal obstruction or increased vascular tone, this pressure is reduced, as depicted in Figure 35-4. The precise degree of reduction is unknown to the clinician. Although the pressure at the end of the circuit is unknown and the subject of controversy,[20] it is convenient and useful to consider ventricular filling pressure (VFP) as this end pressure. Therefore, a low VFP is ideal both in terms of improving perfusion (higher pressure gradient) and in re-

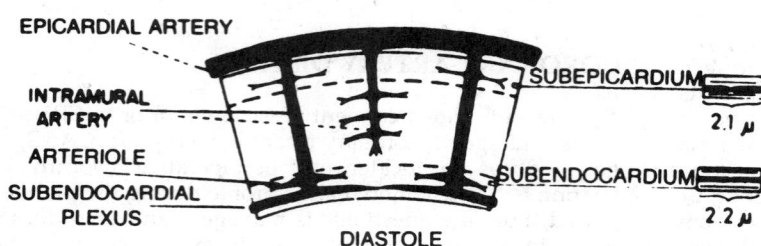

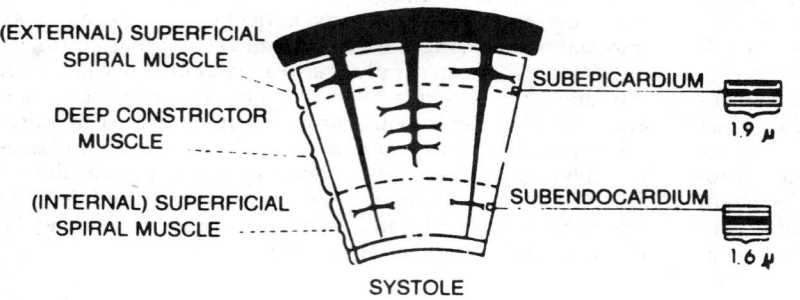

FIG. 35-1. Cross-sectional views of the left ventricular wall during diastole and systole. Numbers at right represent sarcomere length. Vulnerability of the subendocardium to ischemia results from both systolic compression of blood vessels (decreased oxygen supply) and increased systolic shortening (increased oxygen demand) relative to subepicardium. (Reprinted with permission from Bell JR, Fox AC: Pathogenesis of subendocardial ischemia. Am J Med Sci 268:2, 1974.)

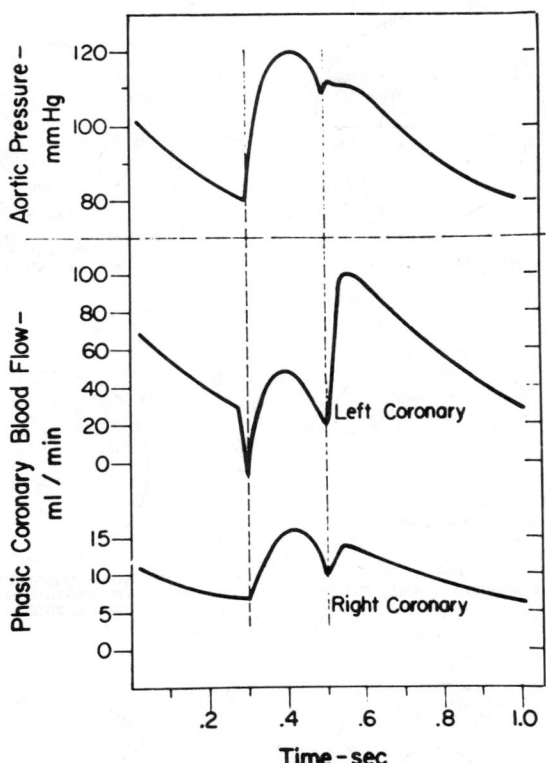

FIG. 35-2. Coronary artery blood flow during a single cardiac cycle. Left ventricular flow via the left coronary artery occurs primarily during diastole, whereas right ventricular perfusion is predominantly systolic. (Reprinted with permission from Berne FM, Levy MN: Cardiovascular Physiology, 5th ed, p 200. St Louis, CV Mosby, 1986.)

FIG. 35-3. The percentage of each cardiac cycle in diastole as a function of heart rate. The time available for subendocardial perfusion decreases in nonlinear fashion as heart rate (and myocardial oxygen demand) increases. (Reprinted with permission from Boudoulas H, Ritter SE, Lewis RP: Changes in diastolic time with various pharmacologic agents: Implications for myocardial perfusion. Circulation 60:165, 1979.)

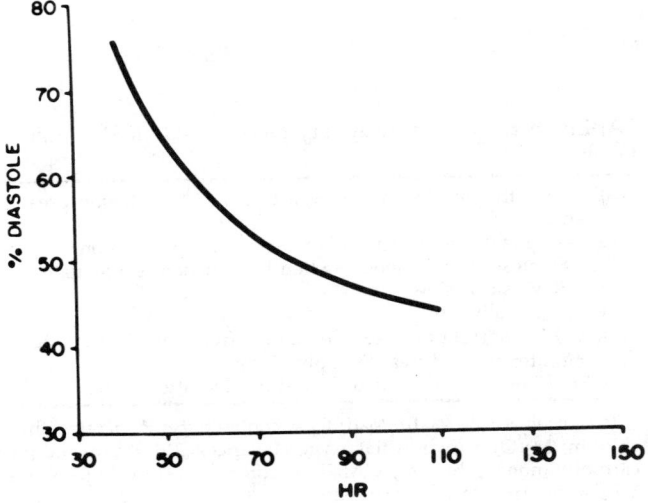

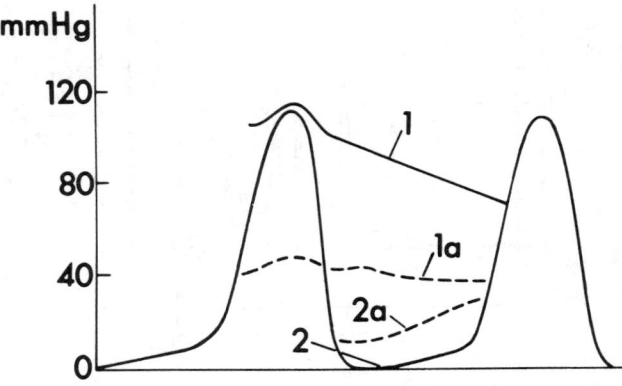

FIG. 35-4. The pressure relationships between the aorta (1) and the left ventricle (2) determine coronary perfusion pressure. In coronary artery disease, myocardial perfusion may be compromised by decreased pressure distal to a significant stenosis (1a) (not quantifiable clinically) and/or by an increase in LVEDP (2a). (Reprinted with permission from Gorlin R: Coronary Artery Disease, p 75. Philadelphia, WB Saunders, 1976.)

ducing MVO₂ (decreased ventricular volume and wall tension). The consequences of altering systemic pressure are more difficult to predict, since the cost of increasing perfusion pressure is increased MVO₂. It has been shown experimentally that at any given heart rate, hypotension is more likely to induce ischemia than is hypertension.[21]

Alterations in tone of the small intramyocardial arterioles regulate diastolic vascular resistance in the absence of flow limiting obstructions in the epicardial vessels. These adjustments, mediated primarily by adenosine, a metabolite of high-energy phosphates, allow matching of oxygen supply and metabolic demand over a wide range of perfusion pressures.[22] The difference between autoregulated supply and the amount available under conditions of maximal vasodilation is coronary vascular reserve, normally 3 to 5 times basal flow. As epicardial stenosis becomes more pronounced, progressive vasodilation of these resistance vessels allows preservation of basal flow, but at the cost of reduced reserve. Whenever demand increases above available reserve, signs, symptoms, and metabolic evidence of ischemia develop (Fig. 35-5).

Prinzmetal et al[23] first described angina and myocardial infarction in patients with angiographically normal coronaries. Subsequently Maseri and colleagues and others have emphasized repeatedly the frequency with which primary reductions in oxygen supply cause ischemia (Fig. 35-5).[8, 23–26] Small adjustments in coronary vascular tone at the site of previous obstructions can cause substantial reductions in luminal cross-sectional area (Fig. 35-6).[27] Alterations in stenosis diameter are possible, because at least two thirds of plaques or atheroma are not concentric.[28] Therefore, a certain portion of normal vessel wall, or at least reactive vessel wall, are present in the stenosis. It is now apparent that anesthesia is not protective against "supply" ischemia, which occurs frequently during surgery. The etiology of this is unclear but may be due to circulating catecholamines, local effects of blood components such as platelets at areas of atherosclerosis,[29] or other, as yet, undetermined factors. It is not uncommon during an anesthetic for a patient to show signs of ischemia without any change in heart rate, blood pressure, or VFP. Drugs such as

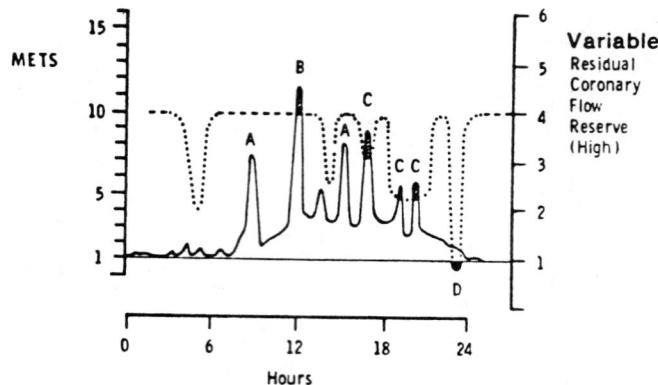

FIG. 35-5. Schematic illustration of mechanisms producing myocardial ischemia. Myocardial oxygen demand is plotted on the left (as multiples of basal oxygen consumption), and oxygen supply on the right. In this example, maximal coronary flow reserve is reduced from 6 to 4 times basal levels by fixed intraluminal obstruction. As long as myocardial oxygen demand remains below this maximal limit, no ischemia occurs (A). Ischemia will develop, however, whenever oxygen demand does maximal supply (B) or when supply is further compromised by coronary vasoconstriction (C). More pronounced coronary vasospasm may produce ischemia at rest (D). (Reprinted with permission from Masseri A, Chierchia S, Kaski JC: Mixed angina pectoris. Am J Cardiol 56:30E, 1985.)

nitroglycerin and the calcium entry blockers may be used to prevent and/or treat such episodes of coronary spasm.[30-32]

Hypotension, vasospasm, and acute thrombosis decrease coronary perfusion pressure, reduce CBF, and limit oxygen delivery to the myocardium. Acute thrombosis generally occurs at the site of a disrupted plaque on which a thrombus has formed. This type of acute thrombosis is thought to be the cause of acute myocardial infarction and sudden death (generally ischemia-induced cardiac dysrhythmias).

Hemodynamic Goals

It is thus apparent that the goal of a successful anesthetic is the prevention of ischemia. Failing that, the prompt identification and treatment of new episodes is essential. As is evident from the previous discussion and from the summary in Table 35-2, anesthetic decisions are designed to reduce and control those factors that increase myocardial oxygen demand, specifically, contractility and wall tension. At the same time, every attempt is made to optimize coronary blood flow—notably, maintaining coronary perfusion pressure and reducing diastolic time. The buzz words for patients with coronary artery disease are "slow, small, and well perfused." Combinations of anesthetics, sedatives, muscle relaxants, and vasoactive drugs are selected to provide this hemodynamic milieu. Techniques to effectively prevent or treat alterations in coronary vascular tone are still evolving and await further clinical trial before definitive recommendations can be made.

Monitoring for Ischemia

ELECTROCARDIOGRAM. The ideal monitoring technique is not yet available. ST-segment analysis in multiple leads (most commonly II and V_5) is currently the standard. In patients likely to develop right ventricular ischemia, the addi-

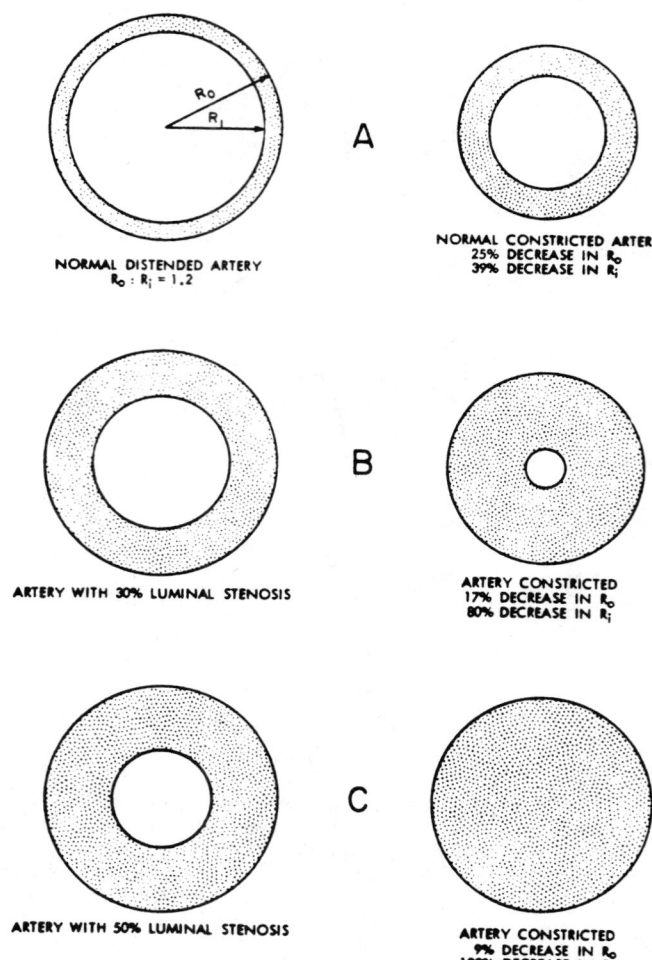

FIG. 35-6. The effect of coronary vasoconstriction on luminal cross-section in normal and stenosed arteries. R_o represents the outer radius, R_i the luminal radius of the vessel. Any reduction in outer radius is associated with a substantially greater decrease in inner radius (A). This effect is magnified by pre-existing stenosis (B). A 9% decrease in R_o in a vessel with 50% stenosis completely occludes the lumen (C). (Reprinted with permission from MacAlpin R: Contribution of dynamic vascular wall thickening to luminal narrowing during coronary arterial constriction. Circulation 60:296, 1980.)

TABLE 35-2.   Coronary Artery Disease—Hemodynamic Goals

P—Keep the heart small; ↓ wall tension; ↑ perfusion pressure
A—Maintain; hypertension is better than hypotension
C—Depression is beneficial when LV function is adequate
R—Slow, slow, slow
Rhy—Usually sinus
MVO_2—Control of oxygen demand is frequently not enough; monitor for and treat "supply" ischemia
CPB—Elevated VFP is usually not needed after CABG

P = preload; A = afterload; C = contractility; R = rate; Rhy = rhythm; MVO_2 = myocardial oxygen balance; CPB = pre- and post-cardiopulmonary bypass; CABG = coronary artery bypass graft; VFP = ventricular filling pressure

tion of V_{5R} might be beneficial.[33] Computerized ST-segment trending and interactive monitors that alarm when the ST segment deviates from the programmed algorithm may aid in the detection of intraoperative events overlooked by even the most astute observer.[34]

HEART RATE AND BLOOD PRESSURE. Multiple attempts have been made to determine ischemic thresholds using commonly measured hemodynamic variables. Among the earliest of these was the rate–pressure product (RPP),[35] obtained by multiplying heart rate by peak systolic pressure. For each patient, ischemia developed when a particular RPP was reached. The RPP was considered an easily determined index of $M\dot{V}O_2$. Although RPP may correlate with oxygen demand, especially during exercise, it is not a sensitive or specific indicator of intraoperative ischemia. Kissin *et al*[36] point out that identical RPPs are possible from multiple combinations of heart rate and blood pressure. Improved conditions for oxygen balance are likely with a low heart rate and high blood pressure compared with the opposite, that is, hypotension and tachycardia.[21]

In an effort to produce a more reliable predictor of ischemia, Buffington[21] devised the rate–pressure ratio. He found that in a canine model, whenever the ratio of heart rate to mean arterial pressure exceeded unity, ischemia developed. This ratio has not yet been validated in the clinical setting.

PULMONARY ARTERY CATHETER. Sudden elevations in pulmonary artery or capillary wedge pressure indicating systolic and/or diastolic dysfunction; large "A" waves, reflecting decreased ventricular compliance; and "V" waves, signaling the development of ischemia-induced papillary muscle dysfunction and mitral regurgitation are signs of ischemia that may be detected with the PA catheter.[37, 38] Although used almost universally in coronary artery bypass surgery, the sensitivity and specificity of these findings, as well as their frequency, has not been quantitated in any large study.

ECHOCARDIOGRAPHY. Transesophageal two-dimensional echocardiography permits on-line evaluation of regional wall motion (RWM) and global ventricular function. Identification of new RWM abnormalities represents a very sensitive indicator of ischemia. More extensive use of this device awaits studies delineating the specificity of these findings,[39] outcome studies demonstrating improved results, and a more inexpensive monitor.

Selection of Anesthetic

Numerous reports documenting the pattern of prebypass hemodynamics and the frequency of prebypass ischemia support the conclusion that there is no "best" anesthetic for patients with coronary artery disease.[40] Nearly every combination of anesthetic and vasoactive drug has both favorable studies and ardent zealots promoting its use. However, the choice of anesthetic should depend primarily upon both the extent of pre-existing myocardial dysfunction and the pharmacologic properties of the drugs themselves. The fit patient who has angina only with heavy exertion and good ventricular muscle profits from having $M\dot{V}O_2$ decreased with a volatile-based technique.[41-43] Conversely, the patient with severe congestive heart failure and a scarred myocardium might be better served by a less depressant technique. Clearly, there are patients who fall all along this spectrum. These examples illustrate the point that myocardial depression is only harmful in the patient whose heart cannot be

further depressed without fear of precipitating overt heart failure. Most patients with mild or even moderate dysfunction may benefit from some degree of myocardial depression decreasing oxygen demand and alleviating or at least decreasing episodes of ischemia.

OPIOIDS. The primary advantages of opioids are lack of myocardial depression, maintenance of a stable hemodynamic state, and reduction of heart rate (except for meperidine). Problems include hypertension and tachycardia during surgical stimulation[44-46] (sternotomy and aortic manipulation), especially in patients with good ventricular function, predictable hypotension when combined with benzodiazepines, lack of titratability when used in high doses, and a small incidence of intraoperative recall.[47, 48] It is apparent that a primary opioid technique may be of value in the patient with severe myocardial dysfunction; in patients with normal ventricles, this may be inadequate as an anesthetic and may need to be combined with other anesthetics or vasoactive drugs.

INHALATIONAL ANESTHETICS. The desirable features of volatile anesthetics include dose dependence, easily reversible and titratable myocardial depression,[49, 50] and reliable suppression of sympathetic responses to surgical stress and cardiopulmonary bypass. Disadvantages include myocardial depression, systemic hypotension (whether induced by decreased contractility or vasodilation), and lack of postoperative analgesia. Combinations of narcotics and volatile anesthetics may produce the advantages of each with minimal untoward effects.

The use of isoflurane in patients with coronary artery disease is still controversial.[51] Isoflurane is a coronary vasodilator, as are the other volatile anesthetics although to a lesser degree.[52-55] This effect is dose-related and appears to be clinically insignificant in doses less than 1 MAC. Clinical studies using isoflurane to clinical rather than pharmacologic end points do not show increased episodes of ischemia or a worsened outcome.[56]

Treatment of Ischemia

Selection of anesthetics or vasoactive drugs that will enable the heart to return to the slow, small, perfused state are frequently required during an anesthetic. The principal vasoactive drugs are nitrates, beta blockers, peripheral vasoconstrictors, and calcium entry blockers. Clinical scenarios for their use are given in Table 35-3. These drugs are discussed extensively in Chapter 7 and will be reviewed only

TABLE 35-3. Treatment of Intraoperative Ischemia

"Demand"	
↑ BP ± ↑ PCWP	TNG, ↑ anesthetic depth
↑ HR	Usual causes, then beta blocker
"Supply"	
↓ BP	Vasoconstrictor, ↓ anesthetic depth
↓ BP and ↑ PCWP	Phenylephrine + TNG, Inotrope
"NL" hemodynamics	TNG, CEB

BP = blood pressure; PCWP = pulmonary capillary wedge pressure; HR = heart rate; NL = normal; TNG = nitroglycerin; CEB = calcium entry blocker

briefly here. Volatile or halogenated anesthetics can also be used to control blood pressure and reduce contractility.

NITRATES. Nitroglycerin is a venodilator and reduces venous return, lessening wall tension and MVO_2, and also a coronary arterial dilator, effective at coronary stenoses and in collateral beds.[57, 58] Nitroglycerin is the drug of choice for the acute treatment of coronary vasospasm. The evidence for the prophylactic use of nitroglycerin for prevention of ischemic episodes is conflicting; further studies are needed to resolve this issue.[59-61] Although nitroglycerin is primarily a venodilator, at higher doses it does dilate arterial beds and may cause systemic hypotension.

VASOCONSTRICTORS. Vasoconstrictors are useful adjuncts in the prevention and treatment of ischemia owing to reduced systemic blood pressure. Administration of an alpha-adrenergic agent such as phenylephrine improves coronary perfusion pressure, although at the expense of increasing afterload and MVO_2. In addition, concomitant vasoconstriction increases venous return and left ventricular preload. In most situations, the increase in coronary perfusion pressure more than offsets any increase in wall tension. Peripheral vasoconstriction is indicated during episodes of systemic hypotension, especially those caused by reduced surgical stimulation or drug-induced vasodilation. Nitroglycerin is sometimes added in order to counteract any increase in preload. Similarly, phenylephrine can be administered to patients in whom nitroglycerin results in decreased ventricular filling pressures but unacceptably low arterial pressure.

BETA BLOCKERS. Beta-adrenergic blockade is often useful in improving myocardial oxygen balance by preventing or treating tachycardias as well as decreasing contractility. Myocardial depression can result in increased volume and wall tension, but clinically this is not a considerable problem. Indications for beta blockers include treatment of sinus tachycardia not resulting from the usual causes (*e.g.*, light anesthesia, hypoxia), slowing the ventricular response to supraventricular dysrhythmias, and decreasing heart rate and contractility in hyperdynamic states. Intravenous preparations include propranolol, metoprolol, labetalol, and esmolol. Propranolol is a nonselective beta blocker with an elimination half-life from 4 to 6 hours. Metoprolol is similar to propranolol but has the advantage of beta-1 selectivity. Labetalol combines alpha-blocking properties with those of beta blockade and is useful in treating hyperdynamic situations and in controlling hypertension. Esmolol is a newly released beta blocker that is cardioselective with a half-life of only 9.5 minutes. It is often useful in treating momentary increases in heart rate owing to episodic sympathetic stimulation.[62, 63]

CALCIUM CHANNEL BLOCKERS. *In vitro*, all calcium entry blockers depress contractility, reduce coronary and systemic vascular tone, decrease sinoatrial node firing rate, and impede atrial-ventricular conduction. Unlike the beta blockers, which are very similar both in structure and in pharmacodynamic effect, the calcium entry blockers vary remarkably in their predominant pharmacologic action. Nifedipine is the most prominent peripheral vasodilator and, when administered sublingually, is useful intraoperatively in treating hypertension or episodes of coronary vasospasm. Verapamil's effect on coronary vascular tone is equal to that of nifedipine, but its peripheral effects are less pronounced, although still present. In addition to treating presumed coronary spasm, verapamil is very useful in the treatment of supraventricular

tachycardia and in slowing the ventricular response to atrial fibrillation or flutter. Some clinicians simultaneously administer phenylephrine to counteract the peripheral vasodilation and hypotension that often accompany the use of verapamil.

VALVULAR HEART DISEASE

Alterations in loading conditions are the initial physiologic burdens imposed by valvular heart lesions, both stenotic and regurgitant. For example, the left ventricle (LV) is pressure overloaded in aortic stenosis (AS) and volume overloaded in aortic insufficiency (AI) and mitral regurgitation (MR). However, in mitral stenosis, the LV is both volume and pressure underloaded, whereas the RV faces the progressively increasing left atrial and pulmonary artery pressures. The mechanisms used to compensate for these additional stresses consist of chamber enlargement, myocardial hypertrophy, and variations in vascular tone and the level of sympathetic activity.[64, 65] These mechanisms in turn induce secondary alterations, including altered ventricular compliance, development of myocardial ischemia, chronic cardiac dysrhythmias, and progressive myocardial dysfunction. Myocardial contractility is often transiently depressed but may progress to irreversible impairment even in the absence of clinical symptoms. This is especially true in MR and AI, where markedly reduced afterload favors ejection and forward flow.[66, 67] Conversely, the patient with AS may complain of dyspnea not because of impaired systolic function, but, rather, because of reduced ventricular compliance, increased LVEDP, and pulmonary pressures.

When a decision for valve replacement or repair is made, we are often presented with a patient with pulmonary hypertension, severe ventricular dysfunction, and chronic rhythm disorders. Anesthetic management is predicated on understanding these altered loading conditions, preserving the compensatory mechanisms, maintaining circulatory homeostasis, and anticipating the problems that may arise during and after valve surgery. In this section, we will briefly describe the pathophysiology, the desirable hemodynamic profile, and other pertinent anesthetic considerations for each valvular lesion.

AORTIC STENOSIS

PATHOPHYSIOLOGY. Progressive calcification and narrowing of the aortic valve orifice is a degenerative process affecting a normal or congenitally bicuspid valve. This results in chronic obstruction to LV ejection. Increased intraventricular systolic pressure, with concomitant increase in wall tension is required in order to maintain forward flow. "Concentric" ventricular hypertrophy, in which the wall gradually thickens but chamber size remains unchanged, is the compensatory response normalizing wall tension.[68] Contractility is preserved and ejection fraction is maintained at a normal range until late in the disease process[69] (Fig. 35-7).

The cost of this concentric hypertrophy is decreased diastolic compliance and a precarious balance between myocardial oxygen supply and MVO_2. The clinical implications of the low compliance ventricle are summarized in Table 35-4. Since the ventricle is so stiff, atrial contraction is often critical for maintenance of ventricular filling and stroke volume. The "atrial kick" may account for up to 40% of left ventricular end diastolic volume (LVEDV). Hypertrophy-induced impairment of diastolic relaxation can further impede LV filling.[70]

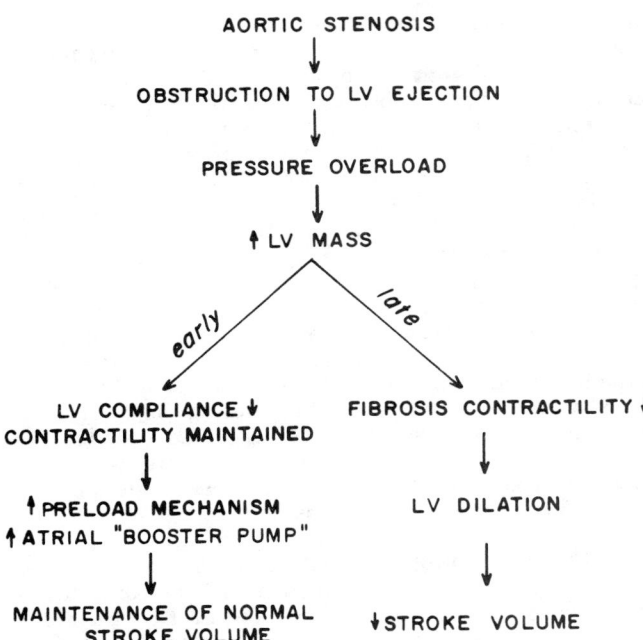

FIG. 35-7. The physiologic consequences of aortic stenosis. (Reprinted with permission from Thomas SJ, Lowenstein E: Anesthetic management of the patient with valvular heart disease. Int Anesth Clin 17:67, 1979.)

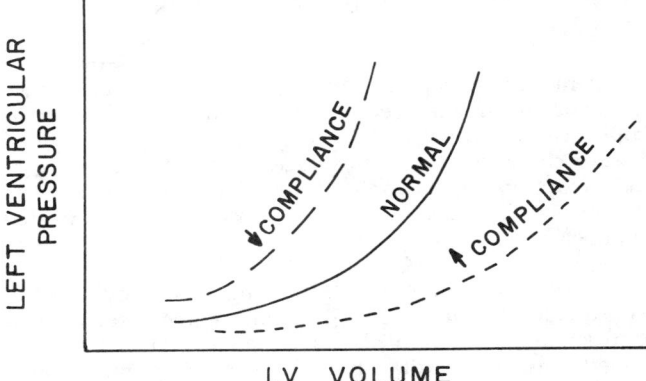

FIG. 35-8. Diastolic pressure–volume relationship (compliance) of the left ventricle. Any increase in the volume of a poorly compliant ventricle as in aortic stenosis or hypertension (left-shifted curve) is associated with increases in intracavitary pressure greater than that seen in a normal ventricle. Conversely, a ventricle with increased compliance (chronic valvular insufficiency right-shifted curve) accommodates large volumes with minimal pressure change. Note also that the normal relationship is curvilinear, and, at increased volumes, compliance is markedly reduced (*e.g.*, acute aortic insufficiency). (Reprinted with permission from Thomas SJ, Lowenstein E: Anesthetic management of the patient with valvular heart disease. Int Anesth Clin 17:67, 1979.)

Ventricular filling pressure is sometimes difficult to interpret, since it may vary widely yet reflect only small changes in ventricular volume (Fig. 35-8).

Hypertrophied myocardium is susceptible to ischemia, even in the absence of concurrent coronary artery disease. The enlarged muscle mass increases basal myocardial oxygen requirements while demand per beat rises owing to the elevated intraventricular systolic pressure.[71] Simultaneously, supply may be impaired, perfusion pressure is reduced (aortic diastolic pressure is decreased, ventricular filling pressure is increased), capillary density is often inadequate in the hypertrophic muscle,[72] and total vasodilator reserve may be impaired.[73] This situation is compounded in the presence of coronary obstruction.

ANESTHETIC CONSIDERATIONS. The ideal hemodynamic environment for the patient with AS is summarized in Table 35-5. Maintenance of adequate ventricular volume and sinus rhythm are crucial. Hypotension must be prevented if at all possible and treated early if it develops. Coronary perfusion pressure must be maintained to prevent the catastrophic cycle of hypotension-induced ischemia, subsequent ventricular dysfunction, and worsening hypotension. Bradycardia is a common clinical etiology for hypotension in the patient with AS. Slowing the heart rate and increasing diastolic time will not increase stroke volume. Therefore, bradycardia will induce a fall in total cardiac output and systemic arterial pressure. This is especially pertinent in the elderly patient, in whom sinus node disease and reduced sympathetic responses[74] may predispose to significant bradycardia.

Ischemia may be difficult to detect since the characteristic changes are often obscured by the electrocardiographic (ECG) signs of left ventricular hypertrophy and strain. Unfortunately, an ideal alternative is not available. Elevated LV filling pressures, although not necessarily reflecting increased volume, often require treatment in order to optimize coronary perfusion pressure. Nitroglycerin is very useful in this regard, but it must be remembered that minimal reductions in ventricular volume are required; therefore, very small doses of nitroglycerin should be used and titrated to effect.

TABLE 35-4. Clinical and Physiologic Implications of a Low Compliance Ventricle

Sensitive to volume depletion
Dependent upon atrial kick for adequate ventricular filling
Wide swings in ventricular filling pressure
PCWP underestimates LVEDP
↑ LVEDP reduces coronary perfusion pressures

PCWP = pulmonary capillary wedge pressure; LVEDP = left ventricular end diastolic pressure

TABLE 35-5. Aortic Stenosis—Hemodynamic Goals

P—Full; adequate intravascular volume to fill noncompliant ventricular chamber
A—Already elevated, but relatively fixed; coronary perfusion pressure must be maintained
C—Usually not a problem; inotropes may be helpful preinduction in end-stage AS with hypotension
R—Not too slow (↓ CO), not too fast (ischemia)
Rhy—Sinus!! Cardioversion if hemodynamic crash from supraventricular dysrhythmia
MVO₂—Ischemia is an everpresent risk; tachycardia and hypotension must be avoided

Abbreviations are spelled out in Table 35-2 footnote.

IDIOPATHIC HYPERTROPHIC SUBAORTIC STENOSIS

Idiopathic hypertrophic subaortic stenosis (IHSS), also known as asymmetric septal hypertrophy (ASH) or hypertrophic cardiomyopathy (HCM), is a genetically determined disease characterized by histologically abnormal myocytes and myocardial hypertrophy developing *a priori* and not in response to pressure or volume overload in a nondilated chamber.[75,76]

PATHOPHYSIOLOGY. The physiologic consequences of IHSS are depicted in Figure 35-9. Some degree of subvalvular obstruction is present in 20–30% of patients. During systole, the left ventricular outflow tract is narrowed by apposition of the hypertrophic intraventricular septum to the anterior leaflet of the mitral valve (Fig. 35-10). Blood is ejected rapidly

FIG. 35-9. The physiologic interrelationships of primary left ventricular hypertrophy in IHSS. LVSP = left ventricular systolic pressure; LVFP = left ventricular filling pressure. (Reprinted with permission from Maron BJ, Bonow RO, Cannon RO *et al*: Hypertrophic cardiomyopathy: Interrelations of clinical manifestations, pathophysiology, and therapy. N Engl J Med 316:344, 1987.)

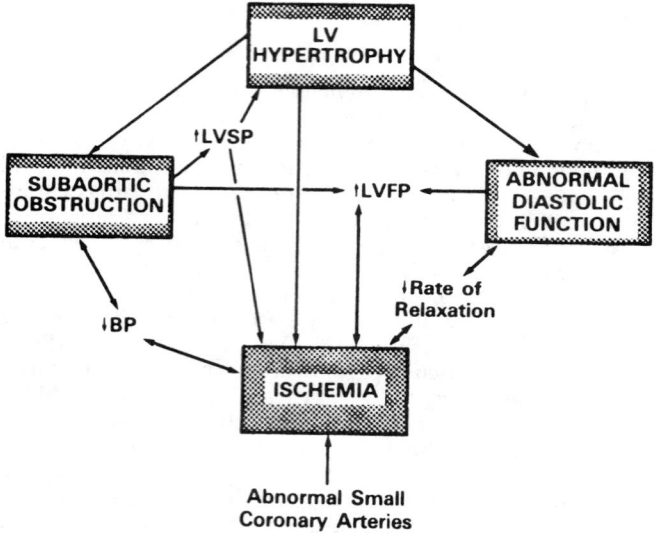

through this area, creating a Venturi effect, pulling the mitral valve leaflet even closer to the septum.[77] The timing and duration of septal–leaflet contact determine the severity and clinical significance of the obstruction.[78] Early prolonged contact can generate pressure gradients greater than 100 mm Hg. If the apposition occurs later, although a pressure gradient may exist, it is of little importance since most of the stroke volume has already been ejected.[79] This obstruction is dynamic and is accentuated by any intervention that reduces ventricular size facilitating septal–leaflet contact. Therefore, increases in contractility or heart rate or decreases in either preload or afterload are detrimental in this regard. This histologically abnormal muscle demonstrates impaired diastolic relaxation and reduced ventricular compliance.[80] The clinical and hemodynamic implications are similar to those detailed for AS.

The ventricles are hypertrophic, even in the absence of a pressure gradient. In addition, there is evidence of alterations in the small intramyocardial vessels.[81] Therefore, as expected, myocardial oxygen balance is tenuous, and the development of ischemia is an everpresent possibility.

ANESTHETIC CONSIDERATIONS. Anesthetic management focuses on maintenance of ventricular filling and on reduction in the factors predisposing to outflow tract obstruction or ischemia (Table 35-6). Myocardial depression is desirable, and volatile anesthetics are useful, although their tendency to cause junctional rhythm is of some concern. Because of the exquisite sensitivity of preload to atrial contraction, these patients often benefit from placement of pulmonary artery catheters with atrial pacing capabilities. This permits the administration of volatile anesthetics without fear of compro-

TABLE 35-6. Idiopathic Hypertrophic Subaortic Stenosis (IHSS)—Hemodynamic Goals

P—Full, full, full; volume is first Rx for hypotension
A—Up, up, up; a pure vasoconstrictor is next Rx for hypotension
C—Depression is fine
R—Not too slow, not too fast
Rhy—Sinus, sinus, sinus; consider pacing PA catheter to better control atrial mechanism
MVO₂—Usual precautions apply
CPB—Avoid inotropes post CPB; the myocardial disease is still present; try vasoconstrictors first

Abbreviations are spelled out in Table 35-2 footnote.

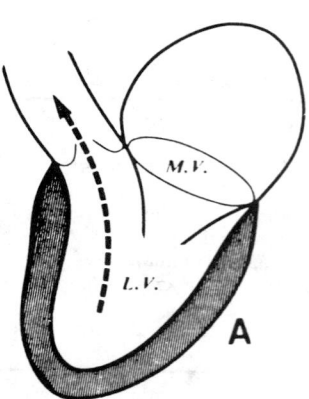
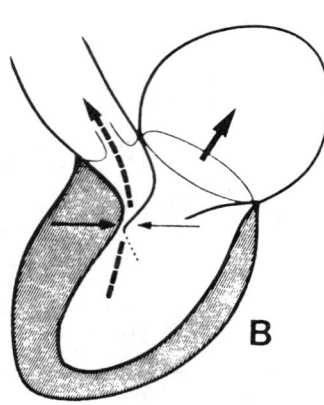

FIG. 35-10. Proposed mechanism for outflow tract obstruction in IHSS. (*A*) The normal outflow tract is ample and offers no impedance to ejection. (*B*) The outflow tract is narrowed by the hypertrophic ventricular septum in IHSS. A Venturi effect is produced as blood is ejected rapidly through this area drawing the anterior mitral leaflet toward the septum. Obstruction to forward flow (owing to mitral-septal contact) as well as mitral regurgitation can occur. (Reprinted with permission from Wigle ED, Sasson Z, Henderson MA *et al*: Hypertrophic cardiomyopathy. The importance of the site and the extent of hypertrophy. A review. Prog Cardiovasc Dis 28:1, 1985.)

mising sinoatrial conduction. In addition, control of atrial rate and rhythm is very beneficial during the prebypass period.

Although infrequent, IHSS occasionally coexists with valvular AS and may explain unanticipated difficulties in separating from bypass following seemingly uncomplicated aortic valve replacement. If this is suspected, measurement of the gradient between the left ventricle and the outflow tract will resolve the dilemma.

AORTIC INSUFFICIENCY

Rheumatic disease, endocarditis, or processes that dilate the aortic root such as ascending aortic aneurysms or collagen vascular diseases are the primary causes of aortic insufficiency.

PATHOPHYSIOLOGY. The fundamental physiologic derangement is chronic volume overload (Fig. 35-11). Chamber size increases gradually, sometimes to massive proportions, increasing wall stress and inducing mural hypertrophy. This pattern of chamber enlargement and increasing ventricular wall thickness is termed *eccentric hypertrophy*. Despite these enormous increases in end diastolic volume, end diastolic pressures are usually within the normal range, evidence of a significant increase in chamber diastolic compliance.[80] In contrast to aortic stenosis, considerable alterations in LV volume can occur with only minimal changes in LV filling pressure (see Fig. 35-8). Although the ventricle may pump three to four

FIG. 35-11. The physiologic consequences of aortic insufficiency. (Reprinted with permission from Thomas SJ, Lowenstein E: Anesthetic management of the patient with valvular heart disease. Int Anesth Clin 17:67, 1979.)

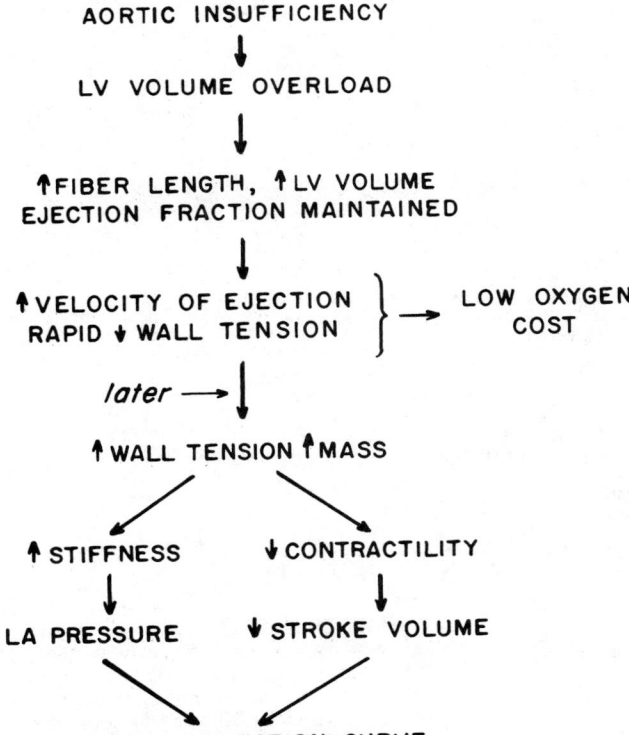

TABLE 35-7. Acute Versus Chronic Aortic Insufficiency

	CHRONIC	ACUTE
LV size	↑	—
LV compliance	↑	—
LVEDP	—	↑
Effective cardiac output	NORMAL	↓
Systemic Vascular Resistance	—	↑
Pulmonary edema	NO	YES
Pulse pressure	↑	↑/—
Heart rate	—	↑

times the normal cardiac output, $M\dot{V}O_2$ does not increase extraordinarily, since the oxygen cost for muscle shortening is quite low. The contractile state of the myocardium is often difficult to discern from clinical signs and symptoms. Ventricular afterload is chronically reduced because of the low diastolic pressure reflecting continuing diastolic run-off as well as a moderately vasodilated state. This will allow patients to be relatively symptom free even in the presence of reduced contractility.[82] This is important in terms of preparing the anesthetic, but perhaps even more so with respect to timing of aortic valve replacement. Ideally, the valve should be replaced just prior to the onset of irreversible myocardial damage. Therefore, continued follow-up of these patients emphasizes repeated noninvasive measurements of contractility, usually after some form of afterload stress, either pharmacologic or exercise induced.

In contrast to chronic AI, acute aortic insufficiency subjects a ventricle with normal diastolic function to sudden volume overload. The chamber is now on the steep portion of the normal pressure volume relationship (see Fig. 35-8). Left ventricular end diastolic pressure increases to alarming levels, and poor myocardial contractility becomes evident. Compensatory mechanisms include tachycardia and peripheral vasoconstriction, but, occasionally, hypotension and low cardiac output ensue (Table 35-7). Some patients are so acutely ill that emergency aortic valve replacement is required, whereas in less severe circumstances, mild systemic vasodilation and inotropic support can return hemodynamics toward normal.

ANESTHETIC CONSIDERATIONS. Full, mildly vasodilated and modestly tachycardic describe the optimal cardiovascular state for patients with AI (Table 35-8). Vasodilation promotes forward flow, although additional intravascular volume may be necessary to maintain preload.[83] The ideal heart rate is still somewhat controversial.[84, 85] It is likely that changes in rate

TABLE 35-8. Aortic Insufficiency—Hemodynamic Goals

P—Normal to sl ↑
A—Reduction beneficial with anesthetics or vasodilators; increases augment rugurgitant flow
C—Usually adequate
R—Modest tachycardia reduces ventricular volume, raises aortic diastolic pressure
Rhy—Usually sinus; not a problem
MVO_2—Not usually a problem
CPB—Observe for ventricular distention (↓ HR, ↑ VFP) when going onto CPB

Abbreviations are spelled out in Table 35-2 footnote.

alone will not alter net forward or regurgitant flow; they will each be proportionately reduced. Tachycardia does reduce diastolic ventricular volume and wall tension and also increases diastolic blood pressure.

Ventricular distention may occur with the onset of CPB if the heart slows or if there is unexpected ventricular fibrillation. Monitoring of the appearance of the heart, the rate and rhythm, and ventricular filling pressure if available is especially important in these patients. If distention occurs, the insertion of a left ventricular vent or the immediate application of aortic crossclamp should relieve the problem.

MITRAL STENOSIS

Stenosis of the mitral valve is usually of rheumatic origin, with clinical disease becoming manifest within 3 to 5 years following initial infection. Debilitating symptoms such as fatigue and dyspnea on exertion do not begin for another decade or two.

PATHOPHYSIOLOGY. The spectrum of physiologic disruption in patients with mitral stenosis (MS) is presented in Figure 35-12. This complicated pathophysiologic profile may be simplified by grouping the changes as either proximal or distal to the obstructing mitral valve.

In MS, unlike other valvular lesions, the LV is not subject to either pressure or volume overload. In fact, it is often relatively underloaded owing to the obstruction preventing LV filling. Although the LV may be small, ventricular function is usually maintained, although one third of patients may demonstrate contractile abnormalities by angiography, presumably as a result of rheumatic carditis or involvement of the subvalvular apparatus.[86] The diminished ventricular volume precludes effective use of vasodilators to improve LV flow.[87]

Increased left atrial pressure (LAP) and volume overload

are inevitable consequences of the narrowed mitral orifice. The relationship between LAP and the size of the valve orifice is expressed in the formula derived by Gorlin and Gorlin

$$\text{Valve area} = (\text{flow}/K) \times \text{pressure gradient}$$

where

$$\text{Flow} = \text{cardiac output}/\text{diastolic filling time,}$$
$$\text{pressure gradient} = \text{left atrial} - \text{LV end diastolic pressures,}$$
$$\text{and } K = \text{hydraulic pressure constant}$$

This calculation assumes no regurgitant flow. Assuming a constant valve area, rearranging terms and eliminating the constant provides us with a more useful expression of the clinical variables determining atrial and ventricular pressures.

$$\text{LAP} - \text{LVEDP} = (\text{cardiac output}/\text{diastolic time})^2$$

Therefore, whenever cardiac output increases or diastolic filling period decreases, the gradient across the mitral valve is altered by the square of the original changes. This explains why tachycardia or increases in forward flow, seen classically with pregnancy, thyrotoxicosis, or infection can precipitate pulmonary edema. In fact, as LAP increases, LV filling pressure may actually decrease. Therefore, the development of atrial fibrillation causes hemodynamic embarrassment, not so much because of the loss of atrial kick, but because of the rapid rate that ensues. We are left with the paradoxical situation of a patient in pulmonary edema with a relatively empty LV. The treatment in this situation is, therefore, not inotropic or vasodilator therapy but, rather, attempts to reduce the heart rate or diagnose and treat the cause responsible for the increased flow.

The pulmonary capillary wedge pressure can be used as an

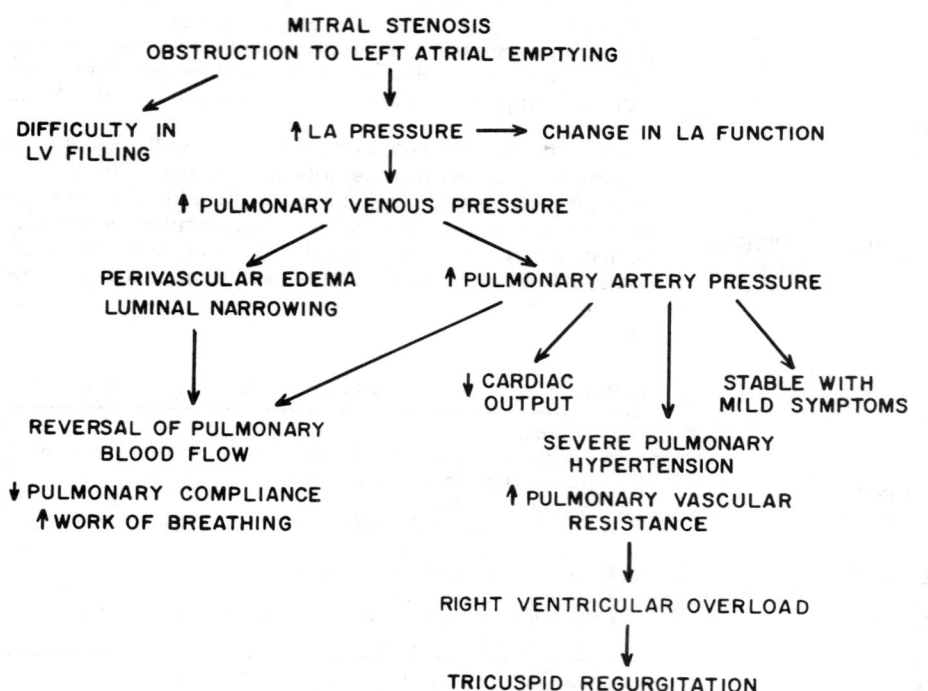

FIG. 35-12. The cardiovascular and pulmonary effects of mitral stenosis. (Reprinted with permission from Thomas SJ, Lowenstein E: Anesthetic management of the patient with valvular heart disease. Int Anesth Clin 17:67, 1979.)

index of LV filling, keeping in mind that it is higher than the true LVEDP, at least by the amount of the pressure gradient. During episodes of tachycardia or increased flow, the wedge pressure *continues* to reflect LAP; however, this is no longer indicative of LV filling pressure.

Persistent elevations in LAP are reflected back through the pulmonary circulation leading to right ventricular (RV) pressure overload with compensatory RV hypertrophy and strain. The progression and severity of pulmonary hypertension are variable and reflect further narrowing of the valve orifice and irreversible reactive changes in the pulmonary vasculature. Right ventricular dysfunction may develop in response to the afterload stress. Tricuspid annular dilatation and insufficiency may climax this hemodynamic nightmare.

Chronically elevated LAP causes perivascular edema in the lung, increased vascular pressure in the dependent portions of the lung, redistribution of blood to the upper lung fields, and a somewhat increased work of breathing.

ANESTHETIC CONSIDERATIONS. Prevention is the cornerstone of prebypass anesthetic management (Table 35-9), because treatment of hemodynamic derangements is sometimes difficult. Avoiding tachycardia precludes episodes of left atrial and pulmonary hypertension with potential RV dysfunction as well as inadequate LV filling with concomitant systemic hypotension. Preoperative maintenance of digitalis and beta-blocking drugs, selection of anesthetics with no propensity to increase heart rate, and attainment of anesthetic levels deep enough to suppress autonomic responses are methods to achieve these laudable goals. Episodes of pulmonary hypertension and potential right heart failure stemming from pulmonary vasoconstriction must also be prevented. Hypoxia, hypercarbia, and acidosis are the classic offenders; follow the ancient internist's classic nostrum and avoid them.

Treatment of hypotension in patients with MS can present a challenging dilemma. Although these patients normally take diuretics, hypovolemia is not usually the cause, and response to volume administration is often disappointing. Use of a vasoconstrictor to offset mild peripheral vasodilation is acceptable, bearing in mind the risk of pulmonary vasoconstriction and possible accentuation of RV dysfunction. It is often prudent to select a drug with some inotropic effect such as ephedrine or epinephrine, rather than rely on a pure vasoconstrictor.

In separating from CPB, although much is made of RV failure (discussed subsequently), more commonly it is the LV that is dysfunctional. This may be due to intraoperative injury or sudden increase in flow to and distention of the chronically underloaded LV. After bypass, prominent "V" waves may be present in the LAP curve. This almost always reflects in-

creased left atrial filling from the right side rather than mitral regurgitation, since cardiac output is increased after bypass when compared with preinduction values.[88]

MITRAL REGURGITATION

Mitral valve prolapse, chronic ischemic heart disease, endocarditis, and annular dilation are causes of mitral regurgitation (MR). Emergency surgery is sometimes required in patients suffering with chordal rupture and/or papillary muscle dysfunction, acute complications of myocardial infarction.

PATHOPHYSIOLOGY. Chronic volume overload similar to that described with AI, is the cardinal feature of MR. Atrial and ventricular chamber enlargement, ventricular wall hypertrophy, and increased blood volume are the compensatory responses. The volume of regurgitant flow is related to the size of the regurgitant orifice, the time available for retrograde flow, and the pressure gradient across the valve.[89] Regurgitant orifice size, in turn, is dependent upon ventricular size. Therefore, both increases in heart rate and preload reduction decrease the amount of regurgitant flow by diminishing ventricular volume.[89] Arteriolar dilators, in contrast, are effective by reducing the ventriculoatrial pressure gradient.[90]

Other similarities to AI include increases in ventricular chamber compliance and difficulty in evaluating LV contractile function. The latter is particularly troublesome, since, in MR, the LV is maximally unloaded. The incompetent valve acts as a low pressure vent for LV ejection. There is no period of isovolumic contraction, since blood is immediately ejected retrograde with the onset of ventricular systole. This explains why many patients have minimal symptoms despite progressive myocardial damage. This also explains why ejection fraction, a measure heavily afterload-dependent, can be misleading in patients with MR. Normal or minimally reduced ejection fractions (EFs) can be present even with severe impairment of contractile function.[67] Repairing or replacing the valve increases afterload, and often the dysfunctional myocardium becomes apparent. Administration of inotropes and/or vasodilators may be necessary to successfully separate from bypass.

When MR is of acute onset, the hemodynamic picture is quite different. Volume overload of the left atrium and ventricle occur in the absence of compensatory ventricular enlargement. Ventricular filling pressures increase dramatically as do pulmonary pressures. Cardiac output decreases, and pulmonary edema develops. If this occurs in the setting of acute myocardial infarction, cardiac performance may be inadequate despite pharmacologic support. Intraaortic balloon assistance as well as emergency surgery may be life saving.

ANESTHETIC CONSIDERATIONS. Selection of anesthetics that promote vasodilation and tachycardia are ideal with the patient with MR (Table 35-10). Active pharmacologic intervention is usually unnecessary, since most patients are not teetering on the brink of myocardial failure. However, in some patients, especially those with acute MR, aggressive pharmacologic management may be required. In the absence of acute deterioration, difficulties in management are usually limited to the postbypass period.

The problem of unmasking depressed myocardial contractility has already been discussed. Paradoxically, after the administration of vasodilators and inotropes, a patient will occasionally deteriorate even further. In these patients, the physiologic and clinical picture is exactly that of IHSS and is

---

TABLE 35-9.   Mitral Stenosis—Hemodynamic Goals

P—Enough to maintain flow across stenosis
A—Avoid ↑ RV afterload (pulmonary vasoconstrictors)
  ? inotropes for systemic hypotension
C—LV usually OK until after CPB; right ventricle may be impaired if there is long-standing pulmonary hypertension
R—slow to allow time for ventricular filling
Rhy—often atrial fibrillation; control ventricular response
MVO$_2$—Not a problem
CPB—Vasodilators may help post CPB RV failure; control of ventricular response may be difficult

Abbreviations are spelled out in Table 35-2 footnote.

TABLE 35-10.   Mitral Regurgitation—Hemodynamic Goals

P—Usually pretty full; may need to keep that way, although preload reduction may reduce regurgitant flow
A—Decreases are beneficial; increases augment regurgitant flow
C—Unrecognized myocardial depression possible; titrate myocardial depressants carefully
R—A faster rate decreases ventricular volume
Rhy—Atrial fibrillation is occasionally a problem
MVO_2—Only if mitral regurgitation is a complication of coronary artery disease; then be careful!!
CPB—Newly competent valve post CPB increases afterload; vasodilators may be helpful; inotropes are frequently required

Abbreviations are spelled out in Table 35-2 footnote.

seen only after valve repair, not replacement. Systolic anterior motion of the anterior mitral leaflet is demonstrable by echocardiography.[91] If this scenario is suspected, a trial of volume expansion and vasoconstrictors is indicated.

CARDIOPULMONARY BYPASS

CIRCUITS

Although there are multiple configurations used for CPB, they all incorporate essential components, including large catheters for venous drainage, an oxygenator/heat exchanger, a pump and tubing and cannula for arterial return[92] (Fig. 35-13). In many institutions, additional components are added to this elementary circuit. These include a filter on the arterial return cannula and often on the suction catheters, alarms to detect low levels of blood in the oxygenator in order to prevent pumping of air, in-line pressure and/or blood gas monitors and a separate circuit for infusion of crystalloid or blood cardioplegia. Vaporizers can be positioned in the gas inflow circuit so that volatile anesthetics can be administered during the bypass period.

Blood is drained into a reservoir from either a large single two-stage cannula (drains the right atrium and the inferior vena cava) inserted into the right atrium or from two separate smaller cannulae placed in the superior and inferior vena cavae. The rate of venous return is dependent upon intravascular volume, the height of the patient above the reservoir, and proper placement of the cannulae. Flow can be reduced by partially or completely clamping these lines either by the surgeon or the perfusionist. Additional blood is returned from the operative field using suction generated by two small roller pumps. The first is the coronary suction that scavenges blood from the operative field, the other is the vent suction used either to decompress the LV or as an additional "coronary sucker." When used to decompress the LV, this suction line is connected to either a catheter inserted across the mitral valve via the left superior pulmonary vein or to a metal or plastic tube inserted directly into the apex of LV. Many surgeons choose not to routinely vent the LV during coronary artery bypass operations.

Most commonly, oxygenated blood is returned to the patient through a cannula placed in the ascending aorta. If this proves technically difficult, if emergency cannulation is necessary, or during partial bypass for surgery on the descending thoracic aorta, the femoral artery is usually selected.

OXYGENATORS

BUBBLE. The more commonly used and somewhat less expensive bubble oxygenators utilize direct contact between fresh gas and blood to effect transfer of oxygen (O_2) and carbon dioxide (CO_2). It is far more difficult to transfer O_2 than CO_2, since the solubility ratio is 1:25. Foaming is an extremely efficient method of oxygenation and, in combination with high oxygen tensions, alleviates this problem. Gas is passed through a ceramic manifold to create bubbles small enough to provide sufficient total surface area for gas exchange but not so small to preclude easy removal. The smaller the bubbles, the greater the surface-to-volume ratio and the greater the oxygen transfer. In bubble oxygenators, CO_2 transfer is proportional to total gas flow, whereas oxygen transport is chiefly dependent upon bubble size. Gas flows do affect oxygen transport, and, at higher flows, CO_2 is sometimes added to the gas mixture in order to prevent unacceptable levels of hypocarbia. Critical to the function of the bubble oxygenator is the ability to reconstitute the perfusate ("defoaming") by passage through spongy polypropylene mesh impregnated with a charged silicon-containing polymer.[93]

Bubble oxygenators are associated with time-dependent trauma to blood because of the direct blood–gas interface. Hemolysis develops with potential capillary plugging and organ damage from red cell debris. Platelet activity is impaired secondary to platelet destruction, induction of aggregation, and adherence to parts of the oxygenator. Decreases in leukocyte counts have also been reported.[94, 95] Additional problems

CARDIOPULMONARY BYPASS CIRCUIT

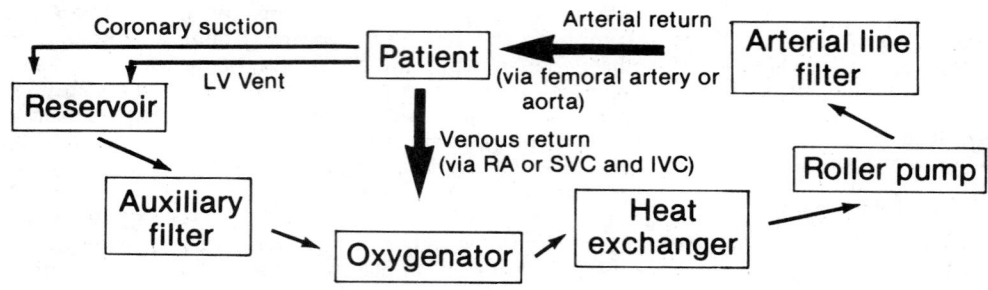

FIG. 35-13. The basic circuit for cardiopulmonary bypass. See text for details. (Reprinted with permission from Tinker JH: Cardiopulmonary bypass: Technical Aspects. In Thomas SJ [ed]: Manual Of Cardiac Anesthesia, p 375. New York, Churchill Livingstone, 1984.)

associated with bubble oxygenators include activation of complement via the alternate pathway, formation of particulate and gaseous microemboli, and denaturation of blood proteins (including those of the coagulation cascade).[96–99]

MEMBRANE. The membrane oxygenator attempts to eliminate or attenuate these problems associated with the blood–gas interface by separating the two phases by a thin silicon, Teflon, or polypropylene gas-permeable membrane.[100] Blood flows in a thin film along the membrane while gas slowly diffuses across it. The oxygen tension is controlled by the F_{IO_2} of the inspired gas, and CO_2 is regulated by total gas flow.

Studies comparing membrane with bubble oxygenators demonstrate less blood trauma with membranes and, in some cases, improved postoperative hemostasis.[101, 102] However, other investigators report that these differences are clinically insignificant as long as perfusion time is less than 2 hours.[99, 102] Differences in performance of the two types of oxygenators are also obscured by the amount of blood scavenged from the operative field, since these cells are the most severely damaged from direct mechanical trauma as well as from the turbulent blood–gas interface.[103]

PUMPS

ROLLER. Two types of pumps are used to generate the pressure required to return the perfusate to the patient (or, in the case of a membrane, to drive blood through the oxygenator and then to the patient). The first and by far the most commonly used is a roller pump. A roller pump consists of a central housing with two arms extending 180 degrees in opposite directions with smooth-faced rollers on each end. Flow is generated by compression of a heavy walled section of Silastic tubing by the rollers. Contact between one arm of the roller and the tubing begins as contact between the second roller ends, thus preventing retrograde flow. Shearing forces that would disrupt cells are minimized by ensuring that contact between the roller and tubing is nonocclusive. The roller pump head is driven by an electric motor that is designed to maintain constant speed and therefore flow despite variations in arterial inflow line resistance or power line voltage. If the motor or its power supply fails, the pump can be hand cranked in an attempt to provide adequate flow rates and systemic pressures.

CENTRIFUGAL. Centrifugal pumps are conical-shaped hardened plastic housings with rapidly rotating cones inside that impart momentum to the blood. This mechanism is pressure sensitive, and flow is determined by both inflow and outflow pressures as well as by pump head speed. An in-line electromagnetic flowmeter is necessary to indicate forward flow, since, in contrast to a roller pump, direct conversion from RPMs to flow rate is inaccurate. The maximal pressure generated with this pump is lower than that with a roller pump, and the likelihood of disconnects following inadvertent cannula obstruction is reduced. These are being used more frequently, especially for long-term mechanical ventricular support, because blood trauma is less than with a roller.

PULSATILE FLOW. Roller pumps generate a sine wave pattern of flow, which, after dampening during transit through the inflow tubing and cannulae, results in a nonpulsatile arterial pressure wave. Selection of a different pump or insertion of additional components into a circuit allows the production of a pulsatile wave form.[92] Theoretically, this sounds attractive and is intuitively more physiologic, but whether or not this is beneficial is controversial.[104–106] Pulsatile flow is thought to provide improved perfusion at the capillary level and is associated with lower systemic vascular resistance during bypass, improved oxygen extraction, and less production of pyruvate and lactate.[107–110] A decrease in the need postbypass for pharmacologic or mechanical support as well as improved mortality has also been reported. Some investigators advocate converting to pulsatile perfusion, especially in those patients with severe preoperative impairment of ventricular function.[111] After extensive review, other investigators remain unconvinced by studies that differ significantly with regard to patient populations, the type of pumps used, and the efficiency of pulse generation.[105, 112] Until noncontroversial studies demonstrate beyond doubt the superiority of pulsatile flow, the convenience and simplicity of nonpulsatility will continue to make it the overwhelming choice for routine CPB.

HEAT EXCHANGER

A heat exchanger adjusts the temperature of the perfusate to provide moderate systemic hypothermia during the period of cardiac repair. Metabolic requirements are reduced approximately 8% per °C decrease in body temperature (about 50% of normal at 28°C).[113] Deliberate hypothermia provides protection during periods of hypoperfusion and potential tissue ischemia. In addition, adequate tissue oxygenation is achieved at lower flow rates, reducing trauma to the blood. Lower systemic flow also decreases flow to the heart via noncoronary collaterals (vessels arising from pericardial reflections), diminishing the rewarming and the rate of washout of cardioplegic solution. Also, by cooling the tissues surrounding the heart, reducing the rate of cardiac rewarming, hypothermia acts as an adjunct to myocardial protection.

PRIME

The prime for most adult perfusions contains a balanced salt solution, since it resembles plasma in terms of osmolality and electrolyte composition. Individual recipes add albumin or hetastarch (increased oncotic pressure), mannitol (to promote diuresis), additional heparin, bicarbonate, calcium, and so on.[114] Blood is infrequently used except in neonates, children, and adults with significant preoperative anemia in whom profound hemodilution might decrease oxygen-carrying capacity below acceptable levels. After mixing of the patient's blood volume with the 1500 to 2500 ml (depending upon oxygenator and circuitry) prime, acute normovolemic hemodilution to hematocrits of 20 to 30% are normal. This offsets the increase in viscosity associated with systemic hypothermia.[115] An asanguineous prime is not associated with metabolic acidosis and is reported to result in improved intra- and postoperative hemostasis and renal function.[116]

ANTICOAGULATION

Prior to cannulation, systemic anticoagulation is mandatory in order to prevent catastrophic thrombus formation triggered by contact between the blood and oxygenator. Heparin, a polyanionic mucopolysaccharide extracted from bovine lung or porcine intestinal mucosa, accelerates the velocity of the reaction between antithrombin III and the activated forms of factors II, X, XI, XII, and XIII, effectively neutralizing these factors.[117] A tertiary complex is formed between heparin, antithrombin III, and these serine proteases.[118] The half-life of heparin's anticoagulant effect is approximately 90 minutes in a normothermic patient, the rate of decay decreasing with hypothermia.[119]

Anticoagulant activity varies between samples of commercially prepared heparin, as does patient response to a given dose. Patients receiving heparin in the period immediately prior to surgery and those with reduced levels of antithrombin III are notably resistant to normal pre-CPB doses.[120] It seems prudent to assess the adequacy of heparinization prior to starting CPB because of the lack of correlation between heparin dosage, blood levels, and clinical effect as well as to ensure that heparin has in fact been given and distributed. Disagreement exists as to whether this is best done by measuring heparin levels or the effect of heparin on the coagulation process. The former utilizes a manual or automated protamine titration test or other assays for heparin level; the latter utilizes a thrombin time (not usually available) or an activated clotting time (ACT). Since heparin levels do not always correlate with effect, many centers opt for the more functional test.

The ACT, introduced by Hattersley,[121] is the most commonly used test for the adequacy of anticoagulation. It is performed either manually or automatically and indicates the time required for thrombus formation, detected visually or magnetically, when blood is mixed with one of a variety of clotting accelerators. The exact ACT value necessary before initiation of CPB to ensure absolute anticoagulation remains controversial. Many use 400 seconds, a value derived from a study in primates that found no fibrin monomer, an indicator of coagulation, as long as ACT was above that level.[122]

The interpatient relationship between heparin concentration and ACT is not linear nor is the sensitivity of the ACT, that is, the change in ACT per unit increase in heparin level.[123] However, the association between the dose of heparin administered and ACT in an individual patient before CPB is somewhat linear.[124] Bull et al[124] have advocated use of such a dose–response curve to determine heparin and protamine requirements. This is often too time consuming; it also overestimates protamine needs because hemodilution and hypothermia alter intrapatient ACT sensitivity.[125] Heparin is usually given in an initial dose of 3 to 4 mg·kg^{-1}; an ACT is measured 5 minutes later, and additional heparin is given as required. The ACT should be rechecked periodically, especially if the interval following inital administration is unduly protracted,[126] or if the rewarming period on CPB is prolonged, since the rate of heparin decay increases.

MYOCARDIAL PROTECTION

A wide variety of methods are used to maintain myocardial cell integrity and energy stores while the coronary circulation is interrupted. Although techniques utilizing cold cardioplegia are the most common, other techniques used include hypothermic fibrillation[127, 128] and intermittent cross-clamping interspersed with periods of reperfusion.[129] The two critical elements with respect to cardioplegia are hypothermia (10–15°C) and hyperkalemia to ensure diastolic electrical arrest. Individual formulas add a variety of other ingredients, including, but not limited to, glucose as an energy substrate, buffering agents, albumin or mannitol for osmotic activity, citrate to reduce the calcium concentration, and nitroglycerin to improve distribution of the cardioplegic mixture. This solution is mixed with either crystalloid or oxygenated blood and is infused into the aortic root after the crossclamp is applied. The cardioplegia may be injected by way of a separate circuit on the bypass machine or manually, using a pneumatic infusion device. Direct injection into the aortic root is not feasible in patients with AI. Here, the aorta must be opened and the cardioplegia injected directly into the coronary ostia with small perfusion cannulae. In patients with severe coronary ostial stenosis or multiple severe lesions preventing adequate distribution, cardioplegia may be injected retrograde via the coronary sinus.[130–132] During the period of cardioplegic arrest, the anesthesiologist should monitor the ECG for return of electrical activity, the wedge pressure and/or the appearance of the heart for evidence of ventricular distention, and the operative field for return of contraction. The atria are often first to show return of contractile activity. Depending upon the duration of ischemia necessary, periodic reinjection may be necessary to maintain hypothermia and diastolic arrest and to wash out metabolic products. The variations of cardioplegic recipes and techniques are staggering. Several recent reviews discuss the physiologic and technologic details of cardioplegia; the interested reader is urged to consult them.[133–137]

PREOPERATIVE EVALUATION

The preoperative visit appropriately concentrates upon the cardiovascular system but should also focus on the assessment of pulmonary, renal, endocrine, and hematologic function. Equally important is a discussion with the patient of the projected events on the day of surgery, including transport to the operating room, preoperative routines (O$_2$ mask, vascular cannulation, anesthetic induction), and, finally, the awakening process in the recovery room or intensive care unit. The importance of communicating to the anesthesiologist any symptoms such as chest pain, shortness of breath, or the need for nitroglycerin during transport or the preinduction period should be stressed. The depth and detail of the explanation depends upon the patient's emotional state and "desire to know."

Data from the history, physical examination, and laboratory investigations are used to delineate cardiovascular anatomy and functional state. Of critical importance is the assessment of severity of LV or RV failure. Pertinent findings suggestive of dysfunction are described in Table 35-11. Increases in the severity or frequency of anginal attacks or the presence of ischemia-induced ventricular dysfunction suggest that there are large areas of myocardium at risk. Integration of this information leads to appropriate selection of monitoring devices and anesthetic techniques.

Conditions commonly associated with heart disease such as hypertension, diabetes mellitus, and cigarette smoking must also be evaluated. The last is extremely important and may be useful in differentiating whether episodes of intraoperative pulmonary hypertension are due primarily to pulmonary or cardiac factors. Higher systemic arterial pressures may be desirable throughout surgery in patients with a history or other evidence of carotid artery disease.[138] Evidence for renal dysfunction must be sought, since the most common cause of postoperative renal failure is pre-existing renal insufficiency.[139] If renal reserve is reduced, intraoperative measures such as diuretics or the use of dopamine may be used, although data showing an improved outcome are still not available.

TABLE 35-11. Preoperative Findings Suggestive of
Ventricular Dysfunction

History
History of MI, intermittent or chronic CHF
Symptoms of CHF: fatigue, DOE, orthopnea, PND, ankle swelling

Physical Examination
Hypotension/tachycardia (severe CHF).
Prominent neck veins, laterally displaced apical impulse, S_3, S_4,
rales, pitting edema, pulsatile liver, ascites (tricuspid regurgitation)

Electrocardiogram
Ischemia/infarction, rhythm, or conduction abnormalities

Chest X-ray
Cardiomegaly, pulmonary vascular congestion/pulmonary edema,
pleural effusion, Kerley B lines

Cardiac Testing
Cath data—LVEDP > 18, EF < 0.4, CI < 2.0 $l \cdot min^{-1} \cdot m^{-2}$
Echocardiography—low EF, multiple regional wall motion abnor-
malities
Ventriculography—low EF, multiple areas of hypo-, a-, or dyskin-
esis.

MI = myocardial infarction; CHF = congestive heart failure;
DOE = dyspnea on exertion; PND = paroxysmal nocturnal dyspnea;
LVEDP = left ventricular end diastolic pressure; EF = ejection frac-
tion; CI = cardiac index

CURRENT DRUG THERAPY

Almost without exception, cardiovascular drugs, including
cardiac antidysrhythmics, beta or calcium channel blockers,
and nitrates are continued until the time of surgery. Interactions between these drugs and anesthetics are rarely detrimental,[140] rather, they are more often beneficial in maintaining hemodynamic control during periods of surgical stress.[45]

The beta-blocking drugs are similar in structure and physiologic effect and differ chiefly in mode of excretion and
therefore in duration of action.[141] Despite the known washout of these drugs during CPB, the very long-acting drugs
(*e.g.*, nadolol) may have persistent effects (either beneficial or
detrimental) in the postbypass period. The calcium entry
blockers have shorter elimination half-lives and somewhat
different pharmacologic actions.[142] Concern about intraoperative hypotension and increased requirement for vasopressor support seems unwarranted.[143] Studies are needed to
assess whether intraoperative administration might be beneficial in terms of reduction of postbypass ischemic episodes
resulting from coronary vasospasm.

Digoxin is prescribed to suppress cardiac dysrhythmias,
control the ventricular response to atrial fibrillation, and improve contractility in patients with congestive heart failure.
The efficacy of this last indication is sometimes difficult to
discern clinically, so that discontinuation of digoxin in order
to avoid digitoxic dysrhythmias seems appropriate. However, in those patients in whom it is being used for rate or
rhythm control, continuation until the time of surgery seems
advisable. Signs or symptoms of digoxin excess, including
ventricular ectopy, atrial tachydysrhythmias, and variable
degrees of atrioventricular (AV) block, should be sought. The
latter is typically manifested by slowing and regularization
of the ventricular response to AF. This represents digoxin-

induced AV blockade with a regular junctional escape
rhythm. Noncardiac symptoms include gastrointestinal distress or visual disturbances. Toxicity is more common in patients concomitantly receiving drugs that increase digoxin
levels (*e.g.*, nifedipine, verapamil, amiodarone) or reduce
potassium levels (*e.g.*, diuretics).

Most cardiac antidysrhythmics should also be continued
to the time of surgery. Their pharamacology is well known
(Chapters 7 and 22), and they usually present little problem
with anesthetic management. A newly available antidysrhythmic, amiodarone, is a notable exception.[144] This drug is
a myocardial depressant with a half-life of 30 days. It can
cause atropine-resistant bradycardia, severe hypotension,
and AV blockade. Discontinuing it the night before surgery is
obviously useless in terms of ameliorating possible side-
effects. Rather, suitable preparations for pacing and cardioactive support should be readily available.

PHYSICAL EXAMINATION

As mentioned previously, the physical examination seeks to
elicit signs of cardiac decompensation such as an S_3 gallop,
jugular venous distention, or pulsatile liver. Routes for vascular access should be assessed, and the status of peripheral
arteries should be evaluated. As always, the airway should be
carefully evaluated with respect to ease of mask ventilation
and intubation of the trachea. Other pertinent points are
described in Table 35-12.

PREMEDICATION

Even the most thorough preoperative psychological preparation is often inadequate to assuage the anxieties and appre-
hensions of a patient facing cardiac surgery. Premedication
will assist in providing a calm, anxiety-free but arousable and
hemodynamically stable patient prepared, if not exactly enthusiastic, for surgery. Selection of drug and dosage is predicated upon the patient's age, cardiovascular state, and level
of anxiety. Heavy premedication is ideal for the fit person
scheduled for coronary artery bypass grafting. Inadequate
sedation may predispose to hypertension, tachycardia, or
coronary vasospasm, all potential causes of myocardial ischemia. The frail, 50-kg cachectic patient with severe valvular
dysfunction fares better with light premedication in order to
avoid possible respiratory depression or loss of endogenous
catecholamine support. Additional sedation can always be
given in the operating room.

Premedication for cardiac surgery often combines the sedative and analgesic properties of an opioid (morphine, 0.1 to
0.2 $mg \cdot kg^{-1}$) with the sedative and amnestic properties of
scopolamine (0.006 $mg \cdot kg^{-1}$) or a benzodiazepine (diazepam,
0.05 to 0.1 $mg \cdot kg^{-1}$, midazolam, 0.07 to 0.1 $mg \cdot kg^{-1}$, or
lorazepam, 0.05 to 0.07 $mg \cdot kg^{-1}$). The possibility of oversedation, hypercarbia, or hypoxia following premedication is
always of concern. However, Hensley *et al*[145] have shown that
morphine and scopolamine when administered in standard
doses do not produce hypoxia. Rather, if hypoxia does occur
after this combination, it is secondary to the additional supplementation administered in the operating room.[145]

The choice of premedication may also affect the hemodynamic response to anesthetics. Thomson *et al*[146] administered a standard high-dose fentanyl anesthetic to patients
premedicated with either morphine and scopolamine or lorazepam. In general, the patients receiving lorazepam were

TABLE 35-12. Preoperative Physical Examination

Vital Signs
Current values and range while hospitalized

Height, Weight
For calculation of drug dosages and pump flows

Airway
Anatomic features that could make mask ventilation or intubation
  difficult

Neck
Jugular venous distension (CHF)
Carotid bruit (cerebrovascular disease)
Landmarks for jugular vein cannulation

Heart
Murmurs characteristic of valve lesions
S_3 (increased LVEDP)
S_4 (decreased compliance)
Click (MVP) or rub (pericarditis)
Lateral PMI displacement (cardiomegaly)
Precordial heave, lift (hypertrophy, wall motion abnormality)

Lungs
Rales (CHF)
Rhonchi, wheezes (COPD)

Vasculature
Sites for venous and arterial access
Peripheral pulses

Abdomen
Pulsatile liver (CHF, tricuspid regurgitation)

Extremities
Peripheral edema (CHF)

Nervous System
Motor or sensory deficits

CHF = congestive heart failure; LVEDP = left ventricular end
diastolic pressure; MVP = mitral valve prolapse; PMI = point of
maximal impulse; COPD = chronic obstructive pulmonary disease

hemodynamically less responsive in that they had less hypertension, more hypotension, and a greater requirement for vasoactive drugs. This suggests that premedication may have a previously unappreciated but profound effect on intraoperative hemodynamics.

MONITORING

We will emphasize only those aspects of monitoring particularly relevant to cardiac surgery. The subject is discussed extensively in Chapter 21, and we have already reviewed techniques for identification of myocardial ischemia.

Pulse Oximeter

The need for multiple vascular cannulations and applications of numerous monitoring devices often prolongs the pre-induction period. The pulse oximeter should be positioned prior to catheter insertion in order to detect clinically unsuspected episodes of hypoxemia, especially if additional intravenous (iv) sedation has been administered. Attention must be focused on the entire patient, even during the exciting thrill and hunt for successful vascular access.

Electrocardiogram

Simultaneous observation of both a precordial lead V_5 and an inferior lead II for the presence of ischemia has been emphasized. If the standard leads prove inadequate for cardiac dysrhythmia detection and analysis, esophageal or epicardial leads may be used. Atrial activity can be amplified by recording bipolar atrial ECGs from two atrial epicardial pacing electrodes. These may prove invaluable in diagnosing supraventricular dysrhythmias after bypass or in the postoperative period.[147] Occasionally, intraoperative myocardial injury causes substantial reductions in QRS voltage. Monitoring an ECG via a surgically placed ventricular pacing wire will provide adequate voltage to facilitate dysrhythmia analysis or to trigger an intraaortic balloon pump, if this be necessary. A strip-chart recorder documents and facilitates detailed analysis of both ST-segment alterations and complex dysrhythmias.

Temperature

Central temperature can be measured with esophageal, tympanic, or Foley catheter probes or with a thermistor from a pulmonary artery catheter. Obviously, this last method is not reliable during the period of aortic cross-clamping when there is no flow through the heart. Rectal and toe probes record peripheral temperatures that lag behind central measurements during both cooling and rewarming.[148]

Arterial Blood Pressure

Systemic arterial pressure is always monitored invasively. The radial or femoral artery is usually cannulated, although the brachial and axillary arteries may also be used. The exact site is often the matter of personal or institutional preference. Criteria include convenience, selection of the fullest or most bounding pulse, or avoidance of the dominant hand. In addition, during dissection of the internal mammary artery (IMA), the ipsilateral pulse is often transiently occluded, so the radial artery opposite a planned IMA is selected.[149] Occasionally, the site of surgery dictates appropriate placement; for example, the right radial artery should be used for any procedure involving the descending thoracic aorta, since the left subclavian artery may be included in the proximal aortic clamp. Following cardiopulmonary bypass, radial artery pressure is often misleading and may be as much as 30 mm Hg lower than central aortic pressure.[150] The mechanism is thought to be peripheral vasodilation during rewarming.[151] Whenever such a discrepancy is suspected, aortic pressure can be estimated by palpation by the surgeon or, if direct measurement is needed, a needle may be placed directly into the aorta. The gradient between aortic and radial pressure usually disappears within 45 minutes of separation from bypass.

Central Venous Pressure/Pulmonary Artery Catheter

Access to the central circulation is mandatory for infusion of cardioactive drugs. In addition, right atrial or central venous pressure (CVP) accurately reflects RV filling pressure and is of critical importance whenever RV dysfunction is suspected. In patients with unimpaired LV function, transduced right atrial pressure is often assumed to be a reliable guide of left-sided filling.[152] This relationship is less predictable in the presence of severe LV dysynergy, pulmonary hypertension, or reduced LV compliance. In these instances, insertion of a pulmonary artery (PA) catheter and measurement of pulmonary capillary wedge pressure (PCWP) provides a more precise index of LV filling. In addition, determination of cardiac output and calculation of derived hemodynamic indices offer additional information to guide hemodynamic and anesthetic management.

Indications for PA catheterization vary greatly among institutions. In some, they are used routinely, whereas in others, they are limited to patients with specific disease states such as severe LV dysfunction or pronounced pulmonary hypertension. Additional indications include combined procedures (valvular plus coronary) or those that require prolonged time for dissection (cardiac reoperations or use of one or both IMAs). Insertion of a pacing PA catheter can be very helpful whenever exact control of rate and rhythm is desirable, for example, during IHSS or significant bradycardia secondary to beta blockade.[153]

When pulmonary artery catheters are used, disagreement still exists as to whether they should be placed before or after the induction of anesthesia.[154, 155] In some patients, early insertion of the catheter and determination of baseline hemodynamic values can beneficially influence anesthetic selection and guide the induction sequence. However, the anxious uncomfortable hypertensive patient is better served by a smooth induction of anesthesia followed by catheter placement. Incremental sedation followed by preinduction placement is a suitable alternative associated with minimal, if any, hemodynamic change.[155]

It must be remembered that the catheter often migrates toward the periphery of the lung with cardiac manipulation before and during CPB.[156] Therefore, it seems wise to pull the catheter back a few centimeters prior to the initiation of bypass in order to prevent permanent wedging.

Despite the controversy concerning the routine use of these catheters, there is no disagreement that the capability to measure both cardiac output and VFPs must be available in any institution performing cardiac surgery. Whether this is done with a PA catheter or with direct cannulation of the left atrium and dye dilution techniques is immaterial. The critically ill patient requires these measurements in order to determine the effectiveness of vasoactive drugs, to adjust dosage, and to evaluate the need for further pharmacologic or mechanical intervention.

Echocardiography

Two-dimensional transesophageal echocardiography (2DTEE) is the newest, most complex, and most expensive diagnostic device. Its role in cardiac anesthesia is still evolving. Detection of ischemia by on-line evaluation of new regional wall motion abnormalities has been mentioned. Other applications specific to cardiac surgical patients may prove even more useful. It is well known that following CPB VFP, irrespective of site of measurement (LVEDP, left atrium [LA], PCWP), is a poor and often misleading indicator of ventricular volume status.[157–159] Direct estimation of LV volume with 2DTEE may more appropriately direct fluid infusion and selection of vasoactive drugs in patients who are difficult to wean from bypass. In addition, residual valve lesions, intracardiac air, or new areas of ischemia are readily identified. Global dysfunction suggesting residual crossclamp effect, inadequate cardioplegia, or reperfusion injury can be detected. 2DTEE has already proved invaluable in detecting residual valvular insufficiency following mitral valve repair.[160]

Central Nervous System Function

Monitoring the brain during extracorporeal bypass is still in its infancy and not yet universally used. Studies correlating postoperative neurologic or psychological outcome with changes in intraoperative "neurodynamics" have not yet been performed. In addition, definition of "normal" changes related to hemodilution or hypothermia is needed before recommendations for interventions based on central nervous system (CNS) measurements can be made. The electroencephalogram (EEG) has demonstrated global cerebral ischemia when perfusion pressure was reduced in order to facilitate surgical exposure.[161] A three-lead EEG was used to assess the adequacy of CNS depression in patients given thiopental to reduce CNS damage after CPB.[162] Here, the EEG was used to detect a therapeutic end point rather than for diagnosis of an intraoperative misadventure. In an attempt to prevent paraplegia, somatosensory evoked potentials have been recommended as a means of monitoring spinal cord integrity during operations on the descending thoracic aorta.[163] Once again, further studies with larger numbers of patients are required to confirm the usefulness of this technique.

SELECTION OF ANESTHETIC DRUGS

The task confronting the anesthesiologist is to render the patient undergoing cardiac surgery analgesic, amnesic, and unconscious while simultaneously suppressing the endocrine and autonomic responses to intraoperative stress. Equally important is preservation of compensatory cardiovascular mechanisms and prevention of perioperative episodes of myocardial ischemia. Although these goals are not unique to the cardiac surgical patient, they are sometimes a bit more difficult to accomplish because of the severity of ischemic and/or valvular disease. Although there tends to be institutional and personal bias with respect to choice of anesthetic (with preponderance favoring high-dose opioid techniques), there are no data that document superiority of any anesthetic for either coronary or valvular surgery.[46, 164–167] As was previously emphasized, the most critical factor governing anesthetic selection is the degree of ventricular dysfunction. Anticipated difficulties during the tracheal intubation sequence, the expected length of surgery, and the anticipated time until extubation of the trachea also influence choice of anesthetic. It is desirable to be able to alter anesthetic depth in order to accommodate the varying intensity of surgical stress. During intubation of the trachea, incision, sternotomy, pericardiotomy, and manipulation of the aorta, there is intense stimulation, and prebypass episodes of ischemia are most likely to follow these events. The period of prepping and draping following intubation of the trachea requires minimal levels of anesthetic, as does the period of hypothermic bypass.

There is no one "best technique." Familiarity with all anesthetics and their physiologic and pharmacologic effects in the patient with severe cardiac disease allows great flexibility in anesthetic selection. In addition, it provides numerous options applicable to the cardiac patient undergoing noncardiac surgery.

Potent Inhalation Anesthetics

These drugs are useful both as primary anesthetic drugs and as adjuvants to treat or prevent "breakthrough" hypertension associated with high-dose opioid techniques.[168–170] The balance of myocardial oxygen supply and MVO_2 is usually altered favorably by reduction in contractility and afterload. Deleterious declines in perfusion must be prevented or treated, and the possibilities of increases in wall tension must be considered. The potential for intracoronary steal has been mentioned previously. These agents have been used successfully in all types of valve surgery without untoward effects, although they are sometimes associated with more hemodynamic variability than is seen with opioids.[88, 171] Use of these drugs involves no more hemodynamic intervention than upfront loading with opioids,[172] and the ability to rapidly increase and decrease concentrations permits easy adjustment to variable levels of surgical stimulation. Volatile anesthetics can be administered during bypass through a vaporizer mounted on the pump; they are also appropriate in the postbypass period assuming that cardiac function is adequate.

Opioids

The opioids lack negative inotropic effects in the doses used clinically and have thus found widespread use as the primary agent for cardiac surgery.[44] This era began in 1969 when high doses of morphine were used to anesthetize patients for aortic valve replacement.[173] However, hypotension, histamine release,[174] increased fluid requirements,[175] and, often, inadequate anesthesia resulted in a decline in the use of morphine in favor of the newer synthetic fentanyl derivatives. Aside from bradycardia, fentanyl and its analogs are relatively devoid of cardiovascular effects and have proved to be effective anesthetics. As a primary anesthetic agent, fentanyl (50 to 100 $\mu g \cdot kg^{-1}$) or sufentanil (10 to 20 $\mu g \cdot kg^{-1}$) and oxygen provide hemodynamic stability, although they do not consistently prevent a hypertensive response to periods of increased surgical stimulation.[176–178] In patients with good ventricular function, although large doses of opioids produce unconsciousness and characteristic EEG slowing, patient recall of intraoperative events remains a potential problem.[47, 48] Adjuvant agents are frequently used to supplement the opioids—benzodiazepines to provide amnesia, and volatile anesthetics or vasodilators to control hypertension. Superiority of any one opioid has not been demonstrated for either coronary or valvular surgery.[46, 167, 179] The use of high-dose opioids prolongs the time until emergence and extubation when compared with techniques primarily based on volatile anesthetics. This is usually inconsequential for cardiac surgical patients, since mechanical ventilation of the lungs is continued for variable periods of time postoperatively. Sufentanil has been reported to result in earlier emergence and extubation of the trachea than either morphine or fentanyl.[180] Alfentanil, with an elimination half-life shorter than that of fentanyl or sufentanil is suitable for infusion techniques and may provide optimal conditions for early extubation of the trachea.[181] Combinations of the fentanyl-type drugs and benzodiazepines, whether given concomitantly or as premedication, result in hypotension secondary to a fall in systemic vascular resistance (SVR).[182, 183] The use of any opioid in high doses can produce excessive bradycardia. Vecuronium or atracurium may magnify this problem,[184] whereas pancuronium is often useful in preventing it. Abdominal and chest wall rigidity commonly occur with high-dose opioids and can be severe enough to render ventilation impossible. A small dose of nondepolarizing muscle relaxant should be given prior to opioid administration.[185]

Nitrous Oxide

In many centers, nitrous oxide is not used at all during cardiac surgery. In addition to the metabolic effects recently emphasized,[186] increases in pulmonary vascular resistance (PVR) have been demonstrated with the greatest response in patients with pre-existing pulmonary hypertension.[187, 188] The drug is also a mild myocardial depressant and elicits a compensatory sympathetically mediated increase in SVR.[164] These minimal changes may not be well tolerated in patients with minimal cardiovascular reserve. It has been reported that nitrous oxide produces coronary ischemia in a dog model of coronary stenosis,[189] but this has yet to be confirmed in clinical studies.[190] In addition, it is well known that nitrous oxide increases the size of any air-filled cavity. The possibility of expansion of air introduced into the circulation either before or during bypass should preclude its use immediately before, during, or immediately after bypass.

Induction Drugs

The benzodiazepines, the barbiturates, and etomidate can be used as supplements to either inhalation or opioid anesthetics and, more importantly, are excellent as sole induction drugs in patients with cardiac disease.[191, 192] Obviously, dosage requirements must be altered to fit the clinical situation, but these are excellent drugs with which to begin an anesthetic.

Neuromuscular Blocking Drugs

Muscle relaxants are usually part of an anesthetic plan for cardiac surgery. Although not essential to surgical exposure of the heart, muscle paralysis facilitates intubation of the trachea, prevents shivering, and attenuates skeletal muscle contraction during defibrillation. In addition, they are necessary to prevent or treat opioid-induced truncal rigidity. The chief criteria for selection are the hemodynamic properties associated with each relaxant,[193] the patient's myocardial function, current pharmacologic regimen, and anesthetic technique. This translates into what is a desirable heart rate and blood pressure for any particular patient.[194–197] Doxecurium and pipecuronium have not yet been released but offer the tantalizing promise of prolonged muscle relaxation without hemodynamic side-effects.[198, 199]

INTRAOPERATIVE MANAGEMENT

In this section, we describe the anesthetic management of a patient undergoing a cardiac surgical procedure from the time of arrival in the operating room until care is transferred to recovery room personnel. Since the physiologic and pharmacologic rationale for anesthetic selection has previously been discussed, this is rather a sequential description of what happens and what is required during surgery. Anticipation of needs specific to each stage of the procedure and ready availability of necessary equipment and drugs will prevent untoward hemodynamic aberrations as well as last minute scrambling and potentially avoidable delays.

Preparation

The operating room must be readied prior to arrival of the patient. Check the anesthesia machine, and have available all supplies necessary for management of a normal airway or any additional equipment if a difficult intubation of the trachea is anticipated. Anesthetic drugs, emergency drugs, and medicated infusions should be prepared and ready for use. Heparin must be drawn up prior to induction of anesthesia in the unlikely event of the need to "crash" onto bypass. All monitoring equipment should be switched on, working, and calibrated. Confirm that typed and crossmatched blood is available in the operating suite. Table 35-13 is a checklist to aid in proper preoperative preparation of the operating room.

Preinduction Period

A brief conversation outside the operating room serves to evaluate the patient's general status and level of anxiety and to assess the effectiveness of premedication. Remind the patient to inform you if chest pain, shortness of breath, or other symptoms occur. Angina should be promptly treated with oxygen, sublingual or iv nitroglycerin, additional sedation,

TABLE 35-13.   Anesthetic Preparation for Cardiac Surgery

Anesthesia Machine
Check in usual manner

Airway Management
Nasal cannula for oxygen supplementation
Laryngoscope/blades, endotracheal tubes, airways, etc
Suction apparatus
Special equipment, if difficult airway is anticipated
Inspired gas humidifier/warmer

Circulatory Access
Intravenous fluids/infusion tubing
Proper catheters for peripheral/central sites
Infusion pumps
Blood/fluid warmers

Monitoring
ECG leads, blood pressure cuff
Pulse oximeter
Esophageal stethoscope
Temperature probes (esophageal, rectal, tympanic membrane)
Central venous and/or pulmonary artery catheters
Transducers calibrated and zeroed
Strip-chart recorder
Cardiac output computer
Heparin monitoring equipment

Medications
Anesthetic and related—Opioids
                       Barbiturates, benzodiazepines
                       Neuromuscular blockers
Heparin (must be drawn up prior to starting case)
Cardioactive drugs

Syringe:	Infusion:
Atropine	Nitroglycerin/nitroprusside
Calcium Chloride	Inotrope
Nitroglycerin	
Phenylephrine or	
ephedrine or	
inotrope	

Antibiotics

Miscellaneous
Pacemaker (standard and A–V sequential)
Warming blanket
Compatible blood in operating suite

or, perhaps if related to anxiety-induced hypertension or tachycardia, the prompt induction of general anesthesia. Supplemental oxygen via nasal cannula should be given to all patients once they have been transferred to the operating table, and peripheral oxygen saturation should be monitored with a pulse oximeter during line placement. Electrocardiographic leads and blood pressure cuff are placed, and initial vital signs are recorded.

One or two large-bore iv cannulae are inserted following local anesthesia (additional routes for infusion are desirable in patients undergoing repeat cardiac surgery). In some centers, anesthesia is then induced, and, following intubation of the trachea, arterial and central venous cannulae are inserted. In most institutions, however, these additional "lines" are inserted prior to anesthesia. Pre- or postinduction insertion of central venous or PA catheters has been discussed previously. Once inserted, however, initial values for all pressures and cardiac output should be recorded, and baseline determinations of arterial blood gases, hematocrit, and ACT should be obtained.

Throughout the preinduction period, the anesthesiologist must never let preoccupation with placement of iv and pressure monitoring catheters divert his or her attention from the patient. In addition to continuously monitoring vital signs, careful observation of the patient with periodic verbal contact facilitates detection of increased anxiety, excessive response to iv sedation, and hemodynamic or ECG abnormality.

Induction and Intubation

The exact choice and sequence of drugs is a subtle combination of art and science. The dose, speed of administration, and specific agents (*e.g.*, sedative, opioid, volatile drug, muscle relaxant) selected depend primarily upon the patient's cardiovascular reserve and desired cardiovascular profile. A smooth transition from consciousness to blissful sleep is desired without untoward airway difficulties (coughing, laryngospasm) or hemodynamic responses (either hypotension—too much drug, loss of sympathetic tone, myocardial depression; or hypertension—insertion of airway, "tugging" on the jaw). A "slow cardiac induction" sometimes creates rather than alleviates these latter problems. On the other hand, a slow, awake, sedated intubation of the trachea technique may be most appropriate in a bull-necked, obese patient who appears both difficult to intubate and ventilate. These examples re-emphasize the necessity for an individual approach to each patient.

Deep planes of anesthesia, brief duration of laryngoscopy, and innumerable pharmacologic regimens have been proposed for eliminating the hypertension and tachycardia associated with intubation of the trachea (Chapter 20).[200] None is uniformly successful, and all drug interventions carry some degree of risk, small though they may be. In addition, in some patients, especially those with a slow heart rate prior to induction of anesthesia, the reflex response to intubation of the trachea is primarily vagal, and severe bradycardia and rarely sinus arrest can occur. Furthermore, recent evidence suggests that intubation of the trachea is a strong stimulus for coronary vasoconstriction irrespective of the anesthetic, since LV blood flow is dramatically altered in the absence of hemodynamic changes.[12] Therefore, the response to tracheal intubation may be varied, although it is usually short-lived. Nevertheless, evidence for persistently abnormal hemodynamics or ischemia should be sought and treated.

After documented successful intubation of the trachea, the

tube is then secured, an esophageal stethoscope is inserted, and the eyes and all pressure points are protected. The importance of frequent checks of all monitors during these busy minutes cannot be overemphasized.

Pre-incision Period

The period of time from intubation of the trachea until skin incision is one of minimal stimulation as the surgical team attends to insertion of a bladder catheter, temperature probe, positioning, prepping, and draping. Hypotension often occurs during this period regardless of the anesthetic technique used. It may be necessary to reduce anesthetic depth or alternatively support systemic pressure with a vasoconstrictor. The potential risks of vasoconstriction in patients with poor LV or RV performance must be remembered. Deeper planes of anesthesia are obviously necessary immediately prior to incision and sternotomy.

Incision to Bypass

As previously emphasized, the pre-bypass period is characterized by periods of intense surgical stimulation that may cause hypertension, tachycardia, or ischemia. Anticipating these events and deepening the anesthetic may be effective, but, often, a vasodilator or other adjuvant is required. This is particularly true in patients with good ventricular function when an opioid–oxygen technique is used.[176, 177, 201] Hypotension can occur during the less stressful moments pre-bypass, but it is more commonly associated with cardiac manipulation in preparation for and during atrial cannulation. This may interfere with venous return or produce episodic ectopic beats or sustained supraventricular dysrhythmias. Atrial fibrillation is not uncommon. Depending upon the blood pressure and heart rate response, appropriate treatment may range from nothing at all, to vasoconstrictors, to cardioversion, to rapid cannulation and institution of bypass. Maintenance of adequate intravascular volume may attenuate the extent of blood pressure fall. This is a critical time; continual observation of the surgical field is essential.

During all cardiac procedures (perhaps more so than with any other type of surgery), hemodynamic change must be immediately correlated with events in the surgical field. Retracting, lifting, and, in general, "mugging" the heart are sometimes necessary; the hemodynamic consequences are unpredictable. This is particularly true following CPB when grafts and suture lines are inspected and repaired if necessary. This is also true during reoperations, when dissection may be difficult, tedious, and time consuming and when continuous retraction of the heart is often necessary. Bleeding, sometimes unexpectedly profuse, will compound the problem. In rare cases in which a cardiac chamber is entered and bleeding is uncontrollable, heparin is administered, the femoral vessels are cannulated, and CPB is begun using coronary suction from the field as a major source of venous return. Communication between the anesthesiologist and the surgeon is necessary to keep both appraised of the situation and to ensure that the heart gets a periodic "rest."

Cardiopulmonary Bypass

After heparin has been administered, the cannulae are inserted and adequate levels of anticoagulation are checked to ensure that the patient is ready for the institution of CPB (Table 35-14). Attention is focused on adequacy of venous drainage, oxygenation, unobstructed arterial return, and pro-

TABLE 35-14.   Checklist Prior to Initiating Cardiopulmonary Bypass

Laboratory Values
    ACT or measure of adequate heparinization
    Hematocrit

Anesthesia/Machine
    Adequate anesthesia and muscle relaxants given
    Nitrous oxide off (if used)

Monitor
    Arterial pressure—initial hypotension and then return
    CVP—indication of inadequate venous drainage
    PCWP—LV distention—inadequate drainage, AI

Patient/Field
    Cannulas in place: no air locks, clamps, or kinks; no bubbles in
        arterial cannula
    Facial appearance
        Suffusion (inadequate SVC drainage)
        Unilateral blanching (innominate artery cannulation)
    Heart
        Signs of distention (especially in AI, ischemia)

Support
Usually not required

The major categories for this table and Tables 35-15 and 35-16 are organized using the mnemonic **LAMPS**.
ACT = activated clotting time; CVP = central venous pressure; PCWP = pulmonary capillary wedge pressure; LV = left ventricle; SVC = superior vena cava; AI = aortic insufficiency

vision of necessary anesthetics and muscle relaxants. Anesthetic requirements will decrease if systemic hypothermia is used.

Once full CPB is established, it is no longer necessary to continue ventilation of the lungs. There is complete agreement on this point. However, there is no such consensus about what exactly to do with the lungs during the period of bypass. Some anesthesiologists completely disconnect the patient from the anesthesia machine; others maintain the lungs slightly inflated with low levels of positive end-expiratory pressure (PEEP) using 100% oxygen or various mixtures of room air. No specific method is associated with superior postoperative pulmonary function.

During the initial minutes of bypass, systemic pressure initially drops to 30 to 40 mm Hg as pulsatile flow ceases and the effect of the dilute prime becomes apparent. Once adequate mixing is obtained, blood pressure increases to levels primarily determined by flow rate (Table 35-15). There is no consensus as to what constitutes the ideal blood pressure or flow rate during bypass for maintenance of adequate vital organ perfusion, especially of the brain. Commonly, flow rates are maintained at approximately 50 to 60 ml $\cdot$ kg^{-1}, with systemic blood pressures in the 50 to 60 mm Hg range. Alternatively, some institutions believe that lower flows are beneficial (less hematologic damage, less rewarming of the heart through noncoronary collaterals) and that the need for higher flows or pressures has not been conclusively demonstrated.[202] Some surgeons believe that a higher perfusion pressure affords better myocardial protection when surgery is performed on the cold fibrillating heart rather than with cardioplegia.[127, 128]

CENTRAL NERVOUS SYSTEM PROTECTION. Of particular concern is preservation of CNS function. The exact etiology of

TABLE 35-15. Checklist During Cardiopulmonary Bypass

Laboratory Values
  ACT or measure of adequate heparinization
  ABGs (uncorrected)—acidosis
  Hematocrit, potassium, calcium

Anesthesia/Machine
  What to do with the lungs??

Monitor
  Arterial pressure
    Hypotension
      Venous cannula—kink, malposition, clamp, air lock
      Inadequate venous return (bleeding, hypovolemia, IVC
        obstruction, table too low)
      Pump—poor occlusion, low flows
      Arterial cannula—misdirected, kinked, partially clamped,
        dissection
      Vasodilation—anesthetics, hemodilution, idiopathic
      Transducer or monitor malfunction, stopcocks the wrong
        way
    Hypertension
      Pump—↑ flow
      Arterial cannula—misdirected
      Vasoconstrict—light anesthesia, response to temperature
        changes
      Transducer or monitor malfunction
  Venous pressure—above level of atrium—obstruction to return
    LV filling pressure—LA, PCW (if available)—any elevation?
  EKG—electrical quiescence (if cardioplegia used)
  EEG
  Adequacy of perfusion?
    Flow and pressure??
    Acidosis
    Mixed venous oxygen saturation
  Urine output
  Temperature

Patient/Field
  Conduct of the operation
  Cyanosis, venous engorgement, skin temperature
  Movement
    Breathing, diaphragmatic movement (hypercarbia, light anesthe-
      sia)

Support
  Vasodilators, anesthetics, or constrictors to control blood pres-
    sure when flow is appropriate

ACT = activated clotting time; ABG = arterial blood gas; IVC =
inferior vena cava; LV = left ventricle; LA = left atrium; PCW =
pulmonary capillary wedge

---

post-CPB neurologic injury is still unclear but probably involves many factors, including age, pre-existing cerebrovascular disease, duration of CPB, hypoperfusion, and emboli. A recent review of the literature suggests that emboli are
foremost on the list, with the role of cerebral hypoperfusion
still to be determined.[203] Govier et al[204] reported preservation
of cerebral autoregulatory activity at systolic pressures above
30 mm Hg. If this is confirmed, it would make cerebral hypoperfusion secondary to hypotension a less likely cause of CNS
injury. The potential for calcium or particulate emboli during
cardiac surgery is enormous, especially during procedures
when a chamber is opened (valve replacement, aneurysmectomy).[205] This problem persists despite the use of arterial
tubing filters and meticulous maneuvers to de-air the heart.
Nussmeier et al[162] reported improved neurologic outcome
after administration of sufficient thiopental to completely
suppress the EEG in a group of patients undergoing open

ventricle procedures with normothermic bypass. The dose
required averaged 40 mg · kg^{-1} and resulted in increased inotropic requirements and a prolonged time to extubation of
the trachea.[162] Further verification of these studies is necessary to delineate cerebral perfusion during CPB and to identify therapeutic options effective in preventing cerebral dysfunction. At this time, the definition of "normal" flow rate
and pressure remains one of institutional habit and convenience.

MONITORING AND MANAGEMENT DURING BYPASS. The
common etiologies of blood pressure changes during CPB are
listed in Table 35-15. Of primary importance is continuous
observation of the surgical field and cannulae to ensure that
nothing mechanical is awry. Attention can then be directed
toward other causes of hypo- or hypertension and their appropriate treatment. Other areas that require periodic monitoring and occasional intervention during bypass are also described in Table 35-15. Maintenance of adequate depths of
anesthesia are obviously important during the bypass run,
although clinical signs are few. Anesthetic requirements are
decreased during the period of hypothermia but return toward normal when the patient is rewarmed. Continued muscle relaxation is helpful to prevent increases in oxygen consumption from shivering or massive muscle movement during defibrillation.

Another area of controversy concerns proper measurement
and interpretation of arterial P_{CO_2} and pH. Two lines of evidence now suggest that arterial P_{CO_2} should *not* be temperature corrected. Carbon dioxide, like other gases, is more
soluble at lower temperatures, and reported values after correction are often below 40 mm Hg. Under such circumstances,
CO_2 is then added to oxygenator gas mixture in order to bring
CO_2 to "normal." When this is done, Murkin et al[206] have
demonstrated that cerebral flow is dependent upon P_{CO_2} and
blood pressure but independent of cerebral metabolic rate.
Conversely, when CO_2 is uncorrected, flow and metabolism
remain linked and flow is autoregulated and, thus, pressure
independent.[206] Such cerebral overperfusion and pressure dependency seems undesirable during bypass. The other issue
concerns the optimal intracellular environment for enzyme
function, which is present when the ratio of hydrogen to hydroxyl ions remains constant. This ratio is maintained as temperature falls despite the change in pH. Therefore, it seems
wise to report arterial blood gases at 37°C, the temperature at
which they are measured, and not to correct them back to the
temperature of the perfusate.[207]

Arterial pH and mixed venous oxygen saturation are often
used to assess the adequacy of perfusion, although changes in
these values probably occur late. Urine output is also monitored, but so many variables influence this, such as arterial
and venous pressure, flow rate, temperature, and diuretic
history, that it is difficult to draw meaningful conclusions
from this measurement. In addition, postoperative renal failure develops from either aggravation of pre-existing renal
dysfunction or persistent low cardiac output following bypass. Although many institutions administer diuretics routinely, they are just as assiduously avoided elsewhere.

REWARMING. When surgical repair is nearly complete,
gradual rewarming of the patient begins. A gradient of approximately 10°C is maintained between the patient and the
perfusate in order to prevent formation of gas bubbles. Patient
awareness becomes a possibility as the anesthetic effects of
hypothermia dissipate. Volatile anesthetics are often avoided
because of residual myocardial depression present at the time

of separation from bypass. If adequate doses of anesthetics have not been given, administration during rewarming should be considered in order to prevent recall of intraoperative events. Upon completion of the surgical repair, a variety of maneuvers are performed to remove any residual air in the ventricles. The anesthesiologist is called upon to vigorously inflate the lungs in order to remove air from the pulmonary veins and aid in filling the cardiac chambers. The heart is defibrillated and allowed to beat and replace some of its oxygen debt. The field is tidied up, and preparations are made to separate from CPB.

Discontinuation of Cardiopulmonary Bypass

Prior to discontinuing CPB, the patient should be warmed, the surgical field dry, appropriate laboratory values checked, pulmonary compliance evaluated, and ventilation of the lungs begun (Table 35-16). Heart rate and rhythm should be regulated either pharmacologically or electrically with appropriate pacing. The venous cannulae are then incrementally occluded as bypass flow is slowly decreased and sufficient pump volume is transfused into the patient. During this time, cardiac function is continually evaluated from monitoring data and direct inspection of the heart; the need for vaso- or cardioactive drugs is assessed. The potential disparity, previously alluded to, between radial artery and aortic pressure must be kept in mind. Contractility, rhythm, and ventricular filling can all be estimated by careful observation of the beating heart. For example, the patient with a low blood pressure but a vigorously contracting, relatively empty ventricle suggests that volume and perhaps a vasoconstrictor are all that is needed to wean from bypass, whereas adequate blood pressure in the presence of a sluggish and overdistended heart may be treated with a vasodilator or small dose of an inotrope.

TABLE 35-16.   Checklist Prior to Separation from Cardiopulmonary Bypass

Laboratory Values
  Hematocrit, ABGs
  Potassium (? ↑ 2° cardioplegia)

Anesthesia/Machine
  Lung compliance evaluated
  Lungs ventilated (mechanical or manual)
  Vaporizers off
  Alarms on

Monitor
  Temperature (37°C nasopharyngeal, esophageal; 35°C rectal)
  ECG—rate, rhythm, ST-segment
  Monitors zeroed and recalibrated
  Arterial pressure, ventricular filling pressures
  Strip-chart recorder on (if avail)

Patient/Field
  Look at the heart, look at the heart
    Deaired—aspiration, ballotment of heart
    Contractility, size, rhythm
  LV vent out, caval snares released—grafts, suture lines, LV vent site
  No major bleeding sites

Support
  As needed

ABG = arterial blood gas; ACT = activated clotting time; LV = left ventricle

TABLE 35-17.   Etiology of Post-CPB Right or Left Ventricular Dysfunction

Ischemia
Inadequate myocardial protection
Coronary spasm
Technical difficulties
Emboli (air, thrombus, calcium)
Intraoperative infarction
Reperfusion injury

Uncorrected Structural Defects
Nongraftable vessels
Kinked or clotted grafts
Residual valve gradient
Idiopathic hypertrophic subaortic stenosis
Shunts

Excess Cardioplegia

Pre-existing Dysfunction
Cardiomyopathy

Inadequate cardiac performance must prompt a search for possible etiologies (Table 35-17); structural defects require more than mere regulation of inotropes or vasodilators. If the clinical picture is suggestive of air emboli with diffuse ST-segment elevation and a hypocontractile heart, continuous support on CPB with a high perfusion pressure and an empty ventricle is indicated.

If pharmacologic support is required, an integration of cardiac physiology (Chapter 34) and pharmacology (Chapter 7) will lead to the rational selection of an appropriate drug or drugs. Numerous algorithms are available to guide decision making; two are described in Tables 35-18 and 35-19. The first algorithm uses arterial pressure and VFP (CVP, palpation of PA pressure, direct left atrial measurement); the second algorithm adds cardiac output to the data base. After integrating

TABLE 35-18.   Diagnosis and Therapy of Cardiovascular Dysfunction (Arterial and Ventricular Filling Pressures)

BP	VFP	DIAGNOSIS	TREATMENT
NL or ↑↑	↑	Too full	Take off fluid or await surgical losses
	NL	All is well	None Wait
	↓	↑ SVR	Anesthesia Vasodilate and gently add volume
↓ or ↓↓	↑	↓↓ Contractility	CaCl₂, inotrope, vasodilator
	NL	↓ Contractility (? low volume)	CaCl₂, inotrope (volume challenge)
	↓	Hypovolemia	Transfuse
		(? right heart failure)	(Check CVP, appearance of right ventricle, inotropes, vasodilators)

(Reprinted with permission from Thomas SJ: Manual of Cardiac Anesthesia. New York, Churchill Livingstone, 1984.)
NL = normal; VFP = ventricular filling pressure; SVR = systemic vascular resistance

TABLE 35-19. Diagnosis and Therapy of Cardiovascular Dysfunction Post CPB (Cardiac Output, Systemic and Ventricular Filling Pressures)

BP	VFP	CO	DIAGNOSIS	TREATMENT
↑	↑	↑	Too full	Take off volume Vasodilators
		↓	↑ SVR ? ↓ Contractility	Slow vasodilation, then remeasure CO, inotrope if necessary
	↓	↑	Hyperdynamic	Anesthetics ? β-blockers
		↓	↑ ↑ SVR	Vasodilate, add volume
↓	↑	↑	Vasodilated Too full—High on Frank–Starling curve	Wait Vasoconstrict gently
		↓	↓ ↓ Contractility	Inotrope Vasodilator IABP LV assist
	↓	↑	↓ SVR	Vasoconstrictor
		↓	Hypovolemia (? right heart failure)	Transfuse (Diagnose, inotropes, vasodilators)

(Redrawn with permission from Thomas SJ: Manual of Cardiac Anesthesia. New York, Churchill Livingstone, 1984.)

VFP = ventricular filling pressure; CO = cardiac output; IABP = intraaortic balloon pump

available data, a diagnosis is made and appropriate treatment is begun. Continual reassessment of the situation is necessary to document the efficacy of treatment or to suggest new diagnoses and therapeutic approaches.

Our approach to patients with inadequate cardiac output is summarized in Table 35-20. Heart rate is adjusted as much as possible. Ventricular filling is then optimized by transfusing blood from the pump. It is important not to overdistend the heart by transfusing to an arbitrary level of filling pressure, since this could precipitate further myocardial dysfunction. Looking at the heart and monitoring the response to small incremental volume infusions is more appropriate. If further therapy is required and systemic pressure is adequate, an

TABLE 35-20. Improving Systemic Flow

1. Appropriate heart rate (pacing—A, V, A/V)
2. Optimize ventricular filling
3. or 4. Reduce afterload if blood pressure is acceptable (arteriolar dilators)
4. or 3. Improve contractility (inotrope)
5. Recheck adequacy of ventricular filling
6. Combination therapy
7. IABP
8. VAD

A = atrial; V = ventricular; IABP = intraaortic balloon pump; VAD = ventricular assist device

arteriolar dilator may improve forward flow. If pressure is too low, precluding use of vasodilators, an inotrope should be selected. Each inotropic drug has a distinct profile with respect to its effects on rate, contractility, systemic and PVR, and cardiac dysrhythmogenic potential. By *first* defining the hemodynamic problem and *then* deciding what needs treatment and in what order, the most suitable drug for that situation may be selected rather than always selecting the standard "institutional inotrope." If these initial therapies are insufficient to promote adequate forward flow, various combinations of drugs may be tested. If systemic perfusion is still inadequate, some form of mechanical circulatory support is required.

A therapeutic approach to RV failure is outlined in Table 35-21. When PA pressure is normal or decreased, the etiology is usually severe RV ischemia owing to intraoperative damage or to air. Initially, treatment is aimed at improving perfusion on bypass and awaiting recovery and improvement in contractility. If this does not occur, inotropic and vasodilator therapy are indicated. Patients who have RV failure secondary to high PVR are approached differently. Reduction of PVR with vasodilators such as prostaglandin E₁ (PGE₁)[208] and inotropic support are the mainstays of therapy. Overdistention of the ventricle must be assiduously avoided. Combination therapy refers to the infusion of inotropes with vasoconstrictive properties into the left side of the circulation in order to maintain systemic perfusion but avoid increasing resistance in the pulmonary circulation.[209] Persistent RV failure precluding separation from CPB may require the insertion of a RV assist device.

INTRAAORTIC BALLOON PUMP. The simplest and most readily mechanical support device is the intraaortic balloon pump (IABP). It consists of a 25-cm sausage-shaped balloon composed of nonthrombogenic polyurethane mounted on a 90-cm stiff vascular catheter. It is usually inserted into the femoral artery either percutaneously or, after surgical exposure, through a graft sutured directly to the artery and advanced so that the tip is distal to the left subclavian artery (in order to prevent emboli to the upper arterial circulation). Occasionally, peripheral vascular disease prevents passage of the balloon via the femoral artery and it must be placed into the ascending aorta.

The IABP does not pump blood. Rather, it utilizes the principle of synchronized counterpulsation to assist a beating, ejecting heart. Aortic blood volume is moved in direction "counter" to normal flow. Immediately prior to systole, the IABP deflates, "removing blood," precipitously reducing blood pressure (afterload reduction), enhancing forward

TABLE 35-21. Right Ventricular Failure

PAP	INCREASED	NORMAL OR DECREASED
Dx	? Poor right ventricular protection	Air, ischemia
Rx	Do not ↑ preload	Volume
	Inotropes	Support on CPB
	Afterload reduction (PGE₁, etc)	High perfusion pressure
	? Differential infusions	?CABG
	RVAD	

RVAD = right ventricular assist device; PAP = pulmonary artery pressure; CPB = cardiopulmonary bypass; CABG = coronary artery bypass graft

flow, and reducing M$\dot{V}O_2$. Proper timing of balloon deflation is necessary to reduce end diastolic pressure as much as possible in order to maximally offload the ventricle. This blood is then "returned" during diastole as the balloon inflates, elevating aortic diastolic blood pressure (diastolic augmentation), increasing the gradient for coronary perfusion. The indications and contraindications for IABP placement are listed in Table 35-22. The primary indications for IABP in the cardiac surgical patient are inability to separate from CPB and poor hemodynamic function following CPB despite increasing drug support. Myocardial function often improves with the IABP, and systemic perfusion and vital organ function are preserved.[210, 211] It is crucial to control heart rate and suppress atrial and ventricular dysrhythmias in order to ensure proper balloon timing. As cardiac function returns, the assist ratio is gradually weaned from every beat to every other beat and, assuming no further cardiac deterioration, finally to 1:8, and then removed.

Complications associated with the IABP are primarily related to ischemia distal to the site of balloon insertion. Direct trauma to the vessel, arterial obstruction, and thrombosis are most common, although aortic perforation and balloon rupture occur rarely.[212, 213]

VENTRICULAR ASSIST DEVICE. Infrequently (<1%), the heart is unable to meet systemic metabolic demands despite maximal pharmacologic therapy and insertion of the IABP. Under these circumstances, devices that actually pump blood and bypass either the RV or LV are required.[214] These devices are effective because the injury producing myocardial dysfunction takes place intraoperatively and, more importantly, is often reversible. Markedly impaired cardiac function after bypass is not necessarily synonymous with cell death but, rather, may represent temporary "stunning" of the myocardium.[215] Survival ranges from 20–30%, many with minimal or no decline in cardiac function.[216, 217]

Pierce[218] has summarized clinical guidelines when using ventricular support. He emphasizes the necessity for adequate monitoring of cardiac function, prompt decision making and progression of therapy, and the necessity for continuously evaluating both ventricles. Very often, mechanical support for one ventricle unmasks previously unrecognized failure in the other ventricle, necessitating additional pharmacologic or mechanical intervention. Pennington et al[219] have emphasized the importance of diagnosing and treating RV failure in patients in cardiogenic shock.

Post Cardiopulmonary Bypass

The procedure is not over when the patient is safely "off pump." Continued vigilance is mandatory during decannulation, protamine administration, "drying up," and chest closure. Anesthetics are administered when clinically indicated. Although removal of the atrial cannula may trigger cardiac dysrhythmias, they are usually transient. In fact, atrial or junctional dysrhythmias often disappear when the cannulae are out. Heparin is reversed with protamine following removal of the atrial cannulae; the arterial return remains in place for continued transfusion of pump contents. When this is completed and bleeding is controlled, the arterial cannula is removed and the chest is closed. During decannulation, the possibility exists for unexpected bleeding from the atrial or aortic suture lines, sometimes requiring rapid transfusion.

REVERSAL OF ANTICOAGULATION. Protamine, a polycationic protein derived from salmon sperm is used to neutralize heparin. The initial and total dose administered vary widely. Some use a fixed ratio of protamine to heparin; others use 2 to 4 mg · kg^{-1}; whereas still others look to automated protamine titrations to suggest the initial dose.[220] Regardless of the method selected, further requirements are assessed by repeated measures of the ACT or other clotting assay, as well as the appearance of the surgical field.

Protamine administration is associated with a broad spectrum of hemodynamic effects.[221] Idiosyncratic responses include Type I anaphylactic reactions and both immediate and delayed anaphylactoid responses. True anaphylaxis, mercifully very rare, is characterized by increased airway pressure, decreased SVR with systemic hypotension, and skin flushing.[222] An increased incidence of reactions has been reported in patients sensitized to protamine from previous cardiac catheterization,[223] hemodialysis,[224] cardiac surgery,[225] or exposure to neutral protein Hagedorn (NPH) insulin.[226] Perhaps the most devastating complication associated with protamine is sudden and profound pulmonary hypertension accompanied by an elevated CVP, a flaccid distended RV, and systemic hypotension.[227] This may occur in approximately 1% of patients and is mediated by release of thromboxane and C5a anaphylatoxin.[228] The reaction is extremely short-lived, and, although reinstitution of bypass has been reported, it is usually not necessary. Whether protamine should be administered via the right atrium, left atrium, or aorta or peripherally remains controversial.[229–231]

POST-BYPASS BLEEDING. Persistent oozing following heparin reversal is not uncommon. The usual causes include inadequate surgical hemostasis and reduced platelet count or function,[232, 233] neither of which is identified by a prolonged ACT. Insufficient doses of protamine, dilution of coagulation

---

TABLE 35-22.   Intraaortic Balloon Pump Indications and Contraindications

INDICATIONS
Complications of Myocardial Infarction
Hemodynamic—cardiogenic shock
Mechanical—mitral regurgitation, ventricular septal defect
Intractable dysrhythmias
Extension—postinfarction angina
?? limitation of infarct size

Acute Cardiac Instability
Unstable angina—preinfarction angina
PTCA misadventure
Pretransplantation
Cardiac contusion
?? septic shock

Open Heart Surgery
Separation from cardiopulmonary bypass
Right or left ventricular failure
Increasing inotropic requirement
Progressive hemodynamic deterioration

CONTRAINDICATIONS
Irreversible brain damage
Severe aortic insufficiency
Inability to insert
Irreversible cardiac disease
   (if not a candidate for transplant)

factors, and, very rarely, "heparin rebound" are also in the differential diagnosis.[234, 235] Definitive diagnosis is frequently difficult, since neither the ACT nor other readily available tests identifies the problem.

After adequate hemostasis is obtained, the chest is closed. This is occasionally associated with transient decreases in blood pressure, which usually respond to volume infusion or "tincture of time." If hypotension persists, the chest should be reopened to rule out cardiac tamponade, a kinked graft, or other serious problems.

As the surgeon completes skin closure, the anesthesiologist prepares for an orderly, unhurried transfer of the patient from the operating room to the recovery room or intensive care unit (ICU). Medicated infusions must be regulated either manually or with portable infusion pumps. Additional syringes with emergency cardiac medications and necessary equipment for airway management should be carried. Blood pressure and ECG are monitored, and adjustments of infusions are made as clinically indicated.

BRING-BACKS. Postoperative re-exploration is needed in 4–10% of cases. The indications are persistent bleeding, excessive blood loss, cardiac tamponade, and, infrequently, unexplained poor cardiac performance (rule out tamponade). Surgery is usually required within the first 24 hours but may be later in cases of delayed tamponade. The possibility of cardiac tamponade must always be included in the differential diagnosis of the postoperative "dwindles," since the classical symptoms and signs (Table 35-23) are often absent.

Cardiac tamponade exists when intrapericardial pressure, not intravascular volume and venous pressure, determines venous return.[236] The ventricle is small and underloaded despite elevations in RV and LV filling pressures. These increases occur because pressures are routinely measured using atmospheric pressure as the zero reference point. Normally, this is acceptable, since the pressure surrounding the heart is within 1 to 3 mm Hg of atmospheric. With tamponade, this pressure is increased, transmural pressure (inside minus outside) is actually decreased, and intracardiac chamber pressures are deceptively elevated. Classically, there is equilibration of diastolic pressures across the heart. Stroke volume is limited, and fixed cardiac output and blood pressure become dependent upon heart rate. Compensatory mechanisms include peripheral vasoconstriction to preserve venous return and systemic blood pressure and tachycardia. Also noteworthy is the potential for concurrent myocardial

ischemia because of the tachycardia and reduced coronary perfusion pressure.

Clinically, patients present with dyspnea, orthopnea, tachycardia, and hypotension. The intubated, sedated, mechanically ventilated patient in the recovery room following cardiac surgery may only manifest hypotension. Ventricular filling pressures are usually elevated but not consistently so. In postoperative cardiac patients, the pericardium is no longer intact, and loculated areas of clot may compress only one chamber, causing isolated increases in filling pressure. Urine output is usually diminished. Serial chest films typically show progressive mediastinal widening.

The cure for cardiac tamponade is surgical; anesthetics can only further depress cardiac function. Therefore, drugs are selected that will preserve the compensatory mechanisms sustaining forward flow. Drugs with vasodilator (either venous or arteriolar) or myocardial depressant properties should be avoided in patients with serious hemodynamic compromise; dosages of induction agents should be appropriately reduced. Ketamine, because of its sympathomimetic effects, may be helpful in preserving heart rate and blood pressure response. It is not, however, a panacea and can induce hypotension in those patients under maximal sympathetic stress. If, upon reopening the chest, there is minimal fluid or if the patient shows little improvement, a thorough search for other causes of inadequate cardiac performance such as clotted or kinked grafts, myocardial ischemia, or valve malfunction is indicated.

CONGENITAL HEART DISEASE

In contrast to the adult with acquired cardiac disease, the anesthetic management of the child with congenital heart disease focuses on understanding those factors that determine where the blood goes, how much goes where, and why. The prevention, detection, and management of myocardial ischemia, although it does occur, is not pivotal to the care of these children. Our discussion will center on classification of these lesions, their anesthetic implications, and important clinical lessons common to any child with congenital heart disease. Other sources are available for detailed analysis of individual lesions.[7, 237]

CLASSIFICATION

Development abnormalities of the heart and great vessels result in a variety of congenital anomalies—some quite complex anatomically and physiologically. The numerous anatomic combinations that occur are best understood if considered in the context of a classification system based on patterns of altered blood flow and resistances to flow (Table 35-24). Simple shunts involve shunting of blood in a left-to-right direction or right-to-left direction. Obstructive lesions introduce an impediment to flow through either the pulmonary or systemic circulation. Complex shunt lesions combine an obstructive lesion with one or more shunts.

SIMPLE SHUNTS. Interruptions in the normal barriers between the pulmonary and systemic circulations (ASD, VSD, patent ductus arteriosus [PDA]) result in simple shunts. Since pressure is higher on the left side of the orifice, blood is shunted from left to right. Pulmonary blood flow is increased, and the RV and pulmonary vasculature become pressure and/or volume overloaded, depending upon the location, size,

TABLE 35-23.   Cardiac Tamponade—Clinical Features

Dyspnea, orthopnea, tachycardia
Beck's triad
  Quiet heart
  Venous pressure
  Arterial pressure
Paradoxical pulse
Equalization of diastolic pressures
  RA = RVEDP = PAEDP = LA = LVEDP
ECG—ST-segment change, electrical alternans
Chest x-ray—silhouette nl or slightly enlarged
Echo—best diagnostic tool

RA = right atrium; RVEDP = right ventricular end diastolic pressure; PAEDP = pulmonary artery end diastolic pressure; LA = left atrium; LVEDP = left ventricular end diastolic pressure

TABLE 35-24.   Classification of Congenital Heart Defects

1. Increased pulmonary blood flow
    Atrial septal defect
    Ventricular septal defect
    Patent ductus arteriosus
    Endocardial cushion defect
    Aortopulmonary windows
2. Decreased pulmonary blood flow
    Tetralogy of Fallot
    Pulmonary atresia
    Tricuspid atresia
    Ebstein's anomaly
3. Complex shunts/mixing of pulmonary and systemic circulation
    Truncus arteriosus
    Transposition of the great arteries
    Total anomalous pulmonary venous drainage
    Common ventricle
4. Obstructive lesions
    Aortic stenosis
    Pulmonary stenosis
    Coarctation of the aorta
5. Airway obstruction
    Double aortic arch
    Anomalous pulmonary artery

and duration of the shunt. The ratio of pulmonary to systemic flow can be calculated using the Fick equation:

$$\dot{Q}_P = \frac{O_2 \text{ consumption}}{\text{Art } Sa_{O_2} - \text{PA } Sv_{O_2}}$$

$$\dot{Q}_s = \frac{O_2 \text{ consumption}}{\text{Art } Sa_{O_2} - \text{SVC } Sv_{O_2}}$$

$$\dot{Q}_P/\dot{Q}_s = \frac{\text{Art } Sa_{O_2} - \text{SVC } Sv_{O_2}}{\text{Art } Sa_{O_2} - \text{PA } Sv_{O_2}}$$

where

$\dot{Q}_P$ = pulmonary blood flow
$\dot{Q}_s$ = systemic blood flow
Sa_{O_2} = arterial oxygen saturation
Sv_{O_2} = venous oxygen saturation
SVC = superior vena cava
PA = pulmonary artery

Increased pulmonary blood flow may delay the normal decrease in PVR that occurs in the neonatal period and may eventually result in morphologic changes in the intimal and medial layers of the pulmonary vasculature.[238-240] The pulmonary hypertension produced is usually reversible with correction of the lesion but may persist after surgery if the increased pulmonary blood flow has been long-standing or very severe. Left untreated, a substantial left-to-right shunt can lead to irreversible destruction of the pulmonary vasculature with progressive reversal of the shunt to a right-to-left direction (Eisenmenger's complex). In these patients, the hemodynamic picture becomes one of inadequate pulmonary blood flow and systemic hypoxemia.

When the orifice of a simple shunt is small, the magnitude of flow across it is almost entirely dependent upon the size of the defect and relatively independent of outflow resistance. These lesions (a small ASD or VSD) are known as restrictive shunts (Table 35-25). The magnitude of shunt flow across a larger ASD or VSD (a nonrestrictive shunt) is less dependent upon orifice size and more dependent upon the relative resistances to RV and LV outflow (PVR and SVR, respectively).[241] At the extreme of this group are lesions characterized by a common chamber (single atrium, single ventricle, truncus arteriosus) in which complete mixing of arterial and venous blood occurs. Shunting in these situations is bidirectional, with the magnitude and direction of net flow entirely dependent upon relative outflow resistances. A marked increase in PVR results in net right-to-left shunting, producing arterial oxygen desaturation and cyanosis.

OBSTRUCTIVE LESIONS. Obstructive lesions include AS or aortic coarctation on the left side of the circulation, pulmonic stenosis on the right. Obstruction results in pressure overloading of the corresponding ventricle. Ventricular hypertrophy is the compensating mechanism, but the immature myocardium deals poorly with pronounced afterload stress.[242] With a purely obstructive lesion, shunting is not a part of the pathophysiologic scenario.

COMPLEX SHUNTS. Complex shunt lesions involve obstruction outflow on one side of the heart with shunting to the opposite side through an associated lesion (ASD, VSD or PDA) (Table 35-25). If partial outflow obstruction exists, the magnitude of shunt flow directed to the unobstructed circulation is somewhat dependent upon the relationship of SVR and PVR; the more severe the obstruction, the less the dependence on relative outflow resistance. With tetralogy of Fallot, for example, partial right outflow tract obstruction results in right-to-left shunting of blood through a VSD. The magnitude of shunt flow increases if PVR is increased or if SVR is allowed to fall. As right-to-left shunting increases, so does arterial oxygen desaturation. If outflow tract obstruction is complete, all blood passes through a shunt to the opposite circulation. The magnitude and direction of shunt flow is fixed. Viability of the patient depends upon the presence of a second more distally located shunt to return blood to the obstructed circulation. If tetralogy of Fallot is accompanied by pulmonary atresia, for example, there is shunting of all venous return across the VSD in a right-to-left direction. Left-to-right flow through the PDA then provides the entire pulmonary blood supply. In patients with mitral or aortic atresia, intracardiac left-to-right shunting occurs through an ASD or VSD. Right-to-left shunting via the patent ductus provides systemic flow. Prostaglandin E_1 is commonly used to maintain ductal patency in patients in whom premature closure would be life threatening.[243]

SYSTEMIC AND PULMONARY VASCULAR RESISTANCE

It is essential to understand each patient's cardiac anatomy and pattern of blood flow in order to predict the effects of SVR and PVR on hemodynamics and arterial oxygenation. When the direction and magnitude of shunt flow are dependent upon relative outflow resistances, hemodynamic management by the anesthesiologist affects the degree and direction of shunting. With simple left-to-right shunting, for example, further increases in pulmonary blood flow are avoided by preventing increases in SVR. Excessive pulmonary vasodilation can result in a marked increase in pulmonary blood flow—in extreme cases, at the expense of systemic flow.[244] This is a particular problem in the patient with

TABLE 35-25.   Classifications of Shunts

| | SIMPLE SHUNTS | | | COMPLEX SHUNTS | |
	Restrictive (small)	Nonrestrictive (large)	Common Chamber (complete mixing)	Partial Obstruction	Total Obstruction
PRESSURE GRADIENT	Large	Small	None	Orifice size and degree of obstruction	Orifice size only
DIRECTION	L→R*	L→R*	Bidirectional	Shunt flow dependent upon obstruction	Away from obstruction circulation
DEPENDENCE UPON PVR/SVR	Independent	Dependent	Totally dependent	Minimally dependent	Independent
EXAMPLES	Small ASD, VSD Blalock	Large VSD, PDA, Waterston	Single ventricle Truncus	TOF VSD with PS	Valvular atresia

(Adapted with permission from Hickey PR, Wessel DL: Anesthesia for treatment of congenital heart disease. In Kaplan JA (ed): Cardiac Anesthesia, 2nd ed. Orlando, Grune and Stratton, 1987.)

* = R→L shunt flow if severe pulmonary hypertension secondary to pulmonary vascular disease

ASD = atrial septal defect; PDA = patent ductus arteriosus; PS = pulmonary stenosis; TOF = tetralogy of Fallot; VSD = ventricular septal defect

a single ventricle, since shunt flow in these situations is bidirectional and entirely dependent upon SVR and PVR. Exacerbation of pre-existing pulmonary hypertension in patients with increased pulmonary blood flow is best prevented by avoiding maneuvers that increase PVR and utilizing for hemodynamic benefit those that decrease it (Table 35-26). Decreasing right-to-left shunting in patients with complex shunt lesions lessens arterial oxygen desaturation. Systemic vascular resistance must be maintained in these patients, because excessive hypotension will result in increased right-to-left flow. Increases in PVR promote right-to-left shunting and hypoxemia. Pulmonary vasodilation should prove beneficial. Note again that PVR/SVR effects are greater with a larger (nonrestrictive) shunt orifice.

PREOPERATIVE EVALUATION

The history and physical examination should determine the presence or absence of congestive heart failure and/or cyanosis, the most significant consequences of congenital heart disease. Pump failure may result from either pressure or volume overload of a ventricle. Due to the close association between ventricles in very young patients, univentricular failure quickly becomes biventricular.[245] The Starling curve of an infant's ventricle plateaus quickly, and heart rate becomes

the primary determinant of cardiac output. Thus, tachycardia, an important compensatory mechanism, is a common finding in children with congestive heart failure. Other findings (Table 35-27) include tachypnea, dyspnea, diaphoresis, recurrent pulmonary infections, decreased exercise tolerance, and developmental delays. Cyanosis occurs with lesions resulting in right-to-left shunting and the inevitable desaturation of arterial blood. Older children with longstanding hypoxemia may develop clubbing of the fingers and toes. Polycythemia occurs in response to systemic hypoxemia as a means of increasing oxygen-carrying capacity. Hematocrits above 60% place the child at risk for cerebral infarction or coagulation abnormalities.[246, 247]

The diagnosis of simple ASD, PDA, or coarctation is often made noninvasively. When a more complicated lesion exists, the most useful data regarding the child's anatomic diagnosis are provided by echocardiography and cardiac catheterization. Echocardiography is used to visualize misalignment of the cardiac chambers or great vessels but will not always demonstrate the presence of septal defects.[248] Cardiac catheterization remains the best available means of assessing the physiologic consequences of congenital cardiac lesions. Pressures and oxygen saturation are measured in the cardiac chambers and great vessels, and the results are used to confirm the location and direction of shunts and the presence of obstructive lesions. A step-up in oxygen saturation from the superior vena cava to the right atrium or ventricle is indicative of left-to-right shunting. Desaturation of LV or aortic blood suggests right-to-left shunting of venous blood into the sys-

TABLE 35-26.   Manipulations Altering PVR

INCREASE PVR	DECREASE PVR
Hypoxia	Oxygen
Hypercarbia	Hypocarbia
Acidosis	Alkalosis
Hyperinflation	Normal FRC
Atelectasis	Blocking sympathetic stimulation
Sympathetic stimulation	
High hematocrit	Low hematocrit
Surgical constriction	

(Reprinted with permission from Hickey PR, Wessel DL: Anesthesia for treatment of congenital heart disease. In Kaplan JA (ed): Cardiac Anesthesia, 2nd ed. Orlando, Grune and Stratton, 1987.)

TABLE 35-27.   Symptoms of Congenital Heart Disease

INFANTS	CHILDREN
Tachycardia	Tachycardia
Tachypnea	Tachypnea/dyspnea
Diaphoresis	Diaphoresis
Feeding difficulties	Poor weight gain
Failure to thrive	Repeated pulmonary infections
Pulmonary infections	Decreased exercise tolerance
Congestive heart failure	Congestive heart failure
Cyanosis	Cyanosis +/- clubbing

temic circulation. Oxygen saturations are also used to calculate relative pulmonary and systemic resistances and flows using the Fick equation.

PREMEDICATION

Premedication is selected considering the child's age, level of activity, and the severity of the lesion. Children younger than 6 months of age and those older but critically ill usually receive no preoperative sedation. Older, active children should be sedated with intramuscular opioids and/or barbiturates prior to transport to the operating room. This is especially important with lesions resulting in right-to-left shunting. Struggling and crying increase right-to-left flow and worsen hypoxemia. The goal of premedication is a hemodynamically stable child, asleep or awake but cooperative. Table 35-28 lists appropriate doses for preoperative medications in children with congenital heart disease.

PREPARATION FOR ANESTHESIA

Since hypoxemia and hypotension can occur quickly, the margin for error in managing critically ill children is slim. Preparedness is essential. The anesthesiologist must have on hand all standard equipment normally used for the pediatric patient. In addition, appropriate cardioactive drugs should be available (Table 35-29). An isoproterenol infusion should be ready in case hypotension secondary to decreased heart rate occurs or if inotropy becomes a problem. It is critical that all iv catheters, injection ports, and stopcocks be meticulously cleared of bubbles to prevent systemic embolization. Aspiration should precede injection of all iv drugs. All patients are at risk regardless of the site or direction of the shunt.

MONITORING

Standard monitoring for all pediatric patients undergoing repair of congenital cardiac lesions includes an ECG, a blood pressure cuff (usually an automated device), a pulse oximeter, and appropriate temperature probes. A precordial stethoscope is essential prior to and during induction of anesthesia and intubation of the trachea. Intraarterial blood pressure monitoring is necessary in patients requiring CPB and in

TABLE 35-28.   Premediction for Children

Anticholinergics		
Scopolamine	$0.01-0.02$ mg·kg^{-1}	IM
Atropine	$0.01-0.02$ mg·kg^{-1}	IM
Sedatives		
Diazepam	0.4 mg·kg^{-1}	IM
	$0.1-0.2$ mg·kg^{-1}	PO
Pentobarbital	$2-6$ mg·kg^{-1}	IM/PO
Diphenhydramine	$0.2-0.5$ mg·kg^{-1}	IM/PO
Hydroxyzine	$0.5-1.0$ mg·kg^{-1}	IM/PO
Midazolam	0.4 mg·kg^{-1}	IM
Analgesics		
Morphine	$0.05-0.15$ mg·kg^{-1}	IM
Meperidine	$1-2$ mg·kg^{-1}	IM

TABLE 35-29.   Commonly Used Drugs for Patients With Congenital Heart Defects

Atropine	$0.01-0.02$ mg·kg^{-1}
Bicarbonate	1 mEq·kg^{-1}
Calcium chloride	10 mg·kg^{-1}
Calcium gluconate	30 mg·kg^{-1}
Lidocaine	1 mg·kg^{-1}
Propranolol	$0.01-0.02$ mg·kg^{-1}
Verapamil	$0.125-0.25$ mg·kg^{-1}
Digoxin	20 μg·kg^{-1} premature
	40 μg·kg^{-1} infant
	20 μg·kg^{-1} child
COMMON INFUSIONS	
Lidocaine	$20-50$ μg·kg^{-1}·min^{-1}
Sodium nitroprusside	$0.5-10$ μg·kg^{-1}·min^{-1}
Prostaglandin E$_1$	0.1 μg·kg^{-1}·min^{-1}
Isuprel	$0.1-0.5$ μg·kg^{-1}·min^{-1}
Epinephrine	$0.1-1.0$ μg·kg^{-1}·min^{-1}
Dopamine	$1-20$ μg·kg^{-1}·min^{-1}
Dobutamine	$1-10$ μg·kg^{-1}·min^{-1}
Norepinephrine	$0.1-0.5$ μg·kg^{-1}·min^{-1}
Phenylephrine	$0.1-0.5$ μg·kg^{-1}·min^{-1}

those undergoing thoracotomy. A central venous catheter (CVP) is necessary when the need for pharmacologic support is anticipated or monitoring of central blood volume will aid in management of the patient. A CVP catheter can be inserted percutaneously after the patient is intubated or an intracardiac catheter can be placed later in the procedure.

ANESTHETIC SELECTION

All patients regardless of age require an anesthetic. Recent evidence documents the perception of pain in even the youngest neonate.[249, 250] As with adults, anesthetic induction and maintenance must be tailored to suit the needs of each patient, with careful regard for depressant effects on the cardiovascular system and on PVR and SVR. Most intramuscular, iv, and inhalational drugs have been used safely in anesthetizing children with congenital heart disease.

INDUCTION

The tracheas of neonates and premature infants are usually intubated awake after administration of atropine and following preoxygenation. Older children arriving with a functioning iv catheter can be induced with iv opioids, barbiturates, benzodiazepines, or ketamine. Atropine and a muscle relaxant can be given prior to intubation of the trachea. An inhalation induction with 1–2% halothane in nitrous oxide and oxygen is safe for patients without an iv provided that excessive myocardial depression is avoided. Intramuscular ketamine (5 to 10 mg·kg^{-1}) is useful in handling frightened or combative children. The drug has sympathetic stimulating properties and does not cause increases in PVR regardless of pre-existing pulmonary hypertension as long as airway patency and adequate oxygenation and ventilation of the lungs are ensured.[251] Theoretically, the speed of anesthetic induction can be affected by the presence of circulatory shunts.[252] The presence of a right-to-left shunt slows the equilibration between alveolar and arterial partial pressures, prolonging an inhalation induction. This effect is most evident when using less-soluble gases such as nitrous oxide.

The presence of concomitant left-to-right shunting attenuates this effect. In the presence of a right-to-left shunt, drugs administered iv reach the brain more quickly and in greater concentrations. Anesthetic effects appear rapidly. Pure left-to-right shunting has little effect on the speed of an inhalation induction provided that cardiac output is maintained. If output falls, as in any low output state, induction occurs more rapidly. The increased pulmonary blood flow associated with left-to-right shunts dilutes any iv agent. The initial peak concentration of the drug is decreased, and the effects are prolonged.

MAINTENANCE

Drugs to be used after induction of anesthesia and airway control are chosen considering the patient's response to the induction sequence, the current hemodynamic status, the length of the procedure, and the plans for postoperative care. High-dose opioid techniques (fentanyl 25 to 50 $\mu g \cdot kg^{-1}$ or sufentanil 5 to 15 $\mu g \cdot kg^{-1}$) provide cardiovascular and pulmonary vascular stability for major procedures involving CPB.[203, 253, 254] They may, however, be inappropriate for simpler repairs, after which early extubation is planned. For relatively healthy children with minimally affected cardiovascular reserve, use of an inhalational agent as the primary anesthetic with or without low-dose opioid supplementation is useful in achieving this goal. Volatile anesthetics may also be useful in sicker children receiving a high-dose opioid technique for controlling intraoperative hypertensive responses. It must be remembered that the immature myocardium and vascular system are very sensitive to the depressant effects of halothane, enflurane, and isoflurane.[255, 256] Hemodynamic deterioration secondary to myocardial depression is an ongoing possibility and the avoidance of the potent inhalational drugs in children with reduced cardiovascular reserve is warranted.

As it does in adults, nitrous oxide administered to children decreases cardiac output, heart rate, and systemic blood pressure.[257] Contrary to findings in adults, however, its use does not increase PVR regardless of the baseline condition of the child's pulmonary vasculature.[257] Additional nitrous oxide does not result in arterial oxygen desaturation in patients with cyanotic lesions, since, with large shunts, Pa_{O_2} becomes relatively independent of FI_{O_2}. Concern does arise over the possibility of increasing the size of systemic air emboli. These are the primary considerations in deciding whether to use or avoid using the drug.

CARDIOPULMONARY BYPASS

The techniques and basic circuit used for CPB in children are similar to those used for adults (components and primes are smaller). Some differences do exist. A sanguinous prime avoids excessive hemodilution in infants. Perfusion is regulated by pump flow and, in the very young, high flows (up to 150 to 175 $ml \cdot kg^{-1} \cdot min^{-1}$) may be required to maintain adequate perfusion. As children grow and their arterial trees mature and become less distensible, flows closer to those used for adults can be used. The presence of previous systemic to pulmonary shunts or significant bronchial collateral flow makes maintenance of adequate perfusion pressure more difficult and ligation of these shunts may be necessary prior to initiation of CPB. Adequacy of perfusion is difficult to assess in children, as in adults, but can be inferred if urine output, mixed venous oxygen saturation, and pH are all normal. The temperature gradient that exists between core and peripheral sites also serves as an indicator of the adequacy of perfusion.

DEEP HYPOTHERMIC CIRCULATORY ARREST

Profound hypothermia to 10 to 15°C with periods of circulatory arrest is used in infants weighing less than 10 kg who are undergoing repair of complex congenital lesions. Topical cooling (ice bags, cooled room temperature) is begun immediately after induction and intubation of the trachea and supplements core cooling provided by the bypass pump and maintains deep hypothermia once the bypass pump is shut off. Deep hypothermic circulatory arrest (DHCA) provides a bloodless field, shortens bypass time, and aids protection of the myocardium by preventing both washout of cardioplegia solution and rewarming of the heart by contiguous organs. Circulatory arrest times are limited by the potential for CNS damage. Detrimental effects to other vital organs are unusual. Most centers using DHCA consider 60 minutes the upper limit of safe continuous arrest.[258] If more time is required for completion of the repair, a 15-minute period of reperfusion separates two 40- to 50-minute periods of arrest.[259] Patients undergoing DHCA should have their temperature monitored at multiple sites (tympanic membrane, esophagus, rectum), since significant temperature gradients between parts of the body may exist. In an attempt to prevent rewarming of the brain during the period of arrest, uniform cooling of the entire body is the goal.[258]

SEPARATION FROM BYPASS

Separation from the bypass pump is done using information obtained from the surgical field and, if necessary, from measurement of intracardiac pressures. Weaning is not usually a problem provided that appropriate surgical correction has occurred and that adequate ventilation and oxygenation are provided. Ischemia and residual problems with contractility are uncommon in pediatric patients, although they can occur. Low cardiac output requiring pharmacologic support postbypass is unusual but is more common when a large ventriculotomy incision has been made or if long bypass or aortic crossclamp times have been used. Prolonged difficulty separating from bypass warrants a search for residual defects or signals a problem with the repair itself.

TIMING OF EXTUBATION

Extubation of the trachea in the operating or early postoperative period is appropriate for patients undergoing repair of a simple ASD, PDA, or aortic coarctation. The anesthesiologist must be certain that surgical hemostasis has been obtained, that the child is warm, that residual narcosis and paralysis are not a problem, and that spontaneous ventilation is adequate. More controversial is the timing of extubation of the trachea after correction of complex shunts. Postoperative respiratory insufficiency or failure are more likely to occur in patients in whom preoperative pulmonary blood flow was markedly increased and in those with significant pulmonary hypertension or pre-existing pulmonary infection, as well as in those born prematurely, neonates, and patients younger than 6 months of age. Postoperative respiratory support is recommended in these incidences. Nasotracheal intubation, because it better maintains endotracheal tube position, is preferred when postoperative ventilation is anticipated. Extubation can be accomplished once the normal criteria have been met.

REFERENCES

1. Keats AS: The Rovenstine Lecture, 1983: Cardiovascular anesthesia: Perceptions and perspectives. Anesthesiology 60:467, 1984
2. Branthwaite MA: Anaesthesia for Cardiac Surgery and Allied Procedures. Oxford, Blackwell Scientific, 1980
3. Kaplan JA: Cardiac Anesthesia, 2nd ed. Orlando, Grune & Stratton, 1987
4. Lake CL: Cardiovascular Anesthesia. New York, Springer-Verlag, 1985
5. Ream AK, Fogdall RP: Acute Cardiovascular Management: Anesthesia and Intensive Care. Philadelphia, J.B. Lippincott, 1982
6. Reves JG, Hall KD: Common Problems in Cardiac Anesthesia. Chicago, Year Book Medical Publishers, Inc, 1982
7. Tarhan S: Cardiovascular Anesthesia and Postoperative Care. Chicago, Year Book Medical Publishers, Inc, 1982
8. Thomas SJ: Manual of Cardiac Anesthesia. New York, Churchill Livingstone, 1984
9. Slogoff S, Keats AS: Does perioperative myocardial ischemia lead to postoperative myocardial infarction? Anesthesiology 62:107, 1985
10. Slogoff S, Keats AS: Further observations on perioperative myocardial ischemia. Anesthesiology 65:539, 1986
11. Isom OW, Spencer FC, Feigenbaum H et al: Prebypass myocardial damage in patients undergoing coronary revascularization: An unrecognized vulnerable period. Circulation 52(supp II): 119, 1975
12. Kleinman B, Henkin RE, Glisson SN et al: Qualitative evaluation of coronary flow during anesthetic induction using Thallium-201 perfusion scans. Anesthesiology 64:157, 1986
13. Buffington CW, Ivey TD: Coronary artery spasm during general anesthesia. Anesthesiology 55:466, 1981
14. Merin RG, Lowenstein E, Gelman S: Is anesthesia beneficial for the ischemic heart? III. Anesthesiology 57:461, 1985
15. Weber KT, Janicki JS: The metabolic demand and oxygen supply of the heart: Physiologic and clinical considerations. Am J Cardiol 44:722, 1979
16. Buffington CW: Impaired systolic thickening associated with halothane in the presence of a coronary stenosis is mediated by changes in hemodynamics. Anesthesiology 64:632, 1986
17. Bell JR, Fox AC: Pathogenesis of subendocardial ischemia. Am J Med Sci 268:2, 1974
18. Hoffman JIE: Transmural myocardial perfusion. Prog Cardiovasc Dis 29:429, 1987
19. Boudoulas H, Rittger SE, Lewis RP: Changes in diastolic time with various pharmacologic agents: Implication for myocardial perfusion. Circulation 60:164, 1979
20. Klocke FJ, Mates RE, Canty JM Jr et al: Coronary pressure–flow relationships. Controversial issues and probable implications. Circ Res 56:310, 1985
21. Buffington CW: Hemodynamic determinants of ischemic myocardial dysfunction in the presence of coronary stenosis in dogs. Anesthesiology 63:651, 1985
22. Feigl EO: Coronary physiology. Physiol Rev 63:1, 1983 (Review)
23. Prinzmetal M, Kennamer R, Merliss R: Angina pectoris: A variant form of angina pectoris. Am J Med 27: 375, 1959
24. Chierchia S, Brunelli C, Simonetti I et al: Sequence of events in angina at rest: Primary reduction in coronary flow. Circulation 61:759, 1980
25. Deanfield JE, Maseri A, Selwyn AP: Myocardial ischemia during daily life in patients with stable angina: Its relation to symptoms and heart rate changes. Lancet 2:753, 1983
26. Maseri A, Chierchia S: Coronary artery spasm, definition, diagnosis and consequences. Prog Cardiovasc Dis 25:169, 1982
27. McAlpin RN: Contribution of dynamic vascular wall thickening to luminal narrowing during coronary arterial constriction. Circulation 60:296, 1980
28. Freudenberg H, Lichtlen PR: The normal wall segment in coronary stenosis—A post-mortem study. Z Cardiol 70:863, 1981
29. VanHoutte PM, Houston DS: Platelets, endothelium, and vasospasm. Circulation 72:729, 1985
30. Nussmeier NA, Slogoff S: Verapamil treatment of intraoperative coronary artery spasm. Anesthesiology 62:539, 1985
31. Humphrey LS, Blanck TJJ: Intraoperative use of verapamil for nitroglycerine—refractory myocardial ischemia. Anesth Analg 64:68, 1985
32. Brown BG, Bolson EL, Dodge HJ: Dynamic mechanisms in human coronary artery stenosis. Circulation 70:917, 1984
33. Hines RL: Monitoring for right ventricular ischemia: Is it necessary? J Cardiothorac Anesth 1:95, 1987
34. Kotrly KJ, Kotter GS, Mortara D et al: Intraoperative detection of myocardial ischemia with an ST segment trend monitoring system. Anesth Analg 63:343, 1984
35. Robinson BF: Relation of heart rate and systolic blood pressure to the onset of pain in angina pectoris. Circulation 35:1073, 1967
36. Kissin I, Reves JG, Mardes M: Is the rate–pressure product a misleading guide? Anesthesiology 52:373, 1980
37. Kaplan JA, Wells PM: Early diagnosis of myocardial ischemia using the pulmonary artery catheter. Anesth Analg 60:789, 1981
38. Waller JL, Johnson SP, Kaplan JA: Usefulness of pulmonary artery catheters during aortocoronary bypass surgery. Anesth Analg 56:219, 1982
39. Smith JS, Cahalan MK, Benefiel DJ et al: Intraoperative detection of myocardial ischemia in high-risk patients: Electrocardiography vs two-dimensional transesophageal echocardiography. Circulation 72:1015, 1985
40. Moffitt EA, Sethna DH: The coronary circulation and myocardial oxygenation in coronary artery disease: Effects of anesthesia. Anesth Analg 65:395, 1986 (Review)
41. Roizen MF, Hamilton WK, Yung JS: Treatment of stress-induced increases in pulmonary wedge pressure using volatile anesthetics. Anesthesiology 55:446,1981
42. Tarnow J, Markschies-Hornung A, Schulte-Sasse U: Isoflurane improves the tolerance to pacing-induced myocardial ischemia. Anesthesiology 64:147, 1986
43. Delaney TJ, Kistner JR, Lake CL et al: Myocardial function during halothane and enflurane anesthesia in patients with coronary artery disease. Anesth Analg 59:240, 1980
44. Bovill JG, Sebel PL, Stanley TH: Opioid analgesics in anesthesia with special reference to their use in cardiovascular anesthesia. Anesthesiology 61:731, 1984
45. de Lange S, Boscoe MJ, Stanley TH et al: Comparison of sufentanil-02 and fentanyl-02 for coronary artery surgery. Anesthesiology 56:112, 1982
46. Howie MB, McSweeny TD, Rao PL et al: A comparison of fentanyl-02 and sufentanil-02 for cardiac anesthesia. Anesth Analg 64:877, 1985
47. Hilgenberg JC: Intraoperative awareness during high-dose fentanyl oxygen anesthesia. Anesthesiology 54:341, 1981
48. Mark JB, Greenberg LM: Intraoperative awareness and hypertensive crisis during high-dose fentanyl–diazepam anesthesia. Anesth Analg 62:698, 1983
49. Bland JHL, Lowenstein E: Halothane-induced decrease in experimental myocardial ischemia in the nonfailing canine heart. Anesthesiology 45:287, 1976
50. Van Trigt P, Christian CC, Fagraeus L et al: Myocardial depression by anesthetic agents (halothane, enflurane and nitrous oxide): Quantitation based on end-systolic pressure-dimension relations. Am J Cardiol 53:243, 1984

51. Becker LC: Is isoflurane dangerous for the patient with coronary artery disease? Anesthesiology 66:249, 1987

52. Reiz S, Balfors E, Sorensen MB et al: Isoflurane—A powerful coronary vasodilator in patients with coronary artery disease. Anesthesiology 59:91, 1983

53. Sill JC, Bove AA, Nugent M et al: Effects of isoflurane on coronary arteries and coronary arterioles in the intact dog. Anesthesiology 66:273, 1987

54. Buffington CW, Romson JL, Levine A et al: Isoflurane induces coronary steal in a canine model of chronic coronary occlusion. Anesthesiology 66:280, 1987

55. Hickey RF, Sybert PE, Verrier ED et al: Effects of halothane, enflurane, and isoflurane on coronary blood flow regulation and coronary vascular reserve in the canine heart. Anesthesiology 68:21, 1988

56. Carson BA, Verrier ED, London MJ et al: Effects of isoflurane and halothane on coronary vascular resistance and collateral myocardial blood flow: Their capacity to induce coronary steal. Anesthesiology 67:665, 1987

57. Brown BG, Bolson EL, Petersen RB et al: The mechanisms of nitroglycerin action: Stenosis vasodilation as a major component of the drug response. Circulation 64:1089, 1981

58. Feldman RL, Joyal M, Conti CR et al: Effect of nitroglycerin on coronary collateral flow and pressure during acute coronary occlusion. Am J Cardiol 54:958, 1984

59. Gallagher JD, Moore RA, Jose AB et al: Prophylactic nitroglycerin infusions during coronary artery bypass surgery. Anesthesiology 64:785, 1986

60. Thomson IR, Mutch WA, Culligan JD: Failure of intravenous nitroglycerin to prevent intraoperative myocardial ischemia during fentanyl–pancuronium anesthesia. Anesthesiology 61:385, 1984

61. Coriat P, Deloz M, Bousseau D et al: Prevention of intraoperative myocardial ischemia during noncardiac surgery with intravenous nitroglycerin. Anesthesiology 61:193, 1984

62. Girard D, Shulman BJ, Thys DM et al: The safety and efficacy of esmolol during myocardial revascularization. Anesthesiology 65:157, 1986

63. Harrison L, Ralley FE, Wynands JE et al: The role of an ultra short-acting adrenergic blocker (esmolol) in patients undergoing coronary artery bypass surgery. Anesthesiology 66:413, 1987

64. Mason DT: Regulation of cardiac performance in clinical heart disease. Am J Cardiol 32:437, 1973

65. Sonnenblick E, Lesch M: Valvular Heart Disease. New York, Grune & Stratton, 1974

66. Ross J: Cardiac function and myocardial contractility: A perspective. J Am Coll Cardiol 1:52, 1983

67. Ross J: Afterload mismatch in aortic and mitral valve disease: Implications for surgical therapy. J Am Coll Cardiol 5:811, 1985

68. Hood WP, Rackley CE, Rolett EL: Wall stress in the normal and hypertrophied human left ventricle. Am J Cardiol 22:550, 1968

69. Sasayama S, Franklin D, Ross J: Hyperfunction with normal inotropic state of the hypertrophied left ventricle. Am J Physiol 232:H418, 1977

70. Horrow JC: Thrombocytopenia accompanying a reaction to protamine sulfate. Can Anaesth Soc J 32:49, 1985

71. Marcus ML: Effects of cardiac hypertrophy on the coronary circulation. In Marcus ML (ed): The Coronary Circulation in Health and Disease. New York, McGraw-Hill, 1983

72. Rakusan K: Quantitative morphology of capillaries of the heart. Number of capillaries in animal and human hearts under normal and pathological conditions. Methods Achiev Exp Pathol 5:272, 1971

73. Marcus ML, Doty DB, Hiratzka LF et al: Decreased coronary reserve: A mechanism for angina in patients with aortic stenosis and normal coronary arteries. N Engl J Med 307:1362, 1982

74. Lakatta EG: Age-related alterations in the cardiovascular response to adrenergic mediated stress. Fed Proc 39:3173, 1980

75. Maron BJ, Bonow RO, Cannon RO 3d et al: Hypertrophic cardiomyopathy. Interrelations of clinical manifestations, pathophysiology, and therapy (2). N Engl J Med 316:844, 1987

76. Maron BJ, Bonow RO, Cannon RO 3d et al: Hypertrophic cardiomyopathy. Interrelations of clinical manifestations, pathophysiology, and therapy (1). N Engl J Med 316:780, 1987

77. Wigle ED, Sasson Z, Henderson MA et al: Hypertrophic cardiomyopathy. The importance of the site and the extent of hypertrophy. A review. Prog Cardiovasc Dis 28:1, 1985 (Review)

78. Pollick C: Unlocking the mystery of systolic anterior motion: The key is timing. Can J Cardiol 1:33, 1985

79. Criley JM, Siegel RJ: Has "obstruction" hindered our understanding of hypertrophic cardiomyopathy? Circulation 72:1148, 1985 (Review)

80. Dodge HT, Hay RE, Sandler H: Pressure–volume characteristics of diastolic left ventricle of man with heart disease. Am Heart J 64:503, 1962

81. Maron BJ, Wolfson JK, Epstein SE et al: Intramural ("small vessel") coronary artery disease in hypertrophic cardiomyopathy. J Am Coll Cardiol 8:545, 1986

82. Gaasch WH, Carroll JD, Levine HJ et al: Chronic aortic regurgitation: Prognostic value of left ventricular end-systolic dimension and end-diastolic radius/thickness ratio. J Am Coll Cardiol 1:775, 1983

83. Stone JG, Hoar PF, Calabro JR: Afterload reduction and preload augmentation improve the anesthetic management of patients with cardiac failure and valvular regurgitation. Anesth Analg 59:737, 1980

84. Firth BG, Dehmer GJ, Nicod P et al: Effect of increasing heart rate in patients with aortic regurgitation. Effect of incremental pacing on scintigraphic, hemodynamic, and thermodilation measurements. Am J Cardiol 49:1860, 1982

85. Judge TP, Kennedy JW, Bennet LJ et al: Quantitative hemodynamic effects of heart rate in aortic regurgitation. Circulation 44:355, 1971

86. Heller SJ, Carleton RA: Abnormal left ventricular contraction in patients with mitral stenosis. Circulation 42:1099, 1970

87. Bolen JL, Lopes MG, Harrison DC et al: Analysis of left ventricular function in response to afterload changes in patients with mitral stenosis. Circulation 52:894, 1975

88. Yared JP, Estafanous FG, Zurick AM: Anesthesia for patients with mitral valve disease secondary to rheumatic and coronary artery disease. Cleve Clin Q 51:59, 1984

89. Yoran C, Yellin EL, Becker RM et al: Dynamic aspects of acute mitral regurgitation: Effects of ventricular volume, pressure, and contractility on the effective regurgitant orifice area. Circulation 60:170, 1979

90. Chatterjee K, Parmley WW, Swan HJC et al: Beneficial effects of vasodilator agents in severe mitral regurgitation due to dysfunction of subvalvular apparatus. Circulation 48:684, 1973

91. Galler M, Kronzon I, Slater J et al: Long-term follow-up after mitral valve reconstruction: Incidence of postoperative left ventricular outflow obstruction. Circulation 74:I99, 1986

92. Taylor RM: Cardiopulmonary Bypass: Principles and Management. Baltimore, Williams & Wilkins, 1986

93. DeWall RA, Warden HE, Gott VL et al: Total body perfusion for open cardiotomy utilizing the bubble oxygenator. J Thorac Surg 32:591, 1956

94. Edmunds LH, Ellison N, Colman RW: Platelet function during cardiac operation—comparison of membrane and bubble oxygenators. J Thorac Cardiovasc Surg 83:805, 1982

95. Kusserow B, Larrow R, Nicholls J: Perfusion- and surface-induced injury in leukocytes. Fed Proc 30:1516, 1971

96. Cavarocchi NC, Pluth JR, Schaff HV et al: Complement activation

during cardiopulmonary bypass. Comparison of bubble and membrane oxygenators. J Thorac Cardiovasc Surg 91:252, 1986

97. Chiu RC, Samson R: Complement (C3, C4) consumption in cardiopulmonary bypass, cardioplegia, and protamine administration. Ann Thorac Surg 37:229, 1984
98. vanOeveren W, Kazatchkine MD, Descamps–Latscha B et al: Deleterious effects of cardiopulmonary bypass—a prospective study of bubble vs membrane oxygenation. J Thorac Cardiovasc Surg 89:888, 1985
99. Clark RE, Beauchamp RA, Magrath RA et al: Comparison of bubble and membrane oxygenators in short and long perfusions. J Thorac Cardiovasc Surg 78:655, 1979
100. Pierce EC: Membrane oxygenation. In Taylor KM (ed): Cardiopulmonary Bypass—Principles and Management, p 184. Baltimore, Williams & Wilkins, 1986
101. van den Dungen JJ, Karliczek GF, Brenken U et al: Clinical study of blood trauma during perfusion with membrane and bubble oxygenators. J Thorac Cardiovasc Surg 83:108, 1982
102. Cosgrove DM, Loop FD: Clinical use of travenol TMO membrane oxygenator. In Ionescu MI (ed): Techniques in Extracorporeal Circulation, pp 85–99. London, Butterworths, 1981
103. Siderys H, Herod GT, Halbrook H et al: A comparison of bubble and membrane oxygenation as used in cardiopulmonary bypass in patients: The importance of pericardial blood as a source of hemolysis. J Thorac Cardiovasc Surg 69:708, 1975
104. Mavroudis C: To pulse or not to pulse. Ann Thorac Surg 25:259, 1978
105. Hickey PR, Buckley MJ, Philbin DM: Pulsatile and nonpulsatile cardiopulmonary bypass: Review of a counterproductive controversy. Ann Thorac Surg 36:720, 1983 (Review)
106. Philbin DM, Hickey PR, Buckley MJ: Should we pulse? J Thorac Cardiovasc Surg 84:805, 1982
107. Trinkle JK, Helton NE, Wood RC et al: Metabolic comparison of a new pulsatile pump and a roller pump for cardiopulmonary bypass. J Thorac Cardiovasc Surg 58:562, 1969
108. Dunn J, Kirsch MM, Harness J et al: Hemodynamic, metabolic, and hematologic effects of pulsatile cardiopulmonary bypass. J Thorac Cardiovasc Surg 68:138, 1974
109. Jacobs LA, Klopp EH, Seamone W et al: Improved organ function during cardiac bypass with a roller pump to deliver pulsatile flow. J Thorac Cardiovasc Surg 58:703, 1969
110. Taylor KM, Bain WH: Comparative clinical study of pulsatile and non-pulsatile perfusion in 350 consecutive patients. Thorax 37:324, 1982
111. Taylor KM: Pulsatile perfusion. In Taylor KM (ed): Cardiopulmonary Bypass—Principles and Management, p 184. Baltimore, Williams & Wilkins, 1986
112. Edmunds LE: Pulseless cardiopulmonary bypass. J Thorac Cardiovasc Surg 84:800, 1982
113. Blair E: Clinical Hypothermia. New York, McGraw-Hill, 1964
114. Tobias MA: Choice of priming fluids. In Taylor KM (ed): Cardiopulmonary Bypass—Principles and Management, pp 221–248. Baltimore, Williams & Wilkins, 1986
115. Utley JR, Wachtel C, Kain RB et al: Effect of hypothermia, hemodilution, and pump oxygenation on organ water content, blood flow and oxygen delivery and renal function. Ann Thorac Surg 31:121, 1981
116. Verska JJ, Ludington LG, Brewer LA: A comparative study of CPB with non-blood prime. Ann Thorac Surg 18:72, 1974
117. Barrowcliffe TW, Johnson EA, Thomas D: Antithrombin III and heparin. Br Med Bull 34:143, 1978
118. Pomerantz MW, Owen WG: A catalytic role for heparin: Evidence for a ternary complex of heparin cofactor, thrombin and heparin. Acta Biochim Biophys 535:66, 1978
119. Cohen JA, Frederickson EL, Kaplan J: Plasma heparin activity and antagonism during cardiopulmonary bypass with hypothermia. Anesth Analg 56:564, 1977

120. Esposito RA, Culliford AT, Colvin SB et al: Heparin resistance during cardiopulmonary bypass. The role of heparin pretreatment. J Thorac Cardiovasc Surg 85:346, 1983
121. Hattersley PG: Activated coagulation time of whole blood. JAMA 1986: 436, 1966
122. Young JA, Kisker CT, Doty DB: Adequate anticoagulation during cardiopulmonary bypass determined by activated clotting time and the appearance of fibrin monomer. Ann Thorac Surg 26:231, 1978
123. Esposito RA, Culliford AT, Colvin SB et al: The role of the activated clotting time in heparin administration and neutralization for cardiopulmonary bypass. J Thorac Cardiovasc Surg 85:174, 1983
124. Bull BS, Korpman RA, Huse WM: Heparin therapy during extracorporeal circulation. I. Problems inherent in existing heparin protocols. J Thorac Cardiovasc Surg 69:674, 1975
125. Culliford AT, Gitel SN, Starr N et al: Lack of correlation between activated clotting time and plasma heparin during cardiopulmonary bypass. Ann Surg 193:105, 1981
126. Gravlee GP, Angert KC, Tucker WY et al: Early anticoagulation peak and rapid distribution after intravenous heparin. Anesthesiology 68:126, 1988
127. Akins CW: Noncardioplegic myocardial preservation for coronary revascularization. J Thorac Cardiovasc Surg 88:174, 1984
128. Akins CW: Resection of left ventricular aneurysm during hypothermic fibrillatory arrest without aortic occlusion. J Thorac Cardiovasc Surg 91:610, 1986
129. Brenowitz JB, Kayser KL, Johnson WD: Results of coronary artery endarterectomy and reconstruction. J Thorac Cardiovasc Surg 95:1, 1988
130. Gundry SR, Kirsch MM: A comparison of retrograde cardioplegia versus anterograde cardioplegia in the presence of coronary artery obstruction. Ann Thorac Surg 38:124, 1984
131. Menasche P, Kural S, Fauchot M et al: Retrograde coronary sinus perfusion: A safe alternative for ensuring cardioplegic delivery in aortic valve surgery. Ann Thorac Surg 34:647, 1982
132. Schaper J, Walter P, Scheld H et al: The effects of retrograde perfusion of cardioplegic solution in cardiac operations. J Thorac Cardiovasc Surg 90:882, 1985
133. Silverman NA, Levitsky S: Intraoperative myocardial protection in the context of coronary revascularization. Prog Cardiovasc Dis 29:413, 1987
134. McGoon DC: The ongoing quest for ideal myocardial protection. J Thorac Cardiovasc Surg 89:639, 1985
135. Lell WA, Huber S, Buttner EE: Myocardial protection during cardiopulmonary bypass. In Kaplan JA (ed): Cardiac Anesthesia, 2nd ed, p 927. Orlando, Grune & Stratton, 1987
136. Schaper J, Scheld HH, Schmidt U et al: Ultrastructural study comparing the efficacy of five different methods of intraoperative myocardial protection in the human heart. J Thorac Cardiovasc Surg 92:47, 1986
137. Buckberg GD: A proposed "solution" to the cardioplegic controversy. J Thorac Cardiovasc Surg 77:803, 1979
138. Gravlee GP, Cordell AR, Graham JE et al: Coronary revascularization in patients with bilateral internal carotid occlusions. J Thorac Cardiovasc Surg 90:921, 1985
139. Hilberman M, Myers BD, Carrie BJ et al: Acute renal failure following cardiac surgery. J Thorac Cardiovasc Surg 77:880, 1979
140. Merin RG: Calcium channel blocking drugs and anesthetics: Is the drug interaction beneficial or detrimental? Anesthesiology 66:111, 1987
141. Prichard BNC: B-adrenoceptor blocking agents. In Abschagen V (ed): Clinical Pharmacology of Antianginal Drugs, pp 385–458. New York, Springer-Verlag, 1985
142. Reves JG, Kissin I, Lell WA et al: Calcium entry blockers: Uses and implications for anesthesiologists. Anesthesiology 57:504, 1982

143. Massagee JT, McIntyre RW, Kates RA et al: Effects of preoperative calcium entry blocker therapy on alpha-adrenergic responsiveness in patients undergoing coronary revascularization. Anesthesiology 67:485, 1987

144. Liberman BA, Teasdale SJ: Anaesthesia and amiodarone. Can Anaesth Soc J 32:629, 1985

145. Hensley FA, Dodson DL, Martin DE et al: Oxygen saturation during preinduction placement of monitoring catheters in the cardiac surgical patient. Anesthesiology 66:834, 1987

146. Thomson IR, Bergstrom RG, Rosenbloom M et al: Premedication and high-dose fentanyl anesthesia for myocardial revascularization: A comparison of lorazepam versus morphine–scopolamine. Anesthesiology 68:194, 1988

147. Waldo AL, MacLean WAH: Diagnosis and Treatment of Cardiac Arrhythmias Following Open Heart Surgery: Emphasis on the Use of Atrial and Ventricular Epicardial Wire Electrodes. Mount Kisco, New York, Futura Publishing Company, Inc, 1980

148. Davis FM, Parimelazhagan KN, Harris EA: Thermal balance during cardiopulmonary bypass with moderate hypothermia in man. Br J Anaesth 49:1127, 1977

149. Kinzer JB, Lichtenthal PR, Wade LD: Loss of radial artery pressure trace during internal mammary artery dissection for coronary artery bypass graft surgery. Anesth Analg 64:1134, 1985

150. Mohr R, Lavee J, Goor DA: Inaccuracy of radial artery pressure measurement after cardiac operations. J Thorac Cardiovasc Surg 94:286, 1987

151. Stern DH, Gerson JI, Allen FB et al: Can we trust the direct radial artery pressure immediately following cardiopulmonary bypass? Anesthesiology 62:557, 1985

152. Mangano DT: Monitoring pulmonary artery pressure in coronary artery disease. Anesthesiology 53:364, 1980

153. Latson TW, Lappas DG: Use of a pacing catheter to control heart rate in a patient with aortic insufficiency and coronary artery disease. Anesthesiology 63:712, 1985

154. Lunn JK, Stanley TH, Webster LR et al: Arterial blood pressure and pulse-rate responses to pulmonary and radial artery catheterization prior to cardiac and major vascular operations. Anesthesiology 51:265, 1979

155. Waller JL, Zaidan JR, Kaplan JA: Hemodynamic responses to preoperative vascular cannulation in patients with coronary artery disease. Anesthesiology 56:219, 1982

156. Johnston WE, Royster RL, Choplin RH et al: Pulmonary artery catheter migration during cardiac surgery. Anesthesiology 64:258, 1986

157. Douglas PS, Edmunds LH, Sutton MS et al: Unreliability of hemodynamic indexes of left ventricular size during cardiac surgery. Ann Thorac Surg 44:31, 1987

158. Hansen RM, Viquerat CE, Matthay et al: Poor correlation between pulmonary arterial wedge pressure and left ventricular end-diastolic volume after coronary artery bypass graft surgery. Anesthesiology 64:764, 1986

159. Ellis RJ, Mangano DT, Van Dyke DC: Relationship of wedge pressure to end-diastolic volume in patients undergoing myocardial revascularization. J Thorac Cardiovasc Surg 78:605, 1979

160. Cahalan MK, Litt L, Botvinick EH et al: Advances in noninvasive cardiovascular imaging: Implications for the anesthesiologist. Anesthesiology 66:356, 1987

161. Levy WJ, Parcella PA: Electroencephalographic evidence of cerebral ischemia during acute extracorporeal hypoperfusion. J Cardiothorac Anesth 1:300, 1987

162. Nussmeier NA, Arlund C, Slogoff S: Neuropsychiatric complications after cardiopulmonary bypass: Cerebral protection by a barbiturate. Anesthesiology 64:165, 1986

163. Cunningham JN, Laschinger JC, Spencer FC: Monitoring of somatosensory evoked potentials during surgical procedures on the thoracoabdominal aorta. J Thorac Cardiovasc Surg 94:275, 1987

164. Moffitt EA, Scovil JE, Barker RA et al: The effects of nitrous oxide on myocardial metabolism and hemodynamics during fentanyl or enflurane anesthesia in patients with coronary disease. Anesth Analg 63:1071, 1984

165. Moffitt EA, Sethna DH, Bussell JA et al: Myocardial metabolism and hemodynamic responses to halothane or morphine anesthesia for coronary artery surgery. Anesth Analg 61:979, 1982

166. Bastard OG, Carter JG, Moyers JR et al: Circulatory effects of isoflurane in patients with ischemic heart disease: A comparison with halothane. Anesth Analg 63:635, 1984

167. Bovill JG, Warren PJ, Schuller JL et al: Comparison of fentanyl, sufentanil, and alfentanil anesthesia in patients undergoing valvular heart surgery. Anesth Analg 63:1081, 1984

168. Hess W, Arnold B, Schulte Sasse U et al: Comparison of isoflurane and halothane when used to control intraoperative hypertension in patients undergoing coronary artery bypass surgery. Anesth Analg 62:15, 1983

169. Heikkila H, Jalonen J, Arola M et al: Low-dose enflurane as adjunct to high-dose fentanyl in patients undergoing coronary artery surgery: Stable hemodynamics and maintained myocardial oxygen balance. Anesth Analg 66:111, 1987

170. Gerson JI, Hickey RF, Bainton CR: Treatment of myocardial ischemia with halothane or nitroprusside–propranolol. Anesth Analg 61:10, 1982

171. Stoelting RK, Reis RR, Longnecker DE: Hemodynamic responses to nitrous oxide—halothane in patients with valvular heart disease. Anesthesiology 37:430, 1972

172. Chester WL, Ranieri T, Grossi EA et al: Isoflurane vs sufentanil for CABG surgery. Anesth Analg 67:S529, 1988

173. Lowenstein E, Hallowell P, Levine FH et al: Cardiovascular response to large doses of intravenous morphine in man. N Engl J Med 281:1389, 1969

174. Rosow CE, Moss J, Philbin DM et al: Histamine release during morphine and fentanyl anesthesia. Anesthesiology 56:93, 1982

175. Stanley TH, Gray NG, Stanford W et al: The effects of high-dose morphine on fluid and blood requirements in open-heart situations. Anesthesiology 38:536, 1973

176. Sebel PS, Bovill JG, Boekhorst RAA: Cardiovascular effects of high-dose fentanyl anesthesia. Acta Anaesthesiol Scand 26:308, 1982

177. Sebel PS, Bovill JG: Cardiovascular effects of sufentanil anesthesia. Anesth Analg 61:115, 1982

178. Sonntag H, Larsen R, Hilfiker O et al: Myocardial blood flow and oxygen consumption during high-dose fentanyl anesthesia in patients with coronary artery disease. Anesthesiology 56:417, 1982

179. de Lange S, Boscoe MJ, Stanley TH: Comparison of sufentanil–02 and fentanyl–02 for coronary artery surgery. Anesthesiology 56:112, 1982

180. Sanford TJ, Smith NT, Dec-Silver H et al: A comparison of morphine, fentanyl, and sufentanil anesthesia for cardiac surgery: Induction, emergence, and extubation. Anesth Analg 65:259, 1986

181. de Lange S, Stanley TH, Boscoe MJ: Alfentanil–oxygen anaesthesia for coronary artery surgery. Br J Anaesth 53:1291, 1981

182. Tomicheck RC, Rosow CE, Philbin DM et al: Diazepam–fentanyl interaction—hemodynamic and hormonal effects in coronary artery surgery. Anesth Analg 62:881, 1983

183. West JM, Estrada S, Heerdt M: Sudden hypotension associated with midazolam and sufentanil. Anesth Analg 66:693, 1987

184. Starr NJ, Sethna DH, Estafanous FG: Bradycardia and asystole following the rapid administration of sufentanil with vecuronium. Anesthesiology 64:521, 1986

185. Jaffe TB, Ramsey FM: Attenuation of fentanyl-induced truncal rigidity. Anesthesiology 66:693, 1987

186. Vina JR, Davis DW, Hawkins RA: The influence of nitrous oxide on methionine, S-adenosylmethionine, and other amino acids. Anesthesiology 64:490, 1986

187. Schulte Sasse U, Hess W, Tarnow J: Pulmonary vascular responses to nitrous oxide in patients with normal and high pulmonary vascular resistance. Anesthesiology 57:9, 1982

188. Hilgenberg JC, McCammon RL, Stoelting RK: Pulmonary and systemic vascular responses to nitrous oxide in patients with mitral stenosis and pulmonary hypertension. Anesth Analg 59:323, 1980

189. de Lange S, Boscoe MJ, Stanley TH et al: Comparison of sufentanil–02 and fentanyl–02 for coronary artery surgery. Anesthesiology 56:112, 1982

190. Cahalan MK, Prakash O, Rulf ENR et al: Addition of nitrous oxide to fentanyl anesthesia does not induce myocardial ischemia in patients with ischemic heart disease. Anesthesiology 67:925, 1987

191. Dauchot PJ, Staub F, Berzina L et al: Hemodynamic response to diazepam: Dependence on prior left ventricular end-diastolic pressure. Anesthesiology 60:499, 1984

192. Kawar P, Carson IW, Clarke RS et al: Haemodynamic changes during induction of anaesthesia with midazolam and diazepam (Valium) in patients undergoing coronary artery bypass surgery. Anaesthesia 40:767, 1985

193. Stoelting RK: Choice of muscle relaxants in patients with heart disease. Semin Anesth 4:1, 1985

194. Estafanous FG, Zurick AM: Hemodynamic effects of sufentanil/metocurine versus sufentanil/pancuronium in patients undergoing coronary artery surgery. Cleve Clin Q 52:391, 1985

195. Zaidan JR, Kaplan JA: Cardiovascular effects of metocurine in patients with aortic stenosis. Anesthesiology 56:395, 1982

196. Thomson IR, Putnins CL: Adverse effects of pancuronium during high-dose fentanyl anesthesia for coronary artery bypass grafting. Anesthesiology 62:708, 1985

197. Heinonen J, Salmenpera M, Suomivuori M: Contribution of muscle relaxant to the haemodynamic course of high-dose fentanyl anaesthesia: A comparison of pancuronium, vecuronium and atracurium. Can Anaesth Soc J 33:597, 1986

198. Caldwar JE, Castagnoli KP, Canfer PC: Pipecuronium and pancuronium: A comparison of their pharmacokinetics and durations of actions. Anesthesiology 67:A-611, 1987

199. Horrow JC: Thrombocytopenia accompanying a reaction to protamine sulfate. Can Anaesth Soc J 32:49, 1985

200. Stoelting RK: Circulatory changes during direct laryngoscopy and tracheal intubation: Influence of duration of laryngoscopy with or without prior lidocaine. Anesthesiology 47:381, 1977

201. Sonntag H, Larsen R, Hilfiker O et al: Myocardial blood flow and oxygen consumption during high-dose fentanyl anesthesia in patients with coronary artery disease. Anesthesiology 56:417, 1982

202. Kolkka R, Hilberman M: Neurologic dysfunction following cardiac operation with low-flow, low-pressure cardiopulmonary bypass. J Thorac Cardiovasc Surg 79:432, 1980

203. Thomson IR: Neurologic aspect of cardiopulmonary bypass. Prob Anesth 1:394, 1987

204. Govier AV, Reves JG, McKay RD et al: Relationship of cerebral blood flow and perfusion pressure during cardiopulmonary bypass. Anesthesiology 59:A-70, 1983

205. Slogoff S, Girgis KV, Keats AS: Etiologic factors in neuropsychiatric complications associated with cardiopulmonary bypass. Anesth Analg 61:903, 1982

206. Murkin JM, Farra JK, Tweed WA et al: Cerebral autoregulation and flow/metabolism coupling during cardiopulmonary bypass: The influence of Pa_{CO_2}. Anesth Analg 66:825, 1987

207. Ream AK, Reitz BA, Silverberg G: Temperature correction of P_{CO_2} and pH in estimating acid-base status: An example of the emperor's new clothes? Anesthesiology 56:41, 1982

208. D'Ambra MN, Laraia PJ, Philbin DM et al: Prostaglandin E_1: A new therapy for refractory right heart failure and pulmonary hypertension after mitral valve replacement. J Thorac Cardiovasc Surg 89:567, 1985

209. Pearl RG, Maze M, Rosenthal MH: Pulmonary and systemic hemodynamic effects of central venous and left atrial sympathomimetic drug administration in the dog. J Cardiothorac Anesth 1:29, 1987

210. Buckley MJ, Craver JM, Gold HK et al: Intra-aortic balloon pump assist for cardiogenic shock after cardiopulmonary bypass. Circulation 97–98: 90, 1973

211. Craver JM, Kaplan JA, Jones EL: What role should the intraaortic balloon have in cardiac surgery? Ann Surg 189:769, 1979

212. Rajani R, Keon WJ, Bedard P: Rupture of intraaortic balloon. J Thorac Cardiovasc Surg 79:301, 1980

213. Sanfelippo PM, Baker NH, Ewe HG et al: Experience with intra-aortic balloon counterpulsation. Ann Thorac Surg 41:36, 1986

214. Dembitsky WP, Daily PO, Raney AA et al: Temporary extracorporeal support of the right ventricle. J Thorac Cardiovasc Surg 91:518, 1986

215. Braunwald E, Kloner RA: The stunned myocardium: Prolonged, postischemic ventricular dysfunction. Circulation 66:1146, 1982

216. Pennington DG, Bernhard WF, Golding LR et al: Long-term follow-up of postcardiotomy patients with profound cardiogenic shock treated with ventricular assist devices. Circulation 72 SII:II216, 1985

217. Rose DM, Laschinger J, Grossi E et al: Experimental and clinical results with a simplified left heart assist device for treatment of profound left ventricular dysfunction. World J Surg 9:11, 1985

218. Pierce WS: Effective clinical application of ventricular bypass. Ann Thorac Surg 39:2, 1985

219. Pennington DG, Merjavy JP, Swartz MT et al: The importance of biventricular failure in patients with postoperative cardiogenic shock. Ann Thorac Surg 39:16, 1985

220. Umlas J, Taff RH, Gauvin G et al: Anticoagulant monitoring and neutralization during open heart surgery—a rapid method for measuring heparin and calculating safe reduced protamine doses. Anesth Analg 62:1095, 1983

221. Horrow JC: Protamine: A review of its toxicity. Anesth Analg 64:348, 1985 (Review)

222. Moorthy SS, Pond W, Rowland RG: Severe circulation shock following protamine (an anaphylactic reaction). Anesth Analg 59:77, 1980

223. Holland CL, Singh AK, McMaster PRB et al: Adverse reactions to protamine sulfate following cardiac surgery. Clin Cardiol 7:157, 1984

224. Anderson JM, Johnson TA: Hypertension associated with protamine sulfate administration. Am J Hosp Pharm 38:701, 1981

225. Doolan L, McKenzie I, Krafchek J et al: Protamine sulfate hypersensitivity. Anaesth Intensive Care 9:147, 1981

226. Stewart WJ, McSweeney SM, Kellet MA et al: Increased risk of severe protamine reactions in NPH insulin-dependent diabetics undergoing cardiac catheterization. Circulation 70:788, 1984

227. Lowenstein E, Johnston WE, Lappas DG et al: Catastrophic pulmonary vasoconstriction associated with protamine reversal of heparin. Anesthesiology 59:470, 1983

228. Morel DR, Zapol WM, Thomas SJ et al: C5a and thromboxane generation associated with pulmonary vaso- and broncho-constriction during protamine reversal of heparin. Anesthesiology 66:597, 1987

229. Kronenfeld MA, Gaguilo R, Weinberg P et al: Left atrial injection of protamine does not reliably prevent pulmonary hypertension. Anesthesiology 67:126, 1987

230. Casthely PA, Goodman K, Fyman PN et al: Hemodynamic changes after the administration of protamine. Anesth Analg 65:78, 1985

231. Frater RWM, Oka Y, Hong Y et al: Protamine-induced circulatory changes. J Thorac Cardiovasc Surg 87:687, 1984

232. Michaelson EL, Torosian M, Morganroth *et al:* Early recognition of surgically correctable causes of excessive mediastinal bleeding after coronary artery bypass graft surgery. Am J Surg 139:313, 1980

233. Harker LA, Malpass TW, Branson HE *et al:* Mechanism of abnormal bleeding in patients undergoing cardiopulmonary bypass: Acquired transient platelet dysfunction associated with selective-granule release. Blood 56:824, 1980

234. Beatty N, Beatty CP, Blake DR *et al:* Heparin rebound studies in patients and volunteers. J Thorac Cardiovasc Surg 67:723, 1974

235. Purandare SV, Parulkar GB, Panday SR *et al:* Heparin rebound— A cause of bleeding following open heart surgery. J Postgrad Med 25:70, 1979

236. Reddy PS, Curtiss EL, O'Toole JD *et al:* Cardiac tamponade: Hemodynamic observations in man. Circulation 58:265, 1978

237. Hickey PR, Wessel DL: Anesthesia for treatment of congenital heart disease. In Kaplan JA (ed): Cardiac Anesthesia, 2nd ed, p 635. Orlando, Grune & Stratton, 1987

238. Haworth SG: Normal pulmonary vascular development and its disturbance in congenital heart disease. In Godman MJ (ed): Paediatric Cardiology, pp 46–55. New York, Churchill Livingstone, 1981

239. Hoffman JIE, Rudolph AM, Heymann MA: Pulmonary vascular disease with congenital heart lesions: Pathologic features and causes. Circulation 64:873, 1981

240. Rabinovitch M, Haworth SG, Castaneda AR *et al:* Lung biopsy in congenital heart disease: A morphometric approach to pulmonary vascular disease. Circulation 58:1107, 1978

241. Berman W: The hemodynamics of shunts in congenital heart disease. In Johansen K, Burggran WW (eds): Cardiovascular Shunts: Phylogenic, Ontogenic, and Clinical Aspects, pp 399–410. New York, Raven Press, 1985

242. Downing SE, Talner NS, Gardner TH: Ventricular function in the newborn lamb. Am J Physiol 208:931, 1965

243. Freed MA, Heymann MA, Lewis AB *et al:* Prostaglandin E_1 in infants with ductus arteriosus–dependent congenital heart disease. Circulation 64:899, 1981

244. Hansen DD, Hickey PR: Anesthesia for hypoplastic left heart syndrome: Use of high-dose fentanyl in 30 neonates. Anesth Analg 65:127, 1986

245. Romero T, Covell J, Friedman WF: A comparison of pressure–volume relations of the fetal, newborn, and adult. Am J Physiol 222:1285, 1972

246. Phornphutkul C, Rosenthal A, Nadas A: Cerebrovascular accidents in infants and children with cyanotic congenital heart disease. Am J Cardiol 32:329, 1973

247. Kontras S, Sirak H, Newton W: Hematologic abnormalities in children with congenital heart disease. JAMA 195:611, 1976

248. Sanders S: Echocardiography and related techniques in the diagnosis of congenital heart defects. Echocardiography 1:185, 1984

249. Anand KJ, Hickey PR: Pain and its effects in the human neonate and fetus. N Engl J Med 317:1321, 1987

250. Berry FA, Gregory GA: Do premature infants require anesthesia for surgery? Anesthesiology 67:291, 1987

251. Hickey PR, Hansen DD, Cramolini GM *et al:* Pulmonary and systemic hemodynamic responses to ketamine in infants with normal and elevated pulmonary vascular resistance. Anesthesiology 62:287, 1985

252. Tanner GE, Angers DG, Barash PG *et al:* Effect of left-to-right, mixed left-to-right, and right-to-left shunts on inhalational anesthetic induction in children. Anesth Analg 64:101, 1985

253. Hickey PR, Hansen DD, Wessel DL *et al:* Blunting of stress responses in the pulmonary circulation of infants by fentanyl. Anesth Analg 64:1137, 1985

254. Hickey PR, Hansen DD, Wessel DL *et al:* Pulmonary and systemic hemodynamic responses to fentanyl in infants. Anesth Analg 64:483, 1985

255. Friesen RH, Lichtor JL: Cardiovascular effects of inhalation induction with isoflurane in infants: A study of three induction techniques. Anesth Analg 61:42, 1982

256. Friesen RH, Lichtor JL: Cardiovascular effects of inhalation induction with isoflurane in infants. Anesth Analg 62:411, 1983

257. Hickey PR, Hansen DD, Strafford M *et al:* Pulmonary and systemic hemodynamic effects of nitrous oxide in infants with normal and elevated pulmonary vascular resistance. Anesthesiology 65:374, 1986

258. Hickey PR, Anderson NP: Deep hypothermic circulatory arrest: A review of pathophysiology and clinical experience as a basis for anesthetic management. J Cardiothorac Anesth 1:137, 1987

259. Tharion J, Johnson DC, Celermajer JM *et al:* Profound hypothermia with circulatory arrest: Nine years clinical experience. J Thorac Cardiovasc Surg 84:66, 1984

Chapter 36   *Michael F. Roizen*

Anesthesia for Vascular Surgery

GOALS OF ANESTHESIA

As in any surgical endeavor, the obvious goal in anesthesia for vascular surgical procedures is to minimize patient morbidity and maximize the surgical benefit. The anesthesiologist may, however, have a greater influence in reducing morbidity in vascular surgery, and perhaps in no other area has morbidity decreased so quickly, from a 6-day mortality rate of more than 25% for major aortic reconstruction in the mid-1960s to 1–2% today. This chapter will discuss the major types (and causes) of morbidity that follow specific surgical procedures.

Despite the fact that the blood flow to many different organs is interrupted, that the stress of clamping and unclamping vessels is different in different operations, and that co-morbid conditions of patients are dissimilar in different operations, the data presented in this chapter suggest that the heart should be the major focus of the anesthesiologist's attention since myocardial dysfunction is the greatest cause of morbidity following surgery for cerebrovascular, visceral, or peripheral vascular insufficiency, or following aortic reconstruction for aneurysm.

CAUSES OF MORBIDITY AFTER OPERATIONS FOR CEREBROVASCULAR INSUFFICIENCY

There are two types of operations for correction of cerebrovascular insufficiency: carotid endarterectomy and cerebral bypass. However, the extracranial-to-intracranial (EC-IC) bypass is not performed with even $^1/_{100}$th the frequency of carotid endarterectomy (see Surgery for Cerebrovascular Insufficiency). The results, morbidity, and mortality following carotid endarterectomy vary directly with the preoperative neurologic and cardiac status of patients. In a Mayo Clinic series,[1] those patients with "strokes in progress" or unstable neurologic status had a 2.5% rate of death from postoperative neurologic deficits, and 1% died of cardiovascular complications. Those patients with a history of coronary artery disease (CAD) had a 1.9% mortality rate from myocardial ischemia. Since more patients in this large Mayo Clinic series had CAD than had unstable neurologic status, the greatest cause of morbidity and mortality following carotid endarterectomy was myocardial (see Table 36-1). In two other surgical series in which routine neurologic and cardiologic examinations were performed, Hertzer and Lees[2] found 60% of the deaths within 60 days of carotid endarterectomy to be due to myocardial dysfunction; and Ennix and colleagues[3] reported an 0.8% rate of myocardial infarctions and a 1.1% rate of severe strokes in those patients without CAD symptoms, a 12.9% myocardial infarction rate and a 2.4% severe stroke rate in those patients with symptomatic CAD, and a 2.6% rate of myocardial infarctions and a 1.3% rate of severe strokes in patients with a history of CAD with prior or simultaneous coronary artery bypass grafting (CABG).

Age undoubtedly also plays a role in morbidity. Glaser[4] has shown a strong correlation between age and both myocardial and central nervous system (CNS) morbidity after carotid endarterectomy. Whereas Ennix *et al*[3] and others[5] have stressed the potential benefits of CABG prior to carotid endarterectomy or other surgical procedures, these studies to date show no significant reduction in mortality when the mortality

1015

TABLE 36-1. Mortality After Carotid Endarterectomy

SENIOR AUTHOR	YEAR OF PUBLICATION	NO. OF PATIENTS STUDIED	% PATIENTS WITH SERIOUS MORBIDITY OR MORTALITY FROM	
			Cardiac Causes	Central Nervous System Causes
Sundt[1]	1981	1145	50	31
Hertzer[2]	1981	355	60	17
Ennix[3]	1979	1546	60	30
Callow[10]	1982	1141	67	33
Gewertz[11]	1986	105	100	0
Smith[12]	1988	60	0	100

due to the CABG is included in the overall mortality rate (Fig. 36-1). Perhaps the reason for the reduced morbidity and mortality after carotid endarterectomy in patients who have undergone CABGs is that those patients at greatest risk experience myocardial and CNS morbidity and mortality during the first (the CABG) procedure. It may be that identification of high-risk patients by noninvasive tests, or better intraoperative monitoring and management of myocardial ischemia, will alter these results.

Patients with symptomatic carotid artery disease appear to be at as much as 17 times higher risk of stroke during coronary artery bypass grafting than are patients without carotid artery disease.[6] Such statistics have led to simultaneous carotid and coronary vascular procedures, with mortality and serious morbidity in the best series at about 10%.[7, 8] However, patients with asymptomatic carotid stenosis do not have a higher stroke rate following coronary artery surgery than do those without carotid stenosis, but they do have a higher mortality

FIG. 36-1. On the basis of coronary angiograms obtained in 1000 patients prior to peripheral vascular surgical procedures, the results are stratified (correctable and inoperative) for major risk factors. For example, 19% (151 of 802) of patients in whom angina pectoris was absent had correctable coronary artery disease (CAD) and 3.5% (28 of 802) had inoperable CAD. The remaining 78% (623 of 802) patients were symptom-free. This and the other enumerated risk factors document the presence of occult CAD in this high-risk population. (Based on data from Hertzer NR, Beven EG, Young JR et al: Coronary artery disease in peripheral vascular patients: A classification of 1000 coronary angiograms and results of surgical management. Ann Surg 199:223, 1984.)

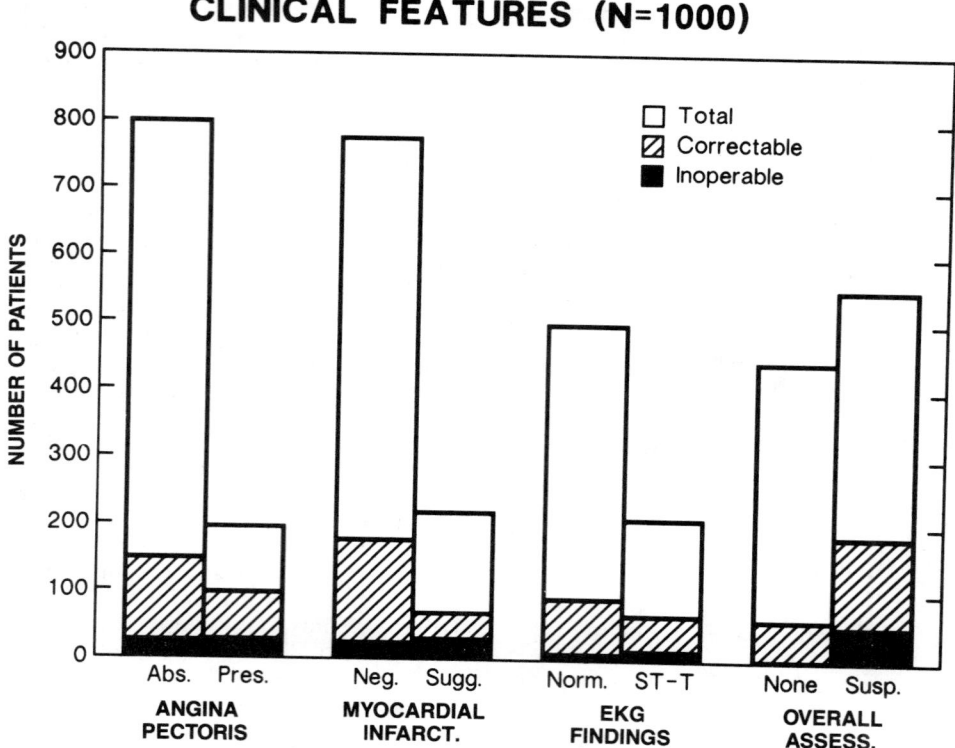

after coronary artery surgery, mostly resulting from myocardial infarction.

Thus, the morbidity and mortality statistics from virtually all series but our own surprisingly show that, even when a vessel to the brain is occluded, the major cause of morbidity and mortality after carotid endarterectomy is myocardial (Table 36-1).[1-4, 9-12] Even in our own series, 34% of the patients evidenced myocardial ischemia intraoperatively, but none went on to suffer myocardial infarcts or death from myocardial events during their hospital stay.[12] Perhaps the reason for the difference between our results and the outcome in other published series is that we focus on the goal of decreasing myocardial insults and on maintaining myocardial well-being perioperatively.

CAUSES OF MORBIDITY AFTER OPERATIONS FOR VISCERAL ISCHEMIA, THORACOABDOMINAL ANEURYSMS, AND AORTIC RECONSTRUCTION FOR ANEURYSM OR ATHEROSCLEROTIC DISEASE

The major cause of morbidity and mortality following these different procedures relates to the heart (Table 36-2). Despite this common cause, distinct pathologic and physiologic patterns exist for the different diseases.

There are three distinct patterns of occlusive peripheral vascular disease:

Type I is isolated aortoiliac disease. This pattern of atherosclerosis is characterized by disease localized to the bifurcation of the aorta and the common iliac vessels. Despite the association of this disease with smoking, the atherosclerosis tends to be absent in coronary vessels and to exhibit symptoms only of thigh and hip claudication. Type I disease is associated with a 5-year survival rate of 90% following surgery.

Type II, aortoiliac disease, has a diffuse atherosclerotic pattern, often involving the coronary and cerebral circulation. As with Types I and III, smoking is common in this group of patients. Diabetes and hypertension are more common than in patients with Type I disease. The 5-year survival rate following surgery is about 80%.

Type III, atherosclerotic peripheral vascular disease, involves femoral-popliteal and tibial atherosclerosis as well as small-vessel disease. The patients have a 60–65% 5-year survival rate following surgery.[15, 16]

Although the associated conditions and prognoses for these three types of occlusive peripheral vascular diseases differ, the mortality in most cases and the limiting factor in patient prognosis are the same and are related to the heart (Table 36-2).[17-32]

Patients undergoing surgery for aneurysmal disease have higher perioperative morbidity and mortality by a factor of 2 and a lower median survival rate (5.8 vs 10.7 years) than do patients undergoing aortic reconstruction for occlusive disease.[33, 34] Should patients, then, be exposed to surgery for asymptomatic aneurysms? This question was answered by Szilagyi et al[17] in 1966 for aneurysms more than 6 cm in diameter, when he showed that such surgery approximately doubled a patient's life expectancy. Since then, perioperative mortality rates have declined from 18 to 25% in the mid-1960s, to 8 to 12% in the early 1970s, to 2 to 4% today. Consequently, even patients with abdominal aortic aneurysms less than 6 cm in diameter are considered candidates for aortic reconstructive surgery. This change is due to three factors: 1) the lessened morbidity of elective repair now *versus* that in the 1960s; 2) the higher mortality (45–90%) associated with emergency aortic reconstruction *versus* elective reconstruction; and 3) the lack of predictability as to which patients' aneurysms will enlarge and rupture (19% of aneurysms less than 6 cm in Szilagyi's[17] series resulted in death from rupture).[35-38]

Other causes of morbidity following vascular surgery include pulmonary infections, graft infections, renal insufficiency and failure, hepatic failure, and spinal cord ischemia resulting in paraplegia. The incidence rates of these other causes of morbidity has declined substantially over the last 20 years, with death from renal failure declining from 25% to less than 1% at present.[17, 22, 26, 39] Much of the improvement toward elimination of renal failure has resulted from better perioperative fluid management.[40-44]

Investigators have used sensory-evoked potentials and electroencephalograms (EEG) to gauge spinal cord and cerebral protection during resection of abdominal or thoracoabdominal aneurysms or coarctation repairs.[45] We have found no evidence in the literature that monitoring of the EEG is of benefit in these procedures, and no evidence that stroke is a predictable consequence of even supraceliac or descending thoracic aortic reconstruction. However, in 1–11% of operations involving repair of the distal descending thoracic aorta, spinal cord ischemia does occur.[46]

The arterial blood supply to the spinal cord is generally divided into superior, midthoracic, and thoracolumbar areas

TABLE 36-2. Percentages of Perioperative Mortality Related to Cardiac Events

AORTIC RECONSTRUCTION SERIES	DEATHS/TOTAL NO. OF PATIENTS	% MORTALITY CAUSED BY CARDIAC DYSFUNCTION
Szilagyi et al[17] (1966)	59/401	48
Young et al[18] (1977)	7/144	100
Hicks et al[19] (1975)	19/225	53
Thompson et al[20] (1975)	6/108	83
Mulcare et al[21] (1978)	14/140	79
Whittemore et al[22] (1980)	1/110	100
Crawford et al[23] (1981)	41/860	54
Hertzer[24] (1983)	22/523	64
Yeager et al[25] (1986)	4/97	100
Benefiel et al[26] (1986)	3/96	67

(Adapted with permission from Roizen MF, Sohn YJ, Stoney RJ: Intraoperative management of the patient undergoing supraceliac aortic occlusion. In Wilson SE, Veith FJ, Hobson RW *et al* [eds]: Vascular Surgery, pp 312–321. New York, McGraw-Hill, 1986.)

(Fig. 36-2). This subdivision is better defined for the anterior spinal cord than for posterior areas, as the posterior arteries show more variation in blood flow from one area to the next.[47, 48] The major radiculomedullary arteries arising from the aorta terminate in three longitudinal trunks that run the length of the cord. The two posterior arteries, which together supply only 25% of the blood to the cord, are formed from the anastomoses of the posterior branch of the vertebral artery and the ascending branch of the bifurcation of the second posterior radicular artery. The anterior spinal artery, which supplies the blood to the anterolateral 75% of the cord, is formed throughout by a series of radicular arteries. Blood does *not flow* from cephalad to caudad in this artery.

Each segment of the spinal cord receives its blood supply from opposing ascending and descending flows.[48] The superior area includes the cervical segment and first two segments of the thoracic cord. The radiculomedullary arteries that supply this segment arise from the branches of the subclavian artery, but there are additional contributions of the vertebral arteries, resulting in a rich blood supply to this region. The midthoracic region, supplied by the anterior spinal artery, usually receives only one afferent vessel, which arises from a left or right intercostal vessel. The afferent arteries to the posterior spinal cord from T-2 to T-8 are also poor in collateralization. The blood supply to the thoracolumbar cord (from T-8 to the conus terminalis) is derived from the radicular artery known as the artery of Adamkiewicz. It arises from the left side in 60% of cases; in 75% of patients, it joins the anterior spinal artery between T-8 and T-12; and, in 10% of patients, it joins between L-1 and L-2. Although other radicular arteries supply this third section, much of the blood flow in the anterior spinal artery is dependent upon the artery of Adamkiewicz.

Because the flow in the spinal arteries is dependent upon collateralization and is often bidirectional, the blood supply to the spinal cord can be "stolen" and "given" to the rest of the body when pressures in the other areas of the body are lower. Such a situation may arise when a single high aorta-occluding clamp is applied. Thus, surgical techniques designed to minimize spinal cord ischemia include bypass shunts to supply blood to the lower extremities, femoral-femoral extracorporeal bypass techniques, double-clamping techniques, cerebrospinal fluid (CSF) drainage techniques, and preservation of the native aorta with its intercostal artery.[48, 49] Nevertheless, only rarely will a patient develop complications from spinal cord ischemia, and this is a rare cause of morbidity and mortality in published series as well as in anecdotes.

Thus, in patients undergoing vascular surgery, the major cause of morbidity, and the factor limiting both perioperative and long-term survival in almost every series, relates to the heart. For this reason, a major theme of this chapter is that the anesthetist should concentrate on factors that prevent myocardial damage perioperatively in patients undergoing major vascular surgery, whether on the aorta or on the carotid, femoral, popliteal, or other vessels. This concentration on the heart should be kept in mind when decisions are made as to how to manage the patient's co-morbid conditions such as hypertension, chronic obstructive lung disease, renal insufficiency, and/or diabetes.

THE PATIENT AND THE PATIENT'S DISORDERS

Many disorders are associated with vascular disease; however, diabetes, smoking and its sequelae, chronic pulmonary disease, hypertension, and ischemic heart disease are the

FIG. 36-2. (*A*) Blood supply to spinal cord. (*B*) Segmental distribution of blood supply to spinal cord. (Reproduced with permission from Romero-Sierra C: Neuroanatomy—A conceptual approach. New York, Churchill Livingstone, 1986.)

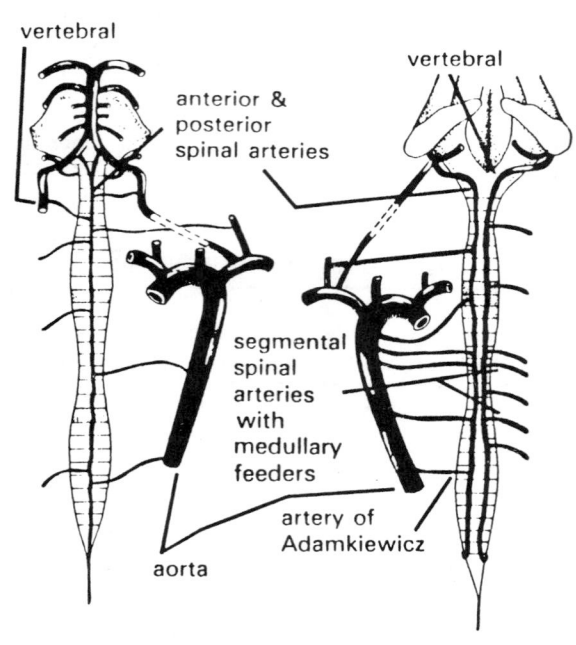

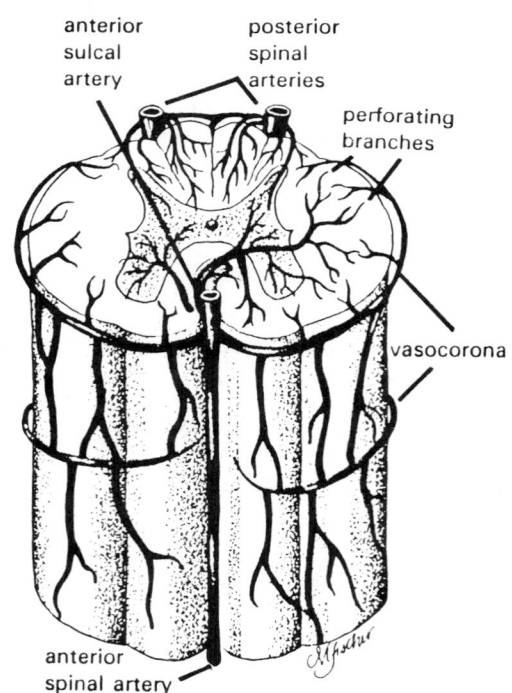

A

B

most common. The management of these diseases is reviewed in Chapters 32, 35, and 44. Perhaps the most important factor in planning the perioperative management of these co-morbid conditions is understanding and searching for the end-organ effects of these diseases and understanding the appropriate drug therapy. Although it would be unusual to administer anesthesia to patients with uncontrolled hypertension, uncontrolled metabolic disease, or untreated pulmonary infections, or to patients 3 to 6 months following a myocardial infarction when other portions of the myocardium are still at risk of infarct,[50, 51] an expanding aneurysm, crescendo transient ischemic attacks (TIAs), or threatened limb loss can force one's hand. Attempts at rapid control of blood pressure or electrolytes may be more hazardous than leaving the condition untreated and trying to control the abnormality slowly. For example, rapid reduction of blood pressure in a patient with TIAs may precipitate cerebral ischemia and should be postponed to the postoperative period (assuming that surgery cannot be delayed to permit gradual preoperative control of blood pressure). Similarly, stopping a drug may be more hazardous than continuing drug therapy and being cognizant of its effects.

Specific attempts have been made to identify, prior to surgical operations, patients at risk of myocardial insult[5, 51]; but, until these procedures gain widespread acceptance, and until extensive trials are shown to reduce the overall mortality, the goal of optimizing care, with the specific focus on doing what is best to minimize myocardial morbidity, seems logical. This goal is based on both the preoperative likelihood, in patients with vascular disorders, of CAD and the fact that the major cause of morbidity and mortality following vascular surgery is related to the heart.

SURGERY FOR CEREBROVASCULAR INSUFFICIENCY

SURGICAL APPROACHES

Two groups of surgical approaches are available for the treatment and prevention of cerebrovascular insufficiency: extracranial-to-intracranial (EC-IC) bypass and carotid endarterectomy. The EC-IC bypass is used to increase the collateral blood flow to a presumably focal ischemic area of the brain. Recent multicenter trials indicated that this operation does not improve the neurologic outcome from either "strokes in evolution" or completed strokes.[52–54] Furthermore, the patients who underwent EC-IC bypass surgery had greater immediate disability and no better long-term prognosis than did those patients treated medically. Thus, it appears that the EC-IC bypass may have few indications, except possibly to prevent a stroke in patients having TIAs thought to be flow- and not embolus-related and who have bilateral carotid occlusions or lesions located so high in the carotid as to preclude extracranial carotid surgery.[55] Since it is thus expected that this operation will be performed only rarely, we will deal briefly with it.

In EC-IC bypass, blood flow to the brain should be interrupted only during the short period of the EC-IC anastomosis to the recipient vessel, and shunting of the flow during such time is usually not an option. Therefore, the monitors used for making judgments about the need for shunting, the adequacy of the shunt, and the adequacy of the repair are not necessary. Otherwise, the basic surgical goals and anesthetic goals, monitoring strategies, and anesthetic techniques are quite similar to those used in carotid endarterectomy, since the patients in both groups have similar medical and surgical problems and present similar challenges.

In carotid endarterectomy, surgical approaches vary by surgical group, but the aim is to gain a "smooth" ulcer- and plaque-free vessel with "smooth" end points and no emboli or intraoperative neurologic ischemia.[56] To reach these goals, most surgeons wish to have some measure of cerebral blood flow or neurologic function, whereas others rely solely on shunting of the carotid blood flow of all patients, and still others rely on skillful general anesthesia and short occlusion times. Each of these choices of technique has been used with success by surgeons experienced in their use.[1, 3, 10–13, 57–59]

Initially, the surgical approach is to isolate the internal carotid artery where the plaque or ulcerative lesion is shown radiographically to be located (usually starting near the bifurcation). Heparin is given in a dose of 2,000–20,000 units/70-kg person. Again, the dose varies according to the surgical group and appears to be based on local custom. The surgeon isolates this diseased carotid segment with clamps or ties placed on the proximal and distal internal carotid artery and on the external carotid artery. After a period of test occlusion during which regional cerebral blood flow, neurologic function, EEG, processed EEG, somatosensory evoked potential (SSEP), stump pressure, or nothing is measured, an incision is made into the artery, a shunt is inserted (usually first in the proximal, then in the distal vessel, often with clamps, sometimes with ties; often with a pressure-measuring side arm to ensure that one or more ends are not crimped or occluded). Since insertion of a shunt is associated with at least a 0.7% embolism-associated stroke rate,[60] routine shunting is not advocated by everyone.

The surgeon then endarterectomizes the ulcerated or plaque-containing area, leaving a smooth intimal surface joining the endarterectomized vessel and native vessel. Occasionally, a long or tortuous region is shortened by resection and reanastomosis, or occasionally, the remaining portion of the intima is too thin, in which case a vein or a Dacron patch is used. Because suturing of the patch requires more time than does suturing of the native vessel, an internal shunt is frequently used during these procedures. Time is of the essence, because, at a stump pressure of 40 mm Hg, neurologic dysfunction can occur in 40 minutes and is common when occlusion times extend beyond 60 minutes.[61] (See Monitoring Techniques, Carotid Stump Pressure.)

In those situations in which it is used, the shunt is removed, and, in all cases, the arteriotomy is closed, usually with a running suture. Shunt placement and removal rarely take less than 1 minute or more than 4 minutes, and the total occlusion time rarely exceeds 40 minutes.

Most surgeons wish to have their patients awaken soon after skin closure, because a new neurologic deficit is thought by some to demand immediate re-exploration, or at least arteriography. A few surgeons do arteriography routinely after restoring blood flow, but most believe that the complications of routine arteriography (emboli, allergic reactions, vasospasm, bleeding from the puncture hole, and stroke) are greater than its benefits (the rare detection of inadequate repairs, suture lines, or flow).

ANESTHETIC GOALS AND MONITORING TECHNIQUES

For minimal morbidity and mortality, the anesthetic goals must be: 1) to protect the heart from ischemia, and 2) to protect the brain from ischemia. Other prominent anesthesiologists believe that the order of priority for these goals should be reversed.[55, 62] However, the major cause of morbidity and the major effect that we as anesthesiologists can have strongly argue for protection of the heart to receive a higher priority than does brain protection in this operation. Unfortunately, the two goals are often in conflict.

To decrease myocardial oxygen requirements, one tries to decrease the heart rate and blood pressure and the contractility of the myocardium.[63] To maintain oxygen delivery to the brain, one tries to increase the cerebral perfusion pressure and to decrease the cerebral metabolic requirements. For increased cerebral perfusion pressure, an attempt is made to increase the arterial blood pressure at least to levels above which the normal brain autoregulates.[12, 60, 64] This usually also means trying to avoid severe bradycardia, or to decrease central venous pressure.

Not only the blood pressure reduction and augmentation but also the heart rate changes lead to conflicts in priority management between the well-being of the heart and that of the head. However, we believe that there are compromise solutions that allow both goals to be met. To decrease the myocardial work, one tries to decrease the heart rate; but sudden bradycardia can occur when the surgeon stretches the baroreceptor nerve endings directly (because of atherosclerosis, these nerve endings are supersensitive, since they usually have not been stretched easily by blood pressure changes over a period of many years). This sudden bradycardia can result in substantial decreases in arterial pressure, which could compromise collateral cerebral perfusion. Injection of the area of the bifurcation with 1% lidocaine 10 to 15 minutes before the carotid artery is to be occluded has united the two goals by allowing or facilitating a stable heart rate of approximately 70 beats·min^{-1}. In addition, the goals of decreasing myocardial contractility and decreasing the cerebral metabolic rate are consonant, regardless of whether thiopental or isoflurane is used as the major anesthetic.

To maintain blood pressure, we usually use "light" anesthesia (without paralysis, so that inadequate anesthesia can be detected), allowing native vasopressor substances to maintain blood pressure. This light-anesthesia technique has been associated with a substantially lower incidence of myocardial ischemia than was possible with deeper anesthesia and administration of phenylephrine.[12] In fact, one of the major benefits of EEG or processed EEG monitoring is that when the EEG is normal or unchanged from pre- to postclamping of the carotid, one can decrease the blood pressure to facilitate protection of the heart.

The hemodynamic and metabolic means for facilitating the goals of protecting the heart and brain from ischemia as previously described in theory should work in practice. It would be reassuring, however, to have monitors to ensure that these goals are actually being met. Unfortunately, the detection of both myocardial and cerebral ischemia by monitors during general or regional anesthesia is imperfect at present, with both false-negative and false-positive results confusing the technicians who perform the monitoring.

Myocardial Ischemia

ST-T SEGMENTS OF THE ELECTROCARDIOGRAM. Lead V_5 is usually selected. However, in a study that we performed, ST segments of even seven leads of the electrocardiogram (ECG) did not enable us to detect 75% of the instances of myocardial ischemia detected by changes in regional wall motion and by wall-thickening defects on two-dimensional echocardiograms (2D-TEE).[65] In another vascular surgery, the ECG had a

40–60% sensitivity rate if systolic wall motion abnormalities (SWMA) and wall-thickening abnormalities were considered the ultimate standard.[66] In addition, lead V_5 was insensitive compared with other leads (notably II) in detecting ischemia during carotid endarterectomy.

ECG MONITORING WITH ST-SEGMENT TREND ANALYSIS (2 OR 3 LEADS). Although these devices are purported to facilitate easier detection of myocardial ischemia than can be obtained with simple oscilloscopic ECG traces, and although they might meet this stated goal,[66, 67] they should not be expected to be as sensitive as an ECG printout or 2D-TEE. In our preliminary study, they were approximately 70–90% as sensitive as a hard-copy ECG.[66]

CHANGES IN PULMONARY CAPILLARY WEDGE PRESSURE (PCWP) OR APPEARANCE OF V WAVES ON PCWP. Although changes in PCWP in the absence of systemic pressure changes or fluid administration may be a sensitive indicator of myocardial ischemia, such changes are not specific. The appearance of v waves on the PCWP may be specific (detection of ischemia where it is present), but v waves are not sensitive (normal where ischemia is not present) detectors of myocardial ischemia.[68] In addition, with the 2% carotid arterial puncture rate during cannulation of the internal jugular vein that has been reported in large series, it is difficult to justify that route during this operation. Most surgeons would postpone the operation to another day after disturbing the contralateral carotid. The risks of pulmonary artery (PA) catheter insertion from subclavian, external jugular, arm, or femoral sites do not justify the benefit. A PA catheter is not justified except in rare cases in which the patient is to undergo general anesthesia and the patient's only documented evidence of myocardial ischemia is that of PCWP changes without ST-segment changes, or in operations in which a 2D-TEE is unavailable or satisfactory echograms cannot be obtained.

ANGINA IN PATIENTS UNDERGOING REGIONAL ANESTHESIA. No reports on the usefulness of this symptom are available; and the incidence of myocardial ischemia and death from myocardial mechanisms after carotid endarterectomy performed during regional anesthesia is similar to that following general anesthesia.[69]

Cerebral Ischemia

REPEATED NEUROLOGIC EVALUATION OF THE CONSCIOUS PATIENT. This evaluation is cited as a major reason for choosing regional anesthesia. If the patient is to cooperate, he or she cannot be heavily sedated. Regional anesthesia thus requires a completely successful blockade and a surgeon who is accustomed to operating under this technique. Usually, the carotid artery is occluded for a 1- to 4-minute trial period; if no deficit is detected by neurologic examination, the surgeon proceeds with the endarterectomy. If a new neurologic deficit occurs, the surgeon releases the clamp. After reperfusion with return of neurologic function, some surgeons immediately proceed to reocclude the vessels and try rapidly to insert a shunt and complete the surgical procedure. However, in our experience, most surgeons prefer to cancel surgery at this point and return on another day to do the procedure under general anesthesia with a shunt. Still other surgeons apparently consider the lack of tolerance for carotid occlusion to be a contraindication for any further carotid surgery on such patients.[61] The disadvantages of the technique include the need for patient cooperation; the possible loss of patient cooperation with the onset of a neurologic deficit because of confusion, panic, or seizures; the possibility that an unexpected delayed deficit will develop at some time after the test period; the inability to administer drugs such as thiopental, which might protect the brain; and the inability to secure the airway if panic, seizure, or oversedation occurs. Those surgeons who revert to general anesthesia in the event of a deficit in response to test occlusion seem to perceive general anesthesia as best for the worst cases; if this is so, as Dr. J. Michenfelder states, "it should be best for most cases."[61]

The techniques for assaying of neurologic function during general anesthesia are discussed next.

ELECTROENCEPHALOGRAM. The scalp-recorded EEG reflects the electrical activity of the underlying cortical tissue. Conventional recording methods provide vast amounts of information, including a voltage value at each instant in time for each pair (16 or more) of electrodes. However, the interpretation of this type of information is unwieldy in the operating room. Data reduction methods have been developed with which the EEG is described in terms of several calculated variables, and the changes in these variables are charted over time.

Various physiologic and anesthetic manipulations have effects on the EEG. Reductions in cerebral blood flow, temperature changes, hypotension, and the administration of anesthetic agents have been shown to have characteristic effects on the EEG. The proper interpretation of EEG changes at surgery depends upon familiarity with the effects of the commonly used anesthetic agents and of temperature on the EEG. It should be remembered, however, that the blood flow threshold for electrical failure (approximately $18\ ml \cdot 100\ g^{-1} \cdot min^{-1}$) is higher than the blood flow threshold for metabolic failure (approximately 10 to $12\ ml \cdot 100\ g^{-1} \cdot min^{-1}$).[70]

The EEG can be viewed in a raw form, or it can be subjected to various transformations. For example, with the development of rapid computer transformation of the EEG by Fourier transform into spectral arrays of power and frequency, on-line assessment of the brain's electrical activity is made simpler. Generally, if focal ischemia occurs, the usual change is a localized decrease in frequency or decrease in amplitude or both.

How well does the EEG do as an early-warning signal of ischemia? How well does it do in improving the outcome after carotid endarterectomy? These are quite different questions. The EEG is a sensitive early-warning device, but it is not very specific (too many false-positive results), and we have no idea whether outcome is improved by its use. However, myocardial well-being may be improved more than cerebral well-being.

In the Mayo Clinic series of 1145 carotid endarterectomies that were monitored with EEG and xenon blood flow measurements, no patient awoke from anesthesia with a new deficit that had not been predicted by the EEG. An analysis of the results of a series of 111 carotid endarterectomies monitored with a single channel of the EEG that was analyzed in real time to produce a density spectral array[71] revealed that among patients with no preoperative neurologic deficit, new postoperative deficits appeared in only the five patients who had ischemic EEG events of 5 or more minutes' duration. However, the EEG was not as predictive of outcome in patients who had an existing preoperative neurologic deficit. One such patient without intraoperative EEG changes developed a new postoperative deficit, and one patient with EEG changes lasting 13 minutes had no demonstrable new deficit postoperatively.

The need for caution when monitoring patients with pre-existing neurologic deficits was emphasized in a report of 125 patients who had had strokes or reversible ischemic neurologic deficits (RIND) and who underwent carotid endarterectomy.[72] Four patients in that study awoke with new deficits, despite unchanged EEGs.

In a study of a series of 172 carotid endarterectomies,[73] EEG monitoring was undertaken in only the last 93 cases. The use of EEG monitoring was associated with a reduction in the use of indwelling shunts (from 49% to 12%) and a reduction of the combined major neurologic morbidity and mortality rates (from 2.3% to 1.1%). However, this study suffers from the use of historic controls and nonrandomization.

Other investigators have shown that EEG monitoring may be of limited use, because 65–95% of neurologic deficits following carotid endarterectomy are due to thromboembolic and not to flow-related events. Although both can easily be detected with the EEG, no major benefit will be achieved from any therapeutic maneuver to the 65–95% of patients in whom neurologic problems are detected. In fact, if more shunts or a higher afterload result, more emboli or worsening of myocardial oxygen balance could ensue. For example, one group[74] reviewed its experience with 176 consecutive patients undergoing carotid endarterectomy without shunt, but with EEG monitoring. The authors concluded that, although the majority of clamp-associated EEG changes were related to lowered regional cerebral blood flow (CBF), postoperative deficits in their series were usually caused by embolism. Other studies have yielded similar results.[75-76]

Other issues that have been raised in the evaluation of the appropriateness of EEG monitoring for carotid endarterectomy include the false-positive and false-negative results and the cost-effectiveness of EEG monitoring. Intraoperative false-positive results, that is, changes in the EEG without accompanying demonstrable deficits, may be related to several factors. First, the brain can tolerate relatively brief periods of ischemia without infarction. Thus, temporary, reversible EEG changes should not be expected in association with postoperative deficits. Second, the EEG must be viewed as a sensitive but nonspecific measure of ischemia. The EEG can be affected by factors such as anesthesia or alterations in temperature and blood pressure in addition to cerebral ischemia. Third, as stated previously, the flow threshold for electrical failure is higher than the flow threshold for metabolic failure. This means that, whereas the EEG may be viewed as an "early-warning system" for cerebral ischemia, not all EEG changes indicate that ischemia is taking place. Fourth, focal embolic events may not be detected by EEG. Except as noted previously, that is, in patients with pre-existing neurologic deficits, strokes in evolution, or recent RINDs, there are relatively few reports of false-negative results.

In general, patients who do not show intraoperative EEG changes do not awaken with new neurologic deficits. Since most neurologic deficits following carotid endarterectomy are not the result of flow-related ischemia, detection of EEG changes does not guarantee reversibility upon shunt placement. In fact, shunt placement is associated with a low, but definite risk of causing emboli.

The evaluation of the cost-effectiveness of EEG monitoring can be thought of as a comparison of the cost of monitoring with the cost of the deficits that monitoring may prevent. Let us assume that 100,000 carotid endarterectomies are performed each year with a deficit rate of 3% (3000 new deficits each year) and that use of monitoring devices might prevent one sixth of these deficits (i.e., 500 deficits per year). One might assume that an additional 15% of patients would receive temporary shunting of their carotid flow because of EEG monitoring and that 0.7% would experience "shunt insertion—associated" neurologic deficits. This would result in an additional 106 deficits related to the monitoring, or a net 394 deficits preventable by the monitoring. If each deficit costs $100,000, on average, in medical care and loss of wages and productivity, the deficits preventable by monitoring cost $39,400,000 per year. The break-even point for monitoring costs would be $394 per patient; at that price, the cost of monitoring would equal the cost of the deficits that monitoring would prevent. If monitoring could be provided for less than $394, it would be cost-effective. This analysis neglects the benefit that EEG monitoring may have in preserving myocardial function. It also neglects factors to which no dollar amount can be assigned, such as human suffering. If different values are assumed for the cost per deficit, for the percentage of deficits preventable by monitoring, and for the deficit rate, or for the shunt insertion—caused deficit rate, the break-even point will be higher or lower. But, as long as the percentage of deficits preventable by EEG monitoring is not zero, the break-even point will also not be zero. This implies that there is some cost below which monitoring is cost-effective for large-scale application, assuming that EEG monitoring is better at prevention than are other strategies of monitoring, such as somato-sensory evoked potentials (SSEP) or stump pressure (see Carotid Stump Pressure).

However, it is entirely possible that EEG monitoring would allow the anesthesiologist to maintain a lower blood pressure during the period of temporary carotid occlusion than would be feasible if only stump pressure was used. Thus, perhaps EEG monitoring provides a benefit in allowing one to decrease the afterload in the patient who is at risk for myocardial ischemic events, as well as permitting an unhurried and technically superior endarterectomy, identifying delayed ischemia, and aiding in the detection of other problems such as shunt malfunction.

Unfortunately, there are no data showing that this method of detection of neurologic dysfunction during carotid endarterectomy results in a better patient outcome than does any other method.

SOMATOSENSORY EVOKED POTENTIAL. Evoked potentials offer a method of processing the neural activity after a stimulus in which activity that is stimulus-related (signal) is separated from activity that is not related to the stimulus (noise). The primary problem with evoked potentials is an unfavorable signal-to-noise ratio. The neural potentials evoked by any sensory stimulus are small compared with the spontaneous activity that is recorded at the same time. When recorded noninvasively from the scalp, evoked cerebral electrical activity (the signal) from electrical stimulation of a peripheral nerve amounts to a few microvolts in amplitude, whereas the spontaneous electrical activity (noise) of the cerebrum can be of the order of 100 or more microvolts. The assumption made for separation of the signal from the noise is that the signal is always found after a certain latency period following the stimulation, whereas the noise bears no temporal relationship to the stimulus. By giving repeated stimuli and summing (or averaging) the resulting responses, one can "average out" the noise.

The most frequently used evoked potential during vascular procedures is the SSEP. This evoked potential is usually elicited by electrical stimulation of a selected peripheral nerve at an intensity sufficient to cause a twitch of the muscles supplied by that nerve. The resulting afferent activity may be recorded from rostral portions of the nerve, the spinal cord and brain stem, and thalamocortical projections. The variables

that describe evoked potentials are the *latency* (related to the conduction velocity characteristics of the pathway) and the *amplitude* (related to the number and synchrony of conducting fibers in the pathway) of the afferent volley recorded at successively higher levels of the nervous system. It has been observed that damage to the pathways mediating these responses is manifested as alterations in these two variables.[76]

Recently, investigators have started to examine the SSEP as a monitor of neurologic function during carotid endarterectomy. A case report on a 69-year-old woman undergoing carotid endarterectomy under general anesthesia without a shunt of the carotid flow is an example.[77] The median nerve was stimulated, and the resulting afferent activity was recorded from a cervical spinous process and from the scalp over the cortical somatosensory receiving area in the parietal cortex. The cortical evoked potential disappeared immediately after carotid cross-clamping, but the potential recorded from the nape of the neck was preserved. Immediately after awakening from anesthesia, the patient was noted to have a paresis and hypesthesia of the contralateral arm, but this effect cleared over the next 24 hours.

A series of 25 carotid endarterectomies was performed under general anesthesia without the use of an intraluminal shunt and with SSEP monitoring.[78] Two patients had no electrical response, one bilaterally and the other unilaterally, following carotid cross-clamping. The patient with the unilateral changes developed a perioperative stroke, the only one that occurred in that series.

Authors[79, 80] who have monitored the SSEP during carotid endarterectomy with both cervical-plexus blockade and general anesthesia reported, without providing critical evidence, that the SSEP is a sensitive measure of cerebral ischemia and of the need for a shunt. The rate of shunt placement based on SSEP was roughly the same as that when selective shunting was based on the EEG, that is, about 10%. However, the fact that the patients in this series had no complications upon awakening limits the conclusions that can be drawn concerning the predictive value of the SSEP in patients undergoing carotid endarterectomy.

Thus, the benefit of SSEP in monitoring of neurologic function during carotid endarterectomy is even more conjectural than is the role of EEG monitoring.

REGIONAL CEREBRAL BLOOD FLOW. Measurement of regional CBF usually involves washout of a radioisotope such as xenon-133 after its injection into a surgically occluded carotid artery.[1] Flows above $24 \ ml \cdot min^{-1} \cdot 100 \text{-} g^{-1}$ brain are regarded as satisfactory, and those below $18 \ ml \cdot min^{-1} \cdot 100 \text{-} g^{-1}$ brain are considered to indicate the potential for cerebral ischemia. These measurements require expensive and highly technical equipment in the operating room. Of the few centers that have such equipment, one has reported an excellent correlation between CBF and outcome, but flow differences representing ischemia were dependent upon the anesthetic agents used.[1, 81] Questions about this method of monitoring involve both its sensitivity and its specificity. As with all the other monitors of neurologic function during carotid endarterectomy, no benefit has yet been shown for it.

CAROTID STUMP PRESSURE. Stump pressure (mean blood pressure distal to the carotid clamp, also sometimes termed back pressure) is widely used for evaluation of the adequacy of cerebral perfusion during carotid surgery. Cerebral ischemia will rarely occur at stump pressures above 60 mm Hg during halothane anesthesia, presumably because of the excellent collateral circulation required for maintaining that pres sure[61, 82] and presumably because of the autoregulation that is present at this level. If the stump pressure decreases below that value, the likelihood of ischemia increases. However, since pressure is not identical to flow, it is possible for stump pressures to be below 60 mm Hg and for the flow to be perfectly adequate.

The major criticism of the use of stump pressure concerns the large number of false-positive results—that is, a stump pressure of less than 60 mm Hg and a regional CBF of more than 24 ml · min^{-1} · 100-g^{-1} brain. Such results occur in about 30% of patients.[82] Thus, a shunt may be placed when none is needed. However, the simplicity of the measurement and its validity when the pressure exceeds 60 mm Hg during anesthesia with volatile anesthetics still render it the most useful clinical method for ensuring adequate perfusion during carotid endarterectomy. The stump pressure must be higher during an opioid-based anesthesia for blood flow to be adequate.[82]

As with all other measures, no benefit has been proved for the use of stump pressure, but logic dictates that monitors that ensure adequate cerebral function at the lowest myocardial work have a role during carotid endarterectomy.

ANESTHESIA FOR SURGERY FOR CEREBROVASCULAR INSUFFICIENCY

Many surgeons have requested general anesthesia in surgery for patients with cerebrovascular insufficiency. If the patient has no medical problem that requires optimization before surgery, the preoperative interview focuses on reducing anxiety, obtaining informed consent, and searching for the status of end-organs likely to be affected by atherosclerosis, hypertension, or other diseases. In addition, multiple blood pressure and heart rate readings are obtained while the patient is in various positions, and the nurses are asked to obtain at least four additional such readings (one every 2 hours while the patient is awake, and one during the night) before surgery.

The preoperative values become important in defining a window of acceptable intraoperative values. To elaborate, such preoperative data are used to determine the individualized range of values considered tolerable for a particular patient during and after surgery; that is, if the blood pressure is 180/100 mm Hg and the heart rate is 96 beats · min^{-1} on admission, with no signs or symptoms of myocardial ischemia, the patient can probably tolerate these levels during surgery. If the blood pressure decreases during the night to 80/50 mm Hg and the heart rate decreases to 48 beats · min^{-1} and the patient does not awaken with signs of a new cerebral deficit, he or she can probably safely tolerate such levels during anesthesia. Thus, from preoperative data, an individualized set of values is derived for each patient. The cardiovascular variables are then kept within that range and, prior to induction of anesthesia, one should decide which therapies to use to accomplish that goal (e.g., administration of more or less anesthesia, nitroglycerin, or nitroprusside/dopamine, dobutamine, phenylephrine, or propranolol/esmolol/isoproterenol, atropine).

This type of planning is especially important for the patient who has suspected cardiovascular disease, such as is usual in the patient undergoing carotid endarterectomy. It is relatively unimportant for the totally healthy patient. It is unknown whether keeping cardiovascular variables within an individualized range of acceptable values improves the surgical outcome, but logic implies that using such a plan would reduce morbidity. For example, in several studies, major intraopera-

tive deviations of the blood pressure from the preoperative level have been correlated with the occurrence of myocardial ischemia.[12, 14, 83]

These acceptable values are listed at the top of the anesthesia record prior to induction of anesthesia. Prior to working with surgeons who routinely use the EEG, I worked with surgeons who wanted the patient's blood pressure to be at the upper end of his ward pressure. This desire on the part of the surgeons was based on data indicating better collateral CBF distal to a carotid occlusion if the systemic blood pressure was higher.[64] On the other hand, such an increase in blood pressure increases the work that the heart has to perform; thus, it increases the likelihood of myocardial ischemia.[12, 62] If the surgeon requires an increase in the patient's blood pressure above his or her upper limits of normal, as they sometimes do for a patient whose carotid flow cannot be shunted because of the anatomy of his lesion, we do so in a test period preoperatively, asking questions about angina and examining seven ECG leads for evidence of ischemia. Only rarely (2 of the approximately 1500 patients to whom I have administered anesthesia for carotid artery surgery) in patients in whom myocardial ischemia is evidenced by PCWP changes without ECG changes will we use a PA catheter during carotid surgery. I have tried to avoid inserting PA catheters during carotid artery surgery for two reasons: 1) There is little fluid shift during these operations, and 2) the rate of complications associated with PA catheters is reported to exceed that from carotid artery surgery at our institution.

Other data obtained during the preoperative visit and assessment are which ECG lead is most likely to reveal ischemia (often found on an exercise ECG study or from evaluation of a thallium redistribution study) and what is the patient's normal Pa_{CO_2} level. Usually, the latter can be assumed to be normal if the patient's bicarbonate level on an electrolyte panel is normal, or if the patient does not have a history suggestive of chronic obstructive pulmonary disease.

There is controversy concerning the optimal intraoperative carbon dioxide level in patients undergoing carotid endarterectomy.[64] Most practitioners now opt for slight hypocarbia or normocarbia.[55, 64] The maintenance of slight hypocarbia has the possible advantage of preferentially diverting CBF to potentially ischemic areas of the brain by constricting the nonischemic, normally reactive vessels.[55]

Historically, we have not given any premedication to patients about to undergo carotid artery surgery, because this might delay awakening and might confuse the results of tests of mental function prior to induction of anesthesia. Although we worried about the possibility of increasing anxiety[84] and causing myocardial ischemia because of this lack of premedication, only one patient among the 1500 whom we "premedicated" with only an interview for this operation has arrived in the preoperative holding area or operating room with angina or ECG evidence of myocardial ischemia. Either the preoperative interview is very effective,[84] or there is a substantial difference between our patients and those of Slogoff and Keats.[83] Thus, local custom as well as logical considerations have biased us in our treatment of such patients to seek the following goals with the techniques indicated:

1. Avoid myocardial ischemia by maintaining normal hemodynamics (especially normal heart rates). For this purpose, we usually monitor lead V_5 and lead II of the ECG for ST-T and heart rate changes and the transesophageal echocardiogram for wall-motion and systolic wall-thickening abnormalities.
2. Avoid cerebral ischemia by maintaining normal or high-

normal blood pressure and by shunting carotid flow if an abnormal EEG develops; maintain slight hypocarbia.

3. Use general anesthesia, but have the patient awake at the end of the operation. To accomplish this, we avoid drug premedication and "premedicate" only by interview, and we use light levels of volatile agents for general anesthesia.

4. Delay operations when there is uncontrolled hypertension, untreated pulmonary disease, myocardial infarction less than 3 months old with areas of myocardium still at risk, and uncontrolled metabolic diseases, unless crescendo TIAs are present.

Obviously, some goals are in conflict and have been modified by study results. For example, we could provide deeper anesthesia and maintain blood pressure with an alpha$_1$-adrenergic drug such as phenylephrine. However, we found that "light" general anesthesia and maintenance of the same systolic pressure is associated with one third the incidence of myocardial ischemia compared with that of "deep" anesthesia and the use of vasopressors to attain that blood pressure.[12] The usual procedure is as follows:

After the preoperative interview, the patient is made NPO after midnight, and an iv infusion is begun through an 18-gauge plastic cannula, ($D_5$0.45 NS) at a maintenance rate of 100 ml·hr^{-1}·70 kg^{-1}. This fluid administration is intended to ensure that the patient is not hypovolemic and thus subject to a large decrease in blood pressure during induction of anesthesia. When the patient arrives in the preoperative holding area, the intravenous (iv) solution is changed to normal saline and an 18-gauge arterial catheter is placed (after iodine prep and lidocaine skin wheal) in the radial artery contralateral to the planned carotid surgery. This arterial catheter is 18-gauge rather than 20-gauge because no greater morbidity ensues[85] and because the 20-gauge catheter tends to have a 5–10% incidence of kinking when surgeons "push" on the arm (with their bellies) during carotid dissection. Normal saline, rather than dextrose or lactated Ringer's solution, is used because lactate is metabolized to dextrose and because recent animal studies indicated that increasing blood glucose may increase neurologic damage after global ischemia.[86] Although some different results have been found for focal CNS ischemia in at least one laboratory,* and some investigators may say that survival is better with fructose than with saline,[87] the most prudent approach at this time seems to be to maintain normoglycemia.

The patient is then brought to the operating room and transferred to an operating table with an already warmed heating mattress. Here, EEG, ECG, blood pressure measurement, pulse oximetry, and other standard monitoring methods are applied, and the data are examined prior to induction of anesthesia. The heating mattress[88] is important for maintaining normothermia, which probably helps to reduce circulatory instability postoperatively.

Induction of anesthesia is then begun with a barbiturate. Some anesthesiologists titrate the dose at this time and during carotid occlusion to achieve burst suppression on the EEG,[55] because this electrical suppression is associated with a reduction of cerebral metabolism to as little as 40–50% of awake levels and, at the same time, decreases the CBF and intracranial pressure. Once burst suppression occurs, barbiturates have no further cerebral metabolic effect or any effet in pro-

*Pearl et al as presented at the meeting of the Association of University Anesthetics, Portland, Oregon, May 1987.

tecting the brain from ischemia.[89] We administer 100% oxygen, and 1 to 2 mg·kg^{-1} of thiopental and 3 mg of curare, followed by thiopental 25–50 mg (70 kg patient) intravenously, along with isoflurane at increasing concentrations in oxygen by mask. When the systolic blood pressure has been reduced by 20–30%, we administer 1.5 mg·kg^{-1} succinylcholine (assuming that the patient has no muscle or lower motor neuron [LMN] dysfunction), or atracurium or vecuronium or nothing if muscle or LMN dysfunction is present (see Chapter 13), and either 100 mg of lidocaine or 100 mg of thiopental (each given iv) to blunt the cardiovascular (blood pressure and heart rate) response to laryngoscopy and tracheal intubation. After the routine checks and after verification of endotracheal intubation by end-tidal capnography, a transesophageal echocardiographic probe is inserted to obtain echocardiographic images of a cross-section of the left ventricle at the level of the papillary muscles.

Controlled ventilation of the lungs is instituted at this time, often with 50% nitrous oxide in oxygen, and at other times with oxygen alone, titrating the concentration of isoflurane or enflurane, and adjusting the table position, to achieve the desired blood pressure. We avoid administering more than 10 ml·kg^{-1} of crystalloid or other fluid in this 2-hour operation, because increasing the fluid administration to these patients may contribute to postoperative hypertension. This results from the absence of baroreceptor function, which such patients usually exhibit.[90] The lack of baroreceptor function may also account for the stability that we find in these patients' heart rates intraoperatively.[12]

During the operation, "light" anesthesia is usually administered, with patient movement as well as hemodynamic changes signaling that the anesthesia is inadequate. If it cannot be ensured that the patient will be anesthetized sufficiently so that he will not move during the period of temporary carotid occlusion, a muscle relaxant is added, the choice of which is dictated by the heart rate response that one wishes to obtain (see Chapter 13).

Although the effects of anesthetics on normal CBF are known, the choice of an anesthetic for this operation appears to have no sound scientific basis. Perhaps the only information suggesting that one should choose isoflurane over other inhalational agents or opioids is that from a nonrandomized study at the Mayo Clinic,[81] it was evident that the CBF associated with ischemic changes in the EEG is 10 ml·min^{-1}·100 g^{-1} during isoflurane anesthesia, as opposed to about 20 ml·min^{-1}·100 g^{-1} with other agents, and that there is a less frequent need to shunt during isoflurane anesthesia than is the case during anesthesia with other agents.

Our preference to avoid opioids in these operations is based on our ability to have patients awaken shortly after the last stitch is placed (although this may now be possible with alfentanil) and the desire to avoid the hemodynamic effects of naloxone and of muscle relaxant reversal, not on the anecdotal evidence that opioids worsen the neurologic outcome after focal or global cerebral ischemia.[91]

Before beginning carotid occlusion, the surgeon infiltrates the carotid at the bifurcation with 1% lidocaine, with the hope of preventing the sudden onset of bradycardia during stretching of the baroreceptor or of the nerve from the varoreceptor. The anesthetic depth is then kept at a minimum, so that the blood pressure increases to the upper ward level. If no EEG evidence of ischemia is found, or if the stump pressure is comfortably above 50 mm Hg, the anesthetic depth is increased somewhat and the systemic blood pressure falls slightly. If myocardial ischemia is indicated by one of our monitors, we treat it by reversing the hemodynamic cause, if any, or by administering nitroglycerin when no obvious hemodynamic cause exists. Such myocardial ischemia occurred between 8 and 35% of the time at this point in the operation in our studies[12]; we do not know the cause of this event at this time, because the hemodynamics did not differ substantially from that just prior to cross-clamping.

After the carotid artery repair is completed and the flow in the carotid is restored, the focus again shifts totally to the patient's myocardial well-being. When the muscle layer is repaired, the patient is allowed to resume spontaneous ventilation. Usually, the surgeons identify the recurrent laryngeal nerve; this enables extubation of the trachea in as light a plane of anesthesia as possible, but before the gag reflex is restored. Usually within 2 to 3 minutes after the last stitch, the patient will respond to pain, and, before leaving the operating room (and usually within 4 to 6 minutes after the last stitch), the patient is able to follow simple commands.

The four problems feared most in the postanesthesia care unit are hemodynamic instability, respiratory insufficiency (usually as a result of vocal cord paresis), hematoma formation, and onset of new neurologic dysfunction.

Circulatory instability is usually evidenced by hypertension, but it is reported in the literature that hypotension also occurs. Since we began hydrating patients starting the night before surgery, giving antihypertensives, including diuretics on the morning of surgery, using a heating blanket to help maintain temperature, and limiting our intraoperative administration of crystalloid to 10 ml·kg^{-1}, the incidence of postoperative hypotension has dropped to zero, and the incidence of postoperative hypertension has decreased to about 10% (from 35%). Although this change is based on historical controls and is anecdotal, any hypertension needs vigorous treatment so that the myocardial work is decreased. We often titrate combinations of nitroprusside or hydralazine and propranolol or esmolol or labetalol to achieve normotension. Such therapies have been found superior to administration of nitroglycerin or trimethaphan in an elegant study on post-CABG patients by Stinson et al.[92] Other causes of hypertension are sought (e.g., pain, a full bladder, myocardial ischemia, hypoxia, hypercarbia). However, the association of hypertension and neurologic deficit postoperatively is too strong (assuming that the patient is neurologically normal) to allow one to let the hypertension persist.[93]

Other authors have stated that hypotension following carotid endarterectomy is due to hypersensitivity of the carotid sinus nerve,[94] but we have found that significant hypotension (<80 mm Hg systolic) is often associated with myocardial ischemia. We routinely obtain a 12-lead ECG soon after the patient's arrival in the postanesthesia care unit, and we monitor the ECG lead(s) most noted or likely to detect ischemia in these patients, which often proves to be lead II following carotid surgery (not lead V$_5$).[65]

Ventilatory insufficiency can appear as stridor owing to unilateral or, more often, bilateral vocal cord paresis (in the patient who has undergone bilateral carotid operations, or a thyroidectomy and a carotid operation), to hematoma, or to deficient carotid-body function in patients who chronically retain CO_2. In the case of stridor, immediate securing of the airway is necessary; treatment of hematomas can consist of opening of the suture line and application of external drainage. (This may need to be done even in the postanesthesia care unit. I have been involved in only one of each of the two previously mentioned procedures in 1500 anesthetics for carotid artery surgery that I have given.) The chemoreceptor function of the carotid body is predictably damaged for up to 10 months following carotid endarterectomy, with complete loss of the ventilatory and circulatory response to hypoxia following bilateral endarterectomy.[90] Such loss results in an increase in the Pa$_{CO_2}$ of 6 mm Hg at rest, and, for this reason, the routine use of supplemental oxygen is justified, at least until the patient ambulates.

Wound hematoma from venous oozing usually accumulates slowly, but both it and arterial hemorrhage can threaten the airway. This is probably the most painful part of most carotid operations. (Pain relief stronger than that provided by acetaminophen is usually not required for most patients.) Re-exploration in the operating room is occasionally necessary, but rapid opening of the wound in the recovery room can be lifesaving in an emergency.

ANESTHESIA FOR EMERGENCY CAROTID ARTERY REVASCULARIZATION

Etiology and Indications

The results of some recent studies indicate that the reluctance to perform emergency carotid endarterectomy in patients who have fluctuating neurologic deficits may be unwarranted.[95, 96] Therefore, anesthesiologists may be presented more frequently than in the past with patients who have crescendo TIAs or stroke in evolution and who are candidates for emergency carotid revascularization. Indications may include tight stenosis (<95%) with or without symptoms, symptomatic occlusion in the first 6 to 10 hours after occlusion sets in, and recent carotid endarterectomy that either led to bleeding or has resulted in new neurologic symptoms.

Anesthetic Management

PREOPERATIVE PREPARATION AND INDUCTION OF ANESTHESIA. A patient undergoing emergency carotid endarterectomy may have a full stomach and thus may require protection against aspiration of gastric contents. The main goal is to minimize the hemodynamic stress of a rapid-sequence anesthesia induction while maintaining adequate perfusion pressure across the stenotic lesion. The patient is allowed to breathe 100% oxygen. Venous access is secured, and peripheral arterial cannulation is performed for direct monitoring of systemic blood pressure and for obtaining blood samples for determination of gas tensions. One should then proceed with a rapid-sequence iv induction with a short-acting barbiturate, a muscle relaxant, and endotracheal intubation. Before intubation of the trachea, a bolus of lidocaine (1.5 mg·kg^{-1}) or sodium nitroprusside (1 to 2 μg·kg^{-1}) may be administered iv for attenuation of the hypertensive response to visualization of the larynx and the intubation. Hypotension is treated by tilting of the table and/or by iv infusion of phenylephrine or methoxamine (direct alpha$_1$-adrenergic agonists). If a PA catheter is desired (the indications for this in the patient requiring emergency exploration of the carotid artery are not common), a peripheral brachial or subclavian vein contralateral to the operative side can be used as the site of insertion. If the patient is believed to have an empty stomach, a gentle titrated induction of anesthesia with barbiturate, followed by inhalation of a volatile anesthetic at increasing concentrations, is often used. The roles of nonparticulate antacids, histamine receptor-blocking drugs, and/or metoclopramide remain controversial.

General anesthesia is maintained with any one of a variety of techniques aimed at attenuating hemodynamic fluctuations, achieving normocarbia (or a CO_2 level slightly below normal as in elective operations), and maintaining adequate carotid artery perfusion pressure. An anesthetic technique similar to that used in elective situations is used.

If a hematoma is noted near the operative site and surgical exploration is anticipated, oxygen is given at high concentration by face mask with a reservoir bag or Ayre's T-piece. A tracheostomy or cricothyroidotomy tray should be immediately available. It may be difficult to visualize the trachea because of edema or because of deviation away from the hematoma, caused by pressure of the hematoma. In the event of acute airway obstruction, a high concentration of oxygen in the functional residual volume of the lung may provide additional protection against hypoxemia until the airway is secured by intubation or until the hematoma is evacuated surgically.

If the hematoma does not obstruct the airway and the patient is not having difficulty breathing spontaneously, induction may be accomplished as in an elective procedure. If the airway appears compromised, topical anesthesia for the lips, tongue, posterior pharynx, and epiglottis is provided. The larynx is then visualized. If no difficulty with endotracheal intubation is anticipated, induction is performed as described previously. However, if difficulty is expected, the wound is opened and drained externally, and endotracheal intubation is performed before general anesthesia is induced.

If a new neurologic deficit occurs in the postanesthesia recovery unit, most surgeons believe that immediate re-exploration is indicated, and logic would dictate utilization of pharmacologic methods of "cerebral protection," but this "logic" is controversial.

Thus, the most common causes of morbidity following carotid endarterectomy dictate the following goals:

1. To protect the heart from ischemia
2. To protect the brain from ischemia
3. To be able to have the patient awaken soon after the operation.

These seemingly diverse goals can result in a consonant monitoring technique (such as the EEG, which may aid both the heart and the CNS by allowing afterload reduction if normal CNS electrical activity is present) and in therapies such as injection of local anesthetic around the carotid sinus nerve for prevention of increases in myocardial oxygen demand and avoidance of sudden bradycardia, and hypotension. As in most aspects of anesthesia, meticulous attention to details such as overnight hydration and the intraoperative use of warming mattresses may be as important as the choice of anesthetic agents or even of monitoring techniques.

I have exposed my biases in both monitoring and anesthetic techniques, but it should be clear that many other techniques can be used for avoiding myocardial and cerebral dysfunction postoperatively. The major postoperative complications that can lead to adverse sequelae include circulatory instability, which may be due to either myocardial or cerebral ischemia or other causes, including respiratory insufficiency resulting from edema, laryngeal nerve trauma, inadequate or too vigorous hydration, inadequate prevention of hypothermia, or deficient carotid chemoreceptor function; wound hematoma, which may compromise the airway; and a new neurologic deficit. Each of these factors may require emergency treatment.

SURGERY FOR VISCERAL ISCHEMIA, THORACOABDOMINAL AORTIC ANEURYSMS, AND INFRARENAL AORTIC RECONSTRUCTION

SURGICAL APPROACHES TO AND PATHOPHYSIOLOGY OF VISCERAL ISCHEMIA AND THORACOABDOMINAL AORTIC ANEURYSMS

In vascular surgery, perhaps more than in other types of surgery, understanding the pathophysiology of the disease and anticipating the surgical approach and techniques can allow the anesthesiologist to serve his or her patient most effectively. The surgical goal in these operations is to create an enduring restoration of the normal circulation to the viscera while, at the same time, minimizing the duration of ischemia to viscera, especially to the renal circulation. Stating this goal is easy, but the performance of it is difficult, because each of the possible surgical approaches leads to compromises in the achievement of some aspects of this goal while optimizing the performance of other aspects.[97] For example, the site of origin of the bypass graft to the celiac axis is an important consideration. Whereas the supraceliac aorta is usually relatively free of atheroma and a graft from this site lies anatomically so that there is antegrade flow at all times, the exposure of this segment of the aorta is more difficult than that of the infrarenal aorta. Most surgeons have limited experience with the supraceliac region and are naturally hesitant about working in unfamiliar areas. Probably the major concern is the need for suprarenal clamping and the subsequent risk of ischemic renal damage. This complication in an elderly patient with arterial disease may prove fatal, and it is this added potential for morbidity that prevents the routine use of supraceliac grafting. On the other hand, although the use of the infrarenal aorta as the site of origin of the bypass graft provides familiar territory for the surgeon, this infrarenal site is often diseased; also, after grafting, flow is not always antegrade, and kinking or twisting of vessels may be likely.

The pathologic conditions giving rise to chronic visceral ischemia include atherosclerotic occlusive disease as well as fibromuscular dysplasia, inflammatory arteriopathies, external compression, and aneurysmal atherosclerotic disease.

In most cases, symptomatic disease of the mesenteric artery is due to atherosclerotic narrowing of the origins of the three major visceral vessels: celiac, superior mesenteric, and inferior mesenteric arteries. This disease is usually an extension of atheroma of the aorta into the origins of its branches. It rarely extends more than 1 to 2 cm into the visceral arteries, and it has a well-defined end point.[98, 99] The distal thoracic aorta is often spared, but concomitant disease of the infrarenal vasculature is common. The lesion in the superior mesenteric artery may be more extensive than the celiac lesion, and propagation of thrombus to the first major collateral vessel (the inferior pancreaticoduodenal artery) often leaves a relatively long occluded segment.

A lateral aortogram is required for demonstration of the origins of the unpaired anterior aortic branches, including the celiac axis, superior mesenteric artery, and inferior mesenteric artery. The extensive collateral network of the gut is usually sufficient to maintain an adequate intestinal blood supply if one of these vessels is occluded. Morris et al,[100] in 1966, was the first investigator to suggest that occlusion or major stenosis of at least two of these three arteries was necessary for compromise of the collateral supply and production of symptoms of visceral ischemia. This two-vessel-disease-requirement-for-symptoms concept is currently accepted, with few cases of single-vessel lesions reported as symptomatic in any series.[101, 102] However, single-vessel lesions may be important when previous intraabdominal surgery has interrupted collateral pathways.

When there is occlusive disease in the celiac and superior mesenteric arteries, the major mesenteric supply often comes from the inferior mesenteric artery via the marginal artery. If the inferior mesenteric artery is not revascularized during infrarenal aortic grafting, the risk of bowel ischemia is present, with a reported incidence of colonic infarction after aortic operations of 1–2% and that of small bowel infarction of 0.15%, and with a mortality of up to 90% after the occurrence of such infarction.[103, 104]

Other, less common causes of visceral ischemia include fibromuscular dysplasia, in association with superior mesenteric insufficiency,[101] Takayasu's arteritis,[103] and external compression of the celiac axis by the median arcuate ligament of the diaphragm.[99] All three of these conditions most commonly occur in women between the ages of 20 and 40 years, as contrasted with chronic ischemia in atherosclerotic arteriopaths or with acute occlusive disease, which occurs in the elderly, who often are hypertensive, and in persons who have smoked cigarettes extensively. Acute mesenteric occlusion is of either embolic or thrombotic origin. If embolic, it commonly has a cardiac source and may follow a recent myocardial infarction. If thrombotic, it may occasionally be due to aortic dissection or trauma but is usually based on progressing atherosclerosis. Sudden occlusion of the superior mesenteric artery, without previous development of collateral vessels, can lead to bowel infarction within a few hours. The diagnosis is often difficult in the early phase. The patient frequently complains of severe pain in the absence of specific signs, until peritonitis develops as a result of intestinal gangrene. The diagnosis must be strongly suspected in patients with prior cardiac disease who suddenly develop central abdominal pain, often severe, but with minimal physical signs in the first 4 to 6 hours.[97] If surgical intervention occurs before gangrene of the bowel develops, revascularization will reduce the otherwise high mortality and morbidity.

An embolus can usually be extracted by Fogarty catheter from the superior mesenteric artery by means of a direct approach to the proximal artery. Surgeons worry that fragmentation of the embolus in the attempt at catheter embolization with occlusion of the distal branches may make full revascularization impossible. However, proponents of this approach believe that clearance of major vessels will limit the extent of bowel infarction. Thrombolytic agents may prove useful for removal of distal embolic fragments, but their use has not yet been established.[105]

More invasive surgery is usually attempted for both acute and chronic visceral ischemia. Long-term results of surgical management of chronic visceral ischemia depend upon the extent of the revascularization that is undertaken.[101] Single-vessel repair is associated with rates of recurrence of symptoms as high as 50%. In contrast, full revascularization is associated with recurrence of symptoms in only 11% of cases. These data lead to the current practice in elective procedures of performing as complete a revascularization as possible.[98, 106–109]

Elective surgery for asymptomatic mesenteric occlusive disease is generally not justified, as the risks of surgery often outweigh the possible gains. The perioperative mortality rates range from 7.5 to 18%.[98, 101, 102, 107] Cardiac disorders, postoperative hemorrhage, and early graft occlusion with bowel infarction are the major causes of perioperative death.

The approach to the visceral arteries is determined by the vessels involved and by the procedure contemplated for restoration of adequate blood flow. The choice may depend upon the surgeon's preference for either endarterectomy or bypass, or a combination of both.[97]

Generous exposure of the thoracic and abdominal aorta and its major branches is obtained with a left thoracoabdominal incision and retroperitoneal dissection. The incision is made over the eighth intercostal space and is extended obliquely across the left abdomen toward the symphysis pubis. A retroperitoneal plane of dissection anterior to the left kidney exposes the abdominal aorta and the diaphragm, which is divided circumferentially close to the rib attachments so that innervation is preserved. Good exposure of the descending aorta to the bifurcations of the iliac arteries is obtained, and all major aortic branches can be controlled with this approach. However, the dissection is more extensive than that with a transabdominal approach, and the left thoracic cavity is entered, with possible added morbidity. The thoracoabdominal approach is favored for complex thoracoabdominal aortic replacement in the presence of stenotic or aneurysmal disease. In these major grafting procedures, the visceral branches are often excised from the parent aorta with a button of aortic wall. If needed, endarterectomy of these branch vessels is performed before they are attached to small openings cut in the graft at appropriate positions.[97, 107] If aortic replacement is not used, endarterectomy of any or all of the major branches of the aorta may be performed with this exposure.

Single-vessel endarterectomy may be carried out for either the celiac axis or the superior mesenteric artery. After exposure of these vessels, and with control of the aorta above and below, the celiac axis is opened transversely at the distal extent of the palpable atheroma. A plane of dissection is found, and retrograde endarterectomy to the aorta is performed. The arteriotomy is then closed directly, and the flow is restored. It is difficult to obtain a clean end point in the distal aortic atheroma, and, for this reason, not many surgeons use this technique.

Two major controversies are still unresolved with respect to bypass options in the presence of mesenteric vascular disease. The first controversy concerns the choice of bypass material (whether it is to be autologous or synthetic), and the second refers to the site of origin of the graft. Synthetic grafts are undesirable in cases of actual or potential bowel contamination but have long-term patency rates equal to those for autologous grafts in the conditions associated with mesenteric disease without bowel contamination.[101, 107] This situation differs from that in femoral-popliteal bypass, in which autologous grafts result in substantially higher patency rates.

As stated previously, the site of origin of the graft is usually selected on the basis of the familiarity of the surgeon; a healthy vessel is chosen, and antegrade flow is preferred. Synthetic grafts require a live tissue buffer between them and the gut (e.g., omentum can be the buffer). The orientation of the graft in an anatomic position provides antegrade flow, which is considered advantageous because turbulence is minimized and development of neointima is lessened. This is best achieved with a supraceliac origin of the graft and end-to-end anastomosis of the recipient vessel(s). If the graft origin is infrarenal, a long, curved course for the graft and an end-to-end anastomosis will allow direct antegrade flow into the superior mesenteric artery.[110] A direct line to the superior mesenteric artery with end-to-side anastomosis is thought to maximize turbulence and graft kinking. An infrarenal graft origin for revascularization of the celiac axis does not allow an easy direct anastomosis to the recipient vessel. Instead, most surgeons choose to anastomose the graft end-to-side to the splenic or common hepatic branch of the celiac axis.[107, 110]

A major problem with revascularization of the superior mesenteric artery from an infrarenal graft origin, with end-to-side anastomosis in the base of the small bowel mesentery, is the mobility of the mesentery and the tendency for such grafts to kink and thrombose. This problem does not arise with supraceliac grafts and end-to-end anastomosis. To overcome the problem of kinking from the infrarenal location, surgeons have used externally supported Goretex grafts.[109] Another approach to this problem involves constructing a very short H-anastomosis from the anterior aortic wall to the proximal superior mesenteric artery in the manner of a portacaval shunt with a very short, but wide (10 mm) graft.[110]

Thus, surgical problems abound in this condition. Symptomatic intestinal ischemia is uncommon because of extensive development of collaterals between the branches of the three major vessels of the mesenteric supply. At least two of these vessels are usually diseased before symptoms develop unless other surgery has been performed that interrupted the collateral network. Patients with chronic ischemia have postprandial abdominal pain, weight loss, and minimal signs apart from an epigastric bruit. Thoracoabdominal aneurysms occur in patients with hypertension or other risk factors for atherosclerotic disease. Acute mesenteric ischemia is often caused by emboli from the heart and is accompanied by acute, severe abdominal pain but minimal signs in the first 4 to 6 hours before bowel infarction and peritonitis develop.

Results of surgery in these conditions are improved if revascularization of all involved mesenteric vessels is performed. A transabdominal approach is satisfactory for most procedures, including supraceliac grafting. A left thoraco-retroperitoneal approach is advantageous for transaortic endarterectomy of the celiac axis and superior mesenteric artery and for thoracoabdominal aneurysms. Surgery is indicated for symptomatic patients and for a small group of asymptomatic patients with proven major occlusive disease of mesenteric vessels who are to undergo a concomitant intraabdominal procedure that is likely to interrupt collateral pathways. Such procedures include aortic reconstruction for occlusive or aneurysmal disease and colonic, smallbowel, or gastric resections.

Controversy exists as to the optimal surgical approach to the creation of enduring revascularizations. Both endarterectomy and grafting techniques are reported to yield satisfactory long-term results. The autogenous vein bypass does not appear to provide a clear advantage in this disease, and many surgeons prefer synthetic conduits because of their lower rate of kinking. In acute situations in which there is potential contamination of the abdominal cavity, endarterectomy or autogenous grafting are the only safe options. Transluminal balloon angioplasty for chronic situations and thrombolytic agents for acute ischemia are potentially useful new options for these patients.

SURGICAL APPROACHES FOR AND PATHOPHYSIOLOGY OF DISEASES NECESSITATING INFRARENAL AORTIC RECONSTRUCTION

Reconstruction of the abdominal aorta is performed either for replacement in the presence of aneurysmal degenerative disease or for increased inflow to and outflow from a vessel with stenosing occlusive disease. Although the natural history of the two diseases is different, the segmental nature of the disease processes, with relatively normal vessels above and below the lesion, provides the basis for reconstruction in each.

Aneurysmal Disease

Aneurysms pose an ever-present threat to the life of the patient because of their unpredictable tendency to rupture or embolize. Therefore, aggressive surgical management is warranted, even in the absence of symptoms.[111–113] Patients with aneurysms of the abdominal aorta who have not been operated on, have an 80% 5-year mortality rate, predominantly owing to rupture.[114–116] A larger diameter of the aneurysm is associated with a higher risk of rupture, with about a 25% 5-year incidence rate of rupture for lesions 4 to 7 cm, 45% for those 7 to 10 cm, and 60% for lesions larger than 10 cm.[116] The larger the aneurysm, the greater the likelihood of early rupture, with 71.8% of fatal ruptures of larger lesions occurring in the first 2 years, compared with 39.1% of fatal ruptures of smaller lesions during that time.[117]

Successful surgical repair of an abdominal aortic aneurysm is associated with prolonged life expectancy.[17, 20, 112, 113, 115] Improvements in surgical and anesthetic management have led to a steady decline in perioperative mortality rate, from approximately 17% prior to 1960 to 2–5% since 1980 in elective cases, despite broadening indications for surgery.[20, 118, 119] During the same period of time, however, mortality rates following surgery of ruptured aneurysms have remained high, ranging from 25 to 75%.[112, 120, 121]

Recommended preoperative evaluations of the patient's anatomy include palpation alone, ultrasound, CT scan, digital subtraction angiography, aortography, and magnetic resonance imaging (MRI). More invasive testing exposes the patient to risks and increases costs but allows determination of the presence of iliac occlusive or aneurysmal disease, juxtarenal or suprarenal extension of the aneurysm, renal artery aneurysmal or occlusive disease, and visceral artery lesions, including the presence of a "meandering mesenteric artery" (a collateral artery), horseshoe kidney, accessory renal arteries, A–V fistula, and disease of other organs.

No single approach has been shown in a randomized clinical trial to yield the best results for the patient. Clinical judgment remains the basis for individualizing tests for each patient with this disease, even when it is asymptomatic.

Occlusive Disease

Occlusive disease tends to be progressive, with compromise of the distal circulation leading to disabling claudication or limb-threatening ischemia. In the case of aneurysmal disease, surgery is indicated whenever the disease is present; in the case of occlusive disease, surgical intervention is indicated only for the relief of disabling symptoms.[111]

In setting out to correct occlusive disease of the aortoiliac segment, the surgeon endeavors to return to near normal the inflow to the limbs at the groin while maintaining flow to the internal iliac and visceral branches. The mean age of patients undergoing aortoiliac reconstruction is 54 years; these patients are more than 10 years younger, on the average, than those with aneurysmal disease of the aorta.[122]

Patients who have critical limb ischemia and stenotic aortoiliac disease commonly have concomitant occlusive lesions of the femoral, popliteal, or tibial vessels. The incidence of distal femoropopliteal occlusive disease in patients undergoing repair of an abdominal aortic aneurysm is approximately 11%; for occlusive aortoiliac procedures, it is much higher (45% or more).[122–125] The patency of an aortobifemoral bypass depends upon the status of distal occlusive disease in the femoral segment.[123, 126] The need for subsequent femoro-popliteal bypass can be reduced greatly if the profunda femoris artery is opened by profundoplasty performed concomitantly with the aortobifemoral bypass.[125, 127]

Surgical Techniques

CHOICE OF EXPOSURE. The most popular surgical exposure for either occlusive or aortic disease is that through a vertical anterior midline abdominal incision, with a transperitoneal approach to the retroperitoneal structures. This approach is versatile, providing access to all major arteries between the diaphragm and pelvis. The other major approach is a retroperitoneal one anterior to the kidney. Such an approach appears to be associated with more limited blood loss and with lower intraoperative fluid requirements. Postoperatively, ileus occurs less often, and oral intake can be resumed after a shorter period of time. Less pain is experienced, as judged by opioid requirements; and fewer pulmonary complications appear to occur with shorter hospital stays.

GRAFT REPLACEMENT. After the relevant portion of the aorta and the iliac arteries are exposed, the segment of the aorta involved by aneurysm is replaced by a graft. Heparin is commonly administered systemically so that the risk of thromboembolic complications is lessened. If the aortic graft is to be preclotted, blood for preclotting is usually harvested before the heparin is given. It is now recognized that distal ischemia complicating aortic surgery is related to the dislodgement of atheroemboli from the diseased aorta. The recognition of the embolic nature of distal ischemic problems prompted Starr et al[128] to perform aneurysm resections without administration of heparin. In their series of 434 procedures, there was only one case of embolism. Thus, in the absence of major distal occlusive disease, systemic heparinization may be unnecessary in the repair of abdominal aortic aneurysms; careful technique is probably a more important factor for avoidance of distal ischemia.[128, 129]

A tube graft (i.e., end-to-end anastomoses on both sides), in which the graft is covered with old aorta, is often used for aneurysmal resection. When the iliac vessels are not aneurysmal or stenotic, a tube graft may be used as replacement for the diseased aorta, thus making the procedure faster, with less blood loss.[129]

The standard graft material, in use since the late 1950s, has been Dacron, in either knitted or woven form.[111] More recently, polytetrafluoroethylene grafts, which are less porous, have become available. Knitted Dacron grafts are quite porous and require preclotting before implantation. These grafts develop a larger pseudointima and, as a result, may have good resistance to late infection.[130] In addition, they are relatively pliable and easy to suture, and they do not fray at the edges when cut. On the other hand, woven Dacron grafts are non-porous and do not require preclotting; this is a considerable advantage in patients with ruptured aneurysms and in those with a bleeding diathesis. A pseudointima does not form as readily, and the incidence of late infection may be greater than that for knitted grafts.[130] If woven Dacron is cut by sharp instruments, its edges tend to fray; but this can be overcome by use of an electrocautery for cutting the graft. Woven grafts are more rigid and not as easily manipulated as are knitted grafts. Both appear to be associated with rare episodes of anaphylactic reactions, which may be related to the stabilizers used in their manufacture.[131]

Since there is no need to exclude a segment of artery from the circulation when aortoiliac occlusive disease is present, the proximal anastomosis of the graft to the aorta is often performed in an end-to-side configuration after an ellipse of anterior aortic wall has been excised. If there is any suggestion of early aneurysmal dilatation, however, this segment must be excluded. Similarly, advanced degenerative changes in the infrarenal aorta may require end-to-end placement of the graft so that subsequent embolization of atheromatous debris can be avoided. In either case, because of the expected progression of disease, the origin of any graft is usually placed as close to the renal arteries as possible.[132]

Occlusive disease may be managed by endarterectomy or angioplasty. The former procedure is now reserved for isolated lesions of iliac origin or for unusual situations in which the use of synthetic material is contraindicated, such as in sepsis. In general, bypass procedures have proved to yield long-lasting and very satisfactory results for treatment of occlusive disease.

In the long term, surgical resection of abdominal aortic aneurysms has been shown to result in approximately double the life expectancy achieved with nonsurgical management. Bypass for occlusions in the aortoiliac region has been shown to provide good long-term patency, and limb salvage rates are high. Increasing severity of distal occlusive disease is associated with poorer patency rates. Sepsis associated with groin incisions and repeat surgery remain major problems for successful treatment.

Arterial reconstructive surgery has been developed based on the principle of anatomic correctness. Although this is usually the easiest and best option, situations do occur that require less advantageous revascularization procedures. Such situations include repeat surgery, surgery for graft infection, the presence of contraindications to transabdominal surgery (e.g., sepsis, adhesions, radiation therapy, malignancy), as well as less traumatic alternatives in frail, usually elderly, high-risk patients. In general, the price paid when alternative techniques are used is reduced long-term patency. Axillofemoral bypass, with the use of synthetic material in a subcutaneous tunnel, is the most popular extraanatomic bypass for aortoiliac reconstruction.[133, 134] Surgery involves exposure of relatively superficial arteries in the axilla and groin, with a long subcutaneous tract between them. The long-term patency of such grafts is significantly poorer than that for aortofemoral grafts, although surgical revision may be performed with good results.[134] The patency rate of the initial graft at 3 years is only 54% with this procedure.[133, 135]

Another option for reconstruction in the presence of unilateral iliac occlusive disease is femorofemoral bypass, either alone or in combination with axillounifemoral or aorto-unifemoral bypass.[133] These procedures are used with the knowledge that long-term patency rates are lower. The current development of forms of transluminal treatment for occlusive disease, including the use of lasers and angioplasty, promises new horizons in this field.

Several situations, both in patients with aneurysmal disease and in those with occlusive disease, may cause the surgeons to change from an infrarenal procedure, which is less risky to the heart and other organs, to a suprarenal procedure. Aneurysms of the abdominal aorta involve the pararenal aorta in up to 20% of cases.[136] Also, significant stenosis of the renal artery may coexist with an abdominal aortic aneurysm in an infrarenal or pararenal site, and correction of these renal artery lesions may well be contemplated in conjunction with aneurysm repair. Significant stenoses of the celiac trunk or superior mesenteric artery may similarly be addressed at the time of aortic reconstruction. Aortic surgery for a patient who has previously undergone aortic surgery will frequently necessitate revision to a higher graft origin; and problems with infection in prosthetic materials may require a clean site for a new graft origin. Ruptured aneurysms often must be controlled initially by supraceliac clamping.

In chronic aortic occlusion, even in the absence of disabling claudication, the risk of embolic disease in the kidneys is high, and surgery should be performed for re-establishment of distal aortic flow. During operative manipulation and clamping, great care must be taken that material is not dislodged into the renal arteries. Many surgeons first clamp the aorta above the level of the renal vessels, open the infrarenal aorta, and clear out the thrombus, then move the aortic clamp to an infrarenal position before proceeding with bypass grafting from the infrarenal aorta.[132]

Thus, many situations may arise that require aortic cross-clamping more cephalad than in the usual infrarenal position. Cardiac and renal function is most at risk in these situations, with patients known to have preoperative renal insufficiency being at greatest risk of developing postoperative renal failure. These and other concerns that the anesthesiologist can assist in managing are discussed in the following section.

ANESTHETIC GOALS IN SURGERY FOR AORTIC AND VISCERAL ARTERY RECONSTRUCTION

For minimal morbidity and mortality, the anesthetic goals are to preserve: 1) myocardial, 2) renal, 3) pulmonary, 4) CNS, and 5) visceral organ function. To meet these goals, one must ensure an adequate oxygen supply to the myocardium commensurate with need, at the same time reducing, if possible, the myocardial requirement for oxygen, and maintain adequate perfusion to all other organs. This latter objective usually requires preservation of adequate intravascular volume so that cardiac output can be maintained.

Pathophysiologic Events

To better understand the monitors that are used and why they are used, it is helpful to be aware of the pathophysiologic events that occur on application and removal of aortic cross-clamps.

Occlusion of the aorta causes hypertension in the proximal segment and hypotension in the distal segment. During resection of a congenitally coarcted aorta, acute occlusion of the thoracic aorta has very little effect on cardiovascular variables because of the normal development, over the years, of extensive collateral vessels around the coarctation. However, in patients who have an aortic aneurysm or atherosclerosis and who have no extensive collateral circulation, aortic occlusion increases afterload and peripheral vascular resistance in proportion to the level of the occlusion. We have found that myocardial stress varies with the level of occlusion.[14]

Myocardial performance and circulatory variables remain within an acceptable range after the aorta is occluded at infrarenal levels.[14] This result is in agreement with many of the findings in previous work. In 1968, Perry[137] demonstrated that the increase in afterload after temporary infrarenal aortic occlusion had little effect on circulatory variables. The use of newer, more sophisticated techniques has shown that deepening anesthesia or administering vasodilating drugs at the time of infrarenal aortic occlusion maintains indices of myocardial performance within an acceptable range,[28–30, 138] even in sick patients (in our series, 25% had severe left ventricular dysfunction before aortic surgery). Abnormalities of ventricu-

lar wall motion and systolic thickening, as well as changes in the ejection fraction, appear to be early signs of myocardial ischemia.[139] However, we did not detect abnormal motion of myocardial walls in any of the patients with infrarenal occlusion.[14] Thus far, the results of only one study contradicted the view that myocardial well-being is preserved after infrarenal aortic occlusion. Attia et al[31] reported a 30% incidence (three of ten patients) of myocardial ischemia following infrarenal occlusion. Investigators from the same institution (Massachusetts General Hospital), however, later described a technique (the vasodilation already described at the time of cross-clamping) that allows infrarenal aortic occlusion without eliciting evidence of myocardial ischemia.[32] Therefore, on the basis of these data, we consider it safe to assume that aortic occlusion at the infrarenal level increases the afterload only slightly and that current techniques prevent much of the stress on the heart that is associated with such occlusion.

There are few data in published reports on myocardial and cardiovascular effects of occluding the aorta at the suprarenal-infraceliac or supraceliac level in humans. After occluding the descending thoracic aorta in eight patients, Kouchoukos et al[34] noted increases of 35, 56, 43, and 90% in mean arterial, central venous, mean pulmonary arterial, and PCWPs, respectively, and a decrease of 29% in cardiac index. These hemodynamic effects are greater than those that we found for supraceliac aortic occlusion and may be attributable to the more proximal level of thoracic aortic occlusion. Occlusion at the supraceliac level causes substantially more myocardial stress, as evidenced by abnormal motion of segments of the left ventricular wall, than does occlusion at the suprarenal-infraceliac or infrarenal level (Table 36-3).[14] Although systemic and PCWPs were kept normal at all times in 10 of 12 patients who underwent occlusion at the supraceliac level, 11 patients had abnormal motion of the left ventricular wall, suggesting ischemia. Some of the factors contributing to this increase in resistance to myocardial ejection may be the more than 100% increase in peripheral vascular resistance, the change in aortic impedance characteristics, the release of vasoactive substances with intestinal ischemia, or the activation of hormonal systems, all of

TABLE 36-3.   Effect of Level of Aortic Occlusion on Changes in Cardiovascular Variables (%)

	LEVEL OF AORTIC OCCLUSION		
	Supraceliac	Suprarenal-Infraceliac	Infrarenal
Mean arterial blood pressure	54	5*	2*
Pulmonary capillary wedge pressure	38	10*	0*
End-diastolic area	28	2*	9*
End-systolic area	69	10*	11*
Ejection fraction	−38	−10*	−3*
Abnormal motion of wall (% of patients)	92	33	0
New myocardial infarctions (% of patients)	8	0	0

* Statistically different ($P < 0.05$) from group undergoing supraceliac aortic occlusion.

(Adapted with permission from Roizen MF, Sohn YJ, Stoney RJ: Intraoperative management of the patient undergoing supraceliac aortic occlusion. In Wilson SE, Veith FJ, Hobson RW et al [eds]: Vascular Surgery, pp 312–321. New York, McGraw-Hill, 1986.)

which lead to ventricular dilation. Despite low ejection fractions, these patients were able to maintain cardiac output and stroke volume via stretch (expansion) of the left ventricle muscle fibers. The PCWP frequently did not reflect this increased left-ventricular end-diastolic volume accurately; however, 2D-TEE made possible the identification and treatment of myocardial dysfunction that was not detected by conventional monitoring techniques.[14, 65] The most important lesson learned from the use of 2D echocardiograms on patients undergoing vascular surgery is that dilating the heart with the administration of fluid (as often requested by surgeons for stimulation of urine output) is a likely precursor of myocardial ischemia.

These pathophysiologic changes in hemodynamic variables could result from the effect that clamping has on normal patterns of flow to the arteries. For example, 22% of the cardiac output usually goes to renal vessels, and 27% to the superior mesenteric vessels and celiac trunk.[140] Thus, the expected decrease in flow and the increase in afterload and peripheral vascular resistance after supraceliac aortic occlusion could cause left ventricular dilation. Other factors that may contribute to myocardial dysfunction during operative supraceliac occlusion include release of vasoactive substances from ischemic areas and the presence of unmetabolized citrate from transfused blood.[141]

Results of studies on animals support the view that myocardial function is altered after occlusion of the descending thoracic aorta. Longo et al[142] studied coronary and systemic hemodynamic changes in dogs during suprarenal and infrarenal aortic clamping and unclamping. On application of the crossclamp to the suprarenal aorta, peripheral resistance increased two- to threefold, with immediate hypertension in the proximal segment, marked increases in CBF and pulse pressure, decreases in aortic blood flow and cardiac output, and little change in the pulse rate. These results were similar to ours.[14] In the study of Longo et al,[142] the canine left ventricles were dilated on application of the crossclamp. Mandelbaum and Webb[143] showed that occluding the descending thoracic aorta in dogs decreased left ventricular function. However, occluding the infrarenal aorta was much less stressful, the cardiovascular consequences being only slight (as they are in human patients with diseased hearts).[14, 143]

In normal dogs, the renal artery can be occluded for an hour before the kidneys are injured even slightly.[144] Data from a study that we performed on human subjects support this observation.[42] Preoperative and postoperative renal function did not differ among patients who underwent less than 40 minutes of suprarenal cross-clamping and those who underwent infrarenal aortic occlusion.[42]

Despite the negligible cardiovascular effects of temporarily applying an infrarenal aortic crossclamp, hypotension ("declamping shock") still occurs on restoration of flow in the aorta. This hemodynamic alteration occurs even when blood flow is restored to only one leg. Although the occurrence of severe hypotension in patients is rare,[32, 34, 39] moderate hypotension (i.e., a decrease in systolic blood pressure of 40 mm Hg) is not uncommon.

Two hypotheses are advanced to account for this hypotension. The first suggests that myocardial depression is caused by the washout of acid, acid metabolites, and vasoactive substances from ischemic extremities when blood flow is restored. This hypothesis has largely been discredited in recent years.[28, 34, 138] Our own work with 2D-TEE supports the second hypothesis, that of a relative depletion of volume. Reactive hyperemia in the freshly revascularized area decreases total vascular resistance, venous return, and blood pressure.

Thus, hypotension can be ameliorated by expansion of volume without a decrease in cardiac output; in fact, the expansion may increase cardiac output. However, if hypotension persists for more than 4 minutes after removal of the clamp, and if blood deficits have been replaced, we believe that other causes should be sought. A 2D-TEE of the left ventricle often reveals in these patients that venous return is still inadequate, sometimes as a result of hidden persistent bleeding or misjudged replacement of blood deficits, or that a rare allergic reaction to graft material has occurred.[137]

Because of these complications, we stress, in our monitoring practices, preservation of myocardial, pulmonary, and renal function as well as intravascular volume. We almost always insert a catheter in the radial artery of the nondominant hand. We also monitor urinary output and some form of ventricular filling pressure, the latter usually via a PA catheter. This catheter allows monitoring of systemic vascular resistance, cardiac output, and PCWP. For its insertion, we prefer the external jugular route, although many anesthesiologists use the internal jugular or subclavian route. We use a modified chest lead to monitor the ECG during the operation, except in those patients who have demonstrated myocardial ischemia in areas other than the anterior myocardial wall. In addition, body temperature is monitored and maintained by warming all fluids (starting preoperatively), and by the use of heating mattresses on the operating room table. If necessary, we humidify the anesthetic gases. We have found 2D-TEE to be an invaluable tool for monitoring of the myocardial consequences of cross-clamping and unclamping of the aorta, and we now use it routinely for such procedures as temporary aortic occlusion at the supraceliac level. A short-axis cross-sectional view of the left ventricle provides an excellent qualitative assessment of left ventricular filling volumes, global ventricular contractility, and regional ventricular function[144] (Fig. 36-3).

FIG. 36-3. Left ventricular echocardiograph obtained from a transesophageal echocardiogram. The transesophageal echocardiogram originates in the esophagus, the small piece of the pie-shaped wedge shown at the top of the picture. The area marked "LV" is the inside of the heart where blood is normally shown. The whiteness surrounding the LV cavity that is not marked "A" or "P" is the endocardium. The "A" and "P" represent the anterior and posterior papillary muscles, respectively. At the bottom of the picture is the anterior wall of the myocardium. To the right is the left ventricular free wall; to the left is the septum; and to the top is the posteroinferior portion wall of the myocardium.

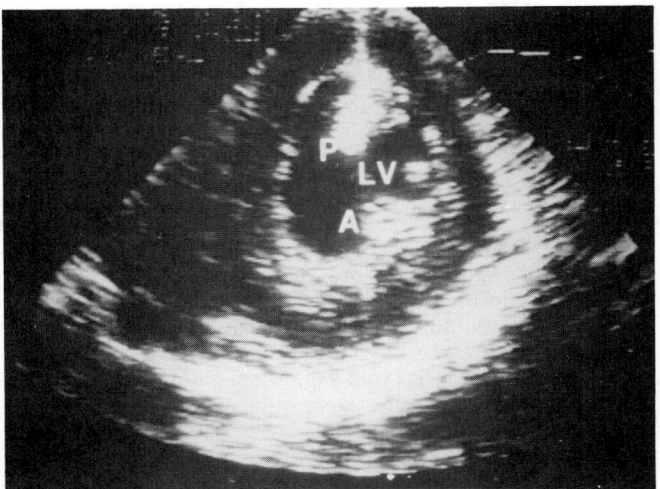

When a discrepancy exists between pulmonary capillary filling pressures and end diastolic dimension (volume) obtained by 2D-TEE, we have found the latter to be more reliable and useful.[14, 145]

To reduce the incidence of organ ischemia and of pulmonary dysfunction, fluid administration is managed with the aim of preventing intraoperative hypotension and minimizing cardiac dilation. Although there are no supporting data at present, it is strongly believed that prehydration of patients undergoing vascular reconstructive surgery minimizes the hemodynamic fluctuations that occur with induction of anesthesia, by ensuring that perfusion of vital organs is adequate. During the early period of dissection, intravascular volume is maintained at normal levels by noting ventricular filling on the 2D-TEE or by sustaining a normal PCWP. To accomplish this, blood losses of less than $10 \text{ ml} \cdot \text{kg}^{-1}$ and insensible losses (assumed to be 5 to $7 \text{ ml} \cdot \text{kg}^{-1}$ during this dissection phase) are replaced with Ringer's lactate or saline solution.

The indicators used for assessing perfusion of the organs before cross-clamping are: 1) for the heart, myocardial contractility as judged by global and regional motion of the wall on the 2D-TEE,[14, 65, 139] by the ST segments on the modified chest lead V of the ECG, and by cardiac output; 2) for the kidney, urinary output (2 ml per half hour per 70 kg is adequate, although with 20 to 30 ml per half hour per 70 kg, it may be easier to convince surgeons of adequacy); urinary flow almost always decreases during dissection around the renal vessels; 3) for the central nervous system, eye signs (although the EEG or sensory evoked potentials or both[45] can be used, we have had little experience with these monitors); and 4) for the lung, gas exchange.

PROTECTION OF MYOCARDIUM. For the half hour immediately before cross-clamping and aortic occlusion, we keep the patient slightly hypovolemic by examining the ventricular volume, using 2D-TEE, or by keeping pulmonary or arterial pressure at 5 to 12 mm Hg. At the time of occlusion, we are prepared to give a vasodilating drug through an iv catheter available specifically for that purpose, to avoid hypotension that is secondary to an accidental bolus of vasodilator. This infusion site is often the third lumen of the PA catheter. The difference in our management of aortic occlusion at different levels (e.g., supraceliac vs infrarenal) is that we are absolutely meticulous in planning our management and in executing that procedure in all occlusions planned at renal vessels or above.

During the early part of the aortic dissection, the heart is protected by trying to maintain hemodynamic variables within the range of the preoperative values.[50] Without evidence to the contrary, it is assumed that a little hypertension is just as harmful as a little hypotension. For example, in extreme cases, we might let the systolic blood pressure of a patient whose preoperative range was 110 to 170 mm Hg fall to a level as low as 90 mm Hg, or rise as high as 190 mm Hg. If values approach or exceed these limits, we have a contingency treatment plan. If the blood pressure reaches 150 mm Hg, the amount of anesthetic is increased; at approximately 160 mm Hg, nitroprusside is infused; at 165 or 175 mm Hg, the table is tilted. If the systolic blood pressure drops to 110 mm Hg, the anesthetic is decreased and the possible causes of hypotension are reviewed. At 105 mm Hg, the amount of anesthetic is decreased even more, and the patient is placed in a head-down position. At 100 mm Hg, more fluid is infused, the patient is tilted in a more steeply head-down position, the possible causes of hypotension are reviewed again, and, if possible, the cause is corrected. At 90 mm Hg, a dilute infusion of phenylephrine (10 mg in 500 ml, infused at a rate that restores systolic blood pressure to approximately 100 mm Hg) is added.

For the heart rate, again, a range of acceptable values is set based on preoperative determinations. If a preoperative range of 60 to 90 beats $\cdot \text{min}^{-1}$ is used as an example, once these limits were exceeded, treatment would be initiated. Here, it is assumed that tachycardia is of greater concern than bradycardia, and it is avoided more aggressively. At 95 beats $\cdot \text{min}^{-1}$, the level of anesthesia might be increased, more opioid may be given, or an iv infusion of a beta-adrenergic receptor blocking drug may be added. At 100 beats $\cdot \text{min}^{-1}$, a bolus is given, or an iv infusion of a beta-adrenergic receptor blocker is begun, assuming that the intravascular fluid volume is acceptable. At 45 beats $\cdot \text{min}^{-1}$, the anesthetic might be decreased or a dilute solution of dopamine (200 mg in 500 ml) might be administered to keep the heart rate within the acceptable range. It is important to re-emphasize that bradycardia is tolerated more than is tachycardia during these operations, because minimizing the myocardial oxygen demand should be of primary importance. Use of 2D-TEE gives some latitude in the range of acceptable values before intervention. However, PA pressures are not allowed to remain abnormal, that is, below 5 or above 15 mm Hg, during this procedure, assuming that these values correlate with the echocardiographic values. Increases in PA pressure are treated aggressively by administering nitroglycerin or nitroprusside, depending upon whether the suspected cause is an increase in preload or an increase in afterload.[146, 147] For low pressures, more fluid is infused except in the 1- or 2-minute interval immediately before application of the aortic crossclamp.

The application of a crossclamp to the supraceliac aorta probably produces the greatest hemodynamic stress ever experienced by a patient. In fact, 92% of the patients whom we studied had ischemia, as evidenced by abnormal motion and thickening of the wall (Table 36-3; Fig. 36-4).[14] More distal levels of temporary occlusion are less stressful hemodynamically. Stabilizing PA pressure and systemic blood pressure by administering vasodilating drugs before and during suprarenal cross-clamping may not be sufficient. When myocardial ischemia was indicated by abnormal global or regional motion of the wall in patients in our study, we gave more vasodilating drugs, to the point of bringing the systolic blood pressure toward the low end of the normal preoperative range. Once the blood pressure is as low as possible (this is achieved by reduction of the afterload with administration of nitroprusside), we often attempt to decrease the preload with nitroglycerin and, if necessary, to decrease the heart rate with iv propranolol or, preferably, with esmolol. If, despite these maneuvers, one sees myocardial dysfunction on placement of the crossclamp (before he has actually incised the aorta or its branches), to unclamp the aorta partially until myocardial function is more stable. In our study, despite myocardial dysfunction in 11 of the 12 patients who underwent supraceliac cross-clamping, only one of the 11 had perioperative myocardial infarction.[14] Therefore, myocardial contractile function seems to be affected most by ventricular size and by maintenance of vital signs within the normal preoperative range.

Administration of exogenous vasoconstrictors is avoided if possible. Although coronary and cerebral vessels are not prominently innervated, alpha$_1$- and alpha$_2$-adrenergic agents can induce cerebral vasoconstriction. In addition, alpha-adrenergic vasoconstriction appears to be important in maintaining an appropriate distribution of flow between the outer and inner myocardium.[148] Perhaps because of this, or perhaps for other reasons, patients who are deeply anesthe-

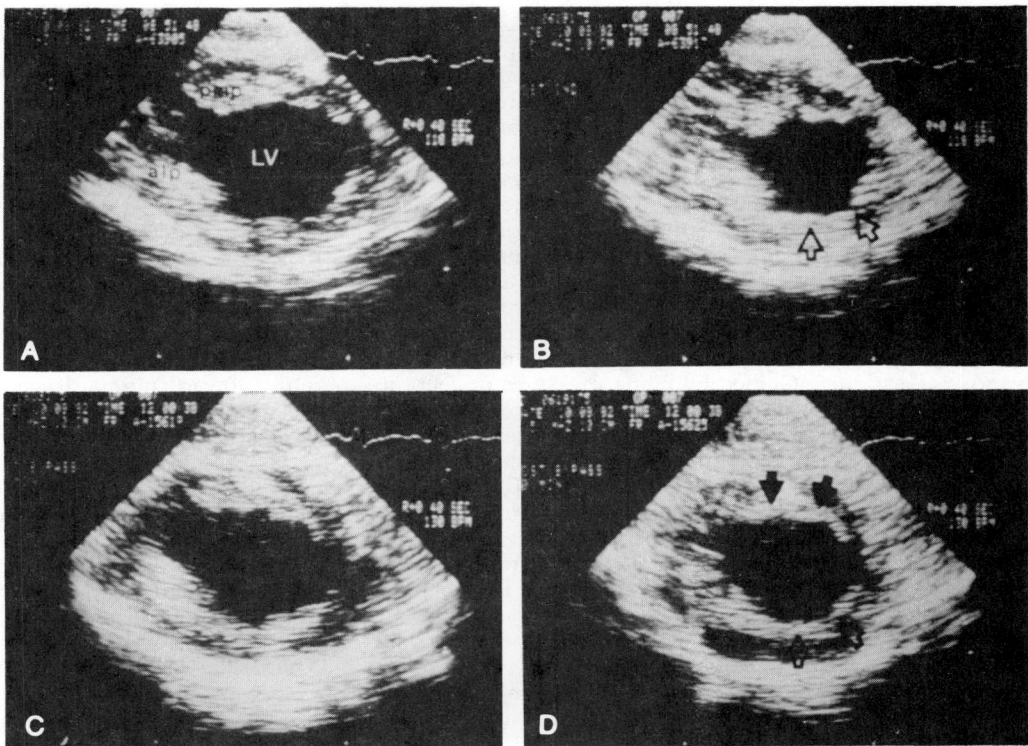

FIG. 36-4. Echocardiographic view of the left ventricle with the papillary muscles on the left side of the figure. The *A* and *C* figures are end-diastolic pictures; the end-systolic views are shown in Figures *B* and *D*. The *arrows* in figure *B* indicate an area of permanent myocardial infarction with no contraction occurring. Note that the placement of the anterior wall or the wall in the bottom part of the picture where the *arrows* are is no different from where it was end-diastole. In figure *D*, one sees that the posterior part or the part toward the uppermost part of that figure is also not moving. That is different than it was in Figure *B* and indicates a new area of ischemia. This wall motion abnormality, coupled with the absence of thickening of the wall in this area, is a sign of myocardial ischemia and depicts a way that the echocardiogram can aid in the diagnosis of myocardial ischemia.

tized and whose systemic pressure is maintained with an infusion of phenylephrine have more than twice the incidence of myocardial ischemia than do patients whose blood pressure is maintained simply by light anesthesia and endogenous vasoconstrictors.[12] This ischemia appears to be related to the myocardial dilation induced by these agents (the problem of a stretched, dilated myocardium).[12]

During unclamping of the aorta, a different set of maneuvers is performed for reaching the same goals. To ensure adequate volume when the crossclamp is removed, blood losses are replaced during occlusion by administering warmed blood, milliliter for milliliter. We normally have only four units of packed cells available during this procedure. The packed cells are diluted with normal saline or lactated Ringer's solution. Although we would prefer to administer whole blood (as that is what is lost), we are unable to obtain it routinely at our institution.

When greater blood loss is anticipated (*e.g.,* for patients previously operated on for the same condition), autotransfusion is often available and a second person to operate it. After the sixth unit of blood has been given and if more blood loss is anticipated, or after eight units of blood have been administered, ten units of platelets are requested for the patient (and occasionally two units of fresh frozen plasma). After giving 8 to 10 units of packed cells, we routinely administer a unit of fresh frozen plasma for each unit of packed cells. When no more blood is at hand, and if it is absolutely necessary (*i.e.,* when colloid or crystalloid cannot be used), the best available type-specific, washed packed cells are administered. For example, if B-negative blood is needed but not available, we give B-positive blood. Blood filters are changed after every two units when the blood for transfusion is more than 10 days old, and after every four units when it is less than 10 days old.

Because a large part of the vascular tree is excluded from circulation during temporary aortic occlusion, blood loss can be considerable during supraceliac cross-clamping without onset of hypotension or tachycardia.

Since maintenance of volume status is so important, more than just PA pressures or PCWP is monitored. Observation of the surgical field is of key importance. When any blood vessel is dissected, the anesthesiologist and surgeon must communicate closely; blood loss can occur with astonishing rapidity, and the attention of the anesthesiologist may not be directed at the operative field. Watching the volumes in the suction bottles supplements the data, as does observation of left ventricular cavity size on 2D-TEE.

Blood loss into the pleural or retroperitoneal cavity may not be detected in the amounts that are measured every 5 to 10 minutes. In addition, evisceration of bowel, often necessary for optimal exposure of the thoracoabdominal aorta, further depletes the intravascular volume. Thus, one must be guided closely by PA pressures or echocardiographic estimates of left ventricular filling volumes, or both. Just before opening of the aorta, we allow blood pressure, PCWP, and filling volumes to go as high as possible without the occurrence of myocardial ischemia (Fig. 36-5). The surgeon then opens the aorta gradually to ensure that overly severe hypotension does not develop and that there is not too much bleeding from the suture line.

Pathophysiologic events on removal of the aortic crossclamp (see previous discussion) are associated with inadequate return of volume to the heart (*i.e.*, inadequate preload). Thus, immediately before and during removal of the crossclamp, we stop infusing nitroprusside and start infusing crystalloid or blood; usually, two units of whole blood are pressured into venous access sites. Guided by filling pressures or echocardiographic estimates of volume, or both, we are careful not to dilate the left ventricle to an abnormal size. Another technique for maintaining normal volumes during crossclamping is controlled volume depletion, that is, the removal of a specific amount of blood from the patient just before or during application of the crossclamp for a short period of time. During the minutes remaining just before the crossclamp is removed, this amount is replaced. Although we have used this technique, we do not advocate its routine use.

A third technique for maintaining normal hemodynamic values involves the use of halothane, enflurane, or isoflurane, rather than nitroglycerin or nitroprusside, as the vasodilating agent. This is an interesting technique that is usually effective,[149] but it requires very close observation of PA pressures,

the echocardiogram, or both, to ensure that myocardial dilation and dysfunction do not occur. This technique is not recommended for routine use.

It is not uncommon for moderate hypotension (*i.e.*, decreases in systolic pressure of 40 to 60 mm Hg) to occur on removal of the aortic crossclamp, regardless of whether the clamp is replaced infrarenally or in such a way that blood flow to only one leg is obstructed. Our anecdotal impressions, gained in work with 2D-TEE, support the view that such hypotension is caused mainly by relative depletion of volume. Reactive hyperemia in the freshly revascularized area decreases vascular resistance, venous return, and systemic blood pressure. If hypotension persists for more than 4 minutes following removal of the clamp and the pressure does not return toward normal levels after blood deficits have been replaced, other causes should be sought. These include myocardial dysfunction caused by inadequate metabolism of the citrate present in replacement blood; such blood has not yet gone to the liver, where citrate is metabolized. This problem can be treated by administration of calcium, which antagonizes the effect of citrate.[141] Other causes include hidden, persistent bleeding or misjudged replacement of blood deficits; on the echocardiogram, the ventricular cavity is devoid of volume, and, on the oscilloscope, filling pressures reflecting PA pressures are low. If necessary, the surgeon can reclamp or occlude the aorta, preferably below the renal arteries. Thus, replacement and maintenance of volume are mainstays of therapy before, during, and immediately after removal of the supraceliac crossclamp. When blood flow is restored to the

FIG. 36-5. Set of echocardiograms with the papillary muscles shown on the right side of the picture. In these pictures, one sees the end-diastolic pictures in *A* and *C* and the end-systolic pictures in *B* and *D*. All the walls of the heart are contracting symmetrically and come in so that there is almost no volume at end-systole in the left ventricular cross-section at the area of the papillary muscles. This picture of hypovolemia can be seen often when one releases the crossclamp.

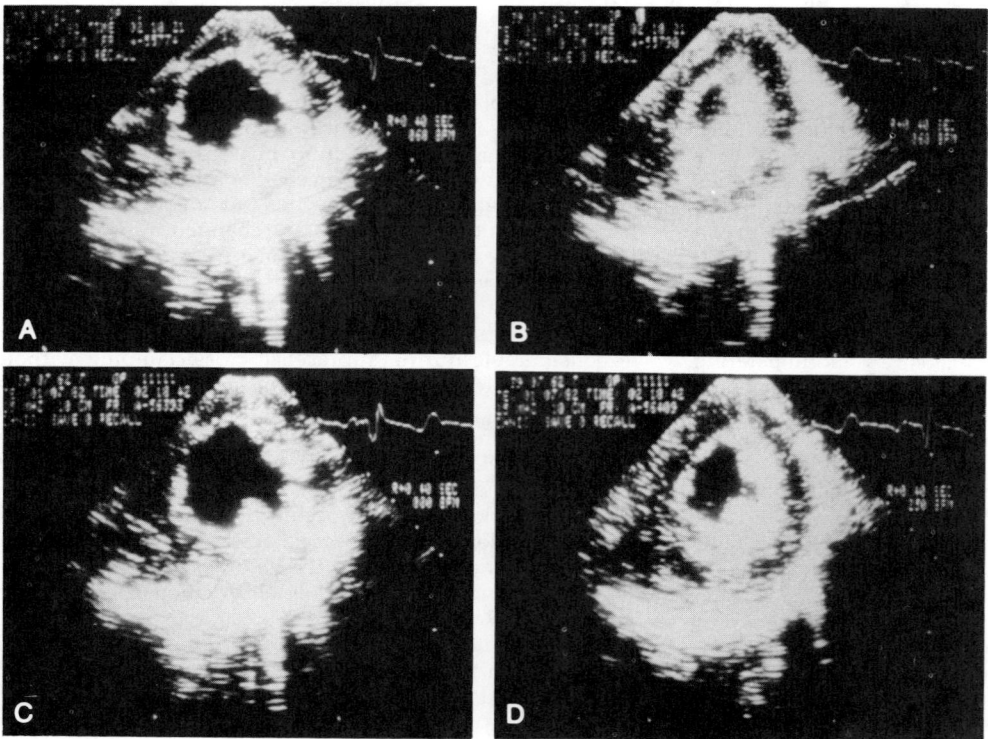

first extremity, replacement of volume should also be considered. Removal of the clamp from the second leg usually causes few hemodynamic effects, presumably because of collateral blood vessels across the pelvis.

CENTRAL NERVOUS SYSTEM PROTECTION. Other investigators have used sensory evoked potentials and the EEG to gauge protection of the spinal cord and cerebrum.[45, 150] We have found no benefit in examining the EEG and no evidence that stroke is a predictable consequence of aortic reconstruction, even of supraceliac aortic reconstruction. However, in rare instances, spinal cord ischemia is a predictable consequence of this procedure. Spinal cord sensory evoked potentials may prove useful, but there has not been much experience in the use of this technique. Experiments on animals indicate that isoflurane may allow longer periods of temporary occlusion of the blood supply to the spinal cord before development of permanent neurologic injury than are possible with other anesthetic agents. Other halogenated anesthetics and iv anesthetics decrease the interval during which the spinal cord can be ischemic before permanent neurologic damage sets in in this animal model.[151]

RENAL PROTECTION. Intraoperative urinary output is not predictive of postoperative renal function.[42] In 137 patients undergoing aortic reconstruction (38 at the supraceliac level), we measured the hourly urine output and calculated each patient's lowest and mean urinary outputs. The PCWP was kept within normal limits in each patient. If urinary output was less than $0.125 \text{ ml} \cdot \text{kg}^{-1} \cdot \text{hr}^{-1}$, patients were given either crystalloid (so that the PCWP was raised to a high-normal level) or furosemide, mannitol, or nothing. For each patient, serum creatinine and blood urea nitrogen (BUN) were assayed on the first, third, and seventh postoperative days. There was no significant correlation between intraoperative mean urinary output, or lowest hourly urinary output, and changes from preoperative to postoperative levels of creatinine or BUN (Fig. 36-6). Thus, urinary output, which is believed to be an index of perfusion and therefore is monitored routinely during surgery, was not predictive of postoperative renal function in normovolemic patients.

When patients who underwent aortic occlusion at the suprarenal level were compared with those who underwent occlusion at the infrarenal level, there was no difference in postoperative renal function.[42]

Our results for patients who underwent aortic reconstruction conflict with those of other studies. In investigations in which a period of renal ischemia was imposed on patients and animal models, pretreatment with mannitol lessened postischemic increases in creatinine.[152–155] Direct infusion of mannitol into the renal artery sustained renal cortical perfusion (as assayed by the xenon washout technique) in mongrel dogs after infrarenal aortic occlusion.[152] In rabbits, pretreatment with mannitol prevented an increase in serum creatinine after 60 minutes of renal artery occlusion.[155] In dogs subjected to aortic clamping and unclamping, adequate replacement of blood with saline prevented a decrease in renal blood flow, an occurrence that is consistent with the findings of Alpert *et al.*[42] In addition, furosemide and ethacrynic acid significantly increase both the total and the cortical components of renal blood flow, as demonstrated by studies of xenon-133 washout.[152] The use of mannitol, furosemide, or ethacrynic acid, however, has not been clearly shown to prevent renal failure. The difference between the results of Alpert *et al*[42] and those of others[152–155] may be due to variations among species, the maintenance of normal intravascular volume by Alpert *et al*, the insensitivity of urinary output as a measure of the adequacy of renal perfusion, or a combination of these factors. We believe that preoperative renal function and the maintenance of an appropriate intravascular volume and of normal myocardial function are the most important determinants of postoperative renal function.

It is important to monitor renal function, because development of acute renal failure after aortic reconstruction is associated with high morbidity and a mortality rate of more than 30%.[156] This complication is most frequent in patients with ruptured aneurysms who have significant hypotensive episodes, and in those for whom suprarenal aortic clamping is required. Despite our aforementioned data, infusion of mannitol prior to clamping of the renal arteries is believed by some to be beneficial and is commonly used.[97, 157] Furosemide, vasodilators, and angiotensin-converting enzyme inhibitors may also have a place before renal artery clamping. If prolonged renal ischemia is anticipated, selective profound hypothermia of the kidneys may decrease the incidence of postoperative renal impairment. Recently, it was suggested that infusion of verapamil into the renal arteries just before reperfusion may also be beneficial,[157] although the question has been raised as to whether anything better than good surgical technique exists.[42] Our management, however, is biased by the results of our own studies. Thus, when intraoperative urinary output is less than $0.125 \text{ ml} \cdot \text{kg}^{-1} \cdot \text{hr}^{-1}$, we ensure that no mechanical problems in urine collection are present and that left-sided cardiac filling volumes or pressures are adequate. We then continue to monitor but do not treat. Urinary output usually returns to acceptable levels within 2 hours. If it does not, or if we are uneasy about low urinary output, 2 to 5 mg of furosemide is administered iv for stimulation of urine production.[42]

Thus, virtually all investigators have concluded that the maintenance of adequate intravascular volume and myocardial function largely prevents renal insufficiency and insufficiency of other organs from being major clinical problems and that it is the key to intraoperative perfusion of critical organs.

FIG. 36-6. Lowest hourly intraoperative urinary output and maximal adverse change in renal function as assayed by change in creatinine from pre- to 7 days postoperatively; there was no correlation between lowest intraoperative urinary output and change in renal function postoperatively. (Modified with permission from Alpert RA, Roizen MF, Hamilton WK *et al:* Intraoperative urinary output does not predict postoperative renal function in patients undergoing abdominal aortic revascularization. Surgery 95:707, 1984.)

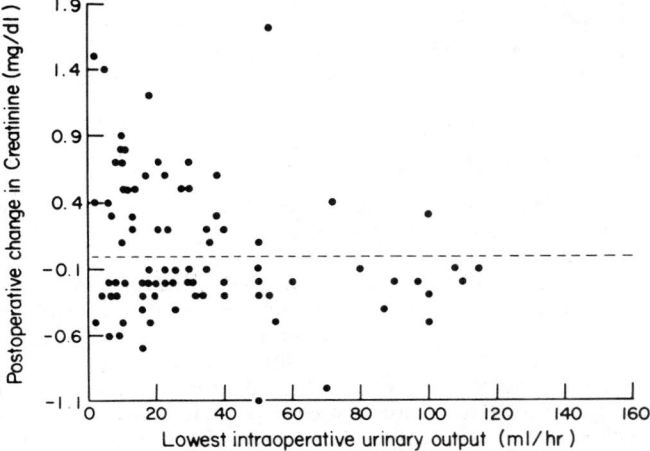

ANESTHETIC AGENTS AND TECHNIQUES FOR AORTIC RECONSTRUCTION

Virtually all anesthetic techniques and drugs have been used for aortic reconstructive surgery. For this operative procedure, as for other types of vascular surgery, the skill of the anesthesiologist in maintaining hemodynamic equilibrium and in attending to detail appears to be more crucial to the outcome than is the choice of drugs.[158] Although it is now believed that the choice of the agent or technique is important to the outcome[26, 159, 160]; however, the quality and attentiveness of the anesthesiologist are much more important than is choice of agent.

Inhalational Anesthetics

Halothane, enflurane, and isoflurane are halogenated hydrocarbons that have negative inotropic properties when they are administered to volunteers not undergoing surgery. However, during surgery, these agents act as vasodilators,[149, 161, 162] isoflurane being the most potent. Vasodilation is both advantageous and disadvantageous. It provides an additional means (besides administration of nitroglycerin or nitroprusside) of controlling afterload and preload but can lead to an increased need for intravascular volume. The resultant increase in intravascular volume can be detrimental at the end of the procedure. As the amount of the anesthetic is decreased, intravascular volume could return to the central compartment and cause relative hypervolemia and even pulmonary edema. To prevent this problem in patients who are still receiving a volatile anesthetic or an epidural anesthetic, the situation of increased central blood volume that occurs with awakening by tilting the patient (head lower than feet) is simulated for the 30 to 45 minutes of closure, and the patient is then slowly returned to the level position while the concentration of the anesthetic agent is gradually being reduced if it is a volatile agent or the effects of the epidural anesthetic are dissipating. The tilting allows one to predict the patient's postanesthetic volume status and make appropriate adjustments.

Volatile drugs have several other advantages. They permit careful, deliberate induction, manipulation and monitoring of hemodynamic variables, and adjustment of dose. In addition, by providing a moderate degree of muscle relaxation, they decrease the need for muscle relaxants and increase the ease of reversing paralysis.

With the use of volatile hydrogen anesthetics, extubation of the trachea is usually accomplished by the end of surgery, and the patient is allowed to breathe spontaneously. Thus, the stressful stimuli and hypertension associated with continued intubation of the trachea are avoided, and early assessment of neurologic function is facilitated, allowing evaluation of motor function and sensation of the limbs before placement of an epidural catheter if one wishes to do so to facilitate postoperative analgesia. Also, because extubation of the trachea occurs at the end of surgery, the patient is able to complain of angina (if it is present), for which nitroglycerin can be administered.

Since the introduction of isoflurane, we have tried to avoid the use of halothane—the reason for this being that occlusion of the aorta at the supraceliac level tends to make the liver hypoxic for a time, and, under this condition, halothane can, in theory, create a hepatitis-like condition.[163] However, 20 of the first 40 patients whom we anesthetized for supraceliac aortic revascularization received halothane without any adverse effect that was attributable to the drug.

Opioids

All commonly used opioids produce similar cardiovascular effects unless they are administered rapidly in large doses.[158] Induction of anesthesia with opioids can be accomplished quickly and decreases the cardiac index by a small, but statistically significant amount. In sufficient doses, opioids produce analgesia and hypnosis, with only slight decreases in cardiac contractility and blood pressure.[158] By continuing to infuse opioids or administer other drugs, one can maintain anesthesia throughout the surgical procedure. Surgical stimulation after such induction significantly increases the heart rate, arterial blood pressure, and systemic vascular resistance. Nitroglycerin, nitroprusside, or a volatile anesthetic can be added to the opioid for manipulation of the circulation during cross-clamping and unclamping.

Nitrous oxide can be used with opioids, as with the inhalational drugs. It increases afterload and myocardial work, while it depresses myocardial inotropic performance and output and decreases renal and splanchnic blood flows.[161, 164] In addition, nitrous oxide may have the potential for producing a long-lasting toxicity by causing nutritional, neurologic, and immunologic deficits.[165] It can also contribute to distention of the bowel.

A disadvantage of using opioids is that they linger in the patient into the postoperative period. Until opioids that provide pain relief without affecting the respiratory drive are produced, the likelihood increases that controlled ventilation of the lungs will be required in the postoperative period. However, in more than 50% of the opioid/nitrous oxide anesthetic techniques used for suprarenal aortic reconstruction, Benefiel et al[26] were able to extubate the trachea in the operating room. An advantage of the use of opioids in high doses as the anesthetic is the continued, excellent postoperative analgesia.

In a prospective controlled study at our institution, patients who consented and were about to undergo aortic reconstruction were randomly assigned to receive either a volatile anesthetic (isoflurane) or an opioid (sufentanil)-based anesthetic.[26] Intraoperatively and postoperatively, systemic and pulmonary capillary blood pressures and heart rates were kept within 20% of mean (baseline) values on the ward before surgery. Sufentanil anesthesia alone was associated with less major morbidity than was isoflurane for patients undergoing aortic reconstruction (Table 36-4). Because published data[17–26] indicate that the rates of complication in patients who underwent aortic reconstruction are as high as or higher than those for the isoflurane group of Benefiel et al,[26] we postulate that sufentanil has a protective effect. Further study is needed for determination of whether all opioids are protective, or whether the combination of sufentanil and isoflurane can produce an outcome as good as, or better than, that with sufentanil alone.

Epidural Anesthetics

Epidural anesthesia has been used successfully for resection of infrarenal aortic aneurysms and aortic reconstruction,[166] and it can be combined with general anesthesia for supraceliac aortic reconstruction. A significant risk with epidural anesthetics is that administration of heparin might create an epidural hematoma and subsequent neurologic deficit.[167] Such a deficit could be confused with that caused by spinal cord ischemia, thereby delaying correct diagnosis, evacuation of the hematoma, and return of neurologic function. Thus, we are reluctant to use epidural anesthesia for supraceliac aortic

TABLE 36-4. Morbidity After Aortic Reconstruction With Either of Two Different Anesthetic Agents

MORBIDITY	ISOFLURANE-BASED ANESTHETIC (n = 50)	SUFENTANIL-BASED ANESTHETIC (n = 46)
Renal insufficiency	16	4*
CHF	13	4*
Ventilation >24 hr	9	4
Pneumonia	2	1
Renal failure	3	1
Stroke	2	0
Myocardial ischemia	0	1
Death	2	1
Important or severe complications	20	9*
Important or severe complications and failure	17	7*

* = $P < 0.05$ by Fisher's Exact Test
n = number of patients
(Modified with permission from Benefiel DJ, Roizen MF, Lampe GH et al: Morbidity after aortic surgery with sufentanil versus isoflurane anesthesia. Anesthesiology 65:A516, 1986.)

reconstruction. In addition, the absence of sensation and movement of the leg postoperatively might create undue worry for the patient. This disadvantage can be ameliorated by the use of concentrations of epidural anesthetic agents at the end of the operation that affect sensory but not motor fibers. Another disadvantage of epidural anesthesia is the possibility of a relative overload of fluid toward the end of the procedure. As with inhalational agents, we tilt the patient (head lower than feet) near the end of the procedure so that the fluid status is normal as the anesthetic wears off. A number of studies, including a large series by Rao et al[167] and a study on use of epidural anesthesia even after full heparinization in cardiac surgery,[168] indicate that this potential problem is of more theoretical than actual concern. Thus, use of heparin does not appear to contraindicate the use of epidural anesthesia, or even continuous epidural anesthesia.

Rao and El-Etr[169] stated that proper patient selection and atraumatic technique for regional anesthesia were important in ensuring a low complication rate. Their protocol included postponement of the planned elective vascular surgery procedure for 24 hours if blood returned from the epidural needle. This protocol was intended to allow clot formation in the epidural space before intraoperative anticoagulation.[169] Other groups use a "single-shot" epidural or intrathecal technique with a 25- or 26-gauge needle to reduce the risk of postponement of surgery and to provide for postoperative pain relief by addition of an opioid.[170] To reduce the incidence of pruritus and respiratory depression from such epidural or intrathoracic analgesia, some anesthesiologists routinely infuse naloxone (2 mg in 250 ml saline, which equals $8 \mu g \cdot ml^{-1}$, given at a rate of 0.5 to 1.5 $\mu g \cdot kg^{-1} \cdot hr^{-1}$ or about 7 $ml \cdot hr^{-1}$).[170, 171] Since most patients who undergo aortic reconstruction have urinary catheters for at least 36 hours following surgery, retention of urine, another side-effect of spinal or epidural opioids, is not a major issue.

Advantages of epidural anesthesia include a potential decrease in myocardial ischemia,[168] although it may also make myocardial ischemia worse;[148] excellent muscle relaxation; a smaller bowel (because of sympathectomy) that tends not to obstruct the operative field; and hemodynamic stability once the blockade is fully achieved. However, most findings suggesting that an advantage of epidural anesthesia is a potential decrease in myocardial ischemia include a comparison group that received a fixed dose of isoflurane, rather than an individualized dose based on the patient's hemodynamic variables.[168] The initiation of epidural anesthesia often causes a decrease in blood pressure, cardiac output, and possibly perfusion to the gut and kidney, which, in the stenotic state, may be pressure-dependent. During cross-clamping and unclamping in a patient under epidural anesthesia, the circulation can be controlled by administration of volatile anesthetics or iv drugs that reduce the afterload.

In addition, Yeager et al[160] compared outcomes after epidural anesthesia with outcomes after general anesthesia for surgical procedures in 48 patients, some of whom underwent vascular operations. They found that patients who received epidural anesthesia and analgesia postoperatively had fewer cardiovascular and infectious disease complications and lower medical care costs than did those receiving general anesthesia. Similar results were obtained for those receiving epidural analgesia postoperatively.[170] Thus, the data may imply that epidural anesthesia is not only not a risky technique, but that it even may be an advantageous one for providing anesthesia for aortic reconstruction.

Muscle Relaxants

The choices of muscle relaxants for use during aortic reconstruction are succinylcholine as a continuous infusion or, in bolus injections, d-tubocurarine, metocurine, pancuronium, vecuronium, or atracurium. The newer neuromuscular relaxants, vecuronium and atracurium, have shorter half-lives and provide more hemodynamic stability than do the other agents. d-Tubocurarine is preferable to metocurine or pancuronium when the degree of hypertension is significant, the vagolytic effect of pancuronium is not desired, or renal insufficiency is great enough to prolong the excretion of metocurine or pancuronium. We routinely titrate the muscle relaxant to the chronotropic cardiovascular effect that we want to achieve.

In view of the small number of patients in general and of vascular patients in particular, and the detail provided about the general anesthesia technique in the study of Yeager et al,[160] another study verifying these findings similar to our study, which showed a benefit for sufentanil compared with inhalational anesthetics, would be helpful.[26]

Anesthesia for Aortic Reconstruction

As soon as the patient assumes an NPO status, prehydration is begun at maintenance rates. Although we are unable to prove this with specific data, we believe that such maintenance of a normal hydration status reduces variations in blood pressure upon induction of anesthesia.

After optimizing a patient's preoperative condition, the range of hemodynamic variables for this particular patient is obtained. Anesthetic management is then planned to keep the patient within 20% of this range, as long as the PCWP does not exceed 15 mm Hg, the heart rate does not exceed 100 beats $\cdot$ min^{-1}, and signs of organ ischemia are absent. Premedication consisting of a benzodiazepine and an opioid is requested (usually 0.015 mg $\cdot$ kg^{-1} of diazepam 1.5 to 2 hours before the planned incision and 0.01 mg $\cdot$ kg^{-1} of morphine sulphate im 1 hour before the planned incision; this is modified downward for old age, debility, pulmonary disease, and so on), in addition to all the patient's usual medications. Any drug therapy that is required before major vascular surgery will most probably also be required during the operative period. Omitting chronic drug therapy can result in a worsened disease condition in the postoperative period, for example, tachycardia, angina, or both, if propranolol is omitted; aspiration if L-dopa is omitted; or accelerated hypertension if clonidine is omitted. The patient should be given antihypertensive medication, including diuretics, before being brought to the operating room.[50] Many diabetic patients who require insulin are given an insulin infusion throughout surgery. Preoperative considerations and drug therapy for diabetic patients are described in Chapters 15 and 44.[50] However, because no particular premedication seems indicated or contraindicated for most patients, the patient's anesthesiologist should determine what is appropriate. The use of anticholinergic drugs might be avoided, because they produce a dry mouth and tachycardia, which increases myocardial oxygen consumption.

In the preoperative holding area and/or in the operating room, those monitors and catheters that are needed for induction of anesthesia are placed—usually, an 18-gauge radial artery catheter in the nondominant hand, a manual blood pressure cuff, pulse oximeter, ECG (leads II and MCL 5), ST-segment trend monitor, precordial stethoscope, 16-gauge iv, and, occasionally, a PA catheter (or central venous polyethylene [CVP] if the patient shows no evidence of myocardial, pulmonary, or renal disease, but usually this last can wait until induction of anesthesia is completed. Then, after giving 3 mg of d-tubocurarine, an infusion of 750 μg of sufentanil in 100 ml of saline at a rate of about 15 to 50 μg $\cdot$ min$^{-1} \cdot$ 70 kg^{-1} is begun, and the patient is coached to breathe 100% oxygen from a face mask. After about 3 minutes, 75 mg of thiopental iv is administered, and 0.1 mg $\cdot$ kg^{-1} pancuronium or 0.5 mg $\cdot$ kg^{-1} metocurine is given over 3 to 5 minutes, depending upon whether one wishes the heart rate to increase or stay the same. Other drugs are chosen if the patient has renal insufficiency with a creatinine level above 2 mg $\cdot$ dl^{-1}.

When the depth of anesthesia is judged adequate by lack of response to Foley catheter insertion or placement of another iv or by pinpoint pupils, and when muscle relaxation is adequate, endotracheal intubation occurs and mechanical ventilation with 0 to 60% N$_2$O in O$_2$ is begun. The remainder of the pre-cross-clamping phase is devoted to meticulous attention to details of maintaining temperature homeostasis (by a heating mattress and heating of all fluids and, if necessary, heating of ventilatory gases), maintaining volume homeostasis as

judged by heart rate, blood pressure, pulmonary capillary or central venous pressure, left ventricular end-diastolic volume as assessed by 2D-TEE, ensuring absence of organ ischemia, monitoring (but usually not treating) urine output, and keeping systemic and pulmonary blood pressures and heart rate in the patient's usual range. Every increase in blood pressure or heart rate is either anticipated or treated as soon as it occurs with 25 to 50 μg of sufentanil. Further increases are treated with repeated doses, or with addition or nitroglycerine or nitroprusside, enflurane, isoflurane, esmolol, or propranolol, depending upon the event and on one's best guess as to its cause. The remainder of the patient's course is managed with the physiologic principles alluded to previously.

For the half hour immediately before cross-clamping and aortic occlusion, the patient is kept slightly hypovolemic by examining the ventricular volume (end diastolic dimension) by means of 2D-TEE or by keeping PCWP at 5 to 12 mm Hg. At the time of occlusion one should be prepared to give a vasodilating drug through an iv line placed specifically for that purpose in order to avoid hypotension secondary to an accidental bolus of vasodilator. This catheter site is often the third lumen of the PA catheter.

Stabilizing of the PA pressure and systemic blood pressure with more sufentanil (25 to 50 μg) and vasodilating drugs before and during cross-clamping may not be enough. When myocardial ischemia is noted by regional wall motion abnormalities (WMA) or ST-segment changes, or by new v waves on PCWP transduction, more vasodilating drugs are given, to the point of bringing the systolic blood pressure toward the low end of the normal preoperative range. Once the blood pressure is made as low as possible (by reduction of afterload with nitroprusside), we often attempt to decrease the preload with nitroglycerin and, if necessary, to decrease the heart rate with propranolol or esmolol given iv. If, despite these maneuvers, one sees myocardial dysfunction on placement of the cross-clamp, the surgeon can be asked to unclamp the aorta partially until myocardial function is more stable before he has incised the aorta or its branches. Close communication with the surgeon and a mutual appreciation of what the other physician is doing are key factors in facilitating the patient's course. We try to avoid the use of exogenous vasoconstrictors at this time.

To ensure adequate volume at the time of crossclamp removal, replace blood lost during occlusion by giving warmed blood, milliliter for milliliter, to keep the hematocrit slightly above 30% it will fall to 30% in the postocclusion period. (This is my personal belief, substantiated by some data, as the minimal acceptable value for patients in this risk group.[172-174]) Much of the transfused blood administered is from either predeposit or autotransfusion of blood salvaged from the operative field. Immediately before and during removal of the crossclamp, we stop infusing the vasodilator and start infusing crystalloid or blood; usually, two units of whole blood are pressured into venous access sites. Guided by filling pressures and/or echocardiographic estimates of volume, we are careful not to dilate the left ventricle to an abnormal size.

It is not uncommon for moderate hypotension (i.e., a decrease in systolic pressure of 40 to 60 mm Hg) to occur upon removal of the aortic crossclamp, regardless of whether the clamp is replaced infrarenally or such that blood flow to only one leg is obstructed. On observations with 2D-TEE, we believe that such hypotension is caused mainly by relative volume depletion. If hypotension persists for more than 4 minutes after removal of the clamp and does not return toward normal levels after blood deficits have been replaced, we search for other causes, including myocardial dysfunction, hidden blood loss, and so on. If necessary, the surgeon can reclamp or occlude the aorta, preferably below the renal arteries. Thus, volume replacement and maintenance are mainstays of therapy before, during, and immediately after removal of the aortic crossclamp. When blood flow to the first extremity is opened up, volume replacement should also be considered.

During closure, again ensure adequate organ perfusion as well as hemodynamic and temperature homeostasis, and we reverse muscle relaxants. Nitroglycerin and/or esmolol infusions should be available at this time, and hemodynamic variations outside the patient's normal range are not allowed. If the patient demonstrates adequate ventilation (as is common 6 hours after our initial dose of sufentanil), the trachea is extubated; otherwise, controlled ventilation is maintained until spontaneous ventilation is judged adequate. If an inhalational anesthetic technique is used, I often place an epidural catheter in the operating room at the end of the operation, after the patient has demonstrated bilateral foot movement (with light anesthesia during closure). Epidural opioids are administered to this group of patients, but rarely is other pain therapy needed for 24 hours when the sufentanil-based technique described here is used. Continuing care into the postoperative period is very important for patient outcome.

The outcome after infrarenal aortic reconstructive surgery has improved. Hicks et al[19] reported a decrease in the rate of mortality from 22% during 1955–1960 (for 41 patients) to 12.5% during 1966–1970, and to 4.2% during 1970–1973. In the series of Scobie and Masters,[175] the rate of perioperative mortality for elective repair of an abdominal aneurysm decreased from 12% during 1961–1969 to 4.1% during 1971–1975, and to 1.8% during 1976–1980. Accompanying this decrease in the rate of mortality was an increase in the use of venous pressure (fluid) monitoring devices—from 13% for 1961–1969 to 100% after 1971. After 1975, the use of pulmonary artery thermodilution catheters also increased.[175] Thus, overall, the rates of mortality and morbidity for aortic reconstructive surgery have decreased greatly over the last 3 decades. Crawford et al[23] attributed most of the reduction in morbidity in patients who had infrarenal resections before 1971 to improvement in operative techniques and, after 1981, to improvements in anesthesia, monitoring, and supportive care. However, the rate of perioperative mortality from supraceliac aneurysms still exceeds 4%.

An 8% incidence rate of myocardial infarction, with no mortality, which occurred in 12 patients who were studied with 2D-TEE is possible in patients who have severe myocardial dysfunction.[14] However, we believe that aiming for the 4% rate of mortality that Crawford et al[23] reported and the even lower rate that Benefiel et al[26] reported is probably as good as one can achieve with current techniques. In patients who have isolated celiac artery disease and little dysfunction in other organs, the occurrence of mortality or morbidity should be negligible.

ANESTHESIA FOR EMERGENCY AORTIC RECONSTRUCTION

Causes and Indications

The most common cause of emergency aortic reconstruction is a leaking or ruptured aortic aneurysm. Patients who have symptoms of acute ischemia are discussed in the following section. Ruptured aneurysms can be atherosclerotic, mycotic, syphilitic, or inflammatory or may occur in patients with the Marfanoid syndrome.[175–186] These ruptures are ten times more common in male than in female patients, as opposed to aortic aneurysms in general, which have a 4:1 male to female preponderance.

Ruptures most commonly occur into the retroperitoneum.[176–183] This site permits tamponade of the hemorrhage; however, retroperitoneal hemorrhage and subsequent hematoma can displace the left renal vein, inferior vena cava, and intestine, possibly leading to damage to these structures during the surgical approach. Venous hemorrhage is often much more difficult to control than is arterial hemorrhage.

Approximately 25% of aneurysms rupture into the peritoneal cavity, a site associated with a great degree of exsanguination. Other sites of rupture include adjacent structures after formation of fistulae with the inferior vena cava, iliac veins, or renal veins.[187–191]

Aortoenteric fistulae most commonly rupture into the fixed third portion of the duodenum.[192] These fistulae usually occur between the overlying bowel and a portion of the aorta that has previously undergone resection and grafting for an existing aneurysm. Mortality rates for these fistulae are high, often exceeding 50%. An abdominal aortic aneurysm may dissect proximally, resulting in hemopericardium.[193] The overall mortality rates vary in published series from 15 to 90%, with the time from the onset of symptoms to control of bleeding the key in determining outcome. This gives credence to the inescapable sense of urgency that accompanies such events. Other factors that adversely affect outcome[180, 181, 186] are a history of chronic hypertension, heart disease, or renal insufficiency, a hematocrit below 32.5% at diagnosis, hypotension at diagnosis, surgery lasting more than 400 minutes, and blood loss greater than 11,000 ml. Factors associated with a poor outcome that may be influenced by anesthetic management are hypotension lasting longer than 110 minutes and a systolic blood pressure below 100 mm Hg at the end of the operation.

The interval from the onset of symptoms to arrival at the hospital ranges from 0.3 to 22.5 hours, the mean interval being approximately 7 hours.[186] Among 100 patients with ruptured abdominal aortic aneurysms, Ottinger[183] found the following distribution of symptoms: pain, 92 patients; collapse, 17 patients; faintness, 13; vomiting, 13; numbness in leg, 3; inability to void, 2; and weakness in leg, 1. For 8 patients, an adequate history could not be obtained. Pain in the back, abdomen, or both was almost always present. This pain resulted from "dissection of the aortic wall and retroperitoneal spaces by blood." Therefore, many surgeons believe that pain in combination with a known abdominal aortic aneurysm or pulsatile abdominal mass indicates dissection or rupture and the immediate need for surgical exploration until proved otherwise.

Shock also frequently accompanies rupture. May et al[182] reported that 56% of patients with ruptured abdominal aortic aneurysms were in shock at the time of admission, with cold and clammy extremities or blood pressures of 100/60 mm Hg or less. However, the absence of hypotension does not rule out the possibility of rupture, and shock may occur suddenly. Patients with dissection may have severe hypertension, which must be controlled immediately if rupture is to be prevented.

Rapid diagnosis with immediate laparotomy and control of the proximal aorta are of the highest priority. If systolic blood pressure is less than 90 mm Hg, some clinicians advocate the administration of oxygen by face mask, with endotracheal intubation only after proximal control of the aorta is achieved.[180] Because experienced anesthesia personnel can usually intubate the trachea rapidly, and because of the substantial threat of aspiration pneumonitis, we usually do not follow the procedure of Lawrie et al.[180, 181] Initially, rapid-sequence endotracheal intubation is performed. We believe that this causes little morbidity, creates only a slight delay, and prevents a potentially serious complication. The probability of rupture into the free peritoneal cavity is high if loss of consciousness and/or mental aberration occurs along with marked hypotension that is unresponsive to rapid volume infusion. In this case, the trachea is immediately intubated in a rapid-sequence fashion, usually with the aid of muscle relaxants and with only small doses of barbiturates or opioids; ventilation with 100% oxygen is also started. Almost simultaneously, laparotomy is begun so that the surgeon can clamp the aorta.

I attempt to replace volume to the point of normalizing the systemic blood pressure (at this time, often the only guide to volume replacement in the patient with an uncontained rupture). A difference from elective surgery is that heparin is not administered before aortic cross-clamping.

The patient is resuscitated quickly (before induction of anesthesia, if possible) with type-specific uncrossmatched blood and crystalloid that are administered via large-bore venous catheters by roller pumps and/or pressured bags. If type-specific blood is not available, O-negative washed red blood cells may be given.

Once the aorta is controlled with a crossclamp and blood pressure and perfusion are restored, additional venous access is obtained if necessary. It is often helpful, indeed necessary, to have a second anesthesiologist secure vascular access while the first is securing the airway, monitoring blood pressure, and administering volume into the iv sites that have been established. Peripheral arterial and PA catheters are then inserted. At this point, volume administration is guided by means of filling pressures obtained from PA catheter readings.

We do not administer diuretics routinely, although many clinicians do. If intraoperative oliguria (urinary output of 0.125 ml·kg^{-1}·hr^{-1} or less) is noted, patency of the urinary catheter and collection system and adequate left-sided cardiac filling pressures are first ensured. In situations in which hypotension secondary to rupture has occurred, and perhaps low-output acute tubular necrosis is present, 12.5 to 25 g of mannitol or 40 to 120 mg of furosemide is administered in an attempt to increase the urinary output.

We do not hesitate to paralyze and administer large doses of opioids to these patients if they are hemodynamically stable, because these patients usually require postoperative mechanical ventilation of the lungs and sedation for minimizing of cardiovascular stress.

A second group of patients has pain and shock that reverses with volume administration. In such a patient, it may be assumed that hemorrhage has been contained at least partially. However, because rapid exsanguination can occur at any time, patients are transported immediately to the operating room for emergency laparotomy, and the same sense of urgency is maintained.

If the blood pressure and heart rate are stable when the patient arrives, sterile preparation of the abdomen is begun. The intravascular volume status may be assessed by observation of the patient for a decrease in systemic blood pressure and/or an increase in the heart rate when the head is raised 10 to 15 degrees. Administration of a 50-mg bolus of thiopental iv may also aid in the assessment of volume. Induction of anesthesia is delayed until the patient's abdomen is prepped and draped and the surgeon is ready. Venous access is ensured, and positive indications of acceptable volume loading are demonstrated by tilt test or small doses of thiopental, or measurements from a PA catheter (rapidly placed) are sought. Thus, in this situation, minimal extra time is spent on insertion and attaching of monitors.

Preoxygenation is followed by rapid-sequence induction of anesthesia, with small doses of fentanyl or sufentanil, small to moderate doses of thiopental (0.5 to 5 mg·kg^{-1}, depending upon the response to the test dose of thiopental), a rapidly acting muscle relaxant, application of cricoid pressure, and endotracheal intubation. To blunt the hemodynamic effects of laryngeal visualization and endotracheal intubation, one may administer an iv bolus of lidocaine, sodium nitroprusside, nitroglycerin, esmolol, or additional fentanyl, sufentanil, or thiopental.

If hypotension occurs following induction, administer 100% oxygen, elevate the patient's legs, and rapidly administer blood and fluids. If these measures fail to produce adequate blood pressure and perfusion, we infuse phenylephrine or dopamine until the aorta can be occluded.

During temporary aortic occlusion, we insert a PA catheter (if it is not already in place) to guide volume administration. High-normal filling pressures are desirable for attenuation of hypotension following removal of the aortic clamp.

Because of the site of aortic occlusion, replacement blood may not pass through the liver in amounts adequate to allow for metabolism of citrate.[141] Therefore, if hypotension owing to poor myocardial contractility or to coagulopathy develops, administration of calcium may be therapeutic.

A third possibility is the patient who was initially treated with a military antishock trouser (MAST) suit. This temporizing measure allows transport of the patient to the operating room with less hemorrhage and, some believe, with clot formation and temporary sealing of the aortic rent. If possible, pressure should be removed in stages (e.g., from the epigastrium, then one leg, and then the other leg) rather than all at once, and only after the surgeons are scrubbed and ready to begin immediately if necessary. Reducing all pressure at once would allow increased blood flow (reactive hyperemia) to occur in all areas simultaneously, thereby causing a large and precipitous decrease in blood pressure and filling volumes of the heart.

We routinely use autotransfusion in patients with actual or suspected aortic aneurysm rupture. However, a separate team is available to set up and operate autotransfusion devices, as the primary anesthesiologist should direct all of his or her attention to the patient's volume status, gas exchange, and depth of anesthesia. Our mnemonic for treatment of such patients is "wovcath," for wonder what anesthetic to give, or wonder whether the patient can tolerate an anesthetic, oxygen, vecuronium, coagulation, acid-base, temperature, and hemodynamics. This mnemonic lists, in reverse order, the important aspects of patient care that we try to remember when everything about these patients invites disorganization.

Whereas, in elective resection, the most important determinant of outcome is the maintenance of cardiac well-being, in that cardiovascular complications account for more than 50% of all mortality in elective aortic reconstruction,[17-26] hypotension because of exsanguination is the primary cause of death if rupture occurs.[175-186] Therefore, when rupture is suspected, rapid control of the proximal portion of the aorta is probably more important than is optimizing of the patient's preoperative condition.

The primary goal of aortic reconstruction is an enduring restoration of normal visceral and limb perfusion. The complications that occur during aortic occlusion can usually be linked to the heart, CNS, or kidneys. I believe that organ dysfunction, which involves the heart, can be minimized by maintenance of intraoperative values for hemodynamic variables within the normal preoperative range, ensuring that cardiac dilation does not occur at any point, and minimizing episodes of tachycardia. Attention to details of preoperative drug therapy, preoperative hydration, and temperature homeostasis may also promote an improved outcome. Further, vigilance must continue into the postoperative period if the risks of morbidity or mortality are to be minimized. As opposed to elective aortic reconstruction in which preserving myocardial function is the primary goal, in emergency resection the crucial factor for patient survival is initial rapid control of blood loss and reversal of hypotension, and then preservation of myocardial function.

SURGERY FOR PERIPHERAL VASCULAR INSUFFICIENCY

There are three clinical indications for elective surgery for chronic peripheral occlusive disease: 1) claudication, 2) ischemic rest pain or ulceration, and 3) gangrene.[194] Patients with claudication have symptoms on walking that are relieved by rest. Such patients are not at significant risk for imminent limb loss. Patients with rest pain, ulceration, and/or gangrene are at variable risk for imminent limb loss and may have severe progressive ischemia. Thus, reconstruction is semiurgent or urgent. Vascular reconstruction procedures are generally categorized as either inflow or outflow procedures. Inflow reconstruction involves bypass of the obstruction in the aortoiliac segment, whereas outflow procedures are those performed distal to the inguinal ligament for bypass of femoropopliteal or distal obstructions.

The most common inflow reconstruction procedure for obstructions in the aortoiliac segment is aortofemoral bypass. This method was discussed in the previous section. The usual vascular reconstruction below the inguinal ligament is a bypass graft that originates in the common femoral artery and extends to the popliteal or tibial artery. Such a bypass may be performed with a reversed saphenous vein, the saphenous vein in situ, or a prosthetic graft.[195] For the vascular surgeon, the differences among these procedures involve different technical aspects of vessel dissection and exposure, of anastomosis, and of tunneling.

The complexity of femoropopliteal and femorotibial bypass varies widely. The site for distal anastomosis and the quality of the outflow vessels are assessed by preoperative angiography. The best short- and long-term results are achieved when the saphenous vein is used[196, 197]; however, this requires longer operative time and greater technical expertise than are needed for prosthetic grafts. The duration and complexity of the operation are usually determined by the quality of the saphenous vein and the quality and size of the distal outflow vessels. Operative arteriography is commonly used for evaluation of the adequacy of the surgical repair. Major blood loss or hemodynamic changes are not usually encountered with distal reconstruction, but the procedure tends to be lengthy, making intraoperative urinary drainage advisable. Since the major morbidity and mortality with this procedure are related to the cardiovascular system, with rates above 8% and 2%, respectively, the noninvasive nature and the absence of hemodynamic alterations should not lull the anesthesiologist into taking a casual attitude.[195–197]

In a reversed saphenous vein bypass, the vein is dissected from its entrance into the common femoral vein to the level of the distal anastomosis. All branches of the saphenous vein are ligated and divided, and the vein is excised and inspected. After exposure of the proximal and distal vessels, the direction of the saphenous vein is reversed to permit blood flow in the direction of the valves, and the vein is tunneled from the femoral artery to the distal vessel. In this process, the surgeon tries to avoid damaging, injuring, or twisting the vein. After the proximal and distal anastomoses are completed, the adequacy of flow is determined from the quality of pulse and ultrasound signals, and from angiographic images obtained upon completion.

The use of the vein in situ offers significant advantages over the reversed-vein bypass. The large proximal saphenous vein is sutured to the large common femoral vein, and the small distal vein is sutured to the small distal artery. The size match is particularly important for tibial artery bypass, which permits the use of small saphenous veins that were previously judged unsuitable. In addition, since the vein is not removed from its bed, it is subjected to little trauma; twisting or kinking is unlikely. These advantages have resulted in improved patency rates.[198, 199]

For bypass procedures in which the saphenous vein in situ is used, the vein in its bed is dissected, and side branches are ligated. The proximal saphenous vein is then sutured end-to-side to the common femoral artery, and arterial flow is introduced into the vein. The valves that obstruct retrograde flow in the saphenous vein are lysed with a valvulotome or valve cutter, which is introduced through side branches. When all valves have been rendered incompetent, blood is seen flowing from the distal end of the vein. This distal end is then anastomosed to the appropriate arterial site. Here, also, the quality of the repair is determined from the pulse quality, doppler ultrasound studies, and completion angiography.

Prosthetic bypasses can be performed more quickly and require less dissection than does saphenous-vein bypass, because it is not necessary to make multiple incisions for vein harvest. Prosthetic bypasses, however, have significantly lower patency rates than do saphenous-vein bypasses, particularly when they extend below the knee.[198] Incisions are made for exposure of the proximal and distal arteries, and a tunneling instrument is used for tunneling of the graft between the incisions. After completion of the proximal and distal anastomoses, the quality of the anastomoses and the blood runoff to the foot are judged by intraoperative angiography. The patient is usually given heparin during the procedure; in most cases, the heparin effect is not antagonized, since bleeding problems are rare.

Emergency surgery for peripheral vascular insufficiency is required when acute arterial occlusion results in severe ischemia and threatens the viability of a limb. Immediate operation and restoration of blood flow are needed if limb loss is to be avoided. Depending upon the etiology of the occlusion, the patient may or may not be at very high risk.

Acute arterial occlusion causes the involved extremity to suddenly become cold and pulseless. Patients usually complain of coldness, pain, numbness, and paresthesias, and they may lose motion and sensation. The severity of ischemia and the urgency of immediate operation can be assessed by examination of leg motion and sensation. Abnormal sensation in the toes, feet, and legs in response to light touch and pin prick, as well as abnormal proprioception and loss of motor function in the feet and toes, are hallmarks of acute ischemia and nonviability. If the ischemia is not reversed in a matter of hours, irreversible loss of viability is likely to result.

Acute arterial occlusion may develop in patients who have pre-existing peripheral occlusive or aneurysmal disease caused by thrombosis of a stenotic or ulcerated atherosclerotic artery. Acute arterial occlusion can also occur in patients with normal peripheral arteries that contain emboli. Such embolism is usually of cardiac origin in patients with cardiac dysrhythmias, recent myocardial infarctions, or ventricular aneurysms.[200, 201]

The cause is important in planning operative treatment. If the cause is an arterial embolus, Fogarty embolectomy through a groin incision under local anesthesia may suffice. However, if the cause is thrombosis of severely diseased atherosclerotic arteries, bypass reconstruction will be required. Preoperative angiography may be of help in the differential diagnosis; often the cause is not uncovered until the vessel is opened. Thus, the anesthesiologist must be prepared for either a simple or a complex, extended procedure.

Patients with acute ischemia (arterial insufficiency) may be very ill. Significant fluid losses can be anticipated when the artery is flushed during thrombectomy, and fluid can be sequestered in edematous revascularized tissue. Serum potassium levels can change quickly, since cell death and release of intracellular potassium into the circulation can be anticipated. Myoglobin may also be released into the circulation, and the development of a compartment syndrome is a possibility.

An incision in the groin is usually made for exposure of the femoral artery. Attempts to pass Fogarty catheters proximally and distally are made in the effort to establish flow and extract the thrombus. If flow is not restored in this manner, more complex reconstructive procedures such as aortofemoral, axillofemoral, or femoropopliteal bypass may be required. Femoral venous drainage on restoration of flow to the femoral artery can aid in management by wasting the initial venous effluent from an acutely ischemic extremity. This may entail significant blood loss.

ANESTHETIC GOALS AND MANAGEMENT

There is perhaps no other disease entity in which the anesthesiologist can be misled so easily. "Oh, it's just a local procedure"; or, "just put a spinal in and let's get on with it, you don't have to read the chart." The latter was a comment used by an experienced vascular surgeon. However, the morbidity and mortality following these distal operations approach those following infraaortic reconstruction and are mainly of cardiac origin. Thus, although I tend to use epidural anesthesia and epidural opioids for pain relief, attention to body temperature, oxygen delivery, and hemodynamic homeostasis should be just as intense here as in aortic procedures that involve much greater hemodynamic fluctuations. The devices and the concerns previously described apply, with special attention to the postoperative period. It is during the postoperative period that most cardiac problems arise, and this is when pain relief and correction of hemodynamic and fluid dysequilibria are most likely to be needed. Care must be taken not to allow overhydration to occur intraoperatively in support of blood pressure, and then to cause congestive heart failure as the epidural sympathectomy wears off. As is done for patients with aortic disease, I routinely tilt the patient's head down (while monitoring gas exchange closely) for the last hour of the planned surgery. Dye loads given for completion angiography also contribute to fluid shifts; I consider monitoring of left ventricular filling volumes to be important for a successful outcome for these patients.

The surgeons' concerns for patients with peripheral vascular insufficiency include not only those involving the cardiovascular system, but also specific problems related to the operative repair. Graft patency is evaluated carefully in the recovery room. Most surgeons believe that the patient's feet should be kept warm and that the patient should be well hydrated so that peripheral vasoconstriction, which may limit outflow from the new graft, is prevented. If graft thrombosis develops in the early postoperative period, the patient is promptly returned to the operating room for graft thrombec-

tomy and for evaluation and correction of the cause of the thrombosis. It can be anticipated that, during graft thrombectomy, significant blood loss will occur with flushing of the graft.

ANESTHESIA FOR EMERGENCY SURGERY FOR PERIPHERAL VASCULAR INSUFFICIENCY

Acute peripheral vascular occlusion must be attended to quickly. Although this problem may appear to be localized in an extremity, it is vitally important to remember that the occluding material may originate in the heart or in major arteries. Therefore, peripheral vascular occlusion may be the result of a more serious cardiovascular problem. In fact, some patients with peripheral vascular occlusion are the sickest patients I have ever anesthetized.

Anticoagulants are commonly administered to patients suspected of having peripheral vascular occlusion. If a patient has received anticoagulants, the appropriateness of using a major conduction block (subarachnoid or epidural block with or without catheter placement) is controversial. Cunningham et al[166] described the effect of continuous epidural anesthesia in 100 patients who underwent resection of abdominal aortic aneurysms and operations for aortoiliac occlusion. No epidural hematoma was encountered. Another group reported on the results of continuous epidural anesthesia in 3,168 patients and continuous subarachnoid anesthesia in 841 patients undergoing peripheral vascular surgery of the lower extremities.[167] Patients who received anticoagulants or who had leukemia, thrombocytopenia, hemophilia, or traumatic insertion of the catheter were given a general anesthetic. In this series, also, no hematomas or neurologic sequelae were reported. If patients with acute peripheral occlusion who are to undergo emergency surgery have received anticoagulants before arriving in the operating room, we avoid giving major conduction blockade anesthesia. This rule is based on anecdotal case reports of epidural hematoma, which caused paraplegia in similar situations.[202-204]

In addition, as previously mentioned, these patients often have hyperkalemia and acidosis, which arise from ischemic extremities, and myoglobin may be released into the circulation. Although the surgical procedure may be only a peripheral one, cardiac causes, generalized atherosclerosis, electrolyte and acid-base balance disturbances, and fluid shifts, as well as the high morbidity and mortality associated with these procedures, will bring the cavalier anesthesiologist to his knees. And getting away with no care, or little care, for such patients is just a matter of luck. Skill and intensive care as meticulous as that given patients with visceral ischemia may also benefit those with peripheral vascular insufficiency.

CONCLUSION

Perhaps in no other subspecialty can anesthesiologists have as great an influence on patient outcome as they do in anesthesia for vascular surgery. Similar considerations for preoperative patient evaluation can be made for patients with cardiac disease undergoing other noncardiac procedures. The patients undergoing vascular reconstruction are generally elderly. Vascular disease is a generalized process; thus, patients having surgery for a specific vascular disorder are likely to have atherosclerotic disease elsewhere in their vascular system. Most of the patients have CAD. Many have a history of smoking, and chronic obstructive pulmonary disease, renal insufficiency, and lipid abnormalities are frequently present. Data presented in this chapter show that, although blood flow to many different organs may be interrupted, the stress of clamping and unclamping of vessels differs in different operations, and co-morbid conditions of patients are not similar in different operations, the major morbidity in each of the operations relates to myocardial well-being; therefore, the heart should be the major focus of the anesthesiologist's attention.

Attempts have been made to segregate patients who have significant CAD by use of dipyridamole-thallium scanning or coronary angiography or other means, and then to have patients at high risk for myocardial events undergo coronary artery bypass surgery before their vascular surgery. However, it has not been proved that such approaches reduce morbidity. Critics claim that such segregation is useful for identification of high-risk patients but that coronary angiography and surgery are simply a survival test preparatory to vascular surgery.

In cerebrovascular surgery, the goals in anesthesia management of ensuring adequate myocardial and brain perfusion and a rapidly arousable patient may be facilitated with the use of the EEG as a guide to afterload reduction. In aortic reconstruction, the available data imply that ensuring intact myocardial function is probably the best way of making certain that spinal cord, visceral, and renal perfusion will be adequate.

In the case of peripheral occlusive disease, the absence of hemodynamic changes should not lull the anesthesiologist into believing that vigilance about the patient's myocardial well-being will not be rewarded. It is also important to remember that vigilance in ensuring that routines such as prehydration and use of a warming mattress is probably more important for the outcome than is occasional brilliance. If given the opportunity I would opt for the diligent, compulsive practitioner rather than the occasionally brilliant one, if I needed vascular surgery.

Perhaps in no circumstance is the mettle of an anesthesiologist determined better than in anesthesia for emergency vascular surgery. The conversion in our mind from being a trauma anesthesiologist to caring for the heart is a difficult challenge that should be undertaken as soon as hemodynamic stability occurs.

In this chapter, I have expressed my biases regarding both monitoring and anesthetic techniques; but it should be clear that many other approaches can be used for avoiding myocardial dysfunction. Perhaps it is most important to remember that the best patient results probably are achieved when the great vigilance shown intraoperatively is also applied preoperatively as well as postoperatively.

REFERENCES

1. Sundt TM, Sharbrough FW, Piepgras DG et al: Correlation of cerebral blood flow and electroencephalographic changes during carotid endarterectomy with results of surgery and hemodynamics of cerebral ischemia. Mayo Clin Proc 56:533, 1981
2. Hertzer NR, Lees CD: Fatal myocardial infarction following carotid endarterectomy; three hundred thirty-five patients followed 6–11 years after operation. Ann Surg 194:212, 1981
3. Ennix CL, Lawrie GM, Morris GC: Improved results of carotid endarterectomy in patients with symptomatic coronary artery disease: An analysis of 1,546 consecutive carotid operations. Stroke 10:122, 1979
4. Glaser RB: Morbidity and mortality resulting from vascular surgery. In Roizen MF (ed): Anesthesia for Vascular Surgery. New York, Churchill Livingstone, 1989
5. Hertzer NR, Beven EG, Young JR et al: Coronary artery disease in peripheral vascular patients: A classification of 1000 coronary angiograms and results of surgical management. Ann Surg 199:223, 1984
6. Kartchner MM, McRae LP: Carotid occlusive disease as a risk factor in major cardiovascular surgery. Arch Surg 117:1086, 1982
7. Dunn EJ: Concomitant cerebral and myocardial revascularization. Surg Clin North Am 66:385, 1986
8. Hertzer NR, Loop FD, Taylor PC et al: Combined myocardial revascularization and carotid endarterectomy—operative and late results in 331 patients. J Thorac Cardiovasc Surg 85:577, 1983
9. Barnes RW, Marsalek PG: Asymptomatic carotid disease in the cardiovascular surgical patient: Is prophylactic endarterectomy necessary? Stroke 12:497, 1981
10. Burke PA, Callow AD, O'Donnell TF et al: Prophylactic carotid endarterectomy for asymptomatic bruit. Arch Surg 117:1222, 1982
11. Graham AM, Gewertz BL, Zarins CK: Predicting cerebral ischemia during carotid endarterectomy. Arch 121:595, 1986
12. Smith JS, Roizen MF, Cahalan MK et al: Does anesthetic technique make a difference: Augmentation of systolic blood pressure during carotid endarterectomy: Effects of phenylephrine versus light anesthesia and of isoflurane versus halothane on the incidence of myocardial ischemia. (submitted)
13. Roizen MF, Ellis JE, Smith JS et al: Anesthesia for major vascular surgery. In Estafanous FG (ed): Anesthesia and the Heart. Stoneham, Massachusetts, Butterworth Publishers, 1988 (in press)
14. Roizen MG, Beaupre PN, Alpert RA et al: Monitoring with two-dimensional transesophageal echocardiography: Comparison of myocardial function in patients undergoing supraceliac, supra-renal-infraceliac, or infrarenal aortic occlusion. J Vasc Surg 1:300, 1984
15. Nevelsteen A, Suy R, Daenen MD et al: Aortofemoral grafting: Factors influencing late results. Surgery 88:642, 1980
16. Martinez BD, Hertzer NR, Beven EG: Influence of distal arterial occlusive disease on prognosis following aortobifemoral bypass. Surgery 88:795, 1980
17. Szilagyi DE, Smith RF, Derusso FJ et al: Contribution of abdominal aortic aneurysmectomy to prolongation of life. Ann Surg 164:678, 1966
18. Young AE, Sandberg GW, Couch NP: The reduction of mortality of abdominal aortic aneurysm resection. Am J Surg 134:585, 1977
19. Hicks GL, Eastland MW, Deweese JA et al: Survival improvement following aortic aneurysm resection. Ann Surg 181:863, 1975
20. Thompson JE, Hollier LH, Patman RD et al: Surgical management of abdominal aortic aneurysms: Factors influencing mortality and morbidity—a 20-year experience. Ann Surg 181:654, 1975
21. Mulcare RJ, Royster TS, Lynn RA et al: Long-term results of operative therapy for aortoiliac disease. Arch Surg 113:601, 1978
22. Whittemore AD, Clowes AW, Hechtman HB et al: Aortic aneurysm repair. Reduced operative mortality associated with maintenance of optimal cardiac performance. Ann Surg 192:414, 1980
23. Crawford ES, Saleh SA, Babb JW III et al: Infrarenal abdominal aortic aneurysm. Factors influencing survival after operation performed over a 25-year period. Ann Surg 193:699, 1981
24. Hertzer NR: Myocardial ischemia. Surgery 93:97, 1983
25. Yeager RA, Weigel RM, Murphy SS et al: Application of clinically valid cardiac risk factors to aortic aneurysm surgery. Arch Surg 121:278, 1986
26. Benefiel DJ, Roizen MF, Lampe GH et al: Morbidity after aortic surgery with sufentanil versus isoflurane anesthesia. Anesthesiology 65:A516, 1986
27. Roizen MF: Anesthesia for vascular surgery. In Benumof JL (ed):

Clinical Frontiers in Anesthesiology, pp 93–104. New York, Churchill Livingstone, 1983

28. Carroll RM, Laravuso RB, Schauble JF: Left ventricular function during aortic surgery. Arch Surg 111:740, 1976

29. Lunn JK, Dannemiller FJ, Stanley TH: Cardiovascular responses to clamping of the aorta during epidural and general anesthesia. Anesth Analg 58:372, 1979

30. Meloche R, Pottecher T, Audet J et al: Haemodynamic changes due to clamping of the abdominal aorta. Can Anaesth Soc J 24:20, 1977

31. Attia RR, Murphy JD, Snider M et al: Myocardial ischemia due to infrarenal aortic cross-clamping during aortic surgery in patients with severe coronary artery disease. Circulation 53:961, 1976

32. Silverstein PR, Caldera DL, Cullen DJ et al: Avoiding the hemodynamic consequences of aortic cross-clamping and unclamping. Anesthesiology 50:462, 1979

33. Plecha FR, Avellone JC, Beven EG et al: A computerized vascular registry: Experience of the Cleveland Vascular Society. Surgery 86:826, 1979

34. Kouchoukos NT, Lell WA, Karp RB et al: Hemodynamic effects of aortic clamping and decompression with a temporary shunt for resection of the descending thoracic aorta. Surgery 85:25, 1979

35. DeBakey ME, Creech O Jr, Morris GC Jr: Aneurysm of thoraco-abdominal aorta involving the celiac, superior mesenteric, and renal arteries. Report of four cases treated by resection and homograft replacement. Ann Surg 144:549, 1956

36. Burham SJ, Johnson G Jr, Gurri JA: Mortality risks for survivors of vascular reconstructive procedures. Surgery 92:1072, 1983

37. Denlin A, Ohlsen H, Swedenborg J: Growth rate of abdominal aortic aneurysms as measured by computed tomography. Br J Surg 72:530, 1985

38. Darling RC: Ruptured arteriosclerotic abdominal aortic aneurysms: A pathologic and clinical study. Am J Surg 119:397, 1970

39. Sabawala PB, Strong MJ, Keats AS: Surgery of the aorta and its branches. Anesthesiology 33:229, 1970

40. Barry KG, Mazze RI, Schwartz FD: Prevention of surgical oliguria and renal-hemodynamic suppression by sustained hydration. N Engl J Med 270:1371, 1964

41. Wheeler CG, Thompson JE, Kartchner MM et al: Massive fluid requirement in surgery of the abdominal aorta. N Engl J Med 275:320, 1968

42. Alpert RA, Roizen MF, Hamilton WK et al: Intraoperative urinary output does not predict postoperative renal function in patients undergoing abdominal aortic revascularization. Surgery 95:707, 1984

43. Bush HL Jr, LoGerfo FW, Weisel RD et al: Assessment of myocardial performance and optimal volume loading during elective abdominal aortic aneurysm resection. Arch Surg 112:1301, 1977

44. Moyer JH, Heider C, Morris GC Jr et al: Renal failure: I. The effect of complete renal artery occlusion for variable periods of time as compared to exposure to subfiltration arterial pressures below 30 mm Hg for similar periods. Ann Surg 145:41, 1957

45. Laschinger JC, Cunningham JN Jr, Catinella FP et al: Detection and prevention of intraoperative spinal cord ischemia after cross-clamping of the thoracic aorta: Use of somatosensory evoked potentials. Surgery 92:1109, 1982

46. Crawford ES, Walker HSJ, Saleh SA et al: Graft replacement of aneurysm in descending thoracic aorta: Results without bypass or shunting. Surgery 89:73, 1981

47. Djindjian R, Hurth RM, Houdart M et al: Arterial supply of the spinal cord. In Angiography of the Spinal Cord, pp 3–13. Baltimore, University Park Press, 1970

48. Connolly JE: Prevention of paraplegia secondary to operations on the aorta. J Cardiovasc Surg 27:410, 1986

49. Wadouh F, Arndt C-F, Oppermann E et al: The mechanism of spinal cord injury after simple and double aortic cross-clamping. J Thorac Cardiovasc Surg 92:121, 1986

50. Roizen MF: Anesthetic implications of concurrent diseases. In Miller RD (ed): Anesthesia, 2nd ed, Vol 1, pp 255–357. New York, Churchill Livingstone, 1986

51. Boucher CA, Brewster DC, Darling RC et al: Determination of cardiac risk by dipyridamole-thallium imaging before peripheral vascular surgery. N Engl J Med 312:389, 1985

52. Samson D, Boone S: Extracranial-intracranial (EC-IC) arterial bypass. Past performance and current concepts. Neurosurgery 3:79, 1978

53. EC/IC Bypass Study Group: Failure of extracranial-intracranial arterial bypass to reduce the risk of ischemic stroke; results of an international randomized trial. N Engl J Med 313:1191, 1985

54. Haynes RB, Mukherjee J, Sackett DL et al: Functional status changes following medical or surgical treatment for cerebral ischemia; result of the extracranial-intracranial bypass study. JAMA 257:2043, 1987

55. Larson CP: Anesthesia for cerebrovascular insufficiency: How I do it in Palo Alto. In Roizen MF (ed): Anesthesia for Vascular Surgery. New York, Churchill Livingstone, 1989

56. Lusby R: Surgery for cerebrovascular insufficiency: What the surgeon is trying to accomplish and how. In Roizen MF (ed): Anesthesia for Vascular Surgery. New York, Churchill Livingstone, 1989

57. Baker WH, Dorner DB, Barnes RW: Carotid endarterectomy: Is an indwelling shunt necessary? Surgery 82:321, 1977

58. Ferguson GG: Intra-operative monitoring and internal shunts: Are they necessary in carotid endarterectomy. Stroke 13:287, 1982

59. West H, Burton R, Roon AJ et al: Comparative risk of operation and expectant management for carotid artery disease. Stroke 10:117, 1979

60. Stundt TM, Houser OW, Sharbrough FW et al: Carotid endarterectomy: Results, complications, and monitoring techniques. Adv Neurol 16:97, 1977

61. Wylie EJ: Is an asymptomatic carotid stenosis a surgical lesion? Presidential Address. Society of Cardiovascular Surgeons, 1982

62. Hamilton WK: Do let the blood pressure drop and do use myocardial depressants! Anesthesiology 45:273, 1976

63. Boysen G, Engell HC, Henriksen H: The effect of induced hypertension on internal carotid artery pressure and regional cerebral blood flow during temporary carotid clamping for endarterectomy. Neurology 22:1133, 1972

64. Ehrenfeld WK, Hamilton WK, Larson CP et al: Effect of CO_2 and systemic hypertension on downstream cerebral arterial pressure during carotid endarterectomy. Surgery 67:87, 1970

65. Smith JS, Cahalan MK, Benefiel DJ et al: Intraoperative detection of myocardial ischemia in high-risk patients: Electrocardiography versus two-dimensional transesophageal echocardiography. Circulation 872:1015, 1985

66. Ellis JE, Roizen MF, Aronson S et al: Frequency with which ST segment trends predict intraoperative myocardial ischemia. Anesthesiology 67:A002, 1987

67. Kotrly KJ, Kotter GS, Mortara D et al: Intraoperative detection of myocardial ischemia with an ST-segment trend monitoring system. Anesth Analg 63:343, 1984

68. Pichard AD, Diaz R, Marchant E et al: Large V waves in the pulmonary capillary wedge pressure tracing without mitral regurgitation; influence of pressure/volume relationship on the V wave size. Clin Cardiol 6:534, 1983

69. Riles TS, Kopelman I, Imparato AM: Myocardial infarction following carotid endarterectomy: A review of 683 operations. Surgery 85:249, 1979

70. McCaffrey MT: EEG and its transformation and meaning. In Roizen MF (ed): Anesthesia for Vascular Surgery. New York, Churchill Livingstone, 1989

71. Rampil IS, Holzer JA, Quest DO et al: Prognostic value of computerized EEG analysis during carotid endarterectomy. Anesth Analg 62:186, 1983

72. Rosenthal D, Stanton PE, Lamis PA: Carotid endarterectomy: The unreliability of intraoperative monitoring in patients having had stroke or reversible ischemic neurological deficit. Arch Surg 116:1569, 1981

73. Cho I, Smullens SN, Streletz LJ et al: The value of intraoperative EEG monitoring during carotid endarterectomy. Ann Neurol 20:508, 1986

74. Blume WT, Ferguson GG, McNeil DK: Significance of EEG changes at carotid endarterectomy. Stroke 17:891, 1986

75. Morawetz RB, Zeiger HE, McDowell HA et al: Correlation of cerebral blood flow and EEG during carotid occlusion for endarterectomy (without shunting) and neurologic outcome. Surgery 96:184, 1984

76. McCaffrey MT: Somatosensory and motor evoked potentials, their interpretation and meaning. In Roizen MF (ed): Anesthesia for Vascular Surgery. New York, Churchill Livingstone, 1989

77. Russ W, Fraedrich G: Intraoperative detection of cerebral ischemia with somatosensory evoked potentials during carotid endarterectomy—presentation of a new method. Thorac Cardiovasc Surg 32:124, 1984

78. Jacobs JA, Brinkman SD, Morrell RM et al: Long latency somatosensory evoked potentials during carotid endarterectomy. Am Surg 49:338, 1983

79. Markand ON, Dilley RS, Moorthy SS et al: Monitoring of somatosensory evoked potentials during carotid endarterectomy. Arch Neurol 41:375, 1984

80. Moorthy SS, Markand ON, Dilley RS et al: Somatosensory evoked responses during carotid endarterectomy. Anesth Analg 61:879, 1982

81. Messick JM, Casement B, Sharbrough FW et al: Correlation of regional cerebral blood flow (rCBF) with EEG changes during isoflurane anesthesia for carotid endarterectomy: Critical rCBF. Anesthesiology 66:344, 1987

82. McKay RD, Sundt TM Jr, Michenfelder JD et al: Internal carotid artery stump pressure and cerebral blood flow during carotid endarterectomy: Modification by halothane, enflurane and innovar. Anesthesiology 45:390, 1976

83. Slogoff S, Keats AS: Further observations on perioperative myocardial ischemia. Anesthesiology 65:539, 1986

84. Egbert LD, Battit GE, Turndorf H et al: The value of the preoperative visit by an anesthetist. JAMA 185:553, 1963

85. Bedford RF: Radial arterial function following percutaneous cannulation with 18- and 20-gauge catheters. Anesthesiology 47:37, 1977

86. Lanier WL, Stangland KJ, Scheithauer BW et al: The effects of dextrose infusion and head position on neurologic outcome after complete cerebral ischemia in primates: Examination of a model. Anesthesiology 66:39, 1987

87. Farias LA, Willis M, Gregory GA: Effects of fructose-1,6-diphosphate, glucose, and saline on cardiac resuscitation. Anesthesiology 65:595, 1986

88. Roizen MF, Sohn YJ, L'Hommedieu CS et al: Operating room temperature prior to surgical draping: Effect on patient temperature in recovery room. Anesth Analg 59:852, 1980

89. Nehls DG, Todd MM, Spetzler RF et al: A comparison of the cerebral protective effects of isoflurane and barbiturates during temporary focal ischemia in primates. Anesthesiology 66:453, 1987

90. Wade JG, Larson CP, Hickey RF et al: Effect of carotid endarterec-

91. Hosobuchi Y, Baskin DS, Woo SK: Reversal of induced ischemic neurologic deficit in gerbils by the opiate antagonist naloxone. Science 215:69,

92. Stinson EB, Holloway EL, Derby G et al: Comparative hemodynamic responses to chlorpromazine, nitroprusside, nitroglycerin, and trimethaphan immediately after open-heart operations. Circulation 53 (suppl I): I-26, 1974

93. Assidoa CB, Donegan JH, Whitesell RC et al: Factors associated with perioperative complications during carotid endarterectomy. Anesth Analg 61:631, 1982

94. Tarlov E, Schmidek H, Scott RM et al: Reflex hypotension following carotid endarterectomy: Mechanism and management. J Neurosurg 39:323, 1973

95. Goldstone J, Effeney DJ: The role of carotid endarterectomy in the treatment of acute neurologic deficits. Prog Cardiovasc Dis 22:415, 1980

96. Mentzer RM Jr, Finkelmeier BA, Crosby IK et al: Emergency carotid endarterectomy for fluctuating neurologic deficits. Surgery 89:60, 1981

97. Lusby RJ: Visceral ischemia: What the surgeons are trying to accomplish and how. In Roizen MF (ed): Anesthesia for Vascular Surgery. New York, Churchill Livingstone, 1989

98. Stoney RJ, Ehrenfeld WK, Wylie EJ: Revascularization methods in chronic visceral ischemia caused by atherosclerosis. Ann Surg 186:468, 1977

99. Stoney RJ, Lusby RJ: Surgery of celiac and mesenteric arteries. In Haimovici H (ed): Vascular Surgery Principles and Techniques. Norwalk, Connecticut, Appleton-Century-Crofts, 1984

100. Morris GC, DeBakey ME, Bernhard V: Abdominal angina. Surg Clin North Am 46:919, 1966

101. Hollier LH, Bernatz PE, Pairolero PC et al: Surgical management of chronic intestinal ischaemia: A reappraisal. Surgery 90:940, 1981

102. Baur GM, Millay DJ, Taylor LM Jr et al: Treatment of chronic visceral ischemia. Am J Surg 148:138, 1984

103. Rogers DM, Thompson JE, Garrett WV et al: Mesenteric vascular problems. A 26-year experience. Ann Surg 195:554, 1982

104. Bergqvist D, Bowald S, Eriksson I et al: Small bowel necrosis after aorto-iliac reconstruction. Br J Surg 73:28, 1986

105. Boley SJ, Borden EB: Acute mesenteric vascular disease. In Wilson SE, Veith FJ, Hobson RW et al (eds): Vascular Surgery—Principles and Practice, pp 659–671. New York, McGraw-Hill, 1987

106. Connolly JE, Kwaan JHM: Management of chronic visceral ischemia. Surg Clin North Am 62:345, 1982

107. Crawford ES, Morris GC Jr, Myhre HO et al: Celiac axis, superior mesenteric artery, and inferior mesenteric artery occlusion: Surgical considerations. Surgery 82:856, 1977

108. Zelenouk GR, Graham LM, Whitehouse WM Jr et al: Splanchnic arteriosclerotic disease and intestinal angina. Arch Surg 115:497, 1980

109. Jaxheimer EC, Jewell ER, Persson AV: Chronic intestinal ischemia. The Lahey Clinic approach to management. Surg Clin North Am 64:123, 1985

110. Eidemiller LR, Nelson JC, Porter JM: Surgical treatment of chronic visceral ischemia. Am J Surg 138:264, 1979

111. DeBakey ME: Changing concepts in vascular surgery. J Cardiovasc Surg 27:367, 1986

112. May AG, DeWeese JA, Frank I et al: Surgical treatment of abdominal aortic aneurysms. Surgery 63:711, 1968

113. Hollier LH, Reigel MM, Kazmier FJ et al: Conventional repair of abdominal aortic aneurysm in the high-risk patient: A plea for abandonment of non-resective treatment. J Vasc Surg 3:712, 1986

114. Estes E: Abdominal aortic aneurysm; a study of one hundred and two cases. Circulation 2:258, 1950

115. Foster JH, Bolashy BL, Gobbel WG Jr: Comparative study of elective resection and expectant treatment of abdominal aortic aneurysm. Surg Gynecol Obstet 129:1, 1969

116. Darling RC, Messian CR, Bewster DC: Autopsy study of unoperated abdominal aortic aneurysms. The case for early resection. Circulation 56(suppl 2):161, 1977

117. Szilagyi DE, Elliott JP: Clinical fate of the patient with asymptomatic abdominal aortic aneurysm and unfit for surgical treatment. Arch Surg 104:600, 1972

118. Thurmond AS, Semler HJ: Abdominal aortic aneurysm: Incidence in a population at risk. J Cardiovasc Surg 27:457, 1986

119. Reigel MM, Hollier LH, Kazmier EJ et al: Late survival in abdominal aortic aneurysm patients: The role of selective myocardial revascularization on the basis of clinical symptoms. J Vasc Surg 5:222, 1987

120. Khaw H, Sottiurai VS, Craighead CC et al: Ruptured abdominal aortic aneurysm presenting as symptomatic inguinal mass: Report of six cases. J Vasc Surg 4:384, 1986

121. Lambert ME, Baguley P, Charlesworth D: Ruptured abdominal aortic aneurysms. J Cardiovasc Surg 27:256, 1986

122. Brewster DC, Darling RC: Optimal methods of aortoiliac reconstruction surgery. Surgery 84:739, 1978

123. Szilagyi DE, Elliott JP Jr, Smith RF et al: A thirty-year survey of the reconstructive surgical treatment of aorto-iliac occlusive disease. J Vasc Surg 3:421, 1986

124. DeBakey ME, Crawford ES, Cooley DA et al: Aneurysm of abdominal aorta: Analysis of results of graft replacement therapy one to eleven years after operation. Ann Surg 160:622, 1964

125. Simma W, Bassiouny H, Haril P et al: Evaluation of profundoplasty in reconstructions of combined aorto-iliac and femoropopliteal occlusive disease. J Cardiovasc Surg 27:141, 1986

126. Sladen JG, Gilmour JL, Wong RW: Cumulative patency and actual palliation in patients with claudication after aorto-femoral bypass. Prospective long-term follow-up of 100 patients. Am J Surg 152:190, 1986

127. Poulias GE, Polemis L, Skoutas B et al: Bilateral aorto-femoral bypass in the presence of aorto-iliac occlusive disease and factors determining results. Experience and long-term follow-up with 500 consecutive cases. J Cardiovasc Surg 26:527, 1985

128. Starr DS, Lawrie GM, Morris GC Jr: Prevention of distal embolism during arterial reconstruction. Am J Surg 138:764, 1979

129. Burnett JR, Gray–Weale AC, Byrne K et al: The place of systemic heparin in elective aortic aneurysm repair. J Cardiovasc Surg 28 (suppl):7, 1987

130. Williams GM, Ricotta J, Zinner M et al: The extended retroperitoneal approach for treatment of extensive atherosclerosis of the aorta and renal vessels. Surgery 88:846, 1980

131. Roizen MF, Rodgers GM, Valone FH et al: Anaphylactoid reaction to vascular graft material (submitted)

132. Wylie EJ, Stoney RJ, Ehrenfeld WK: Aorto-iliac atherosclerosis. In Manual of Vascular Surgery, vol 1, pp 107–157. New York, Springer-Verlag, 1980

133. Donaldson MC, Louras JC, Bucknam CA: Axillofemoral bypass: A tool with a limited role. J Vasc Surg 3:757, 1986

134. Moore WS: Thrombosis of aortofemoral, axillofemoral, or femorofemoral grafts. In Veith FJ (ed): Critical Problems in Vascular Surgery, pp 445–461. Norwalk, Connecticut, Appleton-Century-Crofts, 1982

135. Kazman PG, Hosang M, Cina C et al: Current indications for axillounifemoral and axillobifemoral bypass grafts. J Vasc Surg 5:828, 1987

136. Qvarfordt PG, Stoney RJ, Reilly LM et al: Management of pararenal aneurysms of the abdominal aorta. J Vasc Surg 3:84, 1986

137. Perry MO: The hemodynamics of temporary abdominal aortic occlusion. Ann Surg 168:193, 1968

138. Bush HL Jr, LoGerfo RW, Weisel RD et al: Assessment of myocardial performance and optimal volume loading during elective abdominal aortic aneurysm resection. Arch Surg 112:1301, 1977

139. Pandian NG, Kerber RE: Two-dimensional echocardiography in experimental coronary stenosis. I. Sensitivity and specificity in detecting transient myocardial dyskinesis: Comparison with sonomicrometers. Circulation 66:597, 1982

140. Guyton AC: Textbook of Medical Physiology, 6th ed. Philadelphia, W.B. Saunders, 1981

141. Olinger GN, Hottenrott C, Mulder DG et al: Acute clinical hypocalcemic myocardial depression during rapid blood transfusion and postoperative hemodialysis. A preventable complication. J Thorac Cardiovasc Surg 72:503, 1976

142. Longo T, Marchetti G, Vercellio G: Coronary hemodynamic changes induced by aortic cross-clamping. J Cardiovasc Surg 10:36, 1969

143. Mandelbaum I, Webb MK: Left ventricular function during cross-clamping of the descending thoracic aorta. JAMA 186:229, 1963

144. Schlüter M, Langenstein BA, Polster J et al: Transesophageal cross-sectional echocardiography with a phased array transduced system. Technique and initial clinical results. Br Heart J 48:67, 1982

145. Beaupre PN, Cahalan MK, Kremer PF et al: Does pulmonary artery occlusion pressure adequately reflect left ventricular filling during anesthesia and surgery? Anesthesiology 59:A3, 1983

146. Flaherty JT, Magee PA, Gardner TL et al: Comparison of intravenous nitroglycerin and sodium nitroprusside for treatment of acute hypertension developing after coronary artery bypass surgery. Circulation 65:1072, 1982

147. Gerson JI, Allen FB, Seltzer JL et al: Arterial and venous dilation by nitroprusside and nitroglycerin—is there a difference? Anesth Analg 61:256, 1982

148. Feigl EO: The paradox of adrenergic coronary vasoconstriction. Circulation 76:737, 1987

149. Roizen MF, Hamilton WK, Sohn YJ: Treatment of stress-induced increases in pulmonary capillary wedge pressure using volatile anesthetics. Anesthesiology 55:446, 1981

150. Rampil IJ, Correll JW, Rosenbaum SH et al: Computerized electroencephalogram monitoring and carotid artery shunting. Neurosurgery 13:276, 1983

151. Koike M, Roizen MF, Zivin JA et al: Naloxone ameliorates adverse effects of some anesthetics on CNS injury. Anesthesiology 59:A333, 1983

152. Abbott WM, Austen WG: The reversal of renal cortical ischemia during aortic occlusion by mannitol. J Surg Res 16:482, 1974

153. Barry KG, Cohen A, Knochel JP et al: Mannitol infusion. II. The prevention of acute functional renal failure during resection of an aneurysm of the abdominal aorta. N Engl J Med 264:967, 1961

154. Flores J, DiBona DR, Beck CH et al: The role of cell swelling in ischemic renal damage and the protective effect of hypertonic solute. J Clin Invest 51:118, 1972

155. Hanley MJ, Davidson K: Prior mannitol and furosemide infusion in a model of ischemic acute renal failure. Am J Physiol 241:F556, 1981

156. Ostri P, Mouritsen L, Jorgensen B et al: Renal function following aneurysmectomy of the abdominal aorta. J Cardiovasc Surg 27:714, 1986

157. Miller DC, Myers BD: Pathophysiology and prevention of acute renal failure associated with thoraco-abdominal or abdominal-aortic surgery. J Vasc Surg 5:518, 1987

158. Roizen MF: Does choice of anesthetic (narcotic vs inhalational) significantly affect cardiovascular surgery? In Estafanous FG

(ed): Opioids in Anesthesia, pp 180–189. Boston, Butterworths, 1984

159. Reiz S, Balfors E, Sorensen MB et al: Isoflurane—a powerful coronary vasodilator in patients with coronary artery disease. Anesthesiology 59:91, 1983

160. Yeager MP, Glass DD, Neff RK et al: Epidural anesthesia and analgesia in high-risk surgical patients. Anesthesiology 66:729, 1987

161. Smith NT, Eger EI II, Stoelting RK et al: The cardiovascular and sympathomimetic responses to the addition of nitrous oxide to halothane in man. Anesthesiology 32:410, 1970

162. Smith JS, Cahalan MK, Benefiel DJ et al: Fentanyl versus fentanyl and isoflurane in patients with impaired left ventricular function. Anesthesiology 63:A18, 1985

163. Shingu K, Eger EI II, Johnson BH et al: Effect of oxygen concentration, hypothermia, and choice of vendor on anesthetic-induced hepatic injury to rats. Anesth Analg 62:146, 1983

164. Eisele JH, Smith NT: Cardiovascular effects of 40 percent nitrous oxide in man. Anesth Analg 51:956, 1972

165. Koblin DD, Watson JE, Deady JE et al: Inactivation of methionine synthetase by nitrous oxide in mice. Anesthesiology 54:318, 1981

166. Cunningham FO, Egan JM, Inahara T: Continuous epidural anesthesia in abdominal vascular surgery. A review of 100 consecutive cases. Am J Surg 139:624, 1980

167. Rao TLK, Gorski D, El-Etr AA: Epidural and subarachnoid catheters and anticoagulants. Anesthesiology 53:S213, 1980

168. Reiz S, Balfors E, Sorensen MB et al: Coronary hemodynamic effects of general anesthesia and surgery: Modification by epidural analgesia in patients with ischemic heart disease. Reg Anesth 7:S8, 1982

169. Rao TLK, El-Etr AA: Anticoagulation following placement of epidural and subarachnoid catheters: An evaluation of neurologic sequelae. Anesthesiology 55:618, 1981

170. Isaacson IJ, Berry AJ, Venner DS et al: Beneficial effects of intrathecal morphine on patients for abdominal aortic surgery. Anesthesiology (in press)

171. Jones ROM, Jones JG: Intrathecal morphine: Naloxone reverses respiratory depression but not analgesia. Br Med J 281:645, 1980

172. Lundsgaard–Hansen P: Hemodilution—New clothes for an anemic emperor. Vox Sang 36:321, 1979

173. Most AS, Ruocco NA, Gerwirtz H: Effect of a reduction in blood viscosity on maximal myocardial oxygen delivery distal to a moderate coronary stenosis. Circulation 74:1085, 1986

174. Weisel RD, Charlesworth DC, Mickleborough LL et al: Limitations of blood conservation. J Thorac Cardiovasc Surg 88:26, 1984

175. Scobie TK, Masters RG: Changing factors influencing abdominal aortic aneurysm repair. J Cardiovasc Surg 23:309, 1982

176. Butler MJ, Chant ADB, Webster JHH: Ruptured abdominal aortic aneurysms. Br J Surg 65:839, 1978

177. Darling RC, Messina CR, Brewster DC et al: Autopsy study of unoperated abdominal aortic aneurysms. The case for early resection. Circulation 56 (suppl II):II-161, 1977

178. Friedman SA: The evaluation and treatment of patients with arterial aneurysms. Med Clin North Am 65:83, 1981

179. Gardner RJ, Gardner NL, Tarnay TJ et al: The surgical experience and a one to sixteen year follow-up of 277 abdominal aortic aneurysms. Am J Surg 135:226, 1978

180. Lawrie GM, Crawford ES, Morris GC Jr et al: Progress in the treatment of ruptured abdominal aortic aneurysm. World J Surg 4:653, 1980

181. Lawrie GM, Morris GC Jr, Crawford ES et al: Improved results of operation for ruptured abdominal aortic aneurysm. Surgery 85:483, 1979

182. May AG, DeWeese JA, Frank I et al: Surgical treatment of abdominal aortic aneurysms. Surgery 63:711, 1968

183. Ottinger LW: Ruptured arteriosclerotic aneurysms of the abdominal aorta: Reducing mortality. JAMA 233:147, 1975

184. Sabiston DC Jr: Davis–Christopher Textbook of Surgery. The Biological Basis of Modern Surgical Practice, 10th ed, p 1672. Philadelphia, W.B. Saunders, 1972

185. Thompson JE, Garrett WV: Peripheral-arterial surgery. N Engl J Med 302:491, 1980

186. Wakefield TW, Whitehouse WM Jr, Shu-Chen W et al: Abdominal aortic aneurysm rupture: Statistical analysis of factors affecting outcome of surgical treatment. Surgery 91:586, 1982

187. Merrill WH, Ernst CB: Aorta-left renal vein fistula: Hemodynamic monitoring and timing of operation. Surgery 89:678, 1981

188. Savrin RA, Gustafson R: Spontaneous aorto-vena caval fistula: Hemodynamic monitoring. J Cardiovasc Surg 22:88, 1981

189. Schramek A, Hashmonai M, Better OS et al: Aortocaval fistula due to rupture of abdominal aortic aneurysm. Isr J Med Sci 16:733, 1980

190. Clowes AW, DePalma RG, Botti RE et al: Management of aortocaval fistula due to abdominal aortic aneurysm. Am J Surg 137:807, 1979

191. Cohen LJ, Sukov RJ, Boswell W et al: Spontaneous aortocaval fistula. Radiology 138:357, 1981

192. Connolly JE, Kwaan JHM, McCart PM et al: Aortoenteric fistula. Ann Surg 194:402, 1981

193. Snow N: Hemopericardium from retrograde dissection of an abdominal aortic aneurysm. Am Surg 46:589, 1980

194. Zarins CZ: Surgery for peripheral vascular insufficiency: What the surgeon is trying to accomplish and how. In Roizen MF (ed): Anesthesia in Vascular Surgery. New York, Churchill Livingstone, 1989

195. Veith FJ, Gupta SK, Ascer E: Femoral, popliteal, and tibial occlusive disease. In Wilson SE, Veith FJ, Hobson RW et al (eds): Vascular Surgery—Principles and Practice, pp 353–375. New York, McGraw-Hill, 1987

196. Mannick JA, Jackson BT, Coffman JD: Success of bypass vein grafts in patients with isolated popliteal artery segments. Surgery 61:17, 1967

197. Reichle FA, Tyson R: Comparison of long-term results of 364 femoropopliteal or femorotibial bypasses for revascularization of severely ischemic lower extremities. Ann Surg 182:449, 1975

198. Leather RP, Shah DM, Karmody AM: Infrapopliteal arterial bypass for limb salvage: Increased patency and utilization of the saphenous vein used in-situ. Surgery 90:1000, 1981

199. Buchbinder D, Singh JK, Karmody AM et al: Comparison of patency rate and structural change of in-situ and reversed vein arterial bypass. J Surg Res 30:213, 1981

200. Abbott WM, Maloney RD, McCabe RD et al: Arterial embolism: A 44-year perspective. Am J Surg 143:460, 1982

201. Connett MC, Murray DH Jr, Denneker WW: Peripheral arterial emboli. Am J Surg 148:14, 1984

202. Brem SS, Hafler DA, Van Uitert RL et al: Spinal subarachnoid hematoma: A hazard of lumbar puncture resulting in reversible paraplegia. N Engl J Med 304:1020, 1981

203. DeAngelis J: Hazards of subdural and epidural anesthesia during anticoagulant therapy: A case report and review. Anesth Analg 51:676, 1972

204. Edelson RN, Chernick NL, Posner JB: Spinal subdural hematomas complicating lumbar puncture. Arch Neurol 31:134, 1974

Chapter 37   *Kathryn E. McGoldrick*

Anesthesia and the Eye

Anesthesia for ophthalmic surgery presents many unique challenges (Table 37-1). In addition to possessing technical expertise, the anesthesiologist must have detailed knowledge of ocular anatomy, physiology, and pharmacology. It is essential to appreciate that ophthalmic drugs may significantly alter reaction to anesthesia and that, concomitantly, anesthetic drugs and maneuvers may dramatically influence intraocular dynamics. Patients undergoing ophthalmic surgery may represent extremes of age and coexisting medical diseases (*e.g.,* diabetes mellitus, coronary artery disease, essential hypertension, chronic lung disease), but they are likely to be in the elderly age group. Apprehension is predictable in blind or potentially blind patients awaiting surgery.

It is mandatory to be knowledgeable about the numerous surgical procedures unique to the specialty of ophthalmology. Whereas the list of ocular surgical interventions is lengthy, these procedures may, in general, be classified as extraocular or intraocular. This distinction is critical since anesthetic considerations are different for these two major surgical categories. For example, with intraocular procedures, profound akinesia (relaxation of recti muscles) and meticulous control of intraocular pressure (IOP) are requisite. However, with extraocular surgery, the significance of IOP fades, whereas concern about elicitation of the oculocardiac reflex assumes prominence.

OCULAR ANATOMY

The anesthesiologist should be knowledgeable about ocular anatomy in order to enhance his or her understanding of surgical procedures and to aid the surgeon in the performance of regional blocks when needed (Fig. 37-1).[1, 2] Salient subdivisions of ocular anatomy include the orbit, the eye itself, the extraocular muscles, the eyelids, and the lacrimal system.

The orbit is a bony box, or pyramidal cavity, housing the eyeball and its associated structures in the skull. The walls of the orbit are composed of the following bones: frontal, zygomatic, greater wing of sphenoid, maxilla, palatine, lacrimal, and ethmoid. A familiarity with the surface relationships of the orbital rim is mandatory to the skilled performance of regional blocks.

The optic foramen, located at the orbital apex, transmits the optic nerve, artery, and vein as well as sympathetic nerves from the carotid plexus. The superior orbital fissure transmits the superior and inferior branches of the oculomotor nerve, the lacrimal, frontal, and nasociliary branches of the trigeminal nerve, as well as the trochlear and abducens nerves and the superior and inferior ophthalmic veins. The inferior orbital or sphenomaxillary fissure contains the infraorbital and zygomatic nerves and a communication between the inferior ophthalmic vein and the pterygoid plexus. The infraorbital foramen, located about 4 mm below the orbital rim in the maxilla, transmits the infraorbital nerve, artery, and vein. In the superior temporal orbit, one finds the lacrimal fossa, which contains the lacrimal gland. The supraorbital notch, located at the junction of the medial one third and temporal two thirds of the superior orbital rim, transmits the supraorbital nerve, artery, and vein. The supraorbital notch, the infraorbital foramen, and the lacrimal fossa are clinically palpable and function as major landmarks for administration of regional anesthesia.

The eye itself is actually one large sphere with part of a smaller sphere incorporated in the anterior surface, constituting a structure with two different radii of curvature. The coat of the eye is composed of three layers: sclera, uveal tract, and retina. The fibrous outer layer, or sclera, is protective, providing sufficient rigidity to maintain the shape of the eye. The anterior portion of the sclera, the cornea, is transparent, permitting light to pass into the internal ocular structures. The double spherical shape of the eye exists because the corneal arc of curvature is steeper than the scleral arc of curvature. The focusing of rays of light to form a retinal image commences at the cornea.

The uveal tract, or middle layer of the globe, is vascular and in direct apposition to the sclera. A potential space, known as the suprachoroidal space, separates the sclera from the uveal tract. This potential space, however, may become filled with blood during an expulsive or suprachoroidal hemorrhage, oftentimes associated with surgical disaster. The iris, ciliary body, and choroid compose the uveal tract. The iris includes the pupil, which, by contractions of three sets of muscles, controls the amount of light entering the eye. The iris dilator is

sympathetically innervated; the iris sphincter and the ciliary muscle have parasympathetic innervation. Posterior to the iris lies the ciliary body, which produces aqueous humor. (See the section entitled Formation and Drainage of Aqueous Humor.) The ciliary muscles, situated in the ciliary body, adjust the shape of the lens to accommodate focusing at various distances. Large vessels and a network of small vessels and capillaries known as the choriocapillaris constitute the choroid, which supplies nutrition to the outer part of the retina.

The retina is a neurosensory membrane composed of ten layers that convert light impulses into neural impulses. These neural impulses are then carried through the optic nerve to the brain. Located in the center of the globe is the vitreous cavity, filled with a gelatinous substance known as vitreous humor. This material is adherent to the most anterior 3 mm of the retina as well as to large blood vessels and the optic nerve. The vitreous humor may pull on the retina, thus causing retinal tears and retinal detachment.

The crystalline lens, located posterior to the pupil, refracts rays of light passing through the cornea and pupil to focus images on the retina. The ciliary muscle, whose contractile state causes tautness or relaxation of the lens zonules, regulates the thickness of the lens.

In addition, six extraocular muscles move the eye within the orbit to various positions. The bilobed lacrimal gland provides the majority of the tear film, which serves to maintain a moist anterior surface on the globe. The lacrimal drainage system, composed of the puncta, canaliculi, lacrimal sac, and lacrimal duct, drains into the nose below the inferior turbinate. Blockage of this system occurs not infrequently, necessitating procedures ranging from lacrimal duct probing to dacryo-

TABLE 37-1.   Requirements of Ophthalmic Surgery

Safety
Akinesia
Profound analgesia
Minimal bleeding
Avoidance or obtundation of oculocardiac reflex
Proper control of IOP
Awareness of drug interactions
Smooth emergence

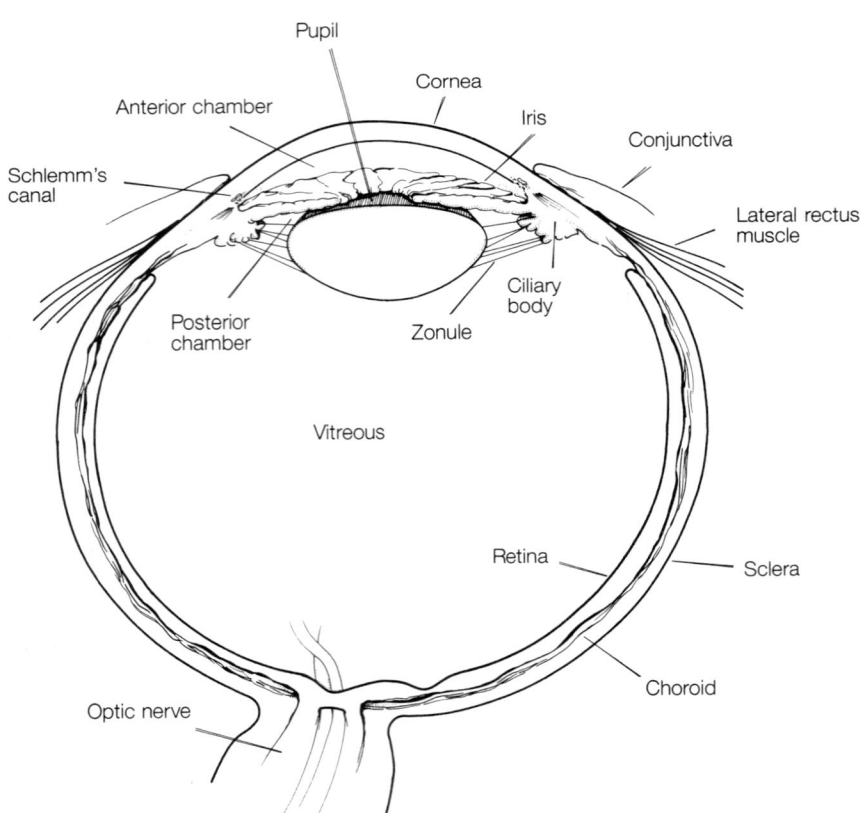

FIG. 37-1. Diagram of ocular anatomy.

cystorhinostomy, which involves anastomosis of the lacrimal sac to the nasal mucosa.

Covering the surface of the globe and lining the eyelids is a mucous membrane called the conjunctiva. Since drugs are well absorbed across the membrane, it is a popular site for administration of ophthalmic drugs.

The eyelids consist of four layers: 1) the conjunctiva; 2) the cartilaginous tarsal plate; 3) a muscle layer composed mainly of the orbicularis and the levator palpebrae; and 4) the skin. The eyelids protect the eye from foreign objects; through blinking, the tear film produced by the lacrimal gland is spread across the surface of the eye, keeping the cornea moist.

Blood supply to the eye and orbit is by means of branches of both the internal and external carotid arteries. Venous drainage of the orbit is accomplished through the multiple anastomoses of the superior and inferior ophthalmic veins. Venous drainage of the eye is achieved mainly through the central retinal vein. All these veins empty directly into the cavernous sinus.

The sensory and motor innervations of the eye and its adnexa are very complex, with multiple cranial nerves supplying branches to various ocular structures. A branch of the oculomotor nerve supplies a motor root to the ciliary ganglion, which in turn supplies the sphincter of the pupil and the ciliary muscle. The trochlear nerve supplies the superior oblique muscle. The abducens nerve supplies the lateral rectus muscle. The trigeminal nerve constitutes the most complex ocular and adnexal innervation. In addition, the zygomatic branch of the facial nerve eventually divides into an upper branch, supplying the frontalis and the upper lid orbicularis, whereas the lower branch supplies the orbicularis of the lower lid.

OCULAR PHYSIOLOGY

Despite its relatively diminutive size, the eye is a complex organ, concerned with many intricate physiologic processes. The formation and drainage of aqueous humor and their influence on IOP in both normal and glaucomatous eyes are among the most important functions, especially from the anesthesiologist's perspective. An appreciation of the effects of various anesthetic manipulations on IOP requires an understanding of the fundamental principles of ocular physiology.

FORMATION AND DRAINAGE OF AQUEOUS HUMOR

Two thirds of the aqueous humor is formed in the posterior chamber by the ciliary body in an active secretory process involving both the carbonic anhydrase and the cytochrome oxidase systems (Fig. 37-2). The remaining third is formed by passive filtration of aqueous humor from the vessels on the anterior surface of the iris.

At the ciliary epithelium, sodium is actively transported into the aqueous humor in the posterior chamber. Bicarbonate and chloride ions passively follow the sodium ions. This active mechanism results in the osmotic pressure of the aqueous being many times greater than that of plasma. And it is this disparity in osmotic pressure that leads to an average rate of aqueous humor production of 2 $\mu l \cdot min^{-1}$.

Aqueous humor flows from the posterior chamber through the pupillary aperture into the anterior chamber where it mixes with the aqueous formed by the iris. During its journey into the anterior chamber, the aqueous humor bathes the

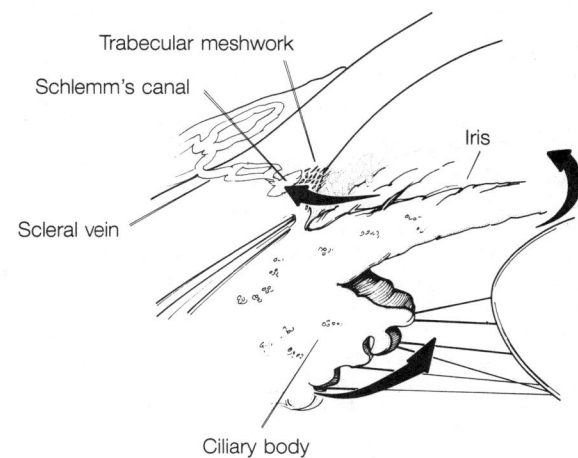

FIG. 37-2. Ocular anatomy concerned with control of intraocular pressure.

avascular lens, providing essential metabolic materials and, additionally, removing metabolic wastes. After arrival in the anterior chamber, the aqueous also bathes the corneal endothelium, maintaining healthy corneal metabolism. Then the aqueous flows into the peripheral segment of the anterior chamber and exits the eye via the trabecular network, Schlemm's canal, and the episcleral venous system. A network of connecting venous channels eventually leads to the superior vena cava and the right atrium. Thus, obstruction of venous return at any point from the eye to the right side of the heart impedes aqueous drainage, elevating IOP accordingly.

MAINTENANCE OF INTRAOCULAR PRESSURE (IOP)

IOP normally varies between 10 and 22 mm Hg and is considered abnormal above 25 mm Hg. This level varies 1 to 2 mm Hg with each cardiac contraction. Also, a diurnal variation of 2 to 5 mm Hg is observed, with a higher value noted upon awakening. This higher awakening pressure has been ascribed to vascular congestion, pressure on the globe from closed lids, and mydriasis—all of which occur during sleep.

IOP far exceeds not only tissue pressure (2 to 3 mm Hg) but also intracranial pressure (7 to 8 mm Hg). Apparently the maintenance of such a relatively high pressure in the eye is demanded by the optical properties of refracting surfaces; the corneal surface should be kept at a constant curvature, and the stroma must be under constant high pressure to maintain a uniform refractive index.[3] However, an abnormally high pressure may result in opacities by interfering with normal corneal metabolism.

During anesthesia, a rise in IOP can produce permanent visual loss. If the IOP is already elevated, a further increase can trigger acute glaucoma. If penetration of the globe occurs when the IOP is excessively high, rupture of a blood vessel with subsequent hemorrhage may transpire. Intraocular pressure becomes atmospheric once the eye cavity has been entered, and any sudden rise in pressure may lead to prolapse of the iris and lens, and loss of vitreous. Thus, proper control of IOP is critical.

Three main factors influence IOP: 1) external pressure on the eye by the contraction of the orbicularis oculi muscle and the tone of the extraocular muscles, venous congestion of orbital veins (as may occur with vomiting and coughing), and conditions such as orbital tumor; 2) scleral rigidity; and 3) changes in intraocular contents that are semisolid (lens, vitreous, or intraocular tumor) or fluid (blood and aqueous humor). Although these factors are significant in affecting IOP, the major control of intraocular tension is by the fluid content, especially the aqueous humor.

Sclerosis of the sclera, not uncommonly seen in the aged, may be associated with decreased scleral compliance and increased IOP. Other degenerative changes of the eye linked with aging can also influence IOP—the most significant being a hardening and enlargement of the crystalline lens. When these degenerative changes occur, they may lead to anterior displacement of the lens–iris diaphragm. A resultant shallowness of the anterior chamber angle may then occur, reducing access of the trabecular meshwork to aqueous. This process is usually gradual, but, if rapid lens engorgement occurs, angle closure glaucoma may transpire.

Changes in the nature of the vitreous that affect the amount of unbound water also influence IOP. Myopia, trauma, and aging produce liquefaction of vitreous gel and subsequent increase in unbound water, which may lower IOP by facilitating fluid removal. However, under different circumstances, the opposite may occur, that is, the hydration of more normal vitreous may be associated with elevation of IOP. Hence, it is often prudent to produce a slightly dehydrated state in the surgical glaucoma patient.

Intraocular blood volume, determined primarily by vessel dilation or contraction in the spongy layers of the choroid, contributes significantly to IOP. Although changes in both arterial or venous pressure may secondarily affect IOP, excursions in arterial pressure have much less importance than do venous fluctuations. In chronic arterial hypertension, ocular pressure returns to normal levels after a period of adaptation brought about by compression of vessels in the choroid as a result of increased IOP. Thus, a feedback mechanism reduces the total volume of blood, keeping IOP relatively constant in patients with systemic hypertension.[4]

However, if venous return from the eye is disturbed at any point from Schlemm's canal to the right atrium, IOP increases substantially. This is due to both increased intraocular blood volume and distention of orbital vessels, as well as to interference with aqueous drainage. Straining, vomiting, or coughing greatly increases venous pressure and will raise IOP as much as 40 mm Hg or greater. The deleterious implications of these activities cannot be overemphasized. Laryngoscopy and tracheal intubation may also elevate IOP, even without any visible reaction to intubation, but especially when the patient coughs. Topical anesthetization of the larynx may attenuate the hypertensive response to laryngoscopy but does not reliably prevent associated increases in IOP.[5] Ordinarily, the pressure elevation from such increases in blood volume or venous pressure dissipates rapidly. However, if situations of coughing or straining arise during ocular surgery when the eye is open, as in cataract extraction or in penetrating keratoplasty, the result may be a disastrous expulsive hemorrhage, at worst, or a disconcerting loss of vitreous, at best.

Despite the significant role of venous pressure, scleral rigidity, and vitreous composition, maintenance of IOP is determined *primarily* by the rate of aqueous formation and the rate of aqueous outflow. The most important influence on formation of aqueous humor is the difference in osmotic pressure between aqueous and plasma.[3] This fact is illustrated by the equation

$$IOP = K<(OPaq - OPpl) + CP> \qquad (37\text{-}1)$$

where

K	=	coefficient of outflow
OPaq	=	osmotic pressure of aqueous humor
OPpl	=	osmotic pressure of plasma
CP	=	capillary pressure

The fact that a small change in solute concentration of plasma can markedly influence formation of aqueous humor and, hence, IOP is the rationale for using hypertonic solutions, such as mannitol, to lower IOP.

Fluctuations in aqueous outflow can also account for a dramatic alteration in IOP. The most significant factor controlling aqueous humor outflow is the diameter of Fontana's spaces[6] as illustrated by the equation:

$$A = \frac{r^4 \times (Piop - Pv)}{8\,\eta\,L} \qquad (37\text{-}2)$$

where

A	=	volume of aqueous outflow per unit of time
r	=	radius of Fontana's spaces
Piop	=	intraocular pressure
Pv	=	venous pressure
η	=	viscosity
L	=	length of Fontana's spaces

When the pupil dilates, Fontana's spaces narrow, resistance to outflow is increased, and IOP rises. Since mydriasis is undesirable in both narrow- and wide-angle glaucoma, miotics such as pilocarpine are applied conjunctively in patients with glaucoma.

GLAUCOMA

Glaucoma is a condition characterized by elevated IOP, resulting in impairment of capillary blood flow to the optic nerve with eventual loss of optic nerve tissue and function. Two different anatomic types of glaucoma exist: 1) open-angle, or chronic simple glaucoma; and 2) closed-angle, or acute glaucoma. (Other variations of these processes occur but are not especially germane to anesthetic management.)

With open-angle glaucoma, the elevated IOP exists with an anatomically open anterior chamber angle. It is thought that sclerosis of trabecular tissue results in impaired aqueous filtration and drainage. Treatment consists of medication to produce miosis and trabecular stretching. Commonly used eyedrops are epinephrine, timolol, dipivefrin, and betaxolol.

Closed-angle glaucoma is characterized by the peripheral iris moving into direct contact with the posterior corneal surface, mechanically obstructing aqueous outflow. People who have a narrow angle between the iris and posterior cornea are predisposed to this condition. In these patients, mydriasis can produce such increased thickening of the peripheral iris that corneal touch occurs and the angle is closed. Another mechanism producing acute, closed-angle glaucoma is swelling of the crystalline lens. In this case, pupillary block occurs with the edematous lens blocking the flow of aqueous from the posterior to the anterior chamber. This situation can also develop if the lens is traumatically dislocated anteriorly, thus physically blocking the anterior chamber.

It was a previously held notion by some clinicians that patients with glaucoma should not be given atropine premedication. However, this claim is untenable. Atropine premedication in the dose range used clinically has no effect on IOP in either open- or closed-angle glaucoma. When 0.4 mg of atropine is given to a 70-kg person, approximately 0.0001 mg is absorbed by the eye.[7] Garde et al[8] reported, however, that scopolamine has a greater mydriatic effect than atropine and recommended not using scopolamine in patients with known or suspected *narrow*-angle glaucoma.

Equation 37-2, describing volume of aqueous outflow per unit of time, clearly demonstrates that outflow is exquisitely sensitive to fluctuations in venous pressure. Since a rise in venous pressure produces an increased volume of ocular blood as well as decreased aqueous outflow, it is obvious that considerable elevation of IOP occurs with any maneuver that increases venous pressure. Hence, in addition to preoperative instillation of miotics, other anesthetic goals for the patient with glaucoma include perioperative avoidance of venous congestion and of overhydration. Furthermore, hypotensive episodes are to be avoided, since these patients are allegedly vulnerable to retinal vascular thrombosis.

Primary congenital glaucoma is classified according to age of onset, with the infantile type presenting any time after birth until 5 years of age. The juvenile type presents between the ages of 6 and 30 years. Moreover, childhood glaucoma may also occur in conjunction with various eye diseases or developmental anomalies such as aniridia, mesodermal dysgenesis syndrome, and retinopathy of prematurity.[9]

Successful management of infantile glaucoma is crucially dependent upon early diagnosis. Presenting symptoms include epiphora, photophobia, blepharospasm, and irritability. Ocular enlargement, termed *buphthalmos*, or "ox eye," and corneal haziness secondary to edema are common. Buphthalmos is rare, however, if glaucoma develops after 3 years of age because, by then, the eye is much less elastic.

Since infantile glaucoma is frequently associated with obstructed aqueous outflow, management of it often requires surgical creation, via goniotomy or trabeculotomy, of a route for aqueous humor to flow into Schlemm's canal. However, advanced disease may be unresponsive to even multiple goniotomies, and the more radical trabeculectomy or some other variety of filtering procedure may be necessary.

The juvenile form of glaucoma, presenting with normal cornea and eye size, is commonly associated with a family history of open-angle glaucoma and is treated similarly to primary open-angle glaucoma.

In cases of pediatric secondary glaucoma, goniotomy and filtering may be unsuccessful, whereas cyclocryotherapy may effect a reduction in IOP, pain, and corneal edema. The ciliary body is destroyed with a cryoprobe, cooled to $-70°$ C, thus dramatically decreasing aqueous formation.

It is essential to appreciate that the high IOP frequently encountered in infantile glaucoma can be reduced by more than 15 mm Hg when surgical anesthesia is achieved. (Some clinicians maintain that ketamine is a useful drug to use for examination under anesthesia when infantile glaucoma is part of the differential diagnosis, since ketamine does not appear to reduce IOP, giving a spuriously low reading.) Moreover, even normal infants will sporadically have pressures in the mid-20s. Hence, diagnosis is not based exclusively on the numerical pressure recorded under anesthesia. Other factors such as corneal edema and increased corneal diameter, tears in Descemet's membrane, and cupping of the optic nerve are considered in making the diagnosis. If these aberrations are noted, surgical intervention may be mandatory, even in the face of a reputedly normal IOP.

EFFECTS OF ANESTHESIA AND ADJUVANT DRUGS ON INTRAOCULAR PRESSURE

CENTRAL NERVOUS SYSTEM DEPRESSANTS

Inhalation anesthetics purportedly cause dose-related decreases in IOP.[10] The exact mechanism(s) is (are) unknown, but postulated etiologies include depression of a central nervous system (CNS) control center in the diencephalon,[4] reduction of aqueous humor production, enhancement of aqueous outflow, or relaxation of the extraocular muscles.[7] Moreover, virtually all CNS depressants, including barbiturates,[11, 12] neuroleptics,[13] opioids,[14] tranquilizers,[7] and hypnotics[15] lower IOP in both normal and glaucomatous eyes. It is interesting that etomidate, despite its proclivity to produce pain upon intravenous (iv) injection and skeletal muscle movement, is associated with a significant reduction in IOP.[16]

Controversy, however, surrounds the issue of ketamine's effect on IOP. Administered iv or intramuscularly (im), ketamine initially was thought to increase IOP significantly, as measured by indentation tonometry.[17] Corssen and Hoy[18] had also reported a slight but statistically significant increase in IOP that appeared unrelated to changes in blood pressure or to depth of anesthesia. However, nystagmus made proper positioning of the tonometer difficult and may have resulted in less than accurate measurements.

Conflicting results arose from a study in which 2 mg·kg^{-1} of ketamine given iv to adults failed to reflect a significant effect on IOP.[19] Furthermore, a pediatric study reported no increase in IOP following an im ketamine dose of 8 mg·kg^{-1}. Indeed, values obtained were similar to those reported with halothane and isoflurane.[20, 21]

Some of the confusion may be based on differences in premedication practices and on use of different instruments to measure IOP. (More recent studies have used applanation tonometry rather than indentation tonometry.) However, even if future studies should confirm that ketamine has minimal, if any, effect on IOP, it is important to appreciate that ketamine's proclivity to cause nystagmus and blepharospasm makes it a less than optimal agent for many types of ophthalmic surgery.

VENTILATION AND TEMPERATURE

Hyperventilation decreases IOP, whereas asphyxia, administration of carbon dioxide, and hypoventilation have been shown to elevate IOP.[3, 22]

Hypothermia lowers IOP. On superficial musing, one might expect a rise in IOP with hypothermia because of the associated increase in viscosity of aqueous humor. However, hypothermia is linked with decreased formation of aqueous humor and with vasoconstriction; hence, the net result is a reduction in IOP.

ADJUVANT DRUGS: GANGLIONIC BLOCKERS; HYPERTONIC SOLUTIONS; ACETAZOLAMIDE

Ganglionic blockers such as tetraethylammonium[23] and pentamethonium both effect a dramatic decrease in IOP. Trimethaphan also significantly lowers IOP in normal subjects, despite mydriasis.

Intravenous administration of hypertonic solutions such as dextran, urea, mannitol, and sorbitol elevate plasma osmotic pressure, thereby decreasing aqueous humor formation and reducing IOP.[24] As effective as urea is in reducing IOP, iv mannitol has the advantage of fewer side-effects. Mannitol's onset, peak (30 to 45 min), and duration of action (5 to 6 hr) are similar to those of urea. Moreover, both drugs may produce acute intravascular volume overload. Sudden expansion of plasma volume secondary to efflux of intracellular water into the vascular compartment places a heavy workload on the kidneys and heart, often resulting in hypertension and dilution of plasma sodium. Furthermore mannitol-associated diuresis, if protracted, may trigger hypotension in volume-depleted persons.

Glycerin has the advantage of being effective orally. However, the ocular hypotensive effect is said to be less predictable than that of mannitol. Onset is usually within 10 minutes of ingestion, and peak action is noted at 30 minutes. Duration of action is 5 to 6 hr. Unfortunately, glycerin may trigger nausea or vomiting, and the presence of gastric fluid trapping causes an increased risk of aspiration.

Intravenous administration of acetazolamide inactivates carbonic anhydrase and interferes with the sodium pump. The resultant decrease in aqueous humor formation lowers IOP. However, the action of acetazolamide is not limited to the eye, and systemic effects include loss of sodium, potassium, and water secondary to the drug's renal tubular effects. Such electrolyte imbalances may then be linked with cardiac dysrhythmias during general anesthesia.

An advantage of acetazolamide is its relative ease of administration. Whereas large volumes of hypertonic solutions must be infused to reduce IOP, acetazolamide is easily given as a typical adult dose of 500 mg dissolved in 10 ml of sterile water. Acetazolamide may also be given orally.

NEUROMUSCULAR BLOCKING DRUGS

Neuromuscular blocking drugs have both direct and indirect actions on IOP. Hence, a paralyzing dose of d-tubocurarine (dTc) directly lowers IOP by relaxing the extraocular muscles.[25] The same is true of equipotent doses of the other nondepolarizing drugs, including pancuronium (Fig. 37-3). However, if paralysis of the respiratory muscles is accompanied by alveolar hypoventilation, the latter secondary effect may supervene to increase IOP.

In contrast to nondepolarizing drugs, the depolarizing drug succinylcholine (SCh) elevates IOP. Lincoff et al[27] reported

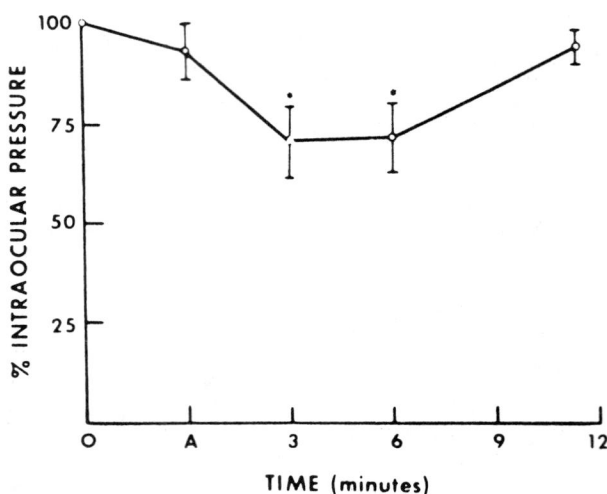

FIG. 37-3. Mean intraocular pressure following administration of thiopental, 3 to 4 mg · kg^{-1}, and pancuronium, 0.08 mg · kg^{-1} at 0. A = loss of lid reflex. *$P < 0.05$. (Reprinted with permission from Litwiller RW, DeFazio CA, Rushia EF: Pancuronium and intraocular pressure. Anesthesiology 42:750, 1975.)

extrusion of vitreous following SCh administration to a patient with an open eye injury. An average peak IOP increase of about 8 mm Hg is produced within 1 to 4 minutes of an iv dose. Within 7 minutes, return to baseline usually transpired.[28] The ocular hypertensive effect of SCh has been attributed to several mechanisms, including tonic contraction of extraocular muscles,[7] choroidal vascular dilatation, and relaxation of orbital smooth muscle.[29] It is interesting to note that ocular muscles differ anatomically from skeletal muscles in having a population of muscle fibers with multiple motor nerve endings. Whereas skeletal muscle responds to depolarizing drugs with flaccid paralysis, the ocular response to SCh is one of sustained tonic contracture. It has been postulated that this action results from a summation of the local depolarizing effects of SCh on the numerous postjunctional membrane areas of these fibers.[30]

A variety of methods have been advocated to prevent SCh-induced elevations in IOP. In truth, although some attenuation of the increase results, none of these techniques consistently and completely blocks the ocular hypertensive response. Prior administration of such drugs as acet-

TABLE 37-2.   Effects of Succinylcholine (SCh) on Intraocular Pressure: Double-Blind d-Tubocurarine (dTc) or Gallamine Pretreatment

PRETREATMENT*	MEAN AGE (yr)	INTRAOCULAR PRESSURE (mm Hg, mean ± SE)		
		Baseline	*3 Minutes after Pretreatment*	*1 Minute after SCh†*
dTc	13.4	13.0 ± 1.0	12.3 ± 1.2	24.0 ± 1.3
Gallamine	8.7	10.9 ± 1.1	10.6 ± 1.0	23.4 ± 2.3

*dTc 0.09 mg · kg^{-1} or gallamine 0.3 mg · kg^{-1}
†1 to 1.5 mg · kg^{-1} iv
(Reprinted with permission from Meyers EF, Krupin T, Johnson M et al: Failure of nondepolarizing neuromuscular blockers to inhibit succinylcholine-induced increased intraocular pressure—a controlled study. Anesthesiology 48:149, 1978.)

azolamide,[31] propranolol, and nondepolarizing neuromuscular blocking drugs has been suggested. The efficacy of pretreatment with nondepolarizing drugs is controversial.

In 1968, Miller et al,[32] using indentation tonometry, reported that pretreatment with small amounts of gallamine or dTc prevented SCh-associated increases in IOP. However, in 1978, Meyers and colleagues,[33] using the more sensitive applanation tonometer, were unable to consistently circumvent the ocular hypertensive response following similar pretreatment therapy (Table 37-2). Additionally, Verma,[34] in 1979, had claimed that a "self-taming" dose of SCh is protective, but Meyers et al[35] in 1980, in a controlled study using applanation tonometry, challenged this claim. Although iv pretreatment with lidocaine 1 to 2 $mg \cdot kg^{-1}$ may blunt the hemodynamic response to laryngoscopy,[5, 36] such therapy does not reliably prevent the ocular hypertensive response associated with SCh and/or intubation.[37]

Certainly, no one would disagree that SCh—if unaccompanied by pretreatment with a nondepolarizing neuromuscular blocking drug—is contraindicated in patients with penetrating ocular wounds and should not be given for the first time after the eye has been opened. Nonetheless, it no longer is valid to recommend that SCh be used only with extreme reluctance in ocular surgery. Clearly, any SCh-induced increment in IOP is usually dissipated before surgery is started. Of concern, however, is Jampolsky's warning that SCh be avoided in patients having repeat strabismus surgery, since the forced duction test does not return to baseline for approximately 30 minutes after administration of the drug.[38] More recent and quantitatively sophisticated studies by France et al[39] have supported this caveat.

OCULOCARDIAC REFLEX

Bernard Aschner and Guiseppe Dagnini first described the oculocardiac reflex in 1908. This reflex is triggered by pressure on the globe and by traction on the extraocular muscles, especially the medial rectus, as well as on the conjunctiva or on the orbital structures. Moreover, the reflex may also be elicited by performance of a retrobulbar block,[40] by ocular trauma, and by direct pressure on tissue remaining in the orbital apex after enucleation.[41] The afferent limb is trigeminal, and the efferent limb is vagal. Although the most common manifestation of the oculocardiac reflex is sinus bradycardia, a wide spectrum of cardiac dysrhythmias may occur, including junctional rhythm, ectopic atrial rhythm, atrioventricular (a-v) blockade, ventricular bigeminy, multifocal premature ventricular contractions, wandering pacemaker, idioventricular rhythm, asystole, and ventricular tachycardia.[42–44] This reflex may present during either local or general anesthesia; however, hypercarbia and hypoxemia are thought to augment the incidence and severity of the problem.

Reports on the alleged incidence of the oculocardiac reflex are remarkable in their striking variability. Berler's study[40] reported an incidence of 50%, but other sources quote rates ranging from 16%–82%.[42, 45] Commonly, those articles disclosing higher incidence involved the pediatric population, who tend to possess more vagal tone.

A variety of maneuvers to abolish or obtund the oculocardiac reflex have been promulgated. None of these methods has been consistently effective, safe, and reliable. Inclusion of im anticholinergic drugs such as atropine or glycopyrrolate in the usual premedication regimen for oculocardiac reflex prophylaxis is ineffective.[46] Nearly complete vagolytic blockade in the adult mandates 2 to 3 mg of atropine or 0.03 to 0.05

$mg \cdot kg^{-1}$.[47] In light of the fact that the peak action of im atropine occurs approximately 30 minutes after administration, it is not surprising that studies of the usual, routine, much smaller doses of atropine administered more than 1 hour prior to surgery have shown inconsistent protection against the oculocardiac reflex.

For the young child who is extremely apprehensive about "shots," giving oral atropine, 0.04 $mg \cdot kg^{-1}$, with a small amount of water 60 to 90 minutes preoperatively is an alternative.[48] However, the oral route has not enjoyed tremendous popularity with anesthesiologists because of its slower absorption and more erratic efficacy.

Atropine given iv within 30 minutes of surgery[45] is thought to effect a reduced incidence of the reflex. However, reports differ concerning dosage and timing. Moreover, it must be pointed out that some anesthesiologists claim that prior iv administration of atropine may yield more serious and refractory cardiac dysrhythmias[49] than the reflex itself. Clearly, atropine may be considered a potential myocardial irritant. A variety of cardiac dysrhythmias[50, 51] and several conduction abnormalities,[52] including ventricular fibrillation, ventricular tachycardia, and left bundle branch block have been attributed to iv atropine.

Although administration of retrobulbar anesthesia may provide some cardiac antidysrhythmic value by blocking the afferent limb of the reflex arc, such a regional technique is not devoid of potential complications, which include, but are not limited to, optic nerve damage, retrobulbar hemorrhage, and stimulation of the oculocardiac reflex arc by the retrobulbar block itself.

It is generally believed that, in adults, the aforementioned prophylactic measures, laced with inherent hazards, are usually not indicated. If a cardiac dysrhythmia appears, initially the surgeon should be asked to cease operative manipulation. Next, the patient's anesthetic depth and ventilatory status are evaluated. Commonly, heart rate and rhythm will return to baseline within 20 seconds following institution of these measures. Moreover, Moonie et al[53] noted that, with repeated manipulation, bradycardia is less likely to recur, probably secondary to fatigue of the reflex arc at the level of the cardioinhibitory center. However, if the initial cardiac dysrhythmia is especially serious or if the reflex tenaciously recurs, atropine should be administered iv, but only after the surgeon stops ocular manipulation.

During pediatric strabismus surgery, however, current popular practice favors administration of iv atropine, 0.02 $mg \cdot kg^{-1}$, prior to commencing surgery.[54] Alternatively, glycopyrrolate 0.01 $mg \cdot kg^{-1}$ administered iv may be associated with less tachycardia than atropine in this setting.

Clearly, considerable controversy surrounds the issues of incidence and prophylaxis of the oculocardiac reflex. Nonetheless, there is consensus that continuous monitoring of the electrocardiogram (ECG) is important during all types of eye surgery in order to detect potentially dangerous cardiac rhythm disturbances.

ANESTHETIC RAMIFICATIONS OF OPHTHALMIC DRUGS

There is considerable potential for drug interactions during administration of anesthesia for ocular surgery. Topical ophthalmic drugs may produce undesirable systemic effects and/or have deleterious anesthetic implications. Systemic absorption of topical ophthalmic drugs may occur from either the conjunctiva or the nasal mucosa following drainage through the nasolacrimal duct. Additionally, some percutaneous absorption, from spillover, through the immature epidermis of the premature infant may transpire.[55]

Some of the potentially worrisome topical ocular drugs include acetylcholine, anticholinesterases, cocaine, cyclopentolate, epinephrine, phenylephrine, and timolol. In addition, intraocular sulfur hexafluoride has important anesthetic ramifications. Furthermore, certain ophthalmic drugs given systemically may produce untoward sequelae germane to anesthetic management. Drugs in this category include glycerol, mannitol, and acetazolamide.

ACETYLCHOLINE

Acetylcholine is commonly used following lens extraction to produce miosis. The local use of this drug may occasionally result in such systemic effects as bradycardia, increased salivation, and bronchial secretions, as well as bronchospasm. The side-effects, including hypotension and bradycardia,[56] that may develop in patients given acetylcholine after cataract extraction may be rapidly reversed with iv atropine. Furthermore, one might anticipate that vagotonic anesthetic agents such as halothane could accentuate the effects of acetylcholine.

ANTICHOLINESTERASE AGENTS

Echothiophate is a long-acting anticholinesterase miotic that lowers IOP by decreasing resistance to the outflow of aqueous humor. Useful in the treatment of glaucoma, echothiophate is absorbed into the systemic circulation after instillation in the conjunctival sac. Any of the long-acting anticholinesterases may prolong the action of SCh,[57] since, after a month or more of therapy, plasma pseudocholinesterase activity may be less than 5% of normal.[58] It is said, moreover, that normal enzyme activity does not return until 4 to 6 weeks after discontinuance of the drug.[59] Hence, the anesthesiologist should anticipate prolonged apnea if these patients are given a usual dose of SCh. In addition, a delay in metabolism of ester local anesthetics should be expected.

COCAINE

Cocaine, introduced to ophthalmology in 1884 by Koller, has limited topical ocular use, as resulting vasoconstriction may injure the cornea. However, as the only local anesthetic that inherently produces vasoconstriction and shrinkage of mucous membranes, cocaine is commonly used in a nasal pack during dacryocystorhinostomy. The drug is so well absorbed from mucosal surfaces that plasma concentrations comparable to those following direct iv injection are achieved.[60] Since cocaine interferes with catecholamine uptake, it has a sympathetic nervous system potentiating effect.[60]

Historically, epinephrine had often been mixed with cocaine in hopes of augmenting the degree of vasoconstriction produced. This practice is both superfluous and deleterious, since cocaine is a potent vasoconstrictor in its own right, and the combination of epinephrine with cocaine may trigger dangerous cardiac dysrhythmias. It has been shown that cocaine used alone, without topical epinephrine, to shrink the nasal mucosa in conjunction with halothane or enflurane does not sensitize the heart to *endogenous* epinephrine during halothane or enflurane anesthesia.[61] However, animal studies

have shown that following pretreatment with *exogenous* epinephrine, cocaine facilitates the development of epinephrine-induced cardiac dysrhythmias during halothane anesthesia.[62]

The usual maximal dose of cocaine used in clinical practice is 200 mg for a 70-kg adult, or $3 \text{ mg} \cdot \text{kg}^{-1}$. However, $1.5 \text{ mg} \cdot \text{kg}^{-1}$ is preferable, since this lower dose has been shown not to exert any clinically significant sympathomimetic effect in combination with halothane.[63] Although 1 g is considered to be the usual lethal dose for a adult, considerable variation occurs. Furthermore, systemic reactions may appear with as little as 20 mg.

Meyers[64] described two cases of cocaine toxicity during dacryocystorhinostomy, underscoring that cocaine is contraindicated in hypertensive patients or in patients receiving drugs such as guanethidine, reserpine, tricyclic antidepressants, or monoamine oxidase inhibitors. Additionally, sympathomimetics such as epinephrine or phenylephrine should not be given with cocaine.

Obviously, before administering cocaine or another potent vasoconstrictor for dacryocystorhinostomy, the physician should carefully search out possible contraindications. In order to avoid toxic levels, doses of dilute solutions should be meticulously calculated and carefully administered. If serious cardiovascular effects occur, a beta-adrenergic antagonist may be given to counteract them.[65]

CYCLOPENTOLATE

Despite the popularity of cyclopentolate as a mydriatic, it is not without side-effects, which include CNS toxicity. Manifestations include dysarthria, disorientation, and frank psychotic reactions. Purportedly, CNS dysfunction is more likely to follow use of the 2% solution, as opposed to the 1% solution.[66] Furthermore, cases of convulsions in pediatric patients following ocular instillation of cyclopentolate have been reported.[67] Hence, for pediatric usage, 0.5%–1.0% solutions are recommended.

EPINEPHRINE

Although topical epinephrine has proved useful in some patients with open-angle glaucoma, the 2% solution has been associated with such systemic effects as nervousness, hypertension, angina pectoris, and tachycardia and with cardiac dysrhythmias.[68]

Some anesthesiologists have maintained that it is unwise to use epinephrine in patients being anesthetized with a halogenated hydrocarbon. However, Smith and colleagues[69] reported on the administration of epinephrine into the anterior chamber of patients undergoing cataract surgery by phacoemulsification and aspiration. They concluded it is safe to administer epinephrine into the anterior chamber in doses up to $68 \text{ } \mu\text{g} \cdot \text{kg}^{-1}$ under these circumstances. It was postulated that the iris, with its rich supply of adrenergic receptors, may be able to capture with extreme rapidity the epinephrine given into the eye. Apparently, there is not much systemic absorption from the globe.

PHENYLEPHRINE

Pupillary dilatation and capillary decongestion are reliably produced by topical phenylephrine. Although systemic effects secondary to topical application of prudent doses are rare,[70] severe hypertension, headache, tachycardia, and tremulousness have been reported.[68]

Persons with coronary artery disease may develop severe myocardial ischemia, cardiac dysrhythmias, and even myocardial infarction following topical 10% eye drops. Those with cerebral aneurysms may be susceptible to cerebral hemorrhage following phenylephrine in this concentration. In general, a safe systemic level follows absorption from either the conjunctiva or the nasal mucosa after drainage by the tear ducts. However, phenylephrine should not be given in the eye after surgery has begun and venous channels are patent.

Pediatric patients are especially vulnerable to overdose and may respond in a dramatic and adverse fashion to phenylephrine drops. Hence, the use of only 2.5%, rather than 10%, phenylephrine is recommended in infants and the elderly, and frequency of application should be strictly limited in these patient populations.

TIMOLOL

Timolol, a nonselective beta-adrenergic blocking drug, is a popular antiglaucoma drug. Since significant conjunctival absorption may occur, timolol should be administered with caution to patients with known obstructive airways disease, congestive heart failure, or greater than first-degree heart block. Life-threatening asthmatic crises have been reported following the administration of timolol drops to some patients with chronic, stable asthma.[71] Not unexpectedly, the development of severe sinus bradycardia in a patient with cardiac conduction defects (left anterior hemiblock, first degree a-v block, and incomplete right bundle branch block) has been reported following timolol.[72] Moreover, timolol has been implicated in the exacerbation of myasthenia gravis[73] and in the production of postoperative apnea in neonates and young infants.[74, 75]

In contrast to timolol, an even newer antiglaucoma drug, betaxolol, is said to be oculospecific and have virtually no systemic effects. However, patients receiving an oral beta blocker and betaxolol should be observed for potential additive effect on known systemic effects of beta blockade. Caution should be exercised in patients receiving catecholamine-depleting drugs. Although betaxolol has produced only minimal effects in patients with obstructive airways disease, caution should be exercised in the treatment of patients with excessive restriction of pulmonary function. Moreover, betaxolol is contraindicated in patients with sinus bradycardia, congestive heart failure, greater than first-degree heart block, cardiogenic shock, and overt myocardial failure.

INTRAOCULAR SULFUR HEXAFLUORIDE

For a patient with a retinal detachment, intraocular sulfur hexafluoride (SF6) may be injected into the vitreous in order to mechanically facilitate reattachment. These recommendations do not apply to open eye procedures during which volume and pressure changes are readily compensated for by fluid and gas leak.

Stinson and Donlon[77] suggest terminating nitrous oxide 15 minutes before gas injection in order to prevent significant changes in the size of the intravitreous gas bubble. The patient is then given virtually 100% oxygen (admixed with a small percentage of volatile agent) for the balance of the operation without adversely affecting intravitreous gas dynamics. Furthermore, if a patient requires reoperation and general anesthesia after intravitreous gas injection, nitrous oxide should be

TABLE 37-3. Differential Solubilities of Gases

	BLOOD GAS PARTITION COEFFICIENTS
Sulfa hexafluoride	0.004
Nitrous oxide	0.468
Nitrogen	0.015

avoided for 5 days subsequent to air injection and for 10 days following SF6 injection (Table 37-3).[78]

SYSTEMIC OPHTHALMIC DRUGS

In addition to topical therapies, various ophthalmic drugs given systemically may result in complications of concern to the anesthesiologist. These systemic drugs include glycerol, mannitol, and acetazolamide. For example, oral glycerol may be associated with nausea, vomiting, and risk of aspiration. Hyperglycemia or glycosuria, disorientation, and seizure activity may occur following oral glycerol.

The recommended iv dose of mannitol is 1.5 to 2 $g \cdot kg^{-1}$ over a 30- to 60-minute interval. However, serious systemic problems are linked with rapid infusion of large doses of mannitol. These complications include renal failure, congestive heart failure, pulmonary congestion, electrolyte imbalance, hypotension or hypertension, myocardial ischemia, and, rarely, allergic reactions. Clearly, the patient's renal and cardiovascular status must be thoroughly evaluated prior to mannitol therapy.

Acetazolamide, with its renal tubular effects, should be considered contraindicated in patients with marked hepatic or renal dysfunction or in those with low sodium levels or abnormal potassium values. As is well known, severe electrolyte imbalances can trigger serious cardiac dysrhythmias during general anesthesia. Furthermore, persons with chronic lung disease may be vulnerable to the development of severe acidosis with long-term acetazolamide therapy.

PREOPERATIVE EVALUATION

ESTABLISHING RAPPORT AND ASSESSING MEDICAL CONDITION

Preoperative preparation and evaluation of the patient begins with the establishment of rapport and communication among the anesthesiologist, the surgeon, and the patient. Most patients realize that surgery and anesthesia entail inherent risks, and they appreciate a candid explanation of potential complications, balanced with information concerning probability, or frequency, of permanent adverse sequelae. Such an approach, furthermore, fulfills the medicolegal responsibilities of the physician to obtain informed consent.

A thorough history of the patient and physical examination are the *sine qua non* of safe patient care. A complete list of medications that the patient is currently taking, both systemic and topical, must be obtained so that potential drug interactions can be anticipated and, additionally, so that essential medication will be administered during the hospital stay. Naturally, a history of any allergies to medicines, foods, or tape should be documented. Clearly, knowledge of any personal or family history of adverse reactions to anesthesia is mandatory. The requisite laboratory data will vary, depending upon the age and physical status of the patient. An ECG is often obtained on patients older than 40 years of age and on younger patients if their medical history suggests the possibility of cardiovascular disease.

The anesthesiologist must be aware of the anesthetic implications of congenital and metabolic diseases with ocular manifestations. Diabetics often present with ocular complications, and the anesthesiologist must be knowledgeable about the systemic disturbances of physiology that affect these patients. Indeed, the list of congenital and metabolic diseases with ocular pathology that have significant anesthetic implications is lengthy. A partial summary includes such syndromes as Crouzon's, Apert's, Goldenhar's (oculoauriculovertebral dysplasia), Sturge–Weber's, Marfan's, Lowe's (oculocerebrorenal syndrome) Down's (Trisomy 21), Wagner–Stickler's, and Riley–Day's (familial dysautonomia). Other diseases in this category are homocystinuria, malignant hyperthermia, myotonia dystrophica, and sickle cell disease.[79]

Furthermore, eye patients are often at the extremes of age—ranging from premature babies to nonagenarians. Hence, special age-related considerations, such as altered pharmacokinetics and pharmacodynamics, apply. In addition, elderly patients not infrequently suffer from thyroid dysfunction and cardiopulmonary and renal diseases.

SELECTION OF ANESTHESIA

Requirements of ophthalmic surgery include safety, akinesia, profound analgesia, minimal bleeding, avoidance or obtundation of the oculocardiac reflex, prevention of intraocular hypertension, awareness of drug interactions, and a smooth emergence devoid of vomiting, coughing, or retching (Table 37-1). Moreover, the exigencies of ophthalmic anesthesia mandate that the anesthesiologist be positioned remote from the patient's airway, and this necessity sometimes creates certain logistic problems.

Most ophthalmic procedures may be performed in adults under either local or general anesthesia. (Obviously, in the pediatric population, general anesthesia is almost always selected.) When local anesthesia is elected, the ophthalmologist usually administers the local or regional blockade, and the anesthesiologist is present to continually monitor the patient's ECG, routinely check vital signs, and administer sedation appropriately. If a mature, cooperative patient and a gentle, communicative surgeon are involved, local anesthesia should provide satisfactory conditions for almost any ophthalmic operation of reasonable length. Local anesthesia is especially popular for anterior segment surgery of 2 hours duration or less. Many retina operations of similar length, however, may also be done under local anesthesia.

Clearly, choice of anesthesia should be individualized according to the nature and duration of the procedure, coagulation status of the patient, the ability of the patient to communicate and cooperate, and the personal preference of the surgeon (Table 37-4). Patients who are deaf or speak a foreign language and those with psychiatric conditions such as claustrophobia or excessive anxiety are poor candidates for local anesthesia. Other relative contraindications include tremors, chronic coughing, and inability to lie flat.

Retrobulbar block is the most practical means to achieve akinesis of the globe. Deep general anesthesia or nondepolarizing muscle relaxants also produce a motionless eye. Retrobulbar block entails injection of local anesthesia behind the eye into the muscle cone. The patient is asked to gaze superonasally; a 25-gauge needle is then introduced through the lower lid, just nasal to the junction of the lateral and

TABLE 37-4.   Factors Influencing Choice of Anesthesia

Nature and duration of procedure
Coagulation status
Patient's ability to communicate and cooperate
Personal preference

inferior rim of the orbit. The needle is advanced approximately 1.5 cm along the inferotemporal wall of the orbit and is then directed upward and nasally toward the orbital apex. The plunger of the syringe is withdrawn to reveal an unwanted intravascular location, and 3 or 4 ml of local anesthetic solution is then injected. The retrobulbar injection should be followed by gentle massage of the globe to enhance dispersion of the local anesthetic. (Sensory innervation of the eye is by way of the nasociliary branch of the ophthalmic nerve. This branch sends the long posterior ciliary nerves to the globe by the ciliary ganglion. These nerves are efficaciously blocked with retrobulbar injection.)

Akinesia of the eyelids is obtained by blocking the branches of the facial nerve supplying the orbicularis muscle. Since first used for ophthalmic surgery by Van Lint[80] in 1914, numerous methods of facial nerve blockade have been described. All these techniques block the facial nerve either proximally or distally to its exit point from the skull by the stylohyoid foramen.

Available data have failed to demonstrate a signficant difference in complications such as iris prolapse or vitreous loss between local and general anesthesia for cataract surgery,[81] and local anesthesia has proved safe for patients with certain types of cardiovascular disease such as a relatively recent myocardial infarction.[82] Nonetheless, use of general anesthesia for intraocular surgery has increased significantly during the past 2 decades.

One must not be lulled into a false sense of security with local anesthesia, because this technique does not necessarily involve less physiologic trespass than does general anesthesia. Complications associated with retrobulbar block may be local or systemic and may result in blindness and even death (Table 37-5). The most common complication is retrobulbar hemorrhage secondary to puncture of vessels within the retrobulbar space. This misadventure is characterized by the simultaneous appearance of an excellent motor block of the globe, closing of the upper lid, proptosis, and a palpable increase in IOP. If this develops, it is prudent to defer the proposed intraocular procedure.

Other complications of retrobulbar block include direct intravascular injection, with all the attendant CNS and cardiovascular effects of excessive drug levels; stimulation of the oculocardiac reflex; inadvertent intraocular injection; inadequate blockade of extraocular muscles with compression of the globe and extrusion of intraocular contents; puncture of the

TABLE 37-5.   Complications of Retrobulbar Blockade

Stimulation of oculocardiac reflex arc
Retrobulbar hemorrhage
Puncture of posterior globe, resulting in retinal detachment
    and vitreous hemorrhage
Central retinal artery occlusion
Penetration of optic nerve
Inadvertent brain stem anesthesia
Inadvertent intraocular injection

posterior segment of the globe, producing a posterior retinal tear resulting in retinal detachment and vitreous hemorrhage; and penetration of the optic nerve. Furthermore, central retinal artery occlusion, a potentially blinding situation, may result either after a retrobulbar hemorrhage or if dura around the optic nerve is penetrated and local anesthetic solution is accidently injected into the subarachnoid space. It is essential to realize that an initially insidious but potentially lethal complication may also develop when accidental access to cerebrospinal fluid during performance of a retrobulbar nerve block occurs secondary to perforation of the meningeal sheaths that surround the optic nerve. One case report[83] described the gradual onset of unconsciousness and apnea over the course of 7 minutes without any accompanying seizures or cardiovascular collapse. Hence, anesthesiologists and ophthalmologists should be exquisitely aware of the possibility of accidental brain stem anesthesia following retrobulbar block. It is axiomatic that persons skilled in airway maintenance and in ventilatory and circulatory support should be immediately available whenever retrobulbar block is administered.

Many advocate the administration of approximately 10 to 30 mg of methohexital iv immediately prior to performance of the retrobulbar block, provided that no contraindications to the use of this drug exist. Such a practice is usually quite satisfactory, affording considerable comfort and amnesia. What should be avoided at all costs, however, is the combination of local anesthesia with heavy sedation in the form of high doses of opioids, benzodiazepines, and hypnotics. This polypharmacology is highly unsatisfactory because of the pharmacologic vagaries in the geriatric population and the attendant risks of respiratory depression, airway obstruction, hypotension, CNS aberrations, and prolonged recovery time. This undesirable technique has all the disadvantages of a general anesthetic in the absence of a tracheal tube without the advantage of controllability that general anesthesia offers. Undersedation should likewise be avoided, because tachycardia and hypertension may have deleterious effects, especially in patients with coronary artery disease. Moreover, patients with orthopedic deformities or arthritis must be meticulously positioned and given comfortable padding on the operating table. Adequate ventilation about the face is essential for all patients, and each must be comfortably warm. (The hazards of shivering in patients with cardiac disease and, for that matter, in any patient having delicate eye surgery are well known.) Continuous ECG monitoring is vital, lest performance of the retrobulbar block, pressure on the orbit, or tugging on the extraocular muscles stimulate the oculocardiac reflex arc and produce dangerous cardiac dysrhythmias.

A question that is frequently asked is whether, for cardiac patients, epinephrine may be safely combined with local anesthetics in order to achieve vasoconstriction and increased anesthetic duration. Donlon and Moss[84] emphasize that release of endogenous catecholamines secondary to suboptimal analgesia may greatly exceed the relatively minute amount of injected exogenous catecholamine. Specifically, they mention that 0.06 mg epinephrine (12 ml of 1:200,000) produces some systemic uptake but no untoward clinical effects.[84]

ANESTHETIC MANAGEMENT OF SPECIFIC SITUATIONS

GENERAL CONCEPTS AND OBJECTIVES

The majority of patients having eye surgery are either younger than 10 years of age or older than 55 years of age. In the pediatric age group, operations on the ocular adnexa, includ-

ing lid surgery, repair of lacrimal apparatus, and adjustment of extraocular muscles, are common. However, surgery on the anterior segment, such as cataract removal, glaucoma procedures, and trauma repair, is definitely not limited to the adult population. Nor are posterior segment operations such as scleral buckling and vitrectomy the exclusive domain of geriatrics.

Most ocular procedures demand profound analgesia but minimal skeletal muscle relaxation. The airway must be protected from obstruction, and the anesthesiologist must distance himself or herself—along with anesthetic apparatus—from the surgical field. Depending upon whether the patient is a child or an adult and various other factors previously discussed, a decision is reached regarding whether to select local or general anesthesia. Additional preparation must include, of course, identification of underlying diseases, such as asthma, diabetes mellitus, or nephropathy. The patient should also be prepared emotionally for the recovery period, when he will awaken with one or both eyes closed by bandages. This is important not only to spare him fear and anxiety but also to prevent much of the thrashing about that fright might produce to the detriment of the eye.

Preoperative sedation is chosen carefully. Except for strabismus correction, retinal detachment surgery, and cryosurgery, ophthalmic procedures are generally associated with little pain. Thus, the routine use of opioid premedication, replete with emetic potential, is ill-advised. Rather, premedication should be prescribed with a view toward amnesia, sedation, and antiemesis. Reasonable selections would include a benzodiazepine for sedative–hypnotic effect or the phenothiazine promethazine or the antihistaminic hydroxyzine for their sedative, antiemetic properties.

Analgesia and akinesis are then secured through either local or general anesthesia, with careful attention paid to proper control of IOP and to the possible appearance of the oculocardiac reflex. The anesthesiologist strives to provide a smooth intraoperative course and to prevent coughing, retching, and vomiting, lest harmful increases in IOP transpire that could hinder successful surgery. If general anesthesia is elected, extubation of the trachea should be accomplished before there is a tendency to cough. The administration of iv lidocaine, 1.5 to 2 mg·kg^{-1}, prior to extubation of the trachea is helpful in attenuating coughing. Likewise, prophylactic iv droperidol, is valuable in reducing the incidence and severity of nausea and vomiting.[85, 86]

"OPEN EYE–FULL STOMACH" ENCOUNTERS

The anesthesiologist involved in caring for a patient with a penetrating eye injury and a full stomach must confront special challenges. He or she has to weigh the risk of aspiration against the risk of blindness in the injured eye that could result from elevated IOP and extrusion of ocular contents.

If time permits, preoperative prophylaxis against aspiration may involve administering H$_2$ receptor antagonists to elevate gastric fluid pH and to reduce gastric acid production.[87, 88] Metoclopramide may be given to induce peristalsis and enhance gastric emptying.

Not infrequently, a barbiturate, nondepolarizing neuromuscular blocking drug technique is described as the method of choice for the emergency repair of an open eye injury, since the nondepolarizing drug pancuronium in a dose of 0.15 mg·kg^{-1} has been shown to lower IOP. However, this method has its disadvantages, including risk of aspiration and death during the relatively lengthy period—ranging from 75 seconds[89] to 150 seconds[90]—that the airway is unprotected. (Performance of the Sellick maneuver during this interval affords some protection.) Furthermore, a premature attempt at intubation of the trachea will produce coughing, straining, and a dramatic rise in IOP, emphasizing the need to confirm the onset of drug effect with a peripheral nerve stimulator. Moreover, the cardiovascular side-effects of tachycardia and hypertension may prove worrisome in patients with coronary artery disease. Also, the long duration of action of intubating doses of pancuronium may mandate postoperative mechanical ventilation of the lungs. Intermediate-acting nondepolarizing drugs such as vecuronium and atracurium have briefer durations of action, less dramatic, if any, circulatory effects, and lack of cumulative tendency, but, nevertheless, have an onset of action similar to that of pancuronium.[91, 92]

However, SCh offers the distinct advantages of swift onset, superb intubating conditions, and brief duration of action. If administered after careful pretreatment with a nondepolarizing drug and an induction dose of thiopental ($4 \text{ mg} \cdot \text{kg}^{-1}$), SCh produces only small increases in IOP.[93, 94] Although the advisability of this technique has vociferously been debated, there are no published reports of loss of intraocular contents from a pretreatment–barbiturate–SCh sequence when used in this setting.[95] Upon completion of surgery and return of spontaneous ventilation, an awake extubation of the trachea may be performed with the patient in a lateral, head-down position.

In managing certain pediatric patients in this situation, a reasonable approach might be to perform an inhalation induction with cricoid pressure and intubation of the trachea under deep halothane anesthesia.[96] In these cases, attempting to start an iv infusion prior to induction of anesthesia can trigger struggling, sobbing, and screaming, and optimal visual outcome may be compromised. Moreover, it is important to keep in mind that much damage to the eye may already have occurred as a result of vomiting owing to pain or as a result of eye-rubbing and eye-squeezing by the child. The anesthesiologist cannot be held accountable for every insult to the eye.

What about the so-called priming principle?[97, 98] This concept involves using approximately one tenth of an intubating dose of nondepolarizing drug, followed 4 minutes later by an intubating dose. Then, after waiting an additional 90 seconds, intubation of the trachea may be performed. However, studies in this area demonstrate wide variability and disconcerting scatter of data. Future investigations should use a randomized, double-blind design, since studies of intubating conditions are notoriously difficult to interpret. Moreover,

priming is not devoid of risk, since a case of pulmonary aspiration after a priming dose of vecuronium was reported.[99]

Perhaps the wisest approach to the management of open eye–full stomach situations is summarized by Baumgarten and Reynolds,[100] who wrote in 1985:

> It may be possible to devise a combination of intravenous anesthetics and nondepolarizing relaxants that totally prevents coughing after rapid intubation. Until this combination is devised and confirmed in a large, controlled double-blind series, clinicians should not apply the priming principle to the open eye–full stomach patient. Use of a blockade monitor to predict intubating conditions may be unreliable, since muscle groups vary in their response to nondepolarizing relaxants. At this time, succinylcholine with precurarization probably remains the most tenable compromise in the open eye–full stomach challenge.

STRABISMUS SURGERY

Approximately 5% of the population have malalignment of the visual axes, which may be accompanied by diplopia, amblyopia, and loss of stereopsis (Table 37-6).[101] Indeed, strabismus surgery is the most common pediatric ocular operation performed in the United States, and it entails a variety of techniques to weaken an extraocular muscle by moving its insertion on the globe (recession) or to strengthen an extraocular muscle by eliminating a short strip of the tendon or muscle (resection).[102]

Infantile strabismus occurs within the first 6 months of life and is often observed in the early neonatal period. Although the majority of patients with strabismus are healthy, normal children, the incidence of strabismus is increased in those with CNS dysfunctions such as cerebral palsy and meningomyelocele with hydrocephalus. Moreover, strabismus may be acquired secondary to oculomotor nerve trauma or to sensory abnormalities such as cataracts or refractive aberrations.

In addition to the well-known propensity of strabismus surgery to trigger the oculocardiac reflex (previously discussed), it is also important to realize that an increased incidence of malignant hyperthermia has been noted in patients with conditions such as strabismus or ptosis. This observation is consistent with the impression that malignant hyperthermia-susceptible persons often have localized areas of skeletal muscle weakness or other musculoskeletal abnormalities.[103, 104] Other aspects of strabismus surgery of interest to anesthesiologists include SCh-induced tonic contracture of the extraocular muscles and an increased incidence of postoperative nausea and vomiting.

In formulating a surgical treatment plan for incomitant strabismus, ophthalmologists often find the forced duction test (FDT) to be exquisitely helpful in differentiating between a paretic muscle and a restrictive force preventing ocular motion. To perform FDT, the surgeon grasps the sclera of the anesthetized eye with a forceps near the corneal limbus and moves the eye into each field of gaze, concomitantly assessing tissue and elastic properties. This simple test provides valuable clues to the presence and site of mechanical restrictions of the extraocular muscles.

France et al[39] quantitated the magnitude and duration of change of the FDT following SCh administration. They demonstrated that quantitation of the force necessary to rotate the globe remained significantly elevated over control for 15 min-

TABLE 37-6.   Concerns with Various Ocular Procedures

PROCEDURE	CONCERNS
Strabismus repair	Forced duction testing
	Oculocardiac reflex
	Oculogastric reflex
	Malignant hyperthermia
Intraocular surgery	Proper control of IOP
	Akinesia
	Drug interactions
	Associated systemic disease
Retinal detachment surgery	Oculocardiac reflex
	Proper control of IOP
	Nitrous oxide interaction with air or sulfur hexafluoride

utes, despite the fact that duration of rise in IOP and skeletal muscle paralysis was less than 5 minutes. Since SCh interferes with FDT, its use is contraindicated less than 20 minutes prior to testing. Hence, France suggests performing FDT on the anesthetized patient either while mask inhalation anesthesia is being administered, prior to intubation of the trachea and then using SCh to expedite intubation; or, after intubation, facilitated by nondepolarizing neuromuscular blocking drugs; or after intubation under moderately deep inhalation anesthesia, unaided by SCh. However, when deep inhalational anesthesia is elected, atropine (0.02 mg·kg^{-1}, administered iv) should be given before, or in the early stage of, induction of anesthesia to prevent the fall in cardiac output that may accompany the significant dose-dependent depression of left ventricular function in children.[106, 107] Additionally, the use of iv atropine at this time affords some protection against elicitation of the oculocardiac reflex. For these reasons, many anesthesiologists administer iv atropine routinely to pediatric patients scheduled for strabismus surgery.

Once intubation of the trachea has been accomplished, anesthesia is commonly maintained with halothane, nitrous oxide, and oxygen. The patient is carefully monitored with a precordial stethoscope, ECG, blood pressure device, pulse oximeter, and temperature probe. If bradycardia occurs, the surgeon is asked to discontinue ocular manipulation, and the patient's ventilatory status and anesthetic depth are quickly assessed. If additional iv atropine is deemed indicated, it is not given while the oculocardiac reflex is active, lest even more dangerous cardiac dysrhythmias be triggered.

Vomiting after eye muscle surgery is common, giving credibility to the existence of the oculogastric reflex. Abramowitz et al[85, 86] reported that prophylactic iv administration of 0.075 mg·kg^{-1} of droperidol, given 30 minutes prior to termination of surgery, was "highly effective" in reducing the frequency and severity of vomiting in pediatric patients undergoing repair of strabismus. (The incidence was decreased from 85% to 43%.) Fortunately, since strabismus surgery is commonly performed on an ambulatory basis, no significant prolongation of recovery time was observed with this protocol. More recently, the administration of droperidol, 0.075 mg·kg^{-1} at induction of anesthesia before manipulation of the eye has been claimed to reduce the incidence of vomiting after strabismus surgery to a more clinically acceptable level of approximately 10%.[108]

INTRAOCULAR SURGERY

Advances in both anesthesia and in technology now permit a level of controlled intraocular manipulation not possible a quarter of a century ago (Table 37-6).

Proper control of IOP is crucial for such intraocular procedures as glaucoma drainage surgery, open eye vitrectomy, penetrating keratoplasty (corneal transplantation), and traditional intracapsular cataract extraction. Prior to scleral incision (when the intraocular pressure then becomes equal to atmospheric pressure), a low-normal IOP is essential, since abrupt decompression of a hypertensive eye could result in iris or lens prolapse, vitreous loss, or expulsive choroidal hemorrhage. Although available data[81] have not demonstrated a major difference in complications such as vitreous loss and iris prolapse between local anesthesia and general anesthesia and although local anesthesia has proved to be a safe technique for eye patients with a recent myocardial infarction,[82] utilization of general anesthesia for intraocular surgery has increased impressively during the past 20 years.

Premedication is selected with a view toward antiemesis.

Furthermore, atropine may be given safely, if desired, for antisialogue properties. In the usual, systemic premedicating dose, atropine is not harmful to glaucoma patients.[109]

Many anesthetic techniques may be safely used for elective intraocular surgery. If general anesthesia is selected, virtually any of the inhalation drugs may be given following iv induction of anesthesia with a barbiturate and neuromuscular blocking drug and topical laryngeal lidocaine. Since complete akinesia is essential for delicate intraocular surgery, nondepolarizing drugs are administered, followed by neuromuscular function monitoring to ensure a 90%–95% twitch suppression level during surgery. Because proper control of IOP is critical, controlled ventilation of the lungs is used, along with end-tidal carbon dioxide monitoring to ensure avoidance of hypercarbia.

Maximal pupillary dilation is important for many types of intraocular surgery and can be induced by continuous infusion of epinephrine 1:200,000 in a balanced salt solution, delivered through a small-gauge needle placed in the anterior chamber. Almost simultaneous with its administration, the drug is removed by aspirating it from the anterior chamber. The iris usually dilates immediately on contact with the epinephrine infusion, and drug uptake is presumably limited by the associated intense vasoconstriction of the iris and ciliary body. However, epinephrine may also be potentially absorbed by drainage through Schlemm's canal into the venous system or by spillover of the infusion into the conjunctival vessels or drainage to the nasal mucosa.

Clearly, the extent of systemic absorption of epinephrine is of concern to the anesthesiologist, especially in view of the drug's cardiac dysrhythmogenic potential when given concomitantly with potent inhalation drugs. However, plasma catecholamine levels during epinephrine infusion into the anterior chamber have not been investigated extensively. Nonetheless, under halothane anesthesia, in both children and adults, Smith et al[69] were unable to show any increased incidence of cardiac dysrhythmias or signs of systemic effects following instillation of 1:1000 epinephrine (0.4 to 68 μg·kg^{-1}) directly into the anterior chamber during cataract surgery. (However, all patients were given lidocaine, 2 mg·kg^{-1}, as topical laryngeal anesthesia.) The authors postulated that the globe is not a fertile site for systemic absorption. Hence, general guidelines for subcutaneous injection may not be germane for intraocular injection.[69]

At completion of surgery, any residual neuromuscular blockade is reversed. Upon resumption of spontaneous ventilation, the patient's trachea is extubated (often in the lateral position) still deeply anesthetized and following iv administration of lidocaine to prevent coughing. Of note is the fact that atropine and neostigmine may be safely used to reverse neuromuscular blockade even in patients with glaucoma, since this combination of drugs, in conventional doses, will have minimal effects on pupil size and IOP.[110]

RETINAL DETACHMENT SURGERY

Surgery to repair retinal detachments involves procedures affecting intraocular volume, frequently using a synthetic silicone band or sponge to produce a localized or encircling scleral indentation (Table 37-6). Furthermore, internal tamponade of the retinal break may be accomplished by injecting the expandable gas SF6 into the vitreous. Owing to blood gas partition coefficient differences, the administration of nitrous oxide may enhance the internal tamponade effect of SF6 intraoperatively only to be followed by a dramatic drop in IOP and volume upon discontinuance of nitrous oxide. The injected SF6 bubble, in the presence of concomitant administration of nitrous oxide, can cause a rapid and dramatic rise in IOP, reaching a peak within 20 minutes.[76-78] (See the section entitled Intraocular Sulfur Hexafluoride.) Since the resultant rise in IOP may compromise retinal circulation, Stinson and Donlon[77] recommend cessation of nitrous oxide administration 15 minutes before gas injection in order to prevent significant changes in the volume of the intravitreous gas bubble. Furthermore, Wolf et al[78] state that if a patient requires anesthesia after intravitreous gas injection, nitrous oxide should be omitted for 5 days following an air injection, and for 10 days following SF6 injection.

Alternatively, silicone oil, a vitreous substitute, may be injected to achieve internal tamponade of a retinal break.

Retinal detachment operations are basically extraocular but may briefly become intraocular if the surgeon elects to perforate and drain subretinal fluid. Furthermore, rotation of the globe with traction on the extraocular muscles may elicit the oculocardiac reflex, so the anesthesiologist must be vigilant about potential cardiac dysrhythmias. Additionally, since it is desirable to have a soft eye while the sclera is being buckled, iv administration of acetazolamide or mannitol is common during retina surgery to lower IOP.

These patients are generally managed in the same manner as those having intraocular surgery except that maintenance of intraoperative skeletal muscle paralysis is not as critical as during intraocular surgery. Hence, inhalational anesthetics need not be accompanied intraoperatively by nondepolarizing neuromuscular blocking drugs.

POSTOPERATIVE OCULAR COMPLICATIONS

Postoperative complications include corneal abrasion, chemical injuries, thermal injury, minor visual disturbances, and serious visual disturbances, including visual loss. The latter, serious misadventures may be due to such diverse conditions as acute corneal epithelial edema,[111] central retinal artery occlusion,[112] ketamine,[113] Valsalva hemorrhagic retinopathy,[114] retinal ischemia, and acute glaucoma.

CORNEAL ABRASION

The most common ocular complication of general anesthesia is corneal abrasion caused by the anesthesia mask or surgical drapes.[115] Ocular injury may also occur owing to loss of pain sensation, obtundation of protective corneal reflexes, and decreased tear production. Taping the eyelids closed, application of protective goggles, and instillation of petroleum-based ointments (artificial tears) into the conjunctival sac provide protection. Disadvantages of ointments include occasional allergic reactions; flammability, which may make their use undesirable during surgery around the face; and blurred vision in the early postoperative period.[116] During general anesthesia for procedures away from the head and neck in the supine position lasting less than 3 hours, closure of the eyelids with tape with or without ointments seems to be sufficient for most patients.[116]

Patients with corneal abrasion usually complain of a foreign body sensation, pain, tearing, and photophobia. The pain is typically exacerbated by blinking and ocular movement. It is wise to have an ophthalmologic consultation immediately. Treatment consists of the prophylactic application of antibiotic ointment and patching the injured eye. Although permanent sequelae are possible, healing usually occurs within 24 hours.

CHEMICAL INJURY

Spillage of solutions during skin preparation may result in chemical damage to the eye. Again, with meticulous attention to detail, this misadventure is preventable. Treatment consists of liberal bathing of the eye with water to remove the offending agent. Postoperatively, it may be desirable to have an ophthalmologist examine the eye to document any residual injury, or lack thereof.

THERMAL INJURY

The potential for thermal injury to the cornea or retina from certain laser beams requires that the patient's eyes be protected with moist gauze pads and metal shields and that operating room personnel wear protective glasses.[117]

MILD VISUAL SYMPTOMS

After anesthesia, mild visual disturbances, such as photophobia or diplopia, are not uncommon.[118] Blurred vision in the early postoperative period may reflect residual effects of petroleum-based ophthalmic ointments or ocular effects of anticholinergic drugs administered in the perioperative period. (See the section entitled Corneal Abrasion.) Dhamee et al[119] reported an incidence (7%-14%) of benign, transient visual disturbances after gynecologic procedures.

By contrast, the complaint of visual loss postoperatively is rare and is cause for alarm. Several of the following conditions may be associated with visual loss after anesthesia and surgery and should be included in differential diagnosis: hemorrhagic retinopathy, retinal ischemia, and acute glaucoma.

HEMORRHAGIC RETINOPATHY

Retinal hemorrhages, occurring in otherwise healthy persons, secondary to hemodynamic changes associated with turbulent emergence from anesthesia or protracted vomiting are termed Valsalva retinopathy.[120] Fortunately, these venous hemorrhages are usually self-limiting, with complete resolution in a few days to a few months.

Since no visual changes occur unless the macula is involved, the vast majority of cases are asymptomatic. However, if bleeding into the optic nerve occurs, resulting in optic atrophy, or, if the hemorrhage is massive, permanent visual impairment may ensue.[121] In some instances of massive hemorrhage, vitrectomy may offer some improvement.

RETINAL ISCHEMIA

Retinal bleeding may also originate from the arterial circulation. This bleeding may be associated with extraocular trauma. Fundoscopic examination shows cotton-wool exudates,[122] and this condition is known as Purtscher's retinopathy. Thus, Purtscher's retinopathy should be ruled out when a trauma patient complains of postanesthetic visual loss. Unfortunately, this condition is associated with a poor prognosis, and the majority of patients afflicted sustain permanent visual impairment.

Retinal ischemia or infarction may also result from direct ocular trauma secondary to pressure exerted by an ill-fitting anesthetic mask, especially in a hypotensive setting, as well as from embolism during cardiac surgery[123] or from the intraocular injection of a large volume of SF6 in the presence of high concentrations of nitrous oxide.

ACUTE GLAUCOMA

Although *topical* application of such mydriatic-inducing drugs as atropine and scopolamine is contraindicated in patients with glaucoma, systemic use of anticholinergics in usual premedicating doses is safe for glaucomatous eyes.[109] Moreover, the use of atropine–neostigmine combination for reversal of neuromuscular blockade is also safe in patients with glaucoma.[110] Topical ophthalmic medications that are being administered to control glaucoma should be continued through the perioperative period.

Acute angle-closure glaucoma, caused by pupillary block, is a serious, multifactorial disease. Risk factors include genetic predisposition,[124] shallow anterior chamber depth,[125] increased lens thickness,[125] small corneal diameter,[125] female gender,[125] and advanced age.[124] A recent study[126] explored possible precipitating events in at-risk persons and found no evidence that the type of anesthetic agent, the duration of surgery, the volume of parenteral fluids, or the intraoperative blood pressure were related to the development of acute angle-closure glaucoma.

Despite its seriousness, acute angle-closure glaucoma may be difficult to recognize. However, physicians should be knowledgeable about this potential complication, since diagnostic delay may detrimentally affect visual outcome. Fazio *et al*[126] recommend, therefore, that preoperative evaluation include a thorough ocular history as well as a penlight examination to detect a shallow anterior chamber. Those patients considered to be at risk should then have a preoperative ophthalmic evaluation as well as perioperative miotic therapy. Postoperatively, these patients should be scrupulously watched for red eye or for complaints of pain and blurred vision.

REFERENCES

1. Bruce RA: Ocular anatomy. In Bruce RA, McGoldrick KE, Oppenheimer P. Anesthesia for Ophthalmology, p 3. Birmingham, Aesculapius, 1982
2. Wolff E: Anatomy of the Eye and Orbit, 7th ed, p 1. Philadelphia, W. B. Saunders, 1976
3. Aboul–Eish E: Physiology of the eye pertinent to anesthesia. In Smith RB (ed): Anesthesia in Ophthalmology, p 1. Boston, Little, Brown and Co, 1973
4. Adler FH: Physiology of the Eye: Clinical Application, 5th ed, p 249. St. Louis, CV Mosby, 1970
5. Stoelting RK: Circulatory changes during direct laryngoscopy and tracheal intubation: Influence of duration of laryngoscopy with or without prior lidocaine. Anesthesiology 47:381, 1977
6. Hill DW: Physics Applied to Anaesthesia, Norwalk, Connecticut, Appleton-Century-Crofts, 1968
7. Duncalf D, Foldes FF: Effect of anesthetic drugs and muscle relaxants on intraocular pressure. In Smith RB (ed): Anesthesia in Ophthalmology, p 21. Boston, Little, Brown and Co, 1973
8. Garde JF, Aston R, Endler GC et al: Racial mydriatic response to belladonna preparations. Anesth Analg 57:572, 1978
9. Lee P: Congenital glaucoma. In Femann SS, Reinecke RD (eds): Handbook of Pediatric Ophthalmology. New York, Grune & Stratton, 1978
10. Al–Abrak MH, Samuel JR: Effects of general anesthesia on intraocular pressure in man. Comparison of tubocurarine and pancuronium in nitrous oxide and oxygen. Br J Ophthalmol 58:806, 1974
11. Joshi C, Bruce DL: Thiopental and succinylcholine: Action on intraocular pressure. Anesth Analg 54:471, 1975
12. Everett WG, Vey EK, Veenis CY: Factors in reducing ocular tension prior to intraocular surgery. Trans Am Acad Ophthalmol 64:286, 1959
13. Presbitero JV, Ruiz RS, Rigor BM et al: Intraocular pressure during enflurane and neuroleptic anesthesia in adult patients undergoing ophthalmic surgery. Anesth Analg 59:50, 1980
14. Leopold IH, Comroe JH: Effect of intramuscular administration of morphine, atropine, scopolamine, and neostigmine on the human eye. Arch Ophthalmol 40:285, 1948
15. Famewo CE, Odugbesan CO, Osuntokun OO: Effect of etomidate on intraocular pressure. Can Anaesth Soc J 24:712, 1977
16. Thompson MF, Brock–Utne JG, Bean P et al: Anaesthesia and intraocular pressure: A comparison of total intravenous anaesthesia using etomidate with conventional inhalational anaesthesia. Anaesthesia 37:758, 1982
17. Yoshikawa K, Murai Y: Effect of ketamine on intraocular pressure in children. Anesth Analg 50:199, 1971
18. Corssen G, Hoy JE: A new parenteral anesthetic–CI581: Its effect on intraocular pressure. J Pediatr Ophthalmol 4:20, 1967
19. Peuler M, Glass DD, Arens JF: Ketamine and intraocular pressure. Anesthesiology 43:575, 1975
20. Ausinsch B, Rayburn RL, Munson ES et al: Ketamine and intraocular pressure in children. Anesth Analg 55:773, 1976
21. Ausinsch B, Graves SA, Munson ES et al: Intraocular pressure in children during isoflurane and halothane anesthesia. Anesthesiology 42:167, 1975
22. Duncalf D, Weitzner SW: Ventilation and hypercapnia on intraocular pressure in children. Anesth Analg 43:232, 1963
23. Drucker AP, Sadove MS, Unna KR: Ocular manifestations of intravenous tetraethylammonium chloride in man. Am J Ophthalmol 33:1564, 1950
24. Galin MA, Aizawa F, McLean JM: Intravenous urea in the treatment of acute angle glaucoma. Am J Ophthalmol 50:379, 1960
25. Agarwal LP, Mathur SP: Curare in ocular surgery. Br J Ophthalmol 36:603, 1952
26. Litwiller RW, Difazio CA, Rushia EL: Pancuronium and intraocular pressure. Anesthesiology 42:750, 1975
27. Lincoff HA, Ellis CH, DeVoe AG et al: Effect of succinylcholine on intraocular pressure. Am J Ophthalmol 40:501, 1955
28. Pandey K, Badolas RP, Kumar S: Time course of intraocular hypertension produced by suxamethonium. Br J Anaesth 44:191, 1972
29. Bjork A, Hallidin M, Wahlin A: Enophthalmus elicited by succinylcholine. Acta Anaesthesiol Scand 1:41, 1957
30. Bach-y-rita P, Lennerstrand G, Alvarado J et al: Extraocular muscle fibers: Ultrastructural identification of iontophoretically labeled fibers contracting in response to succinylcholine. Invest Ophthalmol Vis Sci 16:561, 1977
31. Carballo AS: Succinylcholine and acetazolamide in anesthesia for ocular surgery. Can Anaesth Soc J 12:486, 1965
32. Miller RD, Way WL, Hickey RF: Inhibition of succinylcholine-induced increased intraocular pressure by nondepolarizing muscle relaxants. Anesthesiology 29:123, 1968
33. Meyers EF, Krupin T, Johnson M et al: Failure of nondepolarizing neuromuscular blockers to inhibit succinylcholine-induced increased intraocular pressure—a controlled study. Anesthesiology 48:149, 1978
34. Verma RS: "Self-taming" of succinylcholine-induced fasciculations and intraocular pressure. Anesthesiology 50:245, 1979
35. Meyers EF, Singer P, Otto A: A controlled study of the effect of succinylcholine self-taming on IOP. Anesthesiology 53:72, 1980
36. Stoelting RK: Blood pressure and heart rate changes during

short duration laryngoscopy for tracheal intubation: Influences of viscous or intravenous lidocaine. Anesth Analg 57:197, 1978

37. Smith RB, Babinski M, Leano N: Effect of lidocaine on succinylcholine-induced rise in IOP. Can Anaesth Soc J 26:482, 1979

38. Jampolsky A: Strabismus: Surgical overcorrections. Highlights Ophthalmol 8:78, 1965

39. France NK, France TD, Woodburn JD et al: Succinylcholine alteration of the forced duction test. Ophthalmology 87:1282, 1980

40. Berler DK: Oculocardiac reflex. Am J Ophthalmol 12:56, 954, 1963

41. Kirsch RE, Samet P, Kugel V et al: Electrocardiographic changes during ocular surgery and their prevention by retrobulbar injection. Arch Ophthalmol 58:348, 1957

42. Bosomworth PP, Ziegler CH: The oculocardiac reflex in eye muscle surgery. Anesthesiology 19:7, 1958

43. Alexander JP: Reflex disturbances of cardiac rhythm during ophthalmic surgery. Br J Ophthalmol 59:518, 1975

44. Smith RB, Douglas H, Petruscak J: The oculocardiac reflex and sino-atrial arrest. Can Anaesth Soc J 19:138, 1972

45. Taylor C, Wilson FM, Roesch R et al: Prevention of the oculocardiac reflex in children: Comparison of retrobulbar block and intravenous atropine. Anesthesiology 24:646, 1963

46. Mirakur RK, Clarke RSJ, Dundee JW et al: Anticholinergic drugs in anaesthesia—a survey of their present position. Anaesthesia 33:133, 1978

47. Gaviotaki A, Smith RM: Use of atropine in pediatric anesthesia. Int Anesth Clin 1:97, 1962

48. Joseph MC, Vale RJ: Premedication with atropine by mouth. Lancet 2:1060, 1960

49. Katz RL, Bigger JT: Cardiac arrhythmias during anesthesia and operation. Anesthesiology 33:193, 1970

50. Massumi RA, Mason DT, Amsterdam EA et al: Ventricular fibrillation and tachycardia after intravenous atropine for treatment of bradycardias. N Engl J Med 287:336, 1972

51. Horgan J: Atropine and ventricular tachyarrhythmias. JAMA 223:693, 1973

52. McGoldrick KE: Transient left bundle branch block during local anesthesia. Anesthesiol Rev 8(6):36, 1981

53. Moonie GT, Rees DI, Elton D: Oculocardiac reflex during strabismus surgery. Can Anaesth Soc J 11:621, 1964

54. Steward DJ: Anticholinergic premedication for infants and children. Can Anaesth Soc J 30:325, 1983

55. Nachman RL, Esterly NB: Increased skin permeability in preterm infants. J Pediatr 79:628, 1971

56. Rongey KA, Weisman H: Hypotension following acetylcholine. Anesthesiology 36:412, 1972

57. Humphreys JA, Holmes JH: Systemic effects produced by echothiophate iodide in treatment of glaucoma. Arch Ophthalmol 69:737, 1963

58. DeRoeth A, Detbarn W, Rosenberg P et al: Effect of phospholine iodide on blood cholinesterase levels of normal and glaucoma subjects. Am J Ophthalmol 59:586, 1965

59. Ellis EP, Esterdahl M: Echothiophate iodide therapy in childen; effect upon blood cholinesterase levels. Arch Ophthalmol 77:598, 1967

60. Ritchie JM, Greene NM: Local anesthetics. In Gilman AG, Goodman LS, Rall TW et al (eds): The Pharmacological Basis of Therapeutics, 7th ed, p 302. New York, Macmillan, 1985

61. Chung B, Naraghi M, Adriani J: Sympathetic effects of cocaine and their influence on halothane and enflurane anesthesia. Anesthesiol Rev 5:16, 1978

62. Koehntop DE, Liao J, Van Bergen FH: Effects of pharmacologic alterations of adrenergic mechanisms by cocaine, tropolone, aminophylline, and ketamine on epinephrine-induced arrhythmias during halothane-N$_2$O anesthesia. Anesthesiology 46:83, 1977

63. Barash PG, Kopriva CJ, Langou R et al: Is cocaine a sympathetic stimulant during general anesthesia? JAMA 243:1437, 1980

64. Meyers EF: Cocaine toxicity during dacryocystorhinostomy. Arch Ophthalmol 98:842, 1980

65. Rappolt RT, Gay GR, Inaba DS: Propranolol: A specific antagonist to cocaine. Clin Toxicol 10:265, 1977

66. Binkhorst RD, Weinstein GW, Baretz RM et al: Psychotic reaction induced by cyclopentolate: Results of pilot study and a double-blind study. Am J Ophthalmol 55:1243, 1963

67. Kennerdell JS, Wucher FP: Cyclopentolate associated with two cases of grand mal seizure. Arch Ophthalmol 87:634, 1972

68. Lansche RK: Systemic effects of topical epinephrine and phenylephrine. Am J Ophthalmol 49:95, 1966

69. Smith RB, Douglas H, Petruscak J et al: Safety of intraocular adrenaline with halothane anaesthesia. Br J Anaesth 44:1314, 1972

70. Brown MM, Brown GC, Spaeth GL: Lack of side effects from topically administered 10% phenylephrine eye drops: A controlled study. Arch Ophthalmol 98:487, 1980

71. Jones FL, Eckberg NL: Exacerbation of asthma by timolol. N Engl J Med 301:170, 1979

72. Kim JW, Smith PH: Timolol-induced bradycardia. Anesth Analg 59:301, 1980

73. Shavitz SA: Timolol and myasthenia gravis. JAMA 242:1612, 1979

74. Olson RJ, Bromberg BB, Zimmerman TJ: Apneic spells associated with timolol therapy in a neonate. Am J Ophthalmol 88:120, 1979

75. Bailey PL: Timolol and postoperative apnea in neonates and young infants. Anesthesiology 61:622, 1984

76. Fineberg E, Machemer R, Sullivan P et al: Sulfur hexafluoride in owl monkey vitreous cavity. Am J Ophthalmol 79:67, 1975

77. Stinson TW, Donlon JV: Interaction of SF6 and air with nitrous oxide. Anesthesiology 51:S16, 1979

78. Wolf GL, Capriano C, Hartung J: Effects of nitrous oxide on gas bubble volume in the anterior chamber. Arch Ophthalmol 103:418, 1985

79. McGoldrick KE: Anesthetic implications of congenital and metabolic diseases. In Bruce RA, McGoldrick KE, Oppenheimer P (eds): Anesthesia for Ophthalmology, p 139. Birmingham, Aesculapius, 1982

80. Van Lint: Paralysis palperbrale temporaire provoquee dans l'operation de la cataracte. Ann Occul 151:420, 1914

81. Lynch S, Wolf GL, Berlin I: General anesthesia for cataract surgery: A comparative review of 2217 consecutive cases. Anesth Analg 53:909, 1974

82. Backer CL, Tinker JH, Robertson DM: Myocardial reinfarction following local anesthesia. Anesthesiology 51:S61, 1979

83. Chang J-L, Gonzalez−Abola E, Larson CE: Brain stem anesthesia following retrobulbar block. Anesthesiology 61:789, 1984

84. Donlon JV, Moss J: Plasma catecholamine levels during local anesthesia for cataract operations. Anesthesiology 51:471, 1979

85. Abramowitz MD, Epstein BS, Friendly DS et al: Effect of droperidol in reducing vomiting in pediatric strabismic outpatient surgery. Anesthesiology 55:A329, 1981

86. Abramowitz MD, Oh TH, Epstein BS: Antiemetic effect of droperidol following outpatient strabismus surgery in children. Anesthesiology 59:579, 1983

87. Dobb G, Jordan MJ, Williams JG: Cimetidine in prevention of pulmonary acid aspiration syndrome. Br J Anaesth 51:967, 1979

88. Williams JG: H$_2$ receptor antagonists and anaesthesia. Can Anaesth Soc J 30:264, 1983

89. Brown EM, Krishnaprasad D, Smiler BG: Pancuronium for rapid induction technique for tracheal intubation. Can Anaesth Soc J 26:489, 1979

90. Goudsouzian NG, Liu LMP, Cote CJ: Comparison of equipotent doses of nondepolarizing muscle relaxants in children. Anesth Analg 60:862, 1981

91. Savarese JJ: New neuromuscular blocking drugs are here. Anesthesiology 55:1, 1981

92. Basta SJ, Ali HH, Savarese JJ et al: Clinical pharmacology of atracurium besylate (BW33A): A new nondepolarizing muscle relaxant. Anesth Analg 61:723, 1982

93. Konchiergeri HN, Lee YE, Venugopal K: Effect of pancuronium on intraocular pressure changes induced by succinylcholine. Can Anaesth Soc J 26:479, 1979

94. Smith RB, Leano N: Intraocular pressure following pancuronium. Can Anaesth Soc J 20:742, 1973

95. Libonati MM, Leahy JJ, Ellison N: The use of succinylcholine in open eye surgery. Anesthesiology 62:637, 1985

96. McGoldrick KE: Pediatric anesthesia for ophthalmic surgery. In Bruce RA, McGoldrick KE, Oppenheimer P (eds): Anesthesia for Ophthalmology, p 75. Birmingham, Aesculapius, 1982

97. Foldes FF: Rapid tracheal intubation with nondepolarizing neuromuscular blocking drugs: The priming principle. Br J Anaesth 56:663, 1984

98. Schwarz S, Ilias W, Lackner F et al: Rapid tracheal intubation with vecuronium: The priming principle. Anesthesiology 62:388, 1985

99. Musich J, Walts LF: Pulmonary aspiration after a priming dose of vecuronium. Anesthesiology 64:517, 1986

100. Baumgarten RK, Reynolds WJ: Priming principle and the open eye–full stomach. Anesthesiology 63:561, 1985

101. Reinecke RD: Current concepts in ophthalmology: Strabismus. N Engl J Med 300:1139, 1979

102. Isenberg SJ: New techniques in the treatment of strabismus. Surg Rounds 12, 1980

103. Beasley H: Hyperthermia associated with ophthalmic surgery. Am J Ophthalmol 77:76, 1974

104. Dodd MJ, Phattiyakul P, Silpasuvan S: Suspected malignant hyperthermia in a strabismus patient. Arch Ophthalmol 99:1247, 1981

105. Sessler DI: Malignant hyperthermia. J Pediatr 109:9, 1986

106. Barash PG, Katz JD, Firestone S et al: Cardiovascular performance in children during induction: An echocardiographic comparison of enflurane and halothane. Anesthesiology 51(3S):315, 1979

107. Barash PG, Glanz S, Katz D et al: Ventricular function in children during halothane anesthesia: An echocardiographic evaluation. Anesthesiology 49:79, 1978

108. Lerman MD, Eustis S, Smith DR: Effect of droperidol pretreatment on postanesthetic vomiting in children undergoing strabismus surgery. Anesthesiology 65:322, 1986

109. Schwartz H, de Roeth A, Papper EM: Pre-anesthetic use of atropine in patients with glaucoma. JAMA 165:144, 1957

110. Rawstron RE, Hutchinson BR: Pupillary and circulatory changes at the termination of relaxant anesthesia. Br J Anaesth 35:795, 1963

111. Richardson RB, McBride CM, Berkely RG et al: An unusual ocular complication after anesthesia. Anesthesiology 43:357, 1975

112. Givner I, Jaffe N: Occlusion of the central retinal artery following anesthesia. Arch Ophthalmol 43:197, 1950

113. Fine J, Weissman J, Finestone SC: Side effects after ketamine anesthesia: Transient blindness. Anesth Analg 53:72, 1974

114. Boldner PM, Norton MI: Retinal hemorrhage following anesthesia. Anesthesiology 61:595, 1984

115. Batra YK, Bali M: Corneal abrasions during general anesthesia. Anesth Analg 56:363, 1977

116. Siffring PA, Poulton TJ: Prevention of ophthalmic complications during general anesthesia. Anesthesiology 66:569, 1987

117. Kalhan SB, Cascorbi HF: Anesthetic management of laser microlaryngeal surgery. Anesth Rev 8:23, 1981

118. Conway C: Neurological and ophthalmic complications of anaesthesia. In Churchill–Davidson HC (ed): A Practice of Anaesthesia, 4th ed, p 1021. Philadelphia, WB Saunders, 1978

119. Dhamee MS, Ghandi SK, Callen KM et al: Morbidity after outpatient anesthesia—a comparison of different endotracheal anesthetic techniques for laparoscopy. Anesthesiology 57:A375, 1982

120. DeVoe AG, Norton EWD, Kearns TP et al: Valsalva hemorrhagic retinopathy: Discussion. Trans Am Ophthalmol Soc 70:307, 1972

121. Madsen PH: Traumatic retinal angiopathy. Ophthalmologica 165:453, 1972

122. McLeod D: Reappraisal of the retinal cotton–wool spot. J R Soc Med 74:682, 1981

123. Gutman FA, Zegarra H: Ocular complications in cardiac surgery. Surg Clin North Am 51:1095, 1971

124. Drance SM: Angle-closure glaucoma among Canadian Eskimos. Can J Ophthalmol 8:252, 1973

125. Alsbirk PH: Angle-closure glaucoma surveys in Greenland Eskimos. Can J Ophthalmol 8:260, 1973

126. Fazio DT, Bateman JB, Christensen RE: Acute angle-closure glaucoma associated with surgical anesthesia. Arch Ophthalmol 103:360, 1985

Chapter 38

Robert Feinstein
William D. Owens

Anesthesia for ENT

Like many other areas of medicine, anesthesia has evolved into subspecialties. One might say that otorhinolaryngology (ENT) anesthesia was the parent of all anesthesia, since it was for an ENT procedure that the first public demonstration of anesthesia took place in the ether dome in 1846. Thus, while anesthesia has adapted to the changing needs of surgery and the surgical subspecialties, many of the surgical advances we have come to take for granted today were made possible by comparable adaptations in anesthetic techniques.

Anesthesia for ENT surgery poses many unique problems for the anesthesiologist. The primary intent of this chapter is to examine some of the challenges that are unique to ENT anesthesia. We will examine in some detail the functional anatomy of the head and neck and what insights we may glean so as to better enable us to deal with ENT procedures. We will discuss the implications of a shared airway and how we can best maintain patient safety during such procedures. Laser technology is being applied to various ENT problems, and we will examine how to deal with the special problems created for the anesthesiologist by this technology. Finally, we will examine how mastery of some of the techniques routinely used in anesthesia for ENT surgery can carry over to other areas of anesthetic practice.

ANATOMY OF THE HEAD AND NECK

A discussion of the salient features of head and neck anatomy will be presented to better enable us to conceptually deal with the procedures and problems presented to us by patients' pathology and surgical approaches.[1-4]

The visceral tube consists of the pharynx and larynx. These structures are continuous with the trachea and esophagus. The pharynx is a muscular tube extending from the base of the skull to the esophagus. It serves as a passageway for both air and food. Note that the passage for air is always open except during swallowing. Since this passageway serves the transport of both air and liquids and solids, a very complex control system exists to permit the pharynx to serve as a conduit for the intake of food at one time and for air at another. The pharynx also serves as a modulating chamber for the voice generated by the larynx. Figure 38-1 is a schematic representation of many of the structures of the pharynx and larynx and their relationships.

The pharynx is a midline structure, and, on both sides of the neck, the carotid sheath and its contents (internal jugular vein, common carotid artery, vagus nerve, and internal carotid artery) are located in the neck just lateral to the pharynx throughout its course. The nasal pharynx communicates with the pharynx by the choanae, which are approximately 2.5 cm by 1.25 cm oblong openings.[1] The accessory sinuses all drain into the nasal pharynx. The eustachian tube also opens into the nasal pharynx. Thus, it is easy to understand why patients whose trachea is nasally intubated are prone to sinus infections, especially of the maxillary sinuses, and middle ear infections.

The oropharynx lies posterior to the mouth. The most prominent structure is the base of the tongue, which lies in the posterior part of the mouth. At the same level as the base of the tongue and forming an arch at this level are the palatine tonsils and other lymphoid structures, which form Waldeyer's ring. The palatine tonsils project into the pharynx for a variable

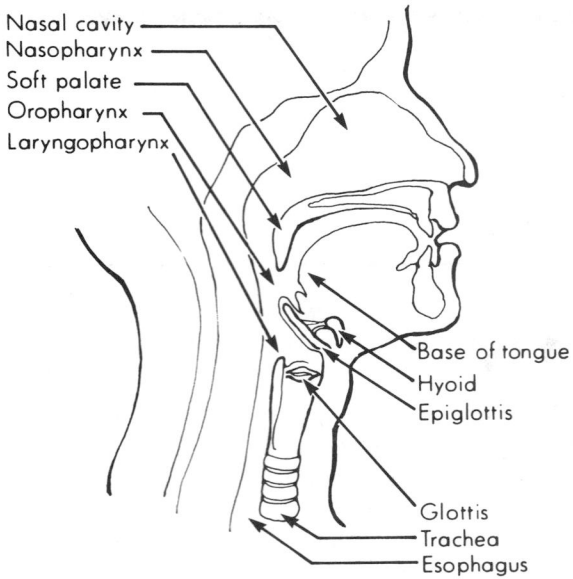

FIG. 38-1. Schematic representation of significant anatomic features of human head and neck anatomy. Note especially the space between the hyoid bone and the mandible.

distance, depending upon their size. This tonsilar bed lies in close relation to the facial artery and the internal carotid artery. The tonsils are richly supplied with blood by branches of the external carotid artery, the maxillary artery, and the facial artery, as well as others. Posterior to and caudal to this lymphoid ring lies the larynx.

The larynx is a hollow organ that serves as a direct connection between the pharynx and the trachea. The larynx is made up of three larger unpaired cartilages: 1) thyroid, 2) cricoid, and 3) epiglottic; and three paired cartilages: 1) arytenoid, 2) corniculate, and 3) cuneiform. The thyroid cartilage forms an open shield, with the shield facing anteriorly. The epiglottic cartilage is a leaf-shaped structure that extends superiorly and posteriorly from the thyroid cartilage. Beneath the thyroid cartilage lies the cricoid cartilage, which is broader posteriorly than anteriorly. The cricoid is the only complete cartilagenous ring found in the respiratory system. This property can be used to compress the esophagus, which lies posterior to the cricoid cartilage, when there is an increased risk of aspiration of oral and/or gastric contents during the induction and intubation phase of anesthesia, that is, cricoid compression.[5]

The arytenoid cartilages attach at the posterior portion of the cricoid cartilage. A membrane connects the arytenoids with the epiglottic cartilage, forming the beginning of the tube that becomes the trachea. The true vocal cords are found at this level in the larynx. The membrane that joins the thyroid and cricoid cartilages anteriorly is a common site for the anesthesiologist to obtain emergency access to the airway. The trachea is located inferior to the true vocal cords. Superior to the thyroid cartilage is the hyoid bone, which, like the thyroid cartilage, is wishbone-shaped, with the open portion facing posteriorly. The membrane connecting the thyroid cartilage and the hyoid bone is called the thyrohyoid membrane, and it is pierced by the superior laryngeal nerve. The junction of the thyroid cartilage and the posterior portion of the hyoid bone serves as a landmark for a superior laryngeal nerve blockade.

The nerve supply to the larynx can be divided into sensory

innervation to the mucous membrane, which is responsible for inducing the cough reflex when something other than air enters the larynx, and the motor nerve supply to the intrinsic muscles. The sensory nerve supply to the mucous membrane from the epiglottis to and including the vocal cords is from the superior laryngeal branch of the vagus nerve. The external branch of the superior laryngeal nerve, which comes off just prior to the nerve piercing the thyrohyoid membrane, provides motor innervation to the cricothyroid muscle and to a portion of the transverse arytenoid muscle. The mucous membrane beneath the vocal cords to the trachea is innervated by the recurrent laryngeal nerve, which also provides motor innervation to all the intrinsic muscles of the larynx for the cricothyroid muscle. The cricothyroid muscle is the only tensor of the vocal cords, and it is also the only intrinsic muscle to lie outside the cartilagenous framework of the larynx. This innervation pattern explains the fact that in humans, the vocal cords tend to close if both recurrent laryngeal nerves are accidentally cut during surgery. Since the only remaining muscles are the cricothyroid muscles, whose action is to tense the vocal cords, and the transverse arytenoid muscle, which will bring the vocal cords closer together, one would predict that if both recurrent laryngeal nerves were cut, the vocal cords would be tensed and approximated. However, in actuality, the vocal cords are flaccid and approximated. This is probably due to the inability of the cricothyroid muscles to tense the cords without resistance from the other intrinsic muscles. This can result in the patient's inability to ventilate through a closed glottis, and a tracheostomy should be done immediately. However, if only one of the inferior laryngeal nerves is cut, one cord is flaccid and midline, whereas the other cord functions normally. The patient is usually hoarse, and aspiration can be a significant problem, since the nonfunctional cord is flaccid and thus sags below the level of the remaining innervated cord, resulting in an incompetent glottis.

In the adult, the vocal cords constitute the most narrow portion of the larynx, whereas in children, usually until the age of 5 years, the cricoid cartilage is the most narrow portion of the larynx. Also, uncuffed tubes may be preferentially selected in children, since the cuff is more likely to cause subglottic edema and damage than in older patients.[6]

It was mentioned earlier that control of the structures of the pharynx and larynx required a complex control system to sort out the appropriate contents for the esophagus and trachea. In order to get food into the esophagus, three openings must be closed: 1) the opening to the nasal pharynx; 2) the opening to the mouth; and 3) the opening to the larynx. The opening to the nose is closed by elevating the soft palate and approximating the walls of the pharynx to meet the raised soft palate. The oral cavity is closed off by elevation of the tongue against the hard palate. The larynx is closed off during swallowing by raising the larynx so that it meets the epiglottis. The larynx actually forces the epiglottis into the base of the tongue. In addition, breath-holding occurs, which results in closing of the vocal cords.[1] Thus, the epiglottis does not serve as a leaflet valve that falls over the laryngeal opening; rather, the larynx is elevated onto it. Recall that this passageway, pharynx–larynx, is open except during swallowing.

Other salient anatomic features that anesthesiologists make use of in their everyday practice should be noted. In Figure 38-1, notice that the tongue lies superior to the hyoid bone. The space between the hyoid and the mandible is commonly used to evaluate the adequacy of a patient's airway.[7–11] It is into this space that the tongue is displaced during laryngoscopy. Thus, the trachea of patients with a short mandible and/

or large tongue, for example, those with Pierre Robin syndrome and those with acromegaly, will be difficult to intubate because there is inadequate room for displacement of the tongue during laryngoscopy.

Notice in Figure 38·1 that if a tube is inserted through the nasal pharynx into the oropharynx, it lies directly above the pharynx and the larynx. If the tube is an endotracheal tube, it would be in an excellent position for a blind nasotracheal intubation, or, if it were a fiberoptic laryngoscope, it would provide a view of the supraglottic structures: epiglottis, vocal cords, and esophagus.

Let us consider the external anatomy of the head and neck as it relates to the practice of ENT anesthesia. The facial nerve runs in a groove that is in close proximity to the middle ear; it then exits the skull through the stylomastoid foramen. Just prior to leaving the skull, it sends forth the chorda tympani, which conveys taste from the anterior two thirds of the tongue. After giving off the posterior auricular nerve, the facial nerve passes over the external carotid artery, where it then enters the posterior median portion of the parotid gland. The nerve then quickly divides into branches, which go on to supply the muscles of facial expression. The trigeminal nerve conveys sensory information from the face and also provides motor innervation to the muscles of mastication. The glossopharyngeal nerve carries somatic sensory information for the base of the tongue and the pharynx. The recurrent laryngeal branches of the vagus nerve run along the posterior lateral portion of the thyroid gland and are intimately associated with the gland and its blood supply. Since many of these nerves are intimately involved with the structures of the head and neck, it is not surprising that the ENT surgeon is always concerned with their identification and preservation. Thus, the use of muscle relaxants, other than transiently, is usually restricted in ENT anesthesia.

ANESTHETIC CONSIDERATIONS FOR COMMON ENT PROCEDURES

The discussion that follows highlights the unique features of anesthesia with regard to ENT procedures. Emphasis is placed on the concept of the "shared airway" and the rapidly changing field of laser laryngoscopy.

LARYNGOSCOPY AND MICROLARYNGOSCOPY

Airway management was discussed in Chapter 20. We now enter into the realm of the so-called shared airway. We shall examine some of the considerations unique to airway endoscopic procedures. Just as in other areas of medicine, endoscopy is used as a diagnostic tool requiring direct visualization of the structures under consideration and, frequently, the obtaining of biopsies for diagnosis or excisional biopsies for therapy. It is vital to remember throughout this discussion that the maintenance of adequate ventilation of the lungs is vital. The advent of pulse oximetry has provided us with a means for assessing oxygenation. Remember that oxygenation can take place in the absence of ventilation and that adequate oxygenation does not equate with adequate ventilation.[12-14] Many patients presenting for endoscopic procedures are hoarse or stridorous or have pharyngeal or laryngeal pathology that is already compromising their airway. Thus, it would be prudent to avoid sedation from preoperative medication in such patients.

In order to facilitate the surgeon's task, a dry immobile field

with minimal intrusion by our implements will provide optimal conditions. Minimization of oral secretions can usually be effectively accomplished with the use of an antisialogogue as a premedicant. Providing an immobile patient for the surgeon can be accomplished in any one of several acceptable ways. It is possible to adequately anesthetize the mouth, pharynx, larynx, and trachea with local anesthetic so that any of the endoscopic procedures can be carried out on cooperative awake patients under local anesthesia supplemented with some sedation. As a matter of fact, with proper patient selection and surgical skill, many of the minor airway procedures, for example, vocal cord stripping; excison of vocal cord nodules; vocal cord biopsies, as well as biopsies of other pharyngeal and laryngeal structures; and Teflon injections, can be accomplished safely under local anesthesia.[15] Local anesthesia can be effected by superior laryngeal nerve blockade, glossopharyngeal nerve blockade and transtracheal injection.[16-18] The gag reflex can be obliterated, and sufficient local anesthesia can be obtained by spraying the appropriate structures with a local anesthetic solution. Lidocaine is the most frequently used anesthetic, with the toxic dose being approximately $5 \ mg \cdot kg^{-1}$ and absorption from mucosal surfaces being almost as rapid as from intravenous (iv) administration.[19] Any contraindication to obliteration of the pharyngeal reflexes would most likely preclude the use of a purely local technique, and patients who have had their airways locally anesthetized should be fasted for at least 2 hours afterward or until their reflexes have returned. Often, for patient's preference, for surgeon's preference, or because of the chance for bleeding and/or gastric reflux (with resultant aspiration), a general anesthetic with a relatively protected and controlled airway is preferred.

Having decided upon a general anesthetic technique, there are several methods available for providing adequate surgical exposure and ventilation of the patient's lungs.[20-24] It is necessary to provide an immobile patient; this can be accomplished with or without the use of muscle relaxants. Immobility is important not only for the surgeon's benefit; coughing can result in a positive feedback condition invoking both airway and cardiovascular reflexes that can be life threatening.[25-28] For laryngoscopy, esophagoscopy, and rigid bronchoscopy, muscle relaxation provides good operating conditions for the surgeon. Induction of anesthesia can be done in any acceptable, safe manner, for example, iv or inhalation. Muscle relaxation can be achieved through the use of intermittent doses or continuous infusions of succinylcholine (SCh) or intermediate-acting muscle relaxants, atracurium, or vecuronium.[29] Neuromuscular blockade must be monitored, and the patient's airway reflexes must be intact prior to leaving the operating room. Maintenance of anesthesia can be accomplished by any acceptable method, keeping in mind that endoscopic procedures are usually of short duration, 5 to 60 minutes, and that the patient's airway reflexes must be intact at the end of the procedure.

Intubation of the trachea with a small diameter endotracheal tube will permit ventilation of the patient's lungs and still provide the surgeon with adequate visualization. A 5- or 6-mm internal diameter cuffed endotracheal tube will provide an adequate airway; however, higher than normal pressures will be required to ventilate the lungs owing to the increased resistance associated with the small bore endotracheal tube.[30] In most instances, the surgeon prefers to have the endotracheal tube taped on the left side of the patient's mouth, because the laryngoscope will be inserted down the right side of the mouth. Since the anesthesiologist and the surgeon will both be working in the patient's airway, it is vital that the anesthesiologist and the surgeon communicate with each other. The surgeon's and anesthesiologist's objectives and concerns are different. Therefore, it is only through adequate communication that both can arrive at a safe means of achieving both sets of objectives. The use of an endotracheal tube will provide adequate ventilation of the lungs and good direct visualization of the glottis in most cases. However, for posterior commissure laryngeal lesions, the endotracheal tube will obstruct the surgeon's field of view, and something other than the standard endotracheal tube must be used. A special endotracheal tube has been developed by Coplans[31] such that it possesses an asymmetric cuff, which makes it possible to have the tube clear of the posterior commissure.

If the endotracheal tube interferes with the surgeon's field of view, an alternate method of ventilating the lungs must be used. These techniques may leave an unprotected airway and do not always ensure adequate ventilation. The Carden tube is a short flexible cuffed tube that is meant to be inserted in its entirety below the level of the vocal cords.[32-34] Gas mixtures can be instilled into the tube through a small diameter tube comparable in size to the tubing used for the endotracheal tube cuff. With the vocal cords above the tube, it is possible to

FIG. 38-2. Mean Pa_{O_2} and Pa_{CO_2} values in 18 adult patients whose lungs were ventilated at a rate of 100 breaths·min^{-1} by a 3.5-mm internal diameter tube placed in the trachea. Because of air entrainment, the inspired concentration of oxygen was less than 100%. Exhalation occurred around the tracheal tube. (Reprinted with permission from Babinski M, Smith RB, Klain M: High-frequency jet ventilation for laryngoscopy. Anesthesiology 52:178, 1980.)

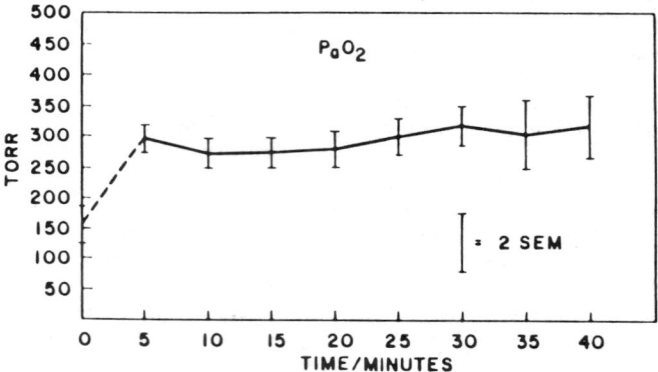

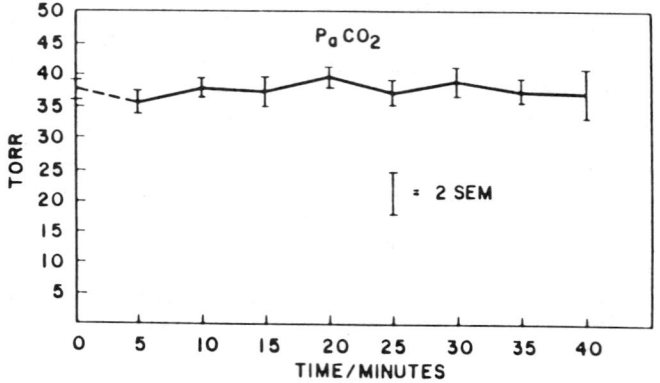

ventilate the patient's lungs through such a device using jet ventilation. Others have used a catheter and tube, connecting the catheter to a gas supply to either ventilate the patient's lungs with both an inspiratory and expiratory phase, or to just insufflate gas mixtures through the catheter. Adequacy of ventilation is assessed by observing the rise and fall of the chest, and adequacy of oxygenation is assessed by using pulse oximetry or an equivalent. Both jet ventilation and constant gas insufflation use the Venturi effect to entrain room air, thereby diluting the delivered gas mixture. For that reason, most investigators use 100% oxygen or at most a 50–50 mixture of nitrous oxide and oxygen. Many of the operating laryngoscopes used by ENT surgeons have side arms that can be used to provide jet ventilation to the patient. By using high pressure gas jets, as high as 60 psi, it is possible to adequately ventilate the lungs.[35-38] Inspiration is achieved through the instillation of a jet of gas, whereas exhalation is accomplished by passive relaxation of the chest wall and lungs. Recent studies have also examined the use of high-frequency jet ventilation for laryngoscopy (Fig. 38-2).[39-42] At present, it is not clear whether high-frequency ventilation techniques possess any advantage over traditional ventilation techniques. The aforementioned techniques are contraindicated in patients in whom an unprotected airway would be contraindicated. All the jet ventilation techniques are not without significant risks. The jets must be directed at or through the glottic opening; otherwise, the patient will not receive the desired gas, and the gas jets will go into structures other than the trachea. Cases of pneumothorax, subcutaneous air, mediastinal air, gastric distention, and respiratory acidosis (hypoventilation) have been reported.[43]

The only significant difference between laryngoscopy and microlaryngoscopy is the use of a microscope in microlaryngoscopy. Often, the laryngoscope will be suspended from a Mayo stand or a specially designed bracket attached to the operating room table. This frees both of the surgeon's hands. Remember that whenever the head is flexed or extended, the relative position of the endotracheal tube with respect to the carina changes. Therefore, after each manipulation of the head and airway by the surgeon, the location of the endotracheal tube should be verified.

LASER LARYNGOSCOPY

The laser (light amplification by stimulated emission of radiation) is now more than 25 years old. The first demonstration of this phenomenon was by T.H. Maiman in 1960, with the development of the ruby laser. Since that time, lasers have been developed that span the electromagnetic spectrum from the infrared to the threshold of the x-ray region. Lasers have been used in medicine almost since their inception.[44] They provide the surgeon with several advantages and are capable of providing very high intensity outputs that can be collimated, resulting in spot sizes on the order of the wavelength of light, having extremely high energy densities. Laser output is monochromatic; thus, substances that absorb at specific wavelengths can be selectively targeted while sparing others. Absorption of the laser's energy is essential; it is the key to all laser tissue interactions. It is possible to precisely control the duration of the laser pulses, and this is critical for the spatial confinement of the heat produced in tissue by the laser, thus sparing surrounding healthy tissue while destroying target tissue. Laser output is either continuous wave or pulsed. The mode used is a function of energy output and the desired result. Most of the time, lasers used in ENT surgery are carbon dioxide lasers, which are run in the continuous wave mode with intermittent bursts delivered to the tissues. Lasers provide the advantages of extreme precision, almost no blood loss (since the heat generated produces immediate coagulation), and minimal edema.

Carbon dioxide lasers emit energy with a wavelength of 10.6 μm, which lies in the infrared portion of the electromagnetic spectrum and is invisible to the unaided eye. Most medical carbon dioxide lasers have a helium–neon laser built into them. The radiation of the helium–neon laser is visible, is not absorbed by tissues, is of low energy, and serves as a means of directing the carbon dioxide laser beam, which is invisible. The wavelength of energy at which carbon dioxide emits energy is strongly absorbed by water. Since tissue is approximately 80% water, the tissue is rapidly heated, boiled, and finally vaporized, resulting in a clean cut through the tissue. Argon lasers, on the other hand, emit radiation at approximately 500 nm, which is in the visible portion of the spectrum and is highly absorbed by hemoglobin and poorly absorbed by water. Thus, the argon laser can be used to coagulate blood vessels in the back of the eye and pass harmlessly through the humors of the eye unattenuated by its passage.

The primary anesthetic consideration in laser surgery is safety of the patient and the operating room personnel. The energy of the laser must be absorbed with sufficient energy density over a long enough period of time to cause tissue damage. If the energy can be dispersed before it encounters viable tissue, or if the dispersed energy is delivered in short bursts, it is possible to greatly reduce the chance of unintentional injury. The operating room should have a sign posted cautioning all who enter that a laser is in use and that protective eyewear should be worn. All operating room personnel should wear goggles that absorb the radiation frequency of the laser being used, since the eye is the most susceptible organ to damage. The goggles should wrap around the face so as to protect the eyes from the side as well as from the front. The patient's eyes should be closed and protected with moistened eye pads. If at all possible, viable tissue within the surgical field should be protected with moistened sponges, so that if the laser beam inadvertently is diverted, it will be absorbed harmlessly. Another means of protecting adjacent tissues and operating room personnel is to dissipate and disperse the laser's energy in case it inadvertently strays from the desired target and strikes a reflective surface (*e.g.*, the laryngoscope or suction). Thus, instruments used for laser surgery should be nonreflective, have rough surfaces that will not act as a mirror for the laser beam, and be nonflammable. These features will serve to disperse the beam and hence reduce the energy density.

The most serious danger during any laser surgery is fire; this is especially true in laser surgery in the airway. There are numerous case reports of endotracheal tube fires in laser surgery in the airway, and there is a recent report of an endotracheal tube fire ignited by electrocautery.[45, 46] When a fire is started in an endotracheal tube, the tube becomes a blowtorch because of the high oxygen content and the high gas flows that occur during ventilation of the lungs. Such a fire can cause great devastation to the tracheobronchial tree. The incidence rate of endotracheal tube fire has been reported to be as high as 1.5% in patients undergoing laryngeal surgery with the carbon dioxide laser.[47] Endotracheal tube fires can be avoided by using other means to ventilate the patient's lungs. Jet and Venturi ventilation have been successfully used for such procedures[48, 49]; however, in addition to all the limita-

tions previously described for these techniques, in laser laryngoscopy procedures these techniques can result in instillation of debris, tumor, and smoke inhalation. In an attempt to provide some degree of protection, several special-purpose endotracheal tubes have been designed, and they all have a similar objective, which is to provide a nonflammable airway capable of either harmlessly absorbing the laser's energy or reflecting and dispersing the energy. Polyvinylchloride (PVC) is the compound most frequently used to make endotracheal tubes. It is highly flammable, and PVC endotracheal tubes should not be used during laser airway surgery, if at all possible. Tubes used especially for laser airway surgery are made of other compounds, ranging from rubber and silicone to metal. All endotracheal tubes not made from metal will ignite in an enriched oxygen atmosphere.[50, 51] Remember that nitrous oxide will also support combustion and thus does not provide any protection. A recent study suggests that the substitution of helium, which is an inert gas, for nitrous oxide will significantly increase the amount of energy required to produce combustion in PVC endotracheal tubes.[52] Thus, many anesthesiologists are substituting helium for nitrous oxide when doing laser laryngoscopy.

A popular method of producing a "laser-proof" tube is to wrap a red rubber tube with an aluminum foil tape. Selection of the correct tape is critical, since some tapes have the aluminized surface on the back layer of the tape so that the laser beam would pass through a clear layer of plastic compound before encountering the reflective surface. Chances are that this plastic compound is flammable. The correct metal tape is actually a metal ribbon with no surface coating, but it has an adhesive coating on the back. Proper technique in wrapping is essential; otherwise, gaps will exist, exposing the underlying endotracheal tube to the laser, and rough edges can damage laryngeal structures.[53] A tube manufactured by Xomed, made from silicone and metallic particles, provides some advantages over the red rubber tube, especially for its cuff. Silicone tube fires have occurred,[54] even though the silicone tube requires substantially more energy for ignition than either PVC or rubber tubes. An all-metal endotracheal tube, Norton tube, is available but has no cuff. The weak link in all cuffed tubes is the vulnerability of the cuff itself to puncture by the laser beam. Another tube has two cuffs, each with a separate pilot, such that if one cuff is made incompetent by laser penetration, there is a back-up cuff beneath it to maintain a sealed airway. Figure 38-3 shows a wrapped red rubber tube and the laser tube with the redundant cuffs. Other special-purpose tubes have been developed for laser laryngoscopy, but no study has shown any clear advantage to any one of them.[47, 55] The cuffs of all tubes should be filled with either saline or water. This will enable them to absorb more energy before becoming hot or disrupted, and, if they do get penetrated by the laser beam, the escaping liquid will help extinguish any fire. Some anesthesiologists have suggested adding methylene blue to the solution used to inflate the endotracheal tube cuff. Thus, if the cuff was pierced by the laser beam, a visible stream of liquid would be seen by the surgeon. Observing these precautions will greatly reduce the risk of endotracheal tube fires. These precautions should also be observed in patients who have tracheostomies. The trachea should be fitted with a protected tube prior to the laser procedure. If the cuff is penetrated in any of the single-cuffed endotracheal tubes, the endotracheal tube should be changed.

In the eventuality that a fire occurs, it is vital that a well-thought-out plan be followed. The first and most important thing to do is to stop ventilation, turn off the oxygen, remove

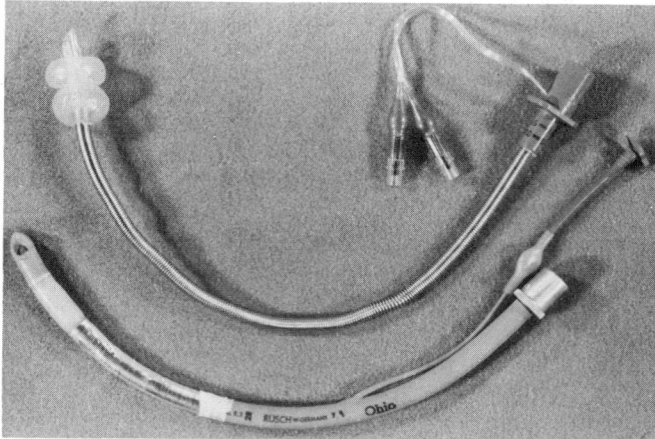

FIG. 38-3. Photograph of two types of endotracheal tubes used for laser laryngoscopy. The lowermost endotracheal tube is the familiar red rubber endotracheal tube, which has been wrapped with aluminum foil tape. The end of the aluminum tape is wrapped with a small piece of silk tape to prevent unraveling. The uppermost endotracheal tube is manufactured by National Catheter Corporation. It is made from a flexible stainless steel spiral tubing with soft silicone tip. Note that this endotracheal tube has two independent cuffs. Thus, if the uppermost cuff is punctured by the laser beam, the lower cuff will still protect the airway.

the flaming endotracheal tube from the airway, and extinguish the fire with sterile water or saline. The water is for the endotracheal tube, not the patient, unless flaming remnants of the tube remain in the patient's airway; in this case, some of the liquid should be used to extinguish these fragments before they are removed. Thus, an ample quantity of sterile water or saline must be kept in the sterile field at all times during laser laryngoscopy. Bronchoscopy, both rigid and flexible, should then be performed to determine the extent of the damage and to remove any debris from the airway. Ventilation of the lungs should be performed during these maneuvers, either with jet ventilation through a ventilating bronchoscope or through an endotracheal tube of as small a diameter as possible to minimize further airway trauma. Depending upon the extent of damage, tracheostomy and assisted ventilation of the lungs may be required. The administration of steroids[56] and humidification of inhaled gases should be accomplished. The patient should have a chest x-ray taken and be admitted to an intensive care unit for observation, even if no significant damage is suspected.

The anesthetic considerations for laser laryngoscopy are the same as those for other forms of laryngoscopy. The only possible exception is that immobility is mandatory to prevent inadvertent laser damage to healthy tissue if the patient moves. This can be accomplished with the use of muscle relaxants or through the use of deep anesthesia. At the end of the procedure, after the patient's trachea is extubated, the endotracheal tube should be inspected to ensure that no piece of foil tape or other protective covering is missing and presumed left in the airway. If something is missing, laryngoscopy and bronchoscopy are mandatory to retrieve it. Recently, some surgeons have started to resect tracheal and bronchial lesions with a laser, using either a rigid scope or a fiberoptic scope. The considerations for the anesthesiologist are the same as

those for any other bronchoscopy. If a fiberoptic bronchoscope is used, a PVC endotracheal tube may be used, since the laser will be active at a point below the end of the endotracheal tube.

ADENOTONSILLECTOMY

Many consider adenotonsillectomy to be an innocuous procedure. The patients, for the most part, are children and young adults who are usually classified as ASA physical status I or II. Many institutions are now performing this procedure on an outpatient basis. Indications for the surgical procedure are varied and controversial.[57] In the mid-1970s, it was estimated that approximately 750,000 young Americans underwent this surgical procedure or a variant thereof. Estimates of mortality associated with various forms of tonsillectomies are difficult to determine, but, in 1963, it was reported as being 1 of 10,000 patients in England.[58] Most of these deaths were associated with hypovolemia or a compromised airway and occurred as a result of postoperative bleeding. The reported incidence of mortality in patients requiring reoperation for postoperative bleeding was approximately 1 of 500 patients.[59, 60] In another study, there were no deaths in 9409 children undergoing adenoidectomy, tonsillectomy, or adenotonsillectomy over a 4 year period.[61]

The population undergoing tonsillectomies is also changing. The operation is now part of a surgical procedure used to alleviate obstructive sleep apnea, of which Pickwickian syndrome patients are a subset. During rapid eye movement sleep, the pharyngeal muscles relax along with the other muscles of the body. In obstructive sleep apnea patients, this relaxation produces airway obstruction, which can lead to episodes of hypoxia, eventually resulting in pulmonary hypertension, cor pulmonale, and congestive heart failure, if left untreated.[62] Adults with this syndrome are usually obese, have short thick necks, relatively large tongues, and redundant soft tissue in the oropharynx. Children with obstructive sleep apnea usually have obstruction secondary to a congenital anomaly such as Pierre Robin or Treacher Collins syndromes. It is also possible to produce obstructive sleep apnea in children with cleft palates who have undergone pharyngeal flap corrections, which have a tendency to decrease the antero-posterior oropharyngeal distance and can result in airway obstruction when the pharyngeal muscles relax during sleep. Sudden death during sleep in sleep apnea patients is probably caused by fatal arrhythmias that are secondary to asphyxia.[63] In adults, this condition can be surgically remedied by performing a uvulopharyngopalatoplasty (UPP), which consists of a tonsillectomy, uvulectomy, and limited pharyngectomy with resection of the redundant soft tissue of the soft palate and oropharynx.[64, 65] In children, in whom the obstruction is secondary to one of the previously mentioned syndromes, correction of the skeletal abnormality will usually correct the obstruction. The tonsils and adenoids sometimes become so hypertrophic in children that they can significantly encroach on the airway, and removal would be indicated to alleviate the obstruction.[66] In extreme cases, or if the patient's medical condition warrants, a tracheostomy can be performed to relieve the obstruction. The tracheostomy can be plugged during the day for normal laryngeal function while the patient is awake.

In all patients being considered for adenotonsillectomy, one must consider whether or not airway obstruction is a significant factor. If it is a factor, sedative/hypnotics should be avoided as preoperative medications. Since it is an intraoral procedure, an antisialogogue would be a good choice for premedication. In children, recurrent tonsillitis is an indication for tonsillectomy; however, the procedure should not be performed on an elective basis if signs and symptoms of upper respiratory infection or tonsillitis are present. This admonition is also true for adults. Adults with obstructive sleep apnea should be in stable condition from a cardiovascular point of view prior to operation. As with any other anesthetic, the anesthesiologist should look for signs and symptoms of cor pulmonale and congestive heart failure preoperatively. These conditions should be optimally managed medically before proceeding surgically.

Induction of anesthesia in patients without a history of airway obstruction and in whom airway assessment indicates normal airway anatomy can take place either by iv or inhalational routes as may be appropriate depending upon the age of the patient. In patients with a history of obstruction during sleep and in whom airway assessment indicates that oral intubation of the trachea should present no significant problem, preoxygenation and an iv induction of anesthesia with an ultrashort acting barbiturate is appropriate. These patients are usually more sensitive to hypnotics, analgesics, and anesthetics, and these drugs should be titrated for effect in each patient. Often, insertion of an oral or nasal airway is all that is required to be able to ventilate the lungs. By providing topical anesthesia to the mouth and nasal passages, it is possible to insert an airway and use a reduced dose of barbiturate, thereby reducing the time required for spontaneous breathing to return in case it is not possible to adequately ventilate the lungs. A lighter plane of anesthesia, however, will increase the likelihood of positive pressure–induced laryngospasm. One should have instruments at one's disposal for difficult tracheal intubations; these instruments include a stylet, an assortment of laryngoscope blades, and a fiberoptic laryngoscope. Equipment should also be available for performing a cricothyrotomy and ventilating through it if necessary. If the assessment of the patient's airway is that it will be difficult to intubate the trachea, an awake intubation should be performed in adults and a spontaneously breathing inhalation induction should be done in children with the maintenance of spontaneous breathing. In all cases, blood oxygen saturation should be measured with a pulse oximeter during the entire procedure.

Once the airway is secured, the surgeon inserts a mouth gag into the patient's mouth. There are a variety of mouth gags in use. They all require that the endotracheal tube be located in the midline, and the endotracheal tube is usually held in place by being pressed between the tongue blade of the mouth gag and the tongue. The most popular gag is a modification of the Crowe–Davis mouth gag. The tongue blade of this gag has a groove in it, so that it will accept an endotracheal tube. The endotracheal tube can be moved while the surgeon is placing the mouth gag, and it can also be compressed to the point of kinking the tube between the tongue blade and the tongue, especially if the endotracheal tube is not entirely within the groove. Thus, it is essential to check breath sounds after gag placement and the pressure required to ventilate the patient. The tube can be taped in place, or a piece of tape can be placed on the tube to serve as a visual marker indicating whether or not the surgeon has inserted or withdrawn the tube during placement of the mouth gag. Maintenance of anesthesia can be accomplished with either additional drugs or solely with the use of inhalation drugs. The use of muscle relaxants is acceptable if indicated. All muscle relaxation should be completely reversed prior to extubation of the trachea. As in laryngoscopy and bronchoscopy, the goal is to have an awake patient at the end of the procedure whose protective airway

reflexes are intact. Thus, the use of long-acting iv drugs is probably unwise in these patients. At the end of the surgical procedure, many surgeons will relax the tension on the mouth gag to determine whether or not the gag itself has been compressing vessels, which will bleed when the tension on the tissues is released. When this is done, be aware that if the endotracheal tube has not been taped in place, it is only loosely held in place by the mouth gag and can easily become dislodged.

It is difficult to determine exactly blood loss during these procedures, since a significant amount of blood can enter the gastrointestinal tract and be undetected. A graduated suction should be used by the surgical team, and blood loss should be adequately replaced with crystalloid or, if sufficient volume is lost, by blood transfusion. Make a habit of requesting that the surgeon insert an orogastric tube at the end of the procedure, and empty the stomach with suction. This will reduce the likelihood of nausea and emesis, since blood in the stomach is a potent stimulus for nausea. Prior to awakening the patient, the anesthesiologist should inspect the mouth for the presence of blood, blood clots, debris, and active bleeding and should take proper action. Carefully suction the nasopharynx through the nares, as a significant amount of blood can be lodged there and can slowly ooze into the oropharynx, resulting in laryngospasm[67, 68] after extubation of the trachea. When the patient is awake, is breathing adequately, and it appears that his airway reflexes are intact, it is appropriate to extubate the trachea. Patients are often transported to the recovery room in the lateral head-down position, the "tonsil position," and kept in this position until they are fully awake. This will help to prevent aspiration of blood from either the nasopharynx or the tonsillar bed and also prevents blood and secretions from dripping on the vocal cords and resulting in laryngospasm. In sleep apnea patients, the use of steroids to help reduce tissue edema is worthy of consideration. Obstructive sleep apnea patients should be admitted to an intensive care unit setting overnight, where their breathing, oxygen saturation, and ECG can be monitored, since relief of the obstruction does not always immediately relieve apnea but may unmask an underlying central apneic component. It may also take several weeks before central mechanisms have readjusted.

As mentioned earlier, the most frequent complication associated with this procedure is postoperative bleeding, with resultant hypovolemia and airway obstruction. There are two likely periods for postoperative bleeding. The first period is in the immediate 4 to 6 hours postoperatively. A study by Crysdale indicated that 76% of postoperative bleeding occured within the first 6 hours, and 87% occurred within 9 hours.[61] Only 0.06% of the patients in his study bled postoperatively, and, of these, only 3% required reoperation. Other studies have reported reoperation rates as high as 0.9% of all patients undergoing one of the variants of adenotonsillectomy. Most of the postoperative bleeding that occurs is of a slow oozing nature, and it is not until the patient vomits a large amount of blood, which he has been swallowing, that anyone realizes the problem. At this point, the patient may be hypovolemic and should be adequately rehydrated so that at least no orthostatic blood pressure changes are present. Airway obstruction may be present, and the presumption of a stomach full of blood should be made. If the surgeon believes that the bleeding cannot be controlled through application of electrocautery, silver nitrate, or topical vasoconstrictors, preparations should be made to return the patient to the operating room. The patient should have an adequate iv, preferably two. An awake intubation of the trachea is often preferable if at all possible. If not, a rapid sequence induction of anesthesia with use of adequate preoxygenation and the Sellick maneuver is indicated. In children, an inhalation induction can be accomplished using halothane in oxygen and adding cricoid pressure as soon as consciousness is lost. With the patient breathing spontaneously, a gentle laryngoscopy can be performed, and only when the glottis is visualized can SCh be administered. If bleeding is active, the head can be held in the lateral position during induction of anesthesia. Laryngoscopy and endotracheal intubation is surprisingly easy in this position, but it should be practiced in patients when it is not necessary so that one can acquire some skill. It is probably wise to avoid thiopental as the induction drug since the patient's intravascular status may be tenuous at best. Ketamine, 1 to 2 mg·kg^{-1}, or etomidate, 0.2 to 0.4 mg·kg^{-1} may be better choices for an induction drug. The important point is to maintain intravascular volume status. Most patients undergoing tonsillectomy will tolerate transient anemia. Obtaining a hematocrit will help determine whether or not a blood transfusion is advisable. After the bleeding has been stopped, the stomach should be emptied with suction through an orogastric tube. The criteria for extubation of the trachea are the same as they were the first time. Through this conservative approach, it is possible to greatly reduce the mortality associated with adenotonsillectomy.

The second common period for postoperative tonsillar bleeding is approximately 5 to 10 days postoperatively and is usually attributable to infection with the persistence of fever and sore throat in the postoperative period.

CANCER OF THE HEAD AND NECK

Most cancers of the head and neck structures are associated with a history of chronic cigarette smoking and alcohol use. As a result, most patients presenting with tumors of the head and neck are in their 5th or 6th decade of life. In addition to their cancer, they have also acquired the other sequellae of heavy smoking and drinking. These patients often have some degree of chronic obstructive pulmonary disease (COPD) and coronary artery disease (CAD). Many of these patients will be hypertensive. There should be high suspicion of alcohol withdrawal, and treatment with a long-acting hypnotic such as diazepam should be accomplished if a history of heavy drinking is elicited. Obviously, this does not apply if any degree of sedation would be contraindicated owing to a compromised airway. If airway compromise prevents preoperative use of delirium tremens precautions, a long-acting hypnotic should be administered once the airway has been secured. Often, the patient's nutritional status will be poor secondary to dysphagia. If the tumor has involved the vocal cords either directly or indirectly, there may be evidence of aspiration pneumonia.

A thorough history and physical examination should be performed with special emphasis placed on the respiratory and cardiac systems. Neoplasms will often cause inflammation and resultant edema. Thus, a careful search for signs and symptoms of airway compromise should be performed. Many of these patients will already have had a course of radiation therapy, which produces fibrosis. A thin patient with normal-appearing external airway anatomy may be difficult to intubate, since the fibrosed tissue is unyielding. In most cases, the surgeon has performed an indirect laryngoscopy and will be able to tell you whether or not, in his or her opinion, you will be able to intubate the patient's trachea. If the surgical procedure will require a tracheostomy, an awake tracheostomy under local anesthesia should be discussed with the surgeon.

An awake tracheostomy should be done if the lesion is considered to be extremely friable or exophytic, thereby avoiding dislodging cancerous tissue into the tracheobronchial tree and the possibility of starting significant bleeding in the airway. If the patient's trachea can be intubated, even though there is airway compromise or distortion, an awake intubation either by direct laryngoscopy or fiberoptic laryngoscopy should be seriously considered. If there is any reservation about the ability to intubate the patient's trachea by direct oral laryngoscopy after induction of anesthesia, it is advisable to be aggressive about awake intubations. Once the airway has been traumatized after several unsuccessful attempts at intubation of the trachea in an anesthetized patient, it is much more difficult to then perform a fiberoptic laryngoscopy with a bloody field added to the already distorted anatomy.

Pulmonary function tests, baseline arterial blood gases, chest x-rays, and computed tomograms of the neck should be obtained. In addition to a routine 12-lead ECG, other tests may be indicated to evaluate the cardiovascular status of these patients, since it is often difficult to differentiate between pulmonary and cardiac etiology for symptoms in these patients. If consultations are indicated, the anesthesiologist should discuss any concerns with the surgeon and the consultant prior to the consult, so that the consultant's response will directly address your (the anesthesiologist's) concerns. The patient's medical condition should be optimized prior to surgery. Unless airway obstruction is imminent, none of the oncology procedures are emergencies. Whether the procedure is a glossectomy, pharyngectomy, or laryngectomy, with or without an accompanying neck dissection, all these procedures will require anywhere from 3 to 8 hours to complete, and significant blood loss of 1000 ml or more is not uncommon. Blood loss is difficult to estimate in these procedures, since much of it is hidden from view, pooling under the patient's head, saturating the surgical sheets, and eventually dripping onto the floor. The choice of an induction drug should be based on the patient's medical condition; for example, a patient with severe coronary artery disease would not likely benefit from an induction of anesthesia with ketamine. Monitoring for these procedures should consist of the routine monitors as well as a Foley catheter to monitor urine output. Depending upon the patient's pulmonary and cardiac status, and also on whether or not a neck dissection will be part of the procedure, monitoring of blood pressure by an arterial catheter may be indicated. Certainly, if for no other reason than repeated arterial blood gas determinations in patients with significant COPD, an arterial line is appropriate. Also, depending upon cardiac function, expected blood loss, and length of procedure, a central venous line or pulmonary artery catheter may be indicated.[6] If central venous access is required, preoperative placement is indicated. Internal jugular vein access is denied by most of the head and neck procedures, since the access line would be in the operative field. Anticubital access can be achieved at the time of the procedure; however, it is frequently difficult to pass the line around the shoulder and into the central circulation. Subclavian access can be accomplished at the time of the surgical procedure; however, after line placement, a chest x-ray may be useful to ensure that no pneumothorax exists prior to induction of anesthesia, positive pressure ventilation of the lungs, and the use of nitrous oxide. Subclavian access can be obtained the night before surgery, and an x-ray can be taken and read by a radiologist before the patient arrives in the operating room the next morning, thus avoiding unnecessary delay in the operating room.

Intraoperative management of these patients requires consideration of their pre-existing medical problems. Several authors have discussed the anesthetic management of specific procedures[69–73]; however, there is no one anesthetic technique that has been shown to be superior to others for any of these procedures. Use of muscle relaxants may be limited by the need of the surgeon to evaluate intactness of nerves during neck dissection or parotid surgery. If the procedure will involve a tracheostomy, it may be useful to avoid muscle relaxants for this portion of the procedure and try to maintain spontaneous respiration. Administration of 100% oxygen prior to the actual tracheotomy is advised, so that if, for any reason, the airway is lost, there will be some oxygen reserve before hypoxia results. During tracheostomy, it is possible to produce a tracheoesophageal fistula, a false passage, damage to the recurrent laryngeal nerve, subcutaneous emphysema, pneumothorax, bleeding, and blood aspiration.[74, 75] If the procedure involves a neck dissection, manipulation of the carotid sinus can result in cardiac dysrhythmias and wide fluctuations of blood pressure. If this occurs, request that the surgeon stop his manipulation and infiltrate the tissues surrounding the carotid sinus with a local anesthetic. Cardiac dysrhythmias associated with a prolonged QT interval and cardiac arrest have been described in patients undergoing radical neck dissection (Fig. 38-4).[76] Open neck veins can serve to entrain air into the venous system and result in significant venous air embolism. Venous air embolism can be reduced, if not eliminated, by keeping the patient in a slight head-down position. Tumor can involve the major vessels of the neck and may require sacrifice of either one or both internal jugular veins. If this occurs, cerebral perfusion pressure may be decreased and the increased intracerebral venous pressure can result in cerebral edema. Some authors have advocated induced hypotension for these procedures to help reduce the blood loss and to aid the surgeon by providing a dryer surgical field. The use of induced hypotension in these patients is controversial. Since most of these patients will have, at best, silent CAD and since the chance of compromising cerebral blood flow is present, it is difficult to a priori predict what degree of hypotension would be tolerated.[77, 78]

Occasionally, a tumor may involve the carotid artery, requiring sacrifice of the carotid artery on the side of the lesion. The radiologist can temporarily occlude the involved vessel with a balloon during angiography in an awake patient to determine whether or not the patient will tolerate loss of blood flow from the involved vessel. Regardless of the outcome of the temporary occlusion, the electroencephalogram (EEG) should be monitored intraoperatively if there is any chance that the surgeon will sacrifice the carotid artery. It would also be prudent to maintain normal systemic blood pressure and normocarbia to preserve cerebral blood flow in these patients. These functions can be facilitated by the use of an arterial pressure monitor, arterial blood gases, and an end-tidal carbon dioxide monitor.

If the patient has had a tracheostomy as part of the procedure, the cuffed tracheostomy tube will serve to help protect the airway. The portion of trachea lying superior to the tracheostomy site should be suctioned prior to changing the temporary tracheostomy tube for a permanent one, since a significant amount of blood can be sequestered there. If it is necessary to ventilate the patient's lungs in the postoperative period, a cuffed tracheal tube can be used. If no tracheostomy was done, the anesthesiologist and the surgeon will have to decide whether or not the surgical procedure produced sufficient edema and distortion to compromise the patient's airway in the immediate postoperative period. If there is any doubt, the patient's trachea should remain intubated in the immediate postoperative period, and one should continue to evaluate

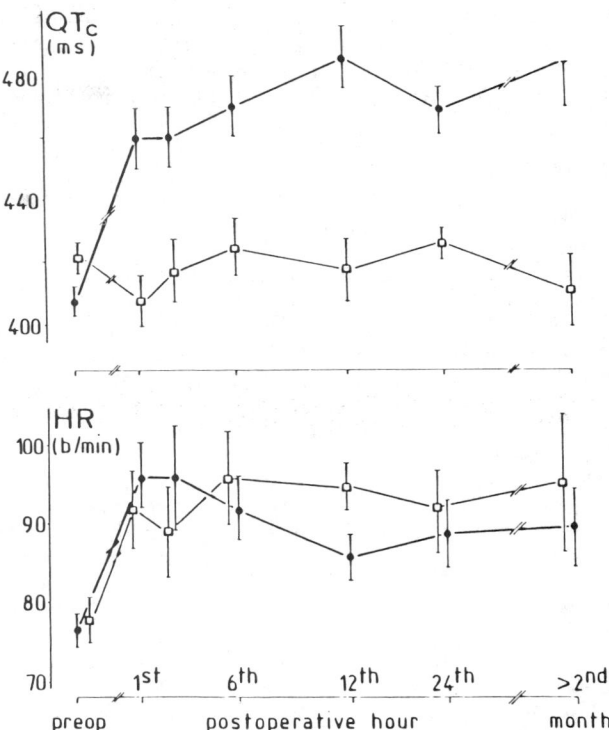

FIG. 38-4. Corrected QT interval (Q-T$_c$) and heart rate (HR) as measured before and after right (*solid symbols*) or left (*clear symbols*) radical neck dissection. Right radical neck dissection increased QT$_c$ when compared with left radical neck dissection ($P < 0.001$). Mean ± SE. (Reprinted with permission from Otteni JC, Pottecher T, Bronner G *et al*: Prolongation of the Q-T interval and sudden cardiac arrest following right radical neck dissection. Anesthesiology 59:358, 1983.)

the airway postoperatively. Administration of steroids early on may help to minimize tissue edema.

SURGICAL PROCEDURES INVOLVING THE EAR

The majority of procedures done on the ear involve the middle ear, its contents, and the mastoid air cells. Usually these procedures are carried out for hearing loss in patients who are, for the most part, young and otherwise healthy. Chronic infection can cause scarring of the tympanic membrane, fibrosis, and cholesteatoma involving the ossicular chain, all resulting in hearing loss. Involvement of the labyrinth will result in vertigo, nystagmus, nausea, and vomiting. The facial nerve is intimately associated with the structures of the ear, and its preservation is always a consideration. Often the disease processes in the middle ear can involve the facial nerve, and surgical procedures expressly for facial nerve decompression are done. There are three aspects of surgery of the ear that are controversial: 1) the use of nitrous oxide; 2) induced hypotension; and 3) the use of muscle relaxants.

The fact that nitrous oxide is approximately 34 times more soluble than nitrogen can present a problem in closed spaces in the body. Since nitrous oxide will enter the closed space at a faster rate than nitrogen can be removed, the volume of any gas contained within a closed space can significantly expand.[79] The middle ear represents an air-filled noncompliant space within the body. Numerous studies have documented the increase in middle ear pressure that occurs during the use of nitrous oxide and the harmful effects associated with its use (Fig. 38-5).[80-87] Cases of actual rupture of the tympanic membrane have been reported and attributed to the use of nitrous oxide.[88] Typanic membrane grafts have been dislodged through the use of nitrous oxide. The other consideration is that when the nitrous oxide is discontinued and a previously open space is closed, the withdrawal of nitrous oxide will produce a negative pressure.

In operative procedures on the middle ear, until the surgeon begins to close the middle ear, there is no closed space. It has been proposed that the use of nitrous oxide be discontinued approximately 30 minutes before the tympanic membrane graft is placed.[89] In practice, if the nitrous oxide is discontinued for approximately 5 minutes before the graft is placed, it usually does not present a problem for the surgeon. If the surgeon packs the middle ear with Gelfoam, this will usually prevent significant retraction of the graft postoperatively. Surgeons have their own individual biases with respect to the use of nitrous oxide and middle ear surgery. At the start of the case, one should ask whether or not the surgeon is concerned about the use of nitrous oxide. If he or she is concerned, the nitrous oxide can be discontinued several minutes before placement of the graft. If for any reason the surgeon appears to be having difficulty with the graft, discontinue the nitrous oxide.

Many surgeons believe that a bloodless operative field is a requirement for them to sucessfully perform microsurgical procedures on the ear. Much of the anesthesia literature supports this position.[6, 77] Profound hypotension has been advocated with systolic blood pressure being reduced to 50 mm Hg for significant periods of time with spontaneous breathing and with no means of monitoring the adequacy of cerebral perfusion other than the regularity of the respiratory pattern.[90, 91] Interestingly, Eltringham and colleagues[91] found no correlation with the degree of hypotension and the surgeon's assessment of the adequacy of the surgical conditions. Many surgeons infiltrate the tissues of the ear with epinephrine-containing solutions to help provide hemostasis. Most patients requiring these procedures are young and healthy, with

FIG. 38-5. Rate of increase of middle ear pressure in children (5 to 12 years of age) during assisted ventilation of the lungs with halothane and nitrous oxide in oxygen (*circles*) compared with children breathing halothane in oxygen (*squares*). (Reprinted with permission from Casey WF, Drake–Lee AB: Nitrous oxide and middle ear pressure. Anaesthesia 37:896, 1982.)

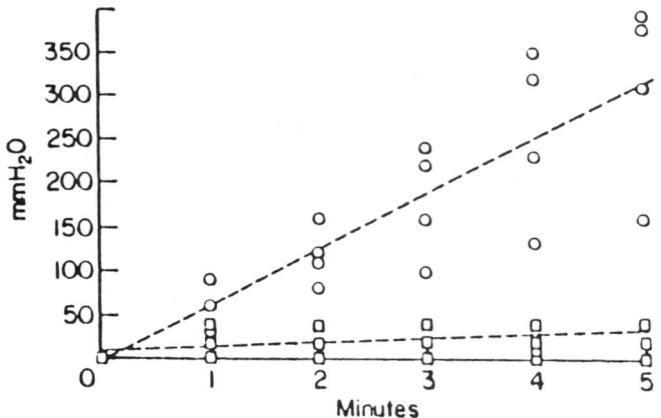

no history or evidence of pulmonary or cardiovascular disease. This group of patients tolerate hypotension well. Adequate measures must be taken to ensure the adequacy of vital organ perfusion during hypotension. An arterial catheter to measure blood pressure and obtain samples for arterial blood gas analysis, end-tidal carbon dioxide measurement, an EEG, and other monitors have been proposed as standards of care during induced hypotension.[67] Spontaneous ventilation has been advocated during the hypotensive anesthetic so as to reduce cerebral venous pressure.[77] It has also been suggested that the operating table be positioned so that the head is elevated 15 to 30 degrees in order to aid in venous drainage and reduce cerebral venous pressure.[67] Elevating the operative field above the level of the heart increases the risk of venous air embolism. Is profound hypotension in addition to the use of potent vasoconstrictors necessary or greatly beneficial in microsurgical procedures of the ear? There is no definitive answer at this time.

Identification and preservation of the facial nerve is always a consideration in surgical procedures on the ear. It is known that different muscle groups possess different sensitivities to muscle relaxants[92] and that it is possible to provide skeletal muscle relaxation without complete paralysis, thus enabling the surgeon to elicit a response from direct nerve stimulation, even though the patient has only a small percentage of neuromuscular function intact. Theoretically, there is no logical reason why neuromuscular blocking drugs cannot be used, even when nerve preservation is a significant consideration. Practically speaking, if for any reason there is facial nerve dysfunction postoperatively and if muscle relaxants were used as other than as an aid to intubation of the trachea, it could create an awkward situation for the anesthesiologist and the surgeon.

As in all surgical procedures, patient safety is the anesthesiologist's prime concern. In microsurgery of the ear, an immobile patient is a requirement for the procedure. This can be accomplished by producing an adequate level of anesthesia without the use of muscle relaxants. Volatile inhalation anesthetics provide some degree of muscle relaxation, can easily produce an adequate level of anesthesia, do not require nitrous oxide for their effective use, and can be used to induce hypotension. Thus, volatile inhalation anesthesia would appear to be a logical choice as a primary anesthetic technique for microsurgery of the ear. In addition, the incidence of nausea is less with a pure inhalation technique than when opioids are used.[93] Nausea and dizziness are always postoperative problems in patients undergoing ear surgery. Avoidance of opioids as well as prophylactic administration of antiemetics such as droperidol or promethazine are useful in these patients.[94, 95]

CONCLUSIONS

In most other areas of anesthesia, the anesthesiologist is at the patient's head and is in control of the airway. This can produce a false sense of security. In anesthesia for ENT procedures, the anesthesiologist is almost never at the head and normally does not have easy access to the airway. In ENT, patients frequently have intraoral lesions that will make direct oral laryngoscopy and intubation of the trachea difficult if not impossible. The anesthesiologist in ENT must learn to accurately assess the patient's airway and, as part of that assessment, to communicate with the surgeon, who has knowledge of the patient's pathology. Communication is the key to safe anesthesia in ENT. It is vital for good patient care that the anesthesiologist know what the surgeon is doing at all times, and it is vital for the surgeon to know what technique the anesthesiologist is using.

REFERENCES

1. Crafts RC: A Textbook of Human Anatomy. New York, Ronald Press Co, 1966.
2. Goss CM: Gray's Anatomy of the Human Body, 28th ed. Philadelphia, Lea & Febiger, 1966
3. Anderson JE: Grant's Atlas of Anatomy, 7th ed. Baltimore, Williams & Wilkins, 1978
4. Clemente CD: Anatomy, A regional atlas of the human body. Philadelphia, Lea & Febiger, 1978
5. Sellick BA: Cricoid pressure to control regurgitation of stomach contents during induction of anaesthesia. Lancet 2:404, 1961
6. Miller RD: Anesthesia, 2nd ed. New York, Churchill Livingstone, 1986
7. Bhagwandas G, McDonald JS. The difficult airway. Hospital Physician 22:65, 1986
8. Spoerel WE: Problems of the upper airway. Int Anesthesiol Clin 10:1,1972
9. Salem MR, Mathrubhutham M, Bennett EJ: Difficult intubation. N Engl J Med 295:879, 1976
10. Ament R: A systemic approach to the difficult intubation. Anesthesiol Rev 5:12, 1978
11. White A, Kander PL: Anatomical factors in difficult laryngoscopy. Br J Anaesth 47:468, 1975
12. Rah KH, Salzberg AM, Boyan CP et al: Respiratory acidosis with small Storz–Hopkins bronchoscopes: Occurrence and management. Ann Thorac Surg 27:197, 1979
13. Eger EI, Severinghaus JW: The rate of rise of Pa_{CO_2} in the apneic anesthetized patient. Anesthesiology 22:419, 1968
14. Neil SG, Lam AM, Turnbull KW et al: Monitoring of oxygen. Can J Anaesth 34:56, 1987
15. Calcaterra TC, House J: Local anesthesia for suspension microlaryngoscopy. Ann Otol 85:71, 1976
16. Moore DC: Regional Block. A Handbook for Use in the Clinical Practice of Medicine and Surgery, 4th ed. Springfield, Illinois, Charles C Thomas, 1965
17. Eriksson E: Illustrated Handbook in Local Anesthesia, 2nd ed. Philadelphia, WB Saunders, 1980
18. Barton S, Williams JD: Glossopharyngeal nerve block. Arch Otolaryngol 93:186, 1971
19. Covino BG, Vassello HG: Local Anesthetics. Mechanisms of Action and Clinical Use. New York, Grune & Stratton, 1976
20. Rajagopalan R, Smith F, Ramachandran PR: Anaesthesia for microlaryngoscopy and definitive surgery. Can Anaesth Soc J 19:83, 1972
21. Raj PP, Forestner J, Watson TD et al: Technics for fiberoptic laryngoscopy in anesthesia. Anesth Analg 53:708, 1974
22. Glenski JA MacKenzie RA, Maragos NE et al: Assessing tidal volume and detecting hyperinflation during Venturi jet ventilation for microlaryngeal surgery. Anesthesiology 63:554, 1985
23. Webster AC: Anesthesia for operations on the upper airway. Int Anesth Clin 10:61, 1972
24. Spoerel WE, Narayanan PS, Singh NP: Transtracheal ventilation. Br J Anaesth 43:932, 1971
25. Strong MS, Vaughan CW, Mahler DL et al: Cardiac complications of microsurgery of the larynx: Etiology, incidence and prevention. Laryngoscope 84:908, 1974
26. Elguindi AS, Harrison GN, Abdulla AM et al: Cardiac rhythm disturbances during fiberoptic bronchoscopy: A prospective study. J Thorac Cardiovasc Surg 77:557, 1979
27. Katz AS, Michelson EL, Stawicki J et al: Cardiac arrhythmias.
28. Pereira W, Kovnat DM, Snider GL: A prospective cooperative study of complications following flexible fiberoptic bronchoscopy. Chest 73:813, 1978
29. Carnie J: Continuous suxamethonium infusion for microlaryngeal surgery. Br J Anaesth 54:11, 1982
30. Bolder PM, Healy TEJ, Bolder AR et al: The extra work of breathing through adult endotracheal tubes. Anesth Analg 65:853, 1986
31. Coplans MP: A cuffed nasotracheal tube for microlaryngeal surgery. Anaesthesia 31:430, 1976
32. Carden E, Schwesinger WB: The use of nitrous oxide during ventilation with the open bronchoscope. Anesthesiology 39:551, 1973
33. Carden E, Vest HR: Further advances in anesthetic technics for microlaryngeal surgery. Anesth Analg 53:584, 1974
34. Carden E, Ferguson GB, Crutchfield WM: A new silicone elastomer tube for use during microsurgery on the larynx. Ann Otol Rhinol Laryngol 83:360, 1974
35. Pybus DA, O'Connor AF, Henville JD: Anaesthesia for laryngoscopy: A technique using the Nuffield anaesthetic ventilator. Br J Anaesth 50:501, 1978
36. Keen RI, Kotak PK, Ramsden RT: Anaesthesia for microsurgery of the larynx. Ann R Coll Sur Eng 64:111, 1982
37. Carden E, Galido J: Foot-pedal control of jet ventilation during bronchoscopy and microlaryngeal surgery. Anesth Analg 54:405, 1975
38. Frederickson JM, Haight JS, Soder CM: Ventilation during laryngoscopy in chronic obstructive lung disease. Laryngoscope 94:1606, 1984
39. Eng UB, Eriksson I, Sjostrand U: High-frequency positive-pressure ventilation (HFPPV): A review based upon its use during bronchoscopy and for laryngoscopy and microlaryngeal surgery under general anesthesia. Anesth Analg 59:594, 1980
40. Eriksson I, Sjostrand U: A clinical evaluation of high-frequency positive-pressure ventilation (HFPPV) in laryngoscopy under general anesthesia. Acta Anaesth Scand 64:101, 1977
41. Rogers RC, Gibbons J, Cosgrave J et al: High-frequency jet ventilation for tracheal surgery. Anaesthesia 40:32, 1985
42. Babinski M, Smith RB, Klain M: High-frequency jet ventilation for laryngoscopy. Anesthesiology 52:178, 1980
43. Chang JL, Meeuwis H, Bleyaert A et al: Severe abdominal distention following jet ventilation during general anesthesia. Anesthesiology 49:216, 1978
44. Walsh JT, Parrish JA: Lasers: The healing tool of the future. IEEE Potentials 4:36, 1985
45. Simpson JI, Wolf GL: Endotracheal tube fire ignited by pharyngeal electrocautery. Anesthesiology 65:76, 1986
46. Sommer RM: Preventing endotracheal tube fire during pharyngeal surgery. Anesthesiology 66:439, 1987
47. Hermens JM, Bennett MJ, Hirshman CA: Anesthesia for laser surgery. Anesth Analg 62:218, 1983
48. Ruder CB, Rapheal NL, Abramson AL et al: Anesthesia for carbon dioxide laser microsurgery of the larynx. Otolaryngology 89:732, 1981
49. Gussack GS, Evans RF, Tacchi EJ: Intravenous anesthesia and jet ventilation for laser microlaryngeal surgery. Ann Otol Rhinol Laryngol 96:29, 1987
50. Hayes DM, Gaba DM, Goode RL: Incendiary characteristics of a new laser-resistant endotracheal tube. Otolaryngology 95:37, 1986
51. LeJeune FE, Guice C, LeTard F et al: Heat sink protection against lasering endotracheal cuffs. Ann Otol Rhinol Laryngol 91:606, 1982
52. Pashayan AG, Gravenstein JS: Helium retards endotracheal tube fires from carbon dioxide lasers. Anesthesiology 62:274, 1985

53. Brown B: Anesthesia and ENT Surgery. Philadelphia, FA Davis, 1987
54. Giffin B, Shapshay SM, Bellack GS et al: Flammability of endotracheal tubes during Nd–YAG laser application in the airway. Anesthesiology 65:54, 1986
55. Patil V, Stehling LC, Zauder HI: A modified endotracheal tube for laser microsurgery. Anesthesiology 51:571, 1979
56. Orkin FK, Cooperman LH: Complicaitions in Anesthesiology. Philadelphia, JB Lippincott, 1983
57. Carden TS: Tonsillectomy—trials and tribulations. JAMA 240:1961, 1978
58. Tate N: Deaths from tonsillectomy. Lancet 2:1090, 1963
59. Keenan RL, Boyan CP: Cardiac arrest due to anesthesia. JAMA 253:2373, 1985
60. Davies DD: Re-anaesthetizing cases of tonsillectomy and adenoidectomy because of persistent postoperative haemorrhage. Br J Anaesth 36:244, 1964
61. Crysdale WS: Complications of tonsillectomy and adenoidectomy in 9409 children observed overnight. CMAJ 135:1139, 1986
62. Hall JB: The cardiopulmonary failure of sleep-disordered breathing. JAMA 255:930, 1986
63. Bradley TD, Phillipson EA: Pathogenesis and pathophysiology of the obstructive sleep apnea syndrome. Med Clin North Am 69:1169, 1985
64. Chung F, Crago RR: Sleep apnea syndrome and anaesthesia. Can Anaesth Soc J 29:439, 1982
65. Tobin MJ, Cohn MA, Sackner MA: Breathing abnormalities during sleep. Arch Intern Med 143:1221, 1983
66. Weinberg S, Kravath R, Phillips L et al: Episodic complete airway obstruction in children with undiagnosed obstructive sleep apnea. Anesthesiology 60:356, 1984
67. Rex MAE: A review of the structural and functional basis of laryngospasm and a discussion of the nerve pathways involved in the reflex and its clinical significance in man and animals. Br J Anaesth 42:891, 1970
68. Suzuki M, Saski CT: Laryngeal spasm: A neurophysiologic redefinition. Ann Otol 86:150, 1977
69. Donlon JV: Anesthetic management of patients with compromised airways. Anesthesiol Rev VII:22, 1980
70. Davies RM, Scott JG: Anaesthesia for major oral and maxillofacial surgery. Br J Anaesth 40:202, 1968
71. Geffin B, Bland J, Grillo HC: Anesthetic management of tracheal resection and reconstruction. Anesth Analg 48:884, 1969
72. Ellis RH, Hinds CJ, Gadd LT: Management of anaesthesia during tracheal resection. Anaesthesia 31:1076, 1976
73. Kamvyssi-dea S, Kritikou P, Exharhos N et al: Anaesthetic management of reconstruction of the lower portion of the trachea. Br J Anaesth 47:82, 1975
74. Kirchner JA: Tracheotomy and its problems. Surg Clin North Am 60:1093, 1980
75. Greenway RE: Tracheostomy: Surgical problems and complications. Int Anesth Clin 10:151, 1972
76. Otteni JC, Pottecher T, Bronner G et al: Prolongation of the Q-T interval and sudden cardiac arrest following right radical neck dissection. Anesthesiology 59:358, 1983
77. Morrison JD, Mirakur RK, Craig HJL: Anaesthesia for Eye, Ear, Nose and Throat Surgery, 2nd ed. Edinburgh, Churchill Livingstone, 1985
78. Enderby GEH: Hypotensive Anaesthesia. Edinburgh, Churchill Livingstone, 1985
79. Eger EI: Anesthetic Uptake and Action. Baltimore, Williams & Wilkins, 1974
80. Shaw JO, Stark EW, Gannaway SD: The influence of nitrous oxide anaesthetic on middle-ear fluid. J Laryngol Otol 92:131, 1978
81. Marshall FPF, Cable HR: The effect of nitrous oxide on middle-ear effusions. J Laryngol Otol 96:893, 1982
82. Patterson ME, Bartlett PC: Hearing impairment caused by intratympanic pressure changes during general anesthesia. Laryngoscope 86:399, 1976
83. Davis I, Moore JRM, Lahiri SK: Nitrous oxide and the middle ear. Anaesthesia 34:147, 1979
84. Matz GJ, Rattenborg CG, Holaday DA: Effects of nitrous oxide on middle ear pressure. Anesthesiology 28:948, 1967
85. Thomsen KA, Terkildsen K, Arnfred I: Middle ear pressure variations during anesthesia. Arch Otolaryngol 82:609, 1965
86. Casey WF, Drake–Lee AB: Nitrous oxide and middle ear pressure. Anaesthesia 37:896, 1982
87. Waun JE, Sweitzer RS, Hamilton WK: Effect of nitrous oxide on middle ear mechanics and hearing acuity. Anesthesiology 28:846, 1967
88. Owens QD, Gustave F, Sclaroff A: Tympanic membrane rupture with nitrous oxide anesthesia. Anesth Analg 57:283, 1978
89. Jahrsdoerfer RA: Anesthesia in otologic surgery. Otolaryngol Clin North Am 14:699, 1981
90. Kerr AR: Anaesthesia with profound hypotension for middle ear surgery. Br J Anaesth 49:447, 1977
91. Eltringham RJ, Young PN, Fairbairn MD et al: Hypotensive anaesthesia for microsurgery of the middle ear. A comparison between enflurane and halothane. Anaesthesia 37:1028, 1982
92. Caffrey RR, Warren ML, Becker KE: Neuromuscular blockade monitoring comparing the orbicularis oculi and adductor pollicis muscles. Anesthesiology 65:95, 1986
93. Clarke RSJ: Nausea and vomiting. Br J Anaesth 56:19, 1984
94. Palazzo MGA, Strunin L: Anaesthesia and emesis. I. Etiology. Can Anaesth Soc J 31:178, 1984
95. Palazzo MGA, Strunin L: Anaesthesia and emesis. II. Prevention and management. Can Anaesth Soc J 31:407, 1984

Chapter 39

Donald S. Prough
Arthur S. Foreman

Anesthesia and the Renal System

ANATOMY AND PHYSIOLOGY OF THE RENAL EXCRETORY SYSTEM

ANATOMY OF THE KIDNEYS, URETERS, AND BLADDER

The kidneys, bilateral, paired organs weighing 115 to 160 g each, are located retroperitoneally just beneath the diaphragm. Medially, the kidneys are bounded by the psoas muscles; superiorly, they lie adjacent to the adrenal glands and the diaphragm; and, anterolaterally, the right kidney borders the liver, the colon, and the ileum, whereas the left kidney borders the stomach, the pancreas, and the ileum. The center of each kidney approaches the level of the second lumbar vertebra. Vasomotor and pain fibers innervating the kidney originate in the fourth through twelfth thoracic segments, the vagus nerves (through the celiac axis), and the splanchnic nerves.

The kidneys' blood supply originates from the aorta via the renal arteries. A single renal artery supplies two out of three kidneys; one third have multiple renal arteries. Each renal artery divides into five interlobar arteries, each an end artery. The interlobar branches divide, at the junction of the renal medulla and cortex, into arcuate arteries, which course at right angles to the interlobar arteries. The interlobular arteries arise at right angles to the arcuate arteries and penetrate through the renal cortex. The afferent arterioles, which arise from the interlobular arteries, divide within the cortical tissue to form the glomerular capillary network (Figure 39-1). The capillaries then reunite to form the efferent arterioles. The subsequent course of the efferent arterioles varies depending upon whether they are located superficially in the cortex or are situated in the cortex adjacent to the renal medulla. Superficial efferent arterioles feed a plexus of peritubular venous capillary vessels, which supply the proximal and distal tubules and portions of the loops of Henle and the collecting ducts before joining the interlobular veins and returning to the inferior vena cava through the arcuate, interlobar, and renal veins. Juxtamedullary efferent arterioles also supply the venous capillary network or form the vasa recta, small diameter vessels that penetrate deeply into the medulla, then return to the arcuate veins. The juxtaglomerular apparatus (JGA) is formed by the angle between the afferent and efferent arterioles and the macula densa, a specialized group of cells in the distal convoluted tubule.

The glomerular capillaries course within Bowman's capsule, the beginning of the tubular system. Bowman's capsule empties into the proximal convoluted tubule, which, in turn, joins the loop of Henle. The loop of Henle feeds the distal convoluted tubule, which empties into the collecting duct. As they pass through the medulla, the collecting ducts from many glomeruli join to form the minor and major calyces prior to emptying into the renal pelvis. Each renal pelvis empties into a ureter, which courses retroperitoneally to join the urinary bladder. The ureters, each about 28 to 30 cm long and 5 mm in diameter, develop cyclic peristaltic waves, which raise intraluminal pressure as high as 30 mm Hg. Because of the highly anastomotic blood supply from multiple sources, the ureters may be extensively mobilized during surgery with minimal risk of ischemic injury.

PHYSIOLOGY OF URINE FORMATION

The kidneys perform three major functions: Filtration, reabsorption, and secretion. One must understand the physiology of filtration and reabsorption in order to appreciate the

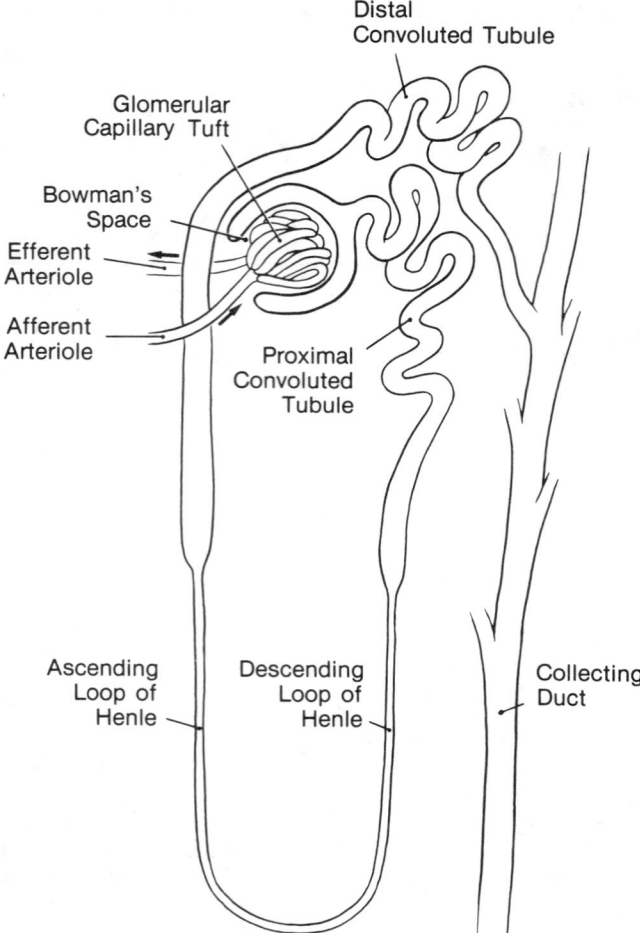

FIG. 39-1. Schematic diagram of renal glomerulus and tubule. Constriction of the afferent arteriole decreases pressure within the glomerular capillary bed, thereby decreasing the glomerular filtration rate (GFR). In contrast, an increase in the efferent arteriolar resistance increases pressure within the glomerular capillary bed, thereby increasing GFR.

effects of surgical stress and anesthesia on renal function. The kidneys receive 20%–25% of the total cardiac output—1,000 ml·min^{-1} to 1,250 ml·min^{-1} in the average adult. Ten per cent of renal blood flow (or about 20% of renal plasma flow) is filtered, producing a glomerular filtration rate (GFR) of 125 ml·min^{-1}. The total filtration volume of approximately 180 l·day^{-1} contrasts strikingly with the final volume of urine excreted, which averages only 1 to 2 l·day^{-1} (Table 39-1). The tubules and collecting ducts of the kidney reabsorb approximately 99% of the filtered solute.

Sodium Filtration and Reabsorption

Urinary sodium excretion decreases if the GFR decreases or if sodium reabsorption increases. The concentration of sodium in the glomerular filtrate approximates that in plasma. Thus, if GFR is normal, the kidneys filter more than 25,000 mEq of sodium per day, of which roughly 65% is reabsorbed by the proximal renal tubule. Because water reabsorption occurs at nearly the same rate, the concentration of sodium remains similar throughout the proximal tubule.

TABLE 39-1. Overview of Renal Function (Euvolemic, Young Adult)

Cardiac output	$\simeq$5000 ml·min^{-1}
Renal blood flow	$\simeq$1250 ml·min^{-1}
Renal plasma flow	$\simeq$750 ml·min^{-1}
Glomerular filtration rate	$\simeq$125 ml·min^{-1}
Urinary flow	$\simeq$2 ml·min^{-1}

An additional 25% of filtered sodium is actively reabsorbed as the filtrate passes through the ascending loop of Henle. Thus, only 10% of the original filtered sodium load enters the distal tubule. Aldosterone regulates the reabsorption of this fraction of filtered sodium. Usually, the distal tubules and collecting ducts reabsorb 90% of the remaining sodium so that only 1% of filtered sodium is ultimately excreted in the urine.

Water Filtration and Reabsorption

As noted previously, the proximal tubular epithelium reabsorbs 65% of filtered water in conjunction with sodium reabsorption. In the loop of Henle, water is reabsorbed to a lesser extent than is sodium. Nonetheless, the fluid leaving the loop remains iso-osmotic, because urea has replaced about half of the total osmolar load originally contributed by sodium and chloride. Subsequently, water is reabsorbed to a variable extent in the distal tubules, the cortical collecting tubules, and the medullary collecting ducts. Antidiuretic hormone (ADH) regulates the amount of water reabsorbed in the collecting ducts.

The countercurrent multiplier system in the loop of Henle is a vital component of the kidney's ability to conserve salt and water. Sodium and water reabsorption critically depend upon the presence of a hypertonic medullary interstitium. Increasing or decreasing blood flow within the vasa recta will diminish the interstitial gradient. The rate of filtrate flow through the loop of Henle also influences the ability of the kidney to produce a concentrated urine, since a high filtrate flow rate (such as is produced by the administration of mannitol) may "wash out" the concentrating gradient. Table 39-2 summarizes urine flow and sodium excretion.

Physiologic Control of Glomerular Filtration and Solute Reabsorption

Glomerular filtration rate (the rate at which fluid is filtered through the glomerular capillaries into Bowman's space) depends upon several factors. The permeability of the glomerular membrane and the surface area of that membrane together constitute the glomerular filtration coefficient (K_f). The hydraulic gradient across the endothelium is determined by the pressure within the glomerular capillary bed (P_{GC}) and by the pressure outside the capillary bed in Bowman's capsule (P_{BC}). The hydraulic gradient works in opposition to the plasma oncotic pressure (π_{GC}), according to the equation

$$GFR = K_f \times (P_{GC} - P_{BC} - \pi_{GC})^1$$

Acute changes in the GFR most commonly result from changes in P_{GC}, although K_f may be reduced by active contraction of glomerular mesangial cells, a physiologic response that decreases glomerular surface area. The P_{GC} will decline if the resistance increases in the afferent arterioles (the input

TABLE 39-2.   Sodium, Water, and Osmolar Excretion (Euvolemic, Young Adult)

	FLOW RATE ($ml \cdot min^{-1}$)	$[NA^+]$ ($mEq \cdot l^{-1}$)	NA^+ ($mEq \cdot min^{-1}$)	UREA ($mg \cdot dl^{-1}$)	OSMOLARITY ($mOsm \cdot l^{-1}$)
Plasma	750	140	105	10	290
Filtrate	125	140	17	10	290
Proximal tubule	44	140	6	15	290
Loop of Henle	25	70	1.7	50	150
Distal tubule	20	10	0.2	50	100
Final urine	2	100	0.2	250	300

TABLE 39-3.   Sodium, Water, and Osmolar Excretion (Maximal Aldosterone Secretion, Minimal ADH Secretion)

	FLOW RATE ($ml \cdot min^{-1}$)	$[NA^+]$ ($mEq \cdot l^{-1}$)	NA^+ ($mEq \cdot min^{-1}$)	UREA ($mg \cdot dl^{-1}$)	OSMOLARITY ($mOsm \cdot l^{-1}$)
Plasma	750	140	105	10	290
Filtrate	125	140	17	10	290
Proximal tubule	44	140	6	15	290
Loop of Henle	25	70	1.7	50	150
Distal tubule	20	0.1	0.002	50	100
Final urine	2	1.0	0.002	250	100

TABLE 39-4.   Sodium, Water, and Osmolar Excretion (Maximal* and Minimal ADH Secretion)

	FLOW RATE ($ml \cdot min^{-1}$)	$[NA^+]$ ($mEq \cdot l^{-1}$)	NA^+ ($mEq \cdot min^{-1}$)	UREA ($mg \cdot dl^{-1}$)	OSMOLARITY ($mOsm \cdot l^{-1}$)
Plasma	750	140	105	10	290
Filtrate	125	140	17	10	290
Proximal tubule	44	140	6	15	290
Loop of Henle	25	70	1.7	50	150
Distal tubule	20	10	0.20	50	50–290
Final urine	0.2*–20	10–300*	0.20	50–1000*	50–1400*

vessels for the glomerulus) and will increase if the resistance in efferent arterioles rises (Fig. 39-1).

Neurohumoral Regulation of Renal Function

The major physiologic influences determining the reabsorption of filtered sodium and water are the hormonal factors aldosterone, antidiuretic hormone, atrial natriuretic factor, and the renal prostaglandins.

ALDOSTERONE. This most important hormonal regulator of sodium reabsorption is produced by the adrenal cortex as a result of a chain of endocrine events: 1) Renin is released from the granular cells of the JGA in response to either activation of the sympathetic nervous system, stimulation of intrarenal baroreceptors, or reduced delivery of sodium chloride to the macula densa.[1] 2) After entering the systemic circulation, renin catalyzes the release of angiotensin I from angiotensinogen. 3) Angiotensin I transformation to angiotensin II then follows, catalyzed by angiotensin-converting enzyme in the lungs. 4) Angiotensin II stimulates the cells of the adrenal cortex to produce aldosterone. Acting primarily in the distal tubules and collecting ducts, aldosterone regulates the excretion of about 2% of the total load of filtered sodium. High concentrations of aldosterone may reduce urinary sodium concentration to nearly zero, while low levels of aldosterone permit excretion of urine high in sodium. Table 39-3 illustrates the effects of maximal aldosterone stimulation.

ANTIDIURETIC HORMONE. Release of ADH from the posterior pituitary occurs in response to stimulation of the osmoreceptors (located primarily in the hypothalamus) by increased blood osmolarity. ADH release is inhibited by increased stretch of atrial baroreceptors when atrial volume is increased. Thus, the secretion of ADH responds both to changes in osmolarity and to changes in intravascular volume. ADH acts primarily on the cortical collecting tubules and medullary collecting ducts to increase water permeability. Hence, high circulating levels of ADH produce rapid reabsorption of water as the urine flows through the collecting ducts, resulting in the excretion of small volumes of highly concentrated urine. Urinary volume may vary 100-fold, depending upon ADH concentration. Table 39-4 summarizes the range of urine flow rates and osmolarities produced by minimal and maximal ADH secretion.

ATRIAL NATRIURETIC FACTOR. The complete physiologic role of this hormone, which is released from the cardiac atria,

TABLE 39-5. Sodium, Water, and Osmolar Excretion ("Average" Perioperative Effects on RBF, GFR, and ADH and Aldosterone Secretion)

	FLOW RATE (ml · min^{-1})	[NA$^+$] (mEq · l^{-1})	NA$^+$ (mEq · min^{-1})	UREA (mg · dl^{-1})	OSMOLARITY (mOsm · l^{-1})
Plasma	750→500	140	105→70	10	290
Filtrate	125→100	140	17→14	10	290
Proximal tubule	44→35	140	6→5	15	290
Loop of Henle	25→20	70	1.7→1.5	50	100
Distal tubule	20→10	10→1.0	0.20→0.01	100	290
Final urine	0.5	100→20	0.20→0.01	500	800

remains unclear. Atrial natriuretic factor (ANF) does have systemic vasodilatory effects and appears to partially regulate the renal excretion of sodium and water.[2] Acute sodium loading significantly increases ANF, in contrast to chronic sodium loading, which does not significantly affect ANF levels.[3] Many of the physiologic effects of ANF appear to be mediated by hemodynamic factors that increase GFR, thus resulting in diuresis.[2]

PROSTAGLANDINS. The kidney also contains large quantities of prostaglandin (PG) metabolites, including PGE$_2$ and thromboxane A$_2$, which appear to modulate the renal effects of other hormones. For instance, the vasodilator PGE$_2$ decreases the contraction of glomerular mesangial cells produced by angiotensin II.[4] Thromboxane A$_2$, in contrast, produces mesangial contraction.[4]

NEUROENDOCRINE RESPONSE TO TRAUMA. The physiologic stress of trauma and surgery is associated with reduced urinary excretion of sodium and water, which occurs in response to changes in intravascular and extracellular volume and to secondary neuroendocrine effects, especially the release of ADH, catecholamines, and aldosterone (Table 39-5).[5,6]

RENAL PHARMACOLOGY

COMPARATIVE RENAL PHARMACOLOGY OF INHALED AND INJECTED ANESTHETICS

Anesthetic drugs may alter renal function by changing renal blood flow, GFR, or renal tubular function. Moreover, anesthetics influence renal function not only by direct renal effects but also by producing changes in cardiovascular function and/or neuroendocrine activity. For example, an anesthetic could alter renal blood flow indirectly by reducing myocardial contractility and changing cardiac output, by activating the sympathetic nervous system to increase renal vascular resistance, or by increasing endogenous secretion of ADH to produce renal vasoconstriction. Conversely, a drug could act directly by modifying renal vascular resistance.

Anesthetic drugs exert diverse cardiovascular effects, many of which could adversely affect renal function. These include myocardial depression, an actual or effective decrease in intravascular volume, or a change in peripheral vascular resistance. Commonly used potent inhalation drugs decrease stroke volume in a dose-dependent fashion. At higher concentrations, these drugs reduce cardiac output sufficiently to decrease renal blood flow. High levels of spinal

or epidural anesthesia can impair venous return, thereby diminishing cardiac output to levels that compromise renal perfusion. Either an increase or a decrease in peripheral vascular resistance may indirectly reduce renal blood flow. Anesthetics such as diethyl ether and cyclopropane stimulate catecholamine secretion, increase total peripheral resistance, and decrease renal blood flow.[7] During anesthesia, other physiologic insults (e.g., hemorrhage) may produce greater renal compromise than would occur in the unanesthetized state.

Surgical stress and anesthesia may also alter autonomic and neuroendocrine function. Norepinephrine and epinephrine, released by sympathetic postganglionic fibers and by the adrenal medulla, respectively, cause both renal vasoconstriction and renin release from the juxtamedullary apparatus. Secretion of renin leads to the production of angiotensin II, a potent renal vasoconstrictor. Renin release is also stimulated by atrial baroreceptors and, in the kidney, by a low ratio of serum sodium to serum potassium. Intrarenal prostaglandins, released in response to various local and systemic factors, serve a variety of functions, including renal vasodilatation and constriction, and release of renin.

Anesthetics are associated with numerous changes in endocrine function. The perioperative period is associated with high circulating levels of ADH and increased secretion of aldosterone. It is unclear whether anesthetics directly cause ADH and aldosterone release or whether the release is due to the changes in hemodynamic function noted previously. It is clear that stress, whether preoperative, intraoperative, or postoperative, triggers ADH and aldosterone secretion.

In addition to the direct and indirect effects of the anesthetic agents themselves, other intraoperative interventions may also directly and indirectly modify renal function. The initiation of mechanical ventilation of the lungs and positive end-expiratory pressure (PEEP) are associated with reduced urinary output. This form of renal dysfunction accompanies decreased cardiac output, increased sympathetic outflow, and the release of renin. During mechanical ventilation of the lungs, volume expansion alone may return renal function to normal despite continued depression of cardiac output.[8] ADH release probably has little effect on renal function during ventilation with PEEP.[9]

A further complicating factor involved in anesthetic-induced alterations in renal function is the extensive capacity of the kidney to adapt to changing conditions. The phenomenon of autoregulation, a physiologic process whereby the kidney maintains nearly constant blood flow despite major changes in perfusion pressure,[10] is an example of the complex intrinsic processes that are superimposed on extrinsic influences.

Measurement of Renal Blood Flow

One of the greatest difficulties involved in the precise description of the renal effects of anesthetics is the accurate measurement of renal blood flow. The technical challenges involved in determining renal blood flow certainly contribute to the conflicting reports of anesthetic effects on renal function.[11] Renal blood flow can be measured either directly or indirectly.[12] Direct experimental measurement techniques, including cannulation of venous vessels and placement of circumferential arterial probes, permit repeated analyses in conscious animals. Potential errors introduced by the techniques of direct measurement include changes in flow caused by the probes themselves as well as the possible effects of inadvertent renal denervation as a consequence of the surgical preparation.

Several techniques measure renal blood flow indirectly by clearance of inert filtered substances, washout of inert gases, and distribution of radioactive microspheres. Para-amino hippurate (PAH) is filtered by the glomeruli and secreted to a limited extent by the tubules. PAH clearance is proportional to renal plasma flow, which, in turn, relates to renal blood flow. Inert gas washout permits some inferences to be made regarding the intrarenal distribution of flow, whereas radioactive microsphere techniques allow more precise quantitation of changes in intraorgan blood flow. These methods, however, also have several limitations. The clinical pharmacology of anesthetic drugs would be markedly enhanced by a minimally invasive measurement of renal blood flow that permitted repeated assessment of renal perfusion.

Effects of Inhaled Anesthetics on Renal Function

Methoxyflurane nephrotoxicity offers a classic example of an alteration in renal function produced by an anesthetic drug. The clinical manifestations of methoxyflurane nephrotoxicity, first described in the mid 1960s, include hypo-osmotic diuresis, azotemia, hypernatremia, and hyperosmolality.[13] In most cases, the impairment resolves in 10 to 20 days; some deficits persist for a year or longer. The toxin responsible for renal dysfunction is inorganic fluoride ion, a methoxyflurane metabolite.[14] The insult caused by fluoride ion is not idiosyncratic but, rather, is dose-related. Greater exposure to methoxyflurane is associated with higher fluoride levels and with greater clinical toxicity, which occurs consistently at serum inorganic fluoride levels greater than 50 $\mu M \cdot l^{-1}$.[15] Likely mechanisms for fluoride ion toxicity include impaired ultratransport in the ascending loop of Henle, increased solute washout by enhanced medullary blood flow, and swelling and destruction of the proximal convoluted tubule mitochondria.[16, 17]

Significant amounts of fluoride ion are also released from enflurane, but not from halothane or isoflurane (Fig. 39-2).[17] Some volunteers receiving enflurane for more than 9.5 hours have peak serum inorganic fluoride levels in the 30–40 $\mu M \cdot l^{-1}$ range.[18] Clinically, this correlates with a decrease in urine concentrating ability (Fig. 39-3).[18] Although probably not significant in healthy patients, it is not known what effects such levels of inorganic fluoride have on renal function in patients with minimal reserve. Concentrations of fluoride ion in excess of 50 $\mu M \cdot l^{-1}$ have been observed in obese patients with prolonged exposure to enflurane. Also, some patients treated with isoniazid have high levels of free fluoride ion following enflurane anesthesia (Fig. 39-4).[19]

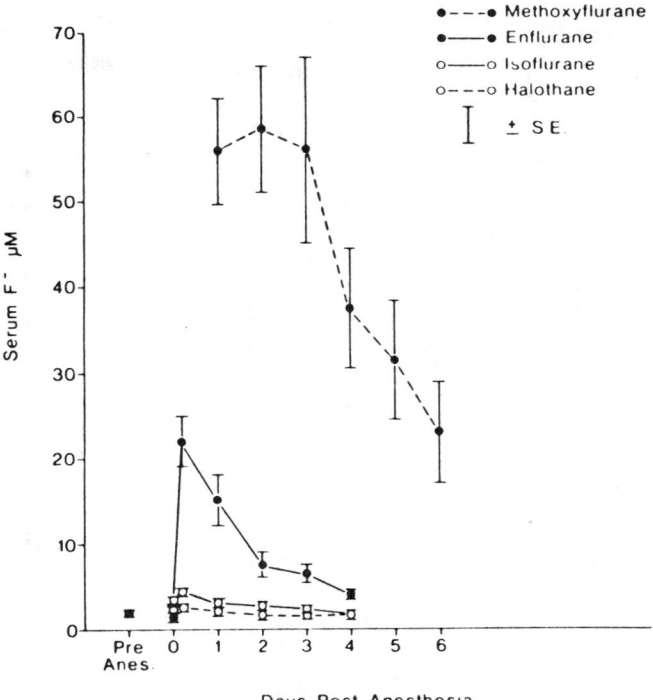

FIG. 39-2. Serum inorganic fluoride (F⁻) concentrations prior to and following administration of methoxyflurane, enflurane, isoflurane or halothane to adult patients (From Cousins MJ, Greenstein LR, Hitt BA, Mazze RI: Metabolism and renal effects of enflurane in man. Anesthesiology 44:44, 1976).

With the possible exception of methoxyflurane, halothane remains the best studied anesthetic agent with regard to effects on renal function. Although most anesthesiologists agree that halothane decreases GFR and urinary output,[20] studies of renal blood flow changes with halothane anesthesia have yielded conflicting results. Reasons for this include difficulty in controlling other factors influencing renal blood flow, such as circulating catecholamine levels, as well as methodologic problems with the measurement of renal blood flow. Initial studies, using techniques based on the clearance of inert filtered substances, concluded that halothane reduces renal blood flow.[21] Later, direct measurement techniques indicated that clinical doses of halothane decrease renal vascular resistance but have little effect on renal blood flow.[22] Low to moderate doses of halothane appear not to change the autoregulation of renal blood flow (Fig. 39-5).[23] Even when administering halothane under conditions of acute hemorrhagic hypovolemia, autoregulation remains intact and decreased renal vascular resistance maintains renal blood flow at normal levels.[24]

Data describing the renal effects of other inhaled anesthetics remain scarce. Enflurane decreases GFR, renal blood flow, and urinary output.[17] Although it produces little change in renal blood flow, isoflurane decreases GFR and urine output.[25, 26] When added to halothane, nitrous oxide potentiates the reduction in urine flow.[27] Nitrous oxide and halothane in combination, however, do not appear to adversely affect the autoregulation of renal blood flow.[28]

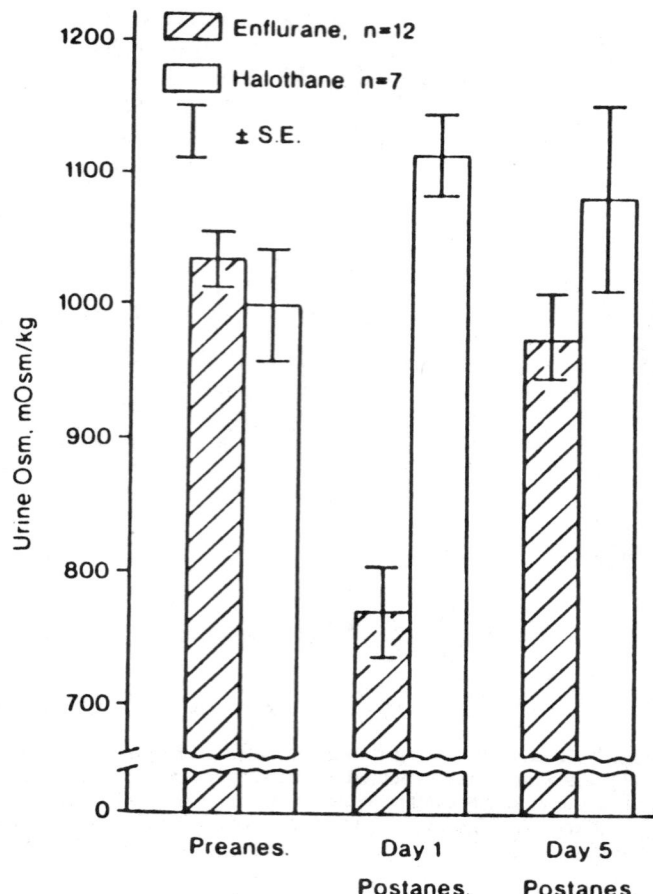

FIG. 39-3. Histogram showing maximum urinary osmolarities before and after administration of vasopressin to volunteers. One group had received enflurane for an average 9.6 MAC hours and the second group had received halothane for 13.7 MAC hours. The ability to concentrate urine was decreased on day 1 following administration of enflurane. (From Mazze RI, Calverley RK, Smith NT: Inorganic fluoride nephrotoxicity: Prolonged enflurane and halothane anesthesia in volunteers. Anesthesiology 46:265–271, 1977.)

Effects of Intravenous Induction Agents on Renal Function

Thiopental, delivered in both high- and low-dose regimens, does not alter renal blood flow. Following low doses, systemic blood pressure, renal resistance, and renal blood flow change little from baseline.[29] Initially, thiopental administration can even produce a transient elevation of systemic blood pressure and a rise in renal blood flow. This may be due to sympathetic nervous system activity, as the subject senses the onset of anesthesia. At high doses, thiopental's cardiovascular depressant properties, which include venodilation, decreased myocardial contractility, and decreased cardiac preload, reduce blood pressure and induce a reflex increase in peripheral vascular resistance.[30] Despite increased systemic vascular resistance and decreased cardiac output, renal blood flow remains unchanged, owing to reduced renal vascular resistance.[30] Local autoregulation, diminished sympathetic tone, or direct renal arteriolar dilation by thiopental may account for the maintenance of renal blood flow.

Most of the data regarding the effects of other intravenous drugs on renal blood flow derive from animal models. One such study found that systemic blood pressure, renal blood flow, and renal vascular resistance increase after ketamine administration.[30] Other animal studies of the effects of ketamine and diazepam on renal blood flow have yielded varied results; some data suggest that renal blood flow decreases, and some data indicate that renal blood flow is well maintained.[31, 32] Variations in measurement techniques and in types of animal preparation are likely explanations for the differences. Morphine, even when given in doses that lower blood pressure, does not reduce renal blood flow.[33] Fentanyl decreases urine flow and GFR while renal blood flow increases or decreases, depending upon whether direct or indirect measurement techniques are used.[34, 35]

The effects of regional anesthesia on renal physiology have been evaluated in moderate detail. Spinal anesthesia only slightly decreases GFR and renal blood flow in humans, despite levels of spinal blockage to the first thoracic dermatome.[36] Thoracic levels of epidural block using epinephrine-containing local anesthetics cause moderate reductions in GFR and renal blood flow that parallel the decrease in mean arterial pressure.[37] Epidural block performed with epinephrine-free solutions generates little change in systemic hemodynamics and only a small decrease in GFR and renal blood flow.[38] Obviously, the pre-existing intravascular volume and the quantity of intravenous fluids strongly influence the renal response to spinal and epidural anesthesia.

In summary, virtually all anesthetic agents and techniques are associated with a decrease in GFR and urinary output. It is less clear what effects most anesthetics have on human renal blood flow. Results vary with respect to subjects studied, anesthetic methods, and measurement techniques. Also, the question of whether renal blood flow autoregulation remains intact during the administration of various anesthetic drugs remains unanswered.

PHARMACOLOGY OF DIURETICS

Diuretics are drugs that increase urinary output. Although all diuretics increase urine flow in patients with functioning kidneys, the sites and mechanisms of action differ markedly among commonly used drugs. In addition, these agents exert diverse effects on electrolyte and water losses. Anesthesiologists daily encounter patients who have received or will receive diuretics as part of their management. For instance, thiazide diuretics commonly serve as the initial treatment for hypertension, loop diuretics are an indispensable component of the management of congestive heart failure, and mannitol is an invaluable tool for acutely reducing intracranial hypertension. During neurosurgical procedures, anesthesiologists use furosemide and/or mannitol to reduce brain bulk and facilitate surgery. Many surgeons and anesthesiologists administer mannitol to "protect" the kidneys during high-risk procedures such as aortic aneurysm resection or cardiopulmonary bypass. Both intraoperatively and postoperatively, patients commonly receive diuretics to relieve acute intravascular overload and, based upon simplistic physiologic reasoning, to increase urinary output. Because these drugs are an ubiquitous part of perioperative management, anesthesiologists must possess an understanding of the use, and the potential for misuse, of these agents.

PEAK SERUM FLUORIDE AFTER ENFLURANE

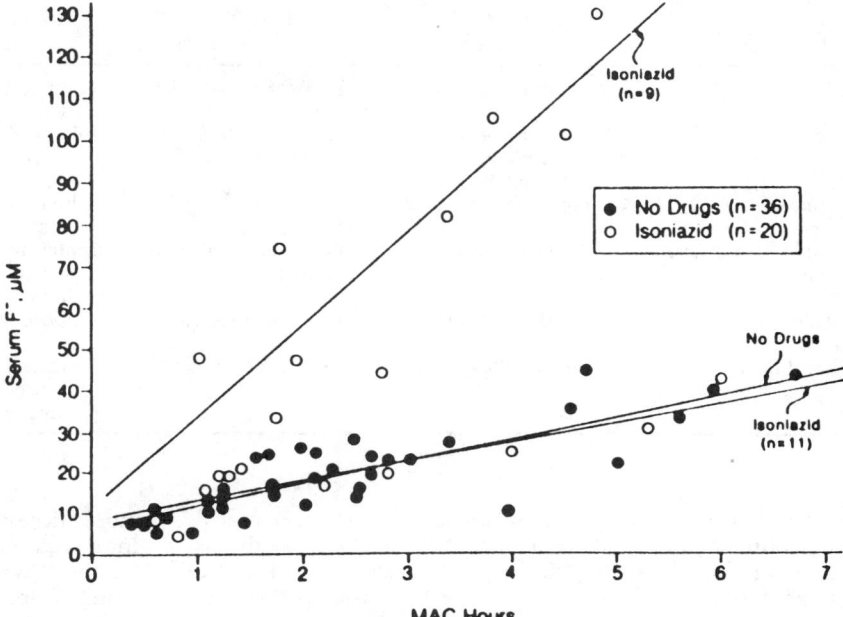

FIG. 39-4. Peak serum fluoride (F⁻) levels for individual patients with or without concomitant treatment with isoniazid. A subgroup of isoniazid-treated patients (n = 9) manifested significant elevations in serum F⁻ concentrations. (From Mazze RI, Woodruff RE, Heerdt ME: Isoniazid-induced enflurane defluorination in humans. Anesthesiology 57:5, 1982.)

Classification of Diuretics

The pharmacologic classification of diuretics (Table 39-6) includes the following: osmotic diuretics, loop or "high-ceiling" diuretics, benzothiadiazides and related agents, carbonic anhydrase inhibitors, aldosterone antagonists, xanthines, other potassium-sparing diuretics, and uricosuric diuretics.[39]

Osmotic diuretics are agents that are filtered at the glomerulus but not reabsorbed in the tubules. Their major effect is to hold water within the tubular lumen, thereby limiting water reabsorption in the loop of Henle and in the distal nephron.[1] *"High-ceiling" diuretics* inhibit sodium chloride reabsorption in the thick ascending limb of the loop of Henle.[39] *Benzothiadiazides* act at the distal tubule to inhibit the reabsorption of sodium.[39] The *carbonic anhydrase inhibitors* are weak diuretics that act by limiting the secretion of hydrogen ions into the proximal tubular lumen, thereby promoting the loss of bicarbonate in the urine.[39] Clinicians rarely use carbonic anhydrase inhibitors as diuretics but, rather, use them for their inhibitory effect on cerebrospinal fluid production and aqueous humor secretion. *Aldosterone antagonists*, as the name implies, exert potassium-sparing effects by opposing the action of aldosterone on the late distal tubule and collecting system.[40] *Xanthines*, such as aminophylline, induce diuresis partly by increasing cardiac output and partly by direct effects on the renal tubules. Other potassium-sparing diuretics include triamterene and amiloride, agents that interfere with ion transport in the distal tubular system to reduce the excretion of potassium. *Uricosuric diuretics*, none of which are currently available, increase the urinary excretion of urate.

Osmotic diuretics, frequently used during anesthesia, reduce brain bulk[41] and, in surgical procedures that threaten renal function, are often used prophylactically or therapeutically, with the hope of attenuating renal ischemic injury. During osmotic diuresis, sodium is lost to a lesser extent than

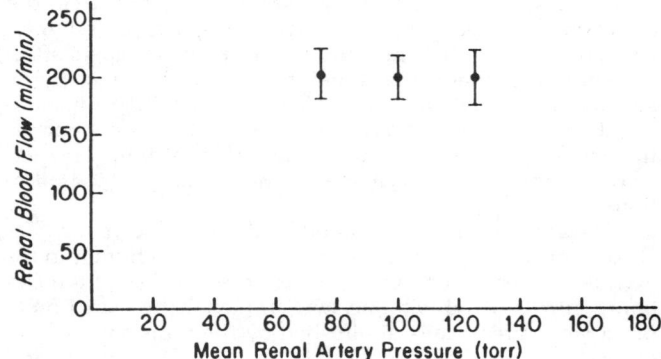

FIG. 39-5. Renal blood flow in dogs remained unchanged in the presence of 0.9% end-expired halothane (From Bastron RD, Perkins, FM, Pyne JL: Autoregulation of renal blood flow during halothane anesthesia. Anesthesiology 46:142, 1977.)

water. Mannitol is usually given in doses of 0.25 – 1.5 g · kg⁻¹ intravenously. The drug is available in the form of 50-ml ampules containing 12.5 g (25% solution) and in 500-ml bottles containing 100 g (20% solution). The smaller dose is appropriate for use in patients with acute oliguria that is unresponsive to volume expansion and other hemodynamic support. Larger doses are given acutely to produce brain dehydration in patients with intracranial hypertension. Administration of an osmotic load has the immediate hemodynamic effect of increasing intravascular volume and cardiac output.[42] Consequently, one should not administer mannitol to patients with congestive heart failure or established oliguric renal failure because of the risk of precipitating acute pulmonary edema.

TABLE 39-6. Classification of Diuretic Drugs

CLASS	EXAMPLES	PRINCIPLE SITE OF ACTION	MECHANISM OF ACTION
Osmotic	Mannitol, glycerol	Loop of Henle, distal nephron	Limit water reabsorption
Loop	Furosemide, ethacrinic acid, bumetanide	Ascending limb of loop of Henle	Inhibit NaCl reabsorption
Thiazide	Hydrochlorothiazide	Distal tubule	Inhibit Na reabsorption
Carbonic anhydrase inhibitors	Acetazolamide	Proximal tubular lumen	Inhibit hydrogen ion secretion into the lumen
Aldosterone antagonists	Spironolactone	Late distal tubule	Oppose aldosterone
Xanthines	Theophylline	Renal blood flow	Increased cardiac output, (some tubular effects)

The loop diuretics, such as furosemide, ethacrynic acid, and bumetanide, limit the reabsorption of NaCl in the ascending loop of Henle.[39] Renal vasodilation is produced to some extent by the acute administration of loop diuretics; however, rapid depletion resulting from excessive diuresis of intravascular volume may lead to a secondary reduction in GFR.

Benzothiadiazides are rarely used during anesthesia but are commonly used for the management of chronic hypertension. Perhaps their most important pharmacologic effect in reference to anesthesia is their tendency to produce hypokalemia and metabolic alkalosis. In addition, the thiazides slightly increase or decrease GFR, especially when given intravenously, and decrease the excretion of calcium.[39] Hyperuricemia and hyperglycemia are other occasional complications.

The carbonic anhydrase inhibitors decrease bicarbonate reabsorption and reduce the secretion of aqueous humor in the eye and cerebrospinal fluid. However, the utility of the carbonic anhydrase inhibitor acetazolamide for the reduction of intracranial pressure is diminished by the transient increase in cerebral blood flow produced by the drug.[43] From a clinical standpoint, anesthesiologists should be aware of the potential for potassium loss and for the production of metabolic acidosis.

Aldosterone antagonists and other potassium-sparing agents are rarely used acutely in the perioperative period. These agents reduce the hypokalemia that otherwise occurs with the chronic use of potassium-wasting diuretics such as the loop diuretics and the benzothiadiazides. Controversy continues regarding whether these agents reduce morbidity when used in this fashion.[44] Spironolactone is also used to counteract the intense hyperaldosteronism that accompanies cirrhosis. Because of the potential for producing hyperkalemia, the anesthesiologist should be wary of rapid administration of potassium to patients who have recently received potassium-sparing diuretics.

CHRONIC RENAL FAILURE

CLINICAL CHARACTERISTICS

Chronic renal failure produces a wide variety of pathophysiologic conditions.[45] In the past few decades, a progressively better understanding of these abnormalities has led to more successful management of patients with renal disease. Improved dialysis techniques have extended life expectancy for those with chronic renal failure. Although renal failure results from a variety of specific disease processes, the common denominator is the progressive loss of nephron function.

Chronic renal failure is not an "all or nothing" phenomenon. As the number of functioning nephrons declines, the signs, symptoms, and biochemical abnormalities pass through several stages (Table 39-7). Until fewer than 40% of normal functioning nephrons remain, there are no signs, symptoms, or laboratory abnormalities. This has been described as a state of decreased renal reserve. When approximately 10%–40% of nephrons are functioning adequately, only mild signs of renal failure exist, such as nocturia, which occurs secondary to a decrease in concentrating capability. This stage represents renal insufficiency, and, although patients seem well compensated when excretory capacity is unstressed, there is little or no renal reserve. The excretion of certain drugs is impaired as is the ability to eliminate an unusually large protein catabolic load. In this stage, the preservation of remaining functional nephrons is at a premium since toxic substances (e.g., aminoglycosides) can worsen renal insufficiency.

As the GFR decreases further, outright renal failure develops. The concentrating and diluting properties of the kidney are severely compromised. Electrolyte, hematologic, and acid–base disturbances are common. The loss of approximately 95% of functioning nephrons culminates in uremia, which leads to all the problems of overt renal failure, including fluid overload and congestive heart failure. The uremic syndrome usually requires dialysis.

The Uremic Syndrome

Patients with dialysis-dependent renal failure have several disease manifestations, including metabolic acidosis, platelet dysfunction, fluid overload, electrolyte disorders, central nervous system (CNS) abnormalities, and gastrointestinal disorders. These components of the uremic syndrome are controlled to a variable extent by dialysis. The accumulation each day of about 50 mEq of hydrogen ion, normally excreted by the kidneys, produces metabolic acidosis. Dialysis returns pH to normal or near-normal values. Renal failure results in the accumulation of waste products that inhibit platelet function by interfering with the process by which platelets release

TABLE 39-7. Stages of Chronic Renal Failure

	GFR (ml·min⁻¹)	SIGNS/SYMPTOMS	LABORATORY ABNORMALITIES
Normal	125	None	None
Decreased renal reserve	50–80	None	None
Renal insufficiency	12–50	Nocturia	Increased BUN; Cr, especially when stressed
Uremia	<12	Uremic syndrome	Multiple

and respond to adenosine diphosphate (ADP).[46] A further qualitative defect in platelet function results from a decline in platelet factor III activity. Although there are other defects in the coagulation cascade, the prothrombin time and the partial thromboplastin time usually remain normal.

Excretory failure results in a wide variety of other complications. Fluid overload occurs, since free water and sodium are not excreted. Resulting signs and symptoms include congestive heart failure, hypertension, and sometimes left ventricular hypertrophy. Several common electrolyte disturbances that accompany renal failure are listed in Table 39-8. Hyperkalemia is one abnormality of paramount anesthetic importance because of the potential for fatal cardiac dysrhythmias. Neurologic complications include central, peripheral, and autonomic dysfunction. Fatigue, malaise, and intellectual impairment are common. Left untreated, uremia encephalopathy progresses to coma. Paresthesiae, burning, and itching of the lower extremities are the most frequent peripheral neuropathic symptoms. Autonomic dysfunction, including postural hypotension, may be present. Orthostasis may be aggravated by the wide swings in hydration status that accompany renal failure. Common gastrointestinal disorders associated with uremia include nausea and vomiting, gastrointestinal bleeding, anorexia, and hiccups. Most of the platelet, fluid and electrolyte, nervous system, and gastrointestinal system manifestations of uremia improve with dialysis. However, dialytic treatment does not adequately resolve some uremic complications. Chronic anemia, with hemoglobin levels of 5–7 g·dl⁻¹, results from decreased production of erythropoietin and diminished red cell survival time. Recently, research has been directed toward the development of human recombinant erythropoietin.[47] Despite the threat of tissue hypoxia from decreased oxygen-carrying capacity, patients usually tolerate such anemia well because of its slow onset and because tissue blood flow increases secondary to decreased blood viscosity and increased stroke volume. Heart rate usually remains in the normal range. The oxyhemoglobin dissociation curve shifts to the right owing to metabolic acidosis and an increased concentration of 2,3 diphosphoglycerate.[48] This aids tissue oxygenation.

In the chronic renal failure patient, an altered immune system imparts greater susceptibility to infection. Sepsis, the leading cause of death in uremic patients, is even more likely in the post-transplant period, owing to immunosuppressive therapy. Additionally, there is a greater incidence of hepatitis B in patients with renal failure.

DIALYTIC TREATMENT

There are 72,000 patients in the United States undergoing chronic dialytic therapy. Of these, a substantial percentage require hospitalization each year; many require surgery, if only for maintenance of dialytic access.

The replacement of renal excretory and homeostatic functions poses a complex technical challenge. The normal kidneys eliminate waste products, especially the waste products of protein catabolism. They also regulate total body water and total body sodium, as well as the serum concentrations of sodium, potassium, phosphate, magnesium, and calcium.

Although even a small percentage of residual renal function is superior to any form of dialytic therapy, much of the function of the normal kidney can be replaced by artificial means. Hemodialysis, peritoneal dialysis, continuous arteriovenous hemofiltration, and continuous arteriovenous hemodialysis are capable of processing large quantities of water and solutes and of eliminating waste products.[49–55]

Hemodialysis

Dialysis refers to a process based on diffusive transport of solute down an osmotic gradient across a semipermeable membrane. Solutes such as urea and potassium that accumulate in the blood in renal failure move across the membrane into a chemically prescribed dialysate. Substances such as the bicarbonate substrate, acetate, move from higher concentrations in the dialysate into blood.

The semipermeable membrane that separates blood from the dialysate during hemodialysis must have a large surface area to be efficient. Blood and dialysate flow rapidly in opposite directions through the dialyzer (blood inside and dialysate outside the hollow fibers) to achieve the maximal effective solute exchange. Both diffusive and convective transport occur during this countercurrent flow.

For removal of a particular substance from the blood, the dialysate should contain little or none of that substance. To maintain the blood concentration of a solute, the dialysate concentration of that solute should be similar to that of blood. To achieve a positive balance, dialysate is prepared with a concentration higher than that present in blood. Solute is transported in direct relationship to the surface area and permeability of the membrane and to the difference in molecular concentrations on either side of the membrane. Mathematically, transport across the dialysis membrane is expressed by the following equation:

$$J_S = DA(C_B - C_D)$$

TABLE 39-8. Common Electrolyte Disturbances in Chronic Renal Failure

Hyperkalemia
Hyponatremia
Hypercalcemia
Hypocalcemia
Hypermagnesemia
Hyperphosphatemia

where

    J_S = solute flux
    D = diffusion coefficient of the membrane for the solute,
         which varies, depending upon size and charge
    A = area of membrane
    C_B = concentration of the solute in blood
    C_D = concentration of the solute in the dialysate

Substances move across the dialyzer membrane in a manner quite different from the transport of substances across the renal glomerular membrane. The glomerulus quantitatively filters substances up to a molecular weight of 7000–10,000 daltons. As molecular weight increases further, the glomerulus filters progressively less, until the upper limit of filtration size (approximately 100,000 daltons) is attained. In contrast, clearance of solute by dialysis relates inversely to molecular weight across the entire range of 0–100,000 daltons. Small molecules, for example, urea, are cleared readily by dialysis, their clearance depending primarily upon blood flow through the dialyzer. The largest discrepancies between filtration by the normal kidney and clearance by the dialyzer occur for molecules with molecular weights of 300–5,000 daltons, the so-called middle molecules.[55]

Anticoagulation during hemodialysis counteracts the activation of the coagulation cascade brought on by contact between blood and the surface of the dialyzer. One may use either systemic or regional heparinization. For the latter, heparin is added to the blood in the arterial line and is neutralized with protamine in the venous line before being returned to the patient, thereby limiting the consequences of systemic heparinization. With either systemic or regional heparinization, careful monitoring of anticoagulation is required.

Hemodialysis requires vascular access sufficient to provide adequate blood flow. Emergency hemodialysis frequently proceeds through a Shaldon catheter inserted percutaneously in a femoral vein. Blood is returned through a peripheral vein or, when necessary, through a second Shaldon catheter inserted in the same or a contralateral femoral vein. Similar catheters, inserted in the subclavian vein, may be superior to femoral catheterization for temporary access for hemodialysis.[56] Acute hemodialysis is now performed only infrequently through arteriovenous shunts. Chronic hemodialysis, in contrast, is usually performed through an arteriovenous fistula such as the Brescia–Cimino fistula, which joins the radial artery and the cephalic vein in the forearm. Patients requiring chronic hemodialysis often undergo numerous surgical procedures to revise or replace failed fistulae, particularly in the first month after the shunt is placed.[57] The necessity for maintaining vascular access represents a major cause of morbidity in patients with chronic renal failure.

Peritoneal Dialysis

This intracorporeal diffusive method utilizes a natural semipermeable membrane consisting of the tissue layers that separate peritoneal capillary blood from the dialysate. Dialysate is infused into and drained from the peritoneal cavity in a tidal fashion. Peritoneal dialysis takes advantage of the large capillary network in the peritoneal cavity to provide contact between blood and dialysate. Peritoneal dialysis clears small molecules such as urea more slowly than hemodialysis and clears larger molecules such as inulin more rapidly. Acute peritoneal dialysis is usually used for correction of severe accumulation of water or solutes. Intermittent peritoneal dialysis is used to maintain chronic renal failure patients. It consists of three to seven treatments per week, each requiring 8 to 12 hours of cyclic infusion and removal of dialysate. Continuous ambulatory peritoneal dialysis (CAPD) is a strategy developed to facilitate the activities of daily living for patients on chronic peritoneal dialysis.[58] Therapy is performed daily throughout the day. Compared to intermittent peritoneal dialysis, dwell time (the duration of time during which the dialysate is permitted to remain in the peritoneal cavity) is much longer. Three to five exchanges are performed daily, generally allowing an uninterrupted night of sleep.

Peritoneal dialysis begins with the surgical placement of an indwelling peritoneal catheter similar to that first described by Tenckhoff.[59] Short-term peritoneal access may be obtained with a percutaneously inserted catheter, but this introduces the risk of bowel perforation, catheter loss, or both. Clearance of solutes during peritoneal dialysis depends upon the volume and composition of the dialysate, the rate of blood flow in the peritoneal capillaries, the permeability of the tissue between blood and dialysate, the area of the peritoneal membrane, and the circulation of the fluid film in the peritoneal cavity.[60] The volume of dialysate infused per exchange in adults is usually 2 l. Higher volumes increase the efficiency of dialysis but may restrict diaphragmatic motion. The composition of the dialysate may be modified to increase or decrease blood concentrations of solute. The tonicity of the dialysate may be increased by increasing the dextrose concentration, which will then increase the rate of ultrafiltration of water and solute out of the capillary bed. Peritonitis remains the major complication of long-term peritoneal access.

Continuous Arteriovenous Hemofiltration

Ultrafiltration is a process whereby water and solutes are transported convectively from blood through a semipermeable membrane by hydrostatic pressure or by the osmotic force exerted by a hypertonic solution on the side of the membrane opposite the blood compartment.

Continuous arteriovenous hemofiltration (CAVH) is an innovative technique for the purely convective removal of fluid and solute.[61–63] The hydraulic driving pressure generated by systemic arterial pressure or by the addition of a blood pump produces continuous ultrafiltration of serum across the membrane. Slow continuous ultrafiltration (SCUF) is a closely related technique. The apparatus consists of an arterial cannula connected to a high solvent flux filter, which empties into a venous return cannula. The rate of ultrafiltration with these devices is described by the following equation:

$$QF = KA(P_{tm} - P_{onc})$$

where

    QF = flow of filtrate
    K = filtration characteristics of the membrane
    A = membrane area
    P_{tm} = transmembrane hydrostatic pressure gradient
    P_{onc} = serum oncotic pressure

The rate of ultrafiltration is directly proportional to the mean arterial pressure and blood flow through the filter and is inversely proportional to the serum oncotic pressure. The addition of a blood pump on the arterial side to raise the hydrostatic pressure may increase formation of ultrafiltrate from 300 to 1000 $ml \cdot hr^{-1}$ to as much as 2400 $ml \cdot hr^{-1}$.[63] The application of negative pressure to the ultrafiltrate line will also improve ultrafiltration by increasing the transmembrane pressure.[62] Thus, CAVH or SCUF may rapidly remove fluid containing solute in roughly the same concentrations as those in serum. The serum concentrations of solutes are not changed by the filtration process itself, but rather by the infusion of replacement fluid that dilutes waste solutes or increases the concentration of desired solutes. Because of its considerable capacity for removing salt and water, CAVH has been used to permit full-calorie, high-protein nutritional support of critically ill patients.[64] Critically ill patients have also undergone CAVH as part of the treatment for acute renal failure associated with sepsis[65] and to speed removal of fluid in those patients with noncardiac pulmonary edema.[66] Continuous arteriovenous hemodialysis (CAVHD), a modification of CAVH, adds the capacity for diffusive transport to the considerable filtrational transport achieved by CAVH.[67]

Table 39-9 lists the relative indications for and limitations of hemodialysis, peritoneal dialysis, and continuous arteriovenous hemofiltration.

PHYSIOLOGIC EFFECTS AND COMPLICATIONS OF DIALYSIS AND ULTRAFILTRATION

In most instances, renal replacement therapy improves the profound physiologic abnormalities induced by renal failure, that is, fluid overload, pericarditis, electrolyte abnormalities, coagulopathy, and uremic encephalopathy. However, despite major advances over the past 25 years, the complications of hemodialysis, peritoneal dialysis, and CAVH still represent problems in the management of patients with acute or chronic renal failure.[68, 69] The most important physiologic effects and complications of renal replacement therapy involve the CNS, the cardiovascular system, the respiratory system, the striated musculature, and nutritional status (Table 39-10).

Central Nervous System Effects

The disequilibrium syndrome is an uncommon but potentially severe complication of acute hemodialysis.[70] Predisposing factors include severe azotemia (blood urea nitrogen concentration greater than 150 mg·dl^{-1}), hypernatremia,

TABLE 39-9. Selection of Renal Replacement Therapy[53, 55]

	INDICATIONS	LIMITATIONS
Hemodialysis	Rapid catabolism Severe volume, electrolyte, or acid–base disorders	Hypotension Anticoagulation risk Need for vascular access
Peritoneal dialysis	Lower cost Anticoagulation risk Difficult vascular access Hypotension Infants and small children	Rapid catabolism Diaphragmatic defects Severe volume, electrolyte, or acid–base disorders
CAVH, SCUF	Hemodynamic instability Inexpensive equipment	Rapid catabolism Severe volume, electrolyte, or acid–base disorders Constant supervision

TABLE 39-10. Complications of Dialysis and Ultrafiltration

Central nervous system
   Disequilibrium syndrome
   Dialysis dementia
Cardiovascular system
   Hypotension
Respiratory system
   Hypoxemia
Neuromuscular
   Cramping
Nutritional
   Protein depletion
   Hyperglycemia
   Peritonitis

profound acidemia, and pre-existing brain disease. The syndrome may be mild or may progress to stupor, coma, and seizures. Proposed mechanisms for the syndrome include transient cerebral intracellular hypertonicity and cerebral intracellular acidosis.[70] Management is primarily prophylactic, that is, the avoidance of rapid simultaneous reduction of urea and sodium concentrations in high-risk patients.

Dialysis dementia, another CNS complication of hemodialysis, occurs in a small number of patients. Mahoney and Arieff[70] list three forms of dialysis dementia: sporadic, epidemic, and the type associated with pediatric renal disease. Elimination of aluminum from the dialysate has been associated with a gradual clearance of symptoms in some but not in all patients.[71] Dialysis dementia does not appear to be due to abnormalities of cerebral perfusion.[72]

Cardiovascular Effects

Symptomatic hypotension complicates 25% of individual hemodialysis treatments.[73] Critically ill septic patients are particularly prone to develop hypotension during dialysis.[74]

The cause of hemodialysis-induced hypotension is multifactorial. Intravascular volume is certainly reduced by dialysis, although mobilization of extravascular volume can help to offset dialytic losses. Hemofiltration alone produces a similar reduction in volume but less hypotension than hemodialysis.[75] The vasoconstrictor response in patients undergoing hemodialysis often cannot adequately compensate for reductions in plasma volume and cardiac output. In healthy nonuremic persons, the response to mild plasma volume reduction consists of venoconstriction; if hypovolemia is more severe, the venoconstriction is followed by the catecholamine-induced effects of arterial constriction and increased myocardial contractility.[76] In contrast, uremic patients appear to have defective carotid and aortic body reflex arcs.[77] Peripheral resistance declines during hemodialysis despite a decreased pulmonary capillary wedge pressure and hypotension.[78] The failure of peripheral resistance to increase in order to compensate for decreasing plasma volume may be due to the presence of acetate in the dialysate. Acetate, which is metabolized in the liver to bicarbonate, is added to dialysate to replace bicarbonate consumed by buffering the hydrogen ions from nonexcreted acids. As a vasodilator, acetate interferes with reflex vasoconstriction.[79] Replacement of acetate with bicarbonate in the dialysate reduces hemodynamic instability, especially in critically ill septic patients.[79, 80]

Dialysis does not reduce myocardial function. Both acetate and bicarbonate dialysis modestly improve left ventricular function,[81, 82] most markedly in those patients with impaired ventricular function before dialysis.[83] Increasing the calcium concentration of dialysate from 5.5 to 7.5 mg · dl^{-1} improves left ventricular function and produces substantially higher intradialytic blood pressure.[84]

The management of hemodialysis-induced hypotension is based on maneuvers designed to decrease the rapidity and extent of plasma volume reduction. Transfusion sufficient to maintain a hematocrit greater than 20% may decrease the incidence of hypotension.[53] Leg elevation, intravenous fluid administration, and, occasionally, vasoconstrictors can be used for the short-term management of hypotension. When hypotension remains a persistent problem despite these maneuvers, substitution of a bicarbonate dialysate for an acetate dialysate will often permit adequate dialytic therapy, even in patients with underlying hemodynamic instability.[74] In general, hypotension occurs less commonly during peritoneal dialysis and CAVH than during hemodialysis.

Respiratory System Effects

Dialytic therapy produces a complex, incompletely understood series of changes in Pa_{O_2}, Pa_{CO_2}, pH, and $[HCO_3^-]$. Although oxygenation may improve because of dialysis, especially if intravascular volume overload is resolved, hemodialysis more commonly results in hypoxemia. Two general mechanisms may contribute to hypoxemia during hemodialysis: ventilation/perfusion mismatch and hypoventilation.

Because neutropenia consistently occurs shortly after the initiation of hemodialysis,[85] some investigators have attempted to explain hypoxemia on the basis of ventilation/perfusion mismatch secondary to leukocyte-mediated pulmonary dysfunction.[86] However, more precise measurements suggest that during dialysis, the alveolar-arterial oxygen gradient may remain unchanged.[85, 87, 88] These data support the hypothesis, first proposed by Aurigemma and colleagues,[89] that patients may hypoventilate during hemodialysis without becoming hypercarbic. Sherlock and colleagues[88] documented a decrease in Pa_{O_2} during hemodialysis, which they attributed to loss of CO_2 across the dialyzer membrane. They explained the resulting effects in terms of the alveolar gas equation:

$$PA_{O_2} = PI_{O_2} - Pa_{CO_2} \left[FI_{O_2} + \frac{1 - FI_{O_2}}{RE} \right]$$

where

PA_{O_2} = alveolar oxygen tension
PI_{O_2} = FI_{O_2} × (barometric pressure − 47)
FI_{O_2} = fractional inspired concentration of oxygen
RE = CO_2 excretion by the lung divided by oxygen consumption.

Under circumstances other than hemodialysis, RE equals the respiratory quotient (RQ), which is carbon dioxide production divided by oxygen consumption. However, when dialysis proceeds against a bath containing acetate, carbon dioxide is both excreted by the lung and transported through the dialyzer membrane into the dialysate. Therefore, carbon dioxide excretion by the lung becomes less than carbon dioxide production, thereby decreasing the numerator of the fraction RE and necessarily decreasing PA_{O_2}. If the $P(A-a)_{O_2}$ remains the same, Pa_{O_2} must fall.

Hypoxemia during hemodialysis is easily treated by increasing the inspired oxygen concentration. In reference to the alveolar gas equation, as FI_{O_2} increases, the term by which Pa_{CO_2} is multiplied progressively decreases toward one, regardless of the value of the RQ (or RE). In rare cases, bicarbonate rather than acetate dialysis may be necessary. Occasionally, a less rapid rate of plasma volume reduction may be used if a decrease in cardiac output is contributing to hypoxemia through the production of a lower mixed-venous oxygen content.

During peritoneal dialysis, hypoxemia occurs if upward displacement of the diaphragm is poorly tolerated or if fluid traverses the diaphragm. Hypoxemia seldom occurs during CAVH.

Muscular Complications

Skeletal muscle cramping occasionally complicates hemodialysis but rarely occurs during other forms of renal replacement therapy. Because approximately 30% of dialysis procedures are associated with skeletal muscle cramping if the dialysate contains only 130 mEq · l^{-1} of sodium,[53] clinicians often prefer to dialyze against a bath containing a higher sodium concentration (132–140 mEq · l^{-1}). When skeletal muscle cramping does occur, treatment consists of slowing the rate of reduction of serum sodium concentration and intravascular volume.

Nutritional Complications

Disease processes that produce chronic or acute renal failure are associated with nutritional depletion. For patients with chronic renal failure, dietary restriction may produce a tasteless diet leading to a decrease in nutritional intake. Patients with acute renal failure frequently have severe catabolic illnesses. Hemodialysis and CAVH produce few additional nutritional complications. To a limited extent, amino acids are lost into the dialysate during hemodialysis,[90] and some filtration of amino acids presumably occurs during CAVH. Usually, however, nutritional status improves during dialysis, because removal of excess fluid permits more aggressive nutritional support.

In contrast, peritoneal dialysis induces marked protein losses into the dialysate.[91] Peritonitis, a frequent complication of peritoneal dialysis, further increases protein-wasting.[91] Although these losses do not preclude effective peritoneal dialytic therapy, they do produce hypoalbuminemia and have been implicated in immunocompromise. In order to prevent progressive protein loss, patients undergoing peritoneal dialysis should consume 1.5 g · kg^{-1} · day^{-1} of protein.

ANESTHETIC MANAGEMENT OF THE PATIENT WITH CHRONIC RENAL FAILURE

PREOPERATIVE EVALUATION

A comprehensive preoperative evaluation of overall physiologic reserve should include an assessment of renal function.[92, 93] Renal function tests are influenced not only by intrinsic renal disease but also by intravascular and extracellular volume, by cardiovascular function, and by neuroendocrine factors. The more severe the expected surgical insult, the greater the likelihood of perioperative renal compromise and the greater the urgency of adequate preoperative identification of risk. The choice of monitoring devices and of anesthetic techniques depends upon these factors.

Unfortunately, there is no simple, inexpensive test that adequately quantitates renal function. The readily available tests fail to accurately reflect the status of the kidneys in a large percentage of patients, especially the elderly, the malnourished, and the dehydrated. The commonly obtained tests of renal function include urinalysis and determination of blood urea nitrogen (BUN), serum creatinine (SCr), and creatinine clearance (CCr).

The urinalysis provides qualitative information that one must interpret with caution. Hematuria (more than 1 to 2 red cells per high power field in a concentrated sediment) suggests glomerular disease or, in a trauma patient, injury to the kidneys or the lower urinary tract. Pyuria (more than four white cells per high power field) suggests urinary tract infection. Although urine may normally contain hyaline and granular casts, cellular casts (either red cell or white cell) represent a pathologic finding. Red cell casts indicate active glomerulonephritis, whereas white cell casts suggest interstitial nephritis, including pyelonephritis. Urinary pH, although difficult to interpret on a spot urine sample, may assist in the diagnosis of some acid–base disturbances. The presence of proteinuria on a routine dipstick examination may be "normal," or it may suggest severe renal disease. In a concentrated urine sample, trace or 1 + proteinuria is a nonspecific finding, whereas 3+ or 4+ proteinuria suggests glomerular disease.

Both BUN and SCr offer rapid but inexact estimates of CCr. The actual measurement of CCr constitutes the best overall indicator of GFR. However, all three measurements require careful interpretation (Table 39-11). BUN, a product of protein metabolism, will be greater in patients receiving a high-protein diet, in those with blood in their gastrointestinal tract, or in those with accelerated catabolism (*e.g.*, traumatized or septic patients). The normal range is between 8.0 and 20 mg·dl^{-1}. Because urea is synthesized in the liver, hepatic dysfunction will result in a decreased production of urea and, therefore, a lower BUN. Most importantly, BUN fails to fulfill the key criterion for a good test of GFR. Although urea is freely filtered at the glomerulus, it is reabsorbed to a large, and variable, extent. The reabsorption of urea is greater (approximately 60% of the filtered load) when urinary flow is low; in comparison, only about 40% is reabsorbed when flow is high.

Creatinine, a product of skeletal muscle protein catabolism, is produced at a lower rate in elderly than in young adults and in females than in males. Consequently, SCr may fail to

accurately reflect the magnitude of nephron loss. Similarly, patients with muscle-wasting owing to chronic disease may manifest misleadingly low SCr measurements. In contrast, heavily muscled or acutely catabolic patients may have SCr values greater than the normal range (0.5 to 1.5 mg·dl^{-1}) because of more rapid muscle breakdown.

Combining the evaluation of BUN and SCr may provide more information than either alone. If the BUN:SCr ratio exceeds the normal range of 10 to 20, one should suspect dehydration or one of the individual factors that alter the serum concentration of the two metabolites.

Measurements of CCr are superior to BUN or SCr alone or to the combination for the estimation of renal reserve. One approximation of CCr is derived from the following equation:

$$GFR = \frac{(140 - age)\ wt^*}{72 \times SCr}$$

where

wt = weight measured in kilograms
*multiplied by 0.8 for women

More precise measurements of CCr require collection of timed urine samples, using the following formula:

$$GFR = \frac{UV}{P}$$

where

U = urinary concentration of Cr (mg·dl^{-1})
V = volume of urine (ml·min^{-1})
P = plasma concentration (mg·dl^{-1})

Although 24-hour specimens are usually used, a 2-hour sample, collected through a urinary catheter, provides acceptable accuracy (Fig. 39-6).[93]

The preoperative evaluation of patients with chronic renal failure should include consideration of the physiologic problems associated with loss of renal function and the adequacy of recent dialytic therapy, in addition to the usual history, physical examination, and laboratory evaluation. Questioning a patient about exercise tolerance can be as important as the absolute hemoglobin concentration in determining whether to transfuse red blood cells preoperatively. It is helpful to ascertain a patient's usual and recent weight. Dialysis is usually advisable shortly before anesthesia and surgery. Blood transfusion, if necessary, can proceed during dialysis without adding to the patient's intravascular volume. Because renal failure produces neuropathy and decreases gastric emptying, a premedicant that decreases gastric pH and volume may prove beneficial. Usually, light premedication with sedatives or opioids is warranted because of the possibility of exaggerated effects.

INTRAOPERATIVE MANAGEMENT

Monitoring

The selection of monitoring techniques for patients with diminished or absent renal function should be based on the same physiologic considerations as would be appropriate if

TABLE 39-11.   Preoperative Assessment, Renal Function

TEST	NORMAL RANGE	LIMITATIONS
BUN	8–20 mg·dl^{-1}	Dehydration Variable protein intake Gastrointestinal bleeding Catabolism
SCr	0.5–1.2 mg·dl^{-1}	Age Muscle mass Catabolic state
CCr (estimated)	120 ml·min^{-1}	Similar to SCr Weight-dependency
CCr (measured)	120 ml·min^{-1}	Inaccurate urine volume measurement

*Multiplied by 0.8 for females

the same patient were to undergo nonrenal surgery (Table 39-12). Frequent recording of the blood pressure and continuous recording of the body temperature, heart rate, and electrocardiogram (ECG) are essential. Electrocardiography will allow early detection of hyperkalemia. Because, in the presence of chronic anemia, a further reduction in oxygen delivery owing to hypoxemia could be extremely hazardous, pulse

2 vs. 22 hr Creatinine Clearance

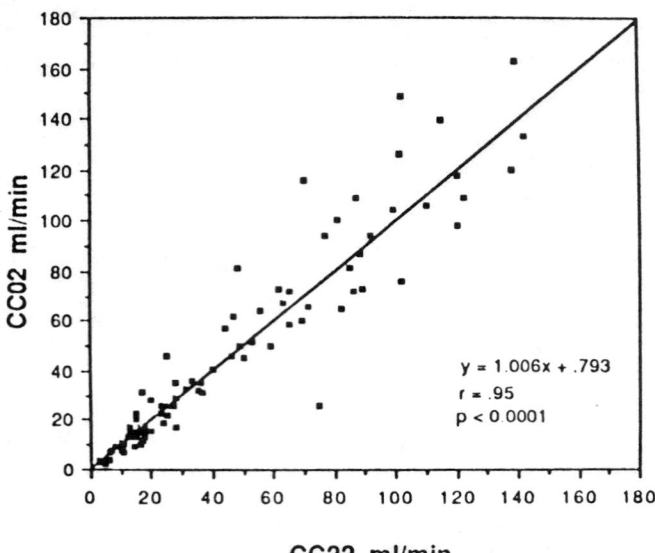

$$y = 1.006x + .793$$
$$r = .95$$
$$p < 0.0001$$

FIG. 39-6. Correlation between the 2-hour creatinine clearance (Cc_{O_2}) and 22-hour creatinine clearance (Cc_{22}). (Reprinted with permission from Sladen RN, Endo E, Harrison T: Two-hour *versus* 22-hour creatinine clearance in critically ill patients. Anesthesiology 67:1013, 1987.)

TABLE 39-12.   Anesthesia for the Anephric Patient-Key Considerations

Preoperative Evaluation
  Adequacy of dialytic therapy
    Volume status
    Acid–base status
  Hemoglobin concentration
  Cardiovascular status
Monitoring
  Blood pressure
  Heart rate
  ECG
  Pulse oximeter
  Capnometer
  Peripheral nerve stimulator
  Invasive cardiovascular monitoring as needed
Fluid Management
  Cautious
  No contraindication to packed rbc's
  If necessary, dialyze postoperatively
Anesthetic Choice
  Lower induction dose of thiopental
  Exaggerated response to benzodiazepines
  Prolonged morphine effect
  Avoid succinylcholine if serum K^+ exceeds 6.0 mEq·l^{-1}
  Delayed excretion of pancuronium, *d*-tubocurarine
  Prolonged effect of anticholinesterase agents

oximetry is especially desirable. Capnometry may also be valuable. Because of the chronic metabolic acidosis present in many patients with chronic renal failure, hypercarbia will reduce pH to a greater extent than in a patient with normal bicarbonate levels. Acid–base assessment will provide sensitive information regarding superimposition of additional disturbances in these fragile patients. The decision to use an arterial catheter or a pulmonary artery catheter depends upon the patient's functional cardiac reserve and the severity of hypertension. These devices may facilitate evaluation of the status of cardiac performance, intravascular volume, and venous capacitance. In the future, the further development of continuous monitors of blood pressure and cardiac output should simplify monitoring decisions. Additionally, one must identify and protect vascular access ports such as shunts and fistulas, because malfunction may occur as a consequence of diminished flow in the perioperative period. Extremities should be well padded.

Perioperative fluid management must take into account the inability of the kidney to excrete free water given to patients as well as water produced by catabolic body processes. Nevertheless, if inadequate volume exists in a patient exposed to vasodilation and cardiac depressants, organ hypoperfusion and frank hypotension will ensue. If intraoperative fluid requirements increase intravascular volume to a level that is unsatisfactory in the postoperative period, or if acid–base or electrolyte problems develop intraoperatively, dialysis can be repeated in the immediate postoperative period.

Selection of Anesthetic Agents

Formulation of a satisfactory intraoperative anesthetic plan for a renal failure patient requires an understanding of pharmacology and the judicious use of anesthetic drugs. The action and elimination of several anesthetic and nonanesthetic drugs can affect a patient's perioperative course.

INTRAVENOUS AGENTS. Highly protein-bound drugs may cause exaggerated and prolonged effects, because renal failure reduces protein binding. For example, intravenous administration of short-acting barbiturates (with a high affinity for protein) to renal failure patients leads to a larger fraction of unbound, bioavailable drug.[94] In addition, the acidemic pH of renal failure increases the proportion of the agent that exists in the nonionized, unbound form, the state in which tissue availability, particularly to the brain, is greatest. Further, uremia alters the blood–brain barrier, which increases the sensitivity to intravenous induction agents such as thiopental. Hence, uremic patients require a lower dose of thiopental for the induction of anesthesia.[95] However, thiopental clearance, after adjusting for the altered protein-binding, volume of distribution, and tissue-binding, is similar in patients with and without renal failure. Although the initial dose should be lower and given more cautiously than in patients with normal renal function, the same total dose of short-acting barbiturate induction agents may be necessary.[96]

Because ketamine and the benzodiazepines are less heavily protein-bound than the barbiturates, induction doses do not need to be altered as much. Ketamine frequently increases blood pressure and cardiac output—effects that may aggravate pre-existing hypertension or decreased left ventricular function. Benzodiazepines, given in doses that usually exert minimal respiratory or cardiovascular effects, may profoundly affect a generally debilitated renal failure patient.

Morphine-induced respiratory depression is prolonged in some renal failure patients.[97] Hepatic glucuronidation by glucuronyl transferase represents the major route of morphine biotransformation. Very little unchanged morphine undergoes urinary excretion, and patients with and without renal disease have similar morphine plasma concentrations.[98] Morphine glucuronides alone can cause analgesia and respiratory depression.[99] Therefore, the increased accumulation of morphine glucuronides accounts for the prolonged respiratory depression observed in patients with renal failure.

The elimination of fentanyl is also largely accomplished through hepatic metabolism, with subsequent renal excretion of metabolites. Whether renal failure can cause prolonged narcosis owing to metabolite activity remains unclear. In theory, low doses of fentanyl should represent a good analgesic choice, because rapid tissue redistribution should preserve the short duration of action observed in normal persons.

INHALATIONAL ANESTHETICS. These drugs offer some advantages in renal failure. Unlike the intravenous drugs, elimination does not rely on adequate renal function, although, to varying degrees, biotransformation may produce renally excreted metabolites. In addition, inhalational agents can be administered without nitrous oxide, permitting high inspired oxygen concentrations. To a limited extent, this may offset the decrease in arterial oxygen content resulting from anemia. Although the direct nephrotoxicity of some of the inhalation agents restricts their selection for patients with remaining renal function, avoidance of nephrotoxic agents is not a major consideration in dialysis-dependent renal failure. Potent inhalational agents may also facilitate neuromuscular blockade, thereby allowing lower doses of neuromuscular blockers.

NEUROMUSCULAR BLOCKING AGENTS. Succinylcholine, administered to normal patients, transiently increases serum potassium by approximately $0.5 \text{ mEq} \cdot l^{-1}$. Serum potassium increases similarly in response to succinylcholine in patients with renal failure.[100] Renal failure is not associated with the larger increases in serum potassium that lead to serious cardiac dysrhythmias in patients with burns, trauma, and neuromuscular disease. Uremic patients with normal serum potassium can receive succinylcholine; however, if the potassium is already elevated, an additional increase of $0.5-0.7 \text{ mEq} \cdot l^{-1}$ may be sufficient to induce cardiac dysrhythmias. If life-threatening cardiac dysrhythmias occur, the general debility of chronic renal failure patients may then render resuscitation more difficult.

Serum cholinesterase levels appear normal in renal failure patients, whether or not they are undergoing dialysis.[101] Repeated doses of succinylcholine in these patients do not incrementally elevate serum potassium or prolong muscle relaxation.

Historically, most nondepolarizing muscle relaxants have had a prolonged elimination half-life in chronic renal failure, because they have been primarily excreted through the kidneys. Some clinicians have preferred to use d-tubocurarine to pancuronium, metocurine, and gallamine in uremic patients, since d-tubocurarine's elimination half-life is less prolonged. Chronic renal failure increases the duration of action of d-tubocurarine slightly in the low-dose range and considerably at higher doses.[102] Although evidence suggests that renal failure accelerates the onset of neuromuscular blockade with d-tubocurarine, this effect is probably not secondary to changes in plasma protein-binding, because binding is approximately 40% in both normal and renal failure patients.[103]

The intermediate-duration nondepolarizing muscle relaxants qualify as suitable adjunctive agents in patients with chronic renal failure. Atracurium has an elimination half-life of less than 30 minutes in patients with and without renal failure.[104] There is little, if any, difference between patients with normal renal function and those with renal impairment with respect to pharmacokinetics and pharmacodynamics of atracurium. Ester hydrolysis and Hoffmann elimination, neither of which depend upon renal function, clear atracurium from the blood. Similarly, renal disease does not alter the duration of action of vecuronium.[105] Because they have a shorter duration of action than d-tubocurarine, atracurium and vecuronium are more easily titrated in fragile patients.

Neostigmine, pyridostigmine, and edrophonium are three commonly used anticholinesterase agents used to reverse nondepolarizing muscle relaxants. Because all three agents undergo elimination primarily through the kidney, renal failure prolongs their duration of action at least 100%.[106-108] Thus, these agents effectively counteract the lingering nondepolarizing effects of d-tubocurarine in renal failure patients, making recurarization theoretically unlikely. Anticholinesterase reversal of atracurium or vecuronium seems especially safe, because the duration of action of these neuromuscular blockers is not prolonged.

Despite the longer half-lives of the anticholinesterases, the clinician must consider several other factors that contribute to the ease of reversal of neuromuscular blockade, such as temperature, the depth of the blockade, the acid–base status, and the concomitant use of potentiating drugs such as diuretics or antibiotics. Because of the marked variability among patients, clinical assessment of depth of neuromuscular blockade should be supplemented by the use of a peripheral nerve stimulator to quantitate the response to train-of-four and tetanic stimulation.

Anesthesia for Renal Transplantation

Renal transplantation has been performed experimentally for nearly a century. Surgeons reported the first successful clinical series of renal homotransplantation in identical twins about three decades ago.[109] Since then, improved surgical and immunosuppressive techniques have resulted in routine transplantation of nonidentical living and cadaveric donors. Developments in the techniques of immunosuppression have led to better graft survival. Since the introduction of cyclosporin A, the long-term survival of cadaveric grafts has nearly equaled that of those obtained from living, related donors.[110] The combination of cyclosporin A and further refinements in immunosuppressive therapy may, in the future, eliminate the need for living, related donors. Although much of the early success of renal transplantation depended upon living, related donors, such selfless persons voluntarily function with decreased renal reserve. Subsequent damage to the remaining kidney can prove devastating. Stresses such as a high protein diet, which are well tolerated by those with normal renal function, may result in renal insufficiency in patients with compromised renal function.[111]

Consequently, in planning the anesthetic management for transplantation from a living, related donor, the anesthesiologist must concentrate intensively on preservation of function in the donor's remaining kidney. In contrast, if the donor kidney is to be acquired from a brain-dead patient, preserving function in the graft should be the highest priority. The preservation of renal function in such circumstances may present difficulties. Many brain-dead organ donors are hypovolemic and require fluid resuscitation. Diabetes insipidus, a common accompaniment of brain death, may produce rapid diuresis, thereby obscuring hypovolemia while worsening it. Adequate replacement of ADH is therefore essential. The loss of sympathetic tone following brain death may produce mild hypotension despite adequate volume resuscitation and control of diabetes insipidus. Consequently, dopamine, continuously infused at a low dose ($1.0–3.0\ \mu g \cdot kg^{-1} \cdot min^{-1}$), may be necessary. However, indiscriminate use of high doses of vasopressors may lead to severe regional vasoconstriction, eventually damaging both the kidneys and other procurable organs. Poor management of the donor kidney prior to harvesting represents one of the most common, and most avoidable, causes of graft malfunction.

Regardless of whether the donor kidney comes from a living, related or cadaveric donor, the transplant recipient should be in the best possible medical condition. Common preoperative problems in the anephric patient include inadequate or excessive intravascular volume, electrolyte disturbances, anemia, hypertension, concurrent drug therapy, and infection. If time permits, dialysis, an invaluable part of patient preparation, improves several abnormalities. For unacceptable anemia, transfusion during dialysis may increase the hematocrit without increasing intravascular volume. Preoperative blood transfusion improves graft survival without sensitizing the immune system.[112] Often, preoperative dialysis will also improve hypertension. As with other preoperative patients, antihypertensive therapy should continue prior to surgery.

Although transplants from living, related donors may be scheduled electively, transplant surgery from cadaveric donors must be performed on an emergency basis. The anesthesiologist must prevent the aspiration of gastric contents, because, in the recipient, the neuropathy of renal failure may impair gastric emptying. One should consider preoperative administration of agents such as H_2 antagonists, which decrease the volume and acidity of gastric contents, and metoclopramide, which speeds gastric emptying. If no contraindications exist, a rapid sequence induction of anesthesia may lessen the likelihood of aspiration.

The selection of monitoring techniques for the recipient should be based on the same physiologic considerations as would be appropriate if the same patient were to undergo nonrenal surgery.

The choice of general or regional anesthesia is subject to the experience of the anesthesiologist; both methods have been successfully used for renal transplantation. Earlier reports of anesthesia for renal transplant describe either spinal or epidural techniques.[113] Regional anesthesia was once considered especially desirable for those patients in whom dialysis had failed to adequately control hypervolemia, hyperkalemia, and acidemia. In addition, regional anesthesia reduced concern regarding the potential for aspiration and the unpredictable response of anephric patients to renally excreted drugs. Since the early days of transplantation, improvements in dialytic techniques and the development of newer anesthetic drugs and adjuvant drugs have reduced the apparent disadvantages of general anesthesia. However, regional anesthesia continues to offer some potential benefits. Theoretically, the necessity for tracheal intubation during general anesthesia may increase the risk of nosocomial pneumonia. Pulmonary infection occurs in 10%–25% of those receiving renal transplants, whether from living, related or cadaveric donors[114] In large part because of concurrent immunosuppression, pulmonary infection in this population is associated with a high mortality rate. In contrast to general anesthesia, regional analgesia can continue into the postoperative period, thereby improving pulmonary toilet and potentially reducing the risk of pulmonary infection.

Regardless of the theoretical considerations, most anesthesiologists choose general anesthesia for renal transplantation. When general anesthesia is used, the pharmacologic principles (outlined previously) determine the selection of agents and adjuvants. One should avoid the potent inhalational agents methoxyflurane and enflurane. Although the serum inorganic fluoride level increases less with enflurane than with methoxyflurane anesthesia, it can still approach levels nearly as great as those that produce nephrotoxicity in normal kidneys.[115] Nevertheless, despite the potential for nephrotoxicity in a newly transplanted kidney, one series of patients receiving enflurane has done well.[116]

As described in the section on the use of intravenous drugs in renal failure patients, short-acting barbiturates should be titrated more slowly and usually in smaller doses than would be used in patients with normal kidneys. Opioids must be administered carefully, in anticipation of an increased magnitude and duration of effect for a given dose. In patients receiving cadaveric transplants for which the cold ischemic time usually exceeds that of kidneys from living, related donors, the effects of morphine are prolonged, presumably because the duration of cold ischemia influences the rate of return of function of the transplanted organ.[117] The introduction of newer muscle relaxants, such as atracurium and vecuronium, that do not undergo extensive renal elimination has improved the safety of anesthesia for renal failure patients undergoing renal transplantation.

Because immunosuppressive therapy will begin in the postoperative period, intraoperative asepsis critically affects the well-being of the recipient. Postoperatively, several potent immunosuppressive drugs decrease the frequency and severity of rejection episodes. Currently, the most common drugs are azathioprine, corticosteroids, and cyclosporin A. Azathioprine causes leukopenia and decreases the effectiveness of the immune system. Corticosteroids suppress the febrile response to infection, thereby delaying diagnosis. Cyclosporin A, although predisposing less to infection than the traditional immunosuppressive drugs, requires caution when given in the postoperative period, since it can cause renal failure.

Despite improved anesthetic techniques, complications continue to occur with renal transplantation. Included are hemodynamic changes, prolonged anesthetic action, complications related to invasive monitoring, and postoperative infection and graft rejection.[118] Although complications can never be completely eliminated in this group of severely compromised persons, careful attention to the details of preoperative preparation and intraoperative monitoring and drug administration should help to minimize these complications.

ACUTE OLIGURIA

Acute renal failure (ARF) is a frequently lethal, distressingly common complication of critical surgical illness. Perioperative ARF accounts for one half of all patients requiring acute dialysis.[119] Despite the rapid development of sophisticated techniques to replace renal function over the past 25 years, ARF is still associated with a mortality in excess of 50%.[120–122] During the intraoperative and acute postoperative management of patients at risk for ARF, the anesthesiologist is confronted with the challenge of reducing the incidence of this lethal complication by applying physiologic and pharmacologic principles.

PATHOPHYSIOLOGY

Oliguric states are conventionally defined as prerenal, renal, and postrenal. Prerenal refers to oliguria produced by hemodynamic and/or endocrine factors; renal refers to parenchymal disease; postrenal denotes obstructive oliguria. In this section, we will discuss only prerenal and renal oliguria. For reference purposes, oliguria will be defined as a urinary output of less than $0.5 \text{ ml} \cdot \text{kg}^{-1} \cdot \text{hr}^{-1}$ in a patient subjected to acute stress. This urinary volume ($30 \text{ ml} \cdot \text{hr}^{-1}$ on the average) exceeds that which defines oliguria in unstressed patients, that is, $17 \text{ ml} \cdot \text{kg}^{-1} \cdot \text{hr}^{-1}$. The higher limit is necessary in acutely stressed patients because many such patients are unable to maximally concentrate urine.

Prerenal Oliguria

The conditions producing this state include an acute reduction in GFR, an acute increase in the reabsorption of salt and water, and both mechanisms acting in concert. Increased circulating levels of exogenous or endogenous alpha-adrenergic agonists, increased concentrations of ADH, and increased concentrations of aldosterone represent major systemic physiologic factors that can decrease urinary output. Frank hypotension need not occur for the production of severe prerenal oliguria. If not treated promptly, prerenal oliguria may progress to parenchymal renal failure.

Experience with military trauma convincingly demonstrates the crucial link between the severity (i.e., magnitude and duration) of prerenal insults and the subsequent development of parenchymal renal failure. In World War II, the overall incidence of ARF was 5% in all wounded combatants and 42% in those with severe wounds. During the Korean War, the overall incidence declined to about 0.12% of all wounded soldiers and to 35% of those severely wounded. The incidence further declined in the Vietnam War to 6% of all those wounded and to 17% of those severely wounded.[123, 124] Rapid, effective resuscitation and transport produced the improvement. For those wounded combatants who did not develop ARF, the mortality decreased from 90% (World War II) to 50% (Vietnam).[124] The introduction of dialytic therapy accounted for this decrease in mortality—an improvement of far less clinical import than the dramatic reduction in incidence.

Renal Oliguria

Acute renal failure, frequently termed acute tubular necrosis, may be produced by a variety of factors that interfere with glomerular filtration and tubular reabsorption. The pathogenesis of ARF may be divided into an initiation period, a maintenance period (Table 39-13), and a recovery period.[125]

Renal hypoperfusion, nephrotoxic insults, or both may initiate ARF. In surgical patients, hypoperfusion, produced either by external or internal fluid loss or sepsis, constitutes a frequent cause. Experimental renal hypoperfusion, whether induced by norepinephrine infusion or hemorrhagic shock, impairs renal function in proportion to the depletion of high-energy phosphates.[126, 127] A recently proposed hypothesis states that the renal medulla, because of its lower baseline flow, is particularly at risk for damage from moderate renal ischemia.[128]

The initiating insult ultimately culminates in the development of one or more of the maintenance factors (e.g., decreased tubular function, tubular obstruction, decreased glomerular filtration, and decreased renal blood flow) that reduce urine flow and osmolar excretion. Although decreased renal blood flow characterizes both the initiation and the maintenance phases, once the maintenance phase begins, pharmacologic improvement in renal blood flow will not reverse ARF. In contrast, the hemodynamic factors that initiate perioperative ARF often prove amenable to acute therapeutic intervention during the period when the anesthesiologist is directly responsible for the patient's welfare.

In general, improved management of acute prerenal oliguria has resulted in both a decreasing incidence of ARF and an increase in the proportion of patients with ARF who remain nonoliguric.[124, 129] Myers and Moran[129] recently proposed a more detailed classification of hemodynamically mediated ARF, dividing it into abbreviated, overt, and protracted ARF on the basis of 1) the pattern of reduction in creatinine clearance, and 2) the increase in serum creatinine. This classification is clinically pertinent because it emphasizes the role of secondary insults, such as sepsis, in protracted ARF. Sepsis often complicates the course of patients with protracted critical illness.[129, 130] Myers and Moran's[129] classification emphasizes the frequency of nonoliguric ARF and provides a useful framework for grouping patients with similar prognoses.

DIAGNOSTIC TESTS

Researchers have expended considerable effort to develop tools to evaluate laboratory tests that could clearly differentiate prerenal from renal oliguria and predict the outcome of acute oliguric states. Unfortunately, none of the tools are sufficiently sensitive or specific to predict which patients will or will not respond to therapy. Consequently, the physician usually must treat the acutely oliguric patient without information that could accurately determine whether a patient has already developed or will develop ARF.

Table 39-14 summarizes typical laboratory findings in patients with prerenal and renal oliguria. Prerenal oliguria is associated with physiologic mechanisms that conserve salt and water, resulting in excretion of waste products in a minimal volume of urine; therefore, patients with prerenal oliguria classically produce urine with high osmolality and low sodium. However, in patients with a chronic reduction in

TABLE 39-13.   Pathogenesis of Acute Renal Failure

INITIATION	MAINTENANCE
Renal hypoperfusion	Tubular dysfunction
Hemodynamic factors	Tubular obstruction
Nephrotoxins	Decreased glomerular filtration
	Decreased renal blood flow

TABLE 39-14.   Diagnostic Tests in Acute Oliguria

	PRERENAL	RENAL
Urine osmolality ($mOsm \cdot l^{-1}$)	>500	<350
Urine/plasma osmolality	> 1.3	< 1.1
Urine sodium ($mEq \cdot l^{-1}$)	< 20	> 40
Urine/plasma urea	> 8	< 3
Urine/plasma creatinine	> 40	< 20
Fractional excretion of sodium (%)	< 1	> 2

concentrating ability owing to pre-existing renal disease, urinary sodium and osmolality may not achieve "prerenal" values during acute prerenal insults. In addition, diuretics increase urinary sodium and decrease urinary osmolality.

In an effort to clarify ambiguous laboratory findings, several investigators have proposed the fractional excretion of sodium as a laboratory guide that can more accurately differentiate patients according to those with prerenal oliguria and those with renal oliguria. The fractional excretion of sodium is calculated by dividing the urine-to-plasma sodium ratio by the urine-to-plasma creatinine ratio, then multiplying by 100.[132] Values less than 1% suggest prerenal azotemia. Despite early enthusiasm for this derived index, it is now apparent that it has limited diagnostic and prognostic use in the acute situation.[133, 134] The most critical limitation of these derived indices is that they may suggest established parenchymal ARF at a time when hemodynamically mediated prerenal factors are still reversible. Moreover, these tests are unreliable in sodium-avid patients (those with liver failure, nephrotic syndrome, and cirrhosis) in whom numerical values may be low despite inexorably progressive renal failure.[135]

EXPERIMENTAL VERSUS CLINICAL ACUTE RENAL FAILURE: THERAPEUTIC IMPLICATIONS

Many therapeutic approaches to ARF have their origins in animal models. These models differ substantially from clinical ARF. The development of clinical ARF involves moderate-to-severe prerenal hemodynamic insults, often in combination with nephrotoxic factors, which progress over a highly variable period of time to acute parenchymal injury. In contrast, experimental renal failure is generated by very severe insults, usually administered over a short period of time. In Table 39-15, the differences between typical clinical and experimental ARF are summarized.

At present, the most widely used experimental models of ARF utilize a 40- to 60-minute interval of complete renal ischemia to produce a lesion physiologically and prognostically similar to human ARF. Ischemia of shorter duration does not cause reproducible ARF; more prolonged ischemia produces irreversible injury.[136] The majority of interventions proved to alleviate experimental ARF have been administered before or immediately following an ischemic insult, the magnitude and duration of which are precisely defined. Clinicians, in interpreting the results of such studies, must bear in mind that the clinical setting, in contrast to the animal laboratory, provides the opportunity to limit the magnitude and duration of the initiating insult by promptly providing adequate hemodynamic resuscitation. Table 39-16 lists potential therapeutic approaches for treating fixed experimental versus variable clinical renal insults. The potential management options are similar except for the critical role of effective hemodynamic management.

The clinician must take care to avoid the uncritical application of results from animal studies to the clinical setting. Experimental data suggesting that the routine administration of dopamine, mannitol, and furosemide is justified may not apply to clinical acute oliguria. The diuresis produced by any of these agents, singly or in combination, may further complicate hemodynamic management, thereby increasing the magnitude and the duration of the prerenal insult.[137] However, one can reasonably conclude from the animal and clinical data that the addition of dopamine, mannitol, or furosemide to appropriate hemodynamic support and monitoring

TABLE 39-15. Comparison of Clinical and Experimental Renal Ischemia

FIXED INSULT	VARIABLE INSULT
ANIMAL MODELS	ANIMAL MODEL
Complete renal ischemia	Profound hemorrhagic shock
Intrarenal norepinephrine	
Renal artery occlusion	CLINICAL MODELS
Nephrotoxin	Shock
Uranyl nitrate	Sepsis
	Multifactorial (often including
CLINICAL INSULT	nephrotoxic antibiotics)
Complete surgical ischemia	
Suprarenal aortic cross-clamp	

may improve the results beyond what could be obtained with hemodynamic management alone.[129, 138–147] The experimental demonstration of the renal protective effects of the calcium entry blockers,[148–150] of various prostaglandins,[151–156] and of ATP-MgCl$_2$[157–159] hold promise. However, the reduction in blood pressure associated with all these interventions suggests that their clinical application may be limited to patients with ensured hemodynamic stability. Potential interventions such as thyroxine administration[160] and inhibition of angiotensin-converting enzyme[161] require further study.

COMPARISON OF OLIGURIC AND NONOLIGURIC ACUTE RENAL FAILURE

Nonoliguric ARF, once uncommon, now appears frequently. In contrast to oliguric ARF, nonoliguric ARF is somewhat easier to manage clinically, since it requires less scrupulous control of fluid and electrolyte intake. The first extensive clinical description of nonoliguric ARF stressed its lower mortality rate.[162] In that study, a larger percentage of patients with

TABLE 39-16. Treatment Strategies for Acute Renal Insults

FIXED EXPERIMENTAL INSULT	VARIABLE CLINICAL INSULT
Increase solute excretion	Limit magnitude and duration
Mannitol[28–31]	Hemodynamic support
Furosemide[31–33]	Increase renal blood flow
Dopamine[33]	Dopamine[34, 35]
Increase renal blood flow	Mannitol[36, 37]
Mannitol[28–31]	Furosemide
Furosemide[31–33]	Increase solute excretion
Dopamine[33]	Dopamine[34, 35]
Decrease substrate consumption	Mannitol[36, 37]
Hypothermia	Furosemide
Antagonize calcium entry	Decrease substrate consumption
Verapamil[38–40]	Hypothermia
Nifedipine[40]	Enhance cellular metabolism
Vasodilatory prostaglandins	ATP-MgCl$_2$[40]
PGI$_2$[41, 42]	
PGE$_1$[43–45]	
PGE$_2$[46]	
Enhance cellular metabolism	
ATP-MgCl$_2$[47–49]	
Thyroxine[50]	
Angiotensin-converting enzyme inhibition	
Captopril[51]	

nonoliguric ARF had a nephrotoxic injury, whereas a larger group of oliguric patients had ARF in association with surgery, with prolonged volume depletion, or with impaired cardiac output.[162] Therefore, it appears that nonoliguric ARF, occurring spontaneously in a hospitalized population, is associated with a lower mortality. Nonoliguric ARF occurring as a complication of trauma may also carry a better prognosis. Shin et al[163] reported on two consecutive groups (groups 1 and 2) of trauma patients. In group 2, more liberal fluid administration and less frequent diuretic administration increased the incidence of nonoliguric ARF and decreased the incidence of oliguric ARF in comparison with group 1, which received fluid in lower volumes and was more frequently chemically diuresed.[163] The mortality and morbidity in group 2 was substantially less than that in group 1.[163]

Because ARF represents a syndrome that includes both oliguric patients and a heterogeneous group of nonoliguric patients, the accurate characterization and classification of clinical ARF should improve prognosis and treatment. Myers and colleagues extensively studied hemodynamically mediated ARF in surgical patients, using a combination of clinical variables and creatinine kinetic modeling to describe the key pathogenetic features.[129, 164–168] They defined three types. The first type, abbreviated ARF, is characterized by an abrupt decrement in creatinine clearance, followed by a steady improvement in renal function. The second type, overt ARF, represents a sustained prerenal insult, recovery from which is contingent upon hemodynamic improvement. Protracted ARF, the third type, represents the net effects of multiple episodes of renal injury. Prognostically, one can anticipate low mortality in abbreviated ARF and high mortality in protracted ARF.[129]

Because of the reported improved mortality and morbidity in patients with nonoliguric ARF, several investigators have attempted to convert established oliguric ARF to nonoliguric ARF using diuretic drugs with or without dopamine. Uncontrolled series emphasize the efficacy of induced diuresis.[169, 170] However, controlled randomized trials have failed to demonstrate that conversion of oliguric ARF to nonoliguric ARF improves mortality, morbidity, the duration of renal failure, or the number of necessary dialyses.[171, 172] In addition, direct intrarenal administration of furosemide (275 mg over 30 minutes) failed to improve renal function or renal blood flow in patients with ARF.[173] The aforementioned data support the conclusion that early, aggressive hemodynamic support of the patient with prerenal oliguria may produce a better outcome, even if nonoliguric ARF develops. Conversely, the chemical conversion of oliguric to nonoliguric ARF does not improve outcome.

THERAPEUTIC CONFLICTS IN THE MANAGEMENT OF ACUTE OLIGURIA

Effective treatment of oliguria requires not only an understanding of the effects of various therapeutic interventions on the kidney but also an assessment of the effects of those interventions on the lungs and the heart.

Kidney/Lung Therapeutic Conflicts

Aggressive expansion of intravascular volume, a common strategy in the hemodynamic management of prerenal oliguria, will increase pulmonary microvascular pressure, thereby potentially increasing pulmonary edema. In a healthy person, clinical pulmonary edema will occur at a pulmonary microvascular pressure exceeding 25 mm Hg. However, in patients with decreased serum oncotic pressure or increased pulmonary capillary permeability, pulmonary edema may occur at lower pulmonary microvascular pressures.[174] Consequently, the clinician treating a patient with prerenal oliguria frequently confronts the question of whether to risk ARF or acute respiratory failure.[175] Several recent series emphasize the frequency with which this important question arises. Approximately 40% of patients with ARF develop pulmonary complications.[162, 176–178] Conversely, more than 50% of patients with the adult respiratory distress syndrome (ARDS) develop ARF.[179] In a broader cross-section of patients with respiratory failure resulting from a variety of medical and surgical illnesses, 11%–33% developed ARF.[180, 181]

In general, the argument in favor of sacrificing pulmonary function to save renal function rests on the ease with which mechanical ventilation can support the patient with deteriorating pulmonary function. One can defend this position by noting that the mortality from ARF ranges from 50%–70%.[120, 175] The counterargument, less often heard, states that it is better to sacrifice renal function, since dialysis can effectively support patients with acute ARF. One can defend this approach by noting that the mortality from ARDS also ranges from 50%–70%.[182]

Certainly, in the course of providing hemodynamic support for the oliguric patient, one should avoid the two extremes of frank hypovolemia and inappropriate overhydration. However, the practical definition of these two terms presents a problem. In everyday terms, the pulmonary artery occlusion pressure (PAOP), though imperfect, may be the best single estimate. In choosing an upper limit for the PAOP, the clinician decides which extreme to risk. The lower the limit, the greater the chance of inadequate resuscitation and the more frequent the need for inotropic support; the higher the PAOP limit, the greater the risk of pulmonary edema. Nevertheless, pulmonary edema does not occur simply because of fluid administration. For example, Shin et al[163] reported that respiratory failure occurred less often in group 2, the group receiving a greater amount of fluid and less frequent diuretics. More thorough resuscitation from shock may limit the pathophysiologic responses that produce ARDS.

Kidney/Heart Therapeutic Conflicts

Just as aggressive volume expansion may worsen pulmonary edema, so may it lead to increased left ventricular end-diastolic pressure and wall tension, thereby increasing myocardial oxygen consumption.[183] Because left ventricular end-diastolic pressure limits left ventricular subendocardial perfusion, increases in filling pressure may also limit myocardial oxygen availability.[184] The production of myocardial ischemia by aggressive volume loading represents a more subtle, less easily appreciated complication of volume resuscitation than does the production of pulmonary edema. Unfortunately, limiting volume expansion to a lower PAOP limit and utilizing positive inotropic agents or vasodilators earlier in the course of hemodynamic resuscitation does not necessarily reduce the cardiac risk. Rather, positive inotropic agents, by increasing heart rate and myocardial contractility, may increase myocardial oxygen consumption.[185] Vasodilators may precipitate sudden hypotension and myocardial ischemia, particularly if used in the setting of inadequate intravascular volume. However, when used with careful augmentation of intravascular volume, vasodilators such as nitroprusside may substantially improve both hemodynamic and renal function.[186]

SUGGESTED MANAGEMENT

No specific guidelines exist that routinely and simultaneously produce the least compromise to the kidneys, lungs, and heart. Instead, therapy needs to be individualized, based on the apparent risk to each of the systems. Lacking an easy "cookbook" approach to preventing the progression from acute prerenal oliguria to ARF, the following generalizations form the basis of a logical approach

1. The most common cause of ARF is prolonged renal hypoperfusion.
2. The prophylaxis of ARF reduces mortality more effectively than does dialytic therapy.
3. The duration and magnitude of the initiating renal insult are critical in determining the severity of ARF.

Based on those generalizations, the following strategies can be applied:

Limit the magnitude and duration of renal ischemic insults that might initiate ARF. This constitutes the key strategy in limiting the incidence of renal failure. In the majority of patients, oliguria signals inadequate systemic perfusion, and carefully monitored efforts to improve perfusion, including volume expansion, pulmonary artery catheterization, inotropic support (ideally with dopamine), and vasodilation should be used (Fig. 39-7).

Promote solute excretion. When aggressive attempts to restore perfusion have failed to establish adequate urinary output, dopamine, mannitol, and/or furosemide should be added. Earlier use, though theoretically attractive, removes the value of urinary output as a monitor of the adequacy of resuscitation. No evidence exists that the administration of small "test" doses of diuretics decreases either morbidity or mortality in patients with uncertain volume status. At best, there will be no effect; at worst, production of short-term increases in urine output will delay effective therapy and potentiate the development of volume deficits.[137] However, in the special circumstance of rhabdomyolysis-induced pigmenturia, early diuresis may limit the incidence of ARF.[187] The use of diuretics earlier in the course of prerenal oliguria would be easier to defend if an appropriate monitor of renal function were available to permit ongoing assessment of changes in renal function.

Consider diagnostic data with caution. Urinary output, although an extremely crude estimate of renal function, offers the most consistently useful diagnostic information in the acute intraoperative management of potential renal failure.[134, 188] Hemodynamic data prove useful in situations where empiric volume expansion does not restore urine flow. In the acute situation, most therapeutic decisions should not rely on urinary sediment, electrolytes, osmolality, or complex formulae derived from urinary and plasma sodium and creatinine measurements. This is not to say that those measurements have no value (although that has been suggested[134]), but rather that their discriminatory value is too limited for application in the perioperative setting. Unfortunately, the readily available tests are insufficiently sensitive and specific, require excessive time for completion, and provide little information that can guide therapy. All acutely oliguric patients at risk for ARF should receive fluids and should undergo monitoring and hemodynamic support in the same fashion, using the same end points, regardless of the results of those tests. The resuscitation of patients with significant perioperative oliguria should be sufficiently aggressive to restore urine flow and systemic perfusion or should be continued until oliguria

CURRENT ALGORITHM

ARF RISK?

↓

EMPIRICAL FLUID CHALLENGE

↓

PA CATHETER

↓

DATA-DIRECTED THERAPY

FLUID
DOPAMINE
DIURETICS

IDEAL ALGORITHM

ARF RISK?

↓

EMPIRICAL FLUID CHALLENGE

↓

(RENAL FUNCTION MONITOR?)
DIURETICS, DOPAMINE

↓

PA CATHETER

↓

DATA-DIRECTED THERAPY

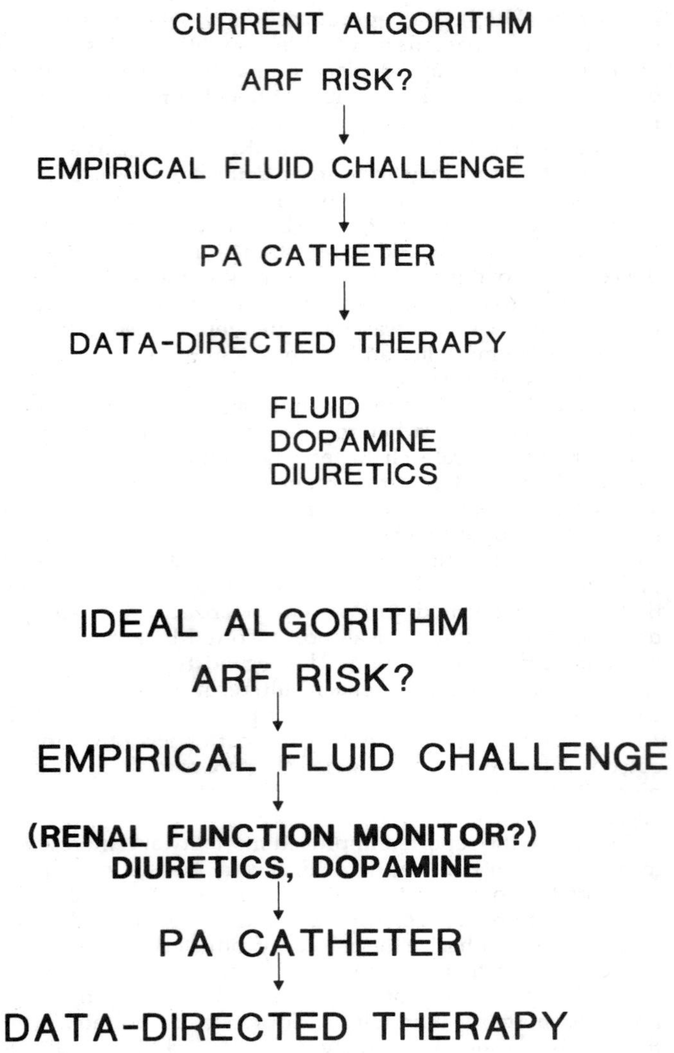

FIG. 39-7. (*Top*) Clinical algorithm for managing acute oliguria. In the current suggested algorithm, diuretic drugs are given when aggressive hemodynamic support has failed. (*Bottom*) Ideally, a future protocol may incorporate a better monitor of renal function, thereby permitting earlier use of diuretic drugs.

persists despite a PAOP of 18 mm Hg or greater following the administration of dopamine and diuretics.

Excessive reliance on the determination of urinary electrolytes, osmolality, or specialized indices may lead to the delay, interruption, or premature termination of appropriate, timely therapy, thereby increasing the chance that a patient will suffer the high morbidity and mortality of ARF.

MANAGEMENT OF ACUTE RENAL FAILURE

When renal replacement therapy proves necessary despite intensive efforts to prevent ARF, several aspects of care deserve special consideration. Occasionally, controversy will exist regarding optimal therapy. The physicians caring for the patient must consider the timing and selection of renal replacement techniques, must review the patient's pharmacologic management, must make careful plans regarding fluid and electrolyte therapy and nutritional support, must intensify surveillance for infection, and must maintain an appropriate level of monitoring.

TIMING AND TECHNIQUE OF RENAL REPLACEMENT THERAPY

After establishing the diagnosis of ARF, the clinician must decide how soon to begin renal replacement therapy and must choose from the various available modalities the most suitable technique for the individual patient. At this point in the patient's care, conflicts are likely. Because many of these patients will have undergone extensive fluid resuscitation for the management of traumatic, surgical, or septic sequestration of sodium and water, the health care team often attempts to aggressively remove fluid. Unfortunately, the processes resulting in fluid sequestration frequently persist at the time when renal failure becomes manifest. Aggressive attempts to remove sodium and water with hemodialysis, peritoneal dialysis, or CAVH will frequently result in intravascular volume depletion. At such times, one should keep in mind the indications for acute dialytic therapy: intravascular volume overload, azotemia, hyperkalemia, and severe acid–base disturbances. In addition, dialysis may facilitate the improvement of white cell function and permit more aggressive nutritional support.[49]

REVIEW PHARMACOLOGIC THERAPY

A large number of drugs are excreted by the kidney. Other drugs are removed by dialytic therapy or by CAVH. At the time of initiation of renal replacement therapy, the clinician should review all pharmacologic therapy and should adjust that therapy appropriately for the patient's acute change in renal status. A recent review comprehensively describes drug dosages for adults with renal failure.[189]

Because of the high incidence of stress gastritis in critically ill patients, particularly in those with ARF, some form of stress ulcer prophylaxis should be considered. The three approaches to the prophylaxis of stress ulceration include aggressive antacid titration,[190] the administration of an H_2 receptor antagonist, and the administration of sucralfate.[191, 192] Although aggressive titration of antacids represents the gold standard for prophylaxis,[190] the frequent requirement for large quantities of antacids has prompted a search for a more convenient form of treatment. H_2 receptor antagonists appear most effective in patients with few risk factors for stress gastritis but are less effective in patients with renal failure.[192–194] Sucralfate, originally introduced for the management of duodenal ulceration, seems to compare favorably with either antacids or cimetidine for the prevention of gastrointestinal bleeding in critically ill patients.[191, 192]

CAREFULLY MONITOR FLUID AND ELECTROLYTE THERAPY

Patients with ARF do not easily tolerate inappropriate intravascular volume expansion. In those who are hemodynamically stable, fluid administration can be restricted to that necessary to provide adequate nutritional intake. Patients with sepsis or multiple system failure, however, often require continued sodium and water administration despite the cessation of renal function. Serum potassium, magnesium, and phosphate levels should be monitored carefully. In general, potassium excretion is a function of urinary flow rate rather than of GFR. Magnesium may accumulate in patients receiving magnesium-containing antacids. Hyperphosphatemia may occur as a consequence of excretory failure; conversely, hypophosphatemia may become a problem in patients receiving aggressive nutritional support and phosphate-binding antacids. Dialysis best manages metabolic acidosis. Some patients with nonoliguric renal failure develop a hyperchloremic acidosis, which responds to the administration of sodium bicarbonate.

NUTRITIONAL SUPPORT

The recovery of patients with ARF may depend, in part, upon the adequacy of their nutritional support. Inadequate nutrition will result in muscle-wasting and immune compromise. One of the goals of renal replacement therapy should be to remove sufficient excess fluid to permit the provision of an adequate number of calories and an adequate amount of protein.

SURVEILLANCE OF INFECTION

Infection remains the most common cause of death in patients with ARF. In addition, ARF constitutes one of the earliest manifestations of multiple system organ failure, the cause of which is usually sepsis and the mortality of which is prohibitively high.[195–197] The control of apparent infection, the search for occult sepsis, and vigilance regarding the development of new infectious complications must be intensive and persistent. The clinician must realize that ARF may be followed by failure of other organ systems, which, in patients with severe infections may, in turn, require aggressive support.

MONITORING

The indications for pulmonary artery catheterization in patients with ARF resemble those indications in other critically ill patients. Hemodynamic monitoring proves especially useful for those patients in whom a conflict exists regarding the need for aggressive dialytic removal of sodium and water. The estimation of PAOP before and during dialysis may assist the dialysis personnel in managing fluid removal during dialysis and in determining appropriate therapy if hypotension develops.

One of the greatest limitations of current monitoring techniques is the lack of an effective means for determining the rate of recovery of renal function in patients with ARF. The inability to accurately estimate renal blood flow and GFR means that dialysis will frequently continue for an unnecessarily long period of time. Myers and Moran[129] suggest that limiting the number of dialyses, and their attendant risk of hypotension, would hasten recovery from renal failure in some patients.

REFERENCES

1. Vander AJ: Renal Physiology, 3rd ed, p 27. New York, McGraw-Hill, 1985
2. Huang C-L, Lewicki J, Johnson LK et al: Renal mechanism of

action of rat atrial natriuretic factor. J Clin Invest 75:769, 1985

3. Salazar FJ, Romero JC, Burnett JC Jr et al: Atrial natriuretic peptide levels during acute and chronic saline loading in conscious dogs. Am J Physiol 251:R499, 1986

4. Scharschmidt LA, Lianos E, Dunn MJ: Arachidonate metabolites and the control of glomerular function. Fed Proc 42:3058, 1983

5. Philbin D, Coggins CH: Plasma antidiuretic hormone levels in cardiac surgical patients during morphine and halothane anesthesia. Anesthesiology 49:45, 1978

6. Sladen RN: Effect of anesthesia and surgery on renal function. Crit Care Clin 3:373, 1987

7. Price HL, Linde HW, Jone RE et al: Sympathoadrenal responses to general anesthesia in man and their relation to hemodynamics. Anesthesiology 20:563, 1959

8. Priebe H-J, Heimann JC, Hedley–Whyte J: Mechanisms of renal dysfunction during positive end-expiratory pressure ventilation. J Appl Physiol 50:643, 1981

9. Payen DM, Farge D, Beloucif S et al: No involvement of antidiuretic hormone in acute antidiuresis during PEEP ventilation in humans. Anesthesiology 66:17, 1987

10. Pitts RF: Physiology of the Kidney and Body Fluids, p 167. Chicago, Year Book Medical Publishers, 1974

11. Sykes BJ, Hoie J, Schenk WG Jr: An experimental study into the validity of clearance methods of measuring renal blood flow. Surg Gynecol Obstet 135:877, 1972

12. Marsh DJ: Renal Physiology. New York, Raven Press, 1983

13. Crandell WB, Pappas SG, Macdonald A: Nephrotoxicity associated with methoxyflurane anesthesia. Anesthesiology 27:591, 1966

14. Mazze RI, Trudell JR, Cousins MJ: Methoxyflurane metabolism and renal dysfunction: Clinical correlation in man. Anesthesiology 35:247, 1971

15. Cousins MJ, Mazze RI: Methoxyflurane nephrotoxicity. A study of dose response in man. JAMA 225:1611, 1973

16. Whitford GM, Taves DR: Fluoride-induced diuresis: Renal-tissue solute concentrations, functional, hemodynamic, and histologic correlates in the rat. Anesthesiology 39:416, 1973

17. Cousins MJ, Greenstein LR, Hitt BA et al: Metabolism and renal effects of enflurane in man. Anesthesiology 44:44, 1976

18. Mazze RI, Calverley RK, Smith NT: Inorganic fluoride nephrotoxicity: Prolonged enflurane and halothane anesthesia in volunteers. Anesthesiology 46:265, 1977

19. Mazze RI, Woodruff RE, Heerdt ME: Isoniazid-induced enflurane defluorination in humans. Anesthesiology 57:5, 1982

20. Mazze RI, Schwartz FD, Slocum HC et al: Renal function during anesthesia in surgery. I. The effects of halothane anesthesia. Anesthesiology 24:279, 1963

21. Blackmore WP, Erwin KW, Wiegand OF et al: Renal and cardiovascular effects of halothane. Anesthesiology 21:489, 1960

22. Theye RA, Maher FT: The effects of halothane on canine renal function and oxygen consumption. Anesthesiology 35:54, 1971

23. Bastron RD, Perkins FM, Pyne JL: Autoregulation of renal blood flow during halothane anesthesia. Anesthesiology 46:142, 1977

24. Priano LL: Effect of halothane on renal hemodynamics during normovolemia and acute hemorrhagic hypovolemia. Anesthesiology 63:357, 1985

25. Lundeen G, Manohar M, Parks C: Systemic distribution of blood flow in swine while awake and during 1.0 and 1.5 MAC isoflurane anesthesia with or without 50% nitrous oxide. Anesth Analg 62:499, 1983

26. Gelman S, Fowler KC, Smith LR: Regional blood flow during isoflurane and halothane anesthesia. Anesth Analg 63:557, 1984

27. Hill GE, Lunn JK, Hodges MR et al: N₂O modification of halothane-altered renal function in the dog. Anesth Analg 56:690, 1977

28. Leighton KM, Macleod BA, Bruce C: Renal blood flow: Differ-

ences in autoregulation during anesthesia with halothane, methoxyflurane, or alphaprodine in the dog. Anesth Analg 57:389, 1978

29. Lebowitz PW, Cote ME, Daniels AL et al: Comparative renal effects of midazolam and thiopental in humans. Anesthesiology 59:381, 1983

30. Priano LL: Alteration of renal hemodynamics by thiopental, diazepam, and ketamine in conscious dogs. Anesth Analg 61:853, 1982

31. Hirasawa H, Yonezawa T: The effects of ketamine and Innovar on the renal cortical and medullary blood flow of the dog. Anaesthesist 8:349, 1975

32. Idvall J, Aronsen KF, Stenberg P: Tissue perfusion and distribution of cardiac output during ketamine anesthesia in normovolemic rats. Acta Anaesth Scand 24:257, 1980

33. Bidwai AV, Stanley TH, Bloomer HA et al: Effects of anesthetic doses of morphine on renal function in the dog. Anesth Analg 54:357, 1975

34. Hunter JM, Jones RS, Utting JE: Effect of anaesthesia with nitrous oxide in oxygen and fentanyl on renal function in the artificially ventilated dog. Br J Anaesth 52:343, 1980

35. Priano LL: Effects of high-dose fentanyl on renal haemodynamics in conscious dogs. Can Anaesth Soc J 30:10, 1983

36. Kennedy WF Jr, Sawyer TK, Gerbershagen HU et al: Simultaneous systemic cardiovascular and renal hemodynamic measurements during high spinal anaesthesia in normal man. Acta Anaesthesiol Scand (Suppl) 37:163, 1970

37. Kennedy WF Jr, Sawyer TK, Gerbershagen HU et al: Systemic cardiovascular and renal hemodynamic alterations during peridural anesthesia in normal man. Anesthesiology 31:414, 1969

38. Sivarajan M, Amory DW, Lindbloom LE: Systemic and regional blood flow during epidural anesthesia without epinephrine in the rhesus monkey. Anesthesiology 45:300, 1976

39. Weiner IM, Mudge GH: Diuretics and other agents employed in the mobilization of edema fluid. In Gilman AG, Goodman LS, Rall TW (eds): Goodman and Gilman's The Pharmacologic Basis of Therapeutics, 7th ed, p 887. New York, Macmillan, 1985

40. Corvol P, Claire M, Oblin ME et al: Mechanism of the mineralocorticoid effects of spironolactones. Kidney Int 20:1, 1981

41. Schettini A, Stahurski B, Young HF: Osmotic and osmotic-loop diuresis in brain surgery: Effects on plasma and CSF electrolytes and ion excretion. J Neurosurg 56:679, 1984

42. Warren SE, Blantz RC: Mannitol. Arch Intern Med 141:493, 1981

43. Hijer–Pedersen E: Effect of acetazolamide on cerebral blood flow in subacute and chronic cerebrovascular disease. Stroke 18:887, 1987

44. Moser M: Diuretics in the management of hypertension. Med Clin North Am 71:935, 1987

45. Bastron RD: Anesthetic considerations for patients with end-stage renal disease. In Barash PG (ed): Refresher Course in Anesthesiology. Philadelphia, JB Lippincott, 1985

46. Dodds A, Nicholls M: Haematological aspects of renal disease. Anaesth Intensive Care 11:361, 1983

47. Eschbach JW, Egrie JC, Downing MR et al: Correction of the anemia of end-stage renal disease with recombinant human erythropoietin. Results of a combined phase I and II clinical trial. N Engl J Med 316:73, 1987

48. Lichtman MA, Murphy MS, Byer BJ et al: Hemoglobin affinity for oxygen in chronic renal disease: Effect of hemodialysis. Blood 43:417, 1974

49. Prough DS, Adams PL, Hamilton RW: Complications of renal replacement therapy. In Lump PD, Bryan–Brown CW (eds): Complications in Critical Care Medicine, p 145. Chicago, Year Book Medical Publishers, 1988

50. Levey AS, Harrington JT: Continuous peritoneal dialysis for chronic renal failure. Medicine 61:330, 1982

51. Nolph KD: Continuous ambulatory peritoneal dialysis. Am J Nephrol 1:1, 1981
52. Kliger AS: Complications of dialysis: Hemodialysis, peritoneal dialysis, CAPD. In Arieff AI, DeFronzo RA (eds): Fluid, Electrolyte, and Acid–Base Disorders, Vol II, p 777. New York, Churchill Livingstone, 1985
53. Cogan MG, Garovoy MR: Introduction to Dialysis. New York, Churchill Livingstone, 1985
54. Drukker W, Parsons FM, Maher JF: Replacement of Renal Function by Dialysis. A Textbook of Dialysis, 2nd ed. Boston, Martinus Nijhoff, 1983
55. Alfred HJ, Cohen AJ: Use of dialytic procedures in the intensive care unit. In Rippe JM, Irwin RS, Alpert JS et al (eds): Intensive Care Medicine, p 562. Boston, Little, Brown and Co, 1985
56. Dorner DB, Stubbs DH, Shadur CA et al: Percutaneous subclavian vein catheter hemodialysis—Impact on vascular access surgery. Surgery 91:712, 1982
57. Palder SB, Kirkman RL, Whittemore AD et al: Vascular access for hemodialysis. Patency rates and results of revision. Ann Surg 202:235, 1985
58. Kurtz SB, Wong VH, Anderson CF et al: Continuous ambulatory peritoneal dialysis. Three years' experience at the Mayo Clinic. Mayo Clin Proc 58:633, 1983
59. Tenckhoff H, Schechter H: A bacteriologically safe peritoneal access device. Trans Am Soc Artif Intern Organs 14:181, 1968
60. Maher JF: Characteristics of peritoneal transport: Physiological and clinical implications. Miner Electrolyte Metab 5:201, 1981
61. Synhaivsky A, Kurtz SB, Wochos DN et al: Acute renal failure treated by slow continuous ultrafiltration. Preliminary report. Mayo Clin Proc 58:729, 1983
62. Kaplan AA, Longnecker RE, Folkert VW: Continuous arteriovenous hemofiltration. A report of six months' experience. Ann Intern Med 100:358, 1984
63. Lauer A, Saccaggi A, Ronco C et al: Continuous arteriovenous hemofiltration in the critically ill patient. Clinical use and operational characteristics. Ann Intern Med 99:455, 1983
64. Bartlett RH, Mault JR, Dechert RE et al: Continuous arteriovenous hemofiltration: Improved survival in surgical acute renal failure? Surgery 100:400, 1986
65. Ossenkoppele GJ, van der Meulen J, Bronsveld W et al: Continuous arteriovenous hemofiltration as an adjunctive therapy for septic shock. Crit Care Med 13:102, 1985
66. Gotleib L, Barzilay E, Shustak A et al: Sequential hemofiltration in nonoliguric high capillary permeability pulmonary edema of severe sepsis: Preliminary report. Crit Care Med 12:997, 1984
67. Geronemus R, Schneider N: Continuous arteriovenous hemodialysis: A new modality for treatment of acute renal failure. Trans Am Soc Artif Intern Organs 30:610, 1984
68. Twardowski ZJ, Nolph KD: Blood purification in acute renal failure. Ann Intern Med 100:447, 1984
69. Freeman RD: Treatment of chronic renal failure: An update. N Engl J Med 312:577, 1985
70. Mahoney CA, Arieff AI: Uremic encephalopathies: Clinical, biochemical, and experimental features. Am J Kidney Dis 2:324, 1982
71. Pierides AM, Edwards WG Jr, Cullum UX Jr et al: Hemodialysis encephalopathy with osteomalacic fractures and muscle weakness. Kidney Int 18:115, 1980
72. Mathew RJ Rabin P, Stone WJ et al: Regional cerebral blood flow in dialysis encephalopathy and primary degenerative dementia. Kidney Int 28:64, 1985
73. Henderson LW: Symptomatic hypotension during hemodialysis. Kidney Int 17:571, 1980
74. Huyghebaert M-F, Dhainaut J-F, Monsallier JF et al: Bicarbonate hemodialysis of patients with acute renal failure and severe sepsis. Crit Care Med 13:840, 1985
75. Wehle B, Asaba H, Castenfors J et al: Hemodynamic changes during sequential ultrafiltration and dialysis. Kidney Int 15:411, 1979
76. Chaudry IH, Baue AE: Overview of Hemorrhagic Shock. In Cowley RA, Trump BF (eds): Pathophysiology of Shock, Anoxia, and Ischemia, p 203. Baltimore, Williams & Wilkins, 1982
77. Lazarus JM, Hampers CL, Lowrie EG et al: Baroreceptor activity in normotensive and hypertensive uremic patients. Circulation 47:1015, 1973
78. Endou K, Kamijima J, Kakubari Y et al: Hemodynamic changes during hemodialysis. Cardiology 63:175, 1978
79. Graefe U, Milutinovich J, Follette WC et al: Less dialysis-induced morbidity and vascular instability with bicarbonate in dialysate. Ann Intern Med 88:332, 1978
80. Leunissen KML, Hoorntje SJ, Fiers HA et al: Acetate versus bicarbonate hemodialysis in critically ill patients. Nephron 42:146, 1986
81. Hung J, Harris PJ, Uren RF et al: Uremic cardiomyopathy: Effect of hemodialysis on left ventricular function in end-stage renal failure. N Engl J Med 302:547, 1980
82. Nixon JV, Mitchell JH, McPhaul JJ Jr, et al: Effect of hemodialysis on left ventricular function. Dissociation of changes in filling volume and in contractile state. J Clin Invest 71:377, 1983
83. Ruder MA, Alpert MA, Van Stone J et al: Comparative effects of acetate and bicarbonate hemodialysis on left ventricular function. Kidney Int 27:768, 1985
84. Maynard JC, Cruz C, Kleerekoper M et al: Blood pressure response to changes in serum ionized calcium during hemodialysis. Ann Intern Med 104:358, 1986
85. Francos GC, Besarab A, Burke JF Jr et al: Dialysis-induced hypoxemia: Membrane dependent and membrane independent causes. Am J Kidney Dis 5:191, 1985
86. Craddock PR, Fehr J, Brigham KL et al: Complement and leukocyte-mediated pulmonary dysfunction in hemodialysis. N Engl J Med 296:769, 1977
87. De Backer WA, Verpooten GA, Borgonjon DJ et al: Hypoxemia during hemodialysis: Effects of different membranes and dialysate compositions. Kidney Int 23:738, 1983
88. Sherlock J, Ledwith J, Letteri J: Determinants of oxygenation during hemodialysis and related procedures. A report of data acquired under varying conditions and a review of the literature. Am J Nephrol 4:158, 1984
89. Aurigemma NM, Feldman NT, Gottlieb M et al: Arterial oxygenation during hemodialysis. N Engl J Med 297:871, 1977
90. Rubini ME, Gordon S: Individual plasma-free amino acids in uremics: Effect of hemodialysis. Nephron 5:339, 1968
91. Blumenkrantz MJ, Gahl GM, Kopple JD et al: Protein losses during peritoneal dialysis. Kidney Int 19:593, 1981
92. Burke JF, Francos GC: Surgery in the patient with acute or chronic renal failure. Med Clin North Am 71:489, 1987
93. Sladen RN, Endo E, Harrison T: Two-hour versus 22-hour creatinine clearance in critically ill patients. Anesthesiology 67:1013, 1987
94. Ghoneim MM, Pandya H: Plasma protein binding of thiopental in patients with impaired renal or hepatic function. Anesthesiology 42:545, 1975
95. Dundee JW, Richards RK: Effect of azotemia upon the action of intravenous barbiturate anesthesia. Anesthesiology 15:333, 1954
96. Burch PG, Stanski DR: Decreased protein binding and thiopental kinetics. Clin Pharmacol Ther 32:212, 1982
97. Don HF, Dieppa RA, Taylor P: Narcotic analgesics in anuric patients. Anesthesiology 42:745, 1975
98. Chauvin M, Sandouk P, Scherrmann JM et al: Morphine pharmacokinetics in renal failure. Anesthesiology 66:327, 1987
99. Yoshimura H, Ida S, Oguri K et al: Biochemical basis for analgesic activity of morphine-6-glucuronide. I. Penetration of mor-

phine-6-glucuronide in the brain of rats. Biochem Pharmacol 22:1423, 1973

100. Miller RD, Way WL, Hamilton WK et al: Succinylcholine-induced hyperkalemia in patients with renal failure? Anesthesiology 36:138, 1972

101. Ryan DW: Preoperative serum cholinesterase concentration in chronic renal failure. Clinical experience of suxamethonium in 81 patients undergoing renal transplant. Br J Anaesth 49:945, 1977

102. Gibaldi M, Levy G, Hayton WL: Tubocurarine and renal failure. Br J Anaesth 44:163, 1972

103. Orko R, Heino A, Rosenberg PH et al: Dose–response of tubocurarine in patients with and without renal failure. Acta Anesthesiol Scand 28:452, 1984

104. Fahey MR, Rupp SM, Fisher DM et al: The pharmacokinetics and pharmacodynamics of atracurium in patients with and without renal failure. Anesthesiology 61:699, 1984

105. Fahey MR, Morris RB, Miller RD et al: Pharmacokinetics of Org NC45 (norcuron) in patients with and without renal failure. Br J Anaesth 53:1049, 1981

106. Cronnelly R, Stanski DR, Miller RD et al: Renal function and the pharmacokinetics of neostigmine in anesthetized man. Anesthesiology 51:222, 1979

107. Cronnellly R, Stanski DR, Miller RD et al: Pyridostigmine kinetics with and without renal function. Clin Pharmacol Ther 28:78, 1980

108. Morris RB, Cronnelly R, Miller RD et al: Pharmacokinetics of edrophonium in anephric and renal transplant patients. Br J Anaesth 53:1311, 1981

109. Vandam LD, Harrison JH, Murray JE et al: Anesthetic aspects of renal homotransplantation in man: With notes on the anesthetic care of the uremic patient. Anesthesiology 23:783, 1962

110. Tilney NL, Milford EL, Araujo JL et al: Experience with cyclosporine and steroids in clinical renal transplantation. Ann Surg 200:605, 1984

111. Brenner BM, Meyer TW, Hostetter TH: Dietary protein intake and the progressive nature of kidney disease: The role of hemodynamically mediated glomerular injury in the pathogenesis of progressive glomerular sclerosis in aging, renal ablation, and intrinsic renal disease. N Engl J Med 307:652, 1982

112. Vincenti F, Amend WJC Jr, Feduska NJ et al: Blood transfusions and kidney transplantation. Arch Intern Med 142:680, 1982

113. Linke CL, Merin RG: A regional anesthetic approach for renal transplantation. Anesth Analg 55:69, 1976

114. Munda R, Alexander JW, First MR et al: Pulmonary infections in renal transplant recipients. Ann Surg 187:126, 1978

115. Wickström I: Enflurane anesthesia in living donor renal transplantation. Acta Anesthesiol Scand 25:263, 1981

116. de Temmerman P, Gribomont B: Enflurane in renal transplantation: Report of 375 cases. Acta Anaesthesiol Scand (Suppl) 71:24, 1979

117. Sear J, Moore A, Hunniset A et al: Morphine kinetics and kidney transplantation: Morphine removal is influenced by renal ischemia. Anesth Analg 64:1065, 1985

118. Heino A, Orko R, Rosenberg PH: Anesthesiological complications in renal transplantation: A retrospective study of 500 transplantations. Acta Anaesthesiol Scand 30:574, 1986

119. Kasiske BL, Kjellstrand CM: Perioperative management of patients with chronic renal failure and postoperative acute renal failure. Urol Clin North Am 10:35, 1983

120. Abreo K, Moorthy AV, Osborne M: Changing patterns and outcome of acute renal failure requiring hemodialysis. Arch Intern Med 146:1338, 1986

121. Lordon RE, Burton JR: Post-traumatic renal failure in military personnel in Southeast Asia. Experience at Clark USAF Hospital, Republic of the Philippines. Am J Med 53:137, 1972

122. Hou SH, Bushinsky DA, Wish JB et al: Hospital-acquired renal insufficiency: A prospective study. Am J Med 74:243, 1983

123. Schrier RW: Acute renal failure. JAMA 247:2518, 1982

124. Tilney NL, Lazarus JM: Acute renal failure in surgical patients. Causes, clinical patterns, and care. Surg Clin North Am 63:357, 1983

125. Wilkes BM, Mailloux LU: Acute renal failure. Pathogenesis and prevention. Am J Med 80:1129, 1986

126. Sinsteden TD, O'Neil TJ, Hill S et al: The role of high-energy phosphate in norepinephrine-induced acute renal failure in the dog. Circ Res 59:93, 1986

127. Ratcliffe PJ, Moonen CTW, Holloway PAH et al: Acute renal failure in hemorrhagic hypotension: Cellular energetics and renal function. Kidney Int 30:355, 1986

128. Brezis M, Rosen S, Silva P et al: Renal ischemia: A new perspective. Kidney Int 26:375, 1984

129. Myers BD, Moran SM: Hemodynamically mediated acute renal failure. N Engl J Med 314:97, 1986

130. Wardle N: Acute renal failure in the 1980s: The importance of septic shock and of endotoxaemia. Nephron 30:193, 1982

131. Miller TR, Anderson RJ, Linas SL et al: Urinary diagnostic indices in acute renal failure. A prospective study. Ann Intern Med 89:47, 1978

132. Espinel CH, Gregory AW: Differential diagnosis of acute renal failure. Clin Nephrol 13:73, 1980

133. Oken DE: On the differential diagnosis of acute renal failure. Am J Med 71:916, 1981

134. Pru C, Kjellstrand CM: The FE_{Na} test is of no prognostic value in acute renal failure. Nephron 36:20, 1984

135. Diamond JR, Yoburn DC: Nonoliguric acute renal failure associated with a low fractional excretion of sodium. Ann Intern Med 96:597, 1982

136. Cronin RE, Erickson AM, de Torrente A et al: Norepinephrine-induced acute renal failure: A reversible ischemic model of acute renal failure. Kidney Int 14:187, 1978

137. Lucas CE, Zito JG, Carter KM et al: Questionable value of furosemide in preventing renal failure. Surgery 82:314, 1977

138. Cronin RE, de Torrente A, Miller PD et al: Pathogenic mechanisms in early norepinephrine-induced acute renal failure: Functional and histological correlates of protection. Kidney Int 14:115, 1978

139. Patak RV, Fadem SZ, Lifschitz MD et al: Study of factors which modify the development of norepinephrine-induced acute renal failure in the dog. Kidney Int 15:227, 1979

140. Burke TJ, Cronin RE, Duchin KL et al: Ischemia and tubule obstruction during acute renal failure in dogs: Mannitol in protection. Am J Physiol 238:F305, 1980

141. Hanley MJ, Davidson K: Prior mannitol and furosemide infusion in a model of ischemic acute renal failure. Am J Physiol 241:F556, 1981

142. de Torrente A, Miller PD, Cronin RE et al: Effects of furosemide and acetylcholine in norepinephrine-induced acute renal failure. Am J Physiol 235:F131, 1978

143. Lindner A, Cutler RE, Goodman WG et al: Synergism of dopamine plus furosemide in preventing acute renal failure in the dog. Kidney Int 16:158, 1979

144. Henderson IS, Beattie TJ, Kennedy AC: Dopamine hydrochloride in oliguric states. Lancet 2:827, 1980

145. Davis RF, Lappas DG, Kirklin JK et al: Acute oliguria after cardiopulmonary bypass: Renal functional improvement with low-dose dopamine infusion. Crit Care Med 10:852, 1982

146. Barry KG, Cohen A, Knochel JP et al: Mannitol infusion. II. The prevention of acute functional renal failure during resection of an aneurysm of the abdominal aorta. N Engl J Med 264:967, 1961

147. Bush HL Jr, Huse JB, Johnson WC et al: Prevention of renal

insufficiency after abdominal aortic aneurysm resection by optimal volume loading. Arch Surg 116:1517, 1981

148. Wait RB, White G, Davis JH: Beneficial effects of verapamil on postischemic renal failure. Surgery 94:276, 1983

149. Goldfarb D, Iaina A, Serban I et al: Beneficial effect of verapamil in ischemic acute renal failure in the rat. Proc Soc Exper Biol Med 172:389, 1983

150. Burke TJ, Arnold PE, Gordon JA et al: Protective effect of intrarenal calcium membrane blockers before or after renal ischemia. Functional, morphological, and mitochondrial studies. J Clin Invest 74:1830, 1984

151. Lifschitz MD, Barnes JL: Prostaglandin I₂ attenuates ischemic acute renal failure in the rat. Am J Physiol 247:F714, 1984

152. Lelcuk S, Alexander F, Kobzik L et al: Prostacyclin and thromboxane A₂ moderate postischemic renal failure. Surgery 98:207, 1985

153. Casey KF, Machiedo GW, Lyons MJ et al: Alteration of postischemic renal pathology by prostaglandin infusion. J Surg Res, 29:1, 1980

154. Tobimatsu M, Konomi K, Saito S et al: Protective effect of prostaglandin E₁ on ischemia-induced acute renal failure in dogs. Surgery 98:45, 1985

155. Mauk RH, Patak RV, Fadem SZ et al: Effect of prostaglandin E administration in a nephrotoxic and a vasoconstrictor model of acute renal failure. Kidney Int 12:122, 1977

156. Mandal AK, Miller J: Protection against ischemic acute renal failure by prostaglandin infusion. Prostaglandins Leukotrienes Med 8:361, 1982

157. Hirasawa H, Odaka M, Soeda K et al: Experimental and clinical study on ATP-MgCl₂ administration for postischemic acute renal failure. Clin Exp Dial Apheresis 7:37, 1983

158. Gaudio KM, Taylor MR, Chaudry IH et al: Accelerated recovery of single nephron function by the postischemic infusion of ATP-MgCl₂. Kidney Int 22:13, 1982

159. Siegel NJ, Glazier WB, Chaudry IH et al: Enhanced recovery from acute renal failure by the postischemic infusion of adenine nucleotides and magnesium chloride in rats. Kidney Int 17:338, 1980

160. Cronin RE, Brown DM, Simonsen R: Protection by thyroxine in nephrotoxic acute renal failure. Am J Physiol 251:F408, 1986

161. Magnusson MO, Rybka SJ, Stowe NT et al: Enhancement of recovery in postischemic acute renal failure with captopril. Kidney Int 24 (suppl 16):S324, 1983

162. Anderson RJ, Linas SL, Berns AS et al: Nonoliguric acute renal failure. N Engl J Med 296:1134, 1977

163. Shin B, Mackenzie CF, McAslan TC et al: Postoperative renal failure in trauma patients. Anesthesiology 51:218, 1979

164. Moran SM, Myers BD: Pathophysiology of protracted acute renal failure in man. J Clin Invest 76:1440, 1985

165. Hilberman M, Derby GC, Spencer RJ et al: Sequential pathophysiological changes characterizing the progression from renal dysfunction to acute renal failure following cardiac operation. J Thorac Cardiovasc Surg 79:838, 1980

166. Hilberman M, Myers BD, Carrie BJ et al: Acute renal failure following cardiac surgery. J Thorac Cardiovasc Surg 77:880, 1979

167. Moran SM, Myers BD: Course of acute renal failure studies by a model of creatinine kinetics. Kidney Int 27:928, 1985

168. Myers BD, Miller DC, Mehigan JT et al: Nature of the renal injury following total renal ischemia in man. J Clin Invest 73:329, 1984

169. Krasna MJ, Scott GE, Scholz PM et al: Postoperative enhancement of urinary output in patients with acute renal failure using continuous furosemide therapy. Chest 89:294, 1986

170. Lindner A: Synergism of dopamine and furosemide in diuretic-resistant, oliguric acute renal failure. Nephron 33:121: 1983

171. Kleinknecht D, Ganeval D, Gonzalez–Duque LA et al: Furosemide in acute oliguric renal failure. A controlled trial. Nephron 17:51, 1976

172. Brown CB, Ogg CS, Cameron JS: High dose furosemide in acute renal failure: A controlled trial. Clin Nephrol 15:90, 1981

173. Epstein M, Schneider NS, Befeler B: Effect of intrarenal furosemide on renal function and intrarenal hemodynamics in acute renal failure. Am J Med 58:510, 1975

174. Prewitt RM, Matthay MA, Ghignone M: Hemodynamic management in the adult respiratory distress syndrome. Clin Chest Med 4:251, 1983

175. Miller SB, Anderson RJ: The kidney in acute respiratory failure. J Crit Care 2:45, 1987

176. McMurray SD, Luft FC, Maxwell DR et al: Prevailing patterns and predictor variables in patients with acute tubular necrosis. Arch Intern Med 138:950, 1978

177. Frankel MC, Weinstein AM, Stenzel KH: Prognostic patterns in acute renal failure: The New York Hospital, 1981–1982. Clin Exp Dial Apheresis 7:145, 1983

178. Bullock ML, Umen AJ, Finkelstein M et al: The assessment of risk factors in 462 patients with acute renal failure. Am J Kidney Dis 5:97, 1985

179. Bell RC, Coalson JJ, Smith JD et al: Multiple organ system failure and infection in adult respiratory distress syndrome. Ann Intern Med 99:293, 1983

180. Bartlett RH, Morris AH, Fairley HB et al: A prospective study of acute hypoxic respiratory failure. Chest 89:684, 1986

181. Kraman S, Khan F, Patel S et al: Renal failure in the respiratory intensive care unit. Crit Care Med 7:263, 1979

182. Montgomery AB, Stager MA, Carrico CJ et al: Causes of mortality in patients with the adult respiratory distress syndrome. Am Rev Respir Dis 132:485, 1985

183. Conahan TJ III: Coronary artery disease—Special anesthetic considerations. In Cardiac Anesthesia, p 180. Palo Alto, California, Addison-Wesley, 1982

184. Calkins JM, Conahan TJ III: Pumps, primes, and perfusion techniques. In Conahan TJ III (ed): Cardiac Anesthesia, p 194. Palo Alto, California, Addison-Wesley, 1982

185. Ream AK: Cardiovascular physiology: Application to clinical problems. In Ream AK, Fogdall RP (eds): Acute Cardiovascular Management: Anesthesia and Intensive Care, p 15. Philadelphia, JB Lippincott, 1982

186. Maseda J, Hilberman M, Derby GC et al: The renal effects of sodium nitroprusside in postoperative cardiac surgical patients. Anesthesiology 54:284, 1981

187. Honda N, Kurokawa K: Acute renal failure and rhabdomyolysis. Kidney Int 23:888, 1983

188. Byrick RJ: Acute renal failure: Update. Can Anaesth Soc J 33:S9, 1986

189. Bennett WM, Aronoff GR, Morrison G et al: Drug prescribing in renal failure: Dosing guidelines for adults. Am J Kidney Dis 3:155, 1983

190. Hastings PR, Skillman JJ, Bushnell LS et al: Antacid titration in the prevention of acute gastrointestinal bleeding. A controlled randomized trial in 100 critically ill patients. N Engl J Med 298:1041, 1978

191. Borrero E, Bank S, Margolis I et al: Comparison of antacid and sucralfate in the prevention of gastrointestinal bleeding in patients who are critically ill. Am J Med 79(suppl 2C):62, 1985

192. Tryba M, Zevounou F, Torok M et al: Prevention of acute stress bleeding with sucralfate, antacids, or cimetidine. A controlled study with pirenzepine as a basid medication. Am J Med 79(suppl 2C):55, 1985

193. Priebe HJ, Skillman JJ, Bushnell LS et al: Antacid versus cimetidine in preventing acute gastrointestinal bleeding. A randomized trial in 75 critically ill patients. N Engl J Med 302:426, 1980

194. Zinner MJ, Zuidema GD, Smith PL et al: The prevention of upper

gastrointestinal tract bleeding in patients in an intensive care unit. Surg Gynecol Obstet 153:214, 1981

195. Tilney NL, Bailey GL, Morgan AP: Sequential system failure after rupture of abdominal aortic aneurysms: An unsolved problem in postoperative care. Ann Surg 178:117, 1973

196. Fry DE, Pearlstein L, Fulton RL *et al:* Multiple system organ failure. The role of uncontrolled infection. Arch Surg 115:136, 1980

197. Knaus WA, Draper EA, Wagner DP *et al:* Prognosis in acute organ-system failure. Ann Surg 202:685, 1985

Chapter 40

Wen-Shin Liu
K.C. Wong

Anesthesia for Genitourinary Surgery

In this decade, important advances have been made in surgery of the genitourinary system. Especially notable is the use of shock wave lithotripsy for the nonsurgical removal of renal stones. With improved health care and diet in the United States, the elderly population is increasing to occupy a quarter of the population of surgical patients. Prostatectomy, a surgical intervention of the elderly male, is being performed with increased frequency. To meet these challenges, sophisticated and invasive monitors have also become more common in the operating room.

An appreciation of the pathology that can alter normal physiologic functions and the surgical procedures to correct the pathology will help the anesthesiologist to optimize preoperative preparation and intraoperative anesthetic management of these patients.

REGIONAL ANESTHESIA IN GENITOURINARY PROCEDURES

Regional anesthesia has a particular place in urologic surgery because the majority of procedures are in the lower abdomen and are thus easily performed under regional anesthetic techniques. Most of the urologic procedures, with the exception of operations on the kidney, can be well managed under regional anesthesia alone. Some require supplement with light general anesthesia in addition to regional anesthesia because of either exaggerated position or prolonged surgery.

The surgical procedures on the kidney in the lateral position with the kidney elevator beneath the twelfth rib can be performed under epidural anesthesia in some selected patients.

But the kidney position may not only be uncomfortable for a conscious patient but may also cause serious cardiovascular and respiratory embarrassment. The anesthesiologist must be wary of the potential problems of accidental injury to the pleura and lung with a subcostal incision in a spontaneously breathing patient.

Deep vein thrombosis of the legs occurs more often in patients undergoing genitourinary surgery. Lumbar epidural anesthesia was significantly better than general anesthesia in reducing the incidence of deep vein thrombosis.[1] It is probable that both the increased circulation produced by epidural anesthesia and the reduced blood loss with a decreased need for blood transfusion of the epidural patients may have contributed to the reduced occurrence of deep vein thrombosis.

It is commonly believed that regional anesthesia causes a higher incidence of postoperative urinary retention and the need for catheterization than does general anesthesia. The mechanism is presumed to be delayed recovery of autonomic and somatic nerve function, eventually leading to overdistention and atony of the bladder under regional anesthesia. The inability to empty the bladder is also exaggerated by overdistention when intravenous fluid therapy is overzealous. The site of operation, however, may be more important than the type of anesthesia in determining whether urinary retention would occur. Operative trauma to the detrusor muscle of the bladder or pelvic nerves, edema around the bladder neck, and pain-induced reflex spasm of the urethral sphincters may contribute to postoperative urinary retention. An indwelling catheter should be prophylactically inserted to minimize urinary retention from bladder dysfunction or vesical neck obstruction following surgery.

POSITIONS IN GENITOURINARY PROCEDURES

The positions required for surgery on the genitourinary system are anatomically unusual. These include the Trendelenburg position (head down and feet up tilt) for intrapelvic surgeries, lithotomy position for cystoscopic procedures, exaggerated lithotomy position for perineal prostatectomy, flank position with the kidney rest elevated, and the semisitting position in a water bath for extracorporeal shock wave lithotripsy. These positions have physiologically disadvantageous effects on patients (see Chapter 10).

ANESTHESIA FOR URETHRAL AND BLADDER PROCEDURES

URETHRAL PROCEDURES

Simple procedures, such as external urethrostomy or dilatation of the urethra, can sometimes be performed with topical anesthesia using 2% lidocaine jelly in addition to premedication or intravenous sedation, especially in older patients with poor risk status and in patients with neurogenic bladder dysfunction owing to spinal injury. Penile blockade also offers good analgesia for the distal urethra and is simple to perform for outpatients.

Internal urethrotomies are procedures that use the lithotomy position and need good sacral block with some lumbar analgesia for muscle relaxation of the legs to keep the legs in stirrups. Caudal or spinal anesthesia is useful for these procedures and, with supplemental intravenous sedation, patients can be kept comfortable. Urethroplasties are generally done in the exaggerated lithotomy position, requiring 3 to 4 hours of surgery; therefore, general anesthesia is preferable. However, regional anesthesia has been used in selected patients. Spinal anesthesia with hyperbaric tetracaine with epinephrine or continuous lumbar epidural anesthesia with 0.5% bupivacaine has been used with success. Supplemental sedation is usually necessary.

BLADDER PROCEDURES

Cystoscopic procedures done for diagnosis or surgical therapy are relatively minor and are generally performed on an outpatient basis. There is wide variation in anesthetic techniques for cystoscopy, including intramuscular opioid premedication, topical anesthetic jelly, intravenous sedation (diazepam or midazolam), regional blocks, and general anesthesia. Sensations aroused by bladder distention are mediated by sensory fibers accompanying the sympathetic and parasympathetic nerves that arise from T9 to L2 segments of the spinal cord. Therefore, a level of block to T9 is usually required. Spinal, lumbar epidural, or caudal anesthesia have all proved satisfactory. All the usual local anesthetics have been used satisfactorily. Quadriplegics or paraplegics are a special group of patients who may undergo repeated cystoscopies and stone manipulations; care must be taken to avoid autonomic hyperreflexia if the injured cord level is above T5.[2] Autonomic hyperreflexia is a disorder limited primarily to spinal cord–injured patients, occurring in 66–85% of quadriplegics and high paraplegics.[3] It is manifested by acute generalized sympathetic hyperactivity (e.g., paroxysmal hypertension, bradycardia, cardiac dysrhythmias) in response to stimuli below the level of transection, such as catheterization or irrigation of the bladder. To develop a full-blown paroxysmal hypertension, the lesion of spinal cord injury has to be above the splanchnic outflow (from T4 or T6). Lesions between T5 and T10 result in mild elevations of blood pressure.[2] General, epidural, or spinal anesthesia is effective in preventing this phenomenon, although it may technically be difficult to perform regional anesthesia in spinal cord–injured patients.[4]

Endoscopic Treatment of Bladder Tumors

Bladder tumors are generally resected by endoscopic transurethral resection. Bladder perforation has been reported from jerking of the patient's legs during surgery. In addition to inadequate anesthesia, electrical stimulation of the obturator nerve from the resectoscope can also cause leg movements, which can be abolished by muscle relaxants under general anesthesia or by regional blockade (spinal caudal or epidural).

Vesicouretal Reflux

Vesicouretal reflux (VUR) is manifested by the reflux of urine into the ureter secondary to an incompetent valve mechanism at the ureterovesicular junction. Vesicouretal reflux is the most frequent urinary tract problem other than urinary tract infection and is usually a congenital anomaly frequently manifested in children. Anesthesia is needed for the diagnostic evaluation or the surgical treatment of these pediatric patients.

The usual diagnostic studies include cystoscopy, retrograde intravenous pyelograms, and various forms of urodynamics, including urethral pressure profile and voiding cystourethrograms. It has been found that sedative and all inhalation anesthetics except nitrous oxide decrease sphincter pressure to such a degree as to invalidate the results.[5] The urodynamic studies are difficult to perform in awake children; therefore, some anesthesia is needed to facilitate the study. Light general anesthesia, however, may lead to laryngospasm associated with instrumentation of the urethra; therefore, the anesthesiologist should be prepared to provide deeper anesthesia to carry out urethral instrumentation and later light anesthesia to perform voiding studies. It has been shown that if urodynamic studies are delayed for an appropriate period of time following induction of anesthesia and if instrumentation is performed under deeper anesthesia, reliable results can be obtained by lightening anesthesia, using nitrous oxide and oxygen only in children.[6] Although atropine may be a desirable antisialogogue drug and is effective in preventing bradycardia during induction of anesthesia in children, it relaxes the smooth muscle of the bladder and invalidates urodynamic studies. Therefore, premedication with atropine should be avoided.

The major medical problems associated with VUR are renal damage and hypertension. These problems have been documented in 10–20% of children with VUR and renal scarring. Hypertension resulting from VUR may occur in the absence of altered renal function because it is associated more with vascular damage than with any particular amount of parenchymal damage. Also, the frequency of urinary tract infection and the need for antibiotics may result in the administration of various antibiotics that could enhance, or by themselves may cause, neuromuscular blockade. The surgical approach of VUR is to reimplant the ureter(s).

Suprapubic Cystostomy

Regional anesthesia in the form of spinal, epidural, caudal, or field blockade can also be performed for suprapubic cystostomy. Field block or local infiltration, which are still performed by some surgeons, may be inadequate because of the limited muscular relaxation and analgesia.

Radical Cystectomy with Ileal Conduit Formation

The removal of the bladder and its replacement by an ileal conduit for bladder cancer is a major operation that carries a high morbidity and mortality. Preoperatively, patients are frequently undernourished and often have undergone radiation therapy, making surgical dissection more difficult. Preoperative nutritional supplement with intravenous hyperalimentation has been advocated. Patients may be dehydrated from extensive bowel preparation and enemas preoperatively; thus, particular care should be taken to hydrate these patients before instituting anesthesia, especially if spinal or epidural anesthesia is used. Notable intraoperative problems include bleeding, prolonged operative time, intravascular fluid loss to "third space," and heat loss frequently associated with bowel surgery. Manipulation of the bowel during surgery can cause significant fluid loss to third-space compartments, and this combined with the inability to measure urine output make the use of a central venous pressure catheter important in monitoring changes in intravascular volume.

Regional anesthesia alone is unsuitable for most of the patients undergoing this surgery because of the long duration and extent of surgery. Continuous epidural anesthesia combined with light general endotracheal anesthesia has been shown to reduce intraoperative blood loss.[7] Other advantages for the use of this technique are early extubation of the trachea and continued postoperative analgesia, which can be achieved by epidural opioids or local anesthetics. Since blood loss can be considerable, hypotensive anesthesia has been advocated to minimize blood loss.

ANESTHESIA FOR OPERATIONS ON THE EXTERNAL GENITALIA

These procedures are done in patients of various age groups. High reflexogenic sensitivity is present in the genital and perineal areas; therefore, when general anesthesia is used, deep planes of anesthesia are generally required to prevent undesirable autonomic reflexes such as laryngospasm and hypertension. Laryngospasm is a common occurrence secondary to urethral instrumentation or dilation of the rectum in a lightly anesthetized patient.[8] Neural blockade in the form of penile, caudal, saddle, or epidural blockade suppresses these responses completely. Another major reason for consideration of regional techniques is to provide postoperative pain relief and obviate the need for analgesics during the immediate postoperative period.

Surgical procedures on the scrotum, testicles, and epididymis and reconstructive operations on the vas deferens can be done under spinal anesthesia or epidural anesthesia, depending upon the duration and extent of surgery. Testicular innervation can be traced up to the T10 segment; thus, a T10 level blockade may be required to prevent pain from testicular traction and/or manipulation. Vasectomies performed in clinics are usually done under local infiltration anesthesia with 1% lidocaine or mepivacaine. Reconstructive surgery on the vas deferens, however, requires longer surgical time, and regional blockade is required. Penile prosthetic surgery requires several hours of analgesia and can be done under spinal anesthesia with hyperbaric tetracaine with epinephrine, continuous lumbar epidural, or caudal anesthesia using 15 to 20 ml of 0.5% bupivacaine.

Hypospadias is one of the most frequent genitourinary anomalies. It is associated with hernias and hydroceles but does not appear to carry an increased risk of upper urinary tract anomalies. The potential psychological difficulty, along with the concerns of toilet training, usually favors surgical repair at the age of 1 year under general anesthesia.

Orchiopexy is increasingly being performed on an outpatient basis.[9, 10] General anesthesia should be used in children, because the procedure may be lengthy, and abdominal musculature relaxation is often helpful. Considerable postoperative pain, associated with a high incidence of nausea and vomiting, occurs with this operation. Caudal anesthesia (0.25% bupivacaine, 0.5 ml·kg^{-1}) or ilioinguinal/iliohypogastric nerve blocks (0.25% bupivacaine, in dosages up to 2 mg·kg^{-1}) have been shown to provide highly effective postoperative analgesia following orchiopexy in children under general anesthesia.[10]

Surgical procedures on the penis, such as circumcision and hypospadias correction are most commonly performed in children. In these patients, postoperative analgesia may be especially important, because agitation and restlessness with pain may cause unwanted manipulation of the operative site by patients resulting in postoperative hemorrhage. Caudal and penile blockade have both been used after children are anesthetized with intravenous drugs or light general anesthesia with mask. These techniques have proved valuable in providing postoperative analgesia.

CAUDAL BLOCKADE

Caudal blockade provides excellent postoperative analgesia following a wide variety of surgical procedures such as hypospadias repair, orchiopexy, and circumcision. The blockade is performed with the child in a lateral or semiprone position after induction of general anesthesia or anesthesia with ketamine or a barbiturate. Bupivacaine 0.25% (1.25 to 1.5 mg·kg^{-1}) can be injected through the sacrococcygeal membrane with a 20-gauge 3.75-cm needle. It has been shown that caudal analgesia (1.25 to 1.5 mg·kg^{-1} bupivacaine) was significantly better than intramuscular morphine (0.15 mg·kg^{-1}) or buprenorphine for immediate postoperative analgesia and had a lower frequency of postoperative vomiting after circumcision in boys.[11, 12]

PENILE BLOCKADE

Penile blockade may be used for most surgical procedures performed on the penis, such as circumcision, and for insertion of a penile prosthesis. It is a simple and safe procedure to perform in adult and pediatric patients, with fewer associated complications compared with caudal blockade. To perform this blockade for penile surgery in adults, a 25- or 27-gauge needle is inserted through the skin at the 2:00 o'clock and 10:00 o'clock positions at the base of the penis until the lower border of the symphysis pubis is contacted. The needle is withdrawn slightly and moved progressively in a caudal direction until bone is no longer contacted. A "pop" may be felt as the deep (Buck's) fascia of the penis is pierced. Local anesthetics are injected, 1 ml of 1% lidocaine at each side. A triangle of local anesthetic (about 10 to 15 ml of 1% lidocaine) is also placed at the base of the penis, with the pubic tubercles and a point just inferior to the undersurface of the penis on the scrotum as the corners of the triangle.[13] A blockade of the dorsal nerves of the penis only (1 to 4 ml of 0.25% bupivacaine) has also been found to provide good postoperative analgesia (lasts more than 6 hours) in 96% of children after circumcision or correction of hypospadias and has proved to be a good alternative to opioid analgesics.[14] For postoperative analgesia, the local anesthetic used most often is 0.25% bupivacaine without epinephrine; volumes range from 0.8 ml in the neonate to 10 ml in the adult. Epinephrine-containing solutions should not be used because of the risk of ischemia of the penis.

Topical analgesia has also been successfully used for pain relief after circumcision in pediatric patients. A thin film of lidocaine spray, 10 to 20 mg of 10% solution, lidocaine ointment (0.5 to 1 ml of a 5% preparation), or lidocaine jelly (0.5 to 1 ml of a 2% preparation) can be applied to the surgical wound postoperatively but before the child is awake. Topical lidocaine has the advantage of being noninvasive and simple and provides an extended period of analgesia.[15]

ANESTHESIA FOR PROSTATIC SURGERY

Benign prostatic hypertrophy is a common disease of the elderly male that requires surgical removal of the prostatic gland when obstruction of urinary outflow through the prostatic urethra becomes symptomatic. This patient population generally carries greater anesthetic risk because its members are likely to have coexisting cardiovascular and/or pulmonary problems. It is estimated that only 4% of the U.S. population were 65 years or older in 1900, but this group had increased to 11% by 1980 and is expected to increase to 12.5% (about 52 million) by the year 2000. Thus, an increasing number of elderly male patients is expected to come to the operating room for surgical resection of their enlarged prostate gland. In addition to the increase in incidence of cardiopulmonary disease in the elderly male, the physiologic changes of aging will reduce the anesthetic or drug requirement for the body as well as contribute to intraoperative and postoperative morbidity and mortality (see Chapter 48).

OPEN PROSTATECTOMY

Open prostatectomy can be performed through a suprapubic (transvesical), a retropubic, or perineal approach. The choice of using an open prostatectomy versus transurethral resection of the prostate is mainly due to an excessively enlarged prostate gland or to the presence of other intravesical pathologic conditions that warrant open exploration. Prostates greater than 80 g are more conveniently removed by open prostatectomy, which reduces the morbidity associated with the transurethral approach.

Open prostatectomy can be performed under either general or regional anesthesia. Considerations that influence the choice of regional or general anesthesia are: 1) the status of the patient's cardiopulmonary system, 2) the position of the patient for the surgery, and 3) the patient's mental status. The patient who has significant cardiopulmonary problems will often not tolerate fluid overload and electrolyte imbalance compared with a more healthy patient. Having control of ventilation of the lungs and ensuring adequate oxygenation will favor general anesthesia for such patients. Uncooperative patients, especially those elderly persons who are mentally confused or disoriented, are also easier managed by general anesthesia. On the other hand, regional anesthesia, especially spinal anesthesia, has the advantage of being simple to administer and allows the patient to be relatively pain-free during the recovery period. Furthermore, this approach lessens postoperative agitation and restlessness, which are frequently associated with general anesthesia in elderly patients during the postoperative period. In addition, the use of epidural or spinal anesthetic technique has been shown to reduce operative blood loss during lower abdominal or transurethral resection of the prostate (TURP) procedures.[16-18] Although spinal anesthesia has the advantage of being simpler to perform than epidural anesthesia and also requires less local anesthetic, it does have the disadvantage of producing a more profound sympathetic blockade, thus often requiring large initial infusions of fluid to prevent hypotension in contrast to epidural anesthesia which is more controllable and produces less hypotension. Since the patient is supine during suprapubic retropubic prostatectomy, spinal or epidural anesthesia with light sedation has good patient acceptance as well as providing adequate anesthesia.

Perineal prostatectomy requires an exaggerated lithotomy position combined with some flexion of the trunk and moderate head down tilt. This position can cause marked impairment of the cardiovascular and respiratory systems. Although a continuous epidural anesthesia combined with a light general anesthesia with endotracheal intubation and controlled ventilation of the lungs using nitrous oxide–oxygen have been successfully used, most anesthesiologists prefer general anesthesia in such patients so that they may better control the cardiopulmonary system and intravascular fluid volume.

TRANSURETHRAL RESECTION OF THE PROSTATE (TURP)

TURP is preferred over suprapubic, retropubic, and perineal approaches which allow better surgical exposure to large prostate glands but carry higher morbidity. TURP carries unique complications because of the necessity to use large volumes of irrigating fluid for the endoscopic resection. Systemic absorption of nonelectrolyte irrigating fluid can produce circulatory overload, hyponatremia, hypoproteinemia, and the presence of the irrigating solute in circulation. Mortality from TURP appears to be significantly higher than the average anesthetic mortality.[20, 21] The anatomy of the pathologic hypertrophic gland, the size of the gland, and the skill of the resectionist all contribute to the morbidity associated with this surgical procedure. Therefore, it is germane to describe the pathologic changes of benign prostatic hypertrophy to better understand the pathophysiology associated with TURP and anesthetic management.

The prostate is a pear-shaped gland surrounding the prostatic urethra at the base of the bladder. Although anatomically the prostate has five lobes (one anterior, two lateral, one median, and one posterior), only the median and lateral lobes are enlarged and surgically excised in primary idiopathic prostatic hypertrophy (Fig. 40-1). In the majority of males older than 50 years of age, the submucosal glands and the smooth muscle of the prostatic urethra undergo glandular and leiomyomatous hyperplasia. This growth is stimulated by testicular hormones and presses the normal prostatic tissue against the fibrous capsule, forming a "surgical capsule" consisting of compressed normal prostatic tissue and veins, infiltrated by nodular new growth. Therefore, it is sometimes unavoidable that these compressed prostatic veins (sinuses) are entered during TURP and that irrigating fluid is absorbed into the intravascular compartment. However, fibrosis can sometimes occur in the hypertrophic prostatic gland and re-

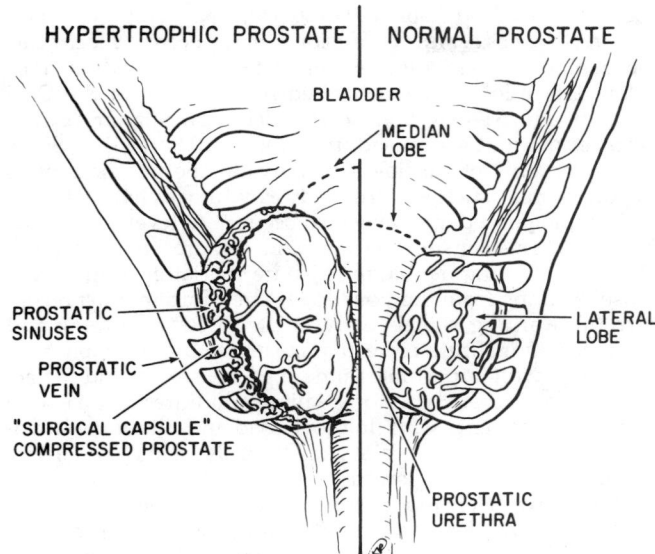

FIG. 40-1. Anatomy of hypertrophic prostate. The hypertrophic gland represents glandular and leiomyomatous hyperplasia of the submucosal glands and the smooth muscle of the prostatic urethra, thus pushing the normal prostatic tissue to create a "surgical capsule." (Reprinted from Stoelting RK, Barash PG, Gallagher TJ: Advances in Anesthesia, vol III, p 379. Chicago, Year Book Medical Publishers, with permission.)

duce the vascularity of the gland. Resection of a fibrotic gland is associated with less bleeding and fluid access into the circulation.

TURP is performed through a resectoscope and consists of excising the hypertrophied lateral and median lobes of the prostate gland with an electrically energized wire loop; bleeding is controlled with a coagulating current. Continuous irrigating fluid is used to distend the bladder and to wash away blood and dissected prostatic tissue. Distilled water provides the least interference with visibility; however, absorption of large quantities of water can lead to excessive dilutional hyponatremia, which results in hemolysis of red blood cells, water intoxication, and central nervous system (CNS) symptoms, ranging from confusion to convulsions and coma. Because of this, distilled water is generally abandoned in favor of non-electrolyte iso-osmotic or near–iso-osmotic solutions for TURP. On the other hand, electrolytic solutions such as normal saline or Ringer's lactate would do least harm when absorbed into the circulation, but they are highly ionized and promote dispersion of high current from the resectoscope. Therefore, non-electrolyte solutions consisting of sorbitol and mannitol (Cytal), or of glycine, 1.5%, which are slightly hypoosmolar to the blood, have been used most often.[22, 23]

Since the prostate gland contains large venous sinuses, it is inevitable that irrigating solution will be absorbed. The amount of absorption is governed mainly by the hydrostatic pressure driving fluid into prostatic veins and sinuses, which is determined by the height of the container of irrigating solution above the surgical table. The amount of irrigating fluid absorbed during TURP is proportional to the duration of resection. On average, 10 to 30 ml of fluid is absorbed per minute of resection time, with as much as 6 to 8 l absorbed in some cases, lasting up to 2 hours.[24, 25] In addition, the number

and sizes of the venous sinuses opened during resection influences vascular absorption.[25] Although water intoxication is not totally preventable, limiting resecting time to less than 1 hour is desirable.[26, 27]

Optimizing the patient's preoperative condition is essential to the anesthetic management. Males older than 60 years of age generally carry greater anesthetic risk because they are more likely to have coexisting cardiovascular and/or pulmonary problems. Common findings in elderly patients are hypertension, angina, congestive heart failure, presence of an artificial cardiac pacemaker, diabetes mellitus, neurologic problems, and renal failure. Since TURP is generally an elective surgery, these patients should be in the best condition possible before surgery.

TURP Syndrome

Near the end of or immediately following TURP, anesthesiologists and urologists infrequently note a reaction that is initially characterized by headache, restlessness, confusion, nausea and vomiting, skeletal muscle twitching, bradycardia, and hypertension. These symptoms may evolve to hypotension, with cyanosis, dyspnea, cardiac dysrhythmias, seizures, and, occasionally, death.[24, 26, 28] A major component of the TURP syndrome is severe hyponatremia. Intravascular absorption of irrigating solution can lead to a significant increase in the blood volume (hypervolemia), dilutional hyponatremia, and decreased serum osmolarity (hypo-osmolarity), and adverse hemodynamic and central venous system changes.[26, 29, 30] A summary of complications of TURP is listed in Table 40-1.

Pathophysiology of Absorption of the Irrigating Fluid

As previously noted, the ideal irrigating solution for TURP should be optically satisfactory, iso-osmolar, nonhemolytic, weakly or nonionized, and inexpensive. Today, glycine and Cytal are the two most commonly used irrigating solutions for TURP. Cytal is a combination of 2.7% sorbitol and 0.54% mannitol, nonelectrolytic, iso-osmolar, and cleared from the plasma rapidly but is more expensive than glycine. Glycine 1.5% in water is most commonly used because of low cost but is a slightly hypo-osmolar solution (230 mOsm $\cdot$ l^{-1}). Nevertheless, it has eliminated hemolysis and reduced sequelae associated with TURP compared with the use of distilled water as the irrigating solution. However, the other major

TABLE 40-1. Complications of TURP of Particular Interest to Anesthesiologists

I. Intravascular absorption of irrigating fluid
   a. Fluid overload
   b. Serum hypo-osmolarity
   c. Hyponatremia
   d. Hyperglycinemia and hyperammonemia
   e. Hemolysis
   f. Hypothermia
   g. Bacteremia
II. Blood loss
III. Perforation of bladder or urethra with extravasation
   a. Extraperitoneal
   b. Intraperitoneal

problem associated with absorption of large volumes of irrigating solution, and overhydration, still remains. Moreover, recent data suggest potential chemical toxicity associated with the absorption of glycine and its metabolic product (ammonia).[31-33]

The irrigation solution used during TURP is absorbed through open venous sinuses of the gland; the amount absorbed varies considerably depending upon the area of raw surface exposed by the surgeon, the hydrostatic pressure exerted by the irrigating solution, and the duration of the procedure.[24] When irrigating fluid rapidly enters the vascular compartment, the load on the circulation as well as myocardial work are increased. The nonelectrolytic solution (glycine, 1.5%) dilutes blood proteins as well as electrolytes. The additive effects of increased intravascular pressure and decreased protein oncotic pressure favor the movement of the fluid from the vascular compartment to the interstitial compartment.[34] Under usual conditions, only 20–30% of a load of crystalloid solution remains in the intravascular space; the remainder enters the interstitial space. For every 100 ml of fluid entering the interstitial compartment, 10 to 15 mEq of sodium also moves with it.[22] Desmond reported a patient who gained 2.2 kg by the end of the operation but whose blood volume increased only 500 ml. The other 1,500 ml of fluid presumably moved into the interstitial compartment and carried with it 100 to 150 mEq of sodium. When intravenous pressure is increased, movement of fluid into the interstitial space and the formation of pulmonary edema are favored. Whether patients will develop symptoms of circulatory overload depends upon their cardiovascular status, the amount and rapidity of absorption of irrigating fluid, and the extent of surgical blood loss. Therefore, it is imperative to monitor the patients carefully. In this regard, spinal or epidural anesthesia, supplemented with only light intravenous sedation, has the advantage of allowing the patient to verbalize potential cardiopulmonary and CNS problems during surgery. In addition, cardiovascular depression associated with administration of potent volatile anesthetics is avoided. Regional anesthesia produces sympathetic blockade and increases venous capacitance, which tends to mitigate against intraoperative fluid overload during TURP. However, a note of caution is needed when the blockade dissipates: Venous capacity acutely decreases, and circulatory overload could occur during postsurgical recovery. In this regard, urinary output must be ensured.

If dilutional hyponatremia develops rapidly, serum osmolarity also falls, promoting efflux of intravascular fluid into other compartments. Signs of cerebral and pulmonary edema may appear. All TURP patients will have some degree of dilutional hyponatremia, but only those in whom the heart is incapable of handling the fluid overload will manifest cerebral edema, increased intracranial pressure, and pulmonary edema. Central nervous system symptoms, including apprehension, irritability, confusion, headache, seizures, transient blindness, and coma, have been usually attributed to hyponatremia and water hypo-osmolarity.

Hyponatremia can disturb electrophysiology. The concentration of extracellular sodium must be in a physiologic range for effective depolarization of excitable cells and for production of action potentials. When brain cells are incapable of producing effective impulses, CNS symptoms ensue. When myocardial cells are incapable of producing effective impulses, cardiac dysrhythmias may develop. Hyponatremia also contributes to negative inotropic effects and hypotension. A serum sodium level of 120 mEq·l⁻¹ appears to be borderline for the development of severe reactions. When extracellular sodium levels drop below 120 mEq·l⁻¹, CNS symptoms, usually restlessness and confusion, may occur. Electrocardiographic changes are seen when the serum sodium falls below 115 mEq·l⁻¹, characterized by widening of the QRS complex and ST elevation on the electrocardiogram (ECG). Seizures occur at serum sodium levels of 102 mEq·l⁻¹. Signs and symptoms of cardiovascular dysfunction secondary to hyponatremia, such as cardiac dysrhythmias, hypotension, and pulmonary edema, may also occur.[35] At levels below 100 mEq·l⁻¹, consciousness is lost and seizures may ensue.[36] However, it is impossible to separate the latter events from those resulting from fluid overload. The clinician must recognize the warning signals early in the TURP syndrome and immediately institute corrective measures by re-establishing isotonicity with hypertonic saline (e.g., 5% saline) and replacing the blood loss. Hypertonic saline and diuretics are useful therapy for patients with fluid overload and dilutional hyponatremia, but the patients' serum electrolytes and osmolarity should be carefully followed.

There have been reports of transient blindness following TURP, and attention has turned to the absorption of glycine, a nonessential amino acid, and its metabolic by-product, ammonia, as possible causes of visual impairment and CNS symptoms associated with TURP.[31, 37] Ovassapian and colleagues[31] suggested glycine as the possible cause of visual impairment. It is possible that both glycine and ammonia,[32] which is a primary metabolite of glycine, can produce CNS symptoms, which vary from mild depression, confusion, and transient blindness to coma. We have demonstrated in laboratory animals[33] and in TURP patients,[38] that pharmacologic doses of glycine can inhibit visual evoked potentials.

Glycine has a distribution in the CNS similar to gamma-aminobutyric acid (GABA), the latter an inhibitory transmitter, acting in the spinal cord and brain stem.[39, 40] Normal plasma glycine levels are 13 to 17 mg·l⁻¹, whereas levels as high as 1029 mg·l⁻¹ were measured during one episode of blindness in one patient.[31] Twelve hours later, the glycine level in this patient had fallen to 143 mg·l⁻¹, by which time vision had returned. It has also been suggested that systemic absorption of glycine may result in CNS toxicity as a result of the oxidative biotransformation of glycine to ammonia.[32, 37] In one report, encephalopathy after TURP was noted in three patients in association with elevated blood ammonia concentrations.[37] Each patient had blood ammonia levels more than 10 times the upper limit of normal. High ammonia concentration in the CNS after neutral amino acid metabolism can result in the production of false neurotransmitters and suppression of norepinephrine and dopamine release. This has been the proposed pathologic etiology of encephalopathy in a subset of patients who develop TURP syndrome.[37] Marked elevation in blood ammonia from metabolism of absorbed glycine solution may enhance or act independently of dilutional hyponatremia to produce encephalopathy common to TURP syndrome.[37] The picture is not yet clear, and the data are far from conclusive, but hyperglycinemia and increased serum concentrations of ammonia could be the potential causes of problems during TURP. In summary, fluid overload, hypo-osmolarity, and hyponatremia are the recognized factors contributing to the TURP syndrome; however, glycine and ammonia may also contribute to this complex clinical problem.

Blood Loss in TURP

Assessment of blood loss is difficult during TURP because of the dilution of blood with the irrigating fluid. The visual estimations of blood loss are often grossly inaccurate,[41, 42] and the usual hemodynamic responses of blood loss (*e.g.*, tachycardia, hypotension) are unreliable owing to the increased circulating volume accompanying absorption of irrigating fluid. Furthermore, a measurement of intraoperative hematocrit may be increased, decreased, or unchanged, depending upon the amount of fluid that is in the intravascular space at the time of measurement. Generally, intraoperative blood transfusion has not been necessary until more reliable indices of blood loss are ascertained in the postoperative period. It has been suggested[43] that given adequate blood bank service with provisions for emergency crossmatching and an experienced surgeon operating on a prostate weighing less than 30 g, preoperative crossmatching should not be required. If the predicted weight of the gland is 30 to 80 g, two units of blood will probably be required for transfusion; if the gland is larger than 80 g, the probable requirement will be four units. Blood transfusion intraoperatively should be based on preoperative hematocrit, duration and difficulty of the resection, and clinical assessment of the patient's condition. Continuous postoperative tendency to bleed may indicate a coagulation problem. Patients undergoing prostatic surgery have a much higher incidence of fibrinolysis.[44] It is postulated that prostatic tissue releases urokinase, which activates the transformation of plasminogen to plasma, which, in turn, lyses fibrin.[44]

Blood loss during TURP is generally related to vascularity of the prostate gland, the surgeon's experience and technique, the weight of the prostate resected, and length of operation (Table 40-2).[18, 43, 45–47] It is believed that a better way of comparing blood loss is to express it in milliliters per gram prostate resected per minute. Abrams et al[18] reported a significant reduction in blood loss when the regional anesthesia group (median 0.25 ml·g^{-1}·min^{-1}) was compared with the general anesthesia group (median 0.38 ml·g^{-1}·min^{-1}). There was no correlation between blood pressure and blood loss during operation. Blood loss is usually less in those patients undergoing TURP for carcinoma of the prostate.

Levin et al[43] showed that the bleeding per gram of resected tissue was fairly constant at about 15 ml·g^{-1}, although the severity of bleeding increased with duration of operation. Surgeons should, therefore, probably not try to undertake single-stage resection of a large prostate that cannot be completed within 1 hour. A two-stage resection or an open operation may be preferable if the feasibility of this time limit is in doubt.

Hypothermia During TURP

Older patients have an age-related decline in the function of the autonomic nervous system, which leads to progressive thermoregulatory impairment.[48] The ability to increase mean body temperature by increasing heat production is negatively correlated to age.[49] Elderly patients tolerate hypothermia poorly. Administration of intravenous fluid at ambient temperature and the constant irrigation of cold fluid through the bladder together with its intravascular absorption will rapidly lower core body temperature of patients undergoing TURP, especially in cold operating rooms. Intraoperative hypothermia is not influenced by the anesthetic technique used.[49, 50] General anesthesia reduces heat production, whereas this is uninfluenced by lumbar epidural analgesia.[49] But after termination of general anesthesia, oxygen uptake and plasma catecholamines increased; no such changes could be detected when epidural analgesia was used. The use of warming mattresses, together with the warming of both intravenous fluid infusions and bladder irrigating fluids, and even warming inspired anesthetic gases, will do much to ameliorate this problem. Hypothermia could be another intraoperative cause of confusion and disorientation in elderly patients. Hypothermia can cause shivering with increased oxygen consumption and cardiac irritability. Nasal administration of oxygen or mask oxygen supplementation should be provided along with regional anesthesia to these elderly patients. Shivering is also a common postoperative sequela, which, in turn, increases venous pressure and promotes hemorrhage. Hypothermia and pain are common causes of postsurgical increases of body metabolism; maintaining body temperature and ensuring postsurgical analgesia are important measures for providing optimal care of TURP patients.

Bacteremia

Bacteremia is a common occurrence following TURP. Infection of the prostate should be controlled prior to surgery. Sudden cardiovascular collapse after TURP is most commonly a manifestation of bacteremia, and no time should be lost in obtaining blood cultures. Broad-spectrum antibiotic therapy is given on the basis of the preoperative urine culture results, which should always be available at the time of TURP.[51]

Perforation of Bladder

Another complication of TURP is perforation of the bladder.[52] Perforations usually occur during difficult resections and are most often made by the cutting loop or knife electrode. Some, however, are made by the tip of the resectoscope or result from overdistention of the bladder with irrigating fluid. Most perforations are extraperitoneal and, in the conscious patient, result in pain in the periumbilical, inguinal, or suprapubic

TABLE 40-2. Intraoperative Blood Loss in TURP

	RELATED TO DURATION OF OPERATION	RELATED TO BLOOD PRESSURE IN OPERATING ROOM	INTRAOPERATIVE BLOOD LOSS (ml·g^{-1}·MIN OF RESECTED TISSUE) General	Regional	CORRELATED WITH SURGEONS SKILLS
Abrams et al[18]	Yes	No	0.38 (median)	0.25 (median)	Yes
McGowan et al[45]	Yes	Yes	Controlled ventilation 0.25 (median); spontaneous ventilation 0.27 (median)	0.21 (median)	Yes
Levin et al[43]	Yes	—	15.1 ± 1.2*	15.1 ± 1.2*	Yes
Madsen and Madsen[47]	Yes	Yes	21.0	14.6	Yes

*Author did not separate general *vs* regional intraoperative blood loss.

regions. Perforation of the prostatic capsule is suspected if the irrigation fluid fails to return as it should. Less often, the perforation is through the wall of the bladder and is intraperitoneal, or a large extraperitoneal perforation may extend into the peritoneum. In such cases, pain may be generalized in the upper abdomen or referred from the diaphragm to the precordial region or the shoulder. Other signs and symptoms such as pallor, diaphoresis, abdominal rigidity, nausea, vomiting, hypotension, and hypertension have been reported; their number and severity depend upon the location and size of the perforation and the type of irrigating fluid. Subdiaphragmatic irritation from intraperitoneal irrigating fluid may induce hiccup and shortness of breath. Generally, intraperitoneal fluid will be eventually excreted by the kidneys without the necessity for aggressive treatment. A small perforation can be managed conservatively with catheter drainage, but, if significant extravasation has occurred, it should be drained suprapubically.[51] When hemodynamic embarrassment occurs, suprapubic drainage is the most efficient manner of eliminating the excess intraperitoneal fluid. The incidence of perforation is estimated at 1.1%.[53]

Choice of Anesthetic Techniques

Choice of anesthetic technique for TURP is a matter for individual assessment. Regional techniques would seem to have the advantages of early warning of fluid overload and possibly decreased blood loss, but difficulties of placement of the local anesthetics because of vertebral disease, and the desire of many patients to be asleep, make general anesthesia just as acceptable.

General anesthesia may mask the early signs and symptoms of TURP syndrome but may be more desirable than regional anesthesia in patients who require pulmonary support, who cannot tolerate intravenous infusion of fluids to compensate for the rapid loss of sympathetic tone from regional anesthesia, or who require invasive monitoring. Provided that 1.5% glycine solution is used, hemolysis is generally avoided, but fluid overload can still occur with hyponatremia. Central venous pressure monitoring is helpful under such situations, and hyponatremia and fluid overload is corrected by administration of hypertonic saline solutions and diuretics.[51] Although increases in systolic and diastolic blood pressures are considered to be the classical signs of hypervolemia, abrupt falls in blood pressure can occur in response to dilutional hyponatremia and hypervolemia.

Spinal anesthesia has been advocated as the anesthetic of choice for TURP, because the patient is awake and capable of aiding the anesthesiologist in early recognition of intravascular absorption of irrigating fluid and can exhibit early signs of fluid overload and water intoxication. Also, the early diagnosis and treatment of inadvertent urinary bladder perforation, with extravasation of irrigating fluid can be recognized promptly. The amount of local anesthetic used for spinal anesthesia is small, and a solid block is generally predictable. Epidural or caudal anesthetics do not offer much advantage over spinal anesthesia because of a generally lower success rate using the extradural approaches. Furthermore, the controllability of continuous epidural anesthesia for the level and duration of anesthesia is usually not necessary for TURP. Since bladder sensation from overfilling can be uncomfortable, a T9–T10 level is desirable, but even a level of S3 is adequate in approximately 25% of patients. If the level is greater than T10, the capsular sign (pain on perforation of the capsule of the prostate) may not be preserved. Spinal anesthesia using isobaric 5% lidocaine or hyperbaric 0.5% tetracaine is

useful for TURP. Sacral segments may be missed with lumbar epidural blockade, and caudal anesthesia may be more suitable if the patient has had previous spine surgery or has an osteoarthritic spine. Recently, it has been reported that TURP can be performed successfully under local anesthesia with intravenous supplementation with sedatives in the majority of patients with small to moderate-sized prostate glands.[54] Local anesthetics (0.25% bupivacaine, 1% lidocaine, or both) were injected into the prostate transurethrally, and transperineal infiltration into the gland was with a lidocaine–bupivacaine mixture.

The use of regional techniques for this surgery is advocated by other anesthesiologists to minimize blood loss compared with general anesthetic techniques.[18] This is, however, debatable, because others found no difference in blood loss with patients under spinal anesthesia compared with those under general anesthesia, either breathing spontaneously or during mechanical ventilation of the lungs.[45] A significant cause of blood loss may be a rise in venous pressure brought about by straining or coughing as a result of a partially obstructed upper airway or from painful stimuli. The abolition of both of these factors by either regional anesthesia or maintenance of a patent upper airway could decrease hemorrhage. There is no place for controlled hypotension as a technique to limit blood loss in these patients. Regardless of whether general or regional anesthesia is selected, a careful evaluation of cardiopulmonary parameters is vital. Anesthesia and surgery for these patients require a high degree of expertise and vigilance.

Postoperatively, these patients benefit from diuresis to prevent clot formation as well as to remove excess water and glycine from the body. To maintain accurate fluid balance is difficult in these patients intraoperatively but should be achieved postoperatively. Analgesia is not usually a problem after patients are fully awake or after their regional blockade has worn off, because there is little discomfort from the operation.

ANESTHESIA FOR OTHER UROLOGIC PROCEDURES

LITHOTRIPSY

Percutaneous ultrasonic lithotripsy and extracorporeal shock wave lithotripsy (ESWL) represent new techniques in urologic surgery. Anesthetic management for these procedures may be different from routine general anesthesia.

Percutaneous Ultrasonic Lithotripsy

A nephroscope is introduced through a small flank incision in percutaneous ultrasonic lithotripsy. A hollow metal probe is inserted through the nephroscope to contact the calculus. The ultrasonic energy, delivered by this metal probe through this percutaneous nephrostomy track into the renal pelvis, is used to fracture renal or upper ureteral stones. The fragments are then flushed out with large quantities of irrigating fluids such as normal saline. This technique is being widely adopted by urologists, and, with the advent of ESWL, it is predicted that open renal surgery for stones will become an uncommon event.[51] Acute hyponatremia, acute hemolysis with hyperkalemia owing to sudden absorption of a bolus of water, and air embolism are possible complications in percutaneous ultrasonic lithotripsy. Because absorption of irrigating fluid is likely, the use of normal saline for irrigation is recommended.[55] In contrast to electroresection of the prostate, electrolytic irrigating solution does not interfere with percutaneous ultrasonic lithotripsy.

General, epidural, and local anesthesia have been successfully used for this procedure.

Extracorporeal Shock Wave Lithotripsy

Extracorporeal shock wave lithotripsy (ESWL) is a technique for pulverizing urinary stones, without surgical intervention, by means of shock waves, so that the disintegrated pieces of stones can be passed in the urine. Shock waves impose mechanical stresses that exceed the strength of brittle material such as kidney stones, and shock waves can be transmitted through water and propagated through the body without energy loss. In conjunction with suitable reflectors, shock waves can be focused and reproduced reliably. Extracorporeal shock wave lithotripsy promises to provide a completely noninvasive method for the treatment of kidney stones, and, since 1980, many patients have been treated by ESWL in many countries. Anesthesia is required for ESWL, because the shock wave causes pain. The shock wave (lasting a fraction of a second per each shock, but up to 2000 shocks occurring per treatment) feels like the prick of a pin when it reaches the skin; the pain is not restricted to the affected area. It also elicits visceral pain when it reaches the peritoneum and the renal capsule. Although local infiltration of the entry site with high doses of local anesthetic and intravenous sedatives has been used effectively in selected patients,[56] in the majority of patients, regional (spinal, epidural) or general anesthesia is required.

In ESWL, anesthesiologists are confronted with the problems of anesthetizing patients who are partly submerged in a stainless steel tank of warm water with only the head and arms out of the bath and the relative inaccessibility of the patient's airway (Fig. 40-2). The patient must be positioned properly so that the shock waves will travel harmlessly through the water until they hit the kidneys and disintegrate the stones, but not reach the lungs. Immersion has been shown to augment cardiac preload as a result of compression of peripheral vessels by hydrostatic pressure and a shift of blood volume into the central vascular compartment. Administration of anesthesia, immersion in water, or ESWL may affect these hemodynamic changes.[57-59] The use of a transesophageal Doppler ultrasonic cardiac output monitor has demonstrated a reduction in cardiac output together with an increase in mean arterial pressure and systemic vascular resistance in patients under general anesthesia for ESWL.[60] All these hemodynamic changes can be detrimental to patients

with cardiac insufficiency and valvular heart diseases. Patients with dilated hearts, dilated left atrium, paroxysmal tachycardia, frequent extrasystoles, or syncope should be properly evaluated and treated preoperatively before subjected to anesthesia and ESWL.

Epidural anesthesia has been used in most cases in many centers. Continuous epidural anesthesia has the following advantages: 1) Many of these patients require cystoscopy with stone manipulations just prior to ESWL, and the same epidural catheter can be used for both procedures. 2) An awake patient can cooperate to a certain extent and facilitate positioning onto the frame; thus, brachial plexus injury owing to positioning can be avoided. Compared with general anesthesia, it also requires less anesthetic equipment attached to the patient in the bath. 3) The length of treatment is often quite variable. Under continuous epidural anesthesia, if necessary, analgesia can be extended as long as desired. In cases in which this regional technique is contraindicated, whether for medical or psychological reasons, general endotracheal anesthesia can be performed. The latter is also preferred for high-risk patients, because it enables closer cardiopulmonary control of patients. Regional anesthesia is not recommended for apprehensive patients who require high doses of sedative drugs. Analgesia to T-6 is required for ESWL, and epidural anesthesia is preferable to spinal anesthesia because of the controllability of it. Spinal anesthesia produces more profound sympathetic blockade than epidural anesthesia and can produce more pronounced circulatory responses during positioning. The epidural catheter site must be immersed in the water, and, to ensure sterile conditions, the site should be covered by an adhesive, water-impermeable dressing. All patients who undergo general anesthesia for ESWL are intubated endotracheally and ventilated at a higher respiratory rate. Using higher rate and smaller tidal volume, the respiratory-induced excursions of the diaphragm and the kidney are minimized, and focuses of the shock waves on the stone are facilitated. High-frequency jet ventilation, at a rate of 100–300 breaths · min^{-1},[61, 62] and high-frequency positive pressure ventilation (HFPPV), using a conventional anesthesia machine at a rate of 80 breaths · min^{-1} with a tidal volume of 3 ml · kg^{-1} have been advocated as methods to improve the efficiency of ESWL by decreasing stone displacement with ventilation and thus keeping the stone in focus.[63] It is common practice to induce anesthesia with thiopental and fentanyl. For skeletal muscle relaxation, an intermediate-acting muscle relaxant, such as vecuronium or atracurium, is administered. Anesthesia is maintained with halothane, enflurane, or isoflurane, supplemented by nitrous oxide. Inspiratory oxygen concentrations

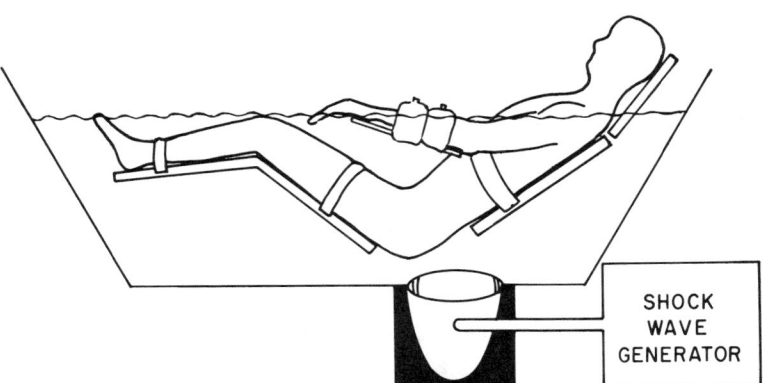

FIG. 40-2. Patient position for ESWL. The patient is positioned in the frame and is partially immersed in or emersed out of water bath by moving frame in and out of the bath. Arm floats are used for arm support.

SHOCK WAVE GENERATOR

are adjusted to the patient's needs. Pulse oximetry is very useful in these patients.

Fluid regimens during ESWL are aimed at adequate urine formation to ensure renal function and passage of disintegrated stones and to maintain acceptable hemodynamics during anesthesia. This goal is complicated by patients who have significant cardiac problems (*e.g.*, coronary artery disease, pump failure, and valvular insufficiency). Continuous arterial and central venous pressure monitoring are needed in critically ill patients in order to carefully monitor changes and to titrate vasopressors for circulatory support.

A problem unique to ESWL is the sudden exaggerated peripheral vasodilatation and hypotension after sympathetic blockade under regional or general anesthesia as the patient is emersing from the bath. Caution should be exercised at the time of transferring the patient out of the bath. During immersion or emersion, cardiac dysrhythmias occasionally occur, even in healthy patients. The cause is acute change in the right atrial and right ventricular wall tensions, which are caused by the rapid increase and decrease in preload.

At present, the following conditions are contraindications to ESWL: aortic aneurysm, hemangioma in the vertebral canal (intra- and extradural), orthopedic implants in the lumbar region, pregnancy, morbid obesity, and presence of an artificial cardiac pacemaker. Coagulation disturbances may also contraindicate the use of ESWL.[64]

Worldwide, ESWL has emerged as the treatment of choice for fragmentation and removal of stones in the kidney and upper ureter. The combined use of percutaneous lithotripsy and ESWL makes open surgical removal of stones in the future an exception in stone treatment.[65] Complications of ESWL include 1) high incidence of cardiac dysrhythmias from the discharge of shock waves independent of the cardiac cycle (cardiac dysrhythmias have been minimized by coupling the lithotriptor to the patient's continuously monitored ECG so that shock waves are triggered by the R waves); 2) renal subcapsular hematoma; 3) myocardial ischemia and infarction; and 4) cerebrovascular accident.

Optimal anesthetic management of patients undergoing ESWL should include the following: 1) If regional anesthesia is administered, all equipment for airway control should be present in the ESWL room. 2) A cardiac defibrillator and a well-stocked emergency cart should be easily accessible. 3) The ECG tracing must be of good quality, since the R wave of the tracing is used to trigger the shock waves. Waterproof ECG pads and properly positioned leads are necessary to prevent complication of burns. 4) The use of a pulse oximeter is essential. 5) Invasive lines, such as radial artery, central venous, and pulmonary artery pressure catheters, may be indicated in some high-risk patients.

LASER PROCEDURES

Lasers, especially the neodymium-YAG laser, have been increasingly used to treat tumors of the bladder and external genitalia.[66] For endoscopic procedures, if extensive or numerous tumors are present, the operation is generally performed under spinal or general anesthesia. For treatment of benign and malignant lesions of the external genitalia, lasers may prove to have a significant advantage over existing methods of treatment. Local infiltration with local anesthetics provides sufficient analgesia for the treatment of small penile or vulvar lesions, but extensive lesions or perianal lesions require regional (spinal or epidural) or general anesthesia.

REFERENCES

1. Hendolin H, Mattila MAK, Poikolainen E: The effect of lumbar epidural analgesia on the development of deep vein thrombosis of the legs after open prostatectomy. Acta Chir Scand 147:425, 1981
2. Guttmann L, Whitteridge D: Effects of bladder distention on autonomic mechanisms after spinal cord injuries. Brain 70:361, 1947
3. Bors E: The challenge of quadriplegia. Bull LA Neurol Soc 21:105, 1956
4. Lambert DH, Deane RS, Mazuzan JE: Anesthesia and the control of blood pressure in patients with spinal cord injury. Anesth Analg 61:344, 1982
5. Doyl PT, Briscoe CE: The effects of drugs and anaesthetic agents on the urinary bladder and sphincters. Br J Urol 48:329, 1976
6. Stehling LC, Patil U, Patil V: Anesthesia for urodynamic studies in children. Anesthesiol Rev 6:13, 1969
7. Ryan DW: Anaesthesia for cystectomy. Anaesthesia 37:554, 1982
8. Stephen CR, Ahlgren EW, Bennett EJ: Elements of Pediatric Anesthesia, p 8. Springfield, Illinois. Charles C Thomas, 1970
9. Cloud DT: Outpatient pediatric surgery. Int Anesthesiol Clin 20:99, 1982
10. Hannallah RS, Broadman LM, Belman AB et al: Comparison of caudal and ilioinguinal/iliohypogastric nerve blocks for control of post-orchiopexy pain in pediatric ambulatory surgery. Anesthesiology 66:832, 1987
11. Lunn JN: Postoperative analgesia after circumcision. Anaesthesia 34:552, 1979
12. May AE, Wandless J, James RD: Analgesia for circumcision in children. Acta Anaesth Scand 26:331, 1982
13. Katz J: Atlas of Regional Anesthesia, pp 138–139. Norwalk, Connecticut, Appleton-Century-Crofts, 1985
14. Soliman MG, Tramblay NA: Nerve block of the penis for postoperative pain relief in children. Anesth Analg 57:495, 1978
15. Tree–Trakarn T, Pirayavaraporn S: Postoperative pain relief for circumcision in children: Comparison among morphine, nerve block and topical analgesia. Anesthesiology 62:519, 1985
16. Moir DD: Blood loss during major vaginal surgery. A statistical study of the influence of general anaesthesia and epidural analgesia. Br J Anaesth 40:233, 1968
17. Donald JR: The effect of anaesthesia, hypotension, and epidural analgesia on blood loss in surgery for pelvic floor repair. Br J Anaesth 41:155, 1969
18. Abrams PH, Shah PJR, Bryning K et al: Blood loss during transurethral resection of the prostate. Anaesthesia 37:71, 1982
19. Peters CA, Walsh PC: Blood transfusion and anesthetic practices in radical retropubic prostatectomy. J Urol 134:81, 1985
20. Melchior J, Valk WL, Foret JD et al: Transurethral prostatectomy: Computerized analysis of 2,223 consecutive cases. J Urol 112:634, 1974
21. Desmond J: Complications of transurethral prostatic surgery. Can Anaesth Soc J 17:25, 1970
22. Desmond J: Serum osmolality and plasma electrolytes in patients who develop dilutional hyponatremia during transurethral resection. Can J Surg 13:116, 1970
23. Nesbitt TE, Carter OW, Tudor JM et al: Complications of transurethral prostatectomy and their management. South Med J 59:361, 1966
24. Marx GF, Orkin LR: Complications associated with transurethral surgery. Anesthesiology 23:802, 1962
25. Hagstrom RS: Studies on fluid absorption during transurethral prostatic resection. J Urol 73:852, 1955
26. Harrison RH, Boren JS, Robinson JR: Dilutional hyponatremia shock: Another concept of the transurethral prostatic resection reaction. J Urol 75:95, 1956

27. Fillman EM, Hanson OL, Gilbert LO: Radioisotopic study of effects of irrigation fluid in transurethral prostatectomy. JAMA 171:1488, 1959
28. Norris HT, Aasheim GM, Sherrard DJ et al: Symptomatology, pathophysiology, and treatment of the transurethral resection of the prostate syndrome. Br J Urol 45:420, 1973
29. Wakim KG: The pathophysiologic basis for the clinical manifestations and complications of transurethral prostatic resection. J Urol 106:719, 1961
30. Hurlbert BJ, Wingard DW: Water intoxication after fifteen minutes of transurethral resection of the prostate. Anesthesiology 50:355, 1979
31. Ovassapian A, Joshi CW, Brunner EA: Visual disturbance: An unusual symptom of transurethral prostatic resection reaction. Anesthesiology 57:332, 1982
32. Roesch RP, Stoelting RK, Lingeman JE et al: Ammonia toxicity resulting from glycine absorption during a transurethral resection of the prostate. Anesthesiology 58:577, 1983
33. Wang JM, Wong KC, Creel DJ et al: Effects of glycine on hemodynamic responses and visual evoked potentials in the dog. Anesth Analg 64:1071, 1985
34. Mani M: Transurethral prostatic surgery revisited. Anesthesiol Rev Nov 1976, p 15
35. Aasheim GM: Hyponatremia during transurethral surgery. Can Anaesth Soc J 20:247, 1973
36. Henderson DJ, Middleton RG: Coma from hyponatremia following transurethral resection of prostate. Urology 15:267, 1980
37. Hoekstra PT, Kahnoski R, McCamish MA et al: Transurethral prostatic resection syndrome—a new perspective: Encephalopathy with associated hyperammonemia. J Urol 130:704, 1983
38. Creel DJ, Wang JML, Wong KC: Transient blindness associated transurethral resection of the prostate. Arch Ophthalmol 105:1537, 1987
39. Apreson MH, Werman R: The distribution of glycine in cat spinal cord and roots. Life Sci 4:2075, 1965
40. Snyder SH, Enna EJ: The role of central receptors in the pharmacologic actions of benzodiazepines. Adv Biochem Psychopharmacol 14:81, 1975
41. Desmond J: A method of measuring blood loss during transurethral prostatic surgery. J Urol 109:453, 1973
42. Jansen H, Berseus O, Johansson JE: A simple photometric method for determination of blood loss during transurethral surgery. Scand J Urol Nephrol 12:1, 1978
43. Levin K, Nyren O, Pompeius R: Blood loss, tissue weight and operating time in transurethral prostatectomy. Scand J Urol Nephrol 15:197, 1981
44. Lambardo LJ: Fibrinolysis following prostatic surgery. J Urol 77:289, 1957
45. McGowan SW, Smith GFN: Anaesthesia for transurethral prostatectomy. Anaesthesia 35:847, 1980
46. Perkins JB, Miller HC: Blood loss during transurethral prostatectomy. J Urol 101:93, 1969
47. Madsen RE, Madsen PO: Influence of anaesthesia form on blood loss in transurethral prostatectomy. Anesth Analg 46:330, 1967
48. Collins KJ, Dore C, Exoton–Smith AN, et al: Accidental hypothermia and impaired temperature homeostasis in the elderly. Br Med J 1:353, 1977
49. Stjerstrom H, Henneberg S, Eklund A et al: Thermal balance during transurethral resection of the prostate: A comparison of general anesthesia and epidural analgesia. Acta Anaesth Scand 29:743, 1985
50. Jenkins J, Fox J, Sharwood–Smith G: Changes in body heat during transvesical prostatectomy. Anaesthesia 38:748, 1983
51. Whitfield HN, Hendry WF: Endoscopic surgery. In Textbook and Genito-Urinary Surgery, Vol 2, Chapter 126, p 1373. Churchill Livingstone, 1985
52. Kenton HR: Perforation in transurethral operations; technic for immediate diagnosis and management of extravasations. JAMA 142:798, 1950
53. Holtgrewe HL, Valk WL: Factors influencing the mortality and morbidity of transurethral prostatectomy: A study of 2015 cases. J Urol 87:450, 1962
54. Sinha B, Haikel G, Lange PH et al: Transurethral resection of the prostate with local anesthesia in 100 patients. J Urol 135:719, 1986
55. Bennett MJ, Smith RW, Fuchs E: Sudden cardiac arrest during percutaneous ultrasonic nephrostolithotomy. Anesthesiology 60:245, 1984
56. Loening S, Karamolowsky EV, Willoughby B: Use of local anesthesia for extracorporeal shock wave lithotripsy. J Urol 137:626, 1987
57. Arborelius M, Balldin Ul, Lilja B et al: Hemodynamic changes in man during immersion with the head above water. Aviat Space Environ Med 43:592, 1972
58. Begin R, Epstein M, Sackner MA et al: Effects of water immersion to the neck on pulmonary circulation and tissue volume in man. J Appl Physiol 40:293, 1976
59. Loellgen H, Von Nieding G, Horres R: Respiratory and hemodynamic adjustment during head out water immersion. Int J Sport Med 1:25, 1980
60. Behnia R, Shanks CA, Ovassapian A et al: Hemodynamic responses associated with lithotripsy. Anesth Analg 66:354, 1987
61. Schulte am Esch J, Kochs E, Meyer WH: Improved efficiency of extracorporeal shock-wave lithotripsy during high frequency ventilation. Anesthesiology 63:A177, 1985
62. Carlson CA, Gravenstein JS, Banner MJ et al: Monitoring techniques during anesthesia and HFJV for extracorporeal shockwave lithotripsy. Anesthesiology 63:A178, 1985
63. Perel A, Hoffman B, Podeh D et al: High frequency positive pressure ventilation during general anesthesia for extracorporeal shock wave lithotripsy. Anesth Analg 65:1231, 1986
64. Drach GW, Dretler S, Fair W et al: Report of the United States Cooperative study of extracorporeal shock wave lithotripsy. J Urol 135:1127, 1986
65. Jocham D, Brandl H, Chaussey C et al: Treatment of nephrolithiasis with ESWL. In Gravenstein JS, Peter K (eds): Extracorporeal Shock-Wave Lithotripsy for Renal Stone Disease, p 35. London, Butterworths, 1986
66. Staehler G, Chaussey C, Jocham D et al: The use of neodymium-YAG lasers in urology: Indications, technique and critical assessment. J Urol 134:1155, 1985

Chapter 41   *F. Peter Buckley*

Anesthesia and Obesity and Gastrointestinal Disorders

OBESITY

Obesity is usually defined in relation to ideal body weight (IBW) derived from actuarial tables, or in relation to height using indices such as body mass index (BMI).* Patients who weigh 20% above IBW or have a BMI of greater than 28 are regarded as obese and constitute 10%–15% of the population.[1,2] The very obese, usually termed the *morbidly obese*, weigh more than 45 kg above IBW or have a BMI of greater than 35.

Obesity is associated with a number of anatomic, physiologic, and biochemical deviations from normality. These abnormalities can affect all body systems and have implications for the health of individuals and for their anesthetic management.[3] Much of the information about obesity and the anesthetic management of the obese has been derived from studies of morbidly obese patients with no systemic clinical disease. Therefore, caution should be applied when applying such information to the less heroically obese and when dealing with the general morbidly obese population, who have a high incidence of systemic clinical disease.

Body fat distribution falls into two broad categories: Android obesity is that which is primarily of truncal distribution (with a waist–hip ratio of 1.0 in men and 0.8 in women) and is associated with a rise in oxygen consumption ($\dot{V}_{O_2}$) and an increased incidence of cardiovascular disease. Fat in the gynecoid distribution, primarily on the buttocks and thighs, is metabolically less active and appears to be less closely associated with cardiovascular disease.

*Body mass index (BMI) is wt (kg) divided by ht^2 (m). Thus, a 1.7 m, 70-kg patient has a BMI of 24.

PATHOPHYSIOLOGY OF OBESITY

Respiratory System

Obese persons have a raised $\dot{V}_{O_2}$ and carbon dioxide production ($\dot{V}_{CO_2}$), but basal metabolic rate (BMR), being related to body surface area (BSA), is usually normal.[4–6] Contributing to the raised $\dot{V}_{O_2}$ are the metabolic activity of fat, an increase in energy expenditure for locomotion, and breathing (to move the mass-loaded chest and abdomen and in order to maintain a high minute volume to remain normocarbic in the face of a raised $\dot{V}_{CO_2}$). On exercising, $\dot{V}_{O_2}$ and $\dot{V}_{CO_2}$ rise more sharply than in persons of normal body weight, as does the oxygen (O_2) cost of respiration, implying respiratory muscle inefficiency.

As a consequence of fat producing mass loading, chest wall compliance is reduced, but lung compliance remains relatively normal. Mass loading also results in a fall in static lung volumes. In the upright position, residual volume (RV) remains normal, but expiratory reserve volume (ERV) and functional residual capacity (FRC) are often reduced so that tidal ventilation may fall within the range of closing capacity (CC) with ensuing ventilation/perfusion (V/Q) abnormalities, or frank right-to-left shunt, with ensuing hypoxemia (Fig. 41-1). As mass loading is increased by adopting the supine position, FRC often falls further within the range of CC with worsening hypoxemia (Fig. 41-1). The usual clinical tests of respiratory function (*e.g.*, forced vital capacity [FVC], forced expiratory volume in 1 sec [FEV$_1$], and peak expiratory flow rate [PEFR]) are usually normal in the healthy obese patient. Although it is likely that android obesity will have more marked effects on lung volumes than will gynecoid obesity, this issue has not been studied.

1117

EFFECT OF POSITION ON LUNG VOLUMES

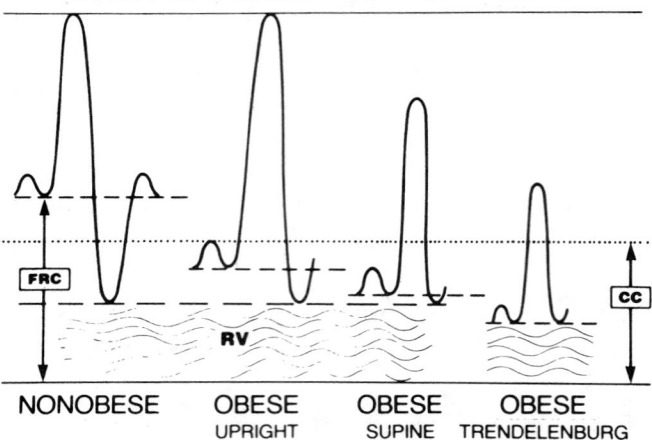

NONOBESE   OBESE   OBESE   OBESE
            UPRIGHT SUPINE   TRENDELENBURG

FIG. 41-1. The effect of change in position upon various lung volumes in nonobese and morbidly obese patients. (FRC = functional residual capacity; RV = residual volume; CC = closing capacity) (Reprinted with permission from Vaughan RW: Pulmonary and cardiovascular derangements. In Brown BR [ed]: Anesthesia and the Obese Patient. Contemporary Anesthesia Practice Series, p 19. Philadelphia, FA Davis, 1982.)

The majority of obese patients maintain a sufficient minute volume of ventilation ($\dot{V}_E$) to remain normocarbic and preserve a normal response to carbon dioxide (CO_2) challenge. However, with advancing obesity, intercurrent lung disease, and the changes wrought by pulmonary hypertension, their condition may deteriorate to the obesity hypoventilation syndrome (loss of hypercarbic drive, sleep apnea, hypersomnolence, and potential or overt airway difficulties) or to the worst end of the spectrum: the Pickwickian syndrome (hypercarbia, hypoxemia, polycythemia, hypersomnolence, pulmonary hypertension, and biventricular failure).[7] A schematic of the interactions of the respiratory and cardiovascular effects of obesity leading to these conditions is given in Figure 41-2.

Cardiovascular System

In obese persons, circulating blood volume (CBV), plasma volume (PV), and cardiac output (CO) increase proportionately with rising weight and $\dot{V}_{O_2}$. Cerebral and renal blood flows are similar to those in normal persons, but splanchnic blood flow is 20% higher than that in normal persons.[6, 8, 9] The rest of the increase in CO is distributed to skin and muscles and to the large fat stores. Blood flow to fat is usually 2–3 ml $\cdot$ 100 g^{-1} tissue $\cdot$ min^{-1}. Thus, for a patient whose fat mass is 50 kg, blood flow to this extra mass will account for an extra CO of 1.5–2.0 l $\cdot$ min^{-1}. The rise in CO parallels the rise in $\dot{V}_{O_2}$; thus, systemic arteriovenous O_2 difference remains normal or slightly above normal. The pulse rate in the obese person is usually within normal limits; thus, with an increased CO, stroke volume is increased.

Arterial hypertension occurs frequently in the morbidly obese, being severe in 5%–10% of the population and moderate in 50%. The rise in CO in response to exercise is more abrupt than in normal persons and may be accompanied by rises in left ventricular end-diastolic pressure and pulmonary capillary wedge pressure. Changes similar to those seen during exercise have been observed in the perioperative period. Thus, patients with any degree of cardiovascular compromise are particularly at risk in the perioperative period.[10]

In 20%–50% of the morbidly obese, cardiac diameter is increased on a chest radiograph, but a substantial proportion of patients maintain normal left ventricular (LV) function in the face of raised CBV, PV, CO, and systemic blood pressure. This is usually achieved by a compensatory increase in LV wall thickness relative to LV chamber size.[9] However, in some patients, such compensation does not occur; in these patients, LV decompensation may occur in the face of cardiac stressors. The two groups—LV compensated and uncompensated—can only be distinguished by studying LV function.

The pulmonary circulation is also vulnerable to the pathophysiologic changes produced by obesity. A rise in pulmonary blood volumes and flows occurs to predispose the patients to pulmonary hypertension, which may be accentuated or precipitated by hypoxic pulmonary vasoconstriction, which, in turn, occurs secondary to the static lung volume changes found in the morbidly obese. A schematic of the

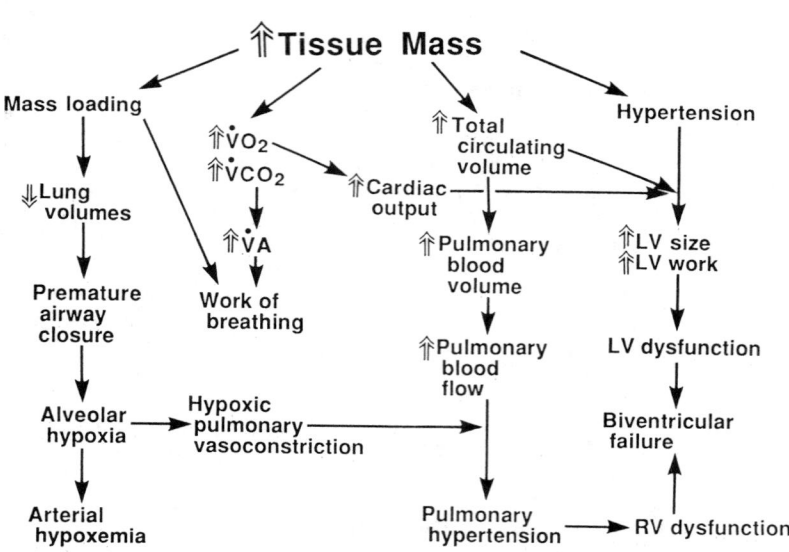

FIG. 41-2. A schema interrelating the cardiovascular and respiratory abnormalities in morbidly obese patients to the pathophysiologic changes found in such patients.

interaction of pulmonary, systemic, and pulmonary vascular changes that occur in morbidly obese persons is given in Figure 41-2.

Endocrine and Metabolic Systems

In order to maintain a stable weight, morbidly obese patients have to maintain a greater than normal caloric intake.[11] But, as with $\dot{V}_{O_2}$, when this intake is related to BSA, the values are similar to those of normal persons. Glucose tolerance is frequently impaired, with pancreatic islet hypertrophy and hyperinsulinemia, irrespective of the state of carbohydrate tolerance, and is reflected in a high incidence of diabetes mellitus in the morbidly obese. Abnormal serum lipid profiles are often found and may be associated with an increased incidence of ischemic heart disease.

Gastrointestinal System

Morbidly obese patients have an increased incidence of hiatal hernia and a linear increase in intraabdominal pressure with increasing weight. At the time of induction of anesthesia, 90% of morbidly obese patients presenting for elective surgery will have a gastric fluid volume in excess of 25 ml, and a gastric fluid pH of less than 2.5.[12] Such volume and pH figures are generally accepted as being indicative of a high risk of acid aspiration pneumonitis if such fluid reaches the airway. Because both intraabdominal pressure and the volume of gastric contents increase during pregnancy, the pregnant morbidly obese patient is at particular risk.

There is an increase in liver fat content in 90% of morbidly obese patients,[11, 13] which may not be reflected by abnormalities in the usual clinical tests of hepatic function.[13] The increase appears to be a reflection of the duration, rather than the degree, of obesity. The incidence of hepatic dysfunction is particularly high among those patients who have undergone intestinal bypass operations. The effect of gastric partitioning operations on hepatic function is uncertain.

Airway

Obesity produces a number of anatomic changes that can affect the airway. Movement of both the cervical spine and the atlantoaxial joint may be limited by numerous "chins" and by thoracic wall or breast fat. Extension of these joints may be limited by low cervical or upper thoracic fat pads. Mouth opening may be restricted by submental fat. Fleshy cheeks, a large tongue, and copious flaps of palatal, pharyngeal, and supralaryngeal soft tissue may narrow the airway. Moreover, the laryngeal aperture may occupy a "high and anterior" infantile position. Patients with a history of sleep apnea syndrome have particularly difficult airways to manage when anesthetized.

PSYCHOLOGY OF THE OBESE

Although the incidence of psychopathology among the general obese population is similar to that in the normal population, it may be somewhat higher in the morbidly obese.[14] Obese patients have a reputation among the medical profession for being difficult to manage, intolerant of discomfort, noncompliant with therapies, and prone to resort to outbursts of anger or hysteria. Whether these characteristics are inherent in the obese or a result of their interaction with their environment and its "thin thinking" inhabitants is uncertain. There is evidence that the obese suffer from prejudices and discriminations from an early age and are characterized as ugly, slothful, lacking in self control, and prone to depression and self-consciousness. Physicians are not exempt from holding such prejudices. The author's bias is that the alleged behavior is largely a consequence of their interactions with those around them, not exempting physicians. Experience with a number of morbidly obese patients about to undergo gastric stapling operations has been that they were compliant with management regimens and conducted themselves in a normal fashion throughout the perioperative period.[15] However, much time and effort were expended with this group, who were obviously highly selected and motivated, having decided on a very dramatic course of action in an attempt to reduce their obesity.

PHARMACOKINETICS IN THE OBESE

While there are few direct data about drug kinetics in the obese, certain inferences may be drawn, based on the known pathophysiologic changes in obesity.[16] Because obese persons have a larger than normal fat compartment, the proportion of body water and muscle mass to total body weight will be less than normal. Drug biotransformation may be altered owing to hepatic disease, diabetes, or changes in splanchnic blood flow. Renal drug excretion may be changed as a result of alterations in glomerular filtration, and biliary excretion may be changed by the presence of gallstones or pancreatitis. Finally, the high incidence of hyperlipoproteinemia may affect drug binding.

Lipophilic drugs such as benzodiazepines[17] and thiopental[18] have an increased volume of distribution, more selective distribution to fat stores, and a longer elimination half-life in obese patients when compared with normal persons, but clearance values are similar in both groups. The implication of these findings is that fat-soluble volatile anesthetic agents may have a prolonged elimination time, with a consequent slow recovery. However, theoretical[19] studies have shown that for prolonged recovery to occur, such agents would have to be administered for periods in excess of 24 hours. Clinical studies of volatile agents administered to morbidly obese patients for commonly encountered operative times, that is, to 2–4 hours, have shown normal recovery times.[20] Fentanyl and sufentanil, relatively fat-soluble drugs, have a similar distribution, elimination half-life, and clearance in both obese and nonobese persons.[21, 22]

Hydrophilic drugs have similar volumes of distribution, elimination half-life, and clearance in obese and nonobese patients. To produce a given degree of neuromuscular blockade, the dose of pancuronium necessary in the morbidly obese is larger than that in normal patients. However, when this dose is related to BSA, it is similar to the normal dose.[23] Larger doses of suxamethonium are necessary, possibly as a consequence of the higher levels of pseudocholinesterase found in the morbidly obese.[24]

PREOPERATIVE EVALUATION

Although obese persons have a reputation for being difficult to handle, this difficulty can be minimized by a suitable preoperative evaluation and visit. The anesthesiologist should be aware of his or her own feelings, attitudes, and prejudices toward the obese and carefully identify and suppress those that could convey an unsympathetic and condescending attitude toward the patient. The patients should be evaluated in a thorough, nonjudgmental fashion, with particular emphasis on the difficulties that obesity presents to the anesthesiologist. Time should be taken to allow the patient to detail previous adverse experiences with anesthetics and operations, as well as their fears and anxieties about the upcoming experience. The various potential difficulties that the patient presents should be enumerated, and the specific anesthesia plan that is to be used to minimize or avoid such difficulties should be discussed with the patient. The likely postoperative course should be discussed with the patient, and the patient should be allowed some degree of input and choice in the management plan.

Cardiovascular System

The evaluation should be directed toward the abnormalities detailed in the pathophysiology section. Hypertension, signs of LV or right ventricular (RV) failure, and signs of pulmonary hypertension should be sought. It is worthwhile to check for potential sites of venous access and to perform an Allen's test to ensure ulnar artery patency if radial artery cannulation is anticipated. The ECGs and chest radiograph should be scrutinized for evidence of ischemic heart disease, LV or RV hypertrophy, increase in cardiac size, and pulmonary congestion. Findings of any of these abnormalities should lead to appropriate detailed investigations such as exercise ECGs, echocardiography, LV ejection fraction, or pulmonary artery catheterization. For patients who have evidence of the obesity hypoventilation syndrome (OHS) or the Pickwickian syndrome, a cardiologist's opinion should be sought, both to define the magnitude of the problem and to advise as how best to optimize the patient's condition prior to operation.

Respiratory System

The clinical history should seek to identify symptoms that are suspicious of severe degrees of respiratory disease (e.g., orthopnea), OHS, or sleep apnea syndrome and of a history of upper airway obstruction, especially if associated with previous anesthesia and surgery. In young morbidly obese patients, the results of routine pulmonary function tests such as FVC, FEV_1, and PEFR are usually normal, but, in older patients and smokers, the results may help identify unsuspected bronchospastic disease. Chest radiographs should be obtained, as should sitting and supine blood gases, to rule out CO_2 retention and to provide guidelines for pre- and postoperative O_2 administration. More detailed pulmonary investigations should be reserved for those with severe disease. Because the degree of respiratory compromise in the postoperative period is often pronounced, it is imperative to optimize the patient's pulmonary status prior to embarking on anesthesia or surgery.

Endocrine, Metabolic, and Gastrointestinal Systems

Fasting blood glucose levels should be obtained, and the urine should be tested for ketones. If gross carbohydrate intolerance, diabetes, or ketosis is found, it should be corrected before either elective or emergency operations are begun. The patient should be closely questioned for symptoms of esophageal reflux and for a previous history of investigations or therapies that might be aimed at such a problem. Routine liver function tests should be obtained.

Airway

A history of airway difficulties during previous anesthetics and operations should be obtained from the patient or previous anesthetic records. The patient should be questioned about symptoms suggestive of obstructive sleep apnea syndrome, such as excessive nocturnal snoring, with or without apneic episodes, because they suggest a potential for mechanical airway obstruction when the level of consciousness is decreased. Patients with such histories and those presenting for operations (tracheostomy, palatoplasty) designed to alleviate such conditions should be scrutinized especially closely, because they often present formidable airway difficulties. Physical examination of the patient should include range of motion of the atlantoaxial joint and cervical spine, the degree to which the mouth can open, and the distance between the tip of the chin and the hyoid cartilage. The interior of the mouth and pharynx should be scrutinized for excessive folds of tissue. Lateral soft-tissue radiographs of the neck in neutral and extended positions and CAT scans of the pharynx, hypopharynx, and the larynx will help to evaluate airway difficulties, as may a consultation with an otolaryngologist for direct or indirect laryngoscopy.

PERIOPERATIVE MANAGEMENT

Premedication

Premedication, if any, should be given intravenously or orally. Attempts to give an intramuscular injection will usually result in an intra-fat injection, absorption from which is unpredictable. Because the effects of central nervous system (CNS) active drugs on the morbidly obese are not predictable and because of the high incidence of respiratory disease in the morbidly obese, premedication should not be administered until the patient is in a safely monitored environment (e.g., the holding area or the operating room). This is particularly true for any patient with a history of airway obstruction or cardiovascular or respiratory disease. Even when such drugs are administered in the operating room, the patient should be monitored diligently. Anticholinergic drugs should always be given in an attempt to reduce secretions if an awake or a fiberoptic intubation of the trachea is anticipated.

Because the risk of gastric regurgitation is high in obese patients, specific measures should be taken to guard against it. If a large volume of gastric contents is suspected (e.g., in an emergent situation), an attempt should be made to empty the stomach with a nasogastric tube. The tube should be removed prior to induction of anesthesia for fear of making a likely difficult tracheal intubation even more difficult. For elective cases, the preoperative administration of a clear antacid, metoclopramide and H_2 histamine blockers is advisable to both lower volume and increase the pH of gastric contents.[25-28] Suggested doses would be metoclopramide 10 mg intravenously (iv),[25-28] cimetidine 300 mg or ranitidine 50 mg iv 1 hour before operation.

Operating Room Preparation

It is important to ensure that equipment such as gurneys, operating tables, and lithotomy stirrups are capable of bearing the load that the obese patient will impose upon them. The heels, buttocks, and shoulders of obese persons are at risk of developing decubitus ulcers; therefore, vulnerable areas should be padded. The distribution of body fat may make the usual operating table positions hazardous to the obese. For example, excessive posterior extension of the shoulder, with the potential for brachial plexus injury may occur when a patient with a large posterior thoracic fat pad is placed supine with arms abducted at 90 degrees to the body. Thus, when the obese patient is placed on the operating table, care should be taken to ensure that the various body parts are placed in positions that will minimize the risk of damage, particularly to neural structures.

Monitoring

If cuff blood pressure monitoring is to be used, the cuff should be of an appropriate size (the bladder should enclose 70% of the arm). Cuff blood pressure monitoring may be both difficult and inaccurate in obese patients, and it is advisable to use intraarterial monitoring for all but the shortest and simplest cases. Paradoxically, although it is often difficult to secure venous access in the obese, intraarterial cannulation is usually no more difficult than in nonobese persons. A V_5 or equivalent ECG lead should be used on all patients. Monitoring of those patients with cardiovascular disease will be dictated by their specific problem. Those with raised pulmonary artery pressure or evidence of LV compromise may necessitate the placement of a pulmonary artery catheter for both pressure and cardiac output determinations.

Perioperative hypoxia is a constant threat in obese patients; therefore, oxygenation should be monitored by pulse oximetry and/or by frequent arterial blood gas measurements. End-tidal CO_2 monitoring should be used to ensure adequacy of artificial ventilation and to confirm correct endotracheal tube placement.

To ensure that any nondepolarizing neuromuscular blockade is adequate intraoperatively and fully reversed at the conclusion of the operation, any such blockade must be monitored with a peripheral nerve stimulator. As considerable amounts of tissue may separate skin electrodes from the relevant nerve, adequate stimulation may be difficult to achieve. This problem can be circumvented by the use of percutaneous needle electrodes.

Because the obese are no less likely than normal persons to lose heat intraoperatively, body temperature should be monitored and maintained. It is particularly important to avoid postoperative shivering in obese patients, because this may produce further mixed venous, and subsequently arterial, desaturation in patients who may be borderline normal in this regard.

INTRAOPERATIVE MANAGEMENT

Airway Maintenance

Other than for the shortest general anesthetics in highly selected patients, general anesthesia should be delivered by an endotracheal tube. This is advocated because

1. It may be difficult or impossible to maintain a gas-tight fit with a mask while maintaining an adequate airway *and* attending to the manual tasks necessary during anesthesia.
2. Obese patients have a high risk of aspiration of gastric contents.
3. Obese patients, if allowed to breathe spontaneously under general anesthesia, will hypoventilate and be-

come undesirably hypoxic and/or hypercarbic. Artificial ventilation via an endotracheal tube is almost mandatory.

Difficulties with endotracheal intubation should be anticipated in all obese patients, and *the person doing the intubation* should thoroughly evaluate the patient and define all risks at the preoperative visit. All appropriate airway management equipment should be available, including a selection of oropharyngeal and nasopharyngeal airways, endotracheal tubes with introducers, intubation stylets, and laryngoscope blades of different patterns and sizes. If chest wall or breast fat is likely to obstruct the usual laryngoscope handles, a "polio blade" laryngoscope, which has a handle in the reverse of the usual direction, may be helpful. Fiberoptic intubation devices or bronchoscopes should also be available.

A carefully considered choice as to whether the patient's trachea should be intubated awake or asleep should be made in each case, bearing in mind the anticipated difficulties and the expertise of the anesthesiologist. With morbidly obese patients, an incidence rate of 13% for difficult tracheal intubations has been quoted.[15] It has been recommended that when a patient is in excess of 75% above IBW, awake tracheal intubation should be the rule,[29] but difficulties can also be encountered at weights below such a cutoff point.

A useful practice is to topically anesthetize the mouth, pharynx, and supralaryngeal area with a local anesthetic and then gently introduce a standard laryngoscope and attempt to visualize the epiglottis and the larynx. If it is possible to see these structures, it is likely that intubation of the trachea after induction of anesthesia can be performed; if not, an awake intubation should be performed. If in doubt, the anesthesiologist should err on the side of caution and perform an awake intubation. Awake intubations should be accomplished with a fiberoptic laryngoscope or bronchoscope after suitable topical anesthesia. Any CNS depressant drug used to provide patient comfort should be kept to a minimum, and its effects should be monitored closely. Supplemental O_2 should be given while performing awake intubations. Although blind nasal intubation has been strongly advocated,[30] it should be used only by those who are very proficient and have a high success rate with this technique. Initiation of epistaxis can make subsequent airway management exceedingly difficult.

Patients with a history suggestive of obstructive sleep apnea syndrome and those who are to undergo operations designed to alleviate such conditions inevitably present formidable endotracheal intubation difficulties. When endotracheal intubation under general anesthesia is attempted, there is a high incidence of failure. The difficulty in bag and mask ventilation subsequent to a failed tracheal intubation and ensuing life-threatening hypoxia dictate that a majority of such patients should be intubated while awake.

If tracheal intubation under general anesthesia is to be performed, it is a useful policy to have two pairs of experienced hands available. If the initial attempt at intubation is not successful and it is necessary to resort to bag and mask ventilation, it may require one person to maintain a gas-tight fit with the mask and an airway. The second pair of hands is then available to squeeze the bag. Moreover, a second pair of educated hands may be useful to cope with other difficulties.

Intubation under general anesthesia should be performed in a manner designed to avoid hypoxia and the aspiration of vomited or regurgitated gastric contents. Cricothyroid pressure (Sellick's maneuver) should be applied in all cases. Thorough preoxygenation/denitrogenation by a conventional

3-minute period or a four-breath technique[31] is essential, because intubation may take longer than usual, and obese patients have smaller than normal O_2 stores in their lungs (low FRC) and a high $\dot{V}_{O_2}$, thus making them particularly at risk of hypoxia during this period. As with all tracheal intubations, the routine use of a pulse oximeter will provide early warning of hypoxia.

Irrespective of the method used to place the endotracheal tube, special care should be taken to ensure its correct placement. Placement within the trachea should be confirmed by capnography, as the usual auscultatory methods of confirming placement may be difficult owing to chest wall fat.

CHOICE OF ANESTHETIC TECHNIQUE

General Anesthesia

The doses of induction drugs used for the obese patient should be larger than for normal patients (*e.g.*, thiopental $7.5 \text{ mg} \cdot \text{kg}^{-1}$ IBW), but allowance should be made for any cardiovascular dysfunction. Nitrous oxide is a logical choice as a maintenance anesthetic, because it is fat insoluble, has a rapid onset and decrement of action, and is subject to little metabolism. However, even in the most fit morbidly obese patients, it may be necessary to use an FI_{O_2} in excess of 0.5 to maintain an adequate Pa_{O_2}[32]; thus, the usefulness of nitrous oxide is limited.

Obese patients metabolize volatile anesthetics to a greater extent than do normal patients. Compared with normal patients, blood levels of fluoride after methoxyflurane, halothane, and enflurane and blood levels of bromide after halothane are higher in the morbidly obese.[11] Moreover, as the incidence of "halothane hepatitis" is allegedly higher in the obese and because the obese metabolize some halothane by a potentially hepatotoxic reductive pathway,[32a] this drug should be used with caution. However, simple tests of hepatic function are similarly marginally impaired after either halothane or enflurane anesthesia. Isoflurane, which is metabolized by normal patients to a lesser extent than are other drugs, would appear to be a logical choice, but its degree of metabolism by the obese has not been studied.

The supposition that a prolonged recovery from fat-soluble volatile anesthetics may occur in the obese, as such drugs may take a long time to leach out of fat stores, has been elegantly disproved in theory[19] and in clinical studies of speed of awakening[20] (see section on pharmacokinetics).

Great care should be exercised when giving opioids to obese patients. Unless the patient's trachea is to be left intubated, with ventilator support, in the immediate postoperative period, it is wise to keep the dose of opioid to a minimum. Maintenance of normal ventilation is already difficult for obese patients, and further respiratory depression with opioids could predispose the patients to hypoxia and/or hypercarbia in the recovery room.

As mentioned previously, the absolute dose requirement for nondepolarizing neuromuscular blocking drugs is larger in obese than in normal persons, but, if the dose is related to BSA, it is similar.[23] The use of short-duration drugs, such as vecuronium and atracurium, may guarantee a more complete and swift reversal of neuromuscular blockade. The degree of neuromuscular blockade and its reversal should always be monitored with a peripheral nerve stimulator.

Paramount among the changes in the physiology of obese patients produced by general anesthesia are respiratory abnormalities. With the induction of anesthesia, there is further disruption of the already altered FRC/CC relationship, with further deterioration in V/Q relations or development of frank right-to-left shunt. In addition, the impairment of pulmonary hypoxic vasoconstriction by volatile agents will contribute further to such changes. All obese patients should be considered at risk of hypoxia under general anesthesia, and their oxygenation should be monitored with a pulse oximeter. Obese patients should not receive an FI_{O_2} of less than 0.5, and, in those with cardiovascular or respiratory disease, an FI_{O_2} of 1.0 is indicated. The FI_{O_2} delivered should be titrated against Sa_{O_2} or Pa_{O_2}, obtained from pulse oximetry or frequent blood gas measurements. The application of positive end-expiratory pressure (PEEP) may improve Pa_{O_2} if it falls to particularly low levels.[33]

Even in fit obese patients, intraoperative events that influence lung volumes may produce changes in oxygenation. The assumption of the Trendelenburg or the lithotomy position and the placement of subdiaphragmatic packs or retractors may lead to further falls in Sa_{O_2} and Pa_{O_2}.[6] Given these findings, it is important that particular attention be paid to oxygenation at the time of positional changes and various surgical maneuvers. Morbidly obese patients may, however, be safely maintained by one-lung anesthesia performed via a double-lumen endobronchial tube during transthoracic operations.[35]

Because of the hypoventilation produced by general anesthesia, spontaneous respiration during general anesthesia is relatively contraindicated. Intermittent positive-pressure ventilation (IPPV) is best accomplished with large tidal volumes* at a rate of 8–10 breaths · min.$^{-1}$ Hypocarbia with a Pa_{CO_2} of less than 30 mm Hg is best avoided, as this may result in a rise in shunt fraction.[34] Ventilation may also be judged by end-tidal CO_2, obtained by capnography, or sampling of arterial blood gases.

It deserves reiteration that the studies concerning general anesthesia and obese patients have been performed in patients who are otherwise fit. It is likely that those patients who have respiratory or cardiovascular disease will have even more marked changes in respiratory parameters during anesthesia and require even more careful attention.

At the conclusion of the operation, it is essential that any neuromuscular blockade be totally reversed, as judged by the response to peripheral nerve stimulation, and that parameters for extubation are fulfilled. Patients' tracheas should not be extubated until the patients are fully awake and in control of their airway in order to avoid hazards of pulmonary aspiration or airway obstruction. It should be ensured, either by pulse oximetry or arterial blood gas measurements, that hypoxia is not present prior to extubation.

Regional Anesthesia

Regional anesthesia would appear to be a useful alternative to general anesthesia, but it brings its own constellation of difficulties. The presence of much body fat and the indistinct nature of bony landmarks make regional anesthesia techniques difficult. For peripheral nerve blockades, this may be

---

*By rearranging the BMI equation (BMI = wt (kg) ht^2 (m) to BMI × ht^2 (m) = wt (kg), one may calculate various body weights for the individual. Thus, a patient with a true body weight of 139 kg and a height of 1.77 m has a BMI of 139/1.77^2 = 44.4. At IBW, BMI = 25, and at low body weight (LBW), BMI = 30. Thus, for this patient, IBW = 25 × 1.77^2 = 78 kg. LBW = 30 × 1.77^2 = 94 kg. IPPV at a rate of 12 ml · kg^{-1} at the LBW at a rate of 8 to 10 breaths · min^{-1} will achieve a Pa_{CO_2} of approximately 30 mm Hg.[36]

circumvented by use of insulated needles and a peripheral nerve stimulator to ensure correct needle and drug placement.

Subarachnoid blockades may be more difficult to perform in the obese than in normal patients, but these difficulties are not insurmountable. The midline of the back in the lumbar region generally does not have as thick a layer of fat as does the more lateral portions, and subarachnoid puncture may be made easier by having the patient sit up. Often needles longer than usual may be needed. For a given age and height of patient, the dose requirement for subarachnoid anesthesia is approximately 75%–80% of that of normal.[37] Evidence from case reports implies that the level of blockade produced by subarachnoid local anesthetics is not very predictable and that the blockade is of slow onset and creeps insidiously higher over the first 30 minutes.[38] Anecdotal reports have implied that a high subarachnoid blockade tends to produce respiratory compromise, especially if patients are sedated.[38] However, in obese patients with a blockade at T5, both respiratory volumes[39] and blood gases[40] show minimal change from baseline. If the blockade does extend higher in the thoracic area than T5 there is a distinct possibility of respiratory compromise, particularly in obese patients with respiratory disease. Moreover, the high extension of the blockade, with the variable extent of the autonomic blockade above the somatic blockade,[41] may lead to cardiovascular compromise, which can also be precipitated by panniculus retraction.[42]

Because it may be difficult to deal with respiratory or cardiovascular emergencies in morbidly obese patients, it is critical that any such potential hazards are detected as early as possible by vigilant monitoring and remedied by vigorous early intervention. Monitoring should be as intensive as for general anesthesia, and supplementary oxygen should be used in all cases. A strong case may be made for using a continuous subarachnoid blockade in morbidly obese patients. This would provide all the benefits of regional anesthesia and yet enable the anesthesiologist to titrate the dose of drug necessary to achieve the desired extent of blockade, and no more.

While technically more exacting than subarachnoid anesthesia, epidural anesthesia has been widely used and described in obese patients,[15, 30, 43, 44] particularly for abdominal operations. The technique usually consists of a high lumbar or thoracic puncture, with the introduction of a catheter and the induction of a segmental block. Catheter placement may be made easier by the use of fluoroscopic assistance.[44] The technique is usually used in combination with a light general anesthetic delivered by an endotracheal tube and IPPV. Such a technique bypasses many of the problems of general anesthesia, reduces the requirement for volatile drug, eliminates the need for neuromuscular blocking drugs and permits rapid postoperative mobilization. As is true for subarachnoid anesthesia, the dose requirement for epidural anesthesia is approximately 75%–80% of that of normal patients.[15, 45] The use of epidural analgesia may confer some benefits on morbidly obese patients intraoperatively and postoperatively (decreased shunt fraction, left ventricular work, A–Vd$_{O_2}$ and V$_{O_2}$).[46, 47] The use of an epidural technique may be made more desirable by the fact that the catheter may be used to provide postoperative analgesia either with local anesthesia[15, 30] or with opioids,[47] which may be particularly beneficial in morbidly obese patients.[15, 47]

The anesthesiologist should not choose regional anesthesia unless he or she is prepared to convert to general anesthesia if the regional anesthesia is unsatisfactory for the surgical procedure or if the patient develops respiratory difficulties.

Irrespective of the regional anesthesia technique used, careful monitoring of no lesser an intensity than that for patients receiving general anesthesia (i.e., ECG, blood pressure, and arterial oxygenation) is essential. Sedation should be used sparingly, supplemental oxygen should be delivered, and respiratory function should be monitored closely.

POSTOPERATIVE CARE

Obese patients with a previous history of respiratory disease, those with the OHS or Pickwickian syndrome, and those having major abdominal and thoracic operations are likely to have a high incidence of respiratory complications. Thus, it may be wise to admit these patients electively to an intensive care unit (ICU). Their management in the ICU will depend upon the individual patient but should include IPPV if necessary and aggressive prophylaxis against the development of respiratory complications. Obese patients are highly immobile postoperatively; measures should be taken to assist them in moving by the provision of an adjustable bed, overhead trapeze, and the availability of sufficient nursing staff.

Respiratory Function

Even in healthy obese patients, postoperative hypoxemia is a universal hazard. Supplemental oxygen should be given during transport from the operating room to the recovery room. Respiratory monitoring should be particularly aggressive in the recovery room and should include pulse oximetry and/or arterial blood gases. Prior to discharge, patients should be carefully reviewed by the use of any appropriate investigations. Patients should not be discharged to the ward until they have been shown not to be hypoxemic, and it may be appropriate to use long-term oxygen therapy on the ward. Following intraabdominal operations, arterial hypoxemia may last 4 to 6 days[48] and is of greater magnitude with vertical than with horizontal incisions. Postoperative hypoxemia can be minimized by nursing patients in the sitting position. There is some evidence that the use of regional anesthesia techniques intra- and postoperatively will reduce the incidence of postoperative respiratory complications.[15, 47]

Immobilization

Obese patients have a high incidence of postoperative deep vein thrombosis and pulmonary emboli. The use of mini–heparin prophylaxis may be appropriate. The use of regional anesthesia techniques may decrease the incidence of deep vein thrombosis and pulmonary emboli.[15, 47]

Analgesia

Obese patients may have lesser need for postoperative analgesics than normal patients.[49] For previously stated reasons, the use of opioid analgesics can be hazardous in obese patients. Moreover, the routine use of intramuscular injections may not provide predictable blood levels of the opioid. If opioids are to be used, they should probably be delivered directly into the intravascular compartment using devices such as patient-controlled analgesia machines, but there are no data to back up this contention.

If the patient has had an epidural catheter placed for operative anesthesia, this may be used as the route for injecting either local anesthetic or opioid to provide analgesia postoperatively. The use of local anesthesia[15] or opioid[47] is associated with a greater speed of postoperative recovery and a lesser incidence of respiratory complications than the use of conventional opioid techniques. The doses of either local anesthetic[15] or opioid[47] necessary to provide postoperative epidural analgesia are similar to those in normal patients. If epidural opioid analgesia is used, it has a potential for delayed respiratory depression, and, given the difficulty of maintaining or securing the airway in obese patients, those receiving epidural opioids should probably be nursed in a closely monitored environment (*e.g.*, an ICU) until the potential for such a complication has passed.

GASTROINTESTINAL SYSTEM

FUNCTIONAL ANATOMY AND PHYSIOLOGY

The mouth and pharyngeal musculature are under voluntary control—boluses of food and fluid being swallowed and delivered to the esophagus. Such boluses are lubricated by saliva, which amounts to approximately 1200 ml · day^{-1}.[50]

Esophagus

The esophageal musculature is under involuntary control and is innervated by the vagus nerve and a sympathetic component derived from segments T6 to T10. Waves of esophageal contraction pass boluses of food down to the gastroesophageal junction, which relaxes to allow them to enter the stomach.

At the gastroesophageal junction, reflux is prevented by a number of means, including the esophagus acting as a flap valve and the diaphragmatic crura pinching off the esophagus. The major barrier to gastroesophageal reflux is now believed to be the lower esophageal sphincter (LES).[51] The LES is histologically similar to the rest of the esophagus but is functionally quite different. It may be identified by gastroesophageal manometry, drawing a series of transducers from the stomach back through the gastroesophageal junction into the esophagus. The LES appears as an area of raised pressure as depicted in Figure 41-3. It is usually 2 to 3 cm in length, extends both above and below the diaphragm, with peak pressure being found just above the diaphragm, and varies with respiration. It relaxes on swallowing, in contrast with the rest of the esophagus, which exhibits peristalsis.

The tendency for esophageal reflux is related to some degree to LES tone but more to the barrier pressure, that is, the difference between the LES pressure and the gastric pressure.[51] Thus, if intragastric pressure is sufficiently high, it may surmount the LES to produce reflux. However, in health, the LES pressure usually rises in response to a rise in intragastric pressure. The LES tends to relax during pregnancy; thus, the tendency for reflux to occur is greater at that time. Patients with hiatal hernia can exhibit a normal LES pressure, although, in such patients, the LES is nearly always above the diaphragm. Patients with gastroesophageal reflux tend to have lower barrier pressures, ranging from low to near normal range rather than exhibiting a distinct cutoff point. The LES is innervated by both the vagus and sympathetic nerves, but the role of the innervation is uncertain; vagal denervation does not affect resting tone or active function. Clinical circumstances associated with reduced LES tone include pregnancy, obesity, and hiatal hernia. Patients with gastroesophageal reflux may also have reduced LES tone. A number of drugs may increase or decrease LES tone (Table 41-1).

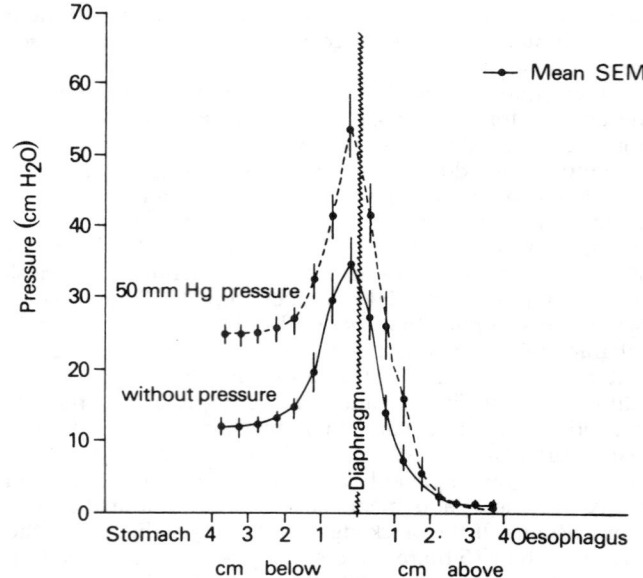

FIG. 41-3. The pressures found by lower esophageal manometry illustrating the relationship of the lower esophageal sphincter to the diaphragm. Note also the effect of increasing intraabdominal pressure causing a concurrent rise in lower esophageal sphincter pressure. (Reprinted with permission from Colton BR, Smith G: The lower esophageal sphincter and anaesthesia. Br J Anesth 56:37, 1984.)

The Stomach

The stomach can be described in the following manner and has these functions: 1) a distensible receptacle allowing the storage of large amounts of food and fluids (it may accept 1 to 1.5 l of fluid with minimal rises in intragastric pressure), 2) a chamber in which ingested food and gastric secretions may be mixed and digestion commenced, and 3) a system for expelling small and manageable amounts of gastric contents into the duodenum.[52]

The proximal part of the stomach is functionally a receptacle, exhibiting little mobility and in which little mixing occurs. Mixing occurs primarily in the distal stomach, with electrical activity originating from a "pacemaker," which is usually sited near the midpoint of the greater curvature. The

TABLE 41-1.   Lower Esophageal Sphincter Effect of Drugs Used in Anesthesia

INCREASE	DECREASE	NO CHANGE
Metoclopramide	Atropine	Propranolol
Domperidone	Glycopyrrolate	Oxprenolol
Prochlorperazine	Dopamine	Cimetidine
Cyclizine	Sodium nitroprusside	Ranitidine
Edrophonium	Ganglion blockers	Atracurium
Neostigmine	Thiopental	?Nitrous oxide
Histamine	Tricyclic antidepressants	
Suxamethonium	Halothane	
Pancuronium	Enflurane	
Metoprolol	Opioids	
Antacids	?Nitrous oxide	

electrical activity and resulting mechanical activity spread circumferentially and longitudinally toward the pylorus. Pyloric relaxation occurs in response to the waves of gastric activity permitting expulsion of small amounts of gastric contents into the duodenum. In health, gastric emptying occurs at a rate that closely approximates an exponential curve, although varying from this curve when the stomach is full or when it is nearly empty.

The rate of gastric emptying can be influenced by physiologic factors such as the type of intake; liquids leaving the stomach more quickly than solids; and the volume, pH, and osmotic qualities of the gastric contents.[52] The customary 4-hour preoperative fast does not guarantee that the stomach is empty, and evidence is accumulating that modest feeding or intake of small amounts of fluid during the preoperative period may be associated with lower volumes of gastric contents.[53, 53a] Certain groups of patients tend to have a high resting gastric content volume, for example, pregnant persons, the obese, and the bedridden (Table 41-2). Pathologic states associated with high resting gastric content volume include pain and trauma. Patients in shock may also be included. Laparotomy will slow the rate of gastric emptying for approximately 24 hours, although this is probably the result of a combination of mechanical effects of bowel handling and postoperative use of opioids. A number of drugs may influence the rate of gastric emptying; these are summarized in Table 41-2.

Gastric secretions are produced at a rate of nearly 2000 ml·day^{-1}. They have a pH of 1.0 to 3.5, are isotonic with extracellular fluid, and consist predominantly of hydrochloric acid, with a higher potassium content than extracellular fluid. The pH of gastric contents may be raised by the administration of antacids or H_2 histamine-blocking drugs.

The Duodenum

In the duodenum, secretions of the pancreas and the biliary tract are mixed with the gastric contents. Secretions of the pancreas and the biliary tract are predominantly alkaline, with pHs in region of 7.8 to 8.3 and daily volumes of 1200 and 700 ml, respectively. The pH of the resultant mix of gastric contents and duodenal secretions will be a function of the respective volumes and pH of gastric contents and pancreatic and biliary tract secretions.

Small Intestine

At rest, activity of the small intestine is governed by what is termed the migrating myoelectric complex (MMC). It has two components: 1) electromyographic, and 2) manometric. Four phases may be seen: Phase I, with slow wave electrical activity with quiescent intestine; Phase II slow wave, with some spikes accompanied by periodic intestinal contractions; Phase III intense spiking, accompanying slow waves electrically with vigorous mechanical contractions; and Phase IV, which reverts from Phase III to Phase I and is associated with rapid subsiding of contractions.[50]

When food is taken, the MMC is disrupted, and there is contractile activity throughout the whole intestine. Postprandial intestinal activity can be divided into a cephalic phase, which may be abolished by vagotomy, a gastric phase promoted by gastric distention, and an intestinal phase provoked by perfusion of the intestine with nutrients.

The mode of control of small intestinal activity is uncertain. The parasympathetic system has a role, as parasympathetic stimulation produces increased activity, and suppression of the parasympathetic system produces a decrease in activity. The sympathetic nervous system also has a role, as sympathetic suppression causes an increase in activity and stimulation, a decrease in activity mediated by both catecholamines and dopaminergic receptors. However, with bowel denervation, there appears to be little change in activity, and it is likely that humoral secretions, especially pancreatic polypeptides and somatostatin, play a major role in mediating activity. Small intestinal activity is suppressed for 24 to 48 hours following laparotomy and may also be decreased by peritonitis and a fall in serum potassium level.

The small intestine secretes 2,000 ml of fluid a day, which has a pH of between 7.0 and 8.0. The small intestine is the site of the majority of the absorption of fluid and nutrients in the gastrointestinal tract. It is presented with 5500 ml of fluid a day (2,000 ml from the stomach, 1500 ml from the pancreas and biliary tract, and 2,000 ml from the small intestine) but passes on only 500 ml to the colon. Thus, the net turnover of fluid in the small intestine is of the order of about 5,000 ml·day^{-1}. The absorptive abilities of the small intestine are impaired for approximately 36 hours following laparotomy.

The Colon

Approximately 500 to 700 ml of bowel contents are presented to the colon each day. The colon expels only 100 to 200 ml·day^{-1}; therefore, its function is predominantly absorptive. The motility of the colon is controlled by a pacemaker located in the transverse colon. Three types of activity can be observed: 1) antiperistalsis from the transverse colon to the cecum, which permits maximal exposure of the feces for absorption of fluid; 2) peristalsis pushing forward feces to the distal parts of the colon; and 3) a powerful peristaltic movement, which is responsible for the evacuation of fecal content, which moves anally in a series of large mass movements.

Parasympathetic neural control of the colon as far as the splenic flexure is furnished by the vagus nerve; beyond that point, it is furnished by the sacral parasympathetic outflow.

TABLE 41-2.   Some Factors Influencing Gastric Emptying Rate

	ACCELERATE	DELAY
Physiologic	Gastric distention Neuroticism	Food Acid High osmotic pressure Posture Pregnancy
Pathologic	Thyrotoxicosis	Shock Trauma and pain Myocardial infarction Pyloric stenosis Crohn's disease Celiac disease Diabetic autonomic neuropathy
Pharmacologic	Metoclopramide Neostigmine Propranolol Sodium bicarbonate Cigarette smoking	Anticholinergics Tricyclic antidepressants Aluminum hydroxide Alcohol Isoprenaline Opioid analgesics

The sympathetic supply is from segments T6 to T10. Parasympathetic stimulation increases motility, whereas sympathetic stimulation decreases activity. Administration of neostigmine increases activity both in terms of activity and tone, whereas morphine decreases activity.[54]

SPLANCHNIC BLOOD FLOW

Splanchnic oxygenation can be influenced by changes in the blood oxygen-carrying capacity (such as anemia), and by changes in blood flow to the bowel. There is anecdotal evidence that anemia may lead to poor rates of wound healing in areas of relatively compromised blood flow such as the colon.[55] The optimal hematocrit is thought to be in the mid-30s.

In normal circumstances of a normal cardiac output, splanchnic blood flow remains relatively stable, being regulated by the splanchnic vascular resistance through mechanisms similar to those regulating hepatic blood flow. Splanchnic vascular resistance is regulated largely by the sympathetic nervous system, sympathectomy decreasing splanchnic vascular resistance, alpha-adrenergic stimulation promoting vasoconstriction, and beta-adrenergic stimulation promoting vasodilation. Dopamine may act in the splanchnic vascular bed through two receptors, with alpha-adrenergic vasoconstriction predominating over the mild vasodilatation produced by beta stimulation. Parasympathetic stimulation results in an increase in blood flow and an increase in motor activity.

In stress states, a number of humoral agents may influence splanchnic blood flow, including catecholamines, vasopressin, and angiotensin II. With hemorrhage, splanchnic vascular resistance rises, presumably as a teleologic mechanism to permit the diversion of cardiac output to organs more vital to survival. Modest hemorrhage of 10%–15% of circulating blood volume, which does not affect systemic arterial pressure, may markedly impair splanchnic blood flow. Restoration of circulating volume does not result in a rapid restoration of splanchnic blood flow, which may remain decreased for several hours. Although blood loss and hypotension are not particularly critical for the blood supply to the stomach and small bowel, which have a liberal vascular supply, such circumstances may be associated with an increased rate of colonic anastomotic dehiscence.[55, 56]

A number of perioperative factors may alter splanchnic blood flow. Post-trauma, there may be an increase in splanchnic blood flow, but laparotomy alone produces little change. Morphine will decrease splanchnic vascular resistance and, therefore, increase splanchnic blood flow. There is almost a linear relationship between splanchnic blood flow and Pa_{CO_2}, with hypocapnia decreasing flow and hypercapnia increasing flow. Halothane and isoflurane decrease splanchnic blood flow.[57] Regional anesthesia with high levels of sympathetic blockade results in an increase in splanchnic blood flow owing to a decrease in splanchnic vascular resistance, both as a consequence of the sympathectomy itself and the fall in catecholamine levels associated with sympathetic blockade.[54] However, if such a sympathectomy results in a fall in cardiac output, splanchnic blood flow may fall. Sympathectomy does not influence the changes in splanchnic blood flow produced by changes in Pa_{CO_2}.[58] Neostigmine will reduce mesenteric blood flow by 30%–50% in association with the exaggerated motor activity of the intestine. Such decreases in blood flow may be somewhat ameliorated by the prior administration of atropine.[56]

GENERAL CONSIDERATIONS FOR ANESTHESIA AND THE GASTROINTESTINAL TRACT

Irrespective of the target of the surgery in the gastrointestinal tract, a number of factors impacting upon patient evaluation and management must be taken into consideration.

Airway Management and Protection

ANATOMIC. The oral, pharyngeal, and hypopharyngeal areas may be distorted by a number of pathologic processes, including tumor, infection, obstruction by an ingested foreign body, thermal or chemical damage, and nonmalignant variations from normal anatomy such as pharyngeal pouches. Thus, it is necessary to carefully evaluate the patient with respect to the site, type and magnitude of distortion, and the pathologic process producing the airway abnormality. The choice of airway management and securing the airway should be based on clinical findings and supplemented where necessary by investigations such as direct or indirect laryngoscopy, soft-tissue x-rays and CAT or magnetic resonance imaging (MRI) scans of the abnormal area (see Chapter 20).

PROTECTION. A major consideration in anesthesia for surgery of the gastrointestinal tract is the reduction in the risk of, and prevention of, inadvertent airway soiling by aspiration of gastrointestinal contents during induction and maintenance of anesthesia. During the maintenance of routine anesthesia, in the absence of risk factors, the incidence of regurgitation of gastric contents into the perilaryngeal area is approximately 8%. In approximately 1% of the total population, gastric contents can be shown to reach the airway.[59] Regurgitation/aspiration is most likely to occur during the induction of anesthesia, when the airway is not securely protected by an endotracheal tube and when active vomiting is most likely.

The consequences of regurgitation and subsequent aspiration of gastric contents into the airway will depend upon the character and volume of the aspirate. Solid matter will produce an anatomic obstruction of the airway, and fluid of neutral pH will produce a near-drowning-like picture, whereas the aspiration of even small amounts of acidic fluid may be associated with the aspiration syndrome (Mendelson syndrome). The incidence of the latter is estimated at 0.05%.[60] It is generally accepted that a gastric content in excess of 25 ml with a pH of less than 2.5 implies a special risk of producing an aspiration syndrome if such fluid is aspirated.[61] However, there is also opinion that acid aspiration syndromes can be produced by aspirates with a higher pH.[62] Therefore, it is incumbent upon anesthesiologists to attempt to reduce the volume and increase the pH of any gastric contents.

If the volume of gastric contents is suspected to be high, this volume may be reduced by attempting to empty the stomach with a nasogastric tube or by the induction of vomiting with apomorphine.[63] Gastric emptying can also be facilitated by using drugs to increase gastric motility. A number of pharmacologic agents that hasten gastric emptying are listed in Table 41-2. However, the use of such maneuvers does not guarantee an empty stomach, and their use should not lull the anesthesiologist into a false sense of security. By no means does the use of these techniques absolve the anesthesiologist of the responsibility of taking other precautions to prevent regurgitation and possibly pulmonary aspiration of gastrointestinal tract contents.

A major thrust in reducing the potential for acid aspiration syndrome has been the raising of the pH of gastric contents.

This may be done effectively with particulate antacids such as aluminum hydroxide or magnesium trisilicate. However, it has been shown that such drugs can potentially cause lung damage if they are aspirated; thus, the trend is toward non-particulate antacids such as sodium citrate (0.3 mM).[61a, 61b] Drugs that will reduce acid secretion, such as the H₂ blockers cimetidine and ranitidine, in iv doses of 300 and 50 mg, respectively, have been shown to effectively raise pH.[27, 28] Ranitidine is probably the drug of choice, as it is associated with fewer side-effects and has a longer duration of action than cimetidine. Some anticholinergics, particularly glycopyrrolate, will also reduce gastric acidity.

Studies of the acid aspiration syndrome have shown that a high proportion of patients who suffer from this problem have a LES dysfunction.[60] Thus, the maintenance of LES function is of importance. Circumstances associated with a lowered LES tone were discussed in an earlier section. Drugs that raise LES tone are listed in Table 41-1.

Thus, prior to induction of anesthesia, the risk of regurgitation and pulmonary aspiration may be reduced by

I. Reducing volume of stomach contents
    A. By the use of nasogastric tubes
    B. By the induction of vomiting
    C. By hastening the speed of gastric emptying with drugs such as metoclopramide
II. Raising gastric content pH with clear antacids and H₂ histamine blockers
III. Increasing LES tone with metoclopramide.

Having attempted to reduce the likelihood of regurgitation and aspiration, the airway should be secured coincident with the induction of anesthesia by the expeditious passage of an endotracheal tube and with the use of maneuvers designed to prevent gastric contents reaching the airway, such as application of cricoid pressure (Sellick's maneuver).

Fluid and Electrolyte Balance

Patients with gastrointestinal disease[64] may be in fluid or electrolyte imbalance for a number of reasons.

1. Inadequate intake. Patients awaiting surgery are often kept NPO for varying periods of time preoperatively. This is especially likely to be a factor in children, small adults, and patients in a hot environment or with pyrexia in whom insensible fluid loss may be high. In the chronically ill patient, there may be a long period of inadequate intake, or oral intake may be prevented by anorexia and/or gastrointestinal tract obstruction.
2. Sequestration of water and electrolytes into abdominal structures, for example, bowel lumen, bowel wall, and peritoneum in patients who have inflammatory bowel disease or intestinal obstruction.
3. Extracorporeal loss of fluid such as from vomiting, diarrhea, or loss by fistulae.

Frequently, the etiology of the fluid deficit will be an amalgam of these three causes. The magnitude of fluid and electrolyte deficit will be determined by the duration of the problem and by the site of the fluid loss. Deficient intake and salivary loss, for example, in a patient with a pharyngeal tumor, is primarily water loss with minimal electrolyte loss.

Loss of fluid that is primarily gastric contents (which, in a patient with pyloric stenosis may reach 2,000 ml · day⁻¹), will result in a hypochloremic alkalosis and hypokalemia. Potas-

sium is not only lost in the gastric fluid but will also be excreted by the kidney in response to the alkalosis.

If fluid is lost externally from the lower gastrointestinal tract, the resulting deficit will be predominantly a metabolic acidosis and hypochloremia. The loss may be up to 3,000 ml · day⁻¹.

When small bowel obstruction occurs, a complex series of events takes place. The segment of bowel proximal to the obstruction dilates and will contain gas (which is primarily swallowed gas) and fluids. The fluids result from bowel contents upstream and an increase in small bowel secretion with a decrease in fluid absorption. As bowel dilation increases, fluid will be lost into the bowel wall and peritoneal cavity. Progressive dilation and edema of the bowel, or of a volvulus, may lead to an impaired bowel blood supply with potential bowel necrosis and perforation. In these circumstances, further rapid fluid loss will occur and the patient may get a bacterial toxemia or septicemia. The usually encountered abnormalities include hemoconcentration, a fall in circulating blood volume, and a fall in total body potassium.

Large bowel obstruction tends to occur more slowly and presents less dramatically than does small bowel obstruction. The effects of the obstruction depend upon the competence of the ileocecal valve. If the valve is competent, the closed obstruction will result in large bowel dilation, particularly of the right colon and cecum, with the potential for progression to impairment of colon blood supply and necrosis and perforation. However, if the ileocecal valve is not competent, the bowel contents will reflux into the small bowel and will ultimately result in feculent vomiting. The speed of progression of symptoms in large bowel obstruction tends to be slower than that for small bowel obstruction, but the fluid and electrolyte disturbance may be just as severe with similar intravascular and extracellular fluid consequences.

Diarrhea may result from impaired intestinal absorption of water and electrolytes, from abnormal bowel motility, or from an increase in the osmotically active substances in the bowel lumen. The fluid and volume deficit reflects the hypotonic, potassium-containing nature of the stools and tends to produce a hypokalemic metabolic acidosis.

Preoperative evaluation of the patient's fluid and electrolyte deficit should be based on assessment of clinical parameters such as skin turgor, peripheral circulation, heart rate, blood pressure, and urine output. Useful laboratory studies include hematocrit, serum electrolytes, and blood urea nitrogen. If necessary, invasive monitoring such as central venous pressure and pulmonary artery pressure should be used to further assess the patient's vascular volume. The speed with which resuscitation and rehydration should be accomplished will depend upon the urgency of the surgical procedure. Small bowel obstruction, which may rapidly progress to bowel ischemia and perforation, necessitates urgent operation. Therefore, resuscitation should be swift and aggressive and aimed at rendering the patient fit for operation in a brief period of time. Resuscitation for large bowel obstruction or for a more chronic fluid loss, from whatever source, may be accomplished in a somewhat more leisurely fashion. The type of fluid resuscitation will depend upon the volume of loss and the clinical and laboratory findings. This subject is also discussed in Chapters 25 and 27.

Malabsorption and Malnutrition

The gastrointestinal tract is responsible for absorbing all nutrients; therefore, bowel abnormalities may be associated with malabsorption of nutrients and consequent malnutrition. The malabsorption may be of one element only, but, more commonly, it is of multiple elements and is usually associated with chronic rather than acute disease.[64]

Gastric lesions and gastric resections are commonly associated with a poorly understood iron deficiency anemia and with megaloblastic vitamin B_{12} deficiency anemia owing to either lack of intrinsic factor or overgrowth of vitamin B_{12}-consuming bacteria in a blind loop. A deficiency of bile salt secretion impairs fat absorption, leading to steatorrhea and deficiencies of the fat-soluble vitamins, A, D, and K and of calcium. Pancreatic insufficiency may lead to protein and fat malabsorption, with steatorrhea and fat-soluble vitamin deficiency. Intestinal malabsorption may occur owing to motility disorders, reduction in absorptive area, mucosal abnormalities, or bacterial overgrowth. The severity of the malabsorption and malnutrition will be related to the magnitude, site, and the duration of the disease and the magnitude of the decrease in absorptive surface. Malabsorption is generally of protein, fats, and vitamins, with carbohydrate absorption being relatively well preserved.

Malnutrition may also result from loss of bowel contents through fistulae or from intestinal loss of protein into the bowel lumen in diseases such as regional enteritis, ulcerative colitis, and allergic enteropathies.

Although the correction of malnutrition in the preoperative period is relatively unimportant for acute diseases, it may be extremely important in chronic disease states. Experience with preoperative elemental diets or hyperalimentation has shown that by correcting malnutrition, both wound healing and the overall outcome of surgical procedures for chronic bowel diseases is improved. Postoperatively, adequate nutrition is also important to improve healing and to reduce the incidence of complications. After abdominal operations, most patients manifest an increase in caloric and protein requirement, particularly in patients with major abdominal infections.

SPECIAL ANESTHESIA CONSIDERATIONS FOR BOWEL SURGERY

Use of Nitrous Oxide

The solubility of nitrous oxide in blood is much greater than that of nitrogen. The blood–gas partition coefficient of nitrous oxide is 34 times that of nitrogen. In consequence, nitrous oxide in the blood stream will enter gas-containing body cavities much faster than the nitrogen in those cavities will be removed by the circulation. If this occurs in the bowel, the gas-containing bowel will distend.[65] The amount of distention will depend upon:

1. *The amount of gas within the bowel.* In health, the bowel contains about 100 ml of gas, the majority of which is swallowed; therefore, distention is relatively unimportant. However, with obstruction or aerophagy, the bowel may contain much larger amounts of gas; therefore, the potential for expansion is much greater.
2. *The duration of administration.* During the initial administraiton of nitrous oxide, there will be a linear increase in bowel gas cavity size. By 100 minutes after the commencement of administration of nitrous oxide, bowel gas cavity size will have increased by 75–100%, and, at that time, the bowel nitrous oxide/end-tidal nitrous oxide ratio is about 0.5.

The distention of bowel by nitrous oxide may produce a number of problems. In a critical situation with an already distended bowel, that is, in bowel obstruction, the increases in size and intraluminal pressure may tip the balance toward bowel ischemia and necrosis. More commonly, the increase in size will cause difficulties for the surgeon intraoperatively, especially during abdominal closure. Therefore, it is best to avoid nitrous oxide when the bowel contains much gas. It is probably safe to use nitrous oxide, limiting its concentration to 50% for a brief period of time, that is, 10 to 15 minutes, at the start of an operation in order to facilitate induction of anesthesia with a volatile drug. The nitrous oxide should be withdrawn thereafter, and anesthesia should be maintained with oxygen and a volatile drug—a technique that leads to little or no increase in size of gas-containing cavities.

Neostigmine

Parasympathetic activity results in increased bowel peristalsis. Thus, drugs that increase parasympathetic effects, for example, cholinesterase inhibitors such as neostigmine, will also increase bowel activity.[54] In normal bowel, neostigmine increases the frequency and magnitude of the pressure waves, particularly in the colon, and this effect is magnified in diseased bowel. Such effects may be reduced by the presence of anesthetic drugs or the previous administration of atropine or glycopyrrolate.[66] There is anecdotal evidence that the administration of neostigmine to patients with a large bowel anastomosis may lead to an increased incidence of anastomotic disruption.[55] Thus, if neostigmine is to be used in these circumstances, it should be used with caution.

Specific Disease States

ESOPHAGEAL PERFORATION. Patients with this anomaly may be extremely ill, fluid depleted, and septic. They may have pneumomediastinum, pneumothorax, and pleural effusions. The patient's inability to swallow may complicate airway management.

ACUTE PANCREATITIS. This is commonly associated with chronic alcohol ingestion; thus, the patient is usually suffering from the effects of that particular disease. The patient may be malnourished with impaired liver function and possibly an alcohol withdrawal syndrome. More acute problems include a fluid deficit, hypocalcemia, hyperglycemia, pleural effusions, and adult respiratory distress syndrome (ARDS).

PANCREATIC CYSTS AND PSEUDOCYSTS. These are usually a consequence of acute or chronic pancreatitis. Patients are usually malnourished and often septic.

CROHN'S DISEASE. Patients with this disease are chronically ill, malnourished, and dehydrated owing to bowel obstruction, malabsorption, or loss of fluids and nutrients via fistulae. They are often very ill, taking large doses of steroids or immunosuppressive therapy.

ULCERATIVE COLITIS. This chronic disease often results in electrolyte and fluid imbalance, vitamin B_{12} and folate deficiency, and extracolonic manifestations such as arthritis, iritis, and hepatitis. Operations in the quiescent phases are often undertaken for precancerous lesions. Acute problems that may necessitate urgent operation include hemorrhage, bowel perforation, bowel obstruction, and toxic megacolon.

Patients undergoing operations in the acute phase are often very ill, on large doses of steroids, and undergoing extensive operations, for example, total colectomy or total procto-colectomy. Careful resuscitation and intensive monitoring may be required.

CARCINOID TUMORS.[68] Although carcinoid tumors may occur at other anatomic sites, the gastrointestinal tract is the source of most of them. The tumors are usually small and frequently multiple. Fifty per cent occur in the appendix, 25% occur in the ileum (these are usually the source of metastatic tumors), and 20% occur in the rectum. The hormones secreted by nonmetastatic carcinoid tumors reach the liver by way of the portal vein and are usually inactivated there. However, once metastases to the liver have occurred, the hormones secreted by the hepatic metastases may have direct access to the systemic circulation to there produce the symptoms and signs of the carcinoid syndrome. Approximately 35% of patients with carcinoid tumors and metastases will have symptoms of the carcinoid syndrome.[69] The classical presentation of the carcinoid syndrome is not evident in all patients: 75% have cutaneous flushing, 70% exhibit an increase in gastrointestinal motility, 40% have cardiovascular symptoms, and 20% experience bronchospasm.

Carcinoid tumors produce a variety of hormones, and the symptoms produced in each person's carcinoid syndrome will probably depend upon the hormone(s) secreted. A summary of the hormones secreted, their physiologic effects, and suggested treatments are given in Table 41-3.

Although carcinoid tumors are relatively rare, those patients with carcinoid tumors presenting for surgery are usually the worst affected and present a number of problems. Carcinoid heart disease occurs in about one third of the patients, but its etiology is somewhat uncertain. The pathologic findings are predominantly right-sided fibrinous plaques deposited on the right ventricular wall and on the tricuspid valve producing incompetence or, less frequently, stenosis or deposition on the pulmonary valve. Such plaques are rarely found on the left side of the heart. Invasive or noninvasive cardiologic evaluation is necessary to determine the magnitude and the effects of heart disease.

It is difficult to give blanket recommendations for the management of all patients with carcinoid syndrome, as it is likely that the extent and proportion of hormonal secretion and the effects that they produce will vary from person to person. The majority of information dealing with patients with carcinoid syndrome comes from anecdotal reports; there are no good published series of large number of patients dealing with overall management. When anesthetizing a patient with a carcinoid syndrome, it may be possible to get clues for likely intraoperative events from the previous history, although this is not necessarily so (*e.g.*, 50% of the patients with intraoperative bronchospasm may have no previous history). Likely problems that one may encounter include:

1. *Bronchospasm*. This may be quite severe. It can be provoked by the use of histamine releasing drugs such as morphine and *d*-tubocurarine. Because adrenergic drugs are likely to cause release of histamine, these should also be avoided. The use of H_1 and H_2 histamine blockers and steroids prophylactically is advised. If the bronchospasm occurs intraoperatively, the use of steroids, diphenhydramine, halothane, ketanserin, and somatostatin have been recommended.
2. *Hypotension*. This may be a consequence of the disease causing a generalized fluid deficit, but, if it occurs acutely, it may be secondary to hormone release. It is important to have the patient adequately volume resuscitated preoperatively. The measurement of central venous pressure or pulmonary artery pressure to assess cardiovascular status may be helpful. Prophylactic measures to minimize hypotension include steroids, H_1 and H_2 histamine blockers, cautious titration of volatile anesthetics, avoiding histamine releasing drugs, such as morphine and *d*-tubocurarine, and the avoidance of succinylcholine, which can cause abdominal wall fasciculations, pressure upon the tumor, and hormone release. If hypotension occurs intraoperatively, it is important to give volume and avoid the use of catecholamines. The use of angiotensin in a dose of 1.5 $mg \cdot kg^{-1}$ may improve the hypotension.
3. *Hypertension*. This is usually an acute intraoperative phenomenon, often associated with bronchospasm, and is probably due to tumor release of serotonin. Prophylactic treatment with ketanserin has been described. If hypertension occurs acutely, the use of

TABLE 41-3. Hormones Released by Carcinoid Tumors and Their Management

		TREATMENT		
	PHYSIOLOGIC EFFECTS	*Inhibiting Synthesis*	*Hormone Depletion*	*Receptor Blockers*
Serotonin	Vasoconstriction Vasodilatation Increased motility Tryptophan depletion	Parachlorophylalamine	Fenluranine	Methysergide Cyproheptadine Ketanserin
Kinins	Vasodilatation Histamine release Bronchoconstriction	Steroids Aprotinin		
Histamine	Vasodilatation H_1 = extravascular smooth muscle contraction H_2 = extravascular smooth muscle relaxation			H_2 antagonists Phenothiazines

methotrimeprazine, conventional vasodilating agents such as sodium nitroprusside and nitroglycerine, or ketanserin has been described.

REFERENCES

1. Rosenbaum S, Skinner RF, Knight AB et al: A survey of height and weight in Great Britain 1980. Ann Hum Biol 12:115, 1985
2. Van Itallie TB: Health implications of overweight and obesity in the United States. Ann Intern Med 103:983, 1985
3. Fisher A, Waterhouse TD, Adams AP: Obesity: Its relation to anaesthesia. Anaesthesia 30:633, 1975
4. Farebrother MJB: Respiratory function and cardiorespiratory response to exercise in obesity. Br J Dis Chest 73:211, 1979
5. Luce JM: Respiratory complications of obesity. Chest 78:626, 1980
6. Vaughan RW: Pulmonary and cardiovascular derangements in the obese patient. In Brown BR (ed): Anesthetics and the Obese Patient, pp 19–39. Contemporary Anesthesia Practice Series, Philadelphia, FA Davis, 1982
7. Burwell CS, Robin ED, Whaley RD et al: External obesity associated with alveolar hypoventilation—A Pickwickian syndrome. Am J Med 21:811, 1956
8. Reisin E, Frolich ED: Obesity—cardiovascular and respiratory pathophysiological alterations. Arch Intern Med 141:431, 1981
9. Alexander JK: The cardiomyopathy of obesity. Prog Cardiovasc Dis 28:325, 1985
10. Paul DR, Hoyt JL, Boutros AR: Cardiovascular and respiratory changes in response to change of posture in the obese. Anesthesiology 45:73, 1976
11. Vaughan RW: Biochemical and biotransformation alterations in obesity. In Brown BR (ed): Anesthesia and the Obese Patient, p 55. Contemporary Anesthesia Practice Series, Philadelphia, FA Davis, 1982
12. Vaughan RW, Bauer S, Wise L: Volume and pH of gastric juice in obese patients. Anesthesiology 43:686, 1975
13. Nomura F, Ohnishi K, Satomura Y et al: Liver function in moderate obesity—study in 536 moderately obese subjects among 4613 male company employees. Int J Obes 10:349, 1986
14. Wadden TA, Stunkard AJ: Social and psychological consequences of obesity. Ann Intern Med 103:1062, 1985
15. Buckley FP, Robinson NB, Simonowitz DA et al: Anesthesia in the morbidly obese. A comparison of anesthetic and analgesic regimes for upper abdominal surgery. Anaesthesia 38:840, 1983
16. Abernathy DR, Greenblatt DS: Pharmacokinetics of drugs in obesity. Clin Pharmacokinet 7:108, 1981
17. Abernathy DR, Greenblatt DS, Divoll M et al: The influence of obesity on the pharmacokinetics of oral alprazolam and triazolam. Clin Pharmacokinet 9:177, 1984
18. Mayersohn M, Calkins JM, Perrier DG et al: Thiopental kinetics in obese patients. Anesthesiology 55:A178, 1981
19. Ladergaard–Pederson MJ: Recovery from general anesthesia in obese patients. Anesthesiology 55:720, 1981
20. Cork RC, Vaughan RW, Bentley JB: General anesthesia for morbidly obese patients—an examination of postoperative outcomes. Anesthesiology 54:310, 1981
21. Bentley JB, Borel JD, Gillespie TS et al: Fentanyl pharmacokinetics in obese and non-obese patients. Anesthesiology 55:A177, 1981
22. Schwartz AE, Matteo RS, Ornstein E et al: Pharmacokinetics of sufentanil in the obese. Anesthesiology 65:A652, 1986
23. Tseueda K, Warren JE, McCafferty LA: Pancuronium bromide requirement during anesthesia for the morbidly obese. Anesthesiology 48:483, 1978

24. Bentley JB, Bond JD, Vaughan RW et al: Weight, pseudocholinesterase activity and succinylcholine requirements. Anesthesiology 57:48, 1982
25. Wilson SL, Manaltea NR, Malvesa JD: Effects of atropine, glycopyrrolate and cimetidine on gastric secretions in markedly obese patients. Anesth Analg 60:37, 1981
26. Goldberg ME, Rosenberg FI, Everts EA Jr et al: Metoclopramide and cimetidine pretreatment does not reduce the risk of acid aspiration in the morbidly obese patient. Anesthesiology 63:A279, 1985
27. Lam AM, Grace DM, Penny FJ et al: Prophylactic IV cimetidine reduces the risk of acid aspiration in morbidly obese patients. Anesthesiology 65:684, 1986
28. Manchikanti L, Roush JR, Colliver JR: Effect of preanesthetic ranitidine and metoclopramide on gastric contents of morbidly obese patients. Anesth Analg 65:195, 1986
29. Lee JJ, Larson RM, Buckley JJ et al: Airway maintenance in the morbidly obese. Anesthesiol Rev 7:33, 1980
30. Bromage PR: Epidural Analgesia, p 502. Philadelphia, WB Saunders, 1980
31. Moyer GA, Rein P: Preoxygenation in the morbidly obese patient. Anesth Analg 65:S106, 1986
32. Vaughan RW, Wise L: Intraoperative hypoxemia in obese patients. Ann Surg 184:35, 1976
32a. Bentley JB, Vaughn RW, Gandolfi J et al: Halothane biotransformation in obese and nonobese patients. Anesthesiology 57:94, 1982
33. Salem MR, Joseph N, Lim R et al: Respiratory and hemodynamic response to PEEP in grossly obese patients. Anesthesiology 61:A511, 1984
34. In-amani M, Kikuta Y, Nagai H et al: The increase in pulmonary venous admixture by hypocapnia is enhanced in obese patients. Anesthesiology 63:A520, 1985
35. Brodsky JB, Wyner J, Ehrenwerth S et al: One lung anesthesia in morbidly obese patients. Anesthesiology 57:132, 1982
36. Ferguson CL, Sivashankaran S, Dauchot PJ: Ventilator settings mitigate hypocarbia in the obese patient. Anesth Analg 65:S53, 1986
37. McCullough WJD, Littlewood DG: Influence of obesity on spinal analgesia with bupivacaine. Br J Anaesth 58:610, 1984
38. Catennacci AJ, Anderson JD, Boersma D: Anesthetic hazards of obesity. JAMA 175:657, 1961
39. Catennacci AJ, Sampathakar DR: Ventilation studies in the obese patient during spinal anesthesia. Anesth Analg 48:48, 1969
40. Blass NM: Regional anesthesia in the morbidly obese. Reg Anesth 5(3):20, 1979
41. Chamberlain DD, Chamberlain BDL: Changes in skin temperature and their relationship to sympathetic blockade during spinal anesthesia. Anesthesiology 65:139, 1986
42. Hodgkinson R, Hussein FJ: Caesarian section associated with gross obesity. Br J Anaesth 52:919, 1980
43. Fox GS, Whalley DG, Bevan DR: Anaesthesia for the morbidly obese. Experience with 110 patients. Br J Anaesth 53:811, 1981
44. Gelman S, Vitek JJ: Thoracic epidural catheter placement under fluoroscopic control in morbidly obese patients. Reg Anesth 4(4):19, 1980
45. Hodgkinson R, Hussein FJ: Obesity and the spread of analgesic following epidural administration of bupivacaine for caesarian section. Anesth Analg 59:89, 1980
46. Gelman S, Laws ML, Potzick J et al: Thoracic epidural vs. balanced anaesthesia in morbid obesity: An intraoperative and postoperative hemodynamic study. Anesth Analg 59:902, 1980
47. Rawal N, Sjostrand V, Christofferson E et al: Comparison of intramuscular and epidural morphine for postoperative analgesia in the grossly obese. Influence on postoperative ambulation and pulmonary function. Anesth Analg 63:583, 1986

48. Vaughan RW, Wise L: Intraoperative hypoxemia in obese patients. Ann Surg 180:872, 1974
49. Rand CSW, Kuldau JM, Yost RL: Obesity and postoperative pain. J Psychosom Res 29:43, 1985
50. Scratcherd T, Grundy O: The physiology of intestinal motility and secretion. Br J Anaesth 56:3, 1984
51. Colton BR, Smith G: The lower oesophageal sphincter and anaesthesia. Br J Anaesth 56:37, 1984
52. Nimmo WS: Effect of anaesthesia on gastric motility and emptying. Br J Anaesth 56:29, 1984
53. Miller M, Wishart MY, Nimmo WS: Gastric contents at induction of anaesthesia—Is a four hour fast necessary? Br J Anaesth 33:1183, 1983
53a. Maltby JR, Sutherland AP, Sace JP et al: Preoperative oral fluids: Is a five-hour fast justified prior to elective surgery? Anesth Analg 65:1112, 1986
54. Aitkenhead AR: Anaesthesia and bowel surgery. Br J Anaesth 56:95, 1984
55. Schrock TR, Deveney CW, Dunphy JE: Factors contributing to leakage of colonic anastomosis. Ann Surg 173:515, 1973
56. Whittaker BL: Observations on the bloodflow in the inferior mesenteric artery and the healing of colonic anastomosis. Ann Surg 43:89, 1968
57. Gelman S, Fowler KC, Smith LR: Regional blood flow during isoflurane and halothane anesthesia. Anesth Analg 63:557, 1986
58. Aitkenhead AR, Gilmour PS, Hothersall AP et al: Effects of subarachnoid nerve block and arterial P_{CO_2} on colon blood flow. Br J Anaesth 52:1071, 1980
59. Blitt CD, Gutman ML, Cohen DD et al: Silent regurgitation and aspiration during general anesthesia. Anesth Analg 49:707, 1970
60. Olsson GL, Hallen B, Hambraeus–Jonzn K: Aspiration during anesthesia: A computer-aided study. Acta Anaesth Scand 30:844, 1970
61. Roberts RB, Shirley MA: Reducing the risk of acid aspiration during caesarian section. Anesth Analg 53:859, 1976
61a. Eyler SW, Cullen BF, Murphy ME et al: Antacid aspiration in rabbits: A comparison of Mylanta and Bicitra. Anesth Analg 61:288, 1982
61b. Viegas OJ, Ravindran RS, Schumaker CA: Gastric fluid pH in patients receiving sodium citrate. Anesth Analg 60:521, 1981
62. Crawford JS: Cimetidine in elective caesarian section. Anaesthesia 36:641, 1981
63. Holdsworth JD, Furness RMB, Rulston RG: A comparison of apomorphine and stomach tubes for emptying the stomach before general anesthesia in obstetrics. Br J Anaesth 46:526, 1974
64. Saik RP, Chadwick MC, Katz J: Gastrointestinal disorders. In Katz J, Benemof J, Kadis LB (eds): Anesthesia and Uncommon Diseases, p 386. Philadelphia, WB Saunders, 1981
65. Eger EI III, Saidman LJ: Hazards of nitrous oxide in bowel obstruction and pneumothorax. Anesthesiology 26:61, 1985
66. Childes CS: Prevention of neostigmine-induced colonic activity. Anaesthesia 39:1083, 1984
67. McCammon RL: The gastrointestinal system. In Stoelting RK, Dierdorf SF (eds): Anesthesia and Coexisting Disease, p 363. New York, Churchill, Livingstone, 1983
68. Longnecker M, Roizen MF: Patient with carcinoid syndrome. Anesthesiol Clin North Am 52:313, 1987
69. Moeretel CA, Sauer WA, Dockerty MG et al: The life history of the carcinoid tumor of the small intestine. Cancer 14:901, 1961

Chapter 42   *Simon Gelman*

Anesthesia and the Liver

INCIDENCE OF POSTOPERATIVE HEPATIC COMPLICATIONS

The incidence of postanesthesia/surgery complications related to hepatic dysfunction varies greatly.[1-9] The differences result not only from the different population of patients but also from the different criteria that the authors use to define postoperative hepatic dysfunction. Most patients who demonstrate postoperative hepatic dysfunction experience only a transient increase in liver enzymes and/or bilirubin. The latter may be related to an excessive load of bilirubin, resulting from blood transfusions rather than hepatic dysfunction. Some studies have demonstrated relatively high incidences (up to 20%) of temporary jaundice without any signs of preoperative liver disease.[7-9] Evans et al[7] analyzed the results of 218 major surgical procedures in a prospective study and found an incidence of 3.7% severe jaundice and 16.5% mild jaundice. The causes of jaundice were varied, but it seems that the primary cause was a bilirubin overload, which resulted mainly from blood transfusions. The bilirubin overload was apparently combined with disturbances in the hepatic cellular metabolism, with a subsequent deterioration of the ability of the liver cells to excrete bilirubin. The authors did not find any correlation between the incidence and severity of jaundice on the one hand, and the incidence and severity of arterial hypotension on the other. It is noteworthy that the majority of their patients did not have any preoperative liver disease; neither could the authors demonstrate a statistically significant association between jaundice and halothane anesthesia. However, it is also interesting to note that the few cases of severe postoperative jaundice and postoperative jaundice accompanied by other abnormal postoperative liver function tests were observed only in patients who received halothane anesthesia. In addition to hyperbilirubinemia, approximately one third of these patients demonstrated a temporary increase in the plasma concentrations of hepatic enzymes. Thus, it appears that hyperbilirubinemia, in a rather large part of the surgical population, is due to blood transfusion and/or resorption of hematomas from the operating field.

Dykes and Walzer[4] concluded in 1967 that the incidence of postoperative hepatic dysfunction varied between 1:239 and 1:1091 administrations of a general anesthetic. Later analysis revealed that approximately 0.15% of completely asymptomatic patients actually had significant liver disease before anesthesia and surgery.[10, 11] It is clear that patients who are scheduled for elective surgical procedures may have unknown hepatic disease or may risk developing hepatic disease, including acute viral hepatitis.

Schemel[10] reported that 1 of 700 patients admitted for elective surgery without any notable symptomatic disease showed unexpected and unexplained abnormalities in liver blood tests during routine preoperative evaluations. One third of these patients had jaundice a short period of time following cancellation of the scheduled surgical operation. If these patients had undergone the elective surgical procedures as planned, the anesthetic administered in these cases—halothane, isoflurane, or anything else—would surely have been deemed guilty of induction of jaundice.

The issue of severe hepatic necrosis following a halothane anesthetic is intriguing. The National Halothane Study reviewed more than 850,000 surgical cases from 1959 to 1962. Massive hepatic necrosis occurred in 0.01% of these cases. The majority of complications could be attributed to shock, prolonged use of vasopressors, infection, congestive heart failure, or pre-existing hepatic disease. Only nine cases of massive hepatic necrosis were of unknown origin.[12]

It is important to realize that a laparotomy with liver biopsy (without major abdominal surgery) in patients with liver disease carries an extremely high mortality rate. The immediate postoperative mortality was rather high two decades ago.[13, 14] With time, despite the rather impressive developments in anesthesia care, the mortality rate has not substantially decreased. A report from Britain documents a 31% and 61% 30-day mortality and morbidity rate, respectively, after laparotomy and liver biopsy.[15] In that study, all patients with viral hepatitis and alcoholic hepatitis died, and the majority of patients with ascites also died (13 of 15).[15] The results in the United States are not very different: the 30-day mortality rate in patients with severe hepatic disease and ascites approaches 83% and prolongation in prothrombin time by more than 2½ sec increased the 30-day mortality rate up to 91%.[16]

ANATOMY AND PHYSIOLOGY OF THE LIVER AND BILIARY TRACT

The liver lies in the right upper quadrant of the abdominal cavity and is attached to the diaphragm. It is the largest gland in the human body, weighing approximately 1.5 kg and representing 2% of body weight in the adult. In the neonate, the liver accounts for approximately 5% of body weight. It is divided into four lobes, which are supplied by right and left branches of the portal vein and hepatic artery; bile drains into the right and left hepatic ducts. The liver is covered by a thin connective tissue capsule called Glisson's capsule. Under normal conditions, the liver contains relatively little connective tissue; however, the connective tissue provides an internal supporting framework for the hepatic parenchyma, vessels, and nerves within the liver.

Hepatic blood flow (portal vein and hepatic artery) equals approximately $100 \, \text{ml} \cdot \text{min}^{-1} \cdot 100\text{g}^{-1}$, which represents about 25% of cardiac output. The liver is supplied by two large vessels: The hepatic artery brings arterial blood to the liver and represents approximately 25% of total hepatic blood flow and approximately 45–50% of hepatic oxygen supply, whereas the portal vein provides 75% of the total hepatic blood supply and only 50–55% of the hepatic oxygen supply. Portal venous blood is partially deoxygenated in the preportal organs and tissues (stomach, intestines, spleen, and pancreas) (Fig. 42-1). In contrast, portal venous blood is rich with nutrients and other substances absorbed in the gastrointestinal tract. Portal venous blood flow is controlled primarily by the arterioles in the preportal splanchnic organs. This flow, combined with resistance to portal flow within the liver, determines portal pressure (7 to 10 mm Hg). Presinusoidal (precapillary) sphincters determine the relatively uniform distribution of flow through the liver and play a certain, although rather limited, role in the regulation of portal blood flow.

FIG. 42-1. Schematic representation of splanchnic circulation. (Reproduced with permission from Gelman S: Effects of anesthetics on splanchnic circulation. In Altura BM, Halevy S [eds]: Cardiovascular Action of Anesthetics and Drugs Used in Anesthesia, p 127. Basel, Karger Publishing Co, 1986.)

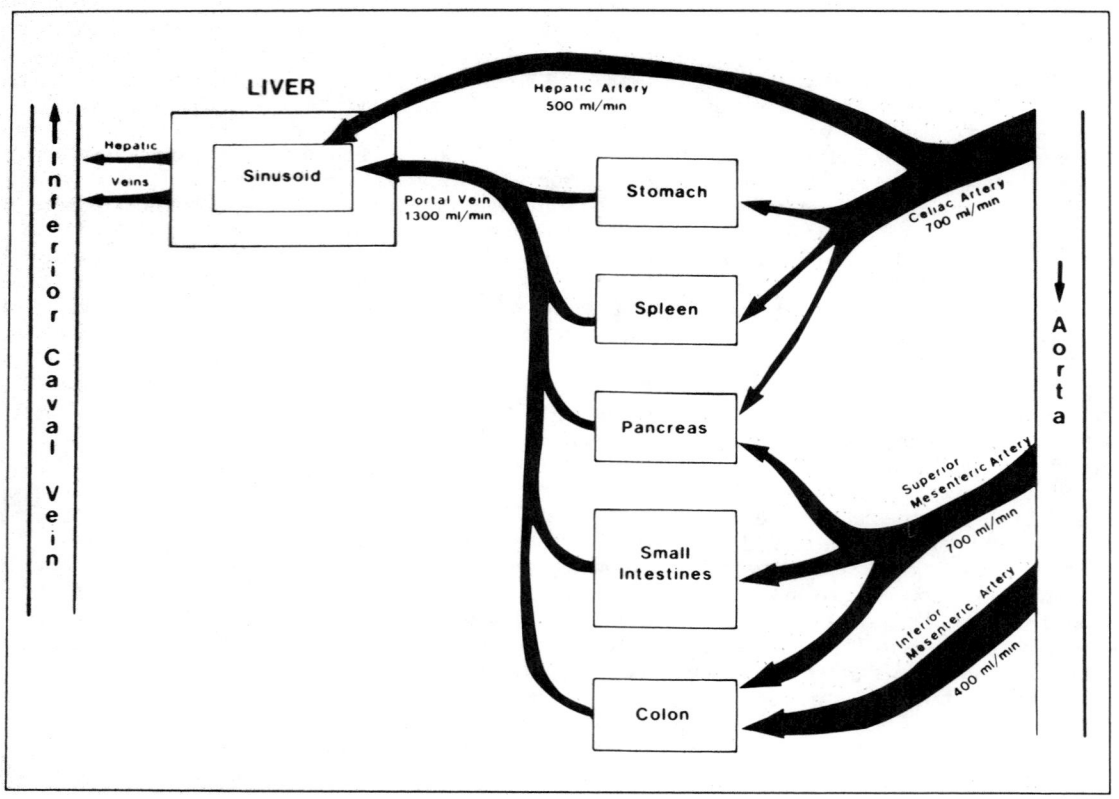

There are data, however, suggesting that the major site of venous resistance within the liver is postsinusoidal. The sinusoidal pressure is determined by the tone of presinusoidal and postsinusoidal sphincters and blood flow. Smooth muscles in the wall of the venules regulate venous compliance and blood volume. Both resistance and compliance are predominately controlled by the sympathetic innervation mediated through alpha-adrenoceptors. Changes in hepatic venous compliance play an essential part in the overall regulation of cardiac output, whereas the myogenic and metabolic intrinsic regulation of hepatic venous compliance play a very small role, if any, in controlling the hepatic venous resistance. The main controlling mechanism seems to be sympathetic innervation mediated through alpha-adrenoceptors. Therefore, the liver vasculature does have a vital role as a blood reservoir. An increase or a decrease in resistance in the hepatic veins is accompanied by rather dramatic changes in blood volume within the liver. This reservoir function is mainly mediated through the sympathetic nervous system. For example, during hemorrhage, the liver may "squeeze" an additional 500 ml of blood into the systemic circulation. Anesthetics that suppress the sympathetic nervous system function may interfere with such compensatory responses and lead to decompensation if blood is not replaced immediately. Patients with liver disease have a decreased sensitivity to catecholamines, probably as a result of an increase in glucagon concentration. Therefore, these patients may have a decreased ability to compensate for hemorrhage and hypovolemia by mechanisms related to the sympathetic nervous system: 1) lack of ability to develop vasoconstriction to divert blood to the heart and brain from the muscles and splanchnic circulation, 2) lack of ability to expel blood from the splanchnic reservoir into the systemic circulation, and 3) lack of ability to constrict the capacitance vasculature.

The major site of resistance in the hepatic arterial vasculature is the arterioles. Regulation of the hepatic arteriolar tone is mainly achieved by local and intrinsic mechanisms that adjust hepatic arterial flow to compensate for changes in portal blood flow. This phenomenon is referred to as the arterial buffer response. The decrease in portal blood flow is usually associated with an increase in hepatic arterial blood flow.[17, 18] This increase in hepatic arterial blood flow may be considered an attempt to maintain hepatic oxygen supply (which is essential for hepatocyte function) and/or total hepatic blood flow (which, in turn, is essential for clearance of exogenous and endogenous compounds with a high hepatic extraction). The mechanisms by which the described hepatic arterial blood flow autoregulation is achieved involve neural, myogenic, and metabolic controls, as well as content of portal blood and washout effect.[17, 18] It has been demonstrated that a decrease in portal blood pH and/or oxygen content is accompanied by an increase in hepatic arterial blood flow, even when portal blood flow is intentionally maintained unaltered.[17] The washout theory suggests that a substance, apparently adenosine, is generated within the liver tissue; when portal blood flow decreases, this vasodilating substance is not washed out but accumulates and subsequently leads to hepatic arterial vasodilation. Increased portal blood flow leads to an effective washout of this substance and a reduction in the vasodilating effect on the hepatic arterial vasculature.

The liver and hepatic vasculature also play an extremely important role in fluid homeostasis. With even small increases in hepatic venous pressure, excessive amounts of fluid transude into the lymph and also leak through the outer surface of the liver capsule into the peritoneal cavity. This fluid contains 80–90% of normal plasma protein.

Bile ducts accompany the hepatic arteries and the portal veins. Bile flows from the bile canaliculi of the liver to enter ductules, larger interhepatic bile ducts, and, finally, the right and left hepatic bile ducts, which form the hepatic duct proper (Fig. 42-2). The common hepatic duct is formed at the porta from the right and left hepatic lobular ducts. It is approximately 3 cm long and is joined by the cystic duct from the gallbladder to form the common bile duct–ductus choledochus, which is approximately 7 cm long and empties into the duodenum. The gallbladder is located under the surface of the right lobe of the liver. It is very distensible and may contain 30 to 50 ml of bile. The cystic artery, which usually arises from

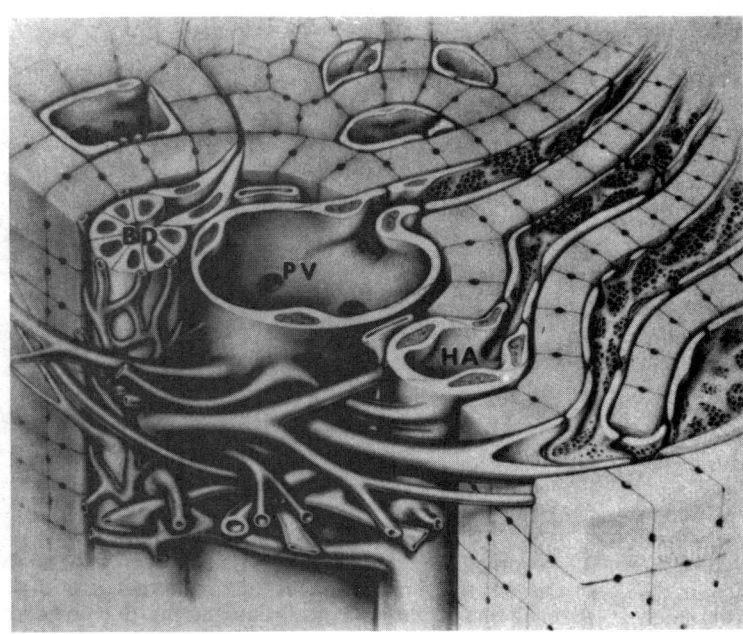

FIG. 42-2. Relationships of branches of the portal vein (PV), hepatic artery (HA), and bile duct (BD). Notice the peribiliary capillary plexus associated with the bile duct. (Reproduced with permission from Jones AL: Anatomy of the normal liver. In Zakim D, Boyer TD [eds]: Hepatology: A Textbook of Liver Disease. Philadelphia, WB Saunders, 1982.)

the right hepatic artery, provides arterial blood supply to the gallbladder.

STRUCTURAL CONCEPTS OF LIVER LOBULATION

Small histologic units or lobules have been identified since the 17th century. Two primary models have been developed to describe these histologic and functional units.

The classic lobule is a polyhedral prism of liver tissue about 1×2 mm in size. The lobule is roughly hexagonal, and, at the angles of the hexagon, there are interlobular portal canals containing some connective tissue and portal triad. The central vein, which is actually the terminal hepatic venule, lies in the center of this lobule. The parenchyma lies between blood-carrying vascular channels of the sinusoids. The parenchymal cells form plates that radiate from the central vein to the portal canals at the periphery of the lobule (Fig. 42-3).

Approximately 30 years ago, Rappaport and colleagues[19] defined the liver lobule as an acinus. According to this concept, parenchymal cells are grouped into zones surrounding the terminal afferent vessels (Fig. 42-4). Zone 1 cells receive blood and oxygen first, are usually last to undergo necrosis, and regenerate first. Cells in Zones 2 and 3, particularly Zone 3, are located more distal to the afferent blood vessels. They receive blood with a lesser amount of oxygen and nutrients and are therefore probably less resistant to hepatotoxins and oxygen deprivation.

The smallest branches of the biliary tree are the bile canaliculi, which are located between a few hepatocytes. Bile proceeds down the bile canaliculi, moving from the centrilobular cells toward the perilobular and interlobular portal triads (from Zone 3 to Zone 1). The canaliculi bile then enters the small terminal bile ductules or canals of Hering. From the terminal ductules, bile enters into the interlobular bile ducts, which then form a continuous passageway with increasing size and complexity of the wall structure.

ULTRASTRUCTURE OF HEPATOCYTES

Hepatocytes, or hepatic parenchymal cells, represent approximately 80% of the cytoplasmic mass within the liver. The cells are relatively large, approximately 20×30 μm in size, and their function is extremely diverse and complex. They absorb digestive material from the portal venous blood; they store proteins, vitamins, carbohydrates, and lipids. They release these compounds into the blood in bound or unbound forms. They excrete bile salts, which facilitate absorption of fat from the intestines. They synthesize plasma proteins, glucose, cholesterol, fatty acids, and phospholipids. These cells also metabolize, detoxify, and inactivate exogenous and endogenous compounds, including drugs, some poisons, as well as steroids and the majority of other hormones. Hepatocytes may also play an important role in the immune system.

It is clear that a system of intracellular organelles is needed to perform multiple and complex functions. Approximately 800 mitochondria can be found in every liver cell. Mitochondria also occupy about 18% of hepatocyte volume and play a crucial role in oxidative phosphorylation and in the oxidation of fatty acids. Lysosomes are usually located in the pericanalicular region and interact in the digestion and catabolism of many exogenous substances. Both rough and smooth endoplasmic reticula are probably involved in essentially every function of the liver cells. It appears that hepatic drug metabolizing activities, as well as the conversion of cholesterol to bile acids and certain steps in cholesterol biosynthesis, occur within the endoplasmic reticulum. The Golgi complex is involved in the production of very low-density lipid proteins, glycoprotein synthesis, and albumin secretion. The Golgi complex may also play a role in bile secretion. Other cellular inclusions contain stores of fat droplets and other compounds, including stores of glycogen that first appear in Zone 1 and disappear from Zone 3 (centrilobular areas) of the liver acinus.

The liver contains large reticuloendothelial Kupffer's cells, which primarily phagocytize bacteria and other foreign matter in the blood. In addition to hepatocytes and Kupffer's cells, the liver also contains endothelial cells, sinusoidal lining cells, and lipocytes.

METABOLIC FUNCTIONS OF THE LIVER

The liver synthesizes and excretes many different substances. Among the most important is *bilirubin*. When cell membranes of erythrocytes rupture, the released hemoglobin is phagocytized by the reticuloendothelial cells where hemoglobin is split into globin and heme. Heme provides a substrate from

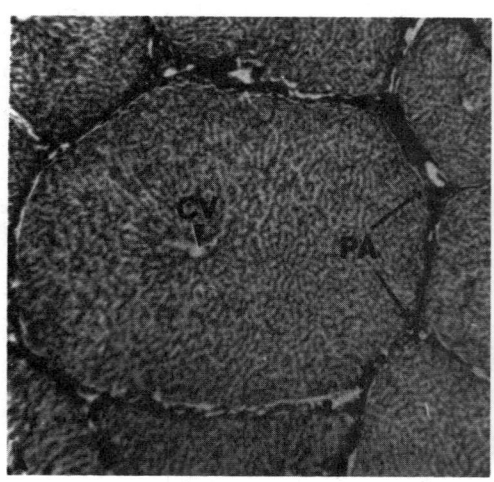 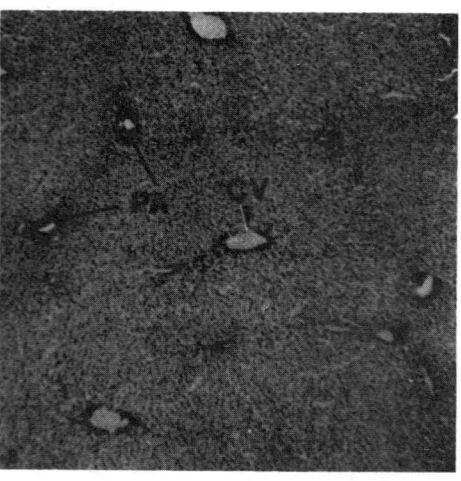

FIG. 42-3. (*A*) Cross-section of a pig liver lobule, illustrating the boundaries of the classic lobule. (*B*) A classic lobule of normal human liver. The human lobular boundaries are poorly visualized because of the absence of connective tissue septa. (PA = portal area; CV = central vein; ≈ × 100. (Reproduced with permission from Jones AL, Schmucker DL: Gastroenterology 73:833, 1977. Copyright 1977 by The American Gastroenterological Association.)

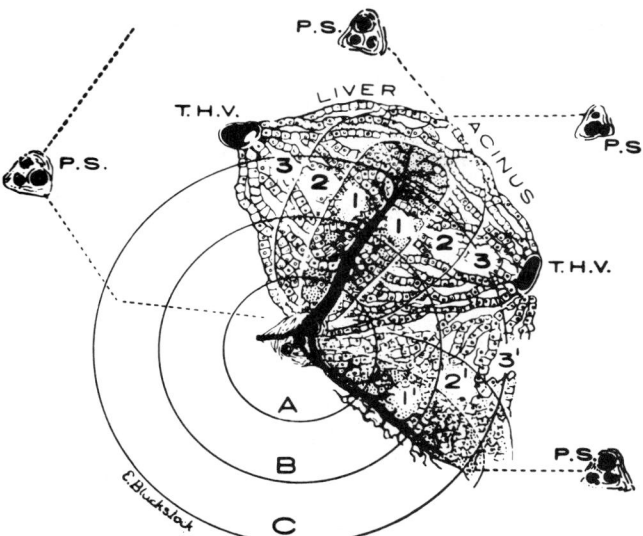

FIG. 42-4. The blood supply of the hepatic structural unit. The structural unit occupies adjacent sectors of neighboring hexagonal fields. Zones 1, 2, and 3 represent areas supplied with blood of first, second, and third quality, respectively, with regard to oxygen and nutrients. These zones cluster about the terminal afferent vascular twigs and extend into the periportal field from which these twigs originate. Zones 1', 2', and 3' designate corresponding areas in a portion of an adjacent structural unit. In Zones 1 and 1', the afferent vascular twigs empty into the sinusoids. The circles A, B, and C delimit concentric bands of the hepatic parenchyma arranged around a small portal field. (Reproduced with permission from Rappaport AM, Borowy ZJ, Lougheed WM et al: Subdivision of hexagonal liver lobules into a structural and functional unit. Anat Rec 119:16, 1954.)

which the bile pigments are formed. The first pigment is the biliverdin, which is reduced to free bilirubin, which is, in turn, released into the plasma. Then, free bilirubin combines strongly with the plasma albumin and is transported throughout the blood and intestinal fluids. Bilirubin is then released from the plasma albumin and subsequently absorbed by hepatocytes. Within the liver cells, bilirubin conjugates with different substances, primarily glucuronic acid. In conjugated forms, bilirubin is excreted by the active transport process into the bile. A small portion of conjugated bilirubin returns to the plasma directly into the sinusoids and indirectly by absorption from the bile ducts and lymphatics. Bilirubin is converted into urobilinogen in the intestine by bacteria. Some of the urobilinogen, being very soluble, is reabsorbed through the intestinal mucosa into the blood and is then re-excreted by the liver into the intestine. About 5% of the urobilinogen is excreted by the kidneys. When exposed to air in the urine, urobilinogen is oxidized to urobilin (or to stercobilin in the feces).

Hyperbilirubinemia can be due to an overproduction of bilirubin (unconjugated hyperbilirubinemia), which results from hemolysis, large hematomas or ineffective erythropoiesis, or defective elimination of bilirubin. The latter can result from a defective hepatobiliary elimination of conjugated bilirubin (conjugated hyperbilirubinemia), which would primarily include cholestatic diseases of the liver and biliary obstruction. Also, defective hepatic removal of bilirubin can result in unconjugated hyperbilirubinemia. These forms of disorders include all diseases interfering with hepatic bil-

irubin uptake or conjugation, such as neonatal hyperbilirubinemia, breast milk jaundice of the newborn, and some syndromes such as Gilbert syndrome and Crigler-Najjar disease.

It is well known that unconjugated hyperbilirubinemia may result in severe neurologic dysfunction, including a rapidly fatal encephalopathy.[20-22] Conjugated hyperbilirubinemia is not accompanied by apparent neurotoxicity.

Bilirubin is toxic for many different enzymes.[23] This effect on the enzyme systems occurs usually in very high concentrations of bilirubin and can be modified with the addition of albumin.[24] Bilirubin may play a role in uncoupling oxidative phosphorylation in mitochondria. However, it seems that such kinds of metabolic disturbances occur only with very high concentrations of bilirubin. Alternative mechanisms, proposed to explain the neurotoxicity of hyperbilirubinemia, include bilirubin-mediated changes in ATPase, inhibition of protein synthesis, and cellular growth. Bilirubin may also interfere with membrane function.[25]

The main function of the liver in *carbohydrate* metabolism consists of storing glycogen, converting galactose to glucose, gluconeogenesis, and forming many intermediate compounds of carbohydrate biotransformation. The liver plays a major role in maintaining normal blood glucose levels, which is termed the *glucose buffer function*.

Specific functions of the liver in *fat* metabolism consist of beta oxidation of fatty acids and formation of acetoacetic acid, formation of lipoproteins, cholesterol, phospholipids, and conversion of carbohydrates and proteins into fat.

The most important liver function in *protein* metabolism consists of deamination of amino acids, formation of urea for removal of ammonia, formation of plasma proteins, and interconversions among the different amino acids and other compounds.

Other metabolic functions of the liver include blood coagulation, storage of iron, vitamins, and some other compounds.

PHARMACOKINETICS AND PHARMACODYNAMICS

Involvement of the liver in pharmacokinetics is reflected by elimination of exogenous, as well as endogenous, compounds by biotransformation or by an excretion of unchanged compounds into the bile.[26, 27] The hepatic elimination of a drug can be affected by different mechanisms. The main mechanisms include changes in hepatic blood flow and changes in the ability of the liver cells to biotransform and/or excrete a given compound. The latter is called *intrinsic clearance*. These two mechanisms, hepatocyte function and hepatic blood flow, have an important role in patients with liver disease, as well as in patients with relatively normal liver function that may temporarily deteriorate during anesthesia and surgery. Other mechanisms of altered pharmacokinetics include changes in the binding of drugs—in other words, changes in the ratio of bound to unbound (free drug), and also changes in volume of distribution. These mechanisms often play an extremely important role in patients with advanced liver disease. Some specific information regarding the pharmacokinetics of certain drugs relative to anesthesia practice is presented later in a discussion of comparative pharmacology of anesthetics and anesthetic management for patients with liver disease.

The *pharmacodynamic* observations in patients with hepatic disease are limited, since, unfortunately, studies related to the pharmacologic effect of drugs in patients with hepatic disease have attracted relatively little attention. The reasons for this are multifactorial; however, some of them are relatively clear. A study of this type would necessitate concurrent pharmacokinetic studies; otherwise, the interpretation of the pharmacologic effects would become impossible, since it would never be clear which effects are related to altered pharmacodynamics and which are the result of changed pharmacokinetics. In other words, a changed response to a drug that resulted from an altered interaction between the drug and corresponding receptors (pharmacodynamics) would not be distinguishable from one that resulted from a change in the concentration of available drug to the receptors (pharmacokinetics).

Despite certain methodologic limitations, some studies suggest that patients with liver cirrhosis, particularly those with histories of hepatic coma, are much more sensitive to morphine[28] and chlorpromazine[29, 30] than are normal persons. It has also been demonstrated that equal plasma concentrations of diazepam resulted in much more pronounced encephalographic alterations in patients with severe hepatic disease compared with normal persons.[31] However, there are reasons to believe that the response to catecholamines in patients who have hepatic cirrhosis and portal hypertension may be substantially decreased. Patients, as well as animals, with portal hypertension have an increased plasma glucagon concentration.[32] Glucagon substantially reduces the response of different vessels to catecholamines.[33] Thus, it is not surprising that patients who have hepatic cirrhosis do not respond to catecholamines as do normal persons. It seems, therefore, that the dose of drugs such as morphine and chlorpromazine should be decreased, whereas the dose of catecholamines, if needed, should be increased, or a different vasopressive drug, such as vasopressin, should be used.

The pharmacokinetic/pharmacodynamic interactions can be rather complex, and an ideal choice of one or another drug may not be possible. As an illustration, it was observed more than 20 years ago that patients with hepatic cirrhosis required higher doses of d-tubocurarine to achieve a similar degree of muscle relaxation than normal persons.[34] This effect seems to be related purely to pharmacokinetic deviations in patients with hepatic cirrhosis: These patients have an increased volume of distribution for d-tubocurarine, which is primarily related to an increased gamma-globulin fraction of the protein with a subsequent increased binding of d-tubocurarine to gamma globulin and a decreased free fraction of the drug. On the other hand, all drugs, including muscle relaxants, excreted with bile are excreted much slower in patients with hepatic cirrhosis or obstructive jaundice/cholestasis. These observations *per se* suggest the use of gallamine or atracurium, since these relaxants are not excreted with bile. However, overall judgment should include not only pharmacokinetics but also the pharmacodynamics of a drug or, in this case, other effects (side-effects) of muscle relaxants. For example, the clearance and half-life of vecuronium in patients with severe liver disease is prolonged compared with that in normal persons, whereas the clearance of gallamine is not significantly altered. This does not mean that one should not use vecuronium in patients with hepatic cirrhosis: If a drug is cautiously titrated against effect, it can be safely used; however, gallamine, which induces tachycardia, may not be a drug of choice.

The lesson is clear. Owing to pharmacodynamic and pharmacokinetic alterations, the response of each patient to a drug in question is virtually unpredictable. Therefore, each drug must be carefully selected and, probably more importantly, carefully titrated to the desirable effect.

PATHOPHYSIOLOGY OF LIVER DISEASE

For practical clinical purposes, anesthesiologists may divide patients with liver disease into two large heterogeneous groups: 1) those with parenchymal liver disease, including acute and chronic viral hepatitis, hepatic cirrhosis with or without portal hypertension, and some other disorders; and 2) those with cholestasis, including obstruction of extrahepatic biliary pathway.

PARENCHYMAL DISEASE (VIRAL HEPATITIS, CIRRHOSIS)

For simplicity, we will discuss the pathophysiology of parenchymal liver disease, with an example of hepatic cirrhosis as it relates to the practice of anesthesia.

The most common clinical features of liver cirrhosis are an enlarged spleen and liver, often ascites, mild to moderate jaundice, weakness, large esophageal varices, spider nevi, anorexia, nausea, vomiting, encephalopathy, and sometimes abdominal pain. Practically, the function of every organ and system is altered in a patient with advanced parenchymal hepatic disease.

Cardiovascular Function in Cirrhosis (Table 42-1)

SYSTEMIC CIRCULATION. Systemic cardiovascular function in patients with liver cirrhosis and portal hypertension is characterized by a hyperdynamic state, including high cardiac output, low peripheral vascular resistance, and normal filling pressures, heart rate, and arterial pressure. Circulating blood volume is usually increased. Peripheral blood flow is substantially increased above the metabolic oxygen requirements. Therefore, oxygen tension and oxygen saturation in peripheral venous and mixed venous blood are usually increased, whereas arteriovenous oxygen content difference is narrowed. This clinical and pathophysiologic syndrome mimics the picture usually observed in patients with peripheral arteriovenous fistula. Patients with liver cirrhosis and portal hypertension have developed arteriovenous collaterals in many organs and tissues, including splanchnic organs, lungs, skin, muscles, and probably others. The reasons for the development of arteriovenous collaterals in these tissues are multifactorial and not completely understood. It has been demon-

TABLE 42-1.   Cardiovascular Function in Hepatic Cirrhosis

1. Decreased vascular resistance (peripheral vasodilation, increased arteriovenous shunting)
2. Increased circulating blood volume
3. Increased cardiac output
4. Maintained arterial blood pressure, filling pressures, and heart rate (deterioration is late)
5. Possible cardiomyopathy
6. Decreased arteriovenous oxygen content difference and increased venous oxygen content
7. Decreased responsiveness to catecholamines
8. Increased splanchnic (except the liver), pulmonary, muscle, and skin blood flow
9. Decreased portal blood flow to the liver
10. Maintained or decreased hepatic arterial blood flow
11. Maintained or decreased renal blood flow

strated in rats with experimentally induced portal stenosis, for example, that an increase in arteriovenous shunting and blood flow in preportal tissues, at least by 40% is due to an increase in glucagon concentration in blood.[32] It is yet to be established which factors are responsible for the remaining 60% increase in arteriovenous shunting and blood flow in the preportal tissues. Other substances such as ferritin and vasoactive intestinal polypeptide may also be responsible for peripheral vasodilation, decreased vascular resistance, and increased arteriovenous shunting.

Arterial vasodilation decreases vascular resistance and aortic pressure, which may increase stroke volume and cardiac output even with certain degrees of cardiomyopathy. Thus, the majority of patients with hepatic cirrhosis have high cardiac output despite some degree of cardiomyopathy. Patients with hepatic cirrhosis have a decreased ability to develop vasoconstriction, as well as tachycardia, in response to appropriate stimuli. This distorted response is probably related to circulating vasodilating factors but may also be due to an impairment in baroreceptor-mediated responses.

The responsiveness of the cardiovascular system to sympathetic discharge or catecholamines is reduced.[28] The mechanism for such decrease in the responsiveness is not completely clear; however, it seems that the increased glucagon concentration in blood plays an important role in this event. Experimentally, it has been shown that glucagon (the concentration is always increased in patients with liver cirrhosis and portal hypertension) decreases the vasculature responsiveness to infused catecholamines and other vasopressors.[35, 36] Clinically, however, patients with liver cirrhosis and portal hypertension who are already decompensated and would not respond well to an infused alpha-adrenoceptor agonist may still respond better to vasopressin.

The decompensation of cardiovascular function in patients with liver cirrhosis often starts with an increase in ventricular filling pressures and/or a decrease in stroke volume, with a subsequent increase in heart rate. This is often associated with a further increase in mixed venous oxygen tension and saturation and a decrease in oxygen consumption. The state of decompensation becomes similar to that observed in decompensated septic shock.

Ascites can be one of the important complications aggravating cardiovascular function in patients with liver cirrhosis. With an increase in intraabdominal pressure and a shift of the diaphragm upward, intrathoracic pressure also increases, with a subsequent reduction in transmural pressure gradient across the heart. As ascites accumulates, venous return and cardiac output decrease. Removal of the intraabdominal fluid decreases intraabdominal pressure, with, often, a subsequent improvement in overall cardiovascular function. Obviously, if paracentesis is performed, the ascitic fluid should be removed slowly while carefully observing cardiovascular function.

Alcohol *per se* decreases myocardial contractile force *in vitro* and myocardial contractility *in vivo*. Alcohol ingestion is usually accompanied by an increase in the concentration of catecholamines. Therefore, the direct depressive effect of alcohol on contractile force is often masked by catecholamine-mediated stimulation of myocardial contractility. Chronic alcoholism is often accompanied by alcoholic cardiomyopathy, which may eventually develop into low-output congestive heart failure. Often, alcoholics develop either alcoholic cardiomyopathy or alcoholic cirrhosis, but normally these two do not coexist. Episodes of disorders in cardiac rhythm are sometimes observed after heavy weekend or holiday drinking and are even called *holiday heart syndrome*.[37]

RENAL CIRCULATION. Renal blood flow is normal and without obvious renal dysfunction in patients with portal hypertension. A decrease in renal cortical blood flow is probably one of the first signs of impairment of renal function. Renal circulatory disturbances play an important role in the pathogenesis of the hepatorenal syndrome, which sometimes complicates liver cirrhosis. Renal blood flow, especially renal cortical blood flow, can be decreased as a result of an increase in renal vascular resistance, despite a relatively high cardiac output and low total peripheral vascular resistance. Other organs and tissues are hyperperfused, whereas the kidneys suffer from hypoperfusion. In fact, blood flow through preportal organs and tissues, as well as through skin, lungs, and muscles (although to a lesser extent) is often increased. An increase in renal vascular resistance is due to an increase in resistance in afferent, more than efferent, arterioles. There are different humoral substances involved in the pathogenesis of renal circulatory disorders in patients with liver cirrhosis and portal hypertension.

HEPATIC CIRCULATION. Portal hypertension is the main feature of splanchnic circulatory disorders in hepatic cirrhosis. Theoretically speaking, portal pressure is determined by one or any combination of these three factors: 1) blood flow into the portal system; 2) resistance to portal flow; and 3) resistance in the portacaval collaterals. The classic, so-called backward theory proposed that fibrotic tissue within the liver, formed during liver cirrhosis, increases resistance to portal flow with a subsequent development of portal hypertension. However, many clinical and experimental observations do not fit the backward theory of portal hypertension. For example, in experimental animals, restriction of transhepatic portal flow does not always produce portal hypertension comparable to that encountered clinically, nor does it produce bleeding from esophageal varices. In addition, acute portal hypertension, induced by specific narrowing of the portal vein, is accompanied by a substantial decrease in splanchnic venous oxygen saturation, an increase in arteriomesenteric venous oxygen content difference, an increase in mesenteric vascular resistance, and a decrease in mesenteric arterial flow. To the contrary, completely opposite changes are observed in patients with hepatic cirrhosis and portal hypertension. To explain the clinical and physiologic features in patients with hepatic cirrhosis that do not fit the backward theory, a "forward theory" has been introduced.[38] The forward theory suggests that certain factors (glucagon and some other vasodilating compounds) lead to vasodilation and formation of arteriovenous fistulas in the intestine and the spleen, which result in a hyperdynamic state with increased splanchnic blood flow and cardiac output. Concerning the hepatic circulation *per se*, portal blood flow to the liver is substantially decreased, whereas hepatic arterial blood flow is maintained or even increased. Therefore, in the majority of situations, hepatic oxygen supply is maintained, while total hepatic blood flow is decreased. A decrease in total hepatic blood flow has certain pharmacokinetic implications: Compounds, exogenous as well as endogenous, with high hepatic clearance are eliminated more slowly than in normal persons.

CIRCULATORY EFFECTS OF SOME MODALITIES OF TREATMENT FOR PORTAL HYPERTENSION. In an attempt to stop acute bleeding from esophageal varices in patients with hepatic cirrhosis and portal hypertension, a triple lumen Sengstaken–Blakemore tube, which has a gastric balloon and an esophageal balloon, can be inflated to compress the varices and very often effectively stop the bleeding. One lumen provides the opportunity to remove gastric contents. Many different surgical procedures have been suggested and are still used to stop or prevent bleeding from esophageal varices. Some procedures such as ligation of varices, portal vein–azygos vein disconnection, or transposition of the spleen are rarely used, whereas other procedures such as sclerosing varices, portasystemic shunts (including portacaval shunt end-to-end or end-to-side) as well as mesocaval, mesorenal, or splenorenal peripheral shunts are used more often. It is important that the anesthesiologist realize certain pathophysiologic changes occur after creation of a *portacaval shunt*. Surgical and pharmacologic treatment of portal hypertension produces important alterations in systemic and regional hemodynamics. Surgical formation of a portacaval shunt leads to immediate redistribution of blood flow from the portal vein through the surgical shunt to the inferior caval vein with an apparent increase in flow in the inferior caval vein and venous return. Surgical portacaval shunts lead to an immediate decrease in resistance to the portal flow, which, in turn, leads to a decrease in arterial resistance in the intestine and spleen with a subsequent increase in flow through these organs. However, this increase in blood flow through the preportal area is associated with an increased flow through the surgical shunt but is also accompanied by a decrease in portal blood flow to the liver. In the majority of patients, this decrease in portal flow to the liver is associated with some increase in hepatic arterial blood flow, which maintains hepatic oxygen supply. Total hepatic blood flow is apparently decreased, which is probably responsible, at least partially, for an increase in the concentrations of circulating glucagon and other vasodilating substances. Total peripheral vascular resistance is decreased, and ejection fraction

may be subsequently increased, which, in combination with an increase in venous return, leads to a further increase in cardiac output (Fig. 42-5).

Many patients with portal hypertension undergoing portacaval shunt surgery are given specific medications to stop or prevent bleeding from esophageal varices. *Vasopressin* is a commonly used drug to control bleeding from esophageal varices in patients with portal hypertension. The beneficial effect of vasopressin is related to vasoconstriction in the preportal area, with a subsequent decrease in portal blood flow and portal pressure. Hepatic arterial blood flow is often slightly increased. However, vasopressin, has certain adverse effects, mainly related to systemic vasoconstriction (including coronary vasoconstriction) with subsequent arterial hypertension. The combination of vasopressin with a vasodilating drug, such as sodium nitroprusside or nitroglycerin, is beneficial, since it produces a further decrease in portal pressure, an increase in hepatic arterial blood flow, and possibly improvement in coronary circulation.[39–41] *Somatostatin* can also be successfully used to control bleeding from esophageal varices. Somatostatin decreases portal blood flow and portal pressure by a substantial reduction in glucagon activity and intestinal motility, resulting in a substantial decrease in mesenteric blood flow.[42]

Propranolol has gained popularity during recent years in attempts to prevent gastrointestinal bleeding in patients with portal hypertension. Experimental data demonstrate that propranolol decreases portal hypertension by both beta$_1$- and beta$_2$-adrenergic blockade. Beta$_1$-adrenergic blockade is associated with a reduction in cardiac output and a subsequent decrease in portal blood flow. Beta$_2$-adrenergic blockade results in splanchnic vasoconstriction and a decrease in blood

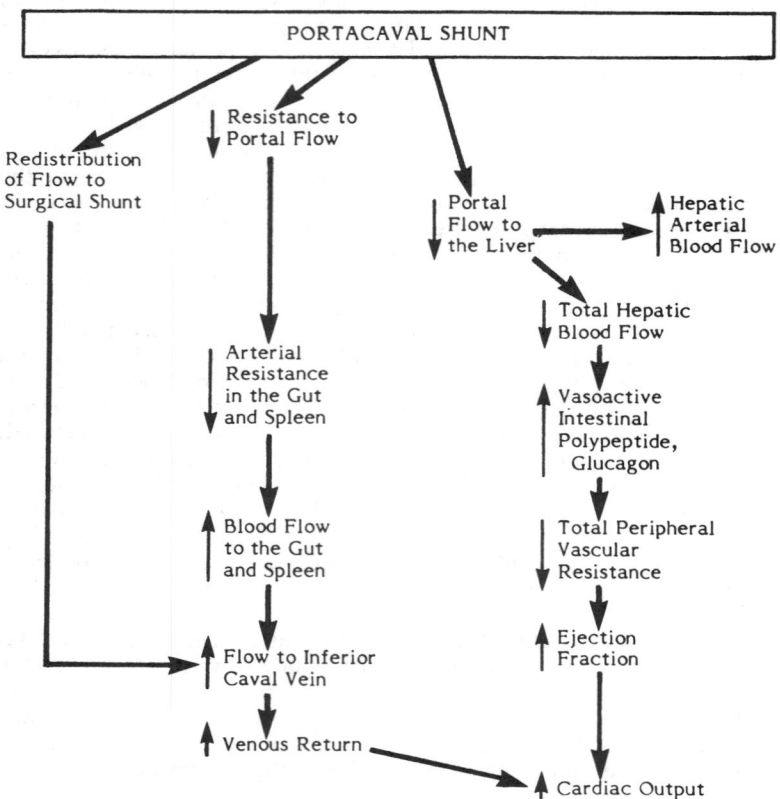

FIG. 42-5. Schematic representation of cardiovascular consequences of portacaval shunt. (Reproduced with permission from Kang YG, Gelman S: Liver transplantation. In Gelman S, [ed]: Anesthesia and Organ Transplantation, p 150. Philadelphia, WB Saunders, 1987.)

flow through portacaval collaterals.[43] The antirenin activity of propranolol probably also plays a role in the effectiveness of this drug. The beneficial effect of propranolol is partially attributed to a decrease in anxiety and degree of alcohol abuse. The adverse effects of propranolol treatment include a decrease in the efficacy of diuretic therapy, an increase in ammonia concentration in blood, with signs of encephalopathy, sometimes hypoglycemia, and decreased clearance of other drugs. Severe withdrawal syndrome and gastrointestinal bleeding may result from termination of propranolol treatment. Conn has stated, "Once treatment with propranolol is begun, it is a lifetime sentence."[44] Some controlled trials were unable to demonstrate that propranolol is effective in the prevention of variceal rebleeding in patients with liver cirrhosis.[45]

Respiratory Function and Pulmonary Circulation in Cirrhosis

Patients with liver cirrhosis and portal hypertension usually have an increased content of 2,3-diphosphoglycerate (2,3DPG) in red blood cells, which is accompanied by a decreased affinity of hemoglobin for oxygen and a shift of the oxyhemoglobin dissociation curve to the right.

Patients with liver cirrhosis commonly demonstrate different degrees of arterial oxygen desaturation. There are many reasons for these observations (Table 42-2). Collaterals between portal venous and pulmonary vasculature systems have been very well documented but they probably do not play a clinically significant role in the development of arterial oxygen desaturation. Intrapulmonary shunting is most likely a result of an increase in the concentration of vasodilating substances (glucagon, vasoactive intestinal polypeptide, ferritin), which apparently play a substantial role in the development of hypoxemia. These and some other vasodilating substances are probably responsible for impaired hypoxic pulmonary vasoconstriction. A decrease in the inspired fraction of oxygen is usually accompanied by an increase in pulmonary vascular resistance in healthy volunteers but not in patients with liver cirrhosis.[46]

In patients with liver cirrhosis complicated by ascites, an increase in closing volume, which may exceed the functional residual capacity, is often observed.[47] This leads to the gas trapping in the lower lung zones and a decrease in ventilation/perfusion ratio with subsequent hypoxemia.

Patients with hepatic cirrhosis sometimes develop pulmonary hypertension. The pathogenesis of pulmonary hypertension observed in these relatively rare events is not clear. The mechanisms probably involve an increased cardiac output and circulating blood volume, which may secondarily involve the pulmonary vasculature with a subsequent development of pulmonary hypertension. An increase in the activity of some circulating vasoconstricting substances may also be involved in the process of developing pulmonary hypertension.

Blood and Coagulation in Cirrhosis

Hematocrit values in patients with liver cirrhosis are usually decreased owing to an increased plasma volume and obviously to blood loss when gastrointestinal bleeding occurs. Megaloblastic anemia, resulting from vitamin B_{12} and other vitamin deficiencies, is not uncommon, especially in alcoholics because of malnutrition. An increased rate of hemolysis also contributes to anemia. Increased hemolytic activity is proportional to the size of the spleen but not to the degree of portal hypertension[48, 49] and is related to reticulocytosis and splenomegaly. Leukopenia and thrombocytopenia, usually related to hypersplenism and ethanol-induced depression of the marrow, are also not uncommon in patients with liver cirrhosis.

The majority of patients with liver cirrhosis have some mild abnormalities in coagulation processes. The most common is a reduction in concentration of Factor VII, and then Factors V, X, and II (prothrombin); the concentration of Factor I (fibrinogen) is also often decreased. Usually, the concentration in fibrin degradation products is not increased; however, an increased fibrinogen consumption may be observed. Occasionally, severe disseminated intravascular coagulation (DIC) develops after LeVeen shunt surgery. Hepatic failure is associated with a substantial decrease in the synthesis of clotting factors, resulting in prolongation of prothrombin time and partial thromboplastin time. Factors II, VII, IX, and X are vitamin K–dependent, whereas Factors I and V are not. Factor VIII, which is not synthesized in the liver, can even be increased in patients with hepatic cirrhosis. Owing to the relatively short half-life of Factor VII, it decreases earlier and to a greater extent than other liver-producing clotting factors.[50] Factor I (fibrinogen) synthesis deteriorates last. Changes in prothrombin time usually reflect well the extent of liver dysfunction.

The plasma concentration of albumin in patients with liver cirrhosis is usually decreased. The reasons for this decrease are relatively complex but are related to a decrease in the rate of albumin synthesis, as well as to an increase in total body water and other factors.

Endocrine Disorders

The growth hormone concentration usually increases in patients with liver cirrhosis, which may be partially responsible for the intolerance of carbohydrates. Many patients have an abnormal glucose utilization; the mechanism of such phenomenon is rather complex and includes an increased plasma concentration of fatty acids, which interfere with the insulin effect on glucose uptake by skeletal muscles. An increased plasma glucagon concentration also plays a role in disorders of carbohydrate metabolism observed in patients with liver cirrhosis.

An abnormal sex hormone metabolism may cause gonadal function disorders in both sexes and feminization in men, as evidenced by microscopic pictures of testicular dystrophy, a decrease in testicular size, frequency of impotence, and hypospermia in those who can still produce and ejaculate. Gynecomastia is not uncommon, and the prostate gland is small. Oligomenorrhea or amenorrhea is common among women.

TABLE 42-2. Hypoxemia in Hepatic Cirrhosis

1. Rightward shift of the oxyhemoglobin dissociation curve
2. Ventilation/perfusion abnormalities (impaired hypoxic pulmonary vasoconstriction)
3. Hypoventilation owing to ascites
4. Decrease in pulmonary diffusing capacity owing to an increase in extracellular fluid
5. Right-to-left shunt across the lungs owing to:
   a. spider angiomas in the lungs
   b. portapulmonary venous communications
   c. humoral factors (vasodilation—glucagon, ferritin, vasointestinal polypeptide, etc.)

Encephalopathy

Patients with hepatic encephalopathy usually appear obtunded and mentally confused. An increase in the blood concentration of nitrogenous compounds, resulting from gastrointestinal bleeding or an overdose of diuretics, can be found in such patients. It is believed that the increased blood ammonia concentration is responsible for the severity of hepatic encephalopathy. However, the severity of encephalopathy does not seem to be directly related to the blood ammonia concentration. Some patients with hepatic encephalopathy do not have an increased blood ammonia concentration, whereas others with an increased blood ammonia concentration might not have detectable encephalopathy.

The pathogenesis of hepatic encephalopathy involves insufficient hepatic elimination of nitrogenous compounds (ammonia is one of them) ingested (e.g., meat) or formed (from the blood during gastrointestinal bleeding) in the gastrointestinal tract. Hepatic encephalopathy may result from inadequate hepatocyte function, as well as from reduced sufficient blood flow and increased collaterals, that is, portacaval blood flow. The portacaval collaterals include the esophageal, rectal, and other areas that usually develop in patients with hepatic cirrhosis, as well as surgically created portacaval shunts. There are some data suggesting that the central nervous system (CNS) of patients with advanced hepatic disease is more sensitive to the nitrogenous compounds than is the neural tissue of normal subjects. The nitrogenous compounds enter the CNS and interfere with its function. Many recent studies have been devoted to revealing the precise role of different substances, including ammonia, in the pathogenesis of hepatic encephalopathy.

It has been suggested that certain mercaptans, short-chain fatty acids, play a significant role in the pathogenesis of hepatic encephalopathy. Further, it has been theorized that in patients with hepatic encephalopathy, biogenic amines are formed within the CNS and then released in response to neural stimulation along with normal neurotransmitters or instead of them. Structurally, they are similar to norepinephrine or dopamine but are much less active in eliciting a response from the effector. Thus, the false neurotransmitter displaces the normal neurotransmitter from the nerve endings, which results in nervous system dysfunction, manifested in hepatic encephalopathy. At present, a false neurotransmitter hypothesis, even though it looks very attractive, still requires more evidence to be accepted. It has been demonstrated that hepatic encephalopathy in certain experimental models may be accompanied by an increased gamma-aminobutyric acid (GABA) concentration. However, the significance of these findings to clinical hepatic encephalopathy is still uncertain and also requires further studies.

The treatment of hepatic encephalopathy mainly includes minimization of factors that lead to worsened hepatic encephalopathy. For example, all attempts should be made to stop gastrointestinal bleeding, to control infection (neomycin is usually the drug of choice), and to carefully titrate diuretic therapy and fluid load. Acid–base and electrolyte balance should be normalized. Specific diet reduces the intake of food containing nitrogen (protein). Lactulose has been successfully used in the treatment of hepatic encephalopathy: Lactulose traps ammonia in the acidified fecal stream and makes it unavailable for absorption. Thus, lactulose would promote ammonia excretion from the body. Dopamine agonists and L-dopa have also been used successfully in the treatment of hepatic encephalopathy. The hypothetical mechanism of action seems to be a displacement of false neurotransmitters in

the CNS by L-dopa. It has also been suggested that L-dopa facilitates renal excretion of ammonia.

The effects of anesthesia on patients with hepatic encephalopathy have not been thoroughly studied. However, some data suggest clinically significant alterations in this regard. Cerebral uptake of benzodiazepines is substantially increased in hepatic encephalopathy. This increase may indicate an increase in the density or affinity of benzodiazepine receptors. Alternatively, the observed increase in cerebral uptake of benzodiazepines may result from the enhanced permeability of the blood–brain barrier.[51] The lesson from this observation is clear: Any drug administered to a patient with advanced hepatic disease must be carefully titrated against effect. The pathogenesis and management of hepatic encephalopathy is described in detail elsewhere.[52]

Renal Function in Patients with Liver Disease

Renal dysfunction and electrolyte imbalance often accompany advanced liver disease. Disorders in sodium, potassium, and water metabolism and in excretion are often observed in patients with severe hepatic disease. Certain forms of glomerulopathy and disorders in renal acidification, as well as acute renal failure and hepatorenal syndrome, are observed in patients with hepatic cirrhosis and other forms of severe liver disease.

Patients with liver disease frequently excrete urine that is virtually free of sodium. It is not surprising that this leads to extracellular fluid accumulation with subsequent ascites and edema. It is important to realize that ascites and edema in patients with liver cirrhosis are mainly related to disturbances in sodium rather than in water excretion. Such patients can excrete very large volumes of dilute urine when a large amount of water without sodium is administered. It is noteworthy that most patients with liver cirrhosis do not excrete sodium sufficiently. The pathogenesis of sodium retention in patients with hepatic cirrhosis is rather complex and is currently explained by a decrease in "effective" blood volume and/or by the so-called overflow theory.[53] Both hypotheses are represented schematically in Figure 42-6. The hypothesis of reduced "effective" blood volume involves an imbalance of Starling forces in the hepatic sinusoids and splanchnic capillaries, resulting in excessive lymph formation. Subsequently, lymph accumulates in the peritoneal cavity as ascites. This, in turn, leads to a reduction in circulating plasma volume. Total plasma volume may be normal or even increased at that time, and the reduction in the "effective" plasma volume is mainly due to a redistribution of fluid. Actually, by "effective" plasma volume, circulating plasma volume is assumed. The reduced effective (circulating) plasma volume is sensed by the renal tubule, resulting in increased sodium and water resorption. Thus, this hypothesis explains renal sodium retention as being a secondary rather than a primary phenomenon.

In contrast, the "overflow" theory assumes that the primary factor in the pathogenesis of sodium retention in patients with liver cirrhosis is inappropriate retention of excessive sodium per se, resulting in increased plasma volume. Conditions of increased hydrostatic pressure (portal hypertension), in conjunction with a reduced plasma colloid osmotic pressure and expanded plasma volume (supposedly owing to sodium retention), lead to formation of ascites. Thus, according to the overflow theory, renal sodium retention and plasma volume expansion, rather than a reduction in plasma volume, are responsible for ascites formation. These two hypotheses are not necessarily exclusive. It is conceivable that the primary defect in sodium excretion plays a more important role in the

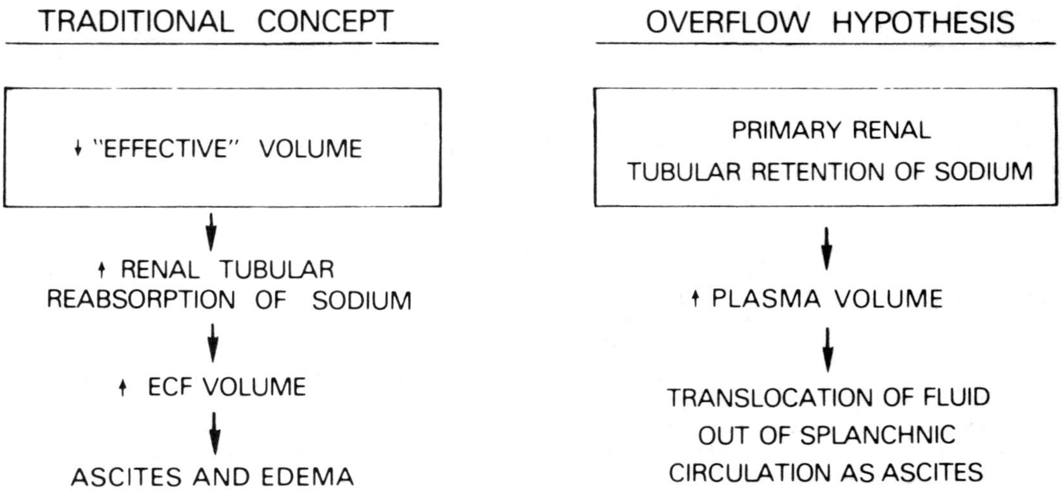

TRADITIONAL CONCEPT

OVERFLOW HYPOTHESIS

FIG. 42-6. The presumed sequences of events resulting in ascites formation according to two alternative theories: 1) the traditional theory; and 2) the "overflow" hypothesis. The primary events are shown within the rectangular boxes. According to the traditional concept, the primary event is a diminution in effective volume attributable to the development of abnormal Starling forces in the portal vein circulation with a maldistribution of circulating volume. The diminished "effective" volume is thought to constitute an afferent signal to the renal tubule to augment renal salt and water reabsorption. The attempt to replenish the diminished effective volume results in an expansion of the total blood volume to values far in excess of normal, with resultant ascites and edema formation.

In contrast, the "overflow" theory of ascites formation holds that retention of excessive sodium by the kidneys is the primary event. In the setting of abnormal Starling forces in the portal venous bed, the expanded plasma volume is sequestered preferentially in the peritoneal sac with ascites formation. (Reproduced with permission from Epstein M: Renal functional abnormalities in cirrhosis: Pathophysiology and management. In Zakim D, Boyer TD [eds]: Hepatology: A Textbook of Liver Disease, p 448. Philadelphia, WB Saunders, 1982)

early stages of cirrhosis, whereas a reduced circulating plasma volume may be more important in patients with advanced liver cirrhosis.[53]

There are quite a few neural, hemodynamic, and hormonal factors that play an important role in the pathogenesis of sodium retention in patients with hepatic cirrhosis. When the "effective" plasma volume is decreased, the sympathetic nervous discharge is increased, most probably through stimulation of volume receptors. This is accompanied by an increase in renin activity, which, through the angiotensin system, increases aldosterone secretion. Both an increase in sympathetic nervous tone and an increase in aldosterone activity lead to an enhanced tubular resorption of sodium. This is also aggravated by a redistribution of intrarenal blood flow, a result of increased vasoconstricting influences such as sympathetic nervous tone and activity of the renin-angiotensin system. Prostaglandins and the kallikrein-kinin system also participate in modulating sodium retention. An interesting study by Perez–Ayuso et al[54] suggests that prostaglandins and the kallikrein-kinin system probably play a compensatory, counteracting role in renal circulation and function. As the concentration of these vasodilating substances ceases to increase further, decompensation occurs and different degrees of renal insufficiency develop.

Diuretics are often used in patients with hepatic cirrhosis and ascites to increase urine output and decrease ascites. However, diuretic therapy is often accompanied by many complications such as hypovolemia, azotemia, sometimes hyponatremia, and encephalopathy. It is conceivable that diuretic therapy without proper fluid volume management may decrease "effective" plasma volume with a subsequent deterioration in renal function and the development of the hepatorenal syndrome.

A peritoneovenous LeVeen shunt is another modality for treating severe ascites in patients with hepatic cirrhosis. The idea behind this treatment is rather simple and logical: If the abnormality in patients with ascites is a maldistribution of excellular fluid, an attempt to reverse such a maldistribution of body fluids between compartments seems to be justified. The shunt between the peritoneal cavity and the central venous system has a one-way valve activated by a pressure gradient that allows the ascites fluid to move into the venous system. Treatment with a LeVeen shunt is mainly used in patients with ascites who are refractory to dietary and diuretic treatment.

The pathogenesis of water retention in patients with hepatic cirrhosis is rather complex, and the mechanisms include an increased secretion of antidiuretic hormone, as well as a reduced delivery of filtrate to the diluting segments of the nephron.[53] Causes for observed hypokalemia include inadequate diet, vomiting, diarrhea, hyperaldosteronemia, and diuretic therapy.

HEPATORENAL SYNDROME. Hepatorenal syndrome usually develops in patients with classic symptoms of hepatic cirrhosis, portal hypertension, and, particularly, ascites. These patients usually maintain urine output, although it is somewhat decreased; however, urine, even concentrated, contains almost no sodium; blood creatinine and BUN concentrations progressively increase. Actually, the characteristics of urine from patients with hepatorenal syndrome are similar to those of patients with hypovolemia. Apparently the renal damage in hepatorenal syndrome is reversible: Kidneys transplanted from patients with hepatorenal syndrome can resume normal function in recipients.[55]

The pathogenesis of hepatorenal syndrome has not been clearly established, but it is believed that renal vasoconstriction, with a subsequent decrease in renal blood flow, is primarily responsible for the development of hepatorenal syndrome. The renin-angiotensin system, sympathetic nervous system, alterations in prostaglandins, and the kallikrein-kinin system, as well as endotoxemia, all play a certain role in the pathogenesis of hepatorenal syndrome.

Since hepatorenal syndrome seems to develop in the hospital, rather than before the patient is admitted, this raises the question of how and what events in the hospital affect the development of hepatorenal syndrome. This coincides with the impression from some studies that hepatorenal syndrome develops after a decreased plasma volume, as in vigorous diuretic therapy, gastrointestinal bleeding, and paracentesis. The majority of patients with hepatorenal syndrome die; therefore, the prevention of this syndrome with very carefully managed diuretic therapy and volume status is mandatory.

Acute renal failure and/or acute tubular necrosis may also develop in patients with hepatic cirrhosis and often complicates arterial hypotension and infection. It has been demonstrated that acute tubular necrosis develops more often during and/or after the release of obstructive jaundice compared with similar operations performed on nonjaundiced patients.[56] It is conceivable that patients with hepatic disease or obstructive jaundice have a very limited ability to mobilize blood from the splanchnic (including hepatic) vasculature to increase central blood volume.[57] Thus, in response to even very moderate hemorrhage, such patients may develop severe hypotension with subsequent development of acute tubular necrosis. Some studies also demonstrated that circulating conjugated bilirubin exercises a toxic effect on the tubule in the kidneys and may be responsible for the development of acute tubular necrosis in jaundiced patients.[58] The differential diagnosis between hepatorenal syndrome and acute tubular necrosis is usually relatively simple (Table 42-3). The treatment of hepatorenal syndrome, as well as that for acute tubular necrosis, is complex and includes a careful search for underlying causes of renal insufficiency, supportive therapy, and careful maintenance of necessary circulating blood volume, particularly when bleeding occurs or when diuretics are used.

It is clear that the pathogenesis of hepatic cirrhosis and portal hypertension is extremely complex and is still not

clearly understood. A schematic representation of the pathogenesis of hepatic cirrhosis is depicted in Figure 42-7.

Ischemic Hepatitis

Respiratory and/or cardiovascular dysfunction may result in a condition termed *ischemic hepatitis,*[59] a relatively rare form of hepatic disease that may be particularly interesting to anesthesiologists. Typically, ischemic hepatitis is diagnosed when a patient with cardiac disease develops acute changes in liver blood tests mimicking acute hepatitis. Usually, there is a moderate increase in bilirubin and alkaline phosphatase concentrations in blood, moderate jaundice, and a very dramatic increase in both aspartate and alanine aminotransferases. Histologically, centrilobular hepatic necrosis might be seen. An interesting feature of ischemic hepatitis is that despite a rather extreme increase in hepatic enzymes, severe hepatic dysfunction does not develop. If cardiovascular function is normalized, ischemic hepatitis resolves by itself without serious sequela. It seems that ischemic hepatitis is associated more with a decrease in hepatic blood and oxygen supply than with hepatic congestion.[60, 61] The concentration of aminotransferases usually decreases and returns to relatively normal values within 5 to 10 days, much faster than in patients with viral hepatitis. Also, patients with ischemic hepatitis usually develop an increase in lactic dehydrogenase, whereas this enzyme changes little in the majority of patients with viral hepatitis.

CHOLESTASIS (OBSTRUCTIVE JAUNDICE)

In most cases of cholestasis, the presence of bile in liver tissue is histologically identifiable. Bile is most often visible in canaliculi in Zone 3 of the liver acinus, the tissue surrounding the terminal hepatic venulae or central vein. Physiologically, cholestasis means a reduction in the hepatic secretion of bile. It is clinically always accompanied by an accumulation of substances in the blood, which are normally excreted with bile. Such substances include bilirubin, cholesterol, bile acids, and some other compounds.

Most cases of cholestasis that require surgical intervention are due to extrahepatic biliary obstruction. On the other hand, there are many forms of cholestasis that result from certain hepatocyte dysfunction. These forms include disorders that result from certain alterations in the structure and enzymatic activity of liver cell membranes, dysfunction of microfilaments and microtubles, alterations in canalicular permeability, and certain interactions between chemical (including bile acids) substances and biliary solutes.

Bilirubin is toxic for many different enzyme systems, in-

TABLE 42-3. Differential Diagnosis of Acute Azotemia in the Patient With Liver Disease—Important Differential Urinary Findings

	PRERENAL AZOTEMIA	HEPATORENAL SYNDROME	ACUTE RENAL FAILURE (ATN)
Urinary sodium concentration	<10 mEq $\cdot$ l^{-1}	<10 mEq $\cdot$ l^{-1}	>30 mEq $\cdot$ l^{-1}
Urine-to-plasma creatinine ratio	$>30:1$	$>30:1$	$<20:1$
Urinary osmolality	At least 100 mOsm $>$ plasma osmolality	At least 100 mOsm $>$ plasma osmolality	Equal to plasma osmolality
Urinary sediment	Normal	Unremarkable	Casts, cellular debris

(Reproduced with permission from Epstein M: Renal functional abnormalities in cirrhosis: Pathophysiology and management. In Zakim D, Boyer TD [eds]: Hepatology: A Textbook of Liver Disease, p 460. Philadelphia, WB Saunders, 1982.)

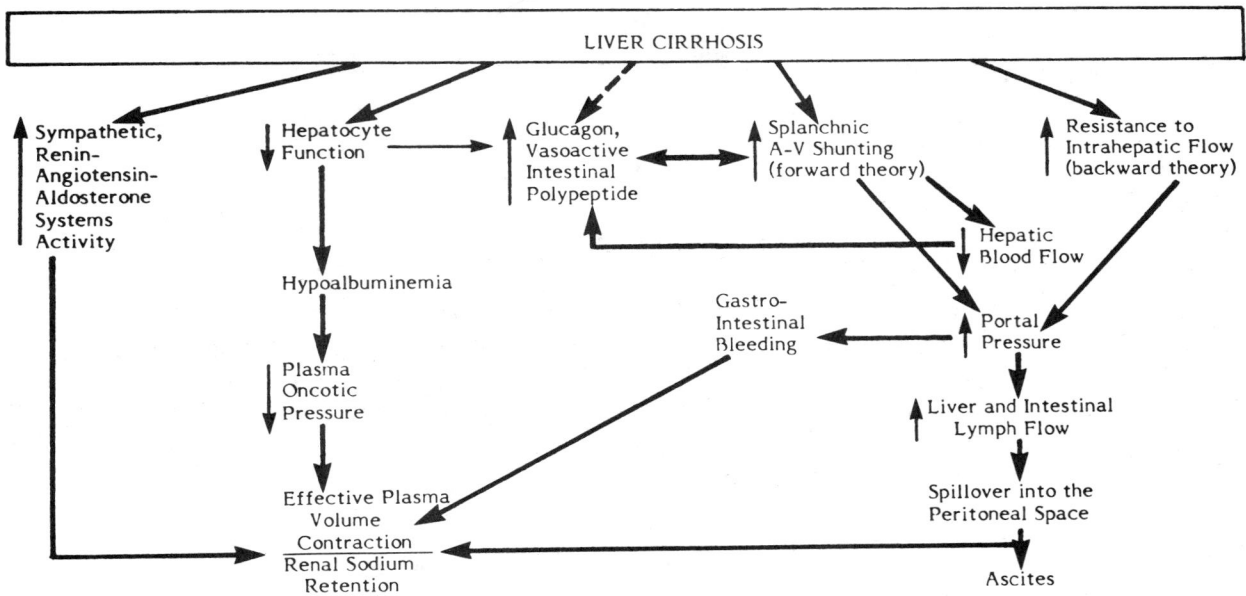

FIG. 42-7. Pathogenesis of liver cirrhosis—schematic representation. (Reproduced with permission from Kang YG, Gelman S: Liver transplantation. In Gelman S [ed]: Anesthesia and Organ Transplantation, p 145. Philadelphia, WB Saunders, 1987.)

cluding respiration and oxidative phosphorylation, glycolysis, glycogenesis, tricarboxylic acid cycle, as well as enzymes involved in heme biosynthesis, and lipid, amino acid, and protein metabolism.[23] This effect on the enzyme system occurs at high concentrations of bilirubin and can be modified with additional albumin.[24] Bilirubin may also interfere with membrane function.[25]

Cardiovascular Function

There are data strongly suggesting that cholemia *per se* impairs myocardial contractility.[62–64] It has also been demonstrated that cholemia blunts the response to isoproterenol, probably by interfering with the binding of these agents to membrane receptors. It has been suggested that bile acids interfere either with the entry of calcium into or with the exit of potassium from the myocardial cells.[64]

Cardiovascular dysfunction in patients with biliary obstruction mimics (but to a lesser extent) the same pattern observed in patients with hepatic cirrhosis, namely, peripheral vascular resistance decreases while cardiac output increases; portal venous blood flow decreases while portal venous pressure increases; hepatic arterial blood flow does not change significantly while portacaval shunting increases substantially.[65]

It has been observed that patients with liver disease, both parenchymal and cholestatic, have decreased sensitivity to vasopressor drugs. The reasons for this resistance have not been clarified. However, experiments *in vitro* and *in vivo* strongly suggest that bile acids *per se* may contribute to the vasodilation and hypotension often observed in patients with biliary obstruction.[64] An increase in blood concentrations of vasoactive substances such as ferritin, vasoactive intestinal polypeptide, and glucagon also contribute to the vasodilating and hyperdynamic state.

It seems conceivable that the decreased sensitivity of patients with biliary obstruction to vasoactive substances, including catecholamines, is responsible for the rather interesting and clinically important observation that these patients do not seem to tolerate even minimal blood loss as well as do normal persons. It has been demonstrated in animals that very moderate blood loss, that is, 10% of the estimated blood volume, does not substantially decrease mean arterial pressure, whereas, in animals with experimentally induced biliary obstruction, such a blood loss led to severe arterial hypotension by approximately 50% (Fig. 42-8). Moreover, this study demonstrated that in intact animals, pulmonary blood volume and splanchnic blood volume decreased by approximately 15% in response to blood loss, but, in animals with biliary obstruction, pulmonary blood volume decreased by only 7%, whereas splanchnic blood volume did not change at all (Fig. 42-9). These observations imply that patients (if we can extrapolate these results to humans) with biliary obstruction would not respond sufficiently to blood loss by expelling blood volume into the systemic circulation to compensate for bleeding as would normal persons. Further, it may be necessary to immediately replace volume losses occurring in these patients during the perioperative period. The anesthesiologist should be aware that biliary decompression may be accompanied by severe cardiovascular collapse.[66]

Blood Coagulation

Patients with biliary obstruction develop certain coagulation disorders. Usually, at least during short-lasting biliary obstruction, coagulopathy is due to a deficiency of vitamin K–dependent coagulation factors, since absorption of vitamin K depends upon the absorption of fat and, therefore, on excretion of bile into the gastrointestinal tract. Later, with long-lasting biliary obstruction, parenchymal component develops with a subsequent deterioration in protein synthesis and synthesis of coagulation factors. Usually, coagulation disorders are moderate and can be restored relatively easily by parenteral vitamin K therapy. However, if this treatment is not effective, which probably would mean that the patient has

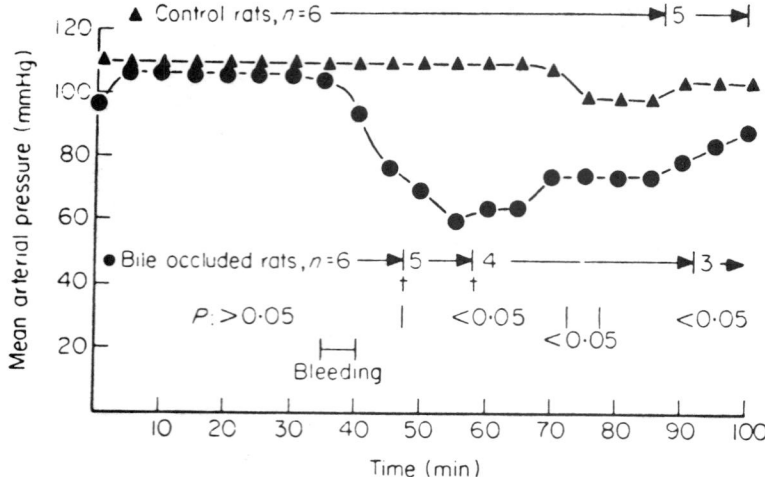

FIG. 42-8. Effect of a 10% blood loss on mean arterial pressure in anesthetized rats. ●, bile duct occluded 7 days previously. ▲, sham-operated. Two of the bile occluded animals died immediately after the blood loss. The level of significant difference between the groups is given. In response to similar blood loss, animals with an occluded bile duct developed more severe arterial hypotension than did control rats. (Reproduced with permission from Aarseth S, Bergan A, Aarseth P: Circulatory homeostasis in rats after bile duct ligation. Scand J Clin Lab Invest 39:93, 1979.)

parenchymal liver disease or parenchymal component in his or her cholestasis, or if surgery is urgent and coagulopathy should be treated immediately, therapy with fresh frozen plasma is indicated. If the prolonged prothrombin time does not respond to vitamin K therapy, it confirms a significant depression of hepatic parenchymal function and coincides with a poor prognosis.

Renal Function

It has been suggested that bilirubin and/or bile salts sensitize the kidneys to hypoxic/ischemic damage.[58, 67] Bile duct ligation actually increases the glomerular filtration rate and renal blood flow in the dog.[68] Some recent studies suggest that intrarenal infusion of dilute bile into the dog increased renal production of prostaglandin E_2 (PGE_2). Moreover, indomethacin abolished both the natriuresis and the increase in renal PGE_2 synthesis associated with intrarenal infusion of bile.[64] It is currently believed that moderate cholemia is not nephrotoxic, nor are even high bilirubin concentrations. However, the increase in jaundice can be considered a prelude to

the hepatorenal syndrome.[64] Deterioration in renal function in patients with biliary obstruction may result from endotoxin produced in the intestines. Some toxemia is related to a reduction in bile salts, with a subsequent change in the intestinal flora in patients with biliary obstruction, as well as to a reduction in reticuloendothelial function of the liver.

BLOOD TESTS FOR PATIENTS WITH LIVER DISEASE

Hepatic function is extremely complex; therefore, it is not surprising that many different biochemical tests are used to evaluate liver function. Generally speaking, some tests characterize liver function and some identify liver damage, whereas others deal with specific markers of hepatic disease (Table 42-4).

Serum Enzymes

High serum concentrations of enzymes such as aspartate aminotransferase (AST or SGOT) and alanine aminotransferase (ALT or SGPT) may be, and usually are, indicative of hepatocellular injury. Both of these enzymes are present in tissues other than the liver, for example, in skeletal muscles, kidneys, and the heart. Therefore, an increase of concentrations in the blood of these enzymes may reflect damage of other tissues, not necessarily the liver. These enzymes are simply released from the cell when a liver cell is damaged or dies. ALT is considered to be a more specific enzyme for the liver than is AST. The degree of increase in these enzyme concentrations in blood reflects acuteness and extent of injury, but by no means characterizes liver function *per se* or prognosis. Moreover, a decrease in the high plasma concentration of the enzymes may not reflect recovery, but, to the contrary, may reflect a decreased ability of hepatocytes to synthesize enzymes and, therefore, possibly implies a poor prognosis. Concentrations of serum aminotransferases in chronic liver disease are often considerably less than those seen in acute liver disease. It is not uncommon to observe a perfectly normal or decreased concentration of these enzymes in patients with severe hepatic parenchymal disease or even liver failure.

Alkaline phosphatase is another serum enzyme frequently measured when hepatic disease is suspected. This enzyme may be released not only from the hepatobiliary system but

FIG. 42-9. Effect of a 10% blood loss on pulmonary (PBV) and splanchnic (SBV) in anesthetized rats. The blood loss resulted in a 15% decrease in both PBV and SBV in control animals, while PBV decreased only 7%, and SBV did not change at all in animals with an occluded bile duct. The observation suggests a decrease in reservoir function (response to hypovolemia) of pulmonary and, particularly, splanchnic vasculature. (Reproduced with permission from Aarseth S, Bergan A, Aarseth P: Circulatory homeostasis in rats after bile duct ligation. Scand J Clin Lab Invest 39:93, 1979.)

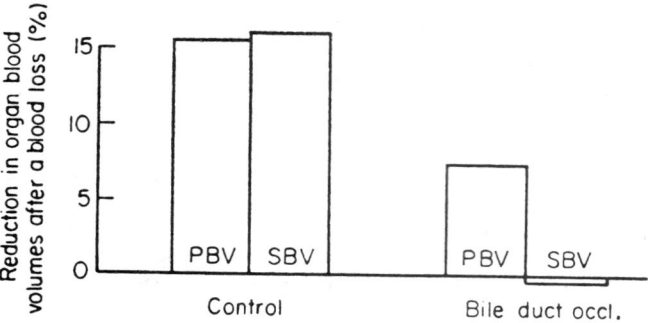

TABLE 42-4.   Blood Tests and the Differential Diagnosis of Hepatic Dysfunction

	BILIRUBIN OVERLOAD (HEMOLYSIS)	PARENCHYMAL DYSFUNCTION	CHOLESTASIS
Bilirubin Aminotransferases	Unconjugated Normal	Conjugated Increased (may be normal or decreased in advanced stages)	Conjugated Normal (may be increased in advanced stages)
Alkaline phosphatase	Normal	Normal	Increased
Prothrombin time	Normal	Prolonged	Normal (may be prolonged in advanced stages)
Serum proteins	Normal	Decreased	Normal (may be decreased in advanced stages)
BUN	Normal	Normal (may be decreased in advanced stages)	Normal
BSP/ICG (dye)	Normal	Retention	Normal or retention

also from the intestinal tract, bones, and placenta. Therefore, the concentration of this enzyme may be increased during normal pregnancy, normal growth (in teenagers), and, in the case of bone metastasis, during certain forms of hepatobiliary diseases, mainly extrahepatic biliary obstruction. Elevation of this enzyme in the blood is not considered a reflection of deterioration in liver function or liver damage. Some other enzymes such as 5'-nucleotidase, leucine aminopeptidase, and gamma-glutamyl transpeptidase are considered to be more specific and better reflections of cholestasis and biliary obstruction.

Serum Bilirubin and Bile Acids

Serum bilirubin concentrations reflect the efficacy of hepatic uptake and excretion relative to the production rate (i.e., hemolysis) of bilirubin. An increase in conjugated versus unconjugated bilirubin in plasma (see metabolism of bilirubin) often helps to differentiate jaundice related to parenchymal disease from jaundice resulting from biliary obstruction. The measurements of serum bile acids seem to be a more accurate and useful test characterizing this hepatic function. It is more sensitive than the dynamics of bilirubin concentration in the blood. Determination of bile acids is especially useful in the diagnosis of the different forms of cholestasis and biliary obstruction. After all, the definition of cholestasis is impaired bile excretion with subsequently increased plasma bile acid concentrations.

Prothrombin Time and Serum Proteins

The serum concentration of proteins synthesized in the liver reflects the protein synthesizing ability of the liver. Therefore, the concentration of different proteins synthesized by the liver reflects this particular hepatic function. One such protein is prothrombin. Prolongation of prothrombin time is not highly specific for hepatic disease. One of the most common reasons other than hepatic disease for prolongation of prothrombin time is vitamin K deficiency, which may result from specific medication for antagonizing the prothrombin complex (bis-hydroxycoumarin). Other reasons for prolongation of prothrombin time include incomplete clearing of activated clotting factors and coagulation inhibitors from the plasma by the liver, impaired plasminogen synthesis by the liver, primarily fibrinolysis and DIC. However, if all these reasons are ruled out (differential diagnosis is seldom difficult and is based on other clinical and laboratory data), the prolongation of prothrombin time is considered a relatively sensitive test characterizing liver function. Prothrombin time is probably one of the most accurate qualitative, rather than quantitative, estimates of hepatic function in patients with hepatic disease. However, "it gives the liver more of a pass or fail than a numerical grade on its performance."[69] Prolongation of prothrombin time confirms a rather significant depression of hepatic parenchymal function.

Albumin is synthesized by the liver; thus, the low plasma albumin concentration may, but not necessarily, reflect depressed hepatic function. Despite certain deficiencies, the determination of albumin concentration in plasma may have a predictive value for survival of patients with advanced hepatic disease, basically hepatic cirrhosis, after major surgery. Many hepatic diseases are accompanied by a decrease in albumin and an increase in different fractions of globulin levels in the blood. Hyperglobulinemia usually indicates a chronic hepatic disease but says very little about hepatic reserves or the degree of hepatic dysfunction.

Metabolizing Function of the Liver

BUN is not considered a blood test characterizing liver function; however, low BUN concentrations in plasma, for example, below 5 mg·dl^{-1}, may indicate a severely depressed hepatic ability to synthesize urea. This test seems to be especially valid in patients with alcoholic cirrhosis. The metabolizing function of the liver can be evaluated not only by urea synthesis but also by galactose elimination and metabolism and excretion of different drugs. The liver removes many lipophilic substances from the plasma and excretes them into bile. Some of these substances are excreted unchanged, whereas others are excreted after conversion to more polar forms. These forms include mainly organic anions and, to a lesser extent, organic cations and neutral organic compounds.

Dyes such as sulfobromophthalein (BSP) and indocyanine green (ICG) are organic anions that characterize the metabolic and excretory function of the liver. The BSP and ICG tests require the injection of dye into the bloodstream and then subsequent evaluation of the rate of disappearance and/or the degree of retention of dye in the blood. There are many different approaches to using these tests. At present, the clinical application of these tests is somewhat limited, since interpretation of the results is difficult and often questionable.

The metabolism of some drugs can be used as an indicator of the metabolizing function of the liver. The most commonly used tests at present are the antipyrine clearance and aminopyrine breath test. However, these tests cannot be considered very sensitive since they become abnormal only with relatively advanced liver disease. Thus, the substantial decrease in the metabolism of these substances would indicate an already very severe hepatic dysfunction, whereas relatively normal test results may be found in patients with very limited hepatic reserves.

The galactose elimination test is even less sensitive in detecting hepatic dysfunction than the BSP and ICG tests. The reason for this is probably because BSP and ICG are distributed mainly in plasma volume, whereas galactose is distributed in the extracellular space. Extracellular volume can vary rather substantially from patient to patient, and this would be reflected in the test results.

Specific Tests

Certain immunologic and serologic tests can be of some value in patients with parenchymal hepatic disease. Antigens and antibodies may help identify viral hepatitis. The diagnosis of halothane hepatitis is sometimes suggested by specific serological tests.[70] There are many other tests that may verify certain common and uncommon hepatic diseases.[71]

In summary, the determination of aminotransferases and alkaline phosphatase is extremely useful in differentiating cholestasis from acute parenchymal disease. Aminotransferases are substantially increased in acute parenchymal hepatic disease, whereas alkaline phosphatase is increased in cholestatic disease.

The severity and prognosis of hepatic disease are best evaluated by determinations of serum albumin and prothrombin time. The diagnosis of hepatobiliary disease, as well as the degree of hepatic dysfunction, is extremely difficult and should be made by an experienced and knowledgeable hepatologist who is probably most qualified to interpret the tests. Detailed information regarding the tests characterizing different hepatic function as well as various hepatic diseases are available in the literature.[71]

ANESTHESIA, SURGERY, AND LIVER FUNCTION

COMPARATIVE PHARMACOLOGY AND HEPATOTOXICITY OF ANESTHETICS

Different anesthetics affect hepatic function in various directions and to different degrees. Perioperative hepatic dysfunction may result from the direct effect of an anesthetic on hepatocyte function or from the indirect effect of decreased oxygen and blood supply to the liver, accumulation of certain hormones and substances that affect liver function, and the initiation of more complex mechanisms such as the formation of antibodies and the involvement of immunologic mechanisms.

HALOTHANE. Halothane is probably the anesthetic most well studied regarding possible hepatotoxicity. The National Halothane Study analyzed approximately 850,000 cases with halothane administered to only 250,000 of these patients.[12] Eighty-two patients had fatal hepatic necrosis. Only nine cases were unexplainable on grounds other than anesthesia; seven of these nine cases received halothane; therefore, the true incidence of unexplained fatal hepatic necrosis following halothane anesthesia is 7 of 250,000 population, or 1 per 35,000 persons. This number is often misquoted and misinterpreted: The number 1 per 10,000 persons is frequently, unjustifiably quoted.[72, 73] Later studies have shown that severe hepatic dysfunction following halothane anesthesia occurs in approximately 1 of 6,000 to 1 of 20,000 halothane administrations.[74, 75] Schemel[10] found that 11 of 7,620 ASA I status patients scheduled for elective surgery had increased plasma concentrations of hepatic enzymes preoperatively. The surgery was postponed in these cases; however, 3 of the 11 patients developed jaundice. If these patients had undergone surgery, the jaundice observed postoperatively would have been attributed to the anesthesia. Moreover, surgery and anesthesia could have aggravated the condition, and these 3 jaundiced patients could have suffered from more severe hepatic dysfunction after anesthesia and surgery than they developed without surgery. It is extremely difficult to differentiate halothane hepatitis from viral hepatitis that develops in the postoperative period.[15] Simple calculations show that approximately 100 of one million anesthetized patients may have unrecognized viral A hepatitis prior to anesthesia and surgery and, subsequently, may develop signs of hepatitis postoperatively.[76]

There is relatively strong evidence in the literature indicating that certain factors substantially enhance the risks of halothane-induced hepatotoxicity. These factors include multiple exposure to halothane, obesity, gender (females are more susceptible to halothane hepatitis than are males), middle-age, and ethnic origin (Mexican–Americans seem to be more susceptible than others).[70] There are data that strongly suggest a familiar constitutional susceptibility factor that predisposes certain persons to halothane hepatitis.[77] A recent study by Japanese investigators posed that genetic susceptibility to halothane hepatitis may be associated with certain alterations in the region of the 6th chromosome.[78]

There are mainly three proposed mechanisms for halothane-induced hepatotoxicity: 1) a direct hepatotoxic effect of intermediates of halothane metabolism. This mechanism assumes that halothane undergoes a reductive metabolism in conditions of hepatic oxygen deprivation and that the products of this biotransformation are toxic for the liver cells; 2) hepatic oxygen deprivation per se, resulting from respiratory, systemic circulatory, and/or regional hepatic circulatory disturbances induced by halothane; and 3) immunologically mediated hepatic necrosis. This mechanism assumes that the oxidative metabolism of halothane, without hepatic oxygen deprivation, results in the formation of haptene, which then reacts with protein and lipoprotein of hepatocyte membranes with a subsequent involvement of autoimmune-mediated injury to liver cells.

METABOLIC THEORY. The metabolic theory of halothane-induced hepatotoxicity assumes that particular animals (rats) and some patients developing halothane-induced liver damage possess an enhanced ability to biotransform halothane by the reductive pathway, thereby producing toxic reactive intermediates.[79] The primary function of the cytochrome P450 oxygenase system is to transfer electrons from nicotinamide-adenine dinucleotide phosphate hydrogenase (NADPH) to oxygen, activating oxygen, which then oxidizes a drug. During hepatic oxygen deprivation, the cytochrome P450 system transfers an electron directly to certain substrates, thereby reducing them. All volatile anesthetics undergo some degree of metabolism, and the cytochrome P450 system plays the main role in this biotransformation. Exposure to many drugs and chemicals may induce the cytochrome P450 system, increasing the amount of enzymes with a subsequent increase in the turnover rate of substrate to product. It has been established and reviewed[80] that enflurane, and particularly isoflurane, undergo very limited metabolism in the liver compared with halothane. The latter can undergo an oxidative metabolism when the oxygen supply is adequate and a reductive metabolism when hepatic oxygen deprivation develops. The reductive metabolism of halothane results in the release of inorganic fluoride and some other intermediates. Free radicals have been proposed as potentially harmful intermediates in the reductive metabolism of halothane.

It is interesting to note that patients with cyanotic congenital heart disease have a greater reductive metabolism of halothane than do acyanotic patients. However, both groups of patients, cyanotic and acyanotic, demonstrated similar postoperative hepatic and renal dysfunction.[81] These observations do not fit the contention that the reductive metabolism of halothane plays a particularly important role in the development of halothane-induced hepatic injury. The supporters of the metabolic theory collected some valuable data that probably better fit this theory than prove it. Many observations, however, are still difficult to explain by the metabolic theory. For example, similar degrees of the reductive metabolism of halothane may be accompanied by different degrees of hepatic injury.[82] The end products of the reductive metabolism of halothane have never been found to be hepatotoxic: Liver damage could not be reproduced by exposure to these end products (fluoride; 2-chloro-1,1,1-trifluoroethane (CTF); and 2-chloro-1,1-difluorethylene (CDF)).[73] Free radical intermediates have also been blamed for halothane-induced hepatic damage; however, the extent of free radical formation is not reflected in hepatotoxicity.[73] The evidence suggests that hepatic injury occurs during exposure, at a time before metabolism takes place and before the binding of reactive metabolites, either to lipids or proteins, is at its peak.[80] It seems that hepatotoxicity is initiated without the full impact of metabolism, suggesting that the reductive metabolism plays only a limited role, if any, in the mechanism of hepatotoxicity. A detailed and critical analysis of the results of experimental studies in this area is described elsewhere.[73, 80, 83]

Some data suggest that even in the model of phenobarbital-pretreated rats exposed to hypoxia and halothane (this model was primarily used to collect the data supporting the metabolic theory of halothane-induced hepatotoxicity), hepatic injury is related not so much to the reductive metabolism of halothane but to hepatic oxygen deprivation.[84, 85] An interesting model for studying anesthesia-induced hepatotoxicity was introduced in Australia.[86] The authors demonstrated that guinea pigs, without pretreatment with phenobarbital and exposure to hypoxia, developed hepatic necrosis after exposure to halothane but not to isoflurane when similar degrees of arterial hypotension (50%) were achieved.[86] These authors assumed that equal degrees of arterial hypotension are accompanied by equal degrees of hepatic oxygen deprivation and that the hepatic injury observed after halothane anesthesia was attributed to the reductive metabolism of halothane. However, a subsequent study in our laboratory demonstrated that equal degrees of arterial hypotension (50%) exactly as in the Australian study[86] was accompanied by very different degrees of hepatic oxygen deprivation: A 50% decrease in arterial blood pressure achieved by halothane was associated with a 65% decrease in hepatic oxygen supply, whereas the same degree of arterial hypotension achieved with isoflurane led to a 35% decrease in hepatic oxygen supply.[87] Thus, the role of the reductive metabolism of halothane in the halothane-induced hepatotoxicity is still questionable.

HEPATIC OXYGEN DEPRIVATION. This might play an important, if not leading, role in some forms of halothane-induced hepatic injury.[84] Many animal experimental observations on halothane-induced hepatotoxicity, explained by the metabolic theory, can be successfully attributed to hepatic oxygen deprivation per se, without direct involvement of reductive biotransformation of halothane. This issue has been thoroughly reviewed.[80, 88] Regarding inhalational anesthetic toxicity, an interesting hypothetical mechanism was proposed by Van Dyke and Madson from the Mayo Clinic.[89] They demonstrated that halothane, enflurane, and isoflurane affect phosphorylase activity in isolated rat hepatocytes. The results of their observations suggest that all three of these anesthetics, even at low concentrations, raise intracellular calcium concentrations, which may result in hepatocellular injury.

IMMUNOLOGIC THEORY. The involvement of hypersensitivity and idiosyncrasy in halothane hepatitis has been based on several important observations.[70, 90] These observations include frequent associations of halothane hepatitis with multiple exposures to halothane, mild fever after the first exposure, followed by severe jaundice on re-exposure, association with fever and eosinophilia, frequent history of drug allergy, positive challenge tests, and demonstration of circulating antibodies to liver microsomes. It was believed that halothane hepatitis does not develop in children; however, recently, five cases were reported among children, one of whom died.[91] The immunologic theory of halothane hepatitis assumes that one of the possible mechanisms of the halothane-induced hepatic injury involves some intermediates produced by the oxidative pathway of halothane metabolism.[92, 93] The intermediates of oxidative halothane biotransformation can bind covalently to liver tissue (proteins or lipoproteins) and form complexes that can potentially act as haptenes and induce an immunologically mediated response in susceptible persons. Thus, it seems that, in part, halothane hepatitis is due to specific cellular susceptibility. Another part of the complex appears to be multifactorial.

It has been suggested that trifluoroacetyl chloride, which is produced by oxidative biotransformation of halothane, covalently binds to the lysine residuals on proteins. This distorted protein may act as an antigen with a subsequent production of antibodies.[94-96] Circulating antibodies, bound to the membrane surface of halothane-altered rabbit hepatocytes, were detected in 9 of 14 samples from 11 patients with halothane hepatitis.[96] The halothane-related antibodies have been detected in other patients with hepatitis following halothane administration.[97, 98] Contrary to the metabolic theory, which implies the involvement of the reductive pathway of halothane metabolism, the halothane-altered membrane antigen is produced by the oxidative pathway of halothane metabolism.[92] Thus, according to the immunologic theory, the role of the reductive metabolism of halothane and/or hepatic oxygen deprivation in the development of halothane hepatitis is probably negligible, if any.

In their recent review, Stock and Strunin[73] have come to the following conclusions: 1) Halothane has a very low risk potential for liver damage in children, even when used repeatedly; 2) there is no contraindication for the use of halothane in the presence of pre-existing compensated liver disease provided that this does not relate to a previous anesthetic—outcome will be determined by the degree of preoperative liver dysfunction and the extent of the surgical procedure; 3) severe liver damage is unlikely to follow a single exposure to halothane; 4) repeated exposure to halothane in adult humans, particularly in obese, middle-aged women, and over a short period of time (probably 4 to 8 weeks), may result in severe liver damage to only a few persons; 5) if repeated halothane anesthesia is contemplated, the anesthesiologist should document the reason for using halothane on the second occasion; 6) the mechanism of hepatitis following halothane is unclear but most probably involves an immunologic response; and 7) at present, there is no reliable, specific test for halothane-induced liver damage.

It is important to focus on the effects of halothane on liver function *per se*, even when halothane hepatitis does not develop, since halothane does affect hepatic function. As an example, halothane suppresses the synthesizing ability of the liver: In experiments with isolated perfused livers, halothane decreased the protein synthesis in a dose-related fashion.[99] Experimental data on the effects of halothane on hepatic function are not very elaborate; however, most of the available data suggest that halothane, compared with other widely used inhalational anesthetics (enflurane and isoflurane), is probably the worst in regard to its influence on liver function. Prolonged enflurane or isoflurane anesthesia in volunteers did not affect BSP elimination, whereas halothane significantly increased BSP retention.[100, 101]

Drug biotransformation is one of the most important and sensitive functions of the liver. It was clearly demonstrated that aminopyrine half-life was prolonged and for a longer duration of time postanesthetically during and after halothane administration than with enflurane or isoflurane. With the latter two agents, the prolongation of aminopyrine half-life was observed for a very short period of time or was not noticed at all.[102] Clinical observations are in agreement with the aforementioned experimental data: Halothane anesthesia is accompanied by a substantial release of hepatic glutathione S-transferase (GST), whereas patients anesthetized with isoflurane do not demonstrate any increase in the blood concentration of this hepatic enzyme.[103] The excretory function of the liver is impaired during halothane, whereas it is well maintained during isoflurane anesthesia, even when both anesthetics are used in equipotent doses according to MAC values, as well as according to the degree of arterial hypotension.[85] The reasons for these differences in impairment of hepatic function during halothane anesthesia compared with other inhalational anesthetics are not clear and may be related to the direct effect of halothane on hepatic function. However, other mechanisms may be involved: Halothane decreases hepatic oxygen supply to a much greater extent than isoflurane or enflurane when used in equipotent doses.[88, 104, 105] Portal blood flow usually decreases parallel with a reduction in cardiac output, while hepatic arterial blood flow compensates for this decrease in an attempt to meet the hepatic oxygen requirement and/or to maintain total hepatic blood flow. Enflurane, and particularly isoflurane, preserve the ability of hepatic arterial blood flow to increase when portal blood flow is decreased; halothane preserves this autoregulation ability to a very limited extent and only when it is used in relatively small doses. This ability is completely abolished when halothane is used in doses that decrease arterial blood pressure by approximately 20–25%.[88, 104]

An appropriate comment on this subject appeared in a recent editorial in the *British Medical Journal*: "the revolution that resulted from the introduction of halothane is likely to be replaced by another—the use of the more expensive but less hazardous enflurane and isoflurane."[91]

ENFLURANE. The incidence of hepatitis following enflurane anesthesia is much lower than with halothane. Lewis et al[106] reviewed observations on hepatic damage following enflurane anesthesia and concluded that enflurane caused the injury in 24 patients. The authors based their conclusions on the following speculations: Enflurane is a halogenated organic compound similar to halothane; therefore, enflurane may, and even should, cause liver injury similar to that observed with halothane. The authors[106] could not find any other obvious explanation for the liver injury. They also believed that clinical and histologic pictures observed in these patients were similar to those seen with halothane hepatitis. These arguments appear to be weak, since enflurane does not undergo biotransformation as does halothane and since the physical and biological properties of these two anesthetics are very different (Table 42-5). In 9 of these 24 cases, rational explanations other than enflurane were suggested.[101, 107] It seems at present that the known incidence of hepatic injury following enflurane anesthesia is too small to suggest any association between enflurane and hepatic injury. Even if enflurane may be hepatotoxic on rare occasions, the toxicity of enflurane is much less than that attributed to halothane. There is no specific histologic picture that exists in patients who develop hepatic injury following enflurane anesthesia.[101] Eger et al[101] examined 88 cases of postoperative liver dysfunction attributed to enflurane and could say that only 15 cases were possibly related to enflurane. This "possible" group did not present any consistent pathology or clinical picture.

Contrary to halothane administration, repeated administrations of enflurane do not increase the incidence of liver blood test abnormalities.[108] The incidence of hepatic damage following halothane anesthesia, as defined by the authors of published case reports, dramatically increased approximately 5 years after halothane was introduced into clinical practice,[109] whereas such an increase has not occurred with enflurane anesthesia (Fig. 42-10).[101] This difference in patterns of hepatic injury following halothane or enflurane anesthesia can be explained by the need to develop a pool of previously exposed patients, that is, patients sensitized to an anesthetic. It happened with halothane but has not happened with enflurane. Within the first 4 years following the introduction of halothane, more than 350 cases of unexplained postoperative jaun-

TABLE 42-5.   Differences Between Inhalational Anesthetics Relevant to a Consideration of Hepatotoxicity

	HALOTHANE	ENFLURANE	ISOFLURANE
Stable in sunlight	No	Yes	Yes
Stable in soda lime	No	Yes	Yes
Toxic breakdown products?	Yes	—	—
Metabolism	15–20%	2.4%	0.2%
Reductive metabolism	Yes	No	No
Metabolism to free radicals	Yes	No	No
Tissue binding of metabolites?	Yes	No	—
Hepatic oxygen delivery	Decreased	Slightly decreased	Unchanged

(Table modified with permission from Eger EI II: IARS Review Course Lectures 116, 1986.)

dice were reported and attributed to halothane. Eight years following the introduction of enflurane, Lewis et al[106] described 24 patients with postoperative liver disorders that were possibly attributed to enflurane. More than 20 million enflurane anesthetics had been administered by that time. If the rate of "enflurane hepatitis" were 1 per 800,000 enflurane administrations, this would still result in a remarkably low rate, even much lower than the spontaneous rate of viral hepatitis. One cannot completely rule out the possibility that enflurane can cause hepatic injury. However, the incidence of such injury, if it occurs at all, is so small that an accurate estimation seems to be impossible. There is no evidence of crossover sensitivity between halothane- and enflurane-induced hepatic injury.

ISOFLURANE.   There have been 45 reports of hepatic injury following isoflurane anesthesia.[110] An estimated incidence of hepatic injury following isoflurane anesthesia is 0.00032%— 45 cases from 14 million anesthetics administered, with an approximate 25% mortality rate. The incidence of viral hepatitis in apparently healthy patients with anesthesia and surgery may be as great as 1 per 1,000[10, 11] which is much higher than the incidence of unexplained hepatic injury following anesthesia. A subcommittee of the Anesthetic and Life Support Advisory Committee of the FDA evaluated all available reports to determine whether an association exists between administration of isoflurane and subsequent hepatic dysfunction. The committee concluded that "current evidence does not indicate a reasonable likelihood of an association between the use of isoflurane and the occurrence of postoperative hepatic dysfunction."[110]

Enflurane and isoflurane undergo minimal to no biotransformation while substantial amounts of halothane are metabolized.[11–113] Halothane undergoes a reductive metabolism, whereas enflurane and isoflurane do not. The metabolism of halothane may be accompanied by the formation of free radicals and also some metabolites that bind to lipids or proteins within the tissue. This is not the case with enflurane or isoflurane. Finally, halothane decreases hepatic blood and oxygen supply to a much greater extent than do either enflurane[105] or isoflurane[85, 87, 104] when used in equipotent doses, titrated by MAC values, or similar decreases in blood pressure or cardiac output. Other hepatic functions seem to be affected by halothane to a greater extent than by enflurane or isoflurane, as mentioned earlier.

NITROUS OXIDE.   Nitrous oxide *per se* is usually not associated with significant changes in blood pressure and cardiac output. Hepatic circulation is not disturbed when nitrous

oxide is used in trained animals without any baseline anesthesia or surgical preparation.[114] However, a significant decrease in both portal and hepatic arterial blood flows, by 15% and 24%, respectively, was observed when nitrous oxide was used in conditions of barbiturate anesthesia and laparotomy.[115] In the rat, nitrous oxide decreased cardiac output, intestinal blood flow, splenic blood flow, and total hepatic blood flow.[116] It has not been proved whether this decrease subjects the liver to ischemic injury.

Nitrous oxide in clinically used concentrations decreases methionine synthetase activity in the livers of animals and humans.[117] This decrease becomes greater with increased time of exposure. It is not clear whether or not this decrease in methionine synthetase activity is detrimental to liver function. One study clearly demonstrated that persons anesthetized with halothane and nitrous oxide showed a significant increase in serum liver enzymes compared with the patient

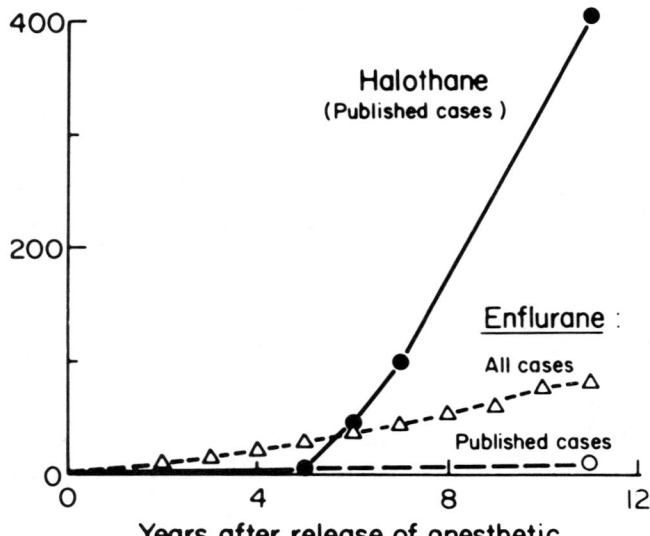

FIG. 42-10.   Total reported cases from release of halothane or enflurane to date of liver injury or jaundice. The number of published reports of hepatic injury after halothane anesthesia dramatically increased about 5 years after the introduction of halothane (●) into clinical practice. No such upturn has appeared in the 11-year period following the release of enflurane (▲ and ○). (Reproduced with permission from Eger EI II, Smuckler EA, Ferrell LD et al: Is enflurane hepatotoxic? Anesth Analg 65:21, 1986.)

anesthetized with halothane in oxygen.[118] The difference can be attributed to a somewhat better hepatic oxygenation in the group of patients who did not receive nitrous oxide, but the difference can also be explained by the absence or presence of nitrous oxide *per se*. Other studies could not demonstrate significant liver dysfunction during nitrous oxide anesthesia supplemented with methohexital.[119] Currently, there is no convincing evidence that nitrous oxide causes hepatotoxicity.[120]

Intravenous Anesthetics

The effect of intravenous anesthetics and opioids on the liver has not been thoroughly studied. A time-related reduction in hepatic arterial blood flow during a constant infusion of etomidate was observed in dogs.[121] These changes, however, probably resulted from systemic hemodynamic disturbances—mainly a decrease in cardiac output: Etomidate and althesin produce dose-dependent reductions in cardiac output and mean arterial pressure.[122] Small doses of etomidate and althesin, doses unaccompanied by significant changes in cardiac output or mean arterial pressure, still led to a significant decrease in hepatic arterial blood flow. These data are partially in agreement with the results observed in experiments with isolated perfused rat livers.[123] In those experiments, althesin and ketamine, when added to the perfusate, caused vasoconstriction of the hepatic arterial vasculature. All three drugs studied by Thomson increased vascular resistance in the hepatic arterial and mesenteric vasculatures when infused at low rates. The higher infusion rates were accompanied by systemic hemodynamic disturbances, with a subsequent decrease in hepatic blood flow.[122]

Liver blood tests were found to be unchanged in patients after minor surgery with etomidate, propofol, thiopental, midazolam, and althesin, whereas similar surgery under ketamine anesthesia was associated with a moderate increase in the serum concentration of some liver enzymes.[124–127] Major surgical procedures under similar kinds of intravenous anesthetics supplemented with nitrous oxide were accompanied by a significant increase in the plasma concentrations of liver enzymes.[119, 128]

Sear,[129] in his review on the toxicity of intravenous anesthetics, concluded that, "it appears that single infusions of all the iv hypnotic agents (with the possible exceptions of thiopentone and ketamine) cause only minimal alterations in plasma concentrations of the routinely measured liver function tests."

Opioids can induce spasm of sphincter Oddi with a subsequent increase in intrabiliary pressure, as well as severe abdominal pain. Such spasms may be responsible for false results on intraoperative cholangiography. It is important to realize that spasm of sphincter Oddi is observed in approximately 3% of patients receiving opioids.[130] It seems that with equipotent doses, the largest increase in intrabiliary pressure is associated with fentanyl and morphine; meperidine and pentazocine are associated with smaller increases (Fig. 42-11).[131–133] Nalbuphine, however, probably does not cause spasm of sphincter Oddi.[134]

PHARMACOKINETICS. Elimination of midazolam is significantly delayed in patients with severe hepatic cirrhosis.[135] Total plasma clearance and total apparent volume of distribution at the steady state for thiopental are unchanged in patients with hepatic cirrhosis. Therefore, the elimination half-life is not prolonged.[136] Thiopental has a low extraction ratio; therefore, its clearance is independent of hepatic blood flow. However, an increase in the unbound fraction of thiopental may enhance the activity of a single dose of the drug and

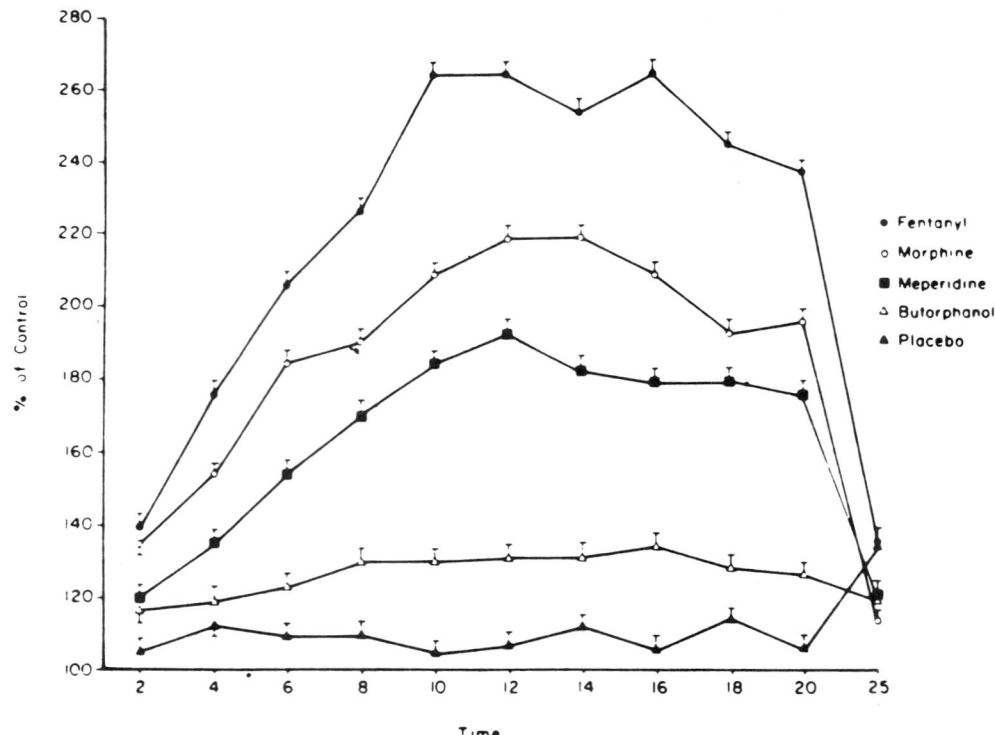

FIG. 42-11. The effect of narcotics and placebo on common bile duct pressure and the response to naloxone administered at 20 minutes. (Reproduced with permission from Radnay PA, Duncalf D, Novakovic M *et al*: Anesth Analg 63:441, 1984.)

therefore may increase the incidence of an acute harmful effect during anesthesia induction.

The plasma clearance of fentanyl is significantly lower in patients with hepatic cirrhosis than in controls. Total apparent volume of distribution is not changed, whereas elimination half-life is prolonged owing to decreased plasma clearance. The plasma free fraction of alfentanil is also increased in patients with hepatic cirrhosis.[137] It is clear that alfentanil exerts a prolonged and pronounced effect in patients with advanced liver disease.

The data regarding morphine pharmacokinetics in patients with hepatic cirrhosis are contradictory. For example, Patwardhan *et al*[138] did not find a significant difference in morphine pharmacokinetics in patients with hepatic cirrhosis compared with healthy persons. The authors suggested that "reported morphine intolerance to the central effects of morphine cannot be explained by impaired drug elimination and increased availability of morphine to cerebral receptors."[138] However, a more recent French study found a somewhat decreased clearance and prolonged half-life of free morphine, as well as morphine metabolites in patients with liver cirrhosis compared with healthy controls.[139]

It seems that opioids and intravenous anesthetics *per se* do not affect hepatic function to any extent provided that they do not jeopardize hepatic blood and oxygen supply. Hepatic function, evaluated by increased serum concentrations of intracellular enzymes, depends much more upon the severity of surgical stress than on the specific anesthetic chosen.[6, 140] The hepatic oxygen supply–demand relationship can be different during different anesthetics when anesthesia is superimposed with surgery. The pertinent question that may be raised is to what extent one or another anesthetic protects the liver from surgical stress. In other words, it is important to know whether the combination of one or another anesthetic with surgical intervention results in different degrees of hepatic dysfunction.

Effects of Anesthetics on Drug Pharmacokinetics

Anesthetics can decrease the elimination of many other drugs, mainly by a decrease in intrinsic clearance (*i.e.*, a decrease in the ability of the liver cells to metabolize and/or excrete the drug) and/or by a decrease in hepatic blood flow (for drugs with a high hepatic extraction ratio). It has been shown, for example, that halothane substantially decreases the intrinsic clearance of diazepam,[141] as well as propranolol.[142] Clearance of lidocaine was also substantially decreased during halothane anesthesia.[143] On the other hand, elimination of aminophylline was not significantly altered by enflurane or halothane.[144] There are approximately three dozen reports demonstrating a reduction of drug clearance by halothane.

Enflurane had no significant effect on the pharmacokinetics of thiopental.[145–147] Isoflurane has not been extensively studied in this regard; however, it has been reported that isoflurane inhibits the oxidative metabolism of halothane.[148] Nitrous oxide prolongs the half-life of etomidate,[149] whereas diazepam prolongs the half-life of ketamine.[150]

EFFECTS OF SURGICAL STRESS ON LIVER FUNCTION

Surgical intervention induces certain, sometimes rather severe, disorders in homeostasis, including alterations in hepatic circulation and function. The general response to stress

has been well studied, and certain responses to surgical stress such as an increase in circulating catecholamines, cortisol, growth hormone, antidiuretic hormone, aldosterone, and activation of the renin-angiotensin system are well known. However, specific effects of stress on hepatic function have been studied to a lesser degree. Available data strongly suggest that laparotomy *per se* reduces blood flow through the intestine and the liver.[151, 152] The mechanisms responsible for such disorders have not been directly studied. Traction and manipulation of the viscera probably play a significant role; however, a general biological response to stress is also very important. For example, laparotomy is associated with marked mesenteric vasoconstriction and a decrease in gastrointestinal blood flow, which can be abolished by hypophysectomy.[153] Surgical stress is usually accompanied by the release of different hormones and substances, including catecholamines, renin-angiotensin, and vasopressin, which can and do disturb the splanchnic circulation. The concentration of these circulating compounds may be increased for many hours and days following surgery.[154, 155]

One study demonstrated that phenobarbital-pretreated (liver enzyme–induced) rats anesthetized with halothane developed liver necrosis after laparotomy alone or after laparotomy with ligation of the hepatic artery.[156] Under similar conditions, halothane anesthesia without laparotomy was not associated with hepatic necrosis. This suggests that laparotomy *per se* may be accompanied by a reduction in the liver oxygen supply severe enough to cause hepatic necrosis in these particular experimental conditions. Actually, this is not surprising considering the sensitivity of the liver to oxygen deprivation.

In patients with chronic lung disease, when oxygen content is decreased below 9 $ml \cdot dl^{-1}$ blood, liver injury developed in all patients without obvious myocardial or cerebral damage.[157] There are experimental and even clinical data substantiating the detrimental effect of oxygen deprivation on the hepatic perioperative function when otherwise similar anesthetic management is provided.[158] There is a specific term, *ischemic hepatitis,* for relatively moderate hepatic injury that results from mild hepatic oxygen deprivation.

Hepatic function may be compromised when hepatic blood flow is reduced; it has been shown that major surgery was associated with a substantial increase in the concentration of enzymes supposedly released from the liver. The degree of such an increase depends upon the type of surgery rather than the anesthesia provided; such an increase is rarely observed during minor surgery, even under the same type of anesthesia.[6, 159] Other studies have also demonstrated that postoperative liver dysfunction mainly results from the operation *per se* rather than from the selected anesthetic technique.[160–162] Thus, surgery, particularly laparotomy, does affect liver function, but usually without detrimental consequences. However, in patients with advanced hepatic disease, laparotomy *per se* is often accompanied by extremely high postoperative morbidity and mortality. In the 1960s, the immediate mortality rate from laparotomy alone in patients with acute hepatitis approached 10–11% in certain groups.[13, 14] During the last 20 years, the situation has not significantly improved: As was mentioned at the beginning of this chapter, British and American literature both report extremely high 30-day postoperative morbidity and mortality after laparotomy and liver biopsy in patients with advanced hepatic disease.[15, 16]

As mentioned previously, all anesthetics, particularly inhalational anesthetics, decrease total hepatic blood flow in a dose-related fashion to a variable degree. When surgical intervention is superimposed, hepatic blood flow is further decreased.[152] The degree of this reduction depends upon the specific type of surgical intervention. Minor peripheral procedures are accompanied by a relatively small reduction in hepatic blood flow, whereas major procedures, especially upper abdominal laparotomy, are associated with a much larger decrease in hepatic blood flow.[152] These data demonstrate that anesthesia may play a modifying role in the complex of surgery and anesthesia: Similar surgical interventions are associated with different degrees of hepatic circulatory disturbances when different types of anesthesia are administered.[152] Therefore, the modifying role of anesthesia in the development of hepatic circulatory disorders, as well as hepatic dysfunction during surgery, can be clinically more important than the effect of one or another anesthetic *per se.* A question that is probably of paramount importance in this regard is, "What kind of anesthesia administered for similar surgical procedures would be accompanied by minimal hepatic circulatory disturbances and hepatic dysfunction?"

During surgical stress, even a 30% reduction in mean arterial pressure induced by isoflurane is not associated with a deterioration in hepatic oxygen supply, whereas a similar degree of arterial hypotension achieved by halothane reduces the hepatic oxygen supply and supply–uptake ratio during severe surgical stress in pigs (thoracotomy, laparotomy, and extensive surgical preparation).[163] It is interesting to note that fentanyl anesthesia in a porcine model maintains hepatic oxygen supply at baseline levels (or even higher) but is accompanied by hepatic oxygen requirements somewhat higher than observed during isoflurane or halothane anesthesia. Therefore, the hepatic oxygen supply–uptake relationship during anesthesia with fentanyl is maintained rather than increased, and halothane is less desirable than isoflurane or fentanyl anesthesia.[163] The reasons for the increase in hepatic oxygen uptake during fentanyl administration are not clear. It seems conceivable that the stress response to surgical intervention is accompanied by an increased metabolism within the liver, yielding a subsequent increase in hepatic oxygen demand. This increase in demand (followed by an increase in supply) was not blocked by fentanyl but was substantially modified by isoflurane as well as halothane.

ANESTHESIA FOR PATIENTS WITH LIVER DISEASE

PREOPERATIVE EVALUATION

During the preoperative visit, the anesthesiologist should determine the current drug therapy, previous and/or present jaundice, history of blood transfusions and gastrointestinal bleedings, previous surgical operations, and anesthetic managements. The physical examination should include, in addition to routine examination of organs and systems, a careful evaluation of the patient's appearance, as well as degree of ascites and encephalopathy. The physical evaluation of a patient with chronic liver disease is particularly valuable: The patient may feel unwell and look unwell a long time before hepatic dysfunction can be revealed by certain changes in liver blood tests. Abnormal values of hepatic blood tests may have somewhat limited importance if the patient feels well, since the tests are relatively nonspecific.[164]

Blood tests should include determinations of hemoglobin and hematocrit; platelet count; serum bilirubin; serum electrolytes, particularly sodium and potassium; creatinine and BUN; arterial blood gases; serum proteins; prothrombin time;

and several enzymes; including aminotransferases, alkaline phosphatase, lactate dehydrogenase, and hydroxybutyrate dehydrogenase (lactate dehydrogenase isoenzyme being more specific for liver function).

The function of the coagulation system should be evaluated and properly treated before surgery. In patients with obstructive jaundice, demonstrating abnormal prothrombin time and partial thromboplastin time, a trial of vitamin K (10 mg im, t.i.d. for a few days) may prove to be beneficial. If a trial of vitamin K treatment is not successful or if there is no time for correction of hypocoagulation with vitamin K, treatment with fresh frozen plasma should be considered. Thrombocytopenia, which often accompanies advanced liver disease, must be corrected, if possible, prior to surgery by an appropriate transfusion of platelet concentrates. The platelet count should be $100,000 \cdot mm^3$; approximately each unit of platelets increases the count approximately $10,000 \cdot mm^3$ in an average adult. The diagnosed coagulopathy must be corrected before spinal or epidural anesthesia.

Blood glucose concentration should be checked and, in the case of hypoglycemia, which sometimes develops in patients with advanced liver disease, glucose solution should be infused with periodic monitoring of blood glucose concentrations.

The surgical procedure that the patient is undergoing is important in planning the anesthetic management. Even surgical procedures that are relatively short and considered to be "safe" for average patients can be extremely dangerous for the patient with advanced liver disease. It has been stated earlier in this chapter that even simple laparotomy without other major interventions is accompanied by extremely high perioperative morbidity and mortality.

If there are no clotting abnormalities for peripheral surgery, a regional blockade can be the anesthetic management of choice. However, for surgical procedures involving the abdomen, and in patients with obvious coagulopathy, regional anesthesia is usually contraindicated. For some relatively minor procedures, such as sclerotherapy, local anesthesia with sedation can be used successfully. Benzodiazepines, for example, midazolam can be a drug of choice for sedation and may be combined with small doses of fentanyl. It is noteworthy that midazolam is a highly protein-bound compound, therefore, if the patient has a decreased protein concentration in blood, a relative overdose can occur. Also, a relative overdose of benzodiazepines may result from greater affinity of the CNS (possibly owing to an increased population of specific receptors to benzodiazepines in patients with advanced hepatic disease compared with normal persons).[51] Therefore, all drugs, including sedatives, should be carefully titrated against their effect.

Preoperative treatment for patients with severe liver disease should be devoted to normalization of coagulopathy; the treatment may be based on changes in prothrombin time. Assurance of adequate hydration and adequate diuresis (approximately $1 \ ml \cdot kg^{-1} \cdot hr^{-1}$) is also of paramount importance. Inadequate diuresis should be treated by appropriate fluid load—both volume and content are equally important. The volume load should be titrated against ventricular filling pressures, central venous pressure if myocardial and pulmonary function is adequate, and/or pulmonary capillary wedge pressure, if needed. Proper fluid content should be ensured by analysis of blood for electrolytes (mainly sodium and potassium as well as ionized calcium), hematocrit, and glucose. Patients with liver disease require infusion of albumin more often than do other patients. Diuretic therapy should include furosemide and/or mannitol and a low dose of dopamine (2 to

$4\ \mu g \cdot kg^{-1} \cdot min^{-1}$) owing to its renal vasodilation and anti-aldosterone effect. In chronic situations, spironolactone may be a diuretic of choice because of its strong antialdosterone activity.

PREMEDICATION

All medications needed to control the diseased state should be administered. Considering the decreased ability of the liver to metabolize drugs, sedatives should be omitted or the dose decreased.

Patients with advanced liver disease may have a full stomach even if they have not taken food/fluid for several hours. This can be related to hiatal hernia, massive ascites, and decreased gastric and intestinal motility; therefore, premedication may include H_2 histamine-receptor blocker (e.g., ranitidine), metoclopramide, as well as sodium citrate.

MONITORING

Routine monitoring, including electrocardiogram, blood pressure, precordial or esophageal stethoscope, temperature, $F_{I_{O_2}}$, end-expired carbon dioxide, and pulse oximeter, should be used. Cannulation of an artery is important for direct arterial blood pressure monitoring, as well as for periodic sampling for determinations of arterial blood gases, electrolytes, hematocrit, and other tests as needed during surgery. Fluid load should be carefully titrated in patients with advanced liver disease. Therefore, insertion of a pulmonary artery catheter, or at least a central venous catheter, is often necessary. Monitoring with a pulmonary artery catheter may be important if, in addition to advanced hepatic disease, the patient has compromised left ventricular function, pulmonary disease, or severe renal dysfunction. Urine output should always be monitored in patients with advanced liver disease who are undergoing surgery longer than 1 or 2 hours. Surgical procedures associated with massive blood loss (e.g., liver transplantation) require monitoring of the blood coagulation status. The monitoring should include periodic determinations of prothrombin time, partial thromboplastin time, and platelet count. Thromboelastography seems to be helpful.[165] A transcutaneous nerve stimulator is helpful in titrating muscle relaxants in every patient, but particularly in patients with advanced liver disease, since the effects of muscle relaxants in this population are unpredictable.

ANESTHESIA INDUCTION

Rapid sequence induction of anesthesia (or awake intubation of the trachea) should be provided if a full stomach is suspected. All widely used intravenous anesthetics for anesthesia induction have been administered in patients with advanced hepatic disease. The chosen drug has to be carefully titrated until the desired effect is achieved. Depolarizing muscle relaxants may be used to facilitate endotracheal intubation. Succinylcholine activity is usually relatively normal, despite some decrease in plasma cholinesterase. In cases with severely decreased cholinesterase activity, the effect of succinylcholine can last longer than it can in normal persons. Nondepolarizing muscle relaxants chosen to facilitate endotracheal intubation have a high affinity to gamma globulin (e.g., d-tubocurarine). The volume of distribution for such a drug can be increased; therefore, the dose required to achieve total relaxation can be higher in patients with liver disease than in normal persons. The volume of distribution of pancuronium is also increased in patients with advanced liver disease, although the reasons for such an increase are not clear and probably differ from those for d-tubocurarine. Pancuronium is poorly bound to plasma protein, and there is no correlation between volume of distribution and plasma gamma-globulin concentrations.[166] The volume of distribution of atracurium is also increased,[167] possibly owing to a substantial increase in extracellular fluid. The volume of distribution of vecuronium, however, is not significantly altered[168]; therefore, a substantial change in the requirement for the effective dose of this muscle relaxant should not be expected. However, the titration of the muscle relaxant using transcutaneous nerve stimulator is still desirable.

MAINTENANCE OF ANESTHESIA

Intraoperative liver injury can develop from hepatic oxygen deprivation, stress response, drug toxicity, blood transfusion, and infection. It is important to realize that the hepatic oxygen supply can be jeopardized at any step of oxygen transport to the liver: 1) Hypoxic hypoxia may result from inadequate $F_{I_{O_2}}$ or hypoventilation. 2) Anemic hypoxia may develop if the appropriate oxygen-carrying capacity of the blood (adequate hematocrit) is not ensured. 3) Circulatory hypoxia may result from systemic (hypovolemia, arterial hypotension, reduction in cardiac output) and/or regional (decrease in hepatic blood and oxygen supply) hemodynamic disorders. The decrease in hepatic blood and oxygen delivery may follow systemic circulatory disturbances and/or may result from surgical manipulations around the liver as well as from the effects of many endogenous vasoconstrictive substances (e.g., renin-angiotensin, catecholamines, antidiuretic hormone). 4) Possible interference of anesthetics with electron transport at the cellular level may lead to a histotoxic hypoxia; however, the clinical relevance of such mechanisms has not been demonstrated.

The concept of the oxygen supply–demand relationship in the liver should be kept in mind. For example, in a recent study in pigs, severe surgical stress under anesthesia with moderate doses of fentanyl was accompanied by a somewhat higher hepatic oxygen supply and uptake than identical stress under isoflurane anesthesia, which resulted in similar values of hepatic oxygen supply–uptake ratio.[163] Taking this into consideration, the main rule is to maintain adequate pulmonary ventilation and cardiovascular function, including cardiac output, blood volume, and perfusion pressures. Arterial hypotension, owing to inadequate blood/volume replacement, relative overdose of inhalational anesthetics, or controlled drug-induced hypotension, should be avoided, because vasodilation and a decrease in perfusion pressure, accompanied by a decrease in blood velocity, would unavoidably lead to an increase in oxygen extraction in all tissues, including the preportal area. Decreased blood velocity and increased oxygen extraction result in a decrease in venous oxygen content—in this case, decreased oxygen content in portal venous blood. A decrease in portal blood oxygen content and/or flow is usually accompanied by a compensatory increase in hepatic arterial blood flow. Thus, hepatic injury after moderate arterial hypotension is a relatively rare event. However, in animals with severe liver dysfunction, the autoregulatory ability of hepatic arterial blood flow to increase is diminished or abolished.[169] Therefore, in such animals, and probably in patients with severe hepatic disease, the hepatic arterial blood flow would not increase when portal blood flow and/or oxygen content in portal venous blood are decreased. This might lead to a decrease in hepatic blood and oxygen supply, with subsequent hepatic oxygen deprivation. Thus, the lesson is clear: Arterial hypotension, as well as states with reduced cardiac output, should be avoided.

Regional anesthesia should be used whenever possible in patients with advanced liver disease. Keeping in mind the comparative pharmacology of inhalational anesthetics, it seems that halothane should be avoided, because this anesthetic is accompanied by the most prominent decrease in hepatic blood and oxygen supply and postoperative hepatic dysfunction; rarely will severe postoperative halothane hepatitis follow halothane anesthesia. Enflurane, particularly isoflurane, seems to be the anesthetic of choice if an inhalational technique is selected. Nitrous oxide has been used in patients with advanced hepatic disease for many years and thus far has not been incriminated in an increased anesthesia-related hepatic postoperative complication. However, a well-known sympathomimetic effect of nitrous oxide and some possibilities of jeopardized oxygenation render the routine use of nitrous oxide in patients with advanced liver disease undesirable according to some experts. It is important to remember that long surgical operations under anesthesia with nitrous oxide may result in the accumulation of nitrous oxide in the intestinal lumen with subsequent intestinal distention.

Opioids can also be used successfully in patients with hepatic disease. Despite certain pharmacokinetic consequences (decreased clearance and prolonged half-life), fentanyl should probably be considered the opioid of choice. Interestingly, fentanyl does not decrease the hepatic oxygen and blood supply; however, neither does it prevent an increase in hepatic oxygen requirements when used in relatively moderate doses. Therefore, the hepatic oxygen supply–demand relationship during anesthesia with fentanyl is not much better than that during anesthesia with isoflurane.[163] It seems at present that anesthetic management using inhalational agents (isoflurane would probably be the drug of choice) alone or in combination with small doses of fentanyl can be considered as the anesthetic management of choice provided that adequate pulmonary ventilation, cardiac output, and arterial pressures are maintained. Other drugs can also be used successfully in patients with advanced hepatic disease.

When administering drugs, one must appreciate the substantially changed pharmacokinetics. For example, the half-life of lidocaine in patients with liver disease may be increased by more than 300%, for benzodiazepines by more than 100% and so on. For drugs binding to albumin, the volume of distribution can be decreased, and, therefore, the dose of the drug should be decreased (e.g., sodium pentothal). On the other hand, the volume of distribution of many drugs can be substantially increased (for different reasons, including an increase in gamma globulin, edema), dictating a necessity to increase the first effective dose of the drug; however, owing to a decrease in hepatic blood flow and the hepatic metabolic and excretory functions, as well as impairment of renal function, the clearance of such drugs can be decreased and therefore the effect can be prolonged (e.g., d-tubocurarine, pancuronium). It seems that advanced hepatic disease does not significantly affect the pharmacokinetics of vecuronium, although dose dependent, some pharmacokinetic alterations have been observed.[168] This is possibly the result of a limited hepatic uptake capacity, which is usually exceeded after doses of vecuronium greater than 0.15 mg·kg⁻¹. With a smaller dose, hepatic dysfunction does not affect the pharmacokinetics or duration of action of vecuronium.[168] Actually, any muscle relaxant can be used in patients with advanced liver disease. Atracurium has a theoretic advantage, because the metabolism of atracurium is not dependent upon liver function. The elimination of atracurium is determined mainly by Hofmann decomposition and therefore is relatively independent of renal or hepatic function. Thus, it is not surprising that the clearance and elimination half-life of atracurium in patients with liver cirrhosis and impaired renal function is not particularly different from that of persons who have normal hepatorenal function. However, volumes of distribution are larger, and, accordingly, the distribution half-lives are shorter in patients with severe hepatorenal dysfunction compared with normal persons.[167] This study also demonstrated that the only situation that prolongs the elimination half-life of atracurium is marked metabolic acidosis, which may decrease the rate of Hofmann decomposition.[167] The pharmacokinetics of many muscle relaxants in conditions of cholestasis/obstructive jaundice may also be altered: Prolonged duration of action has been demonstrated.[170] However, if it is planned to continue controlled ventilation of the lungs postoperatively, vecuronium, atracurium and pancuronium can be used successfully. Titration of any relaxant according to the transcutaneous nerve stimulation monitoring is beneficial. It is noteworthy that pharmacokinetic studies in patients with hepatic cirrhosis provide interesting results that are helpful in understanding the pathogenetic aspects of chronic liver disease. However, the results of such studies do not have significant value for predicting the safety of a drug. The degree of hepatic dysfunction affects the degree of pharmacokinetic disorders; therefore, again, the best way to avoid complications is to titrate drugs against effect.

Renal function must be maintained by administering proper fluid load (volume and content) and diuretics, if needed. It is extremely difficult, if not impossible, to maintain proper fluid load without monitoring filling pressures. Therefore, insertion of a pulmonary artery catheter, or at least a central venous catheter, is often mandatory in patients with advanced hepatic disease. The content of infused solutions should be chosen and often adjusted according to periodic analysis of the blood for electrolytes. For example, normal, or especially high serum concentrations of sodium require an infusion of solution such as D5W, whereas a decrease in sodium concentration below 130 to 135 mEq·l⁻¹ allows an infusion of a solution such as Normosol. Furosemide, particularly mannitol, should be considered an effective diuretic in these patients. A small dose of dopamine (2–4 μg·kg⁻¹·min⁻¹) can be beneficial owing to many different effects, including improvement in renal perfusion and the antialdosterone effect.

The parameters of controlled ventilation should be carefully selected in order to avoid an unnecessary increase in intrathoracic pressure, which may impede venous return, thereby decreasing cardiac output. Hypocarbia should probably be avoided, because it can aggravate hepatic encephalopathy. It has been mentioned previously that opioids can induce spasm of sphincter Oddi (see Fig. 42-11). The incidence of such spasm does not exceed 3%.[130] Spasm of sphincter Oddi induced by opioids can be successfully treated with many different drugs. One of these drugs is atropine[133]; the clinical disadvantage of this treatment is accompanied tachycardia. Another drug that relaxes the sphincter Oddi is naloxone[171, 172]; one of the possible problems with this drug is that the analgesic effect of the opioid is reversed (together with relaxation of sphincter Oddi); some other means of anesthesia/analgesia should be provided. Possible cardiovascular complications observed during naloxone treatment should also be kept in mind. Glucagon is effective in producing relaxation of sphincter Oddi[173, 174]; however, this drug might not be the drug of choice, since it has many different side-effects, including hyperglycemia and a hyperdynamic cardiovascular state. Finally, nitroglycerin is also effective in treating the opioid-induced spasm of sphincter Oddi. It has been demonstrated that volatile anesthetics attenuate the response of sphincter Oddi to opioids.[175]

Coagulopathy can develop during surgery. Monitoring of the coagulation state can be important, particularly during liver transplantation. The treatment should be based on the results of hematologic monitoring and may include administration of platelets, fresh frozen plasma, cryoprecipitate, and sometimes epsilon-aminocaproic acid and protamine sulfate. Interestingly, some coagulopathies that develop during liver transplantation may be related to the washout of heparin sequestered in and then washed out from the transplant when circulation is re-established and the homograft is included in the systemic circulation. Protamine sulfate effectively reverses this effect of heparin.[176] Some authors observed DIC.[177] Sometimes fibrinolysis can also be identified.[176] A detailed description of monitoring and treatment of hepatic coagulopathy during liver transplantation is available elsewhere.[165]

POSTOPERATIVE HEPATIC DYSFUNCTION

There are many different forms of hepatic disorders that may develop during the postoperative period (Table 42-6). Fortunately, most clearly identified postoperative hepatic dysfunctions will resolve without treatment. However, certain precautions should be taken in the event that liver function deteriorates. Gas exchange and cardiovascular function should be optimized, and appropriate viral studies initiated. All medications should be examined, and potential harm to the liver should be weighed against potential benefits. Infection should be treated vigorously. A diagnosis of jaundice, cholestasis versus parenchymal jaundice, should be established. A hepatic biopsy does not always provide answers to questions in such situations. However, to diagnose whether the patient has developed hepatic injury during the perioperative period, this observer agrees with the statement that "most importantly, the patient feels and looks unwell."[164] When a patient develops severe hepatic injury, the symptoms are striking enough to make the diagnosis simple; however, diagnosing the exact cause of injury is difficult. It may be compared to a house that is in flames: It is easy to see that the

TABLE 42-6. Etiology of Postoperative Liver Dysfunction

A. Hepatic O$_2$ deprivation
  1. Hypoxia
  2. Decreased arterial pressure or cardiac output
  3. Decreased hepatic blood flow
B. Viral hepatitis, acute
C. Aggravated chronic hepatitis
  1. Immunity depression by anesthesia and/or surgery
  2. Respiratory/circulatory depression resulting in liver hypoxia
  3. Deteriorated hepatic artery blood flow autoregulation
  4. Relative overdose (altered pharmacokinetics)
D. Fulminant hepatitis with specific halothane-related antibodies
E. Free radicals produced by reductive metabolism of halothane
F. Specific drug therapy
G. Blood transfusion
H. Infection

(Table modified with permission from Kang YG, Gelman S: Liver transplantation. In Gelman S [ed]: Anesthesia and Organ Transplantation, p 152. Philadelphia, WB Saunders, 1987.)

house is burning but impossible to determine the cause and origin of the fire.

Postoperative jaundice, as any other jaundice, can be due to one of three or any combination of the three causes: 1) overproduction/overload of bilirubin; 2) impaired excretion of bilirubin resulting from hepatocellular injury; and 3) biliary obstruction (Fig. 42-12).

An increased load of bilirubin can be due to blood transfusion, resorption of extravasated blood accumulation (*e.g.,* hematomas, hemothorax), hemolytic anemia, and prosthetic heart valve.[1] Excessive blood transfusions, as well as resorption of hemoglobin from hematomas, represent a classic and probably the most common cause of postoperative jaundice related to overproduction/overload of bilirubin. Approximately 10% of transfused stored blood undergoes hemolysis within 24 hours after transfusion. A blood transfusion of 500 ml results approximately in the production of 250 mg of bilirubin. The normal liver excretes this bilirubin load easily, without any increase in the plasma bilirubin concentration. However, if a seriously ill patient undergoing a major surgical procedure receives a transfusion load much higher than 500 ml of blood, the hemolysis of transfused blood follows and is reflected in an increase, mainly in the indirect or unconjugated bilirubin. If

FIG. 42-12. Etiology of postoperative jaundice.

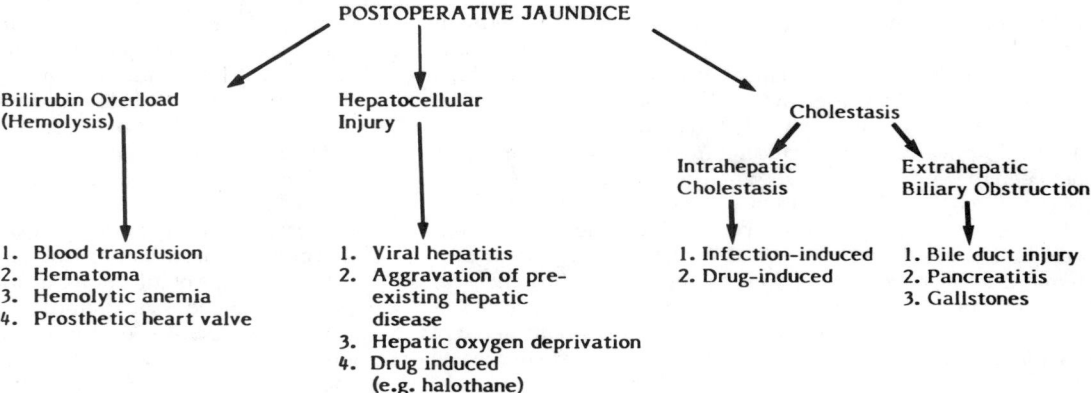

the extrabilirubin pigment is conjugated, but not excreted enough, an increase is also observed in the direct or conjugated fraction of bilirubin. Conjugated hyperbilirubinemia may result in severe neurologic dysfunction, including rapidly developed fetal encephalopathy.[20-22] On the other hand, unconjugated hyperbilirubinemia is not accompanied by apparent neurotoxicity.

Hemolytic anemia, as a cause of postoperative jaundice, is relatively rare but should be considered, especially if the indirect/unconjugated bilirubin represents 90% or more of the total bilirubin. Sickle cell anemia (and maybe some forms of autoimmune hemolytic anemia) is probably the most common cause of hemolytic anemia observed postoperatively. Some patients with congenital deficiencies of glucose-6-phosphate dehydrogenase may develop hemolysis after surgical stress and also after administration of certain drugs such as sulfonamides, chloramphenicol, nitrofurantoin, aspirin, and others. Patients with prosthetic heart valves, particularly aortic valves, develop hemolytic jaundice, apparently as a result of the damage of the erythrocytes, resulting from contact of red cells with the prothesis. Some patients demonstrate a positive Coombs' test, which suggests an autoimmune component in the hemolytic process.

Hepatocellular injury is characterized primarily by an increased concentration of liver enzymes, as well as prolonged prothrombin time, decreased albumin concentrations, increased ammonia concentrations, and different degrees of hepatic encephalopathy. Alkaline phosphatase can also be elevated, even though this is usually a sign of a cholestatic disorder; however, in the case of hepatocellular injury, the primary abnormalities are observed in synthetizing functions of the liver.

Postoperative viral hepatitis can be due to hepatitis that the patient had before surgery—unknown chronic hepatitis or incubation period of acute hepatitis. Postoperative viral hepatitis can also be a complication of blood transfusion, which usually develops somewhere between 30 and 70 days following transfusion.

Pre-existing hepatic disease, known or unknown, probably plays a substantial role in postoperative hepatic dysfunction, including jaundice. The deterioration in pre-existing hepatic disease can result from a stress response to surgery, with an increase in the concentration of hormones and substances affecting hepatic blood and oxygen supply, as well as hepatic cellular function. Hepatic oxygen deprivation may develop in these patients, since they may not be able to increase hepatic arterial blood flow in response to a decrease in portal blood flow and/or portal venous blood content, which is usually accompanied by any severe stress.[152, 178] The inability of hepatic arterial blood flow to increase may jeopardize oxygen supply to the liver.

The most common cause (but fortunately without frequent clinically detrimental consequences) for postoperative hepatic dysfunction is probably hepatic oxygen deprivation, which can be induced by all anesthetics at any step of oxygen transport to the liver tissue. Any kind of hypoxic hypoxia (decrease in FI_{O_2}, hypoventilation, including inadvertent disconnection between the endotracheal tube and the respirator) may lead to hypoxic/ischemic damage to any organ, including the liver. Most commonly, however, hepatic oxygen deprivation develops as a result of a decreased cardiac output and/or systemic arterial pressure, as well as regional disturbances in hepatic blood supply, even when blood pressure is maintained at acceptable levels. Regional (splanchnic and hepatic) circulatory disturbances may result from a decrease in cardiac output, as well as surgical manipulations in the surgical field

near the liver. The role of circulating vasoconstricting substances such as antidiuretic hormones, renin-angiotensin, and catecholamines apparently play a significant role in hepatic circulatory disturbances during surgery. Hepatic oxygen deprivation resulting from hypoxia and hypovolemia is usually associated with a relatively moderate increase in bilirubin concentrations, somewhere up to 20 mg · dl^{-1} within 2 to 12 days after surgery. A moderate increase in the concentration of liver enzymes is often observed. The most common histologic finding in such situations is centrilobular congestion, sometimes with centrilobular necrosis. Often, this type of hepatic dysfunction heals by itself, without additional treatment and apparent sequela.

Severe hepatocellular injury may be induced by different drugs used during anesthesia. Halothane is one of them. "Halothane hepatitis" is rare but is associated with an extremely high mortality rate. It appears that the severity of halothane hepatotoxicity is increased with repeated exposure to halothane within relatively short periods of time. Clinically, "halothane hepatitis" can be manifested by fever, jaundice, an increase in the concentration of liver enzymes, and eosinophilia. It seems that females, as well as obese patients, are more susceptible to halothane hepatitis than are other groups of persons. Children are much less susceptible to halothane hepatitis than are adults. Typically, halothane hepatitis may develop in patients after minor surgery without any episodes of hypoxia. The clinical picture develops a few days after the administration of halothane anesthesia. At the beginning, an increase in hepatic enzymes and bilirubin concentrations are relatively minimal. However, if massive hepatic necrosis follows, it is accompanied by a very dramatic increase in the plasma concentration of hepatic enzymes and bilirubin. Associated coagulation abnormalities and hepatic encephalopathy may follow. Liver biopsy or autopsy often reveals acute yellow atrophy and massive hepatocellular necrosis, practically indistinguishable from fulminant viral hepatitis. Specific serologic tests may help confirm the diagnosis of halothane hepatitis.[70] Mortality fluctuates between 20% and 50%. The mechanism of "halothane hepatitis" has not been clarified. The issue is addressed in a previous section of this chapter.

Cholestasis is another possible cause of postoperative jaundice. Extrahepatic biliary obstruction can be caused by stones in the common duct, postoperative bile duct stricture, or pancreatitis. Postoperative cholestasis can also be intrahepatic in origin and can be induced by drugs or infection. This type of liver dysfunction is primarily characterized by deterioration of excretory function of the liver and is accompanied clinically by a dramatic increase in bilirubin and alkaline phosphatase concentrations in blood, whereas other hepatic enzymes, prothrombin time, and albumin concentrations are relatively normal or just slightly decreased.

Some patients with arterial hypotension and hypoxemia develop postoperative jaundice that clinically mimics biliary obstruction. This condition usually occurs in patients who underwent major surgical procedures, often complicated with episodes of severe hypotension and/or hypoxemia, massive blood transfusion, sometimes cardiac failure, renal failure, or sepsis. Despite the seeming severity of the disorder, it heals by itself without apparent sequela. It has been named "benign postoperative intrahepatic cholestasis."[86, 179] The nature of this type of cholestasis has not been clarified.

Different kinds of infection can and do lead to postoperative hepatic dysfunction with jaundice, being cholestatic in origin. Many drugs such as erythromycin, tetracycline, chloramphenicol, sulfonamides, and others can induce cholestasis. Some other relatively rare disorders such as Gilbert's syndrome and Dubin–Johnson syndrome should also be kept in mind.

The differential diagnosis of postoperative hepatic injury may be extremely difficult. It is usually necessary to go through a rather difficult process, with the final conclusion being based on meticulous attention to small, sometimes seemingly unimportant details related to medical history, physical examination, laboratory tests, and the perioperative course of each patient.

REFERENCES

1. LaMont JT: Postoperative jaundice. Surg Clin North Am 54:637, 1974
2. Craver WL, Johnson G Jr, Beal JM: Alterations in serum glutamic-oxalacetic transaminase activity following operations. Surg Forum 8:77, 1957
3. Dunlap RW, Dockerty MB, Waugh JM: Hepatic changes occurring during upper abdominal operations: Biopsy studies. Surg Gynecol Obstet 99:220, 1954
4. Dykes MHM, Walzer SG: Preoperative and postoperative hepatic dysfunction. Surg Gynecol Obstet 124:747, 1967
5. Morgenstein L: Postoperative jaundice, miscellaneous disorders, Part 2. In Schiff L (ed): Diseases of the Liver, 4th ed, p 1353. Philadelphia, J.B. Lippincott, 1975
6. Clarke RSJ, Doggart JR, Lavery T: Changes in liver function after different types of surgery. Br J Anaesth 48:119, 1976
7. Evans C, Evans M, Pollock AV: The incidence and causes of postoperative jaundice. Br J Anaesth 46:520, 1974
8. Koff RS, Gardner RC, Harinasuta U et al: Profile of hyperbilirubinemia in three hospital populations. Clin Res 18:680, 1970
9. Cahalan MK, Mangano DT: Liver function and dysfunction with anesthesia and surgery. In Zakim D, Boyer TD (eds): Hepatology, A Textbook of Liver Disease, p 1250. Philadelphia, W.B. Saunders, 1982
10. Schemel WH: Unexpected hepatic dysfunction found by multiple laboratory screening. Anesth Analg 55:810, 1976
11. Wataneeywech M, Kelly KA Jr: Hepatic diseases unsuspected before surgery. NY Stage J Med 75:1278, 1975
12. National Research Council (U.S.). In Bunker JP, Forrest WH Jr, Mosteller F et al: National Halothane Study: A Study of the Possible Association Between Halothane Anesthesia and Postoperative Hepatic Necrosis. Washington, D.C., National Institute of General Medical Sciences, U.S. Government Printing Office, 1969
13. Harville DD, Summerskill WHJ: Surgery in acute hepatitis. Causes and effects. JAMA 184:257, 1963
14. Keeri-Szanto M, Lafleur F: Postanaesthetic liver complications in a general hospital: A statistical study. Can Anaesth Soc J 10:531, 1963
15. Powell-Jackson P, Greenway B, Williams R: Adverse effects of exploratory laparotomy in patients with suspected liver disease. Br J Surg 69:449, 1982
16. Aranha GV, Greenlee HB: Intraabdominal surgery in patients with advanced cirrhosis. Arch Surg 121:275, 1986
17. Gelman S, Ernst E: Role of pH, P_{CO_2} and O_2 content of portal blood in hepatic circulatory autoregulation. Am J Physiol 233:E255, 1977
18. Lautt WW: Mechanism and role of intrinsic regulation of hepatic arterial blood flow: Hepatic arterial buffer response. Am J Physiol 249:G549, 1985
19. Rappaport AM, Borowy ZJ, Lougheed WM et al: Subdivision of hexagonal liver lobules into a structural and functional unit. Anat Rec 119:16, 1954
20. Scheidt PC, Mellits ED, Hardy JB et al: Toxicity to bilirubin in

neonates: Infant development during first year in relation to maximum neonatal serum bilirubin concentration. J Pediatr 1:292, 1977
21. Naeye RL: Amniotic fluid infections, neonatal hyperbilirubinemia, and psychomotor impairment. Pediatrics 62:497, 1978
22. Haymaker W, Margoles C, Pentschew A et al: Pathology of kernicterus and posticteric encephalopathy. Presentation of 87 cases, with a consideration of pathogenesis and etiology. In Cerebral Palsy, p 221. Springfield, Illinois, Charles C Thomas, 1961
23. Karp WB: Biochemical alterations in neonatal hyperbilirubinemia and bilirubin encephalopathy: A review. Pediatrics 64:361, 1979
24. Odell GB: The distribution of bilirubin between albumin and mitochondria. J Pediatr 68:164, 1966
25. Sanchez E, Tephly TR: Activation of hepatic microsomal glucuronyl transferase by bilirubin. Life Sci 13:1483, 1973
26. Wilkinson GR, Schenker S: Drug disposition and liver disease. Drug Metabol Rev 4:139, 1975
27. Williams RL, Benet LZ: Hepatic function and pharmacokinetics. In Zakim D, Boyer TD (eds): Hepatology, A Textbook of Liver Disease, p 230. Philadelphia, W.B. Saunders, 1982
28. Laidlaw J, Read AE, Sherlock S: Morphine tolerance in hepatic cirrhosis. Gastroenterology 40:389, 1961
29. Read AE, Laidlaw J, McCarthy CF: Effects of chlorpromazine in patients with hepatic disease. Br Med J 3:497, 1969
30. Maxwell JD, Carrella M, Parkes JD et al: Plasma disappearance and cerebral effects of chlorpromazine in cirrhosis. Clin Sci 43:143, 1972
31. Branch RA, Morgan MH, James J et al: Intravenous administration of diazepam in patients with chronic liver disease. Gut 17:975, 1976
32. Benoit JN, Granger DN: Splanchnic hemodynamics in chronic portal hypertension. Semin Liver Dis 6:287, 1986
33. Bomzon A, Blendis LM: Vascular reactivity in experimental portal hypertension. Am J Physiol 252:G158, 1987
34. Baraka A, Gabali F: Correlation between tubocurarine requirements and plasma protein pattern. Br J Anaesth 40:89, 1968
35. Bomzon A, Blendis LM: Vascular reactivity in experimental portal hypertension. Am J Physiol 252:G158, 1987
36. Richardson PDI, Withrington PG: The inhibition by glucagon of the vasoconstrictor actions of noradrenaline, angiotensin and vasopressin on the hepatic arterial vascular bed of the dog. Br J Pharmacol 57:93, 1976
37. Ettinger PO, Wu CF, DeLaCruz C Jr et al: Arrhythmias and the "holiday heart": Alcohol-associated cardiac rhythm disorders. Am Heart J 95:555, 1978
38. Witte CL, Witte MH: Splanchnic circulatory and tissue fluid dynamics in portal hypertension. Fed Proc 42:1685, 1983
39. Gelman S, Ernst E: Nitroprusside prevents adverse hemodynamic effects of vasopressin. Arch Surg 113:1465, 1978
40. Groszmann RJ, Kravetz D, Bosch J et al: Nitroglycerin improves the hemodynamic response to vasopressin in portal hypertension. Hepatology 2:757, 1982
41. Changler JG: Vasopressin and splanchnic shunting. Ann Surg 195:543, 1982
42. Price BA, Jaffe BM, Zinner MJ: Effect of exogenous somostatin infusion on gastrointestinal blood flow and hormones in the conscious dog. Gastroenterology 88:80, 1985
43. Bosch J, Mastai R, Kravetz D et al: Measurement of azygos venous blood flow in the evaluation of portal hypertension in patients with cirrhosis. J Hepatol 1:125, 1985
44. Conn HO: Propranolol in portal hypertension: Problems in paradise? Hepatology 4:560, 1984
45. Villeneuve JP, Pomier–Layragues G, Infante–Rivard C et al: Pro-

pranolol for the prevention of recurrent variceal hemorrhage: A controlled trial. Hepatology 6:1239, 1986

46. Daoud FS, Reeves JT, Schaefer JW: Failure of hypoxic pulmonary vasoconstriction in patients with liver cirrhosis. J Clin Invest 51:1076, 1972

47. Ruff F, Hughes JMB, Stanley N et al: Regional lung function in patients with hepatic cirrhosis. J Clin Invest 50:2403, 1971

48. Maennl HFK, Matzander U, Tkocz HJ et al: Surgery of portal hypertension in cirrhotics. J Abdominal Surg 18:17, 1976

49. Paumgartner G, Richter H, Brunner H et al: Enterohepatic vascular dimensions and the erythrocyte survival time in patients with cirrhosis of the liver. Wein Z Inn Med 51:278, 1970

50. Dymock IW, Tucker JS, Woolf IL et al: Coagulation studies as a prognostic index in acute liver failure. Br J Haematol 29:385, 1975

51. Samson Y, Bernuau J: Cerebral uptake of benzodiazepine measured by positron emission tomography in hepatic encephalopathy. N Engl J Med 316:414, 1987

52. Black M: Hepatic detoxification of endogenously produced toxins and their importance for the pathogenesis of hepatic encephalopathy. In Zakim D, Boyer TD (eds): Hepatology, A Textbook of Liver Disease, p 397. Philadelphia, W.B. Saunders, 1982

53. Epstein M: Renal functional abnormalities in cirrhosis: Pathophysiology and management. In Zakim D, Boyer TD (eds): Hepatology, A Textbook of Liver Disease, p 446. Philadelphia, W.B. Saunders, 1982

54. Perez–Ayuso RM, Arroyo V, Camps J et al: Renal kallikrein excretion in cirrhotics with ascites: Relationship to renal hemodynamics. Hepatology 4:247, 1984

55. Koppel MH, Coburn JW, Mims MM et al: Transplantation of cadaveric kidneys from patients with hepatorenal syndrome. Evidence for the functional nature of renal failure in advanced liver disease. N Engl J Med 280:1367, 1969

56. Dawson JL: The incidence of postoperative renal failure in obstructive jaundice. Br J Surg 52:663, 1965

57. Aarseth S, Bergan A, Aarseth P: Circulatory homeostasis in rats after bile duct ligation. Scand J Clin Lab Invest 39:93, 1979

58. Baum M, Stirling GA, Dawson JL: Further study into obstructive jaundice and ischaemic renal damage. Br Med J 2:229, 1969

59. Gibson PR, Dudley FJ: Ischaemic hepatitis: Clinical features, diagnosis and prognosis. Aust NZ J Med 14:822, 1984

60. Cohen JA, Kaplan MM: Left-sided heart failure presenting as hepatitis. Gastroenterology 74:583, 1978

61. Bynum TE, Boitnott JK, Maddrey WC: Ischemic hepatitis. Dig Dis Sci 24:129, 1979

62. Garrard CL Jr, Weissler AM, Dodge HT: The relationship of alterations in systolic time intervals to ejection fraction in patients with cardiac disease. Circulation 42:455, 1970

63. Weissler AM, Harris WS, Schoenfeld CD: Systolic time intervals in heart failure in man. Circulation 37:149, 1968

64. Better OS: Renal and cardiovascular dysfunction in liver disease. Kidney Int 29:598, 1986

65. Bosch J, Enriquez R, Groszmann RJ et al: Chronic bile duct ligation in the dog: Hemodynamic characterization of a portal hypertensive model. Hepatology 3:1002, 1983

66. Tamakuma S, Wada N, Ishiyama M et al: Relationship between hepatic hemodynamics and biliary pressure in dogs: Its significance in clinical shock following biliary decompression. Jap J Surg 5:255, 1975

67. Aoyagi T, Lowenstein L: The effect of bile acid and renal ischemia on renal function. J Lab Clin Med 71:686, 1968

68. Levy M, Finestone H: Renal response to four hours of biliary obstruction in the dog. Am J Physiol 244:F516, 1983

69. Galambos JT: Cirrhosis, Vol XVII, p 191. Philadelphia, W.B. Saunders, 1979

70. Brown BR Jr, Gandolfi AJ: Adverse effects of volatile anaesthetics. Br J Anaesth 59:14, 1987

71. Kaplowitz N, Eberle D, Yamada T: Biochemical tests for liver disease. In Zakim D, Boyer TD (eds): Hepatology, A Textbook of Liver Disease, p 583. Philadelphia, W.B. Saunders, 1982

72. Strunin L: The Liver and Anaesthesia. Philadelphia, W.B. Saunders, 1977

73. Stock JGL, Strunin L: Unexplained hepatitis following halothane. Anesthesiology 63:424, 1985

74. Inman WHW, Mushin WW: Jaundice after repeated exposure to halothane: An analysis of reports to the Committee on Safety of Medicines. Br Med J 1:5, 1974

75. Bottinger LE, Dalen E, Hallen B: Halothane-induced liver damage: An analysis of the material reported to the Swedish Adverse Drug Reaction Committee 1966–1973. Acta Anaesthesiol Scand 20:40, 1976

76. Johnstone M: Halothane hepatitis (letter). Lancet 2:526, 1978

77. Farrell G, Prendergast D, Murray M: Halothane hepatitis. Detection of a constitutional susceptibility factor. N Engl J Med 313:1310, 1985

78. Otsuka S, Yamamoto M, Kasuya S et al: HLA antigens in patients with unexplained hepatitis following halothane anesthesia. Acta Anaesthesiol Scand 29:497, 1985

79. McLain GE, Sipes IG, Brown BR: An animal model of halothane hepatotoxicity: Roles of enzyme induction and hypoxia. Anesthesiology 51:321, 1979

80. Van Dyke RA: Halogenated anaesthetic hepatotoxicity—Is the answer close at hand? Clin Anaesthesiol 1:485, 1983

81. Moore RA, McNicholas KW, Gallagher JD et al: Halothane metabolism in acyanotic and cyanotic patients undergoing open heart surgery. Anesth Analg 65:1257, 1986

82. Plummer J, Hall P de la M, Jenner MA et al: Sex differences in halothane metabolism and hepatotoxicity in a rat model. Anesth Analg 64:563, 1986

83. Gelman S: Halothane hepatotoxicity—Again? Anesth Analg 65:831, 1986

84. Shingu KI, Eger EI II, Johnson BH: Hypoxia per se can produce hepatic damage without death in rats. Anesth Analg 61:820, 1982

85. Gelman S, Rimerman V, Fowler KC et al: The effect of halothane, isoflurane, and blood loss on hepatotoxicity and hepatic oxygen availability in phenobarbital-pretreated hypoxic rats. Anesth Analg 63:965, 1984

86. Lunam CA, Cousins MJ, Hall P: Guinea pig model of halothane-associated hepatotoxicity in the absence of enzyme induction and hypoxia. J Pharmacol Exp Ther 232:802, 1985

87. Hursh D, Gelman, Bradley EL Jr: Hepatic oxygen supply during halothane and isoflurane anesthesia in guinea pigs. Anesthesiology 67:701, 1987

88. Gelman S: General anesthesia and hepatic circulation. Can J Physiol Pharmacol 252:G648, 1987

89. Van Dyke RA, Madson TH: Stimulation of phosphorylase activity by volatile anesthetics in isolated rat hepatocytes. Fed Proc 45:699, 1986

90. Klatskin G, Kimberg DV: Recurrent hepatitis attributable to halothane sensitization in an anesthetist. N Engl J Med 280:515, 1969

91. Blogg CE: Halothane and the liver: The problem revisited and made obsolete. Br Med J 292:1691, 1986

92. Neuberger N, Mieli–Vergani G, Tredger JM et al: Oxidative metabolism of halothane in the production of altered hepatocyte membrane antigens in acute halothane-induced necrosis. Gut 22:669, 1981

93. Rice SA, Maze M, Smith CM et al: Halothane hepatotoxicity in Fischer 344 rats pretreated with isoniazid. Toxicol Appl Pharmacol 87:411, 1987

94. Callis AH, Brooks SD, Waters SJ et al: Evidence for a role of the immune system in the pathogenesis of halothane hepatitis. In Roth SH, Miller KW (eds): Molecular and cellular mechanisms of anesthetics. New York, Plenum, 1986

95. Satoh H, Fukada Y, Anderson DK et al: Immunological studies on the mechanism of halothane-induced hepatotoxicity: Immunohistochemical evidence of trifluoroacetylated hepatocytes. J Pharmacol Exp Ther 233:857, 1985

96. Vergani D, Mieli–Vergani G, Alberti A et al: Antibodies to the surface of halothane-altered rabbit hepatocytes in patients with severe halothane-associated hepatitis. N Engl J Med 303:66, 1980

97. Neuberger J, Vergani D, Mieli–Vergani G et al: Hepatic damage after exposure to halothane in medical personnel. Br J Anaesth 53:1173, 1981

98. Lewis RB, Blair M: Halothane hepatitis in a young child. Br J Anaesth 54:349, 1982

99. Flaim KE, Jefferson LS, McGwire JB et al: Effect of halothane on synthesis and secretion of liver proteins. Mol Pharmacol 24:277, 1983

100. Eger EI II, Calverley RK, Smith NT: Changes in blood chemistries following prolonged enflurane anesthesia. Anesth Analg 55:547, 1976

101. Eger EI II, Smuckler EA, Ferrell LD et al: Is enflurane hepatotoxic? Anaesth Analg 65:21, 1986

102. Wood M, Wood AJJ: Contrasting effects of halothane, isoflurane, and enflurane on *in vivo* drug metabolism in the rat. Anesth Analg 63:709, 1984

103. Allan LG, Howie J, Smith AF et al: Hepatic glutathione S-transferase release after halothane anaesthesia: Open randomized comparison with isoflurane. Lancet 1:771, 1987

104. Gelman S, Fowler KC, Smith LR: Liver circulation and function during isoflurane and halothane anesthesia. Anesthesiology 61:726, 1984

105. Hughes RL, Campbell D, Fitch W: Effects of enflurane and halothane on liver blood flow and oxygen consumption in the greyhound. Br J Anaesth 52:1079, 1980

106. Lewis JH, Zimmerman HJ, Ishak KG et al: Enflurane hepatotoxicity. A clinico-pathologic study of 24 cases. Ann Intern Med 98:984, 1983

107. Eger EI II: Anesthetic-induced hepatitis. IARS Review Course Lectures 116, 1986

108. Fee JPH, Black GW, Dundee JW et al: A prospective study of liver enzyme and other changes following repeat administration of halothane and enflurane. Br J Anaesth 51:1133, 1979

109. Zimmerman HJ: Hepatotoxicity: The Adverse Effects of Drugs and Other Chemicals on the Liver, p 370. Norwalk, Connecticut, Appleton-Century-Crofts, 1978

110. Stoelting RK, Blitt CD, Cohen PJ et al: Hepatic dysfunction after isoflurane anesthesia. Anesth Analg 66:147, 1987

111. Rehder K, Forbes J, Alter H et al: Halothane biotransformation in man: A quantitative study. Anesthesiology 28:711, 1967

112. Chase RE, Holaday DA, Fiserova–Bergerova V et al: The biotransformation of Ethrane in man. Anesthesiology 35:262, 1972

113. Holaday DA, Fiserova–Bergerova V, Latto IP et al: Resistance of isoflurane to biotransformation in man. Anesthesiology 43:325, 1975

114. Lundeen G, Manohar M, Parks C: Systemic distribution of blood flow in swine while awake and during 1.0 and 1.5 MAC isoflurane anesthesia with and without 50% nitrous oxide. Anesth Analg 62:499, 1983

115. Thomson IA, Fitch HW, Campbell D: Effects of nitrous oxide on liver haemodynamics and oxygen consumption in the greyhound. Anaesthesia 37:548, 1982

116. Ellis JE, Longnecker DE: Nitrous oxide decreases renal and splanchnic blood flow in rats. Anesthesiology 61:A26, 1984

117. Koblin DD, Waskell L, Watson JE et al: Nitrous oxide inactivates methionine synthetase in human liver. Anesth Analg 61:75, 1982

118. Pratilas V, Pratila MG, Bramis J et al: The hepatoprotective effect of oxygen during halothane anesthesia. Anesth Analg 57:481, 1978

119. Prys–Roberts C, Sear JW, Low JM et al: Hemodynamic and hepatic effects of methohexital infusion during nitrous oxide anesthesia in humans. Anesth Analg 62:317, 1983

120. Brodsky JB: Toxicity of nitrous oxide. In Eger EI II (ed): Nitrous Oxide/N₂O, p 265. New York, Elsevier, 1985

121. Van Lambalgan AA, Bronsveld W, van den Bos GC et al: Cardiovascular and biochemical changes in dogs during etomidate–nitrous oxide anaesthesia. Cardiovasc Res 16:599, 1982

122. Thomson IA, Fitch W, Hughes RL et al: Effects of certain i.v. anaesthetics on liver blood flow and hepatic oxygen consumption in the greyhound. Br J Anaesth 58:69, 1986

123. Sear JW: The metabolism of steroid intravenous anaesthetic agents, and their modification by liver disease. Ph.D. thesis, University of Bristol, 1981

124. Blunnie WP, Zacharias M, Dundee JW et al: Liver enzyme studies with continuous infusion anaesthesia. Anaesthesia 36:152, 1981

125. Kawar PK, Briggs LP, Bahar M et al: Liver enzyme studies with disoprofol (ICI 35868) and midazolam. Anaesthesia 37:305, 1982

126. Robinson FP, Patterson CC: Changes in liver function tests after propofol (Diprivan). Postgrad Med J 61(suppl 3):160, 1985

127. Dundee JW, Fee JPH, Moore J et al: Changes in serum enzyme levels following ketamine infusions. Anaesthesia 35:12, 1980

128. Sear JW, Prys–Roberts C, Dye A: Hepatic function after anesthesia for major vascular reconstructive surgery. A comparison of four anaesthetic techniques. Br J Anaesth 55:606, 1983

129. Sear JW: Toxicity of i.v. anaesthetics. Br J Anaesth 59:24, 1987

130. Jones RM, Detmer M, Hill AB et al: Incidence of choledochoduodenal sphincter spasm during fentanyl-supplemented anesthesia. Anesth Analg 60:638, 1981

131. Economou G, Ward–McQuaid JN: A crossover comparison of the effect of morphine, pethidine, and pentazocine on biliary pressure. Gut 12:218, 1971

132. Tremblay PR, Poncelet P, Dinh DK: Le fentanyl et la pression dans les voies biliaires. Can Anaesth Soc J 20:747, 1973

133. Arguelles JE, Franatovic Y, Romo–Salas F et al: Interbiliary pressure changes produced by narcotic drugs and inhalation anesthetics in guinea pigs. Anesth Analg 58:120, 1979

134. Vatashsky E, Haskel Y: Effect of nalbuphine on intrabiliary pressure in the early postoperative period. Can Anaesth Soc J 33:433, 1986

135. MacGilchrist AJ, Birnie GG, Cook A et al: Pharmacokinetics and pharmacodynamics of intravenous midazolam in patients with severe alcoholic cirrhosis. Gut 27:190, 1986

136. Pandele G, Chaux F, Salvadori C et al: Thiopental pharmacokinetics in patients with cirrhosis. Anesthesiology 59:123, 1983

137. Ferrier C, Marty J, Bouffard Y et al: Alfentanil pharmacokinetics in patients with cirrhosis. Anesthesiology 62:480, 1985

138. Patwardhan RV, Johnson RF, Hoyumpa A Jr et al: Normal metabolism of morphine in cirrhosis. Gastroenterology 81:1006, 1981

139. Maziot JX, Sandouk P, Zerlaoui P et al: Pharmacokinetics of morphine in normal and cirrhotic patients. Anesthesiology 61:A244, 1984

140. Ghoneim MM, Pandya H: Plasma protein binding of thiopental in patients with impaired renal or hepatic function. Anesthesiology 42:545, 1975

141. Bell LE, Slattery JT, Calkins DF: Effect of halothane–oxygen anesthesia on the pharmacokinetics of diazepam and its metabolites in rats. J Pharmacol Exp Ther 233:94, 1985

142. Reilly CS, Wood AJJ, Koshakji RP et al: The effect of halothane on drug disposition: Contribution of changes in intrinsic drug metabolizing capacity and hepatic blood flow. Anesthesiology 63:70, 1985

143. Burney RG, DiFazio CA: Hepatic clearance of lidocaine during N₂O anesthesia in dogs. Anesth Analg 55:322, 1976

144. Berger JM, Stirt JA, Sullivan SF: Enflurane, halothane, and aminophylline—uptake and pharmacokinetics. Anesth Analg 62:733, 1983

145. Duthie DJR, Nimmo WS: The pharmacokinetics of fentanyl by constant rate IV infusion for pain relief after surgery. Anesthesiology 63:A282, 1985

146. Ghoneim MM, van Hamme MJ: Pharmacokinetics of thiopentone: Effects of enflurane and nitrous oxide anaesthesia and surgery. Br J Anaesth 50:1237, 1978

147. Runciman WB, Mather LE: Effects of anaesthesia on drug disposition. In Feldman SA, Scurr CF, Paton SW (eds): Drugs in Anaesthesia: Mechanisms of Action, p 87. Great Britain, Edward Arnold, 1987

148. Fiserova−Bergerova V: Inhibitory effect of isoflurane upon oxidative metabolism of halothane. Anesth Analg 63:399, 1984

149. Sear JW, Walters FJM, Wilkins DG et al: Etomidate by infusion for neuroanaesthesia. Anaesthesia 39:12, 1984

150. Idvall J, Aronsen KF, Stenberg P et al: Pharmacodynamic and pharmacokinetic interactions between ketamine and diazepam. Eur J Clin Pharmacol 24:337, 1983

151. Gelman S: Effects of anesthetics on splanchnic circulation. In Altura BM, Halevy S (eds): Cardiovascular action of anesthetics and drugs used in anesthesia. Basel, Karger Publishing Co, 1986

152. Gelman S: Disturbances in hepatic blood flow during anesthesia and surgery. Arch Surg 111:881, 1976

153. McNeill JR, Pang CC: Effect of pentobarbital anesthesia and surgery on the control of arterial pressure and mesenteric resistance in cats. Role of vasopressin and angiotensin. Can J Physiol Pharmacol 60:363, 1982

154. Johnston IDA: Endocrine aspects of the metabolic response to surgical operation. Ann R Coll Surg Engl 35:270, 1964

155. Oyama T: Endocrine response to general anesthesia and surgery. Monographs in Anaesthesiology 11:1, 1983

156. Harper MH, Collins P, Johnson BH et al: Postanesthetic hepatic injury in rats: Influence of alterations in hepatic blood flow, surgery, and anesthesia time. Anesth Analg 61:79, 1982

157. Refsum HE: Arterial hypoxaemia, serum activity of GO-T, GP-T and LDH, and central lobular liver cell necrosis in pulmonary insufficiency. Clin Sci 25:369, 1963

158. Sims JL, Morris LE, Orth OS et al: The influence of oxygen and carbon dioxide levels during anesthesia upon postsurgical hepatic damage. J Lab Clin Med 38:388, 1951

159. Viegas O, Stoelting RK: LDH₅ changes after cholecystectomy or hysterectomy in patients receiving halothane, enflurane, or fentanyl. Anesthesiology 51:556, 1979

160. Zinn SE, Fairley HB, Glenn JD: Liver function in patients with mild alcoholic hepatitis, after enflurane, nitrous oxide−narcotic, and spinal anesthesia. Anesth Analg 64:487, 1985

161. Loft S, Boel J, Kyst A et al: Increased hepatic microsomal enzyme activity after surgery under halothane or spinal anesthesia. Anesthesiology 62:11, 1985

162. Oikkonen M, Rosenberg PH, Neuvonen PJ: Hepatic metabolic ability during anaesthesia. Anaesthesia 39:660, 1984

163. Gelman S, Dillard E, Bradley EL Jr: Hepatic circulation during surgical stress and anesthesia with halothane, isoflurane, or fentanyl. Anesth Analg 66:936, 1987

164. Strunin L, Davies JM: The liver and anaesthesia. Can Anaesth Soc J 30:208, 1983

165. Kang YG, Gelman S: Liver transplantation. In Gelman S (ed): Anesthesia and Organ Transplantation, p 139. Philadelphia, W.B. Saunders, 1987

166. Duvaldestin P, Agoston S, Henzel D et al: Pancuronium pharmacokinetics in patients with liver cirrhosis. Br J Anaesth 50:1131, 1978

167. Ward S, Neill EAM: Pharmacokinetics of atracurium in acute hepatic failure (with acute renal failure). Surv Anesth 28:364, 1984

168. Arden JR, Cannon JC, Lynam DP et al: Vecuronium pharmacokinetics and pharmacodynamics in hepatocellular disease. Anesth Analg 66:S3, 1987

169. Gelman S, Ernst EA: Hepatic circulation during sodium nitroprusside infusion in the carbon tetrachloride−treated dog. Ala J Med Sci 19:371, 1982

170. Westra P, Houwertjes C, DeLange AR et al: Effect of experimental cholestasis on neuromuscular blocking drugs in cats. Br J Anaesth 52:747, 1980

171. McCammon RL, Viegas OJ, Stoelting RK et al: Naloxone reversal of choledochoduodenal sphincter spasm associated with narcotic administration. Anesthesiology 48:437, 1978

172. Lang DW, Pilon RN: Naloxone reversal of morphine-induced biliary colic. Anesth Analg 59:619, 1980

173. Bordley J, Alson JE: The use of glucagon in operative cholangiography. Surg Gynecol Obstet 149:583, 1979

174. Jones RM, Fiddian−Green R, Knight PR: Narcotic-induced choledochoduodenal sphincter spasm reversed by glucagon. Anesth Analg 59:946, 1980

175. Tigerstedt I, Turunen MT, Hastbacka J: Effect of anaesthesia on fentanyl-induced changes in human intracholedochal pressure. Ann Clin Res 16:204, 1984

176. Belani KG, Estrin JA, Ascher NL et al: Reperfusion coagulopathy during human liver transplantation. Anesth Analg 66:S10, 1987

177. Groth CG: Changes in coagulation. In Starzl TE (ed): Experience in Hepatic Transplantation, p 54. Philadelphia, W.B. Saunders, 1969

178. Boher SL, Rogers EL, Koehler RC et al: Effect of hypovolemic hypotension and laparotomy on splanchnic and hepatic arterial blood flow in dogs. Curr Surg; Sept−Oct:325, 1981

179. Schmid M, Hefti ML, Gattiker R et al: A benign postoperative intrahepatic cholestasis. N Engl J Med 272:545, 1965

Chapter 43

Tamas Kallos
Theodore C. Smith

Anesthesia and Orthopedic Surgery

Orthopedic surgery has undergone a quiet revolution as advances in medicine have influenced changes in the focus of the orthopedist. Diseases previously responsible for large numbers of orthopedic operations have now become uncommon. Rickets and scurvy are usually detected and cured before they reach a stage that requires surgery. Poliomyelitis is now nearly eradicated, and tuberculosis is detected early and effectively treated with drugs. Antibiotics and prompt care have radically changed the character of operations for chronic osteomyelitis and septic arthritis. Early detection often results in effective nonoperative treatment for congenital hip dysplasia, club foot, ideopathic scoliosis, and Legg–Calvé–Perthes disease, or permits simpler surgery, as in slipped femoral capital epiphysis. These factors have acted to decrease certain kinds of orthopedic operations.

Other advances have occurred that broaden the scope of orthopedic interests. Automobile and industrial accidents have resulted in an increase in trauma surgery. As the population ages, there are more age-related orthopedic problems. Oncology and pain clinics are generating increasing demands for orthopedic consultations and collaboration. Rehabilitation after stroke and spinal cord injury demands new and more inventive procedures. The increasing demand for joint replacements for fingers, knees, shoulders, and especially hips has made major contributions to improved function and the relief of pain and suffering.[1] Sports medicine has grown from an occasional interest to a subspecialty in its own right.[2] New materials from space age technology such as carbon ribbons and carbon-reinforced plastics have invited new applications.[3, 4] New sensors and controls from computer technology provide electronic assistance to paralyzed or prosthetic limbs,[5, 6] which, although not yet the equivalent of television's "bionic" Six Million Dollar Man, have certainly progressed beyond Captain Hook's wildest dream. Magnetic and electromagnetic field studies have opened new investigations and new therapies in the field of bone growth and healing.[7] Piezoelectric effects and bone chemistry are adding to detailed knowledge of bone repair and remodeling under strain.

All of these phenomena of the new orthopedics have increased the need for anesthesiologists to understand the patient, the wide variety of problems, and the complicated apparatus and procedures that today's orthopedic surgeon is bringing to the operating room. In this chapter, preoperative, intraoperative, and postoperative factors of importance in orthopedic anesthesia will be discussed, as well as specific operations and procedures in orthopedics.

PREOPERATIVE CONSIDERATIONS

The preoperative period should be used for discovery and planning in orthopedic procedures, as in other areas of anesthesia. First, one should learn as much as possible about the patient and the procedure consistent with the time frame permitted. In the acutely traumatized patient who requires emergency surgery, there is time to do no more than survey the three most important systems: central nervous, circulatory, and respiratory. Some procedures that are true emergencies include dislocated hip,[8] digital replantation, and the compartment syndrome. For elective procedures such as implantation or removal of prostheses, one spends as long as necessary in preoperative preparation. Even in a semi-

1163

emergent situation, for example, an elderly patient with an acute fractured hip, it may be judicious to spend 12 to 48 hours properly preparing the patient for surgery. Careful preoperative evaluation should lead to a rational and safe choice of anesthetic technique. It may also uncover serious systemic disease requiring further diagnostic and therapeutic measures prior to operation.[9]

Some orthopedic patients present special considerations. The pediatric patient, the acutely traumatized patient, the arthritic patient, and the elderly patient are examples of patients in whom there are frequently occurring problems. (Table 43-1)

PEDIATRIC PATIENTS

The special problems of pediatric anesthesia include small airway diameter, high cardiac index and small blood volume, sensitivity to certain drugs and resistance to others, and lack of cooperation in some cases, especially when pain is present (see Chapter 47). These patients may be emotionally distressed either from acute injury or from recollection of recent prior hospitalizations and anesthetics. Although the patient's history is commonly given by another person (the parent or guardian), performance of the physical examination and various laboratory tests is most efficient if rapport can be established with the patient and if cooperation can be achieved. Good rapport is especially important to improve the likelihood that subsequent inductions of anesthesia will be pleasant in children with cerebral palsy, muscular dystrophy, and other diseases that may necessitate multiple procedures.[10] The mentally retarded child may pose particular problems in gaining rapport and cooperation, but no unusual problems exist in sensitivity to anesthetic drugs.[11]

ACUTELY TRAUMATIZED PATIENTS

Patients with acute trauma require careful evaluation of all systems by a multidisciplinary team. Modern traumatology requires institution of emergency treatment for potentially lethal events prior to evaluation of the patient (see Chapter 50).[12] Diagnostic steps are taken in the order that will detect life-threatening injuries first. Entities that require immediate attention such as hypotension, respiratory obstruction or depression, facial and neck lesions that affect airway patency, severed blood vessels, pneumothorax, hemothorax, hemopericardium, ruptured viscus, and peridural hematoma should be detected and treated immediately. In the absence of life-threatening problems, relief of the severe pain that is usually present can be addressed. The possibility of prior administration of opioids should be considered, and dosage should be adjusted if necessary. With resuscitation, a previously ineffective intramuscular (im) dose of a depressant drug may unexpectedly exert its several effects.

After important occult injuries are ruled out, relatively urgent intervention may be necessary for some fractures. Immobilization will act to prevent secondary injury to other organs as well as minimize pain and decrease the incidence of fat embolism. Rapid treatment of femoral, pelvic, and some open fractures can help limit the large amount of bleeding that may occur. If more than 6 hours are allowed to pass between trauma and surgery, the risk of infection may require that an open wound not be primarily closed. Delaying an orthopedic procedure may result in excessive soft tissue swelling, which can make closed reduction of a fracture more difficult or the compartment syndrome more likely.

Under stress, in the presence of severe pain, or after opioids, gastric emptying time may be prolonged several fold. Early treatment with cimetidine (two doses of 300 mg 6 hours apart) helps to decrease hydrogen ion secretion. Antacids are often used to neutralize existing acid. Soluble salts such as sodium citrate are less damaging than particulate suspensions if aspirated. Metoclopramide (10 mg im 1 hour prior to induction, or intravenous [iv] over 1 to 2 minutes), can decrease gastric emptying time.[13] However, even waiting 6 to 8 hours for gastric emptying will not ensure an empty stomach, and precautions against regurgitation and aspiration must be taken.

In patients with cervical vertebral fracture, dislocation, or subluxation, the possibility of spinal cord damage with neck motion must be considered. When the nature of the procedure and the patient permit, regional anesthesia is preferable. When general anesthesia is elected, a clear airway must be ensured prior to induction of anesthesia.

ARTHRITIC PATIENTS

Arthritic patients present with chronic pain and often fixation of joints, making positioning difficult. Since difficulty in intubation of the trachea is frequent, physical examination should include evaluation of the patient's airway, focusing on range of motion of the neck, temporomandibular joint function and jaw motion, and glottic narrowing owing to involvement of the cricoarytenoid joint.[14, 15] A hoarse or weak voice may be a

TABLE 43-1.   Common Patients and Problems in Orthopedics

PATIENT	AIRWAY	CIRCULATION	PAIN	MEDICATION	ALLIED
Pediatric	Narrow diameter	Small blood volume	Uncooperative	Varied tolerance	Congenital anomalies
Traumatized	Facial injury	Blood loss	Severe pain	Prior opioids	Hidden injuries
Arthritic	Difficult intubation	Cardiac dysrhythmia	Chronic pain	Aspirin steroids	Limits to positioning
Elderly	Edentulous sleep apnea	Ischemic diseases	Disorientation	Multiple interactions	Multisystem afflictions

Certain problems such as noted here occur so frequently that experienced anesthesiologists develop a well-thought out approach to their management. Although it is economical timewise to have such routines, the measures should not be applied unless they are appropriate and consistent with the management of other concurrent problems. Common practice may be routine, but routine is never mandatory.

clue to a cricoarytenoid dysfunction. Instability of the first cervical vertebra on the second cervical vertebra may present a problem during positioning and tracheal intubation, warranting lateral spine radiograph or CT scan examination. Tracheal intubation may be difficult in patients with ankylosing spondylitis (Marie– Strümpell disease) because of cervical fixation in flexion.[16] When intubation of the trachea is necessary, special aids (*e.g.,* modified laryngoscopes, lighted stylets, and flexible fiberoptic laryngoscopes) can be helpful (see Chapter 20). In rare cases, tracheostomy under local anesthesia must be performed before anesthesia can safely be induced. If tracheal intubation is not necessary, oral or nasal airways may aid in maintaining unobstructed breathing. Topical anesthesia produced before induction facilitates the introduction of an airway under light anesthesia with decreased respiratory or circulatory consequences.

The specific arthritic condition frequently suggests associated problems that may be of importance to the anesthesiologist. The osteoarthritic patient's problem may be related to obesity or to repetitive occupational stress. The gouty arthritic patient may have renal disease. The traumatic arthritic patient may have other sequelae of the accident. The infected arthritic patient may have bacteremia or metastatic infections. The rheumatoid arthritic patient usually has multiple manifestations, which may include airway limitation, pleural effusion, pulmonary fibrosis with alveolar capillary block syndrome, cardiac dysrhythmias and conduction defects, valvular involvement, coronary insufficiency, renal amyloid disease, and anemia.[17]

The arthritic patient is likely to be taking a variety of medications of significance to the anesthesiologist. Aspirin depresses platelet function with the attendant risk of increased bleeding. Steroid therapy is frequent, with its risk of adrenal cortical insufficiency in the presence of surgical and anesthetic stress. The characteristic thin skin and decreased subcutaneous fat may make venipuncture difficult, and infiltration around even a soft venous catheter is a frequent problem. Although steroids prescribed for arthritis are selected for their anti-inflammatory efficacy and relative lack of mineralocorticoid effect, steroid replacement for several days postoperatively should be chosen to ensure both glucocorticoid and mineralocorticoid aspects of the stress response. A common regimen for a patient undergoing an extensive surgical procedure includes a preoperative dose of hydrocortisone 100 mg, followed by a 100-mg dose every 6 hours for the first postoperative day, tapering off the daily dose by 100 mg each day thereafter.

ELDERLY PATIENTS

Elderly patients have decreased reserve in every body system (see Chapter 48). Even in the absence of disease, there is progressive loss of brain cells, nephrons, alveoli, muscle fibers, and even subcellular organelles, as well as stiffening of heart, skeletal muscle, lung, ligaments, and tendons.[18] Not only is there a general decrease in the number of functioning cells, but the capabilities of the remaining cells and systems also slowly decrease (Fig 43-1). Mental quickness and acuity may be diminished, arterial oxygen tension decreases, cardiac index is diminished, and gastrointestinal motility slows. The special senses are obtunded with presbyopia, presbyacusia, hyposmia, and failing taste. Lack of dentition makes airway maintenance more difficult.

Mental status is an important factor in the evaluation of these patients. There is a great difference between one septuagenarian who broke a hip canvassing door to door during a political campaign and another who broke a hip stumbling to an adjacent bathroom in a nursing home. Disorientation in the elderly can result from pain or from their multiple medications. In addition, the potential interactions of their medica-

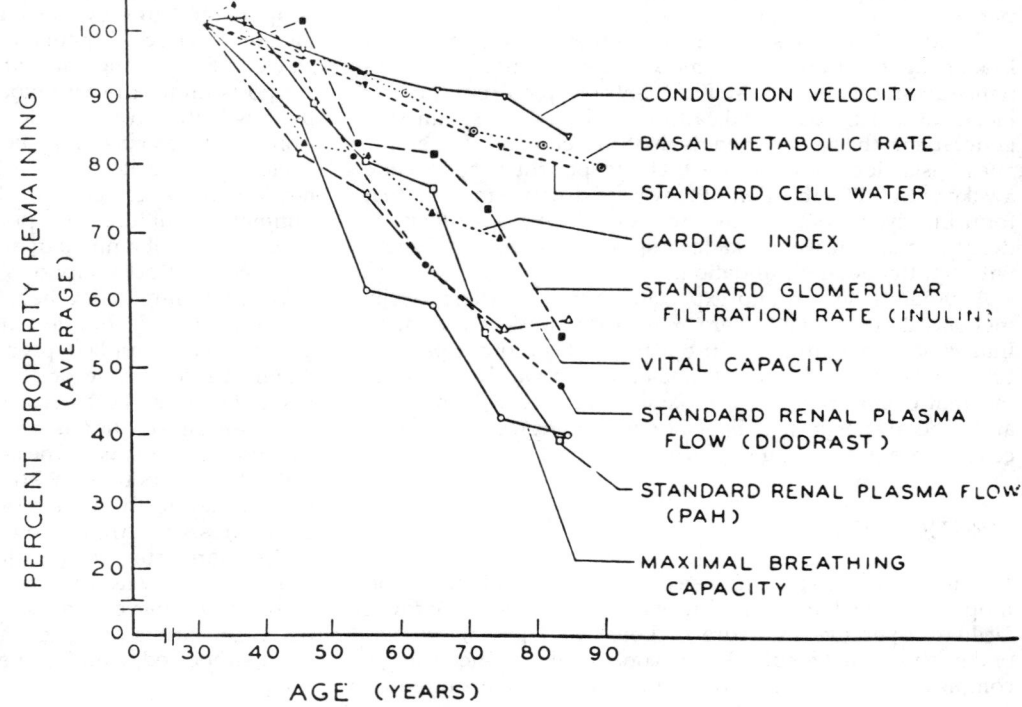

FIG. 43-1. Changes in physiologic functions with aging. For each function, values are expressed as the per cent of the mean value for subjects aged 25 to 35 years. All subjects were males. Whereas deterioration occurs at different rates for different functions, measures of reserve such as maximum breathing capacity (now called maximum voluntary ventilation) fall faster than resting values such as basal metabolic rate. (Reproduced by permission from Jeffers FC [ed]: The science of gerontology. In Proceedings of Seminars 1959–61, p 123. Durham, Duke University Press, 1962.)

tions with anesthetic drugs must be kept in mind. For example, methyldopa alters anesthetic requirements, and droperidol antagonizes the beneficial effects of methyldopa. The induction of anesthesia may increase the incidence or severity of certain drug effects such as phenothiazine-induced hypotension or digitalis-induced cardiac dysrhythmias.

In the elderly, there is a high incidence of degenerative diseases, including Alzheimer's disease, ischemic cerebral and cardiovascular problems, and emphysema. Thus, hypoxia is more likely and more dangerous in these patients.[19] The elderly are also prone to become confused in the postoperative period. Although the incidence does not appear to be related to the choice of anesthetic, a history of depression and premedication with anticholinergic drugs can be contributory factors.[20]

INTRAOPERATIVE MANAGEMENT

CHOICE OF ANESTHETIC TECHNIQUE

Although the final choice of anesthesia depends upon the usual interplay of patient and surgical factors, one can build a strong argument for consideration of specific nerve blockades, iv regional anesthesia, plexus anesthesia, and spinal or epidural blockade in orthopedic anesthesia. Even though there are potential complications of spinal and epidural anesthesia,[21] several studies provide data favoring these methods over general anesthesia in hip procedures.[22-27] In operations in which low regional blockade can be used, abdominal motor power and, hence, cough is preserved and a number of potential advantages may be realized, including profound skeletal muscle relaxation,[24] normal respiratory mechanics,[28] no maldistribution of ventilation/perfusion matching,[29] blockade of the stress response,[30] decreased blood loss,[31] decreased venous thromboembolism without additional anticoagulants,[32-34] decreased serum enzymes,[35] preservation of monocyte function,[36] postoperative analgesia,[37] and lower immediate mortality.[38] Active beneficial effects may even accrue in patients with cardiac problems.[39]

Use of regional anesthesia is sometimes limited because of lack of patient acceptance. Some anesthesiologists feel repugnance about the need to "sell" patients on spinal, epidural, or blockade anesthesia. It takes time and tact to explain that general anesthesia is not equivalent to sleep and that spinal anesthesia does not require that the patient remain wide awake with full perception. It may be instructive to recall that John Lundy, in 1926, coined the term *balanced anesthesia* to describe major nerve blockade or spinal anesthesia combined with light general obtundation.

A patient's desires and expectations may be satisfactorily met only if time and effort are expended to understand them. Inaz et al,[40] in a study of European practice, found patients bring an "out-dated and distorted attitude toward anesthesia, but that overall they are comparably satisfied with regional and general anesthesia." Specific suggestions for specific procedures are given in the following sections.

POSITIONING

No other surgical specialty uses such varied positions as orthopedics (see Chapter 24). The positions, chosen primarily to facilitate operative exposure of bones and joints, are secondarily modified for physiologic considerations. Increasingly complex "fracture tables" with special attachments often re-

place the typical operating room table (Fig. 43-2). Because the patient may be in pain preoperatively or may suffer pain during positioning on the fracture table, anesthetization before final positioning may be necessary. This places additional burdens on the surgeon and anesthesiologist to ensure safety for the unconscious or paralyzed patient during positioning. Surgeons, operating room staff, and anesthesiologists should discuss and agree upon the positioning procedure. A compromise between optimal exposure and optimal circulation and ventilation may be required at times, but the anesthesiologist must be able to protect the airway and monitor ventilation and circulation at all times.

The supine position is usually safe and simple. For some arthroscopies, a leg holder may support the thigh.[41] This should be placed so as not to injure muscle, nerve, or vessels, nor place unusual strain on joints that will be unsupported when anesthesia or paralysis decrease skeletal muscle tone. The leg holder may be tried just before induction of anesthesia to ensure that it is reasonably comfortable. When a fracture table is used, the supine position offers a challenge. The trunk is usually supported by a sacral plate and post, which must be properly padded, and a biscapular shelf. Arm supports must protect against brachial plexus stretch. On many tables, the Trendelenburg position is neither quickly nor easily provided, thus making treatment of vomiting or hypotension more difficult. Two people may be needed to support and elevate the legs when the lock is released to provide head-down tilt. The lock may require a special key or wrench to operate. The vagaries and mechanisms of specific tables must be familiar to the operating room team preoperatively.

The prone position is used primarily for spinal operations. The aim is to preserve thoracic kyphosis and reverse lumbar lordosis without increasing abdominal pressure. Abdominal pressure not only compromises ventilation but can also decrease venous return, thus contributing to hypotension and increased venous bleeding in the wound. Various mattresses, frames, and supports have been devised for these purposes. Ventilation is usually adequate if the chest and abdomen are free to move either laterally or anteriorly. Thus, frames that support the trunk by the sides and can be arched after the patient is placed on them are most useful and are simple and stable.[42] Supporting the patient by upper thoracic rolls or supports under the acromioclavicular joint and by iliac supports is better, in theory, for abdominal pressure and excursion but, in practice, may be less stable.

Flexing the thighs past a 90-degree angle puts sufficient tension on the relaxed gluteal muscles to reverse the lordosis optimally. Dinmore[43] has pointed out that this may be overdone in the Mohammedan praying position; he describes one of several buttocks supports that are safe, comfortable, and effective. Failure to flex the thighs more than 90 degrees leads to instability, allowing for shifts during operation. If a body cast has been applied preoperatively, the anesthesiologist should be certain he or she can remove part or all of it if resuscitation is necessary.

The sitting position is used occasionally for operations on the shoulder and neck. The anesthesiologist should be wary of orthostatic hypotension after induction of anesthesia and should elevate the back slowly, with frequent checking of blood pressure. Application of elastic bandages to the lower limbs before sitting the patient up helps to avoid hypotension. The hips may be flexed 20 to 45 degrees and the knees 15 to 20 degrees to achieve a chaise lounge effect for stability and to decrease venous pooling. Care should be taken to keep the head supported, avoiding neck injuries and airway obstruction.

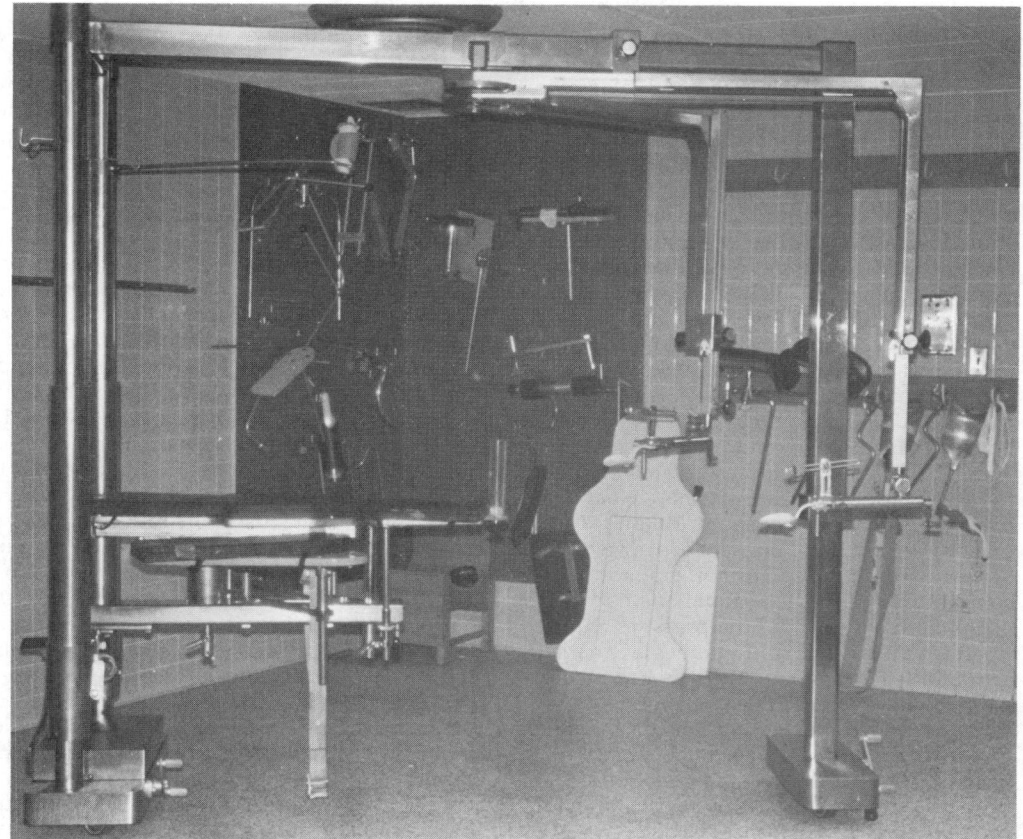

FIG. 43-2. This Orthopaedic Fracture Table is one of many available for complex operative approaches to pelvic, hip, and leg fractures. In this model, a single-foot–operated hydraulic pump raises the two posts at the head and the single post at the foot simultaneously with the back plate and arm board supports. Two buttons release the head and foot pillars separately to allow either tilting or lowering. Two separate foot supports provide adjustable distraction. A hand crank at the head end provides side tilt, while a foot treadle at the other end locks the wheels. In the background are other typical appliances such as a hand table, thigh and knee supports, and weights tourniquets.

Spontaneous ventilation is more effective in the sitting position than in the supine position, and the incidence of air embolism and pneumothorax is small for operations on the shoulder in the sitting position. Air embolism may occur, however, during cervical laminectomy in the sitting position. An esophageal stethoscope, transthoracic Doppler,[44] and end-tidal carbon dioxide monitoring[45] are helpful in diagnosis. In high-risk patients, a right atrial catheter permits removal of air.[46]

The lateral position is commonly used for prosthetic replacement of the hip and occasionally for laminectomy. The problems are primarily comfort for the awake patient and stability for the unconscious patient. Extra mattresses or a layer of "egg crate" foam over the usual mattress are appreciated by the awake patient. Pillows rather than folded sheets or blankets are always more comfortable, especially when the patient must lie on his ear, not moving for hours. The extremities should be moderately flexed at the knees and elbows for comfort. When hypobaric spinal anesthesia is used, a small additional injection of hyperbaric drug will often promote comfort in the dependent parts. The use of ribbed hypo-hyperthermia blankets under the patient is rarely effective in this position because of a decreased area of contact. If body temperature decreases, a smaller water blanket draped over the thorax is more effective for rewarming than one under the patient.

Stability may be promoted with side-to-side 7.5 cm adhesive straps, but these must be applied carefully. The upper arm and elbow may be included in the strapping of the shoulder girdle. Better and safer support comes from appliances attached to the table, which cradle the pelvis and shoulder girdle, or from individually moldable bean bags, which are "set" by vacuum. An axillary roll is often routinely placed, presumably to prevent nerve and vascular compression in this position. However, neurovascular compression is not a problem in the lateral position except in cases in which obesity may cause a roll of fat to compress axillary structures. A palpable pulse and a free-flowing iv infusion in the lower arm are sufficient evidence of adequate circulation. The upper arm is reserved for blood pressure measurement and the starting of a second iv infusion if necessary.

Occasionally, patients may require intubation of the trachea in the lateral position. This can be made easier with the following technique: An assistant should pull the upper shoulder backward and down, so the shoulder girdle rotates the spinal axis about 45 degrees. The laryngoscope should be initially inserted in the superior side of the mouth (the left side in patients in the right lateral decubitus position), so that the tongue falls away from the path of visualization. This may be easier than elevating the tongue. If the anesthesiologist then bends laterally at the waist, the usual view of the larynx is obtained.

PREVENTION OF BLOOD LOSS

Tourniquets

Orthopedic procedures involving tumors or major skeletal muscle and bone dissections may be quite bloody. In these cases, tourniquets can be useful in minimizing blood loss. The pneumatic tourniquet has universally replaced older methods of vascular occlusion. The inflated cuff should be of a width more than half the limb diameter, applied over limited smooth padding or none at all. The danger of padding is that it can promote irritation by wrinkles and folds or by absorbing skin preparation solution such as soap or iodophor. During skin preparation, the cuff may be protected by an absorbent layer of padding just distal to the cuff or by an impermeable plastic drape. The cuff should more than encircle the limb to ensure circumferentially uniform pressure, and the overlap point should be rotated 180 degrees from the neurovascular bundle, because there is some area of decreased compression at the overlap point (Fig. 43-3). Pressure is maintained by compressed gas (air or oxygen), a volatile refrigerant (Freon), or a dedicated pump and must be monitored continually while the tourniquet is in use. Deliberately squeezing the inflated cuff should produce visible oscillations on the cuff pressure monitor, which itself should regularly be checked for accuracy, linearity, hysteresis,[47] and pressure creep from faulty regulators.[48] The limb should be elevated for about 1 minute and tightly wrapped with an Esmarch bandage from distal to proximal immediately before inflating the cuff. Since compressive exsanguination may be unwise when there is infection or an undiagnosed tumor, limb tourniquets are relatively contraindicated in these situations.

Opinions differ about the pressure required in tourniquets to prevent bleeding. Some gauges are marked with "average" arm and leg pressures, but it is irrational to expect that all patients are average. Leg tourniquets are often pressurized more than arm tourniquets on the theory that larger limbs require more pressure than smaller limbs. Shaw and Murray[49] have shown that deep tissue pressure is 70–95% of intracuff pressure, depending mainly upon the diameter of the limb. Femoral systolic pressure is slightly higher than brachial pressure owing to complex hemodynamic factors. If the cuff is applied loosely, there may be a big pressure drop across the noncompliant cuff wall itself. Thus, it seems rational to suggest that a cuff pressure 100 mm Hg above a patient's measured systolic pressure is adequate for the thigh, and 50 mm Hg for the arm, with the understanding that if hypertensive epi-

sodes occur, the cuff pressure should be increased. Continued oozing after cuff inflation may rarely be due to inadequate occlusion of the major arterial inflow, corrected by reapplication and the proper degree of inflation. Oozing may more commonly be due to intramedullary blood flow in the long bones, particularly in the skeletally immature, and to small arterial vessels between the two bones of distal extremities. In neither of these cases will overinflation stop the oozing.

The dangers from a properly maintained, properly applied, and properly monitored pneumatic tourniquet are few. There are reports of a fatal pulmonary embolus apparently caused solely by inflation of a tourniquet on a traumatized limb, and there are several reports of emboli following Esmarch bandaging.[50–52] The duration of safe tourniquet inflation is unknown.[53] Various recommendations range from 30 minutes to 4 hours. Ten minutes of intermittent perfusion between 1- and 2-hour inflations, followed by repeated exsanguination through elevation and compression, does not allow more extended use. Current belief is that reperfusion simply supplies more substrate for free radical production. When tourniquets are used on multiple sites, it is wise to loosen or remove underlying padding at one site before starting at the next site.

There are a few reports of damage to underlying vessels, nerves, and skeletal muscles.[54] As might be expected, the injury is a function of both inflation pressure and duration of inflation.[53, 55] The pressure under the cuff is more damaging than the distal ischemia.[56, 57] Arterial spasm, venous thrombosis, and nerve injury are all demonstrable after many hours, depending upon the technique used to search for injury. Electron microscopy after 1 hour of ischemia shows only depletion of glycogen granules in sarcoplasm with some extracellular edema.[58] After 2 hours, there are lesions of acidosis: mitochondrial swelling, myelin degeneration, and z line lysis[57] (Fig. 43-4). Clinical examination, electromyography, and effluent blood analysis all show completely reversible changes for inflations of 1 to 2 hours.[59, 60] Transient metabolic acidosis and elevation of arterial carbon dioxide after tourniquet deflation does not cause deleterious effects in healthy children, but prolonged inflation and/or simultaneous release of two tourniquets may produce clinically significant acidosis, particularly in previously acidotic patients.[61]

Rarely, neuralgia paresthetica has been reported, which reverses within weeks to months. Sickling of red cells in properly exsanguinated limbs is not a problem.[62] Alteration in clotting factors does not occur. Reactive hyperemia in the limb lasts no more than 30 to 45 minutes after tourniquet deflation. When the tourniquet is released, potassium and acid metabolites, which are washed out, become diluted with the rest of the cardiac output and usually cause no serious systemic changes.[61, 63] However, foreign material administered iv in a Bier block has caused loss of a forearm.[64] Washout of local anesthetic drug may produce rapid return of sensation after lidocaine or toxic blood levels after bupivacaine. Prilocaine is reportedly a suitable compromise, giving long enough analgesia following tourniquet release to permit surgical hemostasis and closure without toxicity.[65] An alternate approach avoiding prilocaine and its risk of methemoglobinemia is the use of low-dose iv regional blockade and repeating the blockade through an indwelling catheter.[66]

When a pneumatic tourniquet is used with regional anesthetic techniques, a number of patients complain of dull aching pain, or they may demonstrate restlessness even though seemingly adequate analgesia exists for the operation itself. The pain usually appears 45 minutes or more after the tourniquet is inflated and becomes more intense with time. No satisfactory explanation for its genesis has been found. Two

FIG. 43-3. Typical modern pneumatic tourniquet. Note the point of overlap (arrow) where the pressure exerted by the cuff on the underlying tissue is uncertain but lower than that opposite it. This area of overlap should be opposite the neurovascular bundle of a limb rather than over it.

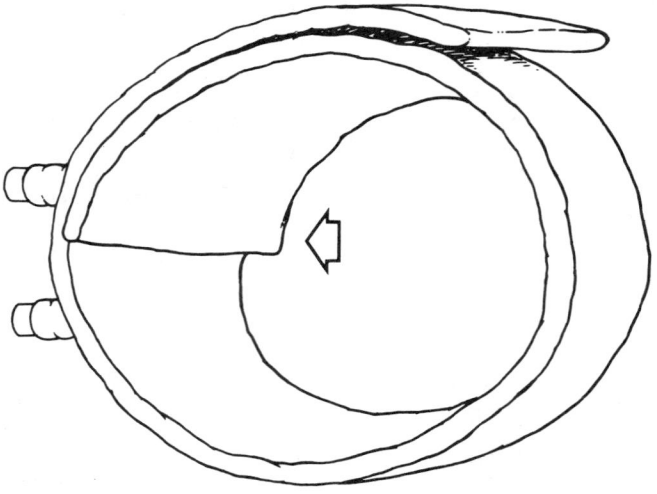

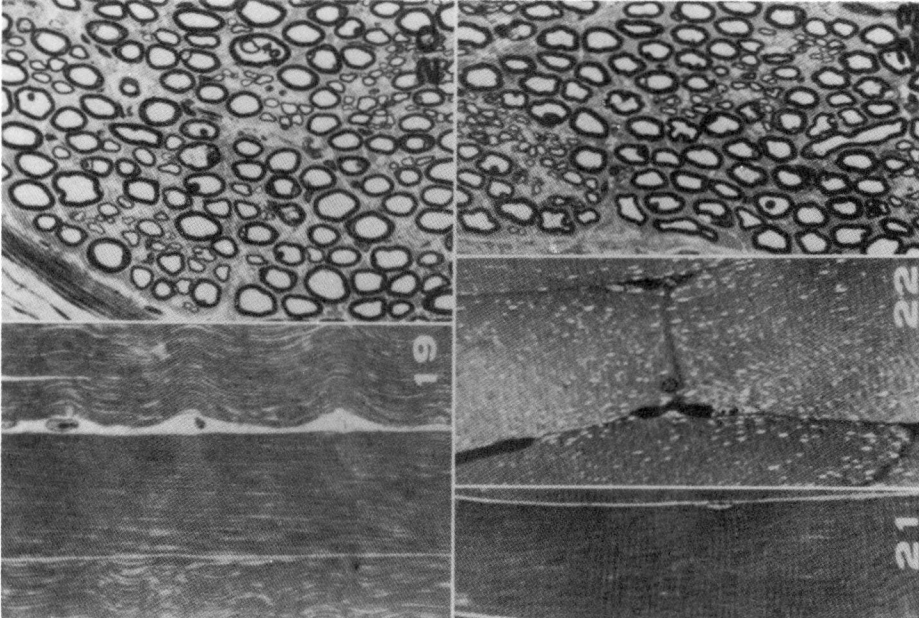

FIG. 43-4. Electron micrograph of nerve *(top)* and muscle *(bottom)*. After 3 hours of ischemia, the muscle was normal in appearance *(left panel)*. After 4 hours, small vacuoles began to appear. Also noted in other sections were swelling of mitochondria and dilation of sarcoplasmic reticulum, but the nerve was normal. (Reprinted with permissiom from Tountas CP, Bergman RA: Tourniquet ischemia: Ultrastructural and histochemical observations of ischemic human muscle and of monkey muscle and nerve. J Hand Surg 2:31, 1977.)

hypotheses have been suggested: 1) the pain is transmitted by large fibers that can be completely blocked only by greater concentrations of local anesthetic than are generally used[67, 68]; 2) the pain is transmitted by small unmyelinated fibers that travel with the sympathetic nerves and enter the spinal cord at a higher segment than that of cutaneous analgesia.[69, 70] Tourniquet pain of the lower extremities is less likely if a "solid" blockade to the mid-thoracic dermatomes is produced. Analogous phenomena may be observed under general anesthesia: Forty-five to 50 minutes after tourniquet inflation, signs of light anesthesia (increase in blood pressure and pulse rate) often appear, even though the same concentrations of anesthetic are being delivered.[71]

The definitive treatment for tourniquet pain is release of the tourniquet. During surgery, however, analgesics and hypnotics are usually administered. Sometimes only a general anesthetic will relieve the patient's discomfort. If excessive iv medications have been given, with or without general anesthesia, the anesthesiologist must be prepared for sudden central depression when the tourniquet is deflated and the afferent arousal ceases.

Deliberate Hypotension

Hypotension as a measure to reduce surgical blood loss has been recommended when the benefits can be expected to outweigh the risks. In hip surgery and in scoliosis surgery, deliberate hypotension has proved to be beneficial.[72] In Jehovah's Witnesses, it may be the only option available.[73] In a comparative study, average blood loss during induced nitroprusside hypotension with nitrous oxide–halothane anesthesia for hip arthroplasty was 1.3 l, whereas neuroleptanalgesia or nitrous oxide–halothane without hypotension yielded blood losses of 2.6 and 2 l, respectively.[25] Epidural anesthesia with no attempt to alter blood pressure was associated with an intermediate blood loss, 1.6 l. In adolescents undergoing scoliosis correction, Knight and colleagues,[74] using ganglionic blockade and propranolol during nitrous oxide–morphine anesthesia, achieved a "dry field" with a mean blood pressure of

40 to 55 mm Hg. There was no tachycardia, near normal cardiac index, and no increase in plasma renin, angiotensin II, norepinephrine, or dopamine. McNeil and colleagues,[75] in another study of scoliosis surgery, found deliberate hypotension achieved with pentolinium or trimethaphan or deep halothane anesthesia associated with a blood loss that was 900 ml less than that during normotension. Hypotension also shortened operative time by 33 minutes. Diltiazem, nitroprusside with and without captopril, and nitroglycerine have been used in other studies.[76, 77]

REPLACEMENT OF BLOOD

Despite efforts to reduce bleeding, some orthopedic procedures can be associated with major blood loss, sometimes approximating the patient's blood volume.[78] This is especially true in patients with rheumatoid arthritis, Paget's disease, and tumor metastases to bone and in patients who had operations performed at the site of previous surgery. In such cases, blood loss should be continually calculated by weighing sponges, measuring the suction bottle contents, estimating the amount of blood on the drapes, and subtracting the amount of irrigating fluid when that is used.

Normal circulating blood volume with adequate amounts of hemoglobin is the aim of intraoperative fluid therapy. The complications of homologous blood transfusion may be avoided by use of autologous blood or hemodilution. Several methods of autologous transfusion have been used: 1) storing the patient's blood removed 1 to 2 weeks preoperatively (earlier if the blood is frozen);[79–81] 2) removing blood from the patient before the procedure and replacing it with crystalline or albumin solutions for reinfusion of the shed blood at the end of the operation;[82] and 3) reinfusing blood removed from the operative field, especially in major trauma surgery.[83] In orthopedic procedures, the presence of marrow fat and bone chips in the lost blood has limited the use of the latter technique, but scoliosis surgeons are increasing their use of these "cell saving" techniques.[84] A theoretically attractive but complicated method for autotransfusion involves removing 1 unit of blood at the beginning of week 1, removing 2 units of blood at week 2 and reinfusing last week's single unit; removing 3 units of blood at week 3 and reinfusing the 2 units from the previous week. Thus, at N + 1 weeks, there are N units of the patient's blood available for transfusion during surgery, all 1 week old!

Moderate hemodilution is emerging as a beneficial, rather than a tolerable, situation. Oxygen transport has been shown to be maximal at hematocrits around 30%. In patients without fixed arterial resistance, for example, those with severe coronary artery disease, peripheral tissue oxygenation is not compromised at even lower hematocrits.[85, 86] Albumin, plasma protein fraction, or other diluents such as cellulose or starch solutions have been found useful in decreasing the number of blood transfusions. Emulsions of fluorocarbons and stroma-free hemoglobin solutions offer the hope for simultaneous maintenance of vascular volume and oxygen-carrying capacity. However, the fluorocarbons have a straight-line hemoglobin dissociation curve requiring very high oxygen tension, and dilute stroma-free hemoglobins have a markedly left-shifted dissociation curve, interfering with tissue unloading of their oxygen content. Dextran solutions find little favor today because of the possibility of bleeding and anaphylaxis,[87] although the use of haptens has reduced the latter markedly.[32]

In choosing among the available fluids, cost, convenience, availability, and personal preference are all factors to be considered. Since full intravascular replacement of 1 ml of shed blood requires 5 to 7 ml of crystalloid solution or 1 ml of colloid, there is little net cost difference between balanced salt solutions and hetastarch. However, an increased incidence of pulmonary edema may be seen after excessive infusion of electrolyte solutions unless the more conservative 3 ml for 1 ml replacement formula is used. Such a 3:1 ratio has been rationalized on the basis of the extracellular fluid to blood volume ratio, which is about 3:1. This neglects the fact that red cell volume is a part of the extracellular space and that the extracellular to plasma volume ratio is between 5:1 and 7:1.

Deliberate isovolemic hemodilution requires careful estimation of continuing loss, concurrent replacement, and maintenance of an adequate level of hematocrit or hemoglobin. Since intraanesthetic oxygen demand is lower than awake convalescing oxygen demand, many anesthesiologists believe that it is safe and in fact preferable to delay transfusion with red cell concentrates to the postoperative period if at all possible. Intraoperative hemoglobin concentrations of 8 g·dl^{-1} are probably adequate in most patients. Postoperative hemoglobin concentrations of 9 to 10 g·dl^{-1} can be achieved by red cell replacement in the recovery room and convalescent ward. It is safer to transfuse an awake patient in whom signs of a blood reaction are more easily identifiable, and it is reasonable to allow loss of relatively low hematocrit blood intraoperatively rather than to lose recently transfused red blood cells.

With continued blood loss, replacement of red blood cells eventually becomes necessary. As with cold fluids, transfusions should be warmed before infusion, and the use of microfilters for multiple transfusions of blood should be considered. The near universal use of red cell concentrates instead of whole blood slows transfusion rates and promotes the misconception that 1 unit can replace 500 ml of loss. The infusion rate may be speeded by dilution of the cells with a less viscous fluid. Saline or calcium-free–balanced salt solutions are usually used. Lactated Ringer's or Hartman's solutions contain insufficient calcium to trigger clotting in CPD anticoagulated blood after separation of cells from most of the plasma but are nonetheless usually avoided. Five per cent dextrose solutions increase viscosity by favoring rouleaux formation and are also best avoided. Unless concentrated red cells are diluted with colloid solutions, they should be considered as replacing no more than 250 ml of intravascular volume per unit.

INTRAOPERATIVE RADIOGRAPHY

Protection from radiation should be available to the anesthesiologist. The internal shields of the x-ray generator are used to cone down the primary beam as much as possible. The secondary (scattered) radiation is inherently softer (longer wave length, less penetrating, and, therefore, absorbed in tissues to a greater extent). A number of practices serve to protect against this exposure: The anesthesiologist should wear the standard lead apron, be positioned as far from the axial beam of the x-ray tube as possible, and turn away at the moment of exposure to minimize thyroid and lens dosage.[88] Leaded eyeglasses and thyroid shields are available for those who are frequently exposed.[89] The greatest protection lies in the inverse square law, which states that doubling the distance from the ionizing radiation source reduces the dose fourfold. The doors and walls in most operating suites provide little additional attenuation. Users of flammable anesthetic agents should be aware that the anode of x-ray machines is usually rotated by an electric motor with sparking commutators.

Intraoperative fluoroscopy and arthroscopy sometimes require darkness in the operating room. The anesthesiologist can use a flashlight to check machine settings and to observe the patient. Often a surgical light can be directed at the anesthesia machine and floor beyond the patient's head, so that the illuminated area is shielded from the surgeon's dark-adapted peripheral vision by the sterile drapes. Even in the dark, the patient's heart tones, peripheral pulse, and electrocardiogram (ECG) may be continuously monitored. The use of anesthesia monitors with a lighted display and use of videofluoroscopic equipment materially reduces the problem of both radiation and patient care in the dark.

CONTROL OF INFECTION

Postoperative infections can be disastrous in orthopedic surgery for several reasons. They may delay healing or destroy the operative repair, resulting in function that may be worse than that prior to the operative procedure. Implanted devices or prostheses may have to be removed if infection occurs. Eradication of an established osteomyelitis is extremely difficult, time consuming, and expensive. Finally, subsequent surgery, even after cure of a deep infection, is more likely to become complicated by infections.[90] Thus, prevention of infections should be constantly kept in mind. Crow and Greene[91] showed that anesthesiologists commit aseptic transgressions at a rate twice that of surgeons.

The most common sources of wound infection include the patient's skin and oropharyngeal bacteria, airborne bacteria originating from the head and neck of operating room personnel, cross-infection from other patients, and bacteria harbored on dust and lint particles. The measures available to reduce infection rates include having patients take preoperative baths and showers, meticulous skin preparation,[92] multilayered draping with impervious sterile materials,[93] use of double gloves,[94] meticulous attention to covering of the head and neck of personnel, and limiting conversation and traffic in the operating room.[95, 96]

There is general acceptance that operating room attire (cap, mask, suit, and shoe covers) should be of nonlinting materials that are effective bacterial barriers, provide maximal skin coverage, are comfortable, provide freedom of movement, transmit heat and water vapor, are nonflammable or flame retardant, and, although not necessarily conductive, do not accumulate static electric charge. Shirt and drawstrings should be tucked into the waistband of trousers. Shoe covers are preferable to operating room–dedicated shoes, because the latter require and do not usually receive frequent cleansing. Face masks worn *inside* head hoods reduce the number of bacterial colony-forming units per cubic foot of air[97] (Fig. 43-5). The prophylactic use of antibiotics when prostheses are implanted lowers infection rates; overuse, however, leads to the development of antibiotic-resistant bacteria.

More extreme measures have been studied and recommended but have not achieved uniform acceptance. These include continuous ultraviolet radiation, high efficiency particulate air filtration combined with laminar flow ventilation, and nearly complete enclosure of the head and/or entire body of operating personnel in a suit supplied with air and communication equipment and aspirated to an exhaust outside the operating room.[98] With each of these measures, added inconvenience is introduced. For example, ultraviolet light at an intensity of 25 μ watt·cm^{-2} at the wound reduces infection rate[99, 100] but requires head gear, goggles, and protective cream to protect personnel from eye and skin damage. Lowell *et al*[101] suggest that it is vital to germicidal effect to control operating room humidity closely—a detail neglected in previous studies of germicidal lamps.

Application of laminar flow ventilation to operating rooms in an effort to reduce infection rates is notable because of the vast literature about it and its remarkable cost.[102–107] High efficiency particle air (HEPA) filters produce a 1,000-fold reduction of airborne particles larger than a half micron in the air supply. By virtue of a great increase in ventilation at the operative site (up to 500 air exchanges per hour as opposed to the 12 to 15 in ordinary operating rooms), particles shed by the operating team are excluded from the wound. Although this procedure can reduce bacterial counts, it is estimated that more than 5,000 matched cases would be required in a clinical study to show real reduction in the incidence of surgical infection caused by a single intervention such as laminar air flow. It is clear that the cost–benefit ratio would be most favorable in patients with prosthetic implants or reduced resistance to infection owing to age, disease, or therapy.

The flow of air in laminar flow rooms may be horizontal or vertical from a plenum (a chamber in which the air is under slight pressure and emitted to the operating room through multiple adjacent orifices). In the horizontal design, the plenum is mounted on one wall with the gas flow sweeping across the operative site horizontally. This is generally cheaper and easier to install in existing operating rooms than the vertical type, but it is, in practice, less easy to ensure

laminar flow at the operative site. The more effective design involves a ceiling plenum providing a high rate of laminar flow over the entire operative field. Large quantities of air must be blown through large surfaces of the HEPA filters and sweep through the room in a single pass. Thus, one might expect noise and drafts. The latter are not serious, as a linear air velocity of approximately 33 m·min^{-1} is perceived as only a gentle zephyr. As an additional feature, the Allander air curtain provides a peripheral frame of still higher flow of filtered air, which tends to entrain bacterial particles from the center of the field, and prevents particles in the rest of the room from entering the operative field when they are stirred up by personnel walking about.[102]

The thoughtless habit of entering a room without a cap and mask is not a serious break in technique in a laminar flow room, but turbulence can be generated by picking objects from the floor and depositing them on anesthesia machines or carts, thereby transiently defeating the laminar flow design. In general, these rooms reinforce good sterile technique rather than obviate the results of carelessness.

Since most rooms recirculate air through the HEPA filters, the anesthesiologist should be sure that the overflow scavengers exhaust by a separate route. The anesthesiologist should also be aware that the increased air flow at the operative site promotes drying of the operative field, increases patient cooling, and may limit or obscure some of the auditory clues that the anesthesiologist relies on subliminally. It is important to also remember that the operating room light may materially interfere with the designed laminar flow, as may operating room microscopes, radiograph machines, and other equipment. There should be regular checks of pressure, temperature, and humidity in laminar flow rooms.

There have been many previous studies of infection rates in operating rooms that are obsolete by present standards. Recent multi-institutional surveys usually disclose a wound infection rate of about 5% in all patients.[108] However, numerous studies of special devices report infection rates lower than 1%. This may be due to the device or to the increased consciousness of sterile technique associated with the study, or both.

AUTONOMIC HYPERREFLEXIA

Patients with spinal cord injuries often require orthopedic intervention for débridement of pressure sores, ischiotomies, osteotomies, or spinal fusions.[109, 110] Depending upon the level and completeness of cord section, the patient may require no anesthesia. However, because completeness of the lesion is not often certain and because of the possibility of autonomic hyperreflexia, anesthesia is often necessary. Autonomic hyperreflexia, a sudden massive sympathetic discharge with severe hypertension, results from reflex stimulation of the sympathetic neurons in the anterolateral column of the cord below the lesion which are not under higher control of the

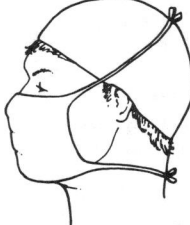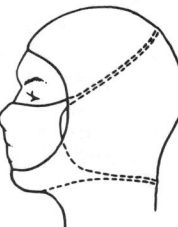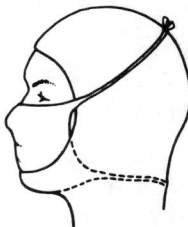

FIG. 43-5. Complete coverage of facial hair is best obtained with a full hood. Although mask-inside-hood *(center)* is recommended rather than mask-over-cap *(left)*, it is difficult to tie the mask directly over hair. An alternate method *(right)* involves tying the top ends over the hood and the bottom ones around the neck under the hood before tying the hood neck bands.

central nervous system.[111, 112] A lesion at or above mid-thoracic segments may be associated with this condition. Autonomic hyperreflexia may be treated by drugs that block the sympathetic system either at the central, ganglionic, or peripheral levels.

Adequate spinal or general anesthesia usually prevents occurrence of the syndrome. Some might think that the obvious central nervous system disease would serve as a contraindication to spinal anesthesia, but most anesthesiologists believe that if the lesion has not been progressing or improving, no harm will result from spinal anesthesia. Gentle handling of the spinal cord–injured patient is necessary to prevent hypotension resulting from a lack of vasomotor control. Massive potassium release may follow the use of succinylcholine; this drug is usually avoided.

POSTOPERATIVE CONSIDERATIONS

POSITIONING AND IMMOBILIZATION

Immobilization is an important part of orthopedic treatment during the weeks necessary for bone and ligament healing. General anesthesia should be maintained until the desired postoperative immobilization is ensured by cast, splint, sling, or bulky dressing. Smooth emergence is important, with avoidance of coughing and bucking during extubation of the trachea. Early use of postoperative analgesics can often be of value. Emergence delirium should be detected and treated early. After a patient has received regional anesthesia, the recovery room staff should be made aware of the patient's motor status and the importance of protecting a paralyzed limb from injury. To minimize postoperative edema and circulatory embarrassment, it is often desirable to keep the operated part of the body elevated. Careful padding and positioning of an extremity may be necessary to avoid nerve damage. The ulnar nerve may be predisposed to injury, augmented by pressure resulting from the Gardner elevator[113] (Fig. 43-6). The recovery room and nursing staff must be apprised of the proper postoperative positioning for each patient.

RELIEF OF PAIN

Postoperative pain is a frequent occurrence in orthopedics. The basic armamentarium for treatment of pain consists of immobilization, systemic analgesics, and local anesthetics. Epidural and intrathecal opioids are possible alternative options.

Immobilization and rest of the affected part is more practical in extremity than in trunk surgery because of the movements associated with ventilation in the latter. In adequate doses, systemic opioids are still the mainstay for postoperative pain relief.[114] With patients of advanced age and infirmity, prudence and caution in dosage are necessary, but it *is* important to ensure that sufficient drug is given to achieve the desired effect.[115] Initial routine orders must be tempered by observation of the patient's response, and the dose should be adjusted accordingly. One major concern in the use of opioid drugs is depression of ventilation. Use of several opioids of the agonist–antagonist type may minimize the risk of severe ventilatory depression, but these drugs (*e.g.*, buprenorphine, butorphanol, nalbuphine) do not always provide total relief for severe pain (see Chapter 14).

Both pharmacokinetic principles and experience suggest that initial loading and frequent multiple small doses are more

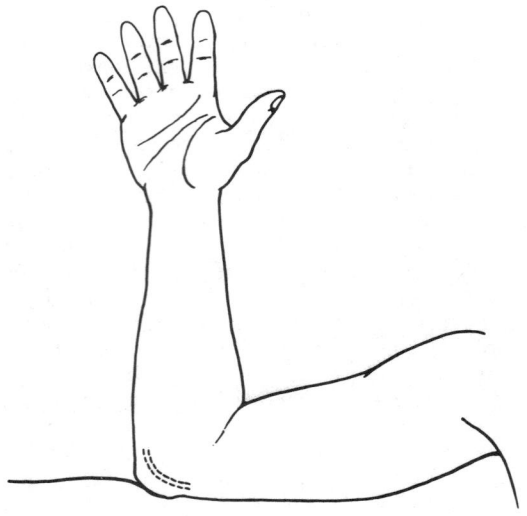

FIG. 43-6. After hand surgery, the forearm is often kept elevated to decrease swelling and pain by suspending it from an iv pole or other device. Care must be taken to either pad the ulnar nerve in the olecranon groove or elevate the hand enough to keep pressure off the nerve. The abducted humerus should be allowed to rotate caudad rather than let the hand go cephalad, to protect both the ulnar nerve and the brachial plexus.

likely to achieve smooth and safe analgesia than q 6-hour administrations. Parenteral administration by continuous infusion and demand injection into a continuous infusion have produced good results.[116–118] Patient-controlled analgesia has been given a firm pharmacokinetic basis by Tamsen *et al*.[119, 120]

Nerve blockade as an alternate to systemic analgesics may be particularly useful in extremity surgery. Epidural and intrathecal administration of opioids can also be useful.[121] Morphine, which is commonly used epidurally, may require 1 or 2 hours to reach peak efficacy.[122] The lipid-soluble drugs such as fentanyl and meperidine act more quickly, but their duration is shorter. Doses from 2 to 10 mg of morphine have been recommended, but good pain relief usually requires doses in the upper half of that range.[123] Despite considerable enthusiasm,[124] not all patients gain adequate relief. In addition to occasional severe respiratory depression, there may be annoying pruritis, distressing nausea and vomiting, and acute urinary retention.[118, 123, 125–128]

EMBOLIC PHENOMENA

Fat Embolism

Fat embolism is an ever-present threat in severely traumatized patients, especially those with long bone fractures.[129–131] The etiology seems to be related to mobilization of marrow fat from the cavity of fractured long bones. An important result of pulmonary fat embolism is hypoxia,[132, 133] often signalled by tachypnea and tachycardia. The affected lungs suffer a number of changes, including blockage of small pulmonary arterioles, interstitial pulmonary edema, epithelial damage permitting leakage of proteins into the interstitial and then the alveolar spaces, decrease in surfactant, and alveolar collapse. There is frequently a diphasic clinical course with initial disability attributed to mechanical effects of the blockade in the lesser circulation. Subsequent effects are caused by hydrolysis of the neutral fat to irritating free fatty acids and by migration of the fat to systemic circulatory beds. Signs include change in consciousness, petechial hemorrhages, fat globules in the urine and sputum, elevation of serum triglycerides and lipase, progressive anemia, and thrombocytopenia. In the late stages, the diseased lung becomes stiff (decreased compliance) and the vital capacity decreases.[130]

Blood gas analysis is a useful diagnostic measure. Oxygen tension below the expected value should make one suspicious of fat embolism. Early correction of hypoxia with increased inspired oxygen to produce a Pa_{O_2} in the range of 70 to 100 mm Hg, intubation of the trachea, and ventilation of the lungs with positive end-expiratory pressure (PEEP) are routine in the respiratory care of this syndrome. Other treatment measures that have been suggested include high doses of corticosteroids and the use of heparin, low–molecular weight dextran, and iv alcohol.[129, 134]

Thromboembolism

Venous thrombosis and pulmonary embolism are common complications in the postoperative period. The mechanism of development of venous thrombosis is not totally clear, but contributing factors include increased platelet adhesiveness, hypercoagulability of blood owing to activation of clotting factors, vessel wall lesions, and stagnation of blood in the venous system. The source of pulmonary emboli is usually the ileofemoral segment or the deep veins of the calf, where thrombosis may develop without obvious signs.

The risk of postoperative thromboembolism is increased with advanced age, immobilization, lack of muscle contraction in the lower extremities, a history of previous thromboembolism, congestive heart failure, decreased arterial flow to the extremities, estrogen therapy, gram-negative sepsis, carcinoma of the lung or pancreas, blood groups other than O, and trauma. It is clear that orthopedic patients share many of these risk factors.

In patients with pre-existing venous thrombosis, the anesthesiologist should avoid succinylcholine fasciculations to prevent mobilization of a thrombus. In the recovery room and throughout the postoperative period, the operated part should be examined to ensure that an immobilizing cast or dressing does not produce pressure and ischemia or cause undue obstruction to venous return.

The treatment of established venous thrombosis consists of elevation, rest, analgesics, anticoagulants, and antiplatelet agents to prevent extension. Administration of thrombolytic substances such as streptokinase or urokinase or surgical removal is sometimes considered.

Attempts to reduce the incidence of thrombosis by early ambulation, limb elevation, bed exercise, and support garments have some, but not complete success. Surprisingly, prolonged or continuous regional anesthesia may be desirable in preventing thromboembolism.[135–137] Other preventive methods include the use of high–molecular weight dextran and aspirin, with varying degrees of success. Reduction of anaphylactic reactions with hapten dextran of 1000 daltons molecular weight is bringing a resurgence of interest in dextran prophylaxis.[32, 138] Coumadin and heparin in low doses have produced good results in general surgical patients but may not be similarly effective in orthopedics. Anticoagulant treatment is probably more effective if initiated before surgery. Some surgeons, however, hesitate to operate on patients who are anticoagulated because of the increased incidence of bleeding and wound hematoma. The anesthesiologist may similarly be loath to administer an otherwise indicated regional anesthetic. Thus, initiation of anticoagulant therapy is often delayed until the postoperative period.

Xenobiotic Gas

Air embolism is largely a theoretical problem, as most orthopedic incisions are below the hydrostatic pressure level of the right atrium. But postoperatively, gas has been found in tissues from several interesting sources. Gas may be forced into tissues in long bone reaming and rodding, in hip arthroplasty from malfunction of nitrogen-powered tools, and even from extensive use of hydrogen peroxide.[139–141] Carbon dioxide used to distend the knee joint can dissect to the abdomen and even to the pericardium[142] (Fig. 43-7).

PAIN

Anesthesiologists' interest in relieving pain and suffering appropriately extends to the postoperative period. Immobilization of the operated part is a major part of such pain relief, but it is in part counterproductive to attempts at early ambulation, and, in some cases, it is impossible, as in lumbar spine operations. Some success has been reported with all the tools of the pain clinic, including opioids and partial opioid agonists, epidural and spinal local anesthetics and opioids, and even the transcutaneous electrical nerve stimulator (TENS).[143–147] Aside from humanitarian indications, pain relief preserving motor function may prevent postoperative muscle atrophy,[148] which may be sufficient reward to attract more anesthesia groups to provide prolonged pain relief. Buprenorphine, a long-acting agent, is increasingly used.[149, 150]

SPECIAL CONSIDERATIONS FOR SPECIFIC PROCEDURES

HIP FRACTURES

Hip fractures occur most often in elderly persons and may result from an apparently minor fall. When hip fractures occur in younger persons, they are usually due to motorcycle, automobile, and other high-impact accidents. In a study of more than 200 patients with fractured hips, Haljamae et al[151] found important nonorthopedic findings in 92% of patients, the majority of which required treatment or correction preoperatively. The average patient had correctable abnormalities in two major organ systems, underlining the importance of careful preoperative evaluation. Whereas adequate preparation of the elderly or the traumatized patient is essential,[152, 153] protracted delay without active therapy is associated with a greater incidence of aseptic necrosis of the head of the femur and a significant increase in mortality, largely owing to respiratory causes.

Preoperative evaluation and preparation of the patient for hip surgery should include careful assessment of blood volume. An apparently normal hemoglobin concentration may be a sign of dehydration, since many elderly patients exhibit low normal values. Hematomas containing more than a liter of blood may be unrecognized after fracture of the hip. In the absence of adequate fluid replacement, such a hematoma may not result in decreased hemoglobin or hematocrit. Evaluation and monitoring of fluid status may be facilitated by central

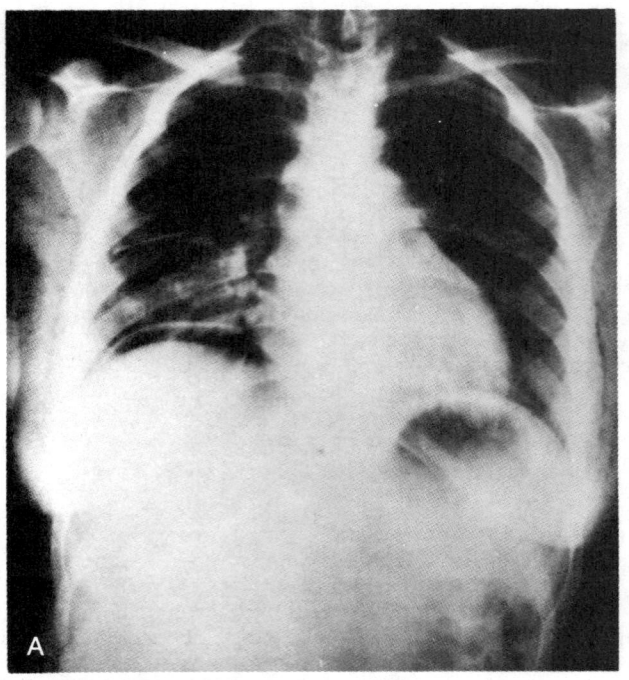
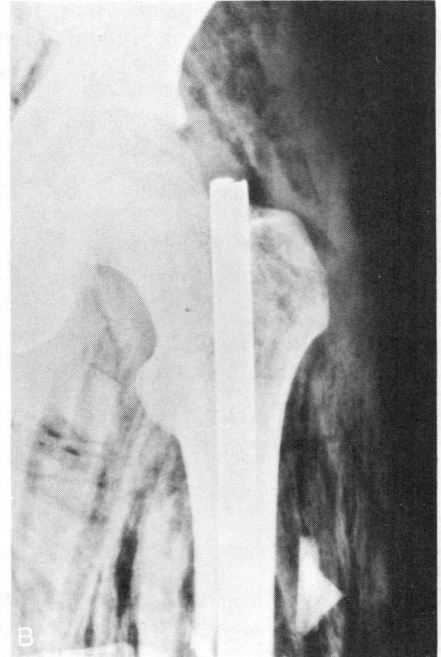
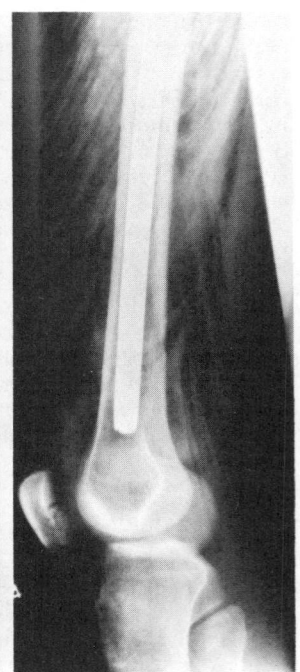
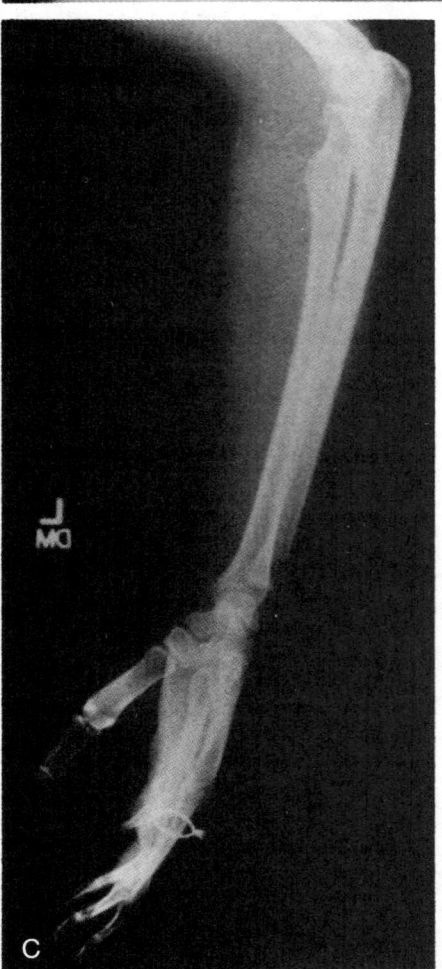

FIG. 43-7. Gas is demonstrable in tissue from three foreign sources. (A) Carbon dioxide is in the chest, dissected from the knee during arthroscopy; (B) nitrogen, which came from the power supply for pneumatically driven instruments; (C) an arm after hydrogen peroxide treatment. (Reprinted by permission from Shupak RC, Shuster H, Funch RS: Airway emergency in a patient during CO₂ arthroscopy. Anesthesiology 60:171, 1984; Whitehall R, Moskal JT, Scully KS et al: Nitrogen–gas injection from a power reamer: A complication of closed intramedullary nailing of the femur. J Bone Joint Surg 65A:860, 1983; Friedman RJ, Gumley GJ: Crepitation stimulating gas gangrene. J Bone Joint Surg 67A:646, 1985.)

venous pressure measurement, orthostatic stress testing, evaluation of urine output, and determination of urine sodium and osmolarity. The frequency of intraoperative hypothermia in these procedures makes temperature monitoring advisable.

Choice of anesthetic technique for urgent hip fractures remains controversial.[154] Some studies recommend spinal or epidural anesthesia,[155] and even femoral nerve blockade is espoused.[156] Wickstrom et al[157] found a lower immediate mortality after regional anesthesia than after dissociative or inhalation anesthesia, but after 1 month there was no difference. Mortality was similar to that reported by others—about 7%.[158] Although the patient's age, physical status, and type of fracture seem to be the most important determinants for survival, careful attention to details intra-and postoperatively (including thrombosis prophylaxis, oxygen therapy, continued hemodilution, and pain relief with nerve blockade) are also important factors.[159] The combination of trauma and age may produce extraordinarily long gastric emptying times, and the possibility of a full stomach must always be considered.

Continuous spinal anesthesia is often useful in such patients.[24, 160] The technical problems of lumbar puncture and insertion of a subarachnoid catheter in the elderly are compounded by the patient's pain, but this can be minimized for the patient in the lateral decubitus position with traction. Immediately after the catheter is inserted, the patient is returned to the supine position, with maintenance of traction of the fractured limb. After the first few milliliters of spinal solution (hypobaric if the fractured hip is up, hyperbaric if down) are injected, there is sufficient relief of pain to permit moving the patient to the fracture table. Once the patient is supine, a hypobaric solution best maintains or augments the blockade. Supine, the lumbar nerve roots are highest in the spinal canal. Isobaric solutions are also useful, as are rapid injections of heavy solutions through a catheter; turbulence minimizes spread "down" the canal to higher spinal levels.

If the lateral decubitus is the desired surgical position, hypobaric spinal anesthesia may be induced with the patient in the operative position, eliminating the need for further movement. Gentle traction on the injured limb and a pillow between the legs will decrease discomfort. Despite the large spinal needle used in these cases, post–lumbar puncture headache is not an important consideration. The incidence of headache is low in elderly people, and this group of patients is rarely nursed in an upright position immediately postoperatively.[24]

Gentle handling is a must, since hypotension may occur with either regional or general anesthesia, especially in debilitated and elderly patients. To lie awake, immobile, for several hours of operation is difficult. Etomidate or other sedatives may be of help.[161] Light planes of general anesthesia may be maintained during positioning. Small iv doses of ketamine (25-mg increments until the sensorium is depressed) usually permit safe and easy positioning without hypotension or airway obstruction.

HIP JOINT REPLACEMENT

This procedure is a common one owing to the frequency of disabling pain and limitation of motion produced by a variety of diseases such as osteoarthritis, traumatic arthritis, rheumatoid arthritis, aseptic necrosis of the femoral head, and congenital hip disease. Smith–Peterson's concept of a mould arthroplasty brought remarkable relief to some patients[162] (Fig. 43-8). The cup, which was originally of glass and later of vitallium, induced the formation of fibrous cartilage, and even a synovium-like lining of a joint space in some patients, after which it was removed. However, unsatisfactory results in some patients included continued pain despite good motion, aseptic necrosis with bone collapse, cup migration, and infection. Moore and Thompson introduced prostheses that were essentially balls on stalks. These implants, however, could result in pain and acetabular erosion.

A number of biomechanical principles were appreciated and applied by Charnley in the 1960s.[163] He pioneered total replacement of the hip joint with a low friction bearing, a small ball so that more material could be placed in the acetabular component to provide for wear, a small neck diameter relative to the ball to improve mobility, flexibility of the shaft to simulate the flexibility of bone, and, in particular, the use of acrylic

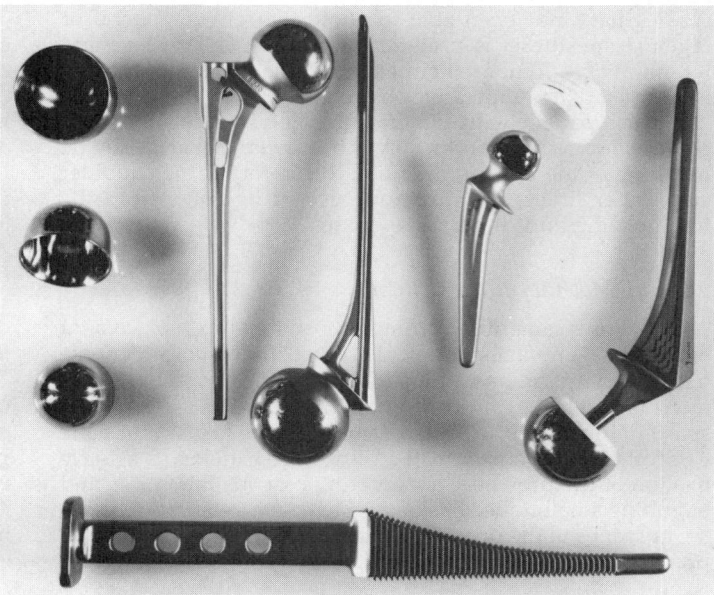

FIG. 43-8. Three generations of hip prostheses: At left are three Smith–Peterson arthroplasty cups, and in the center are two sizes of Austin–Moore nails. At the right are two modern bipolar prostheses, a Charnley with a small ball and plastic acetabular component, and a modification showing the figuring on the humeral stem to aid fixation with cement. Below is a precision reamer.

bone cement to transmit forces from the prosthesis to a broad surface of the femoral cortex, thus minimizing loosening and postoperative failure.[164] It is now recognized that ultimate success or failure of any surgical implant depends upon many elements, including physical, mechanical, and biochemical properties of the implant material; design, construction, and surface finish of the implant; operative technique; and postoperative management of the patient. Charnley further highlighted the importance of measures to prevent infection. His published series show a decrease in the infection rate from 5% to well below 1%.

Attempts to improve on his results with other bearing materials (such as Teflon and nylon, which unfortunately abraded to produce increased tissue reaction) or with different bearing surfaces such as trunion joints (which wore out of round irregularly) have not added substantially to progress in hip prostheses. They have, however, stimulated development of artificial joints for knees, shoulders, and other joint improvement. Currently, materials for implants are chosen with a view to the yield strength, tensile strength, ductility, and resistance to fatigue. The bulk of metal prostheses are cobalt chromium alloys or stainless steel, but titanium, tantalum, and an occasional exotic alloy have been used. The materials and methods of manufacture have been chosen to produce high corrosion resistance, low crevice formation, and little or no local irritation. High-density polyethylene for low friction and silicone elastomers for high flexibility are examples of materials chosen for special properties.

The surgical procedure is generally accomplished in the lateral decubitus position. As with hip fracture, there is no general agreement as to the type of anesthesia that is most appropriate for these procedures. In more than 200 operations, Sculco and Ranawat[27] found that complications were less frequent with spinal anesthesia. In a prospective study of 157 consecutive patients, Roseberg et al[25] found that surgical blood loss could be related directly to blood pressure, with the least loss following general anesthesia with deliberate hypotension, using nitroprusside. Somewhat more blood loss occurred with epidural anesthesia, and the most blood was lost during normotensive general anesthesia.[25] Hole et al[23, 36, 165, 166] found clear-cut advantages for epidural versus general anesthesia in the postoperative course. In regard to postoperative ventilatory function and mental recovery, studies have not been able to show that either general or regional anesthesia is preferable.[20, 167, 168] Similarly, urinary retention may occur after either anesthetic regimen, probably more related to preoperative obstruction than to anesthesia.[124] As in the patient with hip fracture, good management includes slow accurate induction of the anesthetic level, gentle handling of the patient, attention to comfort of the shoulder and upper limbs, and judicious use of iv drugs from the tranquilizing and dissociative classes.

Methyl Methacrylate Cement

Acrylic bone cement is commonly used in hip replacement operations. The anesthesiologist must understand its function, its complications, and their treatment. Acrylic bone cement is a self-polymerizing methyl methacrylate used as a space-filling mortar to transmit compressive loads from bone to prothesis to bone.[168] It is not a glue. It helps to achieve fixation of the prosthesis by entering osseous interstices and engulfing small trabeculae of the bone surface and deliberate irregularities in the prosthesis, producing a tight fit. Available preparations consist of two parts: 1) a powder of spherical granules of polymerized methyl methacrylate with an activator and anti-inhibitor to initiate polymerization, and sometimes other additives such as carbon fibers for strength or barium sulfate for radiopacity[169]; and 2) liquid methyl methacrylate monomer with a polymerization inhibitor such as hydroquinone. The exothermic polymerization process is begun by mixing as little liquid as possible with the powder to achieve a semisolid that can be squeezed or injected into desired cavities. Within minutes after mixing (the time may vary slightly with ambient temperature and humidity), the cement loses its tacky surface and is ready to be implanted. Hardening occurs in the next few minutes with the release of heat, the extent of which depends upon the amount of liquid used. The temperature of a ball of cement with a radius of 1 cm may reach over 100° C in the interior. Thus, there is a potential for tissue necrosis in the vicinity of large globs.

During mixing, the odor of the monomer is perceivable throughout the entire room and is objectionable to some, although it is not known to be a biological hazard. Shrouded mixing bowls attached to suction lines or the scavenging system in the operating room are available to minimize this problem.

Insertion of the cement has sometimes been associated with sudden episodes of hypotension in some, but not all, patients.[170] During N_2O-opioid-muscle relaxant anesthesia, mean rises in pressure were reported, although one fourth of the patients had an initial fall in blood pressure.[171] Hypotension has been attributed to vasodilating effects of the absorbed volatile monomer,[172-176] to emboli forced into the circulation by the force of insertion of the prosthesis into a reamed and curetted medullary bone,[139, 177] to effects of heating of bone marrow and blood cells with release of thrombotic and vasoactive substances,[178] or to hydrolysis of the methyl methacrylate to methacrylate acid.[179]

All the postulated mechanisms probably play a role in one patient or another, judging from the variability in time and extent of hypotension.[180] The degree of hypotension probably depends upon the condition of capacitance vessels in a particular patient. If these vessels are constricted, as is the case in hypovolemic patients, sudden vasodilation results in a significant decrease in arterial blood pressure. If the patient is normovolemic and the vasculature is well filled, or if the vessels are dilated through the use of deliberate hypotension, the decrease in blood pressure may be minimal. The hypotensive effect may appear within 30 to 60 seconds after insertion of the cement, or up to 10 minutes after the prosthesis is inserted. It usually terminates spontaneously in less than 5 minutes. The hypotension may be prevented or treated with vasopressor drugs such as ephedrine. Cardiac arrest with less than a 50% recovery rate has been reported following application of bone cement in the femoral shaft, but this is a grossly higher mortality rate than is currently experienced, albeit not reported. Autopsy reports have revealed severe degrees of pulmonary fat and bone marrow emboli.[134, 181] Such pulmonary embolism results from the high femoral medullary pressure generated during cement insertion and may be prevented by venting the femoral shaft during insertion of the cement and prosthesis.[182]

In addition to hypotension, a sudden decrease in arterial oxygen tension, presumably resulting from fat and marrow emboli, has been observed in some patients.[180, 183] This can be prevented by maximizing alveolar oxygen tension before femoral cement insertion.[184] In one patient, cement intended to stabilize cervical spine surgery extruded anteriorly, obstructing the airway.[185]

The cement used may be subjected to centrifugation to help

eliminate air bubbles in an effort to improve the mechanical strength of the prosthetic–bone interface,[186] but the process is controversial.[187] The cement may have antibiotic added, perhaps useful in infected operative sites.[188] The cement may be replaced, in the future, with prostheses allowing bone growth into the appliance, as with sintered metal coatings, but the latter may have their own sets of problems, usually late post-implantation.[189, 190]

PROCEDURES ON THE EXTREMITIES

Operations on the Upper Limb

Perhaps the most frequent use of regional anesthetic procedures is for surgery of the hand, forearm, elbow, and arm. There are a variety of techniques, described in detail in Chapter 29, including iv (Bier) blockade, specific nerve blockades of digital, ulnar, median, radial, musculocutaneous, intercostobrachialis, and the brachial plexus. There is no substitute for thorough anatomic grounding in performing these blockades. Given that fact, each limb should be individually examined before a final decision has been made as to the approach. The description of axillary blockade by Thompson in Seattle, Winnie in Chicago, and Murphy in Philadelphia are nearly as different as their home cities. All can produce satisfactory working conditions, and the aim should be to reduce failure to a low level.

In that regard, the anesthesiologist should be prepared to "rescue" a blockade by supplementation with another, usually more distal blockade. Early detection of a partial failure by sensory and motor observation will permit "rescue" by a specific blockade of the missed nerve (Fig. 43-9). To do this, the anesthesiologist must have sufficient experience and insistence to differentiate a slow onset of blockade from a missed nerve before the orthopedic prepping and draping is complete. Sensory testing with a sterile needle can continue through the scrub without violating aseptic principles. Motor function may be tested during the prep as well. The anesthesiologist can also arrange to perform the blockade elsewhere to permit 30 minutes or more of "soak" time with reduction in the number of failed blockades. Lidocaine diffuses better through tissue than does mepivacaine or bupivacaine.

The steps in performing the various regional blockades are found elswhere; however, I cannot refrain from noting three factors about axillary approaches to the nerves of the brachial plexus. First, palpating excessively high in the axilla is ill advised. It is harder to feel the axillary artery, and the pressure of the probing finger distorts the anatomy. When the finger is withdrawn, the sheath moves back to the normal position, so that the needle is effectively placed too deep. Second, the nerves as well as vessels can often be easily felt distal to the crossing of the coracobrachialis by the pectoralis major, by having the arm abducted 70 to 80 degrees flat on a table or armboard, with the forearm flexed 90 degrees and pointing upward. The anesthesiologist can then pluck the structures in the sheath much like a guitarist plucks his strings. Third, the sheath is relatively superficial just dorsad (below in this position) to the coracobrachialis. If the tip of the needle is placed subcutaneously and if the skin is moved slightly back and forth as the needle is advanced, one can often appreciate a scratching sensation and the fixation of the point of the needle in the investing facia at a depth about equal to a skin fold pinched at the site—1.5–2.25 cm is the range in the majority. Any insertion much deeper has probably passed through the sheath to provide a solid blockade of the muscle fibers of the triceps.

Closed Reduction of Fractures or Dislocations

These procedures present a special set of considerations. They are usually of short duration, especially reductions of dislocated joints, and usually require analgesia and nearly complete skeletal muscle paralysis. Most closed reductions are performed as emergency procedures to avoid loss of blood supply and aseptic necrosis. Prior attempts to reduce a dislocation under the muscle relaxing effect of diazepam and/or morphine, if unsuccessful, bring a depressed patient to the anesthesiologist. Patients recently may have had a full meal. Thus, Bier (intravenous regional) blockades are useful in distal dislocations,[191] or plexus anesthesia may be used when it is not contraindicated by vascular or nerve damage. When closed reduction is performed as an elective procedure, a brief general anesthetic technique with succinylcholine for skeletal muscle relaxation is efficient. Fasciculations may further dislocate or fracture long bone segments or result in vascular or nerve damage. Although a slow iv drip of succinylcholine or "self-taming" may be used instead of bolus injections to avoid violent muscular movements, more commonly, pretreatment with a nondepolarizing neuromuscular paralysant in a small dose blocks fasciculations.

Operations on the Shoulder

Perhaps the most frequent use of general anesthesia in orthopedic surgery is for shoulder operations. The proximity of the awake patient's head to the operative site suggests that unpleasant sensory inputs will be more annoying than those from more distant operative sites. Furthermore, an adequate regional procedure requires either a supraclavicular blockade such as Winnie's subclavian perivascular approach, or paravertebral plus interscalene blockades, which are relatively unfamiliar to many anesthesiologists.[192] Nonetheless, an anesthesiologist may confidently recommend a blockade secure in the knowledge that any procedure in the orthopedic repertoire for the shoulder can be done painlessly with a regional procedure. Preoperative informative interviews, analgesic

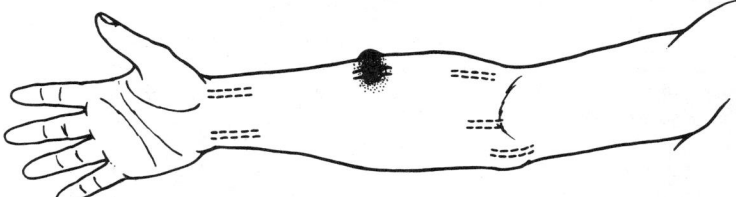

FIG. 43-9. Diagram of arm with suggestions for blockade of radial (at elbow and forearm), ulnar (at elbow and forearm), and median nerve (at elbow and forearm). Either the anesthesiologist or surgeon may be able to forestall a general anesthetic by supplemental blockade of a distal nerve.

and sedative adjuvants, and intraoperative support are solutions to the largely perceptual problems.

Operations on the Knee

A variety of techniques are available for these procedures. Arthroscopy may be done with field blockade and intraarticular local anesthetic,[193] with the "three-in-one-block" plus lateral femoral cutaneous nerve blockade,[194] with a limited epidural, and with hypobaric spinal analgesia. The latter is relatively easy to confine to low thoracic levels (T-9 or T-12) by very slowly (>60 sec) injecting 10 to 12 mg in 5 to 6 ml of sterile water, providing 3 to 4 hours of analgesia. Intraoperative tourniquet pain may be encountered and treated with opioid analgesics (vide supra).

Amputations

Amputation of part of an extremity may be required when insufficient blood supply results in gangrene. The most common causes of gangrene are peripheral vascular disease, especially in diabetics, and trauma with devascularization or gas gangrene. The patient undergoing amputation may present important systemic diseases (diabetes, cardiovascular disease, sepsis) that require careful preoperative evaluation and the cooperation of consultants to ensure optimal preparation. Analgesic drugs are often administered for pain control and should be continued until anesthesia is induced. Cryoanesthesia, achieved by packing the limb in ice for 12 to 24 hours, is an old but still occasionally useful method, conferring pain control, surgical anesthesia, and remission of toxemia as absorption from the gangrenous limb is decreased.

Spinal anesthesia is often preferred for lower extremity amputations if there are no contraindications, although the advantages are demonstrable only in the first 24 hours.[195] A hypnotic dose of a short-acting barbiturate may be given just before sawing of the bone to spare the patient psychological trauma. An amnestic state from diazepam, lorazepam, or midazolam injection is not entirely reliable in this regard, resulting in an incidence of true amnesia of 50–80%. Tourniquets may be used in younger patients for post-traumatic amputation, but they are generally omitted when the surgeon wishes to identify viable tissue or fears damage to sclerotic vessels in elderly patients.

Regional anesthesia in some patients produces a subjective sensation that the blocked extremity occupies a position different from the actual one. This phantom limb syndrome[196] is named after the phantom limb pain that some amputees experience long after their amputation. The patient has the impression that the extremity is floating up, slightly flexed, often in the same position as it was when afferent conduction was interrupted. The phantom sensation disappears after nerve conduction is restored. There is no established explanation for the phantom sensation.

Joint Manipulation and Examination

Joints with limited range of motion are sometimes manipulated in order to break up adhesions. The procedure is short and almost always elective and may be performed under thiopental–nitrous oxide anesthesia. Succinylcholine at 0.5 mg·kg^{-1} suffices, and tracheal intubation is not necessary. Opioid premedication together with reduction of the barbiturate dosage iv is helpful in relieving postmanipulation pain without significantly prolonged emergence.

REPLANTATION OF LIMBS AND DIGITS

Microsurgical anastomosis of vessels and nerves permits remarkable salvage of traumatic amputations. The anesthetic problems are largely related to the extraordinary duration of some of these operations.[197, 198] Interruption of sympathetic innervation is thought to be important, giving rise to use of catheter techniques for continuous blockades. Adequate sedation and analgesia are challenges often best met by light continuous general anesthesia. More than usual attention must be given to positioning in order to avoid necrosis at pressure areas, to humidification of inspired gas, and to fluid intake and output, all because of the prolonged procedures. A team of anesthesiologists may be needed to provide maintained vigilance.[197] Hypothermia should be avoided, since vasoconstriction and shivering postoperatively may jeopardize the reimplanted tissue.

OPERATIONS ON THE SPINE

The most common procedures on the spine include spinal fusion (for scoliosis, vertebral fracture, or spine instability) and operations for herniated intervertebral disc, including laminectomy, microdissectomy, and chemonucleolysis. Common to the majority of these procedures is the necessity for the prone position,[199, 200] although, rarely, surgeons may use the lateral position. The sitting position is used for some posterior cervical laminectomies, and the supine position is used for anterior cervical fusion. Fiberoptic-assisted intubation of the trachea is advantageous in many of these patients with severe or unstable spines.[201] In positioning the patient, one weighs the conflicting needs for surgical exposure, freedom of ventilation and venous return, and patient comfort and safety.

Several methods have been developed for prone positioning. The most commonly used methods include use of the Wilson and Relton frames[42] and the Georgia prone position.[202] Other devices place the weight of the buttocks on a seat or support with the thighs flexed (the Mohammedan praying position),[43] or on a pelvic frame.[203] In most instances, the surgeon's aim is to flatten or reverse the lumbar lordosis and the anesthesiologist's aim is to provide free excursion, either laterally or ventrally for the abdomen. Both are interested in preventing engorgement of the epidural venous system, which results in increased venous oozing. These aims can be accomplished if the iliac crest can be held securely and if the pelvis is allowed to tilt or, more commonly, if flexion of the thigh creates tension in the gluteal muscles accomplishing the same end result.

The neck should be kept in the same plane as the back and slightly flexed to avoid strain and postanesthetic discomfort. The arms should be well padded and pointing cephalad, with the elbows at the level of the head and somewhat anterior. The head must be supported with attention paid to avoid injuring the eyes or kinking the airway. Sufficient help must be available during positioning to avoid exceeding a patient's normal range of motion of the spine and extremities. A useful technique is neuroleptanalgesia plus topical anesthesia for awake intubation, so that the patient may pronate comfortably and safely before losing consciousness.[204]

Spinal Fusion

Scoliosis is a deformity of the thoracolumbar spine and rib cage caused by lateral deviation and rotation of the vertebral bodies. One hemithorax is compressed toward residual volume, and the other is expanded toward total lung capacity. When the angle of the deformity exceeds 65 degrees, there is severe functional change in the respiratory system as both hemithoraces are on flattened (*e.g.*, stiff) portions of their pressure volume curves.[205] A decrease in total lung capacity and residual volume plus mechanical impairments lead to an increase in the work of breathing and alveolar hypoventilation. Ventilation/perfusion mismatch with increased physiologic shunting and dead space increases the functional severity of the deformity. The result is a decrease in arterial oxygen tension, an increase in the alveolar-arterial difference for oxygen, and an increase in arterial carbon dioxide tension (Fig. 43-10).

The kyphoscoliotic patient with chronic hypercapnia responds subnormally to further elevations of carbon dioxide tension, hypoventilates when inhaling a high inspired oxygen concentration, and may be unusually sensitive to depressant drugs (*e.g.*, opioids and barbiturates). Pulmonary vascular resistance is elevated and leads to right ventricular hypertrophy and cor pulmonale. In the patient with respiratory symptoms or with a significant curvature, preoperative pulmonary function testing and arterial blood gas analysis should be performed to determine the severity of the impairment. The ECG is helpful in detecting cor pulmonale. When nonoperative treatment is unsuccessful in arresting the progression of deformity, and when the deformity has progressed to a degree that will predictably cause severe respiratory or cardiovascular embarrassment, surgery becomes mandatory.[206] In these instances, postoperative ventilatory support in an intensive care unit may be necessary, since respiratory deteriora-

FIG. 43-10. Pressure–volume diagram of chest wall and lung *(top)* and approximate position at end-expiratory lung volume of the hyperinflated (convex) and hypoinflated (concave) hemithorax. Note that both are on flattened (less compliant) portions of the PV curve.

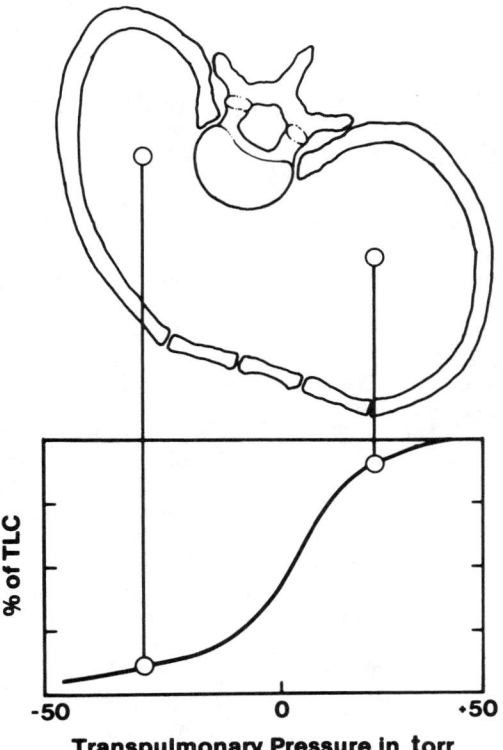

tion in the immediate postoperative period is common.[207] Risk factors include mental retardation, anterior approaches, age over 20 years, preoperative hemoglobin desaturation, and obstructive as well as restrictive lung disease.[208]

Regional and general anesthesia may be used separately or may be combined for scoliosis surgery.[209] It is more important to attend to ventilatory and cardiovascular function than to search for a single best anesthetic, and the anesthesiologist must closely follow estimates of blood loss, fluid requirements, and changing effects of mechanical ventilation of the lungs.

In patients who are having spinal fusions for scoliosis, the anesthesiologist faces problems of blood loss and spinal cord function. Deliberate hypotension has gained widespread acceptance for minimizing blood loss in the procedure. A variety of hypotensive techniques have been used.[74, 75, 210, 211] Hemodynamic and hormonal analysis suggests that sodium nitroprusside produces safe hypotension with preservation of central nervous system blood flow and oxygen consumption, and maintenance of some degree of autoregulation of spinal cord blood flow.[212] Assurance that cord function has not been impaired can be provided by two different techniques. Waldman *et al*[213] have described a wakeup technique before closure to ensure that voluntary motion of the lower extremity remains, but the technique is not foolproof.[213] Grundy *et al*[214] have shown that the somatosensory evoked response can be used in a nearly continuous fashion for the same purpose. A continuous opioid infusion technique has been adapted to either method.[216]

Patients with kyphoscoliosis who may require anesthesia for other surgical procedures (*e.g.*, labor and delivery, abdominal surgery) are prepared for surgery and managed in a similar way.[217] Scoliosis may be associated with a high risk of malignant hyperpyrexia in the patient suffering from myotonia dystrophica. But previous posterior spinal fusion is not a contraindication to lumbar epidural blockade.[218]

Herniated Intervertebral Disc

This problem may be treated with extensive laminectomy, microlaminectomy and dissectomy, or chemonucleolysis. In the first two types of procedures, positioning for optimal surgical exposure without circulatory or ventilatory embarrassment is the major problem.[219] The choice of anesthesia is generally endotracheal inhalational anesthesia with a variety of muscle relaxants and adjuvants, but spinal[26] epidural,[220] and local anesthesia have been successfully applied. Muscle relaxants facilitate surgical exposure in laminectomy but abolish muscle movement upon nerve root stimulation. When this type of response is desired, relaxants must be avoided or the surgeon must be assured that their effect has waned by evidence provided through neuromuscular stimulation elsewhere. Partial paralysis facilitates surgical exposure without deep anesthesia, but total abolition of neuromuscular transmission is not essential.

Blood loss is rarely sufficient to require deliberate hypotension. Cyanotic blood in the surgical field may be due to venous stasis and not to hypoxia.[221] Especially after microdissectomy, stability of the back is rarely compromised, and the patient may be transported and nursed in any position thought desirable.

Smith began testing chemonucleolysis in 1963,[222] but a variety of events slowed approval of chymopapain, the drug used in the procedure,[223] in the United States. Accumulated experience following approval in Canada and England was followed by approval by the U.S. Food and Drug Administration of chymopapain in 1982.[224] This drug lyses mucopolysaccharides, but not the annular ring of the ruptured disc. A rapid decrease in size of the herniated mass is attributed to loss of the mucopolysaccharide's ability to bind water.

With the patient in the lateral decubitus position, a needle is introduced into the disc under fluoroscopic guidance, and a discogram is obtained to demonstrate pathology. It is desirable to avoid cerebrospinal fluid (CSF) puncture and injection of the dye or drug into the epidural space. General anesthesia is most frequently used despite some advantages claimed for local anesthesia.[225] The anesthetic management is uneventful except for the occurrence of uncommon but severe allergic reactions,[226] signs of which include flushing, tachycardia, hypotension, wheezing, and edema of skin, larynx, and lung. The treatment is administration of epinephrine, which aborts degranulation of mass cells and histamine release. Anticipating this treatment, most anesthesiologists avoid the use of halothane and choose enflurane, isoflurane, or a balanced supplement with nitrous oxide. Steroids and aminophylline should be available for immediate parenteral use, but their prophylactic use has not been validated. A rational but also unvalidated treatment would be the use of both histamine$_1$ and histamine$_2$ blockers in premedication (e.g., diphenhydramine, cimetidine).

The final New Drug application to the U.S. Food and Drug Administration contained 909 patients treated with chymopapain, with 9 cases of anaphylaxis. The majority were in women with erythrocyte sedimentation rates greater than 20 mm·hr^{-1}. A multicenter double-blind study demonstrated clinical efficacy of chymopapain with 90% successful outcomes and no anaphylaxis.[227] The surgical procedure was taught in a training course sponsored jointly by the American Academy of Orthopedic Surgeons and the American Association of Neurological Surgeons. The drug produces local capillary dissolution leading to the possibility of hematoma formation in muscle, intrathecally, or in the disc itself. Alpha$_2$ macroglobulins in the plasma inactivate the drug if it is given systemically. The enthusiasm for chemonucleolysis in the early 1980s is now clearly waning, as evidenced by the paucity of published papers since the 1980–1983 period.

REFERENCES

1. Office for Medical Applications of Research, National Institutes of Health: Consensus Conferences. Total Hip-joint Replacement. JAMA 243:1817, 1982

2. Farfan HF: Major sports injury. Clin Orthop 164:2, 1982

3. Merz B: Try a carbon ribbon 'round the old hurt knee (and shoulder). JAMA 248:1681,1982

4. Pilliar RM, Blackwell R, Macnab I et al: A carbon fiber–reinforced bone cement in orthopedic surgery. J Biomed Mater Res 10:893, 1976

5. Law HT: Engineering of upper limb prostheses. Orthop Clin North Am 12:929, 1981

6. Solomonow M: Restoration of movement by electrical stimulation. Orthopedics 7:245, 1984

7. Connelly JF (ed): Clinical application of bioelectrical effects. Clin Orthop 161:2, 1981

8. Pietrafesa CA, Hoffman JR: Traumatic dislocation of the hip. JAMA 249:3342, 1983

9. Banks HH: Symposium on care of the critically ill orthopedic patient. Orthop Clin North Am 9:3, 1978

10. Stehling L: Anesthesia for children requiring orthopedic surgery. Anesthesiol Rev 5:19, 1978

11. Stiles CM: Anesthesia for the mentally retarded. Orthop Clin North Am 12:45, 1981

12. Poticha SM: Management of patients with multiple injuries. In Beal JM (ed): Critical Care for Surgical Patients. New York, Macmillan, 1982

13. Olsson GL, Hallen B: Pharmacologic evacuation of the stomach with metoclopramide. Acta Anaesth Scand 26:417, 1982

14. Marbach JJ, Spiera H: Rheumatoid spondylitis and systemic lupus erythematosus with temporomandibular joint changes. NY State Med J 69:2908, 1969

15. Phelps JA: Laryngeal obstruction due to cricoarytenoid arthritis. Anesthesiology 27:518, 1966

16. Calabro JJ, Maltz BA: Ankylosing spondylitis. N Engl J Med 282:606, 1970

17. Edelist G: Principles of anesthetic management in rheumatoid arthritic patients. Anesth Analg 43:227, 1964

18. Ellison N, Mull TD: Unique anesthetic problems in the elderly patient coming to surgery for fracture of the hip. Orthop Clin North Am 5:493, 1974

19. Sari A, Miyauchi Y, Yamashita S et al: The magnitude of hypoxemia in elderly patients with fractures of the femoral neck. Anesth Analg 65:892, 1986

20. Berggren D, Gustafson Y, Eriksson B et al: Confusion after anesthesia in elderly patients with femoral neck fractures. Anesth Analg 66:497, 1987

21. Katz J, Aidinis SJ: Complications of spinal and epidural anesthesia. J Bone Surg 62:1219, 1980

22. Davis FM, Laurenson VG: Spinal anaesthesia or general anaesthesia for emergency hip surgery in elderly patients. Anaesth Intensive Care 9:352, 1981

23. Hole A, Terjesen T, Breivik H: Epidural versus general anaesthesia for total hip arthroplasty in elderly patients. Acta Anaesth Scand 24:279, 1980

24. Kallos T, Smith TC: Continuous spinal anesthesia with hypobaric tetracaine for hip surgery in lateral decubitus. Anesth Analg 51:766, 1972

25. Rosberg B, Fredin H, Gustafson C: Anesthetic techniques and surgical blood loss in total hip arthroplasty. Acta Anaesth Scand 26:189, 1982

26. Rosenberg MK, Berner G: Spinal anesthesia in lumbar disc surgery: Review of 200 cases, with a case history. Anesth Analg 44:419, 1965

27. Sculco TP, Ranawat C: The use of spinal anesthesia for total hip-replacement arthroplasty. J Bone Joint Surg 57A:173, 1975

28. Mebius C, Hedenstierna G: Airway closure and gas distribution during hip arthroplasty. Acta Anaesth Scand 26:72, 1982

29. Hedenstierna G, Mebius C, Bygdeman S: Ventilation—perfusion relationship during hip arthroplasty. Acta Anaesth Scand 27:56, 1983

30. Engquist A, Brandt MR, Fernandes A et al: The blocking effect of epidural analgesia on the adrenocortical and hyperglycemic responses to surgery. Acta Anaesth Scand 21:330, 1977

31. Davis FM, Laurenson VG: Spinal anaesthesia or general anaesthesia for emergency hip surgery in elderly patients. Anaesth Intensive Care 9:352, 1981

32. Fredin H, Gustafson C, Rosberg B: Hypotensive anesthesia, thromboprophylaxis and postoperative thromboembolism in total hip arthroplasty. Acta Anaesth Scand 28:503, 1984

33. Modig J, Borg T, Bagge L et al: Role of extradural and of general anesthesia in fibrinolysis and coagulation after total hip replacement. Br J Anaesth 55:625, 1983

34. Modig J, Malberg P, Karlstrom G: Effect of epidural versus general anaesthesia on calf blood flow. Acta Anaesth Scand 24:305, 1980

35. Benoni G, Johnell O, Rosberg B: Postoperative course of serum aminotransferases after total hip arthroplast. J Bone Joint Surg 69A:255, 1987

36. Hole A, Unsgaard G, Breivik H: Monocyte functions are depressed during and after surgery under general anaesthesia but

not under epidural anaesthesia. Acta Anaesth Scand 26:301, 1983

37. Scott DB, Schweitzer S, Thron J: Epidural block in postoperative pain relief. Reg Anesth 7:135, 1982

38. McKenzie PJ, Wishart HY, Smith G: Long-term outcome after repair of fractured neck of femur. Br J Anaesth 56:581, 1984

39. Amaranath L, Esfandiari S, Lockrem J et al: Epidural analgesia for total hip arthroplasty in a patient with dilated cardiomyopathy. Can Anaesth Soc J 33:84, 1986

40. Inaz E, Theiss D, Emmerich EA et al: Regional versus general anesthesia: Attitudes and experiences of patients. Reg Anesth 7:S163, 1982

41. Rosenbert TD, Wong HC: Arthroscope knee surgery in a free-standing outpatient center. Orthop Clin North Am 13:277, 1982

42. Relton JES, Hall JE: An operation frame for spinal fusion: A new apparatus designed to reduce hemorrhage during operation. J Bone Joint Surg 49:327, 1957

43. Dinmore P: A new operating position for posterior spinal surgery. Anaesthesia 32:377, 1977

44. Michenfelder JD, Miller RH, Gronert GA: Evaluation of an ultrasonic device (Doppler) for the diagnosis of venous air embolism. Anesthesiology 36:164, 1972

45. Brechner VL, Bethune RWM: Recent advances in monitoring pulmonary air embolism. Anesth Analg 50:255, 1971

46. Michenfelder JD: Central venous catheters in the management of air embolism: Whether as well as where. Anesthesiology 55:339, 1981

47. McEwen JA, Auchinleck GF: Advances in surgical tourniquets. AORN J 36:889, 1982

48. Hurst LN, Weinglein O, Brown WF et al: The pneumatic tourniquet: A biomechanical and electrophysiologic study. Plast Reconstr Surg 67:648, 1981

49. Shaw JA, Murray DG: The relationship between tourniquet pressure and underlying soft-tissue pressure in the thigh. J Bone Joint Surg 64:1148, 1982

50. Hofman AA, Wyatt RWB: Fatal pulmonary embolism following tourniquet inflation. J Bone Joint Surg 67A:633, 1985

51. Pollard BJ, Lovelock HA, Jones RM: Fatal pulmonary embolism secondary to limb exsanguination. Anesthesiology 58:373, 1983

52. San Juan AC, Stanley TH: Pulmonary embolism after tourniquet inflation. Anesth Analg 63:371, 1982

53. Klenerman L: Tourniquet time—how long? Hand 12:231, 1980

54. Hamilton WK, Sokoll MD: Tourniquet paralysis. JAMA 199:37, 1967

55. Hurst LN, Weinglein O, Brown WF et al: The pneumatic tourniquet: A biomedical and electrophysiologic study. Plast Reconstr Surg 67:648, 1981

56. Miller SH, Price G, Buch D et al: Effects of tourniquet ischemia and postischemic edema on muscle metabolism. J Hand Surg 4:547, 1979

57. Patterson S, Klenerman L: The effect of pneumatic tourniquets on ultra-structure of skeletal muscle. J Bone Joint Surg 61B:178, 1979

58. Jozsa L, Renner A, Santha E: The effect of tourniquet ischaemia on intact, tenotomized and motor nerve–injured human hand muscles. Hand 12:235, 1980

59. Heppenstall RB, Balderston R, Goodwin C: Pathophysiologic effects distal to a tourniquet in the dog. J Trauma 19:234, 1979

60. Tountas CP, Bergman RA: Tourniquet ischemia: Ultrastructural and histochemical observations of ischemic human muscle and of monkey muscle and nerve. J Hand Surg 2:31, 1977

61. Lynn AM, Fischer T, Brandford HG, et al: Systemic responses to tourniquet release in children. Anesth Analg 65:865, 1986

62. Stein RE, Urbaniak J: Use of tourniquet during surgery in patients with sickle cell hemoglobinopathies. Clin Orthop 151:231, 1980

63. Klenerman L, Biswas M, Hulands GH et al: Systemic and local effects of the application of a tourniquet. J Bone Joint Surg 62A:385, 1980

64. Luce EA, Mangubat E: Loss of hand and forearm following Bier block: A case report. J Hand Surg 8:280, 1983

65. Tryba M, Zenz M, Hausmann E: Prolonged analgesia after cuff release following IV regional analgesia with prilocaine. Br J Anaesth 55:631, 1983

66. Drexler H, Felman B, Finsterbusch A et al: Low-dose intravenous regional anesthesia in a case of multistaged, bilateral hand surgery. Anesth Analg 65:812, 1986

67. Egbert LD, Deas TC: Cause of pain from a pneumatic tourniquet during spinal anesthesia. Anesthesiology 23:287, 1962

68. Egbert LD: Tourniquet pain. Anesthesiology 25:247, 1964

69. DeJong RH: Tourniquet pain during spinal anesthesia. Anesthesiology 23:881, 1962

70. DeJong RH: Letter to the editor. Anesthesiology 25:248, 1964

71. Valli H, Rosenberg PH: Effects of three anaesthetic methods on haemodynamic responses connected with the use of thigh tourniquets in orthopaedic patients. Acta Anaesth Scand 29:142, 1985

72. Lambert DH, Deane RS, Mazuzan JE: Anesthesia and the control of blood pressure in patients with spinal cord injury. Anesth Analg 61:344, 1982

73. Nelson CL, Bowen WS: Total hip arthroplasty in Jehovah's Witnesses without blood transfusion. J Bone Joint Surg 68A:350, 1986

74. Knight PR, Lane GA, Nichols MG et al: Hormonal and hemodynamic changes induced by pentolinium and propranolol during surgical correction of scoliosis. Anesthesiology 53:127, 1980

75. NcNeil TW, DeWald RL, Kuo KN et al: Controlled hypotensive anesthesia in scoliosis surgery. J Bone Joint Surg 56A:1167, 1974

76. Bernard JM, Pinaud M, Carteau S et al: Hypotensive actions of diltiazem and nitroprusside compared during fentanyl anaesthesia for total hip arthroplasty. Can Anaesth Soc J 33:308, 1986

77. Pilliar RM, Blackwell R, Macnab I et al: A carbon fiber-reinforced bone cement in orthopedic surgery. J Biomed Mater Res 10:893, 1976

78. Gardner RC: Blood loss in orthopedic operations: Comparative studies in 19 major orthopedic procedures utilizing radioisotope labeling and an automatic blood volume computer. Surgery 68:489,1970

79. Cowell HR, Swickard JW: Autotransfusion in children's orthopaedics. J Bone Joint Surg 56A:908, 1974

80. Thompson JD, Callaghan JJ, Savory CG et al: Prior deposition of autologous blood in elective orthopaedic surgery. J Bone Joint Surg 69A:320, 1987

81. Woolson ST, Marsh JS, Tanner JB: Transfusion of previously deposited autologous blood for patients undergoing hip replacement surgery. J Bone Joint Surg 69A:325, 1987

82. Ochsner JL, Mills NL, Leonard GL et al: Fresh autologous blood transfusions with extracorporeal circulation. Ann Surg 177:811, 1973

83. Rakower SR, Worth MH, Lackner H: Massive intraoperative autotransfusion of blood. Surg Gynecol Obstet 137:633, 1973

84. Bailey TE, Mahoney OM: The use of autologous blood in patients undergoing surgery for spinal deformity. J Bone Joint Surg 69A:329, 1987

85. Messmer K, Lewis DH, Sunder–Plassman L et al: Acute normovolemic hemodilution: Changes of central hemodynamics and microcirculatory flow in skeletal muscle. Eur Surg Res 4:55, 1972

86. Messmer K, Sunder–Plassman L, Jesch F et al: Oxygen supply to the tissues during limited normovolemic hemodilution. Res Exp Med 159:152, 1973

87. Kallos T, Smith TC: Replacement for intraoperative blood loss. Anesthesiology 41:293, 1974

88. Cullings HM, Hendee WR: Radiation risks in the orthopaedic operating room. Contemp Orthop 8:48, 1984

89. Miller ME, Davis ML, MacClean CR et al: Radiation exposure and associated risks to operation room personnel during use of fluoroscopic guidance for selected orthopaedic surgical procedures. J Bone Joint Surg 65:1, 1983

90. Nelson JP, Glassburn AR, Talbott RD et al: The effect of previous surgery, operating room environment, and preventive antibiotics on postoperative infection following total hip arthroplasty. Clin Orthop 147:167, 1980

91. Crow S, Greene VW: Aseptic transgressions among surgeons and anesthesiologists: A quantitative study. Arch Surg 117:1012, 1982

92. Alexander JW, Fisher JE, Boyojian M et al: The influence of hair-removal methods on wound infections. Arch Surg 118;347, 1983

93. Ha'eri GB, Wiley AM: Wound contamination through drapes and gowns: A study using "tracer particles." Orthopedics 154:181, 1981

94. McCue SF, Berg EW, Saunders EA: Efficacy of double-gloving as a barrier to microbial contamination during total joint arthroplasty. J Bone Joint Surg 63A:811, 1981

95. Fitzgerald RH, Washington JA: Contamination of the operative wound. Orthop Clin North Am 6:1105, 1975

96. Letts RM, Doemer E: Conversation in the operation theater as a cause of airborne bacterial contamination. J Bone Joint Surg 65A:357, 1983

97. Ha'eri GB, Wiley AM: The efficacy of standard surgical face masks: An investigation using "tracer particles." Clin Orthop 148:160, 1980

98. Rawal N, Sjostrand UH, Dahlstrom B et al: Epidural morphine for postoperative pain relief: A comparative study with intramuscular narcotic and intercostal nerve block. Anesth Analg 61:93, 1982

99. Hart D: Bacterial ultraviolet radiation in the operating room. Twenty-nine-year studies for control of infections. JAMA 172:1019, 1960

100. Howard JM, Barker WF, Culbertson MR et al: Postoperative wound infections: The influence of ultraviolet irradiation on the operating room and various other factors. Ann Surg 160S:1, 1964

101. Lowell JD, Kundsin RB, Schwartz CM et al: Ultraviolet radiation and reduction of deep wound infection following hip and knee orthoplasty. Ann NY Acad Sci 353:285, 1980

102. Allander C, Abel E: Investigation of a new ventilating system for clean rooms. Med Res Engl 7:28, 1968

103. Charnley J: A sterile-air operating theatre enclosure. Br J Surg 51:195, 1964

104. Charnley J, Eftekhar N: Postoperative infection in total prosthetic replacement arthroplasty of the hip joint, with special reference to the bacterial content of the air. Br J Surg 56:641, 1969

105. Coriell LL, Blakemore WS, McGarrity GJ: Medical applications of dust-free rooms: II. Elimination of airborne bacteria from an operating theater. JAMA 203:1038, 1968

106. Ha'eri GB, Wiley AM: Total hip replacement in a laminar flow environment, with special reference to deep infections. Clin Orthop 148:163, 1980

107. Haslam KR: Laminar air-flow air conditioning in the operating room: A review. Anesth Analg 53:194, 1974

108. Cruse RJ, Ford R: A five-year prospective study of 23, 649 surgical wounds. Arch Surg 107:206, 1973

109. Fraser A, Edmonds–Seal J: Spinal cord injuries: A review of the problems facing the anaesthetist. Anaesthesia 37:1084, 1982

110. Rocco AG, Vandam LD: Problems in anesthesia for paraplegics. Anesthesiology 20:348, 1959

111. Caron CF, Bors E: A study of vascular changes during surgery of paraplegic patients. Paraplegia 7:292, 1970

112. Lambert DH, Deane RS, Mazuzan JE: Anesthesia and the control of blood pressure in patients with spinal cord injury. Anesth Analg 61:344, 1982

113. Alvine FG, Schurrer ME: Postoperative ulnar–nerve palsy. J Bone Joint Surg 69A:255, 1987

114. Mather LE: Parenteral opiates for postoperative analgesia. Reg Anesth 7:144, 1982

115. Griffen WO, Bennett RL: Inadequate treatment of pain in hospitalized patients: Letter to the editor. N Engl J Med 307:56, 1982

116. Bennett RL, Batenhorst RL, Bivins B et al: Patient-controlled analgesia: A new concept of postoperative pain relief. Ann Surg 195:700, 1982

117. Check WA: Results are better when patients control their own analgesia. JAMA 247:945, 1982

118. Scott DB: Postoperative pain relief. Reg Anesth 7:S110, 1982

119. Tamsen A, Hartvig P, Fagerlund C et al: Patient–controlled analgesic therapy. Part I. Pharmacokinetics of pethedine in the pre- and postoperative periods. Clin Pharmocokinet 7:149, 1982

120. Dahlstrom B, Tamsen A, Pallzow L: Patient-controlled analgesic therapy. Part IV. Pharmacokinetics and analgesic plasma concentrations of morphine. Clin Pharmacokinet 7:266, 1982

121. Ebert J, Varner PD: The effective use of epidural morphine sulfate for postoperative orthopedic pain. Anesthesiology 53:257, 1980

122. Gustafsson LL, Friberg–Nielson S, Garle M et al: Extradural and parenteral morphine: Kinetics and effects in postoperative pain: A controlled clinical study. Br J Anaesth 54:1167, 1982

123. Martin R, Salbaing J, Blaise G et al: Epidural morphine for postoperative pain relief: A dose–response curve. Anesthesiology 56:423, 1982

124. Rawal N, Sjostrand UH, Dahlstrom B et al: Epidural morphine for postoperative pain relief: A comparative study with intramuscular narcotic and intercostal nerve block. Anesth Analg 61:93, 1982

125. Barron DW, Strong JE, Postoperative analgesia in major orthopaedic surgery: Epidural and intrathecal opiates. Anaesthesia 36:937, 1981

126. Bromage PR, Camporesi EM, Durant PAC et al: Rostral spread of epidural morphine. Anesthesiology 56:431, 1982

127. Busch EK, Stedman PM: Epidural morphine for postoperative pain on medical-surgical wards—A clinical review. Anesthesiology 67:101, 1987

128. Peterson TK, Husted SE, Rubro L et al: Urinary retention during I.M. and extradural morphine analgesia. Br J Anaesth 54:1175, 1982

129. Gossling HR, Ellison LH, Degraff AC: Fat embolism: The role of respiratory failure and its treatment. J Bone Joint Surg 56A:1327, 1974

130. Gossling HR, Pellegrini VD: Fat embolism syndrome: A review of the pathophysiology and physiological basis of treatment. Clin Orthop 165:68, 1982

131. Peltier LF: The diagnosis and treatment of fat embolism: J Trauma 11:661, 1971

132. Weisz GM, Steiner E: The cause of death in fat embolism. Chest 59:511, 1971

133. Wilson RF, McCarthy B, LeBlanc LP et al: Respiratory and coagulation changes after uncomplicated fractures. Arch Surg 106:395, 1973

134. Gresham GA, Kuczynski A, Rosborough D: Fatal fat embolism following replacement arthroplasty for transcervical fractures of femur. Br Med J 2:617, 1971

135. Modig J, Malmberg P, Karlstrom G: Effects of epidural versus general anesthesia on calf blood flow. Acta Anaesth Scand 24:305 1980

136. Modig J, Borg T, Karlstrom G et al: Thromboembolism after total hip replacement: Role of epidural and general anesthesia. Anesth Analg 62:174, 1983

137. Saltzman EW, Harris WM: Prevention of venous thromboembolism in orthopaedic patients. J Bone Joint Surg 58A:903, 1976
138. Consensus Conference: Prevention of venous thrombosis and pulmonary embolism. JAMA 256:744, 1986
139. Anderson KH: Air aspirated from the venous system during total hip replacement. Anaesthesia 38:1175, 1983
140. Friedman RJ, Gumley GJ: Crepitation simulating gas gangrene. J Bone Joint Surg 67A:646, 1985
141. Whitehall R, Moskal JT, Scully KS et al: Nitrogen-gas injection from a power reamer: A complication of closed intramedullary nailing of the femur. J Bone Joint Surg 65A:860, 1983
142. Shupak RC, Shuster H, Funch RS: Airway emergency in a patient during CO₂ arthroscopy. Anesthesiology 60:171, 1984
143. Brady MM, Furness G, Fee JPH: Comparison of the analgesic and sedative effects of nalbuphine and morphine following hip replacement. Br J Anaesth 58:1332P, 1986
144. Allen PD, Walman T, Concepcion M et al: Epidural morphine provides postoperative pain relief in peripheral vascular and orthopedic surgical patients. Anesth Analg 65:165, 1986
145. Rechtine GR, Teinert CM, Bohlman HH: The use of epidural morphine to decrease postoperative pain in patients undergoing lumbar laminectomy. J Bone Joint Surg 66A:113,1984
146. Kalso E: Effects of intrathecal morphine, injected with bupivacaine, on pain after orthopaedic surgery. Br J Anaesth 55:415, 1983
147. Arvidsson I, Eriksson E: Postoperative TENS pain relief after knee surgery: Objective evaluation. Orthopedics 9:1346, 1986
148. Arvidsson F, Ericksson E, Knutsson E et al: Reduction of pain inhibition on voluntary muscle activation by epidural analgesia. Orthopedics 9:1415, 1986
149. Murphy DF, MacGrath P, Stritch M: Postoperative analgesia in hip surgery. Anaesthesia 39:181, 1984
150. Risbo A, Jorgensen BC, Kolby P et al: Sublingual buprenorphine for premedication and postoperative pain relief in orthopaedic surgery. Acta Anaesth Scand 29:180, 1985
151. Haljamae H, Stefansson T, Wickstrom I: Preanesthetic evaluation of the female geriatric patient with hip fracture. Acta Anaesth Scand 26:393, 1982
152. Allen HL, Metcalf DW: Fractured hip: A study of anesthesia in the aged. Anesth Analg 44:408, 1965
153. Davie IT, MacRae WR, Malcom-Smith NA: Anesthesia for the fractured hip: A survey of 200 cases. Anesth Analg 49:165, 1970
154. Davis FM, Woolner DF, Frampton C et al: Prospective, multicentre trial of mortality following general or spinal anaesthesia for hip fracture surgery in the elderly. Br J Anaesth 59:1080, 1987
155. Nightingale PJ, Marstrand T: Subarachnoid anaesthesia with bupivacaine for orthopaedic procedures in the elderly. Br J Anaesth 53:369, 1981
156. Howard CB, Mackie IG, Fairclough J et al: Femoral neck surgery using a local anaesthetic technique. Anaesthesia 38:993,1983
157. Wickstrom I, Holmberg I, Stefansson T: Survival of female geriatric patients after hip fracture surgery: A comparison of five anaesthetic methods. Acta Anaesth Scand 26:607, 1982
158. Valentin N, Lomholt B, Jensen JS et al: Spinal or general anaesthesia for surgery of the fractured hip? A prospective study of mortality in 578 patients. Br J Anaesth 58:284, 1986
159. Groucke CR: Mortality following surgery for fracture of the neck of the femur. Anaesthesia 40:578, 1985
160. Underwood RJ: Experiences with continuous spinal anesthesia in physical status group IV patients. Anesth Analg 47:18, 1969
161. Birks RIS, Edbrooke DL, Mundy JVB: Etomidate as a sedative agent in patients undergoing hip surgery under epidural anaesthesia. Anaesthesia 38:295, 1983
162. Smith-Peterson MN: Evolution of mould arthroplasty of the hip joint. J Bone Joint Surg 30B:59, 1948
163. Charnley J: Acrylic Cement in Orthopaedic Surgery. Baltimore, Williams & Wilkins, 1970
164. Eftekhar N: Low-friction arthroplasty: Indications, contraindications and complications. JAMA 218:705, 1971
165. Hole A: Pre- and postoperative monocyte and lymphocyte function: Effects of combined epidural and general anaesthesia. Acta Anaesth Scand 28:367, 1984
166. Hole A: Unsgaard G: The effect of epidural anaesthesia on lymphocyte functions during and after major orthopaedic surgery, Acta Anaesth Scand 27:135, 1983
167. Hedenstierna G, Lofstrom J: Effect of anaesthesia on respiratory function after major lower extremity surgery. Acta Anaesth Scand 29:55, 1985
168. Riis J, Lomholt B, Haxholdt O et al: Immediate and long-term mental recovery from general versus epidural anaesthesia in elderly patients. Acta Anaesth Scand 27:44, 1983
169. Combs SP, Greenwald AS: The effects of barium sulfate on the polymerization temperature and sheer strength of surgical simplex P. Clin Orthop 145:287, 1979
170. Gooding JM, Smith RA, Weng JT: Is methylmethacrylate safer than previously thought? Anesth Analg 59:542, 1980
171. Svartling N, Lehtinen AM, Tarkkanen L: the effect of anaesthesia on changes in blood pressure and plasma cortisol levels induced by cementation with methylmethacrylate. Acta Anaesth Scan 30:247, 1986
172. Eillis RH, Mulvein J: The cardiovascular effects of methylmethacrylate, J Bone Joint Surg 56:59, 1974
173. Johansen I, Benumof JL: Methylmethacrylate: A myocardial depressant and peripheral dilator. Anesthesiology 51:S77, 1979
174. Peebles DJ, Ellis RH, Stide SDK et al: Cardiovascular effects of methylmethacrylate cement. Br Med J 1:349, 1972
175. Samii K, Elmelik E, Goutalier D et al: Hemodynamic effects of prosthesis insertion during knee replacement without tourniquet. Anesthesiology 52:271, 1980
176. Samii K, Elmelik E, Mourtada MB et al: Intraoperative hemodynamic changes during total knee replacement. Anesthesiology 50:239, 1979
177. Weissman BN, Sosman JL, Braunstein EM et al: Intravenous methylmethacrylate after total hip replacement. J Bone Joint Surg 66A:44, 1984
178. Bengtson A, Larsson M, Gammer W et al: Anaphylatoxin release in association with methylmethacrylate fixation of hip prostheses. J Bone Joint Surg 69A:46, 1987
179. Crout DHG, Corkill JA, James ML et al: Methylmethacrylate metabolism in man: The hydrolysis of methylmethacrylate to methacrylate acid during total hip replacement. Clin Orthop 141:90, 1979
180. Modig J, Busch C, Olerud S et al: Arterial hypotension and hypoxaemia during total hip replacement: The importance of thromboplastic procedures, fat embolism and acrylic monomers. Acta Anaesth Scand 19:28, 1975
181. Sevitt S: Fat embolism in patients with fractured hips. Br Med J 2:257, 1972
182. Kallos T, Enis JE, Gollan F et al: Intramedullary pressure and pulmonary embolism of femoral medullary contents in dogs during insertion of bone cement and a prosthesis. J Bone Joint Surg 56A:1363 1974
183. Mebius C, Heedenstierna G: Airway closure and gas distribution during hip arthroplasty. Acta Anaesth Scand 26:72, 1982
184. Kallos T: Impaired arterial oxygenation associated with use of bone cement in the femoral shaft. Anesthesiology 42:210, 175
185. Cromwell TH: Methylmethacrylate airway obstruction. Anesthesiology 52:89,1980
186. Burke DW, Gates ET, Harris WH: Centrifugation as a method of improving tensile and fatigue properties of acrylic bone cement. J Bone Joint Surg 1984; 66A:1265, 1984

187. Rimnac CM, Wright TM, McGill DL: The effect of centrifugation on the fracture properties of acrylic bone cements. J Bone Joint Surg 68A:281, 1986

188. Trippel SB: Current concept review: Antibiotic-impregnated cement in total joint arthroplasty. J Bone Joint Surg 68A:1297, 1986

189. Buchert PK, Vaughn BK, Mallory TH et al: Excessive metal release due to loosening and fretting of sintered particles on porous-coated hip prostheses. J Bone Joint Surg 68A:606, 1986

190. Turner TM, Sumner DR, Urban RM et al: A comparative study of porous coatings in a weight-bearing total hip arthroplasty model. J Bone Joint Surg 68A:1396, 1986

191. Schiller MG: Intravenous regional anesthesia for closed treatment of fractures and dislocations of upper extremities. Clin Orthop 118:25, 1976

192. Peterson DO: Shoulder block anesthesia for shoulder reconstruction surgery. Anesth Analg 64:373, 1985

193. Ericksson E, Haggmark T, Saartok T et al: Knee arthroscopy with local anesthesia in ambulatory patients. Orthopaedics 9:186, 1986

194. Patel NJ, Flashburg MH, Paskin S et al: A regional anesthetic technique compared to general anesthesia for outpatient knee arthroscopy. Anesth Analg 65:185, 1986

195. Mann RAM, Bisset WLK: Anaesthesia for lower limb amputation. Anaesthesia 38:1185, 1983

196. Bromage PR, Melzack R: Phantom limbs and the body schema. Can Anaesth Soc J 21:267, 1974

197. Bird TM, Strunin L: Anaesthetic considerations for microsurgical repair of limbs. Can Anaesth Soc J 31:51, 1984

198. MacDonald DJF: Anaesthesia for microvascular procedures. Br J Anaesth 57:904, 1985

199. Pearce DJ: The role of posture in laminectomy. Proc R Soc Med 50:109, 1957

200. Taylor AR, Gleadhill CA, Bilsland WL et al: Posture and anaesthesia for spinal operations with special reference to intervertebral disc surgery. Br J Anaesth 28:213, 1956

201. Ovassapian A, Land P, Schafer MF et al: Anesthetic management for surgical correction of severe flexion deformity of the cervical spine. Anesthesiology 58:370, 1983

202. Smith RH, Gramling ZW, Volpitto PP: Problems related to the prone position for surgical operations. Anesthesiology 22:189, 1961

203. Smith RH: One solution to the problem of the prone position for surgical procedures. Anesth Analg 53:221, 1974

204. Lee C, Barnes A, Nagel EL: Neuroleptanalgesia for awake pronation of surgical patients. Anesth Analg 56:276, 1977

205. Bergofsky EH, Turino GM, Fishman AP: Cardiorespiratory failure in kyphoscoliosis. Medicine 38:263, 1959

206. Harrington PR: Treatment of scoliosis. J Bone Joint Surg 44A:591, 1962

207. Levin DB: Pulmonary function in scoliosis. Orthop Clin North Am 10:761, 1979

208. Anderson PR, Puno MR, Lovell SL et al: Postoperative respiratory complications in non-idiopathic scoliosis. Acta Anaesth Scand 29:186, 1985

209. Wills DG: Anaesthetic management of posterior lumbar osteotomy. Can Anaesth Soc J 32:248, 1985

210. Mandel RJ, Brown MD, McCollough NC et al: Hypotensive anesthesia and autotransfusion in spinal surgery. Clin Orthop 154:27, 1981

211. Marshall WK, Bedford RF, Arnold WP et al: Effects of propranolol on the cardiovascular and renin–angiotensin systems during hypotension produced by sodium nitroprusside in humans. Anesthesiology 55:277, 1981

212. Hoffman WE, Albrecht RT, Miletich DJ: Cardiovascular and metabolic effects of SNP-induced hypotension in young and aged hypertensive rats. Anesthesiology 56:427, 1982

213. Waldman J, Kaufer H, Hensinger RN et al: Wake-up technique to avoid neurologic sequelae during Harrington Rod procedure: A case report. Anesth Analg 56:733, 1977

214. Diaz JH, Lockhart CM: Postoperative quadriplegia after spinal fusion for scoliosis with intraoperative awakening. Anesth Analg 66:1039, 1987

215. Grundy BL, Nash CL, Brown RH: Deliberate hypotension for spinal fusion: Prospective random study with evoked potential monitoring. Can Anaesth Soc J 29:452, 1982

216. Pathak KS, Brown RH, Nash CL Jr et al: Continous opioid infusion for scoliosis fusion surgery. Anesth Analg 62:841, 1983

217. Kafer ER: Respiratory and cardiovascular functions in scoliosis and the principles of anesthetic management. Anesthesiology 52:339, 1980

218. Feldstein G, Ramanathan S: Obstetrical lumbar epidural anesthesia in patients with previous posterior spinal fusion for kyphoscoliosis. Anesth Analg 64:83, 1985

219. Fielding JW, Rothman RH (eds:) Symposium on the lumbar spine. Orthop Clin North Am 8:3, 1977

220. Matheson D: Epidural anaesthesia for lumbar laminectomy and spinal fusion. Can Anaesth Soc J 7:149, 1960

221. Brown EM, Gass H, Noe FD et al: Oxygen tension during laminectomy. JAMA 205:882, 1968

222. Smith L, Brown JE: Treatment of lumbar intervertebral disc lesions by direct injection of chymopapain. J Bone Joint Surg 49B:502, 1967

223. Nordby EJ, Brown MD: Present status of chymopapain and chemonucleolysis. Clin Orthop 129:79, 1977

224. Department of Health and Human Services: Chymopapain approved. FDA Drug Bull 12:17, 1982

225. Spencer CW: Chemonucleolysis under local anesthesia. Orthopedics 6:1617, 1983

226. Hall BB, McCulloch JA: Anaphylactic reaction following the intradiscal injection of chymopapain under local anesthesia. J Bone Joint Surg 65A:1215, 1983

227. Javid MJ, Nordby EJ, Ford LT et al: Safety and efficacy of chymopapain (Chymodiactin) in herniated nucleus pulposus with sciatica: Results of a randomized, double-blind study. JAMA 249:2489, 1983

Chapter 44   *George Graf*
Stanley Rosenbaum

Anesthesia and the Endocrine System

THYROID GLAND

The thyroid hormones, thyroxine and 3,5,3'-l-triiodothyronine, are the major regulators of cellular metabolic activity. Thyroid hormones influence a variety of proteolytic reactions by regulating the synthesis and activity of various proteins. They are necessary for proper cardiac, pulmonary, and neurologic function during both health and illness.

THYROID METABOLISM AND FUNCTION

The production of thyroid hormone is initiated by the active uptake and concentration of iodide within the thyroid gland (Fig. 44-1). Iodine is absorbed and reduced to iodide in the gastrointestinal tract. Circulating iodide is taken up and concentrated in the thyroid gland, where the iodide is oxidized by a peroxidase reaction to form iodine. It is then bound to tyrosine residues to form various iodotyrosines. After organification, mono- or diiodotyrosine are coupled enzymatically (thyroid peroxidase) to form either triiodothyronine (T_3) or thyroxine (T_4). These hormones are attached to the thyroglobulin protein and stored as colloid within the gland. The release of T_3 and T_4 from the gland is accomplished through proteolysis from the thyroglobulin and diffusion into the circulation. Thyrotropin (TSH) is produced in the anterior pituitary gland, and its secretion is regulated by thyrotropin-releasing hormone (TRH) produced in the hypothalamus. Thyrotropin is responsible for maintaining the uptake of iodide and proteolytic release of thyroid hormone.[1] Excess iodine inhibits the synthesis and secretion of thyroid hormone.[2]

The thyroid gland is solely responsible for the daily secretion of thyroxine (80 to 100 $\mu g \cdot day^{-1}$).[3] The half-life of T_4 in the circulation is 6 to 7 days.

Approximately 80% of T_3 is produced by the extrathyroidal deiodination of T_4 (20% direct thyroid secretion). The half-life of T_3 is 24 to 30 hours. Most of the effects of thyroid hormones are mediated by the more potent and less protein-bound T_3. The degree to which these hormones are protein-bound in the circulation is the major factor influencing their activity and degradation. T_4 is metabolized by monodeiodination to either T_3 or reverse T_3. T_3 is biologically active, whereas reverse T_3 is inactive. The major fraction of circulating hormone is bound to thyroid binding globulin with a smaller fraction bound to thyroid binding prealbumin. Changes in serum binding protein concentrations have a major effect on total T_3 and T_4 serum concentrations. The plasma normally contains 5 to 12 $\mu g \cdot dl^{-1}$ of T_4 and 80 to 220 $\mu g \cdot dl^{-1}$ of T_3. The secretion of TRH and TSH appears to be regulated by a negative feedback loop, which is dependent upon circulating levels of T_4 and T_3. T_3 probably exerts its numerous effects through interaction with nuclear receptors.[4, 5] This nuclear binding stimulates messenger RNA synthesis, which, in turn, controls protein synthesis.

Although the thyroid hormone is important to many aspects of growth and function, the anesthesiologist is most often concerned with the cardiovascular manifestations of thyroid disease. Thyroid hormones affect tissue responses to sympathetic stimuli and increase the intrinsic contractile state of cardiac muscle.[6, 7] Beta-adrenergic receptors are increased in number,[8, 9] and cardiac cholinergic receptors are decreased by thyroid hormone.[10] It has been proposed that thyroid hor-

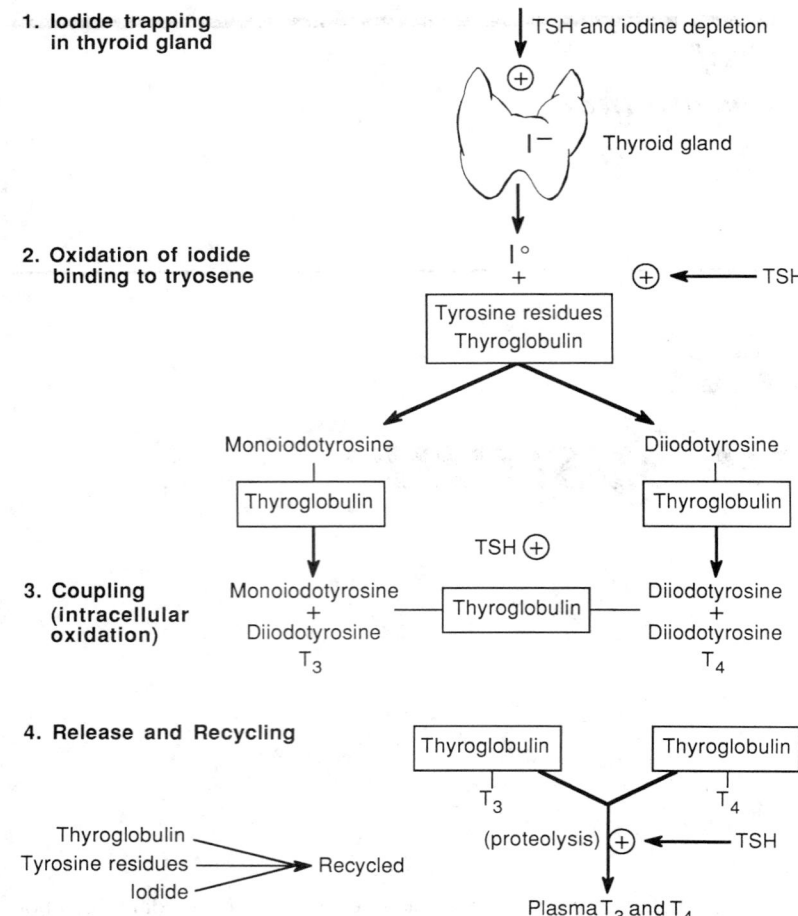

1. Iodide trapping in thyroid gland

TSH and iodine depletion

$\oplus$

I^- Thyroid gland

2. Oxidation of iodide binding to tryosene

I°
+
$\oplus \longleftarrow$ TSH

Tyrosine residues
Thyroglobulin

Monoiodotyrosine   Diiodotyrosine

Thyroglobulin   Thyroglobulin

TSH $\oplus$

3. Coupling (intracellular oxidation)

Monoiodotyrosine   Diiodotyrosine
+   Thyroglobulin   +
Diiodotyrosine   Diiodotyrosine
T_3 T_4

4. Release and Recycling

Thyroglobulin   Thyroglobulin
T_3 T_4

Thyroglobulin
Tyrosine residues $\longrightarrow$ Recycled
Iodide

(proteolysis) $\oplus \longleftarrow$ TSH

Plasma T_3 and T_4

FIG. 44-1. Thyroid hormone biosynthesis consists of four stages: 1) organification; 2) binding; 3) coupling; and 4) release.

mone may modulate the conversion of alpha to beta receptors without affecting the overall affinity of these receptors.[9] Two possible explanations for the "hyperadrenergic" state of thyrotoxicosis or the decreased tone of hypothyroidism are an increased or decreased number of sympathetic receptors or possibly an alteration in the beta-adrenergic signal between hormone and receptor.[11, 12]

TESTS OF THYROID FUNCTION

Total Serum Thyroxine (T_4)

The serum T_4 is the standard screening test for evaluation of thyroid gland function (Table 44-1). The total T_4 will be elevated in about 90% of patients with hyperthyroidism, and it will be low in 85% of those who are hypothyroid.[13] The concentration of T_4 is measured by radioimmunoassay (RIA). The serum T_4 is influenced by thyroid hormone protein-binding capacity. An increase or decrease in thyroid-binding globulin (TBG) levels or protein-binding may therefore alter the total T_4. Elevations in the TBG concentration are the most common cause of hyperthyroxinemia in euthyroid patients. Acute liver disease, pregnancy, or drug-induced increases in TBG (oral contraceptives, exogenous estrogens, clofibrate, opioids) may be responsible. Because a total T_4 can be misleadingly high in

euthyroidism or normal in hypothyroidism, some measure of free thyroid hormone activity (free T_4) must also be used.

Free T_4 (FT$_4$) and Free T_3 (FT$_3$)

The percentage of free T_4 (normal 1.5 to 5.0 ng·dl^{-1}) or T_3 is currently measured by equilibrium dialysis. A small quantity of radiolabeled T_4 or T_3 is added to the patient's serum. The percentage of the labeled hormone that crosses a dialysis membrane represents the percentage of free hormone in the serum. This volume is multiplied by the total serum T_4 or T_3 to give the amount of free hormone in the plasma. A free T_4 by RIA has recently become available and may soon replace this older method of analysis.[15] This test is independent of the plasma concentration of TBG.

Serum Triiodothyronine (T_3)

The serum T_3 is also measured by radioimmunoassay. The normal range is 80 to 200 ng·dl^{-1}. Serum T_3 levels are often determined to detect disease in patients who manifest clinical evidence of hyperthyroidism in the absence of elevations of T_4. T_3 may be the only thyroid hormone produced in excess.[13] T_3 concentrations may be depressed by factors that impair the peripheral conversion of T_4 to T_3 (sick euthyroid syndrome). In

TABLE 44-1. Tests of Thyroid Gland Function

	T_4	RT_3U	T_3	TSH
Hyperthyroidism	Elevated	Elevated	Elevated	Normal or low
Primary hypothyroidism	Low	Low	Low or normal	Elevated
Secondary hypothyroidism	Low	Low	Low	Low
Sick euthyroidism (decreased peripheral conversion T_4 to T_3)	Normal	Normal	Low	Normal
Pregnancy	Elevated	Low	Normal	Normal

T_4 = total serum thyroxine, RT_3U = T_3 resin uptake, T_3 = serum triiodothyronine, TSH = thyroid-stimulating hormone

50% of hypothyroid patients, the T_3 is low; in the remaining 50%, the serum T_3 is normal.[14]

T_3 Resin Uptake (RT$_3$U)

The triiodothyronine resin uptake is an indirect measure of the unbound plasma concentration of thyroxine. Radiolabeled T_3 is added to the patient's serum. Some of this T_3 binds to available protein-binding sites. A resin is then added that binds to the remaining unbound T_3. Resin uptake of radiolabeled T_3 varies indirectly with the number of free binding sites. In normal patients, the T_3 resin uptake is 25-35%. The T_3 resin uptake is not related to serum T_3 levels since the affinity of TBG for T_3 is low compared with that of T_4. The T_3 resin uptake is high in hyperthyroidism, when protein binding sites are occupied by other substances (salicylates) or when TBG is decreased (nephrotic syndrome, chronic liver disease). The T_3 resin uptake is decreased when fewer binding sites are occupied by T_4 (hypothyroidism) or when TBG is increased.

In general, if both the total T_4 and T_3 resin uptake are high or if both are low, the patient probably has hyper- or hypothyroidism, respectively. When the T_4 and T_3 resin uptake are in opposite directions, a binding abnormality is probable.

Free Thyroxine Index

The free thyroxine index (FTI) is calculated by multiplication of the total T_4 and the T_3 resin uptake. Normal values range from 1.6 to 5.7 $\mu g \cdot dl^{-1}$. The free T_4 index is frequently used to distinguish alterations in binding from true metabolic abnormalities.

Thyroid-Stimulating Hormone

The radioimmunoassay for this hormone has proved most useful in detecting patients who are hypothyroid. It is often higher than 20 $\mu IU \cdot ml^{-1}$ in primary hypothyroidism (normal $< 8 \mu IU \cdot ml^{-1}$). Thyroid-stimulating hormone assays are not sensitive enough to discriminate between hyperthyroid and euthyroid states. A low TSH level in the hypothyroid patient indicates disease at the pituitary or hypothalamic level. Starvation, fever, stress, corticosteroids, and T_3, or T_4 can all depress TSH levels.[16]

Thyroid-Releasing Hormone Testing

The administration of TRH (400 μg) increases the serum TSH level within 30 minutes in normal subjects. Hypothyroid pa-

tients have an exaggerated response, whereas hyperthyroid patients have a subnormal response or no response.[17] This illustrates the exquisitely sensitive response of the hypothalamic-pituitary axis to T_3 or T_4. Other conditions that may blunt the response to TRH include fasting glucocorticoid administration, dopamine, some psychiatric disorders, and advanced age.[18-21]

Radioactive Iodine Uptake

The thyroid gland has the ability to concentrate large amounts of inorganic iodide. The oral administration or radioactive iodine (^{131}I) can be used to indicate thyroid gland activity. Thyroid uptake is elevated in hyperthyroidism unless caused by thyroiditis, in which case the uptake is low or absent. Because of overlap in values, it is difficult to distinguish euthyroid from hypothyroid persons. Radioactive iodide uptake (RAIU) may be increased by a variety of factors, including dietary iodine deficiency, renal failure or congestive heart failure. Remembering that uptake is under TSH-control, elevated free T_4 levels, corticosteroids, and dopamine will all decrease RAIU. Functioning thyroid tissue ("hot") is rarely malignant. Nonfunctioning ("cold") tissue may be malignant or benign.

HYPERTHYROIDISM

Hyperthyroidism results from the exposure of tissues to excessive amounts of thyroid hormone. The most common etiology is the multinodular diffuse goiter of Graves' disease (Table 44-2). This typically occurs between the ages of 20 and 40 years and is predominant in females. The majority of these patients demonstrate a syndrome characterized by diffuse glandular enlargement, ophthalmopathy, dermopathy, and clubbing of the fingers. A thyroid-stimulating autoantibody (LATS) may be present.[22] Thyroiditis is another cause of increased thyroid hormone synthesis.[23] Subacute thyroiditis frequently follows a respiratory illness[24] and is characterized by a viral-like illness with a firm painful gland. This type of thyroiditis is frequently treated with anti-inflammatory agents alone. Rarely, subacute thyroiditis may present with a normal-sized painless gland.[25] Hashimoto's thyroiditis is a chronic autoimmune disease,[26] which usually produces hypothyroidism but may occasionally produce hyperthyroidism. Hyperthyroidism may also be associated with pregnancy,[27] thyroid adenoma ^{131}I therapy, thyroid carcinoma, trophoblastic tumors, or solely from a TSH-secreting pituitary adenomas. Iatrogenic hyperthyroidism

TABLE 44-2. Causes of Hyperthyroidism

INTRINSIC THYROID DISEASE
Hyperfunctioning thyroid adenoma
Toxic multinodular goiter

ABNORMAL TSH STIMULATOR
Graves' disease
Trophoblastic tumor

DISORDERS OF HORMONE STORAGE OR RELEASE
Thyroiditis

EXCESS PRODUCTION OF TSH
Pituitary thyrotropin (rare)

EXTRATHYROIDAL SOURCE OF HORMONE
Struma ovarii
Functioning follicular carcinoma

EXOGENOUS THYROID
Iatrogenic
Iodine-induced

may follow thyroid hormone replacement or may occur following iodide exposure[28] (angiography dye) in patients with chronically low iodide intake (Job–Basedow's phenomenon).

The major manifestations of hyperthyroidism are weight loss, diarrhea, skeletal muscle weakness, warm moist skin, heat intolerance, and nervousness. Hypercalcemia, thrombocytopenia, and a mild anemia may be present. Elderly patients may present with heart failure owing to papillary muscle dysfunction, atrial fibrillation, or other cardiac dysrhythmias without other systemic signs or symptoms of hyperthyroidism (apathetic hyperthyroidism).[29, 30] Patients with Graves' disease may have a number of extrathyroidal manifestations, including an ophthalmopathy and clubbing.

"Thyroid storm" is a life-threatening exacerbation of hyperthyroidism seen during periods of stress (e.g., infection, injury, surgery).[31–33] It is manifested by hyperpyrexia, tachycardia, anorexia, extreme anxiety, altered consciousness, and cardiovascular instability. Although free T_4 levels are often markedly elevated, no laboratory test is diagnostic.[34] The potential for significant perioperative morbidity with uncontrolled hyperthyroidism requires postponing elective surgery until the patient has been made clinically euthyroid. Therapy takes several directions: suppression of thyroid hormone synthesis through the use of antithyroid drugs; blocking the release of preformed hormone; inhibition of the peripheral conversion of T_4 to T_3; supportive therapy, including correction of fluid and electrolyte imbalances and, most importantly, when thyroid storm is a consideration in the treatment of the precipitating (nonthyroidal) cause.

Treatment and Anesthetic Considerations

The drugs propylthiouracil (PTU) and methimazole are thiourea derivatives that inhibit the synthesis of thyroid hormone. Propylthiouracil also decreases the peripheral conversion of T_4 to T_3. Both drugs are well absorbed from the gastrointestinal tract. Normal thyroid glands usually contain a store of hormone that is large enough to maintain a euthyroid state for several months even if all synthesis is abolished.[35] Therefore, hyperthyroid patients are unlikely to be regulated to a euthyroid state with antithyroid drugs alone in less than 6 to 8 weeks. Once a euthyroid state is achieved, the dose of these

drugs should be reduced in order to avoid hypothyroidism. Toxic reactions from these drugs are uncommon but include skin rash, nausea, fever, agranulocytosis, hepatitis, and a lupus-like syndrome.

Inorganic iodide inhibits iodide organification and thyroid hormone release.[36] Oral iodide is supplied as a potassium iodide solution (Lugol's), which is usually given about an hour after the administration of antithyroid drugs so that the thyroidal accumulation of iodide may be avoided. Iodide is also effective in reducing the size of the hyperplastic gland.

Beta-adrenergic antagonists are effective in attenuating the manifestations of excessive sympathetic activity. For example, propranolol rapidly (12 to 24 hours) improves tachycardia, heat intolerance, anxiety, and tremor. Beta-adrenergic blockade alone does not inhibit hormone synthesis, but it does impair the peripheral conversion of T_4 to T_3 over a period of 1 to 2 weeks. The combination of propranolol (in doses titered to effect) plus potassium iodide (2 to 5 drops q. 8 h.) is frequently used preoperatively to ameliorate cardiovascular symptoms and reduce circulating concentrations of T_4 and T_3.[37] Preoperative preparation usually requires 7 to 14 days. Beta antagonists should not be used routinely in patients manifesting symptoms of congestive heart failure or bronchospasm. Heart failure, secondary to poorly controlled paroxysmal atrial fibrillation, may improve with slowing of the ventricular rate, but abnormalities of left ventricular function secondary to hyperthyroidism may not be corrected with the use of beta antagonists.[38] If a hyperthyroid patient with clinically apparent disease requires emergency surgery, propranolol is administered in 0.5 mg intravenous (iv) boluses. As an alternative the ultra–short-acting beta antagonist esmolol may be delivered as a continuous infusion, which is adjusted to maintain a heart rate less than 90 beats $\cdot$ min^{-1}.

Other drugs infrequently used to combat the symptoms of hyperthyroidism are the catecholamine-depleting drugs reserpine and guanethidine.[32, 39] Glucocorticoids such as dexamethasone (8 to 12 mg $\cdot$ day^{-1}) reduce thyroid hormone secretion in Graves' disease and reduce the peripheral conversion of T_4 to T_3. The mild hypercalcemia often seen in hyperthyroid patients is also reduced by glucocorticoids through an inhibition in bone resorption.

Radioactive iodine therapy is an effective treatment for some patients with thyrotoxicosis. It should not, however, be administered to pregnant patients, because it crosses the placenta and may destroy the fetal thyroid. A side-effect of RAI therapy includes hypothyroidism (10–60% in the first year, and 2% per year thereafter).[40]

Surgery

Subtotal thyroidectomy, as an alternative to prolonged medical therapy, is used less frequently today. Patients are rendered euthyroid prior to thyroid surgery through the use of a combination of beta blockers plus potassium iodide for 7 to 14 days or antithyroid medication for 6 to 8 weeks.[37] Potassium iodide may be added to the antithyroid medication for the 7 to 10 days prior to surgery in order to facilitate shrinking of the gland. All antithyroid medications are continued through the morning of surgery.

A variety of anesthetic techniques and drugs have been used for hyperthyroid patients undergoing surgery.[41] The key to the management of these patients is delaying the stress of surgery until the patient has been brought to a euthyroid state. The goal of intraoperative management in the hyperthyroid patient is achieving a depth of anesthesia that prevents an exaggerated sympathetic response to surgical stimulation while avoiding the administration of medication that stimulates the sympathetic nervous system. It is best to avoid using ketamine even when a patient is clinically euthyroid.[42] The treatment of hypotension during surgery is best accomplished with direct-acting vasopressors rather than a medication that provokes the release of catecholamines. The appropriate selection of neuromuscular blocking drug deserves mention. Pancuronium has the ability to increase the heart rate and should probably be avoided; drugs that provide greater cardiovascular stability (vecuronium, atracurium) should be used. The incidence of myasthenia gravis is increased in hyperthyroid patients[43]; thus, the initial dose of muscle relaxant should be reduced and a twitch monitor should be used to guide all subsequent administration of neuromuscular blocking agents. Regional anesthesia is an excellent alternative when appropriate; however, epinephrine-containing solutions are avoided.

Complications of surgery in hyperthyroid patients occur more frequently when preoperative preparation has been inadequate. Airway obstruction is a potential problem in the patient with a large goiter. A CT scan of the neck preoperatively provides valuable information about airway anatomy.[44] Thyroid storm, "thyrotoxicosis," may occur intraoperatively or during the immediate postoperative period. Hyperthermia, tachycardia, and dysrhythmias may mimic the onset of malignant hyperthermia.[45] In addition to the use of the various antithyroid medications mentioned previously, supportive measures to control fever and restore intravascular volume should be used. Hemodynamic monitoring (PA catheter, arterial catheter) is especially useful in guiding the treatment of patients with significant left ventricular dysfunction. Once again, it is essential to remove or treat the precipitating event.

The complications following subtotal thyroidectomy include recurrent laryngeal nerve damage, tracheal compression secondary to hematoma or tracheomalacia, and hypoparathyroidism.[46] Hypoparathyroidism secondary to the inadvertent surgical removal of parathyroid glands is most frequently seen after total thyroidectomy. The symptoms of hypocalcemia develop within the first 24 to 48 hours following surgery. Laryngeal stridor progressing to laryngospasm may be one of the first indications of hypocalcemic tetany. The iv administration of calcium chloride or calcium gluconate is warranted in this situation. Bilateral recurrent laryngeal nerve injury is an extremely rare injury and necessitates reintubation. Unilateral nerve injury is more common and often goes unnoticed. Unilateral damage to the recurrent laryngeal nerve is characterized by hoarseness and a paralyzed vocal cord, while bilateral injury causes aphonia. It is wise to evaluate vocal cord function pre- and postoperatively by laryngoscopy or by asking the patient to phonate by saying the letter "e." Postoperative extubation of the trachea should be performed under optimal conditions. Intraoperative laryngeal nerve injury or collapse of the tracheal rings from previous weakening may mandate emergency reintubation.[47]

HYPOTHYROIDISM

Hypothyroidism is a relatively common disease (0.5–0.8% of the adult population) resulting from inadequate circulating levels of T_4 and/or T_3. The development of hypothyroidism is often slow and progressive, making the clinical diagnosis difficult, especially in the more subtle cases. Hypofunctioning of the thyroid gland has many causes (Table 44-3).[10, 48, 49] Primary failure of the thyroid gland refers to a decreased production of thyroid hormone despite adequate TSH production

TABLE 44-3. Causes of Hypothyroidism

PRIMARY HYPOTHYROIDISM
Autoimmune
Irradiation to the neck
Previous ^{131}I therapy
Surgical removal
Thyroiditis (Hashimoto's)
Severe iodine depletion
Medications (iodines, propylthiouracil, methimazole)
Hereditary defects in biosynthesis
Congenital defects in gland development

SECONDARY OR TERTIARY HYPOTHYROIDISM
Pituitary
Hypothalamic

(From Petersdorf RG [ed]: Harrison's Principles of Internal Medicine, 10th ed. New York, McGraw-Hill, 1983, with permission.)

and accounts for 95% of all cases of thyroid dysfunction, the remainder being caused by either hypothalamic or pituitary disease (secondary hypothyroidism).

Clinical Manifestations

A lack of thyroid hormone produces a variety of signs and symptoms. These early findings are often nonspecific and difficult to recognize. A history of RAI therapy, external neck radiation, or the presence of a goiter are all helpful in making a diagnosis. There is a generalized reduction in metabolic activity resulting in lethargy, slow mental functioning, cold intolerance, and slow movements. The cardiovascular manifestations of hypothyroidism reflect the importance of the thyroid hormone on myocardial contractility and catecholamine function. These patients demonstrate bradycardia and depressed myocardial contractility.[50] The accumulation of a cholesterol rich pericardial fluid produces low voltage on the ECG.[51] Impaired myocardial contractility generally correlates with the severity of hypothyroidism, but, interestingly, myxedema rarely produces congestive heart failure in the absence of coexisting heart disease.[52] Autopsy findings of more advanced coronary artery disease in myxedematous hypertensive patients compared with euthyroid hypertensive controls may reflect the abnormal lipid profile of hypothyroidism.[53] Angina pectoris itself is unusual in hypothyroidism and usually appears when thyroid hormone treatment is initiated (catecholamine hypersensitivity).[54] Peripheral vasoconstriction may lead to hypertension and cool dry skin. Hypothyroidism with amyloidosis is associated with cardiac conduction abnormalities, renal dysfunction, and enlargement of the tongue. Zwilich and colleagues[55] have reported that the ventilatory responsiveness to hypoxia and hypercapnia is depressed in hypothyroid patients. This depression is potentiated by sedatives, opioids, and general anesthesia. It should be noted that postoperative ventilatory failure requiring prolonged ventilation is rarely seen in hypothyroid patients in the absence of coexistent lung disease, obesity, or myxedema coma.[55] Other abnormalities found in hypothyroidism include various coagulation abnormalities, reduced platelet adhesiveness, gastrointestinal bleeding, anemia, hypothermia, and impaired renal concentrating ability.[56–58] Basal plasma levels of cortisol are usually normal in hypothyroidism; however, in long-standing or severe disease, the stress response may be blunted and adrenal depression may occur.[59]

In addition to these clinical findings, laboratory analysis is used to confirm the diagnosis of hypothyroidism and aid the clinician in determining the severity of the disease. "Severe" hypothyroidism denotes those patients with extreme clinical abnormalities, including "myxedema coma" and T_4 levels as low as $1 \mu g \cdot dl^{-1}$ or less and TSH levels in the range of 50 to 100 $\mu IU \cdot ml^{-1}$. When the diagnosis of hypothyroidism is suspected, a blood sample is obtained for T_4, TSH, resin T_3 uptake (RT_3U) and cortisol. Thyroid replacement may be started while awaiting results. Primary hypothyroidism is characterized by a low T_4 and RT_3U and an elevated TSH. Secondary hypothyroidism is evidenced by a low T_4, RT_3U, and TSH. A thorough evaluation of other pituitary function should be undertaken when this condition exists (pituitary tumor, postpartum pituitary necrosis).

Treatment and Anesthetic Considerations

Controversy remains regarding the preoperative anesthetic management of the hypothyroid patient. Although it seems logical to recommend that all surgical candidates who are hypothyroid be restored to a euthyroid state prior to surgery, these recommendations are in general based on uncontrolled case reports. There have been few controlled studies to support the position that most hypothyroid patients are unusually sensitive to anesthetic drugs, have prolonged recovery times, or suffer from a higher incidence of cardiovascular instability or collapse.

Two recent controlled studies have investigated the subject of surgery in the hypothyroid patient. Weinberg et al[60] conducted a retrospective analysis of 59 hypothyroid patients who were matched with 59 euthyroid controls. All patients underwent surgery with general anesthesia and endotracheal intubation. The hypothyroid patients were divided into three subsets ($T_4 < 1 \mu g \cdot dl^{-1}$, $T_4 < 3 \mu g \cdot dl^{-1}$, $T_4 \geq 3 \mu g \cdot dl^{-1}$). Of the 59 study patients, 52 were classified as mild or moderately hypothyroid ($T_4 > 1 \mu g \cdot dl^{-1}$). Analysis of the three subsets of hypothyroid patients and their matched controls disclosed no significant differences with regard to fluid and electrolyte imbalances, hemodynamic stability, time to extubation of the trachea, or length of postoperative hospitalization. There were no significant differences in the incidence of complications between the groups. Because the number of patients with severe hypothyroidism was small (seven patients) no conclusions can be drawn with regard to the proper management of this group. The authors did recommend that it was safe to proceed with anesthesia and surgery before thyroid replacement in those patients with mild or moderate hypothyroidism. Ladenson et al[61] retrospectively reviewed 40 hypothyroid patients undergoing surgery and compared them with 80 euthyroid controls. Although 33 of the hypothyroid patients received thyroid replacement preoperatively, all of the test patients had persistent chemical hypothyroidism at the time of surgery. A comparison of partially treated patients with untreated hypothyroid patients showed no significant differences in the frequency of complications. Despite a higher incidence of intraoperative hypotension and postoperative gastrointestinal and neuropsychiatric complications among hypothyroid patients undergoing noncardiac surgery, the authors did not believe that there were compelling clinical reasons to postpone surgery in mild or moderate hypothyroid patients. They further concluded that conventional clinical or biochemical criteria may not accurately define a subgroup of hypothyroid patients with increased operative risk. Their recommendations were that surgery should be postponed when possible in severely hypothyroid patients until these patients are at least partially treated.

The management of hypothyroid patients with symptomatic coronary artery disease has been a subject of controversy. The need for thyroid replacement must be weighed against the risk of precipitating myocardial ischemia. Drucker and Burrow[62] prospectively studied 10 patients with mild to moderate hypothyroidism who underwent cardiac surgery requiring cardiopulmonary bypass. No patient received thyroid replacement preoperatively. There were no significant differences in the frequency of intraoperative or postoperative complications when compared with a large control group. They concluded that there was no justification in postponing coronary artery bypass surgery in the ischemic patient with mild or moderate hypothyroidism. Hay and associates[63] retrospectively reviewed 18 hypothyroid patients with coronary artery disease who underwent coronary artery bypass graft. Nine patients were rendered euthyroid preoperatively, and nine patients received no preoperative treatment. The authors noted no significant differences between the groups with regard to complications or outcome. An extensive literature review by Becker[64] supports the position that cardiac catheterization or coronary artery bypass surgery can be done safely without preoperative thyroid hormone replacement. When dealing with symptomatic patients or unstable patients with cardiac ischemia who are surgical candidates, thyroid replacement should probably be delayed until the postoperative period in order to avoid the risk of precipitating acute myocardial ischemia or infarction.

On the basis of recent investigations, there appears to be little evidence to justify the postponement of elective surgery in patients who have mild or moderate hypothyroidism. In contrast, thyroid replacement is indicated for patients with severe hypothyroidism or myxedema coma and in pregnant patients who are hypothyroid. Untreated hypothyroidism in pregnant patients is associated with an increased incidence of spontaneous abortion and mental as well as physical abnormalities in the offspring.[65]

Myxedema coma represents a severe form of hypothyroidism characterized by stupor or coma, hypoventilation, hypothermia, hypotension, and hyponatremia. This is a medical emergency with a high mortality rate ($> 50\%$) and, as such, requires aggressive therapy. Intravenous thyroid replacement is initiated as soon as the clinical diagnosis is made. An iv loading dose of T_4, sodium levothyroxine, 400 to 500 μg is initially given to be followed by a maintenance dose of T_4, 50 to 200 μg iv daily.[66, 67] Alternatively, an iv loading dose of T_3 (50 to 200 μg bolus) is followed by a maintenance dose.[68] Initial treatment with T_3 is preferred since it has a more rapid onset of activity. Improvements in the heart rate, blood pressure, and body temperature may occur within 24 hours. Because there is an increased likelihood of acute primary adrenal insufficiency in these patients, they receive 100 to 300 mg $\cdot$ day^{-1} of hydrocortisone by infusion. Steroid replacement continues until normal adrenal function can be confirmed.

A number of anesthetic medications have been used without difficulty in hypothyroid patients. Greater than two thirds of the patients in the study of Weinberg et al[60] received an opioid premedication without problems. Although ketamine has been proposed as the ideal induction agent, thiopental has also been used in the hypothyroid patient. The suggestion that thiopental may decrease the peripheral conversion of T_4 to T_3 does not appear to be clinically relevant.[69] The maintenance of anesthesia may be safely achieved with either iv or inhaled anesthetics. To date, there are no controlled studies dealing with the specific questions of increased opioid potency and prolonged depression of ventilation in hypothyroid patients. Inhaled volatile anesthetics have also been used in hypothyroid patients without difficulty. There appears to be little if any decrease in the minimum alveolar concentration (MAC) for volatile agents (Fig. 44-2).[70] Regional anesthesia is a good choice in the hypothyroid patient provided that the intravascular volume is well maintained. Monitoring is directed toward the early recognition of hypotension, congestive heart failure, and hypothermia. Scrupulous attention should be paid to maintaining normal body temperature.

PARATHYROID GLANDS

CALCIUM PHYSIOLOGY

The normal adult body contains approximately 1000 g of calcium (Ca^{++}), of which 99% is in the skeleton and 1% is elsewhere. Plasma calcium is present in three forms: 1) a protein bound fraction (40%); 2) an ionized fraction (50%); and 3) a diffusable, but nonionized fraction (10%), which is complexed with phosphate, bicarbonate, and citrate. This division is of interest, because it is the ionized fraction that is physiologically active and homeostatically regulated. The normal total serum calcium concentration is 8.8 to 10.4 $mg \cdot dl^{-1}$. Albumin binds about 90% of the protein bound fraction of calcium. Total serum calcium is consequently dependent upon albumin levels.[71] In general, an increase or decrease in albumin of 1 $g \cdot dl^{-1}$ is associated with a parallel change in total serum calcium of 0.8 $mg \cdot dl^{-1}$. The serum ionized calcium concentration is affected by temperature and blood pH through alterations in calcium protein binding to albumin.[71, 72] Acidosis decreases protein-binding (increases ionized Ca^{++}), and alkalosis increases protein-binding (decreases ionized Ca^{++}). The concentration of free calcium ion is of

critical importance in regulating skeletal muscle contraction, coagulation, neurotransmitter release, endocrine secretion, and a variety of other cellular functions. As a consequence, the maintenance of serum Ca^{++} concentration is subject to exquisite hormonal control by parathyroid hormone (PTH) and vitamin D (Fig. 44-3).

Parathyroid hormone acts to maintain the extracellular fluid calcium concentration through direct effects on bone resorption and renal calcium reabsorption (distal tubule) and indirectly through its effects on the synthesis of 1, 25-dihydroxyvitamin D.[73, 74] Renal effects of PTH include phosphaturia and bicarbonaturia, in addition to enhanced calcium and magnesium reabsorption.[75] Most evidence suggests that rapid changes in blood calcium levels are primarily due to hormonal effects on bone and to a lesser extent on renal calcium clearance, whereas maintenance of calcium balance is more dependent upon the indirect effects of the hormone on intestinal calcium absorption. The effects of PTH are mediated by specific hormone–target cell membrane interaction.[76] Hormone–receptor activation of adenylate cyclase leads to increased intracellular cyclic AMP (cAMP). Presumably, the rapid rise of cAMP promotes an increase in protein kinase, leading to a phosphorylation of key effector proteins that initiate the hormonal effect. Following the administration of PTH, there is a rise in urinary cAMP. This "nephrogenous-cAMP" leaks from renal tubular cells and provides an index of the biologic activity of PTH.[77]

Parathyroid hormone secretion is primarily regulated by the serum ionized calcium concentration.[78] This negative feedback mechanism is exquisitely sensitive in maintaining calcium levels in a normal range.[79] Release of parathormone is also influenced by phosphate, magnesium, and catecholamine levels.[80–82] Acute hypomagnesemia directly stimulates PTH release, whereas chronic magnesium depletion appears to inhibit proper functioning of the parathyroid gland. The plasma phosphate concentration has an indirect influence on PTH secretion by causing reciprocal changes in the serum ionized calcium concentration.

VITAMIN D METABOLISM

Vitamin D is absorbed from the gastrointestinal tract and can be produced enzymatically by ultraviolet irradiation of the skin.[78, 83] Calciferol is hydroxylated in the liver to 25-hydroxycholecalciferol (25-OHD) and in the kidney is further hydroxylated to 1, 25-dihydroxycholecalciferol (1,25(OH)₂D) or 24,25-dihydroxycholecalciferol (24,25(OH)₂D). 25-OHD is the major circulating form of vitamin D. The synthesis of this hormone is not regulated by a hormone or the Ca^{++} or phosphate level. 1,25(OH)₂D and 24,25(OH)₂D are the major active metabolites of vitamin D, and their production is reciprocally regulated at the kidney. Hypocalcemia and hypophosphatemia cause an increased production of 1,25(OH)₂D and a decreased production of 24,25(OH)₂D. 1,25(OH)₂D stimulates bone, kidney, and intestinal absorption of calcium and phosphate.[78, 83] 24,25(OH)₂D stimulates bone synthesis and mineralization and augments intestinal Ca^{++} absorption. Vitamin D deficiency can lead to decreased intestinal absorption of calcium and secondary hyperparathyroidism.

HYPERPARATHYROIDISM

Primary hyperparathyroidism (HPT) increases with age and female sex, reaching its highest incidence in women older than 60 years of age.[84] Primary HPT is most commonly due to a

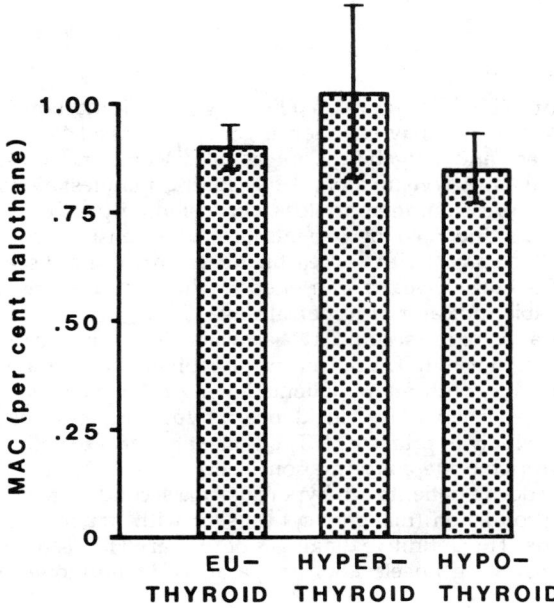

FIG. 44-2. The minimum alveolar concentration of halothane (MAC, mean ± SD) was determined in euthyroid, hyperthyroid, and hypothyroid dogs. There was no significant difference in MAC between euthyroid and either hyperthyroid or hypothyroid animals. MAC in hyperthyroid dogs was greater than the MAC in hypothyroid dogs ($P<0.05$). (Data adapted from Babad AA, Eger EI: The effects of hyperthyroidism and hypothyroidism on halothane and oxygen requirements in dogs. Anesthesiology 29:1087, 1968.)

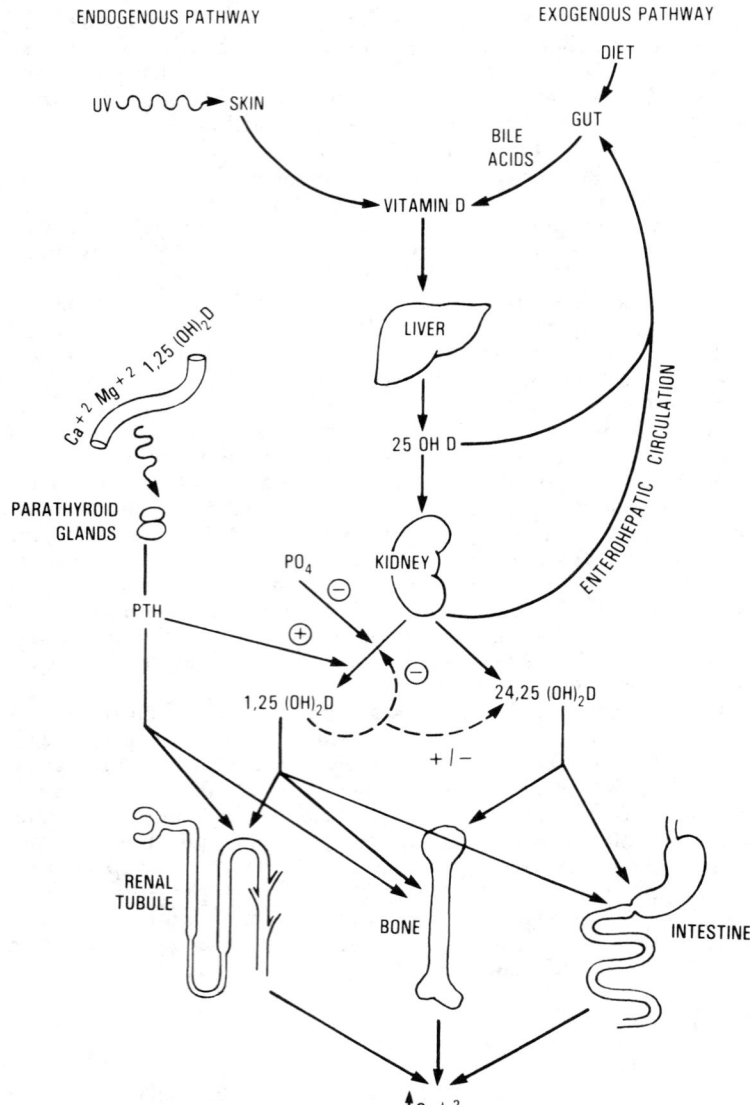

ENDOGENOUS PATHWAY

EXOGENOUS PATHWAY

FIG. 44-3. Parathyroid hormone and vitamin D metabolism and action. (From Geelhoed GW, Chernow B [eds]: Endocrine Aspects of Acute Illness. New York, Churchill Livingstone, 1985, with permission.)

benign parathyroid adenoma (90%) or hyperplasia (9%) and very rarely to a parathyroid carcinoma.[78] Primary HPT may also exist as part of a multiple endocrine neoplastic syndrome. Hyperplasia usually involves all four glands. Although the majority of patients with primary HPT are hypercalcemic, most are asymptomatic at the time of diagnosis.[85] When symptoms occur, they usually result from the hypercalcemia that accompanies the disease. Primary PTH occurring during pregnancy is associated with a high maternal and fetal morbidity (50%). The placenta allows the fetus to concentrate calcium, promoting hypercalcemia in the fetus and leading to hypoparathyroidism in the newborn. Pregnant patients with primary PTH should be treated with surgery.

Hypercalcemia is responsible for a broad spectrum of signs and symptoms. Nephrolithiasis is the most common manifestation, occurring in 60–70% of patients.[86] Polyuria and polydipsia are also common complaints. An increase in bone turnover may lead to generalized demineralization and subperiosteal bone resorption; however, only a small group of

patients (10–15%) develop clinically significant bone disease.[87] Patients may experience generalized skeletal muscle weakness and fatigability, epigastric discomfort, peptic ulceration, and constipation.[88] Psychiatric manifestations include depression, memory loss, confusion, or psychosis. Between 20 and 50% of patients are hypertensive, but this usually resolves with successful treatment of the disease.[89] The ECG may reveal a shortened QT interval, but this is an unreliable indicator of hypercalcemia.[90, 91]

Elevation of the serum Ca^{++} is a valuable diagnostic indicator of primary HPT. The serum phosphate concentration is nonspecific, with many patients having normal or near-normal levels. The reported incidence of hyperchloremic acidosis varies widely in primary HPT, but most patients usually have a serum chloride concentration in excess of 102 $mEq \cdot l^{-1}$.[92] Rarely does a patient with hypercalcemia secondary to ectopic HPT production (malignancy) present with hyperchloremic acidosis. The definitive diagnosis of primary HPT is made by demonstrating an elevation in parathyroid hormone levels

(RIA) in the presence of hypercalcemia. An elevated nephrogenous cAMP is noted in more than 90% of patients with primary HPT.[78]

Hypercalcemia may also result from the ectopic production of PTH or PTH-like substances from lung, genitourinary, breast, gastrointestinal, and lymphoproliferative malignancies.[93, 94] Tumors may also produce hypercalcemia through direct bone resorption or the production of osteoclast activating factor.[95] In the absence of a clinically obvious neoplasm, there may be difficulty in differentiating between PTH-producing malignancies and primary PTH. PTH fragments from malignant tissue differ from native PTH and aid in distinguishing between ectopic HPT and primary HPT.[96] Investigators have found that for any given serum calcium concentration, the serum PTH level is generally higher in patients with primary PTH than in those with malignancy.[97]

Secondary hyperparathyroidism represents an increase in parathyroid function as a result of conditions that produce hypocalcemia or hyperphosphatemia. Chronic renal disease is a common cause of hyperphosphatemia (due to decreased phosphate excretion) and decreased vitamin D metabolism. The hypocalcemia that results leads to an increased production of PTH. Gastrointestinal disorders accompanied by malabsorption may also lead to a secondary increase in parathyroid activity.

Tertiary hyperparathyroidism refers to the development of hypercalcemia in a patient who has had prolonged secondary hyperparathyroidism that is suddenly corrected (renal transplantation). The usually mild and transient hypercalcemia reflects an inability of the hyperactive parathyroid glands to adapt to the normal handling of renal calcium phosphorylate and vitamin D.

Treatment and Anesthetic Considerations

Surgery is the treatment of choice for the patient with symptomatic disease. Considerable controversy, however, surrounds the choice of treatment in the asymptomatic patient.[98] It is not clear that mild, primary HPT decreases longevity. Surgery is often chosen over medical therapy because it offers definitive treatment and is generally safe.

Preoperative preparation focuses on the correction of intravascular volume and electrolyte irregularities. It is particularly important to evaluate the patient with chronic hypercalcemia for abnormalities of the renal, cardiac, or central nervous systems. Emergency treatment of hypercalcemia is undertaken preoperatively when the serum Ca^{++} concentration exceeds 15 $mg \cdot dl^{-1}$ (7.5 $mEq \cdot l^{-1}$).[99] Lowering of the serum Ca^{++} concentration is initially accomplished by expanding the intravascular volume and establishing a sodium diuresis. This is achieved with the iv administration of normal saline and furosemide. Rehydration alone is capable of lowering the serum Ca^{++} level by 2 $mg \cdot dl^{-1}$ or more. Hydration dilutes the serum Ca^{++}, and a sodium diuresis promotes Ca^{++} excretion through an inhibition of sodium and Ca^{++} reabsorption in the proximal tubule. Another element in the treatment of hypercalcemia is the correction of hypophosphatemia. Hypophosphatemia increases the gastrointestinal absorption of Ca^{++},[100] stimulates the breakdown of bone, and impairs the uptake of Ca^{++} by bone. Low serum phosphate levels impair cardiac contractility and may contribute to congestive heart failure.[101] Hypophosphatemia also causes skeletal muscle weakness, hemolysis, and platelet dysfunction.

Other medications that have a role in lowering the serum Ca^{++} include mithramycin, calcitonin, and glucocorticoids. Mithramycin, a cytotoxic agent administered in a dose of 25 $\mu g \cdot kg^{-1}$, inhibits PTH-induced osteoclast activity and can lower the serum Ca^{++} levels by 2 $mg \cdot dl^{-1}$ or more in 24 to 48 hours.[102] Toxic effects include azotemia, hepatotoxicity, and thrombocytopenia. Calcitonin is useful in transiently lowering the serum Ca^{++} level 2 to 4 $mg \cdot dl^{-1}$ through direct inhibition of osteoclastic bone resorption. The advantages of calcitonin are that side-effects are mild (urticaria, nausea) and the onset of activity is rapid.[103] Calcitonin resistance usually develops within 24 to 48 hours.[104] Glucocorticoids are effective in lowering the serum Ca^{++} concentration in several conditions (sarcoidosis, some malignancies, hyperthyroidism, vitamin D intoxication) through its actions on osteoclast bone resorption, gastrointestinal calcium absorption, and the urinary excretion of calcium.[105] Glucocorticoids are usually of no benefit in the treatment of primary HPT. Finally, hemodialysis or peritoneal dialysis can be used to lower the serum Ca^{++} when alternate regimens are ineffective or contraindicated.

There is no evidence that a specific anesthetic drug or technique has advantages over another. A thorough knowledge of the clinical manifestations attributable to hypercalcemia is of the greatest value in choosing an anesthetic technique. Special monitoring is usually not required. In view of the unpredictable response to neuromuscular blocking drugs in the hypercalcemic patient, a conservative approach to muscle paralysis makes sense. Careful positioning of the osteopenic patient is necessary to avoid pathologic bone fractures.

Postoperative complications include recurrent laryngeal nerve injury, bleeding, and transient or complete hypoparathyroidism. Unilateral recurrent laryngeal nerve injury is characterized by hoarseness and usually requires no intervention. Bilateral recurrent laryngeal nerve injury is a rare complication, producing aphonia and requiring immediate endotracheal intubation. Following successful parathyroidectomy, one should observe a decrease in the serum Ca^{++} level within 24 hours. Patients with significant preoperative bone disease may develop hypocalcemia following removal of the PTH-secreting glands. This "hungry bone" syndrome comes as a result of the rapid remineralization of bone. Thus, serum Ca^{++}, magnesium, and phosphorus should be closely monitored until stable. The serum Ca^{++} nadir usually occurs within 3 to 7 days.

HYPOPARATHYROIDISM

An underproduction of parathormone or resistance of the end-organ tissues to PTH results in hypocalcemia (< 8 $mg \cdot dl^{-1}$). The normal physiologic response to hypocalcemia is an increase in PTH secretion and $1,25(OH)_2D$ synthesis with an increase in Ca^{++} mobilization from bone, gastrointestinal absorption, and renal tubule reclamation. The most common cause of acquired parathyroid hormone deficiency is as a result of the inadvertent removal of the parathyroid glands during thyroid or parathyroid surgery. Other causes of acquired hypoparathyroidism include ^{131}I therapy for thyroid disease, neck trauma, granulomatous disease, or an infiltrating process (malignancy or amyloidosis). Idiopathic hypoparathyroidism is rare and may occur as an isolated disease or as part of an autoimmune polyglandular process (hypothyroidism, adrenal insufficiency). Pseudohypoparathyroidism is an inherited disorder in which parathyroid gland function is normal, but the end-organ response to the PTH is deficient.[78] These patients have hypocalcemia and hyperphosphatemia. They are characterized by mental retardation, a short stature, obesity, and shortened metacarpals. Pseudopseudohypoparathyroid patients are characterized by the same physical findings but a normal serum calcium and phosphate. Severe hypomagnesemia (< 0.8 mEq·l^{-1}) from any cause can produce hypocalcemia by suppressing PTH secretion.[106, 107] Renal insufficiency leads to phosphorus retention and impaired 1,25(OH)$_2$D synthesis, and this results in hypocalcemia.[108] These patients are commonly treated with vitamin D, which increases intestinal calcium absorption and suppresses secondary increase in PTH secretion. Hypocalcemia resulting from pancreatitis and burns results from the suppression of PTH and from the sequestration of calcium.[109]

Clinical Features and Treatment

The clinical features of hypoparathyroidism are a manifestation of hypocalcemia. Neuronal irritability and skeletal muscle spasms, tetany, or seizures reflect a reduced threshold of excitation. Latent tetany may be demonstrated by eliciting Chvostek's or Trousseau's signs. Chvostek's sign is a contracture of the facial muscle produced by tapping the facial nerve as it passes through the parotid gland. Trousseau's sign is contraction of the fingers and wrist, following application of a blood pressure cuff inflated above the systolic blood pressure for approximately 3 minutes. Other common complaints of hypocalcemia include fatigue, depression, paresthesias, and skeletal muscle cramps. The acute onset of hypocalcemia following thyroid or parathyroid surgery may manifest as stridor and apnea. Cardiovascular manifestations of hypocalcemia include congestive heart failure, hypotension, and a relative insensitivity to the effects of beta-adrenergic agonists.[110, 111] Delayed ventricular repolarization results in a prolonged QT interval on the ECG. Although prolongation of the QT interval may be a reliable sign of hypocalcemia for an individual patient, the ECG is relatively insensitive for the detection of hypocalcemia.[112]

The treatment of hypoparathyroidism consists of electrolyte replacement. The objective is to have the patient's clinical symptoms under control prior to anesthesia and surgery. Hypocalcemia caused by magnesium depletion is treated by correcting the magnesium deficit. Serum phosphate excess is corrected by the removal of phosphate from the diet and the oral administration of phosphate-binding resins (aluminum hydroxide). The urinary excretion of phosphate can be increased with a saline volume infusion.[113] Ca^{++} deficiencies are corrected with calcium supplements and/or vitamin D analogs. Patients with severe symptomatic hypocalcemia are treated with iv calcium gluconate (10 to 20 ml, 10% solution) given over several minutes and followed with a continuous infusion (1 to 2 mg·kg^{-1}·hr^{-1}) of elemental Ca^{++}. The correction of serum Ca^{++} levels should be monitored by measuring serum Ca^{++} concentrations and following clinical symptoms. When oral or iv calcium is inadequate to maintain a normal serum ionized calcium, vitamin D is added to the regimen.

ADRENAL GLAND

The adrenal cortex functions to synthesize and secrete three types of hormones. Endogenous and dietary cholesterol is utilized in the adrenal biosynthesis of glucocorticoids (cortisol), mineralocorticoids (aldosterone and 11-deoxycorticosterone) and androgens (dehydroepiandrosterone) (Fig. 44-4). Cortisol and aldosterone are the two essential hormones, whereas adrenal androgens are of relatively minor physiologic significance in adults. The major biological effects of adrenal cortical hyper- or hypofunction occur as a result of cortisol or aldosterone excess or deficiency. Abnormal function of the adrenal cortex may render a patient unable to respond appropriately during a period of surgical stress or critical illness.

GLUCOCORTICOID PHYSIOLOGY

Cortisol (hydrocortisone) is the most potent glucocorticoid produced by the inner portions of the adrenal cortex (zona fasciculata, zona reticularis). Cortisone is a glucocorticoid produced in small amounts. Cortisol is produced under the control of adrenocorticotropic hormone (ACTH), a polypeptide synthesized and released by the anterior pituitary gland. Glucocorticoids exert their biological effects by diffusing into the cytoplasm of target cells and combining with specific high-affinity receptor proteins. The steroid receptor protein complex influences the transcription of new RNA by attaching to the nuclear chromatin. The synthesis of new proteins ultimately mediates the expression of the hormone.[115]

The daily production of endogenous cortisol is about 20 mg. Most of the circulating hormone is bound to the alpha globulin transcortin (cortisol-binding globulin).[116] It is the relatively small amount of free hormone that exerts the biological effects.[117] Glucocorticoids such as cortisol are inactivated primarily by the liver and are excreted in the urine as 17-hydroxycorticosteroids. Cortisol is also filtered at the glomerulus and may be excreted unchanged in the urine. Although the rate of cortisol secretion is decreased by about 30% in the elderly patient, plasma cortisol levels remain in a normal range because of a corresponding decrease in hepatic and renal clearance.

Cortisol has multiple effects on intermediate carbohydrate, protein, and fatty acid metabolism. Glucocorticoids enhance gluconeogenesis, elevate blood glucose, and promote hepatic glycogen synthesis.[120, 121] In supraphysiologic amounts, glucocorticoids suppress growth hormone secretion and impair somatic growth. The anti-inflammatory actions of cortisol relate to its effect in stabilizing lysosomes and promoting capillary integrity. Cortisol also antagonizes leukocyte migration inhibition factor (MIF), thus reducing white cell adherence to vascular endothelium and diminishing leukocyte response to local inflammation.[122] Phagocytic activity does not decrease, although the killing potential of macrophage and monocytes is diminished.[123] Other diverse actions include the facilitation of free water clearance, maintenance of blood pressure, a weak mineralocorticoid effect, promotion of appetite, stimulation of hematopoiesis, and induction of liver enzymes.

CONTROL OF GLUCOCORTICOID SECRETION

Cortisol secretion is directly controlled by ACTH, which in turn is regulated by the corticotropin-releasing factor (CRF). ACTH is synthesized in the pituitary gland from a precursor molecule that also produces beta-lipotropin and beta-endorphin. The secretion of ACTH and CRF is governed chiefly by cortisol-like steroids, the sleep–wake cycle, and stress. Cortisol is the most potent regulator of ACTH secretion, acting by a negative feedback mechanism to maintain cortisol levels in a physiologic range. There is some evidence that cortisol may also feed back on higher neuronal centers.[121] ACTH acts within minutes to elicit adrenal secretion by activating adenylate cyclase and the production of cAMP. ACTH release follows a diurnal pattern, with maximal activity occurring soon after awakening. This diurnal pattern of activity

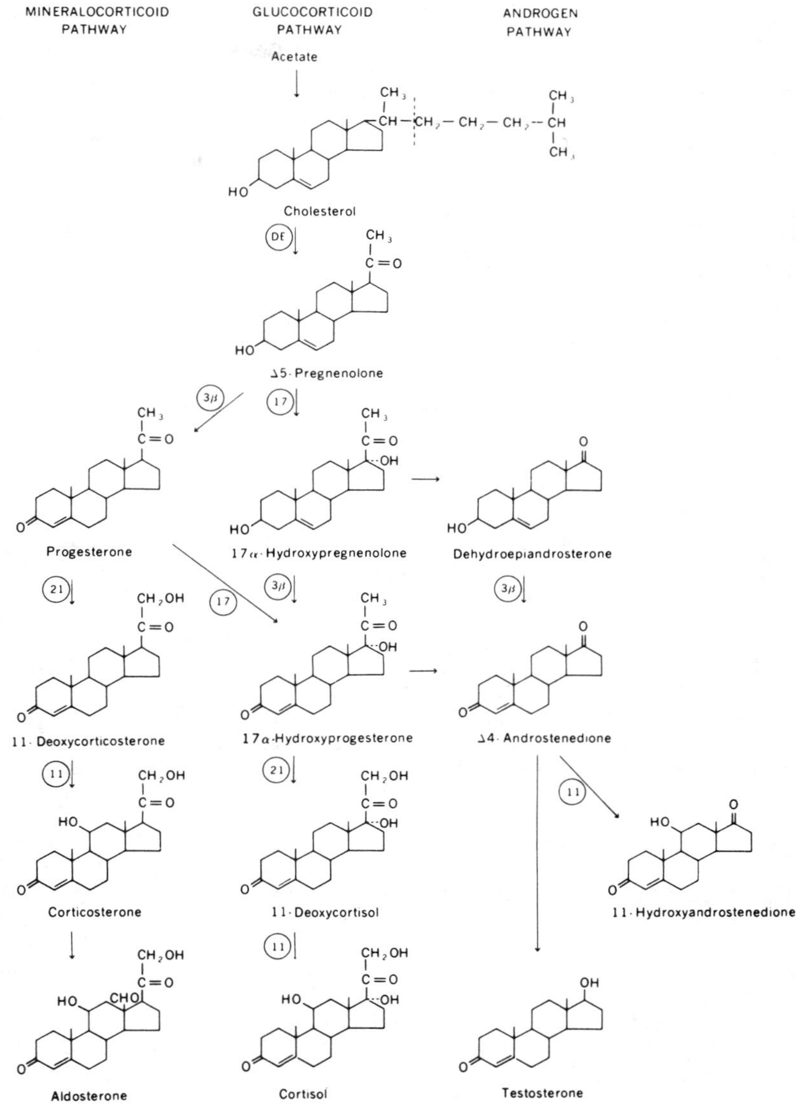

FIG. 44-4. Biosynthetic pathways for adrenal steroid production. Major pathways for mineralocorticoids, glucocorticoids, and androgens. Circled letters and numbers denote specific enzymes DE = debranching enzyme; 3B = 3B-ol-dehydrogenase with 4,5 isomerase; 11 = C-11 hydroxylase; 17 = C-17 hydroxylase; 21 = C-21 hydroxylase. (From Petersdorf RG [ed]: Harrison's Principles of Internal Medicine, 10th ed. New York, McGraw-Hill, 1983, with permission.)

occurs in normal subjects as well as in those with adrenal insufficiency.[124] Psychologic or physical stress (trauma, surgery, intense exercise) also promotes ACTH release regardless of the level of circulating cortisol or the time of day.[125]

MINERALOCORTICOID PHYSIOLOGY

Aldosterone is the most potent mineralocorticoid produced by the zona glomerulosa of the adrenal gland. This hormone binds to receptors in sweat glands, the alimentary tract, and the distal convoluted tubule of the kidney. Aldosterone is a major regulator of extracellular volume and potassium homeostasis through the reabsorption of sodium and secretion of potassium by these tissues.[121, 126] The major regulators of aldosterone release are the renin-angiotensin system, serum potassium, and ACTH[121] (Fig. 44-5). The juxtaglomerular apparatus located surrounding the renal afferent arterioles produces renin in response to decreased perfusion pressures (hypovolemia), sympathetic stimulation, and hypokalemia.[121]

Renin splits the hepatic precursor angiotensinogen to form the decapeptide, angiotensin I, which is then altered enzymatically by converting enzyme (primarily in the lung) to form the octapeptide angiotensin II. Angiotensin II is the most potent vasopressor produced in the body. It directly stimulates the adrenal cortex to produce aldosterone. The renin angiotensin system is the body's most important protector of volume status. Other stimuli that increase the production of aldosterone include hyperkalemia and, to a limited degree, ACTH.[121]

ANDROGEN PHYSIOLOGY

Dehydroepiandrosterone and androstenedione are weak androgens produced in the adrenal cortex. These adrenal androgens are converted outside of the adrenal gland to testosterone, which is inactivated in the liver to form 17-ketosteroids. Dehydroepiandrosterone serves as the major precursor of urinary 17-ketosteroids. There is a progressive

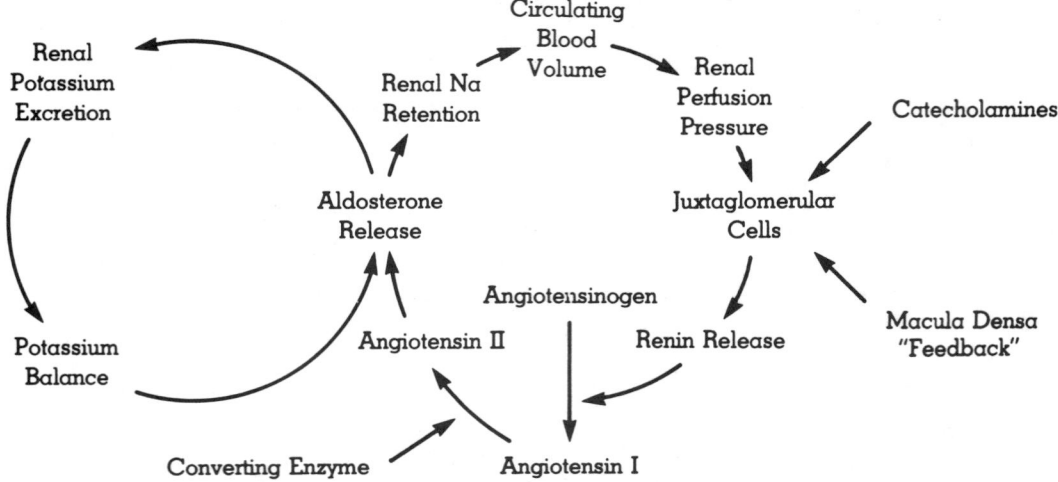

FIG. 44-5. The interrelationship of the volume and potassium feedback loops on aldosterone secretion. (From Petersdorf RG [ed]: Harrison's Principles of Internal Medicine, 10th ed. New York, McGraw-Hill, 1983, with permission.)

decline in adrenal androgen production with age. Some congenital defects in adrenal enzyme activity are associated with alterations in adrenal androgen production and cortisol deficiency.[127] The release of adrenal androgens is stimulated by ACTH, not by gonadotropins.

GLUCOCORTICOID EXCESS

The overproduction of cortisol by the adrenal cortex results in a syndrome characterized by truncal obesity, hypertension, hyperglycemia, increased intravascular fluid volume, hypokalemia, fatigability, abdominal striae, osteoporosis, and muscle weakness.[117, 128, 129] The majority of cases arising spontaneously are due to bilateral adrenal hyperplasia secondary to ACTH produced by an anterior pituitary microadenoma or nonendocrine tumor (lung, kidney, pancreas). The incidence of adrenal hyperplasia secondary to pituitary overproduction of ACTH is three times higher in women than in men.[121, 130] The primary overproduction of cortisol and other adrenal steroids is caused by an adrenal neoplasm in approximately 20–25% of patients with Cushing's syndrome. These tumors are usually unilateral, and about half are malignant.[121] Spontaneously occurring Cushing's disease is more common in younger patients, with a peak incidence occurring during the 3rd decade of life. When Cushing's syndrome occurs in patients older than 60 years of age, the most likely cause is an adrenal carcinoma or ectopic ACTH produced from a nonendocrine tumor. Finally, an increasingly common cause of Cushing's syndrome is the prolonged administration of exogenous glucocorticoids to treat a variety of illnesses.

The signs and symptoms of Cushing's syndrome follow from the known actions of glucocorticoids. Truncal obesity and thin extremities reflect increased muscle wasting and a redistribution of fat in facial, cervical, and truncal areas. Impaired calcium absorption and a decrease in bone formation may result in osteopenia.[131] Sixty per cent of patients have hyperglycemia, but overt diabetes mellitus occurs in less than 20%.[117] Hypertension and fluid retention are seen in a majority of patients. Profound emotional changes ranging from emotional lability to frank psychosis may be present. An in-

creased susceptibility to infection reflects the immunosuppressive effects of corticosteroids.[132] If adrenal androgen secretion is increased, acne and hirsutism are frequent in women. Hypokalemic alkalosis without distinctive physical findings is common when adrenal hyperplasia is caused by ectopic ACTH production from a nonendocrine tumor.[117, 133]

Diagnosis

The biochemical diagnosis of hyperadrenocorticism is based on a variable elevation in plasma and urinary cortisol, urinary 17-hydroxycorticosteroids, and plasma ACTH. The diagnosis can be established by a failure to normally suppress endogenous cortisol secretion following the exogenous administration of dexamethasone. Initial screening is accomplished with a low-dose dexamethasone suppression test (0.5 mg q. 6 h. × 48 h.). As an aid to diagnosing the specific type of Cushing's disease, a high-dose dexamethasone suppression test (2 mg q. 6 h. × 48 h.) may follow. Patients with pituitary adenomas frequently show a marked depression in cortisol and 17-hydroxycorticosteroid levels when a high dose of dexamethasone is administered. The ectopic production of ACTH by a nonendocrine tumor usually shows no suppression with low- or high-dose dexamethasone. The administration of metyrapone, a drug that suppresses cortisol production by inhibiting the conversion of 11-deoxycortisol to cortisol (11β-hydroxylase inhibition), is useful in differentiating adrenal tumors from adrenal hyperplasia. When metyrapone is given to the patient with an adrenal tumor, the suppressed pituitary fails to release ACTH in an appropriate manner. In contrast, patients with adrenal hyperplasia display a normal or hyperactive response.[121] At the current time, computerized tomography is the radiologic technique most commonly used to identify abnormalities of the adrenal glands. Magnetic resonance imaging (MRI) is becoming popular as a method to study the pituitary.

Treatment and Anesthetic Management

Adrenalectomy is the traditional treatment for hyperadrenocorticism. General considerations for the preoperative preparation of the patient include regulating hypertension and diabetes and normalizing intravascular fluid volume and electrolyte concentrations. Diuresis with the aldosterone antagonist spironolactone helps to mobilize fluid and normalize the potassium concentration. Careful positioning of the osteopenic patient is very important. Intraoperative monitoring is planned after evaluation of the patient's cardiac reserve and consideration of the site and extent of the proposed surgery. In general, excision of a pituitary tumor carries less morbidity than either unilateral or bilateral adrenalectomy. The incidence of postoperative complications and perioperative mortality is highest in the patient undergoing bilateral adrenalectomy.[134, 135] When unilateral or bilateral adrenalectomy is planned, glucocorticoid replacement is initiated during surgery at the rate of 100 mg of hydrocortisone succinate q. 8 h. A continuous hydrocortisone infusion (10 mg·hr^{-1}), administered on the day of surgery, is an alternative regimen. The total dosage is reduced by about 50% per day until a maintenance dose of daily steroids is achieved (20 to 30 mg·day^{-1}). Hydrocortisone given in doses of this magnitude exerts significant mineralocorticoid activity, and additional exogenous mineralocorticoid is generally not necessary during the perioperative period. The oral administration of mineralocorticoid is usually started on day 5. Following bilateral adrenalectomy, most patients require 0.05–0.1 mg·day^{-1} of fludrocortisone (9-alpha-fluorohydrocortisone). Slightly higher doses may be needed if prednisone is used for glucocorticoid maintenance (little intrinsic mineralocorticoid activity). The fludrocortisone dose is reduced if congestive heart failure, hypokalemia, or hypertension develops. For the patient with a solitary adrenal adenoma, unilateral adrenalectomy may be followed by a normalization of function in the contralateral gland over time. Treatment plans should therefore be individualized, and adjustments in dosage may be necessary. The production of glucocorticoids or ACTH by a neoplasm may not be eliminated if the tumor is unresectable. These patients often require continuous medical therapy with steroid inhibitors (metyrapone or O,P^1-DDD[2,2 bis(2-chlorophenyl-4-chlorophenyl)-11-dichloroethane]) to control their symptoms.

There are no recommendations regarding the use of a particular anesthetic technique or medication in patients with hyperadrenocorticism. When significant skeletal muscle weakness is present, a conservative approach to the use of muscle relaxants is warranted.

MINERALOCORTICOID EXCESS

Hypersecretion of the major adrenal mineralocorticoid aldosterone increases the renal tubular exchange of sodium for potassium and hydrogen ions. This leads to potassium depletion, skeletal muscle weakness, fatigue, and hypokalemic alkalosis.[136, 137] Approximately 1% of unselected hypertensive patients have primary hyperaldosteronism. The increase in renal sodium reabsorption and extracellular volume expansion is in part responsible for the high incidence of diastolic hypertension in these patients.[138] Patients with primary hyperaldosteronism (Conn's syndrome) characteristically do not have edema; however, in long-standing cases, a nephropathy may occur, and, in rare instances, it is associated with congestive heart failure and pretibial edema. The majority of cases are caused by a unilateral adenoma; however, bilateral adrenal hyperplasia is another possible etiology.[121] The diagnosis of primary or secondary hyperaldosteronism should be entertained in the nonedematous hypertensive patient with persistent hypokalemia who is not receiving potassium-wasting

diuretics. The hyposecretion of renin that fails to increase appropriately during volume depletion is an important finding in primary aldosteronism. Secondary aldosteronism results from an elevation in renin production. The measurement of plasma renin levels is useful in distinguishing these two from one another; however, it is of limited value in differentiating patients with primary aldosteronism from those with other causes of hypertension, because suppressed renin activity also occurs in about 25% of patients with essential hypertension. The hypersecretion of aldosterone that is not suppressed during volume expansion (salt loading) is the final diagnostic criteria.[139, 140] The most common diagnostic problem is distinguishing between an adenoma and bilateral adrenal hyperplasia as a cause of the hypersecretion. Although patients with bilateral adrenal hyperplasia tend to have lower aldosterone levels and less severe hypokalemia, differentiation is impossible on clinical or biochemical grounds. Computerized tomography is useful in this situation.[141] This distinction is particularly important since the hypertension associated with an adenoma is usually markedly improved or cured following surgical excision of the tumor. In contrast, hypertension associated with bilateral hyperplasia is usually not benefited by bilateral adrenalectomy. Surgery is indicated only when symptomatic hypokalemia cannot be controlled with medical therapy.

Anesthetic Considerations

Preoperative preparation for the patient with primary aldosteronism is directed toward restoring the intravascular volume and the electrolyte concentrations to normal. Hypertension and hypokalemia may be controlled by restricting sodium intake and administration of the aldosterone antagonist spironolactone. This diuretic works slowly to produce an increase in potassium levels, with doses in the range of 25 to 100 mg q. 8 h.[136, 137] Total body potassium deficits are difficult to estimate and may be in excess of 300 mEq. Whenever possible, potassium is replaced over a 24- to 48-hour period in order to allow equilibration between intra- and extracellular potassium stores. Extended medical management is possible, but chronic therapy with spironolactone is limited by the occurrence of gynecomastia and impotence.

ADRENAL INSUFFICIENCY

The undersecretion of adrenal steroid hormones may develop as the result of a primary inability of the adrenal gland to elaborate sufficient quantities of hormone or a secondary deficiency in the production of ACTH.

Clinically, primary adrenal insufficiency is usually not apparent until at least 90% of the adrenal cortex has been destroyed. The predominant cause of primary adrenal insufficiency during the early part of the century was tuberculosis; however, at the present time, the most frequent cause of Addison's disease is idiopathic adrenal insufficiency secondary to an autoimmune destruction of the gland (Table 44-4).[142] The autoimmune destruction of the adrenal cortex causes both a glucocorticoid and a mineralocorticoid deficiency. A variety of other conditions presumed to have an autoimmune pathogenesis may also occur concomitantly with idiopathic Addison's disease. Hashimoto's thyroiditis in association with autoimmune adrenal insufficiency is termed Schmidt's syndrome.[143] Other possible causes of adrenal gland destruction include certain bacterial or fungal infections, cancer, or hemorrhage.[121, 144]

TABLE 44-4.   Classification of Adrenal Insufficiency

PRIMARY ADRENAL INSUFFICIENCY
Anatomic destruction of gland (chronic and acute)
"Idiopathic" atrophy (autoimmune)
Surgical removal (metastatic breast cancer)
Infection (tuberculosis, fungus)
Hemorrhage
Invasion: metastatic

METABOLIC FAILURE IN HORMONE PRODUCTION
Congenital adrenal hyperplasia
Enzyme inhibitors (metyrapone)
Cytotoxic agents (OP1–DDD)

SECONDARY ADRENAL INSUFFICIENCY
Hypopituitarism due to pituitary disease
Suppression of hypothalamic-pituitary axis
    Exogenous steroid
    Endogenous steroid from tumor

Secondary adrenal insufficiency occurs when the anterior pituitary fails to secrete sufficient quantities of ACTH. The most important cause of hypothalamic-pituitary-adrenal suppression confronting the anesthesiologist occurs as a result of the exogenous administration of glucocorticoids.[121] Pituitary failure may also result from tumor, infection, surgical ablation, or radiation therapy.[121, 145]

Clinical Presentation

Several important differences exist between primary adrenal insufficiency and hypopituitarism. The cardinal symptoms of idiopathic Addison's disease include asthenia, weight loss, anorexia, abdominal pain, nausea, vomiting, diarrhea, and constipation.[146] Hypotension is almost always encountered in the disease process.[144, 147] Diffuse hyperpigmentation occurs in most patients with primary adrenal insufficiency and is secondary to the compensatory increase in ACTH and beta-lipotropin.[121, 148] These hormones stimulate an increase in melanocyte production. Mineralocorticoid deficiency is characteristically present in primary adrenal disease, and, as a result, there is a reduction in urine sodium conservation and a decreased pressure response to circulating catecholamines. Hyperkalemia may be a cause of life-threatening cardiac dysrhythmias. Female patients may exhibit decreased axillary and pubic hair growth owing to the loss of adrenal androgen secretion. Adrenal insufficiency secondary to pituitary suppression is not associated with cutaneous hyperpigmentation or mineralocorticoid deficiency. Salt and water balance are usually maintained unless severe fluid and electrolyte losses overwhelm the subnormal aldosterone secretory capacity. Organic lesions of pituitary origin require a diligent search for coexisting hormone deficiencies.

It is important to recognize the patient with adrenal insufficiency secondary to exogenous steroid therapy, because it is possible for acute adrenal crisis to occur if high-dose glucocorticoids are abruptly withdrawn or if deficient patients are subjected to even minor stress.[149–151] Because patients who have received exogenous glucocorticoids may exhibit pituitary-adrenal suppression for up to 12 months following cessation of therapy, these patients receive supplemental glucocorticoid coverage during periods of increased stress (e.g., trauma, surgery, infection).[152] Patients receiving inhaled or topical steroids may also exhibit pituitary-adrenal suppression for up to 9 months following the cessation of therapy.[153]

Diagnosis

A determination of the patient's pituitary adrenal responsiveness should be obtained when the diagnosis of primary or secondary adrenal insufficiency is first suspected. Biochemical evidence of impaired adrenal or pituitary secretory reserve will unequivocally confirm the diagnosis. Patients who are clinically stable may undergo testing before treatment is initiated. Those patients suspected of having acute adrenal insufficiency should receive immediate therapy.

Plasma cortisol levels are obtained before and after (30 and 60 minutes) the iv administration of 250 µg of synthetic ACTH. Patients with adequate adrenal reserve will demonstrate an elevation in plasma cortisol of at least 7 $\mu g \cdot dl^{-1}$ or a total greater than 18 $\mu g \cdot dl^{-1}$ 60 minutes following the injection of the synthetic ACTH.[121, 154] Patients with adrenal insufficiency usually demonstrate little or no adrenal response. When extended ACTH testing is used, both plasma ACTH (radioimmunoassay) and urinary metabolites (17-hydroxycorticosteroids) are measured to avoid diagnostic errors. Endogenous pituitary ACTH reserve may be further tested through the administration of metyrapone. Patients with primary adrenal insufficiency exhibit elevated ACTH levels, whereas those with secondary adrenal insufficiency demonstrate either a subnormal or absent ACTH response to the administration of metyrapone.[121] The value of metyrapone testing is limited in many clinical settings (e.g., exogenous steroids, hypothyroidism pregnancy)[155] and has largely been replaced by ACTH stimulation tests. In addition, the metyrapone test may precipitate adrenal crisis in a patient with primary adrenal insufficiency.

Treatment

Normal adults secrete 20 mg of cortisol (hydrocortisone) and 0.1 mg of aldosterone per day. Glucocorticoid therapy is usually given twice daily in sufficient dosage to meet physiologic requirements. A typical regimen may consist of prednisone, 5 mg in the morning and 2.5 mg in the evening, or hydrocortisone, 20 mg q.A.M. and 10 mg q.P.M. The daily glucocorticoid dosage is typically 50% higher than basal adrenal output in order to cover the patient for mild stress. Replacement dosages are adjusted in response to the patient's clinical symptoms or to the occurrence of intercurrent illnesses. Addisonian patients should be instructed to increase glucocorticoid medication to three or four times their usual daily dosage during periods of increased stress. Mineralocorticoid replacement is also administered on a daily basis; most patients require 0.05 to 0.1 $mg \cdot day^{-1}$ of fludrocortisone. The mineralocorticoid dose may be reduced if severe hypokalemia, hypertension, or congestive heart failure develop or increased if postural hypotension is demonstrated. Children with Addison's disease receive lesser amounts of daily steroids. Twelve milligrams of cortisol per square meter of the body surface area is usually sufficient.

Secondary adrenal insufficiency often occurs in the presence of multiple hormone deficiencies. A decrease in ACTH production results in the decreased secretion of cortisol and adrenal androgens, but aldosterone control by more dominant mechanisms remains intact. A liberal salt diet is encouraged. Glucocorticoid substitution follows the same guidelines previously outlined for primary adrenal insufficiency.

Acute Adrenal Insufficiency

Acute adrenal insufficiency is usually precipitated by sepsis, trauma, or surgical stress in the setting of hypovolemic shock and severe electrolyte imbalance.[121] Immediate therapy is mandatory regardless of the etiology. Minimal therapy consists of fluid and electrolyte resuscitation and steroid replacement.

Initial therapy begins with the rapid iv administration of an isotonic crystalloid solution (D5NS). When emergency ACTH testing is being carried out, methylprednisolone (20 mg) is initially given. (Methylprednisolone is not detected by either RIA or protein displacement methods for steroid measurements.) If ACTH testing is not being performed, 200 to 300 mg hydrocortisone is administered as an iv bolus over several minutes. Steroid replacement is continued during the first 24 hours with 100 mg iv hydrocortisone q. 6 h. Provided that the patient is stable, the steroid dose is reduced starting on the second day. Following adequate fluid resuscitation, if the patient continues to be hemodynamically unstable, inotropic support may be necessary. Invasive monitoring is extremely valuable as a guide to both diagnosis and therapy. When primary adrenal insufficiency is diagnosed, mineralocorticoid replacement is also initiated. Once again, it is important to individualize therapy.

MINERALOCORTICOID INSUFFICIENCY

Isolated mineralocorticoid insufficiency has been reported as a congenital biosynthetic defect following unilateral adrenalectomy for removal of an aldosterone-secreting adenoma, during protracted heparin therapy, and in patients with a deficiency in renin production.[156-158] This syndrome is commonly seen in patients with mild renal failure and long-standing diabetes mellitus.[121] A feature common to all patients with hypoaldosteronism is a failure to increase aldosterone production in response to salt restriction or volume contraction.

Most patients present with hyperkalemia and a metabolic acidosis that is out of proportion with the degree of coexisting renal impairment. Most patients are hypotensive, and the hyperkalemia may be life threatening. Patients with low renin secretion, hypoaldosteronism, and renal dysfunction will respond to ACTH stimulation. Nonsteroidal anti-inflammatory drugs, which inhibit prostaglandin synthesis, may further inhibit renin release and exacerbate the condition.[159] Patients

with isolated hypoaldosteronism are given fludrocortisone orally in a dose of 0.05 to 0.1 mg·day^{-1}. Patients with low renin secretion usually require higher does to correct the electrolyte abnormalities. Caution should be observed in patients with hypertension or congestive heart failure. An alternative approach in these patients is the administration of furosemide alone or in combination with mineralocorticoid.[121]

EXOGENOUS GLUCOCORTICOID THERAPY

The therapeutic utilization of supraphysiologic doses of glucocorticoids has expanded, and, as a consequence, the clinical implications of such therapy are important. The relative glucocorticoid and mineralocorticoid properties of the various preparations is listed in Table 44-5. Dexamethasone, methylprednisolone, and prednisone have less mineralocorticoid effect than do cortisone and hydrocortisone. The anti-inflammatory activity of a glucocorticoid depends upon the hydroxyl group at the carbon 11 position. Therefore, glucocorticoids such as cortisone and prednisone must undergo hepatic conversion from 11-keto compounds to 11 beta-hydroxyl compounds before anti-inflammatory activity can occur. Consequently, prednisone and cortisone should probably be avoided in the presence of severe liver disease. Since most side-effects from steroids are related to the dose and duration of administration, the smallest effective dose is used for the shortest period of time.

Patients at particular risk for developing complications related to steroid therapy include those with diabetes mellitus, pre-existing infection, hypertension, or congestive heart failure. Aseptic necrosis of the bones, subscapular cataracts, pancreatitis, benign intracranial hypertension, and glaucoma are complications associated with exogenous steroid administration.[160-162] Although the overall incidence of steroid-associated peptic ulceration is small (2%), patients receiving exogenous steroids have approximately twice the risk of developing peptic ulceration or gastrointestinal hemorrhage than do controls.[163, 164]

Steroid Replacement During the Perioperative Period

The normal adrenal gland secretes somewhat less than 200 mg cortisol per day during the perioperative period.[164] During periods of extreme stress, the adrenal gland may be exog-

TABLE 44-5.   Glucocorticoid Preparations

GENERIC NAME	TRADE NAME	RELATIVE POTENCY* ANTI-INFLAMMATORY	RELATIVE POTENCY* MINERALOCORTICOID	APPROXIMATE EQUIVALENT DOSE MG
SHORT-ACTING				
Hydrocortisone (cortisol)	Cortef	1.0	1.0	20.0
Cortisone	Cortigen	0.8	0.8	25.0
Prednisone	Deltasone	4.0	0.25	5.0
Prednisolone	Hydeltrasol	4.0	0.25	5.0
Methylprednisolone	Medrol	5.0	±	4.0
INTERMEDIATE-ACTING				
Triamcinolone	Aristocort	5.0	±	4.0
LONG-ACTING				
Dexamethasone	Decadron	30.0	±	0.75

*Relative milligram comparisons with cortisol. The glucocorticoid and mineralocorticoid properties of cortisol are set as 1.

enously stimulated to secrete between 200 and 500 mg·day^{-1} of cortisol.[165] The pituitary-adrenal axis is generally considered to be intact if plasma cortisol greater than 22 µg·dl^{-1} is measured during acute stress.[166] Plumpton et al[167] have correlated the degree of adrenal responsiveness with the duration of surgery and the extent of surgical trauma. The mean maximal plasma cortisol level measured during major surgery (colectomy, hip osteotomy) was 47 µg·dl^{-1}. Minor surgical procedures (herniorrhaphy) resulted in mean, maximal plasma cortisol levels of 28 µg·dl^{-1}. Adrenal activity may also be affected by the anesthetic technique used. Engquist et al[168] demonstrated the effectiveness of regional anesthesia in postponing the elevation of cortisol levels for surgery of the lower abdomen and extremities. Deep general anesthesia may also suppress the elevation of stress hormones such as ACTH and cortisol during the surgical procedure.[169-172] Although symptoms indicative of clinically significant adrenal insufficiency have been reported during the perioperative period, these clinical findings have rarely been documented in direct association with glucocorticoid deficiency.[149-151, 172, 173] Since occurrence of acute adrenal crisis is life threatening, and since there is relatively little risk in providing "stress" steroid coverage, supplemental steroids are empirically administered to all patients who have received daily steroid replacement for at least 1 week in the year prior to surgery.[152]

A controlled study by Udelsman et al[174] recently demonstrated the life-threatening consequences of inadequate glucocorticoid replacement during a period of surgical stress. Primates were maintained on physiologic doses of glucocorticoids for 4 months following bilateral adrenalectomy. The adrenalectomized animals were then separated into three groups receiving, respectively, subphysiologic, physiologic, and supraphysiologic doses of steroid replacement. After 4 days, the animals underwent cholecystectomy. Those primates receiving subphysiologic doses of steroid during the perioperative period were hemodynamically unstable and had a significantly higher mortality rate than did sham-operated controls. Those monkeys receiving physiologic or supraphysiologic replacement doses of steroids had similar hemodynamic profiles and mortality rates when compared with sham-adrenalectomized controls. Wound healing and metabolic profiles were no different for animals receiving physiologic or supraphysiologic doses of steroids. Although there was no apparent advantage in providing supraphysiologic coverage, it was clear from the results that subphysiologic corticosteroid replacement was associated with an increase in cardiovascular instability and a higher mortality.

Symreng et al[175] advocate the iv infusion of 25 mg of cortisol before the induction of anesthesia, followed by a continuous infusion of cortisol (100 mg) during the following 24 hours. This "low-dose" cortisol replacement program was used in patients with proven adrenal insufficiency and resulted in plasma cortisol levels that were as great as the values seen in healthy control subjects subjected to a similar operative stress (Fig. 44-6). Although this "low-dose" approach appears logical, many clinicians are unwilling to adopt this regimen until further trials are undertaken in patients receiving physiologic steroid replacement. A popular regimen calls for the administration of 200 to 300 mg·70 kg^{-1} body weight of hydrocortisone in divided doses on the day of surgery. The lower dose is adjusted upward for longer and more extensive surgical procedures. Patients who are using steroids at the time of surgery receive their usual dose on the morning of surgery and are supplemented at a level that is at least equivalent to the usual daily replacement.[176] Glucocorticoid coverage is reduced to the patient's normal maintenance dosage during the

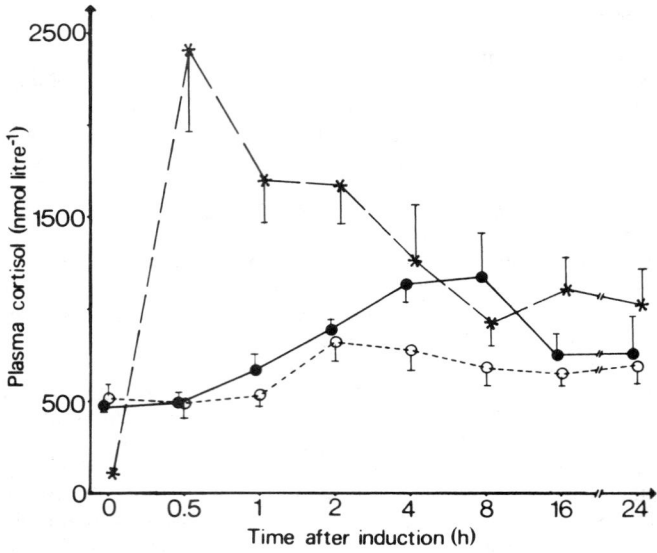

FIG. 44-6. Plasma cortisol concentrations (mean ± SEM) were measured in three groups of patients undergoing elective surgery. Group I, control patients n = 8 (●—●), had never received corticosteroids. Group II, n = 8 (○—○), patients received corticosteroids preoperatively with a normal response to ACTH (corticotropin) stimulation testing preoperatively. These patients and controls received no corticosteroid substitution during the perioperative period. Group III, n = 6 (*—*), consisted of patients receiving long-term corticosteroid therapy with an abnormal response to ACTH stimulation testing during the perioperative period. These patients (Group III) received intravenous cortisol, 25 mg, following the induction of anesthesia plus a continuous intravenous infusion of cortisol, 100 mg, during the next 24 hours. Plasma cortisol levels in Group III were significantly lower than in the other two groups before the induction of anesthesia. Following intravenous administration of cortisol to Group III patients, plasma concentrations were significantly higher compared with Groups I and II for the next 2 hours (P<0.01). Thereafter, the mean plasma concentrations were similar for all groups. There were no clinical signs of circulatory insufficiency in any group. (From Symreng T, Karlberg BE, Kagedol B, Schildt B: Physiological cortisol substitution of long-term steroid-treated patients undergoing major surgery. Br J Anesth 53:949, 1981, with permission.)

postoperative period. Although there is no conclusive evidence supporting an increased incidence of infection or abnormal wound healing when supraphysiologic doses of supplemental steroids are used acutely, the goal of therapy is to use the minimal drug dosage necessary to adequately protect the patient.

ADRENAL MEDULLA

The adrenal medulla is derived embryologically from neuroectodermal cells. As a specialized part of the sympathetic nervous system, the adrenal medulla synthesizes and secretes the catecholamines epinephrine (80%) and norepinephrine (20%). Preganglionic fibers of the sympathetic nervous system bypass the paravertebral ganglia and pass directly from the spinal cord to the adrenal medulla. The adrenal medulla is analogous to a postganglionic neuron, although the catecholamines secreted by the medulla function as hormones, not as neurotransmitters.

The biosynthetic pathway for catecholamines produced in the adrenal medulla is outlined in Figure 44-7. The synthesis of norepinephrine begins with hydroxylation of tyrosine to DOPA. This rate-limiting step in catecholamine biosynthesis is regulated so that synthesis is coupled to release. In the adrenal medulla and in those rare central neurons utilizing epinephrine as a neurotransmitter, the majority of norepinephrine is converted to epinephrine by the enzyme phenylethanolamine-N-methyltransferase. It is likely that the capacity of the adrenal medulla to synthesize epinephrine is influenced by the flow of glucocorticoid-rich blood from the adrenal cortex through the intraadrenal portal system, since it is known that high concentrations of glucocorticoid are able to induce the enzyme phenylethanolamine-N-methyltransferase.[121]

In the adrenal medulla, catecholamines are stored in chromaffin granules complexed with ATP and Ca^{++}. The normal adrenal releases epinephrine and norepinephrine by exocytosis in response to stimulation by preganglionic cholinergic fibers. The circulatory half-life (10 to 30 sec) of these catechols is considerably longer compared with the brief receptor activity of norepinephrine released as a neurotransmitter from postganglionic sympathetic nerve endings. Biotransformation of circulating norepinephrine and epinephrine is accomplished chiefly by the enzyme catechol-o-methyltransferase located in the liver and kidney. Monoamine oxidase is of less importance in the metabolism of circulating catechols. Metanephrines and vanillylmandelic acid (VMA) are the major end products of catecholamine metabolism. These metabolites and a small amount of unchanged catecholamine (less than 1%) appear in the urine.

The outflow of postganglionic sympathetic neurotransmitters and circulating catecholamine from the adrenal medulla is coordinated by higher cortical centers connected to the brain stem. The intrinsic activity of the brain stem sympathetic areas is modulated by higher cortical functions, emotional reactions (anger, fear), and various physiologic stimuli, including changes in the physical and chemical properties of the extracellular fluid (hypoglycemia, hypotension). The adrenal medulla and sympathetic nervous system are often stimulated together in a generalized fashion, although many physiologic conditions exist where they act independently.

PHEOCHROMOCYTOMA

The only important disease process associated with the adrenal medulla is pheochromocytoma. These tumors produce, store, and secrete catecholamines. Most pheochromocytomas secrete both epinephrine and norepinephrine, with the percentage of secreted norepinephrine being greater than the normal gland. Although pheochromocytomas occur in fewer than 0.1% of hypertensive patients, it is important to aggressively evaluate the patient with clinically suspicious symptoms, because surgical extirpation is curative in more than 90% of patients[177, 178] and because complications are often lethal in undiagnosed cases. Postmortem series have reported high perioperative mortality rates in undiagnosed patients undergoing relatively minor surgical procedures.[179, 180] The majority of deaths are from cardiovascular causes. Of particular importance to the anesthesiologist is the fact that anesthetic drugs can exacerbate the life-threatening cardiovascular effects of the catecholamines secreted by these tumors.

The majority (85–90%) of pheochromocytomas are solitary tumors localized to a single adrenal gland, usually the right. Approximately 10% of adults and 25% of children have bilateral tumors. The tumor may originate in extraadrenal sites (10%) anywhere along the paravertebral sympathetic chain; however, 95% are located within the abdomen, and a small percentage are located in the thorax, urinary bladder, or neck. Malignant spread of these highly vascular tumors occurs in about 10% of cases.[181, 182]

In about 5% of cases, this tumor is inherited as a familial autosomal dominant trait. It may be part of the polyglandular syndrome referred to as multiple endocrine neoplasia (MEN) Type IIA or IIB. Type IIA includes medullary carcinoma of the thyroid, parathyroid hyperplasia, and pheochromocytoma; Type IIB consists of medullary carcinoma of the thyroid, pheochromocytoma, and neuromas of the oral mucosa. Pheochromocytomas may also arise in association with von Recklinghausen's neurofibromatosis or von Hippel–Lindau disease (retinal and cerebellar angiomatosis). Pheochromocytoma of the familial syndromes is rarely extraadrenal or malignant. Bilateral tumors occur in approximately 75% of cases. When these patients present with a single adrenal pheochromocytoma, the chances of subsequent development of a second adrenal pheochromocytoma are sufficiently high to consider bilateral adrenalectomy. Every member of a MEN family should be screened periodically for pheochromocytoma.

Clinical Presentation

Pheochromocytoma may occur at any age, but it is most common in young to mid–adult life. The clinical manifestations are mainly due to the pharmacologic effects of the catecholamines released from the tumor. These tumors are not innervated, and catecholamine release is independent of neurogenic control. Although most patients (90%) are hypertensive, the blood pressure profile is labile in half of these cases. Forty per cent have paroxysmal hypertension, which occurs only during an attack. When true paroxysms occur, the blood pressure may rise to alarmingly high levels, placing the pa-

FIG. 44-7. The synthesis and metabolism of endogenous catecholamines. (From Stoelting RK, Dierdorf SF [eds]: Anesthesia and Co-Existing Disease. New York, Churchill-Livingstone, 1983, with permission.)

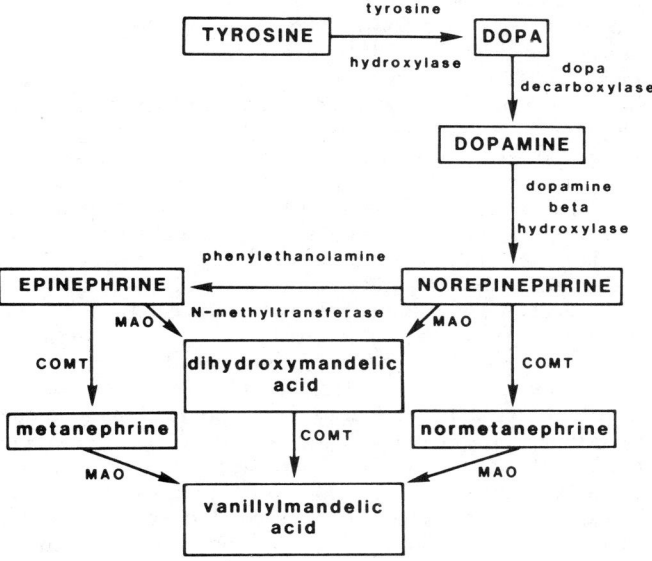

tient at risk for cerebrovascular hemorrhage, heart failure, dysrhythmias, or myocardial infarction. Headache, palpitations, tremor, profuse sweating, and either pallor or flushing may accompany an attack. Orthostatic hypotension, probably resulting from a reduction in plasma volume, is a frequent finding. Physical examination of the patient with pheochromocytoma may be unrevealing during the period between attacks unless the patient presents with symptoms and signs of sequelae related to long-standing hypertension. A well-described catecholamine-induced cardiomyopathy may present as myocarditis accompanied by heart failure and cardiac dysrhythmias. Paroxysms are commonly not associated with clearly defined events but may be precipitated by displacement of the abdominal contents or, in the case of bladder tumor, by micturition.

Diagnosis

Biochemical determination of free catecholamine concentration and catecholamine metabolites in the urine is the most common screening test used to establish the diagnosis of pheochromocytoma. Urinary VMA and unconjugated norepinephrine and epinephrine are measured in a 24-hour urine collection and are expressed as a function of the creatine clearance (Table 44-6). The level of VMA is elevated in most cases.[181, 183] Urinary metanephrine is not quantified, because it is not predictably elevated in pheochromocytoma. Free catecholamines represent < 1% of the originally released hormone, and urine levels are not always elevated to a significant degree. Hence, differentiation from normals may be difficult. A change in the ratio of unconjugated epinephrine to norepinephrine may be the only biochemical finding. In addition, certain drugs interfere with urinary assays,[184] and some patients with paroxysmal hypertension have normal values between attacks. The sensitivity of the urine assay has been greatly increased through the use of high-pressure liquid chromatography. The yield is further improved when multiple 24-hour urine specimens are collected. Although the distinction between "normal" and pheochromocytoma levels of urinary catecholamines may be difficult, provocative (glucagon, histamine) or suppression (clonidine) testing is seldom utilized. The determination of plasma catecholamine levels (RIA) has been advocated by some investigators as a more reliable diagnostic tool than urine assays.[185] It is their contention that plasma norepinephrine measurements are invariably elevated in these patients, irrespective of blood pressure (even between paroxysms).[186] Plasma catecholamine determinations have not gained widespread acceptance because of problems with the interpretation of results. It is extremely difficult to adequately control for the many physiologic and pharmacologic variables that affect plasma catecholamine levels.

Standardized imaging methods such as computerized tomography and MRI are used in the noninvasive localization of these tumors. Ultrasound and MRI are especially useful in pregnancy. ^{131}I-metaiodobenzylguanidine ([131]IMIBG) scintigraphy is also effective in localizing recurrent or extraadrenal masses. This guanidine analog has a molecular structure similar to that of norepinephrine and is concentrated in catecholamine storage vesicles. Arteriography must be carried out with extreme care in these patients, because a pressor crisis can be precipitated.

Anesthetic Considerations

PREOPERATIVE PREPARATION. The reduction in perioperative mortality from a high of 45% to between 0 and 3% with the excision of pheochromocytoma followed the introduction of alpha-antagonists for preoperative therapy. Perioperative blood pressure fluctuations, myocardial infarction, congestive heart failure, cardiac dysrhythmias, and cerebral hemorrhage all appear to be reduced in frequency when the patient has been treated preoperatively with alpha-blockers and the intravascular fluid compartment has been reexpanded.[187, 188] Extended treatment with alpha antagonists is also effective in treating the clinical manifestations of catecholamine myocarditis.[189] A list of drugs frequently used in the management of pheochromocytoma is found on Table 44-7.

Alpha-adrenergic blockade is initiated once the diagnosis of pheochromocytoma is established. The patient receives phenoxybenzamine, a long-acting (24 to 48 hr) noncompetitive presynaptic (alpha$_2$) and postsynaptic (alpha$_1$) blocker, at doses of 10 mg q. 8 h. Increments are added until the blood pressure is controlled and paroxysms disappear. Most patients require between 80 and 200 mg $\cdot$ day^{-1}. The absorption following oral administration is variable, and side-effects are common. Certain cardiovascular reflexes are blunted (baroreceptor), and postural hypotension is common. Alpha-blockade also causes nasal stuffiness and impairs ejaculation. Prazosin, a postsynaptic (alpha$_1$) blocking agent, with a shorter half-life than phenoxybenzamine, has also been used effectively. Because postural hypotension can be pronounced with the commencement of therapy, the initial dose is given at bedtime (1 mg). Postural changes are also seen with maintenance therapy (6 to 10 mg per day). A comparison of patients receiving phenoxybenzamine and prazosin has shown both drugs to be equally effective in controlling the blood pressure of patients with pheochromocytoma. A case report of severe hypertension in a prazosin-treated patient following the initiation of beta-blocker therapy suggested that a less selective blockade of both alpha$_1$ and alpha$_2$ receptors (phenoxybenzamine) might be preferable in patients with severe hypertension.[190] Although the optimal period of preoperative treatment has not been established, most clinicians recommend beginning alpha-blockade therapy at least 10 to 14 days before the proposed surgery. During this time, the contracted intravascular volume returns toward normal and the blood pressure is stabilized. Despite the real possibility of hypotension following vascular isolation of the tumor, we continue alpha-blockers up until the morning of surgery.

Beta-adrenergic blockade is often added after alpha-blockade has been established. This addition is considered in patients with persistent tachycardia or cardiac dysrhythmias that may be exacerbated by alpha-blockade. Beta-blockers should not be given until adequate alpha-blockade is ensured in order to avoid the possibility of unopposed alpha-mediated vasoconstriction. There is no clear advantage of one beta-antagonist over another. We have effectively used both propranolol and atenolol. Labetolol, a beta-antagonist with alpha-blocking activity, is effective as a second line medication, but there are reports of an increase in blood pressure when this

TABLE 44-6.   Reference Values for Normal Daily Urinary Excretion of Catecholamines and Catecholamine Metabolites

Vanillylmandelic acid	less than 5.0–6.0 mg $\cdot$ 24 hr^{-1}
Norepinephrine	less than 80 mg $\cdot$ 24 hr^{-1}
Epinephrine	less than 20 mg $\cdot$ 24 hr^{-1}
Total catecholamines	less than 100 mg $\cdot$ 24 hr^{-1}

TABLE 44-7. Drugs Used in the Management of Pheochromocytoma

| Drug | Action | PRESSOR CRISIS | | PREOPERATIVE BLOOD PRESSURE CONTROL | | |
		Route	Dose	Route	Dose	Comment
Phentolamine	Alpha-blocker	IV	2–5 mg	—	—	Rapid onset, short-acting; give bolus every 5 mins or infuse initially 1 mg · min^{-1}
Phenoxybenzamine	Alpha-blocker	—	—	Oral	30 mg · day^{-1} increasing daily dosage by 30 mg	Long half-life; may accumulate; give twice or three times daily
Prazosin	Alpha-blocker	—	—	Oral	1.0 mg single dose, increasing to t.i.d. regimen	First dose phenomenon; may cause syncope, so start with low dose before bedtime
Propranolol	Beta-blocker	IV	1.0 mg bolus to total of 10 mg	Oral	40 mg b.i.d.; increase to 480 mg · day^{-1}	When used alone may cause syncope, so start with low dose
Atenolol	Beta-blocker	—	—	Oral	50 mg · day^{-1} initially; may increase to 100 mg · day^{-1}	Long-acting selective beta$_1$ antagonist eliminated unchanged by kidney
Esmolol	Beta-blocker	IV	500 μg · kg^{-1} · min^{-1} loading followed by maintenance infusion	—	—	Ultra short-acting selective beta$_1$ antagonist may be used during anesthesia
Labetalol	Alpha- and beta-blocker	IV	10 mg bolus to 150 mg	Oral	200 mg t.i.d.	A much weaker alpha-blocker than beta-blocker; may cause pressor response in pheochromocytoma
Nitroprusside	Vasodilator	IV	Infusion initially 0.5–1.5 μg · kg^{-1} · min^{-1}	—	—	Powerful vasodilator; short-acting; may be used during anesthesia
Alpha-methyl-tyrosine	Inhibitor of biosynthesis of catecholamines	—	—	Oral	1–4 g · day^{-1}	Suitable for patients not amenable to surgery; may be nephrotoxic

drug is used alone.[191] In our opinion, inadequate postsynaptic alpha-blocking properties disqualify this medication as a first choice in the preoperative preparation of the patient.

Acute hypertensive crises are treated with iv infusions of nitroprusside or phentolamine. Phentolamine is a short-acting alpha-antagonist that may be given as an iv bolus (2–5 mg) or a continuous infusion. Tachydysrhythmias are controlled with iv boluses of propranolol (1-mg increments) or a continuous infusion of the ultra–short-acting selective beta$_1$ antagonist esmolol.

Alpha-methyl tyrosine is an agent that inhibits the enzyme tyrosine hydroxylase, the rate-limiting step in catecholamine biosynthesis. This medication is currently reserved for patients with metastatic disease or for those situations in which surgery is contraindicated and long-term medical therapy is required. When alpha-methyl tyrosine is used in combination with alpha-adrenergic blocking agents, there is a significant reduction in catecholamine biosynthesis.[184]

Unrecognized pheochromocytoma during pregnancy may be life threatening to the mother and fetus. Although the safety of adrenergic-blocking agents during pregnancy has not been established, these agents probably improve fetal survival in pregnant patients with pheochromocytoma.[192] There is no reason to terminate an early pregnancy, but the patient should be aware of the risk of spontaneous abortion resulting from abdominal surgery to remove the tumor. When pheochromocytoma is diagnosed during the third trimester, the mother is treated in the usual manner, and, when the fetus is sufficiently mature, the child is electively delivered by cesarean section, and the tumor is excised.

PERIOPERATIVE ANESTHETIC MANAGEMENT. Symptomatic patients continue to receive medical therapy until tachycardia, cardiac dysrhythmias and paroxysmal elevations in blood pressure are well controlled. Occasionally, a patient with pheochromocytoma unaccompanied by hypertension is referred for consultation prior to surgery. These patients are difficult to manage with alpha-blockade therapy on an outpatient basis because of the fear of clinically significant orthostatic hypotension. These patients are admitted to the hospital at least 24 hours before surgery in order to institute bedrest, "prophylactic" alpha-adrenergic blockade (prazosin), and fluid therapy. Central venous and peripheral artery pressure monitoring is routinely used to guide preoperative intervention. Owing to the unpredictable and potentially lethal nature of the patient response to the stress of anesthesia and surgery, all patients presenting for pheochromocytoma surgery should receive preoperative anesthesiology consultation and alpha-blocker therapy. Experience suggests that pretreated patients have fewer cardiac dysrhythmias and less fluctuation in blood pressure and heart rate during the induction of anesthesia compared with other "normotensive" patients who do not receive preoperative alpha-blockade. If it is not possible to initiate alpha-blocking therapy prior to surgery, or if the patient has received less than 48 hours of intensive treatment, it is frequently necessary to infuse phentolamine or nitroprusside during the induction of anesthesia. A low-dose "prophylactic" infusion is often initiated in anticipation of the marked blood pressure elevations that can occur with laryngoscopy and surgical stimulation.

Although there is no clear advantage of one anesthetic

technique over another, drugs that are known to liberate histamine are avoided. Because of the potential for ventricular irritability, halothane is not administered. Pulmonary artery and peripheral artery pressure monitoring are used in all adult patients. A well-sedated patient facilitates the placement of these monitoring devices before the induction of anesthesia. A potent sedative hypnotic in combination with an opioid analgesic is used for induction. It is extremely important to achieve an adequate depth of anesthesia before proceeding with laryngoscopy in order to minimize the sympathetic nervous system response to this maneuver. Maintenance is provided with an opioid analgesic and either isoflurane or enflurane. Manipulation of the tumor may produce marked elevations in the blood pressure, which are controlled with nitroprusside and, if necessary, phentolamine. Tachydysrhythmias are treated with iv beta blockers (*e.g.*, propranolol, labetalol, esmolol). The reduction in blood pressure that may occur following ligation of the tumor's venous supply should be anticipated through close communication with the surgical team. The restitution of any intravascular fluid deficit is the initial therapy in this situation. Following replenishment of the intravascular volume, if the patient remains hypotensive, phenylephrine is administered. Postoperatively, catecholamine levels return to normal over several days. Approximately 75% of patients become normotensive within 10 days.

DIABETES MELLITUS

Diabetes mellitus is the most commonly occurring endocrine disease found in surgical patients.[193–195] It has a broad spectrum of severity, and its manifestations can be altered in reaction to the patient's metabolic stress. Although the most serious complications of diabetes mellitus are related to its character as a chronic disease, it can cause difficulties in the short-term management of acute illness. Occasionally, diabetes will have been clinically inapparent until exacerbated by the stress of trauma or surgery.

The principles of the treatment of diabetes will be easier to understand if we review the physiology of glucose metabolism and the stress response and then consider some of the specific pathologic entities that make up the clinical picture of diabetes mellitus. The reader is also referred to Chapter 15.

CLASSIFICATION

Diabetes mellitus is primarily a disease of carbohydrate metabolism; however, it has numerous manifestations and interactions with a large range of hormonal and endocrinologic functions. Despite a variety of etiologic factors, its hallmark is a deficiency, either absolute or relative, in the amount of insulin available to the tissues.

Diabetes is often divided into two broad types.[196] Type I, or insulin-dependent diabetes mellitus (IDDM) is distinguished from Type II, or noninsulin-dependent diabetes mellitus (NIDDM). The patient with IDDM typically has had onset of the disease early in life. Consequently, this form is also referred to as juvenile onset diabetes. Generally, the patient with IDDM is not obese, had an abrupt onset of the disease, and has very low levels of circulating insulin. These patients cannot be controlled with diet or oral hypoglycemic agents and require insulin therapy. Patients in this group are often difficult to maintain in good glucose balance, are more likely to become ketotic, and are likely to develop the end-organ complications of diabetes if they live long enough.

Patients with NIDDM, also called maturity onset diabetes, typically have had a gradual onset of the disease later in life. They are often obese and have some degree of resistance to the effects of insulin. They may have normal or even elevated levels of insulin. In milder forms, this version of diabetes can often be treated with diet and/or oral hypoglycemic agents. Since these patients are relatively resistant to ketosis, their disease may be clinically inapparent until exacerbated by the stress of surgery or intercurrent illness.

This classification of diabetes mellitus is only a generalization. Occasionally, a younger person will have the disease in the milder NIDDM form, and there are many older adults who develop a severe and brittle form of IDDM. Diabetes can also be a secondary result of a disease that damages the pancreas and thus impairs insulin secretion. Pancreatic surgery, chronic pancreatitis, cystic fibrosis, and hemochromatosis can damage the pancreas and thus impair insulin secretion to produce clinical diabetes. Diabetes can result from one of the endocrine diseases that produces a hormone that opposes the action of insulin. Hence, a patient with a glucagonoma, pheochromocytoma, or acromegaly may be diabetic. An increased effect of glucocorticoids, either from Cushing's disease or steroid therapy, may also oppose the effect of insulin enough to elicit clinical diabetes and would certainly complicate the management of pre-existing diabetes. Patients with circulating anti-insulin receptor antibodies in association with other autoimmune processes are also diabetics. Finally, there is a clinical triad of severe insulin resistance in young hirsute women with polycystic ovaries who have decreased insulin receptors.

PHYSIOLOGY

Insulin has multiple and complex interactions with lipid, protein, and glucose metabolism.[197–199] For the present purpose, it is easiest to regard the effects of insulin on glucose metabolism as primary and to view its effects on other metabolic functions only as they relate to glucose.

Insulin is a small protein produced by the beta cells of the islets of Langerhans in the pancreas. Normal production in the adult human is about 40 to 50 units·day^{-1}. Insulin acts through receptor sites on cells. The half-life of insulin in the circulation is only a few minutes. However, it may clinically appear to have a longer duration of action owing to delays in binding and release from the cellular receptors. These facts lead us to the important principle that once a high level of insulin saturates all the binding sites, insulin will not have a more potent effect, just a more long-lasting effect. This is key to the understanding of insulin therapy, to be discussed in the following paragraphs.

Insulin is metabolized in the liver and kidney. In patients with hepatic dysfunction, the loss of gluconeogenesis as well as a prolongation of insulin effect increases the risk of hypoglycemia. Renal disease is another risk factor for hypoglycemia and is an important factor in managing the use of exogenous insulin in diabetic patients.

Insulin release is related to a number of events. First is the direct effect of glucose (and amino acids) to stimulate insulin release. The mechanism involves interaction with hormones from the gastrointestinal tract released during enteral feeding. The autonomic nervous system, also via vagal stimulation, will increase insulin release, as will beta-adrenergic stimulation and alpha-adrenergic blockade.

The most fundamental action of insulin is to cause increased uptake of glucose into the cells. This is particularly important in skeletal muscle cells, where muscle activity will also increase glucose uptake and is an important variable in the management of the physically active diabetic. (The brain and liver are exceptional areas where insulin does not affect glucose transport). Hence, the diabetic patient has hyperglycemia because of inadequate cellular uptake of glucose. Along with glucose, potassium enters the cells under the influence of insulin. So the diabetic patient is also likely to have an imbalance of potassium concentrations across the cell membranes.

Other important metabolic functions of insulin include the stimulation of glycogen formation and the depression of gluconeogenesis and lipolysis. The patient with insulin deficiency will have low glycogen stores and active gluconeogenosis. This implies that, in the diabetic, owing to an absence of glycogen, protein will have to be broken down to make glucose. Insulin also increases the uptake of amino acids into muscle cells. Hence, an insulin deficiency will lead to catabolism and negative nitrogen balance.

Fat metabolism is also abnormal in the diabetic state, with acceleration of lipid catabolism and increased formation of ketone bodies.[200] A deficiency of insulin leads to increased fatty acid liberation from adipose tissue. These fatty acids have multiple metabolic effects, including an interference with carbohydrate phosphorylation in muscle, which leads to further hyperglycemia. Low concentrations of insulin, which may be inadequate to prevent hyperglycemia, are often sufficient to block lipolysis. This effect explains the common clinical situation in which a patient is hyperglycemic without being ketotic.

Glucagon is a polypeptide released from the alpha cells of the pancreas and has actions both to stimulate the release of insulin and to oppose some of the effects of insulin. Hence, it has both a direct and an indirect ability to increase circulating glucose levels. In some patients, after total pancreatic resection, glucose balance is not as poor as might be expected because of the concomitant absence of glucagon. Glucagon release is stimulated by hypoglycemia as well as epinephrine and cortisol and is suppressed by glucose ingestion.[201]

DIABETES AND STRESS

The metabolic effects of stress are intricately involved with the same pathways as those involved in diabetes mellitus (Fig. 44-8).[202] During stress, elevations in the circulating levels of cortisol, glucagon, catecholamines, and growth hormones all act to cause hyperglycemia at the tissue level. In addition, glucagon and epinephrine exert a suppressive effect on insulin release. Hyperglycemia is common in the stressed patient who does not have diabetes mellitus. In the diabetic patient, stress will make the diabetes more difficult to control. In a patient with minimal or subclinical diabetes prior to the stressful episode, the glucose balance may become quite difficult to manage during the stress-related event. Thus, in the stressed diabetic patient, the catabolic effects of the stress may not be adequately countered by the anabolic effects of an inadequate insulin response.

The induction of anesthesia will increase the levels of circulating catecholamines and is a form of metabolic stress. Regional anesthesia may block part of the metabolic stress response during surgery, probably by blockade of the neural communications from the surgical area. It is theorized that the persistently high levels of circulating catecholamines in trauma and critical illness lead to stress hyperglycemia through a direct inhibition of insulin release. The bypass of the gastrointestinal hormonal actions in patients receiving iv glucose feedings, especially if given in large amounts, contributes to the impairment of insulin release during illness and can create a particularly difficult management problem for diabetics.

HYPERGLYCEMIA

Many diabetic patients, especially those with NIDDM, have circulating levels of insulin that in normal patients would be considered adequate or even excessive. Since insulin resistance at the cellular level is typical of diabetics, such patients have difficulty with glucose homeostasis and have elevated concentrations of blood sugar. Nevertheless, they often have enough insulin effect present to prevent ketosis. Such patients, especially with a therapeutic boost from sulfonylureas, diet, or exercise, are often able to control their metabolism enough to avoid severe swings in blood glucose concentrations and to avoid ketoacidosis. With more severe disease or with added stress, their metabolism may become quite disarrayed; insulin plus aggressive therapy of the concomitant disease may be required.

The insulin-dependent diabetic may have enough endogenous insulin present after the initial boost provided by a therapeutic dose of exogenous insulin. In such circumstances, the patient is likely to remain in good diabetic control, avoiding large swings in blood sugar and ketosis. However, when the amount of endogenous insulin available continues to be much less than what is metabolically required, additional therapeutic dosing is required to match the body's varying needs. The use of computerized insulin pumps with continuously reading glucose meters is more precise than other approaches to insulin therapy.

FIG. 44-8. Ketone production is increased in diabetes by augmented release (1) of free fatty acids (FFA) from adipose tissue, and beta oxidation of these FFA into ketones in the liver (2). (Illustration from McGarry JD, Foster DW: Arch Intern Med 137:496, 1977, with permission. Copyright 1977, American Medical Association.)

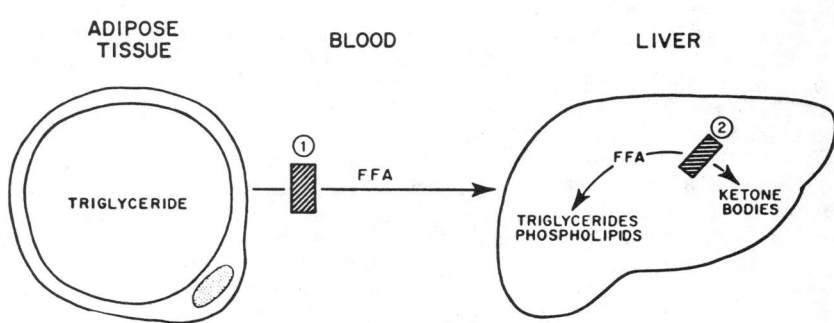

HYPOGLYCEMIA

Hypoglycemia is the clinical occurrence most feared when dealing with diabetic patients.[203] The precise level at which symptomatic hypoglycemia occurs is variable. The normal, fasted patient may have blood sugars lower than 50 mg · dl^{-1} without symptoms. However, the diabetic patient who has a chronically elevated blood sugar may be symptomatic quite above this glucose concentration. Hypoglycemia is almost impossible to diagnose clinically in the unconscious patient.

In the awake patient, hypoglycemia will often produce central nervous system (CNS) changes. These can range from light-headedness to coma with seizures. Often, the patient has learned to recognize the symptoms and can tell that his blood sugar is low before there are any clinical signs that an observer would be aware of. With hypoglycemia, there is a reflex catecholamine release that produces overt sympathetic hyperactivity causing tachycardia, lacrimination, diaphoresis, and hypertension. In the anesthetized patient, these signs of sympathetic hyperactivity can easily be misinterpreted as inadequate or "light" anesthesia. In the anesthetized, sedated, or seriously ill patient, the mental changes of hypoglycemia will also be unrecognizable. Furthermore, in patients being treated with beta-adrenergic blocking agents or with advanced diabetic autonomic neuropathy, the sympathetic hyperactivity of hypoglycemia may be obscured. Thus, the clinical diagnosis of hypoglycemia in the surgical patient may be quite difficult.

Hypoglycemia is more likely to occur in the diabetic surgical patient under certain circumstances. With renal insufficiency, the action of insulin and oral hypoglycemic agents is prolonged. This is a common problem due to the prevalence of renal disease in the diabetic. Since the effect of some of the oral agents, especially chlorpropamide, can be long-lasting, an accurate medical history with attention to medications taken in the past day or two is essential. A frequent, and totally avoidable, cause for inadvertent hypoglycemia is the administration of insulin to a patient who is not receiving sufficient oral or iv caloric input. For the purpose of preventing hypoglycemia, transfused blood has a low glucose concentration (even with CPD added, it contains only about 2 g of glucose per unit); lactated Ringer's solution is also inadequate (the lactate is metabolized to produce about 9 kcal · l^{-1}).

The anesthesiologist must recognize that hypoglycemia in the critically ill or anesthetized patient is a serious hazard that may be difficult to diagnose. It is therefore quite reasonable to aim for mild hyperglycemia as the goal in diabetes management in these patients. There is considerable discussion by endocrinologists as to how close to normal blood sugar should be maintained (chronic management) in long-standing diabetes in order to avoid the end-organ damage that diabetes can produce in the eyes, kidneys, nerves, and blood vessels.[204] In the perioperative period it is unlikely that such chronic damage is exacerbated by mild hyperglycemia.

Patients with chronic diabetes will often develop autonomic neuropathies that can cause bladder atony, postural hypotension, impotence, and delayed gastric emptying. There have also been rare reports of sudden death under anesthesia that are associated with autonomic cardiac dysfunction.[205, 206] Although all these phenomena are of concern, there is no reason to believe that they are effected by short-term glucose fluctuations.

Even if mild hyperglycemia is the "ideal" for the perioperative patient, the clinician should be alert to problems associated with hyperglycemia. There is a potential for increased risk of infection. Owing to osmotic changes in the lens, the alert patient may complain of some changes in vision. An osmotic diuresis is likely to result that leads to hypovolemia and a washout of potassium. If hyperglycemia is severe, the plasma will be hyperosmolar, and stupor or even coma could occur. Therefore, even if hyperglycemia is the intended goal, blood sugars above 500 to 600 mg · dl^{-1} are to be avoided. Hyperglycemia is likely if, in an overly eager attempt to avoid hypoglycemia, all the replacement fluids given to a perioperative patient contain dextrose. Such therapy will result in a large dextrose load that will cause significant hyperglycemia.

HYPEROSMOLAR NONKETOTIC COMA

Occasionally, an elderly patient with minimal or mild diabetes may present with remarkably high blood glucose levels and profound dehydration.[207] Such patients usually have enough endogenous insulin activity to prevent ketosis; even with blood sugar concentrations above 1000 mg · dl^{-1}, they are not in ketoacidosis. Presumably, it is the combination of an impaired thirst response and mild renal insufficiency that allows such hyperglycemia to develop. This marked hyperosmolarity may lead to coma and seizures, with the increased plasma viscosity producing a tendency to intravascular thrombosis. It is characteristic of this syndrome that the metabolic disturbance responds quickly to rehydration and small doses of insulin. With rapid correction of the hyperosmolarity, cerebral edema is a risk, and the recovery of mental acuity may be delayed after the blood glucose and circulating volume have been normalized.

DIABETIC KETOACIDOSIS

If the diabetic patient has insufficient insulin effect to block the mobilization and metabolism of free fatty acids, the metabolic by-products acetoacetate and beta-hydroxybutyrate will accumulate (Fig. 44-9).[208] These ketone bodies are organic acids and will cause a metabolic acidosis with an increased unmeasured anion "gap." Clinically, the patient often presents because of intercurrent illness, trauma, or the untoward cessation of insulin therapy. Although hyperglycemia is almost always present, the degree of hyperglycemia does not correlate with the severity of the acidosis. Blood sugar levels are often in the 300 to 500 mg · dl^{-1} range. The patient is always dehydrated because of the combination of the hyperglycemia-induced osmotic diuresis and the nausea and vomiting typical of this syndrome. Because leukocytosis, abdominal pain, gastrointestinal ileus, and mildly elevated amylase are all common in ketoacidosis, occasionally a patient will be misdiagnosed as having an intraabdominal surgical problem.

Potassium replacement is a key concern in patients with diabetic ketoacidosis. Owing to the diuresis, the total body potassium stores are reduced. However, acidosis by itself causes a shift of potassium ions out of the cell. Thus, the serum potassium concentration may be normal or even slightly elevated while the patient is acidotic. As soon as the metabolic acidosis is corrected, the potassium ions shift back into the cells. Consequently, the serum potassium concentration can decline acutely. Therefore, early and vigorous potassium replacement is required in these patients—the exception being those patients with renal failure. Hypophosphatemia also occurs with the correction of the acidosis and, if severe, may cause impairment of ventilation resulting from skeletal muscle weakness in the vulnerable patient. Instead of diabetic ketoacidosis, the diabetic patient with a meta-

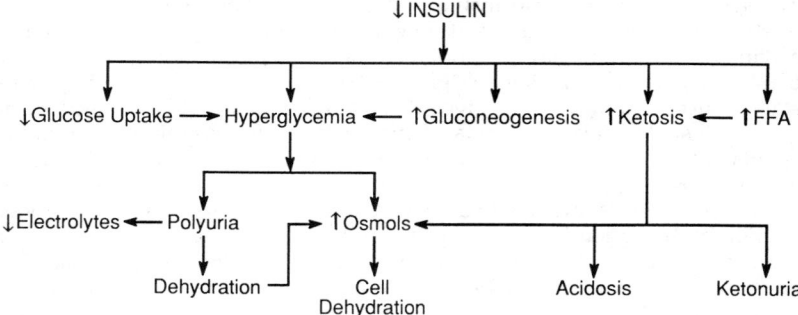

FIG. 44-9. Pathophysiology of diabetic ketoacidosis starting from relative insulin deficiency. (Illustration adapted with permission from Olefsky JM: In Wyngaarden JB, Smith LH [eds]: Cecil Textbook of Medicine, Philadelphia, p 1375. WB Saunders, 1988.)

bolic acidosis may have lactic acidosis, which results from poor tissue perfusion or sepsis. It is diagnosed by the presence of an increased serum lactate without an elevated concentration of ketones.

Diabetic ketoacidosis must also be distinguished from the syndrome of alcoholic ketoacidosis.[209] This typically occurs in the poorly nourished alcoholic following acute intoxication. Except for the presence of chemical ketoacidosis, alcoholic ketoacidosis is not clinically related in any way to diabetes mellitus. The alcoholic patient may be hypoglycemic or mildly hyperglycemic. The predominant ketone in this syndrome is beta-hydroxybutyrate, which tends to react less sensitively in the standard laboratory nitroprusside reaction measurement of ketones. Hence, the diagnosis may be obscured. Dextrose and parenteral fluids are the specific treatment for alcoholic ketoacidosis; insulin is not indicated (except in the rare circumstance in which the patient also has clear-cut diabetes mellitus). Although unrelated to the ketoacidosis, early thiamine supplementation to prevent the development of Wernicke–Korsakoff syndrome may be the most important part of the therapy of any poorly nourished alcoholic.

PERIOPERATIVE MONITORING

The anesthesiologist must usually determine in advance the types of physiological monitoring that will be used during surgery.[210] For the diabetic patient, fluid output and metabolic measurements are likely to be particularly important. It is reasonable to request that all diabetic surgical patients have preoperative determinations of blood glucose and potassium, urine glucose and ketones and that these tests be repeated immediately after surgery. For operations of short duration in nonbrittle patients, it is unlikely that much metabolic dysfunction can occur. However, for longer surgical procedures, changes may be very significant, and blood glucose measurements should be obtained every 2 to 4 hours. A urinary catheter allows for frequent testing for glucose and ketones. Another argument for the use of a urinary catheter is to prevent bladder distention, which can cause serious bladder dysfunction in the diabetic who may already have a neurogenic bladder. This is further potentiated by the presence of a large urine output caused by a hyperglycemic osmotic diuresis. The urinary catheter may, however, cause a bladder infection in the susceptible diabetic.

On the basis of a preoperative osmotic diuresis, the diabetic patient may present to the operating room with clinically significant dehydration. In addition to the usual principles of perioperative fluid management, it is important to note the amount of glucose administered iv to avoid a massive over-dose of glucose. The standard amount of glucose for an adult patient is 5 to 10 g·hr^{-1} (100 to 200 ml of 5% dextrose solution hourly). It is best to monitor and record the dextrose administration separately from the fluids given. It would be wrong to give large amounts of dextrose (contained in the iv solutions) just because that patient required vigorous fluid replacement. If this happens, the patient is likely to be very hyperglycemic in the Post Anesthesia Care Unit. It is difficult to determine the proper dose of insulin to correct this iatrogenic hyperglycemia, and prolonged observation and therapy may be required.

Management of the patient who presents to the operating room with significant metabolic impairment, such as diabetic ketoacidosis, is very similar to that in the medical intensive care unit, including hourly determinations of blood glucose, arterial pH, electrolytes, and fluid balance. Frequent reassessments with medical consultation, if required, guide the use of fluids, electrolytes (especially potassium), insulin, phosphate, and glucose.[211, 212]

Another area of patient monitoring that is extremely important in the diabetic patient is the positioning on the operating table. Injuries to the limbs or nerves is more likely in the patient who comes to the operating room already suffering from diabetic peripheral vascular disease or neuropathy. The peripheral nerves may already be partly ischemic and, therefore, particularly vulnerable to pressure or stretch injuries.[213]

MANAGEMENT REGIMENS

There are several different regimens that can be used to provide an appropriate balance of insulin and glucose in the diabetic patient undergoing anesthesia and surgery.[214–217] These approaches use different combinations of iv and subcutaneous insulin and seem, in general, to be equally satisfactory in the hands of experienced clinicians. However, regardless of the approach used, the basic principles of diabetic management must be recognized. Firstly, and most obviously, it is important to avoid hypoglycemia. Secondly, since hypoglycemia may develop insidiously and be difficult to detect quickly, insulin and glucose therapy is administered to result in a mild transient hyperglycemia that can be corrected gradually in the postoperative period. Mild hyperglycemia is not an acute problem, and there is no need for it to be corrected rapidly. It is never simple to determine what is the precise dose of insulin required to correct hyperglycemia. Attempts at excessively rapid correction may lead to glucose instability and fluctuations that can persist for many hours and days.

For some diabetic patients, the best method of diabetic

management is to give no insulin. For short procedures in unstressed patients, especially if they are not chronically receiving insulin, there may be enough endogenous production of insulin to maintain reasonable glucose balance in the unfed state. Glucose should still be given during surgery as protection against the delayed effects of prior oral hypoglycemic agents or long-acting insulin and to prevent the occurrence of mild ketosis.

Another common method of management is to administer a fraction of the patient's usual morning NPH insulin dose the morning of the day of surgery. Often, half the usual NPH dose will suffice to maintain the patient through the day. It is critical for the patient who is NPO and receiving insulin to also receive an iv infusion of a dextrose solution. If 5 to 10 g · hr^{-1} of dextrose (100 to 200 ml · hr^{-1} of 5% dextrose solution) is administered to the adult, the risk of hypoglycemia is small. Nevertheless, the patient's usual dosage depends upon caloric intake and physical activity, which are very different in the hospital setting.

The "sliding scale" regimen for insulin administration is one that is very popular and easy to use. Varying doses of regular insulin are administered on a 4- to 6-hr schedule, depending upon a determination of blood or urine glucose levels and the patient's prior responses to insulin. This method of management guarantees that frequent checks are made of the patient's glucose levels. Large fluctuations in blood glucose can occur if insulin is administered in the presence of high glucose levels and no insulin is given for normal or intermediate levels. This can be avoided if some insulin is always present. Small doses of insulin can be prescribed for all but the lowest levels of blood glucose, or the sliding scale can be combined with a small morning dose of long-acting NPH insulin.

Although regular insulin may also be given intramuscularly (im),[218, 219] a continuous infusion of insulin may be the only method that is effective in the hypotensive or hypothermic patient. Intravenous boluses of insulin will have a rapid onset of action but will have a short duration because of the rapid clearance of insulin from the blood (10 units of iv insulin will have an effect lasting about an hour). Except in the patient with renal failure, in whom insulin effects are difficult to predict, the continuous infusion method has the advantage of rapidly adjusting the insulin effect by changing the rate of infusion. If the insulin is mixed with a 5% dextrose solution, the balance of insulin and dextrose can be maintained. In the adult with normal renal function, 7 to 10 units of regular insulin in 1 l of 5% dextrose, infused at 75 to 100 ml · hr^{-1}, provides 0.5 to 1 unit · hr^{-1} of insulin. This tends to be a low dose, and many patients will require more insulin, which can be given as either increased insulin concentration in the infusion, or in a sliding scale subcutaneous regimen.[220] This regimen must also have added in the standard amount of water and electrolytes needed for maintenance and replacement. A small amount of iv insulin will be lost by adherence to the wall of the tubing and containers, but this is not clinically significant and should not be a deterrent to this route of administration.[221]

PITUITARY GLAND

The pituitary gland is located below the base of the brain in a bony structure referred to as the sella turcica. The pituitary gland together with the hypothalamus form a central unit that regulates the release of various hormones. The pituitary gland is divided into two components. The anterior pituitary (adenohypophysis) secretes prolactin, growth hormone, go-

nadotropins (luteinizing hormone and follicle-stimulating hormone), thyroid-stimulating hormone, and ACTH. The posterior pituitary (neurohypophysis) secretes the hormones vasopressin and oxytocin. Hormone release from the anterior and posterior pituitary is regulated by the hypothalamus. Regulatory peptides or preformed hormone from the hypothalamus is transported to the pituitary gland through vascular or tissue connections.

Hyposecretion of anterior pituitary hormones is usually due to compression of the gland by tumor. This may begin as an isolated deficiency, but it usually develops into multiglandular dysfunction. Male impotence or secondary amenorrhea in the female is an early manifestation of panhypopituitarism. Panhypopituitarism following postpartum hemorrhagic shock (Sheehan's syndrome) is due to necrosis of the anterior pituitary gland.[222] Radiation therapy delivered to the sella turcica or nearby structures and surgical hypophysectomy are other causes of panhypopituitarism. Treatment of panhypopituitarism is with specific hormone replacement.

The hypersecretion of various anterior pituitary hormones is usually caused by an adenoma. Excess prolactin secretion with galactorrhea is a common hormonal abnormality associated with pituitary adenoma.[223] Cushing's disease may occur secondary to excess ACTH production, and giantism or acromegaly may occur as a consequence of excess growth hormone production in the child or adult, respectively. Excessive secretion of TSH is rare.

Acromegaly in the adult patient may present several problems for the anesthesiologist. Excess hypertrophy occurs in skeletal connective and soft tissues.[224] The tongue and epiglottis are enlarged, making the patient susceptible to upper airway obstruction. Hoarseness may reflect thickening of the vocal cords or paralysis of a recurrent laryngeal nerve owing to stretching. Dyspnea or stridor is associated with subglottic narrowing. Peripheral nerve and/or artery entrapment, hypertension, and diabetes mellitus are other common findings. The anesthetic management of these patients is complicated by distortion of the facial anatomy and upper airway. The induction of general anesthesia may put the patient at increased risk if mask placement or vocal cord visualization is impaired. When the preoperative history suggests upper airway or vocal cord involvement, it is prudent to consider intubation of the trachea while the patient is awake.

POSTERIOR PITUITARY

The posterior pituitary or neurohypophysis is composed of terminal nerve endings that extend from the ventral hypothalamus. Vasopressin (ADH) and oxytocin are the two principle hormones secreted by the posterior pituitary. Both hormones are synthesized in the supraoptic and paraventricular nuclei of the hypothalamus. They are bound to inactive carrier proteins, neurophysins, and transported by axons to membrane-bound storage vesicles located in the posterior pituitary. Antidiuretic hormone (vasopressin) is a nonapeptide that circulates as a free peptide after its release. The primary functions of ADH are the maintenance of extracellular fluid volume and regulation of the plasma osmolality. Oxytocin elicits contraction of the uterus and promotes milk secretion and ejection by the mammary glands.

Vasopressin

ADH promotes reabsorption of solute free water by increasing cell membrane permeability to water alone. Target sites for ADH are the collecting tubules of the kidneys. A decrease in free water clearance causes a fall in serum osmolality and a corresponding increase in circulating blood volume. Under normal conditions, the primary stimulus for the release of ADH is an increase in serum osmolality.[225] Osmoreceptors located in the hypothalamus are sensitive to changes in the normal serum osmolality of as little as 1% (normal osmolality about 285 mOsm $\cdot$ l^{-1}). Stretch receptors in the left atrium and perhaps pulmonary veins, which are sensitive to moderate reductions in the blood volume, are also capable of stimulating ADH secretion. The need to restore plasma volume may at times override osmotic inhibition of ADH release. Various physiologic and pharmacologic stimuli also influence the secretion of ADH. Positive pressure ventilation of the lungs, stress, anxiety, hyperthermia, beta-adrenergic stimulation, and any histamine-releasing stimulus can promote the release of ADH.

ADH also has other actions. ADH can increase blood pressure by constricting vascular smooth muscle.[226] This activity is most significant in the splanchnic, renal, and coronary vascular beds and provides the rationale for administering exogenous vasopressin in the management of hemorrhage owing to esophageal varices (decreased portal venous pressure).[227] Caution must be observed when using this drug in patients with coronary artery disease. ADH can precipitate myocardial ischemia (even in small doses) through vasoconstriction of the coronary arteries. It is unclear whether selective arterial infusion is safer than systemic administration with regard to cardiac and vascular side-effects.[228]

ADH also promotes hemostasis through an increase in the level of circulating von Willebrand factor and factor VIII. Desmopressin (DDAVP), an analog of ADH, administered to patients following cardiopulmonary bypass in a dose of 0.3 μg $\cdot$ kg^{-1} significantly decreased blood loss and reduced transfusion requirements in comparison to a group of patients who did not receive the drug.[229] ADH may also have a place in the management of mild hemophiliacs undergoing surgery.

Diabetes Insipidus

This disorder results from an inadequate secretion of ADH or resistance on the part of the renal tubules to the ADH hormone (nephrogenic diabetes insipidus). Failure to secrete adequate amounts of ADH results in polydipsia, hypernatremia, and a high output of poorly concentrated urine. Hypovolemia and hypernatremia may become so severe as to be life threatening. This disorder usually occurs following destruction of the pituitary gland by intracranial trauma, infiltrating lesions, or surgery. Patients who develop diabetes insipidus (DI) secondary to head trauma usually recover after a short period of time. The treatment of DI is dependent upon the extent of the hormonal deficiency. Intraoperatively, the patient with complete DI receives an iv infusion of aqueous ADH (100 to 200 milliunits $\cdot$ hr^{-1}) combined with the administration of an isotonic crystalloid solution. The serum sodium and plasma osmolality are measured on a regular basis, and therapeutic changes are made accordingly. ADH may also be given im (vasopressin tannate in oil). DDAVP administered intranasally has prolonged antidiuretic activity (12 to 24 hr) and a low incidence of pressor effects. As a consequence of the large outpouring of ADH in response to surgical stress, patients with residual functioning gland usually do not require parenteral ADH during the perioperative period unless the plasma osmolality rises above 290 mOsm $\cdot$ l^{-1}. Nonhormonal agents that have efficacy in the treatment of incomplete DI include the oral hypoglycemic chlorpropamide (200 to 500 mg $\cdot$ day^{-1}). This drug stimulates the release of ADH and sensitizes the renal tubules to the hormone. Hypoglycemia is a serious side-effect that limits the usefulness of the drug. Clofibrate, a hypolipidemic agent, is also capable of stimulating ADH release and has been used in the outpatient setting. None of these medications are effective in the patient with nephrogenic diabetes insipidus. Paradoxically, the thiazide diuretics exert an antidiuretic action in patients with this disorder.

Inappropriate Secretion of ADH

The inappropriate and excessive secretion of ADH may occur in association with a number of diverse pathologic processes, including head injuries, intracranial tumors, pulmonary infections, small cell carcinoma of the lung, and hypothyroidism. The clinical manifestations occur as a result of a dilutional hyponatremia, decreased serum osmolality, and a reduced urine output with a high osmolality. Weight gain, skeletal muscle weakness, and mental confusion or convulsions are presenting symptoms. Peripheral edema and hypertension are rare. The diagnosis of syndrome of inappropriate antidiuretic hormone (SIADH) is one of exclusion, and other causes of hyponatremia must first be ruled out. Prognosis is dependent upon the underlying cause of the syndrome.

The treatment of patients with mild or moderate water intoxication is restriction of fluid intake to 800 ml $\cdot$ day^{-1}. Patients with severe water intoxication associated with hyponatremia and mental confusion may require more aggressive therapy, with the iv administration of a hypertonic saline solution. This may be administered in conjunction with furosemide. Isotonic saline is substituted for hypertonic solutions once the serum sodium is brought into a safe range. Caution must be observed in patients with poor left ventricular function. Other drugs that may be used in the patient with SIADH are demeclocycline and lithium. Demeclocycline interferes with the ability of the renal tubules to concentrate urine and is frequently used in the outpatient. Lithium is generally not used because of the high incidence of toxicity.

The Endocrine Response to Surgical Stress

Anesthesia and surgery elicit a generalized endocrine metabolic response characterized by an increase in the plasma levels of cortisol, ADH, renin, catecholamines, endorphins, and metabolic changes such as hyperglycemia and a negative nitrogen balance. Various neural and humoral factors (e.g., pain, anxiety, acidosis, local tissue factors, hypoxia) play a role in activating this stress response.

Endorphins are a group of endogenous peptides with opioid activity that have been isolated from the CNS. It is well documented that beta-endorphin is released from the anterior pituitary, where it is contained as part of beta-lipoprotein, a 91-chain amino acid, which is a cleavage product of the precursor peptide for ACTH. Large elevations in the CNS and plasma concentration of endorphins in response to emotional or surgical stimuli suggest that these substances play a role in the body's response to stress. These substances modulate painful stimuli by binding to opiate receptors located throughout the brain and spinal cord.

Numerous experiments have focused on the stress response and its relationship to the depth of anesthesia. Regional and general anesthesia appear to blunt the release of various stress hormones during the period of surgical stimulation in a dose-dependent fashion.[230-233] Historically, anesthesiologists have relied on the indirect measurement of hemodynamic variables such as blood pressure and heart rate to evaluate the level of autonomic activity in response to anesthesia and surgery. It is assumed that the physiologic manifestations of stress are potentially harmful, especially in patients with limited functional reserve. As such, our anesthetic techniques and pain management strategies are designed to limit this neurohormonal response, with the hope of providing the patient with some benefit. Further investigations are needed to assess the impact of these efforts on perioperative morbidity and mortality.

REFERENCES

1. Larsen PR: Thyroid-pituitary interaction. N Engl J Med 306:23, 1982
2. Sherwin JR, Tong W: The actions of iodide and TSH on thyroid cells showing a dual control system for the iodide pump. Endocrinology 94:1465, 1974
3. Brennan MD: Thyroid hormones. Mayo Cl Proc 55:33, 1980
4. Catt KJ, Dufau ML: Hormone action: Control of target cell function by peptide, thyroid and steroid hormones. In Felig P, Baxter JD, Broadus AE et al (eds): Endocrinology and Metabolism, pp 100–102. New York, McGraw-Hill, 1981
5. Eberhardt NW, Apulette JW, Baxter JB: The molecular biology of thyroid hormone action. In Litwok G (ed): Biochemical Action of Hormones, Vol 7, p 311. New York, Academic Press, 1980
6. Chernow B, O'Brien JT: Overview of catecholamines in selected endocrine disorders. In Lake CR, Ziegler M (eds): Norepinephrine, Vol 2. Baltimore, Williams & Wilkins, 1984
7. Buccins RA, Spann JF, Pool PE et al: Influence of the thyroid state on the intrinsic contractile properties and energy stores of the myocardium. J Clin Invest 46:1669, 1967
8. Baneyie SP, King LS: Beta-adrenergic receptors in rat heart; Effects of thyroidectomy. Eur J Pharmacol 43:207, 1977
9. Williams LT, Lefkowitz RJ, Watanabe AM: Thyroid hormone regulation of beta-adrenergic receptor number. J Biol Chem 252:2787, 1977
10. Spaulding SW, Utiger RD: In Felig P, Baxter JD, Broadus AE et al (eds): Endocrinology and Metabolism, p 281. New York, McGraw-Hill, 1981
11. Malbon CL, Moreno FJ, Cobelli RJ et al: Fat cell adenylate cyclase and β-adrenergic receptors in altered thyroid states. J Biol Chem 253:671, 1978
12. Sterling K: Thyroid hormone action at the cell level. N Engl J Med 300:173, 1979
13. Abuid J, Larsen PR: Triiodothyronine and thyroxine in hyperthyroidism: Comparison of the acute changes during therapy with antithyroid agents. J Clin Invest 54:201, 1974
14. Melmed S, Geola FL, Reed AW et al: A comparison of methods for assessing thyroid function in non-thyroidal illness. J Clin Endocrinol Metab 54:300, 1982
15. Sterling K, Brenner MA, Newman ES et al: The significance of triidothyronine in maintenance of euthyroid status after treatment of hyperthyroidism. J Clin Endocrinol 33:729, 1971
16. Morley JE: Neuroendocrine control of thyrotropin secretion. Endocrinol Rev 2:396, 1981
17. Jackson IMD: Thyrotropin releasing hormone. N Engl J Med 306:145, 1982
18. Snyder PJ, Utiger RD: Response to thyrotropin releasing hormone in normal man. J Clin Endocrinol Metab 34:380, 1972
19. Prange AJ, Lipton MA, Nemeroff CB et al: The role of hormones in depression. Life Sci 20:1305, 1977
20. Dussault JH: The effect of dexamethasone in TSH and prolactin secretion after TRH stimulation. Can Med Assoc J 111:1195, 1974
21. Spaulding SW, Burrow GN, Donabedian R et al: L-Dopa suppression of thyrotropin releasing hormone in man. Clin Endocrinol Metab 35:182, 1972
22. McKenzie JM, Zakarija M, Soto A: Humoral immunity in Graves' disease. Clin Endocrinol Metab 7:31, 1978
23. Volpe R: Thyroiditis: Current views of pathogenesis. Med Clin North Am 59:1163, 1975
24. Greene JW: Subacute thyroiditis. Am J Med 51:97, 1971
25. Woolf PD, Daly R: Thyrotoxicosis with painless thyroiditis. Am J Med 60:73, 1976
26. Doniach D, Roitt IM: Autoimmunity in Hashimoto's disease and its implications. J Clin Endocrinol Metab 17:1293, 1957
27. Amino N, Morik H, Iwantani Y et al: High prevalence of transient post partum thyrotoxicosis and hypothyroidism. N Engl J Med 306:849, 1982
28. Fradkin JE, Wolff J: Iodide induced thyrotoxicosis. Medicine 62:1, 1983
29. Channick BJ, Aldin EV, Marks AD et al: Hyperthyroidism and mitral valve prolapse. N Engl J Med 305:497, 1981
30. Davis PJ, Davis FB: Hyperthyroidism in patients over the age of 60 years. Clinical features in 85 patients. Medicine 53:161, 1974
31. Carter JN, Eastman CJ, Kilham HA et al: Rational therapy for thyroid storm. Aust NZ J Med 5:458, 1975
32. Mackin JE, Canary JJ, Pittman CS: Thyroid storm and its management. N Engl J Med 291:1396, 1974
33. Mazzaferri EL, Skillman TG: Thyroid storm. Arch Intern Med 124:684, 1969
34. Brooks MH, Waldstein SS: Free thyroxine concentration in thyroid storm. Ann Intern Med 93:694, 1980
35. Greer MA: Antithyroid drugs in the treatment of thyrotoxicosis. Thyroid Today 3:1, 1980
36. Wartofsky L, Ransil BJ, Ingbar SH: Inhibition by iodine of the release of thyroxine from the thyroid glands of patients with thyrotoxicosis. J Clin Invest 49:78, 1970
37. Feek CM, Sawers JS, Irvine WJ et al: Combination of potassium iodide and propranolol in preparation of patients with Graves' disease for thyroid surgery. N Engl J Med 302:883, 1980
38. Eriksson M, Rubenfeld S, Garber AJ et al: Propranolol does not prevent thyroid storm. N Engl J Med 296:263, 1977
39. Dillon PT, Baba J, Meloni CR et al: Reserpine in thyrotoxic crisis. N Engl J Med 283:1020, 1970
40. Dunn JT, Chapman EM: Rising incidence of hypothyroidism after radioactive iodine therapy in thyrotoxicosis. N Engl J Med 271:1037, 1964
41. Stehling LC: Anesthetic management of the patient with hyperthyroidism. Anesthesiology 41:585, 1974
42. Kaplan JA, Cooperman LH: Alarming reactions to ketamine in patients taking thyroid medication treatment with propranolol. Anesthesiology 35:229, 1971
43. Swanson JW, Kelly JJ, McConahey WM: Neurologic aspects of thyroid dysfunction. Mayo Clin Proc 56:504, 1981
44. Wade JSH: Respiratory obstruction in thyroid surgery. Ann Coll Surg Engl 62:15, 1980
45. Peters KR, Nance P, Wingard DW: Malignant hyperthyroidism or malignant hyperthermia? Anesth Analg 60:613, 1981
46. Waldstein SS: Medical complications of thyroid surgery. Otolaryngol Clin North Am 13:99, 1981
47. Green WER, Sheppard HWH: Tracheal collapse after thyroidectomy. Br J Surg 66:544, 1979
48. Capiferri R, Evered D: Investigation and treatment of hypothyroidism. Clin Endocrinol Metab 8:39, 1979
49. Hall R, Scanlon MF: Hypothyroidism: Clinical features and complications. Clin Endocrinol Metab 8:29, 1979
50. Amidi M, Leon DF, de Groot WJ et al: Effect of the thyroid state on myocardial contractility and ventricular ejection rate in man. Circulation 38:229, 1968
51. Zondek H: The electrocardiogram in myxedema. Br Heart J 26:227, 1964
52. Aber CP, Thompson GS: Factors associated with cardiac enlargement in myxedema. Br Heart J 25:421, 1963
53. Kannel WB, Dowler TR: Factors of risk in the development of coronary heart disease. Ann Intern Med 55:33, 1961

54. Ingbar SH, Woeber KA: The thyroid gland. In Williams RH (ed): Textbook of Endocrinology, 5th ed, pp 117–247. Philadelphia, W.B. Saunders, 1981

55. Zwilich CW, Pierson DJ, Hofeldt FD et al: Ventilatory control in myxedema and hypothyroidism. N Engl J Med 292:662, 1975

56. Edson JR, Feeber DR, Doc RP: Low platelet adhesiveness and other hemostatic abnormalities in hypothyroidism. Ann Intern Med 82:342, 1975

57. Tudhope GR, Wilson GM: Anemia in hypothyroidism: Incidence, pathogenesis, and response to treatment. Q J Med 29:513, 1960

58. Goldberg M, Rervich M: Studies on the mechanism of hyponatremia and impaired water excretion in myxedema. Ann Intern Med 56:120, 1962

59. Ridgway EC, McCammon JA, Benotti J et al: Acute metabolic responses in myxedema to large doses of intravenous L-thyroxine. Ann Intern Med 77:549, 1972

60. Weinberg AD, Brennan MD, Gorman CA et al: Outcome of anesthesia and surgery in hypothyroid patients. Arch Intern Med 143:893, 1983

61. Ladenson PW, Levin AA, Ridgway EC et al: Complications of surgery in hypothyroid patients. Am J Med 77:261, 1984

62. Drucker DJ, Burrow GN: Cardiovascular surgery in the hypothyroid patient. Arch Intern Med 145:1585, 1985

63. Hay ID, Duick DS, Vlietstra RE et al: Thyroxine therapy in hypothyroid patients undergoing coronary revascularization: A retrospective analysis. Ann Intern Med 95:456, 1981

64. Becker C: Hypothyroidism and atherosclerotic heart disease: Pathogenesis, medical management, and the role of coronary artery bypass surgery. Endocr Rev 6:432, 1985

65. Cohen SE, Wyner J: Endocrine disease. In James F III, Wheeler AS (eds): Obstetric Anesthesia: The Complicated Patient, pp 160–161. Philadelphia, FA Davis Co, 1982

66. Baaverman LB: Treatment of hypothyroidism: A practical guide. Thyroid Today 2:1, 1979

67. Blum M: Myxedema Coma. Am J Med Sci 264:432, 1972

68. Chernow B, Burman KD, Johnson DL et al: T_3 may be a better agent than T_4 in the critically ill hypothyroid patient. Crit Care Med 11:99, 1983

69. Murkin JM: Anesthesia and hypothyroidism: A review of thyroxine physiology, pharmacology and anesthetic implications. Anesth Analg 61:371, 1982

70. Babad AA, Eger EI: The effects of hyperthyroidism and hypothyroidism on halothane and oxygen requirements in dogs. Anesthesiology 29:1087, 1968

71. Robertson WG: Measurement of ionized calcium in body fluids/ A review. Ann Clin Biochem 13:540, 1976

72. Moore EW: Ionized calcium in normal serum. Ultrafiltrates and whole blood determined by ion-exchange electrodes. J Clin Invest 49:318, 1987

73. Habener JF, Potts JT: Biosynthesis of parathyroid hormone. N Engl J Med 299:580 (Part I), 635 (Part II), 1978

74. Martin KJ, Hruska KA, Freitag JJ et al: The peripheral metabolism of parathyroid hormone. N Engl J Med 301:1092, 1979

75. Nordin BEC, Peacock M: Role of kidney in regulation of plasma calcium. Lancet ii: 1280, 1969

76. Spiegel AM, Marx SJ: Parathyroid hormone and vitamin D receptors. Clin Endocrinol Metab 12:221, 1983

77. Broadus AE, Mahaffey JE, Bartter FC et al: Nephrogenous cyclic adenosine monophosphate as a parathyroid function test. J Clin Invest 60:771, 1977

78. Broadus AE: Mineral metabolism. In Felig P, Baxter JD, Broadus AE, Frohman LA (eds): Endocrinology and Metabolism, pp 953–1079. New York, McGraw-Hill, 1981

79. Blum JW, Mayer GP, Potts JT: Parathyroid hormone response during spontaneous hypocalcemia and induced hypercalcemia in cows. Endocrinology 95:84, 1974

80. Buckle RH, Care AD, Cooper CW et al: The influence of plasma magnesium concentration on parathyroid hormone secretion. J Endocrinol 42:529, 1968

81. Anast CF, Winnacker JL, Forte LR et al: Impaired release of parathyroid hormone in magnesium deficiency. J Clin Endocrinol Metab 42:707, 1976

82. Kukreja SC, Hargis GK, Bowser EN et al: Role of adrenergic stimuli in parathyroid hormone secretion in man. J Clin Endocrinol Metab 46:478, 1975

83. Haussler MR, McCain TA: Basic and clinical concepts related to vitamin D metabolism and action. N Engl J Med 297:974, 1041–1050, 1977

84. Heath H, Hodgson SF, Kennedy MA: Primary hypoparathyroidism: Incidence, morbidity, and potential economic impact in a community. N Engl J Med 302:89, 1980

85. Tsang RC, Donovan EF, Steichen JJ: Calcium physiology and pathology in the neonate. Pediatr Clin North Am 23:611, 1976

86. Mazzaferri EL: The parathyroid glands, calcium metabolism, and disorders of calcium homeostasis. In Mazzaferri EL (ed): Endocrinology. New York, Medical Examination Publishing Company, 1974

87. Fogelman I, Bessent RG, Beastall G: Estimation of skeletal involvement in primary hypoparathyroidism. Ann Intern Med 92:65, 1980

88. Dent PI, James JH, Wang CA et al: Hypoparathyroidism, gastric acid secretion, and gastrin. Ann Surg 176:360, 1972

89. Mallette LE, Bilezikian JP, Heath DA et al: Primary hypoparathyroidism; Clinical and biochemical features. Medicine 53:127, 1974

90. Ellman H, Dembin H, Seriff N: The rarity of the QT interval in patients with hypercalcemia. Crit Care Med 10:320, 1982

91. Weidmann P, Massry SG, Coburn WJ et al: Blood pressure effects of acute hypercalcemia. Ann Intern Med 76:741, 1972

92. Wills MR: Value of plasma chloride concentration and acid base status in the differential diagnosis of hyperparathyroidism from other causes of hypercalcemia. J Clin Pathol 24:219, 1971

93. Buckle R: Ectopic PTH syndrome, pseudohyperparathyroidism, hypercalcemia of malignancy. J Endocrinol Metab 3:237, 1974

94. Stewart AF, Horst R, Deftos LJ et al: Biochemical evaluation of patients with cancer associated hypercalcemia. N Engl J Med 303:1377, 1980

95. Mundy GR, Raisz LG, Cooper RA et al: Evidence for the secretion of an osteoclast stimulating factor in myeloma. N Engl J Med 291:1041, 1974

96. Benson RC, Riggs BL, Pickard BM et al: Immunoreactive forms of circulating parathyroid hormone in primary end ectopic hyperparathyroidism. J Clin Invest 54:175, 1974

97. Riggs BI, Arnaud OD, Reynolds, JC et al: Immunologic differentiation of primary hypoparathyroidism from hyperparathyroidism due to nonparathyroid cancer. J Clin Invest 50:2079, 1971

98. Purnell DC, Scholz DA, Smith LH et al: Treatment of primary hyperparathyroidism. Am J Med 56:800, 1974

99. Heath DA: Emergency treatment of disorders of calcium and magnesium. Clin Endocrinol Metab 9:487, 1980

100. Lotz M, Zisman E, Bartter FC: Evidence of phosphorus-depletion syndrome in man. N Engl J Med 278:409, 1968

101. Chopra RA, Janson P, Sawin CT: Insensitivity to digoxin associated with hypocalcemia. N Engl J Med 296:917, 1977

102. Perlia CP, Gubisch NJ, Wolter J et al: Mythramycin treatment of hypercalcemia. Cancer 25:389, 1970

103. West TET, Joffe M, Sinclair L et al: Treatment of hypercalcemia with calcitonin. Lancet 1:675, 1971

104. Deftos LJ, First BP: Calcitonin as a drug. Ann Intern Med 95:192, 1981

105. Bell NH, Stern PH, Pantzer E et al: Evidence that increased circulating 1, 25-dihydroxy vitamin D is a probable cause of

abnormal calcium metabolism in sarcoidosis. J Clin Invest 64:210, 1975

106. Chase LR, Slatopolsky E: Secretion and metabolic efficacy of parathyroid hormone in patients with severe hypomagnesemia. J Clin Endocrinol Metab 38:363, 1974

107. Rude RK, Oldham SB, Sharp CF et al: Parathyroid hormones secretion in magnesium deficiency. J Endocrinol Metab 47:800, 1978

108. Coburn JW, Coppel MH, Brickman AF et al: Study of intestinal absorption of calcium in patients with renal failure. Kidney Int 3:264, 1973

109. Condon JR, Ives D, Knight MJ et al: The etiology of hypocalcemia in acute pancreatitis. Br J Surg 62:115, 1975

110. Brenton DP, Pollard AB, Gonzales J: Hypocalcemic cardiac failure. Postgrad Med 54:633, 1978

111. Chaimowitz C, Abinader E, Benderly A et al: Hypocalcemic hypotension. JAMA 22:86, 1972

112. Rumancik WM, Denlinger JK, Nahrwold ML et al: The QT interval and serum ionized calcium. JAMA 240:366, 1978

113. Zaloga GP, Chernow B: Calcium magnesium and other minerals. In Chernow B, Lake CR (eds): The Pharmacologic Approach to the Critically Ill Patient, pp 530–561. Baltimore, William & Wilkins, 1983.

114. Kumar R, Riggs BL: Vitamin D in the therapy of disorders of calcium and phosphorus metabolism. Mayo Clin Proc 56:327, 1981

115. McPartland RP: Metabolic and pharmacologic actions of glucocorticoids. In Mulrow PJ (ed): The Adrenal Gland, pp 85–116. New York, Elsevier, 1986

116. DeMoor P, Heyns W: Cortisol binding affinity to plasma transcortin (CBA) as studied by competitive absorption. J Clin Endocrinol Metab 28:1281, 1968

117. Ruder HJ: Hypercortisolism. In Hare JW (ed): Signs and Symptoms in Endocrine and Metabolic Disorders, pp 106–120. Philadelphia, JB Lippincott, 1986

118. West CD, Brown H, Simons EL et al: Adrenocortical function and cortisol metabolism in old age. J Clin Endocrinol Metab 21:1197, 1961

119. Wolfsen AR: Aging and the adrenals. In Korenman SG (ed): Endocrine Aspects of Aging, pp 55–79. New York, Elsevier, 1982

120. Baxter JD, Forsham PH: Tissue effects of glucocorticoids. Am J Med 53:573, 1972

121. Petersdorf RG (ed): Harrison's Principles of Internal Medicine. New York, McGraw-Hill, 1983

122. Fauci AS, Dale DC, Balow JE: Glucocorticosteroid therapy: Mechanisms of action and clinical consideration. Ann Intern Med 84:304, 1976

123. Hirsch JG, Church AB: Adrenal steroids and infection: The effect of cortisone administration on polymorphonuclear leukocyte functions and on serum opsonins and bacteriocidins. J Clin Invest 40:794, 1961

124. Graber AL, Givens JR: Persistence of diurnal rhythmicity in plasma ACTH concentrations in cortisol-deficient patients. J Clin Endocrinol Metab 25:804, 1965

125. Williams RH: (ed): Textbook of Endocrinology, 6th ed. Philadelphia, W.B. Saunders, 1981

126. Hollenberg NK, Williams GH: Hypertension the adrenal and the kidney: Lessons from pharmacologic interruption of the renin-angiotensin system. Adv Intern Med 25:327, 1980

127. Kaplan SA: Diseases of the adrenal cortex. II. Congenital adrenal hyperplasia. Pediatr Clin North Am 26:77, 1989

128. Gold EM: The Cushing-syndromes: Changing views of diagnosis and treatment. Ann Intern Med 90:829, 1979

129. Soffer LJ, Iannaccone A, Gabrilove JL: Cushing's syndrome. Am J Med 30:129, 1961

130. Neville AM: The Human Adrenal Cortex, pp 1–341. New York, Springer-Verlag, 1982

131. Avioli LV: Effects of chronic corticosteroid therapy on mineral metabolism and calcium absorption. Adv Exp Biol Med 171:80, 1984

132. Dale DC, Fauci AS, Wolff SM: Alternate day prednisone. Leukocyte kinetics and susceptibility to infections. N Engl J Med 291:1154, 1974

133. Narins RG, Jones ER, Stom MC et al: Diagnostic strategies in disorders of fluid, electrolyte and acid-base homeostasis. Am J Med 72:496, 1982

134. Ernest I, Ekman H: Adrenalectomy in Cushing's disease. A long-term follow-up. Acta Endocrinol (Copenhägen) (Suppl) 160:3, 1972

135. Welbourne RB, Montgomery DAD, Kennedy TL: The natural history of treated Cushing's syndrome. Br J Surg 58:1, 1971

136. Herf SM, Teates DC, Tegtmeyer CJ et al: Identification and differentiation of surgically correctable hypertension due to primary aldosteronism. Am J Med 67:397, 1979

137. Weinberger MH, Grim CE, Hollifield JW et al: Primary aldrosteronism: Diagnosis, localization, and treatment. Ann Intern Med 90:386, 1979

138. Izenstein BZ, Dluhy RG, Williams GH: Endocrinology. In Vandam LD (eds): To Make the Patient Ready for Anesthesia: Medical Care of the Surgical Patient, pp 112–146. Menlo Park, California, Addison-Wesley, 1980

139. Arteaga E, Klein R, Biglieri EG: Use of the saline infusion test to diagnose the cause of primary aldosteronism. Am J Med 79:722, 1985

140. Holland OB, Brown H et al: Further evaluation of saline infusion for the diagnosis of primary aldosteronism. Hypertension 6:717, 1984

141. White EA, Schambelan M et al: The use of computed tomography in diagnosing the cause of primary aldosteronism. N Engl J Med 303:1503, 1980

142. Nerup J: Addison's disease—clinical studies. A report of 108 cases. ACTA Endocrinol 76:127, 1974

143. Anderson P: Familial Schmidt's syndrome. JAMA 244:2068, 1980

144. Levin J: Endotoxemia and adrenal hemorrhage. J Exp Med 121:247, 1965

145. Moore T: Adrenal insufficiency. In Hare JW (ed): Signs and Symptoms in Endocrine and Metabolic Disorders, pp 121–134. Philadelphia, J.B. Lippincott, 1986

146. Rowntree LG, Snell AM: A clinical study of Addison's disease. Mayo Clin Monographs, Philadelphia, W.B. Saunders, 1931

147. Dunlop D: Eighty-six cases of Addison's disease. Br Med J 2:887, 1963

148. Hirata Y, Matsukura F, Imura H et al: Size heterogeneity of B-MSH in ectopic ACTH-producing tumors. Presence of B-LPH-like peptides. J Clin Endocrinol Metab 42:33, 1976

149. Sampson PA, Brooke BN, Winstone NE: Biochemical confirmation of collapse due to adrenal failure. Lancet 1:1377, 1961

150. Sampson PA, Winstone NE, Brooke BN: Adrenal function of surgical patients after steroid therapy. Lancet 2:322, 1962

151. Knudsen L, Christiansen LA, Lorentzen JE: Hypotension during and after operation in glucocorticoid-treated patients. Br J Anesth 53:295, 1981

152. Meakin J: Pituitary-adrenal function following long-term steroid therapy. Am J Med 29:459, 1960

153. Carruthers JA, August PJ, Staughton RCD: Observations on the systemic effect of topical clobetasol propionate (Dermovate). Br Med J 4:203, 1975

154. Graber AL, Ney RL, Nicholson WE et al: Natural history of pituitary adrenal recovery following long-term suppression with corticosteroids. J Clin Endocrinol Metab 25:11, 1965

155. Chernow B: Hormonal and metabolic considerations in critical care medicine. In Thompson WL (ed): Critical Care: State of the Art, Vol 3. Fullerton, California, Society of Critical Care Medicine, 1982

156. Schambelan M: Prevalence, pathogenesis, and functional significance of aldosterone deficiency in hyperkalemic patients with chronic renal insufficiency. Kidney Int 17:89, 1980
157. Schambelan M, Sebastian A: Hyporeninemic hypoaldosteronism. Adv Intern Med 24:385, 1979
158. Bondy PK (ed): Metabolic Disease and Control, 8th ed. Philadelphia, W.B. Saunders, 1980
159. Zusman RM: Prostaglandins and water excretion. Annu Rev Med 32:359, 1981
160. David DS, Berkowitz JS: Ocular effects of topical and systemic corticosteroids. Lancet 2:149, 1961
161. Heimann GW, Freiberger RN: Avascular necrosis of the femoral and humoral heads after high-dose corticosteroid therapy. N Engl J Med 263:672, 1960
162. Ragan C: Corticotropin, cortisone and related steroids in clinical medicine: Practical considerations, Bull NY Acad Med 29:355, 1953
163. Spiro HM: Is the steroid ulcer a myth? N Engl J Med 309:45, 1983
164. Knowlton AI: Addison's disease: A review of its clinical course and management. In Christie NR (ed): The Human Adrenal Cortex, pp 329–358. New York, Harper & Row, 1971
165. Wyngaarden JB (ed): Cecil Textbook of Medicine, 17th ed. Philadelphia, W.B. Saunders, 1982
166. Byyny RL: Preventing adrenal insufficiency during surgery. Postgrad Med 67:219, 1980
167. Plumpton FS, Besser GM, Cole PV: Corticosteroid treatment and surgery. I. An investigation of the indications for steroid cover. Anesthesia 24:3, 1969
168. Engquist A, Brandt MR, Fernandes A et al: The blocking effect of epidural analgesia on the adrenocortical and hyperglycemic responses to surgery. ACTA Anesth Scand 21:330, 1977
169. Cooper GM, Paterson JL, Ward ID et al: Fentanyl and the metabolic response to gastric surgery. Anesthesiology 36:667, 1981
170. Lehtinen AM, Fyhrquist F, Kivalo I: The effect of fentanyl on arginine vasopressin and cortisol secretion during anesthesia. Anesth Analg 63:25, 1984
171. Namba Y, Smith JB, Fox GS et al: Plasma cortisol concentrations during cesarean section. Br J Anesth 52:1027, 1980
172. Oyama T, Taniguchi K, Jin T et al: Effects of anesthesia and surgery on plasma aldosterone concentration and renin activity in man. Br J Anesth 51:747, 1979
173. Oyama T: Hazards of steroids in association with anesthesia. Can Anesth Soc J 16:361, 1969
174. Udelsman R, Ramp J, Gallucci WT et al: Adaptation during surgical stress: A reevaluation of the role of glucocorticoids. J Clin Invest 77:1377, 1986
175. Symreng T, Karlberg BE, Kagedal B et al: Physiological cortisol substitution of long-term steroid-treated patients undergoing major surgery. Br J Anesth 53:949, 1981
176. Axelrod L: Glucocorticoid therapy. Medicine 55:39, 1976
177. Scott HW Jr, Oates JA, Nies AS et al: Pheochromocytoma: Present diagnosis and management. Ann Surg 183:587, 1976
178. Manger WN, Gifford RW: Current concepts of pheochromocytoma. Cardiovasc Med 3:289, 1978
179. St. John Sutton N, Sheps SG, Lie JT: Prevalence of clinically unsuspected pheochromocytoma. Review of a 50-year autopsy series. Mayo Clin Proc 56:354, 1981
180. Cross DA, Meyer JS: Postoperative deaths due to unsuspected pheochromocytoma. South Med J 70:1320, 1977
181. Manger WN, Gifford RW: Pheochromocytoma. New York, Heidelberg, Berlin, Springer-Verlag, 1977
182. ReMine WH, Chong GC, vanHeerden JA et al: Current management of pheochromocytoma. Ann Surg 179:740, 1974
183. Engelman K: Pheochromocytoma. Clin Endocrinol Metab 6(3):769, 1977
184. Ram CVS, Engelman K: Pheochromocytoma—recognition and

185. Henry DT, Starman BJ, Johnson DG et al: A sensitive radio enzymatic assay for norepinephrine in tissues and plasma. Life Sci 16:375, 1975
186. Bravo EL, Tarazi RC, Gifford RW et al: Circulating and urinary catecholamines in pheochromocytomas. N Engl J Med 301:682, 1979
187. Desmonts JM, LeHouelleur J, Remond P et al: Anesthetic management of patients with pheochromocytoma. A review of 102 cases. Br J Anesth 49:991, 1977
188. Roizen MF, Horrigan RW, Koike M et al: A perspective randomized trial of four anesthetic techniques for resection of pheochromocytoma. Anesthesiology 57:A43, 1982
189. Roizen MF, Hunt TK, Beaupre PN et al: The effect of alpha adrenergic blockade on cardiac performance and tissue oxygen delivery during excision of pheochromocytoma. Surgery 94:941, 1983
190. Knapp HR, Fitzgerald GA: Hypertensive crisis in prazosin-treated pheochromocytoma. South Med J 77:535, 1984
191. Briggs RSJ, Birtwell AJ, Pohl JEF: Hypertensive response to labetalol in pheochromocytoma. Lancet 1:1045, 1978
192. Schaffer MS, Zuberbuhler P, Urlson G et al: Catecholamine cardiomyopathy: An unusual presentation of pheochromocytoma in children. J Pediatr 99:276, 1981
193. Gusberg RJ, Moley J: Diabetes and abdominal surgery. Yale J Biol Med 56:285, 1983
194. Alberti KGMM, Thomas DJB: The management of diabetes during surgery. Br J Anaesth 51:693, 1979
195. Walts LF, Miller J, Davidson MB: Perioperative management of diabetes mellitus. Anesthesiology 55:104, 1981
196. National Diabetes Group: Classification and diagnosis of diabetes mellitus and other categories of glucose intolerance. Diabetes 28:1039, 1979
197. Allison SP, Tomlin PJ, Chamberlain MJ: Some effects of anaesthesia and surgery on carbohydrate and fat metabolism. Br J Anaesth 41:588, 1969
198. Clarke RSJ, Johnston H, Sheridan B: The influence of anaesthesia and surgery on plasma cortisol, insulin and free fatty acids. Br J Anaesth 42:295, 1970
199. Stevens A, Roizen MF: Patients with diabetes mellitus and disorders of glucose metabolism. Anesth Clin North Am 5:339, 1987
200. McGarry JD, Foster DW: Ketogenesis and its regulation. Am J Med 61:9, 1976
201. Unger RH, Orci L: Glucagon and the A cell (two parts). N Engl J Med 304:1518; 304:1575, 1981
202. Cryer PE, Gerich JE: Glucose counter-regulation, hypoglycemia, and intensive insulin therapy in diabetes mellitus. N Engl J Med 313:232, 1985
203. Fischer KF, Lees JA, Newman JM: Hypoglycemia in hospitalized patients. N Engl J Med 315:1245, 1986
204. Raskin P, Rosenstack J: Blood glucose control and diabetic complications. Ann Intern Med 105:254, 1986
205. Page MM, Watkins PJ: Cardiorespiratory arrest and diabetic autonomic neuropathy. Lancet 1:14, 1978
206. Bhatnagar SK, Al–Yusuf AR, Al–Asfoor AR: Abnormal autonomic function in diabetic and non-diabetic patients after first acute myocardial infarction. Chest 92:5, 1987
207. Foster DW: Insulin deficiency and hyperosmolar coma. Adv Intern Med 19:159, 1974
208. Foster DW, McGarry JD: The metabolic derangements and treatment of diabetic ketoacidosis. N Engl J Med 309:159, 1983
209. Fulop M, Hoberman HD: Alcoholic ketosis. Diabetes 24:785, 1975
210. Loughran PG, Giesecke AH: Diabetes mellitus—Anesthetic considerations. Seminars in Anesthesia 3:207, 1985

management. In Harvey P (ed): Current Problems in Cardiology, Vol 4, No 1. Chicago, Year Book Medical Publishers, Inc, 1979

211. Kriesberg RA: Diabetic ketoacidosis—New concepts and trends in pathogenesis and treatment. Ann Intern Med 88:691, 1978

212. Morris LR, Murphy MB, Kitabchi AE: Bicarbonate therapy in severe diabetic ketoacidosis. Ann Intern Med 105:836, 1986

213. Harati Y: Diabetic peripheral neuropathies. Ann Intern Med 107:546, 1987

214. Rossini AA, Hare JW: How to control the blood glucose level in the surgical diabetic patient. Arch Surg 111:945, 1976

215. Woodruff RE, Lewis SB, McLeskey CH et al: Avoidance of surgical hyperglycemia in diabetic patients. JAMA 244:166, 1980

216. Podolsky S: Management of diabetes in the surgical patient. Med Clin North Am 66:1361, 1982

217. Meyers EF, Alberts D, Gordon MD: Perioperative control of blood glucose in diabetic patients—A two-step protocol. Diabetes Care 9:40, 1986

218. Taitelman U, Reece EA, Bessman AN: Insulin in the management of the diabetic surgical patient. JAMA 237:658, 1977

219. Barnett AH, Robinson MH, Harrison JH et al: Mini-pump method of diabetic control during minor surgery under general anesthesia. Br Med J 280:78, 1980

220. Bowen DJ, Proctor EA, Norman J: Perioperative management of insulin dependent diabetic patients. Anaesthesia 37:852, 1982

221. Weisenfeld S, Podolsky S, Goldsmith L et al: Adsorption of insulin to infusion bottles and tubing. Diabetes 17:766, 1968

222. Sheehan HL, Stanfield JP: A pathogenesis of post-partum necrosis of the anterior lobe of the pituitary gland. ACTA Endocrinol Scand 37:479, 1961

223. Kleinberg DL, Noel GL, Frantz AG: Galactorrhea: A study of 235 cases including 48 with pituitary tumors. N Engl J Med 296:589, 1977

224. Kitahata LM: Airway difficulties associated with anesthesia in acromegaly. Br J Anesth 43:1187, 1971

225. Dunn FL, Brennan TJ, Nelson AE et al: The role of blood osmolality and volume in regulating vasopressin secretion in the rat. J Clin Invest 52:3212, 1973

226. Corliss RJ, McKenna DH, Sialer S et al: Systemic and coronary hemodynamic effects of vasopressin. Am J Med 256:293, 1968

227. Edmunds R, West JB: A study on the effect of vasopressin on portal and systemic blood pressure. Surg Gynecol Obstet 114:458, 1962

228. Getzen LC, Brink RR, Wolfman EF: Survival following infusion of pitressin into the superior mesenteric artery to control bleeding esophageal varices in cirrhotic patients. Ann Surg 187:337, 1978

229. Solzman EW, Weinstein MJ, Weintraub RM et al: Treatment with desmopressin acetate to reduce blood loss after cardiac surgery: A double-blind randomized trial. N Engl J Med 314:1402, 1986

230. Dubois M, Picker D, Cohen M et al: Plasma beta-endorphin immunoreactivity is raised by surgical stress but not anesthetic induction. Anesthesiology 55:A244, 1981

231. Cork RC, Finley J, Hameroff SR et al: Plasma beta-endorphin during cardiac anesthesia: Halothane versus fentanyl. Anesthesiology 57:A300, 1982

232. Abboud TK, Sarkis F, Goebelsmann U et al: Effects of epidural anesthesia during labor on maternal plasma beta-endorphin levels. Anesthesiology 57:A382, 1982

233. Thomas TA, Fletcher JE, Hill RG et al: Influence of medication, pain and progressive labor on plasma beta-endorphin-like immunoreactivity. Br J Anesth 54:401, 1982

Chapter 45

Hilda Pedersen
Alan C. Santos
Mieczyslaw Finster

Obstetric Anesthesia

THE PHYSIOLOGIC CHANGES OF PREGNANCY

During pregnancy, with the increasing metabolic and nutritional demands of the growing fetus, there are major alterations in nearly every maternal organ system. These changes are initiated by hormonal secretions from the corpus luteum and placenta. The mechanical effects of uterine size and compression of surrounding structures play an increasing role in the second and third trimesters. This "altered physiologic state" has important implications for the anesthesiologist in treatment of the pregnant patient. The most pertinent changes, involving hematologic, cardiovascular, ventilatory, metabolic, and gastrointestinal functions, will be considered here (Table 45-1).

HEMATOLOGIC ALTERATIONS

Increased mineralocorticoid activity during pregnancy produces sodium retention and increased body water content and plasma volume.[1] Thus, under hormonal influence, plasma volume begins to increase between the 6th and 12th gestational weeks, resulting in a total increase of 40%–50% and a 25%–40% increase in total blood volume at term. The relatively lesser increase in red blood cell volume (20%) accounts for a reduction in hemoglobin (to 11–12 $g \cdot dl^{-1}$) and hematocrit (to 35%).[2] The leukocyte count remains 8,000–10,000 mm^3 throughout pregnancy, whereas the platelet count shows no remarkable change. Plasma fibrinogen concentrations increase during normal pregnancy by about 50%, whereas some clotting factor activities increase and others decrease.[3]

Serum cholinesterase activity declines to a level of 20% below normal at term and into the puerperium.[4] However, there is no structural malformation of the enzyme molecule, and it is doubtful that moderate succinylcholine doses can lead to prolonged apnea in otherwise normal circumstances.[5]

Plasma proteins show changes similar to those seen in erythrocytes, namely their total concentration declines (to less than 6 $g \cdot dl^{-1}$ at term), whereas the total amount in the circulation increases.[6] The albumin–globulin ratio declines because of the relatively greater reduction in albumin concentration. As stated above, fibrinogen increases in both absolute and relative concentrations. During gestation, alterations in protein content, especially albumin, may be clinically significant, in that the free fractions of protein-bound drugs can be expected to increase.[7]

In the first two to three weeks after delivery, the blood volume slowly decreases, whereas the hematocrit increases to nonpregnant levels.[1]

CARDIOVASCULAR CHANGES

As oxygen consumption increases during pregnancy, the maternal cardiovascular system adapts to meet the metabolic demands of the growing fetus.[8] Decreased vascular resistance may be the initiating factor. For example, the administration of various estrogens to nonpregnant ewes leads to increased cardiac output and reduced vascular resistance, whereas the decrease in vascular resistance and vasodilation in normal human pregnancy may also be related, in part, to the increased production of prostacyclin.[9, 10]

Lowered resistance is found in the uterine, renal and other

1215

TABLE 45-1. Summary of Physiologic Changes of Pregnancy at Term

Total blood volume	Increase	25%–40%
Plasma volume	Increase	40%–50%
Fibrinogen	Increase	50%
Serum cholinesterase activity	Decrease	20%–30%
Cardiac output	Increase	30%–50%
Minute ventilation	Increase	50%
Alveolar ventilation	Increase	70%
Functional residual capacity	Decrease	20%
Oxygen consumption	Increase	20%
Arterial carbon dioxide tension	Decrease	10 mm Hg
Arterial oxygen tension	Increase	10 mm Hg
Minimum alveolar concentration	Decrease	32%–40%

vascular beds; at term the heart rate (92–95 beats · min⁻¹), cardiac output, and blood volume are increased. Arterial blood pressure decreases slightly because the decrease in peripheral resistance exceeds the increase in cardiac output. Cardiac output, increasing from the 8th week, reaches its plateau of 30%–50% above the normal nonpregnant state at approximately the 30th–34th weeks. Additional increases occur during labor (when cardiac output may reach 12–14 l · min⁻¹) and in the immediate postpartum period.

From the second trimester, aortocaval compression by the enlarged uterus becomes progressively more important. Studies of cardiac output, measured with the patient in the supine position during the last weeks of pregnancy, have indicated a decrease to nonpregnant levels, which did not occur while they were in the lateral decubitus position.[11, 12] In another group of patients reductions were seen while they were in the supine, sitting, or lateral decubitus positions, the greatest occurring when they were supine.[13] Vena caval compression can develop from the second trimester and becomes maximal at 36–38 weeks, after which it may decrease as the fetal head descends into the pelvis. Roentgenograms have shown complete vena caval obstruction in as many as 90% of supine pregnant women at term, venous blood being shunted to the superior vena cava by the intervertebral plexus and the azygos vein.[12] Despite this, most women maintain a normal, or near-normal, brachial artery pressure by increasing peripheral resistance, although this may indirectly be harmful to the fetus through a reduction in utero-placental blood flow.[14] As has been known for a long time, obstructed venous return can lead to maternal tachycardia, arterial hypotension, faintness, and pallor, the so-called "supine hypotensive syndrome," which occurs in approximately 10% of pregnant patients near term when placed supine.[15] Compression of the lower aorta with this position, as demonstrated by aortography, may also lead to decreased uteroplacental perfusion and fetal distress.[16] Therefore, left uterine displacement, or lateral pelvic tilting, should be used during the second and third trimesters of pregnancy, regardless of the lack of maternal arterial hypotension. Shortly after delivery, the increased cardiac output probably results from the addition of 500–600 ml of blood to the central circulation by contraction of the evacuated uterus; cardiac output gradually decreases over the next 24–72 hours.

Changes in the electrocardiogram (ECG) result from the shift in the position of the heart (left axis deviation), resulting from the upward displacement of the diaphragm by the gravid uterus. There is also a tendency toward premature contractions, sinus tachycardia, and paroxysmal supra-

ventricular tachycardia, the cause of which is unknown. In the absence of organic heart disease, these cardiac dysrhythmias do not alter the normal course of pregnancy, and there is no significant hazard to the mother.

VENTILATORY CHANGES

The increased extracellular fluid and vascular engorgement, typical of gestation, may not only lead to edema of the extremities, but may also compromise the upper airway. Many pregnant women complain of difficulty in nasal breathing, and the friable nature of the mucous membranes can cause severe bleeding, especially on insertion of nasopharyngeal airways or nasogastric and endotracheal tubes.[17] Airway edema may be particularly severe in patients with preeclampsia, in patients with prolonged placement in the Trendelenburg position, or with the use of tocolytic agents. It is also difficult to perform laryngoscopic examination in obese, short-necked, parturients with enlarged breasts. Use of a short-handled laryngoscope has proved helpful.[18]

The level of the diaphragm rises as the uterus increases in size, but diaphragmatic breathing remains unimpeded.[19] The upward shift is compensated by an increase in the anteroposterior and transverse diameters of the thoracic cage, through flaring of the ribs.

Progesterone-induced relaxation of bronchiolar smooth muscle decreases airway resistance, whereas lung compliance remains unchanged.[20] This, in turn, paves the way for the increase in minute ventilation ($\dot{V}_E$) necessary to meet the increasing metabolic demand for oxygen. $\dot{V}_E$ increases from the beginning of pregnancy to a maximum of 50% above normal at term.[21] This is accomplished by an approximate 40% increase in tidal volume and an approximate 15% increase in respiratory rate. Because dead space does not change significantly, alveolar ventilation is increased by 70% at term.

With enlarging uterine size, lung volumes change. From the 5th month, the expiratory reserve volume (ERV), residual volume (RV), and functional residual capacity (FRC) decrease, the latter to 20% less than that of the nonpregnant state.[22] However, there is a concomitant increase in inspiratory reserve volume (IRV), so that total lung capacity (TLC) remains unchanged. In most parturients decreased FRC does not cause problems, but those with preexisting alterations in closing volume (CV), resulting from smoking, obesity, or scoliosis, may experience early airway closure leading to hypoxemia as pregnancy advances. The Trendelenburg and supine positions also exacerbate the abnormal relationship between CV and FRC.[23] RV and FRC quickly return to normal after delivery. As blood progesterone levels decline, ventilation returns to normal within 1–3 weeks.[22]

METABOLISM

The fetus depends upon the mother for nutritional substances such as amino acids, glucose, and iron. Basal oxygen consumption increases during early pregnancy, with an overall increase of 20% at term.[8] However, increased alveolar ventilation—probably resulting from the effects of progesterone—leads to a reduction in Pa_{CO_2} to 32 mm Hg and an increase in Pa_{O_2} to 106 mm Hg.[21] The plasma buffer base decreases from 47 to 42 mEq · l⁻¹ so that pH practically remains unchanged.[24]

Increased alveolar ventilation, along with the decreased FRC, enhances maternal uptake and elimination of inhalational anesthetics.[25] On the other hand, the decreased FRC and increased metabolic rate predispose the mother to hypoxemia during endotracheal intubation or airway obstruction.[26]

Human placental lactogen (HPL) and cortisol increase the tendency to hyperglycemia and ketosis, which may unmask or exacerbate preexisting diabetes mellitus. The patient's ability to handle a glucose load is decreased, and the transplacental passage of glucose may stimulate fetal secretion of insulin, leading in turn to neonatal hypoglycemia in the immediate postpartum period.[27]

GASTROINTESTINAL CHANGES

Enhanced progesterone production causes decreased gastrointestinal motility, slower absorption of food, and a lower volume of intestinal secretions.[28, 29] The gastric juice is more acidic, and lower esophageal sphincter (LES) tone is decreased.[30] Uterine growth leads to upward displacement and rotation of the stomach, with increased pressure and delayed gastric emptying. By the 34th week, evacuation of a watery meal may be prolonged by 60%.[31] Pain, anxiety, and administration of opioids and belladonna alkaloids may further exacerbate this delay.

In patients near term, the lithotomy and Trendelenburg positions will increase intragastric pressure. The risk of regurgitation, leading to aspiration pneumonitis on induction of general anesthesia, depends on the gradient between the intragastric and LES pressures. In most patients the gradient increases after succinylcholine administration, because the increase in LES pressure exceeds that in intragastric pressure.[32] However, in parturients with "heartburn," the LES tone is greatly reduced.[33] The current requirement for consideration as being "at risk" for aspiration is gastric juice with a pH less than 2.5 and volume greater than 25 ml. The efficacy of prophylactic nonparticulate antacids is reduced by inadequate mixing with gastric contents, improper timing of administration, and the tendency for antacids to increase gastric volume. Administration of H_2 receptor antagonists, such as cimetidine and ranitidine requires careful timing and dose schedules. There are many drug interactions and side-effects, including aplastic anemia, anaphylaxis, bradycardia, hypotension, cardiac dysrhythmias, cardiac arrest, and inhibition of cytochrome P_{450}, with impaired elimination of many drugs currently used in anesthesia, e.g., diazepam, theophylline, and amide local anesthetics.[34] A good case can be made for the administration of intravenous metoclopramide before elective cesarean section. This dopamine antagonist hastens gastric emptying and increases resting LES tone in both nonpregnant and pregnant women.[35] However, conflicting reports have appeared on its efficacy as well as side-effects such as extrapyramidal reactions and postoperative neurologic dysfunction.[36–38.] It seems that no routine prophylactic regimen can be recommended, although the available agents may all be useful. A rapid-sequence induction of anesthesia, with cricoid pressure, and intubation of the trachea with a cuffed tube are necessary for all pregnant patients receiving general anesthesia from the second trimester.

There is some doubt as to when the gastric volume of the postpartum patient has returned to normal; a nonparticulate antacid and a rapid-sequence induction of anesthesia should be used in women having general anesthesia within 48 h after delivery.

ALTERED DRUG RESPONSES

In pregnancy many anesthetic drugs have a reduced dose requirement. The minimum alveolar concentration (MAC) for halothane, isoflurane, and methoxyflurane is decreased by 32%–40% in pregnant ewes, which may be related to the gestational increase in endorphin levels.[39] It has also been noted that lower doses of local anesthetics were needed per segment of epidural or spinal block. This was originally attributed to venous engorgement reducing the volume of the epidural and subarachnoid spaces. However, more recent investigations of conduction blockade induced in the vagus nerve, excised from pregnant and nonpregnant rabbits, indicate that in pregnancy there is a greater sensitivity to local anesthetics.[40] This explains the reduced local anesthetic requirement found as early as the first trimester.[41]

FETAL EXPOSURE TO DRUGS USED IN OBSTETRIC ANESTHESIA

It is generally accepted that most drugs, including anesthetic agents, readily cross the placenta. We have learned more about this area from the development of highly sensitive and specific techniques for drug analysis in biologic fluids and tissues, as well as from a better understanding of the fetal circulation.

PLACENTAL TRANSFER

Several factors influence the placental transfer of drugs, including the physicochemical characteristics of the drug itself, maternal drug concentrations in the plasma, properties of the placenta, and hemodynamic events within the fetomaternal unit.

Drugs cross biologic membranes by simple diffusion, the rate of which is determined by the Fick principle, which states that

$$Q/t = \frac{K\ A\ (Cm - Cf)}{D}$$

where

Q/t = rate of diffusion
K = diffusion constant
A = surface area available for exchange
Cm = concentration of free drug in maternal blood
Cf = concentration of free drug in fetal blood
D = thickness of diffusion barrier

The diffusion constant (K) of the drug depends on physicochemical characteristics such as molecular size, lipid solubility, and degree of ionization.

Compounds with a molecular weight less than 500 are unimpeded in crossing the placenta, whereas those with molecular weights of 500 to 1,000 are more restricted. Most drugs commonly used by the anesthesiologist have molecular weights that permit easy transfer.

Drugs that are highly lipid-soluble cross biologic membranes more readily, and the degree of ionization is important because the un-ionized moiety of a drug is more lipophilic than the ionized one. Local anesthetics and opioids are weak bases, with a relatively low degree of ionization and considerable lipid solubility. In contrast, muscle relaxants are less lipophilic and more ionized. Their placental transfer is more limited.[42, 43]

The relative concentrations of drug existing in the un-ionized and ionized forms can be predicted from the Henderson-Hasselbalch equation:

$$pH = pK_a + \log \frac{(base)}{(cation)}$$

The ratio of base to cation becomes particularly important with local anesthetics because the un-ionized form penetrates tissue barriers, whereas the ionized form is pharmacologically active in blocking nerve conduction.

The pK_a is the pH at which the concentrations of free base and cation are equal. For the amide local anesthetics, the pK_a values (7.7–8.1) are sufficiently close to physiologic pH that changes in maternal or fetal biochemical status may significantly alter the proportion of ionized and un-ionized drug present (Fig. 45-1). At equilibrium, the concentrations of un-ionized drug in the fetal and maternal plasma are equal. In the case of the acidotic fetus, a greater tendency for drug to exist in the ionized form, which cannot diffuse back across the placenta into the maternal plasma, causes a larger total amount of drug to accumulate in the fetal plasma. This is the mechanism for the phenomenon described as "ion trapping."[44] It also causes enhanced accumulation of local anesthetic in the tissues of acidotic fetuses (Fig. 45-2).[45] Fetal acidosis should also increase the uptake of other basic drugs such as opioids.

The effects of maternal plasma protein binding on the rate and amount of drug transferred to the fetus are not understood as well. One would assume that highly bound drugs, having a lesser fraction in the unbound form, would be more restricted in crossing the placenta. Animal studies have shown that the transfer rate is slower for drugs that are extensively bound to maternal plasma proteins, such as bupiva-

caine, but if enough time is allowed for the fetomaternal equilibrium to be approached, substantial accumulation can occur in the fetus.[46–48] Indirect evidence in humans was provided by the observation that neonates exposed in utero to the drug administered for epidural anesthesia had measurable plasma concentrations and urinary excretion of bupivacaine for at least 3 days after delivery.[49]

As already stated, the driving force for placental drug transfer is the concentration gradient of free drug between the maternal and fetal blood. On the maternal side there is an interaction of the following factors: the dose administered, the mode and site of administration, and, in the case of local anesthetics, the use of vasoconstrictors. The rate of distribution, metabolism, and excretion of the drug, which may vary at different stages of pregnancy, as well as interactions with other drugs, such as cimetidine, are equally important.

Generally speaking, higher doses result in higher maternal blood concentrations. This effect is illustrated by a study in which thiamylal was administered by intravenous injection to mothers having elective cesarean section while under general anesthesia.[50] In the group of patients receiving thiamylal, 4 mg·kg^{-1}, the peak maternal arterial and umbilical vein barbiturate concentrations at the time of birth were approximately 50 mg·l^{-1} and 14 mg·l^{-1} respectively. Doubling the dose resulted in an almost double maternal drug concentration (84 mg·l^{-1}) and an increase in the umbilical vein concentration of thiamylal (18 mg·l^{-1}).

The absorption rate varies with the site of drug injection. Compared with other forms of administration, an intravenous bolus results in the highest blood concentrations. This was documented in a study comparing maternal and fetal plasma levels of meperidine after intravenous, intramuscular, or epidural injection (2 mg·kg^{-1} over 60 s) to pregnant ewes.[51] A mean peak concentration of 1,623 ng·ml^{-1} was measured in the maternal plasma 2 min after intravenous injection, whereas a mean peak concentration of 500 ng·ml^{-1}

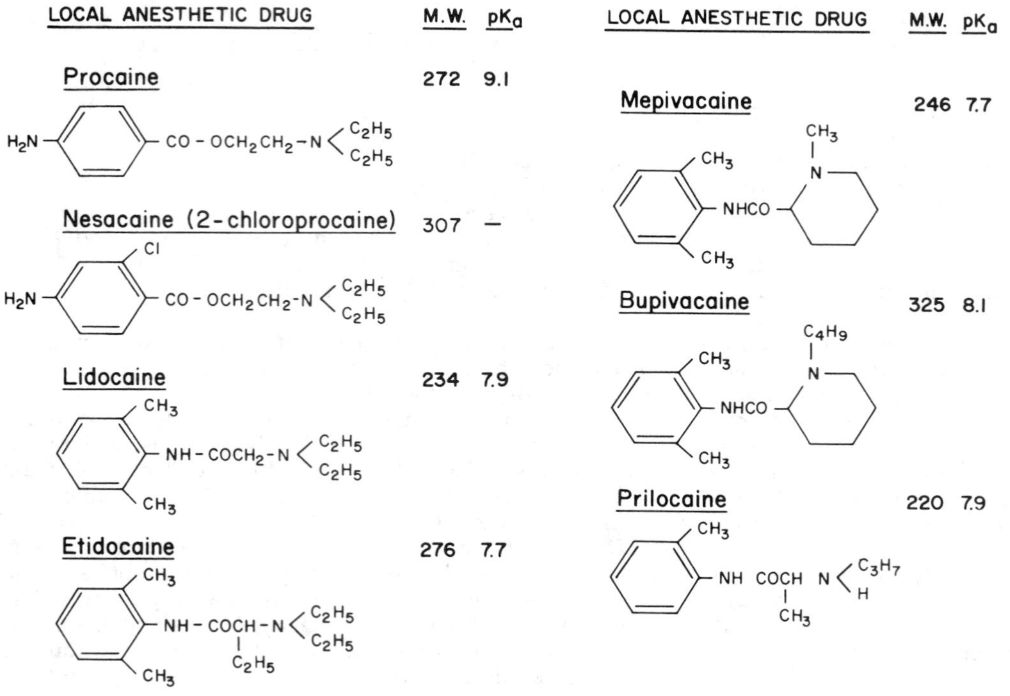

FIG. 45-1. Chemical structures, pK_a, and molecular weights of commonly used local anesthetics. (Reprinted with permission. Finster M, Pedersen H: Placental transfer and fetal uptake of local anesthetics. Clin Obstet Gynecol 556, 1975.)

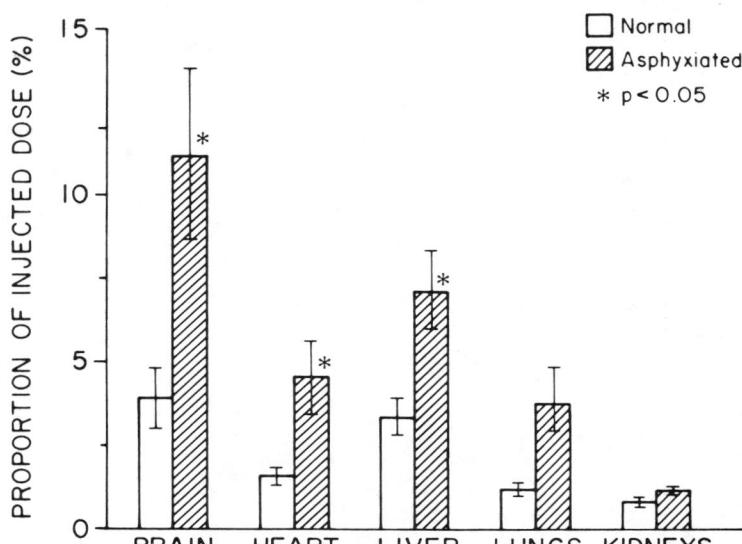

FIG. 45-2. Mean (±SE) values for the proportions of injected lidocaine dose found in the brain, heart, liver, lungs, and kidneys in nonasphyxiated and asphyxiated fetuses. (Reprinted with permission. Morishima HO, Covino BG: Toxicity and distribution of lidocaine in nonasphyxiated and asphyxiated baboon fetuses. Anesthesiology 54:182, 1981.)

occurred at 15 min after intramuscular or epidural administration. Fetuses whose mothers received the drug intravenously had significantly higher plasma concentrations of meperidine for at least 30 min compared with those whose mothers received the drug by the other two routes. It has also been shown that, after an intravenous injection of meperidine during labor, a greater proportion of the dose administered is transferred to the fetus when compared with that after an intramuscular injection.[52]

It was believed that intrathecal administration of local anesthetics resulted in negligible plasma concentrations because of the small doses used and the relatively poor vascularity of this area. However, in a recent study involving pregnant patients having cesarean section with spinal anesthesia (induced with lidocaine 75 mg), maternal plasma concentrations of the drug were similar to those reported by others after epidural anesthesia.[53] Furthermore, significant levels of the drug were found in the umbilical vein at birth.

Increased maternal blood concentrations after repeated administration of a drug greatly depend on the dose and frequency of reinjection, as well as on the kinetic characteristics of the drug. The elimination half-life of amide local anesthetic agents is relatively slow, so that repeated injection may lead to accumulation in the maternal plasma[54] (Fig. 45-3). On the other hand, 2-chloroprocaine, an ester local anesthetic, undergoes rapid enzymatic hydrolysis in the presence of pseudocholinesterase. In vitro studies have shown the half-life of this drug to be 21 sec in the maternal serum.[55] After epidural injection, the mean half-life in the mother was 3.1 min.[56] After reinjection, 2-chloroprocaine could be detected in the maternal plasma for only 5–10 min, and no accumulation of this drug was evident (Fig. 45-4).[57] The discrepancy in the half-life between in vivo and in vitro studies can be ascribed to continued absorption of 2-chloroprocaine from the epidural space.

Pregnancy is associated with physiologic changes that may influence maternal pharmacokinetics and the action of anesthetic drugs. Furthermore, these changes are progressive during the course of gestation. Kinetic studies after thiopental injection for induction of anesthesia at cesarean section showed a greater volume of distribution and plasma clearance and longer elimination half-life than were obtained by the same authors in a group of nonpregnant women.[58] When methohexital was administered by intravenous injection to pregnant and nonpregnant ewes, plasma clearance was significantly higher in the former group.[59]

Alterations in ventilation and lung volumes have a significant effect on the rate of uptake and excretion of inhalation agents. Of most concern to the anesthesiologist is a 20% reduction in FRC. As a result, the equilibration time between the alveolar and inspired concentrations of inhalation agents is shortened.

PLACENTA

Maturation of the placenta can affect the rate of drug transfer to the fetus, as the thickness of the trophoblastic epithelium decreases from 25 μm to 2 μm at term. In pregnant mice, diazepam and its metabolites are transferred more rapidly in late than in early pregnancy.[60]

Uptake and biotransformation of anesthetic drugs by the placenta would decrease the amount transferred to the fetus. However, the placental drug uptake is limited, and there is no evidence to suggest that this organ metabolizes any of the agents commonly used to produce anesthesia or analgesia in pregnant women.

HEMODYNAMIC FACTORS

Any factor decreasing placental blood flow—such as aortocaval compression, hypotension resulting from sympathetic blockade, or hemorrhage—can decrease drug delivery to the fetus. During labor, uterine contractions intermittently reduce perfusion of the placenta. If a uterine contraction coincides with the rapid decline in plasma drug concentration after an intravenous bolus injection, by the time perfusion has returned to normal, the concentration gradient across the placenta will have been greatly reduced. When women were

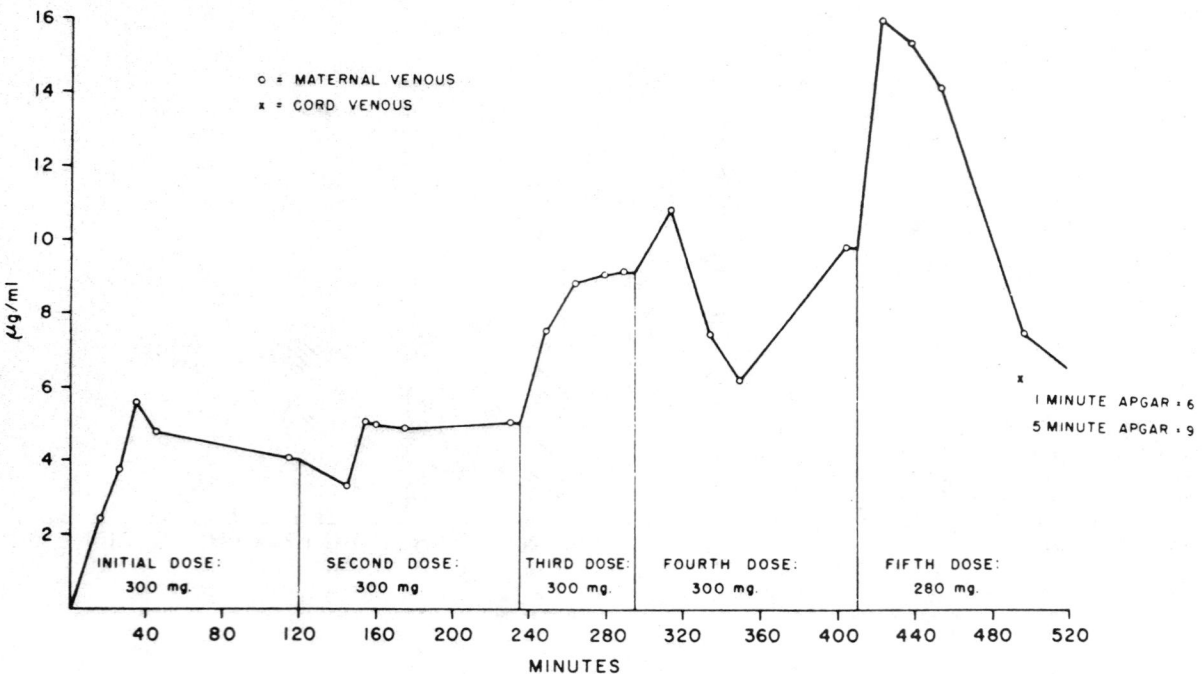

FIG. 45-3. Increased levels of mepivacaine with each reinforcing dose in a patient receiving continuous caudal anesthesia during parturition. (Reprinted with permission. Moore DC, Bridenbaugh LD, Bagdi PA *et al*: Accumulation of mepivacaine hydrochloride during caudal block. Anesthesiology 29:585, 1968.)

given an intravenous injection of diazepam—administered at the onset of contraction in one group and during uterine diastole in the other—less drug was found in infants born to mothers in the former group.[61]

Several characteristics of the fetal circulation delay the equilibration between the fetal arterial and venous blood and thus delay the depressant effects of anesthetic drugs (Fig. 45-5). The liver is the first fetal organ perfused by the umbilical vein blood, which carries drug to the fetus. Substantial uptake by this organ has been demonstrated for a variety of drugs such as thiopental, lidocaine, and halothane. During its transit to the arterial side of the fetal circulation, the drug is progressively diluted as blood in the umbilical vein becomes admixed with fetal venous blood from the gastrointestinal tract, the lower extremities, the head and upper extremities, and, finally, the lungs. Because of this unique pattern of the fetal circulation, administration of anesthetic concentrations of nitrous oxide or cyclopropane during elective cesarean sections caused newborn depression only if the induction-to-delivery interval exceeded 5–10 min. On the other hand, because of the rapid decline of maternal plasma drug concentrations, administration of thiopental or thiamylal, not in excess of 4 mg · kg^{-1}, results in fetal arterial concentrations of barbiturate below a level that would result in neonatal depression (Fig. 45-6).[50]

Fetal regional blood flow changes can also affect the amount of drug taken up by individual organs. For example, it has been shown that during asphyxia and acidosis, a greater proportion of the fetal cardiac output perfuses the fetal brain, heart, and placenta. Infusion of lidocaine to asphyxiated baboon fetuses resulted in increased drug uptake in the heart, brain, and liver as compared with that in non-asphyxiated controls.[45]

FETUS AND NEWBORN

Any drug that reaches the fetus will be subjected to metabolism and excretion. In this respect the fetus has an advantage over the newborn in that it can excrete the drug back to the mother once the concentration gradient of the free drug across the placenta has been reversed. With the use of local anesthetics, this may occur even though the total plasma drug concentration in the mother may exceed that in the fetus, because there is lower protein binding in fetal plasma.[47] One drug, namely 2-chloroprocaine, is metabolized in the fetal blood so rapidly (t ½ = 43 s) that substantial accumulation in the fetus is avoided even in acidosis.[55, 57]

In the term as well as preterm newborn, the liver contains enzymes essential for the biotransformation of amide local anesthetics.[62] A study, comparing the pharmacokinetics of lidocaine among adult ewes and fetal and neonatal lambs, showed that the metabolic clearance in the newborn was similar to, and renal clearance greater than, that in the adult.[63] Nonetheless, the elimination half-life was more prolonged in the newborn. This was attributed to a greater volume of distribution and tissue uptake of the drug, so that at any given time the neonate's liver and kidneys are exposed to a smaller fraction of lidocaine accumulated in the body. Similar results were obtained in another study involving lidocaine administration to human infants in a neonatal intensive care unit.[62] Prolonged elimination half-lives in the newborn

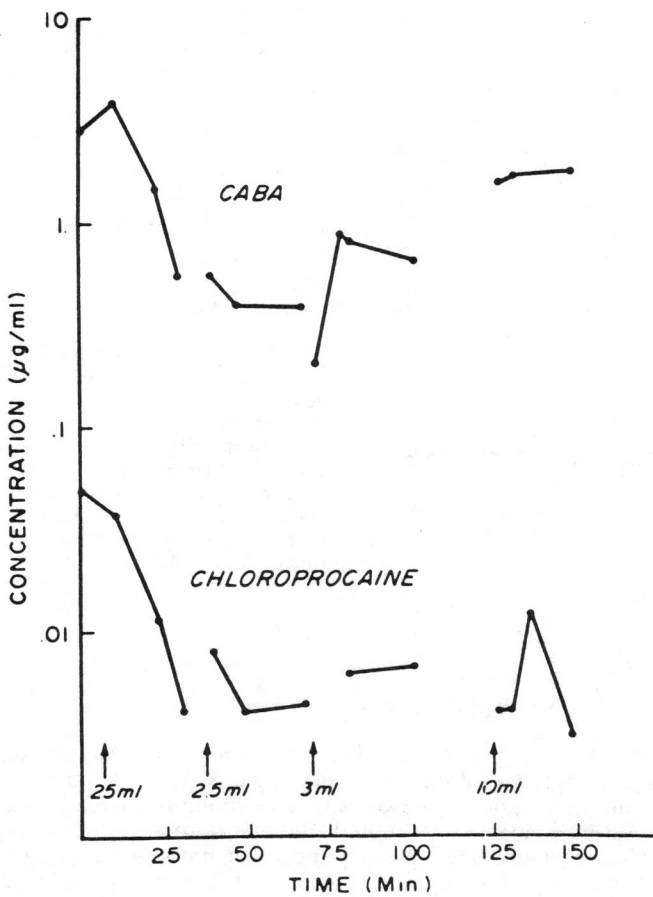

FIG. 45-4. Plasma concentrations of chloroprocaine and chloro-aminobenzoic acid (CABA) in a typical patient after epidural anesthesia (multiple injections) for vaginal delivery. (Reprinted with permission. Kuhnert BR, Kuhnert PM, Prochaska AL *et al:* Plasma levels of 2-chloroprocaine in obstetric patients and their neonates after epidural anesthesia. Anesthesiology 53:21, 1980.)

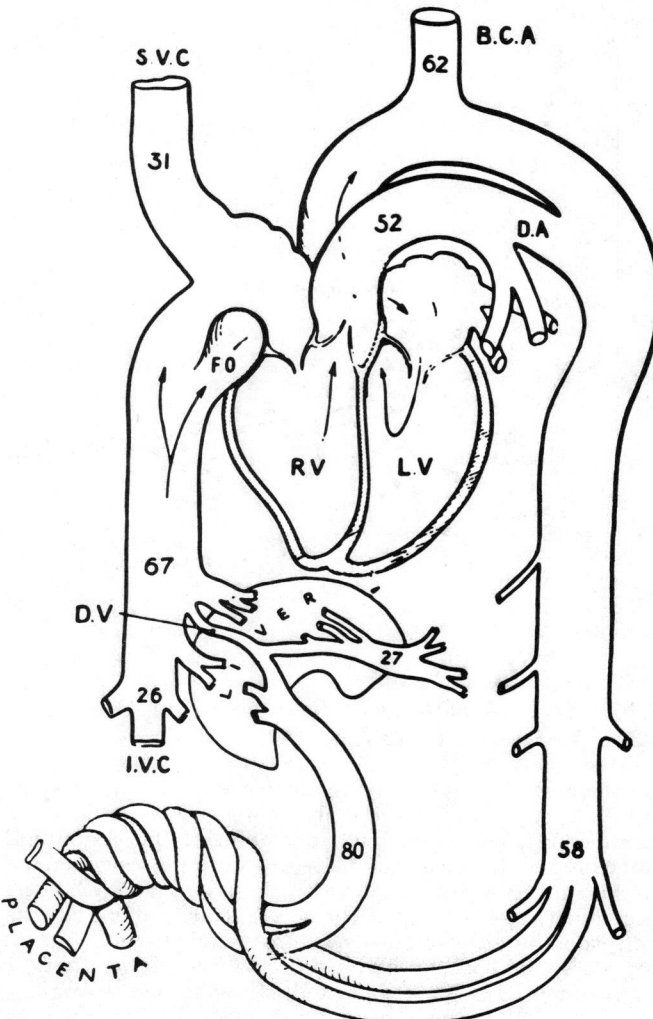

FIG. 45-5. Diagram of the circulation in the mature fetal lamb. The numerals indicate the mean oxygen saturation (%) in the great vessels of six lambs: right ventricle (RV); left ventricle (LV); superior vena cava (SVC); brachiocephalic artery (BCA); foramen ovale (FO); ductus arteriosus (DA); ductus venosus (DV). (Reprinted with permission. Born GVR, Dawes GS, Mott JC, *et al:* Changes in the heart and lungs at birth. Cold Spring Harbor Symp Quant Biol 19:103, 1954.)

compared with the adult have been noted for other amide local anesthetics.

The question remains whether the fetus and newborn are more sensitive to the depressant and toxic effects of drugs than is the adult. Laboratory investigations have shown that the newborn is, in fact, more sensitive to the depressant effects of opioids. With local anesthetics, neonatal depression occurred at blood concentrations of mepivacaine or lidocaine that were approximately 50% less than those producing toxic manifestations in the adult. However, infants accidentally injected with mepivacaine in utero (intended for maternal caudal anesthesia) stopped convulsing when the drug concentration decreased below the threshold level for convulsions in the adult.[64] The relative central nervous and cardiorespiratory toxicity of several local anesthetics has been studied in adult ewes and fetal and newborn lambs.[65, 66] The sequence of toxic manifestations was similar in the three groups: convulsions, followed by hypotension, apnea, and circulatory collapse. The doses required to produce toxicity in the fetus and newborn were significantly higher than those required in the adult. In the fetus this difference was attributed to placental clearance of drug into the mother and better

maintenance of blood gas tensions during convulsions. In the newborn, the larger volume of distribution is probably responsible for the higher doses required to induce toxicity.

Bupivacaine has been implicated as a possible cause of neonatal jaundice.[67] It was postulated that high affinity of the drug for fetal erythrocyte membranes leads to a decrease in filterability and deformability, rendering red blood cells more prone to hemolysis.[68] However, a recent study failed to show increased bilirubin production in newborns whose mothers received bupivacaine for epidural anesthesia during labor and delivery.[69]

Lastly, neurobehavioral studies revealed subtle changes in newborn neurologic and adaptive function. In the case of most anesthetic agents, these changes are minor and transient, lasting for only 24–48 h.[70, 71]

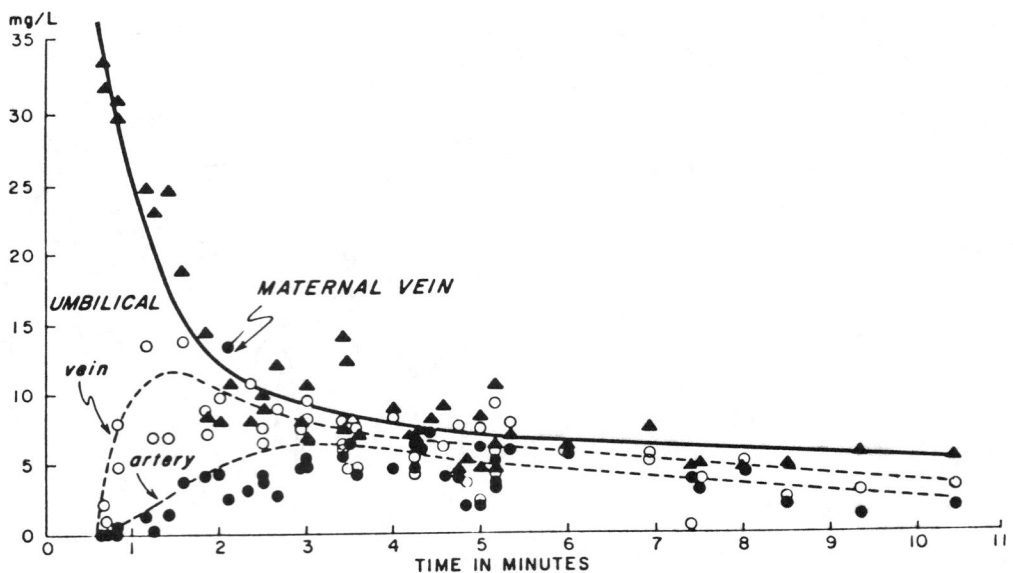

FIG. 45-6. Cesarean section. Thiamylal concentrations in maternal vein (Δ—Δ), umbilical vein (O—O), umbilical artery (●—●). Curves drawn by inspection. (Reprinted with permission. Kosaka Y, Takahashi T, Mark LS: Intravenous thiobarbiturate anesthesia for cesarean section. Anesthesiology 31:489, 1969.)

ANESTHESIA FOR LABOR AND VAGINAL DELIVERY

Most women experience moderate to severe pain during parturition. In the first stage of labor it is caused by uterine contractions, associated with dilatation of the cervix and stretching of the lower uterine segment. Impulses generated in this process are carried in visceral afferent "Type C" fibers accompanying the sympathetic nerves. Pain is referred to the corresponding dermatomal segments where these fibers enter the spinal cord. In early labor, only the lower thoracic dermatomes (T11–12) are affected, but with progressing cervical dilatation in the transition phase, adjacent dermatomes may be involved and pain referred from T-10 to L-1. In the second stage because of the descent of the fetal presenting part, additional impulses arise from distention of the vaginal vault and perineum. These impulses are carried by the pudendal nerves composed of lower sacral fibers (S2–4).

Well-conducted obstetric analgesia, in addition to relieving pain and anxiety, may benefit the mother. For instance, in animal models pain has been shown to result in maternal hypertension and reduced uterine blood flow.[72,73] During the first and second phases of labor, epidural analgesia blunts the increases in maternal cardiac output, heart rate, and blood pressure, which occur with painful uterine contractions and "bearing-down" efforts.[74] In reducing maternal secretion of catecholamines, epidural analgesia may convert a previously dysfunctional labor pattern to normal.[75] Maternal analgesia may also benefit the fetus. It may eliminate maternal hyperventilation, which often leads to a reduced fetal arterial oxygen tension consequent to the leftward shift of the maternal oxygen–hemoglobin dissociation curve.[76]

The most frequently chosen methods for relieving the pain of parturition are psychoprophylaxis, the administration of systemic medications, and epidural or spinal analgesia. Inhalation analgesia, intrathecal opioids, or paracervical blockade are less commonly used. General anesthesia is rarely necessary but may be indicated for uterine relaxation in some deliveries.

PSYCHOPROPHYLAXIS

The philosophy of prepared childbirth maintains that lack of knowledge, misinformation, fear, and anxiety can heighten a patient's response to pain and consequently increase the need for analgesics. Although there is no question that an informed patient is better equipped for the stresses of parturition, few women are able to withstand labor without some pharmacologic analgesia.[77] The most popular method of prepared childbirth is that introduced by Lamaze. It provides an educational program on the physiology of parturition and attempts to diminish cortical pain perception by encouraging responses such as specific patterns of breathing and focused attention on a fixed object. This approach is usually successful through the latent and early active phase but not if labor is prolonged or augmented with the use of oxytocin. However, the advantage of the method is that well-prepared patients generally require less medication.[78] Neonatal outcome appears to be similar for women who deliver babies solely with the Lamaze technique compared with those who receive appropriate supplementary analgesia. A realistic attitude is to encourage the mother in the Lamaze method, recognizing individual variations in pain tolerance and need for medication. Of course, this should not be withheld if required.

SYSTEMIC MEDICATION

Advantages of systemic analgesics include ease of administration and patient acceptability. However, the drug, dose, time, and method of administration must be chosen carefully, so as to avoid maternal and/or neonatal depression. Drugs used for that purpose are opioids, tranquilizers, and, occasionally, ketamine.

Opioids

Meperidine is the most commonly used and is reasonably effective in ameliorating pain during the first stage of labor.

It has virtually replaced morphine, because in equianalgesic doses morphine appears to cause greater neonatal ventilatory depression.[79] Meperidine can be administered by intravenous injection (effective analgesia in 5–10 min) or intramuscularly (peak effect 40–50 min). The major side-effects of this drug are a high incidence of nausea and vomiting, dose-related depression of ventilation, and orthostatic hypotension. Placental transmission is rapid, and fetal blood and tissue levels depend on the dose, mode, and frequency of administration.[52] Meperidine may cause transient alterations of the fetal heart rate, such as decreased beat-to-beat variability and tachycardia. Among other factors, the risk of neonatal depression is related to the last drug injection-to-delivery interval.[80] The placental transfer of active metabolite, normeperidine, has also been implicated in contributing to neonatal depression.[81] Subtle neonatal neurobehavioral dysfunction may be related to the long elimination half-life of normeperidine in the neonate (62 h).[82]

Experience with the newer synthetic opioids, such as fentanyl and alfentanil, has been limited. Although they are potent, their use during labor is restricted by the short duration of analgesia consequent to a very brief distribution phase. An intravenous injection of fentanyl, up to $1 \mu g \cdot kg^{-1}$, results in prompt pain relief without severe neonatal depression.[83] These drugs offer an advantage in situations in which analgesia of rapid onset but short duration is necessary (such as with forceps application).

Opioid agonists–antagonists, such as butorphanol and nalbuphine, have also been used for obstetric analgesia. Those drugs have the proposed benefits of a lower incidence of nausea, vomiting, and dysphoria, as well as a "ceiling effect" on depression of ventilation. However, studies, for the most part, have not demonstrated a clear advantage in parturition.[84] Butorphanol is probably most popular; unlike meperidine, it is biotransformed into inactive metabolites and has a "ceiling effect" on depression of ventilation in doses exceeding 2 mg. A potential disadvantage is the high incidence of maternal sedation. The recommended dose is 1–2 mg by iv or im injection. Nalbuphine, 10 mg iv or im, is an alternative to butorphanol.

Naloxone, a pure opioid antagonist, should not be administered to the mother shortly before delivery in an attempt to prevent neonatal ventilatory depression. Although the technique is effective in this regard, it reverses analgesia at a time when it is most needed and, in some instances, has caused maternal pulmonary edema and cardiac arrest.[85] If necessary, the drug should be given directly to the newborn (10 $mg \cdot kg^{-1}$).

Patient-Controlled Analgesia

The patient can regulate the iv administration of opioids with a device that she can trigger to release a preset dose. Patients accept this method, and the total amount of drug used is less than during conventional analgesia with iv or im injections.[86] The high cost of the device may preclude its routine application.

Tranquilizers

Tranquilizers are principally used during labor to control maternal anxiety and as adjuvants to opioids. Promethazine is most commonly used to provide sedation and diminish nausea and vomiting. Its addition to meperidine resulted in no greater neonatal depression than when meperidine was given alone.[87] Barbiturates are no longer popular because of their antianalgesic effects and neonatal depression. Diazepam should not be used routinely because it results in transient hypotonia and impaired thermoregulation of the newborn.[88]

Ketamine

Ketamine is a potent analgesic capable of producing profound amnesia. The latter is a disadvantage in routine obstetrics, because most mothers want to remember the birthing process. However, ketamine is a useful adjuvant to incomplete regional analgesia during vaginal delivery or obstetric manipulations. In low doses, 0.2–0.4 $mg \cdot kg^{-1}$, ketamine provides adequate analgesia without causing neonatal depression.[89]

REGIONAL ANESTHESIA

The following techniques of regional anesthesia are used in obstetrics: continuous lumbar or sacral (caudal) epidural block, paracervical and pudendal block, and spinal anesthesia. Regional blocks have several advantages that make them preferable to other modalities of analgesia during labor and delivery. They can provide excellent pain relief without obtunding mother or fetus and, if properly applied, should not affect the progress of labor or the mother's ability to "bear down" during the second stage.

Spinal and Epidural Anesthesia

Because of the profound motor paralysis it produces, the use of spinal anesthesia is limited to delivery itself. It is particularly useful to provide rapid, reliable anesthesia for operative delivery, such as midforceps or vacuum extraction, and for perineal repair. To reduce the incidence of postdural puncture headache, 25- or 26-gauge spinal needles should be used routinely. Local anesthetics, prepared as hyperbaric solution, are lidocaine 5% (30–50 mg), tetracaine 0.5% (4–5 mg), and bupivacaine 0.75% (5–6 mg). Lidocaine is the drug of choice because of its shorter duration of action.

In contrast to spinal anesthesia, segmental epidural analgesia can be provided for labor as well as delivery. For adequate pain relief with the smallest amount of drug, only T10–L1 segments need to be blocked during the first stage of labor. For the second stage, the block should be extended to the S2–4 segments. Unless the patient receives oxytocin stimulation, epidural block is usually induced when labor has been well established and the cervix is dilated to 5–6 cm in the primipara and 3–4 cm in a multipara. In the absence of cephalopelvic disproportion, epidural anesthesia does not impede the progress of labor. This applies equally to the first and second stages.[90, 91]

The most frequent complication of spinal and epidural anesthesia is maternal hypotension (systolic blood pressure of less than 100 mm Hg, or a 20% decrease in systolic pressure). Therefore, maternal blood pressure and heart rate must be checked frequently, i.e., every 2–5 min for 15–20 min immediately after induction of the block and every 5–10 min thereafter. In most instances, hypotension can be prevented by acute plasma volume expansion (prehydration) and proper positioning of the parturient to avoid aortocaval compression. Prehydration should be accomplished by rapid intravenous infusion of a balanced salt solution, 500–1,000 ml. Unless the mother is hypoglycemic, use of glucose-containing solutions is better avoided to prevent neonatal hypoglycemia.[27] If hypotension occurs, the intravenous infusion rate should be increased. If the blood pressure is not restored within 1–2 min, ephedrine should be administered intravenously in 5–10-mg increments.

Spinal or epidural anesthesia can be induced with the patient in the lateral decubitus or sitting position. We prefer to use the sitting position because the midline of the back is easier to identify in pregnant women, who frequently have sacral edema, and because, with the common use of narrow-gauge spinal needles, cerebrospinal fluid flows more readily in this position. For epidural anesthesia, the "loss of resistance" is more reliable than the "hanging drop" technique, because epidural pressures tend to be positive during parturition. Once the catheter has been threaded, its placement should be carefully determined to rule out intrathecal or intravenous penetration. Aspiration of the catheter may not be diagnostic because the thin-walled epidural veins are easily collapsed. A more reliable method is to inject 0.5–1.0 ml of saline through the catheter to distend the vessel if the placement was indeed intravenous, hold the catheter in the dependent position, and observe for back flow of blood. Thereafter, a test dose must be administered. Bupivacaine, 7.5 mg; lidocaine, 45 mg; or 2-chloroprocaine, 60 mg, is effective when detecting intrathecal injection. The inclusion of 15 μg of epinephrine, with careful blood pressure and heart rate monitoring (ECG), may be a marker for intravascular injection because it causes a transient increase in both parameters within 30–90 s.[92] However, the use of epinephrine is controversial in obstetrics because false-positive tests do occur with uterine contractions, and the drug may reduce uteroplacental perfusion.[93, 94] After a test dose with negative results, adequate first-stage analgesia is usually achieved with an additional injection of 5 ml of lidocaine 1.0%, bupivacaine 0.25%, or 2-chloroprocaine 2%. The dose may be repeated as necessary or be followed immediately by a continuous epidural infusion of a more dilute solution: 0.33% lidocaine, 10–15 ml · h^{-1}; 0.125% bupivacaine, 8–12 ml · h^{-1}; or 1.0% 2-chloroprocaine, 20–25 ml · h^{-1}. For the second stage of labor, analgesia can be extended to include the sacral segments by administration of an additional 5–10 ml of the originally used local anesthetic solution with the patient in a semirecumbent position. Significant motor blockade should be avoided.

Mepivacaine and etidocaine are other local anesthetics currently available for epidural anesthesia. Neither has been popular in obstetrics because of untoward effects of mepivacaine on neonatal neurobehavioral adaptation and because of the profound motor blockade caused by etidocaine in the mother.[95, 96] However, a recent study refutes the untoward effects of mepivacaine on the neonate.[97]

Caudal anesthesia is used infrequently. It does not allow for a selective blockade of thoracic segments in the first stage of labor. Consequently, larger doses of local anesthetics are necessary from the outset. However, caudal may be preferable to epidural block when rapid onset of perineal anesthesia is desired, as with midforceps delivery. To avoid accidentally injecting the fetus, the mother's rectum must be examined when the needle is still in place and before administration of the test dose.[64]

Spinal and epidural (lumbar or sacral) blocks are generally contraindicated in the presence of coagulopathy, acute hypovolemia, or infection at the site of needle puncture.

Paracervical Block

Although paracervical block effectively relieves pain during the first stage of labor, the technique has fallen out of favor because it is associated with a high incidence of fetal distress and poor neonatal outcome, particularly with the use of bupivacaine. This may be related to uterine artery constriction or increased uterine tone.[98, 99] The technique is basically simple and involves a submucosal injection of local anesthetic at the vaginal fornix, in the proximity of those fibers innervating the uterus. All local anesthetics, except bupivacaine, may be used for that purpose.

Pudendal Nerve Block

The pudendal nerves, derived from the lower sacral nerve roots (S2–4), supply the vaginal vault, perineum, and rectum and parts of the bladder. The nerves are easily anesthetized transvaginally because they loop around the ischial spines. Ten milliliters of local anesthetic deposited behind each sacrospinous ligament provides adequate anesthesia for outlet forceps delivery and episiotomy repair.

Epidural and Intrathecal Opioids

The use of epidural opioids to relieve labor pain has been disappointing. Although morphine, 4–5 mg, provides prolonged and intense analgesia after cesarean section, it is not as consistently beneficial during labor.[100, 101] Better pain relief may be obtained with higher drug doses (7.5 mg), but the risk of delayed depression of ventilation and the fetal effects after placental transfer preclude its routine use.[102] However, addition of fentanyl 3–5 μg · ml^{-1} or butorphanol 0.2 mg · ml^{-1} to a dilute solution of bupivacaine (0.125%) has been quite valuable.[103] This combination achieves a solid block with a greatly reduced dose of local anesthetic. In contrast, opioids very effectively relieve the pain of uterine contractions when injected intrathecally (morphine 0.5–1.5 mg, fentanyl 37.5–50 μg).[104, 105] A pudendal block or local infiltration of the perineum may be required at delivery. Intrathecal opioids are particularly useful in parturients with severe heart disease in whom sympathetic blockade should be strongly avoided. Complications of epidural and intrathecal opioids in obstetric patients are the same as in the general surgical population, viz., pruritus, urinary retention, and delayed ventilatory depression.

INHALATION ANALGESIA

Inhalation analgesia is easy to administer, and, although it does not relieve pain completely, it makes uterine contractions more tolerable. During delivery, a combination of inhalation analgesia with a pudendal block or infiltration of the perineum with a local anesthetic can be very satisfactory. A particular advantage of inhalation analgesia pertains to the uptake and excretion of the drugs. The desired level of analgesia can be easily and rapidly achieved or terminated. The neonate can also excrete inhalation agents through the lungs. A serious disadvantage is the need for a scavenging system. The potential for fluoride nephrotoxicity is greatest with methoxyflurane and much less so with enflurane. However, nephrotoxicity with methoxyflurane has not been a problem in laboring patients so long as the total dose does not exceed 15 ml of the agent.[106] Use of either drug should probably be avoided with compromised renal function.

Inhalation drugs can be administered by trained personnel or by the patient herself, with adequate supervision. A conventional anesthesia circuit can be used, and a methoxyflurane inhaler is commercially available for self-administration. The system must be able to deliver a precise concentration of the agent over a wide range of inspiratory flow rates. The parturient is instructed to breathe deeply from the inhaler when she detects the onset of uterine contraction, so that analgesia will be established at its peak. Commonly used inhalation drugs for analgesia during labor are nitrous oxide, up to 50 vol%, methoxyflurane, 0.25–0.4 vol%, or enflurane, 0.5–1.0 vol%. A mixture of either potent drug in nitrous oxide and oxygen has also been used. The inspired concentration of oxygen in nitrous oxide–containing mixtures should be monitored. Halothane is a poor analgesic.[107]

GENERAL ANESTHESIA

General anesthesia is rarely used for vaginal delivery and always with precautions against aspiration. It may be required when time constraints prevent induction of regional anesthesia, as in acute fetal distress. If uterine relaxation is necessary for obstetric maneuvers, potent inhalation drugs can provide a dose-related response.[108] This may be at delivery of the second twin or breech or after delivery, for manual removal of a retained placenta. An inhaled concentration of 2 MAC is usually adequate. In all cases, preoxygenation and rapid intravenous induction of anesthesia with the use of cricoid pressure and placement of a cuffed tube in the trachea are mandatory. High inspiratory flows ensure quick delivery of the drug. The mother must not be overdosed during controlled ventilation of the lungs. Immediately after the obstetric procedure is completed, the potent drug should be discontinued, or its concentration reduced, to minimize the risk of hemorrhage resulting from continued uterine relaxation. Oxytocin, 20–30 units, should be added to the intravenous infusion. The patient's trachea should not be extubated until she is awake and airway reflexes have returned.

ANESTHESIA FOR CESAREAN SECTION

The frequency of cesarean section has steadily increased in recent decades, reaching the high incidence of 20%–25% of all deliveries. The most frequent indications include failure to progress, fetal distress, cephalopelvic disproportion, malpresentation, prematurity, and prior uterine surgery. The choice of anesthesia should depend on the urgency of the procedure, as well as on the condition of the mother and fetus. In the absence of specific indications, the mother's wishes should be seriously considered.

REGIONAL ANESTHESIA

A recent survey of obstetric anesthesia practices in the United States revealed that most patients having cesarean section do so under spinal or epidural anesthesia.[109] Regional techniques have several advantages: a lessened risk of gastric aspiration, fulfillment of the mother's wish to remain awake, and avoidance of depressant anesthetic drugs. It has also been suggested that operative blood loss is less with regional than general anesthesia.[110] The time required for induction of regional anesthesia makes the technique less suitable for urgent cesarean section. Induction-to-delivery interval averages

15–20 min with spinal anesthesia and 30–40 min with epidural anesthesia. In elective cesarean sections, the duration of antepartum anesthesia does not affect the neonatal outcome, as long as there is no protracted aortocaval compression or hypotension.[111] The risk of hypotension is greater than during vaginal delivery because the block must extend to the T-4 segment. Therefore, proper positioning and prehydration are critical. At least 1,500–2,000 ml of a crystalloid solution is required. In this regard, epidural anesthesia is advantageous, because of its slower onset and progression. Prophylactic intramuscular injection of 50 mg ephedrine 10–15 min before induction has been efficacious in decreasing the incidence and severity of hypotension resulting from spinal anesthesia.[112] If hypotension occurs despite these measures, left uterine displacement should be increased, the rate of intravenous infusion augmented, and ephedrine, in 10–15 mg increments, administered by intravenous injection.

Spinal Anesthesia

Subarachnoid block is the more commonly administered regional anesthetic for cesarean delivery.[109] It is popular partially because of the simplicity and reliability of the technique, as well as the relative rapidity with which adequate anesthesia can be established. In fact, it has been suggested as a reasonable alternative to general anesthesia for emergency cesarean section.[113]

Solutions of lidocaine 5%, tetracaine 1.0%, or bupivacaine 0.75% are available. The doses and duration of action of these local anesthetics are listed in Table 45-2.

Blood pressure, ventilation, and ECG should be monitored throughout, and hemoglobin oxygen saturation (pulse oximeter) should be monitored when possible. Before delivery, oxygen should be routinely administered by face mask to improve fetal oxygenation.[114]

Despite a block extending to the T-4 segment, patients experience varying degrees of visceral discomfort, particularly with exteriorization of the uterus, and traction on abdominal viscera. Supplementary analgesia may be provided by the incremental intravenous injection of 2–3 mg morphine, 20–30 mg meperidine, or 25 μg fentanyl. The patient can be sedated by addition of 2.5–5 mg diazepam. Midazolam is a less desirable sedative in the obstetric setting because of its strong amnestic properties. Nausea and vomiting may be alleviated by the administration of a small dose of droperidol or metoclopramide.[115, 116] One should take care not to oversedate the mother and blunt her airway reflexes. The addition of as little as 0.1 mg of preservative-free morphine to the local anesthetic solution can provide prolonged postoperative analgesia.[117, 118]

Lumbar Epidural Anesthesia

Lumbar epidural anesthesia is also popular for use with cesarean sections. In contrast to spinal anesthesia, more time and drug are required to establish an adequate sensory block. The advantages are the lessened risk of postdural puncture headache and the ability to titrate the dose of local anesthetic through an indwelling epidural catheter. The usual precautions must be taken to ensure proper placement of the needle and catheter to prevent inadvertent intrathecal or intravascular injection. This is especially important because drug requirements for cesarean section are greater compared with those for labor and vaginal delivery.

The most commonly used agents are 2-chloroprocaine 3%, bupivacaine 0.5%, and lidocaine 2% with epinephrine

TABLE 45-2. Local Anesthetics Commonly Used
for Cesarean Section with Subarachnoid Block

	LIDOCAINE 5% IN 7.5% DEXTROSE	TETRACAINE 1% IN EQUAL VOLUME OF 10% DEXTROSE	BUPIVACAINE 0.75% IN 8.25% DEXTROSE
Dosage (mg) according to height (cm)			
150–160	65	8	8
160–182	70	9	10
182 and taller	75	10	12
Onset of action (min)	1–3	3–5	2–4
Duration of action (min)	45–75	120–180	120–180

1:200,000. Adequate anesthesia is usually achieved with 15–25 ml of the solution, given in divided doses. The patient should be monitored as with spinal anesthesia.

Because of its extremely high rate of metabolism in the maternal and fetal plasma, 2-chloroprocaine provides a rapid-onset, reliable block with minimal risk of systemic toxicity.[55] It is the local anesthetic of choice in the presence of fetal acidosis and when a preexisting block is to be rapidly extended for an urgent cesarean section.[119] Reports of transient neurologic deficits after massive inadvertent intrathecal administration of the drug have somewhat diminished enthusiasm for its use.[120, 121] The formulation containing a relatively high concentration of sodium bisulfite, at a low pH, has been implicated as being neurotoxic.[122] A new formula, in which ethylene diamino tetra acetate (EDTA) has been substituted for sodium bisulfite, is currently on the market.

Bupivacaine 0.5% provides profound anesthesia for cesarean section, of slower onset but longer duration than the other two drugs. Considerable attention has focused on the drug since it was reported that unintentional intravascular injection could result not only in convulsions, but also in an almost simultaneous cardiac arrest, often refractory to resuscitation.[123] The greater cardiotoxicity of bupivacaine (and etidocaine) in comparison with other amide local anesthetics has been well demonstrated in various animal models.[66, 124] Pregnancy itself appears to enhance the cardiotoxic effects of the drug.[125]

Lidocaine has an onset and duration intermediate to 2-chloroprocaine and bupivacaine. The need to include epinephrine (1:200,000) in the local anesthetic solution, to ensure adequate lumbosacral anesthesia, limits its use in the presence of maternal hypertension and reduced uteroplacental perfusion.

With epidural anesthesia, prolonged pain relief also can be provided in the postoperative period by intraspinal administration of an opioid. The following opioids have been used successfully: 5 mg morphine, 2 mg butorphanol, 1 mg hydromorphone, 50 μg fentanyl, and 20–30 μg sufentanil.[100, 126–130] All were diluted to a volume of 10 ml with normal saline. Because delayed depression of ventilation may occur, particularly with the use of morphine, the patient must be monitored carefully in the postoperative period.[131]

GENERAL ANESTHESIA

The advantages of general anesthesia are the rapidity and reliability with which the patient can be prepared for surgery. It is the technique of choice for emergency cesarean section

and when substantial hemorrhage is anticipated (placenta previa, fibromyomata). We also prefer to use general anesthesia in situations in which uterine relaxation will facilitate delivery, as in prematurity, breech presentation, and transverse lie, and in patients with multiple gestation or polyhydramnios, who frequently have dyspnea and supine hypotension syndrome. General anesthesia should be used cautiously in patients with asthma, upper respiratory infection, or a history of difficult tracheal intubation. The airway should be evaluated carefully during the preoperative visit, because inability to intubate the trachea is one of the leading causes of maternal death.[132] If difficulties are anticipated, one should consider using a regional technique, an awake tracheal intubation, or a fiberoptic bronchoscope. Preoperative medication is usually not necessary, except for oral administration of 15–30 ml of a nonparticulate antacid within 30 min of induction of anesthesia. On the operating table, the patient's pelvis should be tilted to prevent aortocaval compression. Routine monitoring is the same as with regional anesthetic techniques, with the addition of a capnometer, pulse oximeter, nerve stimulator, inspired oxygen concentration monitor, and temperature probe.

Preoxygenation is an important step that should be carried out for 3–5 min with the use of a tight-fitting mask. In an emergency situation, four deep breaths with 100% oxygen will suffice.[133] A "defasciculating" dose of a nondepolarizing muscle relaxant is not necessary. Rapid induction of anesthesia is achieved with an intravenous injection of thiopental (4 mg · kg^{-1}), ketamine (up to 1 mg · kg^{-1}), or a combination of thiopental (2–3 mg · kg^{-1}) and ketamine (0.5 mg · kg^{-1}). If the patient is in labor, and time constraints permit, induction drugs should be administered at the onset of uterine contraction to decrease fetal drug exposure.[61] Succinylcholine (1–1.5 mg · kg^{-1}) is then injected, while cricoid pressure is applied by a trained assistant until the airway is properly secured with a cuffed endotracheal tube. If there is difficulty in securing the airway, cricoid pressure should be maintained throughout and the mother ventilated with 100% oxygen before a subsequent attempt at tracheal intubation. It is safer to permit the mother to awaken and to reassess the method of induction, than to persist with traumatic efforts at tracheal intubation, which may result in loss of the airway because of edema and bleeding. Once the endotracheal tube placement is confirmed, preferably with a capnometer, the obstetrician may proceed with skin incision. In the predelivery interval, anesthesia is maintained with a 50:50 mixture of nitrous oxide in oxygen and 0.5 MAC of a potent agent. An infusion of succinylcholine may only be added when there is evidence that neuromuscular function has returned. Severe maternal hyperventilation should be avoided, because it may reduce uterine blood flow. A study performed in pregnant sheep established that placental hypoperfusion results from the mechanical effect of hyperventilation, because it could not be corrected by restoring Pa_{CO_2} to normal or above-normal levels.[134] A few minutes before delivery is anticipated, the concentration of the potent agent may be increased temporarily to 2 MAC, when uterine relaxation is desired.

Newborn condition after cesarean section with general anesthesia is comparable to that with regional techniques.[135] The uterine incision-to-delivery interval seems to be more important to neonatal outcome than induction of anesthesia-to-delivery interval. Lower Apgar scores at 1 minute and acidosis were reported in cases in which the uterine incision-to-delivery time interval exceeded 180 sec, whereas anesthesia for up to 30 min before delivery appears to have no adverse effects on the infant.[136, 137] This is in contrast to the earlier practice of using 70%–75% nitrous oxide in oxygen, which resulted in neonatal depression within approximately 10 min of anesthesia.[138] The increase to 50% in the oxygen concentration inhaled by the mother also benefits the fetus by increasing its Pa_{O_2}.[139]

After delivery of the infant, 20 units oxytocin is added to the infusion, and anesthesia is deepened with adjuvants such as an opioid. At the end of the procedure, the mother's trachea is extubated once she is awake. The usual blood loss at a cesarean section is 750–1,000 ml, and transfusion is rarely necessary.

MANAGEMENT OF HIGH-RISK PARTURIENTS

Pregnancy or parturition are considered "high risk" when accompanied by conditions unfavorable to the well-being of the mother or fetus or both. Maternal problems may be related to pregnancy, such as preeclampsia–eclampsia and other hypertensive disorders of pregnancy, or antepartum hemorrhage resulting from placenta previa (literally "the placenta going ahead") or abruptio placentae ("breaking away of the placenta"). Diabetes mellitus; cardiac, chronic renal, neurologic, or sickle cell disease; asthma, obesity, and drug abuse are not related to pregnancy but often are affected by it. Prematurity (gestation of less than 37 weeks), postmaturity (42 weeks or longer), intrauterine growth retardation, and multiple gestation are fetal conditions associated with high risk. During labor and delivery, fetal malpresentation (breech, transverse lie), placental abruption, compression of the umbilical cord (prolapse, nuchal cord), precipitous labor, or intrauterine infection (prolonged rupture of membranes) may enhance the risk to the mother or the fetus.

In general, the anesthetic management of the high-risk parturient is based on the same maternal and fetal considerations as the management of healthy mothers and fetuses. These include maintenance of maternal cardiovascular function and oxygenation; maintenance, and possibly improvement, of the uteroplacental blood flow; and creation of optimal conditions for a painless, atraumatic delivery of an infant without significant drug effects. However, there is less room for error, because many of the above functions may be compromised before the induction of anesthesia. For example, significant acidosis is prone to develop in fetuses of diabetic mothers when delivered by cesarean section with spinal or epidural anesthesia complicated by even brief maternal hypotension.[140] Because the high-risk parturient may have received a variety of drugs, anesthesiologists must be familiar with potential interactions between these drugs and the anesthetic drugs they plan to administer.

PREECLAMPSIA–ECLAMPSIA

Hypertensive disorders that occur in approximately 7% of all late pregnancies are among the major causes of maternal mortality, accounting for approximately one-fifth of maternal deaths, and have been estimated to result in 30,000 neonatal deaths and stillbirths per year in the United States alone. Preeclampsia is diagnosed on the basis of development of hypertension with proteinuria or edema, or both. The added appearance of convulsions and coma makes for the diagnosis of eclampsia.

Preeclampsia–eclampsia is a disease unique to human pregnancy, occurring predominantly in young nulliparas. Symptoms usually appear after the 20th week of gestation, occasionally earlier than that if in association with a hydatidiform mole. Thus, the condition requires the presence of a trophoblast but not a fetus.

The origin of preeclampsia–eclampsia is unknown. One proposed theory invokes immunologic rejection of fetal tissues by the mother, which causes a placental vasculitis and ischemia.[141] This theory explains why the disease is more common among nulliparas (no previous exposure to a trophoblast) and in conditions associated with an abnormally large mass of trophoblastic tissues, as in hydatidiform mole, multiple pregnancy, diabetes, and Rh incompatibility. Various studies have demonstrated an abnormal maternal immune responsiveness in preeclampsia. Placental ischemia would result in a release of uterine renin and an increase in angiotensin activity (Fig. 45-7).[142] This would lead to a widespread arteriolar vasoconstriction, causing hypertension, tissue hypoxia, and endothelial damage. Adherence of platelets at sites of endothelial damage would result in coagulopathies, occasionally in disseminated intravascular coagulation (DIC). Enhanced angiotensin-mediated aldosterone secretion would lead to an increased sodium reabsorption and edema. Proteinuria, another symptom of preeclampsia, may also be attributed to placental ischemia, which would lead to local tissue degeneration and a release of thromboplastin with subsequent deposition of fibrin in constricted glomerular vessels and increased permeability to albumin and other plasma proteins. Furthermore, there is thought to be a decreased production of prostaglandins E, potent vasodilators secreted in the trophoblast, which normally would balance the hypertensive effects of the renin-angiotensin system.

A recent study has suggested that many of the symptoms associated with preeclampsia, including placental ischemia, systemic vasoconstriction, and increased platelet aggregation, may result from an imbalance between the placental production of prostacyclin and thromboxane (Fig. 45-8).[143] During normal pregnancy the placenta produces equivalent quantities of these prostaglandins, whereas in preeclamptic pregnancy there is seven times more thromboxane than prostacyclin. In another study, a significant correlation was found between intervillous blood flow and the ratio of placental productions of thromboxane and prostacyclin.[144]

Preeclampsia is classified as severe if associated with any of the following:

1. Systolic blood pressure of 160 mm Hg or greater
2. Diastolic blood pressure of 110 mm Hg or greater
3. Proteinuria of 5 g or more per 24 h
4. Oliguria (400 ml or less per 24 h)
5. Cerebral or visual disturbances
6. Pulmonary edema or cyanosis
7. Epigastric pain

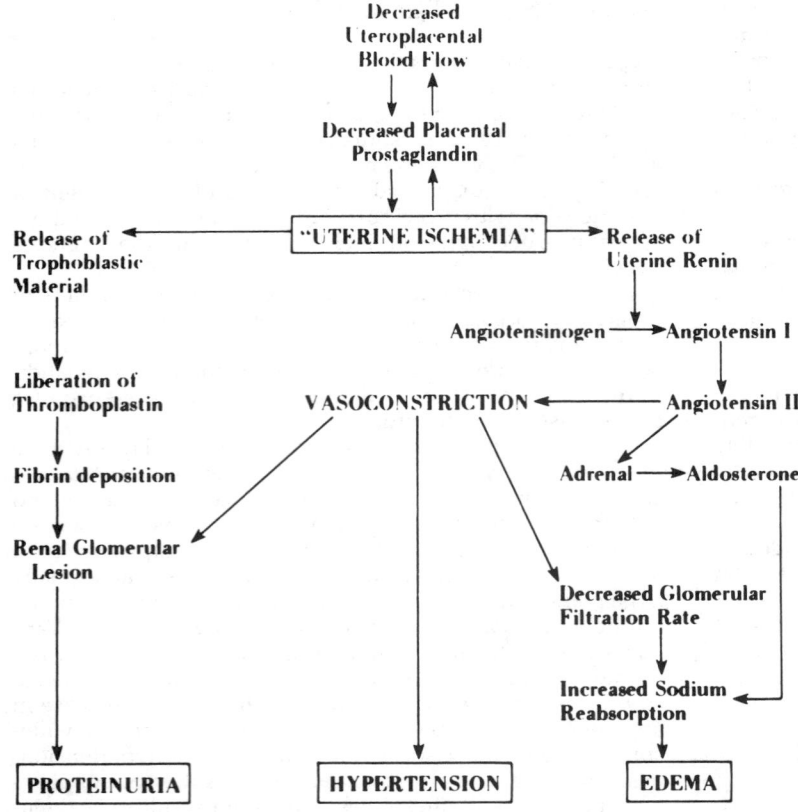

FIG. 45-7. Proposed scheme of pathophysiologic changes in toxemia of pregnancy. (Reprinted with permission. Speroff L: Toxemia of pregnancy: Mechanism and therapeutic management. Am J Cardiol 32:582, 1973.)

In severe preeclampsia–eclampsia, all major organ systems are affected because of widespread vasospasm. Overall cerebral blood flow is not diminished, but focal hypoperfusion cannot be ruled out. Indeed, postmortem examination has revealed hemorrhagic necrosis in the proximity of thrombosed precapillaries, suggesting intense vasoconstriction. Edema and small foci of degeneration have been attributed to hypoxia. Petechial hemorrhages are common after the onset of convulsions. Symptoms related to the above changes include headache, vertigo, cortical blindness, hyperreflexia, and convulsions. The extent of blood pressure elevation correlates poorly with the incidence of seizures, which are commonly generalized. In a recent study, 50% of preeclamptic and 75% of eclamptic women were found to have abnormal electroencephalograms (EEGs) consisting of diffuse slowing in the form of theta and delta waves.[145] Cerebral hemorrhage and edema are the leading causes of death with preeclampsia–eclampsia, together accounting for approximately 50% of deaths.[146]

In the eyes, intense arteriolar constriction may result in blurred vision, even temporary blindness.

Heart failure may occur in severe cases as a result of peripheral vasoconstriction and increased blood viscosity secondary to hemoconcentration. Changes described in autopsy specimens include left ventricular hypertrophy, subendocardial hemorrhages, cloudy swelling, and fatty and hyaline degeneration.

Decreased blood supply to the liver may result in periportal necrosis of variable extent and severity. Subcapsular hemorrhages account for the epigastric pain encountered in severe cases. Rarely, there is a rupture of the overstretched liver capsule and massive hemorrhage into the abdominal cavity.

Hepatic function tests have shown elevated plasma levels of serum glutamic-oxalocetic transaminase (SGOT), lactic dehydrogenase (LDH), and alkaline phosphatase, whereas bilirubin levels were unaltered.[147]

In the kidneys, swelling of glomerular endothelial cells and deposition of fibrin leading to a constriction of the capillary lumina have been described. Renal blood flow and glomerular filtration rate decrease, resulting in reduced uric acid clearance and, in severe cases, reduced clearance of urea and creatinine.[147] As already stated, oliguria and proteinuria are among the characteristic symptoms of severe preeclampsia. The severity of renal involvement is reflected in the degree of proteinuria, which may reach nephrotic levels of $10–15 \ g \cdot 24 \ h^{-1}$.

A mild degree of pulmonary ventilation–perfusion imbalance has been reported in severe cases. It is not believed to be clinically important because the arterial oxygen tension was within normal limits.[148] In contrast, airway edema, which may also occur in severe preeclampsia, is of great concern because it may lead to respiratory embarrassment and difficulty in endotracheal intubation. Pulmonary edema is commonly found at autopsy in fatal cases. It may result from heart failure, circulatory overload, or aspiration of gastric contents during convulsions.

In the placenta, a reduction in the intervillous blood flow may result from vasoconstriction or the development of occlusive lesions in decidual arteries, despite the elevated maternal blood pressure. Histologic examination of the placenta often reveals nodular ischemia and varying stages of infarction. Necrosis of the supporting tissues may lead to a rupture of fetal cotyledonary vessels and hemorrhage. If the hemorrhage is extensive, it may rupture retroplacentally, ini-

NORMAL PREGNANCY

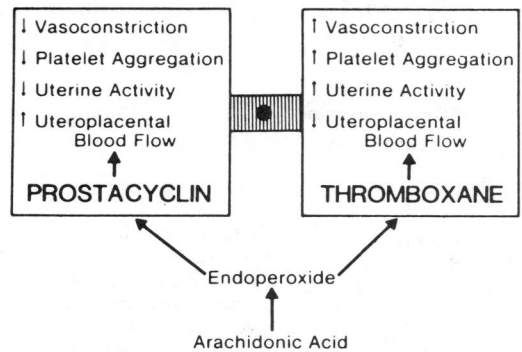

PREECLAMPSIA

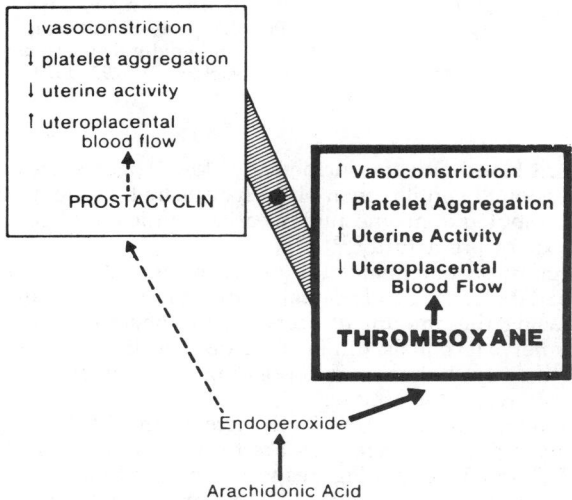

FIG. 45-8. Comparison of the balance in the biologic actions of prostacyclin and thromboxane in normal pregnancy with the imbalance of increased thromboxane and decreased prostacyclin in preeclamptic pregnancy. (Reprinted with permission. Walsh SW: Preeclampsia: An imbalance in placental prostacyclin and thromboxane production. Am J Obstet Gynecol 152:335, 1985.)

tiating the process of abruption. Reduced placental blood flow leads to chronic fetal hypoxia and malnutrition. The risks of intrauterine growth retardation, premature birth, and perinatal death are substantially higher than in normal pregnancies and correlate with the severity of preeclampsia.[149]

Although preeclampsia is accompanied by exaggerated retention of water and sodium, the shift of fluid and proteins from the intravascular into the extravascular compartment may result in hypovolemia, hypoproteinemia, and hemoconcentration. This phenomenon may be further aggravated by proteinuria. The risk of uteroplacental hypoperfusion and poor fetal outcome has been shown to correlate with the degree of maternal plasma and protein depletion.[150] The mean plasma volume in women with preeclampsia was found to be 9% less than normal, and in those with severe disease it was as much as 30%–40% below normal.[151] The inverse relationship between the intravascular volume and

the severity of hypertension was confirmed more recently with measurements of central venous pressure (CVP) (Fig. 45-9).[152] Patients with a diastolic pressure of 110 mm Hg or greater may have a CVP as low as -4 cmH$_2$O and may require an infusion of approximately 3 liters volume to increase the CVP to the normal range. It has also been shown that a significant reduction in the maternal plasma volume may precede the clinical appearance of preeclampsia in previously normotensive patients.[153]

Earlier studies involving the use of a pulmonary artery flow–directed catheter suggested that patients with severe preeclampsia were in a hyperdynamic state.[154] However, these investigations were performed when patients were in labor or in the postpartum period, after treatment had been instituted. More recently, hemodynamic data were obtained in 10 preeclamptic and four healthy pregnant women near term.[155] None were in labor. In the preeclamptic women, measurements were made before treatment, after volume expansion, and, finally, after vasodilation was achieved with a continuous intravenous infusion of dihydralazine (Table 45-3). The initial measurements revealed a low pulmonary capillary wedge pressure, a low cardiac index, a high systemic vascular resistance, and an increased heart rate, indicating the existence of a low output state in untreated preeclamptic women. Volume expansion resulted in a significant increase in pulmonary capillary wedge pressure and cardiac index, whereas the systemic vascular resistance and maternal heart rate decreased. The mean arterial pressure was significantly reduced, mainly because of a decrease in systolic pressure. Others have also documented this beneficial effect of volume expansion on systemic blood pressure.[152] Subsequent infusion of dihydralazine did not alter the capillary wedge pressure but led to an additional increase in cardiac index and a decrease in systemic vascular resistance. These data indicate that volume expansion may improve maternal tissue perfusion in severe preeclampsia.

Simultaneous determinations of CVP and pulmonary capillary wedge pressure were obtained in another group of 18 patients with severe preeclampsia.[156] In approximately half of cases, there was a linear relation between the two modalities, but even in these women it was impossible to predict the pulmonary capillary wedge pressure from CVP because of wide interindividual variations.

Adherence of platelets at sites of endothelial damage may result in consumption coagulopathy, which develops in approximately 20% of patients with preeclampsia. Thrombocytopenia is the most frequent finding. It is usually mild, with the platelet count in the range of 100,000–150,000 mm^3. Elevated levels of fibrin degradation products are found less frequently, and plasma fibrinogen concentrations remain normal unless there is a placental abruption. Prolongation of prothrombin and partial thromboplastin times indicates consumption of procoagulants. Bleeding time may be the most reliable test of clotting in preeclampsia because it was prolonged in approximately 25% of patients with normal platelet counts.[157]

General Management

Because the origin of preeclampsia–eclampsia is not known, management is symptomatic. Its goals are to prevent or control convulsions, improve organ perfusion, normalize blood pressure, and correct clotting abnormalities. Delivery is indicated in refractory cases or if the pregnancy is close to term. In severe cases, aggressive management should continue for at least 24–48 h after delivery.

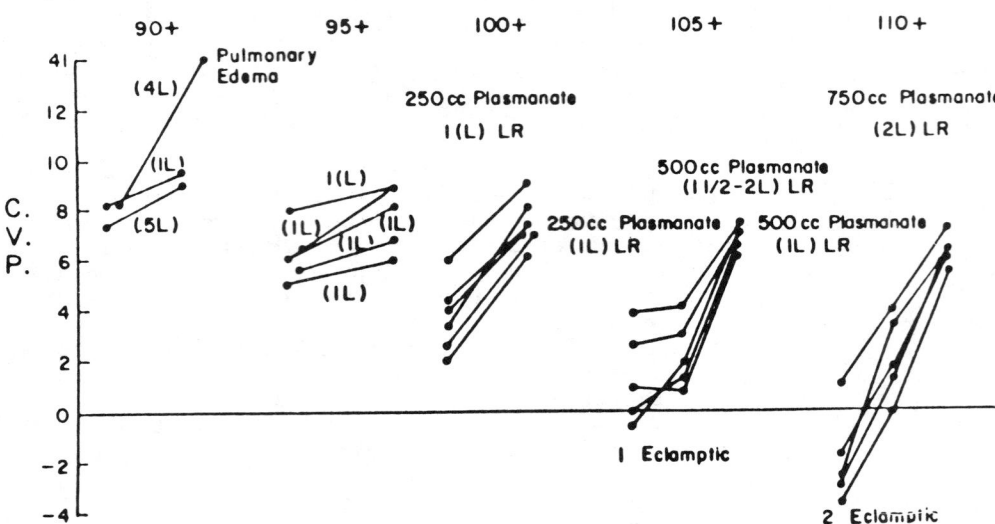

FIG. 45-9. Initial central venous pressure measurements (three or more recordings of maternal diastolic pressure) and intravenous volume replacement required to attain the range of 6–8 cm H₂O in five groups of women with preeclampsia classified according to the severity of the disease. (Reprinted with permission. Joyce TH III, Debnath KS, Baker, EA: Preeclampsia—Relationship of CVP and epidural analgesia. Anesthesiology 51:S297, 1979.)

The mainstay of anticonvulsant therapy in the United States is magnesium sulfate. Although its efficacy in preventing seizures has been well substantiated, its mechanism of action remains controversial. In preeclamptic–eclamptic patients who had serial EEG recordings, the EEG abnormalities noted during an intravenous infusion of magnesium sulfate were similar to those occurring in the absence of magnesium sulfate therapy.[145] The patient usually receives an intravenous loading dose of 4 g in a 20% solution, administered over 5 min. Therapeutic blood levels are maintained by continuous infusion of $1–2 \text{ g} \cdot \text{h}^{-1}$. In addition to its anticonvulsant properties, by causing peripheral arterial vasodilation, magnesium sulfate may affect the maternal hemodynamic state.[158] Magnesium ions cross the placenta readily and may lead to fetal and neonatal hypermagnesemia. There is a poor correlation between magnesium concentrations in the umbilical cord blood and the incidence of low Apgar scores and depression of ventilation at birth. It appears that the depression attributed to magnesium in earlier studies resulted from asphyxia or prematurity.[159]

Magnesium potentiates the duration and intensity of action of depolarizing and nondepolarizing muscle relaxants by decreasing the amount of acetylcholine liberated from the motor nerve terminals, diminishing the sensitivity of the endplate to acetylcholine, and depressing the excitability of the skeletal muscle membrane.

The aim of fluid therapy is to increase the CVP and pulmonary capillary wedge pressure to the normal range (4–6 cm H₂O and 5–10 mm Hg, respectively) and to increase the urine output to $1 \text{ ml} \cdot \text{kg}^{-1} \cdot \text{h}^{-1}$. As already mentioned, this has been shown to improve the cardiac index and, interestingly, to decrease the mean systemic arterial pressure as

TABLE 45-3. Hemodynamic Variables (mean and range) in Preeclamptic Patients and Control Subjects

	PREECLAMPTIC PATIENTS (n = 10)					CONTROL SUBJECTS (n = 4)
	Initial	After Volume Expansion	P*	After Vasodilatation	P†	
Diastolic blood pressure (mm Hg)	106 (100–120)	102 (90–120)	NS‡	85 (75–100)	<0.01	77 (70–90)
Mean arterial pressure (mm Hg)	121 (113–136)	116 (103–136)	<0.02	102 (97–116)	<0.01	95 (93–106)
Heart rate (beats · min⁻¹)	100 (90–130)	81 (60–110)	<0.01	82 (70–100)	NS	84 (70–90)
Pulmonary capillary wedge pressure (mm Hg)	3.3 (1–5)	8 (7–10)	<0.01	8 (7–9)	NS	9 (6–12)
Systemic vascular resistance (dynes · s⁻¹ · cm⁻⁵)	1,943 (1,480–2,580)	1284 (1,073–1,600)	<0.01	947 (782–1,028)	<0.01	886 (805–1,021)
Cardiac index (1 · min⁻¹ · m⁻²)	2.75 (1.97–3.33)	3.77 (3.26–4.05)	<0.01	4.40 (3.94–5.00)	<0.01	4.53 (3.96–4.97)

Wilcoxon signed-rank test (two-tailed).
* As compared with initial values.
† As compared with values after volume expansion.
‡ NS = not significant.
(Groenendijk R, Trimbos MJ, Wallenberg HCS: Hemodynamic measurements in preeclampsia: Preliminary observations. Am J Obstet Gynecol 150:232, 1984.)

well as systemic vascular resistance.[155] Approximately one-third of the fluid infused may consist of 5% albumin solution to correct the decreased colloid osmotic pressure. The infusion should be administered slowly, over a period of several hours, to avoid fluid overload. In severe cases, careful monitoring of arterial pressure, central venous pressure, pulmonary artery and pulmonary capillary wedge pressure, urine output, and specific gravity should be started as soon as possible. Monitoring should be carried out in the postpartum period as well, preferably in the recovery room or intensive care setting. In patients with blood clotting abnormalities, the risk of inadvertent puncture of the carotid artery associated with internal jugular cannulation may be averted by inserting the line in the basilic or external jugular vein.

The antihypertensive therapy in preeclampsia is used to lessen the risk of cerebral hemorrhage in the mother while maintaining, even improving, tissue perfusion. Plasma volume expansion combined with vasodilation will fulfill these goals.[155] Hydralazine is the most commonly used vasodilator in preeclampsia because it increases uteroplacental and renal blood flows. It can be given orally, intramuscularly, or intravenously. Nitroprusside, a potent vasodilator of resistance and capacitance vessels, having an immediate but evanescent action, is useful in preventing dangerous elevations in systemic and pulmonary blood pressure during laryngoscopy and intubation and is ideal for treatment of hypertensive emergencies. Its infusion can be decreased gradually in the interim when a longer-acting agent, such as hydralazine, is beginning to take effect. Infusion rates of nitroprusside less than $5-10~\mu g \cdot kg^{-1} \cdot min^{-1}$, depending on the length of administration, can be maintained without undue risk of cyanide toxicity in the mother and fetus.[160] Trimethaphan, a ganglionic blocking agent, is particularly useful in hypertensive emergencies when cerebral edema and increased intracranial pressure are of particular concern, because it will not cause vasodilation in the brain. Other agents used less frequently to control maternal blood pressure in preeclampsia include alpha-methyldopa and clonidine (acting in the central nervous system), as well as nitroglycerin, ketanserin (a serotonin receptor antagonist), atenolol (a beta-adrenoreceptor antagonist), and labetalol (a nonselective beta blocker with some alpha₁-blocking effects).

Consumption coagulopathy may require corrective measures involving infusion of fresh whole blood, platelet concentrates, fresh frozen plasma, and cryoprecipitate. The administration of conduction anesthesia is contraindicated in patients with coagulation failure because of the increased risk of formation of an epidural hematoma, leading to permanent neurologic damage.

Anesthetic Management

Epidural anesthesia for labor and delivery should no longer be considered contraindicated, providing there is no clotting abnormality or plasma volume deficit. In volume-repleted patients positioned with left uterine displacement, epidural anesthesia does not cause unacceptable reduction in blood pressure and leads to a significant improvement in placental perfusion.[152, 161] With the use of radioactive xenon, it was shown that the intervillous blood flow increased by approximately 75% after the induction of epidural analgesia (10 ml of bupivacaine 0.25%).[162] However, the total maternal body clearance of amide local anesthetics is prolonged in preeclampsia, and repeated administration of these drugs can lead to higher blood concentrations than in normotensive patients.[163] Spinal anesthesia should be used with great

caution, if at all, because it produces severe alterations in cardiovascular dynamics resulting from sudden sympathetic blockade.

For cesarean section, the sensory level of regional anesthesia must extend to T3–T4, making adequate fluid therapy and left uterine displacement even more vital. If hypotension occurs, its correction will require a reduced dose of ephedrine in view of the increased sensitivity to vasopressors.

General anesthesia in preeclamptic patients has its particular hazards. The rapid-sequence induction of anesthesia and intubation of the trachea necessary to avoid aspiration are occasionally difficult because a swollen tongue, epiglottis, or pharynx distort the anatomy. In patients with impaired coagulation, laryngoscopy of the trachea may provoke profuse bleeding. Marked systemic and pulmonary hypertension occurring at intubation and extubation enhance the risk of cerebral hemorrhage and pulmonary edema (Fig. 45-10).[164, 165] However, these hemodynamic changes can be minimized with appropriate antihypertensive therapy, such as administration of a trimethaphan or nitroprusside infusion. Use of ketamine and ergot alkaloids should be avoided. As already mentioned, magnesium sulfate may prolong effects of all muscle relaxants through its actions on the myoneural junction. Therefore, relaxants should be administered with caution (using a nerve stimulator) to avoid overdosage. General anesthesia is indicated in acute emergencies, such as abruptio placentae, and in patients who do not meet the criteria for epidural anesthesia.

ANTEPARTUM HEMORRHAGE

Antepartum hemorrhage occurs most commonly in association with placenta previa (abnormal implantation on the lower uterine segment, and partial-total occlusion of the internal cervical os) and abruptio placentae.

Placenta previa occurs in 0.1%–1.0% of all pregnancies, resulting in up to a 0.9% incidence of maternal and 17%–26% incidence of perinatal mortality.[166] Its presence occasionally leads to an abnormality in fetal presentation, such as transverse lie or breech. Placenta previa should be suspected in a patient presenting with painless, bright red bleeding, usually after the 7th month of pregnancy. The diagnosis is confirmed by ultrasonography. Obstetric management is conservative if the bleeding is not profuse and the fetus is immature, in order to prolong pregnancy. In severe cases, or if the fetus is mature at the onset of symptoms, prompt delivery is indicated, usually by cesarean section. Hemorrhage may be severe even after delivery of the placenta because of poor contractility of the lower uterine segment, occasionally necessitating an emergency hysterectomy.

Abruptio placentae occurs in 0.2%–2.4% of pregnant women, usually in the final 10 weeks of gestation. Approximately 50% of the women are hypertensive.[167] Complications include Couvelaire uterus (i.e., when extravasated blood dissects between the myometrial fibers), renal failure, DIC, and anterior pituitary necrosis (Sheehan syndrome). The maternal mortality rate is high, 1.8%–11.0%, and the perinatal mortality rate is even higher, in excess of 50%.[166] Diagnosis of abruptio placentae is based on the presence of uterine tenderness and hypertonus and vaginal bleeding of dark, clotted blood. Bleeding may be concealed if the placental margins have remained attached to the uterine wall. If the blood loss is severe (2 l or more), there may be changes in the maternal blood pressure and pulse rate indicative of hypovolemia. Fetal movements may increase in acute hypoxia or decrease if hypoxia is grad-

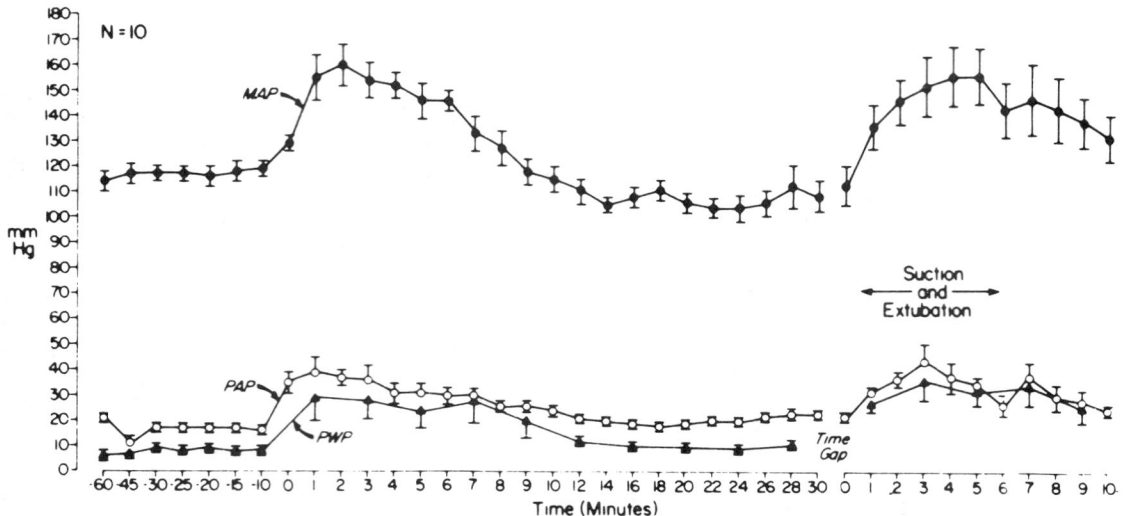

FIG. 45-10. Mean and SE of mean arterial pressure (MAP), mean pulmonary artery pressure (PAP), and pulmonary wedge pressure (PWP) in patients with severe preeclampsia receiving thiopental and nitrous oxide (40%) anesthesia with 0.5% halothane for cesarean section. (Reprinted with permission. Hodgkinson R, Husain FJ, Hayashi RH: Systemic and pulmonary blood pressure during cesarean section in parturients with gestational hypertension. Can Anaesth Soc J 27:389, 1980.)

ual. Fetal bradycardia and death may ensue, usually if maternal blood loss exceeds 2.5 l.[168] Management of milder cases of abruptio includes artificial rupture of amniotic membranes and oxytocin augmentation of labor, if required. In the presence of fetal distress, an emergency cesarean section should be performed.

The anesthesiologist plays a dual role in acute hemorrhage. He or she acts as a resuscitator of the mother. This may include the establishment of invasive monitoring (an arterial and central venous catheter are usually adequate) and blood volume replacement, preferably through 14- or 16-gauge cannulae. To correct clotting abnormalities, blood components such as fresh-frozen plasma, cryoprecipitate, and platelet concentrates may be required. The anesthesiologist also plays a traditional role of providing appropriate anesthesia for a cesarean section or, occasionally, a hysterectomy. General anesthesia is indicated in all cases, in view of the high risk of postpartum hemorrhage and clotting disorders. As usual, it should be preceded by adequate denitrogenation. In hypovolemic patients, induction should be accomplished with ketamine, 0.75–1.0 mg·kg^{-1}. As in all obstetric patients, proper precautions should be taken to prevent aspiration of gastric contents. These include the administration of a clear antacid, rapid-sequence induction of anesthesia, and tracheal intubation with the application of cricoid pressure.

HEART DISEASE

Heart disease during pregnancy occurs in 0.4%–4.1% of patients and is the leading nonobstetric cause of maternal mortality, ranging from 0.4% among patients in Class I or II of the New York Heart Association's functional classification, to 6.8% among those in Classes III and IV.[169–171] The following

lesions present the greatest risk for the mother: pulmonary hypertension, particularly in Eisenmenger's syndrome; mitral stenosis with atrial fibrillation; tetralogy of Fallot; Marfan's syndrome; and coarctation of the aorta. Cardiac decompensation and death occur most commonly at the time of maximum hemodynamic stress, i.e., in the third trimester of pregnancy, during labor and delivery, and during the immediate postpartum period. During labor, cardiac output increases above antepartum levels. Between contractions this increase is approximately 15% in the early first stage, about 30% during the late first stage, about 45% during the second stage, and after delivery, 30%–50%.[74] With each uterine contraction about 200 ml of blood is squeezed out of the uterus into the central circulation. Consequently, stroke volume, cardiac output, and left ventricular work increase, and each contraction consistently increases cardiac output by 10%–25% above that between contractions.[172] The greatest increase occurs immediately after delivery of the placenta, when cardiac output increases to an average of 80% above that prepartum, and in some patients it may increase by as much as 150%. These changes in cardiac output can be reduced by administration of regional anesthesia. In patients managed with continuous caudal anesthesia, cardiac output increased only 24% above prepartum control values during the second stage and 59% immediately postpartum.[74]

Until 1960, rheumatic fever was responsible for almost 90% of the heart disease encountered in pregnant women.[173] Since that time, with improved medical care and surgical techniques, more patients with congenital disease survive to reach the childbearing age. Simultaneously, better living conditions and antibiotic treatment have reduced the incidence of rheumatic heart disease, and the ratio of rheumatic to congenital heart disease among the parturients has declined to 3:1.[173]

Rheumatic Heart Disease

Mitral stenosis is the sole or predominant valvular lesion in most parturients with rheumatic heart disease. The primary defect is obstruction to the diastolic blood flow from the left atrium to the left ventricle. This becomes hemodynamically significant when the valve orifice is diminished or the rate of blood flow through the constricted orifice is increased sufficiently to raise left atrial pressure and, consequently, pressure in the pulmonary veins and capillaries.

The physiologic changes of pregnancy usually aggravate the problems of mitral stenosis. The increased pulse rate necessitates a higher diastolic flow rate across the mitral orifice to maintain cardiac output. The flow rate is also augmented by the increased cardiac output that pregnancy demands. In the presence of significant mitral stenosis, these increases in flow rate can only be accomplished by an increase in left atrial and pulmonary venous pressure. The increased blood volume within the lungs, which occurs in pregnancy, may also add to the distention of pulmonary capillaries. Atrial fibrillation may occur in the presence of an enlarged left atrium, leading to pulmonary edema with an associated maternal mortality as high as 17%.[174] Cardioversion should be undertaken if drug therapy does not decrease the ventricular rate.[175] Mitral commissurotomy may be necessary because of symptoms of congestive heart failure or, less frequently, because of hemoptysis or emboli. When performed in the second or early third trimester, closed as well as open commissurotomies have been reported to be well tolerated by the mother and were accompanied by fetal survival in excess of 80%.[176] Fortunately, 90% of pregnant women with mitral stenosis are in functional Classes I and II. These patients generally tolerate childbearing well. The relatively small number in functional Classes III and IV account for most maternal cardiac deaths.

Other valvular diseases, namely mitral regurgitation, aortic stenosis, or regurgitation, are much less frequent in pregnant cardiac patients. Together they account for 10%–35% of all cases. Pure mitral regurgitation is rarely a problem. Properly managed patients can have repeated pregnancies without serious complications.[173] Similarly, pure aortic insufficiency rarely causes disability in the absence of bacterial endocarditis. Aortic stenosis is frequently associated with aortic insufficiency and mitral stenosis. Myocardial failure secondary to pure aortic stenosis is rare in patients of childbearing age because symptoms develop in most patients when they are in their fifth or sixth decades. Left ventricular hypertrophy and a relatively fixed stroke volume develop in those with significant aortic stenosis. These changes reduce their tolerance to decreases in systemic vascular resistance, bradycardia, and decreased venous return (and left ventricular filling).[177]

Continuous epidural block offers particular advantages to the pregnant cardiac patient. It not only eliminates pain and tachycardia throughout labor and delivery, but it also prevents the progressive increase in cardiac output and stroke volume that normally occurs in parturition.[74] It also abolishes the "bearing-down" reflex. In view of these advantages, continuous lumbar epidural analgesia is recommended for most pregnant women with rheumatic valvular diseases, whether they are to have vaginal or cesarean section deliveries, except for those with severe, symptomatic aortic stenosis. In patients with this condition, even transient episodes of hypotension may cause serious coronary hypoperfusion, arrhythmias, and even cardiac arrest. Intrathecal opioids have been used in an attempt to provide adequate obstetric analgesia without the risk of hypotension.[104, 178] Morphine, 0.5–1.5 mg, or fentanyl, 37.5–50 μg, relieve the pain of uterine contractions. Pudendal

block will be needed for delivery. Should general anesthesia be deemed necessary for cesarean section, the standard thiopental–nitrous oxide–halogenated anesthetic–muscle relaxant technique is recommended. In cases of severe mitral stenosis, etomidate, 0.2–0.3 mg·kg^{-1}, or a slow induction with halothane or intravenous fentanyl is preferred. In patients with severe aortic stenosis and evidence of left ventricular compromise, use of halogenated agents should be avoided.[177]

Congenital Heart Diseases

Patent ductus arteriosus, atrial septal defect, and ventricular septal defect are the more common congenital cardiovascular abnormalities. In all these conditions, anomalous communicating channels exist between the cardiac chambers or the great vessels. Normally, pressures on the left side of the circulation are higher than those on the right and there is a left-to-right shunt. Late in the natural history of these diseases, pulmonary hypertension may develop, causing a reversal of the shunt (Eisenmenger's syndrome).[179] Patients with Eisenmenger's syndrome rarely live beyond the age of 40. Pregnancy is poorly tolerated, because the gestational decrease in systemic vascular resistance, in the presence of fixed pulmonary vascular resistance, results in a significant increase in the right-to-left shunt.[180] Changes in systemic and pulmonary pressures are also likely to occur with the aortocaval compression near the end of pregnancy, hypotension caused by epidural or spinal anesthesia, and bearing-down efforts of parturition. Severe shunt disturbances induced by these changes may lead to further cyanosis, even death.

Tetralogy of Fallot is the most common cyanotic congenital heart defect.[179] It consists of an interventricular septal defect, pulmonary stenosis, displacement of the aortic orifice so that it overlies the ventricular septal defect, and right ventricular hypertrophy. The pulmonary stenosis leads to increases in right ventricular systolic pressure with dilation and hypertrophy of that chamber. Blood from the right ventricle is shunted through the septal defect, and the overriding aorta receives venous blood from this source and oxygenated blood from the left ventricle. Reduced arterial oxygenation leads to cyanosis, polycythemia, and clubbing. Symptoms develop in patients during the first few months of life, their severity being related to the degree of the pulmonic stenosis. However, introduction of cardiac surgery has increased the number of patients surviving to childbearing age.

Anesthesia for parturients with cyanotic heart disease should provide effective pain relief, while avoiding hypotension, struggling, or coughing, and eliminating bearing-down efforts, all of which could increase the right-to-left shunt. For labor, intrathecal opioids rather than epidural anesthesia should be administered. Light planes of general anesthesia are usually well tolerated for cesarean section.[177]

PRETERM DELIVERY

Preterm labor and delivery present a significant challenge to the anesthesiologist, because the mother and the infant may be at risk.

The definition of prematurity was altered recently to distinguish between the preterm infant, born before the 37th week of gestation is completed, and the "small for gestational age" (SGA) infant, who may be born at term but whose weight is more than two standard deviations below the mean. Although preterm deliveries occur in 8%–10% of all births, they constitute approximately 80% of early neonatal deaths.[181] In general, the mortality and morbidity is greater among the preterm infants than among the SGA babies of comparable weight.

Severe problems, including the respiratory distress syndrome, intracranial hemorrhage, hypoglycemia, hypocalcemia, and hyperbilirubinemia, are prone to develop in preterm infants. Fortunately, with improved neonatal intensive care, severe lasting impairment, such as cerebral palsy, mental retardation, or chronic lung disease, has become infrequent among the survivors.[182]

Obstetricians frequently try to inhibit preterm labor to enhance fetal lung maturity. Delaying delivery by even 24–48 h may be beneficial if glucocorticoids are administered to the mother. Various agents have been used to suppress uterine activity (tocolysis), including ethanol, magnesium sulfate, prostaglandin inhibitors, beta sympathomimetics, and calcium channel blockers. Beta-adrenergic drugs, such as ritodrine and terbutaline, are the most commonly used tocolytics. These agents are initially administered by an intravenous infusion at the rate of $0.05–0.1 \ mg \cdot min^{-1}$ for ritodrine and $0.01 \ mg \cdot min^{-1}$ for terbutaline.[183] Their predominant effect is beta$_2$-receptor stimulation, resulting in myometrial inhibition, vasodilation, and bronchodilation. Numerous maternal complications have been reported: hypotension, hypokalemia, hyperglycemia, myocardial ischemia, pulmonary edema, and death.[184] Complications also may occur because of interactions with anesthetic drugs and techniques. With the use of regional anesthesia, peripheral vasodilation caused by beta-adrenergic stimulation enhances the risk of hypotension. Acute prehydration must be managed carefully to avoid pulmonary edema. General anesthesia may be risky in the presence of preexisting tachycardia, hypotension, and hypokalemia. It is better to avoid using halothane (cardiac dysrhythmias) as well as atropine and pancuronium (tachycardia). In nonemergency situations, delay of anesthesia by at least 3 h from the cessation of tocolysis will allow beta-mimetic effects to dissipate. Potassium supplementation is not necessary.[185]

It has become axiomatic that the premature infant is more vulnerable than the term newborn to the effect of drugs used in obstetric analgesia and anesthesia. However, there have been few systematic studies to determine the maternal and fetal pharmacokinetics and dynamics of drugs throughout gestation. There are several postulated causes of enhanced drug sensitivity in the preterm newborn: less protein available for drug binding; higher levels of bilirubin, which may compete with the drug for protein binding; greater drug access to the central nervous system because of poorly developed blood-brain barrier; greater total body water and lower fat content; and decreased ability to metabolize and excrete drugs. However, these deficiencies of the preterm infant should not be as serious as we have been led to believe. Although the serum albumin and alpha$_1$-acid glycoprotein concentrations are lower in the preterm fetus, this would primarily affect drugs that are highly bound to these proteins. However, most drugs used in anesthesia exhibit only low to moderate degrees of binding in the fetal serum: approximately 50% for etidocaine and bupivacaine, 25% for lidocaine, 52% for meperidine, and 75% for thiopental.

The placenta efficiently eliminates fetal bilirubin. Thus, the hyperbilirubinemia of prematurity normally occurs in the postpartum period. With the exception of diazepam, bilirubin will not compete with anesthetic drugs because most are bound to other serum proteins, e.g., meperidine and local anesthetics to alpha$_1$-glycoproteins, d-tubocurarine to gamma globulin.

It seems likely that the human blood-brain barrier develops

substantially in early gestation.[186] Thus, factors such as tissue affinity changes may account for differences between immature and mature animals in brain uptake of highly lipid-soluble drugs.

Greater total body water in the preterm fetus results in a greater volume of distribution for drugs. Thus, to achieve equal blood concentrations, the immature fetus will have to receive a greater amount of drug transplacentally than will the mature fetus. A study of age-related toxicity of lidocaine in sheep showed that the greater the volume of distribution, the greater the dose required to achieve toxic blood concentrations of the drug.[65]

Decreased ability to metabolize or excrete drugs, associated with prematurity, is certainly not a universal phenomenon. In a study comparing the pharmacokinetics of lidocaine in preterm newborns and adults, plasma clearance was similar in both groups.[62] Neonates excreted much more unchanged lidocaine than did adults. Similarly, although meperidine metabolism is more limited in the neonate, as compared with that in the adult, urinary excretion of the unchanged drug is greater in the neonate.

Another factor is gestational changes in maternal serum albumin and alpha$_1$-acid glycoprotein concentrations, which tend to decrease. Serial determinations of protein binding of diazepam, phenytoin, and valproic acid in the maternal serum, performed in early (8–16 weeks), mid- (17–32 weeks), and late pregnancy, showed a progressive increase in the unbound fraction of these drugs.[187] That would increase drug availability for placental transfer. Placental permeability itself increases as pregnancy progresses because of the increased area and decreased thickness of tissue barriers.[60]

In a largely ignored, prospective study of more than 1,000 premature labors, during which mothers received meperidine alone or with scopolamine, medication had no effect on the perinatal death rate, incidence of respiratory distress syndrome (RDS), Apgar scores, need for resuscitation, and incidence of severe neurologic defects within 1 yr.[188]

Therefore, it appears that in selection of the anesthetic drugs and techniques for delivery of a preterm infant, concerns regarding drug effects on the newborn are far less important than prevention of asphyxia and trauma to the fetus. For labor and vaginal delivery, well-conducted epidural anesthesia is advantageous in providing good perineal relaxation. Preterm infants with breech presentation are usually delivered by cesarean section. General anesthesia with uterine relaxation, provided by a halogenated drug, will facilitate delivery of the aftercoming head.

FETAL AND MATERNAL MONITORING

The development of biophysical and biochemical monitoring of the fetus during labor and delivery has had a tremendous impact on obstetric practice over the last 20 yr. Monitoring procedures are now performed routinely, and it is important that the anesthesiologist understand the basic principles of the technology, as well as the interpretation of results, because they relate to both mother and fetus.

During the same period there has been an explosion in monitoring technology in the fields of anesthesiology and intensive care. The mother with serious medical problems requiring intensive care or the one whose baby is delivered in an operating room under an anesthesiologist's care is subject to the same standards of monitoring as any other surgical patient. It is generally agreed that the use of intensive peripartum monitoring is appropriate in "high-risk" pregnancy. In contrast, patients with routine labor are frequently observed in the same way that patients were many generations ago, *i.e.,* with intermittent blood pressure readings. With the growing sophistication of electronic devices, and specifically the science of telemetry, we can look forward to better surveillance of both mother and fetus, without the loss of freedom and activity that monitoring currently entails.

The importance of maternal ECG and blood pressure recording during induction and maintenance of epidural anesthesia has already been discussed. Noninvasive maternal oxygen saturation monitoring (pulse oximetry) during labor and delivery is applied easily and should provide useful information about the degree of pain and adequacy of analgesia.[189]

The early reports of continuous fetal heart rate monitoring came from Hon in 1958, who also recognized variable decelerations associated with umbilical cord compression. In 1971 and 1972, those working in this field met at two international conferences and agreed on nomenclature and standards that are still in use today.[190]

BIOPHYSICAL MONITORING

A fetal monitor is a two-channel recorder of fetal heart rate and uterine activity. In the direct system, the fetal ECG is obtained from an electrode attached to the presenting part. Intrauterine pressure is measured continuously with a transducer connected to a saline-filled catheter, which is inserted transcervically. Direct monitoring is quantitative, but it requires rupture of the membranes and a cervical dilation of at least 1.5 cm. In addition, the presenting part must dip into the true pelvis. Indirect fetal monitoring uses data obtained from transducers secured to the mother's abdomen with adjustable straps. The following three systems can be used to obtain fetal heart signals: electrocardiography, phonocardiography, and ultrasound cardiography. The first two approaches are impractical. Fetal QRS complexes obtained with abdominal electrodes are too small to distinguish from the maternal tracing, whereas phonocardiography provides a poor signal-to-noise ratio. Thus, the ultrasound cardiography is the most commonly used indirect method today. Uterine activity is monitored with a tocodynamometer, which is triggered by the changing shape of the uterus during the contraction. Indirect monitoring is mostly quantitative. Its advantage is that it can be applied without rupture of membranes, even before the onset of labor.

The following variables are taken into account when fetal well-being is determined: baseline heart rate, beat-to-beat variability, periodic patterns, and uterine activity.

The baseline fetal heart rate is measured between contractions. It is 120–160 beats · min^{-1} in the normal fetus. Persistently elevated rates may be associated with chronic fetal distress, maternal fever, or administration of drugs such as ephedrine and atropine. Abnormally low rates may be encountered in fetuses with congenital heart block or as a late occurrence during the course of fetal hypoxia and acidosis.

The baseline fetal heart rate tracing normally is not flat. The variability reflects the beat-to-beat adjustments of the parasympathetic and sympathetic nervous systems to a variety of internal and external stimuli. When these divisions of the nervous system are functioning normally, variability is also normal, with the fetus being in good condition. Fetal central nervous system depression by asphyxia may decrease baseline variability. Therefore, a smooth fetal heart rate tracing may be an ominous finding. Studies comparing beat-to-beat variability with fetal acid–base analysis indicate a good correlation between the two parameters.[191] However, drugs can also decrease fetal heart rate variability by depressing mechanisms in the central nervous system integrating cardiac control (tranquilizers, opioids, barbiturates, anesthetics) or by blocking the transmission of control impulses to the cardiac pacemaker (atropine). In contrast, ephedrine administration increases beat-to-beat variability.[192]

Periodic fetal heart rate patterns consist of decelerations or accelerations, of relatively brief duration, in association with uterine contractions (Fig. 45-11). There are three major forms of fetal heart rate deceleration: early, late, and variable. Early decelerations are U-shaped, with the heart rate usually not decreasing to less than 100 beats · min^{-1}. The fetal heart begins to slow with the onset of the contraction; the low point coincides with the peak of the contraction; and the rate generally returns to the baseline as the uterus relaxes. This type of deceleration has been attributed to fetal head compression, leading to increased vagal tone. It is not ameliorated by increasing fetal oxygenation but is blocked by atropine administration. Early decelerations are transitory and well tolerated by the fetus because there is no systemic hypoxemia or acidosis.[193]

Late decelerations are also U-shaped. They begin 20–30 s or more after the onset of uterine contraction, and the low point of the deceleration occurs well after the peak of the contraction. Myocardial ischemia resulting from uteroplacental insufficiency is believed to cause this pattern. The pattern of late deceleration can be corrected by improving fetal oxygenation, which may be accomplished with oxygen administration to the mother, correction of maternal hypotension, or aortocaval compression, or by taking measures that decrease uterine activity. If this pattern is repetitive, continuous, and progressive in severity, there is a significant correlation with fetal acidosis. Uncorrectable late decelerations, or late decelerations that worsen despite corrective measures, are indications for prompt delivery.[190]

Variable decelerations, which result from umbilical cord compression, are the most common periodic patterns observed in the intrapartum period. They are variable in shape and onset, the rate usually decreasing to less than 100 beats · min^{-1}. Although the initial fetal heart rate changes are of reflex origin, if the cord compressions are frequent or prolonged, fetal asphyxia may result in direct myocardial depression.

Cervical dilatation and descent of the presenting part during the first stage of labor result primarily from uterine contractions. During the active phase, contractions should occur every 2–3 min, with peak intrauterine pressures of 50–80 mm Hg and resting pressures of 5–20 mm Hg. Uterine activity may be abnormally elevated in association with abruptio placentae or injudicious use of oxytocics. Tetanic uterine contractions have been reported after the use of methoxamine, a pure alpha agonist.[194] In the first and second trimester of pregnancy, increased uterine tone may be induced with ketamine in a dose-dependent manner. At term, ketamine does not appear to have this effect.[195]

Poor uterine contractility may result from overdistention (polyhydramnios, multiple pregnancy) or maintenance of the supine position.[196] During early labor, administration of opioids, sedatives, or regional anesthesia may delay the onset of the active phase by diminishing uterine activity. However, in large, well-controlled studies, regional anesthesia instituted during the active phase has been shown to have no untoward effects on uterine activity as long as hypotension and the supine position are avoided.[197] Addition of epinephrine to a local anesthetic solution may have an inhibitory effect on uterine activity.[198]

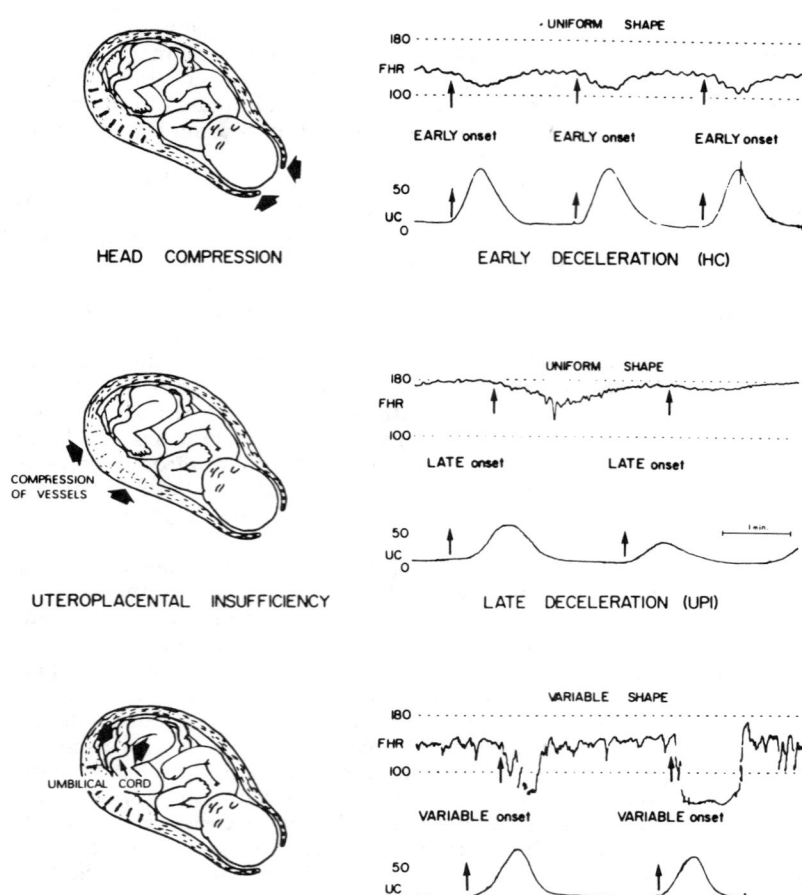

FIG. 45-11. Classification and mechanism of fetal heart rate patterns. (Reprinted with permission. Hon EH: An Introduction to Fetal Heart Rate Monitoring, p 29. New Haven, Harty Press, 1969.)

BIOCHEMICAL MONITORING

Before labor, the normal fetus is neither hypoxic nor acidotic. During labor many events, including uterine contractions, cord compression, aortocaval compression, and maternal hypotension, from any cause, may decrease uteroplacental blood flow sufficiently to produce fetal hypoxia and acidosis. Acidosis associated with short-term placental hypoperfusion primarily results from carbon dioxide accumulation ("respiratory acidosis"). In prolonged asphyxia, hypercarbia is accompanied by metabolic acidosis resulting from anaerobic metabolism. Thus, fetal acid–base indices, such as P_{CO_2} and base deficit, usually reflect the degree and duration of asphyxia.

Assessment of acid–base status of the fetus became possible in the early 1960s, when Saling developed a fetal capillary blood-sampling technique.[199] Blood is usually obtained from the scalp but may also be sampled from the breech. It is collected into a heparinized glass capillary tube, and pH, P_{CO_2}, P_{O_2}, and base deficit are determined immediately with an appropriate electrode system adapted to small sample size.

This technique has been validated in animal and clinical studies. It has been shown in fetal monkeys that the blood values obtained from the scalp are closely correlated with those in simultaneously obtained samples from the carotid artery and jugular vein.[200] A fetal capillary blood pH of 7.25 is the lowest limit of normal. Values between 7.24 and 7.20 are

considered "preacidotic," whereas a pH below 7.20 indicates fetal acidosis. Several studies correlated the last predelivery fetal pH with the Apgar score at 1 or 2 min after birth.[201, 202] Ninety-two per cent of infants scored 7 or better when the pH was above 7.25. With the pH below 7.16, 80% of babies scored 6 or less.[201] In general, when the pH is normal immediately before delivery, one can assume that the baby will be in good condition. However, there is a small incidence of false-positive and false-negative results. In one study, normal pH was associated with low Apgar scores (false-positive results) in approximately 10% of cases (Fig. 45-12).[202] In approximately 8% of cases (false-negative results), a vigorous infant was born despite a low capillary scalp pH. The major factors contributing to false-positive outcomes are administration of sedative drugs or anesthetics, infection, airway obstruction, and congenital anomalies. False-negative outcomes are usually associated with maternal acidosis, which may occur after prolonged labor, excessive muscular activity, or inadequate fluid and caloric intakes. Obtaining a maternal sample (arterial or free-flowing venous) for the evaluation of the acid–base status helps identify this group. If the fetal acidosis is of maternal origin, the mother's blood will show a large base deficit value, and the difference between the fetal and maternal base deficit values (ΔBD) will be small. In contrast, fetal acidosis resulting from prolonged asphyxia is reflected in a large fetal but a normal maternal base deficit value; consequently, ΔBD will be

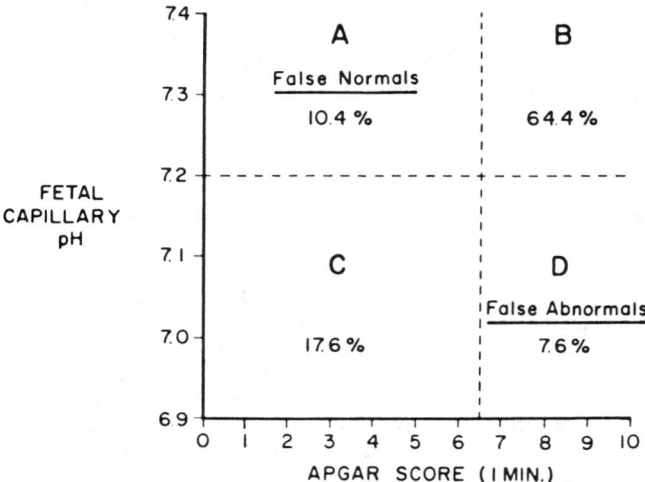

FIG. 45-12. Fetal *p*H as an index of infant's condition at birth in 355 patients during labor. Segment A: depressed infants with normal *p*H; segment B: vigorous infants with normal *p*H; segment C: depressed infants with low *p*H; segment D: vigorous infants with low *p*H. (Reprinted with permission. Bowe ET, Beard RW, Finster M *et al*: Reliability of fetal blood sampling. Am J Obstet Gynecol 107:279, 1970.)

large. Fetal acidosis of maternal origin can be treated by correcting the maternal acid–base imbalance.

COMPLICATIONS

There are data correlating direct fetal monitoring with maternal infection.[203, 204] However, conclusions from these reports are tenuous because most of the affected patients had prolonged rupture of membranes. A less frequent complication of internal monitoring is uterine perforation. The firm plastic cannula, which is used to introduce the intraamniotic pressure catheter, has been implicated.

Fetal complications related to scalp electrodes are ecchymoses, lacerations, leakage of cerebrospinal fluid, osteomyelitis of the skull, sepsis, scalp abscesses, and a case of meningitis, with ventriculitis and hydrocephalus. The overall incidence of these complications is unknown. Scalp abscess is the most commonly reported. One publication indicates that with the use of a coil electrode, it occurs in 5.4% of cases.[205] In most reviews the incidence is less than 1%.[206]

Scalp capillary blood sampling can also lead to fetal complications. The two major ones are hemorrhage and abscess formation. Bleeding from the sampling site is usually self-limited, but massive hemorrhage resulting in severe anemia, and, rarely, neonatal death, has been reported. After a sample has been obtained, pressure should be applied to the scalp with a sponge through at least two contractions. Occasionally, prolonged pressure or a skin clip may be necessary to achieve hemostasis. Prenatal and postnatal bleeding from a sampling incision may be the first manifestation of a severe coagulation disorder.[207] Excessive bleeding from the vagina after scalp capillary blood sampling may be of fetal origin. Thus, testing for fetal hemoglobin is advised in these circumstances.

The costs and benefits of fetal monitoring are still being questioned. There is a conflict between the desire for a "natural" childbirth experience and the physician's concern for maternal and fetal safety. It is generally agreed that the use of intensive intrapartum monitoring is appropriate in high-risk pregnancies. Debate continues concerning the benefits of these methods to low-risk fetuses. A recent large randomized controlled trial comparing continuous electronic fetal monitoring with traditional intermittent auscultation of the fetal heart (with an option to measure fetal scalp capillary blood *p*H) showed that cases of neonatal seizures and abnormal neurologic signs were twice as frequent in the group with intermittent auscultation. In addition, the study showed no difference in the cesarean section rate between the two groups.[208]

ANESTHETIC COMPLICATIONS

GENERAL ANESTHESIA

The changes in the respiratory tract associated with pregnancy, such as lowered FRC and mucosal congestion, may enhance problems in the patient awakening from anesthesia. These may include laryngeal spasm or edema after extubation, rapid desaturation secondary to soft tissue airway obstruction or opioid depression of respiration, and the ever-present chance of vomiting or regurgitation, with aspiration of gastric contents. The anesthesiologist may be deceived by the patient's restlessness and agitation on emergence from anesthesia when she is frequently anxious, in pain, and relatively unsedated. Before extubation of the trachea she should be observed carefully until she is conscious and pharyngeal and laryngeal reflexes have fully returned.

Pulmonary Aspiration

As already described, aspiration of gastric contents contributes seriously to maternal complications and deaths. To decrease the incidence of this complication, efforts should be directed at careful preoperative assessment of obstetric patients, emphasis on the training and experience of obstetric anesthesia personnel, and the use of regional anesthesia where appropriate, as well as the measures already outlined in the section on physiologic changes of pregnancy.[209]

REGIONAL ANESTHESIA

Complications of regional anesthesia can be separated into those that occur concurrently with the block, such as hypotension, total spinal anesthesia, convulsions induced by local anesthetics, nausea, vomiting, and breathing difficulties, and those arising later, such as headache or effects of nerve injury.

Hypotension

This is the most likely side-effect to occur on induction of either spinal or epidural anesthesia, although the rapidity of onset and severity are more controllable in the case of epidural block, with which a test dose and subsequent slow incremental injections of drug are usually used. The best method of decreasing the incidence and morbidity of this complication is careful attention to preventive measures before induction, such as prehydration, left uterine displacement, and administration of ephedrine. Treatment includes improved displacement of the uterus, rapid intravenous infusion of fluids, small intravenous doses of ephedrine (5–10 mg), oxygen given by face mask, as well as placement of the patient in the Trendelenburg position. Rapid reversal of hypotension usually prevents serious sequelae in either mother or neonate.[210]

Total Spinal Anesthesia

High or total spinal anesthesia is relatively rare, occurring after excessive spread of local anesthetic in the subarachnoid or epidural space. Accidental puncture of the dura during attempted or continuous epidural block (catheter migration) may also lead to this complication, especially when the aberrant catheter position is not recognized. Most important is prompt diagnosis and treatment, which mandates the presence of trained personnel in the labor suite. The airway should be quickly established and protected by means of an endotracheal tube while ventilation with oxygen is applied. Left uterine displacement and the Trendelenburg position should be used and fluids and ephedrine given to maintain normal blood pressure. With proper management, the outcome for mother and baby should be good.

Convulsions

High blood levels of local anesthetics may result from accidental intravascular injection (though a needle or catheter), accumulation of drugs after repeated epidural or caudal injection, or rapid absorption of local anesthetic from a highly vascular site of injection. Thus, paracervical and pudendal blocks can be implicated, as well as epidural techniques.

When any major nerve block is undertaken, the equipment and drugs needed for resuscitation (including means for establishing the airway and administering positive-pressure ventilation with 100% oxygen, a laryngoscope, endotracheal tubes, oral airways, an oxygen source, and an ambu bag with mask) should always be available. In addition, a suction device should be on hand, as well as the following drugs: thiopental or diazepam, atropine, and succinylcholine. It is necessary to establish a venous access for these drugs before the local anesthetic is injected. The best way of preventing systemic toxic reactions is to adhere strictly to recommended dosages and avoid intravascular injection, as outlined previously. Despite precautions, a few patients may have life-threatening convulsions and, more rarely, cardiovascular collapse. Convulsions should be treated by protecting the airway and establishing effective ventilation of the lungs, because hypoxia and acidosis develop very rapidly. If thiopental or diazepam is administered intravenously to stop convulsions, very small doses (50–100 mg and 5–10 mg, respectively) are adequate and will help avoid cardiorespiratory depression. If cardiovascular collapse occurs, cardiopulmonary resuscitation and cesarean delivery should be started immediately, the latter to relieve aortocaval compression and ensure the effectiveness of cardiac massage.[211]

Headache

Unfortunately, later development of headache, resulting from puncture of the dura mater and subsequent leakage of cerebrospinal fluid from the subarachnoid space, is quite common in parturients. The incidence is related to the diameter of the puncture hole, being very high after use of a 16-gauge needle (more than 70%) and as little as 1% with a small spinal needle (25 or 26-gauge). Bed rest, hydration, and analgesics are beneficial when the discomfort is mild to moderate, but severe headaches that do not respond to conservative measures are best treated by an autologous blood patch in the epidural space. With an aseptic technique, 10–15 ml of the patient's blood is injected epidurally, near the site of the dural tear. This procedure has a success rate of more than 90%.[212] Intravenous injection of caffeine sodium benzoate, in doses of 500 mg, has

been shown to alleviate headache in 70% of cases.[213] When an epidural catheter is in place after delivery, 40–60 ml of preservative-free saline may be injected through it, before its removal. This effectively lowers the incidence of severe headache.[214]

Nerve Injury

Although rare, neurologic sequelae have been reported after administration of major regional blocks with all the known local anesthetics. Pressure by a needle or catheter on spinal roots produces immediate pain, and the irritant should be withdrawn quickly. Infections such as epidural or caudal abscess or meningitis are very rare and may be secondary to infection at another site. Epidural hematoma can occur as a result of coagulation defects. Unfortunately, recovery from trauma to the nerve roots may be very prolonged, involving weeks or months. Other causes of nerve injury, resulting from fetal compression of the lumbosacral trunk or prolonged use of the lithotomy position for bearing down in the second stage of labor, should be kept in mind.

NEWBORN RESUSCITATION IN THE DELIVERY ROOM

Of the approximately 3.5 million babies born in the United States each year, 6% require resuscitation in the delivery room. Among those weighing 1,500 g or less, the incidence is approximately 80%.[215]

The following factors may contribute to depression of the newborn: drugs used in labor or during delivery, including anesthetic agents; trauma of precipitate labor and operative obstetrics; and birth asphyxia, meaning hypoxia and hypercapnea with acidosis.

FETAL ASPHYXIA

Fetal asphyxia, the best-studied cause of neonatal depression, generally develops as a result of interference with maternal or fetal perfusion of the placenta. As stated previously, the normal fetus is neither hypoxic nor acidotic before labor. Experimental data have revealed that transplacental gradients for pH and P_{CO_2} are approximately 0.05 pH units and 5 mm Hg, respectively.[216] Although oxygen tension is low, oxygen saturation is relatively high (80%–85%) by virtue of the shift to the left of the fetal dissociation curve for hemoglobin.

During labor, uterine contractions decrease the blood flow through the intervillous space of the placenta or may stop it completely. On the fetal side, cord compression occurs during the final stages of approximately one-third of vaginal deliveries. Thus, mild degrees of hypoxia and acidosis occur even during normal labor and delivery and play an important role in initiation of ventilation.[217] On the average, healthy vigorous infants (at birth) have an oxygen saturation of 21%, a pH of 7.24, and a P_{CO_2} of 56 mm Hg in their arterial blood.

Severe fetal asphyxia occasionally develops as a result of fetal and maternal complications such as a tight nuchal cord, prolapsed cord, premature separation of the placenta, uterine hyperactivity, or maternal hypotension.

During asphyxia, changes in blood gases and hydrogen-ion concentration are rapid. Investigations performed on newborn animals have shown that the oxygen content of arterial blood decreases to near zero in 2.5 min, whereas pH declines by nearly 0.1 pH unit·min^{-1}.[218] The decrease in pH results from accumulation of carbon dioxide as well as of end products of anaerobic glycolysis. After oxygen stores are exhausted, the documented ability of fetal brain and myocardium to derive energy from anaerobic metabolism is essential for survival. However, anaerobic glycolysis is *pH* dependent, and its rate is greatly diminished when the *pH* decreases below 7.0.[219] Other untoward effects of severe hypoxia and acidosis include depression of the myocardium resulting from a decrease in its responsiveness to catecholamines; shift to the right of the fetal dissociation curve for hemoglobin, resulting in reduced oxygen-carrying capacity; and increase in pulmonary vascular resistance, which plays an important role during circulatory readjustment after birth.

Ventilatory and cardiovascular responses to controlled experimental asphyxia have been investigated extensively in newborn monkeys (Fig. 45-13).[220] During the initial phase of asphyxia, the unanesthetized animal exhibits respiratory efforts that increase in depth and frequency for up to 3 min. This period, called primary hyperpnea, is followed by primary

FIG. 45-13. Schematic diagram of changes in rhesus monkeys during asphyxia and with resuscitation by positive-pressure ventilation. Brain damage was assessed by histologic examination some weeks or months later. (Reprinted with permission. Dawes GS: Foetal and Neonatal Physiology: A Comparative Study of the Changes at Birth, p. 149. Chicago, Year Book Medical Publishers, 1968.)

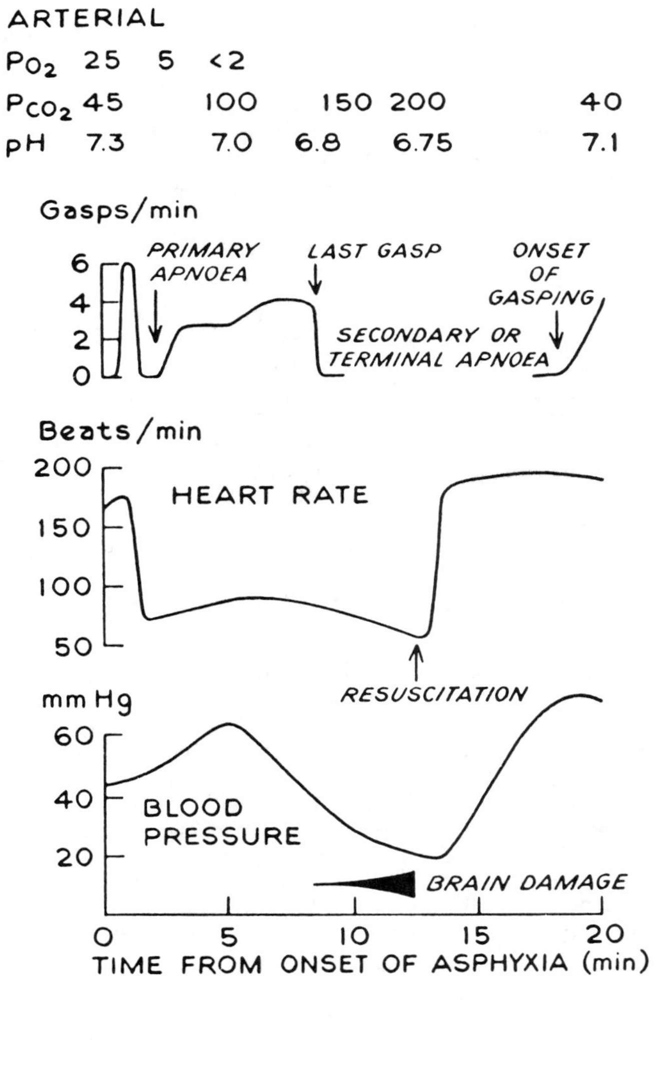

apnea, which lasts for approximately 1 min. Rhythmic gasping then begins and is maintained at a fairly constant rate of about 6 gasps·min^{-1} for 4–5 min. Thereafter, the gasps become weaker and slower. Their cessation at approximately 8.5 min after the onset of asphyxia marks the beginning of secondary apnea. Administration of opioids and systemic anesthetic agents to the mother can abolish the period of primary hyperpnea and prolong primary apnea.

There is a linear relationship between the duration of asphyxia and the onset of gasping and rhythmic spontaneous breathing. In the newborn monkey, for each minute of asphyxia beyond the last gasp, 2 additional minutes of artificial ventilation are required before gasping begins again and 4 min before rhythmic breathing is established.[221] This indicates that the longer artificial ventilation of the lungs is delayed during secondary apnea, the longer it will take to resuscitate the infant. Furthermore, in the newborn monkey, prolongation of asphyxia for 4 min beyond the last gasp is accompanied by extensive damage to brain-stem nuclei, whereas animals resuscitated before the last gasp show little or no brain damage. Thus, a relatively short delay in resuscitation can have serious sequelae.

NEONATAL ADAPTATIONS AT BIRTH

During this period, and through the early hours and days of life, many morphologic and functional changes take place, with the cardiovascular and ventilatory systems undergoing the most dramatic alterations. In the normal newborn, two events occur almost simultaneously, and within seconds of delivery: the arrest of umbilical circulation through the placenta and expansion of the lungs. These events change the fetal circulation toward the adult type. Survival of the neonate depends primarily upon prompt expansion of the lungs and establishment of effective ventilation.

The onset of ventilation and expansion of the lungs opens up the pulmonary vascular bed, resulting in decreased resistance and a significant increase in pulmonary blood flow. A fetal pulmonary blood flow of 30–40 ml·kg^{-1}·min^{-1} increases to approximately 300 ml·kg^{-1}·min^{-1} shortly after birth, not only because of the mechanical effects of lung expansion, but also the direct effects of oxygen and carbon dioxide on the blood vessels. Pulmonary vascular resistance decreases as oxygen tension increases and carbon dioxide levels decrease. As soon as pulmonary perfusion increases, the foramen ovale, which constitutes a communication between the inferior vena cava (IVC) and the left atrium (LA), undergoes functional closure because of pressure changes across the valve of the foramen (Fig. 45-5). Cessation of the umbilical circulation reduces pressure in the IVC and right atrium, whereas the increase in pulmonary blood flow increases venous return and pressure in the LA. The ductus arteriosus (DA) does not constrict completely or abruptly after birth; functional closure may take hours, even days. Thus, shunting still occurs in the neonatal period, its direction depending on relative resistances in the pulmonary and systemic vascular beds. The smooth muscle of the DA constricts in response to increased oxygen tension in the newborn's blood. Catecholamines, which exist in increased concentrations in the newborn, particularly during the first 3 h of life, also constrict the DA. In contrast, prostaglandins PGI$_2$ and PGE$_2$, produced by the wall of the DA, relax the ductal smooth muscle. Administration of prostaglandin synthesis inhibitors to fetal animals promotes constriction of the DA. Thus, control of the DA involves a balance between constricting and relaxing substances.[222]

Cardiac output and its distribution also increase; left ventricular output increases from approximately 150–400 ml·kg^{-1}·min^{-1}, whereas right ventricular output increases less significantly. Cardiac output changes closely parallel the increase in oxygen consumption.[223] The redistribution of cardiac output also leads to increases in myocardial, renal, and gastrointestinal blood flow, while decreasing cerebral, adrenal, and carotid flows.

During fetal life, respiratory gas exchange takes place through the placenta. Delivery of the infant's trunk relieves thoracic compression, occurring within the birth canal, and the thorax and the lungs expand. Most infants initiate respiratory efforts a few seconds after birth. After the first inspiration, a cry usually results, as the infant exhales against a partially closed glottis, thus increasing intrathoracic pressure significantly. Negative pressures in excess of 40 cm H_2O bring about the initial entry of air into fluid-filled alveoli. In the mature, normal neonate, the lungs expand almost completely after the first few breaths, and pressure volume changes achieved with each respiration resemble those of the adult. After lung expansion, the FRC approximates 70 ml in the term newborn and changes little over the first 6 days of life. The tidal volume varies between 10 and 30 ml, the breathing frequency ranges from 30 to 60 breaths·min^{-1}, and the minute ventilation exceeds 500 ml.

It has been difficult to evaluate the factors responsible for the initial respiratory efforts to achieve expansion of the lungs and for the subsequent maintenance of rhythmic respiration because many stimuli contribute simultaneously. Asphyxia is considered the principal driving force.

After delivery and prompt lung expansion, reoxygenation is rapid, but it takes 2 or 3 h to achieve a relatively normal acid–base balance, primarily by pulmonary excretion of carbon dioxide. By 24 h the healthy newborn infant has reached the same acid–base state as that of the mother before labor.

RESUSCITATION

The delivery room must be prepared for adequate and prompt treatment of severe depression at birth. All members of the delivery room team should be trained in resuscitation methods because both mother and baby may have difficulty at the same time. Every piece of apparatus necessary for emergency resuscitation should be checked carefully before delivery (Table 45-4).

Initial Treatment and Evaluation of All Infants

Immediately after delivery, the baby should be held head down while the cord is clamped and cut. The infant should then be placed supine on a table, the head kept low with a slight lateral tilt. A nurse or assistant should listen to the heart beat immediately, indicating the rate by finger movement. If help is not available, the rate can be detected from pulsation of the umbilical cord. At the same time, the resuscitator should aspirate the mouth, pharynx, and nose with a catheter. This suction should be brief. The time interval from birth to completion of suctioning should be about 1 min. Slapping the infant's soles lightly frequently aids in initiating a deep breath and crying.

The initial appraisal of the newborn should start from the moment of birth, with particular attention being paid to the first few breaths and the evenness and ease of respiration. The scoring system introduced by Apgar is a useful method of

TABLE 45-4. Resuscitation Equipment in the Delivery Room

Radiant warmer
Suction with manometer and suction trap
Suction catheters
Wall oxygen with flow meter
Resuscitation bag (≤750 ml)
Infant face masks
Infant oropharygeal airways
Endotracheal tubes, 2.5, 3.0, 3.5, and 4.0 mm
Endotracheal tube stylets
Laryngoscope(s) and blade(s)
Sterile umbilical artery catheterization tray
Needles, syringes, three-way stopcocks
Medications and solutions
  1 : 10,000 epinephrine
  Naloxone hydrochloride (neonatal)
  Sodium bicarbonate
  Volume expanders

clinically evaluating the baby (Table 45-5).[224] Most infants are vigorous, with scores of 7–10, and cough or cry within seconds of delivery. The administration of oxygen or oxygen-enriched air by a tight-fitting mask will rapidly improve their oxygenation and decrease pulmonary vascular resistance. To maintain thermal homeostasis, the infant's skin should be dried promptly and the baby should be placed under a radiant heater.

Mildly to moderately depressed infants constitute the largest group requiring some form of resuscitation at birth. These infants are pale or cyanotic at 1 min after delivery; they have not established sustained respiration and may be nearly flaccid. However, their heart rate and reflex irritability are good. Their scores may be 4, 5, or 6. The severely depressed infant is flaccid, unresponsive, and pale; its Apgar score is 0, 1, 2, or 3.

Treatment of Moderately Depressed Infants (Apgar Scores 4–6)

If initial resuscitative methods have produced no response by 1–2 min after delivery, the progressing asphyxia usually leads to diminished skeletal muscular tone and decreased heart rate. A small plastic oropharyngeal airway should then be inserted into the mouth and oxygen applied under pressure of 16–20 cm H_2O for 1–2 s. Although this pressure is insufficient to expand the alveoli, some oxygen will reach the respiratory bronchioles. The increase in intrabronchial pressure stimulates pulmonary stretch receptors. This stimulus, added to that of the chemoreceptors, initiates a gasp in about 85% of the infants.

If there is no respiratory effort and the heart rate continues to decrease, with the infant becoming visibly flaccid, the larynx should be visualized with the laryngoscope. If foreign material, such as small blood clots, meconium-stained mucus, or vernix, obstructs the larynx, quick, brief suction is indicated. When the glottis is seen to be patent, a curved endotracheal tube is inserted through the cords. Ventilation through the tube with enough force to cause the lower chest to rise gently will usually start spontaneous respiration. Pressures between 25 and 35 cm H_2O are necessary to expand the alveoli initially and can be applied safely for 1–2 s. With the first or second application of positive pressure, the infant usually makes an effort to breathe. The endotracheal tube may be withdrawn after the infant has taken five or six breaths.

TABLE 45-5.   Apgar Scores

SIGN	0	1	2
Heart rate	Absent	Less than 100 beats · min^{-1}	More than 100 beats · min^{-1}
Respiratory effort	Absent	Slow, irregular	Good, crying
Muscle tone	Limp	Some flexion of extremities	Active motion
Reflex irritability	No response	Grimace	Cough, sneeze, or cry
Color	Pale, blue	Body pink, extremities blue	Completely pink

Treatment of Severely Depressed Infants (Apgar Scores 0–3)

Ventilation should be established without delay. The glottis should be inspected immediately with the laryngoscope. If meconium or thick meconium-stained mucus has been aspirated into the trachea, it must be suctioned out at once before the lungs are inflated. It is usually possible to accomplish this within 1–2 min of delivery. Severely depressed infants may require 3–8 min of artificial ventilation before a spontaneous gasp is taken. The endotracheal tube can be removed as soon as quiet and sustained respiration is established.

Use of Cardiac Massage

If the blood pressure is unduly low at the beginning of resuscitation, positive-pressure ventilation is unlikely to be successful unless cardiac massage is employed. The technique preferred by the authors consists of intermittent compression of the middle third of the sternum 120 times per minute with the index and middle fingers. Massage is interrupted every 5 s to permit three to four inflations of the lungs. It should be used if a heartbeat cannot be detected or if the heart rate does not increase promptly after the lungs have been well expanded. Cardiac massage and ventilation should be maintained until the heart rate exceeds 100 beats · min^{-1}.

Rapid Correction of Acidosis

Experiments on newborn monkeys have shown that maintenance of a normal pH during asphyxia by rapid infusion of base together with glucose prolongs gasping and delays cardiovascular collapse.[218] Furthermore, the rapid correction or maintenance of pH during asphyxia can reduce or prevent morphologically detectable brain damage. Resuscitation is also facilitated if alkali and glucose are infused when artificial ventilation is started; oxygen consumption is greater and the time needed to establish spontaneous breathing is shorter.[221] In clinical practice, severe acidosis (pH less than 7.0 or a base deficit in excess of 15 mEq · l^{-1}) should be corrected promptly to improve pulmonary perfusion and oxygenation.[225] For that purpose, a 3.5 or 5 French catheter should be inserted, under sterile precautions, into the umbilical artery and advanced just above the bifurcation of the aorta. The umbilical vein may be used, if arterial catheterization has not been immediately successful, and the catheter advanced through the ductus venosus into the inferior vena cava. A dose of sodium bicarbonate, 1–2 mEq · kg^{-1}, diluted with equal parts of sterile water to reduce the osmolality of the solution, is then infused over 3–5 min. Adequate pulmonary ventilation should be assured during the infusion.

Other Drugs and Fluids

If it is believed that persistent depression has resulted from maternal opioid medication, naloxone should be given after adequate ventilation has been established. The recommended dose of 10 mg · kg^{-1} may be injected intravenously, intramuscularly, or subcutaneously. The initial dose may be repeated every 2–3 min as needed. Use of naloxone should be avoided in infants born to opioid addicted mothers in order not to precipitate acute withdrawal. A severely asphyxiated newborn might require cardiotonic drugs during early resuscitation. Epinephrine should be used to treat asystole or persistent bradycardia despite adequate ventilation and external cardiac massage. A dose of 0.1–0.3 ml · kg^{-1} of 1:10,000 solution should be injected intravenously, or by the endotracheal tube, and repeated every 5 min if necessary.

Hypovolemia frequently follows severe birth asphyxia, because a greater than normal portion of fetal blood remains in the placenta. The infant appears pale and has low arterial pressure, tachycardia, and tachypnea. Acute blood volume expansion may be accomplished with the intravenous administration of the following solutions over 5–10 min: O-negative blood, crossmatched with mother's blood, 10 ml · kg^{-1}; 5% albumin, 10 ml · kg^{-1}; and normal saline or Ringer's lactate, 10 ml · kg^{-1}.

Diagnostic Procedures

After the neonate is successfully resuscitated and stabilized, several diagnostic procedures are indicated. To rule out choanal atresia, each nostril should be obstructed. Because newborn babies must breathe through their noses, occlusion of the nostril on the patent side would cause respiratory obstruction. To rule out esophageal atresia, a suction catheter is inserted into the stomach. Gastric contents are aspirated: volume in excess of 12 ml after vaginal delivery and 20 ml after cesarean section may result from an abnormality of the upper gastrointestinal tract.

ANESTHESIA FOR INTRAUTERINE FETAL SURGERY

Development of invasive as well as noninvasive procedures, involving amniocentesis, amniography, fetoscopy, fetal blood sampling, and real-time ultrasonography, has enabled physicians to diagnose and, in some cases, treat fetal anomalies. Neonatal morbidity and mortality may be improved by surgical procedures performed while the fetus is still *in utero* when there is a correctable anatomic lesion or deficiency state impairing normal organ growth and development. At present, intrauterine surgery on a fetus can be justified for obstructive lesions, such as hydronephrosis or hydrocephalus, or in a fetus with conditions resulting from failure of normal embryonic tissues to close, *e.g.*, diaphragmatic hernia, gastroschisis, and neural tube defects.[226–229]

In addition to the usual concerns for maternal safety and fetal well being, anesthetic considerations for prenatal fetal surgery must include fetal anesthesia and adequate relaxation of the uterus. The fetus has the sensitivity and ability to respond to varying stimuli with increases in motor and sympathetic activity.[230] The anesthetic drug effect in the fetus is greater than that in the mother. Determination of the MAC of halothane in chronically instrumented pregnant ewes and their fetuses has shown that it is lower in the fetus, 0.33 vol% compared with 0.69 vol% in the mother.[231] As already described, because of the unique pattern of the fetal circulation, accumulation of effective anesthetic concentrations is delayed in the fetal brain. Neonatal depression was seen after cesarean sections with general anesthesia only when anesthetic concentrations of nitrous oxide were used for approximately 10 min.[138] An anesthetic agent with a higher lipid solubility than nitrous oxide may take longer to anesthetize the fetus.[232, 233]

The use of nondepolarizing neuromuscular blocking agents as adjuvants to fetal anesthesia has recently been investigated. Because these drugs do not cross the placenta readily, d-tubocurarine, 1.5 mg·kg^{-1} of estimated fetal weight, or pancuronium, 0.3 mg·kg^{-1}, were injected into the fetal buttocks under ultrasonic guidance.[234] Paralysis was achieved approximately 5 min after d-tubocurarine blockade, and 4 min after pancuronium administration. The mean duration of neuromuscular d-tubocurarine, estimated from maternal perception of the return of fetal movements, was 3.8 and 6.8 h in the d-tubocurarine and pancuronium-treated groups, respectively. For minor surgical procedures on the fetus that involve minimal pain but require fetal immobilization (*e.g.*, fetal transfusion), maternal sedation combined with fetal paralysis may be adequate.

Fetal surveillance during intrauterine surgical procedures has been difficult because invasive monitoring techniques often are not feasible. At present, continuous fetal heart rate monitoring in conjunction with determination of blood *p*H and gas tensions appear to be good indicators of fetal well-being. Continuous oxygen saturation monitor (pulse oximeter) may also be applied to an accessible fetal extremity.[235]

Intraoperative management should include techniques that induce uterine relaxation. In this respect, the use of potent halogenated agents is advantageous, not only in inducing and maintaining fetal anesthesia, but also in providing dose-related inhibition of uterine tone and contractions. Because the onset of preterm labor is a major complication of intrauterine procedures, postoperative administration of tocolytic agents, such as ritodrine, terbutaline, or magnesium sulfate, is recommended. In some reported cases, indomethacin, a prostaglandin synthetase inhibitor, was given with preoperative medication to prevent early labor.[227, 236]

NONOBSTETRIC SURGERY IN THE PREGNANT WOMAN

Frequently, pregnant women have surgery for reasons unrelated to parturition, the rate being estimated at 1.6%–2.2%.[237, 238] Apart from trauma, the most common emergencies are abdominal, involving torsion or rupture of ovarian cysts and acute appendicitis, but breast tumors are not uncommon, and serious conditions such as intracranial aneurysms, cardiac valvular disease, and pheochromocytoma have been described.[239, 240] Surgery to correct an incompetent cervix with Shirodkar or McDonald sutures is more related to the pregnancy itself.

When the necessity for surgery arises, anesthetic considerations are related to the alterations in maternal physiologic condition with advancing pregnancy, the teratogenicity of anesthetic drugs, the indirect effects of anesthesia on uteroplacental blood flow, and the potential for abortion or premature delivery. The risks must be balanced to provide the most favorable outcome for mother and child.

Four major studies have attempted to relate surgery and anesthesia during human pregnancy to fetal outcome, as determined by anomalies, premature labor, or intrauterine death.[237, 238, 241, 242] Although they failed to correlate surgery and anesthetic exposure with congenital anomalies, all of them demonstrated an increased incidence of fetal deaths particularly after operations during the first trimester. No particular anesthetic agent or technique was implicated, and it seemed that the condition that necessitated surgery was the most relevant factor, being highest after pelvic surgery.

A report in 1963 on a large population of pregnant women, of whom 67 had operations during pregnancy, showed a fetal mortality of 11.2%, survival being poorest when the procedure was performed for cervical incompetence.[241] In 1965, a study among approximately 9,000 parturients, of whom 1.6% had surgery, found an 8.8% incidence of premature labor (and perinatal mortality of 7.5%) in the surgical group, compared with only 2% in the control group.[237] More recently, pregnancy outcome after surgery in 287 women of a population of approximately 13,000 dental assistants or dentists' wives, showed that surgery during pregnancy was associated with a significant increase in spontaneous abortion rates compared with those not having surgery (8% *vs.* 5.1%).[238] In an attempt to answer the questions raised by these findings, a review was taken of the entire population of the province of Manitoba between the years 1971–1978.[242] State health insurance records were used to identify approximately 2,500 pregnant women who had surgery during this period. Each patient was matched with a woman of similar age, living in the same area, with a pregnancy-related condition but no surgical intervention. As in earlier studies, there was no increase in the incidence of congenital anomalies in the offspring of mothers who had surgery. However, there was an increased risk of spontaneous abortion in women who received general anesthesia during the first or second trimesters. This was most evident after gynecologic operations. Few of the surgical group had procedures to treat cervical incompetence, suggesting that factors other than the obstetric condition itself might be important. Results also might have been influenced by the fact that a small number of gynecologic procedures were performed with anesthesia other than general, so that the effect of the surgical site alone could not be evaluated. The authors emphasize the multiplicity of factors other than choice of anesthetic agent (*e.g.*, diagnostic roentgenograms, antibiotics, analgesics, infection, decreased uterine perfusion, and stress) that might be responsible for the increased risk of abortion.

The study of the effects of chronic exposure to subanesthetic concentrations of inhalation agents on pregnancy offers a different approach to the question of outcome. Evidence originates from animal studies and from epidemiologic surveys performed on operating room personnel and their children. A nationwide survey conducted by the American Society of Anesthesiologists found a higher incidence of cancer among female anesthesia personnel as well as increased rates of abortion and congenital abnormalities in their infants.[243]

Furthermore, the last of these misfortunes also applied, although to a lesser degree, to unexposed wives of male operating room personnel. Another study, involving nurse anesthetists, suggested a higher than expected incidence of cancer.[244] These studies have been disputed because of possible statistical inaccuracies and inappropriate choices of control groups.[245, 246] Another survey conducted among dentists and their female assistants compared the incidence of spontaneous abortions and congenital abnormalities among those exposed to inhalation anesthetics and those using only local anesthetics in their daily practices.[247] A significant increase in these complications occurred among assistants and wives of dentists exposed to inhalation drugs. Because of the controversy surrounding this issue, the American Society of Anesthesiologists commissioned an independent review by a team of epidemiologists.[248] This group found the data from most of the surveys to be flawed for a variety of reasons. These included responder bias, inappropriate control groups, failure to document exposure levels or verify medical data, and inability to ascertain which of the many environmental factors present in operating rooms might be blamed. The group concluded that, although exposed women appeared to have an increased risk of abortion (and to a much lesser extent, congenital anomalies), the increase was small enough to be accounted for by bias and uncontrolled variables. Some of these problems are absent in two subsequent studies in which questionnaire information was matched with information obtained from medical records or registries of abortions, births, and congenital malformations.[249, 250] Neither of these studies found significant deviations from expected rates of threatened abortion in exposed women. In addition, no differences in birth weight distribution, perinatal mortality, or congenital malformations between exposed and nonexposed women were detected.[250] The authors point out that their results do not indicate that there is no reproductive hazard relating to working in operating rooms; effects that might have been missed include very early abortions not requiring hospitalization, congenital abnormalities not apparent at birth, and infertility.

PHYSIOLOGIC CHANGES IN PREGNANCY

Because these changes have been described earlier in the chapter, only a few points will be emphasized. The lesser increase in red blood cell volume relative to total blood volume leads to a decline in red blood cell count, hemoglobin, and hematocrit.[2] Serum cholinesterase activity declines moderately.[4] Cardiac output and heart rate gradually increase to a peak of 30%–50% above normal at 30%–34 weeks. From this time on, inferior vena caval compression becomes increasingly important.[15] Drug requirement for regional anesthesia may be reduced by 25%–30%. Capillary engorgement throughout the respiratory tract makes nasal breathing more difficult and intubation of the trachea more hazardous.[17] From the 5th month, FRC decreases, and, at term, alveolar ventilation exceeds that of the nonpregnant state by about 70%.[21, 22] These two factors enhance maternal uptake and elimination of inhalation anesthetics.[25] The low FRC and increased metabolic rate predispose the mother to hypoxemia, especially during airway obstruction or endotracheal intubation.[26] The stomach and intestines are gradually pushed upward by the enlarging uterus. Evacuation of a watery meal may be delayed by as much as 60% from the 34th week onward.[31] Pain and opioids will potentiate this delay. The administration of general anesthesia enhances the risk of regurgitation and aspiration during pregnancy, making rapid induction with cricoid pressure and endotracheal intubation mandatory in all patients having general anesthesia during the last two trimesters.

DIRECT EFFECTS OF ANESTHETIC AGENTS ON EMBRYO AND FETUS

The idea that surgical anesthesia, although deemed necessary for the patient, might have detrimental effects on the growth and development of the human fetus has led to a great deal of investigation, both *in vitro* and in experimental animals. These studies present difficulties in interpretation because the concentrations of anesthetic and duration of exposure are frequently far in excess of what is clinically used and because most of them were performed in lower animals. The first test of embryotoxicity of an anesthetic agent (nitrous oxide) was made in the chick embryo.[251] Subsequent studies mostly have been on mammalian models, such as the rat, in which pregnancy lasts for a few weeks and organogenesis only for a few days.

Animals exposed to toxic substances and anesthetics show a dose-related response, the first change being decreased fertility and increased fetal death. With increasing dose, the number of surviving fetuses with anomalies begins to increase, the peak incidence occurring at a dose that causes a 50% incidence of fetal death.[252] The teratogenic effects between species and also within the same species vary significantly. The developmental stage is crucial, with dramatic sensitivity to exposure at certain times and little or no effect at a later time.[252, 253] The period of organogenesis is most critical. In humans it corresponds to the 15th–56th days of gestation.

Several experiments have demonstrated that brief intrauterine exposure of rats to halothane adversely affected postnatal learning behavior and caused central nervous system cellular degeneration and decreased brain weight; the findings with enflurane have been inconsistent.[254–256]

Many congenital malfunctions show a pattern of multifactorial inheritance. In this mode, maldevelopment may result from a combination of factors within one person, such as hereditary predisposition, sensitivity to a given drug, and exposure at a vulnerable time in development. There are numerous other factors contributing to the potential teratogenicity of anesthesia. The cytotoxicty of anesthetic agents is closely associated with biodegradation, which, in turn, is influenced by oxygenation and hepatic blood flow. Thus, the complications associated with anesthesia, such as maternal hypoxia, hypotension, administration of vasopressors, hypercarbia, hypocarbia, electrolyte disturbances, *etc.*, may possibly be a greater cause for concern as regards teratogenesis than the use of the agents themselves.[257–259] Hypoxia is certainly a well-documented teratogen in the incubating chick embryo.[260] The role of maternal carbohydrate metabolism on embryonic development is also very important. For example, the effects of 48 h of fasting and administration of insulin to pregnant rats have included a large number of skeletal deformities.[261]

Experimental evidence on exposure to specific drugs and agents will be highlighted very briefly, with the consideration that it is difficult to extrapolate laboratory data to the clinical situation as seen in humans. Very large numbers of patients must be exposed to a suspected teratogen before its safety can be ascertained. Complicating factors include the frequency of maternal exposure to a multiplicity of drugs; the difficulty in separating the effects of the underlying disease process and surgical treatment from those of the drug administered; differing degrees of risk with stage of gestation; and the variety, rather than the consistency, of anomalies that appear in association with one agent. Of the premedicants, anticholinergics have not been found to be teratogenic, whereas tranquilizers and sedatives such as phenothiazines and barbiturates produce anomalies in some species.[253, 262, 263, 264] Several reports have described a specific relationship between diazepam and oral clefts, but another study has not confirmed this.[265–267] Intravenous agents such as thiopental, methohexital, and ketamine, in doses normally used in the operating room, have not been associated with birth defects. Only one study has shown musculoskeletal deformities involving the joints after infusion of a muscle relaxant (d-tubocurarine) in the chick embryo between the 7th and 15th day of incubation.[268] Although local anesthetics have not been shown to be teratogenic in animals or humans, procaine, lidocaine, and bupivacaine affected cultures of hamster lung fibroblasts by decreasing cell survival with ED_{50} values at concentrations as low as one-tenth of those used clinically.[269] Halogenated inhalation drugs have produced conflicting results. Pregnant rats exposed to halothane 0.8% for 12 h at various times during gestation have increased incidences of anomalous skeletal development and fetal death.[270] Other investigations have failed to show teratologic effects of halothane in rats, rabbits, and mice exposed to subanesthetic concentrations for brief periods. Subanesthetic concentrations of enflurane do not appear to be teratogenic. However, mice exposed to 1% enflurane for 4 h·day^{-1} on days 6–15 of gestation showed an increased incidence of cleft palates and minor skeletal and visceral abnormalities.[271] In a subsequent study by the same authors, teratogenic changes after exposure to 0.6% isoflurane in mice were similar to those found with enflurane, but the incidence of cleft palate was six times more frequent (12% vs. 1.9%).[272] Because cleft palate readily develops in mice, its occurrence as an isolated finding suggests that this might be a species-specific response. So that the results from earlier studies could be clarified, rats were exposed to 0.75 MAC halothane, isoflurane, or enflurane; 0.55 MAC nitrous oxide; or a known teratogen, retinoic acid, for two 6-h periods at three different stages of pregnancy.[273] No major morphologic abnormalities occurred in any of the anesthetic-exposed groups.

Nitrous oxide has been the most extensively investigated agent since the 1955 observation that patients with tetanus had developed leukopenia after inhaling nitrous oxide for several days. Numerous studies have demonstrated significant effects on fetal growth, skeletal development, and death rate in both pregnant rats and incubating chicks exposed to concentrations of from 50% to 80% for periods ranging from hours to days.[274, 275] The question arises whether adverse effects at such high doses resulted from the anesthetic itself or from the accompanying physiologic derangements. After prolonged exposure of rats to subanesthetic concentrations of nitrous oxide or room air, 1,000 ppm of nitrous oxide resulted in a higher incidence of fetal resorptions, skeletal malformations, and smaller fetuses than did air.[276] Because these concentrations do not produce anesthesia, this study supports the conclusion that nitrous oxide itself may be teratogenic. In contrast to the above findings with high dosage or prolonged exposure, concentrations of 50% or less for periods of less than 24 h resulted in no adverse fetal effects.[277, 278]

Although the mechanism of the teratogenic effect of nitrous oxide has not been determined, it may be related to the inhibitory effect of the agent on methionine synthetase activity.[279] Vitamin B_{12}, a cofactor of this enzyme, is irreversibly oxidized to an inactive form. Inhibition of methionine synthetase has

been detected in liver biopsy specimens obtained from surgical patients after exposure to 50%–70% nitrous oxide for 1.25–2.75 h.[280] A dose-dependent decrease in both maternal and fetal methionine synthetase activity occurred in pregnant rats receiving 10% or 50% nitrous oxide for periods ranging from 60 to 240 min.[281] It is possible that failure of this enzyme to convert homocysteine to the essential amino acid methionine may lead to abnormalities of myelination of nerve fibers (Fig. 45-14). Furthermore, inhibition of methionine synthesis results in decreased thymidine production, which in turn can lead to decreased DNA synthesis and inhibition of cell division. Because there is evidence that nitrous oxide adversely affects methionine synthetase activity, it has been recommended that it not be administered to pregnant women in the first two trimesters.[282, 283] However, a recent human study demonstrated no significant changes in plasma methionine concentrations after anesthesia with 60%–70% nitrous oxide for up to 4 h.[284] Two other reviews of exposure to this agent, this time for cervical cerclage procedures, showed no effects on the fetal outcome.[285, 286] Further, in rats, the teratogenic effects of nitrous oxide could be prevented by the concomitant administration of isoflurane or halothane.[287] It is controversial whether pretreatment with folinic acid, the concentration of which is reduced when methionine synthetase is inhibited, affords protection against the effects of nitrous oxide.[287, 288] Because a single exposure to anesthetic agents seems unlikely to result in fetal abnormality, the selection of agent should be based on specific surgical requirements.

INDIRECT EFFECTS OF AGENTS AND TECHNIQUES

The adequacy of the uteroplacental circulation, so vital to the well-being of the fetus, is easily affected by drugs and anesthetic procedures. As discussed previously, perfusion of the intervillous space of the placenta may be diminished consequent to maternal systemic hypotension, which, in turn, may result from the use of epidural or spinal anesthesia, from aortocaval compression with the patient in the supine position, or from hemorrhage. Similarly, increased uterine activity may result in reduced placental perfusion. Thus, the use of alpha-adrenergic drugs to correct maternal hypotension and anesthetics such as ketamine (in doses above 1 mg·kg^{-1}) may produce increased uterine tone sufficient to endanger the fetus.[194, 289] If severe, hyperventilation of the mother may also reduce uterine blood flow.[134] Finally, it has been shown in experimental animals that epinephrine or norepinephrine infusion results in decreased uterine blood flow and deterioration of fetal condition. Maternal pain and apprehension or administration of local anesthetic solutions containing epinephrine may similarly affect the fetus.[290, 291]

PRACTICAL SUGGESTIONS

It is generally agreed that only emergency surgery should be performed during pregnancy, particularly in the first trimester. The possibility of pregnancy should be considered in all female surgical patients of reproductive age. Based on the maternal and fetal hazards already described, the following approach to anesthesia seems indicated:

1. The patient's apprehension should be allayed as much as possible by personal reassurance during the preanesthetic visit and by adequate sedation and premed-

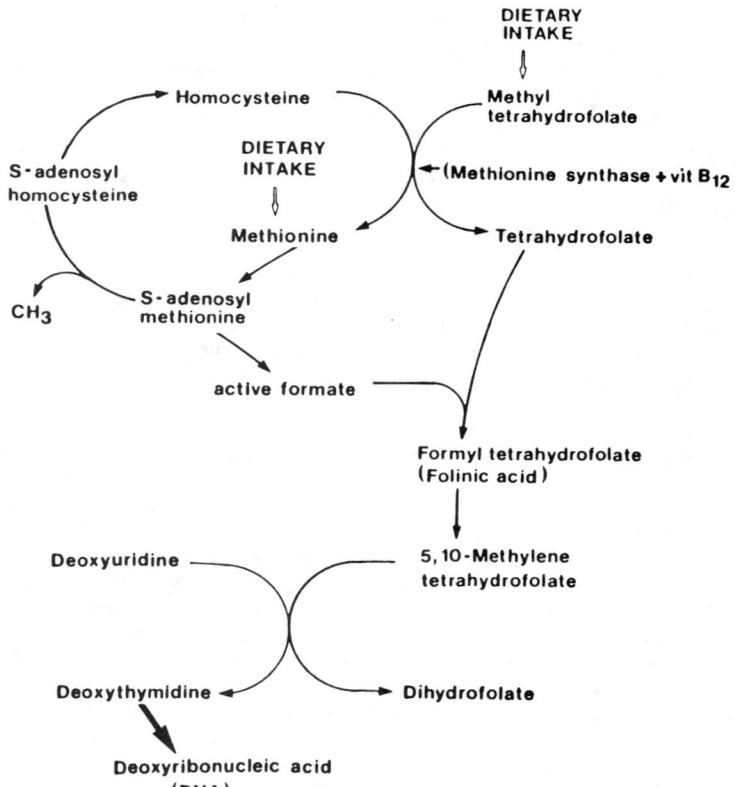

FIG. 45-14. Abridged metabolic map showing the relationship between methionine and deoxythymidine syntheses. (Reprinted with permission. Nunn JF: Interaction of nitrous oxide and vitamin B_{12}. Trends Pharmacol Sci 5:225, 1984.)

ication. It is important to discuss the hazards of anesthesia with the patient and her family, because they are likely to have many fears for the unborn baby.

2. Pain should be relieved whenever present.

3. Administration of an antacid, 15–30 ml, within half an hour before induction of anesthesia will usually increase the *p*H of the gastric fluid above the critical level. Ranitidine and metoclopramide may be useful.

4. Beginning in the second trimester, mothers should not be transported or placed in the supine position on the operating table. The lateral decubitus, or left uterine displacement, will minimize the risk of aortocaval compression.

5. Hypotension related to spinal or epidural anesthesia should be prevented as much as possible by rapid intravenous infusion of crystalloid solution before induction. If the mother becomes hypotensive despite this pretreatment, a predominantly beta-adrenergic vasopressor, such as ephedrine, should be promptly administered intravenously.

6. Administration of general anesthesia should be preceded by careful denitrogenation.

7. The risk of aspiration should be minimized by application of cricoid pressure and rapid tracheal intubation with a cuffed tube.

8. To reduce fetal hazard, particularly during the first trimester, it appears preferable to choose drugs with a long history of safety, which include thiopental, morphine, meperidine, muscle relaxants, and low concentrations of nitrous oxide. However, ketamine, 0.5–0.75 mg · kg^{-1}, might be preferable to thiopental as an induction agent in the face of severe hypovolemia. Halo-

thane or other volatile drugs may offer the specific advantage of relaxing the uterus during procedures involving the pelvic organs, particularly the uterus itself, *e.g.*, cervical cerclage (Shirodkar or McDonald procedure).

9. To avoid maternal hyperventilation, one should monitor end-expiratory P_{CO_2} or arterial blood gases.

10. Fetal heart rate should be monitored continuously throughout surgery and anesthesia, providing that the placement of the transducer does not encroach upon the surgical field.[292, 293] Using the directional Doppler apparatus, this monitoring becomes technically feasible from the 16th week of pregnancy. Uterine tone may also be monitored with an external tocodynamometer if the uterus has grown enough to reach the umbilicus or above.

11. Monitoring of uterine activity should be continued after operation, and tocolytic agents should be administered, if necessary, to inhibit uterine contractions.

12. Special procedures, such as hypothermia and induced hypotension, might be necessary to facilitate surgery, despite the potential fetal hazard. It is reassuring to know that there was successful fetal outcome after both procedures for intracranial operations.[294, 295] There are numerous reports of cardiopulmonary bypass being performed during pregnancy, with generally good maternal and fetal results.[176, 296–298] A frequent finding was a persistent fetal bradycardia and loss of beat-to-beat variability throughout the period of bypass, despite acceptable maternal oxygenation and acid–base balance. One survey reported only one maternal death in 86 procedures using extracorporeal cir-

culation and a more than 80% survival rate of fetuses.[176] It was suggested that the procedures might be safer when fetal heart and uterine monitoring were used and perfusion hypothermia avoided. At this time, little work has been done to determine the fetal effects of cardiopulmonary bypass.

REFERENCES

1. Ueland K: Maternal cardiovascular dynamics. VII. Intrapartum blood volume changes. Am J Obstet Gynecol 126:671, 1976
2. Lund CJ, Donovan JC: Blood volume during pregnancy. Am J Obstet Gynecol 98:393, 1967
3. Williams: Obstetrics. In Pritchard JA, Macdonald PC (eds): Maternal Adaptation to Pregnancy, p 236. New York, Appleton-Century-Crofts, 1980
4. Hazel B, Monier D: Human serum cholinesterase: Variations during pregnancy and post-partum. Can Anaesth Soc J 18:272, 1971
5. Wildsmith JAW: Serum pseudocholinesterase, pregnancy and suxamethonium. Anaesthesia 27:90, 1972
6. De Alvarez RR, Afonso JF, Sherrard DJ: Serum protein fractionation in normal pregnancy. Am J Obstet Gynecol 82:1096, 1961
7. Levy G: Protein binding of drugs in the maternal-fetal unit and its potential clinical significance. In Krauer B, Krauer F, Hytten FE et al (eds): Drugs and Pregnancy, p 29. London, Academic Press, 1984
8. Pernoll ML, Metcalf J, Schlenker TL et al: Oxygen consumption at rest and during exercise in pregnancy. Respir Physiol 25:285, 1975
9. Ueland K, Parer JT: Effects of estrogens on the cardiovascular system of the ewe. Am J Obstet Gynecol 96:400, 1966
10. Goodman RP, Killom AP, Brash AR et al: Prostacyclin production during pregnancy—Comparison of production during normal pregnancy and pregnancy complicated by hypertension. Am J Obstet Gynecol 142:817, 1982
11. Hamilton HFH: Cardiac output in normal pregnancy. J Obstet Gynaecol Br Commonw 56:548, 1949
12. Kerr MG, Scott DB, Samuel E: Studies of the inferior vena cava in late pregnancy. Br Med J 1:532, 1964
13. Ueland K, Novy MJ, Peterson EN: Maternal cardiovascular dynamics. IV. The influence of gestational age on the maternal cardiovascular response to posture and exercise. Am J Obstet Gynecol 104:856, 1969
14. Humphrey MD, Chang A, Wood EC et al: A decrease in fetal pH during the second stage of labour when conducted in the dorsal position. J Obst Gynaecol Br Commonw 81:600, 1974
15. Howard BK, Goodson JH, Mengert WF: Supine hypotensive syndrome in late pregnancy. Obstet Gynecol 1:371, 1953
16. Bieniarz J, Crottogini JJ, Curuchet E et al: Aortocaval compression by the uterus in late human pregnancy. II. An angiographic study. Am J Obstet Gynecol 100:203, 1968
17. Bonica JJ: Principles and Practice of Obstetric Analgesia and Anesthesia, p 21. Philadelphia, FA Davis, 1967
18. Datta S, Briwa J: Modified laryngoscope for endotracheal intubation of obese patients. Anesth Analg 60:120, 1981
19. Kruttgen HG, Emerson K Jr: Physiological response to pregnancy at rest and during exercise. J Appl Physiol 36:549, 1974
20. Gee JBL, Packer BS, Miller JE et al: Pulmonary mechanics during pregnancy. J Clin Invest 46:945, 1967
21. Andersen GJ, James GB, Mathers NP et al: The maternal oxygen tension and acid-base status during pregnancy. J Obstet Gynaecol Brit Commonw 76:16, 1969
22. Cugell DW, Frank NR, Gaensler EA et al: Pulmonary function in pregnancy. I. Serial observations in normal women. Ann Rev Tuberc 67:568, 1953
23. Bevan DR, Holdcroft A, Loh L et al: Closing volume and pregnancy. Br Med J 1:13, 1974
24. Prowse CM, Gaensler EA: Respiratory and acid-base changes during pregnancy. Anesthesiology 26:381, 1965
25. Moya F, Smith BE: Uptake, distribution and placental transport of drugs and anesthetics. Anesthesiology 26:465, 1965
26. Archer GW, Marx GF: Arterial oxygenation during apnaea in parturient women. Br J Anaesth 46:358, 1974
27. Datta S, Kitzmiller JL, Naulty JS et al: Acid-base status of diabetic mothers and their infants following spinal anesthesia for cesarean section. Anesth Analg 61:662, 1982
28. Murray FA, Eskine JP, Fielding J: Gastric secretions in pregnancy. Journal of Obstetrics and Gynaecology of the British Commonwealth 64:313, 1957
29. Taylor G, Pryse-Davies J: The prophylactic use of antacids in the prevention of the acid-pulmonary aspiration syndrome (Mendelson's syndrome). Lancet 1:288, 1966
30. Lind JF, Smith AM, McIver DR et al: Heartburn in pregnancy—A manometric study. Can Med Assoc J 98:571, 1968
31. Davison JS, Davison MC, Hay DM: Gastric emptying time in late pregnancy and labour. J Obstet Gynaecol Brit Commonw 77:37, 1970
32. Smith G, Dalling R, Williams TIR: Gastro-oesophageal pressure gradient changes produced by induction of anaesthesia and suxamethonium. Br J Anaesth 50:1137, 1979
33. Brock-Utne JG, Dow TGB, Dimopoulos GE et al: Gastric and lower oesophageal sphincter (LOS) pressures in early pregnancy. Br J Anaesth 53:381, 1981
34. Coombs DW: Editorial: Aspiration pneumonia prophylaxis. Anesth Analg 62:1055, 1983
35. Wyner J, Cohen SE: Gastric volume in early pregnancy: Effect of metoclopramide. Anesthesiology 57:209, 1982
36. Cohen SE, Woods WA, Wyner J: Antiemetic efficacy of droperidol and metoclopramide. Anesthesiology 60:67, 1984
37. Murphy DF, Nally B, Gardiner J et al: Effect of metoclopramide on gastric emptying before elective and emergency cesarean section. Br J Anaesth 56:1113, 1984
38. Scheller MS, Sears KL: Post-operative neurologic dysfunction associated with preoperative administration of metoclopramide. Anesth Analg 66:274, 1987
39. Palahniuk RJ, Shnider SM, Eger EI: Pregnancy decreases the requirements for inhaled anesthetic agents. Anesthesiology 41:82, 1974
40. Datta S, Lambert DH, Gregus et al: Differential sensitivities of mammalian nerve fibers during pregnancy. Anesth Analg 62:1070, 1983
41. Fagraeus L, Urban BJ, Bromage PR: Spread of epidural analgesia in early pregnancy. Anesthesiology 58:184, 1983
42. Drabkova J, Crul JF, Van Der Kleijn E: Placental transfer of ^{14}C labelled succinylcholine in near-term Macaca mulatta monkeys. Br J Anaesth 46:1087, 1973
43. Duvaldestin P, Demetriou M, Henzel D et al: The placental transfer of pancuronium and its pharmacokinetics during caesarean section. Acta Anaesth Scand 22:327, 1978
44. Brown WU, Bell GC, Alper MH: Acidosis, local anesthetics and the newborn. Obstet Gynecol 48:27, 1976
45. Morishima HO, Covino BG: Toxicity and distribution of lidocaine in nonasphyxiated and asphyxiated baboon fetuses. Anesthesiology 54:182, 1981
46. Hamshaw-Thomas A, Rogerson N, Reynolds F: Transfer of bupivacaine, lignocaine and pethidine across the rabbit placenta: Influence of maternal protein binding and fetal flow. Placenta 5:61, 1984
47. Kennedy RL, Miller RP, Bell JU et al: Uptake and distribution of bupivacaine in fetal lambs. Anesthesiology 65:247, 1986
48. Morishima HO, Pedersen H, Santos A et al: Maternal and fetal

uptake of bupivacaine vs. lidocaine at steady state plasma drug concentrations. Anesthesiology 67:A437, 1987

49. Kuhnert PM, Kuhnert BR, Stitts BS et al: The use of a selected ion monitoring technique to study the disposition of bupivacaine in mother, fetus and neonate following epidural anesthesia for cesarean section. Anesthesiology 55:611, 1981

50. Kosaka Y, Takahashi T, Mark LC: Intravenous thiobarbiturate anesthesia for cesarean section. Anesthesiology 31:489, 1969

51. Finster M, Morishima HO, Pedersen H et al: Meperidine: Placental transfer after epidural, intramuscular, and intravenous injection. Anesthesiology 55:A321, 1981

52. Crawford JS, Rudofsky S: The placental transmission of pethidine. Br J Anaesth 37:929, 1965

53. Kuhnert BR, Philipson EH, Pimental R et al: Lidocaine disposition in mother, fetus, and neonate after spinal anesthesia. Anesth Analg 65:139, 1986

54. Morishima HO, Daniel SS, Finster M et al: Transmission of mepivacaine hydrochloride (Carbocaine) across the human placenta. Anesthesiology 27:147, 1966

55. O'Brien JE, Abbey V, Hinsvark O et al: Metabolism and measurement of 2-chloroprocaine, an ester type local anesthetic. J Pharm Sci 68:75, 1979

56. Kuhnert BR, Kuhnert PM, Philipson EH et al: The half-life of 2-chloroprocaine. Anesth Analg 65:273, 1986

57. Kuhnert BR, Kuhnert PM, Prochaska AL et al: Plasma levels of 2-chloroprocaine in obstetric patients and their neonates after epidural anesthesia. Anesthesiology 53:21, 1980

58. Morgan DJ, Blackman GL, Paul JD et al: Pharmacokinetics and plasma binding of thiopental. II. Studies at cesarean section. Anesthesiology 54:474, 1981

59. Santos A, Morishima HO, Pedersen H et al: Pharmacokinetics of methohexital in pregnant and nonpregnant ewes. Anesthesiology 63:A441, 1985

60. Idanpaan-Heikkila JE, Taska RJ, Allen HA et al: Placental transfer of diazepam—¹⁴C in mice, hamsters and monkeys. J Pharmacol Exp Ther 176:752, 1971

61. Haram K, Bakke OM, Johannessen KH et al: Transplacental passage of diazepam during labor: Influence of uterine contractions. Clin Pharmacol Ther 24:590, 1978

62. Mihaly GW, Moore RG, Thomas J et al: The pharmacokinetics and metabolism of the anilide local anaesthetics in neonates. Eur J Clin Pharmacol 13:143, 1978

63. Morishima HO, Finster M, Pedersen H et al: Pharmacokinetics of lidocaine in fetal and neonatal lambs and adult sheep. Anesthesiology 50:431, 1979

64. Finster M, Poppers PJ, Sinclair JC et al: Accidental intoxication of the fetus with local anesthetic drug during caudal anesthesia. Am J Obstet Gynecol 92:922, 1965

65. Morishima HO, Pedersen H, Finster M et al: Toxicity of lidocaine in adult, newborn and fetal sheep. Anesthesiology 55:57, 1981

66. Morishima HO, Pedersen H, Finster M et al: Etidocaine toxicity in the adult, newborn and fetal sheep. Anesthesiology 58:342, 1983

67. Campbell N, Harvey D, Norman AP: Increased frequency of neonatal jaundice in a maternity hospital. Br Med J 2:548, 1975

68. Clark DA, Landaw SA: Bupivacaine alters red blood cells properties: A possible explanation for neonatal jaundice associated with maternal anesthesia. Pediatr Res 19:341, 1985

69. Gale R, Ferguson JE II, Stevenson D: Effect of epidural analgesia with bupivacaine hydrochloride on neonatal bilirubin production. Obstet Gynecol 70:692, 1987

70. Hodgkinson R, Marx GF, Kim SS et al: Neonatal neurobehavioral tests following vaginal delivery under ketamine, thiopental and extradural anesthesia. Anesth Analg 56:548, 1977

71. Amiel-Tison C, Barrier G, Shnider SM et al: A new neurologic and adaptive capacity scoring system for evaluating obstetric medications in full term newborns. Anesthesiology 56:340, 1982

72. Morishima HO, Yeh M-N, James LS: Reduced uterine blood flow and fetal hypoxemia with acute maternal stress: Experimental observation in the pregnant baboon. Am J Obstet Gynecol 134:270, 1979

73. Shnider SM, Wright RG, Levinson G et al: Uterine blood flow and plasma norepinephrine changes during maternal stress in the pregnant ewe. Anesthesiology 50:524, 1979

74. Ueland K, Hansen JM: Maternal cardiovascular dynamics. III. Labor and delivery under local and caudal analgesia. Am J Obstet Gynecol 103:8, 1969

75. Moir DD, Willocks J: Management of incoordinate uterine action under continuous epidural analgesia. Br Med J 2:396, 1967

76. Miller FC, Petrie RH, Arce JJ et al: Hyperventilation during labor. Am J Obstet Gynecol 120:489, 1974

77. Melzack R, Taenzer P, Feldman P et al: Labour is still painful after prepared childbirth training. Can Med Assoc J 125:357, 1981

78. Scott JR, Rose NB: Effect of psychoprophylaxis (Lamaze preparation) on labor and delivery in primiparas. N Engl J Med 294:1205, 1976

79. Way WL, Cortley EC, Way EL: Respiratory sensitivity of the newborn infant to meperidine and morphine. Clin Pharmacol Ther 6:454, 1965

80. Shnider SM, Moya F: Effects of meperidine on the newborn infant. Am J Obstet Gynecol 89:1009, 1964

81. Kuhnert BR, Kuhnert PM, Philipson EH et al: Disposition of meperidine and normeperidine following multiple doses during labor. II. Fetus and neonate. Am J Obstet Gynecol 151:410, 1985

82. Kuhnert BR, Linn PL, Kennard MJ et al: Effect of low doses of meperidine on neonatal behavior. Anesth Analg 64: 335, 1985

83. Eisele JH, Wright R, Rogge P: Newborn and maternal fentanyl levels at cesarean section. Anesth Analg 61:179, 1982

84. Maduska AL, Hajghassemali M: A double blind comparison of butorphanol and meperidine in labor: Maternal pain relief and effect on newborn. Can Anaesth Soc J 25:398, 1978

85. Clark RB: Transplacental reversal of meperidine depression in the fetus by naloxone. J Arkansas Med Soc 68:128, 1971

86. Evans JM, Rosen M, MacCarthy J et al: Patient-controlled intravenous narcotic administration during labor. Lancet 1:906, 1976

87. Powe CE, Kiem IM, Fromhagen C et al: Propiomazine hydrochloride in obstetrical analgesia. JAMA 181:280, 1962

88. Cree IE, Meyer J, Hailey DM: Diazepam in labour: Its metabolism and effect on the clinical condition and thermogenesis of the newborn. Br Med J 4:251, 1973

89. Akamatsu TJ, Bonica JJ, Rehmet R et al: Experiences with the use of ketamine for parturition. I. Primary anesthetic for vaginal delivery. Anesth Analg 53:284, 1974

90. Schellenberg JC: Uterine activity during lumbar epidural analgesia with bupivacaine. Am J Obstet Gynecol 127:26, 1977

91. Chestnut DH, Bates JN, Choi WW: Continuous infusion epidural analgesia with lidocaine: Efficacy and influence during the second stage of labor. Obstet Gynecol 69:323, 1987

92. Moore DC, Batra MS: The components of an effective test dose prior to epidural block. Anesthesiology 55:694, 1984

93. Cartwright PD, McCarroll SM, Antzaka C: Maternal heart rate changes with plain epidural test dose. Anesthesiology 65:226, 1986

94. Hood DD, Dewan DM, James FM III: Maternal and fetal effects of epinephrine in gravid ewes. Anesthesiology 64:610, 1986

95. Scanlon JW, Brown WV Jr, Weiss JB et al: Neurobehavioral responses of newborn infants after maternal epidural anesthesia. Anesthesiology 40:121, 1974

96. Bromage PR, Datta S, Dunford LA: Etidocaine: An evaluation in epidural analgesia for obstetrics. Can Anaesth Soc J 21:535, 1974

97. Abboud TK, Kern S, Jacobs J et al: The neonatal neurobehavioral

effects of mepivacaine for epidural anesthesia during labor. Regional Anesthesia 11:143, 1986

98. Baxi LV, Petrie RH, James LS: Human fetal oxygenation following paracervical block. Am J Obstet Gynecol 135:1109, 1979

99. Thiery M, Vroman S: Paracervical block analgesia during labor. Am J Obstet Gynecol 113:988, 1972

100. Kotelko DM, Dailey PA, Shnider SM et al: Epidural morphine analgesia after cesarean delivery. Obstet Gynecol 63:409, 1984

101. Husemeyer RP, O'Connor ML, Davenport HT: Failure of epidural morphine to relieve pain in labour. Anaesthesia 35:161, 1980

102. Hughes SC, Rosen MA, Shnider SM et al: Maternal and neonatal effects of epidural morphine for labor and delivery. Anesth Analg 63:319, 1984

103. Cohen SE, Tan S, Albright GA et al: Epidural fentanyl/bupivacaine mixtures for obstetric analgesia. Anesthesiology 67:403, 1987

104. Baraka A, Noueihid R, Hajj S: Intrathecal injection of morphine for obstetric analgesia. Anesthesiology 54:136, 1981

105. Abboud TK, Shnider SM, Dailey PA et al: Intrathecal administration of hyperbaric morphine for the relief of pain in labour. Br J Anaesth 56:1351, 1984

106. Creasser CW, Stoelting RK, Krishna G et al: Methoxyflurane metabolism and renal function after methoxyflurane analgesia during labor and delivery. Anesthesiology 41:62, 1974

107. Dundee JW, Moore J: Alterations in response to somatic pain associated with anaesthesia. IV. The effects of sub-anaesthetic concentrations of inhalation agents. Br J Anaesth 32:453, 1960

108. Munson ES, Embro WJ: Enflurane, isoflurane and halothane and isolated human uterine muscle. Anesthesiology 46:11, 1977

109. Gibbs CP, Krischer J, Peckam BM et al: Obstetric anesthesia: A national survey. Anesthesiology 65:298, 1986

110. Gilstrap LC III, Hauth JC, Hankins GDV et al: Effect of type of anesthesia on blood loss at cesarean section. Obstet Gynecol 69:328, 1987

111. Shnider SM, Levinson G: Anesthesia for cesarean section. In Shnider SM, Levinson G (eds): Anesthesia for Obstetrics, 2nd ed, p 159. Baltimore, Williams & Wilkins, 1987

112. Gutsche BB: Prophylactic ephedrine preceding spinal anesthesia for cesarean section. Anesthesiology 45:462, 1976

113. Marx GF, Luykx WM, Cohen S: Fetal-neonatal status following cesarean section for fetal distress. Br J Anaesth 56:1009, 1984

114. Ramanathan S, Gandhi S, Arismendy J et al: Oxygen transfer from mother to fetus during cesarean section under epidural anesthesia. Anesth Analg 61:576, 1982

115. Santos A, Datta S: Prophylactic use of droperidol for control of nausea and vomiting during spinal anesthesia for elective cesarean section. Anesth Analg 63:85, 1984

116. Chestnut DH, Vandewalker GE, Owen CL et al: Administration of metoclopramide for prevention of nausea and vomiting during epidural anesthesia for elective cesarean section. Anesthesiology 66:563, 1987

117. Abboud TK, Dror A, Mosaad P et al: Mini-dose intrathecal morphine for the relief of post-cesarean section pain: Safety, efficacy and ventilatory responses to CO$_2$. Anesthesiology 67:A464, 1987

118. Abouleish E, Rawal N, Fallon K et al: Combined intrathecal morphine and bupivacaine for cesarean section. Anesthesiology 67:A619, 1987

119. Philipson EH, Kuhnert BR, Syracuse CD: Fetal acidosis, 2-chloroprocaine, and epidural anesthesia for cesarean section. Am J Obstet Gynecol 151:322, 1985

120. Ravindran RS, Bond VK, Fasch MD et al: Prolonged neural blockade following regional analgesia with 2-chloroprocaine. Anesth Analg 59:447, 1980

121. Reisner LS, Hochman BN, Plumer MH: Persistent neurologic deficit and adhesive arachnoiditis following intrathecal 2-chloroprocaine injection. Anesth Analg 59:452, 1980

122. Gissen AJ, Datta S, Lambert D: The chloroprocaine controversy: Is chloroprocaine neurotoxic? Reg Anesth 9:135, 1984

123. Albright GA: Cardiac arrest following regional anesthesia with etidocaine or bupivacaine. Anesthesiology 51:285, 1979

124. Tanz RD, Heskett T, Loehning RW et al: Comparative cardiotoxicity of bupivacaine and lidocaine in the isolated perfused mammalian heart. Anesth Analg 63:549, 1984

125. Morishima HO, Pedersen H, Finster M et al: Bupivacaine toxicity in pregnant and nonpregnant ewes. Anesthesiology 63:134, 1985

126. Chambers WA, Mowbray A, Wilson J: Extradural morphine for the relief of pain following caesarean section. Br J Anaesth 55:1201, 1983

127. Abboud TK, Moore M, Zhu J et al: Epidural butorphanol or morphine for the relief of post-cesarean section pain: Ventilatory responses to carbon dioxide. Anesth Analg 66:887, 1987

128. Chestnut DH, Choi WW, Isbell TJ: Epidural hydromorphone for post-cesarean analgesia. Obstet Gynecol 68:65, 1986

129. Naulty JS, Datta S, Ostheimer GW et al: Epidural fentanyl for post-cesarean delivery pain management. Anesthesiology 63:694, 1985

130. Madej TH, Strunin L: Comparison of epidural fentanyl with sufentanil. Analgesia and side effects after a single bolus dose during elective caesarean section. Anaesthesia 42:1156, 1987

131. Leicht CH, Hughes SC, Dailey PA et al: Epidural morphine sulphate for analgesia after cesarean section: A prospective report of 1000 patients. Anesthesiology 65:A366, 1986

132. Morgan M: Anaesthetic contribution to maternal mortality. Br J Anaesth 59:842, 1987

133. Norris MC, Dewan DM: Preoxygenation for cesarean section: A comparison of two techniques. Anesthesiology 81:A400, 1984

134. Levinson G, Shnider SM, deLorimier AA et al: Effects of maternal hyperventilation on uterine blood flow and fetal oxygenation and acid-base status. Anesthesiology 40:340, 1974

135. James FM III, Crawford JS, Hopkinson R et al: A comparison of general anesthesia and lumbar epidural analgesia for elective cesarean section. Anesth Analg 56:228, 1977

136. Datta S, Ostheimer GW, Weiss JB et al: Neonatal effect of prolonged anesthetic induction for cesarean section. Obstet Gynecol 58:331, 1981

137. Crawford JS, James FM, Crawley M: A further study of general anaesthesia for caesarean section. Br J Anaesth 48:661, 1976

138. Finster M, Poppers PJ: Safety of thiopental used for induction of general anesthesia in elective cesarean section. Anesthesiology 29:190, 1968

139. Marx GF, Mateo CV: Effects of different oxygen concentrations during general anaesthesia for elective caesarean section. Can Anaesth Soc J 18:587, 1971

140. Datta S, Brown WU: Acid-base status in diabetic mothers and their infants following general or spinal anesthesia for cesarean section. Anesthesiology 47:272, 1977

141. Willems J: The etiology of preeclampsia: A hypothesis. Obstet Gynecol 50:495, 1977

142. Speroff L: Toxemia of pregnancy: Mechanism and therapeutic management. Am J Cardiol 32:582, 1973

143. Walsh SW: Preeclampsia: An imbalance in placental prostacyclin and thromboxane production. Am J Obstet Gynecol 152:335, 1985

144. Makila U-M, Jouppila P, Kirkinen P et al: Placental thromboxane and prostacyclin in the regulation of placental blood flow. Obstet Gynecol 68:537, 1986

145. Sibai BM, Spinnato JA, Watson DL et al: Effect of magnesium sulfate on electroencephalographic findings in preeclampsia-eclampsia. Obstet Gynecol 64:261, 1984

146. Hibbard LT: Maternal mortality due to acute toxemia. Obstet Gynecol 42:263, 1973

147. Sibai BM, Anderson GD, McCubbin JH: Eclampsia II. Clinical significance of laboratory findings. Obstet Gynecol 59:153, 1982

148. Wright JP: Anesthetic considerations in preeclampsia-eclampsia. Anesth Analg 63:590, 1983

149. Lin CC, Lindheimer MD, River P et al: Fetal outcome in hypertensive disorders of pregnancy. Am J Obstet Gynecol 142:255, 1982

150. Soffronoff EC, Kaufmann BM, Connaughton JF: Intravascular volume determinations and fetal outcome in hypertensive diseases of pregnancy. Am J Obstet Gynecol 127:4, 1977

151. Chesley LC: Plasma and red cell volumes during pregnancy. Am J Obstet Gynecol 112:440, 1972

152. Joyce TH III, Debnath KS, Baker EA: Preeclampsia—relationship of CVP and epidural analgesia. Anesthesiology 51:S297, 1979

153. Hays PM, Cruickshank DP, Dunn LJ: Plasma volume determination in normal and preeclamptic pregnancies. Am J Obstet Gynecol 151:958, 1985

154. Rafferty TD, Berkowitz RL: Hemodynamics in patients with severe toxemia during labor and delivery. Am J Obstet Gynecol 138:263, 1980

155. Groenendijk R, Trimbos MJ, Wallenburg HCS: Hemodynamic measurements in preeclampsia: Preliminary observations. Am J Obstet Gynecol 150:232, 1984

156. Cotton DB, Gonik B, Dorman K et al: Cardiovascular alterations in severe pregnancy-induced hypertension. Relationship of central venous pressure to pulmonary capillary wedge pressure. Am J Obstet Gynecol 151:762, 1985

157. Kelton JG, Hunter DJS, Neame PB: A platelet function defect in preeclampsia. Obstet Gynecol 65:107, 1985

158. Cotton DB, Gonik B, Dorman KF: Cardiovascular alterations in severe pregnancy-induced hypertension: Acute effects of intravenous magnesium sulfate. Am J Obstet Gynecol 148:162, 1984

159. Green KW, Key TC, Coen R et al: The effects of maternally administered magnesium sulfate on the neonate. Am J Obstet Gynecol 146:29, 1983

160. Shoemaker CT, Meyers M: Sodium nitroprusside for control of severe hypertensive disease of pregnancy: A case report and discussion of potential toxicity. Am J Obstet Gynecol 149: 171, 1984

161. Newsome LR, Bramwell RS, Curling PE: Severe preeclampsia: Hemodynamic effects of lumbar epidural anesthesia. Anesth Analg 65:31, 1986

162. Jouppila P, Jouppila R, Hollmen A et al: Lumbar epidural analgesia to improve intervillous blood flow during labor in severe preeclampsia. Obstet Gynecol 59:158, 1982

163. Ramanathan J, Botorff M, Jeter JN et al: The pharmacokinetics and maternal and neonatal effects of epidural lidocaine in preeclampsia. Anesth Analg 65:120, 1986

164. Hodgkinson R, Husain FJ, Hayashi RH: Systemic and pulmonary blood pressure during cesarean section in parturients with gestational hypertension. Can Anaesth Soc J 27:389, 1980

165. Connell H, Dalgleish JG, Downing JW: General anaesthesia in mothers with severe pre-eclampsia/eclampsia. Br J Anaesth 59:1375, 1987

166. Abdul-Karim RW, Chevli RN: Antepartum hemorrhage and shock. Clin Obstet Gynecol 19:533, 1976

167. Pritchard JA, Mason R, Corley M et al: Genesis of severe placental abruption. Am J Obstet Gynecol 108:22, 1970

168. Pritchard JA: Haematological problems associated with delivery, placental abruption, retained dead fetus and amniotic fluid embolism. Clin Haematol 2:562, 1973

169. Perloff JK: Pregnancy and cardiovascular disease. In Braunwald E (ed): Heart Disease: Textbook of Cardiovascular Medicine, 2nd ed, p 1763. Philadelphia, WB Saunders, 1984

170. Hibbard LT: Maternal mortality due to cardiac disease. Clin Obstet Gynecol 18:27, 1975

171. Sugrue D, Blake S, MacDonald D: Pregnancy complicated by maternal heart disease at the National Maternity Hospital, Dublin, Ireland, 1969–1978. Am J Obstet Gynecol 139:1, 1981

172. Ueland K, Hansen JM: Maternal cardiovascular dynamics. II. Posture and uterine contractions. Am J Obstet Gynecol 103:1, 1969

173. Szekely P, Snaith L: Heart Disease and Pregnancy, p 29. London, Churchill Livingstone, 1974

174. Sullivan JM, Ramanathan KB: Management of medical problems in pregnancy—Severe cardiac disease. N Engl J Med 313:304, 1985

175. Schroeder JS, Harrison DC: Repeated cardioversion during pregnancy: Treatment of refractory paroxysmal atrial tachycardia during 3 successive pregnancies. Am J Cardiol 27:445, 1971

176. Becker RM: Intracardiac surgery in pregnant women. Ann Thorac Surg 36:453, 1983

177. Mangano DT: Anesthesia for the pregnant cardiac patient. In Shnider SM, Levinson G (eds): Anesthesia for Obstetrics, 2nd ed, p 345. Baltimore, Williams & Wilkins, 1987

178. Abboud TK, Raya J, Noueihid R et al: Intrathecal morphine for relief of labor pain in patients with severe pulmonary hypertension. Anesthesiology 59:477, 1983

179. Campbell M: The incidence and later distribution of malformations of the heart. In Watson H (ed): Paediatric Cardiology, p 71. London, Lloyd-Luke, 1968

180. Jones AM, Howitt G: Eisenmenger's syndrome in pregnancy. Br Med J 1:1627, 1965

181. Rush RW, Davey DA, Segall ML: The effect of pre-term delivery on perinatal mortality. Br J Obstet Gynaecol 85:806, 1978

182. Allen MC, Jones MD: Medical complications of prematurity. Obstet Gynecol 67:427, 1986

183. Dailey PA: Anesthesia for preterm labor. In Shnider SM, Levinson G (eds): Anesthesia for Obstetrics, 2nd ed, p 243. Baltimore, Williams & Wilkins, 1987

184. Benedetti TJ: Maternal complications of parenteral beta-sympathomimetic therapy for premature labor. Am J Obstet Gynecol 145:1, 1983

185. Young DC, Toofanian A, Leveno KJ: Potassium and glucose concentration without treatment during ritodrine tocolysis. Am J Obstet Gynecol 145:105, 1983

186. Saunders NR: Development of blood-brain barrier in the fetus. In Bossart H (ed): Perinatal Medicine, p 54. Bern, Hans Huber, 1973

187. Krauer B, Krauer F, Hytten F: Drug Prescribing in Pregnancy, Vol 7, Current Reviews in Obstetrics and Gynaecology, p 44. Edinburgh, Churchill Livingstone, 1984

188. Kaltreider DF: Premature labor and meperidine analgesia. Am J Obstet Gynecol 99:989, 1967

189. Deckardt R, Fembacher PM, Schneider KTM et al: Maternal arterial oxygen saturation during labor and delivery: Pain-dependent alterations and effects on the newborn. Obstet Gynecol 70:21, 1987

190. Freeman RK, Garite TJ: Fetal Heart Rate Monitoring, p 1. Baltimore, Williams & Wilkins, 1981

191. Martin CB, Gingerich B: Factors affecting the fetal heart rate: Genesis of FHR patterns. JOGN (Nurs) 5(suppl):30S, 1976

192. Wright RG, Shnider SM, Levinson G et al: The effect of maternal administration of ephedrine on fetal heart rate and variability. Obstet Gynecol 57:734, 1981

193. Finster M, Petrie RH: Monitoring of the fetus. Anesthesiology 45:198, 1976

194. Vasicka A, Hutchinson HT, Eng M et al: Spinal and epidural anesthesia, fetal and uterine response to acute hypo- and hypertension. Am J Obstet Gynecol 90:800, 1964

195. Oats JN, Vasey DP, Waldron BA: Effects of ketamine on the pregnant uterus. Br J Anaesth 51:1163, 1979

196. Caldeyro-Barcia R, Noriega-Guerra L, Cibils LA et al: Effect of position changes on the intensity and frequency of uterine contractions during labor. Am J Obstet Gynecol 80:284, 1960

197. Ralston DH, Shnider SM: The fetal and neonatal effects of regional anesthesia in obstetrics. Anesthesiology 48:34, 1978

198. Matadial L, Cibils LA: The effect of epidural anesthesia on uterine activity and blood pressure. Am J Obstet Gynecol 125:846, 1976

199. Goodlin RC: History of fetal monitoring. Am J Obstet Gynecol 133:323, 1979

200. Adamsons K, Beard RW, Cosmi EV et al: The validity of capillary blood in the assessment of the acid-base state of the fetus. In Adamsons K (ed): Diagnosis and Treatment of Fetal Disorders, p 175. New York, Springer-Verlag, 1968

201. Beard RW. Fetal blood sampling. Br J Hosp Med 3:523, 1970

202. Bowe ET, Beard RW, Finster M et al: Reliability of fetal blood sampling. Am J Obstet Gynecol 107:279, 1970

203. Gibbs RS, Listwa HM, Read JA: The effect of internal monitoring on maternal infection following cesarean section. Obstet Gynecol 48:653, 1976

204. Gassner CB, Ledger WJ: The relationship of hospital-acquired maternal infection to invasive intrapartum monitoring techniques. Am J Obstet Gynecol 126:33, 1976

205. Sola A, Bednarek FJ, Davidson R et al: Meningitis, ventriculitis, and hydrocephalus: A complication of fetal monitoring. Obstet Gynecol 56:663, 1980

206. Lang-Gee C, Ledger WJ: Maternal and fetal morbidity associated with intrapartum monitoring. JOGN (Nurs) 5:(suppl)65S, 1976

207. Modanlou HD, Linzey M: An unusual complication of fetal blood sampling during labor. Obstet Gynecol 51(suppl):7S, 1978

208. MacDonald D, Grant A, Sheridan-Pereira M et al: The Dublin randomized controlled trial of intrapartum fetal heart rate monitoring. Am J Obstet Gynecol 152:524, 1985

209. Cohen SE: The aspiration syndrome. Clin Obstet Gynaecol 9:235, 1982

210. Brizgys RV, Dailey PA, Shnider SM et al: The incidence and neonatal effects of maternal hypotension during epidural anesthesia for cesarean section. Anesthesiology 67:782, 1987

211. Kasten GW, Martin ST: Resuscitation from bupivacaine-induced cardiovascular toxicity during partial inferior vena cava occlusion. Anesth Analg 65:341, 1986

212. DiGiovanni AJ, Galbert MW, Wahle WM: Epidural injection of autologous blood for postlumbar puncture headache. II. Additional clinical experiences and laboratory investigation. Anesth Analg 51:226, 1972

213. Jarvis AP, Greenwalt JW, Fagraeus L: Intravenous caffeine for postdural puncture headache. Anesth Analg 65:313, 1986

214. Brownridge P: The management of headache following accidental dural puncture in obstetric patients. Anaesth Intensive Care 11:4, 1983

215. Standards and guidelines for cardiopulmonary resuscitation (CPR) and emergency cardiac care (ECC). Part VI: Neonatal advanced life support. JAMA 255:2969, 1986

216. Adamsons K, James LS, Towell ME et al: Physiologic observations during induced anemia in utero in the rhesus monkey. J Pediatr 67:1042, 1965

217. James LS, Weisbrot IM, Prince CE et al: The acid-base status of human infants in relation to birth asphyxia and the onset of respiration. J Pediatr 52:379, 1958

218. Adamsons K, Behrman R, Dawes GS et al: The treatment of acidosis with alkali and glucose during asphyxia in foetal rhesus monkey. J Physiol 169:679, 1963

219. Birmingham MK, Elliot KAC: Effects of pH, bicarbonate and cofactors on the metabolism of brain suspensions. J Biol Chem 189:73 1951

220. James LS, Adamsons K: Respiratory physiology of the fetus and newborn. N Engl J Med 271:1352, 1964

221. Adamsons K, Behrman R, Dawes GS et al: Resuscitation by positive pressure ventilation and Tris-hydroxymethylaminomethane of rhesus monkeys asphyxiated at birth. J Pediatr 65:807, 1964

222. Heymann MA, Iwamoto HS, Rudolph AM: Factors affecting changes in the neonatal systemic circulation. Ann Rev Physiol 43:371, 1981

223. Klopfenstein HS, Rudolph AM: Postnatal changes in the circulation and responses to volume loading in sheep. Circ Res 42:839, 1978

224. Apgar V: A proposal for a new method of evaluation of the newborn infant. Anesth Analg 32:260, 1953

225. Rudolph AM, Yuen S: Response of the pulmonary vasculature to hypoxia and H$^+$ ion concentration changes. J Clin Invest 45:399, 1966

226. Harrison MR, Golbus MS, Filly RA et al: Fetal surgical treatment. Pediatr Ann 11:896, 1982

227. Harrison MR, Golbus MS, Filly RA et al: Fetal surgery for congenital hydronephrosis. N Engl J Med 306:591, 1982

228. Clewell WH, Johnson ML, Meier RR et al: A surgical approach to the treatment of fetal hydrocephalus. N Engl J Med 306:1320, 1982

229. Harrison MR, Golbus MS, Filly RA: Management of the fetus with a correctable congenital defect. JAMA 246:774, 1981

230. Anand KJS, Hickey PR: Pain and its effects in the human neonate and fetus. N Engl J Med 317:1321, 1987

231. Gregory GA, Wade JG, Biehl DR et al: Fetal anesthetic requirement (MAC) for halothane. Anesth Analg 62:9, 1983

232. Marx GF, Joshi CW, Orkin LR: Placental transmission of nitrous oxide. Anesthesiology 32:429, 1970

233. Siker ES, Wolfson B, Dubnonsky J et al: Placental transfer of methoxyflurane. Br J Anaesth 40:588, 1968

234. Moise KJ, Carpenter RJ, Deter RL et al: The use of fetal neuromuscular blockade during intrauterine procedures. Am J Obstet Gynecol 157:874, 1987

235. Rosen MA: Anesthesia for fetal surgery. In Shnider SM, Levinson G (eds): Anesthesia for Obstetrics, 2nd ed, p 206. Baltimore, Williams & Wilkins, 1987

236. Harrison MR, Anderson J, Rosen MA et al: Fetal surgery in the primate. I. Anesthetic, surgical and tocolytic management to maximize fetal-neonatal survival. J Pediatr Surg 17:115 1982

237. Shnider SM, Webster GM: Maternal and fetal hazards of surgery during pregnancy. Am J Obstet Gynecol 92:891, 1965

238. Brodsky JB, Cohen EN, Brown BW Jr et al: Surgery during pregnancy and fetal outcome. Am J Obstet Gynecol 138:1165, 1980

239. Levine W, Diamond B: Surgical procedures during pregnancy. Am J Obstet Gynecol 81:1046, 1962

240. Babaknia A, Parsa H, Woodruff JD: Appendicitis during pregnancy. Obstet Gynecol 50:40, 1977

241. Smith BE: Fetal prognosis after anesthesia during gestation. Anesth Analg 42:521, 1963

242. Duncan PG, Pope WDB, Cohen MM et al: Fetal risk of anesthesia and surgery during pregnancy. Anesthesiology 64:790, 1986

243. Ad hoc Committee on the Effect of Trace Anesthetics on the Health of Operating Room Personnel, American Society of Anesthesiologists: Occupational disease among operating room personnel: A national study. Anesthesiology 41:321, 1974

244. Corbett TH, Cornell RG, Lieding K et al: Incidence of cancer among Michigan nurse-anesthetists. Anesthesiology 38:260, 1973

245. Walts LF, Forsythe AB, Moore JG: Critique: Occupational disease among operating room personnel. Anesthesiology 42:608, 1975

246. Fink BR, Cullen BF: Anesthetic pollution: What is happening to us? Anesthesiology 45:79, 1976

247. Cohen EN, Brown BW, Wu M: Anesthetic health hazards in the dental operatory. Anesthesiology 51:S256, 1976

248. Buring JE, Hennekens CH, Mayrent SL: Health experiences of operating room personnel. Anesthesiology 62:325, 1985

249. Axelsson G, Rylander R: Exposure to anesthetic gases and spontaneous abortion: Response bias in postal questionnaire study. Int J Epidemiol 11:250, 1982

250. Ericson HA, Källén AJB: Hospitalization for miscarriage and

delivery outcome among Swedish nurses working in operating rooms, 1973–1978. Anesth Analg 64:981, 1985

251. Rector GHN, Eastwood DW: The effects of nitrous oxide and oxygen on the incubating chick. Anesthesiology 25:109, 1964

252. Smith BE: Teratogenicity of inhalation anesthetics. Progress in Anesthesiology, p. 589. London, Excerpta Medica, 1970

253. Smith BE: Teratogenic capabilities of surgical anesthesia. Adv Teratol 3:127, 1968

254. Chalon J, Hillman D, Gross S et al: Intrauterine exposure to halothane increases murine postnatal autotolerance to halothane and reduced brain weight. Anesth Analg 62:565, 1983

255. Chalon J, Tang C-K, Ramanathan S et al: Exposure to halothane and enflurane affects learning function of murine progeny. Anesth Analg 60:794, 1981

256. Peters MA, Hudson PM: Postnatal development and behavior in offspring of enflurane exposed pregnant rats. Arch Int Pharmacodyn Ther 256:134, 1982

257. Hienonen OP, Slone O, Shapiro S: Birth Defects and Drugs in Pregnancy, p 516. Littleton, MA, Publishing Sciences Group, 1977

258. Hodach RJ, Gilbert EF, Fallon JF: Aortic arch anomalies associated with administration of epinephrine in chick embryos. Teratology 9:203, 1974

259. Haring OM: Cardiac malformations in rats induced by exposure of the mother to carbon dioxide during pregnancy. Circ Res 8:1218, 1960

260. Grabowski CT, Paar JA: The teratogenic effects of graded doses of hypoxia on the chick embryo. Am J Anat 103:313, 1958

261. Hannah RS, Moore KL: Effects of fasting and insulin on skeletal development in rats. Teratology 4:135, 1971

262. Shepard TH: Catalog of Teratogenic Agents, 3rd ed. Baltimore, Johns Hopkins University Press, 1980

263. Roux C: Action tératogène de la prochlorpérazine. Arch Fr Pediatr 16:968, 1959

264. Hartz SC, Heinonen OP, Shapiro S et al: Antenatal exposure to meprobamate and chlordiazepoxide in relation to malformations, mental development and childhood mortality. N Engl J Med 292:726, 1975

265. Sáxen I, Sáxen L: Association between maternal intake of diazepam and oral clefts. Lancet 2:498, 1975

266. Safra MJ, Oakley GP: Association between cleft lip with or without cleft palate and prenatal exposure to diazepam. Lancet 2:478, 1975

267. Rice SA, Pellegrini M: Teratology of fixed agents. In Baden JM, Brodsky JB (eds): The Pregnant Surgical Patient, p 53. Mt Kisco, NY, Futura Publishing, 1985

268. Drachman DB, Coulombre AJ: Experimental clubfoot and arthrogryposis multiplex congenita. Lancet 2:523, 1962

269. Sturrock JE, Nunn JF: Cytotoxic effects of procaine, lignocaine and bupivacaine. Br J Anaesth 51:273, 1979

270. Basford AB, Fink BR: The teratogenicity of halothane in the rat. Anesthesiology 29:1167, 1968

271. Wharton RS, Mazze RI, Wilson AI: Reproduction and fetal development in mice chronically exposed to enflurane. Anesthesiology 54:505, 1981

272. Mazze RI, Wilson AI, Rice SA et al: Effects of isoflurane on reproduction and fetal development in mice. Anesth Analg 63:249, 1984

273. Mazze RI, Fujinaga M, Rice SA et al: Reproductive and teratogenic effects of nitrous oxide, halothane, isoflurane and enflurane in Sprague-Dawley rats. Anesthesiology 64:339, 1986

274. Fink BR, Shepard TH, Blandau RJ: Teratogenic activity of nitrous oxide. Nature 214:146, 1967

275. Smith BE, Gaub MI, Moya F: Teratogenic effects of anesthetic agents: Nitrous oxide. Anesth Analg 44:726, 1965

276. Vieira E, Cleaton-Jones P, Austin JC et al: Effects of low concentrations of nitrous oxide on rat fetuses. Anesth Analg 59:175, 1980

277. Pope WDB, Halsey MJ, Lansdown ABG et al: Fetotoxicity in rats following chronic exposure to halothane, nitrous oxide or methoxyflurane. Anesthesiology 48:11, 1978

278. Mazze RI, Wilson AI, Rice SA et al: Reproduction and fetal development in mice chronically exposed to nitrous oxide. Teratology 26:11, 1982

279. Chanarin I: Cobalamins and nitrous oxide: A review. J Clin Pathol 33:909, 1980

280. Koblin DD, Waskell L, Watson JE, et al: Nitrous oxide inactivates methionine synthetase in human liver. Anesth Analg 61:75, 1982

281. Baden JM, Serra M, Mazze RI: Inhibition of fetal methionine synthase by nitrous oxide. Br J Anaesth 56:523, 1984

282. Nunn JF, Chanarin I: Nitrous oxide inactivates methionine synthetase. In Eger EI II (ed): Nitrous Oxide/N$_2$O, p 221. New York, Elsevier-Dutton, 1985

283. Eger EL II: Should we not use nitrous oxide? In: Eger EI II (ed): Nitrous Oxide/N$_2$O, p 339. New York, Elsevier-Dutton, 1985

284. Nunn JF, Sharer NM, Battiglieri T et al: Effect of short-term administration of nitrous oxide on plasma concentration of methionine, tryptophan, phenylalanine, and S-adenosyl methionine in man. Br J Anaesth 58:1, 1986

285. Crawford JS, Lewis M: Nitrous oxide in early human pregnancy. Anaesthesia 41:900, 1986

286. Aldridge LM, Tunstall ME: Nitrous oxide and the fetus: A review and the results of a retrospective study of 175 cases of anaesthesia for insertion of Shirodkar suture. Br J Anaesth 58:1348, 1986

287. Fujinaga M, Baden JM, Yhap EO et al: Halothane and isoflurane prevent the teratogenic effects of nitrous oxide in rats, folinic acid does not. Anesthesiology 67:A456, 1987

288. Nunn JF, Chanarin I, Tanner AG et al: Megaloblastic bone marrow changes after repeated nitrous oxide anaesthesia. Reversal with folinic acid. Br J Anaesth 58:1469, 1986

289. Galloon S: Ketamine for obstetric delivery. Anesthesiology 44:522, 1976

290. Adamsons K, Mueller-Heubach E, Myers RE: Production of fetal asphyxia in the rhesus monkey by administration of catecholamines to the mother. Am J Obstet Gynecol 109:148, 1971

291. Rosenfeld CR, Barton MD, Meschia G: Effects of epinephrine on distribution of blood flow in the pregnant ewe. Am J Obstet Gynecol 124:156, 1976

292. Katz JD, Hook R, Barash PG: Fetal heart rate monitoring in the pregnant patients under surgery. Am J Obstet Gynecol 125:267, 1976

293. Liu PL, Warren TM, Ostheimer GW et al: Foetal monitoring in parturients undergoing surgery unrelated to pregnancy. Can Anaesth Soc J 32:525, 1985

294. Hehre RW: Hypothermia for operations during pregnancy. Anesth Analg 44:424, 1965

295. Kofke WA, Wuest HP, McGinnis LA: Cesarean section following ruptured cerebral aneurysm and neuroresuscitation. Anesthesiology 60:242, 1984

296. Estafanous FG, Buckley S: Management of anesthesia for open heart surgery during pregnancy. Cleve Clin Q 43:121, 1976

297. Trimakas AP, Maxwell KD, Berkay S et al: Fetal monitoring during cardiac pulmonary bypass for removal of a left atrial myxoma during pregnancy. Johns Hopkins Med J 144:156, 1979

298. Bahary CM, Ninio A, Gorokesky IG et al: Tococardiography in pregnancy during extracorporeal bypass for mitral valve replacement. Isr J Med Sci 16:395, 1980

Chapter 46

Frederic A. Berry

Neonatal Anesthesia

PHYSIOLOGY OF THE INFANT AND THE TRANSITION PERIOD

The first year of life is characterized by an almost miraculous growth in size and maturity. The body weight alone changes by a factor of three, and there is no other period in extrauterine life when changes occur so rapidly. Before birth, fetal growth and development depend upon the genetic composition of the fetus, the mother's placental function, and potential exposure to chemicals or infectious agents that can affect mother, fetus, or both. The journey down the birth canal (or through the abdominal wall)—called the most dangerous trip in a person's life—ends the fetal period, and the newborn must adapt to extrauterine life. This change from fetal to extrauterine life is called the period of transition or adaptation

The newborn infant is an infant in the first 24 h of life. This chapter focuses upon the neonatal period, which is defined as the first 30 days of extrauterine life, and includes the newborn period. The most significant part of transition occurs within the first 24–72 h after birth. All systems of the body change during transition, but the most important to the anesthesiologist are the circulatory, pulmonary, and renal systems. For purposes of discussion, the circulatory system refers to the systemic and pulmonary circulation. The pulmonary system refers to the ventilatory system. The circulatory and pulmonary systems are so interdependent that they will be discussed together.

TRANSITION OF THE CARDIOPULMONARY SYSTEM

FETAL CIRCULATION

Fetal circulation is characterized by the presence of three main shunts, as seen in Figure 46-1A. These shunts are the placenta, foramen ovale, and ductus arteriosus. The relatively low pressure in the left atrium and the high pressure in the right atrium result in the foramen ovale being open. The pulmonary vascular bed has a high vascular resistance because the alveoli are relatively closed and filled with fluid and the blood vessels are compressed. In addition, the low Pa_{O_2} and pH increase pulmonary vascular resistance. On the other hand, the ductus arteriosus represents a low-resistance system because it is dilated secondary to a low Pa_{O_2}, therefore, the blood that leaves the right ventricle by the pulmonary artery is shunted preferentially (90%) through the ductus arteriosus and down the descending aorta, whereas only 10% of the output of the right ventricle flows through the pulmonary artery into the pulmonary vascular bed. The pulmonary vascular bed requires only enough blood flow to assure growth and development of the pulmonary tissue, which includes surfactant production.

The placenta oxygenates the blood, which then courses up the inferior vena cava into the right atrium. The right atrium is divided by a structure called the crista dividends, so that this relatively well-oxygenated blood is shunted from the right atrium through the foramen ovale into the left atrium, thereby bypassing the right ventricle and the pulmonary vascular bed. This blood is the best oxygenated in the fetus, and its course progresses from the left atrium to the left ventricle, out the ascending aorta, to provide oxygenation for the brain and upper extremities. Blood returns from the upper body to the right heart by the superior vena cava. Blood in the right atrium is directed by the crista dividends into the right ventricle, where it is then pumped out the pulmonary artery. The pulmonary vascular resistance is high, however, so 90% of the blood is shunted by the ductus arteriosus to the descending aorta.

The clamping of the umbilical cord and the initiation of ventilation produce enormous circulatory changes in the newborn, which are illustrated in Figure 46-1B. The transition of the alveoli from a fluid- to an air-filled state has a mechanical effect on the pulmonary circulation, resulting in a reduced

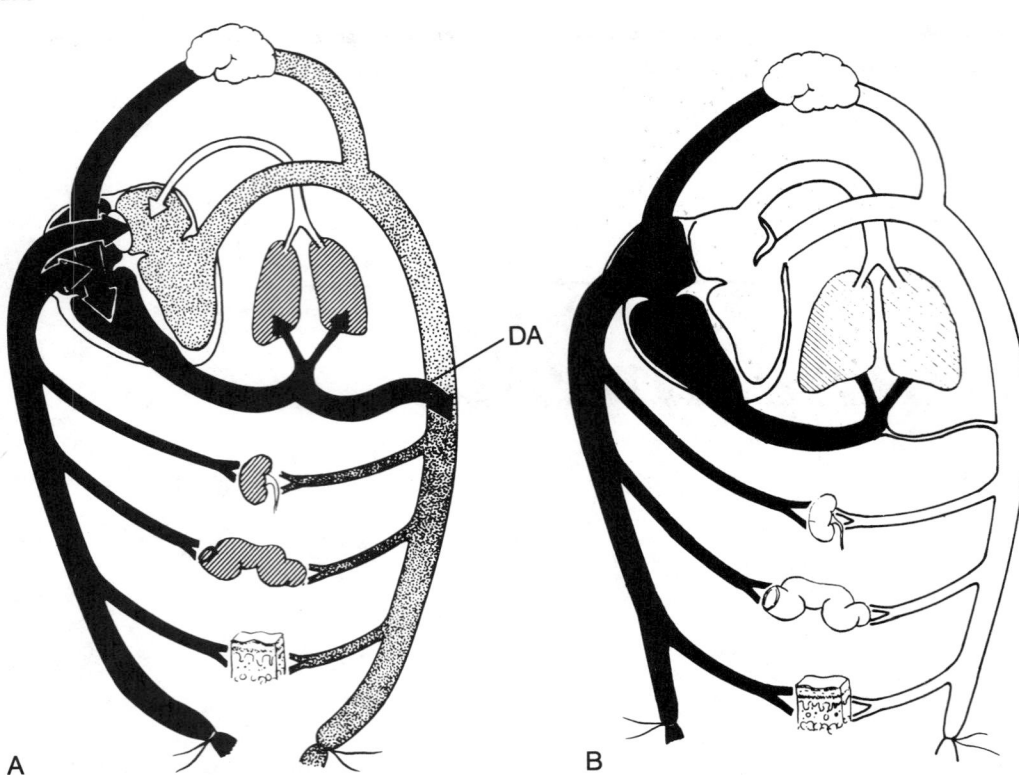

A

B

FIG. 46-1. (*A*) Schematic representation of the fetal circulation. Oxygenated blood leaves the placenta in the umbilical vein (*vessel without stippling*). Umbilical vein blood joins blood from the viscera (*represented by kidney, gut and skin*) in the inferior vena cava. Approximately half of the inferior vena cava flow passes through the foramen ovale to the left atrium, where it mixes with a small amount of pulmonary venous blood, and this relatively well oxygenated blood (*light stippling*) supplies the heart and brain by way of the ascending aorta. The other half of the inferior vena cava stream mixes with superior vena cava blood and enters the right ventricle (blood in the right atrium and ventricle has little oxygen, which is denoted by *heavy stippling*). Because the pulmonary aterioles are constricted, most of the blood in the main pulmonary artery flows through the ductus arteriosus (DA), so that the descending aorta's blood has less oxygen (*heavy stippling*) than does blood in the ascending aorta (*light stippling*). (Reprinted with permission. Phibbs R: Delivery room management of the newborn. In Avery GB [ed]: Neonatology, Pathophysiology and Management of the Newborn. Philadelphia, JB Lippincott, 1981.) (*B*) Schematic representation of the circulation in the normal newborn. After expansion of the lungs and ligation of the umbilical cord, pulmonary blood flow and left atrial and systemic arterial pressures increase. When left atrial pressure exceeds right atrial pressure, the foramen ovale closes so that all the inferior and superior vena cava blood leaves the right atrium, enters the right ventricle, and is pumped through the pulmonary artery toward the lung. With the increase in systemic arterial pressure and decrease in pulmonary artery pressure, flow through the ductus arteriosus becomes left-to-right and the ductus constricts and closes. The course of circulation is the same as in the adult. (Reprinted with permission. Phibbs R: Delivery room management of the newborn. In Avery GB [ed]: Neonatology, Pathophysiology and Management of the Newborn, p. 184. Philadephia, JB Lippincott, 1981.)

compression of the pulmonary alveolar capillaries with a reduction in pulmonary vascular resistance, however, the decrease in pulmonary vascular resistance is relatively slow. It takes 3–4 days for the pulmonary vascular resistance to decrease to the eventual level that it will achieve during the neonatal period. The moderate decrease in pulmonary vascular resistance is accompanied by constriction of the ductus arteriosus secondary to oxygenation. This results in an increase in pulmonary blood flow and an increase in left atrial pressure, so that the foramen ovale functionally closes. Closure of these two neonatal shunts (*i.e.*, the ductus arteriosus and the foramen ovale), is initially only a functional closure.

They usually close permanently by the time the infant is 2–3 months of age. However, approximately 20% of adults have a persistent patent foramen ovale, which may be clinically significant if air emboli occur during surgery.

TRANSITION OF THE PULMONARY SYSTEM

The pulmonary system transition occurs more quickly than the circulatory system transition. The primary event of the pulmonary system transition is the initiation of ventilation, which changes the alveoli from a fluid-filled to an air-filled

TABLE 46-1. Normal Blood Gas Values in the Newborn

SUBJECT	AGE	P_{O_2} (mm Hg)	P_{CO_2} (mm Hg)	pH
Fetus (term)	Before labor	25	40	7.37
Fetus (term)	End of labor	10–20	55	7.25
Newborn (term)	10 min	50	48	7.20
Newborn (term)	1 h	70	35	7.35
Newborn (term)	1 week	75	35	7.40
Newborn (preterm, 1,500 g)	1 week	60	38	7.37

state. During the first 5–10 min of extrauterine life, normal ventilatory volumes develop and a normal tidal ventilation is established. The initial negative intrathoracic pressures that the newborn generates are often in the range of 40–60 cm H_2O. By 10–20 min, the newborn has achieved its near normal functional residual capacity and the blood gases are well stabilized. Table 46-1 lists the normal blood gases for the various periods of life.

PERSISTENT PULMONARY HYPERTENSION (PERSISTENT FETAL CIRCULATION)

The major pulmonary system transition occurs over the first hour of life, whereas the major transition of the circulatory system occurs over the first 2 or 3 days of life. Figure 46-2 illustrates the correlation of the mean pulmonary artery pressure with age during the first 3 days of life. The pulmonary circulation is extremely sensitive to oxygenation and pH changes. Hypoxia and acidosis, along with unknown factors, either may cause pulmonary artery pressure to persist at a

high level, or, after having been at a low level, to increase. The result is termed "persistent pulmonary hypertension." It was previously called persistent fetal circulation, but this is obviously a misnomer, because the fetal circulation is characterized by the presence of a placental shunt that is no longer present. The pathophysiologic characteristics of persistent pulmonary hypertension are a spectrum, ranging from normal pulmonary vasculature that maintains the pulmonary pressures present *in utero* to completely abnormal pulmonary vasculature that is characterized by extension of smooth muscle into the distal respiratory units. There are all degrees in between. In some situations, the pulmonary vessels initially appear to vasodilate normally and later they vasoconstrict. This situation is seen in some infants after repair of a congenital diaphragmatic hernia in which the initial "honeymoon period" during and immediately after operation is followed by episodes of vasoconstriction that may or may not be amenable to therapy. This results in pulmonary hypertension with a right-to-left shunt through the foramen ovale and the ductus arteriosus, as is depicted in Figure 46-3. The persistence of pulmonary hypertension occurs in three main situations in

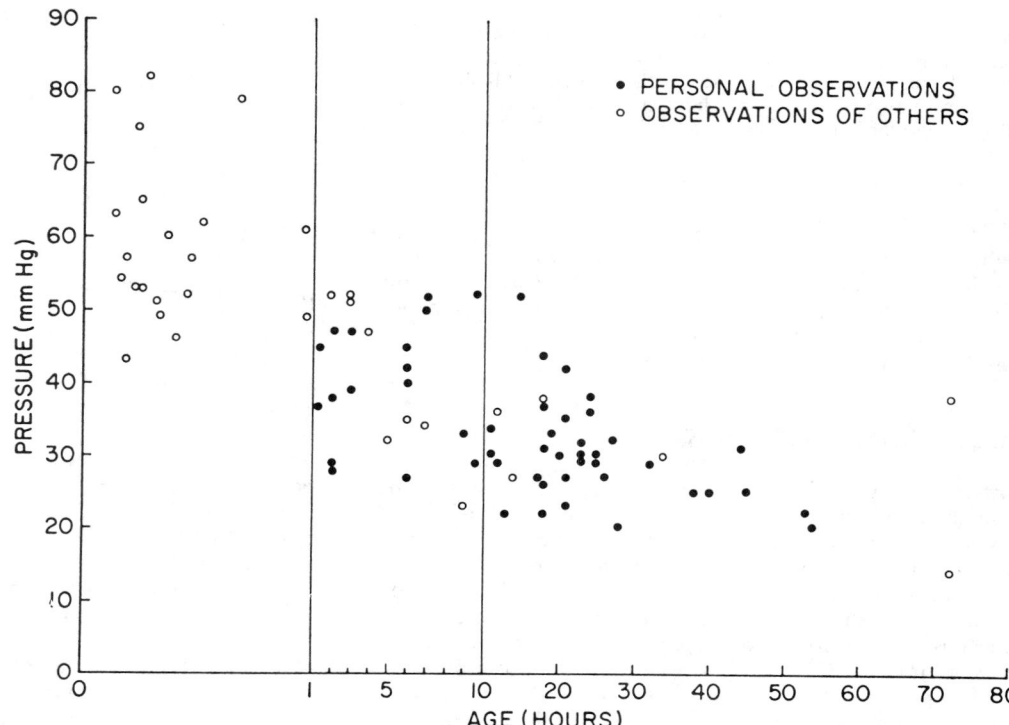

FIG. 46-2. Correlation of mean pulmonary arterial pressure with age in 85 normal term infants studied during the first 3 days of life. (Reprinted with permission. Emmanouilides GC *et al*: Pulmonary arterial pressure changes in human newborn infants from birth to 3 days of age. J Pediatr 65:327, 1964.)

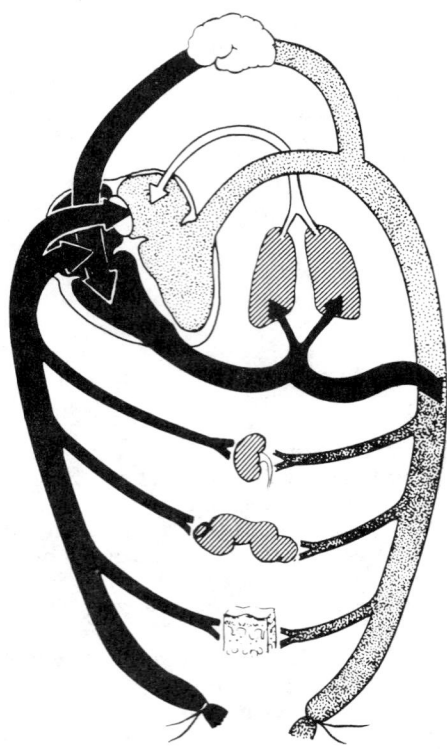

FIG. 46-3. Schematic representation of the circulation in an asphyxiated newborn with incomplete expansion of the lungs. Pulmonary vascular resistance is high, pulmonary blood flow is low (see small caliber of pulmonary vein), and flow through the ductus arteriosus is high. With little pulmonary venous flow, left atrial pressure decreases below right atrial pressure, the foramen ovale opens, and vena cava blood flows through the foramen into the left atrium. This partially venous blood flows to the brain by the ascending aorta. The descending aorta blood that flows to the viscera has less oxygen than that of the ascending aorta (*heavy stippling*) because of the right-to-left flow through the ductus arteriosus. The circulation is the same as in the fetus except that there is no oxygenated blood in the inferior vena cava from the umbilical vein. (Reprinted with permission. Phibbs R: Delivery room mangement of the newborn. In Avery GB [ed]: Neonatology, Pathophysiology and Management of the Newborn. Philadelphia, JB Lippincott, 1981.)

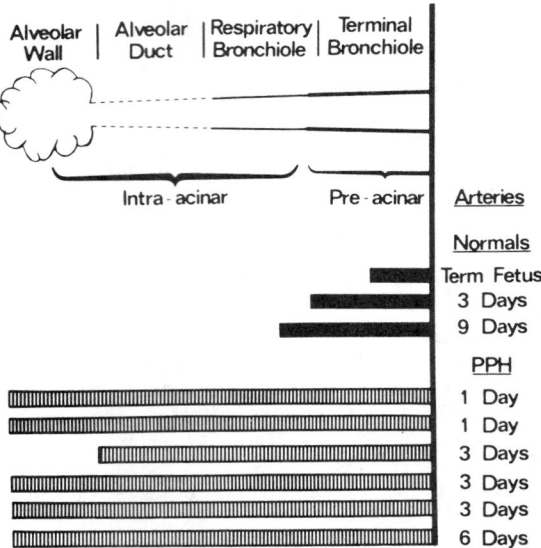

FIG. 46-4. Diagram of muscle location in the walls of the intra-acinar arteries. In normal infants younger than 1 week of age, no muscular arteries are found within the acinus. All the patients with persistent pulmonary hypertension have "extension" of muscle into the small intraacinar arteries. (Reprinted with permission. Murphy JD *et al*: J Pediatr 98:964, 1981.)

which the anesthesiologist may become involved: meconium aspiration, respiratory failure of the neonate, and congenital diaphragmatic hernia (CDH). The pathophysiologic characteristics and treatment of CDH will be discussed in the section on "Congenital Diaphragmatic Hernia."

MECONIUM ASPIRATION

Interference with the normal maternal placental circulation in the third trimester may cause chronic fetal hypoxia. Fetal hypoxia can result in an increase in the amount of muscle in the blood vessels of the distal respiratory units.[1] Figure 46-4 illustrates the muscle increase found in blood vessels of a series of 11 infants who died from persistent pulmonary hypertension. Chronic fetal hypoxia leads to the passage of meconium *in utero*. The fetus swallows the meconium, which ends up in the pulmonary system. It is thought that the meconium, *per se*, does not cause the extension of the muscle

of the pulmonary vascular system but that fetal hypoxia results in the extension of the vascular muscle and that the passage of meconium and the resultant meconium aspiration is a marker of chronic fetal hypoxia in the third trimester. This condition is quite different than the meconium aspiration that occurs during delivery, when, again, fetal hypoxia leads to the passage of meconium. However, this meconium is quite thick and tenacious and mechanically obstructs the tracheobronchial system. It is evident that the presence of meconium may be a marker of chronic fetal hypoxia, cause acute airway obstruction of the tracheobronchial system, or be a combination of the first two factors. At any rate, because it may be difficult to differentiate which condition exists, tracheal intubation and suctioning should be performed on all infants who have meconium present in the amniotic fluid at the time of birth.

PERSISTENT PULMONARY HYPERTENSION AND RESPIRATORY FAILURE

Any infant who has respiratory failure for whatever reason and in whom hypoxia, carbon dioxide retention, and acidosis develop may have persistent pulmonary hypertension. Persistent pulmonary hypertension and respiratory failure have been treated in several ways.[2] There was initial enthusiasm for the use of hyperventilation to reduce the P_{CO_2} levels to between 20 and 30 mm Hg.[3] These infants often require inflating pressures of 40–50 cm of H_2O, with rates of 100–150 breaths · min.[-1] However, there has been some recent controversy over this therapeutic technique, the concern being that it will cause barotrauma and increase the incidence of residual lung disease. Alternate treatments have been used. One of these is based on the belief that oxygenation of the infant is the major concern and carbon dioxide control is secondary.[4] Therefore, if the infant can maintain Pa_{O_2} between 50 to 70 mm Hg, with 5–8 cm H_2O positive end-expiratory pressure (PEEP), then Pa_{CO_2} levels of up to 60–70 mm Hg were accepted. This therapeutic approach has apparently increased the number of survivors and decreased the incidence of residual lung disease. But, the issue has yet to be settled.

An increasing number of reports have discussed the use of extracorporeal membrane oxygenation (ECMO) to treat persistent pulmonary hypertension.[5, 6] The therapy is aimed at resting the infant's lungs while providing adequate oxygenation for survival and lung repair. It is hoped that the rested lung will be able to recover its function by repairing the pulmonary parenchyma and restructuring the pulmonary vascular bed. The lung is ventilated with low pressures, i.e., 20 cm H_2O pressure with 5 cm H_2O of PEEP. As the infant's pulmonary function improves, evidenced by increasing Pa_{O_2} levels, the ECMO is reduced accordingly. This is an extremely expensive and high-risk technique that requires an experienced and talented team. The vascular shunt is performed either through a veno–veno or a veno–arterial circuit. Heparin must be administered to the infants, and this may increase the chance of intracranial bleeding.[7] Some infants have been treated with ECMO for as long as 7–8 days and have survived without apparent complications. As with all new therapies, ECMO represents the last step, and perhaps some of the complications or poor results that occur from ECMO are caused by a prolonged period of hypoxia before therapy is instituted. On the other hand, use of ECMO too early might lead to the use of a major invasive technique in an infant who would have survived with more conservative therapy. It is hoped that the answer will be determined in the future.

TRANSITION AND MATURATION OF THE RENAL SYSTEM

The fetal kidneys and the fetal lungs have certain similarities. During the fetal period, both have a relatively low blood flow compared with that during the newborn and neonatal periods

because both organs need only enough blood flow for growth and development. The maternal placenta removes fetal waste material. The major function of the fetal kidneys is the passive production of urine, which contributes to the formation of amniotic fluid, which is important for the normal development of the fetal lung and acts as a shock absorber for the fetus. The fetal kidney is characterized by a low renal blood flow (RBF) and glomerular filtration rate (GFR). There are four major reasons for the low RBF and GFR: low systemic arterial pressure, high renal vascular resistance, low permeability of the glomerular capillaries, and the small size and number of glomeruli. The low systemic arterial pressure and high renal vascular resistance are the two characteristics that are similar to those found in the fetal lung. This results in a low renal blood flow, which in turn results in a low GFR. Transition changes the first two factors: the systemic arterial pressure increases and the renal vascular resistance decreases. Again, this is similar to what occurs in the lung. The other two factors are changed through maturation. The limited ability of the newborn's kidney to concentrate or dilute urine results from the low GFR at birth. However, during the first 3–4 days, the circulatory changes increase renal blood flow and GFR and improve the neonate's renal function. By 3–4 days, there is a significant improvement in the ability to concentrate and dilute the urine. The maturation continues, and by the time the normal full-term infant is 1 month of age, the kidneys are approximately 70% mature. This is sufficient renal function to handle almost any contingency. The neonatal kidney does have certain limitations. It is an "obligate sodium loser." The renin–angiotensin–aldosterone system is the primary compensatory system for the reabsorption of sodium and water to compensate for the loss of plasma, blood, gastrointestinal tract fluid, and third-space fluid (Fig. 46-5). Although the neonate has a normal renin–angiotensin–aldosterone system, the neonatal kidney cannot completely conserve sodium, even with a severe sodium deficit. Aldosterone facilitates the reabsorption of sodium in the distal tubule. The immature tubular cells cannot completely reabsorb sodium under the stimulus of aldosterone, therefore, the neonate will continue to excrete

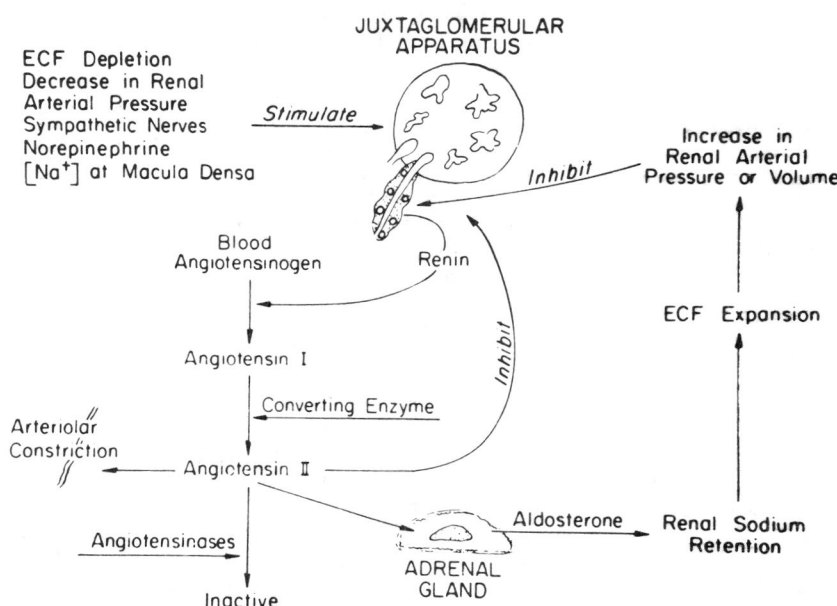

FIG. 46-5. The juxtaglomerular apparatus and control of renin secretion. (Reprinted with permission. Mulrow PJ, Siegel NJ: Mechanisms in hypertension. In Edelmann CM Jr [ed]: Pediatric Kidney Disease. Boston, Little, Brown and Co, 1978.)

sodium in the urine despite what may be a severe sodium defect. For this reason, the neonate is considered an "obligate sodium loser." In the mature state, the distal tubule can reabsorb essentially all of the sodium, so the urine will have less than 5–10 mEq of sodium per liter of urine. In the neonate, this figure may be as high as 20–25 mEq·l^{-1} of urine.

FLUID AND ELECTROLYTE THERAPY IN THE NEONATE

The neonatal kidney matures rapidly. In the mature state, the kidney's ability to fully conserve sodium and water compensates for fluid and electrolyte deficits. The inability of the neonatal distal tubule to fully respond to aldosterone results in the obligatory sodium loss in the urine. Therefore, fluids given intravenously to the neonate must contain sodium. Most operations on neonates involve loss of blood and extracellular fluid, which must be replaced with a fluid of similar electrolyte content. This type of fluid is referred to as balanced salt solution and comes in many forms, such as lactated Ringer's solution. Sometimes infants also lose enough blood that the blood must be replaced. The neonate needs a higher hematocrit (approximately 35%) because of a high oxygen demand and relatively limited ability to increase cardiac output, whereas the 3-month-old infant can easily tolerate a hematocrit of 25%. The other problems of the neonate are those of appropriate glucose administration. Infants of diabetic mothers and those small for gestational age have particular problems with hypoglycemia. Therefore, it is helpful to have a separate intravenous line to administer glucose. Glucose administration should be monitored with blood glucose determinations.

Premature infants and neonates must have full-strength, balanced salt solution for the replacement of third-space and blood losses during the perioperative period. There is a misconception that these infants cannot tolerate the salt load, therefore, they are often given hypotonic fluids. It is not unusual to see premature infants with postoperative sodium values of 125–130 mEq·l^{-1}. Alone, these levels may not be a major problem, but when added to the residual effects of muscle relaxants and antibiotics and with a sick infant, they may result in depression of neuromuscular function.

Premature infants and those with bronchopulmonary dysplasia have problems with increased pulmonary lung water, and furosemide has been shown to acutely decrease airway resistance in chronic bronchopulmonary dysplasia.[9] Fluid therapy should be administered conservatively, i.e., 2–3 ml·kg^{-1}·h^{-1} of maintenance requirement plus the replacement fluid for trauma and blood loss.[10] These infants need balanced salt solution for replacement fluid and more than the usual dose if being treated with a diuretic. Lung function will improve in these infants as they age and mature.[11]

ATRIAL NATRIURETIC FACTOR

There has been recent interest in the role of atrial natriuretic factor (peptide) in sodium homeostasis of the infant.[12, 13] Atrial natriuretic factor (ANF) reduces sodium overload in the body.[14] ANF affects renal function by altering renal hemodynamics and increasing urinary sodium and water excretion; it also increases GFR, which results in a significant natriuresis without an alteration of total renal blood flow. In addition, ANF opposes the renin system. The renin–angiotensin–aldosterone system is a tightly controlled system that imme-

diately activates when there is a challenge to arterial blood pressure as well as a deficit of sodium. Sometimes there is an overshoot of this system and the patient acquires an excessive sodium load. ANF is released from the atria, which causes significant natriuresis as well as inhibition of the renin system. ANF inhibits the renin system at four points: 1) ANF inhibits renin secretion; 2) its natriuretic action opposes aldosterone in the distal tubule; 3) it opposes the vasoconstrictor action of angiotensin II; and 4) it blocks the angiotensin stimulation of aldosterone release from the adrenal cortex. There has been some question about blood levels of ANF and the function of ANF in the neonate. It has been found that in the first several days of life, the neonate has elevated ANF levels. ANF has also been found to be present in the premature infant, and it may provide a sensitive and important system for the control of sodium balance in the premature and full-term infant and play a role in reducing the extracellular fluid volume to normal. Water and sodium balance are usually negative in the early neonatal period. The role of ANF in this fluid shift is unknown. The newborn infant, and particularly the premature infant, has a relatively high extracellular fluid volume. This volume is reduced from 50% of body weight in the premature infant and 40% of body weight in the newborn to approximately 20% of body weight in the 18-month-old infant.

ANATOMIC AND MATURATIONAL FACTORS OF NEONATES AND THEIR CLINICAL SIGNIFICANCE

The neonate has anatomic and maturational factors that have far-reaching clinical implications (Fig. 46-6). The anatomic differences of the neonatal head and airway are as follows: narrow naries, a large tongue, a high glottis, slanting vocal cords, a narrow cricoid ring, and a large occiput. Neonates must breathe through their noses because they cannot coordinate the usual swallowing and breathing mechanics. There-

FIG. 46-6. Complicating anatomic factors in infants. (Modified with permission. Smith RM: Anesthesia for Infants and Children, 4th ed. St Louis, CV Mosby, 1980.)

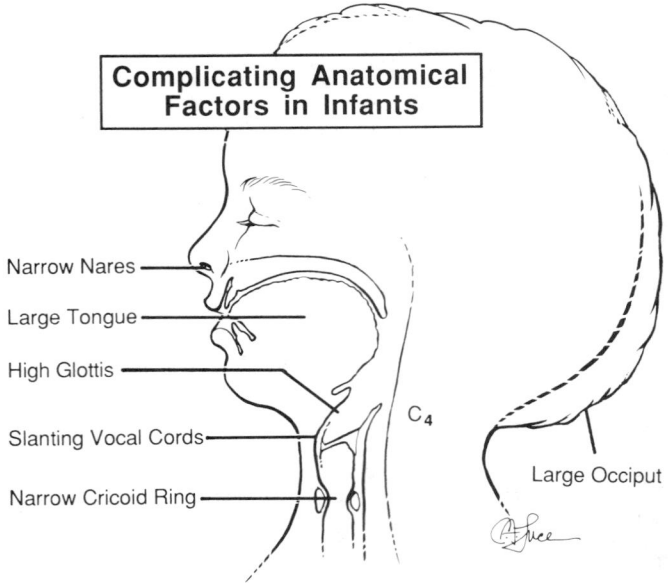

Complicating Anatomical Factors in Infants

Narrow Nares

Large Tongue

High Glottis

Slanting Vocal Cords

Narrow Cricoid Ring

C$_4$

Large Occiput

fore, anything that obstructs the naries will compromise the neonate's ability to breathe. This is why the presence of choanal atresia is a life-threatening surgical problem for the infant. The large tongue occupies space in the infant's airway and makes it difficult to use the laryngoscope and intubate the infant's trachea. In the normal adult, the glottis is at the level of C5. In the full-term infant, the glottis is at the level of C4, whereas in the premature infant it is at the level of C3. The combination of the large tongue and the relatively high glottis means that with laryngoscopic examination it is more difficult to establish a line of vision between the mouth and larynx. There is relatively more tissue in less distance. Therefore, the infant's larynx appears to be "anterior." When combined with the anterior slanting vocal cords, the result is a more difficult laryngoscopic examination and intubation. Application of cricoid pressure by the anesthesiologist or an assistant will help one to see the neonate's larynx. If the anesthesiologist's hand is large enough, he or she can apply cricoid pressure with the little finger (Fig. 46-7). This is more effective than having an assistant apply pressure because the anesthesiologist can determine the best position for intubation.

The presence of a narrow cricoid ring is significant because it means that narrowest portion of the neonate's airway is not the vocal cords but the cricoid ring. In the mature state, the airway from the vocal cords down the trachea is of equal dimensions (Fig. 46-8). If the endotracheal tube will pass comfortably through the vocal cords, it also will not be tight within the cricoid cartilage. On the other hand, the neonate's laryngeal structures resemble a funnel; even though the endotracheal tube may pass through the vocal cords, which are at the midpoint of the funnel, the endotracheal tube may be tight within the cricoid ring.[15] This tight fit may cause either temporary or permanent damage to the cricoid cartilage, resulting in either short-term or long-term airway difficulties. When the infant has a large occiput, this results in the head being flexed forward onto the chest when the infant is lying in the supine position with the head in the midline (Fig. 46-9A). Extreme extension can also obstruct the airway so that a midposition of the head with slight extension is preferred for airway maintenance. This is accomplished by placing a small roll at the base of the neck and shoulders (Fig. 46-9B).

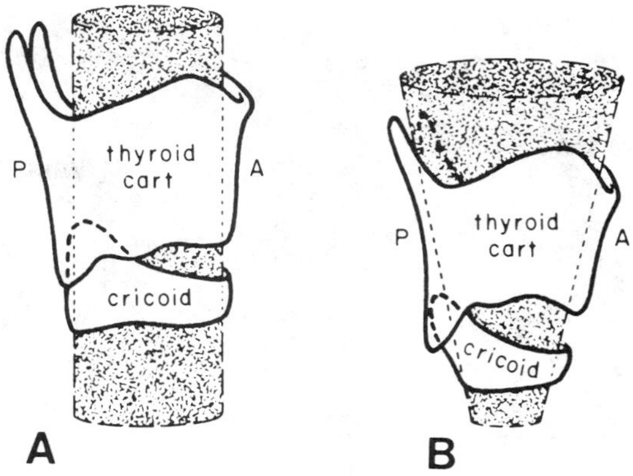

FIG. 46-8. Configuration of the adult (A) versus the infant larynx (B). (A) The adult larynx has a cylindric shape. (B) The infant larynx is funnel shaped because of narrow, undeveloped cricoid cartilage. (Reprinted with permission. Ryan JF, Todres ID, Cote, CJ et al [eds]: A Practice of Anesthesia for Infants and Children. Orlando, Grune & Stratton, 1986.)

ANATOMIC AND PHYSIOLOGIC FACTORS OF THE PULMONARY SYSTEM

The neonate's pulmonary system has at least four anatomic and physiologic differences from that of the mature infant: a high oxygen consumption, high closing volumes, a high minute ventilation to functional residual capacity (FRC) ratio, and pliable ribs. The oxygen consumption of the infant is $7-9$ ml·kg^{-1}·min^{-1}, whereas in the mature state it is 3 ml·kg^{-1}·min.$^{-1}$ Therefore, varying degrees of airway obstruction have more impact on oxygen delivery and reserve for the neonate. The neonate, infant, and child require high oxygen consumption for growth and development, but in terms of supplying oxygen during periods of airway compromise, it is a distinct disadvantage. Because of the high oxygen consump-

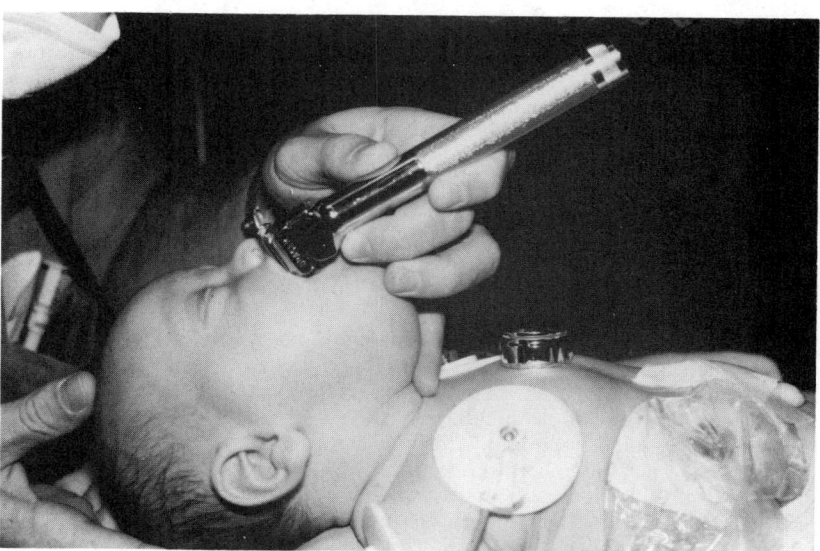

FIG. 46-7. Cricoid pressure applied with little finger. (Reprinted with permission. Berry FA [ed]: Anesthetic Management of Difficult and Routine Pediatric Patients. New York, Churchill Livingstone, 1986.)

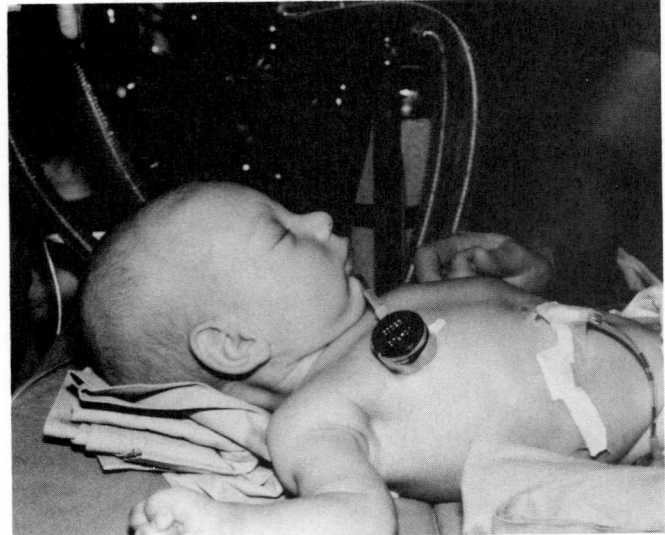

A

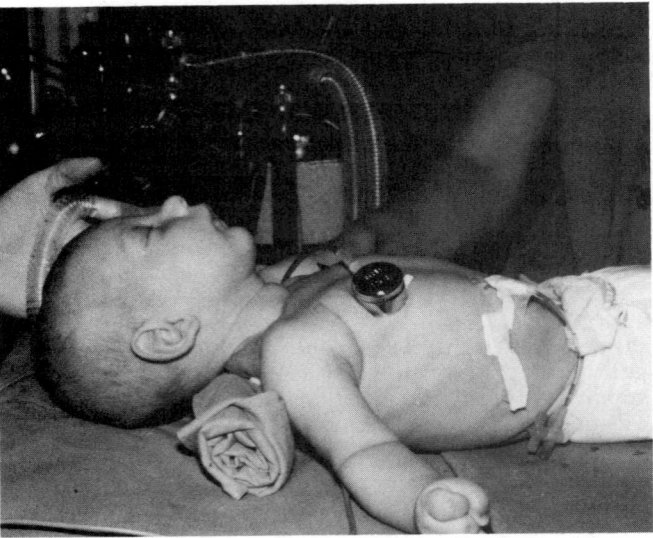

B

FIG. 46-9. (A) Pad under occiput in an attempt to obtain the "sniffing" position obstructs the infant's airway. (Reprinted with permission. Berry FA [ed]: Anesthetic Management of Difficult and Routine Pediatric Patients. New York, Churchill Livingstone, 1986.) (B) Pad is placed under infant's neck to improve the airway patency and for laryngoscopic examination. (Reprinted with permission. Berry FA [ed]: Anesthetic Management of Difficult and Routine Pediatric Patients. New York, Churchill Livingstone, 1986.)

tion, apnea in an infant uses up the residual oxygen in the lungs much more quickly than in the older child and adult.

The high closing volumes of the neonate's lungs are within the lower range of the normal tidal volume (Fig. 46-10). This is also true of the elderly patient. Closing volumes are the lung volumes at which alveoli close, resulting in the shunting of blood by a closed alveolus. If an infant experiences mild laryngospasm and a reduction in lung volume, the larger closing volumes will contribute to shunting of blood and rapid desaturation. When a high oxygen consumption is combined with high closing volumes in the presence of laryngospasm, the rapidity with which desaturation occurs is not only breathtaking for the infant but also for the anesthesiologist. When coughing, breathholding, and so on occur when an endotracheal tube is in place, the situation is not much different, because there is an inability to ventilate the alveoli. Positive pressure will ventilate the large airways, but there will be no oxygen delivery to the closed alveoli. Therefore, even though an endotracheal tube may be in the appropriate anatomic location, severe desaturation can occur in infants who are lightly anesthetized and are coughing on the endotracheal tube. At times, because of the inability to oxygenate the infant, it might be incorrectly believed that the endotracheal tube has come out of the trachea. Management of the patient in this situation should involve deepening the anesthetic or paralysis. The bottom line is that the infant needs either depression of the central nervous system or paralysis of the muscles. This can be done with either small intravenous doses of succinylcholine $0.5 \text{ mg} \cdot \text{kg}^{-1}$ or intravenous lidocaine $1.5 \text{ mg} \cdot \text{kg}^{-1}$.

The third unique pulmonary feature of the neonate is the high minute ventilation to FRC ratio, which is similar to that of the term pregnant woman, but which occurs for different reasons. The pregnant patient has a reduction in FRC because of the elevation of the diaphragm by the uterus. The neonate has an increased alveolar ventilation because of the need to increase oxygen delivery secondary to the high oxygen consumption. Table 46-2 gives the normal respiratory values for the newborn compared with those for the adult.

It is important to remember that the tidal ventilation for an infant is the same in $\text{ml} \cdot \text{kg}^{-1}$ as for the adult; therefore, with an oxygen consumption that is three times greater, a respiratory rate is needed that is three times greater, which results in an alveolar ventilation that is three times greater. The result is that the ratio of minute ventilation to FRC is 5:1 in the neonate, whereas in older patients it is 1.5:1. The clinical implication of the high minute ventilation to FRC ratio is that there is a much more rapid induction of inhalation anesthesia, as well as more rapid awakening from inhalation anesthesia. The more rapid induction of anesthesia also results from a higher percentage of the neonate's body weight consisting of vessel-rich tissues.[16] Figure 46-11 compares the predicted versus observed ratio of end-tidal to inspired halothane in infants and adults. The practical implication of Figure 46-11 is that clinicians who use the adult curve and the usual overpressure of halothane (approximately 3% inspired) for induction will find the neonate more rapidly induced and perhaps at risk for an overdose of anesthetic. This will be discussed later in the chapter, under Uptake and Distribution of Anesthetic Agents.

The fourth anatomic difference of the neonate is a pliable rib cage. Normal, quiet ventilation in the neonate has similar physical appearances to that of the older child. However, if there is a need for increased minute ventilation, requiring an increase in respiratory frequency or tidal volume, the pliable ribs of the neonate will be a disadvantage. The neonate's diaphragm is the major ventilatory muscle. In order to increase oxygen delivery by either an increase in frequency or excursion, the contraction of the diaphragm results in greater negative intrathoracic pressures. In mature patients with a fixed rib cage, this results in an increase in air movement. However, with a pliable rib cage, the resulting increases in negative intrathoracic pressure result in retractions of ribs as well as retraction in the subcostal and supraclavicular area. This results in less efficient ventilation and a high energy price for the effort involved. This is one of the reasons why neonates are susceptible to fatigue with airway obstruction, pneumonia, and any other condition that results in interference

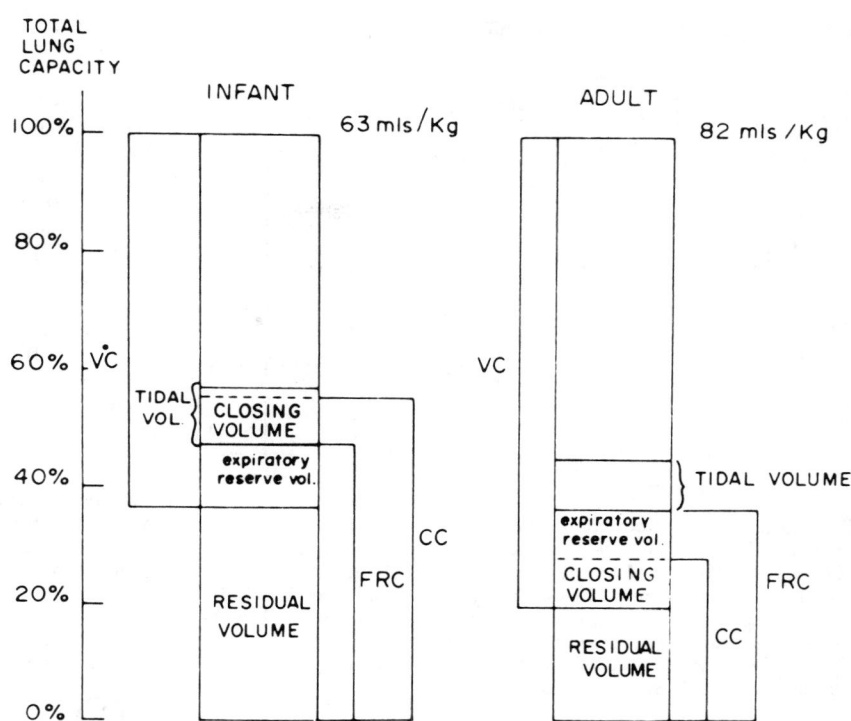

FIG. 46-10. Static lung volumes of infants and adults. (Reprinted with permission. Smith CA, Nelson NM: Physiology of the Newborn Infant, 4th ed. Springfield, IL, Charles C Thomas, 1976.)

TABLE 46-2. Comparison of Normal Respiratory Values of Infant *Versus* Adult

	INFANT	ADULT
Respiratory frequency	30–50	12–16
Tidal volume (ml · kg^{-1})	7	7
Dead space (ml · kg^{-1})	2–2.5	2.2
Alveolar ventilation (ml · kg^{-1} · min^{-1})	100–150	60
Functional residual capacity (ml · kg^{-1})	27–30	30
Oxygen consumption (ml · kg^{-1} · min^{-1})	7–9	3

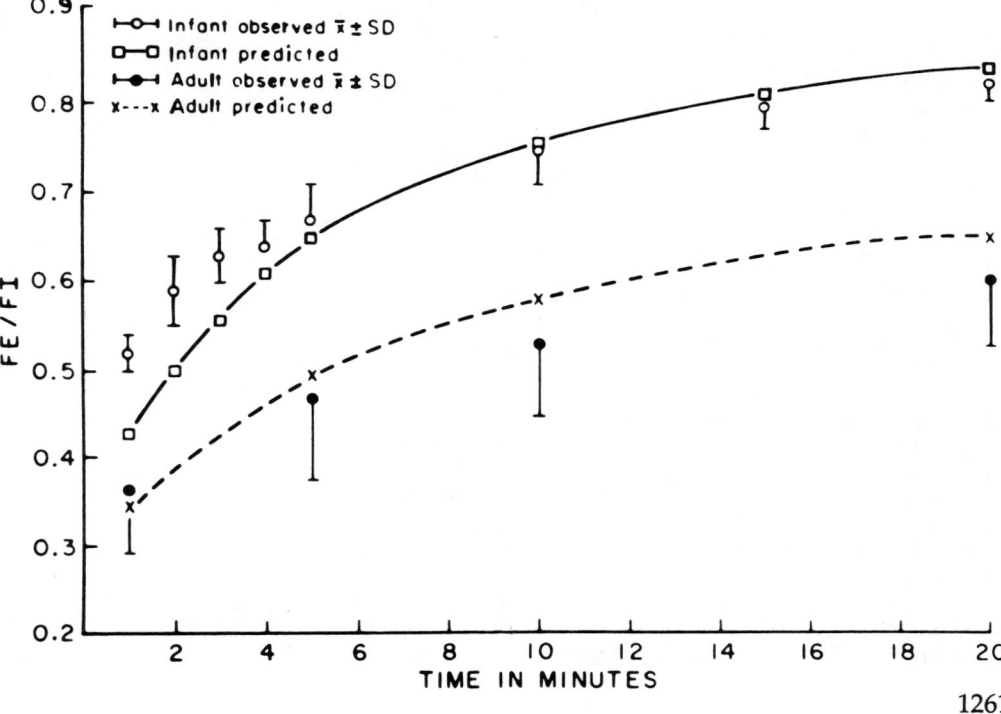

FIG. 46-11. Predicted *versus* observed FE/FI for halothane in infants and adults. Predicted FE/FI values are those generated by a computer program of anesthetic uptake and distribution. In infants, the minute ventilation averaged 1.9 l; in adults, 6.9 l. The inspired fraction of halothane was 0.5% in both cases. (Reprinted with permission. Brandom BW, Brandom RB, Cook DR: Uptake of halothane in infants. Anesth Analg 62:404, 1983.)

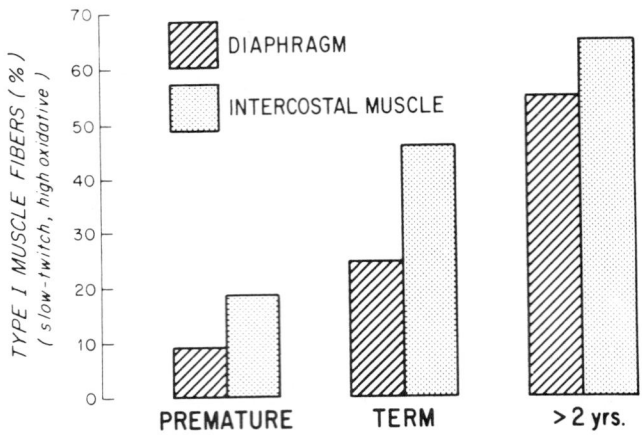

FIG. 46-12. Muscle fiber composition of diaphragm and intercostal muscles related to age. The premature infant's diaphragm and intercostal muscles have fewer type 1 fibers compared with those of newborns and older children. The data suggest a possible mechanism for early fatigue in premature and term infants when the effort of breathing is increased. (Reprinted with permission. Ryan JF, Todres ID, Cote CJ et al [eds]: A Practice of Anesthesia for Infants and Children. Orlando, Grune & Stratton, 1986.)

with pulmonary function; another reason is the immaturity of the muscles.

MATURATION OF RESPIRATORY MUSCLES

There are two types of muscles: Type 1, slow-twitch, high oxidative muscles, which are necessary for sustained muscle activity; and Type 2, fast-twitch, low oxidative muscles, which have an immediate but short activity.[17] The development of Type 1 muscles is necessary for sustained ventilatory activity. The premature infant has 10% Type 1 and the newborn 25% Type 1 muscles in the diaphragm, which is the primary muscle for ventilation (Fig. 46-12). The infant achieves maturity of Type 1 muscles at approximately 8 months of age. At that point, he or she will have approximately 55% Type 1 muscles. The intercostal muscles are the other ventilatory muscles. The premature infant has 20% Type 1 intercostal muscles and the newborn, 46%. The age of maturity for these muscles is 2 months, when there will be 65% Type 1 muscles.

MATURATION OF THE CARDIOVASCULAR SYSTEM

THE HEART AND SYMPATHETIC NERVOUS SYSTEM

The ability of the neonate's immature cardiovascular system to respond to stress is limited by the relatively low contractile mass per gram of cardiac tissue, which results in a limited ability to increase myocardial contractility, as well as a reduction in the compliance of the ventricle.[18] The clinical implication of this limited stretchability or compliance of the ventricle means that, although there may be some ability to increase stroke volume, it is extremely limited. Therefore, any need to increase cardiac output must be accomplished by an increase in heart rate. For this reason, the infant is said to be "rate dependent" for its cardiac output. Thus, any slowing of the heart rate is reflected in a reduction in cardiac output. This is why bradycardia has such serious consequences for the infant. The major cause of bradycardia in an infant is hypoxia. The second major cause is vagal stimulation. Even in the absence of stress, the neonatal heart has a limited ability to increase cardiac output as compared with the mature heart (Fig. 46-13). The resting cardiac output of the immature heart is very close to the maximal cardiac output, so there is a very limited reserve.[19] The mature heart can increase cardiac output by 300%, whereas the immature heart can only increase cardiac output by 30%–40%.

In summary, the neonatal heart has some significant limitations and disadvantages. The resting cardiac output is much

FIG. 46-13. Schema of reduced cardiac reserve in fetal and newborn animal hearts compared with adult hearts. (A) In the newborn infant, resting cardiac muscle performance is close to a peak of ventricular function because of limitations in diastolic, systolic, and heart rate reserve. (B) Similarly, pump reserve early in life is limited by these factors as well as by much higher resting cardiac output relative to body weight, compared with that in adults. (Reprinted with permission. Friedman G: J Pediatr 106:700, 1985.)

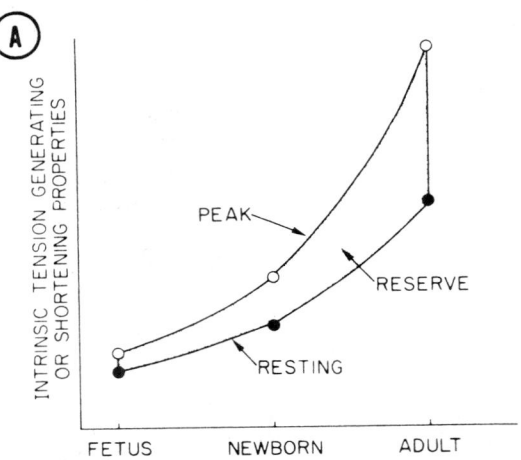

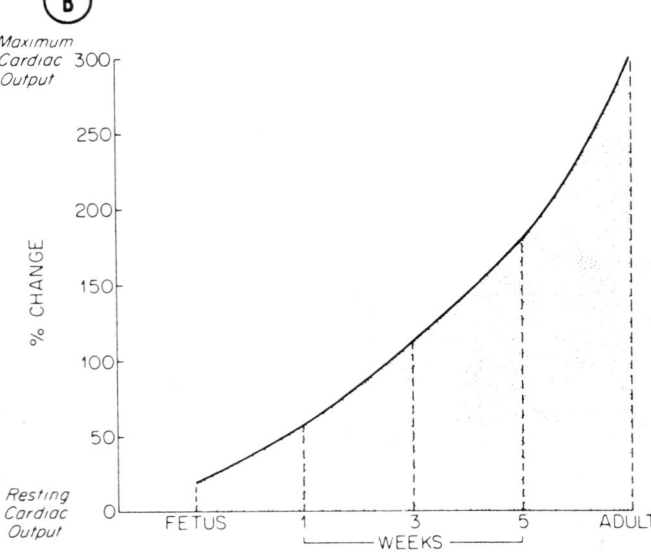

higher relative to body weight. The neonatal heart is less able to handle a volume or pressure change. Stimulation of the myocardium produces a limited increase in contractility and cardiac output. The sympathetic nervous system, which usually provides the important chronotropic and inotropic support to the mature circulation during stress, due to its immaturity, is severely limited in the neonate.

THE BARORESPONSE

An immaturity of the baroresponse, a reflex tachycardia in response to hypotension, has been demonstrated in baby rabbits.[20] Therefore, the immaturity of this reflex would limit the neonate's ability to compensate for hypotension. In addition, the baroresponse of the neonate is more depressed than that of the adult at the same level of anesthesia.

ANESTHESIA FOR THE NEONATE

PREMEDICATION

There is controversy about the need for premedication with anticholinergics. Some people believe that the administration of atropine will override the warning of bradycardia that accompanies hypoxia. This concern has been somewhat reduced by the recent development of the pulse oximeter, which is a reasonably accurate and dependable indicator of oxygen saturation. There are also those who believe that anticholinergics should be administered to prevent reflex bradycardia. Some anesthesiologists also prefer to give anticholinergics to prevent bradycardia after the intravenous administration of succinylcholine, particularly if a repeat injection of the muscle relaxant is required.

One of the major indications for anticholinergics is to reduce secretions. The management of the combination of a difficult infant airway and excessive secretions can be simplified by reducing secretions. The dose of atropine in the neonate is $0.02 \text{ mg} \cdot \text{kg}^{-1}$ and glycopyrrolate $0.01 \text{ mg} \cdot \text{kg}^{-1}$ im.

There is very little indication for premedicating a neonate with sedatives or opioids. If used, it is important to note that the neonate, as compared with older patients, has an increased sensitivity to the central nervous system and respiratory depressant effects of these drugs.[21, 22]

ENDOTRACHEAL INTUBATION

One of the frequently asked questions about the anesthetic management of neonates is whether or not their tracheas need to be intubated routinely. The answer to this question depends upon the skill of the anesthesiologist and the surgical procedure, but in most clinical situations, the neonate's trachea needs to be intubated because of various anatomic and physiologic considerations. If the anesthesiologist is skilled and the surgery is short, intubation may not be necessary. This is a clinical judgment that must be determined individually for each anesthesiologist and situation. Another question is whether or not to control ventilation of all neonates. If the overall condition of the neonate is healthy and the procedure is short, then spontaneous ventilation is certainly acceptable. However, if the neonate is debilitated, has had a relatively long-standing illness, has circulatory instability, and requires muscle relaxation for the surgery, then intraoperative controlled ventilation of the lungs is certainly indicated.

The view of whether or not to perform awake tracheal intubation in the neonate has changed in the last several years. There is concern that awake tracheal intubation causes hypertension and that the hypertension can rupture the fragile intercerebral vessels, particularly in premature infants. There are times when awake tracheal intubation would seem to be the technique of choice, *i.e.*, in neonates who are critically ill and need resuscitation. Neonates who are persistently vomiting and in whom the stomach cannot be emptied should have an awake tracheal intubation if at all possible. An awake tracheal intubation can be accomplished with topical anesthesia of the oropharynx and intravenous lidocaine $1.5 \text{ ml} \cdot \text{kg}^{-1}$ iv in order to blunt the response of the intubation. If problems of a full stomach and the resulting concern for aspiration are not present, the current trend is for endotracheal intubation after the induction of anesthesia. This will be discussed more fully under the topic of anesthetic techniques. The question of extubation of the trachea is considerably easier to answer. The awake state is associated with control of the airway reflexes. Therefore, the trachea of the neonate should be extubated when awake and reacting on the endotracheal tube. Partially anesthetized infants are susceptible to laryngospasm and its associated apnea. Laryngospasm, apnea, and a high oxygen consumption are a devastating combination that is best avoided.

DOES THE NEONATE NEED ANESTHESIA?

There was some question in past years about whether the premature infant needed anesthesia for surgery. However, the state-of-the-art today is such that the neonate and premature infant should be considered as any other patient who needs anesthesia.[23] Infants perceive pain, and they react to pain.[24–27] There is a concern that the hypertensive response to pain may cause intracranial bleeding in susceptible infants. The selection of anesthetic techniques for the neonate is based on the same criteria as for any patient, while at the same time recognizing the pharmacokinetic and pharmacodynamic differences, such as the volume and cardiovascular status of the patient, and so on. Patients who are in shock and are extremely unstable are resuscitated, and the anesthetic agents are titrated according to the patients response. At times, because of the presence of shock and circulatory instability, it may be that no anesthetic agent is administered and that the initial anesthetic management is that of resuscitation. As the patient stabilizes, the anesthetics are titrated in appropriate doses. This is the art and science of anesthesia that applies to patients of all ages.

WHICH ANESTHETIC TECHNIQUE IS BEST?

Which anesthetic technique is best: nitrous oxide and relaxant; opioid and relaxant; volatile agent, opioid, and relaxant; or any combination thereof? The answer depends upon the knowledge, skills, and experience of the anesthesiologist and the surgical needs of the patient. Rarely is a situation encountered in which one anesthetic agent or technique is indicated to the exclusion of all others. On the other hand, all anesthetic agents and techniques are not the same, and careful thought should be given to selection of the best anesthetic for each patient and operation.

THE IMPACT OF SURGICAL REQUIREMENTS UPON ANESTHETIC TECHNIQUE

Blood loss and muscle relaxation are two areas of concern for the surgeon and anesthesiologist. Parents and health care workers also have an appropriate, enormous concern about the transmission of acquired immunodeficiency syndrome (AIDS) and hepatitis by blood and blood products. The use of blood and blood products should be minimized whenever possible. One of the techniques to minimize blood replacement is to minimize blood loss. This can be accomplished through the control of blood pressure by the various anesthetics and muscle relaxants. The anesthetic techniques used can be directed either at preventing hypertension, which often occurs with the use of nitrous oxide or low-dose opioid plus muscle relaxant, or inducing controlled normovolemic hypotension. Therefore, it is extremely important for the anesthesiologist and surgeon to discuss the impact of blood pressure upon the surgical procedure, as well as the potential for loss of blood. Blood replacement is indicated if the neonate has demonstrated circulatory instability and considerable blood loss (i.e., 10%–20% of the blood volume) is anticipated. However, if the neonate is basically healthy and anticipated blood loss is less than 25%–30% of the blood volume, then blood transfusion probably can be avoided. This will be discussed more fully under the section on fluid and blood therapy. The anesthesiologist can tailor the anesthetic to control the blood pressure and thereby reduce blood loss. This requires an appreciation of the cardiovascular effects of anesthetics and muscle relaxants.

THE CARDIOVASCULAR EFFECTS OF MUSCLE RELAXANTS

Although d-tubocurarine (dTc) does have a dose-related histamine release that causes peripheral vasodilation, the incremental administration of dTc will minimize, if not eliminate, any effect upon the blood pressure. The same is true for atracurium. Pancuronium has vagolytic and sympathomimetic actions that will cause a tachycardia and an increase in blood pressure (Table 46-3).[28] If a neonate is moribund, or in shock, or there is concern about the volume status, then pancuronium may well be the muscle relaxant of choice. However, in a relatively normal neonate with a normal blood pressure and normal blood volume, the use of pancuronium may result in hypertension, which has the potential to increase

blood loss. In this type of infant, atracurium would be a more logical choice of muscle relaxant for short surgical cases, or perhaps dTc for longer cases. Atracurium has certain advantages over vecuronium in the infant younger than 1 year of age. The duration of action of vecuronium is approximately twice that observed in older children, either because of liver immaturity or an increased volume of distribution.[29–31] The length of action of atracurium in the neonate is similar to that in the older infant or child. The infant's neuromuscular junction may be more sensitive to muscle relaxants, and the infant has a larger volume of distribution because of a large extracellular fluid volume. These two effects tend to balance each other, so that, roughly speaking, the dose of a muscle relaxant in the infant is quite similar to that of the child on a $mg \cdot kg^{-1}$ basis. The major difference in neonates is the great variability of response to the nondepolarizing muscle relaxants so that dose response effects must be carefully observed to avoid either overdose or underdose.

However, there is some increase in succinylcholine requirement in the infant compared with the older child.[32, 33] The intramuscular dose of succinylcholine is $5 \ mg \cdot kg^{-1}$ in the infant, whereas the dose for children is $4 \ mg \cdot kg^{-1}$. The intravenous dose of succinylcholine in the infant and child is $2 \ mg \cdot kg^{-1}$, and it is $1 \ mg \cdot kg^{-1}$ in the adolescent if there has been no pretreatment with a nondepolarizer. There is a difference of opinion about the use of nondepolarizing muscle relaxants before succinylcholine administration. Prevention of succinylcholine-induced fasciculations will reduce postoperative skeletal muscle pain. In addition, it has been shown in the malignant hyperthermia–susceptible pig that pretreatment with dTc before succinylcholine administration can prevent fasciculations and the development of malignant hyperthermia resulting from succinylcholine administration.[34] For that reason, this author routinely administers a pretreatment dose of atracurium, $0.025 \ mg \cdot kg^{-1}$, or gallamine, $0.3 \ mg \cdot kg^{-1}$, before the administration of succinylcholine, starting when patients are 1 year old.[35] Fortunately, development of malignant hyperthermia is extremely rare in patients younger than the age of 18 months.

A concern about the administration of succinylcholine in the neonate is the development of bradycardia. Bradycardia will develop in a small number of infants and children with the first dose of intravenous succinylcholine. Intramuscular succinylcholine is not associated with muscle fasciculation or cardiovascular effects. The bradycardia is self-limited and of no consequence unless the patient is hypoxic at the time. However, some believe that atropine should be administered before intravenous succinylcholine.

TABLE 46-3.   Cardiovascular Effects of Muscle Relaxants

DRUG	MECHANISM OF ACTION ON CIRCULATION	CIRCULATORY CHANGES
Curare	Histamine release	Slow administration—minimal Rapid administration—20–30% decrease in blood pressure
Atracurium	Histamine release	Rapid administration, high dose—20% decrease in blood pressure
Metacurine	None	Minimal change
Vecuronium	None	No change
Pancuronium	Vagal blockade, indirect adrenergic stimulation	Increased pulse and blood pressure

Atracurium appears to be the drug of choice among the intermediate-acting, nondepolarizing muscle relaxants. As already mentioned, it does not have a prolonged effect in the neonate. Its metabolism is by Hofmann elimination, ester hydrolysis, and the liver and kidney.[36] Atracurium must be metabolized to be excreted. The metabolites laudanosine and a related quaternary acid are eliminated in the bile and urine. There is some controversy about the dose of atracurium for tracheal intubation. The recommended doses have varied from 0.6 to 0.9 $mg \cdot kg^{-1}$. The recovery time from the action of atracurium depends upon whether or not a volatile drug is used along with the atracurium, because the volatile drugs will increase the neuromuscular blocking effects of atracurium. The use of nondepolarizing muscle relaxants should be guided by monitoring of neuromuscular function with a nerve stimulator. There is some controversy about the routine reversal of nondepolarizing muscle relaxants, because a nerve stimulator indicates only 75%–80% return of function.[33, 37] One opinion is that if the usual time period for the spontaneous reversal of neuromuscular function has been exceeded by a factor of 2, and if neuromuscular function is determined to be normal, there is no need for reversal. The other opinion is that, regardless of time, there is relatively little risk in administering neuromuscular reversal drugs.

REVERSAL OF NONDEPOLARIZING NEUROMUSCULAR BLOCKING AGENTS

In a dose of 1 $mg \cdot kg^{-1}$, edrophonium will achieve a 90% reversal of a neuromuscular block in 2 min, whereas neostigmine in a dose of 0.06 $mg \cdot kg^{-1}$ will require 10 min for a 90% reversal of neuromuscular block.[38, 39] This difference in time to peak effect allows the anesthesiologist to decide which agent is needed. A word of caution: in reversing neuromuscular blockade with edrophonium, the effect is so rapid that atropine should be administered before the edrophonium; and there is some opinion that atropine is superior to glycopyrrolate for this reversal. The dose of atropine is 0.01–0.02 $mg \cdot kg^{-1}$. Neostigmine is a suitable alternate for reversal of nondepolarizing muscle relaxants in neonates. The muscarinic effects of neostigmine can be blocked with glycopyrrolate (0.01 $mg \cdot kg^{-1}$), and the two can be given concurrently. The two advantages of edrophonium over neostigmine are a more rapid reversal and fewer muscurinic side-effects.

CARDIOVASCULAR EFFECTS OF THE ANESTHETIC DRUGS

Opioids are vasodilators but have little effect upon cardiac function. If the neonate is hypovolemic, the administration of opioids may well decrease blood pressure. On the other hand, if the infant is adequately volume resuscitated, then the administration of opioids should have little if any effect upon the blood pressure.[40–43] Ketamine has mild alpha-adrenergic agonist activity and may cause tachycardia and a mild degree of vasoconstriction. Ketamine is a useful agent for the infant who has an unstable cardiovascular system or in whom there is some question about volume repletion.[44–46] The intravenous induction dose of ketamine is 1–2 $mg \cdot kg^{-1}$ in titrated doses and then 0.5–1 $mg \cdot kg^{-1}$ every 15–30 min.

Nitrous oxide usually is considered a reasonably benign anesthetic drug from the standpoint of the cardiovascular system. However, it has been shown in adult patients that when nitrous oxide is combined with opioids, cardiac index and arterial pressure decrease because of myocardial depression.[47–50] A recent study has documented the pulmonary and systemic hemodynamic effects of nitrous oxide in infants.[51] The conclusion of the study was that nitrous oxide did have mild depressant effects on systemic hemodynamics in sedated infants similar to those reported in adults, but that nitrous oxide does not produce the elevations in pulmonary artery pressure and pulmonary vascular resistance that are seen in adults. Therefore, it would appear that nitrous oxide is a reasonable drug in neonates if there is no concern for expanding gas pockets within the body (i.e., pneumoencephalograms, intestinal obstruction, pneumothorax, etc.) or no need for a high FI_{O_2} to maintain saturation.

All of the volatile anesthetics are myocardial depressants.[52] Halothane has little effect on peripheral vascular resistance; therefore, the decrease in blood pressure that accompanies the administration of halothane results from myocardial depression. On the other hand, isoflurane decreases systemic vascular resistance so that the major effect on blood pressure is a decrease in peripheral vascular resistance. The decrease in arterial blood pressure with isoflurane does not result from a decrease in cardiac output but from a decrease in afterload. On the other hand, in the presence of heart disease or a compromised circulation, all of the volatile drugs may have a profound effect upon myocardial contractility and their administration should be monitored carefully.

ANESTHETIC DOSE REQUIREMENTS OF NEONATES

Gregory et al showed that the minimal alveolar concentration (MAC) of halothane decreases with age, but there were only two infants younger than 6 months of age in the original study.[53] Recent work has expanded this information to demonstrate that neonates and premature infants have decreased anesthetic requirements relative to older children.[54] A study by Lerman et al demonstrated that the MAC of halothane in neonates is 0.87% ± 0.03 standard error of the mean (SEM).[55] Infants 1 to 6 months of age have a MAC of halothane of 1.20% ± 0.06 SEM. The MAC of halothane for the premature infant is 0.6%, for full-term neonates 0.89%, and for 2–4-month-old infants 1.12%.[54, 55] The reasons for the lower MAC requirements are thought to be an immature nervous system, progesterone, and elevated blood levels of endorphins, coupled with an immature blood–brain barrier. The neonate has an immature central nervous system with attenuated responses to nocioceptive cutaneous stimuli. These responses rapidly mature in the first several months of an infant's life, along with an increase in the MAC requirements for anesthesia. Progesterone has been shown to reduce the MAC requirements of the pregnant mother. The newborn infant has elevated progesterone levels similar to those of the mother. In a study in lambs, Gregory et al showed that MAC levels increased progressively over the first 12 h of life, whereas the progesterone levels decreased concomitantly.[56] Elevated levels of β-endorphin and β-lipotropin have been demonstrated in newborns and in the first few days of postnatal life. The levels return to adult concentrations by the time the infant is 24 days of age. Endorphins do not cross the blood–brain barrier in adults; however, it is thought that the neonate's blood–brain barrier is more permeable and that the endorphins might well pass into the central nervous system, thus elevating the pain threshold and reducing the MAC requirement.

ANESTHETIC MANAGEMENT OF THE NEONATE

The anesthesiologist has a host of anesthetic drugs and muscle relaxants from which to choose and can tailor the anesthetic drugs to the requirements for surgery and the condition of the neonate. The neonate who is moribund or has a severely compromised cardiovascular status needs resuscitation. If muscle relaxants are needed, pancuronium is the relaxant of choice. As the neonate's status improves, anesthetic drugs may be titrated in. The neonate who has a questionable cardiovascular and volume status needs anesthetic drugs such as ketamine or an opioid. On the other hand, in neonates who have a stable cardiovascular state, the choice of drugs depends upon the type of surgery and the anticipated blood loss. If maintaining a normal blood pressure or controlled hypotension is indicated, a combination of a volatile drug and a nondepolarizing muscle relaxant, such as atracurium, appears to be the technique of choice in the neonate. Nitrous oxide and low-dose fentanyl ($1-3 \mu g \cdot kg^{-1}$) can also be added to reduce the concentration of the volatile drug that is needed.

The administration of high inspired oxygen concentrations to the neonate, especially with low birth weight (less than 1,500 g) and low gestational age (younger than 44 weeks), poses a risk of producing blindness from retrolental fibroplasia. Arterial hyperoxia causes vasoconstriction of immature retinal vessels, neovascularization, and scarring. For neonates at risk, the arterial P_{O_2} should be kept between 50 and 80 mm Hg.

Nitrous oxide can be added so long as oxygenation is closely monitored and expansion of any gas pockets within the body is considered. In the case of intestinal obstruction, the use of air along with appropriate concentrations of oxygen and the volatile drug is indicated. The normal full-term neonate has a systolic blood pressure between 60 and 70 mm Hg. For purposes of controlled hypotension, a blood pressure of 40–50 mm Hg is desired. If there is any problem with oxygen saturation or the development of metabolic acidosis, blood pressure should be increased and a fluid bolus of $10 ml \cdot kg^{-1}$ of lactated Ringer's solution should be given. All neonates with an arterial pressure below 40 mm Hg should be vigorously resuscitated (*i.e.*, with fluids, controlled ventilation, oxygenation, relaxation with pancuronium), and when the patient responds to the resuscitation with an increase in blood pressure, ketamine should be administered in titrated doses of 0.5 $mg \cdot kg^{-1}$. As the blood pressure increases further, opioids can be administered incrementally. The use of opioids and a muscle relaxant can be advantageous when caring for the hemodynamically unstable infant. A recent study on the dose response of fentanyl in neonates having surgery demonstrated that, in doses of $10-12.5 \mu g \cdot kg^{-1}$, fentanyl produced a stable hemodynamic state and reliable anesthesia as determined by the heart rate and blood pressure.[43] The muscle relaxant used was metocurine, because it was believed that pancuronium with its tachycardia would mask the autonomic response to pain. The doses were given in increments of 2.5 $\mu g \cdot kg^{-1}$. In all infants in the study, heart rate and systolic blood pressure decreased with the administration of fentanyl. One of the concerns with the administration of opioids to neonates is the altered pharmacokinetics and pharmacodynamics.[57, 58] In a recent study, $25-50 \mu g \cdot kg^{-1}$ of fentanyl was given to infants, which resulted in an unpredictable effect and postoperative respiratory depression.[57] Four of 14 neonates studied, none of whom had any respiratory impairment secondary to surgery or disease, needed ventilatory support for 11–40 h after operation. All infants had a rebound of fentanyl blood levels. There was a prolonged metabolism of the fentanyl, particularly in

those with an increase in intraabdominal pressure. It was believed that there might be a reduction in liver blood flow and hence metabolism of fentanyl. This is evidence of altered pharmacokinetics. In addition, it also appeared that newborns were more sensitive at the same plasma level to the respiratory depressant effects of fentanyl. This is evidence of altered pharmacodynamics.

Care should be taken in determining which muscle relaxant to use in conjunction with opioids. The reason for this is that the new opioids, such as fentanyl, sufentanil, and alfentanil, will have a cholinergic response leading to a decreased heart rate.[59] Vecuronium, for example, has minimal, if any, effects on heart rate, and when it is used with the new opioids, bradycardia may develop. Because heart rate determines cardiac output, any decrease reduces blood pressure and cardiac output. Pretreatment with atropine to minimize the cholinergic effect or the use of a muscle relaxant such as pancuronium, which has a vagolytic and a sympathomimetic effect, will help offset the bradycardia associated with the opioids. Caution must be used to avoid profound tachycardia (heart rate greater than 180 $beats \cdot min^{-1}$) because this can cause hypertension, increased bleeding, and so on.

POSTOPERATIVE VENTILATION

The choice of an anesthetic drug should also be determined by the concerns for postoperative management of ventilation, as well as the effects on circulation. If the surgical procedure or the neonate's condition is such that postoperative ventilation of the lungs is indicated, the prolonged respiratory effects of opioids or any other drug are of little concern. However, if the surgical procedure is to be relatively short and by itself would not require postoperative ventilation, one should carefully select drugs and doses of anesthetic drugs and relaxants that will not necessitate prolonged postoperative ventilation of the lungs or intubation of the trachea. Postoperative ventilation places the neonate at added risk, from the standpoint of the technical aspects of a ventilator and for the trauma to the subglottic area and the development of postoperative subglottic stenosis or edema.[60] On the other hand, after any anesthetic in a neonate, if there is any question about the neonate's ability to maintain his protective airway reflexes or maintain normal ventilation, he should be returned to the recovery room or newborn intensive care unit with his trachea intubated, and either ventilated or treated with a small amount of PEEP ($2-4$ cm H_2O).

UPTAKE AND DISTRIBUTION
OF ANESTHETICS IN NEONATES

Rapid induction of anesthesia with volatile drugs can cause a greater degree of hypotension in young infants than in older infants and children.[61-63] However, no adverse effects from this blood pressure were reported. There are several possible reasons for this observation. One reason for the hypotension may be that younger infants have a higher end-tidal halothane or isoflurane concentration than may be appreciated, because if has been shown that the uptake of anesthetic drugs is more rapid in infants than in adults.[64, 65] Brandom *et al* reported a study of both computer-simulated and measured halothane concentrations in infants (Fig. 46-11).[66] Whereas in the adult it takes 15–20 min to arrive at approximately a 50%–60% equilibration of the end-tidal to the inspired halothane concentration, the infant will be 70%–80% equilibrated in the same period. The computer simulation likewise documents a higher concentration of halothane in the heart of infants (Fig. 46-14). The same anesthetic concentration would also be present in the brain.

Various reasons for this more rapid uptake of anesthetics in infants have been given: 1) the ratio of alveolar ventilation to FRC is 5:1 in the infant and 1.5:1 in the adult. 2) In the neonate, more of the cardiac output goes to the vessel-rich group of organs that includes the heart and brain. 3) The neonate has a greater cardiac output per kilogram of body mass. 4) The infant has a lower blood gas partition coefficient for volatile anesthetics. In addition neonates have lower anesthetic requirements than older patients.[54, 55] An appreciation of the lower MAC requirements of neonates, along with recognition of the more rapid uptake, suggests that care must be taken not to overpressure the concentration of the volatile drugs to as great a degree or for as long before intubation as would be done with an older infant or adult. The use of the mass spectrometer to determine both inspired and end-tidal anesthetic concentrations of the various volatile drugs can be helpful.

SURGICAL PROCEDURES IN NEONATES

For purposes of discussion, surgical procedures in neonates will be divided into two time periods: the first week and the first month. This time difference is somewhat arbitrary because most of the procedures during the first week are performed in the first 24–48 h, but postoperative care, when the

FIG. 46-14. Predicted concentration of halothane in the heart. The values were derived from a computerized model of anesthetic uptake and distribution. The model infant weighed 4 kg; the model adult weighed 70 kg. In both cases normal ventilation and a constant inspired fraction of 0.5% halothane were used. Tissue levels are given in milligrams per 100 ml of tissue. (Reprinted with permission. Brandom BW, Brandom RB, Cook DR: Uptake of halothane in infants. Anesth Analg 62:404, 1983.)

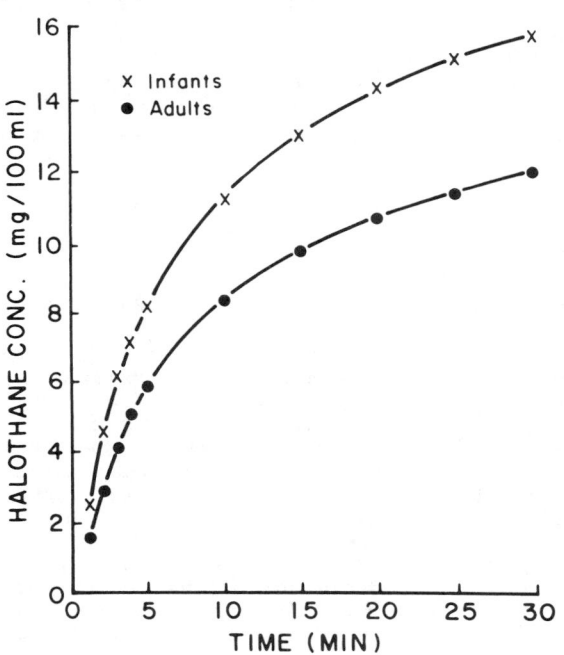

anesthesiologist is often still involved, may extend for several days.

SURGICAL PROCEDURES OF THE FIRST WEEK OF LIFE

The five most frequent major surgical procedures of the first week of life are for congenital diaphragmatic hernia (CDH), omphalocele and gastroschisis, tracheoesophageal fistula (TEF), intestinal obstruction, and meningomyelocele. Some of these conditions are obvious at birth, such as CDH, omphalocele and gastroschisis, and meningomyelocele. It may take hours or days for a TEF or intestinal obstruction to become manifest.

Two confounding factors in neonatal surgery are prematurity and associated congenital anomalies. The presence of one congenital anomaly increases the likelihood of another congenital anomaly. In conditions such as tracheoesophageal fistula, the mortality from the associated congenital anomaly may be far higher than the mortality from the surgical correction of the TEF.[67, 68] Prematurity, particularly when associated with the respiratory distress syndrome, may adversely affect surgical outcome.[69] A neonatologist should be consulted for all neonates with a congenital defect who present for surgery. All of these neonates need a chest radiograph and an echocardiogram. The most serious associated congenital lesion is that of the cardiovascular system. Twenty-five to 30% of infants with a CDH will have a cardiac anomaly.[70] From 15% to 25% of infants with TEF will have an associated congenital cardiac anomaly, and the congenital heart defect is the major cause for death in neonates with a TEF.[71]

Congenital Diaphragmatic Hernia (CDH)

CDH has an incidence of approximately one in 4,000 live births. Despite intensive and often heroic postoperative measures, the mortality in CDH remains in the range of 40%–50% because of the severe underdevelopment of the lung. A brief discussion of the embryologic characteristics of CDH will be given to help the clinician understand the potentially enormous postoperative problems that may be encountered. It will become evident that the defect is more than a hernia of the diaphragm.

Early in fetal development, the pleuroperitoneal cavity is a single compartment. The gut is herniated or extruded to the extraembryonic coelom during the fifth to 10 weeks of fetal life (Fig. 46-15). During this time period, the diaphragm develops to separate the thoracic and abdominal cavities (Fig. 46-16). The development of the diaphragm is usually completed by the seventh fetal week, thereby separating the thoracic from the abdominal cavity. In the ninth to 10th weeks, the developing gut returns to the peritoneal cavity. If there is delay or incomplete closure of the diaphragm or if the gut returns early and prevents normal closure of the diaphragm, a diaphragmatic hernia will develop with varying degrees of herniation of the intestinal contents into the chest. The left side of the diaphragm closes later than the right side, which results in the higher incidence of left-sided diaphragmatic hernias (foramen of Bochdalek). Approximately 90% of hernias presenting in the first week of life are on the left side.

The spectrum for the clinical presentation and outcome from a diaphragmatic hernia is very broad. At one end of the spectrum, the diaphragmatic hernia may develop early in fetal life so that the abdominal contents compress the developing lung bud, resulting in an extremely small hypoplastic lung with no chance for survival. At the other end of the spectrum, a moderately small diaphragmatic hernia may develop late in fetal life, so that the lung is normal but compressed by the abdominal viscera. In between is a great spectrum of possibilities; at the mild end of the scale the infant might have a relatively normal pulmonary vascular bed that develops varying degrees of persistent pulmonary hypertension that may revert to normal. On the more serious end of the spectrum would be abnormal pulmonary parenchyma and abnormal pulmonary vasculature with a very low chance for survival.[72]

After closure of the pleuroperitoneal membrane, muscular development of the diaphragm occurs. Incomplete muscularization of the diaphragm results in the development of a hernia sac because of intraabdominal pressure. The condition

is known as eventration of the diaphragm, and the diaphragm may extend well up into the thoracic cavity. The other possibility is that the innervation of the diaphragm is incomplete and the muscle, atonic. Eventration of the diaphragm usually does not present in the first week of life.

ANTENATAL DIAGNOSIS. Increased awareness of the potential of congenital defects has resulted in intrauterine diagnosis of many congenital defects. Because 30% of the cases of diaphragmatic hernia are associated with polyhydramnios, one can suspect it while the fetus is *in utero*. Also, with the increasingly sophisticated diagnostic capabilities of ultrasound, some diaphragmatic hernias are being diagnosed in this manner as well.

CLINICAL PRESENTATION. Because the infant's status immediately at birth is determined primarily by the oxygenation of the placenta, the 1-min Apgar score may well be normal. The occurrence of symptoms depends upon the degree of the hernia and the interference with pulmonary function. At times, the degree of interference is so great that the neonate's clinical condition begins to deteriorate immediately, whereas in other situations it may be several hours before the infant's condition is fully appreciated. In the severely involved newborn, the initial clinical findings are usually classical. The infant presents with a scaphoid abdomen secondary to the absence of intraabdominal contents, which have herniated into the chest (Fig 46-17). Breath sounds on the affected side will be reduced or absent. The diagnosis can be confirmed by an immediate radiograph. The immediate supportive care is for endotracheal intubation and control of the airway, along with decompression of the stomach. Excessive airway pressure carries a high risk for pneumothorax and worsening of a bad situation.

ANESTHETIC CONSIDERATIONS FOR CDH. There is some difference of opinion about the timing of surgery for CDH. However, all efforts should be directed toward preparing the neonate for the operating room. Whenever possible, the neonate's condition should be stabilized before operation. The anesthetic choices depend upon the neonate's condition. At times, the condition of the neonate is so borderline that only small amounts of anesthetic drugs are tolerated. In this situation, small doses of ketamine, 0.5–1 mg·kg^{-1}, or titrated doses of fentanyl, 1–3 µg·kg^{-1}, are administered. As the infant responds to resuscitation, the anesthetic can be in-

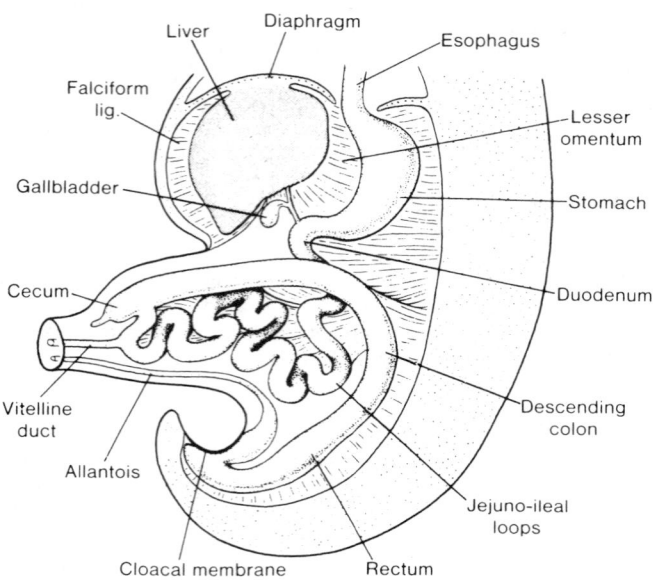

FIG. 46-15. Umbilical herniation of the intestinal loops in an embryo of approximately 8 weeks gestation, (crown–rump length, 35 mm). Coiling of the small intestinal loops and formation of the cecum occur during the herniation. (Reprinted with permission. Sadler TW: Langman's Medical Embryology, 5th ed. Baltimore, Williams & Wilkins, 1985.)

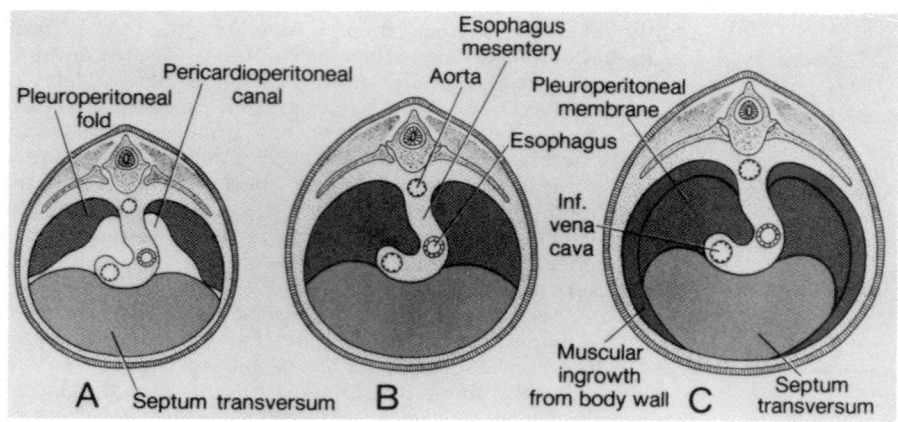

FIG. 46-16. Schematic drawings illustrating the development of the diaphragm. (A) The pleuroperitoneal folds appear at the beginning of the 6th week. (B) The pleuroperitoneal folds have fused with the septum transversum and the mesentery of the esophagus in the 7th week, thus separating the thoracic cavity from the abdominal cavity. (C) In a transverse section at the 4th month of development, an additional rim derived from the body wall forms the most peripheral part of the diaphragm. (Reprinted with permission. Sadler TW: Langman's Medical Embryology, 5th ed. Baltimore, Williams & Wilkins, 1985.)

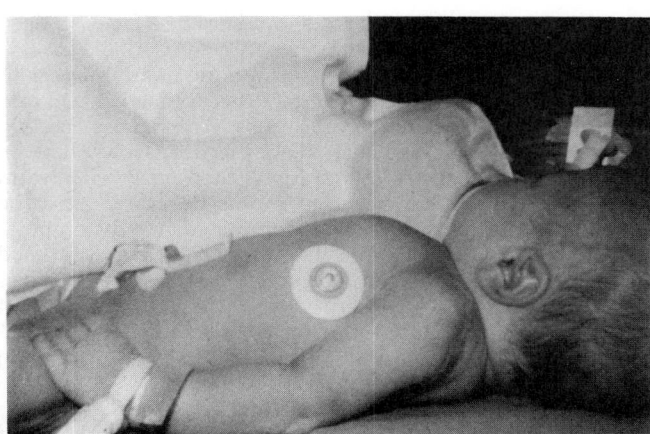

FIG. 46-17. Infant with CDH, demonstrating scaphoid abdomen. (Reprinted with permission. Berry FA [ed]: Anesthetic Management of Difficult and Routine Pediatric Patients. New York, Churchill Livingstone, 1986.)

creased accordingly. After repair of the diaphragmatic hernia, it may be difficult to return all of the abdominal contents to the abdominal cavity. For that reason, use of nitrous oxide should be avoided. After the intestinal contents have been removed from the chest, the lung should be gently reexpanded under direct vision using pressures no greater than 30 cm H_2O. It should be remembered that the involved lung may not reexpand because it is so hypoplastic that it cannot expand. High-pressure attempts to expand the lung may cause a contralateral pneumothorax. This condition should be suspected in any infant in whom a sudden decrease in oxygen saturation or vital signs develops after the application of positive pressure ventilation.

POSTOPERATIVE CARE. Intensive postoperative care of the diaphragmatic hernia patient is critical. Not only will infants have had CDH, but postoperative difficulty can arise, resulting from prematurity or an associated congenital cardiac anomaly. After surgical repair of a CDH, infants will have various types of recovery, depending upon the condition of the lung and the pulmonary vasculature. For purposes of discussion, these infants will be placed into three groups: infants in Group 1 have normal lungs and pulmonary vasculature and will do quite well; those in Group 2 have mildly hypoplastic lungs and reactive pulmonary vasculature and may go through episodic periods of decreased oxygenation; those in Group 3 have severely hypoplastic lungs and abnormal vasculature; these infants have severe problems with oxygenation and hypercarbia from the outset. Infants in the last two groups are candidates for persistent pulmonary hypertension in the postoperative period.

Group 2 infants may have a "honeymoon period," during surgery and in the immediate postoperative period, when oxygenation is improved. However, for unknown reasons, these infants may have episodes of pulmonary vascular constriction leading to a decrease in oxygen saturation. Various attempts have been made to treat infants in both Groups 2 and 3. Vacanti et al described the use of "chronic anesthesia" for infants who demonstrated persistent pulmonary hypertension in the postoperative period.[73, 74] By inserting a pulmonary artery catheter immediately after surgery, they could evaluate the response of the pulmonary vascular bed to pharmacologic and ventilatory manipulation. Infants with an elevated pulmonary artery pressure were paralyzed with pancuronium and given small doses of fentanyl to establish a state of "chronic anesthesia." They found basically two different groups of infants: responders, in whom it was felt the problems were primarily those of vasoconstriction, and nonresponders, in whom the problems were anatomic, i.e., the extension of muscle into the terminal blood vessels of the pulmonary system. In the group of infants determined to be nonresponders, additional therapy consisted of the use of ECMO.[75, 76] The object of ECMO is to rest the lung. Vascular access is accomplished either through a veno–veno shunt or an arteriovenus shunt. There is concern of intracranial hemorrhage because of the need for heparinization. However, in selected patients the early results appear to be promising, particularly in light of the otherwise 100% mortality in these infants. However, the technology is expensive, invasive, and extremely high risk.

Omphalocele–Gastroschisis

Although omphalocele and gastroschisis may appear to be similar, which may cause the clinician to confuse the two conditions, they have entirely different origins and associated congenital anomalies.[77] During the fifth to tenth weeks of fetal life, the abdominal contents are extruded into the extraembryonic coelom, and the gut returns to the abdominal cavity at approximately the tenth week (Fig. 46-15). Failure of part or all of the intestinal contents to return to the abdominal cavity results in an omphalocele that is covered with a membrane called the amnion. The amnion protects the abdominal contents from infection and the loss of extracellular fluid. The umbilical cord is found at approximately the apex of the sac (Fig. 46-18). On the other hand, gastroschisis develops later in fetal life, after the intestinal contents have returned to the abdominal cavity. It results from interruption of the omphalomesenteric artery, which results in dissolution of the various layers of the abdominal wall at the base of the umbilical cord.[78] The gut then herniates through this tissue defect (Fig. 46-19). The degree of herniation may be slight, or almost all of the abdominal viscera may be found outside the peritoneal cavity. The umbilical cord is found to one side of the intestinal contents. The intestines and viscera are not covered

FIG. 46-18. Omphalocele. (Reprinted with permission. Berry FA [ed]: Anesthetic Management of Difficult and Routine Pediatric Patients. New York, Churchill Livingstone, 1986.)

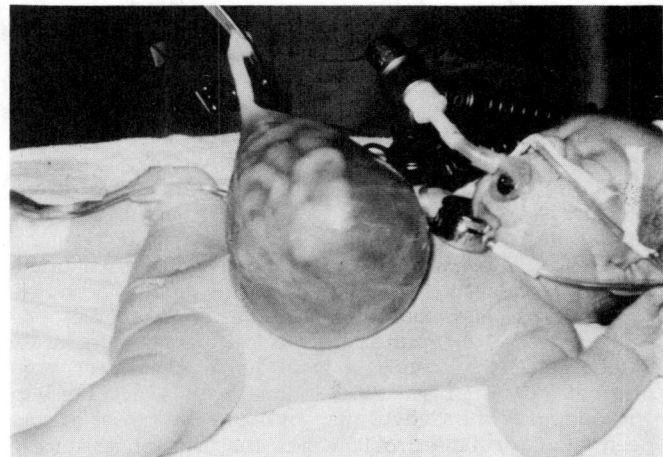

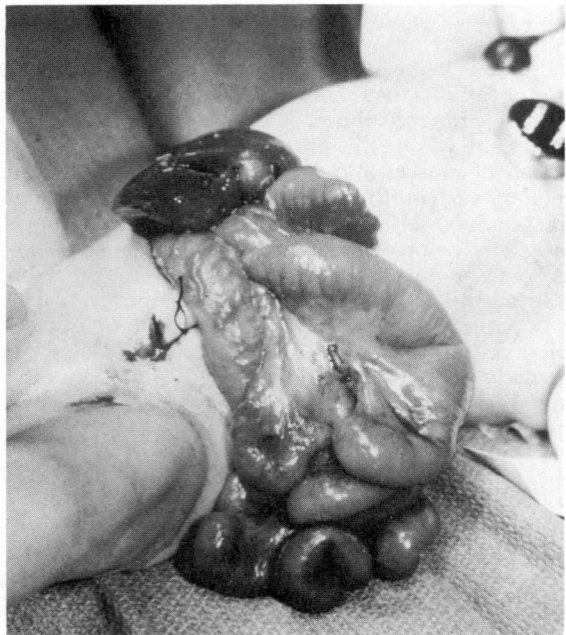

FIG. 46-19. Gastroschisis. (Reprinted with permission. Berry FA [ed]: Anesthetic Management of Difficult and Routine Pediatric Patients. New York, Churchill Livingstone, 1986.)

by any membrane and, therefore, are highly susceptible to infection and loss of extracellular fluid. There is a high incidence of associated congenital anomalies with omphalocele but not with gastroschisis. The Beckwith-Wiedemann syndrome is a collection of problems consisting of mental retardation, hypoglycemia, congenital heart disease, a large tongue, and an omphalocele. Congenital heart lesions are found in approximately 20% of infants with omphalocele. Other associated congenital defects are found with gastroschisis and omphalocele; most involve the gastrointestinal tract and consist primarily of intestinal atresia or stenosis and malrotation.

ANTENATAL DIAGNOSIS. Alpha-fetoprotein (AFP) is a protein present in fetal tissues during fetal development. Closure of the abdominal wall and the neural tube (see section on Meningomyelocele) prevents release of large quantities of this protein into the amniotic fluid. High levels of AFP in the amniotic fluid can cross the placenta and be detected in maternal blood. Thus, abnormal levels of AFP in the mother raise concerns over the possibility of either an abdominal wall defect or a neural tube defect in the fetus, as do high levels of AFP in fluid obtained during amniocentesis. Ultrasonography is reliable in helping to diagnose either condition.

DELIVERY ROOM MANAGEMENT. There is controversy over the issue of mode of delivery, vaginal *versus* caesarean section, in parturients in whom the antenatal diagnosis has been made. Those who advocate operative delivery maintain that it is necessary to prevent trauma to the exposed bowel and that it allows better coordination of the various medical specialities needed for immediate surgical management of the defect. Those who choose vaginal delivery, however, point out that most infants with abdominal wall defects are born without prior knowledge, that injury to the bowel has not been shown to be a problem, and that the convenience of

surgeons and anesthesiologists should not be a factor in decisions regarding mode of delivery.

The aspect of delivery room care unique to an infant with gastroschisis is the need to protect the exposed bowel and minimize fluid and temperature loss. This is best accomplished by "bagging" the neonate, by placing its lower body in a sterile, clear plastic bag. The bag is then filled with warm saline, and a drawstring is used to seal the bag against the infant's body. This fluid must be maintained at body temperature to prevent hypothermia. Use of a protective fluid-filled bag helps protect against infection and the massive fluid loss that can occur with exposed bowel. This procedure is not necessary with omphalocele because the bowel is still enclosed by amnion.

PERIOPERATIVE CONCERNS. The perioperative concerns are fluid loss, infection, associated congenital anomalies, and postoperative hypertension and ventilation. The preoperative preparation of the infant with gastroschisis primarily focuses on controlling infection and ensuring that the infant has a normal extracellular fluid volume. The fluid volume management of the infant often requires enormous amounts of full-strength balanced salt solution. The adequacy of the peripheral circulation and urine output is an indicator of the adequacy of the volume resuscitation. Both conditions may present an intraoperative challenge to the anesthesiologist, because with an omphalocele, after the amniotic membrane is removed, the potential is present for the transudation and exudation of large volumes of fluid from the exposed abdominal viscera. The fluid that is being lost is extracellular fluid, which should be replaced with full-strength balanced salt solution.

If the defect in the abdominal wall is small, a primary repair of the deficit can be accomplished. However, it may be difficult to return the abdominal viscera to the peritoneal cavity. For this reason, nitrous oxide should not be used because of the concern for the increase in the volume of gas in the intestine. Excellent skeletal muscle relaxation is required to allow closure of the abdomen. With moderate-sized abdominal wall defects, it may not be possible to close the peritoneum, but there may be sufficient skin to close the defect. With large defects, the peritoneal cavity may be too small to contain the viscera, and attempted closure can impair circulation to the bowel and lower extremities as well as compromise respiration. A Doppler ultrasound device over an artery in the foot is a useful intraoperative monitor. If primary closure is impossible, a Dacron silo is incorporated into the abdominal wall to contain and cover the abdominal viscera (Fig. 46-20). The repair is then staged from this point onward. Every two or three days the size of the silo is reduced in a fashion similar to squeezing a tube of toothpaste. The infant may feel some degree of discomfort as the peritoneum and skin are stretched. Small doses of ketamine, 0.5–1.0 mg·kg,$^{-1}$ are titrated as the silo is reduced in size. The infant is allowed to breathe spontaneously and without intubation. Oxygen saturation should be monitored with a pulse oximeter, and the infant's pulse and blood pressure are also monitored. These help the surgeon and anesthesiologist to determine the appropriate silo reduction that allows adequate ventilation and circulation. This is a situation that requires clinical judgment. After several stages of silo reduction, the final operation is complete closure of the abdominal wall defect. This requires a full anesthetic with complete muscle relaxation.

POSTOPERATIVE CARE. The postoperative care of these infants is critical. Some require tracheal intubation and ventila-

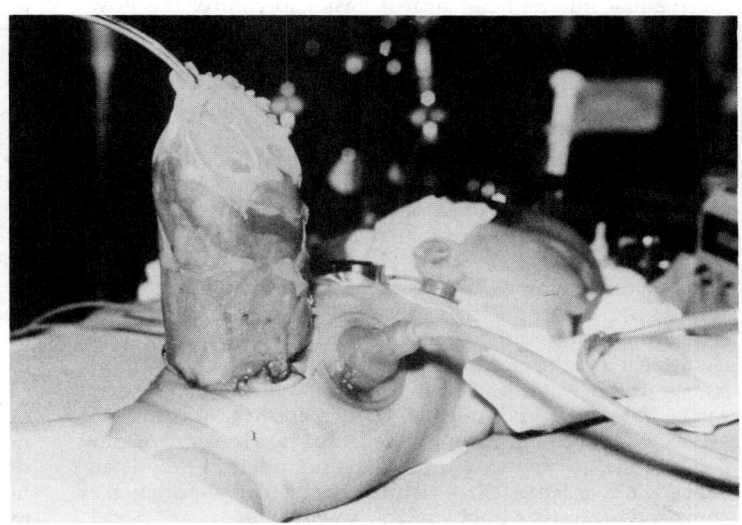

FIG. 46-20. Dacron silo for extruded viscera. (Reprinted with permission. Berry FA [ed]: Anesthetic Management of Difficult and Routine Pediatric Patients. New York, Churchill Livingstone, 1986.)

tion of the lungs for as long as 3–7 days. Additional complications include postoperative hypertension and edema of the extremities.[79–82] The increased abdominal pressure can reduce the circulation to the kidneys, which results in a release of renin. Renin activates the renin–angiotensin–aldosterone system, which is thought to cause the hypertension. The obstruction of the venous circulation of the lower body may cause a large amount of edema of the legs. Monitoring of a central venous pressure is quite useful. These infants require large amounts of extracellular fluid resuscitation.

Tracheoesophageal Fistula (TEF)

The treatment of esophageal atresia and TEF can be both challenging and satisfying for the anesthesiologist. Death in the perioperative period in most patients results from either the infant being premature or having an associated congenital heart defect. TEF occurs in approximately 1 in 3,000 live births. Approximately 85% consist of a fistula from the distal trachea to the esophagus and a blind proximal esophageal pouch. Ten per cent of cases consist of a blind proximal esophageal pouch with no tracheoesophageal fistula. The embryologic defect results from imperfect division of the foregut into the anteriorly positioned larynx and trachea and the posteriorly positioned esophagus, which occurs between the fourth and fifth weeks of intrauterine life. Fifty percent of these infants have associated congenital anomalies, with approximately 15%–25% involving the cardiovascular system.

CLINICAL PRESENTATION. Atresia of the esophagus leads to the inability of the fetus to swallow amniotic fluid and the subsequent development of polyhydramnios. For that reason, if polyhydramnios is present, attempts should be made to pass a nasogastric tube shortly after delivery. Passing a nasogastric tube is not routine in the delivery room, therefore, the diagnosis may not become apparent until the infant is fed. Cyanosis and choking with oral feedings should raise suspicion.

There are two major complications of esophageal atresia with a distal tracheal fistula: aspiration pneumonia and dehydration. The presence of a distal TEF increases the likelihood of reflux of gastric juice up the esophagus and into the pulmonary system. Dehydration results from the fact that the proximal esophagus does not communicate with the stomach. Therefore, preoperative preparation of these infants is aimed at evaluation and treatment of the pulmonary system and ensuring adequate hydration and electrolyte balance. At times the degree of reflux and pneumonia is so great that a gastrostomy must be performed to protect the pulmonary system, and a period of several days is needed to improve the general condition of the infant. However, if the infant is in good condition, an immediate primary repair can be performed. This consists of ligation of the fistula and a primary repair with approximation of the two ends of the esophagus.

ANESTHETIC CONSIDERATIONS. The presence of a gastrostomy reduces the potential for reflux of gastric juice during the surgical procedure. If a gastrostomy is present, the gastrostomy tube should be open to air and left at the head of the table under the anesthesiologist's observation to avoid kinking and obstruction. Not all patients need a gastrostomy, however.[83] There is a difference of opinion concerning the technique for intubation of the trachea. There are some who prefer to intubate the trachea with the patient awake, whereas others prefer intubation after induction of anesthesia. The important issue is to avoid positive-pressure ventilation, which will distend the stomach, thereby increasing the risk for reflux and ventilatory compromise. If an awake tracheal intubation is used, it can be facilitated by the topical administration of lidocaine and with the use of 1 mg·kg^{-1} of lidocaine intravenously 1–2 min before laryngoscopic examination.

There are two approaches for tracheal intubation after induction of anesthesia. One is to use an inhalation induction, then the infant's trachea is intubated after topical anesthesia with lidocaine while he or she is breathing spontaneously. The other technique is to use an intravenous or inhalation induction and intubate the trachea after muscle paralysis. This technique may lead to distension of the fistula and stomach with positive-pressure ventilation. With either technique, topical anesthesia of the larynx may be accomplished by use of 3–5 mg of 1% lidocaine sprayed on the larynx and vocal cords. One per cent lidocaine is preferred to higher concentrations in these small infants because it is easier to control the dose. When controlled ventilation of the lungs is used, attempts must be made to minimize the distention of the stomach and the potential for reflux. If a gastrostomy tube is in place, the point is moot. Alternatively, because the fistula is usually located just above the carina on the posterior wall of the trachea, the endotracheal tube can be placed just distal to the tracheoesophageal fistula.[83] To do this, the endotracheal tube can be inserted until it enters one or the other mainstem bronchi. This is judged by unilateral expansion of the chest and unilateral breath sounds. The endotracheal tube is then slowly withdrawn until bilateral chest movement and breath sounds are present. Or, if there is a gastrostomy in place, constant pressure can be placed on the rebreathing bag while it is attached to the endotracheal tube. The gastrostomy tube is placed under water seal so that the gas bubbles can be seen easily. While the endotracheal tube is above the fistula, the excess gas will course through the fistula into the gastrostomy and out the gastrostomy tube. The endotracheal tube is advanced and, as it passes the fistula, there will be a reduction or stoppage in the gas bubbles (Fig. 46-21).

There is a fear of introducing the endotracheal tube into the fistula. This can occur either during the initial tracheal intubation of the infant or later, when the infant is turned or with surgical manipulation. The clinical indications that this may have happened are increased difficulty in ventilation of the lungs and decreased oxygen saturation. Because these findings are also present when the lung is packed away to perform the surgery, and because there are other explanations for these findings, intubation of the fistula should always be included in the differential diagnosis. Any time ventilation is difficult and desaturation is occurring, the surgeon must stop the procedure and the lungs should be ventilated. The surgeon will be able to palpate the tip of the tube in the fistula if this is the problem.

TEF may occur in a premature infant with the respiratory distress syndrome for whom tracheal intubation and ventilation of the lungs may be necessary. Treatment of the pulmonary condition can be greatly complicated by the presence of TEF. The relatively low compliance of the pulmonary system, coupled with the high compliance of the fistula and the stomach, may result in the anesthetic gas preferentially traversing the fistula into the stomach and upper gastrointestinal sys-tem. The result is both a decrease in ventilation, as well as the possibility of regurgitation and aspiration and the potential for gastric and intestinal distension and perforation. Presence of the gastrostomy will reduce the chances of the latter problem occurring. At times, however, these infants may require ligation of the fistula in order to improve ventilation for the respiratory distress syndrome. A technique has been described for placement of a Fogarty catheter in the fistula until ligation can be accomplished.[84]

POSTOPERATIVE CARE. Although there have been great advances in the treatment of TEF and esophageal atresia, postoperative care can be complicated by associated congenital heart disease, respiratory distress syndrome, and a need for continued postoperative ventilation. The anesthetic techniques often consist of the use of muscle relaxants and opioids, and both of these can have prolonged effects in the newborn because of altered pharmacokinetics and pharmacodynamics. In addition, the compression of the lung for several hours, along with the preexisting aspiration pneumonia that many of these infants have, suggests the need in the more difficult cases for a short period of postoperative ventilation, or at least intubation with PEEP, as the most conservative technique for postoperative airway management. If extubation of the trachea is planned for the end of surgery, the anesthetic technique must be tailored accordingly.

A very high percentage of infants with esophageal atresia have residual difficulties of the tracheobronchial tree and esophagus for many years.[85] These include tracheomalacia, gastroesophageal reflux, and esophageal stricture.[86]

Intestinal Obstruction

For purposes of discussion, obstruction of the gastrointestinal system arbitrarily can be divided into upper gastrointestinal tract (i.e., duodenum) and lower gastrointestinal tract obstruction (i.e., terminal ileum, colon, imperforate anus). Obstruction of the upper gastrointestinal system usually becomes manifest within the first 24 h of life, with the institution of feedings, whereas obstruction of the lower gastrointestinal tract becomes manifest somewhere between 2 and 7 days of age, as the infant becomes progressively distended, little or no stool is passed, and there is vomiting.

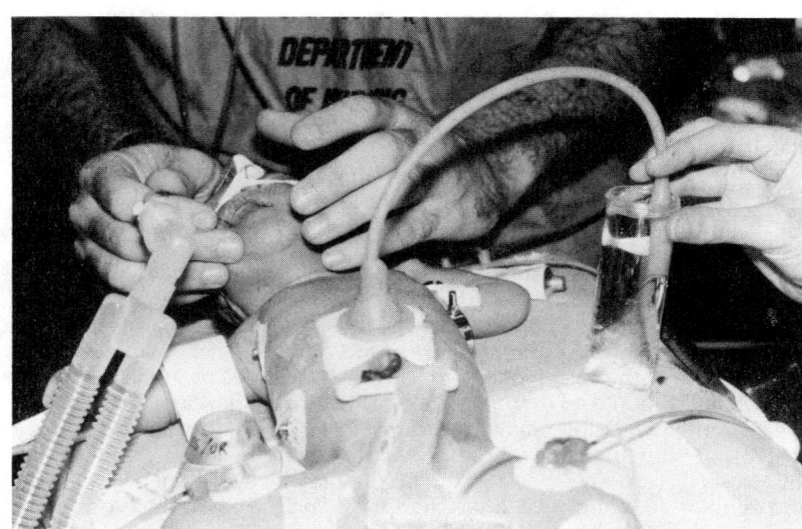

FIG. 46-21. Gastrostomy tube under water seal. (Reprinted with permission. Berry FA [ed]: Anesthetic Management of Difficult and Routine Pediatric Patients. New York, Churchill Livingstone, 1986.)

UPPER GASTROINTESTINAL TRACT OBSTRUCTION. If there has been persistent vomiting, upper intestinal obstruction usually means that a major deficit of fluids or electrolytes will develop in the infant. The stomach contains approximately 100–130 mEq·l^{-1} of sodium and 5–10 mEq·l^{-1} of potassium. The greatest deficit will be for sodium. The major concern in the infant with upper gastrointestinal tract obstruction is aspiration of gastric contents. Therefore, awake tracheal intubation is often preferred. Because of concern that awake tracheal intubation will cause hypertension, and intracranial hemorrhage in premature infants with immature cerebral blood vessels, several techniques have been described for modifying the discomfort and ensuing hypertension of awake intubation. These techniques include topical anesthesia and intravenous lidocaine. Topical anesthesia of the tongue and hypopharynx with lidocaine will reduce, but not eliminate, the discomfort of awake intubation. Intravenous administration of lidocaine in a dose of 1 mg·kg^{-1} also acts as a central nervous system depressant and reduces the stimulation associated with awake tracheal intubation. There is the theoretic concern that any amount of sedation or topical anesthesia will increase the incidence of aspiration of gastric contents. This appears to be more of a theoretic than practical concern.

The anesthetic management of these patients is directed toward assuring adequate relaxation for abdominal exploration, repair of the congenital defect, and closure of the abdomen. Nitrous oxide can be used in high intestinal obstruction because there is essentially no gas in the gastrointestinal tract. The next concern is whether or not the infant's trachea should be extubated at the end of surgery. If the infant is robust and the incision relatively small, extubation of the trachea at the end of surgery can be anticipated. On the other hand, if the infant is moderately debilitated or the surgical incision extensive, a period of postoperative tracheal intubation with PEEP may well be indicated, particularly if moderate doses of opioids have been used.

LOWER GASTROINTESTINAL TRACT OBSTRUCTION. The problems usually develop from 2 to 7 days after birth. It may take this long for the lesion to become manifest because it is low in the gastrointestinal tract. An imperforate anus should be recognized shortly after birth. Some of these infants may have vomiting secondary to the obstruction and present a problem with fluid and electrolyte management. An enormous amount of fluid can be sequestered within the intestinal tract. This fluid is essentially extracellular fluid and has a high sodium content. Therefore, these infants should be prepared carefully for surgery and have a serum sodium level greater than 130 mEq·l^{-1} and a urine volume of 1–2 ml·kg^{-1}·h^{-1}.

The trachea of these infants may need to be intubated while awake. If the infant has had minimal or no vomiting, rapid-sequence induction of anesthesia and tracheal intubation can be done. Rapid-sequence induction in an infant is the same as an adult, with intravenous barbiturate, muscle relaxant, cricoid pressure, oxygenation, etc. If the infant has had vomiting, the most conservative approach would be that of an awake tracheal intubation after gastric decompression. Although a nasogastric tube is in place, there is no guarantee that the stomach is empty. Therefore, in the face of vomiting, an awake tracheal intubation is the usual technique of choice, which is performed as described above. Although there is little difference in choice between anesthetic drugs for upper and lower gastrointestinal tract obstruction, it is evident that nitrous oxide should not be used in any infant who has a gaseous distension of the intestine. This is easily determined by the preoperative radiograph. Providing adequate muscle relax-

ation for the surgery is also a consideration. This can be done with various anesthetic techniques.

The criteria for tracheal extubation at the end of surgery are the same as those described for upper gastrointestinal tract obstruction. In general, however, these infants may have a greater degree of debilitation because they have had intestinal obstruction for a longer period of time. The caveat about timing of tracheal extubation is, "When in doubt, leave the endotracheal tube in place and ventilate the lungs with PEEP." This is not to suggest that prolonged endotracheal intubation is benign. It is not. There is a small, but significant, risk for the development of subglottic stenosis; but this is a situation in which the risk of subglottic stenosis and other airway trauma must be weighed against the risk of too early tracheal extubation with vomiting and aspiration, airway obstruction, fatigue, *etc.*

Meningomyelocele

Although the incidence of meningomyelocele has decreased over the past 20 years, it still occurs in a significant number of infants. There are five major concerns with a meningomyelocele: infection, fluids, positioning for tracheal intubation, the presence of the Arnold-Chiari malformation, and hydrocephalus. The meningomyelocele is very susceptible to trauma, leakage, and, hence, infection. Positioning alone can cause enough trauma to the meningomyelocele to cause this problem. The delivery process may also cause rupture and leakage of fluid. Spinal fluid is extracellular fluid with serum levels of sodium and potassium. Leakage of this fluid can create a preoperative and intraoperative volume and electrolyte problem. Replacement of spinal fluid with full-strength, balanced salt solution is indicated. If the surgical procedure is extensive because of a large meningomyelocele, there can be additional intraoperative third-space and blood loss.

A second concern is appropriate positioning for tracheal intubation. Use of the supine position required for intubation of the trachea necessitates the use of padding, which will prevent contact of the meningomyelocele with the operating table. The trachea of infants can be intubated while on their sides with the left side down, but it is more difficult than in a supine intubation. If a lateral approach to intubation is attempted, provision must be made to immediately turn the infant into the supine position if it is unsuccessful.

Virtually all infants with a meningomyelocele also have an associated anomaly of the brainstem known as the Arnold-Chiari malformation. The Arnold-Chiari malformation is characterized by a caudal displacement of the brainstem and the cerebellar tonsils into the cervical spinal canal. This is associated with an obliteration of the normal exit foramina of the fourth ventricle and in more than 90% of cases will result in progressive hydrocephalus necessitating a shunting procedure. This is usually not a problem at the time the meningomyelocele is repaired but may occur in the postoperative period. Any unusual breathing or blood pressure patterns should immediately raise one's suspicion of increased intracranial pressure.

SURGICAL PROCEDURES IN THE FIRST MONTH

Surgical procedures in the first month also are considered emergency, or at least urgent, surgery. The six most frequent surgical procedures in the first month are exploratory laparotomy for necrotizing enterocolitis (NEC), inguinal hernia repair, correction of pyloric stenosis, patent ductus arteriosus ligation, a shunt procedure for hydrocephalus, and placement of a central venous catheter.

Necrotizing Enterocolitis (NEC)

NEC is a disease of premature infants. The exact origin of NEC has yet to be determined.[87-89] Kosloske proposed the hypothesis that NEC occurs by the coincidence of two of three pathologic events: intestinal ischemia, colonization by pathogenic bacteria, and excess protein substrate in the intestinal lumen. NEC is more likely to appear after quantitative extremes (*i.e.*, severe ischemia, highly pathogenic flora, or significant excess of substrate). NEC develops only if a threshold of injury sufficient to initiate intestinal necrosis is exceeded and is characterized by a cascade of pathologic events. It begins with an immature intestine that has a decreased absorption of substrate, leading to stasis. Stasis encourages bacterial proliferation, which leads to local infection. The picture is complicated by further pooling of fluid. There is ischemia and infection, which may lead to necrosis of the intestinal mucosa, which is followed by perforation. The perforation leads to gangrene, fluid loss, peritonitis, and septicemia. The first signs that NEC may be developing are distension, irritability, and the development of metabolic acidosis. NEC is primarily a medical disease and is treated by cessation of oral intake and administration of antibiotics and supportive care, particularly fluid and electrolyte therapy. At times, however, the condition worsens, the infant becomes more septic with severe peritonitis, and the only solution is to perform an exploratory laparotomy to remove the gangrenous bowel and perform an ileostomy.[90]

The preoperative problems are an acute abdomen with severe peritonitis, necrosis and gangrene of the intestine, septicemia, metabolic acidosis, and hypovolemia. Preparation of the patient must include stabilization of the circulation. Often the septicemia, coupled with the distended abdomen as well as the overall clinical deterioration of the infant, also necessitates the use of intubation and ventilation in the nursery. The anesthetic requirements are continuation of resuscitation, provision of excellent abdominal relaxation for the surgery, and careful titration of anesthetic drugs. These infants are often so critically ill that they tolerate minimal anesthesia. One choice is to start with small doses of ketamine, $0.5-1 \text{ mg} \cdot \text{kg}^{-1}$. This can be administered every 20–30 min. If the condition improves, fentanyl, $2-3 \text{ μg} \cdot \text{kg}^{-1}$, can be administered up to a total dose of $10-12 \text{ μg} \cdot \text{kg}^{-1}$. If the infant's condition improves dramatically, small doses of volatile drug can be added as well. Use of nitrous oxide should be avoided because of the gas pockets within the abdomen.

These infants represent one of the most challenging cases in all of pediatric anesthesia. Monitoring of intraarterial pressure, central venous pressure, and arterial blood gases is usually indicated. The fluid loss can be enormous.[91] They need full-strength, balanced salt solution for maintenance of blood pressure and urine output. If the hematocrit level is below 30%–35%, whole blood should be administered. These infants must be returned to the intensive care unit, with their tracheas intubated and lungs ventilated, and their postoperative care must be coordinated carefully with the surgeon, neonatologist, or pediatrician.

Inguinal Hernia Repair in the Neonate

The development of a hernia in the premature infant or neonate is a different clinical problem than the development of a hernia in an infant older than 1 year of age.[92-94] Of 100 infants younger than 2 months of age who needed inguinal hernia repair,[93] 30% were premature, 42% had a history of respiratory distress syndrome, 16% had been ventilated, and 19% had congenital heart disease. Furthermore, 31% of the infants had incarcerated hernias, 9% had an intestinal obstruction, and 2% had gonadal infarction. These data should preclude the possibility of waiting until a premature infant or neonate is 6 months or 1 year old in order to perform "elective" surgery. The potential for emergency or urgent intervention is so great that surgical repair should be accomplished within a reasonable amount of time after an inguinal hernia is discovered. The "reasonable" amount of time depends upon the infant's condition. If the infant is normal and has no other medical problems, repair can be done within several days or weeks. If the infant has another problem such as respiratory distress syndrome, the waiting period should be longer, in order to maximally improve the infant's status.

Perioperative complications are frequent in these infants.[95-98] In the 100 patients reported by Rescorla and Grosfeld, two had apnea and bradycardia, four required postoperative ventilatory support, one had a cardiac arrest resulting from digoxin toxicity, and one patient developed Klebsiella sepsis.[93] It has long been recognized that the premature infant having elective surgery has a predisposition to a higher incidence of complications than the full-term infant having the same type of surgery. Steward reported that 13 of a group of 33 premature infants having elective inguinal hernia repair had complications, whereas only 1 of 38 full-term infants having the same type of surgery had complications.[95] Five of the complications were intraoperative and eight were postoperative.

One of the major concerns in the premature infant is the development of apnea in the postoperative period. The presence of an endotracheal tube in any infant leads to the development of short periods of apnea, however, the apnea that develops in premature infants can be quite prolonged and associated with bradycardia. Most of the time this apnea and bradycardia can be treated by conservative methods, such as the administration of oxygen and stimulation. Rarely the condition may alarm the clinician to the point where the infant's trachea is reintubated or remains intubated after operation. There are individual case reports of apnea developing as long as 12 h after operation.[98] Therefore, questions arise as to whether or not these infants are candidates for same-day surgery, what type of monitoring they need, and how long they need to be monitored. The consensus today is that infants who were born prematurely and who are still younger than 50–55 weeks conceptual age should not be operated on as ambulatory surgical patients. They should be admitted to the hospital and monitored with an apnea monitor and a cardiac monitor until the morning after surgery.[97, 98]

Premature infants at particular risk are those who have a history of apnea, although premature infants who have had no history of apnea have had apneic episodes after anesthesia. The exact origin of postoperative apnea is not known, although it may involve lingering effects of anesthetics. A study in adult volunteers showed that subanesthetic concentrations of halothane (0.15% inspired) profoundly depressed the peripheral chemoreflex pathway.[99] There is no reason to think that the premature infant and the neonate might not respond in the same way. Subjects were somewhat drowsy, but they remembered everything and were coherent and talked to the investigators. The peripheral chemoreflex pathway protects the body from hypoxia through the carotid bodies, which, when stimulated, initiate a cascade of protective physiologic defense mechanisms. These mechanisms include an increase in minute ventilation, hypertension, a favorable redistribution of cardiac output, and an arousal of the patient. It becomes evident, then, that the anesthetic implication of this study combined with the anatomic and physiologic handicaps of the infants, suggests that infants should remain intubated until completely awake and active at the end of surgery and that they should be monitored very carefully. In addition, because the premature infant and neonate are particularly susceptible to laryngospasm, oral feedings should be delayed for at least 2–3 hr after tracheal extubation. Laryngospasm is a protective reflex of the airway. The closure of the glottic opening is accompanied by apnea.

ANESTHETIC TECHNIQUES FOR HERNIA REPAIR. Surgical procedures below the umbilicus can be performed with either general or regional anesthesia. There is no consensus about which is preferred. Local or regional anesthesia can be used entirely for the surgery or as an adjunct to reduce general anesthetic requirements and produce postoperative analgesia.[100–102] The bottom line is that the anesthesiologist must always be prepared to manage the airway. There is also a very easy technique for providing postoperative analgesia in patients with hernias. Ileoinguinal–ileohypogastric nerve block with 0.5% bupivacaine, 3 mg·kg^{-1}, with epinephrine can be administered, either shortly after the induction of anesthesia or at the end of surgery, and it provides excellent postoperative analgesia without the need for opioids.[103]

There remains considerable debate regarding when to operate on graduates of the premature nursery as ambulatory patients, what types of postoperative monitors to use, the length of time they should be monitored, the anesthetic techniques, and whether or not surgery should be delayed for some length of time. The current consensus is that ambulatory surgery is appropriate for infants who are at least 50 conceptual weeks of age (gestational age + postnatal age). If an infant is younger than 50 conceptual weeks, he or she should be hospitalized and postoperative apnea monitoring should be used for approximately 18 hr.

Pyloric Stenosis

Pyloric stenosis is a relatively frequent surgical disease of the neonate and infant. It can appear as early as the second week of life. The pathologic characteristics include hypertrophy of the pyloric smooth muscle with edema of the pyloric mucosa and submucosa. This process develops over a period of days and sometimes weeks, so that there is progressive obstruction of the pyloric valve, causing persistent vomiting. The vomiting leads to varying losses of fluids and electrolytes. Pediatricians are now adept at diagnosing pyloric stenosis, so it is rare to find an infant with severe fluid and electrolyte derangements. It is discovered so early in some infants that only minimal defects are present. However, an infant is occasionally seen whose problem has developed slowly over a period of weeks, resulting in severe fluid and electrolyte derangements. The stomach contents contain sodium, potassium, chloride, hydrogen ions, and water. The infant may have a hyponatremic, hypokalemic, hypochloremic metabolic alkalosis, with a compensatory respiratory acidosis. The anesthesiologist, as well as the pediatrician and surgeon, is responsible for preparing these infants before operation. This condition is a medical emergency and should not be converted into an anesthetic nightmare by premature surgical repair before adequate fluid and electrolyte homeostasis. The infant should have normal skin turgor, and the correction of the electrolyte imbalance should produce a sodium level that is greater than 130 mEq·l^{-1}, a potassium level that is at least 3 mEq·l^{-1}, a chloride level that is greater than 85 mEq·l^{-1} and increasing, and a urine output of at least 1–2 ml·kg^{-1}·hr^{-1}. These patients need a resuscitation fluid of full-strength, balanced salt solution, and, after the infant begins to urinate, the addition of potassium chloride.

ANESTHETIC MANAGEMENT. The major concern in the anesthetic management of patients with pyloric stenosis is the aspiration of gastric contents. These infants are usually older and stronger than those in whom an intestinal obstruction appears in the first day or so of life. For that reason, a slightly different approach is used. A large orogastric tube is passed and the stomach contents aspirated. Then, 5–7 ml of sodium bicarbonate (the intravenous solution will suffice) is administered down the orogastric tube. The infant is gently agitated to distribute the fluid. The tube is suctioned and removed. This procedure greatly reduces the quantity of gastric fluid and increases the pH to 6–7. Intubation of the trachea can be done while the patient is awake or after induction of anesthesia. I prefer to first anesthetize these infants. If the infant does not have an intravenous line and one cannot be started with reasonable ease, then, after the above regimen is followed to adequately prepare the stomach, an inhalation induction of anesthesia is done with nitrous oxide and halothane. Use of nitrous oxide should be discontinued as soon as the infant loses the lid reflex. If a vein becomes evident, an intravenous line is started and a rapid intubation of the trachea accomplished with the use of succinylcholine or atracurium and cricoid pressure. If an intravenous line still cannot be started easily, one of two options exists: one should either deepen inhalation anesthesia with 3%–4% halothane, perform laryngoscopic examination, topically anesthetize the vocal cords with 2–3 mg·kg^{-1} of lidocaine, and intubate the trachea; or administer 5 mg·kg^{-1} of succinylcholine intramuscularly before intubation. If intravenous access has already been obtained, a rapid-sequence tracheal intubation technique is preferred. The infant is preoxygenated with high-flow oxygen; atropine, 0.01 mg·kg^{-1}, is given, followed by thiopental, 3–4 mg·kg^{-1}, and succinylcholine, 2 mg·kg^{-1}, or atracurium, 0.8 mg·kg^{-1}. Cricoid pressure is applied as soon as tolerated and the infant's trachea intubated. Anesthesia can be maintained by almost any technique that the clinician prefers. The point to remember is that surgeons will need skeletal muscle relaxation at two times: when they deliver the pylorus at the beginning of surgery and when they replace the pylorus into the abdomen at the end of surgery shortly before closing the peritoneum. Atracurium, as both an intubating relaxant and a maintenance relaxant, seems to be a useful drug. I also prefer to use a volatile drug plus 70% nitrous oxide, along with controlled ventilation of the lungs. Use of halothane or isoflurane is discontinued as soon as the peritoneum is closed. The atracurium is reversed and the nitrous oxide discontinued as the last two or three skin sutures are placed. The infant's trachea should remain intubated until he or she is awake with eyes opened and is reaching for the endotracheal tube.

Ligation of a Patent Ductus Arteriosus (PDA)

As the number of small premature infants that are surviving has increased, so has the number of infants who have PDA with heart failure and respiratory failure. Prostaglandins (PGE$_2$ and PGI$_2$) relax the smooth muscle of the ductus so that it cannot constrict. Indomethacin, a prostaglandin synthetase inhibitor, is administered to encourage closure of the ductus. However, indomethacin is often unsuccessful in the small premature infant because of the lack of muscle within the ductus. Infants with a PDA and heart failure require maximal medical management with fluid restriction and diuretics. These infants represent a special risk because of the reduced blood volume and precarious cardiopulmonary system. Fentanyl with pancuronium is a frequent choice for anesthesia. The clinician must be prepared to rapidly augment volume with 10–15 ml·kg^{-1} of lactated Ringer's solution. If the lactated Ringer's solution accompanies the administration of 20–25 ug·kg^{-1} of fentanyl and pancuronium, the pressure changes will be minimal and the infant will be appropriately anesthetized.[104] The tracheas of these infants usually remain intubated and the lungs ventilated in the postoperative period, so concern about the length of action of muscle relaxants and opioids is minimized.

Hydrocephalus

Hydrocephalus may be seen after closure of a meningomyelocele because of the Arnold-Chiari malformation. The cranium of the neonate is characterized by the presence of open sutures, so intracranial pressure increases are blunted or minimized by the open sutures. However, these infants eventually have an increase in head size and sometimes in intracranial pressure, resulting in lethargy, vomiting, and cardiorespiratory problems. The anesthetic approach and the technique for tracheal intubation depend upon the infant's condition. The major concern is protection of the airway and control of intracranial pressure. Awake tracheal intubation, crying, struggling, and straining can increase intracranial pressure, but this increase will be blunted by the open sutures. I prefer to perform a rapid-sequence induction of anesthesia in order to control the airway and intracranial pressure. A rapid-sequence induction with 4–5 mg·kg^{-1} of thiopental, 2 mg·kg^{-1} succinylcholine, and cricoid pressure can lead to rapid control of the airway. Hyperventilation, along with the barbiturate, will rapidly control intracranial pressure. Volatile drugs, nitrous oxide, and opioids are all reasonable choices for maintenance anesthesia. Noninvasive intracranial pressure measurements in neurologically normal preterm neonates have shown a decrease in intracranial pressure with all drugs, a 10% decrease after ketamine, a 10% decrease after fentanyl, a 11% decrease after isoflurane, and a 9% decrease after halothane.[105] The blood pressure decreased with the volatile drugs but not with ketamine or fentanyl. The failure of volatile anesthetics and ketamine to increase intracranial pressure as in adults, is attributed to the compliance of the neonate's open-sutured cranium.

After operation, the trachea of these infants should remain intubated and be on PEEP for a period of time, if they were experiencing periods of apnea or bradycardia before operation because of the intracranial abnormalities. If not, the trachea can be extubated as soon as the protective reflexes are recovered.

Placement of a Central Venous Catheter

The use of a central venous catheter for monitoring central venous pressure, serum electrolytes, blood gases, *etc.*, for hyperalimentation, and for administering medications is increasing. It can be done either as part of another surgical procedure or at some other time as a separate procedure. The three major concerns in central venous line placement are airway management, pneumothorax, and bleeding. The airway must be secured by an endotracheal tube in these small infants because of the difficulty in sharing the head, neck, and upper chest with the surgeon and as an adjunct for treating complications such as pneumothorax and bleeding. The anesthetic technique depends upon the infant's condition, but the neonate must be motionless for the procedure. A pneumothorax may occur with attempts at subclavian vein puncture. The first signs of trouble may be a decreasing oxygen saturation or difficulty with ventilation of the lungs. Because a fluoroscope is often used for central venous line placement, it can be used to rapidly diagnose a pneumothorax. If not, the chest must be rapidly aspirated for both diagnostic and therapeutic reasons. Bleeding is an unusual but serious complication of central venous line placement. It usually becomes manifest in the postoperative period as a hemothorax or as hypovolemia with a decreasing hematocrit.

SIGNIFICANCE OF A HISTORY OF RESPIRATORY DISTRESS SYNDROME

Because of the enormous technical ability of the neonatologist and the resources of newborn intensive care units, many very small infants will survive who need surgery. One of the frequent problems of these infants is the occurrence of the respiratory distress syndrome, secondary to a deficiency of surfactant. Respiratory distress syndrome is not an all-or-none disease. There are varying degrees of the disease, and there are varying techniques for the treatment of the disease. Respiratory distress syndrome can progress to a chronic form of respiratory disease called bronchopulmonary dysplasia (BPD). The exact cause or causes for BPD are thought to be barotrauma, oxygen, and infection. A survey of eight centers caring for these infants revealed that there were differences in the techniques of care, in outcome, and in incidence of chronic lung disease.[2] The group with the best outcome and the lowest incidence of chronic lung disease used some different management techniques from some of the other institutions. One difference was the use of nasal prongs to institute continuous positive airway pressures at an approximate pressure of 5 cm H_2O. This was done soon after birth in all infants who showed signs of respiratory distress, with tachypnea and retractions. The Pa$_{CO_2}$ value was allowed to increase as high as 60 mm Hg before endotracheal intubation was performed. Hyperventilation was avoided, and muscle relaxants were not used.

However, despite the advances, there are still infants who need tracheal intubation and ventilation of the lungs and who have a higher incidence of residual lung disease, characterized by a decrease in compliance and a reactive airway.[106, 107] For that reason, a careful history must be obtained for any infant, particularly as pertains to respiratory distress syndrome and whether or not the infant's trachea was intubated or lungs ventilated. This may affect the infant's response to anesthesia. These infants should be premedicated with anticholinergics, and a more difficult induction of anesthesia and awakening should be anticipated because of the potential for residual airway disease and the complicating factors of decreased compliance and reactive airways. Extubation of the trachea may be complicated at the end of surgery because of the reactive airway disease, and, for that reason, the endotracheal tube should be left in longer so that the infant is completely awake and in control of his or her airway reflexes. If the infant has a problem with airway reactivity and the trachea cannot yet be extubated, intravenous lidocaine in a dose of 1 mg·kg^{-1} can be used. This dose can be repeated up to a total dose of 3 mg·kg^{-1} in 10 min. Infants who have residual lung disease have a higher incidence of sudden infant death syndrome (SIDS).[108]

SUDDEN INFANT DEATH SYNDROME (SIDS)

Prematurity and congenital defects cause most infant deaths in the first month of life. SIDS is the most frequent cause of death in infants between the ages of 1 month and 1 yr.[109] Death from SIDS is relatively rare in the first month of life, with the peak occurring at the third to fourth months of life. SIDS remains a mystery in many ways; its exact causes are unknown. There is some information, however, that certain groups of infants may be more at risk for development of SIDS, such as premature infants, infants who have had bronchopulmonary dysplasia, and infants with the "infant apnea syndrome."[108] The infant apnea syndrome is the new designation for what was previously termed the "near-miss sudden infant death syndrome."[110] It was previously believed that SIDS might be more frequent among siblings of SIDS victims, but a report by Peterson et al suggests that the risk of SIDS in siblings of SIDS victims is inflated.[111] There are reports that infants who have had episodes of the infant apnea syndrome have a defect in the regulation of alveolar ventilation.[112] They have slightly increased levels of carbon dioxide, and they have an impaired response to carbon dioxide breathing. Elevated levels of beta endorphin have also been observed in the cerebrospinal fluid of infants with the infant apnea syndrome.[110] This syndrome should not be confused with apnea resulting from prematurity, however, which disappears as the infant matures. There is currently no evidence that general anesthesia might trigger SIDS or the infant apnea syndrome.[109] Premature infants with or without a history of apnea have an increased risk for development of apnea in the postoperative period, which may last until the infant is 50 weeks of conceptual age (gestational age plus the postnatal age). For that reason, these infants who need surgery should be admitted to the hospital after surgery and monitored with an apnea and cardiac monitor for approximately 18 h. Families of SIDS victims also are reported to have a higher incidence of malignant hyperthermia and other serious reactions to anesthetics.[113, 114]

POSTOPERATIVE MANAGEMENT OF THE NEONATE

Neonates undergoing surgery still have the handicaps of immature skeletal muscles, an immature nervous system, and an immature cardiovascular system. In addition, they may have severe physiologic derangements secondary to congenital defects. For that reason, the postoperative care of these infants requires a great deal of teamwork between surgeon, anesthesiologist, pediatrician, or neonatologist. The anesthetics should be tailored for one of two situations: immediate tracheal extubation in the perioperative period and postoperative intubation of the trachea with varying length and needs for ventilation. If the infant has a surgical problem that does not impair ventilation to any great extent and the infant is in good condition, attempts should be made to extubate the trachea, either at the end of surgery or in the immediate postoperative period. In this situation, the anesthetics should be tailored so that the infant recovers his or her protective reflexes, has full neuromuscular function, and is awake. The endotracheal tube should be left in place until the infant makes purposeful attempts to remove it. When older infants and children move their extremities, it is usually a sign that the trachea can be extubated. This may not be true with the neonate. For that reason, a purposeful move toward the endotracheal tube and opening of the eyes signifies that the infant will be able to maintain spontaneous ventilation without laryngospasm.

If the trachea of the infant is to remain intubated with or without assisted or controlled ventilation of the lungs, the anesthesiologist must transfer the care and responsibility of this patient to the pediatrician or neonatologist. This is best documented on the anesthesia record and progress notes.

TRANSFER OF PATIENTS—WHAT TO DO WITH THE PATIENT WHO EXCEEDS THE ANESTHESIOLOGIST'S ABILITY. Because the practice of anesthesia includes a wide range of cases, the anesthesiologist sometimes has infrequent experience with neonates. Therefore, on occasion, the hospital or surgical staff may place certain demands on the anesthesiologist for neonatal anesthesia care when the anesthesiologist may not believe that he or she has the appropriate knowledge or experience to manage the ill neonate. Unless the surgical procedure is a life-or-death emergency, the anesthesiologist has two options: to refer the patient to a colleague who is qualified to manage the anesthesia, or to insist that the neonate be transferred to an appropriate medical center where there are facilities available for the anesthetic and postoperative management of the neonate. The emergency transport facilities for neonates (and other patients) are well developed in this country. The medicolegal climate is so pernicious that appropriate patient care and legal questions should not be risked. The transfer of patients is often difficult for the physician to accept, particularly with the increasing competition for patients, as well as the enormous financial pressures being brought upon the medical care system by the government and insurance companies. Government and insurance company health care administrators are mainly interested in cost. The concepts of quality care and safety have almost been forgotten. It is up to the physician to maintain quality and safety. There is no other choice.

REFERENCES

1. Murphy JD, Vawter GF, Reid LM: Pulmonary vascular disease in fetal meconium aspiration. J. Pediatr 104:758, 1984
2. Avery ME, Tooley WH, Keller JB et al: Is chronic lung disease in low birth weight infants preventable? A survey of eight centers. Pediatrics 79:26, 1987
3. Fox WW, Duara S: Persistent pulmonary hypertension in the neonate: Diagnosis and management. J Pediatr 103:505, 1983
2. Avery ME, Tooley WH, Keller JB et al: Is chronic lung disease in low birth weight infants preventable? A survey of eight centers. Pediatrics 79:26, 1987
3. Fox WW, Duara S: Persistent pulmonary hypertension in the neonate: Diagnosis and management. J Pediatr 103:505, 1983
4. Wung J-T, James LS, Kilchevsky E et al: Management of infants with severe respiratory failure and persistence of the fetal circulation, without hyperventilation. Pediatrics 76:488, 1985
5. Kirkpatrick BV, Krummel TM, Mueller DG et al: Use of extracorporeal membrane oxygenation for respiratory failure in term infants. Pediatrics 72:872, 1983
6. Andrews AF, Nixon CA, Cilley RE et al: One- to three-year outcome for 14 neonatal survivors of extracorporeal membrane oxygenation. Pediatrics 78:692, 1986
7. Cilley RE, Zwischenberger JB, Andrews AF et al: Intracranial hemorrhage during extracorporeal membrane oxygenation in neonates. Pediatrics 78:699, 1986
8. Berry FA: The renal system. In Gregory GA (ed): Pediatric Anesthesia, Vol 1, p 63. New York, Churchill Livingstone, 1983
9. Kao LC, Warburton D, Sargent CW et al: Furosemide acutely decreases airway resistance in chronic bronchopulmonary dysplasia. J Pediatr 103:624, 1983

10. Berry FA: Practical aspects of fluid and electrolyte therapy. In Berry FA (ed): Anesthetic Management of Difficult and Routine Pediatric Patients, Vol 6, p 107. New York, Churchill Livingstone, 1986

11. Gerhardt T, Hehre D, Feller R et al: Serial determination of pulmonary function in infants with chronic lung disease. J Pediatr 110:448–456, 1987

12. Tulassay T, Rascher W, Seyberth HW et al: Role of atrial natriuretic peptide in sodium homeostasis in premature infants. J Pediatr 109:1023, 1986

13. Shaffer SG, Geer PG, Goetz KL: Elevated atrial natriuretic factor in neonates with respiratory distress syndrome. J Pediatr 109:1028, 1986

14. Laragh JH: Atrial natriuretic hormone, the renin-aldosterone axis, and blood pressure-electrolyte homeostasis. N Engl J Med 313:1330, 1985

15. Cote CJ, Todres ID: The pediatric airway. In Ryan JF, Todres ID, Cote CJ et al (eds): A Practice of Anesthesia for Infants and Children, p 35. New York, Grune & Stratton, 1985

16. Cook DR: Pharmacology of pediatric anesthesia. In Katz J, Steward DJ (eds): Anesthesia and Uncommon Pediatric Diseases, p 12. Philadelphia, WB Saunders, 1987

17. Keens TG, Bryan AC, Levison H et al: Developmental pattern of muscle fiber types in human ventilatory muscles. J Appl Physiol 44:909, 1978

18. Friedman WF: The intrinsic physiologic properties of the developing heart. Prog Cardiovasc Dis 15:87, 1972

19. Friedman WF, George BL: Treatment of congestive heart failure by altering loading conditions of the heart. J Pediatr 106:697, 1985

20. Wear R, Robinson S, Gregory GA: The effect of halothane on the baroresponse of adult and baby rabbits. Anesthesiology 56:188, 1982

21. Mirkin BL: Perinatal pharmacology. Anesthesiology 43:156, 1975

22. Way WL, Costley EL, Way EL: Respiratory sensitivity of newborn infants to meperidine and morphine. Clin Pharmacol Ther 6:454, 1965

23. Berry FA, Gregory GA: Do premature infants require anesthesia for surgery? Anesthesiology 67:3, 1987

24. Levine JD, Gordon NC: Pain in prelingual children and its evaluation by pain-induced vocalization. Pain 14:85, 1982

25. Williamson PS, Williamson ML: Physiologic stress reduction by a local anesthetic during newborn circumcision. Pediatrics 71:36, 1983

26. Owens ME, Todt EH: Pain in infancy: Neonatal reaction to a heel lance. Pain 20:77, 1984

27. Anand KJS, Brown MJ, Causon RC et al: Can the human neonate mount an endocrine and metabolic response to surgery? J Pediatr Surg 20:41, 1985

28. Cabal LA, Siassi B, Artal R et al: Cardiovascular and catecholamine changes after administration of pancuronium in distressed neonates. Pediatrics 75:284, 1985

29. Fisher DM, O'Keeffe C, Stanski DR et al: Pharmacokinetics and pharmacodynamics of d-tubocurarine in infants, children and adults. Anesthesiology 57:203, 1982

30. Miller RD, Rupp SM, Fisher DM et al: Clinical pharmacology of vecuronium and atracurium. Anesthesiology 61:444, 1984

31. Fisher DM, Miller RD: Neuromuscular effects of vecuronium (ORG NC45) in infants and children during N_2O, halothane anesthesia. Anesthesiology 58:519, 1983

32. Liu LMP, DeCook TH, Goudsouzian NG et al: Dose response to intramuscular succinylcholine in children. Anesthesiology 55:599, 1981

33. Goudsouzian NG: Relaxants in paediatric anaesthesia. In Sumner E, Hatch DJ (eds): Clinics in Anaesthesiology, Vol 3, p 539, 1985

34. Hall GM, Lucke JN, Lister D: Porcine malignant hyperthermia. IV: Neuromuscular blockade. Br J Anaesth 48:1135, 1976

35. Berry FA: General philosophy of patient preparation, premedication, and induction of anesthesia; and inhalation anesthetic agents. In Berry FA (ed): Anesthetic Management of Difficult and Routine Pediatric Patients, p 35. New York, Churchill Livingstone, 1986

36. Fisher DM, Canfell PC, Fahey MR et al: Elimination of atracurium in humans: Contribution of Hofmann elimination and ester hydrolysis versus organ-based elimination. Anesthesiology 65:6, 1986

37. Cook DR: Muscle relaxants in infants and children. Anesth Analg 60:335, 1981

38. Meakin G, Sweet PT, Bevan JC et al: Neostigmine and edrophonium as antagonists of pancuronium in infants and children. Anesthesiology 59:316, 1983

39. Fisher DM, Cronnelly R, Miller RD et al: Neuromuscular pharmacology of neostigmine in infants and children. Anesthesiology 59:220, 1983

40. Robinson S, Gregory GA: Fentanyl-air-oxygen anesthesia for patent ductus arteriosus in preterm infants. Anesth Analg 60:331, 1981

41. Hickey PR, Hansen DD, Wessel DL et al: Pulmonary and systemic hemodynamic responses to fentanyl in infants. Anesth Analg 64:483, 1985

42. Hickey PR, Hansen DD, Wessel DL et al: Blunting of stress responses in the pulmonary circulation of infants by fentanyl. Anesth Analg 64:1132, 1985

43. Yaster M: The dose response of fentanyl in neonatal anesthesia. Anesthesiology 66:433, 1987

44. Morray JP, Lynn AM, Stamm SJ et al: Hemodynamic effects of ketamine in children with congenital heart disease. Anesth Analg 63:895, 1984

45. Hickey PR, Hansen DD, Gramolini GM et al: Pulmonary and systemic hemodynamic responses to ketamine in infants with normal and elevated pulmonary vascular resistance. Anesthesiology 62:287, 1985

46. Greeley WJ, Bushman GA, Davis DP et al: Comparative effects of halothane and ketamine on systemic arterial oxygen saturation in children with cyanotic heart disease. Anesthesiology 65:666, 1986

47. McDermott RW, Stanley TH: The cardiovascular effects of low concentration of nitrous oxide during morphine anesthesia. Anesthesiology 41:89, 1974

48. Lunn JK, Stanley TH, Eisele J et al: High dose fentanyl anesthesia for coronary artery surgery: Plasma fentanyl concentrations and influence of nitrous oxide on cardiovascular responses. Anesth Analg 58:390, 1979

49. Lappas GD, Buckley MJ, Daggett WM et al: Left ventricular performance and pulmonary circulation following addition of nitrous oxide during coronary artery surgery. Anesthesiology 43:61, 1975

50. Maretoja OA, Takkunen O, Heikkila H et al: Haemodynamic response to nitrous oxide during high-dose fentanyl pancuronium anaesthesia. Acta Anaesthesiol Scand 29:137, 1985

51. Hickey PR, Hansen DD, Strafford M et al: Pulmonary and systemic hemodynamic effects of nitrous oxide in infants with normal and elevated pulmonary vascular resistance. Anesthesiology 65:374, 1986

52. Berry FA: Inhalation agents in paediatric anaesthesia. In Sumner E, Hatch DJ, (eds): Clinics in Anaesthesiology, Vol 3, p 515. London, WB Saunders, 1985

53. Gregory GA, Eger EI, Munson EA: The relationship between age and halothane requirements in man. Anesthesiology 30:488, 1969

54. LeDez KM, Lerman J: The minimum alveolar concentration (MAC) of isoflurane in preterm neonates. Anesthesiology 67:301, 1987

55. Lerman J, Robinson S, Willis MM et al: Anesthetic requirements for halothane in young children 0–1 month and 1–6 months of age. Anesthesiology 59:421, 1983

56. Gregory GA, Wade JG, Beihl DR et al: Fetal anesthetic requirement (MAC) for halothane in adults and children. Anesthesiology 62:9, 1983

57. Koehntop DE, Rodman JH, Brundage DM et al: Pharmacokinetics of fentanyl in neonates. Anesth Analg 65:227, 1986

58. Davis PJ, Cook R, Stiller RL et al: Pharmacodynamics and pharmacokinetics of high-dose sufentanil in infants and children undergoing cardiac surgery. Anesth Analg 66:203, 1987

59. Starr NJ, Sethna DH, Estafanous FG: Bradycardia and asystole following the rapid administration of sufentanil with vecuronium. Anesthesiology 64:521, 1986

60. Jones R, Bodnar A, Roan Y et al: Subglottic stenosis in newborn intensive care unit graduates. Am J Dis Child 135:367, 1981

61. Friesen RH, Lichtor JL: Cardiovascular depression during halothane anesthesia in infants: A study of three induction techniques. Anesth Analg 61:42, 1982

62. Diaz JH, Lockhart CH: Is halothane really safe in infancy? Anesthesiology 51:S313, 1979

63. Friesen RH, Lichtor JL: Cardiovascular effects of inhalation induction with isoflurane in infants. Anesth Analg 62:411, 1983

64. Salanitre E, Rackow M: The pulmonary exchange of nitrous oxide and halothane in infants and children. Anesthesiology 30:388, 1969

65. Steward DJ, Creighton RE: The uptake and excretion of nitrous oxide in the newborn. Can Anaesth Soc J 25:215, 1978

66. Brandom BW, Brandom RB, Cook DR: Uptake and distribution of halothane in infants: In vivo measurements and computer simulations. Anesth Analg 62:404, 1983

67. Koop CE, Schnaufer L, Broeule AM: Esophageal atresia and tracheoesophageal fistula: Supportive measures that affect survival. Pediatrics 54:558, 1974

68. Louhimo I, Lindahl H: Esophageal atresia: Primary results of 500 consecutively treated patients. J Pediatr Surg 18:217, 1983

69. Holmes SJK, Kiely EM, Spitz L: Tracheoesophageal fistula and respiratory distress syndrome. Pediatric Surgery International 2:16, 1987

70. Greenwood RD, Rosenthal A, Nadas AS: Cardiac anomalies associated with congenital diaphragmatic hernia. Pediatrics 57:92, 1976

71. Greenwood RD, Rosenthal A: Cardiovascular malformations associated with tracheoesophageal fistula and esophageal atresia. Pediatrics 57:87, 1976

72. Geggel RL, Murphy JD, Langleben D et al: Congenital diaphragmatic hernia: Arterial structural changes and persistent pulmonary hypertension after surgery. J Pediatr 107:457, 1985

73. Vacanti JP, Crone RK, Murphy JD et al: The pulmonary hemodynamic response to perioperative anesthesia in the treatment of high risk infants with congenital diaphragmatic hernia. J Pediatr Surg 19:672, 1984

74. Crone RK, O'Rourke PP, Vacanti JP et al: Survival of infants with congenital diaphragmatic hernia treated by perioperative anesthesia. Anesthesiology 63:A481, 1985

75. O'Rourke PP, Crone RK, Vacanti JP et al: The use of extracorporeal membrane oxygenation (ECMO) in infants with congenital diaphragmatic hernia (CDH) who have a 100% predicted mortality. Anesthesiology 63:A482, 1985

76. Bartlett RH, Roloff DW, Cornell RG et al: Extracorporeal circulation in neonatal respiratory failure: A prospective randomized trial. Pediatrics 76:479, 1985

77. Grosfeld JL, Weber TR: Congenital abdominal wall defects: Gastroschisis and omphalocele. Curr Probl Surg 19:158, 1982

78. Hoyme HE, Higginbottom MC, Jones JL: The vascular pathogenesis of gastroschisis: Intrauterine interruption of the omphalomesenteric artery. Pediatrics 98:228, 1981

79. Masey SA, Buck JR, Koehler RC et al: Effects of increased intraabdominal pressure of regional blood flow in newborn lambs. Anesthesiology 59:A425, 1983

80. Masey SA, Buck JR, Koehler RC: Cardiovascular and metabolic effects of increased intra-abdominal pressure in newborn lambs. Anesthesiology 59:A426, 1983

81. Harman PK, Kron IL, McLachlan HD et al: Elevated intra-abdominal pressure and renal function. Ann Surg 196:90, 1982

81a. Kron IL, Harman PK, Nolan SP: The measurement of intra-abdominal pressure as a criterion for abdominal re-exploration. Ann Surg 199:28, 1984

82. Salem MR, Wong AY, Lin YH et al: Prevention of gastric distention during anesthesia for newborns with tracheoesophageal fistulas. Anesthesiology 38:82, 1973

84. Filston HC, Chitwood WR, Schkolne B et al: The Fogarty balloon catheter as an aid to management of the infant with esophageal atresia and tracheoesophageal fistula complicated by severe RDS or pneumonia. J Pediatr Surg 17:149, 1982

85. Leendertse-Verloop K, Tibboel D, Hazebroek FWJ et al: Postoperative morbidity in patients with esophageal atresia. Pediatric Surgery International 2:2, 1987

86. Jolley SG, Johnson DG, Roberts CC et al: Patterns of gastroesophageal reflux in children following repair of esophageal atresia and distal tracheoesophageal fistula. J Pediatr Surg 15:857, 1980

87. Ostertag SG, LaGamma EF, Reisen CE et al: Early enteral feeding does not affect the incidence of necrotizing enterocolitis. Pediatrics 77:275, 1986

88. Milner ME, de la Monte SM, Moore GW et al: Risk factors for developing and dying from necrotizing enterocolitis. J Pediatr Gastroenterol Nutr 5:359, 1986

89. Kosloske AM: Pathogenesis and prevention of necrotizing enterocolitis: A hypothesis based on personal observation and a review of the literature. Pediatrics 74:1086, 1984

90. Buras R, Guzzetta P, Avery G et al: Acidosis and hepatic portal venous gas: Indications for surgery in necrotizing enterocolitis. Pediatrics 78:273, 1986

91. Buntain WL, Conner E, Emrico J et al: Transcutaneous oxygen (tcPO$_2$) measurements as an aid to fluid therapy in necrotizing enterocolitis. J Pediatr Surg 14:728, 1979

92. Puri P, Guiney EJ, O'Donnell B: Inguinal hernia in infants: The fate of the testis following incarceration. J Pediatr Surg 19:44, 1984

93. Rescorla FJ, Grosfeld JL: inguinal hernia repair in the perinatal period and early infancy: Clinical considerations. J Pediatr Surg 19:832, 1984

94. Peevy KJ, Speed FA, Hoff CJ: Epidemiology of inguinal hernia in preterm neonates. Pediatrics 77:246, 1986

95. Steward DJ: Preterm infants are more prone to complications following minor surgery than are term infants. Anesthesiology 56:304, 1982

96. Gregory GA, Steward DJ: Life-threatening perioperative apnea in the ex-"preemie." Anesthesiology 59:495, 1983

97. Liu LMP, Cote CJ, Goudsouzian NG et al: Life-threatening apnea in infants recovering from anesthesia. Anesthesiology 59:506, 1983

98. Kurth CD, Spitzer AR, Broennle AM et al: Postoperative apnea in former premature infants. Anesthesiology 63:A475, 1985

99. Knill RL, Clement JL: Site of selective action of halothane on the peripheral chemoreflex pathway in humans. Anesthesiology 61:121, 1984

100. Melman E, Pennelas J, Maruffo J: Regional anesthesia in children. Anesth Analg 54:387, 1975

101. Berkowitz S, Greene BA: Spinal anesthesia in children: Report based on 350 patients under 13 years of age. Anesthesiology 12:376, 1951

102. Abajian JC, Mellish P, Browne AF et al: Spinal anesthesia for surgery in the high risk infant. Anesth Analg 63:359, 1984

103. Shandling B, Steward DJ: Regional anesthesia for postoperative pain in pediatric outpatient surgery. J Pediatr Surg 15:477, 1980

104. Robinson SR, Gregory GA: Fentanyl-air-oxygen anesthesia for ligation of patent ductus arteriosus in preterm infants. Anesth Analg 60:331, 1981

105. Friesen RH, Thieme RE, Honda AT et al: Changes in anterior fontanel pressure in preterm neonates receiving isoflurane, halothane, fentanyl, or ketamine. Anesth Analg 66:431, 1987

106. Bryan MH, Hardie MJ, Reilly BJ et al: Pulmonary function studies during the first year of life in infants recovering from the respiratory distress syndrome. Pediatrics 52:169, 1973

107. Smyth JA, Tabachnik E, Duncan WJ et al: Pulmonary function and bronchial hyperreactivity in long-term survivors of bronchopulmonary dysplasia. Pediatrics 68:336, 1981

108. Werthammer J, Brown ER, Neff RK et al: Sudden infant death syndrome in infants with bronchopulmonary dysplasia. Pediatrics 69:301, 1982

109. Steward DJ: Is there a risk of general anesthesia triggering SIDS? Possibly not! Anesthesiology 63:326, 1985

110. Orlowski JP: Cerebrospinal fluid endorphins and the infant apnea syndrome. Pediatrics 78:233, 1986

111. Peterson DR, Sabotta EE, Daling JR: Infant mortality among subsequent siblings of infants who died of sudden infant death syndrome. Pediatrics 108:911, 1986

112. Shannon DC, Kelly DH, O'Connell K: Abnormal regulation of ventilation in infants at risk of sudden-infant-death syndrome. N Engl J Med 297:747, 1977

113. Denborough MA, Galloway GJ, Hopkinson KC: Malignant hyperpyrexia and sudden infant death. Lancet 2:1068, 1982

114. Peterson DR, Davis N: Malignant hyperthermia diathesis and sudden infant death syndrome. Anesth Analg 65:209, 1986

Chapter 47   D. Ryan Cook

Pediatric Anesthesia

Pediatric anesthesia involves the anesthetic management of patients in the process of rapid growth and development. The anatomic, physiologic, pharmacologic, and psychologic characteristics of the infant or child influence anesthetic care. Thus, appropriate anesthetic management of the pediatric surgical patient must be considered within the context of the patient's maturity and the severity of the surgical problem.

Rapid growth, development, and maturation of organ function occur during the first several months of life.[1-3] Circulatory and ventilatory adaptation are completed, thermoregulation processes change, the sizes of body fluid compartments are shifting to adult values, skeletal muscle mass is developing, hepatic enzyme systems responsible for the metabolism of drugs are developing, and renal function is maturing (Table 47-1).[4-14] By the time an infant is 3 months of age, the major tasks of maturation have been accomplished. Over the next 1–1.5 yr the infant gradually is physically transformed into a miniature adult; psychologic maturation may take years. Between 6 months and 1 yr of age, the infant begins to show sufficient awareness of his or her surroundings so that the psychologic aspects of hospitalization and surgery must be considered. At this age, therefore, sedative drugs may be used in preoperative preparation. The preschool child (2–6 yr of age) presents relatively few technical problems to the anesthesiologist. However, the child's fear, apprehension, and lack of cooperation are of particular concern to the anesthesiologist. For good anesthetic management, children at this age need to be prepared psychologically by both parent and anesthesiologist and may need preoperative medication. Children of school age (6–18 yr of age) may be considered to be small adults from a physiologic and, to a lesser extent, a psychologic point of view. Fear and apprehension are still problems, but children of this age will usually be cooperative.

PREANESTHETIC EVALUATION AND PREPARATION

The anesthesiologist should visit the patient and, when possible, the patient's parents. The primary purpose of the visit should be to obtain information about the surgical problem and medical history and make an estimate of the patient's personality and response to hospitalization. Parental anxieties and fears concerning the surgical procedure may be profound and may be transmitted to the child. These fears and anxieties, whether seemingly rational (realistic) or irrational (unrealistic), may stress or threaten the family unit. In addition, children may have age-related fears of their own.[15-17] To prepare the child psychologically for elective surgery educational booklets, movies, slide shows, puppet shows, and preoperative hospital tours may be useful. The anesthesiologist and other health care workers should also reinforce the information. Unified, coherent, noncontradictory teaching materials and information should be developed. Outpatient surgery or same-day surgery programs, in addition, minimize separation anxieties of the younger child. Such programs provide support to the parents and child. Ordinarily, it is best to give a simple explanation of what the patient can expect before induction of anesthesia; this reduces the element of surprise. This period can be used to reinforce preoperative teaching materials. In the older child the preoperative visit allows the anesthesiologist to establish a personal rapport, which aids in

TABLE 47-1.   Body Composition During Growth

BODY COMPARTMENT	PERCENTAGE OF BODY WEIGHT	
	Infant	Adult
Total body water	73	60
Extracellular fluid	44	15–20
Blood volume	8–10	7
Intracellular water	33	40
Muscle mass	20	50
Fat	12	18

a smoother anesthetic induction. Some children who have had previous hospitalizations or whose parents or friends have told them about operations may show interest in or anxiety about the anesthesia. These children deserve a frank explanation without too many details and forthright answers to their questions.

MINIMUM HEMOGLOBIN VALUES

There is controversy as to what constitutes the minimum acceptable hemoglobin value for elective pediatric surgery and if, indeed, such a minimum should be considered at all.[18] The arbitrary figure of 10 g·dl^{-1} has been used extensively for patients older than 3 months, with appropriately higher values for the younger infant. The use of an arbitrary value as a minimum requirement for elective surgery is useful as a simple screening procedure, but it should not be used as the final criterion for deciding if a patient may be anesthetized for elective surgery. Anemia is defined dynamically in infants and children because a normal "physiologic" anemia occurs within the first several months. Cardiac output, oxygen-carrying capacity, type of anesthesia, and type of surgery are factors other than hematocrit that help one define allowable blood loss. Neonates have 60–90% hemoglobin F, and it is not until they are 6 months of age that the adult hemoglobin A/hemoglobin F ratio is achieved. Hemoglobin F has a high affinity for oxygen, and the oxygen dissociation curve is shifted to the left. Thus, oxygen delivery to the tissues at a given oxygen tension is decreased. As the infant matures from 1 to 6 months, the arterial to venous difference in oxygen content and tissue oxygen delivery progressively increase. A full-term infant's hematocrit rarely decreases below 50% during the first several weeks of life. It takes about 3 months for the hematocrit to reach its nadir at 30%. This decrease in hematocrit results from decreased erythropoietin production, a shorter red blood cell survival time, and increased plasma volume.

Patients whose hemoglobin values are found to be below the arbitrary standard should be investigated and the cause of the anemia determined. The decision to proceed with surgery and anesthesia should then be based on the findings and not merely on a numeric value. Patients with low hemoglobin values that result from chronic dietary iron deficiency present less anesthetic risk than do those whose anemia results from blood loss. There seems little reason not to proceed with elective surgery in patients with low hemoglobin values of the iron-deficiency type if the anticipated surgical procedure is to be short and no significant blood loss is anticipated. Major surgical procedures in which transfusion is planned also may be started in this type of patient, provided there is no hypovolemia. Elective major surgery in which transfusion is not anticipated is better postponed until the anemia has been corrected by medical treatment. In elective procedures, preoperative blood transfusion is never justified simply to treat uncomplicated iron-deficiency anemia or to increase a hemoglobin value to some arbitrary standard.

Patients with sickle cell anemia (SS) require special preoperative preparation. These patients run the risk of intravascular sickling and thrombosis if subjected to hypoxia, hypothermia, acidosis, and so on. Therefore, blood should be transfused, over a period of several days if possible, so that the sickle hemoglobin may be replaced by enough hemoglobin A (approximately 7 g·dl^{-1}) to carry such patients through the period of anesthesia, operation, and recovery. Blood should be available during surgery as well.

HYDRATION AND RESTRICTION OF FLUIDS

The safety of an anesthetic depends to a large extent on the patient's stomach being empty. On the other hand, it is desirable that the patient have anesthesia and surgery under conditions of optimal hydration. These two goals are not incompatible or difficult to achieve.

The patient who is normally fed at the usual meal times and sleeps through the night presents no particular problems. The preoperative orders should include the scheduled time of operation, the instruction that food or fluids be offered or encouraged until a specific time 8 h before the scheduled surgery, and the instruction that the patient have "nothing by mouth" after that hour. The traditional "nothing by mouth after midnight" then applies only to early morning cases. Infants and younger children scheduled for later surgery may have clear liquids 4 h before their operation.

In the case of the infant who is fed more frequently or still has fourth-hour feedings, the preoperative orders should distinguish between solid food and clear liquids. (The term solid food includes not only the usual foods but also milk and pulp-containing fruit juices—in short, anything other than clear liquids.) The preoperative orders should include the time of the scheduled surgery, the instruction that no solid food or milk be allowed after a specific time 4 h before the scheduled surgery, the instruction that glucose water be offered until a specific time 2 h before surgery, and the instruction that the patient have "nothing by mouth" after that hour.

If these details are not clearly stated in a positive, itemized fashion with stated hours, the child, particularly the infant, inadvertently may not be given fluids for excessively long periods. Although these facts are well known to surgeons and anesthesiologists, pediatric patients nevertheless are occasionally subjected to unnecessarily long periods without fluid intake. This sometimes arises from improper case scheduling and delays in the surgical schedule, but it results most often from carelessly written preoperative orders. In general, the youngest infant should be first on the operating schedule or at least should be scheduled and operated on at a specific time. Both the surgeon and the anesthesiologist must be alert to delays and make sure that the infant's fluid restriction is revised accordingly.

PREANESTHETIC MEDICATION

Preanesthetic medication can play an important part in the anesthetic care of infants and children. It is unclear whether sedation is a substitute for or a supplement to rapport. Key reasons for the use of preanesthetic medications are to help allay fear and apprehensiveness; to induce quiescence; to control secretions in the airway; to prevent vagal reflexes, which may be stimulated by the anesthetic agent or by surgical maneuvers; and to reduce gastric volume and increase gastric pH. Sedative–hypnotics, opioids, or ataractic drugs, either alone or in combination, are generally used for the first two objectives; anticholinergic drugs for the next two; and antacids, H_2 histamine blockers, and metoclopramide for the last reason. It is not necessary and sometimes not desirable to achieve all these goals. The relative importance of each one varies with the age and condition of the patient and the type of anesthesia to be used.

It is desirable to induce sleep (or quiescence) and freedom from apprehension for the child who is to have anesthesia and surgery; however, such states are achieved at the price of some degree of respiratory depression or hypoxemia.[19] Anesthesiologists must decide not only the degree of sedation they desire for their patients, but also how much sedation patients can "afford." The type of anesthesia to be used and the quality of the postanesthetic care must be considered. The heavily sedated patient will have no memory of the surgical experience and may have an uneventful induction of anesthesia, but may be severely depressed after anesthesia. Return of protective reflexes and consciousness certainly will be delayed.

Atropine and Scopolamine

Certain drugs, particularly halothane and succinylcholine, have a cholinergic effect and may cause vagally induced bradycardia. This effect is most prominent in infants, especially those younger than 3 months. Atropine is superior to scopolamine dose for dose (0.15 mg) in controlling bradycardia and other cardiac dysrhythmias in infants younger than 6 months of age.[20,21] A vagolytic dose of atropine (0.03 $mg \cdot kg^{-1}$) provides complete protection against a cholinergic challenge in infants; relatively smaller doses of atropine provide adequate protection in older infants and children. These seemingly large doses are well tolerated by the infant and may be used safely. In general, we prefer to administer atropine in the operating room rather than as a preanesthetic medication.

At the age when sedative drugs are added to the preanesthetic medication, we prefer scopolamine to atropine because it contributes additional sedation, amnesia, and effective suppression of secretions in the airway. Because we usually combine scopolamine with an opioid, we seldom see delirium. Flushing of the face and restlessness are more common with scopolamine. These symptoms have little significance and usually can be avoided by careful dosage; the usual dose is approximately half that of atropine. In our experience, hyperthermia does not occur with these doses. In fact, an elevated temperature after scopolamine administration in this dosage almost certainly indicates infection or dehydration.

Sedatives and Opioids

Many drugs and combinations of drugs have been tried, but in our view none is better than the combination of opioid, barbiturate, and scopolamine. Table 47-2 shows a dosage schedule that may be used as a guide. The doses of barbiturate and opioid on this table are quite conservative. With scopolamine they provide adequate sedation in most situations. However, either the opioid or the barbiturate may safely be increased several degrees or even doubled for the particularly apprehensive child or if heavier sedation is needed.

Route and Time of Administration

Preanesthetic medication may be administered orally, by rectum, or by intramuscular injection. A number of commonly used barbiturates and sedatives are available as suppositories or flavored syrups. Absorption from the rectum is uneven and unpredictable, and oral preparations may be refused or vomited. Unless the child has an intense fear of needles or requires frequent injections, the intramuscular route does not appear to be unduly traumatic and is by far the most reliable.

Both atropine and scopolamine are most frequently administered intramuscularly, although either drug may be given intravenously if necessary. Oral administration is used only in rare circumstances; the effect by the oral route is generally less certain, and much larger doses must be used.

Sedative drugs can be effective only if sufficient time is allowed for the full effect to be achieved. The various drugs reach their maximum effect at different times and, therefore, theoretically, should be given separately. However, in most cases this is impractical, and usually all drugs are administered at the same time. They should be given at least 45 min to 1 h before anesthesia. Atropine and scopolamine ideally should be given 30–50 min before anesthesia. The vagolytic

TABLE 47-2. Preoperative Medication

AGE	WEIGHT		MORPHINE (mg)	ATROPINE OR SCOPOLAMINE (mg)	SECO-BARBITAL (mg)
	Kilograms	Pounds			
Premature	Less than 2.5	Less than 5½		Atropine 0.075	
0–1 mo	2.5–3.0	5½–7		Atropine 0.1	
1–3 mo	3.0–5.5	7–12		Atropine 0.15	
3–6 mo	5.5–7	12–15		Atropine 0.2	
6–12 mo	7–9	15–20	0.6	Scopolamine 0.1	20
12–18 mo	9–11	20–25	0.8	Scopolamine 0.15	25
18–24 mo	11–14	25–30	1.0	Scopolamine 0.15	30
2–3 yr	14–16	30–35	1.5	Scopolamine 0.15	40
3–5 yr	16–20	35–45	2.0	Scopolamine 0.15	50
5–8 yr	20–30	45–65	3.0	Scopolamine 0.2	75
8–10 yr	30–40	65–80	4.0	Scopolamine 0.2	75
10–12 yr	40–45	80–100	5.0	Scopolamine 0.3	100
12–14 yr	45–60	100–130	8.0	Scopolamine 0.3	100
Older than 14 yr	More than 60	More than 130	10.0	Scopolamine 0.3	100

effect of atropine does not last much more than 1 h; hence, the full dose should be repeated if induction is delayed more than 1 h after injection.

It is our practice that each patient is called twice: 1 h before surgery, for medication, and a second time just before anesthesia is begun. This requires planning and the cooperation of the surgical, nursing, and anesthesia staffs, but it is well worth the effort because the sedation is more effective and anesthetic inductions are made easier for both patient and anesthesiologist.

Antacids, H₂-blockers, and Metoclopramide

Children may be at slightly greater risk than adults for acid aspiration syndrome because they have a greater gastric residual volume and nearly all have a gastric pH of less than 2.5.[22] Specific H₂ receptor antagonists such as cimetidine or ranitidine, clear antacids, or metoclopramide may have an important role in reducing the likelihood of gastric aspiration in patients having elective or emergent surgery.[23–25]

ANESTHETIC DRUGS AND RELATED DRUGS

The choice of anesthetic drugs for infants and children is not strikingly different from that for adults. There appears to be no specific contraindication to any of the commonly used anesthetic drugs on the basis of age alone. Likewise, no contraindications on the basis of age alone have been demonstrated for any of the commonly used anesthetic induction techniques—inhalation, intravenous, or rectal. Selection of drugs and techniques is based on the individual anesthesiologist's experience, preference, and skill. Nevertheless, the anesthesiologist should use special care in choosing the optimal method for each patient. Nitrous oxide reinforced by potent inhalation drugs or intravenous drugs is frequently used to maintain anesthesia in pediatric patients; muscle relaxants are common adjuncts.

In some clinics it is common to have parents actively participate in the anesthetic induction process.[26, 27] For some parents and preschool children, this joint experience attenuates a multitude of fears and anxieties and is, thus, a positive experience. However, for other parents participation is emotionally traumatic. The psychodynamics of these experiences are poorly understood. One is constantly amazed at how well many preschool children adapt to so-called stressful situations if provided with information in advance. This adaptation does not necessarily require active parental participation but most likely is a complex reflection of general parenting. For example, pediatric dentists commonly perform routine dental care with limited or no fuss in preschool children without the parents present; for many children this is an immense source of pride. This issue is obviously complex and is not resolved by evangelism.

INHALATION AGENTS

Induction of general anesthesia in the infant may be difficult no matter what technique is selected. Inhalation inductions are frequently complicated by breath-holding, laryngospasm, and distension of the stomach with anesthetic gases. Difficulty in maintaining a good mask fit is common. The procedure must be performed gently, cautiously, and with close attention to vital signs and indications of deepening anesthesia.

Young infants usually are not upset at induction of anesthesia with a loosely applied facemask. With increasing age, the induction process becomes progressively easier. Older children may prefer to hold the mask for themselves if they have chosen an inhalation method over a "shot." In general, halothane allows the most rapid and smooth induction compared with enflurane and isoflurane. The ether anesthetics are pungent and produce airway irritation. For example, there is a high incidence of laryngospasm during an inhalation induction in infants. Flavored lip gloss or food oils can be used to hide the pungency of these agents. A "single-breath" method for induction of anesthesia with halothane has been described: the patient exhales to residual volume and then takes a full inspiration from a reservoir bag containing 5% halothane in 70% nitrous oxide with oxygen. The halothane concentration is then reduced to continue the induction process.

The incidence of bradycardia, hypotension, and cardiac arrest during induction of inhalation anesthesia is higher in infants and small children than in adults.[28, 29] This greater incidence of untoward effects from potent drugs can be attributed to age-related differences in uptake, anesthetic requirements, and sensitivity of the cardiovascular system. The uptake of inhalation anesthetics is more rapid in infants and small children than in adults because of major differences in blood–gas solubility coefficients, blood–tissue solubility coefficients, body composition, the ratio of alveolar ventilation to functional residual capacity, and the distribution of cardiac output.[30–36] Thus, early in anesthetic induction the infant has higher tissue concentrations of anesthetic than the adult (e.g., in brain, heart, muscle).[37]

Intracardiac shunts, common in infants and children, can also alter the uptake of inhalation anesthetics.[38, 39] A right-to-left shunt slows the uptake of anesthetic as the anesthetic tension or concentration in the arterial blood increases more slowly; induction of anesthesia is prolonged. The influence of a left-to-right shunt on anesthetic uptake depends on the size of the shunt and on whether a right-to-left shunt exists. A large (greater than 80%) left-to-right shunt increases the rate of anesthetic transfer from the lungs to the arterial blood; smaller shunts (less than 50%) have a negligible effect on uptake. A left-to-right shunt may speed induction when it coexists with a large right-to-left shunt. Increases in pulmonary vascular resistance or decreases in systemic vascular resistance occasionally can reverse left-to-right shunts.

The anesthetic requirements for various inhalation anesthetics (e.g., cyclopropane, halothane, isoflurane, and enflurane) generally are related inversely to age (Fig. 47-1).[40–44] Thus, higher inspired concentrations (over-pressure) are often used early in an anesthetic induction to compensate for the age-related differences in anesthetic requirements.

Isoflurane has fewer adverse cardiovascular effects than equally potent halothane concentrations.[45–51] Although the drugs similarly reduce contractility and heart rate, isoflurane reduces peripheral resistance several fold, but halothane does not. The resulting reduction in cardiac index with isoflurane is only half that with halothane. Isoflurane may, thus, permit greater hemodynamic stability than halothane. The alarming reduction in blood pressure caused by isoflurane may reflect only a decrease in peripheral resistance with near-normal cardiac output. Anesthetic drugs blunt baroreceptor reflexes in a concentration-dependent manner to a greater degree in infants than in older patients.[52–55] The reasons why anesthetics depress the baroreceptor reflexes more in infants are unknown. Most likely they are related to developmental differences in the autonomic nervous system. The separation between MAC and the lethal concentration of a potent inhala-

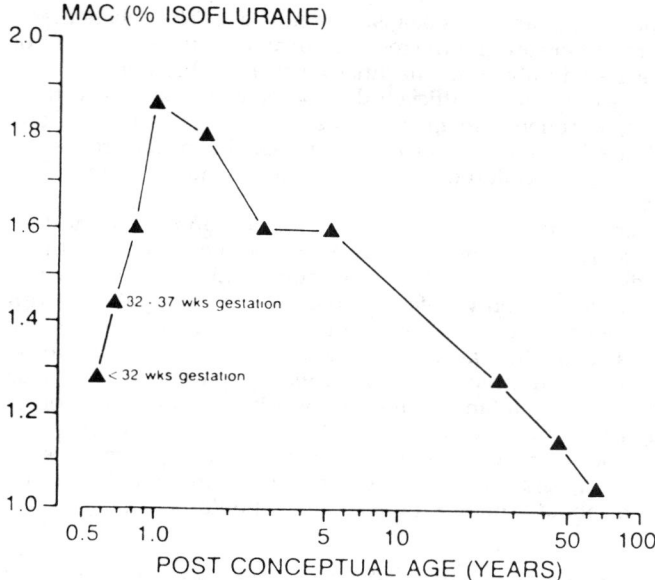

FIG. 47-1. The MAC of isoflurane and postconceptual age. (Data from LeDez KM, Lerman J: The minimum alveolar concentration [MAC] of isoflurane in preterm neonates. Anesthesiology 67:301, 1987.)

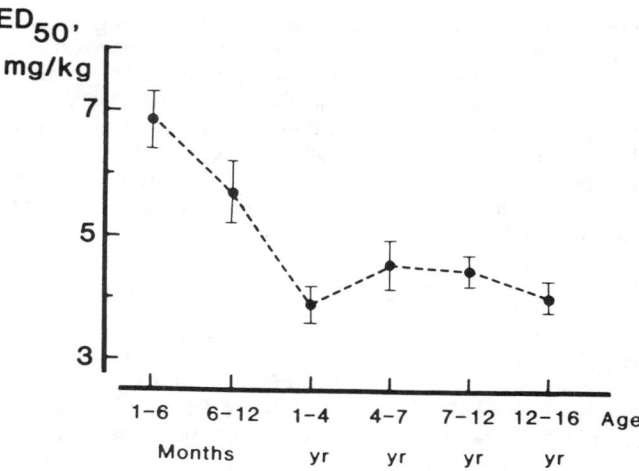

FIG. 47-2. Estimated ED$_{50}$ of thiopental in various age groups of children. (Data from Jonmarker C, Westrin P, Larsson S *et al*: Thiopental requirements for induction of anesthesia in children. Anesthesiology 67:104, 1987.)

tion anesthetic defines the safety margin or therapeutic ratio. Isoflurane has a higher therapeutic ratio than does halothane in older animals, but not in young animals.

INTRAVENOUS DRUGS

In older children, intravenous infusions are more readily started, and induction with an intravenous anesthetic is frequently used. Intravenous drugs can be administered to small infants with very little discomfort if a skilled, "concealed" technique using a fine (27 gauge) needle is used. Dermal lidocaine patches (EMLA) may facilitate intravenous catheter insertion.[56] Intravenous inductions may be preferred for older children because the psychologic sequelae may be less than with inhalation induction. Thiopental, methohexital, and ketamine may be used for intravenous induction of anesthesia. Rarely, each may be given intramuscularly. Infants generally need more thiopental than older children or adults to minimize the reaction to application of a facemask or intubation of the trachea; however, "sleep" doses may be little different (Fig. 47-2).[57–60] Midazolam may be unreliable as an intravenous induction drug.[61]

Both thiopental and methohexital have been used by the rectal route to induce anesthesia in pediatric patients. Methohexital (15–25 mg·kg^{-1}) is now more commonly used and is probably the drug of choice in view of its more rapid metabolism.[62] Hiccough is a common side-effect. Clinical recovery from rectal methohexital occurs in 30–40 min and shows some correlation with plasma concentrations of the drug.

A variety of sedative–hypnotic drugs appear to have increased duration of effects in the infant; in older children higher doses may be needed. The mechanism of this change in sensitivity has been elucidated for some of the barbiturates and benzodiazepines.[63–66] The dose of ketamine (µg·kg^{-1}) required to prevent gross movements is four times greater in infants younger than 6 months than in 6-yr-old children.[67]

Acute studies show little metabolism of ketamine by the newborn. In the "anesthetic" state associated with ketamine, respiration and blood pressure are usually well maintained. However, use of ketamine in infants, particularly at the high doses required for lack of movement, has been associated with depression of ventilation and apnea, generalized extensor spasm with opisthotonus, an increase in intracranial pressure in infants with hydrocephalus, and acute increases in pulmonary artery pressure in infants with congenital heart disease.[68–71] Recent studies suggest that pulmonary vascular resistance is not changed by ketamine in infants with either normal or elevated pulmonary vascular resistance as long as the airway and ventilation are maintained.[72, 73]

OPIOIDS

Meperidine (0.5–1 mg·kg^{-1}), morphine (0.05–0.1 mg·kg^{-1}), or fentanyl (3–5 µg·kg^{-1}), sufentanil (1–2 µg·kg^{-1}), or alfentanil (20–50 µg·kg^{-1}) is used to reinforce nitrous oxide–oxygen anesthesia in the infant or small child. Such doses attenuate the cardiovascular responses to surgical stress. High-dose morphine (1.0 mg·kg^{-1}), fentanyl (25–50 µg·kg^{-1}), or sufentanil (10–15 µg·kg^{-1}) anesthesia is given with oxygen–air to critically ill infants or children, particularly those requiring palliative heart surgery. The cardiovascular effects of these opioids seem minimal.

Bradycardia and chest wall rigidity are potential features of high-dose opioid anesthesia. Therefore, it is common to administer muscle relaxants with desired cardiovascular side-effects (*i.e.*, pancuronium or gallamine) to ameliorate the effects of fentanyl. The cardiovascular effects of fentanyl at doses of 30–75 µg·kg^{-1} (with pancuronium) are minimal.[74–76] The cardiovascular and ventilatory effects of fentanyl (without relaxant) depend on concentration. The dose of fentanyl needed to guarantee satisfactory anesthesia for infants is unknown. Age-related differences in the kinetics and sensitivity to fentanyl and changes in kinetics associated with profound pathophysiologic conditions make generalizations difficult.[77, 78] However, fentanyl clearance in the infant seems comparable to that in the older child or adult; it is significantly reduced in the premature infant. Sufentanil is approximately seven times more potent than fentanyl and has minimal cardiovascular effects. Bradycardia is an uncommon feature.[79, 80] Alfentanil is one-third as potent as fentanyl and has a shorter duration of action. Because of its relatively short duration of action, alfentanil may be particularly useful in anesthesia for infants and children, particularly for short surgical procedures.[81–83]

MUSCLE RELAXANTS

Muscle relaxants are common adjuncts to nitrous oxide–opioid anesthesia. Throughout infancy and early childhood, the neuromuscular junction matures physically and biochemically, the contractile properties of skeletal muscle change, the amount of muscle in proportion to body weight increases, and the neuromuscular junction is variably sensitive to relaxants.[84, 85] In addition, the apparent volume of distribution of relaxants, their redistribution and excretion (clearance), and possibly their rate of metabolism change throughout life. These factors influence the dose–response relationship to relaxants and the duration of neuromuscular blockade. When allowance is made for differences in the volume of distribution and for the type and concentration of anesthetic, infants appear relatively resistant to succinylcholine and relatively sensitive to nondepolarizing relaxants; the response of children to relaxants differs little from that of the adult.[86–105]

ENDOTRACHEAL INTUBATION

The advantages of endotracheal intubation for any patient having anesthesia are beyond question. The endotracheal tube has become an indispensable part of all intrathoracic, neurosurgical, and other surgical procedures involving unusual positions or distortion of the airway or in which the anesthesiologist does not command access to the airway. In a number of other situations, endotracheal intubation is not absolutely necessary but facilitates airway maintenance and ventilation of the lungs. In such cases tracheal intubation is elective and may be considered an aid to both the anesthesiologist and the surgeon. In patients presenting little or no difficulty with the airway, endotracheal intubation is probably unjustified or at least unnecessary.

INDICATIONS

The indications for tracheal intubation are the same for patients of any age, but the infant's anatomic and physiologic problems raise the question of whether infancy itself may not be an indication for endotracheal intubation. At this age the airway is difficult to maintain, mask fit is difficult, and assisted or controlled ventilation of the lungs is essential in view of the poor respiratory reserve of the infant. These problems are all greatly simplified by endotracheal anesthesia.

The suggestion that all infants younger than 1 yr (or some other arbitrary age) should have endotracheal anesthesia has led to controversy among anesthesiologists. All agree that a finite morbidity accompanies endotracheal intubation and that this morbidity and its potential consequences are greater in the infant. There is also agreement that endotracheal intubation in the infant requires special knowledge and skills that

the average anesthesiologist may not have. The debate therefore centers around the relative advantages *versus* the risks of tracheal intubation. The final answer to this question will come only when sufficient data become available. Nevertheless, experience in many thousands of cases in numerous clinics has shown that routine intubation of the trachea of infants and children can be achieved with an exceedingly low morbidity.

Over a number of years we have used endotracheal anesthesia virtually routinely in all patients younger than 9 months of age, except in very short procedures and when elective tracheal intubation was felt to be unsafe (*e.g.*, in patients with histories of recent upper respiratory infections or asthmatic episodes). There are many advantages in standardizing not so much the technique, but the philosophy of good anesthetic care of small infants. When endotracheal intubation becomes a part of standard care, the skill with which the technique is performed by the various members of the department is increased, and there is no need for debate in borderline situations about whether the technique should be used.

SAFETY AND PREVENTION OF COMPLICATIONS

Despite the greater indications for tracheal intubation in very young patients, many surgeons and anesthesiologists have been unenthusiastic about its use because of the danger, real or imagined, of sequelae. Complications of tracheal intubation can and do arise, but for the most part they can be prevented.

Intubation of the infant's trachea is not more difficult than that of the adult, but the anesthesiologist must be familiar not only with the anatomic differences of the infant larynx, but also with the specialized equipment required. Trauma can be minimized in tracheal intubation by working gently and by ensuring adequate relaxation either with a sufficiently deep plane of anesthesia or with muscle relaxants. At least three tube sizes should be available for each case. The tube should pass the glottis and cricoid without resistance, and air should leak around the tube when positive pressure of approximately 20 cm H_2O is applied to the airway (Table 47-3).

Use of cuffed endotracheal tubes in children younger than 10 yr is neither necessary nor good practice: a suitably large tube in patients younger than this age will make sufficiently good contact at the level of the cricoid to prevent significant air leak. If a cuffed tube is used, a smaller size with correspondingly higher air flow resistance may be necessary. Finally, there is an increased likelihood of trauma to the tracheal mucosa from the pressure of the inflated cuff.

Tube selection also is important in controlling the complications of endotracheal intubation. Tubes should be sterile and free of any material that might be irritating or toxic to the mucosa. Sterile, prepackaged, disposable vinyl plastic tubes are recommended. Lubricants must be used carefully. Tubes of ointment or jelly may become contaminated, and those containing local anesthetics may be irritant or allergenic. Sterile water is usually an adequate lubricant except for nasal or cuffed tubes.

PEDIATRIC BREATHING CIRCUITS

An optimal breathing circuit system for the pediatric patient provides minimal dead space and minimal resistance to breathing and permits accurate, rapid control of anesthetic depth, inspired oxygen concentration, and inspired carbon dioxide concentration. Such systems should be small, light,

TABLE 47-3. Approximate Sizes of Endotracheal Tubes for Infants and Children*

AGE	WEIGHT (kg)	INTERNAL DIAMETER (mm)†	FRENCH†
6 mo	6	4.0	16
9 mo	9	4.5	18
1 yr	12	5.0	20
2 yr	14	5.5	22
4 yr	16	6.0	24
6 yr	20	6.5	26
8 yr	28	7.0	28
10 yr	30	7.5	30

* These suggested endotracheal tube sizes will produce a snug fit with a minimal leak during positive-pressure ventilation. Smaller sizes may be used if a moderate leak is desired.

† French size is the outside circumference of the endotracheal tube; Fr = π outside diameter.

and as free from possible malfunction as possible. Although many types of pediatric devices have been developed, modifications of the simple T-piece are the most popular for infants. For older children, modified or traditional circle systems with a carbon dioxide absorber are more reasonable.

In its most elemental form, the T-piece is simply a short length of rigid tubing that is attached to an endotracheal tube at one end and left open to the atmosphere at the distal end.[107] Fresh anesthetic gases are introduced into the tube, midway at right angles. When the open limb is very short (or has no length at all), it functions as a nonrebreathing device. To prevent air dilution on inspiration and facilitate control of ventilation, the volume of the expiratory limb is increased by adding a length of tubing at least equivalent to the tidal volume with a rebreathing bag.[106] Rebreathing can now occur; the amount of rebreathing becomes a function of the fresh gas flow. An additional increase in the volume of the expiratory limb beyond an amount equivalent to the tidal volume, however, does not further affect the rebreathing characteristics of the system. When flows of fresh gas equivalent to 2.5–3 times the minute volume are used, no rebreathing occurs. The addition of a rebreathing bag into the expiratory limb is possible and greatly facilitates the use of assisted or controlled ventilation (e.g., Jackson-Rees system).

A number of combinations of T-piece tubing, breathing bag, and sites of fresh gas entry and overflow are possible. Mapleson classified the various combinations into five types (Fig. 47-3).[108] The rebreathing characteristics of each type were later investigated by Waters and Mapleson. Mapleson's Type A is the so-called Magill system, popular in England but seldom used in this country. Its principal advantage is that during spontaneous ventilation alveolar gas is preferentially vented. Thus, large fresh-gas flows are not needed to prevent rebreathing. The Jackson Rees modification is functionally identical to the Mapleson Type D. Types B and C are not used clinically. Carbon dioxide is removed more effectively in the D configuration when controlled ventilation is used.

In recent years the Mapleson D device has emerged in a new guise, the coaxial circuit.[109] It is virtually identical in principle but much different in design. The light-weight disposable inspired and expired gas conduits are usually arranged coaxially with the inspiratory tubing running within the expiratory tubing. The rebreathing bag and expiratory pop-off valve are permanently mounted on a bracket clamped to the gas ma-

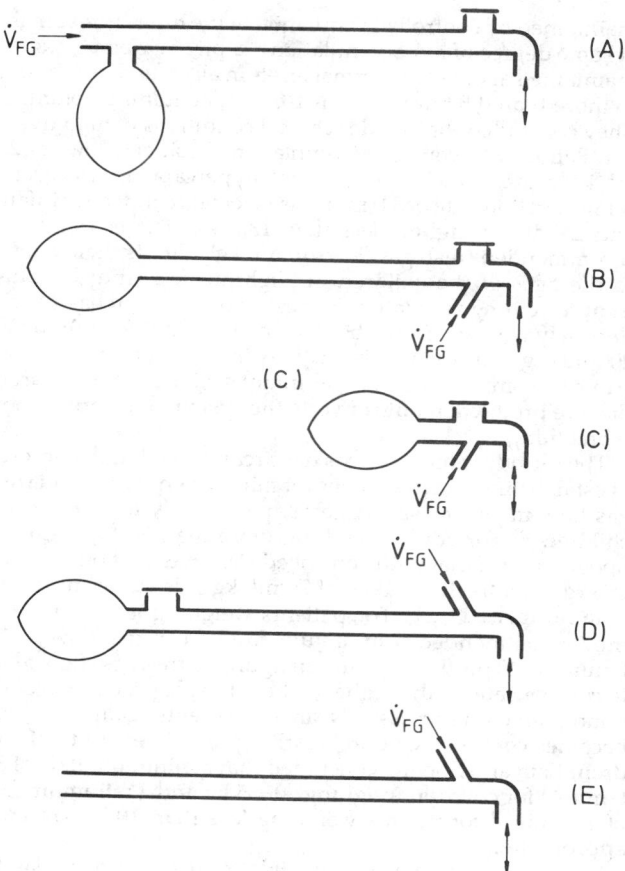

FIG. 47-3. Mapleson classification (A–E) of some rebreathing systems. $\dot{V}_{FG}$ is the fresh gas flow. (From Mushin WW, Jones PL: Physics for the Anesthetist, 4th ed, Chap 17, p 375. Boston, Blackwell Scientific, 1987. By permission of the publisher.)

chine. Scavenging of expired and excess gases is thus easily accomplished. The unit can be used for patients of any size and age, provided suitable volumes of fresh gases are chosen. The coaxial arrangement permits some heat exchange between the warm expired and unwarmed inspired gases, thus preventing some degree of heat loss from the airway.

The T-piece systems, although they incorporate neither directional valves nor soda lime, were originally conceived of as nonrebreathing systems. Thus, early attention was directed toward removal of expired carbon dioxide from the *system* rather than from the *patient*. In the spontaneously breathing patient, a fresh gas flow of three times the minute volume is necessary to flush the expiratory limb completely (regardless of its volume) and thus prevent rebreathing.[109, 110]

With controlled ventilation of the lungs, it is not necessary to completely eliminate expired carbon dioxide from the expiratory limb to maintain eucapnia. When minute volume ventilation is maintained at near normal levels, alveolar carbon dioxide tension (PA_{CO_2}) can be determined by fresh gas flow. Because reduced minute volume ventilation results in increasing arterial carbon dioxide tensions (Pa_{CO_2}) or PA_{CO_2} as well, Pa_{CO_2} is primarily a function of either fresh gas flow or minute volume ventilation, whichever is the lesser of the two.

Nightingale *et al* demonstrated that with the minute volume maintained by controlled ventilation of the lungs (presumably at some degree of hyperventilation), expired carbon dioxide is maintained at or below normal levels in all cases at flows equal to more than 0.5 but less than 1 times the minute volume.[111] They concluded that, under clinical conditions of mild hyperventilation with controlled ventilation, fresh gas flows of 220 ml·kg^{-1} are sufficient to prevent hypercapnia. However, a minimum flow rate of 3 l·min^{-1} was recommended for infants and children weighing less than 13.5 kg. The expression of recommended fresh gas flows in ml·kg^{-1} limits their validity to the ages of the children in Nightingale's study, because minute volume ventilation expressed on a weight basis varies inversely with age from about 90 ml·kg^{-1} in the adult to over 200 ml·kg^{-1} in the newborn.[111] A fixed minimum flow of 3 l·min^{-1} compensates for the infant's higher rate of carbon dioxide production but converts the system to complete nonrebreathing.

The introduction of the coaxial circuit has rekindled interest in establishing suitable values for minute ventilation and fresh gas flow in semiclosed systems, particularly for infants and children.[112] For adults weighing more than 50 kg, Bain and Spoerel found that with controlled hyperventilation (120–140 ml·kg^{-1}), a fresh gas flow of 70 ml·kg^{-1} is sufficient to provide normal Pa$_{CO_2}$.[108] For patients weighing less than 50 kg they recommended a minimum fixed fresh gas flow of 3.5 l·min^{-1}.[113] This fixed minimum figure for fresh gas flow tends to compensate for the higher carbon dioxide production of the infant, but with successively smaller patients again the system becomes completely nonrebreathing. In a later study of children, Bain and Spoerel concluded that a minimum flow of 3.5 l·min^{-1} for children weighing 10–35 kg and a minimum flow of 2 l·min^{-1} for infants weighing less than 10 kg are more appropriate.

These analyses make it possible to arrive at formulas for suitable values of fresh gas flow and minute volume ventilation that can be used for infants and children. Complete nonrebreathing occurs with fresh gas flows two to three times the minute volume. Maximum permissible rebreathing occurs with fresh gas flows in the range of 0.6 to 1 times the minute volume. With increasing rebreathing maintenance of sufficient minute volume ventilation becomes increasingly critical. In large children an obvious advantage of the partial rebreathing approach is the economy of fresh gas flow. Another advantage for patients of all ages is the ability to set fixed ventilatory volumes (on a mechanical ventilator, for instance) and to control Pa$_{CO_2}$ simply by adjustment of fresh gas flow. Dangers of the rebreathing approach for infants are implicit in the "safe" minimum fresh gas flow settings recommended by several authors. In the smallest patients the accuracy of flow meters is critical and the risk of hypercarbia acute unless there is scrupulous Pa$_{CO_2}$ monitoring.

CIRCLE ABSORPTION

The circle absorption system potentially eliminates the problems of carbon dioxide control, humidification, and scavenging of waste gases seen with Mapleson D systems. High-resistance valves, the large dead space of the chimney Y-pieces, and the large, heavy tubing make the standard adult circle system unsuitable for infants and small children. With improved low-resistance valves infants can maintain normal blood gas values even with spontaneous ventilation.[113] With controlled ventilation of the lungs, resistance across valves is moot.

The Foregger-Bloomquist and Ohio infant absorbers were developed in attempt to design a circle absorption system tailored specifically to the needs of the very small patient.[114] The canisters and tubing are reduced in size. Better-designed directional valves and chimney Y-pieces with minimal dead space are substituted. The Ohio and the Foregger-Bloomquist absorbers became quite popular, especially among anesthesiologists who wanted to use closed or semiclosed techniques. The presence of directional valves, however, always raised the specter of possible incompetence or increased airway resistance. More practically, the nuisance of setting up a separate absorber and finding a suitable location for these extra pieces of equipment on or around the anesthesia machine discouraged many anesthesiologists from using these systems.

For the anesthesiologist who only occasionally anesthetizes infants, the possibility of easily adapting an "adult" circle absorber system for infant use has much appeal. The Columbia circle absorber is an adult absorber modifiable for pediatric use by interchangeable smaller canister tubing and fittings and, most important, an especially designed low-resistance and low-dead-space (concentric) valve mount (Fig. 47-4). Smaller tubing and fittings are the most important. The Revell "cirqulator" can reduce the dead space and valve resistance of the standard absorber (Fig. 47-5). As the name implies, a gas- or vacuum-driven pump is incorporated into a standard adult circuit to produce constant circulation and mixing of the gases within the circuit, independent of ventilatory flow. A septate Y-piece is used in conjunction with the circulator to direct the moving gases into the mask to provide better mixing and thus reduce dead space. The constant flow of gases within the

FIG. 47-4. Divided airway adapter. The Columbia Pediatric Circle Valve is shown. Deadspace is 0.5 ml, significantly less than the 40-ml deadspace of a conventional airway adapter. (Reprinted with permission. Rackow H, Salanitre E: A new pediatric circle valve. Anesthesiology 29:833, 1968.)

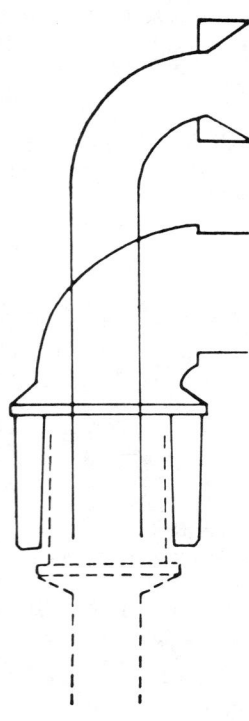

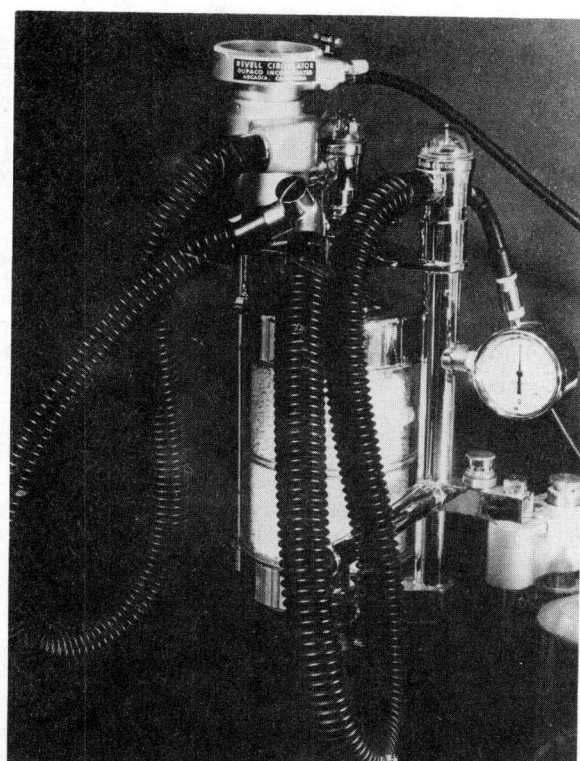

FIG. 47-5. The Revell "Cirqulator" and Septate "Y" piece are used in conjunction to reduce deadspace of the face mask. Circuit diagram: The patient and the rebreathing bag are not included in the circulation. The bag moves normally, reflecting the tidal exchange between the patient and the bag.

circuit tended to keep the directional valves unseated and thus reduce airflow resistance by reducing or eliminating opening pressures.

REGIONAL ANESTHESIA

Regional anesthetic techniques (*e.g.*, axillary block, combined ilioinguinal and iliohypogastric block, penile block, epidural block, and spinal block), are becoming more popular for infants and children to supplement general anesthesia, as the sole anesthetic, or for postoperative analgesia.[116-130] In general, the anatomy and principles of regional anesthesia are the same in infants and children as in adults. Regional anesthesia provides good relaxation; a reduction in the amount of potent anesthetic needed; safe, rapid recovery; early prolonged pain relief; and minimal complications. The use of regional anesthesia is limited, however, because of the lack of cooperation, the child's fear of needles, and the conscious child's apprehension in the atmosphere of the operating room. Heavy sedation or even light general anesthesia may be needed in preschool-age children to maintain the necessary quiescence while the block is in progress; in infants little or no sedation may be needed; in school-age children light sedation is required. Despite the potential problems, the anesthesiologist who is skilled in nerve blocks will find many occasions in which this type of anesthesia is useful.

BRACHIAL PLEXUS BLOCK AND INTRAVENOUS REGIONAL BLOCK

The axillary approach to the brachial plexus block is the most popular one in children. However, the selection of the site of the block should depend on the location of the operation. For operations on the forearm and outer upper arm, including reduction of dislocated shoulders, a supraclavicular technique, usually interscalene, is indicated. The axillary approach is indicated for operations on the forearm and hand. Continuous brachial plexus analgesia has been recommended to follow revascularization procedures of the hands or digits.[131, 132] A simplified dose schedule to calculate the dose of local anesthetics is useful (Table 47-4). Intravenous regional techniques also may be used.[133-135]

ILIOINGUINAL AND ILIOHYPOGASTRIC NERVE BLOCK

The ilioinguinal and iliohypogastric nerves eventually pierce the internal oblique muscle just below and 1–2 cm medial to the anterior superior spine and come to lie between the internal oblique and the aponeurosis of the external oblique muscle. They supply the skin of the lower abdomen and the inguinal region. Thus, the combined block is useful to provide intraoperative or postoperative analgesia for inguinal surgery. If the block is to be used for surgery as well as postoperative analgesia, it is also necessary to infiltrate the hernia sac.[116] Bupivacaine (0.5%) is used for this purpose at a dose of 0.5 ml per year of age.

PENILE BLOCK

The penile block is a useful alternative to caudal anesthesia for providing intraoperative and postoperative analgesia for circumcision.[106, 137] This block can be applied with the patient lying in the supine position. The dorsal nerves of the penis enter from under the symphysis pubis and run below the deep (Buck's) fascia and superficial to the corpora cavernosa. The nerves are blocked just at their point of entry before they divide to also supply the anterior parts. Bupivacaine (0.5%) is used at a dose of $1 \text{ ml} \cdot \text{kg}^{-1}$. Epinephrine-containing solutions must never be used because of the risk of ischemia of the

TABLE 47-4. Simplified Dosage for Brachial Plexus Blocks

AGE (yr)	FORMULA FOR DETERMINING VOLUME (ml)	CONCENTRATION (%)	
		Lidocaine Mepivacaine	Bupivacaine
0–4	$\dfrac{\text{Height (cm)}}{12}$	1	0.25
5–8	$\dfrac{\text{Height (cm)}}{10}$	1	0.25
9–16	$\dfrac{\text{Height (cm)}}{7}$	1	0.25

(Adapted from Lanz E: Blockaden des Plexus brachialis im Kindesalter. In Kuhn K, Hausdorfer J [eds]: Regional Anaesthesie im Kindesalter, p 24. Berlin, Springer Verlag, 1984.)

penis. The only complications of penile block are intravascular injection or extensive hematoma.

SPINAL ANESTHESIA

The patient's size and age do not contraindicate the use of spinal anesthesia. In older, cooperative children and adolescents, the indications for its use are identical to those for adults. Its use for infants and young children was initially limited to those who had liver, kidney, or pulmonary disease and were having surgical procedures below the diaphragm; its use is now advocated for more healthy, fit infants.[138-141] The spinal cord may end as low as L-3 in the infant. Thus, spinal punctures should be performed at the L4-5 or L5-S1 level. With spinal anesthesia the circulation of infants or children tends to be more stable than that of adults. Therefore, use of vasopressor drugs is seldom necessary to maintain the blood pressure.

Although any of the accepted spinal anesthetic drugs may be used, tetracaine has been the most popular. The duration of action of any given spinal anesthetic agent is somewhat less in the infant than in the adult, and, for this reason, epinephrine is nearly always added to the injected mixture of drugs. The dose of tetracaine may be estimated at roughly $0.4\ mg \cdot kg^{-1}$ or at 1 mg per year of age. A minimum dose of 1.5 mg to 2 mg is usually required for even the smallest infant.

EPIDURAL ANESTHESIA

Caudal anesthesia for perineal or lower abdominal procedures has been effective and relatively easy to administer in infants and small children.[142-158] Caudal blocks placed after induction of general anesthesia reduce the amount of potent anesthetic agent required and, more important, reduce postoperative agitation and opioid requirements. Bupivacaine (0.25%) with epinephrine (1:200,000) provides adequate postoperative analgesia; a maximum dose of $3\ mg \cdot kg^{-1}$ is used. Takasaki et al have described formulae for calculating the dose of lidocaine and other local anesthetics for caudal analgesia in infants and children.[150] Because infants and children have limited epidural fat, caudal catheters may be positioned easily at the lumbar or thoracic level. Alternatively, lumbar or thoracic epidural catheters can be inserted for intraoperative and postoperative pain control.

MONITORING

Although most pediatric surgical patients can be monitored adequately by the intelligent use of a few simple devices, the advent of more sophisticated equipment allows moment-to-moment monitoring of blood pressure, oxygenation, electrocardiogram (ECG), central venous pressure, intracranial pressure, and end-tidal gases for the patient having major surgery.[159]

The infant or child should be monitored continuously with a precordial or esophageal stethoscope.[160] The anesthesiologist can thus detect changes in the rate, quality, and intensity of the heart sounds, which may be helpful in evaluating blood loss, depth of anesthesia, or failing circulation or in diagnosing air emboli. Plethysmographic monitors attached to the finger or toe are helpful but are subject to artifacts and are frequently unreliable in the very young. Doppler monitors are the most reliable audible pulse indicators. Electrocardio-

graphic monitoring is useful in determining pulse rate and the presence of cardiac arrhythmias. The value of the ECG tracing in evaluating cardiac function is limited, however, because it indicates only electrical activity and gives no indication of cardiac output.

BLOOD PRESSURE

Systolic blood pressure may be determined in virtually all patients by the oscillometric method with use of a suitable cuff and an aneroid manometer. However, several relatively simple electronic devices have greatly facilitated the indirect determination of blood pressure in small patients. The first of these entails the use of Doppler ultrasound to detect the equivalent arterial wall motion or red blood cell (RBC) movement of the Korotkoff sounds. A transducer containing two lead zirconate crystals is placed over a peripheral artery. Ultrasonic waves are generated at one of the crystals by an electrical signal at 2–8 MHz and directed at the artery. The second crystal receives the waves reflected from the wall of the artery (or RBCs). The frequency differential between transmitted and reflected waves is proportional to the velocity of the arterial wall motion or RBCs (Doppler principle). Amplification of the shift frequencies produces characteristic audible high and low sounds as the arterial wall expands (systolic) and contracts.

Electronic oscillometers (e.g., Dinamap) detect transmitted pulsatile oscillation of the pressure cuff itself.[161, 162] By electronic analysis of serial oscillations, it can be shown that the amplitude of the oscillations in cuff pressure changes at different pressures. At intervals selected by the operator, the cuff is inflated above systolic pressure and deflated automatically in 3-mm Hg decrements. Two successive beats are compared for oscillatory amplitude at each pressure level. At suprasystolic pressures of the cuff, low amplitude oscillations are detected. When systolic pressure is reached, amplitude suddenly increases. As cuff pressure is further reduced, amplitude decreases with succeeding beats until a plateau is reached. Mean pressure corresponds to the lowest level at which maximum oscillations are detected. With continuing deflation, a large abrupt decrease in oscillations occurs at the diastolic pressure. Because oscillations of the cuff itself are being detected, careful positioning of the cuff is not necessary, but a loose fit or residual air severely attenuates the signal. Motion renders the device useless. Long deflation and cycle times are necessary with this technique and, because inflation occurs automatically by means of an electric pump, unrecognized runaway or prolonged inflation may cause ischemic nerve damage.[163, 164]

Cannulation of the radial artery or dorsalis pedis artery allows continuous measurement of blood pressure and permits frequent serial determinations of blood gases and pH, hematocrit, serum solids, electrolytes, and osmolality. With a translumination technique, either 22- or 24-gauge plastic cannulae can be placed percutaneously in infants; rarely, a cutdown may be necessary.

CENTRAL VENOUS PRESSURE

Central venous pressure catheters can be used to estimate mean intrathoracic pressure during mechanical ventilation, estimate adequacy of blood replacement or venous return, and extract air embolism from the right heart. Catheters can be inserted from the antecubital fossa, external jugular, or internal jugular vein. Because the position of the catheter is critical if the catheter is to be used to extract air (venous air embolus), a chest roentgenogram must be taken to confirm its position. Monitoring changes in the P-waves of the ECG can assist in correct placement of a right atrial catheter.

VENTILATION

The anesthesiologist has few direct aids to measure tidal volume in infants and must depend to a large extent on clinical observation. Standard ventilation meters such as the Wright Respirometer are useful for older children, but they either do not respond or are grossly inaccurate in the ranges required for infants. When available, arterial pH, Pa_{CO_2}, and Pa_{O_2} determinations are the most reliable indexes of adequate ventilation.

PULSE OXIMETRY

Continuous noninvasive monitoring of arterial oxygen saturation can be accomplished by pulse oximetry.[165] The probe incorporates two elements: one contains two low-intensity light-emitting diodes, the other a photo-cell detector. It is usually placed on the patient's finger or toe, but any site may be chosen in which a pulsating vascular bed can be imposed between the two elements. Two wavelengths of light chosen for the relative reflectance with oxygenated *versus* reduced hemoglobin illuminate the tissue under the probe. By expanding and contracting, the pulsating vascular bed creates a change in the light path length, which modifies the amount of light detected. The result is a characteristic plethysmographic wave form. The amplitude of this constantly varying detected light depends on the magnitude of the pulse, wavelength, and oxygen saturation of the arterial hemoglobin. Artifact from blood, skin, connective tissue, or bone is completely eliminated. The technique has been shown to be accurate with oxygen saturations from 70 to 100%. Reduction in vascular pulsation diminishes the instrument's ability to calculate saturations, for example, in hypothermia, in hypotension, or with use of vasoconstrictive drugs. In addition to continuous indication of arterial oxygen saturation, the pulse oximeter provides a continuous readout of pulse rate and amplitude. There are several obvious advantages of pulse oximetry over transcutaneous oxygen measurement in the patient having anesthesia: no special site preparation is necessary and application is extremely simple. The risk of burns is eliminated because it is not necessary to heat the sensor.

CAPNOGRAPHY AND MASS SPECTROMETRY

End-tidal carbon dioxide monitors (capnographs) can be used to assess the adequacy of ventilation.[166] Most modern capnographs display the carbon dioxide waveform as well as the numeric readings. The adaptation of the mass spectrometer as a clinical respiratory monitor can now provide continuous on-line analysis of respiratory gases of the anesthetized or acutely ill patient. Heretofore these data were unavailable or available only in part through serial analysis of arterial blood gases. The mass spectrometer also can identify not only the gases present in a given sample, but their percentage composition as well. Almost any gas can be detected, and the purchaser of the equipment can choose the gases to be detected. The list usually includes oxygen, carbon dioxide, nitrogen, nitrous oxide, and the major volatile anesthetic drugs. The mass spectrometer can be used as a sensitive detector of air emboli.

A capnographic tracing is usually displayed as well as an alpha-numeric reading of inspired and end-tidal values of each gas expressed in volumes percent or torr, the respiratory rate, and I:E ratio. Trending can be displayed as well. A computer interprets as inspired and end-tidal values those occurring at the instants of minimal and maximal carbon dioxide concentrations, respectively. Thus, the accuracy of the displayed inspired and end-tidal values depends crucially upon the faithfulness of the capnographic tracing. Mapleson D circuits, particularly coaxial circuits, provide continuous fresh gas flow near the airway. Mixing of this fresh gas with expired gases may dilute the end-tidal concentrations, degrade the capnograph tracing, and yield inaccurately low results.[167-169] These problems can be minimized by using an elbow connector and sampling near the endotracheal tube. In essence, the elbow connector separates the jet stream of the breathing circuit from the expired gases.

TEMPERATURE

The thermistor thermometer and heat-sensitive strips have greatly facilitated continuous temperature determination during anesthesia. Temperature monitoring should be routine in virtually all surgical patients. Its importance is unquestioned in the management of all infants and in major cases with patients any age.

PEDIATRIC FLUID THERAPY

MAINTENANCE FLUIDS

Various calculations involving body weight, surface area, or caloric expenditure have been used to determine fluid therapy for infants and children.[170-172] Body weight, caloric expenditure, and estimates of insensible water loss, renal water requirements, stool water loss, and water needed for growth determine the volume of fluid needed for maintenance.[170, 171] Caloric expenditure is size related. Infants 1–10 kg require 100 calories $\cdot$ kg^{-1} $\cdot$ day^{-1}; small children (10–20 kg) require 1,000 calories $\cdot$ day^{-1} plus 50 calories $\cdot$ kg^{-1} $\cdot$ day^{-1} over 10 kg; older children (weighing more than 20 kg) require 1,500 calories $\cdot$ day^{-1} plus 25 calories for each kg $\cdot$ day^{-1} over 20 kg. For every 100 calories consumed, 67 ml of water is needed for solute excretion; an additional 50 ml $\cdot$ 100 calories^{-1} is associated with insensible loss but 17 ml $\cdot$ 100 calories^{-1} produced by oxidation. Thus, the infant needs 100 ml of water for 100 calories. This simple relationship can be used to calculate the maintenance fluid needed by healthy full-term infants and children; the simplicity may explain the popularity of the method.

If one assumes that each day is 25 h, the hourly fluid needs of the infant can be estimated at 4 ml $\cdot$ kg^{-1} $\cdot$ h^{-1}. For every 100 ml of water, the infant needs 3 mEq Na$^+$, 2 mEq K$^+$, 2 mEq Cl$^-$, and 5 g glucose. It is more convenient to equalize the sodium and chloride requirements at 3 mEq. For routine use, 5% dextrose in 0.25 normal saline adequately provides this.

INTRAOPERATIVE FLUIDS AND BLOOD LOSS REPLACEMENT

Intraoperative fluid therapy may involve the initiation of fluid management or alternatively may be a continuation of ongoing fluid therapy. It can be as simple as replacing the deficits from the preoperative fast and providing maintenance fluids or as complex as correcting preoperative abnormal deficits, intraoperative translocated fluids, and variable blood loss in addition to providing maintenance fluids. It is best to consider each of these factors separately before discussing general guidelines.

FASTING DEFICIT

Because infants have a high metabolic rate and water turnover, significant hypoglycemia and dehydration may occur in those who are allowed to fast for prolonged periods of time. The fasting period before induction of anesthesia should be adjusted by timing feeding and surgery to minimize both the risk of dehydration and the risk of aspiration. However, delays in the surgical schedule may place the infant at risk for hypoglycemia and dehydration. In these instances intravenous administration of fluids is prudent. The fluid deficit incurred during fasting should be replaced during anesthesia. Assuming that a healthy infant is in water and electrolyte balance at the time oral feedings stop, the fluid deficit at the start of anesthesia can be estimated by multiplying the infant's hourly maintenance fluid requirement (MFR) by the number of hours since the last feeding. This deficit may be replaced by giving half of the calculated volume during the first hour of anesthesia and the other half over the next 2 h, in addition to intraoperative maintenance fluids.[173]

Thus, in the first 3 h, in an infant having a superficial surgical procedure with minimal or no third-space losses, fluid would be given as follows:
Estimated fluid deficit (EFD) = hours NPO × MFR $(ml \cdot kg^{-1} \cdot h^{-1})$

First hour fluids	= MFR + 1/2 EFD
Second hour fluids	= MFR + 1/4 EFD
Third hour fluids	= MFR + 1/4 EFD

Five per cent dextrose in quarter-normal saline (5% dextrose/0.25 normal saline or 2.5% 0.5 normal saline) is frequently used for maintenance fluid. Currently, there is a trend to using 2.5% glucose in 0.5 normal saline or lactated Ringer's solution as the maintenance fluid.[174, 175] Minimal deficits can be replaced more rapidly during short surgical procedures.

"THIRD-SPACE" INTRAOPERATIVE LOSSES

Surgical trauma, blunt trauma, burns, infections, and a host of surgical conditions are associated with isotonic transfer of fluids from the extracellular fluid compartment and to a lesser extent from the intracellular compartment to a nonfunctional interstitial compartment.[176–180] This acute sequestration of edema fluid to a nonfunctional compartment has been called third-space loss. Plasma volume may be decreased. The magnitude of third-space loss varies with the surgical procedure and is usually highest in infants having intraabdominal, intestinal surgery. In addition, failure to cover the exposed intestine and the use of heat lamps may increase evaporative loss. In infants, estimated third-space loss during intraabdominal surgery varies from 6 to 10 $ml \cdot kg^{-1} \cdot h^{-1}$; in intrathoracic surgery it is less (4–7 $ml \cdot kg^{-1} \cdot h^{-1}$); in superficial surgery or neurosurgery it is trivial (1–2 $ml \cdot kg^{-1} \cdot h^{-1}$). Translocated fluids are a finite functional loss and contribute to the magnitude of dehydration. Thus, clinical signs of the extent of dehydration may be used to estimate needed fluid replacement. Generally, lactated Ringer's solution is used to restore third-space losses. In cases of massive volume replacement, some

advocate using 5% albumin to restore one-third to one-fourth of the loss. The end point of third space replacement therapy is sustained adequate blood pressure (appropriate for the patient's age and weight), tissue perfusion, and urine volume.

Isotonic fluid also may be translocated in hypovolemic shock. When blood is lost, some interstitial fluid moves into the central circulation to restore plasma volume, but some moves intracellularly, perhaps because of altered membrane permeability. In severe shock, intracellular fluid volume expands to as much as 6% of body weight. Maintenance of adequate circulating volume and avoidance of hypoperfusion during periods of massive volume replacement may prevent these intracellular shifts.

Conceptually, two types of fluids may be indicated for long procedures with moderate to extensive third-space loss: 2.5% dextrose/0.5 normal saline or 5% dextrose/0.25 normal saline should be used for normal maintenance, and balanced salt solution should be used to compensate for third-space losses. For short surgical procedures with minimal to moderate third-space losses, one type of fluid usually suffices (e.g., 5% dextrose/lactated Ringer's solution or 5% dextrose/.9 normal saline). These relatively hypertonic fluids are used for a dual purpose, but large volumes of 5% dextrose/lactated Ringer's solution, especially given over a long time, can lead to profound hyperglycemia and hyperosmolality; an osmotic diuretic effect is common. This diuresis may cause cellular dehydration in the brain leading to intracranial hemorrhage. These problems are more common in stressed infants. To avoid these problems, one can limit the volume of 5% dextrose/lactated Ringer's solution to 15–20 $ml \cdot kg^{-1}$ and switch to lactated Ringer's solution for maintenance, or alternate fluids, or insert a second intravenous catheter for replacement therapy. To mix types of fluids, one should consider 5% dextrose/lactated Ringer's solution a substitute for the usual 5% dextrose/0.25 normal saline used for maintenance and then add volume of lactated Ringer's solution to achieve a total of 7–10 $ml \cdot kg^{-1} \cdot h^{-1}$. Glucose should be maintained between 100–150 $mg \cdot dl^{-1}$; balanced salt solution used as a substitute for blood or packed red blood cells should not contain glucose.

BLOOD REPLACEMENT

All blood loss in infants and children should be replaced in some way. Accurately measuring blood loss and assessing the acceptable blood loss in the infant are vital to any replacement regimen. Weighing sponges, using calibrated miniaturized suction bottles, and visually estimating (combined with a "guess factor") will define the magnitude of the blood loss. "Davenport's Law," which states that intraoperative blood loss of less than 10% requires no replacement and that loss of more than 20% must be replaced, is unsatisfactory in that it does not consider the starting blood volume, hemoglobin, or hematocrit of the patient. The concept of allowable RBC loss or allowable blood loss is a preferable guide to blood replacement.[173, 181] Normovolemic hemodilution to a predetermined hematocrit can be achieved with crystalloid or, more rarely, with colloid solutions.

ESTIMATING ALLOWABLE BLOOD LOSS

Several methods have been proposed for estimating allowable blood loss (ABL) from the blood volume, weight, and hematocrit. The formulae range from the simple to the complex, but all involve an estimate of blood volume. Blood volume is about 100 $ml \cdot kg^{-1}$ in the infant and about 80 $ml \cdot kg^{-1}$ in the older child. These estimates can be used with the following method to calculate ABL. In this equation, H0 is the original hematocrit, H1 is the lowest acceptable hematocrit, and $\overline{H}$ is the average hematocrit (H0 + H1)/2; all hematocrits are decimal values (*i.e.*, 0.6, 0.5, *etc.*). Equation 47-1 assumes that blood loss and replacement were gradual and exponential. This equation has general applicability for all age groups, but the lowest acceptable hematocrit should be age adjusted.

This method can be illustrated by estimating the ABL for a 6-kg infant with a 100 ml · kg^{-1} blood volume and an original hematocrit of 50%; H1 was 40%.

Simplified exponential:

$$ABL = Wt \times EBV \times \frac{[H0 - H1]}{\overline{H}}$$

$$ABL = 6 \text{ kg} \times \frac{100 \text{ ml}}{\text{kg}} \times \frac{[0.5 - 0.4]}{[0.5 + 0.4]/2} = 133 \qquad (47\text{-}1)$$

There is controversy over how the blood volume should be supported while the hematocrit is being allowed to decrease. Data are nonexistent, and several approaches are possible. If ongoing blood loss is replaced milliliter for milliliter with 5% colloid (*i.e.*, albumin, fresh-frozen plasma [FFP]), with the use of equation 47-1 the hematocrit will be within 1–3 vol % · dl^{-1} of the desired level; others replace blood loss with three to four times the volume of lactated Ringer's solution. Although this volume of clear fluid may be needed in patients in shock, it seems excessive in patients with well-perfused tissues. Hypoproteinemia may result. We replace gradual blood loss with volumes of crystalloid 1.5 times the measured or calculated loss.

In major surgery involving one to two body cavities, intravascular albumin may be transiently depleted or translocated. If 25% salt-poor albumin is used to replace these losses, its hypertonicity will mobilize fluids from the extracellular compartment; if the patient's "third space" is depleted, fluid will be mobilized from the intracellular compartment, leading to intracellular dehydration. Therefore, serum albumin should be replaced with 5% albumin.

Blood component therapy depends on the clinical setting and the availability of various blood products. Fresh whole blood (less than 4 h old) has a limited availability. The septic infant benefits from its clotting factors, platelets, and white blood cells. If predicted blood loss is greater than or equal to 40% of blood volume, it is helpful in supplying platelets and clotting factors. However, component therapy is usually the rule.[182] Packed RBCs have a hematocrit between 70 and 80%. On the average, 1 ml · kg^{-1} of packed cells will increase the hematocrit by 1.5%. Units of packed cells can be subdivided into pediatric packs of 80–100 ml. The fluid of these cells is relatively hyperkalemic (K ± 15–20 mEq · l^{-1}), acidotic (*pH* < 7.0), and low in ionized calcium. With rapid administration of packed RBCs, each of these factors is significant.

When blood loss approaches one blood volume, labile clotting factors are greatly reduced; normal clotting requires 5–20% of factor V and 30% of factor VIII. All the coagulation factors except platelets are present in normal quantities in FFP. We prefer to provide near equal volumes of FFP and packed cells to patients (hematocrit = 35–40%) with massive blood loss (*i.e.*, greater than or equal to one blood volume). The ratio of cells and plasma can be varied to produce any desired hematocrit. The intraoperative need for platelets may be predicted from the postoperative platelet count. Platelets can be mobilized from the spleen and bone marrow as bleeding occurs. An infant with a high preoperative count (greater than

250,000 mm^3) may not need a platelet transfusion until two to three blood volumes are lost, whereas an infant who has a low count (less than 150,000 mm^3) may need platelets after only one blood volume is lost. One platelet pack/10 kg is usually adequate. Rapid administration of cold, citrated blood products can be hazardous; obviously, all such products should be warmed before infusion. FFP contains the greatest amount of citrate per unit volume of any blood product; rapid infusion of FFP should cause the greatest change in ionized calcium. Under most circumstances, the mobilization of calcium and hepatic metabolism of citrate are sufficiently rapid to prevent precipitous decreases in ionized calcium. However, because infants' stores of calcium are small and a larger fraction of their blood volume can be replaced more rapidly, they are at special risk for hypocalcemia. For example, transient decreases in ionized calcium are seen in infants with jaundice during exchange transfusion. Coté *et al* demonstrated that FFP infusion at rates of 1–2.5 ml · kg^{-1} · min^{-1} was associated with transient decreases in ionized calcium and occasional significant decreases in arterial blood pressure.[183] Equipotent doses of calcium chloride (2.5 mg · kg^{-1}) or calcium gluconate (7.5 mg · kg^{-1}) effectively increased calcium and ameliorated the hemodynamic changes. Empiric buffering of blood may lead to profound metabolic alkalosis as citrate loads are metabolized.

OUTPATIENT AND SAME-DAY SURGERY

Many pediatric surgical procedures are brief, and the patients require little preoperative preparation. The rapidity with which healthy young patients recover from the effects of anesthesia and surgery has been mentioned already. For these reasons, many procedures are handled easily and safely on an outpatient basis. There are many advantages to this approach. Children need not spend one or more nights away from their home and family, and their exposure to hospital cross-infections is reduced. The convenience to parents of small children is considerable and much appreciated, especially if there are other children in the family. In many cases, the hospital costs for outpatient surgery are less than for inpatients. The surgeon and the patient benefit from quicker and easier scheduling. Finally, outpatient surgery keeps hospital beds available for more seriously ill patients.

SELECTION OF PATIENTS

The types of operation to be managed on an outpatient basis must be chosen and agreed upon by the surgeon, anesthesiologist, and hospital administration. There are no universal criteria, although, in general, only procedures that can reasonably be completed within an hour are permitted. Patients with major medical problems such as juvenile diabetes or cystic fibrosis are best excluded, as well as those who will require blood transfusion or other special preoperative preparation. Limitations of health insurance are another possible deterrent to outpatient status.

PREOPERATIVE PREPARATION

The preoperative history, physical examination, and laboratory work should be completed before the day of surgery. Special forms may be developed to facilitate this aspect of preparation. A hematocrit or hemoglobin determination is the only routine laboratory study required. At the last clinic or office visit, the parents should be given information (preferably printed) on time, place, and administrative details, and, most important, instructions for withholding food and fluids.

On the patient's admission to the outpatient unit, a nurse or clerk determines that all necessary paperwork is completed, including the history, physical examination, laboratory work, and operative permit. Parents are questioned about the possibility of fever or upper respiratory infection within the past few days and about when the patient has last ingested food or drink.

Of course, preoperative psychologic preparation is just as desirable for outpatients as for inpatients, but sedatives and opioids should be used with caution. Their effect continues long after completion of the surgery, thus prolonging recovery time and delaying discharge. We do not use any preoperative medication. Allowing parents to remain with children until they go to the operating room allays the children's apprehension to some extent, especially because they know they may return immediately to their parents after operation and will not have to remain in the hospital.

ANESTHESIA

The type of anesthesia used for outpatients does not differ significantly from that already described for inpatients. Nitrous oxide–halothane is most common, and ketamine may be used if repeated doses are not required. We use endotracheal intubation if it is indicated. In the event tracheal intubation is required, discharge is delayed for 4 h to assure that there are no complications. If there is any question about the airway, the patient is admitted overnight.

RECOVERY AND DISCHARGE

Outpatients receive the same immediate postoperative care as do other patients in the recovery room. After recovery from anesthesia, they are returned to the outpatient unit, where they rejoin their parents. They are discharged when they are fully awake, have retained fluids, have no respiratory problems, and can walk.

To be successful, an outpatient surgery program primarily must be designed to ensure patient safety. The quality of medical care must not be sacrificed for expediency. Preoperative preparation, anesthesia, the surgical procedure, and postoperative care must meet the same standards as for hospitalized patients. Time is the only factor that is altered. The other requirements are good organization and communication between all concerned parties—the parents, surgeon, surgeon's office, hospital business office, outpatient unit, operating room, and, of course, the anesthesiologist.

ANESTHESIA FOR PEDIATRIC NEURORADIOLOGY

Children and infants, unlike their adult counterparts, frequently require general anesthesia or heavy sedation for neuroradiologic diagnostic and therapeutic procedures. Although some of these procedures are painful, at least during part of the procedure, the principal indication for anesthesia is the inability of the young patient or combative patient to cooperate and to maintain the necessary immobility for extended periods; rigid restraints are strong stimuli for struggling and movement in infants and semiconscious and otherwise uncooperative patients.

A major problem common to all these procedures is that they must be performed in a location not usually designed for the administration of anesthesia and that is remote from the operating rooms and recovery facilities. Anesthesia for nuclear magnetic resonance studies is particularly taxing. All or most of the equipment must be transported to the radiology department. The situation is often further complicated by the fact that, in many institutions, these facilities are shared by both adult and pediatric patients, and generally it is the pediatric patient who is the exception; thus, the radiology staff is less likely to be able to deal with the special needs of infants and children. Finally, at the conclusion of the procedures, the anesthetized infant or child must be transported over long distances to the recovery area. Portable oxygen equipment, including a bag-mask/valve unit and a portable ECG monitor, must be available during transportation to the recovery area.

ANESTHESIA OR SEDATION

Because the anesthetic requirement for most of these procedures is minimal, the question frequently arises as to whether sedation may be substituted for formally administered general anesthesia. In our experience sedation has been effective in only a small percentage of these patients—generally the older, cooperative children who are having angiography or those studies that require immobility for only short periods of time. There have been numerous difficulties encountered with sedation as a substitute for general anesthesia. Even moderately heavy sedation with a combination of opioids and sedatives has not provided adequate quiescence and immobility when the child was firmly restrained or placed in an unnatural position. There has been a wide and unpredictable variation in the effectiveness of the drugs even at comparable ages and dosages. The large doses of these drugs by either the intramuscular or intravenous route (or a combination of both) required to achieve quiescence have led to respiratory depression and increased arterial carbon dioxide tension and cerebrovascular dilatation. Dilatation in turn increased intracranial pressure and interfered with successful angiography. Sedation—effective or not—that was "heavy" enough to induce unconsciousness and respiratory depression became a form of general anesthesia in which the anesthesiologist had no direct control of airway or ventilation. The effects of the sedative drugs, not all of which could be satisfactorily reversed, far outlasted the duration of the procedure. For all of these reasons, endotracheal inhalation anesthesia has proved to be far safer, more flexible, and more predictable in our experience. The rare exception is the case of the older, already cooperative child for whom "continuous sedation" may be all that is necessary.

TECHNIQUE OF ANESTHESIA

The type of anesthesia used for these procedures differs little in principle from that for neurosurgical patients of comparable age. The choice of anesthetic drugs and muscle relaxants is usually of secondary importance. Endotracheal intubation is mandatory because the anesthesiologist may not have access to the head and the patient may be turned into one or more difficult positions.

Routine monitoring of heart rate, ventilation, oxygenation, blood pressure, ECG, and temperature is essential. Special efforts to maintain normal body temperature, particularly in the very young, are essential but may prove difficult because it is frequently impossible to regulate the room temperature and the use of the circulating warm water mattress may interfere with radiography. Use of radiant heat lamps, wrapping of the extremities, a plastic bag about the head (when possible), and heated, humidified anesthetic gases effectively combat heat loss.

CEREBRAL ANGIOGRAPHY

The anesthesiologist must be aware of the volume and type of fluids used in conjunction with angiography and adjust fluid administration accordingly. In general, the total volume of Hypaque Sodium (Winthrop Laboratories, New York, New York) should be limited to 4–6 ml·kg^{-1}.

After use of hyperosmolar contrast materials, there is an initial increase in blood viscosity and a decrease in hematocrit followed by translocation of fluid that increases circulating blood pressure, cardiac output, and, usually, urine flow. Occasionally, anaphylactoid reactions with angioneurotic edema, hypotension, and bronchospasm may occur. In addition, severe dehydration has occurred in some patients receiving contrast material. Mass lesions of the brain associated with loss of autoregulation may be managed by hyperventilation, which decreases cerebral blood flow to normal brain tissue; in general, however, hyperventilation facilitates angiography.

AIR STUDIES

The introduction of gas into the ventricles or subarachnoid space for air myelographic, pneumoencephalographic, and ventriculographic studies complicates the use of general anesthesia. Nitrous oxide, which is often used for this type of procedure, is contraindicated; because of its relatively greater solubility in blood than that of nitrogen, it will accumulate in the closed gas-filled compartments and increase their pressure. The exception is, of course, when the radiologist uses nitrous oxide itself as the contrast gas instead of air–oxygen.

The anesthesiologist must be aware and informed of the volumes of cerebrospinal fluid removed and the volumes of gas injected. Changes in pulse and blood pressure as fluid and gas are exchanged must be detected, recorded, and communicated immediately to the radiologist. In all of these procedures, but particularly during pneumoencephalographic studies, it may be necessary to place the patient in a variety of unnatural positions that may affect the circulation and present technical problems with anesthetic and monitoring equipment attached to the patient.

RADIATION THERAPY

The greatest number of technical problems for the anesthesiologist are seen with the infant or child who is to have radiation therapy. These include those common to the infant and the neurologic disease, the need for absolute immobility, lack of access to the patient, and, in addition, the need for daily serial anesthetics, frequently administered on an outpatient basis. Use of sedation, regardless of the combinations and doses of drugs or their route of administration, has proved unsatisfactory for radiation therapy because it does not ensure the absolute immobility required and because the drugs used have a long duration of action. Inhalation anesthetics are unsatisfactory because of the hazards of airway obstruction without intubation or of multiple intubations. The technical difficulties inherent in securing an intravenous infu-

sion in a small infant on so many successive occasions virtually preclude the use of intravenously administered drugs.

The following technique, which involves a degree of compromise, has proved successful. On each treatment day, the fasting infant, preferably accompanied by a parent, is brought to a quiet room adjacent to the radiation laboratory a few minutes before the scheduled treatment. When the radiation team is completely ready, the infant is given a single intramuscular injection containing atropine 0.02 mg·kg^{-1} and ketamine 5 mg·kg^{-1}. Upon becoming quiescent, the infant is quickly taken to the laboratory and positioned by the radiation therapist and anesthesiologist. Monitoring equipment is attached, supplemental oxygen is begun, and the patient is carefully observed for adequate airway and respiration. Radiation treatment is then started without delay. An intravenous catheter with a heparin lock is inserted for subsequent treatments. Ketamine can then be administered intravenously. After treatment, the anesthesiologist takes the infant to the recovery room.

The success of this deceptively simple technique depends on careful prior planning and communication, which are absolutely essential. All necessary equipment must be available. Because the anesthesiologist must leave the patient during the therapy, special arrangements must be available for remote monitoring and unobstructed viewing of the patient. The radiation and anesthesia teams must thoroughly understand each other's problems. The short duration of effective anesthesia necessitates that delays be avoided once the injection is given. A plan must be agreed upon for abortion of therapy in the event of complications.

Slight increases in ketamine dosage usually will be necessary with successive treatments. However, in a few cases the infant seems to adapt to the daily routine and will remain quiescent with progressively smaller dosages. In addition to the usual anesthetic record, a simple tabular log showing date, dosage, effect, and complications should be kept to indicate these trends.

NUCLEAR MAGNETIC RESONANCE STUDIES

Infants and small children may need sedation or general anesthesia for nuclear magnetic resonance (NMR) studies. The scanner employs strong electromagnetic fields to produce detectable nuclear magnetic resonance signals from nuclear components within the body. Therefore, caution must be used in bringing any ferro-magnetic materials within proximity of the scanner.[184] This creates obvious problems in providing anesthesia and monitoring patients in NMR scanners. In general, one may use nonferrous anesthesia equipment within the scanner or ferrous anesthesia equipment outside the scanner. For example, we use a modified Mapleson D circuit with noncompliant 10-M tubing with nonferrous connectors and a traditional ventilator outside the scan room. Blood pressure is measured by Doppler; a pulse oximeter with a 10-M cable is used. Others have tried other similar approaches.[185–187]

POSTANESTHETIC CARE

Infants and children generally recover more quickly from the stress of anesthesia and surgery, have less postoperative pain, and are less disturbed by minor complications than are adults. Nevertheless, the immediate postoperative period may be as hazardous as the operation and anesthetic. The end of the operation should not signal the end of the intensive minute-to-minute observation and care that the patient received while under anesthesia. More and more attention is being directed toward continuing intensive care in the postoperative period; to a large extent, such care is the anesthesiologist's responsibility.

CONCLUSION OF SURGERY

Recovery from anesthesia involves many factors, including the restoration of normal body temperature, return of protective reflexes and neuromuscular function if muscle relaxants have been used, ability to maintain a patent airway without dependence on a mechanical device, and reestablishment of adequate spontaneous ventilation, in addition to regaining of consciousness. Stringent criteria should be used in evaluating infants' recovery. The incompletely reacted infant may appear to breathe adequately when stimulated but may fall asleep again and have very shallow respirations or apnea. Infants should be kept in the operating room until fully conscious and active as indicated by a lusty cry.

IMMEDIATE POSTANESTHETIC CARE

The airway should be maintained and the anesthesiologist should monitor pulse and respiration during transportation from the operating room. In some patients this may entail the continued use of a precordial or esophageal stethoscope and positive-pressure ventilation with oxygen and self-inflating bag.

On the patient's arrival in the recovery room or intensive care unit, attention should first be directed to the assurance of adequate ventilation, either spontaneous or by artificial means if necessary. The vital signs should be ascertained by recovery room personnel and reported to the anesthesiologist as soon as possible. The anesthesiologist, in turn, should report any special problems. Only after these precautions are observed should attention be directed to other aspects of the patient's care.

It is generally believed that the infant or child does not experience postoperative pain to the same extent as does the adult, although this may not be an accurate observation. It appears that in most instances pain can simply be controlled with nonopioid analgesics. However, if necessary, one should not withhold judicious use of more potent opioid analgesics.

Emergence delirium is occasionally seen in children, particularly in those in whom scopolamine has been used for premedication. A dose of 0.01–0.02 mg·kg^{-1} of physostigmine salicylate (Antilirium) has been dramatically effective in treating this condition.[188]

MANAGEMENT OF SUBGLOTTIC EDEMA

Croup or subglottic edema after endotracheal intubation usually is manifested within 2–4 h; in severe cases the signs occur earlier. In most cases only a brassy cough and stertorous respirations are observed. With more severe edema there may be labored respirations, suprasternal retractions, tachypnea, restlessness, and sweating.

Mild cases require little or no therapy other than high concentrations of humidified oxygen. The most effective treatment of subglottic edema is that described by Jordan et al.[189] Racemic epinephrine (0.5 ml of a 2% solution diluted to a volume of 3.5 ml) is administered in a nebulizer with intermittent positive-pressure breathing apparatus (IPPB). The ration-ale of this treatment is that the IPPB relieves the hypoxia and the vasoconstrictor (as opposed to a bronchodilator) tends to relieve the airway obstruction. Our experience with this technique tends to bear out the effectiveness claimed by Jordan et al.

As yet, there is no clear-cut evidence that steroids are effective in the management of postintubation croup, but they seem to be so in some cases. There appears to be no harm in a single large dose, so we have not hesitated to use dexamethasone intravenously in single doses of 4 mg for infants younger than 1 yr of age and 8 mg for older children.

When it results from trauma, untreated subglottic edema reaches its peak in 6–8 h. If the process does not respond to treatment, the patient must be watched very closely. Preparations necessary for tracheostomy should be made, and tracheostomy should not be delayed if airway obstruction is severe or rapidly progressing. If the edema is infectious in origin, the recovery process is much slower and respiratory difficulty may continue for 48 h or more.

REFERENCES

1. Eckenhoff JE: Some anatomic considerations of the infant larynx influencing endotracheal anesthesia. Anesthesiology 12:401, 1951
2. Avery ME, Fletcher BA: The Lung and Its Disorders in the Newborn Infant. Philadelphia, WB Saunders, 1974
3. Motoyama EK, Cook DR: Respiratory physiology. In Smith RM (ed): Anesthesia for Infants and Children, p 38. St Louis, CV Mosby, 1980
4. Goudsouzian NG, Morris RH, Ryan JF: The effects of a warming blanket on the maintenance of body temperatures in anesthetized infants and children. Anesthesiology 39:351, 1973
5. Sereni F: Developmental pharmacology. Annu Rev Pharmacol Toxicol 8:453, 1968
6. Jusko WJ: Pharmacokinetic principles in pediatric pharmacology. Pediatr Clin North Am 1:81, 1972
7. Brown TCK: Pediatric pharmacology. Anaesth Intensive Care 1:473, 1973
8. Cook DR: Neonatal anesthetic pharmacology: A review. Anesth Analg 53:544, 1974
9. Yaffe SJ, Juchau MR: Perinatal pharmacology. Annu Rev Pharmacol Toxicol 14:219, 1974
10. Cook DR: Pediatric anesthesia: Pharmacological considerations. Drugs 12:212, 1976
11. Rylance G: Clinical pharmacology: drugs in children. Br Med J 282:50, 1981
12. Gladtke E, Heimann G: The rate of development of elimination functions in kidney and liver of young infants. In Morselli PC, Garattini S, Sereni F (eds): Basic and Therapeutic Aspects of Perinatal Pharmacology, p 337. New York, Raven Press, 1975
13. Brown AK, Zwelzin WW, Burnett HH: Studies on the neonatal development of the glucuronide conjugating system. J Clin Invest 37:332, 1968
14. Yaffe SJ: Neonatal pharmacology. Pediatr Clin North Am 13:527, 1966
15. Herbert W, Hammond D: Preoperative evaluation of the anemic child. Am Surg 29:660, 1963
16. Visintainer MA, Wolfer JA: Psychological preparation for surgical pediatric patients: The effect on children's and parent's stress responses and adjustment. Pediatrics 56:187, 1975
17. Wolfer JA, Visintainer MA: Prehospital psychological preparation for tonsillectomy patients: Effects on children's and parent's adjustment. Pediatrics 64:646, 1979

18. Ferguson BF: Preparing young children for hospitalization: A comparison of two methods. Pediatrics 64:656, 1979
19. de Bock TL, Petrilli RL, Davis PJ et al: Effect of premedication of preoperative arterial oxygen saturation in children with congenital heart disease. Anesthesiology 67:A492, 1987
20. Bachman L, Freeman A: Cardiac rate and rhythm in infants during induction with cyclopropane: Atropine versus scopolamine as preanesthetic medication. J Pediatr 59:922, 1961
21. Gaviotaki A, Smith RM: Use of atropine in pediatric anesthesia. Int Anesthesiol Clin 1:97, 1962
22. Coté CJ, Goudsouzian NG, Liu LMP et al: Assessment of risk factors related to the acid aspiration syndrome in pediatric patients—Gastric pH and residual volume. Anesthesiology 56:70, 1982
23. Goudsouzian N, Coté CJ, Liu LMP et al: The dose-response effects of oral cimetidine on gastric pH and volume in children. Anesthesiology 55:533, 1981
24. Manchikanti L, Marrero TC, Roush JR: Preanesthetic cimetidine and metoclopramide for acid aspiration prophylaxis in elective surgery. Anesthesiology 61:48, 1984
25. Henderson JM, Spence DG, Clarke WN et al: Sodium citrate in paediatric outpatients. Can Anaesth Soc J 34:560, 1987
26. Berry FA: Preoperative assessment and general management of outpatients. Int Anesthesiol Clin 20:3, 1982
27. Hannallah RS, Rosales JK: Experience with parent's presence during anesthesia induction in children. Can Anaesth Soc J 30:286, 1983
28. Friesen RH, Lichtor JL: Cardiovascular depression during halothane anesthesia in infants: A study of three induction techniques. Anesth Analg 61:42, 1982
29. Rackow H, Salanitre E, Green LT: Frequency of cardiac arrest associated with anesthesia in infants and children. Pediatrics 28:697, 1961
30. Salanitre E, Rackow H: The pulmonary exchange of nitrous oxide and halothane in infants and children. Anesthesiology 30:388, 1969
31. Rackow H, Salanitre E: The pulmonary equilibration of cyclopropane in infants and children. Br J Anaesth 46:35, 1974
32. Steward DJ, Creighton RE: The uptake and excretion of nitrous oxide in the newborn. Can Anaesth Soc J 25:215, 1978
33. Eger EI II, Bahlman SH, Munson ES: The effect of age on the rate of increase of alveolar anesthetic concentration. Anesthesiology 35:365, 1971
34. Brandom BW, Brandom RB, Cook DR: Uptake and distribution of halothane in infants: In vivo measurements and computer simulations. Anesth Analg 62:404, 1983
35. Gibbs CP, Munson ES, Tham MK: Anesthetic solubility coefficients for maternal and fetal blood. Anesthesiology 43:100, 1975
36. Lerman J, Gregory GA, Willis MM et al: Age and solubility of volatile anesthetics in blood. Anesthesiology 61:139, 1984
37. Cook DR, Brandom BW, Shiu G et al: The inspired median effective dose, brain concentration at anesthesia, and cardiovascular index for halothane in young rats. Anesth Analg 60:182, 1981
38. Stoelting RK, Longnecker DE: Effect of right-to-left shunt on rate of increase in arterial anesthetic concentration. Anesthesiology 36:352, 1972
39. Tanner G, Angers D, Barash PG et al: Does a left-to-right shunt speed the induction of inhalational anesthesia in congenital heart disease? Anesth Analg 64:101, 1985
40. Gregory GA, Eger EI II, Munson ES: The relationship between age and halothane requirements in man. Anesthesiology 30:488, 1969
41. Nicodemus HF, Nassiri-Rahimi C, Bachman L: Median effective dose (ED50) of halothane in adults and children. Anesthesiology 31:344, 1969
42. Lerman J, Robinson S, Willis MM et al: Anesthetic requirements for halothane in young children 0–1 month and 1–6 months of age. Anesthesiology 59:421, 1983
43. Gregory GA, Wade JG, Beihl DR et al: Fetal anesthetic requirement (MAC) for halothane. Anesth Analg 62:9, 1983
44. LeDez KM, Lerman J: The minimum alveolar concentration (MAC) of isoflurane in preterm neonates. Anesthesiology 67:301, 1987
45. Rao CC, Bayer M, Krishna G et al: Effects of halothane, isoflurane and enflurane on the isometric concentration of the neonatal isolated rat atria. Anesthesiology 61:A424, 1984
46. Boudreaux JP, Schieber RA, Cook DR: Hemodynamic effects of halothane in the newborn piglet. Anesth Analg 63:731, 1984
47. Bailie MD, Alward CT, Sawyer DC et al: Effect of anesthesia on cardiovascular and renal function in the newborn piglet. J Pharmacol Exp Ther 208:298, 1979
48. Wolfson B, Kielar CM, Lake C et al: Anesthetic index—A new approach. Anesthesiology 38:583, 1973
49. Wolfson B, Hetrick WD, Lake C et al: Anesthetic indices—Further data. Anesthesiology 48:187, 1978
50. Kissen I, Morgan PL, Smith LR: Comparison of isoflurane and halothane safety margins in rats. Anesthesiology 58:556, 1983
51. Murray D, Vandewalker G, Matherne GP et al: Pulsed doppler and two-dimensional echocardiography: Comparison of halothane and isoflurane on cardiac function in infants and small children. Anesthesiology 67:211, 1987
52. Gootman PM, Gootman N, Buckley BJ: Maturation of central autonomic control of the circulation. Fed Proc 42:1648, 1983
53. Gregory GA: The baroresponses of preterm infants during halothane anesthesia. Can Anaesth Soc J 29:105, 1982
54. Duncan P, Gregory GA, Wade JA: The effects of nitrous oxide on the baroreceptor response of newborn and adult rabbits. Can Anaesth Soc J 18:339, 1981
55. Wear R, Robinson S, Gregory GA: The effect of halothane on the baroresponse of adult and baby rabbits. Anesthesiology 56:188, 1982
56. Maunuksela EL, Korpela R: Double-blind evaluation of a lignocaine-prilocaine cream (EMLA) in children. Br J Anaesth 58:1242, 1986
57. Coté CJ, Goudsouzian NG, Liu LMP et al: The dose response of intravenous thiopental for the induction of general anesthesia in unpremedicated children. Anesthesiology 55:703, 1981
58. Jonmarker C, Westrin P, Larsson S et al: Thiopental requirements for induction of anesthesia in children. Anesthesiology 67:104, 1987
59. Brett CM, Fisher DM: Thiopental dose-response relations in unpremedicated infants, children, and adults. Anesth Analg 66:1024, 1987
60. Purcell-Jones G, Yates A, Baker JR et al: Comparison of the induction characteristics of thiopentone and propofol in children. Br J Anaesth 59:1431, 1987
61. Salonen M, Kanto J, Iisalo E et al: Midazolam as an induction agent in children: A pharmacokinetic and clinical study. Anesth Analg 66:625, 1987
62. Liu LMP, Goudsouzian NG, Liu PL: Rectal methohexital premedication in children, a dose-comparison study. Anesthesiology 53:343, 1980
63. Boreus LO, Jalling B, Kallberg N: In Morselli PL, Garattini S, Sereni F (eds): Basic and Therapeutic Aspects of Perinatal Pharmacology, p 331. New York, Raven Press, 1975
64. Morselli PL, Mandelli M, Tognoni G et al: In Morselli PL, Garattini S, Cohen SN (eds): Drug Interactions, p 320. Raven Press, New York, Drug Interactions, 1974
65. Knauer B, Draffen GA, Williams FM: Elimination kinetics of amobarbital in mothers and their newborn infants. Clin Pharmacol Ther 14:442, 1973

66. Sorbo S, Hudson RJ, Loomis JC: The pharmacokinetics of thiopental in pediatric surgical patients. Anesthesiology 61:666, 1984

67. Lockhart CH, Nelson WL: The relationship of ketamine requirements to age in pediatric patients. Anesthesiology 40:507, 1974

68. Eng M, Bonica JJ, Akamatsu TJ et al: Respiratory depression in newborn monkeys at cesarean section following ketamine administration. Br J Anaesth 47:917, 1975

69. Radney PA, Badola RP: Generalized extensor spasm in infants following ketamine anesthesia. Anesthesiology 39:459, 1973

70. Lockhart CH, Jenkins JJ: Ketamine-induced apnea in patients with increased intracranial pressure. Anesthesiology 37:92, 1972

71. Gasser S, Cohen M, Aygen M: The effect of ketamine on pulmonary artery pressure. Anaesthesia 29:141, 1974

72. Morray JP, Lynn AM, Stamm SJ et al: Hemodynamic effects of ketamine in children with congenital heart disease. Anesth Analg 63:895, 1984

73. Hickey PR, Hansen DD, Cranolini GM: Pulmonary and systemic hemodynamic responses to ketamine in infants with normal and elevated pulmonary vascular resistance. Anesthesiology 61:A438, 1984

74. Hickey PR, Hansen DD: Fentanyl- and sufentanil-oxygen-pancuronium anesthesia for cardiac surgery in infants. Anesth Analg 63:117, 1984

75. Hickey PR, Hansen DD, Wessell D: Responses to high dose fentanyl in infants: Pulmonary and systemic hemodynamics. Anesthesiology 61:445, 1984

76. Koren G, Goresky G, Crean P et al: Pediatric fentanyl dosing based on pharmacokinetics during cardiac surgery. Anesth Analg 65:577, 1984

77. Koehntop D, Rodman J, Brundage D et al: Pharmacokinetics of fentanyl in neonates. Anesth Analg 65:227, 1986

78. Singleton MA, Rosen JI, Fisher DM: Pharmacokinetics of fentanyl for infants and adults. Anesthesiology 61:A440, 1984

79. Davis PJ, Cook DR, Stiller RL et al: Pharmacodynamics and pharmacokinetics of high-dose sufentanil in infants and children undergoing cardiac surgery. Anesth Analg 66:203, 1987

80. Greeley WJ, de Bruijn NP, Davis DP: Sufentanil pharmacokinetics in pediatric cardiovascular patients. Anesth Analg 66:1067, 1987

81. Roure P, Jean N, Leclerc AC et al: Pharmacokinetics of alfentanil in children undergoing surgery. Br J Anaesth 59:1437, 1987

82. Goresky GV, Koren G, Sabourin MA et al: The pharmacokinetics of alfentanil in children. Anesthesiology 67:654, 1987

83. Meistelman C, Saint-Maurice C, Lepaul M et al: A comparison of alfentanil pharmacokinetics in children and adults. Anesthesiology 66:13, 1987

84. Goudsouzian NG: Maturation of neuromuscular transmission in the infant. Br J Anaesth 52:205, 1980

85. Crumrine RS, Yodlowski EH: Assessment of neuromuscular function in infants. Anesthesiology 54:29, 1981

86. Cook DR, Fischer CG: Neuromuscular blocking effects of succinylcholine in infants and children. Anesthesiology 42:662, 1975

87. Cook DR, Fischer CG: Characteristics of succinylcholine neuromuscular blockade in infants. Anesth Analg 57:63, 1978

88. Walts LF, Dillon JB: The response of newborns to succinylcholine and d-tubocurarine. Anesthesiology 31:35, 1969

89. Goudsouzian NG, Liu LMP: The neuromuscular response of infants to a continuous infusion of succinylcholine. Anesthesiology 60:97, 1984

90. Goudsouzian NG, Donlon JV, Savarese JJ et al: Re-evaluation of dosage and duration of action of d-tubocurarine in the pediatric age group. Anesthesiology 43:416, 1975

91. Goudsouzian NG, Ryan JF, Savarese JJ: The neuromuscular effects of pancuronium in infants and children. Anesthesiology 41:95, 1974

92. Goudsouzian NG, Liu LMP, Savarese JJ: Metocurarine in infants
and children: Neuromuscular and clinical effects. Anesthesiology 49:266, 1978

93. Goudsouzian NG, Liu LMP, Coté CJ: Comparison of equipotent doses of nondepolarizing muscle relaxants in children. Anesth Analg 60:862, 1981

94. Goudsouzian NG, Martyn JJA, Liu LMP: The dose response effect of long-acting non-depolarizing neuromuscular blocking agents in children. Can Anaesth Soc J 3:246, 1984

95. Cook DR: Clinical use of muscle relaxants in infants and children. Anesth Analg 60:335, 1981

96. Fisher DM, O'Keefe C, Stanski DR et al: Pharmacokinetics and pharmacodynamics of d-tubocurarine in infants, children, and adults. Anesthesiology 57:2030, 1982

97. Brandom BW, Rudd GD, Cook DR: Clinical pharmacology of atracurium in pediatric patients. Br J Anaesth 55:117S, 1983

98. Brandom BW, Woelfel SK, Cook DR et al: Clinical pharmacology of atracurium in infants. Anesth Analg 63:309, 1984

99. Brandom BW, Cook DR, Stiller RL et al: Pharmacokinetics of atracurium in infants and children. Clin Pharmacol Ther 62:404, 1983

100. Goudsouzian NG, Liu L, Coté CJ et al: Safety and efficacy of atracurium in adolescents and children anesthetized with halothane. Anesthesiology 60:97, 1984

101. Goudsouzian NG, Liu LMP, Gionfriddo M et al: Neuromuscular effects of atracurium in infants and children. Anesthesiology 62:75, 1985

102. D'Hollander AA, Luyckx C, Barvais L et al: Clinical evaluation of atracurium besylate requirement for a stable muscle relaxation during surgery: Lack of age-related effects. Anesthesiology 59:2327, 1983

103. Fisher DM, Miller RD: Neuromuscular effects of vecuronium (ORG NC45) in infants and children during N₂O, halothane anesthesia. Anesthesiology 58:519, 1983

104. Rupp SM, Miller RD, Gencarelli PJ: Vecuronium-induced neuromuscular blockade during enflurane, halothane, and isoflurane in humans. Anesthesiology 60:102, 1984

105. Fisher DM, Castagnoli K, Miller RD: Vecuronium kinetics and dynamics in anesthetized infants and children. Clin Pharmacol Ther 37:402, 1985

106. Ayre P: Endotracheal anesthesia for babies with special reference to harelip and cleft palate operations. Anesth Analg 16:330, 1937

107. Harrison GA: Ayre's T-piece: A review of its modifications. Br J Anaesth 36:115, 1964

108. Mapleson WW: The elimination of rebreathing in various semi-closed anaesthetic systems. Br J Anaesth 26:323, 1954

109. Mapleson WW: Theoretical considerations of the effect of rebreathing in two semi-closed anaesthetic systems. Br Med Bull 14:64, 1958

110. Onchi Y, Hayashi T, Ueyama H: Studies on the Ayre T-piece technique. Far East Journal of Anesthesiology 1:30, 1957

111. Nightingale DA, Richards CC, Glass A: An evaluation of rebreathing in a modified T-piece system during controlled ventilation of anaesthetized children. Br J Anaesth 37:762, 1965

112. Wolfson B: Fresh gas inflow requirements in anesthesia circuits. Weekly Anesthesia Update 2:25, 1979

113. Bain JA, Spoerel WE: Flow requirements for a modified Mapleson D system during controlled respiration. Can Anaesth Soc J 20:629, 1973

114. Hickey RF, Graf PD, Nadel JA et al: The effects of halothane and cyclopropane on total pulmonary resistance in the dog. Anesthesiology 31:334, 1969

115. Bloomquist ER: Pediatric circle absorber. Anesthesiology 18:787, 1957

116. Shandling B, Steward DJ: Regional analgesia for postoperative pain in pediatric outpatient surgery. J Pediatr Surg 15:447, 1980

117. Shapiro LA, Jedeikin RJ, Shaley D et al: Epidural morphine and analgesia in children. Anesthesiology 61:210, 1984

118. Jones SEF, Beasley JM, MacFarlane DWR et al: Intrathecal morphine in postoperative pain relief in children. Br J Anaesth 56:137, 1984

119. Tree-Trakarn T, Pirayavaraporn S: Postoperative pain relief for circumcision in children: Comparison among morphine, nerve block, and topical analgesia. Anesthesiology 62:519, 1985

120. Broadman LM, Hannallah R: Regional anesthesia in children. Regional Anesthesia 10:33, 1985

121. Blaise GA, Roy WL: Postoperative pain relief after hypospadius repair in pediatric patients: Regional analgesia versus systemic analgesics. Anesthesiology 65:84, 1986

122. Dalens B, Tanguy A, Haberer JP: Lumbar epidural anesthesia for operative and postoperative pain relief in infants and young children. Anesth Analg 65:1069, 1986

123. Hannallah RS, Broadman LM, Belman AB et al: Comparison of caudal and ilioinguinal/iliohypogastric nerve blocks for control of post-orchiopexy pain in pediatric ambulatory surgery. Anesthesiology 66:832, 1987

124. Hinkle AJ: Percutaneous inguinal block for the outpatient management of post-herniorrhaphy pain in children. Anesthesiology 67:411, 1987

125. Tree-Trakarn T, Pirayavaraporn S, Lertakyamanee J: Topical analgesia for relief of post-circumcision pain. Anesthesiology 67:395, 1987

126. Broadman LM, Hannallah RS, Belman AB et al: Post-circumcision analgesia—A prospective evaluation of subcutaneous ring block of the penis. Anesthesiology 67:399, 1987

127. Warner MA, Kunkel SE, Offord KO et al: The effects of age, epinephrine, and operative site on duration of caudal analgesia in pediatric patients. Anesth Analg 66:995, 1987

128. Desparmet J, Meistelman C, Barre J et al: Continuous epidural infusion of bupivacaine for postoperative pain relief in children. Anesthesiology 67:108, 1987

129. Murat I, Delleur MM, Esteve C et al: Continuous extradural anaesthesia in children. Br J Anaesth 69:1441, 1987

130. Krane EJ, Jacobson LE, Lynn AM et al: Caudal morphine for postoperative analgesia in children: A comparison with caudal bupivacaine and intravenous morphine. Anesth Analg 66:647, 1987

131. Miranda DR: Continuous brachial plexus block. Acta Anaesthesiol Belg 4:323, 1977

132. Selander D: Catheter technique in axillary plexus block. Acta Anaesthesiol Scand 21:316, 1977

133. Carell ED, Eyring EJ: Intravenous regional anesthesia for childhood fractures. Trauma 11:301, 1971

134. Fitzgerald B: Intravenous regional anaesthesia in children. Br J Anaesth 48:485, 1976

135. Stark RA: A review of intravenous regional anesthesia. Anesthesiology Reviews 9:15, 1982

136. Armitage EN: Block of dorsal nerves of penis (penile block). Regional Anaesthesia Paediatr, Clin Anesthesiol 3:535, 1985

137. Yeoman PM, Cooke R, Hain WR: Penile block for circumcision? Anaesthesia 38:862, 1983

138. Dohi S, Seino H: Spinal anesthesia in premature infants: Dosage and effects of sympathectomy (correspondence). Anesthesiology 65:559, 1986

139. Harnik EV, Hoy GR, Potolicchio S et al: Spinal anesthesia in premature infants recovering from respiratory distress syndrome. Anesthesiology 64:95, 1986

140. Blaise GA, Roy WL: Spinal anesthesia for minor paediatric surgery. Can Anaesth Soc J 33:227, 1986

141. Abajian JC, Melish RWP, Browne AF et al: Spinal anesthesia for surgery in the high risk infant. Anesth Analg 63:359, 1984

142. Ruston FG: Epidural anaesthesia in paediatric surgery: Present status in the Hamilton General Hospital. Can Anaesth Soc J 11:12, 1964

143. Schulte-Steinberg O, Rahlfs WR: Caudal anaesthesia in children and spread of 1 percent lignocaine. Br J Anaesth 42:1093, 1970

144. Touloukian RJ, Wugmeister M, Pickett LK et al: Caudal anesthesia for neonatal anoperineal and rectal operations. Anesth Analg 50:565, 1971

145. Lourey CJ, McDonald IH: Caudal anesthesia in infants and children. Anaesth Intensive Care 1:547, 1973

146. Kay B: Caudal blockade for postoperative pain relief in children. Anaesthesia 29:610, 1974

147. Melman E, Peneulas J, Marrufo J: Regional anesthesia in children. Anesth Analg 54:387, 1975

148. Hassan SZ: Caudal anesthesia in infants. Anesth Analg 56:686, 1977

149. Schulte-Steinberg O, Rahlfs WR: Spread of extradural analgesia following caudal injection in children. Br J Anaesth 49:1027, 1977

150. Takasaki M, Dohi S, Kawabata Y et al: Dosage of lidocaine for caudal anesthesia in infants and children. Anesthesiology 47:527, 1977

151. Soliman MG, Ansara S, Laberge R: Caudal anaesthesia in paediatric patients. Can Anaesth Soc J 25:226, 1978

152. McGown RG: Caudal analgesia in children. Anaesthesia 37:806, 1982

153. Bramwell RGB, Bullen C, Radford P: Caudal block for postoperative analgesia in children. Anaesthesia 37:1024, 1982

154. Eyres RL, Bishop W, Oppenheim RC et al: Plasma bupivacaine concentrations in children during caudal epidural analgesia. Anaesth Intensive Care 11:20, 1983

155. Satoyoski M, Kamiyama Y: Caudal anesthesia for upper abdominal surgery in infants and children: A simple calculation of the volume of local anaesthetic. Acta Anaesth Scand 28:57, 1984

156. Melman E, Arenas JA, Tandazo WE: Caudal anesthesia for pediatric surgery: An easy and safe method for calculating dose requirements. Anesthesiology 63:A463, 1985

157. Ecoffey C, Desparmet J, Maury M et al: Bupivacaine in children: Pharmacokinetics following caudal analgesia. Anesthesiology 63:447, 1985

158. Matsumiya N, Dohi S, Takahashi H et al: Cardiovascular collapse in an infant after caudal anesthesia with lidocaine-epinephrine solution. Anesth Analg 65:1074, 1986

159. Ward CF: An update on pediatric monitoring. Journal of Clinical Monitoring 1:172, 1985

160. Dornette WHL: Spinal anesthesia in premature infants: Dosage and effects of sympathectomy (correspondence). Anesthesiology 65:559, 1986

161. Zmyslowski WP, Lena DM: Dinamap adaptation for neonatal blood pressure determination. Anesthesiology 58:583, 1983

162. Kochansky SW: Potential deficiencies in modifying the Dinamap for use in the neonate. Anesthesiology 60:171, 1984

163. Sy WP: Ulnar nerve palsy possibly related to use of automatically cycled blood pressure cuff. Anesth Analg 60:687, 1981

164. Showman A, Betts EK: Hazard of automatic non-invasive blood pressure monitoring. Anesthesiology 55:717, 1981

165. Yelderman M: Evaluation of pulse oximetry. Anesthesiology 59:349, 1983

166. Coté CJ, Liu LMP, Szytelbein SK et al: Intraoperative events diagnosed by expired carbon dioxide monitoring in children. Can Anaesth Soc J 33:315, 1986

167. Gravenstein N, Lampotang S, Beneken JEW: Factors influencing capnography in the Bain Circuit. Journal of Clinical Monitoring 1:6, 1985

168. Beneken JEW, Gravenstein N, Gravenstein JS et al: Capnography and the Bain Circuit I: A computer model. Journal of Clinical Monitoring 1:103, 1985

169. Schieber RA, Namnoum A, Sugden A et al: Accuracy of expira-

tory carbon dioxide measurements using the coaxial and circle breathing circuits in small subjects. Journal of Clinical Monitoring 1:149, 1985

170. Roy RN, Sinclair JC: Hydration of the low-birth-weight infant. Clin Perinatol 2:393, 1975

171. Bell EF, Oh W: Fluid and electrolyte balance in very low birth weight infants. Clin Perinatol 6:139, 1979

172. Holliday MA, Segar WE: The maintenance need for water in parenteral fluid therapy. Pediatrics 19:823, 1957

173. Furman EB, Roman DG, Lemmer LAS et al: Specific therapy in water, electrolyte and blood-volume replacement during pediatric surgery. Anesthesiology 42:187, 1975

174. Sieber FE, Smith DS, Traysman RJ et al: Glucose: A re-evaluation of its intraoperative use. Anesthesiology 67:72, 1987

175. Welborn LG, Hannallah RS, McGill WA et al: Glucose concentrations for routine intravenous infusion in pediatric outpatient surgery. Anesthesiology 67:427, 1987

176. Shires T, Williams J, Brown F: Acute changes in extracellular fluids associated with major surgical procedures. Ann Surg 154:810, 1961

177. Rowe MI, Arango A: The neonatal response to massive fluid infusion. J Pediatr Surg 6:365, 1971

178. Bennett EJ: Fluid balance in the newborn. Anesthesiology 43:210, 1975

179. Rowe MI, Arango A: The choice of intravenous fluid in shock resuscitation. Pediatr Clin North Am 22:269, 1975

180. Rowe MI, Arango A: Colloid versus crystalloid resuscitation in experimental bowel obstruction. J Pediatr Surg 11:635, 1976

181. Bourke DL, Smith TC: Estimating allowable hemodilution. Anesthesiology 41:609, 1974

182. Buchholz DH: Blood transfusion: Merits of component therapy. J Pediatr 84:1, 1974

183. Coté CJ, Drop LJ, Daniels AL et al: Calcium chloride versus calcium gluconate: Comparison of ionization and cardiovascular effects in children and dogs. Anesthesiology 66:465, 1987

184. Fawler JR, TerPenning B, Syverud SA et al: Magnetic field hazard. N Engl J Med 314:1517, 1986

185. Geiger RS, Cascorbi HF: Anesthesia in an NMR scanner. Anesth Analg 63:622, 1984

186. Roth JL, Nugent M, Gray JE et al: Patient monitoring during magnetic resonance imaging. Anesthesiology 62:80, 1985

187. Nixon C, Hirsch NP, Ormerod IEC et al: Nuclear magnetic resonance. Anaesthesia 41:131, 1986

188. Greene LT: Physostigmine treatment of anticholinergic drug depression in postoperative patients. Anesth Analg 50:222, 1971

189. Jordan WS, Graves CL, Elwyn RA: A new therapy for postintubation laryngeal edema and tracheitis (croup) in children. JAMA 212:585, 1970

Chapter 48

Charles H. McLeskey

Anesthesia for the Geriatric Patient

What is a geriatric patient? An absolute definition is not possible because arbitrary limits constantly change. For example, many studies of surgery in the elderly have been published since the early 1900s, but the definition of "elderly" has changed continually. An early report in 1907 described 167 operations performed on patients older than age 50 and described this advanced age as a contraindication to surgery.[1] Twenty years later, Ochsner suggested that "an elective operation for inguinal hernia in a patient older than 50 yr was not justified."[2] In 1937, Brooks reported a series of 293 operations in patients older than age 70, and subsequently most authors have considered patients older than the ages of 65 to 70 yr as being elderly.[3] For convenience in this chapter, geriatric patients will be considered those 65 yr of age or older. However, with the not infrequent recent reports of anesthesia and surgery performed on patients older than the age of 80, there is no consensus today as to the definition of "geriatric" in medical practice, and very likely the arbitrary age defining a geriatric patient will be increasing in the near future. For example, Djokovic and Hedley-Whyte have reported the prediction for outcome after surgery in 500 patients older than age 80.[4] Miller *et al* have described anesthesia and surgery in 147 patients ranging in age from 90 to 102 yr.[5] In 1985, Catlic reported on six patients older than the age of 100 who had anesthesia and surgery.[6] He reflected on the changed mood of medicine today when he stated that "elective surgery should not be deferred nor emergency surgery denied [even for] centenarians on the basis of chronologic age."

Nevertheless, far more important than chronologic age is the patient's physiologic age. Because the aging process varies from person to person and from one organ system to another within a given person, elderly patients do not present to us as a homogeneous entity. There is little correlation between chronologic age and biologic age. People appear to reach their peak physiologic function in their late 20s or early 30s and from then on it is, in general, a "down-hill course" (Fig. 48-1).[7] The amount of physiologic function that remains varies among people with advancing age. Physiologically, some patients may appear as relatively young octogenarians compared with others who appear physiologically as relatively old septuagenarians. Rowe and Kahn have defined this concept more elegantly.[8] They suggest that persons who age with minimal impairment of physiologic function undergo what is known as "successful aging," whereas other persons, who have a deterioration of physiologic function (that which we have grown to associate with the aging process in many persons), are labeled as having undergone "usual aging." Again, those elderly persons who have aged while retaining most physiologic functions associated with youth are regarded as having aged successfully.

Figure 48-2 illustrates that in 1900 only 4% of Americans were 65 yr of age or older. Today, people older than 65 yr of age constitute approximately 11% of the United States population, which is the fastest growing segment of our society.[9] Interestingly, from Figure 48-3 we can see that a subset of the population older than 65, those persons older than age 75 (sometimes referred to as the "old old"), is growing at an even faster rate than the geriatric group as a whole.[10]

Five thousand Americans reach age 65 yr of age every day. A truly remarkable statistic revealed by Alastair Wood in 1986 was that "50% of all humans to have ever attained the age of 65 are alive today." If life spans continue to lengthen in our

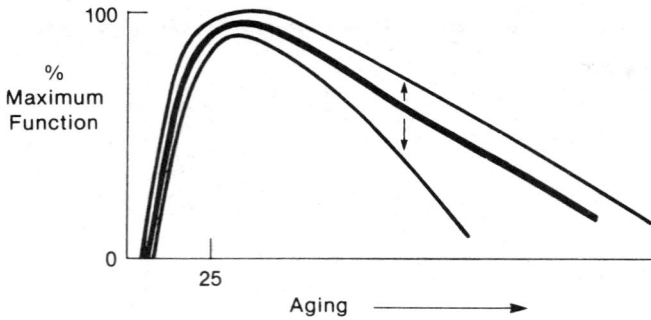

%
Maximum
Function

25

Aging ⟶

FIG. 48-1. The age-related change in physiologic function. Maximum physiologic capacity is usually achieved when someone is in the late 20s or early 30s. The physiologic function that remains becomes increasingly variable as people advance in age. (Reprinted with permission. McLeskey CH: Anesthesia for the geriatric patient. In Stoelting RK, Barash PG, Gallagher TJ [eds]: Advances in Anesthesia, p 31. Chicago, Year Book Medical Publishers, 1985.)

society at the current rate, it is projected that the elderly segment will increase to 13% of the population by the year 2000 and that, by the year 2030, fully 52,000,000 Americans, or 17% of the population, will be older than age 65 (Fig. 48-2).[11, 12] This dramatic increase in the numbers of geriatric Americans has not occurred without social consequence. For example, an article in the November 1985 issue of *Money Magazine* stated that in 1945 there were 50 times as many working Americans contributing to the Social Security system as there were elderly persons deriving pension benefits from it. In 1985 the ratio decreased to only 3.3 working Americans contributing for each person receiving pension benefits, and it was projected that by the year 2030 each beneficiary would be receiving benefits from a system in which contributions will be made by only two working Americans per beneficiary. Legislative changes regarding the Social Security system must be made if the system is to survive.

Why has the average American's life expectancy increased so dramatically? In Figure 48-4, Fries and Crapo have illustrated the gains in life expectancy that have been made from 1900 to 1980 in United States citizens and how the life span of the average American has advanced toward the proposed "ideal."[13] In the described ideal curve of survival for a society, the death rate is low and life is extended until approximately age 85, when death is preceded by a very short period of illness. The progress that has been made in the United States in extending the average life expectancy of our citizens probably results from a combination of improved medical care and improved nutrition of our society as a whole. However, it can be seen in Figure 48-4 that most improvement in life expectancy has resulted from a dramatic improvement in reducing the effects of childhood diseases. Perhaps this improvement can be attributed to advances such as the development of antibiotics and childhood immunizations. Significantly fewer gains have been made in curing the diseases of old age, such as heart disease and cancer. Although it appears that the average life expectancy of an American from 1900 to 1980 has increased, the maximum length of life has not been prolonged nearly as dramatically. It has been suggested, however, that modest improvement has also been made in this area. For example, in 1980 the United States Census Bureau reported that 32,194 people were at least 100 yr of age or older.[14] Rowe and Kahn now encourage health care practitioners to attempt to match the past gains in life span by improving health span, defined as the allowance for maintenance of unchanged physiologic function as near as possible to the end of life.[8]

Because the average life expectancy has been extended, increasing numbers of elderly patients are having surgery. It is estimated that at least 50% of Americans older than the age of 65 will have at least one operative procedure before death. This chapter summarizes the risks of anesthesia and surgery in the elderly patient, identifies the physiologic changes that occur during the aging process, and suggests how these changes affect anesthetic management of these patients. It is hoped that the risk of age, *per se*, in increasing the hazards of anesthesia and surgery, may be minimized by a better under-

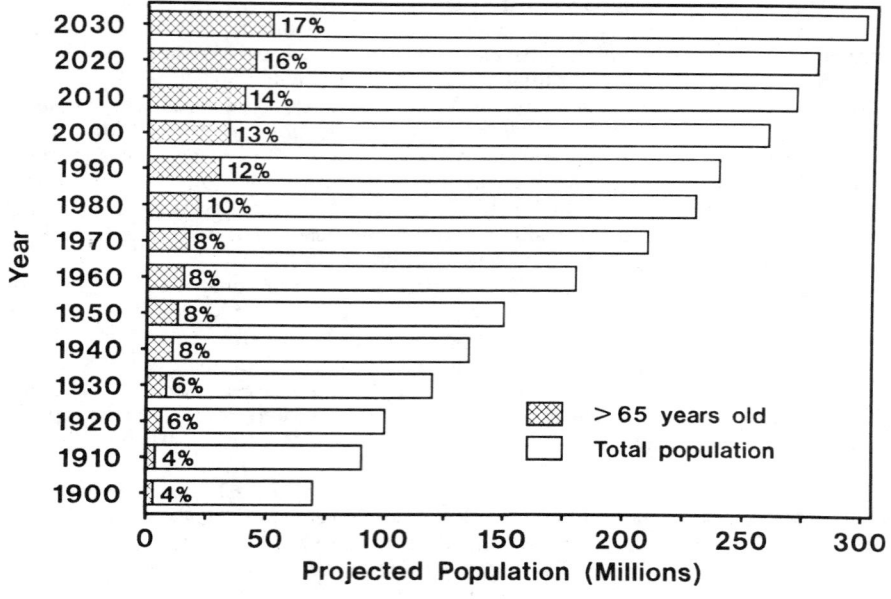

FIG. 48-2. The increasing population in the United States from the year 1900 to present, with projections to the year 2030. People who are now older than 65 (*left portion of bars*) represent approximately 11–12% of the overall population. This portion of the population is expected to increase to 17–18% by the year 2030. (Reprinted with permission. U.S. Census Bureau.)

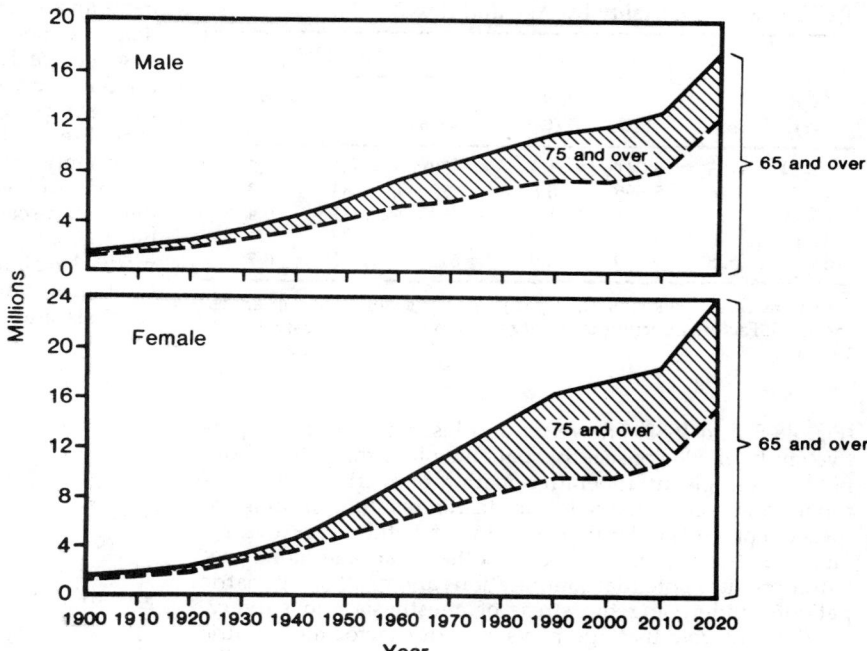

FIG. 48-3. Growth from 1900 to 2020 of the population age 65 yr and older. (Reprinted with permission. Bureau of the Census: Current Population Reports, series P-23, no. 43.)

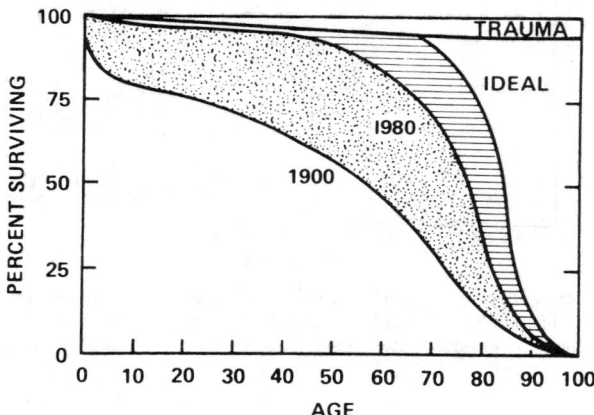

FIG. 48-4. A comparison of the survival curve of Americans observed in the years 1900 and 1980 *versus* the "ideal" survival curve. By the year 1980, more than 80% improvement toward the "ideal" had occurred. (Reprinted with permission. Fries JF, Crapo LM: The sharp downslope of natural death. In Fries JF, Crapo LM [eds]: Vitality and Aging, p 73. San Francisco, WH Freeman and Company, 1981.)

TABLE 48-1. Mortality Within 7 Days of Anesthesia in Consecutive Surgical Patients

AGE (yr)	PATIENTS	DEATHS No.	DEATHS (%)
<1	3,396	56	(1.6)
1–10	3,650	30	(0.8)
11–20	5,608	25	(0.45)
21–30	5,192	41	(0.8)
31–40	3,962	55	(1.4)
41–50	4,129	97	(2.3)
51–60	4,063	126	(3.1)
61–70	2,941	130	(4.4)
71–80	1,162	79	(6.8)
>81	73	6	(8.2)
Total	34,140	645	(1.9)

(Marx GF, Mateo CV, Orkin LR: Computer analysis of post-anesthetic deaths. Anesthesiology 39:54, 1973.)

standing of the physiologic changes occurring during the aging process.

ANESTHESIA RISKS

It is widely believed that, compared with younger patients, elderly patients (even those free of concomitant disease) having major surgery have a significantly higher incidence of complications or death.[15] In an English survey, approximately 50% of intraoperative deaths occurred in geriatric patients, although this group of patients represented only 5% of the overall surgical population.[16] As shown in Table 48-1, age,

per se, appears to predict increased perioperative morbidity and mortality.[17] Similarly, in a large clinical series of patients, Mircea *et al* found that the three most important factors leading to pulmonary complications after operation were duration of surgery, obesity, and a patient age greater than 70 yr.[18] A large study from Cardiff of 108,878 anesthetics between the years 1972 and 1977 also supported the concept of a higher mortality for both men and women of older age groups (Table 48-2).[19]

However, not all studies concur with the notion that patients who are older will necessarily have a higher complication rate during the perioperative period. For instance, in a series of 500 patients having anesthesia and surgery, Djokovic and Hedley-Whyte found no consistent increase in the incidence of death as patients' ages increased from 80 to 95 yr

TABLE 48-2.   Mortality by Age and Sex

AGE (yr)	MALES			FEMALES		
	Deaths	Total	Mortality (%)	Deaths	Total	Mortality (%)
0–14	105	8,041	1.3	59	4,601	1.3
15–24	46	5,695	0.8	27	9,683	0.3
25–44	121	9,488	1.3	94	22,411	0.4
45–64	428	14,174	3.0	331	15,925	2.1
>65	578	9,749	5.9	612	9,111	6.7

(Farrow SC., Fowkes FGR, Lunn JN *et al*: Epidemiology in anaesthesia. II: Factors affecting mortality in hospital. Br J Anaesth 54:811, 1982.)

(Fig. 48-5).[4] In 1983, Filzweiser and List reported a prospective study of 500 consecutive patients older than 70 and did not find a single intraoperative death.[20] Similarly, Hatton *et al* reported an actual reduction in deaths resulting from anesthesia in patients older than 80.[21] In view of this controversy, one wonders if there is a factor other than age alone that better predicts potential complications and deaths in geriatric patients undergoing the stress of anesthesia and surgery.

When the role that age plays as a risk factor for geriatric patients having anesthesia and surgery is examined, the distinction between physiologic age and chronologic age becomes important. Compared with younger patients, elderly patients may be at greater risk for perioperative complications and deaths because of two factors: first, an increased prevalence of age-related, concomitant disease, and, second, a decline in basic organ function (independent of disease) resulting from aging, *per se*. Let us examine each of these factors.

EFFECTS OF CONCOMITANT DISEASE

Multiple concomitant diseases are the rule, rather than the exception, in elderly patients. A current surgical illness is likely to be present in patients in whom old injuries, prior illnesses, past operations, and a variety of chronic disorders,

including cataracts, osteoarthritis, anemia, osteoporosis, and diabetes mellitus, may be observed. Malignancy, cerebral vascular accidents, Parkinsonism, dementia, and fractures of the femur are observed with increased frequency in this patient group. Figure 48-6 illustrates the incidence of four common disease states by patient age and shows how much more commonly these disease processes occur as people become age 65 or older.[22] A similar, significant increase in the incidence of diseases in many organ systems has been confirmed by others. For instance, pathologic findings were observed on medical examination in 92% of patients 81 yr of age or older.[23] Of these, cardiovascular abnormalities, including arteriosclerosis and hypertension, were seen in 78% of patients,

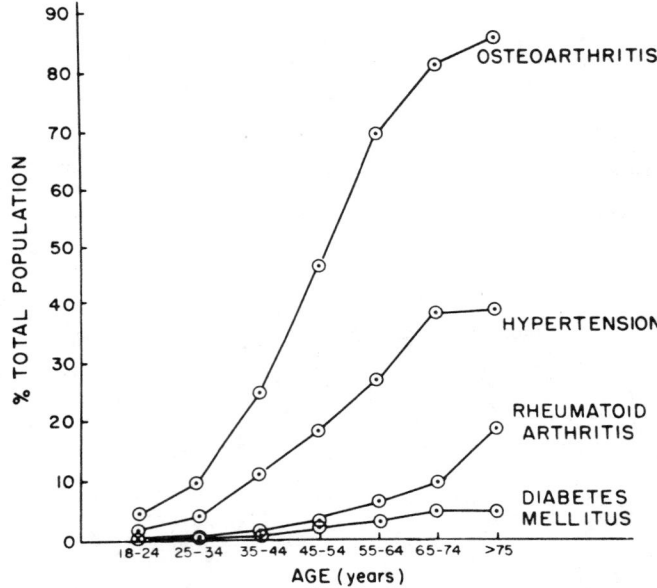

FIG. 48-6. Comparison of the prevalance of four common diseases by age of United States citizens. (Reprinted with permission. Ellison N: Problems in geriatric anesthesia. Surg Clin North Am 55:929, 1975.)

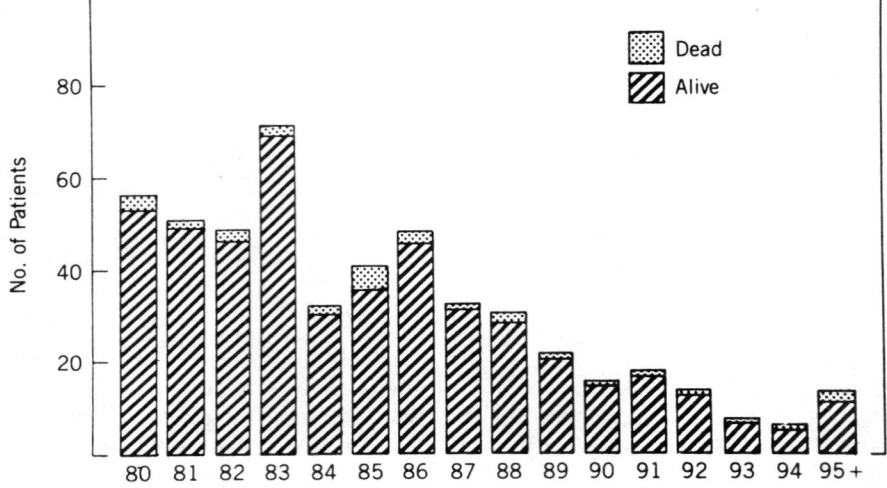

FIG. 48-5. Mortality in patients having anesthesia and surgery who range in age from 80 to older than 95 yr. (Reprinted with permission. Djokvic JL, Hedley-Whyte J: Prediction of outcome of surgery and anesthesia in patients over 80. JAMA 242:2301, 1979. Copyright 1979, American Medical Association.)

TABLE 48-3. Preanesthetic Complications Encountered in 1,000 Elderly Patients

COMPLICATIONS	INCIDENCE (%)
Hypertension	46.6
Renal disease	31.4
Atherosclerosis	26.9
Myocardial infarction	18.5
Chronic obstructive pulmonary disease	14.0
Cardiomegaly	13.6
Diabetes	9.2
Liver disease	8.5
Congestive heart failure	7.5
Angina	6.4
Cerebrovascular accident	5.8

(Stephen CR: The risk of anesthesia and surgery in the geriatric patient. In Krechel SE [ed]: Anesthesia and the Geriatric Patient, p 231. New York: Grune & Stratton, 1984.)

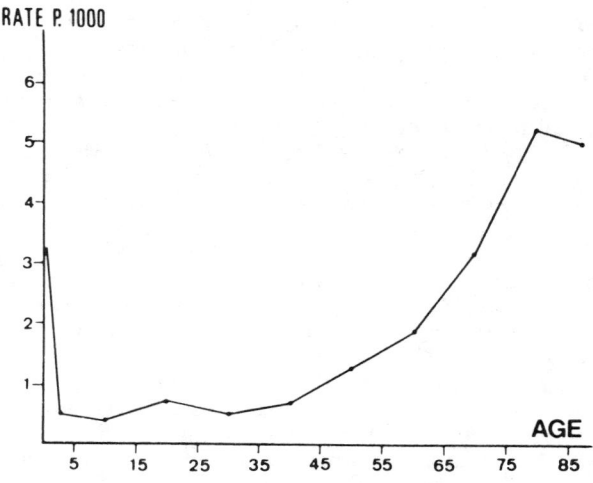

FIG. 48-7. Complication rate per 1,000 anesthetics, related to patient age from age 5 to 85. (Reprinted with permission. Tiret L, Demonts JM, Hatton F et al: Complications associated with anaesthesia—A prospective study in France. Can Anaesth Soc J 33:336, 1986.)

whereas mental dysfunction occurred in 30% and pulmonary, endocrine, and neurologic abnormalities were observed in 14%, 12%, and 10% of patients, respectively. Stephen has reported on the frequency of abnormalities encountered in 1,000 patients older than age 70 (Table 48-3).[24] Once again, hypertension, atherosclerosis, and renal disease led the list of concomitant disease states in patients interviewed before operation.

Which of the common preexisting conditions correlate most closely with an increased risk of perioperative complications and death in elderly patients? Rowe et al found that ischemic heart disease, dementia, and diabetes mellitus seem to correlate most closely with an increased risk.[25] On the other hand, Farrow et al found that cardiac failure, impaired renal function, and angina were the preoperative conditions most indicative of a high risk of perioperative death.[19] These conditions were associated with mortality 10–30 times greater than the overall 0.5% mortality observed in patients without preoperative medical conditions (Table 48-4).

The number of associated diseases also may be important in determining the rate of perioperative complications. A prospective French survey of 198,103 anesthetics appeared to once again demonstrate that the rate of anesthesia-related complications correlates directly with patients' ages (Fig. 48-7).[26] However, on closer examination (Fig. 48-8), it is clear that the complication rate relates far more closely to the number of associated diseases with which the patient presented rather than to the patient's age. The greater incidence of

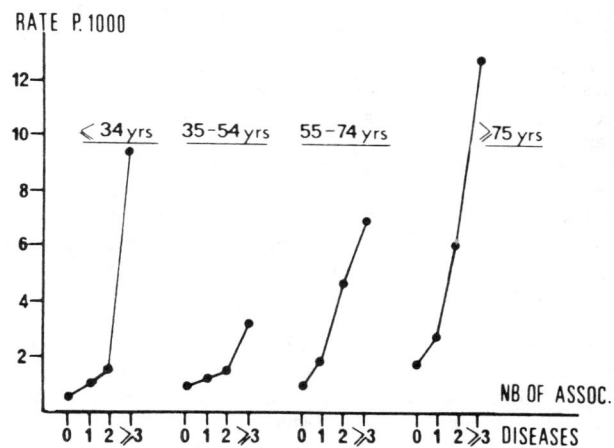

FIG. 48-8. Complications rate per 1,000 anesthetics, related to number of associated diseases in patients of four different age groups. (Reprinted with permission. Tiret L, Desmonts JM, Hatton F et al: Complications associated with anesthesia—A prospective survey in France. Can Anaesth Soc J 33:336, 1986.)

TABLE 48-4. Mortality by Selected Preoperative Condition

CONDITION	DEATHS	OPERATIONS	MORTALITY (%)
Cardiac failure	186	1,175	15.8
Impaired renal function	84	779	10.8
Angina, arteriosclerosis, or ischemic heart disease	544	7,776	7.0
Diabetes	82	1,452	5.7
Chronic lower respiratory tract infection	408	8,060	5.1
No preoperative condition	206	43,483	0.5

(Farrow SC, Fowkes FGR, Lunn JN et al: Epidemiology in anaesthesia. II: Factors affecting mortality in hospital. Br J Anaesth 54:811, 1982.)

complications and death in older patients most likely reflects the fact that these patients are more commonly seen with a greater number of associated preexistent diseases. Stephen observed the same phenomenon.[24] Although he reported an overall mortality of 5.8% in elderly patients, of those who died, 84% had more than three preexistent medical conditions. Likewise, Denney and Denson reported a mortality of 29% among patients older than age 90 who had disease in multiple organ systems, compared with a mortality of 4.9% in a group of healthy persons of similar age.[27] The Goldman study of cardiac risk factors also suggests that the preexistent medical condition is more important than a patient's age when attempting to predict the risks associated with anesthesia and surgery.[28] As outlined in Table 48-5, "points" in the Goldman risk index are assigned to patients before operation, with greater point values given to those criteria more likely to result in perioperative complications and death. Age greater than 70 yr is assigned a point value, indicating that age, *per se*, may be a risk. However, it is a lesser value than that assigned to certain preoperative medical conditions, such as a recent myocardial infarction or signs of congestive heart failure.

The American Society of Anesthesiologists (ASA) physical status classification is not affected by patients' ages but rather by the number and severity of preexistent medical conditions. The ASA classification system predicts with reasonable accuracy the risks of elderly patients having anesthesia and surgery. For instance, in a study of 500 patients older than 80 yr of age, only one of 187 ASA Class II patients died in the perioperative period, whereas 14 of 56 (25%) ASA Class IV patients died (Fig. 48-9).[4] Similarly, a prospective French study of almost 200,000 anesthetics demonstrated an incidence of complications that related very closely to the patient's ASA physical status (Fig. 48-10).[26] Del Guercio and Cohn have also shown in patients older than age 65 that ASA physical status relates directly to perioperative mortality.[29] In their patients, preoperative assignment of a patient to ASA Class II resulted in a mortality of less than 10%. However, ASA Class III patients had an increased mortality between 10 and 15% and ASA Class IV patients had a mortality greater than 20%. From all of the information presented, it appears that the presence of age-related disease probably plays a greater role than does age itself in contributing to perioperative complications and death.

EFFECTS OF EMERGENCY PROCEDURES

The risk of perioperative complications and death is greatly increased in the elderly if surgery must be performed on an

TABLE 48-5.   Cardiac Risk Index

CRITERIA	"POINTS"
Congestive heart failure	11
Myocardial infarction in previous 6 months	10
Rhythm other than sinus on ECG	7
Greater than 5 PVCs/min	7
Age greater than 70 yr	5
Emergency operation	4
General status	3
Intraperitoneal or intrathoracic operation	3
Valvular aortic stenosis	3

(Goldman L, Caldera DL, Nussbaum SR *et al*: Multifactorial index of cardiac risks in non-cardiac surgical procedures. N Engl J Med 297:845, 1977.)

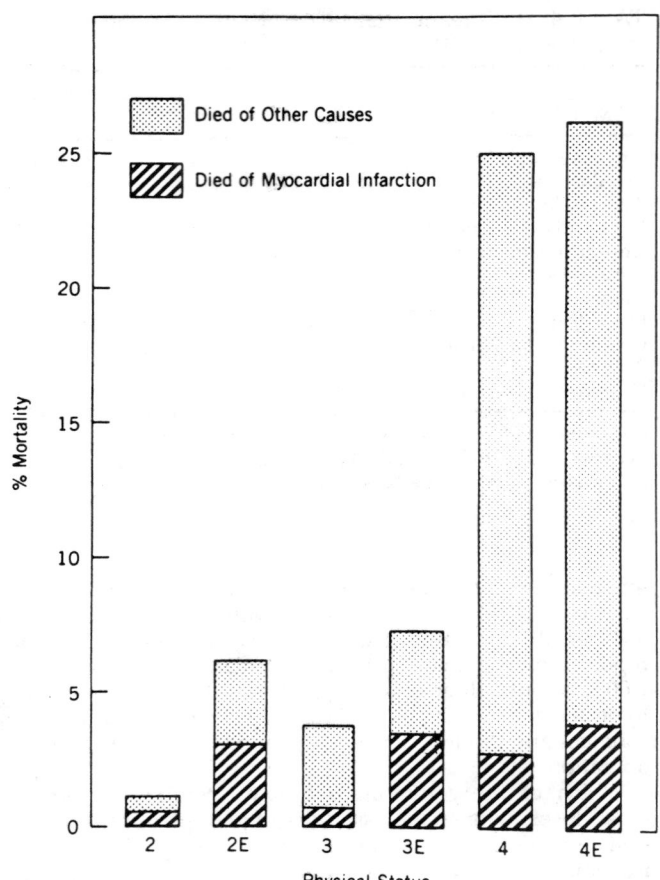

FIG. 48-9. The relationship of ASA physical status to percentage deaths after anesthesia and surgery in patients older than age 80. Perioperative mortality increases significantly as physical status increases. In patients of the same physical status, emergency procedures are generally associated with a higher incidence of death. (Reprinted with permission. Djokovic JL, Hedley-Whyte J: Prediction of outcome of surgery and anaesthesia in patients over 80. JAMA 242:2301, 1979. Copyright 1979, American Medical Association.)

emergency basis.[29-31] Gibson *et al* suggested that death is four times more frequent in the elderly patient with coexistent disease compared with the healthy elderly patient and 20 times more frequent in those requiring emergency surgery.[32] Farrow *et al* also showed that the crude mortality in a large series of patients increased 3.5-fold if the procedures were performed on an emergency rather than an elective basis.[19] Table 48-6 lists findings in three separate studies that illustrate in elderly patients the dramatic increase in mortality associated with emergency herniorrhaphy compared with the mortality when the same procedures were performed electively.[33-35] A large French study has also demonstrated that performing surgical procedures in elderly patients (ASA classification III or greater) on an emergency basis significantly increases the risks of perioperative complications and death (Fig. 48-10).[26]

Perhaps the best explanations for why elderly patients requiring emergency surgery have a higher incidence of perioperative complications and death are that they may have delayed seeking health care and may have more advanced pathologic conditions. Also, presentation for emergency surgery allows little time for control of preexisting disease.

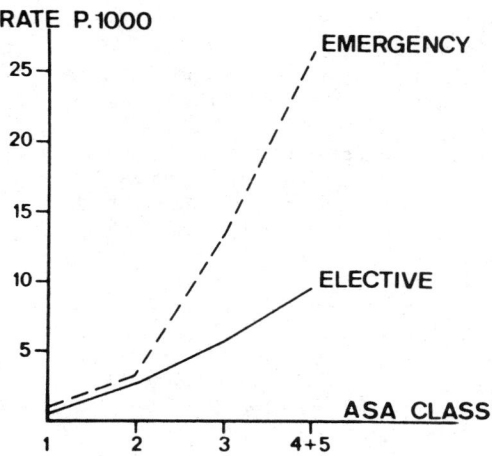

FIG. 48-10. Complications rate per 1,000 anesthetics related to ASA physical status (class) for elective and emergency surgical procedures. Higher ASA classes of surgical patients and surgical procedures performed on an emergency basis exaggerate the risks of perioperative complications and death. (Reprinted with permission. Tiret L, Desmonts JM, Hatton F et al: Complications associated with anaesthesia—A prospective survey in France. Can Anaesth Soc J 33:336, 1986.)

Although apparently healthy elderly patients may tolerate an elective operation, the additional stress of an emergency procedure, because of an acute exacerbation of preexistent disease or an unexpected complication, can tax their limited physiologic reserve and lead to disastrous consequences. In general, it is wise to adequately prepare an elderly patient for elective surgery but unwise to defer surgery simply because of age. An unnecessary delay may result in complications that necessitate surgery under even more adverse emergency conditions, with a significantly increased risk of associated perioperative complications and death.

In this section we have discussed the increased risk associated with surgery on elderly patients if they have preexistent medical conditions that affect their ASA status and if they are to have surgery on an emergency basis. Both of these factors are believed to be more important in contributing to perioperative complications and death than advanced age alone. However, should age, *per se*, influence perioperative morbidity and mortality in elderly patients, it likely does so as a result of the gradual decline in physiologic reserve in a variety of organ systems that occurs during the aging process.

PATHOPHYSIOLOGY OF AGING

We have previously discussed the increased risks that age-related diseases produce. In this section we will discuss the pathophysiologic changes of aging that affect major organ systems and that subsequently influence our anesthetic techniques.

CARDIOVASCULAR SYSTEM

Perhaps the most important age-related physiologic changes that affect the anesthetic management of the elderly patient are those that occur in the cardiovascular system. Many of these physiologic changes that were once thought to reflect the aging process itself now appear rather to be manifestations of age-related disease or a lifestyle resulting in prolonged deconditioning. Because major lifestyle changes occur and the prevalence of disease increases sharply with advancing age, it is difficult to determine the effects of the aging process alone on the cardiovascular system. All three processes are closely interrelated (Fig. 48-11).[36]

Cardiovascular changes associated with aging are summarized in Table 48-7. These changes include the concept that with aging there may be impaired myocardial pump function and reduced cardiac output. For example, variable degrees of myocardial fiber atrophy occur during aging with replacement by connective tissue. When this process develops in an area of the myocardium adjacent to the sinoatrial pacemaker site, the heart rate may be affected in elderly patients. Increasing fibrosis of the endocardial lining of the cardiac chambers and valves leads to progressive endocardial thickening and rigidity. Calcification of valves, especially in the region of

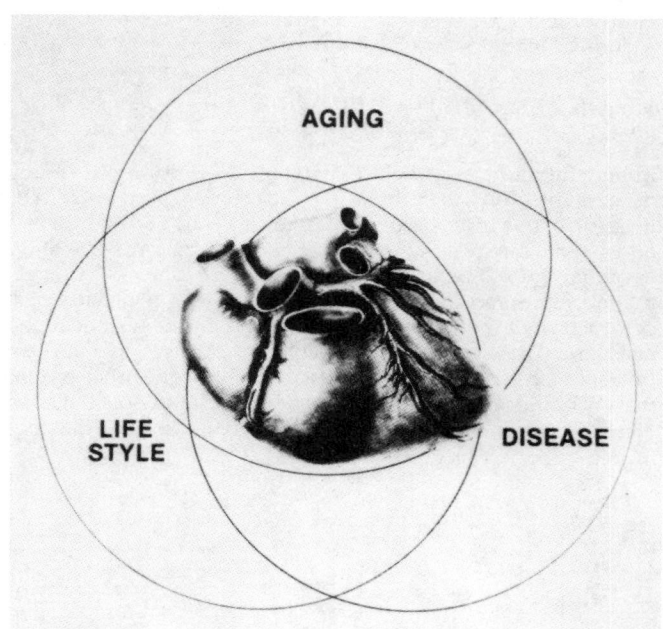

FIG. 48-11. Interrelationship of the effects of lifestyle, age-related disease, and aging on the physiologic changes of the cardiovascular system as people age. (Reprinted with permission. Lakatta EG, Fleg JL: Aging of the adult cardiovascular system. In Stephen CR, Assaf RAE [eds]: Geriatric Anesthesia: Principles and Practices, p 1. Boston, Butterworth, 1986.)

TABLE 48-6. Mortality in Elderly Patients Having Herniorrhaphy

STUDY	ELECTIVE		EMERGENCY	
	Percentage	*Total No.*	*Percentage*	*Total No.*
Nehme[33]	1.3	1,044	7.5	235
Williams and Hale[34]	2		16	
Tingwald and Cooperman[35]	0	44	22	18

TABLE 48-7. Cardiovascular Changes Associated with Aging

SIGN	CHANGE
Maximum coronary blood flow	Decrease
Cardiac index	No change or a decrease
Resting heart rate	No change
Maximum heart rate	Decrease
Arterial distensibility	Decrease
Peripheral vascular resistance	Increase
Impedance to left ventricular output	Increase
Systolic blood pressure	Increase
Stroke volume	No change or an increase
Ejection fraction	No change or a decrease

the annulus, may produce distortion of valvular leaflets, resulting in progressive valvular incompetence. In addition, loss of elasticity throughout the vascular tree with age produces a progressive loss of arterial distensibility and increased impedance to left ventricular output, resulting in a progressive compensatory hypertrophy of the left ventricle. With age-induced diminished caliber and elasticity of coronary arteries as well, maximum coronary perfusion decreases. Not surprisingly, many of these factors combine to contribute to an increased incidence of hypertension and ischemic heart disease in elderly patients.

Vascular Elasticity and Blood Pressure Changes During Aging

In general, large artery elasticity is reduced during the aging process, resulting in stiffening of the arterial vasculature. The histologic and morphologic changes seen in the aging aorta and arterial tree resemble those of younger patients who have essential hypertension.[36] Consequently, there is an age-related increased impedance to ejection of blood with each contraction of the heart, resulting in increased systolic blood pressure. Probably as an adaptive mechanism to maintain normal wall stress, an approximately 30% concentric hypertrophy of the left ventricular wall develops in people between 30 and 80 years of age. Further, the decrease in early diastolic

filling rate and the increase in left atrial dimension observed with advanced age may be consequences of a thicker-walled, less-compliant left ventricle. The thoracic aorta is thought to contribute approximately half of the total capability of the arterial tree to buffer the energy released with each ejection of the heart. Partial compensation for the age-related arterial stiffening is provided by an approximate 6% aortic dilatation that develops between the fourth and eighth decades of life.[37] Despite this partial compensation by the elderly, long-term longitudinal studies of patients, such as that reported in the Framingham study, demonstrated an increased systolic blood pressure of 25–35 mm Hg (Fig. 48-12).[38] Hypertension in the elderly is frequently inadequately treated, and if diastolic blood pressure is chronically greater than 100–110 mm Hg, plasma volume depletion is likely.[39] Pre-existent hypovolemia in poorly treated elderly hypertensive patients makes intraoperative blood pressure lability likely and also renders the patient less tolerant of sudden changes in posture, intrathoracic pressure, or blood loss.

Coronary Artery Disease

The age-associated replacement of elastic tissue by less resilient fibrous connective tissue occurs not only in the peripheral vascular system, but in the coronary arteries as well, reducing maximum available coronary flow. Coronary artery disease progressively increases in severity over the entire adult age span, but clinical symptoms may not be seen until a critical threshold is reached. Although a high percentage of elderly persons have coronary stenosis at autopsy, a much lower percentage demonstrate clinical manifestations such as angina pectoris or myocardial infarction. Thus, coronary artery disease may be occult in many elderly persons. As illustrated in Figure 48-13, an estimate of the prevalence of coronary artery disease in men ages 51–90 will be significantly low and inaccurate if one relies only on resting criteria, such as a history of angina pectoris or previous myocardial infarction or an abnormal ECG.[36] On the other hand, with more intensive evaluation of coronary perfusion, such as with the use of radionuclide imaging of the myocardium, coupled with ECG monitoring during a treadmill stress test, many more cases of significant coronary artery disease may be identified. In fact, it appears that people who are 70 yr of age or older have at

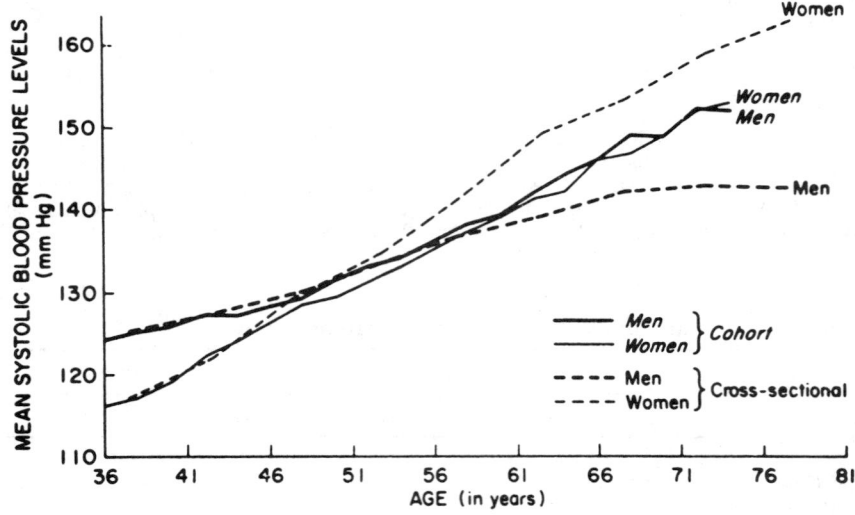

FIG. 48-12. Increases in systolic blood pressure of 25–35 mm Hg occur in both men and women during the aging process. (Reprinted with permission. Kannel WB, Gordon T: Evaluation of cardiovascular risk in the elderly: The Framingham study. Bull NY Acad Med 54:573, 1978.)

least a 50% chance of development of significant coronary artery disease, whether or not they have symptoms.

Cardiac Output

Cardiac output is thought to decrease by approximately 1% per year beyond age 30 (Fig. 48-14).[40] As a consequence, in elderly patients it should take longer for intravenously administered drugs to reach receptor sites, thus delaying the

FIG. 48-13. Estimate of the prevalence of coronary artery disease in men ages 51–90. Resting criteria represent a history of angina pectoris or myocardial infarction, or an abnormal ECG. Stress criteria represent an abnormal exercise ECG or a thallium scan perfusion defect during exercise. (Reprinted with permission. Lakatta EG: Health, disease, and cardiovascular aging. In the Aging Society: The Burden of Long-term Illness and Disability. Washington DC, National Academy Press, 1986.)

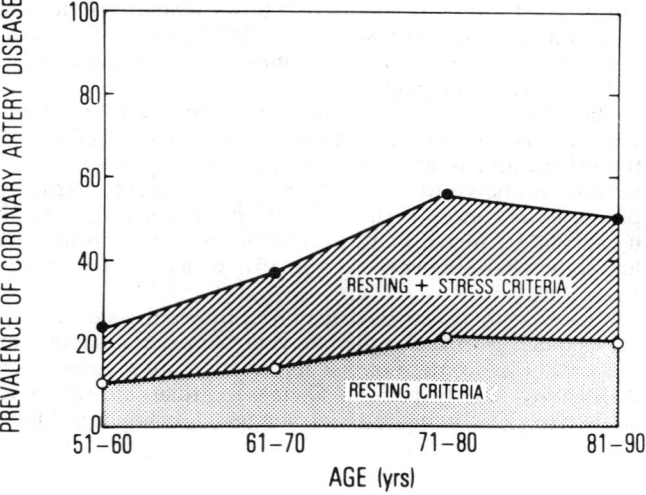

FIG. 48-14. The classically held concept is that various physiologic functions decline as a person ages. Most functions decrease by approximately 1–1.5% per year after age 30. (Reprinted with permission. Evans TI: The physiological basis of geriatric general anaesthesia. Anaesth Intensive Care 1:319, 1973.)

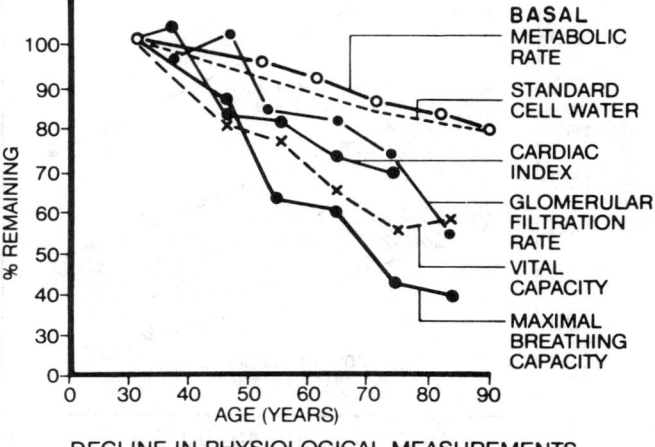

DECLINE IN PHYSIOLOGICAL MEASUREMENTS
WITH AGE

onset of pharmacologic action. An example of this might be the patient's response to the administration of a test dose of thiopental (approximately 50 mg) before a complete induction dose is administered. Some believe that administration of a test dose of thiopental is a useful technique in elderly patients because it allows one to assess the patient's sensitivity to the drug and enables one to estimate the eventual proper dose required to complete the induction of anesthesia. However, allowing 30–45 s for observation of a response to this test dose (which may be an adequate time in a younger patient) may not be an adequate time in an elderly patient with a reduced cardiac output and a prolonged circulation time. Reduced cardiac output and a slower circulation time in the elderly will also affect induction of inhalation anesthesia. A faster induction of anesthesia with inhalation drugs would be expected. If cardiac output is slow, uptake of inhalation drugs from the alveoli will be reduced and will result in a higher partial pressure of anesthetic in the alveoli. This higher partial pressure will, in turn, be reflected as a higher partial pressure of the agent in the blood, the heart, and, in turn, the brain. Profound hypotension may result.

Succinylcholine may theoretically be less effective in the elderly in the presence of a reduced cardiac output. A slower circulation time would permit a longer exposure of the injected drug to plasma pseudocholinesterase, allowing greater metabolism and reduced effectiveness of the drug before its eventual delivery to the effector sites at the neuromuscular junction.

Many studies support the belief that cardiac output gradually declines about 1% per year beyond age 30. A typical example is a study by Brandfonbrener et al, in which a 50% decline in cardiac index from ages 20 to 80 was observed.[41] Unfortunately, the population tested in many of these classic studies was composed of patients who were housed on hospital wards and were being treated for acute or chronic disease. A large percentage of these patients may have been sedentary and may have been convalescing from a variety of illnesses. Thus, it may have been lifestyle or age-associated disease that produced the observed decrease in cardiac output, and it may be incorrect to conclude that aging itself produces a predetermined obligatory decline in cardiac output.

The Baltimore Longitudinal Study on Aging is a program that, on a longitudinal basis, follows volunteer subjects who are carefully screened and are viewed to be healthy and not affected by disease or deconditioning. These subjects return to Baltimore every other year for a complete physical evaluation. Recently, data from this study have yielded a divergent view of the change that has classically been thought to occur in resting cardiac output as a result of age. Rodeheffer et al demonstrated that there is no significant age-associated decline in cardiac output at rest or during exercise in healthy adults between the ages of 25 and 79 yr (Fig. 48-15).[42] Therefore, it appears that elderly people may have a decline in cardiac output with age if they have maintained a sedentary lifestyle or if they are affected by age-related disease. On the other hand, healthy elderly people who have maintained an active lifestyle do not necessarily have a predetermined obligatory decline in cardiac output with age.

Cardiac Reserve

It has been believed for a long time that elderly patients have a reduced myocardial reserve, making them less capable of responding to stress. Traditional studies in exercise physiology have shown that maximum exercise performance is

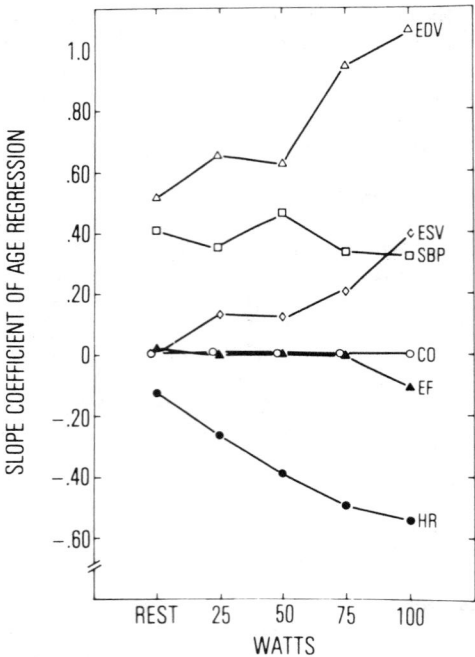

FIG. 48-15. The slope coefficients of the regression functions of age for cardiac parameters in persons tested at rest and at four different exercise workloads. An increase or decrease in the slope coefficient with increasing workloads indicates a respective increasing or decreasing age effect. During exercise, older persons demonstrate a reduced heart rate (HR) and ejection fraction (EF) compared with younger subjects. Despite this, when older persons exercise, they generate a cardiac output (CO) similar to that of youth. This is accomplished by increasing end-diastolic volume (EDV) to a greater extent than the increase in end-systolic volume (ESV), resulting in an age-related increase in stroke volume during increased workloads. (Reprinted with permission of the American Heart Association, Inc. Rodeheffer RJ, Gerstenblith G, Becker LC et al: Exercise cardiac output is maintained with advancing age in healthy human subjects: Cardiac dilatation and increased stroke volume compensate for a diminished heart rate. Circulation 69:203, 1984.)

reduced with age. Specifically, declines have been identified in maximum aerobic capacity, heart rate, stroke volume, and cardiac output. For example, when tested with the stress of exercise, healthy young subjects increased their ejection fraction and stroke volume 10–24% compared with resting values.[43] However, elderly people did not respond with an increase in ejection fraction and many actually had a reduced ejection fraction in response to this stress. Another study suggesting reduced cardiovascular reserve in elderly people demonstrated a diminished cardiovascular response to the stress of acute hemodilution.[44] More specifically, during neurolept anesthesia, acute normovolemic hemodilution from a hematocrit of 38% to 28% resulted in a significant increase in cardiac output in young patients. However, no such increase was observed in elderly patients; rather, oxygen extraction from hemoglobin increased, resulting in a diminished central venous oxygen tension. This study suggests that acute hemodilution does not seem to trigger appropriate reflex mechanisms in the elderly but instead results in a reduced oxygen transport capacity. Caution should be used when this technique is used to reduce surgical blood loss during surgical procedures in geriatric patients.

Newer data from the Baltimore Longitudinal Study on Aging have suggested that the older notion that the elderly have a reduced myocardial reserve in response to stress may be incorrect. When carefully screened in order to exclude coronary disease and other age-associated cardiac diseases, elderly subjects demonstrated no decrease in cardiac output in response to the stress of exercise when compared with younger subjects (Fig. 48-15).[42]

However, physiologic differences in elderly patients allow an increase in cardiac output in response to exercise (and presumably to other stresses as well) by a mechanism different from that observed in younger subjects. For example, the maximum heart rate generated by an elderly person is less than that of younger subjects.[45] Maximum attainable heart rate in persons of different ages is predicted by the following equation:

$$\text{Maximum heart rate} = 220 - \text{age} \qquad (48\text{-}1)$$

Thus, 20-yr-old people have an approximate maximal heart rate of 200 beats · min^{-1}, whereas those who are 60 have an approximate maximal heart rate of 160 beats · min^{-1}. Rodeheffer et al confirmed this observation in the Baltimore Longitudinal Study on Aging.[42]

The principle of reduced maximum attainable heart rate with age is well known and used in exercise facilities. A typical example of an exercise chart posted in many exercise facilities is shown in Figure 48-16. Many exercise instructors promote the concept that an aerobic benefit is achieved only if heart rate is increased by exercise to the "target zone" that lies somewhere between 70 and 85% of maximal attainable heart rate.

If exercise increases cardiac output in healthy elderly people as much as in young people, yet maximal attainable heart rate and enhancement of ejection fraction are reduced, how do healthy elderly patients increase cardiac output in response to exercise or other challenges? As shown in Figure

FIG. 48-16. An exercise chart typical of that posted in many exercise facilities demonstrates the decrease in maximum heart rate observed at an increased age. The maximum heart rate may be determined by this formula: maximum heart rate = 220 − age.

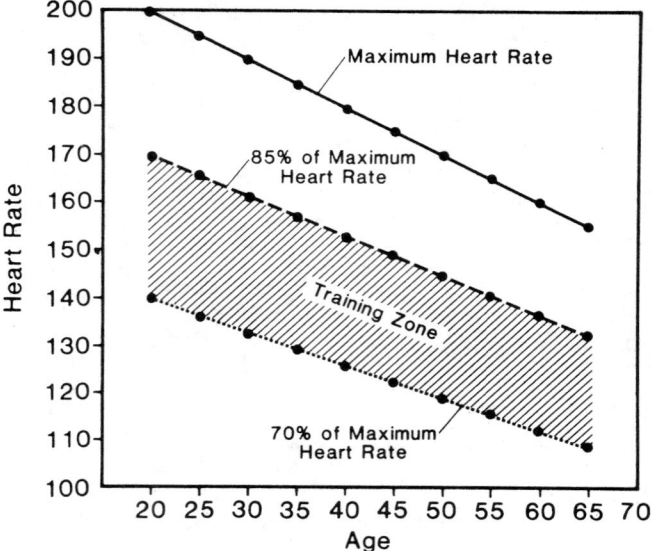

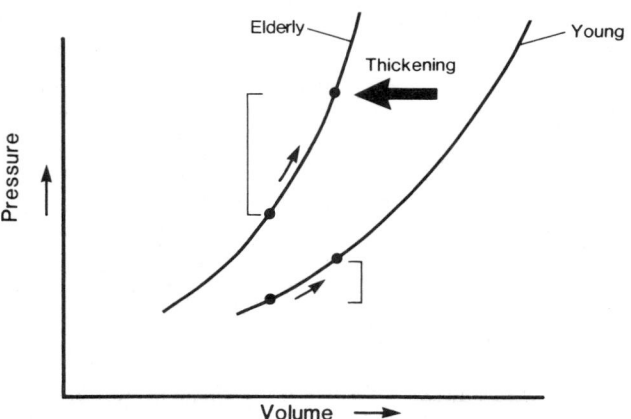

FIG. 48-17. The aged myocardium, after years of pumping against an increased afterload, hypertrophies, resulting in a steeper pressure/volume slope. As a result, when elderly persons increase cardiac output during exercise (primarily by increasing filling volumes of the left ventricle), a much greater filling pressure is required than that for younger persons. Therefore, this compensatory mechanism is more limited in elderly persons and predisposes them to congestive heart failure if large filling volumes are required.

48-15, the major mechanism by which older people enhance cardiac output when demands are placed upon them is by an increased reliance on the Frank-Starling mechanism. An increase in end-diastolic volume, which becomes more pronounced as exercise levels increase, results in a larger stroke volume.[42] Although end-systolic volume also increases to some extent, the increase in end-diastolic volume is significantly greater, resulting in an augmentation of stroke volume. Thus, despite the age-associated attenuation in maximal heart rate and a sluggish enhancement of ejection fraction in response to stress, healthy, nonsedentary elderly patients are able to enhance cardiac output when demands are placed upon them primarily by an enhancement of stroke volume resulting from an increase in end-diastolic volume.

This compensatory increase in end-diastolic volume necessarily requires an increase in filling pressure. As shown in Figure 48-17, the elevation in left ventricular filling pressure necessary to produce an increase in end-diastolic volume in elderly people may be even more dramatic than in young people because older people have a steeper pressure/volume curve as a result of the progressive myocardial hypertrophy that accompanies age. Thus, the primary compensatory mechanisms that healthy elderly people use to improve cardiac output in response to stress may make them less able to tolerate fluid loads and predispose them to congestive heart failure.

Heart Rate and Adrenoreceptor Responsiveness of the Elderly Cardiovascular System

Although the resting heart rate and heart rate response to submaximal exercise loads in the elderly are similar to those of younger patients, the maximum heart rate that can be generated by an elderly patient is considerably less (see Equation 48-1).[45] Regulation of chronotropic and inotropic cardiac function depends partly on a catecholamine effect. During exercise, serum catecholamine levels in elderly subjects exceed those seen in younger subjects.[46] Thus, failure to elaborate and release catecholamines during stress cannot explain

the elderly patient's apparent diminution in adrenergic response, manifested by a reduced maximal heart rate and ejection fraction. Instead, an age-related decrease in target organ responsiveness, whether resulting from a reduced number of receptors or a reduced receptor sensitivity, has been suggested.[47, 48] The number of adrenergic receptors decreases in the aging heart.[47] Thus, catecholamine effects that enhance calcium ion transport in the myocardium and improve calcium ion availability are less pronounced in elderly patients, partly explaining the reduced myocardial contractility and the reduced maximum heart rate in elderly subjects.

Many studies in the elderly have also demonstrated a reduced chronotropic response to a variety of exogenously administered drugs. For example, older patients have a reduced tachycardic response to atropine in comparison with younger patients.[49] When a person is age 50 or older, the heart rate is increased by only 4–5 beats $\cdot$ min^{-1} after atropine administration, whereas the same dose produces a far more dramatic response in younger subjects. Similarly, a multicenter clinical study demonstrated a greater increase in the heart rates of younger patients compared to the elderly in response to the administration of similar concentrations of isoflurane (Fig. 48-18).[50]

Chronotropic and inotropic effects of beta-agonist drugs are also significantly reduced in elderly patients. The decrease in beta-receptor–mediated responsiveness suggests an alteration in beta-receptor numbers or affinity, or an alteration in the dose–response curve of the beta-receptor-adenylate cyclase system, resulting in the generation of less cyclic adenosine monophosphate (cAMP) after beta-receptor stimulation.[47, 48, 51] Isoprenaline produces a far greater increase in heart rate in young subjects compared with older subjects.[52] Terbutaline, another beta-adrenoreceptor agonist with relative beta-2 selectivity, also produces less tachycardia in elderly patients compared with younger patients.[53] Interestingly, the sensitivity of elderly patients to the beta-blocker propranolol is also reduced, as shown by a greater reduction in heart rate in patients younger than age 35 as compared with those older than age 50.[54]

The response of the autonomic nervous system to stress is less effective in the elderly, making stress-related cardiac decompensation more likely in this patient population.[55, 56] For example, healthy elderly subjects in whom blood pressure was reduced by the administration of the alpha-1 antagonist, prazosin, demonstrated significantly less tachycardia in response to the associated hypotension.[57] Younger subjects responded with a heart rate increase to 103 beats $\cdot$ min^{-1}, whereas there was no change observed in the heart rate in elderly patients from the resting rate of 80 beats $\cdot$ min^{-1}. We have also previously seen that elderly patients respond to the stress of acute hemodilution with far less of a compensatory increase in heart rate and cardiac output than that observed in young patients.[44] This reduced compensatory cardiac response to hypotension or hemodilution is compatible with the phenomenon of reduced responsiveness of cardiac beta-receptors and reduced baroreflex mechanisms in elderly patients.

Responsiveness of the vascular adrenoreceptors also seems to be reduced in the elderly. For example, the dose of the alpha-1 agonist phenylephrine required to increase mean arterial pressure by 20 mm Hg is almost twice as great in the elderly as that required in younger patients (Fig. 48-19).[57] When injected intraarterially, isoprenaline produces a lesser increase in forearm blood flow in older subjects compared with that seen in young subjects (Fig. 48-20).[52] Younger

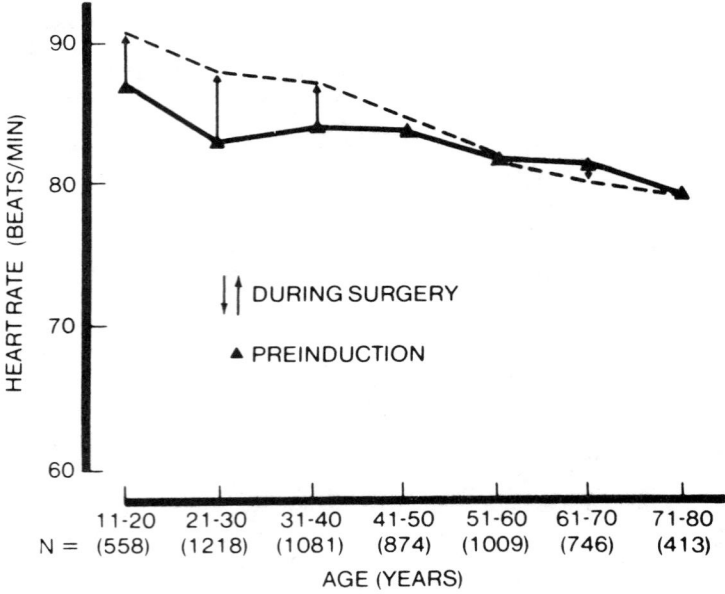

FIG. 48-18. Heart rate response to isoflurane anesthesia during surgery related to age. (Reprinted with permission. Forrest JB: Clinical evaluation of isoflurane: Pulse and blood pressure. Can Anaesth Soc J 29:S15, 1982.)

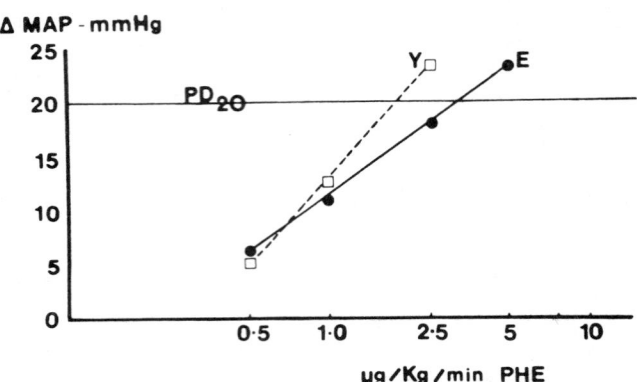

FIG. 48-19. Comparison of the dose of phenylephrine required to produce a 20 mm Hg increase in mean arterial pressure (PD_{20}) in young (Y) and elderly (E) subjects. The responsiveness of vascular adrenoreceptors appears reduced in the elderly because greater drug doses are required to produce the same effect as that produced by smaller doses in younger subjects. (Reprinted with permission of Raven Press, New York. Elliott HL, Sumner DJ, McLean K et al: Effect of age on the responsiveness of vascular alpha-adrenoceptors in man. J Cardiovasc Pharmacol 4:388, 1982.)

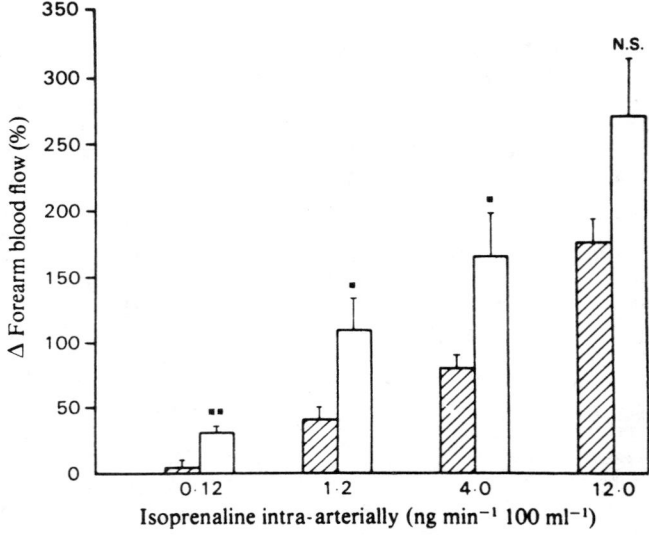

FIG. 48-20. Mean increase in forearm blood flow after intraarterial infusion of isoprenaline in young subjects (▢) *versus* old (▨) subjects. *$P < 0.05$. (Van Brummelen P, Buhler FR, Kiowski W et al: Age-related decrease in cardiac and peripheral vascular responsiveness to isoprenaline: Studies in normal subjects. Clin Sci 60:571, 1981. Copyright 1981 The Biochemical Society, London.)

patients also demonstrate a greater plasma renin response to the administration of beta-agonists.[52] Thus, there appears to be an age-related parallel reduction in cardiac, peripheral vascular, and renal beta-adrenoreceptor-mediated responses. All of these studies indicate a generalized diminution of adrenoreceptor sensitivity in elderly patients. An attractive hypothesis to explain the hemodynamic profiles of a decreased maximum heart rate, increased preload, and reduced ejection fraction at maximum effort, despite elevated levels of circulating catecholamines, is an age-associated decrease in end-organ response, similar to progressive, non-pharmacologically induced beta-adrenergic blockade.

Arrhythmias

The prevalence of cardiac dysrhythmias at rest, during normal routine activity, and during vigorous exercise has been shown to increase with age. With continuous ECG monitoring, isolated supraventricular and ventricular ectopic beats, usually less than 1 every hour, were found in 88 and 78% of elderly men and women, respectively.[58] Seventeen per cent of the subjects demonstrated more than 100 ventricular ectopic beats over a 24-h period, and supraventricular tachyarrhythmias were observed in 33% of subjects. The incidence of ventricular dysrhythmias in elderly patients is also greater than that observed in the young.[59] Other common ECG abnormalities in elderly patients include decreased T-wave amplitude and T-wave inversions, especially in leads I, aV_L, V_5, and V_6. First-degree heart block, left anterior hemiblock, and right bundle-branch block are also commonly seen.

In summary, it may be difficult to determine on an initial examination if an elderly patient has maintained his or her cardiac function during the aging process. To make this decision, a skilled anesthesiologist should try to determine if an elderly patient has age-related cardiac diseases or has allowed a sedentary lifestyle to interfere with the maintenance of long-term cardiovascular fitness. It is reassuring to know that a significant percentage of our population of elderly patients may have surprisingly well maintained cardiac function and will be able to compensate to meet demands of stressful situations, primarily by increasing end-diastolic volume. However, it is unnerving to realize that it is difficult to determine on superficial evaluation what sort of cardiac reserve the average elderly patient may have. More than half of elderly people have significant coronary artery disease, regardless of whether they have symptoms.

VENTILATORY SYSTEM

In general, aging is associated with reduced ventilatory volumes and decreased efficiency of gas exchange. From age 20 to age 70, total lung capacity is reduced by approximately 10%, in part as a consequence of narrowing of the intervertebral disk spaces with shortening of overall body height. Stiffening of cartilage and replacement of elastic tissue in the costal, intercostal, and intervertebral areas produces rigidity of the thoracic cage which impairs the bellows function of the lung. Progressive kyphosis or scoliosis produces upward and anterior rotation of the ribs and sternum, which leads to increased anteropostero chest diameter, further restricting chest expansion. The gradual loss of skeletal muscle mass with aging results in diaphragm and intercostal muscle wastage, further reducing an elderly person's ability to ventilate. All of these changes contribute to an age-related reduction in vital capacity, total lung capacity, and maximum breathing capacity (Figs. 48-14, 48-21, and 48-22).[61, 62]

As seen in Figure 48-21, at age 20 maximum voluntary ventilation is approximately $100\ l\cdot min^{-1}$ or 12–15 times that needed to meet basal metabolic needs. However, at age 80 maximum voluntary ventilation decreases to approximately 30–$40\ l\cdot min^{-1}$, representing a ventilatory reserve of approximately sevenfold. This is more than adequate to meet ventilatory needs for the average nonstressed healthy elderly person. However, if other age-related diseases or the effects on ventilation of anesthesia and surgery are superimposed on this pattern, ventilatory reserve may, in fact, be quite limited. For instance, following an emergency abdominal operation, a patient with pre-existent pulmonary infection and postoperative pain is predisposed to respiratory failure. Residual effects of anesthetic drugs and muscle relaxants may further reduce the patient's ventilatory capability. Similarly, a patient who is septic, with increased ventilatory requirements to meet the needs of an increased basal metabolic rate, who arrives in the recovery room hypothermic and shivering is

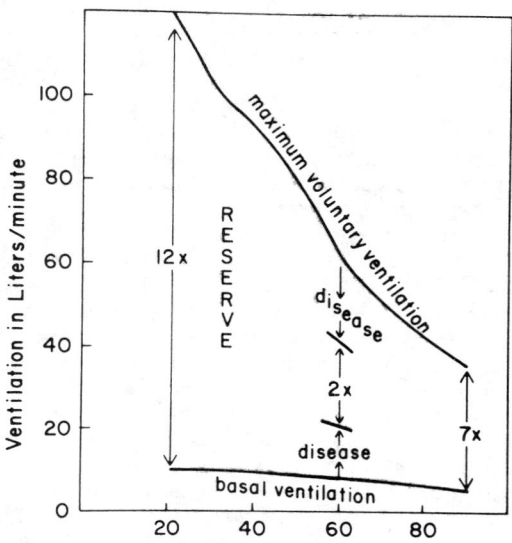

FIG. 48-21. Basal ventilation needs decrease with age primarily because of a reduction in basal metabolic rate. Maximum voluntary ventilation at age 20 is 12–15 times that needed to meet basal metabolic needs. During aging, with loss of elasticity of the chest cage and lung parenchyma, maximum voluntary ventilation declines steeply. Although a healthy elderly person has a ventilatory reserve of approximately sevenfold, this reserve is quickly eroded if disease processes reduce a person's ability to ventilate or increase ventilatory requirements to meet increased metabolic needs. As a result, elderly persons will more likely require postoperative ventilatory support compared with their younger counterparts. (Reprinted with permission. Smith TC: Respiratory effects of aging. Seminars in Anesthesia 5:14, 1986.)

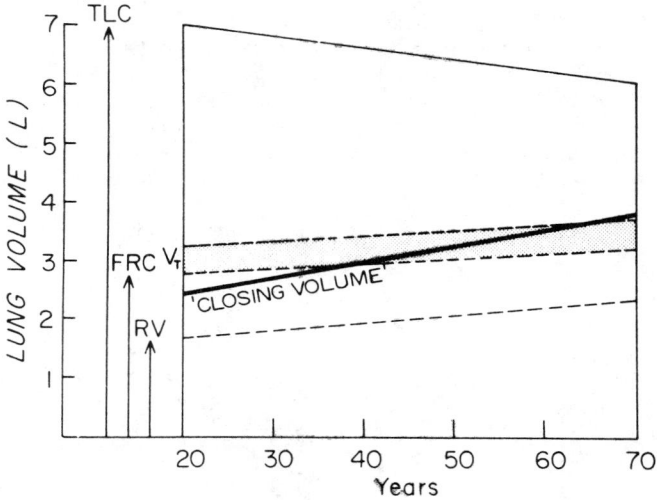

FIG. 48-22. A comparison of pulmonary capacities and volumes at different ages. Total lung capacity (TLC) decreases with age. The reduction in alveoli and alveolar septi reduce tethering of terminal bronchioles and result in an increase in closing volume with advancing age. As closing volume increases with age, greater portions of tidal ventilation occur at lung volumes below closing volume resulting in air trapping, V/Q mismatch, and an associated decrease in resting Pa_{O_2}. (Reprinted with permission. Pontoppidan H, Geffins B, Lowenstein A: Acute respiratory failure in the adult. N Engl J Med 287:690, 1972.)

also at risk for ventilatory failure. Therefore, it is easy to understand why elderly patients with reasonably adequate ventilatory reserve under normal preoperative conditions may have inadequate pulmonary reserves after operation. Not surprisingly, therefore, elderly patients will more commonly require ventilatory support after operation until their metabolic needs are reduced and their ability to ventilate returns toward preoperative levels.

Age-induced parenchymal changes of the lung mimic those of emphysema.[63] With aging, the pores of Kohn enlarge and coalesce into fenestrae, alveolar septi are lost, and alveolar spaces expand, producing decreased alveolar surface area and diminished pulmonary capillary bed density.[62] The progressive diminution in functional alveoli with age reduces elastic recoil of the lung, resulting in an increase in the ratio of residual volume to total lung capacity and the ratio of functional residual capacity to total lung capacity. In addition, because alveolar septi produce radial traction or tethering of the terminal bronchioles, a reduction in their quantity during aging makes the support framework for the terminal bronchioles less stable in geriatric patients. Thus, small airways will collapse at greater and greater lung volumes, producing an age-related increase in the "closing volume" of the lung (Fig. 48-22).[62] As closing volume increases with age, greater portions of tidal ventilation occur at lung volumes below closing volume, thus producing air trapping and ventilation perfusion ratio (V/Q) mismatch. Other major contributors to the decline in gas exchange efficiency during aging include the reduced surface area of alveoli, increased alveolocapillary membrane thickness, reduced membrane permeability, and reduced pulmonary capillary blood volume. As a result, resting Pa_{O_2} normally declines with age at a rate described by the following equation:[64–66]

$$Pa_{O_2} = 100 - (0.4 \times age\ [yr])\ mm\ Hg \qquad (48-2)$$

The normal decline in Pa_{O_2} with age is described by the "pre-op" line in Figure 48-23.[65] For the reasons described above, patients of all ages demonstrate a lower Pa_{O_2} value after operation compared with preoperative levels. As shown in Figure 48-23, this difference becomes more exaggerated as people age. The problem is particularly evident after upper abdominal and thoracic operations, in which there is significant postoperative splinting, causing an exaggeration in V/Q

mismatch and dramatic decreases in Pa_{O_2} after operation.[65] A change in position from sitting to supine will cause a 10 mm Hg decline in Pa_{O_2} because of a reduced functional residual capacity and increased V/Q mismatch. The assumption of a supine posture after operation may partially explain the reduced P_{O_2} values observed in elderly patients after operation. In addition, the response to hypoxia or hypercapnia in healthy geriatric patients is approximately half that seen in younger persons.[68] This is further impaired by opioid premedication and by anesthetic drugs in a dose-related fashion.[69]

For all of these reasons, elderly patients must be observed more closely after operation because their protective mechanisms against hypoxia and hypercapnia are less effective than those of younger patients. Elderly patients may require higher inspired intraoperative concentrations of oxygen because of their lower resting Pa_{O_2} values and reduced efficiency of ventilatory exchange. Supplemental inspired oxygen should be considered for as long as 24 h after operation or until adequate oxygenation is assured while the patient is breathing room air.

CENTRAL NERVOUS SYSTEM

Classically, it has been thought that the physiologic function of most organs, including the central nervous system (CNS), undergoes a gradual decline during the aging process. Cross-sectional comparisons between age groups have shown significantly lower scores in many cognitive capacities for older age groups, commonly interpreted as reflecting a decline in CNS performance with advancing age. However, in a separate longitudinal study in which the same subjects were tested after 7 yr of aging, no age-related decline in cerebral function was determined. It now appears likely that a decline in mental function with age, should it occur, may be related more to nutritional or educational differences that occur as people age, rather than as a result of the aging process itself. Much of the loss of cognitive function in later life that has been considered intrinsic to aging may, in fact, be caused by extrinsic factors and therefore may be preventable with better nutrition and stimulation of mental function in the elderly population.[70]

On the other hand, age-related CNS disease is not uncom-

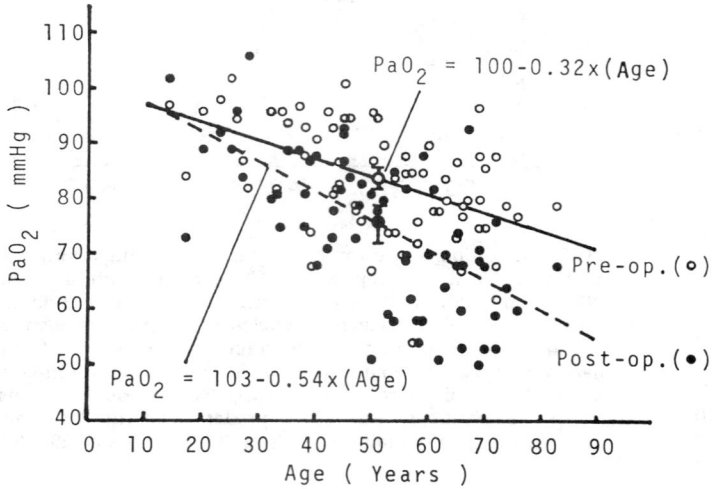

FIG. 48-23. Relationship between Pa_{O_2} and age during room air breathing. (Reprinted with permission. Kitamura H, Sawa T, Ikezono E: Postoperative hypoxemia: The contribution of age to the maldistribution of ventilation. Anesthesiology 36:244, 1972.)

mon in elderly patients. Dementia may result from localized areas of microemboli or from organic brain syndrome (a neuropsychiatric disorder associated with impaired brain tissue function). A common variety of this, Alzheimer's disease, is associated with cerebral atherosclerosis, which results in a gradual reduction of cerebral blood flow and CNS activity.

Although the presence of an obligatory age-induced decline in cerebral cognitive function remains controversial, it is generally agreed that geriatric patients have a reduced requirement for anesthetic agents. This may not be distinguishable in any given patient, but it is observed in cross-sectional studies comparing elderly patients with younger people and is believed to result, at least in part, from a reduction in preexistent CNS activity. Muravchick suggests that we think of anesthetic requirement as resistance to loss of consciousness and that elderly people may have a reduced anesthetic requirement because of a decrement in this resistance.[71] An example of reduced CNS activity in the elderly is the age-dependent reduced sensitivity to painful stimuli (e.g., electrical stimulation).[72] A corollary to this is reported in a double-blind study of 712 patients in which the magnitude of pain relief after administration of either 10 mg morphine or 20 mg pentazocine correlated with age.[73]

Evidence of an age-related reduced anesthetic requirement is the reduced minimum alveolar concentration (MAC) necessary to produce anesthesia in elderly patients with cyclopropane, halothane, or isoflurane.[74-76] The requirement for these inhalational agents decreases linearly with patient age. Munson et al reported that the requirements for all three agents closely parallel each other when age comparisons are made (Fig. 48-24).[76]

The reduced anesthetic requirement for geriatric patients applies not only to inhalation anesthetics, but also to local anesthetics, opioids, barbiturates, benzodiazapines, and other intravenous anesthetic agents. Elderly patients achieve

FIG. 48-24. The relationship between anesthetic requirement (MAC) and age. MAC values are noted for persons of different ages receiving either isoflurane, halothane, or cyclopropane. The parallelism of the three slopes indicates similar age-related effects on anesthetic requirements for all three inhalational agents. (Reprinted with permission of the International Anesthesia Research Society. Munson ES, Hoffman JC, Eger EI: Use of cyclopropane to test generality of anesthetic requirement in the elderly. Anesth Analg 63:998, 1984.)

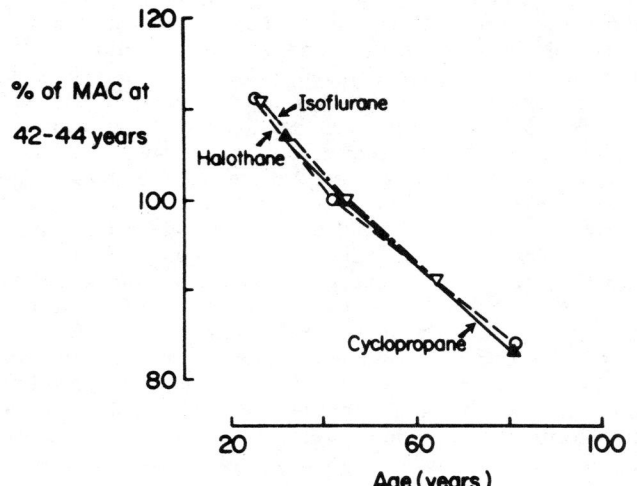

a comparable level of sedation at diazepam plasma concentrations significantly lower than those required in young adults. Equivalent EEG suppression occurs at lower plasma concentrations of both fentanyl and alfentanil in elderly patients.[77] As with opioids, the induction dose of barbiturates required in 70-yr-old adults is approximately 30% less than that required for patients 4–5 decades younger. Arden et al found that the dose of etomidate required to reach a uniform EEG end-point, indicative of anesthesia, decreased significantly with patients of increased age.[78] However, for the barbiturates and etomidate, it has been suggested that elderly patients' increased sensitivity to the drugs may relate more to differences in pharmacokinetics than to pharmacodynamics. For example, Christensen et al found that, in elderly patients, thiopental left the central compartment and entered the peripheral compartment at a slower rate.[79] This might allow the blood brain barrier to be exposed to a greater concentration of drug for a longer period of time, thus permitting greater drug availability at receptor sites in the brain, producing enhanced pharmacologic action. Homer and Stanski, using the "spectral edge" determination of EEG frequencies as a measure of anesthetic depth, found that the serum concentration of thiopental required to induce anesthesia in elderly patients was no different from that of younger patients.[80] They explained elderly patients' greater sensitivity to a given dose of thiopental on the basis of a reduced volume of distribution, resulting in a higher plasma concentration. Similarly, for etomidate, a comparison of plasma concentrations of the drug to depth of anesthesia, as measured by EEG, demonstrated no increased brain sensitivity in the elderly when contrasted to the young. Rather, a greater response in elderly patients to a given dose of etomidate was explained by a decreased volume of distribution for this drug.[78]

Elderly patients may also demonstrate greater sensitivity to drugs on the basis of pharmacodynamic factors associated with aging. The CNS and peripheral nervous system undergo progressive anatomic and functional changes during the aging process that may influence the dose–response relationship to anesthetic agents. Multiple observations have been proposed to explain the enhanced responsiveness of elderly patients to anesthetic drugs.

First, there is a continual loss of neuronal substance with advancing age. On average, a daily attrition of perhaps as many as 50,000 neurons from an initial neuron pool of approximately 10,000,000,000 occurs during a person's life span. Cortical regions of the brain representing the peak of evolutionary development and those subcortical regions responsible for synthesis of neurotransmitters appear to have the most severe degree of age-related loss.[70, 81] The gray matter fraction of human brain decreases from 45 to 35% of total brain weight during the time span between the ages of 20 to 80 yrs, and neuronal density of the occipital cortex decreases 48% during this time period.[82, 83] By the time people reach age 80, brain weight has declined at least 15% from its maximal value of approximately 1,400 g achieved at age 30, to a weight of between 1,100 and 1,200 g. Sapolsky et al reported a similar loss of neurons in the hippocampus of rats, a loss they believe eventually results in functional impairments typical of senescence.[84] Interestingly, their study revealed that exposure to corticosteroids accelerated the process of neuronal loss. They therefore concluded that age-related loss of neurons, resulting in an acceleration of the process of senescence, is exaggerated by stress or exposure to chronically elevated levels of corticosteroids. The reduction in neuronal density that occurs with age is accompanied by a parallel reduction in cerebral blood flow and cerebral oxygen consumption ($CMRO_2$) (Fig. 48-25).[85-87] Regional cerebral blood flow remains as tightly coupled to cerebral metabolic activity in the healthy elderly person as it does in young adults. The absence of a quantitative relationship between age-related brain atrophy (accompanied by reduced cerebral blood flow) and general level of mental function, however, suggests that at the time of maximum brain weight, there is considerable redundancy of neuronal function within each cortical, subcortical, and spinal region.

Peripherally, in nerve axons there is a loss of myelin, a reduction in the number of axons and synapses, and a diminished number of fibers in each tract. The reduction in axonal population may explain the decrease in nerve conduction velocity reported with increased age.[88] This, in turn, may be partially responsible for decreased function of feedback mechanisms that control hormone and enzyme release in response to various stimuli and also reduced baroreflex capability in elderly patients.

A second and closely related explanation for the greater sensitivity of elderly patients to anesthetics is a reduced number of receptor sites or a decrease in receptor affinity for hormones and drugs in the brain. For example, the pharmacologic characteristics of the autonomic nervous system are altered, necessitating increased plasma norepinephrine levels in elderly patients to produce the same effects as lower levels in younger patients.[89] Beta-receptor density has also been observed to decrease in the cerebrum and cerebellum of rats and humans. The reduced sensitivity of the elderly to beta-adrenergic agents has been suggested to result from a functional alteration in beta-receptor affinity or uncoupling of the beta-receptor–adenylate cyclase system.[51] These age-related observations in the CNS parallel the changes in the cardiovascular system of the elderly that have been mentioned previously (see Cardiovascular System).

A third theory proposed for the reduced anesthetic requirements of the elderly involves the rate of synthesis of neurotransmitters. A progressive and significant decrease in the concentration of enzymes that synthesize neurotransmitters is consistently seen in aging neural tissues.[90] Corresponding reductions in brain levels of neurotransmitters have been observed. In a primate model, Gibson and Peterson noted that acetylcholine synthesis in elderly animals is 60% of that seen in young animals.[91] Reduced brain levels of dopamine, norepinephrine, tyrosine, and serotonin have also been observed.[92]

Although the exact explanation for why elderly people may be more sensitive to anesthetics remains unclear, the observation of their greater sensitivity to most agents is not in doubt. The anatomic and functional changes occurring in the CNS with aging that result in a reduced anesthetic requirement may also increase patients' risk for postoperative deterioration of mental function. This may be an issue of equal or even greater importance affecting the quality of an elderly patient's perioperative experience and will be discussed more fully in the section Regional Anesthesia *Versus* General Anesthesia.

CHANGE IN BODY COMPARTMENTS

Important age-related changes in body composition include a loss of skeletal muscle (lean body mass), an increase in percentage of body fat, and intracellular dehydration (Fig. 48-26).[71] The gradual decline in intracellular water content with aging simultaneously occurs with a comparable and slightly greater increase in percentage of body fat (Fig. 48-27).[7] These changes are more exaggerated in women. The reduction in total body water primarily represents intracellular dehydration and a reduction of blood volume. It has been suggested that a 20–30% reduction in blood volume occurs by age 75 (see Standard Cell Water, Fig. 48-14). Therefore, injection of anesthetic drugs will initially be dispersed in a contracted blood volume in the elderly patient, producing a higher-than-expected initial plasma drug concentration (Fig. 48-28).

There is an approximate 10% decline in skeletal muscle mass (lean body mass) with aging. The average loss of muscle mass with age is estimated to be 6 kg at age 80, with more dramatic changes observed in women. Therefore, one might predict that the requirement for muscle relaxants would also be reduced and a smaller initial dose might be required. However, in a variety of experimental studies, this has not been found to be the case. It has been proposed that, although there are reduced numbers of skeletal muscles available, there is similarly a reduced number of muscle receptors present to bind with exogenous muscle relaxants, which, on the whole, makes elderly patients' sensitivity to muscle relaxants no different from that of younger patients. There are pharmacokinetic changes that affect the elimination of muscle relaxants, suggesting that the total dose of muscle relaxants should be reduced, but the initial sensitivity of elderly patients to muscle relaxants seems to be no different from that of a younger patient population.

The increase in percentage of body fat that occurs with age results in an increased availability of lipid-storage sites and a greater reservoir for deposition of lipid-soluble anesthetic drugs (Fig. 48-27). The sequestration of anesthetics in lipid tissues of the elderly slows the elimination of drugs, results in greater residual plasma concentrations of drug, and prolongs anesthetic effects. The retention of anesthetics in lipid also increases the possibility that they will be subject to biotransformation. For this reason, anesthetics that undergo minimal metabolism have theoretic advantages for geriatric patients.

FIG. 48-25. Cerebral blood flow (CBF), cerebral metabolic rate of oxygen consumption ($CMRO_2$), and cortical neuron density expressed as percentage of control values at age 25 yr. (Reprinted with permission. Hilgenberg JC: Inhalation and intravenous drugs in the elderly patient. Seminars in Anesthesia 5:44, 1986.)

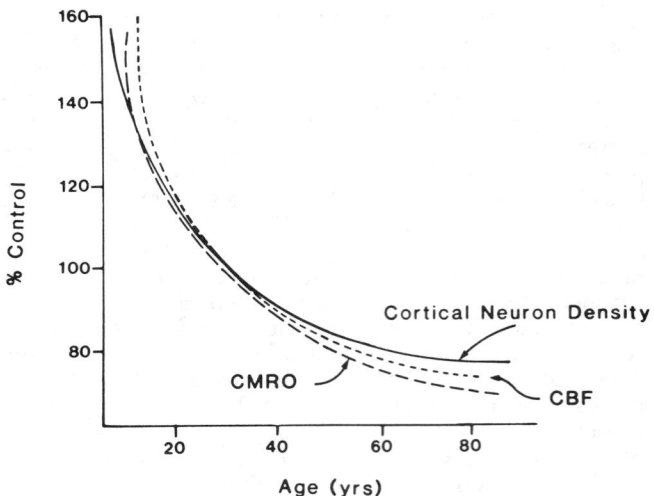

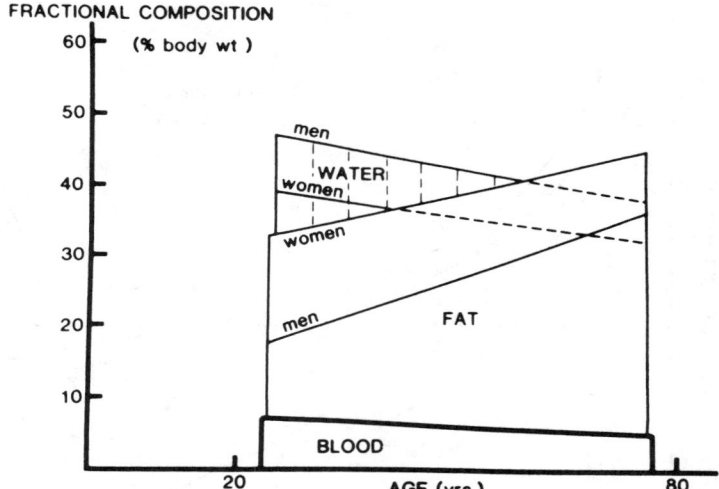

FIG. 48-26. Change in fractional body composition with age. (Reprinted with permission. Muravchick S: Current concepts: Anesthetic pharmacology in geriatric patients. Progress in Anesthesiology I:2, 1987.)

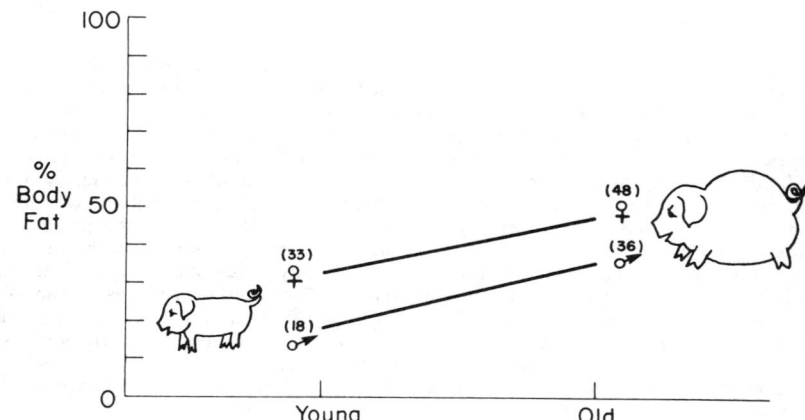

FIG. 48-27. Age-related changes in percentage body fat in nonobese subjects. At all ages, women tend to have a higher percentage body fat than do men. The percentage of body weight that is fat increases with age. (Reprinted with permission. McLeskey CH: Anesthesia for the geriatric patient. In Stoelting RK, Barash PG, Gallagher TJ [eds]: Advances in Anesthesia, p 31. Chicago, Year Book Medical Publishers, 1985.)

PROTEIN BINDING

All anesthetic agents are bound to plasma proteins to some extent. Not all drugs or classes of drugs are equally bound. For instance, of the opioids, fentanyl is 80% protein bound, whereas morphine and meperidine are only 30–40% bound. In contrast, alfentanil and sufentanil are approximately 90% protein bound. The portion of the drug that is bound to protein is unable to cross membranes, including the blood brain barrier, and to produce an effect. The binding between drugs and plasma proteins is reversible and produced by ionic, hydrogen, or van der Waals bonds.

Protein binding of anesthetic drugs is reduced in the elderly. As illustrated in Figure 48-28, a theoretic, highly lipid-soluble drug (that can cross the blood brain barrier readily and be measured in cerebrospinal fluid [CSF]) has been administered in the same intravenous bolus dose to a typical elderly person and a typical young adult. As discussed in the section Change in Body Compartments, the smaller initial volume of distribution of elderly patients results in a higher initial plasma concentration. Also, because protein binding of anesthetic drugs is less in elderly patients, the CSF or brain concentration more closely approaches the plasma concen-

tration. Thus, for a given plasma concentration, one would predict a higher CSF or brain level of anesthetic in elderly patients and a more profound anesthetic effect. The reduced protein binding of anesthetic drugs by elderly patients not only affects the distribution of those drugs but also their elimination. For the period of time a drug is bound to plasma protein, it is not available for metabolism or excretion. Thus, a decrease in binding of anesthetics to plasma proteins with aging should make more drug available for elimination and would have a minor effect in enhancing drug clearance.

Four factors may explain the reduced drug binding to serum protein in elderly patients. First, with aging, the circulating level of serum protein, especially albumin, decreases in quantity, reducing available protein binding sites. Second, qualitative changes may occur in circulating protein, which reduce the binding effectiveness of the available protein. Third, coadministered drugs may interfere with the ability of anesthetic drugs to bind to available serum protein–binding sites. Fourth, certain disease states may inhibit plasma protein binding of anesthetic drugs.

As mentioned above, during the aging process the circulating level of serum protein, especially albumin, and the binding effectiveness of those proteins are gradually re-

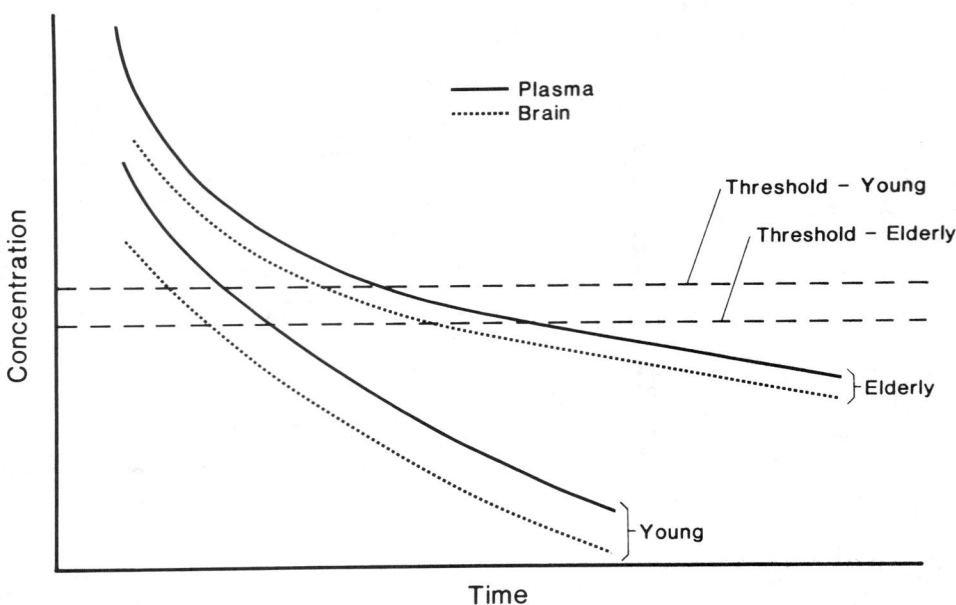

FIG. 48-28. Pharmacokinetic and pharmacodynamic differences resulting from age-related physiologic changes. The curves represent the theoretic processes occurring in a typical young *versus* elderly patient after receiving an identical intravenous bolus dose of an anesthetic. Elderly persons will, in general, have a higher initial plasma concentration because of a contracted intravascular volume decreasing the initial volume of distribution of injected drugs. Elderly persons will also, in general, have brain concentrations more closely approaching plasma concentrations because of less effective protein binding. The enhanced protein binding of anesthetic drugs in younger persons keeps more of the drug in the plasma, making it unavailable for transfer across the blood–brain barrier, and results in a lower brain concentration for a given plasma concentration. It is believed for many drugs, such as opioids, that a reduced plasma concentration and, in turn, a reduced brain concentration produces the same CNS effect in the elderly patient as that resulting from higher plasma and brain concentrations in the young. This is represented as a reduced "threshold" concentration in elderly persons. The end result of all these changes is that, for the same dose of a drug administered to an elderly person, a more profound and more prolonged drug effect may be expected compared with that of young patients.

duced. Most drugs are bound to serum albumin, although other plasma proteins and erythrocytes contribute protein binding sites to a lesser degree. Although at one time controversial, it is now well documented that the concentration of plasma albumin gradually declines during the aging process. For instance, in subjects younger than 50 yr of age, the average plasma albumin concentration is $4.0 \text{ g} \cdot \text{dl}^{-1}$, whereas in subjects older than 50 yr of age, the albumin concentration is reduced to only $3.4 \text{ g} \cdot \text{dl}^{-1}$.[93] In a study by Wallace *et al*,[94] young patients had an albumin concentration of $4.2 \text{ g} \cdot \text{dl}^{-1}$, which reduced to $3.6 \text{ g} \cdot \text{dl}^{-1}$ in healthy older patients. In a large, tightly controlled study, Greenblatt demonstrated a gradual decrease in plasma albumin concentration from approximately $4.0 \text{ g} \cdot \text{dl}^{-1}$ in patients younger than 40 yr of age to approximately $3.6 \text{ g} \cdot \text{dl}^{-1}$ in patients 80 yr of age or older.[95]

With the age-related quantitative decline in serum protein concentration, is there a simultaneous decrement in qualitative binding characteristics? Many authors believe that age is not associated with a major qualitative defect in the binding capacity of serum proteins.[93] In most studies in which there has been a reduced qualitative binding of drugs observed during aging, there has also been a simultaneous, parallel decrease in plasma albumin concentration, which explains the bulk of the observed decrement in protein binding.[96] A notable exception to this was observed for etomidate, where a qualitative difference in its binding by serum albumin exists

between young adults and elderly patients. Old patients were observed to bind 4.1 mol of etomidate/mmol of albumin, whereas young patients bound almost 4.5 mol of etomidate/mmol of albumin, a decrease in the affinity constant for binding of etomidate to plasma protein in elderly patients.[97]

Although acid drugs are bound primarily to albumin, basic drugs may be preferentially bound to a different protein, alpha-1 acid glycoprotein, which increases in concentration with age.[98] Basic drugs, such as lidocaine and propanolol, are thus increasingly bound and less available in free form in the plasma of elderly patients. On the other hand, most acid drugs, such as meperidine, thiopental, and diazepam, are bound to albumin and less highly protein bound on average in the elderly patient.[99]

The presence of one or more exogenous drugs decreases the protein binding of salicylates, sulfadiazine, and phenylbutazone.[94] Elderly patients consume more drugs than do younger patients and therefore may be more susceptible to this type of drug–drug interaction.

Because the incidence of concomitant diseases significantly increases in the elderly patient population (see Effects of Concomitant Disease), the effect of these diseases on plasma protein binding should be considered. For example, Andreason demonstrated that the reduced protein binding of many drugs to the plasma proteins of patients with acute renal failure was explained only partially by the reduced albumin concentration present.[100] He suggested that renal failure caused a structural change in plasma protein or resulted in an accumulation of bound substances to the protein, either of which would interfere with the qualitative effectiveness of albumin for drug binding.[101] Uremic patients generally have less effective binding of acidic drugs, whereas patients with hypoproteinemia resulting from any cause will demonstrate reduced binding of both acidic and basic drugs.[102, 103]

To summarize, because elderly patients have reduced quantities of circulating protein, may have qualitative defects in the binding capacity of their circulating proteins, are susceptible to drug interactions because of increased drug consumption, and may have an increased incidence of age-related pathologic conditions, an exaggerated clinical effect may be expected when drugs are administered that are highly protein bound. As an example, consider a theoretic drug that is 98% protein bound in a young healthy patient. Let us assume, because of the effects of aging on serum albumin, that protein binding decreases to 90% in an elderly patient. This seemingly minor 8% reduction in the amount of drug bound actually results in an increase in free drug availability from 2% to 10%, or a fivefold increased availability. Thus, an exaggerated clinical effect may be expected from anesthetics that are highly protein bound, if delivered to an elderly patient.

RENAL FUNCTION

As other organ functions deteriorate, the number of effective renal glomeruli decreases with age. The glomerular filtration rate is reduced about 1 ml·min^{-1}·yr^{-1}, or about 1–1.5% per year (Fig. 48-14).[104] In addition to reductions in glomerular function (filtration), tubular function (excretion) also shows a parallel decline during aging. As a result, renal clearance of drugs and their metabolites is adversely affected.

The decrease in glomerular filtration rate is far more dramatic than the modest age-associated loss of renal tissue mass (Fig. 48-29), suggesting that reduced renal plasma flow may be the primary explanation for loss of renal function with age.[105] The reduced renal plasma flow associated with increased age may result from an overall age-associated decrease in cardiac output or, more importantly, from a reduction in the magnitude of the renal vascular bed. There is a disproportionately large loss of cortical renal tissue mass (glomeruli) with aging.

Creatinine, a normal metabolic byproduct of muscle creatine, is excreted less efficiently in elderly patients, measured as a decrease in creatinine clearance rate (Table 48-8).[106] However, healthy geriatric patients will have approximately the same circulating level of serum creatinine as do younger patients because there is less skeletal muscle and less creatinine production.[25] Measurement of serum creatinine levels in an attempt to determine renal function is therefore inaccurate; clearance of creatinine or another substance is a more appropriate test for accurately assessing renal function. Elevated serum creatinine levels in an elderly patient imply a decrement in renal function even greater than that normally observed with aging. The reduced capacity for renal clearance in elderly people also affects their ability to clear some anesthetic drugs and may contribute to a longer duration of action of these drugs.

There is sufficient residual renal function to prevent gross uremia, but renal functional reserve needed to withstand gross water or electrolyte imbalance is minimal in elderly patients. In addition, alterations in renal blood flow produced by dehydration, congestive heart failure, or excess

FIG. 48-29. Age-related loss of organ mass and organ blood flow for the liver, kidneys, and brain. Reduction in hepatic metabolism with age results from loss of hepatic tissue and from reduced hepatic blood flow. (Reprinted with permission. Muravchick S: The aging patient and age related disease. ASA Annual Refresher Course Lecture 151, 1987.)

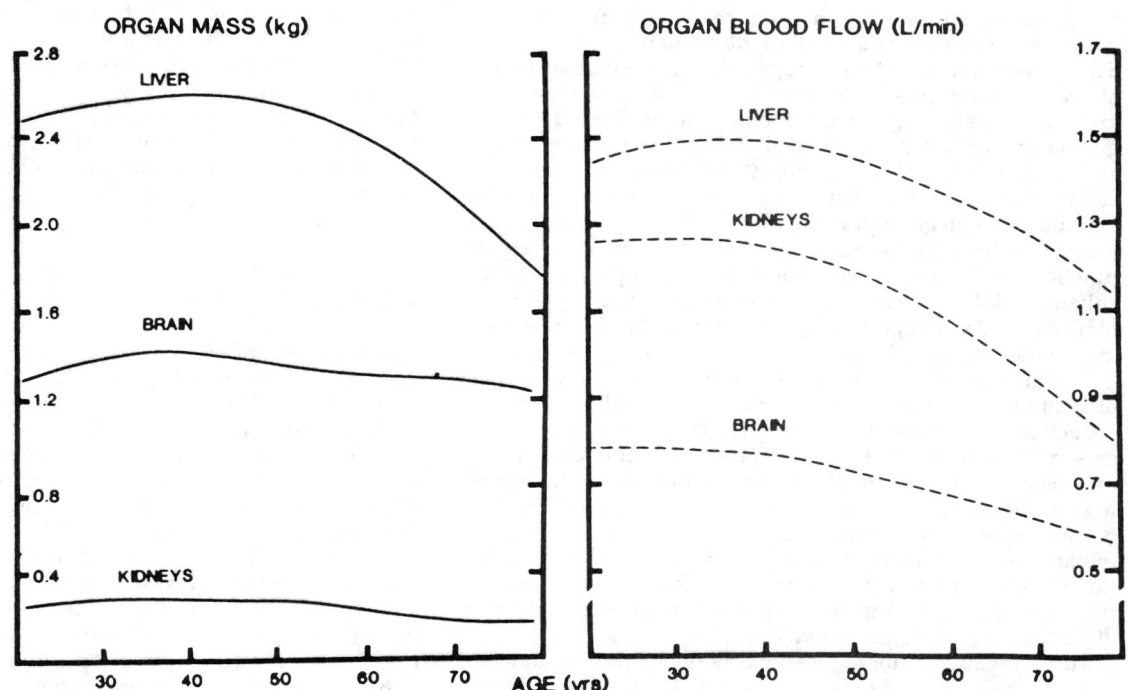

TABLE 48-8.   Creatinine Clearance as a Function of Age

AGE (yr)	CREATININE CLEARANCE (ml·min⁻¹·1.73 m⁻²)	
	Men	Women
20	120	110
30	113	104
40	107	98
50	193	93
60	87	87
70	80	81
80		76

(Hicks R, Dysken MW, Davis JM *et al*: The pharmacokinetics of psychotropic medication in the elderly: A review. J Clin Psychiatry 42:374, 1981.)

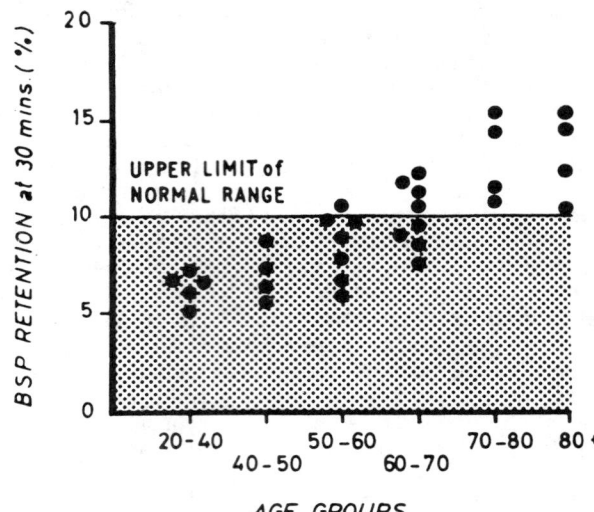

FIG. 48-30. Percentage of administered bromsulphalein (BSP) retained after 30 min in patients of different ages. Increased BSP retention indicates reduced hepatic ability to clear this material and indicates a decline in hepatic function in patients older than age 50. (Reprinted with permission. Thompson EN, Williams R: Effect of age on liver function with particular reference to bromosulphalein excretion. Gut 6:266, 1965.)

sodium or water loads can easily lead to renal failure. Acute renal failure is responsible for a very high percentage of perioperative mortality seen in elderly surgical patients. The best way to protect the kidney during operation is to monitor and maintain urine output at a level of at least 0.5 ml·kg⁻¹·h⁻¹. It is interesting that, because of the reduced renal blood flow of aging, the renal threshold for serum glucose that results in glycosuria is also elevated in elderly patients. Two factors determine if glucose will spill from plasma to urine: the plasma glucose concentration and the amount of renal blood flow. In situations in which there is a reduced renal blood flow (such as that which occurs with aging), a higher plasma glucose concentration is required to reach the renal threshold, which will result in glycosuria. As a result, glycosuria, when present in an elderly patient, implies a far higher blood glucose concentration than that of younger glycosuric patients.

HEPATIC FUNCTION

Lipid-soluble anesthetics filtered by the glomerulus are readily reabsorbed by the renal tubules and not excreted. The liver converts lipid-soluble drugs into water-soluble metabolites by many processes, including conjugation and oxidation. A water-soluble metabolite that is filtered by the glomerulus will be minimally reabsorbed through the tubules and, as a result, will be significantly excreted. Although results of standard liver function tests, notably serum bilirubin, albumin, and alkaline phosphatase levels, may be normal in geriatric patients, other tests reveal the decrement in hepatic function that parallels age. For example, impaired bromosulfaline (BSP) excretion may first be observed in patients older than 50 yr of age and become progressively worse with increasing age (Fig. 48-30).[107]

The most likely explanation for reduced hepatic clearance of a variety of substances in elderly patients is the significant reduction in hepatic size that occurs with the aging process.[12, 105] As shown in Figure 48-29, 40–50% of hepatic tissue may be lost by the age of 80, with a proportional reduction in hepatic blood flow. Hepatic blood flow is particularly important when considering drugs with extensive first pass metabolism, such as propranolol. Compared with young patients, the elderly have been observed to have fivefold greater plasma levels of propranolol despite a lack of clinical evidence of hepatic, renal, or cardiac disease.[108]

Microsomal and nonmicrosomal hepatic enzyme concentration or function appear to be maintained with aging. How-

ever, there are isolated reports that microsomal enzyme activity is reduced.[109] Age-related decreases in hepatic microsomal mixed function oxidase enzymes, especially cytochrome P450, have been observed in aging rats.[110] These enzymes stimulate metabolism of toxic or potentially toxic substances to which all of us are exposed. The age-associated changes in this enzyme system may be partially responsible for the age-related increase in the incidence of tumors and deaths from cancer in our society.[111]

The effect of an age-associated reduction of hepatic blood flow and a potential reduction in microsomal enzyme function impairs the liver's ability to metabolize anesthetics and nondepolarizing muscle relaxants. This, combined with the reduced filtration and excretory capability of the aging kidney, results in a more gradual decline in plasma concentration of drugs used in anesthesia in elderly patients (a prolonged beta elimination half-life) and contributes to a longer duration of effect (Fig. 48-28).

BASAL METABOLIC RATE AND THERMOREGULATION

As seen in Figure 48-14, basal metabolic rate declines approximately 1% per year beyond age 30. Thus, drugs may be expected to be metabolized and excreted more slowly in elderly patients. In addition, the incidence of intraoperative hypothermia is explained at least in part by the decrease in metabolic rate with aging. Goldberg and Roe, in a study of 101 adult surgical patients, have shown that the difficulty in maintaining normothermia during general anesthesia is age related.[112] Elderly patients had a greater decrease in rectal temperature than did young patients, even during short and relatively minor surgical procedures (Fig. 48-31). Not surprisingly, the development of intraoperative hypothermia also correlated with the length of operation. The ability of young patients to maintain intraoperative body temperature has

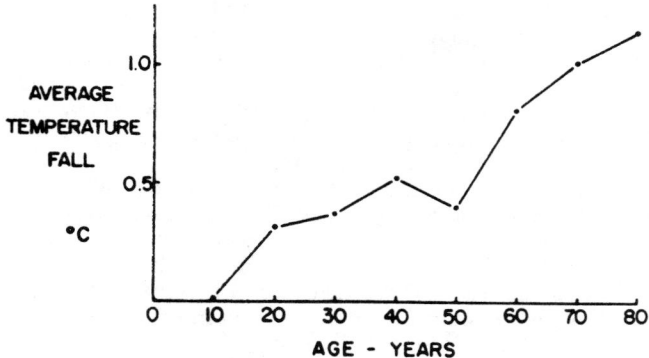

FIG. 48-31. The relationship between patient age and intraoperative decline in rectal temperature. (Reprinted with permission. Goldberg MJ, Roe F: Temperature changes during anesthesia and operations. Arch Surg 93:365, 1966. Copyright 1966, American Medical Association.)

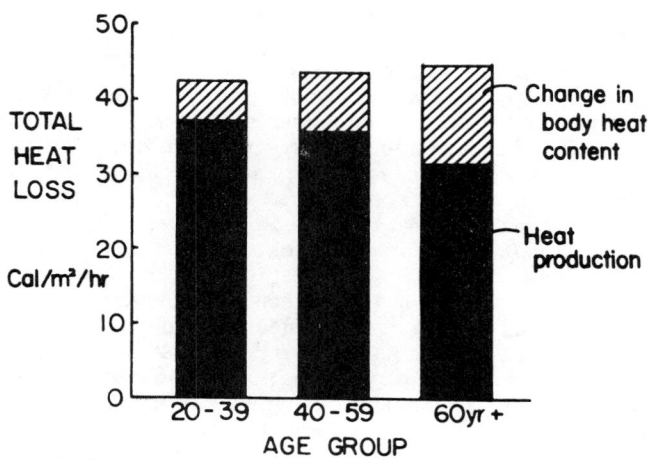

FIG. 48-32. Intraoperative heat loss per unit time is slightly greater in older subjects. This is explained by a reduced basal heat production (*solid bars*), primarily resulting from a reduced basal metabolic rate in the elderly, and a greater change in body heat content (*hatched bars*) as a result of lesser ability to vasoconstrict when placed in a cool environment (reduced autonomic neuronal function). When combined, these changes lead to a greater total intraoperative heat loss in elderly patients. (Reprinted with permission. Goldberg MJ, Roe F: Temperature changes during anesthesia and operations. Arch Surg 93:365, 1966. Copyright 1966, American Medical Association.)

been attributed, in part, to their higher basal metabolic rate and greater endogenous heat production (Fig. 48-32).

Elderly patients also experience more intraoperative hypothermia because of an impaired thermoregulatory system, which includes decreased heat production (as discussed above); increased heat loss; and deficient thermostat control. Heat loss is common in all patients during general anesthesia because anesthetics alter thermoregulation, prevent shivering, and produce peripheral vasodilation. Healthy younger persons, exposed to a cold environment, reduce their heat loss to the environment by intense cutaneous vasoconstriction. The reduced autonomic peripheral vascular control of the elderly may lessen the effectiveness of this protective ability during anesthesia.

Thus, because of elderly patients' impaired heat production and reduced ability to thermoregulate, it is not surprising that Vaughn *et al* have shown that patients older than 60 yr of age are admitted to and discharged from the postanesthesia care unit (PACU) with a lower measured body temperature compared with that of younger patients (Fig. 48-33).[114] The lower temperatures in elderly patients on discharge from the PACU relate to the fact that there is no

difference in the rate of temperature rise in older compared with younger patients. Older subjects thus demonstrated a longer duration of hypothermia in the PACU than that seen in young patients.

Several adverse effects can result from hypothermia. The first problem is shivering.[114, 115] Postoperative shivering may represent a particular risk to the elderly patient because it significantly increases basal metabolic rate. Oxygen consumption must increase, perhaps as much as 400–500%, which increases demands on the cardiac and pulmonary systems.[116, 117] In the elderly patient, if either system cannot adequately compensate for the increased demand produced by shivering, arterial hypoxemia may result. In addition, shiv-

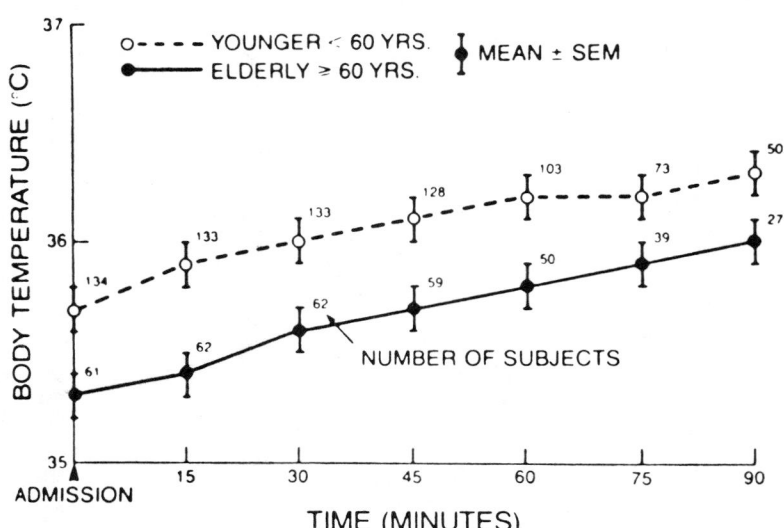

FIG. 48-33. Tympanic membrane temperature in 198 patients measured at time of admission to the PACU and at 15-min intervals thereafter. (Reprinted with permission of the International Anesthesia Research Society. Vaughn MS, Vaughn RW, Cork RC: Postoperative hypothermia in adults: Relationship of age, anesthesia and shivering to rewarming. Anesth Analg 60:746, 1981.)

ering may cause myocardial ischemia in geriatric patients (who frequently have occult coronary artery disease) because of the requirement for an increased cardiac output in the presence of peripheral vasoconstriction. It is fortunate to some extent that hypothermic patients between the ages of 60 and 80 yr cannot increase their oxygen demands to the same degree by shivering as do younger patients.[116] However, this increases the time period required for elderly patients to return to normothermia. Protracted postoperative hypothermia will also reduce elimination of anesthetics and prolong awakening.

Another and longer-lasting adverse effect of intraoperative hypothermia has been demonstrated by Carli et al.[118] In this study, urinary protein loss during the first 48 h after operation was determined to quantitate postoperative catabolism. Elderly patients in whom normothermia was maintained during the intraoperative period had only minimal protein catabolism after operation. However, a similar group of elderly patients having a similar anesthetic, but who were allowed to become hypothermic during operation, spilled significantly greater amounts of urinary nitrogen after operation, indicating dramatically larger degrees of postoperative catabolism.

It is important to concentrate on maintaining intraoperative body temperature in all patients, but it is especially crucial in geriatric patients. Methods to reduce temperature loss—such as warming intravenous fluids, administering humidified and warmed inspired gases, reducing radiation losses by providing adequate blankets, and maintaining a warm room temperature—obviously are beneficial.

AIRWAY REFLEXES

Laryngeal, pharyngeal, and airway reflexes are less effective in older patients.[119] Pontoppidan and Beecher have illustrated the gradual decline in protective airway reflexes that accompanies the aging process (Fig. 48-34). In their study, elderly patients had to inhale a much larger volume of an irritant gas, ammonia vapor, before airway protection was demonstrated. Thus, the blunting of laryngeal and airway reflexes in older patients makes these patients less able to protect their airways from foreign material and makes pulmonary aspiration more likely. A clinical corollary is that a patient who requires endotracheal intubation to facilitate surgical anesthesia should have tracheal extubation delayed during emergence until airway reflexes are as close to normal as possible.[120] Older patients also have fewer cilia in their tracheobronchial tree and are less able to mobilize secretions. Coughing is less efficient in terms of volume, force, and flow rate compared with that of younger patients. For all of these reasons, anesthesia and recovery room personnel must be very attentive to an elderly person's airway to reduce the likelihood of pulmonary aspiration.

ENDOCRINE SYSTEM

It has been known for more than 60 yr that advancing age is associated with progressive impairment in the capacity to metabolize a glucose load.[121] After patients with fasting hyperglycemia indicative of diabetes mellitus were excluded, elderly patients demonstrated an age-related increase in the 2-h postprandial blood glucose level after oral or intravenous glucose administration. The same glucose intolerance has been demonstrated in a study in which intravenous infusion of glucose at a rate of 4 $mg \cdot kg^{-1} \cdot min^{-1}$ produced a blood sugar level of approximately 200 $mg \cdot dl^{-1}$ in elderly patients, compared with 150 $mg \cdot dl^{-1}$ in young patients.[122]

It has been thought that pancreatic function declines during aging, explaining the increased incidence of glucose intolerance and diabetes mellitus that is observed in patients 60–70 yr of age. The variability of insulin responsiveness and glucose tolerance increases substantially in people in successive age groups. In elderly patients, insulin liberation is sluggish in response to hyperglycemia. However, resistance to the effect of insulin at peripheral sites appears to play the major role in the genesis of glucose intolerance among older people without diabetes.[123] As with other insulin-resistant states, aging is associated with progressive increases in postprandial insulin levels.[124] As observed in other organ systems, much of the carbohydrate intolerance of older people may be caused by factors other than biologic aging. It has therefore been suggested that dietary or exercise modifications may substantially blunt the emergence with age of carbohydrate intolerance and insulin resistance.[125]

The greater incidence of diabetes mellitus and glucose intolerance in geriatric patients necessitates the administration of exogenous insulin and limitation of glucose administration in many surgical patients. It is also necessary to measure intraoperative blood glucose levels frequently.

A variety of other endocrine changes occur during aging. For example, plasma renin concentration or activity is diminished 30–50% in elderly patients, which, in turn, results in a reduction in the plasma concentration of aldosterone. Alterations in the renin–aldosterone system contribute to an elderly person's increased risk of development of hyperkalemia in a variety of clinical settings, especially when potassium salts are administered intravenously. Van Brummelen et al have provided evidence of an age-related reduction in renin response to beta-adrenergic agents.[52] It is suggested that a less responsive beta-adrenoreceptor contributes to the decrease in plasma renin activity with age.

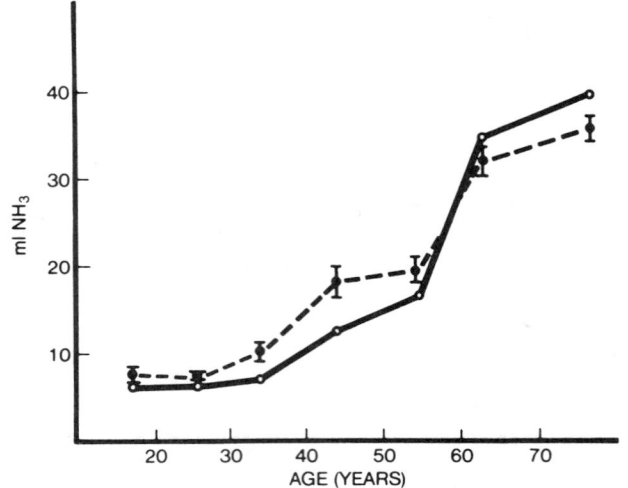

FIG. 48-34. The volume of inhaled ammonia vapor required to cause volunteers of varying ages to hold their breath. Required volumes increase after age 30, indicating an age-related gradual decline in protective airway reflexes. (Reprinted with permission. Pontoppidan H, Beecher HK: Progressive loss of protective reflexes in the airway with the advance of age. JAMA 174:2209, 1960. Copyright 1960, American Medical Association.)

PHARMACOKINETICS AND PHARMACODYNAMICS RELATIVE TO AGING

Pharmacokinetic variables determine the relationship between the dose of a drug administered and the concentration delivered at the site of action. Pharmacodynamic variables determine the relationship between the concentration of drug at the site of action and the intensity and duration of effect produced. Pharmacokinetics has been described as what the body does to the drug, whereas pharmacodynamics has been described as what the drug does to the body. As illustrated in Figure 48-35, pharmacokinetic factors include the physiologic processes of drug absorption (uptake), tissue distribution, metabolism (primarily hepatic), and elimination (primarily renal).[126] The physiologic results produced by a drug concentration at the effector site describe the patient's pharmacodynamic response to a given drug.

Aging significantly changes anesthetic drug distribution and elimination such that the elimination half-life ($T_{1/2}$ beta) for a drug may be significantly increased in an elderly patient. The primary factors affecting $T_{1/2}$ beta are the volume of distribution (V_D) and clearance (Cl), as described by the following equation:

$$T_{1/2} \text{ beta} = \frac{0.693 \times V_D}{Cl} \qquad (48\text{-}3)$$

Volume of distribution relates to protein binding and, for a lipid-soluble drug, to the percentage of body weight that is lipid. Because elderly patients have increased body fat, as shown in Figure 48-27, they have a larger volume of distribu-

tion for lipid-soluble anesthetics. This can delay emergence from anesthesia. As illustrated in Figure 48-36, volume of distribution can be viewed as a reservoir of drugs that is in equilibrium with the plasma. With a larger volume of distribution and greater drug sequestration, the plasma concentration of a lipid-soluble anesthetic will decrease more slowly at the end of a surgical procedure because of constant movement of drug from the storage site into the bloodstream, even if clearance is rapid. Thus, according to Equation 48-3, the increased volume of distribution of anesthetic drugs in elderly patients will significantly prolong beta elimination half-life, assuming no change in clearance occurs, and the prolonged beta elimination half-life will contribute to an overall extended duration of action of anesthetics. Once the storage sites for a lipid-soluble anesthetic are saturated, elution of drugs from this storage site will be relatively constant. In this situation, if a fixed plasma concentration of a drug is desired, it can be given by incremental administrations at greater intervals or by a continuous infusion at a slower rate. Thus, any of the highly lipid-soluble anesthetic drugs, *e.g.*, barbiturates, benzodiazepines, and opioids, will have an increased steady-state plasma concentration in elderly patients, resulting from a prolonged beta elimination half-life.

On the other hand, clearance of a drug, expressed in units of volume per unit time, represents the hypothetical volume of blood from which a drug would be completely cleared in a given period of time. Clearance is inversely related to the beta elimination half-life of drugs (Equation 48-3). Clearance thus indicates a person's ability to remove or eliminate a drug

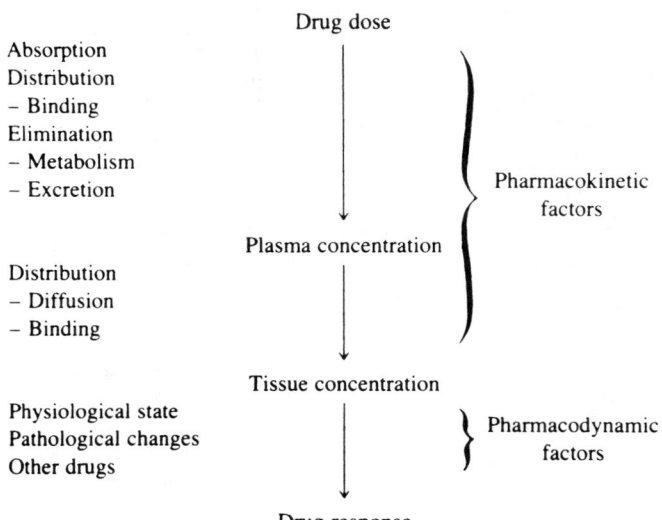

FIG. 48-35. Factors affecting the relationship between the administered dose of drug and the eventual drug response. Pharmacokinetic factors are those that determine the relationship between administered drug dose and the resultant drug concentration at the effector site (tissue concentration). Pharmacodynamic factors are those that determine the eventual response of the effector site to the tissue concentration presented. (Reprinted with permission. Mitenko PA: Geriatric anesthesia: Changes in drug disposition. Can J Anaesth 34:159, 1987.)

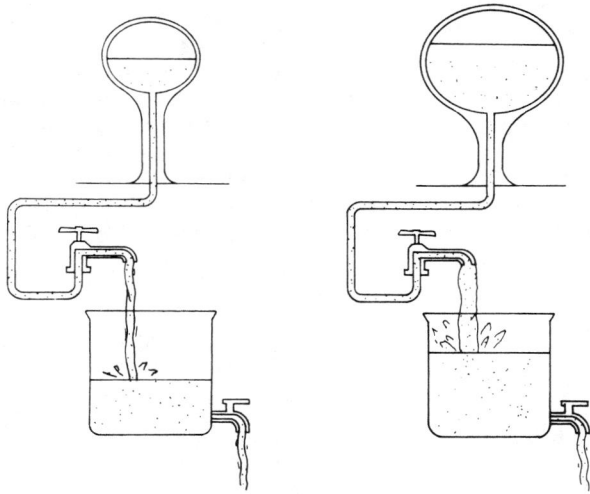

FIG. 48-36. Relationship of volume of distribution of lipid-soluble drugs to emergence from anesthesia. The volume of distribution of these drugs can be viewed as a reservoir that is in equilibrium with the plasma. In the figure, the level of fluid in the beaker represents the plasma concentration of a given lipid-soluble drug. The *left panel* represents the clinical situation of young patients, whereas the *right panel* represents that of older patients. Elderly persons, with a greater percentage of body weight that is fat, may be thought of as having a larger reservoir for lipid-soluble drugs. These drugs administered to elderly persons will be sequestered to a greater extent than in younger patients by filling to a greater capacity a larger reservoir. At the completion of an anesthetic, greater elution of drugs from larger lipid-storage sites in elderly patients tends to result in higher plasma concentrations for longer periods of time, producing delayed emergence from anesthesia.

and usually relates to the efficiency of hepatic metabolism and renal elimination. For the inhalation anesthetics, clearance relates primarily to the efficiency of the cardiovascular system in delivering stored anesthetics to the lung and, in turn, to the efficiency of the pulmonary system in their removal to the atmosphere.

As illustrated in Figure 48-14, hepatic and renal function are reduced about 1% per year beyond age 30. The effect of these age-related changes on hepatic clearance of drugs is complex. A useful scheme categorizing the biotransformation reactions in the liver characterizes reactions as either Phase I (preparative) or Phase II (synthetic). Phase I activity includes reactions such as oxidation, reduction, and hydrolysis. These preparative reactions generally constitute minor molecular modifications, yielding products that may be slightly more water soluble than the parent compound but that may retain part of its pharmacologic activity. Phase II reactions involve conjugation or attachment of a drug molecule to a larger component, such as glucuronide, making the compound more polar and more available for renal excretion. Aging appears to have little effect on Phase II reactions but impairs Phase I reactions, leading to a reduced total drug clearance and higher steady-state plasma concentration of drugs. As discussed above, hepatic function is impaired because of loss of cellular function and reduced hepatic blood flow (Figure 48-29). Hepatic blood flow declines with age partly because of reduced cardiac output but primarily because of a reduced mass of hepatocytes, with an overall 40–50% reduction in hepatic mass and hepatic perfusion in the elderly. For drugs that are metabolized readily by the liver, hepatic blood flow is the major factor determining clearance rate.

Renal blood flow similarly decreases by about 1% per year beyond age 30 and is accompanied by a gradual loss of functioning glomeruli. The combination of these changes produces a predictable decline in glomerular filtration rate in older people that is only 60% of that found in younger people. Because of these renal changes, elderly patients have a reduced ability to excrete drugs and their metabolites.

Pharmacodynamics describes the responsiveness of receptors at the effector site. It is quantitated by determining the plasma concentration–drug response relationship when equilibrium has been achieved between the drug and the receptor. The pharmacodynamics of anesthetic drugs in elderly patients are difficult to determine and have not been extensively studied. The age-associated decline in CNS function, accompanied by a decrease in neuronal and synaptic density, would likely cause elderly patients to be more sensitive to anesthetics and, in turn, to have reduced anesthetic requirements (see Central Nervous System).

Although it is generally agreed that geriatric patients require reduced quantities of anesthetics compared with younger patients, the overlap between pharmacokinetics and pharmacodynamics makes it difficult to substantiate a primary pharmacodynamic explanation for this difference. The next section will address the pharmacokinetic and pharmacodynamic differences of the elderly patient regarding specific anesthetic drugs.

INTRAVENOUS AGENTS

Barbiturates

Barbiturates are among the most commonly used drugs in anesthetic practice today. Numerous studies have shown that the dose of thiopental required to induce anesthesia in elderly patients is less than that for younger patients.[78–80] The smallest dose of thiopental necessary to produce loss of consciousness (failure to "open eyes" on command) in 100% of geriatric patients is only 1.26 mg · kg^{-1} compared with 2.24 mg · kg^{-1} in young adult patients.[78] The dose required to abolish the ciliary reflex in elderly patients (3.9 mg · kg^{-1}) is significantly less than that for younger patients (5.3 mg · kg^{-1}).[79] Similarly, as shown in Figure 48-37, the dose of thiopental required to produce early burst suppression on the EEG (Stage III) decreases with advancing age.[80] Instead of the age-related decrease in thiopental dose requirements shown by others, Christensen and Andreason found that most adult patients premedicated with diazepam, meperidine, and atropine required about the same dose of thiopental for induction of anesthesia until they reached age 60. At that age, a terminal step change occurred whereby the dose requirement for anesthesia in patients older than age 60 was significantly less.[127]

Several authors have determined that the arterial plasma concentration of thiopental required to induce anesthesia is not different between elderly patients and younger patients.[80, 128] Using a 50% decrease in "spectral edge" EEG frequency as a measure of anesthetic depth, Homer and Stanski found that despite a reduced dose of thiopental required to produce this response in elderly patients, the serum concentration of thiopental was no different in the two groups.[80] Thus, it appears that the smaller dose of thiopental required in elderly patients has a pharmacokinetic rather than pharmacodynamic explanation. Elderly people have a reduced initial volume of distribution, a larger volume of distribution at steady state, and reduced clearance. Very likely, the smaller initial volume of distribution results in a higher plasma concentration in the elderly after any given thiopental dose.

In addition, barbiturates have a longer duration of effect in elderly patients. For example, rats receiving hexobarbital at 3

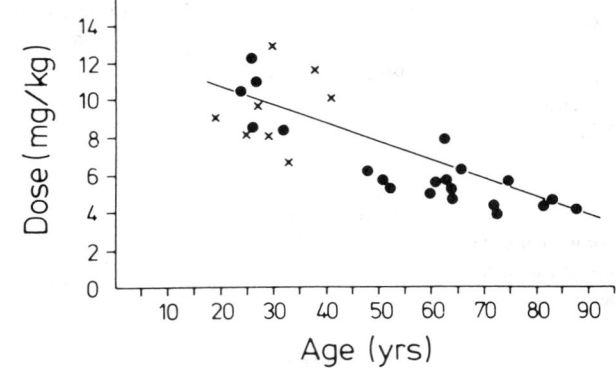

FIG. 48-37. The dose of thiopental required to induce anesthesia (quantitated by burst suppression on EEG) decreases with age. Because the arterial plasma concentration of thiopental required to produce this effect is not different in elderly patients when compared with younger patients, the reduced dose requirement for thiopental in elderly patients must reflect a pharmacokinetic difference. Elderly patients have a reduced initial volume of distribution, which results in a higher plasma concentration after any given administered thiopental dose. Thus, a smaller dose is required in these patients to achieve the same anesthetic effect. (Reprinted with permission. Homer, TD, Stanski DR: The effect of increasing age on thiopental disposition and anesthetic requirement. Anesthesiology 62:714, 1985.)

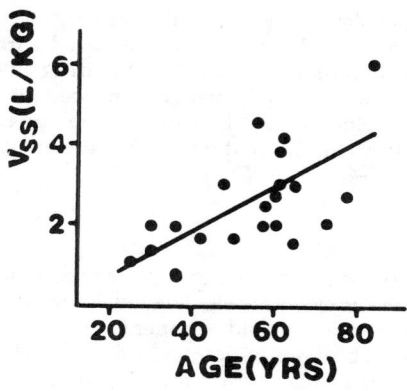

FIG. 48-38. Relationship between the volume of distribution at steady state (Vss) for thiopental *versus* patient age. The greater percentage of body weight that is fat in elderly patients explains the greater volume of distribution of the lipid-soluble drug thiopental in this age group. (Reprinted with permission. Jung D, Mayersohn M, Perrier D *et al*: Thiopental disposition as a function of age in female patients undergoing surgery. Anesthesiology 56:263, 1982.)

month intervals have a duration of hypnosis that increases linearly with age.[129] In humans, recovery from thiopental anesthesia requires 28.5 min in young patients compared with more than 45 min in elderly patients.[130] The age-related increased duration of hypnosis with barbiturates may result from a decline in hepatic enzyme function but more likely results from age-related changes in volume of distribution.[129] The steady-state volume of distribution of the lipid-soluble drug thiopental increases 35% in geriatric patients (Fig. 48-38), largely explaining the 20% increase in beta elimination half-life (see Equation 48-3).[131]

The onset of action of barbiturates is also delayed in the elderly. Muravchick demonstrated that loss of eyelash reflex after thiopental administration to geriatric patients required 48 s compared with 39 s in younger patients.[132] This may be a consequence of a decreased cardiac index and prolonged circulation time seen with advancing age. Also, it may result from the fact that the cardiovascular system of elderly patients is more sensitive to thiopental.[128] After an intravenous barbiturate induction technique, cardiac output, determined by impedance cardiography, was reduced 6% in young patients and 13% in elderly patients. This effect of barbiturates on cardiac output can contribute both to a delay in onset of action and a prolonged clinical effect because of reduced clearance.

Benzodiazepines

The elderly patient is pharmacodynamically more sensitive to benzodiazepines.[133,134] The initial dose and resultant plasma concentration of diazepam preventing response to verbal stimulation, before cardioversion, is significantly lower in elderly patients. In addition, the dose of diazepam producing sedation (grip relaxation) for endoscopic and dental procedures averages 10 mg in 80-yr-old patients and 30 mg in 20-yr-old patients.

Age also affects the pharmacokinetics of benzodiazepines. An age-related impairment of hepatic microsomal oxidation of benzodiazepines results in a prolonged beta elimination half-life for these drugs in elderly patients. As shown in Figure 48-39, a rule of thumb for diazepam is that the beta elimination half-life in hours is approximately the same as the patient's age in years.[135] This is borne out by clinical observations of prolonged sedative effects after relatively small doses

of diazepam in the elderly. Because diazepam impairs performance for almost 24 h in healthy young patients, its prolonged beta elimination half-life in elderly patients emphasizes the need to administer this drug very carefully to older patients.[87]

Newer benzodiazepines have the advantage of a more rapid metabolism to inactive metabolites, resulting in a shorter beta elimination half-life and a shorter duration of pharmacologic action. For this reason, midazolam may have potential advantage in elderly patients, but, as with other benzodiazepines, it also has greater pharmacodynamic activity in this group. In a dose of $0.3 \text{ mg} \cdot \text{kg}^{-1}$, midazolam induces sleep in 100% of unpremedicated elderly patients (62–76 yr), whereas a larger dose of $0.5 \text{ mg} \cdot \text{kg}^{-1}$ successfully induces anesthesia in only 60% of younger adults (29–40 yr).[136] Reports of adverse reactions to midazolam in elderly patients (as a result of an enhanced sensitivity to this drug) have prompted a change in its product labeling, with more conservative dosage recommendations for elderly patients.

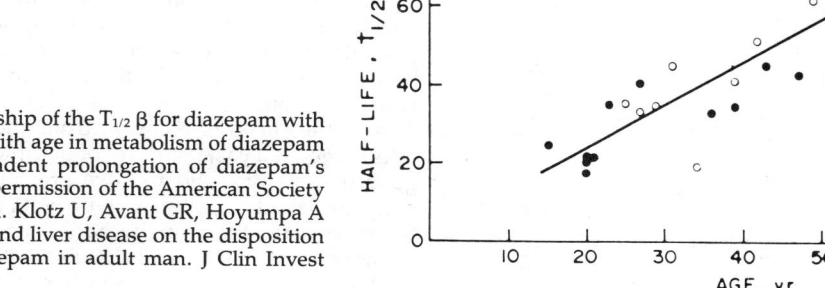

FIG. 48-39. The relationship of the $T_{1/2}\,\beta$ for diazepam with age. The deterioration with age in metabolism of diazepam results in an age-dependent prolongation of diazepam's effect. (Reprinted with permission of the American Society for Clinical Investigation. Klotz U, Avant GR, Hoyumpa A *et al*: The effects of age and liver disease on the disposition and elimination of diazepam in adult man. J Clin Invest 55:347, 1975.)

Because midazolam is also metabolized by hepatic microsomal oxidation, its clearance rate is reduced with age. As a result, the elimination half-life for this drug is more than twice as long in elderly patients compared with that for young, male volunteers.[137] In women, the age-related prolongation of the beta elimination half-life of midazolam is less evident (Fig. 48-40).

Opioids

Age-related pharmacokinetic and pharmacodynamic differences exist for opioids as well. The beta elimination half-life of morphine is 4.5 h in older patients, significantly longer than the 2.9 h observed in younger adults.[138] This primarily results from an increased volume of distribution and only secondarily from decreased clearance. Reduced protein binding with age also has importance for the opioids, especially meperidine. For example, the unbound fraction of meperidine increases from 30% at age 30 to approximately 70% at age 70. This may result in an exaggerated drug effect in elderly patients.[73, 139]

Of all the currently available opioids, fentanyl and its analogues may be best suited for geriatric patients. These drugs have a shorter beta elimination half-life compared with their predecessors and they appear to be better able to blunt the cardiovascular and hormonal responses to intraoperative noxious stimuli.[140] In addition, they are less depressant to myocardial function and cardiac output. However, as with most other drugs, the beta elimination half-life for fentanyl, alfentanil, and other newer opioids is also prolonged in elderly patients. For example, fentanyl has a beta elimination half-life of 265 min in young patients compared with 945 min in elderly patients, whereas alfentanil has an extension of its 83-min beta elimination half-life in young patients to 137 min in the elderly.[141, 142]

As with the barbiturates and benzodiazepines, elderly patients also demonstrate a greater sensitivity to opioids. Scott and Stanski have shown that the dose requirement for fentanyl or alfentanil is decreased approximately 50% in elderly patients.[143] They observed only minor pharmacokinetic differences in this age group and concluded that brain sensitivity (as determined by the "spectral edge" on an EEG) was significantly enhanced in the elderly because of pharmacodynamic factors. Thus, unlike with barbiturates, pharmacodynamic factors appear to explain why fentanyl and its analogues may have a greater effect in elderly patients.

Etomidate

Etomidate, an imidazole intravenous hypnotic drug, is associated with hemodynamic stability, which may offer an advantage for induction of anesthesia in elderly patients, especially those with limited cardiovascular reserve. However, pharmacokinetic differences also exist for this drug in elderly patients. Plasma clearance is reduced 37% and beta elimination half-life is increased 61% in elderly patients.[78] Reduced hepatic blood flow and metabolism explain this alteration. The dose of etomidate required to reach uniform EEG depression, an end point of anesthesia, significantly decreases with age.[78] Thus, etomidate is similar to thiopental. There is no change in the drug's pharmacodynamics in elderly people, but a smaller initial volume of distribution results in the development of a higher initial plasma concentration and the need for a reduced dosage requirement in elderly patients.

INHALATION DRUGS

The MAC of potent inhalation drugs decreases with advancing age (Fig. 48-24).[76] A rough estimate for the true MAC value in elderly patients may be obtained by decreasing the published MAC values approximately 4% for each decade of life over age 40. Age-related changes in cerebral metabolism correspond to changes in MAC requirements, emphasizing the pharmacodynamic correlation between cerebral metabolic function and anesthetic requirements for inhalation drugs (Fig. 48-41).[87]

Many of the physiologic changes of aging discussed earlier suggest that isoflurane has a number of advantages for geriatric patients compared with other inhalation drugs. Because geriatric patients metabolize drugs less readily, any anesthetic that requires metabolism to terminate its activity would be expected to have a more prolonged effect in the elderly. Isoflurane is less metabolized than other potent inhalation anesthetics. Similarly, potentially toxic metabolites, such as fluoride, will exist in lower concentration after isoflurane anesthesia than after enflurane or methoxyflurane anesthesia. This may be even more important in obese elderly patients, in whom (like the obese patient) the percentage of body fat is increased. Isoflurane's low solubility in blood, relative to other potent inhaled anesthetics, not only increases the speed of recovery from anesthesia, but also permits somewhat easier control of depth of anesthesia. Because geriatric patients tend to have greater intraoperative blood pressure lability compared with younger normotensive patients, a drug that can be added and removed rapidly is advantageous. All inhalation anesthetics reduce myocardial contractility and produce peripheral vasodilation. However,

FIG. 48-40. The relationship of age to midazolam's elimination half-life in men and women. Because midazolam is metabolized by hepatic microsomal oxidation, its clearance rate is reduced with age. As a result, the elimination half-life of this drug is more than twice as long in elderly men as it is in younger volunteers. The age-related prolongation of midazolam's elimination half-life is less dramatic, although quite variable, in women. (Reprinted with permission. Reves JG, Fragen RJ, Vinik HR et al: Midazolam: Pharmacology and uses. Anesthesiology 62:310, 1985.)

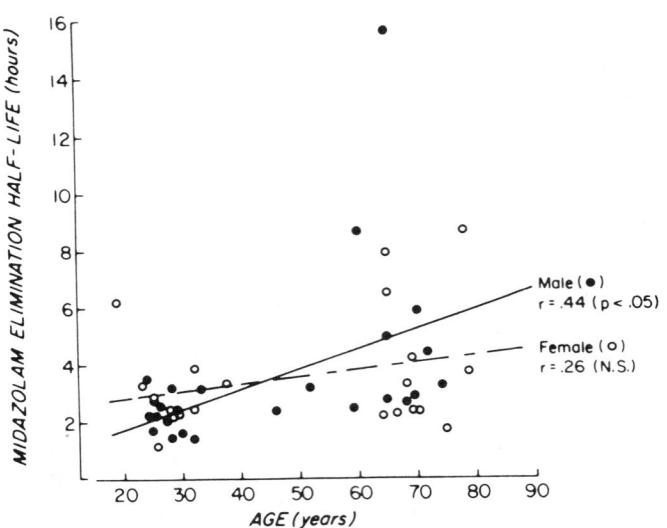

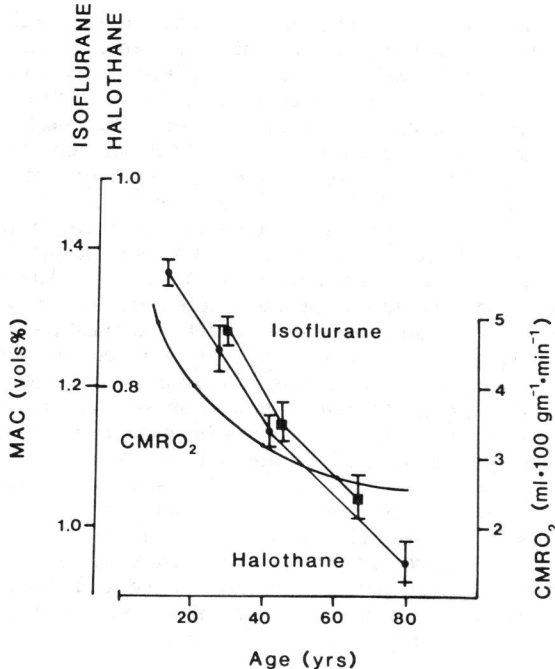

FIG. 48-41. Alveolar concentrations of inhalation anesthetics required to produce anesthesia (MAC) decrease with age. Age-related changes in cerebral metabolism reflected as changes in cerebral metabolic requirements for oxygen (CMRO$_2$) are similar to changes in MAC requirements, emphasizing the pharmacodynamic correlation of cerebral metabolic function to anesthetic requirement. (Reprinted with permission of Grune & Stratton, Orlando. Hilgenberg JC: Inhalation and intravenous drugs in the elderly patient. Seminars in Anesthesia 5:44, 1986.)

studies in human volunteers suggest that isoflurane produces substantially less depression of myocardial contractility and left ventricular ejection fraction than does either halothane or enflurane.[144] Preexisting congestive heart failure exaggerates the myocardial depression produced by inhalation anesthetics.[145] In young adults, the decreased stroke volume produced by isoflurane is offset by a compensatory increase in heart rate such that cardiac output is not significantly altered. In contrast, isoflurane reduces cardiac output in elderly patients because there is a smaller compensatory increase in heart rate (Fig. 48-18).

A decreased cardiac output in elderly patients would be expected to produce a more rapid increase in the alveolar, arterial, and tissue concentrations of inhalation anesthetics

during induction of anesthesia. The increased V/Q mismatch that occurs with aging should accelerate the rate of rise of end-tidal partial pressures of inhalation anesthetics, whereas the rate of increase of arterial partial pressures should be retarded. However, very little pharmacokinetic investigation of inhalation anesthetics in elderly patients has been performed. One study by Lerman et al has shown that, with aging, volatile anesthetic drugs are more soluble in blood and body tissues, which tends to delay induction of anesthesia with inhalation agents.[146, 147] Overall, however, there appear to be no obvious clinically significant differences in the pharmacokinetics of inhalation drugs resulting from age-related changes.

MUSCLE RELAXANTS

Skeletal muscles, the neuromuscular junction, and nerves deteriorate with age. As a result, the volume of distribution for metocurine, d-tubocurarine, and vecuronium are all decreased in elderly patients (Table 48-9). Because elderly patients have a reduced skeletal muscle mass compared with younger patients, one might expect that the initial requirements for neuromuscular blocking agents would be reduced. However, these results have not been obtained in clinical studies. For example, the potency of d-tubocurarine was no different in patients older than 66 yr of age compared with younger patients.[150] The response of elderly patients (older than 75 yr of age) to a given pancuronium dose was comparable to that of patients younger than 60 yr of age.[151] Similarly, no correlation has been observed between age and maximum effect from a given dose of vecuronium.[152, 153] Thus, in general, there is no difference in original dosing requirements for nondepolarizing muscle relaxants in elderly patients compared with younger patients.

Nondepolarizing muscle relaxants (with the exception of atracurium) are usually highly polarized, relatively fat insoluble, and dependent on urinary excretion for elimination from the body. Metabolism and direct biliary excretion, although important, play lesser roles. Because elderly patients metabolize and eliminate most drugs more slowly, a longer duration of action of nondepolarizing relaxants may be expected in elderly patients. With the exception of atracurium, there is a reduction in clearance and an increase in elimination half-life for most nondepolarizing relaxants.

Pancuronium clearance has been shown to be significantly reduced in a geriatric group, necessitating its administration at less frequent intervals than with younger patients. When administered by continuous infusion, pancuronium is effective at lower infusion rates in elderly patients. The time for recovery of twitch tension to 25% of control after pancuro-

TABLE 48-9. Pharmacokinetics of Nondepolarizing Relaxants in Elderly Patients

	VOLUME OF DISTRIBUTION ($l \cdot kg^{-1}$)	PLASMA CLEARANCE ($ml \cdot kg^{-1} \cdot min^{-1}$)	ELIMINATION HALF-LIFE (min)	REFERENCE
Alcuronium	0.29	1.2	182	148
Metocurine	0.26	0.4	530	149
Pancuronium	0.26	1.28	204	150
d-Tubocurarine	0.22	0.8	268	149
Vecuronium	0.18	3.7	58	151
Atracurium	0.16	5.5	20	152, 153

nium administration was prolonged from 44 to 73 min in elderly patients. This is principally due to a 35% decrease in plasma clearance, resulting in an elimination half-life of 204 min, compared with 107 min in younger adult patients.[151]

Vecuronium clearance, as judged by steady-state infusion requirements, is also less in elderly patients. As might be expected, recovery time after vecuronium administration correlates directly with age.[153] After steady-state infusion, elderly patients require 45 min for recovery as compared to 17 min in young adults.[152] In general, in the elderly, the reduction in requirements for nondepolarizing relaxants administered by infusion is explained on a pharmacokinetic basis (reduced clearance) rather than on a pharmacodynamic basis.

The time to onset of action with nondepolarizing muscle relaxants is also age related, as is the time for maximal effect. This implies that there is a slower circulation time in elderly people or that receptor site sensitivity is reduced.[153]

Atracurium is different from other nondepolarizing relaxants in that its action and elimination in elderly patients are very similar to that in younger patients.[154, 155] No significant age-related changes in steady-state dose requirements have been found for atracurium, indicating that inactivation of this drug by Hoffmann elimination or plasma ester hydrolysis is independent of age.[156]

With aging there is the suggestion that trophic support for the neuromuscular junction decreases. There is a loss of peripheral nerve axons, resulting in a net proliferation of muscle end-plates and an increase in the number of acetylcholine receptors. This fact, along with the observation of a reduced level of plasma cholinesterase in elderly patients, may explain why the same degree of muscle blockade can be produced in the elderly from a lower dose of succinylcholine.[157, 159] On the other hand, if cardiac output is reduced significantly in elderly patients, succinylcholine may be less effective because a slower circulation time would permit a longer exposure of succinylcholine to plasma cholinesterase and allow greater metabolism and inactivation of the drug before its delivery to the neuromuscular junction. Overall, the pharmacokinetic and pharmacodynamic differences observed in elderly people produce minimal clinical differences in succinylcholine dose requirements.

LOCAL/REGIONAL ANESTHESIA TECHNIQUES

Controversy surrounds the question of reduced local anesthetic requirements for epidural, spinal, and regional anesthesia techniques in elderly patients compared with younger patients. There are anatomic changes that occur with aging that suggest a generalized reduction in the requirement for local anesthetic drugs in a variety of regional techniques. For example, there is a decrease in the quantity and a change in the configuration of myelinated fibers in the dorsal and ventral roots of the spinal cord. By age 90, only approximately one-third of the original neuronal population remains.[158] In general, the number of axons in peripheral nerves decreases, similar to the decline in CNS neuronal concentration.[159] Functional changes also occur that result in increased permeability of extraneural tissues with advanced age.[160] As myelin sheaths deteriorate and nerve fibers decrease in number, it is reasonable to postulate a reduced requirement for local anesthetics.

Because there is a narrowing of intervertebral spaces and osteophytic growth in elderly patients, Bromage suggested

that local anesthetics injected during epidural anesthesia would be less likely to spread outward (transforaminal escape) and would be more likely to spread upward in the spinal canal, producing an increased level of block.[161] Park et al confirmed this concept when they found that local anesthetic requirements declined from $0.69 \ ml \cdot segment^{-1} \cdot m^{-1}$ of patient height to a dose of $0.62 \ ml \cdot segment^{-1} \cdot m^{-1}$ in patients older than age 40.[162] Although not all authors agree, two studies also suggest greater segmental spread of analgesia in elderly patients with epidural anesthesia produced either by bupivacaine or lidocaine (Fig. 48-42).[163, 164] Although similar to that for epidural anesthesia, the correlation between age and dose requirements for subarachnoid anesthesia may be more closely related to change in vertebral column height with age, rather than to age itself. Veering et al observed that the onset of analgesia with epidural anesthesia was more rapid in elderly patients.[163] This is believed to result from increased permeability of extraneural tissues to local anesthetics. Although not achieving statistical significance, higher plasma concentrations of local anesthetics after epidural anesthesia have been observed in elderly people.[163, 164] This may reflect reduced plasma clearance with age and a prolonged elimination half-life. Because of reduced clearance, toxic plasma concentrations may result from lower doses of local anesthetic drugs in elderly patients.

FIG. 48-42. The relationship between age and the upper level of analgesia achieved after epidural administration of 0.5% bupivacaine. Greater segmental spread of analgesia appears to occur in elderly patients after epidural administration of local anesthetic drugs. (Reprinted with permission of the International Anesthesia Research Society. Veering BT, Burm AGL, van Kleef JW et al: Epidural anesthesia with bupivacaine: Effects of age on neural blockade and pharmacokinetics. Anesth Analg 66:589, 1987.)

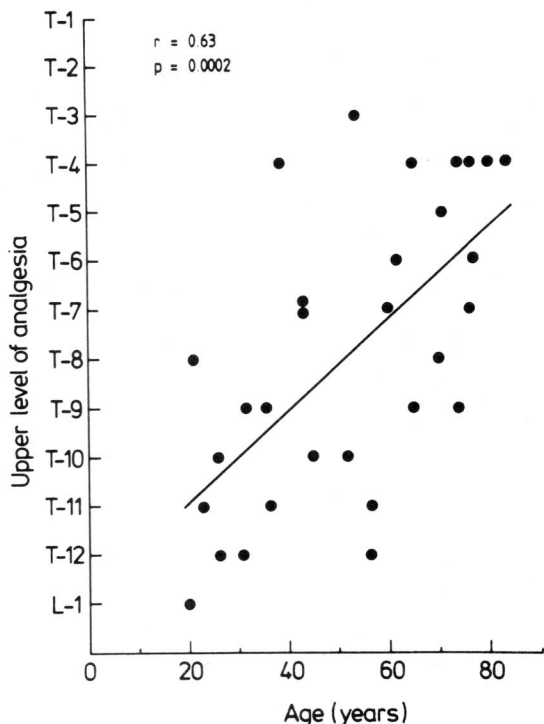

UNIQUE ANESTHETIC CONSIDERATIONS

PREMEDICATION

When visiting elderly patients before operation, the anesthesiologist need not alter his or her normal practice. Elderly people generally have emotions under good control and are frequently placid. Having seen many of life's problems over a long life span, these patients generally are less intimidated by the threat of upcoming surgery than are younger patients. Nevertheless, verbal reassurance is still important for allaying anxiety.

In general, premedicant drugs must be administered with caution to elderly patients, who will manifest a greater sensitivity and a longer duration of drug effect compared with their younger counterparts. Normal adult premedication doses may produce an exaggerated effect in elderly patients and can create unwanted confusion and agitation. If there is doubt, premedication should be light or omitted.

No single premedication regimen is ideal for all elderly patients. Temazepam, triazolam, and diphenhydramine have been suggested as effective premedicant agents for elderly patients.[165] Compared with diazepam, triazolam's far shorter beta elimination half-life of 1.5–5 h has a theoretic advantage in elderly people. Also, in contrast to diazepam, temazepam has been shown to not delay postoperative recovery and not produce excessive sedation 2 h after operation in elderly patients.[165] Diphenhydramine, an antihistamine, exerts sedative and hypnotic effects but minimal psychomotor effects in adults. Kinetic analysis in elderly people has demonstrated a volume of distribution, clearance, and plasma elimination half-life similar to that of younger patients.[166] In general, drugs that have minimal sedative effects or whose sedative effects are short-lived have advantages when used as premedicants in elderly patients.

MONITORING

Because of limited physiologic reserves and a reduced margin for error in elderly patients, monitoring generally should be more intense for this patient group than for younger patients. Del Guercio et al have shown that preoperative invasive monitoring helped predict the elderly patients' tolerance to major operations.[29] Frequently, intensive preoperative monitoring revealed a much worse physical status than suspected on the basis of standard clinical observations. Djokovic et al concluded that invasive monitoring allowed earlier recognition and treatment of intraoperative problems in elderly patients, which resulted, in turn, in a lower mortality rate than previously reported.[4] Although these studies demonstrate positive results with enhanced invasive monitoring, it is not mandatory to monitor every geriatric patient invasively; each patient must be evaluated individually. However, it is likely that older people who have more major and more emergent operations will more frequently benefit from invasive monitoring.

In deciding on the intensity of monitoring for any given elderly patient, it is important to weigh the fact that complications from invasive monitoring are also more likely to be observed in elderly people. For instance, ischemic complications from invasive arterial monitoring are more likely in an elderly person when atherosclerosis reduces the luminal diameter of the artery. Similarly, cardiac dysrhythmias associated with flow-directed pulmonary artery catheters are observed more frequently in elderly patients who more likely have myocardial ischemia and irritability. Thus, every monitoring technique has a cost–benefit relationship that must be assessed individually in view of the patient's age, physical status, and proposed surgical procedure. Inserting invasive monitoring devices before induction of anesthesia allows the establishment of baseline values before induction and surgical stimulation and enhances proper intraoperative interpretation of monitored values. If patients are adequately informed and sedated, invasive devices can be inserted before induction of anesthesia without untoward hemodynamic alterations.[167]

ENDOTRACHEAL INTUBATION

Placement of an endotracheal tube is frequently difficult in elderly patients. If not edentulous, remaining teeth may be loose with poor supportive structure because of resorption of the alveolar ridges of the jaws. Facial shape is also altered by alveolar bone resorption and loss of dentition, leading to concave cheeks. Because of these changes, it may be difficult to adequately ventilate the lungs of an elderly patient by mask. The use of an oropharyngeal airway may partially restore the shape of the face and alleviate this problem. Markedly loose teeth should be removed before laryngoscopic examination is attempted. Temporomandibular joint dysfunction, which reduces anterior advancement of the mandible and mouth opening, combined with cervical arthritis, makes exposure of the larynx more difficult in the elderly patient. Care should be taken during laryngoscopic examination to avoid overextension of the neck because of the increased likelihood of vertebrobasilar arterial insufficiency. In addition, when rapid-sequence endotracheal intubation is performed, cricoid pressure should be applied directly over the cricoid cartilage and not lateral to it, where contact with the carotid artery can loosen an atherosclerotic plaque and possibly result in a cerebrovascular accident.

It is well known that laryngoscopic examination and tracheal intubation are accompanied by tachycardia and hypertension if performed in a lightly anesthetized patient. These changes are normally of short duration and are usually well tolerated by patients who do not have cardiovascular disease. However, myocardial ischemia, ventricular ectopy, left ventricular failure, and cerebral hemorrhage have been reported in response to the stresses of laryngoscopic examination and tracheal intubation. Geriatric patients with preexistent symptomatic or asymptomatic coronary artery disease may be at particular risk for these side-effects and may benefit from efforts taken to blunt these responses. Administration of opioids, local anesthetics, or short-acting vasodilators and antihypertensive agents immediately before induction of anesthesia lessens the severity of cardiovascular responses to placement of an endotracheal tube.

REGIONAL ANESTHESIA VERSUS GENERAL ANESTHESIA

No single anesthetic technique has been shown to be superior for elderly patients. In addition to the significant cardiopulmonary complications associated with anesthesia and surgery, the risk of postoperative mental deterioration in this patient group may be of equal or even greater importance in affecting their quality of life after operation.

Selection of the anesthetic technique should be influenced not only by the patient's clinical condition and surgical requirements, but also by the anesthesiologist's skill and experience. In general, a fragile geriatric patient should be handled gently and the anesthetic achieved in as simple a fashion as possible. Evidence suggests that geriatric patients have an improved prognosis if their surgical procedure is performed with local anesthesia rather than general anesthesia or major regional anesthesia.[33, 168] During certain surgical procedures, regional anesthesia in elderly patients may have the advantages of reduced postoperative negative nitrogen balance, amelioration of endocrine stress responses to surgery, reduction in blood loss, and a reduced incidence of postoperative thromboembolic complications.[169-172]

During hip surgery, regional anesthesia is associated with a reduced incidence of deep vein thrombosis (Table 48-10).[173] A potential explanation for this phenomenon is that sympathectomy produced by spinal anesthesia produces vasodilation and increases lower limb blood flow, whereas general anesthesia reduces cardiac output and peripheral blood flow. Further, stress hormones released during general anesthesia may enhance the coagulation process. As observed in Table 48-10, use of regional anesthesia also resulted in reduced intraoperative blood loss and less postoperative hypoxemia. Deaths occurring within 4 weeks of surgery happened less often in patients receiving regional anesthesia. In a similar study, greater hypoxemia was observed after operation in patients receiving general anesthesia compared with epidural anesthesia for total hip arthroplasty.[170] The development of V/Q mismatch and pulmonary shunt appeared to be greater in patients who required general anesthesia with controlled ventilation *versus* those who maintained spontaneous ventilation with epidural anesthesia. Intraoperative pulmonary changes may have been exaggerated after operation by splinting and reduced coughing in patients receiving general anesthesia.

Mental changes lasting months or years after administration of general anesthesia to elderly patients having major surgery have been reported.[174] Possible explanations for this deterioration in mental function include the stress of the operation, intraoperative or perioperative episodes of hypoxemia, perioperative episodes of hypotension, and prolonged action of administered drugs. As shown in Table 48-11, Hole *et al* have observed persistent postoperative mental changes in more than 20% of patients receiving general anesthesia, whereas no patients receiving epidural anesthesia demonstrated this problem. Five of 31 patients receiving general anesthesia observed a change in quality of life for as long as 3 months after the date of surgery.[174] If it could be reproducibly shown that mental dysfunction occurred in elderly patients to a greater extent after general anesthesia, regional

anesthetic techniques would be of obvious benefit. However, comparison of groups of elderly patients who have had the same surgical procedure with general anesthesia compared with regional or local anesthesia are not universal in this conclusion. For example, Riis *et al* found identical patterns of altered mental function in elderly patients, regardless of type of anesthesia for hip arthroplasty, and concluded that the transient mental impairment that occurred during the first postoperative week was caused by factors other than the selection of anesthesia.[175] Similarly, Karhunen and Jonn found a comparable incidence of postoperative memory loss after cataract extraction whether general or local anesthesia was used.[176] Mann and Bisset have shown no difference in postoperative mental dysfunction whether general or spinal anesthesia was used for surgery of the lower limbs.[177] Berggren *et al* demonstrated no difference in the incidence of postoperative confusion in patients receiving general or epidural anesthesia for repair of femoral neck fractures.[178] Instead, they correlated postoperative confusion with the patient's history of mental depression and use of anticholinergic medication.

In summary, it is difficult to recommend regional anesthesia over general anesthesia for all kinds of surgical procedures in the geriatric patient group. The selection of anesthesia must be based on the patient's individual circumstances. Spinal anesthesia has particular advantages for certain types of surgery, including transurethral resection of the prostrate, during which the patient remains awake and can give early warning of surgical complications. Similarly, allowing a patient to remain conscious during regional anesthesia permits patient recognition of an anginal attack or acute cerebral changes resulting from a variety of causes. Spinal anesthesia

TABLE 48-11. Complications of Total Hip Arthroplasty

PARAMETER	EPIDURAL (0.75% Bupivacaine) ($n = 29$)	GENERAL ANESTHESIA ($n = 31$)
Pa$_{O_2}$ first postoperative day (mm Hg)	75	68
Patients describing persistent mental changes 3 months after operation	0	7
Patients describing change in quality of life 3 months after operation	0	5

(Hole A, Terjesen T, Breivik H: Epidural versus general anaesthesia for total hip arthroplasty in elderly patients. Acta Anaesthesiol Scand 24:279, 1980.)

TABLE 48-10. Complications of Emergency Hip Surgery

PARAMETER	SUBARACHNOID BLOCK ($n = 37$)	GENERAL ANESTHESIA ($n = 39$)
Incidence deep vein thrombosis (%)	46	77
Intraoperative blood loss (ml)	304	468
Total blood loss (ml)	513	714
Postoperative decrease in Pa$_{O_2}$ (mm Hg)	1.2	6.5
Deaths within 4 weeks of surgery (no.)	3	9

(Davis FM, Laurenson VG: Spinal anaesthesia or general anaesthesia for emergency hip surgery in elderly patients. Anaesth Intensive Care 9:352, 1981.)

also has a lower incidence of postpuncture headaches in older patients (Table 48-12).[179] This is thought to result from age-related anatomic changes in the intervertebral foramina, which inhibits leakage of cerebrospinal fluid from the dural rent produced by the spinal needle.

For older patients who are cooperative, regional techniques, especially subarachnoid and epidural blockade, can be used effectively and safely for procedures requiring anesthesia below the T-8 dermatome. Regional blockade also may be used effectively for various procedures on the extremities. However, use of a regional anesthetic in an elderly patient who becomes agitated, excited, or uncomfortable because of awkward positioning tempts the anesthesiologist to provide supplemental sedation. Injudicious use of supplemental drugs may actually result in a pseudo-general anesthetic for a patient that obviates some of the advantages of a regional anesthetic technique. Oversedation of a patient may lead to hypoventilation, an unprotected airway, and the possibility of mental changes after operation resembling those with general anesthesia.[175]

POSITIONING

Aging is associated with a progressive decrease in bone density in both men and women after maturity. Losses in bone density so severe as to result in fractures after minimal trauma define the disease of osteoporosis, which accounts for more than one million fractures in the United States each year.[8] Osteoporosis is of staggering importance in the elderly and contributes to the observation that, by age 65, one-third of women will have had vertebral fractures and, by age 81, one-third of women and one-sixth of men will have had a hip fracture. This loss of bony matrix not only explains many of the orthopedic injuries for which elderly patients are seen for surgery but also emphasizes the fragility of elderly patients and indicates the importance of positioning patients gently for surgical procedures. After receiving either regional or general anesthesia, elderly patients must be placed in a neutral position, with consideration of their decreased range of motion. If possible, the patient's neck should be kept in a position that was comfortable when he or she was awake in order to avoid compromising cerebral blood flow. Great care must be used when turning elderly patients in order to prevent pathologic fractures. Placing elderly patients in the lithotomy position is known to produce postoperative back pain. For example, after a spinal anesthetic is administered to an elderly man for transurethral surgery, it is very easy to place his legs in a position very much more exaggerated

TABLE 48-12.   Incidence of Spinal Headache in Relation to Age

AGE (yr)	PATIENTS (no.)	INCIDENCE OF HEADACHES (%)
20–29	23	17
30–39	36	11
40–49	32	9
50–59	29	7
60–69	14	0
70–79	8	0

(Benzon HT, Linde HW, Molloy RE *et al*: Postdural puncture headache in patients with chronic pain. Anesth Analg 59:772, 1980. Reprinted with permission of the International Anesthesia Research Society.)

than he would have permitted had analgesia and relaxation not been produced as a result of the spinal anesthetic. A postoperative backache incorrectly attributed to the spinal technique more likely results from inadequate attention to positioning.

Senile atrophy, with loss of subcutaneous elastic tissue, makes the skin of elderly patients sensitive to injury from adhesive tape or application of monitoring electrodes. Because elderly patients have fragile skin and decreased subcutaneous elastic tissue, careful padding is essential. Bony prominences such as elbows, ankles, and trochanters must be padded with sheepskin, foam, or other suitable padding. Tape should be removed very carefully.

DRUG INTERACTIONS

Geriatric patients have more illnesses and invariably take more medications than do younger patients, thus exposing them to an increased risk of adverse drug reactions. Although patients 65 yr of age and older make up only 12% of the United States population, 30% of all prescriptions are written for people of this age group.[11] Almost 70% of elderly patients regularly use over-the-counter (OTC) drugs, compared with approximately 10% of the general adult population.[180] OTC drugs account for approximately 40% of all drugs taken by elderly patients.[181]

Because of the larger number and variety of drugs prescribed for and consumed by elderly patients, these patients have an approximate threefold increased potential for adverse drug reactions. For example, in a study of 714 hospitalized patients at Johns Hopkins University, patients ages 41–50 had an 11.8% incidence of adverse drug reactions, whereas patients ages 80 or greater had a 24.9% incidence.[182] Similarly, in a study by Hurwitz, patients ages 40–49 yr had a 7% incidence of adverse drug effects, whereas patients ages 70–79 yr had an incidence three times as great.[183]

Many of these problems with drug interaction in the elderly population simply reflect polypharmacy, resulting from the additive or synergistic action of multiple drugs. However, they also may reflect discrepancies in duration of drug action or may represent the decreased clearance of one drug because of the hepatic effects of another. This last situation has been described for the interaction of cimetidine with beta-blocking drugs, and benzodiazepines.[184]

Before operation, one must inquire into corticosteroid, antihypertensive, anticoagulant, beta-blocker, monoamine oxidase inhibitor, tricyclic antidepressant, and antidiabetic drug use. Also, elderly patients use alcohol in greater quantities than do young patients, with a significant percentage of elderly patients reported as being alcoholics. To minimize the risks of hazardous drug interactions, the anesthetic should be kept simple in elderly patients.

OUTPATIENT ANESTHESIA FOR ELDERLY PATIENTS

In our current system of health care, cost containment has been greatly emphasized. Of course, this has brought the geriatric patient into the outpatient setting. As discussed in the section Regional Anesthesia *Versus* General Anesthesia, postoperative confusion and mental dysfunction are of great concern in the elderly patient. These side-effects may be reduced by allowing elderly patients to have surgery in an ambulatory setting, where they will be given fewer medications and they can return more quickly to normal surroundings with their relatives and friends nearby. As Rowe and Kahn have suggested, the maintenance of control or autonomy for elderly patients (where they make decisions regarding choice of activity, timing, pace, and so on) is very important.[8] Lack of control has adverse effects on their emotional state, performance, subjective well-being, and physiologic function. As a result, it may be beneficial for elderly patients to have surgery in an outpatient setting, where there is a lesser loss of autonomy and control.

Obviously, not all geriatric patients should have surgery in an ambulatory setting. Many of these patients have more than one disease or a significant physiologic decrement in function that prevents them from being candidates for ambulatory surgery. However, if elderly patients pass routine preoperative screening visits, there is no reason why age alone should prevent them from being considered candidates for outpatient procedures. Meridy found that age does not affect the duration of recovery from anesthesia nor the rate of complications after outpatient surgery.[185] However, others have observed that more time was required for older patients to successfully complete a manipulative skill test when they were emerging from thiopental, halothane, and nitrous oxide anesthesia for cervical dilatation and curettage.[130]

The anesthesiologist's preoperative screening visit before surgery is of prime importance and should take place before the day of surgery. This enables anesthesia personnel to make rational judgments as to the patient's acceptability for surgery as an outpatient, permits treatment of preexistent diseases, contributes to more efficient scheduling, allows appropriate laboratory testing to be performed, enhances the visibility of the anesthesiologist in the overall medical practice scheme, and enables an interview of the "responsible adult" who will not only ensure the patient's delivery from the hospital back home, but who will also stay with the patient and assist with recovery in the home setting. In a special study sponsored by the Federated Ambulatory Surgery Association, Natof reviewed 87,492 patients having outpatient procedures and found a relationship between the incidence of complications and the length of the surgical procedure (Table 48-13).[186] As a result, the type and difficulty of the surgical procedure should be taken into consideration before a complex and protracted surgical procedure is allowed to be performed on an elderly patient on an outpatient basis. Similarly, the relationship of complication rate to preexistent disease demonstrates again the importance of preanesthesia screening in determining whether elderly patients with one or more preexistent medical conditions should be allowed to have their surgical procedures on an outpatient basis (Table 48-14). Finally, the selection of anesthesia for the geriatric

patient depends on the anticipated surgical procedure, the patient's state of health, and the anesthesiologist's skill and experience. Many elderly patients fear general anesthesia more than regional or local anesthesia and believe that they have a greater sense of control if they do not receive a general anesthetic. Again, in the large study of the Federated Ambulatory Surgery Association, a much lower incidence of complications was observed in patients who received local anesthesia or regional techniques. A higher incidence of complications was observed in those who received local anesthesia with sedation or general anesthesia (Table 48-15).[186]

Not all elderly patients have multiple medical problems. Physiologic age is obviously more important than chronologic age, and a profile of the patient's medical history and current level of physical activity far better indicates his or her ability to tolerate a surgical procedure as an outpatient than does age alone. A patient should not be denied ambulatory surgery solely on the basis of age.

POSTOPERATIVE MANAGEMENT

The elderly patient needs special attention immediately after operation. Elderly patients have increased V/Q mismatch after operation, which contributes to a greater degree of postoperative hypoxemia compared with that in young patients.[65] Because even young patients are known to experience reduced oxygenation during transfer from the operating room to the postanesthesia care unit (PACU), elderly patients are at greater risk for hypoxia both during transfer to the PACU and during the recovery room stay. For this reason, supplemental oxygen is useful during transport to the PACU and while the patient is in the PACU. Monitoring oxygen saturation with a pulse oximeter enables one to make a rational decision as to the need for supplemental oxygen. Frequently, ventilatory depression from residual anesthetic, ventilatory compromise

TABLE 48-14. Complications Related to Preexisting Disease

PREEXISTING DISEASE	INCIDENCE
Cardiac disease	1/74 patients
Hypertension	1/87 patients
Chronic lung disease	1/112 patients
Asthma	1/139 patients
None	1/156 patients

(Natof HE: FASA Special Study I. Alexandria, VA: Federated Ambulatory Surgery Association, 1985.)

TABLE 48-13. Complications Related to Operating Room Time

OPERATING ROOM TIME	PATIENTS	COMPLICATIONS	INCIDENCE
1 h or less	69,461	449	1/155 patients
1–2 h	11,971	142	1/84 patients
2–3 h	2,481	46	1/54 patients
More than 3 h	729	21	1/35 patients

(Natof HE: FASA Special Study I. Alexandria, VA: Federated Ambulatory Surgery Association, 1985.)

TABLE 48-15. Complications Related to Anesthetic Technique

TECHNIQUE	INCIDENCE
Local and sedation	1/106 patients
General	1/120 patients
Local only	1/268 patients
Regional blockade	1/277 patients

(Natof HE: FASA Special Study I. Alexandria, VA: Federated Ambulatory Surgery Association, 1985.)

(from splinting), or preexistent pulmonary disease necessitates the administration of supplemental oxygen for the first 24 h. Like other patients, elderly patients need to be encouraged to breathe deeply and cough and may benefit from elevation of the head of the bed. As discussed in the section on Airway Reflexes, because of a reduction in airway protective reflexes, elderly patients require greater observation to protect them from passive aspiration.

Because elderly patients lose more body heat during operation and arrive in the PACU cooler than do their younger counterparts (Fig. 48-33), it may be necessary to apply exogenous heat to speed rewarming.[114] Placing them in a warm environment during their recovery room stay reduces the likelihood for shivering with its associated problems. Elderly patients also benefit from reassurance and additional measures to assist them with orientation to reality. They may need to be reminded at frequent intervals with statements such as "your operation is over and you are doing fine" or "you are not at home; you are in the hospital." These comments help them to regain their sense of awareness and a presence of their surroundings. In addition, when they are provided with their dentures, glasses, hearing aids, and other personal items, they gain additional psychologic security while remaining in the PACU.

SUMMARY

Aging is an all-encompassing, multifactorial process that results in a decreased capacity for adaptation and produces a gradual decrease in functional reserve of many of the body's organ systems. Aging itself is not a disease process but, instead, a reminder of the potential for development of many age-related disease states. There is probably no ideal anesthetic drug or technique for all elderly patients. A thorough understanding of the physiologic changes that occur with aging, and the altered pharmacokinetic and pharmacodynamic responses to a variety of anesthetic drugs, is necessary when designing an optimal anesthetic technique for a given elderly patient. Appropriate anesthetic management must therefore be based on a thorough medical evaluation before operation, with correction, if possible, of any detected abnormality. Intensity of monitoring during and after anesthesia will likely be greater than that selected for younger patients but should be determined on an individual basis with consideration of the patient's condition and proposed surgical procedure. Because elderly patients are not only pharmacologically but also physically fragile, they must be positioned and moved very carefully.

The public is becoming more informed on the positive aspects of aging and the uniqueness of older adults. Part of our goal is to prevent feelings of hopelessness and dependency in order that older patients will be able to retain their sense of independence and individuality. By offering them the safest anesthetic possible, we can contribute to the revolutionary increase in average life span of members of our society and help to maintain their full physiologic function as near to the end of life as possible.

REFERENCES

1. Smith OC: Advanced age as a contraindication to operation. Med Rec (NY) 72:642, 1907
2. Ochsner A: Is risk of operation too great in the elderly? Geriatrics 22:121, 1927
3. Brooks B: Surgery in patients of advanced age. Ann Surg 105:481, 1937
4. Djokovic JL, Hedley-Whyte J: Prediction of outcome of surgery and anesthesia in patients over 80. JAMA 242:2301, 1979
5. Miller R, Marlar K, Silvay G: Anesthesia for patients aged over 90 years. NY State J Med 77:1421, 1977
6. Catlic MR: Surgery in centenarians. JAMA 253:3139, 1985
7. McLeskey CH: Anesthesia for the geriatric patient. In Stoelting RK, Barash PG, Gallagher TJ (eds): Advances in Anesthesia, p 31. Chicago, Year Book Medical Publishers, 1985
8. Rowe JW, Kahn RL: Human aging: Usual and successful. Science 237:143, 1987
9. Schneider EL, Butler RN: Geriatrics. JAMA 245:2190, 1981
10. Hayflick L: The cell biology of human aging. In Morin RJ, Bing RJ (eds): Frontiers in Medicine, p 236. New York, Human Sciences Press, 1985
11. Thompson TL, Moran MG, Nies AS: Psychotropic drug use in the elderly. N Engl J Med 308:134, 1983
12. Vestal RE: Drug use in the elderly: A review of problems and special consideration. Drugs 16:382, 1978
13. Fries JF, Crapo LM: The sharp downslope of natural death. In Fries JF, Crapo LM (eds): Vitality and Aging, p 73. San Francisco, WH Freeman and Company, 1981
14. 1980 Census of Population: General population characteristics, p 26. Washington, DC, United States Census Bureau, 1983
15. Renck H: The elderly patient after anaesthesia and surgery. Acta Anaesthesiol Scand [Suppl] 13:9, 1969
16. Davenport HT: Anesthesia for the geriatric patient. Can Anaesth Soc J 30:S51, 1983
17. Marx GF, Mateo CV, Orkin LR: Computer analysis of post-anesthetic deaths. Anesthesiology 39:54, 1973
18. Mircea N, Constantinescu C, Jianu E et al: Risk of pulmonary complications in surgical patients. Resuscitation 10:33, 1982
19. Farrow SC, Fowkes FGR, Lunn JN et al: Epidemiology in anaesthesia. II: Factors affecting mortality in hospital. Br J Anaesth 54:811, 1982
20. Filzweiser G, List WF: Morbidity and mortality in elective geriatric surgery. In Vickers MD, Lunn JN (eds): Mortality and Anaesthesia, p 75. Berlin, Springer-Verlag, 1983
21. Hatton F, Tiret L, Vourc'h G: Morbidity and mortality associated with anesthesia—French survey: Preliminary results. In Vickers MD, Lunn JN (eds): Mortality and Anaesthesia, p 25. Berlin, Springer-Verlag, 1983
22. Ellison N: Problems in geriatric anesthesia. Surg Clin North Am 55:929, 1975
23. Haljamae T, Stefannsson T, Wickstrom I: Preanesthetic evaluation of the female geriatric patient with hip fracture. Acta Anaesthesiol Scand 26:393, 1982
24. Stephen CR: The risk of anesthesia and surgery in the geriatric patient. In Krechel SE (ed): Anesthesia and the Geriatric Patient, p 231. New York, Grune and Stratton, 1984
25. Rowe JW, Adres R, Tobin JD et al: The effect of age on creatinine clearance in man: A cross-sectional and longitudinal study. J Gerontol 31:155, 1976
26. Tiret L, Desmonts JM, Hatton F et al: Complications associated with anaesthesia—A prospective survey in France. Can Anaesth Soc J 33:336, 1986
27. Denney JH, Denson JS: Risk of surgery in patients over 90. Geriatrics 27:115, 1972
28. Goldman L, Caldera DL, Nussbaum SR et al: Multifactorial index of cardiac risks in non-cardiac surgical procedures. N Engl J Med 297:845, 1977
29. Del Guercio LRN, Cohn JD: Monitoring operative risk in the elderly. JAMA 243:1350, 1980
30. Johnson JC: The medical evaluation and management of the elderly surgical patient. J Am Geriatr Soc 31:621, 1983

31. Goldman L, Caldera DL, Southwick FS et al: Cardiac risk factors and complications in non-cardiac surgery. Medicine 57:357, 1978

32. Gibson JR, Mendelhall MK, Axel NJ: Geriatric anesthesia: Minimizing the risk. In Brindly GU (eds): Clinics in Geriatric Medicine, p 313. Philadelphia, WB Saunders, 1985

33. Nehme AE: Groin hernias in elderly patients. Am J Surg 146:257, 1983

34. Williams JS, Hale HW: The advisability of inguinal herniorrhaphy in the elderly. Surg Gynecol Obstet 122:100, 1966

35. Tingwald GR, Cooperman M: Inguinal and femoral hernia repair in geriatric patients. Surg Gynecol Obstet 154:704, 1982

36. Lakatta EG, Fleg JL: Aging of the adult cardiovascular system. In Stephen CR, Assaf RAE (eds): Geriatric anesthesia: Principles and Practices, p 1. Boston, Butterworths, 1986

37. Ensor RE, Fleg JL, Kim YC et al: Longitudinal chest x-ray changes in normal men. J Gerontol 38:307, 1983

38. Kannel WB, Gordon T: Evaluation of cardiovascular risk in the elderly: The Framingham study. Bull NY Acad Med 54:573, 1978

39. Tarazi RC, Frohlich ED, Dustan HP: Plasma volume in men with essential hypertension. N Engl J Med 278:762, 1968

40. Evans TI: The physiological basis of geriatric general anesthesia. Anaesth Intensive Care 1:319, 1973

41. Brandfonbrener M, Landowne M, Shock NW: Changes in cardiac output with age. Circulation 69:557, 1955

42. Rodeheffer RJ, Gerstenblith G, Becker LC et al: Exercise cardiac output is maintained with advancing age in healthy human subjects: Cardiac dilatation and increased stroke volume compensate for a diminished heart rate. Circulation 69:203, 1984

43. Port S, Cobb FR, Coleman RE et al: Effect of age on the responses of the left ventricular ejection fraction to exercise. N Engl J Med 303:1133, 1980

44. Rosberg B, Wulff K: Hemodynamics following normovolemic hemodilution in elderly patients. Acta Anaesthesiol Scand 25:402, 1981

45. Skinner JS: The cardiovascular system with aging and exercise. In Brunner D, Jake E (eds): Medicine and Science in Sport, Vol 4, p 100. Baltimore, University Park Press, 1970

46. Tuzankoff ST, Fleg JL, Norris AH et al: Age-related increase in serum catecholamine levels during exercise and healthy adult men. Physiologist 23:50, 1980

47. Shocken DD, Roth GS: Reduced beta-adrenergic receptor concentrations in aging man. Nature 267:856, 1977

48. Dillon N, Chung S, Kelly J et al: Age and beta adrenoceptor mediated function. Clin Pharmacol Ther 27:769, 1980

49. Grollman A, Grollman EF: Pharmacology and therapeutics, 7th ed, p 269. Philadelphia, Lea & Febiger, 1970

50. Forrest JB: Clinical evaluation of isoflurane: Pulse and blood pressure. Can Anaesth Soc J 29:S15, 1982

51. Feldman RD, Limbird LE, Nadeau J et al: Alterations in leukocyte-receptor affinity with aging: A potential explanation for altered-adrenergic sensitivity in the elderly. N Engl J Med 310:815, 1984

52. Van Brummelen P, Buhler FR, Kiowski W et al: Age-related decrease in cardiac and peripheral vascular responsiveness to isoprenaline: Studies in normal subjects. Clin Sci 60:571, 1980

53. Kendall MJ, Woods KL: Responsiveness to alpha-adrenergic receptor stimulation: The effects of age are cardioselective. Br J Clin Pharmacol 14:821, 1982

54. Conway J, Wheeler R, Sannerstedt R: Sympathetic nervous activity during exercise in relation to age. Cardiovasc Res 5:577, 1971

55. Lakatta EG: Age-related alterations in the cardiovascular response to adrenergic mediated stress. Fed Proc 39:3171, 1980

56. Kennedy RD, Claird FI: Physiology of aging of the heart. Cardiovasc Clin 12:1, 1981

57. Elliott HL, Sumner DJ, McLean K et al: Effect of age on the responsiveness of vascular alpha-adrenoceptors in man. J Cardiovasc Pharmacol 4:388, 1982

58. Fleg JL, Kennedy HL: Cardiac arrhythmias in a healthy elderly population: Detection by 24-hour ambulatory monitoring. Chest 81:302, 1982

59. Levy W: Clinical evaluation of isoflurane: Cardiac arrhythmias. Can Anaesth Soc J 29:S28, 1982

60. Goldman HL, Becklake MR: Respiratory function tests: Normal values at median altitudes and the prediction of normal results. Am Rev Tuberculosis 79:457, 1959

61. Smith TC: Respiratory effects of aging. Seminars in Anesthesia 5:14, 1986

62. Pontoppidan H, Geffins B, Lowenstein A: Acute respiratory failure in the adult. N Engl J Med 287:690, 1972

63. Pump KK: Emphysema and its relation to age. Am Rev Respir Dis 114:5, 1976

64. Raine JM, Bishop MJ: A-a difference in O_2 tension and physiological dead space in normal man. J Appl Physiol 18:284, 1963

65. Kitamura H, Sawa T, Ikezono E: Postoperative hypoxemia: The contribution of age to the maldistribution of ventilation. Anesthesiology 36:244, 1972

66. Wahba W: Body build and preoperative arterial oxygen tension. Can Anaesth Soc J 22:653, 1972

67. Ward RJ, Tolas AG, Benveniste RJ et al: Effect of posture on normal arterial blood gas tensions in the aged. Geriatrics 21:139, 1966

68. Kronenberg RS, Drage GW: Attenuation of the ventilatory and heart rate responses to hypoxia and hypercapnia with aging in normal man. J Clin Invest 52:1812, 1973

69. Hickey RF, Severinghaus JW: Regulation of breathing: Drug effects. In Hornbein TF (ed): Regulation of Breathing, part II, p 1251. New York, Marcel Dekker, 1981

70. Labouvie-Vief G: Intelligence and cognition. In Birren JE, Schaie KW (eds): Handbook of the Psychology of Aging, p 500. New York, Van Nostrand Reinhold, 1985

71. Muravchick S: Current concepts: Anesthetic pharmacology in geriatric patients. Progress in Anesthesiology 1:2, 1987

72. Hess GD, Joseph JA, Roth GS: Effect of age on sensitivity to pain and brain opiate receptors. Neurobiology of Aging 2:49, 1981

73. Bellville JW, Forrest WH, Miller E: Influence of age on pain relief from analgesics: A study of postoperative patients. JAMA 217:1835, 1971

74. Gregory GA, Eger EI II, Munson ES: The relationship between age and halothane requirement in man. Anesthesiology 30:488, 1969

75. Stevens WC, Dolan WM, Gibbons RT et al: Minimum alveolar concentrations (MAC) of isoflurane with and without nitrous oxide in patients of various ages. Anesthesiology 42:197, 1975

76. Munson ES, Hoffman JC, Eger EI: Use of cyclopropane to test generality of anesthetic requirement in the elderly. Anesth Analg 63:998, 1984

77. Kaiko RF, Wallenstein SL, Rogers AG et al: Narcotics in the elderly. Med Clin North Am 66:1079, 1982

78. Arden JR, Holley FO, Stanski DR: Increased sensitivity to etomidate in the elderly: Initial distribution versus altered brain response. Anesthesiology 65:19, 1986

79. Christensen F, Andreasen F, Jansen JA: Influence of age and sex on the pharmacokinetics of thiopentone. Br J Anaesth 53:1189, 1981

80. Homer TD, Stanski DR: The effect of increasing age on thiopental disposition and anesthetic requirement. Anesthesiology 62:714, 1985

81. Lytle LD, Altar A: Diet, central nervous system, and aging. Fed Proc 38:2017, 1979

82. Naritomi H, Meyer JS, Sakai F *et al*: Effect of advancing age on regional cerebral blood flow. Arch Neurol 36:410, 1979
83. Devaney KO, Johnson HA: Neuron loss in the aging visual cortex of man. J Gerontol 35:836, 1980
84. Sapolsky RM, Krey LC, McEwen BS: Prolonged glucocorticoid exposure reduces hippocampal neuron number: Implications for aging. J Neurosci 5:1222, 1985
85. Melamed E, Lavy S, Bentin S *et al*: Reduction in regional cerebral blood flow during normal aging in men. Stroke 11:31, 1980
86. Kety SS: Human cerebral blood flow and oxygen consumption as related to aging. J Chronic Dis 3:478, 1956
87. Hilgenberg JC: Inhalation and intravenous drugs in the elderly patient. Seminars in Anesthesia 5:44, 1986
88. Dorfman LJ, Bosley TM: Age-related changes in peripheral and central nerve conduction in men. Neurology 29:38, 1979
89. Lake CR, Ziegler MG, Coleman MD *et al*: Age-adjusted plasma nor-epinephrine levels are similar in normotensive and hypertensive subjects. N Engl J Med 296:208, 1977
90. McGeer EG, McGeer PL: Age changes in the human for enzymes associated with metabolism of catecholamine, GABA, and acetylcholine. Advances in Behavioral Biology 16:287, 1975
91. Gibson GE, Peterson C: Aging decreases oxidative metabolism and the release and synthesis of acetylcholine. J Neurochem 37:978, 1981
92. McGeer EG, McGeer PL: Neurotransmitter metabolism in the aging brain. In Terry RD, Gershon S (eds): Neurobiology of Aging, p 389. New York, Raven Press, 1976
93. Bender AD, Post A, Meier JP *et al*: Plasma protein binding of drugs as a function of age in adult human subjects. J Pharm Sci 64:1711, 1975
94. Wallace S, Whiting B, Runcie J: Factors affecting drug binding in plasma of elderly patients. Br J Clin Pharmacol 3:3270, 1976
95. Greenblatt DJ: Reduced serum albumin concentration in the elderly: A report from the Boston collaborative drug surveillance program. J Am Geriatri Soc 27:20, 1979
96. Hayes MJ, Langman MJS, Short AH: Changes in drug metabolism with increasing age. 1. Warfarin binding and plasma proteins. Br J Clin Pharmacol 2:69, 1975
97. Carlos R, Calvo R, Erill S: Plasma protein binding of etomidate in different age groups and in patients with chronic respiratory insufficiency. Int J Clin Pharmacol Ther Toxicol 19:1714, 1981
98. Taxton JW, Briant RH: Alpha-1 acid glycoprotein concentration and propranol binding in elderly patients with acute illness. Br J Clin Pharmacol 18:806, 1984
99. Chan K, Kendall MJ, Wells WD *et al*: Factors influencing the excretion and relative physiological availability of pethidine in man. J Pharm Pharmacol 27:235, 1975
100. Andreasen F: Protein binding of drugs in plasma from patients with acute renal failure. Acta Pharmacol Toxicol 32:417, 1973
101. Andreasen F: The effect of dialysis on the protein binding of drugs in the plasma of patients with acute renal failure. Acta Pharmacol Toxicol 34:284, 1974
102. Reidenberg MM: The binding of drugs to plasma proteins from patients with poor renal function. Clin Pharmacokinet 1:121, 1976
103. O'Malley K, Velasco M, Pruitt A *et al*: Decreased plasma protein binding of diazoxide in uremia. Clin Pharmacol Ther 18:53, 1975
104. Hollenberg NK, Adams DF, Solomon HS *et al*: Senescence and the renal vasculature in normal man. Circ Res 34:309, 1974
105. Muravchick S: The aging patient and age related disease. ASA Annual Refresher Course Lecture #151, 1987
106. Hicks R, Dysken MW, Davis JM *et al*: The pharmacokinetics of psychotropic medication in the elderly: A review. J Clin Psychiatry 42:374, 1981
107. Thompson EN, Williams R: Effect of age on liver function with particular reference to bromosulphalein excretion. Gut 6:266, 1965
108. Castleden CM, Kaye CM, Parsons RL: The effect of age on plasma levels of propranolol and practolol in man. Br J Clin Pharmacol 2:303, 1975
109. Greenblatt DJ, Sellers EM, Shader RI: Drug disposition in old age. N Engl J Med 306:1081, 1982
110. McMartin DN, O'Connor JA, Fasco MJ *et al*: Influence of aging and induction on rat liver and kidney microsomal mixed function oxidase systems. Toxicol Appl Pharmacol 54:411, 1980
111. Baird MB, Birnbaum LS: Increased production of mutagenic metabolites of carcinogens by tissues from senescent rodents. Cancer Res 39:4752, 1979
112. Goldberg MJ, Roe F: Temperature changes during anesthesia and operations. Arch Surg 93:365, 1966
113. Collins KJ, Exton-Smith AN: Thermal homeostasis in old age. American Geriatric Society 31:519, 1983
114. Vaughn MS, Vaughn RW, Cork RC: Postoperative hypothermia in adults: Relationship of age, anesthesia and shivering to re-warming. Anesth Analg 60:746, 1981
115. Jones HB, McLaren CAB: Postoperative shivering and hypoxaemia after halothane, nitrous oxide, and oxygen anaesthesia. Br J Anaesth 37:35, 1965
116. Roe CG, Goldberg MJ, Blair CS *et al*: Influence of shivering on early post-operative oxygen consumption. Surgery 60:85, 1966
117. Bay J, Nunn JF, Prys-Roberts C: Factors influencing arterial PO$_2$ during recovery from anaesthesia. Br J Anaesth 40:398, 1968
118. Carli F, Clark MM, Woollen JW: Investigation of the relationship between heat loss and the nitrogen excretion in elderly patients undergoing major abdominal surgery under general anaesthesia. Br J Anaesth 54:1023, 1982
119. Pontoppidan H, Beecher HK: Progressive loss of protective reflexes in the airway with the advance of age. JAMA 174:2209, 1960
120. Stoelting RK, Longnecker BE, Eger EI: Minimal alveolar concentrations on awakening from methoxyflurane, halothane, ether, and fluroxene in man: MAC awake. Anesthesiology 33:5, 1970
121. Minaker KL, Meneilly GS, Rowe JW: Endocrine systems. In Finch CE, Schneider EL (eds): Handbook of the Biology of Aging, p 433. New York, Van Nostrand Reinhold, 1985
122. Robert JJ, Cummins JC, Wolfe RR *et al*: Quantitative aspects of glucose production and metabolism in healthy elderly subjects. Diabetes 31:203, 1982
123. Defronzo RA: Glucose intolerance and aging: Evidence for tissue insensitivity to insulin. Diabetes 28:1095, 1979
124. Davidson MB: The effects of aging on carbohydrate metabolism: A review of the English literature and a practical approach to the diagnosis of diabetes mellitus in the elderly. Metabolism 28:688, 1979
125. Tonino RP, Nedde WH, Robbins DC *et al*: Effect of physical training on the insulin resistance of aging. Clin Res 34:557, 1986
126. Mitenko PA: Geriatric anesthesia: Changes in drug disposition. Can J Anaesth 34:159, 1987
127. Christensen JH, Andreason F: Individual variation in response to thiopental. Acta Anaesthesiol Scand 22:303, 1978
128. Christensen JH, Andreason F, Jansen JA: Pharmacokinetics and pharmacodynamics of thiopentone: A comparison between young and elderly patients. Anaesthesia 37:398, 1982
129. Baird MB: A longitudinal study of the relationship between aging and the duration of hexobarbital hypnosis in male CFN rats. Exp Gerontol 18:47, 1983
130. Sear JW, Cooper GM, Kumar V: The effect of age on recovery. Anaesthesia 38:1158, 1983
131. Jung D, Mayersohn M, Perrier D *et al*: Thiopental disposition as a function of age in female patients undergoing surgery. Anesthesiology 56:263, 1982

132. Muravchick S: Effect of age and premedication on thiopental sleep dose. Anesthesiology 61:333, 1984

133. Reidenberg MM, Levy M, Warner H et al: Relationship between diazepam dose, plasma level, age, and central nervous system depression. Clin Pharmacol Ther 23:371, 1978

134. Kanto J, Aaltone L, Himberg JJ et al: Midazolam as an intravenous induction agent in the elderly. A clinical and pharmacokinetic study. Anesth Analg 65:15, 1986

135. Klotz U, Avant GR, Hoyumpa A et al: The effects of age and liver disease on the disposition and elimination of diazepam in adult man. J Clin Invest 55:347, 1975

136. Reves JG, Fragen RJ, Vinik HR et al: Midazolam: Pharmacology and uses. Anesthesiology 62:310, 1985

137. Greenblatt DJ, Abernathy DR, Locniskar A et al: Effect of age, gender, and obesity on midazolam kinetics. Anesthesiology 61:27, 1984

138. Stanski DR, Greenblatt DJ, Lowenstein E: Kinetics of intravenous and intramuscular morphine. Clin Pharmacol Ther 24:52, 1978

139. Mather LE, Tucker GT, Pflug AE et al: Meperidine kinetics in man: Intravenous injection in surgical patients and volunteers. Clin Pharmacol Ther 17:21, 1975

140. Bennett GM, Stanley TH: Human cardiovascular responses to endotracheal intubation during morphine-N_2O and fentanyl-N_2O anesthesia. Anesthesiology 52:520, 1980

141. Bentley JB, Borel JE, Nenad RE: Influence of age on the pharmacokinetics of fentanyl. Anesth Analg 61:171, 1982

142. Helmers H, Van Peer A, Woestenborghs R et al: Alfentanil kinetics in the elderly. Clin Pharmacol Ther 36:239, 1984

143. Scott JC, Stanski DR: Decreased fentanyl and alfentanil dose requirements with age. A simultaneous pharmacokinetic and pharmacodynamic evaluation. J Pharmacol Exp Ther 240:159, 1987

144. Merin IG, Basch S: Are the myocardial functional and metabolic effects of isoflurane really different from those of halothane and enflurane? Anesthesiology 55:398, 1981

145. Kemmosetsu O, Hasimoto Y, Shimosata S: Inotropic effects of isoflurane on mechanics of contraction in isolated cat papillary muscles from normal and failing hearts. Anesthesiology 39:470, 1973

146. Lerman J, Gregory GA, Willis MM et al: Age and solubility of volatile anesthetics in blood. Anesthesiology 61:139, 1984

147. Lerman J, Schmitt-Bantel BI, Gregory GA et al: Effect of age on the solubility of volatile anesthetics in human tissues. Anesthesiology 65:307, 1986

148. Stephens ID, Ho PC, Holloway AM et al: Pharmacokinetics of alcuronium in elderly patients undergoing total hip replacement or aortic reconstructive surgery. Br J Anaesth 56:465, 1984

149. Matteo RS, Backus WW, McDaniel ZD et al: Pharmacokinetics and pharmacodynamics of d-tubocurarine and metocurarine in the elderly. Anesth Analg 64:23, 1965

150. Dundee JW: Relationship of dosage of d-tubocurarine chloride and laudolissin to body weight, sex and age. Br J Anaesth 26:174, 1954

151. Duvaldestin P, Saada J, Berger JL et al: Pharmacokinetics, pharmacodynamics, and dose-response relationships of pancuronium in control and elderly subjects. Anesthesiology 56:36, 1982

152. Rupp SM, Fisher DM, Millers RD et al: Pharmacokinetics and pharmacodynamics of vecuronium in the elderly. Anethesiology 59:A270, 1983

153. d'Hollander AA, Nevelsteen M, Barvais L et al: Effect of age on the establishment of muscle paralysis induced in anaesthetized adult subjects by ORG NC 45. Acta Anaesthesiol Scand 27:108, 1983

154. deBros FM, Lai A, Scott R et al: Pharmacokinetics and pharmacodynamics of atracurium under isoflurane anesthesia in normal and anephric patients. Anesth Analg 64:207, 1985

155. Fahey MR, Rupp SM, Fisher DM et al: Pharmacokinetics and pharmacodynamics of atracurium in patients with and without renal failure. Anesthesiology 61:699, 1984

156. d'Hollander AA, Luyckx C, Barvais L et al: Clinical evaluation of atracurium besylate requirement for a stable muscle relaxation during surgery: Lack of age-related effects. Anesthesiology 59:237, 1983

157. Shanor SP, Van Hees GR, Baart N et al: The influence of age and sex on human plasma and red cell cholinesterase. Am J Med Sci 242:357, 1961

158. Rexed B: Contributions to the knowledge of the postnatal development of the peripheral nervous system in man. Acta Psychiatr Scand 31(Suppl):33, 1944

159. LaFratta CW, Canestrani RE: A comparison of sensory and motor nerve conduction velocities as related to age. Arch Phys Med Rehabil 47:286, 1966

160. Kirk JR, Laursen TJS: Diffusion coefficients of various solutes for human aortic tissue with special reference to variation to tissue permeability with age. J Gerontol 10:288, 1955

161. Bromage PR: Aging and epidural dose requirements. Br J Anaesth 41:1016, 1969

162. Park WY, Massengale M, Kim S et al: Age and the spread of local anesthetic solutions in the epidural space. Anesth Analg 59:768, 1980

163. Veering BT, Burm AGL, van Kleef JW et al: Epidural anesthesia with bupivacaine: Effects of age on neural blockade and pharmacokinetics. Anesth Analg 66:589, 1987

164. Finucane BT, Hammonds WD, Welch MB: Influence of age on vascular absorption of lidocaine from the epidural space. Anesth Analg 66:843, 1987

165. Clark G, Erwin D, Yate P et al: Temazepam as premedication in elderly patients. Anaesthesia 37:421, 1982

166. Berlinger WG, Goldberg MJ, Spector R et al: Diphenhydramine: Kinetics and psychomotor effects in elderly women. Clin Pharmacol Ther 32:387, 1982

167. Waller JL, Zaidan SR, Kaplan JA et al: Hemodynamic responses to preoperative vascular cannulation in patients with coronary artery disease. Anesthesiology 56:219, 1982

168. Backer CL, Tinker JH, Robertson DM et al: Myocardial reinfarction following local anesthesia for ophthalmic surgery. Anesth Analg 59:257, 1980

169. Brandt MR, Fernandes A, Mordhorst R et al: Epidural analgesia improves postoperative negative nitrogen balance. Br Med J 1:1106, 1978

170. Kehlet H: Influence of epidural analgesia on endocrine metabolic response to surgery. Acta Anaesthesiol Scand [Suppl] 70:39, 1978

171. Keith I: Anaesthesia and blood loss in total hip replacement. Anaesthesia 32:444, 1977

172. Modig J, Malmberg P: Pulmonary and circulatory reactions during total hip replacement surgery. Acta Anaesthesiol Scand 19:219, 1975

173. Davis FM, Laurenson VG: Spinal anaesthesia or general anaesthesia for emergency hip surgery in elderly patients. Anaesth Intensive Care 9:352, 1981

174. Hole A, Terjesen T, Breivik H: Epidural versus general anaesthesia for total hip arthroplasty in elderly patients. Acta Anaesthesiol Scand 24:279, 1980

175. Riis J, Lomholt B, Haxholdt O et al: Immediate and long-term mental recovery from general versus epidural anesthesia in elderly patients. Acta Anaesthesiol Scand 23:44, 1983

176. Karhunen U, Jonn G: A comparison of memory function following local and general anaesthesia for extraction of senile cataracts. Acta Anaesthesiol Scand 26:291, 1982

177. Mann RAM, Bisset WIK: Anaesthesia for lower limb amputation. Anaesthesia 38:1185, 1983

178. Berggren D, Gustafson Y, Eriksson B et al: Postoperative con-

fusion after anesthesia in elderly patients with femoral neck fractures. Anesth Analg 66:497, 1987

179. Benzon HT, Linde HW, Molloy RE *et al:* Postdural puncture headache in patients with chronic pain. Anesth Analg 59:772, 1980

180. Guttman D: Patterns of legal drug use by older Americans. Addict Behav 3:337, 1977

181. Chien CT, Townsend EJ, Ross-Townsend A: Substance use and abuse among the community elderly: The medical aspect. Addict Behav 3:357, 1978

182. Seidl LG, Thornton GF, Smith JW *et al:* Studies on the epidemiology of adverse drug reactions: III. Reactions in patients on a general medical service. Bulletin of Johns Hopkins Hospital 119:299, 1966

183. Hurwitz N: Predisposing factors in adverse reactions to drugs. Br Med J 1:536, 1969

184. Divoll M, Greenblatt DJ, Abernathy DR *et al:* Cimetidine impairs clearance of antipyrine and desmethyldiazepam in the elderly. American Geriatric Society 30:684, 1982

185. Meridy HW: Criteria for selection of ambulatory surgical patients and guidelines for anesthesia management. A retrospective study of 1553 cases. Anesth Analg 61:921, 1982

186. Natof HE: FASA Special Study I. Alexandria, VA: Federated Ambulatory Surgery Association, 1985

187. Tyler IL, Tantisira B, Winter PM *et al:* Continuous monitoring of arterial oxygen saturation with pulse oximetry during transfer to the recovery room. Anesth Analg 64:1108, 1985

Chapter 49 — Bernard V. Wetchler

Outpatient Anesthesia

The 20th century should be viewed as the time when outpatient surgery became viable, when it slowly came into acceptance, when we realized that hospitalization was not the only method of providing quality care, and when, within its last decade, we will see at least 50% of all operations performed on an outpatient basis. We no longer try to determine why this has happened; physicians and the public now accept outpatient surgery readily. There may well be a time in the not too distant future when the number of outpatient surgical procedures with which anesthesiologists are involved exceeds the number of inpatient procedures.

BACKGROUND

Many events have led us to this point:

1909: J. H. Nicoll first documented the practice of outpatient surgery when he presented to the British Medical Association the results of 8,988 operations on outpatients performed at the Glasgow Royal Hospital for Sick Children between the years 1899 and 1909.[1]

1916: R. M. Waters opened a "Down-Town Anesthesia Clinic" in Sioux City, Iowa, for minor surgery and dental cases. His was the prototype of the modern freestanding center. He stated, "When the war is over, I trust many of you may develop down-town minor surgery and dental clinics of much larger scope."[2]

1937: G. Hertzfeld reported on more than 1,000 outpatient pediatric hernia repairs performed with the use of general anesthesia.[3]

1959: Webb and Graves reported their experiences with outpatient surgery.[4]

1962: A formal outpatient surgical program was initiated at the University of California at Los Angeles.*

1966: George Washington University opened its outpatient surgical facility.†

1968: The Dudley Street Ambulatory Surgical Center opened in Providence, Rhode Island. Lacking support from the State Health Department, which considered it to be no more than a physician's office, and finding no support from third-party insurance carriers, the Dudley Street facility could not maintain itself financially.

1970: The Phoenix Surgicenter (a freestanding facility) opened in Phoenix, Arizona. Ralph Waters' message had been heard. A plaque in its lobby proclaims, "Dedicated to the principle that high quality outpatient surgical care can be provided in a caring, personal environment, in a free-standing ambulatory facility at a lower cost than other alternatives."

1974: Society for Advancement of Freestanding Ambulatory Surgical Centers (FASC) was established. It is now known as the Federated Ambulatory Surgery Association (FASA).

1983: Porterfield and Franklin advocated office outpatient surgery. Of 18,000 procedures, 5,038 were performed with the use of general anesthesia.[5]

1984: Society for Ambulatory Anesthesia (SAMBA) was organized. Outpatient anesthesia was becoming recognized as a subspecialty.

*Dillon JB: Personal communication, 1987.
†Levy M-L: Personal communication, 1987.

1985: Five hundred twenty-nine freestanding outpatient surgery centers performed 783,864 surgical operations.

1985: Hospital-affiliated ambulatory surgery accounted for 7.3 million or 34% of all operations performed within a hospital setting.

1987: There were 682 Medicare-participating, freestanding outpatient surgery centers in the United States.

SELECTION

Are lists generated by government, industry, and third-party payors of appropriate outpatient procedures being provided only to inform us that reimbursement for a given procedure may be limited or nonexistent unless the procedure is performed on an outpatient basis? Are we being deprived of our right to exercise sound, flexible medical judgment in determining the appropriateness of our patients for outpatient surgery? As we continue to gain experience in outpatient surgery, are our selection criteria becoming too liberal? All three questions can be answered with a qualified "no."

The determination of suitable patients and procedures for outpatient surgery still generates discussion more than 70 years after the reports of Nicoll and Waters. Selection of appropriate patients and procedures will limit the number of unanticipated hospitalizations after an outpatient surgical procedure.

PATIENT

The surgeon should provide the patient with information about the outpatient procedure, the type of facility in which the procedure will be performed (hospital or freestanding center), laboratory studies that will be ordered, and diet restrictions. The patient must understand that he or she will be going home on the day of surgery, must want to have surgery on an outpatient basis, and must be willing to follow instructions.[6]

Diet Restrictions

Preoperative fasting with the use of conventional guidelines (Table 49-1), even for prolonged periods (13–15 h), does not result in hypoglycemia in healthy outpatients who are 5 yr old or younger.[7] Jensen et al measured blood glucose concentrations in a group of children 6 months to 9 yr of age who were to have inpatient and outpatient anesthesia.[8] They reported only one case (1%) of hypoglycemia in an inpatient who fasted

TABLE 49-1. NPO Orders at Childrens Hospital National Medical Center (Washington, D.C.)

AGE	INTERVAL BETWEEN FEEDINGS OF SOLID FOOD*	INTERVAL BETWEEN FEEDINGS OF† CLEAR LIQUIDS
<1 yr	6 h	4 h
1–6 yr	MN	6 h
>6 yr	MN	8 h

* Includes milk or milk products.
† Includes breast milk.
(Epstein BS, Hannallah RS: The pediatric patient. In Wetchler BV [ed]: Anesthesia for Ambulatory Surgery, p 124. Philadelphia, JB Lippincott, 1985, with permission.)

overnight. Welborn et al measured the effect of preoperative fasting on 446 children, 1 month to 6 yr of age, scheduled for outpatient surgical procedures.[9] Two patients were found to by hypoglycemic at the time of induction of anesthesia: a 6-yr-old boy scheduled for afternoon surgery who had fasted for 17 h and a 15-month-old boy, also scheduled for afternoon surgery, who had fasted for 19 hours. Both patients had no symptoms. Redfern et al measured blood glucose levels immediately after induction of anesthesia in 26 children who fasted overnight for operations in the morning and 28 children who fasted from 8:00 A.M. for afternoon surgery.[10] The mean postinduction glucose concentration of the group that had afternoon surgery was significantly lower than that of the morning group. However, no child in either group was hypoglycemic. The small diurnal variation in fasting blood glucose levels in pediatric patients was similar to that found in other studies.[11, 12] Meakin et al determined the effects of decreasing the traditional period of fasting and of giving oral premedicants before anesthesia to 224 healthy children.[13] Fasting for less than 4 h increased the volume of gastric aspirate. Oral premedicants and their vehicles (capsule vs. elixir) significantly affected the increase in gastric volume. A positive correlation was noted between duration of fast and pH (the longer the fast, the more alkaline the contents) when volume of gastric contents was measured after anesthesia induction in patients scheduled for either morning or afternoon surgery.[14]

In adult patients, Maltby et al examined the effect on residual gastric fluid volume and pH of 150 ml of water taken orally between 2 and 3 h before operation with or without ranitidine.[15] Their study demonstrated that prolonged fasting did not provide a safe gastric environment and the ingestion of 150 ml of water actually reduced residual gastric volume, probably by the reflex contraction of the stomach when it was stimulated by a bolus of liquid. The addition of oral ranitidine 150 mg further reduced residual gastric volume and acidity. In a follow-up study, 2–3 h before the scheduled time of surgery, patients received the following: Group 1—coffee or orange juice 150 ml with oral ranitidine 150 mg; Group 2—coffee or orange juice 150 ml with placebo; Group 3—ranitidine 150 mg; Group 4—placebo. The effect of ranitidine on gastric volume and pH appeared to override all other variables investigated. The authors concluded that prolonged fasting appears to have no benefit in the patient having elective surgery, and they raise the question of whether "NPO after midnight" is justified.[16]

Preoperative Screening

Each outpatient facility should develop its own method of preoperative screening for a time before the day of surgery. The patient can visit the facility or staff members of the facility can call the patient by telephone. Screening allows facility staff members to obtain necessary information about the patient, including complete medical and family history, and information about medications the patient may be taking and problems the patient or his or her family may have had with anesthesia. The process also provides the staff with an opportunity to remind patients of their arrival time, clothes to wear, and restrictions (i.e., nothing to eat or drink since the previous midnight, no jewelry or makeup). Staff members can determine if there is a problem with transportation or whether there will be a responsible person who can escort the patient to and from the facility and care for the patient at home after surgery. The anesthesiologist can review the questionnaire and determine whether laboratory studies in addition to those already ordered must be completed; whether the patient's physical status is medically stable and what precautions must be taken; and whether the patient's medical or family history (problems with anesthesia) warrants an anesthesiologist's evaluation several days before surgery or if it can be done on the day of surgery. Preoperative screening provides staff members with the opportunity to reassure the patient, answer questions, and determine whether any support services are needed (*i.e.*, transportation, visiting nurse, etc.).[17]

The following are simple questions whose answers correlated with a consensus of fitness for anesthesia.[18]

1. Do you feel sick?
2. Have you had any serious illnesses?
3. Do you get more short of breath on exertion than others of your age?
4. Do you have a cough?
5. Do you have a wheeze?
6. Do you have chest pain on exertion?
7. Do you have ankle swelling?
8. Have you taken medications in the last 3 months?
9. Have you allergies?
10. Have you had an anesthetic in the past 2 months?
11. Have you or your relatives had problems with anesthesia?

Wilson *et al* concluded, "Patients who are thought to be perfectly fit on the basis of simple questions, usually prove to be so after the traditional preoperative history and investigations," and suggested that a questionnaire could be developed to aid in selecting appropriate patients for ambulatory surgery.[18] Examples of telephone screening interviews are seen in Tables 49-2 and 49-3.

Additional factors in patient acceptability include the distance the patient lives from the hospital as well as the length of time it will take to get care if problems arise. The term "reasonable," when applied to both distance and time, is not easily defined, and both these areas must be addressed by each facility on an individual patient basis.

Physical Status

Outpatient surgery is no longer restricted to patients of physical status 1 and 2. Patients of physical status 3 (or 4) are appropriate candidates if their systemic disease(s) are medi-

TABLE 49-2.   Pediatric Telephone Interview

Discussed with the Parent in a Telephone Interview for a Pediatric Patient Having Ambulatory Surgery:
1. Breath-holding spells
2. Cardiac, respiratory, or other problems
3. History of prematurity:
   If yes:
   • Was oxygen used?
   • Was the child's trachea intubated?
   • Any lasting effects?
4. Muscular problems
5. Developmental delays
6. Asthma or frequent colds
7. Sickle cell disease/trait
8. Medications
9. Recent exposure to contagious disease

(Children's Hospital National Medical Center, Washington, D.C. Wetchler BV: Patient selection criteria 1987. AORN Journal 45:30, 1987, with permission.)

TABLE 49-3.   Adult Telephone Interview

Discussed with an Adult Patient Having Ambulatory Surgery:
1. Serious past illness
2. Heart problems
3. High blood pressure
4. Chest pain
5. Asthma/emphysema
6. Allergies
7. Diabetes
8. Medications
9. Problems with anesthesia in the past
10. Possibility of pregnancy (where applicable)

(The Methodist Medical Center of Illinois Ambulatory SurgiCare, Peoria. Wetchler BV: Patient selection criteria 1987. AORN Journal 45:30, 1987, with permission.)

cally stable (*i.e.*, chronic obstructive pulmonary disease (COPD), median nerve decompression, regional anesthesia). In seeking information from the patient's primary physician, we want to know if the patient's medical problem is in optimal control; we don't want to hear "maintain blood pressure, monitor ECG, give plenty of oxygen."

Does physical status classification predict complications after an outpatient procedure? Is there a relationship between physical status and unanticipated hospitalization? In 1980 the Phoenix Surgicenter reported their overall hospital transfer rate of 0.2% increased to 0.59% for patients older than age 64 and increased to 1.41% for patients of ASA physical status 3.[19] Natof monitored the correlation of complications to patients with preexisting medical problems.[20, 21] The incidence of major complications (1.12%) in patients with no preexisting disease was comparable to the incidence of major complications (1.16%) in patients having preexisting disease.

In a study encompassing a total of 87,492 patients, FASA concluded the following: Certain surgical procedures have a higher established incidence of complication; there appeared to be little or no cause-and-effect relationship between preexisting disease and the incidence of complication; the longer a patient was in the operating room, the higher the incidence of complication.[22] With the exception of patients having preexisting coronary artery disease, the reason for admission among patients with medical disease was unrelated to their underlying medical problems.* In a 5-year period (1981–1985), Methodist Ambulatory SurgiCare noted an unanticipated admission rate of 1.1% for patients older than 60 compared with an overall unanticipated admission rate of 0.8%. For patients older than age 60 receiving inhalation anesthesia, the admission rate was 4.1% compared with the 1.5% admission rate for all patients receiving inhalation anesthesia.[23]

Geriatric

The acceptability of the very old and the very young for an outpatient surgical procedure is well documented. For the geriatric patient, chronologic age is not a deterrent. The modifying factors in determining the acceptability of a geriatric patient for outpatient surgery are physiologic age, physical status, surgical procedure, anesthetic technique, and quality of care provided at home.[23]

More than half of hospitalized geriatric patients experience some transient confusional state after operation.[24] Because of a

*Gold BS: Personal communication, 1987.

quicker return to normal surroundings, as well as a significant decrease in the number of medications the patient will be subjected to during a shorter stay in the outpatient facility, this high incidence is decreased when elderly patients are managed on an outpatient basis. The older patient is less able to cope with a new environment and frequently has fewer psychologic and physiologic defenses for coping with stress. It is important that the staff members actively try to engage and relate to the geriatric patient.

The geriatric patient has more numerous and totally different problems than do younger patients. Elderly patients show significantly poorer comprehension of consent information. They must be treated with gentle patience; they should not be rushed or made to feel as though they are keeping everyone waiting.

Pediatric

Infants considered at risk are best handled as inpatients. An infant presenting with a hemoglobin or hematrocrit level below the low limits of normal for its particular age group is at risk and needs further medical workup before one proceeds with an elective anesthetic. If an infant with a history of respiratory distress syndrome (RDS) was intubated and required ventilatory support, it may take up to a year to outgrow symptoms and have normal blood gases. If bronchopulmonary dysplasia (BPD) developed in the patient, the at-risk period extends until the patient has no symptoms. The patient with BPD is more likely to die of sudden infant death syndrome (SIDS). A history of prematurity, apnea, or aspiration with feeding places the infant at risk. Should we consider an infant at risk if a sibling has died of SIDS? When one is faced with this situation, a prudent decision would be to monitor the infant for apnea on an inpatient basis for 24 h after surgery.[17]

When is the infant who was born prematurely considered acceptable for outpatient surgery? Several studies have documented an increased incidence of apnea in ex-premature infants for 12 h after anesthesia. Steward found preterm infants of less than 10 weeks postnatal age had apnea develop during anesthesia and up to 12 h after operation, compared with no incidence of apnea in full-term infants.[25] Liu et al discovered an increased incidence of apneic episodes after anesthesia in preterm infants younger than 41–46 weeks postconceptual age.[26] Kurth et al suggested postoperative apnea monitoring (12–24 h) in patients younger than 60 weeks postconceptual age.[27] Welborn et al studied infants younger than 12 months postnatal age having general anesthesia for herniorrhaphy.[28] Premature infants younger than 44 weeks postconceptual age were found to be at high risk for development of postoperative ventilatory dysfunction. They concluded that it is probably best to delay nonessential surgery for preterm infants until they are older than 44 weeks postconceptual age; herniorrhaphy can be performed safely on an outpatient basis in infants older than 44 weeks postconceptual age who do not have major cardiac, neurologic, endocrine, or metabolic diseases.

Although there is no universal agreement as to what constitutes an acceptable postconceptual age (gestation plus postnatal age) for the outpatient infant who was born prematurely, it is agreed that caution must be exercised before he or she is considered acceptable for an ambulatory surgical procedure.

Inappropriate Patient

There are no published guidelines and few data to categorize the inappropriate ambulatory surgery patient. In almost every instance we must individualize; with few exceptions, we must address a combination of the following factors: the patient, surgical procedure, anesthetic technique, and anesthesiologists' comfort level. At Methodist Ambulatory SurgiCare, we have established medical and social reasons that classify a patient as inappropriate. Patients who present with abnormal laboratory values that may cause postponement are viewed as a separate entity.

I. Medical
  A. The infant at risk.
    1. A healthy infant who was born prematurely and is younger than 45 weeks postconceptual age is unacceptable.
    2. An infant still experiencing apneic episodes, difficulty with feeding, displays difficulty with growth and development (failure to thrive) is unacceptable.
    3. An infant who had RDS and was intubated and on ventilatory support: The infant should have no wheezing or bronchospasm at the time of surgery. It may take 6 months or more before the infant has no symptoms and can have surgery. Obtaining blood gases as an indicator of being asymptomatic is an individual preference (Children's Hospital National Medical Center in Washington, D.C., does not routinely check blood gases*). There should have been no recent or recurrent episodes (previous 2–3 months) of wheezing, bronchospasm, or apnea, and no wheezing or bronchospasm that are not precipitated by upper respiratory infection (URI). It should be considered whether the infant manages well if a URI develops. The patient should be symptom free at the time of surgery and when discharged from the facility (no wheezing).* Pulse oximetry may be a useful indicator of patient's status in the postanesthesia care unit (PACU).
    4. An infant in whom BPD developed: The patient must be symptom free before surgery and when discharged from the facility. Again, drawing of blood for blood gases is an individual decision. The infant who had BPD has an increased incidence of SIDS.
    5. An infant with a family history (sibling) of SIDS is not an acceptable candidate when younger than 6 months (with a more conservative approach, possibly up to 1 yr of age).
  B. Patients with malignant hyperthermia (MH) or who are susceptible to malignant hyperthermia (MHS). Most facilities take the position that an MHS patient requires overnight observation. Observation usually involves a 24-h stay, but this time period has not been substantiated by specific data. Overnight hospitalization is indicated if MH is documented or there is a history of MHS with concomitant evidence of skeletal muscle disease. When a patient has only a history (masseter spasm or an MHS episode in the family), some facilities administer a trigger-free anesthetic, watch the patient for 6–8 h, and consider discharge that evening.
  C. Patient with uncontrolled seizure activity. Patients with uncontrolled seizure activity are considered inappropriate by some; however other facilities do not consider this an absolute contraindication (patient is observed for 4–8 h and may be sent home if seizure free).
  D. Medically unstable ASA physical status 3 (or 4) patient.
  E. Morbidly obese patient with other systemic diseases.

*Hannallah RS: Personal communication, 1987.

The obese patient is acceptable if there is no systemic disease that would cause a patient to be classified as physical status 3.[29]
F. Patient being treated with monoamine oxidase (MAO) inhibitors. The patient must have stopped taking medication for 2 weeks. The need for this has been questioned.[30]
G. Acute substance abuse.

II. Social
A. Uncooperative patient.
1. Patient refuses to have procedure done as an outpatient
2. Patient is unwilling to follow instructions
B. No responsible person at home.

PROCEDURE

Parameters established in the early 1970s for procedure selection included the following: The procedure should take less than 90 min; risk of postoperative complications should be reliably low; transfusion should not be anticipated; and the surgeon should be skillful and speedy because outpatient procedures do not lend themselves to resident teaching or performance by a trainee.[31] Are these parameters still appropriate today? Prohibition relating to duration of surgery no longer appears warranted, particularly because the relationship between anesthesia time and recovery time is weak. The length of time for a procedure is a consideration, but one must also look at many variables (*i.e.*, the patient's physical status, the surgeon's ability, whether the procedure is superficial or deep, the type of anesthesia, whether there will be local anesthesia supplementation of inhalation technique).

We should still be interested in performing procedures with reliably low postoperative complications. However, today's definition of a reliably low incidence of postoperative complications appears to depend upon the relative aggressiveness of the facility, surgeon, patient, and payor, as we hear of cholecystectomy, vaginal hysterectomy, reduction mammoplasty, and open arthrotomy with ligament repair being performed on an outpatient basis.

The potential need for a transfusion is no longer an absolute contraindication to outpatient procedure acceptability; autologous blood transfusion is being used in a small percentage of patients having extensive liposuction procedures.*

When it was stated that procedures should take less than 90 min, it was with the belief that skillful and speedy surgeons were essential to the success of a same-day procedure and there was no time for resident training. Today, more than 7 million outpatient surgical procedures are performed each year by qualified surgeons and residents in training.

Three statements can serve as the basis of procedure acceptability as we approach the 21st century:

1. Procedures cannot stand alone as to their acceptability. The procedure cannot be separated from the patient having the procedure. Pediatric inguinal hernia surgery is a good example; it is a perfectly acceptable procedure for outpatient surgery, but one must be aware of the high-risk patient. This is a good reason why procedure lists cannot be allowed to undermine medical judgment.[32]
2. Dawson and Reed stated: "Any procedure which does

*Reed WA: Personal communication, 1987.

not require a major intervention in the cranial vault, abdomen or thorax can be considered acceptable."[19]
3. Orkin wrote: "The actual list of acceptable procedures in a given ambulatory unit is established in an evolutionary process . . . . On a daily basis, the medical director of the unit must decide which procedures (and which patients) are appropriate for the unit, given its equipment, staff and their capabilities, ability and reliability of the given surgeon and medical condition of the particular patient."[33]

FACILITY

Outpatient surgery occurs in a variety of settings, both within the confines of the hospital and in freestanding facilities. Should we look at the appropriateness of the facility, as well as patient and procedure, as we establish our selection process? Outpatient surgery has matured to a level where we should address whether a facility attached to or within a hospital can be more liberal in its selection process compared with a freestanding facility because of the ease with which a patient can be transferred to a hosptial bed if the need arises. Some believe that hospital facilities can be more liberal in their selection process than can freestanding facilities because of the ease of consultation as well as of obtaining inpatient services should the need arise.

ANESTHESIA MANAGEMENT

Standaert stated that "Everyone involved with therapeutic agents, patient, physician, medicinal chemist, wants a magic bullet, a drug that does exactly what is expected of it and does nothing else."[34] As we continue our search for the magic bullet, we should keep those drugs that are useful and cast aside those with adverse effects; this is also how it should be with the drugs we use in outpatient anesthesia.

PREMEDICATION

Although preoperative medication is discussed in Chapter 18, there are special considerations that anesthesiologists should be aware of when managing the outpatient. Outpatient surgery and outpatient anesthesia are a break from tradition; this is also so with outpatient premedication. We must tailor both our psychologic and pharmacologic preparation to be a part of the compacted perioperative care the outpatient receives. We should use medications, dosages, and routes of administration that are practical and do not prolong length of stay in the postanesthesia care unit.

Meridy found that the use of premedicants other than opioids did not prolong recovery.[35] Premedication had a marginal effect on recovery time, with patients given opioids (morphine, meperidine) having a significantly longer recovery time than nonmedicated patients (Table 49-4).

Preanesthesia medication is based on tradition, which is influenced by one's training, clinical experience, and inpatient medication routine. When an outpatient is managed, tradition dictates the use of no or limited premedication. Is this appropriate today? Can we modify our choice of drugs, doses, and routes of administration to limit the outpatients' apprehension without significantly increasing length of stay? Can new drugs supplant old favorites?

In 1967, Dillon stated, "We find that a great deal of premed-

TABLE 49-4.   Relationship Between Premedication Received by 1,553 Patients and Recovery Time

TYPE	NO.	RECOVERY TIME (min)*
No premedication	1,015	179 ± 113
Diazepam	98	168 ± 104
Pentobarbital	25	231 ± 88
Opioids (meperidine and morphine)	388	208 ± 101†
Hydroxyzine	92	192 ± 120

* Values are means ± SD.
† Differs significantly from patients not receiving any premedication ($P < 0.001$).
(Meridy HW: Criteria for selection of ambulatory surgical patients and guidelines for anesthetic management: A retrospective study of 1553 cases. Anesth Analg 61:921, 1982, with permission.)

ication is unnecessary. We frequently give our premedication intravenously, which assures its prompt action in a predictable time and in a predictable manner."[36]

In 1974, Epstein stated, "Minimal or no premedication is advisable. All physicians recognize that the greater the dose and the more long-acting the depressant medication, the greater the chance of prolongation of recovery and coincident drowsiness, dizziness, hypotension, or vomiting. At George Washington University Hospital no premedication is used. In some centers only belladonna drugs are administered."[31]

According to Reed, "heavy, long-lasting premedication, an additional 100 mg to 200 mg of barbiturate, or extra depth with an inhalation drug may cause no deleterious effect in the healthy patient. The resulting increase in recovery time, however, will have an unfavorable impact on the surgical outpatient who would otherwise safely ambulate; it could even create an anesthetic inpatient out of what was meant to be an outpatient surgical procedure."[37]

Levy and Weintraub stated that the outpatient is frequently more apprehensive about the anesthetic, which is perceived as major, compared with "minor surgery," which is thought to be non–life-threatening.[38] They recommended that the anesthesiologist have a frank discussion with the patient and explain the anesthetic, monitoring, and after-effects of anesthesia and surgery to help relieve patient apprehension.

During the preanesthesia interview, the intelligent, well-informed patient will understand and accept the rationale of foregoing traditional methods of providing premedication.

Patient apprehension can be minimized by:

Limited waiting time before surgery
An attractive waiting room with reading materials and television
Games for children
Limited separation time from family or friends
The change to hospital gown as close to the time of surgery as possible

The outpatient wants to maintain an active role in his or her own health care. In an outpatient environment, we are not providing care for the ill, hospitalized patient; wellness should be promoted. The philosophy of outpatient surgery should promote the patient's self-image as that of an otherwise healthy, intact, socially active person with special needs.[39]

The routine of using little or no premedication is advisable.[19, 31] However, others believe the patients' time in the

holding unit can be made more pleasant with the use of premedicant drugs.[40, 41] Premedicant drugs may be used if needed by the patient and if drug and dosage are chosen carefully. Drugs used as premedicants for outpatients include anticholinergics, H_2 receptor antagonists and antacids, opioids, sedative–hypnotics, and gastrokinetics.

Anticholinergics

Tradition dictates the use of anticholinergic drugs as a part of preanesthetic medication for their antisialogogue and vagolytic actions. More satisfactory conditions during inhalation anesthesia resulting from decreased secretions are likely when an anticholinergic is administered as a premedicant, particularly when an endotracheal tube is in place.[42]

Currently used inhalation drugs are considerably less irritating than anesthetics used earlier (diethyl ether), and routine anticholinergic premedication is not needed for the outpatient. Furthermore, drying of mucous membranes by anticholinergics can contribute to postoperative sore throat and complaints of dry mouth.[40] Elderly patients have decreased salivary gland production and do not need antisialogogues. The blocking of vagal reflexes requires larger doses than those given during premedication. Vagal reflexes are best treated by intravenous administration of an appropriate anticholinergic if and when they occur. Glycopyrrolate may have limited use for short outpatient procedures because of its more prolonged and intense drying effect compared with that of atropine.[43]

Clarke and Hurtig found a combination of meperidine (1 $mg \cdot kg^{-1}$) and atropine (0.01 $mg \cdot kg^{-1}$), given intramuscularly as a premedicant, did not prolong recovery in an outpatient population.[40]

For the pediatric outpatient, oral diazepam (0.1 $mg \cdot kg^{-1}$), hydroxyzine (0.5 $mg \cdot kg^{-1}$), or a combination of diazepam (0.2 $mg \cdot kg^{-1}$), meperidine (1.5 $mg \cdot kg^{-1}$), and atropine (0.02 $mg \cdot kg^{-1}$) did not prolong recovery in pediatric outpatients.[44, 45]

H_2 Receptor Antagonists and Antacids

Outpatients and inpatients have the potential for aspiration pneumonitis. This potential is increased in patients who are obese or pregnant (second and third trimesters), have peptic ulceration, hiatal hernia or diabetes mellitus, or have had upper abdominal procedures. The Trendelenberg and prone positions and fasciculation after use of succinylcholine may increase regurgitation.[46]

Does the outpatient have greater potential for acid aspiration than the inpatient? With risk potential considered as a pH less than 2.5 and a gastric volume greater than 25 ml, Ong et al found pH values to be similar in both groups, but 86% of outpatients had volumes greater than 0.4 $ml \cdot kg^{-1}$ compared with only 57% of inpatients.[47] Although an initial study did not find an increased potential for aspiration in outpatients, a more recent study by Manchikanti and Roush reported a significant number of outpatients to have a decreased pH and an increased gastric volume.[48, 49] Wyner and Cohen found no significant difference in residual gastric volume between pregnant (mean gestational age 15 ± 3 weeks) and nonpregnant outpatients at induction of anesthesia.[50]

There is an increased risk for aspiration in patients having emergency surgery. In a computer-assisted study of 185,358 anesthetics, 87 cases of aspiration were identified; frequency of aspiration was six times higher during the night than during the day.[51]

In a multicenter (181 outpatient facilities) study, there were 90 documented cases of aspiration (1.7 per 10,000).* Of 266 suspected cases during the past decade reported by the survey respondents, 54.1% required hospital admission and 27.4% were hospitalized more than 1 day; there were no reported deaths. Natof prospectively reviewed the cases of 32,001 outpatients after their surgical procedures, finding only one case of suspected aspiration and no deaths.[52]

Of the various drug therapies suggested, suspension antacids are no longer recommended because they may cause significant pulmonary damage if aspirated. Antacids reduce gastric acidity but they also increase gastric fluid volume. Martin et al studied the effects of oral Bicitra and intramuscular cimetidine in patients having outpatient breast biopsy.† The potential for aspiration pneumonitis was as follows: control 80% (pH 1.68 ± 0.30, volume 44.67 ± 14.1 ml); Bicitra 26% (pH 3.20 ± 1.00, volume 61.80 ± 25.4 ml); cimetidine 0% (pH 6.3 ± 1.06, volume 12.33 ± 8.5 ml). In this study, Bicitra (15 ml) was administered orally 15 min before induction and cimetidine (300 mg) was administered intramuscularly 30 min before induction of anesthesia.

Oral administration of cimetidine (300 mg) 1–4 h before anesthesia induction resulted in a pH greater than 2.5 in 84% of patients and a gastric volume less than 20 ml in 88% of patients.[48] Glycopyrrolate alone had no effect on volume or acidity, and the addition of glycopyrrolate to cimetidine added no protective effect. Despite convincing evidence that cimetidine increases gastric fluid pH, there are no data to demonstrate that there will be no pulmonary damage if gastric contents are inhaled by patients pretreated with cimetidine or that the use of cimetidine reduces anesthetic mortality from aspiration.[53, 54] Oral administration of ranitidine (150 mg) the evening before and the morning of surgery decreased the incidence of risk from 47 to 0% for outpatients.[55] An oral regimen of either ranitidine 150 mg, cimetidine 400 mg, or placebo approximately 5 h before induction of anesthesia showed both H2 blockers to be significantly better than placebo at reducing gastric acidity and volume. Potential for acid aspiration in the group treated with placebo was 100%, cimetidine 46%, and ranitidine 15%.[56] Oral ranitidine appears to be as effective as oral cimetidine in reducing the number of patients with potential for aspiration pneumonitis without the side-effects and adverse drug interactions associated with cimetidine.[57, 58]

Somori and Kallar administered cimetidine syrup orally (7.5 mg·kg^{-1}) to pediatric outpatients 1 h before surgery.[59] Cimetidine-treated patients had a pH of 5.06 ± 0.35 and a volume of 4.5 ml ± 0.35; the control group had a pH of 1.55 ± 0.09 and volume of 9.5 ml ± 2.00. When ranitidine (2.0 mg·kg^{-1}) was administered orally 1 h before surgery, patients had a pH of 5.1 ± 0.5 and a volume of 0.10 ml·kg^{-1} ± 0.05. A control group had a pH of 2.0 ± 0.3 and a volume of 0.31 ml·kg^{-1} ± 0.07.[60] Oral administration of sodium citrate 0.4 ml·kg^{-1} to pediatric patients 30 min before induction of anesthesia was equally as effective as oral administration of cimetidine (10 mg·kg^{-1}) 60 min before induction of anesthesia in increasing gastric pH.[61]

Both ranitidine and cimetidine appear to be effective agents for reducing the incidence of patient potential for aspiration pneumonitis. Ranitidine can be considered slightly superior to cimetidine because of its longer duration of action.

Cohen et al did not find any significant antiemetic effect when metoclopramide was administered to outpatients.[62] Rao

*Kallar SK, Keenan RL: Personal communication, 1987.
†Martin C, Kallar SK, Ciresi S: Personal communication, 1984.

et al froound that outpatients who received the combination of a 300-mg cimetidine tablet and a 10-mg metoclopramide tablet with 20 ml of water 2 h before induction had both a significantly lower gastric volume and a significantly higher pH than those who received cimetidine alone or metoclopramide alone or the patients in the control group.[63]

Alka Seltzer Effervescent (two tablets dissolved in 20 ml of water), a non–aspirin-containing preparation will increase gastric pH as well as, if not better than, magnesium trisilicate or sodium citrate. The solution should not be administered until all effervescence has ceased.[64]

Antacids, anticholinergics, gastrokinetics, and H2 blocking drugs have been used to limit the potential for aspiration pneumonitis in the outpatient. The use of any of these drugs individually or in combination does not eliminate the need for careful anesthetic technique to protect the airway during induction, maintenance, and emergence from anesthesia.

Opioids

Long-acting opioids such as meperidine and morphine are not recommended for premedication in outpatients.[35] In comparing the use of fentanyl 1.5 μg·kg^{-1} intravenously and meperidine 1 mg·kg^{-1} intravenously 2–5 min before induction for outpatient dilatation and extraction, White and Chang found recovery times decreased by opioid premedication because of the decreased requirement of intravenous induction agent.[65] Neither drug significantly increased the incidence of postanesthetic side-effects. Although the use of opioid premedication in its traditional form has been questioned, opioid premedication just before anesthesia induction can be advantageous in the outpatient setting.

Epstein et al evaluated a group of patients having voluntary interruption of pregnancy or dilatation and currettage (D&C).[66] Patients were given thiopental, nitrous oxide, oxygen, or thiopental, nitrous oxide, oxygen with supplemental fentanyl. Fentanyl-treated patients recovered statistically earlier than those who did not receive opioid premedication. Hunt added a single dose of fentanyl (75–125 μg) intravenously immediately before induction of anesthesia in a group of outpatients.[67] The addition of fentanyl significantly reduced the frequency of pain in the PACU and during the first evening at home. In outpatients having suction termination of pregnancy, Sanders et al found that patients receiving alfentanil as a supplement to their intravenous inhalation anesthesia recovered statistically earlier than those receiving intravenous inhalation anesthesia alone.[68]

Pandit and Kothary compared the use of equianalgesic intravenous premedicant doses of morphine, meperidine, fentanyl, and sufentanil with normal saline, administered 15–30 min before induction, for their effects on anxiety, sedation, ease of anesthetic induction and maintenance, requirement for postoperative analgesic, recovery time, and frequency of side-effects.[69] Opioid premedication generally provided more satisfactory induction and maintenance compared with placebo premedication. Opioid premedication did not prolong recovery time significantly; incidence of side-effects in the PACU was comparable in all groups (Table 49-5).

Sedative–Hypnotics

Diazepam, lorazepam, and midazolam are the currently available benzodiazepines; lorazepam and diazepam are available in oral preparation. The duration of action of lorazepam is too long for it to be useful for the ambulatory surgical patient, and when it is given parenterally it can produce prolonged amne-

TABLE 49-5.   Recovery Time (min)

PREMEDICANT	ORIENTATION	AMBULATION	DISCHARGE
Morphine	21.4 ± 6.63	148.4 ± 49.33	210.3 ± 65.84
Meperidine	19.2 ± 6.54	135.2 ± 30.02	187.0 ± 50.87
Fentanyl	19.9 ± 7.41	145.8 ± 51.73	187.9 ± 67.73
Sufentanil	19.7 ± 8.19	134.2 ± 44.05	181.5 ± 62.01
Placebo	20.2 ± 7.69	156.0 ± 54.04	200.0 ± 69.12

ANOVA—No significant differences between groups.
(Pandit SK, Kothary SP: Should we premedicate ambulatory surgical patients? Anesthesiology 65:A352, 1986, with permission.)

sia for 6 to 8 h. Because of its prolonged sedative and amnesic effect, lorazepam should not be used by any route to premedicate the outpatient.

In the nonpremedicated outpatient, the incidence of awareness after general anesthesia has been reported to be as high as 9%.[41] Epstein found that diazepam 0.15 mg·kg^{-1} (up to a total dose of 5 mg), given intravenously 2–3 min before induction of anesthesia, significantly reduced the incidence of awareness experienced with a balanced anesthetic technique for laparoscopy.* Without diazepam, 4.9% of patients could recall conversation, 2.1% extubation of the trachea, and 0.7% pain. Oral administration of diazepam (0.25 mg·kg^{-1}) significantly decreased preoperative discomfort and apprehension without extending length of stay for outpatients having a variety of surgical procedures.[70] Jansen et al objectively measured postural stability after oral diazepam premedication (0.2 mg·kg^{-1}). Because patients demonstrated a decreased stability with a tendency for falling, the authors believed patients should not be allowed to walk after administration of this premedication dose.[71]

Other benzodiazepines were tried as oral premedicants for outpatients. Temazepam, 20 mg, 1 h before surgery resulted in satisfactory sedation and anxiolysis in outpatients.[72] Recovery was more rapid than that found after use of diazepam 10 mg.[73]

Intramuscular midazolam is a satisfactory premedicant in both adult and pediatric outpatients. Fragen et al compared the effects of midazolam (0.08 mg·kg^{-1}) and hydroxyzine (1.5 mg·kg^{-1}) as intramuscular premedicants.[74] Midazolam produced quicker onset of action, greater anxiolysis for the first hour, greater amnesia, less local irritation, and a higher overall rating by the patients. Drowsiness, while also greater after administration of midazolam, was neither significant nor prolonged. When midazolam was given intramuscularly, sedative effects were seen within 15 min but started to wear off between 60 to 90 min after injection. In comparing midazolam (0.07 mg·kg^{-1}) or hydroxyzine (1.0 mg·kg^{-1}) with a placebo, Vinik et al found midazolam and hydroxyzine reduced anxiety more significantly than did the placebo, with peak onset appearing between 30 to 60 min after drug administration in both groups.[75] There was significantly less evidence of tissue irritation at the injection site in the midazolam-treated patients compared with the hydroxyzine-treated patients. Rita et al compared intramuscular midazolam premedication (starting with 0.04 mg·kg^{-1} and increasing at 0.01 mg·kg^{-1} increments until a dose of 0.1 mg·kg^{-1} was reached) in a wide dosage range for pediatric patients.[76] The 0.08 mg·kg^{-1} dose produced the highest percentage of drowsy or sleeping pa-

*Epstein BS: Personal communication, 1982.

tients in the holding area, smooth induction of anesthesia, calm awakening in the PACU and overall satisfactory ratings from anesthesia staff. All children appeared drowsy within 15 min of receiving the intramuscular injection; the degree and duration of drowsiness were dose dependent. Experience with midazolam as an oral premedicant (oral route of administration is not approved by the Food and Drug Administration) has been limited to outside the United States.

Hydroxyzine, a nonphenothiazine (antihistamine) tranquilizer, does not prolong recovery from anesthesia. In addition to its sedative effects, it has antihistaminic, antiemetic, and antisialagogic effects.

Careful use and appropriate timing of administration of sedative hypnotics and analgesic premedications in outpatients can relieve anxiety without prolonging a patient's length of stay in the PACU.

TECHNIQUES AND DRUGS

Anesthetic techniques and drugs are discussed fully in other chapters within this book. The sections that follow, on regional, conscious sedation, injectable, and inhalation anesthesia, will be discussed only from the perspective of how they impact upon or apply directly to the outpatient.

Regional

Local and regional anesthesia have long been used for ambulatory surgery; at the University of California, Los Angeles, during 1963 and 1964, 56% of ambulatory procedures were performed with the use of these techniques.[77] Mulroy believes that successful outpatient anesthesia depends upon four postanesthesia and postsurgical requirements: alertness, ambulation, analgesia, and alimentation.[78] Although regional anesthetic techniques have a reputation for prolonged induction time and delay in recovery, these techniques can offer significant advantages for outpatients. Additional time needed to perform many regional blocks, as well as time to allow the anesthetic to take effect, is a potential drawback when procedures are short and turnover time between cases usually is rapid. Use of a regional technique that requires more time than the procedure itself (i.e., epidural for dilatation and curettage) should be limited to situations in which it is the indicated technique for the patient. Meridy and Bridenbaugh and Soderstrom found significantly shorter recovery times after local and regional anesthesia compared with general anesthesia.[35, 79]

If use of regional anesthesia is contemplated, it is important that the surgeon be aware of this because he or she must encourage the patient in use of the regional technique. Of 116 appropriately chosen patients who received good preoperative instructions, 98% could complete their laparoscopic examination while under local anesthesia.[80] When preanesthesia education and premedication are often limited, anxiety may be a major drawback to performing a regional anesthetic technique. Small doses of short-acting sedative drugs can be used to overcome simple anxieties without prolonging PACU stay after the procedure. A satisfactory outpatient regional anesthesia experience depends upon appropriate selection of the patient, sedatives, local anesthetics, and specific regional technique and also upon the anesthesiologist's skill.

Sedatives must be selected carefully, whether they are used for premedication or intraanesthetic sedation. Small doses of short-acting drugs should be used.[81] Midazolam is an excellent sedative for the moderately anxious patient; it is a superior choice to diazepam because of its shorter duration of action and lack of venous irritation.[82, 83] The amnesia it produces does not correlate with the apparent level of sedation; fully conscious patients may have no awareness of perianesthetic events. "Awake" patients have completely failed to recall talking to the surgeon or anesthesiologist during the operation.[84]

The analgesic properties of a short-acting opioid (i.e., fentanyl, alfentanil) are especially useful if paresthesias are sought during a regional technique, when obtundation is undesirable. Either of these opioid analgesics can be combined with midazolam (adding potential for amnesia) and allow excellent cooperation with blocks.[78] The combination must be used carefully to avoid oversedation, which blunts or delays the response to paresthesia.

Verbal reassurance and explanation should continue throughout the operation; thereby, the need for supplemental medications will be decreased. Philip and Covino frequently used music through headphones to supplement regional anesthesia, asking the patient to bring in tapes of preferred music.[85]

Although inpatient regional anesthesia may require the longest possible local anesthetic block to provide postoperative analgesia, outpatient surgery necessitates careful selection of shorter-acting agents (i.e., chloroprocaine or lidocaine) for most blocks, particularly for those cases starting late in the day.[78] Reliance on local wound infiltration with long-acting local anesthetic will provide prolonged postoperative analgesia.

Certain block techniques in themselves may be inappropriate in an outpatient setting: sciatic–femoral block may delay discharge because of prolonged loss of motor strength and coordination in the affected lower extremity; supraclavicular or intrascalene brachial plexus block may be contraindicated because of a potential for pneumothorax; spinal anesthesia may be relatively contraindicated because of the potential for postdural puncture headache after discharge. For example, this would pose a disadvantage for patients living a great distance from the hospital or contemplating air travel shortly after surgery.[86]

When a hand or foot is still numb after a peripheral nerve block and the patient is ready for discharge, the patient must be carefully instructed on care of the extremity and warned that there is no normal sensation that protects against injury. The patient should be reassured that sensation will return after discharge and that it is not a problem to be concerned about.

Lumbar epidural anesthesia is suitable for pelvic, lower abdominal, and lower extremity surgery. Epidural anesthesia may delay a patient's ability to walk because of motor block of the legs, however, the use of a short-acting local anesthetic in a continuous catheter technique will reduce this problem to a minimum while it allows the duration of anesthesia to match the sometimes unpredictable duration of surgery. At the Mason Clinic, epidural anesthesia is administered to 50% of patients having a laparoscopic procedure.[78] In a series of patients receiving lumbar epidural compared with general anesthesia for laparoscopy, the incidence of nausea and vomiting was reduced from 38% (general) to 4% (epidural).[79] Mulroy states that not all patients having laparoscopic procedures are suitable for epidural block.[78] Some are limited by anxiety about the procedure, whereas others cannot tolerate the respiratory compromise of abdominal distention in the head-down position. When epidural anesthesia is used for laparoscopic examination, the patient should be forewarned that she may experience shoulder pain. This referred diaphragmatic irrita-

tion can be minimized by appropriate explanation and sedation.

For the outpatient, spinal anesthesia is superior to an epidural technique for lower extremity and perianal surgery because of the absence of sacral nerve root sparing. Use of longer acting agents such as tetracaine is best avoided because of prolonged recovery time and a greater potential for urinary retention.

Major concerns have been expressed regarding postdural puncture headache in outpatients, but we know of no evidence that its incidence is likely to be increased by allowing a patient who has recovered from a spinal block to return home on the same day.[87, 88] Bedrest does not reduce the frequency of headache.[89–91] With good technique, appropriate choice of needle (25 or 26 gauge), and direction of bevel, the incidence of PDPH should be less than 2% in most outpatient facilities.[92] The patient should be advised to avoid straining at home and to maintain good oral fluid intake. If a headache occurs, it can be readily treated on an outpatient basis with an epidural blood patch. Cohen instructs the patient to rest quietly for 1 h after injection of 10 ml of blood before being discharged.[93] Electrolyte infusion is not started before the procedure nor is the patient encouraged to drink large quantities of fluid afterward; this does little to increase cerebrospinal fluid production, "while necessitating multiple, uncomfortable expeditions to urinate."[93]

Conscious Sedation

Conscious sedation is an art not easily learned.[94] Originally developed by dentists and oral surgeons as a part of their office practice, conscious sedation is quickly becoming an important technique in our outpatient anesthesia armamentarium. As defined by the American Dental Association Council on Dental Education, use of conscious sedation emphasizes that the patient must be able to respond rationally to commands and to maintain his or her own airway patency.[95] Shane described his "intravenous amnesia" technique, using a combination of opioid, anticholinergic, ataractic, and barbiturate medications in small incremental doses.[94, 96] The term "conscious sedation," first used by Bennett, described the administration of intravenous agents as supplements to regional and local anesthetics, which minimally depressed consciousness while protective reflexes were maintained intact.[97] The challenge is selection of appropriate drugs and titration of appropriate doses.

The numbers and types of outpatient cases that are being managed with varying drug and dosage modifications of this technique are increasing rapidly. At the Medical College of Virginia Ambulatory Surgery Center, conscious sedation was used in more than 5,000 outpatient procedures from 1981–1986 to supplement local or regional anesthesia for removal of external skeletal fixation, removal of percutaneous Kirschner wire, excision of Morton's neuroma, laser coninization of the cervix, cervical dilatation and evacuation of the uterus, diagnostic dilatation and currettage, myringotomy with tube insertion in adults, laparoscopic tubal sterilization, knee arthroscopic examination (in selected patients), breast biopsy, and a variety of plastic surgical procedures.[98]

During conscious sedation, the anesthesiologist primarily concentrates on monitoring patient awareness or level of consciousness, speaking to the patient frequently, being reassuring, responding to any evidence of distress or discomfort, and warning of stimulating events about to take place (i.e., injection of local anesthetic, insertion of laparoscope, inflation of tourniquet). The expected event will be less stimulating than when the same event is not announced. Patient responsiveness can best be evaluated by his or her ability to obey frequent simple commands that do not require verbal response (*i.e.*, take a deep breath). Verbal response by the patient requires a higher general level of arousal than a mere nod or finger movement or the passive obeying of a command.[97]

The use of digital pulse oximetry is an objective means of assessing oxygenation during conscious sedation and has become standard practice in many institutions for all outpatients. Kallar *et al* found transient but significant hypoxia (Sa$_{O_2}$ less than 90% by digital pulse oximetry) in 28% of patients having elective termination of pregnancy, but no significant clinical sequelae were observed.[99] There were no deaths or serious complications reported when conscious sedation was used during a 6-yr period at the Medical College of Virginia Ambulatory Surgery Center.*

Ceravolo *et al* reported no major complications in 10,000 patients having periodontal surgery with conscious sedation over an 11-yr period.[100, 101] Minor complications included mild, transient phlebitis (4.1%), nausea with or without vomiting (0.37%), and dysphoric reactions (0.42%). Shane *et al* reviewed 10,500 cases during a 7-yr period with a similar incidence of complications.[102]

The potential for serious complications cannot be ignored, which may include idiosyncratic drug reactions, anaphylaxis, malignant hyperthermia, respiratory depression, airway obstruction, hypoxemia, aspiration of gastric contents, bronchospasm, severe hypertension, and cardiac arrhythmias.[103, 104] The risk of death from intravenous sedation is reported as 1 in 314,000 cases in patients having dental procedures and oral surgery.[103]

The low incidence of complications associated with conscious sedation in oral surgical patients is attributed to the following:[101]

- Proper patient preparation (physical and psychologic)
- Proper patient selection
- Use of small-gauge catheters in large veins
- Slow titration of small drug increments to produce desired affects
- Adequate local analgesia
- Proper discharge criteria and postoperative instructions

Injectable Drugs

The injectable drugs we choose play a greater role in determining whether adult patients can go home on the same day as their surgery than does our choice of inhalation agents. The properties of an ideal injectable agent are found in Table 49-6.

THIOPENTAL/METHOHEXITAL. Despite a long elimination half-life (10–12 h) that can contribute to a prolonged recovery time, thiopental is the standard against which other intravenous induction drugs are measured. In studying the pharmacokinetics of thiopental and methohexital in patients having short surgical procedures, Hudson *et al* evaluated the following: disposition of a single intravenous bolus of methohexital followed by other agents for maintenance of anesthesia; comparison of the pharmacokinetics of thiopental and methohexital in surgical patients; and the relative importance of metabolism compared with redistribution in the recovery process after use of both intravenous induction agents.[105]

Although the distribution phase kinetics of thiopental and methohexital appear similar, redistribution is a major factor

*Kallar SK: Personal communication, 1987.

TABLE 49-6. Physical and Pharmacologic Properties of an Ideal Intravenous Agent

1. High therapeutic (safety) index
2. Water-soluble, stable in solution, and long shelf-life
3. Nonirritating after intramuscular or intravenous administration
4. No hypersensitivity (or anaphylactoid) reactions
5. Rapid, smooth onset of action after intramuscular or intravenous administration
6. No depression of cardiovascular and respiratory systems
7. Rapid degradation to inactive, nontoxic metabolites
8. Short elimination half-life (t$_{1/2}\beta$) value
9. Analgesia at subanesthetic levels
10. Rapid, smooth emergence without side-effects

(White PF, Shafer AS: Clinical pharmacology and uses of injectable anesthetic and analgesic drugs. In Wetchler BV (ed): Outpatient Anesthesia, vol 2, p 38. Philadelphia, JB Lippincott, 1988, with permission.)

determining the duration of sedation after a single bolus dose of either drug. The more rapid recovery of complete psychomotor function seen after use of methohexital probably results from its more rapid metabolism. The authors concluded that methohexital would be preferable to thiopental whenever more rapid recovery from anesthesia is desired, particularly after use of large or repeated doses. Others have found methohexital to be associated with a shorter awakening and recovery time than was associated with thiopental.[106, 107]

Elliott *et al* assessed coordination in methohexital-treated patients compared with thiopental-treated patients. Not only did coordination return more quickly in the methohexital-treated patients, but the subjects themselves reported being less sedated and clearer mentally compared with those in the thiopental-treated group.[108]

After patients were given a single intravenous bolus dose of thiopental, EEG studies showed a rapid return to consciousness, however, at 2.5 h and 3.5 h after induction, drowsiness appeared, and at 4.5 h a sleep tracing appeared on the EEG that lasted up to 12 h.[109] The outpatient should be made aware of this probable return of drowsiness before he or she is discharged.

Although there is a more rapid return to consciousness, stability in solution, and less tissue irritation and there are shorter periods of hypotension with methohexital compared with thiopental, Dundee found that it produced a higher incidence of excitatory phenomenon, cough, and hiccough when used as an induction agent.[110]

ETOMIDATE. A short-acting intravenous hypnotic drug without any analgesic action, etomidate is associated with remarkable cardiovascular stability and lacks histamine release.[111–113] Pain on injection (in up to 50% of patients) and involuntary myoclonic movements (in up to 70% of patients) are two of the major side-effects of this drug.[112] Pain can be severe enough that patients refuse a second etomidate induction.[111] Involuntary movements are minimized by the intravenous administration of midazolam 0.07 mg·kg^{-1} or diazepam 0.15 mg·kg^{-1} and fentanyl 1.5 μg·kg^{-1}, or by a preinduction dose of alfentanil (7 μg·kg^{-1}).[114–116] Melnick *et al* completely abolished pain on injection related to etomidate.[117] Just before induction, 25–100 mg of lidocaine is administered through an injection port attached directly to the intravenous catheter; the intravenous drip is turned off for 30 s; etomidate is then injected.

TABLE 49-7. Recovery Times and Side-Effects after Continuous Infusions of Thiopental, Methohexital, or Etomidate

GROUP	RECOVERY TIMES (min)*			POSTOPERATIVE SIDE-EFFECTS (%)			
	Awake	Oriented	Ambulatory	Nausea	Dizzy	Drowsy	Pain
Thiopental	8 ± 7	12 ± 9	84 ± 9	15	10	50	25
Methohexital	2 ± 2†	3 ± 2†	45 ± 4†	10	10	5†	20
Etomidate	5 ± 3	6 ± 4	67 ± 8	45†	5	20	15

*Mean values ± SD.
†Significantly different from thiopental-treated group, $P < 0.05$.
(White PF: Continuous infusions of thiopental, methohexital or etomidate as adjuvants to nitrous oxide for outpatient anesthesia. Anesth Analg 63:282, 1984, with permission.)

Fragen and Caldwell found no difference in quality of patient recovery when comparing etomidate with thiopental induction; however, etomidate-treated patients had a threefold increase in nausea and vomiting.[112] White compared PACU time and side-effects in outpatients receiving thiopental, methohexital, or etomidate continuous infusions as adjuvants to nitrous oxide for outpatient anesthesia (Table 49-7).[118] The methohexital-treated patients were awake, oriented, and discharged significantly faster than those in the other two groups. The incidence of nausea was significantly higher in the etomidate-treated patients.

A single induction dose can produce transient postoperative suppression (approximately 8 h in duration) of adrenocortical function; however, this does not necessitate steroid supplementation.[119] Etomidate does not appear to offer any advantage over barbiturates for outpatient anesthesia.

KETAMINE. The role of ketamine in adult outpatient anesthesia is questionable. In comparing ketamine with thiopental as induction agents for outpatient anesthesia, Thompson et al found that ketamine-treated patients were less alert, had more headaches and dizziness, and complained of "weird dreams" when discharged.[41] Two-thirds of the ketamine-treated patients in this study reported that their unpleasant dreams were frightening; none of the thiopental-treated patients had strange dreams. Although the administration of diazepam or droperidol can decrease the incidence of unpleasant dreams, the addition of these drugs may further delay the patient's recovery. In the PACU, ketamine-treated patients had a significant increase in nausea and vomiting. Ketamine-treated patients also reported an increased awareness for perianesthetic events (9%) compared with thiopental-treated patients (4%). As with other rapid and short-acting intravenous drugs, continuous infusion of ketamine may offer considerable advantages over traditional intermittent bolus technique for the outpatient setting.[120] Ketamine appears to fall short of the requirements for an ideal outpatient anesthetic drug and has not found wide acceptance in the management of adult patients in an ambulatory setting. Its main role may be as a pediatric induction agent in doses of 2–3 mg·kg^{-1} intramuscularly.[121] This technique is useful for the 1–5 yr-old age group and will provide satisfactory conditions for a mask induction within 4–7 min. When pediatric patients receive low-dose intramuscular ketamine as an induction drug, hallucinations and nightmares do not appear to be a problem.[122] Koka compared four induction techniques in nonpremedicated pediatric outpatients: ketamine intramuscularly (2 mg·kg^{-1} deltoid area), halothane by mask, methohexital rectally (25 mg·kg^{-1}), and thiopental intravenously (4–5

mg·kg^{-1}).* Early recovery was faster with halothane; at 1 hour in the PACU recovery was comparable regardless of the induction technique used.

PROPOFOL. A member of the sedative hypnotic group, propofol produces dose-dependent central nervous system, cardiovascular, and ventilatory depression very similar to that produced by the barbiturate induction drugs. Onset of action is almost identical to that of thiopental or methohexital; in the PACU, recovery from propofol is much faster and is associated with few postanesthetic side effects (Table 49-8).[123-125] Pain on injection depends on site of administration (dorsal hand veins) and is minimized if forearm or larger anticubital veins are used.[123, 126] Thrombophlebitis does not appear to be a problem after intravenous administration of this agent. Elimination half-life of propofol (1–3 h) is shorter than that of methohexital (6–8 h) or thiopental (10–12 h). Although Youngberg et al, Doze and White, and Johnston et al concluded that cardiovascular depressant activities of propofol were similar to those of thiopental, others have found it to produce greater cardiovascular depression, typically manifested by decreases in arterial pressure and cardiac index without a significant change in heart rate.[127-132]

When equivalent doses of propofol (2.5 mg·kg^{-1}), methohexital (1.5 mg·kg^{-1}), and thiopental (5 mg·kg^{-1}) were compared as induction agents, propofol induction was smoother but was associated with greater cardiorespiratory depression; speed and quality of recovery was superior with propofol.[123, 133] The propofol induction dose should be decreased in patients aged 60 years or older. Pain on injection (dorsal hand veins) was significantly less with propofol than with methohexital. Postanesthetic recovery was superior for propofol, with virtual absence of side-effects and rapid recovery with little impairment of psychomotor function 30 min after anesthesia.[123] The use of intravenous lidocaine immediately before propofol injection only partially reduced the incidence of pain when dorsal hand veins were used.[124]

When propofol and methohexital were administered by continuous infusion, recovery times were similar for short surgical procedures (less than 50 min); for longer procedures (more than 50 min), recovery times were prolonged in the methohexital-treated group.[134] There was a lower incidence of recovery complications (i.e., nausea, confusion, drowsiness, and restlessness) after propofol infusion. Propofol is a potentially useful new drug for outpatient anesthesia; however, the dose must be carefully titrated in patients with cardiovascular disease to avoid significant cardiovascular depression.[114]

*Koka BV: Personal communication, 1987.

TABLE 49-8.   Patient Response After Administration of Propofol, Methohexitone, or Thiopentone

	PROPOFOL	METHOHEXITONE	THIOPENTONE
Time to open eyes (min)	4.8 ± 0.45	5.6 ± 0.54	9.6 ± 0.74*
Time to repeat date of birth (min)	5.8 ± 0.34	7.2 ± 0.58‡	10.6 ± 0.74*
Sequelae			
Headache	0	3	7†
Nausea/vomiting	0	3	2
Drowsiness	0	0	7†
Venous problems	0	0	0

Crude recovery times (mean ± SEM) and postoperative sequelae (number of patients).
*, † Significance values: propofol *versus* thiopentone—*$P < 0.001$, †$P < 0.01$.
‡ Significance values: propofol *versus* methohexitone: $P < 0.05$.
(Mackenzie N, Grant IS: Comparison of the new emulsion formulation of propofol with methohexitone and thiopentone for induction of anaesthesia in day cases. Br J Anaesth 57:725, 1985, with permission.)

SUCCINYLCHOLINE. Many short outpatient procedures require no neuromuscular blocking drug, whereas some require an ultra-short-acting agent to facilitate tracheal intubation, and other procedures require muscle relaxation during the procedure. Succinylcholine, a depolarizing relaxant, is the relaxant used most widely in outpatient anesthesia to facilitate tracheal intubation and provide a short period of profound relaxation. For the outpatient, a significant drawback to using succinylcholine is the occurrence of postanesthesia skeletal muscle aches and pains. Myalgia may occur up to the fourth postoperative day and may be more painful than the surgery itself. The incidence of myalgia is significantly higher in patients who walk shortly after surgery (66%) compared with inpatients who remain resting in bed (13.9%).[135] Pretreatment with a variety of drugs (d-tubocurarine 0.05 mg·kg^{-1}, diazepam 0.05 mg·kg^{-1}, calcium gluconate 1,000 mg, succinylcholine 10 mg) has been reported to lessen and even eliminate myalgia after use of succinylcholine. In an outpatient study comparing the varying pretreatment regimens, the incidence of moderate to severe complaints of postanesthesia myalgia were never less than 8% in any group (d-tubocurarine 0.05 mg·kg^{-1}).[136] Although d-tubocurarine has been shown to be a better defasciculant than atracurium, postanesthesia myalgia was significantly less in patients pretreated with atracurium (0.025 mg·kg^{-1}).[137] In the healthy outpatient having an elective procedure, onset time of skeletal muscle relaxation to facilitate intubation of the trachea or surgery is less important than eliminating postanesthesia myalgia and the potential problem of prolonged apnea after succinylcholine administration. Short duration of effect after intubation of the trachea is more important. Succinylcholine is far from being an ideal muscle relaxant for the outpatient.

ATRACURIUM/VECURONIUM. These intermediate-acting drugs provide valuable new clinical options, with greater flexibility and safety than we have ever had before; they have an important place in outpatient anesthesia for procedures lasting longer than 20 min. Atracurium has the shortest elimination half-life of all clinically available nondepolarizing relaxants, but the duration of effect after an initial dose is similar to that of vecuronium. Although the recommended intubating dose of 0.4–0.5 mg·kg^{-1} produces good intubating conditions (2.5–3 min), its duration of action (50–70 min to 95% recovery) may be too long for some of the shorter outpatient procedures. Sokoll *et al* found 0.3 mg·kg^{-1} of atracurium produced a block lasting 44 min with an opioid anesthetic compared with 67 min with isoflurane.[138] Stirt *et al* consider atracurium an acceptable alternative to succinylcholine when speed of tracheal intubation is not critical.[139] The volatile anesthetics potentiate atracurium (20%) and vecuronium (20–40%). Enflurane (1.25 MAC) potentiates both muscle relaxants more than isoflurane or halothane.[140, 141]

The duration of effect of these intermediate-acting drugs is dose dependent, and it can be lengthened or shortened, depending on the dose chosen. The lowest dose of atracurium compatible with adequate intubating conditions is 0.25 mg·kg^{-1}.[142] In 18 patients having oral surgery, intubating conditions were excellent in 10, good in seven, and inadequate in one. Fragen and Shanks administered vecuronium (0.045 mg·kg^{-1}) for outpatient gynecologic laparoscopic procedures.[143] Time to maximum blockade (condition suitable for intubation of the trachea) was approximately 5 min. Duration of action was longer when vecuronium was used with inhalation agents than when it was used with opioids. With opioid anesthesia, recovery to 50% depression of twitch height was seen at 15 min, and with isoflurane anesthesia at 20 min.

When desirable, the time to intubation of the trachea after administration of vecuronium or atracurium can be shortened by use of the priming principle (Francis Foldes is associated with its development).[144] The technique consists of a subclinical "priming" dose of relaxant (atracurium 0.05–0.075 mg·kg^{-1}, vecuronium 0.01–0.015 mg·kg^{-1}), followed in approximately 2–2.5 min by the induction dose of anesthetic and immediately thereafter by a slightly smaller than usual intubating dose of the relaxant (atracurium 0.25–0.3 mg·kg^{-1}, vecuronium 0.04–0.05 mg·kg^{-1}). Induction of anesthesia should continue (*i.e.*, nitrous oxide, oxygen, major inhalation drug); satisfactory intubation of the trachea can be performed 2–2.5 min after administration of the intubating dose.[145]

Patient variability and sensitivity (skeletal muscle weakness evidenced by diplopia, difficulty in swallowing, and difficulty in breathing) can occur with the priming dose.[146] The longer one waits after the priming dose, the more likely symptoms will occur. By applying the priming principle to the outpatient, time to intubation of the trachea, as well as length of action, can be shortened (*i.e.*, vecuronium 0.05 mg·kg^{-1} provides 15–25 min of surgical muscle relaxation where 0.1 mg·kg^{-1} provides 30–45 min). The reversal of these nondepolarizing relaxants must be complete at the conclusion of the procedure.

MIVACURIUM. This nondepolarizing relaxant has been under clinical investigation since 1985. The ED_{95} dose of 0.1 mg·kg^{-1} produces maximum blockade in approximately 4 min; recovery to 95% requires about 25 min. The recommended intubating dose of 0.2–0.25 mg·kg^{-1} shortens time to maximum blockade to approximately 2.5 min; recovery to 95% takes only 30 min.[147] Intubating doses of mivacurium are about twice as long acting as those of succinylcholine and half as long acting as those of atracurium or vecuronium.[148] If a priming dose of 0.03 mg·kg^{-1} is followed by an intubating dose of 0.2 mg·kg^{-1} in a well-anesthetized patient, intubation time can be shortened to 90 s.[149] At the completion of surgery, residual blockade, if present, is easily antagonized.

FENTANYL. A preinduction intravenous dose of an opioid analgesic immediately before induction of anesthesia can reduce sedative–hypnotic and inhalation anesthesia requirements and lessen postsurgical analgesia requirement with a resultant decrease of PACU length of stay. However, small preinduction doses of opioid analgesic drugs can increase the incidence of PACU emesis.[65, 113] Although longer acting opioid analgesics (i.e., morphine and meperidine) have been used for outpatient anesthesia, neither is as acceptable as the more potent and shorter-acting opioid analgesics fentanyl, sufentanil, and alfentanil. As a supplement to thiopental, nitrous oxide, oxygen anesthesia, fentanyl not only provided a smoother intraanesthetic course, but decreased postoperative pain and PACU length of stay.[66] Fentanyl 1–3 µg·kg^{-1} is highly effective when included as part of the anesthetic regimen. It decreased the incidence of involuntary movement and hiccoughing when added to a methohexital, nitrous oxide, oxygen anesthetic.[150]

Pollard compared the clinical differences between an intravenous technique using fentanyl–droperidol and an inhalation technique using isoflurane in procedures lasting 30 min or less.[151] The fentanyl–droperidol-treated group had a more rapid recovery to consciousness and orientation and less need for postoperative analgesics. Although there may be a return of depressant effects approximately 4–6 h after the initial intravenous administration of fentanyl, this is of questionable consequence when one uses an acceptable ambulatory anesthesia dose.

SUFENTANIL. The optimal preinduction dose of sufentanil for short outpatient procedures is 10–15 µg iv.[152] At equipotent doses with fentanyl (sufentanil 10 times more potent), it produces shorter lasting depression of ventilation and longer lasting analgesia.[153] When compared with the use of isoflurane, sufentanil-treated patients were significantly more awake on arrival in the PACU and had less need for postoperative pain medication; after 90 min the level of recovery was the same.[154] The incidence of nausea was approximately the same for both groups. After outpatient arthroscopic surgery, awakening was more rapid with sufentanil than isoflurane, although after 2 h there was no difference between the groups.[155] Both anesthetic techniques provided satisfactory operating conditions, but the sufentanil-treated group showed a higher incidence of nausea and vomiting (45%) than the isoflurane-treated group (15%). For outpatients who had laparoscopic examination (sufentanil vs. isoflurane), the opioid compound significantly decreased PACU analgesia requirements and length of stay.[154] In 50 outpatients having D&C who received either fentanyl or sufentanil infusion as an adjuvant to thiopental, nitrous oxide, oxygen anesthesia, the incidence of nausea and pain requiring analgesics was significantly less in the sufentanil-treated group.[156]

ALFENTANIL. White and others believe the potency ratio (fentanyl:alfentanil), based on administered dose, is 8:1.[157, 158] Alfentanil may offer advantages over fentanyl in the outpatient surgery setting; an equianalgesic dose of alfentanil may be associated with less depression of ventilation.[159] Awakening from anesthesia was more rapid with alfentanil than with isoflurane after outpatient arthroscopic procedures and short urologic and gynecologic procedures.[160, 161] When compared with use of halothane or enflurane, alfentanil-treated patients recovered more rapidly; postanesthesia side-effects (nausea, vomiting, drowsiness) were the same for each group.[162] DeChene found alfentanil to be well suited as an adjunct to nitrous oxide and thiopental in short surgical procedures.[163] Minor chest wall rigidity was a consistent side-effect that was eliminated by pretreatment with d-tubocurarine. Coe et al see alfentanil as a clinically superior intravenous adjuvant for ambulatory anesthesia.[164] Comparing fentanyl and alfentanil in patients who had termination of pregnancy, they found a higher incidence of chest wall rigidity and ventilatory depression in the fentanyl-treated group, a higher incidence of mild bradycardia and moderate hypotension in the alfentanil-treated group, and no significant difference in the incidence of nausea, vomiting, dizziness, or excessive drowsiness. The fentanyl:alfentanil potency ratio was 6:1, based on total dose administered. Kallar and Keenan compared recovery times after use of alfentanil and fentanyl in 43 patients in whom pregnancies were terminated.[165] The median time to establish alertness was significantly shorter for the alfentanil-treated group (16 min), than for the fentanyl-treated group (25 min). Although the percentage of completely recovered alfentanil-treated patients was significantly greater than fentanyl-treated patients at 20 and 30 min after operation, at 60 min after anesthesia recovery room scores indicating alertness were the same in both groups. White compared recovery time in outpatients who received fentanyl bolus, fentanyl infusion, alfentanil bolus, and alfentanil infusion.[158] The patients who had alfentanil bolus and infusion were awake, oriented, and able to walk significantly sooner than the fentanyl-treated patients (Table 49-9). There appears to be no return of depressant effects (4–6 h after intravenous administration) when alfentanil is used.

BUTORPHANOL. Discharge time from the PACU and the most common side-effects after anesthesia were compared in a series of outpatients who received fentanyl (3 µg·kg^{-1}), butorphanol (60 µg·kg^{-1}), or nalbuphine (300 µg·kg^{-1}) as part of a balanced anesthesia technique.[166] Fentanyl-treated patients had the shortest awakening time and no admissions into the hospital, whereas there was one admission in the nalbuphine-treated group and three in the butorphanol-treated group because of excessive drowsiness. In comparing butorphanol (40 µg·kg^{-1}) and fentanyl (2 µg·kg^{-1}), the butorphanol patients were more drowsy but also had less pain in the PACU.[167] The incidence of nausea and vomiting was comparable in both groups. When used as preinduction intravenous drugs (butorphanol 20 µg·kg^{-1} and 40 µg·kg^{-1} vs. fentanyl 2 µg·kg^{-1}), there were no significant differences between butorphanol 20 µg·kg^{-1} and fentanyl 2 µg·kg^{-1}.* Statistically significant variation ($P < 0.05$) was found in both length of recovery time and the symptoms of nausea and dizziness when butorphanol 40 µg·kg^{-1} was compared with fentanyl.

*Wetchler BV, Alexander CD, Shariff MS et al: Personal communication, 1985.

TABLE 49-9. Postoperative Recovery Times and Side-Effects After the Use of Either Fentanyl or Alfentanil as an Adjuvant to Nitrous Oxide

	RECOVERY TIMES (min)*			SIDE-EFFECTS (%)			
GROUP	*Awake*	*Oriented*	*Ambulatory*	*Nausea*	*Vomiting*	*Dizziness*	*Drowsiness*
Fentanyl bolus (FB)	5.2 ± 0.9	7.7 ± 1.1	67 ± 5	60	48	52	36
Fentanyl infusion (FI)	3.7 ± 0.8†	6.1 ± 1.2	55 ± 5	68	60	24	28
Alfentanil bolus (AB)	2.5 ± 0.3‡	3.5 ± 0.4‡	48 ± 4‡	52	36	24	16
Alfentanil infusion (AI)	1.2 ± 0.1†,‡	2.6 ± 0.3†,‡	41 ± 3‡	68	60	28	8‡

*Means values ± SEM.
† AI or FI group significantly different from AB or FB group ($P < 0.05$), respectively.
‡ AB or AI group significantly different from FB or FI group ($P < 0.05$), respectively.
(White PF, Coe V, Shafer A *et al:* Comparison of alfentanil with fentanyl for outpatient anesthesia. Anesthesiology 64:99, 1986, with permission.)

TABLE 49-10. Recovery Time (min) after Thiopental or Midazolam

	AWAKE	ORIENTED	AMBULATORY	COGNITIVE
Thiopental (4 $mg \cdot kg^{-1}$)	5.7	14.7	52	33
Midazolam (0.2 $mg \cdot kg^{-1}$)	14.4*	49.9*	108*	125*
Fentanyl–thiopental	7.3	13.3	65	73
Fentanyl–midazolam	12.0*	37.9*	80	104*

*Significantly different from thiopental-treated group: $P < 0.05$.
(Fragen RJ, Caldwell NJ: Awakening characteristics following anesthesia induction with midazolam for short surgical procedures. Arzneim Forsch 31:2261, 1981, with permission.)

NALBUPHINE. Garfield *et al,* in comparing nalbuphine 300 $\mu g \cdot kg^{-1}$ or 500 $\mu g \cdot kg^{-1}$ with fentanyl 1.5 $\mu g \cdot kg^{-1}$, found a significantly longer recovery phase for both nalbuphine-treated groups (three patients in the nalbuphine-treated groups were admitted because of excessive disorientation and sedation), a higher degree of anxiety in the 500 $\mu g \cdot kg^{-1}$ group at time of discharge, and a significantly higher incidence of unpleasant dreams in the nalbuphine-treated groups.[168] For day surgery patients, there were no significant differences in recovery times, levels of nausea and vomiting, or patient acceptance when either nalbuphine (150 $\mu g \cdot kg^{-1}$ or 300 $\mu g \cdot kg^{-1}$) or fentanyl (1.5 $\mu g \cdot kg^{-1}$ or 3 $\mu g \cdot kg^{-1}$) were given.* In response to specific directed questioning, the nalbuphine-treated patients reported having "bad" dreams. In both studies, those having unpleasant dreams ranged from 20 to 38% of nalbuphine-treated patients compared with 0–6% of fentanyl-treated patients.

BENZODIAZEPINES. Diazepam, lorazepam and midazolam have already been discussed in the sections on premedication, regional anesthesia, and conscious sedation. Lorazepam is not acceptable for the outpatient; use of injectable diazepam may well be limited now that we have injectable midazolam.

Does midazolam have a role as an induction drug for outpatient anesthesia? Concerns have been raised regarding delayed recovery and residual amnesia.[167, 170] Midazolam 0.15 $mg \cdot kg^{-1}$ was not sufficient to induce anesthesia reliably in healthy unpremedicated volunteers.[171] Anterograde amnesia (40 ± 3 min duration) and drowsiness (lasting 128 ± 23 min) were observed in all subjects. In a randomized study of 100 women having pregnancies terminated on an outpatient basis, the combination of midazolam, fentanyl, nitrous oxide was compared with thiopental, fentanyl, nitrous oxide.[172] Midazolam (0.2–0.3 $mg \cdot kg^{-1}$) intravenous induction of anesthesia resulted in a lesser degree of awareness 30 min after the termination of anesthesia; at 60 and 180 min the scores were equal. Fragen and Caldwell, when comparing midazolam (0.2 $mg \cdot kg^{-1}$) with thiopental (4 $mg \cdot kg^{-1}$) for induction and maintenance of anesthesia along with 67% nitrous oxide for short gynecologic procedures, found prolongation to orientation and cognition in the midazolam-induced group.[173] Midazolam produced a profound period of amnesia for 1–2 h; important instructions could not be given to patients during that time. Vomiting was less frequent after use of midazolam. All patients were awake enough to be discharged from the hospital 200 min after the last dose of hypnotic was given (Table 49-10).

Use of midazolam for the induction of anesthesia in outpatient surgery may depend entirely on how long the outpatient surgical procedure lasts and the dose of the drug to be given.[174] For very short outpatient procedures it may be best not to use midazolam, because not only will patients be drowsy in the postoperative period, but they will be very amnesic and not likely to remember any instructions given them during that period.

Flumazenil, a specific benzodiazepine antagonist, can reverse benzodiazepine-induced sedation without producing toxic side-effects. Sixty women who had laparoscopic surgery were treated with flumazenil or placebo after the surgical procedure. Flumazenil reversed the hypnotic effect of midazolam within a few minutes.[175] The patients were alert, cooperative, and oriented and had good recall of events after awakening; effects were statistically better than with placebo for up to 30 min after administration. The duration of action of flumazenil is shorter than that of most benzodiazepines, and in

*Robinson DM, Kitz DS, Conahan TJ *et al:* Personal communication, 1987.

the outpatient setting patient observation must be of sufficient length to preclude the recurrence of significant sedation in a noncontrolled setting (*i.e.*, during transport home or at home).

Inhalation

Apfelbaum stated, "In theory, therefore, if all other factors are held constant (inspired partial pressure, ventilation, blood flow, cardiac output, etc.), inhalation agents with low blood/gas partition coefficients (*i.e.*, low solubility) would be preferable for outpatient anesthesia because these agents achieve equilibrium with the brain most rapidly, allowing for fast induction and emergence."[176]

NITROUS OXIDE. Lacking pungency and having a pleasant odor, nitrous oxide is used as an adjunct for starting inhalation induction of anesthesia in both pediatric and adult outpatients who dislike needles. The use of nitrous oxide as a maintenance adjunct can significantly decrease MAC, substantially reducing requirements for other anesthetic drugs, thereby resulting in more rapid emergence from anesthesia.[177] The combination of nitrous oxide plus halothane, enflurane, or isoflurane appears to produce less depression at a given MAC level than either of the potent drugs alone.[178–180] This can be of particular importance in the anesthetic management of an outpatient with a physical status of 3.

A major drawback in using nitrous oxide for the outpatient is the still unresolved question of its role as a causative factor in the incidence of postoperative nausea and vomiting (Table 49-11). Alexander *et al* found a significantly higher incidence of nausea and vomiting after operation (laparoscopic procedures) in patients receiving nitrous oxide as part of their anesthetic management.[181] The findings of Lonie and Harper suggest that an anesthetic technique that avoids use of nitrous oxide may be especially indicated in patients having laparoscopic procedures.[182] Only 17% of the patients not treated with nitrous oxide vomited after operation compared with 49% of patients who received nitrous oxide. These studies have caused some anesthesiologists to advocate elimination of nitrous oxide from outpatient anesthesia. Others (inpatient studies not involving laparoscopic procedures) have challenged this conclusion, having been unable to demonstrate an increase in the incidence or severity of postoperative emesis in patients receiving nitrous oxide compared with those in a control group.[183, 184] Despite any potential drawback, nitrous oxide continues to be the mainstay of inhalation anesthesia in the ambulatory setting.

HALOTHANE. Halothane is the most commonly used potent inhalation drug in pediatric outpatient anesthesia; it offers a smooth mask induction with the lowest incidence of excitement.[185, 186] Halothane or isoflurane was used to induce anesthesia in children scheduled for outpatient surgical procedures.[187] Anesthesia induction, as well as time to intubation of the trachea, was protracted in patients who received isoflurane. Recovery times were similar for both anesthetic drugs. Induction and maintenance of anesthesia were satisfactory when isoflurane was compared with halothane for outpatient dental extractions in 80 children, although there was a higher incidence of coughing, salivation, and laryngospasm in the group receiving isoflurane.[188] Immediate recovery was slower in patients who received isoflurane. Recovery from halothane anesthesia is usually rapid and uneventful, although postoperative shivering, headache, and nausea and vomiting have been reported and may affect time to discharge in outpatients.[189, 190] Compared with use of enflurane or isoflurane, during halothane anesthesia ventricular cardiac dysrhythmias are far more likely, especially in female and younger outpatients.[104, 191–193]

ENFLURANE. Unlike halothane, enflurane can provide skeletal muscle relaxation sufficient for most outpatient surgical procedures. Additionally, enflurane enhances the effect of many nondepolarizing neuromuscular blocking agents. Theoretically, use of less muscle relaxant should provide additional safety after operation and allow the surgical outpatient to return more rapidly to "street fitness."[176]

After 7 min of 2-MAC enflurane or halothane for dilatation and curettage, patients who received enflurane could respond after 5.7 min when their names were spoken as compared with 7.6 min for those who received halothane.[194] Postoperative physical complaints and intellectual or perceptual-motor function appear comparable between groups treated with the two anesthetic agents.[195–197] Jellicoe evaluated recovery time in 60 outpatients receiving either alfentanil, halothane, or enflurane.[162] The alfentanil-treated group recovered more rapidly, but there was no difference between halothane and enflurane in terms of recovery time. In comparing enflurane, isoflurane, and continuous fentanyl infusion for outpatient anesthesia, all three provided satisfactory intraoperative conditions.[198] There was no difference between groups regarding PACU time. The isoflurane and enflurane techniques were equal and were superior to the fentanyl infusion technique regarding incidence of postoperative nausea and vomiting.

In patients having outpatient procedures, recovery appears to be quicker after use of enflurane *versus* halothane.[194, 199] Azar *et al* have shown that awakening times are not significantly different in patients who have had short outpatient procedures with either isoflurane or enflurane.[200]

ISOFLURANE. In high enough concentrations, isoflurane, like enflurane, can produce profound skeletal muscle relaxation as well as substantially potentiate the effects of many nondepolarizing muscle relaxants.[201–203] This effect is reversible when isoflurane is withdrawn and allows the anesthesiologist to use lower intraoperative doses of relaxant.

Because of its pungent smell and irritating airway effects, isoflurane produces a higher incidence of excitement, breath holding, coughing, and laryngospasm than either enflurane or halothane.[186, 204, 205]

TABLE 49-11.   Nitrous Oxide: A Factor in Nausea and Vomiting?

STUDY	PERCENTAGE OF PATIENTS HAVING NAUSEA AND VOMITING	
	Received Nitrous Oxide	*Did Not Receive Nitrous Oxide*
Alexander *et al**[181]	61%	27.5%
Lonie and Harper*[182]	29%	4%
Korttila *et al*†[183]		
Nausea	60%	60%
Vomiting	29.1%	23.6%
Muir *et al*‡[184]	11.1%	9.7%

* Laparoscopic procedures.
† Abdominal hysterectomies.
‡ Variety of procedures, excluding otologic, neurologic, intra-abdominal, and ophthalmologic procedures.

Short *et al* evaluated unpremedicated patients having brief urologic and gynecologic procedures.[161] Although the alfentanil-treated group opened their eyes and gave their names and dates of birth significantly faster after operation than those in the isoflurane-treated group, there were no significant differences between the groups in results of later tests of recovery. Zuurmond and van Leeuwen compared alfentanil by continuous intravenous infusion with isoflurane as anesthetic drugs for outpatient arthroscopic procedures.[155] Although awakening from anesthesia was more rapid with the alfentanil-treated patients, both anesthetic techniques provided satisfactory anesthesia and rapid recovery. The patients who received isoflurane scored better in all early recovery tests, but after 3 h there was no difference between the groups. The alfentanil-treated group had a higher incidence of nausea and vomiting (45%) compared with the isoflurane-treated group (14%). Rising *et al*, in comparing isoflurane *versus* fentanyl for outpatient laparoscopic procedures, found immediate recovery more rapid in the fentanyl-treated group, although reaction times in the isoflurane-treated patients returned to levels of control patients by 3 h whereas fentanyl-treated patients were still 10% slower than control patients at 4 h after anesthesia.[206] Nausea and vomiting were more frequent in the fentanyl-treated group. Both anesthetic techniques provided satisfactory operating conditions, but isoflurane appeared to provide a better recovery with fewer side-effects than did fentanyl.

Korttila *et al* demonstrated that lengthy enflurane anesthesia (longer than 90 min) was associated with significantly slower recovery than shorter enflurane anesthesia (less than 40 min).[207] Rapidity of recovery did not depend on duration of anesthesia when isoflurane was used, suggesting that isoflurane may provide significant advantages with regard to rapidity of recovery in patients having ambulatory surgical procedures lasting longer than 90 min.

Sixty unpremedicated outpatients having D&C were allocated randomly to receive one of three inhalation agents (halothane, enflurane, or isoflurane) to supplement 67% nitrous oxide and oxygen after induction of anesthesia with methohexital.[208] After anesthesia there was no difference between the drugs in the time to when patients could open their eyes or regain a preoperative level of manipulative skill. The p-deletion test, which indicates the subject's ability to concentrate, was completed more quickly by patients in the isoflurane-treated group. The differences among the three inhalation drugs (after intravenous induction) when used for short procedures are insufficient to allow recommendation of one over the other two.

No single agent or technique allows us to provide ideal anesthetic conditions for outpatient surgery. Apfelbaum believes "unless specific circumstances require or exclude a specific technique, most anesthesiologists combine the advantages of several types of drugs (intravenous induction agents, narcotics, potent inhaled agents, nitrous oxide); this approach typically requires smaller amounts of each agent."[176]

POSTANESTHESIA CARE UNIT MANAGEMENT

Managing common PACU problems quickly and effectively is equal in importance to appropriate patient selection and choice of anesthetic technique if our patient is to return home on the same day that surgery is performed. Unanticipated admission rates after an outpatient procedure vary from 0.1 to 5%.[19, 35, ,209, 210] Depending upon the type of surgery, pain

(*i.e.*, after orchiopexy) or nausea and vomiting (*i.e.*, after strabismus correction) can be the significant reason a patient spends the first surgical evening in the hospital rather than at home.

PAIN

Postsurgical pain must be treated quickly and effectively. Medications given in the PACU should be monitored closely and given in small, immediately effective doses. Intramuscular opioid analgesic injection for pain control in the PACU is probably more a custom than a thoroughly considered process.[211] Appropriate control of postoperative pain includes the following:

1. Supplementation of inhalation anesthesia with opioid analgesics
2. Supplementation of inhalation anesthesia with local or regional block
3. Administration of opioid analgesics in the PACU

Epstein *et al* found a significantly higher incidence of pain and a slightly higher incidence of excitement during recovery in outpatients who did not receive an opioid analgesic intra-anesthetically compared with those who did.[66] Although there was a higher incidence of nausea in the fentanyl-treated group, patients recovered statistically sooner than those who did not receive opioid supplementation during anesthesia. The opioid-supplemented patients had a shorter time to walk without support and stand with negative Romberg and they spent less time in the PACU. The use of a longer-acting opioid, meperidine ($1-1.5$ mg $\cdot$ kg^{-1}), when compared with fentanyl (2 µg $\cdot$ kg^{-1}), administered intraoperatively did not delay recovery from anesthesia or patient discharge.[212] Anesthesia techniques that provided the best pain relief in the first 2 h after surgery had a lower incidence of overall complications and more rapid recovery. Sanders *et al* administered alfentanil or halothane to patients who had either etomidate or methohexital, nitrous oxide, oxygen anesthesia for termination of pregnancy. Faster recovery was seen in patients receiving alfentanil.[68] In short urologic and gynecologic procedures, alfentanil-treated patients recovered more rapidly than halothane-, enflurane-, or isoflurane-treated patients.[161, 162] Late recovery scores as well as subjective feelings of drowsiness and unsteadiness were the same.

A decrease in pain, analgesic requirements, and minor complications in the PACU; earlier home readiness; and more rapid return to normal activity can be achieved by combining many simple (sensory) nerve blocks with inhalation anesthesia.[213]

Shandling and Steward believe that children older than 6 months of age almost invariably require some postoperative analgesics after inguinal hernia repair.[214] When ilioinguinal and iliohypogastric nerves were infiltrated with bupivacaine during surgery, pain and vomiting were decreased during the recovery period. The extended duration of action of bupivacaine can produce postoperative analgesia for 8–12 h.

The incidence of postoperative complications after laparoscopic tubal sterilization is low and is primarily related to pain. There is minimal incisional pain, but abdominal discomfort, shoulder pain, and nausea and vomiting frequently delay discharge. The level of discomfort will vary, depending upon the type of sterilization performed; there is less pain and cramping after cautery compared with Yoon fallopian ring sterilization.[215, 216] Infiltration of the mesosalpinx with 0.5% bupivacaine in the area of the Yoon placement at the conclusion of surgical sterilization significantly decreases patients' pain while they are in the PACU.[217, 218]

McGlinchy *et al* supplemented general anesthesia with regional block of the dorsal nerve of the penis (0.5% bupivacaine) in a group of adult outpatients having circumcision.[219] None of the patients required analgesia in the 6 h after surgery, unlike a control group in which all patients required strong opioid analgesic supplementation during the recovery stage. Topical anesthesia (lidocaine spray, 10–20 mg of 10%; lidocaine jelly, 0.5–1 ml of 2%; lidocaine ointment 0.5–1 ml of 5%) has provided postoperative pain relief after pediatric circumcision.[220] The duration of analgesia (4–5 h) approximated that produced by supplemental dorsal nerve block or intramuscular morphine. Pain relief was comparable with all topical techniques; however, children preferred lidocaine spray if repeated application was necessary. Subcutaneous ring block of the penis with 0.25% bupivacaine is another simple and effective method of providing postcircumcision analgesia without delaying discharge from the hospital.[221]

Caudal block supplementation has been used to limit postsurgical pain not only after pediatric circumcision, but also after correction of hypospadias and orchiopexy.[222, 223] Caudal block performed with 0.25% bupivacaine containing epinephrine 1:200,000 produces effective postoperative analgesia. There does not appear to be any advantage to using more concentrated solutions.[224] Nonepinephrine-containing solutions of bupivacaine may provide comparable levels and duration of analgesia.[225] The key to the safety of caudal analgesia is knowledge of children's anatomy and of how it differs from that of adults (the dural sac extends more caudad in children), meticulous attention to detail in site selection and preparation, and careful aspiration to be certain that neither a vessel nor a subarachnoid space has been entered.[226]

Caudal analgesia has consistently been shown to be superior to systemic opioid analgesics administered at the time of surgery in respect to a more tranquil early recovery period, superior analgesia during the early postoperative period, a significantly lower incidence of vomiting, and a swifter resumption of normal activities.[227–230] Dorsal nerve block, when compared with caudal analgesia, provided good pain relief after circumcision and micturition occurred earlier, patients stood unaided sooner, and it had a lower incidence of vomiting.[231] Ilioinguinal nerve block provides a satisfactory alternative to caudal block for patients having herniorrhaphy or orchiopexy.[232]

When the anesthesiologist and postanesthesia care nurse communicate problem-solving techniques to the surgeon, patients can be provided with a smoother course in the PACU and the immediate postoperative period at home.

Although the choice of opioid analgesic is usually a matter of individual judgment, drugs such as morphine and meperidine are generally believed to be too long acting for outpatient use. Potent opioid analgesics given in the PACU may contribute significantly to postoperative drowsiness, nausea and vomiting, and delay in discharge home. A delicate balance must be struck in order to provide a postoperative period as free of pain as possible.

At Methodist Ambulatory SurgiCare, pain in both adults and children is managed with a short-acting opioid analgesic. Intravenous fentanyl (0.35 $\mu g \cdot kg^{-1}$) is given at the first sign of discomfort and repeated at 5-min intervals until pain is controlled. For our pediatric patients, we also use an elixir of acetaminophen containing codeine (acetaminophen 120 mg, codeine 12 mg in each 5 ml of solution). Five milliliters is administered to children between the ages of 3 and 6, and 10 ml to children between the ages of 7 and 12. Our pediatric patients are returned to parent care as soon as they are awake.

At the Children's Hospital National Medical Center (Washington, D.C.), infants younger than 6 months of age usually only need to be reunited with their parents and be nursed (or fed from a bottle) after a procedure not associated with severe pain. For older infants and young children, acetaminophen, 60 mg per year of age (orally or rectally), is one of the drugs most commonly given to relieve mild pain while they are in the PACU. Intravenous fentanyl (up to a dose of 2 $\mu g \cdot kg^{-1}$) is the drug of choice for more severe pain. Meperidine (0.5 $mg \cdot kg^{-1}$) and codeine (1–1.5 $mg \cdot kg^{-1}$) can be used intramuscularly if an intravenous route is not established.[233]

Outpatient facilities should establish a minimum length of time that patients must be observed in the PACU before discharge after administration of any depressant medication.

NAUSEA AND VOMITING

Protracted vomiting (36%) is the leading reason for patient admission to the hospital from the short-stay recovery unit (SSRU) at Children's Hospital National Medical Center (Table 49-12).[234] Nausea (30%) and vomiting (20%) are the most common complications occurring in the PACU at the Phoenix Surgicenter.[34] Contributing factors are history of motion sickness, sudden movement or position changes, pain, administration of opioid analgesic drugs, obesity, and site of surgical procedure.

A relationship between postoperative pain and the frequency of nausea in the early postsurgical period has been established.[235] Relief of pain without relief of nausea was unusual regardless of the analgesic used for pain control. Nausea often accompanies pain in the postoperative period and can be relieved in many patients when pain relief is achieved by the intravenous use of opiates. Using traditional Chinese acupuncture, Dundee *et al* significantly reduced postoperative nausea and vomiting.[236]

An important part of the preanesthesia interview is identification of the nausea-susceptible patient. During the preanesthesia interview, eliciting a history of motion sickness or emesis after prior anesthetics should alert the anesthesiologist to establish an "anesthesia game plan." When faced with this

TABLE 49-12.   Reasons for Admission to the Hospital

REASONS	CASES	
	No.	*Percentage*
Protracted vomiting	26	36%
Croup	8	11%
Family request	6	8%
Fever	6	8%
Bleeding	3	4%
Complicated surgery	3	4%
Sleepiness	2	2%
Other reasons	18	25%
Total	72	

(Patel RI, Hannallah RS, Murphy LS *et al*: Pediatric outpatient anesthesia—A review of postanesthetic complications in 8995 cases. Anesthesiology 65:A435, 1986, with permission.)

type of patient, one must carefully prioritize use of the following: antiemetics, gastrokinetics, nitrous oxide, opioid analgesics, regional block supplementation, or regional anesthesia.

Nausea-susceptible patients should:

Receive positive reassurance by all members of the staff to alleviate anxiety

Be moved slowly at all times to avoid motion sickness

Have a warm blanket placed over them to add to their sense of security

Have limited suction at the conclusion of the procedure (to avoid stimulation of gag reflex)

Be allowed to wake up slowly in the PACU

Antiemetics

Benzquinamide, trimethobenzamide, prochlorperazine, and hydroxyzine have all been used with limited success in an attempt to control postanesthetic nausea and vomiting.[237, 238] Droperidol has been found to be an effective antiemetic in intravenous doses as low as 0.25 mg in a group of ambulatory surgery patients having D&C.* When droperidol (0.625–1.25 mg) was administered intravenously immediately after intubation of the trachea, it proved to be an effective antiemetic in outpatients having laparoscopic tubal surgery.[239] The patients who received droperidol during anesthesia had a lower incidence of nausea and vomiting in the PACU, resulting in a shorter length of stay than that of the control group.

Valanne and Korttila administered droperidol 0.014 mg·kg^{-1}, 5 min after induction of anesthesia. Droperidol-treated patients had less nausea (18%) or vomiting (7%) in comparison with patients given saline (27% and 11%, respectively).[240]

Droperidol can potentiate drowsiness and, if administered during the final phases of recovery care, may increase the patient's length of stay. In an outpatient setting, the maximum antiemetic dose of droperidol should not exceed 2.5 mg; as the dose is increased above 1.25 mg, drowsiness becomes more noticeable.

Cohen et al reported limited effectiveness of prophylactic low-dose droperidol when compared with metoclopramide in patients having outpatient anesthesia.[241] A lack of antiemetic effect was noted for metoclopramide, but these patients could sit and walk and were ready for discharge sooner than control or droperidol-treated groups. A combination of droperidol (0.5–1.0 mg intravenously 3–6 min before induction of anesthesia) and metoclopramide (10–20 mg intravenously 15–30 min before droperidol) was more effective in preventing nausea and vomiting than droperidol alone, and these patients spent a significantly shorter time in the PACU.[242] Rao et al found that outpatients who had laparoscopic procedures and received metoclopramide (10 mg alone or in combination with cimetidine 300 mg) had a significant decrease in nausea and vomiting compared with the control group or the group treated with cimetidine alone.[243] Patients were instructed to fast from midnight and take their tablets with a sip of water on the day of surgery just before starting from home to the outpatient facility. Metoclopramide, 20 mg by mouth 2 h before anesthesia, effectively reduced postoperative nausea and vomiting in a nonoutpatient study.[244] Rao et al believe that metoclopramide, 10 mg administered intravenously, relieves postoperative nausea and vomiting within 5–10 min and does not prolong PACU length of stay. In the PACU, we administer

*Shelley ES, Brown HA: Personal communication, 1978.

droperidol intravenously (10–25 μg·kg^{-1}) to patients who have persistent nausea or after a second emesis.

Nausea and vomiting after outpatient laparoscopic procedures can affect PACU length of stay and cost. Eleven per cent of all patients experienced nausea, and an additional 18% of all patients experienced both nausea and vomiting. PACU stay was extended by 19 min for patients with nausea and by 47 min for patients with nausea and vomiting when compared with asymptomatic patients.[245]

There is a significantly higher incidence of postoperative nausea and vomiting (up to 85%) in pediatric patients who have strabismus surgery.[246–249] In separate studies, droperidol 75 μg·kg^{-1} has been found to be more effective in reducing poststrabismus vomiting than 50 μg·kg^{-1}.[246, 247, 249] When droperidol was given intravenously 30 min before the termination of surgery, 75 μg·kg^{-1} reduced vomiting to 43% compared with 85% in the control group. When droperidol 75 μg·kg^{-1} was administered during induction of anesthesia and before manipulation of the extraocular muscles, the incidence of vomiting was reduced from 75% in the control group to 10% in the droperidol-treated group.[248] Twenty-five μg·kg^{-1} of droperidol effectively lessened the incidence of nausea and vomiting during the time the patient was in the facility; once the patient returned home, there appeared to be an increased incidence of nausea and vomiting in this group compared with the groups treated with 50 and 75 μg·kg^{-1} (Fig. 49-1).[250]

When using doses of 75 μg·kg^{-1}, one should be prepared for a PACU length of stay of several hours. A recovery time of 4–6 h after surgery would be considered prolonged in children after myringotomy or herniotomy, but, because of nausea and vomiting, is not an unusual length of stay after strabismus or orchiopexy surgery. Intraoperative use of droperidol is recommended for these patients. After orchiopexy, up to 5% of patients may have to be admitted because of drowsiness or nausea and vomiting, or because surgery was more extensive than planned.[210]

Nitrous Oxide

As mentioned earlier in this chapter, the role of nitrous oxide in postoperative nausea and vomiting has not been fully established. Studies implicating nitrous oxide as a causative factor in postoperative nausea and vomiting are matched by those refuting it as a potential cause (Table 49-11).[181–184]

FIG. 49-1. Incidence of vomiting after strabismus repair. (Modified with permission. Eustis S, Lerman J, Smith D: Droperidol pretreatment in children undergoing strabismus repair: The minimal effective dose. Can Anaesth Soc J 33:116, 1986.)

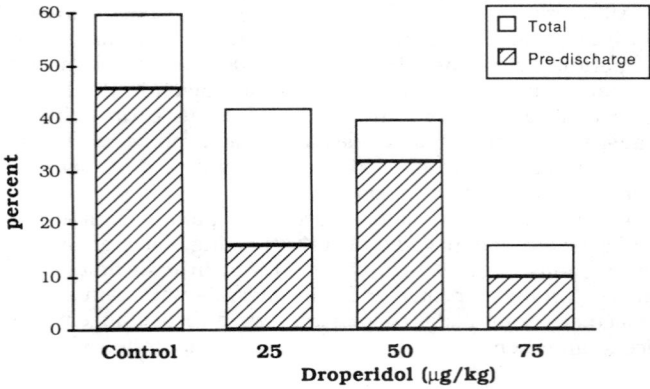

Transdermal Scopolamine

When evaluating this method of preventing or treating nausea and vomiting, we are faced with many anecdotal comments but lack significant outpatient studies. In a nonoutpatient study, a 72-h application of transdermal scopolamine effectively limited postoperative nausea and emesis.[251] The scopolamine dot was applied to the posterior auricular skin 12 h before surgery and removed 48 h after surgery. Insignificant benefits were seen in reducing postoperative emesis after pediatric eye surgery.[252] An unacceptable incidence of behavioral side-effects (hallucination, extreme agitation) was reported. Routine use of scopolamine as a transdermal preparation for the prophylaxis of vomiting in the patient having pediatric eye surgery is not recommended.

DISCHARGE CRITERIA*

Surgery has been completed; the patient has reacted after anesthesia; problems have been managed effectively. How do we determine when the patient can safely leave the outpatient facility? Outpatient surgical facilities must develop practical criteria for patient discharge that in no way compromise patient safety. Although the varying psychomotor tests can provide us with information that can be used in developing practical criteria, most tests are too complex, time consuming, and cumbersome to be used in a busy clinical setting.

To be ready for the ride home, Phoenix Surgicenter patients, in addition to having a responsible person being present, must have the following[253]:

1. Stable vital signs for at least 30 min
2. No new signs or symptoms after operation that may threaten a safe recovery (e.g., the patient with mild shoulder pain after a laparoscopic procedure will be released home, but a patient with more than mild abdominal pain after a diagnostic D&C will be detained for further observation)
3. Cessation of oozing or bleeding when bleeding was a feature of the operation
4. No nausea or emesis for 30 min or evidence that it is waning
5. Good circulation in and return of sensation to the operated extremity when a tourniquet has been used
6. No evidence of swelling or impaired circulation in an extremity when a cast has been applied
7. Voided clear urine after cystoscopic examination
8. The ability to recognize time and place
9. Little or no dizziness after changing clothes and sitting for 10 min
10. No pain not controllable by oral analgesics

After a state of home readiness has been established, the responsible nurse notifies the anesthesiologist and together they make sure that the applicable requirements of the Surgicenter's postoperative checklist and satisfied. This is known as informed discharge.[253]

1. Dietary instructions are given. Clear liquids are allowed until the patient's stomach is settled; then he or she can progress to regular feedings. The patient should not have alcohol (unless by physician's order) for at least 12 h.
2. Pain is provided for with medication appropriate to the need.
3. Prescriptions are checked. The patient or responsible person has prescriptions for all medications ordered by the surgeon.
4. Surgeon's instructions are reviewed, which concern limitation of activity, elevation of operated extremity, when to return to office, anticipated complications, whom to call in event of unanticipated complications.
5. The anesthesiologist's instructions are given:
   a. "You may feel sleepy and somewhat sluggish for several hours." "Don't drive until tomorrow." "Postpone important decisions until tomorrow."
   b. "You may have a sore throat for a few hours" (if patient's trachea was intubated). Patient should be instructed in use of salt-water gargles, humidifying devices, aspirin, or acetaminophen and advised to call if soreness persists more than a day.
   c. "You may have some muscular soreness for a day or two" (soreness, which follows the use of succinylcholine, may be more pronounced than any other discomfort). It is often, but not always, relieved by the medication prescribed to relieve pain at the operative site. Aspirin is recommended to relieve this soreness, and a warm bath is suggested if not contraindicated by the surgical procedure.
6. Dentures, valuables, and clothes are returned.
7. The patient is reassured that he or she has behaved properly. The patient should be informed that dreaming often occurs, and an opportunity should be afforded for the patient to discuss any dream that may be remembered.
8. The patient is informed that a follow-up call is routine and is to be expected.

Methodist Ambulatory SurgiCare patients must meet predetermined discharge criteria[254]:

1. Stable vital signs: Temperature, pulse, respiration, and blood pressure must be stable when appropriate. Vital signs should remain stable (i.e., blood pressure ±20 mm Hg) for a period of at least 30 min and should be consistent with patient's age and preanesthesia levels.
2. Ability to swallow and cough: The patient must demonstrate ability to swallow fluids and be able to cough.
3. Ability to walk: The patient must demonstrate ability to move consistent with age and development level (sit, stand, and walk).
4. Minimal nausea, vomiting, and dizziness:
   a. Minimal nausea: There is absence of nausea or, if nausea is present, patient can still swallow and retain some fluids
   b. Minimal vomiting: Vomiting is either absent or, if present, does not require treatment. After vomiting that requires treatment, patient should be able to swallow and retain fluids.
   c. Minimal dizziness: Dizziness is either absent or present only upon sitting, and patient can still move consistent with his or her age.
5. Absence of respiratory distress: The patient exhibits no signs of snoring, obstructed respiration, stridor, retractions, or croupy cough.
6. Alertness and orientation: The patient is aware of surroundings and what has taken place and is interested in returning home.

*Adapted from Wetchler BV: Problem solving in the postanesthesia care unit. In Wetchler BV (ed): Anesthesia for Ambulatory Surgery p 275. Philadelphia, JB Lippincott, 1985.

When is it safe to permit patients to walk after spinal or epidural anesthesia? The sequence of return of function generally accepted is motor, then sensory, and finally sympathetic. Several studies examining the sequence of return of function have found recovery of sympathetic activity to occur before complete regression of the subarachnoid block.[255-257] Pflug et al considered the ability to urinate a final indication of reversal of sympathetic paralysis because an intact functioning sympathetic nerve supply to bladder and urethra is necessary for this function.[256]

Suitable criteria for walking after spinal anesthesia include normal perianal (S4-5) pinprick sensation, plantar flexion of the foot, and proprioception of the big toe. Discharge criteria after spinal anesthesia include normal sensation, ability to walk (return of strength and proprioception), and ability to urinate (return of sympathetic nervous function).

As mentioned earlier in the section on regional anesthesia, after going home, there is no reason for patients who have had spinal anesthesia to remain flat in bed for 24 h as a means of preventing postdural puncture headache. After discharge, our patients who have had spinal anesthesia are instructed to rest in bed for 24 h; they may be propped up on pillow, sit up to eat, have bathroom privileges but are to wait until the next day before resuming appropriate normal activities. They are instructed to call the facility if they have a headache not relieved by acetaminophen, a stiff neck, or an elevated temperature. Similar instructions are given to patients who have epidural anesthesia, but we are more liberal in allowing them to be up and out of bed.[254] At the outpatient facilities of both the Brigham and Women's Hospital and the Virginia Mason Hospital, patients are instructed not to lift heavy objects or strain, but walking, activity, and position are not otherwise limited.

Before discharge, patients should have their dressings checked and an attempt should be made to have them urinate. Only patients having had spinal or epidural anesthesia must urinate before leaving the facility. It is wise to include the responsible person in all discharge instructions, and these instructions are best made available on printed forms. Patients and responsible parties should be reminded that the patient should not drive a car, operate power tools, or be involved in major business decisions for up to 24 h after sedation or inhalation anesthesia.

Before being discharged home, patients should be informed that they may experience pain, headache, nausea, vomiting, dizziness, and muscle aches and pains not related to the incision (if succinylcholine was used) for at least 24 h after surgery and anesthesia. The well-informed patient will be less stressed if any of the above symptoms occur after return to home.

In 100 consecutive outpatients who were given no written instructions at discharge, Ogg found 31% of patients went home unaccompanied by a responsible adult; 73% of car owners drove within 24 h of surgery, with 30% driving within 12 h; 9% of patients drove themselves home, and a bus driver returned to work on the same day, driving a bus load of passengers a distance of 95 miles.[258] Patients in this study reported postoperative symptoms of headache (27%), drowsiness (26%), nausea (22%), and dizziness (11%). Fifty per cent of medical outpatients do not follow physicians' instructions, but the addition of written and verbal education techniques at discharge has a significant impact on improving compliance.[259]

For patients with whom there is a language barrier (i.e., in a population with a high percentage of immigrants), consent forms, procedural explanation, and discharge information may have to be written in appropriate languages and the services of an interpreter may be necessary.

Nursing staff should assess the adult who will take the patient home to determine whether he or she is in fact a responsible person. The term responsible person refers to someone physically and intellectually capable of taking care of the patient at home.

The Joint Commission on Accreditation of Healthcare Organizations (JCAHO) has adopted new and revised standards that are included in the 1988 edition of the *Accreditation Manual for Hospitals* (AMH). The standards previously read as follows: "Any patient who has received other than local anesthesia is examined before discharge and is accompanied home by a designated person. The examination is performed by a physician or, when appropriate, by a qualified oral surgeon." The new standards no longer require a physician to examine the patient just before discharge. The 1988 standards state as follows: "A licensed independent practitioner who has appropriate clinical privileges and who is familiar with the patient is responsible for the decision to discharge a patient from a postanesthesia recovery area or, when the surgical or anesthesia services are provided on an ambulatory basis, from the hospital. When the responsible licensed independent practitioner is not personally present to make the decision to discharge or does not sign the discharge order, the name of the licensed independent practitioner responsible for the discharge is recorded in the patient's medical record; and relevant discharge criteria are rigorously applied to determine the readiness of the patient for discharge. The discharge criteria are approved by the medical staff."

Facilities should develop a method of follow-up after the patient has been discharged. Staff members at some facilities telephone the patient the next day to determine how they are recovering from surgery and anesthesia, whereas others use follow-up postcards.

INNOVATIVE APPROACHES TO POSTOPERATIVE CARE

Whenever we become innovative in the management of our outpatients, we must carefully assess how different and more compacted care impacts on patient safety. We must determine what we can do for the patient who lives alone, the patient whose responsible person is unable to manage his or her needs, the patient without any means of transportation, and the patient with limited insurance coverage. Some innovative approaches to postoperative care are listed below:

A 23-h observation bed in hospital: Patients going into an observation bed for less than 24 h after an ambulatory surgical procedure are still considered outpatients.

Hospital hotel/medical motel services: Hospitals are establishing in-hospital hotel guest services or are joining with management firms to have a hospital hotel or medical motel built and managed close to the hospital itself. The ambulatory hotel, usually a nonmedical facility, offers the outpatient a comfortable, inexpensive, and convenient place to recuperate while they are cared for by family or health care nurses.

Home health care nursing: After surgical procedures such as reduction mammoplasty, abdominalplasty, vaginal hysterectomy, and major open ligament repairs of the knee, Texas Outpatient Surgicare (Houston) uses home health care nursing services. Patients are transported home in an ambulance with a registered nurse who stays with the patient (administering iv fluids, antibiotics, opioid analgesics) for periods of 12-48 h.

Surgical recovery facility: In Phoenix, Arizona, the freestanding Surgical Recovery Center accepts patients transferred directly from hospital PACUs, freestanding outpatient centers, and physicians' offices and patients from hospitals on the first or second postoperative day for additional nursing care.

The varying outpatient observation and home health care services stand today where outpatient surgery stood in the health care delivery system 20 yr ago. Prospective studies must be done to assess quality of care and the effect these innovative approaches have on patient safety.

Patient, procedure, availability (including quality) of after care, and anesthetic technique must be individually and collectively assessed in determining acceptability for ambulatory surgery. A definite balance exists between physical status of patient, proposed surgical procedure, and appropriate anesthetic technique, never forgetting the comfort level of the anesthesiologist involved in caring for that patient.

REFERENCES

1. Nicoll JH: The surgery of infancy. Br Med J 2:753, 1909
2. Waters RM: The down-town anesthesia clinic. Am J Surg (Anesth-Suppl) 33:71, 1919
3. Herzfeld G: Hernia in infancy. Am J Surg 39:422, 1938
4. Webb E, Graves H: Anesthesia for the Ambulant Patient. Philadelphia, JB Lippincott, 1966
5. Porterfield HW, Franklin LT: The use of general anesthesia in the office surgery facility. Clin Plast Surg 10:292, 1983
6. Wetchler BV: Outpatient general and spinal anesthesia. Urol Clin North Am 14:31, 1987
7. Stafford M, Jeon A, Pascucci R: Pre- and post-induction blood glucose concentrations in healthy fasting children. Anesthesiology 63:A350, 1985
8. Jensen BH, Wernberg M, Adersen M: Preoperative starvation and blood glucose concentrations in children undergoing inpatient and outpatient anesthesia. Br J Anaesth 54:1071, 1982
9. Welborn LG, McGill WA, Hannallah RS et al: Perioperative blood glucose concentrations in pediatric outpatients. Anesthesiology 65:543, 1986
10. Redfern N, Addison GM, Meakin G: Blood glucose in anaesthetised children. Anaesthesia 41:272, 1986
11. Thomas DKM: Hypoglycaemia in children before operation: Its incidence and prevention. Br J Anaesth 46:66, 1974
12. Graham IFM: Preoperative starvation and plasma glucose concentrations in children undergoing outpatient anaesthesia. Br J Anaesth 51:161, 1979
13. Meakin G, Dingwall AE, Addison GM: Effect of fasting and oral premedication in the pH and volume of gastric aspirate in children. Br J Anaesth 59:678, 1987
14. Hutchinson BR, Merry AF, Wild CJ: The relationship of duration of fast to the volume and pH of gastric contents. Anaesth Intensive Care 14:128, 1986
15. Maltby JR, Sutherland AD, Sale JP et al: Preoperative oral fluids: Is a five-hour fast justified prior to elective surgery? Anesth Analg 65:1112, 1986
16. Maltby JR, Sutherland AD, Sale JP et al: Preoperative oral fluids: Is "NPO after midnight" justified? Anesthesiology 65:A244, 1986
17. Wetchler BV: Patient and procedure selection. In Wetchler BV (ed): Outpatient Anesthesia. Problems in Anesthesia, vol 2, p 9. Philadelphia, JB Lippincott, 1988
18. Wilson ME, Williams NB, Baskett PJF et al: Assessment of fitness for surgical procedures and the variability of anaesthetists' judgments. Br Med J 1:509, 1980
19. Dawson B, Reed WA: Anaesthesia for adult surgical outpatients. Can Anaesth Soc J 27:409, 1980
20. Natof HE: Complications associated with ambulatory surgery. JAMA 244:1116, 1980
21. Natof HE: Ambulatory surgery: Patients with pre-existing medical problems. Ill Med J 166:101, 1984
22. FASA Special Study 1. Alexandria, VA, Federated Ambulatory Surgery Association, 1987
23. Wetchler BV: The geriatric outpatient. In Wetchler BV (ed): Outpatient Anesthesia. Problems in Anesthesia, vol 2, p 128. Philadelphia, JB Lippincott, 1988
24. Vandam LD: To make the patient ready for anesthesia: Medical care of the surgical patient, 2nd ed. Reading, MA, Addison-Wesley, 1983
25. Steward DJ: Preterm infants are more prone to complications following minor surgery than are term infants. Anesthesiology 56:304, 1982
26. Liu LMP, Cote CJ, Goudsouzian NG et al: Life-threatening apnea in infants recovering from anesthesia. Anesthesiology 59:506, 1983
27. Kurth CD, Spitzer AR, Broennle MD et al: Postoperative apnea in former premature infants. Anesthesiology 63:A475, 1985
28. Welborn LG, Ramirez N, Oh TH et al: Postanesthetic apnea and periodic breathing in infants. Anesthesiology 65:658, 1986
29. Jensen S, Wetchler BV: The obese patient: An acceptable candidate for outpatient anesthesia. AANA J 50:369, 1982
30. El-Ganzouri AR, Ivankovich AD, Braverman B et al: Monoamine oxidase inhibitors: Should they be discontinued preoperatively? Anesth Analg 64:592, 1985
31. Epstein BS: Outpatient anesthesia. ASA Refresher Courses in Anesthesiology 2:81, 1974
32. Wetchler BV: Patient and procedure selection. In Wetchler BV (ed): Outpatient Anesthesia. Problems in Anesthesia, vol 2, p 13. Philadelphia, JB Lippincott, 1988
33. Orkin FK: Selection. In Wetchler BV (ed): Anesthesia for Ambulatory Surgery, p 77. Philadelphia, JB Lippincott, 1985
34. Standaert FG: Magic bullet, science and medicine. Anesthesiology 63:577, 1985
35. Meridy HW: Criteria for selection of ambulatory surgical patients and guidelines for anesthetic management: A retrospective study of 1,553 cases. Anesth Analg 61:921, 1982
36. Dillon JB: Anesthetic management of the outpatient. Ayrest Anesthesia Rounds 2:3, 1967
37. Reed WA: Recovery from anesthesia and discharge. In Shultz R (ed): Outpatient Surgery, p 45. Philadelphia, Lea & Febiger, 1979
38. Levy ML, Weintraub HD: Premedication: Yes or no? In Wetchler BV (ed): Outpatient Anesthesia. Problems in Anesthesia, vol 2, p 23. Philadelphia, JB Lippincott, 1988
39. Dean AF: Fundamentals for success. In Wetchler BV (ed): Anesthesia for ambulatory surgery, p 433. Philadelphia, JB Lippincott, 1985
40. Clark AJM, Hurtig JB: Premedication with meperidine and atropine does not prolong recovery to street fitness after outpatient surgery. Can Anaesth Soc J 28:390, 1981
41. Thompson GE, Remington JM, Millman BS et al: Experiences with outpatient anesthesia. Anesth Analg 52:881, 1973
42. Falick YS, Smiler BG: Is anticholinergic premedication necessary? Anesthesiology 43:472, 1975
43. Wyant GM, Kao E: Glycopyrrolate methobromide: Effect on salivary secretion. Can Anaesth Soc J 21:230, 1974
44. Desjardins R, Ansara S, Charest J: Preanaesthetic medication in paediatric day-care surgery. Can Anaesth Soc J 28:141, 1981
45. Brzustowicz RM, Nelson DA, Betts EK et al: Efficacy of oral premedication for pediatric outpatient surgery. Anesthesiology 60:475, 1984
46. Miller RD, Way WL: Inhibition of succinylcholine-induced in-

creased intragastric pressure by non-depolarizing muscle relaxants and lidocaine. Anesthesiology 34:185, 1971

47. Ong BY, Palahniuk RJ, Cumming M: Gastric volume and pH in outpatients. Can Anaesth Soc J 25:36, 1978

48. Manchikanti L, Roush JR: Effect of pre-anesthetic glycopyrrolate and cimetidine on gastric fluid pH and volume in outpatients. Anesth Analg 63:40, 1984

49. Manchikanti L, Canella MG, Hohlbein LJ et al: Assessment of effect of various modes of premedication on acid aspiration risk factors in outpatient surgery. Anesth Analg 66:81, 1987

50. Wyner J, Cohen SE: Gastric volume in early pregnancy—Effect of metoclopramide. Anesthesiology 57:209, 1983

51. Olsson GL, Hallen B, Hambraeus Jonzon K: Aspiration during anaesthesia: A computer aided study of 185,358 anaesthetics. Acta Anaesth Scand 30:84, 1986

52. Natof HE: Complications. In Wetchler BV (ed): Anesthesia for Ambulatory Surgery, p 344. Philadelphia, JB Lippincott, 1985

53. Stoelting RK: Gastric fluid pH in patients receiving cimetidine. Anesth Analg 57:675, 1978

54. Manchikanti L, Marrero TC: Effect of cimetidine and metoclopramide on gastric contents in outpatients. Anesth Rev 10:9, 1983

55. Manchikanti L, Colliver JA, Marrero TC et al: Ranitidine and metoclopramide for prophylaxis of aspiration pneumonitis in elective surgery. Anesth Analg 63:903, 1984

56. Gonzalez ER, Butler SA, Jones MK et al: Cimetidine versus ranitidine: Single-dose, oral regimen for reducing gastric acidity and volume in ambulatory surgery patients. Drug Intelligence and Clinical Pharmacy 21:192, 1987

57. Gillett GB, Watson JD, Langford RML: Ranitidine and single-dose antacid therapy as prophylaxis against acid aspiration syndrome in obstetric practice. Anaesthesia 39:638, 1984

58. Zeldis JE, Friedman LS, Isselbacher KJ: Ranitidine: A new H_2 receptor antagonist. N Engl J Med 309:1368, 1983

59. Somori GJ, Kallar SK: The effects of cimetidine on gastric pH and volume in pediatric patients in an ambulatory surgical center. Anesthesiology 61:3A, 1984

60. Young ET, Goudsouzian NG, Shah A: Effect of ranitidine on intragastric pH in children. Anesth Analg 65:S170, 1986

61. Solamki DR, Nicholas DA, Williams KR: Comparative effects of oral sodium citrate and oral cimetidine on gastric pH in pediatric patients. Anesth Analg 65:S147, 1986

62. Cohen SE, Woods WA, Wyner J: Antiemetic efficacy of droperidol and metoclopramide. Anesthesiology 60:67, 1984

63. Rao TLK, Madhavareddy S, Chinthagada M et al: Metoclopramide and cimetidine to reduce gastric fluid pH and volume. Anesth Analg 63:1014, 1984

64. Murrell GC, Rosen M: In vitro buffering capacity of alka seltzer effervescent. Anesthesiology 41:138, 1986

65. White PF, Chang T: Effect of narcotic premedication on the intravenous anesthetic requirement. Anesthesiology 61:A389, 1984

66. Epstein BS, Levy ML, Thein MH et al: Evaluation of fentanyl as an adjunct to thiopental-nitrous oxide-oxygen anesthesia for short surgical procedures. Anesth Rev 2(3):24, 1975

67. Hunt TM, Plantevin OM, Gilbert JR: Morbidity in gynaecological day-case surgery: A comparison of two anaesthetic techniques. Br J Anaesth 51:785, 1979

68. Sanders RS, Sinclair ME, Sear JW: Alfentanil in short procedures. Anaesthesia 39:1202, 1984

69. Pandit SK, Kothary SP: Should we premedicate ambulatory surgical patients? Anesthesiology 65:A352, 1986

70. Jakobsen H, Hertz JB, Johansen JR et al: Premedication before day surgery: A double-blind comparison of diazepam and placebo. Br J Anaesth 57:300, 1985

71. Jansen EC, Wachowiak-Andersen G, Munster-Swendsen J et al: Postural stability after oral premedication with diazepam. Anesthesiology 63:557, 1985

72. Greenwood BK, Bradshaw EG: Preoperative medication for day-case surgery. Br J Anaesth 55:933, 1983

73. Clark G, Erwin D, Yate P et al: Temazepam as premedication in elderly patients. Anaesthesia 37:421, 1982

74. Fragen RJ, Funk DI, Avram MJ et al: Midazolam versus hydroxyzine as intramuscular premedicant. Can Anaesth Soc J 30:136, 1983

75. Vinik HR, Reves JG, Wright D: Premedication with intramuscular midazolam: A prospective randomized double-blind controlled study. Anesth Analg 61:933, 1982

76. Rita L, Seleny FL, Goodarzi M et al: Dose-finding study of intramuscular midazolam in children. Anesth Rev 12:40, 1985

77. Cohen DD, Dillon JB: Anesthesia for outpatient surgery. JAMA 196:98, 1966

78. Mulroy MF: Regional anesthesia: When, why, why not? In Wetchler BV (ed): Outpatient Anesthesia. Problems in Anesthesia, vol 2, p 82. Philadelphia, JB Lippincott, 1988

79. Bridenbaugh LD, Soderstrom RM: Lumbar epidural block anesthesia for outpatient laparoscopy. J Reprod Med 23:85, 1979

80. Coupland GAE, Townsend DM, Martin CJ: Peritoneoscopy—Use in assessment of intraabdominal malignancy. Surgery 89:645, 1981

81. Philip BK: Supplemental medication for ambulatory procedures under regional anesthesia. Anesth Analg 64:1117, 1985

82. Reeves JG, Fragen RJ, Vinik HR et al: Midazolam: Pharmacology and uses. Anesthesiology 62:310, 1985

83. White PF: The role of midazolam in outpatient anesthesia. Anesth Rev 12:55, 1985

84. Philip BK: Hazards of amnesia after midazolam in ambulatory surgical patients. Anesth Analg 66:97, 1987

85. Philip BK, Covino BG: Local and regional anesthesia. In Wetchler BV (ed): Anesthesia for Ambulatory Surgery, p 225. Philadelphia, JB Lippincott, 1985

86. Mulroy MF: Spinal headache and air travel. Anesthesiology 51:479, 1979

87. Flaaten H, Raeder J: Spinal anaesthesia for outpatient surgery. Anaesthesia 40:1108, 1985

88. Atkinson RS, Lee JA: Spinal anaesthesia and day case surgery? Anaesthesia 40:1059, 1985

89. Carbaat P, van Crevel H: Lumbar puncture headache: Controlled study on the preventive effect of 24 hours' bed rest. Lancet 2:1131, 1981

90. Jones RJ: The role of recumbency in the prevention and treatment of postspinal headache. Anesth Analg 53:788, 1974

91. Vandam LD, Dripps RD: Long-term follow-up of patients who received 10,098 spinal anesthetics: Syndrome of decreased intracranial pressure. JAMA 161:586, 1956

92. Burke RK: Spinal anesthesia for laparoscopy: A review of 1,063 cases. J Reprod Med 21:59, 1978

93. Cohen SE: Epidural blood patch in outpatients: A simpler approach. Anesth Analg 64:458, 1985

94. Shane SM: Conscious-Sedation for Ambulatory Surgery, p 1. Baltimore, University Park Press, 1983

95. McCarthy FM, Solomon AL, Jastak JT et al: Conscious sedation: Benefits and risk. J Am Dent Assoc 109:546, 1984

96. Shane SM: Intravenous amnesia for total dentistry in one sitting. J Oral Surg 24:27, 1966

97. Bennett CR: Conscious-Sedation in Dental Practice, 2nd ed, p 12. St Louis, CV Mosby, 1978

98. Kallar SK, Dunwiddie WC: Conscious sedation. In Wetchler BV (ed): Outpatient Anesthesia. Problems in Anesthesia, vol 2, p 93. Philadelphia, JB Lippincott, 1988

99. Kallar SK, Pope BW, Dunwiddie WC et al: Hypoxemia in patients

undergoing conscious sedation techniques in the ambulatory surgery center. Personal communication, 1987

100. Ceravolo FJ, Meyers HE, Baraff LS et al: Full dentition periodontal surgery using intravenous conscious-sedation: A report of 5,000 cases. J Periodontal 51:462, 1980

101. Ceravolo FJ, Meyers HE, Michael JJ et al: Full dentition periodontal surgery using intravenous conscious-sedation: A report of 10,000 cases. J Periodontal 57:462, 1986

102. Shane SM, Carrel R, Vandenberge J: Intravenous amnesia—An appraisal after seven years and 10,500 administrations. Anesth Progr 21:36, 1974

103. Campbell RL: Prevention of complications associated with intravenous sedation and general anesthesia. J Oral Maxillofac Surg 44:289, 1986

104. Miller JR, Redish CH, Fisch C et al: Factors in arrhythmia during dental outpatient general anesthesia. Anesth Analg 49:701, 1970

105. Hudson RJ, Stanski DR, Burch PG: Pharmacokinetics of methohexital and thiopental in surgical patients. Anesthesiology 59:215, 1983

106. Carson IW: Recovery from anaesthesia—A review of methods for evaluation of recovery from anaesthesia. Proc R Soc Med 68:108, 1975

107. Hannington-Kiff JG: Measurement of recovery from outpatient general anaesthesia with a simple ocular test. Br Med J 3:132, 1970

108. Elliott CJR, Green R, Howells TH et al: Recovery after intravenous barbiturate anaesthesia. Lancet 1:68, 1962

109. Doneicke A, Kugler J, Laub M: Evaluation of recovery and "street-fitness" by EEG and psychodiagnostic tests after anaesthesia. Can Anaesth Soc J 14:567, 1967

110. Dundee JW: Clinical studies of induction agents. VII. A comparison of eight intravenous anaesthetics as main agents for a standard operation. Br J Anaesth 35:784, 1963

111. Lees NW, Hendry JGB: Etomidate in urological outpatient anaesthesia. Anaesthesia 32:592, 1977

112. Fragen RJ, Caldwell N: Comparison of a new formulation of etomidate with thiopental—Side effects and awakening times. Anesthesiology 50:242, 1979

113. Horrigan RW, Moyers JR, Johnson BH et al: Etomidate vs. thiopental with and without fentanyl—A comparative study of awakening in man. Anesthesiology 52:362, 1980

114. White PF, Shafer A: Clinical pharmacology and uses of injectable anesthetic and analgesic drugs. In Wetchler BV (ed): Outpatient Anesthesia. Problems in Anesthesia, vol 2, p 37. Philadelphia, JB Lippincott, 1988.

115. Giese JL, Stanley TH, Pace NL: Fentanyl pretreatment reduces side effects associated with etomidate anesthesia induction. Anesthesiology 59:A320, 1983

116. Collin RIW, Drummond GB, Spence AA: Alfentanil supplemented anaesthesia for short procedures. A double-blind study of alfentanil used with etomidate and enflurane for day cases. Anaesthesia 41:477, 1986

117. Melnick BM, Phitayakorn P, McKenzie R: Abolishing pain on injection of etomidate. Anesthesiology 66:444, 1987

118. White PF: Continuous infusions of thiopental, methohexital, or etomidate as adjuvants to nitrous oxide for outpatient anesthesia. Anesth Analg 63:282, 1984

119. Wagner RL, White PF: Etomidate inhibits adrenocortical function in surgical patients. Anesthesiology 61:647, 1984

120. White PF: Use of continuous infusion versus intermittent bolus administration of fentanyl or ketamine during outpatient anesthesia. Anesthesiology 59:294, 1983

121. Wetchler BV: For ambulatory surgery patients, use ketamine with caution. Same-Day Surgery 8, No. 1:11, 1984

122. Krantz EM: Low-dose intramuscular ketamine and hyal-

uronidase for induction of anesthesia in nonpremedicated children. S Afr Med J 58:506, 1983

123. Mackenzie N, Grant IS: Comparison of the new emulsion formulation of propofol with methohexitone and thiopentone for induction of anaesthesia in day cases. Br J Anaesth 57:725, 1985

124. Jones DF: Recovery from day-care anaesthesia—Comparison of a further four techniques including the use of the new induction agent diprivan. Br J Anaesth 54:629, 1982

125. Doze VA, Westphal LM, White PF: Comparison of propofol with methohexital for outpatient anesthesia. Anesth Analg 65:189, 1986

126. McCulloch MJ, Lees NW: Assessment and modification of pain on induction with propofol (Diprivan). Anaesthesia 40:1117, 1985

127. Youngberg JA, Texitor MS, Smith DE: A comparison of induction and maintenance of anesthesia with propofol to induction with thiopental and maintenance with isoflurane. Anesth Analg 66:S191, 1987

128. Doze VA, White PF: Comparison of propofol with thiopental-isoflurane for induction and maintenance of outpatient anesthesia. Anesthesiology 65:A544, 1986

129. Johnston RG, Anderson BJ, Noseworthy TW: Diprivan versus thiopentone for outpatient surgery. Can Anaesth Soc J 33:S106, 1986

130. Henricksson BA, Carlsson P, Hallen B et al: Propofol versus thiopentone as anaesthetic agents for short operative procedures. Acta Anaesthesiol Scand 31:63, 1987

131. Dundee JW, McCollum JSC, Milligan KR et al: Thiopental and propofol as induction agents. Anesthesiology 65:A545, 1986

132. Fahy LT, van Mourik GA, Utting JE: A comparison of the induction characteristics of thiopentone and propofol. Anaesthesia 40:939, 1985

133. O'Toole DP, Milligan KR, Howe JP et al: A comparison of propofol and methohexitone as induction agents for day case isoflurane anaesthesia. Anaesthesia 42:373, 1987

134. Sampson IH, Lefkowitz M, Kohen M et al: A comparison of propofol and methohexital for anesthesia by continuous infusion. Anesth Analg 66:S150, 1987

135. Churchill-Davidson HC: Suxamenthonium chloride and muscle pains. Br Med J 1:74, 1954

136. Perry J, Wetchler BV: Outpatient anesthesia: The effects of diazepam pretreatment of succinylcholine on fasciculation and postoperative myalgia. AANA J 52:48, 1984

137. Sosis M, Broad T, Larijani GE et al: Comparison of atracurium and d-tubocurarine for prevention of succinylcholine myalgia. Anesth Analg 66:657, 1987

138. Sokoll MD, Gergis SD, Mehta M et al: Safety and efficacy of atracurium (BW33A) in surgical patients receiving balanced or isoflurane anesthesia. Anesthesiology 58:450, 1983

139. Stirt JA, Katz RL, Murray AL et al: Intubation with atracurium in man. Anesthesiology 59:A266, 1983

140. Rupp SM, McChristian JW, Miller RD: Neuromuscular effects of atracurium during halothane-nitrous oxide and enflurane-nitrous oxide in humans. Anesthesiology 63:16, 1985

141. Rupp SM, Miller RD, Gencarelli PJ: Vecuronium-induced neuromuscular blockade during enflurane, isoflurane and halothane anesthesia in humans. Anesthesiology 60:102, 1984

142. Pearce AC, Williams JP, Jones RM: The use of atracurium for short surgical procedures in day-case patients. Anesthesiology 59:A265, 1983

143. Fragen RJ, Shanks CA: Neuromuscular recovery after laparoscopy. Anesth Analg 63:51, 1984

144. Gergis SD, Sokoll M, Mehta O et al: Intubation conditions after atracurium and suxamethonium. Br J Anaesth 55:835, 1983

145. Lichtiger M, Wetchler BV, Philip BK: The adult and geriatric

patient. In Wetchler BV (ed): Anesthesia for Ambulatory Surgery, p 175. Philadelphia, JB Lippincott, 1985

146. Glass P, Wilson W, Mace J et al: Assessment of the optimal priming dose for atracurium, pancuronium and vecuronium to obtain rapid onset muscle relaxation. Anesth Analg 66:S69, 1987

147. Basta SJ, Savarese JJ, Ali HH et al: The neuromuscular pharmacology of BW B1090U in anesthetized patients. Anesthesiology 63:A318, 1985

148. Ali HH, Savarese JJ, Embree PB et al: Clinical pharmacology of BW B1090U continuous infusion. Anesthesiology 65:A282, 1986

149. Savarese JJ, Ali HH, Basta SJ et al: Clinical conditions with and without priming after fentanyl-thiopental induction. Anesthesiology 65:A283, 1986

150. Goroszeniuk T, Whitwam JG, Morgan M: Use of methohexitone, fentanyl and nitrous oxide for short surgical procedures. Anesthesiology 32:209, 1977

151. Pollard J: Clinical evaluation of intravenous vs inhalational anesthesia in the ambulatory surgical unit: A multicenter study. Curr Therap Res 36:617, 1984

152. White PF, Sung ML, Doze VA: Use of sufentanil in outpatient anesthesia—Determining an optimal preinduction dose. Anesthesiology 63:A202, 1985

153. Bailey PL, Streisand JB, Pace NL et al: Sufentanil produces shorter lasting respiratory depression and longer lasting analgesia than equipotent doses of fentanyl in human volunteers. Anesthesiology 65:A493, 1986

154. Wasudev G, Kambam JR, Hazlehurst WM et al: Comparative study of sufentanil and isoflurane in outpatient surgery. Anesth Analg 66:S186, 1987

155. Zuurmond WWA, van Leeuwen L: Recovery from sufentanil anaesthesia for outpatient arthroscopy: A comparison with isoflurane. Acta Anaesthesiol Scand 31:154, 1987

156. Phitayakoran P, Melnick BM, Vicinie AF: Comparison of continuous sufentanil and fentanyl infusions for outpatient anesthesia. Can J Anaesth 34:242, 1987

157. Andrews CJH, Sinclair M, Prys-Roberts C et al: Ventilatory effects during and after continuous infusion of fentanyl or alfentanil. Br J Anaesth 55:S211, 1983

158. White PF, Coe V, Shafer A et al: Comparison of alfentanil with fentanyl for outpatient anesthesia. Anesthesiology 64:99, 1986

159. Scamman FL, Ghoneim MM, Korttila K: Ventilatory and mental effects of alfentanil and fentanyl. Acta Anaesthesiol Scand 28:63, 1984

160. Zuurmond WWA, van Leeuwen L: Alfentanil v. isoflurane for outpatient arthroscopy. Acta Anaesthesiol Scand 30:329, 1986

161. Short SM, Rutherfoord CF, Sebel PS: A comparison between isoflurane and alfentanil supplemented anaesthesia for short procedures. Anaesthesia 40:1160, 1985

162. Jellicoe JA: A comparison of alfentanil, halothane and enflurane for day-case gynaecological surgery. Anaesthesia 40:810, 1985

163. Dechene JP: Alfentanil as an adjunct to thiopentone and nitrous oxide in short surgical procedures. Can Anaesth Soc J 32:346, 1985

164. Coe V, Shafer A, White PF: Techniques for administering alfentanil during outpatient anesthesia—A comparison with fentanyl. Anesthesiology 59:A347, 1983

165. Kallar SK, Keenan RL: Evaluation and comparison of recovery time from alfentanil and fentanyl for short surgical procedures. Anesthesiology 61:A379, 1984

166. Fine J, Finestone SC: A comparative of the side-effects of butorphanol, nalbuphine and fentanyl. Anesth Rev 8:13, 1981

167. Pandit SK, Kothary SP, Pandit UA et al: Comparison of fentanyl and butorphanol for outpatient anaesthesia. Can J Anaesth 34:130, 1987

168. Garfield JM, Garfield FB, Philip B et al: A comparison of clinical and psychologic effects of fentanyl and nalbuphine in ambulatory surgical patients. Anesth Analg 66:1303, 1987

169. Berggren L, Eriksson I: Midazolam for induction of anaesthesia in outpatients—A comparison with thiopentone. Acta Anaesthesiol Scand 25:492, 1981

170. Verma R, Ramasubramanian R, Sachar RM: Anesthesia for termination of pregnancy: Midazolam compared with methohexital. Anesth Analg 64:792, 1985

171. Forster A, Gardaz JP, Suter PM et al: I.V. midazolam as an induction agent for anaesthesia: A study in volunteers. Br J Anaesth 52:907, 1980

172. Crawford ME, Andersen CP, Mikkelson BO: Comparison between midazolam and thiopentone-based balanced anaesthesia for day-case surgery. Br J Anaesth 56:165, 1984

173. Fragen RJ, Caldwell NJ: Awakening characteristics following anesthesia induction with midazolam for short surgical procedures. Arzneim Forsch 31:2261, 1981

174. Fragen RJ: The uses of midazolam. Anesth Rev 12:29, 1986

175. Alon E, Baitella L, Hossli G: Double-blind study of the reversal of midazolam-supplemented general anaesthesia with Ro15-1788. Br J Anaesth 59:455, 1987

176. Apfelbaum JL: Inhalational agents in anesthesia for ambulatory surgery. In Wetchler BV (ed): Outpatient Anesthesia. Problems in Anesthesia, vol 2, p 55. Philadelphia, JB Lippincott, 1988

177. Saidman LJ, Eger EI II: Effect of nitrous oxide and of narcotic premedication on the alveolar concentration of halothane required for anesthesia. Anesthesiology 25:302, 1964

178. Bahlman SH, Eger EI II, Smith NT et al: The cardiovascular effects of nitrous oxide-halothane anesthesia in man. Anesthesiology 35:274, 1971

179. Smith NT, Calverley RK, Prys-Roberts C et al: Impact of nitrous oxide on the circulation during enflurane anesthesia in man. Anesthesiology 48:345, 1978

180. Dolan WM, Stevens WC, Eger EI II et al: The cardiovascular and respiratory effects of isoflurane-nitrous oxide anesthesia. Can Anaesth Soc J 21:557, 1974

181. Alexander GD, Skupski JN, Brown EM: The role of nitrous oxide in postoperative nausea and vomiting. Anesth Analg 63:175, 1984

182. Lonie DS, Harper NJN: Nitrous oxide anaesthesia and vomiting. Anaesthesia 41:703, 1986

183. Korttila K, Hovorka J, Erkola O: Omission of nitrous oxide does not decrease the incidence or severity of emetic symptoms after isoflurane anesthesia. Anesth Analg 66:S98, 1987

184. Muir JJ, Warner MA, Buck CF et al: Role of nitrous oxide and other factors in postoperative nausea and vomiting: A randomized and blinded prospective study. Anesthesiology 66:513, 1987

185. Hannallah RS: Pediatric outpatient anesthesia. Urol Clin North Am 14:51, 1987

186. Fisher DM, Robinson S, Brett CM et al: Comparison of enflurane, halothane and isoflurane for diagnostic and therapeutic procedures in children with malignancies. Anesthesiology 63:647, 1985

187. Kingston HGG: Halothane and isoflurane anesthesia in pediatric outpatients. Anesth Analg 65:181, 1986

188. McAteer PM, Carter JA, Cooper GM et al: Comparison of isoflurane and halothane in outpatient paediatric dental anaesthesia. Br J Anaesth 58:390, 1986

189. Jones HD, McLaren AB: Postoperative shivering and hypoxaemia after halothane, nitrous oxide, oxygen anaesthesia. Br J Anaesth 37:35, 1965

190. Tyrell MF, Feldman S: Headache following halothane anaesthesia. Br J Anaesth 40:99, 1968

191. Ryder W, Wright PA: Halothane and enflurane in dental anaesthesia. Anaesthesia 36:492, 1981

192. Johnston RR, Eger EI II, Wilson C: A comparative interaction of epinephrine with enflurane, isoflurane, and halothane in man. Anesth Analg 55:709, 1976

193. Sigurdsson GH, Lindahl S: Cardiac arrhythmias in intubated children during adenoidectomy. A comparison between enflurane and halothane anesthesia. Acta Anaesthesiol Scand 27:484, 1983

194. Stanford BJ, Plantevin OM, Gilbert JR: Morbidity after day-case gynaecological surgery—Comparison of enflurane with halothane. Br J Anaesth 51:1143, 1979

195. Kreienbuhl G: Subjektive beschwerden nach halothan-lund nach enfluraneanaesthesie bei ambulanten (tagesklinik-) patienten. Anaesthetist 27:533, 1978

196. Tracey JA, Holland AJC, Unger L: Morbidity in minor gynaecological surgery: A comparison of halothane, enflurane and isoflurane. Br J Anaesth 54:1213, 1982

197. Storms LH, Stark AH, Calverley RK et al: Psychological functioning after halothane or enflurane anesthesia. Anesth Analg 59:245, 1980

198. Melnick BM, Chalasani J, Hy NTL: Comparison of enflurane, isoflurane and continuous fentanyl infusion for outpatient anesthesia. Anesth Rev 11:36, 1984

199. Padfield A: Recovery comparison between enflurane and halothane technique. A study of outpatients undergoing cystoscopy. Anaesthesia 35:508, 1980

200. Azar I, Karambelkar DJ, Lear E: Neurologic state and psychomotor function following anesthesia for ambulatory surgery. Anesthesiology 60:347, 1984

201. Miller RD, Eger EI II, Way WL et al: Comparative neuromuscular effects of forane and halothane alone and in combination with d-tubocurarine in man. Anesthesiology 35:38, 1971

202. Rupp SM, Fahey MR, Miller RD: Neuromuscular and cardiovascular effects of atracurium during nitrous oxide-fentanyl and nitrous oxide-isoflurane anaesthesia. Br J Anaesth 55:67S, 1983

203. Rupp SM, Miller RD, Gencarelli PJ: Vecuronium-induced neuromuscular blockade during enflurane, isoflurane, and halothane anesthesia in humans. Anesthesiology 60:102, 1984

204. Homi J, Konchigeri HN, Eckenhoff JE: A new anesthetic agent—Forane: Preliminary observation in man. Anesth Analg 41:439, 1972

205. Buffington CW: Clinical evaluation of isoflurane. Reflex actions during isoflurane anesthesia. Can Anaesth Soc J 29:S35, 1982

206. Rising S, Dodgson MS, Steen PA: Isoflurane v fentanyl for outpatient laparoscopy. Acta Anaesthesiol Scand 29:251, 1985

207. Korttila K, Valanne J: Recovery after outpatient isoflurane and enflurane anesthesia. Anesth Analg 64:239, 1985

208. Carter JA, Dye AM, Cooper GM: Recovery from day-case anaesthesia. The effect of different inhalational agents. Anaesthesia 40:545, 1985

209. Faculty expert explains steps to low hospital admission rates. Same-Day Surgery 6:136, 1982

210. Caldamone AA, Rabinowitz R: Outpatient orchiopexy. J Urol 127:286, 1982

211. Aldrete JA: Are intramuscular injections obsolete in the recovery room? Curr Rev: Recovery Room Nurses 5:147, 1983

212. Soni V, Burney R: Anesthetic techniques for laparoscopic tubal ligation. Anesth 55:A145, 1981

213. Wetchler BV: Managing pain in the postanesthesia care unit. J Post Anesth Nurs 1:52, 1986

214. Shandling B, Steward D: Regional analgesia for post-operative pain in pediatric outpatient surgery. J Pediatr Surg 15:477, 1980

215. Yoon F: Fallope ring offers safety, limited tubal damage. Same-Day Surgery 4:85, 1980

216. Burnhill MS: Pitfalls of the fallope ring. Same-Day Surgery 4:86, 1980

217. Thompson RE, Wetchler BV, Alexander CD: Infiltration of the mesosalpinx for pain relief after laparoscopic tubal sterilization with yoon rings. J Reprod Med 32:537, 1987

218. Alexander CD, Wetchler BV, Thompson RE: Bupivacaine infil-

tration of the mesosalpinx in ambulatory surgical laparoscopic tubal sterilization. Can J Anaesth 34:362, 1987

219. McGlinchey J, McLean P, Walsh A: Day case penile surgery with penile block for postoperative pain relief. Ir Med J 76:319, 1983

220. Tree-trakarn T, Pirayavaraporn S: Postoperative pain relief for circumcision in children: Comparison among morphine, nerve block, and topical analgesia. Anesthesiology 62:519, 1985

221. Elder PT, Belman AB, Hannallah RS et al: Postcircumcision pain—A prospective evaluation of subcutaneous ring block of the penis. Regional Anesthesia 9:48, 1984

222. Hannallah RS, Broadman LM, Belman AB et al: Control of post-orchidopexy pain in pediatric outpatients: Comparison of two regional techniques. Anesthesiology 61:A429, 1984

223. Takasaki M, Dohi S, Kawahata Y et al: Dosage of lidocaine for caudal anesthesia in infants and children. Anesthesiology 47:527, 1977

224. Broadman LM, Hannallah RS, Norrie WC et al: Caudal analgesia in pediatric outpatient surgery: A comparison of three different bupivacaine concentrations. Anesth Analg 66:S19, 1987

225. Sharpe TD, Goresky GV, Sabourin MA et al: Do epinephrine-containing solutions decrease the risk of using bupivacaine for caudal anaesthesia in children? Can Anaesth Soc J 33:S114, 1986

226. Broadman LM, Hannallah RS, Norden JM et al: Kiddie caudals: Experience with 1,154 consecutive cases without complications. Anesth Analg 66:S18, 1987

227. Lunn JW: Post-operative analgesia after circumcision. Anaesthesia 34:552, 1979

228. Bramwell RGB, Bullen C, Radford P: Caudal block for postoperative analgesia in children. Anaesthesia 37:1024, 1982

229. May AE, Wandless J, James RH: Analgesia for circumcision in children. Acta Anaesthesiol Scand 26:331, 1982

230. Yeoman PM, Cooke R, Hain WR: Penile block for circumcision. Anaesthesia 38:862, 1983

231. Vater M, Wandless J: Caudal or dorsal nerve block? A comparison of two local anaesthetics for postoperative analgesia following day case circumcision. Acta Anaesthesiol Scand 29:175, 1985

232. Markham SJ, Tomlinson J, Hain WR: Ilioinguinal nerve block in children: A comparison with caudal block for intra- and postoperative analgesia. Anaesthesia 41:1098, 1986

233. Epstein BS, Hannallah RS: The pediatric patient. In Wetchler BV (ed): Anesthesia for Ambulatory Surgery, p 124. Philadelphia, JB Lippincott, 1985

234. Patel RI, Hannallah RS, Murphy LS et al: Pediatric outpatient anesthesia—A review of post-anesthetic complications in 8,995 cases. Anesthesiology 65:A435, 1986

235. Anderson R, Crohg K: Pain as a major cause of postoperative nausea. Can Anaesth Soc J 23:366, 1976

236. Dundee JW, Chestnutt WN, Ghaly RG et al: Traditional chinese acupuncture: A potentially useful antiemetic. Br Med J 293:583, 1986

237. Wheaton NE: Comparison of benzquinamide hydrochloride and droperidol in preventing postoperative nausea and vomiting following general outpatient anesthesia. AANA J 53:322, 1985

238. McKenzie R, Wadhwa RK, Uy NTL et al: Antiemetic effectiveness of intramuscular hydroxyzine compared with intramuscular droperidol. Anesth Analg 60:783, 1981

239. Wetchler BV, Collins IS, Jacob L: Antiemetic effects of droperidol on the ambulatory surgery patient. Anesth Rev 9:23, 1982

240. Valanne J, Korttila K: Effect of a small dose of droperidol on nausea, vomiting and recovery after outpatient enflurane anaesthesia. Acta Anaesthesiol Scand 29:359, 1985

241. Cohen SE, Woods WA, Wyner J: Antiemetic efficacy of droperidol and metoclopramide. Anesthesiology 60:67, 1984

242. Doze VA, Shafer A, White PF: Nausea and vomiting after outpatient anesthesia—Effectiveness of droperidol alone and in combination with metoclopramide. Anesth Analg 66:S41, 1987

243. Rao TLK, Madhavareddy S, Chinthagada M et al: Meto-

clopramide and cimetidine to reduce gastric fluid pH and volume. Anesth Analg 63:1014, 1984

244. Diamond MJ, Keeri-Szanto M: Reduction of postoperative vomiting by preoperative administration of oral metoclopramide. Can Anaesth Soc J 27:36, 1980

245. Meeter SE, Kitz DS, Young ML et al: Nausea and vomiting after outpatient laparoscopy: Incidence, impact on recovery room stay and cost. Anesth Analg 66:S116, 1987

246. Abramowitz MD, Oh TH, Epstein BS et al: The antiemetic effect of droperidol following outpatient strabismus surgery in children. Anesthesiology 59:579, 1983

247. Abramowitz MD, Epstein BS, Friendly DS et al: The effect of droperidol in reducing vomiting in pediatric strabismic outpatient surgery. Anesthesiology 55:A329, 1981

248. Lerman J, Eustis S, Smith DR: Effect of droperidol pretreatment on postanesthetic vomiting in children undergoing strabismus surgery. Anesthesiology 65:322, 1986

249. Hardy JF, Charest J, Girouard G et al: Nausea and vomiting after strabismus surgery in preschool children. Can Anaesth Soc J 33:57, 1986

250. Eustis S, Lerman J, Smith D: Droperidol pretreatment in children undergoing strabismus repair: The minimal effective dose. Can Anaesth Soc J 33:S115, 1986

251. Jackson SH, Schmidt MN, McGuire J et al: Transdermal scopolamine as a preanesthetic drug and postoperative antinauseant and antiemetic. Anesthesiology 57:A330, 1982

252. Gibbons PA, Nicolson SC, Betts EK et al: Scoplamine does not prevent post-operative emesis after pediatric eye surgery. Anesthesiology 61:A435, 1984

253. Reed WA: Recovery from anesthesia and discharge. In Shultz R (ed): Outpatient Surgery, p 45. Philadelphia, Lea and Febiger, 1979

254. Wetchler BV: Problem solving in the postanesthesia care unit. In Wetchler BV (ed): Anesthesia for Ambulatory Surgery, p 275. Philadelphia, JB Lippincott, 1985

255. Daos FG, Virtue RW: Sympathetic block persistence after spinal or epidural analgesia. JAMA 183:285, 1963

256. Pflug AE, Aasheim GM, Foster C: Sequence of return of neurological function and criteria for safe ambulation following subarachnoid block (spinal anaesthetic). Can Anaesth Soc J 25:133, 1978

257. Roe CF, Cohn FL: Sympathetic blockade during spinal anesthesia. Surg Gynecol Obstet 136:265, 1973

258. Ogg TW: An assessment of post-operative outpatient cases. Br Med J 4:573, 1972

259. Blackwell B: Treatment adherence. Br J Psychiatry 129:510, 1976

Chapter 50

Lawrence L. Priano

Trauma

The prominence of trauma as a major health hazard cannot be argued. Trauma is the leading cause of death in the United States in people 38 years of age and younger.[1, 2] Because trauma injuries occur during the victims' peak productivity years, this is the leading cause of lost years of life and lost income to families.[1, 2] Approximately 175,000 people die from trauma annually in the United States and for every death there are two permanent disabilities.[1, 2] Since 1960, while deaths from cancer, heart disease, and stroke have decreased, deaths from trauma have increased.[2, 3]

Death following an accident usually occurs during one of three periods. Fifty per cent of deaths from trauma are "immediate" at the scene and cannot, with a few exceptions, be prevented. Causes of immediate death include lacerations of the brain, brainstem, spinal cord, heart, and great vessels. Thirty per cent of trauma deaths are classified as "early" and occur within 3 hours of the accident. Causes of death after these one or two "golden" hours include an expanding intracranial mass, exsanguination, and hypoxia secondary to airway obstruction, tension pneumothorax, *etc.* Twenty per cent of trauma deaths are classified as "late," that is, they occur days to weeks after injury. These result primarily from sepsis and multiple organ failure. The organ systems most commonly involved are the renal, pulmonary, and coagulation systems.[3]

Improved prehospital care of the trauma victim has contributed to a reduction in mortality.[4] Highly trained paramedical personnel can establish an airway, ventilate the patient's lungs, and perform a number of other life-saving measures at the scene of an accident.[5-6] The efficacy of such intervention by paramedics has been debated, with some people advocat-

ing a "scoop and run" approach, and others advocating a delay in transport until the patient has been stabilized in the field. For critically ill trauma victims, endotracheal intubation, vigorous fluid resuscitation, immobilization of the spine, and rapid transport by paramedics have proven effective.[7] Many emergency personnel apply military antishock trousers (MAST) but they are probably helpful only in tamponading wounds, stabilizing long bone or pelvic fractures, and in preventing hypotension with spinal cord injury.[3, 8]

Transport of a patient directly to a regional center for trauma, rather than to the nearest hospital, results in improved outcome for the trauma victim.[9] A trauma center can most simply be defined as an institution that has made a commitment of personnel and facilities to the care of trauma victims. Functionally, this involves the in-house, immediate availability of trauma surgeons, anesthesiologists, emergency room (ER), operating room (OR), and critical care nurses, as well as the availability of ER, OR, ICU, diagnostic x-ray facilities and blood bank support at all times. The specifics of acceptable variations in the availability of such personnel and facilities have been spelled out by the American College of Surgeons' Committee on Trauma.[10]

Proper care of the trauma victim at the hospital requires detailed, advanced planning, an orderly protocol, and efficiency. A team of physicians, nurses, and technicians must be capable of rapid mobilization and each member of the team should have pre-assigned duties, under the direction of a team leader. In addition, the radiology department must have portable equipment and personnel who are immediately available for the ER, and a CT scan. A stat laboratory must be ready for determination of a complete blood count, coagulation screen,

TABLE 50-1. Suggested Anesthesia Supplies
for the Trauma Emergency Room

1. Laryngoscopes with assorted adult and pediatric blades
2. Assorted face masks
3. Assorted endotracheal tubes and stylets
4. Oral and nasal airways
5. Suction, with a rigid, large orifice tip
6. A source of 100% oxygen
7. A means of providing positive pressure ventilation with 100% oxygen, such as with a self-inflating resuscitation bag or an Ayre's T-piece circuit with a Jackson–Rees modification
8. A large needle, catheter and knife for emergency cricothyrotomy
9. Succinylcholine, vecuronium, pancuronium, thiopental, etomidate
10. Assorted catheters and "cutdown" equipment for establishment of large bore intravenous access
11. Pre-warmed bags of crystalloid solutions
12. Pressurized intravenous infusion devices
13. Monitor and transducer for arterial pressure

TABLE 50-2. Suggested Anesthesia Supplies
and Equipment for the Trauma Operating Room

1. Airway equipment as detailed in items #1–#7 in Table 50-1
2. Properly checked out anesthesia machine with tubing and rebreathing bag attached
3. A mechanical ventilator, capable of delivering PEEP and tidal volume at high inspiratory pressures, preset to normal adult values (e.g., TV = 800 ml, F = 10 breaths · min^{-1})
4. Heated humidifier
5. Warming blanket
6. Primed blood infusion sets in blood warmers
7. Pressurized fluid/blood infusion devices
8. Physiologic monitor with transducers attached, filled, and calibrated (infection potential is small[98])
9. Prefilled and labeled syringes
10. Defibrillator and resuscitation drugs in the room
11. Extra supplies (catheters, tubing, etc.)
12. Supplies for placement of arterial, central venous, and pulmonary artery catheters
13. Capability for increasing the OR temperature

blood gas analysis, toxicology, ethanol levels, and serum electrolytes. The blood bank must be well supplied and be able to perform a crossmatch expediently. Finally, the anesthesiologist must have available, prepared, and checked-out, an assortment of supplies and equipment for the ER and OR (Tables 50-1 and 50-2).

INITIAL ASSESSMENT AND MANAGEMENT OF THE TRAUMA PATIENT

GENERAL

Depending on the circumstances at a particular hospital, the anesthesiologist may play a major role in assessing the trauma victim. Even if the anesthesiologist does no more than place an endotracheal tube, he or she must be knowledgeable about acute trauma and how it may impact on his or her perioperative management. Many anesthesiologists have become certified in Advanced Trauma Life Support (ATLS), a course developed by the Committee on Trauma of the American College of Surgeons.[11] While some of the principles taught may be controversial, the course presents a highly organized and practical approach to the diagnosis and management of trauma.

When first notified of the impending arrival of a trauma victim, it is desirable to know the patient's Trauma Score (Table 50-3).[12] Perhaps the most valuable aspect of the scoring system is that it forces the trauma team to periodically assess the patient's circulatory, ventilatory, and neurologic function. The neurologic portion of this score is based on the Glasgow Coma Scale which examines eye opening, and verbal and motor functions. A high score is positive, whereas a low score signals a poor condition and possible poor outcome.

Upon the patient's arrival, the airway, breathing, circulation, and neurologic status (ABCN) must be quickly assessed. This initial assessment can be done in less than a minute. A first step is to ask the patient to take a deep breath. If no breath is taken, ventilate the patient's lungs and prepare to secure the airway with an endotracheal tube. Simultaneously, palpate a radial pulse for fullness and rate, and obtain a blood pressure as soon as possible. A conscious, normotensive, moving patient with a lack of stridor, tachypnea, tachycardia, or neck

pain is temporarily stable and a slower, more thorough diagnostic approach may be undertaken.

AIRWAY

All trauma victims must be considered to have a full stomach and to be at high risk for vomiting and aspiration. In an unconscious but spontaneously breathing patient with a patent airway, it is probably wise to take time to obtain a radiograph of the cervical spine to rule out a fracture before proceeding with tracheal intubation. In situations where the patient is not ventilating adequately, one needs to establish an airway and ventilate the lungs prior to obtaining a radiograph of the neck.

Early endotracheal intubation has been a major factor in reducing mortality from trauma. Indications for intubation of the trachea include protection of the airway, airway obstruction, positive pressure ventilation, tracheal toilet, coma, and shock. If a patient is semiconscious, combative, or uncontrollable, skeletal muscle paralysis and tracheal intubation may be necessary to facilitate diagnosis and/or treatment.

When performing oral tracheal intubation, an assistant should apply axial head/neck traction, being careful to leave the neck in a neutral position. The intubation should be done in rapid sequence fashion. That is, after pre-oxygenation, muscle paralysis, and application of cricoid pressure, an endotracheal tube (with a stylet inserted) should be placed under direct vision. Nasotracheal intubation is rarely indicated in the acute management of an unconscious trauma patient. Blind attempts are particularly dangerous in an unconscious patient because of the risk of vomiting from stimulation of the gag reflex. Tubes placed through the nose may also penetrate the brain in patients with certain skull or facial fractures.[13–16] Administration of muscle relaxants for tracheal intubation should only be done by those skilled in bag and mask ventilation of the lungs, in the unusual event that intubation of the trachea cannot be accomplished. Rarely, needle or surgical cricothyroidotomy may be necessary. The administration of sedative/hypnotic drugs prior to tracheal intubation should be reserved only for those patients who are awake and hemodynamically stable, or for some patients with an elevated intracranial pressure.

TABLE 50-3.   Trauma Score

TRAUMA SCORE	VALUE	POINTS	SCORE
A. Respiratory rate Number of respirations in 15 sec, multiply by four	10–24 25–35 >35 <10 0	4 3 2 1 0	A. _____
B. Respiratory effort Shallow—markedly decreased chest movement or air exchange Retractive—use of accessory muscles or intercostal retraction	Normal Shallow, or retractive	1 0	B. _____
C. Systolic blood pressure Systolic cuff pressure—either arm-auscultate or palpate No carotid pulse	>90 70–90 50–69 <50 0	4 3 2 1 0	C. _____
D. Capillary refill Normal—forehead, lip mucosa or nail bed color refill in 2 sec Delayed—more than 2 sec of capillary refill None—no capillary refill	Normal Delayed None	2 1 0	D. _____

E. Glasgow coma scale
1. Eye opening
   Spontaneous _____ 4
   To Voice _____ 3
   To Pain _____ 2
   None _____ 1
	Total
	GCS Points
	14–15
	11–13
	8–10
	5–7
	3–4
		Score
		5
		4
		3
		2
		1
			E. _____

2. Verbal response
   Oriented _____ 5
   Confused _____ 4
   Inappropriate words _____ 3
   Incomprehensible words _____ 2
   None _____ 1			

3. Motor response
   Obeys commands _____ 6
   Purposeful movement (pain) _____ 5
   Withdraw (pain) _____ 4
   Flexion (pain) _____ 3
   Extension (pain) _____ 2
   None _____ 1			

Total GCS points (1 + 2 + 3) _____		Trauma score _____ (Total points A + B + C + D + E)	

(Champion HR, Sacco WJ, Carnazzo AJ et al: Trauma score. Crit Care Med 9:673, 1981.)

Initial management of the airway depends on the clinical situation at hand. There are some situations in conscious or unconscious patients where endotracheal intubation is contraindicated or not possible. Examples of this include massive facial trauma and laryngeal or tracheal trauma. If external tracheal or laryngeal damage is not obvious, it should be suspected if hoarseness, stridor, dysphagia, subcutaneous emphysema, or dyspnea in the recumbent position are present.[17,18] Alternate methods for airway management, other than direct oral tracheal intubation, include blind oral intubation, use of a flexible fiberoptic bronchoscope, use of a catheter guide placed retrograde through the larynx, jet ventilation by way of a cricothyroid catheter, and tracheostomy. The use of an esophageal obturator airway should be discouraged.[19] The device, which is similar in appearance to an endotracheal tube, is placed blindly into the esophagus and a cuff is inflated to prevent reflux of gastric contents into the pharynx. Complications of the device include accidental tracheal intubation, esophageal perforation, an inability to provide adequate ventilation, difficulty in performing tracheal intubation around the esophageal tube, and nearly 100% incidence of emesis on removal of the tube.

CERVICAL SPINE AND NECK

Injury to the cervical spinal cord should be suspected when one observes flaccidity (especially of the rectal sphincter), diaphragmatic breathing, priapism, or hypotension with a slow pulse and warm extremities. Complete evaluation of the cervical spine may require a CT scan or multiple radiographs. However, a lateral view of the cervical spine is quick and reveals most unstable fractures (Fig. 50-1). Anesthesiologists should know how to interpret these studies. All seven cervical vertebrae must be seen, as C-7 is the most common site of injury.[20] The cervical spine should be lordotic in attitude. Kyphosis is indicative of spasm and should raise suspicion of injury. Prevertebral soft tissues should be less than 7 mm at C-3 and less than 20 mm at C-5. These tissue thicknesses cannot be evaluated with nasogastric or nasotracheal tubes in place. The disc interspaces should be similar at all levels and narrowing should raise suspicion of an injury. One should check for vertical alignment along the pre- and postvertebral and spinolaminar lines. Although a single normal lateral radiograph does not "clear" the neck, given a careful approach it makes neck injury from tracheal intubation very unlikely. Lack of neck pain and an ability to move all extremities also makes a cervical spine injury unlikely, although not ruled out. Until complete "clearance" is obtained, a rigid collar should be left in place.

The patient should also be evaluated for trauma to the anterior neck, because a number of structures can be damaged.[21] Blunt or penetrating trauma to the anterior neck can lead to a high likelihood for damage. In order of decreasing frequency of injury are veins, arteries, larynx/trachea, pharynx/esophagus, brachial plexus, cranial nerves, and the spinal cord.[22] Arterial hemorrhage in the neck can produce rapid and severe airway obstruction requiring immediate tracheal intubation and/or decompression of the hematoma. Cervical sub-

cutaneous air, pneumothorax, and pneumomediastinum can result from tracheal or laryngeal injury, whereas dysphagia is more common with pharyngeal and esophageal trauma. If airway damage or a hematoma is compromising the airway, it may be advisable not to paralyze the patient with muscle relaxants prior to securing the airway. Neither tracheal intubation nor mask ventilation may be possible.

HEAD INJURIES

Brain damage resulting from an injury to the head is a common cause for mortality and morbidity. With early institution of ventilation, restoration of cerebral perfusion, and reduction of an elevated intracranial pressure, the outcome is much more favorable. The hallmark of a closed head injury is loss of consciousness. With severe scalp lacerations, significant bleeding may have occurred and the patient may be obtunded due to hypovolemia. Examination of the pupils is important; however, anisocoria can be a normal variant in a small percentage of the population and can also occur with an isolated eye injury without intracranial pathology. Knowledge about the mechanism of injury can be helpful when assessing a possible head injury. If the patient is conscious, a thorough neurologic examination should be done. For an unconscious patient, CT scanning is necessary as soon as adequate ventilation has been assured and causes for severe hypotension have been cor-

FIG. 50-1. *A.* Lateral radiograph of the cervical spine. *B.* Diagram. Anatomy of the spine, lateral and superior view. (Blaisdell FW, Trunkey DD: Cervicothoracic Trauma. Trauma Management series, Vol III. New York, Thieme Medical Publishers, 1985.)

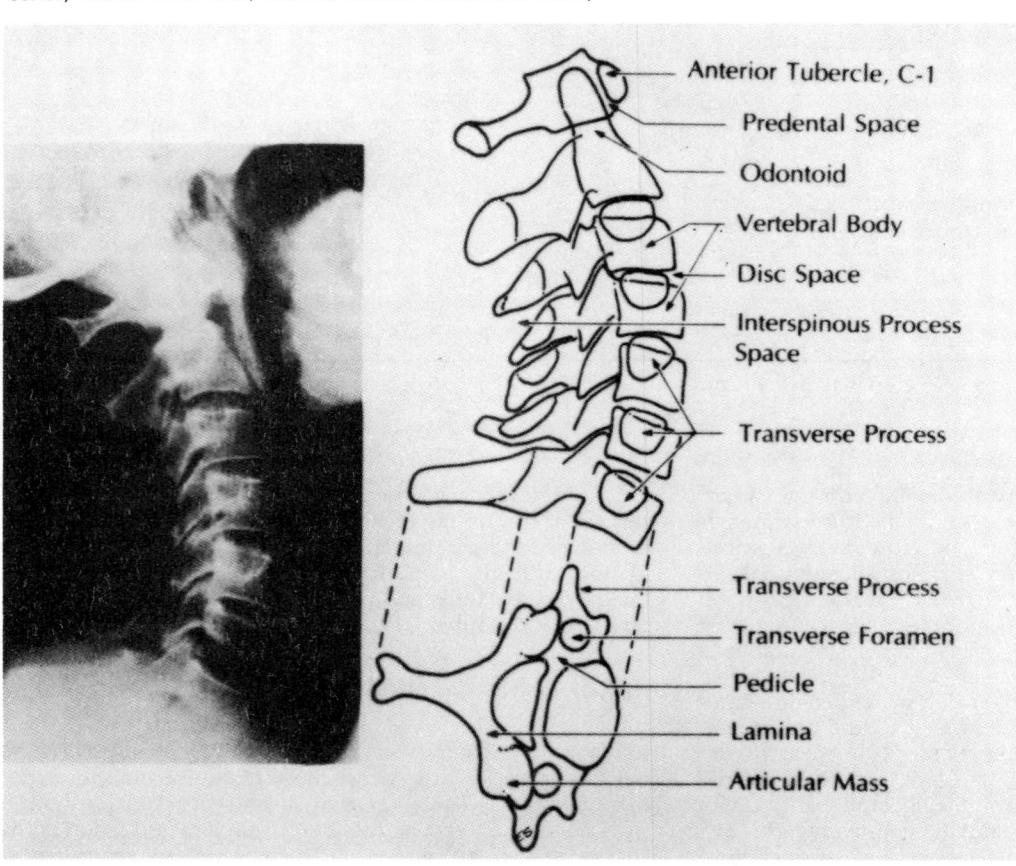

rected. Time is of the essence as intracranial hemorrhage can have devastating effects. Severe closed head injury has a very poor prognosis in multiple trauma patients. In one series of trauma victims who had a thoracotomy and open cardiac massage in the ER, the survival was only 25%. There were no survivors when there was coexistent severe closed head injury.[23]

INJURIES INVOLVING THE THORAX AND ABDOMEN

With penetrating trauma the primary site of injury is usually obvious. Blunt trauma presents a greater diagnostic dilemma because external examination may reveal nothing. While this is true for all injuries, it is particularly so for trauma to the thorax and abdomen. In blunt trauma, rib fractures are the most common injury with hemothorax, pneumothorax and flail chest following in order. With penetrating injury, a hemopneumothorax is most common with isolated hemothorax or pneumothorax seen less frequently.[24]

With thoracic trauma it is necessary to decide if the major injury involves the lungs, the cardiovascular system, or both. Because the majority of intrathoracic volume is air, it is not surprising that a high percentage of chest injuries can be treated conservatively with a tube thoracostomy and observation. If treating only a pneumothorax, a 26–32 Fr tube is adequate. For a hemo or hemopneumothorax, a larger (30–40 Fr) tube should be placed. In either case, the tube should be placed in the 4th or 5th interspace in the midaxillary line and directed posteriorly. The tubes should be placed to minus 15 to 20 cm H_2O suction until there has been no leak and/or less than 100 ml blood evacuated for 24 hours. If 1000 ml of blood is obtained after initial chest tube placement, or if bleeding exceeds 1500 ml in 24 hr, surgical exploration is indicated.

A severe chest injury, penetrating or blunt, is the primary cause of death in approximately 50% of trauma victims who die. In those patients who die, the most common findings are rib fractures, hemothorax, lung lacerations, and great vessel rupture. There is a lower incidence of lung contusion, lacerated diaphragm, or trachea and myocardial injury. Signs that frequently correlate with severe pulmonary or vascular injuries include fracture of 1st or 2nd ribs (15%–20% incidence of vascular injury), a widened mediastinum (33% incidence of vascular injury), flail chest (almost 100% incidence of lung contusion), and massive hemothorax (surgical bleeding requiring immediate thoracotomy). Although the injury may appear to be limited to the thorax, if it is below the 6th rib the major pathology is most likely intra-abdominal.[25]

A chest radiograph is an essential diagnostic tool for thoracic trauma. An upright inspiratory film is preferred (although expiratory films show pneumothorax better) because there is better overall contrast between structures. More common is an anteroposterior supine film, but be aware that significant pneumothoraces can be missed. Cross table laterals may be used to help find free fluid in the pleural space, but decubitus films are contraindicated if pelvic or spinal fractures are suspected. Angiography may be necessary to diagnose a widened mediastinum or clinically apparent vascular injuries, that is, a pulseless arm. Angiograms are contraindicated if shock or expanding head injuries coexist.

Contusions of the lung are not uncommon and are usually associated with multiple rib fractures, with or without flail chest. These result from high force blunt trauma with subsequent hemorrhage into lung tissue. Changes appear on radiograms within the first few hours. Thus, if the initial chest

radiograph is clear and a new radio-opacity appears late, it is most likely aspiration pneumonitis, atelectasis, or pneumonia. The most life threatening aspect of a lung contusion is severe hypoxia. Ventilation and oxygenation need to be supported mechanically with high FI_{O_2}s and PEEP, if necessary. A pulmonary artery catheter may be needed to optimize tissue oxygenation and oxygen transport. Chest tubes are also often necessary either therapeutically or prophylactically. Contusions usually begin to resolve in 2 to 5 days if other pulmonary complications are not superimposed.[26]

Direct cardiac trauma can be either blunt or penetrating. With the exception of high force missiles, penetrating trauma to the heart usually has a better prognosis than blunt trauma as there is less tissue damage. The three most common cardiac injuries are tamponade, contusion, and rupture. Patients with myocardial tamponade can demonstrate hypotension, neck vein distention, and muffled heart sounds (Beck's triad) and, in addition, tachycardia, paradoxical pulse, and a narrowed pulse pressure. If the patient is hypotensive, immediate treatment should consist of fluids, inotropic drugs, and open surgical drainage. Patients with myocardial contusions can develop cardiac dysrhythmias and angina pectoris that do not respond to nitrates. Diagnosis can be difficult. Any patient with a suspected myocardial contusion, who has abnormal ventricular function and is unstable, should probably be managed with a pulmonary artery catheter. Myocardial ruptures usually result in death at the scene, although isolated knife injuries have a better prognosis. About 70% of penetrating cardiac injuries are lethal in the prehospital period.

Aortic injuries are rare, yet it is important to have a high index of suspicion for this injury when other associated conditions exist, that is, sternal, clavicular, and upper rib fractures; rightward shifted trachea, blunting of the aortic knob; or head, cervical, or thoracic spine trauma. The ultimate diagnostic tool is an arch aortogram, although a high percentage of aortograms for widened mediastinum will be negative for arterial injury. In monitoring patients with suspected aortic injuries, radial artery cannulation should be on the right side as the survivable injuries are usually distal to the left subclavian artery.

ABDOMEN

Injury to organs in the peritoneal cavity can be difficult to diagnose when there is blunt trauma. The most common injuries are splenic rupture or laceration of the liver, resulting in significant hemorrhage. Bowel perforation can occur with blunt or penetrating injuries. As radiographs of the abdomen are unreliable, diagnosis of intraabdominal hemorrhage is done with peritoneal lavage or CT scan.[27, 28]

Urinary and pelvic injuries can be difficult to evaluate. If there is bleeding from the urethra, a retrograde urethrogram is indicated prior to insertion of a bladder catheter. After the catheter has been inserted, continued hematuria indicates a possible bladder injury and the need for a cystogram or intravenous pyelogram. Pelvic fractures are present in 10 to 12% of blunt torso injury. These can have a mortality rate of 20 to 30% due to hemorrhage.[29]

Fortunately, vascular injuries of the abdomen (aorta, vena cava, portal vein) are unusual. However, abdominal aortic injuries carry a 50% mortality. Abdominal vascular injuries result primarily from gunshot and stab wounds and occur less often with blunt trauma.[27] They are detected by deterioration of vital signs, by positive peritoneal lavage, or at laparotomy. Peritoneal lavage is considered by some to be too sensitive, giving false-positive results. In addition, it is not organ specific, does not evaluate the retroperitoneum, and is probably contraindicated in patients that have undergone prior abdominal surgery.[28] However, it does have a place in unstable patients where rapid diagnosis of a hemorrhagic abdominal injury may be preferred.[30]

EXTREMITIES

Perhaps the most important aspect of evaluation of the injured extremity is to realize that significant hemorrhage (1000–1500 ml of blood) can occur and not be obvious. This is particularly true with proximal leg injuries. Pay attention to distal pulses, visual symmetry of two extremities, and feel for distention or tightness of the skin, especially in the thigh areas after femur fractures. Early immobilization of obvious fractures is indicated.

BURNS

Care of the burn patient places tremendous demands on the medical team and is costly. Each year about 100,000 patients are hospitalized for a total of 2 million days.[31] The severity of a burn depends on the body surface area involved and the thickness of the burn. Partial thickness burns may only involve the superficial dermis, are exquisitely painful, and usually heal in 2 to 3 weeks without skin grafting. Full thickness burns involve destruction of all dermal appendages and do not heal properly unless the destroyed skin is excised and replaced with grafts. Mortality from burns increases with the severity of the burn and with advancing age. The prognosis of patients with a greater than 50% body surface area (BSA) full thickness burn is poor, but patients have survived a 90% BSA burn.

As is true for any patient who sustains trauma, initial treatment of the burned patient should involve attention to the airway, breathing, and circulation. If the patient is apneic, the face is burned, the patient has stridor or is hoarse, or the patient inhaled steam, smoke, or toxic fumes, the trachea should be intubated immediately. Intubation of the trachea is much easier when first considered, as compared to later when there is glottic and/or facial edema. Oral or nasotracheal intubation is preferable to tracheostomy in the burned patient, as the latter is associated with a high mortality rate.[32]

Inhalation of carbon monoxide is a frequent cause for hypoxia in burned patients. Carbon monoxide has 200 times more affinity for hemoglobin than oxygen, and although the patient's arterial P_{O_2} may be normal, the oxygen content of the blood may be quite low. Measurement of oxygen content and/or carboxyhemoglobin levels is indicated. Treatment of carbon monoxide should be with inhalation of 100% oxygen by mask or via an endotracheal tube. Hyperbaric oxygen is generally not indicated because transport of a severely burned patient to a chamber is hazardous. Damage to the subglottic airway is rare, unless the patient has inhaled live steam. If sloughing of the tracheal epithelium occurs, bronchoscopy may be necessary.[33]

After the airway has been secured and other life-threatening injuries have been treated, the burn patient must be resuscitated with large volumes of fluid. A burn causes a generalized increase in capillary permeability, with a considerable loss of fluid and protein into the interstitial tissue, plus an increase in evaporative losses. Fluid loss is greatest in the first

12 hours and subsists after about 24 hours.[34] One of several formulae to determine replacement needs was developed for adults at Parkland Hospital and calls for administration of 4 $ml \cdot kg^{-1}$ of balanced salt solution for every % BSA burned in the first 24 hours[34] (considerations with burned children differ[37]). However, volume replacement should be determined more by urine output and hemodynamic variables than by a fixed formula.

Within hours after a burn and until it has nearly healed, the patient is hypermetabolic. This is manifested by hyperthermia, increased catabolism, increased oxygen consumption, tachypnea, tachycardia, and increased serum catecholamine levels. As a result, the patient should be given oxygen, ventilation proportionate to the increase in carbon dioxide production, and parenteral nutrition.

Mortality, morbidity, and cosmetic outcome following thermal injury have improved considerably with the introduction of early excision of burned tissue and skin grafting.[35] Providing anesthesia for this operation is challenging and should involve the following considerations[35, 36, 38]:

Access for monitoring can be difficult. Needle electrodes may be required for the electrocardiogram (ECG) and nerve stimulator. A blood pressure cuff can be applied over burned tissue, but an arterial catheter is probably preferable in patients with large burns.

Accurate measurement and maintenance of body temperature is essential. Because of hypermetabolism, evaporative fluid loss, and exposure, the burned patient is particularly susceptible to hypothermia. As a consequence, the OR should be warmed to 28°C to 30°C, intravenous solutions should be warmed, and a heated humidifier should be placed in the anesthetic circuit.

Blood loss can be prodigious. This loss should be anticipated, pressurized infusion devices should be available, and the anesthesiologist should be prepared to encounter all the complications associated with massive transfusion (such as a loss of clotting factors).

The selection of anesthetic drugs is not critical as long as they are used rationally. Opioids should usually be a part of any technique as excruciating pain can be expected in the postoperative period. Halothane may not be a good choice because epinephrine-soaked pads are applied after excision of the burn and cardiac dysrhythmias may result. Ventilation of the lungs should usually be controlled as increased carbon dioxide production and/or respiratory failure may exist. Common anesthesia ventilators may not deliver a sufficient minute volume to maintain normocarbia.

Burned patients do not respond normally to muscle relaxants.[39] After about 24 hours following the burn, until the wound has healed, succinylcholine administration can result in a rapid rise in the serum potassium level and a cardiac arrest. On the other hand, burned patients are resistant to nondepolarizing muscle relaxants and doses must be adjusted upward and administered more frequently. The mechanism for this altered response to muscle relaxants is not known, although a proliferation of receptors is suspected.[39, 40]

The principles for the care of a patient with an electrical burn are, with two exceptions, similar to those for patients with a thermal burn. First, the extent of burn can be misleading. Small cutaneous lesions may overlie extensive areas of devitalized skeletal muscle and other deep tissues. Consequently, the patient should be watched for myoglobinuria and renal failure. Second, patients may suffer spinal cord injury with an electrical burn.

SHOCK

Shock may be defined as a state of generalized inadequate tissue perfusion.[41] Although hypotension usually accompanies shock, shock can be present with a normal blood pressure, and hypotension can exist without shock. Shock can result from hypovolemia, poor cardiac function, sepsis, and blood flow obstruction (e.g., pulmonary embolism). Anaphylactic and neurogenic (spinal) shock are variants of hypovolemic shock. Hypovolemic shock is characteristic of the trauma patient immediately after injury, whereas septic shock develops after several days of hospitalization.

The clinical manifestations of shock include pallor, cyanosis, sweating, disorientation, tachycardia, cardiac dysrhythmias, pump failure, tachypnea, increased wasted ventilation, venous admixture, low cardiac output, hypotension, oliguria, sludging of blood, disseminated intravascular coagulation (DIC), and acidosis.[41, 42]

Hypovolemic shock is usually the result of hemorrhage. The body's normal homeostatic reflexes are geared to vigorously defend blood pressure and vital organ perfusion. As hemorrhage ensues, there is an elevation of plasma renin levels, antidiuretic hormone secretion, and sympathetic nervous system activity to produce tachycardia and arteriolar vasoconstriction. These mechanisms maintain blood pressure until about 30 to 40% of the blood volume has been lost. Thus, a patient may be severely hypovolemic yet have reasonably normal blood pressure. Significant hypovolemia should be suspected if tachycardia, diaphoresis, pallor, and other signs of shock are present, or if there is evidence of orthostatic hypotension. Testing for orthostatic changes is best accomplished with a tilt test on the OR table.[43] With the patient supine, baseline blood pressures and heart rate are recorded. With a safety belt firmly secured across the pelvis, the table and patient are then turned to a 45 to 60° head-up position. After 60 seconds these variables are again measured. Normovolemic patients will show no change or a slight increase (5 mm Hg) in diastolic pressure, no change or a slight decrease (10 mm Hg) in systolic pressure and a 10–15 beat·min^{-1} increase in heart rate.[44] The tilt test only shows significant changes if blood loss of greater than 1000 ml has occurred.[43] Central venous pressure is more sensitive to hypovolemia, with a decline of more than 5 mm Hg (7 cm H$_2$O), or to values below zero, indicative of substantial hypovolemia. Once blood loss exceeds 40% of the blood volume, compensatory mechanisms fail and shock may become "irreversible." Prolonged inadequate tissue perfusion results in vital organ ischemia, loss of membrane integrity, and progressive cellular death.

The key to treatment of hypovolemic shock is aggressive intravenous fluid therapy.[45] Large bore intravenous catheters should be placed and warm, crystalloid solutions and/or blood infused. Although the subject remains controversial, colloid solutions are probably of little advantage in the resuscitation of hypovolemic patients.[46] If type-specific blood is not available, type O, Rh negative, blood can be given on a temporary basis.

Spinal shock is seen with high spinal cord injuries and results from mechanical disruption of sympathetic nervous system outflow. These patients feel warm and dry to the touch and have slow pulses despite being relatively hypotensive. They are functionally hypovolemic; that is, intravascular capacity is greater than intravascular volume, because of an inability to venoconstrict. The pulse is slow because sympathetic supply to the heart is also interrupted. Organ perfusion may or may not be normal in this state. Systemic vascular resistance is low, offering little impedance to flow; however, if venous return is inadequate, cardiac output and organ perfusion may be inadequate. The patient should be left flat with slight leg elevation. Intravenous fluids should be given to restore adequate intravascular volume, venous return, and cardiac output. If arterial pressure is so low that vital organ perfusion is threatened, mixed inotropic/vasoconstrictor type drugs can be used, that is, ephedrine, epinephrine, or metaraminol. Because these patients cannot vasoconstrict to conserve body heat, they are very susceptible to hypothermia. Finally, if the muscles of respiration are involved, administration of oxygen, tracheal intubation, and positive pressure ventilation of the lungs may be needed.[47]

Septic shock is a late complication of trauma. The presence of microorganisms, or their products, in blood produces circulatory insufficiency and defects in oxygen exchange. There is a reduction in peripheral resistance to flow and a maldistribution of blood flow to tissues.[48] Myocardial depression may also exist. Patients with septic shock have enormous fluid requirements caused by vasodilation and capillary leak. Patients may respond early to fluids and vasopressors, but if progress of the disease is not halted, renal, hepatic, and cerebral failure may ensue. A normal cardiac output predicts reversal of septic shock and a favorable outcome.[41]

MONITORING AND FLUID RESUSCITATION

Patients who have sustained a major injury and who are about to undergo an emergent surgical procedure should have at least two large bore intravenous catheters and a urinary catheter in place. If time permits, an arterial and central venous catheter are also indicated. When the patient is unstable, the anesthesiologist should not be distracted to place these additional monitors. It is far preferable to call for additional help so that the anesthesiologist's attention can be directed to assuring the adequacy of ventilation, sorting out lines, giving drugs, monitoring the patient, and infusing fluids. A pulmonary artery catheter is rarely indicated in the acute management of trauma, although it may be placed at the end of surgery to facilitate postoperative care. The preferred site for monitoring central venous pressure is the internal jugular vein as there is a lower incidence of pneumothorax compared to the subclavian approach. However, this may vary with individual skills. When severe neck, upper rib, or clavicular injuries prevent proper positioning for internal jugular vein cannulation, the antecubital or femoral veins are alternate sites. An arterial catheter not only facilitates continuous and instantaneous assessment of blood pressure, but it is invaluable for frequent blood sampling (such as for serial hematocrits, blood gases, electrolytes, and coagulation studies.)

Providing adequate access for rapid infusion of fluids is crucial. Poisseuille's law states that the flow of fluid is proportional to the 4th power of the radius of the vein and, more importantly, the intravenous catheter. Venous catheters should be at least 16 gauge or larger. Introducers for pulmonary artery catheters, particularly if in a central vein,[49] or placement of intravenous tubing in an antecubital or saphenous vein by surgical cutdown, are also effective. The infusion of large volumes of fluid and blood can be facilitated by pressurizing the container. In addition to the traditional hand-inflated blood transfusion pumps, there are now several automated devices available that can infuse up to 1000 ml of fluid or blood per minute. However, damage to blood cells can result if infused at high pressure through too small a catheter.

ADMINISTERING THE ANESTHETIC

ASPIRATION OF GASTRIC CONTENTS

If the trachea has not been intubated prior to the patient's arrival in the ER or OR, it is necessary to protect the patient from pulmonary aspiration of gastric contents while inducing anesthesia. Several measures can be taken to achieve this goal. One is to attempt to empty the stomach by inducing emesis or inserting a large nasogastric tube. However, the stomach cannot ever be completely emptied. Induced vomiting can be achieved by the simultaneous intravenous administration of $0.1 \text{ mg} \cdot \text{kg}^{-1}$ apomorphine and $0.01 \text{ mg} \cdot \text{kg}^{-1}$ atropine. This should not be done in the presence of eye, head/neck, thoracic, or abdominal injuries. There is a small risk of esophageal laceration. Passing a large nasogastric tube can decompress the stomach by drainage of fluid and gas, but it is ineffective for solid material.

To prevent pulmonary damage should the patient aspirate, one can attempt to neutralize gastric contents with 30 to 45 ml of a nonparticulate antacid, such as a 0.3 molar solution of sodium citrate given orally 15 to 20 minutes prior to induction of anesthesia.[50] Alternatively, gastric contents can be neutralized and the volume reduced with H_2 histamine blockers[51] and/or gastric motility-stimulating drugs.[52] The use of gastric motility-stimulating drugs is contraindicated in a patient with an acute abdomen. Recommended doses of H_2 blockers are 300 mg of cimetidine or 50 mg of ranitidine given intravenously 30 to 60 minutes prior to induction. A gastric motility-stimulating agent, such as 10 mg intravenous metoclopramide, can be given 30 to 60 minutes prior to induction of anesthesia. Even if there is not enough time for these drugs to have an effect prior to induction of anesthesia, they probably should be given if extubation of the trachea is anticipated immediately postoperatively. Anticholinergic drugs such as atropine and glycopyrrolate should not be used as they decrease gastroesophageal sphincter tone and thereby facilitate gastric reflux and silent regurgitation.[53] If a nasogastric tube is in place it is best to remove it prior to induction of anesthesia as it serves as a wick to allow passive reflux of gastric contents and is a mechanical hindrance during tracheal intubation.

Endotracheal intubation in the presence of a full stomach can be done awake or with a rapid sequence technique using anesthetics and muscle paralysis. Awake tracheal intubations can be done either orally or nasally. For the oral approach the base of the tongue should be topically anesthetized with a local anesthetic. Benzocaine is a good choice because of its rapid onset. The patient is coached to breathe rapidly and to continue to do so during laryngoscopy. Breathing and gagging are mutually exclusive and if the patient focuses on breathing rapidly he will not gag. If the vocal cords can be exposed, an endotracheal tube is placed between them and an induction drug given rapidly after inflation of the cuff. For the nasal approach, the nasal passage should be topically anesthetized and a small, warmed, lubricated tube passed into the pharynx and then positioned either blindly, or under direct vision with a laryngoscope (after topicalization of the base of the tongue), into the trachea. Recall, that passage of tubes through the nose is not safe if there are facial fractures or a basilar skull fracture. Oral or nasal awake tracheal intubations

can be attempted with a fiberoptic bronchoscope; however, this is frequently ungratifying under emergency conditions. Success is limited because of the lack of proper patient preparation and the presence of secretions that blur the field. The provision of adequate topical anesthesia of the lower airway that is so essential to successful fiberoptic bronchoscopy, that is, superior laryngeal nerve and/or transtracheal blocks, is contraindicated in patients with full stomachs, as is heavy sedation. As a final comment, awake tracheal intubations should be attempted with caution if there is evidence of a brain injury or penetrating eye and/or neck injuries.

The rapid sequence induction technique with muscle paralysis and oral tracheal intubation, is preferred in most acute trauma situations. The patient may breathe 100% oxygen for 3 to 5 minutes, at normal tidal volumes, to denitrogenate the functional residual capacity of the lungs. If time is limited, almost the same degree of preoxygenation can be accomplished with 3 to 5 vital capacity breaths of 100% oxygen. An induction dose of one of several intravenous anesthetic drugs is then given rapidly, followed immediately by an appropriate dose of a rapid-acting muscle relaxant. After the patient loses consciousness, cricoid pressure (Sellick's maneuver)[54] is applied and held until the trachea is intubated and the cuff inflated. It is important not to apply cricoid pressure too early as it may stimulate a gag reflex and result in vomiting and aspiration.

INDUCTION

Induction of anesthesia is one of the more critical aspects of management of the trauma patient. A short-acting intravenous anesthetic is normally used which can be from one of several pharmacologic categories. Most common is thiopental, in a usual dose of 3 to 4 $\text{mg} \cdot \text{kg}^{-1}$. It can cause venodilation with a subsequent decrease in venous return, cardiac output and blood pressure. In the presence of moderate hypovolemia, thiopental has been shown to increase renal blood flow.[55] Thiopental can also be a cardiac depressant when the myocardium is compromised and can depress baroreceptor function.[56] Therefore, in hypovolemic patients one may want to decrease the dose or use an alternate drug. Ketamine is one of the few drugs in the anesthesiologist's armamentarium that is a cardiovascular stimulant. It normally raises blood pressure secondary to a rise in heart rate and cardiac output, mediated by a central anticholinergic mechanism.[57] When using this drug to induce anesthesia in severely hypovolemic patients, the normal intravenous dose of 1 to 2 $\text{mg} \cdot \text{kg}^{-1}$ should be reduced to 0.25 to 0.5 $\text{mg} \cdot \text{kg}^{-1}$. The drug can be a myocardial depressant in patients whose sympathetic nervous system is already maximally stressed. Ketamine also has excellent amnestic properties. It should be avoided, however, in patients with elevated intracranial pressure or open eye injury. Benzodiazepines have been used for induction of anesthesia after trauma; however, diazepam can cause hypotension if hypovolemia exists. Midazolam may have less effect on the cardiovascular system[58] but it has not been adequately tested in severe hypovolemic states.

Perhaps the safest drug from a hemodynamic standpoint is etomidate. This drug, in intravenous doses of 0.1 to 0.3 $\text{mg} \cdot \text{kg}^{-1}$, produces minimal change in cardiovascular variables.[59, 60] It has three drawbacks, none of which should contraindicate its use as a single bolus in a hemodynamically unstable patient. It can produce a transient burning on intravenous administration, it can produce myoclonus, and it can, after a single bolus, produce up to 4 hours of adrenal cortical suppression.[61] Though noteworthy, this latter effect has not been demonstrated to be detrimental to patient outcome. Supplemental cortisol can be used, if necessary.

A major decision in performing a rapid sequence induction of anesthesia is the selection of a muscle relaxant. The drug of choice is succinylcholine, 1 to 1.5 mg·kg^{-1}, unless otherwise contraindicated. Succinylcholine is not recommended if the cornea is lacerated, if there is a risk of massive potassium release, if there is a history of malignant hyperthermia, or in certain neuromuscular disorders. Vecuronium is the preferred alternate to succinylcholine, because it is relatively devoid of hemodynamic effects.[62] However, it is not as rapid in onset as succinylcholine unless large doses are used (0.15–0.2 mg·kg^{-1}) or a priming principal is followed. Both approaches make vecuronium almost as fast in onset as succinylcholine.[63] If one desires to increase the heart rate with the muscle relaxant, pancuronium in intravenous doses of 0.12 to 0.15 mg·kg^{-1} can be employed with an onset time almost as fast as succinylcholine. When doing a rapid sequence induction, an important principle of practice should be observed; that is, "never paralyze someone you do not know you can ventilate." If endotracheal intubation does not appear to be easy, then an awake intubation of the trachea or tracheostomy under local anesthesia should be entertained. Despite our best efforts to assess the airway, the law of averages occasionally places us under circumstances, after proceeding with induction of anesthesia, where tracheal intubation cannot be accomplished. If this occurs, and if succinylcholine has been used, gentle mask ventilation of the lungs, with maintenance of cricoid pressure, should be instituted. At that point, repeat attempts at tracheal intubation can be undertaken, or the patient can be allowed to awaken. If the endotracheal tube has inadvertently been placed into the esophagus, it can be left in place with the cuff inflated and the patient's lungs ventilated with a mask around the esophageal tube. The patient can then be allowed to awaken or repeated attempts at tracheal intubation performed with another endotracheal tube. If repeat tracheal intubation is attempted, flaccid skeletal muscle paralysis and cricoid pressure should be maintained. As a last measure, if the patient is hypoxic due to an inability to intubate the trachea or ventilate the lungs, an emergency cricothyroidotomy or tracheostomy should be performed.

There are few indications for the use of double lumen endotracheal tubes in the acute management of a trauma patient. The greater technical difficulties associated with their placement may predispose the patient to aspiration of gastric contents. If a double lumen tube is necessary, such as for a large broncho-pleural fistula, a single lumen tube can be placed initially, and then changed when adequate visualization of the larynx is assured.

Once the patient's airway has been secured, the essential monitors placed, and induction of anesthesia accomplished, the anesthesiologist must remember several issues of importance during the maintenance phase of anesthesia. The mnemonic "CATHUR" may be helpful in that process (Table 50-4).

The first priority in anesthetizing the trauma patient continues to be respiration (R). With a few exceptions, such as with tracheal injuries, it is best to mechanically control ventilation of the lungs. This permits the anesthesiologist to have an extra hand for infusing blood, drugs, etc. It is also advisable to have a ventilator available that is capable of generating high inspiratory pressure (e.g., greater than 60 cm H_2O) and PEEP. An ordinary anesthesia ventilator may not be effective if there has been pulmonary aspiration or a severe lung contusion. Throughout the anesthetic, frequent monitoring of arterial blood gases is advisable.

TABLE 50-4.   "CATHUR"*

Order of Importance
R—Respiration (airway/ventilation/oxygenation)
H—Hemodynamics
A—Acid/base balance
U—Urine output
T—Temperature
C—Coagulation

*Mnemonic for prioritization of care in trauma patients.

The next important priority is preservation of hemodynamic (H) stability. This can be influenced by a number of factors, but two main ones are the anesthetic drug and the patient's intravascular volume.

There is no perfect anesthetic drug or technique for trauma. Regional anesthesia may be useful for some isolated limb injuries, but techniques associated with major sympathetic nervous system blockade are relatively contraindicated in the face of hypovolemia.[64] Use of regional anesthesia does not obviate the need for concern about aspiration and the full stomach.

In most instances, general anesthesia is preferred. When severe hypovolemic shock and/or a reduced level of consciousness exists, there may be no need for administration of an anesthetic drug. Skeletal muscle paralysis and ventilation of the lungs will suffice. However, when the patient is awake and an anesthetic is necessary, the choice of drugs is less important than titrating their administration carefully. There is a natural tendency to choose an anesthetic for patients in shock that is an adrenergic agonist and associated with the least hypotension when administered to healthy people. Thus, the sympathetic nervous system stimulation associated with cyclopropane made it a popular choice several years ago, and ketamine is popular now. However, there are limited data to support the efficacy of these drugs in hypovolemic shock. Studies have shown that cyclopropane, in comparison to halothane or isoflurane, shortens the survival time and causes excess lactate production when given to hemorrhaged dogs.[65] Ketamine is a potent analgetic and amnestic agent, but when given to hypovolemic pigs, its cardiovascular effects are not different than those of thiopental, and it causes a metabolic acidosis.[66] Similarly, nitrous oxide offers no hemodynamic advantage over halothane, when given to hypovolemic pigs.[67] Because trauma patients frequently have pulmonary contusions, increased venous admixture, and other causes for a large arterial-alveolar oxygen gradient, nitrous oxide should probably not be used unless the adequacy of oxygenation is confirmed by blood gas analysis or pulse oximetry. It should also be used with caution whenever there may be a pneumothorax.[68]

To minimize the hypotension produced by anesthetics in the presence of hypovolemia, it is common practice to administer only small quantities and to prevent patient movement by administration of a muscle relaxant. Unfortunately, patients may not be completely anesthetized and may have recall of events during surgery. In a series of 14 severely injured patients who were given no anesthetic for endotracheal intubation and for at least 20 minutes during a subsequent operation, 6 (43%) had recall of intraoperative events. Conditions that might normally be expected to reduce anesthetic requirements, such as alcohol in the blood, acidosis, hypothermia, and hypotension, did not reliably prevent recall.[69] To establish amnesia, in the face of shock, one might consider administration of small intravenous doses of scopolamine (0.1–0.2 mg), midazolam (1 mg) or ketamine (0.25 mg·kg⁻¹).

Some general guidelines for the administration of anesthetics to severely injured patients include the following:

1. For conscious, hypovolemic patients, induce anesthesia with small doses of ketamine, etomidate, a benzodiazepine, or thiopental.
2. Avoid prolonged use of drugs that stimulate the sympathetic nervous system. Continued use of vasopressors should be interpreted as hypovolemia or cardiac tamponade until proven otherwise.
3. Avoid nitrous oxide until the adequacy of oxygenation is assured.
4. Use opioids if necessary for analgesia.
5. Titrate volatile anesthetics as soon as feasible.
6. Recognize that blood pressure alone is an unreliable index of blood volume, tissue perfusion, or the level of consciousness.
7. Resort to oxygen and skeletal muscle paralysis, alone, only if the patient will not tolerate any anesthetic drugs.

Hemodynamic stability also results from control of surgical bleeding by the surgeon and restoration of blood volume by the anesthesiologist. Several choices of fluids are available for use by the anesthesiologist. With hemorrhage there is a contraction of extracellular volume as the patient attempts to autotransfuse their intravascular compartment with their own interstitial fluid.[70, 71] Initially, administration of a physiologic salt solution, such as lactated Ringers, restores this depletion and also expands intravascular volume to help maintain venous return and cardiac output. Physiologic salt solutions remain intravascularly for only 30 to 60 minutes before they redistribute throughout the entire extracellular fluid volume.[72] Other plasma expanders, such as colloid solutions, maintain intravascular volume for 2 to 5 hours but are fraught with certain hazards. Protein solutions can impair pulmonary function if they extravasate into a damaged lung,[73] and they can cause vasodilation.[74] Dextran solutions can cause bleeding disorders and severe allergic reactions.[75] Fresh frozen plasma should be reserved for treatment of specific, documented, coagulation disorders.[76] Hydroxyethyl starch, a glucose polymer in a 6% solution, has proven useful as a volume expander. It has a long plasma half-life (1.5 days) and does not affect coagulation when given in recommended doses. The dose should be limited to no more than 20 ml·kg⁻¹.[77–79] Finally, hypertonic saline has been effective as a volume expander in preliminary studies with animals[80, 81] and humans.[82] Despite the availability of all of these forms of intravascular volume expansion, and the continuation of a "colloid vs crystalloid" controversy,[83, 84] the mainstay of therapy should be lactated Ringers solution.

Most trauma victims are young, with good cardiac and renal function, so that severe degrees of anemia can be well tolerated if intravascular volume is supported. Nevertheless, with extreme blood loss, red cells eventually must be given. Fresh whole blood (less than 6 hours old) is preferable, if available. After 1 day of storage, only 12% of the original platelets remain in whole blood.[85] Regardless of its age, whole blood is preferable to packed red blood cells. Trauma patients need cells and volume. If there is no time for a crossmatch, type specific whole blood, type specific red cells, or as a last resort, type O negative red cells will suffice.

The "C" of the CATHUR mnemonic refers to coagulation. When whole blood or red cells are given as a massive transfusion (defined as replacement of one or more patient blood volumes), platelets may be necessary to correct a dilutional thrombocytopenia.[86] It is best to obtain coagulation studies at regular intervals, but as a general rule, one should administer 10 to 20 units of platelets per 10 units of replaced blood. Stored whole blood is deficient in Factors V and VIII, but whole blood usually contains adequate levels of these clotting factors for the coagulation process to occur. This may not be the case if most of the replaced blood has been packed red blood cells with the plasma components removed. In that case, fresh frozen plasma (2–3 units), in addition to platelets, may be needed for each 10 units of transfused red cells.

Two other coagulation disorders can be seen in shock—DIC, a consumption coagulopathy with secondary fibrinolysis, and primary fibrinolysis. DIC can also occur after a hemolytic transfusion reaction. In both conditions, serum fibrinogen is decreased, with an elevation of fibrin split products, prothrombin time, and partial thromboplastin time. Thrombocytopenia exists with DIC, but not primary fibrinolysis. If DIC is diagnosed, small doses of heparin can be tried (50 units·kg⁻¹) while also replacing clotting factors and platelets. If the diagnosis of primary fibrinolysis is secure, epsilon aminocaproic acid can be given to inhibit fibrinolysis. However, this will aggravate DIC and if doubt exists as to which pathology exists, it should not be used.[86] In acute trauma the large majority of clotting disorders are secondary to dilutional thrombocytopenia. If a more complicated picture is encountered, testing the patient's coagulation profile is indicated and consultation with a hematologist should be considered.

Although citrate is the anticoagulant in most stored blood, clinically significant citrate intoxication and hypocalcemia is not seen unless blood is infused exceedingly fast and in vast quantities. Serum ionized calcium can decrease during massive transfusion,[87] but should not be clinically significant unless the volume of infused blood exceeds 100 ml·min⁻¹ in the adult patient.[88] Hyperventilation can exacerbate hypocalcemia.[89] The clinical signs of hypocalcemia are those of poor myocardial function.

Assessment of blood loss and the adequacy of replacement can be very difficult when caring for the trauma patient. Lost blood can be on the floor, under drapes, on sponges and gowns as well as in the suction canisters. In such a situation, one must rely on the patient's vital signs, urine output, acid-base balance, and serial hematocrits as a means of achieving satisfactory replacement. Signs of success will be a reasonable heart rate (less than 100 beats·min⁻¹), a reasonable pulse pressure (greater than 30 mm Hg), urine output greater than 0.5–1 ml·kg⁻¹·hr⁻¹, no metabolic acidosis, and a lack of large swings in heart rate and blood pressure with positive pressure ventilation of the lungs.

The standard pore size of filters on blood administration sets is 170 microns. These filters catch a significant portion of the cellular debris from blood products but some of this material does bypass the filter, enter the patient and lodge in the lung. It has been suggested that this may be one of the contributing factors to "shock lung" or adult respiratory distress syndrome (ARDS).[90] Micropore filters, with 20 to 40 micron pore size, can be placed in line and filter out a significantly greater percentage of cellular debris. Some data indicate a pulmonary benefit from the use of micropore filters[90] while others do not.[91] If transfusions are massive, some benefit probably results. The trade-off is that the finer filters offer a great deal of in-line resistance to flow and can make it difficult to keep up with intravascular volume if blood loss is swift. Platelets probably should not be infused through a micropore filter.

The "A" of CATHUR refers to acid/base and electrolyte balance. Not uncommonly, trauma victims have a metabolic acidosis due to shock, hypothermia, hypoxia, and generalized stress. Mechanical ventilation of the lungs can be used to normalize blood pH over the short term by manipulation of Pa_{CO_2}. With time, restoration of tissue perfusion and renal and hepatic function should resolve the problem. However, if the metabolic acidosis does not resolve, or is so severe that ventilatory mechanisms are inadequate, it should be treated with sodium bicarbonate. A reasonable dose is calculated as follows: normal serum bicarbonate ($24\ mEq \cdot l^{-1}$) minus present serum bicarbonate × extracellular fluid volume in liters (body weight × 20%) = bicarbonate deficit (mEq). After replacing one-half to two-thirds of the calculated deficit, blood gases should be rechecked in 10 to 15 minutes. Treatment with bicarbonate should be reserved only for those instances where the acidosis is severe. Studies in dogs suggest that bicarbonate may be detrimental in the treatment of lactic acidosis, as it leads to a deterioration of blood pressure and cardiac output.[92] The most important treatment for metabolic acidosis is fluid resuscitation, ventilation, and re-warming. Although stored blood has a pH of approximately 6.5, a potassium concentration of almost $30\ mEq \cdot l^{-1}$, and a P_{CO_2} of 150 mm Hg or more, hyperkalemia and metabolic acidosis from the rapid administration of blood is not a problem.[93] It is not necessary to prophylactically administer sodium bicarbonate in these situations. Patients with normal liver function who have received a large volume of lactated Ringers solution and/or blood products containing citrate, often develop a metabolic alkalosis 6 to 24 hours later.[94]

The "T" of CATHUR is for temperature. A maximum effort must be made to maintain patient body temperature at normal values. Hypothermia is associated with a number of undesirable effects such as reduced glomerular filtration, poor platelet function, lowered glucose utilization, postoperative shivering with increased oxygen demand, postoperative vasoconstriction with increased peripheral and pulmonary vascular resistance, metabolic acidosis, and decreased metabolism of drugs. Because of exposure and shock, trauma victims are usually hypothermic. This can be compounded if cool resuscitation fluids are also administered. All fluids must be warm, by using pre-warmed, non–glucose-containing crystalloid solutions, or blood warmers. Not only does warming help maintain patient temperature, but it reduces blood viscosity and improves tissue blood flow. Blood should not be warmed beyond 39°C or damage to cells is likely to occur. When selecting blood warming devices be sure they are capable of efficient warming at high rates of infusion.[95] Of perhaps equal benefit in maintaining blood temperature is a warm operating room particularly at the outset until the patient is draped.[96] A warming blanket under the patient is not beneficial, especially if the patient is already hypothermic, because an inadequate area of well perfused body surface is in contact with it. Because the body loses heat by having to warm and humidify inspired gases, the use of a humidifier in the anesthetic circuit helps to maintain normothermia.

The final letter to recall from the mnemonic CATHUR is "U" for urine. Maintenance of good urine output after trauma is important for several reasons. The greatest concern is the prevention of acute oliguric renal failure which can result from hypoperfusion and hypotension. Unfortunately, there is no formula to predict how much hypoperfusion or hypotension, for how long, will result in renal failure. Certainly acute renal failure can occur without apparent hypotension and sometimes does not occur despite the presence of hypotension. If a closed head injury has occurred, maintenance of urine output is important for control of intracranial pressure. If skeletal muscle crush injuries or electrocution have occurred, myoglobinuria must be treated with a vigorous diuresis. Mannitol is the diuretic of choice in all of the above cases. The same concerns apply to the hemoglobinuria seen after a hemolytic transfusion reaction. The initial dose should be $0.25\ g \cdot kg^{-1}$ as a drip, or as a bolus, and the total dose should be limited to 1 to $1.5\ g \cdot kg^{-1}$. If the patient has had angiography, renal function must be preserved to avert the toxic effects of contrast media on the kidney. Mannitol or fluids also work well for this. A healthy renal system contributes significantly to the favorable outcome of patients who survive severe trauma. This concern becomes greater in the postoperative period when primary parenchymal renal failure can occur from toxins (antibiotics) and/or sepsis.[97] It is helpful if a prior prerenal insult has been avoided.

In conclusion, the diagnostic and therapeutic ramifications of trauma patient management are challenging because of the simultaneous involvement of multiple organs, each with its own physiologic priority. For example, it is not uncommon to see a blunt trauma patient with a closed head injury, ruptured spleen, lung contusion, and muscle crush injuries with myoglobinuria. Treatment of the head and lung injuries should entail fluid restriction, whereas hemorrhage and the potential renal injury should not. Such dilemmas in management are common. Thus, it it important for the anesthesiologist to have a clear understanding, from the outset, regarding mechanism of injury and diagnostic considerations, particularly as they relate to anesthesia management. The "bottom line" of care is maintenance of physiologic homeostasis for the uninjured organs, plus mechanical and pharmacological interventions on behalf of the injured organs.

REFERENCES

1. Trunkey DD: The nature of things that go bang in the night. Surgery 92:123, 1982
2. Trunkey DD: Trauma. Sci Am 249:28, 1983
3. Trunkey DD: Shock trauma. Canad J Surg 27:479, 1984
4. Klauber MR, Marshall LF: Cause of decline in head-injury mortality rate in San Diego County, California. J Neurosurg 62:528, 1985
5. Jacobs LM, Berrizbeitia LD, Bennett B et al: Endotracheal intubations in the prehospital phase of emergency medical care. JAMA 250:2175, 1983
6. Smith JP, Bodai BI: The urban paramedic's scope of practice. JAMA 253:544, 1985
7. Copass MK, Oreskovich MR, Bladengroen MR et al: Prehospital cardiopulmonary resuscitation of the critically injured patient. Am J Surg 148:20, 1984
8. Mattox KL, Bickell WH, Pepe PE et al: Prospective randomized evaluation of antishock MAST in post-traumatic hypotension. J Trauma 26:779, 1986
9. West JG, Cales RH, Gazzaniga AB: Impact of trauma regionalization: The Orange County experience. Arch Surg 118:740, 1983
10. American College of Surgeons Committee on Trauma: Hospital resources for optimal care of the trauma patient. Bull Am Coll Surg 64(8):43, 1979
11. American College of Surgeons Committee on Trauma: Advanced trauma life support course for physicians. Student Manual 1984
12. Champion HR, Sacco WJ, Carnazzo AJ et al: Trauma score. Crit Care Med 9:672, 1981
13. Bouzarth WF: Intracranial nasogastric tube insertion. J Trauma 18:819, 1978
14. Fremstad JD, Martin SH: Lethal complication for insertion of a

nasogastric tube after severe basilar skull fracture. J Trauma 18:820, 1978

15. Gregory JA, Tarter PT, Reynolds AF: A complication of nasogastric intubation: Intracranial penetration. J Trauma 18:822, 1978

16. Tintinali JE, Claffey J: Complications of nasotracheal intubation. Ann Emerg Med 10:142, 1981

17. Butler RM, Moser FH: The padded dash syndrome: Blunt trauma to the larynx and trachea. Laryngoscope 78:1172, 1968

18. Green R, Stark P: Trauma of the larynx and trachea. Radiol Clin North Am 16:309, 1978

19. Smith JP, Bodai BI, Seifkin A et al: The esophageal obturator airway. A review. JAMA 250:1081, 1983

20. Parks RE, Livoni JP: Detection of cervical spine injury in the multitrauma patient. In Blaisdell FW, Trunkey DD (eds): Trauma Management III: Cervical Thoracic Trauma, p 56. New York, Thieme, 1986

21. Campbell FC, Robbs JV: Penetrating injuries of the neck: A prospective study of 108 patients. Br J Surg 67:582, 1980

22. Goodnight JE, Jr: Cervical injury. In Blaisdell FW, Trunkey DD (eds): Trauma Management III: Cervical Thoracic Trauma, p 94. New York, Thieme, Inc, 1986

23. Baker CC, Coronna JJ, Trunkey DD: Neurologic outcome after emergency room thoracotomy for trauma. Am J Surg 139:677, 1980

24. Blaisdell FW: Initial assessment of thoracic injuries. In Blaisdell FW, Trunkey DD (eds): Trauma Management III: Cervical Thoracic Trauma, p 1. New York, Thieme, 1986

25. Blaisdell FW: Pneumothorax and hemothorax. In Blaisdell FW, Trunkey DD (eds): Trauma Management III: Cervical Thoracic Trauma, p 150. New York, Thieme, 1986

26. Wiot JF: The radiologic manifestations of blunt chest trauma. JAMA 231:500, 1975

27. Brinton M, Miller SE, Lim RC et al: Acute abdominal aortic injuries. J Trauma 22:481, 1982

28. Trunkey DD, Federle MP: Computed tomography in perspective. J Trauma 26:660, 1986

29. Trunkey DD: Torso trauma. In Ravitch RM (ed): Current Problems in Surgery, 24:211. Chicago, Year Book Medical Publishers, 1987

30. Federle MP, Crass RA, Jeffrey RB et al: Computed tomography in blunt abdominal trauma. Arch Surg 117:645, 1982

31. Lamb JD: Anaesthetic considerations for major thermal injury. Can Anaesth Soc J 32:84, 1985

32. Eckhauser FE, Billote J, Burke JF: Tracheostomy complicating massive burn injury—A plea for conservation. Am J Surg 127:418, 1974

33. Trunkey DD: Inhalation injury. Surg Clin North Am 58:1133, 1978

34. Baxter CR, Shires T: Physiological responses to crystalloid resuscitation of severe burns. Ann NY Acad Sci 150:874, 1968

35. Heimbach D, Engrav L: Surgical Management of the Burn Wound. New York, Raven Press, 1984

36. Szyfelbein SK: Anesthetic considerations for major burn surgery. ASA Refresher Courses in Anesthesiology 8:201, 1980

37. Caravajal HF: A physiologic approach to fluid therapy in severely burned children. Surg Gynecol Obstet 150:379, 1980

38. De Campo T, Aldrete JA: Anesthetic management of the severely burned patient. Intensive Care Med 7:55, 1981

39. Martyn J: Clinical pharmacology and drug therapy in the burned patient. Anesthesiology 65:67, 1986

40. Gronert GA, Theye RA: Pathophysiology of hyperkalemia induced by succinylcholine. Anesthesiology 43:89, 1975

41. Houston MC, Thompson WL, Robertson D: Shock. Diagnosis and management. Arch Intern Med 144:1433, 1984

42. Moss GS, Saletta JD: Traumatic shock in man. N Engl J Med 290:724, 1974

43. Knopp R, Claypool R, Leonardi D: Use of the tilt test in measuring acute blood loss. Ann Emerg Med 9:72, 1980

44. Currens JH: A comparison of blood pressure in lying and standing positions: A study in 500 men and women. Am Heart J 35:646, 1948

45. Shires GT: Management of hypovolemic shock. Bull NY Acad Sci 55:139, 1979

46. Gallagher TJ, Banner MJ, Barnes PA: Large volume crystalloid resuscitation does not increase extravascular lung water. Anesth Analg 64:323, 1985

47. Fraser A, Edmonds-Seal J: Spinal cord injuries. A review of problems facing the anaesthetist. Anaesthesia 37:1084, 1982

48. Parker MM, Parillo JE: Septic shock. Hemodynamics and pathogenesis. JAMA 250:3324, 1983

49. Richey JV, Wilson RE: IV equipment for massive transfusions. Anesthesiology Rev 7:36, 1980

50. Viegas OJ, Ravindran RS, Shumacker CA: Gastric fluid pH in patients receiving sodium citrate. Anesth Analg 60:521, 1981

51. Stoelting RK: Gastric fluid pH in patients receiving cimetidine. Anesth Analg 57:675, 1978

52. Solanki DR, Suresh M, Ethridge HC: The effects of intravenous cimetidine and metoclopramide on gastric volume and pH. Anesth Analg 63:599, 1984

53. Brock-Utne JG, Rubin J, Welman S: The effect of glycopyrrolate on lower esophageal sphincter. Canad Anaesth Soc J 25:144, 1978

54. Sellick BA: Cricoid pressure to control the regurgitation of stomach contents during induction of anesthesia. Lancet 2:404, 1961

55. Priano LL: Renal hemodynamic alterations following administration of thiopental, diazepam or ketamine in conscious hypovolemic dogs. Advances in Shock Research 9:173, 1983

56. Bernards C, Marrone B, Priano L: Effect of anesthetic induction agents on baroreceptor function. Anesthesiology 63:A31, 1985

57. Traber DL, Wilson RD, Priano LL: A detailed study of the cardiopulmonary response to ketamine and its blockade by atropine. South Med J 63:1077, 1970

58. Reeves JG, Fragen RJ, Vinik HR et al: Midazolam: Pharmacology and uses. Anesthesiology 62:310, 1985

59. Gooding JM, Corssen G: Effect of etomidate on the cardiovascular system. Anesth Analg 56:717, 1977

60. Kettler D, Sonntag H, Donath U: Hemodynamic myocard mechanic sowrstuff bedard and sowrstuff versorgum des menshen hurzens unter narco sienlitung mit etomidate. Anaesthetist 23:116, 1974

61. Fragen RJ, Shanks CA, Molteni A et al: Effects of etomidate on hormonal responses to surgical stress. Anesthesiology 61:652, 1984

62. Lennon RL, Olson RA, Gronert GA: Atracurium or vecuronium for rapid sequence endotracheal intubation. Anesthesiology 64:510, 1986

63. Miller RD, Rupp SM, Fisher DM et al: Clinical pharmacology of vecuronium and atracurium. Anesthesiology 61:652, 1984

64. Kennedy WF, Bonica JJ, Akamatsu TJ et al: Cardiovascular and respiratory effects of subarachnoid block in the presence of acute blood loss. Anesthesiology 29:29, 1968

65. Theye RA, Perry LB, Brzica SM: Influence of anesthetic agent on response to hemorrhagic hypotension. Anesthesiology 40:32, 1974

66. Weiskopf RB, Bogetz MS, Roizen MF et al: Cardiovascular and metabolic sequelae of inducing anesthesia with ketamine or thiopental in hypovolemic swine. Anesthesiology 60:214, 1984

67. Weiskopf RB, Bogetz MS: Cardiovascular action of nitrous oxide on halothane in hypovolemic swine. Anesthesiology 63:509, 1985

68. Eger EI, Saidman LJ: Hazards of nitrous oxide anesthesia in bowel obstruction and pneumothorax. Anesthesiology 26:61, 1965

69. Bogetz MS, Katz JA: Recall of surgery for major trauma. Anesthesiology 61:6, 1984

70. Shires T: The role of sodium containing solutions in the treatment of oligemic shock. Surg Clin North Amer 45:365, 1965

71. Shires T, Coln D, Carrico J et al: Fluid therapy and hemorrhagic shock. Arch Surg 88:688, 1964

72. Cervera LA, Moss G: Crystalloid distribution following hemorrhage and hemodilution. J Trauma 14:506, 1974

73. Holcroft JW, Trunkey DD, Carpenter MA: Sepsis in the baboon: Factors affecting resuscitation and pulmonary edema in animals resuscitated with Ringer's lactate versus plasmanate. J Trauma 17:600, 1977

74. Bland JHL, Laver MB, Lowenstein E: Vasodilator effect of commercial 5% plasma protein fraction solutions. JAMA 224:1721, 1973

75. Giesecke AH, Jenkins MT: Fluid therapy. Clin Anesth 11:57, 1976

76. Bove JR: Fresh-frozen plasma: Too few indications, too much use. Anesth Analg 64:849, 1985

77. Lee WH, Cooper N, Weidner MG et al: Clinical evaluation of a new plasma expander, hydroxyethyl starch. J Trauma 8:381, 1968

78. Solanke TF, Khwaja MS, Madojemu EI: Plasma volume studies with four different plasma volume expanders. J Surg Res 11:140, 1971

79. Munoz E, Raciti A, Dove DB et al: Effect of hydroxyethyl starch versus albumin on hemodynamic and respiratory function in patients in shock. Crit Care Med 8:255, 1980

80. Velasco IT, Pontieri V, Rocha E et al: Hyperosmotic sodium chloride and severe hemorrhagic shock. Am J Physiol 239:H664, 1980

81. Layon J, Duncan D, Gallager TJ et al: Hypertonic saline as a resuscitation solution in hemorrhagic shock. Anesth Analg 66:154, 1987

82. De Felippe J, Timenor J, Velasco IT et al: Treatment of refractory hypovolemic shock by 7½% sodium chloride injections. Lancet 2:1002, 1980

83. Shoemaker WC, Schluchter M, Hopkins JA et al: Comparison of the relative effectiveness of colloids and crystalloids in emergency resuscitation. Am J Surg 142:73, 1981

84. Virgilio RW, Rice CL: Crystalloid vs colloid resuscitation: Is one better? A randomized clinical study. Surgery 85:129, 1979

85. Baldini M, Costea N, Dameshek W: The viability of stored human platelets. Blood 16:1669, 1960

86. Miller RD: Complications of massive blood transfusions. Anesthesiology 39:82, 1973

87. Carpenter MA, Trunkey DD, Holcroft J: Ionized calcium and magnesium in the baboon: Hemorrhagic shock and resuscitation. Circ Shock 5:163, 1978

88. Denlinger JK, Nahrwold ML, Gibbs PS et al: Hypocalcemia during rapid blood transfusion in anaesthetized man. Br J Anaesth 48:995, 1976

89. Hinkle JE, Cooperman LH: Serum ionized calcium changed following citrated blood transfusions in anesthetized man. Br J Anaesth 43:1108, 1971

90. Reul GJ, Greenberg SD, Lefrak EA et al: Prevention of post-traumatic pulmonary insufficiency with fine screen filtration of blood. Arch Surg 106:386, 1973

91. Grindlinger GA, Vegas AM, Churchill WH et al: Is respiratory failure a consequence of blood transfusion? J Trauma 20:627, 1980

92. Graf H, Leach W, Arieff AI: Evidence for a detrimental effect of bicarbonate therapy in hypoxic lactic acidosis. Science 227:754, 1985

93. Miller RD, Tong MJ, Robins TO: Effects of massive transfusion of blood on acid-based balance. JAMA 216:1762, 1971

94. Wilson RF, Gibson D, Percinel AK et al: Severe alkalosis in critically ill surgical patients. Arch Surg 105:197, 1972

95. Russell WJ: A review of blood warmers for massive transfusion. Anaesth Intensive Care 2:109, 1974

96. Priano LL, Solanki D: Operating room temperature. Anesth Analg 60:226, 1981

97. Mazze RI: Critical care of the patient with renal failure. Anesthesiology 47:138, 1977

98. Tenold R, Priano L, Kim K et al: Infection potential of nondisposable pressure transducers prepared prior to use. Crit Care Med 15:582, 1987

Chapter 51   *Jerrold H. Levy*

The Allergic Response

The immune system represents a series of complex cellular and humoral elements that can interact with many different types of foreign molecular structures called antigens to provide host defense against foreign substances. These foreign substances (antigens) represent molecular configurations located on cells, bacteria, viruses, circulating proteins, or complex macromolecules. Immunologic mechanisms have two major characteristics: 1) they involve interaction of both antigens with antibodies and/or specific effector cells; and 2) they are reproducible when rechallenged with specific antigens. In addition, they are specific and adaptive, capable of distinguishing between a host of foreign substances and amplifying its reactivity to produce a specific immunologic memory.

The immune system functions to protect the body against external microorganisms and toxins and internal threats from neoplastic cells. The immune system can also respond inappropriately and cause *hypersensitive (allergic) reactions.* Life-threatening allergic reactions to drugs and other foreign substances observed perioperatively may represent different aspects of the immune response.[1, 2] Therefore, basic immunologic principles are reviewed here to understand the complex interplay of cells and molecules.

BASIC IMMUNOLOGIC PRINCIPLES

Host defense systems of the immune organs are usually divided into both cellular and humoral elements.[3] The humoral system includes the circulating protein antibodies, complement, and other serum proteins that provide host defense against most bacteria. Cellular immunity, on the other hand, is mediated by specific lymphocytes of the T-cell series and provides a host defense against intracellular organisms, viruses, fungi and tumor cells. Lymphocytes represent components of the cellular immune system. They have highly specific receptors that distinguish between antigens of normal host origin and those that are foreign. When lymphocytes react with foreign antigens, they respond to orchestrate immunosurveillance, regulate immunospecific antibody synthesis, and destroy foreign invaders. Individual aspects of the immune response and their importance are considered separately.

ANTIGENS

Molecules capable of stimulating an immune response when injected (immunospecific antibody production or lymphocyte stimulation) are called *antigens.* The specificity of the immunologic response to producing antibodies directed against the chemical structure represents an important characteristic.[4] A molecule's ability to act as an antigen to stimulate an immune response is called its immunogenicity and antigens are often referred to as immunogens. Only a few drugs in use by anesthesiologists such as large polypeptides (chymopapain) and other large macromolecules (dextrans) are complete antigens (Table 51-1). Most commonly used drugs are simple organic compounds of low molecular weight, usually less than 1000 daltons. For such a small molecule to become immunogenic, it must form a stable bond with circulating albumin or tissue micromolecules to result in a complete antigen (hapten-macromolecular complex). Small molecular weight substances

TABLE 51-1. Agents Administered During Anesthesia Acting as Antigens

HAPTENS	MACROMOLECULES
Penicillin and its derivatives	Blood products
Anesthetic drugs(?)	Chymopapain
	Colloid volume expanders
—Protamine(?)—	

such as drugs or drug metabolites that bind to host proteins or cell membranes to sensitize patients are called *haptens*. Haptens are not antigenic by themselves. Often, a reactive drug metabolite (*e.g.*, penicilloyl derivative of penicillin) is thought to bind with macromolecules to become antigens but for most drugs this has not been proven.

THYMUS-DERIVED LYMPHOCYTES (T-CELL LYMPHOCYTES)

The thymus of the fetus influences the differentiation of immature lymphocytes into thymus derived cells (T-cells). T-cells are the most abundant type of circulating lymphocytes in the adult. On the surface of T-cells are specific receptors that are activated by binding with foreign antigens. Once activated, these cells secrete specific mediators that regulate the immune response. Subpopulations of T-cells exist in man including helper, suppressor, cytotoxic, and killer cells.[5] The two types of regulatory T-cells are helper (OKT4) and suppressor cells (OKT8). Helper cells are important for normal antibody production and for key effector cell response. Suppressor cells, on the other hand, retard both of these functions. For instance, the acquired immunodeficiency syndrome (AIDS) that is produced by infection of helper T-cells with a retrovirus known as human immunodeficiency virus (HIV) (also known as human T-cell lymphotropic virus type III and the lymphadenopathy virus), produces a specific increase in the number of suppressor cells. Another important function of T-cells is their destruction of foreign cells including mycobacteria, fungi, and viruses by cytotoxic T-cells, activated by antigen from these pathogens. Other lymphocytes called natural killer cells do not require specific antigen stimulation to initiate their function. Both the cytotoxic T-cells and natural killer cells participate in defense against tumor cells as well as the rejection of transplanted tissues. T-cells produce a spectrum of mediators that influence the response of other cell types involved in the recognition and destruction of foreign substances. T-cells activated by antigenic exposure synthesize molecules called lymphokines that regulate the immune response by 1) communicating with other lymphocytes (both T- and B- cells), 2) inducing inflammation and mononuclear cell infiltration, and 3) modulating phagocytic function.

BURSA-DERIVED LYMPHOCYTES (B-CELL LYMPHOCYTES)

B-cells represent a specific lymphocyte cell line that can differentiate, when activated, into specific plasma cells that synthesize antibodies. The differentiation of B-cells to plasma cells is controlled by both helper and suppressor T-cell lymphocytes.[5] B-cells are also called bursa-derived cells because in birds the bursa of Fabricius is important in producing cells responsible for antibody synthesis.

ANTIBODIES

Antibodies represent specific proteins called immunoglobulins that can recognize and bind to a specific antigen.[6] The basic structure of the antibody molecule is illustrated in Figure 51-1. Each antibody has at least two heavy chains and two light chains that are bound together by disulfide bonds. The Fab fragment has the ability to bind antigen while the Fc or crystallisable fragment is responsible for the unique biological properties of the different classes of immunoglobulins (cell binding and complement activation).

Antibodies function as specific receptor molecules located on different immune cell surfaces. When antigen binds covalently to the Fab fragment on the cell, the antibody undergoes conformational changes to activate the Fc receptor. The results of antigen-antibody binding depends on the cell type which causes a specific type of activation (*e.g.*, lymphocyte proliferation and differentiation into antibody secreting cells, mast cell degranulation, and complement activation).

Five major classes of antibodies occur in man that include the IgG, IgA, IgM, IgD, and IgE. The heavy chain determines the structure and the function of each molecule. The basic properties of each antibody are listed in Table 51-2.

EFFECTOR CELLS AND PROTEINS OF THE IMMUNE RESPONSE

Monocytes, neutrophils (polymorphonuclear leukocytes), and eosinophils represent important effector cells that migrate into areas of inflammation in response to specific chemotactic factors including lymphokines, bacterial products, and complement derived mediators. Foreign organisms or cells are recognized specifically by circulating antibody to their component protein system. The deposition of antibody or complement fragments on the surface of foreign cells is called *opsoni-*

FIG. 51-1. Simplified basic structural configuration of the antibody molecule representing human immunoglobulin G (IgG). Immunoglobulins are composed of 2 heavy chains and 2 light chains bound by disulphide linkages (represented by *crossbars*). Papain cleaves the molecule into 2 Fab fragments and 1 Fc fragment. Antigen binding occurs on the Fab fragments whereas the Fc segment is responsible for membrane binding or complement activation. (Levy JH: Anaphylactic Reactions in Anesthesia and Intensive Care. Boston, Butterworths, 1986.)

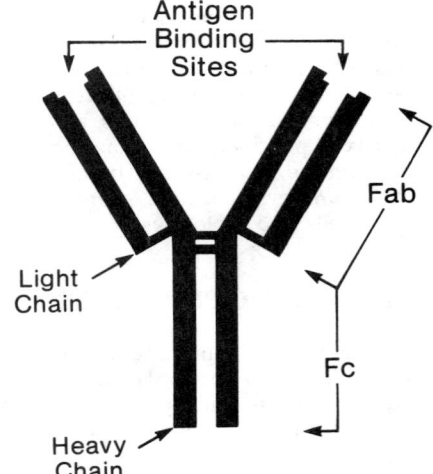

TABLE 51-2. Biologic Characteristics of Immunoglobulins

	IgG	IgM	IgA	IgE	IgD
Heavy Chain	γ	μ	α	ε	δ
Molecular weight	160,000	900,000	170,000	188,000	184,000
Subclasses	1,2,3,4	1,2	1,2		
Serum concentration mg·dl^{-1}	6–14	0.5–1.5	1–3	$< -.5 \times 10^3$	<0.1
Complement activation	all but IgG$_4$	+	–	–	–
Placental transfer	+	–	–	–	–
Serum half-life (days)	23	5	6	1–5	2–8
Cell binding	mast cells (IgG$_4$) neutrophils lymphocytes mononuclear cells platelets	lymphocytes		mast cells basophils lymphocytes	neutrophils lymphocytes

(Modified from Levy J: Anaphylactic Reactions in Anesthesia and Intensive Care. Boston, Butterworths, 1986.)

zation, a process that facilitates phagocytic ingestion. Subsequently, a series of metabolic processes are activated that enable the phagocytes to kill the foreign cell. In addition, lymphokines and other mediators released from lymphocytes produce chemotaxis of other inflammatory cells as follows. Individual roles of each cell type in effecting the immune response are considered separately.

Monocytes and Macrophages

Macrophages play a central role in regulating immune responses by processing and presenting antigens to T-cell lymphocytes, but also in effecting inflammatory, tumoricidal, and microbicidal functions. Macrophages arise from circulating monocytes or may be confined to specific organs such as the lung. They are recruited and activated by lymphokines produced by response to either microorganisms or other causes of tissue injury. Macrophages ingest antigens before they interact with receptors on the lymphocyte surface to regulate their action. In addition, macrophages synthesize mediators to facilitate both B-cell and T-cell lymphocyte response. Macrophages and lymphocytes are the predominant cells at sites of chronic inflammation and their interaction seems important for defense mechanisms.

Neutrophils

The first cells to appear in acute inflammatory reaction are probably neutrophils (polymorphonuclear leukocytes). These cells contain specific lysosomal granules that fuse with ingested material or are extruded into the extracellular environment. The granules contain a variety of enzymes including acid hydrolases, neutral proteases, and lysosomes. In addition, activated neutrophils produce hydroxyl radicals, superoxide, and hydrogen peroxide which aid in microbial killing.

Eosinophils

The exact function of the eosinophil in host defense is unclear; however, these cells are associated with parasitic infections. Mast cells, basophils, and lymphocytes synthesize eosinophilic chemotactic factors to recruit eosinophils to accumulate at sites of parasitic infections, tumors, and allergic reactions. Eosinophils secrete enzymes such as arysylfatase and histaminase that may limit the response of other inflammatory cells including basophils and mast cells.[7]

Basophils

Basophils comprise less than 0.5% to 1% of circulating granulocytes in the blood.[7] On the surface of basophils are IgE receptors that release a spectrum of physiologically active mediators following activation. Basophils function similarly to mast cells but have the capacity for chemotactic migration in response to other stimuli.

Mast Cells

Mast cells are important mediators of immediate hypersensitivity responses. They are tissue fixed, located in the perivascular spaces of the skin, lung, and intestine.[7] Also on the surface of mast cells are IgE receptors that bind to specific antigens. Once activated, these cells release a spectrum of physiologically active mediators important to immediate hypersensitivity responses (see Anaphylactic Reactions—IgE Mediated).

Complement

The primary humoral response to antigen and antibody binding is activation of the complement system.[8] Analogous to the clotting cascade, the complement system consists of approximately 20 different proteins that bind to activated antibodies, other complement proteins, and cell membranes. The complement system is an important effector system of inflammation.

Two pathways activate the complement system, either with or without the aid of antibodies. Activation can be initiated by IgG or IgM binding to antigen, by plasmin through the classical pathway, by endotoxin or by drugs through the alternate (properdin) pathway (Fig. 51-2).[8] Specific fragments released during complement activation of the native complement proteins are important in host defense and hypersensitivity reactions. Breakdown products include C3a, C4a, C5a that have important humoral and chemotactic properties (see Non-IgE Mediated Reactions). The major function of the system is to

COMPLEMENT CASCADE

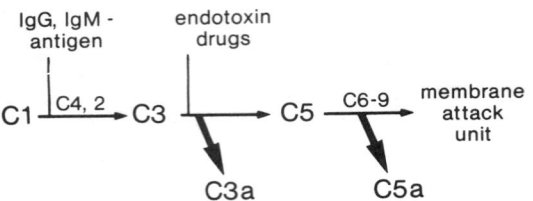

FIG. 51-2. Schematic diagram of complement activation. Complement system can be activated by either the classical pathway (IgG, IgM-antigen interaction) or the alternate (endotoxin, drug interaction) pathways. Small peptide fragments of C3 and C5 called anaphylatoxins (C3a, C5a) released during activation are potent vasoactive mediators. Formation of the complete complement cascade produces a membrane attack unit that lyses cell walls and membranes.

recognize bacteria both directly and indirectly by the attraction of phagocytes (chemotaxis), as well as the increased adherence of phagocytes to antigens (opsonization), and cell lysis by activation of the complete cascade.

As with most biological systems, a series of inhibitors regulate activation to ensure that the complement system is turned off most of the time. Hereditary (autosomal dominant) or acquired (associated with lymphoma, lymphosarcoma, chronic lymphatic leukemia, macroglobulinemia) angioneurotic edema is an example where an inhibitor of the C_1 complement system is deficient (C_1 esterase deficiency). This syndrome is characterized by recurrent increased vascular permeability of specific subcutaneous and serosal tissues (angioedema) producing laryngeal obstruction and respiratory and cardiovascular abnormalities following tissue trauma and surgery, or even without any obvious precipitating factor.[9]

EFFECTS OF ANESTHESIA ON IMMUNE FUNCTION

Exposure to both anesthesia and surgery depress both T-cell and B-cell responsiveness as well as nonspecific host resistance mechanisms including phagocytosis.[6] Various anesthetic drugs depress immune responses; however, the effects are shortlived and may be modified by multiple other factors occurring perioperatively. Immune competence during surgery can be affected by direct and hormonal effects of anesthetic drugs, immunologic consequences of other drugs used, types of surgery, and coincident infections. Although multiple studies demonstrate *in vitro* alterations of immune function, no studies have ever demonstrated the actual importance.[6] Furthermore, they are likely of minor importance when compared with the hormonal aspects of stress responses.

HYPERSENSITIVITY RESPONSES (ALLERGY)

In 1963, Gell and Coombs first proposed a scheme for classifying immune responses. Although this classification is almost 25 years old, it still provides a useful basis for understanding specific diseases mediated by immunologic processes. The immune pathway functions as a protective mechanism but can also react inappropriately to produce a hypersensitivity or allergic response. The Gell and Coombs scheme defines four basic types of hypersensitivity, Types I through IV. It is useful first to review all four mechanisms to understand the different immune reactions that occur in man.

TYPE I REACTIONS

Type I reactions are also known as anaphylactic or immediate type hypersensitivity reactions and are discussed in more detail in the following section (Fig. 51-3). They are produced by the release of physiologically active mediators released primarily from mast cells and basophils following specific antigen binding IgE antibodies bound to the membranes of these cells. Clinically recognized Type I hypersensitivity reactions include anaphylaxis, extrinsic asthma, and allergic rhinitis.

TYPE II REACTIONS

Type II reactions are also known as antibody dependent cytotoxic hypersensitivity or cytotoxic reactions (Fig. 51-4). These are mediated by either IgG or IgM antibodies which are directed against antigens on the surface of foreign cells. These antigens may either be integral cell membrane components (A or B blood group antigens in ABO incompatibility reactions) or haptens which absorb to the surface of a cell stimulating the production of antihapten antibodies (autoimmune hemolytic anemia). The actual damage in Type II reactions can be produced by different mechanisms that include 1) direct cell lysis following complete complement cascade activation, 2) increased phagocytosis by macrophages, or 3) killer T-cell lymphocytes producing antibody dependent cell mediated cytotoxic effects. Systemic effects associated with Type II reactions are produced by release of complement anaphylatoxins. Common examples of Type II reactions in man are ABO incompatible transfusion reactions, drug induced immune hemolytic anemia and heparin-induced thrombocytopenia.

TYPE III REACTIONS (IMMUNE COMPLEX REACTIONS)

Type III reactions result from circulating soluble antigens and antibodies that bind to form insoluble complexes that are subsequently lodged in the microvasculature of different or-

FIG. 51-3. Type I immediate hypersensitivity reactions (anaphylaxis) involve IgE antibodies binding to mast cells or basophils by way of their Fc receptors. On encountering immunospecific antigens, the IgE becomes cross-linked inducing degranulation, intracellular activation, and release of mediators. This reaction is independent of complement.

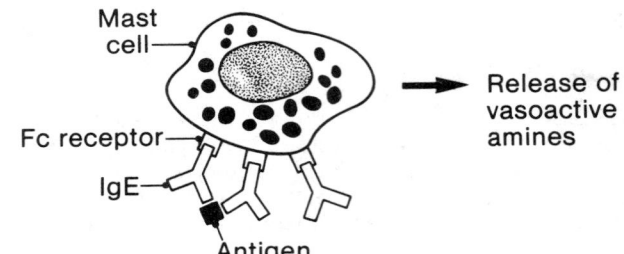

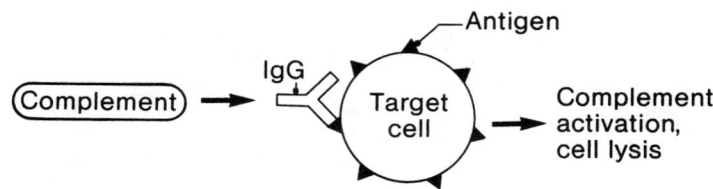

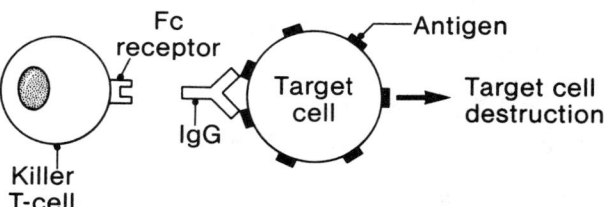

FIG. 51-4. Type II or cytotoxic reactions. Antibody of an IgG or IgM class is directed against antigens on an individual's own cells (target cell). The antigens may be integral membrane components or foreign molecules that have been absorbed. This may lead to complement activation including cell lysis *(upper figure)*, or to cytotoxic action by killer T-cell lymphocytes *(lower figure)*.

gan systems (Fig. 51-5). Complement is subsequently activated which produces leukocyte chemotaxis to the site of the inflammatory stimulus. The polymorphonuclear leukocytes localized to the site of complement deposition release potent inflammatory mediators producing tissue damage. Examples of Type III reactions include classic serum sickness observed following snake antisera or antithymocyte globulin, and immune complex nephritis (poststreptococcal infections).

TYPE IV REACTIONS (DELAYED HYPERSENSITIVITY REACTION OR CELL MEDIATED IMMUNITY)

Type IV reactions result following the interactions of sensitized lymphocytes to specific antigens (Fig. 51-6). The reactions result without complement or antibody involvement. The delayed hypersensitivity reactions are predominantly mononuclear in character and are slow to develop, first appearing in 18 to 24 hours, reaching a maximum in approximately 40 to 80 hours and disappearing in 72 to 96 hours. The antigen binding to specific key lymphocytes produces lymphokine synthesis, lymphocyte proliferation and generation of cytotoxic T-cells. These activated lymphocytes stimulate the migration of macrophages and other mononuclear and polymorphonuclear leukocytes to the site of inflammatory stimulus. In addition, cytotoxic T-cells are generated to specifically kill target cells that bear antigens identical to those that triggered the reaction. This form of immunity is important in tissue rejection, graft *vs* host reactions, contact dermatitis (*i.e.,* poison ivy), and tuberculin immunity.

INTRAOPERATIVE ALLERGIC REACTIONS

The anesthesiologist represents one of the few physicians who personally administers a variety of drugs including anesthetic drugs, antibiotics, and blood products, or monitors patients during radiocontrast dye or chymopapain injection. Because any parenterally administered drugs can cause death from an allergic reaction, anesthesiologists must diagnose and treat the acute cardiovascular and pulmonary changes that occur in *anaphylaxis,* the most severe form of an allergic reaction.

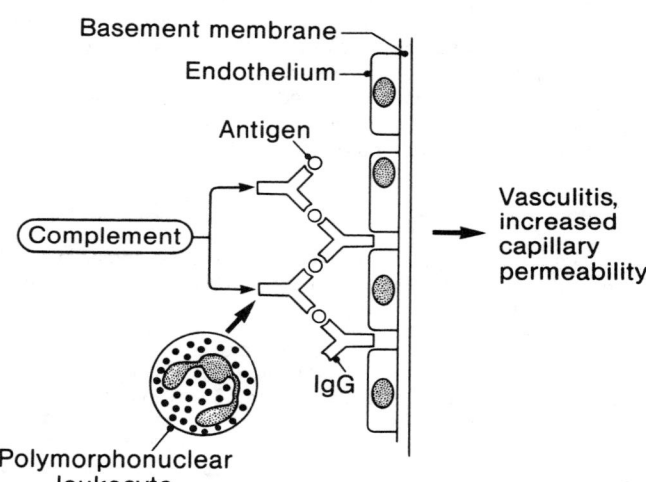

FIG. 51-5. Type III immune complex reactions. Antibodies of an IgG or IgM type bind to the antigen in the soluble base and subsequently are deposited in the microvasculature. Complement is activated producing chemotaxis and activation of polymorphonuclear leukocytes to the site of antigen-antibody complexes and subsequent tissue injury.

FIG. 51-6. Delayed hypersensitivity or cell mediated immunity. Antigen binds to sensitized T-cell lymphocytes to release lymphokines following a second contact with the same antigen. This reaction is independent of circulating antibody or complement activation. Lymphokines induce inflammatory reactions and activate as well as attract macrophages and other mononuclear cells to produce delayed tissue injury.

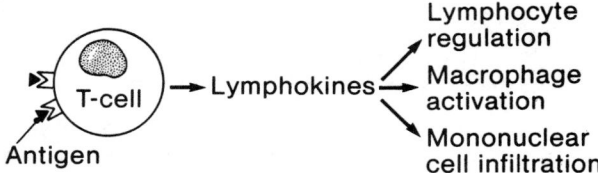

Studies suggest approximately one in every 2700 hospitalized patients experiences drug induced anaphylaxis.[10]

Portier and Richet first used the word anaphylaxis (ana—against, prophylaxis—protection) to describe the profound shock and subsequent death that sometimes occurred in dogs immediately following a second challenge with a foreign antigen.[11] When life-threatening allergic reactions mediated by antibodies occur, they are defined as "anaphylactic." When antibodies are not responsible for the reaction or when we are unable to prove antibody involvement in the reaction, the reaction is called *anaphylactoid*.[12] One cannot distinguish between anaphylactic or anaphylactoid reactions on the basis of clinical observation.

ANAPHYLACTIC REACTIONS: IgE MEDIATED

Pathophysiology

Antigen binding to IgE antibodies initiates anaphylaxis (Fig. 51-7). Prior exposure to the antigen or to a substance of similar structure is required to produce sensitization, although an allergic history may be unknown to the patient. On reexposure, the binding of the antigen to bridge two immunospecific IgE antibodies located on the surfaces of mast cells and basophils liberates histamine and chemotactic factors of anaphylaxis.[13, 14] These preformed mediators are released by a calcium- and energy-dependent process.[15] Other chemical mediators, including arachidonic acid metabolites (leuko-

trienes and prostaglandins) and kinins, subsequently are synthesized and released in response to cellular activation.[16] The liberated mediators produce a symptom complex of bronchospasm and upper airway edema in the respiratory system, vasodilatation and increased capillary permeability in the cardiovascular system, and urticaria in the cutaneous system. Different mediators are released from mast cells and basophils following activation.

Chemical Mediators of Anaphylaxis

HISTAMINE. Histamine, a beta-imidazolethylamine, stimulates H_1 and H_2 receptors. H_1 receptor activation causes increased capillary permeability, bronchoconstriction, and smooth muscle contraction.[17, 18] H_2 receptor activation causes gastric secretion and inhibits mast cell activation.[17] Vasodilation results from stimulation of both H_1 and H_2 receptors. When injected into skin, histamine produces the classic wheal (increased capillary permeability producing tissue edema) and flare (cutaneous vasodilatation) response in man (Fig. 51-8).[19] Histamine undergoes rapid metabolism in humans by the enzymes histamine N-methyltransferase and diamine oxidase located in endothelial cells.[1]

CHEMOTACTIC FACTORS OF ANAPHYLAXIS. Factors are released from mast cells and basophils that cause granulocyte migration (chemotaxis) and collection at the site of the inflammatory stimulus.[16] Eosinophilic chemotactic factor of anaphylaxis (ECF-A) is a small molecular-weight peptide chemo-

FIG. 51-7. *(1)* During anaphylaxis (Type 1 immediate hypersensitivity reaction) antigen enters a patient during anesthesia through a parenteral route. *(2)* It bridges two IgE antibodies on the surface of mast cells or basophils. In a calcium- and energy-dependent process, cells release various substances—histamine, eosinophilic chemotactic factor of anaphylaxis, leukotrienes, prostaglandins, and kinins. *(3)* These released mediators produce the characteristic effects in the pulmonary, cardiovascular, and cutaneous systems. The most severe and life-threatening effects of the vasoactive mediators occur in the respiratory and cardiovascular systems. (Levy JH: Identification and Treatment of Anaphylaxis: Mechanisms of Action and Strategies for Treatment Under General Anesthesia. Chicago, Smith Laboratories.)

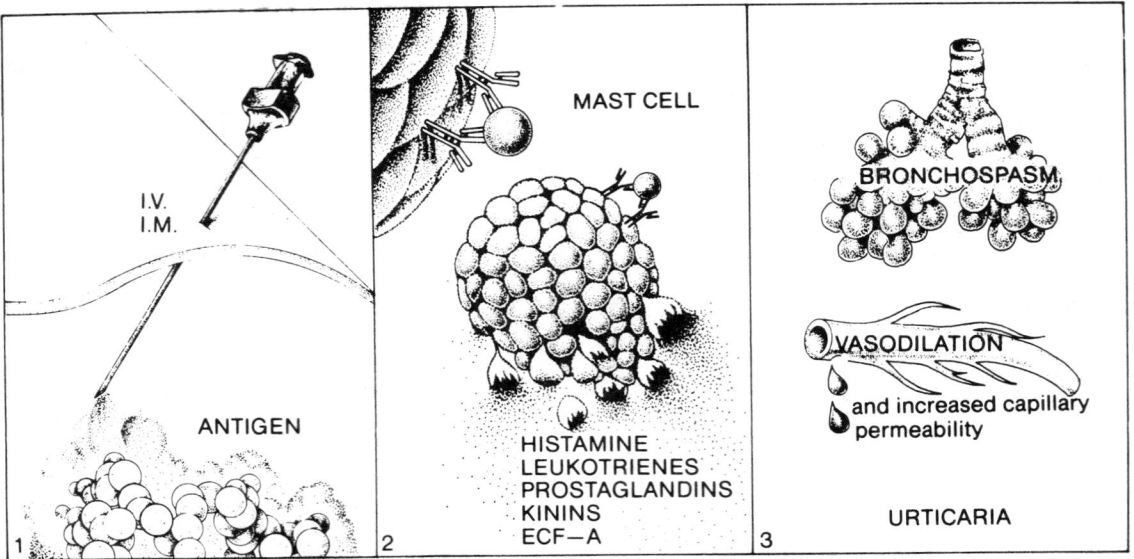

**Anaphylaxis
(Type I Immediate Hypersensitivity Reaction)**

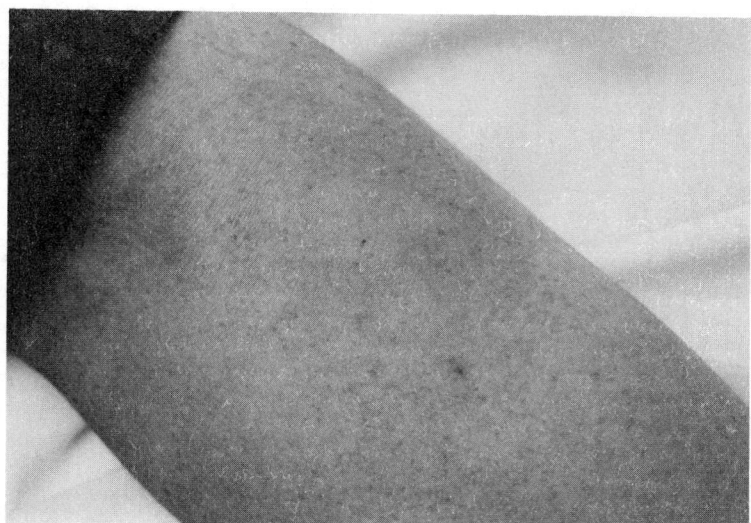

FIG. 51-8. Histamine induced wheal and flare response in man. The injection of a small dose of histamine, 10 μg, produces a profound wheal or localized tissue edema caused by an increased capillary permeability as well as a flare response, characterized by erythema due to cutaneous vasodilatation. This patient demonstrated a profound wheal of 14 mm and a larger flare of 28 mm following the injection of 10 μg of histamine intradermally.

tactic for eosinophils.[20] Although the exact role of ECF-A or the eosinophil in the acute allergic response is unclear, eosinophils release enzymes that can inactivate histamine and leukotrienes.[16] In addition, a neutrophilic chemotactic factor is released that causes chemotaxis and activation.[16, 21] Granulocyte activation may be responsible for recurrent manifestations of anaphylaxis.

LEUKOTRIENES (SLOW-REACTING SUBSTANCE OF ANAPHYLAXIS). Various leukotrienes are synthesized following mast cell activation from arachidonic acid metabolism of phospholipid cell membranes via the lipoxygenase pathway.[22] The slow-reacting substance of anaphylaxis is a combination of leukotrienes C4, D4, and E4.[23] Leukotrienes produce bronchoconstriction, increased capillary permeability, vasodilatation, coronary vasoconstriction, and myocardial depression.[23]

PROSTAGLANDINS. Prostaglandins are the products of arachidonic acid metabolism by way of the cylclooxygenase pathway.[23] Prostaglandins represent potent mast cell mediators that produce vasodilatation, bronchospasm, pulmonary hypertension, and increased capillary permeability.[16, 23] Prostaglandin D_2, the major metabolite of mast cells, produces bronchospasm and vasodilation.[23] Elevated plasma levels of thromboxane B_2 (the metabolite of thromboxane A_2), also a prostaglandin synthesized by mast cells as well as polymorphonuclear leukocytes, have been demonstrated following protamine reactions associated with pulmonary hypertension.[24, 25]

KININS. Small peptides called kinins are synthesized in mast cells and basophils to produce vasodilatation, increased capillary permeability, and bronchoconstriction.[16, 26]

PLATELET-ACTIVATING FACTOR. Platelet-activating factor (PAF), an unstored lipid synthesized in activated human mast cells, is an extremely potent biologic material, producing physiologic effects at concentrations as low as 10^{-10} molar.[16] PAF aggregates and activates human platelets, and perhaps leukocytes, to release inflammatory products. PAF causes a profound wheal and flare response, smooth muscle contraction, and increased capillary permeability.[16]

Recognition of Anaphylaxis

The onset and severity of the reaction relate to the mediator's specific end organ effects. Antigenic challenge in a sensitized individual usually produces immediate clinical manifestations of anaphylaxis, but the onset may be delayed 2 to 20 minutes.[27, 28] The reaction may include some or all of the symptoms and signs listed in Table 51-3. Individuals vary greatly in their manifestations and course of anaphylaxis.[29, 30] A spectrum of reactions exist, ranging from minor clinical changes to

TABLE 51-3.   Recognition of Anaphylaxis During Regional and General Anesthesia

SYSTEMS	SYMPTOMS	SIGNS
Respiratory	Dyspnea Chest discomfort	Coughing Wheezing Sneezing Laryngeal edema Decreased pulmonary compliance Fulminant pulmonary edema Acute respiratory distress
Cardiovascular	Dizziness Malaise Retrosternal oppression	Disorientation Diaphoresis Loss of consciousness Hypotension Tachycardia Dysrhythmias Decreased systemic vascular resistance Cardiac arrest Pulmonary hypertension
Cutaneous	Itching Burning Tingling	Urticaria (hives) Flushing Periorbital edema Perioral edema

(Levy JH: Anaphylactic Reactions in Anesthesia and Intensive Care. Boston, Butterworths, 1986.)

the "full blown" syndrome, leading to death.[29, 31] The enigma of anaphylaxis is the unpredictability of occurrence, the severity of the attack, and the lack of a prior allergic history.

NON-IgE MEDIATED REACTIONS

Other immunologic and nonimmunologic mechanisms liberate many of the mediators previously discussed independent of IgE, creating a clinical syndrome identical to anaphylaxis. Specific pathways important in producing the same spectrum of clinical manifestations are considered later.

Complement Activation

Complement activation follows both immunologic (antibody mediated, i.e., classic pathway) or nonimmunologic (alternative) pathways to include a series of multimolecular, self-assembling proteins that liberate biologically active complement fragments of C3 and C5.[8, 32] C3a and C5a are called anaphylatoxins because they release histamine from mast cells and basophils, contract smooth muscle, and increase capillary permeability (Table 51-4). In addition, C5a interacts with specific high-affinity receptors on white blood cells and platelets, initiating leukocyte chemotaxis, aggregation, and activation.[33] Aggregated leukocytes embolize to various organs producing microvascular occlusion and liberation of inflammatory products such as arachidonic acid metabolites, oxygen-free radicals, and lysosomal enzymes (Fig. 51-9). Antibodies of the IgG class directed against antigenic determinants or granulocyte surfaces can also produce leukocyte aggregation.[34] These antibodies are called leukoagglutinins. Investigators have implicated complement activation and polymorphonuclear leukocyte aggregation in producing the clinical manifestations of transfusion reactions,[34, 35] pulmonary vasoconstriction following protamine reactions,[25] adult respiratory distress syndrome,[36] and septic shock.[36]

Nonimmunologic Release of Histamine

Many diverse molecular structures of the different agents administered during the perioperative period release histamine in a dose-dependent, nonimmunologic fashion (Table 51-5).[37–41] Intravenous administration of morphine or d-tubocurarine can release histamine, producing vasodilatation and urticaria along the vein of administration.[37, 38] These self-limiting reactions can be treated effectively with intravascular volume administration or vasoconstrictors (Fig. 51-10).

The mechanisms involved in nonimmunologic histamine release are not well understood but appear to represent noncytotoxic degranulation of mast cells but not basophils (Fig. 51-11).[39, 41] Human cutaneous mast cells are postulated to have multiple opioid receptors that respond to kappa, beta en-

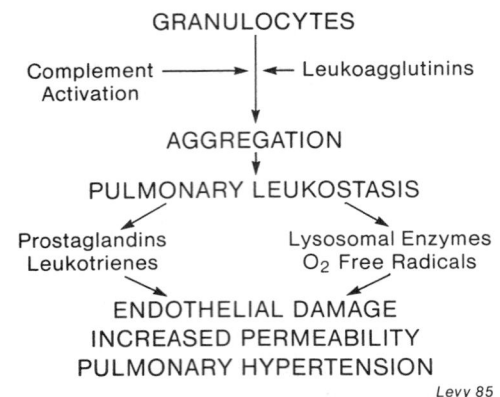

FIG. 51-9. Sequence of events producing granulocyte aggregation, pulmonary leukostasis, and cardiopulmonary dysfunction. (Levy JH: Anaphylactic Reactions in Anesthesia and Intensive Care. Boston, Butterworths, 1986.)

dorphin, delta, and mu agonists.[42] The mu-receptor agonists, morphine, meperidine, and codeine release histamine in human skin equipotently.[42] However, sufentanil, fentanyl, and alfentanil, all mu-receptor agonists, do not appear to release histamine when administered intravenously.[37] A spectrum of different molecular structures release histamine in man, suggesting both opioid and nonopioid receptors are involved.[42]

Antihistamine pretreatment (e.g., H₁ blockers—diphenhydramine, H₂ blockers—cimetidine) prior to administering drugs that are known to release histamine in man do not inhibit histamine release but rather compete with histamine at the receptor and may attenuate decreases in systemic vascular resistance.[43] However, the effect of any drug on systemic vascular resistance may be dependent on other factors in addition to histamine release.[44, 45]

TREATMENT PLAN

A plan for the treatment of anaphylactic or anaphylactoid reactions must be established before the event. Airway maintenance, 100% oxygen administration, intravascular volume expansion, and epinephrine are essential to treat the hypotension and hypoxia that result from vasodilatation, increased capillary permeability, and bronchospasm.[1] Table 51-6 lists a protocol for management of anaphylaxis during general anesthesia, with representative doses for a 70-kg adult. The treatment plan is the same for life-threatening anaphylactic or anaphylactoid reactions. Therapy must be titrated to desired effects with careful monitoring. Severe reactions require aggressive therapy and may be protracted with persistent hypo-

TABLE 51-4.   Biologic Effects of Anaphylatoxins

BIOLOGIC EFFECTS	C3a	C5a
Histamine release	+	+
Smooth muscle contraction	+	+
Increased vascular permeability	+	+
Chemotaxis		+
Leukocyte and platelet aggregation		+

TABLE 51-5.   Drugs Capable of Nonimmunologic Histamine Release

Antibiotics—vancomycin, pentamidine
Basic compounds
Hyperosmotic agents
Muscle relaxants—D-tubocurarine, metocurine, atracurium
Opioids—morphine, meperidine, codeine
Thiobarbiturates

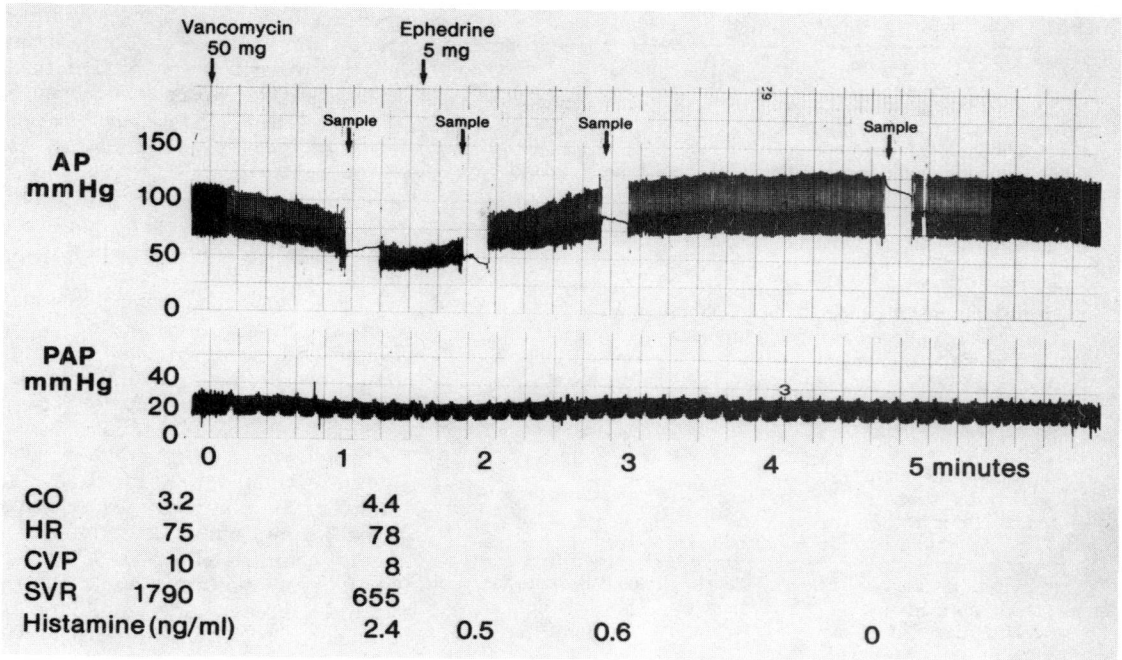

FIG. 51-10. Example of an anaphylactoid reaction following rapid vancomycin administration in a patient. Hypotension is associated with an increased cardiac output and decreased calculated systemic vascular resistance. Plasma histamine levels one minute after the vancomycin administration were 2.4 ng·ml^{-1} and subsequently decreased to zero. The patient was given ephedrine, 5 mg, and blood pressure returned to baseline values. (Levy JH: Anesthesiology, 67:122, 1987.)

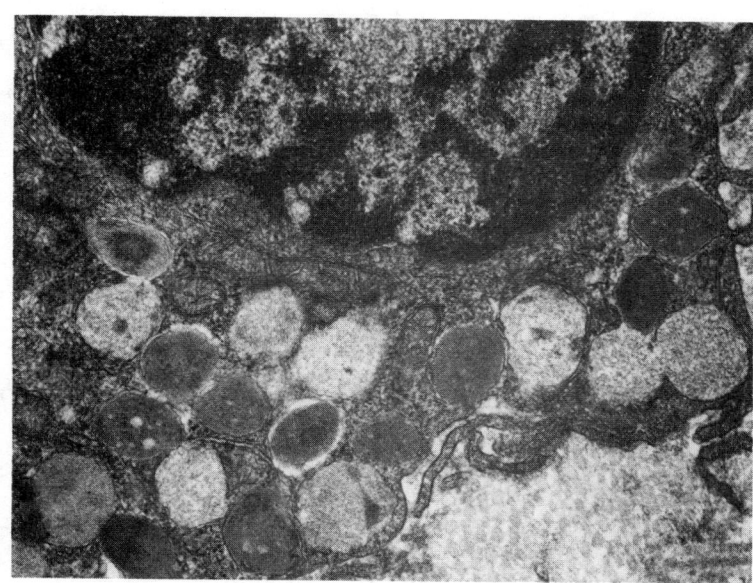

FIG. 51-11. Electron micrograph of human cutaneous mast cell after injection of dynorphin, a Kappa opioid agonist. The cell outline is rounded and the majority of the cytoplasmic granules are swollen, demonstrating varying degrees of decreased electron density and flocculence consistent with ongoing degranulation. The perigranular membranes of the adjacent granules at the periphery of the cell are fused to each other and to plasma membrane. (Original magnification × 72,000; Casale TB: J Allergy Clin Immunol 73:778, 1984.)

tension, pulmonary hypertension, lower respiratory obstruction, or laryngeal obstruction that persist 5 to 32 hours despite vigorous therapy.[46] All patients following an anaphylactic reaction should be admitted to an intensive care unit for 24 hours of monitoring as they may develop recurrence of manifestations following successful treatment.

Initial Therapy

STOP ADMINISTRATION OF ANTIGEN. From a practical perspective, this may not always be possible. Limiting antigen administration may prevent further recruitment of activated mast cells and basophils.

TABLE 51-6. Management of Anaphylaxis

Initial Therapy

1. Stop administration of antigen
2. Maintain airway with 100% O_2
3. Discontinue all anesthetic agents
4. Start intravascular volume expansion (2–4 l of crystalloid with hypotension)
5. Give epinephrine (4–8 μg iv bolus with hypotension, titrate as needed; 0.1 to 0.5 mg iv with cardiovascular collapse)

Secondary Treatment

1. Antihistamines (0.5–1 mg·kg^{-1} diphenhydramine)
2. Catecholamine infusions (starting doses: epinephrine 2–4 μg·min^{-1}, norepinephrine 2–4 μg·min^{-1}, or isoproterenol 0.5–1 μg·min^{-1} as a drip, titrated to desired effects)
3. Aminophylline (5–6 mg·kg^{-1} over 20 min with persistent bronchospasm)
4. Corticosteroids (0.25–1 g hydrocortisone; alternately 1–2 g methylprednisolone)*
5. Sodium bicarbonate (0.5–1 mEq·kg^{-1} with persistent hypotension or acidosis)
6. Airway evaluation (prior to extubation)

* Methylprednisolone may be the drug of choice if the reaction is suspected to be mediated by complement.
(Levy JH: Anaphylactic Reactions in Anesthesia and Intensive Care, p 104. Boston, Butterworths, 1986.)

AIRWAY MAINTENANCE WITH 100% OXYGEN. Profound ventilation-perfusion abnormalities producing hypoxemia can occur with anaphylactic reactions.[47] Always administer 100% oxygen along with ventilatory support as needed. Arterial blood gases should be drawn and followed during resuscitation.

DISCONTINUE ALL ANESTHETIC DRUGS. Inhalational anesthetic drugs are not the bronchodilators of choice in treating bronchospasm following anaphylaxis, especially during hypotension. These drugs interfere with the body's compensatory response to cardiovascular collapse. Furthermore, halothane sensitizes the myocardium to catecholamines, which must be administered in severe reactions.

VOLUME EXPANSION. Hypovolemia rapidly ensues during anaphylactic shock.[48] Fisher has reported an up to 40 per cent loss of intravascular fluid into the interstitial space during reactions, as demonstrated by hemoconcentration.[48] Therefore, volume expansion is extremely important in conjunction with epinephrine in correcting the acute hypotension. Initially, 2 to 4 l of lactated Ringer's solution or normal saline should be administered, keeping in mind that an additional 25 to 50 ml·kg^{-1} may be necessary with persistent hypotension. Refractory hypotension following volume and epinephrine administration requires additional hemodynamic monitoring including pulmonary and radial arterial catheterization for accurate assessment of intravascular volume and to guide rational therapeutic interventions. Fulminant noncardiogenic pulmonary edema with loss of intravascular volume can occur following anaphylaxis. This condition requires intravascular volume repletion with careful hemodynamic monitoring until the capillary defect improves. Colloid volume expansion has not been proven to be more effective than crystalloid volume expansion for treating anaphylactic shock.

EPINEPHRINE. Epinephrine is the drug of choice when resuscitating patients during anaphylactic shock. Alpha-adrenergic effects vasoconstrict to reverse hypotension; beta$_2$ receptor stimulation bronchodilates and inhibits mediator release by increasing cyclic AMP in mast cells and basophils.[30] *The route of epinephrine administration and the dose depends upon the patient's condition. Rapid and timely intervention with common sense must be used when treating anaphylaxis.* Furthermore, during general anesthesia patients may have altered sympathoadrenergic responses to acute anaphylactic shock while the patient during spinal or epidural anesthesia may be partially sympathectomized, requiring even larger doses of catecholamines.[49]

In hypotensive patients, 4–8 μg boluses of epinephrine should be titrated for restoring blood pressure.* Additional volume and incrementally increased doses of epinephrine should be administered until hypotension is corrected. Although an epinephrine infusion represents an ideal method of administering epinephrine, it is usually impossible to infuse the drug through peripheral intravenous access during acute volume resuscitation. With cardiovascular collapse, full intravenous cardiopulmonary resuscitative doses of epinephrine, 0.1 to 0.5 mg, should be administered and repeated until hemodynamic stability occurs. Patients with laryngeal edema without hypotension should receive subcutaneous epinephrine. Epinephrine should not be administered intravenously to patients with normal blood pressures.[50]

Secondary Treatment

ANTIHISTAMINES. Since H$_1$ receptors mediate many of the adverse effects of histamine, the intravenous administration of 0.5 to 1 mg·kg^{-1} of an H$_1$ antagonist such as diphendydramine may be useful in treating acute anaphylaxis. Antihistamines do not inhibit anaphylactic reactions or inhibit histamine release but compete with histamine at receptor sites. H$_1$ antagonists are indicated in all forms of anaphylaxis. The H$_1$ antagonists presently available for parenteral administration may have antidopaminergic effects and should be given slowly to prevent precipitous hypotension in potentially hypovolemic patients.[1] The indication for administering an H$_2$ antagonist once anaphylaxis has occurred remains unclear.

CATECHOLAMINES. Epinephrine infusions may be useful in patients with persistent hypotension or bronchospasm after initial resuscitation.[1] Epinephrine infusions should be started at 2 to 4 μg·min^{-1} and titrated to correct hypotension.

Norepinephrine infusions may be required in patients with refractory hypotension due to decreased systemic vascular resistance. It may be started at 2 to 4 μg·min^{-1} and adjusted to correct hypotension.

Isoproterenol infusions can be used in patients with refractory bronchospasm, pulmonary hypertension, or right ventricular dysfunction. The usual starting dose is 0.5 to 1 μg·min^{-1}. Isoproterenol has profound beta$_2$-adrenergic effects that can produce systemic vasodilatation; therefore, it must be used cautiously in hypotensive or hypovolemic patients.

AMINOPHYLLINE. Aminophylline, a phosphodiesterase inhibitor, bronchodilates and decreases histamine release from mast cells or basophils by effectively increasing intracellular cyclic AMP. In addition, it increases right and left ventricular contractility and decreases pulmonary vascular

*This dose of epinephrine can be obtained with the use of a 1:10,000 dilution (100 μg·ml^{-1}) or by mixing 2 mg epinephrine with 250 ml of fluid to yield an 8 μg·ml^{-1} solution.

resistance. Aminophylline is indicated in patients with persistent bronchospasm and hemodynamic stability. An intravenous loading dose of 5 to 6 mg · kg^{-1} of aminophylline given over 20 minutes should be followed by an infusion of 0.9 mg · kg^{-1} · hr^{-1}.

CORTICOSTEROIDS. Indications for corticosteroid administration during anaphylaxis are not well defined. Experimental evidence suggests that they will decrease arachidonic acid metabolites by inducing synthesis of nuclear regulatory proteins to inhibit phospholipid membrane breakdown.[51] In addition, they may alter the activation and migration of other inflammatory cells (*i.e.*, polymorphonuclear leukocytes) following an acute reaction.[52] Corticosteroids may require 12 to 24 hours to work and, despite their unproven usefulness in treating acute reactions, they often are administered as adjuncts to therapy when refractory bronchospasm or refractory shock occur following resuscitative therapy.[53] Although the exact corticosteroid dose and preparation are unclear, investigators have recommended 0.25 to 1 g of hydrocortisone in IgE-mediated reactions. Alternately, 1 to 2 g of methylprednisolone (30 to 35 mg · kg^{-1}) may be useful in reactions thought to be complement-mediated such as catastrophic pulmonary vasoconstriction following protamine transfusion reactions.[54] Administering corticosteroids after an anaphylactic reaction may also be important in attenuating the late phase reactions reported to occur 12 to 24 hours after anaphylaxis.[46]

BICARBONATE. Acidosis rapidly develops in patients with persistent hypotension. This diminishes the effect of epinephrine on the heart and systemic vasculature. Therefore, with refractory hypotension or acidemia, sodium bicarbonate, 0.5 to 1 mEq · kg^{-1}, should be given and repeated every 5 minutes or as dictated by arterial blood gases.

AIRWAY EVALUATION. Because profound laryngeal edema may be the sequela of anaphylactic reactions, the airway should be evaluated before extubation of the trachea.[27] Persistent facial edema suggests airway edema. The tracheas of these patients should remain intubated until the edema subsides. The development of a significant air leak after endotracheal tube cuff deflation before extubation of the trachea is useful in assessing airway patency. If there is any question of airway edema, then direct laryngoscopy should be performed before extubation of the trachea.

PERIOPERATIVE MANAGEMENT OF THE PATIENT WITH ALLERGIES

ALLERGIC DRUG REACTIONS

Allergic drug reactions account for 6% to 10% of all adverse reactions.[55] DeSwarte suggests the risk of an allergic drug reaction is approximately 1% to 3% for most drugs and approximately 5% of adults in the United States may be allergic to one or more drugs.[56] Unfortunately, patients often refer to adverse drug effects as being allergic in nature. For example, opioid administration can produce nausea, vomiting, or even local release of histamine along the vein of administration. Patients will say they are allergic to a specific drug when in fact their adverse reaction is independent of allergy. Approximately 15% of the adults in the United States believe they are allergic to specific medication(s), and therefore may be denied treatment with an indicated drug. To understand allergic reac-

tions, the spectrum of adverse reactions to drugs needs to be considered.

Predictable adverse drug reactions are 1) often dose-dependent, 2) related to the known pharmacologic actions of the drug, 3) occur in otherwise normal patients, and 4) account for approximately 80% of adverse drug effects. Most serious predictable adverse drug reactions are toxic in nature and either directly related to the amount of drug in the body (overdosage) inadvertent route of administration (*i.e.*, lidocaine-induced seizures). Side-effects are the most common adverse drug reactions and are undesirable but often unavoidable pharmacologic actions of the drugs occurring at usual prescribed dosages. Most anesthetic drugs exhibit multiple side-effects that can produce precipitous hypotension. For example, morphine dilates the venous capacitance bed to decrease preload, releases histamine from cutaneous mast cells to produce arterial and venodilatation, slows the heart rate, and decreases sympathetic tone. However, the net effects of morphine administration on blood pressure and myocardial function depends on the patient's blood volume, sympathetic tone, and ventricular function. A volume depleted patient in pain following an auto accident who receives morphine rapidly develops hypotension. In addition, drug interactions represent important predictable adverse drug reactions. Intravenous fentanyl or sufentanil administration to a patient who has just received intravenous benzodiazepines or other sedative/hypnotic drugs may produce precipitous hypotension that results from decreased sympathetic tone (Fig. 51-12).[57] This represents dose dependent, predictable adverse drug reactions, independent of allergy.

Unpredictable adverse drug reactions are 1) usually dose-independent, 2) usually not related to the drugs' pharmacologic actions, and 3) often related to the immunologic response (allergy) of the individual. On occasion, adverse reactions can be related to genetic differences (*i.e.*, idiosyncratic) occurring among susceptible individuals who possess an isolated genetic enzyme deficiency. The most common example of an idiosyncratic reaction is the hemolytic anemia occurring among patients whose erythrocytes lack the enzyme glucose-6-phosphate dehydrogenase, when exposed to chloramphenicol, sulfonamides, or other oxidant drugs. Allergic reactions are also quantitatively aberrant and cannot be explained in terms of the normal pharmacology of the drug given in the usual therapeutic doses but are related to the individual's immune response.

Most allergic drug reactions are those in which an immunologic mechanism is present or, more often, presumed. Such a mechanism may be impossible to establish with most anesthetic drugs. Proving that the initiating event involves a reaction between the drug or drug metabolites with drug-specific antibodies or sensitized T-lymphocytes is often costly, time consuming, and may be inaccurate. Even in the absence of direct immunologic evidence, criteria that may be helpful in distinguishing an allergic reaction from other adverse reactions are as follows.

Allergic reactions occur in only a small percentage of patients receiving the drug. In addition, the observed clinical manifestations do not resemble known pharmacologic actions of the drug. In the absence of prior drug exposure, allergic symptoms rarely appear after less than one week of continuous treatment. Following sensitization, even years previously, the reaction will develop rapidly upon re-exposure to the drug. In general, drugs that have been administered without complications for several months or longer are rarely responsible for producing drug allergy. The time span between exposure to the drug and noticed manifestations is often the

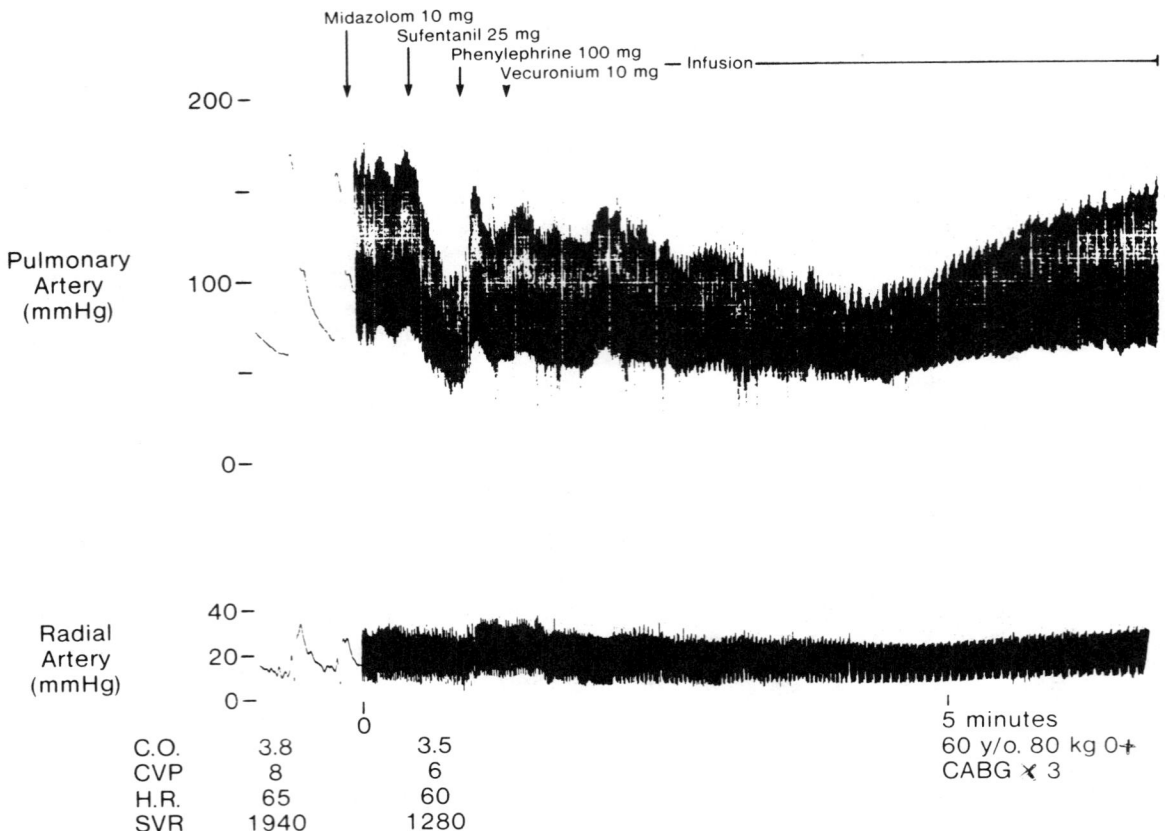

FIG. 51-12. Effects of sufentanil and midazolam on blood pressure. Anesthetic drugs administered alone or in combinations may produce synergistic effects to produce precipitous hypotension. Small doses of intravenous sufentanil (25μg) administered to a patient who has previously received intravenous midazolam can develop precipitous hypotension from decreased sympathetic tone. This interaction also occurs with fentanyl and diazepam. These adverse effects are predictable, dose-dependent, occur in otherwise healthy patients, and can be treated with the administration of a vasoconstrictor such as phenylephrine.

most vital information in determining which drugs administered were the cause of a suspected allergic reaction. While the reaction may produce a life-threatening response in the cardiopulmonary system (anaphylaxis), a variety of cutaneous manifestations, fever, and pulmonary reactions have been attributed to drug hypersensitivity. Usually the reaction may be reproduced by very small doses of the suspected drug or other agents possessing similar or cross reacting chemical structures. On occasion, drug-specific antibodies or lymphocytes have been identified that react with the suspected drug although this is seldom diagnostically useful in practice. Even when an immune response to a drug is demonstrated, it may not be associated with a clinical allergic reaction. As with adverse drug reactions in general, the reaction usually subsides within several days following discontinuation of the drug.

IMMUNOLOGIC MECHANISMS OF DRUG ALLERGY

Different immunologic responses to any antigen can occur. Drugs have been associated with all of the immunologic mechanisms proposed by Gell and Coombs. Although more than one mechanism may contribute to a particular reaction, any one can in fact occur. Penicillin may produce different reactions in different patients, or possibly a spectrum of reactions in the same patient. In one patient penicillin can produce anaphylaxis (Type I reaction), hemolytic anemia (Type II reaction), serum sickness (Type III reaction), as well as contact dermatitis (Type IV reaction).[56] Therefore, any one antigen has the ability to produce a diffuse spectrum of allergic responses in man. Why some patients develop localized rashes to penicillin or angioneurotic edema, while others develop complete cardiopulmonary collapse is unknown.

Most anesthetic drugs and agents administered perioperatively have been reported in the literature to produce anaphylactic/anaphylactoid reactions (Table 51-7).[29, 37–43, 58–77]

Life-threatening allergic reactions are more likely to occur in patients with a history of allergy, atopy, or asthma. Nevertheless, because the incidence is low, the presence of such a history is not a reliable predictor that an allergic reaction will occur and does not mandate that such patients should be investigated, pretreated, or specific drugs be selected or avoided.[58] Although different mechanisms have been proposed, no one hypothesis has been proven.[1] The drugs and

TABLE 51-7.   Agents Implicated in Allergic Reactions During Anesthesia

Anesthetic Agents Implicated in Allergic Reactions

Induction agents
    cremophor solubilized drugs, barbiturates, etomidate
Local anesthetics
    para-aminobenzoic ester agents
Muscle relaxants
    succinylcholine, gallamine, pancuronium, d-tubocurarine, metocurine, atracurium
Opioids
    meperidine, morphine, fentanyl

Other Agents Implicated in Allergic Reactions

Antibiotics
    cephalosporins, penicillin, vancomycin
Blood products
    whole blood, packed cells, fresh frozen plasma, platelets, cryoprecipitate
Bone cement
Chymopapain
Cyclosporin
Drug additives
Mannitol
Methylmetracrylate
Protamine
Radiocontrast dye
Colloid volume expanders
    dextrans, protein fractions, albumin, hydroxyethyl starch

(Levy JH: Anaphylactic Reactions in Anesthesia and Intensive Care. Boston, Butterworths, 1986.)

foreign substances listed may have both immunologic and nonimmunologic mechanisms for adverse drug reactions in man.

EVALUATION OF PATIENTS WITH ALLERGIC REACTIONS

Identifying the drug responsible for a suspected allergic reaction still depends on circumstantial evidence indicating the temporal sequence of drug administration. Conventional *in vivo* and *in vitro* methods to diagnose allergic reactions to most anesthetic drugs are unavailable or not applicable for supporting an allergic reaction. The most important factor in diagnosis is the awareness of the physician that an untoward event may be related to a drug that the patient received. The physician must always be aware of the ability of any drug to produce an allergic reaction. The history is extremely important when evaluating whether an adverse drug reaction is allergic and whether the drug can be readministered. Although a prior allergic reaction to the drug in question is important, this is rarely the case. Direct challenge of a patient with a test dose of drug is the only way to establish reaction, but this is potentially hazardous and not recommended. While the anesthesiologist commonly administers small "test" doses of anesthetic drugs, these are pharmacologic test doses and have nothing to do with immunologic dosages.

The demonstration of drug specific IgE antibodies is generally accepted as evidence that the patient may be at risk for anaphylaxis if the drug is administered.[56] Different clinically available tests to confirm or diagnose drug allergy have been reported and are individually considered as follows.

TESTING FOR ALLERGY

For the patient following anaphylactoid reaction it is important to identify the causative agent to prevent readministration. When one particular drug has been administered and there is a clear correlation between time of administration and occurrence of reaction then testing may be unnecessary and general avoidance of the drug should occur. However, when patients have simultaneously received multiple drugs (*i.e.*, an opioid, muscle relaxant, hypnotic, and antibiotic), it is often difficult to designate which particular drug caused the reaction. Furthermore, the reaction could have been caused by either the vehicle by which the drug was administered or perhaps one of the preservatives. In patients who desire to know which drug was designed or when patients are scheduled for multiple other procedures, then some degree of allergy evaluation should be undertaken to evaluate the drug at risk. Unfortunately, very few *in vitro* tests exist to anesthetic drugs, therefore the presently available allergy tests are discussed.

Leukocyte Histamine Release

Leukocyte histamine release simulates an *in vivo* anaphylactoid reaction by incubating the patient's own leukocytes with different concentrations of the offending drug in measuring histamine release as a marker for basophil activation. Similar to intradermal testing, a positive test identifies the causative agent, suggesting a potential IgE mechanism, but false-positive tests can occur.[29] However, in some instances it is possible to sensitize leukocytes from a nonallergic patient, then challenged in with the drug, thereby identifying the reaction as IgE. This test is not easy to perform and requires large quantities of fresh leukocytes and tedious isolation techniques. Modifications of this test have been made by using whole blood instead of isolated polymorphonuclear leukocytes.[72, 78]

Radioallergosorbent Test (RAST)

The RAST allows *in vitro* detection of specific IgE directed toward particular antigens.[79] In this test, antigens are linked to insoluble material such as cellulose or paper to make an immunoabsorbent.[79, 80] When incubated with the serum in question, antibodies of different classes directed toward the antigen bind to it. After washing, the antigen-antibody complex on the immunoabsorbent is incubated with radio labelled antibodies directed against human IgE. With the anti-IgE bound human complex, the complex may be easily counted in a scintillation counter. A numerical value reflects the concentration of specific IgE in the patient's serum directed toward the allergen. The RAST uses a blood sample to give similar information as the skin test. The RAST is more quantitative than skin tests and avoids the potential of reexposure of an antigen to a patient who had had a life-threatening anaphylactic reaction.[80] Furthermore, it avoids the discomfort of skin testing. However, it is more expensive and the antigens available for these agents to anesthetic drugs are limited. RAST testing has been used to detect the presence of antibodies to meperidine,[47] succinylcholine,[81] and thiopental.[82] Two major limitations to this test include the commercial availability of the drug prepared as an antigen, and false-positive test results in patients with elevated IgE levels.[83]

Enzyme-linked Immunosorbent Assay (ELISA)

The ELISA measures antigen specific antibodies. The basis of the ELISA is similar to the RAST; however, immunospecific

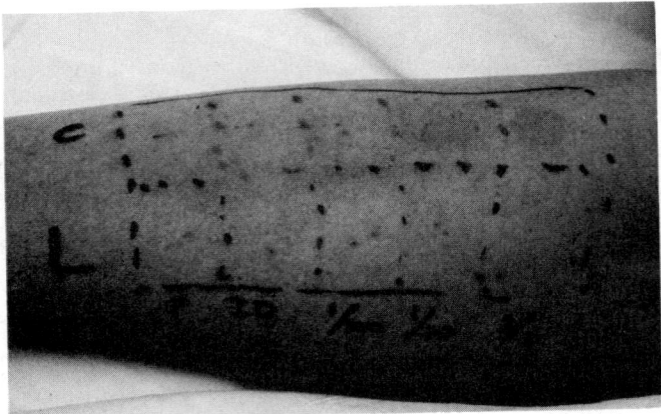

FIG. 51-13. Skin testing in a man with a suspected history of a local anesthetic reaction. Skin testing is used to identify what agents a patient may be allergic to as well as what agents he may safely receive. C represents procaine and L for lidocaine tested without preservatives. The patient developed a positive wheal and flare response to procaine at a 1/10 dilution, but no response to lidocaine. (P = prick test, ID = intradermal, 1/100, 1/10, 1/1 = local anesthetic drug dilutions.)

IgE directed against the antigen in question is determined by the addition of an anti-IgE coupled to an enzyme such as peroxidase that acts as a chromogen.[5] A colorless substrate is acted on by peroxidase to produce a colored byproduct. The ELISA has been used to demonstrate IgE antibodies to chymopapain and protamine and has been developed to screen patients for other antibodies to diverse agents such as the human T-cell lymphotrophic virus Type III (the AIDS virus). At present, there are no clinically available ELISA tests for anesthetic drugs.

Intradermal Testing (Skin Testing)

Skin testing is the method generally used to confirm specific sensitivity in patients following anaphylactic reaction to anesthetic drugs after the history has suggested the relevant antigens for testing.[84-86] Within minutes after antigen introduction, histamine released from cutaneous mast cells causes vasodilatation (flare) and localized edema from increased vascular permeability (wheal). Fisher suggests this to be a simple, safe, and useful method in establishing a diagnosis in most cases of anaphylactoid reactions occurring in the perioperative period.[84, 85] Using strict protocols established by Fisher, intradermal reactions can be very helpful.[84] Intradermal testing is of no value in reactions with contrast media or colloid volume expanders. Furthermore, cross sensitivity between drugs of similar structures can often be evaluated on the basis of skin testing. Skin testing to local anesthetics is considered a direct challenge or provocative dose testing.[87] Local anesthetic drugs are injected in increasing quantities under controlled circumstances. This testing determines if the individual can safely receive amide derivatives (*i.e.*, lidocaine) and can also be used to determine if the individual is sensitive to the para-aminobenzoic ester agents (*i.e.*, procaine; Fig. 51-13).

SUMMARY

Although the immune system functions to provide host defense, it can respond inappropriately to produce hypersensitivity or allergic reactions. A spectrum of life threatening allergic reactions to any drug or agent can occur in the perioperative period. The enigma of these reactions is their unpredictable nature. However, with a high index of suspicion, prompt recognition with appropriate and aggressive therapy can help to avoid a disastrous outcome.

REFERENCES

1. Levy J: Anaphylactic Reactions in Anesthesia and Intensive Care. Boston, Butterworths, 1986
2. Watkins J: Hypersensitivity response to drugs and plasma substitutes used in anesthesia and surgery. In Watkins J, Salo M (eds): Trauma, Stress and Immunity in Anaesthesia and Surgery, p 254. London, Butterworth & Co, 1982
3. Gell PGH, Coombs RRA, Lachmann PJ (eds): Clinical aspects of Immunology, 3rd ed. Oxford, Blackwell Scientific Publications, 1975
4. Butler VP Jr, Beiser SM: Antibodies to small molecules. Biologic and clinical applications. Adv Immunol 17:255, 1973
5. Roitt I, Brostoff J, Male D (eds): Immunology. St Louis, CV Mosby, 1985
6. Walton B: Anaesthesia, surgery, and immunology. Anaesthesia 33:322, 1978
7. Metcalf DD: Effector cell heterogeneity in immediate hypersensitivity reactions. Clin Rev Allergy 1:311, 1982
8. Ruddy S, Gigli I, Austen KF: The complement system of man. N Engl J Med 287:489-, 592-, 642-, 1972
9. Razes PA, Coulson IH, Gould TR et al: Acquired C_1 esterase inhibitor deficiency. Anaesthesia 41:838, 1986
10. Porter J, Jick H: Drug-induced anaphylaxis, convulsions, deafness, and extrapyramidal symptoms. Lancet 1:587, 1977
11. Portier MM, Richet C: De l'action anaphylactique de certains venins. C R Soc Biol 54:170, 1902
12. Watkins J: Anaphylactoid reactions to I.V. substances. Br J Anaesth 51:51, 1979
13. Ishizaka T: Analysis of triggering events in mast cells for immunoglobulin E-mediated histamine release. J Allergy Clin Immunol 67:90, 1981
14. Kazimierczak W, Diamant B: Mechanisms of histamine release in anaphylactic and anaphylactoid reactions. Prog Allergy 4:295, 1978
15. Winslow CM, Austen KF: Enzymatic regulation of mast cell activation and secretion by adenylate cyclase and cyclic AMP-dependent protein kinases. Fed Proc 41:22, 1982
16. Wasserman SI: Mediators of immediate hypersensitivity. J Allergy Clin Immunol 72:101, 1983
17. Reinhardt D, Borchard V: H_1 receptor antagonists: Comparative pharmacology and clinical use. Klin Wochenschr 60:983, 1982
18. Ginsburg R, Bristow MR, Stinson EB et al: Histamine receptors in the human heart. Life Sci 26:2245, 1980
19. Majno G, Palade GE: Studies on inflammation. I. The effect of histamine and serotonin on vascular permeability: An electron microscopic study. J Biophys Biochem Cytol 11:571, 1961
20. Wasserman SI, Goetzl EJ, Austen KF: Preformed eosinophil chemotactic factor of anaphylaxis (ECF-A). J Immunol 112:351, 1974
21. Mathe AA, Hedqvist P, Strandberg K et al: Aspects of prostaglandin function in the lung. N Engl J Med 296:850-, 910-, 1977
22. Parker CW: Leukotrienes: Their metabolism, structure, and role in allergic responses. In Samuelsson B, Paoletti R (eds): Leukotrienes and other lipoxygenase products, pp 115-126. New York, Raven Press, 1982
23. Stenson WF, Parker CW: Metabolites of arachidonic acid. Clin Rev Allergy 1:369, 1983
24. Schulman ES, Newball HH, Demers LM et al: Anaphylactic release of thromboxane A_2, prostaglandin D_2, and prostacyclin from human lung parenchyma. Am Rev Respir Dis 124:402, 1981

25. Morel DR, Zapol WM, Thomas SJ *et al:* C5a and thromboxane generation associated with pulmonary vaso- and bronchoconstriction during protamine reversal of heparin. Anesthesiology 66:597, 1987

26. Meier HL, Kaplan AP, Lichtenstein LM *et al:* Anaphylactic release of a prekallikrein activator from human lung in vitro. J Clin Invest 72:574, 1983

27. Delage C, Irey NS: Anaphylactic deaths: A clinicopathologic study of 43 cases. J Forensic Sci 17: 525, 1972

28. Smith Laboratories: Chymodiactin post marketing surveillance report, 1984

29. Laxenaire MC, Moneret-Vautrin DA, Vervloet D *et al:* Accidents anaphylactoides graves peranesthesiques. Ann Fr Anesth Reanim 4:30, 1985

30. Kelly JF, Patterson R: Anaphylaxis. Course, mechanisms and treatment. JAMA 227:1431, 1974

31. Pavek K, Wegmann A, Nordström L *et al:* Cardiovascular and respiratory mechanisms in anaphylactic and anaphylactoid shock reactions. Klin Wochenschr 60:941, 1982

32. Atkinson JP, Frank MM: Role of complement in the pathophysiology of hematologic disease. Prog Hematol 10:211, 1977

33. Jacob HS, Craddock PR, Hammerschmidt DE *et al:* Complement-induced granulocyte aggregation—An unsuspected mechanism of disease. N Engl J Med 302:789, 1980

34. Dubois M, Lotze MT, Diamond WI *et al:* Pulmonary shunting during leukoagglutinin-induced noncardiogenic pulmonary edema. JAMA 244:2186, 1980

35. Teissner B, Brandslund I, Grunnet N *et al:* Acute complement activation during an anaphylactoid reaction to blood transfusion and the disappearance rate of C3c and C3d from the circulation. J Clin Lab Immunol 12:63, 1983

36. Hammerschmidt DE, Weaver LJ, Hudson LD *et al:* Association of complement activation and elevated plasma-C5a with adult respiratory distress syndrome. Lancet 1:947, 1980

37. Rosow CE, Moss J, Philbin DM *et al:* Histamine release during morphine and fentanyl anesthesia. Anesthesiology 56:93, 1982

38. Moss J, Philbin DM, Rosow CE *et al:* Histamine release by neuromuscular blocking agents in man. Klin Wochenschr 60:891, 1982

39. Hirshman CA, Edelstein RA, Eastman CL: Histamine release by barbiturates in human mast cells. Anesthesiology 63:353, 1985

40. Levy JH, Kettlekamp N, Goertz P *et al:* Histamine release by vancomycin: A mechanism for hypotension in man. Anesthesiology, 67:122, 1987

41. Hermens JM, Ebertz JM, Hanifin JM *et al:* Comparison of histamine release in human skin mast cells by morphine, fentanyl, and oxymorphone. Anesthesiology 62:124, 1983

42. Casale TB, Bowman S, Kaliner M: Induction of human cutaneous mast cell degranulation by opiates and endogenous opioid peptides: Evidence for opiate and nonopiate receptor participation. J Allergy Clin Immunol 73:775, 1984

43. Philbin DM, Moss J, Akins CW *et al:* The use of H_1 and H_2 histamine antagonists with morphine anesthesia: A double-blind study. Anesthesiology 55:292, 1981

44. Levy JH, Hug CC: Cardiopulmonary bypass as a model to study the effects of drugs on myocardial function. Br J Anaesth 60:35S, 1988

45. Hirshman CA, Downes H, Butler J: Relevance of plasma histamine levels to hypotension. Anesthesiology 57:424, 425, 1982

46. Stark BJ, Sullivan TJ: Biphasic and protracted anaphylaxis. J Allergy Clin Immunol 78:76, 1986

47. Levy JH, Rockoff MR: Anaphylaxis to meperidine. Anesth Analg 61:301, 1982

48. Fisher MM: Blood volume replacement in acute anaphylactic cardiovascular collapse related to anaesthesia. Br J Anaesth 49:1023, 1977

49. Barnett A, Hirshman CA: Anaphylactic reaction to cephapirin during spinal anesthesia. Anesth Analg 58:337, 1979

50. Levy JH: Intravenous epinephrine in anaphylaxis. JAMA 249:3173, 1983

51. Austen KF: Tissue mast cells in immediate hypersensitivity. Hosp Pract 17:98, 1981

52. Hammerschmidt DE, White JG, Craddock PR *et al:* Corticosteroids inhibit complement-induced granulocyte aggregation. A possible mechanism for their efficacy in shock states. J Clin Invest 63:798, 1979

53. Halevy S, Altura BM, Altura BM: Pathophysiological basis for the use of steroids in the treatment of shock and trauma. Klin Wochenschr 60:1021, 1982

54. Sheagren JN: Editorial: Septic shock and corticosteroids. N Engl J Med 305:456, 1981

55. Borda IT, Slone D, Jick H: Assessment of adverse reactions within a drug surveillance program. JAMA 205:645, 1968

56. De Swarte RD: Drug allergy—Problems and strategies. J Allergy Clin Immunol 74:209, 1984

57. Tomicheck RC, Rosow CG, Philbin DM *et al:* Diazepam-fentanyl interaction—Hemodynamic and hormonal effect in coronary artery surgery. Anesth Analg 62:881, 1983

58. Fisher M McD, Outhred A, Bowey CJ: Can clinical anaphylaxis to anaesthetic drugs be predicted from allergic history? Br J Anaesth 59:690, 1987

59. Christman D: Immune reaction to propanidid. Anaesthesia 39:470, 1984

60. Watkins J, Clarke SJ: Report of a symposium: Adverse responses to intravenous agents. Br J Anaesth 50:1159, 1978

61. Driggs RL, O'Day RA: Acute allergic reaction associated with methohexital anaesthesia: Report of six cases. J Oral Surg 30:906, 1972

62. Watkins J, Salo M: Incidence of immediate adverse response to intravenous anaesthetic drugs. In Trauma, Stress and Immunity in Anaesthesia and Surgery, p 272. London, Butterworth & Co, 1982

63. Schwartz HJ, Sher TH: Bisulfite sensitivity manifesting as allergy to local dental anaesthesia. J Allergy Clin Immunol 75:525, 1985

64. Brown DT, Beamins D, Wildsmith JAW: Allergic reaction to an amide local anesthetic. Br J Anaesth 53:435, 1981

65. Fisher M McD, Munro I: Life-threatening anaphylactoid reactions to muscle relaxants. Anesth Analg 62:559, 1983

66. Laxenaire MC, Moneret-Vautrin DA, Watkins J: Diagnosis of the causes of anaphylactoid anaesthetic reactions. Anaesthesia 38:147, 1983

67. Vervloet D, Nizankowska E, Arnaud A *et al:* Adverse reactions to suxamethonium and other muscle relaxants under general anesthesia. J Allergy Clin Immunol 71:552, 1983

68. Assesm ESK, Frost PG, Levis RD: Anaphylactoid-like reaction to suxamethonium. Anaesthesia 36:405, 1981

69. Bennet MJ, Anderson LK, McMillan JC *et al:* Anaphylactic reaction during anesthesia associated with positive indraderaml skin test to fentanyl. Can Anaesth Soc J 33:75, 1986

70. Hilgard P: Immunological reactions to blood and blood products. Br J Anesth 51:45, 1979

71. Sheffer AL, Pennoyer DS: Management of adverse drug reactions. J Allergy Clin Immunol 74:580, 1984

72. Levy JH, Zaidan JR, Faraj B: Prospective evaluation of risk of protamine reactions in NPH insulin-dependent diabetics. Anesth Analg 65:739, 1986

73. Doolan L, McKenzie I, Krafchek J *et al:* Protamine sulphate hypersensitivity. Anesth Intensive Care 9:147, 1981

74. Goldberg M: Systemic reactions to intravascular contrast media. A guide for the anesthesiologist. Anesthesiology 60:46, 1984

75. Isbister JP, Fisher M McD: Adverse effects of plasma volume expanders. Anesth Intensive Care 8:145, 1980

76. Colman WR: Paradoxical hypotension after volume expansion with plasma protein fraction. N Engl J Med 299:97, 1978

77. Ring K, Messmer K: Incidence and severity of anaphylactoid to colloid volume substitutes. Lancet 1:466, 1977

78. Grant JA, Cooper JR, Arens JF et al: Anaphylactic reactions to protamine in insulin-dependent diabetics during cardiovascular surgery. Anesthesiology 59:A74, 1983

79. Berg TLO, Johansson SGO: Allergy diagnosis with the radio-allergosorbent test. A comparison with the results of skin and provocation tests in an unselected group of children with asthma and hay fever. J Allergy Clin Immunol 54:209, 1974

80. Johansson SGO: *In vitro* diagnosis of reagin-mediated allergic diseases. Allergy 33:292, 1978

81. Baldo BA, Fisher MM: Detection of serum IgE antibodies that react with alcuronium and tubocurarine after life-threatening reactions to muscle relaxants. Anaesth Intensive Care 11:194, 1983

82. Harle DG, Baldo BA, Smal MA *et al:* Detection of thiopentone-reactive IgE antibodies following anaphylactoid reactions during anesthesia. Clin Allergy 16:493, 1986

83. Dueck R, O'Connor RD: Thiopental: False positive RAST in patient with elevated serum IgE. Anesthesiology 61:337, 1984

84. Fisher MM: Intradermal testing after anaphylactoid reaction to anaesthetic drugs: Practical aspects of performance and interpretation. Anaesth Intensive Care 12:115, 1984

85. Fisher MM, Munro I: Life threatening, anaphylactoid reactions to muscle relaxants. Anesth Analg 62:559, 1983

86. Sage D: Intradermal drug testing following anaphylactoid reactions during anesthesia. Anaesth Intensive Care 9:381, 1981

87. Shatz M: Skin testing and incremental challenge in the evaluation of adverse reactions to local anesthetics. J Allergy Clin Immunol 74:606, 1984

Part V

Postanesthesia and Consultant Practice

Chapter 52

Roger S. Mecca

Postanesthesia Recovery

GENERAL CONSIDERATIONS

Individualized, problem-oriented monitoring and assessment are essential to assure appropriate postoperative support with minimum risk, inconvenience, and expense to patients recovering from anesthesia and surgery. Information concerning facility design, staffing, and equipment required for a state-of-the-art Post Anesthesia Care Unit (PACU) is widely available.[1-4]

ADMISSION CRITERIA

To decide whether a patient requires specialized postoperative care, one must consider severity of underlying illness, physiologic impact of the surgical procedure and anesthetic, and likelihood of anticipated postoperative complications. Patients undergoing superficial procedures under local infiltration or peripheral regional anesthetics (*i.e.*, ankle, finger, or field blocks) and mild sedation can often safely recover in less intensive settings. Risk of bypassing PACU increases with greater intensity or complexity of surgery and anesthesia. A patient should be admitted to a PACU whenever doubt exists concerning ability to safely recover in an unmonitored floor or ambulatory setting. Level of postoperative care should be determined by intensity, duration, and complexity of surgery and anesthesia and by potential for complication, regardless of whether surgery is performed on an ambulatory or an inpatient basis.

Once a patient is admitted to a PACU, a minimum level of monitoring coverage and evaluation should be instituted. All patients should have ventilatory rate and character, heart rate, and systemic blood pressure recorded initially and at intervals that depend on condition. (I prefer assessment every 5 minutes for the first 15 minutes, and every 15 minutes thereafter as a minimum.) Qualitative assessment of level of consciousness, airway patency, and skin color often yield valuable clinical information. Axillary or oral temperature should be recorded at least on admission and discharge, and more frequently if appropriate. Rectal or esophageal routes should be used if assessment of core temperature is important. All patients requiring PACU admission should be monitored with a single lead, continuous electrocardiogram (ECG) to assess rate, rhythm, and dysrhythmia. Invasive intraoperative monitors should also be monitored during recovery, so equipment and personnel necessary for transduced measurement of central venous, systemic arterial and pulmonary arterial, and intracranial pressure should be readily available. All patients should receive supplemental oxygen unless waived by an anesthesiologist. Patients at risk of compromised pulmonary function should be monitored with pulse oximetry, capnography, or repeated arterial blood gas (ABG) determinations as appropriate.[5]

Assessment of postoperative requirements and possible complications should begin before transferring the patient from the operating room. Anesthesiology personnel should maintain control of the patient until PACU staff have secured appropriate admission vital signs (at least systolic and diastolic blood pressure, heart rate, and ventilatory rate). A succinct and relevant report should be recorded on every PACU record (Table 52-1), including pertinent history and physical examination, operation and surgeon, anesthetic technique, fluid administration, blood loss, neuromuscular status, and other appropriate information about anesthetic course.[6] Plans to achieve specific therapeutic endpoints during recovery should be clearly outlined. Responsibility should not be turned over to PACU personnel until hemodynamic, ventilatory, and airway status are secure. Function of supportive equipment, intravenous catheters, and invasive monitoring devices must be checked prior to leaving the patient. Means of contacting the responsible anesthesiologist should be clearly communicated.

TABLE 52-1. Components of a PACU Admission Report

Preoperative History
Medication allergies or reactions
Pertinent earlier surgical procedures
Underlying medical illness
Chronic medications
Acute problems (ischemia, acid-base, dehydration)
Premedications
NPO status

Intraoperative Factors
Surgical procedure
Surgeon
Type of anesthetic
Relaxant/reversal status
Time/amount opioid administration
Type/amount intravenous fluids
Estimated blood loss
Urine output
Unexpected surgical or anesthetic events
Intraoperative vital sign ranges
Intraoperative laboratory findings
Drugs given (*e.g.*, steroids, diuretics, antibiotics, vasoactive medications)

Assessment and Report of Current Status
Heart rate and heart rhythm
Systemic pressure
Airway patency
Ventilatory adequacy
Level of consciousness
Intravascular volume status
Endotracheal tube position
Function of invasive monitors
Size and location of intravenous catheters
Anesthetic equipment (*e.g.*, epidural catheters)
Overall impression

Postoperative Instructions
Acceptable vital sign ranges
Anticipated cardiovascular problems
Expected airway and ventilatory status
Location of responsible physician
Diagnostic tests to be secured
Acceptable urine output and blood loss
Orders for therapeutic interventions
Surgical instructions (positioning, wound care)
Therapeutic goals and endpoints prior to discharge

POSTOPERATIVE PAIN MANAGEMENT

Achieving maximum attenuation of postoperative pain with minimum side-effects is a primary clinical goal in postoperative care. Before instituting therapy, a careful analysis of postoperative pain should be performed. Nature and degree of pain vary with anesthetic technique, as well as with operative procedure.[7] Assuring that pain seems appropriate for the operation performed avoids masking valuable diagnostic symptoms of an unrelated condition or surgical complication. Central nervous system effects of severe hypoxemia, hypotension, or respiratory acidemia can closely mimic clinical presentation of postoperative pain, especially in patients emerging from general anesthesia. Administration of parenteral analgesics can acutely worsen underlying hypotension, hypoventilation or airway obstruction, causing sudden deterioration and arrest. Usually, evaluating the level of consciousness and orientation as well as cardiovascular and pulmonary status identifies such patients.

A wide divergence exists between cognitive appreciation of postoperative pain and sympathetic nervous system (SNS) response among patients, probably related to psychological, cultural, and cardiovascular variations. Some patients manifest severe hypertension, tachycardia, and cardiac dysrhythmias with minimal complaint of discomfort, while others perceive severe pain without evidence of autonomic nervous system activation. Attenuation of pain often reduces SNS response dramatically, helping to control postoperative hypertension and tachycardia. However, hypoventilation or hypotension may occur in patients relying on SNS activity for arousal or cardiovascular hemostasis. Side-effects of analgesics such as histamine release, peripheral sympathectomy, or sedation can accentuate these conditions. Hypovolemic patients are at especially high risk for cardiovascular complications after elimination of painful stimuli. Careful assessment of a normotensive or hypotensive patient complaining of severe postoperative pain is essential, especially if tachycardia is also present.

One should always eliminate or minimize causes of pain through relatively innocuous interventions such as repositioning, reassurance, extubation of the trachea, or Foley catheter removal. If pain is clearly incisional in nature, intermittent or continuous intravenous administration of long-acting opioids such as morphine or meperidine can be quite effective. Intravenous administration allows titration to a desired level of analgesia with assessment of incremental respiratory or cardiovascular depression. Peak effect occurs rapidly (3–4 min). Sufficient control of pain should be achieved, even if large doses of opioids are necessary in patients addicted to opioids or alcohol. Disadvantages of intramuscular administration include requirement for larger doses, unpredictable uptake in hypothermic patients, delayed onset, and unnecessary tissue trauma. Oral analgesics have little role in immediate postoperative recovery, but can be useful for ambulatory patients in a predischarge recovery setting. Rectal administration of analgesics is useful in selected pediatric patients.

Fear, anxiety, confusion, or disorientation often accompany postoperative pain, especially during emergence from general anesthesia. Incremental administration of a mild intravenous sedative such as diazepam or midazolam attenuates this psychogenic component of postoperative discomfort. It is important to differentiate between requirement for analgesia and for sedation. Although highly touted, sedative properties of opioids are relatively weak compared to those of more specific sedative medications. Similarly, analgesic effects of most sedatives are very poor.

In selected patients, other modalities can effectively reduce postoperative pain, improve postoperative ventilatory function, and control SNS activity. Placement of unilateral percutaneous intercostal blocks can markedly reduce analgesic requirements after thoracic or high abdominal incision or injury (thoracotomy, cholecystectomy, chest tube placement, gastrostomy, multiple rib fractures).[8,9] An analgesic interscalene block can render almost complete relief after painful shoulder and upper extremity procedures, with only mild motor paralysis. In patients suffering from morbid obesity or severe chronic obstructive pulmonary disease (COPD), injection of local anesthetic through an indwelling epidural catheter can assist in weaning from mechanical ventilation after major abdominal surgery.[10,11] Intraoperative local anesthetic infiltration in joints or soft tissues can also somewhat attenuate intensity of postoperative pain.

Intermittent or continuous injection of opioids into the epidural space is a relatively new and promising analgesic intervention.[12–16] Interaction of opioids with spinal cord opioid receptors can generate prolonged analgesia to peripheral pain with minimal adverse side-effects. However, both immediate and delayed ventilatory depression can occur, probably related to vascular uptake and caudad spread in cerebral spinal fluid respectively. Use of epidural opioids may mandate extended ventilatory monitoring. Postinjection nausea and pruritus can also be bothersome side-effects. Other modalities for pain relief, such as transcutaneous nerve stimulation, "white noise," and hypnosis have relatively limited immediate postoperative utility.

DISCHARGE CRITERIA

Prior to discharge, a patient should be sufficiently oriented to assess his physical condition and summon assistance if nec-

TABLE 52-2. Guidelines for Discharge Evaluation from a PACU*

General Condition
Oriented to time, place, and surgical procedure
Responds to verbal input and follows simple instructions
"Acceptable" color without cyanosis, splotchiness, paleness
Adequate muscular strength and mobility for minimal self-care
Absence or control of specific acute surgical complications (*e.g.*, bleeding, edema, neurologic weakness, diminished pulses)
Suitable control of nausea and emesis
Destination unit appropriate for patient's status

Systemic Blood Pressure Heart Rate and Rhythm
Within ±20% resting preoperative value
Relatively constant for at least 30 min
Resolution of any new dysrhythmia
Acceptable intravascular volume status
Any suspicion of myocardial ischemia rectified

Ventilation and Oxygenation
Ventilatory rate greater than 10, less than 30
Forced vital capacity approximately twice tidal volume
Adequate ability to cough and clear secretions
Qualitatively acceptable work of breathing

Airway Maintenance
Protective reflexes (swallow, gag) intact
Absence of stridor, retraction, or partial obstruction
No further need for artificial airway support

Control of Pain
Ability to localize and identify intensity of surgical pain
Adequate analgesia, at least 15 min since last narcotic
Safe, appropriate orders for postdischarge analgesics

Renal Function
Urine output greater than 30 ml · hr^{-1} (catheterized patients)
Appropriate color and appearance of urine, evaluation of hematuria
Followup orders re output if spontaneous voiding has not occurred

Metabolic/Laboratory
Acceptable hematocrit level in view of hydration, blood loss, and potential for future losses
Suitable control of blood glucose
Appropriate electrolyte homeostasis
Evaluation of CXR, ECG, and other tests as appropriate

Ambulatory Patients
Ability to ambulate without dizziness, hypotension, or support
Suitable control of nausea and vomiting after ambulation

---

* All criterion will not be satisfied by every patient, especially if discharge is to a critical care unit. Clinical judgement must always supercede established guidelines if condition is less than optimal in a given area. Whenever doubt exists about diagnosis or patient safety, discharge should be delayed.

essary. Airway reflexes, awareness, and motor function sufficient to recognize and expel vomitus or secretions from the airway should be evident. Ventilation, oxygenation, and ability to cough should be appropriate, with sufficient functional reserve to cover minor deterioration in unmonitored settings. Intravascular volume, systemic blood pressure, and peripheral perfusion need to be adequate and relatively constant for at least one-half hour. Cessation of shivering and an acceptable body temperature are necessary prior to discharge, although requirement for normal temperature is not absolute. Possibility of bleeding, loss of pulses, pneumothorax, or other adverse surgical sequelae should be ruled out. Danger of acute postoperative complications related to underlying conditions like coronary artery disease, diabetes, hypertension, or asthma should be minimal, and results of postoperative diagnostic tests should be reviewed.

It is important to assess nature and degree of postoperative discomfort and to achieve an acceptable level of analgesia before transfer. Patients should be observed for a minimum of 20 to 30 minutes after the last dose of intravenous sedative or opioid, to assess impact of peak effects. Longer periods of observation may be prudent after reinforcement of regional anesthetic techniques. Also, patients should be observed for 15 to 20 minutes after discontinuation of supplemental oxygen to detect unexpected hypoxemia.

If these generic criterion cannot be met, postponement of discharge or transfer to a specialized area where appropriate care and monitoring are available is essential. In my opinion, using fixed discharge criterion in a PACU setting requires great caution, as variability among patients is tremendous. Ideally, an anesthesiologist should evaluate each patient individually for discharge, with a consistent set of general criterion in mind (Table 52-2). Type and severity of underlying disease, surgical procedure, anesthetic and recovery course, and postoperative destination should be carefully considered. Assessment of ambulatory patients must be meticulous, given a low level of care and observation available outside the medical facility (see Chapter 49). Scoring systems that attempt to quantify physical status may be useful to assure thorough assessment, but should not replace individual bedside evaluation.[17, 18] Thresholds for vital signs or blood test results must never replace assessment of specific values with respect to a given patient's condition.

CARDIOVASCULAR COMPLICATIONS

POSTOPERATIVE HYPOTENSION

Systemic hypotension is a common postoperative complication[19] that causes hypoperfusion and inadequate delivery of oxygen and substrates to systemic organs. Consequent tissue hypoxia promotes inefficient anaerobic metabolism and accumulation of lactic acid. (Unexplained metabolic acidemia is a reliable indicator of inadequate postoperative systemic perfusion.) Autoregulation in vital organs maintains adequate blood flow with reduced systemic perfusion pressures. Minimum tolerable pressures are higher in patients with arteriosclerotic disease, fixed stenotic vascular lesions, chronic hypertension, increased intracranial pressure, renal failure, or other diseases that interfere with effectiveness of autoregulation. During hypotension, the autonomic nervous system preferentially maintains blood flow to critical organs such as brain, heart, and kidneys. Symptoms of hypotension referable to these organs (disorientation, nausea, loss of consciousness, angina pectoris, reduced urine output) indicate critical failure of compensatory mechanisms.

Complications of hypotension include cerebral ischemia or stroke, myocardial ischemia or infarction, acute renal failure, bowel infarction, and spinal cord ischemia or paralysis. Reduced venous flow velocities can increase risk of deep vein thrombosis and pulmonary embolism. Decreased hepatic oxygen delivery may change metabolic pathways for drugs, causing accumulation of toxic metabolites and hepatic damage. Systemic blood pressure at which risk of complications increases depends in part on preoperative blood pressure.[20] A 20% to 30% reduction of systemic arterial systolic pressure from chronic preoperative levels, or symptoms of vital organ hypoperfusion are indications for intervention.

Spurious Hypotension

Blood pressure cuffs that are too large yield falsely low values (cuff width should equal approximately two-thirds of arm circumference). An arterial catheter transducer system that is improperly zeroed, poorly calibrated, or excessively damped by air bubbles or catheter obstruction also yields artifactually low readings. Hypothermic patients or those receiving alpha-adrenergic-receptor agonist medications can exhibit arterial constriction and low radial or brachial blood pressure readings, although central aortic pressure may be higher. Ruling out spurious hypotension in postoperative patients avoids unnecessary treatment and risk of serious iatrogenic hypertension.

Hypovolemia

A decrease of circulating intravascular volume ("absolute" hypovolemia) reduces ventricular filling and cardiac output. Compensatory mechanisms mediated by the SNS (tachycardia, increased systemic vascular resistance [SVR], venoconstriction) can usually maintain blood pressure despite a 15% to 20% loss of circulating volume. Greater volume deficits cause hypotension.

Failure to adequately replace preoperative maintenance fluids, evaporative losses during surgery, and blood loss frequently cause postoperative hypovolemia.[21, 22] If intraoperative hypothermia reduces venous capacitance, relatively low intravascular volume may be sufficient to sustain cardiac output on PACU admission. Rewarming can increase venous capacity and cause profound hypovolemia and hypotension.[23] Ongoing internal or external hemorrhage, sweating, insensible losses and "third space losses" (exudation of fluid into tissues) exacerbate postoperative hypovolemia. One must suspect occult internal hemorrage (loss into muscle after trauma or orthopedic procedures, retroperitoneal bleeding) and diffuse oozing related to coagulopathy (disseminated intravascular coagulation [DIC], dilutional coagulopathy, severe thrombocytopenia, residual anticoagulation).[24] Third space losses can persist for 24 to 48 hours after surgery and can be massive during reaccumulation of ascites, high permeability pulmonary edema, or anaphylactic episodes.

Often, even a "normal" intravascular volume is inadequate to maintain postoperative blood pressure (relative hypovolemia). Interference with SNS regulation of venous tone caused by sympathectomy from spinal or epidural anesthesia increases venous capacitance and reduces venous return. Ability to constrict veins in response to changes in position, mild volume deficits, discontinuation of pressors, and warming is also attenuated. Other factors reduce postoperative venous tone. Medications mimic alpha-adrenergic-receptor blockade (droperidol, chlorpromazine), release histamine (d-tubocurarine, morphine), or directly dilate veins (nitrates). Rapid administration of blood, fresh-frozen plasma, low molecular weight dextrans, or platelets may cause venodilation, probably secondary to histamine release. Sudden decreases in endogenous SNS activity caused by removal of stimulus (extubation of the trachea, relief of pain) or vasovagal responses can also increase venous capacity.

Hypotension associated with mechanical ventilation of the lungs or tension pneumothorax is partly caused by compression of thoracic veins by positive airway pressure that impedes venous return. Inferior vena caval compression is common in pregnant patients, and in patients with increased intraabdominal pressure from large intraabdominal tumors or tense ascites. Reverse Trendelenburg, sitting, or upright positions can precipitate serious hypovolemia caused by orthostatic changes, especially in patients with impaired SNS venous regulation. Constrictive pericarditis and acute pericardial tamponade also impede ventricular filling and cause postoperative hypotension.

Ventricular Dysfunction

Postoperative hypotension caused by ventricular dysfunction usually occurs in patients with impaired baseline ventricular contractility which necessitates high ventricular filling pressures and elevated SNS activity to maintain cardiac output.[25] Demand for increased performance can precipitate ventricular dilation, elevate left ventricular end-diastolic pressure (LVEDP), and decrease output and blood pressure.

In patients with poor ventricular dynamics, excessive fluid administration is a common cause of postoperative ventricular failure and hypotension, often complicated by pulmonary edema and hypoxemia. Overhydration may not be evident in patients recovering from spinal or epidural anesthetics. If sympathetic blockade is treated only with fluid administration, ventricular filling pressures can be normal despite "relative" hypervolemia. When the SNS blockade resolves, characteristically high levels of SNS outflow cause large volumes of fluid to be mobilized to the central circulation, precipitating left ventricular failure in vulnerable patients. Right ventricular dysfunction caused by pulmonary thromboembolism or air embolism also presents with systemic hypotension. Sudden reduction of myocardial contractility as seen during myocardial ischemia can cause sudden, profound hypotension. Recovering patients may still exhibit significant alveolar partial pressures of inhalation anesthetics that reduce ventricular contractility and decrease SNS outflow. Resulting myocardial depression may limit ability to increase output in response to hypotension from other causes. Administration of beta-receptor-blocking drugs may further attenuate catecholamine enhancement of myocardial contractility, but usually causes hypotension only in patients with severe myocardial disease who rely on maximal SNS activity for cardiovascular stability. Toxic local anesthetic blood levels from intravascular injection or uptake in highly vascular tissues might cause severe myocardial depression and hypotension during postoperative regional analgesic techniques. Low ionized calcium levels caused by dilution, chelation by citrate preservatives in banked blood, or acute respiratory or metabolic alkalemia can decrease ventricular contractility, although clinical impact is usually minor. Although metabolic or respiratory acidemia initially elicits profound SNS activity and augmented contractility, very low pH levels interfere with catecholamine-receptor interaction and depress cerebral SNS outflow, dramatically decreasing ventricular performance.[22]

Myocardial Ischemia

Postoperative myocardial ischemia or infarction is often caused by unrecognized hypotension from another cause. Inadequate aortic diastolic blood pressure can be unrecognized, especially if systemic pressure decreases to a low normal range. Elevation of LVEDP and LV wall tension from overhydration or increased SNS activity can also initiate ischemia, even with an adequate aortic diastolic pressure. Increased myocardial oxygen consumption caused by shivering or severe hypertension can precipitate ischemia, as can a decrease in diastolic filling time during tachycardia caused by pain, hypovolemia, acidemia, anxiety, or medication. Severe hypoxemia caused by pulmonary dysfunction or hypoventilation precipitates ischemia in spite of adequate coronary perfusion.[25, 26]

Ventricular dysfunction and hypotension indicate severe progression of an ischemic episode toward a point of irreversible infarction. Unfortunately, hypotension is sometimes the first clinical sign of ischemia noted. Close evaluation of hemodynamic responses to stimuli, ST segments and T-wave morphology on ECG, or pulmonary artery pressures often reveals ischemia before hypotension occurs (Fig. 52-1). Aggressive monitoring of patients at risk, control of precipitating factors, early detection, and timely therapy are important to decrease morbidity from intraoperative and postoperative myocardial ischemia.[27]

Cardiac Dysrhythmia

Underlying myocardial disease or previous rhythm disturbances increases risk of postoperative hypotension caused by a cardiac dysrhythmia. (Also see Postoperative Cardiac Dys-

FIG. 52-1. Physiologic consequences of myocardial ischemia. Note that changes in ventricular pressure and compliance may precede electrocardiographic changes (ST segment). LVEDP = left ventricular end diastolic pressure, LVEDV = left ventricular end diastolic volume, EF = ejection fraction, STΔ = ST segment change, CHF = congestive heart failure. (Barash PG: Monitoring myocardial oxygen balance: Physiologic basis and clinical application. In Barash PG, Deutsch S, Tinker J [eds]: Refresher Courses in Anesthesiology, vol 13, p 21. Philadelphia, JB Lippincott, 1985.)

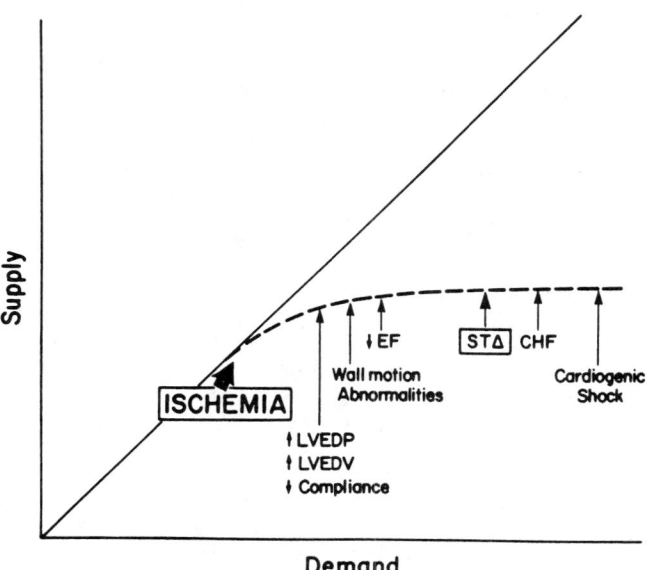

rhythmias.) Sinus or nodal bradycardia can decrease cardiac output and blood pressure, as can slow ventricular rhythms associated with sinus node disease or complete heart block. Tachyarrhythmias (e.g., paroxysmal atrial tachycardia, atrial fibrillation or flutter, fast ventricular tachycardia) that generate ventricular rates greater than 140 to 150 beats $\cdot$ min^{-1} may not allow adequate diastolic intervals for ventricular filling. Interference with ventricular filling can markedly decrease stroke volume, cardiac output, and systemic blood pressure. Ventricular fibrillation, asystole, or electromechanical dissociation cause obvious, life-threatening reductions in output.

Cardiac rhythm disturbances caused by wide swings in postoperative autonomic nervous system activity place patients with valvular abnormalities at particular risk of hypotension.[28] Increased heart rate in patients with aortic stenosis reduces systolic ejection time, promoting increased LVEDP, ventricular dilation, and hypotension. Tachycardia in patients with mitral stenosis impedes ventricular filling, causing marked increase of left atrial pressure and profound decrease of cardiac output and systemic pressure. Augmented contractility and increased heart rate with hypertrophic subaortic stenosis causes similar problems. Increased systemic vascular resistance can also compromise cardiac output and systemic blood pressure by increasing regurgitant fraction in patients with mitral regurgitation.

Decreased Systemic Vascular Resistance

Postoperative hypotension associated with regional anesthesia, alpha-receptor blocking drugs, vasoactive blood components, and warming is caused by decreased SVR as well as reduced venous return. Systemic sepsis may interfere with arteriolar constriction, generating a high output, low resistance hypotension. (In endstage sepsis, myocardial depression is usually superimposed upon very low SVR). Severe systemic acidemia decreases SVR through a direct vasodilatory effect and by interfering with action of catecholamines at alpha-receptors. Antihypertensive medications such as hydralazine and nitroprusside interfere with arteriolar constriction, and can cause profound postoperative hypotension in hypovolemic patients.

Postoperative hypotension can also be caused or accentuated by surgical or anesthetic interference with baroreceptor function,[29, 30] or by intracranial pathology.[31] Rarely, postoperative hypotension can occur as a late manifestation of acute steroid deficiency if the pituitary axis is suppressed by prolonged administration of exogenous steroids. Hypotension, second to steroid deficiency, is often preceded by lethargy, fever, somnolence or nausea, and accompanied by hyponatremia, hyperkalemia, and hypoglycemia. Response to administration of supplemental steroids is often dramatic.

Treatment of Postoperative Hypotension

Upon admission to PACU, intravascular volume status must be assessed in terms of preoperative fluid status, type, and duration of surgery, estimated blood loss, intraoperative fluid replacement, and level of hemostasis. In patients at risk for hypotension, acceptable limits for pressure and heart rate should also be assessed.

If hypotension occurs, supplemental oxygen should be administered. Blood pressure determination should then be validated. Carotid or femoral pulses and auscultation of heart sounds are useful qualitative indicators of central blood pressure. Intravenous infusion rate should be increased to maximum, as hypovolemia is by far the most common etiology. (If hypotension is spurious or caused by reduced SVR or ischemia, amount of fluid infused while these diagnoses are considered will usually be inconsequential.) Trendelenburg position may also be helpful. Cardiac rate and rhythm, and breath sounds should be checked. Infusions that might cause vasodilation should be stopped and recent drug administration noted. A 12-lead ECG, an ABG sample, and a chest x-ray may be indicated. If pulses or ventilation are absent, cardiopulmonary resuscitation with endotracheal intubation should immediately be instituted.

Assessment of postoperative intravascular volume is critical. Monitoring urine output as an index of intravascular volume can be misleading, as surgery and anesthesia interfere with renal function, and osmotic diuresis caused by glycosuria can generate profuse urine output and false security that intravascular volume is adequate. If intravascular volume status is uncertain, invasive evaluation with central venous or pulmonary arterial catheterization is indicated.

Therapy for postoperative hypotension should be directed toward a specific abnormality reducing systemic blood pressure, with repeated reassessment of diagnosis. Simple maneuvers such as reducing airway pressure, lateral tilt in pregnant patients, or supine positioning of patients with orthostatic changes should be used when appropriate. Infusion of crystalloid solutions is usually sufficient to treat hypovolemia, although plasma expanders or blood can facilitate more rapid volume expansion. Sympathomimetic (vasopressor) drugs that increase SVR and venous return can be judiciously used to maintain pressure until sufficient volume can be infused. Increased venous capacity or obstruction to venous return can be treated with an alpha-adrenergic drug such as phenylephrine in conjunction with fluid therapy. Ephedrine is effective but less desirable as increasing heart rate and contractility is usually unnecessary. Tension pneumothorax must be immediately evacuated.

If fluid administration (300–500 ml) does not improve pressure, myocardial dysfunction should be considered. For dysfunction not related to ischemia, drugs that augment contractility (dopamine, ephedrine, calcium chloride, digoxin) in conjunction with systemic vasodilators[32] often restore cardiac output and systemic pressure. If hypotension is caused by ischemia, resolution of ischemia usually restores baseline myocardial function. Support of aortic diastolic pressure with an alpha-receptor agonist such as phenylephrine and reduction of LVEDP with nitroglycerine can be useful to maximize coronary artery pressure gradient.[33] Control of heart rate with analgesics for pain, sedatives for anxiety, or beta-receptor blockers is essential. An accurate diagnosis of ischemia is critical, because therapy for ischemia can worsen hypotension caused by hypovolemia, decreased SVR, or nonischemic ventricular dysfunction. Hypotension caused by ventricular dysfunction is an indication for pulmonary artery catheterization to measure cardiac output (facilitating calculation of SVR), and pulmonary capillary wedge pressure (indicative of LVEDP).

If hypotension occurs coincident with severe metabolic acidemia, bicarbonate should be given intravenously while the cause is identified and remedied. Severe hypoxemia or respiratory acidemia mandates tracheal intubation and mechanical ventilation of the lungs with supplemental oxygen. Sinus bradycardia unrelated to hypoxemia usually responds to intravenous administration of atropine, glycopyrrolate, or ephedrine. Refractory bradycardia caused by sinus node disease or complete heart block must be managed with intravenous administration of epinephrine or isoproterenol, or

with artificial cardiac pacing. Digitalization or calcium channel blockade reduces ventricular rate from acute onset atrial fibrillation, whereas paroxysmal atrial tachycardia often disappears with maneuvers or drugs that change cardiac conduction rates. If hypotension from a tachydysrhythmia is severe, immediate low energy direct current (DC) cardioversion (50 joules) is indicated.

Hypotension caused by low SVR in spite of high cardiac output is treated with an alpha-adrenergic agent. SNS from regional anesthesia usually responds to low levels of alpha stimulation. However, during advanced sepsis or catecholamine depletion norepinephrine infusions may be required to restore SVR. If decreased SVR is caused by acidemia, correction of pH is necessary before pressor therapy is effective.

POSTOPERATIVE HYPERTENSION

Elevation of systemic blood pressure is common in the immediate postoperative period.[34] However, marked hypertension carries significant risk of morbidity, and should be aggressively evaluated and treated. Hypertension can increase postoperative hemorrhage and third space losses from either arterial or venous sources. Disruption of major vascular suture lines is possible. High ventricular intracavitary pressures can cause myocardial fiber stretch with appearance of ventricular dilation or cardiac dysrhythmias. Increases in myocardial oxygen consumption and wall tension may precipitate myocardial ischemia. Intracerebral hemorrhage, exacerbation of intracranial pressure increases or cerebral edema, and elevated intraocular pressure are also possible.

The level of systemic pressure at which risk of complication increases varies among patients. A systolic or diastolic pressure greater than 20% to 30% above resting blood pressure, signs or symptoms of complications (headache, bleeding, ocular changes, angina, ST-segment depression) or unusual risk of morbidity (increased intracranial pressure, open eye injury, mitral regurgitation) are indications for treatment.

An inappropriately small blood pressure cuff yields erroneously high readings, especially in obese patients. An improperly zeroed or calibrated transducer, or a pressure transducing system with an excessive amount of resonance and electronic "overshoot" can grossly overestimate systolic pressure (overshoot does not significantly affect accuracy of diastolic readings assuming proper calibration and zeroing).

Patients with preexisting hypertension often manifest exaggerated postoperative blood pressure responses. Noncompliant arteriosclerotic vasculature, elevated peripheral vascular tone mediated by the renin-angiotensin system, or high levels of baseline endogenous SNS activity can all be contributory, as can preeclampsia. Maintenance of systemic pressures near reasonable preoperative baseline levels is appropriate, as "normal" systemic pressures may promote hypoperfusion of vital organs.

Enhanced SNS activity is a frequent cause of postoperative hypertension. Peripheral arteriolar and venous constriction mediated by alpha-receptor stimulation increases SVR and venous return respectively, whereas increased beta-1-receptor stimulation increases ventricular contractility and heart rate. Increased SNS activity most often reflects an appropriate CNS response to noxious stimuli or adverse physiologic conditions (Table 52-3). SNS activity may be inappropriate with respect to usual cardiovascular homeostatic mechanisms (e.g., administration of exogenous sympathomimetics, pheochromocytoma, enzyme inhibition, drug in-

TABLE 52-3.   Factors that Increase Postoperative Cardiac Sympathetic Influence

INCREASED SYMPATHETIC ACTIVITY	DECREASED PARASYMPATHETIC ACTIVITY

Noxious stimuli
    Pain, anxiety, carinal stimulation, full
    bladder, endotracheal intubation
Adverse physiologic conditions
    Hypercarbia/acidosis, hypoxemia,
    hypotension, hypoglycemia, congestive
    heart failure, increased intracranial
    pressure, myocardial ischemia
Medications
    Beta-mimetic pressors (ephedrine,
    isoproterenol, epinephrine, dopamine,
    dobutamine)
    Bronchodilators (terbutaline,
    aminophylline)
    Anesthetics (ketamine, isoflurane)
    Antihypertensives (hydralazine,
    nitroprusside)
	Medications
	    Parasympatholytics (atropine, glycopyrrolate)
	    Relaxants (pancuronium, gallamine)

teractions). Inappropriate expansion of intravascular volume can increase ventricular filling pressures, stroke volumes, and cardiac output in spite of compensatory decreases in SVR and heart rate, especially if hypothermia causes coincident arteriolar and venous constriction.[35] Hypervolemia and hypothermia are usually more contributory than causative in evolution of postoperative hypertension. Abnormal baroreceptor function after carotid endarterectomy also generates significant postoperative hypertension.[36] Cerebral vascular accidents, hypoxic encephalopathy, increased intracranial pressure, or severe osmotic changes can interfere with central SNS regulation, causing autonomic dysfunction and severe hypertension.[31]

Treatment of postoperative hypertension should first be directed at causes of increased SNS activity by using analgesics for pain or sedatives for anxiety, correcting acidemia or hypoxemia, and assuring ability to void. If hypertension persists once factors promoting SNS activity have been eliminated, administration of antihypertensive medications may be necessary. Parenteral administration avoids uptake problems characteristic of oral or intramuscular routes. A combination of intravenous hydralazine and propranolol for rate control is useful for short-term pressure control, as is intravenous labetolol. Intravenous administration of alphamethyldopa yields longer lasting control that can easily be switched to an oral regimen. Potent intravenous vasodilators (nitroprusside, nitroglycerine, trimethaphan) should probably be reserved to treat refractory or profound hypertension. Of these, nitroprusside seems most effective for systemic pressure control.

CARDIAC DYSRHYTHMIAS IN THE POSTOPERATIVE PERIOD

Asymptomatic ECG Abnormalities

After general anesthesia, a significant number of patients exhibit ECG changes indicative of abnormal myocardial physiology, without clinical signs of symptoms of actual cardiac pathology (see Chapter 22)[36] Changes in P and T wave morphology, repolarization, ST segments, axis, and intra-

ventricular conduction occur,[37] but almost always resolve spontaneously over 3 to 6 hours. ECG changes are most likely caused by myocardial effects of potent anesthetics, autonomic nervous system imbalance, mild electrolyte abnormalities, and hypothermia. Whenever ECG changes indicative of ischemia appear, it is important to optimize factors governing myocardial oxygen supply and demand, and to follow up with repeated ECGs, enzyme determinations, and prolonged monitoring if appropriate.

Bradycardia

Many factors promote sinus bradycardia in the postoperative period.[38] An increase in parasympathetic nervous system (PNS) activity can reduce spontaneous depolarization rates in supraventricular pacemakers, as can a decrease in SNS influence (Table 52-4). "Sick sinus syndrome," or severe hypoxemia can also reduce sinus rate. In most patients, sinus bradycardia does not cause hypotension until rate falls below 40 to 45 beats · min^{-1}. Therapy involves elimination of factors causing autonomic nervous system imbalance or restoration of SNS or PNS tone to normal. Bradycardia caused by excess PNS activity usually responds to muscarinic blocking drugs such as atropine or glycopyrrolate. If decreased SNS activity is the cause, administration of a beta-mimetic drug such as ephedrine can be effective.

Emergence of a dominant pacemaker focus located in either the lower AV node or the bundle of His is also usually caused by postoperative autonomic imbalance. Increased PNS activity sometimes seems to slow a dominant sinus pacemaker more than other suppressed pacemaker cells, allowing a lower focus to emerge. Appearance of nodal rhythms is quite common intraoperatively, as various anesthetic drugs promote emergence of nodal rhythms (*e.g.*, halothane/pancuronium). Factors that stop sinus impulses from reaching the ventricle (SA nodal exit block or AV nodal block) also promote emergence of nodal rhythm.

Nodal rhythms are benign unless low ventricular rate reduces cardiac output and blood pressure. Lack of coordinated atrial contraction can also decrease cardiac output by 10% to 15%. If hypotension requires restoration of sinus rhythm, administration of atropine or beta-mimetic medications can restore the SA node as the dominant pacemaker. However, these measures may only increase nodal rate, especially when the cardiac dysrhythmia is caused by anesthetic drugs. Such dysrhythmias are often difficult to convert, requiring support of blood pressure until spontaneous resolution occurs.

Idioventricular bradycardias almost always indicate life-threatening acidemia, hypoxemia, or myocardial ischemia. Seldom does a slow idioventricular rhythm generate adequate cardiac output and blood pressure. Emergency treatment hinges upon assessing and eliminating underlying conditions while supporting the patient. If acute third degree AV nodal block occurs secondary to digitalis toxicity or ischemia, atropine may improve AV nodal conduction and allow supraventricular impulses to depolarize the ventricles. Atropine does not increase depolarization rates of ventricular pacemakers, since they lack PNS innervation. Addition of epinephrine, isoproterenol, or artificial cardiac pacing may be necessary to accelerate ventricular rate.

Tachycardia

Sinus tachycardia is undoubtedly the most common rhythm change encountered in the postoperative period. Excessive sinus rate is nearly always associated with an increase in SNS influence. (See Table 52-3). Sinus tachycardia is a normal physiologic response and is usually harmless. However, sinus tachycardia can precipitate acute myocardial ischemia in patients with coronary artery disease by decreasing diastolic filling time. Sinus tachycardia seldom causes hypotension by interfering with ventricular filling, but output can be severely compromised in patients with stenotic valvular lesions. Tachycardia can also exacerbate postoperative hypertension. Identification of an underlying stimulus is important, for tachycardia may reflect a life-threatening condition (acidemia, hypoxemia, malignant hyperthermia).

Postoperative sinus tachycardia is best treated by controlling an underlying cause. Administration of analgesics for postoperative pain, IV fluids to counteract hypovolemia or hypotension, sedatives to calm anxiety, or catheterization to relieve a full bladder are usually sufficient. Tachycardia caused by sympathomimetic drugs resolves as serum levels fall. If SNS activity is beyond control or if tachycardia presents a threat to well being, beta-blockade can be useful to control rate.

Sudden onset atrial fibrillation can generate ventricular rates in excess of 150 beats · min^{-1}, which can cause significant hypotension or myocardial ischemia. Untreated atrial fibrillation can appear as a fast, nearly regular supraventricular tachycardia on the ECG. Patients recovering from thoracic surgical procedures, or those with atrial dilation from mitral valvular disease or pulmonary embolic phenomenon exhibit a higher incidence of fibrillation postoperatively. Treatment of atrial fibrillation involves administration of digoxin or calcium channel blockers to decrease the number of impulses that can traverse the AV node per minute. If hemodynamic compromise is too serious to wait for drug effects to decrease ventricular rate, DC cardioversion may convert atrial fibrillation back to sinus rhythm.[38]

As with atrial fibrillation, rapid ventricular rate is the major clinical manifestation of atrial flutter. Ventricular rate tends to be more regular, reflecting a fraction of atrial rate. Atrial flutter is relatively rare in postoperative patients. Treatment is directed toward regularizing atrial electrical activity and decreasing ventricular rate.

Paroxysmal atrial tachycardias (PAT) are usually caused by circus reentry in a loop of conduction tissue, although 10% to 15% are caused by discrete, rapidly firing islands of atrial cells. Emergence of PAT during recovery is relatively uncommon, probably because of depressant effects of anesthetic medications on conduction. When PAT does occur, excessive ventricular rate often precludes ventricular filling between beats, compromising cardiac output. Treatment of PAT involves manipulating conduction velocities of cardiac impulses. Slowing conduction interrupts reentrant synchrony of a PAT, allowing a dominant pacemaker to re-emerge at a slower rate. Often PAT can be "broken" by increasing PNS influence on the heart (Table 52-4). Digoxin or calcium channel blockers can also be useful. PATs caused by a rapidly firing atrial pacemaker focus may slow with beta-blockade or other interventions to decrease spontaneous depolarization rates.[39]

Postoperative ventricular tachycardia or fibrillation almost always reflects severe myocardial ischemia, systemic acidemia or hypoxemia, although reentrant ventricular tachycardia does occur. Cardiopulmonary resuscitation, control of ventilation and oxygenation, manipulation of serum pH, cardioversion, and administration of beta-mimetic medications may be useful in restoring a more synchronized rhythm.

Premature Contractions

An aberrant impulse arising in the atrium, AV node, or upper bundle of His usually generates an atrial premature contraction (APC), manifested by an early but otherwise normal QRS complex on ECG which is often not preceded by a P wave. APCs in postoperative patients are almost always benign, seldom result in hemodynamic compromise, and usually appear during periods of increased SNS activity. Control of stimuli causing increased SNS activity is usually sufficient to eliminate these ectopic impulses (See Table 52-3).[38]

Appearance of large amplitude, wide, bizarre complexes on ECG is quite common in postoperative patients. Peculiar QRS complexes are often categorically considered premature ventricular complexes (PVCs), referring to origination of an impulse peripherally in ventricular conducting tissue. Actually,

TABLE 52-4.   Factors that Increase Postoperative Parasympathetic Influence

INCREASED PARASYMPATHETIC ACTIVITY	DECREASED SYMPATHETIC ACTIVITY

Vagal reflexes
  Carotid sinus massage, Valsalva, gagging, rectal exam, increased ocular pressure, bladder distention, pharyngeal stimulation
	"High" spinal or epidural anesthesia
	Withdrawal of stimulus
	  Extubation, emptying bladder

	Severe acidemia/hypoxemia

Parasympathomimetic medications
  Acetylcholinesterase inhibitors (neostigmine, edrophonium)
  Alpha adrenergic drugs (neosynephrine, norepinephrine)
  Narcotics (morphine, fentanyl)
  Succinylcholine
	Sympatholytic medications
	  Beta-receptor blockers (propranolol)
	  Narcotics/sedatives/general anesthesia
	  Ganglionic blockers
	  Local anesthetics

the majority of these complexes are caused by other electrophysiologic mechanisms which seldom indicate serious physiologic abnormality.[39] ECG complexes generated by actual premature ventricular contractions usually occur at varying intervals from a previous normal QRS. Also, the interval between previous and subsequent normal QRS complexes is often twice the normal interval between sinus complexes (compensatory pause; Fig. 52-2A.) In postoperative patients, spontaneous depolarization in ventricular conducting tissue is almost always associated with either excessive PNS or excessive SNS influence. Increased PNS influence reduces spontaneous depolarization rates in supraventricular pacemakers, allowing emergence of ventricular escape beats. Ventricular escape beats are best treated by accelerating supraventricular pacemaker rates with vagolytic or sympathomimetic medications. An increase in SNS activity accelerates spontaneous Phase 4 depolarization rates in ventricular automatic cells, allowing depolarization between supraventricular impulses. Increased SNS activity also promotes emergence of parasystolic foci. Treatment hinges on analyzing and eliminating autonomic nervous system imbalance, although beta-receptor blockade can also be effective. Failure to eliminate ventricular depolarizations with control of autonomic nervous system imbalance may implicate myocardial ischemia with bizarre, nonphysiologic depolarization mechanisms.[40] Intravenous administration of cardiac antidysrhythmics such as lidocaine, procainamide, and bretylium can be useful to control automaticity in ischemic ventricular conducting tissue. However, mechanical stimulation from central

catheters, stretch of myocardial fibers during hypertension or failure, digitalis toxicity, and electrolyte disturbances might also be responsible.[41]

If a supraventricular impulse enters the ventricular conduction system before all tissues have recovered excitability, asynchronous ventricular depolarization generates wide, high amplitude ECG complexes that are difficult to distinguish from true PVCs. These aberrantly conducted, premature supraventricular depolarizations are sometimes preceeded by a P wave that may not resemble dominant P waves. The interval between a previous and subsequent normal QRS is usually less than twice a normal interval (a noncompensatory pause; Fig. 52-2B). Also, the aberrant QRS often resembles normal complexes in general shape, being merely wider and higher in amplitude.

Increased SNS activity is usually responsible for generating premature supraventricular impulses with aberrant conduction. However, delayed recovery of excitability in conducting tissues caused by general anesthetics, electrolyte abnormalities, or ischemia also favors aberrant conduction.

If a sinus impulse is delayed in one ventricular conduction pathway long enough to encounter tissue that has recovered excitability, the impulse can depolarize this tissue a second time and spread throughout the entire heart.[42] This "reentrant" depolarization generates a wide, high amplitude complex very similar to a true PVC. Reentrant ECG complexes are usually uniform in configuration, follow a preceding normal complex by a constant interval (fixed coupling), and often manifest full compensatory pauses (Fig. 52-2C). Many dis-

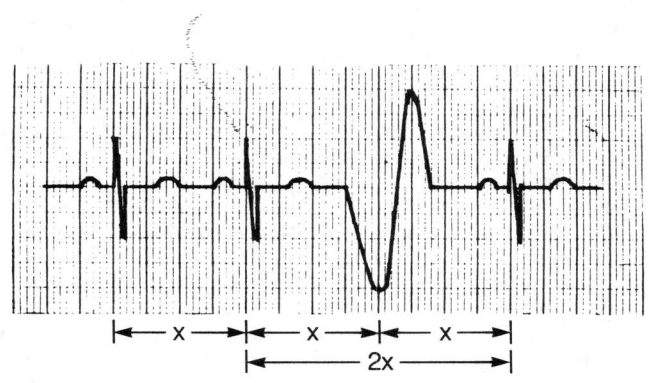

A

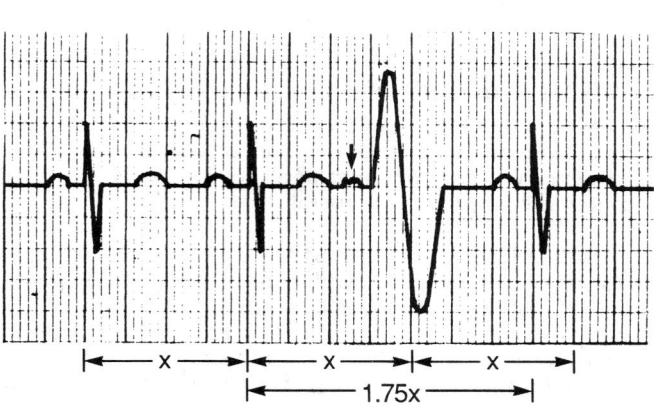

B

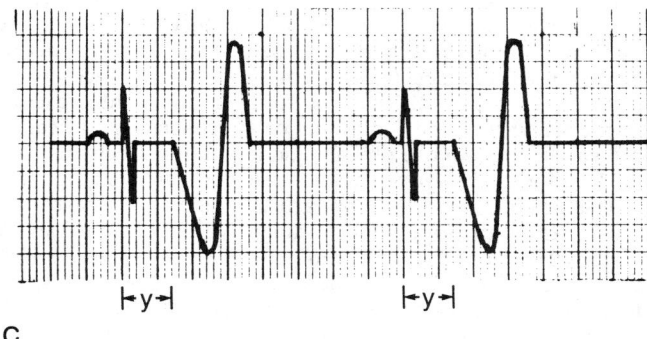

C

FIG. 52-2. Premature ventricular complexes. (A) Actual ventricular depolarization. Note wide, high amplitude configuration, reverse initial deflection, compensatory pause between previous and subsequent normal QRS. (x = normal R-R interval, 2x = full compensatory pause). (B) Aberrantly conducted atrial premature depolarization. Note initial deflection and general configuration similar to normal QRS, presence of abnormal preceding P wave (arrow), noncompensatory pause between previous and subsequent normal QRS. (x = normal R-R interval, 2x = full compensatory pause, 1.75x = noncompensatory pause). (C) Reentry with fixed coupling. Note uniform configuration of abnormal QRS, and fixed interval (y) between preceding normal QRS and abnormal complex.

eases, medications, and environmental influences can create viable reentrant loops. Postoperative reentry is often related to increased SNS activity, especially in conjunction with anesthetic drugs such as halothane.

A high percentage of abnormal ventricular complexes encountered in postoperative patients represent aberrantly conducted supraventricular complexes or reentrant dysrhythmias rather than actual PVCs. Differentiation is important, because aberrant conduction and reentry are almost always benign and seldom require treatment. If aberrantly conducted impulses are so frequent that cardiac output is compromised, control of autonomic nervous system imbalance can be effective to restore a regular rhythm. Cardiac antidysrhythmics are usually unnecessary, although beta-receptor blockade may be useful. Treatment of reentrant impulses should be based on elimination of factors that promote conduction delay or nonuniform recovery of excitability, and on control of SNS activity. Administration of antidysrhythmic medication is seldom indicated and often ineffective.

POSTOPERATIVE PULMONARY DYSFUNCTION

Postoperative pulmonary dysfunction can be caused by mechanical, pharmacologic, and hemodynamic influences related to surgery and anesthesia.[43–45] Division of pulmonary function into ventilation, arterial oxygenation, and maintenance of airway patency and protection facilitates identification of factors causing postoperative dysfunction and simplifies selection of appropriate treatment.

INADEQUATE POSTOPERATIVE VENTILATION

Effective alveolar ventilation can be defined as bulk delivery of fresh gas to perfused alveoli. Adequacy of effective ventilation depends on whether volume of CO_2 removed per unit time matches peripheral CO_2 production, allowing maintenance of normal Pa_{CO_2} and pH. Ventilation distributed to nonperfused alveoli (*i.e.*, dead space ventilation) cannot participate in gas exchange. Effective alveolar ventilation is primarily regulated by medullary centers that are sensitive to pericellular pH in cerebrospinal fluid (CSF). During hypercarbia and CSF acidosis, neural output to muscles of ventilation increases rate and tidal volume, increasing total minute and effective alveolar ventilation. Consequent negative feedback facilitates maintenance of a constant Pa_{CO_2}. Peripheral chemoreceptors in carotid bodies can also increase minute ventilation when carotid P_{O_2} falls, protecting against hypoxemia caused by hypoventilation. Respiratory rate, depth, and pattern are modulated by feedback from various neural elements within lung parenchyma (*e.g.*, stretch receptors, J receptors) which probably monitor pulmonary intravascular or interstitial volume. Volitional or subconscious cortical input can override more physiologic regulation mechanisms.[46]

Elevation of Pa_{CO_2} does not indicate ventilatory inadequacy unless accompanied by respiratory acidemia. A reasonable diagnosis of postoperative ventilatory inadequacy can be made when 1) hypercarbia causes a reduction of arterial pH below 7.30 from whatever cause 2) hypercarbia and respiratory acidemia occur coincident with tachypnea >20 beats · min^{-1}, anxiety, dyspnea, labored ventilation, or increased SNS activity, and 3) a progressive increase in Pa_{CO_2} is noted with an appropriate decrease in arterial pH.

Inadequate Respiratory Drive

In the immediate postoperative period, patients recovering from general anesthesia exhibit a blunted response to hypercarbia and CSF acidosis, caused by residual CNS effects of intravenous or inhalational anesthetics.[47–50] Some degree of respiratory acidemia is therefore expected and acceptable. Medullary centers which regulate sympathetic nervous system activity are also affected. Lack of significant hypertension, tachycardia, cardiac dysrhythmias, agitation, or other SNS responses to acidemia may allow inadequate ventilation to go unnoticed.

Respiratory center depression caused by intraoperative drug administration is most profound on admission to the PACU and wanes thereafter. However, if an intravenous opioid is given just prior to admission, peak depressant effect will occur in the PACU. Time, amount, and route of respiratory depressant medication given intraoperatively must be clearly recorded on admission to recovery. Certain neuroleptic or opioid anesthetic techniques may exhibit a biphasic pattern of respiratory depression, causing delayed hypoventilation.[51] Sedatives can also directly depress ventilation, synergistically augment depression from opioids and anesthetics, or ablate the conscious will to ventilate (sometimes a significant component of ventilatory drive).[52] A cautious balance must be struck between acceptable degree of pain or agitation and acceptable level of postoperative ventilatory depression.

Abrupt diminution of noxious stimuli can upset a balance between depressant effects of medication and excitatory effects of stimuli, generating a dangerous level of postoperative CNS depression. Withdrawal of airway stimulation after extubation of the trachea can promote progressive obtundation as unbalanced depressant effects of residual anesthetics emerge. Trauma or surgical manipulation sometimes interferes with ventilatory feedback and drive. Intracranial hemorrhage or edema after posterior fossa craniotomy often initially manifests as apnea.[31] Bilateral damage to carotid sinuses or neural pathways (as can occur after bilateral carotid endarterectomy) may ablate peripheral hypoxic responses.[29, 53] Chronic respiratory acidemia (as seen with carbon dioxide retention in COPD) alters CNS sensitivity to pH changes. Although supplemental oxygen might eliminate peripheral hypoxic drive and cause intermittent hypoventilation and progressive acidemia, this problem rarely appears in surgical populations. Patients suffering from abnormal CO_2/pH responses associated with morbid obesity, chronic upper airway obstruction, or "sleep apnea" disorders are often very sensitive to respiratory depressants, and are at increased risk of inadequate postoperative ventilation.

Ventilatory Mechanics

Increased work of breathing from high airway resistance, decreased pulmonary compliance, or reduced mechanical efficiency of neuromuscular or skeletal systems can significantly interfere with postoperative ventilation.

INCREASED AIRWAY RESISTANCE. An increase in airway resistance increases both work of breathing and CO_2 production. If inspiratory muscles cannot generate sufficient pressure gradients along airways to overcome resistance, or if effective alveolar ventilation is so reduced that CO_2 removal cannot be maintained, progressive respiratory acidemia and ventilatory failure occurs.

Increased airway resistance during recovery is often attributable to upper airway obstruction in the pharynx (posterior tongue displacement, soft tissue collapse), in the larynx (laryngeal edema, laryngospasm, foreign body obstruction) or in large airways (tracheal stenosis, severe extrinsic compression from hematoma or tumor, foreign body obstruction). Relief of obstruction and elimination of cause are essential. Assuming an airway is clear of vomitus or foreign bodies, simple airway manuevers such as jaw lift, mandible elevation, lateral positioning or placement of an oropharyngeal or nasopharyngeal artificial airway usually relieves pharyngeal obstruction by tongue or soft tissues. (A nasopharyngeal airway may be better tolerated if gag reflexes are functional.) Improving level of consciousness can be equally useful. Edema of vocal cords, tracheal mucosa, or subglottic structures after bronchoscopy or intubation of the trachea sometimes reduces airway caliber and increases airway resistance, especially in children. Obstruction is often ameliorated with inhaled, nebulized racemic epinephrine in oxygen. Complete obstruction is rare.

During emergence, stimulation of pharyngeal tissues or vocal cords by secretions or foreign matter generates tight apposition of vocal cords by laryngeal constrictor muscles, termed laryngospasm.[54] Most episodes of laryngospasm can be overcome with positive pressure in the oropharynx. If laryngospasm is prolonged and severe, a very small dose of succinylcholine (e.g., 0.1 mg · kg^{-1}) usually yields sufficient relaxation to allow ventilation of the lungs.

Extrinsic upper airway compression must be relieved when possible (e.g., evacuation of a carotid hematoma). Intubation of the trachea may be necessary if tissue edema or airway obstruction is severe, as occurs with epiglottitis, retropharyngeal abscess, or tumors encroaching upon the airway. Administration of sedatives to facilitate laryngoscopy and intubation of the trachea may promote further obstruction by eliminating volitional efforts directed toward airway maintenance. Use of muscle relaxants eliminates spontaneous ventilation and ablate muscular tone necessary to keep the airway patent. On occasion, both intubation of the trachea and facemask ventilation are impossible after paralysis, creating an acute airway emergency. When upper airway obstruction is caused by edema or extrinsic compression, trauma from tracheal intubation attempts may convert a marginal airway into one that is totally obstructed. Equipment and personnel necessary for emergency cricothyroidotomy or tracheostomy

and positive pressure ventilation of the lungs with 100% oxygen should be readily available. Cricothyroidotomy using a #14-gauge intravenous catheter (Fig. 52-3) permits oxygenation with 100% oxygen and marginal ventilation until the airway can be secured. (Fig. 52-4).[55]

Reduction of cross sectional area in small airways generates a marked increase in overall airway resistance, as airway resistance varies inversely with a fourth power of airway radius during laminar flow and a fifth power during turbulent flow. Decreased airway caliber in smokers with reactive airway disease or in asthmatics may be caused by diffuse bronchospasm or airway wall edema. Chronic obstructive pulmonary disease or decreased lung volume caused by obesity, surgical manipulation, hypoexpansion during splinting against a painful incision, or excessive lung water can also reduce effective airway cross sectional area. Pharyngeal, tracheal, or carinal stimulation by secretions, suctioning, aspiration, or endotracheal intubation often triggers a reflex increase of bronchial smooth muscle tone, especially as bronchodilatory effects of inhalation anesthetics wane. Histamine release precipitated by

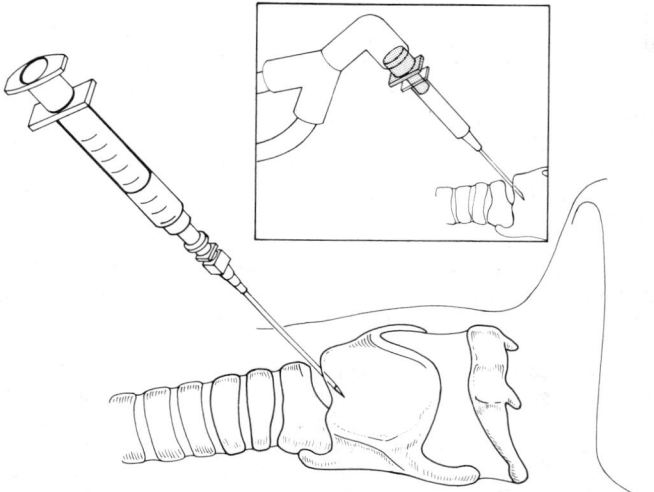

FIG. 52-3. Cricothyroidotomy using large-bore (14-gauge) intravenous catheter attached to syringe.

FIG. 52-4. The effects of apneic oxygenation (Ao) and oxygen flow at 0.2, 0.5, and 2.0 l·min^{-1} through a small bore tracheal catheter in an anesthetized canine preparation. Pa$_{O_2}$ was well maintained (Ao) and improved with low flow oxygen. Despite marked changes in Pa$_{CO_2}$ and pH, no dog exhibited signs of circulatory instability. (Slutsky AS, Watson J, Leith DE et al: Tracheal insufflation of oxygen [TRIO] at low flow rates sustain life several hours. Anesthesiology 63:278, 1985.)

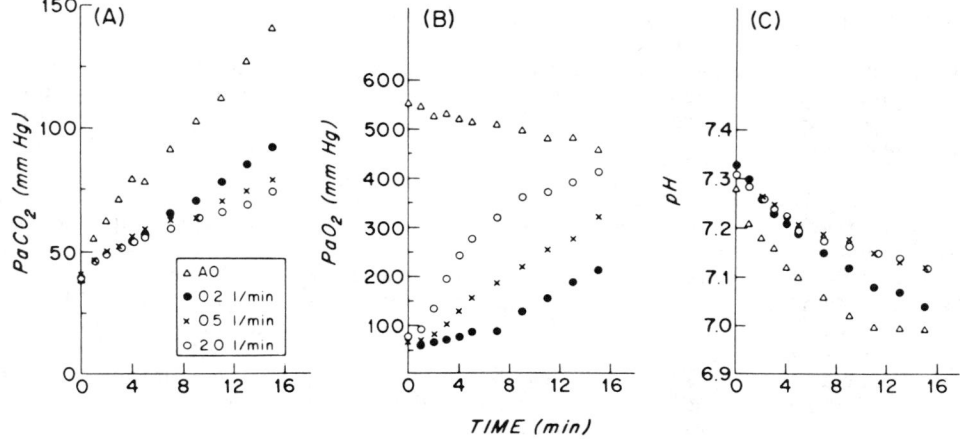

medications or allergic reactions may also increase airway smooth muscle tone. Increased postoperative ventilatory requirements caused by warming, emergence, work of breathing, or pain accentuate resistance by increasing flow rates in small airways and converting normal, low resistance laminar flow to chaotic, high resistance turbulent flow.[56]

Absence of audible turbulent airflow (wheezing) does not rule out increased airway resistance in postoperative patients, because flow may be so impeded that no sound is produced. Generation of a forced vital capacity expiration can be useful to unmask high overall airway resistance. (Resistance is usually highest during expiration because intermediate diameter airways are compressed by positive intrathoracic pressure.) Signs of increased small airway resistance can mimic those of decreased pulmonary compliance. Spontaneously ventilating patients exhibit markedly increased work of breathing with either condition, as evidenced by accessory muscle recruitment and labored ventilation. Mechanically ventilated patients manifest elevation of peak inspiratory pressure required for delivery of a given tidal volume.

Treatment of increased small airway resistance during recovery should be directed toward an underlying etiology. Laryngeal or airway stimulation should be eliminated if possible. Administration of isoetharine or metaproterenol nebulized in oxygen followed by intramuscular or sublingual terbutaline if necessary resolves postoperative bronchospasm in most cases, with minimal tachycardia or agitation. If ventilation of the lungs is still compromised or unduly labored, an aminophylline loading dose and maintenance infusion should be administered. When bronchospasm is life threatening, intravenous epinephrine administration usually yields profound bronchodilation. Blood levels of epinephrine are easily and rapidly reduced or terminated if unwanted side-effects appear. An occassional patient exhibiting bronchospasm resistant to beta-2 sympathomimetic medication may benefit from a trial of parasympatholytic medication such as atropine.[57]

Increased small airway resistance caused by "mechanical" factors (e.g., loss of lung volume, pulmonary edema) does not usually respond well to bronchodilators. Restoration of lung volume with incentive spirometry or deep tidal ventilation increases external radial traction on small airways and decreases overall resistance. Reduction of left ventricular filling pressures and improvement of left ventricular function may be beneficial if airway resistance is caused by increased lung water. Sometimes reduction of pulmonary microvascular filtration pressure does little to acutely ameliorate symptoms, because airway wall edema and interstitial fluid accumulation require time to resolve. Patients with long standing bronchospasm often seem resistant to bronchodilator therapy. Prolonged increases in airway smooth muscle tone cause venous and lymphatic obstruction in airway walls, with persistent edema and reduction of cross sectional area even after smooth muscle relaxation.

DECREASED COMPLIANCE. Factors that reduce pulmonary compliance (change in lung/chest wall volume per unit change in transthoracic pressure) increase work of breathing. Low compliance may preclude generation of adequate alveolar ventilation by respiratory muscles, causing progressive respiratory acidemia.

Postoperative pulmonary compliance depends to a degree on preoperative status. Obesity decreases pulmonary compliance,[58, 59] especially in supine or lateral positions when adipose tissues compress the thoracic cage. Increased intra-abdominal pressure caused by abdominal fat impedes diaphragmatic excursion and promotes reduction of functional residual capacity (FRC), closure of small airways, and collapse of distal lung tissue. Reopening closed airways and reexpansion of atelectatic parenchyma requires additional energy expenditure. Analgous reductions of compliance are encountered in patients with large intraabdominal tumors, ascites, bowel obstruction, intraabdominal hemorrhage, and pregnancy.[60] Thoracic or upper abdominal trauma can cause pulmonary contusion, atelectasis, consolidation, or hemorrhage which interfere with lung expansion, reduce compliance, and accentuate work of breathing.[61] Restrictive lung diseases, musculoskeletal abnormalities, pneumonias, intrathoracic tumors, thoracic aortic aneurysms, and massive cardiomegaly can all cause marked decreases in baseline pulmonary compliance.[62]

Pulmonary compliance is reduced by intraoperative accumulation of abdominal "third space" fluid and gas in the stomach or bowel. Atelectasis caused by intraoperative packing, retraction, steep Trendelenburg position, mainstem tracheal intubation, excessive airway suctioning, or leaning on the abdomen also decrease compliance. In addition, compression of lung tissue by hemo- or tension pneumothorax also reduces compliance.[63] Lateral positioning allows the mediastinum to compress dependent lung, especially when the upper hemithorax is opened to ambient pressure. Loss of lung volume and fluid accumulation caused by gravity and lymphatic obstruction leave the dependent lung with low compliance. (A "down lung syndrome" often appears as unilateral pulmonary edema on chest x-ray film.)[64]

Patients with hydrostatic pulmonary edema (caused by fluid overload, left ventricular failure, or mitral valve dysfunction) or high permeability pulmonary edema (caused by sepsis, aspiration, transfusion reaction, or other causes of adult respiratory distress syndrome) often exhibit very serious reductions in compliance which lead to ventilatory failure. Interstitial fluid and pulmonary blood volume increase lung weight and inertia, rendering the lung more difficult to expand.[65] Accumulation of fluid or secretions in airspaces interferes with effectiveness of pulmonary surfactant in minimizing surface tension and causes small airway obstruction and atelectasis.

Restoration of lung volume using positive airway pressure often improves compliance and decreases work of breathing.[66] However, hyperexpansion can move rib cage and diaphragms toward the limits of their respective excursions, accentuating muscular effort required to achieve further increases in thoracic volume. Hyperexpansion often reduces spontaneous effective minute alveolar ventilation or interferes with weaning from mechanical ventilation. This problem frequently occurs in patients with severe COPD and highly compliant lungs who are treated with positive end expiratory pressure (PEEP) or continuous positive airway pressure (CPAP).[67] Chest wall or abdominal dressings may reduce pulmonary compliance and impede ventilation of the lungs, as can severe cellulitis, extensive scar tissue on thoracic or upper abdominal walls, or other restrictive conditions.

NEUROMUSCULAR AND SKELETAL PROBLEMS. Inadequate postoperative ventilation is frequently related to incomplete reversal of intraoperative muscle relaxation, caused by insufficient administration of anticholinesterese drugs. Reversal drugs also require sufficient time to exert their full effect, especially when hypothermia limits access of drug to neuromuscular junctions. Marginal reversal can be more dangerous than near total paralysis. A gasping, agitated patient exhibiting discoordinate movements and airway obstruction is easily identified. However, marginal neuromuscular function in a somnolent patient exhibiting only minor stridor and mild abdominal rocking motions is easily overlooked. Insidious hypoventilation and progressive respiratory acidemia may occur well into the recovery period, when patients may be less closely observed. Risk of regurgitation and aspiration is also increased.

Patients with preoperative neuromuscular abnormalities such as myasthenia gravis, Eaton–Lambert syndrome, periodic paralysis, or a variety of muscular dystrophies can exhibit exaggerated or prolonged responses to administration of muscle relaxants. Even without relaxant administration, such patients can exhibit postoperative ventilatory insufficiency from inadequate neuromuscular reserve.[68] Certain medications potentiate neuromuscular relaxants or interfere with reversal (e.g., antibiotics, furosemide, propranolol), as do hypocalcemia or hypermagnesemia.[69] Duration of paralysis after administration of succinylcholine can be markedly increased in patients with absent or atypical pseudocholinesterase.[70]

Strength and coordination of diaphragmatic contraction is probably compromised in some postoperative patients, forcing more reliance on intercostal muscles to overcome decreased compliance or to meet increased ventilatory demands.[71] Administration of morphine may compromise intercostal function as well, further compounding ventilatory inadequacy.[72] Postoperative diaphragmatic fatigue may improve with aminophylline infusion.[73]

Thoracic spinal or epidural blockade interferes with external intercostal function and reduces ventilatory ability, especially in patients with COPD. Damage to phrenic nerves from trauma or thoracic and neck operations will paralyze one or even both diaphragms. Adequate ventilation can be maintained with only one functional diaphragm, while marginal ventilation can often be maintained by external intercostal muscles alone. However, in a patient with underlying lung disease, increased work of breathing, or increased ventilatory demands, a nonfunctional diaphragm significantly impedes ventilation.[74] Patients with abnormal motor neuron function (e.g., Guillain–Barré, cervical spinal cord trauma) can certainly exhibit postoperative ventilatory insufficiency.[75,76] Severe kyphosis or scoliosis may markedly reduce ventilatory capacity. Multiple rib fractures that allow paradoxical inward movement of chest wall during inspiration can impede thoracic cavity expansion to such a degree that ventilatory failure supervenes. Loss of compliance from pulmonary contusion underlying such a flail segment is probably of greater significance with respect to ventilatory impairment.[77]

Several simple bedside tests can be useful to assess mechanical ability to ventilate. Forced vital capacity greater than 10 to 12 ml · kg^{-1} usually indicates sufficient strength of ventilatory muscles to achieve lung expansion and sustain ventilation. Observation of expiratory time can also yield qualitative information on airway resistance. Inspiratory pressure more negative than −25 cm H_2O also indicates adequate strength of ventilatory muscles, as does ability to hold the head elevated from a supine position. (Often patients are resistant to lifting the head because of abdominal incisional discomfort, but do sustain head lift if assisted into position). Hand grip, pedal extension, and other maneuvers are less reliable. It is important to realize that these tests indicate

likelihood that a patient will sustain adequate spontaneous ventilation. Failure does not necessarily indicate need for assisted ventilation of the lungs, as many patients with chronic lung diseases cannot meet these criteria preoperatively.

Occasionally, a clinical picture characteristic of postoperative ventilatory insufficiency appears when ventilation is adequate. Ventilation with small tidal volumes caused by thoracic restriction or reduced compliance generates afferent input from pulmonary stretch receptors. Dyspnea, labored ventilation, and accessory muscle recruitment occur in spite of appropriate minute ventilation and Pa_{CO_2}. (This also occurs during mechanical ventilation with low inspired volumes.) Achieving a large, "satisfying" lung expansion often relieves these symptoms. Voluntary limitation of chest cavity expansion in response to pain from an upper abdominal or thoracic incision generates a labored, rapid, shallow breathing pattern, sometimes indicative of inadequate ventilation. However, seldom does hypercarbia or respiratory acidemia appear. Ventilatory pattern usually regularizes merely with repositioning or analgesic administration. Finally, hyperventilation necessary to compensate for metabolic acidemia may require a level of ventilation beyond that which a patient can easily generate. Tachypnea and labored ventilation can easily be mistaken for primary ventilatory insufficiency, especially if one evaluates only arterial pH and ignores Pa_{CO_2}.

Increased Dead Space

Ventilation distributed to air spaces that are not perfused (e.g., dead space ventilation) cannot participate in removal of CO_2. Similarly, if ventilation is distributed to alveoli with high $\dot{V}/\dot{Q}$ ratios, it is less effective in removing CO_2 and proportionally reduces total effective alveolar ventilation per breath.[78] If anatomic or physiologic dead space volume increases without a change in tidal volume, the fraction of each breath wasted in dead space (V_D/V_T) increases. Reduction of tidal volume also increases V_D/V_T. Greater demand for effective alveolar ventilation requires a proportionately larger increase in total minute ventilation if V_D/V_T is high. Many conditions that increase dead space also interfere with ventilatory mechanics, limiting ventilatory reserve. Patients with large dead space volume are therefore at greater risk for postoperative ventilatory failure. If postoperative V_D/V_T is between 0.55 and 0.60 (normal approximately 0.3), patients usually require mechanical assistance to maintain adequate effective alveolar ventilation. If the ratio is greater than 0.60 to 0.65, adequate ventilation often cannot be delivered by conventional volume ventilation. High frequency ventilation may allow adequate CO_2 removal at higher V_D/V_T's.

Occasionally, postoperative hypercarbia and respiratory acidemia are caused by acute increase in dead space. Upper airway dead space is reduced by approximately 75% after endotracheal intubation, and almost eliminated by tracheostomy. However, addition of excessive tubing volume, inappropriate connections, valve reversal or unauthorized modification in breathing circuits can add to anatomic dead space, promoting rebreathing of expired gas rich in CO_2. Increases of anatomic dead space can also occur if airway volume is expanded after application of PEEP or CPAP,[79] especially in patients with high pulmonary compliance. Dead space volume may appear to be increased if expiration is interrupted by a subsequent inspiration before spent alveolar gas is completely exhaled. Consequent "gas trapping" and CO_2 retention occur especially if improper inspiratory to expiratory time ratios or excessive ventilatory rates are used during mechanical ventilation, and when high airway resistance lengthens time required for complete expiration.

Pulmonary embolization with air, thrombus, cellular debris, or foreign matter interferes with blood flow in the lung and can generate significant ventilation—perfusion ($\dot{V}/\dot{Q}$) mismatching. An increase in "physiologic" dead space results. Impact of resulting high $\dot{V}/\dot{Q}$ units on CO_2 excretion is often masked by large increases in minute ventilation mediated by hypoxic drive or reflex responses to emboli.[80, 81] Real time evaluation of end expired P_{CO_2} by capnography is useful to detect air embolization. Pulmonary hypotension can also upset $\dot{V}/\dot{Q}$ matching and increase $\dot{V}_D/\dot{V}_T$.[82] Irreversible increases in physiologic dead space occur postoperatively whenever pathologic processes progressively disrupt or destroy pulmonary microvasculature. For example, elevation of V_D/V_T is often encountered in adult respiratory distress syndrome related to sepsis, massive transfusion, severe hypotension, trauma, or hypoxemia. Increased dead space usually manifests with progressive hypercarbia and difficulty in maintaining adequate levels of mechanical ventilation several days into a postoperative ICU course.

Increased Carbon Dioxide Production

Total body CO_2 production varies directly with metabolic rate, body temperature, and substrate availability. Intraoperatively, CO_2 production can fall by 20% to 40% of normal (approximately 2.3 ml $\cdot$ kg^{-1} $\cdot$ min^{-1}) as hypothermia lowers metabolic activity and neuromuscular relaxation reduces tonic muscle contraction. In the postoperative period, warming returns metabolic rate, oxygen consumption, and CO_2 production toward normal. Shivering, increased work of breathing, infection, SNS activity, or rapid carbohydrate metabolism during intravenous hyperalimentation can markedly accelerate CO_2 production.[35, 83] Even mild postoperative augmention of CO_2 production can precipitate respiratory acidemia and ventilatory failure if decreased compliance, increased airway resistance, or residual neuromuscular paralysis interfere with ventilatory capacity. More pronounced increases in CO_2 production generate ventilatory insufficiency even with normal ventilatory capacity. An episode of malignant hyperthermia can trigger in the postoperative period and cause CO_2 production many times greater than normal. Production rapidly exceeds ventilatory reserve, resulting in severe hypercarbia and respiratory acidemia.[84, 85]

There are few indications for manipulation of CO_2 production during recovery, with the exception of adjusting hyperalimentation or treating malignant hyperthermia. However, if increased dead space precludes mechanical delivery of adequate alveolar ventilation, deliberate hypothermia and paralysis can be employed to reduce CO_2 production in the hope that increased V_D/V_T is partially reversible.

INADEQUATE POSTOPERATIVE OXYGENATION

Maintenance of systemic arterial oxygenation through oxygen transfer from alveolar gas to pulmonary venous blood does not guarantee arterial perfusion pressure, cardiac output, and distribution of blood flow required to maintain adequate tissue oxygenation. Marked tissue ischemia can exist with totally normal pulmonary oxygenation (peripheral shunts, sepsis, severe hypotension, anemia, hemoglobin dissociation curve shifts, carbon monoxide, arsenic, or cyanide poisoning.) The most accessible index of oxygenation as a pulmonary function is Pa_{O_2}. Noninvasive analysis of arterial

hemoglobin saturation (pulse oximetry) will establish adequacy of oxygenation, but is affected by hemoglobin dissociation curve shifts and is far less quantitative.[5] Evaluation of metabolic acidemia, mixed venous oxygen content, or venous hemoglobin saturation yields more insight into peripheral oxygen delivery than pulmonary oxygen transfer.

In the postoperative period, each patient must be individually evaluated when defining an "acceptable" Pa_{O_2} for a given FI_{O_2} (i.e., an acceptable A-a oxygen gradient), or when selecting a minimally acceptable PaO_2. During recovery, little advantage is gained elevating Pa_{O_2} above 100 to 110 mm Hg, because hemoglobin is fully saturated and additional dissolved oxygen at higher Pa_{O_2} is negligible. Reduction of Pa_{O_2} below 70 mm Hg may cause significant arterial hemoglobin desaturation, although tissue oxygen delivery can be maintained at lower levels. I prefer to maintain Pa_{O_2} between 80 and 100 mm Hg, in order to insure adequate oxygen delivery yet minimize therapeutic intervention. One must also assess efficiency of oxygenation relative to FI_{O_2} and positive airway pressure required to maintain Pa_{O_2}. In routine postoperative settings, patients can usually maintain oxygenation after tracheal extubation if Pa_{O_2} is above 80 mm Hg during mechanical ventilation with 40% inspired oxygen and 5 cm H_2O PEEP or CPAP.

Distribution of Ventilation

Ventilation-perfusion mismatch caused by loss of volume in dependent lung parenchyma is probably the most common cause of postoperative arterial hypoxemia. Reduction of FRC decreases radial traction on airways, promoting small airway collapse, distal atelectasis, and $\dot{V}/\dot{Q}$ mismatch that can progressively worsen for 24 to 36 hours after surgery. Reduction of dependent lung volume is particularly damaging, as gravitational effects direct a significant proportion of pulmonary blood flow to dependent areas.[86–89]

Certain patients are at increased risk for reduction of FRC during and after surgery. Older patients normally exhibit some degree of airway closure at end expiration. Reduction of small airway support caused by COPD promotes severe airway closure that can be markedly exacerbated by even small reductions in FRC.[90] Obesity, immobility, or increased intraabdominal pressure limit diaphragmatic excursion, decrease lung volume, and generate $\dot{V}/\dot{Q}$ mismatching. Patients exhibiting reduced pulmonary compliance caused by increased lung water, actelectasis, consolidation, pleural effusions, and restrictive pulmonary or chest wall disorders are also at increased risk.

Retraction, packing, and manipulation during upper abdominal surgery reduce FRC, as do gastric and bowel distention, intraabdominal third space accumulation, and external abdominal compression from leaning of surgical assistants. Prone, lithotomy or Trendelenburg positions are disadvantageous, especially in obese patients. Splinting against pain from an upper abdominal incision inhibits deep inspiration, discouraging restoration of lung volume in the postoperative period[91–93] (Figs. 52-5 and 52-6).

Significant reduction of FRC and profound $\dot{V}/\dot{Q}$ mismatching frequently occur during intrathoracic surgery, especially when endobronchial intubation and one lung anesthesia are employed in a lateral position. Direct surgical compression, weight of unsupported mediastinal contents, and weight of abdominal contents forcing the paralyzed dependent diaphragm high into the chest cavity all reduce dependent lung volume.[64, 94] Augmentation of blood flow to dependent lung worsens intrapulmonary shunting, es-

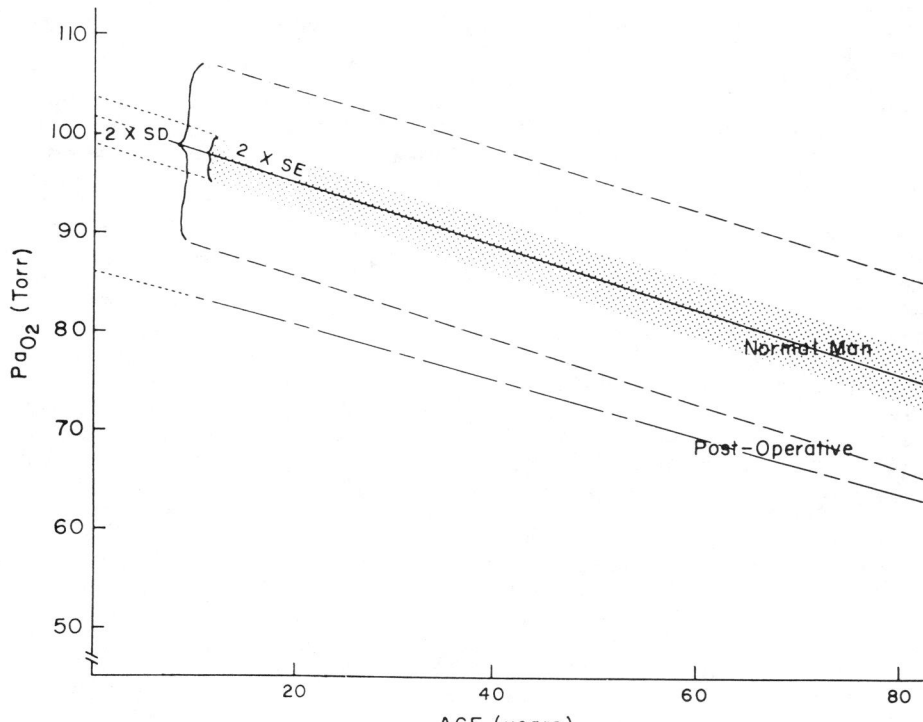

FIG. 52-5. The influence of age on Pa_{O_2}. For any given age the Pa_{O_2} is lower in the postoperative period. The *dashed line* indicates range of normal individual values and the *shaded area*, the range of normal mean values. (Marshall BE, Wyche MQ Jr: Hypoxemia during and after anesthesia. Anesthesiology 37:178, 1972.)

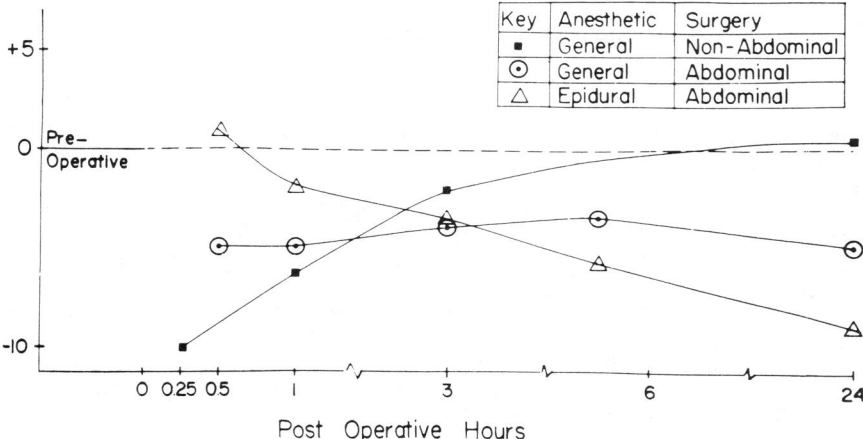

FIG. 52-6. Effect of anesthetic technique on early and late hypoxemia. General anesthesia administered for nonabdominal procedures has maximal decrease in Pa_{O_2} upon emergence, and returns to normal within 3 hours. In contrast, general anesthesia for abdominal surgery is followed by similar early changes, but Pa_{O_2} does not return to baseline value within 3 hours. Regional anesthesia for abdominal operations results in a late decrease in Pa_{O_2}. (Marshall BE, Wyche MQ Jr: Hypoxemia during and after anesthesia. Anesthesiology 37:178, 1972.)

pecially when hypoxic pulmonary vasoconstriction is rendered relatively ineffective by general anesthesics.[95] Accumulation of interstitial fluid caused by lymphatic obstruction and gravity also accentuates V/Q mismatching.

Accumulation of fluid in air spaces caused by overhydration, elevated ventricular filling pressures, or increased capillary permeability interferes with both diffusion of oxygen and V/Q matching.[65] Pneumothorax or hemothorax, tumor mass, expanding pulmonary blebs, cardiomegaly, vascular engorgement, pulmonary contusion or intrapulmonary hemorrhage also upset V/Q matching and promote hypoxemia. Retention of secretions, bronchospasm, and airway wall edema or inflammation promote hypoventilation of distal airspace, as will obstruction of larger airways by foreign body aspiration, mainstem intubation or external compression by tumor or vascular abnormalities. Right upper lobe collapse caused by partial right mainstem intubation is a frequently overlooked cause of significant postoperative hypoxemia. Also, strong inspiratory efforts against an obstructed airway can both decrease FRC and promote hydrostatic pulmonary edema.[96]

During recovery, conservative measures aimed at restoring lung volume often produce marked and lasting improvement in arterial oxygenation.[97] Obese patients should recover in a semisitting rather than supine position whenever possible, to reduce pressure of abdominal contents on the diaphragm. Deep tidal ventilation, vigorous cough, chest physiotherapy, and suction when required may help mobilize secretions and accustom a patient to minor incisional discomfort during deep inspiration. Application of incentive spirometry techniques can be particularly helpful to maintain FRC. Some authorities advocate intermittent positive pressure breathing techniques although effectiveness is questionable.[98, 99]

Adequate postoperative analgesia is pivotal to ensure restoration and maintenance of FRC, especially with upper abdominal or chest wall incisions. Pain with ventilatory motion encourages rapid, shallow breathing which may provide adequate minute ventilation but does little to maintain expansion. Analgesia can be provided with parenteral opioids, or with selected regional anesthetic techniques. Intercostal blocks can provide relief of pain from thoracotomy and cholecystectomy incisions, whereas continuous lumbar or thoracic epidural techniques can be helpful for upper abdominal incisions. Continuous postoperative regional analgesia can also be invaluable in weaning patients with limited pulmonary reserve from postoperative ventilatory support.[9, 11, 100]

Supplemental oxygen often improves Pa_{O_2} to some degree, but does little to rectify whatever underlying problem is causing poor $\dot{V}/\dot{Q}$ matching. Effectiveness of a given FI_{O_2} in elevating Pa_{O_2} is highly variable. Actual inspired concentration is difficult to predict with commonly used face masks, tents, or nasal prongs, as ambient gas is entrained with each inspiration.[101] In addition, if hypoxemia is caused by "shunting", supplemental oxygen should have a negligible effect on Pa_{O_2}. (Shunted blood is not exposed to increased FI_{O_2}, whereas blood passing ventilated alveoli is already fully saturated.) However, if hypoxemia is caused by "low $\dot{V}/\dot{Q}$ units", increasing concentration of oxygen in a limited amount of ventilation to a group of alveoli can improve saturation of passing blood.

Risk of supplemental oxygen is almost negligible, although high FI_{O_2} (probably greater than 0.8) may promote resorption atelectasis as inert nitrogen in low $\dot{V}/\dot{Q}$ units is replaced with oxygen.[102] Inspiration of 100% oxygen for 24 to 36 hours can generate early signs of pulmonary oxygen toxicity, characterized by alveolar epithelial degeneration and evolution of capillary leak pulmonary edema.[103] Development of oxygen toxicity is faster in patients undergoing hyperbaric oxygen therapy. Administration of supplemental oxygen perhaps accelerates pulmonary damage associated with bleomycin therapy,[104] although controversy exists concerning actual risk.[105] Alveolar P_{O_2} should probably be maintained as near to "room air" values as possible in patients exposed to bleomycin, with careful monitoring of Pa_{O_2} or oxygen saturation.

If loss of lung volume is significant, continuous positive airway pressure is very effective for restoring and maintaining FRC in the postoperative period. CPAP (5–7 cm H_2O) can be delivered effectively by face mask for several hours to maintain Pa_{O_2} within acceptable limits until factors promoting loss of lung volume resolve.[106] However, if arterial hypoxemia is severe or if patient acceptance of mask CPAP is poor, endotracheal intubation is usually required. Intubation of the trachea for delivery of CPAP does not indicate need for positive pressure ventilation. Ventilatory requirements should be assessed independently, considering Pa_{CO_2}, arterial pH, and work of breathing.

In most patients, 5 to 10 cm of CPAP or PEEP is sufficient to restore lung volume and Pa_{O_2} without significant transmission to thoracic veins and hypotension or increase in intracranial pressure.[107, 108] Risk of barotrauma is minimal, even when positive airway pressure is administered as PEEP with positive pressure ventilation. If improvement of Pa_{O_2} is not achieved with 5 to 10 cm H_2O positive pressure, one should reevaluate the etiology of low Pa_{O_2}, for higher positive pressure is seldom helpful in routine postoperative settings. In an occasional patient with severe pulmonary pathology (e.g., adult respiratory distress syndrome, severe pulmonary contusion), higher levels of pressure may yield improvement of both oxygenation and compliance. However, pressures greater than 10 to 15 cm H_2O are more transmitted to thoracic veins, and probably associated with an increased incidence of barotrauma.[109, 110] In addition, high positive pressure can increase vascular resistance in well ventilated, more compliant portions of lung and actually divert blood toward poorly ventilated areas, worsening $\dot{V}/\dot{Q}$ matching. This phenomenon is rare at more conservative levels of positive pressure.[111]

Endotracheal intubation eliminates a patient's ability to create expiratory resistance and "physiologic PEEP" (2–5 cm H_2O), which may be very useful in maintaining lung volume during spontaneous ventilation. Exposing an intubated trachea to ambient airway pressure in the postoperative period can cause a gradual, progressive reduction of FRC, significant $\dot{V}/\dot{Q}$ mismatch, and arterial hypoxemia. Generally, a patient whose trachea is intubated should exhale against some degree of CPAP. Young, slender patients left intubated for short periods (0.5–1 hour) are usually able to spontaneously restore any reduction of FRC after tracheal extubation.

Distribution of Perfusion

Poor distribution of pulmonary perfusion also interferes with $\dot{V}/\dot{Q}$ matching and postoperative oxygenation. Distribution of pulmonary blood flow is primarily determined by mechanical factors (pulmonary arterial and venous pressures, arteriolar and capillary resistance), which are in turn affected by gravity, airway pressure, lung volume, and overall cardiovascular status. Gross distribution of blood flow is further modulated by hypoxic pulmonary vasoconstriction, which diverts flow away from air spaces that are poorly ventilated and exhibit low alveolar P_{O_2}.[112]

Pain, agitation, hypoxemia, or acidemia increase SNS activity, cardiac output, and pulmonary vascular resistance, generating significant elevations of pulmonary artery pressure. Pulmonary vascular resistance can also be increased by positive airway pressure, accumulation of interstitial fluid, and a change in lung volume either above or below functional residual capacity.[113] Elevation of pulmonary venous pressures caused by left ventricular dysfunction (as seen with ischemia, anesthetic depression, and chronic cardiomyopathy) or increased filling pressures (as seen with hypervolemia or increased systemic venous return) necessitate an increase in pulmonary arterial pressures to maintain output.

Increased pulmonary artery pressure can redistribute blood flow to less dependent areas of lung, interfering with $\dot{V}/\dot{Q}$ matching. Flow through the bronchial circulation and pulmonary arteriovenous anastomoses can also increase, augmenting right to left shunting. Recruitment of pulmonary vessels can interfere with effectiveness of hypoxic pulmonary vasoconstriction in regulating localized distribution of blood flow.[114] All of these changes can reduce arterial oxygenation.

Significant reduction of pulmonary artery pressure may also significantly change $\dot{V}/\dot{Q}$ matching. Pulmonary artery pressure can decrease to a point that perfusion against gravity to uppermost parenchyma is compromised. If loss of dependent lung volume simultaneously causes redistribution of fresh ventilation to nondependent lung, regional $\dot{V}/\dot{Q}$ mismatch results. Also, hypoxic pulmonary vasoconstriction depends on differences in arteriolar resistance among areas of the vascular bed. Reduction of pulmonary artery pressure decreases the "tendency" for blood to flow down lower resistance pathways, reducing effectiveness of hypoxic pulmonary vasoconstriction.

Position changes affect oxygenation by changing distribution of blood flow, especially when gravity directs flow to areas with reduced ventilation. Placing a patient with severe unilateral ventilatory abnormality (*e.g.*, pneumonitis, mainstem intubation) lateral with the poorly ventilated lung dependent can cause serious reductions in PaO_2, while placing unventilated lung in a nondependent position can improve $\dot{V}/\dot{Q}$ matching and arterial oxygenation. Great caution should be exercised with such a manuever, because placing a diseased lung in a nondependent, "up" position can promote drainage of purulent or obstructing material to the unaffected dependent lung, creating a more global problem. Alterations in position can also effect oxygenation by way of changes in venous return and filling pressures.

Pulmonary vascular resistance and distribution of blood flow are markedly affected by changes in lung volume. Positive pressure lung inflation can increase resistance in both intraalveolar and extraalveolar vessels, whereas spontaneous "negative pressure" inspiration probably decreases extraalveolar vascular resistance.[115] Reduction of dependent lung volume can decrease capillary transmural pressure gradients, and may promote an increase in dependent vascular resistance. Because reduction of lung volume and ventilation usually occurs in dependent lung tissue, resulting decreases in blood flow to dependent lung could cause a beneficial redistribution of blood flow and an improvement in $\dot{V}/\dot{Q}$ matching. However, significant redistribution of blood flow to nondependent lung can also worsen matching. Net effects of changes in lung volume on $\dot{V}/\dot{Q}$ matching are difficult to predict.

Postoperative $\dot{V}/\dot{Q}$ matching is affected by various medications. Changes in ventricular function caused by inhalation anesthetics or sympathomimetics can markedly alter pulmonary arterial and venous pressure and change distribution of pulmonary blood flow.[116] Anesthetic drugs may also affect pulmonary vascular tone directly. Nitrous oxide, ketamine, and pentazocine may cause pulmonary vascular constriction, whereas pentolinium, phentolamine, and nitroprusside appear to cause pulmonary vasodilation. Inhalation anesthetics and nitroprusside also significantly impair hypoxic pulmonary vasoconstriction,[117] at least partially explaining a well documented increase in A-a oxygen gradient associated with general anesthesia. (Changes in lung volume and distribution of ventilation probably also contribute.) Effects of anesthetics on hypoxic pulmonary vasoconstriction persist well into recovery. Other ancillary medications such as antihypertensives and beta-mimetic drugs also probably interfere with $\dot{V}/\dot{Q}$ matching and oxygenation.[118]

Several other factors are suspected to interfere with postoperative $\dot{V}/\dot{Q}$ matching. Circulating endotoxin can impair hypoxic pulmonary vasoconstriction, perhaps contributing to difficulties encountered in maintaining PaO_2 in patients with systemic sepsis.[119] Patients with cirrhosis of the liver often exhibit poor $\dot{V}/\dot{Q}$ matching and arterial hypoxemia,[120] perhaps caused by circulating humoral substances related to inappropriate hepatic metabolism. Increased FIO_2 has also been shown to interfere with $\dot{V}/\dot{Q}$ matching in patients with acute lung disease. Whether this is due to interference with hypoxic pulmonary vasoconstriction or to resorption atelectasis is unclear.

Few therapeutic interventions are useful to regulate pulmonary blood flow and improve $\dot{V}/\dot{Q}$ matching. Occasionally, positioning a patient to avoid placing severely diseased lung tissue in a dependent position improves oxygenation. Although eliminating beta-mimetic or vasodilatory medications may improve PaO_2, therapeutic benefit of the medication usually outweighs drawbacks of impaired hypoxic pulmonary vasoconstriction. With respect to cardiovascular dynamics, maintenance of pulmonary artery pressure within acceptable limits is probably the best approach to optimize $\dot{V}/\dot{Q}$ matching. In short, $\dot{V}/\dot{Q}$ abnormalities are more easily resolved by improving distribution of ventilation than by manipulating perfusion.

Inadequate Alveolar P_{O_2}

Occasionally, postoperative hypoxemia is caused by a reduction of alveolar partial pressure of oxygen (PA_{O_2}), usually due to a ventilatory problem that interferes with delivery of fresh gas to alveoli. Whenever uptake of oxygen from alveoli exceeds delivery of oxygen, PA_{O_2} and arterial oxygenation decreases. Many factors interfere with postoperative ventilation, causing variable degrees of respiratory acidemia. However, hypoventilation must be severe for hypoxemia to appear based solely on a reduction of oxygen delivery.

Hypoxemia can occur when severe hypoventilation is caused by excessive opioid administration and respiratory center depression. Significant arterial desaturation can also occur during periodic apnea or obstruction.[121] Opioids and residual anesthetic levels interfere with hypoxic respiratory drive.[122] With the central nervous system insensitive to both respiratory acidemia and hypoxemia, apnea can easily supervene. Apnea caused by supplemental oxygen administered to patients with severe COPD represents another example of hypoxemia related to hypoventilation. (Death in such circumstances is probably related more to progressive respiratory acidemia than to hypoxemia.)

Complete airway obstruction caused by foreign bodies, soft tissue edema, or laryngospasm rapidly depletes alveolar oxygen, as do severe increases in airway resistance that preclude effective ventilation. However, partial obstruction or moderate increases in airway resistance do not usually interfere with ventilation enough to reduce PA_{O_2}, especially in postoperative patients receiving supplemental oxygen. Increasing oxygen content in the FRC to safeguard against hypoxemia from hypoventilation or airway obstruction is an excellent rationale for supplemental oxygen in the postoperative period.

Occasionally, excessive concentrations of a second gas in alveoli can reduce PA_{O_2} to a point that clinically significant hypoxemia occurs. For example, when relatively insoluble nitrous oxide is discontinued at the end of a general anesthetic, a very rapid outpouring of nitrous from pulmonary arterial blood into alveoli causes volume displacement of alveolar gas.[123] High alveolar partial pressures of nitrous oxide can lower PA_{O_2} to dangerous levels, especially if a patient is hypoventilating or breathing ambient air. Danger of this "diffusion hypoxia" can be minimized by administration of 100% oxygen during emergence to dilute alveolar nitrous and maintain PA_{O_2} within acceptable limits. Volume displacement of oxygen by carbon dioxide can also occur if severe hypoventilation markedly elevates partial pressure of carbon dioxide in a patient breathing ambient air or nitrous oxide. Usually, severe respiratory acidemia is a more significant problem than hypoxemia.

Reduced Mixed Venous P_{O_2}

Systemic mixed venous P_{O_2} ($P\bar{v}_{O_2}$) is affected by arterial oxygen content, cardiac output, and tissue oxygen extraction. If

PA_{O_2} decreases or tissue extraction increases, $P\bar{v}_{O_2}$ may fall depending on proportional contributions of different tissue beds. Venous blood with low $P\bar{v}_{O_2}$ that is shunted or distributed to low $\dot{V}/\dot{Q}$ units causes a larger decrease of Pa_{O_2} than if $P\bar{v}_{O_2}$ were normal. Reduction of $P\bar{v}_{O_2}$ therefore amplifies impact of shunt or $\dot{V}/\dot{Q}$ mismatch on PA_{O_2}. Reduction of $P\bar{v}_{O_2}$ also necessitates extraction of larger volumes of oxygen from alveolar gas in order to saturate hemoglobin. Increased alveolar extraction might reduce PA_{O_2} if hypoventilation or airway obstruction reduce delivery of fresh gas. Supplemental oxygen again offsets reduction of PA_{O_2} caused by increased alveolar extraction, and attenuates exaggerated impact of low $\dot{V}/\dot{Q}$ units on Pa_{O_2}. Very low $P\bar{v}_{O_2}$ can also increase risk of resorption atelectasis in poorly ventilated alveoli.

In the postoperative period, shivering, infection, or hyperalimentation can significantly increase peripheral oxygen extraction and lower $P\bar{v}_{O_2}$. Reduction of cardiac output and/or systemic blood pressure caused by hypovolemia, myocardial depression, or arteriolar dilation can also lower $P\bar{v}_{O_2}$ by decreasing tissue oxygen delivery. However, actual impact of reduced $P\bar{v}_{O_2}$ on PA_{O_2} is usually small, assuming that recovering patients at risk for $\dot{V}/\dot{Q}$ mismatching are placed on supplemental oxygen.

ASPIRATION

In recovering patients, upper airway reflexes are vital to preserve airway patency and protect against aspiration of foreign matter. Inability to maintain these two functions can cause severe postoperative pulmonary morbidity. (Problems encountered with maintenance of upper airway patency in postoperative patients are discussed in the section on Airway Resistance.)

Aspiration during induction of anesthesia or recovery generates postoperative pulmonary complications of varying severity, depending on type and volume of aspirate. Although aspiration of gastric contents is most widely feared, surgical patients are at risk for other aspiration syndromes as well.

Aspiration of clear oral secretions during induction of anesthesia, extubation of the trachea or face mask ventilation of the lungs is undoubtedly common and of relatively little significance. Cough, transient laryngospasm, and mild irritation are usual sequelae, although chronic or large volume aspiration might predispose to small airway obstruction, infection, or pulmonary edema.[124]

Aspiration of solid foreign matter (unswallowed food, small objects, pieces of teeth or dental appliances) can cause persistent cough, airway obstruction with distal atelectasis, diffuse reflex bronchospasm, and pneumonia. Unless airway obstruction is massive and life-threatening, complications are often localized to a small portion of lung, and easily treated with antibiotics and supportive pulmonary care once foreign matter is either expelled or removed by bronchoscopy. Secondary thermal, chemical, or traumatic airway injury from aspiration of hot, caustic or sharp objects can cause more significant damage, and may require later surgical intervention.[125]

Aspiration of blood secondary to trauma, epistaxis, or surgical manipulations in the oropharynx or large airways often generates frightening changes on the chest radiograph, which are far out of proportion with clinical symptoms. Aspirated "sterile" blood causes minor airway obstruction, but is rapidly cleared from airspaces by phagocytotic processes and resorption. Massive blood aspiration severely impedes gas exchange and causes pulmonary hemochromatosis from iron

accumulation in phagocytic cells. Accumulation of fibrinous material in airspaces can also occur. Secondary infection is always a possibility, especially if bits of soft tissue, purulent matter, or foreign bodies are aspirated as well.

Aspiration of acidic gastric contents during vomiting or regurgitation causes a serious chemical pneumonitis characterized initially by diffuse bronchospasm, hypoxemia, and atelectasis. Subsequent airway epithelial degeneration, interstitial and alveolar edema, and hemorrhage into airspaces rapidly progress to acute adult respiratory distress syndrome with high permeability pulmonary edema. Destruction and sloughing of Types I and II pneumocytes, decreased surfactant activity, accumulation of fibrinous exudates, hyaline membrane formation, and destruction of parenchyma with atelectasis or emphysematous changes can all occur after severe aspiration. Occlusion or destruction of pulmonary microvasculature is often evident, causing increases in pulmonary vascular resistance, pulmonary arterial pressure, and V_D/V_T.[126]

Severity and eventual resolution of pathologic changes depend on both volume and pH of acid aspirate.[127, 128] Morbidity rate sharply increases when pH of aspirate is below 2.5. Morbidity also increases with aspirate volumes greater than 0.4 to 1 $ml \cdot kg^{-1}$. Aspiration of fluid with pH greater than 2.5 is less damaging, but still interferes with surfactant activity and disrupts cellular function through osmotic or chemical interactions.[129] Presence of partially digested food particles in aspirate both worsens and prolongs aspiration pneumonitis. Food particles cause mechanical airway obstruction and serve as an excellent nidus for secondary bacterial infection. Aspirated vegetable matter is particularly resistant to phagocytosis, and causes chronic granulomatous process resembling that caused by miliary tuberculosis.[130]

Risk of aspiration is particularly high in surgical patients, so a high index of suspicion and caution is necessary.[131] Interference with protective airway reflexes by central depressant medications (inhalation anesthetics, barbituates, opioids), and muscle relaxants represents the greatest risk factor for perioperative aspiration. Airway trauma, laryngeal nerve blocks, or complications of regional anesthetic placement (seizures, high spinal, cervical plexus involvement) also seriously compromise airway reflexes. Large volumes of intragastric food and fluid in patients requiring emergency surgery increases risk. Delayed gastric emptying caused by ileus, bowel or outlet obstruction, pain, anxiety, opioid administration, salt depletion, or peristaltic abnormalities accentuate gastric accumulation. Pregnant or morbidly obese patients exhibit increased gastric volume and acidity, as well as interference with gastroesophageal sphincter function related to mechanical displacement.[132] Hiatal hernia, achalasia, esophageal diverticuli, esophageal tumors, amyotrophic lateral sclerosis or other abnormalities affecting gastroesophageal function or swallowing also increase risk of regurgitation and aspiration.

Prevention of aspiration is critical, as effectiveness of therapy is limited. A traditional recommendtion is that surgery should be delayed for at least 8 to 12 hours in patients with a "full stomach" to allow gastric emptying, even if a regional anesthetic technique is planned. In patients at risk for acid aspiration, administration of nonparticulate antacids such as sodium citrate will increase pH of existing gastric fluid without excessive increase in volume. Particulate antacids should be avoided because subsequent aspiration of this medication can cause additional chronic granulomatous reactions.[133] Administration of H_2 histamine-receptor blockers (cimetidine or ranitidine) reduce rate of accumulation and increase pH of secretions. Addition of metoclopramide increases gastro-esophageal sphincter tone and accelerates gastric empty-ing.[134, 135] Introduction of a nasogastric tube for gastric empty-ing is often ineffective in removing particulate matter, and interferes with gastroesophageal sphincter integrity.[136]

Induction of general anesthesia in patients at risk for regurgitation and aspiration requires endotracheal intubation using an awake oral or nasal approach, or a "rapid sequence" technique (oxygenation, cricoid pressure, obtundation, rapid paralysis without fasciculation, and oral intubation). Wide bore suction should always be available during any anesthetic induction. Once intubation of the trachea is accomplished, every effort should be made to empty gastric contents. Pres-ence of an endotracheal tube does not preclude aspiration of acidic fluid around the cuff.[137] If cuff deflation occurs, the rigid tube holds the vocal cords open, increasing risk of aspiration. One should avoid cuff deflation, and minimize the time the airway is unguarded if deflation is necessary. Frequent pharyngeal suctioning helps guard against silent aspiration.

Risk of aspiration persists into the postoperative period. During emergence from general anesthesia, function and in-tegration of protective reflexes is often lacking. Incidence of postoperative nausea and emesis is significant, especially with accumulation of gas in the stomach from inadvertent esophageal ventilation or nitrous oxide diffusion. Hypoten-sion, hypoxemia, acidemia, or other serious postoperative complications can cause both emesis and obtundation, in-creasing risk of serious aspiration. Persistent effects of laryn-geal nerve blocks, topical local anesthetics, or other intra-operative interventions used to reduce airway irritability decrease postoperative airway protection. Residual neuro-muscular paralysis reduces ability to generate laryngospasm or cough. The trachea of patients at high risk of aspiration should not be extubated until complete restoration of airway reflexes is assured. Care must be exercised to completely suction the pharynx and extubate the trachea at end inspira-tion or with positive airway pressure, to avoid aspiration of regurgitated material trapped above an inflated endotracheal tube cuff.

Anatomic distortion can mechanically interfere with airway clearance and protection in patients recovering from surgery for mandibular fractures or soft tissue trauma. Mandibular fixation makes expulsion of vomitus, blood, or secretions from the mouth almost impossible. Equipment for immediate release of mandibular fixation should be at hand throughout the postoperative period. Also, patients recovering with mandibular fixation should be awake and able to demonstrate cognitive and physical ability to clear the airway prior to tracheal extubation. Careful observation is essential after tra-cheal extubation because airway reflexes can be rendered transiently ineffective after prolonged intubation.

Appearance of gastric secretions in the pharynx mandates immediate lateral head positioning, clearance by suction, and endotracheal intubation if airway reflexes are absent or com-promised. Although Trendelenburg position may promote regurgitation, head down positioning aids in clearance of secretions once regurgitation or vomiting has occurred. (Head elevation in obtunded patients establishes a gravita-tional gradient from pharynx to lung, makes airway manage-ment difficult, and should be avoided.) Suctioning the trachea through the endotracheal tube prior to instituting positive pressure ventilation of the lungs is critical to avoid widely disseminating aspirated material to distal airways. Instillation of saline or alkalotic solutions is not recom-mended. Assessment of pH on tracheal aspirate is of little

use, because buffering is almost immediate. Determination of pH on pharyngeal aspirate may yield more reliable results, but is of little practical use.

Suspicion of intraoperative or postoperative aspiration mandates careful observation over 24 to 48 hours for devel-opment of aspiration pneumonitis, to include serial tempera-ture checks, white blood cell counts with differential, serial chest x-ray films, ABG determinations, and pulmonary func-tion testing if appropriate. Fluffy infiltrates may appear on the chest x-ray film immediately or within 24 hours of an event. Hypoxemia develops quickly, or may evolve insidi-ously as lung pathology progresses. Aggressive chest phys-iotherapy, incentive spirometry, and reinstitution of med-ications used to treat preexisting pulmonary conditions minimizes loss of lung volume, ventilation-perfusion mis-matching, and infection secondary to aspiration. In cases in which likelihood of significant aspiration is small, followup may be done on an outpatient basis if the chest x-ray film is clear 4 to 6 hours after the event. However, explicit in-structions must be given to contact a medical facility at first appearance of malaise, fever, cough, or other symptoms in-dicative of pneumonitis.

If significant aspiration causes hypoxemia, increased air-way resistance, consolidation, or pulmonary edema with re-duced compliance, institution of ventilatory support with PEEP or CPAP, assisted ventilation, and supplemental oxy-gen is often necessary. Criteria for selection of therapy are similar to those for treatment of ARDS. Pulmonary edema is usually secondary to increased capillary permeability, and should not be treated with diuretics to decrease intravascular volume unless high filling pressures or hypervolemia exist. In fact, hypovolemia from fluid losses into the lung often requires aggressive fluid management.

Although still somewhat controversial, administration of high dose steroids after aspiration has occurred probably yields little real benefit or improvement of long-term out-come.[138-140] Because bacterial infection is not necessarily a component of aspiration pneumonitis, prophylactic antibiotic administration merely promotes colonization by resistant or-ganisms. If evidence of secondary bacterial infection appears, specific antibiotic therapy should be instituted. Sputum sam-ples should be obtained for Gram stain and culture prior to initiating antibiotic therapy. If culture results cannot be ob-tained or are equivocal, broad-spectrum antibiotics should be chosen, with coverage for gram-negative rods and anaerobes including *Bacteroides fragilis*.[141-143]

POSTOPERATIVE RENAL COMPLICATIONS

MONITORING

Evaluation of renal function is important to reduce post-operative morbidity, especially after surgery involving large intravascular volume losses and in patients with marginal cardiovascular status or underlying renal disease. Using urine output as an index of intravascular volume status or renal viability can be misleading, because many surgical and anesthetic factors interfere with renal regulatory mechanisms in postoperative patients.

Ability to spontaneously void should be routinely recorded in all recovering patients, because sympatholytic or parasym-pathomimetic effects of regional anesthetics or opioids inter-fere with sphincter relaxation and promote urinary retention. Patients with indwelling catheters should have urine output recorded hourly.

Postoperative analysis of urine character can yield valuable information concerning renal tubular function.[144] Observation of urine color is relatively useless to estimate renal concentrating ability, but can signal hematuria, hemoglobinuria, or pyuria. Urine osmolarity (affected by number of particles in solution) is more reliable as an index of tubular function than specific gravity, which varies with number of molecules and molecular weight. An osmolarity greater than 450 $mOsm \cdot l^{-1}$ indicates reasonable tubular concentrating ability. (Inorganic fluoride ions released during metabolism of potent inhalation anesthetics such as enflurane may cause a transient, reversible decrease in maximum concentrating ability.) A urine sodium concentration far below or a urine potassium above serum concentrations also indicates renal tubular viability.[145] Osmolarity and electrolyte values close to those in serum may indicate poor tubular function related to acute tubular necrosis. Evaluation of urine pH is also useful, as acidification and alkalinization of urine require intact tubular function.

OLIGURIA

Oliguria (<0.5 ml $\cdot$ kg $\cdot$ hr^{-1}) is frequently encountered during recovery. Usually, postoperative oliguria reflects an appropriate kidney response to real or "perceived" hypovolemia or systemic hypotension. However, decreased urine output occasionally indicates a critical abnormality of renal function. Acceptable degree and duration of oliguria varies with underlying renal status, surgical procedure, and anticipated postoperative course. Oliguria in patients experiencing surgical manipulations or intraoperative events that might jeopardize renal function (i.e., possible inadvertent ureteral ligature, aortic cross clamping, severe hypotensive episodes, massive transfusion) must be aggressively evaluated.

When assessing oliguria in uncatheterized patients, urge to void, bladder fullness, and interval since last voiding should be checked to differentiate between inability to void and oliguria. Catheterization is sometimes necessary. Indwelling catheters should be checked for patency, as obstruction from kinking, blood clots, or debris mimic oliguria. Position changes such as Trendelenburg positioning can force the catheter tip above urine level in the bladder.

Assuring that systemic pressure is adequate for renal perfusion (based on preoperative pressures) is critical in an oliguric patient. To assess possibility of a renal response to hypovolemia, a 300 to 500 ml intravenous crystalloid bolus should be given after specimens are sent for urine electrolytes and osmolarity, even if intraoperative fluid replacement seems adequate. If output does not improve after fluid infusion, one might consider a larger bolus, or a diagnostic trial of 5 mg furosemide. Furosemide overcomes tubular resorption and increases output if oliguria is caused by retention of fluid by the kidneys. Patients on chronic diuretic therapy who require diuretic effect to maintain brisk postoperative urine output also usually respond to a furosemide challenge.

Persistence of oliguria in spite of adequate perfusion pressure, hydration and a low-dose furosemide challenge increases the possibility of acute tubular necrosis, renal artery or vein occlusion, ureteral obstruction, or inappropriate ADH secretion. Cystoscopy, intravenous pyelogram, angiography, or radioisotope imaging may help clarify renal status, whereas pulmonary artery catheterization can clarify cardiovascular function. Although controversial, administration of osmotic or loop diuretics, and low-dose dopamine or dobutamine are probably useful to attenuate renal damage.[146, 147]

POLYURIA

Profuse postoperative urine output is a common occurrence, usually related to generous intraoperative fluid administration. However, sustained polyuria (>4 to 5 ml $\cdot$ kg $\cdot$ hr^{-1}) can indicate abnormal regulation of fluid clearance, especially if urinary losses compromise intravascular volume and systemic blood pressure.

Osmotic diuresis caused by hyperglycemia and glycosuria is a frequent cause of postoperative polyuria. Output can be massive if glucose containing crystalloid solutions are used to replace urinary losses. Diagnosis is made by urine and serum glucose determination. Therapy other than glucose restriction is unnecessary because the process is self-limited. Polyuria might also reflect persistent effects of intraoperative diuretic administration. Polyuria related to diabetes insipidus can occur secondary to intracranial surgery, pituitary ablation, head trauma, increased intracranial pressure, or inadvertent omission of preoperative vasopressin administration. Diagnosis is made by comparison of urine and serum electrolytes and osmolarity. Diagnostic or therapeutic administration of vasopressin can also be useful.[31] Possibility of high output renal failure should also be considered.

METABOLIC COMPLICATIONS

POSTOPERATIVE ACID BASE ABNORMALITIES

Respiratory Acidemia

Respiratory acidemia is probably the most common postoperative acid base abnormality, as potent inhalation anesthetics, opioids, and some sedative medications decrease CNS sensitivity to pH and promote hypoventilation. Hypercarbia and acidemia are usually insignificant in awake, spontaneously ventilating patients. However, deeply anesthetized or sedated patients can suffer serious acidemia without supplemental ventilation. Administration of additional opioid or sedative medications accentuate ventilatory depression.

Postoperative patients are sometimes unable to sustain adequate ventilation in spite of appropriate CNS drive to ventilate. Increased airway resistance, decreased pulmonary compliance, or residual neuromuscular paralysis can severely impede ventilation and generate progressive respiratory acidemia, especially in patients with increased deadspace. An increase in minute production of CO_2 caused by hyperthermia, shivering, hyperalimentation, or malignant hyperthermia contributes to postoperative respiratory acidemia.[83-85]

Acute postoperative respiratory acidemia often causes agitation, dyspnea, and tachypnea as well as hypertension, tachycardia, cardiac dysrhythmias, and other signs of increased SNS activity.[148] Consequently, risk of myocardial ischemia, postoperative bleeding, or cerebrovascular accident may be increased. (Symptoms of respiratory acidemia related to respiratory center depression are often less pronounced, because central autonomic nervous system responses are depressed as well.) Respiratory acidemia increases cerebral blood flow, which can increase intracranial pressure in patients with head injury, intracranial tumors, or cerebral edema. At very low pH, catecholamines no longer effectively interact with adrenergic receptors, so heart rate and blood pressure may decrease precipitously.

Natural compensatory mechanisms for acute respiratory

acidemia are very limited because the kidneys require many hours to generate a compensatory metabolic alkalosis. Therapy of respiratory acidemia must be directed at correcting imbalance between effective alveolar ventilation and CO_2 production through arousal and stimulation, reversal of neuromuscular relaxants or narcotics, relief of airway obstruction, reduction of airway resistance, or improvement of ventilatory mechanics. Occasionally, reduction of CO_2 production by controlling fever or shivering, decreasing work of breathing, or eliminating high glucose loads in hyperalimentation can be employed. (Extreme measures such as core cooling or paralysis are seldom useful in a recovery setting.) If CO_2 elimination cannot be maintained with spontaneous ventilation, then tracheal intubation and mechanical ventilation of the lungs are necessary.

Metabolic Acidemia

Differential diagnosis of postoperative metabolic acidemia is relatively limited. Patients suffering from renal failure, poorly controlled diabetes, severe diarrhea, small bowel drainage, or renal tubular acidosis exhibit some degree of preoperative metabolic acidemia, which persists into the postoperative period. Overdose with certain drugs (phenformin, aspirin) or ingestion of toxic substances (methanol) can also increase metabolic acid load. Postoperative metabolic acidemia is occasionally caused by ketoacidosis in patients with severe diabetes. Serum glucose levels are usually elevated, and ketones are detectable in blood or urine.

In the absence of preexisting metabolic acidemia or ketoacidosis, postoperative metabolic acidemia is almost always caused by lactic acid accumulation related to insufficient delivery or utilization of oxygen in peripheral tissues.[149] In surgical patients, lactic acidemia usually indicates poor peripheral perfusion caused by hypotension from low cardiac output (hypovolemia, cardiac failure, dysrhythmia) or decreased SVR (sepsis, catecholamine depletion). Intense arteriolar constriction from severe hypothermia or inappropriate pressor administration can also reduce perfusion to peripheral tissues. Severe hypoxemia, decreased oxygen carrying capacity of blood (severe anemia, carbon monoxide poisoning), interference with release of oxygen from hemoglobin (alkalemia, hypothermia), or inability of tissues to utilize oxygen (cyanide or arsenic poisoning) can also generate lactic acidemia.

Presentation of metabolic acidemia is similar to that of respiratory acidemia, as signs and symptoms reflect physiologic responses to abnormal pH. However, CNS response to acute metabolic acidemia is often somewhat milder, because hydrogen and bicarbonate ions cross the blood-brain barrier more slowly than CO_2. Similarly, chronic acidemias often generate less dramatic clinical symptoms because CNS bicarbonate concentrations adjust with time to restore brain pH toward normal.

Compensation for postoperative metabolic acidemia through hyperventilation and generation of respiratory alkalosis is rapid, assuming spontaneous ventilation and intact ventilatory drive.[148] Therapy of postoperative metabolic acidemia should be directed at underlying conditions causing accumulation of metabolic acid. Ketoacidosis is treated using intravenous insulin, potassium, and sometimes glucose. Improvement of hypotension or low cardiac output can markedly reduce lactic acid production, as can warming. If conditions causing accumulation of lactic acid are improving and metabolic acidemia are mild, one can allow acidemia to resolve spontaneously through lactic acid metabolism and renal excretion of excess hydrogen ions. However, if acidemia is severe or progressive, intravenous bicarbonate administration is advisable to maintain pH near normal.

Respiratory Alkalemia

Respiratory alkalemia is less frequently encountered during recovery, and is usually less severe than respiratory acidemia. Hyperventilation caused by excessive operative pain or anxiety during emergence from anesthesia is a common cause of postoperative respiratory alkalemia. (Pain from attempts at ABG sampling frequently generates iatrogenic alkalemia). Pathologic causes of central hyperventilation include systemic sepsis, cerebrovascular accident, or paradoxical CNS acidosis (a temporary condition caused by differences in bicarbonate concentration across the blood-brain barrier after chronic mechanical hyperventilation). Delivery of excessive mechanical ventilation frequently causes postoperative respiratory alkalemia, especially in hypothermic or paralyzed patients exhibiting decreased CO_2 production.[148]

Acute respiratory alkalemia usually generates vague clinical symptoms like confusion or dizziness. Atrial dysrhythmias or mild cardiac conduction abnormalities sometimes appear. In patients with cerebrovascular disease, marked respiratory alkalemia may promote cerebral hypoperfusion and even stroke by decreasing cerebral blood flow. Reduction of serum ionized calcium ion concentration can precipitate muscle fasciculation or even hypocalcemic tetany if alkalemia is severe. At very high pH, CNS activity, catecholamine-receptor interaction, and cardiovascular function are all severely affected. Severe iatrogenic alkalemia from excessive hyperventilation or administration of intravenous bicarbonate can preclude resuscitation after cardiopulmonary arrest.

Metabolic compensation for acute respiratory alkalemia is also very limited. Correction of alkalemia necessitates reduction of effective alveolar ventilation, either by control of pain and anxiety using analgesics and sedatives or by reduction in mechanical ventilation. Warming and reversal of paralysis usually have minimal impact on alkalemia. Addition of CO_2 to inspired gases or rebreathing of exhaled CO_2 have little clinical application during recovery.

Metabolic Alkalemia

Acute metabolic alkalemia is rarely a problem in PACU patients, unless intraoperative bicarbonate administration has been excessive or alkalemia existed prior to surgery. (Prolonged vomiting or gastric suctioning, pyloric stenosis, severe dehydration, previous large infusions of Ringer's lactate or blood products containing citrate, excessive administration of alkaline substances, or chronic use of potassium wasting diuretics can generate preoperative metabolic alkalemia that can persist into recovery.)

Respiratory compensation for metabolic alkalemia through retention of CO_2 is rapid but somewhat limited as decrease of ventilation beyond a certain point causes hypoxemia. Treatment of metabolic alkalemia is directed toward resolving conditions causing the acid-base abnormality, in conjunction with hydration and correction of hypochloremia and hypokalemia. Seldom is administration of acid advisable, although intravenous hydrochloric acid drip through central venous catheter can be effectively used to treat severe, life-threatening metabolic alkalemia.

In postoperative patients, characteristic rapid evolution of pathophysiology can often generate two or more primary acid-base disorders. Categorization of postoperative disorders into discrete primary and compensatory couplets is sometimes difficult. Providing appropriate hemodynamic, ventilatory, and metabolic support usually restores postoperative acid-base homeostasis without quantitative diagnosis.

ELECTROLYTES AND GLUCOSE

Hypokalemia

Hypokalemia caused by intraoperative urinary and hemorrhagic losses frequently occurs in postoperative patients, especially those with chronic total body potassium deficits from diuretic administration or starvation.[150, 151] Hypokalemia can be severe after prolonged nasogastric suctioning or diarrhea, massive volume replacement, insulin therapy, or during postoperative respiratory alkalemia. Though generally inconsequential, the risk of serious cardiac dysrhythmias is real, especially in patients taking digitalis preparations. Usually addition of supplemental potassium to intravenous fluids initiates sufficient potassium replacement and maintains serum concentration within acceptable ranges. In selected cases, infusion of concentrated solutions through a central catheter may be necessary. Care should be taken to avoid hyperventilation. Patients should be closely observed during infusion of calcium or beta-mimetic medications, or during periods of excess SNS activity.[152]

Hyperkalemia

Serious postoperative hyperkalemia is occasionally encountered coincident with chronic renal failure, malignant hyperthermia, transfusion of "old" blood, or inadvertent excessive potassium administration.[150] Administration of succinylcholine for intubation of the trachea in the PACU might increase serum potassium to dangerous levels in patients suffering from burns, multiple trauma, neurologic injuries, or neurologic diseases. Acute exacerbation of hyperkalemia occurs if acidemia develops secondary to hypoventilation or hypoperfusion.[153] One should suspect spurious hyperkalemia caused by hemolyzed specimens or sampling near an intravenous infusion containing potassium or banked blood whenever serum potassium is unusually high for no apparent reason. In acute postoperative settings, intravenous insulin and glucose is most efficacious to treat hyperkalemia, while intravenous calcium can temporarily counter myocardial effects. Beta-mimetic medications may also have some role in reduction of serum potassium levels.

Hyponatremia

Postoperative hyponatremia is sometimes seen after transurethral prostatic resection if large amounts of sodium free irrigating solution have been taken up through prostatic venous sinuses.[154] Symptoms include nausea, agitation, visual disturbances, disorientation and hyperactive reflex activity, which can progress to grand mal seizures. Increased serum ammonia levels caused by metabolism of absorbed glycine might exacerbate symptoms.[155] Severe reduction of sodium concentration causes confusion, obtundation, seizures, and decreased effectiveness of airway reflexes. Free water retention and hyponatremia can also be caused by inappropriate ADH secretion, prolonged labor induction with oxytocin, excessive administration of intravenous hypotonic solutions, and respiratory uptake of nebulized droplets.[156] Therapy includes administration of intravenous furosemide to promote renal wasting of free water in excess of sodium and infusion of normal saline. In severe cases, calculation of sodium deficit and administration of hypertonic saline may be necessary, with careful monitoring of serum sodium concentration and osmolality.

Hypocalcemia

Total body and ionized calcium can be decreased after massive fluid replacement, or in patients with underlying parathyroid disease. Though often discussed, symptomatic hypocalcemia caused by extensive transfusion of blood containing chelating agents is rare. Routine postoperative administration of calcium is usually not warranted. However, severe reduction of the critical ionized calcium fraction by metabolic or respiratory alkalemia may cause tetany, conduction abnormalities, reduced myocardial contractility, and decreased vascular tone. Although significant postoperative hypocalcemia seldom occurs, administration of calcium chloride in hypocalcemic patients improves cardiovascular dynamics and "responsiveness" to intravenous fluid administration after major surgical cases.

Hyperglycemia

Elevation of serum glucose caused by infusions and stress response is very common in patients recovering from surgery. Moderate hyperglycemia (<250 to $300\ mg \cdot dl^{-1}$) is generally inconsequential and resolves spontaneously without treatment. (It is doubtful whether transient elevation of serum glucose has any significant effect on wound healing). Higher glucose levels cause glycosuria and osmotic diuresis, interfere with accuracy of serum electrolyte determinations, and increase serum osmotic load. Severe hyperglycemia increases serum osmolality to a point that cerebral dysequilibrium and "hyperosmolar coma" may supervene. In diabetic patients, hyperglycemia may also indicate severe insulin deficiency and evolution of diabetic ketoacidosis. Treatment when necessary includes intravenous regular insulin through small, incremental doses or continuous infusion, potassium replacement, and monitoring of serial blood glucose levels. Intravenous administration of "short-acting" regular insulin allows careful titration of blood glucose, and eliminates delay in peak effect or uptake problems associated with longer acting preparations or subcutaneous administration. Followup with appropriate therapy after discharge from recovery is critical.

Hypoglycemia

Postoperative hypoglycemia is always a serious threat, especially because obtundation or excessive SNS activity in recovering patients may mask signs and symptoms. Hypoglycemia in the PACU can be caused by excessive preoperative or intraoperative administration of long acting insulin, by excessive endogenous insulin secretion, or by inadvertent postoperative insulin administration. Fortunately, serious postoperative hypoglycemia is rare and easily treated by intravenous administration of 50% dextrose in conjunction with infusion of glucose containing solutions.

Repeated accurate monitoring of serum glucose is important in managing postoperative hyperglycemia or hypoglycemia. Urine glucose measurement is inferior to serum glucose determination for blood sugar maintenance. However, urine glucose concentration should be evaluated to assess osmotic diuretic effects and to help estimate renal Tm by comparison with serum levels.

MISCELLANEOUS COMPLICATIONS

A host of postoperative complications unique to anesthesic or surgical manipulations are encountered in the PACU. Although generally minor, incidental complications can have major psychological or physical impact for individual patients.

NAUSEA AND VOMITING

Postoperative nausea and vomiting occurs in a significant percentage of patients recovering from general anesthetics.[157] Risk of postoperative nausea seems higher in females, younger patients, and those with an individual predisposition to nausea or previous postoperative emesis. Obese patients and those undergoing surgical procedures involving middle ear manipulation, peritoneal irritation, or gastrointestinal trauma also probably manifest increased risk. Most likely, several mechanisms are involved in postanesthetic nausea, including direct actions of anesthetics on chemotactic centers, starvation, and autonomic nervous system imbalance. Presence of swallowed blood or secretions and gastric distention often accentuate degree and frequency of vomiting. Use of nitrous oxide has been anecdotally associated with increased incidence of postoperative nausea, although importance of this relationship is questionable.[158] Intraoperative and postoperative administration of opioids undoubtedly contributes to postoperative nausea, especially that occurring after discharge from the PACU. Although conflicting literature exists, meperidine seems to generate a higher incidence of postoperative nausea than morphine.

Aside from unpleasantness for patient and staff, straining and motion during vomiting can increase postoperative pain or jeopardize abdominal or inguinal suture lines. Autonomic nervous system responses to emesis often increase heart rate and systemic blood pressure, increasing risk of cardiovascular, ocular, or intracranial morbidity in selected patients. However, PNS predominance with bradycardia and hypotension can also occur during gagging and retching. Risk of aspiration is obviously increased during postoperative emesis, especially in patients with marginal airway reflexes or those in oral fixation.

Although there is no universally recognized preventative measure for postoperative nausea and vomiting, several interventions seem to reduce incidence. Inclusion of low-dose intravenous droperidol in an anesthetic regimen may decrease incidence and severity of postoperative nausea,[159] especially in ambulatory patients receiving short-acting opioids for one day surgery. Repeating intravenous droperidol in the PACU for breakthrough nausea is also effective, although excessive sedation or hypotension in hypovolemic patients is possible. Other antiemetics are usually less successful. When assessing a patient it is important to rule out other serious causes of nausea and emesis such as hypotension, hypoglycemia, gastric bleeding or bowel obstruction prior to instituting treatment. Limitation of postoperative vestibular stimulation by avoiding brisk head motion may also be efficacious. In patients with a history of severe postoperative nausea, use of regional anesthetic techniques when feasible for intraoperative and postoperative analgesia can reduce parenteral opioid administration and decrease severity and frequency of nausea.

INCIDENTAL TRAUMA

Anesthetized patients in an operating room environment are at risk for incidental trauma related to positioning, nonsurgical manipulations, and equipment.[160] Corneal injury caused by drying or inadvertent eye injury often presents during recovery with tearing, decreased visual acuity, pain, and photophobia. Abrasion is diagnosed with fluoroscein staining and usually heals spontaneously over 24 to 72 hours, leaving no permanent damage. However, severe injury can cause cataract formation and impairment of vision. Treatment with application of artificial tears and eye closure is primarily symptomatic.[161]

Oral soft-tissue trauma secondary to laryngoscopy, indwelling airways, or biting is frequently encountered. Lip, tongue, or gum abrasions generally heal quickly with no therapy other than an icepack, although penetrating injuries caused by entrapment between teeth and laryngoscope blade or airway may require topical antibiotic ointment. After markedly traumatic or difficult tracheal intubations, possibility of upper airway edema or hematoma and obstruction must be considered prior to extubation. Severe airway edema secondary to trauma may respond to administration of nebulized racemic epinephrine. Discovery of loosened or broken dental appliances or teeth in the PACU should be carefully documented and dental consultation obtained. Comparison with preoperative status should be made whenever possible. Observation for fever, cough, or other signs indicating possible aspiration of dental material is important for 48 hours after the event.

Sore throat and hoarseness after endotracheal intubation occur in 20% to 50% of patients, depending on degree of trauma during laryngoscopy, duration of tracheal intubation, and type of tube. Mucosal irritation often presents with a sensation of unquenchable dryness in mouth and throat. Use of local anesthetic ointments probably does not appreciably decrease incidence, and may cause additional irritation to tracheal mucosa.[162] Topical viscous lidocaine attenuates irritation from indwelling nasogastric tubes during recovery. Risk of aspiration secondary to airway anesthesia and interference with reflexes must be balanced against benefit. Other acute complications of laryngoscopy and tracheal intubation include cervical spine injury, hypoglossal or lingual nerve damage, laryngeal or tracheal trauma (e.g., vocal cord evulsion, tracheal tearing or perforation), desquamation of tracheal and laryngeal mucosa, airway wall edema, or ulceration.[163] A small percentage of patients complain of sore throat even without tracheal intubation, related to drying from unhumidified gases or trauma from oral airways or suctioning.

Compression injuries caused by improper positioning during general or regional anesthesia sometimes generate serious, long-term complications.[164] Retinal artery or venous occlusion from unrecognized ocular compression causes postoperative visual disturbances ranging from loss of acuity to permanent blindness. Peripheral nerve compression against metal or other hard surfaces can cause postoperative sensory and motor deficits, as can stretch injuries from inadvertent hyperextension of an extremity. Whenever bruising or skin breakdown related to unnoticed pressure is noted, possible underlying nerve damage should also be considered. Spinal cord injury during positioning or intubation of the trachea is a real possibility, as is nerve injury or accumulation of compressive hematomas related to placement of regional anesthetics. One should carefully evaluate any incidental complaint of pain, numbness, or weakness from a postoperative patient. Soft tissue ischemia and necrosis can occur during long surgical procedures, especially if "pressure points" are improperly padded. Prolonged scalp pressure may cause localized alopecia. Entrapment and necrosis of breasts, genitalia, ears, skin folds, and other superficial soft tissues can also occur, especially during prone or lateral positioning. Regional ischemia secondary to arterial pressure occlusion is possible, though rare. Excess intraoperative joint or muscle extension causes postoperative pain, stiffness, backache, and even joint instability if severe.[165, 166] Thermal, electrical, or chemical burns caused by cautery equipment, preparatory solutions, adhesives or other substances occasionally occur. Extravasation of intravenous medications into tissues may cause severe sloughing or localized chemical neuropathy.

Each patient admitted to a PACU should be carefully evaluated for likely incidental traumatic complications. Incidental injury also occurs in the PACU, especially with thrashing or disorientation during emergence. Possibilities include bruising caused by contact with bedrails, hematoma or drug extravasation caused by dislocation of indwelling catheters, damage to dental appliances caused by biting on rigid airways, and corneal injury caused by rigid disposable facemasks. Discovery or suspicion of a complication necessitates careful documentation, notification of primary physicians responsible for extended postoperative care, arrangement of consultations when appropriate, and assiduous followup. Unfortunately, therapy for most incidental traumatic complications is supportive and expectant.

SKELETAL MUSCLE PAIN

Postoperative skeletal muscle pain is variable in degree, and undoubtedly caused by a variety of intraoperative factors. Prolonged lack of motion or unusual muscle stretch during positioning often contribute to muscle stiffness and aching in the PACU. Administration of succinylcholine has been implicated in causing postoperative myalgias, perhaps related to fasciculation during depolarizing blockade. It is controversial whether administration of a subparalyzing dose of nondepolarizing relaxant to attenuate fasciculation reduces incidence or severity of postoperative myalgia.[167–169] Some patients complain of delayed onset "muscle fatigue" that appears days after surgery and resolves spontaneously. Incidence, etiology, and importance of this problem is unclear.

INADVERTENT HYPOTHERMIA

Many patients undergoing general or regional anesthetics manifest postoperative hypothermia. Intraoperative cooling is caused by low ambient temperature in operating rooms, anesthetic interference with central or peripheral temperature regulating mechanisms, heat loss from surgical wounds, evaporative losses during prepping and respiratory humidification, lack of intraoperative shivering, and administration of cold intravenous fluids.[170] Infants are at increased risk of intraoperative hypothermia because body mass is relatively low when compared to surface area. Elderly, cachectic, traumatized, and burned patients are also more prone to serious reduction of core body temperature. Little difference is noted in amount or rate of heat loss between general and regional anesthetics. However, patients receiving regional anesthetics rewarm more slowly, since residual paralysis of striated musculature and vasodilation interfere with heat generation and retention.

In most cases, reduction of core temperature is less than 2°C to 3°C, and well tolerated. However, patients undergoing prolonged, major surgical procedures with significant blood loss and fluid replacement can arrive in recovery with core temperature below 32°C. Such severe hypothermia can cause serious physiologic changes. Increased SNS activity, elevated SVR, decreased venous capacitance, and hypertension are often evident. Severe hypothermia interferes with cardiac rhythm generation and impulse conduction. Lengthening of the PR, QRS, or QT intervals, and appearance of J waves can appear on ECG. Danger of ectopic impulse generation and dysrhythmia during mechanical stimulation of the myocardium is increased, and spontaneous ventricular fibrillation can occur if temperature falls below 28°C. Hypoperfusion of peripheral tissues promotes tissue hypoxia and metabolic acidemia. Avidity of hemoglobin for oxygen also increases, contributing to poor oxygenation of hypothermic tissues. Reduced peripheral perfusion and decreased rate of drug biotransformation may increase duration of action for muscle relaxants, sedatives, or hypnotics. Similarly, minimum alveolar concentration of inhalation anesthetics decreases approximately 7% per 1°C decrease in core temperature, accentuating sedation from residual alveolar partial pressures. Mild coagulopathy can occur secondary to visceral sequestration of platelets, decreased platelet function, and reduced activity of clotting factors. Moderate to severe hyperglycemia is common during hypothermia.

During emergence from general anesthesia, hypothalamic regulating mechanisms increase metabolic activity and generate shivering in order to increase endogenous heat production and core temperature. However, at less than 32°C, the central shivering response is attenuated, markedly impeding rewarming. Severe postoperative shivering is very uncomfortable, increases risk of incidental trauma, and makes routine postoperative care more difficult to deliver. Accentuated oxygen consumption, cardiac output and CO_2 production markedly increase demands on cardiac and ventilatory reserve. Myocardial ischemia or ventilatory failure can supervene in patients with coronary artery disease or limited ventilatory capacity, because severe shivering can increase peripheral oxygen consumption by 400% to 500%. Intensity of postoperative shivering is sometimes accentuated by postpartum or inhalation anesthetic related "rigors."

Intraoperative maintenance of temperature through warming of ambient air, appropriate covering of body and head surfaces, heated humidification of inspired gases, use of surface or radiant warmers, and warming of intravenous fluids or irrigating solutions minimizes postoperative hypothermia. All hypothermic patients should receive supplemental oxygen in recovery. Patients with oral temperatures above 35°C will passively rewarm during routine recovery, although moderate shivering often occurs. Temperature below 35°C is an indication for assisted rewarming with radiant lighting, heating blankets, reflecting covering, or heated nebulization of inspired gas for intubated patients.[171]

As temperature rises, patients must be carefully observed for hypotension related to increasing venous capacitance, and for posthypothermic hyperthermia.[172] Resolution of metabolic acidemia usually corresponds with rewarming, although bicarbonate administration may be required after prolonged hypothermia. Administration of morphine, meperidine, droperidol, chlorpromazine, magnesium sulfate, or methylphenidate has been advocated to suppress shivering if dangerous cardiopulmonary stress occurs.[173–175] Withholding reversal of intraoperative muscle relaxants in intubated, ventilated patients can also attenuate postoperative shivering, although rewarming time is increased.[176] Wisdom of administering additional muscle relaxants in recovery just to eliminate shivering is questionable.

PERSISTENT OBTUNDATION

Differential diagnosis of prolonged obtundation after general anesthesia requires aggressive and organized evaluation. Level of preoperative responsiveness should be assessed to rule out preexisting obtundation. It is important to check time and amount of all medications with sedative properties or potentiating side-effects. Evaluation of an obtunded patient must include firm tactile stimulus, which is often more effective than verbal stimulus to elicit arousal.

Residual sedation from general anesthetic medications is the most frequent cause of postoperative obtundation and requires no specific therapy.[177] Prolonged postoperative obtundation is especially likely after long surgical procedures, or if high inspired concentrations of inhalation anesthetics are continued through the end of surgery to facilitate a smooth "deep" extubation of the trachea. Long-acting sedatives used for premedication contribute to postoperative somnolence (e.g., pentobarbital, hydroxyzine, promethazine, droperidol, lorazepam, scopolamine) as does excessive intraoperative opioid or sedative administration. Sedative effects of a reasonably conducted anesthetic usually wane within 60 to 90 minutes of admission to the PACU, even in patients who are highly susceptible to sedation. If obtundation persists, low-dose intravenous naloxone (0.04 mg increments every 2 minutes up to 0.2 mg) can be administered.[178] If significant increase in spontaneous ventilation and arousal are not noted, it is unlikely that sedation is related to residual opioid effect unless massive overdose has occurred. Administration of intravenous physostigmine (1.25 mg) may counteract sedative effects of inhalation anesthetics and other sedative medications.[179, 180]

Profound neuromuscular paralysis might rarely mimic prolonged obtundation. This could occur after gross overdosage with relaxants, if reversal agents are inadvertently omitted, or in patients with pseudocholinesterase deficiency or Phase II blockade from excessive succinylcholine administration. Spontaneous ventilation, purposeful motion, reflex activity, or other evidence of neuromuscular function automatically eliminates this possibility.

Once residual anesthetic effects and paralysis have been ruled out, various causes of postoperative coma should be evaluated. The possibility that a patient may be feigning unresponsiveness should be considered. Body temperature should be assessed, because hypothermia below 33°C directly impairs consciousness. Intensity and duration of depressant medication affects are also accentuated. Progressive evolution of coma, fixed dilation of pupils, and absence of reflexes can occur at core temperatures below 30°C. Serum glucose should be checked to rule out severe hypoglycemia or hyperglycemic, hyperosmolar coma. (Suspicion that obtundation may be caused by hypoglycemia is an indication for an immediate empiric trial of intravenous 50% dextrose.) Serum electrolyte concentrations and osmolarity should also be checked to rule out hyponatremia, hypocalcemia, hypercalcemia, hypomagnesemia, or hypoosmolar states. Unrecognized preoperative overdose with depressant oral medication is possible in emergency patients, even if response to naloxone and physostigmine is absent.

A thorough neurological evaluation should be performed, with careful documentation of findings. Consultation with a neurologist might be helpful at this point. Untoward intraoperative influences such as severe hypotension or hypertension, cardiac dysrhythmias, hypoxemia or hypercarbia must be considered as possible causes. Possibility of unrecognized preoperative head trauma and evolving increased intracranial pressure should be assessed. Likelihood of intraoperative cerebral thromboembolism should be considered, especially in patients recovering from cardiac, proximal major vascular, or invasive neck surgery[181, 182], or those who have undergone internal jugular, subclavian, or intraarterial cannulation. Patients with a history of atrial fibrillation or hypercoagulable states are also at increased risk. Paradoxical air embolism through a right to left intracardiac shunt, or intracerebral hemorrhage are also possible.[183] Of course, in patients recovering from intracranial surgery, increased intracranial pressure from bleeding, edema, or pneumocephalus must also be considered.[184]

REFERENCES

1. Willock MM, Willock GM: Design of the recovery room. In Israel JS, Dekornfeld TJ (eds): Recovery Room Care, p 6. Chicago, Year Book Medical Publishers, 1987
2. Finch JS: Equipment and monitoring. In Israel JS, Dekornfeld TJ (eds): Recovery Room Care, p 25. Chicago, Year Book Medical Publishers, 1987
3. Willock MM: Management and staffing: In Israel JS, Dekornfeld TJ (eds): Recovery Room Care, p 84. Chicago, Year Book Medical Publishers, 1987
4. Drain CB, Shipley SB: The Recovery Room. Philadelphia, WB Saunders, 1979
5. Yelderman MH, New W: Evaluation of pulse oximetry. Anesthesiology 59:349, 1983
6. Orkin LR, Shapiro G: Admission, assessment and general monitoring. In Frost EAM, Andrews IC (eds): Recovery Room Care. International Anesthesiology Clinics, p 1. Boston, Little, Brown & Co., 1983
7. Henderson JJ, Parbrook GD: Influence of anaesthetic technique on postoperative pain. Br J Anaesth 48:587, 1976
8. Bridenbaugh PO, Du Pen SL, Moore DC: Postoperative intercostal nerve block analgesia versus narcotic analgesia. Anesth Analg 52:81, 1973
9. Toledo-Pereyra LH, DeMeester TR: Prospective randomized evaluation of intrathoracic intercostal nerve block with Dupicaine on postoperative ventilatory function. Ann Thorac Surg 27(3):203, 1979
10. Shuman RL, Peters RG: Epidural anesthesia following thoracotomy in patients with chronic obstructive airway disease. J Thorac Cardiovasc Surg 71:82, 1976
11. Pflug AE, Murphy TM, Butler SH: The effects of postoperative peridural analgesia in pulmonary therapy and pulmonary complication. Anesthesiology 41:8, 1974
12. Chrubasik J, Wiemers K: Continuous-plus-on-demand epidural infusion of morphine for postoperative pain relief by means of a small, externally worn infusion device. Anesthesiology 62:263, 1985
13. Lanz E, Kehrberger E, Theiss D: Epidural morphine: A clinical double blind study of dosage. Anesth Analg 64:786, 1985
14. Cuschieri, RJ, Morran CG, Howie JC et al: Postoperative pain

and pulmonary complications: Comparison of three analgesic regimens. Br J Surg 72:495 1985

15. Chayen MS, Rudick V, Borvine A: Pain control with epidural injection of morphine. Anesthesiology 53:338, 1980

16. Cousins MJ, Mather LE: Intrathecal and epidural administration of opioids. Anesthesiology 61:276, 1984

17. Aldrete JA, Kroulik D: A postanesthetic recovery score. Anesth Analg 49:924, 1970

18. Steward DJ: A simplified system for the postoperative recovery room. Can Anaesth Soc J, 22:111, 1975

19. Farman JV: The work of the recovery room. Br J Hosp Med 19:606, 1978

20. Lindrop MJ: Complications and morbidity of controlled hypotension. Br J Anaesth 47:799, 1975

21. Kirklin JW, Theye RA: Cardiac performance after open intracardiac surgery. Circulation 28:1061, 1963

22. Southorn PA, March HM: Postoperative care of the cardiac surgical patient: Cardiovascular care. In Tarhan S (ed): Cardiovascular Anesthesia and Postoperative Care, p 475. Chicago, Year Book Medical Publishers, 1982

23. Ivanov J, Weisel RD, Mickleborough LL et al: Rewarming hypovolemia after aortocoronary bypass surgery. Crit Care Med 12:1049, 1984

24. Ellison N: Diagnosis and management of bleeding disorders. Anesthesiology 47:171, 1977

25. Barash PG: Monitoring myocardial oxygen balance: Physiologic basis and clinical application. In Barash PG, Deutsch S, Tinker J (eds): Refresher Courses in Anesthesiology, vol 12, p 21. Philadelphia, JB Lippincott, 1985

26. Coriat P: Left ventricular dysfunction after non-cardiac surgical procedures in patients with ischemic heart disease. Acta Anaesthesiol Scand 29:804, 1985

27. Slogoff S, Keats AS: Does perioperative myocardial ischemia lead to postoperative myocardial infarction? Anesthesiology 62:107, 1985

28. Chambers DA: Acquired valvular disease. In Kaplan JA (ed): Cardiac anesthesia, p 197. New York, Grune & Stratton, 1979

29. Wade JG, Larson CP Jr, Hickey RF: Effect of carotid endarterectomy on carotid chemoreceptor and baroreceptor function in man. N Engl J Med 282:823, 1977

30. Bove EL, Fry WJ, Gross WS et al: Hypotension and hypertension as consequences of baroreceptor dysfunction following carotid endarterectomy. Surgery 86:633, 1979

31. Marsh ML, Marshall LF, Shapiro HM: Neurosurgical intensive care. Anesthesiology 47:149, 1977

32. Cohn JN, Franciosa JA: Drug therapy: Vasodilator therapy of cardiac failure. N Engl J Med 297:27, 254, 1977

33. Myers RW: Effects of nitroglycerine and nitroglycerine-methoxamine during acute myocardial ischemia in dogs with pre-existing multivessel coronary occlusive disease. Circulation 51:632, 1975

34. Gal TJ, Cooperman LH: Hypertension in the immediate postoperative period. Br J Anaesth 47:70, 1975

35. Sladen RN: Temperature and ventilation after hypothermic cardiopulmonary bypass. Anesth Analg 64:816, 1985

36. Satiani B, Vasko JS, Zarins CK: Hypertension following carotid endarterectomy. Arch Surg 117:1073, 1982

37. Breslow MJ, Miller CF, Parker SD et al: Changes in T-wave morphology following anesthesia and surgery: A common recovery room phenomenon. 64:398, 1986

38. Atlee JL: Causes for perioperative cardiac dysrhythmias. In Atlee JL (ed): Perioperative cardiac dysrhythmias: Mechanisms recognition and treatment, p 151. Chicago, Year Book Medical Publishers, 1985

39. Pratila MG, Pratila V: Anesthetic agents and cardiac electromechanical activity. Anesthesiology 49:338, 1978

40. Cranefield PF, Wit AL, Hoffman BF: Genesis of cardiac arrhythmias. Circulation 47:408, 1973

41. Fisch C: Relation of electrolyte disturbances to cardiac arrhythmias. Circulation 47:408, 1973

42. Wit AL, Rosen MR, Hoffman BF: Electrophysiology and pharmacology of cardiac arrhythmias II: Relationship of normal and abnormal electrical activity of cardiac fibers to genesis of arrhythmias. B: Reentry. Am Heart J 88:664, 1974

43. Beard K, Jick H, Walker AM: Adverse respiratory events occurring in the recovery room after general anesthesia. Anesthesiology 64:269, 1986

44. Epstein BS: Recovery from anesthesia. Anesthesiology 43:285, 1975

45. Hewlett AM, Branthwaite MA: Postoperative pulmonary function. Br J Anaesth 47:102, 1975

46. Mitchell RA, Berger AJ: Neural regulation of respiration. Am Rev Respir Dis 111:206, 1975

47. Harper MH, Hickey RF, Cromwell TH: The magnitude and duration of respiratory depression produced by fentanyl and fentanyl plus droperidol in man. J Pharm Exp Ther 199:464, 1976

48. Jordan C: Assessment of the effects of drugs on respiration. Br J Anaesth 54:763, 1982

49. Hudson HE, Harber PI, Smith TC: Respiratory depression from alkalosis and opioid interaction in man. Anesthesiology 40:543, 1974

50. Knill RL, Gelb AW: Ventilatory responses to hypoxia and hypercarbia during halothane sedation and anesthesia in man. Anesthesiology 49:244, 1978

51. Becker LD, Paulson BA, Miller RD: Biphasic respiratory depression after fentanyl-droperidol or fentanyl alone used to supplement nitrous oxide anesthesia. Anesthesiology 44:291, 1976

52. Fink BR: Influence of cerebral activity in wakefulness on regulation of breathing. J Appl Physiol 16:15, 1961

53. Lugliani R, Whipp BJ, Seard C: Effect of bilateral carotid body resection on ventilatory control at rest and during exercise in man. N Engl J Med 285:1105, 1971

54. Suzuki M, Sasaki CT: Laryngeal spasm: A neurophysiologic redefinition. Annals of Otolaryngology 86:150, 1977

55. Slutsky AS, Watson J, Leith DE et al: Tracheal insufflation of oxygen (TRIO) at low flow rates sustains life for several hours. Anesthesiology 63:278, 1985

56. Aviado DM: Regulation of bronchomotor tone during anesthesia. Anesthesiology 42:68, 1975

57. Ingram RA, Wellman JS, McFadden ER: Relative contributions of large and small airways to flow limitation in normal subjects before and after atropine and isoproterenol. J Clin Invest 59:696, 1977

58. Hedenstierna G, Santesson J: Breathing mechanics, deadspace and gas exchange in the extremely obese. Acta Anaesthesiol Scand 20:248, 1976

59. Paul DR, Hoyt JL, Boutros AR: Cardiovascular and respiratory changes in response to change of posture in the very obese. Anesthesiology 45:73, 1976

60. Weinberg JSE, Weiss ST, Cohen WR et al: Pregnancy and the lung. Am Rev Respir Dis 121:559, 1980

61. Miller HAB, Taylor GA, Harrison AW et al: Management of flail chest. Ann Thorac Surg 129:1104, 1984

62. Bergofsky EH: Respiratory failure in disorders of the thoracic cage. Can Med Assoc J 119:643, 1979

63. Ali J, Weisel RD, Layug AB: Consequences of postoperative alterations in respiratory mechanics. Am J Surg 128:376, 1974

64. Kerr JH, Crampton Smith AC, Prys-Roberts C: Observations during endobronchial anaesthesia II: Oxygenation Br J Anaesth 46:84, 1974

65. Robin ED, Cross CE, Zelis R: Pulmonary edema. N Engl J Med 288:239, 1973

66. Katz JA, Marks JD: Inspiratory work with and without continuous positive airway pressure in patients with acute respiratory failure. Anesthesiology 63:598, 1985

67. Nunn JF: Elastic resistance to ventilation. In JF Nunn (ed): Applied Respiratory Physiology, p 63. London, Butterworths, 1977

68. d'Empaire G, Hoaglin DC, Perlo VP et al: Effect of prethymectomy plasma exchange on postoperative respiratory function in myasthenia gravis. J Thorac Cardiovasc Surg 89:592, 1985

69. Burkett L, Bikhazi GB, Thomas KC: Mutual potentiation of the neuromuscular effects of antibiotics and relaxants. Anesth Analg 58:107 1976

70. Miller RD, Savarese JJ: Pharmacology of muscle relaxants, their antagonists, and monitoring of neuromuscular function. In RD Miller (ed): Anesthesia, p 487. New York, Churchill Livingstone, 1981

71. Ford GT, Whitelaw WA, Rosenal TW et al: Diaphragm function after upper abdominal surgery in humans. Am Rev Respir Dis 127:431, 1983

72. Rigg RA, Rondi P: Changes in rib cage and diaphragm contribution in ventilation after morphine. Anesthesiology 55:507, 1981

73. Dureuil B, Desmonts JM, Mankikian B et al: Effects of aminophylline on diaphragmatic dysfunction after upper abdominal surgery. Anesthesiology 62:242, 1985

74. Loh L, Hughes JMB, Newson Davis J: The regional distribution of ventilation and perfusion in paralysis of the diaphragm. Am Rev Respir Dis 119:121, 1979

75. Troyer AD, Heilporn A: Respiratory mechanics in quadriplegia: The respiratory function of the intercostal muscles. Am Rev Respir Dis 122:591 1980

76. Gibson GJ, Pride NB, Davis JN: Pulmonary mechanics in patients with respiratory muscle weakness. Am Rev Respir Dis 115:389, 1977

77. Richardson JD, Adams L, Flint LM: Selective management of flail chest and pulmonary contusion. Ann Surg 128:481, 1982

78. Nuhn JF: Respiratory dead space. In JF Nunn (ed): Applied Respiratory Physiology, p 213. London Butterworths, 1977

79. Suter PM, Fairley HB, Isenberg MD: Optimum end expiratory airway pressure in patients with acute pulmonary failure. N Engl J Med 292:284, 1975

80. Adornato DC, Gildeenberg PL, Ferrario CM et al: Pathophysiology of intravenous air embolism in dogs. Anesthesiology 49:120, 1978

81. Moser KM: Pulmonary embolism. Am Rev Respir Dis 115:829, 1977

82. Khambatta HJ, Stone JG, Matteo RS: Effect of sodium nitroprusside-induced hypotension on pulmonary deadspace. Br J Anaesth 54:1197, 1982

83. Askanazi J, Mordenstraum J, Rosenbaum SH et al: Nutrition for the patient with respiratory failure. Anesthesiology 54:373, 1981

84. Steward DJ: Malignant hyperthermia—The acute crisis. In Britt BA (ed): Malignant Hyperthermia Int Anesthesiol Clin 17(4):1, 1979

85. Grinberg R, Edelist G, Gordon A: Postoperative malignant hyperthermia episodes in patients who received "safe" anesthetics. Can Anaesth Soc J 30:273, 1983

86. Meyers JR, Lambeck L, O'Kane H: Changes in functional residual capacity of the lung after operation. Arch Surg 110:576, 1975

87. Ali J, Weisel RD, Layug AB: Consequences of postoperative alterations in respiratory mechanics. Am J Surg 128:376, 1974

88. Craig DB: Postoperative recovery of pulmonary function. Anesth Analg 60:46, 1981

89. Tokics L, Hedenstierna G, Strandberg A et al: Lung collapse and gas exchange during general anesthesia: Effects of spontaneous breathing, muscle paralysis, and positive end expiratory pressure. Anesthesiology 66:157, 1987

90. Rehder K, Marsh HM, Rodarte JR: Airway closure. Anesthesiology 47:40, 1977

91. Parfrey PS, Harte PJ, Quinlan JP: Pulmonary function in the early postoperative period. Br J Surg 64:384, 1977

92. Marshall BE, Wyche MQ Jr: Hypoxemia during and after anesthesia. Anesthesiology 37:178, 1972

93. Don HF, Wahbe WM, Craig DB: Airway closure, gas trapping and the functional residual capacity during anesthesia. Anesthesiology 36:533, 1972

94. Larsson A, Malmkvist G, Werner O: Variations in lung volume and compliance during pulmonary surgery. Br J Anaesth 59:585, 1987

95. Benumof JL: One lung ventilation and hypoxic pulmonary vasoconstriction. Anesth Analg 64:821, 1985

96. Jackson FN, Rowland V, Corssen G: Laryngospasm induced pulmonary edema. Chest 78:819, 1980

97. Bartlett RH, Gazzaniga AB, Geraghty TR: Respiratory maneuvers to prevent postoperative pulmonary complications. JAMA 224:1017, 1973

98. Inverson LIG, Ecker RR, Fox HE et al: A comparative study of IPPB, the incentive spirometer, and blow bottles: The prevention of atelectasis following cardiac surgery. Ann Thoracic Surg 25:197, 1978

99. Craven JL, Evans GA, Davenport PJ et al: The evaluation of the incentive spirometer in the management of postoperative pulmonary complications. Br J Surg 61:793, 1974

100. Spence AA, Smith G: Postoperative analgesia and lung function: A comparison of morphine with extradural block. Br J Anaesth 43:144, 1971

101. Gibson RL, Comer PB, Beckman RW: Actual tracheal oxygen concentrations with commonly used oxygen equipment. Anesthesiology 44:71, 1976

102. McAslan TC, Matjasko-Chiu J, Turney SZ et al: Influence of inhalation of 100% oxygen on intrapulmonary shunt in severely traumatized patients. J Trauma 13:811, 1973

103. Miller JN, Winter PM: Clinical manifestations of pulmonary oxygen toxicity. In Brodsky JB (ed): Clinical aspects of oxygen. Int Anesthesiol Clin 19(3):179, 1981

104. Goldiner PG, Carlon GC, Cvifkovic E: Factors influencing postoperative morbidity and mortality in patients treated with bleomycin. Br J Med 1:1664, 1978

105. LaMantia KR, Glick JH, Marshall BE: Supplemental oxygen does not cause respiratory failure in bleomycin treated patients. Anesthesiology 60:65, 1984

106. Greenbaum DM, Millen JE, Eross B: Continuous positive airway pressure without tracheal intubation in spontaneously breathing patients. Chest 69:615, 1976

107. Feeley TW, Saumarez R, Klick JM et al: Positive end expiratory pressure in weaning patients from controlled ventilation. Lancet 2:725, 1975

108. Quist J, Pontoppidan H, Wilson R: Hemodynamic responses to PEEP. Anesthesiology 42:45, 1975

109. Cullen DJ, Caldera DL: The incidence of ventilator-induced pulmonary barotrauma in critically ill patients. Anesthesiology 50:185, 1979

110. Huseby JS, Pavlin EG, Butler J: Effect of PEEP on intracranial pressure. J Appl Physiol 44:225, 1978

111. Ellman H, Dembin H: Lack of adverse hemodynamic effects of PEEP in patients with acute respiratory failure. Crit Care Med 10:706, 1982

112. West JB: Blood flow to the lung and gas exchange. Anesthesiology 41:124, 1974

113. Roos A, Thomas LJ, Nagel EL: Pulmonary vascular resistance as

determined by lung inflation and vascular pressures. J Appl Physiol 16:77, 1961

114. Benumof JL, Wahrenbrock EH: Blunted hypoxic pulmonary vasoconstriction by increasing lung vascular pressure. J Appl Physiol 38:846, 1975

115. Fung YC, Sobin SS: Pulmonary alveolar blood flow. Circ Res 30:470, 1972

116. Mathers J, Benumof JL, Wahrenrock EA: General anesthetics and regional hypoxic pulmonary vasoconstriction. Anesthesiology 46:111, 1977

117. Benumof JL: Hypoxic pulmonary vasoconstriction and sodium nitroprusside perfusion. Anesthesiology 50:481, 1979

118. Hales CA, Kazemi H: Hypoxic pulmonary response of the lung: Effect of aminophylline and epinephrine. Am Rev Respir Dis 110:126, 1974

119. Reeves JT, Grover RF: Blockade of acute hypoxic pulmonary hypertension by endotoxin. J Appl Physiol 36:328, 1974

120. Daoud FS, Reeves JT, Schaefer JW: Failure of hypoxic pulmonary vasoconstriction in patients with liver cirrhosis. J Clin Invest 51:1076, 1972

121. Catley DM, Thornton C, Jordan C et al: Pronounced episodic oxygen desaturation in the postoperative period: Its association with ventilatory pattern and analgesic regimen. Anesthesiology 63:20, 1985

122. Weil JV, McCullough RE, Kline JS: Diminished ventilatory response to hypoxia and hypercapnia after morphine. N Engl J Med 292:1103, 1975

123. Fink BR, Carpenter SL, Holaday DA: Diffusion anoxia during recovery from nitrous oxide/oxygen anesthesia. Fed Proc 13:354, 1954

124. Davidson JT, Rubin S, Eyal Z: A comparison of the pulmonary response to the endotracheal instillation of 0.1 N hydrochloric acid and Hartmann's solution in the rabbit. Br J Anaesth 46:127, 1974

125. Bartlett JG, Gorbach SL: The triple threat of aspiration pneumonia. Chest 68:560, 1975

126. Patterson AR: Pulmonary aspiration syndromes. In Kirby RR, Taylor RW (eds): Respiratory Failure, p 245. Chicago, Year Book Medical Publishers, 1986

127. Teabeaut JR. Aspiration of gastric contents: An experimental study. Am J Pathol 28:51, 1951

128. Greenfield LJ, Singleton RP, McCaffree DR: Pulmonary effects of experimental graded aspiration of hydrochloric acid. Ann Surg 170:74, 1969

129. Schwartz DJ, Wynne JW, Gibbs CP: The pulmonary consequences of aspiration of gastric contents at pH values greater than 2.5. Am Rev Respir Dis 121:119, 1980

130. Vidyarthi SC: Diffuse miliary granulomatosis of the lungs due to aspirated vegetable cells. Arch Pathol 83:215, 1967

131. Laxmaiah M, Colliver JA, Marrero TC et al: Assessment of age related acid aspiration risk factors in pediatric, adult and geriatric patients. Anesth Analg 64:11, 1985

132. James CF, Gibbs CP, Banner T: Postpartum perioperative risk of aspiration pneumonia. Anesthesiology 61:756, 1984

133. Gibbs CP, Schwartz DJ, Wynne JW: Antacid pulmonary aspiration in the dog. Anesthesiology 51:380, 1979

134. Solanki DR, Suresh M, Ethridge HC: The effects of intravenous cimetidine and metoclopramide on gastric volume and pH. Anesth Analg 63:599, 1984

135. Manchikanti L, Colliver J, Marrero T et al: Ranitidine and metoclopramide for prophylaxis of aspiration pneumonitis in elective surgery. Anesth Analg 63:903, 1984

136. Tryba M, Zenz M, Mlasowsky B et al: Does a stomach tube enhance regurgitation during general anesthesia? Anaesthetist 32:407, 1983

137. Petring OU, Adelhoj B, Jensen BN et al: Prevention of silent aspiration due to leaks around cuffs of endotracheal tubes. Anesth Analg 65:777, 1986

138. Chapman RL, Downs JB, Modell JH: The ineffectiveness of steroid therapy in treating aspiration of hydrochloric acid. Arch Surg 108:858, 1974

139. Winne JW, DeMarco FJ, Hood CI: Physiologic effects of corticosteroids in foodstuff aspiration. Arch Surg 116:46, 1981

140. Gates S, Huang T, Cheney FW: Effects of methylprednisolone on resolution of acid aspiration pneumonitis. Arch Surg 118:1262, 1983

141. Bynum LJ, Pierce AK: Pulmonary aspiration of gastric contents. Am Rev Respir Dis 114:1129, 1976

142. Lewis RT, Burgess JH, Hampson LG: Cardiorespiratory studies in critical illness. Arch Surg 103:335, 1971

143. Bartlett JG, Gorbach SL, Finegold S: The bacteriology of aspiration pneumonia. Am J Med 56:202, 1974

144. Berns AS, Linas SL, Miller TR: Urinary diagnostic indices in acute renal failure. Kidney Int 10:495, 1976

145. Espinel CH: The FE$_{Na}$ test: Use in the differential diagnosis of acute renal failure. JAMA 236:579, 1976

146. Levinsky NG, Bernard DB, Johnson TA: Mannitol and loop diuretics in acute renal failure. In Brenner BM, Lazarus JM (eds): Acute Renal Failure, p 462. Philadelphia, WB Saunders, 1983

147. Hilberman M, Maseda J, Stinson EB et al: The diuretic properties of dopamine in patients after open heart operation. Anesthesiology 61:489, 1984

148. Cohen JJ, Madias NE: Acid base disorders of respiratory origin. In Brenner BM, Stein JH (eds): Acid base and potassium homeostasis. p 137. New York, Edinburgh, London, Churchill Livingstone, 1978

149. Relman AS: Lactic acidosis. In Brenner BM, Stein JH (eds): Acid base and potassium homeostasis, p 65. New York, Edinburgh, London, Churchill Livingstone, 1978

150. Kliger AS, Hayslett JB: Disorders of potassium balance. In Brenner BM, Stein JH (eds): Acid base and potassium homeostasis, p 168. New York, Edinburgh, London, Churchill Livingstone, 1978

151. Vitez TS, Soper LE, Wong KC et al: Chronic hypokalemia and intraoperative dysrhythmias. Anesthesiology 63:130, 1985

152. Brown MJ, Brown DC, Murphy MB: Hypokalemia from beta-2 receptor stimulation by circulating epinephrine. N Engl J Med 309:1414, 1983

153. Scribner BH, Fremont-Smith K, Burnell JM: The effect of acute respiratory acidosis on the internal equilibrium of potassium. J Clin Invest 34:1278, 1975

154. Desmond J: Complications of transurethral prostatic surgery. Can Anaesth Soc J 17:25, 1970

155. Roesch RP, Stoelting RK, Lingeman JE: Ammonia toxicity resulting from glycine absorption during a transurethral resection of the prostate. Anesthesiology 58:577, 1983

156. Bancroft ML: Problems with humidifiers. In Rendell-Baker L (ed): Problems with anesthetic and respiratory equipment. International Anesthesiol Clin 20(3):95, 1982

157. Palazzo MGA, Strunin L: Anesthesia and emesis: Etiology. Can Anaesth Soc J 31:178, 1984

158. Muir JJ, Warner MA, Offord KP et al: Role of nitrous oxide and other factors in postoperative nausea and vomiting: A randomized and blinded prospective study. Anesthesiology 66:513, 1987

159. Cohen SE, Woods WA, Wyner J: Antiemetic effects of droperidol and metaclopramide. Anesthesiology 60:67, 1984

160. Cullen DJ, Cullen BL: Post anesthetic complications. Surg Clin North Am 55:987, 1975

161. Batra KY, Bali ML: Corneal abrasion during general anesthesia. Anesth Analg 56:363, 1977

162. Stock MC, Downs JB: Lubrication of tracheal tubes to prevent sore throat from intubation. Anesthesiology 57:418, 1982

163. Keane WM, Denneny JC, Rowe LD et al: Complications of intubation. Ann Otol Rhinol Laryngol 91:584, 1982

164. Dornette WHL: Compression neuropathies: Medical aspects and legal implications. In Hindman BJ (ed): Neurological and psychological complications of surgery and anesthesia, p 201. Boston, Little, Brown & Co, 1986

165. Lincoln JR, Sawyer HP: Complications related to body position during surgical procedures. Anesthesiology 22:800, 1961

166. O'Donnovan N, Healy TEJ, Faragher EB et al: Postoperative backache: The use of an inflatable wedge. Br J Anaesth 58:280, 1986

167. Brodsky JB, Brock-Unte JG, Samuels SI. Pancuronium pretreatment and post-succinylcholine myalgias. Anesthesiology 51:259, 1979

168. Jansen EC, Hansen PH: Objective measurement of succinylcholine-induced fasciculation and the effect of pretreatment with pancuronium or gallamine. Anesthesiology 51:159, 1979

169. Manchikanti L, Grow JB, Colliver JA et al: Atracurium pretreatment for succinylcholine induced fasciculations and postoperative myalgia. Anesth Analg 64:1010, 1985

170. Morris RH, Wilkey BR: The effect of ambient temperature during surgery not involving body cavities. Anesthesiology 32:102, 1970

171. Lilly RB: Inadvertent hypothermia, a real problem. In Barbash PG, Deutsch S, Tinker J (eds): Refresher Courses in Anesthesiology, vol 15, p 93. Philadelphia, JB Lippincott, 1987

172. Martyn JW: Diagnosing and treating hypothermia. Can Med J 125:1089, 1981

173. Rodriguez JL, Weissman C, Damask MC: Morphine and postoperative rewarming in critically ill patients. Circulation 68:1238, 1983

174. Liem ST, Aldrette JA: Control of post anaesthetic shivering. Can Anaesth Soc J 21:506, 1974

175. Claybon LE, Hirsch RA: Meperidine arrests postanesthetic shivering. Anesthesiology 59(3A):S180, 1983

176. Rodriguez JL, Weissman JC, Damask MC et al: Physiologic requirements during rewarming: Suppression of the shivering response. Crit Care Med 11:490, 1983

177. Denlinger JK: Prolonged emergence and failure to regain consciousness. In Orkin FK, Cooperman LH (eds): Complications in Anesthesiology, p 368. Philadelphia, JB Lippincott, 1983

178. Longnecker DE, Grazis PA, Eggers GWN: Naloxone for antagonism of morphine induced respiratory depression. Anesth Analg 52:447, 1973

179. Bourke DI, Rosenberg M, Allen P: Physostigmine: Effectiveness as an antagonist of respiratory depression and psychomotor effects caused by morphine or diazepam. Anesthesiology 61:523, 1984

180. Hill GE, Stanley TH, Seutker CR: Physostigmine reversal of postoperative somnolence. Can Anaesth Soc J 51:256, 1977

181. Skillman JJ: Neurologic complications of cardiovascular surgery: I. Procedures involving the carotid arteries and abdominal aorta. In Hindman BJ (ed): Neurological and psychological complications of surgery and anesthesia, p 135. Boston, Little, Brown & Co, 1986

182. Shaw PJ: Neurologic complications of cardiovascular surgery: II. Procedures involving the heart and thoracic aorta. In Hindman BJ (ed): Neurological and psychological complications of surgery and anesthesia, p 159. Boston, Little, Brown & Co, 1986

183. Hindman BJ: Perioperative stroke: The noncardiac surgical patient. In Hindman BJ (ed): Neurological and psychological complications of surgery and anesthesia, p 101. Boston, Little, Brown & Co, 1986

184. Toung TJ, McPherson RW, Ahn H et al: Pneumocephalus: Effects of patient position on the incidence and location of aerocele after posterior fossa and upper cervical cord surgery. Anesth Analg 65:65, 1986

Chapter 53

Stephen E. Abram

Pain—Acute and Chronic

PAIN PATHWAYS AND MECHANISMS

Pain is most often experienced as a result of injury. Its survival value to an organism is based on the fact that it is initiated by tissue injury or by stimuli that threatens damage,[1] and it produces sufficient arousal and distress that it is unlikely to be ignored. It is tempting to envision pain as a straightforward receptive system with transducers that respond to intense, tissue-threatening stimuli and neurons that project to areas of the brain capable of processing pain information. Unfortunately, such a view of pain perception fails to explain the tremendous variation in pain sensitivity between individuals or the major changes in sensitivity that can occur in a single individual. It also fails to explain chronic pain that is experienced without any noxious stimulation. Oversimplified anatomic concepts also predispose to simplistic therapeutic interventions, such as neurectomy or rhizotomy, which may aggravate rather than relieve pain.

In reality, the nociceptive system is highly complex and highly adaptable. Sensitivity of most of its components can be reset by a variety of physiological conditions. Injury to neural elements may result in loss of ability to perceive pain or may cause spontaneous pain or heightened pain sensitivity.

An understanding of acute pain perception requires a knowledge of the physiology of receptors that respond to tissue-threatening stimuli, the anatomy of peripheral and central nervous system (CNS) neural pathways that are activated by noxious stimulation, and the mechanisms by which various components of the pain projection system can be modulated or sensitized. Mechanisms of chronic pain are even more complex. Chronic injury may lead to marked alterations in nociceptor sensitivity or to spontaneous firing of peripheral or central pain projection fibers. To further complicate matters, a variety of psychological and behavioral alterations frequently occur in patients with long-standing pain. This chapter provides an overview of the anatomic pathways, the physiological modulating mechanisms, and the pathological alterations that are important to the perception of pain.

ANATOMIC PATHWAYS

NOCICEPTORS

The existence of receptors that respond exclusively to intense, potentially tissue-damaging stimuli is now well accepted. Cutaneous nociceptors have been extensively studied and are now fairly well characterized. Receptors responsive to intense stimuli have been studied in deep somatic structures, but considerably less is known about their response characteristics and function, and still less is known about the physiology of visceral pain.

CUTANEOUS NOCICEPTORS

There are two principle groups of cutaneous nociceptors—high threshold mechanoreceptors (HTMs), which have thinly myelinated axons and respond only to intense mechanical stimuli, and polymodal nociceptors (PMNs), which have unmyelinated (C) fibers and respond to intense mechanical or thermal stimuli and to a variety of chemical irritants.[1] The receptors themselves are morphologically free nerve endings.

HTM axons conduct mainly in the A-delta range, although velocities into the alpha-beta range have been recorded.[2] They respond to strong pressure applied to several discrete points within a receptive field that can cover 1 cm² of skin or more. HTMs do not ordinarily respond to noxious heating of the skin, but may become responsive to heating following a period of sensitization by high temperatures.[3] The receptors of HTMs have been recently described through electron microscopic studies.[4] Fine myelinated fibers were shown to send non-myelinated processes into the epidermis, terminating near keratinocytes in the basal layer. Myelinated mechanical nociceptors are generally believed to subserve fast, well localized, pricking pain.

PMN units respond with slow adaptation to strong pressure. They respond rapidly to noxious heat and are excited by a range of irritant chemicals.[2] Receptive fields may be over 1 cm wide in primates.[5] Firing frequency increases in a roughly linear fashion as skin temperature is increased within the noxious range. Some units demonstrate sensitization by prior strong heating of the receptive field. Heat sensitization is probably related to release of several peptides and amines from local tissues.[2]

Small myelinated axons that respond to noxious heat, strong pressure, and chemical irritation have been found in humans[6] and nonhuman primates.[7] These rapidly conducting polymodal nociceptors may be responsible for rapid reactions to intense heating of the skin. Some fibers that appear to be insensitive or poorly responsive to strong mechanical stimuli have been described. These units have been termed thermal nociceptors, but are probably best characterized as polymodal units that occupy the most insensitive end of the mechanical sensitivity range.[2] Likewise, some C fibers have been found that respond to strong pressure but not to heat.[8] It is not clear whether these structures represent a separate group from the PMNs.

NOCICEPTORS IN OTHER SOMATIC STRUCTURES

A large number of A-delta and C fibers may be found in skeletal muscle, fascia, and tendon, which are poorly responsive to normal stretching or contraction and are probably nociceptive in function. Many of the C fibers are responsive to chemical irritants, heat, and strong pressure.[2] A few respond to strong contraction, and to ischemia, whereas others fire in response to muscle stretching.[9] Some A-delta fibers in muscle have relatively low sensitivity to mechanical stimuli and respond best to chemicals, such as bradykinin. Others that tend to be arranged near muscle-tendon junctions respond to local pressure, stretch, and contractions.[2]

It is obvious from clinical experience that joints are well endowed with nociceptors. Small myelinated and unmyelinated fibers terminate in free nerve endings in joints, and A-delta fibers form a widespread plexus in capsule, fat-pads and ligaments.[10] Some of the A-delta axons respond to noxious stimuli.[11] Moncada has reported generalized nociceptive responses to intracapsular bradykinin injections in anesthetized dogs.[12] The responses were enhanced by prostaglandin injection.

Corneal sensitivity serves a primarily protective function, and most stimuli to corneal epithelium are sensed as pain. Innervation is mainly from A-delta fibers with fine terminals devoid of Schwann cell covering.[2] These fibers have response characteristics similar to PMNs. Tooth pulp afferents respond to a variety of chemical stimuli, strong heating, cooling, and pressure. Electrical stimulation almost always produces painful sensations.[2]

VISCERAL PAIN RECEPTORS

Because of the infrequency with which visceral structures are exposed to potentially damaging events, it is not efficient to provide these structures with receptors designed solely to detect intense stimuli in the environment. Although severe pain of visceral origin is a common clinical phenomenon, there is little evidence that specialized pain receptors exist in visceral structures. Many damaging stimuli, such as cutting, burning or clamping, produce no pain when applied to visceral structures. On the other hand, inflammation, ischemia, mesenteric stretching, or dilation or spasm of hollow viscera may produce severe pain. These stimuli are usually associated with pathological processes, and the pain they induce may serve a survival function by promoting immobility.

For almost all intrathoracic, intraabdominal, and pelvic viscera, pain perception is a function of sympathetic afferent fibers.[2] These neurons accompany sympathetic efferent axons in the sympathetic chain and intraabdominal and intrathoracic plexuses, but most, like other afferent fibers, have their cell bodies in the dorsal root ganglia, and synapse with dorsal horn neurons.

PAIN PERCEPTION IN THE INTESTINE

It is widely accepted that nociceptive-specific fibers do not exist in the intestine.[13] Pain is felt as a result of intense activation of afferent fibers that serve other functions, such as stretch receptors. High-frequency activation of these visceral afferents in turn activates dorsal horn pain projection neurons, producing pain perceived within cutaneous referral sites. This referred pain is probably the result of viscerosomatic convergence, the phenomenon of a single spinothalamic tract neuron that can be activated by visceral or somatic stimuli.[14] Bahr reports another type of convergence based on the existence of afferent neurons with two sensory branches, one visceral (sympathetic afferent) and one somatic.[15] It is not possible to locate the site of a painful stimulus to the gut with any accuracy, because stimulation of widely distant sites can give rise to the same referred sensations.[16]

CARDIAC PAIN

The phenomenon of cardiac pain, or at least the behavioral manifestations of pain, in response to intracoronary injection of bradykinin,[17] strongly suggests the presence of a nociceptor. Cardiac afferent fibers, conducting in the C and A-delta range, have been shown to fire at high rates in response to coronary occlusion or to intracoronary bradykinin.[18] However, to designate these nerves as nociceptors, they should respond only to noxious stimuli and should exhibit no background discharge.[19] Malliani has shown that these putative nociceptors are tonically active, demonstrate mechanosensitivity, and respond to normal hemodynamic events.[18] It is likely that cardiac afferents that are responsive to tissue-threatening stimuli have physiological functions under normal circumstances, but give rise to volleys of activity that can cause poorly localized pain referred to somatic structures. Viscerosomatic convergence probably occurs with these fibers.

OTHER VISCERAL STRUCTURES

Pain from the upper portions of the esophagus is most likely caused by activation of vagal afferents.[2] Heartburn pain may be a vagally-mediated phenomenon, but little study of the activation of pain by acids in the esophagus has been carried out.

Distension of the renal pelvis or ureters is known to produce pain, but few studies have characterized afferent responses from the urinary tract. Pain of urethral origin is probably transmitted through sacral nerve roots rather than through sympathetic afferents.

Little is known about pain of hepatic origin. Stretching of the bile ducts and gallbladder activates two populations of afferent fibers, one responding to small changes in pressure, the other responding only to high pressures (>25 mm Hg).[20] The high threshold stretch receptors may have a nociceptive function.

PEPTIDES INVOLVED IN NOCICEPTION

Painful cutaneous stimulation results in local vasodilation that is independent of central mechanisms as well as activation or dorsal horn neurons. There is now abundant evidence that substance P (SP), an 11-amino acid peptide, plays a role in both phenomena. It may have a role in the function of the nociceptor's transducer mechanism. In response to axonal transmission centrally, SP is released in the dorsal horn, serving as the sensory neurotransmitter and activating spinothalamic and other pain projection neurons. Anatomically, SP axons are not simple structures that connect a few receptors to a synapse in the dorsal horn. It appears that there is branching near the cutaneous end that sends fibers to nearby blood vessels, mast cells, hair follicles and sweat glands.[21] More centrally, but distal to the dorsal root ganglion, further branching occurs. These more central collaterals are thought to go by way of rami communicantes to the paravertebral sympathetic chain and ganglia and to visceral structures[21] (Fig. 53-1).

Following relatively mild painful stimulation, activation of a simple orthodromic mechanism may be the only pathway involved. When stimulation is intense, activation of cutaneous branches occurs, with release of substance P causing vasodilation and release of histamine from mast cells. High intensity activation of substance P containing nociceptors may also antidromically activate branches to the sympathetic chain and viscera, causing postganglionic sympathetic discharge, and perhaps alterations in visceral function. Thus, such a network could cause dramatic changes in vasomotor, autonomic, and visceral function independent of any spinal cord effect of sensory stimulation. Visceral branches of substance P containing neurons may be activated to high firing rates by distension, spasm, ischemia or inflammation. Intense activation of the visceral branch may, in turn, cause antidromic activation of the cutaneous branch of the axon, producing cutaneous vasodilation and histamine release as well as pain perception within that cutaneous distribution.

NOCICEPTOR SENSITIZATION

As a result of inflammation or repeated tissue injury, nociceptors may become sensitized, responding to innocuous stimuli. It is generally believed that the sensitized or hyperalgesic state is mediated by several endogenous chemical substances. Two vasoactive amines, 5-hydroxytryptamine and histamine, and

a widely distributed peptide, bradykinin, have been shown to produce pain under certain circumstances or to lower nociceptor thresholds,[22] and there is evidence that all of these substances are important sensitizers.

Prostaglandins are complex fatty acids whose precursors are found in cell membranes. They are released in response to noxious stimuli. They do not themselves produce pain, but markedly potentiate the algesic action of bradykinin, and probably act as sensitizers of nociceptors. They are formed from cell membrane phospholipids in a stepwise fashion. Cell membrane phospholipids are acted upon by phospholipase A_2 to form arachidonic acid, which is transformed by cyclo-oxygenase to form cyclic endoperoxides. Cyclic endoperoxides are transformed to prostacyclin or to prostaglandin E_2 and F_{2a}. Prostacyclin potentiates bradykinin or histamine induced edema, whereas PGE_2 potentiates pain induced by these substances.[22] Corticosteroids exert at least part of their anti-inflammatory effect by inhibition of phospholipase A_2, whereas aspirin and other nonsteroid antiinflammatory drugs are cyclo-oxygenase inhibitors.

DORSAL HORN MECHANISMS

The spinal dorsal horn and its analog in the medulla are exceedingly complex sensory processing areas. They contain the central terminals of peripheral afferent fibers, projection neurons of spinothalamic and other ascending tracts, local neurons that activate or inhibit projection neurons, and axon terminals of descending brainstem fibers.

As nerve roots approach the dorsal horn, segregation of fibers according to size takes place, with large myelinated afferents becoming arranged medially, and small, unmyelinated and thinly-myelinated fibers arranged laterally. Most large myelinated fibers enter the cord medial to the dorsal horn. Many of these axons bifurcate, sending one branch rostrally in the dorsal columns. The other branch enters deeper layers of the dorsal horn, sending terminals into laminae IV and V and extensive arborizations into the substantia gelatinosa (laminae II and III) (Fig. 53-2).

Most unmyelinated or thinly-myelinated afferents pass directly through the outer layer of lamina I, where they synapse with marginal layer cells and send a few branches into the underlying substantia gelatinosa. Some axons pass ventrally through these outer layers to terminate in laminae V and X.[23]

There are two groups of cells in the dorsal horn that respond to noxious stimulation in the periphery. One group, located mainly in lamina I, responds exclusively to noxious stimulation.[24] Most of these nociceptive specific (NS) cells have relatively limited receptive fields, confined to some fraction of a dermatome. The second group of cells, wide dynamic range (WDR) neurons, can be activated by either tactile or noxious stimuli. Most of these cells are located in lamina V. They have large, complex receptive fields that often have a central area of responsiveness to either noxious or tactile stimulation surrounded by an area of responsiveness only to noxious stimulation. Stimulation just outside the entire receptive field may produce inhibition.[25] It is generally accepted that WDR neurons contribute to pain perception and that their selective activation is sufficient to cause pain.[25] It is likely that many of the neurons in lamina I and lamina V that respond to noxious stimuli are spinothalamic tract (STT) neurons.

There are several systems capable of suppressing activity in STT neurons. Substantial evidence indicates that both descending and segmental neuronal inputs can inhibit activation of NS and WDR neurons.

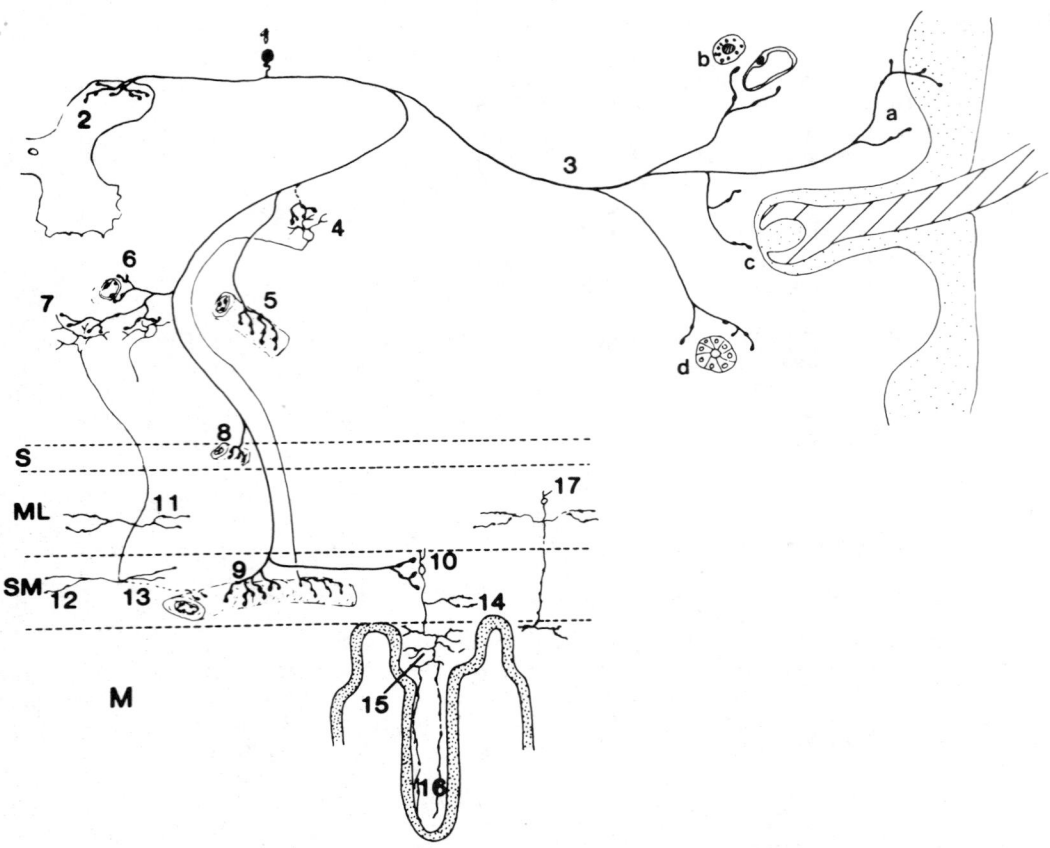

FIG. 53-1. Proposed organization of the distribution of substance P-containing fibers innervating the skin and the alimentary tract and its blood vessels. Tentative or putative nerve connections are indicated by broken lines. Sensory SP immunoreactive neurones of dorsal root ganglia, here presented as a single cell (1), send their central processes into laminae I and II of the spinal cord (2) and their peripheral processes pass either to the somatic territory including the skin (3) or toward the visceral territory. In the skin, SP immunoreactive fibers terminate as free endings (a) in the dermis and deepest stratum of the epidermis. In the dermis, SP-containing fibers are closely associated with blood vessels and mast cells (b) that are involved in histamine release, with hair follicles (c), and with sweat glands (d). Peripheral processor SP-containing fibers enter the visceral territory by passing, through rami communicantes, through the paravertebral sympathetic ganglia, where SP immunoreactive collaterals may be given off. The postganglionic territory of these ganglia includes the major blood vessels of the region, which receive also an SP immunoreactive innervation at this level (5). The SP immunoreactive fibers pass on, by way of splanchnic nerves, through the prevertebral ganglia (6, 7), where there is evidence that collaterals of the SP immunoreactive sensory fibers form the basis of the intraganglionic varicose SP immunoreactive nerve works (7). The postganglionic territory of the prevertebral ganglia includes the myenteric and submucous plexuses of the alimentary tract (11, 12) and to some extent the intramural blood vessels (13). The SP immunoreactive enteric sensory fibers pass from the prevertebral ganglia to the gut, supplying SP immunoreactive nerve networks to its blood vessels, including mesenteric and serosal (8) vessels and the submucosa (9), and contributing large boutons to the submucous plexus (10). Intrinsic SP immunoreactive neurons in the myenteric (17) and submucous plexuses (10) provide dense SP immunoreactive meshworks of fine caliber locally throughout the plexuses and in the muscle coats (14, 17) and in the mucosa form pericryptal (15) and subepithelial villous (16), and SP immunoreactive networks, including SP immunoreactive nerve strands in the muscularis mucosae. s = serosa, ML = muscular layer, SM = submucosa, M = mucosa (Cuello AC, Matthews MR: Peptides in peripheral sensory nerve fibers. In Melzack R, Wall PD [eds]: Textbook of Pain, p 77. Edinburgh. Churchill-Livingstone, 1984.)

The amino acids glycine and gamma-aminobutyric acid (GABA) are known to be inhibitors of synaptic transmission and there is some speculation that they are important mediators of segmental inhibition of nociception,[26] such as the analgesia induced by transcutaneous electrical stimulation (TENS). Little pharmacological investigation of their role in antinociception has been done.

Two pentapeptides, leucine enkephalin and methionine enkephalin, appear to be important spinal cord inhibitors of nociception. STT neurons in lamina I and V receive input from

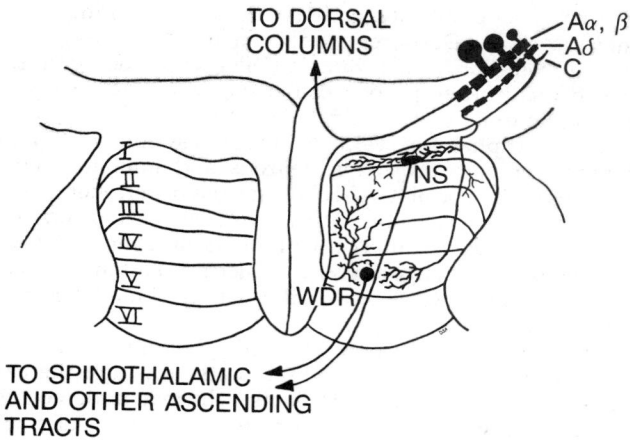

FIG. 53-2. Simplified scheme of sensory input to the dorsal horn. Large non-nociceptive afferents (A alpha, beta) enter through the medial aspect of the dorsal root, send a branch cephalad in the dorsal columns and a branch ventrally to enter the deeper layers of the dorsal horn. They synapse with wide dynamic range (WDR) neurons, lamina V, and send extensive arborizations into the substantia gelatinosa (laminae II and III). A-delta mechanical nociceptors, arranged more laterally in the dorsal root, enter the dorsal horn directly through lamina I, synapse with nociceptive-specific (NS) neurons in lamina I and WDR neurons in lamina V. C polymodal nociceptors also enter through the lateral aspect of the dorsal root directly into lamina I, where they synapse with NS neurons. Both A-delta and C fibers send a few arborizations into the substantia gelatinosa.

enkephalin-containing cells in the dorsal horn. It has been proposed that enkephalins are released in proximity to primary afferent terminals in the dorsal horn, activating presynaptic opioid receptors that prevent release of SP. However, the presence of direct synaptic contact between enkephalin-containing cells and STT neurons suggests that their inhibitory mechanism is, at least in part, postsynaptic. Enkephalins are found in highest concentrations in lamina I and II, but are also present in deeper laminae. Most dorsal horn enkephalin originates from local neurons.

It is not clear whether dorsal horn enkephalins function in a tonic fashion or whether their activity is stimulated primarily by descending or peripheral segmental activity. If there is significant tonic inhibition by enkephalins, then administration of naloxone should markedly increase activity in STT neurons. There is only equivocal evidence for such disinhibition.[26] Release of enkephalins in response to descending neural activity has not been well documented. There is, however, evidence of enkephalin release in response to segmental activity.[27]

Both 5-hydroxytryptamine (serotonin, 5HT) and norepinephrine (NE) produce analgesia when injected intrathecally, and their antagonists (methysergide for 5HT, phentolamine and phenoxybenzamine for NE) attenuate the analgesia produced by certain pharmacologic interventions.[25] It is likely that both of these neurotransmitters are involved in descending control mechanisms that originate in the midbrain and medulla.

In summary, the dorsal horn functions as a relay center for nociceptive and other sensory activity. The degree of activation of spinothalamic and other pathways with nociceptive function depends on the degree of activation of inhibitory neurons in the dorsal horn as well as the number of nocicep-

tors that are firing and frequencies at which they discharge. Intense activation of inhibitory neurons by descending pathways or by segmental inputs markedly attenuates STT excitation by noxious peripheral stimuli.

ASCENDING PATHWAYS

The spinothalamic tract is considered to be the most important pathway transmitting nociceptive stimuli to the brain. Although it is important to normal perception of pain, it is by no means the only pathway with that function. The ability of patients to perceive pain following spinothalamic tractotomy provides evidence that other pathways are involved.

Many of the neurons in laminae I and V that respond to noxious stimulation are probably cells of origin of the STT. The majority of STT fiber cross near their level of origin. There are thought to be two functionally distinct divisions of the STT—the neospinothalamic tract, whose fibers tend to be more lateral, and the paleospinothalamic tract, which is located in the medial portion of the pathway. The phylogenetically newer neospinothalamic tract projects to posterior nuclei of the thalamus, such as the ventral posterolateral nucleus, and is thought to be involved with discriminative functions, (e.g., location, intensity, and duration of noxious stimulation).[28] The paleospinothalamic tract projects to medial thalamic nuclei, and its activation is probably associated with autonomic and unpleasant emotional aspects of pain. This older portion of the STT is likely to be important in pain associated with denervation dysesthesia. Stimulation of the thalamic projections of the paleospinothalamic tract in patients with denervation dysesthesia reproduces the burning pain these patients experience spontaneously.[29]

The spinoreticular tract is likely to play a role in pain perception. Its cells of origin are unknown. It is thought to produce arousal associated with pain perception, and probably contributes to neural activity underlying motivational-affective and autonomic responses to pain.[30] The spinomesencephalic tract projects to the midbrain reticular formation. It probably evokes nondiscriminative painful sensations and may be important in the activation of descending antinociceptive pathways.[30]

Following bilateral spinothalamic tractotomy, it is still possible for patients to perceive pain from peripheral stimulation. There must be pathways in the dorsal portions of the spinal cord that are capable of producing pain perception. The spinocervical tract is a likely candidate for such a function. It is located in the dorsolateral funiculus. Its fibers ascend uncrossed to the lateral cervical nucleus, which serves as a relay, sending fibers to the contralateral thalamus.[30] There is also evidence that some fibers in the dorsal columns are responsive to noxious stimuli.

The distinction between ascending pathways is not entirely clearcut. For instance, some spinothalamic neurons projecting to the ventrobasal portion of the thalamus also send collaterals to the periaqueductal gray and midbrain reticular formation. Some spinothalamic fibers are therefore also spinomesencephalic. Similarly, collateralization exists between spinothalamic and spinoreticular fibers.[30]

DESCENDING CONTROL

In the early 1970s several reports showed that electrical stimulation of the periaqueductal gray (PAG) area of the midbrain could produce widespread analgesia in animals and in humans.[25] The PAG was later found to have high concentrations of endogenous opioids and to be rich in opioid receptors. Microinjection of small quantities of morphine into that area could also produce generalized analgesia.[31] Anatomic connections from the PAG to the nucleus raphe magnus (NRM) and to the medullary reticular formation were subsequently described. From the NRM, serotoninergic fibers descend through the dorsolateral funiculus (DLF) to spinal cord dorsal horn cells. It is not clear whether serotoninergic fibers produce a direct, postsynaptic inhibition of STT neurons or whether they act by activation of inhibitory neurons that release enkephalins or GABA.[32]

There are also adrenergic fibers that descend in the DLF that are thought to be pain-inhibitory. The relationship of these fibers to analgesia-inducing CNS sites is not as well defined as in the case of serotoninergic pathways. The role of adrenergic pathways in producing analgesia is complex. There is substantial evidence for analgesic effects of adrenergic agonists in the spinal cord, but adrenergic agents appear to inhibit analgesic mechanisms in the medulla.[32]

Multiple environmental factors appear to be able to activate descending pain-control mechanisms. Nociceptive inputs and various types of stress can produce generalized increases in pain threshold. Anxiety, depression, and emotional distress can reduce pain threshold. The descending control mechanisms described may respond to such factors.

DEAFFERENTATION PAIN

The preceding discussions have concentrated on mechanisms of pain perception in normal individuals. When damage to the nervous system occurs, pathological changes occur in the peripheral and central nervous system that can give rise to pain in the absence of potentially tissue-injuring stimuli. Deafferentation pain may result from peripheral nerve injury, from spinal cord lesions, or from lesions in the brain. The common factor in all of these situations is spontaneous activity or heightened sensitivity of neurons in the pain projection system.

Spontaneous discharge of injured peripheral nerves was demonstrated by Wall and Gutnick, who reported spontaneous neural activity originating from experimentally induced neuromas.[33] It was later demonstrated that sympathetic stimulation or norepinephrine infusion could increase such abnormal firing.[34, 35] Devor proposed that sodium and calcium channel proteins and adrenergic receptor proteins are transported to abnormal areas of nerve membrane (neuroma sprouts, demyelinated segments).[36] Spontaneous depolarization takes place at these areas and is enhanced by stimulation of the alpha receptors.

Another possible mechanism for chronic pain following peripheral nerve lesions involves short-circuiting of action potentials (ephaptic transmission) across demyelinated segments. Several possible types of interaction might exist. Demyelination of large afferent fibers could cause activation of nociceptors at the site of injury in response to stimulation of mechanoreceptors by non-noxious stimuli. Injury of motor fibers could cause nociceptor activation in response to motoneuron activation. Loss of Schwann cell protection of postganglionic sympathetics could produce nociceptor firing in response to sympathetic discharge. Little physiologic evidence for these interactions has been reported.

In addition to impulse generation originating from the site of injury, there is considerable evidence that impulse generation occurs at points of membrane instability proximal to the injury. Wall and Devor reported spontaneous discharge originating from dorsal root ganglia (DRG) in sciatic nerve sectioned rats.[37] They proposed that the DRG impulses could contribute to pain after peripheral nerve injury.

Intact peripheral nerve pathways are essential for normal function of pain projection neurons and inhibitory interneurons in the dorsal horn. Following loss of peripheral nerve activity there may be an increase in sensitivity or onset of spontaneous activity in STT neurons. It has been postulated that disruption of large afferents, which send extensive arborizations into the SG, decreases the activity of inhibitory neurons in those areas.

Spontaneous activity or heightened sensitivity of neurons is thought to occur at more central locations within the pain projection system as well. Thalamic cells may undergo such changes following cord injury or some cerebrovascular accidents. Sensitization of central neurons may also occur some time after peripheral nerve injuries.

SYMPATHETICALLY MAINTAINED PAIN

There are several mechanisms by which the sympathetic nervous system influences the perception of pain. Interactions between sympathetic outflow and spontaneous depolarization of injured nerve segments has already been discussed. Following trauma, surgery, and certain illnesses a syndrome of pain, hyperalgesia, autonomic dysfunction, and dystrophy, usually referred to as reflex sympathetic dystrophy (RSD) can occur. The usual explanation is that there is interference with the normal regulatory function of the sympathetics to the affected area induced by pain or injury. Periods of heightened sympathetic activity result in vasoconstriction, ischemia, changes in interstitial environment and, perhaps, release of prostaglandins, bradykinin, and other pain sensitizing substances. Experimental evidence for interference with sympathetic regulatory function following injury is provided by Blumberg and Janig, who demonstrated loss of the normal reciprocity between skin and muscle vasoconstrictors following peripheral nerve lesions in animals.[38]

Another possible interaction between sympathetic nervous system activity and pain perception involves ephaptic transmission, or "crosstalk" between different fiber types at injured nerve segments. Segmental loss of myelin or Schwann cell protection of axons could lead to depolarization of nociceptor fibers by efferent sympathetic transmission. While such segmental demyelination has been demonstrated anatomically, physiologic evidence for the phenomenon is scant.

Another proposal is the direct sensitization of nociceptor nerve endings by sympathetic nerve terminals. While such interactions have not been demonstrated, there is considerable evidence that sympathetic fibers are in direct contact with mechanoreceptors and that sympathetic nervous system activity can sensitize mechanosensitive afferents.[39] Roberts has proposed that a combination of sensitization of mechanoreceptors plus disinhibition of WDR neurons could occur in certain posttraumatic states.[39] Such a situation would lead to high frequency firing of spinothalamic tract neurons and pain perception in response to non-noxious mechanical stimulation. Anatomic contact of adrenergic fibers with cell bodies in the dorsal root ganglia has been demonstrated.[40] Such contact may represent a mechanism of regulation of afferent sensitivity. However, no physiological correlates to this phenomenon have been shown.

ACUTE PAIN MANAGEMENT

Acute pain that requires medical intervention is most often the result of surgery or trauma. It is generally nociceptive, *i.e.*, caused by activation of high threshold pain receptors. Pain that persists into the recovery phase following injury may have some survival benefit in nature, as it promotes immobility, thereby encouraging rest, healing, and recuperation.[41] However, there are several negative aspects to postinjury pain that far outweigh the potential benefits, the patient's suffering being the most obvious. Immobility following injury predisposes to thrombophlebitis. Substantial reduction in vital capacity and FEV_1, particularly following abdominal or thoracic surgery or injury, has been documented.[42] Persistent acute pain may trigger reflex myofascial and autonomic nervous system changes that can produce pathological changes persisting well beyond the usual recovery period. Pain-induced alterations in mood and appetite may also lead to physical changes that can delay recovery.

An increasingly diverse list of treatment modalities is available for acute pain management. Oral and intramuscular analgesics are the simplest and most widely used, and are reasonably effective for the majority of patients. Intravenous infusions and patient-controlled infusion techniques allow for more rapid adjustment of dosage and less fluctuation in blood levels. Intraspinal opioids can produce more profound regional analgesia, often with less sedation or confusion. TENS has the advantage of providing analgesia with essentially no systemic effects.

SYSTEMIC ANALGESICS

In the early postoperative period, intravenous or intramuscular opioids are the most frequently used means of pain control. Morphine is the most commonly used drug in many centers. Intramuscular administration results in peak plasma levels in about 20 minutes, and absorption is nearly complete in 45 minutes.[43] Analgesia from a single intramuscular dose lasts 3 to 4 hours. Intravenous administration results in more rapid peak blood levels but shorter duration (90 minutes). Other short-acting opioid analgesics have very similar response characteristics. The dosages for oral and parenteral administration and the durations of analgesia are shown for a number of drugs in Table 53-1.

Intramuscular administration of opioids on a PRN basis invariably results in gaps in analgesia. When meperidine is administered intramuscularly every 3 to 4 hours, blood levels equal or exceed the minimal analgesic concentration through only 35% of the dosing interval (Fig. 53-3).[44] In addition, there are often delays between analgesic requests and administration. Nurses may be busy at the time of the request, or may delay administration in a misguided effort to reduce the risk of addiction (creation of addiction in previously nonaddicted patients is rare). One way to eliminate the gaps in analgesia is to give opioids on a time-contingent basis. If doses are given by the clock, timed to peak as the previous dose falls below the therapeutic level, constant relief can be achieved. Still less fluctuation in blood level can be achieved by the use of long-acting agents such as levorphanol and methadone. Methadone has an elimination half life of 18 to 30 hours. A relatively large intramuscular or intravenous dose given intraoperatively can produce prolonged postoperative analgesia, then subsequent analgesia can be achieved with twice a day dosing.[45]

Addiction and depression of ventilation are the most common fears associated with opioid administration. Drugs with mixed agonist-antagonist properties, such as pentazocine, nalbuphine, butorphanol and buprenorphine, have been introduced in an effort to reduce these risks. The price for the added safety is a ceiling on the efficacy of these preparations. Increasing the dose beyond the usual amounts results in only slight increase in analgesic efficacy, a definite drawback for patients with severe pain.[46] Care must be taken not to use these mixed agonist-antagonists in addicted patients, as physiologic withdrawal symptoms may ensue.

Once postoperative or posttraumatic patients are able to take medications orally, they can be shifted to oral opioids, even when pain is fairly severe. It is even more important to use oral analgesics on a time-contingent basis, as the onset is even more prolonged, and significant periods of inadequate analgesia occur if the patient waits until the pain returns to request the next dose. The oral availability of morphine was shown to be quite variable, ranging from 15% to 64%.[47] In general, three times the intramuscular dose given orally every 4 hours produces satisfactory analgesia. Because there is such variability in oral bioavailability, however, one must be prepared to go up to six times the parenteral dose. Timed-release morphine, available in 30 mg tablets, produces sustained blood levels for up to 12 hours. It was developed for cancer pain management, but, in my experience, is it has been extremely effective for postoperative pain. Dosage is calculated by determination of the patient's 24-hour morphine requirement and multiplying by three to obtain the 24-hour oral morphine requirement. That dose is divided in half to determine the twice daily dose. One may wish to start slightly below the calculated dose to reduce the risk of depression of ventilation. Breakthrough pain can be treated with small intramuscular or intravenous morphine doses while the timed-release dose is being adjusted.

Methadone can also be used orally for postoperative pain. Like timed-release morphine, it can be administered twice daily. However, it may take up to 48 hours to achieve stable blood levels. By that time many patients can be shifted to less potent opioids or to nonopioid analgesics. Several short-acting drugs besides morphine are effective for moderate to severe pain. These include hydromorphone, oxycodone, and meperidine. Meperidine is often ordered orally in the same doses used parenterally. Oral bioavailability is less than 50%, with considerable first pass liver metabolism, and two to three times the parenteral dose is needed.[46] Oral doses of several opioids are shown in Table 1. As pain becomes less severe, some of the less efficacious opioids, such as codeine and propoxyphene, may provide adequate analgesia. These drugs are frequently combined with nonopioid analgesics, such as aspirin or acetaminophen. The combination of opioid and nonsteroid anti-inflammatory drugs (NSAID) is a rational one, because the NSAIDs reduce excitability of nociceptors and opioids raise firing thresholds of pain projection cells in the CNS.

PATIENT-CONTROLLED ANALGESIA

Intravenous infusion of opioids has been used to achieve stable, adequate blood levels and a more constant degree of analgesia. Because of the great variability of dosage requirements, an average starting dose would be grossly inadequate for some patients and greatly excessive for others. The technique requires close supervision because of the need for fre-

TABLE 53-1. Oral and Parenteral Narcotic Analgesics for Severe Pain

	ROUTE*	EQUIANALGESIC DOSE (mg)†	DURATION (hr)	PLASMA HALF-LIFE (hr)	COMMENTS
Narcotic Agonists					
Morphine	IM	10	4–6	2–3.5	Standard for comparison; also available in slow-release tablets
	PO	60	4–7		
Codeine	IM	130	4–6	3	Biotransformed to morphine; useful as initial narcotic analgesic
	PO	200†	4–6		
Oxycodone	IM	15		—	Short acting; available alone or as 5-mg dose in combination with aspirin and acetaminophen
	PO	30	3–5		
Heroin	IM	5	4–5	0.5	Illegal in U.S.; high solubility for parenteral administration
	PO	60	4–5		
Levorphanol (Levo-Dromoran)	IM	2	4–6	12–16	Good oral potency, requires careful titration in initial dosing because of drug accumulation
	PO	4	4–7		
Hydromorphone (Dilaudid)	IM	1.5	4–5	2–3	Available in high-potency injectable form (10 mg/ml) for cachectic patients and as rectal suppositories; more soluble than morphine
	PO	7.5	4–6		
Oxymorphone (Numorphan)	IM	1	4–6	2–3	Available in parenteral and rectal-suppository forms only
	PR	10	4–6		
Meperidine (Demerol)	IM	75	4–5	3–4 Normeperidine	Contraindicated in patients with renal disease; accumulation of active toxic metabolite normeperidine produces CNS excitation
	PO	300†	4–6	12–16	
Methadone (Dolophine)	IM	10		15–30	Good oral potency; requires careful titration of the initial dose to avoid drug accumulation
	PO	20			
Mixed Agonist-Antagonist Drugs					
Pentazocine (Talwin)	IM	60	4–6	2–3	Limited use for cancer pain; psychotomimetic effects with dose escalation; available only in combination with naloxone, aspirin, or acetaminophen; may precipitate withdrawal in physically dependent patients
	PO	180†	4–7		
Nalbuphine (Nubain)	IM	10	4–6	5	Not available orally; less severe psychotomimetic effects than pentazocine; may precipitate withdrawal in physically dependent patients
	PO	—			
Butorphanol (Stadol)	IM	2	4–6	2.5–3.5	Not available orally; produces psychotomimetic effects; may precipitate withdrawal in physically dependent patients
	PO	—			
Partial Agonists					
Buprenorphine (Temgesic)	IM	0.4	4–6	?	Not available in U.S.; no psychotomimetic effects; may precipitate withdrawal in tolerant patients
	SL	0.8	5–6		

*IM denotes intramuscular, PO oral, PR rectal, and SL sublingual.
†Based on single-dose studies in which an intramuscular dose of each drug listed was compared with morphine to establish the relative potency. Oral doses are those recommended when changing from a parenteral to an oral route. For patients without prior narcotic exposure, the recommended oral starting dose is 30 mg for morphine, 5 mg for methadone, 2 mg for levorphanol, and 4 mg for hydromorphone.
(Foley KM: The treatment of cancer pain. N Engl J Med 313:84, 1985.)

quent changes in dosage in the initial phase. As the patient's analgesic requirements diminish with time, the dose must be reduced. The usual technique involves initial rapid titration until analgesia is achieved. A relatively low infusion rate is then started. If the patient experiences pain during the infusion, an additional small bolus is given and the infusion is increased slightly. The process continues until an infusion rate that keeps the patient comfortable is achieved. As the patient recovers, the rate is reduced as tolerated by the patient. The process is quite labor intensive, requiring close observation and frequent intervention.

Over the past 20 years analgesic researchers have worked on

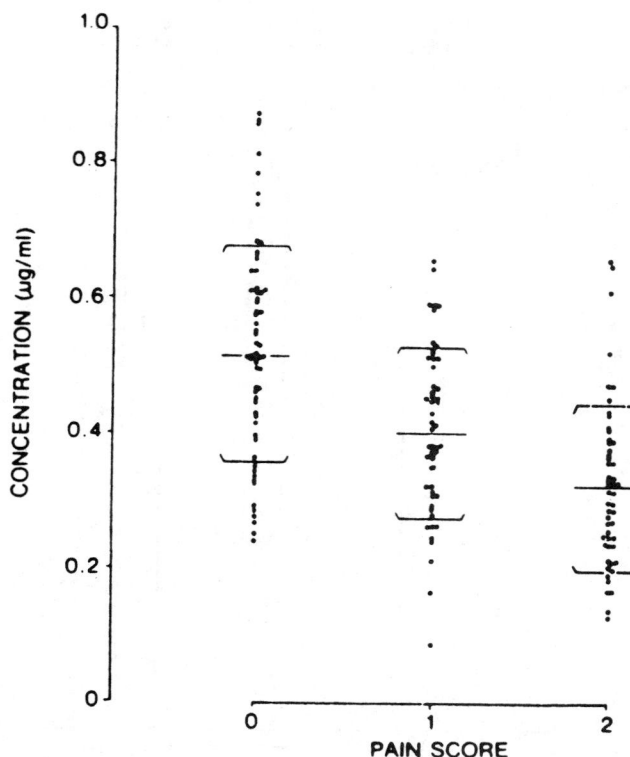

FIG. 53-3. Individual plasma concentrations of meperidine and associated pain scores. *Bars* and *horizontal square brackets* depict mean ± SD. (Austin KL, Stapleton JV, Mather LE: Multiple intramuscular injections. A major source of variability in analgesic response to meperidine. Pain 8:47, 1980. Reproduced with permission of the authors and publisher.)

TABLE 53-2.   Guidelines Regarding Bolus Dosages and Lockout Intervals for Various Parenteral Analgesics when Using a PCA System

DRUG	BOLUS DOSE (mg or μg)	LOCKOUT INTERVAL (min)
Agonists		
Morphine	0.5–3.0	5–20
Methadone	0.5–3.0	10–20
Hydromorphone	0.1–0.5	5–15
Meperidine	5–30	5–15
Fentanyl	15–75	3–10
Sufentanil	2–10	3–10
Agonist-Antagonists		
Pentazocine	5–30	5–15
Nalbuphine	1–5	5–15
Buprenorphine	0.03–0.2	5–20

(White PF: Patient-controlled analgesia: A new approach to the management of postoperative pain. Seminars in Anesthesia 4:255, 1985.)

the development of devices that would allow patients to regulate the dose of opioids administered (*i.e.*, patient-controlled analgesia, PCA). Basically, the device allows the patient to self administer small bolus doses of opioid. The dose is preset by the nurse or physician, and is delivered when the patient presses a button at the bedside. After the dose is administered, a preselected interval (the lockout interval) must elapse before another dose can be administered. The lockout feature ensures that the administered dose has time to produce an analgesic effect before the next dose is given. A typical regimen involves initiation of analgesia with a bolus dose of morphine ranging from 2 to 10 mg. Patient initiated boluses range from 0.5 to 3 mg with lockout intervals of 5 to 20 minutes[48] (Table 53-2). The times of patient dosing attempts, both successful and unsuccessful, are recorded by the device and can be displayed. Very frequent dosing indicates a need for increasing the bolus dose. With most devices, access to the controls requires a key, precluding patient adjustment of dose. Some devices allow for continuous infusion of drug at a preset rate with the patient triggering administration of small additional bolus doses. Another method designed to smooth out opioid blood levels involves splitting the dose. Half the dose is given as a bolus on demand, while the remainder of the dose is infused over the next hour.

The drug selected for patient-controlled analgesia (PCA) administration should have a rapid onset, should not have a ceiling effect, and should have a reasonably long duration, so that frequent dosing is not necessary.[48] Fentanyl and sufen-

tanil have a rapid onset, but the short duration requires frequent activation by the patient unless a background infusion is used. Methadone's duration is perhaps too long, and risk of drug accumulation is higher than for shorter acting drugs.

One study of postoperative PCA administration of morphine showed a wide range in patient requirements.[48] Median hourly requirements ranged from 1.1 to 2.6 mg · hr^{-1}, with the maximum recorded at 16.5 mg · hr^{-1}. Over 70% of patients reported no significant discomfort during the period of PCA use. Most studies indicate that the incidence of clinically significant depression of ventilation is extremely low. However, attention should be given to the possibility of the occurrence of such problems. Rosenberg *et al* reported a higher incidence of mildly elevated capillary CO_2 levels in patients who received PCA following abdominal surgery than in patients treated with intramuscular or epidural opioids.[49] The higher incidence of depression of ventilation in these patients may have been related to the use of fentanyl in this study.

INTRASPINAL OPIOIDS FOR ACUTE PAIN

After Wang[50] reported prolonged and profound relief of cancer pain following intrathecal injections of 0.5 to 1 mg morphine, intrathecal and epidural opioids began to be applied frequently for postoperative pain. Unfortunately, the lack of side-effects reported by Wang for cancer patients was not the usual experience for postoperative patients, who, unlike the cancer patients, had not been on systemic opioids chronically. Nausea and vomiting, pruritus, and urinary retention occurred frequently, and occasional cases of ventilatory depression were reported.

The majority of reports of depression of ventilation associated with intraspinal opioids have occurred with intrathecal morphine. Early reports cited depression lasting up to 18 hours. However, most of these involved high doses (3 to 15 mg intrathecal). The incidence of depression from more modest intrathecal doses is still higher than that for epidural morphine. In a survey of cases in Sweden, Gustafsson[51] reported clinically significant depression of ventilation in 22 of 6000 patients (0.33%) who received epidural morphine postoperatively and in 6 of 90 patients (5.5%) who received intrathecal morphine. Most cases appeared within 6 hours of injection. The incidence of depression of ventilation was considerably higher in patients over age 70 and when injection was in the thoracic epidural space. The incidence of depression of ventilation with more lipid soluble drugs appears to be considerably lower. Brownridge[52] reported only one case among 2000 post-cesarean-section patients who received a total of 9000 doses of epidural meperidine 50 mg. Highly lipid soluble drugs, such as fentanyl and sufentanil, appear to have a very low potential for producing depression of ventilation, probably because of the very low potential for drug accumulation in the cerebrospinal fluid (CSF). A list of factors that may increase risk of respiratory depression following intraspinal opioid administration is provided in Table 53-3.

Nonventilatory side-effects (nausea and vomiting, pruritus, and urinary retention) also have a higher incidence in patients receiving intrathecal rather than epidural opioids. All of the side-effects are at least partially reversible with naloxone. It is possible to reverse the adverse effects without affecting analgesia, and some authors advocate the concomitant use of an intravenous naloxone drip. Intramuscular agonist-antagonist analgesics, such as nalbuphine, may be effective in reducing the incidence of ventilatory and nonventilatory side-effects of intraspinal opioid agonists.

Despite the risk of life-threatening depression of ventilation, many reports appeared documenting the efficacy of epidural opioids for postoperative pain. Morphine has been the most popular opioid for intraspinal use, probably because of its long duration (up to 24 hrs). It has a somewhat prolonged latency (generally 30 to 60 min to achieve profound analgesia). A large number of studies have documented that more profound and longer lasting analgesia occurs with epidural as opposed to systemic morphine.[53] Pulmonary function in the postoperative period has been shown to be better in abdominal surgery patients receiving epidural morphine than in those receiving intravenous opioid[54, 55] or intercostal blocks (Fig. 53-4).[55]

Intrathecal doses of 0.5 to 1 mg morphine appear to be uniformly effective for postoperative pain. Little experience with doses below 0.5 mg has been published. Several studies have sought to establish dose response curves for epidural morphine. Most studies suggest that 2 mg is relatively ineffective, while doses of 5 mg or more are almost uniformly efficacious. There is some evidence that abdominal operations, particularly those with upper abdominal incisions, require higher doses of epidural opioids than is needed for extremity surgery. When bolus dosing is employed, higher doses appear to provide somewhat longer duration of analgesia.

Several investigators have studied the efficacy of shorter-acting, more lipid soluble opioids, hoping to reduce the incidence of side-effects by using drugs that have less tendency to

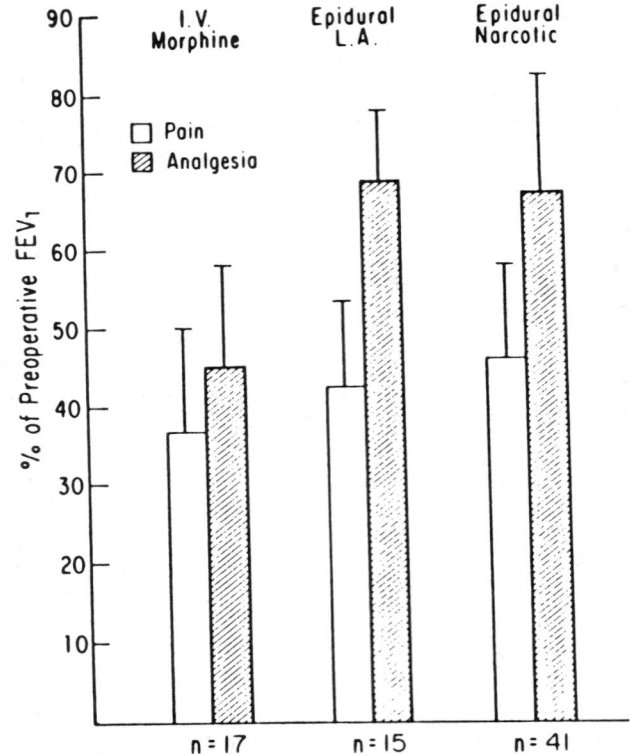

FIG. 53-4. Forced exhaled volume in 1 second (FEV₁) as a per cent of preoperative values after upper abdominal surgery, prior to and after relief of pain with intravenous morphine, epidural local anesthetic, or epidural opioid (narcotic). Mean ± SD. (Bromage PR, Camporesi E, Chestnut D: Epidural narcotics for postoperative analgesia. Anesth Analg 59:473, 1980. Reproduced with permission of the authors and publisher.)

TABLE 53-3.   Factors that May Increase Risk of Respiratory Depression from Intraspinal Narcotic Administration

Advanced age
Water-soluble narcotic (morphine)
Increased abdominal or thoracic pressure
Lack of opioid tolerance
Concomitant systemic administration of opioids or other CNS
  depressants
Intrathecal route of administration (vs epidural)
High doses
Thoracic level of administration (epidural)

accumulate in the CSF. Epidural meperidine in doses of 50 to 100 mg produces analgesia lasting about 6 hrs. Hydromorphone 1 mg epidurally produces about 12 hours of analgesia, has a more rapid onset than morphine, but does not seem to have an appreciably lower incidence of nausea or pruritis.[56] Methadone produces postoperative analgesia for 6 to 8 hours. It may be hazardous to use this drug epidurally for long periods, because the frequent dosing required leads to systemic accumulation because of the drug's extremely long half life.[53] Epidural fentanyl produces prompt but relatively short duration analgesia (2–4 hrs) in 50 to 100 μg doses. It is often used as a continuous infusion. Rates of 50 to 100 μg·hr⁻¹ are usually required to produce satisfactory postoperative analgesia. Sufentanil has similar characteristics. With both drugs, analgesia appears to be more profound with epidural application when compared to intravenous infusion of the same dose. However, the epidural doses required for effective postoperative analgesia do have substantial analgesic and ventilatory effects when administered systemically.

Agonist-antagonist drugs have been used intraspinally in several studies. Epidural butorphanol was reported to provide up to 5 hours of analgesia in doses of 1 to 4 mg, and had a lower incidence of pruritis than morphine.[57] Lanz reported up to 12 hours of postoperative analgesia following 0.3 mg epidural buprenorphine.[58] The incidence of urinary retention, pruritis, nausea, and vomiting was the same as that for patients receiving no epidural opioids. In my experience with epidural buprenorphine for post-cesarean section pain, a substantial number of patients experienced considerably less than 12 hours of relief following a single injection of 0.3 mg.

There are very few reports on the use of intraspinal opioids for posttraumatic pain. Epidural morphine 2 mg, delivered at the level of injury, was found to be effective for managing pain of fractured ribs.[59] Duration ranged from 6 to 24 hours.

LOCAL ANESTHETIC BLOCKADE

The use of either intermittent or continuous local anesthetic blockade considerably predates the use of intraspinal opioids. Continuous epidural blockade provides a convenient means of providing profound analgesia for abdominal and lower extremity surgery. There is potential benefit to prolonging sympathetic nervous system blockade into the postoperative period in patients undergoing vascular surgery or in patients undergoing lower extremity surgery who are prone to development of reflex sympathetic dystrophy. The obvious drawbacks of the technique are hypotension from sympathetic blockade, urinary retention, and interference with ambulation by motor and sensory blockade.

Postoperative epidural analgesia with local anesthetics can be carried out with on-demand bolus injections, timed-bolus injections, or continuous infusions. Scott et al were able to achieve good analgesia following lower abdominal surgery with hourly injections of 5 ml 0.5% bupivacaine or with 2 hourly injections of 6 to 10 ml 0.5% bupivacaine.[60] Using on-demand dosing for postthoracotomy pain, Shuman was able to provide 48 hours of analgesia with 0.25% to 0.5% bupivacaine with epinephrine, giving doses up to 6 hours apart.[61] Griffiths et al found on-demand dosing to be at least as effective as continuous infusion for postthoracotomy pain.[62]

There are two major concerns with continuous epidural infusion of local anesthetics. First, intrathecal migration of the epidural catheter could result in high or total spinal anesthesia. Such cases are unusual but occasionally occur, necessitating close patient monitoring. The second concern is for cumulative toxicity from systemic absorption of local anesthetic. Denson et al studied 50 normal patients (without renal or hepatic disease) who received bupivacaine infusions at several sites, including epidural, for 5 days or more. They found no relationship of blood levels to injection site. No toxic blood levels were encountered, even at 5 days, using doses at or below 30 mg·hr^{-1}.[63] Continuous epidural bupivacaine infusion produced over 80% success in a study by Raj et al.[64] Infusions were begun at 20 mg·hr^{-1} and were reduced to 13 to 15 mg·hr^{-1} by the third postoperative day.

Intercostal block provides substantial analgesia for postoperative thoracotomy and abdominal surgical pain. Unilateral intercostal blockade was shown to markedly reduce postoperative opioid requirements for 48 hours after cholecystectomy.[65] The analgesic effects often seem to outlast the sensory blocking duration of the anesthetic. Pulmonary function in the postoperative period has been shown to be better after intercostal block than after systemic opioids.[55]

An innovative regional analgesic technique was described by Reiestad to provide pain relief after cholecystectomy, renal surgery, or unilateral breast surgery.[66] Small epidural type catheters were inserted into the ipsilateral pleural space through a Tuohy needle placed at the eighth intercostal space. Twenty ml of 0.5% bupivacaine was injected intrapleurally during surgery and whenever pain was experienced post-

operatively. All but 3 of 81 patients so treated required no other analgesics for the first 48 hours. It was postulated that analgesia resulted from diffusion across the parietal pleura to multiple intercostal nerves.

TRANSCUTANEOUS ELECTRICAL NERVE STIMULATION

The application of pulsed electrical current to the skin was initially employed in the treatment of chronic pain. It was originally used prognostically to attempt to predict which patients would be likely to benefit from implanted peripheral nerve stimulators.[67] It was soon discovered that some patients could control their pain repeatedly with TENS and did not need surgical implantation of perineural electrodes. The original applications of TENS involved devices that delivered regularly-spaced pulses in the 20 to 100 Hz range, with maximum currents ranging from 100 to 200 mA. Addition of other modes, such as low frequencies (2–4 Hz) delivered at higher amplitudes, "burst" mode (short trains of high frequency stimulation) and modulation of frequency and pulse width at 0.5 to 1 second intervals increased the percentage of patients responding to the modality.

TENS is felt by many investigators to work by a mechanism of selective large afferent fiber activation, which has been shown to occur at currents too low to activate C or α-delta fibers.[68] Selective large afferent stimulation is thought to stimulate inhibitory dorsal horn neurons. Initial suggestions that TENS might act through release of endogenous opioids have had only partial support. While low frequency, high intensity acupuncture-like TENS appears to produce analgesia that is partially reversible by naloxone,[69] analgesia resulting from conventional high frequency TENS is not affected by opioid antagonist administration.[70, 71]

Despite its lack of side effects and demonstrated efficacy, TENS has had limited application for postoperative and post-traumatic analgesia. For postoperative pain, sterile, disposable, self-adhering electrodes are available for placement on either side of the wound at the time of dressing application. As soon as the patient is awake and responsive, the current is turned on and increased until the patient feels fairly strong paresthesias. For patients with pain from rib fractures, electrodes are placed on either side of the site of injury. Some patients find that increasing the current to the point of skeletal muscle contraction produces additional relief by internally splinting the injured ribs.

Efficacy of TENS has been documented in several acute pain studies. Hymes compared 115 patients who received postoperative TENS to 154 patients, reviewed retrospectively, who had similar operations but who did not receive TENS treatment.[72] Although no statistical comparison was made, the TENS patients had a lower incidence of ileus and atelectasis, and had shorter hospital stays. All demonstrated that patients treated with TENS postoperatively had significantly better vital capacities, FRCs and Pa$_{O_2}$s than patients treated with sham TENS or no stimulation.[73] In another study, patients treated with TENS following thoracotomy had significant improvement in pulmonary function following institution of treatment.[74] Several studies have demonstrated significant reductions in postoperative opioid use when TENS was used.[73, 75, 76] Another study found that patients using TENS used significantly less opioid analgesic medication in the first 3 hours postoperatively, but did not have reduced analgesic requirements during the ensuing 21 hours.[77]

Few studies have documented the effects of TENS on post-traumatic pain. Woolf *et al* showed that TENS provided good analgesia for patients with rib fracture.[71] An anecdotal report relates some benefit from TENS for athletic injuries.[78]

MANAGEMENT OF CHRONIC PAIN

Unlike acute pain, chronic pain is frequently unrelated to activation of nociceptors. Neuropathological processes lead to spontaneous activity or hyperalgesic states in which pain occurs without noxious stimuli. Autonomic nervous system dysfunction and myopathic states are also associated with pain that can occur without potentially tissue damaging stimulation. Psychological factors can alter sensitivity to somatic stimuli and can lead to intense suffering in response to relatively mild sensory inputs.

Therapeutic methods that are highly successful for managing acute pain are often inappropriate for managing chronic pain. Long-term use of opioids leads to dependency and tolerance in many patients, and may diminish the effectiveness of endogenous opioid mechanisms. Local anesthetic techniques are inappropriate for use outside the hospital setting.

There is a bewildering variety of chronic pain conditions. This chapter discusses several painful conditions that are likely to respond to regional analgesic techniques or other modalities that anesthesiologists are likely to use.

LUMBOSACRAL RADICULOPATHY

The increasing acceptance of the use of epidural steroid injections for managing lumbosacral radiculopathy in recent years has encouraged many anesthesiologists to become involved with pain management outside of the operating suite. As many low back pain referrals do not respond to epidurals, many anesthesiologists began to seek other methods of dealing with the difficult and complex back pain problems referred to them. In addition to development of other interventional modalities, physical and psychological modalities have been incorporated into many former nerve block clinics.

After Mixter and Barr reported on the relationship between sciatica and lumbar disk protrusion in 1934, surgical intervention became the accepted treatment for lumbosacral radiculopathy.[79] Unfortunately, it took nearly 20 years for the literature to reflect the fact that outcomes from laminectomy and nerve root decompression were not entirely satisfactory. Even after disappointing results were published, laminectomy has continued to be performed frequently and, in many cases indiscriminantly. One study published in 1952[80] and another published in 1963[81] reported that long-term success after surgery for sciatica was achieved in fewer than one-third of patients. Subsequent studies indicate that more than 75% of patients with acute lumbosacral radiculopathy who are treated nonsurgically experience complete or nearly complete pain relief.[82, 83, 84]

Mechanical nerve root compression was originally presumed to be the cause of pain in discogenic radiculopathy. The lack of uniform success with surgical decompression and the fact that many asymptomatic patients demonstrate substantial disk protrusion on myelography[85] or on subsequent postmortem examination,[86] suggests that other mechanisms must be operative as well. Following a period of mechanical nerve root compression an acute inflammatory process may ensue, leading to intraneural accumulation of serum protein and fluid, raised intraneural pressure, ischemia, and axonal de-

generation.[87] It has also been proposed, on the basis of animal experimentation, that intense inflammation of the nerve root may result from exposure to degenerating glycoprotein material from the nucleus pulposus.[88]

It has been proposed that epidural or subarachnoid injection of corticosteroids provides beneficial effects by reducing the inflammation initiated by either mechanical or chemical insult to the nerve root.[89] The earliest use of epidural steroids was published by Lievre in 1957, who reported good to excellent results in 50% of patients following injection of cortisone acetate plus radiographic dye.[90] Most subsequent series of epidural steroid injections used a combination of local anesthetic and insoluble steroids. In order to determine whether local anesthetic alone provided benefit for patients with sciatica, Coomes[91] compared patients receiving bedrest plus epidural injections of procaine to patients treated with bedrest alone. He found that patients treated with procaine became ambulatory in 11 days, while it took the noninjected patients an average of 31 days to regain ambulation. In a nonrandomized study, Swerdlow found consistently better results among chronic pain patients treated with epidural lidocaine and methylprednisolone than for patients treated with caudal saline or lidocaine injections.[92] There was no difference in success rates among the three treatment groups for patients with acute or recurrent sciatica. Winnie *et al* compared patients treated with epidural methylprednisolone to patients treated with local anesthetic combined with the steroid.[93] Success was close to 100% in both groups.

Unfortunately, very few controlled studies of the efficacy of epidural steroid injections have been published. Dilke *et al* reported that patients treated with epidural steroids had a lower incidence of severe pain, were less likely to take analgesics, and were more likely to have returned to work than patients treated with placebo.[94] Breivik *et al*,[95] in a randomized, crossover designed study, reported that patients treated with caudal steroid plus bupivacaine had an initial success rate of 56%, while only 26% of patients treated with bupivacaine alone responded to initial therapy.[95] They also noted that 73% of patients who failed to respond to bupivacaine improved when crossed over to steroid treatment. A few studies failed to document that epidural steroid injections were more effective than epidural local anesthetics alone. Two such studies[96, 97] compared results 24 to 48 hours after injection, before response to steroids is usually seen, and one of the studies employed injections at the L3–4 level, well above the usual level of radiculopathy.[97] Despite the scant and somewhat ambiguous results from the literature, many orthopedic surgeons and neurosurgeons have become convinced of the efficacy of the procedure because of their patients' responses, and a growing number of sciatica patients are treated with epidural steroids.

The L-5 and S-1 nerve roots are most commonly affected by disk disease, probably because those roots pass through a narrow lateral bony recess as they exit the spinal canal, a circumstance which increases the likelihood of root compression or irritation.[98] Symptoms of lumbosacral radiculopathy consist of varying degrees of low back pain, pain radiating a varying distance into the lower extremity, and, in more severe cases, motor and sensory loss consistent with damage to the affected root. Typical signs and symptoms are listed in Table 53-4.

If bowel and bladder dysfunction are present, indicative of a large midline disk, prompt surgical intervention may be indicated. Otherwise, initial treatment of acute discogenic radiculopathy consists of immobilization and mild analgesics. Most patients are able to tolerate the pain reasonably well when

TABLE 53-4.   Pain Distribution and Physical Signs Associated with Acute Disk Herniation

LEVEL OF HERNIATION	PAIN DISTRIBUTION	NUMBNESS	WEAKNESS	REFLEX CHANGES
L3-4 disk (L4 root)	Low back, buttock, lateral thigh, anterior calf, ankle, and occasionally big toe	Lower anterior thigh and patella	Mild (quadriceps)	Diminished (knee jerk)
L4-5 disk (L5 root)	Low back, buttock, lateral thigh, and calf, big toe	Lateral calf, web space of first and second toe	Foot (dorsiflexion)	None
L5-S1 disk (S1 root)	Low back, buttock, posterior thigh, and calf	Posterior calf, lateral heel, and foot	Foot (plantar flexion)	Diminished or absent (ankle jerk)

(Abram SE: Management of pain. In Cottrell JE, Turndorf H (eds): Anesthesia and Neurosurgery, p 496. St Louis, CV Mosby, 1986.)

placed on bedrest. If severe pain persists after reasonable trials of conservative management, epidural steroids may be used.

Triamcinolone diacetate or methylprednisolone acetate are the most commonly used steroid preparations. Injection should be performed as close to the affected nerve root as possible. Placing the patient in the lateral position with the involved side down may increase the amount of steroid reaching the affected root. Addition of a small volume (3–4 ml) of local anesthetic produces considerable analgesia if it reaches the affected nerve root, confirming proper drug placement. In occasional patients, particularly those with S-1 pathology, the drug does not spread adequately to the affected root. Placement of the epidural laterally in the L-5–S-1 interspace or caudal injection sometimes results in better drug access to the injured nerve. Reassessment should be carried out 1 to 2 weeks after the initial treatment. If the patient has little or no pain at the time of the return visit, there is no point in repeating the injection. If symptoms are improved, but some pain is still present, it is likely that a repeat injection will produce further improvement. A third block can be performed 1 to 2 weeks later if some symptoms persist. There is some controversy regarding the advisability of repeating injections when no benefit is evident at the end of 1 to 2 weeks. In my experience few patients obtain relief from subsequent injections if the first epidural was of no help at all.

Intrathecal steroid injection has been advocated for patients who obtain minimal or no benefit from epidural steroids. A study that evaluated response of such patients to intrathecal injections of methylprednisolone acetate or triamcinolone diacetate failed to demonstrate any benefit to intrathecal steroids in patients who were totally unresponsive to epidural steroid injections.[99] Patients who had experienced partial improvement from epidural injections were likely to experience some further improvement from intrathecal injections. However, the study was terminated early because of the fairly high incidence of symptoms consistent with aseptic meningitis that appeared in the first 48 hours after intrathecal injection.

Patients with chronic radicular low back pain are much less likely to benefit from epidural steroid injections. Abram and Anderson reported that patients with long-standing symptoms were much less likely to experience even transient relief form epidural steroid injections.[100] Patients who had undergone previous back surgery also had a much lower success rate. Several mechanisms may lead to chronic radicular pain that is unresponsive to steroid injections. Spontaneous activity or ephaptic transmission may occur from the injured, demyelinated root. Scarring of the root, with replacement of neural elements with fibrous tissue causes inelasticity of the nerve. The nerve root can no longer stretch with leg motion, and chronic mechanical irritation ensues.[87] Loss of large afferent fibers may lead to disruption of dorsal horn gating mechanisms and disinhibition of spinothalamic projection cells. Loss of disk height following herniation can lead to narrowing of intervertebral foramina, with subsequent root irritation laterally, or may cause redundancy and buckling of the ligamentum flavum, which can effectively narrow the spinal canal. Loss of disk height can also produce facet joint subluxation and degeneration, producing pain from the joint itself and osteophyte formation, which can narrow foramina or the central canal. Injury to the vertebral plate, the bony portion of the vertebral body adjacent to the disk, often accompanies disk disease and may lead to osteophytic growth into the central canal[101] (Fig. 53-5).

With increasing duration of symptoms, the emphasis of therapy should be shifted away from medical types of intervention (injections, analgesic medications, surgery) and toward rehabilitation and psychological approaches. Programs that teach patients new ways of coping with pain, which reduce dependency on chemical substances, and actively work to develop strength, range of motion, and physical conditioning are more likely to be of benefit to chronic low back pain patients.

LUMBOSACRAL ARTHROPATHIES

Degeneration and inflammation of the lumbar facet joints and sacroiliac joints can produce low back pain that is often difficult to distinguish from radicular pain. Both conditions may cause pain that radiates to the lower extremities. CT scanning is a fairly reliable method of demonstrating pathology in these joints.[102, 103] Bone scans, particularly SPECT scanning, may also be useful diagnostically.

When facet arthropathy is the suspected cause of low back pain, the diagnosis can be confirmed by injection of local anesthetic into the facet joint. The procedure can be done easily under fluoroscopic control. The patient is placed prone and the affected side is tilted upward until the joint space is visualized. Proper needle placement can be confirmed by injection of 0.5 to 1 ml of contrast media. The injection should transiently reproduce the patient's pain, and the dye will outline the extent of the capsule. Occasionally herniation of the capsule into the foramen, which can produce radiculopathy, can be documented. Injection of 1 ml local anesthetic should produce dramatic relief of arthropathic pain. Injection of a small volume of insoluble corticosteroid into an affected joint produces analgesia that lasts 6 months or longer in about 25% of patients who experience relief from the local anesthetic.[102] NSAID may be of some benefit. Resistant cases have been treated with radiofrequency coagulation of the nerves

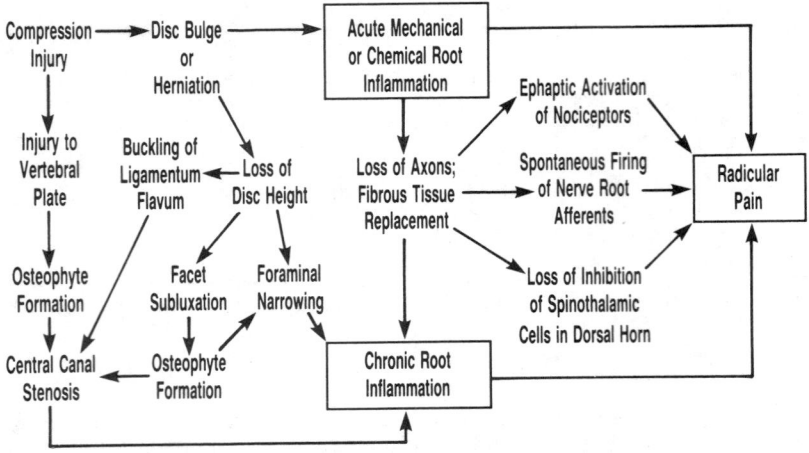

FIG. 53-5. Pathophysiologic processes involved in the production of acute and chronic radicular pain.

supplying the facet joints, but long-term success is generally low with that technique. More recently, cold lesioning (cryoanalgesia) of the facet nerves has been reported to be helpful. Long-term followup data are not yet available, however.

When sacroiliac pathology is demonstrated, injection of the joint with local anesthetic helps confirm the diagnosis. By using a technique similar to that described by Bonica, [104] (Fig. 53-6) I have found that 25 of 35 patients with suspected sacroiliac disease had pain relief from local anesthetic injection of the joint. After injection of triamcinolone diacetate, 7 of 20 patients who were followed long term experienced at least 6 months of moderate to complete pain relief (unpublished data).

MYOFASCIAL PAIN

The myofascial syndrome is an extremely common cause of somatic pain. It is associated with marked tenderness of discrete points, (trigger points) within affected skeletal muscles, pain which is referred to areas some distance from the trigger point, and the appearance of tight, ropy bands of skeletal muscle. Autonomic changes, such as vasoconstriction and skin conductivity changes may occur some distance from the affected muscle. [105] Biopsies of trigger points have been reported to show little or no change or to show degenerative changes, the severity of which corresponds to the intensity of the symptoms. [105] Although the pathophysiology of the condition has not been clearly defined, Travell and Simons propose the following explanation: Acute muscle strain causes disruption of sarcoplasmic reticulum and release of calcium, which, in turn produces sustained or repeated skeletal muscle contraction and fatigue. Blood flow becomes inadequate for the degree of metabolic activity occurring locally. Adenosine triphosphate (ATP) becomes depleted, preventing release of myosin from actin, causing sarcomeres to become rigid, and affected skeletal muscles become taut. Nociceptor sensitizing substances, such as prostaglandins, bradykinin and serotonin are released from platelets and mast cells, causing increased firing of muscle nociceptors. [105]

Many of the commonly affected skeletal muscles, the site of their trigger points and their zones of referred pain have been mapped out. [106] Scapulocostal syndrome, one of the most common patterns of myofascial pain, is characterized by a trigger point located just medial and superior to the upper portion of the scapula and pain that can radiate to the occipital region,

the shoulder, the medial aspect of the arm, or to the anterior chest wall. [107] Myofascial pain involving gluteal muscles produces pain referred into the posterior thigh and calf, mimicking S-1 radiculopathy. Myofascial pain involving the piriformis muscle, which overlies the sciatic nerve, can produce sciatic irritation and, occasionally, hypesthesia, again resembling radiculopathy.

The most important aspect of treatment for myofascial pain is to regain skeletal muscle length and elasticity. This is best done by maneuvers that gently stretch affected muscles. Because of the sensitization of muscle afferents, appropriate physical therapeutic maneuvers are often painful, and may reinitiate muscle contraction. Therapy aimed at reducing skeletal muscle pain and sensitivity should therefore be employed prior to stretching exercises. Trigger point injections, infiltration of local anesthetic directly into the trigger point, is a valuable initial therapy. Pain relief following injection confirms the diagnosis of myofascial syndrome, and a series of several injections performed daily or every several days can markedly reduce skeletal muscle sensitivity. Fairly vigorous therapy can be carried out during the analgesic period after each injection. Ultrasound therapy applied over the affected skeletal muscle may also produce periods of analgesia.

Trigger point injections and ultrasound require the participation of trained personnel, precluding their use on a frequent regular basis (e.g., several times per day). Several treatment modalities can be used by the patient alone or with the help of family members. TENS applied directly over the trigger points, may produce analgesia during stimulation and often for some time afterward. Stimulation should be carried out for 20 to 30 minutes prior to stretching exercises. Some patients who do not respond to the usual high frequency TENS may benefit from a brief period (about 5–10 minutes) of low frequency (2 to 4 Hz) high intensity TENS. The current should be high enough to cause skeletal muscle contraction and mild discomfort. Vapocoolant spray (e.g., Fluorimethane) sprayed over the affected skeletal muscle may produce transient analgesia sufficient to facilitate physical therapy. Massage of the affected skeletal muscle with ice may also be of some benefit.

Many physicians feel that myofascial pain often develops in patients whose response to stress is increased muscle tone. Surface measurement of electromyogram (EMG) in such patients often demonstrates extremely high activity at rest. EMG biofeedback is a useful added therapy for such patients, and appears to be helpful in preventing future painful episodes for patients with recurrent problems.

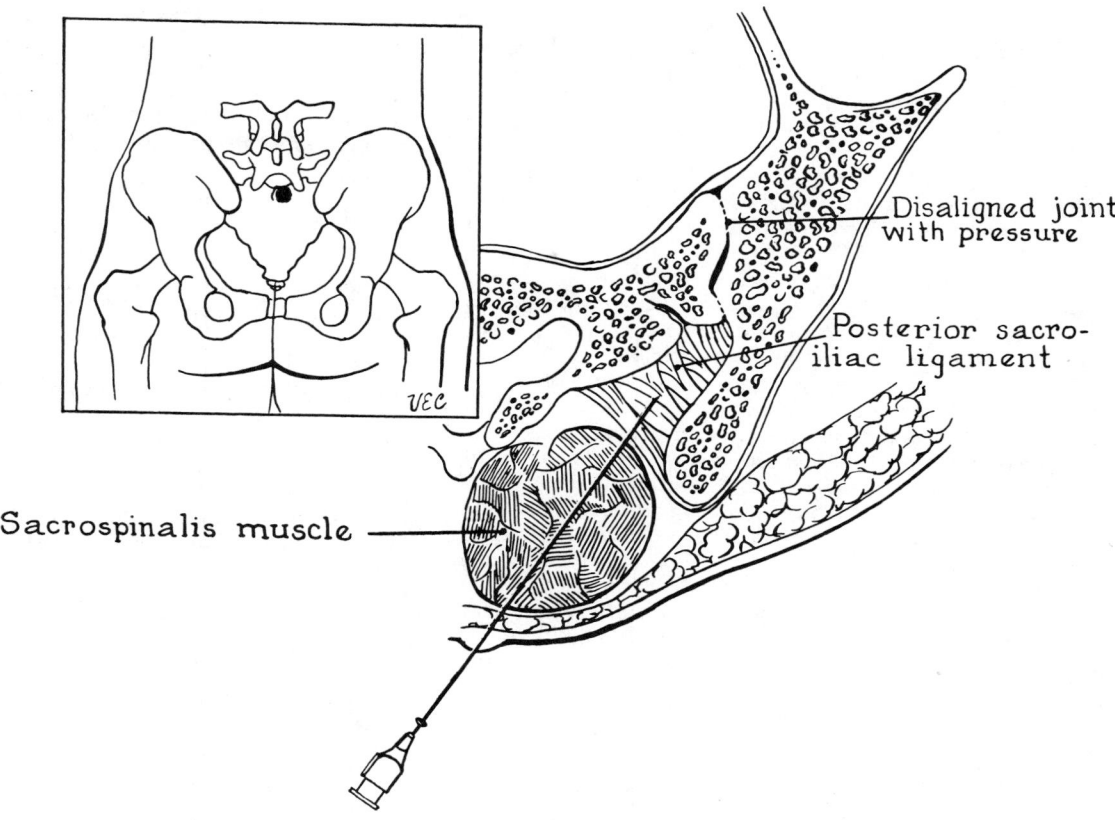

FIG. 53-6. Techniques for sacroiliac joint injection (Bonica JJ: The Management of Pain, p 1200. Philadelphia, Lea and Febiger. 1953.)

SYMPATHETICALLY MAINTAINED PAIN

There is a tendency to consider all painful conditions associated with autonomic nervous system dysfunction or with sympathetic nervous system contributions to pain perception as a single entity. There are in fact several distinct pathological states in which autonomic nervous system contributions are important, and it is necessary to recognize these different pathological processes in order to provide patients with optimal care. Unfortunately, the differences between syndromes are often indistinct.

Though there may be a larger number of sympathetically-mediated pain conditions, it is convenient to divide the group into three entities—reflex sympathetic dystrophy (RSD), causalgia, and sympathetically aggravated neuralgia. RSD refers to conditions in which autonomic dysfunction triggered by injury or illness plays a major role in the pathophysiology of the painful condition. Causalgia is specific term that refers to a syndrome of pain and autonomic nervous system dysfunction resulting from major nerve trunk injury. Sympathetically aggravated neuralgia refers to conditions in which pain arises from an injured peripheral nerve and is increased in intensity by sympathetic stimulation, but sympathetic dysfunction is not the major cause of the pain. Obviously, there can be considerable overlap between these syndromes.

Reflex Sympathetic Dystrophy

RSD describes a syndrome consisting of pain, autonomic nervous system dysfunction, and dystrophic changes, usually occurring after trauma or surgery. Crush injuries, lacerations, fractures, sprains, and burns have all been reported to precipitate the syndrome.[108] Many postoperative cases occur after surgery involving the median nerve distribution, such as carpal tunnel release or palmar fasciectomy.[108] The syndrome occasionally occurs after cerebrovascular accident or myocardial infarction. The pain is usually burning in quality, and is often accompanied by diffuse tenderness and pain on light touch. Hands and feet are commonly the major sites of pain. The pain and hyperalgesia often spread beyond the original sites of pain.

Autonomic nervous system dysfunction is manifested as changes in skin temperature, cyanosis, edema, and hyperhydrosis. Early in the course of the disease, the skin may be warm and erythematous with occasional to frequent bouts of intense vasoconstriction. As the process becomes more chronic, the involved extremity is usually cool and pale or cyanotic. The vascular phase of bone scanning often demonstrates differences in flow between the normal and the affected extremity. Thermography or local measurement of skin temperature using surface thermistors are also useful in documenting differences in regional blood flow.

Dystrophic changes become increasingly evident with time if the condition is untreated. Skin of the affected area becomes smooth and glossy. Bone demineralization takes place to a much greater extent than would be expected on the basis of reduced activity. Joints in the affected extremity become stiff and painful as a result of synovial edema, hyperplasia, fibrosis, and perivascular inflammation.[109]

Local anesthetic blockade of the sympathetic chain is useful diagnostically, particularly when only a portion of the spectrum of possible symptoms are present. Cervicothoracic sympathetic block is usually carried out by injection of local anesthetic on the anterior tubercle of C-6 or on the transverse process of C-7. Lumbar sympathetic block is performed by injecting local anesthetic at the anterolateral aspect of the L-2 vertebral body. Once the diagnosis is confirmed, treatment consists of a series of local anesthetic sympathetic blocks. If lumbar sympathetic block is technically difficult or is particularly painful to the patient, repeated or continuous lumbar epidural blockade can be used instead. Injections are generally continued until symptoms are minimal. Three to seven blocks are usually sufficient, but occasionally the series must be longer. Physical therapy, consisting of active or active-assisted range of motion, is usually indicated, and should be carried out immediately after each sympathetic block. Vigorous passive range of motion and heavy weights should be avoided, as they may retrigger RSD symptoms.

Patients whose condition is diagnosed and treated early are very likely to respond to sympathetic blocks. Success rates of 90% or more have been reported.[110, 111] In one of a very few controlled studies of outcome for RSD, Wang reported that, at 3-year followup, 65% of patients treated with sympathetic blockade were considered to have satisfactory results, while only 41% of patients who did not receive blocks were doing well.[112] Patients treated with sympathetic blockade within 1 month of the onset of symptoms had a success rate of 87%, while the long-term success for patients treated 6 months to a year after the onset of symptoms was 50%.

Hannington-Kiff described an alternative technique for producing temporary sympathetic blockade using intravenous regional injection of guanethidine.[113] The technique has been shown to be as effective as local anesthetic blockade in some reports,[114, 115] and has the advantage of being safer in anticoagulated patients. Reports have not yet shown the technique to be superior to local anesthetic blocks. I treated 32 RSD patients with one to four intravenous guanethidine blocks. Most of the patients had experienced symptoms for at least 6 months, and all had experienced only transient relief (up to 48 hours) from local anesthetic sympathetic blocks. Most patients in the series experienced one to several days of relief from the guanethidine blocks, but only three patients had relief for 3 months or more (unpublished data). A major limitation to the use of intravenous guanethidine is the fact that the injectable preparation is not FDA approved for use in the United States at the time of this writing.

Kozin et al reported substantial benefit from treatment of RSD with a brief course of high dose corticosteroids.[116] Their success rate was 82%, which is particularly impressive because many of their patients had experienced long-term symptoms. Unfortunately, their criteria for diagnosing RSD were somewhat vague and did not include response to sympathetic block, hyperpathia, or burning pain. Side-effects from high-dose systemic steroids are often troublesome. An alternative treatment is the intravenous regional injection of soluble steroids in the affected limb.[117] TENS is often a useful adjunctive treatment for RSD. Increased skin temperature during stimulation has been documented in patients who experience pain relief following treatment,[118] and TENS has been reported to provide substantial clinical benefit when used as the sole therapy for RSD.[119]

Patients with long-standing symptoms of RSD who develop dystrophic changes and, frequently, the behavioral and psychological profiles typical of chronic pain patients, are extremely resistant to the types of intervention described above. Surgical or neurolytic sympathectomy has been suggested as a treatment for RSD patients who respond only transiently to sympathetic blocks.[111] It has been my experience, however, that most patients with chronic RSD get no relief or only a few days to weeks of benefit from sympathetic ablation. Therapy instead should be directed toward extinguishing pain behavior, increasing strength and mobility, and developing coping strategies.

Causalgia

The term causalgia (Greek, meaning burning pain) has been used interchangeably with RSD and a variety of other terms that denote pain syndromes with autonomic nervous system findings. More recently, causalgia has been used to indicate a specific syndrome of burning pain and autonomic nervous system dysfunction associated with major nerve trunk injury.[111] Most cases of causalgia are caused by gunshot wounds. Rapid, violent deformation of the nerve seems to play a major pathophysiologic role. Most cases involve partial injury to the brachial plexus, the median nerve proximal to the elbow or the tibial division of the sciatic nerve proximal to the knee. Pain often begins immediately after injury and may spread to involve previously unaffected areas. There is usually severe burning pain and hyperpathia, often accompanied by deep shooting, crushing, or stabbing pains. The pain is aggravated by movement or any physical stimulation, such as light touch or pressure. Stimuli that increase sympathetic nervous system activity, such as a loud noise, a flash of light, or anxiety, often increase the severity of the pain. Pain may persist for many years in inadequately treated patients.[120] There is usually evidence of reduced sympathetic nervous system activity in the affected extremity, which is generally warm, dry, and venodilated. Vasoconstriction, hyperhydrosis, cyanosis, and edema are occasionally seen. Dystrophic changes of skin, bone, and joints, similar to those encountered in RSD patients, often begin early.

Reports on the therapy of causalgia from the early 1900s described surgical destruction of peripheral nerves, which was uniformly unsuccessful. Opioid analgesics were likewise ineffective. In 1930, Spurling published encouraging results of treatment with sympathetic ganglionectomy.[121] Since then, numerous reports have documented the efficacy of such treatment. Mayfield reported complete relief of symptoms in 91% of 105 causalgia victims treated with surgical sympathectomy.[122] In a review of over 500 cases, Bonica found that over 80% of patients responded to sympathectomy.[111]

More recently, less invasive therapy has been undertaken in the management of causalgia. Neurolytic lumbar sympathetic block has been proposed as an alternative to surgical lumbar sympathectomy, and has been shown to produce long-term sympathetic denervation in the large majority of patients.[123] Aggressive treatment with local anesthetic sympathetic blockade has met with some success. Bonica reported success in 10 of 17 causalgia patients managed with frequent local anesthetic blocks. I have treated three patients with early, severe causalgia who responded dramatically to continuous infusion lumbar epidural blockade or continuous infusion brachial plexus block that was maintained for 5 to 7 days (unreported findings).

PSYCHOGENIC FACTORS

When a painful disorder becomes chronic, a number of psychological responses to the pain become evident. In many patients, the consequences of the psychological changes that occur become a major source of disability, and with time may become more disabling than the original somatic pain.

Depression is a frequent consequence of chronic pain, and is often readily evident from the history. Loss of appetite, inability to concentrate, difficulty sleeping, and loss of interest in social, recreational, and sexual activity are common signs. Several psychological tests have depression scales or ratings, and can be helpful in assessing the presence and degree of depression. Psychotherapy specifically directed towards the depressive aspects of the problem may be warranted. Antidepressant medications may be helpful in this situation.

Pain tends to alter behavior in fairly predictable ways. It leads to reduction in activity, including avoidance of social and vocational obligations, grimacing, moaning, complaining, assuming certain postures, visiting health-care professionals, and taking analgesics. When such behaviors result in pleasurable consequences or in avoidance of unpleasant situations, those behaviors become reinforced, and may be perpetuated long after the original pain has diminished.[124] For example, taking opioid analgesics may produce euphoria as well as pain relief, and patients may continue to seek these medications long after they are needed for pain. Complaining about pain to family members may lead to solicitous attention and avoidance of some unpleasant obligations. Pain may allow the patient to avoid a job that he does not like. Therapy of such operant pain mechanisms is directed toward cessation of rewards for pain behaviors. Patients may need to be placed in an environment where analgesics are unavailable. Family members are instructed to ignore verbal complaints and to actively discourage inactivity and overutilization of the health-care system. Physical, social, and recreational activity is gradually increased. Vocational counseling is undertaken to encourage return to employment that is within the patient's physical capability. Group therapy is a useful tool for dealing with these operant mechanisms. Reinforcement of "well behavior" by fellow patients is often more effective than efforts of staff personnel. Unfortunately, financial reinforcers of pain behavior work against goals of therapy. Patients may perceive that continued compensation for an injury is contingent on continued manifestation of symptoms. When litigation is planned, it is unusual for the patient's pain complaints to subside prior to the court settlement.

One group of patients encountered occasionally in pain clinics was termed *dissatisfied pain patients* by Swanson *et al.*[125] These patients typically have a long, complicated medical and surgical history, tend to be unresponsive to any type of treatment, and are often disruptive to treatment programs. They often have a poor work record, a history of analgesic abuse and accident proneness, and were often abused as children. It is important to recognize such patients, mainly so that they can be excluded from interaction with other patients. Any type of treatment, including psychiatric intervention, is unlikely to be of benefit.

CANCER PAIN

In assessing patients with malignant disease who seek treatment for pain, it is essential to determine the specific site and mechanism of their pain. It is not enough to make a diagnosis of "cancer pain." The entire range of acute and chronic pain mechanisms is encountered among patients with malignancy. It is also essential to know the stage of the patient's malignant disease. The approach to a given pain for a terminal patient may vary greatly from the approach to the same type of pain in a patient whose cancer is curable.

It is useful to determine whether the patient's pain is acute or chronic, and whether it is related to tumor progression, to therapeutic intervention, or as is occasionally the case, to factors unrelated to the patient's malignant disease (arthritis, herniated disk, etc.).[126] It is also useful to know whether the patient has a history of chronic pain or drug abuse predating the onset of malignant disease.[127] Pain caused by tumor progression can result from compression or infiltration of peripheral nerves, nerve root or spinal cord, infiltration of bone and soft tissue, obstruction or distension of visceral structures, and vascular occlusion. Surgical intervention may lead to scar pain, neuroma formation, sympathetic dystrophy, and venous or lymphatic obstruction. Chemotherapy may be associated with peripheral neuropathies. Therapy with steroids can cause aseptic bony necrosis or rheumatoid-like symptoms when therapy is withdrawn. Herpes zoster is associated with agents that suppress immune function. Radiation therapy sometimes results in esophagitis, plexopathy and myelopathy, and bone necrosis.[127]

There is a substantial range of therapeutic options that are available to the cancer patient. A major consideration in approaching the patient with severe pain is when to institute a particular modality. It is generally advisable to consider less invasive, lower-risk options initially, progressing to procedures that are more invasive, more painful to perform and carry a higher risk of complications only when the more benign procedures are ineffective. Occasionally, it is prudent to select a more invasive procedure early in the course of management if it is felt that it will provide the patient maximum comfort or if the patient's pain level has progressed to a crisis state.

Pharmacological Therapy

The use of oral analgesic agents is the mainstay of treatment for cancer pain. Adequate analgesia can be achieved in the large majority of patients with cancer-related pain if sound pharmacological principles are employed. Several guidelines such as the ones listed below are essential to cancer pain management:

1. Use drugs appropriate for the nature and severity of the patient's pain. Weaker opioids such as codeine may be adequate for mild to moderate pain. For severe pain, potent opioids such as morphine, hydromorphone, or methadone should be employed. Agonist-antagonist opioids such as pentazocine have a ceiling effect on their analgesic efficacy and are generally effective only for relatively mild pain. Meperidine is a poor drug for repetitive dosing, because accumulation of its metabolite normeperidine can cause CNS stimulation manifested as anxiety, tremors, or seizures.[128] Be aware of the oral bioavailability of the drug used (see Table 53-1). The oral dose of morphine, for instance, is about three times the parenteral dose. When peripheral nociceptive processes are involved (such as bony or soft tissue invasion), the addition of NSAID may be very helpful.
2. Use adequate doses. The dose of opioid analgesic should be escalated until satisfactory analgesia occurs (usually the case) or until problematic side-effects occur. The potent agonists, *e.g.*, morphine, do not have a ceiling on analgesic effect. The dose required varies tremendously. It is not unusual for cancer patients to require 100 to 200 mg oral morphine or more every 3 to 4 hours. As patients become tolerant or as tumor spreads, dose requirements increase.

3. Maintain steady blood and tissue levels of analgesic. All analgesics should be given by the clock. Administration of drugs on a PRN basis invariably results in periods of inadequate relief. The time interval for administration should be consistent with the duration of action of the drug. When possible, use long-acting drugs. Methadone, whose plasma half-life is 24 to 36 hours, can be given twice a day, avoiding the need for nighttime awakening for analgesic administration. Morphine is now available in a time-release form that can be administered twice a day.

4. Consider the use of adjuvant drugs. Tricyclic antidepressants are frequently of benefit for postherpetic neuralgia, may be helpful for some patients with other types of neuralgic pain or denervation dysesthesia, and can be very effective for treating concomitant depression. Some anticonvulsants may be beneficial for neuralgic pain. Phenothiazines or butyrophenones have been shown to reduce symptoms of nausea, agitation, and pain when used in conjunction with narcotic analgesics.[129] Corticosteroids should be considered for increased intracranial pressure, cord compression, severe bone pain or pain from liver metastases. Calcitonin is being investigated for treatment of bone pain.

5. Anticipate and promptly treat side-effects. Constipation, which may become a major problem, occurs in most patients on opioids. Prophylactic management is essential. Nausea is a common opioid side-effect and concomitant administration of antiemetics may be necessary. Depression of ventilation should be treated with small incremental doses of naloxone (e.g., 0.05–0.1 mg) until respiratory rate increases to an acceptable range. Large doses precipitate withdrawl and reverse all of the patient's analgesia.

Patients who are unable to take analgesics orally can often be satisfactorily managed with parenteral opioid administration. Some patients who do not achieve satisfactory analgesia with oral drugs have adequate control with parenteral drugs, possibly because enteric absorption is poor. When the parenteral route is chosen, a constant infusion technique is usually superior to intermittent intramuscular injections. Many cancer patients have long-term venous access ports for chemotherapy that can be used for opioid infusion.

When beginning opioid infusions, it is generally prudent to begin with a relatively low-dose bolus injection and a modest infusion rate. If analgesia is inadequate after 1 to 2 hours, a small bolus is repeated and the infusion rate is increased. The process is repeated until the infusion rate is adequate. An alternative, less labor intensive method is to use a patient-controlled analgesia device.[130] Once the daily opioid requirement is established, the patient can be switched to a portable, battery-powered constant infusion device. When venous access is not available, portable external infusion devices can be used to deliver opioids subcutaneously through a "butterfly" type needle.[131] The infusion site is changed every few days or when screness occurs. When large doses are required, the use of a concentrated preparation of hydromorphone (10 mg·ml^{-1}) allows for longer intervals between refilling the portable infusion pump and reduces the mass of fluid injected.

Intraspinal Opioids

Some cancer patients do not achieve satisfactory analgesia with systemic opioids without increasing the doses to the point of marked sedation or confusion. Less conventional methods of opioid administration may be effective for some of those patients. The discovery of spinal cord opioid receptors led to speculation regarding feasibility of intraspinal administration of opioids. In 1979 Wang et al reported profound analgesia lasting up to 24 hours after intrathecal injection of 0.5 to 1 mg morphine in 8 patients with cancer pain (Table 53-5).[50] Since then, the chronic administration of epidural opioids for the treatment of cancer pain has come into fairly widespread use.

Most experience with chronic intraspinal opioid administration has been with morphine, probably because it has a long duration, allowing bolus as well as continuous administration, and because it has been FDA approved for intraspinal use. Wang reported essentially no side-effects or complications in his initial series of cancer patients treated with intrathecal morphine.[50] Subsequent use of intraspinal opioids in patients who had not previously been on systemic opioids, e.g., postoperative patients and volunteers, was associated with nausea and vomiting, urinary retention, pruritus, and depression of ventilation. As more experience with cancer patients accumulated, it became evident that these problems were, indeed, uncommon in this population, probably because the patients had been on systemic opioids chronically, and had become tolerant to these side-effects.

Intraspinal opioids have been chronically administered by both the epidural and intrathecal routes. Intrathecal administration has the advantage of allowing use of much lower doses, potentially minimizing systemic side-effects, but carries the risks of CSF leak, headache, meningitis, and arachnoiditis. With either epidural or intrathecal administration, drug may be administered as a bolus, by infusion using an external pump, or by infusion using a totally implanted pump.

Percutaneous placement of an epidural catheter followed by bolus administration of opioid constitutes the simplest method of administration. The principle drawback of this technique is the risk of infection, which may spread to the epidural space. Such a technique is useful as a temporary measure to evaluate efficacy of epidural opioids and is a reasonable method of administration for patients whose life expectancy is very short. The simple expedient of tunneling the catheter subcutaneously to the flank minimizes the risk of epidural infection and allows the patient access to the catheter exit site to facilitate dressing changes.

The decision to use an external pump is based on pharmacokinetic, technical, and financial considerations. There is some evidence that lower doses of morphine can be employed when using a continuous infusion. Coombs was able to provide good analgesia for a group of cancer pain patients using a mean dose of 2 mg·day^{-1} initially and 6.6 mg·day^{-1} at the end of 12 weeks.[132] Reports of studies that use bolus injection describe much higher daily doses. Bolus injection produces much higher peak CSF levels,[133, 134] which may predispose to more cephalad migration of the drug. Another advantage to continuous infusion techniques is the lower incidence of catheter occlusion. Inability to inject is a fairly common problem with bolus injection technique. When an obstructed catheter is removed, it is common to find fibrin material in the lumen. The use of large bore silicone rubber catheters should minimize that possibility, however. Patients with epidural metastases may have severe pain with bolus injection, but tolerate continuous infusion quite well. Perhaps the biggest drawback to continuous infusion techniques is the expense. Portable pumps cost up to several thousand dollars, and the use of implantable systems adds several thousand dollars in additional physician and operating room expenses.

The totally implantable infusion pump is the most elegant and most expensive drug delivery system. The Infusaid pump

TABLE 53-5.   Clinical Results with Intrathecally Applied Morphine

	AGE (years), SEX	NUMBER OF INJECTIONS	AGENT AND DOSE (mg)	PAIN	
				Mean Change in Intensity (scale of 0 to 10)	Mean Duration of Relief (hr)
Patient 1	56, M	3	Morphine (0.5)	7, 1	18
		2	Saline solution	6, 1	6
Patient 2	60, M	2	Morphine (0.5)	7, 1	12
		2	Saline solution	8, 8	No relief
Patient 3	57, F	2	Morphine (0.5)	5, 0	22
		1	Saline solution	6, 5	No relief
Patient 4	68, M	2	Morphine (1.0)	5, 0	20
		2	Saline solution	5, 4	No relief
Patient 5	66, M	2	Morphine (0.5)	5, 1	14
		1	Saline solution	6, 7	No relief
Patient 6	71, M	2	Morphine (0.5)	3, 1	10
		1	Saline solution	3, 1	8
Patient 7	51, M	3	Morphine (1.0)	4, 0	24
		2	Saline solution	5, 4	No relief
Patient 8	62, M	1	Morphine (0.5)	4, 0	21
		1	Saline solution	5, 5	No relief

(Wang JK, Nauss LA, Thomas JE: Pain relief by intrathecally applied morphine in man. Anesthesiology 50:149, 1979.)

is a Freon driven device with a 50 ml, percutaneously filled drug chamber and a constant infusion rate.[135] Pumps with a 2 to 3 ml · day^{-1} flow rate run for 15 to 20 days between refills. Daily dose is adjusted by changing the morphine concentration. A separate drug injection septum allows injection directly into the epidural space, bypassing the drug chamber. The technique is most appropriate for patients with a relatively long life expectancy (months rather than weeks).

Perhaps the most frustrating problem associated with intraspinal opioid administration is the development of marked resistance or tolerance to the medication. While most patients develop tolerance slowly and to a limited degree, some demonstrate rapid escalation of doses. Woods reported a patient who had been on 280 mg morphine intravenously and 90 mg methadone orally each day prior to starting epidural opioids. He was initially comfortable on 5 mg epidural morphine per day (Fig. 53-7). However, by the fifth day of epidural morphine administration, the dose had increased to 7 to 10 mg · hr^{-1}.[136] Greenberg et al reported a patient who initially experienced 17 hrs relief from 1 mg intrathecal morphine, but after several weeks, required an intrathecal infusion of 96 mg · day^{-1} plus modest oral doses of levorphanol.[137] I have treated a patient who required 60 mg epidural morphine every 6 hours plus an intravenous morphine infusion of 300 mg · hr^{-1}.

Various efforts to overcome the massive tolerance occasionally seen with intraspinal opioids have been undertaken. Limited trials of the alpha-2 agonist clonidine injected epidurally and intrathecally have proven at least temporarily effective (Fig. 53-8).[138] There is some evidence that patients who are highly tolerant to mu-receptor agonists (morphine, fentanyl, meperidine, etc) may experience good relief from intraspinal delta-receptor agonists, e.g., D-Ala-D-Leu-enkephalin (DADL).[139] However, it now appears that tolerance to delta agonists also develops rapidly, and there is some cross tolerance between mu- and delta-receptor agonists. Another approach is to provide several days of analgesia with intraspinal local anesthetics, allowing the opioid receptors to again become sensitive to their ligands, or to use combinations of opioids and dilute local anesthetics. The combined use of these agents makes sense, as the local anesthetic, even at subblocking concentrations, can reduce the maximum firing rates of nociceptor fibers, and the opioid reduces the sensitivity of WDR and nociceptive specific neurons in the dorsal horn to activation by nociceptors. Other substances which may have promise in either reversing tolerance or producing analgesia when injected intraspinally are somatostatin, baclofen, and ketamine.

One potential problem that can arise when instituting treatment with intraspinal opioids is the occurrence of withdrawl symptoms, particularly if the total daily opioid dose is reduced sharply.[140] Withdrawal symptoms can be minimized by the use of oral clonidine or maintenance doses of oral methadone.

Non-Neurolytic Nerve Blocks

The anesthesiologist is often called upon to perform neurodestructive nerve blocks to control intractable pain from advanced malignancy. These procedures carry a significant risk of paresis, bowel and bladder dysfunction, and painful neuritis. There are several conditions encountered in patients with cancer that are likely to respond to less dangerous nerve block procedures. RSD occurs fairly often in cancer patients. Severe burning pain following surgery, particularly if accompanied by any symptom of autonomic nervous system dysfunction, should arouse suspicion. Occasionally tumor invasion of soft tissues may trigger RSD. Sympathetic blocks should be performed diagnostically if the diagnosis is entertained, and blocks should be repeated if there is substantial improvement in symptoms.

Myofascial pain is common among cancer patients. It is

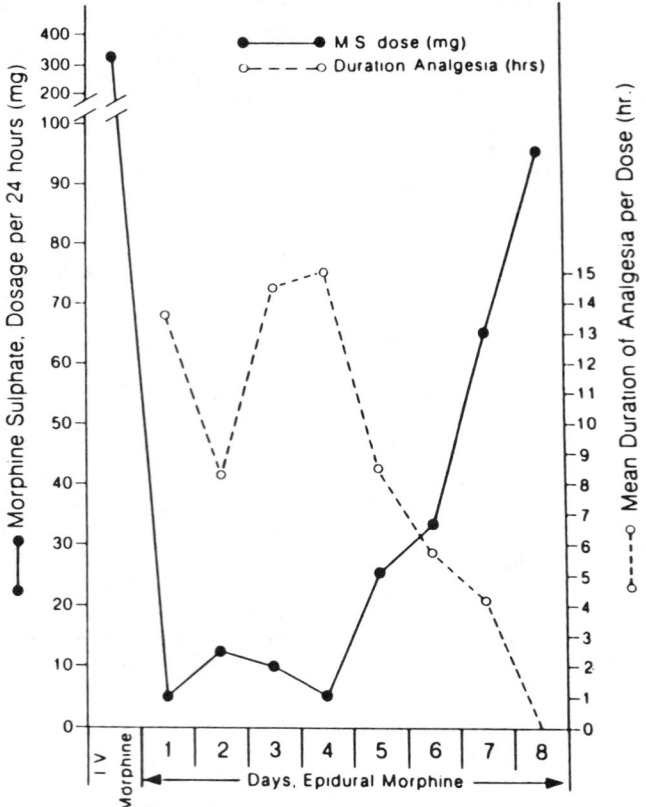

FIG. 53-7. Daily dose of morphine (oral and intravenous) and duration of analgesia produced by epidural morphine (2.5 to 15 mg). After fifth day, even the large dose of morphine produced only a few hours of analgesia (Woods WA, Cohen SE: High-dose epidural morphine in a terminally ill patient. Anesthesiology 56:311, 1982. Reproduced with permission of the authors and publisher.)

FIG. 53-8. Mean daily visual analogue pain score reported by a patient before and for 45 days during treatment with intrathecal infusion of clonidine and morphine (Coombs DW, Saunders RL, Lachance D et al: Intrathecal morphine tolerance: Use of intrathecal clonidine, DADLE, and intraventricular morphine. Anesthesiology 62:358, 1985.)

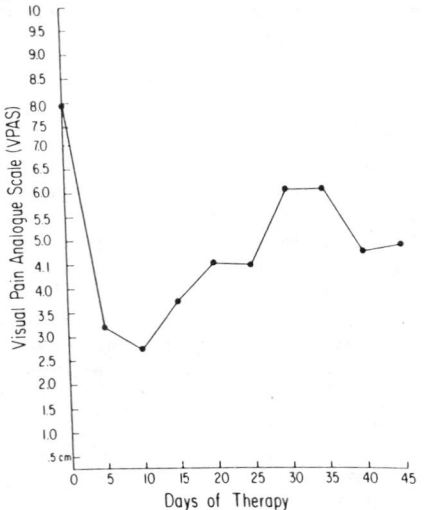

often associated with bony infiltration, neural compression, or visceral pain. Local anesthetic injections of trigger points may be surprisingly effective. Fluorimethane spray of trigger points combined with gentle stretching of affected skeletal muscles can be very helpful. TENS is also very likely to be of benefit.

Tumor compression of nerve roots, brachial or femoral plexus, or peripheral nerves sometimes responds dramatically to perineural injection of insoluble steroids. I have found that pain relief can be achieved for up to 1 month in many instances. When radicular pain is caused by epidural tumor spread, epidural injections of triamcinolone diacetate are likely to be of benefit. Tumor compression of the brachial plexus may respond to brachial plexus block with a combination of depo steroid and local anesthetic. The interscalene, supraclavicular, infraclavicular, or axillary approaches may all be used, depending on the site of pathology. Femoral plexopathy can be treated with a paravertebral approach (psoas compartment block) to the femoral plexus, again using triamcinolone diacetate and local anesthetic. Steroid-local anesthetic blocks of involved peripheral nerves are occasionally beneficial, particularly if they are performed reasonably soon after the onset of pain. Patients with severe neurogenic pain should be warned that, if the injections are successful in producing pain relief, they are likely to be left with some numbness, not from the injections but from the already present neural pathology.

Acute herpes zoster is a relatively common and often debilitating source of pain in patients with malignancy. There is some evidence that local anesthetic blockade of sympathetic fibers, using either paravertebral sympathetic blocks or epidurals, promptly relieves pain, may shorten the acute phase of the illness, and may reduce the incidence of postherpetic neuralgia.[141] Even if the overall course of the illness is not dramatically affected, patients are usually extremely grateful for any respite from the severe pain associated with this condition.

Occasionally patients with severe cancer pain are refractory to any opioid analgesic intervention. These patients may progress to psychological decompensation without reasonably prompt intervention. The use of continuous infusion local anesthetic blockade may be the best answer for patients who reach such a crisis situation. Continuous epidurals with dilute local anesthetics can be performed at any level of the neuraxis. When upper thoracic or cervical approaches are used, close monitoring of blood pressure and ventilation is necessary.

Neurolytic Blocks

There is a much greater willingness among anesthesiologists to perform neurolytic blocks for terminal cancer patients with pain than for patients with nonmalignant causes of pain. Reluctance to use neurolytic blocks for noncancer pain is certainly justified. The extent and duration of analgesia from neurodestructive procedures is limited by regrowth of axons and by development of central pain mechanisms (denervation dysesthesia). While neurolytic blocks can produce dramatic relief for some cancer pain patients, there are some serious potential drawbacks to the technique, and therefore, overzealous use of neurodestructive procedures should be avoided.

The principle disadvantage of neurolytic blocks is the inability to precisely control the spread of the destructive agents. Loss of motor function or inability to control bowel or bladder function following neurolysis can be devastating to a patient, and can greatly impair the quality of remaining life. The expected analgesia may not always result from destruction of the intended neural structures, even when prognostic local anesthetic blocks have been performed. If central nervous system mechanisms play a major role in a patient's pain, neurolysis is unlikely to be of benefit. In some cases, tumor progression rapidly produces pain beyond the confines of the block. With the advent of improved methods of cancer therapy, more patients survive well beyond the efficacy of the block. Overall, the incidence of fair to good results following neurolytic blockade is estimated at 50% to 60%.[142]

Alcohol and phenol are the agents most commonly used for prolonged interruption of neural function. There is relatively little difference in overall efficacy between these agents, but there are major differences in the initial responses. Phenol produces no pain on injection, has an initial local anesthetic effect and takes about 15 minutes to exert its neurolytic effect. Alcohol causes significant pain on injection, and produces neurolysis promptly. When used for intrathecal neurolysis, alcohol is hypobaric, whereas phenol in glycerine, the usual intrathecal preparation, is hyperbaric.

Intrathecal neurolysis with small volumes of alcohol or phenol requires careful positioning to place the affected sensory root uppermost (for alcohol) or in the most dependent position (for phenol). In such a way, only the involved sensory roots are affected. Patient movement during or shortly after injection can produce spread of drug to the cord, to other dermatomes, or to motor roots. Papo and Visca published results in a large series of patients who underwent phenol rhizotomy.[143] They reported good results (pain free until death) in 40% of 290 patients and fair results (reduced analgesic requirements or temporary complete relief) in 35%. Patients with localized pain to sacral dermatomes had the best results, while patients with pain in the upper thoracic area or upper or lower extremities had poor analgesia and more frequent complications. Swerdlow reviewed 13 reports of the results of phenol and alcohol rhizotomies and found good relief of pain in about 60% of patients.[144] In reviewing results on his own patients, he found that analgesia lasted less than 2 months in half the patients and less than 1 month in 25% of patients. Complications lasting longer than a week occurred in 15% of patients.

Patients with severe, localized perineal pain are very likely to experience relief with intrathecal blocks with phenol in glycerine. I use 7% phenol in glycerine, injected in 0.25 ml increments up to a maximum of 2 ml with the patient in the sitting position. This treatment is limited to patients who have undergone fecal and urinary diversion procedures.

Bladder pain and spasm has been successfully treated with transsacral phenol injections.[145] If blocks are confined to one or two roots there is little risk of disrupting bladder function. There are several reports of gasserian ganglion alcohol injection for severe facial pain.[146] Unfortunately most of these reports constitute a description of the procedure, and little data about efficacy are available.

Celiac plexus block for pain associated with upper abdominal malignancy is the most successful and rewarding of the neurolytic blocks. Thompson et al reported that 94 of 97 patients who underwent celiac plexus block for pain of upper abdominal cancer had good to excellent pain relief.[147] Injections were performed with 50 ml of 50% alcohol. Survival from the cancer ranged form 2 days to 14 months. Fourteen patients required repeat injections for recurrent pain. Ten patients experienced transient orthostatic hypotension and one patient had partial motor loss in one leg.

The classical technique for percutaneous injection of the celiac plexus involves bilateral placement of block needles just anterior to the body of L-1 and posterior to the aorta and diaphragmatic crura.[148] Recently techniques have been described that involve more anterior positioning of the needle tip with computed tomography (CT) assistance so that it lies anterior to the diaphragmatic crura.[149, 150] The injected solution can be seen to spread more anteriorly, surrounding the aorta. There is much less tendency of the injected solution to spread posteriorly to the paravertebral nerve roots or sympathetic chain, minimizing risk of paresis or orthostatic hypotension. Using this technique, Ischia et al reported 93% success in relieving pain in 28 patients with cancer pain.

Because celiac ganglion neurolysis is highly effective and carries a relatively low incidence of complications, it may be reasonable to consider implementing it early in the course of the patient's pain. When tumor becomes more widespread late in the course of the disease, it becomes more difficult to completely block the appropriate visceral afferent fibers with neurolytic solution. Systemic or epidural opioids may be a better choice in far advanced disease.

Other Modes of Therapy

There are a number of therapeutic options that are relatively specific for the type of malignancy being dealt with. When dealing with tumors that are extremely radiosensitive, radiation therapy is often the most effective form of intervention. If chemotherapeutic options are available, they may provide analgesia through reduction of tumor mass. Pain caused by hormonally sensitive tumors may be best treated by appropriate manipulation of the patient's hormonal environment. Surgical debulking of a large tumor sometimes relieves pain of obstruction or abdominal distension. Stabilization of an isolated pathological fracture can be an extremely effective pain relieving procedure. Certain neurosurgical procedures, such as spinal cord stimulation and cordotomy, may afford months of profound relief in certain types of cases. Some patients benefit considerably with psychological interventions such as hypnosis or other cognitive strategies. With the complexity of the disease processes involved with cancer related pain and the number of pain mechanisms and therapeutic interventions that are possible, it is essential that the full range of medical and behavioral science disciplines be made available to cancer patients.

ORGANIZATION OF A PAIN CLINIC

The successful management of the entire group of pain problems encountered in clinical practice requires an extensive array of physician specialties, diagnostic facilities, therapeutic modalities, nonphysician health-care professionals, research capabilities, and office support staff. Ideally, each patient should have access to the full range of facilities and professional expertise. In order to support such staff and facilities, a pain treatment center must have a considerable and diverse case load. Obviously, our ideal pain clinic must be located in a large metropolitan area or must be located at a substantial tertiary care center. Unfortunately, the need for effective pain management is not confined to larger population centers, and modifications of the ideal approach must be accepted where more extensive facilities cannot be supported. This section describes the relatively new multidisciplinary approach to pain management and discusses some alternative organizational plans that may be more appropriate for smaller medical centers and for specific conditions.

The number of pain facilities in the United States has recently been estimated at over 400.[151] They are generally categorized as multidisciplinary (implying ability to manage a diverse group of disorders and using a wide range of modalities), syndrome-oriented or modality-oriented clinics. The multidisciplinary clinic is the ideal pain management facility defined in the previous paragraph. The syndrome-oriented clinic is organized to treat a specific type of pain problem, such as low back pain, headache, or facial pain. The most successful syndrome-oriented clinics are organized in a multidisciplinary fashion. They have the advantage of needing fewer specialties and may function with more limited physical facilities than the diverse multidisciplinary clinic. A physician staffing a syndrome-oriented clinic has a better chance of developing an in-depth understanding of the entire range of problems likely to be encountered. Modality-oriented clinics are organized around a single type of treatment, such as nerve blocks, biofeedback, acupuncture, or hypnosis. In order for such clinics to be productive, the referring physician must be aware of the clinic's capability and must know which patients are likely to benefit from the treatment offered. The practitioner operating such a clinic must confine his efforts to patients with a high likelihood of responding to their therapy, and must coordinate his treatment with other appropriate therapeutic interventions.

A fourth type of organization that does not fit clearly into any of the previously described categories is seen frequently. It is organized around a small group of specialists who have a fairly wide understanding of the pain conditions they encounter, but they are limited to a restricted range of modalities that are directly provided in the clinic. Such a clinic functions, however, effectively, by using consultation mechanisms within their medical center. Perhaps the best title for such a clinic is "oligodisciplinary." A typical composition might be an anesthesiologist, a clinical psychologist or psychiatrist, a physical therapist, and a nurse. While a substantial percentage of referrals may be successfully managed by such a team, consultation by other disciplines are invariably needed for some patients, and patients with certain conditions (e.g., headache) might be better managed by a clinic with a somewhat different composition. The composition of a pain clinic is determined by the interest, expertise, and availability for pain clinic practice of the health-care professionals in that community.

THE MULTIDISCIPLINARY MODEL

Setting

Both inpatient and outpatient facilities have a role in chronic pain management. Initial screening and most therapy can be adequately managed on an outpatient basis. Inpatient treatment should be used for very chronic patients who require drug detoxification, intensive behavior modification, which may require total removal from the home environment, or invasive therapeutic interventions.

The outpatient facility should have examination rooms adequately stocked with appropriate physical diagnosis equipment and examining tables. Treatment rooms should be equipped with OR-type tables, adequate lighting, patient monitoring equipment (BP, ECG, skin temperature), intravenous equipment, and resuscitation drugs and equipment (including defibrillator and "crash cart"). Adequate storage facilities for nerve block equipment, TENS equipment, linen and gowns, and resuscitation drugs and equipment must be furnished. Oxygen, suction, adequate counter space and a

sink are needed in each treatment room. Separate facilities allow more rapid turnover of treatment areas.

The clinic area should have pleasant waiting facilities and should provide patients with space for filling out questionnaires, for psychological testing instruments, and for viewing educational materials. A quiet treatment area is needed for biofeedback training and other cognitive strategies and for psychiatric interviews and treatment. Clinic staff should have office space and conference facilities that are physically separated from patient reception, waiting, and treatment areas. View boxes and appropriate audiovisual equipment should be available in the conference areas. Office staff should have space within the clinic for reception, patient files, and transcription facilities.

Ideally, inpatient facilities for chronic pain patients should be separated from conventional medical, surgical, psychiatric, or rehabilitation floors. It is important that pain clinic inpatients not think of their problems in conventional medical model terms. They should be provided with facilities where they can meet and socialize during nontherapy times. Extensive exercise and physical therapy equipment and space must be provided. Space for group and individual pscyhotherapy and for educational sessions should be available. A nursing station, with around-the-clock staffing, is required for detoxification protocols, for administration of maintenance non-analgesic drugs, and for monitoring medical problems that may arise during periods of increased physical activity.

STAFFING

The composition of the pain clinic staff depends on the interest and availability of personnel with chronic pain management skills and the needs of the population served. The director must be a physician, as a wide variety of medical problems will be encountered among clinic patients. According to a Pain Clinic/Center Directory published by the American Society of Anesthesiologists, anesthesiologists served as directors of 61% of 251 pain clinics listed.[152] Regardless of specialty, the director should have a broad range of knowledge and experience with chronic pain management. At least one integral member of the team should specialize in behavioral sciences. There are advantages to having both Psychiatry and Clinical Psychology directly involved with the clinic. Psychologists generally have expertise and interest in psychometrics, cognitive strategies, behavior modification protocols, and group therapy, while psychiatrists are needed for assessment and therapy of major psychiatric disorders that are often seen in the pain clinic population. Obviously, there is some overlap in the interests and abilities of these practitioners.

The composition of the remainder of the physician staff depends on the emphasis and philosophy of the clinic. If the goals are predominantly rehabilitative, a physical therapist is an essential member. If a large number of relatively acute problems are encountered, anesthesiologists and orthopedic surgeons should be actively involved. For cancer pain patients, anesthesiology, radiation therapy, and oncology should provide staffing. If a large number of headache patients are seen, a neurologist should be an active team member. To treat facial pain, a neurologist and a dentist should be included on the staff. Services of specialties that are not members of the pain clinic team should be readily available on a consultation basis.

Services that should be available on a regular and continuing basis are physical therapy, nursing, pharmacy, social services, dietetics, vocational services, occupational therapy, and exercise physiology. Diagnostic radiology and laboratory services must be readily accessible. Reception and secretarial services should be solely dedicated to the pain clinic rather than shared with other services.

ADMISSION CRITERIA

The types of the patients admitted to the pain clinic depends on the emphasis and philosophy of the clinic staff. Treatment outcomes are greatly influenced by the kinds of patients admitted and some centers may admit as few as one-third of their referrals in an effort to maintain high success rates. Although there has been increased public awareness of the value of multidisciplinary pain management, third-party payers, particularly government funded programs, are often reluctant to cover the cost of comprehensive pain management programs, and many centers must limit admissions to patients with adequate health insurance.

In order to maximize benefit to the patients evaluated by the pain clinic, certain guidelines should be followed strictly. 1) All patients must be referred by a physician. Patients referred by lawyers or insurance representatives are almost invariably being sent to collect information that may be helpful to the patient's case or the insurance company's case. Referrals from an emergency room or walk-in clinic are inappropriate. Patients from these facilities have been inadequately evaluated and often present with problems that are better managed by other types of clinics. 2) Referring physicians must send enough historical, physical examination, and laboratory data prior to the first visit to provide a reasonable working diagnosis and to rule out conditions that require specific medical or surgical intervention. Patients with an inadequate data base should be referred to an appropriate diagnostic service or sent back to the referring physician for further evaluation. The pain clinic should not be the initial facility to evaluate the patient's condition. 3) Referred patients should have an understanding of the purpose of the referral and of the nature of the proposed pain clinic treatment. Patient brochures, provided by referring physicians or sent directly to the patient, are helpful in providing such information. It is useful to explicitly describe clinic policy on opioid prescriptions in order to discourage drug-seeking behavior at the time of the initial visit.

INITIAL VISIT

An extensive pain questionnaire is an extremely valuable tool in the evaluation of the pain patient, and should be completed before the physician's history and physical. It should ask about the onset, duration, location, and intensity of the pain, associated symptoms, previous treatment, and analgesic and other medications. A pain diagram and pain intensity scales should be included. Other questions should inquire about effects of the pain on sleep, employment, social, recreational, and sexual activity and interpersonal relationships. Financial consequences of the painful condition (compensation for injuries, present income sources, pending litigation) should be explored.

Psychological testing is generally carried out on the first visit. It is helpful for detecting psychopathology that may initiate or aggravate pain complaints and for determining the psychological impact of chronic pain and illness. Several types of testing instruments have proven useful for assessing pain patients. The State-Trait Anxiety Inventory is a self-administered test that evaluates the patient's level of anxiety or distress. Very high scores correlate with suicidal intent. Several depression scales have been used for pain clinic populations. The McGill Pain questionnaire is a checklist of words describing the patients symptoms. Certain pain problems, *e.g.*, radiculopathy, are typically associated with particular descriptors. Selection of descriptors not typical of that condition might raise doubts concerning the diagnosis. Selection of a large number of descriptors or of predominantly affective descriptors, would suggest a strong psychological component to that patient's pain. The Dartmouth Questionnaire combines the McGill checklist with an assessment of the effect of pain on the patient's daily activity. It asks the patient to compare the way they feel now to the way they felt before their pain started.

A personality assessment is often a part of the initial psychological screening procedure. The Minnesota Multiphasic Personality Inventory (MMPI) has been widely used in pain clinics, but has several drawbacks. It is lengthy, often taking over an hour to complete, and has a number of questions that patients find insulting or objectionable. Investigators have found relatively little qualitative difference in results between patients with acute pain and those with chronic pain. The SCL (system checklist) 90 is a computer-scored personality inventory that pain clinic patients find more palatable.

A psychologist's behavioral assessment, looking for the character and frequency of verbal complaints and evaluating nonverbal complaints (moaning, grimacing, posturing) is a helpful addition to psychological testing. A psychological interview helps to assess the degree of psychological distress associated with the patient's pain.

On the first visit, the patient is assigned to a physician, sometimes termed *pain manager* who is primarily responsible for making decisions regarding that patient's care. Although that physician does not necessarily directly provide most of the patient's care, he/she does direct the diagnostic and therapeutic intervention. In a teaching institution a resident or fellow may act as a patient's pain manager, consulting with staff physicians prior to making decisions regarding that patient's care. The pain manager usually conducts the initial history and physical examination.

The patient's history should complement the pain questionnaire. In addition to a detailed history of the pain complaint, a complete history and review of systems should be carried out. The social, psychological, and vocational aspects of the history are particularly important in these patients. A complete physical examination should be carried out. Major emphasis should be placed on the painful area. Maneuvers to test neurological function, including procedures for evaluating radicular or peripheral nerve sensitivity, are done routinely. A systematic search for myofascial trigger points should be carried out. Evaluation of autonomic nervous system function (skin color, temperature, moisture, edema) and peripheral pulses are important components of the evaluation. Range of motion must be evaluated. When motion of a joint is limited it should be noted whether limitation is secondary to pain or to mechanical conditions.

Attempts at measurement of the patient's pain may be carried out on the first visit. A 10-cm long visual analog scale (VAS) with two anchors (no pain, worst pain imaginable) is commonly used. It has proven to be reliable and valid, and is useful in assessing the degree of improvement following intervention. The ischemic tourniquet test was developed for evaluating efficacy of analgesic medications, but has been adapted for pain clinic use. Following mild exercise of an upper extremity under ischemic conditions, time elapsed until pain begins (pain threshold) is determined. The tourniquet remains inflated, and time to patient request to terminate the ischemia (pain tolerance) is measured. The patient is also asked to acknowledge the point in time when the ischemic pain equals the clinical pain. If the clinical pain is perceived as mild, it will be close to the threshold. If it is severe it should be close to the tolerance time.

If, following the first day's evaluation, the pain manager determines that the patient's pain is fairly straightforward and that a particular course of treatment is warranted, that treatment would be initiated at that time. If further evaluation is needed, the appropriate evaluations are scheduled. The patient may be asked to keep a pain diary, noting times of the day that the pain is most severe, when analgesics are taken, and what physical activities are done.

SUBSEQUENT VISITS

Once the assessment is complete, members of the pain team meet to discuss the patient and to decide on treatment options. Once the pain team has decided on a course of therapy, it is discussed with the patient and the patient's family. Often family members are given important roles in the patient's rehabilitation. At this time the patient should be made aware of the goals of the therapy. If physical or medical interventions are planned, what is the chance that they will reduce the patient's pain. If treatment is aimed at developing coping skills, reducing analgesic use, and increasing physical activity, those goals should be made clear, and should be acceptable to the patient before treatment is started.

When treatment consists of progressive increases in activity, giving up pain behaviors, and decreasing medication use, goals should be spelled out in writing. It is particularly useful to list behaviors or activities that will not be tolerated by the treatment team, such as requesting replacement of medications that were "lost" or "stolen," or "accidentally flushed down the toilet." These expectations of the patient can be expressed as a written contract, with notice that flagrant disregard for contractural obligations will result in dismissal from the program.

When physical modalities such as nerve blocks, TENS, or physical therapy are employed, it is important to document the degree of analgesia achieved by the procedure and to follow the patient's progress from one visit to the next. Immediate changes can be assessed with VAS and with objective changes in range of motion or tenderness. Changes occurring over days to weeks can be assessed with VAS and with pain diaries or activity scales. When treatment is behavioral or operant, pain diaries and activity levels are much more important assessment tools than are subjective pain ratings.

THE MODALITY-ORIENTED CLINIC

Many Departments of Anesthesia and individual practitioners have organized pain clinics whose function is based on the use of nerve blocks for the management of difficult pain problems. It is well established that certain regional anesthetic techniques can provide dramatic benefit for certain intractable pain problems, most of which are relatively acute, such as RSD, sciatica, and some types of cancer pain. Nerve blocks also serve important diagnostic functions, such as differentiation between somatic and visceral pain, and are of prognostic use. However, the usefulness of nerve blocks in the management of chronic pain is not clear cut. While regional block techniques may be useful adjuncts in managing chronic pain,[153] success rates of nerve blocks used as the sole modality in treating noncancer pain of long duration are very low.[154]

For a modality-oriented clinic to serve a worthwhile function, it is extremely important that the director be aware of the limitations of the modality employed. When therapeutic techniques are used for conditions that are unlikely to respond, the added costs, risks, and frustrations to the patient are considerable. When procedures are performed unnecessarily on a large scale, insurance carriers become reluctant to reimburse for those services, even when used appropriately.

For physicians who staff modality-oriented clinics, frequent referrals of patients who are unlikely to respond to the modality offered become a major source of frustration. In order to better serve the population of referred patients, those physicians may choose one of two options. The first option is to expand the clinic services to include modalities that many referred patients require. The addition of psychological services, pharmacological management (including drug detoxification), and physical therapy, for instance, can markedly increase the range of patients who can be successfully managed in a nerve block clinic. The second option involves integration with other pain management facilities. If a Psychology-Rehabilitation Medicine pain program is already in existence in the community, patients who need the services of such a program can be evaluated and treated by that facility simultaneously. Establishment of a common data base between various separate components of the pain program minimizes referral delays and reduces duplication of services. Anesthesia services can be integrated with rehabilitation and psychological services in a productive way. For instance, nerve blocks or trigger point injections can be scheduled prior to physical therapy sessions that are ordinarily painful to the patient.

ACUTE PAIN SERVICE

The development of new, invasive, and potentially hazardous techniques for postoperative and posttraumatic pain has created a need for an organized approach to acute pain management. An acute pain service must be able to provide needed analgesic techniques around the clock and to provide continuous, or at least frequent, monitoring of ventilatory, cardiovascular, and CNS function.

The use of constant infusion regional anesthesia techniques, intraspinal opioids, and intravenous opioid infusions create the risk of sudden, profound depression of ventilation, respiratory muscle paralysis, cardiovascular collapse, and local anesthetic toxicity. These techniques mandate frequent or continuous surveillance coupled with prompt availability of anesthesia personnel. Such techniques are contraindicated in settings where anesthesia personnel are not available in house 24 hours a day. An intensive care setting is the ideal environment for patients placed at increased risk by regional analgesic procedures. The cost of intensive care unit care for patients who would not otherwise need such attention is prohibitive, however. A sensible alternative is the establishment of a multiple bed monitoring unit staffed by a small number of nurses with frequent visual surveillance but little else in the way of additional care compared to the surgical ward. Telemetered monitoring of ECG, blood pressure, and breathing rate for patients in private rooms is another alternative. The frequency of false-positive events with apnea monitoring has been somewhat of a problem when such alternatives have been employed.

The acute care team should be fully integrated with the operating room anesthesiologists. Planning for postoperative analgesic care should be done preoperatively, when the patients needs and preferences can be best assessed. Early planning allows regional analgesic techniques to be incorporated into the intraoperative management as well.

CANCER PAIN SERVICE

The concept of an interdisciplinary approach to cancer pain management is belatedly finding application in many centers. The need for a team approach is most critical in this field. The severity of the pain, the complexity of the medical care needed, and the desperation of the patient and the family do not permit leisurely approach to the cancer pain patient. Sequential use of consultants results in inexcusable delays in starting appropriate therapy. A modality-oriented approach leaves the majority of patients with grossly suboptimal care.

The oncologist is usually (and appropriately) the central physician member of the cancer pain team. The oncologist's familiarity with the course of the disease, the definitive and palliative chemotherapeutic management, and management of nonpain complications is essential to rational patient care. Most oncologists are reasonably skilled in conventional pharmacological approaches to cancer pain (the use of oral and parenteral opioids, nonopioid analgesics, psychotropics, steroids, etc.). The radiation oncologist is a critical member of the team. The appropriate use of radiation in the palliation of certain cancer pain problems can greatly reduce the use of depressant medications and high-risk procedures. Anesthesiology is another critical discipline. The advent of intraspinal opioids has greatly strengthened the anesthesiologist's armamentarium. Neuroablative techniques can be performed with neurolytic agents with less trauma than most neurosurgical procedures. Local anesthetic block techniques can sometimes provide lasting relief, and continuous blocks can provide periods of respite from crisis situations when prolonged, severe pain has caused a state of desperation. Psychological services are essential. While the psychological contributions to pain in cancer differ to some extent from those associated with non-cancer pain, they are nevertheless exceedingly important, and the services of a psychiatrist or psychologist who is familiar with the psychodynamics of cancer pain are very important. Neurosurgery consultation is certainly not needed on all patients with cancer pain, but neuroablation or CNS stimulation may be the best option for some patients. The neurosurgeon must, therefore, be readily available for consultation.

Without the services of a skilled oncology nurse, any cancer pain management program is sure to fail. Without the nurse's input, recognition of problems may not occur. The nurse must provide feedback to the physician when treatment is inadequate or when side-effects are becoming intolerable. The nurse must be resilient and able to adapt to new or innovative treatment protocols. The nurse's role as interface between patient and physician is nowhere more critical than in cancer pain management. With the increasing complexity of analgesic techniques, it is essential that the pharmacist be intimately involved with the cancer pain team. The use of infusion pumps for drug administration requires the pharmacist's familiarity with a variety of systems. Maintenance of analgesic infusions outside the hospital setting requires close cooperation of pharmacy and visiting nurse programs.

Most new cancer pain problems are encountered in an inpatient setting. They occur in two different settings, the first involving patients who are receiving definitive treatment for their cancer. It is often not clear whether these patients are curable. Patients and their oncologists may wish to use their pain symptoms as a measure of treatment success, and do not always seek major intervention for pain control. Such motives are occasionally taken to extremes, however, and patients may

be deprived of appropriate analgesic management. The second setting involves the terminal patient. These patients may be in the hospital or hospice specifically for management of intractable pain. It is critical that their pain be addressed promptly and as aggressively as the situation warrants. Humanitarian considerations must be kept in mind, however. It may be far more humane, for instance to push opioid analgesics to the point of marked sedation to relieve pain than to risk loss of bowel or bladder function in a near terminal patient. Such ethical questions are common in these cases and often need to be discussed with the patient and the family.

The format of the cancer pain management service may vary greatly, but certain elements are necessary 1) input by the needed services listed above, 2) prompt and frequent staffing conferences on new pain problems by members of those services, 3) prompt institution of measures decided upon by the team, and 4) quick recognition of treatment inadequacy or side-effects and institution of alternative measures. Ward rounds on patients selected by the oncology nurse as having significant pain problems serves as a very useful tool. A relatively small nucleus of the pain team may be involved in initial rounds, with other members being called in as needed. Less frequent staffing involving the entire team should be carried out for the most difficult patients.

REFERENCES

1. Burgess PR, Perl ER: Cutaneous mechanoreceptors and nociceptors. In Iggo A (ed): Handbook of Sensory Physiology, vol 2, p 29, Berlin, Springer Verlag, 1973
2. Lynn B: The detection of injury and tissue damage. In Melzack R, Wall PD (eds): Textbook of Pain, p 19. New York, Churchill Livingstone, 1984
3. Campbell JN, Meyer RA, LaMotte RH: Sensitization of myelinated nociceptive afferents that innervate the monkey hand. Neurophysiology 42:1669, 1979
4. Kruger L, Perl ER, Sedivic MJ: Fine structure of myelinated mechanical nociceptor endings in cat hairy skin. J Comp Neurol 198:137, 1981
5. Torebjork HE: Afferent C units responding to mechanical, thermal and chemical stimuli in human non-glabrous skin. Acta Phys Scand 92:374, 1974
6. Adriaensen H, Gybels J, Handwerker HO et al: Latencies of chemically evoked discharges in human nociceptors and the concurrent subjective sensations. Neurosci Lett 20:55, 1980
7. Georgopoulos AP: Functional properties of primary afferent units probably related to pain mechanisms in primate glabrous skin. J Neurophysiol 39:71, 1976
8. Bessou P, Perl E: Response of cutaneous sensory units with unmyelinated fibers to noxious stimuli. J Neurophysiol 32:1025, 1969
9. Kniffki K-D, Mense S, Schmidt RE: Muscle receptors with fine afferent fibers which may evoke circulatory reflexes. Circ Res 48:I, 25, 1981
10. Freeman MAR, Wyke B: The innervation of the knee joint. An anatomical and histological study of the cat. J Anat 101:505, 1967
11. Burgess PR, Clark FJ: Characteristics of knee joint receptors in the cat. J Physiol 203:317, 1969
12. Moncada S, Ferreira SH, Vane JR: Inhibition of prostaglandin biosynthesis as the mechanism of analgesia of aspirin-like drugs in the dog knee joint. Eur J Pharmacol 31:250, 1975
13. Kendall GPN: Visceral Pain. Br J Surg (suppl):s4:72, 1985
14. Milne RJ, Foreman RD, Giesler GJ et al: Viscerosomatic convergence onto primate spinothalamic neurones: An explanation for referral of pelvic visceral pain. In Bonica JJ (ed): Advances in Pain Research and Therapy, vol 5, p 131. New York, Raven Press, 1983

15. Bahr R, Blumberg H, Janig W: Do dichotomizing afferent fibers exist which supply visceral organs as well as somatic structures? Neurosci Lett 24:25, 1981

16. Moriarty KJ, Dawson AM: Functional abdominal pain: Further evidence that the whole gut is affected. Br Med J 284:1670, 1982

17. Guzman F, Braun C, Lim RKS: Visceral pain and the pseudoaffective response to intra-arterial injection of bradykinin and other algesic agents. Arch Int Pharmacodyn Ther 136:353, 1962

18. Malliani A: Cardiovascular sympathetic afferent fibers. Rev Physiol Biochem Pharmacol 94:11, 1982

19. Perl ER: Is pain a specific sensation? J Psychiatr Res 8:273, 1971

20. Cervero F: Afferent nerve activity evoked by natural stimulation of the biliary system in the ferret. Pain 13:137, 1982

21. Cuello AC, Matthews MR: Peptides in peripheral sensory nerve fibers. In Melzack R, Wall PD (eds): Textbook of Pain, p 65. New York, Churchill Livingstone, 1984

22. Terenius L: Biochemical mediators in pain. Triangle 20:19, 1981

23. Light AR, Perl ER: Spinal termination of functionally identified primary afferent neurons with slowly conducting myelinated fibers. J Comp Neurol 168:133, 1979

24. Wall PD: The dorsal horn. In Melzack R, Wall PD (eds): Textbook of Pain, p 80. New York, Churchill Livingstone, 1984

25. Dubner R, Bennett GJ: Spinal and trigeminal mechanisms of nociception. Ann Rev Neurosci 6:381, 1983

26. Duggan AW: Transmitters involved in central processing of nociceptive information. Anaesth Intens Care 10:133, 1982

27. Yaksh TL, Elde RP: Factors governing release of methionine enkephalin-like immunoreactivity from mesencephalon and spinal cord of the cat in vivo. J Neurophysiol 46:1056, 1981

28. Yaksh TL, Hammond DL: Peripheral and central substrates involved in the rostrad transmission of nociceptive information. Pain 13:1, 1982

29. Tasker RR: Deafferentation. In Melzack R, Wall PD (eds): Textbook of Pain, p 119. New York, Churchill Livingstone, 1984

30. Willis WD: The origin and destination of pathways involved in pain transmission. In Melzak R, Wall PD (eds): Textbook of Pain, p 88. New York, Churchill Livingstone, 1984

31. Fields HL: Brainstem mechanisms of pain modulation. In Kruger L, Liebeskind JC (eds): Advances in Pain Research and Therapy, vol 6, p 241. New York, Raven Press, 1984

32. Basbaum AI, Fields HL: Endogenous pain control systems: Brainstem spinal pathways and endorphin circuitry. Ann Rev Neurosci 7:309, 1984

33. Wall PD, Gutnick M: Ongoing activity in peripheral nerves: The physiology and pharmacology of impulses originating from a neuroma. Exp Neurol 43:580, 1974

34. Blumberg H, Janig W: Discharge pattern of afferent fibers from a neuroma. Pain 20:335, 1984

35. Devor M, Janig W: Activation of myelinated afferents ending in neuroma by stimulation of the sympathetic supply in the rat. Neurosci Lett 24:43, 1981

36. Devor M: Nerve pathophysiology and mechanisms of pain in causalgia. J Auton N Syst 7:371, 1983

37. Wall PD, Devor M: Sensory afferent impulses originate from dorsal root ganglia as well as from the periphery in normal and nerve injured rats. Pain 17:321, 1983

38. Blumberg H, Janig W: Changes in vasoconstrictor neurons supplying cat hindlimb following chronic nerve lesions: A model for studying mechanisms of reflex sympathetic dystrophy? J Auton Nerv Syst 7:399, 1983

39. Roberts WJ: A hypothesis on the physiological basis for causalgia and related pains. Pain 24:297, 1986

40. Owman C, Santini M: Adrenergic nerves in the spinal ganglia of the cat. Acta Physiol Scand 67:127, 1966

41. Wall PD, On the relation of injury to pain. Pain 6:253, 1979

42. Bromage PR, Camporesi EM, Chestnut D: Epidural narcotics for postoperative analgesia. Anesth Analg 59:473, 1980

43. Stanski DR, Greenblatt DJ, Lowenstein E: Kinetics of intravenous and intramuscular morphine. Clin Pharmacol Ther 24:52, 1978

44. Austin KL, Stapleton JV, Mather LE: Multiple intramuscular injections—A major source of variability in analgesic response to meperidine. Pain 8:47, 1980

45. Gourlay GK, Wilson PR, Glyn CJ: Methadone produces prolonged postoperative analgesia. Br Med J 284:630, 1982

46. Boas RA, Holford NHG, Villiger JW: Opiate drug choice and drug use. Clinical Journal of Pain 1:117, 1985

47. Sawe J, Dahlstrom B, Paalzow L et al: Morphine kinetics in cancer patients. Clin Pharmacol Ther 30:629, 1981

48. White PF: Patient-controlled analgesia: A new approach to the management of postoperative pain. Seminars in Anesthesia 4:255, 1985

49. Rosenberg PH, Heino A, Scheinin B: Comparison of intramuscular analgesia, intercostal block, epidural morphine and on-demand IV fentanyl in the control of pain after upper abdominal surgery. Acta Anaesthesiol Scand 28:603, 1984

50. Wang JK, Nauss LA, Thomas JE: Pain relief by intrathecally applied morphine in man. Anesthesiology 50:149, 1979

51. Gustafsson LL, Schildt B, Jacobsen KJ: Adverse effects of extradural and intrathecal opiates: Report of a nationwide survey in Sweden. Br J Anaesth 54:479, 1982

52. Brownridge PR: Epidural and intrathecal opiates for postoperative pain relief. Anaesthesia 38:74, 1983

53. Cousins MJ, Mather LE: Intrathecal and epidural administration of opioids. Anesthesiology 61:276, 1984

54. Behar M, Olshwang D, Magora F et al: Epidural morphine in treatment of pain. Lancet 1:527, 1979

55. Rawal N, Sjostrand UH, Dahlstrom B et al: Epidural morphine for postoperative pain relief: A comparative study with intramuscular narcotic and intercostal block. Anesth Analg 61:93, 1982

56. Matthew EB, Henderson SK, Avram MJ et al: Epidural hydromorphone versus epidural morphine for postcesarean section analgesia. Anesth Analg 66:S112, 1987

57. Palacios QT, Jones MM, Tessem J et al: Comparison of epidural butorphanol and morphine for analgesia cesarean section. Anesth Analg 66:S133, 1987

58. Lanz E, Simko G, Theiss D et al: Epidural buprenorphine—a double-blind study of postoperative analgesia and side effects. Anesth Analg 63:593, 1984

59. Johnston JR, McCaughey W: Epidural morphine: A method of management of fractured ribs. Anaesthesia 35:155, 1980

60. Scott DB, Schweitzer S, Thorn J: Epidural block in postoperative pain relief. Reg Anesth 7:135, 1982

61. Shuman PL, Peters RM: Epidural anesthesia following thoracotomy in patients with chronic obstructive airway disease. J Thorac Cardiovasc Surg 71:82, 1976

62. Griffiths DPG, Diamond AW, Cameron JD: Postoperative extradural analgesia following thoracic surgery. A feasibility study. Br J Anaesth 47:48, 1975

63. Denson DD, Raj PP, Saldahna F et al: Perineural infusions of bupivacaine for prolonged analgesia: Pharmacologic considerations. Int J Clin Pharmacol Ther Toxicol 21:591, 1983

64. Raj PP, Knarr D, Hartrick CT et al: Efficacy of continuous epidural bupivacaine infusion for postoperative pain relief. Anesthesiology 61:A186, 1984

65. Nunn JF, Slavin G: Posterior intercostal nerve block for pain relief after cholecystectomy, Br J Anaesth 52:253, 1980

66. Reiestad F, Stromskag KE: Interpleural catheter in the management of postoperative pain. A preliminary report. Reg Anesth 11:89, 1986

67. Long DM, Hagfors N: Electrical stimulation in the nervous system: The current status of electrical stimulation of the nervous system for pain relief. Pain 1:109, 1975

68. Eriksson MBF, Sjolund BH, Nielzen S: Long term results of conditioning stimulation as an analgesic measure in chronic pain. Pain 6:335, 1979
69. Chapman CR, Benedetti C: Analgesia following transcutaneous electrical stimulation and its partial reversal by a narcotic antagonist. Life Sci 21:1645, 1977
70. Abram SE, Reynolds AR, Cusick JF: Failure of naloxone to reverse analgesia from transcutaneous electrical stimulation in patients with chronic pain. Anesth Analg 60:81, 1981
71. Woolf CJ, Mitchell D, Myers RA et al: Failure of naloxone to reverse peripheral transcutaneous electroanalgesia in patients suffering from acute trauma. S Afr Med J 53:179, 1978
72. Hymes AC, Raab DE, Yonohiro EG et al: Acute pain control by electrostimulation: A preliminary report. In Advances in Neurology, vol 4, p 761. New York, Raven Press, 1974
73. Ali J, Yaffe CS, Serette C: The effect of transcutaneous electric nerve stimulation on postoperative pain and pulmonary function. Surgery 89:507, 1981
74. Stratton SA, Smith MM: Post-operative thoracotomy: Effect of transcutaneous electrical nerve stimulation on forced vital capacity. Phys Ther 60:45, 1980
75. Rosenberg M, Curtis L, Bourke DL: Transcutaneous electrical nerve stimulation for the relief of postoperative pain. Pain 5:129, 1978
76. Solomon RA, Viernstein MC, Long DM: Reduction of postoperative pain and narcotic use by transcutaneous electrical nerve stimulation. Surgery 87:142, 1980
77. Baker SBC, Wong CC, Wong PC et al: Transcutaneous electrostimulation in the management of postoperative pain: Initial report. Can Anaesth Soc J 27:150, 1980
78. Roeser WM, Meeks LW, Venis R et al: The use of transcutaneous nerve stimulation for pain control in athletic medicine. A preliminary report. Am J Sports Med 4:210, 1976
79. Mixter WJ, Barr JS: Rupture of the intervertebral disc with involvement of the spinal cord. N Engl J Med 211:210, 1934
80. Aitken AP: Rupture of the intervertebral disc in injury: Further observations and results. Am J Surg 84:261, 1952
81. Hirsch C, Nachemson A: The reliability of lumbar disc surgery. Clin Orthop 29:189, 1963
82. Hakelius A: Prognosis in sciatica. Acta Orthop Scand 129(suppl):1, 1970
83. Green LN: Dexamethosone in the management of symptoms due to herniated lumbar disc. J Neurol Neurosurg Psychiat 38:1211, 1975
84. Friedenberg ZB, Shoemaker RC: The results of non-operative treatment of ruptured lumbar discs. Am J Surg 88:933, 1954
85. Hitzelberger WE, Witten RM: Abnormal myelograms in asymptomatic patients. J Neurosurg 28:204, 1968
86. McRae DL: Asymptomatic intervertebral disc protrusions. Acta Radiol (Stockholm) 46:9, 1956
87. Murphy RW: Nerve roots and spinal nerves in degenerative disc disease. Clin Orthop 129:46, 1977
88. Marshall LL, Trethwie ER: Chemical irritation of nerve roots in disc prolapse. Lancet ii:230, 1973
89. Benzon HT: Epidural steroid injections for low back pain and lumbosacral radiculopathy. Pain 24:277, 1986
90. Lievre JA, Block-Michael H, Attali P: L'injection transsacree. Étude Clinique et Radiologique. Bull Soc Med 73:1110, 1957
91. Coomes EN. A comparison between epidural anesthesia and bedrest in sciatica. Br Med J 1:20, 1961
92. Swerdlow M, Sayle-Creer W: A study of extradural medication in the relief of the lumbosciatic syndrome. Anaesthesia 25:341, 1970
93. Winnie AP, Hartman JT, Myers HL et al: Pain clinic II: Intradural and extradural corticosteroids for sciatica. Anesth Analg 51:990, 1972
94. Dilke TFW, Burry HC, Grahame R: Extradural corticosteroid

95. Breivik H, Hesia PE, Molnar I et al: Treatment of chronic low back pain and sciatica: Comparison of caudal epidural steroid injections of bupivacaine and methylprednisolone with bupivacaine followed by saline. In Bonica JJ, Albe-Fessard D (eds): Advances in Pain Research and Therapy, vol 1, p 927. New York, Raven Press, 1976
96. Snoek W, Weber H, Jorgensen B: Double blind evaluation of extradural methylprednisolone for herniated lumbar discs. Acta Orthop Scand 48:635, 1977
97. Cuckler JM, Bernini PA, Wiesel SW et al: The use of epidural steroids in the treatment of lumbar radicular pain. J Bone Joint Surg 67A:63, 1985
98. Finneson BE: Low Back Pain. Philadelphia, JB Lippincott, 1973
99. Abram SE: Subarachnoid corticosteroid injection following inadequate response to epidural steroids for sciatica. Anesth Analg 57:313, 1978
100. Abram SE, Anderson RA: Using a pain questionnaire to predict response to steroid epidurals. Reg Anesthesia 5:11, 1980
101. Keim HA, Kirkaldy-Willis WH: Low back pain. Clin Symp 32:2, 1980
102. Carrera GF: Lumbar facet joint injection in low back pain and sciatica. Radiology 137:665, 1980
103. Carrera GF, Foley WD, Kozin F et al: CT of sacroiliitis. Am J Radiol 136:41, 1981
104. Bonica JJ: The Management of Pain, p 1200. Philadelphia, Lea and Febiger, 1953
105. Travell JG, Simons DG: Myofascial Pain and Dysfunction. Baltimore, Williams and Wilkins, 1983
106. Travell JG, Rinzler SH: The myofascial genesis of pain. Postgrad Med 11:425, 1952
107. Berges PV: Myofascial pain syndromes. Postgrad Med 53:161, 1953
108. Kleinert HE, Cole NM, Wayne L et al: Post-traumatic sympathetic dystrophy. Orthop Clin North Am 4:917, 1973
109. Genant NK, Kozin F, Bekerman C et al: The reflex sympathetic dystrophy syndrome. Radiology 117:21, 1975
110. Carron H, Weller RM: Treatment of post-traumatic sympathetic dystrophy. In Advances in Neurology, vol 4, p 485. New York, Raven Press, 1974
111. Bonica JJ: Causalgia and other reflex sympathetic dystrophies. In Bonica JJ, Albe-Fessard D (eds): Advances in Pain Research and Therapy, vol 1, p 141. New York, Raven Press, 1979
112. Wang JK, Johnson KA, Ilstrup DM: Sympathetic blocks for reflex sympathetic dystrophy. Pain 23:13, 1985
113. Hannington-Kiff JG: Intravenous regional sympathetic block with guanethidine. Lancet 1:1019, 1974
114. Boneli S, Conoscente F, Movilia PG et al: Regional intravenous guanethidine vs stellate block in reflex sympathetic dystrophies: A randomized trial. Pain 16:297, 1983
115. Eriksen S: Duration of sympathetic blockade. Anaesthesia 36:768, 1981
116. Kozin F, Ryan LM, Carrera GF et al: The reflex sympathetic dystrophy syndrome (RSDS) III. Scintigraphic studies, further evidence for the therapeutic efficacy of systemic corticosteroids, and proposed diagnostic criteria. Am J Med 70:23, 1981
117. Poplawski ZJ, Wiley AM, Murray JF: Post-traumatic dystrophy of the extremities. J Bone Joint Surg 65A:642, 1983
118. Abram SE, Asiddao CB, Reynolds AC: Increased skin temperature during transcutaneous electrical stimulation. Anesth Analg 59:22, 1980
119. Stilz RJ, Carron H, Sanders DB: Reflex sympathetic dystrophy in a 6 year old: Successful treatment by transcutaneous nerve stimulation. Anesth Analg 56:438, 1977
120. Abram SE, Lightfoot R: Treatment of long-standing causalgia with prazosin. Reg Anesth 6:79, 1981

121. Spurling RG: Causalgia of the upper extremity: treatment by dorsal sympathetic ganglionectomy. Arch Neurol Psychiatry 23:784, 1930

122. Mayfield FH: Causalgia. Springfield IL, Charles C. Thomas, 1951

123. Boas RS, Hatangdi VS, Richards EG: Lumbar sympathectomy— A percutaneous technique. In Bonica JJ, Albe-Fessard D (eds): Advances in Pain Research and Therapy, vol 1, p 485, New York, Raven Press, 1976

124. Fordyce WE: Learning processes in pain. In Sternbach RA (ed): The Psychology of Pain. New York, Raven Press, 1978

125. Swanson DW, Swenson WW, Maruta T et al: The dissatisfied patient with chronic pain. Pain 4:367, 1978

126. Foley KM: The treatment of pain in the patient with cancer. CA 36:194, 1986

127. Payne R, Foley KM: Recent advances in cancer pain management. Cancer Treat Rep 68:173, 1984

128. Kaiko RF, Foley KM, Grabinski PY et al: Central nervous system excitatory effects of meperidine in cancer patients. Ann Neurol 13:180, 1983

129. Walsh TD, Saunders CM: Heroin and morphine in advanced cancer. N Engl J Med 31:599, 1984

130. Baumann TJ, Batenhorst RL, Graves DA et al: Patient-controlled analgesia in the terminally ill cancer patient. Drug Intell Clin Pharm 20:297, 1986

131. Miser AW, Davis DM, Hughes CS et al: Continuous subcutaneous infusions of morphine in children with cancer. Am J Dis Child 137:383, 1983

132. Coombs DW, Saunders RL, Gaylor MS et al: Relief of continuous chronic pain by intraspinal narcotics infusion via an implanted reservoir. JAMA 250:2336, 1983

133. Jorgensen BC, Andersen HB, Engquist A: CSF and plasma morphine after epidural and intrathecal application. Anesthesiology 55:714, 1981

134. Coombs DW, Fratkin JD, Meier FA et al: Neuropathologic lesions and CSF morphine concentrations during chronic continuous intraspinal morphine infusion. A clinical and post-mortem study. Pain 22:337, 1985

135. Coombs DW, Saunders RL, Gaylor M et al: Epidural narcotic infusion reservoir: Implantation technique and efficacy. Anesthesiology 56:469, 1982

136. Woods WA, Cohen SE: High-dose epidural morphine in a terminally ill patient. Anesthesiology 56:311, 1982

137. Greenberg HS, Taren J, Ensminger WD et al: Benefit from and tolerance to continuous intrathecal infusion of morphine for intractable cancer pain. J Neurosurg 57:360, 1982

138. Coombs DW, Saunders RL, Lachance D et al: Intrathecal morphine tolerance: Use of intrathecal clonidine, DADLE and intraventricular morphine. Anesthesiology 62:358, 1985

139. Moulin DE, Max MB, Kaiko RF et al: The analgesic efficacy of D-Ala-D-Leu-enkephalin in cancer patients with chronic pain. Pain 23:213, 1985

140. Messahel FM, Tomlin PJ: Narcotic withdrawal syndrome after intrathecal administration of morphine. Br Med J 283:471, 1981

141. Tenicela R, Lovasik D, Eaglestein W: Treatment of herpes zoster with sympathetic blocks. Clinical Journal of Pain 1:63, 1985

142. Swerdlow M: Relief of Intractable Pain. Amsterdam, Excerpta Medica, 1974

143. Papo I, Visca A: Phenol subarachnoid rhizotomy for the treatment of cancer pain: A personal account of 290 cases. In Bonica JJ, Ventafridda V (eds): Advances in pain research and therapy, vol 2, p 339, New York, Raven Press, 1979

144. Swerdlow M: Subarachnoid and extradural neurolytic blocks. In Bonica JJ, Ventafridda V (eds): Advances in Pain Research and Therapy, vol 2, p 325, New York, Raven Press, 1979

145. Simon DL, Carron H, Rowlingson JC: Treatment of bladder pain with transsacral nerve block. Anesth Analg 61:46, 1982

146. Madrid JL, Bonica JJ: Cranial nerve blocks. In Bonica JJ, Ventafridda V (eds): Advances in Pain Research and Therapy, vol 2, p 347. New York, Raven Press, 1979

147. Thompson GE, Moore DC, Bridenbaugh LD et al: Abdominal pain and alcohol celiac plexus nerve block. Anesth Analg 56:1, 1977

148. Moore DC: Regional Block. Springfield IL, Charles C. Thomas, 1975

149. Singler RC: An improved technique for alcohol neurolysis of the celiac plexus. Anesthesiology 56:137, 1982

150. Ischia S, Luzzani A, Ischia A et al: A new approach to the neurolytic block of the celiac plexus: The transaortic technique. Pain 16:333, 1983

151. Kroening RJ: Pain clinics structure and function. Seminars in Anesthesia 4:231, 1985

152. Moya F, Mayne GE: Organization of a pain clinic. In Raj PP (ed): Practical Management of Pain, p 20. Chicago, Year Book, 1986

153. Carron H: Management of the patient with chronic pain. Resident and Staff Physician 6:46, 1981

154. Abram SE, Anderson RA, Maitra D'Cruze AM: Factors predicting short-term outcome of nerve blocks in the management of chronic pain. Pain 10:323, 1981

Chapter 54   *Morris Brown*

ICU–Critical Care

Critical care medicine is now a clearly recognized specialty of the practice of medicine. It is a multidisciplinary specialty based in the intensive care unit, with its primary concern being care of the patient with a critical illness. Critical care medicine crosses traditional departmental and specialty lines and requires a physician whose knowledge is broad, involving all aspects of management of the critically ill patient.[1]

HISTORY OF CRITICAL CARE MEDICINE

The Society of Critical Care Medicine (SCCM), founded in 1970, was the first formal organization established in the United States to represent physicians and ancillary personnel devoted to the care of critically ill patients. In 1977 the American Board of Medical Specialties allowed recognition for physicians with expertise in critical care medicine. Thereafter, the American Board of Anesthesiology (ABA) received approval to issue a certificate of special qualifications in critical care medicine to their diplomates. Anesthesiologists were the first specialists to be issued certificates of special qualifications in critical care medicine by virtue of an examination administered in September 1986. Since that time the American Boards of Internal Medicine, Pediatrics, and Surgery have offered examinations for their diplomates. The American Society of Critical Care Anesthesiologists (ASCCA) was formed to organize anesthesiologists interested in the practice of critical care

medicine. The ASCCA maintains liaison with the American Society of Anesthesiologists (ASA) and the SCCM.

ANESTHESIOLOGISTS AND CRITICAL CARE MEDICINE

Critical care medicine has always been an integral part of the practice of anesthesiology. Anesthesiologists have been intimately involved, indeed instrumental, in the development of critical care medicine as a specialty. Many consider the practice of operating room anesthesiology the practice of critical care medicine limited to the operative period. The anesthesiologist is involved daily with rapid alterations in physiologic status that requires prompt recognition and early intervention—the hallmark of critical care medicine. By virtue of training, experience, competence, and interest, the anesthesiologist brings skills and knowledge that uniquely qualify him to care for critically ill patients. This expertise has been recognized by the ABA, which included critical care medicine in its definition of anesthesiology, and by the ASA, which included critical care medicine in its standards of practice. Further, training in critical care medicine is an integral part of the curriculum for residents in anesthesiology. Advanced training in this specialty following completion of residency training is required to be eligible to receive a certificate of special qualifications in critical care medicine by the ABA. Recommendations for the content of fellowship training programs in critical care medicine, as well as recommendations for the qualifications of a director of these programs have been developed by a task force on guidelines from the SCCM.[2, 3]

HISTORY OF INTENSIVE CARE UNITS

Intensive Care Units (ICU) have been in existence for over 30 years.[4, 5] They evolved from postanesthesia care units and surgical recovery rooms. The earliest ICUs developed in this country were multidisciplinary medical-surgical units.[6] In the 1960s there was a proliferation of cardiac care units when lifesaving detection and treatment of cardiac dysrhythmias was noted.[7] This led to the proliferation of other organ-specific intensive care units, such as, respiratory, neurologic, and cardiothoracic ICUs. However, it appears that interdisciplinary ICUs have both patient care and economic advantages over segregated departmental or specialty organ-oriented units.[8] Certainly, staffing is easier and the ability to share resources is a distinct advantage. However, some units such as neonatal ICU, burn units, and spinal cord centers may justify special designation established on a regional basis.[9] Current estimates indicate that 60% of hospitals with intensive care facilities have only one identifiable ICU. If coronary units are excluded, then 82% of hospitals with intensive care facilities have only a single unit.

The numbers of ICU beds required for an institution varies between 3% and 25% of the total hospital beds with an average of 12% for major adult and general hospitals.[10] In children's hospitals the per cent of special care beds averages over 23% and may be as high as 46%. Currently, ICU beds comprise 7% to 8% of all hospital beds.[11] The number of beds required for any institution varies depending on the patient population served. It appears, however, that with changes in the political climate and only the very sickest of patients being admitted to the hospital, there will be a need in the future for more critical care beds and fewer beds for elective admissions.

COST AND OUTCOME OF INTENSIVE CARE

There is increasing concern about the cost of medical care, especially associated with critical illness. ICU beds are growing at approximately 6% annually, while other beds are closing.[12] ICU care consumes 20% of total hospital charges. In addition, because of the intensity and stress placed on the personnel working in ICUs there is a disproportionally high loss of personnel from these areas.[13] It has been estimated the annual turnover of nurses from critical care units approaches 50% and it is common to not be able to use all resources because of inadequate staffing.[14]

It is still uncertain whether ICU care decreases patient morbidity and mortality. Reports in the literature are conflicting. Several early studies demonstrated a significant benefit of ICU care when specialty units were reviewed.[15–18] For example, in a review of coronary ICUs, a reduction in mortality was noted and attributed to these units.[19] Similarly, the national burn information exchange noted a reduction in mortality and in the length of hospitalization in burned patients due to improvement in the critical care aspects of burn management.[17] Likewise, other studies have shown a reduction in mortality in noncardiac surgical patients, trauma patients, and other selected surgical groups after the introduction of a surgical ICU teaching service and computer-based approach to patient monitoring and therapy.[20] However, these studies and many

in the literature have used historical controls. Unfortunately, this does not consider differences in treatment modalities and other factors that may have contributed to the change in morbidity and mortality. Indeed, several studies have failed to show any benefit from hospitalization in critical care units.[21–22] More carefully designed, rigorously controlled trials are necessary to assess the true efficacy of ICUs.

PATIENT ASSESSMENT SYSTEMS

Because intensive care is so expensive and consumes so many resources, several attempts have been made at methods to predict patient outcome. In this way patient care could be optimized by limiting admission to only those patients who would benefit from intensive care and withholding or removing therapy from patients who would not. This clearly would be a means of significantly reducing medical cost and providing optimal use of available resources. Unfortunately, the systems introduced to assess the severity of illness of patients and their need for intensive care, as well as predict outcome, have met with limited success.

Illness severity scoring systems have been devised on an anatomical, therapeutic, and physiological basis.[23] The Clinical Classification System was introduced as a means to assess severity of illness along with a therapeutic intervention scoring system (TISS) to measure the amount of therapy given.[24] TISS serves as an indirect measure of illness severity with the greater number of interventions occurring with sicker patients. The clinical classification system along with the TISS has been used to assist in appropriate use of facilities, provide information on nurse staffing ratios, and relate costs to extent of care given in both the adult and pediatric population. In addition, it was an attempt to be able to compare treatment and outcome in different ICUs.[24–27]

The acute physiology and chronic health evaluation (APACHE) system relates the severity of a patient's illness to the degree of physiologic derangement of a series of physiologic measurements. With an assigned weight given to each measurement, it is then possible to assess preadmission health status and probability of survival.[28] It also has been used to compare patient populations in different institutions.[29, 30] Attempts to simplify the APACHE system resulted in the simplified acute physiology score and APACHE II.[31, 32] The physiologic stability index (PSI) is an adaptation of the APACHE system for use in the pediatric population.[33] Other scoring systems have been developed for patients following trauma,[34] myocardial infarction,[35] adult respiratory insufficiency,[36] shock,[37] and neonatal resuscitation.[38] Unfortunately, to date none of these systems can unequivocally predict outcome or benefit from intensive care.

CENTRAL NERVOUS SYSTEM

Assessment and treatment of critically ill patients with central nervous system disorders requires a thorough knowledge of cerebral blood flow and metabolism, as well as cerebral pharmacology, neurophysiology, and pathophysiology.

DETERMINANTS OF CEREBRAL BLOOD FLOW

Control of cerebral perfusion is essential in maintaining neurologic function in pathologic states. Cerebral blood flow is regulated by intracerebral and extracerebral factors. Intracerebral blood flow regulation is controlled by chemical and metabolic influences including hydrogen ion concentration, cyclooxygenase, products of phospholipid membrane metabolism and adenosine. In addition, neurogenic and myogenic components contribute to the regulation of cerebral blood flow.[39]

The extracerebral determinants of blood flow include the arterial partial pressure of carbon dioxide (Pa_{CO_2}) and oxygen (Pa_{O_2}), arterial blood pressure, venous blood pressure, and pharmacologic effects of drugs. There is a linear correlation between cerebral blood flow and Pa_{CO_2} with progressive hypercarbia. Similarly, there is a marked reduction in cerebral blood flow during hypocarbia through a pH-mediated change in arteriolar tone that results in vasoconstriction and reduced intracranial pressure (ICP).[40, 41] Taken to extremes, hypocarbia provides no additional benefit and may be detrimental.[42] Therefore, current recommendations suggest maintaining Pa_{CO_2} between 25 mm Hg and 30 mm Hg. However, prolonged hypocarbia is ineffective, because cerebrospinal fluid (CSF) bicarbonate adapts to the change in Pa_{CO_2}. Therefore, the long-term value of hyperventilation of the lungs for reducing ICP is offset by the normalization of CSF pH which occurs in 6 hours.[43]

Arterial oxygenation has a lesser effect on cerebral blood flow than carbon dioxide. When the Pa_{O_2} falls below 50 mm Hg, cerebral vasodilation and an increase in cerebral blood flow results which may exacerbate intracranial hypertension.[44] Hyperoxia generally results in very small changes in cerebral blood flow until Pa_{O_2} exceeds 300 mm Hg.

AUTOREGULATION

Autoregulation, the ability of the brain to maintain cerebral blood flow constant despite alterations in mean arterial pressure, is functional over a mean arterial pressure range of 50 to 150 mm Hg. At levels below 50 mm Hg, symptoms of cerebral ischemia may appear. If the upper limit of autoregulaton is exceeded, cerebral blood flow increases which may result in cerebral edema. It is important to note that the autoregulatory curve may be shifted in the presence of chronic hypertension, intracranial tumors, head trauma, and shock states which render the brain more susceptible to ischemic effects.[45]

INTRACRANIAL PRESSURE MONITORING

ICP can normally range up to 15 mm Hg and beyond that point any increase in ICP can result in a decrease in cerebral perfusion pressure (CPP). Once CPP falls below 40 to 60 mm Hg, ischemic injury to nerve cells may occur. There is a close correlation between clinical outcome and the level of ICP elevation after acute injury.[46] Aggressive treatment of elevated ICP in the ICU is essential. The symptoms associated with increased ICP are variable, though they generally reflect effects of compression of structures around the tentorial opening. If left untreated, raised ICP leads to global cerebral ischemia, coma, and death.

Continuous monitoring of ICP can be accomplished through a ventriculostomy, a subdural bolt or an epidural transducer.[47] Advantages and disadvantages of each technique are outlined in Table 54-1. The intraventricular catheter is inserted through a burr hole through the coronal suture. It provides an accurate and reliable reading of ICP, as well as withdrawing CSF for pressure control and culture. Disadvan-

TABLE 54-1. Techniques of Direct ICP Monitoring

ICP MONITOR	ADVANTAGE	DISADVANTAGE
Ventriculostomy	Very accurate Access to CSF for pressure control and culture	Must pass through brain tissue Infection
Subarachnoid bolt	Easily performed Bedside procedure	Infection Less accurate
Epidural transducer	Easy to place Little risk of infection	Questionable accuracy and reliability

tages to this technique include the necessity to pass through brain tissue in order to introduce the catheter into the ventricle. This may be very difficult when the brain is distorted from trauma and edema. Further, the risk of infection is greatest with this technique as compared to the others. Indeed, positive CSF culture have been reported to occur in approximately 9% of patients monitored with intraventricular catheters.[48] The possibility of infection is reduced if catheterization is limited to 3 days and prophylactic antibiotics are administered.

The subarachnoid bolt is a less invasive means of monitoring ICP. This device is inserted into the skull after the dura and arachnoid have been opened. It is easily inserted, does not require penetration of brain tissue, and can be performed at the bedside. As with all invasive procedures, insertion of a subarachnoid bolt carries the risk of infection.

The epidural transducer used to monitor intracranial pressure is placed between the inner table of the skull and the dura. This device is easy to place and monitors pressures exerted by the CSF and brain on the dura. Although this technique carries little risk of infection, its accuracy and reliability for monitoring ICP are questionable.[47]

CONTROL OF ELEVATED INTRACRANIAL PRESSURE

Treatment of increased ICP is generally recommended when levels exceed 20 mm Hg. Certainly, treatment may be indicated at a lower pressure if evidence of impaired cerebral perfusion is present. Modalities available to treat increased ICP include diuretics and fluid restriction, hyperosmotic agents, hyperventilation of the lungs, corticosteroids, barbiturates, positioning, and removal of CSF.

Once surgicaly correctable causes of increased ICP have been eliminated, treatment should be initiated with hyperventilation to maintain Pa_{CO_2} between 25 and 30 mm Hg. Additional measures include drainage of CSF if an intraventricular catheter has been placed and elevation of the head to 30 degrees which encourages venous drainage from the brain and hence lowers ICP. Mannitol may be added in an attempt to remove brain water. This osmotic agent helps draw water from the tissues because of the transient increase in plasma osmolarity. The onset of action following intravenous administration of mannitol is 30 minutes with a maximum lowering of ICP occurring within 1 to 2 hours and lasting 6 hours. Diuretics such as furosemide may also be used to lower ICP and are especially useful in patients with increased intravascular volume. Corticosteroids are effective in lowering ICP due to localized cerebral edema surrounding intracranial tumors. Dexamethasone is the most commonly used steroid preparation and generally causes improvement in neurologic status within 12 to 36 hours of therapy. Barbiturate administration can also assist in lowering ICP by a dose-related reduction in cerebral metabolic oxygen requirement, as well as decreasing cerebral blood volume. Some authors suggest barbiturate coma for cerebral protection in patients with elevated ICP.[49, 50, 51]

Fluid and electrolyte abnormalities including hyponatremia, hypokalemia, and hypochloremia with fluid retention are common accompaniments of CNS disease. Other complications include acute respiratory failure, gastrointestinal bleeding, hypertension, cardiac dysrhythmias and disseminated intravascular coagulation (DIC).[52] These related complications must be recognized and treated, should they occur.

SEIZURES

The etiology of a seizure generally depends on the age of the patient and the type of seizure.[53] Young children frequently present with seizures associated with febrile illness. In adolescent and young adults, head trauma is a major cause of focal seizure disorders, while generalized seizures tend to be associated with drug or alcohol withdrawal in this age group. Brain tumors are the most common cause of seizures in patients between 30 and 50 years of age, and over 50 years of age, cerebral vascular disease is the most common cause of focal or generalized seizure disorders.[52] The initial evaluation of the patient with a seizure consists of assuring adequate ventilation and perfusion, as well as stopping the seizure. A full history and examination must be obtained. It is important to differentiate the kind of seizure to aid in determining the etiology. Treatment is directed at eliminating the cause and suppressing the seizure.[53] Certainly, metabolic disturbances such as hypoglycemia or hypocalcemia should be sought and corrected. Structural brain lesions must be removed. Most seizure disorders are amenable to anticonvulsion medication.[54] However, neurosurgical treatment should be considered if a structural lesion causes recurrent seizures and removal of that lesion and nearby affected brain will make them easier to control or eliminate them entirely. In addition, neurosurgical ablation of epileptogenic foci may prove a valuable treatment modality.

CENTRAL NERVOUS SYSTEM TRAUMA

Head injuries are a significant cause of morbidity and mortality with over 2 million injuries causing brain damage yearly. In order to quantitate the severity of head injury an objective clinical scale was developed. The Glasgow Coma Scale evaluates motor response, verbal response, and eye opening (Table 54-2).[55] It provides an estimate of the severity of neurologic dysfunction and predicts an 85% mortality within 24 hours after injury.[56] Evoked potentials are another means of assessing prognosis in patients following head injury. The accuracy of evoked potentials is greater than clinical observation and ICP measurements. Somatosensory evoked potentials are the most useful and can predict death or a vegetative state in approximately 90% of patients if bilaterally absent.[57]

Any patient who presents with severe head injury should have the airway protected and secured, ventilation and blood pressure stabilized, as well as attention given to life-threatening non-cranial injuries, followed by full neurologic evaluation. As with any head injury, the possibility of cervical spine injury should be considered and the cervical spine should be

TABLE 54-2.   Glasgow Coma Scale

PARAMETER	RESPONSE	SCORE
Eye opening	No response	4
	Spontaneously	3
	To verbal command	2
	To pain	1
Motor response	Obeys verbal command	6
	Localizes pain	5
	Flexion-withdrawal	4
	Decorticate rigidity	3
	Decerebrate rigidity	2
	No response	1
Verbal response	Oriented and converses	5
	Disoriented and converses	4
	Inappropriate words	3
	Incomprehensible sounds	2
	No response	1

immobilized until full evaluation is possible. Surgically treatable causes of increased ICP should be sought including epidural or subdural hematoma, as well as intracerebral hemorrhage. Aggressive surgical intervention may dramatically improve outcome.[58, 59] If, however, there are no surgically treatable lesions on CT scan, attention should be directed towards reducing increased ICP.[60] Direct intracranial pressure monitoring should be considered.[61] Hypoxia, hyperthermia, hypercarbia, malpositioning of the endotracheal tube and high mean airway pressures may exacerbate the intracranial hypertension. Persistent elevation in ICP despite conservative therapy generally portends a poor prognosis. Fluid and electrolytes should be monitored closely. Anticonvulsants and prophylaxis to prevent gastrointestinal bleeding are generally administered.

It must be remembered that patients who sustain head trauma have other associated problems. Indeed, medical complications generally dominate the intermediate term intensive care of head trauma patients. Fluid and electrolyte balance can be a major problem following head injury.[62] Indeed, over half of the patients who have persistent coma develop abnormalities of fluid and electrolyte balance. It is important to monitor serum osmolarity and sodium concentrations as treatment of intracranial hypertension may cause marked alterations in these parameters. Coagulation parameters must also be monitored as DIC may accompany head trauma in 5% to 10% of cases.[63]

CARDIOVASCULAR SYSTEM

CARDIOGENIC SHOCK

Cardiogenic shock is a syndrome that results directly from severely impaired left ventricular pump function. This may result from end-stage cardiac disease or as a catastrophic complication of acute myocardial infarction. With improvement in cardiac dysrhythmia monitoring and treatment, cardiogenic shock has emerged as the most common cause of death among patients in coronary care units. Indeed, cardiogenic shock occurs in 10% to 15% of patients who suffer an acute myocardial infarction.[64] Mortality remains high despite advances in hemodynamic monitoring and newer pharmacologic drugs. Cardiogenic shock, like hypovolemic or septic shock, manifests as inadequate oxygen delivery to tissues with failure of mitochondrial oxidative metabolism and accumulation of lactic acid. Inadequate organ perfusion in cardiogenic shock is caused by a marked reduction in the quantity of contracting myocardium. The initial insult leads to a decrease in arterial pressure with a resultant decrease in coronary blood flow. This fall in coronary perfusion pressure further compromises myocardial function leading to progressive circulatory deterioration. The clinical consequences of the decrease in myocardial contractility manifest as either circulatory insufficiency, (forward failure), or as circulatory congestion, (backward failure).

Typical signs and symptoms of patients in cardiogenic shock include restlessness and mental confusion with skin that is cool, moist, and cyanotic. Peripheral pulses are usually weak and rapid and arterial blood pressure is decreased. However, shock can occur without severe hypotension, a relatively late indicator of inadequate reflex vasoconstriction. Nonetheless, the syndrome is usually defined by a systolic arterial pressure less than 80 mm Hg, with a cardiac index of less than $2 \, l \cdot min^{-1} \cdot m^{-2}$ with an increase in left ventricular end diastolic pressure or pulmonary capillary wedge pressure greater than 18 mm Hg.[65]

Because prognosis is poor and mortality is high, close monitoring and early aggressive invention is essential for successful outcome. Certainly, any patient in shock should have continuous monitoring of arterial pressure and left ventricular filling pressures. Measurement of central venous pressure (CVP) alone is inadequate and may actually be misleading because the CVP often fails to reliably reflect left ventricular pressures.[66] Close monitoring of urinary output is important as it gives an indication of renal artery perfusion and provides a monitor of the progress of treatment.

Successful treatment of cardiogenic shock depends on early restoration of adequate tissue perfusion to meet metabolic demands. To achieve this goal, initial resuscitation and general supportive measures should be instituted immediately. Specific pharmacological therapy to maintain adequate blood pressure, cardiac output, and oxygenation should be initiated. Consideration should then be given to mechanical cardiac assist devices or cardiac surgical intervention including transplantation and implantation of an artificial heart.[67]

Drugs with positive inotropic properties improve the contractile performance of the failing heart. Sympathomimetic amines are potent positive inotropic drugs that exert their effects through action on alpha- and beta-adrenergic receptors. Isoproterenol is rarely used in the treatment of shock. Though it increases contractility, it does so at an increase in myocardial oxygen consumption and reduction of coronary perfusion pressure. Norepinephrine is a combined alpha- and beta agent, with alpha properties generally dominant, causing intensive vasoconstriction. It can be useful in raising blood pressure, but the increase in afterload causes a marked increase in myocardial oxygen consumption. Dopamine has been used successfully as a positive inotropic drug with varying effects at different dosage ranges.[68, 69] At low doses the drug has positive chronotropic and inotropic effects, but at higher doses vasoconstriction occurs through an alpha-mediated response. Dobutamine is a synthetic, sympathomimetic amine with positive inotropic effects without the chronotropic or peripheral vasoconstrictive properties of dopamine.[70] It therefore, should be used in patients without profound hypotension. Dopamine and dobutamine may also be used in combination.[71] Amrinone is a newer inotropic drug that causes a dose-dependent increase in cardiac output while reducing systemic vascular resistance and left ventricular fill-

ing pressures. In addition, it increases renal blood flow and improves renal function.[72] Other new phosphodiesterase inhibitors such as milrinone, enoximone, and piroximone are currently under investigation.

Mechanical circulatory assist devices, most commonly the intra-aortic balloon pump, have gained wide-spread clinical use since first introduced by Moulopoulus in 1962.[73] The balloon pump assist device results in a reduction in myocardial oxygen consumption and therefore myocardial ischemia. In addition, by decreasing left ventricular volume and pressure, and augmenting coronary perfusion there is a positive balance established between myocardial oxygen demand and supply. The intra-aortic balloon pump has been shown in experimental models to improve hemodynamics,[74] augment myocardial perfusion, and enhance impaired contractile function,[75-77] as well as potentially limit infarct size.[78-79] Indeed, it has been shown that an increase in coronary blood flow is seen in patients in cardiogenic shock.[80] Unfortunately, although myocardial ischemia is relieved and heart failure lessened in most patients with intra-aortic balloon pump assist, long-term survival has not been established. In recent clinical experience, intra-aortic balloon pumping alone was associated with an overall survival rate of less than 30% when used in patients with cardiogenic shock. The addition of emergency cardiac surgical revascularization has improved survival rates.[81]

Although, intra-aortic balloon pumping is generally a simple and relatively safe procedure, serious complications occur in 10% of patients.[82] Complications include aortic and arterial trauma, vascular insufficiency in the catheterized limb distal to the insertion site, infection, embolic phenomena, balloon rupture with gas embolization, and thrombocytopenia. With newer assist devices on the horizon,[83] and the success of percutaneous transluminal coronary angioplasty, temporary assistance may provide support until definitive therapy can be undertaken.

With refractory cardiogenic shock, heart transplantation should be considered. The one year survival for heart recipients exceeds 80% with a five year survival of 50% to 60%.[67] Certainly, surgical approaches should be explored when cardiogenic shock cannot otherwise be managed.

CARDIAC TAMPONADE

The accumulation of fluid or blood in the pericardial space resulting in a fall in cardiac output due to insufficient inflow of blood to the ventricles results in tamponade. The amount of fluid necessary to cause pericardial tamponade is variable depending on the rapidity of accumulation. Rapid accumulation of as little as 250 ml can result in tamponade; whereas, over 1000 ml can accumulate in the pericardial space without tamponade if accumulated slowly. The most common cause of tamponade is blood in the pericardial space following cardiac surgery, trauma, tuberculosis or tumor. However, other etiologies include acute viral or idiopathic pericarditis, postradiation pericarditis, and renal failure. Clinical manifestations of tamponade include dyspnea, jugular venous distention, and low arterial blood pressure with very distant heart sounds. Electrical alternans may be seen on the electrocardiogram and distention of the jugular veins on inspiration (Kussmaul's sign) may also be noted. Another finding suggestive of pericardial tamponade is a paradoxical occurrence of greater than 10 mm Hg inspiratory decrease in systolic arterial pressure. Equalization of pulmonary artery wedge, right atrial, right ventricular, and pulmonary artery diastolic pressures with low cardiac output may also be seen.

Treatment of cardiac tamponade must be initiated immediately because pericardiocentesis may be life-saving. A small catheter advanced over a needle inserted in the pericardial space allows drainage of pericardial fluid and return of cardiac function.

PULMONARY EMBOLISM

Pulmonary embolism is a leading cause of morbidity and mortality in the United States. It has been estimated that pulmonary embolism accounts for over 50,000 deaths annually, though most pulmonary emboli are nonfatal. The vast majority of pulmonary emboli arise in the deep venous system of the lower extremities. The three primary etiologic factors in the development of deep vein thrombosis and subsequent pulmonary embolism are venous stasis, abnormalities of the vessel wall, and alterations in blood coagulation.[84]

Pulmonary embolism should be suspected in any patient with sudden onset of unexplained dyspnea in association with venous thrombosis.[85] Other symptoms may include substernal chest pain, syncope, cardiac dysrhythmias, worsening of congestive heart failure, or sudden worsening of chronic obstructive lung disease. Pleuritic chest pain and hemoptysis may be present, but only when pulmonary infarction has occurred. Physical examination may be remarkably normal. Rales or wheezing may be noted on auscultation of the lungs. A pleural friction rub or effusion may be present if infarction has occurred. Findings on auscultation of the heart may include tachycardia, right ventricular gallop, wide splitting of the second heart sound, or systolic ejection murmur in the pulmonic area.

Laboratory studies may assist with the diagnosis of pulmonary embolism.[85, 86] The electrocardiogram is generally normal aside from tachycardia. However, there may be evidence of right axis deviation, tall peaked P waves, or ST-T wave changes consistent with right ventricular strain. Chest x-ray film findings may be very subtle. Indeed, a normal chest x-ray film does not exclude the possibility of pulmonary embolism and is a common finding. Arterial blood gases associated with pulmonary embolism generally reveal arterial hypoxemia with hypocapnia and respiratory alkalosis. However, normal ABG analysis does not exclude the possibility of thromboembolic disease.

The diagnosis of pulmonary embolism can be confirmed by radioisotope-tagged and microaggregated albumin perfusion scan along with a xenon ventilation scan. The definitive diagnosis, however, is with pulmonary angiography, which is the only means for providing anatomic information about the pulmonary vasculature.[86] Heparin administration is the initial treatment of PTE. Fibrinolytic agents also have been used to dissolve venous thrombi in the pulmonary vasculature. Surgical therapy with formal thoracotomy and thrombectomy has uniformly poor results.

THROMBOLYTIC THERAPY

Streptokinase, urokinase, and tissue plasminogen activator (t-PA) are pharmacologic activators used to accelerate fibrinolysis in patients with massive pulmonary emboli, acute arterial and coronary thrombi, and peripheral venous thrombi. Streptokinase is an indirect activator that forms a complex with plasminogen and initiates fibrinolysis. Urokinase, like t-PA, can directly convert plasminogen to plasmin. Tissue plasminogen activator peripherally activates plasminogen when it is absorbed to fibrin clots.[87] The major complication of fibrinolytic therapy is hemorrhage due to severe hypofibrinogenemia and intense systemic fibrinolysis. Therefore, fibrinolytic therapy is not recommended for patients with recent surgery, indwelling cannulas, history of neurologic lesions, or gastrointestional bleeding. Indications for fibrinolytic therapy include massive pulmonary emboli, acute peripheral arterial embolism, and extensive iliofemoral thrombophlebitis. The fibrinolysis begins immediately after vascular injury, though clot lysis and vessel recannulation may not be complete for 7 to 10 days.[88] Fibrinolytic therapy has also gained wide-spread clinical use in treatment of intracoronary lytic therapy to restore arterial patency and reduce myocardial damage during acute coronary occlusion.[88, 89] In particular, t-PA has been used successfully with improved left ventricular function.[90] Additionally, t-PA can lyse fibrin clots without causing systemic fibrinolysis and bleeding.

RESPIRATORY SYSTEM

ACUTE RESPIRATORY FAILURE

Acute respiratory failure in the critically ill patient is often synonymous with the adult respiratory distress syndrome (ARDS). This is a descriptive term applied to many acute diffuse infiltrative lung lesions with diverse etiology. However, severely diminished lung compliance, refractory hypoxemia, and diffuse radiographic abnormalities are a common denominator. Regardless of the initiating event, this form of acute respiratory failure is associated with increased lung water. This type of pulmonary edema is associated with relatively normal cardiac function and "leaky" pulmonary capillaries and has been termed *high permeability pulmonary edema*.[91] The precise incidence of ARDS is difficult to determine, though it appears to be increasing.[92] One-third of adult deaths from shock and trauma following severe injury results from progressive respiratory failure.[93] Although ARDS may be precipitated by many different causes (Table 54-3), the resulting clinical syndrome is the same. The mortality rate remains greater than 50% despite current supportive therapy and treatment modalities.[92, 94]

Pathophysiology

Following injury to the lung with damage of the alveolar capillary membrane, there is an increased permeability of the capillary endothelium and alveolar epithelium with leakage of plasma and erythrocytes into the interstitial and alveolar spaces. In addition, there is proliferation of Type II pneumocytes which probably aid in the restoration of the integrity of the capillary-endothelial lining.[95]

Although platelet aggregation occurs, the major alterations in lung function relate to leukoaggregation on endothelial surfaces.[96] Indeed, bronchoalveolar lavage fluid from patients

TABLE 54-3.   Conditions Associated with ARDS

Shock	Fat or air embolism
Aspiration	Burns
Sepsis	Drug ingestion
Trauma	Uremia
Pancreatitis	Massive blood transfusion
Head injury	Cardiopulmonary bypass
Radiation of thorax	Drowning

with ARDS contains an accumulation of neutrophils and leukocyte elastase.[97] These cells release mediators of inflammation such as leukotrienes, thromboxanes, and prostaglandins. These leukoagglutinins are caused by activation of complete Factor C5a.[98] Thus, complement activation, a frequent accompaniment of trauma, sepsis, and other predisposing clinical insults, may explain the leukoaggregates commonly found in the lungs of patients with ARDS.[99] With release of toxic oxygen radicals and lysosomal proteases, these aggregated neutrophils damage the endothelial cells by destruction of structural protein and promotion of local inflammatory reactions.[94]

In addition to leukoaggregrates, microemboli are commonly found in patients with ARDS at autopsy.[100] Indeed, platelet and coagulation abnormalities have been implicated in the pathogenesis of the syndrome. Trauma, sepsis, and other predisposing conditions can activate the coagulation system, either by release of thromboplastin from soft tissue injury or through complement activation of the coagulation cascade. This results in platelet adhesiveness and aggregation which, along with the generation of fibrin, produces microemboli that are washed into the pulmonary vasculature.[101] These defects have been clearly demonstrated by wedge angiography and correlated with the severity of lung injury.[102]

Clinical Manifestations

Patients may be asymptomatic immediately following insult. The earliest signs are frequently tachypnea followed by dyspnea. Arterial blood gas analysis generally reveals a respiratory alkalosis due to hyperventilation and mild hypoxemia. At this time, administration of supplementation oxygen frequently improves arterial oxygenation. As the disease progresses, however, hypoxemia cannot be corrected by increasing inspired oxygen concentrations because hypoxemia is the result of right to left shunting of blood through collapsed or fluid filled alveoli. Mechanical ventilatory support with positive airway pressure therapy is then required to maintain adequate oxygenation.[103]

Treatment

Certainly, early recognition and prompt initiation of therapy are essential. The cornerstone of therapy is to assure adequate tissue oxygenation. An indwelling arterial cannula is useful to monitor arterial blood pressure and allow access for measurement of arterial blood gases and other laboratory values. A pulmonary artery catheter aids immeasurably in optimizing fluid management. A Foley catheter is important to assure close and accurate measurement of urine output. Bronchial hygiene is an important aspect of the management of these patients. Antibiotics should be used only if evidence of infection is present and treatment should be guided by the results of cultures and antibiotic sensitivity testing. Prophylactic antibiotics are not indicated and may cause a drug resistant infection. The use of high dose corticosteroids in the treatment of ARDS remains controversial despite wide-spread clinical use. Theoretical advantages of steroids include inhibition of complement-induced granulocyte aggregation, disaggregation of neutrophils, and limitation of the increase in lung microvascular permeability. However, a recent prospective double-blind, placebo-controlled trial of methylprednisolone therapy found no difference in mortality.[104]

Fluid management in patients with ARDS presents a clinical dilemma. Fluid is constantly lost through the alveolar capillary membrane into the lung parenchyma. Yet, adequate circulatory volume is essential to restore the perfusion important

in reversal of lung damage. Therefore, it is crucial that fluid administration be judicious and is best guided by the use of a balloon-tipped, flow-directed pulmonary artery catheter. Diuretics and vasoactive agents can be used to maximize tissue oxygen delivery. Fluid replacement with crystalloid or colloid solution remains controversial.[105, 106] Regardless of the choice, meticulous attention must be given to fluid balance.

If adequate oxygenation cannot be maintained with an increased inspired oxygen concentration, mechanical ventilatory support should be instituted. The supportive benefits of positive end-expiratory pressure (PEEP) therapy are well documented.[107] The clinical goals include improvement in arterial oxygenation, decrease in the work of breathing, and improvement in ventilation-perfusion inequality. With diffuse lung injury, PEEP improves functional residual capacity, compliance, and arterial oxygenation. In addition, PEEP decreases shunting and dead space ventilation, and decreases venous admixture. This allows adequate arterial oxygenation with a lower inspired oxygen concentration.[81]

Several criteria have been applied in attempting to define the clinical end point for PEEP therapy.[108] Indices used include arterial oxygen tension, alveolar-arterial oxygen gradient, shunt fraction, compliance, and oxygen delivery.[109, 110] The usual clinical approach is to increase PEEP in increments of 3 cm H_2O to 5 cm H_2O and obtain appropriate measurements. Certainly, the optimal PEEP level chosen for any individual must fulfill the oxygenation as well as hemodynamic needs of that patient.[111] The appropriate level depends on the degree of hypoxemia, the type of lung disorder, the functional residual capacity of the lungs, the presence of pre-existing pulmonary disease, lung compliance, the state of hydration, and the status of left ventricular function.

While PEEP therapy is an integral part of the treatment of acute respiratory failure, it causes complex hemodynamic effects. Changes in airway pressure can be anticipated to impact on the heart and great vessels within the thorax. Potential adverse effects of PEEP include impaired venous return,[112] decreased ventricular filling,[113] increased pulmonary vascular resistance,[114] interference with subendocardial blood flow,[115] reduced left ventricular afterload and altered configuration and compliance of the right and left ventricles.[116] In addition to hemodynamic alterations, PEEP may cause interstitial emphysema, pneumothorax, and pneumomediastinum.[117] Other effects of PEEP therapy include changes in ICP,[118] alterations in renal function,[119] and abnormalities in hepatic and gastrointestinal function.[120, 121]

Research on ARDS has emphasized the mechanism of lung injury in the hope of identifying a marker that would facilitate early recognition. Current investigation is directed at altering the pathogenic sequence of increased alveolar capillary permeability and destruction of pulmonary structure.[122, 123] Some experimental therapeutic interventions including anticoagulation, extracorporeal membrane oxygenation[124] cyclooxygenase inhibitors, oxygen free-radical scavenger therapy, antiendotoxin antibody therapy, and prostaglandin E therapy have not yet proven to be of definite benefit to patients with ARDS and await further prospective, controlled clinical trials.

MECHANICAL VENTILATION

Types of Ventilators

There are three kinds of mechanical ventilators. The simplest mechanical ventilators are those that substitute for diaphragmatic function such as the pneumobelt or rocking bed. These devices have limited utility and are used only in patients with neuromuscular disease and normal lung function. A second kind of mechanical ventilator is the intermittent negative pressure ventilator. These devices artificially produce a negative extrathoracic pressure during inspiration to substitute for the pleural and airway pressures normally produced by contraction of the respiratory muscles. Examples of this form of mechanical ventilation include the chest cuirass and iron lung. These devices are best suited for patients with respiratory muscle dysfunction and normal lungs.

The third kind of mechanical ventilator, and the one most commonly used today, is the intermittent positive pressure ventilator (IPPV). In this system, gas is directed under positive airway pressure into the lungs. The major advantages of IPPV are the ability to ventilate the lungs adequately despite increased airway resistance or decreased lung compliance, patient accessibility, and access for bronchial hygiene. The mean airway pressure is positive with IPPV, so that venous return is compromised and cardiac performance may be impaired.[125] Most of the positive pressure ventilators in common clinical use today are volume ventilators that deliver a preset volume to the patient's lungs. Cycling of standard ventilators occurs whenever a certain volume or pressure is reached or at a preset time interval. When positive PEEP is added to IPPV, it is called continuous positive ventilation (CPPV).

In recent years, mechanical ventilators have become very sophisticated and complex.[126] The current microprocessor-based new generation of mechanical ventilators are a logical extension of their earlier counterparts. The newest generation of adult mechanical ventilators offer more modes of ventilation, intrinsic microprocessors, computer compatible monitoring or control, and extensive patient data monitoring and collection in a highly versatile and flexible ventilating device.[127] However, many of the new methods of ventilation available must await the results of rigorously controlled, objective, double-blinded, randomized studies. The most common ventilatory modes available today with standard positive pressure ventilators, are controlled-mode ventilation (CMV), assist CMV, and intermittent or synchronized intermittent mandatory ventilation. Newer ventilatory modalities include, pressure support ventilation, (PSV), high frequency ventilation (HFV), extended mandatory minute ventilation (EMMV), and airway pressure release ventilation (APRV).

CONTROLLED MECHANICAL VENTILATION. Controlled mechanical ventilation of the lungs is the oldest mode of IPPV. The ventilator obligatorily delivers a gas at a preset rate and volume independent of patient effort or response. The patient is unable to alter or influence any portion of the ventilatory cycle. Thus, a patient with an intact ventilatory drive often must be hyperventilated or given sedatives or muscle relaxants to diminish the tendency to breathe asynchronously with the ventilator. In addition, mean airway pressure is highest with this form of IPPV.[128]

ASSIST CONTROL VENTILATION. Assist mechanical ventilation, or assist control, is an IPPV mode in which the patient creates a sub-baseline pressure in the inspiratory limb of the ventilator circuit that triggers the ventilator to deliver a predetermined tidal volume. If the patient's ventilatory rate falls below a preset level, the machine automatically enters the control mode.[128]

INTERMITTENT MANDATORY VENTILATION. Intermittent mandatory ventilation is a mode of IPPV in which the ventilator delivers a preset volume at a specified interval while also providing a continuous flow of gas for spontaneous ventilation. The patient spontaneously breathes gas with the same temperature, humidity, and oxygen concentration as the ventilator provides, while the ventilator delivers a preset tidal volume at predetermined intervals through a parallel ventilatory circuit.

SYNCHRONIZED INTERMITTENT MANDATORY VENTILATION. Synchronized intermittent mandatory ventilation is a mode using a combination of assist control with a mechanism and circuitry that allows for independent spontaneous ventilation. In this mode the patient may spontaneously breathe through the circuit while at a predetermined interval, the spontaneous breath is assisted by the machine. Therefore, a positive pressure breath is always in synchrony with the patient's spontaneous ventilatory pattern. In this system a pressure sensing device is located near the patient's airway that detects the initiation of a spontaneous breath, which activates the ventilator or the demand flow device. The major disadvantage of the demand flow system is the delay in providing adequate gas flow, that can result in an increased work of breathing.

PRESSURE SUPPORT VENTILATION. PSV is a form of ventilation that aids normal breathing with a predetermined level of positive airway pressure. PSV is similar to IPPV, but PSV differs in that airway pressure is held constant throughout the inspiratory period. PSV differs from conventional volume-cycled ventilation since the clinician selects only the inspiratory pressure. The patient controls ventilatory timing and interacts with the delivered pressure to determine the inspiratory flow and tidal volume. The unique wave forms of pressure and flow produced by PSV may have an advantage by providing better support of spontaneous tidal volume, and also by decreasing the overall work of breathing.[129] The objective of PSV is to increase the patient's spontaneous tidal volume by delivering airway pressure to achieve volumes equal to 10 ml·kg^{-1} to 12 ml·kg^{-1}. PSV may also decrease airway resistance by increasing airflow during inspiration and thereby decrease the work of breathing and delay muscle fatigue. Unfortunately, to date there are few clinical studies documenting the efficacy of this new ventilatory mode, though theoretical advantages and safety of the mode in appropriately monitored patients support its use. Further studies are required to better evaluate the complex process of ventilatory reflexes and muscle conditioning during mechanical ventilation in order to fully establish the proper role of PSV.

EXTENDED MANDATORY MINUTE VENTILATION. Extended mandatory minute ventilation provides a preset minute volume of gas either from a positive pressure breath or from spontaneous breathing. The clinician determines the minimal accepted minute volume and selects the appropriate rate and volume. As the patient's ability to spontaneously breathe improves, less assisted ventilation is provided.[130] Application of EMMV may enhance the weaning process by encouraging spontaneous breathing and enabling the patient to adjust to short-term changes in oxygen demand.[131] EMMV may also prove useful in tailoring tidal volume and respiratory rate more closely to meet patient needs. It may encourage patients who have become ventilator-dependent to use their respiratory muscles.

AIRWAY PRESSURE RELEASE VENTILATION. Airway pressure release ventilation was designed to augment ventilation for those patients with decreased lung compliance.[132, 133] The system is designed to provide alveolar ventilation as an adjunct to continuous positive airway pressure (CPAP) by intermittent and transient release of positive pressure, followed by restoration of pressure back to the CPAP level. The duration and frequency of CPAP release provide whatever level of ventilation is required. Because the peak airway pressure during APRV equals the level of CPAP, cardiovascular depression, barotrauma, and ventilation-perfusion mismatch associated with conventional forms of ventilatory support may be expected to decrease. Theoretical advantages of APRV over conventional positive pressure ventilatory techniques include its lower peak and mean airway pressures, improved arterial oxygenation and smaller physiologic dead space ventilation.[133] These advantages may lead to less depression of cardiac function as well as a decreased incidence of barotrauma. It differs from inverse inspiratory to expiratory ratio (I:E) ventilation in that with APRV, the patient breathes in an unrestricted manner during all parts of the ventilatory cycle. In contradistinction, an inverse I:E ratio requires skeletal muscle paralysis, sedation, or hyperventilation, because no gas flow is available for spontaneous breathing during mechanical inspiration. Certainly, further study is necessary to better define the role of APRV.

HIGH FREQUENCY VENTILATION. High frequency ventilation (HFV) was originally used as a technique to provide adequate oxygenation and alveolar ventilation for rigid bronchoscopy and laryngeal surgery.[134] Since that time, the literature is replete with clinical applications of HFV. It is important to note there are several different modalities to provide HFV. These ventilatory modes include high frequency positive pressure ventilation (HFPPV),[135] high frequency jet ventilation (HFJV),[136] high frequency flow interrupters (HFFI),[137] and high frequency oscillation (HFO).[138] Several reviews of HFV are available.[139–143] The common characteristic of all forms of HFV is ventilation at small tidal volumes (less than deadspace) with high rates (60–3000 breaths·min^{-1}). These systems enhance diffusive transport, minimize bulk transport, and improve intrapulmonary gas distribution. Problems described with HFV include inadequate humidification, barotrauma, necrotizing tracheobronchitis, hepatocellular injury, bronchospasm, and inadequate monitoring capabilities.[143] Thus, while HFV is effective in maintaining pulmonary gas exchange at lower mean airway pressures, its precise role is yet to be determined.

Have all of the advances in technology and new ventilatory modalities had an impact on the outcome of critically ill patients in the ICU? Clearly, for select patient populations ventilatory support has improved survival. For example, in the infant respiratory distress syndrome this has been accomplished by the use of CPAP.[144] Outcome has been similarly affected in patients with neuromuscular paralysis by the use of simple mechanical ventilation. However, despite all the newer ventilatory modalities available, little impact has been made on many other patient groups. The adult form of ARDS has not shown the documentable increase in survival obtained in infant respiratory distress syndrome. Further, in patients with multiple organ system failure, including respiratory failure requiring mechanical support, outcome is determined more by the underlying cause than the technique of mechanical ventilatory support. Despite an increasingly sophisticated array of mechanical support devices and detailed physiologic methodologies for augmenting support, little or no further increment of survival has been demonstrated in patients whose lungs are commonly ventilated with underlying sepsis and multiple organ failure. Certainly, ventilatory support has

a place in effecting outcome in critical illness, though newer ventilatory techniques and technology must await further evaluation.

CYSTIC FIBROSIS

Cystic fibrosis (CF) is an inherited multisystem disorder characterized by abnormalities in exocrine gland function. The most common cause of morbidity and mortality in patients with CF is pulmonary dysfunction.[145] Pancreatic dysfunction is also a common accompaniment, as is hepatobiliary and genitourinary disease. The median survival for patients with CF is about 20 years. However, with improvements in diagnosis and treatment many patients survive through the third and fourth decades.

All levels of the respiratory tract can be involved with CF. Nasal polyposis, sinusitis, and lower respiratory tract disease are common findings in patients with CF. The common denominator is the alteration in mucous secretion. These patients have large amounts of secretion that predispose them to bacterial pneumonia, particularly with pseudomonas aeruginosa.

Other organ systems involved with CF include the gastrointestinal and genitourinary systems and the sweat glands.[146] Pancreatic insufficiency leading to protein and fat malabsorption is common, and recurrent pancreatitis may occur. Hepatobiliary disease is common in older patients with chronic cholestasis, inflammation, fibrosis, and even cirrhosis. Extrahepatic disease of the biliary system and abnormalities of the genitourinary tract are also common.

Abnormality in sweat gland function is the most reliable diagnostic test for CF. Examination of sweat of patients with CF reveals elevations of sodium, potassium, and chloride levels.[147] This increase in electrolyte content results from a failure of reabsorption in the sweat duct.

Treatment of patients with CF is primarily directed at the respiratory system. Every attempt must be made to increase mechanical drainage and clear secretions with chest physiotherapy and exercise programs. Control of bacterial infection with antibiotic therapy is essential. Bronchodilators should be used to reverse any bronchospastic component to the lung disease. Fluid management and general supportive measures are essential to successful treatment.[148]

RENAL SYSTEM

ACUTE RENAL FAILURE

Acute renal failure (ARF) is impairment of the normal homeostatic functions of the kidney resulting in retention of nitrogenous wastes. It is a comon problem occurring in 5% of all hospitalized patients.[149] It is particularly problematic in critically ill patients where the incidence of ARF is approximately 23%.[150] Despite advances in understanding the disease process, mortality remains high.[149–151] Sixty per cent of all cases of ARF are related to surgery or trauma. The most common cause is renal ischemia with sepsis, hypovolemic shock, and nephrotoxic agents as major etiologic factors. The site of interference with renal function may be prerenal, renal, or postrenal.

Prerenal Causes

Prerenal causes of ARF result from hypoperfusion of the kidneys, most commonly from extracellular fluid volume contraction. Reduced renal perfusion results from decreased effective circulating volume by hypovolemia or redistribution of circulating volume. Reduction in cardiac output can also result in prerenal failure because of inadequate perfusion to the kidneys. This may result from primary myocardial disease, valvular heart disease, constrictive pericarditis, or cardiac tamponade. Decreased perfusion to the kidneys may also result from vascular disease of both large and small vessels. Certainly, bilateral renal artery stenosis can cause prerenal azotemia. However, although most prerenal causes of renal failure are accompanied by hypotension, renal artery stenosis is usually associated with hypertension.

Intrinsic Renal Causes

Intrinsic renal causes of ARF can be divided by the component of the kidney most affected *i.e.*, the glomeruli, blood vessels, and the tubulointerstitial region. Glomerular diseases account for 5% to 10% of all cases of ARF,[152] and may be caused by direct immunologically mediated injury or decreased renal perfusion. Vascular disease can result in intrinsic renal failure primarily due to either thromboembolic injury or systemic diseases.

Acute tubular necrosis (ATN) is the most common cause of ARF in critically ill patients, and accounts for over 75% of the renal causes of kidney failure. The two major causes of ATN are ischemia and nephrotoxins.[153] Renal ischemia is the most common cause of ARF and may be caused by a variety of clinical conditions including volume depletion, shock, and operations that interrupt the renal circulation. It appears that prostaglandins play an important role in maintaining renal perfusion, so patients taking drugs that inhibit prostaglandin synthesis may be predisposed to renal injury with hypoperfusion.

Nephrotoxic agents may also cause ATN. Categories of toxins include antibiotics, contrast material, anesthetic drugs, heavy metals, and organic solvents. In the past heavy metals, organic solvents, and glycols were a common cause of ARF. However, today aminoglycosides have supplanted them as the major nephrotoxic cause of ARF.[154] All aminoglycosides have nephrotoxic potential. Clinical nephrotoxicty, defined as a decrease in glomerular filtration rate, occurs in 5% to 25% of patients receiving aminoglycosides. The toxicity of these antibiotics is enhanced by advanced age, pre-existing renal dysfunction, concomitant administration of other nephrotoxic agents, and hypotension. Renal toxicity can also occur with antibiotics other than aminoglycosides including cephalosporins, penicillins, and amphotericin B.

Toxic ARF associated with the use of radiocontrast media is the second most common cause of nephrotoxic ATN. Patients particularly at risk for radiocontrast-induced renal failure include patients with diabetes mellitus, the elderly, and those with pre-existing renal insufficiency. Dehydration compounds the risk in susceptible patients.

Methoxyflurane is the most common of the anesthetic drugs described to precipitate ARF. Anesthetic induced nephrotoxicity is generally due to fluoride toxicity. Because toxicity results from high free fluoride levels in the plasma, prolonged duration of anesthesia and pre-existing renal dysfunction appear to put patients at risk for methoxyflurane nephrotoxicity.[151] Several common chemotherapeutic drugs can also cause ATN including cisplatin and high dose methotrexate.[151] Adequate extracellular fluid volume expansion and concomitant use of diuretics may significantly lessen nephrotoxic affects of cisplatin, and alkalinization of the urine may decrease toxicity of high dose methotrexate. Rhabdomyolysis has become an important cause of ARF described in association with crush injuries, extensive burns, muscle inflammation and a variety of settings in which muscle blood flow and metabolism are disturbed or muscle energy production is increased. The toxic effect of myoglobin causes ATN with rhabdomyolysis just as hemoglobin is the toxic pigment in ATN associated with hemolysis from mismatched blood.

An increasing number of drugs have been associated with acute interstitial nephritis (AIN) and subsequent ARF.[155] The most common cause of AIN is an acute drug induced hypersensitivity reaction. Drugs commonly implicated include beta-lactam antibiotics (especially methicillin), nonsteroidal anti-inflammatory agents, and diuretics. AIN is associated with an increased eosinophil count in blood and urine.

Postrenal Causes

Postrenal causes of ARF may be asymptomatic and must be considered in any patient with renal failure. This form of acute deterioration of renal function is often reversible and occurs in up to 10% of patients with decreasing renal function.[156] Obstruction to urine flow may occur at any level from the kidney to the bladder. Ureteral obstruction from calculi, clots, tumor, stricture, retroperitoneal fibrosis, or malignancy may cause ureteral obstruction, whereas bladder tumors or a neurogenic bladder can result in obstruction at the level of the bladder. Urethral obstruction can be caused by prostate disorders, urethral stricture, cervical carcinoma, or meatal stenosis. In most cases of possible obstruction, a combination of a flat abdominal film, renal scan, and ultrasonogram can supply as much information as excretory urography with much less risk.[156] However, if the clinical history is suggestive of obstruction, even if the noninvasive studies are negative, cystoscopy and retrograde pyelography should be considered.

OLIGURIC vs NONOLIGURIC ACUTE RENAL FAILURE

In the past ARF was often defined by oliguria, the production of less than 400 ml $\cdot$ day^{-1} of urine. However, nonoliguric ARF is now recognized as a distinct clinical entity with a more favorable prognosis.[157] Hospitalization time, complications, and mortality are less in nonoliguric patients. Drugs that increase solute excretion such as mannitol and furosemide may have the capacity to convert oliguric acute renal failure to the nonoliguric type. Some authors suggest large doses of intravenous furosemide be given to attenuate the course of ARF, whereas others claim that furosemide responders simply may have less severe renal impairment. The results are still controversial and the efficacy of furosemide may depend on its administration in the initiation phase of ARF. Nonetheless, after prerenal and postrenal factors contributing to azotemia have been corrected, a trial of furosemide 2 to 10 mg $\cdot$ kg^{-1} can be given in an attempt to convert an incipient oliguric renal failure to a nonoliguric state with restoration of blood volume if diuresis ensues.[156]

URINARY INDICES

Urine sediment is almost never normal in ARF.[158] A chemical profile of the urine aids immeasurably in assessing the cause of ARF. In prerenal azotemia, tubular function remains relatively intact and sodium and water resorption results. There is an increase in sodium loss in the urine in patients with ATN

TABLE 54-4. Diagnostic Urinary Indices

PARAMETER	PRERENAL	RENAL
Urinary osmolality	>500 mosm	<350 mosm
Urine/plasma creatinine	>30	<20
Urine sodium concentration	<20 mEq·l^{-1}	>40 mEq·l^{-1}
Fractional excretion of sodium	<1%	>2%
Renal failure index	<1%	>2%

because tubular function is impaired (Table 54-4).[159] In acute oliguric renal failure, daily increases of blood urea nitrogen (BUN) and serum creatinine average 10 mg·dl^{-1} to 20 mg·dl^{-1}, and 0.5 mg·dl^{-1} to 1 mg·dl^{-1}, respectively. If creatinine is elevated out of proportion to the BUN it suggests that rhabdomyolysis may be the etiology of acute renal failure. The rapid rise in serum creatinine with rhabdomyolysis is due to the release of creatine from skeletal muscle which is converted by nonenzymatic hydrolysis to creatinine.[160]

COMPLICATIONS OF ACUTE RENAL FAILURE

Hyponatremia, edema and pulmonary congestion can occur with oliguric acute renal failure due to salt and water overload. In addition, serum potassium may rise because of the decreased elimination of potassium associated with ARF. The usual rate of increase in serum potassium in the noncatabolic, oliguric patient is 0 meq to 0.5 meq 24 hr^{-1}. If potassium increases at a greater rate, other contributing factors should be sought and treated. Other electrolyte abnormalities present in acute renal failure include hyperphosphatemia, hypocalcemia, and mild hypermagnesemia. These abnormalities must be monitored closely and treated accordingly.

Because the kidneys can no longer eliminate the daily production of nonvolatile acid, there is a daily decrease of 1 meq to 2 meq in plasma bicarbonate with a resultant anion gap metabolic acidosis. Still other complications include anemia, platelet abnormalities, and altered host defenses leading to an increased incidence of infection. Gastrointestinal complications include nausea, vomiting and, most commonly, gastrointestinal hemorrhage that occurs in 10% to 30% of patients.

TREATMENT

Mortality rates of patients with ARF vary from 30% to 60%. However, if ARF follows surgery or trauma, the mortality may be as high as 70%. The first step in the management of ARF is to exclude remedial causes of renal failure. Specifically, identification and correction of prerenal and postrenal factors is essential. The treatment of ARF includes diuresis and control of the extracellular fluid volume, treatment of hyperkalemia and acidosis, prophylaxis against infection and gastrointestinal bleeding, nutritional support, and dialysis. Since the prognosis is better with polyuria than anuria, efforts should be made to produce and maintain a polyuric state. Intake and output must be monitored closely.

Conservative therapy is frequently ineffective for critically ill patients with ARF, so some form of dialytic therapy is usually indicated. The absolute indications for dialysis include symptomatic uremia, development of resistant hyperkalemia, severe acidemia or fluid overload not responsive to conservative therapy, and pericarditis. In addition, many advocate maintaining a BUN less than 100 mg·dl^{-1} and a creatinine

less than 8 mg·dl^{-1}. Inadequate nutrition has recently been recognized as a reason for dialysis. Both hemodialysis and peritoneal dialysis have been used to manage ARF and survival data are similar.[161] Each method has unique advantages and disadvantages.

Recently, several modifications of hemodialysis have been applied to patients with ARF. These include slow continuous ultrafiltration (SCUF), with intermittent hemodialysis, continuous arterial venous hemodialysis (CAVHD), and continuous arterial venous hemofiltration (CAVH). All of these methods provide excellent hemodynamic stability. Access to blood is obtained either by percutaneous cannulation of the femoral artery and vein or by way of an arteriovenous shunt. No blood pump is used in this system because blood is driven by the patient's own arterial pressure. In CAVH, large amounts of ultrafiltrate are removed through a porous filter with the ultrafiltrate replaced by sterile intravenous fluid.[162] In SCUF, much smaller volumes of ultrafiltrate are removed to correct any extracellular fluid volume expansion. However, intermittent dialysis is required to control uremia, hyperkalemia, and acidemia.[163] With CAVHD dialysate flows through the dialysate compartment at approximately 20 ml·min^{-1} which is sufficient to achieve a low, steady-state BUN and creatinine levels.[164] Unfortunately, the various improvements in resuscitative techniques and technical advances in dialytic therapy have not reduced the mortality of ARF.

HEPATORENAL SYNDROME

Acute renal failure in the presence of severe advanced liver disease in the absence of clinical, laboratory, or anatomic evidence of other causes of renal dysfunction, is known as hepatorenal syndrome. It is usually an oliguric form of renal failure with low urinary sodium concentrations. The picture appears similar to a prerenal azotemia; however, it occurs in the setting of advanced liver disease. The precise mechanism for the renal failure is unknown. Currently, there is no effective treatment for hepatorenal syndrome.

INFECTIOUS DISEASES

NOSOCOMIAL INFECTIONS

Advances in technology and the use of a greater number of monitoring devices and therapeutic interventions have led to an increased number of infections. Indeed, hospital acquired infections have emerged as the leading cause of death in most critical care units. These infections are often polymicrobial, involve multiple resistant strains of bacteria and do not respond to simple therapy. The incidence of nosocomial infections in ICUs is commonly 40% to 50%, many of which are preventable.[165] The cost implications of prolonged hospitalization and treatment of infection are apparent.[166]

The major determinants of the incidence and outcome of nosocomial infections include patient age, underlying disease, integrity of mucosal and integumentary surfaces, and the status of the immunologic defenses. Common sources of hospital-acquired infections in critically ill patients include the urinary tract, surgical wounds, pneumonia, intravascular devices, and sinusitis. Immunocompromised patients with a deficiency in any of the multi-faceted host defenses are particularly prone to these infections and to other unusual infections. In particular, patients with acquired immunodeficiency syndrome (AIDS) commonly present with opportunistic infections caused by viruses, bacteria, parasites, and fungi. These patients invariably die despite transiently effective antimicrobial therapy and current attempts at immune reconstitution.[167]

Urinary Tract Infections

Urinary tract infections account for approximately 40 percent of hospital-acquired infections.[168] Because most critically ill patients have an indwelling Foley catheter, it is not surprising that the urinary tract is a common source of infection. It is the most common site resulting in gram-negative bacteremia. The urinary tract should be considered a possible source of infection if the patient has bacteriuria and a clinical picture consistent with infection.

Wound Infections

Most surgical wound infections are caused by the introduction of bacteria directly into the tissue at the time of operation. They account for 10% of all infections in postsurgical ICU patients.[169] Wounds should be observed for any signs of infection and any purulent material should be sampled and sent for gram stain and culture. Most wound infections are evident 3 to 7 days following surgical intervention. Wounds infected within 24 hours are generally fulminant infections due to clostridium or beta-hemolytic streptococci. Later surgical wound infections are generally caused by gram-negative bacilli, anaerobic bacteria, and staphylococci. The administration of prophylactic antibiotics has aided immeasurably in reducing the postoperative wound infection rate.

Pneumonia

The most serious complication among hospital-acquired infections is lower respiratory tract infection. Hospital-acquired pneumonia occurs in up to 15% of ICU patients and is the leading cause of mortality in this group.[170] The major organisms causing pneumonia in the critically ill patient population are gram-negative bacilli and staphylococcus aureus.[171] The diagnosis of pneumonia in critically ill patients who are maintained on mechanical ventilatory support can be difficult.[170] Physical examination by itself is not an adequate screening procedure.[172, 173] Bacterial colonization of the upper airway is common[174, 175] and may not reflect lower respiratory tract disease.[176, 177] Nosocomial pneumonia is generally diagnosed by signs and symptoms of infection with bacteriologic verification, in addition to a new pulmonary infiltrate that is unchanged by physical therapy. Unfortunately, gram stain and culture of aspirated material through the endotracheal tube may not be a reliable indicator of true lower respiratory tract infection.[178, 179] Antibody coating and quantitative cultures have not significantly improved diagnostic efficacy. Protected brush catheter bronchoscopy has recently been advocated as an effective adjunct to the diagnosis of pneumonia for patients maintained on mechanical ventilatory support.[180]

Intravascular Devices

With advances in technology and invasive monitoring, intravascular device-related bacteremia has become a common problem accounting for over 25,000 cases of bacteremia annually.[181] Contamination of intravascular devices may occur anywhere along the line from the infusate bottle to the skin entry site. Predisposition to intravascular device-related bacteremia is determined by both patient factors and hospital factors. The patient-related factors generally reflect the severity of underlying disease. Hospital-related factors are more controlled and include the type of catheter, the site of insertion, the technique of placement and the duration of cannulation.[182] Recommendations for prevention of intravascular-device related infections should be based on the Center for Disease Control guidelines.[183]

Intra-abdominal Infections

Abdominal infections generally occur in patients who have undergone prior intra-abdominal procedures. Risk factors for infection include prolonged operative time, use of foreign substances, inadequate drainage, presence of devitalized tissue, hematoma formation, and fecal contamination at the time of surgery.[184] Acalculus cholecystitis is another potential etiology of abdominal infection in the postoperative period. Stress ulceration with significant GI bleeding and perforation, or perforation due to mechanical causes, such as nasogastric drainage, can result in intra-abdominal infection in the absence of prior surgical intervention. The diagnosis of intra-abdmonial infection relies primarily on physical examination with adjunctive radiologic evaluation including CT scan, ultrasonography, and abdominal roentgenograms.

Sinusitis

One of the recognized complications of nasotracheal intubation is the development of sinusitis. Nosocomial sinusitis accounts for 5% of all nosocomial infections in the critically ill patient population.[185] However, this infection is frequently difficult to diagnose and often goes unrecognized. Patients may present with fever and leukocytosis, but with few other signs or symptoms of overt infection. Fewer than half of the patients have purulent nasal drainage. The diagnosis of sinusitis relies on x-ray films of the paranasal sinuses. Unfortunately, these are frequently of suboptimal quality taken in the critical care unit with a portable apparatus. However, if opacification of the sinuses is present or an air fluid level is noted and aspiration reveals purulent material, the endotracheal tube should be removed and replaced using the oral route along with initiation of antibiotic therapy. Patients generally respond well and rarely require surgical drainage.

Central Nervous System Infections

Nosocomial central nervous system infections are uncommon in critically ill patients unless there are predisposing conditions such as neurosurgical procedures or central nervous system trauma. All pyogenic infections of the cranial contents originate either by hematogenous spread or extension from contiguous sites. Acute meningitis is a medical emergency that requires high level diagnostic and therapeutic skills because it has a significant mortality rate. Patients frequently present with headache, stiff neck, seizures, and altered mental status. In order to differentiate bacterial meningitis from an aseptic meningitis syndrome, analysis of the CSF is necessary. All febrile patients with lethargy, headache, or confusion of sudden onset, even if only low-grade temperature is present, should be subjected to a lumbar puncture.

Brain abscess has occurred with a constant incidence even with the introduction of broad-spectrum antibiotic coverage. It is associated with a high morbidity and mortality. The most common age of patients for a brain abscess to occur is between 30 and 40 years of age, and is frequently associated with sinusitis or otitis. Streptococci are the most common etiologic organisms. Treatment is both medical and surgical with anaerobic antibiotic coverage and surgical drainage. Although mortality has improved, there is still a significant incidence of neurologic residual, primarily seizure disorders.

Fungal Infections

With the use of broad-spectrum antibiotic therapy, organ transplantation, prosthetic cardiac valves and immunosuppression from neoplasm, transplants, burns, and drugs, there has been an increased incidence of fungal infections. Clinical manifestations range from thrush to disseminated candidiasis. Organs involved with systemic disease include the kidneys, brain, myocardium, and eyes. The hallmark, pathologically, is diffuse microabscesses with a combined suppurative and granulomatous reaction. The diagnosis of candidemia may be difficult as serum antibodies have been uniformly disappointing, and cultures are often negative. Though not all patients with candidemia require antifungal therapy, if treatment is indicated, Amphotericin B is the drug of choice.

SEPTIC SHOCK

Septic shock is a form of circulatory shock that usually develops as a complication of an overwhelming infection. As with any form of shock, it is a state in which the supply of blood to the tissues of the body is inadequate to meet the body's metabolic demands. It has been estimated there are over 300,000 gram-negative bacteremias in the United States each year. When bacteremia is caused by gram-negative bacteria, shock intervenes in up to 40% of these patients with a 40% to 90% mortality.[186] *Escherichia coli* is the most common causative organism followed by Klebsiella, Enterobacter, Proteus, Pseudomonas, and Serratia. As is evident from the causative agents, the sites of infection are usually the urinary, intestinal, biliary, and female genital tracts. There is a predominance of males over 40 years of age and females between 20 and 45 years of age who are affected.[187] Nonspecific predisposing afflictions are quite common including diabetes mellitus, cirrhosis of the liver, burns, and neoplasms, as well as drug therapy including chemotherapy and steroids.

Unfortunately, it has become very commonplace to label septic shock as gram-negative shock or endotoxin shock. It appears that gram-negative bacillary endotoxin is only one of the potential culprits in the pathogenesis of the clinical manifestations of the shock syndrome.[188] Indeed, it has been extremely difficult to clinically differentiate between gram-positive and gram-negative infection.[189] The gram-negative bacilli have a complex three-layered cell wall structure.[188] The lipopolysaccharide component of the outermost layer has been of particular interest because of its association with endotoxin properties.[190, 191]

Endotoxin is a complex molecule consisting of an outer core of repetitive sugar moieties, an O-antigen-specific side chain conferring serologic specificity, and an inner core linked to a structure termed lipid A.[192] Endotoxin and other bacterial products activate cell membrane phospholipases to liberate arachidonic acid and initiate synthesis and release of leukotrienes, prostaglandin, and thromboxanes.[193] It is these inflammatory mediators that primarily influence vasomotor tone, microvascular permeability, leukoaggregation, and the aggregation of platelets. Bacterial endotoxin can trigger a cascade of enzymatic processes, which leads to the release of vasoactive kinins, kallikreins in particular.[194] The micro-organisms activate the classic complement pathway while endotoxin activates the alternate pathway. Complement activation, leukotriene generation, and the direct effect of endotoxin on neutrophils leads to accumulation of inflammatory cells in the lung. This has been proposed as the underlying mechanism for initiation of ARDS, which is a common accompaniment of septic shock.[195] In addition, activation of the intrinsic coagulation cascade via a direct effect on Hageman factor leads to activation of the fibrinolytic system that can lead to DIC, which may accompany the shock syndrome.

Hemodynamic alterations in septic shock generally take two forms.[186, 191, 196–198] Early in shock, the patient may present with an increase in cardiac output, vasodilatation, decrease in systemic vascular resistance, decrease in CVP, and an increase in stroke volume. As shock progresses, the predominant picture is one of vasoconstriction with an increase in systemic vascular resistance and a decrease in cardiac output, CVP, and in stroke volume.

Organ systems involved by septic shock include the cardiac, renal, respiratory, and hemologic systems. Cardiac failure may develop in the setting of sepsis, primarily related to a myocardial depressant factor.[199] DIC is not uncommon in septic shock. The pathogenesis probably involves the activation of the intrinsic clotting system by Hageman factor leading to activation of kallikrein. This in turn activates the potent vasodilator, bradykinin, which promotes pooling of blood in peripheral tissues, as well as increases in capillary permeability and localized tissue damage. Respiratory failure is probably the most important cause of death in patients with shock. Septic shock is an important cause of ARDS and severe respiratory failure.[195] The kidneys are also target organs in septic shock with resultant ARF. Oliguria occurs early and probably results from inadequate renal perfusion.

Clinically, gram-negative bacteremia usually begins abruptly with chills, fever, nausea, vomiting, diarrhea, and prostration. When septic shock develops, there is in addition tachycardia, tachypnea, hypotension, cool pale extremities with peripheral cyanosis, mental obtundation, and oliguria. Laboratory data vary greatly and depend on both the cause and extent of the shock syndrome.

Laboratory data are variable. There is usually leukocytosis. However, the white blood cell count may be normal or even depressed. Serum bicarbonate is usually low and blood lactate level elevated. Electrolyte pattern may vary considerably, though there is a tendency to hyponatremia and hypochloremia.

Treatment of septic shock is directed at two primary therapeutic goals—1) rapid reversal of perfusion failure and 2) identification and control of infection. Certainly, every effort should be made to identify the cause of infection. However, treatment must be initiated early if it is to be successful. Indeed, antibiotic therapy should be initiated immediately and not await blood culture results. Early aggressive intervention including antibiotics, fluid resuscitation, vasoactive drug support, mechanical ventilatory support, and surgical drainage of any infected site is essential for successful treatment. Certainly, surgical drainage of closed space infections is mandatory and a vigorous search for the infectious site is indicated in all patients.

Fluid resuscitation is the mainstay in treatment of septic shock. The fluid of choice for volume repletion remains controversial.[200] Regardless of the fluid infused, however, it appears that survival can be improved if stroke volume or cardiac output improves in response to fluid challenge. If volume resuscitation and other supportive measures are inadequate in restoring perfusion, then vasoactive drug support may be indicated. Because in the low flow state of hypodynamic septic shock, peripheral vascular resistances increase, drugs with predominantly alpha-adrengic efforts should be avoided. Dopamine and dobutamine have been used successfully in treating septic shock. These drugs have predominantly beta-adrenergic effects and result in an increase in cardiac output due to both an increase in contractility and heart rate. It is also important to maintain urine flow in an attempt to prevent renal failure. Urine output should ideally be kept greater than 30 ml $\cdot$ hr^{-1} to 40 ml $\cdot$ hr^{-1} with fluid resuscitation and if necessary diuretic therapy.

Corticosteroids have been advocated in the past as adjunctive therapy to the treatment of septic shock.[201–203] However, more recent studies suggest the use of high dose corticosteroids provide no benefit in the treatment of severe sepsis and septic shock and are no longer recommended.[204, 205] Efforts are now being directed at developing techniques to facilitate early diagnosis of the septic syndrome, identify markers of causative organisms and discover more promising pharmacologic or immunologic drugs to reduce the still unacceptably high mortality from systemic sepsis.

NUTRITION

Adequate nutrition is essential to replace the nutrients used to meet the energy needs of tissues and to repair tissues being catabolized. In the critically ill or injured patient, nutrition is an essential part of treatment.[206, 208] For patients undergoing surgical procedures, malnutrition is well documented to be a risk factor and perioperative nutritional support can reduce complications, mortality, morbidity, and length of hospital stay.[209, 210]

NUTRITIONAL ASSESSMENT

Assessment of nutrition is the first step in assuring adequate support for the critically ill patient. Adequacy of nutrition can be assessed by anthropomorphic measurements, delayed cutaneous hypersensitivity to several antigens, and laboratory measurements reflecting severe protein and calorie malnutrition.[211–214] Nitrogen balance is an important measure of nutritional status. The relationship between urea nitrogen excretion and metabolic rate is due to the obligatory oxidation of body cell mass that occurs with stress and starvation. Therefore, the extent of hypermetabolism can be predicted from a simple clinical determination of urea nitrogen collected in a timed urine specimen.

ESTIMATION OF ENERGY REQUIREMENT

The Harris-Benedict equation derived from indirect calorimetry measurements provides a reasonable estimate of basal caloric requirements (Table 54-5). Basal energy expenditure calculated in this manner correlates well with values obtained by contemporary techniques of continuous expired air analysis.[215] The goal of nutritional support in nondepleted postoperative patients is to prevent excessive loss of lean tissue, whereas in nutritionally depleted patients it is restoration of lean tissue with concomitant restoration of fat reserves.[216] Calculated basal energy needs should be increased by 30% with sepsis.

ENTERAL vs PARENTERAL NUTRITION

The gastrointestinal tract is the route of choice for nutritional supplementation whenever possible.[217] There are a variety of commercially available enteral feeding formulas. With near normal proteolytic and lipolytic activity in the gastrointestinal tract, meal replacement formulas can be used. These formulas are polymeric mixtures containing proteins, fats, and carbohydrates in high molecular weight forms. The lactose content is generally low, and fat content represents approximately 30% of the calories. Elemental diets use aminoacids as the nitrogen source, and usually contain little fat and no lactose. These diets also have a low viscosity that make them particularly useful for infusion through needle catheter jejunostomy tubes. Feeding modules are concentrated sources of one nutrient that can yield a small volume, high caloric mixture when added to a formula diet. This is particularly useful for patients on fluid restriction. A continuous-drip infusion of enteral feedings through a feeding tube is the preferred technique. The most common complication of enteral feedings is diarrhea. Other potential hazards include malpositioning of the feeding tube, hyperglycemia, and abnormalities in liver function tests.

When the enteral route is unavailable or provides inadequate intake for the depleted patient, parenteral nutrition support should be undertaken. Certainly, critically ill patients who are hypercatabolic, nutritionally depleted, or have multiple organ system failure should have total parenteral nutrition administered through a central line.

It is not only important that adequate calories be supplied to critically ill patients, but distribution of calories provided as carbohydrates, fats, and protein is equally important. Historically, caloric requirements for total parenteral nutrition were given primarily as carbohydrates, which has a respiratory quotient (RQ) of 1 resulting in a large increase in carbon dioxide production and oxygen consumption. In recent years an appreciation has been gained that fat emulsions supply essential fatty acids in a concentrated source of calories.[218] Because fat emulsions are oxidized with an RQ of 0.7, carbon dioxide production and ventilatory requirements are reduced.[219]

While nutritional support has been shown to improve wound healing, decrease morbidity and mortality, and assist in immunocompetence, many complications have been described. Technical complications relate primarily to insertion of the central venous catheter used for access.[220] Other complications of hyperalimentation include sepsis, metabolic abnormalities, electrolyte disturbances, acid-base disorders, hepatic dysfunction, hypercalcemia and pancreatitis, metabolic bone disease, and fluid overload.[221]

DISORDERS OF COAGULATION

There are three essentials for a normal clotting mechanism: 1) vascular integrity, 2) normal platelet function, and 3) normal coagulation factors. The initial step in normal coagulation is

TABLE 54-5. Harris-Benedict Equations for Estimation of Basal Energy Expenditure (BEE)

Women BEE = 655 + (9.6 × Wt) + (1.8 × Ht) − (4.7 × Age)
Men BEE = 66 + (13.7 × Wt) + (5 × Ht) − (6.8 × Age)

Wt = weight in kilograms; Ht = height in centimeters;
Age = age in years.

compensatory reduction in intravascular pressure of the severed ends of blood vessels, followed by platelets covering the damaged surfaces. They accumulate at the site to ultimately form a hemostatic plug. The coagulation cascade is then activated with the formation of fibrin. Two distinct pathways operate to form thrombin, which then converts fibrinogen into fibrin. The intrinsic pathway produces thrombin from factors present only in the plasma, while the extrinsic pathway uses extraplasma tissue factors, as well as plasma factors. The final step in the normal coagulation scheme is removal of the fibrin and platelet clot by the fibrinolytic system. The end result of the activation of these pathways is the conversion of plasminogen into plasmin which cleaves both fibrinogen and fibrin. There is an ongoing equilibrium between the activation of the coagulation system and activation of the fibrinolytic system.

Disorders in the coagulation system lead either to bleeding or thrombosis. Clinical evaluation of disorders of coagulation is based on history, physical examination, and laboratory studies. A history of abnormal bleeding or evidence of bleeding on physical examination may assist in making a definitive diagnosis. Laboratory screening tests for hemostatic profile are essential.[222] Such a profile of test should include a platelet count, bleeding time, prothrombin time (PT), partial thromboplastin time (PTT), and review of the peripheral blood smear. The PT is a measure of the efficiency of thrombin formation by the extrinsic pathway. Abnormalities in the PT can be caused by absence or impairment of any coagulation factor in the intrinsic or extrinsic clotting system. The PTT is used to assess the efficiency of the intrinsic clotting system. Prolongation of the PTT generally represents deficiency or inhibition of Factors I, II, V, VIII, IX, X, XI, or XII. Qualitative abnormalities in platelets are manifested by prolongation of the bleeding time. If platelet function is intact, bleeding abnormalities usually do not occur unless the platelet count is below $100,000 \cdot mm^3$.

Disorders of hemostasis in critically ill patients are generally complex and represent multiple acquired deficiencies. Indeed, in most critically ill patients a bleeding disorder is but one manifestation of a complex series of failing organ system interactions. Common acquired deficiencies of hemostasis include DIC, liver disease, vitamin K deficiency, anticoagulants, and massive blood transfusion.

DISSEMINATED INTRAVASCULAR COAGULATION

DIC is a syndrome and not a primary disease state that reflects severe underlying pathology. The coagulation cascade is activated, resulting in the deposition of small thrombi and emboli throughout the microvasculature. This phase is then followed by secondary fibrinolysis. Repetition of this cycle leads to depletion of coagulation proteins and platelets and the antihemostatic effects of fibrin degradation products. Clinical manifestations of DIC can result in thrombosis or hemorrhage. Most commonly bleeding is manifest from multiple sites including venipuncture sites, nasogastric tubes, urinary catheters, or endotracheal tubes. Laboratory manifestations of DIC include thrombocytopenia, hypofibrinogenemia, and prolongation of the PT. Abnormalities of these indicators confirm DIC. If all are not abnormal, then additional studies including PTT, thrombin time and fibrin degradation products should be ordered.[222] In addition, review of the peripheral smear may reveal a microangiopathic hemolytic anemia from cell trapping and damage within fibrin thrombi.

The treatment of DIC is the treatment of the underlying cause. Some authors have suggested the use of heparin as supportive therapy in order to reduce thrombin generation and prevent further consumption of clotting proteins until the underlying disease process could be controlled.[223] Although it remains controversial, current recommendations do not support the use of routine heparin therapy, but rather, the administration of fresh frozen plasma and cryoprecipitate to replace depleted clotting factors and platelet concentrates to correct thrombocytopenia.[224]

An unusual cause of bleeding can result from defects in the fibrinolytic system. Patients with alpha-2 plasmin inhibitor deficiency, cirrhosis of the liver, or malignancy may develop diffuse bleeding from primary fibrinolysis rather than DIC. Laboratory data reveals relatively normal PT and PTT with a normal platelet count and a disproportionally low fibrinogen level. Patients with clearly established primary fibrinolysis should receive epsilon aminocaproic acid (EACA) and not heparin. However, if concomitant DIC is suspected, EACA should be avoided as it can cause massive, often fatal thrombosis.

POISONING

Despite preventive health programs and increased public awareness, poisoning remains a common and serious medical problem. Accidental poisonings account for approximately 5000 deaths per year, with suicides by chemical agents causing an additional 6000 deaths per year.[225] Poisoning is of particular importance in the pediatric population. As many as 2 million children in the United States accidentally swallow toxic material and approximately one ingestion of 1000 is fatal. However, poisoning is by no means a problem limited to children. One half of all poisoned patients are over the age of twenty.

The causative agents in poisoning vary with age. Children less than 5 years of age tend to ingest household products, whereas older patients are more likely to choose drugs. Aspirin accounts for 25% of all ingestions and is reported as the most common medicine involved in poisoning.

Prompt recognition and early intervention is essential to the successful treatment of poisoning. The diagnosis of poisoning can be very difficult because the toxic effects of many agents are nonspecific. Certainly, a high index of suspicion must be maintained when confronted with a patient presenting with seizures, coma, psychosis, acute renal or hepatic insufficiency, or bone marrow depression. However, most poisoning syndromes manifest nonspecific symptoms. Similarly, it is uncommon for the physical examination to show characteristic toxic effects of chemical substances.

Identification of the toxic agent should be attempted in every case of poisoning. Gastric fluid, urine, and blood samples should be sent to screen for possible poisons. Modalities available to identify the offending agents include thin-layer chromatography, gas-liquid chromatography, high-performance liquid chromatography, and spectrometry. Patients poisoned with drugs frequently take more than one agent which can lead to drug interactions and difficulty in interpreting test results.

TREATMENT

Treatment of poisoning should not await toxicologic determinations. Supportive care should begin immediately including the essentials of basic cardiopulmonary support. In addition, symptomatic treatment of neurologic, renal, and hepatic dysfunction is mandatory. Attention should then be directed to minimizing absorption of the poison. For ingested poisons this means prevention of absorption from the gastrointestinal tract by lavage, emetics, and adsorbents such as charcoal. Cathartics generally have no role in treating poisoning.[226]

Attempts should also be made to hasten elimination of absorbed poisons. Techniques available to increase elimination of poisons include diuresis, dialysis, chelation, hemoperfusion, exchange transfusion, and antibodies. Glomerular filtration and dialysis are generally effective only with substances found in plasma water and not protein bound poisons. Hemoperfusion is most effective if used immediately after ingestion of the poison. Exchange transfusion may be especially useful in small children when hemoperfusion may be technically difficult. Antibodies can also be used as a high affinity adsorbent in the patient's blood stream to hasten elimination.

COMMON POISONS

Application of the principles used for the management of acute poisonings can be exemplified by several common agents.

Acetaminophen

This aspirin substitute is a frequent cause of poisoning. Clinical manifestations are generally nonspecific. Patients may initially present with pallor, lethargy, nausea, vomiting, and diaphoresis. Hepatotoxicity may become evident 1 to 2 days after ingestion and can be fatal. Liver damage results when the normal metabolic pathways become saturated so that an increased fraction of drug is inactivated by the P-450 system, glutathione stores are depleted, and the reactive intermediates bind to liver macromolecules. Treatment of acetaminophen intoxication is initiated by induction of emesis or gastric lavage followed by administration of activated charcoal. Attention is next directed towards increasing sulfhydryl donors such as glutathione to allow greater binding of the toxic acetaminophen metabolites and therefore reduce liver damage. Early administration of n-acetylcystine can significantly reduce the incidence of acetaminophen-induced hepatotoxicity.[227]

Alcohols

Although the low molecular weight alcohols, methanol, ethanol, ethylene glycol, and isopropanol are relatively weak poisons, the result of their metabolism can be fatal. Ethanol depresses ventilation, decreases myocardial contractility, predisposes to hypothermia and causes hypoglycemia, especially in children. Although there is no antidote to ethanol and no way to hasten its metabolism, it is readily removed by hemodialysis.[228] However, usually critical care support with assisted ventilation of the lungs suffices in the treatment of ethanol intoxication. It is as important to treat associated illnesses in the patient with an ethanol overdose as it is to support the patient for the drug poisoning.

Methanol and ethylene glycol poisonings are common, yet frequently undetected. It is important to detect poisoning with these agents early because the metabolites are potent poisons and may lead to irreversible toxicity if they go unrecognized.[229, 230] Methanol is present in windshield washer antifreeze and solvents, and in organic synthetic processes, while ethylene glycol is the major automotive antifreeze. Treatment of methanol and ethylene glycol poisoning is systemic alkalinization to decrease ocular and renal toxicity followed by hemodialysis to accelerate elimination of the alcohols and their metabolites.

Carbon Monoxide

Carbon monoxide (CO) is a colorless, odorless, tasteless, non-irritating gas produced by the incomplete combustion of carbonaceous material. It is the major cause of death in patients exposed to smoke inhalation from fires. CO is responsible for approximately 3500 accidental and suicidal deaths per year in the United States. It exerts its toxic effects through tissue hypoxia.[231] The hemoglobin molecule has an affinity for carbon monoxide that is over 200 times greater than for oxygen. The combination of CO with hemoglobin forms carboxyhemoglobin which is incapable of carrying oxygen. It also interferes with the release of oxygen from oxyhemoglobin which decreases the amount of oxygen available to the tissues. In addition, because the rate of dissociation of CO from hemoglobin is extremely low, carboxyhemoglobin produces an acute decrease in blood oxygen content that is not readily reversed. The amount of carboxyhemoglobin present in blood depends on the concentration of CO in the inspired air and on the time of exposure.[232]

Symptomatology depends on the amount of carboxyhemoglobin present and the patient's activity level, tissue oxygen demands, and hemoglobin concentration. Exposure to low concentrations of CO cause irritability, altered visual and motor skills, headache, nausea, vomiting, and predisposition to angina pectoris. Severe poisoning may result in seizures, coma, respiratory failure, and death. The classic cherry red color of the skin and mucous membranes of patients with CO poisoning results from the bright red cast of carboxyhemoglobin. However, in patients with severe poisoning, cyanosis may be predominant over the cherry red color.

Treatment of CO poisoning is to remove the offending agent and provide a high oxygen enriched environment. The half time of CO elimination can be shortened from 4 hours to 40 minutes by hyperventilation of the lungs with 100% oxygen. Ventilation may require mechanical support. Other treatment modalities include hyperbaric oxygen, transfusion therapy, as well as diuretics and steroids for the treatment of complicating cerebral edema.[231]

LEGAL AND ETHICAL ISSUES

BRAIN DEATH

Brain death is defined as the irreversible cessation of all functions of the entire brain.[233] This clinical definition is confirmed by autopsy studies revealing destruction of the entire brain in both the cerebral hemispheres and the brain stem. The primary insult leads to brain edema with increases in intracranial pressure. In the vast majority of brain death cases, the ICP exceeds systolic blood pressure within 12 to 24 hours. Currently, most states recognize brain death as sufficient criteria for declaration of death. There have been many definitions offered of brain death. However, the broadly held consensus opinion was reflected in *Defining Death*, a report issued in 1981 by the President's Commission for the Study of Ethical Problems in Medicine and Biomedical and Behavioral Research.[234] In response to a congressional mandate, the commission recommended a statute, The Uniformed Determination of Death

Act (UDDA), which has become the most widely accepted legal formulation of the standards for determining human death. In addition, it also provided an update formulation of the medical criteria for applying the standard.[235] Representatives of the American Bar Association, American Medical Association, National Conference of Commissioners on Uniform State Laws, and the Academy of the American Encephalographers Society agreed on the UDDA definition as follows: An individual who has sustained either 1) irreversible cessation of circulatory and respiratory functions, or 2) irreversible cessation of all functions or the entire brain, including the brain stem, is dead. A determination of death must be made in accordance with accepted medical standards. These guidelines are now widely accepted by physicians and hospitals for clinical decision making. This formulation of brain death is based on a clinical diagnosis with certain preconditions and confirmatory tests.[236, 237]

With advances in technology and medical capability, even seemingly clear-cut definitions, such as death, become complex and difficult to translate into law and policy. Indeed, for many years courts were slow to modify the common law definition of death, i.e., cessation of all vital functions including respiration and circulation, in order to accept the determination of death based on irreversible cessation of all functions of the brain. The most common and familiar criteria for the diagnosis of whole brain death are the Harvard criteria published in 1968[238] by an Ad Hoc Committee of the Harvard Medical School. Tests generally used to determine brain death rely on response to stimuli, the presence of reflexes and spontaneous movements, and the electroencephalogram. There must be no evidence of hypothermia or drugs that depress brain function. The findings must persist over 24 hours. These Harvard criteria are now widely accepted by the medical profession and can be recognized legally as defining death in many states.

Indeed, organ transplantation was a major impetus for focusing public attention on the need to update standards for determining death, even though only approximately 15% of patients who are declared brain dead become organ donors. A special standard only for organ donors would fail to address the overwhelming majority of comatose ventilator supported cases. This could create a separate standard of death for donors that could lead to abuse and confusion.[239] Thus, along with the clinical diagnosis confirmatory tests are generally required and can be dependent on normal function or intracranial blood flow.

DO NOT RESUSCITATE ORDERS

Few areas in clinical medicine generate as much controversy and debate as does the decision to withdraw or withhold treatment of critically ill patients.[240, 241] Certainly, the opinion in the Joseph Saikewicz case issued by the Massachusetts Supreme Judicial Court in November 1977, was the most controversial judicial decision in the health law field in recent years.[242] In this case a profoundly retarded institutionalized 67-year-old man with acute myeloblastic monocytic leukemia was appointed a guardian and the court was asked to decide if treatment should be undertaken. It was understood that treatment would be painful and carry potential hazards with very little hope for recovery. The County Probate Court recommended withholding therapy and the Supreme Court affirmed this order. However, the Supreme Court further stated that the decision to withhold or withdraw the life-support measures in a terminally ill, incompetent patient was not within the jurisdiction of any hospital committee or panel, but rather the ultimate decision-making responsibility rested with the courts. Justice Paul J. Liacos, the author of the Saikewicz decision, offered a different approach to do not resuscitate (DNR) orders when he suggested they present a case for physician discretion, and the principles of Saikewicz are inapplicable.[243]

In a subsequent court opinion, in the matter of Dinnerstein, the legality of DNR orders was addressed. In this case, the patient was a 67-year-old woman with Alzheimer's disease, a massive stroke, and left hemiparesis. She was left in a persistent vegetative state, immobile, speechless, unable to swallow without choking and barely able to cough. The patient's physician recommended no resuscitation in the event of cardiopulmonary arrest and the patient's family concurred. Because of the legal uncertainty surrounding "no code" orders, the physician, hospital, and family asked the court to rule about the legality of the order. The Massachusetts Appeal Court held that a DNR order in these circumstances was lawful and advance judicial approval was not necessary to write such orders. Resuscitation was not "a treatment offering hope of restoration to normal integrated functioning cognitive existence. Attempts to apply resuscitation if successful will do nothing to cure or relieve the illness, which will have brought the patient to the threshold of death."[244] A second Massachusetts case upholding DNR orders involved a 5-month old infant abandoned at birth who suffered from profound congenital cardiopulmonary disease with little hope of survival. The patient's physician recommended a DNR order be entered on the patient's medical chart, but the guardian, the department of social services, refused to consent. In this case the Massachusetts Supreme Judicial Court found that a full resuscitation effort would not serve the child's interest and if the child were competent to decide would reject full resuscitation.[245]

The right to reject resuscitative or any life-saving medical treatment was best outlined in the Karen Ann Quinlan case.[246] The court stated that the constitutional right to privacy encompasses the freedom of the terminally ill but competent individual to decline medical treatment when such treatment will only prolong suffering needlessly and denigrate the quality of life.

The practice of critical care medicine frequently requires decisions regarding the level of care to be provided to patients. These decisions are generally under highly stressful situations and carry significant medical, legal, psychological, ethical, and economical ramifications. They are very complex, emotional, and controversial areas that must be confronted when treating critically ill patients.

Should families dictate medical therapy? Is withdrawing therapy different than withholding it? What are the legal ramifications of these kinds of decisions? There is a fine line distinguishing prolonging life and prolonging the dying process. There are many complex and difficult issues that confront the critical care practitioner that still await further clarification.

REFERENCES

1. Grenvik A, Leonard JJ, Arens JR et al: Critical care medicine. Certification as a multidisciplinary subspecialty. Crit Care Med 9:2, 1981
2. Bekes CE, Greenbaum DM, Fein A et al: Recommendations for program content for fellowship training in critical care medicine. Crit Care Med 15:971, 1987

3. Bekes CE, Greenbaum DM, Fein A *et al:* Recommendations for the qualifications of a director of a fellowship training program in critical care medicine. Crit Care Med 15:977, 1987

4. Sadove MS, Kritchmer HE, Wyant GM *et al:* An ideal recovery room. Modern Hospital 76:88, 1951

5. Ibsen B: The anesthetist's viewpoints on treatment of respiratory complications during the epidemic in Copenhagen. Proc Roy Soc Med 47:72, 1954

6. Safar P, DeKornfeld T, Pearson J *et al:* Intensive Care Unit. Anaesthesia 16:275, 1961

7. American Heart Association: Coronary care unit (1) and (2). A specialized intensive care unit for acute myocardial infarction. Mod Concepts Cardiovasc Dis 34:23, 1965

8. Safar P, Grenvik A: Critical care medicine, organizing and staffing intensive care units. Chest 59:535, 1971

9. Safar P, Grenvik A: Organization and physician education in critical care medicine. Anesthesiology 47:82, 1977

10. Weil MH, Shubin H: Symposium on care of the critically ill. Mod Med 39:83, 1971

11. Greenbaum DM: Standards for critical care medicine. In Shoemaker WC, Thompson WL, Holbrook PR (eds): Textbook of Critical Care Medicine, p 1004. Philadelphia; WB Saunders, 1984

12. Lave JR, Knaus WA: The economics of intensive care units. In Abramson NS, Grenvik A (eds): Medicolegal Aspects of Critical Care, p 87 Maryland, Aspen, 1986

13. Greenbaum DM: Physician manpower in critical care medicine. Crit Care Med 10:407, 1986

14. Wagner KD: Exodus of the ICU nurse: The cause is the cure. Focus on AACN 9:4, 1982

15. Rogers RM, Weiler C, Ruppenthal B: Impact of the respiratory intensive care unit in survival of patients with acute respiratory failure. Chest 77:501, 1972

16. Klaus AP, Sarachek NS, Greenberg D *et al:* Evaluating coronary care units. Am Heart J 79:471, 1970

17. Feller I, Tholen D, Cornell RG: Improvements in burn care, 1965–1979. JAMA 244:2074, 1980

18. Sinclair JC, Torrance GW, Boyle MH *et al:* Evaluation of neonatal intensive care programs. N Engl J Med 305:489, 1981

19. Stern MP: The recent decline in ischemic heart disease mortality. Ann Intern Med 91:630, 1979

20. Siegel JH, Cerra FB, Moody EA *et al:* The effect on survival of critically ill and injured patients of an ICU teaching service organized about a computer-based physiologic CARE system. J Trauma 20:558, 1980

21. Mather HJ, Morgan DC, Pearson NG *et al:* Myocardial infarction: A comparison between home and hospital care for patients. Br Med J 1:925, 1976

22. Hill JD, Hampton JR, Mitchell JRA: A randomized trial of home-*versus*-hospital management for patients with suspected myocardial infarction. Lancet 2:837, 1978

23. Baldock GJ, Marshal C: Illness severity scoring in the general intensive care unit. Intensive Care World 4:54, 1987

24. Cullen DJ, Civetta JM, Briggs BA *et al:* Therapeutic intervention scoring system: A method for quantitive comparison of patient care. Crit Care Med 2:57, 1974

25. Cullen DJ: Results and costs of intensive care. Anesthesiology 47:203, 1977

26. Rothstein P, Johnson P: Pediatric intensive care: Factors that influence outcome. Crit Care Med 10:34, 1982

27. Yeh TS, Pollack MM, Holbrook PR *et al:* Assessment of pediatric intensive care—Application of the therapeutic intervention scoring system. Crit Care Med 10:497, 1982

28. Knaus WA, Zimmerman JE, Wagner DP *et al:* APACHE—Acute physiology and chronic health evaluation: A physiologically based system. Crit Care Med 9:591, 1981

29. Draper EA, Wagner DP, Knaus WA: The use of intensive care: A comparison of a university and community hospital. Health Care Financing Rev 3:49, 1981

30. Wagner DP, Knaus WA, Draper EA: Statistical validation of a severity of illness measure. Am J Public Health 73:878, 1983

31. LeGall JR, Loirat P, Alperovitch A *et al:* A simplified acute physiology score for ICU patients. Crit Care Med 12:975, 1984

32. Knaus WA, Draper EA, Wagner DP *et al:* APACHE II: A severity of disease classification system. Crit Care Med 13:818, 1985

33. Pollack MM, Yeh TS, Ruttiman VE *et al:* Development of the physiologic stability index (PSI) for use in critically ill infants and children. Pediatr Res 16:187A, 1982

34. Champion HR, Sacco WJ, Lesper RL *et al:* An anatomic index of injury severity. J Trauma 20:197, 1980

35. Mulley AG, Thibault GE, Hughes RA *et al:* The course of patients with suspected myocardial infarction. N Engl J Med 302:943, 1980

36. Bartlett RH, Gazzaniga AB, Wilson AF *et al:* Mortality prediction in adult respiratory insufficiency. Chest 67:680, 1975

37. Ledingham IM, Cowan BN, Burns HJ: Prognosis in severe shock. Br Heart J 284:443, 1982

38. Apgar V: A proposal for a new method of evaluation of the newborn infant. Anesth Analg 32:260, 1953

39. Siesjo BK. Cerebral circulation and metabolism. J Neurosurg 60:883, 1984

40. Michenfelder JD, Theye RA: The effect of profound hypocapnia and dilutional anemia on canine cerebral metabolism and blood flow. Anesthesiology 31:449, 1969

41. Harp JR, Wollman H: Cerebral metabolic effects of hyperventilation and deliberate hypotension. Br J Anaesth 45:256, 1973

42. Sounsen SC: Theoretical considerations on the potential hazards of hyperventilation during anesthesia. Acta Anaesthesiol Scand (suppl) 67:106, 1978

43. Plum F, Siesjo BK: Recent advances in CSF physiology. Anesthesiology 42:708, 1975

44. Cohen PJ, Alexander SC, Smith TC *et al:* Effects of hypoxia and normocarbia on cerebral blood flow and metabolism in man. J Appl Physiol 23:183, 1967

45. Defalque RJ, Musunuru VS: Disease of the nervous system. In Stoelting RK, Dierdorf SF (eds): Anesthesia and Coexisting Disease, p 239. New York, Churchill-Livingstone, 1983

46. Miller JD, Becker DP, Ward JD *et al:* Significance of intracranial hypertension in severe blood injury. J Neurosurg 47:503, 1977

47. Zierski J: Extradural, ventricular, and subdural pressure recording: Comparative clinical study. In Shulman K, Marmarou A, Miller JD *et al:* (eds): Intracranial pressure IV, p 371. Berlin, Springer-Verlag, 1980

48. Mayball CG, Archer NH, Lamb VA *et al:* Ventriculostomy-related infections: A prospective epidemiologic study. N Engl J Med 310:553, 1984

49. Marshall LF, Smith RW, Shapiro HM: Outcome with aggressive treatment in severe head injuries: Acute and chronic barbiturate administration in the management of head injury, Part II. J Neurosurg 50:26, 1979

50. Rockoff M, Marshall L, Shapiro H: High dose barbiturate therapy in humans: A clinical review of 60 patients. Am Neurol 6:194, 1979

51. Woodcock J, Ropper AH, Kennedy SK: High dose barbiturates in non-traumatic brain swelling: ICP reduction and effect on outcome. Stroke 13:785, 1982

52. Ropper AH: Trauma on the head and spinal cord. In Braunwald E, Isselbacher, KJ, Peterdorf RG *et al:* (eds): Harrison's Principles of Internal Medicine, p 1960. New York, McGraw-Hill, 1987

53. Engel J Jr, Troupin AS, Crandall PH *et al:* Recent developments in the diagnosis and treatment of epilepsy. Ann Intern Med 97:584, 1982

54. Leppik IE: Drug treatment of epilepsy. In Johnson RT (ed):

Current Therapy in Neurologic Disease, p 41. Philadelphia, BC Decker, 1986

55. Jennett B, Teasdale G: Aspects of coma after severe head injury. Lancet 1:878, 1977

56. Jennett B, Teasdale G, Braakman R et al: Predicting outcome in individual patients after head injury. Lancet 1:1081, 1976

57. Narayan RK, Greenberg RP, Miller JD et al: Improved confidence of outcome prediction in severe head injury. A comparative analysis of the clinical examination, multimodality evoked potentials, CT scanning, and intracranial pressure. J Neurosurg 54:751, 1981

58. Miller JD, Becker DP, Ward JD et al: The outcome of severe head injury with early diagnosis and intensive management. J Neurosurg 47:491, 1977

59. Marshall LF, Smith RW, Shapiro HM: The outcome with aggressive treatment in severe head injuries. J Neurosurg 48:679, 1978

60. Marshall LF, Shapiro HM: Examination by computerized axial tomography. Int Anesthesiol Clin 17:391, 1979

61. Narayan RK, Greenberg RP, Miller JD et al: Intracranial pressure: To monitor or not to monitor? J Neurosurg 56:650, 1982

62. Kern KB, Meislin HW: Diabetes insipidus: Occurrence after minor head trauma. J Trauma 24:69, 1984

63. Ropper AH, Kennedy SK, Zervas NT (eds): Neurological and Neurosurgical Intensive Care. Baltimore, University Park Press, 1983

64. Thompson JA, Ayres SM, Hess ML: Cardiogenic shock: Causes, diagnosis and management. J Crit Ill 2:22, 1987

65. Pasternak RC, Braunwald E, Alpert JS: Acute myocardial infarction. In Braunwald E, Isselbacher KJ, Peterdorf RG, et al: (eds): Harrison's Principles of Internal Medicine. New York, McGraw-Hill, 982, 1987

66. Forrester JS, Diamond G, Chatterjee K: Medical therapy for acute myocardial infarction by application of hemodynamic subsets. N Engl J Med 295:1356, 1976

67. Schroeder JS, Hunt S: Cardiac transplantation. JAMA 258:3142, 1987

68. Goldberg LI: Cardiovascular and renal effects of dopamine: Potential clinical applications. Pharmacol Rev 24:1, 1972

69. Mueller HS, Evan R, Ayres SM: Effect of dopamine on hemodynamics and myocardial metbolism in shock following acute myocardial infarction in man. Circulation 27:271, 1978

70. Bourdarias JP, Dubourg O, Gveret P et al: Inotropic agents in the treatment of cardiogenic shock. Pharmacol Ther 22:53, 1983

71. Richard C, Ricome JL, Rimailho A et al: Combined hemodynamic effects of dopamine and dobutamine in cardiogenic shock. Circulation 67:620, 1983

72. Bennotti JR, Grossman W, Braunwald E et al: Effects of amrinone on myocardial energy metabolism and hemodynamics in patients with severe congestive heart failure due to coronary artery disease. Circulation 62:28, 1980

73. Moulopoulus SD, Topaz S, Kolff WJ: Diastolic balloon pumping with carbon dioxide in the aorta—A mechanical assistance to the failing circulation. Am Heart J 63:669, 1962

74. Qvist J, Pontoppidan H, Wilson RS et al: Hemodynamics responses to mechanical ventilation with PEEP: The effect of hypervolemia. Anesthesiology 42:45, 1975

75. Gill CC, Wechsler AS, Newman GE et al: Augmentation and redistribution of myocardial blood flow during acute ischemia by intraaortic balloon pumping. Ann Thorac Surg 16:455, 1973

76. Limet RR, Freola M, Glick G et al: Effects of intraaortic balloon counterpulsation (IABCP) on the distribution of coronary blood flow in experimental ischemic left ventricular failure. J Cardiovasc Surg 22:305, 1971

77. Saini VK, Hood WB Jr, Hechtman HB et al: Nutrient myocardial blood flow in experimental myocardial ischemia. Circulation 52:1086, 1975

78. Maroko PR, Bernstein EF, Libby P et al: Effects of intraaortic balloon counterpulsation on the severity of myocardial ischemic injury following acute coronary occlusion. Circulation 45:1150, 1972

79. Roberts AJ, Alonso DR, Combes JR et al: Role of delayed intraaortic balloon pumping in treatment of experimental myocardial infarction. Am J Cardiol 41:1202, 1978

80. Mueller HS, Evan R, Ayres SM et al: Effect of isoproterenol, 1-neopinephrine, and intraaortic counterpulsation on hemodynamics and myocardial metabolism in shock following acute myocardial infarction. Circulation 45:335, 1972

81. Brown, M: Immediate postresuscitation care: Part I. Emergency Med Clin North Am 3:671, 1983

82. Amsterdam EA, Awan NA, Lee G et al. Intra-aortic balloon counterpulsation: rationale, application and results. Cardiovasc Clin 11:79, 1981

83. Ream AK, Portner PM: Cardiovascular assist devices and the artificial heart. In Ream AK, Fogdall RP (eds): Acute Cardiovascular Management: Anesthesia and Intensive Care, p 852. Philadelphia, JB Lippincott, 1982

84. Goldhaber SZ (ed): Pulmonary Embolism and Deep Venous Thrombosis. Philadelphia, WB Saunders, 1985

85. Bell WR, Simon TL. Current status of pulmonary thromboembolic disease: Pathophysiology, diagnosis, prevention and treatment. Am Heart J 103:239, 1982

86. Hull RD, Raskob GE, Hirsh J: The diagnosis of clinically suspected pulmonary embolism: Practical approaches. Chest 89:417S, 1986

87. Sobel BE: Pharmacologic thrombolysis: Tissue-type plasminogen activator. Circulation 76:39, 1987

88. Laffel GL, Braunwald E: Thrombolytic therapy: A new strategy for the treatment of acute myocardial infarction. N Engl J Med 311:710, 1984

89. The TIMI study group: The thrombolysis in myocardial infarction (TIMI) trial: Phase I findings. N Engl J Med 312:932, 1985

90. Guerci AD, Gerstenblith G, Brinker JA et al: A randomized trial of intravenous tissue plasminogen activator for acute myocardial infarction with subsequent randomization to elective coronary angioplasty. N Engl J Med 317:1613, 1987

91. Robin ED: Permeability pulmonary edema. In Fishman AP, Renkin EM (eds): Pulmonary Edema. Bethesda, American Physiologic Society, 1979

92. Hudson LD: Adult respiratory distress syndrome. Semin Respir Med 2:99, 1981

93. Michaelis LL: Pulmonary changes in shock and trauma. Review course, general surgery. Cook County Graduate School of Medicine, 1982

94. Shapiro BA, Cane RD: Acute lung injury and positive end expiratory pressure. Anesth Clin North Am 5:797, 1987

95. Demling RH: The pathogenesis of respiratory failure after trauma and sepsis. Surg Clin North Am 60:1373, 1980

96. Rinaldo JE, Rogers RM: Adult respiratory distress syndrome—Changing concepts of lung injury and repair. N Engl J Med 306:900, 1982

97. Lee CT, Fein AM, Lippmann M et al: Elastolytic activity in pulmonary lavage fluid from patients with adult respiratory distress syndrome. N Engl J Med 304:192, 1981

98. Hammerschmidt D, White JG, Craddock PR: Corticosteroids inhibit complement-induced granulocyte aggregation. J Clin Invest 63:798, 1979

99. Hammerschmidt D, Hudson LD, Weaver LJ et al: Association of complement activation and elevated plasma C5a with adult respiratory distress syndrome—Pathophysiological relevance and possible prognostic value. Lancet 1:947, 1980

100. Bone RC, Francis PB, Pierce AK: Intravascular coagulation asso-

ciated with adult respiratory distress syndrome. Am J Med 61:585, 1976

101. Blaisdell FW, Lim RC, Stallone RJ: The mechanism of pulmonary damage following traumatic shock. Surg Gynecol Obstet 130:15, 1970

102. Greene R, Zapol W, Snider M et al: Early bedside detection of pulmonary vascular occlusion during acute respiratory failure. Am Rev Respir Dis 124:593, 1981

103. Shapiro BA, Crane RD, Harrison RA: Positive end-expiratory pressure therapy in adults with special reference to acute lung injury: A review of the literature and suggested clinical correlations. Crit Care Med 12:127, 1984

104. Bernard GR, Luce JM, Sprung CL et al: High dose corticosteroids in patients with the adult respiratory distress syndrome. N Engl J Med 317:1565, 1987

105. Vergilio RW, Rice CL, Smith DE et al: Crystalloid vs colloid resuscitation: Is one better? Surgery 85:129, 1979

106. Lowe RJ, Moss GS, Jilek J et al: Crystalloid vs colloid in the etiology of pulmonary failure after trauma: A randomized trial in man. Surgery 81:676, 1977

107. Brown M: Immediate post-resuscitative care: Part I. Emerg Med Clin North Am 1:671, 1983

108. Mathru M: The therapeutic application of positive end-expiratory pressure. Anesth Clin North Am 5:789, 1987

109. Gallagher TJ, Civetta JM, Kirby RR: Terminology update: Optimal PEEP. Crit Care Med 6:323, 1978

110. Suter PM, Fairley HB, Isenberg MD: Optimum end-expiratory airway pressure in patients with acute pulmonary failure. N Engl J Med 292:284, 1975

111. Marini JJ: Hemodynamic assessment and management of patients with respiratory failure. Clin Crit Care Med 14:179, 1988

112. Quist J, Pontoppidan H, Wilson RS et al: Hemodynamic responses to mechanical ventilation with PEEP: The effect of hypervolemia. Anesthesiology 26:754, 1975

113. Jarden F, Farcot JC, Boisante L et al: Influence of positive end-expiratory pressure on left ventricular performance. N Engl J Med 304:387, 1981

114. Roos A, Thomas LJ Jr, Nagel EL et al: Pulmonary vascular resistance as determined by lung inflation and vascular pressure. J Appl Physiol 16:77, 1961

115. Buda AJ, Pinsky MR, Ingels NB Jr, et al: Effect of intrathoracic pressure on left ventricular performance. N Engl J Med 301:453, 1979

116. Rowbotham JL, Lixfeld W, Holland L et al: The effects of positive end-expiratory pressure on right and left ventricular performance. Am Rev Respir Dis 121:677, 1980

117. Hillman KM: Pulmonary barotrauma. Clin Anaesthesiol 3:877, 1985

118. Luce JM, Huseby J, Kirk W et al: Mechanism by which positive-end expiratory pressure increases cerebrospinal fluid pressure in dogs. J Appl Physiol 52:231, 1982

119. Annat G, Viale JP, Xuan BB et al: Effect of PEEP ventilation on renal function, plasma renin, aldosterone, neurophysins, urinary ADH and prostaglandins. Anesthesiology 136:141, 1983

120. Beyer J, Beckenlechner P, Messmer K: The influence of PEEP ventilation on organ blood flow and peripheral oxygen delivery. Int Care Med 8:75, 1982

121. Brendenberg CE, Paskanik A, Fromm D: Portal hemodynamics in dogs during mechanical ventilation with positive end-expiratory pressure. Surgery 90:817, 1981

122. Petty TL: Adult respiratory distress syndrome. Semin Respir Med 3:219, 1982

123. Niedermyer ME, Brigham KL: Prospects for therapeutic interventions in acute respiratory failure. Respir Ther 14:15, 1984

124. Zapol WM, Snider MT, Schneider RC: Extracorporeal membrane oxygenation for acute respiratory distress syndrome. Am J Med 61:585, 1976

125. Luce JM: The cardiovascular complications of mechanical ventilation and positive end-expiratory pressure. JAMA 252:807, 1984

126. Brown M, Smith PC: Special requirements of perioperative airway pressure support. In Shapiro BA, Cane RD (eds): Anesthesiology Clin North Am 126:857, 1987

127. Spearman CB, Sanders HG: The new generation of mechanical ventilators. Resp Care 32:403, 1987

128. Cane RD, Shapiro BA: Mechanical Ventilatory Support. JAMA 254:87, 1985

129. MacIntyre NR. Respiratory function during pressure support ventilation. Chest 89:677, 1986

130. Hewlett AM, Platt AS, Terry G: Mandatory minute volume: A new concept in weaning from mechanical ventilation. Anaesthesia 32:163, 1977

131. Willatts SM: Alternatives for mechanical ventilation. Intensive Care Med 11:51, 1985

132. Downs JB, Stock MC: Editorial: Airway pressure release ventilation: A new concept in ventilatory support. Crit Care Med 15:459, 1987

133. Stock MC, Downs JB: Airway pressure release ventilation: A new approach to ventilatory support during acute lung injury. Resp Care 32:517, 1987

134. Eng UB, Eriksson I, Sjostrand U: High frequency positive pressure ventilation: A review based upon its use during bronchoscopy and for laryngoscopy and microlaryngeal surgery under general anesthesia. Anesth Analg 59:594, 1980

135. Sjostrand U: High-frequency positive-pressure ventilation (HFPPV): A review. Crit Care Med 8:345, 1980

136. Gallagher J: Clinical use of high-frequency jet ventilation in intensive care. In Carlon GC, Howland WS (eds): High Frequency Ventilation in Intensive Care and During Surgery, p 159. New York, Marcel Dekker, 1985

137. Gettinger A, Glass DD: High frequency positive pressure ventilation use in neonatal and adult intensive care. In Carlon GG, Howland WS (eds): High Frequency Ventilation in Intensive Care and During Surgery, p 63. New York, Marcel Dekker, 1985

138. Kolton M: A review of high frequency oscillation. Can Anaesth Soc J 31:416, 1984

139. Drazen JM, Kamm RD, Slutsky AS: High-frequency ventilation. Physiol Rev 64:505, 1984

140. Froese AB: High-frequency ventilation: A critical assessment. In Shoemaker WC (eds): Critical Care: State of the Art, Vol 5, (A)1. Fullerton, CA, Society of Critical Care Medicine, 1984

141. Froese AB, Bryan AC: State of the art: High frequency ventilation. Am Rev Respir Dis 135:1363, 1987

142. Smith RB: Ventilation at high respiratory frequencies. Anaesthesia 37:1011, 1982

143. McCulloch PR, Froese AB: High frequency ventilation. In Shapiro BA, Cane RD (eds): Positive Airway Pressure Therapy: PPV and PEEP, Vol 5, p 873. Philadelphia, WB Saunders 1987

144. Gregory GA, Kitterman JA, Phibbs RH et al: Treatment of the idiopathic respiratory distress syndrome with continuous positive airway pressure. N Engl J Med 284:1333, 1971

145. Matthews LW, Dearborn DG, Tucker AS: Cystic fibrosis. In Fishman AP (ed): Pulmonary Diseases and Disorders, p 600. New York, McGraw-Hill, 1980

146. Park RW, Grand RJ: Gastrointestinal manifestations of cystic fibrosis: A review. Gastroenterology 81:1143, 1981

147. Shwachman H, Mahmoodian A, Neff RK et al: The sweat test: Sodium and chloride values. J Pediatr 98:576, 1981

148. Davis PB: Cystic fibrosis. Semin Resp Med 6:243, 1985

149. Hou SH, Bushinsky DA, Wish JB et al: Hospital-acquired renal insufficiency: A prospective study. Am J Med 74:243, 1983

150. Wilkins RG, Faragher EB: Acute renal failure in an intensive care unit. Incidence, prediction, and outcome. Anaesthesia 38:628, 1983

151. Brenner BM, Lazarus JM (eds): Acute renal failure. Philadelphia, WB Saunders, 1983

152. Glassock RJ, Adler SG, Ward HJ: Primary glomerular disease—rapidly progressive glomerulonephritis. In Brenner BM, Rector FL (eds): The Kidneys, p 939. Philadelphia, WB Saunders 1986

153. Jindal K, Goldstein MB: Acute renal failure in critically ill patients. J Crit Illness 2:13, 1987

154. Cronin RE: Aminoglycoside nephrotoxicity: Pathogenesis and prevention. Clin Nephrol 11:251, 1979

155. Linton AL, Clark WF, Driedger AA et al: Acute interstitial nephritis due to drugs. Ann Intern Med 93:735, 1980

156. Schrier RW: Acute renal failure: Pathogenesis diagnosis and management. Hosp Practical 93:112, 1981

157. Anderson RJ, Lines SL, Burns AS et al: Non-oliguric acute renal failure. N Engl J Med 296:1134, 1977

158. Miller TR, Anderson RJ, Linas SL et al: Urinary diagnostic indices in acute renal failure—prospective study. Ann Intern Med 89:47, 1978

159. Goldstein MB: Acute renal failure. Med Clin North Am 61:1325, 1983

160. Bastl CP, Rudnick MR, Narins RG: Diagnostic approaches to acute renal failure. In Brenner BM, Stein JH (eds): Acute Renal Failure, p 17. New York, Churchill-Livingstone, 1980

161. Kleinknecht D, Jungers P, Chanard J et al: Uremic and non-uremic complications of acute renal failure: Evaluation of early and frequent dialysis on prognosis. Kidney Int 1:190, 1972

162. Kramer P: Continuous arteriovenous hemofiltration of physiologic and effective kidney replacement therapy. Contrib Nephrol 44:236, 1985

163. Paganini EP, O'Hara P, Nakamoto S: Slow continuous ultrafiltration in hemodialysis-resistant oliguric acute renal failure patients. Trans Am Soc Artif Intern Organs 30:173, 1984

164. Geronemus R, Schneider N: Continuous arteriovenous hemodialysis: A new modality for the treatment of acute renal failure. Trans Am Soc Artif Intern Organs 30:610, 1984

165. Farber BF: Nosocomial infections: An introduction. In Farber BF (ed): Infection Control in Intensive Care, p 1. New York, Churchill-Livingstone, 1987

166. Farber BF: Reimbursement for nosocomial infections under prospective payment plan: The future or decline of infection control. Infect Control 5:425, 1984

167. Fauci AS, Lane HC: The acquired immunodeficiency syndrome: an update. Ann Intern Med 102:800, 1985

168. Centers for Disease Control: Nosocomial infection surveillance. 1983. In CDC Surveillance Summaries 33 (No. 2ss):9ss, 1984

169. de Jongh CA, Caplan ES, Schimpff SC: Infections in the critical care patient. In Shoemaker WC, Thompson WL, Holbrook PR (eds): Textbook of Critical Care, p 505. Philadelphia, WB Saunders, 1984

170. Lambert RS, Geroge RB: Diagnosing nosocomial pneumonia in mechanically ventilated patients. J Crit Illness 2:57, 1987

171. Sanford JP, Pierce AK: Lower respiratory tract infections, p 255. In Bennett J, Brachtman P, (eds): Hospital Infections. Boston, Little Brown & Co, 1979

172. Jay SJ: Nosocomial infections. Med Clin North Am 67:1251, 1984

173. Bell R, Coalson JJ, Smith JD et al: Multiple organ system failure and infection in adult respiratory distress syndrome. Ann Intern Med 99:293, 1983

174. Johanson WG Jr, Pierce AK, Sanford JP: Changing pharyngeal bacterial flora of hospitalized patients. N Engl J Med 281:1137, 1969

175. Johanson WG Jr, Higuchi JH, Chadhuri TR et al: Bacterial adherence to epithelial cells in bacillary colonization of the upper respiratory tract. Am Rev Respir Dis 121:55, 1980

176. Andrews CP, Coalson JJ, Smith JD et al: Diagnosis of nosocomial bacterial pneumonia in acute diffuse lung injury. Chest 80:254, 1981

177. Berger R, Arango L: Etiologic diagnosis of bacterial nosocomial pneumonia in seriously ill patients. Crit Care Med 13:833, 1985

178. Guckian JC, Christensen WD: Quantitative culture and Gram stain of sputum in pneumonia. Am Rev Respir Dis 118:997, 1978

179. Barrett-Connor E: The nonvalue of sputum culture in the diagnosis of pneumococcal pneumonia. Am Rev Respir Dis 103:845, 1971

180. Baughman RP, Thorpe JE, Staneck J et al: Use of the protected specimen brush in patients with endotracheal or tracheostomy tubes. Chest 91:233, 1987

181. Henderson DE: Bacteremia due to percutaneous intravascular devices. In Mandell GL, Douglas RG, Bennett JE (eds): Principle and Practice of Infectious Diseases. New York, p 1612. John Wiley, 1985

182. Maki DG: Infections associated with intravascular lines. In Remington JA, Swartz MA (eds) Current Topics in Infectious Diseases, Vol 3, p 309. New York, McGraw-Hill, 1982

183. Centers for Diease Control Working Groups: Guidelines for prevention of intravascular infections. In Guidelines for the Prevention and Control of Nosocomial Infections. VSDHHS-PHS, 1981

184. Nichols RL, Smith JW, Klein DB et al: Risk of infection after penetrating abdominal trauma. N Engl J Med 311:1065, 1984

185. Caplan ES, Hoyt NJ: Nosocomial sinusitis. JAMA 647:639, 1982

186. Parker MM, Parrillo JE: Septic Shock: Hemodynamics and pathogenesis. JAMA 250:3324, 1983

187. Kreger BE, Craven DE, Carling PC et al: Gram-negative bacteremia: III. Reassessment of etiology, epidemiology, and ecology in 612 patients. Am J Med 68:332, 1980

188. Young LS, Martin WJ, Myer RD et al: Gram-negative rod bacteremia: Microbiologic, immunologic and therapeutic considertions. Ann Intern Med 86:456, 1977

189. Wiles JB, Cerra FB, Siegel JH et al: The systemic septic response: Does the organism matter? Crit Care Med 8:55, 1980

190. McCabe WR, Treadwell TL, DeMaria A Jr, Pathophysiology of bacteremia. Am J Med 75:225, 1983

191. Root RK, Sande MM: Septic Shock. New York, Churchill-Livingstone, 1985

192. Shine KI: Aspects of the management of shock. Ann Intern Med 93:723, 1980

193. Bernton EW, Long JB, Holaday JW et al: Opiods and neuropeptides: Mechanisms in circulatory shock. Fed Proc 44:290, 1985

194. O'Donnell TF Jr, Clowes GH Jr, Talamo RC et al: Kinin activation in the blood of patients with sepsis. Surg Gynecol Obstet 539, 1976

195. Raffin TA: Novel approaches to ARDS and sepsis. In Chernon B, Shoemaker WC (eds): Critical Care State of Art, Vol 7, p 247. Fullerton, CA, Society of Critical Care Medicine, 1986

196. Sibbald WJ, Driedger AA: Specific organ function/dysfunction in sepsis and septic shock: Cardiovascular. In Sibbald WJ, Sprung CL (eds): Perspectives on sepsis and septic shock. p 125. Fullerton, CA, Society of Critical Care Medicine, 1986

197. Goldfarb RD: Cardiac mechanical performance in circulatory shock: A critical review of methods and results. Circ Shock 9:633, 1982

198. Hess ML, Hastills A, Greenfield LJ: Spectrum of cardiovascular function during gram-negative sepsis. Prog Cardiovasc Dis 23:279, 1981

199. Lefer A: Blood-borne humoral factors in the pathophysiology of circulatory shock. Circ Res 33:129, 1973

200. Demling RH: Colloid or crystalloid resuscitation in sepsis. In Sibbald WJ, Sprung CL (eds) Perspectives on Sepsis and Septic Shock. Fullerton, CA, p 275. Society of Critical Care Medicine, 1986

201. Sprung CL, Caralis PV, Marcial EH et al: The effects of high-dose corticosteroids in patients with septic shock. N Engl J Med 311:1137, 1984

202. Sheagren JN: Septic shock and corticosteroids. N Engl J Med 305:456, 1981
203. Shumer W: Steroids in the treatment of clinical septic shock. Ann Surg 184:333, 1976
204. Bone RC, Fisher CJ Jr, Clemmer TP: A controlled clinical trial of high-dose methylprednisolone in the treatment of severe sepsis and septic shock. N Engl J Med 317:653, 1987
205. Henshaw L, Peduzzi P, Young E et al: Effect of high-dose glucocorticoid therapy on mortality in patients with clinical signs of systemic sepsis. N Engl J Med 317:659, 1987
206. Moldawer LL, Bistrian BR, Sobrado J et al: Muscle proteolysis in sepsis and trauma. N Engl J Med 309:494, 1983
207. Lundholm KG: Nutritional problems in trauma. Acta Chir Scand (suppl) 522:183, 1985
208. Cuthbertson DP: Post-traumatic metabolism: A multidisciplinary challenge. Surg Clin North Am 58:1045, 1978
209. Corman LC: The relationship between nutrition, infection and immunity. Med Clin North Am 69:519, 1985
210. Blackburn GL, Maini BS, Pierce EC: Nutrition in the critically ill patient. Anesthesiology 17:101, 1977
211. Blackburn GL, Bistrian BR, Maini BS et al: Nutritional and metabolic assessment of the hospitalized patient. J Parenter Enteral Nutr 1:11, 1977
212. Bistrian BR, Blackburn GL, Sherman M et al: Therapeutic index of nutritional depletion in hospitalized patients. Surg Gynecol Obstet 141:512, 1975
213. Shetty PS, Watrasiewicz KE, Jung RT et al: Rapid turnover transport proteins: An index of subclinical protein-energy malnutrition. Lancet 2:230, 1979
214. Ingenbleck Y, Van Den Schrieck HG, De Nayer P et al: The role of retinol-binding protein in protein-calorie malnutrition. Metabolism 24:633, 1975
215. Long CL, Schaffel N, Geiger JW et al: Metabolic response to injury and illness: Estimation of energy and protein needs from indirect calorimetry and nitrogen balance. JPEN 3:452, 1979
216. Elevyn DH: Nutritional requirements of adult surgical patients. Crit Care Med 8:9, 1980
217. Cerra FB: Nutrition in the critically ill: Modern metabolic support in the intensive care unit. In Chernon B, Shoemaker WC (eds) Critical Care State of the Art. Vol 7, p 1. Fullerton, CA, Society of Critical Care Medicine, 1986
218. Wretlind A: Current status of intralipid and other fat emulsions. In Meng HC, Wilmore DW (eds): Fat Emulsions in Parenteral Nutrition, p 109. Chicago, American Medical Association, 1976
219. Askanazi J, Nordenstrom J, Rosenbaum SH et al: Nutrition for the patient with respiratory failure: Glucose vs fat. Anesthesiology 54:373, 1981
220. Ryan JA Jr, Abel RM, Abbott WM et al: Catheter complications in total parenteral nutrition: A prospective study of 200 consecutive patients. N Engl J Med 290:757, 1974
221. Michel L, Serrano A, Malt RA: Nutrition support of hospitalized patients. N Engl J Med 304:1147, 1981
222. Giddings JC, Peake IR: Laboratory support in the diagnosis of coagulation disorders. Clin Haematol 14:571, 1985
223. Lasch HG, Heene DH: Heparin therapy of DIC Thromb Diath HAEM 33:105, 1974
224. Mant MJ, King EG: Severe acute disseminated intravascular coagulation: A reappraisal of its pathophysiology, clinical significance and therapy based on 47 patients. Am J Med 67:557, 1979
225. Friedman PA: Poisoning and its management. In Harrison's Principles of Internal Medicine, p 883. New York, McGraw-Hill Book Company, 1987
226. Powell SH, Van De Graaff WB, Thompson WI et al: Charcoals, emetics, and cathartics in care of poisoned patients. Crit Care Med 8:233, 1980
227. Rumack BH, Peterson RG: Acetaminophen overdose: Incidence, diagnosis and management in 416 patients. Pediatrics 62(Suppl):898, 1978
228. Levy R, Elo T, Hanenson IB: Intravenous fructose treatment of acute alcohol intoxication: Effects on alcohol metabolism. Arch Intern Med 137:1175, 1977
229. DaRoza R, Henning RJ, Sunshine I et al: Acute ethylene glycol poisoning. Crit Care Med 12:1003, 1984
230. Kaplan K: Methyl alcohol poisoning. Am J Med Sci 244:170, 1982
231. Dolan MC: Carbon monoxide poisoning. Can Med Assoc J 133:392, 1985
232. Turino GM: Effect of carbon monoxide on the cardiorespiratory system. Circulation 63:253A, 1981
233. Black PM: Brain death (2 parts). N Engl J Med 299:338, 1978
234. President's commission for the study of ethical problems in medicine and biomedical and behavioral research. Defining Death. US Government Printing Office, 1981
235. President's Commission for the study of ethical problems in medicine and biomedical and behavioral research. Guidelines for the determination of death. JAMA 246:2184, 1981
236. Black PM: Brain death in the intensive care unit. J Intensive Care Med 2:177, 1987
237. Powner DJ: The diagnosis of brain death in the adult patient. J Intensive Care Med 2:181, 1987
238. Ad Hoc Committee of Harvard Medical School: A definition of irreversible coma. JAMA 205:337, 1968
239. Cranford RE: Brain death and the presistent vegetative state. In Doudera AE, Petus JD (eds): Legal and Ethical Aspects of Treating Critically and Terminally Il Patients, p 63. Ann Arbor, AUPHA Press, 1982
240. Ruark JE, Raffin TA: Initiating and withdrawing life support: Principles and practice in adult medicine. N Engl J Med 318:25, 1988
241. Tomlinson T, Brody H: Ethics and communication in do-not-resuscitate orders. N Engl J Med 318:43, 1988
242. Curran WJ: The Saikewicz Decision. N Engl J Med 298:499, 1978
243. Liacos PJ: Dilemma of dying. In Doudera AE, Peters JD (eds): Legal and Ethical Aspects of Treating Critically and Terminally Ill Patients, p 149. Ann Arbor, AUPHA Press 1982
244. In the matter of Shirley Dinnerstein, 380 NE 2nd 134 (Mass App 1978)
245. Custody of A Minor 385 Mass 697, 434 Ne 2d 601 (1982)
246. In the matter of Karen Quinlan, 70 NJ 10, 355 A 2d 647, 1976

Chapter 55

Alan Jay Schwartz
Frederick W. Campbell

Cardiopulmonary Resuscitation

HISTORY OF CARDIOPULMONARY RESUSCITATION

Cardiopulmonary resuscitation (CPR) seems synonymous with the growth of modern medicine. The public and professional perception of CPR as a young discipline is not totally accurate.[1] Development of CPR is not a recent "dramatic achievement . . . comparable to the conquest of Mt. Everest."[2] The currently accepted CPR procedures evolved over years of slow, stepwise progress, and many concepts initially relegated to obscurity that were then rediscovered and applied to clinical practice.

The earliest reference to CPR is found in the biblical story of creation, where God created Adam " . . . and breathed into his nostrils the breath of life." Other biblical references to mouth-to-mouth rescue breathing appear in the Book of Kings I and II in accounts of both Elijah and his student Elisha successfully resuscitating children who were apparently dead.[3]

Use of an artificial airway was suggested by Vesalius, and tracheal intubation was popularized at the end of the 18th century. A connection between use of an airway and mouth-to-mouth rescue breathing was not made until the late 19th and early 20th centuries.[4–7] In 1744, the surgeon William Tossach reported successful mouth-to-mouth ventilation for a victim who had suffered cardiac arrest.[9] In 1754, John Fothergill, a physician from Edinburgh, friend of Ben Franklin, and force in the establishment of the first medical school in the United States at the University of Pennsylvania, reported Tossach's success and provided the procedure with some respectability in the medical community.[10] Clinicians used

other methods of resuscitation such as barrel rolling and bellows insufflation of the lungs, and mouth-to-mouth ventilation did not become popular. Interestingly enough, laboratory physiologists often used rescue breathing as early as the 1850s.[7]

Use of mouth-to-mouth rescue breathing in the clinical setting did not become a possibility until the 1940s. Ralph Waters taught his students that the active rescue breathing technique should be considered in emergency care of the arrest victim.[7] Subsequently, Robert Dripps passed this concept to one of his own students, David Cooper.[6, 7] Later, Cooper was in the U.S. Army faced with solving the problem of life support for soldiers poisoned with nerve gas. The accepted but remarkably ineffective method for artificial ventilation commonly employed during those days was the Schafer prone-pressure method. Compression of the lower portion of the thoracic cage posteriorly was thought to effect pulmonary gas exchange. Cooper and his colleagues proved that a modification of the gas mask could be used effectively for mask-to-mask ventilation.[7] Pulmonary gas exchange was analyzed and data provided to show that the use of exhaled air from the rescuer could benefit a nonbreathing victim.[10] James Elam combined the data of clinical effectiveness and respiratory physiology and began to popularize the mouth-to-mouth technique with the help of Gordon.[11–15] Safar, an anesthesiologist, made the final contribution to the adoption of the active rescue breathing technique by making everyone aware of the fact that airway patency was much easier to establish with the new technique and almost impossible with the older passive resuscitation methods.[16] The anesthesiologist was needed to make the connection between what was known about the effectiveness of mouth-to-mouth rescue breathing and the fact that an open airway was essential for any breathing technique. Thus, from Tossach's report in 1744 to Safar's contribution in 1960, more than 200 years elapsed before the modern rescue breathing technique was defined.

Development of the technique for producing artificial circulation and defibrillation has also required an extended time.[17] In the late 1800s and early 1900s, laboratory animals were resuscitated by chest massage.[18] In 1899 Prevost and Battelli reported that electrical countershock stopped ventricular fibrillation.[19] An influential factor in the development of both of these techniques was the common public use of electricity.[17] As public utility companies developed in the early 1900s, more and more electrocutions were reported. When linemen became the victims of electrocution, compensation became very costly for the electric companies. Under the sponsorship of the Consolidated Edison Electric Company, a major research effort was launched in the 1920s at the Rockefeller Institute and Johns Hopkins University to solve the electrocution problem. The modern defibrillator is a direct result of this effort.

In 1947 the first success at human open-chest defibrillation was reported,[20] and a few years later Kouwenhoven developed a closed-chest defibrillation device.[21] Throughout the 1950s the alternating current (AC) defibrillator was used repeatedly and successfully in animal studies. Recognition of the need for a portable defibrillator spurred the development of the direct current (DC) defibrillator. By the late 1950s, a portable defibrillator was available that was effective without damaging the heart, and did not require an open chest for current delivery.

In 1954, during the development of the defibrillator, Guy Knickerbocker, who was working with Kouwenhoven, observed that when defibrillator paddles were applied to the chest cage of experimental animals, the external chest pressure resulted in a rise in blood pressure.[22] This led to the rediscovery of the effective production of artificial cardiac output by external chest compression, a technique described first in the 1920s.[17] In 1958, after extensive animal studies and clinical trials of the external chest massage technique, a 2-yr-old child was successfully resuscitated.[17] As the 1960s began, closed-chest cardiac compression, artificial mouth-to-mouth rescue breathing, and the portable DC defibrillator, three essential ingredients for modern-day CPR, were clinically available. It would take another 10 to 15 years of application and discussion before the development of standard CPR protocols using these techniques and equipment.

THE NEED FOR CPR

The American Heart Association (AHA) CPR program was initiated specifically to develop the treatment of the major complications of coronary artery disease, myocardial infarction and lethal cardiac dysrhythmias. In the United States, cardiovascular disease affects an estimated 39 million individuals.[23] The number of patients in the United States with the clinical diagnosis of coronary artery disease is 6 million. Deaths due to diseases of the heart numbered 978,000 in 1984, 540,000 of which were attributed to ischemic disease. Of the leading causes of death, diseases of the heart rank first, accounting for 40% of the deaths.

More than one-half of the deaths attributed to ischemic heart disease occur outside a hospital setting within the first several hours after the onset of symptoms. Patients with chest pain often deny the presence of a serious problem. Denial

delays the initiation of measures that might prevent more lethal events resulting from the ischemic heart disease.

The AHA developed their program to cope with those otherwise healthy individuals in whom coronary artery disease progresses to a critical point, producing sudden lethal cardiac dysrhythmias or an acute myocardial infarction with heart failure or dysrhythmias as later sequelae. The AHA reasoned that many of these people should not die under these circumstances. The goal of the program is to educate the public to 1) recognize the disease process and symptoms; 2) seek help immediately; and 3) provide resuscitation, at the scene, to victims without respiration or cardiac output.

Several studies have documented the success of this approach.[24-27] Teaching basic resuscitative procedures to the lay public, who then apply these techniques to victims in the community within a short time (4 min or less) after a cardiac arrest, and adding to this the provision of more advanced CPR within yet another brief interval (a total elapsed time of 8–10 min), results in approximately 40% overall survival.[28, 29] When the same approach is tried in selected groups of patients, the success can be improved to approximately 60%. Delay in either the basic or advanced life-support maneuvers results in a significant decrease in survival.

The same basic and advanced life-support system can and should be applied in all situations requiring life support. In 1979, accidents accounted for 103,400 or 5% of deaths in the United States,[30] while cerebrovascular disease was associated with 175,629 deaths.[23] Many stroke victims are not salvage-

TABLE 55-1. Component Parts of CPR

BCLS: Temporary Oxygen Delivery to the Cardiac Arrest Victim by a Rescuer

Diagnoses
1. Stupor or Coma
2. Presence of Breathing
3. Presence of Circulation

Therapy
1. Rescue Breathing
2. Artificial Circulation

ACLS: Therapy Directed Toward Reestablishment of Spontaneous Oxygen Delivery by the Victim

Diagnoses
1. Dysrhythmias
2. Cardiovascular Instability
3. Acid–Base Derangements

Therapy
1. Cardioversion/Defibrillation
2. Intravascular Access/Monitoring/Volume Replacement
3. Pharmacologic Therapy for Hemodynamic/Acid–Base Derangements

PRLS: Definition of the Primary Cause of the Cardiac Arrest and Maintenance of What Has Been Salvaged During BCLS–ACLS

Diagnoses
1. Cause of the Cardiac Arrest
2. Consequences of the Cardiac Arrest

Therapy
1. General Intensive Care
2. Specific Intensive Care—Pulmonary/Cardiovascular/Renal/Metabolic/Brain Resuscitation

---

BCLS = basic cardiac life support; ACLS = advanced cardiac life support; PRLS = postresuscitation life support.

able, but some may experience full neurologic return if given the chance provided by the basic and advanced CPR life-support measures.

Life support provided as CPR is a specific application of intensive care medicine. Mobile intensive care, a concept and technique introduced in the late 1960s, is CPR provided in the field setting where cardiac arrest so often occurs.[31] Highly developed community-based health-care delivery systems have been established in many locations throughout the country with clearly documented success.[26-29]

A key CPR concept is that the cardiac arrest event most often occurs in the community and, therefore, requires response from and within the community. In its 1980 CPR standards, the AHA emphasized this point, stating " . . . it is clear that the community deserves to be recognized as the ultimate coronary care (or life support) unit."[32]

CPR: THE PROBLEM AND ITS SOLUTION

Deficiency of oxygen delivery is the source of all cardio-pulmonary arrests, irrespective of the initial cause. Basic cardiac life support (BCLS) solves the problem by providing oxygen delivery to the lungs with rescue breathing and oxygen transport from the lungs to the body tissues with cardiac compression (Table 55-1, Fig. 55-1A). BCLS is the procedure used by the rescuer or rescue team to provide the patient with temporary oxygen delivery.[33] BCLS is only a temporizing measure, however, as long-term survival depends on the return of spontaneous oxygenation on the part of the arrest victim. Only when patients can ventilate and perfuse their own tissues with oxygenated blood will successful resuscitation be achieved.

Advanced cardiac life support (ACLS) provides the necessary supportive maneuvers such that the patients can maintain their own adequate cardiac output.[33] ACLS implies that expert BCLS is provided during the establishment of the self-sufficient state by the patient.[33] The prerequisites for spontaneous oxygen delivery (cardiac output) by the patient include a relatively normal cardiac rate, rhythm, and contractility, and relatively normal vascular volume and tone. The recommended components of ACLS (Table 55-1, Fig. 55-1B) directly or in a supportive manner contribute to the return and continuation of spontaneous cardiac output.

If spontaneous oxygen delivery by the victim can be reestablished, the CPR effort is termed a short-term success. To maintain this status, the post-resuscitative life support (PRLS) phase of CPR must be activated[33] (Table 55-1, Fig. 55-1C). Airway, hemodynamic, and pharmacologic supportive therapy is employed where indicated to allow the victim to continue adequate spontaneous oxygen delivery and not revert to another cardiac-arrest state. Brain resuscitation is a specific and vital part of this PRLS phase that is designed to salvage as much normally functioning central nervous system (CNS) tissue as possible. A major task during PRLS is determining the underlying malady that resulted in the cardiac arrest and correcting it. Only through PRLS intensive care and monitoring can long-term survival result from a CPR effort.

BASIC CARDIAC LIFE SUPPORT

The temporary delivery of oxygen to vital tissues is accomplished by providing effective airway management, ventilation, and artificial circulation, with and without supportive equipment.

AIRWAY MANAGEMENT DURING CPR

Opening the Airway

An open airway is a prerequisite to effective oxygen administration. Obstruction of the hypopharynx by the base of the tongue is the most common cause of airway obstruction in the unconscious individual. With loss of consciousness, relaxation of the head and neck muscles supporting the mandible occurs when tone is decreased in the muscular attachments of the tongue to the mandible. The unsupported tongue falls against the posterior pharyngeal wall, obstructing the airway. In a group of 80 anesthetized, uncurarized, spontaneously breathing adults, Safar found an unobstructed airway in only 10% with the head in a neutral position and airway unsupported.[34] Hypopharyngeal obstruction by the base of the tongue can occur regardless of whether the patient is prone, lateral, or supine. While gravity will aid drainage of liquid from the pharynx of an individual lying in the lateral or prone position, it does not assure airway patency.[35, 36]

The cardinal principle of opening the airway is anterior displacement of the mandible and elevation of the tongue from the posterior pharyngeal wall. This may be accomplished by chin lift, neck lift, jaw thrust, or head hyperextension.[34-39] Head tilt extends the head at the atlantooccipital joint and indirectly elevates the mandible and lifts the tongue from the posterior pharyngeal wall. Safar et al found they could maintain a patent airway in nearly one-half of their anesthetized patients with maximal hyperextension of the head alone.[34] Neck lift is combined with head tilt to assist and augment the hyperextension of the head. In many patients, however, head-tilt—neck-lift may be insufficient, and a technique that further displaces the mandible and tongue will be necessary. Two maneuvers that support the mandible directly and elevate the base of the tongue are the chin lift and the jaw thrust.

Heat-tilt—chin-lift (Fig. 55-2) provides support of the jaw by lifting the mentum of the mandible with the fingers of one hand while the other hand continues to apply head-tilt at the forehead. Care must be taken not to compress the soft tissue under the chin, thereby obstructing the airway. Further anterior displacement of the mandible may be obtained by use of the jaw thrust. This is accomplished by lifting the jaw at the angles of the mandible and displacing the jaw forward. Guildner compared the three techniques for opening the airway in anesthetized adults who were either apneic or completely obstructed and making spontaneous respiratory efforts.[40] The head-tilt—chin-lift and head-tilt—jaw-thrust were superior to the head-tilt—neck-lift in both situations. In apneic patients receiving mouth-to-mouth ventilation, the patency of the airway was judged to be good in 91% with the chin-lift technique, and 78% with the jaw-thrust method as compared with 39% with the neck-lift technique. Tidal volumes achieved by the initially obstructed, spontaneously breathing patients were used to gauge the effectiveness of the three techniques. Tidal volumes greater than 400 ml were achieved in 7% with the neck lift, 63% with the jaw thrust, and 70% with the chin lift. Thus, since it is more effective in opening the airway than the previously taught head-tilt—neck-lift, head-tilt—chin-lift is currently the first-line recommended technique. The jaw thrust is a technically difficult and fatiguing procedure for the lay person to apply and is, therefore, taught as an ancillary technique for professional rescuers.

The jaw thrust without head tilt is the preferred method for opening the airway in a patient with a suspected cervical spine

CARDIOPULMONARY-CEREBRAL RESUSCITATION

(CPCR)

PHASE I

EMERGENCY OXYGENATION BASIC LIFE SUPPORT

(BLS)

IF UNCONSCIOUS

Airway

Tilt head back

IF NOT BREATHING

Breathe

Inflate lungs rapidly 3–5 times
mouth-to-mouth, mouth-to-nose,
mouth-to-adjunct, bag-mask

MAINTAIN HEAD TILT
■ Feel carotid pulse
■ If pulse present, continue 12 lung inflations
  per minute

IF PULSE ABSENT
        pupils dilated and
        deathlike appearance,

Circulate

ONE OPERATOR:
Alternate 2 quick lung inflations with 15 sternal
compressions

TWO OPERATORS:
Interpose one inflation after every fifth
compression

Depress lower sternum 1½–2" (4–5 cm)
CONTINUE RESUSCITATION until spontaneous pulse returns

A

CARDIOPULMONARY-CEREBRAL RESUSCITATION

(CPCR)

PHASE II

ESTABLISHMENT OF NORMAL ARTERIAL OXYGEN TRANSPORT

(RESTART SPONTANEOUS CIRCULATION)

ADVANCED LIFE SUPPORT

(ALS)

DO NOT INTERRUPT CARDIAC COMPRESSIONS AND LUNG VENTILATION
INTUBATE TRACHEA WHEN POSSIBLE

Drugs and fluids, I.V. lifeline

EPINEPHRINE
0 5–1 0 mg IV repeat larger dose as necessary

SODIUM BICARBONATE
1 mEq/kg IV
Repeat dose every 10 minutes until pulse returns.
Monitor and normalize arterial pH

I V FLUIDS as indicated

E.K.G. Ventricular fibrillation? Asystole? Bizarre complexes?

Fibrillation treatment

EXTERNAL DEFIBRILLATION
D C 100–400 W/sec
Repeat shock as necessary

LIDOCAINE
1–2 mg/kg IV if necessary

IF ASYSTOLE
repeat step D–calcium and vasopressors as needed
CONTINUE RESUSCITATION until good pulse
is maintained

D C 100–400 W sec

B

1480

CARDIOPULMONARY-CEREBRAL RESUSCITATION

(CPCR)

PHASE III

POST-RESUSCITATIVE LIFE SUPPORT

(PLS)

Gauging

Determine and treat cause of demise
Determine salvageability

Human mentation--Cerebral resuscitation

Support perfusion pressure, oxygenation, ventilation
If arrest > 5 min , coma > 5 min after reperfusion
    --clinical trials (e g , thiopental)

Intensive care

PaCO$_2$ 25-35	Art , CV, (PA) catheters
PaO$_2$ >100	Temp Control, EKG
pHa 7 3-7 6	(Curarization)

ICP (osmotherapy, hypothermia)
Suppress convulsions
Steroid, Dextrose 5-10%, electrol , IV Fluids, alimentation
Hct , plasma COP, serum osm
Outcome

C

FIG. 55-1. (A) Basic life support: emergency oxygenation, a temporizing measure provided by a rescuer or rescuers. (B) Advanced life support: techniques to aid restoration of spontaneous oxygen delivery by the cardiac arrest victim. (C) Postresuscitative life support: critical care therapies to support and maintain the resuscitated victim with particular emphasis on the cause of the cardiopulmonary arrest, its treatment and prevention, and the post-CPR cardiopulmonary, neurologic, and renal status. (Reproduced with permission from Safar P: Cardiopulmonary-cerebral resuscitation including emergency airway control. In Schwartz GR, Safar P, Stone JH et al [eds]: Principles and Practice of Emergency Medicine, p 177. Philadelphia, WB Saunders, 1978.)

injury. This may provide a patent airway without hyperextension of the head and neck. When applying the jaw thrust, mouth-to-mouth ventilation, if required, can be administered while the patient's nostrils are occluded by the rescuer's cheek pressed tightly against them.

If the patient has dentures, they can be left in place to help maintain a normal facial contour, facilitating adequate lip seal and mouth-to-mouth ventilation. Dentures are removed only if they obstruct the airway. Loose dentures are best held in position by opposing the teeth with the head-tilt–chin-lift or head-tilt–jaw-thrust technique.

Establishing the Diagnosis of Breathlessness

The rescuer places his ear over the patient's mouth *looking* toward the patient's chest for movement, *listening* for exhaled air, and *feeling* for the flow of air on his cheek. Breathlessness may be due to apnea as occurs in circulatory arrest or it may be due to airway obstruction. The absence of respiratory effort does not rule out the possibility of foreign-body airway obstruction causing the patient's collapse.

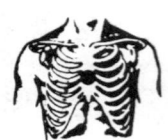
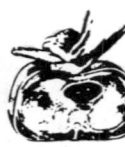
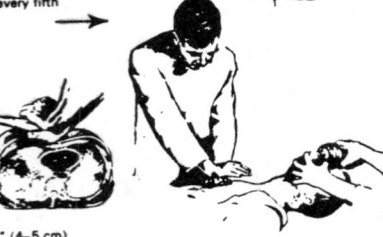
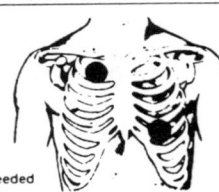

Mouth-to-Mouth Ventilation

Research on mouth-to-mouth rescue breathing has documented the superiority of this active process of intermittent positive pressure ventilation (IPPV) using the rescuer's exhaled air over manual passive artificial respiration protocols, such as the back-pressure–arm-lift or chest-pressure–arm-lift methods.[35, 36] The failure of passive manual methods of artificial ventilation is due to the inability of the rescuer to control the patient's airway patency, resulting in inadequate ventilation of the lungs. Rescue breathing is intended to maintain airway patency and, if necessary, reinflate atelectatic alveolar units. In so doing, this rescue breathing permits alveolar–capillary oxygen transfer and reduces alveolar–arterial oxygen difference. The advantages of mouth-to-mouth artificial ventilation include: 1) the rescuer maintains control of the patient's airway at the same time ventilation of the lungs is provided; 2) normal tidal volumes may be easily delivered; 3) thoracopulmonary compliance can be easily estimated; 4) adequacy of ventilation can be easily sensed; 5) the procedure can be instituted quickly without the use of adjunctive equipment; and 6) it is simple to perform and easily taught to both medical and lay persons.

Mouth-to-nose artificial ventilation is an alternative to the mouth-to-mouth technique employed when it is impossible to ventilate a patient *via* the mouth, *i.e.*, in cases of trauma to the mouth and jaw, and also when it is extremely difficult to establish a tight seal around the mouth. Mouth-to-stoma ventilation may be performed in the tracheotomized or laryngectomized patient.

Successful resuscitation depends on the rescuer ensuring adequate ventilation with every breath by using criteria such as observing the patient's chest rise and fall, feeling the patient's pulmonary compliance during lung inflation, and hearing and feeling the air escape during exhalation. Inadequate ventilation may be due to airway obstruction, air leak at the lip seal or nostrils, or inadequate force of the rescuer's ventilation. Inability to ventilate the patient's lungs can be the result of failure to open the airway, but also may be due to airway obstruction by an unsuspected foreign-body airway obstruction.

Gastric inflation may occur during rescue breathing when inspiratory airway pressures exceed esophageal opening pressures, approximately 15 cm H_2O. High pharyngeal pressures are likely to result from ventilation using excessive tidal volumes or rapid inspiratory flow rates.[41–43] The previously taught techniques of "staircasing" breaths required the rescuer to deliver excessive inspiratory flow rates to the patient. Current recommendations for ventilation provide a 1–1.5-sec inspiratory time for the delivery of each exhaled air breath. The patient is then allowed to exhale after each breath. By providing a deliberately slower inspiratory flow rate, avoiding air trapping in the lungs between breaths, and limiting the tidal volume to that which results in observable chest expansion, an adequate (800–1200 ml) tidal volume will be delivered and the probability of gastric inflation is minimized. Gastric distention is more likely to occur if an adequate airway has not been established because partial airway obstruction necessitates the use of higher inflation pressure to deliver an adequate tidal volume. Distention of the stomach should be managed by repositioning the airway and attempting to ventilate the patient again using a longer inspiratory time. Adjunctive equipment to help open the airway should be used if available. The risks associated with regurgitation and aspiration of gastric contents contraindicate any attempt to relieve gastric distention with manual pressure to the patient's epigastrium

unless distention is so severe that it results in inadequate ventilation.

In single-rescuer CPR, two 1–1.5-sec full breaths are delivered after each cycle of 15 cardiac compressions. One breath every 5 sec is performed for apneic patients with a pulse (*rescue breathing*). During two-rescuer CPR, a breath is interposed during a short pause between the fifth and first chest compressions of two 5:1 cycles.

Exhaled air ventilation provides fractional inspired oxygen concentration (FI_{O_2}) of 0.15 to 0.18 and, therefore, an alveolar oxygen tension (PA_{O_2}) less than 80 mm Hg. The arterial oxygen tension (Pa_{O_2}) will be considerably less as a result of cardiopulmonary arrest factors such as reduced cardiac output and increased venous admixture contributing to an increased alveolar–arterial oxygen difference. In anesthetized adults, exhaled air ventilation is also associated with mild hypercarbia, P_{CO_2} 56 ± 6.5 mm Hg during 15:2 compression:ventilation cycles and 50 ± 3.5 mm Hg during 5:1 cycles.[44] Because some hypoxemia and hypercarbia occur during exhaled air ventilation, the use of adjunctive airway equipment should be instituted as soon as it is available to provide a high FI_{O_2} and allow augmented ventilation.

Foreign-Body Airway Obstruction

In 1984, The National Safety Council reported 3100 deaths due to foreign-body airway obstruction,[45] a number that has remained relatively unchanged over the past decade. Accurate numbers are difficult to obtain, and most certainly more than 3100 deaths have occurred from foreign-body airway obstruction, although this is still an infrequent cause of death compared with cardiovascular diseases. Haugen first reported a series of adults who died suddenly in restaurants, some of whose deaths were ascribed to myocardial infarction until autopsies revealed the true cause of death, *i.e.*, foreign-body airway obstruction.[46] He coined the term *cafe coronary* and concluded that the only effective treatment was immediate tracheostomy.

Foreign-body obstruction of the airway in adults usually occurs while eating and is associated with elevated blood alcohol levels, poor dentition, dentures, and large, poorly

FIG. 55-2. Management of the airway in the unconscious victim. (*Top*) When a victim is unconscious, the tongue recedes into the posterior pharynx, causing airway obstruction. (*Bottom*) This is managed by anterior displacement of the mandible using the chin-lift/head-tilt technique. (Reproduced with permission. Textbook of Advanced Cardiac Life Support, p 27. Dallas, American Heart Association, 1987.)

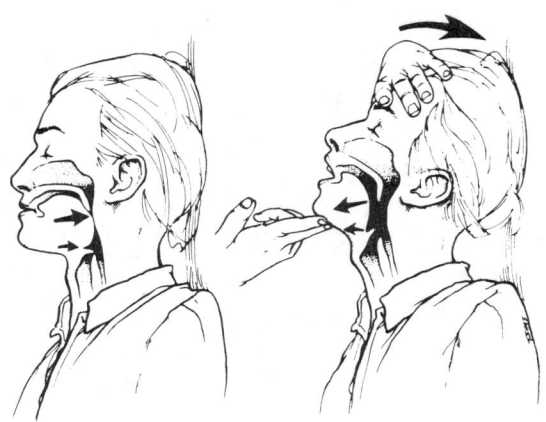

chewed pieces of food. In addition to food, children can choke on a variety of small foreign bodies while playing.

Early recognition of foreign-body airway obstruction is essential so the appropriate therapeutic maneuvers can be applied. Differential diagnosis of this emergency from other conditions that cause sudden cardiorespiratory arrest is important. The conscious victim may be using the *universal distress signal for choking* (Fig. 55-3). In the unconscious victim whose collapse was unwitnessed, foreign-body obstruction should be suspected upon observing paradoxical respiratory efforts and chest wall retractions despite airway opening maneuvers, or noting an inability to perform ventilation despite proper airway positioning.

Foreign bodies may cause either partial or complete airway obstruction. Partial obstruction will be associated with either adequate or poor air exchange. Because the rescuer's course of action will be determined by this diagnosis, it is crucial to differentiate partial airway obstruction with adequate air exchange from both partial obstruction with poor air exchange and complete airway obstruction. The former is recognized when the victim is acyanotic and can speak and generate an effective cough despite some respiratory distress. As long as adequate oxygenation continues, a rescuer should not interfere with the victim's own efforts to expel the foreign body. Artificial coughs are considerably less effective than natural coughs. In anesthetized human subjects with obstructed airways, Gordon *et al* demonstrated that artificial cough procedures such as back blows and manual thrusts produce one-half and one-fourth to one-fifth, respectively, of the airway pressure produced by a normal cough starting from resting lung volume (functional residual capacity, FRC) in the same subjects when awake.[47] This discrepancy is more marked when the artificial coughs are compared with normal coughs at end inspiration. Additionally, there is a grave danger that an interfering rescuer will convert a partial airway obstruction

with maintained oxygenation to complete obstruction with inadequate oxygenation.

Partial obstruction with poor air exchange and complete airway obstruction are characterized by an inefficient or absent cough or an inability to speak. Management must be initiated immediately. Early recommendations for clearing foreign-body airway obstructions included back blows and finger probes of the throat. In 1974, Heimlich introduced a simple manual method for relieving airway obstruction, the abdominal thrust. He theorized that as aspiration of a foreign body occurred during inspiration, there will be air trapped in the lungs behind the obstruction.[48] With rapid inward and upward compression of the victim's epigastrum, the diaphragm is forced cephalad, compressing this trapped air volume. The rapid increase in airway pressure and air flow generated should move the foreign body from its obstructing position in the airway. In conscious adult volunteers, application of this maneuver at mid-exhalation produced airway pressures of 18–40 mm Hg, (average 31 mm Hg) with peak flow rates of 130–310 $l \cdot min^{-1}$ (average 205 $l \cdot min^{-1}$).[48] Substantially lower peak flow rates were measured during application of the abdominal thrust at end-exhalation, thus demonstrating the role of lung volume in the effectiveness of this technique. Guildner *et al* found that in adult volunteers, manual thrusts applied to the middle or lower chest (*chest thrusts*) produced slightly better airway pressures and peak flow rates[49] (Table 55-2). Chest thrusts are preferred to abdominal thrusts in specific instances, *i.e.*, in infants, obese patients, and pregnant women, for reasons of effectiveness and potential intraabdominal complications.

Early recommendations for the treatment of foreign-body airway obstruction were based on laboratory and clinical data obtained during comparison of the various methods of producing an artificial cough. Gordon *et al*[47] and Ruben and McNaughton[50] compared several artificial-cough maneuvers in adult subjects measuring peak airway pressure, exhaled volume, and peak flow rates in complete and partially obstructed airways (Table 55-3). Back blows generated greater airway pressures but lower volumes and flow rates than manual thrusts applied to the abdomen or chest (Table 55-4). The rate of airway pressure rise was also examined (Figure 55-4).[47] Back blows produced instantaneous pressure pulses while the pulses developed by manual thrusts were slower developing and sustained. In the same report, Gordon *et al* attempted to clear pieces of meat from the airways of anesthetized animals using back blows and manual thrusts. They found that the combination of back blows followed by abdominal or chest thrusts was more effective than either alone. A series of blows

FIG. 55-3. Conscious victims of foreign-body airway obstruction can indicate their problem by using the universal distress signal represented in this drawing. (Reproduced with permission. Standards and Guidelines for Cardiopulmonary Resuscitation and Emergency Cardiac Care. JAMA 255:2841. Copyright 1986, American Medical Association.)

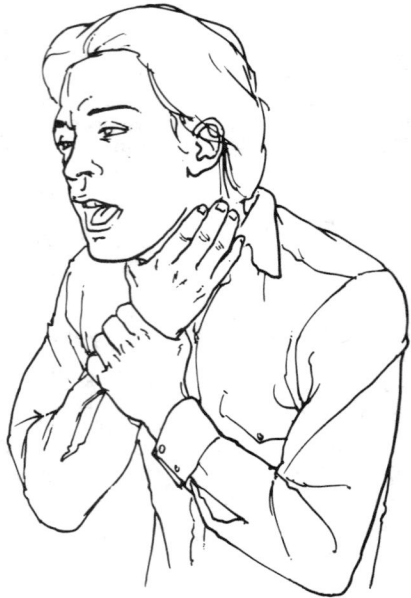

TABLE 55-2.   Comparison of Abdominal and Chest Thrusts in Supine, Anesthetized, Apneic Adults*

	PEAK AIRWAY PRESSURE (mm Hg)	PEAK FLOW RATE ($l \cdot min^{-1}$)
Abdominal thrust	17	55
Low-chest thrust†	25	68
Mid-chest thrust‡	19	60

* Mean values for 6 human volunteers.
† Thrust applied 2–3 finger-breadths above xiphoid.
‡ Thrust applied at level of nipple line.
(Modified with permission. Guildner CW, Williams D, Subitch T: Airway obstruction by foreign material: The Heimlich maneuver. JACEP 5:675, 1976.)

TABLE 55-3. Comparison of Artificial Cough Techniques at Different Lung Volumes in Anesthetized Apneic Adults*

TECHNIQUE	PEAK AIRWAY PRESSURE (cm H_2O)	
	Resting Lung Volume	+600 ml Tidal Volume
Abdominal thrust	10	16
Chest thrust	20	30
Back blow	25	32

*Mean values for 12 patients.
(Modified with permission. Ruben H, McNaughton FI: The treatment of food choking. Practitioner 221:725, 1978.)

and a series of thrusts, four to six of each, were required to move the meat.

The AHA compiled anecdotal clinical data from 225 cases of actual foreign-body airway obstruction.[51] The artificial-cough methods used included back blows, abdominal thrusts, chest thrusts, and finger probes. There were 386 trials of various maneuvers, alone and in combination, with successes and failures attributed to each of the maneuvers. When used alone, back blows were successful in 20% of trials; abdominal thrusts, 44%; chest thrusts, 36%; and finger probes, 17%. When used in combination with other maneuvers, back blows were successful in 49% of trials; abdominal thrusts, 79%; chest thrusts, 64%; and finger probes, 58%. Each method was sometimes given credit for success after another method had failed, and it was not possible to determine whether a maneuver marked unsuccessful might have contributed to the successful result of another following. Redding concluded that in the emergency management of the obstructed airway, a combination of maneuvers is more likely to be effective than any single maneuver.[51]

Subsequently, Day et al used an accelerometer to measure the inertial forces generated in the airway of subjects receiving back blows.[52] When struck on the back, the head and neck of their subjects were rapidly propelled in a cephalad direction. They inferred that, as a consequence, a foreign object within the airway may actually be impacted further into the airway rather than expelled by back blows. Transmission of inertial forces directly to the foreign body, as well as to the head and neck, was not measured by these investigators. The degree to which the expulsive intrathoracic pressure pulse produced by the back blow would counteract the potentially deleterious cervical inertial forces also remains unstudied. Thus, the theoretical basis supporting the efficacy of back blows as an artificial-cough technique is unsettled.

Current recommendations for the management of the obstructed airway in the adult (Table 55-5) and child are based on the theoretical and clinical observations supporting the effectiveness of the Heimlich maneuver. Until more data are available, the Heimlich maneuver and its variation, the chest thrust, appear to be at least as effective as any other airway-clearing technique. It is thought that teaching a single therapeutic technique instead of two may simplify CPR instruction and improve skill retention by the lay public.

Alternating series of chest thrusts and back blows in combination are recommended for the infant with foreign-body airway obstruction. When back blows are delivered to an infant whose head and torso are supported by the opposite hand or thigh of the rescuer, intrathoracic pressure increases most likely as a result of both the direct blow and compression

of the thorax (analogous to the isolated chest thrust). The inertial forces propelling the head and neck in a cephalad direction are likely minimized when the infant's head and torso are restrained.

Complications have been reported following the use of each airway-clearing maneuver. Manual thrusts have resulted in rupture of the stomach, esophageal laceration, regurgitation, fractured ribs, retinal detachment, and abdominal aortic rupture. Complications resulting from finger probes include pharyngeal abrasion, regurgitation, and impacting a foreign body further into the larynx. Each of the techniques, if misapplied, can turn a partial airway obstruction into a lethal complete obstruction.

As the patient becomes more hypoxic and unconscious, profound skeletal muscle relaxation occurs, and maneuvers that were previously ineffective may dislodge the foreign object. With muscular relaxation it may also become possible both to ventilate around the obstruction with slow, forceful breaths and to remove the obstructing object with a finger sweep of the posterior pharynx. The finger sweep is administered to unconscious victims in conjunction with a tongue–jaw-lift maneuver. By firmly grasping the patient's tongue and mandible between the thumb and fingers of one hand, this block of tissue may be pulled anteriorly, thereby dislodging supraglottic foreign bodies or, at least, providing more space in the hypopharynx for the rescuer's probing fingers. Care must be taken during blind probing of the pharynx to avoid impaction of an object deeper into the airway. Endoscopy or other instrumentation techniques of the airway should be employed by those rescuers proficient in their application, i.e., anesthesiologists. The Kelly clamp and Magill or Kolodney

TABLE 55-4. Comparison of Artificial Cough Techniques in Anesthetized, Apneic Adults*

TECHNIQUES AND VICTIM POSITION (RESCUER AT VICTIM'S SIDE)	PARTIAL AIRWAY OBSTRUCTION† PEAK FLOW RATE ($l \cdot min^{-1}$)	COMPLETE OBSTRUCTION‡ PEAK AIRWAY PRESSURE (mm Hg)
Normal Cough		
From end-exhalation	108	72
From end-inspiration	162	115
Artificial Cough BACK BLOWS		
Sitting	12	35
Lateral horizontal	11	30
ABDOMINAL THRUSTS		
Sitting	120	15
Supine	132	12
CHEST THRUSTS		
Sitting	132	19
EXTERNAL CARDIAC COMPRESSION	120	17

*Mean values for 6 human volunteers. Normal cough measurements were made prior to induction of general anesthesia.
†Airway pressure not reported.
‡No air flow when airway completely obstructed.
(Modified with permission. Gordon A, Belton M, Ridolpho P: Emergency management of foreign body airway obstructions. In Safar P, Elam JO [eds]: Advances in Cardiopulmonary Resuscitation, p 43. New York, Springer Verlag, 1977.)

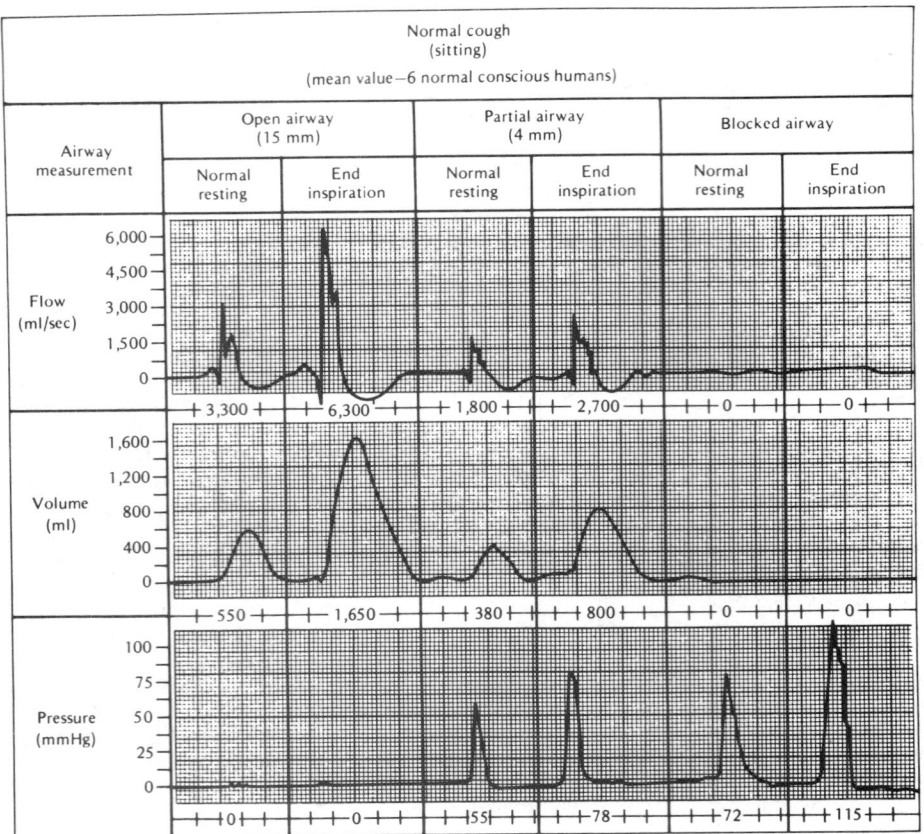

A

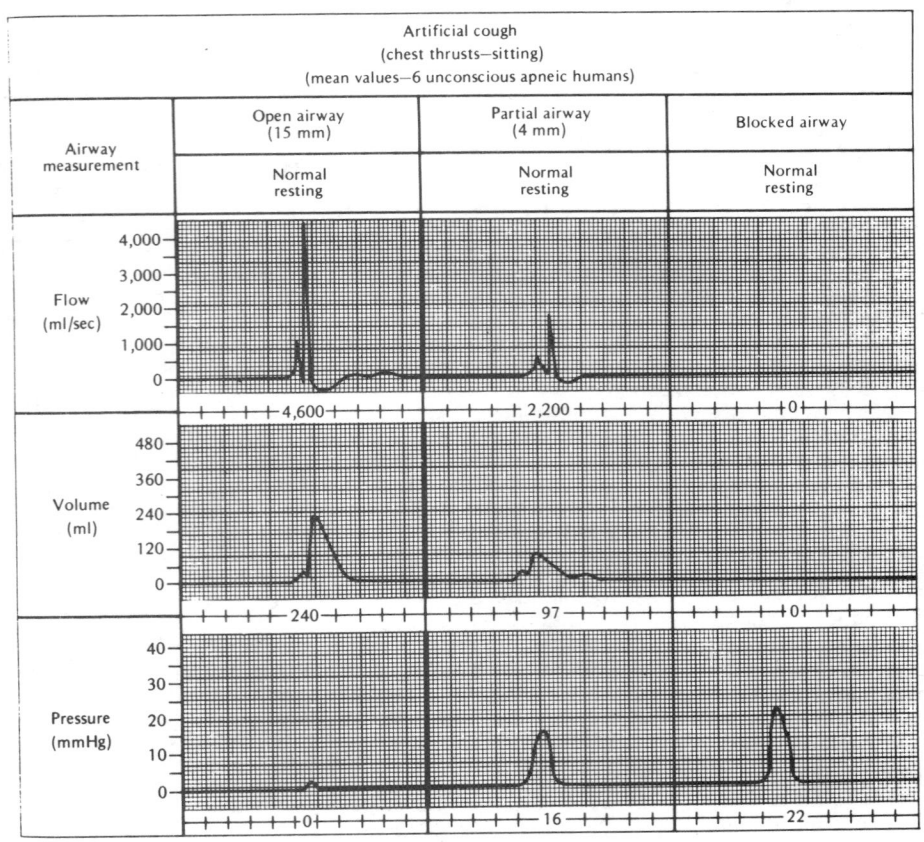

FIG. 55-4. (A) Air flow, volume of air moved, and pressure generated within a totally open airway, partially obstructed airway, or a totally obstructed (blocked) airway in conscious individuals with a normal cough. (B) Air flow, volume of air moved, and pressure generated within a totally open airway, partially obstructed airway, or a totally obstructed (blocked) airway in unconscious apneic individuals with an artificial cough. (Reproduced with permission. Safar P [ed]: Advances in Cardiopulmonary Resuscitation, p 44. New York, Springer-Verlag, 1977.)

B

TABLE 55-5.   Recommended Sequence for Management of an Adult with Foreign-Body Airway Obstruction

A. For the conscious choking victim, with poor or no air exchange:
   1. Identify airway obstruction
   2. Apply Heimlich maneuver manual thrusts, abdominal or chest, until effective or the victim becomes unconscious

B. For the choking victim becoming unconscious, or the victim of a cardiopulmonary arrest, etiology undetermined, who cannot be ventilated:
   1. Open the airway with head-tilt–chin-lift, finger-sweep the posterior oropharynx, and attempt to ventilate
   2. If unsuccessful, apply step 2 above
   3. If step 2 is unsuccessful, reposition the airway and attempt to ventilate; repeat the sequence

forceps are acceptable extraction devices, but they should be used only with direct visualization of the foreign body. Once the patient is unconscious, direct visualization can be accomplished with a laryngoscope, tongue blade or spoon, and flashlight. Devices such as the Choke Saver (Salvita Corporation, Fort Lauderdale, FL), used blindly, must be avoided. Cricothyrotomy should be performed by a properly trained individual after failure of the other maneuvers (see below).

Adjuncts for Airway Control

The supplemental oxygen that must be administered to all seriously ill patients may be delivered to spontaneously breathing individuals by nasal cannulas, venturi masks, or plastic face masks with and without reservoirs. In the absence of adequate spontaneous ventilation, artificial ventilation with oxygen may be accomplished with the pocket mask, bag-valve devices, oxygen-powered breathing devices, and mechanical respirators.

Airway patency, ventilation, and protection may be facilitated by the use of pharyngeal airways, the pocket mask, esophageal obturator airway, and tracheal intubation.

PHARYNGEAL AIRWAYS. Airway obstruction during cardiac arrest can be alleviated in most cases by noninvasive maneuvers that move the tongue away from the posterior pharyngeal wall. Head tilt with chin lift and jaw thrust should be attempted before use of an adjunct to open the airway because instrumentation of the airway may be associated with a myriad of potential complications. When necessary, an oropharyngeal or nasopharyngeal airway may be used to open an occluded airway.

The oropharyngeal airway holds the base of the tongue away from the posterior pharyngeal wall and keeps the mouth open and lips apart. It is not tolerated by responsive patients with an intact gag reflex and may induce vomiting. Additionally, improper insertion can exacerbate upper airway obstruction by pushing the tongue backward into the posterior pharynx.

The nasopharyngeal airway opens the airway by creating a groove in the tongue. It is not as effective as the oropharyngeal airway in relieving airway obstruction, but it is more likely to be accepted by responsive patients without inducing the gag reflex or vomiting. The nasopharyngeal airway may cause epistaxis, especially when used in children with adenoidal hypertrophy that impedes its insertion. Proper head and neck position of the patient must be maintained during the use of these adjuncts if the airway is to remain patent.

MOUTH-TO-MASK VENTILATION. A simple and esthetic means to deliver oxygen and ventilate the lungs of the victim of cardiopulmonary arrest is the pocket mask. The pocket mask can be used for exhaled-air mouth-to-mask ventilation, or bag-valve–mask ventilation. When mouth-to-mask ventilation is performed, the jaw-thrust maneuver will hold the mask in place and airway open. Untrained rescuers will achieve ventilation with this apparatus more easily than by bag-valve–mask because exhaled air ventilation provides larger tidal volumes to overcome mask leakage and both hands are free for airway control and mask fit. An inlet nipple with one-way valve may be incorporated into the pocket mask for oxygen administration. During mouth-to-mask ventilation with an oxygen inflow of $10 \, l \cdot min^{-1}$, an FI_{O_2} of 0.5 can be expected. If an oxygen flow of $30 \, l \cdot min^{-1}$ is feasible, a victim's lungs may be ventilated with 100% oxygen by intermittent occlusion of the mask port with the thumb. Increasing concerns about the risk of infection transmission from patient to rescuer will likely lead to the widespread use of mouth-to-mask ventilation and the incorporation of nonrebreathing valves in these devices to protect the rescuer from exhaled respiratory droplets.

CRICOID PRESSURE. Gastric inflation during mouth-to-mouth or bag-valve–mask ventilation may be minimized by the application of cricoid pressure (Sellick maneuver). This maneuver increases the resistance to air flow into the stomach and is accomplished in unconscious victims by application of pressure to the cricoid cartilage, pushing it posteriorly to compress the esophagus between the cricoid ring and cervical spine. A second rescuer will be required to perform this maneuver while ventilation is provided by the first. Cricoid pressure may be released once tracheal intubation is accomplished.

ESOPHAGEAL OBTURATOR AIRWAY. When airway protection from regurgitation of gastric contents is desired, the esophageal obturator airway (EOA) may be effectively used by the lay person, paramedical personnel, and physicians unskilled in laryngoscopy. The technique of esophageal intubation with the EOA is simply taught and in contrast to tracheal intubation, direct visualization of the larynx is not required. EOA insertion does not require the temporary cessation of chest compression, while tracheal intubation often does. In addition, the EOA may be inserted in any patient position and without neck extension in patients with cervical injury.

The EOA was introduced by Don Michael et al[53] and later modified by Gordon.[54] The EOA is a 9.5-mm ID tube with multiple air outlets along its proximal portion, and a 30 ml inflatable cuff just proximal to its blind distal tip (Fig. 55-5). The tube snaps into a transparent face mask and is inserted into a patient's esophagus with the mask in place on the tube. The mask is identical to a pocket mask with the tube attached to the fresh-gas inlet. Using a jaw lift, the obturator is inserted into the mouth and passed blindly into the esophagus. Complications are minimized by advancing the tube in the midline and without force. Slight flexion of the neck is used to facilitate esophageal intubation. The EOA must be inserted maximally so that the mask seats properly on the victim's face and ensures a sealed external airway. The length of the tube (37 cm) has been standardized so that in the adult, the cuff of the tube in the esophagus will rest below the carina. Properly inserted, the inflated cuff will not compress the posterior membranous wall of the trachea and, therefore, not obstruct the airway. Esophageal intubation is confirmed by the observation of chest expansion and by the auscultation of breath sounds. Unintentional tracheal intubation must be promptly recognized to prevent asphyxia.

INSERTION OF ESOPHAGEAL AIRWAY

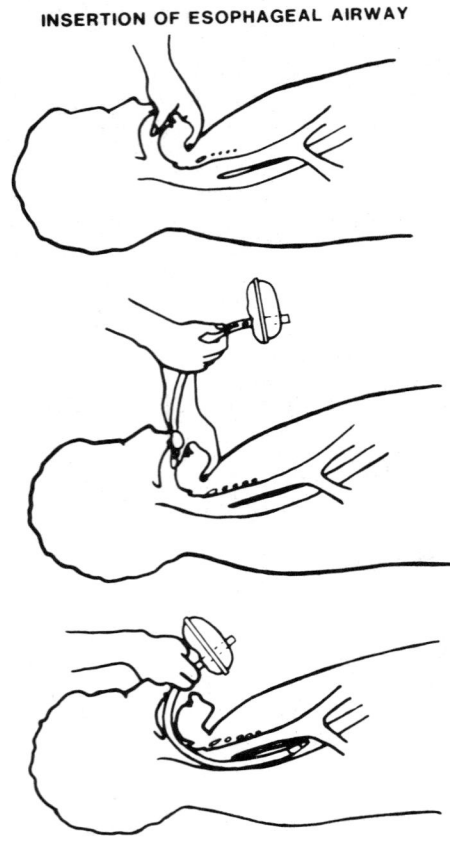

A

FINAL POSITION OF ESOPHAGEAL AIRWAY AND MASK

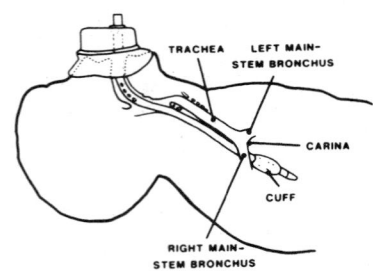

B

FIG. 55-5. *(A)* Insertion of an esophageal obturator airway. *Top:* The rescuer elevates the mandible. *Middle.* Maintaining elevation of the mandible, the rescuer inserts the obturator airway. *Bottom.* The obturator airway is positioned with the mask seated upon the face. *(B)* The esophageal obturator airway, properly positioned. (Reproduced with permission. Textbook of Advanced Cardiac Life Support, p 29. Dallas, American Heart Association, 1987.)

In such situations, the tube is repositioned properly. After inflation of the cuff with 30 ml of air or until the pilot balloon becomes tense, ventilation of the lungs may be provided by mouth, bag-valve devices, or O_2-powered breathing devices attached to the EOA. Because the esophagus is occluded, inspiratory flow passes through the multiple openings of the EOA at the level of the pharynx into the trachea. The esophageal balloon precludes air entry into the stomach and the mask precludes air leak from the mouth or nose.

The usefulness of the EOA in resuscitation from cardiopulmonary arrest has been illustrated in two reviews[55, 56] of studies that compare its use in humans with other airway opening adjuncts. Ventilation of victims of cardiac arrest *via* an EOA produced Pa_{O_2} levels similar to those achieved when the airway was maintained with an oropharyngeal airway alone.[57] Oxygenation improved after tracheal intubation in both EOA and oropharyngeal airway groups; however, the EOA protected patients from tracheal aspiration of gastric contents while the oropharyngeal airway failed to do so. Ventilation and oxygenation (gauged by arterial blood-gas analysis) achieved *via* the EOA have been compared with those obtained with a tracheal airway in patients with cardiac arrest in emergency room settings. EOA ventilation was most commonly observed to be inferior to that accomplished *via* a tracheal airway.[58-61] In one study, ventilation with the two airway devices was comparable.[62] EOA oxygenation was similarly inferior[58, 59] or, at best, comparable[60-62] with that obtained when ventilation was performed *via* an endotracheal tube. In anesthetized adults, ventilation with the EOA produced inferior exhaled tidal volume and was associated with a greater occurrence of supraglottic obstruction and operator fatigue when compared with mask and oropharyngeal airway.[63] One edentulous patient could not be ventilated. Without a good mask fit, effective ventilation of the lungs cannot be achieved with the EOA.

Tracheal intubation, rather than the use of EOA, is the preferred technique for provision of airway patency and protection during CPR. The EOA is considered an alternative to tracheal intubation in situations where the rescuer cannot, or is not permitted to, intubate the trachea; when equipment for tracheal intubation is not available; and in patients in whom tracheal intubation is not technically possible or desirable.

Esophageal perforation due to the use of the EOA has been reported, often associated with forceful insertion, overinflation of the cuff, or failure to deflate the cuff completely prior to extubation of the esophagus. The EOA can be used in unconscious patients, but use in semiconscious patients with an active gag reflex will induce vomiting. The EOA is not designed for use in children less than 16 years of age and should not be used in patients with known esophageal disease.

Passive regurgitation or active vomiting of gastric contents should be assumed to follow removal of the EOA. The EOA, therefore, should be removed only after the patient has awakened and regained protective airway reflexes, or in the unconscious patient, after the airway has been secured with a cuffed endotracheal tube. The EOA must be left in place during tracheal intubation in order to prevent regurgitation and aspiration. Laryngoscopy can be performed easily with the EOA moved to the left side of the mouth. Once endotracheal position is confirmed and the tracheal tube cuff inflated, the esophageal cuff may be deflated and the EOA removed.

The esophageal gastric tube airway (EGTA) is a modification of the EOA introduced by Gordon.[64] In this modification the tube is used for orogastric suction. The distal end of the tube is open and connected to a port above the mask. This allows passage of a size-16 gastric tube to decompress the stomach while the esophagus is still occluded. This reduces the opportunity for regurgitation and aspiration of gastric contents but never assures a totally empty stomach. A second port on the mask is used for ventilation. A spring-loaded pop-off valve inside the proximal end of the tube prevents inflation of the stomach if the incorrect port is used for ventilation.

TRACHEAL INTUBATION. Tracheal intubation is the preferred technique for airway control during ACLS. Bag-valve—mask ventilation may result in gastric distention due to the high inflation pressures generated during CPR and inadequate ventilation when used by inexperienced personnel. Adequate ventilation and oxygenation are more consistently achieved *via* an endotracheal tube than an EOA. Tracheal intubation reliably provides a patent airway and a means for oxygen supplementation; facilitates IPPV of the lungs; prevents tracheal aspiration of gastric contents; and allows tracheal suctioning.

Attempts at tracheal intubation should not delay oxygenation of the patient. Ventilation by exhaled-air methods or using simple airway adjuncts should precede attempts at tracheal intubation in most settings. As soon as convenient, intubation of the trachea may then be performed in a preoxygenated patient. A variety of endotracheal tube sizes and laryngoscope blades, a stylet, and strong suction should be available prior to instrumentation of the airway. The technique of tracheal intubation and associated complications are discussed in Chapter 20.

CRICOTHYROTOMY AND TRANSTRACHEAL CATHETER VENTILATION.

Emergency percutaneous cricothyrotomy and transtracheal catheter ventilation (TTCV) are techniques that allow rapid institution of oxygenation and ventilation under circumstances in which the insertion of an EOA or endotracheal tube may be impossible. These may include upper airway obstruction due to foreign-body aspiration, epiglottitis, croup, anaphylaxis, burns, tumors, maxillofacial and laryngeal trauma, or conditions such as congenital mandibulofacial dysostosis, severe cervical arthritis, and cervical fractures. Subsequent tracheostomy, controlled tracheal intubation, or panendoscopic examination may be performed while TTCV continues.

TTCV is provided by a high-flow (100 l·min^{-1}), low-pressure (50 psi) oxygen source *via* an airway inserted through the cricothyroid membrane (Fig. 55-6). The ventilation system consists of any airway such as a 12- or 14-gauge plastic intravenous cannula connected by a length of intravenous extension tubing to a hand-operated release valve. The release valve (time cycled) is, in turn, connected by tubing to a source that delivers 100% oxygen at 50 psi. The source may be a standard wall oxygen outlet (50–60 psi), an anesthesia machine, or an oxygen tank with a pressure-regulating valve.

The relatively avascular cricothyroid membrane is identified as a palpable transverse indentation between the thyroid and cricoid cartilages. The 12- or 14-gauge intravenous catheter (catheter-over-needle extracatheter) is inserted percutaneously into the middle of the trachea through the cricothyroid membrane. The tracheal lumen is recognized by aspiration of air into an attached syringe. The needle is then withdrawn as the catheter is advanced caudally into the trachea. Cricothyrotomy may also be accomplished surgically with a short, horizontal incision made over the cricothyroid membrane that is then stabbed and spread apart. A small-bore, hollow cannula must be inserted into the trachea to keep the opening patent.

If effective ventilation and oxygenation are to be achieved through a cricothyrotomy, insertion of a transtracheal cannula of adequate size and use of an appropriate ventilating device are mandatory. A 12-, 14-, or 16-gauge intravenous catheter (length 5 cm) can be used to provide effective ventilation in adults and children in conjunction with high-flow, jet oxygen-ventilation systems. These specialized ventilation systems are not likely to be available to most rescuers. A bag-valve device, coupled to a 15-mm endotracheal tube connector attached to the intravenous catheter will not provide effective ventilation *via* large-bore intravenous catheters.[65] Adequate ventilation and oxygenation with a bag-valve device can be achieved in

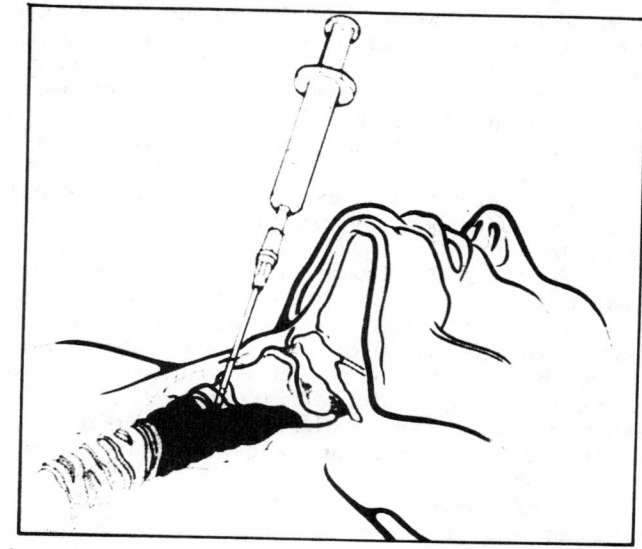

A

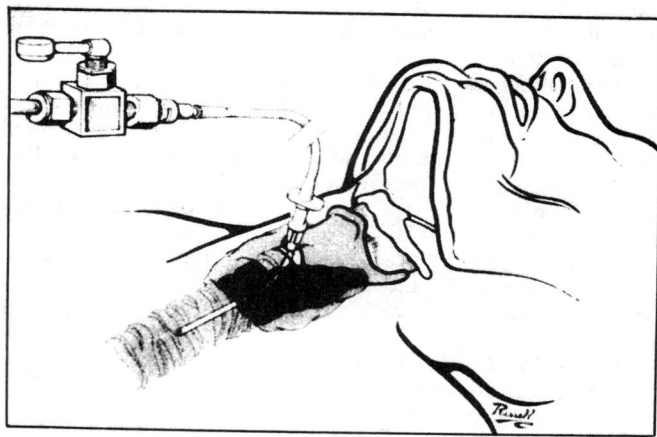

B

FIG. 55-6. *(A)* Establishment of a transtracheal airway by percutaneous insertion of a large-bore intravenous catheter through the cricothyroid membrane. Upon syringe aspiration of air, indicating catheter entry into the trachea, the intravenous catheter is threaded into the airway. *(B)* Having properly positioned the intravenous catheter in the trachea, an oxygen-powered ventilation device can be attached to facilitate mechanical ventilation. (Reproduced with permission. Textbook of Advanced Cardiac Life Support, p 34. Dallas, American Heart Association, 1987.)

children and small adults provided a 3-mm ID or larger transtracheal cannula is used.[66] Cannulation devices (4.5 mm and larger ID) for percutaneous cricothyrotomy are available commercially.

Once cricothyrotomy has been performed and the catheter is connected to the extension tubing, a jet of oxygen is introduced into the trachea by pressing the pressure-release valve. Lung inflation occurs despite a retrograde oral leak that may be present. When the patient's chest is visibly inflated, the valve is released and exhalation occurs passively through the upper airway, if open. Because exhalation during TTCV occurs passively through the upper airway, complete airway obstruction at or above the glottis will prevent exhalation from occurring and may produce dangerously high airway pressures. If the upper airway is obstructed, exhalation must occur through the ventilating catheter that is intermittently disconnected from the oxygen source and opened to the atmosphere. Chest excursion must be observed carefully to avoid overinflation of the lungs. In cases of partial airway obstruction, slow ventilation rates must be used to allow for complete passive exhalation between breaths and to prevent overinflation of the lungs.

TTCV may also be accomplished with simplified equipment, *i.e.*, using an ordinary wall oxygen flowmeter set at the flush position and a piece of standard oxygen tubing with a side hole cut near its distal end.[67] This end is connected to the transtracheal catheter. Lung inflation occurs when the side hole in the tubing is occluded by the rescuer's thumb, and exhalation occurs passively when the thumb is removed.

TTCV provides adequate arterial oxygenation and ventilation in critically ill or anesthetized adults[68–70] and children.[71, 72] During CPR, however, Pa_{O_2} deterioration and carbon dioxide retention occur[73] because external chest compression impedes the flow of oxygen into the lungs and increases the retrograde oral leak. Inadequate ventilation resulting in carbon dioxide retention occurs during TTCV in patients with reduced lung compliance, *e.g.*, pneumonia, pulmonary aspiration, and pulmonary edema.

A transtracheal catheter may be used for apneic oxygenation of victims with spontaneous circulation by insufflation of oxygen to meet basal metabolic requirements (6–8 $ml \cdot kg^{-1} \cdot min^{-1}$ in infants and 3–4 $ml \cdot kg^{-1} \cdot min^{-1}$ in adults). Although marked hypercarbia will develop, arterial oxygenation will be maintained[74, 75] while tracheostomy is performed.

Complications of TTCV include subcutaneous and mediastinal emphysema if the catheter tip is not properly placed in the tracheal lumen, and pneumothorax if excessive airway pressures are generated.[76]

BAG-VALVE DEVICES. Bag-valve devices consist of a hand-powered, self-inflating bag with a nonbreathing valve (Fig. 55-7). These devices may be used to provide ventilation in conjunction with a mask, EOA, or endotracheal tube and will deliver room air unless oxygen is supplemented. The FI_{O_2} delivered by a simple resuscitation bag (without oxygen reservoir) is limited to between 0.4 and 0.6 (oxygen inflow at 10 $l \cdot min^{-1}$), depending on the rate of bag reinflation. If bag reinflation is rapid and exceeds the oxygen inflow rate, the FI_{O_2} is decreased by entraining room air.

Higher concentrations of oxygen can be delivered with currently available self-inflating bags fitted with oxygen reservoirs. With flow rates of 10 $l \cdot min^{-1}$ and 15 $l \cdot min^{-1}$, inspired oxygen concentrations of 75% and greater than 90% are delivered, respectively. Ideal features of bag-valve devices include a transparent mask that permits recognition of regurgitated gastric contents and a nonrebreathing valve that can be quickly cleared of vomitus. Pop-off valves are not desirable because pressures required for ventilation during CPR may exceed those that open the pop-off mechanism. Complications with bag-valve–mask devices are most often related to the rescuer's skill. Inadequate ventilation due to mask leakage, airway obstruction, and gastric distention are the most common problems.

OXYGEN-POWERED BREATHING DEVICES. Chest compression may prematurely terminate inspiration provided by pressure-cycled mechanical ventilators. Volume-cycled machines may not be able to deliver adequate tidal volumes during external cardiac massage if the pressure limits are set too low. Manually triggered, oxygen-powered breathing devices (O_2 PBD) that provide instantaneous oxygen flow rates of 100 $l \cdot min^{-1}$ or more are often used during CPR to overcome the problems associated with the other types of mechanical ventilators. O_2PBD devices are time cycled and enable one rapidly to interpose breaths between compressions, inflating the lungs with 100% oxygen at a pressure not exceeding 50 psi for as long as the control button is depressed. Intrathoracic pressure generated by chest compression will not turn the O_2PBD off. The chest excursions, however, must be observed carefully for overinflation during inspiration. Problems associated

FIG. 55-7. A self-inflating bag-valve ventilation device. *(A)* Detailed diagram of the valve mechanism that couples the ventilating bag to the patient. Supplemental oxygen can be supplied (see O_2 delivery site). Rebreathing is prevented by the closure of the inflation port by the ball valve. *(B)* Generalized view of the bag-valve unit for use on a patient. (Reproduced with permission. Safar P [ed]: Advances in Cardiopulmonary Resuscitation, p 74. New York, Springer-Verlag, 1977.)

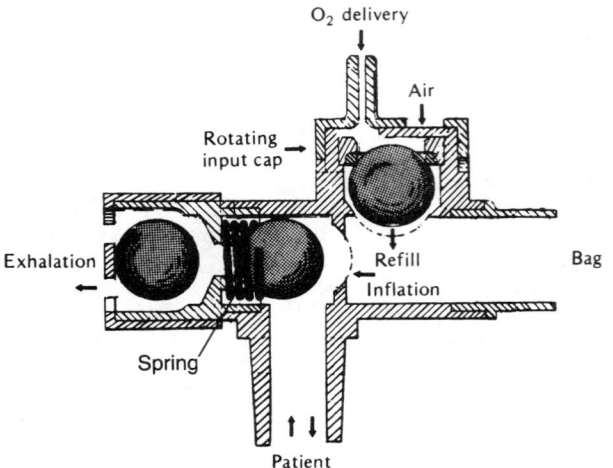

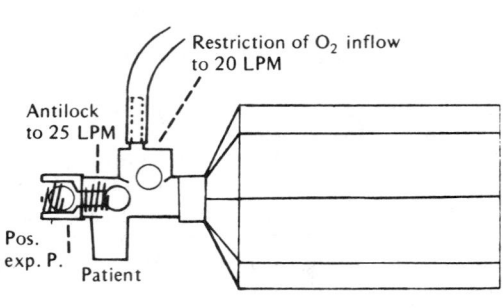

with the O_2PBD demand valves are related to the high airway pressures that may develop. Gastric distention may occur when the O_2PBD is used with an inadequately opened airway; therefore, use of this device with either the EOA or endotracheal tube is preferred. The device is not recommended for ventilation of children under 12 years of age because the high pressures may result in pulmonary barotrauma and gastric distention.

SUCTION DEVICES. Suction may be obtained from a wall vacuum outlet, or a portable, battery-operated or electrically powered suction device. Wall outlets should generate an air flow greater than $300\,l \cdot min^{-1}$ and, when occluded, a vacuum greater than 300 mm Hg. Portable suction devices do not meet these criteria. Suction equipment should be available at all resuscitations prior to airway instrumentation and should include rigid tonsil suction tips capable of suctioning large particulate matter often contained in regurgitated gastric contents.

When suctioning, it must be remembered that gas as well as liquid or particles may be removed from the airway. Hyperoxygenation prior to suctioning, and a technique of suctioning only on removal, not insertion, of the suction catheter will minimize hypoxemia and its sequelae.

ARTIFICIAL CIRCULATION DURING CPR

External Chest Compression

An absent pulse is the indication for initiating artificial circulation by external chest compression. Pulselessness is determined by palpating the carotid or femoral artery as these central pulses persist when more peripheral pulses are no longer palpable. Patients who are in shock with marked peripheral vasoconstriction and absent peripheral pulses are best treated with such measures as fluids and drugs that augment circulation. These patients do not require external chest compression because they have a functioning circulation.

In 1960 Kouwenhoven et al introduced closed-chest cardiac compression, providing artificial circulation in dogs and in five patients with cardiac arrest.[77] Prior to this, thoracotomy and internal cardiac massage were the only means to support the circulation during cardiac arrest. The report by Kouwenhoven et al, together with the development of the portable DC defibrillator, meant that resuscitation from circulatory arrest could be performed outside the hospital and by the non-physician.

External chest compression can produce a systolic blood pressure of 100 mm Hg and greater. Diastolic blood pressures, however, do not exceed 10–40 mm Hg.[44, 78–83] Mean carotid arterial blood pressure is generally less than 40 mm Hg and carotid artery blood flow is usually less than one-third of normal in animals[78–80, 84, 85] and humans.[86] As a result of the low aortic diastolic blood pressures, coronary artery blood flow during external chest compression in animal models seldom exceeds 5% of normal levels.[83, 85, 87, 88] While these blood flow levels will temporarily sustain cerebral viability, prompt restoration of spontaneous circulation and coronary perfusion by advanced cardiac life support techniques is critical for survival.

Circulation of unoxygenated blood will not sustain cerebral or myocardial viability, and sternal compression alone produces minimal ventilation. External cardiac compression must always be accompanied by effective airway management and oxygenation. Essential for effective externally produced artificial circulation are proper rescuer hand position; adequate depth of compression; proper ratio of compression time to relaxation time (at least 50% systolic time) during each compression cycle; and accompanying ventilation.

Proper hand position is found using the patient's costal margins and epigastric notch as landmarks. The heels of the rescuer's hands should lie on top of one another on the lower one-half of the sternum 1 finger-breadth above the xiphoid. The rescuer's shoulders should be directly over his hands with elbows locked such that the vector of compression force is applied straight downward onto the sternum. Improper application of pressure is less effective and will produce complications. While the rescuer must release the pressure completely during the relaxation phase to allow the heart to fill and intrathoracic pressure to return toward zero, the hand must not lose contact with the chest because correct hand position may be lost.

The sternum of an adult must be depressed 4–5 cm to produce adequate chest compression. The depth achieved by chest compression must exceed a threshold value in order to effect blood flow.[89] Above this threshold blood flow appears to be linearly related to compression depth.

The importance of the correct ratio of compression to relaxation time in each compression cycle was demonstrated by Taylor et al using a computer-driven chest-compression device for patients with cardiac arrest undergoing CPR.[90] Transcutaneous carotid or femoral artery blood flow velocities were measured with an ultrasonic Doppler flow-meter. During chest compression at a rate of 60 compressions $\cdot min^{-1}$, increasing compression duration from 40% of cycle length to 50–60% increased flow velocity 34% and 85%. The authors indicated that to achieve the necessary prolongation of compression at a rate of 60 compressions $\cdot min^{-1}$, there must be a distinct pause at maximal compression. If a compression duration of 60% of cycle length was maintained, flow velocity and arterial pressure were not significantly different at compression rates of 40, 60, or 80 compressions $\cdot min^{-1}$. The study concluded that the major emphasis during instruction of cardiac compression should be on proper compression duration rather than precise compression rate. If the optimal rate for external chest compression is that which most easily brings compression duration to 50% of the cycle time, this rate is likely to be 80–90 compressions $\cdot min^{-1}$ or greater.[91] At this rate, natural body movement during compression and release of the chest brings systolic duration near 50%.

Complications resulting from external cardiac compression may be minimized by attention to proper performance. Nonetheless, even properly performed CPR may cause injuries to some patients. These complications include rib fractures, sternal fracture, costochondral separation, blunt traumatic injuries to the intrathoracic and intraabdominal organs, and pneumothorax.

Mechanisms of Blood Flow

Understanding the mechanism by which blood flow is generated during external chest compression may permit the development of modifications in technique to improve oxygen delivery. Presently, the mechanism of blood flow during CPR is controversial. The concept that blood flows during external chest compression as a result of direct compression of the heart between the sternum and vertebral column has been widely taught and accepted. This "cardiac-pump" theory of blood flow during CPR was originally proposed by Kouwenhoven in 1960 when he introduced external cardiac compression (Fig. 55-8). This theory of blood flow is a logical inference from the mechanism of cardiac pumping during open-chest cardiac massage, the predecessor of external chest compression.

In the cardiac-pump model, if the degree of sternal displacement is relatively constant and venous return to the arrested heart unlimited, stroke volume is fixed and cardiac output will be directly related to compression rate. This theory is supported by data from a study of high-impulse (brief compression duration and moderate force) manual external chest compression in animals.[92] There is evidence of direct compression of ventricular dimensions and a linearly proportional relationship between compression rate and cardiac output. Another study reports direct cardiac-chamber compression with mitral valve closure and aortic valve opening during the initial 5 min of CPR.[93]

Efforts to explain blood flow during cough CPR and observations made during experiments to define proper compression duration led investigators to question the cardiac-pump concept. In 1976, Criley et al reported 3 patients undergoing coronary angiography who developed ventricular fibrillation but maintained arterial blood pressure and consciousness for 24–39 sec by repetitive coughing.[94] Cough CPR is a form of self-administered artificial circulation that requires previous patient training and prompt institution prior to loss of consciousness. During a cough, contraction of the diaphragm and intercostal and abdominal muscles against a closed glottis produces an abrupt increase in intrathoracic pressure. Aortic blood flow and systolic aortic pressure greater than 100 mmHg are generated as a result of the increase in intrathoracic pres-sure. Direct compression of the heart does not occur during coughing. While self-induced cough CPR is possible, its application is limited to patients who are at high risk for sudden life-threatening cardiac dysrhythmias, have a cardiac monitor in place, possess the ability to cough forcibly on command, and in whom arrest is recognized before loss of consciousness. The ability of cough CPR to produce blood flow suggests that phasic changes in intrathoracic pressure may be an alternative explanation of the mechanism generating cardiac output during external chest compression.[95]

In experiments studying compression duration, Rudikoff observed that during CPR in instrumented dogs, chest compression immediately following ventilation results in higher arterial pressure and blood flow than subsequent compressions.[96] With the lung inflated, the sternum is farther from the vertebral column, and there should be less direct compression of the heart. Rudikoff et al postulated that blood flow during CPR might be related to increase in intrathoracic pressure. To characterize this relationship, intracardiac, intrathoracic, and major vascular pressures as well as common carotid and jugular venous blood flows during external chest compression were measured. Intracardiac and intrathoracic vascular pressures rose simultaneously to equal levels during external systole. This is a physiologic circumstance that precludes blood flow because no pressure gradients are developed across the heart and great vessels to open the cardiac valves. The intracardiac and intrathoracic vascular pressures produced with each compression were equal to the intrathoracic pressure measured in the esophagus and were transmitted to the extrathoracic arterial system (carotid artery) but not the extra-

FIG. 55-8. *(A)* Cardiac pump mechanism for generating blood flow during closed-chest compression of CPR. During artificial systole, central chest compression squeezes the heart against the spine, forcing blood out. Air is vented from the thorax *via* the trachea *(top, right)*. During artificial diastole, chest resiliency creates negative pressure for filling. The site of application of force *(broad arrow)* is critical. For simplicity, only one pumping chamber is shown. *(B)* Thoracic pump mechanism for generating blood flow during closed-chest compression of CPR. During artificial systole, thoracic compression or cough generates intrathoracic pressure, which is vented by arterial outflow to peripheral tissues. During artificial diastole, release of intrathoracic pressure allows for filling. Site of application of force is not important. (Reproduced with permission from Babbs CF: New versus old theories of blood flow during CPR. Crit Care Med 8:191, 1980.)

ARTIFICIAL SYSTOLE

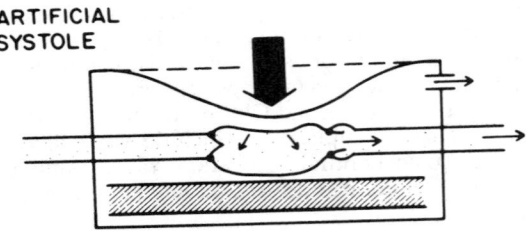

ARTIFICIAL SYSTOLE

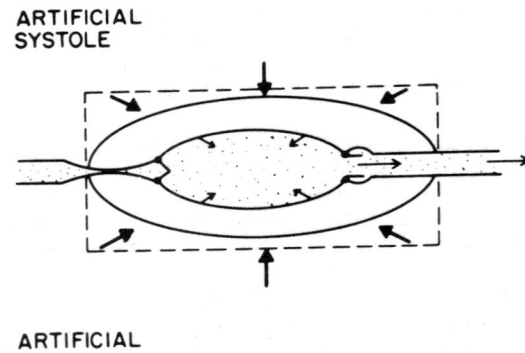

ARTIFICIAL DIASTOLE

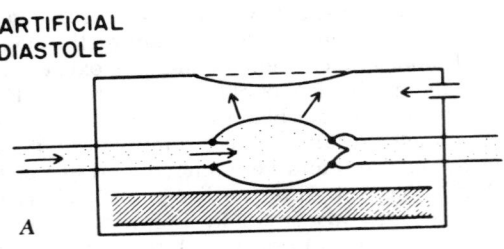

A

ARTIFICIAL DIASTOLE

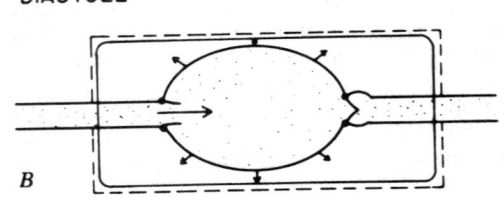

B

thoracic venous system (jugular vein). The unequal transmission of the intrathoracic pressure to the extrathoracic arterial and venous systems results in a lower pressure in the peripheral venous system (jugular vein) than peripheral arterial system (carotid artery) and, thus, establishes an extrathoracic arteriovenous pressure gradient that permits forward blood flow (Fig. 55-9). When chest compression is released, intrathoracic pressure decreases below venous pressure and blood from the extrathoracic venous system flows into the chest.

Unequal transmission of intrathoracic pressure to the extrathoracic arterial and venous systems is crucial to this theory. Systolic intrathoracic pressure is not transmitted to the extrathoracic jugular veins because of the greater capacitance of the peripheral venous than arterial system and the anatomic and functional venous valves at the thoracic inlet.[96] The thin-walled veins function as Starling resistors, collapsing on chest compression, while the stiffer-walled arteries are resistant to collapse, permitting transmission of intrathoracic arterial pressure to the carotid artery and the arterioles it supplies. There are no valves in the inferior vena cava and, therefore, intrathoracic pressures are transmitted in a retrograde direction into the extrathoracic veins of the abdomen and lower extremities. Blood flow to organs below the diaphragm, including the kidneys, is extremely low during external cardiac compression.

Further studies[78, 96] performed with this animal model at higher intrathoracic pressure obtained by occluding the airway at end-inspiration, simultaneous ventilation and chest compression, and abdominal binding, resulted in greater arterial pressures and improved carotid blood flow velocity during chest compression until sufficient elevation of intrathoracic pressure resulted in collapse of the carotid artery and cessation of all extrathoracic blood flow. This data support the concept that blood flow during external chest compression results from pulses of intrathoracic pressure, not direct cardiac compression. This explanation of blood flow during CPR has been coined the *"thoracic-pump" mechanism* (Figs. 55-8 and 55-9).

In contrast to the cardiac-pump model in which blood flow is compression-rate dependent, in the thoracic-pump model, blood flow should be sensitive to the degree and duration of rise in intrathoracic pressure.[97] The finding that cardiac output during external chest compression is improved by use of a prolonged compression time (50–60% of cycle time) and is not changed by a two-fold variation in compression rate[90] supports the thoracic pump concept.

Echocardiography during CPR in humans[98] and cineangiograms obtained during CPR in dogs[99] demonstrate that both left heart valves are open during external compression, the mitral leaflets moving further apart during maximum compression, and the left ventricular chamber size remains unchanged. The pulmonary valve closed with compression and opened with relaxation. These studies suggest that blood flow during CPR does not rely on a mechanism requiring mitral valve closure during compression, *i.e.,* the cardiac-pump theory; rather, the heart merely serves as a conduit through which blood flows to and from the pulmonary circuit.

An array of new techniques to improve blood flow and oxygen delivery during external chest compression has been studied. Many of these methods aim to increase blood flow by augmenting the rise in intrathoracic pressure occurring during compression. Levels of intrathoracic pressure generated have been elevated by 1) pressurizing the airway during chest compression (simultaneous compression–ventilation CPR (SCV-CPR),[78, 84, 85, 100] 2) binding the abdomen to restrict diaphragmatic motion during compression (CPR with continuous abdominal binding);[101–103] CPR with military antishock trousers (MAST)[104] 3) circumferential compression of the thorax (pneumatic vest CPR);[83] and 4) combinations of these modalities (abdominal compression with synchronized ventilation,[105] synchronized pneumatic chest–abdominal binder ventilation CPR).[106]

Interposed abdominal-compression CPR is another alternative to conventional CPR in which an additional rescuer compresses the abdomen in the diastolic interval between chest compressions.[107] This produces diastolic augmentation of blood flow in the same manner provided by intraaortic balloon counterpulsation.

Each of these investigational CPR techniques has been shown to improve hemodynamics (arterial blood pressure, aortic or carotid artery blood flow), and SCV-CPR[84, 85] and pneumatic vest CPR[83] provide more cerebral blood flow (measured by radiolabeled microsphere technique) when compared with conventional external chest compression.

Coronary artery blood flow is a major determinant of successful resuscitation from cardiac arrest.[101, 102, 106, 108] Coronary perfusion pressure and myocardial blood flow (meas-

FIG. 55-9. Intrathoracic and extrathoracic hemodynamic variables during closed-chest compression *(top)*, which explain forward blood flow during CPR *(bottom)*. (Reproduced with permission from Weisfeldt ML, Chandra N, Tsitlik JE *et al:* New attempts to improve blood flow during CPR. In Schluger J, Lyon AF [eds]: CPR and Emergency Cardiac Care Looking to the Future, p 20. New York, EM Books.)

How blood flows in CPR

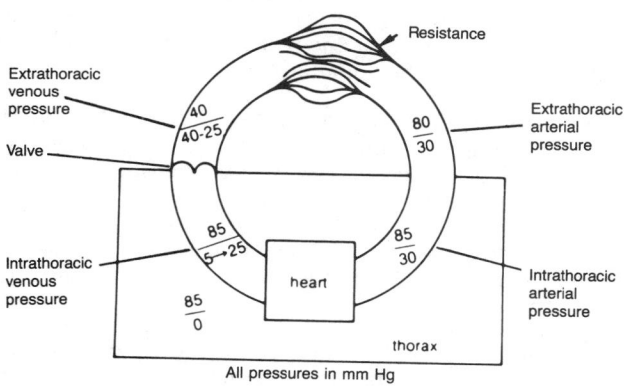

All pressures in mm Hg

Mechanism of forward carotid blood flow during CPR in dogs

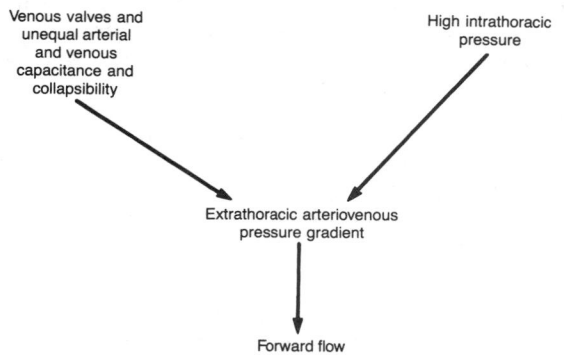

ured by radiolabeled microsphere technique) are not enhanced by SCV-CPR[82, 84, 85] or CPR augmented with MAST garments.[104] Studies of coronary perfusion during pneumatic vest CPR report improved myocardial perfusion (measured by radiolabeled microsphere technique)[83] or no difference in coronary perfusion pressure[109] when compared with conventional CPR. Failure to enhance myocardial perfusion may occur because the augmented aortic blood pressure produced by these methods does not persist into the diastolic phase when coronary flow takes place, or the intrathoracic pressure generated during artificial systole is also transmitted to the intracardiac chambers and maintained into diastole, thus compromising the pressure gradient driving blood across the coronary circulation.

Conventional CPR is unlikely to be replaced by a new method until an alternative technique can be demonstrated consistently to improve both myocardial perfusion, increasing the likelihood of resuscitation from cardiac arrest, and cerebral perfusion, enhancing neurologic recovery following resuscitation. Currently, there is a lack of comparable studies that analyze outcome after resuscitation, including complications, accomplished using different methods of external artificial circulation. In one report, pneumatic vest CPR produced significantly better 24-h survival and neurologic function when compared with conventional CPR,[83] while no differences were measured in another comparison of conventional CPR, SCV-CPR, and pneumatic vest CPR.[109] Additionally, many of the proposed methods require the use of devices (e.g., tracheal intubation, programmable mechanical compressors, pneumatic vests) that are not available to the rescuer performing out-of-hospital CPR.

The cardiac-pump and thoracic-pump theories are not mutually exclusive, and both may explain aspects of the generation of blood flow during external chest compression. Which one is predominant in a particular victim may depend on patient-related factors (heart size, anterior–posterior chest diameter, thoracic compliance, and duration of cardiac arrest) and technique-related variables (manual vs. mechanical compression, compression duration and depth).

Current recommendations for the performance of external cardiac compression are consistent with both the cardiac-pump and thoracic-pump theories of blood flow. An increase in compression rate to 80–100 compressions $\cdot$ min^{-1} from previous recommendations should improve blood flow as a result of increasing the duration of compression to 50% of cycle time (thoracic pump) or producing a rate-dependent increase in cardiac output (cardiac pump). Adequate depth of chest compression is essential to achieve direct cardiac compression (cardiac pump) or produce a substantial increase in intrathoracic pressure (thoracic pump). Early provision of ACLS to restore spontaneous cardiac function is essential to survival because the low levels of myocardial and cerebral blood flow produced by artificial circulation techniques limit the capability of external chest compression to sustain heart and brain viability for more than a few minutes.

Adjuncts for Artificial Circulation

CARDIAC BACK BOARD. Cardiac output is produced when the relatively immovable objects (sternum and spine) squeeze the movable objects (heart and lungs) in sandwich-like fashion. To insure that the bony structures effectively squeeze the soft tissues, the spine must be anchored. If the spine is not fixed in position, compression of the sternum toward the vertebrae results in displacement of the entire thoracic cage rather than compression of the intrathoracic contents. This commonly occurs when chest compression is being performed on a patient lying on a soft mattress. Inability to perform cardiac compression on a victim in water is also accounted for in this way. A more rigid foundation under the spine is required to anchor and limit its displacement. Such a rigid surface is always available by placing the patient on a walking surface such as the floor. A back board serves the same purpose and obviates the need to move the victim out of bed onto the floor. Ideally, the back board or bed board is made of material rigid enough to serve as a resistive surface on which to compress the chest. A bed board should be located in all areas where life-support equipment is available. A reasonable compromise can often be found in most hospital patient rooms by using a food tray that, while smaller than ideal, is usually large enough and rigid enough for cardiac compression. Modern-day design of dental chairs and other similar medical devices must take into account the potential need to do cardiac compression and should be manufactured with materials adequate for producing a rigid back rest.

CARDIAC PRESS. A lever acts to provide a mechanical advantage in performance of a physical task. A cardiac press is a device that provides such a lever advantage. With a cardiac press, a plunger replaces the hands upon the chest, displacing the sternum toward the spine. Movement of the plunger is produced with an attached lever. In this fashion, manual cardiac-compression endurance is enhanced. There is a fatigue factor that must still be considered, however, because movement of the lever and plunger is accomplished manually.

The major advantage of the cardiac press is in permitting one operator greater ability to do cardiac compression. The disadvantages of the cardiac press include the time and expertise required to set up the press on a patient being given BCLS, and the need for constant surveillance of the plunger so that it compresses only the lower one-half of the sternum and in fact displaces it toward the spine the proper distance.

OXYGEN-POWERED MECHANICAL COMPRESSION DEVICE. The ultimate in adjuncts for cardiac compression is the mechanical chest-compression device consisting of a back board and oxygen-powered plunger. Cardiac compression can be regulated without fatigue by a rescuer who need only monitor correct position of the plunger and adequacy of sternal motion. The "thumper," as it is often called, will consistently provide cardiac compression as long as there is sufficient gas supply. While the gas-driven compression devices permit longer periods of CPR when used in some transport settings, i.e., air transport rescue, the oxygen tank size (oxygen quantity) is limited and, therefore, time is a factor. Extremes in temperature also alter gas-powered mechanical compressors by changing gas volumes and pressures as well as gas valve function.

Integral in the design of the oxygen-driven mechanical chest compressor is a volume-cycled ventilator delivering 100% oxygen. The use of a volume-cycled ventilator rather than the ideal CPR time-cycled ventilator derives from the limited amount of oxygen that may be available. The time-cycled breathing device uses an oxygen flow rate of 120–150 l $\cdot$ min^{-1} and is thus able to interpose rapidly ventilations between cardiac compressions without requiring a pause in compression for ventilation. When a volume-cycled ventilator with a lower oxygen flow rate of approximately 40–60 l $\cdot$ min^{-1} is used, a longer time is required to produce adequate tidal volumes. Cardiac compression must be stopped long enough to permit ventilation of the lungs with this type of ventilator. The compromise of accepting a pause in compression is required to permit using the lower oxygen flow rates. Because oxygen serves as the driving force for both the compressor and ventilator, the oxygen flow rate for the ventilating portion of the device must be limited so as not to deplete the gas source. It is unclear whether the slower heart rate that is produced is really detrimental in view of the fact that with the thoracic pump mechanism of blood flow, slower rates are adequate if compression duration is 50–60% of cycle time.

Safe and effective use of the oxygen-powered mechanical chest compressor requires considerable knowledge by the rescuer. As with the cardiac press, placement of the compression device and monitoring of its use is essential for effective CPR.

MILITARY ANTISHOCK TROUSERS (MAST) GARMENTS. MAST garments[110, 111] (pneumatic antishock garments, G suits) aid production of blood pressure principally by increasing peripheral vascular resistance in the lower one-half of the body. They may also improve cardiac output by displacing pooled blood into a more central venous location to restore venous return to the heart. MAST garments have one abdominal and two lower-extremity compartments, each of which can be inflated independently. Inflation of the leg and abdominal chambers of the garment forces venous blood out of the extremities and abdominal viscera and restricts arterial blood flow to the abdomen and periphery. The autotransfusion that results from inflation of the antishock trousers may be remarkably beneficial for the hypovolemic patient, but may be devastating for the cardiogenic shock patient. Monitoring the clinical effect of garment inflation is essential. A distinct advantage of this device is the possibility of rapid reversal of a detrimental effect by chamber deflation. Adequacy of fluid resuscitation can be assessed by monitoring graded deflation of the individual compartments of the garment.

In addition to producing hemodynamic effects that are readily reversible, the antishock device stabilizes fractures and tamponades intraabdominal, retroperitoneal, and extremity bleeding. Application of the garment to the lower one-half of the body, however, may conceal injuries. Rapid but thorough survey of the body should be made prior to covering the abdomen and legs with the trousers.

The principle clinical indication for MAST garment application is hypovolemic shock due to traumatic injury. Individuals with pelvic and lower-extremity injuries may particularly benefit from the vasopressor-like and hemostatic effects of garment inflation. The device is useful only as a temporary measure until definitive therapy, e.g., fluids or blood transfusion, and surgical repair is accomplished.

There are several major concerns with the use of antishock garments. Premature deflation in a patient who still has a marginal blood volume will result in sudden recurrence of shock. Excessive and prolonged pressure applied to the lower one-half of the body may result in tissue hypoxia and local acidosis. Upon deflation of the trousers, metabolic acid may be released systemically. Improperly positioned antishock garments may hinder ventilation by the limitation of lower thoracic cage motion. Properly positioned, the trousers will still decrease ventilatory efficiency by limiting diaphragmatic descent.

There appears to be little need for MAST garment use in normovolemic patients in cardiac arrest during CPR. While their use raises arterial blood pressure during external chest compression, central venous pressure is increased as well; coronary and cerebral perfusion are, therefore, not improved.[104] Survival is not increased by the application of MAST suits during CPR.[112]

OPEN-CHEST CARDIAC COMPRESSION. Historically, open-chest cardiac compression was the first method used to provide cardiac output during cardiac arrest. Kouwenhoven's report of the effectiveness of closed-chest cardiac compression, however, obviated the need to continue the more complicated and dangerous open-chest method. While closed-chest compression has replaced direct cardiac compression during CPR, it is apparent that direct cardiac massage produces superior arterial blood pressure, cardiac output, and coronary perfusion compared with external compression.[86, 108, 113, 114] Coronary perfusion and survival in animal models are improved when direct cardiac compression is instituted within 15 min of cardiac arrest.[108, 109] If open-chest CPR is delayed 20 min or more, outcome is not improved despite the superior hemodynamics. In a report of patients with out-of-hospital cardiac arrest, open-chest CPR failed to improve survival when applied after 30 min of arrest time and external cardial compression.[115]

Although early thoracotomy and direct cardiac compression have been recommended by some in instances of unsuccessful resuscitation employing external CPR,[116] it is impractical for use on most patients with out-of-hospital arrest and is inappropriate for unskilled rescuers. The results of early open-chest CPR are unstudied. There are, however, indications for open-chest cardiac compression in a hospital setting, including:

1. Cardiac arrest occurring in the operating room during intrathoracic procedures
2. Cardiac arrest associated with penetrating or blunt injuries to the chest where thoracotomy may allow control of hemorrhage or eliminate the underlying pathology. Flail chest may preclude effective thoracic compression
3. Cardiac tamponade
4. Cardiac arrest associated with major mediastinal shifts, e.g., tension pneumothorax, massive pleural effusion, or the postpneumonectomy patient
5. Anatomic deformities of the chest, e.g., severe kyphoscoliosis, and severely emphysematous, barrel-chested patients with inelastic chest walls that preclude adequate thoracic compression
6. In the patient who cannot assume the supine position, e.g., patients undergoing neurosurgical procedures in an upright position
7. Massive air embolism where thoracotomy allows needle aspiration of the air from the heart under direct vision
8. Massive pulmonary embolism where thoracotomy allows direct access to the obstructing embolus
9. Cardiac arrest associated with exsanguination below the diaphragm, e.g., ruptured abdominal aortic aneurysm—thoracotomy facilitates clamping of the aorta proximal to the diaphragm before instituting cardiac compression
10. Refractory ventricular fibrillation in a victim of hypothermic cardiac arrest—pericardial lavage with warm saline may warm the heart to a temperature permitting defibrillation

CARDIOPULMONARY BYPASS. Emergency cardiopulmonary bypass has been employed in canine models of cardiac arrest without thoracotomy using the femoral artery and vein for access to the circulation. When instituted after 12 min of cardiac arrest in place of BCLS and ACLS[117, 118] or following 30 min of arrest and external chest compression,[119] cardiopulmonary bypass improved immediate resuscitability and short-term survival when compared with conventional resuscitation techniques. Neurologic outcome was not consistently improved in all studies. Emergent cardiopulmonary bypass is useful for the rapid rewarming of victims of hypothermic cardiac arrest.

ADVANCED CARDIAC LIFE SUPPORT

The establishment of spontaneous oxygen delivery by the victim of cardiac arrest depends on the efficient and effective implementation of the BCLS protocols outlined above with, in many cases, the addition of the recognition of cardiac dysrhythmias and the institution of indicated antidysrhythmic and cardiovascular pharmacology. Special cardiac arrest situations will indicate other specific therapies such as fluid resuscitation for exsanguination.

RECOGNITION OF DYSRHYTHMIAS

Sudden death frequently results from sudden, severe cardiac dysrhythmias. These dysrhythmias occur commonly in individuals with ischemic heart disease. Hypertensive cardiovascular disease, cardiomyopathies, valvular heart disease, and other cardiac conditions are additional underlying causes of sudden dysrhythmic death. In situations in which a disturbance in cardiac rhythm is not the primary cause of arrest, *e.g.*, ventilatory arrest, dysrhythmias may occur as secondary events. The rapid recognition and treatment of cardiac rhythm disturbances is central to the process of resuscitation. In addition, early detection and correction of life-threatening, although acutely nonlethal, dysrhythmias may prevent the occurrence of cardiac arrest.

ECG monitoring should be established immediately on all patients with symptoms of myocardial ischemia. During myocardial infarction most sudden deaths are due to dysrhythmias, and approximately 60% occur within the first 2 h after onset of symptoms. ECG monitoring of these patients allows recognition and treatment of prodromal dysrhythmias and immediate intervention in case of lethal dysrhythmias.

In victims of sudden collapse, ECG monitoring should begin as soon as possible after the initiation of CPR, primarily to differentiate ventricular fibrillation or ventricular tachycardia from the other dysrhythmias such as asystole and electromechanical dissociation (EMD). Definitive therapy for cardiac arrest is specific for the cause of the arrest. In the case of ventricular fibrillation (VF) or ventricular tachycardia, immediate defibrillation and cardioversion, respectively, are indicated. In a study of 352 instances of prehospital cardiac arrest, ventricular fibrillation was the initial rhythm observed in 62%, ventricular tachycardia in 7%, and severe bradydysrhythmia or asystole in 31%.[120]

The cardiac rhythm can be most rapidly determined using defibrillator paddles that incorporate "quick-look" ECG electrodes. This rapid-diagnosis feature should be provided with all modern defibrillators. When the paddles are applied to the patient's chest, the rhythm is displayed on the defibrillator oscilloscope and in the presence of a dysrhythmia, the unit can be charged and electrical therapy administered immediately.

During a prolonged resuscitation, it is desirable to place stick-on or strap-on ECG monitoring electrodes that allow uninterrupted external cardiac compression. Limb placement of the ECG electrodes will not interfere with subsequent defibrillation attempts or central venous access. External chest compression may be interrupted for a few seconds at a time to record an ECG rhythm without artifact. Either a conventional ECG recording machine or a portable ECG monitoring–defibrillator unit with ECG electrodes may be used.

ECG monitoring systems should include a monitor screen, recording system (to transcribe the rhythm signal onto paper), a heart-rate meter, and the capacity to select a variety of leads. Detailed dysrhythmia diagnosis can be made during CPR using the six standard limb leads and an exploratory electrode for precordial or special leads. ECG leads used for dysrhythmia recognition should show P waves and clearly demonstrate the relationship between the P wave and QRS complex. Lead II is generally adequate for P-wave identification. During some tachydysrhythmias, however, P waves may be clearly demonstrable only in the MCL_1, esophageal, or intraatrial leads. The differential diagnosis of tachycardias with wide QRS complexes is facilitated by the V_1 and MCL_1 leads, which characterize the QRS morphology.

Dysrhythmias must be evaluated with respect to both their electrical instability and their hemodynamic consequences. Electrically, a dysrhythmia may be a precursor of more serious rhythm disturbance. Ventricular premature beats may trigger the development of ventricular tachycardia or ventricular fibrillation. Bradycardias may be associated with inadequate cardiac output or more serious dysrhythmias. Heart block may lead to asystole or ventricular fibrillation. Hemodynamically, tachycardia may lead to ischemia or cause pump failure due to inadequate ventricular filling, while hypotension and heart failure may result from the loss of properly timed "atrial kick" in atrioventricular (AV) dissociation.

The lethal dysrhythmias, ventricular fibrillation and asystole, are always associated with pulselessness, *i.e.*, absent perfusion. The life-threatening dysrhythmias, ventricular tachycardia and complete heart block, generally result in inadequate cardiac output and hypotension, and are electrically unstable rhythms that may degenerate to lethal dysrhythmias. The significance of third-degree heart block depends on the level at which the AV block occurs. When it occurs at the level of the AV node, a junctional escape pacemaker with a rate of 40–60 beats $\cdot$ min^{-1} will initiate ventricular depolarization. Because the site of origin of this dysrhythmia is located above the bifurcation of the bundle of His, ventricular depolarization occurs in the normal sequence, resulting in a normal QRS. This type of block is usually transient and associated with a favorable prognosis. Infranodal third-degree AV block, on the other hand, usually indicates extensive disease of the conduction system. The ventricular escape pacemaker initiating ventricular depolarization in situations of infranodal third-degree AV block produces a wide QRS and has an inherent firing rate less than 40 beats $\cdot$ min^{-1}. This is not a stable pacemaker, and asystole or ventricular fibrillation may occur.

Other dangerous prodromal dysrhythmias include ventricular premature beats and Mobitz type II second-degree AV block. Traditionally, ventricular premature beats have been considered malignant harbingers of more serious dysrhythmias, ventricular tachycardia and ventricular fibrillation when they occur frequently (greater than 5 beats $\cdot$ min^{-1}), are multifocal in origin, are occurring in salvos of two or more in rapid succession, or when a ventricular premature beat falls on the T wave (vulnerable period) of the preceding beat (R on T phenomenon).[121, 122] Ventricular fibrillation, however, is infrequently preceded by these premonitory dysrhythmias and may occur in their absence.[123, 124]

Mobitz type I second-degree AV block (Wenckebach phenomenon) is generally a transient conduction block occurring at the level of the AV node and rarely progresses to complete heart block. On the other hand, Mobitz type II second-degree AV block occurs at the level of His bundle or below, *i.e.*, infranodal, and sudden progression to complete heart block should be anticipated. A pacemaker must be inserted prophylactically in these patients. Often a temporary pacemaker is inserted into a patient with myocardial ischemia and a newly occurring Wenckebach rhythm until myocardial oxygen balance is restored.

In the patient with a tachydysrhythmia and wide QRS complex, differentiation between supraventricular and ventricular sites of origin may be difficult. Supraventricular tachycardia with aberrant ventricular conduction is usually not life threatening in the absence of myocardial ischemia, aortic stenosis, or mitral stenosis. Ventricular tachycardia, on the other hand, is a more serious dysrhythmia requiring treatment. Premature atrial contractions with aberration may be identified by the presence of a premature P wave preceding the initial wide QRS complex. In the case of a premature junctional complex, the P wave may be difficult to identify. In patients with tachycardia and wide QRS complex, certain features favor the presence of ventricular tachycardia:[125]

1. Atrioventricular dissociation—the occurrence of fusion or capture beats is diagnostic of ventricular tachycardia
2. A QRS duration greater than 0.14 s (in the absence of preexisting conduction system disease)
3. Left-axis deviation in the frontal plane during the tachycardia, which is not present in the absence of tachycardia
4. Monophasic or biphasic right bundle branch block (BBB)-shaped QRS complexes in the right precordial leads; Triphasic right BBB-shaped complexes in V_1 or MCL_1 are found in both supraventricular and ventricular tachycardia, but a classic triphasic right BBB RSR′ pattern strongly suggests supraventricular origin; a triphasic "rabbit-ear" QRS complex with left ear taller than right ear suggests ventricular origin

Other criteria for differentiation of aberration from ventricular ectopy have been described. Although not diagnostic, these criteria may confirm the diagnosis of a supraventricular rhythm with aberrant ventricular conduction:

1. Ashman phenomenon (long-short cycle sequence): In atrial fibrillation, the occurrence of a wide QRS complex in V_1 or MCL_1 with RSR′ configuration closely following a normally conducted beat preceded by a long R–R interval favors aberrant conduction.
2. Absence of a compensatory pause following a wide QRS—Supraventricular premature beats conducted retrograde may depolarize the sinus node, resetting the pacemaker so the next beat follows the premature complex by normal R–R interval. Ventricular premature beats are usually followed by a compensatory pause because retrograde conduction is blocked and the sinus node is not reset.

For the ACLS provider, this challenging differential diagnosis is often a luxury afforded only in the case of a hemodynamically stable patient. The patient who is hemodynamically compromised by a tachydysrhythmia cannot afford the time for definitive assessment, but must be treated immediately. Whether the dysrhythmia is ventricular or supraventricular, the treatment of choice is synchronized cardioversion.

ECG lead disconnection and artifact due to patient movement or 60-cycle interference may occur and must be distinguished from asystole and ventricular fibrillation.

The presence of a stable ECG rhythm does not assure circulation. A patient with an organized ECG pattern but no pulse has EMD. EMD may be a terminal phenomenon, the result of extensive myocardial damage. EMD may also be produced by conditions that interfere with venous return to the heart or ventricular output. These include among others, cardiac tamponade, tension pneumothorax, massive pulmonary embolus, severe hypovolemia, and inhalational anesthetic overdose. In the presence of EMD a high index of suspicion of these conditions is crucial because prompt intervention may restore cardiac output and be lifesaving.

DEFIBRILLATION

Restoration of cardiac output requires the resumption of a relatively normal electrical impulse pattern in the heart. Pharmacologic therapy may be used to restore normal electrical impulse pattern, but often requires a significant amount of time for an effect to occur. Many dysrhythmias alter hemodynamic stability in such a drastic fashion that they require more rapid intervention. Electrical therapy using a defibrillator is often the only practical therapy available to treat these rhythm disturbances.[126]

The defibrillator delivers a prescribed dose of electrical current through the heart. This current uniformly depolarizes the myocardium, which subsequently repolarizes in a coordinated fashion. Electrical current administered to the heart, however, may result in myocardial cell damage.[127, 128] Minimizing the electrical current administered minimizes myocardial destruction.[129] Dispersion of the current over a greater area by use of larger defibrillator paddles,[130] and less frequent delivery of repetitive shocks with greater recovery time between shocks, also reduce the amount of myocardial damage.

The ideal defibrillation dose is not known even though many factors have been outlined that affect defibrillation success.[131-135] Study of the dose needed for defibrillation on a $watt \cdot s^{-1} \cdot kg^{-1}$ basis has failed to demonstrate clearly a dose–weight relationship or a need for high-dose defibrillators. High-dose repetitive defibrillation attempts are hazardous, resulting in a higher incidence of postdefibrillation AV block. Several important factors apart from dose have been identified as crucial in defibrillation success. The more rapidly defibrillation therapy is administered after the onset of cardiac arrest, the better the outcome (Fig. 55-10). A critical mass of myocardial tissue must be defibrillated to be successful. The exact quantity of tissue is unknown, but the concept of a sufficient mass of tissue being affected by the electric shock is strongly supported by the poor result from improper defibrillation technique. The initial rhythm at the time of defibrillation is related to success. Supraventricular rhythms and ventricular fibrillation are more responsive than idioventricular rhythms or asystole.

Reduction of transthoracic impedance to electrical current flow enhances defibrillation success. Transthoracic impedance or resistance to current flow is reduced by use of electrically conductive interface materials linking the defibrillator paddles with the chest wall. Saline-soaked gauze pads and electrode paste or gel increase chest wall conductance. Alcohol-soaked pads risk burns and fire with the application of electrical therapy and should be strictly avoided.

Chest wall and cardiac resistances to current flow are reduced with repetitive shocks.[136] Experimental studies have

Delay Before First Defibrillation

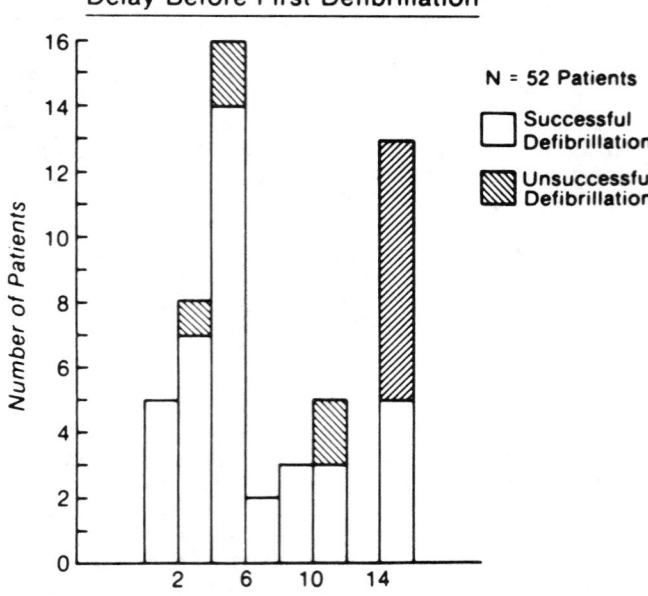

FIG. 55-10. The relationship of the delay before the first defibrillating dose and the success of defibrillation shows the beneficial effect of rapid defibrillation therapy on resuscitation. (Reproduced with permission from Kerber RE, Sarnat W: Factors influencing the success of ventricular defibrillation in man. Circulation 60:226, 1979.)

demonstrated that while the first defibrillation may be ineffective, subsequent shocks at the exact same dose may be successful because of better current flow. Effective defibrillation occurs best when the electrical shock is delivered during the expiratory phase of the respiratory cycle—less air is in the lungs during expiration. Because air is a poor conductor of electrical current flow, the smaller air barrier between the paddles and heart during end-expiration results in better success with defibrillation.

The recommended procedure for defibrillation includes BCLS measures that are continuously provided for all victims of cardiac arrest while a defibrillator is brought to the scene. The defibrillator should have an integral ECG monitor. As mentioned earlier, defibrillator paddles capable of "quick-look" ECG monitoring are very desirable. Because asystole or some other dysrhythmias without a pulse may not be treated best by defibrillation, it is desirable to diagnose the cardiac rhythm before an electrical shock is delivered. The diagnosis of asystole must be made cautiously. Low-voltage ventricular fibrillation may masquerade as asystole. An additional reason for an apparent asystolic ECG tracing is inaccurately low calibration of the monitor oscilloscope. These two circumstances must be kept in mind to avoid withholding electrical shock therapy when the true, but unrecognized rhythm is ventricular fibrillation. In more than one-half of the instances of cardiac arrest, the rhythm disturbance is ventricular fibrillation.

When the diagnosis of ventricular fibrillation is made, the paddles are applied to the chest with adequate electrode–gel interface and the defibrillator capacitor is charged. An appropriate initial dose for the average adult patient is 200 watt·s⁻¹ (joules). When the paddles are fully charged to the selected dose, the electrical shock is delivered. Ideally, the operator

who is holding the paddles should be able to operate and discharge the device without the need for additional personnel. This eliminates potential miscommunication and incorrect charging and discharging of the paddles, with resultant complication to the patient or injury to the rescuers.

The ECG must be reevaluated immediately after the initial defibrillation. If an organized rhythm is apparent, hemodynamic status should be assessed by feeling for the pulse and measuring blood pressure. If ventricular fibrillation persists, the paddles should be recharged immediately to a dose of 200–300 joules and discharged in the same way as before. If after the second electrical defibrillation, the rhythm disturbance and pulselessness persist, a third electrical discharge at 360 joules is administered. If still unsuccessful and the patient remains pulseless, other ACLS measures must be instituted. Correction of acidosis, administration of epinephrine to enhance the fibrillation pattern and ability to defibrillate, and the use of antidysrhythmics may be indicated. Subsequent defibrillation should be conducted using the maximum electrical charge available.

Pulselessness may be associated with rhythm disturbances other than ventricular fibrillation, i.e., supraventricular and ventricular tachycardias. Defibrillation is used only for ventricular fibrillation. Other rhythms are cardioverted (in synchronized fashion). Ventricular fibrillation can be precipitated by delivering an electrical shock to a supraventricular or ventricular tachycardia during the late systolic period of vulnerability immediately prior to the appearance of the T wave. The defibrillator discharge can be synchronized to the ECG (the QRS deflection can be sensed and discharge of the paddles timed accordingly) to avoid delivery of electrical shock at this vulnerable time. To synchronize electrical discharge, a defibrillator must have an integrated ECG monitor that is activated for cardioversion. The synchronization mechanism must be deactivated for defibrillation. Ventricular fibrillation has no QRS deflection to be sensed, and the energy, therefore, will never be discharged if the synchronization mechanism is and remains activated.

In situations where a defibrillator does not have an ECG monitor, the device is used as a defibrillator, irrespective of the dysrhythmia, and if ventricular fibrillation is unintentionally produced when another rhythm is being treated, it is then defibrillated.

Hemodynamic consequences of rhythm disturbances other than ventricular fibrillation vary. If blood pressure and perfusion are maintained adequately, drug therapy may be more appropriate than cardioversion, or if electrical therapy is selected, it will be provided as a controlled elective procedure. If blood pressure and perfusion are diminished, the choice of drugs or cardioversion and the rapidity of treatment depend on the magnitude of organ compromise. Judgment will dictate how emergent the situation is and how rapidly therapy should be instituted. If blood pressure and perfusion are absent, emergency electrical therapy is indicated.

Dose for synchronized cardioversion is decided based on the hemodynamic status described. Elective cardioversion is performed starting at one-tenth to one-fifth the normal defibrillating dose. Selecting a dose for emergency cardioversion in a pulseless victim is approached as if the victim were being defibrillated. The semi-emergency situation requires judgment as to how much hemodynamic compromise exists and how rapidly the victim is deteriorating. Dose in this situation can range from that for elective cardioversion to defibrillation. Low doses may be ineffective and are doubled on repeat shocks until effective.

Internal defibrillation is provided when the chest cage or

pericardiac sac is open and internal defibrillation paddles are available. Lower energy is required when the paddles are placed directly on the heart. The dose for internal defibrillation is the same as for elective external cardioversion, *i.e.*, one-tenth to one-fifth the dose used for external defibrillation.

INTRAVENOUS THERAPY DURING CPR

Drug and fluid administration, blood sampling, and cardiovascular monitoring all require placement of intravascular catheters. Intravenous, and in some instances, intraarterial, and pulmonary artery cannulation is essential in the precardiac-arrest and postcardiac-arrest period.

In the acute cardiac arrest setting, it may not be possible to adhere to rigid aseptic technique when inserting catheters. Nosocomial infections are a real threat. Any attempts to observe sterile precautions and reduce the number of local or systemic bacteremias produced are worthwhile. In the postarrest period invasive devices introduced during the acute arrest should be evaluated with respect to need for replacement or for treatment of potential infection.

The hollow steel needle and its variant, the butterfly needle, can be used during resuscitation if they are already in place when a cardiac arrest occurs. As soon as possible a needle should be replaced with some form of plastic catheter.

Intravenous catheters can be placed in peripheral or central veins. A catheter placed in a peripheral vein is acceptable for administration of fluids or drugs during CPR. Drugs given *via* these peripheral catheters will circulate and be effective, although the circulation time may be slower during cardiac compression than during normal cardiac output. It is inappropriate to withhold indicated medications for administration through an as-yet unestablished central catheter when a peripheral catheter is operational. Central venous catheters are the preferred route for drug therapy during CPR as this better guarantees that drugs will reach and potentially affect the heart, brain, and kidneys. The preferred route for central venous cannulation is that most familiar to the operator.

The femoral vein has been suggested as the preferred central venous route during CPR, because establishing a catheter in this area does not interfere with airway management and cardiac compression. It may be difficult to identify the femoral vein if a femoral arterial pulse is not palpable. The infection potential in the femoral region must always be kept in mind. The internal jugular, subclavian, and supraclavicular venous routes for central catheter placement are effective, but require knowledge of the cervical and thoracic anatomy. Cannulation of these veins often requires a pause in BCLS.

When intravenous catheters are employed, either a minimal amount of fluid is given to keep the lumen patent for drug administration or large amounts of fluid are given to resuscitate intravascular volume. Choice of fluid depends on the cause of the cardiac arrest. Salt-containing solutions will be avoided in myocardial infarction situations, while salt-containing solutions and other volume expanders are used in hypovolemic settings.

DRUG THERAPY

Initial pharmacologic therapy during CPR is directed at the correction of hypoxemia and acid–base disturbances, and the elevation of coronary and cerebral perfusion pressure during external chest compression. Oxygen, bicarbonate, and epinephrine, when combined with adequate BCLS, serve these purposes and are the mainstays of drug therapy during CPR. These three drugs, in addition to defibrillation, may be used rationally during CPR in the absence of a specific diagnosis (Table 55-6). Other drugs with actions directed at the mechanism of arrest are also used to restore spontaneous circulation. Once spontaneous circulation has been achieved, drugs with specific actions on cardiac rate, rhythm, contractility, and vascular tone may be used to provide a stable cardiac output and blood pressure.

Pharmacology of CPR in the Absence of a Specific Diagnosis (Pharmacology of BCLS)

OXYGEN. A basic critical defect in any patient suffering cardiac arrest, or near-arrest, is a deficiency of oxygen delivery to the myocardium and brain. This deficiency can be the end result of a wide variety of causes such as hypotension secondary to hypovolemia, a low Pa_{O_2} secondary to an obstructed airway, or occlusion of a branch of a coronary artery serving a segment of myocardium. Regardless of the etiology, delivery of oxygen is an essential first management step.

Oxygen is a drug in that it can be administered, titrated, and produce a measurable response. Under the best of circumstances, mouth-to-mouth exhaled-air ventilation can provide a Pa_{O_2} of not more than 80 mm Hg. The low cardiac output generated during CPR and the large degree of venous admixture resulting from atelectasis, pulmonary edema, or aspiration intensify the magnitude of arterial hypoxemia. During resuscitation, 100% oxygen should be administered as soon as available to not only enhance oxygen content and delivery where organ blood flow is less than optimal, but also reverse anaerobic metabolism and repay oxygen debts that have accu-

TABLE 55-6.   Drug Therapy in the Absence of a Diagnosis (Pharmacology of BCLS)

DRUG	DOSE	REMARKS
Oxygen	100%	Never withhold; support ventilation as required
Sodium bicarbonate	1 mEq · kg^{-1} iv Repeat as dictated by pH, or use 0.5 mEq · kg^{-1} every 10 min	Need determined by duration of arrest Do not mix with catecholamines or calcium salts
Epinephrine 1 : 10,000 (100 µg · ml^{-1})	5–10 ml (10 µg · kg^{-1}) iv; 10 ml (1 mg) endotracheal	Repeat dose every 5 min May use peripheral iv if central venous route not available Avoid intracardiac injection

mulated. Ventilation devices used during resuscitation should have the capability to deliver 100% oxygen.

Oxygen should never be withheld for fear that a patient breathing on the basis of hypoxic drive will become apneic. The administration of oxygen is essential to raise the Pa_{O_2}, and if hypoventilation or apnea ensues, assisted or controlled ventilation can be provided.

ACID–BASE THERAPY. The acidemia occurring in the patient in cardiopulmonary arrest is the result of combined respiratory and metabolic acidosis. Ventilatory failure, as a primary event or secondary to hypoperfusion of the respiratory control center in the medulla, results in carbon dioxide retention. At the same time, hypoxia-induced anaerobic metabolism results in the generation of lactic acid.

Carbon dioxide rapidly diffuses into myocardial cells, resulting in intracellular acidosis and depression of contractile performance.[137, 138] The negative inotropic action of hydrogen ions is much slower in onset.[139] Myocardial and vasomotor responsiveness to catecholamines is inhibited during respiratory and metabolic acidosis.[140]

While metabolic acidosis lowers the threshold for induction of ventricular fibrillation it has no effect on the defibrillation threshold.[141, 142] In a study in which arterial pH was shown to be a determinant of successful defibrillation (mean pH values: successful defibrillation, 7.36 ± 0.22 *vs.* unsuccessful defibrillation, 7.23 ± 0.12)[143] the relative contributions of carbon dioxide tension and metabolic acid to the acidemia were unknown. The patients not defibrillated were significantly more hypoxemic than those who were resuscitated. Administration of sodium bicarbonate has not been shown to facilitate ventricular defibrillation or survival in cardiac arrest.[144, 145]

Correction of acidemia is accomplished primarily by ventilation of the lungs that eliminates carbon dioxide and provides oxygen. Effective ventilation, most easily achieved *via* an endotracheal tube and when combined with properly performed chest compression, retards the development of metabolic acidemia. Animal studies have shown that during ventricular fibrillation, when ventilation with 100% oxygen that produces hypocarbia is combined with external chest compression, significant pH depression is delayed, *i.e.*, the pH at 15 min is 7.4 and at 30 min is 7.2.[146] When effective BCLS is instituted immediately following cardiac arrest, significant acidosis is not an immediate problem, and bicarbonate administration is not indicated as an initial pharmacologic intervention.

Carbon dioxide is generated during acid neutralization by bicarbonate ($HCO_3 + H^+ \rightarrow H_2CO_3 \rightarrow H_2O + CO_2$). Thus, when sodium bicarbonate is administered without concomitant effective ventilation, carbon dioxide accumulates and blood pH decreases, thereby exacerbating central venous acidosis.[147–150] Rapid diffusion of carbon dioxide into myocardial cells and across the blood–brain barrier occurs. Because the bicarbonate ion crosses into cells more slowly, a paradoxical intracellular acidosis and cerebrospinal fluid acidosis may occur when arterial blood pH is normal. These disturbances may account for cardiac and cerebral dysfunction after resuscitation. This further emphasizes the need for adequate ventilation in the management of acidemia during cardiopulmonary arrest.

Excessive use of bicarbonate results in hyperosmolality,[151] hypernatremia, and alkalosis. Alkalosis lowers serum potassium levels with a resulting propensity for dysrhythmia. Reduced plasma ionized calcium levels occur, decreasing myocardial contractility. Alkalosis shifts the oxyhemoglobin curve to the left, resulting in impaired tissue oxygen delivery.

The uncertain benefits and significant side-effects that result from the administration of sodium bicarbonate have prompted an ongoing reappraisal of its role in resuscitation. Current recommendations reserve the use of bicarbonate until more definitive and better substantiated resuscitation measures (defibrillation, effective chest compression, tracheal intubation, hyperventilation with 100% oxygen, epinephrine) have been applied. Thereafter, bicarbonate therapy should be directed by a specific diagnosis (*e.g.*, preexisting acidosis, hyperkalemia) or based on arterial blood gas and acid–base determinations. Bicarbonate doses may be calculated from knowledge of the measured base deficit and the patient's extracellular volume of distribution for the bicarbonate ion (approximately, the extracellular fluid volume). Commonly, during resuscitation, the drug is given empirically, 1 mEq $\cdot$ kg^{-1} initially followed by 0.5 mEq $\cdot$ kg^{-1} at 10-min intervals, when metabolic acidemia is suspected.

THAM (tris hydroxy amino methane) has been used in lieu of, and in the same dosage (mg $\cdot$ kg^{-1}) as sodium bicarbonate. THAM has the advantages of being sodium free and not producing carbon dioxide during acid neutralization. Its use is not recommended, however, because its dilution, 0.3 M, requires the administration of large volumes. Extravasation of THAM may lead to skin sloughing, and its use must be restricted to patients receiving controlled ventilation because it is readily transferred intracellularly, thus raising the intracellular pH of ventilatory control neurons in the brain stem leading to apnea.

EPINEPHRINE. During external chest compression the maximal cardiac output is one-third of normal. Pharmacologic maneuvers that increase cardiac output are essential for successful resuscitation. Epinephrine administration increases cerebral and coronary perfusion pressure and blood flow during external chest compression. The improved hemodynamics are associated with greater rates of successful resuscitation in animal models of cardiac arrest due to ventricular fibrillation[152, 153] and asystole.[154–157] Epinephrine is widely accepted as the drug of choice to be administered during cardiac arrest, including those situations in which a specific diagnosis is unknown.

Epinephrine is an endogenous catecholamine with both α- and β-adrenergic actions. The relative benefits of α and β agonists during CPR have been studied in a number of resuscitation models. Results of drug studies in asphyxiated dogs in asystole or EMD, where resumption of spontaneous circulation was the endpoint, strongly support the efficacy of α-adrenergic stimulation[153–157] (Fig. 55-11). Epinephrine, phenylephrine, metaraminol, and methoxamine were equally effective. Beta-receptor stimulation by isoproterenol or dobutamine had little or no beneficial effect in this model.

In an animal model of ventricular fibrillation, administration of epinephrine was more effective than phenylephrine or isoproterenol in increasing blood flow to the brain and heart during CPR.[158] When myocardial blood flow was assessed in a fibrillating heart supported by cardiopulmonary bypass, α-adrenergic effects resulted in an improved perfusion of intramyocardial blood flow.[159] Thus, it is epinephrine's α-adrenergic (α-1 and α-2) effects, and not β-adrenergic actions, that are responsible for the return of spontaneous circulation from asystolic cardiac arrest and that render the fibrillating myocardium more susceptible to defibrillation.[160] The improved perfusion and oxygenation of vital organs result from epinephrine's ability to 1) increase vascular tone, thereby preventing arterial collapse during thoracic compression; and 2) produce peripheral vasoconstriction to elevate aortic blood pressure and limit blood flow to nonvital tissues.[161–163]

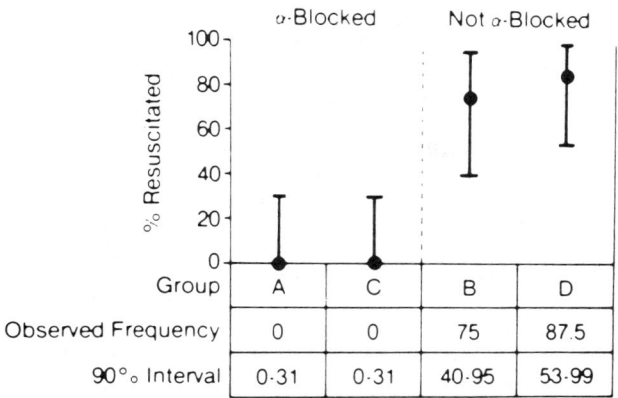

FIG. 55-11. Beneficial effect of α-adrenergic activity on resuscitation. Animals in group A received phenoxybenzamine; group B received propranolol; group C received phenoxybenzamine and propranolol; group D received no drug. The 90% confidence intervals are reported for the sample size and observed resuscitation success. The lack of overlap between the α- and non-α-blocked groups indicates a significant benefit ($P \leq 0.01$) during resuscitation when α-adrenergic activity is intact. (Reproduced with permission from Otto CW, Yakaitis RW, Blitt CO: Mechanism of action of epinephrine in resuscitation from asphyxial arrest. Crit Care Med 9:321, 1981.)

Pure α- adrenergic agonists (*e.g.*, phenylephrine, methoxamine) may have a theoretical advantage over epinephrine during CPR because the desired vascular effects may be obtained without a concomitant increase in myocardial oxygen demand. While these drugs have been shown to be as effective as epinephrine in restoring spontaneous circulation[156, 159, 164, 165] and improving cerebral perfusion,[166] another report indicates that epinephrine produces a greater improvement in coronary perfusion and higher rate of successful resuscitation than achieved by three different doses of methoxamine.[167] The use of α-adrenergic agonists as alternatives to epinephrine during CPR must await more complete evaluation of their efficacy and definition of their dose–response relationships.

The optimal dose of epinephrine to enhance coronary and cerebral perfusion during CPR is unknown. Data from animal studies suggest that improvements in aortic diastolic blood pressure[168] and myocardial blood flow[169] are directly related to epinephrine dose. A ceiling dose may exist, above which further increases in the dose of epinephrine administered do not result in greater improvements in hemodynamics. Epinephrine (15 $\mu g \cdot kg^{-1}$) given to dogs in cardiac arrest did not increase aortic diastolic blood pressure, but doses of ≥ 45 $\mu g \cdot kg^{-1}$, sustained an elevated diastolic pressure for up to 5 min. Myocardial blood flow during CPR was significantly improved in arrested swine treated with epinephrine 200 $\mu g \cdot kg^{-1}$ in contrast to those receiving 20 $\mu g \cdot kg^{-1}$. No further improvement was observed when epinephrine dose was increased to 2 $mg \cdot kg^{-1}$. The currently recommended initial adult dose, 1 mg (approximately 15 $\mu g \cdot kg^{-1}$ for a 70-kg adult) when given intravenously and repeated at 5 min intervals, may not produce the augmentation in perfusion that may be achieved with larger doses. In the near-arrest situation, much smaller doses, as low as 2–4 μg by iv bolus, or infusions initiated at 2–4 $\mu g \cdot min^{-1}$ titrated to the patient's response, may be all that is required.

Ideally, when cardiac output is low, epinephrine should be administered *via* the central venous route to insure delivery.

Effective cardiac massage can circulate drugs from a peripheral venous access site, although the circulation time is delayed. Three other routes can be used. If intravenous access is delayed, epinephrine can be instilled directly into the endotracheal tube. When epinephrine is administered intratracheally to anesthetized dogs[170, 171] or primates[172] with spontaneous circulation or to dogs in cardiac arrest during CPR,[173] peak plasma drug concentration and onset of pressor effect are achieved at a rate comparable to intravenous injection. Plasma drug levels are sustained following endotracheal administration. This reflects gradual intravascular absorption from the airway. Ten times the intravenous dose was administered *via* the endotracheal airway to achieve equivalent hemodynamic effects.[170, 171, 173] However, when equal doses of drug are administered by each route, there is a two-fold to three-fold increase in the pressor response to the intravenous route compared with the endotracheal route.[170] In humans, endotracheal injection produces lower and slightly delayed peak plasma epinephrine concentrations.[174] While it is evident from these findings that a dose larger than that injected intravenously is required to achieve an equivalent hemodynamic action, the dose to be administered *via* tracheal tube has not been established. Drug dilution enhances drug effect after endotracheal administration by reducing the effect of droplet formation in the tracheal tube and promoting peripheral intrapulmonary dispersion.[170, 175] Drugs to be given to the adult *via* the endotracheal route can be diluted in normal saline or sterile water to obtain a volume of injectate of at least 10 ml. Hyperventilation following endotracheal injection will also promote distribution of drugs throughout the lung. Lidocaine, isoproterenol, atropine, propranolol, and naloxone have also been administered by endotracheal route.

Intraosseous administration of fluids and drugs, including epinephrine, is advocated for temporary use in pediatric patients when intravenous access cannot be achieved.[176] The anterior surface of the tibia below the tibial tuberosity is pierced with a needle sized 18-gauge or larger. Crystalloid solutions, blood, catecholamines, lidocaine, atropine, calcium, bicarbonate, digitalis, morphine,and insulin have been delivered *via* this route. Gravity-driven or pressurized infusion systems attached to the needle are used to flush the drug into the marrow cavity. The rate of onset and dose–response obtained *via* the intraosseous route are comparable to peripheral venous injection.

The least desirable route for administration of epinephrine, or any drug during CPR is transthoracic intracardiac injection. While direct intracardiac injection has been employed, often with success, blind transthoracic intracardiac injection is currently recommended as a low-priority procedure due to the availability of other safer techniques of drug administration and the recognition of the many complications associated with its use. Cardiac muscle and coronary artery laceration, pneumohemopericardium, pneumothorax, and intramyocardial deposition of a potent vasoactive or cardioactive drug are all possible when a needle is blindly inserted into the chest and heart. When an intravenous, endotracheal, or intraosseous route is not available, intracardiac injection may be the only alternative.

Pharmacology of ACLS

Once the etiology of the cardiac arrest has been established, specific drugs may be used in ACLS for specific indications in addition to those common to all CPR efforts (Table 55-7). Antidysrhythmic drugs, for example, may facilitate cardioversion of tachydysrhythmias. Once resuscitation is successful, other drugs are used to stabilize the circulation by increasing heart rate, controlling cardiac rhythm, improving myocardial contractility, or altering vascular tone.

CHRONOTROPIC DRUGS. ATROPINE. The cardiac effects of atropine include acceleration of sinus node discharge and improvement of AV conduction resulting from competitive antagonism of cardiac muscarinic receptors. Atropine, in doses of 0.3–0.5 mg intravenously, is indicated in the treatment of severe sinus or nodal bradycardia when accompanied by hypotension or frequent ventricular escape beats. In higher doses, atropine may be effective in treating high-degree AV block at the nodal level, pulseless idioventricular rhythm, and ventricular asystole.[177] While the use of atropine in the treatment of cardiac arrest from asystole improves the likelihood of immediate resuscitation, it has not increased the rate of survival to hospital discharge.[178–180] In cardiac arrest, atropine 1 mg is injected intravenously or 1–2 mg diluted in 10 ml of saline or sterile water is instilled endotracheally. Under usual circumstances, no further chronotropic effect will be seen from a total intravenous dose exceeding 2 mg. There is evidence that this is a complete vagolytic dose in humans.[181]

In the prearrest setting, cautious administration of atropine in the presence of myocardial ischemia is recommended to avoid tachycardia, which increases myocardial oxygen demand and may precipitate myocardial ischemia. Ventricular tachycardia and ventricular fibrillation have occurred following intravenous atropine administration.

ISOPROTERENOL. Isoproterenol is a sympathetic amine with a pure β-adrenergic action, resulting in increased heart rate and contractility and decreased peripheral vascular resistance. The price paid for these effects is an increase in myocardial oxygen demand. The usefulness of isoproterenol in emergency cardiac care is limited to the treatment of hemodynamically significant atropine-refractory bradycardias.

Because tachydysrhythmias and myocardial ischemia may occur, careful titration of the isoproterenol infusion, starting with doses of 2 μg·min^{-1}, is recommended. Isoproterenol is not indicated in the pulseless patient in cardiac arrest because it induces peripheral vasodilation. Epinephrine is preferable to isoproterenol during resuscitation from asystole and EMD because it produces peripheral vasoconstriction and is more likely to maintain a higher coronary perfusion pressure during chest compression and result in a higher frequency of successful resuscitation.[156, 157, 182]

Electrical pacing should be instituted as soon as available in lieu of isoproterenol in the treatment of severe bradycardia. Pacing provides better heart rate control without an inordinate increase in myocardial oxygen consumption.

ANTIDYSRHYTHMIC DRUGS. LIDOCAINE. Lidocaine suppresses dysrhythmias of ventricular origin and may act by decreasing automaticity, elevating the fibrillation threshold, and by terminating reentrant mechanisms. In addition to the treatment of existing ventricular ectopy, it has been recommended that prophylactic lidocaine be given to the prearrest myocardial infarction patient.[183, 184] Lidocaine lowers the incidence of primary ventricular fibrillation in patients with acute myocardial infarction.[185–187] The drug is also used in the treatment of ventricular fibrillation and ventricular tachycardia refractory to initial countershock therapy. Lidocaine and bretylium are equally effective in this regard;[188, 189] however, lidocaine's faster onset of peak effect makes it the preferred drug.

The pharmacokinetics of lidocaine in patients in cardiac arrest are not well understood, but data in animals suggest

high plasma drug levels are achieved and maintained as a result of the low cardiac output seen during CPR.[190] During cardiac arrest, lidocaine should be given by intermittent intravenous bolus only. Initially, 1 mg·kg^{-1} may be injected, followed by injections of 0.5 mg·kg^{-1} every 8–10 min, if needed, to a total dose of 3 mg·kg^{-1}. After termination of ventricular fibrillation or ventricular tachycardia, a continuous infusion of 30–50 μg·kg^{-1}·min^{-1} (approximately 2–4 mg·min^{-1} for the average adult) should be maintained for at least 24 h.

The pharmacokinetics of intravenous lidocaine in the nonarrested human have been studied extensively.[191–193] To achieve therapeutic blood levels (1.5–6 μg·ml^{-1}) in view of the short half-life (8 min) of lidocaine, a bolus of 1 mg·kg^{-1} must be followed by an infusion of 2–4 mg·min^{-1}. Additional 0.5 mg·kg^{-1} boluses at 8–10-min intervals may be given up to a total loading dose of 225 mg if ventricular ectopy persists.

Lidocaine dosage should be reduced by 50% for patients with congestive heart failure, impaired hepatic function, reduced hepatic blood flow (e.g., shock) and advanced age. Lidocaine levels higher than 9 μg·ml^{-1} are likely to be associated with clinical toxicity, usually confined to the CNS. CNS symptoms vary from drowsiness or disorientation to grand mal or focal seizures. In therapeutic doses, lidocaine has minimal effects on myocardial contractility, AV or intraventricular conduction, and systemic blood pressure. Lidocaine should be used with caution, however, in patients with known disorders of the conduction system. Administration of lidocaine during complete AV block may result in ventricular arrest.

PROCAINAMIDE. Procainamide, like lidocaine, is an amide-type local anesthetic that suppresses dysrhythmias of ventricular origin. Unlike lidocaine, procainamide undergoes hydrolysis by plasma esterases. This permits, with relative safety, mixing the two drugs in the same patient in rapid succession. Procainamide has been known to be safe and effective in patients with acute myocardial infarction whose ventricular ectopy was not controlled by lidocaine. Procainamide is rarely used in the treatment of cardiac arrest due to ventricular fibrillation or ventricular tachycardia because it produces vasodilation and requires a long duration to achieve effective plasma drug levels.

Complications following administration of procainamide include conduction disturbances, hypotension from depression of cardiac contractility, and peripheral vasodilation. Procainamide administration is guided by blood pressure and ECG monitoring. Adverse ECG effects include widening of the QRS complex by 50% of its original width and lengthening of the PR and QT intervals. The drug is given in 100-mg divided intravenous boluses every 5 min, or as an intravenous infusion of 20 mg·min^{-1}, until the dysrhythmia is suppressed, hypotension or ECG toxicity occurs, or a total of 1 g of drug has been injected.[194] Maintenance infusion rates of 1–4 mg·min^{-1} are used to achieve therapeutic levels of 4–10 μg·ml^{-1}. Alternatively, a loading dose of 17 mg·kg^{-1} is infused over 1 h, followed by a maintenance infusion of 2.8 mg·kg^{-1}·h^{-1}.[195] In the patient with cardiac failure, the loading dose is reduced to 12 mg·kg^{-1}. The maintenance dose is lowered to 1.4 mg·kg^{-1}·h^{-1} in the presence of severely impaired cardiac or renal function.

BRETYLIUM. Bretylium is an antidysrhythmic drug with both autonomic nervous system and membrane-active effects. The autonomic nervous system effects of bretylium are biphasic: an initial transient increase in heart rate and arterial pressure due to release of norepinephrine from the adrenergic nerve terminal is followed by a decrease in pressure and pulse rate while cardiac output remains unchanged. The subsequent decline in arterial blood pressure is due to blockade of norepinephrine release from peripheral postganglionic adrenergic nerve terminals. The final autonomic effect of bretylium is blockade of the adrenergic terminal reuptake mechanism.

The membrane effects of the drug are less completely understood. Bretylium is known to elevate the fibrillation threshold[196] and reduce the disparity in action potential durations and refractory periods between normal and infarcted cardiac muscle, thereby reducing the ability for reentry dysrhythmias to occur.[197]

Bretylium is used in refractory or recurrent ventricular fibrillation and ventricular tachycardia when countershock and first-line antidysrhythmic therapy have not controlled the rhythm disturbance. In cardiac arrest due to ventricular fibrillation or ventricular tachycardia, $5-10 \text{ mg} \cdot \text{kg}^{-1}$ bretylium is given intravenously and defibrillation attempted again. If the dysrhythmia persists in spite of this dose and countershock, additional doses of $10 \text{ mg} \cdot \text{kg}^{-1}$ can be repeated every $15-30$ min up to a total dose of $30 \text{ mg} \cdot \text{kg}^{-1}$. Ten to fifteen minutes may be required after administration to permit bretylium to be maximally effective and allow successful defibrillation. In recurrent ventricular tachycardia with pulse, $5-10 \text{ mg} \cdot \text{kg}^{-1}$ is injected intravenously over a period of $8-10$ min. A second dose of $5-10 \text{ mg} \cdot \text{kg}^{-1}$ can be given in $1-2$ h and, if necessary, the same repeated every $6-8$ h. Alternatively, the drug can be administered as a continuous infusion at a rate of $1-2 \text{ mg} \cdot \text{min}^{-1}$. Following administration of bretylium to a patient with an effective cardiac rhythm, the initial release of norepinephrine may lead to an increase in blood pressure and pulse rate and a transient exacerbation of some dysrhythmias.

The major side-effects of bretylium are nausea, vomiting, and postural hypotension. Hypotension is more likely following rapid infusion and closely spaced additional doses. Because the decrease in blood pressure is usually small, and related to vasodilation due to peripheral adrenergic blockade rather than depressed cardiac function, the hypotension is responsive to placing the patient in the recumbent position and administering fluids. If vasopressors are used, they should be given cautiously to avoid exaggerated responses in these patients with blockade of the adrenergic reuptake mechanism.

VERAPAMIL. The calcium ion plays an important role in the production of both the cardiac action potential and the myocardial contractile state. AV conduction is primarily dependent on slow-channel calcium influx rather than sodium movement. The clinical effects of verapamil, a slow-channel blocking drug, are a result of the inhibition of the inward flux of calcium ions into cardiac tissue and vascular smooth muscle. By blocking calcium influx to the cardiac contractile mechanism, verapamil exerts a direct depressant effect on the inotropic state and, therefore, myocardial oxygen requirement. It reduces contractile tone in vascular smooth muscle, resulting in coronary and peripheral vasodilation. The antidysrhythmic action of verapamil is the result of slowing conduction and prolonging the refractory period in the AV node.

In emergency cardiac care, verapamil is used primarily in the treatment of paroxysmal supraventricular tachydysrhythmias that do not require electrical cardioversion but compromise cardiac output or increase myocardial oxygen demand. The drug is highly effective in the treatment of paroxysmal supraventricular tachycardia, most commonly an AV nodal reentrant dysrhythmia, where the incidence of suc-

cessful termination approaches 90%.[198, 199] The drug is also useful in slowing the ventricular response to atrial flutter and atrial fibrillation. Verapamil should be used cautiously, if at all, in patients with Wolff-Parkinson-White syndrome and atrial fibrillation or paroxysmal supraventricular tachycardia because dysrhythmias may be accelerated or ventricular fibrillation may result.[200-202]

The dose of intravenous verapamil for adults is $0.075-0.15 \text{ mg} \cdot \text{kg}^{-1}$ (maximum 10 mg) administered over several min (children $0.1-0.3 \text{ mg} \cdot \text{kg}^{-1}$). Effects are seen within $3-5$ min of a bolus injection. The dose may be repeated in 30 min if the initial response is inadequate. Arterial blood pressure may decrease transiently following injection of the drug due to the effects on peripheral vascular resistance. In patients with normal cardiac function, the vasodilator action compensates for the negative inotropic effect, and cardiac output is maintained. In patients with severe left ventricular dysfunction, however, intravenous verapamil has produced congestive heart failure. Verapamil should be avoided or given cautiously with concomitantly administered β-adrenergic blocking drugs and in patients with sick sinus syndrome, AV block, and decompensated cardiac failure. The drug has been used safely and effectively in patients on digitalis therapy.

BETA-ADRENERGIC RECEPTOR BLOCKING DRUGS. These drugs available for intravenous injection are propranolol, metoprolol, and esmolol. These drugs have little place in resuscitation from cardiac arrest but may be useful for control of recurrent ventricular tachycardia, ventricular fibrillation, and supraventricular tachydysrhythmias refractory to first-line therapy.

INOTROPES. EPINEPHRINE. Epinephrine, a major drug in this class, has been discussed earlier.

CALCIUM. Calcium ions increase myocardial contractile force, prolong duration of systole, increase vascular tone, and enhance ventricular automaticity. Based on these actions, calcium has been used to restore cardiac output during cardiac arrest caused by EMD and to generate electrical rhythm in cases of ventricular asystole. Anecdotal observations from CPR situations and an apparent beneficial effect in patients during cardiac surgery had positioned calcium therapy into the standard resuscitation protocols; however, there is no reported evidence that calcium administration is beneficial in asystolic cardiac arrest[203-205] and data are inconclusive regarding its efficacy in instances of EMD.[205-207] To the contrary are reports of dangerously elevated plasma calcium levels following boluses of intravenous calcium chloride in accordance with previous AHA recommendations.[208, 209] In addition, the effective use of calcium antagonists in patients with ischemic heart disease suggests that the administration of calcium to the ischemic heart during cardiac arrest may be detrimental. Calcium therapy may precipitate myocardial ischemia by elevating myocardial oxygen demand and increasing coronary vascular resistance.

While the role of calcium in the acute management of cardiac arrest is questionable, the drug is clearly beneficial in many near-arrest situations in which hypotension occurs with low serum ionized calcium levels. Hypocalcemia may develop following rapid transfusion of citrated blood or large volumes of colloid solutions and in critically ill septic or burned patients. The low ionized calcium levels are readily corrected and blood pressure restored by the administration of intravenous calcium. Calcium may be useful when cardiac arrest occurs in the setting of hypocalcemia, acute hyperkalemia, and calcium channel blocker toxicity.

Calcium chloride is the salt of the calcium ion preferred during resuscitation because it has been shown to produce higher and more predictable levels of ionized calcium than the gluconate or gluceptate salts.[210] Calcium chloride (10 ml of 10%) contains 13.6 mEq calcium. In contrast, calcium gluconate (10 ml of 10%) contains 4.6 mEq calcium. Calcium chloride 10% may be administered in a bolus of 5–10 mg·kg^{-1}. The dose may be repeated at 10-min intervals in view of the rapid decrease in ionized calcium levels following bolus administration. Injection of calcium chloride into a peripheral vein may cause intense local reaction, including skin slough. The local reaction is not a problem with the gluconate or gluceptate preparations. Administration of the chloride salt through a central venous catheter is preferred, but when calcium administration is indicated and only the chloride preparation is available, this should be injected into the first established intravenous catheter, even if that is peripherally located.

While the calcium ion may enhance ventricular automaticity, when injected rapidly it may slow sinus node impulse formation and result in bradycardia. Administration of calcium to a patient receiving digitalis may produce signs of digitalis toxicity, which usually can be treated with administration of potassium chloride. Care must be taken to see that calcium and bicarbonate are not simultaneously injected into the intravenous catheter because they will form an insoluble precipitate.

DOPAMINE, DOBUTAMINE, AND AMRINONE. These drugs (Table 55-7) are inotropic drugs used primarily in the near-arrest or postresuscitation situation to treat hypotension resulting from low cardiac output. These drugs are not commonly employed during initial resuscitation from cardiac arrest although dopamine in high doses mimics epinephrine and produces peripheral vasoconstriction, augments coronary perfusion, and improves resuscitatibility.[153] Dobutamine and amrinone cause peripheral vasodilation and should not be administered during resuscitation from cardiac arrest.

VASOPRESSORS. The α-adrenergic activity of epinephrine and dopamine places these drugs in this category.

Norepinephrine is a naturally occurring catecholamine with α- and β-adrenergic receptor activity. Its strong α-adrenergic effects increase peripheral vascular resistance. Blood pressure is elevated as a result of the increase in peripheral vascular resistance and the β-adrenergic-mediated positive inotropic effect. Effects on cardiac output are variable and depend on the functional state of the left ventricle, the extent of increase in peripheral vascular resistance, and the degree of carotid baroreceptor-mediated cardiac slowing. In cases of significant hypotension, regardless of etiology, norepinephrine will increase coronary and cerebral blood flow by increasing perfusion pressure, at the expense of splanchnic and renal blood flow.

Norepinephrine is indicated for transient use in the treatment of hemodynamically significant hypotension in near-arrest situations when peripheral vascular resistance is known to be low. Two precautions are essential in the use of norepinephrine. First, administration should be *via* a central vein because necrosis and tissue sloughing may result if extravasation from a peripheral vein occurs. Phentolamine, 5–10 mg in 10–15 ml of saline, should be infiltrated into an area of extravasation as soon as possible to reduce the amount of tissue injury. Second, measurement of blood pressure in the presence of intense vasoconstriction may be difficult. The precaution may apply to peripherally placed intraarterial lines as well as to detection of Korotkoff sounds.

VASODILATORS. The short-acting vasodilators, sodium nitroprusside, nitroglycerin, and trimethaphan (Table 55-7), have no place in the arrest situation, but may be useful in peri-resuscitation periods. Following resuscitation, vasodilators may be used to control hypertension, treat pulmonary edema, increase cardiac output by unloading the decompensated left ventricle, and reduce myocardial oxygen demand by lowering ventricular volume and pressure. Like nitroglycerin, morphine exerts its beneficial effects in the settings of angina pectoris and pulmonary edema by dilating venous capacitance beds and reducing venous return to the thorax and ultimately to the heart.

INVASIVE THERAPEUTIC TECHNIQUES DURING CPR

Cardiac pacing, pericardiocentesis, and treatment of tension pneumothorax are invasive procedures that may be life saving during CPR.

Cardiac Pacing

Bradydysrhythmias and asystole are associated with diminished or absent cardiac output. Rhythmic electrical stimulation of the heart with a pacing catheter is indicated in these situations to restore a more normal heart rate and perfusion. Prophylactic insertion of pacing catheters is also indicated in certain instances of myocardial infarction likely to be associated with bradycardia and heart block. Occasionally, a pacing catheter is used to override a tachycardia. Overdrive pacing, a paced rate more rapid than the dysrhythmia, may control impulse generation and allow subsequent slowing of the rate with elimination of the dysrhythmia.

External thoracic pacing devices are occasionally used; however, the most reliable method for cardiac pacing is use of an internal pacing electrode. A central venous insertion route is required through which a pacing catheter is positioned in the right heart, *i.e.*, right atrium, coronary sinus, or right ventricle. Heart block, in which conduction of the electrical impulse from atrium to ventricle is absent, requires placement of the electrode in the right ventricle. A pacing catheter or other catheter with pacing capability, such as pacing pulmonary artery catheter, may be used. A pulse generator is connected to the properly positioned pacing electrode. Amperage, rate, and fixed *versus* demand pacing mode are set according to the rhythm disturbance and its consequences on the hemodynamics of the patient.

Pericardiocentesis

The pericardial sac is a relatively fixed space containing the heart, and a small amount of pericardial fluid. Blood added to the pericardial fluid can be accommodated up to the compliance limits of the pericardial sac. When the contents of the sac (cardiac volume, pericardial fluid, and blood) exceed this limit, increased pressure within the sac results. A traumatic cardiac injury allows blood to enter the pericardial space and compress the heart. Diminished diastolic filling and cardiac output result from increased volume and pressure within the sac. A slow accumulation of pericardial fluid is compensated for, and 800–1200 ml may be tolerated with minimal impairment of cardiac output. Rapid accumulation of pericardial

TABLE 55-7. Drug Therapy for ACLS

DRUG	DOSE	INFUSION RATE	REMARKS
CHRONOTROPES			
Atropine sulfate	0.3–1 mg iv or endotracheal		Total dose 2 mg
Isoproterenol		2–$20\ \mu g \cdot min^{-1}$ Titrate to effect	Beware of tachydysrhythmias and myocardial ischemia
ANTIDYSRHYTHMICS			
Lidocaine	$1\ mg \cdot kg^{-1}$ iv or endotracheal Repeat $0.5\ mg \cdot kg^{-1}$ every 10 min as needed to total dose 225 mg	2–$4\ mg \cdot min^{-1}$ Titrate	Use with caution in presence of high-grade AV block
Procainamide	100 mg iv Repeat every 5 min to total dose 1 g	$20\ mg \cdot min^{-1}$ for loading infusion Titrate 1–$4\ mg \cdot min^{-1}$ for maintenance infusion	Beware of hypotension and ECG toxicity
Bretylium tosylate	5–$10\ mg \cdot kg^{-1}$ iv Repeat dose every 15–30 min as needed to total dose $30\ mg \cdot kg^{-1}$	1–$2\ mg \cdot min^{-1}$	Beware of postural hypotension
Propranolol	0.1–1 mg iv Titrate cautiously as needed to total dose $0.1\ mg \cdot kg^{-1}$		Beware of heart failure, bradydysrhythmias, and bronchospasm
Verapamil	0.075–0.15 mg iv (maximum 10 mg) Repeat dose in 30 min as needed		Beware of hypotension; use with caution in presence of beta blockade, supraventricular conduction disease, heart failure
INOTROPES			
Dopamine		Initial rate 2–$5\ \mu g \cdot kg^{-1} \cdot min^{-1}$ Titrate to effect	Beware of tachydysrhythmias and myocardial ischemia; Vasoconstrictor at $20\ \mu g \cdot kg^{-1} \cdot min^{-1}$
Dobutamine		Initial rate 2–$5\ \mu g \cdot kg^{-1} \cdot min^{-1}$ Titrate to effect	Beware of tachydysrhythmias and myocardial ischemia Vasoconstrictor at $20\ \mu g \cdot kg^{-1} \cdot min^{-1}$
Epinephrine	10–$15\ \mu g \cdot kg^{-1}$ for arrest situation 2–4 μg iv for near arrest situation	Initial rate 2–$4\ \mu g \cdot min^{-1}$ Titrate to effect	Beware of tachydysrhythmias and myocardial ischemia
Calcium chloride 10%	5–$10\ mg \cdot kg^{-1}$ iv Repeat dose every 10 min as needed		Central venous route
VASOPRESSORS			
Norepinephrine		Initial rate 0.1–$0.5\ \mu g \cdot kg^{-1} \cdot min^{-1}$ Titrate to effect	Central venous route
VASODILATORS			
Sodium nitroprusside	50–100 μg iv	Initial rate $0.5\ \mu g \cdot kg^{-1} \cdot min^{-1}$ Titrate to effect Maximum rate $8\ \mu g \cdot kg^{-1} \cdot min^{-1}$	Beware of cyanide toxicity
Trimethaphan	1–2 mg iv	Initial rate 1–$2\ mg \cdot min^{-1}$ Titrate to effect	
Nitroglycerin	50–100 μg iv	Initial rate $0.5\ \mu g \cdot kg^{-1} \cdot min^{-1}$ Titrate to effect	

fluid, however, is poorly tolerated, and as little as 150–300 ml may cause cardiac compression and marked hypotension. The process is rapidly reversible by acute removal of pericardial fluid.

Subxyphoid insertion of a spinal needle, guided by attachment to and monitoring of the ECG, allows safe withdrawal of pericardial fluid. After the acute removal of fluid and stabilization of the hemodynamic status, it may be desirable to insert a continuously draining pericardial catheter or create an open pericardial window for drainage. The major disadvantage of pericardiocentesis is that associated with transthoracic needle insertion into the heart.

Decompression of a Tension Pneumothorax

Air can accumulate within the pleural space as a result of pulmonary rupture and air leak from the lung or a break in the integrity of the thoracic wall and air leak from the atmosphere into the chest. This tension pneumothorax not only compromises alveolar gas exchange, but by its mediastinal shift, compromises venous return to the heart and ultimately cardiac output.

Emergency treatment of a tension pneumothorax requires converting it to an open, simple pneumothorax. A large-bore needle or catheter over needle is inserted into the second or third intercostal space in the anterior chest wall. Insertion at the midclavicular line and no further medially avoids internal mammary artery puncture. Insertion of the needle over the top of the rib avoids intercostal artery puncture. A gush of air indicates that tension has been relieved and hemodynamic stability should rapidly return. Intravenous extension tubing can be attached to the needle or catheter, and an underwater seal provided with a cup partly filled with water. Subsequently, a standard chest tube can be inserted electively.

SPECIAL SITUATIONS IN CPR

MONITORED (WITNESSED) ARREST

A number of therapeutic maneuvers may be considered in the management of witnessed cardiac arrest prior to initiation of the standard recommended CPR sequence. These include cough-CPR, precordial thump, and empiric defibrillation in the absence of an ECG tracing.

Cough CPR may be initiated by those patients previously trained in its performance (Fig. 55-12). Cough CPR occurs when a conscious individual who has a cardiac rhythm that would normally not support adequate cardiac output (*e.g.*, ventricular fibrillation) is able to maintain needed perfusion by repetitive coughing with diaphragmatic motion creating a thoracic pump (see Artificial Circulation During CPR: Mechanisms of Blood Flow). If instituted within seconds of a cardiac arrest, prior to unconsciousness, cough CPR may maintain arterial blood pressure and consciousness for a short period of time. This form of self-administered thoracic compression provides temporary coronary perfusion and may shorten the ischemic interval preceding the delivery of ACLS, rendering definitive care more successful.

The precordial thump consists of a single sharp blow delivered to the midportion of the sternum with the fist from a height of 20–30 cm above the patient's chest.[211] The role of the precordial thump in CPR continues to be a controversial matter. There is clinical experimental evidence that one precordial thump can convert sudden ventricular tachycardia to normal sinus rhythm. In early phases of complete heart block with ventricular asystole, repetitive thumping (fist pacing) may produce a QRS complex and cardiac contraction, which may serve to maintain perfusion until drug therapy or a pacemaker is available. It is questionable, however, whether the electrical current produced in the heart by the precordial thump is of sufficient magnitude to terminate ventricular fibrillation. Indeed, the thump applied to a patient in any rhythm other than ventricular fibrillation may unexpectedly induce ventricular fibrillation.

Currently, the precordial thump is recommended for use in only two monitored arrest settings:

1. At the onset of ventricular tachycardia or ventricular fibrillation in an attempt to convert the heart to normal sinus rhythm
2. At the onset of ventricular asystole due to heart block where rhythmic thumps produce myocardial contraction—BCLS should be instituted if thumping fails to produce a pulse

The thump cannot be expected to generate cardiac contraction in anoxic asystole, nor to cardiovert a long-standing ventricular fibrillation. A single thump delivered quickly will not significantly delay the institution of subsequent BCLS and ACLS. The precordial thump is not recommended in pediatric patients.

The earliest possible delivery of definitive care, particularly defibrillation, has been demonstrated to be crucial to the successful resuscitation of patients from cardiac arrest. In the case of monitored arrest where a defibrillator is available, immediate defibrillation or synchronized cardioversion should be attempted simultaneously with BCLS and without delay for venous access. Such early defibrillation is likely to be effective as long as the heart remains oxygenated, *i.e.*, approximately 30–60 s after the onset of pulselessness. If three countershocks in rapid succession are not successful, BCLS and ACLS should be initiated (see Defibrillation).

When cardiac arrest occurs in the absence of ECG monitoring but a defibrillator is available, empiric "blind" defibrillation may be successful. The basis of blind defibrillation stems from the likelihood of the dysrhythmia being ventricular fibrillation and the importance of early defibrillation for successful resuscitation from ventricular fibrillation. Defibrillation of an asystolic heart will do little harm and does not preclude subsequent definitive care. Defibrillation of ventricular tachycardia or other supraventricular dysrhythmias as opposed to synchronized cardioversion may restore an effective rhythm or produce ventricular fibrillation. If the latter occurs, defibrillation can be immediately repeated.

EXSANGUINATION CARDIAC ARREST

Exsanguination reduces venous return to the chest and precludes effective closed- or open-chest cardiac compression. Artificial circulation requires the restoration of intravascular volume. Successful resuscitation from exsanguination necessitates control of hemorrhage and massive infusion of fluid instituted simultaneously with BCLS. Hemorrhage may be controlled by tourniquet, by direct compression of external wound, or by MAST garment in instances of intraabdominal, pelvic, or lower-extremity bleeding. Uncontrolled intraabdominal hemorrhage may require laparotomy or thoracotomy with clamping of the descending thoracic aorta to gain proximal control. Rapid replacement of intravascular volume through large-bore intravenous catheters with the most immediately available plasma substitute should continue until cardiac compression generates an adequate pulse. The α-adrenergic-mediated vasoconstriction action of epinephrine will temporarily enhance venous return and augment coronary perfusion pressure during fluid resuscitation and cardiac compression. While sufficient vascular volume is being restored in conjunction with the provision of effective BCLS to provide coronary perfusion, ECG monitoring, defibrillation, and appropriate drug therapy are instituted to restore spontaneous circulation. Intraarterial and central venous catheters may be inserted to facilitate further volume replacement. In the setting of thoracoabdominal trauma, difficulty generating a reasonable cardiac output despite massive volume infusion and properly performed cardiac compression suggests the presence of cardiac tamponade, myocardial rupture, injury to the great vessels, or tension pneumothorax. Under these situations it is essential to open the thoracic cavity to make the diagnosis and initiate therapy.

DROWNING AND NEAR-DROWNING

The primary pathophysiologic consequence of drowning is hypoxia resulting initially from asphyxiation due to submersion, and secondarily, from the pulmonary edema that occurs in 75% of near-drowning victims. Pulmonary edema is induced by the aspiration of both salt and fresh water.

Establishing effective ventilation and oxygenation is the primary goal of the initial rescue effort. When attempting to rescue a near-drowning victim, a rescuer must, above all, avoid becoming a second victim. It is important to reach the victim with some conveyance or flotation device. Because outcome is primarily determined by the duration of asphyxia, rescue breathing should be initiated in the water in preference to efforts aimed exclusively at getting the victim out of the water. Mouth-to-mouth ventilation is difficult to perform in deep water unless the rescuer has a type of flotation device,

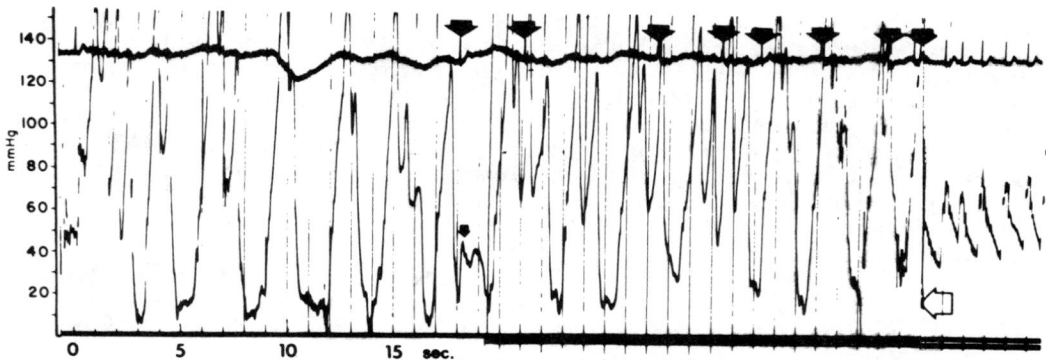

FIG. 55-12. Aortic pressure trace of the effective production of cardiac output in the absence of cardiac rhythm, using cough CPR during prolonged ventricular asystole after coronary arteriographic injection. An 18-s period of asystole after a right coronary arteriographic injection is depicted. During this period, the patient coughed every 2 s, generating peak aortic pressures of over 140 mm Hg. *Large arrows* mark the intrinsic QRS complexes after the 18-s period of asystole and the *small arrow*, the resultant aortic pressure from the first intrinsic beat. The patient continued to cough until the cardiac rhythm stabilized 40 s later. (Reproduced with permission from Niemann JT, Rosborough J, Hausknecht M *et al:* Cough-CPR. Crit Care Med 8:141, 1980.)

but can be initiated once shallower depths allow the rescuer to stand.

In drowning, BCLS should be performed according to the usual protocol. The victim's airway should be cleared of water and vomitus. Rolling the victim onto the side will permit passive drainage of water from the pharynx and trachea. Humans do not inhale large volumes of water as they drown. It is unusual to aspirate more than 200 ml during submersion, and 10–15% of victims are shown at autopsy to have inhaled no water at all.[212] Large volumes of water, however, are swallowed, contributing to the high incidence of regurgitation occurring during resuscitation. Manual attempts to drain fluid from the victim's tracheobronchial tree, *e.g.*, epigastric compression and the Heimlich maneuver, have been recommended by some, but should be discouraged because these maneuvers contribute to the risk of regurgitation and aspiration and delay the initiation of CPR. Airway obstruction during resuscitation from drowning is more likely to result from the aspiration of vomitus or sand. Cervical spine injury should be suspected following diving into shallow water. These victims require appropriate care to maintain cervical stability during removal from the water and airway management.

Drowning consists of a primary ventilatory arrest followed by secondary cardiac arrest. Circulation continues many minutes following cessation of breathing; therefore, the brain continues to be perfused in the apneic victim. During this time, the brain is somewhat protected by the reduced cerebral metabolic demands following unconsciousness, hypothermia in cold water, and possibly by the effects of the diving reflex. It is important that rescuers recognize that cardiac activity may be present in victims after long periods of submersion and the palpation of the pulse may be difficult due to bradycardia, hypotension, and peripheral vasoconstriction. Inappropriate initiation of chest compression may interfere with the victim's own cardiac output, and may precipitate ventricular fibrillation in the hypothermic asphyxiated individual.

Near-drowning victims may recover completely despite extended periods under water, often exceeding 4–5 min, the commonly accepted upper limit for cerebral survival. In 57 reported episodes of near-drowning, average submersion time for survivors was more than 11 min, and for one child, as long as 40 min.[213] The temporary preservation of cerebral perfusion and reduced cerebral metabolic rate account for the reports of successful outcome after prolonged periods of submersion in cold water. Persistent efforts at the resuscitation of drowning victims are indicated despite documented submersion of 30 min or more.

ACCIDENTAL HYPOTHERMIA

Hypothermia is defined as a core body temperature less than 35° C. Mild hypothermia, core temperature between 30 and 35° C, is characterized by shivering, lethargy, increases in heart rate and blood pressure, peripheral vasoconstriction, and hyperventilation.[214, 215]

Moderate to severe hypothermia occurs when body temperature falls below 30° C. Coma, hyporeflexia, dilated pupils, bradycardia, cardiac dysrhythmias, hypotension, hypoventilation, and marked vasoconstriction result. The risk of ventricular fibrillation or asystole, the usual causes of death from hypothermia, increases as the temperature decreases below 28° C. Metabolic acidosis occurs due to decreased hepatic perfusion and increased lactate production emanating from poorly perfused and anaerobically active shivering skeletal muscle.

Vasoconstriction occurs to conserve core temperature. This makes the detection of pulse and blood pressure quite difficult. The hypothermic patient may appear dead. The only way the potential viability of the apparently pulseless hypothermic patient may be established is to attempt active rewarming and resuscitation.

The moderately to severely hypothermic patient with spontaneous circulation should be monitored closely because of the risk of serious cardiac dysrhythmia. Intravenous access and oxygen should be provided. Tracheal intubation may be necessary to correct hypercarbia or hypoxemia, or to protect the airway. External warming devices, *e.g.*, blankets or hot water bottles, are ineffective when hypothermia and vasoconstriction are marked. Core rewarming is accomplished using warmed intravenous fluids, ventilation of the lungs with heated humidified oxygen, and warm lavage of the stomach or urinary bladder.

If cardiac arrest occurs, routine ACLS maneuvers should be

attempted. The hypothermic heart may be unresponsive to cardioactive drugs, pacing and defibrillation until the core temperature is raised. If definitive resuscitation efforts are unsuccessful, BCLS should be continued while a combination of techniques are employed to rewarm the core rapidly, with periodic attempts at definitive therapy as the temperature rises. Open-chest cardiac massage with warmed pericardial lavage,[216] peritoneal lavage,[217] and cardiopulmonary bypass[216] have been used successfully to treat patients with hypothermic cardiac arrest.

ELECTROCUTION

Cardiac arrest due to ventricular fibrillation, ventricular tachycardia, or asystole may occur as a direct result of electric shock. Prolonged apnea may follow electrocution and result in secondary asphyxial cardiac arrest. In attempting to rescue the victim of electric shock, it is imperative that the rescuer not be placed in danger of electrocution, becoming a second victim. If the victim remains in contact with the current source, attempts should be made to shut it off. Otherwise, the victim should be dislodged from the energized source using a nonconductive implement. BCLS and ACLS should then be instituted in the usual manner. Tetanic muscle spasm occurring during current exposure may have resulted in long bone or vertebral fractures. Electric shock can also cause tissue burns. The magnitude of internal tissue damage may not be gauged on the basis of external burns.

Lightning deaths generally result from electrical cardiac arrest.[218] Lightning acts as a massive DC countershock, depolarizing the entire myocardium, following which a normal cardiac rhythm may resume.[219] Apnea often persists longer than asystole and the victim may die if CPR is not started promptly. Victims who do not suffer cardiac arrest immediately have an excellent chance of recovery.

CARBON MONOXIDE POISONING

Sources of carbon monoxide poisoning include smoke inhalation from all types of fires, and improperly maintained or ventilated automobile exhaust systems, industrial furnaces, and home heating systems. Carbon monoxide competes with oxygen 1) for binding sites on hemoglobin, impairing oxygen delivery; 2) on myoglobin, reducing tissue oxygen reserves; and 3) in the cytochrome chain, impairing oxygen utilization. Tissues with the highest oxygen demand, the brain and myocardium, are most susceptible to these effects. Clinically, headaches develop once carboxyhemoglobin saturation exceeds 10%. At 30%–40% carboxyhemoglobin, severe headaches are accompanied by generalized weakness, confusion, dizziness, nausea and vomiting, and diminished visual and auditory acuity. Tachycardia, cardiac dysrhythmias, and syncope occur at carboxyhemoglobin levels greater than 40%. Once carboxyhemoglobin saturation exceeds 50%, coma and seizures occur and myocardial and ventilatory depression become life threatening. Airway obstruction due to unconsciousness, ventilatory depression, cardiac dysrhythmias, or cardiopulmonary arrest each require the institution of appropriate BCLS and ACLS techniques.

Definitive treatment consists of the displacement of carbon monoxide from O_2 binding sites by the maintenance of an elevated Pa_{O_2}. The delivery of 100% O_2 to the patient should be instituted as early as possible. Tracheal intubation and IPPV may be necessary to ensure adequate ventilation and O_2 delivery. In a patient breathing room air, the elimination half-life of carbon monoxide is 5–6 h. Breathing 100% O_2 reduces the carbon monoxide elimination half-life to approximately 1.5 h. Hyperbaric oxygen at 3 atmospheres absolute pressure further reduces the elimination half-life less than 30 min. Once carboxyhemoglobin levels are reduced, attention should be focused on control of cardiac dysrhythmias and amelioration of postanoxic brain damage.

POSTRESUSCITATION LIFE SUPPORT

GENERAL MANAGEMENT PLAN

All patients resuscitated from cardiopulmonary arrest should be closely monitored in an intensive care environment. Unless the cardiac arrest occurred in a special care unit, postresuscitation care begins with transport to a special-care facility. Adequate patient support during transport includes continuous monitoring for rearrest, support of oxygenation and ventilation, maintenance of venous access, and availability of a defibrillator and resuscitation drugs.

The patient who responds optimally to resuscitation, *i.e.*, who is awake and breathing spontaneously, should be continuously monitored and receive supplemental oxygen, intravenous catheterization for fluid and drug therapy, and appropriate diagnostic investigation for the cause of the arrest. The patient should ingest nothing by mouth for a period of 6 h or until cardiopulmonary stability is ensured. Prophylactic continuous infusion of lidocaine after injection of a loading dose is indicated following resuscitation from ventricular fibrillation or ventricular tachycardia to reduce the likelihood of recurrence of the dysrhythmia. The arrest victim who remains unresponsive with the trachea intubated, and has unstable cardiovascular function following resuscitation has hypoxia-related multiple organ system failure. Postresuscitation management of this patient entails stabilization of cardiorespiratory function and support of the postischemic CNS.

Pulmonary problems existing after CPR may have been: 1) the cause of the arrest; 2) secondary to a primary cardiac event; or 3) the result of the resuscitation process itself. Careful physical and radiographic examination of the chest should follow all resuscitations. Rales due to pulmonary edema or aspiration of gastric contents, unilateral breath sounds suggesting right mainstem bronchial intubation, pneumothorax, or hemothorax, and flail chest may be present.

Restoring and maintaining cardiovascular function is central to postresuscitation care and involves the prevention and treatment of life-threatening cardiac dysrhythmias and the treatment of cardiogenic shock. In addition to continuous ECG surveillance and prophylactic lidocaine by infusion following ventricular fibrillation or ventricular tachycardia, anti-dysrhythmic therapy or pacing may be required if serious dysrhythmias occur. The management of cardiogenic shock may require control of heart rate and rhythm disturbances, judicious preload augmentation or diuresis, inotropes, vasopressors, vasodilators, or intraaortic balloon counterpulsation. Therapy should be guided by invasive hemodynamic monitoring of intraarterial, pulmonary artery, and central venous pressures and of cardiac output.

Restoration of adequate intravascular volume and renal perfusion will generally prevent renal failure after cardiopulmonary arrest. Oliguria following successful CPR requires augmentation of cardiac output and renal perfusion pressure. If oliguria persists despite optimization of cardiovascular function, laboratory tests to confirm the diagnosis of renal failure should be obtained and dialysis instituted when indicated. Prophylaxis against gastrointestinal stress bleeding, nasogastric drainage for adynamic ileus, and the provision of enteric or intravenous calories are also features of postresuscitation gastrointestinal and metabolic care.

POSTRESUSCITATION CARE FOR ISCHEMIC–ANOXIC CEREBRAL INJURY

Cessation of cerebral circulation due to circulatory arrest results in depletion of oxygen stores and unconsciousness within 15 s, depletion of glucose and glycogen stores within 4 min, and exhaustion of high-energy phosphate compounds, stopping all energy-requiring reactions within 5 min.[220] When oxygen is depleted, anaerobic glycolysis continues as long as glucose or glycogen are available. This results in lactate production and intracellular acidosis. Lactate production is greater and cellular pH is lower if hyperglycemia is present at the time of arrest. Failure of the energy-dependent cell membrane sodium–potassium pump occurs. Efflux of potassium, influx of sodium, and intracellular edema result. A sudden influx of calcium ions occurs, presumably because voltage-dependent calcium channels are open. A series of events leading to cell death including free fatty acid release from membrane lipids, proteolysis, and lipid peroxidation are triggered, in part, by the high intracellular calcium concentrations that develop. The intracellular influx of sodium and calcium ions may result from the action of glutamine, an excitatory neurotransmitter that is released with cerebral ischemia.[221]

It is unknown exactly when irreversible cerebral injury precluding normal functional recovery occurs. Complete circulatory arrest for 5–7 min or more results in histologic changes, including scattered neuronal necrosis.[222] Studies in monkeys, however, suggest that the temporal threshold for permanent brain damage may be 14–15 min.[223, 224] For ischemic anoxia to disrupt the blood–brain barrier, circulatory arrest for 30–60 min or longer is necessary.[225]

While biochemical events occur during cerebral ischemia, initiating cell injury, the reactions that ultimately cause cell destruction are associated with reperfusion. Restoration of blood flow after more than 5–10 min of circulatory arrest leads to secondary brain injury characterized by regional hypoperfusion and scattered areas of ischemia and neuronal damage. The precise mechanisms have yet to be established, but this nonhomogeneous restoration of cerebral blood flow may be due to vascular obstruction by edematous glial and endothelial cells, sludging by aggregates of red blood cells, vasospasm, or disseminated intravascular coagulation. Regional differences in metabolic rate, capillary density, collateral circulation, and specific sensitivity of neurons to ischemia–anoxia also contribute to the multifocal nature of postischemic brain injury.[226] Lipid peroxidation of cell membranes is accelerated by the generation of free-radical compounds, which occurs upon reperfusion and reoxygenation of the ischemic brain.

With the occurrence of cerebral ischemia, cerebral blood flow autoregulation, and CO_2 response are lost. Cerebral blood flow becomes dependent on the effective cerebral perfusion pressure. Intracranial compliance may be reduced by intracerebral edema; however, intracranial pressure usually remains normal or near normal unless the ischemic–anoxic insult is severe or of long duration and a critical mass of brain tissue has become edematous. Intracranial hypertension compromising cerebral perfusion pressure is more commonly a feature of head injury, cerebral surgery, or inflammatory insults than following global ischemia–anoxia.

Cerebral injury is the result of the primary ischemic insult and secondary postischemic changes that begin with reperfusion and reoxygenation. While postresuscitative management cannot alter the primary insult, it can modify the secondary changes occurring with reperfusion. General therapeutic measures are aimed at optimizing cerebral blood flow and controlling cerebral metabolic demands. In contrast to the cardiovascular aspects of ACLS, there are no standards for cerebral care during and after cardiopulmonary arrest. Investigations of various cerebral therapies have been largely inconclusive or contradictory.

Restoring homeostasis of vital extracranial organ systems is essential to provide the postischemic brain an opportunity for recovery. Continued hypotension, hypoxemia, hypercarbia, and acidosis following resuscitation merely potentiate reperfusion injury to the brain. Restoration of spontaneous circulation and adequate oxygen transport should be accomplished as rapidly as possible. Several groups have demonstrated that animals who experienced normotension following resuscitation from complete ischemia had a better neurologic outcome than animals who were hypotensive after arrest.[227–229] In fact, a brief period of mild hypertension may be of value, but severe, prolonged hypertension is associated with poor neurologic outcome.[229] Hypertension promotes vasogenic cerebral edema and increases intracranial pressure especially in those situations where the blood–brain barrier has been compromised.

Moderate hyperventilation (Pa_{CO_2} 25–35 mm Hg) has been recommended[230] as it tends to normalize brain pH and, through a reverse steal effect, may improve regional cerebral perfusion by shifting blood flow from reactive to vasoparalyzed (injured) vascular beds. However, the value of hyperventilation in postresuscitation care is unproven.[231] Marked hypocapnia may further reduce a cerebral blood flow that is already low. Hyperventilation may be used to control intracranial pressure if severe cerebral edema exists. Pa_{O_2} should be maintained above 100 mm Hg. This may require the use of positive end-expiratory pressure (PEEP) which should be titrated to optimize Pa_{O_2} without marked elevations of central venous and intracranial pressure. Immobilization and controlled ventilation with the aid of partial neuromuscular blockade provides the principle advantage of more reliable oxygenation and prevention of respiratory acidemia; however, this has not been shown to improve neurologic outcome alone.[232]

Normothermia should be maintained with the aid of body temperature monitoring, external cooling, and pharmacologic vasodilation if necessary, because hyperthermia increases cerebral metabolic rate, promoting cerebral ischemia. Moderate hypothermia does not require treatment. Seizures, which elevate cerebral oxygen consumption, should be controlled with anticonvulsant medications. Shivering should be controlled with use of neuromuscular blockade, as this increases ventilation and oxygenation needs.

Intracranial pressure monitoring may be indicated after prolonged cardiac arrests and whenever initial neurologic stabilization is followed by secondary deterioration with signs suggestive of intracranial hypertension. Hyperventilation, neuromuscular blockade, osmotherapy, barbiturates, cerebrospinal fluid drainage, elevation of the head of the bed 30°, and moderate hypothermia may be used to treat elevations in intracranial pressure.

Hyperglycemia at the time of cerebral ischemic insult in dogs[233] and humans[234, 235] is clearly related to a less favorable neurologic outcome when compared with those who are normoglycemic. Elevated blood glucose levels may contribute to development of more severe cerebral intracellular lactic acidosis. Whether it is prudent to limit infusion of dextrose-containing solutions or to monitor blood glucose levels following resuscitation from cardiac arrest is uncertain.

A number of controversial and investigational therapeutic modalities may have a role in brain resuscitation after cardiac arrest. Reduction of cerebral metabolic rate by the administration of moderate and large doses of barbiturates has been shown to ameliorate neurologic injury in animal[236-238] and human[239] models of regional cerebral ischemia if given before or soon after the insult. Data reporting protection from cerebral injury afforded animals given barbiturates prior to global ischemia are contradictory,[240-242] and evidence that high-dose barbiturates given following a global ischemia episode improve neurologic outcome is lacking. Bleyaert et al claimed amelioration of neurologic deficit in a primate model given thiopental ($90 \text{ mg} \cdot \text{kg}^{-1}$) following 16 min of global cerebral ischemia,[243] but these results could not be reproduced by the same investigating group.[244] Furthermore, a multi-institutional study of high-dose barbiturates after cardiac arrest in humans demonstrated no difference in outcome due to barbiturate treatment.[245]

In another animal model of barbiturate cerebral resuscitation, thiopental ($60 \text{ mg} \cdot \text{kg}^{-1}$) given following resuscitation from 12–16 min of ventricular fibrillation did not improve the neurologic function of survivors; however, mortality was reduced in the thiopental-treated animals.[246] The improved survival resulted from the suppresion of abnormal postarrest electroencephalograph (EEG) patterns. These results suggest that postarrest EEG monitoring may be beneficial and that other anticonvulsants, including phenytoin, benzodiazapines, and etomidate, may be equally effective.

Slow calcium channel blocking drugs have been studied in animal models of cerebral resuscitation from global ischemia with conflicting results.[247-251] Theoretically, inhibition of the intracellular accumulation of calcium ions in cerebral vascular endothelium and neurons might be beneficial by decreasing cerebral vascular resistance and ameliorating the cascade of lethal cellular events initiated by high concentrations of calcium within the neuron.[252]

Hemodilution and heparinization have been used in animals to improve cerebral perfusion after global cerebral injury, but this therapy has been unsuccessful.[253] Reduction of blood viscosity by dextran administration has been beneficial for patients recovering from ischemic stroke[254] but is unstudied in patients resuscitated from cardiac arrest.

Desferoxamine, an iron chelating drug currently under investigation, may retard free-radical generation during reperfusion and reduce lipid peroxidation. Inhibition of thromboxane A_2-mediated cerebral vasoconstriction is another potentially useful therapy under study.

Corticosteroids are effective in reducing cerebral edema associated with intracranial mass lesions; however, there is no evidence they reduce neuronal injury or improve neurologic outcome after cardiac arrest. Hypothermia is unquestionably protective if induced prior to or during a hypoxic or ischemic insult. There is no evidence, though, that postischemic hypothermia improves neurologic outcome following global cerebral ischemia–anoxia.

PEDIATRIC CPR

The principles of resuscitation delineated for adult patients apply as well for pediatric patients. The causes of cardio-pulmonary arrest may be quite different in the pediatric population, but oxygen deficit as a result of an oxygen delivery problem remains the common denominator for all cardiac arrests.[255] Airway management, production of effective cardiac output, stabilization of cardiovascular parameters, and continued postresuscitative evaluation and support are the fundamental elements of pediatric as well as adult CPR.

There are specific anatomic, physiologic and pathophysiologic variations in the pediatric population that must be recognized. An understanding of how these variants impact on the fundamental processes of CPR is essential for appropriate tailoring of CPR to pediatric patients.

The first minutes of life are a transition period from intrauterine to extrauterine existence when oxygen deficit may be present and oxygen delivery impaired. Airway obstruction from blood or meconium, respiratory depression from maternally administered and placentally transferred sedatives, hypovolemia, acidosis from marginal placental blood supply during labor and delivery, and congential anomalies are some of the common causes of a depressed newborn in need of resuscitation. Use of the Apgar score to evaluate the adequacy of oxygenation in the newborn, and resuscitation therapy are described in Chapters 45 and 46. This discussion will therefore be confined to non-newborn pediatric CPR.

BASIC CPR FOR PEDIATRIC RESUSCITATION

Mouth (of rescuer) to mouth and nose (of infant or small child) or mouth (of larger child), and bag-valve–mask or endotracheal methods of ventilation may be used. Oxygen supplementation is essential. O_2PBDs are not recommended in pediatric resuscitation, as dangerously high airway pressure may be generated, potentially damaging the lungs. An EOA for pediatric use does not exist.

Cardiac compression for the infant is provided either by 1) the method where the rescuer's hands encircle the thorax, allowing the fingers to serve as the back board and the thumbs as the piston on the sternum; or 2) the standard method of having the rescuer positioned at the infant's side, placing two fingers on the sternum. Body structures are slightly more cephalad in the infant and small child; therefore, the compression point over the ventricles is located 1 finger-breadth below the midsternum.[256] Compression of the lower sternum in the infant can result in liver laceration and fatal hemorrhage. It might be wise to loosen the diaper of an infant receiving cardiac compression as this will allow better diaphragmatic descent with cardiac compression, and minimize trauma to intraabdominal contents. The normal infant heart rate (approximately $100 \text{ beats} \cdot \text{min}^{-1}$) is faster than the adult's and cardiac compression should, therefore, be more rapid.

ADVANCED CPR FOR PEDIATRIC RESUSCITATION

Most newborn and pediatric cardiopulmonary arrests are the result of an airway and ventilation problem, and the resultant hypoxia is the prime concern of therapy. Additional therapy directed at the cardiovascular problems of hypovolemia; poor cardiac contraction, rate or rhythm; and acidosis may also have to be treated.

Vascular access, essential in pediatric resuscitation, is accomplished using a peripheral or central venous route. The same routes, techniques, and precautions observed in adults apply to the insertion of venous catheters in pediatric patients, but equipment specific for children should be employed.

When intravenous access is absent, intraosseous injection into the anterior tibial bone marrow is used. Arterial and pulmonary artery cannulation, and other invasive therapeutic procedures used in adults apply to the appropriate situations in pediatric resuscitation.

Drug therapy for pediatric resuscitation is fundamentally the same as for adults. Oxygen, bicarbonate, and epinephrine are the mainstays of therapy. Bicarbonate is administered to infants in a 1:1 dilution to reduce the tonicity of the solution and minimize the chances of resultant intracranial hemorrhage.

Defibrillation is less commonly needed in pediatric resuscitation as atherosclerotic cardiovascular disease is not present. Ventricular fibrillation and ventricular tachycardia are less commonly seen because ventilatory problems which are usually the etiology of pediatric cardiopulmonary arrests produce hypoxia that often results in asystole. Congenital cardiac lesions do result in dysrhythmias that may require defibrillation or cardioversion. It is most desirable in pediatric patients to monitor the ECG and make the correct diagnosis to determine if pulselessness is the result of a rhythm disturbance amenable to defibrillation or cardioversion.

If electrical therapy is indicated in children, the same basic principles apply as in the adult therapy. Particular attention should be paid to proper paddle size so that the largest paddle surface making full contact with the thoracic wall is utilized. The concerns outlined in the adult defibrillation section with regard to electrical doses also apply in pediatrics. To avoid myocardial damage and postshock dysrhythmias, the recommended dose for pediatric defibrillation is 2 joules $\cdot$ kg^{-1}.[257] The dose, if unsuccessful, is doubled until effective.

The postresuscitative care of infants and children requires the same intensive/critical care facilities as outlined for adults. It may be necessary to transport a resuscitated and stabilized child to a pediatric referral center that can provide pediatric intensive care for postresuscitative treatment.

MEDICOLEGAL CONSIDERATIONS

Over the last 15 years, CPR has developed into an effective set of sophisticated medical techniques that often results in survival from cardiac arrest. This fact raises many medicolegal questions with regard to the delivery of CPR; i.e., the provider's responsibility to provide CPR, the standard of care, definitions of death, termination of CPR, "do not resuscitate" orders, and discontinuation of life-support systems. The consideration of all of these issues balances the provision of the best of CPR available against provision of reasonable care to any individual's medical status and psychological desires.[258]

Once physicians begin the treatment of a patient, they have an implied contractual responsibility to complete such care. A similar situation exists in an emergency facility such as a life-support unit or hospital emergency room. Physicians working in such units must provide CPR in the patient's best interest, even when the patient is unable to request treatment and establish a normal physician–patient relationship. At present in the United States (in distinction to some European countries), there is no legal obligation for a physician to provide CPR to an unknown victim on the street so long as the physician is not acting as a part of a mobile life-support unit. The moral and ethical reasons to initiate CPR in the field are compelling, but no legal obligation to respond exists in the United States for the physician, paramedical person, or lay person. It must be recognized, however, that if field delivery of CPR is initiated by the "good samaritan" (physician or nonphysician), then the victim cannot be abandoned and the

care must be performed up to the level of expertise of the rescuer. Many states have "good samaritan" statutes to protect those who render such aid.

The standard of care for CPR is defined in a rather uniform manner throughout the United States. The AHA CPR protocols are one acceptable standard of care, although not the only to be applied to the definition. The implied standard of care for CPR within the confines of a hospital requires that a cardiac arrest team be defined and readily available to render immediate resuscitative efforts.

One of the major issues that is still not totally resolved is that of an acceptable definition of death. Until this concern is addressed, it is difficult to make rational decisions about the timing of, or even the need for CPR in any of its phases. The traditional definition of death had been based on the absence of cardiovascular function: if the heart stopped and was refractory to return of function, death was present. A more recent perspective on death focuses on the brain. Criteria for brain death have been established, the most famous being the Harvard Criteria. Both medical and legal sanction has been given to the concept of brain death. The definition of death by criteria for absence of both cardiac and brain viability is required for CPR decisions. On the one hand, CPR is begun and often maintained because of the probability of brain viability or even the lack of proof of brain death. On the other hand, CPR may be terminated because it is obvious that cardiovascular unresponsiveness is present and brain viability is in jeopardy.

Decisions to begin or end CPR must consider cardiac and brain function and responsiveness to therapy.[259, 260] In general, CPR is initiated in all instances where brain viability is assumed and no other overriding consideration (e.g., patient's desire not to be resuscitated) precludes this action. It must be remembered that a prospective diagnosis of irreversible brain damage is almost impossible to make. Many cases have been reported where neurologic recovery occurred months after the initial insult. Additionally, hypothermia or medications may depress CNS function and mimic brain death that is not truly present. CPR is often begun to evaluate cardiovascular responsiveness. Often, it is only by a trial of CPR that the heart can be diagnosed as irreversibly damaged and unresponsive to further therapy. A major difficulty in deciding brain and cardiac viability is deciding when the cardiac arrest occurred. Many cardiopulmonary disasters occur totally unwitnessed. It is virtually impossible to determine the length of time of absent oxygen delivery when a rescuer arrives at the scene of the arrest or the patient is delivered to a life-support facility. "Dead on arrival" (DOA) diagnosis is clearly harder to make accurately than was once thought.

In the past several years the personal wish of individuals not to be resuscitated has been a major legal issue. A number of court cases have upheld the desires of mentally competent adults who believe that they have terminal illness and, therefore, do not want CPR, a technique designed for prevention or treatment of sudden, unexpected death. "Do not resuscitate" orders are less clear, however, when a mentally incompetent patient is involved. Under these circumstances as well as in situations where life-support systems might be discontinued, if brain death is documented, then CPR and other life-support methods can be stopped. When strict brain death criteria cannot be met, however, each case should be decided on its own merits with the assistance of the courts.

It behooves all who may be involved with CPR or life-support procedures to be aware of the medicolegal ramifications of their actions or lack of action so that reasonable care may be provided to all who require it and excessive care or excessive lack of care can be avoided.

ROLE OF THE ANESTHESIOLOGIST IN CPR

The professional responsibilities of an anesthesiologist include CPR. The American Board of Anesthesiology in its *Booklet of Information,* and the U.S. Department of Labor in its definition of the specialty of anesthesiology, *i.e.,* its job description, cite, as tasks of the anesthesiologist, clinical care in and teaching of life support and cardiac and pulmonary resuscitation. In addition, CPR research and administrative functions are often delegated to the anesthesiologist.

The practice of operating room anesthesia and critical care medicine give the anesthesiologist considerable expertise in acute life-support practices. A deficiency may exist with anesthesiologists and physicians in general, however, in their field delivery of CPR. Anesthesiologists have been shown to lack CPR knowledge and skill,[261, 262] which can be easily corrected through continuing education. As important members of the team delivering CPR, anesthesiologists must remain current with accepted CPR practice.

Teaching CPR is an important activity for the anesthesiologist. Guiding a student through procedures of tracheal intubation or concepts of pharmacologic intervention can be best accomplished by the anesthesiologist. Rewards for the anesthesiologist CPR tutor include: knowledge that the student becomes competent; the anesthesiologist becomes a respected educator at the medical school or hospital; and a future anesthesiologist may have been recruited.

The administrative duties of the anesthesiologist include review of CPR equipment and its function and establishment of anesthesia response to and collaboration with the total CPR and emergency medical service effort within the community.

CPR research is an activity anesthesiologists have participated in throughout the years. Only by continued investigative effort can basic science rationale be uncovered for the clinical practice of CPR.

REFERENCES

1. Bartecchi CE: Cardiopulmonary resuscitation—An element of sophistication in the 18th century. Am Heart J 100:580, 1980
2. Comroe JH, Dripps RD: Ben Franklin and open heart surgery. Circ Res 35:661, 1974
3. Resen Z, Davidson JT: Respiratory resuscitation in ancient Hebrew sources. Anesth Analg 51:502, 1972
4. Vesalius A: De humani corporis fabrica, libu system, Bosel, Oporinus, 1543, 661
5. Dill DB: Background on manual artificial respiration and mouth-to-mouth resuscitation. Physiologist 23:33, 1980
6. Gordon AS: Background on cardiopulmonary resuscitation. Physiologist 23:35, 1980
7. Cooper DY: Mouth-to-mouth resuscitation: Influence of alcohol on revival of an old technique. Life Sci 16:487, 1975
8. Comroe JH: "...In comes the good air." Part II, mouth-to-mouth method. Am Rev Respir Dis 119:1025, 1979
9. Tossach W: Medical Essays and Observations. Edinburgh, 1744
10. Fothergill J: Philadelphia Transactions. 1754
11. Elam JO, Brown ES, Elder JD: Artificial respiration by mouth-to-mouth method. A study of respiratory gas exchange of paralyzed patients ventilated by operator's expired air. N Engl J Med 250:749, 1954
12. Elam JO, Green DG: Mission accomplished: Successful mouth-to-mouth resuscitation. Anesth Analg 40:578, 1961
13. Elam JO. Clements JA, Brown ES *et al:* Artificial respiration for nerve gas casualty. US Armed Forces Med J 7:797, 1950
14. Gordon AS, Frye CW, Gittelson L *et al:* Mouth-to-mouth versus manual artificial respiration for children and adults. JAMA 172:320, 1960
15. Gordon AS: The principles and practice of heart-lung resuscitation. Acta Anaesthesiol Scand 9 (Suppl): 134, 1961
16. Safar P: Ventilatory efficacy of mouth-to-mouth artificial respiration: Airway obstruction during manual and mouth-to-mouth artificial respiration. JAMA 172:335, 1960
17. Kouwenhoven WB, Langworth OR: Cardiopulmonary resuscitation. JAMA 226:877, 1973
18. Jude JR, Kouwenhoven WB, Knickerbocker GG: Cardiac arrest. JAMA 178:1063, 1961
19. Prevost J, Battelli F: La mort par les courants electrique. J Gen Physiol 1:1085, 1899
20. Beck CS, Pritchard WH, Feil HS: Ventricular fibrillation of long duration abolished by electric shock. JAMA 135:985, 1947
21. Kouwenhoven WB, Milnor WR, Knickerbocker GG *et al:* Closed chest defibrillation. Surgery 42:550, 1957
22. Kouwenhoven WB, Jude JR, Knickerbocker GG: Closed chest cardiac massage. JAMA 173:1064, 1960
23. Heart Facts 1981. American Heart Association (55-005-E). Dallas, Texas, 1980
24. Lemire JG, Johnson AL: Is cardiac resuscitation worthwhile? A decade of experience. N Engl J Med 286:970, 1972
25. Copley DP, Mantle JA, Rogers WJ *et al:* Improved outcome for prehospital cardiopulmonary collapse with resuscitation by bystanders. Circulation 56:901, 1977
26. Eisenberg MS, Bergner L, Hallstrom A: Cardiac resuscitation in the community. JAMA 241:1905, 1979
27. Eisenberg MS, Hallstrom A, Bergner L: Long-term survival after out-of-hospital cardiac arrest. N Engl J Med 306:1340, 1982
28. Eisenberg M, Bergner L, Hallstrom A: Paramedic programs and out-of-hospital cardiac arrest: 1. Factors associated with successful resuscitation. AJPH 69:30, 1979
29. Eisenberg M, Hallstrom A, Bergner L: The ACLS score. JAMA 246:50, 1981
30. Accident Facts 1980. National Safety Council, Chicago, 1980
31. Pantridge JF, Geddes JS: A mobile intensive-care unit in the management of myocardial infarction. Lancet 2:271, 1967
32. Standards and guidelines for cardiopulmonary resuscitation (CPR) and emergency cardiac care (ECC). JAMA 244:453, 1980
33. Safar P: Cardiopulmonary-cerebral resuscitation including emergency airway control. In Schwartz GR, Safar P, Stone JH *et al* (eds): Principles and Practice of Emergency Medicine, Philadelphia, WB Saunders, 1978
34. Safar P, Escarraga LA, Chang F: Upper airway obstruction in the unconscious patient. J Appl Physiol 14:760, 1959
35. Safar P: Failure of manual respiration. J Appl Physiol 14:84, 1959
36. Safar P: Ventilatory efficacy of mouth-to-mouth artificial respiration: Airway obstruction during manual mouth-to-mouth artificial respiration. JAMA 167:335, 1958
37. Green DG, Elam JO, Dobkin AB *et al:* Cinefluorographic study of hyperextension of the neck and upper airway patency. JAMA 176:570, 1961
38. Morikawa S, Safar P, DeCarlo J: Influence of the head-jaw position upon upper airway patency. Anesthesiology 22:265, 1961
39. Ruben HM, Elam JO, Ruben AM *et al:* Investigation of upper airway problems in resuscitation. Anesthesiology 22:271, 1961
40. Guildner CW: Resuscitation-opening the airway: A comparative study of techniques for opening an airway obstructed by the tongue. J Am Coll Emerg Phys 5:588, 1976
41. Ruben H, Knudsen EJ, Carugati G: Gastric inflation in relation to airway pressure. Acta Anaesthesiol Scand 15:107, 1961
42. Melker R: Asynchronous and other alternative methods of ventilation during CPR. Ann Emerg Med 13:758, 1984
43. Melker R: Recommendations for ventilation during cardio-

pulmonary resuscitation. Time for change? Crit Care Med 13:882, 1985

44. Harris LC, Kirimli B, Safar P: Ventilation-cardiac compression rates and ratios in cardiopulmonary resuscitation. Anesthesiology 28:806, 1967

45. Accident Facts. National Safety Council, Chicago, 1984

46. Haugen RK: The cafe coronary: Sudden deaths in restaurants. JAMA 186:142, 1963

47. Gordon AS, Belton MK, Ridolpho PF: Emergency management of foreign body airway obstruction, In Safar P, Elam JO, (eds): Advances in Cardiopulmonary Resuscitation, p 39. New York, Springer Verlag, 1977

48. Heimlich HJ, Hoffman KA, Canestri FR: Food-choking and drowning deaths prevented by external subdiaphragmatic compression: Physiological basis. Ann Thorac Surg 20:188, 1975

49. Guildner CW, Williams D, Subitch T: Airway obstructed by foreign material: The Heimlich maneuver. J Am Coll Emerg Phys 5:675, 1976

50. Ruben H, MacNaughton FI: The treatment of food choking. Practitioner 221:725, 1978

51. Redding JS: The choking controversy: Critique of evidence of the Heimlich maneuver. Crit Care Med 7:475, 1979

52. Day RL, Crelin ES, DuBois AB: Choking: The Heimlich abdominal thrust *vs* back blows: An approach to measurement of inertial and aerodynamic forces. Pediatrics 70:113, 1982

53. Don Michael TA, Lambert EH, Mehran A: "Mouth-to-lung airway" for cardiac resuscitation. Lancet 2:1329, 1968

54. Gordon AS: Adjunctive techniques and equipment for cardiopulmonary resuscitation. In Stephenson H (ed): Cardiac Arrest and Resuscitation, p 634. St. Louis, CV Mosby, 1974

55. Don Michael TA: Comparison of the esophageal obturator airway and endotracheal intubation in prehospital ventilation during CPR. Chest 87:814, 1985

56. Smith JP, Bodai BI, Seifkina AS et al: The esophageal obturator airway: A review. JAMA 250:1081, 1983

57. Donen N, Tweed WA, Dashfsky et al: The esophageal obturator airway: An appraisal. Can Anaesth Soc J 30:194, 1983

58. Auerbach PS, Geehr EC: Inadequate oxygenation and ventilation using the esophageal gastric tube airway in the prehospital setting. JAMA 250:3067, 1983

59. Smith JP, Bodai BI, Aubourg R et al: A field evaluation of the esophageal obturator airway. J Trauma 23:317, 1983

60. Schofferman J, Oill P, Lewis AJ: The esophageal obturator airway: A clinical evaluation. Chest 69:67, 1976

61. Meislin HW: The esophageal obturator airway: A study of respiratory effectiveness. Ann Emerg Med 9:54, 1980

62. Hammargren Y, Clinton JE, Ruiz E: A standard comparison of esophageal obturator airway and endotracheal tube ventilation in cardiac arrest. Ann Emerg Med 14:953, 1985

63. Bryson TK, Benumof JL, Ward CF: The esophageal obturator airway: A clinical comparison to ventilation with a mask and oropharyngeal airway. Chest 74:537, 1987

64. Gordon AS: Improved esophageal obturator airway (EOA) and new esophageal gastric tube airway (EGTA). In Safar P, Elam JO (eds): Advances in Cardiopulmonary Resuscitation, p 58. New York, Springer Verlag, 1977

65. Yearly DM, Stewart RD: Translaryngeal cannula ventilation: continuing misconceptions (letter). Anesthesiology 67:445, 1987

66. Neff CC, Pfister RC, Van Sonnenberg E: Percutaneous transtracheal ventilation: Experimental and practical aspects. J Trauma 23:84, 1983

67. Levinson MM, Scuderi PE, Gibson RL et al: Emergency percutaneous transtracheal ventilation (PTV). J Am Coll Emerg Phys 8:396, 1979

68. Spoerel WE, Narayanan PS, Singh NP: Transtracheal ventilation. Br J Anaesth 43:932, 1971

69. Jacobs HB: Emergency percutaneous transtracheal catheter and ventilator. J Trauma 12:50, 1972

70. Smith RB: Transtracheal ventilation during anesthesia. Anesth Analg 53:225, 1974

71. Smith RB, Myers EN, Sherman H: Transtracheal ventilation in paediatric patients. Br J Anaesth 46:313, 1974

72. Miyaska K, Sloan IA, Forese AB: An evaluation of the jet injector (Sanders) technique for bronchoscopy in pediatric patients. Can Anaesth Soc J 27:117, 1980

73. Dunlap LB: A modified simple device for the emergency administration of percutaneous transtracheal ventilation. J Am Coll Emerg Phys 7:42, 1978

74. Eger EI: Rate of rise of Pa_{CO_2} in the apneic anesthetized patient. Anesthesiology 22:419, 1961

75. Smith RB, Babinski M, Klain M et al: Percutaneous transtracheal ventilation. J Am Coll Emerg Phys 5:765, 1976

76. Smith RB, Schaer WB, Pfaeffle H: Percutaneous transtracheal ventilation for anaesthesia and resuscitation: A review and report of complications. Can Anaesth Soc J 22:607, 1975

77. Kouwenhoven WB, Jude JR, Knickerbocker GG: Closed-chest cardiac massage. JAMA 173:1064, 1960

78. Chandra N, Weisfeldt ML, Tsitlik J et al: Augmentation of carotid flow during cardiopulmonary resuscitation by ventilation at high airway pressure simultaneous with chest compression. Am J Cardiol 48:1053, 1981

79. MacKenzie GJ, Taylor SH, McDonald AH et al: Hemodynamic effects of external cardiac compression. Lancet 1:1342, 1964

80. Pappelbaum S, Lang T, Bazika V et al: Comparative hemodynamics during open *vs* closed cardiac resuscitation. JAMA 193:659, 1965

81. Redding JS, Cozine RA: A comparison of open-chest and closed-chest cardiac massage in dogs. Anesthesiology 22:280, 1961

82. Niemann JT, Rosborough JP, Ung S et al: Coronary perfusion pressure during experimental cardiopulmonary resuscitation. Ann Emerg Med 11:127, 1982

83. Halperin HR, Guerci AD, Chandra N et al: Vest inflation without simultaneous ventilation during cardiac arrest in dogs: Improved survival from prolonged cardiopulmonary resuscitation. Circulation 74:1407, 1986

84. Koehler RC, Chandra N, Guerci AD et al: Augmentation of cerebral perfusion by simultaneous chest compression and lung inflation with abdominal binding after cardiac arrest in dogs. Circulation 67:266, 1983

85. Luce JM, Ross BK, O'Quin RJ et al: Regional blood flow during cardiopulmonary resuscitation in dogs using simultaneous and nonsimultaneous compression and ventilation. Circulation 67:258, 1983

86. DelGuercio LR, Feins NR, Cohn JD et al: Comparison of blood flow during external and internal cardiac massage in man. Circulation 31:I171, 1965

87. Ditchey RV, Winkler JV, Rhodes CA: Relative lack of coronary blood flow during closed-chest resuscitation in dogs. Circulation 66:297, 1982

88. Bellamy RF, DeGuzman LR, Pedersen DC: Coronary blood flow during cardiopulmonary resuscitation in swine. Circulation 69:174, 1984

89. Babbs CF, Voorhees WD, Fitzgerald KR et al: Relationship of blood pressure and flow during CPR to chest compression amplitude: Evidence for an effective compression threshold. Ann Emerg Med 19:527, 1983

90. Taylor GJ, Tucker WM, Green HL et al: Importance of prolonged compression during cardiopulmonary resuscitation in man. N Engl J Med 296:1515, 1977

91. Weisfeldt ML, Halperin HR: Cardiopulmonary resuscitation: Beyond cardiac massage. Circulation 74:443, 1986

92. Maier GW, Tyson GS, Olsen CO et al: The physiology of external

massage: High impulse cardiopulmonary resuscitation. Circulation 70:86, 1984

93. Deshmukh H, Weil MH, Swindall A et al: Echocardiographic observations during cardiopulmonary resuscitation: A preliminary report. Crit Care Med 13:904, 1985

94. Criley JM, Blaufuss AH, Kissel GL: Cough-induced cardiac compression: Self-induced form of cardiopulmonary resuscitation. JAMA 236:1246, 1976

95. Nieman JT, Rosborough J, Hausknecht M et al: Cough CPR. Documentation of systemic perfusion in man and in an experimental model: A "window" to the mechanism of blood flow in external CPR. Crit Care Med 8:141, 1980

96. Rudikoff MT, Maughan WL, Effron M et al: Mechanisms of blood flow during cardiopulmonary resuscitation. Circulation 61:345, 1980

97. Halperin HR, Tsitlik JE, Guerci AD et al: Determinants of blood flow to vital organs during cardiopulmonary resuscitation in dogs. Circulation 73:539, 1986

98. Werner JA, Green HL, Janko CL: Visualization of cardiac valve motion in man during external chest compression using two-dimensional echocardiography: Implications regarding the mechanism of blood flow. Circulation 63:1417, 1981

99. Niemann JT, Garner D, Rosborough J et al: The mechanism of blood flow in closed-chest cardiopulmonary resuscitation. Circulation 60:II, 1979

100. Chandra N, Rudikoff M, Weisfeldt ML: Simultaneous chest compression and ventilation at high airway pressure during cardiopulmonary resuscitation. Lancet I:175, 1980

101. Harris LC, Kirimli B, Safar P: Augmentation of artificial circulation during cardiopulmonary resuscitation. Anesthesiology 28:730, 1967

102. Redding JS: Abdominal compression in cardiopulmonary resuscitation. Anesth Analg 50:668, 1971

103. Niemann JR, Rosborough JP, Ung S et al: Hemodynamic effects of continuous abdominal binding during cardiac arrest and resuscitation. Am J Cardiol 53:269, 1984

104. Bircher N, Safar P, Steward R: A comparison of standard, MAST-augmented, and open-chest CPR in dogs: A preliminary investigation. Crit Care Med 8:147, 1980

105. Rosborough JP, Niemann JT, Criley JM et al: Lower abdominal compression with synchronized ventilation: A CPR modality. Circulation 64:303, 1981

106. Niemann JT, Criley JM, Rosborough JP et al: Predictive indices of successful cardiac resuscitation after prolonged arrest and experimental cardiopulmonary resuscitation. Ann Emerg Med 14:521, 1985

107. Ralston SH, Babbs CF, Niebauer MJ: Cardiopulmonary resuscitation with interposed abdominal compression in dogs. Anesth Analg 61:645, 1982

108. Sanders AB, Keru KB, Atlas M et al: Importance of the duration of inadequate coronary perfusion pressure on resuscitation from cardiac arrest. J Am Coll Cardiol 6:113, 1985

109. Kern KB, Carter AB, Showen RL et al: Comparison of mechanical techniques of cardiopulmonary resuscitation: Survival and neurologic outcome in dogs. Am J Emerg Med 5:190, 1987

110. Kaback KR, Sanders AB, Meislin HW: MAST suit update. JAMA 252:2598, 1984

111. Gaffney FA, Thal ER, Taylor WF et al: Hemodynamic effects of medical anti-shock trousers (MAST garment). J Trauma 21:931, 1981

112. Mahoney BD, Mirick MJ: Efficacy of pneumatic trousers in refractory prehospital cardiopulmonary arrest. Ann Emerg Med 12:8, 1983

113. Weiser FM, Adler LN, Kuhn LA: Hemodynamic effects of closed and open chest cardiac resuscitation in normal dogs and those with acute myocardial infarction. Am J Cardiol 10:555, 1962

114. Bircher N, Safar P: Comparison of standard and "new" closed-chest CPR and open chest CPR in dogs. Crit Care Med 9:384, 1981

115. Geehr EC, Lewis FR, Auerbach PS: Failure of open-heart massage to improve survival after prehospital nontraumatic cardiac arrest (letter). N Engl J Med 314:1189, 1986

116. Bircher N, Safar P: Open-chest CPR: An old method whose time has returned. Am J Emerg Med 2:568, 1984

117. Pretto E, Safar P, Saito R et al: Cardiopulmonary bypass after prolonged cardiac arrest in dogs. Ann Emerg Med 16:611, 1987

118. Martin GB, Nowak RM, Carden DL et al: Cardiopulmonary bypass vs CPR as treatment for prolonged canine cardiopulmonary arrest. Ann Emerg Med 16:628, 1987

119. Levine R, Gorayeb M, Safar P et al: Emergency cardiopulmonary bypass after cardiac arrest and prolonged closed-chest CPR in dogs. Ann Emerg Med 16:620, 1987

120. Myerberg RJ, Conde CA, Sung RJ et al: A clinical electrophysiologic and hemodynamic profile of patients resuscitated from prehospital cardiac arrest. Am J Med 68: 568, 1980

121. DeSanctis RW, Block P, Hutter AM Jr: Tachyarrhythmias in myocardial infarction. Circulation 45:681, 1972

122. Kimball JT, Killip T: Aggressive treatment of arrhythmias in acute myocardial infarction: Procedures and results. Prog Cardiovasc Dis 10:483, 1968

123. Lie KI, Wellens HJ, Downar E et al: Observations on patients with primary ventricular fibrillation complicating acute myocardial infarction. Circulation 52:755, 1975

124. Dhurandhar RW, MacMillan RL, Brown KW: Primary ventricular fibrillation complicating acute myocardial infarction. Am J Cardiol 27:347, 1971

125. Wellens HJ, Bar FW, Lie KI: The value of the electrocardiogram in the differential diagnosis of tachycardia with a widened QRS complex. Am J Med 64:27, 1978

126. Cobb LA, Hallstrom AP: Community-based cardiopulmonary resuscitation: What have we learned? Ann NY Acad Sci 382:330, 1982

127. Dahl CF, Ewy GA, Warner ED et al: Myocardial necrosis from direct current countershock. Circulation 50:956, 1974

128. Warner ED, Dahl C, Ewy GA: Mycardial injury from transthoracic defibrillator countershock. Arch Pathol Lab Med 99:55, 1975

129. Weaver WD, Cobb LA, Copass MK et al: Ventricular defibrillation: A comparative trial using 175-J and 320-J shocks. N Engl J Med 207:1101, 1982

130. Thomas ED, Ewy GA, Dahl CF et al: Effectiveness of direct current defibrillation: Role of paddle electrode size. Am Heart J 93:463, 1977

131. Adgey AA: Electrical energy requirements for ventricular defibrillation. Br Heart J 40:1197, 1978

132. Crampton JA, Crampton RS, Sipes JN et al: Energy levels and patient weight in ventricular defibrillation. JAMA 242:1380, 1979

133. Gasch JA, Crampton RS, Cherwek ML et al: Determinants of ventricular defibrillation in adults. Circulation 60:231, 1979

134. Lown B, Crampton RS, DeSilva RA et al: The energy for ventricular fibrillation—Too little or too much? N Engl J Med 298:1252, 1978

135. Kerber RE, Jensen SR, Gascho JA et al: Determinants of defibrillation: Prospective analysis of 183 patients. Am J Cardiol 52:739, 1983.

136. Dahl CF, Ewy GA, Ewy MD et al: Transthoracic impedance to direct current discharge: Effect of repeated countershocks. Med Instrum 10:151, 1976.

137. Cingolani HE, Faulkner SL, Mattiazzi AR et al: Depression of human myocardial contractility with "respiratory" and "metabolic" acidosis. Surgery 77:427, 1975

138. Cingolani HE, Mattiazzi AR, Blesa ES et al: Contractility in iso-

lated mammalian heart muscle after acid base changes. Circ Res 26:269, 1970

139. Weisfeldt ML, Bishop RL, Green HL: Effects of pH and P_{CO_2} on performance of ischemic myocardium. In Roy PE, Rona G (eds): Recent Advances in Studies on Cardiac Structure and Metabolism, Vol 10, p 355. Baltimore, University Park Press, 1975

140. Houle DB, Weil MH, Brown EB et al: Influence of respiratory acidosis on ECG and pressor response to epinephrine, norepinephrine, and metaraminol. Proc Soc Exp Biol Med 94:561, 1957

141. Gerst PH, Fleming WH, Malm JR: Increased susceptibility of the heart to ventricular fibrillation during metabolic acidosis. Circ Res 19:63, 1966

142. Kerber RE, Pandian NE, Hoyt R et al: Effect of ischemia, hypertrophy, hypoxia, acidosis and alkalosis on canine defibrillation. Am J Physiol 244:H825, 1983

143. Kerber BE, Sarnat W: Factors influencing the success of ventricular defibrillation in man. Circulation 60:226, 1979

144. Minuck M, Sharma GP: Comparison of THAM and sodium bicarbonate in resuscitation of the heart after ventricular fibrillation in dogs. Anesth Analg 56:38, 1977

145. Guerci AD, Chandra N, Johnson E et al: Failure of sodium bicarbonate to improve resuscitation from ventricular fibrillation in dogs. Circulation 74 (suppl IV): IV75, 1986

146. Bishop RL, Weisfeldt ML: Sodium bicarbonate administration during cardiac arrest. Effect on arterial pH P_{CO_2}, and osmolality. JAMA 235:506, 1976

147. Grundler W, Weil MH, Yamaguchi M et al: The paradox of venous acidosis and arterial alkalosis during open-chest CPR. Chest 86:282, 1984

148. Weil MH, Rackow EC, Trevino R et al: Difference in acid-base state between venous and arterial blood during cardiopulmonary resuscitation. N Engl J Med 315:153, 1986

149. Martin GB, Carden DL, Nowak RM et al: Comparison of central venous and arterial pH and P_{CO_2} during open-chest CPR in the canine model. Ann Emerg Med 14:529, 1985

150. Berenyi KG, Wolk M, Killip T: Cerebrospinal fluid acidosis complicating therapy of experimental cardiopulmonary arrest. Circulation 52:319, 1975

151. Mattar JA, Weil MH, Shubin H et al: Cardiac arrest in the critically ill. II. Hyperosmolal states following cardiac arrest. Am J Med 56:162, 1974

152. Redding JS, Pearson JW: Resuscitation from ventricular fibrillation. JAMA 203:255, 1968

153. Otto CW, Yakaitis RW, Redding JS et al: Comparison of dopamine, dobutamine, and epinephrine in CPR. Crit Care Med 9:640, 1981

154. Pearson JW, Redding JS: Epinephrine in cardiac resuscitation. Am Heart J 66:210, 1963

155. Redding JS, Pearson JW: Evaluation of drugs for cardiac resuscitation. Anesthesiology 24:203, 1963

156. Yakaitis RW, Otto CW, Blitt CD: Relative importance of alpha and beta adrenergic receptors during resuscitation. Crit Care Med 7:293, 1979

157. Otto CW, Yakaitis RW, Blitt CD: Mechanism of action of epinephrine in resuscitation from asphyxial arrest. Crit Care Med 9:321, 1981

158. Holmes HR, Babbs CF, Voorhees WD et al: Influence of adrenergic drugs upon vital organ perfusion during CPR. Crit Care Med 8:137, 1980

159. Livesay JJ, Follette DM, Fey KM et al: Optimizing myocardial supply/demand with alpha-adrenergic drugs during cardiopulmonary resuscitation. J Thorac Cardiovasc Surg 76:244, 1978

160. Otto CW, Yakaitis RW: The role of epinephrine in CPR: A reappraisal. Ann Emerg Med 13:840, 1984

161. Michael JR, Guerci AD, Koehler RC et al: Mechanisms by which

162. Koehler RC, Michael JR, Guerci AD et al: Beneficial effect of epinephrine infusion on cerebral and myocardial blood flows during CPR. Ann Emerg Med 14:744, 1985

163. Otto CW, Yakaitis RW, Ewy GA: Spontaneous ischemic ventricular fibrillation in dogs: A new model for the study of cardiopulmonary resuscitation. Crit Care Med 11:883, 1983

164. Ralston SH: Alpha agonist usage during CPR. Ann Emerg Med 13:786, 1984

165. Brilliman J, Sanders A, Otto CW et al: Comparison of epinephrine and phenylephrine for resuscitation and neurologic outcome of cardiac arrest in dogs. Ann Emerg Med 16:11, 1987

166. Brown CG, Werman HA et al: The effect of high-dose phenylephrine versus epinephrine on regional cerebral blood flow during CPR. Ann Emerg Med 16:743, 1987

167. Brown CG, Katz SE, Werman HA et al: The effect of epinephrine versus methoxamine on regional myocardial blood flow and defibrillation rates following a prolonged cardiorespiratory arrest in a swine model. Am J Emerg Med 5:362, 1987

168. Kosnik JW, Jackson RE, Keats S et al: Dose-related response of aortic diastolic pressure during closed-chest massage in dogs. Ann Emerg Med 14:204, 1985

169. Brown CG, Werman HA, Davis EA et al: The effects of graded doses of epinephrine on regional myocardial blood flow during cardiopulmonary resuscitation in swine. Circulation 75:491, 1987

170. Roberts JR, Greenberg MI, Knaub M et al: Comparison of the pharmacological effects of epinephrine administred by the intravenous and endotracheal routes. J Am Coll Emerg Phys 7:260, 1978

171. Roberts JR, Greenberg MI, Knaub M et al: Blood levels following intravenous and endotracheal epinephrine administration. J Am Coll Emerg Phys 8:53, 1979

172. Chernow B, Holbrook P, D'Angona DS et al: Epinephrine absorption after intratracheal administration. Anesth Analg 63:829, 1984

173. Ralston SH, Tacker WA, Showen L et al: Endotracheal versus intravenous epinephrine during electromechanical dissociation with CPR in dogs. Ann Emerg Med 14:1044, 1985

174. Hasegawa EA: The endotracheal administration of drugs. Heart Lung 15:60, 1986

175. Mace SE: Effect of technique of administration on plasma lidocaine levels. Ann Emerg Med 15:522, 1986

176. Rosetti VA, Thompson BM, Miller J et al: Intraosseous infusion: An alternative route of pediatric vascular access. Ann Emerg Med 14:885, 1985

177. Brown DC, Lewis AJ, Criley JM: Asystole and its treatment: The possible role of the parasympathetic nervous system in cardiac arrest. J Am Coll Emerg Phys 8:448, 1979

178. Stueven HA, Tonsfeldt DJ, Thompson BM et al: Atropine in asystole: Human studies. Ann Emerg Med 13:815, 1984

179. Iseri LT, Humphrey SB, Siner EJ: Pre-hospital bradysystolic cardiac arrest. Ann Intern Med 88:741, 1978

180. Coon GA, Clinton JE, Ruiz E: Use of atropine for bradysystolic prehospital cardiac arrest. Ann Emerg Med 10:462, 1981

181. O'Rourke GW, Greene NM: Autonomic blockade and the resting heart rate in man. Am Heart J 80:469, 1970

182. Niemann JT, Haynes KS, Garner D et al: Post-countershock pulseless rhythms: Response to CPR, artificial cardiac pacing, and adrenergic agonists. Ann Emerg Med 15:112, 1985

183. Carruth JE, Silverman ME: Ventricular fibrillation complicating acute myocardial infarction: Reasons against the routine use of lidocaine. Am Heart J 104:545, 1982

184. Dunn HM, McComb JM, Kinney CD et al: Prophylactic lidocaine

in the early phase of suspected myocardial infarction. Am Heart J 110:353, 1985

185. Lie KI, Wellens NJ, van Capelle FJ: Lidocaine in the prevention of primary ventricular fibrillation. A double-blind, randomized study of 212 consecutive patients. N Eng J Med 291:1324, 1974

186. DeSilva RA, Lown B, Hennekens CH et al: Lidocaine prophylaxis in acute myocardial infarction. An evaluation of randomized trials. Lancet II:855, 1981

187. Koster RW, Dunning AJ: Intramuscular lidocaine for prevention of lethal arrhythmias in the prehospitalization phase of acute myocardial infarction. N Engl J Med 313:1105, 1985

188. Haynes RE, Chinn TL, Copass MK et al: Comparison of bretylium tosylate and lidocaine in management of out-of-hospital ventricular fibrillation: A randomized clinical trial. Am J Cardiol 48:353, 1981

189. Olson DW, Thompson BM, Darin JL et al: A randomized comparison study of bretylium tosylate and lidocaine in resuscitation of patients from out-of-hospital ventricular fibrillation in a paramedic system. Ann Emerg Med 13:807, 1984

190. Chow MMS, Ronfeld RA, Hamilton RA et al: Effect of external cardiopulmonary resuscitation on lidocaine pharmacokinetics in dogs. J Pharmacol Exp Ther 224:531, 1983

191. Benowitz NL: Clinical applications of the pharmacokinetics of lidocaine. In Melmon KL (ed): Cardiovascular Drug Therapy, p 77 Philadelphia, FA Davis, 1976

192. Stargel WW, Shand DG, Routledge PA et al: Clinical comparison of rapid infusion and multiple injection methods for lidocaine loading. Am Heart J 102:872, 1981

193. Wyman MG, Lalka D, Hammersmith L et al: Multiple bolus technique for lidocaine administration during the first hours of an acute myocardial infarction. Am J Cardiol 41:313, 1978

194. Giardina EGV, Heissenbuttel RH, Bigger JT: Intermittent intravenous procainamide to treat ventricular arrhythmias. Ann Intern Med 78:183, 1973

195. Lima JJ, Conti DR, Goldfarb AL et al: Safety and efficacy of procainamide infusions. Am J Cardiol 43:98, 1979

196. Chow MSS, Kluger J, DiPersio DM et al: Antifibrillatory effects of lidocaine and bretylium immediately post-cardiopulmonary resuscitation. Am Heart J 110:938, 1985

197. Cardinal R, Sasyniuk BI: Electrophysiological effects of bretylium tosylate on subendocardial Purkinje fibers from infarcted canine hearts. J Pharmacol Exp Ther 204:159, 1978

198. Weiss AT, Lewis BS, Halon DA et al: The use of calcium with verapamil in the management of supraventricular tachyarrhythmias. Int J Cardiol 275, 1983

199. Waxman HL, Myerburg RJ, Appel R et al: Verapamil for control of ventricular rate in paroxysmal supraventricular tachycardia and atrial fibrillation or flutter: A double-blind randomized crossover study. Ann Intern Med 94:1, 1981

200. Gulamhusein S, Ko P, Carruthers SG et al: Acceleration of the ventricular response during atrial fibrillation in the Wolff-Parkinson-White syndrome after verapamil. Circulation 65:348, 1982

201. Harper RW, Whitford E, Middlebrook K et al: Effects of verapamil on the electrophysiologic properties of the accessory pathway in patients with the Wolff-Parkinson-White syndrome. Am J Cardiol 50:1323, 1982

202. McGovern B, Garan H, Ruskin JN: Precipitation of cardiac arrest by verapamil in patients with Wolff-Parkinson-White syndrome. Ann Intern Med 104:791, 1986

203. Stueven HA, Thompson BM, Aprahamian C et al: Calcium chloride: Reassessment of use in asystole. Ann Emerg Med 13:820, 1984

204. Stueven HA, Thompson BM, Aprahamian C et al: Lack of effectiveness of calcium chloride in refractory asystole. Ann Emerg Med 14:630, 1985

205. Stueven HA, Thompson BM, Aprahamian C et al: Use of calcium in prehospital cardiac arrest. Ann Emerg Med 12:136, 1983

206. Harrison EE, Amey BD: use of calcium in electromechanical dissociation. Ann Emerg Med 13:844, 1984

207. Stueven HA, Thompson B, Aprahamian C et al: The effectiveness of calcium chloride in refractory electromechanical dissociation. Ann Emerg Med 4:626, 1985

208. Carlon GC, Howland WS, Kahn RC et al: Calcium chloride administration in normocalcemic critically ill patients. Crit Care Med 8:209, 1980

209. Dembo DH: Calcium in advanced life support. Crit Care Med 9:358, 1981

210. White RD, Goldsmith RS, Rodriquez R et al: Plasma ionic calcium levels following injection of chlorine, gluconate and gluceptate salts of calcium. J Thorac Cardiovasc Surg 71:609, 1976

211. Pennington JE, Taylor J, Lown B: Chest thump for reverting ventricular tachycardia. N Engl J Med 283:1192, 1970

212. Ornato JP: The resuscitation of near-drowning victims. JAMA 256:75, 1986

213. Siebke H, Rod T, Breivik H et al: Survival after 40 minutes of submersion without cerebral sequelae. Lancet I:1275, 1975

214. Edlich RF, Silloway KA, Feldman PS et al: Cold injuries and disorders. Current Concepts Trauma Care 4, 1986.

215. Reuler JB: Hypothermia: Pathophysiology, clinical settings, and management. Ann Intern Med 89:519, 1978

216. Althaus U, Aeberhard P, Schupbach P et al: Management of profound accidental hypothermia with cardiorespiratory arrest. Ann Surg 195:492, 1982

217. Southwick FS, Dalglish PH Jr: Recovery after prolonged asystolic cardiac arrest in profound hypothermia. JAMA 243:1250, 1980

218. Cooper MA: Lightning injuries: Prognostic signs for death. Ann Emerg Med 9:134, 1980

219. Golde RH, Lee WR: Death by lightning. Proc Inst Electric Eng 123:1163, 1976

220. Siesjo BK, Wieloch T: Cerebral metabolism in ischemia: Neurochemical basis for therapy. Br J Anaesth 57:47, 1985

221. Rothman SM, Olney JW: Glutamate and the pathophysiology of hypoxic-ischemic brain damage. Ann Neurol 19:105, 1986

222. Brierly JB, Meldrum BS, Brown AW: The threshold and neuropathology of cerebral anoxic-ischemic cell change. Arch Neurol 29:367, 1973

223. Miller JR, Myers RE: Neuropathology of systemic circulatory arrest in adult monkeys. Neurology 22:888, 1972

224. Wolin LR, Masssopust LC, Taslitz N: Tolerance to arrest of cerebral circulation in the rhesus monkey. Exp Neurol 30:103, 1971

225. Hossman KA, Zimmerman V: Resuscitation of the monkey brain after 1H complete ischemia. I. Physiological and morphological observations. Brain Res 81:59, 1974

226. Nemoto EM: Pathogenesis of cerebral ischemia-anoxia. Crit Care Med 6:203, 1978

227. Cantu RC, Ames A III, Dixon J et al: Reversibility of experimental cerebrovascular obstruction induced by complete ischemia. J Neurosurg 31:429, 1969

228. Fischer EG, Ames A: Studies on mechanisms of impairment of cerebral circulation following ischemia: Effects of hemodilution and perfusion pressure. Stroke 3:538, 1972

229. Bleyaert AL, Sands PA, Safar P et al: Augmentation of postischemic brain damage by severe intermittent hypertension. Crit Care Med 8:41, 1980

230. Todd MM, Tommasino C, Shapiro HM: Cerebrovascular effects of prolonged hypocarbia and hypercarbia after experimental global ischemia in cats. Crit Care Med 13:720, 1985

231. Safar P, Nemoto EM: Brain resuscitation. Acta Anaesth Scand 70:60, 1978

232. Gisvold SE, Safar P, Rao G et al: Prolonged immobilization and controlled ventilation do not improve outcome after global brain ischemia in monkeys. Crit Care Med 12:171, 1984

233. D'Alecy LG, Lundy ER, Barton KJ et al: Dextrose-containing

intravenous fluid impairs outcome and increases death after eight minutes of cardiac arrest and resuscitation in dogs. Surgery 100:505, 1986

234. Longstreth WT Jr, Inui TS: High blood glucose level on hospital admission and poor neurological recovery after cardiac arrest. Ann Neurol 15:59, 1984

235. Pulsinelli WA et al: Increased damage after ischemic stroke in patients with hyperglycemia with or without established diabetes mellitus. Am J Med 74:540, 1983

236. Hoff JT, Smith Al, Hankinson HL et al: Barbiturate protection from cerebral infarction in primates. Stroke 6:28, 1975

237. Michenfelder JD, Milde JH, Sundt TM: Cerebral protection by barbiturate anesthesia: Use after middle cerebral artery occlusion in Java monkeys. Arch Neurol 33:345, 1976

238. Smith Al, Hoff JT, Nielsen SL et al: Barbiturate protection in acute focal cerebral ischemia. Stroke 5:1, 1974

239. Nussmeier N, Arlund C, Slogoff S: Neuropsychiatric complications after cardiopulmonary bypass: Cerebral protection by a barbiturate. Anesthesiology 64:165, 1986

240. Goldstein A Jr, Wells BA, Keats AS: Increased tolerance to cerebral anoxia by pentobarbital. Arch Int Pharmacodyn Ther 161:138, 1966

241. Secher O, Wilhjelm B: The protective action of anesthetics against hypoxia. Can Anaesth Soc J 15:423, 1968

242. Steen PA, Milde JH, Michenfelder JD: No barbiturate protection in a dog model of complete cerebral ischemia. Ann Neurol 5:343, 1979

243. Bleyaert AI, Nemoto EM, Safar P et al: Thiopental amelioration of brain damage after global ischemia in monkeys. Anesthesiology 49:390, 1978

244. Gisvold SE, Safar P, Hendricks HHL et al: Thiopental treatment after global brain ischemia in pigtailed monkeys. Anesthesiology 60:88, 1984

245. Brain Resuscitation Clinical Trial I Study Group: Randomized clinical study of thiopental loading in comatose survivors of cardiac arrest. N Engl J Med 314:397, 1986

246. Todd MM, Chadwick HS, Shapiro HM et al: The neurological effects of thiopental therapy following experimental cardiac arrest in cats. Anesthesiology 57:76, 1982

247. Steen PA, Gisvold SE, Milde JH et al: Nimodipine improves

248. Milde LN, Milde JH, Michenfelder JD: Delayed treatment with nimodipine improves cerebral blood flow after complete cerebral ischemia in the dog. J Cereb Blood Flow Metab 6:332, 1986

249. Dean JM, Hoehner PJ, Rogers MC et al: Effects of lidoflazine on cerebral blood flow following twelve minutes total cerebral ischemia. Stroke 15:531, 1984

250. Newburg LA, Steen PA, Milde JH et al: Failure of flunarizine to improve cerebral blood flow or neurologic recovery in a canine model of complete ischemia. Stroke 15:666, 1984

251. Steen PA, Newberg LA, Milde JH et al: Cerebral blood flow and neurologic outcome when nimodipine is given after complete cerebral ischemia in the dog. J Cereb Blood Flow Metab 4:82, 1984

252. Schanne FAX, Kane AB, Young EE et al: Calcium dependence of toxic cell death: A final common pathway. Science 206:700, 1979

253. Bleyaert A, Safar P, Nemoto E et al: Effect of postcirculatory arrest life-support on neurological recovery in monkeys. Crit Care Med 8:153, 1980

254. Strand T et al: A randomized controlled trial of hemodilution therapy in acute ischemic stroke. Stroke 15:980, 1984

255. Torphy DE, Minter MG, Thompson BM: Cardiorespiratory arrest and resuscitation of children. Am J Dis Child 138:1099, 1984

256. Orlowski JP: Optimal position for external cardiac massage in infants and children. Crit Care Med 12:224, 1984

257. Chameides L, Brown GE, Raye JR et al: Guidelines for defibrillation in infants and children: Report of the American Heart Association target activity group: Cardiopulmonary resuscitation in the young. Circulation 56(suppl):502A, 1977

258. American Heart Association: Textbook of Advanced Cardiac Life Support (70-1004 [CP]), p 271. Dallas, 1987

259. Ruark JE, Raffin TA et al: Initiating and withdrawing life support. N Engl J Med 318:25, 1988

260. Tomlinson T, Brody H: Ethics and communication in do-not-resuscitate orders. N Engl J Med 318:43, 1988

261. Schwartz AJ, Orkin FK, Ellison N: Anesthesiologists' training and knowledge of basic life support. Anesthesiology 50:191, 1979

262. Schwartz AJ, Ellison N, Ominsky AJ et al: Advanced CPR—Student, teacher, administrator, researcher (Editorial). Anesth Analg 61:629, 1982

outcome when given after complete cerebral ischemia in primates. Anesthesiology 62:406, 1985

Index

ISBN 0-397-50836-0

90000

9 780397 508365